LIPPINCOTT

MANUAL OF NURSING PRACTICE

12th Edition

SANDRA M. NETTINA, MSN, ANP-BC
Nurse Practitioner and Founder
Prime Care House Calls
West Friendship, Maryland

CHRISTINE NELSON-TUTTLE, DNS, APRN, PNP-BC
Associate Professor of Nursing
Niagara University
Lewiston, New York
Nurse Practitioner
Division of Adolescent Medicine, Department of Pediatrics, UBMD
Oishei Children's Hospital of Buffalo
Buffalo, New York

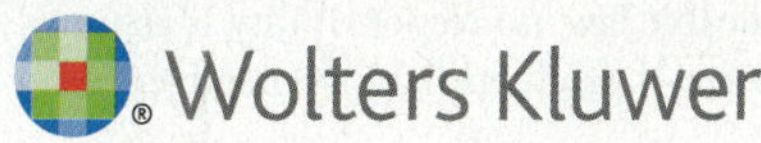

Philadelphia • Baltimore • New York • London
Buenos Aires • Hong Kong • Sydney • Tokyo

Vice President and Segment Leader, Health Learning & Practice: Julie K. Stegman
Director, Nursing Education and Practice Content: Jamie Blum
Senior Acquisitions Editor: Susan Hartman
Senior Development Editor: Meredith L. Brittain
Freelance Development Editor: Rose G. Foltz
Editorial Coordinator: Janet Jayne
Marketing Manager: Amy Whitaker
Editorial Assistant: Sara Thul
Manager, Graphic Arts and Design: Stephen Druding
Art Director, Illustration: Jennifer Clements
Production Project Manager: Alicia Jackson
Manufacturing Coordinator: Bernard Tomboc
Prepress Vendor: S4Carlisle Publishing Services

12th Edition

9 8 7 6 5 4 3 2 1

Printed in Mexico

Library of Congress Cataloging-in-Publication Data

ISBN-13: 978-1-975219-67-3
ISBN-10: 1-975219-67-8

Cataloging in Publication data available on request from publisher.

---

shop.lww.com

QUADM0824

This book is also dedicated to Elyse S. Borsuk MSN, APRN, CPCP-PC (1961-2024),

a long-time contributor for the pediatric primary care content for this text.

She made an impact in the lives of many pediatric patients and mentored many

nurse practitioner students who continue to care for the health of children everywhere.

Contributors and Reviewers

CONTRIBUTORS

CHAPTER 1 Adult Physical Assessment
Sandra M. Nettina, MSN, ANP-BC
Nurse Practitioner and Founder
Prime Care House Calls
West Friendship, Maryland

CHAPTER 2 Intravenous Therapy
Courtney Edwards, DNP, MPH, RN, CCRN, CEN, TCRN, NEA-BC
Director of Nursing
Trauma Community Outreach and BioTel EMS
Parkland Health
Dallas, Texas

CHAPTER 3 Perioperative Nursing
Claudia G. King, RN, BSN, RNFA, CNOR
Clinical Mentor/Educator
The Learning Center
Carroll Hospital Center
LifeBridge Health
Westminster, Maryland

CHAPTER 4 Cancer Nursing
Carol DeClue Riley, RN, MSN, CRNP
Nurse Practitioner, Breast and Gynecological Malignancy Program
The Johns Hopkins Skip Viragh Outpatient Cancer Building
Johns Hopkins University
Baltimore, Maryland

CHAPTER 5 Care of the Older Adult or the Person With a Disability
Elizabeth Galik, PhD, CRNP, FAAN, FAANP
Professor and Chair
Department of Organizational Systems and Adult Health
Editor in Chief, *Caring for the Ages*
University of Maryland School of Nursing
Baltimore, Maryland

CHAPTER 6 Respiratory Function and Therapy
Lori Dambaugh DNP, CNS, RN, ACCNS-AG
Associate Dean, Undergraduate Affairs
St. John Fisher University
Rochester, New York

CHAPTER 7 Respiratory Disorders
Lori Dambaugh, DNP, CNS, RN, ACCN-AG
Associate Dean, Undergraduate Affairs
St. John Fisher University
Rochester, New York

CHAPTER 8 Cardiovascular Function and Therapy
Ann Marie Cullen, MSN, APRN, CCNS
Lead Clinical Nurse/Clinical Nurse Specialist
Department of Medicine
Johns Hopkins Hospital
Baltimore, Maryland

Mary Grace Nayden, RN, BSN, CCRN
Lead Clinical Nurse, CCU
Johns Hopkins Hospital
Baltimore, Maryland

CHAPTER 9 Cardiac Disorders
Ann Marie Cullen, MSN, APRN, CCNS
Lead Clinical Nurse/Clinical Nurse Specialist
Department of Medicine
Johns Hopkins Hospital
Baltimore, Maryland

Mary Grace Nayden, RN, BSN
Nurse Clinician III, Discharge Planner
Johns Hopkins Hospital
Baltimore, Maryland

CHAPTER 10 Vascular Disorders
Ann Marie Cullen, MSN, APRN, CCNS
Lead Clinical Nurse/Clinical Nurse Specialist
Department of Medicine
Johns Hopkins Hospital
Baltimore, Maryland

Pamela S. Moss, MSN, MPH, APRN-CNS, ACCNS-AG, CCRN-CSC
Clinical Nurse Specialist
Department of Cardiac Surgery
The Johns Hopkins Hospital
Baltimore, Maryland

CHAPTER 11 Neurologic Disorders
Donna Avanecean, DNP, FNP-BC, CNRN, FNAP
APRN Epilepsy
Ayers Neuroscience Institute
Director of Advance Practice, HHCMG Specialty Care
Hartford Healthcare Medical Group

Nancy E. Villanueva PhD, CRNP. ANPBC, AGACNP-BC, CNRN
Nurse Practitioner
Department of Neurology
Temple University
Philadelphia, PA

CHAPTER 12 Eye Disorders
Agueda A. Lara-Smalling, MPH, BSN, RN-C
VA Surgical Quality Improvement Program Surgical Quality Nurse
Operative Care Line
Michael E. DeBakey VA Medical Center
Houston, Texas

CHAPTER 13 Ear, Nose, and Throat Disorders
Joy DuGan, DNP, MSN, RN
Retired
Commonwealth University of Pennsylvania
Bloomsburg, Pennsylvania

CHAPTER 14 Gastrointestinal Disorders
Tanya Seymour, DNP, RN, CCRN
Assistant Chair
Breiner School of Nursing
Commonwealth University- Mansfield
Mansfield, Pennsylvania

CHAPTER 15 Hepatic, Biliary, and Pancreatic Disorders
Natalie Masco Dixon, DNP, APRN, FNP-C, CNE
Associate Professor
Wegmans School of Nursing
St. John Fisher University
Rochester, New York

CHAPTER 16 Nutritional Problems
Karen M. Flanders, MSN, CNP, CBN
Metabolic and Bariatric Surgery Nurse Practitioner and Coordinator
Mass General Weight Center, Massachusetts General Hospital
Boston, Massachusetts

CHAPTER 17 Renal and Urinary Disorders
Justin D. Wagner, MSN, RN
Assistant Professor
Department of Undergraduate Nursing
Commonwealth University of Pennsylvania
Bloomsburg, Pennsylvania

CHAPTER 18 Gynecologic Disorders
Alison H. Simpson, PhD, WHNP-BC, RN, CNE
Assistant Professor
Wegmans School of Nursing
St. John Fischer University
Rochester, New York

CHAPTER 19 Breast Conditions
Nelli Zafman, MSN, CRNP, AOCNP
The Sidney Kimmel Comprehensive Cancer Center
Johns Hopkins Medicine
Baltimore, Maryland

CHAPTER 20 Endocrine Disorders
Lori Dambaugh, DNP, CNS, RN, ACCN-AG
Associate Dean, Undergraduate Affairs
St. John Fisher University
Rochester, New York

CHAPTER 21 Diabetes Mellitus and Related Disorders
Adeola Akindana, DNP, CRNP, CDCES
Family Nurse Practitioner, Diabetes Specialist
Professional Practice: Inpatient Glycemic Management Services
University of Maryland Capital Region Medical Center
Largo, Maryland

Claudia Tilley, MSN, RN, APRN-CNS, AGCNS-BC
Patient Education Specialist
Inpatient Diabetes Educator
UM SRH Resiliency in Stressful Events (RISE) Lead
Professional Nursing Practice Department
University of Maryland Shore Regional Health
Easton, Maryland

CHAPTER 22 Hematologic Disorders
Rebekah M. Zonozy, APRN, MSN, CPNP-PC
Pediatric Nurse Practitioner and Founder
Childhood Upstream/Rooted Well
Dallas, Texas

CHAPTER 23 Transfusion Therapy and Blood and Marrow Stem Cell Transplantation
Rebekah M. Zonozy, APRN, MSN, CPNP-PC
Pediatric Nurse Practitioner and Founder
Childhood Upstream/Rooted Well
Dallas, Texas

CHAPTER 24 Asthma and Allergy
Lori Dambaugh, DNP, CNS, RN, ACCN-AG
Associate Dean of Undergraduate Affairs
St. John Fisher University
Rochester, New York

CHAPTER 25 HIV Infection and AIDS

Lisa M. Wolf, RN, BSN, JD
Clinical Nurse
Department of Medicine
Johns Hopkins Hospital
Baltimore, Maryland

CHAPTER 26 Connective Tissue Disorders

Elizabeth Kirchner, DNP
Department of Rheumatic and Immunologic Diseases
Cleveland Clinic
Cleveland, Ohio

CHAPTER 27 Infectious Diseases

Anne M. Caston-Gaa, MPH, MSN, RN
Nurse Clinician III
Department of Psychiatry
Johns Hopkins Hospital
Baltimore, Maryland

Melanie Gavin Ponce, MPH, CIC, M (ASCP)
Independent Contractor
Medical University of South Carolina
Charleston, South Carolina

CHAPTER 28 Musculoskeletal Disorders

Rebecca Toothaker, PhD, RN
Director, *Nursing Living Learning Community*
Assistant Professor of Clinical Practice
School of Nursing
University of West Florida
Pensacola, Florida

CHAPTER 29 Dermatologic Disorders

Lisa S Ball, PhD, APRN, FNP-BC
Dermatology Nurse Practitioner & Owner
Lisa S Ball FNP PLLC
Williamsville, New York

CHAPTER 30 Burns

Tara L. Sacco, PhD, RN, CCRN, ACCNS-AG
Assistant Professor
Wegmans School of Nursing
St. John Fisher University
Rochester, New York

CHAPTER 31 Emergent Conditions

Rebecca Roloff, DNP, FNP-BC, APRN, SANE-A/P, CHSE
Director, FNP Program
Assistant Professor
College of Nursing
Niagara University
Lewiston, New York

CHAPTER 32 Maternal and Fetal Health

Kylene Abraham, DNP, CNS, RNC-OB
Associate Professor of Nursing
Wegmans School of Nursing
St. John Fisher University
Rochester, New York

Susan M. McCarthy, DNP, APRN, RNC-MNM, EFM, CLC
University of Rochester–Thompson Health
Rochester, New York

CHAPTER 33 Nursing Management During Labor and Delivery

Kylene Abraham, DNP, CNS, RNC-OB
Associate Professor of Nursing
Wegmans School of Nursing
St. John Fisher University
Rochester, New York

Susan M. McCarthy, DNP, APRN, RNC-MNM, EFM, CLC
University of Rochester–Thompson Health
Rochester, New York

CHAPTER 34 Maternal and Neonatal Care During the Postpartum Period

Kylene Abraham, DNP, CNS, RNC-OB
Associate Professor of Nursing
Wegmans School of Nursing
St. John Fisher University
Rochester, New York

Susan M. McCarthy, DNP, APRN, RNC-MNM, EFM, CLC
University of Rochester–Thompson Health
Rochester, New York

CHAPTER 35 Complications of the Childbearing Experience

Kylene Abraham, DNP, CNS, RNC-OB
Associate Professor of Nursing
Wegmans School of Nursing
St. John Fisher University
Rochester, New York

Susan M. McCarthy, DNP, APRN, RNC-MNM, EFM, CLC
University of Rochester–Thompson Health
Rochester, New York

CHAPTER 36 Pediatric Growth and Development

Christine Nelson-Tuttle, DNS, APRN, PNP-BC
Associate Professor of Nursing
Niagara University
Lewiston, New York
Nurse Practitioner
Division of Adolescent Medicine, Department of Pediatrics, UBMD
Oishei Children's Hospital of Buffalo
Buffalo, New York

CHAPTER 37 Pediatric Physical Assessment

Christine Nelson-Tuttle, DNS, APRN, PNP-BC
Associate Professor of Nursing
Niagara University
Lewiston, New York
Nurse Practitioner
Division of Adolescent Medicine, Department of Pediatrics, UBMD
Oishei Children's Hospital of Buffalo
Buffalo, New York

CHAPTER 38 Pediatric Primary Care
In memoriam:
Elyse S. Borsuk, MSN, APRN, CPCP-PC
Pediatric Nurse Practitioner Specialty Program
Yale University School of Nursing
Orange, Connecticut

CHAPTER 39 Care of the Sick or Hospitalized Child
Dana Lorber, RN, MS, CPN
Clinical Nurse Specialist, Pediatrics and Pediatric Intensive Care Unit
Nursing Professional Development
Maria Fareri Children's Hospital
Member of the Westchester Medical Center Health Network
Valhalla, New York

CHAPTER 40 Pediatric Respiratory Disorders
Mary Beth Lyons, RN,MS,CPN
Clinical Nurse Specialist
PICU and Pediatrics
Maria Fareri Children's Hospital
Valhalla, New York

CHAPTER 41 Pediatric Cardiovascular Disorders
Wendy K. Hou, DNP, RN, CNS
Assistant Director, Pediatric Nursing
Golisano Children's Hospital
Rochester, New York

CHAPTER 42 Pediatric Neurologic Disorders
Pamela Mapstone, DNP, CPNP
Associate Professor of Nursing
Wegmans School of Nursing
St. John Fisher University
Rochester, New York

CHAPTER 43 Pediatric Eye and Ear Disorders
Cheryl Drabik, MS, RN, CPNP-BC
Nurse Practitioner
Division of Emergency Medicine, UBMD
Oishei Children's Hospital of Buffalo
Buffalo, New York

CHAPTER 44 Pediatric Gastrointestinal and Nutritional Disorders
Christine Nelson-Tuttle, DNS, APRN, PNP-BC
Associate Professor of Nursing
Niagara University
Lewiston, New York
Nurse Practitioner
Division of Adolescent Medicine, Department of Pediatrics, UBMD
Oishei Children's Hospital of Buffalo
Buffalo, New York

CHAPTER 45 Pediatric Renal and Genitourinary Disorders
Alexandra Eden-Walker, NP-PHC, MScN
Nurse Practitioner and Adjunct Lecturer
University of Toronto
Division of Nephrology
The Hospital for Sick Children
Toronto, Ontario, Canada

CHAPTER 46 Pediatric Metabolic and Endocrine Disorders
Christine Nelson-Tuttle, DNS, APRN, PNP-BC
Associate Professor of Nursing
Niagara University
Lewiston, New York
Nurse Practitioner
Division of Adolescent Medicine, Department of Pediatrics, UBMD
Oishei Children's Hospital of Buffalo
Buffalo, New York

Natalie Bellini, DNP, FNP-BC, BC-ADM, CDCES
Endocrine Nurse Practitioner
Clinical Associate Professor of Medicine
Case Western Reserve University
Program Director for Diabetes Technology
University Hospitals
Cleveland, Ohio

CHAPTER 47 Pediatric Oncology
Karen Wolownik, MSN, RN, CPNP-PC, CPHON
Pediatric Nurse Practitioner
Division of Pediatric Hematology, Oncology, Cell Therapy
Maria Fareri Children's Hospital
Valhalla, New York

CHAPTER 48 Pediatric Hematologic Disorders
Barbara Ehrenreich, MSN, CPNP, ACHPN, RN
Pediatric Nurse Practitioner
Tribeca Pediatrics
Ardsley, New York

CHAPTER 49 Pediatric Immunologic Disorders
Holly Convery, RN, BScN
Division of Rheumatology
The Hospital for Sick Children
Toronto, Ontario, Canada

Brenda Reid, RN, MN
Director of Patient Education and Advocacy
Immunodeficiency Canada
Toronto, Ontario, Canada

Audrey Bell-Peter, MN, RN
Division of Rheumatology
The Hospital for Sick Children
Toronto, Ontario, Canada

CHAPTER 50 Pediatric Orthopedic Disorders
Pamela Mapstone, DNP, CPNP
Associate Professor of Nursing
Wegmans School of Nursing
St. John Fisher University
Rochester, New York

CHAPTER 51 Pediatric Integumentary Disorders
Lisa S Ball, PhD, APRN, FNP-BC
Dermatology Nurse Practitioner & Owner
Lisa S Ball FNP PLLC
Williamsville, New York

Kara Sher, BSN, RN, CPN, CCRN
Nurse Manager
Inpatient Unit
Shriners Hospital
Boston, Massachusetts

Tammy Noble, MSN
Staff Nurse, Inpatient Unit
Shriners Children's Boston
Boston, Massachusetts

CHAPTER 52 Developmental Disabilities

Christine Nelson-Tuttle, DNS, APRN, PNP-BC
Associate Professor of Nursing
Niagara University
Lewiston, New York
Nurse Practitioner
Division of Adolescent Medicine, Department of Pediatrics, UBMD
Oishei Children's Hospital of Buffalo
Buffalo, New York

CHAPTER 53 Problems of Mental Health

Catherine Calder Fettig, MSN, RN
Nursing Education and Behavioral Health Practice Specialist
Clinical Practice Support
Legacy Health System
Portland, Oregon

Joseph B. Gundlach, MSN, RN, PMH-BC
Professional Practice Leader
Center for Nursing Excellence and Innovation
Oregon Health and Science University
Portland, Oregon

REVIEWERS

Amanda Brock, BSN, RN, CEN
Senior Burn Nurse Clinician
Parkland Health and Hospital System
Dallas, Texas

Lauren Fischer, BSN
Registered Nurse
Medicine/CCU
The Johns Hopkins Hospital
Baltimore, Maryland

Jennifer Korkosz, DNP, WHNP-BC
Associate Professor
University of Delaware
College of Health Sciences–School of Nursing
Newark, Delaware

Tim Madeira, DNP
Nurse Practitioner
Cardiac Surgery
Johns Hopkins Hospital
Baltimore, Maryland

Anna Manalad, BSN, RN, CCRN
RN III-CVIL/EP
Johns Hopkins Hospital
Baltimore, Maryland

Cheryl Wolf, BSN, RN-BC
General Staff Nurse Pediatrics
Maria Fareri Children's Hospital
Valhalla, New York

Preface

Health care continues to evolve today due to advancements in science and technology. The rate of change has escalated as decades pass. Nursing has evolved from its foundation in 1860 with the founding of the first nursing school by Florence Nightingale at St. Thomas Hospital in London. Although it seems rudimentary in our time, the innovation of strict sanitation practices that Nightingale demanded during the 1850s not only reduced the death rate in military hospitals during the Crimean War but also launched the science of nursing. The idea of nursing care influencing patient outcomes was born.

Additionally, Nightingale introduced reform of inhumane conditions. She was compelled to reduce human suffering through compassionate, patient-centered care. Although procedures and technology may change, caring will never change. Just as Nightingale recognized each patient's own dignity and that each patient deserves respect, so do nurses today. Nurses care for people in all settings, all stages of life, through all aspects of illness and wellness. The patient is the one we serve, at the center, whether we are working in a hospital, an outpatient facility, a long-term care facility, or the home.

With our combined 75+ years of practice, we have found it empowering to advance our own knowledge base through formal education, advanced degrees, countless continuing education programs, and much professional reading and networking. We have always been thankful to have high-quality nursing literature available to shape our practices. We have also learned much through our day-to-day encounters with patients and families.

Now we present the 12th edition of the *Lippincott Manual of Nursing Practice*, with knowledge and caring as its focus. This manual is meant to guide students and nurses across all care settings, and to provide high-quality standardized care, while not forgetting the caring personal interactions that nurses do so well.

Organization

This edition continues to be presented in a basic outline format for easy readability and access to information. The subheadings continue to follow a medical model—Pathophysiology and Etiology, Clinical Manifestations, Diagnostic Evaluation, Management, and Complications—and a nursing process model—Nursing Assessment, Nursing Interventions, Patient Education and Health Maintenance, and Evaluation: Expected Outcomes. Medical model information is presented because nurses need to understand the medical disorder, diagnostic workup, and treatment that are the basis for nursing care. The nursing process section provides a practical overview of step-by-step nursing care for almost any patient scenario. Nursing interventions are grouped by patient problem, which may be related to medical diagnoses or the individual response to illness.

This edition is divided into four parts to present a comprehensive reference for all types of nursing care. Part One encompasses Medical–Surgical Nursing. General topics are presented in Unit I, including Adult Physical Assessment, Intravenous Therapy, Perioperative Nursing, Cancer Nursing, and Care of the Older Adult or the Person With a Disability. Units II through XII cover body system function and dysfunction and the various disorders seen in adult medical and surgical nursing.

Part Two covers Maternity and Neonatal Nursing. Chapters include Maternal and Fetal Health, Nursing Management During Labor and Delivery, Maternal and Neonatal Care During the Postpartum Period, and Complications of the Childbearing Experience. Chapters reflect the routine childbearing experience as well as frequently encountered high-risk situations and maternal and neonatal problems that may arise.

Part Three focuses on Pediatric Nursing. Chapters are divided into two units. Unit XIII covers General Practice Considerations, comprising Pediatric Growth and Development, Pediatric Physical Assessment, Pediatric Primary Care, and Care of the Child Who Is Sick or Hospitalized. Unit XIV covers body system function and dysfunction and the various disorders seen in pediatric nursing.

Part Four consists of a chapter on Psychiatric Nursing. Entries follow the *Diagnostic and Statistical Manual of Mental Disorders*, Fifth Edition, Text Revision (*DSM-5-TR*), classification of mental illness. Treatment and nursing management for each are discussed.

Updated Material

This edition has been extensively updated. You will find updated information on diagnostic tests and medical care for almost every entry. Nursing care has also been updated to reflect new treatments, new medications, and best practice information. In addition, many figures, boxes, and tables have been added or updated.

Areas with especially extensive updates include intravenous therapy (Chapter 2), survivorship care (Chapter 4), updated immunization and other preventative recommendations for older adults (Chapter 5), ischemic disorders (Chapter 9), anticoagulation (Chapter 10), eating disorders (Chapter 16), breast cancer risk and management (Chapter 19), American Diabetes Association updates (Chapter 21), four added disorders (Chapter 26), reorganization of dermatitis (Chapter 29), risk factors for eustachian tube dysfunction (Chapter 43), pediatric immunodeficiency (Chapter 49), and reclassification of disorders according to the *DSM-5-TR* (Chapter 53).

Alerts in the 12th Edition

The 12th edition highlights the following types of important information in its alert features:

- **Clinical Judgment Alerts** emphasize critical observations and actions that require the nurse to quickly incorporate the clinical judgment process and to act.
- **Population Awareness Alerts** highlight information related to variations in care and the need for sensitivity to specific populations based on age, ethnicity, religious and cultural beliefs, and gender and sexual orientation.
- **Drug Alerts** present important nursing considerations when administering certain medications.

Inclusive Language

A note about the language used in this book: Wolters Kluwer recognizes that people have a diverse range of identities, and we are committed to using inclusive and nonbiased language in our content. Please note that whenever "male" is used in this book, it refers to a person assigned male at birth, and whenever "female" is used, it refers to a person assigned female at birth. In line with the principles of nursing, we strive not to define people by their diagnoses, but to recognize their personhood first and foremost, using as much as possible the language diverse groups use to define themselves, and including only information that is relevant to nursing care.

We strive to better address the unique perspectives, complex challenges, and lived experiences of diverse populations traditionally underrepresented in health literature. When describing or referencing populations discussed in research studies, we will adhere to the identities presented in those studies to maintain fidelity to the evidence presented by the study investigators. We follow best practices of language set forth by the *Publication Manual of the American Psychological Association*, 7th Edition, but acknowledge that language evolves rapidly, and we will update the language used in future editions of this book as necessary.

Resources for Readers

Procedural Guidelines, Patient Education Guidelines, and Nursing Care Plans

Procedural Guidelines, Patient Education Guidelines, and Nursing Care Plans referred to in the printed book can be accessed at http://thePoint.lww.com/Nettina12e using the code printed in the front of the textbook.

Ebook

An ebook is available for separate purchase. The Procedural Guidelines, Patient Education Guidelines, and Nursing Care Plans mentioned earlier are included in this product.

It is our pleasure to have prepared the 12th edition of the *Lippincott Manual of Nursing Practice* for you. We hope that it will serve you well in providing high-quality patient-centered care across all settings.

Sandra M. Nettina, MSN, ANP-BC
Christine Nelson-Tuttle, DNS, APRN, PNP-BC

Acknowledgments

We would like to thank past and present reviewers and contributors and the entire Wolters Kluwer team for their contribution to the *Lippincott Manual of Nursing Practice*, 12th Edition. Susan Hartman, senior acquisitions editor, was instrumental in guiding and supporting us in this project. Meredith Brittain and Rose Foltz, development editors, carefully edited the book content. Janet Jayne, editorial coordinator, was invaluable in directing the day-to-day logistics and activities behind the scenes. Alicia Jackson kept the chapters, and all of us involved, moving through production. Lori Dambaugh, DNP, CNS, RN, ACCNS-AG, as our associate clinical editor, provided invaluable updating and editing of medical–surgical and mental health chapters as well as additional help with project vision and planning. Everyone involved has come to respect the enormity of the task and how each step affects the next. We are proud of our accomplishment.

Contents

PART FOUR PSYCHIATRIC NURSING

APPENDICES

Part One

Medical-Surgical Nursing

UNIT

I GENERAL HEALTH CONSIDERATIONS

1 Adult Physical Assessment*

THE PATIENT HISTORY

General Principles

1. The first steps in caring for a patient are to establish a relationship and gather information.
2. In all patient encounters, the assessment process begins with thorough and accurate history taking, thorough review of the patient record, interviewing the patient, and obtaining information from other individuals.
3. Use good communication skills to elicit comprehensive health history and establish rapport with the patient simultaneously.

Interviewing Techniques

1. Provide privacy in as quiet a place as possible and see that the patient is comfortable.
2. Begin the interview with a courteous greeting and an introduction. Ask how the patient (and advocate, if present) would like to be addressed. Explain who you are and the reason for your presence.
3. Make sure that facial expressions, body movements, and tone of voice are pleasant, unhurried, and nonjudgmental and that they convey the attitude of a sensitive listener so the patient will feel free to express thoughts and feelings.
4. Use open-ended questions and avoid narrowing the discussion or reassuring the patient prematurely (before you have adequate information about the problem). This only cuts off discussion; the patient may then be unwilling to expand on a problem causing concern.
5. Be alert for cues or suggestions by the patient that may require you to explore more by asking more pointed questions.
6. Guide the interview so the necessary information is obtained in a timely manner. For those people who have difficulty expressing historical information clearly and concisely, use summarization to clarify and advance the interview in a patient and respectful manner.

Components

Identifying Information

1. Supply date and time of the interview. Review data about the patient if already in the record or obtain patient's demographic data and emergency contact information.
2. Obtain name of referring practitioner, insurance data, and name and contact information of informant(s) other than the patient. Note reliability of an informant if necessary.
3. Explain the reasons why the information is needed to help put the patient at ease.

Chief Complaint

1. Obtain a brief statement of the patient's primary problem or concern in the patient's own words, including the duration of the complaint, for example, "hacking cough for 3 weeks."
2. Purpose is to allow the patient to describe their own problems and expectations with little or no direction from the interviewer and to identify the overriding problem for which the patient is seeking help (there may be numerous complaints).
3. To obtain information, ask the patient a direct question, such as, "For what reason have you come to the facility?" or "What is your primary health concern at this time?"
   a. Avoid confusing questions, such as "What brings you here?" ("The bus.") or "Why are you here?" ("That's what I came to find out.")

*Please note that the term "male" in this chapter refers to a person assigned male at birth, and the term "female" in this chapter refers to a person assigned female at birth.

b. Ask how long the concern or problem has been present, for example, whether it has been hours, days, or weeks. If necessary, establish the time of onset precisely by offering such clues as "Did you feel this way a month (6 months or 2 years) ago?"

4. Write down what the patient says using quotation marks to identify patient's words.

History of Present Illness

1. Obtain a detailed chronologic picture, beginning with the time the patient was last well (or, in the case of a problem with an acute onset, the patient's condition just before the onset of the problem) and ending with a description of the patient's current condition.
2. If there is more than one important problem, describe each in a separate, chronologically organized paragraph in the written history of present illness.
3. Investigate the chief complaint by eliciting more information through the use of the mnemonic "OLD CARTS":
   a. **O**nset (setting, circumstances, rapidity, or manner in which it began).
   b. **L**ocation (exact place where the symptom is felt, radiation pattern).
   c. **D**uration (how long; if intermittent, the frequency and duration of each episode).
   d. **C**haracter/course (nature or quality of the symptom, such as sharp pain, interference with activity, how it has changed or evolved over time; ask to describe a typical episode).
   e. **A**ggravating/associated factors (medications, rest, activity, diet; associated nausea, fever, and other symptoms).
   f. **R**elieving factors (lying down, having bowel movement).
   g. **T**reatments tried (pharmacologic and nonpharmacologic methods attempted and their outcomes).
   h. **S**everity (the quantity of the symptom, e.g., how severe on a scale of 1 to 10).
4. Alternatively, use the mnemonic PQRST: **p**rovocative/palliative factors, **q**uality/quantity, **r**egion/radiation, **s**everity, **t**iming.
5. Obtain OLD CARTS data for all the major problems associated with the present illness, as applicable.
6. Clarify the chronology of the illness by asking questions and summarizing the history of the present illness for the patient to comment on.

Past Medical History

1. Determine the background health status of the patient, including present status, recent health conditions, and past health conditions, that will serve as a basis for nursing care planning for holistic patient care.
2. Childhood illnesses, such as infectious diseases (if applicable).
3. Immunizations—childhood vaccines (see Chapter 38); adult vaccines including hepatitis, human papillomavirus, influenza, tetanus/pertussis, varicella zoster, pneumococcal, and coronavirus vaccines.
4. Operations—surgical procedure, indication, approximate date, any complications.
5. Previous hospitalizations—facility, approximate date, diagnosis, treatment.
6. Injuries—approximate date, treatment, outcome.
7. Major acute and chronic illnesses (any serious or prolonged illnesses not requiring hospitalization)—dates, symptoms, course, treatment.
8. Medications—prescription drugs from all providers (including ophthalmologist and dentist); nonprescription drugs including vitamins, supplements, and herbal products; include dosage, length of use, and adherence.
9. Allergies—environmental allergies, food allergies, drug reactions; give type of reaction (hives, rhinitis, local reaction, angioedema, anaphylaxis). Also note intolerance or adverse reactions to certain drugs that may not be due to allergy.
10. Obstetric history (may appear in review of systems):
    a. Pregnancies, miscarriages, abortions.
    b. Describe course of pregnancy, labor, and delivery; date, place of delivery.
11. Psychiatric history (may appear in review of systems)—treatment by a mental health provider, diagnosis, date, medications.

Family History

1. Purpose is to present a picture of the patient's family health, including that of biologic grandparents, caregivers, siblings, aunts, and uncles because some diseases show a familial tendency or are hereditary.
2. Include age and health status (or age at and cause of death) of biologic grandparents, caregivers, and siblings.
3. History, in immediate and close relatives, of heart disease, hypertension, stroke, diabetes, gout, kidney disease or stones, thyroid disease, pulmonary disease, blood problems, cancer (types), epilepsy, mental illness, arthritis, alcohol use disorder, obesity.
4. Genetic disorders, such as hemophilia or sickle cell disease.

Review of Systems

1. Purpose is to obtain detailed information about the current state of the patient and significant past symptoms, or lack of symptoms, patient may have experienced related to a particular body system.
2. May give clues to diagnosis of multisystem disorders or progression of a disorder to other areas.
3. Include subjective information about what the patient feels or sees with regard to the major systems of the body.
   a. General constitutional symptoms—fever, chills, night sweats, malaise, fatigability, recent weight loss or gain.
   b. Skin—rash, itching, change in pigmentation or texture, sweating, hair growth and distribution, condition of nails, skin care habits, protection from sun.
   c. Skeletal—problems of joints, muscles, or bones including pain, stiffness, deformity, restriction of motion, swelling, redness, heat, cramping.
   d. Head—headaches, dizziness, syncope, head injuries.
   e. Eyes—vision, pain, diplopia, photophobia, blind spots, itching, burning, discharge, glaucoma, cataracts, glasses or contact lenses worn, date of last eye appointment.
   f. Ears—hearing acuity, earache, discharge, tinnitus, vertigo, history of tubes or infection.
   g. Nose—sense of smell, frequency of colds, obstruction, epistaxis, postnasal discharge, sinus pain or therapy, use of nose drops or sprays (type and frequency).
   h. Teeth—pain; bleeding, swollen or receding gums; recent abscesses, extractions; dentures; dental hygiene practices, last dental examination.
   i. Mouth and tongue—soreness of tongue or buccal mucosa, ulcers, swelling.
   j. Throat—sore throat, tonsillitis, hoarseness, dysphagia.

k. Neck—pain, stiffness, swelling, enlarged glands or lymph nodes.
l. Endocrine—goiter, thyroid tenderness, tolerance to heat and cold, changes in skin pigmentation, libido, polyuria, polydipsia, polyphagia, hormone therapy, unexplained weight change.
m. Respiratory—pain in the chest with breathing, dyspnea, wheezing, cough, sputum, hemoptysis, risk factors, and testing for tuberculosis.
n. Cardiovascular—chest pain, palpitations, dyspnea, orthopnea (note number of pillows required for sleeping), history of heart murmur, edema, cyanosis, claudication, varicose veins, exercise tolerance, blood pressure (if known), history of blood clots.
o. Hematologic—anemia, tendency to bruise or bleed, any known abnormalities of blood cells.
p. Lymph nodes—enlargement, tenderness, drainage.
q. Gastrointestinal—appetite, food intolerance, belching, heartburn, nausea, vomiting, hematemesis, bowel habits, diarrhea, constipation, flatulence, stool characteristics, hemorrhoids, jaundice, use of laxatives or antacids, history of ulcers or other conditions, previous diagnostic tests such as colonoscopy.
r. Urinary—dysuria, pain, urgency, frequency, hematuria, nocturia, oliguria, hesitancy, dribbling, decrease in size or force of stream, passage of stones, incontinence.
s. Reproductive—puberty onset, sexual activity, use and type of contraception, libido, sexual dysfunction, history of sexually transmitted infections (STIs), menstrual cycle, pregnancies.
t. Breasts—pain, tenderness, discharge, lumps, mammograms, breast self-examination.
u. Neurologic—loss of consciousness, seizures, confusion, memory, cognitive function, incoordination, weakness, numbness, paresthesia, tremors.
v. Psychiatric—how patient views self, mood, sadness, depression, anxiety, irritability, obsessive thoughts, compulsions, suicidal or homicidal thoughts, hallucinations.

Personal and Social History

1. Explore the patient's family structure and habits to identify resources an individual has to aid in coping with the situation and determine what health promotion activities may improve health.
2. Determine personal status—birthplace, education, position in the family, education level, job status, satisfaction with life situations, personal concerns.
3. Identify habits and lifestyle patterns:
   a. Sleeping pattern, number of hours of sleep, difficulty sleeping.
   b. Exercise, activities, recreation, hobbies.
   c. Nutrition and eating habits (diet recall for a typical day).
   d. Alcohol—frequency, amount, type; CAGE questionnaire—positive response may indicate problem drinking:
      i. Have you ever thought you should **C**ut down on your drinking?
      ii. Have you ever been **A**nnoyed by criticism of your drinking?
      iii. Have you ever felt **G**uilty about your drinking?
      iv. Do you drink in the morning (i.e., an **E**ye-opener)?
   e. Caffeine—type and amount per day.
   f. Recreational or illicit drugs (illegal or improperly used controlled substances).
   g. Tobacco—past and present use, type (cigarettes, cigars, chewing, snuff), pack-years.
   h. Sexual habits (can be part of genitourinary history)—relationships, frequency, satisfaction, number of partners in past year and lifetime, STI and pregnancy prevention.
4. Home conditions.
   a. Marital status, nature of family relationships.
   b. Financial—source of income, health insurance.
   c. Living arrangements, type of housing.
   d. Support systems.
   e. Involvement with agencies (name, caseworker).
   f. History of abuse—physical, intimate partner, sexual.
5. Environmental exposure—through work or other activities, including exposure to stress, noise, chemicals, pollution.
6. Culture—important in coping and health practices.
7. Religion/faith—may affect some treatment decisions.

Ending the History

When you have completed the history, it is often helpful to say, "Is there anything else you would like to tell me?" or "What additional concerns do you have?" This allows the patient to end the history by saying what is on the patient's mind and what concerns the patient the most.

PHYSICAL EXAMINATION

General Principles

1. Conduct a complete or partial physical examination following a careful comprehensive or problem-related history.
2. Make sure the exam takes place in a quiet, well-lit room with consideration for patient privacy and comfort.

Approaching the Patient

1. When possible, begin with the patient in a sitting position so both the front and back can be examined.
2. Completely expose the part to be examined, but drape the rest of the body appropriately.
3. Conduct the examination systematically from head to foot so as not to miss observing any system or body part.
4. While examining each region, consider the underlying anatomic structures, their function, and possible abnormalities.
5. Because the body is bilaterally symmetric for the most part, compare findings on one side with those on the other.
6. Explain all procedures to the patient while the examination is being conducted to avoid alarming or worrying the patient and to encourage cooperation.

Techniques of Examination and Assessment

Use the following techniques of examination, as appropriate, for eliciting findings.

Inspection

1. Begin your first encounter with the patient to observe behavior and physical appearance in a systematic manner.
2. Use your eyes to inspect each part of the body with the appropriate light and exposure for characteristics such as symmetry, color, enlargement or swelling, and deformity.

Palpation

1. Use your fingertips or palms to touch the region or body part just observed for temperature, texture, tenderness, and moisture in a systematic manner.
2. With experience, you will be able to determine abnormal consistency and pinpoint tender areas.

Percussion

1. By setting underlying tissues in motion, percussion helps in determining the density of the underlying tissue and whether it is air-filled, fluid-filled, or solid.
2. Audible sounds and palpable vibrations are produced, which you can distinguish as five basic notes of percussion, differing in sound, pitch, duration, and intensity (see Table 1-1).
3. To perform percussion, follow these steps (see Figure 1-1):
   a. Hyperextend the middle finger of your left hand, pressing the distal portion and joint firmly against the surface to be percussed.
      i. Other fingers touching the surface will damp the sound.
      ii. Be consistent in the degree of firmness exerted by the hyperextended finger as you move it from area to area or the sound will vary.
   b. Cock the right hand at the wrist, flex the middle finger upward, and place the forearm close to the surface to be percussed. The right hand and forearm should be as relaxed as possible.
   c. With a quick, sharp, relaxed wrist motion, strike the extended left middle finger with the flexed right middle finger, using the tip of the finger, not the pad. Aim at the end of the extended left middle finger (just behind the nail bed) where the greatest pressure is exerted on the surface to be percussed.
   d. Lift the right middle finger rapidly to avoid damping the vibrations.
   e. The movement is at the wrist, not at the finger, elbow, or shoulder; use the lightest touch capable of producing a clear sound.

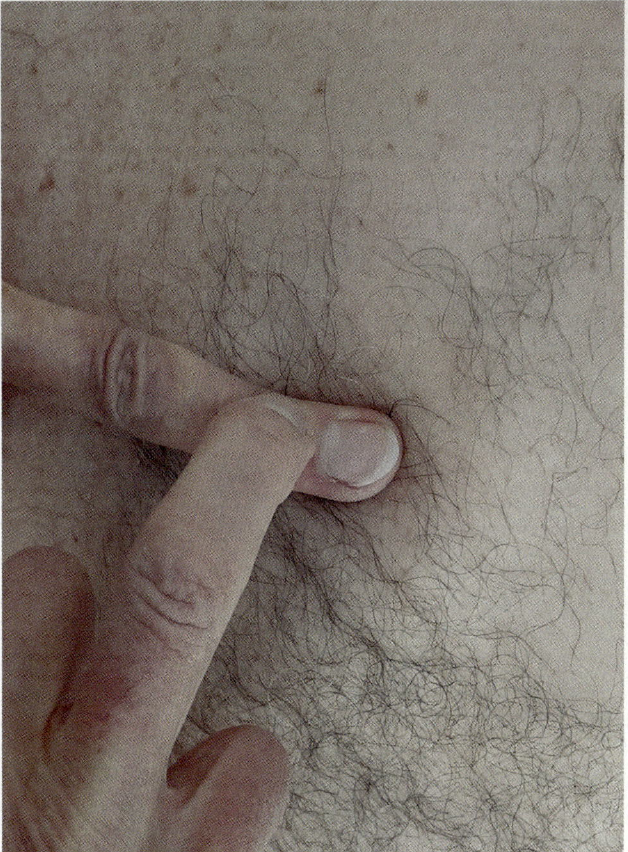

Figure 1-1. Percussion of the posterior chest.

Auscultation

1. You will use a stethoscope to augment your sense of hearing. Earpieces should be comfortable, the length of the tubing should be 10 to 15 in (25 to 38 cm), and the head should have a diaphragm and a bell.
2. Use the bell to detect low-pitched sounds such as certain heart murmurs.
3. Use the diaphragm for high-frequency sounds such as breath sounds.
4. Try to minimize extraneous sounds produced by clothing, hair, and movement of the head of the stethoscope.

Table 1-1 Five Basic Notes Produced by Percussion

	RELATIVE INTENSITY	RELATIVE PITCH	RELATIVE DURATION	EXAMPLE LOCATION
Flatness	Soft	High	Short	Thigh
Dullness	Medium	Medium	Medium	Liver
Resonance	Loud	Low	Long	Normal lung
Hyperresonance	Very loud	Lower	Longer	Emphysematous lung
Tympany	Loud	High[a]	Longer	Gastric air bubble

[a]*Distinguished mainly by its musical timbre.*

Adapted with permission from Bickley, L. S., Szilagyi, P. G., Hoffman, R. M., & Soriano, R. P. (2024). Bates' guide to physical examination and history taking (13th ed., Box 15-3). Wolters Kluwer.

ADULT PHYSICAL ASSESSMENT

Equipment

- Cotton applicator stick
- Flashlight
- Gauze sponges
- Gloves
- Lubricant
- Nasal speculum
- Oto-ophthalmoscope
- Reflex hammer
- Safety pin
- Scented items such as cinnamon and coffee
- Snellen chart
- Sphygmomanometer
- Stethoscope
- Tape measure
- Thermometer
- Tongue blade
- Tuning fork

VITAL SIGNS

Technique	Findings
Important: Many major therapeutic decisions are based on the vital signs; therefore, accuracy is essential.	
Temperature	
Oral, axillary, and rectal temperature are measured routinely as a substitute for core body temperature. Tympanic membrane (ear), temporal artery, and noncontact infrared thermometer readings do not correlate well with core temperature, according to research.	Temperature—may vary with the time of day and method used (axillary slightly lower); 98.6°F (37°C) has long been considered normal oral temperature, but recent research has shown 98.0°F (36.6°C) to be the new average normal oral temperature (Ley et al., 2023). Temporal artery thermometers are widely used in many settings; interpret the results with caution.
A rectal temperature is the most accurate but may be contraindicated with some rectal problems and cardiac arrhythmias.	Rectal temperature is higher than oral by 0.7°F–0.9°F (0.4°C–0.5°C).
Pulse	
Palpate the radial pulse and count for at least 30 sec. If the pulse is irregular, count for a full minute and note the number of irregular beats per minute. Note whether the beat of the pulse against your finger is strong or weak, bounding or thready.	Pulse—normal adult pulse is 60–80 beats/min; regular in rhythm. Elasticity of the arterial walls, blood volume, and mechanical action of the heart muscle are some of the factors that affect the strength of the pulse wave, which normally is full and strong.
Respiration	
Count the number of respirations for 15 sec and multiply by 4. Count longer for better accuracy if abnormality detected. Note rhythm and depth of breathing.	Respiration—normally 12–20 respirations per minute.
Blood pressure	
Measure the blood pressure (BP) in both arms. Document the patient's position. Feet should be supported and legs should not be crossed.	Normal BP is 120/80 mm Hg or less. A difference of 5–10 mm Hg between arms is common.
Palpate the radial artery for return of pulse indicating the systolic pressure, in addition to using the stethoscope to detect an auscultatory gap.	Auscultatory gap: The first sound of blood in the artery is usually followed by continuous sound until nothing is audible with the stethoscope. Occasionally, the sound is not continuous and there is a gap after the first sound, after which the sound of blood in the vessel is heard again. If one uses only the auscultatory method and pumps the cuff up until the sound is no longer heard, it is possible, when there is a gap in the sound or when the sound is not continuous, to get a falsely low systolic reading.
Apply the cuff firmly to exposed upper arm supported at level of the heart; if the cuff is too loose, it will give a falsely high reading. The cuff should be approximately 1 in (2.5 cm) above the antecubital fossa.	Wrist BP readings are not as accurate as upper arm readings; only a validated automated electronic (oscillometric) device should be used.

ADULT PHYSICAL ASSESSMENT *(continued)*

Technique	Findings
Use an appropriate-sized cuff: a pediatric cuff for children; a large cuff or a leg cuff for people with obesity. Obtain readings in lying, sitting, and standing positions if indicated.	Going from a recumbent to a standing position can cause the systolic pressure to fall 10–15 mm Hg and the diastolic pressure to rise slightly (by 5 mm Hg).

BODY MEASUREMENTS

Technique	Findings
Determine the patient's height and weight. Use a measuring device rather than asking the patient for recent measurements.	Height and weight can be used to determine body mass index, which signifies overall health and fitness.
Determine waist circumference by using tape measure just above the umbilicus at the narrowest point.	Waist circumference is an independent risk factor for cardiovascular disease. Normal is ≤40 in (102 cm) for males and ≤35 in (88 cm) for females.
Determine neck circumference by using a tape measure wrapped firmly around the neck just above the larynx.	Neck circumference >17 in (43 cm) for males, and >16 in (40.6 cm) for females may be associated with sleep apnea.

GENERAL APPEARANCE

Technique	Findings
Begin observation on first contact with the patient; continue throughout the interview systematically.	
Inspection	
Observe for: general physical development, nutritional state, mental alertness, affect, evidence of pain, restlessness, body position, clothes, apparent age, hygiene, grooming. Use smell and hearing as well as sight.	Careful observation of the general state of the individual provides many clues about a person's body image, how they behave, and also some idea of how well or ill they are.

SKIN

Technique	Findings
Examine the skin as you proceed through each body system.	
Inspection	
Observe for: skin color, pigmentation, lesions (distribution, type, configuration, size), jaundice, cyanosis, scars, superficial vascularity, hydration, edema, color of mucous membranes, hair distribution, nails.	"Normal" varies considerably depending on racial or ethnic background, exposure to sun, complexion, and pigmentation tendencies (such as freckles). Nails are present and smooth and cared for in some way.
Palpation	
Examine skin for temperature, texture, elasticity, turgor, and superficial tenderness.	The skin is normally warm, slightly moist, and smooth and returns quickly to its original shape when picked up between two fingers and released.

HEAD

Technique	Findings
Inspection	
Observe for: symmetry of face, configuration of skull, hair color and distribution, scalp.	Normally, the skull and face are symmetric, with distribution of hair varying from person to person. (However, determine by history if there has been any change.)
Palpation	
Examine: hair texture, masses, swelling or tenderness of scalp, configuration of skull.	The scalp should be free of flaking, with no signs of nits (small, white louse eggs), lesions, deformities, or tenderness.

(continued)

ADULT PHYSICAL ASSESSMENT (continued)

EYES AND VISION (Figure 1-2)

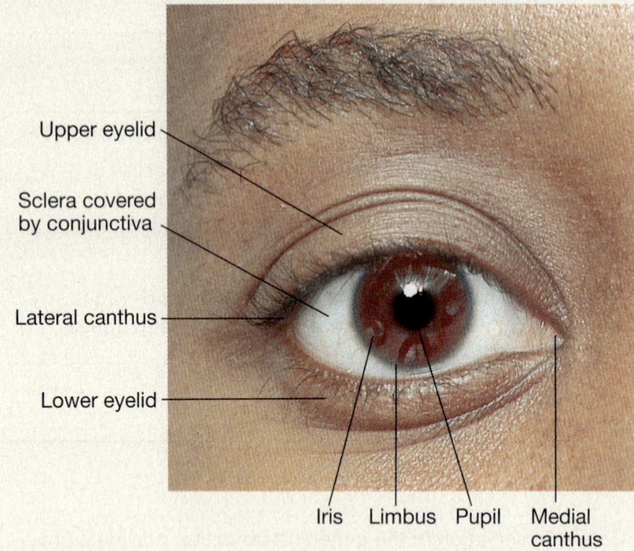

Figure 1-2. Surface anatomy of the eye and eyelids. (Reprinted with permission from Bickley, L. S., Szilagyi, P. G., Hoffman, R. M., & Soriano, R. P. [2024]. *Bates' guide to physical examination and history taking* [13th ed., Fig. 12-1]. Wolters Kluwer).

Technique	Findings
Inspection	
1. Globes (eyeballs)—for protrusion.	
2. Palpebral fissures (oval opening between the upper and lower eyelids)—for width and symmetry.	2. Palpebral fissures—appear equal when eyes open. Normally, upper lid covers small portion of iris and lower lid margin is just below the junction of cornea and sclera (limbus). Ptosis—drooping of the upper eyelid.
3. Lid margins—for scaling, secretions, erythema, position of lashes.	3. Lid margins—clear; the lacrimal duct openings (puncta) are evident at the nasal ends of the upper and lower lids. Eyelashes—normally are evenly distributed and turn outward.
4. Bulbar and palpebral conjunctivae—for congestion and color. Bulbar conjunctiva—membranous covering of the sclera (contains blood vessels). Palpebral conjunctiva—membranous covering of the inside of the upper and lower lids (contains blood vessels).	4. Bulbar conjunctiva—normally, transparent blood vessels may become dilated and produce the characteristic "bloodshot" eye. Palpebral conjunctivae—pink and clear. Conjunctivitis—inflammation of the conjunctival surfaces.
5. Sclerae and iris—for color.	5. Sclerae—should be white and clear.
6. Pupils—for size, shape, symmetry, reaction to light and accommodation (ability of the lens to adjust to objects at varying distances).	6. Pupils—normally constrict with increasing light and accommodation. Pupils are normally round and can range in size from very small ("pinpoint") to large (occupying the entire space of the iris).
7. Eye movement—(Also see neurologic system, p. 29.) a. Extraocular movements—movement of the eyes in conjugate fashion b. Convergence—the eyes turn inward toward each other when focusing on a near object c. Nystagmus—rapid oscillation of the eyes horizontally, vertically, or in a rotary pattern	7. a. Deviation of one eye from the expected position may indicate eye muscle paralysis or hereditary strabismus. b. Inability of the eyes to follow an object to within 5–8 cm of the nose may occur with eye muscle weakness or hyperthyroidism. c. Nystagmus—may be seen briefly on lateral movement as a result of eye fatigue; however, vertical nystagmus or prolonged nystagmus may occur in a variety of neurologic or inner ear disorders.
8. Gross visual fields—by confrontation. (See neurologic system, p. 29.)	8. Peripheral vision—is full (medially and laterally, superiorly and inferiorly) in both eyes.

ADULT PHYSICAL ASSESSMENT *(continued)*

Technique	Findings
9. Visual acuity—check with a Snellen chart for distance vision and a handheld card (Jaeger chart) for near vision (with and without glasses).	9. Normal vision—20/20. Myopia—nearsightedness (reduced distance vision; i.e., 20/30, 20/40, etc.). Hyperopia (presbyopia)—farsightedness (reduced near vision).
Palpation	
1. Determine the strength of the upper lids by attempting to open closed lids against resistance.	1. The examiner should not be able to open the lids when the patient is squeezing them shut.
2. Palpate globes through closed lids for tenderness and tension.	2. Globes normally are not tender when palpated.

EARS AND HEARING

Technique	Findings
Inspection	
1. Pinna—examine for size, shape, color, symmetry, lesions, and masses.	
2. External canal—examine with a flashlight or otoscope for discharge, impacted cerumen, inflammation, masses, or foreign bodies.	2. External canal—is normally clear with perhaps minimal cerumen.
Palpation	
1. Examine all parts of the external ear for tenderness, consistency of cartilage, warmth, and swelling. a. Pinna—outer ear. b. Tragus—cartilage anterior to ear canal. c. Mastoid process—bony area behind the ear.	1. Pain with manipulation of the pinna or pressure on the tragus may indicate external otitis. Tenderness of the mastoid process may indicate extension of middle ear infection.
Otoscopic Examination	
Advanced assessment technique, which visualizes the entire external canal and tympanic membrane.	
Mechanical tests	
1. Test each ear for gross hearing acuity using the whisper test. Ask the patient to occlude the ear not being tested by placing pressure on the tragus, while you stand at arm's length away and slightly behind the patient, facing the ear being tested. After exhaling to lower your voice, whisper two syllables, such as nine-four.	1. A person with normal hearing can accurately hear three out of six whispered word combinations. Failure requires audiometry for further testing.
2. Weber test—test for lateralization of vibration. Tap the tuning fork against your hand to make it vibrate. Then, place the tuning fork in the center of the scalp near the forehead (see Figure 1-3). (Also see Chapter 13.)	2. Sound should be heard equally in both ears.

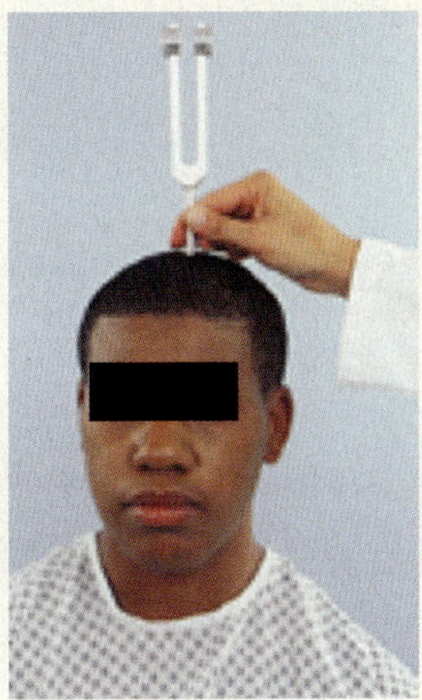

Figure 1-3. The Weber test. (Reprinted with permission from Weber, J., & Kelley, J. [2009]. *Health assessment in nursing* [4th ed.]. Lippincott Williams & Wilkins. Photographs by Barbara Proud.)

(continued)

ADULT PHYSICAL ASSESSMENT (continued)

3. Rinne test—compares air and bone conduction.
   a. Place the vibrating tuning fork on the mastoid process behind each ear and have the patient tell you when the vibration stops (see Figure 1-4, first part).
   b. Then, quickly hold the buzzing end of the tuning fork near the ear canal and ask if patient can hear it (see Figure 1-4, second part).

3. Sound should be heard after vibration can no longer be felt; that is, air conduction is greater than bone conduction. Lateralization and conduction findings are altered by damage to the cranial nerve VIII and damage to the ossicles in the middle ear.

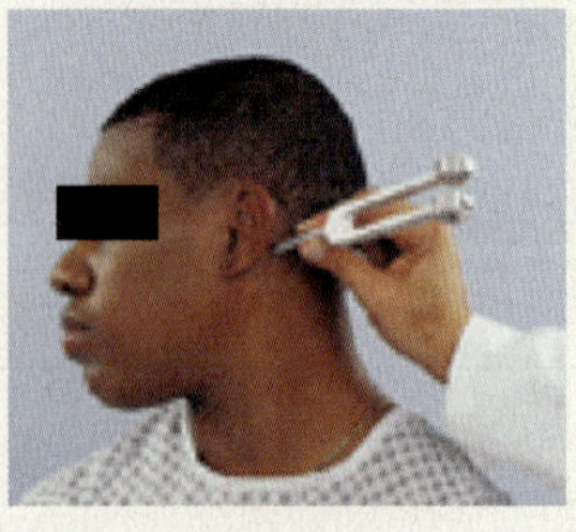

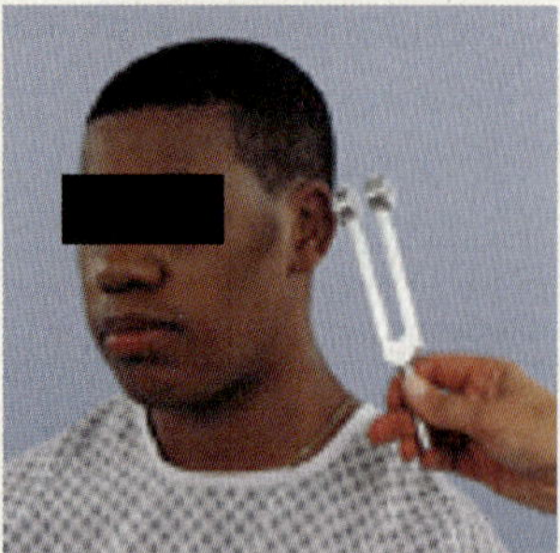

Figure 1-4. The Rinne test. (Reprinted with permission from Weber, J., & Kelley, J. [2009]. *Health assessment in nursing* [4th ed.]. Lippincott Williams & Wilkins. Photographs by Barbara Proud.)

NOSE AND SINUSES

Technique	Findings
Inspection	
1. Observe for general deformity.	1. External features vary but are generally symmetrical.
2. With nasal speculum or otoscope, examine for:	
a. Nasal septum (position and perforation)	a. Nasal septum—is normally straight and not perforated.
b. Discharge (anteriorly and posteriorly)	b. Discharge—none should be present.
c. Nasal obstruction and airway patency	c. Airways—are patent.
d. Mucous membranes for color	d. Mucous membranes—are normally pink.
e. Turbinates for color and swelling (see Figure 1-5)	e. Turbinates—three bony projections on each lateral wall of the nasal cavity covered with well-vascularized, mucous-secreting membranes. They warm the air going into the lungs and may become swollen and pale with colds and allergies.

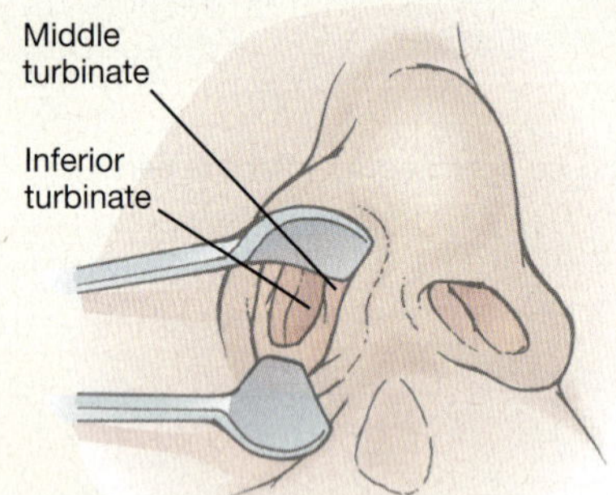

Figure 1-5. Normal internal nose. (Reprinted with permission from Weber, J., & Kelley, J. [2022]. *Health assessment in nursing* [7th ed., Fig. 18-19]. Wolters Kluwer.)

Technique	Findings
Palpation	
Sinuses (frontal and maxillary)—for tenderness (see Figure 1-6).	The patient may identify pressure, but pain or tenderness may indicate sinusitis.
Frontal—direct manual pressure upward toward the wall of the sinus. Avoid pressure on eyes.	
Maxillary—with thumbs, direct pressure upward over lower edge of maxillary bones.	

ADULT PHYSICAL ASSESSMENT *(continued)*

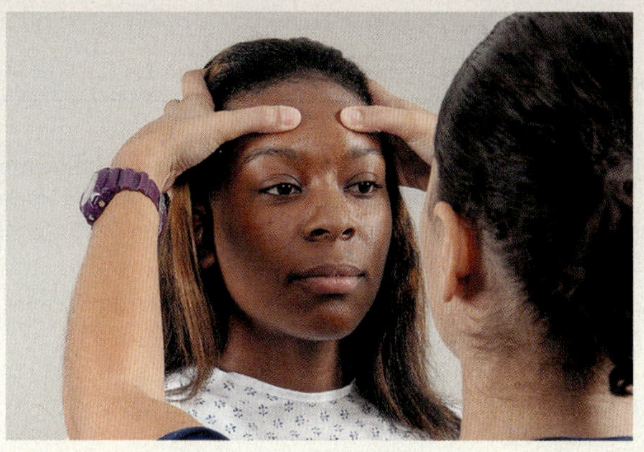
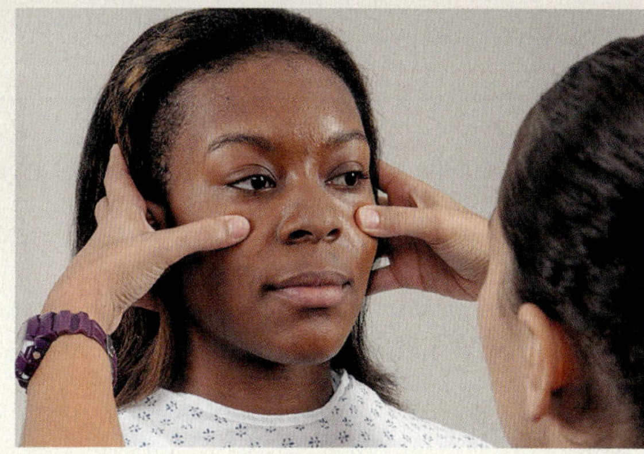

Figure 1-6. Tenderness of sinuses may indicate sinusitis. (Reprinted with permission from Weber, J., & Kelley, J. [2022]. *Health assessment in nursing* [7th ed., Figs. 18-21 and 18-22] Wolters Kluwer.)

MOUTH

Technique	Findings
Inspection	
1. Observe lips for color, moisture, pigment, masses, ulcerations, fissures.	
2. Use tongue blade and penlight to examine:	
a. Teeth—number, arrangement, general condition.	a. Teeth—an adult normally has 32 teeth.
b. Gums—for color, texture, discharge, swelling, retraction.	b. Gums—commonly recede in adults. Bleeding is fairly common and may result from trauma, gingival disease, or systemic problems (less common).
c. Buccal mucosa—for discoloration, vesicles, ulcers, masses.	c. Buccal mucosa and pharynx are pink to reddish brown with some color variation.
d. Pharynx—for inflammation, exudate, masses.	d. Color should be pink to reddish without exudate or swelling (see Chapter 13).
e. Tongue (protruded)—for size, color, thickness, lesions, moisture, symmetry, deviations from midline, fasciculations.	e. Tongue—is normally midline and covered with papillae, which vary in size from the tip of the tongue to the back. (The circumvallate papillae are large and posterior.)
f. Salivary glands—for patency.	
i. Parotid glands	i. Parotid glands—open in the buccal pouch at the level of the upper teeth halfway back.
ii. Sublingual and submaxillary glands	ii. Sublingual and submaxillary glands—open underneath the tongue.
g. Uvula—for symmetry when patient says "ah."	g. Uvula—should be midline.
h. Tonsils—for size, ulceration, exudates, inflammation.	h. Lingual tonsils—can often be seen on the posterior portion of the tongue.
i. Breath—for odor.	i. Odor of breath—may indicate dental caries.
j. Voice—for hoarseness.	j. Hoarseness may indicate laryngeal strain, inflammation, infection, or other disorder.
Palpation	
1. Examine the oral cavity with a gloved hand for masses and ulceration. Palpate beneath the tongue and laterally explore the floor of the mouth.	1. Entire oral cavity should be pink and without ulcers, deep-red color, lesions, palpable masses, or swelling. An indurated mass raises the suspicion of malignancy.
2. Grasp the tongue with a gauze sponge to retract it; inspect the sides and undersurface of the tongue and the floor of the mouth.	

(continued)

ADULT PHYSICAL ASSESSMENT (*continued*)

NECK

Technique	Findings
Inspection	
1. Inspect all areas of the neck anteriorly and posteriorly for muscular symmetry, masses, unusual swelling or pulsations, and range of motion.	1. Range of motion—normally, the chin can touch the anterior chest, and the head can be extended at least 45 degrees from the vertical position and can be rotated 90 degrees from midline to side.
2. Thyroid—ask the patient to swallow and observe for movement of an enlarged thyroid gland at the suprasternal notch.	2. Thyroid—is not usually visible, except in extremely thin people.
3. Muscular strength. a. Cervical muscles—have the patient turn their chin forcefully against your hand. b. Trapezius muscles—exert pressure on the patient's shoulders while they shrug the shoulders.	3. Strength—see "Findings, cranial nerve XI," page 30.
Palpation	
1. Palpate the 10 areas for cervical lymph nodes as shown in Figure 1-7.	1. Cervical nodes—in the adult, the cervical lymph nodes are not normally palpable unless the patient is very thin, in which case the nodes are felt as small, freely movable masses. Tender nodes suggest inflammation; hard, fixed nodes suggest malignancy.

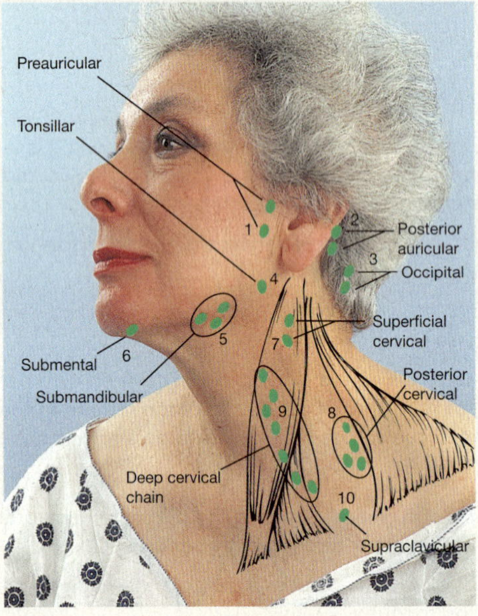

Figure 1-7. Areas for cervical lymph node palpation. (Reprinted with permission form Timby, B. K., & Smith, N. E. [2022]. *Introductory medical-surgical nursing* [13th ed., Fig. 30-9A]. Wolters Kluwer. Photograph by Barbara Proud.)

Technique	Findings
2. Trachea—palpate at the sternal notch. Place one finger along the side of the trachea and note the space between it and the sternomastoid. Compare to the other side.	2. Trachea—should be midline. Spaces measured by fingers should be symmetrical. Tracheal deviation may be caused by neck mass or problems within the chest.

ADULT PHYSICAL ASSESSMENT *(continued)*

3. Thyroid—palpate for size, symmetry, tenderness, and consistency. (See Figure 1-8.)
   a. Stand behind the patient and have them flex the neck slightly to relax the muscles.
   b. Place the fingertips of both hands on either side of the trachea just below the cricoid cartilage. Have the patient swallow and feel for any glandular tissue rising under your fingertips.
   c. Palpate the area over the trachea for the isthmus and laterally for the right and left lobes.
   d. Note any enlargement, nodules, masses, or consistency.

3. If the thyroid is palpable, it is normally smooth, without nodules, masses, or irregularities. Enlargement, asymmetry, tenderness, or nodules require further evaluation.

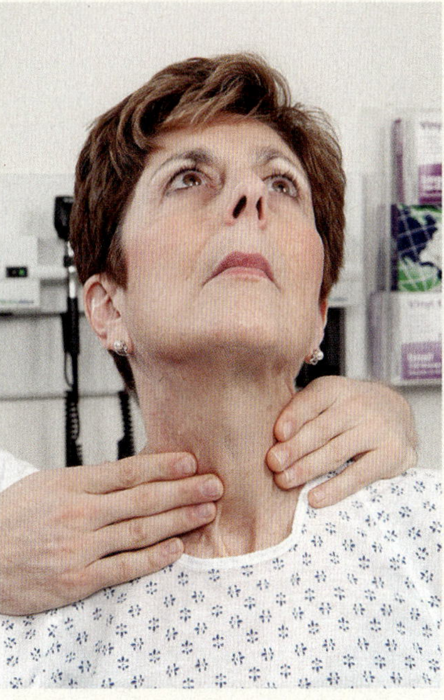

Figure 1-8. Palpating the thyroid gland. (Reprinted with permission from Weber, J., & Kelley, J. [2022]. *Health assessment in nursing* [7th ed., Fig. 15-12]. Wolters Kluwer.)

4. Carotid arteries:
   a. Palpate the carotids one side at a time.
   b. The carotids lie anterolaterally in the neck—avoid palpating the carotid sinuses at the level of the thyroid cartilage just below the angle of the jaw because this may cause slowing of the heart rate.
   c. Note the symmetry of pulsations, strength, and amplitude, as well as any abnormal thrill.

4. A thrill (humming-like vibration) usually indicates arterial narrowing.

Auscultation

1. Use the diaphragm of the stethoscope to listen for bruits (murmur-like sound) over the carotid arteries.

1. A bruit may indicate arterial narrowing with turbulent blood flow. A cardiac murmur may also be referred to the carotid arteries.

LYMPH NODES

Technique	Findings
Additional lymph nodes are examined when the region of the body is examined; for example, the inguinal nodes are inspected when the abdomen is examined.	Lymph nodes are normally not visualized and are nonpalpable, or may be felt as small, nontender, freely movable masses.
Inspection	
Observe size and shape in the expected area.	Lymph nodes are usually not visible unless enlarged or inflamed.

(continued)

ADULT PHYSICAL ASSESSMENT *(continued)*

Palpation

Technique	Findings
1. Supraclavicular and infraclavicular nodes (usually palpated during neck or chest exam). Palpate for size, shape, mobility, consistency, tenderness, and warmth.	1. Supraclavicular and infraclavicular nodes—not normally palpable. Enlargement may indicate a thoracic problem.
2. Axillary nodes (usually done during breast exam). (See Figure 1-9.) a. Examine the patient while they are sitting. b. Place the patient's arm at their side and examine the apex of the patient's axilla. (Use the fingers of your right hand to examine the left axilla and vice versa.) c. Rotate the examining hand so the fingers can palpate the anterior and posterior axillary fossae, pressing against the chest wall. Press against the humerus bone in the axilla to examine the lateral fossa for nodes. Conclude the axillary examination by moving the fingers from the apex of the axilla downward in the midline along the chest wall.	2. Axillary nodes—normally nonpalpable. Enlargement may occur with a breast or arm problem.

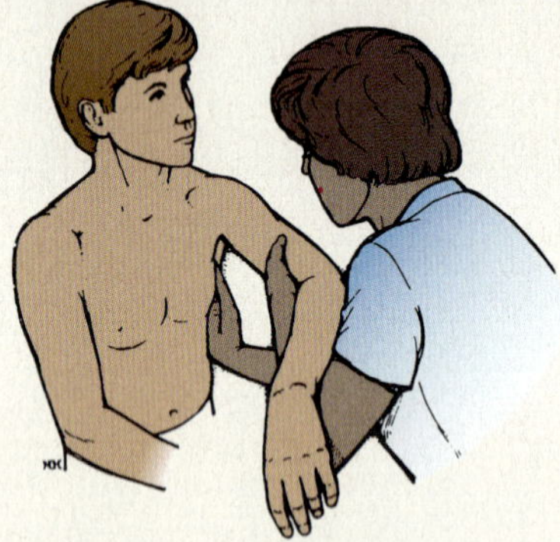

Figure 1-9. Palpating the axillary nodes.

Technique	Findings
3. Inguinal nodes—are located in the groin just below the inguinal ligament and are usually examined when the abdomen is examined.	3. Inguinal nodes—a few may be felt. Enlargement and acute tenderness may indicate a genital or lower extremity problem.
4. Epitrochlear nodes—are palpated just above the medial epicondyle, between the biceps and triceps muscles. (See Figure 1-10.)	4. Epitrochlear nodes—not normally palpable. Enlargement may indicate an arm or systemic problem.

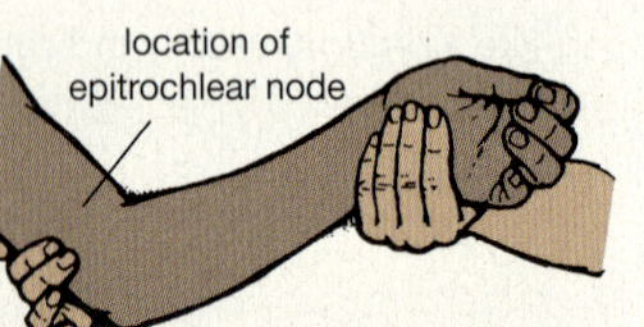

Figure 1-10. Location of epitrochlear node.

BREASTS (MALE AND FEMALE)

Technique	Findings
Female Breast	
Inspection	
(With the patient sitting, arms relaxed at sides.)	
1. Inspect the areolae and nipples for position, pigmentation, inversion, discharge, crusting, and masses. Extra, or supernumerary, nipples may occur normally, most commonly in the anterior axillary region or just below the normal breasts.	1. The *nipples* should be at the same level and protrude slightly. An *inverted nipple* (one that turns inward), if present since puberty, may be normal. A *supernumerary nipple* usually consists of a nipple and a small areola and may be mistaken for a mole.

ADULT PHYSICAL ASSESSMENT (continued)

2. Examine the breast tissue for size, shape, color, symmetry, surface, contour, skin characteristics, and level of breasts. Note any retraction or dimpling of the skin.

2. Breast size—in the female, it is not uncommon to find a difference in the size of the two breasts. Normal asymmetry has usually been present since puberty and is not a recent phenomenon.

3. Ask the patient to elevate hands over head; repeat the observation.

3. If there is a mass attached to the pectoral muscles, contracting the muscles will cause retraction of the breast tissue.

4. Have the patient press hands to hips; repeat the observation.

Palpation

(This is best done with the patient in a recumbent position [see Figure 1-11].)

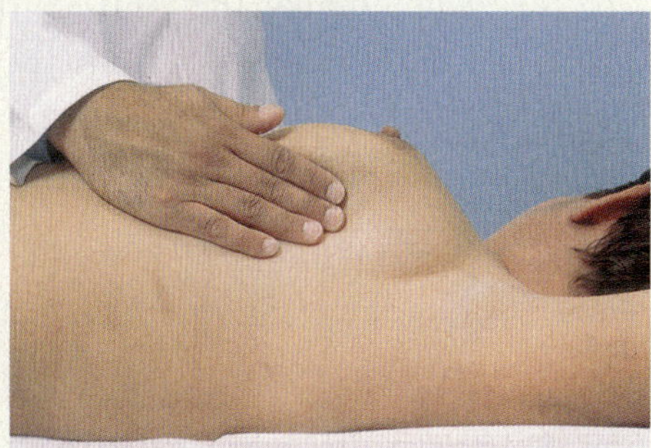

Figure 1-11. Palpating the breast.

1. The patient with pendulous breasts should be given a pillow to place under the ipsilateral scapula of the breast being palpated, so the tissue is distributed more evenly over the chest wall.
2. The arm on the side of the breast being palpated should be raised above the patient's head.
3. Palpate one breast at a time, beginning with the "asymptomatic" breast if the patient complains of symptoms.

3. This allows the examiner to palpate the "normal" breast first and then compare the "symptomatic" breast to it.

4. To palpate, use the palmar aspects of the fingers in a rotating motion, compressing the breast tissue against the chest wall. Don't forget to include the "tail" of the breast tissue, which extends into the axillary region in the upper outer quadrant of the breast.

4. Breast texture—varies according to the amount of subcutaneous tissue present.
   a. In young females, tissue is fairly soft and homogeneous; in females who are postmenopausal, tissue may feel nodular or stringy.
   b. Consistency also varies with menstrual cycle, being more nodular and edematous just prior to menstruation.

5. Note skin texture, moisture, temperature, or masses.

5. Masses—if a mass is palpated, its location, size, shape, consistency, mobility, and associated tenderness are reported.

6. Gently squeeze the nipple and note any expressible discharge.

6. Discharge—in the typical female who is nonpregnant or nonlactating, there is usually no nipple discharge.

7. Repeat the examination on the opposite breast and compare findings.

Male Breast

Examination of the male breast can be brief but may be important.

1. Observe the nipple and areola for ulceration, nodules, swelling, or discharge.

1. There should be no discharge.

2. Palpate the areola for nodules and tenderness.

2. Enlargement of glandular tissue is gynecomastia, related to hormone imbalance.

(continued)

ADULT PHYSICAL ASSESSMENT (continued)

THORAX AND LUNGS

Technique	Findings
Use anatomic landmarks to perform and document assessment of the thorax, keeping in mind the underlying structures of the lungs and heart (see Figures 1-12, 1-13, and 1-14).	

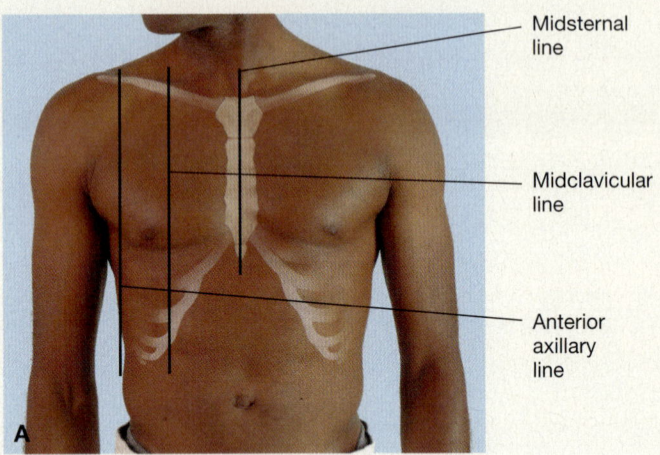

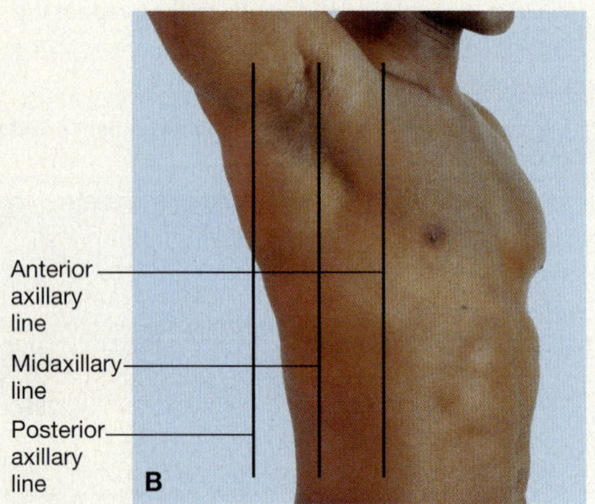

Figure 1-12. Anatomic landmarks of the thorax. **(A)** Midsternal and midclavicular lines. **(B)** Anterior axillary, midaxillary, and posterior axillary lines. (Reprinted with permission from Bickley, L. S., Szilagyi, P. G., Hoffman, R. M., & Soriano, R. P. [2024]. *Bates' guide to physical examination and history taking* [13th ed., Figs. 15-4 and 15-5]. Wolters Kluwer.)

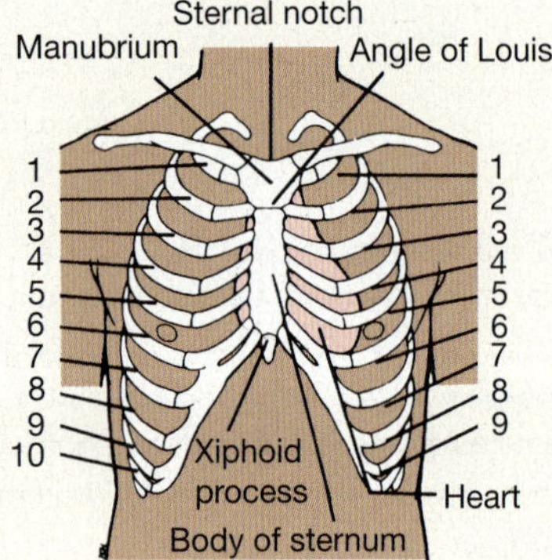

Figure 1-13. Bony thorax, landmarks, and intercostal spaces (anterior).

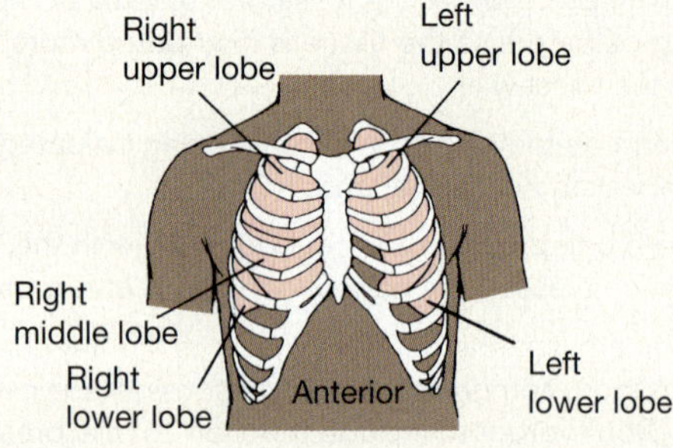

Figure 1-14. Location of lung lobes of anterior thorax.

Posterior Thorax and Lungs

Begin the examination with the patient seated; examine posterior chest and lungs.

Inspection

Technique	Findings
1. Inspect the spine for mobility and any structural deformity.	
2. Observe the symmetry of the posterior chest and the posture and mobility of the thorax on respiration. Note any bulges or retractions of the costal interspaces on respiration or any impairment of respiratory movement.	2. The thorax is normally symmetric; it moves easily and without impairment on respiration. There are no bulges or retractions of the intercostal spaces, which may indicate respiratory distress.
3. Note the anteroposterior diameter in relation to the lateral diameter of the chest.	3. The anteroposterior diameter of the thorax in relation to the lateral diameter is approximately 1:2.

ADULT PHYSICAL ASSESSMENT (*continued*)

Palpation

1. Palpate the posterior chest with the patient sitting; identify areas of tenderness, masses, and inflammation.
2. Palpate the ribs and costal margins for symmetry, mobility, and tenderness and the spine for tenderness and vertebral position. See Figure 1-15.

2. On palpation, there should be no tenderness; chest movement should be symmetric and without lag or impairment. Tenderness may indicate musculoskeletal strain, fracture, or other problems.

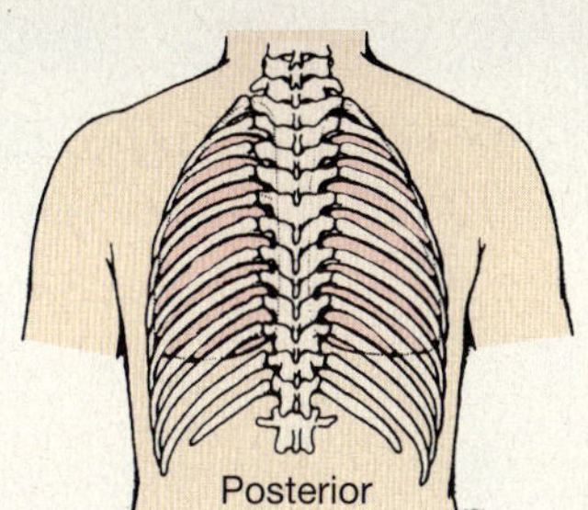

Figure 1-15. Bony thorax (posterior).

3. To assess respiratory expansion, place thumbs at the level of the 10th vertebra. With hands held parallel to the 10th ribs as they grasp the lateral rib cage, ask the patient to inhale deeply and observe movement of the thumbs.

3. Thumbs should move apart and hands move symmetrically with normal expansion.

4. To elicit tactile *fremitus* (palpable vibrations transmitted through the bronchopulmonary system on speaking):
   a. Ask the patient to say "99"; palpate and compare symmetric areas of the lungs with the ball of one hand. Begin at the upper lobes and move downward.
   b. Note any areas of increased or decreased fremitus.
   c. If fremitus is faint, ask the patient to speak louder and in a deeper voice.

4. Posteriorly, fremitus is generally equal throughout the lung fields. It may be increased near the large bronchi because of consolidation of tissue resulting from pneumonia. It may be decreased or absent anteriorly and posteriorly when vocal loudness is decreased, when posture is not erect, or when excessive tissue or underlying structures are present or in cases of pneumothorax and other pathology.

Percussion

As with palpation, the posterior chest is optimally percussed with the patient sitting. Refer to Figure 1-16.

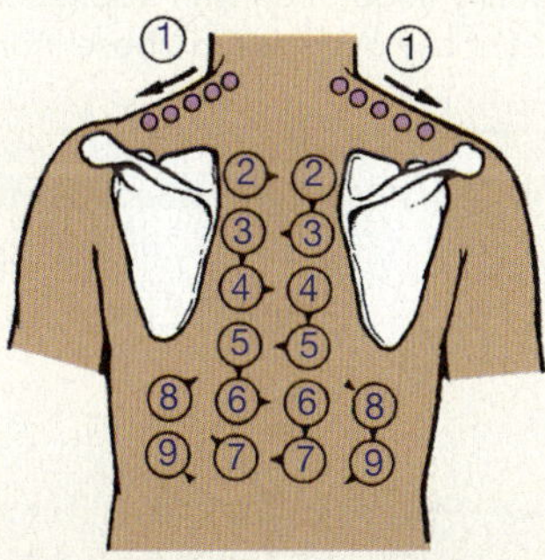

Figure 1-16. Percussion of the posterior chest.

1. Percuss symmetric areas, comparing sides.

1. Percussion normally reveals resonance over symmetric areas of the lung. Percussion sound may be altered by poor posture or the presence of excessive tissue.

2. Begin across the top of each shoulder and proceed down between the scapulae and then under the scapulae, both medially and laterally in the axillary lines.
3. Note and localize any abnormal percussion sound.

3. Dullness may indicate mass or consolidation because of pneumonia.

(*continued*)

ADULT PHYSICAL ASSESSMENT (*continued*)

4. For diaphragmatic excursion, percuss by placing the pleximeter (stationary) finger parallel to the approximate level of the diaphragm below the right scapula. (See Figure 1-17.)
   a. Ask the patient to inhale deeply and hold their breath; percuss downward to the point of dullness. Mark this point.
   b. Let the patient breathe normally, and then, ask patient to exhale deeply; percuss upward from the mark to the point of resonance.
   c. Mark this point and measure between the two marks—normally 2–2½ in (5–6 cm).
   d. Repeat this procedure on the opposite side of the chest.

4. The lower border of the lungs is approximately at the level of the 10th thoracic spinous process on normal respiration. Unilateral abnormality of decreased excursion may indicate pleural effusion, atelectasis, or paralysis of one side of the diaphragm.

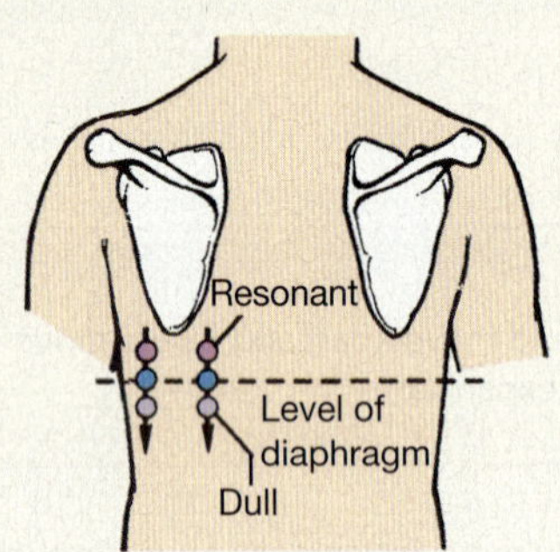

Figure 1-17. Diaphragmatic excursion.

Auscultation

Aids in assessing airflow through the lungs, the presence of fluid or mucus, and the condition of the surrounding pleural space.

1. Have the patient sit erect. (If the patient is unable to sit without assistance for examination of the posterior chest and lungs, position them first on one side and then on the other as you examine the lung fields.)
2. With a stethoscope, listen to the lungs as the patient breathes more deeply than normally with the mouth open. (Let the patient pause, as needed, to avoid hyperventilation.)
3. Place the stethoscope in the same areas on the chest wall as those percussed, and listen to a complete inspiration and expiration in each area.
4. Compare symmetric areas methodically from the apex to the lung bases.
5. It should be possible to distinguish three types of normal breath sounds as indicated in the following table.

On auscultation, breath sounds vary according to proximity of the large bronchi.

- They are louder and coarser near the large bronchi and over the anterior.
- They are softer and much finer (vesicular) at the periphery over the alveolae.

Breath sounds also vary in duration with inspiration and expiration. Sounds may normally decrease in obese individuals.

5. Pathology will alter the normal bronchial, bronchovesicular, and vesicular breath sounds. Adventitious sounds include crackles, wheezes, and rhonchi.

Auscultation Location	Type of Breath Sound	Intensity	Pitch	Other Characteristic
Anterior neck, over the trachea	Tracheal	Very loud	High	Tubular quality; length of inspiration equals expiration.
Manubrium (larger proximal airways)	Bronchial	Loud	High	Hollow quality; length of expiration is greater than inspiration.
1st and 2nd intercostal spaces anterior and between the scapulae posterior	Bronchovesicular	Medium	Medium	Length of inspiration equals expiration.
Lobes of the lungs	Vesicular	Soft	Low	Rustling quality; length of inspiration equals expiration.

ADULT PHYSICAL ASSESSMENT *(continued)*

Technique	Findings
Anterior Thorax and Lungs	
The patient should be recumbent with arms at sides and slightly abducted.	
Inspection	
1. Inspect the chest for any structural deformity.	
2. Note the width of the costal angle.	2. The angle at the tip of the sternum is determined by the right and left rib margins at the xiphoid process. Normally, the angle is less than 90 degrees.
3. Observe the rate and rhythm of breathing, any bulging or retraction of intercostal spaces on respiration, and use of accessory muscles of respiration (sternocleidomastoid and trapezius on inspiration and abdominal muscles on expiration).	3. There are no bulges or retractions of the intercostal spaces.
4. Note any asymmetry of chest wall movement on respiration.	4. The thorax is normally symmetric and moves easily without impairment on respiration.
Palpation	
1. To assess expansion, place your hands along the costal margins and note symmetry and degree of expansion as the patient inhales deeply.	1. Hands should separate slightly on inspiration.
2. Palpate for tactile fremitus with the ball of the hand anteriorly and laterally. (Underlying structures [heart, liver] may damp, or decrease, fremitus.)	2. Vibration should be felt somewhat symmetrically. It may be necessary to displace the female breast gently.
Percussion	
1. With patient's arms resting comfortably at sides, percuss the anterior and lateral chest (see Figure 1-18). Begin just below the clavicles and percuss downward from one interspace to the next, comparing the sound from the interspace on one side with that of the contralateral interspace.	1. Resonance is heard over most of the lungs.

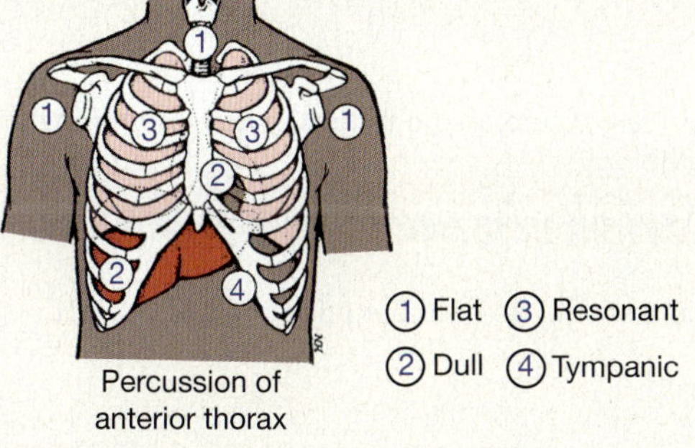

Figure 1-18. Percussion of the anterior and lateral chest.

Technique	Findings
2. Displace the female breast so breast tissue does not damp the vibration. Continue downward, noting the intercostal space where hepatic dullness is percussed on the right and cardiac dullness on the left.	2. A tympanic sound is produced over the gastric air bubble on the left somewhat lower than the point of liver dullness on the right.
3. Note the effect of underlying structures.	3. Percussion over heart will produce a dull sound. The upper border of the liver will be percussed on the right side, producing a dull note.
Auscultation	
Listen to the chest anteriorly and laterally for air flow and any abnormal or adventitious sounds.	Similar airflow should be heard bilaterally, except, perhaps, over the heart.

(continued)

ADULT PHYSICAL ASSESSMENT (continued)

HEART

Technique	Findings
1. Landmarks in relation to the sternum and the ribs are used during examination to yield the most information about function of the heart and its valves (see Figure 1-19).	

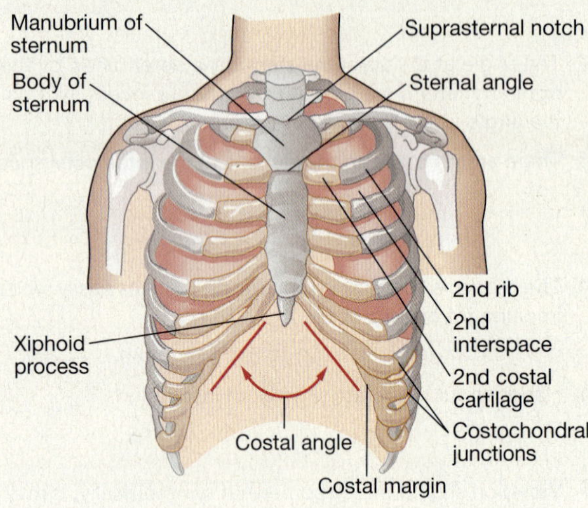

Figure 1-19. Landmarks used when assessing the heart.

a. In locating the intercostal spaces, begin by identifying the angle of Louis, which is felt as a slight ridge approximately 1 in (2.5 cm) below the sternal notch, where the manubrium and the body of the sternum are joined.

b. The 2nd ribs extend to the right and left of this angle.

c. Once the 2nd rib is located, palpate downward and obliquely away from the sternum to identify the remaining ribs and intercostal spaces.

Inspection

Technique	Findings
1. Inspect the precordium for any bulging, heaving, or thrusting.	1. Normally, there are no bulges or heaves; these indicate pathology.
2. Look for the apical impulse in the 5th or 6th intercostal space at or just medial to the midclavicular line.	2. An apical impulse may or may not be observable.
3. Note any other pulsations. Tangential lighting is most helpful in detecting pulsations.	3. There should be no other pulsations.

Palpation

Technique	Findings
1. Use the ball of the hand to detect vibrations, or "thrills," which may be caused by murmurs. (Use the fingertips or palmar surface to detect pulsations.)	1. There should be no thrills or other pulsations. (Thrills are vibrations caused by turbulence of blood moving through valves that are transmitted through the skin, which feels similar to a purring cat.)
2. Proceed methodically through the examination so no area is omitted. Palpate for thrills and pulsations in each area (aortic, pulmonic, tricuspid, mitral).	
a. Begin in the aortic area (2nd right intercostal space, close to the sternum) and proceed to the pulmonic area (2nd left intercostal space) and then downward to the apex of the heart. (The mitral area is considered the apex of the heart.)	
b. In the tricuspid area, use the palm of the hand to detect any heaving or thrusting of the precordium (tricuspid area—5th intercostal space next to the sternum).	Ordinarily, no heaving of the ventricle is felt except, possibly, in the pregnant person.

ADULT PHYSICAL ASSESSMENT *(continued)*

c. In the mitral area (5th intercostal space, at or just medial to the midclavicular line), palpate for the apical beat; identify the point of maximal impulse (PMI) and note its size and force.

The apical pulse should be felt approximately in the 5th intercostal space, at or just medial to the midclavicular line. In a young, thin person, it is a sharp, quick impulse no larger than the intercostal space. In an older person, the impulse may be less sharp and quick. An apical impulse displaced laterally may indicate left ventricular hypertrophy.

Auscultation

1. Place the stethoscope in the pulmonic or aortic area (see Figure 1-20).

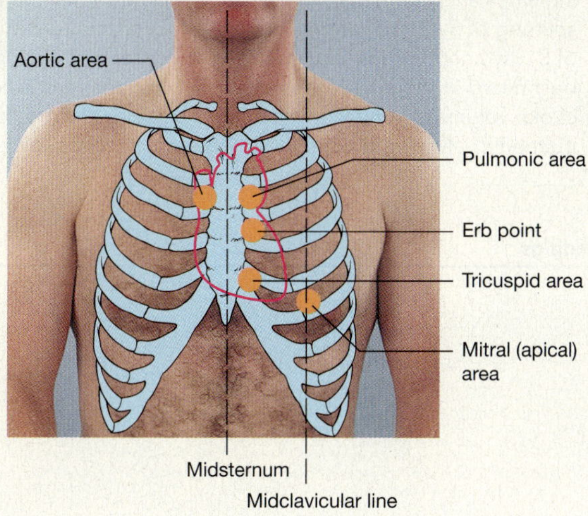

Figure 1-20. Areas of auscultation.

2. Begin by identifying the first (S_1) and second (S_2) heart sounds.
   a. S_1 is caused by the closing of the tricuspid and mitral valves.
   b. S_2 results from the closing of the aortic and pulmonic valves.

2. The two sounds are separated by a short systolic interval; each pair of sounds is separated from the next pair by a longer, diastolic interval. Normally, two sounds are heard—"lub, dub." (See Figure 1-21.)
   - In the aortic and pulmonic areas, S_2 is usually louder than S_1. In this way, each of the paired sounds can be distinguished from the other.
   - In the tricuspid area, S_1 and S_2 are of almost equal intensity and, in the mitral area, S_1 is often slightly louder than S_2.

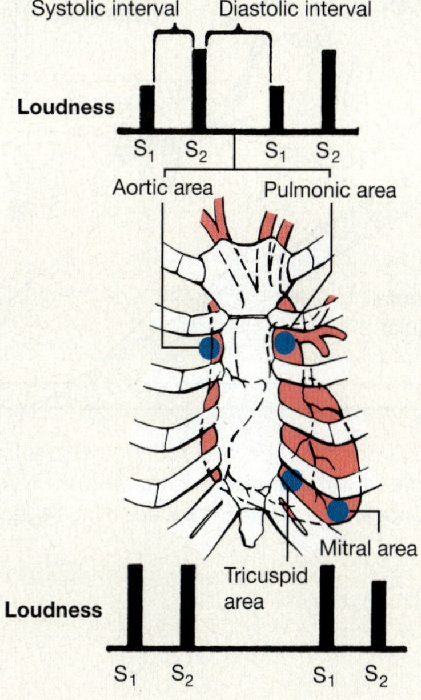

Figure 1-21. Identifying heart sounds.

(continued)

ADULT PHYSICAL ASSESSMENT (*continued*)

Technique	Findings
3. Once the heart sounds are identified, count the rate and note the rhythm as discussed under vital signs. If there is an irregularity, try to determine whether there is any pattern to the irregularity in relation to the intervals, heart sounds, or respirations.	3. Normally, the heart sounds are regular, with a rate of 60–80 beats/min (in the adult). In the athlete or jogger, the resting pulse may be between 40 and 60 beats/min.
4. Once rate and rhythm are determined, listen in each of the four areas and at Erb point (3rd left interspace, close to the sternum) systematically, first with the diaphragm (detects higher-pitched sounds) and then with the bell (detects lower-pitched sounds). In each area, listen to S_1 and then to S_2 for intensity and splitting.	4. An extra "woosh" sound between S_1 and S_2 indicates systolic murmur; between S_2 and S_1 indicates a diastolic murmur. Note the area of its greatest intensity (aortic, pulmonic, mitral, tricuspid). An extra sound of short duration usually indicates an S_3 or S_4 gallop. Occasionally, there may be a splitting of S_2 in the pulmonic area. This is normal. Splitting of S_2 (two contiguous sounds are heard instead of one) is best heard at the end of inspiration, when right ventricular stroke volume is sufficiently increased to delay closure of the pulmonic valve *slightly* behind closure of the aortic valve.

PERIPHERAL CIRCULATION

Technique	Findings
Jugular Veins	
Evaluation of jugular venous distention is most useful in patients with suspected compromise of cardiac function.	
Inspection	
1. Inspect neck for internal jugular venous pulsations (they differ from carotid pulsations in that they are rarely palpable, they can be obliterated by light pressure, and they vary with position).	
2. Note the highest point at which pulsations are seen and measure the vertical line between the point and the sternal angle. With the head raised 30 degrees, the internal jugular venous pulsations should not be visible more than 1 in (2.5 cm) above the sternal angle. (Refer to Figure 1-22.)	2. Increased level of internal jugular pulsations indicates right heart failure.

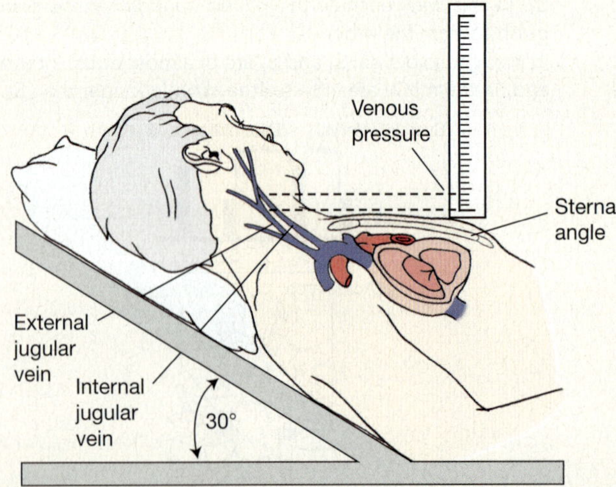

Figure 1-22. Inspecting the neck for internal jugular venous pulsations. (Reprinted with permission from Morton, P. G., & Fontaine, D. K. [2024]. *Critical care nursing* [12th ed., Fig. 14-2]. Wolters Kluwer.)

ADULT PHYSICAL ASSESSMENT *(continued)*

Extremities

Inspection

1. Observe skin over extremities for color, hair distribution, pallor, rubor, and swelling.

1. Extremities should be symmetrically even in color, warmth, and moisture, without swelling. Swelling of feet may occur after prolonged standing or sitting but will disappear when extremity is elevated (dependent edema).

2. Inspect for any visible vessels.

2. Faint veins may be visible, but tortuous and bulging veins may be abnormal.

Palpation

1. Note the temperature of the skin over extremities, comparing one side to the other.

1. Temperature varies but should not be very warm or very cool.

2. Palpate pulses (radial, femoral, posterior tibial [see Figure 1-23], dorsalis pedis [see Figure 1-24]), comparing symmetry from side to side.

2. Absence of peripheral pulses indicates peripheral vascular disease.

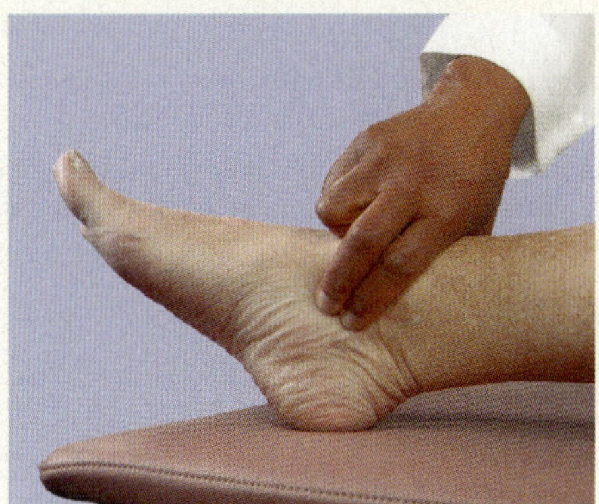

Figure 1-23. Palpating the posterior tibial pulse. (Reprinted with permission from Bickley, L. S., Szilagyi, P. G., Hoffman, R. M., & Soriano, R. P. [2024]. *Bates' guide to physical examination and history taking* [13th ed., Fig. 17-23]. Wolters Kluwer.)

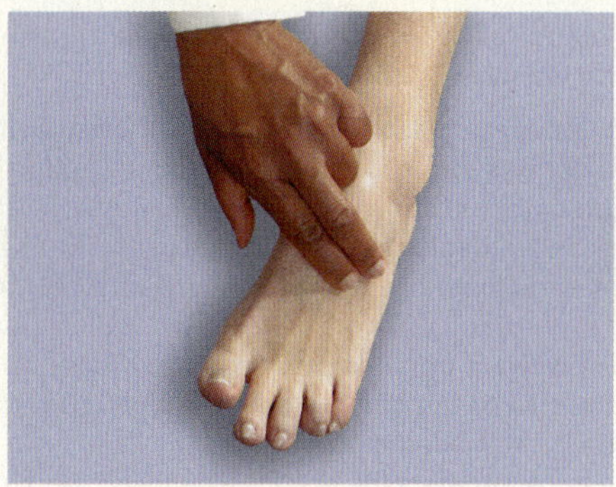

Figure 1-24. Palpating the dorsalis pedis pulse. (Reprinted with permission from Bickley, L. S., Szilagyi, P. G., Hoffman, R. M., & Soriano, R. P. [2024]. *Bates' guide to physical examination and history taking* [13th ed., Fig. 17-22]. Wolters Kluwer.)

3. Palpate the skin over the tibia for edema by applying pressure on the skin for 30–60 sec and note any indentation. If indentation is noted, repeat the procedure, moving up the extremity, and note the point at which no more swelling is present.

3. Edema is usually graded from trace to 4+ pitting. Trace is a slight indentation that disappears in a short time. Grade 3+ or 4+ is deep pitting that does not disappear readily.

ABDOMEN

1. Make sure the patient has an empty bladder and is lying comfortably with arms at sides. Bend the knees to help relax the abdominal muscles if necessary.
2. Expose the abdomen fully. Make sure your hands and the stethoscope diaphragm are warm.
3. Be methodical in visualizing the underlying organs as you inspect, auscultate, percuss, and palpate each quadrant or region of the abdomen (see Figure 1-25).

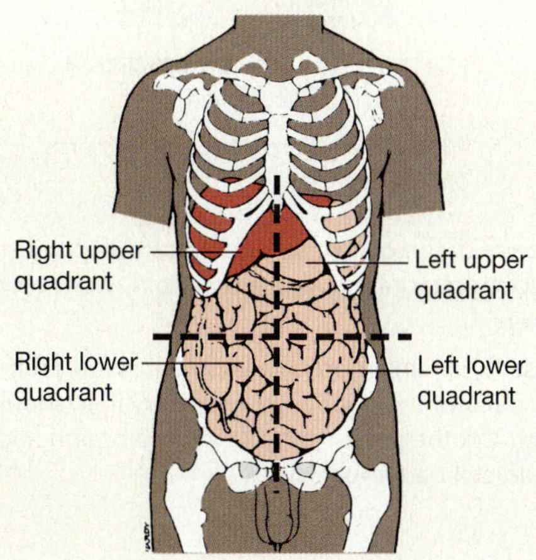

Figure 1-25. The quadrants of the abdomen.

(continued)

ADULT PHYSICAL ASSESSMENT *(continued)*

Inspection

1. Observe the general contour of the abdomen (flat, protuberant, scaphoid, or concave; local bulges). Also, note symmetry, visible peristalsis, and aortic pulsations.
2. Check the umbilicus for contour or hernia and the skin for rashes, striae, and scars.

1. The abdomen may or may not have any scars and should be flat or slightly rounded in the person who is not obese. Slight pulsation may be noted.

Auscultation

1. This is done before percussion and palpation because palpation may alter the character of bowel sounds.
2. Note the frequency and character of bowel sounds (pitch, duration).
3. Listen over the aorta, renal arteries (upper quadrants), and iliac arteries (lower quadrants) for bruits.

2. Anywhere from 5 to 35 bowel sounds per minute may have familiar sound of "growling."
3. Bruits indicate arterial narrowing.

Percussion

1. Percussion provides a general orientation to the abdomen.
2. Proceed methodically from quadrant to quadrant, noting tympany and dullness.
3. In the right upper quadrant (RUQ) in the midclavicular line, percuss the borders of the liver. (Refer to Figure 1-26.)
   a. Begin at a point of tympany in the midclavicular line of the right lower quadrant (RLQ) and percuss upward to the point of dullness (the lower liver border); mark the point.
   b. Percuss downward from the point of lung resonance above the RUQ to the point of dullness (the upper border of the liver); mark the point.
   c. Measure in centimeters the distance between the two marks in the midclavicular line (the liver span).

2. Tympany usually predominates, possibly with scattered areas of dullness because of fluid and feces.
3. Percussion of the liver should help guide subsequent palpation. The liver border in the midclavicular line should normally range from 2½ to 4½ in (6–11 cm).

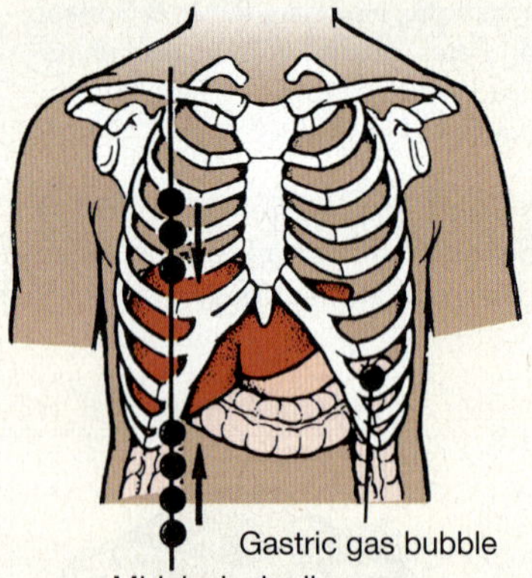

Figure 1-26. Percussing the borders of the liver.

4. Tympany of the gastric air bubble can be percussed in the left upper quadrant over the anterior lower border of the rib cage.
5. Assess for an enlarged spleen by percussing the lowest interspace of the right anterior axillary line (should be tympanic). Ask the patient to take a deep breath and repeat (should still be tympanic).

5. Change in percussion note to dullness on inspiration indicates an enlarged spleen.

ADULT PHYSICAL ASSESSMENT *(continued)*

Palpation

1. Perform light palpation in an organized manner to detect any muscular resistance (guarding), tenderness, or superficial organs or masses.
   1. Tenderness and involuntary guarding indicate peritoneal inflammation.
2. Perform deep palpation to determine location, size, shape, consistency, tenderness, pulsations, and mobility of underlying organs and masses.
   2. Rebound tenderness (pain on quick withdrawal of the fingers following palpation) suggests peritoneal irritation, as in acute appendicitis.
3. Move slowly and gently from one quadrant to the next to relax and reassure the patient.
   3. Palpate painful areas last.
4. Use two hands if the abdomen is obese or muscular, with one hand on top of the other. The upper hand exerts pressure downward, whereas the lower hand feels the abdomen.

Liver

1. Palpate the liver by placing the left hand under the patient's lower right rib cage and the right hand on the abdomen below the level of liver dullness. Press gently inward and upward with your fingertips while the patient takes a deep breath.
   1. A normal liver edge may be palpable as a smooth, sharp, regular surface. An enlarged liver will be palpable and may be tender, hard, or irregular.

Spleen

1. Place your left hand around and under the patient's left lower rib cage and press your right hand below the left costal margin inward toward the spleen while the patient takes a deep breath.
   1. A normal spleen is usually not palpable. Be sure to start low enough so as not to miss the border of an enlarged spleen.

Kidney

1. Next, palpate for the left and right kidneys.
   1. The kidney is usually felt only in people with very relaxed abdominal muscles (the very young, the aged, and multiparous females). The right kidney is slightly lower than the left.
   a. Place the left hand under the patient's back between the rib cage and the iliac crest.
   b. Support the patient while you palpate the abdomen with the right palmar surface of the fingers facing the left side of the body.
   c. Palpate by bringing the left and right hands together as much as possible slightly below the level of the umbilicus on the right and left.
   d. If the kidney is felt, describe its size and shape and note any tenderness.
      d. The kidney is felt as a solid, firm, smooth elastic mass.
2. Costal vertebral angle tenderness is palpated with the patient sitting, usually during the examination of the posterior chest. Locate the costal vertebral angle in the flank region and strike firmly with the ulnar surface of your hand. Note any tenderness over the area.
   2. There should be no costal vertebral angle tenderness. If found, it may indicate kidney infection.

Aorta

1. Palpate for the aorta with the thumb and index finger.
   1. The aorta is soft and pulsatile.
2. Press deeply in the epigastric region (roughly in the midline) and feel with the fingers for pulsations, as well as for the contour of the aorta.

Other Findings

1. Palpation of the RLQ may reveal the part of the bowel called the *cecum*.
   1. The cecum will be soft.
2. The sigmoid colon may be palpated in the lower left quadrant.
   2. The sigmoid colon is ropelike and vertical and, if filled with feces, may be quite firm.
3. The inguinal and femoral areas should be palpated bilaterally for lymph nodes.
   3. Often, small inguinal nodes are present; they are nontender, freely movable, and firm.

(continued)

ADULT PHYSICAL ASSESSMENT *(continued)*

MALE GENITALIA AND HERNIAS

This part of the examination requires wearing gloves and is best done with the patient standing. (A hernia is the protrusion of a portion of the intestine through an abnormal opening.)

Inspection

1. With the groin and genitalia exposed, inspect the pubic hair distribution and the skin of the penis.
2. Retract the foreskin, if present.

   2. The foreskin of the penis, if present, should be easily retractable.
3. Observe the glans penis and the urethral meatus. Note any ulcers, masses, or scars.

   3. The skin of the glans penis is smooth, without ulceration.
4. Note the location of the urethral meatus and any discharge.

   4. The urethral meatus normally is located ventrally on the end of the penis. Normally, there is no discharge from the urethra.
5. Observe the skin of the scrotum for ulcers, masses, redness, or swelling. Note size, contour, and symmetry. Lift the scrotum to inspect the posterior surface.

   5. The scrotum descends approximately 1½ in (4 cm) in the adult; the left side is often larger than the right side.
6. Inspect the inguinal areas and groin for bulges (with and without the patient bearing down, as though having a bowel movement).

Palpation

1. Palpate any lesions, nodules, or masses, noting tenderness, contour, size, and induration. Palpate the shaft of the penis for any induration (firmness in relation to surrounding tissues).

   1. There should be no nodules or tenderness.
2. Palpate each testis and epididymis separately between the thumb and first two fingers, noting size, shape, consistency, and undue tenderness (pressure on the testis normally produces pain).

   2. The testes are usually rubbery and of approximately equal size. The epididymis is located posterolaterally on each testis and is most easily palpable on the superior portion of the testis.
3. Palpate the spermatic cord, including the vas deferens within the cord, from the testis to the inguinal ring.

   3. There should be no nodules or tenderness.
4. Palpate for inguinal hernias, using the left hand to examine the patient's left side and the right hand to examine the patient's right side.

   4. Normally, there is no palpable herniating mass in the inguinal area.

   a. Insert the right index finger laterally, invaginating the scrotal sac to the external inguinal ring (see Figure 1-27).

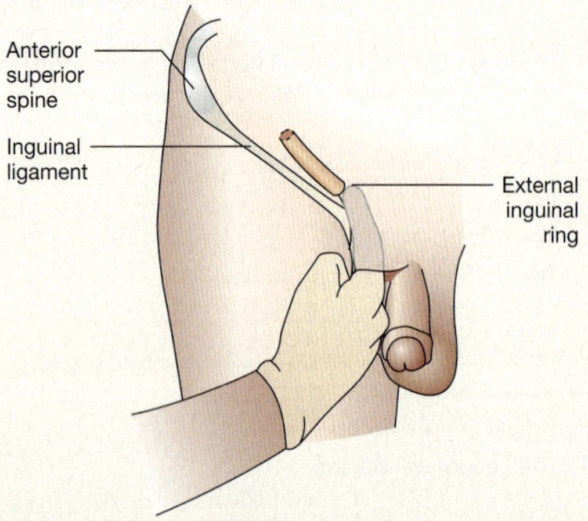

Figure 1-27. Palpating the external inguinal ring. (Adapted with permission from Bickley, L. (2003). *Bates' guide to physical examination and history taking* (8th ed.). Lippincott Williams & Wilkins.)

ADULT PHYSICAL ASSESSMENT (*continued*)

b. If the external ring is large enough, insert the finger along the inguinal canal toward the internal ring, and ask the patient to strain down, noting any mass that touches the finger.

5. Palpate the anterior thigh for a herniating mass in the femoral canal. Ask the patient to strain down. (The femoral canal is not palpable; it is a potential opening in the anterior thigh, medial to the femoral artery below the inguinal ligament.)

5. Ordinarily, there is no palpable mass in the femoral area.

FEMALE GENITALIA

Wearing gloves, observe the external genitalia for abnormalities such as lesions, discharge, or bulging of the vagina. Gently separate the labia to continue visual inspection, noting any tenderness. See Chapter 18 for additional information.

RECTUM

Position patient on the left side with knees drawn up toward chest and drape so that buttocks are exposed. Males may also stand and bend over the edge of the exam table with toes pointed inward. Females may be examined in lithotomy position at the end of a pelvic examination. (Change gloves to prevent cross-contamination.)

Inspection

Spread the buttocks and inspect the anus, perianal region, and sacral region for inflammation, nodules, scars, lesions, ulcerations, or rashes. Ask the patient to bear down; note any bulges.

The perianal and sacrococcygeal areas are dry, with varying amounts of hair covering them. Anal and perianal lesions include hemorrhoids, abscesses, skin tags, and sexually transmitted genital lesions.

Palpation

1. Palpate any abnormal area noted on inspection.

1. Identify any fissures, abnormal masses, or tenderness.

2. Lubricate the index finger of the gloved hand. Rest the finger over the anus as the patient bears down, and as the sphincter relaxes, insert your finger slowly into the rectum (see Figure 1-28).

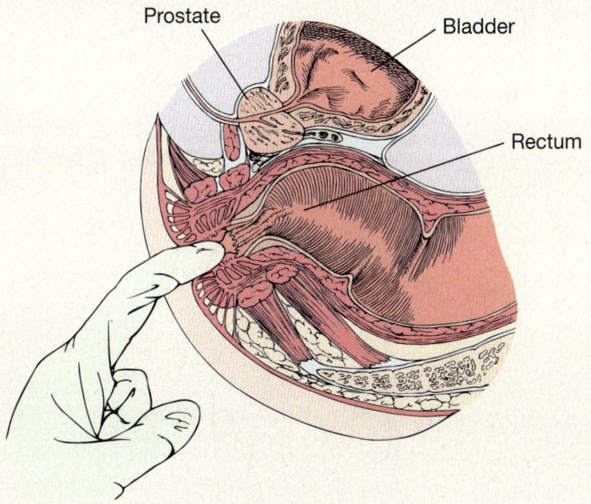

Prostate
Bladder
Rectum

Figure 1-28. Palpating the anus. (Reprinted with permission from Weber, J., & Kelley, J. [2022]. *Health assessment in nursing* [7th ed., Fig. 27-18]. Wolters Kluwer.)

3. Note sphincter tone, any nodules or masses, or tenderness.

3. The anal canal is approximately 1 in (2.5 cm) long; it is bordered by the external and internal anal sphincters, which are normally firm and smooth.

4. Insert the finger further and palpate the walls of the rectum laterally and posteriorly while rotating your index finger. Note irregularities, masses, nodules, tenderness.

4. The wall of the rectum is smooth and moist.

(*continued*)

ADULT PHYSICAL ASSESSMENT (continued)

Technique	Findings
5. Anteriorly, palpate the two lateral lobes of the prostate gland in males and its median sulcus for irregularities, nodules, swelling, or tenderness.	5. The male prostate gland is approximately 1 in (2.5 cm) long, smooth, regular, nonmovable, nontender, and rubbery.
6. If possible, palpate the superior portion of the lateral lobe, where the seminal vesicles are located. Note induration, swelling, or tenderness.	6. The seminal vesicles are generally not palpable unless swollen.
7. Just above the prostate anteriorly, the rectum lies adjacent to the peritoneal cavity. If possible, palpate this region for peritoneal masses and tenderness.	7. No masses or tenderness should be palpable.
8. In the female, anteriorly, the cervix, and perhaps a retroverted uterus, may be felt.	8. Anteriorly, the cervix is round and smooth.
9. Continue to insert the finger as far as possible and have the patient bear down so more of the bowel can be palpated.	
10. Gently withdraw your finger. Any fecal material on the glove should be tested for occult blood.	10. There is normally no occult blood in the stools.

MUSCULOSKELETAL SYSTEM

Technique	Findings
General approach	
1. Examine the muscles, bones, and joints, keeping in mind the structure and functions of each.	
2. Observe posture, gait, and signs of pain on movement.	
Inspection	
1. Inspect the upper and lower extremities for size, symmetry, swelling, deformity, and muscle mass.	
2. Inspect the joints for range of motion (in degrees), enlargement, and redness.	2. Full range of motion may be 90–180 degrees, but varies by joint.
3. Observe the spine for range of motion, lateral curvature, or any abnormal curvature.	3. Note scoliosis or kyphosis.
4. Observe the patient for signs of pain during the examination.	
Palpation	
1. Palpate the joints of the upper and lower extremities and the neck and back for tenderness, swelling, warmth, any bony overgrowth or deformity, and crepitus.	
2. Hold the palm of your hand over the joint as it moves, or move the joint through the fullest range of motion and note any crepitation (crackling feeling within the joint).	
3. Palpate the muscles for size, tone, strength, any contractures, and tenderness.	
4. Palpate the spine for bony deformities and crepitation. Gently tap the spine with the ulnar surface of your fist from the cervical to the lumbar region and note any pain or tenderness. (See Figure 1-29.)	

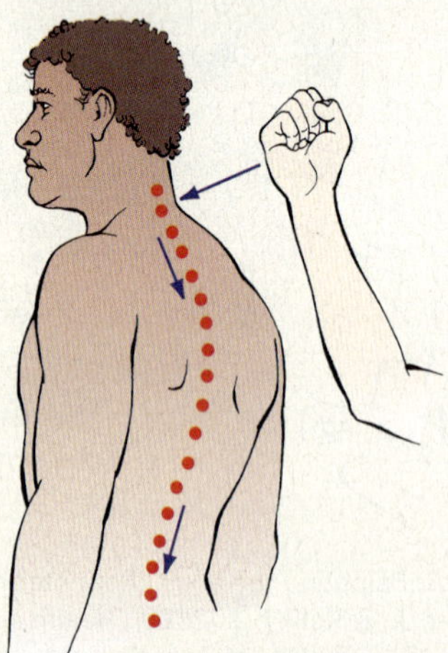

Figure 1-29. Gently tap the spine for tenderness.

ADULT PHYSICAL ASSESSMENT (*continued*)

NEUROLOGIC SYSTEM

The screening neurologic exam or any of its components can be performed with the patient in either the sitting or supine position and may be incorporated into examination of other regions of the body. Rather than using palpation, percussion, and auscultation, the examiner uses inspection and special testing to assess the components of mental status, cranial nerves (CNs), cerebellar function, motor function, sensation, and deep tendon reflexes. Additional equipment that may be necessary includes reflex hammer, tuning fork, cotton, safety pins, and scented items.

Mental Status

1. Determine level of consciousness by speaking the patient's name loudly and gently shaking the patient, if necessary.
   - Normally, the individual is alert, knows who they are and where they live, and can tell you the date.
2. The patient's ability to remember is also evaluated as the history is taken; ask about past medical history (long-term memory) and dietary habits: "What did you eat for breakfast?" (short-term memory).
   - The patient remembers recent and past events consistently and willingly admits forgetting something. Older adults may show slower processing but should be oriented to time, person, and place.
3. Cognition and ideational content are evaluated throughout the history by what the patient says and by articulateness, consistency, and reliability in reporting events.
   - There is no evidence of delusions or hallucinations.
4. Affect or mood is evaluated by observing the patient's verbal and nonverbal behavior in response to questions asked, sudden noises, and interruptions. For example, does the patient laugh or smile when talking about normally sad events, or is the patient easily startled by unexpected noises?
   - Mood should be appropriate to the content of the conversation.

Cranial Nerves

1. Test the olfactory nerve (1st CN) by occluding one nostril and having the patient (with eyes closed) identify a common substance by smell; repeat on the opposite side.
   - The patient should be able to identify common smells such as cinnamon and coffee.
2. Evaluate the optic nerve (2nd CN) by testing visual acuity via a Snellen chart and testing visual fields.
   a. Have the patient cover right eye with the right hand. (You cover your left eye with your left hand.)
   b. Stand approximately 2 feet (60 cm) from the patient and have the patient fix gaze on your nose.
   c. Bring two wagging fingers in from the periphery (in a plane equidistant from the patient and you) in all quadrants of the visual field and ask the patient to tell you when your wagging fingers are seen.
   - Normal vision (with glasses or contact lenses) is at or near 20/20. Assuming your visual fields are grossly normal, the patient and you should see the wagging fingers approximately simultaneously. (The patient's peripheral vision should approximate the examiner's.)
3. Test the oculomotor (3rd CN), trochlear (4th CN), and abducens (6th CN) together. They control the movements of the extraocular muscles of the eye—the superior and inferior oblique and the medial and lateral rectus muscles. The oculomotor nerve also controls pupillary constriction.
   a. Hold your index finger approximately 1 foot (30 cm) from the patient's nose. Ask the patient to hold head steady.
   b. Ask the patient to follow your finger with the eyes.
   c. Move your finger to the right as far as the patient's eye moves. Before bringing your finger back to the center, move it up and then down so that the patient glances up and peripherally and then down and peripherally.
   d. Repeat the test, moving your finger to the left.
   - Eyes should move smoothly through the six cardinal directions of gaze (see Figure 1-30), in a conjugate fashion.

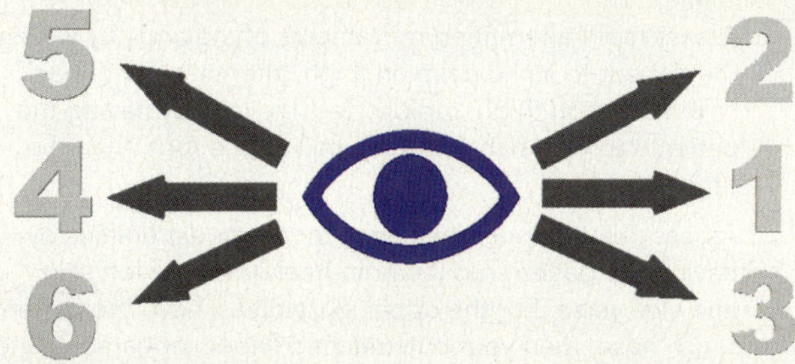

Figure 1-30. The six cardinal directions of gaze.

(continued)

ADULT PHYSICAL ASSESSMENT *(continued)*

4. Test the trigeminal nerve (5th CN) that controls muscles of mastication and has a sensory component that controls sensations of the face.	4. Describing testing beforehand may allay anxiety and encourage participation for accurate results.
a. Test the motor component by having the patient clench teeth while palpating the temporal and masseter muscles of the jaws with both hands.	a. Muscle strength in the face should be present and should be symmetric.
b. Test the sensory component by having the patient close eyes and touch one side of the face then the other (forehead, cheek, chin). Use a safety pin or sharp object for pain sensation, and a gauze sponge or cotton ball for light touch.	b. Sensation should be present and symmetrical.
c. Test corneal reflex by asking patient to look away and approaching from the other side. Gently touch the cornea with a wisp of cotton or gauze.	c. Blink of the eyes indicates normal sensory function of 5th CN, as well as normal motor function of 7th CN.
5. Test the facial nerve (7th CN) by observing facial expression and symmetry of facial movement. Ask the patient to frown, raise eyebrows, close eyes, and smile.	5. The facial muscles should look symmetric when the patient frowns, closes eyes, and smiles. Notice particularly the symmetry of the nasolabial folds.
6. Evaluate the acoustic nerve (8th CN) cochlear branch by testing hearing (see pp. 9–10) and vestibular branch by testing for nystagmus (see p. 8).	6. Hearing should be equal, with air conduction greater than bone conduction; no prolonged nystagmus should be present.
7. Test the glossopharyngeal (9th CN) and vagus nerve (10th CN) together (they both have a motor portion innervating the pharynx).	
a. Ask the patient to say "ah" and observe the movement of the uvula and palate (10th CN).	a. The palate and uvula should move symmetrically without deviation.
b. Gently use a tongue blade to check the presence of the gag reflex (9th CN).	b. The gag reflex should be present, and there should be no difficulty in swallowing.
8. Evaluate the spinal accessory nerve (11th CN), which mediates the sternocleidomastoid and upper portion of the trapezius muscles.	8. Neck and shoulder muscle strength should be symmetric.
a. Ask the patient to turn head to the side against resistance while you apply pressure to the jaw and observe contraction of the sternocleidomastoid muscle on the opposite side.	a. You should feel the force of movement against your hand and see some contraction of patient's neck muscle on the opposite side.
b. Have the patient shrug shoulders while you place your hands on the patient's shoulders from behind and apply slight pressure.	b. Contraction of trapezii can be observed directly and felt through force of shoulder movement.
9. Evaluate the hypoglossal nerve (12th CN), which innervates muscles of the tongue by noting articulation and by having the patient stick out the tongue, noting any deviation or asymmetry.	9. The patient should speak clearly and tongue should be symmetric and should not deviate.

Cerebellar Function

1. Observe posture and gait.	1. The patient should be able to walk forward and backward in a straight line, heel-to-toe; and walk on toes and heels.
2. Assess rapid alternating movements of the arms by asking the patient to strike palm on thigh, alternating with back of the hand on thigh, rapidly. Test the legs by having the patient tap your hand with the ball of one foot, then the other, rapidly.	2. The patient should be able to perform the tests described with smooth, even movement.
3. Assess point-to-point testing in the lower extremities by having the patient run the right heel down the left shin and vice versa. For the upper extremities, have the patient touch nose, then your outstretched finger, repeatedly, and then with eyes closed.	3. Movements should be fairly smooth and accurate, even with eyes closed.
4. Test for cerebellar ataxia by asking the patient to stand with feet together, eyes open.	4. Patient should be able to stand unsupported with eyes open with minimal swaying for 20 to 30 seconds. Ability to stand with eyes open, but losing balance with eyes closed, is a problem of position sense rather than cerebellar function.

ADULT PHYSICAL ASSESSMENT (*continued*)

Motor Function

1. Evaluate muscle mass, tone, strength, and any abnormal movements (tics, fasciculations, twitching). May be done with musculoskeletal exam.

   1. Normally, abnormal movements are not present either at rest or with movement.

   a. Test muscle tone by noting the resistance the muscle offers to movement on passive motion.

   a. Generally, there is slight resistance to passive movement of muscles as opposed to flaccidity (no resistance) or rigidity (increased muscle tone).

   b. Test muscle strength by asking the patient to actively resist your movement to flex or extend their various muscle groups. Grade muscle strength as follows: 0 = no muscle contraction, 1 = faint muscle contraction, 2 = active movement of body part with gravity eliminated, 3 = active movement against gravity, 4 = active movement against gravity and some resistance, 5 = active movement against full resistance without fatigue.

   b. Strength will vary from person to person, but 5 on a scale of 0–5 is considered normal. It should be equal bilaterally. Some symmetric muscle atrophy may be noted with aging.

Sensory Function

1. Test sensitivity to pain and temperature (spinothalamic tracts), position and vibration (posterior columns), light touch (both tracts), and discrimination (spinal tracts and the cerebral cortex). Compare both sides of the body.

   1. Sensation should be equal bilaterally.

   a. Ask the patient to close eyes. Brush the skin with a piece of gauze or cotton on areas of the arms, legs, and trunk. Ask the patient to indicate when they feel the cotton.

   a. Patient should feel light touch bilaterally.

   b. Use a safety pin; touch the skin as lightly as possible to elicit a sharp sensation.

   b. Pain should be felt bilaterally.

   c. Test temperature sensation by using tubes filled with warm and cold water, touching them to body areas.

   c. The patient can discriminate warm and cold bilaterally.

   d. Test vibration sense by placing a vibrating tuning fork on a distal interphalangeal joint of the finger, then of the great toe, and ask if vibration can be felt. If not, move proximally to the next bony prominence.

   d. The patient should be able to detect vibration if there is no peripheral neuropathy. (If the patient is unsure, touch the fork to stop vibration and ask the patient to tell you when it stops).

   e. Test position sense by grasping the great toe and moving it in an upward or downward position.

   e. The patient can determine position of the toe bilaterally.

   f. Test discrimination (which also depends on an intact cortex) by placing a small object such as a paper clip in the hand (stereognosis), using the blunt end of a pen to draw a number in the palm (graphesthesia), or using an open paper clip to touch the skin with 1 or 2 points alternately (two-point discrimination).

   f. The patient should be able to identify object, number, or one- or two-point stimulation when the sensory pathways are intact and the cerebral cortex can interpret sensations.

Deep Tendon Reflexes

1. Make sure the patient is relaxed and extremity is supported for all reflex testing. If the patient is not relaxed and you cannot elicit reflexes, have the patient grasp hands and contract arm muscles to relax the lower extremities or tap feet on the floor to relax the upper extremities.

   1. Amplitude of the reflex may vary for different tendons but is equal bilaterally.

2. Test biceps reflex by striking indirectly (see Figure 1-31).

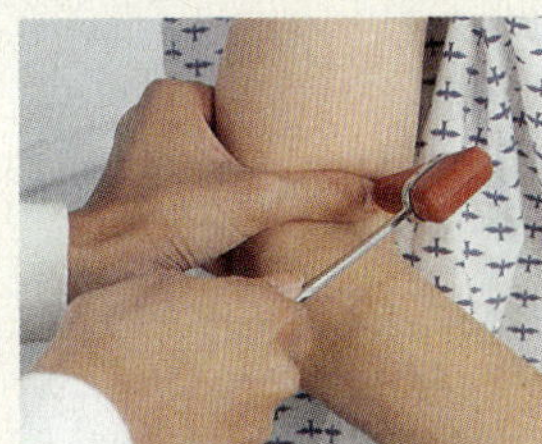

Figure 1-31. Assessing the biceps reflex.

(*continued*)

ADULT PHYSICAL ASSESSMENT (continued)

a. Place your right thumb on the patient's right biceps tendon (located in the antecubital fossa) with the patient's arm slightly flexed.

b. Strike your thumb with the pointed end of the hammer head. Hold the hammer loosely so it pivots in your hand when it is moved with a wrist action.

c. Strike your thumb with the least amount of pressure needed to elicit the reflex.

c. The forearm may flex and you should see and feel contraction of the biceps.

3. Test the triceps tendon by using the pointed end of the hammer. Refer to Figure 1-32.

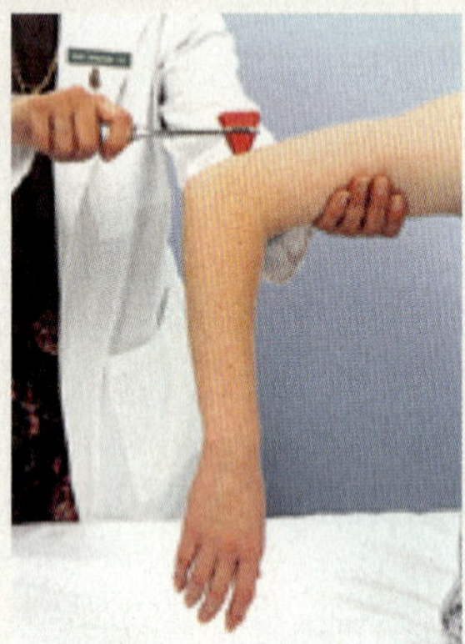

Figure 1-32. Assessing the triceps tendon.

a. Have the patient hang arm freely while you support it with your nondominant hand or rest the slightly flexed arm in the patient's lap.

b. With the elbow flexed, strike the tendon directly.

b. The forearm may extend and you should see contraction of the triceps.

4. Test the brachioradialis tendon by striking the forearm (partially pronated) with the flat end of the hammer about 1 in (2.5 cm) above the wrist over the radius. Refer to Figure 1-33.

4. There should be slight flexion and supination of the forearm.

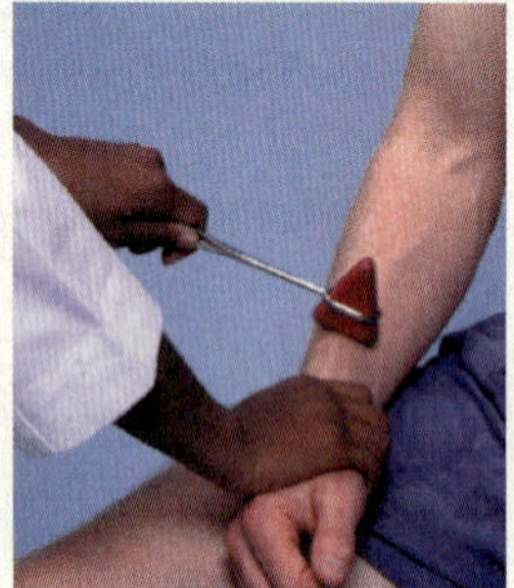

Figure 1-33. Assessing the brachioradialis reflex.

5. Test the quadriceps reflex by having the patient sit with legs hanging over the edge of the table or lay down while you support the legs at the knee (slightly bent), and strike the tendon with the pointed end of the hammer just above the patella.

6. Test the Achilles reflex by supporting the foot in dorsiflexed position and tapping the Achilles tendon with the flat end of the hammer.

6. The foot should move downward into your hand.

7. Stroke the sole of the patient's foot with a flat object such as a tongue blade to test the plantar reflex (L5, S1).

7. Toes normally flex. Dorsiflexion of the great toe and fanning of the other toes is known as a positive Babinski response and indicates a central nervous system problem.

SELECTED READINGS

Bickley, L. S., Szilagyi, P. G., Hoffman, R. M., & Soriano, R. P. (2024). *Bates' guide to physical examination and history taking* (13th ed.). Wolters Kluwer.

Dieterle, T., Battegay, E., Bucheli, B., & Martina, B. (1998). Accuracy and "range of uncertainty" of oscillometric blood pressure monitors around the upper arm and the wrist. *Blood Pressure Monitoring, 3*(6), 339–346.

Ewing, J. A. (1984). Detecting alcoholism: The CAGE questionnaire. *Journal of the American Medical Association, 252*(14), 1905–1907. https://doi.org/10.1001/jama.1984.03350140051025

Fitzwater, J., Johnstone, C., & Schippers, M. (2019). A comparison of oral, axillary, and temporal artery temperature measuring devices in adult acute care. *Medsurg Nursing, 28*(1), 35–41.

Hinkle, J. L., Cheever, K. H., & Overbaugh, K. J. (2021). *Brunner & Suddarth's textbook of medical-surgical nursing* (15th ed.). Wolters Kluwer.

Kario, K., Shimbo, D., Tomitani, N., Kanegae, H., Schwartz, J. E., & Williams, B. (2022). The first study comparing a wearable watch-type blood pressure monitor with a conventional ambulatory blood pressure monitor on in-office and out-of-office settings. *Journal of Clinical Hypertension, 22*(2), 135–141. https://doi.org/10.1111/jch.13799

Khan, S., Saultry, B., Adams, S., Kouzani, A. Z., Decker, K., Digby, R., & Bucknall, T. (2020). Comparative accuracy testing of non-contact infrared thermometers and temporal artery thermometers in an adult hospital setting. *American Journal of Infection Control, 49*(5), 597–602. https://doi.org/10.1016/j.ajic.2020.09.012

Ley, C., Heath, F., Hastie, T., Gao, Z., Protsiv, M., & Parsonnet, J. (2023). Defining usual oral temperature ranges in outpatients using an unsupervised learning algorithm. *JAMA Internal Medicine, 183*(10), 1128–1135. https://doi.org/10.1001/jamainternmed.2023.4291

Lippincott Williams & Wilkins. (2022). *Lippincott nursing procedures.* Wolters Kluwer.

Naccarato, A., & Wilson, C. (2022). Assessment of vision and hearing in older adults. *Home Healthcare Now, 40*(5), 279–280. https://doi.org/10.1097/NHH.0000000000001108

Nirenberg, M., & Ansert, E. (2020). Vascular assessment of the foot surgery patient. *Orthopedic Nursing, 39*(2), 114–118. https://doi.org/10.1097/NOR.0000000000000642

Pirozzo, S., Papinczak, T., & Glasziou, P. (2003). Whispered voice test for screening for hearing impairment in adults and children: Systematic review. *British Medical Journal, 327*(7421), 967. https://doi.org/10.1136/bmj.327.7421.967

Stergiou, G. S., Palatini, P., Parati, G., O'Brien, E., Januszewicz, A., Lurbe, E., Persu, A., Mancia, G., Kreutz, R., & European Society of Hypertension Council and the European Society of Hypertension Working Group on Blood Pressure Monitoring and Cardiovascular Variability. (2021). 2021 European Society of Hypertension practice guidelines for office and out-of-office blood pressure measurement. *Journal of Hypertension, 39*(7), 1293–1302. https://doi.org/10.1097/HJH.0000000000002843

Taylor, C. R., Lynn, P. S., & Bartlett, J. L. (2022). *Fundamentals of nursing: The art and science of person-centered care.* Wolters Kluwer.

Weber, J. R., & Kelly, J. H. (2021). *Health assessment in nursing* (7th ed.). Wolters Kluwer.

Wodwaski, N., & Webber, E. (2022). Cardiovascular assessment. *Home Healthcare Now, 40*(5), 238–244. https://doi.org/10.1097/NHH.0000000000001097

2 Intravenous Therapy

GENERAL CONSIDERATIONS

Purpose

The purpose of intravenous (IV) therapy is to:

1. Provide hydration and correction of electrolyte imbalances in the patient who is unable to maintain adequate oral intake.
2. Administer medications safely and effectively.
3. Administer blood components and blood products.
4. Provide for invasive patient hemodynamic monitoring.
5. Provide nutrition while resting the gastrointestinal (GI) tract.

Physiologic Assimilation of Infusion Solutions

Principles

1. Tissue cells (such as epithelial cells) are surrounded by a semipermeable membrane.
2. Cell membrane permeability refers to the ability of the cellular membrane to allow substances such as water to pass freely, whereas charged ions, such as sodium, cannot cross the membrane and are trapped on one side.
3. Osmotic pressure is the "pulling" pressure demonstrated when water moves through the semipermeable membrane of tissue cells from an area of weaker concentration to stronger concentration of solute (e.g., sodium ions and glucose). The end result is dilution and equilibration between the intracellular and extracellular compartments.
4. Total body water (TBW) is the sum of intracellular fluid volume (about 2/3 TBW) and extracellular fluid volume (EFV; about 1/3 TBW). EFV is the composition of interstitial fluid (about 2/3 of EFV) and intravascular volume (about 1/3 of EFV).
5. Extracellular compartment fluids primarily include plasma and interstitial fluid. Extracellular fluid impacts the movement of electrolytes, delivery of oxygen to the cells, and clearance of metabolic waste.

Types of IV Fluids

IV fluids include colloids and crystalloids. See Table 2-1.

1. Colloid solutions contain large proteins or molecules that cannot pass through the cellular semipermeable membrane. Colloids increase intravascular volume by drawing fluid into the intravascular space via oncotic pressure. Common natural colloids include red blood cells, plasma, and albumin. Common synthetic colloids include dextran, hyperoncotic starch, or gelatin.
2. Crystalloid fluid contains electrolytes but lacks large proteins and molecules. Crystalloid fluid flows easily across the semipermeable membrane. Classified according to their "tonicity," crystalloids are isotonic, hypotonic, or hypertonic solutions.

Isotonic

A solution that exerts the same osmotic pressure as that found in plasma. This fluid will distribute evenly between the extracellular and intracellular space. This type of fluid is typically administered to expand intravascular volume.

1. 0.9% sodium chloride solution (normal saline, NS).
2. Lactated Ringer (LR) solution.
3. Dextrose 5% in water (D_5W) (as dextrose is metabolized, shifts to more hypotonic).

Hypotonic

A solution that exerts less osmotic pressure than that of plasma. Administration of this fluid generally causes a decreased concentration of dissolved solutes in the plasma, forcing water to move into cells to reestablish intracellular and extracellular equilibrium; cells will then rehydrate.

1. 0.45%, 0.33%, or 0.225% sodium chloride solution (half NS, one-third NS, or one-quarter NS).

Hypertonic

A solution that exerts a higher osmotic pressure than that of plasma. Administration of this fluid increases the solute concentration of plasma, drawing water out of the cells and into the extracellular compartment to restore osmotic equilibrium; cells will then shrink.

1. D_5W in LR solution (D_5LR).
2. D_5W in NS solution.

Table 2-1 Composition of Selected Intravenous Solutions

SOLUTION	TONICITY	NA⁺ (MEQ/L)	K⁺ (MEQ/L)	CL⁻ (MEQ/L)	CA⁺⁺ (MEQ/L)	BUFFER	PH
Lactated Ringer (LR)[a]	Isotonic	130	4	109	3	28 lactate	6.5
0.9% normal saline (NS)	Isotonic	154	0	154	0	0	–
D_5W	Isotonic	0	0	0	0	0	4.5
D_5LR	Slightly hypertonic	130	4	109	3	28 lactate	5
D_5NS	Hypertonic	154	0	154	0	0	4
3% NS	Hypertonic	513	0	513	0	0	–
0.45% NS	Hypotonic	77	–	7	–	0	5.3
5% D and 0.45% NS[b]	Slightly hypertonic	77	–	77	–	0	4

D_5W, dextrose 5% in water.
[a]Lactate converts to bicarbonate in the liver.
[b]5% dextrose metabolizes rapidly in the blood and produces minimal osmotic effects.

3. D_5W in 0.45% (half normal) saline solution (only slightly hypertonic because dextrose is rapidly metabolized and renders only temporary osmotic pressure).
4. Dextrose 10% in water ($D_{10}W$).
5. Dextrose 20% in water ($D_{20}W$).
6. 3% or 5% sodium chloride solution.
7. Hyperalimentation solutions.

Uses and Precautions With Common Types of Infusions

See Table 2-2 for signs and symptoms of water excess or deficit.

1. D_5W:
   a. Used to replace water (hypotonic fluid) losses, supply some caloric intake, or as a carrying solution for numerous medications.
   b. Should be used cautiously in patients at risk for increased intracranial pressure or patients with cardiac or renal dysfunction. Dextrose-containing solutions should not be used as a resuscitation fluid because of the risk for hyperglycemia.
   c. Should not be used as concurrent solution infusion with blood or blood components.
2. NS solution (0.9% NS or NaCl):
   a. Commonly used resuscitative crystalloid used to replace extracellular fluid losses (e.g., dehydration, hypovolemia, sepsis) or administer with blood components.
   b. Should be used cautiously in patients at risk for volume overload such as patients with heart or renal failure or patients at risk for pulmonary edema; monitor for hyperchloremic acidosis with resuscitation uses.
3. LR solution:
   a. Commonly used resuscitative crystalloid to replace extracellular fluid losses (e.g., hemorrhage and burn injuries), replenish specific electrolyte losses and moderate metabolic acidosis.
   b. Use cautiously in patients with liver failure.
4. 0.45% NS (half NS):
   a. Commonly used crystalloid in the treatment of hypernatremia or diabetic ketoacidosis.
   b. Can cause hemolysis of red blood cells with rapid infusion.
5. Hypertonic saline solution (3% NS or NaCl):
   a. Acts as a plasma volume expander by increasing the movement of intracellular and interstitial water into the intravascular space.
   b. Risk of hypernatremia and requires careful monitoring, particularly of patient's neurologic status.

Table 2-2 Signs and Symptoms of Water Excess or Deficit

SITE	WATER EXCESS	WATER DEFICIT
Central nervous system	• Muscle twitching • Hyperactive tendon reflexes • Convulsions • Increased intracranial pressure, coma • Headache	• Sleepiness • Apathy • Restlessness • Weakness • Delirium • Coma
Cardiovascular	• Elevated venous pressure, full distended neck veins • Increased cardiac output • High pulse pressure • Heart gallop • Rales, pulmonary edema	• Tachycardia, thready pulse • Orthostatic hypotension, hypotension • Flat neck veins • Cool, clammy skin
Gastrointestinal	• Anorexia, nausea, and vomiting • Edema of stomach, colon, and mesentery	• Anorexia • Thirst • Silent ileus, decreased bowel sounds
Tissues	• Increased salivation, tears • Watery diarrhea • Subcutaneous pitting edema	• Decreased saliva and tears • Dry, sticky mucous membranes • Flushed skin • Decreased skin turgor • Decreased urinary output • Sunken eyes

INTRAVENOUS MEDICATION ADMINISTRATION

General Considerations for Intravenous Medication Administration

1. Before medication administration, confirm patient identification (ID), allergies, and review the order and indication for the selected medication or solution.
2. Use aseptic nontouch technique when preparing and administering intravenous (IV) medications and accessing the vascular device.
3. Perform an appropriate assessment of the patient. This includes an evaluation of the prescribed therapy for the patient's age and clinical condition, rights of medication administration (right patient, medication, dose, route, time), and reason for medication or solution treatment. Assess the vascular site and ensure patency of the vascular device by aspirating for positive blood return and encountering no resistance when manually flushing. Do not force if resistance is felt. Ascertain the dwell time of the catheter.
4. If your facility uses barcode technology, scan your ID badge, the patient's ID bracelet, and the medication or solution barcode.
5. Needleless connectors protect health care providers by eliminating the need for needles and subsequent needlestick injuries when attaching syringes or administration sets to the vascular access device.
6. Educate patient/family about the purpose of the medication or solution, emphasize immediately reporting any adverse signs/symptoms to the health care team. Monitor the patient's reaction to the medication or solution during and after administration.
   a. Be alert for major adverse effects, such as anaphylaxis, respiratory distress, tachycardia, bradycardia, or seizures. If this occurs, stop the medication or solution and notify the health care provider. Institute emergency procedures as necessary.
   b. Assess for minor adverse effects, such as nausea, flushing, skin rash, or confusion. If this occurs, stop the medication or solution and notify the health care provider.
   c. Monitor the vascular access site for any signs of infiltration or extravasation.
7. Document medication or solution administration in the patient's medical record and plan of care as appropriate, completing the sixth right of medication administration.

There are three IV routes of administration: bolus or "IV push," intermittent infusion, and continuous infusion.

IV "Push" (Bolus)

IV "push" (or *IV bolus*) refers to the administration of a medication from a syringe directly into an ongoing IV infusion or may be given directly into a vein by way of an intermittent access device (Luer-locking needleless connector, "saline lock").

Indications

1. When a rapid concentration (e.g., adenosine) or a quicker response (e.g., diuretics or antihypertensives) from a medication is required.
2. To administer "loading" doses of a medication that will be continued by way of infusion (e.g., heparin, pain medications).
3. To reduce patient discomfort by limiting the need for intramuscular injections.
4. To avoid incompatibility problems that may occur when several medications are mixed in one bottle/bag.
5. To deliver medications or solutions to patients unable to take them orally (e.g., patients who are unresponsive) or intramuscularly (e.g., coagulation disorder).

Precautions and Recommendations

1. Be familiar with facility policies and guidelines regarding how, where, and by whom IV push medications or solutions may be administered.
2. Determine the correct (safest) rate of administration. Consult the pharmacy or pharmaceutical text. When administering the medication or solution, use a timer with a second hand to inject according to facility procedures and manufacturer recommendations. Use a push–pause method as indicated. Too rapid administration may result in serious adverse effects. Dilute the medication only when indicated by manufacturer or pharmacy references with the appropriate diluent. Some medications are irritating to veins and require sufficient dilution. Caution during this process because of the associated increased risk for medication errors and contamination of sterile IV medications or solutions.
3. If withdrawing IV push medications from a glass ampule, use a filter needle or straw unless the specific drug precludes their use.
4. Unless the medication or solution is prepared at the patient's bedside for immediate administration without any break in the process, appropriately label all nurse-prepared syringes of IV push medications or solutions.
5. If IV push is to be given with an ongoing IV infusion or to follow another IV push medication, check pharmacy for possible incompatibility. It is recommended to flush the IV tubing or cannula with saline before and after administration of a medication.
6. Use a needleless connector that is closest to the patient to allow the medication or solution to reach the central circulation as soon as possible with a minimal amount of flushing.

CLINICAL JUDGMENT Unless its use would result in a clinically significant delay and potential patient harm (e.g., medication administration during cardiopulmonary resuscitation), barcode scanning or similar technology is recommended immediately prior to medication or solution administration as an effective error reduction strategy.

Intermittent Infusions

Intermittent intravenous infusions are a medication or solution administered over a set period of time at prescribed intervals. An intermittent infusion may be given through an intermittent access device (Luer-locking needleless connectors, "saline lock") or "piggybacked" to a continuous IV infusion as a secondary medication.

Intermittent Access Device (Luer-Locking Needleless Connector, "Saline Lock")

1. This intermittent infusion device permits the administration of periodic IV medications and solutions without continuous fluid administration.

2. After administration of the medication or solution, flush the Luer-locking needleless connector with normal saline at the same rate as the medication administration to ensure that all medication remaining in the Luer-locking needleless connector or extension tubing is administered at the appropriate rate and to prevent future contact incompatibilities.

CLINICAL JUDGMENT Medication errors are often a result of calculation errors, drug preparation errors, human errors, and prescribing errors. Unusual dosages or unfamiliar medication or solutions should always be confirmed with the health care provider and pharmacist before administration. Ultimately, the nurse is accountable for the medication or solutions administered.

Secondary Medication Administration ("Piggyback")

1. Means of administering a medication or solution by way of an established primary infusion line.
2. Verify compatibility between the medication or solution contained within the piggyback and primary infusion.
3. Prime the secondary tubing and use the extension hook.
   a. If using gravity infusion, hang the secondary medication higher than the primary IV solution bag. Use the roller clamp or flow regulators to calculate infusion rate.
   b. If using an infusion pump, set an appropriate rate.
4. When a backcheck valve is present on the primary tubing, it:
   a. Permits the primary infusion to flow after the medication has been administered.
   b. Prevents air from entering the system.
   c. Prevents secondary fluid from "running dry."
   d. Permits less mixing of primary fluid with secondary solution.
5. Always select the access port closest to the insertion site of the vascular access device.
6. Use of an electronic infusion pump with dose-error technology or flow regulator will permit rate changes between primary and secondary infusions.
7. Never administer a solution or medication through a continuous IV line that is infusing blood, blood products, heparin IV, insulin IV, cytotoxic medications, or parenteral nutrition solutions.
8. A volume-controlled intermittent set is a device attached below the primary infusion to regulate the secondary medication or solution. These devices are used most often for children, older adults, or patients who are critically ill where fluid volume is a concern.
9. Secondary medication infusion tubing is considered a primary intermittent IV set when disconnected from the primary IV tubing; it should be changed in accordance with facility protocol.

CLINICAL JUDGMENT For infusion of vesicants, a peripheral catheter placement of 24 hours or less is advisable while avoiding infusion times of 30 to 60 minutes.

Continuous Infusion

Continuous infusion is the IV infusion of a medication or solution over several hours to days to achieve constant plasma concentration. Use of an electronic infusion pump with dose-error technology is recommended.

1. Continuous infusion tubing administration sets should be changed no more frequently than every 96 hours.

Use of Infusion Control Devices

Infusion control devices allow for the infusion of large and small volumes of IV solution or medication with accuracy over a determined time period at prescribed intervals, reducing the risk of rapid infusion or accidental free flows. Use of infusion control devices should be based on the needs and factors of the patient, type of vascular access device, and health care setting. Electronic infusion pumps with dose-error reduction systems are preferred. The nurse must be competent in the use of all available equipment.

Types

Manual Control Flow Regulator

1. Delivers a more precise fluid volume per hour than built-in roller clamps on IV tubing.
2. To be used for lower-risk infusions. Confirm appropriate use with any organizational procedures, policies, or practice guidelines.
3. Nonautomated and requires manual adjustment of a regulator clamp to administer correct flow rate. Manual control flow regulators may be integrated as part of the IV tubing or added on individually.

Electronic Infusion Pumps

1. Deliver a prescribed fluid volume per hour.
2. Often, incorporate dose-error reduction technologies to minimize adverse patient situations. Additional safety features include alarms and other operator alerts (e.g., when air or blockage is detected, risk of adverse drug interaction). Infusion pumps with comprehensive libraries of medications and dose calculation software serve as another safety check that programming is within preestablished organizational limits.
3. Divided into large-volume and small-volume devices.
4. Indicated for continuous infusions of chemotherapy, hyperalimentation, fluid and electrolytes in patients at risk for fluid overload, infant and pediatric therapies, and most medications.
5. Some electronic infusion devices are designed to be used at a patient's bedside, whereas others, called ambulatory infusion pumps, are designed to be portable or wearable.
6. Most common adverse events related to electronic infusion pumps include software defects, device design issues and engineering failure, mechanical or electrical failures, or user interface issues.

Blood and Fluid Warmers

Used when attempting to avoid or treat hypothermia, during cardiopulmonary bypass, when the patient is known to have cold agglutinins, or during replacement of large blood volumes.

Power Injectors

1. Used to deliver specific amounts of contrast media at a specified rate/time during radiologic diagnostic procedures. Radiologic contrast media are to be considered vesicant solutions with the potential to cause severe tissue injury in the setting of infiltration/extravasation.
2. Vascular access device must be able to withstand pressure of 300 psi or greater to be compatible with power injectors.

Nursing Responsibilities

1. Continuous or intermittent infusions must be monitored by the nurse to ensure accurate delivery.
2. Adhere to all manufacturers' guidelines regarding product use.
3. Eliminate all air from the administration tubing set before connecting it to the patient's vascular access device.
4. Continue to check the patient regularly for complications, such as infiltration/extravasation or infection; do not rely solely on device alarms.
5. Ensure that infusion therapy is initiated, changed, or discontinued based on the order of the prescribing health care provider.
6. Explain the purpose of the equipment and the alarm system to the patient and caregivers. Added machines in the room can evoke greater anxiety in the patient and family.
7. For rapid administration of solutions and blood or blood products, avoid using needleless connectors. Instead connect directly to the hub of the vascular access device because needleless connectors can greatly reduce flow rates.

Vascular Access Device Selection

Selecting the appropriate vascular access device is based on the needs of the patient, particularly the prescribed therapy and duration of therapy, as well as characteristics of the patient including age, comorbidities, and vascular characteristics.

Short Peripheral Catheters

1. These catheters are intended for short-term therapy—typically less than 4 days. The time in which short peripheral catheters remain in situ with no orders for infusion therapy should be severely limited.
2. In general, distal extremity sites should be used first, saving more proximal sites for subsequent cannulation. Preferential selection of forearm vessels reduces the risk of adverse outcomes. Upper extremity placement is preferred to lower extremity placement because of an increased risk of thrombosis and thrombophlebitis, with the exception of neonates and infants or emergent insertion. Caution with areas that increase the risk of complications such as areas of flexion, or using dominant upper extremity because of an increased risk of catheter dislodgment and catheter damage due to bending. Contraindications include presence of an arteriovenous fistula, presence of lymphedema with a history of lymph node dissection, veins firm to palpation indicating they may be sclerosed, or where a prior attempt resulted in a hematoma formation.
3. Therapies not appropriate for short peripheral catheters include continuous vesicant therapy, parenteral nutrition, and infusions with a pH less than 5 or greater than 9 or with an osmolality greater than 600 mOsm/L.

Midline Catheters

1. These catheters are intended for short-term therapy—typically 5 to 30 days.
2. These catheters are inserted into the basilic, cephalic, or brachial veins and extend 3 to 8 in (7.5 to 20 cm) up the arm with the proximal tip resting distal to the shoulder, terminating just distal to the axillary vein. For neonates, in addition to arm veins, midline catheters may be inserted via a scalp vein with the distal tip located in the jugular vein above the clavicle, or in the lower extremity with the distal tip located below the inguinal crease.
3. Midline catheters are not appropriate for continuous vesicant therapy such as hyperosmolar solutions, parenteral nutrition, and some antibiotics, such as erythromycin and nafcillin, as well as infusions with a pH less than 5 or greater than 9 or with an osmolality greater than 600 mOsm/L. If known irritants and vesicants are intermittently infused via midline catheters, increase vascular site assessments due to an increased risk of phlebitis or extravasation.
4. Avoid use in patients with a history of thrombosis, hypercoagulability, and decreased venous flow or in the setting of vein preservation such as with end-stage renal disease.

CLINICAL JUDGMENT Caution when placing vascular access devices in extremities with sensory or motor deficits. Anecdotal evidence suggests an increased risk of developing a deep vein thrombosis; however, there is no clear evidence that placement of a short peripheral or midline catheter increases this baseline risk, especially with upper extremity placement. Close assessment of vascular device by the nurse is required, looking for signs and symptoms of complications.

Central Venous Access Devices

Indications

1. Physiologic instability of the patient or complexity of infusion therapies.
2. Continuous vesicant or irritant therapy, chemotherapy, or parenteral nutrition medication.
3. Invasive hemodynamic monitoring.
4. History of difficult peripheral venous access where vascular site selection is limited and the use of ultrasound guidance has failed.
5. Long-term IV therapy—weeks, months, or years.

Types

See Figure 2-1.

CLINICAL JUDGMENT Prior to the initiation of medication or solution therapy, ensure the appropriate placement of all central vascular catheters radiographically or by other imaging technology (ultrasound or transesophageal echocardiography) in the emergent setting.

1. Central catheter—nontunneled; commonly called *percutaneous*; multilumen, single lumen, or venous sheath:
   a. Generally placed for urgent or emergent indications to administer medications at higher risk of peripheral vein thrombophlebitis or extravasation injury, large-volume resuscitation or blood transfusions, aid in hemodynamic monitoring, or to facilitate insertion of emergency transvenous pacing lead.
   b. Dwell time is generally limited to 2 weeks.
   c. May be inserted in the femoral, jugular, or subclavian veins with the catheter tip intended to lie in the superior or inferior vena cava using sterile technique. Sterile technique is recommended even in the setting of emergent placement.
2. Central catheter—tunneled:
   a. A tunneled catheter is inserted into a central vein (usually the subclavian, then the superior vena cava) and subcutaneously tunneled to an exit site approximately 4 in (10 cm) from the insertion site.
   b. A Dacron cuff is located approximately ¾ to 1 in (2 to 3 cm) from the exit site, providing a barrier against microorganisms.

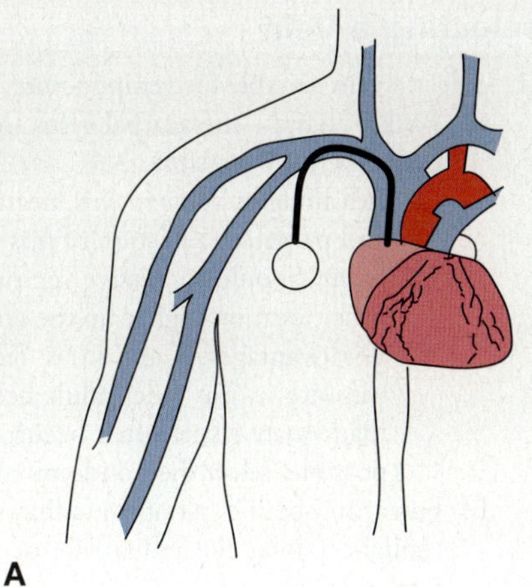

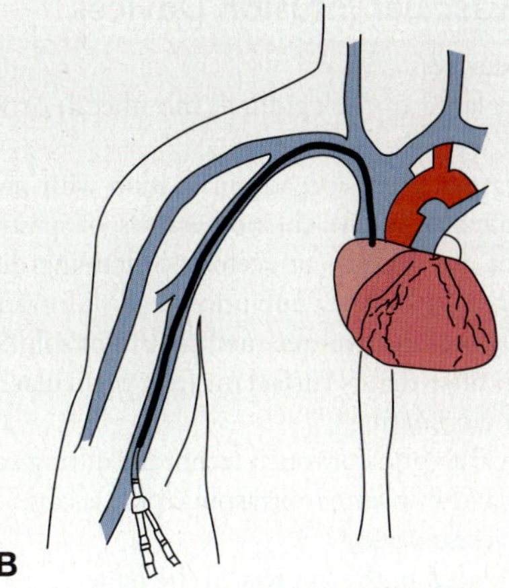

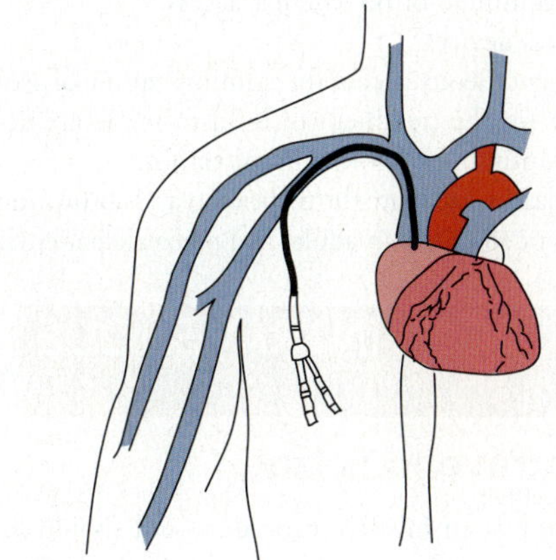

Figure 2-1. Types of central venous catheters for long-term venous access. **(A)** Implantable venous access port. **(B)** Peripherally inserted central catheter (PICC). **(C)** Tunneled central venous catheter.

c. Examples of tunneled catheters in current use are Hickman, Broviac, and Quinton-Mahurkar.

d. Tunneled catheters are generally associated with lower rates of catheter-related bloodstream infections compared to nontunneled central catheters.

3. Peripherally inserted central catheter (PICC):

a. Inserted in basilic, brachial, or cephalic veins in adult patients; additional sites are available in neonate and pediatric patients including axillary, temporal, or saphenous vein. Tip placement should terminate in the proximal superior vena cava or cavoatrial junction; tip placement in subclavian or innominate vein is contraindicated for hyperosmolar solutions (hyperalimentation).

b. Used in patients in acute, long-term, and home care settings for medium-term venous access, usually anywhere from several weeks to 6 months.

c. Many organizations maintain dedicated teams of nurses trained in the placement of PICCs, demonstrating increased success rates for catheter placement with reduced complications.

d. Measure upper arm circumference before and after insertion and as clinically indicated to assess for edema and possible infiltration/extravasation or deep vein thrombosis. Take this measurement 10 cm above the antecubital fossa.

e. Positive pressure flushing will keep PICC from clotting.

4. Central implanted vascular device:

a. A subcutaneous pocket is formed and a reservoir is placed; a catheter is attached to the reservoir and tunneled subcutaneously and inserted into a central vein (usually, the catheter tip is in the superior vena cava). This device cannot be seen exteriorly.

b. Central implanted vascular devices are typically used in patients who require intermittent long-term infusion therapy such as with chemotherapy and can remain in place for 5 years or more.

c. Examples of implanted devices in current use include the Port-A-Cath, Mediport, Infuse-A-Port, Bard Port systems, and PowerPort.

CLINICAL JUDGMENT If central catheters are placed too deeply and extend into the right atrium, an irregular heartbeat may result. Monitor heart rhythm and notify the health care provider immediately.

CLINICAL JUDGMENT The use of chlorhexidine-containing dressings is considered an essential practice to reduce central line–associated bloodstream infections.

EVIDENCE BASE Gorski, L. A., Hadaway, L., Hagle, M. E., Broadhurst, D., Clare, S., Kleidon, T., & Alexander, M. (2021). Infusion therapy standards of practice. *Journal of Infusion Nursing*, *44*(1S), S1–S224. https://doi.org/10.1097/NAN.0000000000000396

Alternative Nonvascular Infusion Devices

1. Intraspinal access devices
   a. Access devices placed in the epidural, intrathecal, or ventricular spaces.
   b. Anticipate intraspinal infusion administration with medications for pain management, chemotherapies, or spasticity control. Do not use alcohol- or acetone-containing disinfectants to cleanse the catheter hub prior to administration.
   c. Administer only preservative-free medications or solutions using a 0.2-µm filter that is surfactant free, particulate retentive, and air eliminating.
   d. Maintain surgical aseptic nontouch technique during catheter placement and implanted intraspinal port access.
2. Intraosseous (IO) access devices
   a. Access devices placed in the marrow of the bone.
   b. Anticipate IO infusion for emergent and nonemergent use in patients with limited or no vascular access.
3. Subcutaneous access devices
   a. Anticipate subcutaneous access for administration of isotonic solutions for the treatment of mild-to-moderate dehydration or continuous opioid administration.
   b. Use hyaluronidase to facilitate the dispersion and absorption of medications or solutions in adults and pediatric patients.

NURSING ROLE IN INTRAVENOUS THERAPY

Initiating an Intravenous Line

Intravenous (IV) therapy is an invasive procedure and should be ordered only when necessary. Nurses must be familiar with the procedure as well as the equipment involved in initiating an IV to provide effective therapy and prevent complications. See Standards of Care Guidelines 2-1, page 40.

See additional online content: Procedure Guidelines 2-1 through 2-4.

Selecting a Vein

1. Select a vein suitable for venipuncture.
   a. Back of hand—metacarpal veins (see Figure 2-2A). Avoid digital veins, if possible.
      i. Advantages: Veins in this location are easily visualized and palpated. Selection of this site permits arm movement. Should successive venipuncture be needed, another location higher up the arm may be utilized.
      ii. Disadvantages: Caution is required when selecting this site in the older adult because of thin skin and inadequate tissue often occurring in this area. When possible, select the nondominant hand.
   b. Forearm—basilic (along the ulnar side of the forearm) or cephalic (along the radial side of the forearm) vein (see Figure 2-2B).
      i. Advantages: These larger veins are usually visualized and palpable, allowing for more rapid infusion. Hand can be used freely.
      ii. Disadvantages: None.
   c. Inner aspect of elbow, antecubital fossa—intermediate median basilic and intermediate median cephalic; used for relatively short-term infusion; not a primary choice for nonemergent IV access.
      i. Advantages: Large, well supported by subcutaneous tissue preventing vein mobility; deeper and more tolerant to caustic substances.
      ii. Disadvantages: Prevents bending of arm; greater risk of infiltration; median basilic and cephalic veins are not recommended for chemotherapy because of the potential for extravasation and poor healing, resulting in impaired joint movement.
   d. Lower extremities—great saphenous vein at the ankle, superficial dorsal plexus, dorsal venous arch, or medial marginal vein of the foot.
      i. Advantages: The lower division of the great saphenous vein is frequently used in infants and toddlers.
      ii. Disadvantages: May require explicit orders from the health care provider because thrombosis occurs more

STANDARDS OF CARE GUIDELINES 2-1

Intravenous (IV) Therapy

To prevent adverse effects of IV therapy, perform the following assessments and procedures:

- Before starting IV therapy, consider the indication for IV therapy including duration of therapy, type of infusion, condition of veins, and medical condition of the patient to assist in choosing IV site and type of catheter.
- Ensure competence in initiating the type of IV therapy to be utilized and familiarity with facility policy and procedure before initiating therapy.
- Perform skin antisepsis prior to venipuncture or placement of a vascular access device. Aseptic nontouch technique should be maintained throughout the procedure.
- Following successful placement of vascular access device, appropriately secure the device to avoid dislodgment and reduce the risk of thrombophlebitis.
- Educate the patient and caregiver regarding the rationale for the vascular access device and expectations during and after the procedure.
- After initiation of IV therapy, monitor the patient frequently for:
  - Signs of infiltration or sluggish flow.
  - Signs of phlebitis or infection.
  - Correct solution, medication, volume, and rate.
  - Dwell time of catheter and need to be replaced.
  - Condition of catheter dressing and frequency of change.
  - Fluid and electrolyte balance.
  - Signs of fluid overload or dehydration.
  - Patient satisfaction with mode of therapy.

This information should serve as a general guideline only. Each patient situation presents a unique set of clinical factors and requires nursing judgment to guide care, which may include additional or alternative measures and approaches.

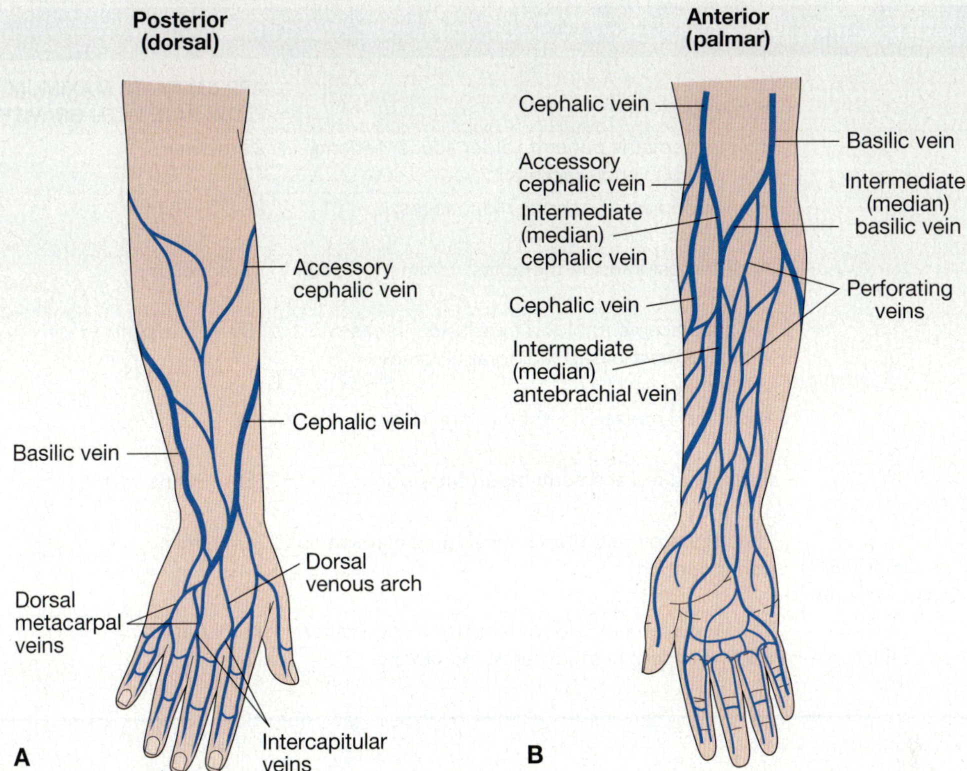

Figure 2-2. **(A)** Superficial veins, dorsal aspect of the hand. **(B)** Superficial veins, forearm. (Reprinted with permission from Smeltzer, S., & Bare, B. [2000]. *Brunner and Suddarth's textbook of medical-surgical nursing* [9th ed.]. Lippincott Williams & Wilkins.)

frequently than in veins of the upper extremities; irregular absorption may occur due to the increased number of valves present in the lower extremities causing infusions to potentially pool.

CLINICAL JUDGMENT Avoid selecting areas of flexion for placement of intravascular access. Areas of flexion are at an increased risk for adverse events because of the superficial presentation of arteries and nerves and are more likely to result in infiltration/extravasation, thrombophlebitis, arterial puncture, and nerve injury.

CLINICAL JUDGMENT Selection of lower extremity sites for venipuncture in patients with diabetes or peripheral vascular disease is not recommended because of the increased risk of phlebitis, thrombosis, infection, and potential for poor healing.

CLINICAL JUDGMENT Vascular visualization technologies (e.g., near-infrared, ultrasound) should be used to identify and select the most appropriate vessel and aid in placement to improve first-attempt success and decrease adverse events.

Methods of Distending a Vein

1. Apply a tourniquet (soft, nonlatex) at least 2 to 6 in (5 to 15 cm) above the planned insertion site, fastening it with a slipknot or hemostat, in a manner to impede venous flow but allowing for arterial circulation. Alternatively, apply a blood pressure cuff (keep pressure just below systolic pressure).
2. Apply manual compression above the site where the cannula is to be inserted.
3. Position the extremity lower than the level of the heart, having the patient open and close their fist, and lightly stoke the vein downward.
4. Lightly tap the vein site; this is to be done gently so the vein is not injured.
5. Apply warmth to site by using a warm dry towel or heat pack.

Selecting Needle or Catheter

1. Use the smallest gauge catheter suitable for the type and location of the infusion to minimize trauma to the vein.
2. Refer to Table 2-3 to assist in selecting the most appropriate catheter type. If a blood transfusion is to be given, use a larger-bore catheter, preferably 18G or larger.
3. Consider local anesthetic agents to minimize pain while obtaining vascular access.
   a. Agents include topical vapocoolant sprays, topical transdermal agents, intradermal lidocaine, and pressure-accelerated lidocaine.
   b. May cause collapse of desired veins, allergic reactions, and increase cost of the procedure.
   c. Warm compresses can mitigate the vasoconstrictive effects of local anesthetics.
4. Do not leave steel-winged devices in place; they are for single-dose administration only.
5. Use catheters manufactured with protective devices to guard against needlestick injuries (see Figure 2-3).

Table 2-3 Types of Short Peripheral Cannulas

CANNULA TYPE	PURPOSE	APPROXIMATE MAXIMUM FLOW RATE WITH GRAVITY	VOLUMES
24 gauge Yellow/lime	Infants; pediatric patients; older adults; patients with difficult venous access	23 mL/min	Small
22 gauge Blue	Infants; pediatric patients; older adults; small veins	22–50 mL/min	Small
20 gauge Pink	Adults; most infusion therapies; commonly used	55–80 mL/min	Medium
18 gauge Green	Fluid replacement; blood transfusion; for use with a contrast-based radiographic study; commonly used	100–120 mL/min	Large
16 gauge Gray	Rapid fluid replacement; blood transfusion	150–240 mL/min	Large
14 gauge Orange/brown	Rapid fluid replacement; blood transfusion	250–300 mL/min	Extra large
18 gauge Medial (blue) and proximal (white) lumen of a triple-lumen catheter	Fluid replacement; blood transfusion; medication administration	26 mL/min	Large
16 gauge Distal (brown) lumen of the triple-lumen catheter	Fluid replacement; blood transfusion; medication administration; hemodynamic monitoring	52 mL/min	Large

Cleaning the Infusion Site

EVIDENCE BASE Buetti, N., Marschall, J., Drees, M., Fakih, M., Hadaway, L., Maragakis, L., Monsees, E., Novosad, S., O'Grady, N. P., Rupp, M. E., Wolf, J., Yokoe, D., & Mermel, L. (2022). Strategies to prevent central line–associated bloodstream infections in acute-care hospitals: 2022 Update. *Infection Control & Hospital Epidemiology, 43*(5), 553–569. https://doi.org/10.1017/ice.2022.87

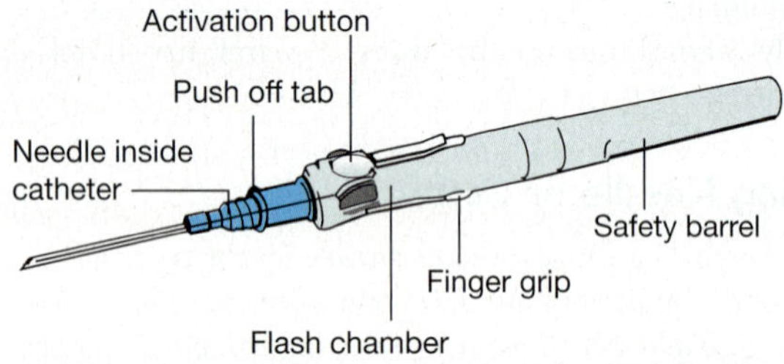

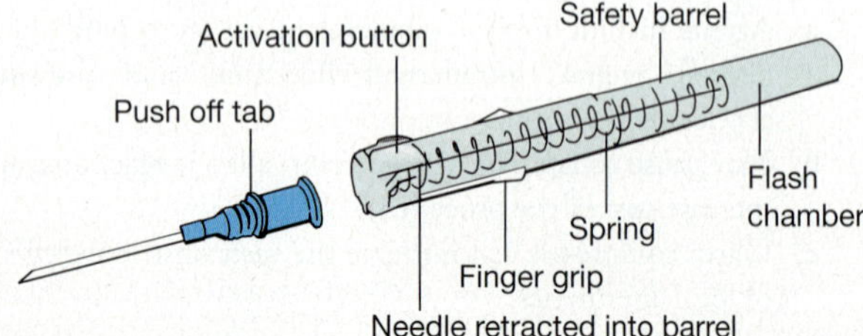

Figure 2-3. The activation button is pressed after the catheter is in the vein so that the needle will retract into the safety barrel while the catheter remains in the vein.

1. Use aseptic nontouch technique according to institutional protocols.
2. Clean the IV site with an effective topical antiseptic according to facility protocol.
   a. The preferred skin antiseptic is chlorhexidine solution used in an outward, circular scrubbing manner following manufacturer's instructions. Allow to dry completely.
   b. Caution with chlorhexidine in neonates and infants younger than 2 months because of increased risks of skin irritation and chemical burns. Avoid the use of tincture of iodine in neonates because of adverse effect on the thyroid gland.
   c. Alcohol swabs, povidone–iodine, or tincture of iodine may be used in the same outward circular scrubbing manner where chlorhexidine is contraindicated. Allow to dry completely.

Use of Stabilization Devices

Stabilizing vascular access devices, such as joint stabilization devices like an arm board, can prevent unintentional dislodgment and adverse complications. Do not rely on vascular access device dressings such as a transparent semipermeable membrane or gauze as a means for stabilization.

Infusion Tubing

1. Drip chambers:
   a. A "microdrip" system delivers 60 drops/mL and is used when small volumes are being delivered (e.g., <50 mL/h); this reduces the risk of clotting the IV line because of slow infusion rates.
   b. The "macrodrip" system delivers 10 to 20 drops/mL and is used to deliver solution in large quantities or at fast rates.
2. Vented tubing should be used with standard glass bottles; this permits air to enter the vacuum in the bottle and displace solution as it flows out. Nonvented tubing should be used for IV bags and glass bottles that have a built-in air vent.

3. Filters help minimize the risk of contamination from certain microorganisms and particulate matter.
   a. Filters are found "inline" on conventional IV, blood, and parenteral nutrition tubing and are preferred because they reduce the risks of contamination. An additional filter is needed for mannitol and may be needed for other solutions based on facility protocol.
   b. "Add-on" filters should be located as close to the insertion site as possible and be changed with administration set changes.
4. Most electronic infusion pumps require specialized tubing to fit their particular pumping chamber. Need for such a device should be determined before initiating infusion therapy.
   a. If extra tubing length is required (especially for children and patients who are restless), extension tubing is available; this should be added at the time of IV setup.
   b. Secondary administration tubing sets are used for administration of intermittent, "piggyback," medications that are connected to the port closest to the drip chamber.
   c. Special-coated tubing, designed to prevent leaching of polyvinyl chloride, is used for delivering medications, such as nitroglycerin, paclitaxel, and cyclosporine.
   d. Add-on devices such as single- and multilumen extension sets, extension loops, needleless connectors, inline filters, manual flow control devices, and stopcocks should be used only when clinically indicated. Use systems that minimize the manipulation and reduce multiple components to limit potential contamination and change with each new administration set.
5. Administration tubing set change—label with date, time opened, and initials.
   a. Continuous tubing administration sets used for medications and solutions should be changed no more frequently than every 96 hours but at least every 7 days.
   b. Intermittent tubing administration sets should be changed every 24 hours.
   c. Tubing administration sets used for parenteral nutrition solutions should be replaced every 24 hours or with each new container.
   d. Tubing administration sets used for IV fat emulsions should be replaced every 12 hours or with each new container.
   e. Tubing administration sets used for blood or blood products should be changed every 2 to 4 units of blood or every 4 hours.

Adjusting Rate of Flow

Three factors are involved in determining a medication or solution flow rate: the concentration of the medication diluted in a given volume, the dose of the medication to be administered over a length of time, or the stated volume of solution or medication to be delivered over a length of time. The health care provider prescribes the flow rate. The nurse is responsible for regulating and maintaining the proper rate.

CLINICAL JUDGMENT When initiating an infusion, consider using electronic infusion pumps with dose-error reduction software and dose calculation software, comprehensive libraries of medications, and safety alarms as an effective error-reducing strategy.

Patient Determining Factors

When determining flow rates, consider patient factors such as age, acuity and severity of the illness/injury, type of therapy, dosing considerations, and health care setting.

1. Age—fluids should be administered slowly in the very young and in older adults.
2. Condition—a patient in hypovolemic shock requires greater amounts of fluids, whereas the patient with heart or renal failure should receive fluids judiciously.
3. Tolerance to solutions—fluids containing medications causing potential allergic reactions or intense vascular irritation (e.g., potassium chloride) should be well diluted or given slowly.
4. Prescribed fluid composition—efficacy of some drugs is based on speed of infusion (e.g., antibiotics); rate for other solutions is titrated to the patient's response to them (e.g., dopamine, nitroprusside, heparin).

System Determining Factors

1. Gauge of IV catheter.
2. Pressure gradient—the difference between two levels in a fluid system.
3. Friction—the interaction between fluid molecules and surfaces of inner wall of tubing.
4. Diameter and length of tubing.
5. Height of column of fluid.
6. Characteristics of fluid.
   a. Viscosity.
   b. Temperature—refrigerated fluids may cause diminished flow and vessel spasm; bring fluid to room temperature before infusion.
7. Vein trauma, clots, plugging of vents, venous spasm, and vasoconstriction.
8. Flow control clamp derangement.
   a. Some clamps may slip and loosen, resulting in a rapid, or "free-flow," infusion. Many tubings now have safety clamps to prevent this rapid infusion.
   b. Plastic tubing may distort, causing "creep" or "cold flow"—the inside diameter of tubing will continue to change long after the clamp is tightened or relaxed.
   c. Marked stretching of tubing may cause distortions of tubing and render clamp ineffective (may occur when patient turns over and pulls on a short tubing).
9. If there is any question about the rate of fluid administration, confirm with the health care provider.

POPULATION AWARENESS Be aware that veins are more likely to roll within the loose tissue beneath the skin, collapse, and become irritated in older adults. Also, fluid overload may be more pronounced, making IV therapy more difficult and potentially dangerous.

Calculation of Flow Rate

1. Most infusion rates are given at a certain volume per hour.
2. Delivery of the prescribed volume is determined by calculating necessary drops per minute to deliver the volume.
3. Calculate the infusion rate using the following formula:

$$\text{Drop/minute} = \frac{\text{Total volume} \times \text{Infused drops/mL}}{\text{Total time for infusion in minutes}}$$

Example: Infuse 150 mL of dextrose 5% in water (D_5W) in 1 hour (set indicates 10 drops/mL)

$$\frac{150 \times 10}{60 \text{ minutes}} = 25 \text{ drops/minute}$$

4. The nurse hanging a new IV solution should write the date, time, and their initials on the container label. To avoid leaks, never write directly on the IV bag. Do not use markers because they are absorbed into the plastic bag and possibly into the solution. Write on the label or tape using a regular pen.

Vascular Access Maintenance and Removal

Maintaining Patency

1. Flush vascular access device with normal saline and aspirate blood prior to each infusion to assess catheter function as well as after each infusion to clear the infused medicine from the catheter lumen and to prevent potential contact of incompatible medicines.
2. Flushing intermittent peripheral catheters with normal saline is equivalent to flushing with heparin in maintaining catheter patency and complication rates. If using bacteriostatic 0.9% sodium chloride, limit volume to less than 30 mL per 24-hour period to reduce potential toxic effects of benzyl alcohol, the preservative used.
3. Prefilled syringes are preferred when flushing. Do not use IV solution bags as a "flush" bag. Recommended flush volume is two times the volume of the catheter and add-on device, usually 10 mL, to remove fibrin deposits, drug precipitate, and other debris from the lumen to ensure patency.
4. Use a push–pause method to inject. Do not force if resistance is met, rather evaluate for patency or complications of the vascular access.
5. Assess vascular access frequently for signs of infiltration, infection, phlebitis, and other complications. See Table 2-4.

Removal of Vascular Access Device

1. Assess vascular access at least daily as part of the patient's overall plan of care, with the goal of removal as soon as possible.
2. Vascular access devices should be removed with any signs and symptoms of complications; work in coordination with the health care team to avoid delays in medically necessary treatments.
3. Ensure appropriate personnel and organizational procedures are followed for the removal of any vascular device.

Evaluation, Documentation, Patient Education, and Quality Improvement

Documentation and Patient Education

1. Documentation must contain accurate, factual, and complete information regarding the initial and ongoing assessment, nursing diagnosis or problems, interventions, and patient's response to those interventions.
2. Documentation specific to IV therapy should include, but is not limited to, the following:
   a. Date and time of cannula insertion.
   b. Site (include anatomic description, laterality), preparation of insertion, and infection prevention precautions taken.
   c. Number of cannulation attempts.
   d. Size and type of inserted cannula.
   e. Dressing and catheter securement.
   f. Tolerance of the procedure.
   g. Monitoring of the site.
   h. Date and time of cannula removal.
   i. Identification and management of complications.
3. The nurse is responsible for educating the patient and caregiver about IV therapies. This education should include such topics as the plan of care, purpose and goals of treatment, intravascular device–related care, and potential complications. The teaching methods and any learning materials provided should be sensitive to the preferred learning style of the patient considering such factors as developmental and cognitive level, health literacy, cultural influences, or readiness to learn.

Table 2-4 Visual Infusion Phlebitis Scale

Intravenous (IV) site appears healthy	0	No signs of phlebitis **OBSERVE CANNULA**
One of the following is evident: ✓ Slight pain near IV site or ✓ Slight redness near IV site	1	Possibly first signs of phlebitis **OBSERVE CANNULA**
Two of the following are evident: ✓ Pain at IV site ✓ Erythema ✓ Swelling	2	Early stage of phlebitis **RESITE CANNULA**
All of the following signs are evident: ✓ Pain along path of cannula ✓ Erythema ✓ Induration	3	Medium stage of phlebitis **RESITE CANNULA** **CONSIDER TREATMENT**
All of the following signs are evident and extensive: ✓ Pain along path of cannula ✓ Erythema ✓ Induration ✓ Palpable venous cord	4	Advanced stage of phlebitis or the start of thrombophlebitis **RESITE CANNULA** **CONSIDER TREATMENT**
All of the following signs are evident and extensive: ✓ Pain along path of cannula ✓ Erythema ✓ Induration ✓ Palpable venous cord ✓ Pyrexia	5	Advanced stage of thrombophlebitis **RESITE CANNULA** **INITIATE TREATMENT**

Adapted with permission from Gallant, P., & Schultz, A. A. (2006). Evaluation of a visual infusion phlebitis scale for determining appropriate discontinuation of peripheral intravenous catheters. Journal of Infusion Nursing, 29(6), 338–345. https://doi.org/10.1097/00129804-200611000-00004; Adapted with permission from Jackson, A. (2003). Reflecting on the nursing contribution to vascular access. British Journal of Nursing, 12(11), 657–665. https://doi.org/10.12968/bjon.2003.12.11.11315, permission conveyed through Copyright Clearance Center, Inc.

Evaluation and Quality Improvement

1. Quality improvement programs should be implemented to advance quality of care with vascular access devices and infusion administration, incorporating surveillance, aggregation, analysis, and reporting of IV-related quality indicators to establish a just culture to improve practice, processes, and systems.
2. Adverse events must be recognized and documented to minimize health care–associated infections related to IV therapy.

Complications of IV Therapy

Infiltration/Extravasation

Cause

1. Dislodgment of the IV cannula from the vein. Infiltration is the unintentional infusion of nonvesicant medications or solutions into the surrounding tissue, whereas extravasation is the unintentional infusion of a vesicant into the surrounding tissues.

Clinical Manifestations

1. Discomfort or pain, depending on the nature of the solution.
2. Swelling, redness or blanching, and coolness of surrounding skin and tissues.
3. Fluid flowing more slowly or ceasing. Fluid noticed from the puncture site.
4. Absence of blood backflow in IV catheter and tubing.

Preventive Measures

1. Select the most appropriate vascular access device and insertion site.
2. Make sure that the IV and distal tubing are secured sufficiently to prevent movement.
3. Splint the patient's arm or hand as necessary.
4. Assess the vascular access device for functionality routinely and prior to use.

Nursing Interventions

1. Stop infusion immediately and remove the IV needle or catheter.
2. In the event of infiltration/extravasation of a short peripheral or midline catheter, stop the infusion immediately and detach all administration sets. Aspirate from the catheter hub or while removing the vascular access device to remove as much of the medication or solution from the catheter lumen and subcutaneous tissue as possible. Aspiration is not recommended with extravasation of contrast media.
3. Notify the health care provider and initiate emergency local treatment as directed to limit the potential damage to subcutaneous tissue by the medication or solution. Serious tissue injury, necrosis, and sloughing may result if actions are not taken.
4. Avoid application of pressure to the area. Elevate the extremity. To localize the medication or solution in the tissues and reduce inflammation, apply dry, cold compresses to the area; or to increase blood flow and disperse the medication, apply dry warm compresses per facility protocol according to the medication or solution exposure.
5. Document assessments and interventions.

Phlebitis

Causes

1. Injury to the vein that occurs during venipuncture (e.g., using too large of a catheter for the selected vein), catheter movement, or caused from prolonged needle or catheter use.
2. Poor aseptic technique.
3. Irritation to vein because of rapid infusions or irritating solutions (e.g., hypertonic glucose solutions, cytotoxic agents, strong acids or alkalis, potassium, antibiotics, and others); smaller veins are more susceptible.
4. Clot formation at the end of the needle or catheter because of slow infusion rates or inadequate hemodilution of medications or solutions—then called "thrombophlebitis."

Clinical Manifestations

1. Pain, tenderness, or swelling to palpation at IV site that may extend along the path of the cannula and vein.
2. Redness, swelling, warmth, induration, or purulence at IV site; the vein may appear as a red streak above the insertion site.
3. Palpable venous cord.

Preventive Measures

1. Routinely assess the vascular access site with a standardized tool for signs and symptoms of phlebitis. See Table 2-4 as an example.
2. Anchor the needle or catheter securely at the insertion site.
3. Sufficiently dilute irritating agents before infusion.

Nursing Interventions

1. Apply warm compresses to stimulate circulation and promote absorption, counteracting venoconstriction caused by phlebitis.
2. Elevate the extremity.
3. Consider removal of the vascular access device.
4. Consider other pharmacologic interventions such as analgesics, anti-inflammatory agents, or corticosteroids as necessary.
5. Document assessments and interventions.
6. Participate in facility quality improvement activities regarding phlebitis occurrence rates. One formula that can be used is:

$$\frac{\text{Number of phlebitis incidents}}{\text{Total number of IV peripheral catheters}} \times 100 = \%\ \text{peripheral phlebitis}$$

Catheter-Associated Bloodstream Infections

Causes

1. Contaminated equipment or infused solutions (see Figure 2-4).
2. Prolonged placement of an IV device (catheter or needle, tubing, solution container).
3. Contaminated IV insertion or dressing change.
4. Cross-contamination by the patient with other infected areas of the body.
5. A patient who is critically ill or immunosuppressed is at greatest risk of bacteremia.

Clinical Manifestations

1. Possible signs of local infection at vascular access insertion site (e.g., redness, pain or tenderness, edema, foul drainage).
2. Elevated temperature, chills.
3. Nausea, vomiting.
4. Elevated white blood cell (WBC) count.
5. Malaise, increased pulse.
6. Backache, headache.
7. May progress to septic shock with profound hypotension.

Preventive Measures

1. Follow the same measures as outlined for thrombophlebitis.
2. Strict adherence to hand hygiene and the use of aseptic non-touch techniques with maximal barrier precautions during

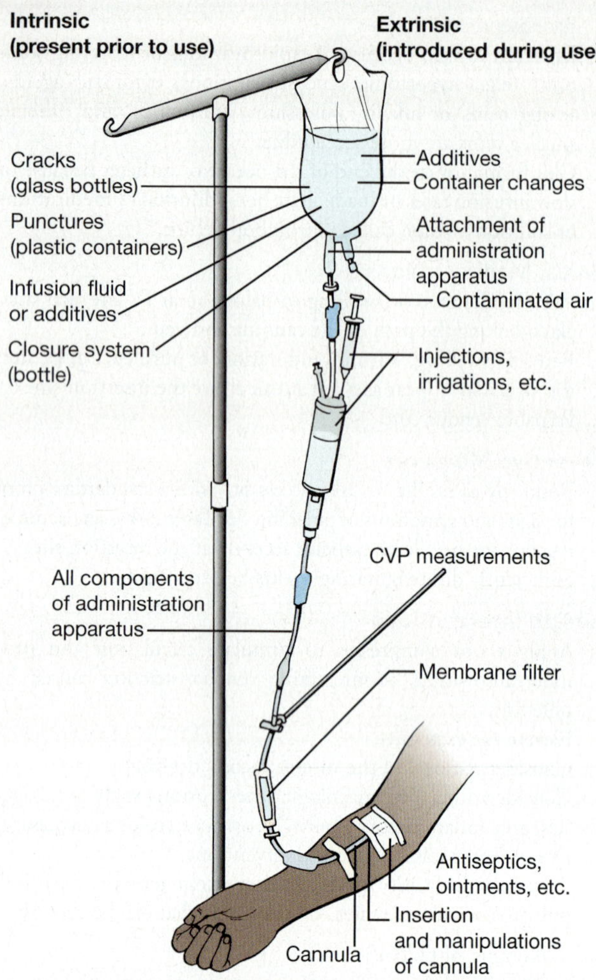

Figure 2-4. Potential mechanisms for contamination of intravenous infusion systems. CVP, central venous pressure.

insertion and dressing changes remain the most important measure for the prevention of catheter-associated bloodstream infections (CABSIs).

3. Ensure appropriate cleaning products are used to cleanse the skin prior to insertion of the cannula. Chlorhexidine is preferred and has been shown to reduce the rate of infections.
4. Choose appropriate sites for catheter insertion.
5. Replacing IV catheters when clinically indicated, rather than routine replacement every 72 to 96 hours, demonstrates no increased patient risk of thrombophlebitis or infection. An exception to this is when adherence to aseptic technique cannot be ensured (e.g., insertion during a medical emergency), at which time, the catheter should be replaced as soon as possible but no longer than 48 hours after insertion.
6. Use antimicrobial-impregnated central venous catheters in patients with high risk of infections such as those with neutropenia, burn injuries, or critical illness.
7. Change catheter administration sets at appropriate intervals. Refer back to "Infusion Tubing" on page 42.
8. Medications and solutions should be administered within 24 hours or should then be replaced with a new container. Lipid-containing solutions should be completed within 24 hours of hanging the solution. Lipid emulsions should be completed within 6 to 12 hours of hanging the solution. Blood or other blood products should be completed within 4 hours of hanging the solution. Maintain integrity of the infusion system at all times.
9. Ensure proper vascular access site assessment and care. Change the IV dressing on a routine basis and immediately if it becomes damp, loosened, or soiled.
   a. Gauze dressing that prevents visualization of the site should be changed every 48 hours.
   b. Transparent semipermeable dressing should be changed every 7 days. In neonatal patients, perform dressing changes when disrupted to reduce the risk of catheter dislodgment, patient discomfort, or skin injury.
   c. Use chlorhexidine-impregnated dressings for all adult patients with short-term, nontunneled central vascular devices.
10. When accessing the port of a vascular access device, vigorously scrub—not wipe—the hub of the catheter for 15 seconds with alcohol or chlorohexidine solution. Use passive disinfection caps containing disinfecting agents (e.g., isopropyl alcohol), which result in reduced intraluminal microbial contamination and decreases the rates of CABSI.
11. Ensure removal of catheters when no longer essential.
12. Hand hygiene, personal protective equipment, and safe injection practices using aseptic nontouch technique form the basis of standard precautions. Appropriate infection control measures with implementation of care bundles and a culture of safety are essential in preventing complications and ensuring the delivery of efficient, high-quality care across care settings.

Nursing Interventions

1. Discontinue infusion and consider removal of vascular access device. A peripheral venous device with signs and symptoms of infection, including erythema extending at least 1 cm from the insertion site, induration, exudate, and fever with no other source of infectious process, should be removed. Collaboration with the health care team is needed to determine whether a central venous access device can be salvaged or necessitates removal.
2. If purulent exudate is present, obtain a sample for culture and Gram staining.
3. With removal of the vascular access device in a suspected CABSI, cut off the tip of the catheter with sterile scissors; place in a dry, sterile container; and immediately send it to the laboratory for culture and Gram staining.
4. Start appropriate antibiotic therapy immediately after receiving orders and obtaining all additional specimens for culture and Gram staining.
5. Document assessments and interventions.

Circulatory Overload

Cause

1. Delivery of excessive amounts of IV fluid (greater risk exists for older patients, infants, or patients with cardiac or renal insufficiency).

Clinical Manifestations

1. Increase in body weight of at least 5% to 10%, or a positive fluid balance of 5% to 10% when intake and output are measured.
2. Increased blood pressure (BP) and pulse.
3. Increased central venous pressure (CVP), venous distention (engorged jugular veins).
4. Headache, anxiety.
5. Shortness of breath, tachypnea, coughing, pulmonary crackles.
6. Peripheral edema.
7. Chest pain (if history of coronary artery disease).

Preventive Measures

1. Assess patient for existing heart or kidney condition. Be particularly vigilant in patients at high risk.
2. Closely monitor the infusion flow rate, and use electronic infusion pumps.
3. Keep accurate intake and output records.
4. Splint the arm or hand if the IV flow rate fluctuates too widely with movement.

Nursing Interventions

1. If circulatory overload is suspected, notify health care provider, sit patient up for easier breathing, and anticipate reduced IV infusion rate and additional medication therapy.
2. Monitor closely for worsening clinical condition.

Air Embolism

Causes

1. A greater risk exists in central venous lines, when air enters catheter during tubing changes (air sucked in during inspiration because of negative intrathoracic pressure).
2. Air in tubing delivered by IV push or infused by infusion pump.

Clinical Manifestations

1. Sudden onset of dyspnea, breathlessness, elevated respiratory rate.
2. Chest pain, hypotension, elevated heart rates.
3. Altered mental status, altered speech.
4. Changes in facial appearance, paralysis.

Preventive Measures

1. Clear all air from any administration device (e.g., tubing, extension sets, syringes, add-on devices) before connecting to patient.
2. Prevent solution containers from emptying entirely.
3. Ensure that all connections are secure. Use Luer-lock connections or administration sets with air-eliminating filters unless contraindicated.
4. Use appropriate technique with removal of central venous access devices.
5. When removing a central venous access device, place the patient in supine or Trendelenburg position so that the insertion site is at or below the level of the heart. Instruct the patient to bear down (Valsalva maneuver) during catheter withdrawal unless contraindicated.

Nursing Interventions

1. Immediately prevent additional air from entering the bloodstream by closing, kinking, clamping, or covering the existing vascular access device or insertion site with an air-occlusive dressing.
2. Immediately turn the patient on their left side and lower the head of the bed; in this position, air will become trapped in the right side of the heart.
3. Notify the health care provider immediately.
4. Administer oxygen as needed and support the medical stability of the patient.
5. Document assessments and interventions.

Mechanical Failure (Sluggish Flow or Occlusion)

Causes

1. Malposition of the catheter including the cannula lying against the side of the vein, cutting off fluid flow, or infiltration of the catheter.
2. Clot at the end of the catheter or needle.
3. External mechanical causes such as kinking of the tubing or catheter, clogged filter, or needless connector.

Clinical Manifestations

1. Inability to withdraw blood or sluggish blood return.
2. Sluggish IV flow, resistance to flushing the lumen, or frequent occlusion alarms on electronic infusion pumps.
3. Signs of infiltration/extravasation.

Preventive Measures

1. Assess the functionality of the vascular access device routinely.
2. Use appropriate flushing procedures.
3. Secure the IV well to prevent catheter dislodgment.
4. Avoid incompatible mixtures of IV solutions and medications.

Nursing Interventions

1. Assess/resolve mechanical causes of occlusion including entire administration set and functionality of the electronic infusion pump if applicable.
2. Assess catheter placement. Consider repositioning the catheter by pulling back on the cannula slightly because it may be lying against the vein wall valve or bifurcation or repositioning the patient's extremity in which the vascular access device is placed.
3. Consider the need for a catheter-clearing agent or thrombolytic agent in collaboration with the health care team.
4. Consider the need to remove the vascular access device.

Hemorrhage

Causes

1. Loose connection of tubing or injection port.
2. Inadvertent removal of vascular access device.
3. Anticoagulant therapy.

Clinical Manifestations

1. External bleeding with visible oozing or trickling of blood from IV site or catheter.
2. Internal bleeding is more difficult to identify; may be identified with hematoma formation or presence of a new hemothorax.

Preventive Measures

1. Maintain integrity of the vascular access device, keeping all access points capped with Luer-locking needleless connectors.
2. Secure catheters using appropriate resources to prevent dislodgment.
3. Keep pressure on sites where catheters have been removed—a minimum of 10 minutes for a patient taking anticoagulants.

Catheter-Associated Venous Thrombosis

Causes

1. Infusion of irritating solutions (e.g., potassium chloride, diazepam, antibiotics, chemotherapy agents).
2. Infection along catheter.
3. Fibrin sheath formation with eventual clot formation around the catheter. (This clot will eventually occlude the vein.)
4. Stasis of blood in and around the IV catheter. Larger diameter, centrally placed catheters are at greater risk.
5. Patient factors including a medical history of a hypercoagulable state (e.g., cancer, diabetes, or end-stage renal failure), history of deep vein thrombosis, surgical or trauma patients, critical care patients, and extremes of age.

Clinical Manifestations

1. Swelling and pain in the area of catheter or in the extremity proximal to the insertion site.
2. Slowing of IV infusion or inability to draw blood from the central line.
3. Palpable lump in the cannulated vessel.

Preventive Measures

1. Select appropriate vascular access device and site location.
2. Ensure proper dilution of irritating substances.
3. Ensure proper placement of vascular access device.
4. Institute nonpharmacologic strategies for thrombosis prevention if possible, such as early patient mobility and adequate hydration.
5. Prophylaxis with anticoagulant therapies as ordered by the health care team.

Nursing Interventions

1. Immediately prevent additional bleeding by closing, kinking, clamping, or applying direct pressure to the existing vascular access device or insertion site.
2. Notify the health care provider immediately.
3. Support the medical stability of the patient.

SELECTED READINGS

Agency for Healthcare Research and Quality. (2021, March 12). *Medication administration errors.* Patient Safety Network. https://psnet.ahrq.gov/primer/medication-administration-errors

Broadhurst, D., Cooke, M., Sriram, D., & Gray, B. (2020). Subcutaneous hydration and medications infusions (effectiveness, safety, acceptability): A systematic review of systematic reviews. *PLoS One, 15*(8), e0237572. https://doi.org/10.1371/journal.pone.0237572

Chopra, V. (2022). Central venous access: Device and site selection in adults. *UpToDate.* Retrieved October 14, 2023, from https://www.uptodate.com/contents/central-venous-access-device-and-site-selection-in-adults

Food & Drug Administration. (2018, August 22). *Infusion pumps.* General Hospital Devices and Supplies. https://www.fda.gov/medical-devices/general-hospital-devices-and-supplies/infusion-pumps#:~:text=An%20infusion%20pump%20is%20a,homes%2C%20and%20in%20the%20home

Guanche-Sicilia, A., Sánchez-Gómez, M. B., Castro-Peraza, M. E., Rodríguez-Gómez, J. Á., Gómez-Salgado, J., & Duarte-Clíments, G. (2021). Prevention and treatment of phlebitis secondary to the insertion of a peripheral venous catheter: A scoping review from a nursing perspective. *Healthcare (Basel, Switzerland), 9*(5), 611. https://doi.org/10.3390/healthcare9050611

Jose, M. D., Marshall, M. R., Read, G., Lioufas, N., Ling, J., Snelling, P., & Polkinghorne, K. R. (2017). Fatal dialysis vascular access hemorrhage. *American Journal of Kidney Disease, 70*(4), 570–575. https://doi.org/10.1053/j.ajkd.2017.05.014

Lv, L., & Zhang, J. (2020). The incidence and risk of infusion phlebitis with peripheral intravenous catheters: A meta-analysis. *The Journal of Vascular Access, 21*(3), 342–349. https://doi.org/10.1177/1129729819877323

Malbrain, M. L. N. G., Langer, T., Annane, D., Gattinoni, L., Elbers, P., Hahn, R. G., De Laet, I., Minini, A., Wong, A., Ince, C., Muckart, D., Mythen, M., Caironi, P., & Van Regenmortel, N. (2020). Intravenous fluid therapy in the perioperative and critical care setting: Executive summary of the International Fluid Academy (IFA). *Annals of Intensive Care, 10*(1), 64. https://doi.org/10.1186/s13613-020-00679-3

Paterson, R. S., Chopra, V., Brown, E., Kleidon, T. M., Cooke, M., Rickard, C. M., Bernstein, S. J., & Ullman, A. J. (2020). Selection and insertion of vascular access devices in pediatrics: A systematic review. *Pediatrics, 145*(Suppl. 3), S243–S268. https://doi.org/10.1542/peds.2019-3474H

Pittiruti, M., Van Boxtel, T., Scoppettuolo, G., Carr, P., Konstantinou, E., Ortiz Miluy, G., Lamperti, M., Goossens, G. A., Simcock, L., Dupont, C., Inwood, S., Bertoglio, S., Nicholson, J., Pinelli, F., & Pepe, G. (2023). European recommendations on the proper indication and use of peripheral venous access devices (the ERPIUP consensus): A WoCoVA project. *The Journal of Vascular Access, 24*(1), 165–182. https://doi.org/10.1177/11297298211023274

Ray-Barruel, G., Xu, H., Marsh, N., Cooke, M., & Rickard, C. M. (2019). Effectiveness of insertion and maintenance bundles in preventing peripheral intravenous catheter-related complications and bloodstream infection in hospital patients: A systematic review. *Infection, Disease & Health, 24*(3), 152–168. https://doi.org/10.1016/j.idh.2019.03.001

Swaminathan, L., Flanders, S., Horowitz, J., Zhang, Q., O'Malley, M., & Chopra, V. (2022). Safety and outcomes of midline catheters vs peripherally inserted central catheters for patients with short-term indications: A multicenter study. *JAMA Internal Medicine, 182*(1), 50–58. https://doi.org/10.1001/jamainternmed.2021.6844

Takahashi, T., Murayama, R., Abe-Doi, M., Miyahara-Kaneko, M., Kanno, C., Nakamura, M., Mizuno, M., Komiyama, C., & Sanada, H. (2020). Preventing peripheral intravenous catheter failure by reducing mechanical irritation. *Scientific Reports, 10*(1), 1550. https://doi.org/10.1038/s41598-019-56873-2

3 Perioperative Nursing

OVERVIEW AND ASSESSMENT

See additional online content: Patient Education Guidelines 3-1.

Introduction

Perioperative nursing is a term used to describe the nursing care provided during the total surgical experience of the patient: preoperative, intraoperative, and postoperative.

Preoperative phase—from the time the decision is made for surgical intervention to the transfer of the patient to the operating room.
Intraoperative phase—from the time the patient is received in the operating room until admission to the postanesthesia care unit (PACU).
Postoperative phase—from the time of admission to the PACU to the follow-up evaluation.

An *anesthesia care provider* is a professional who can administer and monitor anesthesia during a surgical procedure; they may be a licensed physician board certified in anesthesia (anesthesiologist) or a certified registered nurse anesthetist.

Types of surgery include the following:

Elective—the scheduled time for surgery is at the convenience of the patient; failure to have surgery is not catastrophic (e.g., superficial cyst).
Required—the condition requires surgery within a few weeks (e.g., cataract).
Urgent—necessitates surgery as soon as possible but may be delayed for a short amount of time (e.g., internal fixation of fracture).
Emergent—the situation requires immediate surgical attention without delay (e.g., intestinal obstruction). This must be done to save life or limb or functional capacity.

Common abdominal incisions are pictured in Figure 3-1.

Perioperative Safety

The safety and welfare of patients during surgical intervention is a primary concern. Patients entering the perioperative settings are at risk for infection, impaired skin integrity, altered body temperature, fluid volume deficit, and injury related to positioning and chemical, electrical, and physical hazards.

The Surgical Care Improvement Project (SCIP), National Safety Goals for Surgery, and Enhanced Recovery After Surgery (ERAS) programs have resulted in major improvements in clinical outcomes. Care protocols are developed based on evidence of best practice. Examples include practices as apparent as proper identification and early mobilization, as well as proper antibiotic use, minimally invasive surgery, and multimodal approaches to resolving issues.

EVIDENCE BASE The Joint Commission. (2022). *National patient safety goals effective January 2023 for the hospital program.* https://www.jointcommission.org/standards/national-patient-safety-goals/hospital-national-patient-safety-goals/

The Joint Commission. (2018). *Surgical care improvement project.* https://www.jointcommission.org/surgical_care_improvement_project

Surgical Care Improvement Project

1. The SCIP, a national quality partnership interested in improving surgical care by significantly reducing surgical complications, is a coalition of health care organizations that has developed evidence-based interventions that have proven effective.
   a. The goal is to reduce surgical complications by 25%.
   b. Implementing nursing interventions at the earliest stage possible of a developing complication is also of utmost importance.

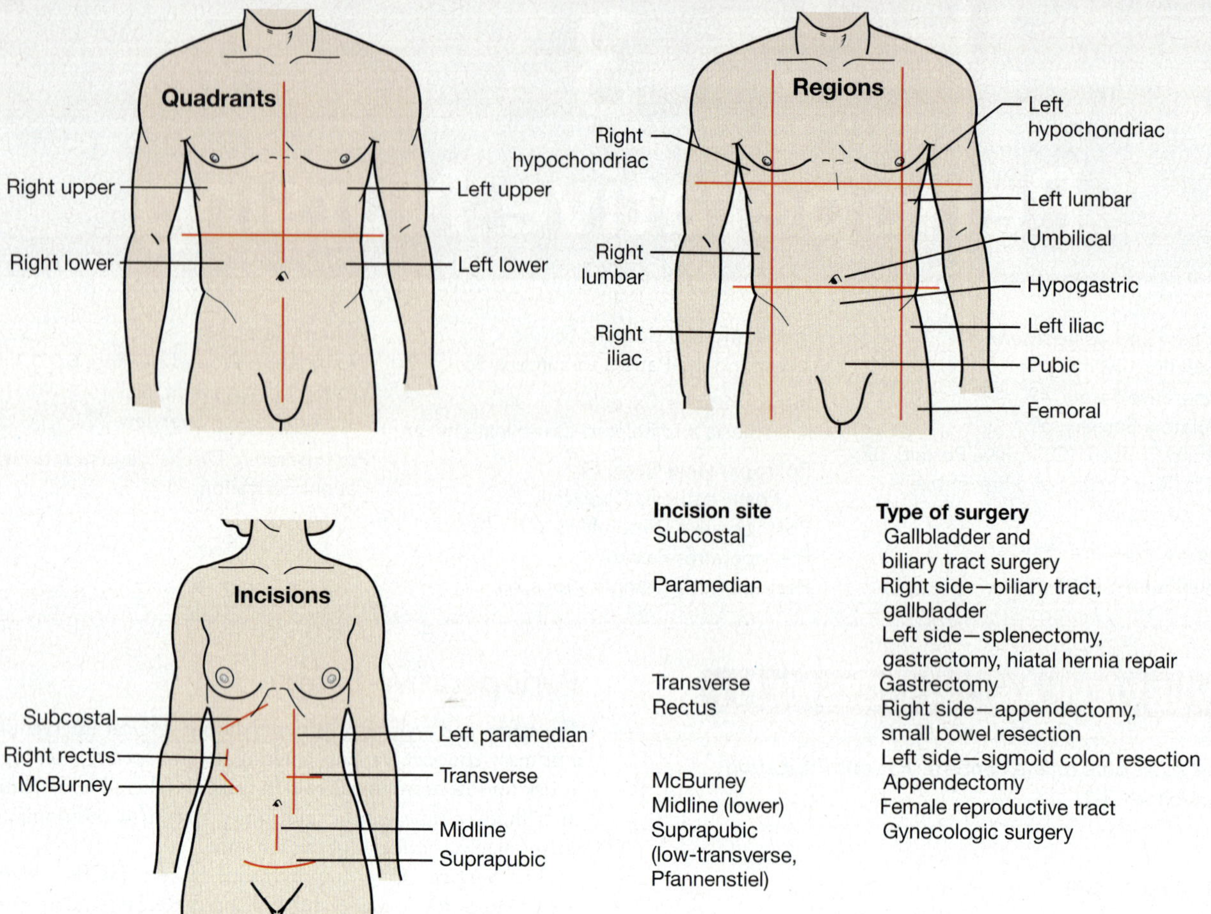

Figure 3-1. Regions and incisions of the abdomen.

2. SCIP measures that have been shown to be effective include the following:
   a. Prophylactic antibiotic received within 1 hour prior to surgical incision.
   b. Prophylactic antibiotic discontinued within 24 hours after surgery end time.
   c. Patients undergoing cardiac surgery with controlled postoperative serum glucose.
   d. Patients undergoing surgery with appropriate hair removal.
   e. Urinary catheter removed on postoperative day 1 or postoperative day 2 with day of surgery being day 0.
   f. Patients continue beta-blockers on day of surgery.
   g. Appropriate venous thromboembolism prophylaxis and treatment.

National Patient Safety Goals

1. Prevent infection—use hand cleaning guidelines from the Centers for Disease Control and Prevention (2023) or the World Health Organization.
   a. Use proven guidelines to prevent infections that are difficult to treat.
   b. Use proven guidelines to prevent infection of the blood from central lines.
   c. Use proven guidelines to prevent infection after surgery.
   d. Use proven guidelines to prevent infections of the urinary tract caused by catheters.
2. Prevent mistakes in surgery—make sure the correct surgery is done on the correct patient at the correct place on the patient's body.
   a. Mark the correct place on the patient's body where the surgery is to be done.
   b. Pause before surgery to make sure a mistake is not being made.

Enhanced Recovery After Surgery

ERAS refers to multimodal perioperative care pathways designed to achieve early recovery after surgical procedures by maintaining preoperative organ function and reducing the profound stress response following surgery.

Ambulatory Surgery

Ambulatory surgery (same-day surgery, outpatient surgery) is a common occurrence for certain types of procedures. Nurses who work in the outpatient setting are in a key position to assess patient status, plan the perioperative experience, and monitor, instruct, and evaluate these patients.

Advantages

1. Reduced cost to the facility and insurance and governmental agencies.
2. Reduced psychological stress to the patient.

3. Less incidence of hospital-acquired infections.
4. Less time lost from work by the patient and minimal disruption of the patient's activities and family life.

Disadvantages

1. Less time to assess the patient and perform preoperative teaching.
2. Less time to establish rapport between the patient and health care personnel.
3. Less opportunity to assess for late postoperative complications (this responsibility is primarily with the patient, although telephone and home care follow-up is possible).

Patient Selection

Criteria for selection include the following:

1. Surgery of short duration (varies by procedure and facility).
2. Noninfected conditions.
3. Type of operation in which postoperative complications are predictably low.
4. Age usually not a factor, although too risky in a premature neonate.
5. Examples of commonly performed procedures but not limited to:
   a. Ear–nose–throat (tonsillectomy, adenoidectomy).
   b. Gynecology (diagnostic laparoscopy, tubal ligation, dilation and curettage).
   c. Orthopedics (arthroscopy, fracture, or tendon repair).
   d. Oral surgery (wisdom teeth extraction, dental restorations).
   e. Urology (circumcision, cystoscopy, vasectomy).
   f. Ophthalmology (cataract).
   g. Plastic surgery (mammary implants, reduction mammoplasty, liposuction, blepharoplasty, face-lift).
   h. General surgery (laparoscopic hernia repair, laparoscopic cholecystectomy, biopsy, cyst removal).

Nursing Management

Initial Assessment

1. Develop a nursing history for the outpatient; this may be initiated in the health care provider's office. The history should include the patient's physical and psychological status. You will also inquire about allergies, tobacco, alcohol, and drug use; disabilities or limitations; current medications (including over-the-counter drugs, vitamins, supplements, and herbal products); current health conditions (focus should be on cardiovascular and respiratory problems, diabetes, and kidney impairments); and any past surgeries or problems with anesthesia.
2. Ensure availability of a signed and witnessed informed consent that includes correct surgical procedure and site.
3. Explain any additional laboratory studies needed and state why.
4. Begin health education with the following instructions:
   a. Notify the health care provider and surgical unit immediately if you get a cold, have a fever, or have any illness before the date of surgery.
   b. Arrive at the specified time.
   c. Restrict food and fluid before surgery according to facility protocol to prevent aspiration of gastric contents. Based on scientific evidence, the American Society of Anesthesiologists has issued guidelines for elective procedures recommending the following:
      i. Clear liquids—minimum fasting of 2 hours.
      ii. Breast milk—minimum fasting of 4 hours.
      iii. Infant formula—minimum fasting of 6 hours.
      iv. Nonhuman milk—minimum fasting of 6 hours.
      v. Light meal—minimum fasting of 6 hours.
   d. Do not wear makeup or nail polish.
   e. Wear comfortable, loose clothing and low-heeled shoes.
   f. Leave valuables or jewelry at home.
   g. Brush your teeth in the morning and rinse but do not swallow any liquid.
   h. Shower the night before or day of the surgery.
   i. Follow the health care provider's instructions for taking medications, including over-the-counter medications and supplements. Medications may be reduced or held prior to surgery including insulin and some oral antidiabetic drugs, anticoagulant and antiplatelet drugs, nonsteroidal anti-inflammatory agents, monoamine oxidase (MAO) inhibitors, among others.
   j. Have a responsible adult accompany you and drive you home; have someone stay with you for 24 hours after the surgery.

EVIDENCE BASE Joshi, G. P., Abdelmalak, B. B., Weigel, W. A., Harbell, M. W., Kuo, C. I., Soriano, S. G., Stricker, P. A., Tipton, T., Grant, M. D., Marbella, A. M., Agarkar, M., Blanck, J. F., & Domino, K. B. (2023). 2023 American Society of Anesthesiologists Practice Guidelines for Preoperative Fasting: Carbohydrate-containing clear liquids with or without protein, chewing gum, and pediatric fasting duration—A modular update of the 2017 American Society of Anesthesiologists Practice Guidelines for Preoperative Fasting. *Anesthesiology, 138*(2), 132–151. https://doi.org/10.1097/ALN.0000000000004381

Centers for Disease Control and Prevention (gov.). (2023). 2024 NHSN Patient Safety Component Manual. *Infection Control and Hospital Epidemiology, 44*, 695-720. https://www.cdc.gov.nhsns pdf

CLINICAL JUDGMENT Minimum fasting times must be followed to reduce the risk of aspiration, but patients are often instructed to fast after midnight because schedule changes the morning of surgery are possible due to cancellations, which can cause surgery time to be moved forward. Be aware that prolonged fasting before surgery may result in undue thirst, hunger, irritability, headache, and possibly dehydration, hypovolemia, and hypoglycemia.

Preoperative Preparation

1. Conduct a nursing assessment, focusing on cardiovascular and respiratory status. Determine if patient has diabetes and, if so, follow glucose control measures. Obtain baseline vital signs, including an oxygen saturation level and current pain score.
2. Review the patient's chart for witnessed and informed consent, laterality (right or left, if applicable), laboratory work, and history and physical.
3. Verify correct patient, correct site, and correct procedure. Consider "time-out" and SCIP measures, including marking of incision.
4. Make sure the patient has followed food and fluid restrictions, has removed all jewelry and dentures, and is appropriately dressed for surgery.
5. Perform medication reconciliation. Certain home meds may be taken, especially beta-blockers. Check with health care provider and have patient take with a sip of water.
6. Inform anesthesia provider if patient is taking any herbal supplements.
7. Administer preprocedural medication, if applicable.

Postoperative Care

1. Check vital signs, including oxygen saturation, temperature, and pain score.
2. Administer oxygen, if necessary.
3. Change the patient's position and gradually progress activity—head of bed elevated, dangling, and walking. Watch for dizziness or nausea.
4. Ascertain, using the following criteria, that the patient has recovered adequately to be discharged:
   a. Vital signs stable and returned to preoperative level.
   b. Stands without excessive dizziness and able to walk short distances.
   c. Pain score within tolerable level (usually less than 3 required).
   d. Able to drink fluids.
   e. Oriented to time, place, and person.
   f. No evidence of respiratory distress.
   g. Has the services of a responsible adult who can escort the patient home and remain with the patient.
   h. Understands postoperative instructions and takes an instruction sheet home.

Informed Consent (Operative Permit)

Informed consent (operative permit) is the process of informing the patient about the surgical procedure—that is, risks and possible complications of surgery and anesthesia. Consent is obtained by the surgeon. This is a legal document. Hospitals usually have a standard operative permit form approved by the hospital's legal department.

Purposes

1. To ensure that the patient understands the nature of the treatment, including potential complications and alternative treatment or procedures.
2. To indicate that the patient's decision was made without pressure.
3. To protect the patient against unauthorized procedures and to ensure that the procedure is performed on the correct body part.
4. To protect the surgeon and facility against legal action by a patient who claims that an unauthorized procedure was performed.

Adolescent Patient and Informed Consent

1. An emancipated minor is usually recognized as one who is not subject to parental control. Regulations vary by jurisdiction but generally include:
   a. Married minor.
   b. Those in military service.
   c. Minor who has a child.
2. Most states have statutes regarding treatment of minors.
3. Standards for informed consent are the same as for adults.

Procedures Requiring Informed Consent and Time-Out

1. Any surgical procedure whether major or minor.
2. Entrance into a body cavity, such as colonoscopy, paracentesis, bronchoscopy, cystoscopy, or lumbar puncture.
3. Radiologic procedures, particularly if a contrast material is required (such as myelogram, magnetic resonance imaging with contrast, angiography).
4. All procedures requiring any type of anesthesia, which includes cardioversion.

Obtaining Informed Consent

1. Before signing an informed consent document, the patient should:
   a. Be told in clear and simple terms by the surgeon what is to be done, the risks and benefits, as well as any alternatives to the surgery or procedure. The anesthesia care provider will explain the anesthesia plan and possible risks and complications.
   b. Have a general idea of what to expect in the early and late postoperative periods.
   c. Have a general idea of the time involved from surgery to recovery.
   d. Have an opportunity to ask any questions.
   e. Sign a separate form for each procedure or operation.
2. Written permission is required by law and a witness may be required according to facility policy.
3. Signature is obtained with the patient's complete understanding of what is to occur; it is obtained before the patient receives sedation and is secured without pressure or duress.
4. For a minor (or a patient who is unconscious or declared incompetent), permission is required from a responsible family member—caregiver, legal guardian, or court-appointed guardian.
5. For a married emancipated minor, permission from the spouse is acceptable when the patient is declared incapable.
6. If the patient is unable to write, an "X" is acceptable.
7. In an emergency, permission by way of telephone is acceptable with two witnesses.

Surgical Risk Factors and Preventive Strategies

Obesity

Danger

1. Increases the difficulty involved in the technical aspects of performing surgery; risk for wound dehiscence is greater.
2. Increases the likelihood of infection because of compromised tissue perfusion.
3. Increases the potential for postoperative pneumonia and other pulmonary complications because patients with obesity chronically hypoventilate.
4. Increases demands on the heart, leading to cardiovascular compromise.
5. Increases the risk for airway complications.
6. Alters the response to many drugs and anesthetics.
7. Decreases the likelihood of early ambulation.

Therapeutic Approach

1. Encourage weight reduction if time permits.
2. Anticipate postoperative obesity-related complications.
3. Be extremely vigilant for respiratory complications.
4. Carefully splint abdominal incisions when moving or coughing.

5. Be aware that some drugs should be dosed according to ideal body weight versus actual weight (owing to fat content) to prevent toxicity, including digoxin, lidocaine, aminoglycoside antibiotics, and theophylline.
6. Be aware that patients with obesity require higher doses of antibiotics to achieve effective tissue levels.
7. Avoid intramuscular (IM) injections in individuals with morbid obesity (IV or subcutaneous routes preferred).
8. Never attempt to move an impaired patient without assistance or without using proper body mechanics.
9. Obtain a dietary consultation early in the patient's postoperative course.

Poor Nutrition

Danger

1. Greatly impairs wound healing (especially protein and calorie deficits and a negative nitrogen balance).
2. Increases the risk of infection.

Therapeutic Approach

1. Any recent (within 4 to 6 weeks) weight loss of 10% of the patient's normal body weight or decreased serum albumin should alert the health care staff to poor nutritional status and the need to investigate as to the cause of the weight loss.
2. Attempt to improve nutritional status before and after surgery. Unless contraindicated, provide a diet high in proteins, calories, and vitamins (especially vitamins C and A); this may require enteral and parenteral feeding.
3. Review a serum prealbumin level to determine recent nutritional status.
4. Recommend repair of dental caries and proper mouth hygiene to prevent infection.

Fluid and Electrolyte Imbalance

Danger

Can have adverse effects in terms of general anesthesia and the anticipated volume losses associated with surgery, causing shock and cardiac dysrhythmias.

CLINICAL JUDGMENT Patients undergoing major abdominal operations (such as colectomies and aortic repairs) often experience a massive fluid shift into tissues around the operative site in the form of edema (as much as 1 L or more may be lost from circulation). Watch for the fluid shift to reverse (from tissue to circulation) around the third postoperative day. Patients with heart disease may develop failure because of the excess fluid load.

Therapeutic Approach

1. Assess the patient's fluid and electrolyte status.
2. Rehydrate the patient parenterally and orally as prescribed.
3. Monitor for evidence of electrolyte imbalance, especially Na^+, K^+, Mg^{++}, and Ca^{++}.
4. Be aware of expected drainage amounts and composition; report excess and abnormalities.
5. Monitor the patient's intake and output; be sure to include all body fluid losses.

Aging

Danger

1. Potential for injury is greater in older adults.
2. Be aware that the cumulative effect of medications is greater in the older patient.
3. Medications in the usual dosages, such as morphine, may cause confusion, disorientation, and respiratory depression.

Therapeutic Approach

1. Consider using lesser medication doses for desired effect.
2. Anticipate problems from chronic disorders such as anemia, obesity, diabetes, and hypoproteinemia.
3. Adjust nutritional intake to conform to higher protein and vitamin needs.
4. When possible, accommodate older patients' set patterns in activities such as sleeping and eating.

Presence of Cardiovascular Disease

Danger

1. May compound the stress of anesthesia and the operative procedure.
2. May result in impaired oxygenation, cardiac rhythm, cardiac output, and circulation.
3. May also produce cardiac decompensation, sudden arrhythmia, thromboembolism, acute myocardial infarction (MI), or cardiac arrest.
4. Holding cardiac medications, particularly beta-blockers, may have negative impact on cardiac status.

Therapeutic Approach

1. Frequently assess heart rate and blood pressure (BP) and hemodynamic status and cardiac rhythm.
2. Avoid fluid overload (oral, parenteral, blood products) because of possible MI, angina, heart failure, and pulmonary edema.
3. In adherence to SCIP measures, make sure the patient has not held beta-blocker prior to surgery. Administer with a sip of water.
4. Prevent prolonged immobilization, which results in venous stasis. Monitor for potential deep vein thrombosis (DVT) or pulmonary embolus.
5. Encourage position changes but avoid sudden exertion.
6. Use antiembolism stockings or sequential compression device intraoperatively and postoperatively.
7. Note evidence of hypoxia and initiate therapy.

EVIDENCE BASE American Society of PeriAnesthesia Nurses. (2022). *2023-2024 Perianesthesia nursing: Standards, practice recommendations, and interpretive statements.* Author.

Presence of Diabetes Mellitus

Danger

1. Hypoglycemia may result from food and fluid restrictions and anesthesia.
2. Hyperglycemia and ketoacidosis may be potentiated by increased catecholamines and glucocorticoids because of surgical stress.

3. Chronic hyperglycemia results in poor wound healing and susceptibility to infection.
4. Research has shown that patients who underwent surgery have better outcomes when glucose levels are well controlled throughout the surgical process.

Therapeutic Approach

1. Recognize the signs and symptoms of ketoacidosis and hypoglycemia, which can threaten an otherwise uneventful surgical experience. Dehydration also threatens renal function.
2. Monitor blood glucose and be prepared to administer insulin, as directed, or treat hypoglycemia.
3. Confirm what medications the patient has taken and what has been held. Facility protocol and provider preference vary, but the goal is to prevent hypoglycemia. If the patient is NPO (nothing by mouth), oral agents are usually withheld and insulin may be ordered at 75% of the usual dose. Metformin is usually held 48 hours before surgery and restarted when full food and fluid intake has restarted and normal kidney function has been confirmed.
4. Reassure the patient with diabetes that when the disease is controlled, the surgical risk is no greater than it is for the patient without diabetes.

Presence of Alcohol Use Disorder

Danger

Malnutrition may be present in the presurgical patient with alcohol use disorder. The patient may also have an increased tolerance to anesthetics.

Therapeutic Approach

1. Note that the risk of surgery is greater for the patient who has chronic alcohol use disorder.
2. Anticipate the acute withdrawal syndrome within 72 hours of the last alcoholic drink.

Presence of Pulmonary and Upper Respiratory Disease

Danger

1. Chronic pulmonary illness may contribute to hypoventilation, leading to pneumonia and atelectasis.
2. Surgery may be contraindicated in the patient who has an upper respiratory infection because of the possible advance of infection to pneumonia and sepsis.
3. Sleep apnea in the perioperative patient provides a great risk to anesthesia and must be noted and assessed prior to surgery.

Therapeutic Approach

1. Patients with chronic pulmonary problems, such as emphysema or bronchiectasis, should be evaluated and treated prior to surgery to optimize pulmonary function with bronchodilators, corticosteroids, and conscientious mouth care, along with a reduction in weight and smoking and methods to control secretions.
2. Patients with obstructive sleep apnea should be evaluated by an anesthesia provider prior to surgery. General anesthesia should be avoided if possible. Patients should bring continuous positive airway pressure (CPAP) machines to the hospital for use postanesthesia.
3. Opioids should be used cautiously to prevent hypoventilation. Patient-controlled analgesia is preferred.
4. Oxygen should be administered to prevent hypoxemia (low liter flow in chronic obstructive pulmonary disease).

Concurrent or Prior Pharmacotherapy

Danger

Hazards exist when certain medications are given concomitantly with others (e.g., interaction of some drugs with anesthetics can lead to hypotension and circulatory collapse). This also includes the use of many herbal substances. Although herbs are natural products, they can interact with other medications used in surgery.

Therapeutic Approach

1. An awareness of drug therapy is essential.
2. Notify the health care provider and anesthesia provider if the patient is taking any of the following drugs:
   a. Certain antibiotics.
   b. Antidepressants, particularly MAO inhibitors, and St. John's wort, an herbal product.
   c. Phenothiazines.
   d. Diuretics, particularly thiazides.
   e. Corticosteroids.
   f. Anticoagulants, such as warfarin or heparin, or medications or herbals that may affect coagulation, such as aspirin, feverfew, Ginkgo biloba, nonsteroidal anti-inflammatory drugs, ticlopidine, and clopidogrel.

PREOPERATIVE CARE

Patient Education

Patient education is a vital component of the surgical experience. Preoperative patient education may be offered through conversation, discussion, the use of audiovisual aids, demonstrations, and return demonstrations. It is designed to help the patient understand the surgical experience to minimize anxiety and promote full recovery from surgery and anesthesia. The educational program may be initiated before hospitalization by the physician, nurse practitioner or office nurse, or other designated personnel. This is particularly important for patients who are admitted on the day of surgery or who are to undergo outpatient surgical procedures. The perioperative nurse can assess the patient's knowledge base and use this information in developing an interdisciplinary plan of care (IPOC), for an uneventful perioperative course.

Teaching Strategies

Obtain a Database

1. Determine what the patient already knows or wants to know. This can be accomplished by reading the patient's chart, interviewing the patient, and communicating with the health care provider, family, and other members of the health care team.
2. Ascertain the patient's psychosocial adjustment to impending surgery.
3. Determine cultural or religious health beliefs and practices that may have an impact on the patient's surgical experience, such as refusal of blood transfusions, burial of amputated limbs within 24 hours, or special healing rituals.

Plan and Implement Teaching Program

1. Begin at the patient's level of understanding and proceed from there.
2. Plan a presentation, or series of presentations, for an individual patient or a group of patients.
3. Include family members and significant others in the teaching process.

4. Encourage active participation of patients in their care and recovery.
5. Demonstrate essential techniques; provide the opportunity for patient practice and return demonstration.
6. Provide time for and encourage the patient to ask questions and express concerns; make every effort to answer all questions truthfully and in basic agreement with the overall therapeutic plan.
7. Provide general information and assess the patient's level of interest in or reaction to it.
   a. Explain the details of preoperative preparation and provide a tour of the area and view the equipment when possible.
   b. Offer general information on the surgery. Explain that the health care provider is the primary resource person.
   c. Notify the patient when surgery is scheduled (if known) and approximately how long it will take; explain that afterward the patient will go to the postanesthesia care unit (PACU). Emphasize that delays may be attributed to many factors other than a problem developing with this patient (e.g., previous case delays).
   d. Let the patient know that their family will be kept informed and that they will be told where to wait and when they can see the patient; note visiting hours.
   e. Explain how a procedure or test may feel during or afterward.
   f. Describe the PACU and what personnel and equipment the patient may expect to see and hear (specially trained personnel, monitoring equipment, tubing for various functions, and a moderate amount of activity by nurses and health care providers).
   g. Stress the importance of active participation in postoperative recovery.
8. Use other resource people: health care providers, therapists, chaplain, and interpreters.
9. Document what has been taught or discussed as well as the patient's reaction and level of understanding.
10. Discuss with the patient the anticipated postoperative course (e.g., length of stay, immediate postoperative activity, follow-up visit with the surgeon).

Use Multimedia Aids If Available

1. Multimedia electronic programs are effective in giving basic information to a single patient or group of patients. Many facilities provide a television channel dedicated to patient instruction.
2. Booklets, brochures, and models, if available, are helpful.
3. Demonstrate any equipment that will be specific for the particular patient. Examples:
   a. Drains and drainage bags.
   b. Monitoring equipment for electrocardiogram (ECG), blood pressure (BP), pulse oximetry, capnography.
   c. Incentive spirometer, flutter valves.
   d. Sequential compression device.

General Instructions

Preoperatively, the patient will be instructed in the following postoperative activities. This will allow a chance for practice and familiarity.

Incentive Spirometry

Preoperatively, the patient uses a spirometer to measure deep breaths (inspired air) while exerting maximum effort. The preoperative measurement becomes the goal to be achieved as soon as possible after the operation.

1. Postoperatively, the patient is encouraged to use the incentive spirometer about 10 to 12 times per hour.
2. Deep inhalations expand alveoli, which prevents atelectasis and other pulmonary complications.
3. There is less pain with inspiratory concentration than with expiratory concentration such as with coughing.

Coughing

Coughing promotes the removal of chest secretions. Instruct the patient to:

1. Interlace fingers and place hands over the proposed incision site; this will act as a splint during coughing and not harm the incision.
2. Lean forward slightly while sitting in bed.
3. Breathe, using the diaphragm.
4. Inhale fully with the mouth slightly open.
5. Let out three or four sharp "hacks."
6. Take in a deep breath with the mouth open and quickly give one or two strong coughs.
7. Clear secretions readily from the chest to prevent respiratory complications (pneumonia, obstruction).

CLINICAL JUDGMENT Be aware that incentive spirometry, deep breathing, and coughing, as well as certain position changes, may be contraindicated after some surgeries (e.g., craniotomy and eye or ear surgery).

Turning

Changing positions from back to side-lying (and vice versa) stimulates circulation, encourages deeper breathing, and relieves pressure areas.

1. Help the patient to move onto their side if assistance is needed.
2. Place the uppermost leg in a more flexed position than that of the lower leg, and place a pillow comfortably between the legs.
3. Make sure that the patient is turned from one side to the back and onto the other side every 2 hours.

Foot and Leg Exercises

Moving the legs improves circulation and muscle tone.

1. Have the patient lie supine; instruct the patient to bend a knee and raise the foot—hold it a few seconds, and lower it to the bed. Alternately, have the patient do ankle pumps by flexing and pointing feet 20 times.
2. Repeat step 1 about five times with one leg and then about five times with the other. Repeat the set five times every 3 to 5 hours.
3. Then, have the patient lie on one side and exercise the legs by pretending to pedal a bicycle.
4. Suggest the following foot exercise: trace a complete circle with the great toe.

Evaluation of Teaching Program

1. Observe the patient for correct demonstration of expected postoperative behaviors, such as foot and leg exercises and special breathing techniques.
2. Ask pertinent questions to determine the patient's level of understanding.
3. Reinforce information when necessary.

Preparation for Surgery

EVIDENCE BASE Ahuja, S., Peiffer-Smadja, N., Peven, K., White, M., Leather, A. J. M., Singh, S., Mendelson, M., Holmes, A., Birgand, G., & Sevdalis, N. (2022). Use of feedback data to reduce surgical site infections and optimize antibiotic use in surgery: A systematic scoping review. *Annals of Surgery, 275*(2), e345–e352. https://doi.org/10.1097/SLA.0000000000004909

Skin Antisepsis

1. Human skin normally harbors transient and resident bacterial flora, some of which are pathogenic. Skin cannot be sterilized without destroying skin cells.
2. The attributes of an appropriate surgical skin antiseptic require the ability to significantly reduce microorganisms, provide broad-spectrum activity, be fast acting, and have a persistent effect.
   a. Preoperative bathing with chlorhexidine reduces pathogenic organisms on the skin. Using multiple showers or showering immediately before coming to the operating room substantially reduces skin organisms.
   b. Cleansing with a bactericidal-impregnated sponge just before operation will provide additional reduction in skin bacteria.
3. The Centers for Disease Control and Prevention recommends that hair not be removed near the operative site unless it will interfere with surgery. The skin is easily injured during shaving that often results in a higher rate of postoperative wound infection.
4. If required, hair removal should be done by clipping, not shaving, and should be performed within 2 hours of surgery. Scissors may be used to remove hair greater than 3 mm in length.
5. For head surgery, obtain specific instructions from the surgeon concerning the extent of shaving.

Gastrointestinal Tract

1. Preparation of the bowel is imperative for patients undergoing intestinal surgery because escaping bacteria can invade adjacent tissues and cause sepsis.
   a. Cathartics and enemas remove gross collections of stool (e.g., GoLYTELY).
   b. Oral antimicrobial agents (e.g., neomycin, erythromycin) suppress the colon's potent microflora.
   c. Enemas "until clear" are generally not necessary. If ordered, they are given the night before surgery. Notify the health care provider if the enemas never return clear.
2. Solid food is withheld from the patient for 6 hours before surgery. Patients having morning surgery are kept NPO (nothing by mouth) overnight. Clear fluids (water) may be given up to 4 hours before surgery depending on facility protocols.

Genitourinary Tract

A medicated douche may be prescribed preoperatively if the patient is to have a gynecologic or urologic operation.

Preoperative Medication

1. Administration of systemic prophylactic perioperative antibiotics is one of the most important steps in preventing surgical site infection, which are the most common and costly type of hospital-acquired infections. It is estimated that 60% of hospital-acquired infections are preventable through evidence-based protocols.
2. Redosing of antibiotics during long procedures and when there is excessive blood loss, and discontinuation within 24 hours after surgery end time (48 hours for cardiac surgeries) is recommended.
3. There is a risk, however, of an increase in *Clostridium difficile* diarrheal infections because of antibiotic use.

DRUG ALERT Antibiotics should be administered just before surgery—preferably 1 hour (2 hours for vancomycin and fluoroquinolones) before an incision is made—to be effective when bacterial contamination is expected.

Administering "On-Call" Medications

1. Have the medication ready and administer it as soon as the call is received from the operating room.
2. Proceed with the remaining preparation activities.
3. Indicate on the chart or preoperative checklist the time when the medication was administered and by whom.

Admitting the Patient to Surgery

Final Checklist

The Comprehensive Surgical Checklist from the Association of periOperative Registered Nurses (AORN) combines the World Health Organization and The Joint Commission measures for patient preparedness. It may be customized for use in any setting or may be used in addition to a facility's specific checklist that the nurse is also responsible for.

Identification and Verification

This includes verbal identification by the perioperative nurse while checking the identification band on the patient's wrist and written documentation (such as the chart) of the patient's identity, the procedure to be performed (laterality, if indicated), the specific surgical site marked by the surgeon with indelible ink, the surgeon, and the type of anesthesia. These are all patient safety goals as outlined by The Joint Commission.

Review of Patient Record

Check for inclusion of the fact sheet; allergies; history and physical; completed preoperative checklist; laboratory values, including most recent results; pregnancy test, if applicable; ECG and chest x-rays, if necessary; preoperative medications; and other preoperative orders by either the surgeon or anesthesia care provider.

Consent Form

All nurses involved with patient care in the preoperative setting should be aware of the individual state laws regarding informed consent and the specific facility policy. Obtaining informed consent is the responsibility of the surgeon performing the specific procedure. Consent forms should state the procedure, various risks, and alternatives to surgery, if any. It is a nursing responsibility to make sure the consent form has been obtained with the patient or guardian's signature and that it is in the chart.

Patient Preparedness

1. NPO status.
2. Proper attire (clean gown and hair covering) and clean linen.
3. Skin preparation, if ordered.
4. IV line started with correct gauge needle.
5. Dentures or plates removed.

6. Jewelry, piercings, contact lenses, and glasses removed and secured in a locked area or given to a family member.
7. Allow the patient to void.

Transporting the Patient to the Operating Room

1. Adhere to the principle of maintaining the comfort and safety of the patient.
2. Accompany operating room attendants to the patient's bedside for introduction and proper identification.
3. Assist in transferring the patient from bed to stretcher (unless the bed goes to the operating room floor).
4. Complete the chart and preoperative checklist; include laboratory reports and x-rays as required by facility policy or the health care provider's directive.
5. Make sure that the patient arrives in the operating room at the proper time.

The Patient's Family

1. Direct the patient's family to the proper waiting room where magazines, television, and beverages may be available.
2. Tell the family that the surgeon will probably contact them there after surgery to inform them about the operation.
3. Inform the family that a long interval of waiting does not mean the patient is in the operating room the whole time; anesthesia preparation and induction take time, and after surgery, the patient is taken to the PACU.
4. Tell the family what to expect postoperatively when they see the patient—tubes, monitoring equipment, and blood transfusion, suctioning, and oxygen equipment.

INTRAOPERATIVE CARE

Nursing competencies for intraoperative care include advanced cardiac life support/pediatric advanced life support (ACLS/PALS), moderate sedation, intralipid protocol, recognition of signs and symptoms of toxicity including cardiac arrhythmias and seizures, pharmacology of local anesthetic agents, and neurovascular/neurologic checks. Nurses should be familiar with each type of block performed, its therapeutic effects, associated side effects, possible adverse reactions associated with the specific block performed, and any indicated emergency interventions. These competencies are necessary to ensure the patient's optimal safety during the perioperative patient experience.

Anesthesia and Related Complications

The goals of anesthesia are to provide analgesia, sedation, and muscle relaxation appropriate for the type of operative procedure as well as to control the autonomic nervous system.

Common Anesthetic Techniques

Moderate Sedation

EVIDENCE BASE Association of periOperative Registered Nurses. (2022). *Recommended practice for managing the patient receiving moderate sedation/analgesia.* Author.

1. Moderate sedation is a specific level of sedation that allows patients to tolerate unpleasant procedures by reducing the level of anxiety and discomfort, previously known as conscious sedation.
2. The patient achieves a depressed level of consciousness (LOC) and altered perception of pain while retaining the ability to respond appropriately to verbal and tactile stimuli.
3. Cardiopulmonary function and protective airway reflexes are maintained by the patient.
4. Knowledge of expected outcomes is essential. These outcomes include, but are not limited to:
   a. Maintenance of consciousness.
   b. Maintenance of protective reflexes.
   c. Alteration of pain perception.
   d. Enhanced cooperation.
5. Adequate preoperative preparation of the patient will facilitate achieving the desired effects.
6. Nurses caring for patients receiving moderate sedation should be specially trained in the agents used for moderate sedation, such as midazolam and fentanyl, and should be skilled in advanced life support. Many facilities have strict regulations and training requirements for staff handling such patients.
7. Nurses working in this setting should also be aware of the regulations from the board of nursing in the state they are practicing concerning the care of patients receiving anesthesia and should be compliant with state advisory opinions, declaratory rules, and other regulations that direct the practice of the registered nurse.
8. Patients who are not candidates for conscious sedation and require more complex sedation should be managed by anesthesia care providers.

Monitored Anesthesia Care

1. Light to deep sedation that is monitored by an anesthesia care provider.
2. The patient is asleep but arousable.
3. The patient is not intubated.
4. The patient may receive local anesthesia and oxygen, is monitored, and receives sedation and analgesia. Midazolam, fentanyl, alfentanil, and propofol are frequently used in monitored anesthesia care procedures.

General Anesthesia

1. A reversible state consisting of complete loss of consciousness. Protective reflexes are lost.
2. With the loss of protective reflexes, the patient's airway needs to be maintained. This can be done by endotracheal (ET) intubation or insertion of a laryngeal mask airway (LMA).
   a. For certain, short, and uncomplicated surgeries (e.g., myringotomies), the insertion of a breathing tube may not be necessary, and the airway is maintained manually with a jaw thrust/chin lift.
   b. ET intubation is facilitated by the use of a laryngoscope. The ET tube is inserted into the trachea and passed through the vocal cords. A cuff is then inflated, thus ensuring a secure airway where no secretions from the oral cavity can enter the lungs.
   c. LMA does not require a laryngoscope for insertion and is inserted only to the entrance of the trachea. Although LMA does not provide a totally protected airway, it is noninvasive and more gentle on the tissue.
3. General anesthesia consists of three phases: induction, maintenance, and emergence.
4. Induction can be accomplished by either the parenteral or the inhalation route. Common agents for IV induction are propofol and phenobarbital. In addition to the induction

agent, a potent analgesic is also often added (e.g., fentanyl) to potentiate the induction agent as well as provide analgesia. Patients can also reach an unconscious state by inhaling a potent, short-acting volatile gas, such as sevoflurane. Once the patient is asleep, and if the surgical procedure so requires, a muscle relaxant is given and the ET tube is inserted.

5. Maintenance is accomplished through a continuous delivery of the inhalation agent, or an IV infusion of an agent, such as propofol, to maintain an unconscious state. Intermittent doses of an analgesic are given as needed as well as intermittent doses of a muscle relaxant for longer surgeries.
6. Emergence occurs at the end of the surgery when the continuous delivery of either the gas or the IV infusion is stopped and the patient slowly returns to a conscious state. If muscle relaxants are still in effect, they can be reversed with neostigmine to allow for adequate muscle strength and return of spontaneous ventilations. A nerve stimulator can be used to assess if adequate muscle control has returned before extubation of the trachea.

CLINICAL JUDGMENT Be aware that during emergence, the patient is very sensitive to any stimuli. Keep noise levels to a minimum, and refrain from manipulating the patient during this stage.

Regional Anesthesia

1. Anesthesia block is achieved by injecting a local anesthetic, such as lidocaine or bupivacaine, in proximity to appropriate nerves. It may be spinal, epidural, or peripheral block.
2. Nursing responsibilities include being familiar with the drug used and maximum dose that can be given, knowing signs and symptoms of toxicity, and maintaining a comfortable environment for the conscious patient.
3. *Spinal anesthesia* is the injection of a local anesthetic into the lumbar intrathecal space. The anesthetic blocks conduction in spinal nerve roots and dorsal ganglia, thereby causing paralysis and analgesia below the level of injection.
4. *Epidural anesthesia* involves injecting a local anesthetic into the epidural space. Results are similar to spinal analgesia but with a slower onset.
   a. Often, a catheter is inserted for continuous infusion of the anesthetic to the epidural space.
   b. The catheter may be left in place to provide postoperative analgesia as well.
5. *Peripheral nerve block* is achieved by injecting a local anesthetic into a bundle of nerves (e.g., axillary plexus) or into a single nerve to achieve anesthesia to a specific part of the body (e.g., hand or single finger).

Intraoperative Complications

1. Hypoventilation and hypoxemia—because of inadequate ventilatory support.
2. Oral trauma (broken teeth, oropharyngeal or laryngeal trauma)—because of difficult ET intubation.
3. Hypotension—because of preoperative hypovolemia or untoward reactions to anesthetic agents.
4. Cardiac dysrhythmia—because of preexisting cardiovascular compromise, electrolyte imbalance, or untoward reactions to anesthetic agents.
5. Hypothermia—because of exposure to a cool ambient operating room environment and loss of normal thermoregulation capability from anesthetic agents.
6. Peripheral nerve damage—because of improper positioning of the patient (e.g., full weight on an arm) or use of restraints.
7. Malignant hyperthermia:
   a. This is a rare reaction to anesthetic inhalants (notably sevoflurane, enflurane, isoflurane, and desflurane) and the muscle relaxant succinylcholine.
   b. It is caused by abnormal and excessive intracellular accumulations of calcium with resulting hypermetabolism, increased muscle contraction, and elevated body temperature.
   c. Treatment consists of discontinuing the inhalant anesthetic, administering IV dantrolene, and applying cooling techniques (e.g., cooling blanket, iced saline lavages).
8. Local anesthetic systemic toxicity (LAST):
   a. This is an adverse outcome that occurs when the serum level of local anesthesia increases to an unsafe level.
   b. It is important for the nurse to recognize signs and symptoms. Central nervous system (CNS) symptoms usually present first (patient has metallic taste, numbness of the tongue and lips, tinnitus, confusion, agitation, and seizures) followed by cardiac symptoms.
   c. Lipid emulsion (20%) therapy must be administered intravenously bolus 100 mL over 2 to 3 minutes for patient >70 kg, bolus 1.5 mL/kg for patient >70 kg, and bolus 0.25 ml/kg/min for 30-60 minutes. Learn more about LAST protocol at *www.lipidrescue.org*.

EVIDENCE BASE Davidson, V. L., McGrath, M. C., & Navarro, S. (2024). Preventing Local Anesthetics Systemic Toxicity After Administration of Long-Acting Local Anesthetics. *AORN Journal, 119*(2), 164-168. https://doi.org/10.1002/aorn.14085

Fencl, J. L. (2015). Local anesthetic systemic toxicity: Perioperative implications. *AORN Journal*, *101*(6), 697–700. https://doi.org/10.1016/j.aorn.2015.03.002

CLINICAL JUDGMENT Recognize malignant hyperthermia immediately so that inhalant anesthesia can be discontinued and treatment measures started, to prevent seizures and other adverse effects.

POSTOPERATIVE CARE

Postanesthesia Care Unit

To ensure continuity of care from the intraoperative phase to the immediate postoperative phase, the circulating nurse or anesthesia care provider gives a thorough report to the postanesthesia care unit (PACU) nurse. See Standards of Care Guidelines 3-1 (page 59). This report should include the following:

1. Type of surgery performed and any intraoperative complications.
2. Type of anesthesia (e.g., general, local, sedation).
3. Drains and type of dressings.
4. Presence of endotracheal (ET) tube or type of oxygen to be administered (e.g., nasal cannula, T piece).
5. Types of lines and locations (e.g., peripheral IV, central line, arterial line).
6. Catheters or tubes, such as a urinary catheter or T-tube.
7. Administration of blood, colloids, and fluids and electrolytes.
8. Drug allergies and pertinent medical history.
9. Preexisting medical conditions.
10. Intraoperative course, including any complications or instability in the patient's vital signs.

STANDARDS OF CARE GUIDELINES 3-1

Postanesthesia Care Unit Care

Postanesthesia care unit (PACU) care is geared toward recognizing the signs of distress and anticipating and preventing postoperative difficulties. Carefully monitor the patient coming out of general anesthesia, and monitor frequently for the following:

- Vital signs are stable and are within normal range.
- The patient has no signs of respiratory distress and can maintain their own airway.
- Reflexes have returned to normal.
- Pain is under control and at a tolerable level for the patient.
- The patient is responsive and oriented to time and place.

This information should serve as a general guideline only. Each patient situation presents a unique set of clinical factors and requires nursing judgment to guide care, which may include additional or alternative measures and approaches.

Initial Nursing Assessment

Before receiving the patient, note the proper functioning of monitoring and suctioning devices, oxygen therapy equipment, and all other equipment. The following initial assessment is made by the nurse in the PACU:

1. Verify the patient's identity, the operative procedure, and the surgeon who performed the procedure.
2. Obtain vital signs, including pulse oximetry and temperature.
3. Evaluate airway status, noting any stridor or snoring respirations. Capnography may be used to assess adequate ventilation as well.
4. Evaluate respiratory status, including rate and effort, and auscultate breath sounds.
5. Assess circulatory status, noting skin color, peripheral pulses, and electrocardiogram (ECG) monitor.
6. Observe level of consciousness (LOC) and orientation to time and place.
7. Evaluate condition of surgical dressings and drains, and check IV lines and infusing fluids or IV medications. Initial surgical dressing is usually maintained for 48 hours.
8. Determine patient's pain level using a 1 to 10 scale.
9. Review the health care provider's orders.

CLINICAL JUDGMENT It is important to communicate effectively with the patient in order to provide an accurate assessment. Obtain an interpreter when necessary.

Initial Nursing Interventions

Maintaining a Patent Airway

1. Closely monitor the patient arriving with an oral or nasal airway in place until fully awake.
2. Monitor for return of cough and gag reflex. When the patient is awake and able to protect their own airway, the oral or nasal airway can be discontinued.
3. Early initiation of continuous positive airway pressure (CPAP) in the PACU is beneficial for patients exhibiting hypoxemia, apnea, and frequent severe airway obstruction because of obstructive sleep apnea.

Maintaining Adequate Respiratory Function

1. Encourage the patient to take deep breaths to aerate the lungs fully and prevent atelectasis; use an incentive spirometer to aid in this function.
2. Assess lung fields frequently through auscultation.
3. Periodically evaluate the patient's LOC—response to name or command. *Note:* Alterations in cerebral function may suggest impaired oxygen delivery.
4. Administer humidified oxygen to reduce irritation of airways and facilitate secretion removal.

Maintaining Glycemic Control

1. Check serum glucose on arrival to PACU and monitor as indicated.
2. For patients with diabetes, administer insulin and follow protocols to keep serum glucose levels between 120 and 160 mg/dL. Studies show that normalizing blood glucose for the first 2 to 3 days postoperatively reduces the incidence of deep wound infections comparable to that in patients who do not have diabetes.

Promoting Tissue Perfusion

1. Monitor vital signs (blood pressure [BP], pulse, respiratory rate, and oxygen saturation) according to protocol, normally every 15 minutes while in the PACU. Monitor ECG tracing for arrhythmias.
   a. Report variations in BP, heart rate, respiratory rate, and cardiac arrhythmias.
   b. Evaluate pulse pressure to determine status of perfusion. (A narrowing pulse pressure indicates impending shock.)
2. Monitor intake and output closely.
3. Recognize the variety of factors that may alter circulating blood volume, such as blood loss during surgery and fluid shifts after surgery.
   a. Recognize early symptoms of shock or hemorrhage: cool extremities, decreased urine output (less than 30 mL/h), slow capillary refill (greater than 3 seconds), decreased BP, narrowing pulse pressure, and increased heart rate.
4. Intervene to improve tissue perfusion.
   a. Initiate oxygen therapy or increase fraction of inspired oxygen of existing oxygen delivery system.
   b. Increase parenteral fluid infusion, as prescribed.
   c. Place the patient in the shock position with the feet elevated (unless contraindicated).
   d. See section "Postanesthesia Care Unit" on page 58 for more detailed consideration of shock.

Stabilizing Thermoregulatory Status

1. Monitor temperature every 15 minutes and be alert for development of both hypothermia and hyperthermia.
2. Report a temperature more than 101.5°F (38.6°C) or less than 95°F (35°C).
3. Monitor for postanesthesia shivering that, although common in patients with hypothermia, may also occur in patients who are normothermic, especially those who received inhalants during anesthesia. It represents a heat-gain mechanism, which drastically increases oxygen demand.
4. Provide warm blankets for patients feeling cold.
5. Provide active warming with forced warm air for patients who are hypothermic.

Maintaining Adequate Fluid Volume

1. Administer IV, as ordered.
2. Monitor intake and output.
3. Monitor electrolytes and recognize evidence of imbalance, such as nausea, vomiting, and weakness.
4. Evaluate mental status and skin color and turgor.
5. Recognize signs of fluid imbalance.
   a. Hypovolemia—decreased BP, decreased urine output, decreased central venous pressure (CVP), and increased pulse.
   b. Hypervolemia—increased BP; changes in lung sounds, such as crackles in the bases; changes in heart sounds (e.g., S_3 gallop); and increased CVP.
6. Evaluate IV sites to detect early infiltration. Restart lines immediately to maintain fluid volume.

Promoting Comfort

1. Assess pain by observing behavioral and physiologic manifestations (change in vital signs may be a result of pain); have the patient rate pain on a scale of 1 to 10.
2. Administer analgesics and document efficacy.
3. Position the patient to maximize comfort.

Minimizing Complications of Skin Impairment

1. Perform handwashing before and after contact with the patient.
2. Inspect dressings routinely and reinforce them, if necessary.
3. Record the amount and type of wound drainage (see "Wound Management" section, page 68).
4. Turn the patient frequently and maintain good body alignment.

Maintaining Safety

1. Keep the side rails up until the patient is fully awake.
2. Protect the extremity into which IV fluids are running so that the needle will not become accidentally dislodged.
3. Avoid nerve damage and muscle strain by properly supporting and padding pressure areas.
4. Be aware that patients who have received regional anesthesia may not be able to complain of an injury, such as the pricking of an open safety pin or a clamp that is exerting pressure.
5. Check the dressing for constriction.
6. Determine the return of motor control following regional anesthesia—indicated by how the patient responds to a request to move a body part.

Ensuring Safety by Minimizing Sensory Deficits

1. Know that the ability to hear returns more quickly than other senses as the patient emerges from anesthesia.
2. Avoid saying anything in the patient's presence that may be disturbing; the patient may appear to be sleeping but still consciously hears what is being said.
3. Explain procedures and activities at the patient's level of understanding.
4. Minimize the patient's exposure to emergency treatment of nearby patients by drawing the curtains and lowering your voice and noise levels.
5. Treat the patient as a person who needs as much attention as the equipment and monitoring devices.
6. Respect the patient's feeling of sensory deprivation and overstimulation; make adjustments to minimize this fluctuation of stimuli.
7. Demonstrate concern for and an understanding of the patient and anticipate the patient's needs and feelings.
8. Tell the patient repeatedly that the surgery is over and that they are in the PACU.

Evaluation: Expected Outcomes

- Absence of respiratory distress.
- Lung sounds clear to auscultation.
- Glucose less than 160 mg/dL.
- Vital signs stable and within preoperative ranges.
- Body temperature more than 95°F (35°C) and less than 101.5°F (38.6°C).
- IV infusion patent; urine output 50 to 60 mL/h.
- Adequate pain control.
- Wound/dressing intact without excessive drainage.
- Side rails up; positioned carefully; moving extremities appropriately.
- Quiet, reassuring environment maintained; no injury.

Transferring the Patient From the PACU

Each facility may have an individual checklist or scoring guide used to determine a patient's readiness for transfer. The above evaluation criteria must be met before transfer.

Transfer Responsibilities

1. Relay appropriate information to the unit nurse regarding the patient's condition. Use an approved method of communication such as SBAR (situation, background, assessment, and recommendations). Point out significant needs, vital signs (trends and most recent set), fluid therapy, incision and dressing requirements, intake needs, urine output, and color and amount of any drainage.
2. Physically assist in the transfer of the patient.
3. Orient the patient to the room, attending nurse, call light, and therapeutic devices.

Postoperative Discomforts

Most patients experience some discomforts postoperatively. These are usually related to the general anesthetic and the surgical procedure. The most common discomforts are nausea, vomiting, restlessness, sleeplessness, thirst, constipation, flatulence, and pain.

Postoperative Nausea and Vomiting

Causes

1. Occurs in many postoperative patients.
2. Most commonly related to inhalation anesthetics (nitrous oxide) and opioid use.
3. Can result from an accumulation of fluid or food in the stomach before peristalsis returns.
4. May occur as a result of abdominal distention, which follows manipulation of abdominal organs.

Preventive Measures

EVIDENCE BASE Association of periOperative Registered Nurses. (2023). *Guidelines for perioperative practice*. Author.

1. Insert a nasogastric (NG) tube intraoperatively for operations on the gastrointestinal (GI) tract to prevent abdominal distention, which triggers vomiting.

2. Evaluate patient preoperatively for risk factors for postoperative nausea and vomiting (PONV), such as being a person assigned female at birth, being a person who does not smoke, and having a history of motion sickness.

Nursing Interventions

1. Encourage the patient to breathe deeply to facilitate elimination of anesthetic.
2. Support the wound during retching and vomiting; turn the patient's head to the side to prevent aspiration.
3. Discard vomitus and refresh the patient—provide mouthwash and clean linens.
4. Provide small sips of a carbonated beverage such as ginger ale, if tolerated or permitted.
5. Report excessive or prolonged vomiting so the cause may be investigated.
6. Maintain an accurate intake and output record and replace fluids as ordered.
7. Detect the presence of abdominal distention or hiccups, suggesting gastric retention.
8. Administer antiemetic agents such as ondansetron or promethazine as directed; be aware that some of these drugs may potentiate the hypotensive effects of opioids.

DRUG ALERT Suspect idiosyncratic response to a drug if vomiting is worse when a medication is given (but diminishes thereafter).

Thirst

Causes

1. Inhibition of secretions by medication with atropine.
2. Fluid lost by way of perspiration, blood loss, and dehydration because of NPO (nothing by mouth) status.

Preventive Measures

Unfortunately, postoperative thirst is a common and troublesome symptom that is usually unavoidable due to anesthesia. The immediate implementation of nursing interventions is most helpful.

Nursing Interventions

1. Administer fluids parenterally or orally, if tolerated and permitted.
2. Offer ice chips.
3. Apply a moistened gauze square over lips occasionally to humidify inspired air.
4. Allow the patient to rinse mouth with mouthwash.

Constipation and Gas Cramps

Causes

1. Trauma and manipulation of the bowel during surgery as well as opioid use.
2. More serious causes: peritonitis or abscess.

Preventive Measures

1. Encourage early ambulation to aid in promoting peristalsis.
2. Provide adequate fluid intake to promote soft stools and hydration.
3. Advocate proper diet to promote peristalsis.
4. Encourage the early use of nonopioid analgesia because many opiates increase the risk of constipation.
5. Assess bowel sounds frequently.

Nursing Interventions

1. Ask the patient about any usual remedy for constipation and try it, if appropriate.
2. Insert a gloved, lubricated finger and break up the fecal impaction manually, if necessary.
3. Administer an oil retention enema (180 to 200 mL), if prescribed, to help soften the fecal mass and facilitate evacuation.
4. Administer a return flow enema (if prescribed) or a rectal tube to decrease painful flatulence.
5. Administer GI stimulants, laxatives, suppositories, and stool softeners, as prescribed.

Postoperative Pain

Pain is a subjective symptom, in which the patient exhibits a feeling of distress; stimulation of, or trauma to, certain nerve endings causes pain. Pain is one of the earliest symptoms that the patient expresses on return to consciousness. Maximal postoperative pain occurs directly after surgery and usually diminishes significantly by 48 hours.

Clinical Manifestations

1. Autonomic:
   a. Elevation of BP.
   b. Increase in heart and pulse rate.
   c. Rapid and irregular respiration.
   d. Increase in perspiration.
2. Skeletal muscle:
   a. Increase in muscle tension or activity.
3. Psychological:
   a. Increase in irritability.
   b. Increase in apprehension.
   c. Increase in anxiety.
   d. Attention focused on pain.
   e. Complaints of pain.
4. The patient's reaction depends on:
   a. Previous experience.
   b. Anxiety or tension.
   c. State of health.
   d. Ability to be distracted.
   e. Meaning that pain has for the patient.

Preventive Measures

1. Reduce anxiety because of anticipation of pain.
2. Teach patient about pain management.
3. Review analgesics with patient and reassure that pain relief will be available quickly.
4. Establish a trusting relationship and spend time with the patient.

Nursing Interventions

Use Basic Comfort Measures

1. Provide therapeutic environment—proper temperature and humidity, ventilation, and visitors.
2. Massage patient's back and pressure points with soothing strokes—move patient gently and with prewarning.
3. Offer diversional activities, soft music, or favorite television program.
4. Provide for fluid needs by giving a cool drink; offer a bedpan.
5. Investigate possible causes of pain, such as bandage or adhesive that is too tight, full bladder, a cast that is too snug, or elevated temperature indicating inflammation or infection.

6. Instruct the patient to splint the wound when moving.
7. Keep bedding clean, dry, and free from wrinkles and debris.

Recognize the Power of Suggestion

1. Provide reassurance that the discomfort is temporary and that the medication will aid in pain reduction.
2. Clarify patient's fears regarding the perceived significance of pain.
3. Assist patient in maintaining a positive, hopeful attitude.

Assist in Relaxation Techniques

1. Teach controlled breathing as a first-line technique for relaxation.
2. Guide the patient through imagery, using multiple sensory images, or meditation, as desired.
3. Discuss the use of progressive muscle relaxation, autogenic training, and provide resources, as needed.

Apply Cutaneous Counter-stimulation

1. Employ vibration—a vigorous form of massage that is applied to a nonoperative site. It lessens the patient's perception of pain. (Avoid applying this to the calf because it may dislodge a thrombus.)
2. Apply heat or cold to the operative or nonoperative site as prescribed. This works best for well-localized pain. Protect the underlying skin and limit contact time to avoid thermal injury.

Give Analgesics as Prescribed in a Timely Manner

1. Instruct the patient to request an analgesic before the pain becomes severe.
2. If pain occurs consistently and predictably throughout a 24-hour period, analgesics should be given around the clock—avoiding the usual "demand cycle" of dosing that sets up eventual dependency and provides less adequate pain relief.
3. Administer prescribed medication to the patient before anticipated activities and painful procedures (e.g., dressing changes).
4. Monitor for possible adverse effects of analgesic therapy (e.g., respiratory depression, hypotension, nausea, skin rash). Have naloxone on hand to relieve significant opioid-induced respiratory depression.
5. Assess and document the efficacy of analgesic therapy.

Pharmacologic Management

Oral and Parenteral Analgesia

1. Surgical patients are commonly prescribed a parenteral analgesic for 2 to 4 days or until the incisional pain abates. At that time, an oral analgesic, opioid, or nonopioid will be prescribed.
2. Although the health care provider is responsible for prescribing the appropriate medication, it is the nurse's responsibility to make sure the drug is given safely and assessed for efficacy.

CLINICAL JUDGMENT The patient who remains sedated because of analgesia is at risk for complications such as aspiration, respiratory depression, atelectasis, hypotension, falls, and poor postoperative course.

DRUG ALERT Opioid "potentiators," such as hydroxyzine, may further sedate the patient.

Patient-Controlled Analgesia

1. Benefits:
   a. Patient-controlled analgesia (PCA) bypasses the delays inherent in traditional analgesic administration (the "demand cycle").
   b. Medication is administered by IV, producing more rapid pain relief and greater consistency in patient response.
   c. The patient retains control over pain relief (added placebo and relaxation effects).
   d. Nursing time is decreased in frequent delivery of analgesics.
2. Contraindications:
   a. Generally, patients younger than age 10 or 11 (depends on the weight of the child and facility policy).
   b. Patients with cognitive impairment (delirium, dementia, mental illness, hemodynamic or respiratory impairment).
3. A portable PCA device delivers a preset dosage of opioid (usually morphine). An adjustable "lockout interval" controls the frequency of dose administration, preventing another dose from being delivered prematurely. An example of PCA settings might be a dose of 1 mg morphine with a lockout interval of 6 minutes (total possible dose is 10 mg/h).
4. Patient pushes a button to activate the device.
5. Instruction about PCA should occur preoperatively; some patients fear being overdosed by the machine and require reassurance.

Epidural Analgesia

1. Requires injections of opioids into the epidural space by way of a catheter inserted by an anesthesiologist under aseptic conditions (see Figure 3-2).
2. Benefit: provides for longer periods of analgesia.
3. Disadvantages:
   a. The epidural catheter's proximity to the spinal nerves and spinal canal, along with its potential for catheter migration, makes correct injection technique and close patient assessment imperative.
   b. Adverse effects include generalized pruritus (common), nausea, urinary retention, respiratory depression, hypotension, motor block, and sensory or sympathetic block. These adverse effects are related to the opioid used (usually, a preservative-free morphine or fentanyl) and catheter position.
4. Strict sterile technique is necessary when inserting the epidural catheter.

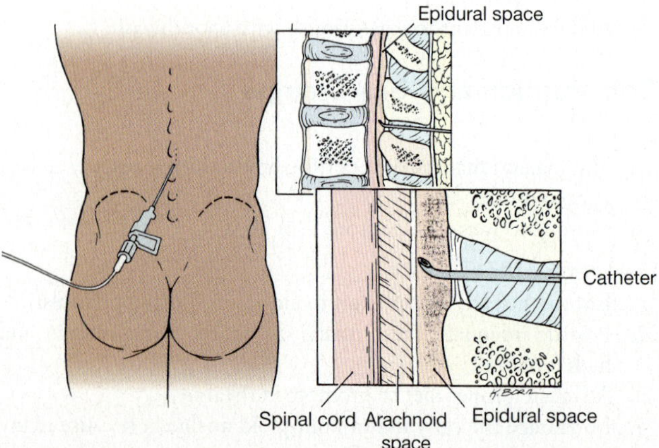

Figure 3-2. Epidural catheter placement.

5. Opioid-related adverse effects are reversed with naloxone.
6. The nurse ensures proper integrity of the catheter and dressing.

Postoperative Complications

Postoperative complications are a risk inherent in surgical procedures. They may interfere with the expected outcome of the surgery and may extend the patient's hospitalization and convalescence. The nurse plays a critical role in attempting to prevent complications and in recognizing their signs and symptoms immediately.

CLINICAL JUDGMENT Be alert for any deviation from the normal expected outcomes postoperatively; notify the appropriate provider with a full assessment.

Shock

Shock is a response of the body to decreased tissue perfusion, culminating, eventually, in cellular hypoxia and death. (See section "Deep Vein Thrombosis" on page 63 for classification and emergency management of shock.)

Preventive Measures

1. Have blood available if there is any indication that it may be needed.
2. Accurately measure any blood loss and monitor all fluid intake and output.
3. Anticipate the progression of symptoms on earliest manifestation.
4. Monitor vital signs per facility protocol until they are stable.
5. Assess vital sign deviations; evaluate BP in relation to other physiologic parameters of shock and the patient's premorbid values. Orthostatic pulse and BP are important indicators of hypovolemic shock.
6. Prevent infection (e.g., indwelling catheter care, wound care, pulmonary care) to minimize the risk of septic shock.

Hemorrhage

Hemorrhage is the escape of blood from a ruptured blood vessel. Hemorrhage from an arterial vessel may be bright red in color and may come in spurts, whereas blood from a vein is dark red and comes in a steady flow. Hemorrhage may be external or internal (concealed).

Clinical Manifestations

1. Apprehension; restlessness; thirst; cold, moist, pale skin; and circumoral pallor.
2. Pulse increases, respirations become rapid and deep ("air hunger"), and temperature drops.
3. With progression of hemorrhage:
   a. Decrease in cardiac output and narrowed pulse pressure.
   b. Rapidly decreasing BP, as well as hematocrit and hemoglobin (if hypovolemic shock is due to hemorrhage).

Nursing Interventions and Management

1. Treat the patient as described for shock (see "Pulmonary complications", point 3 and "Pulmonary Embolism", point 1 on page 64).
2. Inspect the wound as a possible site of bleeding. Apply pressure dressing over an external bleeding site.
3. Increase the IV fluid infusion rate and administer blood as directed and as soon as possible.
4. Administer oxygen.

CLINICAL JUDGMENT Numerous, rapid blood transfusions may induce coagulopathy and prolonged bleeding time. Monitor closely for signs of increased bleeding tendencies after transfusions.

Deep Vein Thrombosis

Deep vein thrombosis (DVT) occurs in pelvic veins or in the deep veins of the lower extremities in postoperative patients. The incidence of DVT varies between 10% and 40% depending on the complexity of the surgery or the severity of the underlying illness. DVT is most common after hip surgery, followed by retropubic prostatectomy and general thoracic or abdominal surgery. Venous thrombi located above the knee are considered the major source of pulmonary emboli. Also see page 168.

Causes

1. Injury to the intimal layer of the vein wall.
2. Venous stasis.
3. Hypercoagulopathy and polycythemia.
4. High risks include obesity, prolonged immobility, cancer, smoking, estrogen use, advancing age, varicose veins, dehydration, splenectomy, and orthopedic procedures.

Clinical Manifestations

1. Most patients with DVT are asymptomatic.
2. Pain or cramp in the calf or thigh, progressing to painful swelling of the entire leg.
3. Slight fever, chills, and perspiration.
4. Marked tenderness over the anteromedial surface of the thigh.
5. Intravascular clotting without marked inflammation may develop, leading to phlebothrombosis.
6. Circulation distal to the DVT may be compromised if sufficient swelling is present.

Preventive Measures and Management

1. Hydrate patient adequately postoperatively to prevent hemoconcentration.
2. Encourage leg exercises and ambulate patient as soon as permitted by the surgeon.
3. Avoid restricting devices, such as tight straps, that can constrict and impair circulation.
4. Avoid rubbing or massaging calves and thighs.
5. Instruct the patient to avoid standing or sitting in one place for prolonged periods and crossing legs when seated.
6. Refrain from inserting IV catheters into legs or feet of adults.
7. Assess distal peripheral pulses, capillary refill, and sensation of lower extremities.
8. Check for positive Homans sign—calf pain on dorsiflexion of the foot, present in nearly 30% of patients with DVT.
9. Prevent the use of bed rolls or knee gatches in patients at risk because there is danger of constricting the vessels under the knee.
10. Initiate anticoagulant therapy IV, subcutaneously, or orally as prescribed.
11. Prevent swelling and stagnation of venous blood by applying appropriately fitting compression stockings or wrapping the legs from the toes to the groin with compression bandage.
12. Apply external pneumatic compression intraoperatively to patients at highest risk of DVT. Pneumatic compression can reduce the risk of DVT by 30% to 50% (see Figure 3-3).

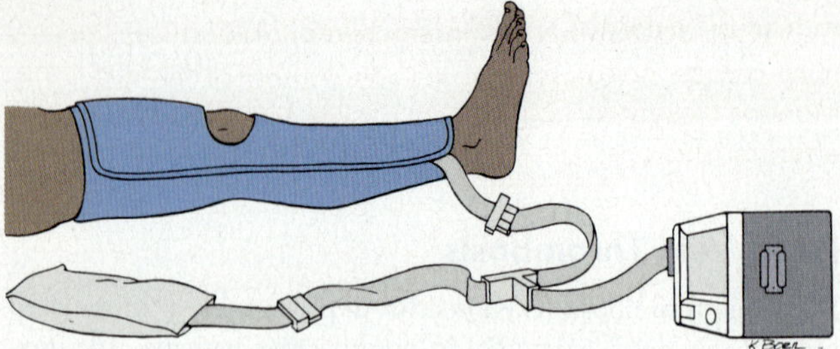

Figure 3-3. Pneumatic compression. Pressures of 35 to 20 mm Hg are sequentially applied from the ankle to the thigh, producing an increase in blood flow velocity and improved venous clearing.

13. Mechanical prophylaxis by having the patient perform foot pumps also provides an alternative to chemical agents in the prevention of thromboembolic disease. The use of foot pumps is safe and patient adherence may be enhanced.

Pulmonary Complications

Causes and Clinical Manifestations

1. Atelectasis:
   a. Incomplete expansion of the lung or portion of it occurring within 48 hours of surgery.
   b. Attributed to the absence of periodic deep breaths.
   c. A mucus plug closes a bronchiole, causing the alveoli distal to the plug to collapse.
   d. Symptoms are typically absent but may include mild to severe tachypnea, tachycardia, cough, fever, hypotension, and decreased breath sounds and chest expansion of the affected side.
2. Aspiration:
   a. Caused by the inhalation of food, gastric contents, water, or blood into the tracheobronchial system.
   b. Anesthetic agents and opioids depress the central nervous system (CNS), causing inhibition of gag or cough reflexes.
   c. Nasogastric (NG) tube insertion renders upper and lower esophageal sphincters partially incompetent.
   d. Gross aspiration has 50% mortality.
   e. Symptoms depend on the severity of aspiration and may be silent or become evident within minutes, including tachypnea, dyspnea, cough, bronchospasm, wheezing, rhonchi, crackles, hypoxia, and frothy sputum.
3. Pneumonia. Also see page 162.
   a. An inflammatory response in which cellular material replaces alveolar gas.
   b. In the postoperative patient, most commonly caused by gram-negative bacilli because of impaired oropharyngeal defense mechanisms.
   c. Predisposing factors include atelectasis, upper respiratory infection, copious secretions, aspiration, dehydration, prolonged intubation or tracheostomy, history of smoking, and impaired normal host defenses (cough reflex, mucociliary system, alveolar macrophage activity).
   d. Symptoms include dyspnea, tachypnea, pleuritic chest pain, fever, chills, hemoptysis, cough (rusty or purulent sputum), and decreased breath sounds over the involved area.

Preventive Measures

1. Report evidence of upper respiratory infection to the surgeon.
2. Suction nasopharyngeal or bronchial secretions if the patient cannot clear their own airway.
3. Use proper patient positioning to prevent regurgitation and aspiration.
4. Recognize the predisposing causes of pulmonary complications:
   a. Infections—mouth, nose, sinuses, and throat.
   b. Aspiration of vomitus.
   c. History of heavy smoking and chronic pulmonary disease.
   d. Obesity.
5. Avoid oversedation.

Nursing Interventions and Management

1. Monitor the patient's progress carefully on a daily basis to detect early signs and symptoms of respiratory difficulties.
   a. Slight temperature, pulse, and respiration elevations.
   b. Apprehension and restlessness or a decreased LOC.
   c. Complaints of chest pain, signs of dyspnea, or cough.
2. Promote full aeration of the lungs.
   a. Turn the patient frequently.
   b. Encourage the patient to take 10 deep breaths hourly, holding each breath to a count of five and exhaling.
   c. Use a spirometer or other device that encourages the patient to ventilate more effectively.
   d. Assist the patient in coughing to bring up mucus secretions. Have patient splint chest or abdominal wound to minimize discomfort associated with deep breathing and coughing.
   e. Encourage and assist the patient to ambulate as early as the health care provider will allow.
3. Initiate specific measures for particular pulmonary problems.
   a. Provide cool mist or heated nebulizer for the patient exhibiting signs of bronchitis or thick secretions.
   b. Encourage the patient to take fluids to help "liquefy" secretions and facilitate expectoration (in pneumonia).
   c. Elevate the head of the bed and ensure proper administration of prescribed oxygen.
   d. Prevent abdominal distention—NG tube insertion may be necessary.
   e. Administer prescribed antibiotics for pulmonary infections.

Pulmonary Embolism

Causes

1. Pulmonary embolism (PE) is caused by the obstruction of one or more pulmonary arterioles by an embolus originating somewhere in the venous system or in the right side of the heart. Also see page 168.
2. Postoperatively, most emboli develop in the pelvic or iliofemoral veins before becoming dislodged and traveling to the lungs.

Clinical Manifestations

1. Sharp, stabbing pains in the chest.
2. Anxiousness and cyanosis.
3. Pupillary dilation and profuse perspiration.
4. Rapid and irregular pulse becoming imperceptible—leads rapidly to death.
5. Dyspnea, tachypnea, and hypoxemia.
6. Pleural friction rub (occasionally).

Nursing Interventions and Management

1. Administer oxygen with the patient in an upright sitting position (if possible).
2. Reassure and calm the patient.
3. Monitor vital signs, ECG, and arterial blood gases.
4. Treat for shock or heart failure, as needed.

5. Give analgesics or sedatives, as directed, to control pain or apprehension.
6. Prepare for anticoagulation or thrombolytic therapy or surgical intervention. Management depends on the severity of the PE.

Urinary Retention

Causes

1. Occurs postoperatively, especially after operations of the rectum, anus, vagina, or lower abdomen.
2. Often seen in patients having epidural or spinal anesthesia.
3. Caused by spasm of the bladder sphincter.
4. More common in patients assigned male at birth because of inherent increases in urethral resistance to urine flow.
5. Can lead to urinary tract infection and possibly kidney failure.

Clinical Manifestations

1. Inability to void or voiding small amounts at frequent intervals.
2. Palpable bladder.
3. Lower abdominal discomfort.

Preventive Measures and Management

1. Help patient to sit or stand (if permissible) because many patients are unable to void while lying in bed.
2. Provide patient with privacy.
3. Run tap water—frequently, the sound or sight of running water relaxes spasm of bladder sphincter.
4. Use warmth to relax sphincters (e.g., a sitz bath or warm compresses).
5. Notify health care provider if the patient does not urinate regularly after surgery.
6. Administer antispasmodic as directed to reduce painful bladder spasm.
7. Catheterize only when all other measures are unsuccessful. The Surgical Care Improvement Project (SCIP) recommends removing an indwelling catheter within 24 hours. Use of bladder scanner can reduce the need for catheterization by checking for residual urine noninvasively.

CLINICAL JUDGMENT Recognize that when a patient voids small amounts (30 to 60 mL every 15 to 30 minutes), this may be a sign of an overdistended bladder with "overflow" of urine.

Intestinal Obstruction

Intestinal obstructions result in a partial or complete impairment to the forward flow of intestinal contents. Most obstructions occur in the small bowel, especially at its narrowest point—the ileum. (Also see page 496.)

Preventive Measures and Management

1. Monitor for adequate bowel sound return after surgery. Assess bowel sounds and the degree of abdominal distention (may need to measure abdominal girth); document these findings every shift.
2. Monitor and document characteristics of emesis and nasogastric (NG) drainage.
3. Relieve abdominal distention by passing a nasoenteric suction tube as ordered.
4. Replace fluid and electrolytes.
5. Monitor fluid, electrolyte (especially potassium and sodium), and acid–base status.
6. Administer opioids judiciously because these medications may further suppress peristalsis.
7. Prepare the patient for surgical intervention if the obstruction continues unresolved.
8. Closely monitor the patient for signs of shock.
9. Provide frequent reassurance to the patient; use nontraditional methods to promote comfort (touch, relaxation, imagery).

Wound Infection

Wound infections are the second most common health care–related infection. The infection may be limited to the surgical site (60% to 80%) or may affect the patient systemically.

Causes

1. Exposed tissues during long operations, operations on contaminated structures, gross obesity, old age, chronic hypoxemia, and malnutrition are directly related to an increased infection rate.
2. The patient's own flora is most commonly implicated in wound infections (*Staphylococcus aureus*).
3. Other common culprits in wound infection include *Escherichia coli*, *Klebsiella*, *Enterobacter*, and *Proteus*.
4. Wound infections typically present 5 to 7 days postoperatively.
5. Factors affecting the extent of infection include:
   a. Type, virulence, and quantity of contaminating microorganisms.
   b. Presence of foreign bodies or devitalized tissue.
   c. Location and nature of the wound.
   d. Amount of dead space or presence of hematoma.
   e. Immune response of the patient.
   f. Presence of adequate blood supply to wound.
   g. Presurgical condition of the patient (e.g., age, dependency on alcohol, diabetes, malnutrition).

Clinical Manifestations

1. Redness, excessive swelling, tenderness, and warmth.
2. Red streaks in the skin near the wound.
3. Pus or other discharge from the wound.
4. Tender, enlarged lymph nodes in the axillary region or groin closest to the wound.
5. Foul smell from the wound.
6. Generalized body chills or fever.
7. Elevated temperature and pulse.
8. Increasing pain from the incision site.

POPULATION AWARENESS Older adults do not readily produce an inflammatory response to infection, so they may not present with fever, redness, and swelling. Increasing pain, fatigue, anorexia, and mental status changes are signs of infection in older patients.

CLINICAL JUDGMENT Mild, transient fevers appear postoperatively as a result of tissue necrosis, hematoma, or cauterization. Be alert for higher sustained fevers that may arise with the following four most common postoperative complications: atelectasis (within the first 48 hours), wound infections (in 5 to 7 days), urinary infections (in 5 to 8 days), and thrombophlebitis (in 7 to 14 days).

Preventive Measures and Management

1. Preoperative:
   a. Encourage the patient to achieve an optimal nutritional level. Enteral or parenteral alimentation may be ordered preoperatively to reduce hypoproteinemia with weight loss.
   b. Reduce preoperative hospitalization to a minimum to avoid acquiring nosocomial infections.
2. Operative:
   a. Follow strict sterile technique throughout the operative procedure.
   b. When a wound has exudate, fibrin, desiccated fat, or nonviable skin, it is not approximated by primary closure but through secondary (delayed) closure.
3. Postoperative:
   a. Keep dressings intact, reinforcing if necessary, until prescribed otherwise.
   b. Use strict sterile technique when dressings are changed.
   c. Monitor and document the amount, type, and location of drainage. Ensure that all drains are working properly. (See Table 3-1 for expected drainage amounts from common types of drains and tubes.)
4. Postoperative care of an infected wound:
   a. The surgeon removes one or more stitches, separates the wound edges, and looks for infection using a hemostat as a probe.
   b. A culture is taken and sent to the laboratory for bacterial analysis.
   c. Wound irrigation may be done; have an aseptic syringe and saline available.
   d. A drain may be inserted or the wound may be packed with sterile gauze.
   e. Antibiotics are prescribed.
   f. Wet-to-dry dressings may be applied (see section "Intestinal Obstruction" on page 65).
   g. If deep infection is suspected, the patient may be taken back to the operating room.

Table 3-1 Expected Drainage From Tubes and Catheters

DEVICE	SUBSTANCE	DAILY DRAINAGE
• Foley catheter • Ileal conduit • Suprapubic catheter	Urine	500–700 mL/24 h for first 48 h; then 1,500–2,500 mL/24 h
• Gastrostomy tube	Gastric contents	Up to 1,500 mL/24 h
• Chest tube	Blood, pleural fluid, air	Varies: 500–1,000 mL first 24 h
• Ileostomy	Small bowel contents	Up to 4,000 mL in first 24 h; then <500 mL/24 h
• Miller-Abbott tube	Intestinal contents	Up to 3,000 mL/24 h
• Nasogastric tube	Gastric contents	Up to 1,500 mL/24 h
• T-tube	Bile	500 mL/24 h

Wound Dehiscence and Evisceration

Causes

1. Commonly occurs between the fifth and eighth day postoperatively when the incision has weakest tensile strength; greatest strength is found between the first and third postoperative day.
2. Chiefly associated with abdominal surgery.
3. This catastrophe is commonly related to:
   a. Inadequate sutures or excessively tight closures (the latter compromises blood supply).
   b. Hematomas and seromas.
   c. Infections.
   d. Excessive coughing, hiccups, retching, and distention.
   e. Poor nutrition and immunosuppression.
   f. Uremia and diabetes mellitus.
   g. Steroid use.

Preventive Measures

1. Apply an abdominal binder for heavy or older adult patients or those with weak or pendulous abdominal walls.
2. Encourage the patient to splint the incision while coughing.
3. Monitor for and relieve abdominal distention.
4. Encourage proper nutrition with emphasis on adequate amounts of protein and vitamin C.

Clinical Manifestations

1. Dehiscence is indicated by a sudden discharge of serosanguineous fluid from the wound.
2. Patient complains that something suddenly "gave way" in the wound.
3. In an intestinal wound, the edges of the wound may part and the intestines may gradually push out. Observe for drainage of peritoneal fluid on dressing (clear or serosanguineous fluid).

Nursing Interventions and Management

1. Stay with patient and have someone notify the surgeon immediately.
2. If the intestines are exposed, cover with sterile, moist saline dressings.
3. Monitor vital signs and watch for shock.
4. Keep patient on absolute bed rest.
5. Instruct the patient to bend the knees, with head of the bed elevated in semi-Fowler position to relieve abdominal tension.
6. Assure patient that the wound will be properly cared for; attempt to keep patient calm and relaxed.
7. Prepare patient for surgery and repair of the wound.

Psychological Disturbances

Depression

1. Cause—perceived loss of health or stamina, pain, altered body image, various drugs, and anxiety about an uncertain future.
2. Clinical manifestations—withdrawal, restlessness, insomnia, nonadherence to therapeutic regimens, tearfulness, and expressions of hopelessness.
3. Nursing interventions and management:
   a. Clarify misconceptions about surgery and its future implications.
   b. Listen to, reassure, and support the patient.
   c. If appropriate, introduce the patient to representatives of ostomy, mastectomy, or amputee support groups.
   d. Involve the patient's family and support people in care; psychiatric consultation is obtained for severe depression.

Delirium

1. Cause—prolonged anesthesia, cardiopulmonary bypass, drug reactions, sepsis, alcohol use disorder (delirium tremens), electrolyte imbalances, and other metabolic disorders.
2. Clinical manifestations—disorientation, hallucinations, perceptual distortions, paranoid delusions, reversed day–night pattern, agitation, and insomnia; delirium tremens often appears within 72 hours of last alcoholic drink and may include autonomic overactivity—tachycardia, dilated pupils, diaphoresis, and fever.
3. Nursing interventions and management:
   a. Assist with the assessment and treatment of the underlying cause (restore fluid and electrolyte balance, discontinue the offending drug).
   b. Reorient the patient to environment and time.
   c. Keep surroundings calm.
   d. Explain in detail every procedure done to the patient.
   e. Sedate the patient, as ordered, to reduce agitation, prevent exhaustion, and promote sleep. Assess for oversedation.
   f. Allow extended periods of uninterrupted sleep.
   g. Reassure family members with clear explanations of the patient's aberrant behavior.
   h. Have contact with the patient as much as possible; apply restraints to the patient only as a last resort if safety is in question and if ordered by the health care provider.

WOUND CARE

See additional online content: Procedure Guidelines 3-1 and 3-2.

Wounds and Wound Healing

A *wound* is a disruption in the continuity and regulatory processes of tissue cells; *wound healing* is the restoration of that continuity. Wound healing, however, may not restore normal cellular function.

Wound Classification

Mechanism of Injury

1. Incised wounds—made by a clean cut of a sharp instrument, such as a surgical incision with a scalpel.
2. Contused wounds—made by blunt force that typically does not break the skin but causes considerable tissue damage with bruising and swelling.
3. Lacerated wounds—made by an object that tears tissues, producing jagged, irregular edges; examples include glass, jagged wire, and blunt knife.
4. Puncture wounds—made by a pointed instrument, such as an ice pick, bullet, or nail.

Degree of Contamination

1. Clean—an aseptically made wound, as in surgery, that does not enter the alimentary, respiratory, or genitourinary tracts.
2. Clean-contaminated—an aseptically made wound that enters the respiratory, alimentary, or genitourinary tracts. These wounds have slightly higher probability of wound infection than do clean wounds.
3. Contaminated—wounds exposed to excessive amounts of bacteria. These wounds may be open (avulsive) and accidentally made or may be the result of surgical operations in which there are major breaks in sterile techniques or gross spillage from the gastrointestinal tract.
4. Infected—a wound that retains devitalized tissue or involves preoperatively existing infection or perforated viscera. Such wounds are often left open to drain.

Physiology of Wound Healing

The phases of wound healing—inflammation, reconstruction (proliferation), and maturation (remodeling)—involve continuous and overlapping processes.

Inflammatory Phase (Lasts 1 to 5 Days)

1. Vascular and cellular responses are immediately initiated when tissue is cut or injured.
2. Transient vasoconstriction occurs immediately at the site of injury, lasting 5 to 10 minutes, along with the deposition of a fibrinoplatelet clot to help control bleeding.
3. Subsequent dilation of small venules occurs; antibodies, plasma proteins, plasma fluids, leukocytes, and red blood cells leave the microcirculation to permeate the general area of injury, causing edema, redness, warmth, and pain.
4. Localized vasodilation is the result of direct action by histamine, serotonin, and prostaglandins.
5. Polymorphic leukocytes (neutrophils) and monocytes enter the wound to engage in destruction and ingestion of wound debris. Monocytes predominate during this phase.
6. Basal cells at the wound edges undergo mitosis; resultant daughter cells enlarge, flatten, and creep across the wound surface to eventually approximate the wound edges.

Proliferative Phase (Lasts 2 to 20 Days)

1. Fibroblasts (connective tissue cells) multiply and migrate along fibrin strands that are thought to serve as a matrix.
2. Endothelial budding occurs on nearby blood vessels, forming new capillaries that penetrate and nourish the injured tissue.
3. The combination of budding capillaries and proliferating fibroblasts is called *granulation tissue.*
4. Active collagen synthesis by fibroblasts begins by the fifth to seventh day, and the wound gains tensile strength.
5. By 3 weeks, the skin obtains about 30% of its preinjury tensile strength, intestinal tissue about 65%, and fascia about 20%.

Remodeling Phase (21 Days to Months or Years)

1. Scar tissue is composed primarily of collagen and ground substance (mucopolysaccharide, glycoproteins, electrolytes, and water).
2. From the start of collagen synthesis, collagen fibers undergo a process of lysis and regeneration. The collagen fibers become more organized, aligning more closely to each other and increasing in tensile strength.
3. The overall bulk and form of the scar continue to change once maturation has started.
4. Typically, collagen production drops off; however, if collagen production greatly exceeds collagen lysis, keloid (greatly hypertrophied, deforming scar tissue) will form.
5. Normal maturation of the wound is clinically observed as an initial red, raised, hard immature scar that molds into a flat, soft, and pale mature scar.
6. The scar tissue will never achieve greater than 80% of its preinjury tensile strength.

Types of Wound Healing

See Figure 3-4.

First Intention Healing (Primary Closure)

1. Wounds are made sterile by minor debridement and irrigation, with a minimum of tissue damage and tissue reaction; wound edges are properly approximated with sutures.
2. Granulation tissue is not visible and scar formation is typically minimal (keloid may still form in susceptible people).

Secondary Intention Healing (Granulation)

1. Wounds are left open to heal spontaneously or are surgically closed at a later date; they need not be infected.
2. Examples in which wounds may heal by secondary intention include burns, traumatic injuries, ulcers, and suppurative infected wounds.
3. The cavity of the wound fills with a red, soft, sensitive tissue (granulation tissue), which bleeds easily. A scar (cicatrix) eventually forms.
4. In infected wounds, drainage may be accomplished using special dressings and drains. Healing is thus improved.
5. In wounds that are later sutured, the two opposing granulation surfaces are brought together.
6. Secondary intention healing produces a deeper, wider scar.

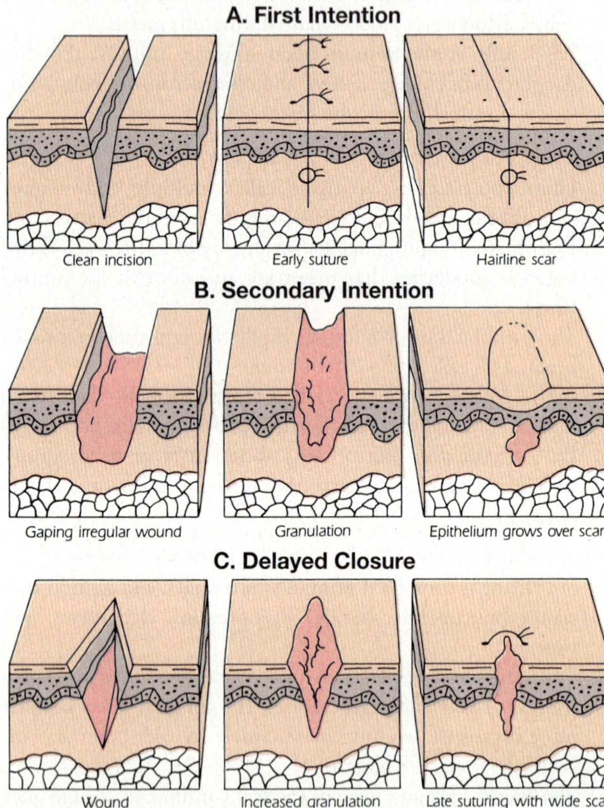

Figure 3-4. Classification of wound healing. **(A)** First intention: A clean incision is made with primary closure; there is minimal scarring. **(B)** Second intention: The wound is left open so that granulation can occur; a large scar results. **(C)** Delayed closure: The wound is initially left open and later closed when there is no further evidence of infection. (Reprinted with permission from Smeltzer, S., & Bare, B. [2000]. *Brunner and Suddarth's textbook of medical-surgical nursing* [9th ed.]. Lippincott Williams & Wilkins.)

Wound Management

Many factors promote wound healing, such as adequate nutrition, cleanliness, rest, and position, along with the patient's underlying psychological and physiologic state. Of added importance is the application of appropriate dressings and drains.

Dressings

Purpose of Dressings

1. To protect the wound from mechanical injury.
2. To splint or immobilize the wound.
3. To absorb drainage.
4. To prevent contamination from bodily discharges (feces, urine).
5. To promote hemostasis, as in pressure dressings.
6. To debride the wound by combining capillary action and the entwining of necrotic tissue within its mesh.
7. To inhibit or kill microorganisms by using dressings with antiseptic or antimicrobial properties.
8. To provide a physiologic environment conducive to healing.
9. To provide mental and physical comfort for the patient.
10. To encourage healing by applying localized subatmospheric pressure at site of wound as in negative pressure dressings.

Advantages of Not Using Dressings

When the initial dressing on a clean, dry, and intact incision is removed, it is often not replaced; this may occur within 24 hours after surgery.

1. Permits better visualization of the wound.
2. Eliminates conditions necessary for growth of organisms (warmth, moisture, and darkness).
3. Minimizes adhesive tape reaction.
4. Aids bathing.

Types of Dressings

1. Dry dressings:
   a. Used primarily for wounds closing by primary intention.
   b. Offers good wound protection, absorption of drainage, and aesthetics for the patient and provides pressure, if needed, for hemostasis.
   c. Disadvantage—they adhere to the wound surface when drainage dries. (Removal can cause pain and disruption of granulation tissue.)
2. Wet-to-dry dressings:
   a. These are useful for infected wounds that must be debrided and closed by secondary intention.
   b. Gauze saturated with sterile saline (preferred) or an antimicrobial solution is packed into the wound, eliminating dead space.
   c. The wet dressings are then covered by dry dressings (gauze sponges or absorbent pads).
   d. As drying occurs, wound debris and necrotic tissue are absorbed into the gauze dressing by capillary action.
   e. The dressing is changed when it becomes dry (or just before). If there is excessive necrotic debris on the dressing, more frequent dressing changes are required.
3. Wet-to-wet dressings:
   a. Used on clean open wounds or on granulating surfaces. Sterile saline or an antimicrobial agent may be used to saturate the dressings.

b. Provides a more physiologic environment (warmth, moisture), which can enhance the local healing processes as well as ensure greater patient comfort. Thick exudate is more easily removed.
c. Disadvantage—surrounding tissues can become macerated, there is an increased risk for infection, and bed linens become damp.

Types of Surgical Dressing Supplies

1. Hydrophobic occlusive (petroleum gauze):
   a. This is an impermeable, nonadhering dressing that protects wounds from air- and moisture-borne contamination.
   b. It is used around chest tubes and any fistula or stoma that drains digestive juices.
   c. It is relatively nonabsorptive.
2. Hydrophilic permeable (oil-based gauze, Telfa pads):
   a. Allows drainage to penetrate the dressing but remains somewhat nonadhering.
   b. For wounds with light to moderate exudate.
   c. Oil-based gauze used on abraded and open ulcerated or granulating wounds.
   d. May also be used to pack "caverns and sinuses" of large open wounds.
   e. Telfa pads are generally reserved for simple, closed, stable wounds.
3. Dressing sponges (general-use gauze sponges):
   a. Gauze sponges come in various sizes (most commonly 2″ × 2″, 4″ × 4″) and may be used for simple dry dressings, wet-to-dry dressings, or wet-to-wet dressings. Gauze allows for better absorption of drainage and necrotic wound debris.
4. All-absorbent combined dressing:
   a. Large (5″ × 9″, 8″ × 10″) cotton-filled dressing that is typically used as an "overdressing," covering gauze or hydrophilic dressings for added wound protection, stabilization of dressings, and drainage absorption.
   b. May also be used unaccompanied over intact surgical wounds.
5. High-bulk gauze bandage ("fluffs")—primarily used for packing large wounds that are undergoing healing by secondary intention.
6. Drain sponge—a gauze sponge with a premade slit, which makes the dressing highly suitable for drain sites and tracheostomy sites.
7. Transparent film dressing:
   a. Highly elastic dressing, adjusts exceptionally well to body contours. It is permeable to oxygen and water vapor but generally impermeable to liquids and bacteria.
   b. Controversies (related to incidence of infection) have reduced its use.
   c. Most common indications include covering arterial and venous catheter sites as well as protecting vulnerable skin exposed to shearing forces.
   d. Commonly used for surgical wounds over gauze dressing to replace tape.
8. Silver-impregnated dressing:
   a. Highly effective for difficult-to-heal wounds. They are available in many sizes and should be placed directly on the wound without any topical ointment.
   b. These may replace need for wet-to-dry or wet-to-wet dressings.
9. Negative pressure wound therapy (NPWT) promotes healing by applying a vacuum through a special sealed dressing.
   a. Evacuates wound fluid, stimulates granulation tissue, and decreases bacterial colonization.
   b. Contraindicated on patients with active bleeding or taking anticoagulants.
   c. NPWT has different interface materials, safety features, and recommended applications by manufacturers. The use is dependent on wound type, provider's preference for gauze or foam packing, and product available.

Drains

Purpose of Drains

1. Drains are placed in wounds only when abnormal fluid collections are present or expected to decrease pooling of body fluids in wound.
2. Drains are usually placed in compartments (e.g., joints and pleural space) that are intolerant to fluid accumulation and have large blood supply (e.g., neck and kidney), in areas of large superficial tissue dissection (e.g., the breast), or in infected wounds.
3. Collection of body fluids in wounds can be harmful in the following ways:
   a. Provides culture media for bacterial growth.
   b. Causes increased pressure at surgical site, interfering with blood flow to area.
   c. Causes pressure on adjacent areas.
   d. Causes local tissue irritation and necrosis (because of fluids such as bile, pus, pancreatic juice, and urine).

Wound Drainage

1. Drains are commonly made of latex, polyvinyl chloride, or silicone and placed within either wounds or body cavities.
2. Drains placed within wounds are typically attached to portable (or, rarely, wall) suction with a collection container.
   a. Examples include the Hemovac, Jackson-Pratt, and Surgivac drainage systems.
3. Drains may also be used postoperatively to form hollow connections from internal organs to the outside to drain a body fluid, such as the T-tube (bile drainage), nephrostomy, gastrostomy, jejunostomy, and cecostomy tubes.
4. Drains create a portal for entry and exit of infectious microorganisms; therefore, the risk of infection exists.
5. Drains within wounds are removed when the amount of drainage decreases over a period of days or, rarely, weeks.
6. Body fluid drains are often left in for longer periods of time.
   a. Careful handling of these drains and collection bags is essential.
   b. Accidental early removal may result in caustic drainage leaking within the tissues.
   c. The risk is reduced within 7 to 10 days when a wall of fibrous tissue has been formed.
7. The amount of drainage varies with the procedure. Drains are commonly not needed on some surgical procedures (e.g., appendectomy, cholecystectomy, abdominal hysterectomy), which usually have minimal wound drainage.

CLINICAL JUDGMENT The greatest amount of drainage is expected during the first 24 hours. Closely monitor dressing and drains and notify provider if persistent or increased drainage occurs.

Nursing Process Overview

EVIDENCE BASE Leaper, D., & Edmiston, C. (2017). World Health Organization: Global guidelines for the prevention of surgical site infection. *Journal of Hospital Infection, 95*(2), 135–136. https://doi.org/10.1016/j.jhin.2016.12.016

Nursing Assessment

The wound should be assessed every 15 minutes while the patient is in the postanesthesia care unit (PACU). Thereafter, the frequency of wound assessment is determined by the nature of the wound, the degree of drainage, and the facility protocol. Assessment and documentation of the wound's status should occur at least every shift until the patient is discharged.

Determine the following, which will affect wound healing:

1. What type of surgery did the patient have?
2. Was hemostasis in the operating room effective?
3. Has the patient received blood to sustain an adequate hematocrit (and promote perfusion to wound)?
4. What is the patient's age?
5. What is the patient's nutritional status? What was it preoperatively?
   a. Is current intake of protein and vitamin C adequate?
   b. Does the patient have obesity or cachexia?
6. What underlying medical conditions does the patient have, and what medications is the patient taking that could affect wound healing (e.g., diabetes mellitus, steroids)?
7. How long has the patient been hospitalized preoperatively? (Longer preoperative facility stays can increase complications.)
8. How is the wound held together?
   a. Staples, nylon sutures, adhesive strips, tension sutures, surgical skin glue.
   b. If the wound is left open, how is it being treated? Is granulation tissue present?
9. Are drains in place? What kind? How many?
   a. Is portable suction being used?
   b. Is the amount of drainage consistent with the nature of surgery?
10. What kinds of dressings are being used?
    a. Are they saturated?
    b. Is the amount and type of drainage consistent with nature of the surgery?
11. How does the wound appear?
    a. Is there evidence of edema, irritation, inflammation?
    b. Are the wound edges well approximated?
    c. Is the wound clean and dry?
12. How does the patient appear?
    a. Are there signs of wound pain or discomfort?
    b. Is fever or elevated white blood cell count present?
    c. Does the patient express concern about the wound and potential disfigurement?
13. Does the patient understand the purpose of wound therapies, and can the patient or family effectively carry out discharge instructions about wound care?

Nursing Interventions

Preventing Infection

1. Prior to the first dressing change (usually performed by the surgeon), reinforce the dressing when saturated.
2. Gather supplies (dressings, tape, scissors, sterile saline solution, cotton swabs, extra gauze, and culture materials if indicated).
3. Explain procedure to the patient. Provide privacy and comfort by premedicating for pain.
4. Wash your hands thoroughly and don gloves. Ensure strict aseptic technique during dressing changes.
5. Remove the old dressings and assess the wound. Loosen all tapes gently. Place dressings in disposable bag. Assess the wound for future documentation noting any redness, swelling, exudate, warmth, bleeding, swelling, or discoloration.
6. Culture the wound if necessary, using sterile technique. Wear sterile gloves. Aspirate a generous amount of drainage liquid into the syringe; inject it into an anaerobic tube. If liquid material is unobtainable, swab the desired area with a cotton-tipped culture swab, attempting to get maximum saturation, and place it in the tube. Prepare and label this specimen and send it to the laboratory.
7. Using sterile gloves, clean around the wound edges with saline moist gauze. Do not go over the area with the same gauze. Repeat as necessary with a fresh gauze until all the areas are clean.
8. Dress the wound with sterile gauze and secure with tape. Use minimal amount of tape to ensure adhesion.
9. Discard contaminated items, ensure the patient's comfort, and document the procedure.

Enhancing Tissue Integrity Through Healing

1. Assess the patient's nutritional intake; consult with the patient's health care provider if supplemental nutritional intake is required.
2. Minimize strain on the incision site:
   a. Use appropriate tape, bandages, and binders.
   b. Have the patient splint abdominal and chest incision when coughing.
   c. Instruct the patient in the proper way to get out of bed while minimizing incision strain (e.g., for abdominal incision, have the patient turn on one side and push self up with the dependent elbow and the opposite hand).
3. Assess and accurately document the condition of the incision site each shift.

Relieving Pain

1. Give the patient prescribed medication before painful dressing changes.
2. Continue to assess for pain at incision site.
3. Consider nonpharmacologic pain relief, such as use of music therapy, relaxation exercises, and acupressure, as indicated.

Patient Education

Before discharge, instruct the patient and family on techniques and rationale for wound care.

1. Report immediately to the health care provider if the following signs of infection occur:
   a. Redness, marked swelling, tenderness, and increased warmth around wound.
   b. Pus or unusual discharge and foul odor from wound.
   c. Red streaks in the skin near wound.
   d. Chills or fever (over 100°F [37.8°C]).
2. Follow the directives of the health care provider regarding activity allowances.
3. Keep the wound clean (the patient may shower unless contraindicated by the health care provider; avoid tub bathing until

sutures or staples are removed); never vigorously rub near the suture line; pat dry.

   a. Sutures that have been placed need to be removed or may be absorbable. Gently cleanse one to two times daily. Dab dry.
   b. Staples if used will need to be removed after 7 to 14 days. Keep the site clean and dry.
   c. Skin glue, which may be used, allows for good approximation of tissue. Keep the wound clean, and remove glue with medical adhesive removing wipes according to your doctor's instruction.

4. Contact your health care provider for follow-up appointment.
5. Report to the health care provider if after 2 months the incision site continues to be red, thick, and painful to pressure (probable beginning of keloid formation).

Evaluation: Expected Outcomes

- No signs of infection.
- Wound edges well approximated without gaping.
- Pain at level 1 or 2.

POSTOPERATIVE DISCHARGE INSTRUCTIONS

It is of primary importance that the nurse makes sure that the patient has been given specific and individualized discharge instructions. These should be written by a provider and reinforced verbally by the nurse. A provider telephone contact should be included as well as information regarding follow-up care and appointments. The instructions should be signed by the patient, provider, and nurse, and a copy becomes part of the patient's chart. Forms and procedures for discharge instructions may vary per facility.

Patient Education

Rest and Activity

1. It is common to feel tired and frustrated about not being able to do all the things you want; this is normal.
2. Plan regular naps and quiet activities, gradually increasing your exercise over the following weeks.
3. When you begin to exercise more, start by taking a short walk two or three times per day. Consult your health care provider if more specific exercises are required.
4. Climbing stairs in your home may be surprisingly tiring at first. If you have difficulty with this activity, try going upstairs backward ("scooching") on your "bottom" until your strength has returned.
5. Consult your health care provider to determine the appropriate time to return to work.

Eating

1. Follow dietary instructions provided at the facility before your discharge.
2. Your appetite may be limited or you may feel bloated after meals; this problem should lessen as you become more active. (Some prescribed medications can cause this.) If symptoms persist, consult your health care provider.
3. Eat small, regular meals and make them as nourishing as possible to promote wound healing.

Sleeping

1. If sleeping is difficult because of wound discomfort, try taking your pain medication at bedtime.
2. Attempt to get sufficient sleep to aid in your recovery.

Wound Healing

1. Your wound will go through several stages of healing. After initial pain at the site, the wound may feel tingling, itchy, numb, or tight (a slight pulling sensation) as healing occurs.
2. Do not pull off any scabs because they protect the delicate new tissues underneath. They will fall off without any help when ready. Change the dressing according to the surgeon's instructions.

Bowels

1. Irregular bowel habits can result from changes in activity and diet or the use of some drugs.
2. Avoid straining because it can intensify discomfort in some wounds; instead, use a rocking motion while trying to pass stool.
3. Drink plenty of fluids and increase the fiber in your diet through fruits, vegetables, and grains, as tolerated.
4. It may be helpful to take a mild laxative. Consult your health care provider if you have any questions.

Bathing and Showering

1. You may get your wound wet 3 days after your operation if the initial dressing has already been changed (unless otherwise advised).
2. Showering is preferable because it allows for thorough rinsing of the wound.
3. If you are feeling too weak, place a plastic or metal chair in the shower so you can be seated during showering.
4. Be sure to dry your wound thoroughly with a clean towel and dress it as instructed before discharge.

Clothing

1. Avoid tight belts and underwear and other clothes with seams that may rub against the wound.
2. Wear loose clothing for comfort and to reduce mechanical trauma to wound.

Driving

1. Ask your health care provider when you may resume driving. Safe driving may be affected by your pain medication. In addition, any violent jarring from an accident may disrupt your wound.

Bending and Lifting

1. How much bending, stretching, and lifting you are allowed depends on the location and nature of your surgery.
2. Typically, for most major surgeries, you should avoid lifting anything heavier than 5 lb for 4 to 8 weeks.
3. It is ideal to obtain home assistance for the first 2 to 3 weeks after discharge.

SELECTED READINGS

Alverdy, J. C., Hyman, N., & Gilbert, J. (2020, March). Re-examining causes of surgical site infections following elective surgery in the era of asepsis. *The Lancet Infectious Diseases, 20*(3), e38–e43. https://doi.org/10.1016/S1473-3099(19)30756-X. PMID: 32006469; PMCID: PMC8019154.

American Society of PeriAnesthesia Nurses. (2022). *Evidence based clinical practice guidelines for the promotion of normothermia.* www.aspan.org/Clinical-Practice/Clinical-Guidelines for the ASPAN Clinical Practice Guidelines

Association of periOperative Registered Nurses. (2016). Guideline at a glance: Skin antisepsis. *AORN Journal, 104*(3), 273–276. https://doi.org/10.1016/S0001-2092(16)30508-7

Association of periOperative Registered Nurses. (2022). *AORN recommended practices for monitoring the patient receiving intravenous sedation.* Author.

Bardia, A., Treggiari, M. M., Michel, G., Dai, F., Tickoo, M., Wai, M., Schuster, K., Mathis, M., Shah, N., Kheterpal, S., & Schonberger, R. B. (2021, December). Adherence to guidelines for the administration of intraoperative antibiotics in a nationwide US sample. *JAMA Network Open, 4*(12), e2137296. https://doi.org/10.1001/jamanetworkopen.2021.37296. PMID: 34905007; PMCID: PMC8672234.

Chetter, I., Arundel, C., Martin, B. C., Hewitt, C., Fairhurst, C., Joshi, K., Mott, A., Rodgers, S., Goncalves, P. S., Torgerson, D., Wilkinson, J., Blazeby, J., Macefield, R., Dixon, S., Henderson, E., Oswald, A., Dumville, J., Lee, M., Pinkney, T., … Wilson, L. (2021, October). Negative pressure wound therapy versus usual care for surgical wounds healing by secondary intention (SWHSI-2 trial): Study protocol for a pragmatic, multicentre, cross surgical specialty, randomised controlled trial. *Trials, 22*(1), 739. https://doi.org/10.1186/s13063-021-05662-2. PMID: 34696784; PMCID: PMC8543414.

Dhatariya, K., Corsino, L., & Umpierrez, G. E. (2020). Management of diabetes and hyperglycemia in hospitalized patients. In K. R. Feingold, B. Anawalt, A. Boyce, et al. (Eds.), *Endotext (Internet).* MDText.com. https://www.ncbi.nlm.nih.gov/books/NBK279093

Gan, T. J., Belani, K. G., Bergese, S. D., Chung, F., Diemunsch, P., Habib, A. S., Jin, Z., Kovac, A. L., Meyer, T. A., Urman, R. D., Apfel, C. C., Ayad, S., Beagley, L., Candiotti, K., Englesakis, M., Hedrick, T. L., Kranke, P., Lee, S., Lipman, D., … Philip, B. K. (2020). Fourth Consensus Guidelines for the Management of Postoperative Nausea and Vomiting. *Anesthesia and Analgesia, 131,* 411–448. https://api.semanticscholar.org/CorpusID:218983784

Ghanei, G. R., Parizad, N., Ebrahimi, A., & Baghi, V. (2023). Nurses' knowledge on the prevention of surgical site infection: A systematic review and meta-analysis study. *Nursing and Midwifery Journal, 21*(1), 58–65. http://unmf.umsu.ac.ir/article-1-4823-en.html

Joshi, G. P., Abdelmalak, B. B., Weigel, W. A., Harbell, M. W., Kuo, C. I., Soriano, S. G., Stricker, P. A., Tipton, T., Grant, M. D., Marbella, A. M., Agarkar, M., Blanck, J. F., & Domino, K. B. (2023). 2023 American Society of Anesthesiologists Practice Guidelines for Preoperative Fasting: Carbohydrate- containing clear liquids with or without protein, chewing gum, and pediatric fasting duration—A modular update of the 2017 American Society of Anesthesiologists Practice Guidelines for Preoperative Fasting. *Anesthesiology, 138*(2), 132–151. https://doi.org/10.1097/ALN.0000000000004381

Irani, J. L., Hedrick, T. L., Miller, T. E., Lee, L., Steinhagen, E., Shogan, B. D., Goldberg, J. E., Feingold, D. L., Lightner, A. L., & Paquette, I. M. (2023). Clinical practice guidelines for enhanced recovery after colon and rectal surgery from the American Society of Colon and Rectal Surgeons and the Society of American Gastrointestinal and Endoscopic Surgeons. *Surgical Endoscopy, 37*(1), 5–30. https://doi.org/10.1007/s00464-022-09758-x

Karuppaiah, I. (2017). Role of prophylactic antibody to prevent the surgical site infections—A study in a tertiary care hospitals. *Journal of Medical Science And clinical Research, 5*(6), 23698–23706. https://doi.org/10.18535/jmscr/v5i6.149

Korte, M., Wheeler, K., Cooper, E., Kalivoshko, N., Gopal, K., Wells, V., Norman, T., & Sykes, S. (2020, August 20). *American Society of Perianesthesia Nurse: Enhanced Recovery After Surgery (ERAS®): Process and continuous improvement methodology.* Summa Health System–Akron Campus.

Link, T. (2022). Guidelines in Practice: Preoperative Patient Skin Antisepsis. *AORN J. 115*(2), 156–166. http://doi.org/10.1002/aorn.13605. PMID: 35084763.

Ljungqvist, O., Scott, M., & Fearon, K. C. (2017). Enhanced recovery after surgery: A review. *JAMA Surgery, 152*(3), 292–298. https://doi.org/10.1001/jamasurg.2016.4952

Manivannan, B., Gowda, D., Bulagonda, P., Rao, A., Raman, S. S., & Natarajan, S. V. (2018). Surveillance, auditing, and feedback can reduce surgical site infection dramatically: Toward zero surgical site infection. *Surgical Infections, 19*(3), 313–320. https://doi.org/10.1089/sur.2017.272

Neal, J. M., Neal, E. J., & Weinberg, G. L. (2021). American Society of Regional Anesthesia and Pain Medicine local anesthetic systemic toxicity checklist: 2020 version. *Regional Anesthesia & Pain Medicine, 46*(1), 81–82. https://doi:10.1136/rapm-2020-101986

Nie, P., & Zhang, C. (2022). Effect of vacuum sealing drainage on soft tissue injury of traumatic fracture and its effect on wound recovery. *Evidence Based Complementary and Alternative Medicine, 2022,* 7107090. https://doi.org/10.1155/2022/7107090

Norman, G., Dumville, J., Mohapatra, D., Owens, G. L., & Crosbie, E. J. (2016). Antibiotics and antiseptics for surgical wounds healing by secondary intention. *Cochrane Database of Systematic Reviews,* (3), CD011712. https://doi.org/10.1002/14651858.CD011712.pub2

Rauch, S., Miller, C., Bräuer, A., Wallner, B., Bock, M., & Paal, P. (2021, August). Perioperative hypothermia—A narrative review. *International Journal of Environmental Research and Public Health, 18*(16), 8749. https://doi.org/10.3390/ijerph18168749. PMID: 34444504; PMCID: PMC8394549.

Ri, M., Aikou, S., & Seto, Y. (2017). Obesity as a surgical risk factor. *Annals of Gastroenterologic Surgery, 2*(1), 13–21. https://doi.org/10.1002/ags3.12049

Scott, A., Stonemetz, J., Wasey, J., Johnson, D. J., Rivers, R. J., Koch, C. G., & Frank, S. M. (2016). Compliance with surgical care improvement project for body temperature management (SCIP Inf-10) is associated with improved clinical outcome. *Survey of Anesthesiology, 60*(2), 82–83. https://doi.org/10.1097/SA.0000000000000212

Sharma, S., & Arora, L. (2020, March). Anesthesia for the morbidly obese patient. *Anesthesiology Clinics, 38*(1), 197–212. https://doi.org/10.1016/j.anclin.2019.10.008. PMID: 32008653.

Steenhagen, E. (2016). Enhanced recovery after surgery: It's time to change practice! *Nutrition in Clinical Practice, 31*(1), 18–29. https://doi.org/10.1177/0884533615622640

Talec, P., Gaujoux, S., & Samama, C. (2016). Early ambulation and prevention of post-operative thrombo-embolic risk. *Journal of Visceral Surgery, 153*(6), S11–S14. https://doi.org/10.1016/j.jviscsurg.2016.09.002

Williams, K. (2022). Guidelines in practice: Moderate sedation and analgesia. *AORN Journal, 115*(6), 553–564. https://doi.org/10.1002/aorn.13690

Ye, J. (2023). Patient safety of perioperative medication through the lens of digital health and artificial intelligence. *JMIR Perioperative Medicine, 6,* e34453. https://doi.org/10.2196/34453

Zens, Y., Barth, M., Bucher, H. C., Dreck, K., Felsch, M., Groß, W., Jaschinski, T., Kölsch, H., Kromp, M., Overesch, I., Sauerland, S., & Gregor, S. (2020, October). Negative pressure wound therapy in patients with wounds healing by secondary intention: A systematic review and meta-analysis of randomised controlled trials. *Systematic Reviews, 9*(1), 238. https://doi.org/10.1186/s13643-020-01476-6. PMID: 33038929; PMCID: PMC7548038.

4 Cancer Nursing*

OVERVIEW AND ASSESSMENT

Cancer is a large group of diseases with the following traits: (a) sustained proliferation of abnormal cells and the ability to replicate indefinitely; (b) uncontrolled growth and cell division and deregulation of repair of defective DNA; (c) ability to grow new blood vessels (angiogenesis); (d) ability to spread to distant sites (metastasize); (e) evasion of normal protective mechanisms of growth suppression, immunologic suppression, and programmed cell death (apoptosis); (f) genetic instability, inflammation, and fibrosis that enable malignant cell transformation.

Etiology, Detection, and Prevention

Epidemiology

EVIDENCE BASE American Cancer Society. (2022). *Cancer facts & figures 2022.* www.cancer.org/research/cancer-facts-statistics/all-cancer-facts-figures/2024-cancer-facts-figures.html

American Cancer Society. (2022). *Global facts and figures.* https://www.cancer.org/research/cancer-facts-statistics/global.html

1. According to the American Cancer Society (ACS), There will be slightly over 1 million predicted cases of invasive cancer diagnosed in the United States in 2023. This does not include basal and squamous cell skin cancers as well as noninvasive cancers or ductal carcinoma in situ (DCIS).
2. Due to the COVID-19 pandemic that began in 2020, the diagnoses and treatment of cancers were delayed, resulting in more advanced stages of cancer at diagnosis. This led to a short-term drop in the number of cases reported.
3. Although the death rate continues to decline, cancer is the second leading, after heart disease, cause of death in the United States with 611.720 predicted for 2024.
4. Multiple factors can lead to the development of cancer, including:
   a. Spontaneous transformation of the cell where no causative agent is identified.
   b. Exposure to a chemical or other carcinogen.
   c. Genetic mutations or alterations.
   d. Exposure to virus.
5. Age is the most outstanding risk factor for cancer.
   a. Cancer incidence increases progressively with age.
   b. Approximately 87% of people diagnosed with cancer are over age 50.
   c. The leading cause of death among females ages 49 to 79 and males ages 60 to 79 is cancer.
   d. Prostate, lung and bronchus, and colorectal cancers account for 47% of all cases in males. For females, the three most commonly diagnosed cancers are breast, lung and bronchus, and colorectal, representing one half of all cases; breast cancer alone is expected to account for 31% all new cancer diagnoses in females.

POPULATION AWARENESS For most cancers, African American/Black individuals have a higher cancer burden, including the highest mortality and the lowest survival of any racial/ethnic group.

6. Forty-two percent of all cancers in the United States are related to lifestyle habits (e.g., smoking, alcohol consumption, diet, physical activity) and environmental carcinogens.
   a. Tobacco is the single greatest cause of cancer-related deaths and is attributed to more than 480,000 deaths annually from various cancers and 42,000 from secondhand smoke.
   b. Excessive alcohol intake is associated with cancers of the mouth, larynx, throat, esophagus, and liver, especially when combined with smoking. In addition, regular consumption of alcohol is associated with an increased risk of breast cancer. This may be due to alcohol-induced increases in circulating estrogens.
   c. Being overweight or obese is clearly linked with an increased risk of many cancers, including cancers of the breast (in postmenopausal females), colon and rectum, endometrium, esophagus, kidney, and pancreas. Overweight and obesity may also be associated with increased risk of gallbladder, liver, cervical, and ovarian cancer, non-Hodgkin lymphoma, and multiple myeloma.
   d. Exposure to carcinogens, such as asbestos, benzene, and radiation, increases the risk of developing certain types of cancer.
   e. Solar ultraviolet radiation exposure is related to an increased risk of skin cancers.

*Please note that the term "male" in this chapter refers to a person assigned male at birth, and the term "female" in this chapter refers to a person assigned female at birth.

7. Most cancers are not inherited. Only about 5% of cancers are linked to an inherited gene. Some examples include: BRCA1 and BRCA2 in breast, prostate, and ovarian cancers; MLH1, MSH2, MSH6, and PMS2 in uterine, ovary, stomach, prostate, and bladder cancers; and many others.
8. Infections and viruses are associated with an increased risk of certain forms of cancer:
   a. Human papillomavirus (HPV)—cervical cancer, anal cancer, head and neck cancers.
   b. Epstein-Barr virus—lymphoma, nasopharyngeal cancers, gastric cancer, Kaposi sarcoma.
   c. Cytomegalovirus—Kaposi sarcoma, colon cancer.
   d. HIV—Kaposi sarcoma, lymphoma.
   e. Human T-lymphocyte virus—T-cell lymphoma/leukemia.
   f. Hepatitis B and C—hepatocellular cancer.
   g. *Helicobacter pylori*—gastric cancer.
9. Five-year survival rates are increasing with improved therapy and earlier detection.
10. Ongoing genetic research is searching for the ability to correct and modify hereditary susceptibility.
11. Patterns of incidence and death rates vary with sex (Table 4-1), age, ethnicity, and geographic location.

Nutrition, Physical Activity, and Cancer

EVIDENCE BASE American Cancer Society. (2020). *American Cancer Society guidelines on nutrition and physical activity for cancer prevention: Reducing the risk of cancer with healthy food choices and physical activity*. www.cancer.org/cancer/risk-prevention/diet-physical-activity/acs-guidelines-nutrition-physical-activity-cancer-prevention/guidelines.html

U.S. Department of Health and Human Services and U.S. Department of Agriculture. (2020). *2020-2025 Dietary guidelines for Americans* (9th ed.). http://health.gov/dietaryguidelines/2020/guidelines

1. Lifestyle does influence the risk of cancer. Among those who do not smoke, dietary choices and physical activity are the most important modifiable risks of cancer. The ACS and the U.S. Department of Health and Human Services have established guidelines on nutrition and physical activity to promote optimal health and prevent cancer.
2. Achieve and maintain a healthy weight.
   a. Be as lean as possible throughout life.
   b. Avoid excessive weight gain at all ages.
   c. Limit the consumption of high-calorie foods and beverages.
3. Adopt a physically active lifestyle.
   a. Adults should engage in 150 to 300 minutes of moderate-intensity or 75 minutes of vigorous-intensity activity each week. Exceeding 300 minutes is ideal.
   b. Children and adolescents should engage in 60 minutes of moderate to vigorous physical activity each day.
   c. Limit sedentary behavior such as sitting, lying down, and watching TV and other forms of screen-based entertainment.
4. Consume a healthy diet, with emphasis on plant sources.
   a. Choose foods and drinks in amounts that help achieve and maintain a healthy weight.
   b. Eat at least 2½ to 3 cups of vegetables and fruits daily.
   c. Choose whole grains over processed (refined) grains.
   d. Limit intake of processed and unprocessed red meats.
   e. Limit calories from added sugars and saturated fat, specifically to less than 10% of total daily calories.
   f. Avoid/limit processed foods.
   g. Limit alcoholic beverages to no more than 2 drinks per day for males and 1 drink per day for females.
5. ACS recommendations for community action:
   a. Increase access to affordable nutritious foods in schools, worksites, and communities.
   b. Changes in public policy and community environment help individuals make smart food choices and portion sizes to help maintain a healthy weight.

Table 4-1 Leading New Cancer Cases and Deaths: 2023 Estimates

ESTIMATED NEW CASES[a]		ESTIMATED DEATHS	
MALE	**FEMALE**	**MALE**	**FEMALE**
Prostate 288,300	Breast 297,790	Lung and bronchus 67,160	Lung and bronchus 59,910
Lung and bronchus 117,550	Lung and bronchus 120,790	Colon 28,470	Breast 43,170
Colon and rectum 81,860	Colon and rectum 71,160	Prostate 34,700	Colon and rectum 24,080
Urinary bladder 62,420	Uterine corpus 66,200	Pancreas 26,620	Pancreas 23,930
Melanoma of the skin 58,120	Thyroid 31,180	Liver and intrahepatic bile duct 19,000	Ovary 13,270
Kidney and renal pelvis 81,800	Melanoma of the skin 15,870	Leukemia 35,670	Uterine corpus 13,030
Non-Hodgkin lymphoma 44,880	Non-Hodgkin lymphoma 35,670	Esophagus 12,920	Leukemia 9,810
Leukemia 35,670	Leukemia 23,940	Urinary bladder 12,160	Liver 10,380
Oral cavity and pharynx 39,290	Pancreas 30,920	Non-Hodgkin lymphoma 11,780	Non-Hodgkin lymphoma 8,400
Liver 27,980	Kidney 29,440	Brain and other nervous system 11,020	Brain and other nervous system 7,970
All sites 1,010,310	All sites 948,800	All sites 322,080	All sites 287,740

[a]*Excludes basal and squamous cell skin cancers and in situ carcinoma except urinary bladder.*

Adapted with permission from Siegel, R. L., Miller, K. D., Wagle, N. S., & Jemal, A. (2023). Cancer statistics, 2023. CA: A Cancer Journal for Clinicians, 73(1), 17–48. https://doi.org/10.3322/caac.21763

c. Provide safe, enjoyable spaces for physical activity in schools.
d. Provide for safe, physically active transportation (such as biking and walking) and recreation in communities.

Detection and Prevention

Primary prevention and secondary prevention are effective measures in decreasing mortality and morbidity of many cancers. Most cancers, however, are diagnosed after reported symptoms. The ACS recommends specific primary and secondary prevention measures to reduce an individual's risk of cancer death.

Primary Prevention

The assessment or reduction of risk factors before the disease occurs:

1. Make appropriate lifestyle changes.
2. Stop smoking.
3. Limit alcohol intake.
4. Eat a healthy diet as outlined earlier.
5. Be physically active: maintain a healthy weight and follow exercise guidelines outlined earlier.
6. Avoid sun exposure, especially during the hours of 10 a.m. and 4 p.m., and cover exposed skin with sunscreen with a skin protection factor of 15 or higher.
7. Those at high risk for certain cancers should consider genetic counseling and testing.
8. Chemoprevention—the use of natural or synthetic substances to reduce the risk of developing cancer.
   a. Aspirin and nonsteroidal anti-inflammatory drugs (NSAIDs)—can decrease the risk of colorectal cancer.
   b. Tamoxifen and raloxifene—can reduce the risk of breast cancer in females who are at high risk by nearly 50%.
   c. Metformin—may decrease the risk of breast, colon, and possibly other cancers.
   d. Statins—may reduce the risk of prostate, lung, colorectal, and breast cancers.
9. Vaccinations—HPV causes most cervical, vulvar, vaginal, anal, and oropharyngeal cancers in females and most oropharyngeal, anal, and penile cancers in males. These could be prevented by HPV vaccinations. The Advisory Committee on Immunization Practices in conjunction with the Centers for Disease Control and Prevention has established guidelines on the use of this vaccine.
   a. Routine HPV vaccination is recommended for males and females ages 11 to 13 in two doses; may begin as early as age 9.
   b. For persons initiating vaccination on or after their 15th birthday, three doses are recommended.
   c. HPV vaccination is not currently recommended for persons over age 27.
   d. Screening for cervical cancer should continue in both vaccinated and unvaccinated females according to current ACS early detection guidelines.

EVIDENCE BASE Centers for Disease Control and Prevention. (2023). *ACIP Vaccine Recommendations and Guidelines.* www.cdc.gov/vaccines/hcp/acip-recs

Secondary Prevention

EVIDENCE BASE American Cancer Society. (2023, February 24). *American Cancer Society Guidelines for the early detection of cancer.* https://www.cancer.org/cancer/screening/american-cancer-society-guidelines-for-the-early-detection-of-cancer.html

1. The goal of screening is early detection to improve overall outcome and survival. Performing routine screening tests should be based on whether these tests are adequate to detect a potentially curable cancer in an otherwise asymptomatic person and are also cost-effective.
2. Screening should be based on an individual's age, sex, family history of cancer, ethnic group, previous iatrogenic factors (prior radiation therapy or drugs such as diethylstilbestrol [DES]), and history of exposure to environmental carcinogens. See Table 4-2 for ACS recommendations for screening.

Table 4-2 ACS Recommendations for the Early Detection of Cancer in Average-Risk, Asymptomatic Individuals

CANCER SITE	POPULATION	TEST OR PROCEDURE	FREQUENCY
Breast	Females, ages 40–54 yr Females, age >55 yr	Mammography Mammography	• Females should undergo regular screening mammography starting at age 45 yr • Females ages 45–54 yr should be screened annually • Females should have the opportunity to begin annual screening between ages 40 and 44 yr • Females ages ≥55 should transition to biennial screening or have the opportunity to continue screening annually • Females should continue screening mammography as long as their overall health is good and they have a life expectancy of ≥10 yr
Cervix	Females, ages 25–65 yr Females, >65 yr Females who have had a total hysterectomy	Primary HPV test every 5 yr Cotesting with HPV and Pap test every 5 yr Pap test alone every 3 yr	Cervical cancer screening should begin at age 25 yr For females ages 25–65 yr, screening should be done every 5 yr with primary HPV testing. Primary HPV tests are those that have been approved by the FDA. As an alternative, cotesting with a Pap test and HPV test may be performed every 5 yr, or a Pap test alone every 3 yr • Females ages >65 yr with normal results of screening over the past 10 yr and without CIN2 should stop screening, and females who have had a total hysterectomy (for a benign condition) should stop cervical cancer screening • Females of any age should not be screened annually by any screening method.

(continued)

Table 4-2 ACS Recommendations for the Early Detection of Cancer in Average-Risk, Asymptomatic Individuals (*continued*)

CANCER SITE	POPULATION	TEST OR PROCEDURE	FREQUENCY
Colorectal	All persons, ages ≥45 yr, for all tests listed	gFOBT with at least 50% test sensitivity for cancer, or FIT with at least 50% test sensitivity for cancer, or	• Annual: Testing stool sampled from regular bowel movements with adherence to manufacturer's recommendation for collection techniques and number of samples is recommended • "Throw in the toilet bowl" FOBTs are also not recommended; compared with guaiac-based tests for the detection of occult blood, immunochemical tests are more patient friendly and are likely to be equal or better in sensitivity and specificity; there is no justification for repeating FOBT in response to an initial positive finding; patients should be referred to colonoscopy
		Multitarget stool DNA test, or	Every 3 yr, per manufacturer's recommendation
		FSIG	Every 5 yr. FSIG can be performed alone, or consideration can be given to combining FSIG performed every 5 yr with a highly sensitive gFOBT or FIT performed annually.
		Colonoscopy	Every 10 yr
		CT colonography	Every 5 yr
Endometrial	Females, at menopause		At the time of menopause, females at average risk should be informed about the risks and symptoms of endometrial cancer and strongly encouraged to report any unexpected bleeding or spotting to their providers.
Lung	Those who currently smoke or did formerly ages 55–74 yr in good health with at least a 30-pack-yr history	LDCT	Clinicians with access to high-volume, high-quality lung cancer screening and treatment centers should initiate a discussion about annual lung cancer screening with apparently healthy patients ages 55–74 yr who have at least a 30-pack-yr smoking history and who currently smoke or have quit within the past 15 yr; a process of informed and shared decision-making with a clinician related to the potential benefits, limitations, and harms associated with screening for lung cancer with LDCT should occur before any decision is made to initiate annual lung cancer screening; smoking cessation counseling remains a high priority for clinical attention in discussions with those who currently smoke, who should be informed of their continuing risk of lung cancer; screening should not be viewed as an alternative to smoking cessation.
Prostate	Males, ages ≥50 yr	DRE and PSA	Males who have at least a 10-yr life expectancy should have an opportunity to make an informed decision with their health care provider about whether to be screened for prostate cancer, after receiving information about the potential benefits, risks, and uncertainties associated with prostate cancer screening. Prostate cancer screening should not occur without an informed decision-making process.

ACS, American Cancer Society; CIN, cervical squamous intraepithelial neoplasia 2; CT, computed tomography; DRE, digital rectal examination; FDA, Food and Drug Administration; FIT, fecal immunochemical test; FOBT, fecal occult blood test; FSIG, flexible sigmoidoscopy; gFOBT, guaiac-based toilet bowl FOBT tests; HPV, human papillomavirus; LDCT, low-dose helical CT; Pap, Papanicolaou; PSA, prostate-specific antigen.

American Cancer Society. (2023, February 24). American Cancer Society guidelines for the early detection of cancer. *https://www.cancer.org/cancer/screening/american-cancer-society-guidelines-for-the-early-detection-of-cancer.html*

Diagnostic Evaluation

1. Complete medical history and physical examination, radiographic evaluation based on the affected body system, laboratory evaluation, and biopsy.
2. Biopsy of tumor site to determine pathologic diagnosis. Biopsy results are used to determine the histology and/or grade of a tumor, which is a prerequisite for planning definitive therapy. Additional cellular and genetic features are also used to form a final diagnosis and guide treatment.
   a. Fine-needle aspiration (FNA)—technique in which cells are aspirated from the tumor using a needle and syringe. FNA cannot distinguish invasive from noninvasive malignancy. Negative results do not rule out malignancy. However, it is inexpensive, causes little discomfort, and can be performed in an outpatient or office setting.
   b. Needle core—needle biopsies are performed with a large-bore needle. This technique retrieves a small piece of intact tumor tissue, which yields enough tissue to adequately diagnose most tumor types. It is highly accurate and can be performed in an office or outpatient setting.
   c. Open biopsy—may be required for some lesions to determine a definitive diagnosis. This is done in the operating room, is more expensive, and requires a longer period of

recovery. The biopsy may be incisional, sampling only part of the tumor, or excisional, removing the total tumor.
3. Classification of tumor type is based on tissue and cellular staining. Differences in cytoplasmic and nuclear staining distinguish one cell type from another and identify their stage of differentiation. The grade of the tumor (rating of 1 to 4) is based on how well differentiated the tissue or cells appear or how closely tumor cells resemble normal cells. The higher the grade, the less differentiated it is, which is associated with poorer prognosis.
4. Flow cytometry testing of tumor tissue determines the DNA content and indicates potential risk of recurrence.
5. Special stains are performed to determine specific markers or proteins that may help guide treatment (i.e., estrogen and progesterone receptors for breast cancer).
6. Laboratory tests—including complete blood count (CBC) with differential; platelet count; and blood chemistries, including liver function tests, blood urea nitrogen (BUN), and creatinine—are done to determine baseline values.
   a. Further testing depends on cancer diagnosis.
7. Blood markers (carcinoembryonic antigen, prostate-specific antigen [PSA], cancer antigen [CA] 15-3, CA 125) may be appropriate to follow response to therapy.
8. Imaging procedures—chest x-ray, nuclear medicine scan, computed tomography (CT) scan, magnetic resonance imaging (MRI), and positron emission tomography (PET)—are used to determine evidence or extent of metastasis.

Staging

Staging is necessary at the time of diagnosis to determine the extent of disease (local vs. metastatic), to determine prognosis, and to guide proper management.

1. The American Joint Committee on Cancer (AJCC) has developed a simple classification system that can be applied to all tumor types. It is a numeric assessment of tumor size (T), presence or absence of regional lymph node involvement (N), and presence or absence of distant metastasis (M) (see Box 4-1).
2. No standard evaluation exists for all cancers. Workup depends on the patient, tumor type, symptoms, and medical knowledge of the natural history of that cancer.

BOX 4-1 AJCC Classification System of Tumors

T—PRIMARY TUMOR
Tx—primary cannot be evaluated
T0—no evidence of primary tumor
Tis—carcinoma in situ
T1, T2, T3, T4—increasing size and/or local extent of primary tumor

N—PRESENCE OR ABSENCE OR REGIONAL LYMPH NODE INVOLVEMENT
Nx—regional lymph nodes are unable to be assessed
N0—no regional lymph node involvement
N1, N2, N3—increasing involvement of regional lymph nodes

M—ABSENCE OR PRESENCE OF DISTANT METASTASIS
Mx—unable to assess
M0—absence of distant metastasis
M1—presence of distant metastasis

American Joint Committee on Cancer. (n.d.). Cancer staging systems. https://www.facs.org/quality-programs/cancer-programs/american-joint-committee-on-cancer/cancer-staging-systems/

PROCEDURES AND TREATMENT

The method of treatment depends on the type of malignancy, the specific histologic cell type, stage, presence of metastasis, and condition of the patient. It is important to have ongoing discussions with the patient regarding the goals of therapy and whether those goals are achievable. The four modalities of treatment are surgery, chemotherapy/hormonal therapy, radiation therapy, and biologic therapy or a combination of these modalities. Many clinical trials are available to evaluate the effectiveness of a new drug or other therapy.

Surgical Management

Surgical management may be curative to remove all or a portion of the primary tumor, it may be the only treatment a patient requires or it may be used in conjunction with other modalities, or it may be used in the palliative setting to alleviate symptoms.

Types of Surgical Procedures

The role of surgery can be divided into several approaches: preventive, primary surgery, cytoreductive, salvage treatment, palliative treatment, and reconstructive.

1. Preventive/prophylactic surgery—removal of lesions that, if left in the body, are at risk of developing into cancer; for example, resection of polyps in the rectum or mastectomy in females who are at high risk.
2. Primary surgery—complete surgical removal of a malignant tumor and may include regional lymph nodes and neighboring structures. This can be performed laparoscopically in some cases.
3. Cytoreductive surgery—partial removal of bulk of disease. This is performed when the spread of tumor precludes the removal of all disease. In some cases, this approach improves survival when used in combination with chemotherapy (i.e., ovarian cancer).
4. Salvage treatment—use of an extensive surgical approach to treat a local recurrence.
5. Palliative treatment—attempts to relieve the complications of cancer (e.g., obstruction of the gastrointestinal [GI] tract, pain produced by tumor extension into surrounding nerves).
6. Reconstructive/rehabilitative surgery—repair of defects from previous radical surgical resection; can be performed early (breast reconstruction) or delayed (head and neck surgery).

Chemotherapy

Chemotherapy is the use of antineoplastic drugs given systemically that may promote tumor cell destruction by interfering with cellular function and reproduction.

Principles of Chemotherapy Administration

1. The intent of chemotherapy is to destroy as many tumor cells as possible with minimal effect on healthy cells.
2. Cancer cells depend on the same mechanisms for cell division as normal cells. Damage to those mechanisms leads to cell death.
3. Chemotherapy is utilized in different clinical settings:
   a. Adjuvant chemotherapy is the use of systemic treatment following surgery and/or radiation therapy. Adjuvant therapy is given to patients who have no evidence of residual disease but who are at high risk for relapse. The justifications for adjuvant chemotherapy are the high recurrence rate after surgery for apparently localized tumors, the inability to identify cured patients at the time of surgery, and the failure of therapy to cure these patients after recurrence of disease.

   b. Neoadjuvant chemotherapy is the use of systemic treatment prior to primary surgery or radiation. The goal is to shrink or downstage the primary tumor to improve the effectiveness of surgery as well as control/eradicate microscopic cancer cells. For example, patients with large breast tumors can preserve the breast and undergo lumpectomy instead of mastectomy. The goal of therapy is to decrease the amount of tissue that needs to be removed as well as to attempt to maximize cure potential.
   c. High-dose/intensive therapy is the administration of high doses of chemotherapy, usually in association with growth factor support before bone marrow transplant/stem cell rescue.
   d. Palliative chemotherapy is used when a cure is not possible to control the cancer and minimize side effects from the disease.
4. Chemotherapeutic agents can be effective on any stage of the cell life cycle. This is the reproductive process in both normal and malignant cells. The cell cycle is divided into five stages:
   a. G0 (gap 0) resting phase: Cells are not dividing in this stage and, for the most part, are refractory to chemotherapy.
   b. G1 (gap one) postmitotic phase: RNA and proteins (enzymes for DNA synthesis) are manufactured.
   c. S (synthesis) phase: DNA is replicated in preparation for cell division.
   d. G2 (gap two) premitotic phase: This is a short period; protein and RNA synthesis occur, and the mitotic spindle apparatus is formed.
   e. M (mitosis) phase: In an extremely short period, the cell divides into two identical daughter cells.
5. Routes of administration:
   a. Oral
   b. Subcutaneous (SC)
   c. Intravenous (IV) push (bolus) or infusion over a specified period
   d. Intramuscular (IM)
   e. Intrathecal/intraventricular—given by injection via an Ommaya reservoir or by lumbar puncture
   f. Intra-arterial
   g. Intraperitoneal cavity
   h. Intravesical—into uterus or bladder
   i. Topical
6. Most drug dosage is based on surface area (mg/m^2) in both adults and children. Some agents are based on area under the curve (AUC), which refers to the amount of drug exposure over time or the total drug concentration in plasma over a period of time.
7. Most chemotherapeutic agents have dose-limiting toxicities that require nursing interventions (see Table 4-3, pp. 79–81). Chemotherapy predictably affects normal, rapidly growing cells (e.g., bone marrow, GI tract lining, hair follicles). It is imperative that these toxicities be recognized early by the nurse. Patient education is very important to minimize hospital admission and readmissions.

Chemotherapy Administration Safety Standards

EVIDENCE BASE LeFebvre, K. B., Olsen, M. K. M., & Dunphy, E. (2023). *Chemotherapy and immunotherapy guidelines and recommendations for practice* (2nd ed.). Oncology Nursing Society.

1. Specialized education, preparation, and training of the oncology nurse who administers chemotherapy and biotherapy are essential and ensure a safe level of care for patients. The Oncology Nursing Society (ONS) offers the ONS/Oncology Nursing Credentialing Center (ONCC) Chemotherapy Biotherapy Certificate Course and provides up-to-date resources. See Standard of Care Guidelines 4-1 (p. 82) for a checklist of the competency required by the ONS.
2. The American Society of Clinical Oncology's (ASCO) quality oncology practice initiative certification program requires that hospitals, infusion centers, and provider practices adhere with safety standards for chemotherapy administration.
3. Check with your hospital/institutional policy on handling and administering antineoplastic drugs.
4. Cytotoxic drugs are considered hazardous to health care workers. A safe level of occupational exposure is unknown. It is important to adhere to practices to minimize occupational exposure.

Guidelines for Personal Protective Equipment

1. Gloves—wear two pairs of disposable gloves that are powder free and have been tested for use with hazardous drugs. Avoid latex gloves because of potential latex sensitivity. Remove outer gloves first, turning them inside out to prevent contaminated outer surfaces from touching the inner gloves. Remove the inner gloves last after discarding all contaminated items. Do not reuse gloves.
2. Gowns—wear a disposable, lint-free gown made of low-permeability fabric. The gown should have a solid front, long sleeves, tight cuffs, and back closure. The inner glove should be worn under the gown cuff and the outer glove should extend over the gown to protect the skin. Gown and gloves are meant for single use only.
3. Respirators—wear a National Institute for Occupational Health and Safety–approved respirator mask when there is a risk of aerosol exposure, such as when administering chemotherapy or cleaning a spill. Surgical masks do not provide adequate protection.
4. Eye and face protection—wear a face shield and/or mask that provides splash protection whenever there is a possibility of splashing.
5. Wear personal protective equipment (PPE) whenever there is a risk of chemotherapy being released into the environment such as preparation or mixing of chemotherapy, spiking/priming IV tubing, administering the drug, and when handling body fluids or chemotherapy spills.

Personal Safety to Minimize Exposure

1. Prepare cytotoxic drugs in a vertical laminar flow hood.
2. Wash hands before donning PPE and change gloves after each use, tear, puncture, or medication spill or after every 60 minutes of wear. Wash hands after removing PPE.
3. Vent vials with filter needle to equalize the internal pressure or use negative-pressure techniques.
4. Wrap gauze or alcohol pads around the neck of ampules when opening to decrease droplet contamination.
5. Wrap gauze or alcohol pads around injection sites when removing syringes or needles from IV injection ports.
6. Use puncture- and leak-proof containers for noncapped, nonclipped needles.
7. Prime all IV tubing with normal saline or other compatible solution to reduce exposure.

Table 4-3 Frequently Used Chemotherapeutic Agents

CLASSIFICATION	MEDICATION NAME	ROUTE OF ADMINISTRATION	COMMON THERAPEUTIC USES	COMMON TOXICITIES	NURSING CONSIDERATIONS
Alkylating Agents	Altretamine	PO	Ovarian cancer	Nausea, vomiting, peripheral neuropathy, myelosuppression	Do not open capsules
	Cyclophosphamide	IV or PO	Lymphomas, leukemias, and a variety of solid tumors	Nausea, vomiting, diarrhea, myelosuppression, alopecia, lethargy, hemorrhagic cystitis	Ensure adequate hydration (2–3 L/d). Have patients void frequently to avoid hemorrhagic cystitis
	Busulfan	IV or PO	Chronic myelocytic leukemia, bone marrow transplantation	Pulmonary fibrosis, hypertension, tachycardia, myelosuppression, alopecia, skin pigmentation	Instruct patients to take on an empty stomach to decrease nausea/vomiting. Monitor blood counts
	Carboplatin	IV or IP	Ovarian cancer	Myelosuppression particularly platelets, alopecia, hypersensitivity reaction	Have emergency medications available for possible hypersensitivity reactions
	Chlorambucil	PO	Chronic lymphocytic leukemia, Hodgkin disease	Myelosuppression, nausea, vomiting, skin reactions, seizures	Contraindications in patients with a history of seizures
	Cisplatin	IV	Ovarian, testicular, bladder, cervical, non–small cell lung, esophageal cancer	Nausea, vomiting, myelosuppression, nephrotoxicity, hypersensitivity reactions, low electrolytes	Monitor renal function and electrolytes. Have emergency medications available for possible hypersensitivity reactions
	Dacarbazine	IV or IM	Malignant melanoma, Hodgkin lymphoma, sarcomas	Nausea, vomiting, myelosuppression, alopecia, rash	Irritant—may cause tissue necrosis if extravasated
	Ifosfamide	IV	Testicular, lymphoma, sarcomas, ovarian, bone	Hemorrhagic cystitis, nausea, vomiting, myelosuppression, confusion, encephalopathy	Always given in conjunction with mesna to decrease risk of hemorrhagic cystitis
	Melphalan	IV or PO	Multiple myeloma, ovarian, malignant melanoma	Myelosuppression, nausea, vomiting	Vesicant—avoid extravasation
	Oxaliplatin	IV	Colorectal cancers	Nephrotoxicity, hypersensitivity reactions, peripheral neuropathy, nausea, vomiting, myelosuppression	Monitor for peripheral neuropathy. Instruct patients to avoid consuming cold beverages for 3–4 d to avoid laryngopharyngeal dysesthesias
	Temozolomide	PO	Glioblastoma, astrocytoma, melanoma	Myelosuppression, nausea, vomiting, headache, photosensitivity	Contraindicated in patients with sensitivity to dacarbazine. Instruct patients to avoid sun exposure for several days
	Thiotepa	IV, IM, SC, IT	Breast, ovarian, bladder, lymphomas, bone marrow transplantation	Myelosuppression, nausea, vomiting, rash, fever	
Antibiotics	Bleomycin	IV, SC, IM	Head and neck cancers, squamous carcinomas including penis, cervix and vulva, Hodgkin's and non-Hodgkin's lymphoma and testicular cancers	Skin reaction, pulmonary fibrosis, fever, allergic reaction, alopecia, stomatitis	Administer a test dose in patients with lymphoma as they seem to have a higher incidence of allergic reactions
	Dactinomycin	IV	Ewing sarcoma, Wilms tumor, testicular	Myelosuppression, nausea, vomiting, alopecia, veno-occlusive disease of the liver, skin rash, and fever	Vesicant—avoid extravasation
	Daunorubicin	IV	Leukemias	Myelosuppression, nausea, vomiting, alopecia, cardiomyopathy, red urine, radiation recall	Vesicant—avoid extravasation. Monitor cardiac function

(continued)

Table 4-3 Frequently Used Chemotherapeutic Agents *(continued)*

CLASSIFICATION	MEDICATION NAME	ROUTE OF ADMINISTRATION	COMMON THERAPEUTIC USES	COMMON TOXICITIES	NURSING CONSIDERATIONS
	Doxorubicin	IV	Breast, ovarian, prostate, thyroid, lung, head and neck cancers, leukemia	Cardiomyopathy, alopecia, red urine, radiation recall, nausea, vomiting	Vesicant—avoid extravasation 550 mg/m^2 lifetime dose
	Doxorubicin liposomal	IV	Ovarian, breast, AIDS-related sarcoma	Myelosuppression, nausea, vomiting, mucositis, diarrhea, alopecia, radiation recall	Similar to Adriamycin, less cardiotoxic
	Epirubicin	IV	Breast cancer	Myelosuppression, nausea, vomiting, alopecia, heart failure, radiation recall, red urine	Vesicant—avoid extravasation
	Mitomycin	IV	Pancreatic, stomach, colon, lung, bladder, esophageal	Delayed myelosuppression, nausea, vomiting, alopecia, mucositis, renal and pulmonary dysfunction	Vesicant—avoid extravasation
	Mitoxantrone	IV	Prostate, acute myelocytic leukemia	Myelosuppression, tachycardia, mucositis, nausea, vomiting, alopecia	May turn urine blue-green
Camptothecins	Irinotecan	IV	Colorectal	Diarrhea, myelosuppression	Monitor for severe diarrhea that may require delays or dose reduction
	Topotecan	IV	Ovarian, cervical, small cell lung cancer	Myelosuppression, alopecia, diarrhea, headache, fatigue	
Plant alkaloids (vinca alkaloids)	Vinblastine	IV	Hodgkin lymphoma, Kaposi sarcoma, testicular, bladder, prostate, renal cell	Myelosuppression, alopecia, peripheral neuropathy, bone pain	Vesicant—avoid extravasation
	Vincristine	IV	Lymphoma, acute leukemia, neuroblastoma, multiple myeloma, testicular	Constipation, nausea, vomiting, alopecia, bone pain	Vesicant—avoid extravasation; monitor for severe constipation
	Vinorelbine	IV	Non–small cell lung, breast, cervical, ovarian cancer	Alopecia, diarrhea, nausea, neuropathy	Distal neuropathies, extravasation, and necrosis; should consider central access
	Etoposide	IV or PO	Small cell lung, testicular cancer	Myelosuppression, nausea, alopecia, mucositis	Monitor renal function
	Teniposide	IV	Childhood acute lymphocytic leukemia, adult neuroblastoma	Myelosuppression, nausea, vomiting, diarrhea, alopecia	Can cause hypersensitivity reactions
Antimetabolites	Azacitidine	SC, IV	MDS	Myelosuppression, nausea, vomiting, elevated serum creatinine	Administration should occur within 1 h of reconstitution
	Methotrexate	IV, IM, IT, or PO	Lymphoma, acute lymphoblastic leukemia, breast, bladder, sarcoma	Mucositis, diarrhea, myelosuppression, acute renal failure, pneumonitis	High doses require concomitant use of leucovorin and IV fluids
	Cytarabine	IV, SC, IT, IM	Hodgkin and non-Hodgkin lymphoma, acute myelogenous leukemia, acute lymphoblastic leukemia	Nausea, vomiting, myelosuppression, cerebellar ataxia, lethargy	Side effects are dose dependent; higher doses are associated with profound myelosuppression, GI toxicity, and neurotoxicity

	5-Fluorouracil	IV or topical	Breast, colorectal, anal, gastroesophageal, hepatocellular, pancreatic, head and neck cancer	Nausea, vomiting, diarrhea, mucositis, myelosuppression, neurotoxicity, photosensitivity	Instruct patients to avoid sun exposure, use sunscreen. Leucovorin may be used concomitantly
	6-Mercaptopurine	PO	Acute lymphoblastic leukemia	Myelosuppression, nausea, vomiting, diarrhea, hepatotoxicity	Instruct patients to take on an empty stomach
	Thioguanine	PO	Acute myelogenous leukemia, acute lymphoblastic leukemia	Myelosuppression, nausea, vomiting, mucositis, diarrhea, hepatotoxicity	Instruct patients to take on an empty stomach
	Fludarabine	IV or PO	Chronic lymphocytic leukemia, non-Hodgkin lymphoma	Myelosuppression, mild nausea, vomiting, fever, interstitial pneumonitis	Monitor pulmonary function tests
	Pemetrexed	IV	Non–small cell lung cancer	Myelosuppression, renal, and liver toxicities	Must be given with folic acid starting 1 wk prior to infusion
	Gemcitabine	IV	Pancreatic, non–small cell lung, breast, bladder, ovarian sarcoma, Hodgkin lymphoma	Nausea, vomiting, myelosuppression, flulike syndrome, fever	Warn patients of flulike symptoms that can occur the day following treatment
Taxanes	Paclitaxel	IV	Breast, ovarian, non–small cell lung, bladder, esophagus, cervical, gastric, head and neck sarcoma	Myelosuppression, peripheral neuropathy, myalgias, alopecia, fatigue	Observe closely for hypersensitivity reaction; premedication required with dexamethasone, diphenhydramine, and H2 blocker requires non-PVC IV tubing
	Docetaxel	IV	Breast, gastric, head and neck, prostate, non–small cell lung, ovarian cancer	Myelosuppression, edema, alopecia, nail changes, peripheral neuropathy	Treatment with dexamethasone prior to and for 2 d after can minimize edema
	Ixabepilone	IV	Breast cancer	Myelosuppression, fatigue, neuropathy, nausea, vomiting, diarrhea, myalgias	Observe closely for hypersensitivity reaction; premedication required with dexamethasone, diphenhydramine, and H2 blocker requires non-PVC IV tubing
Miscellaneous	Asparaginase	IM	ALL	Anaphylaxis, nausea, vomiting, hypercalcemia, fever, renal toxicity	Observe closely for anaphylaxis
	Hydroxyurea	PO	CML, myeloma	Myelosuppression, nausea, vomiting, fever	Do not open capsules
	Eribulin	IV	Breast cancer	Neutropenia, peripheral neuropathy	Not compatible with D5W
	Ixabepilone	IV	Breast cancer	Peripheral neuropathy, myelosuppression, fatigue	Avoid St. John's wort. Monitor for hypersensitivity reaction

ALL, acute lymphoblastic leukemia; CML, chronic myelocytic leukemia; GI, gastrointestinal; IM, intramuscular; IP, intraperitoneal; IT, intrathecal; IV, intravenous; MDS, myelodysplastic syndrome; PO, by mouth; PVC, polyvinyl chloride; SC, subcutaneous.

STANDARD OF CARE GUIDELINES 4-1

Administering IV Chemotherapy

ONS Chemotherapy Administration Competency Evaluation

PRIOR TO ADMINISTRATION

1. Coordinates time of administration with pharmacy and others as needed.
2. Verifies signed consent for treatment.
3. Verifies laboratory values are within acceptable range and reports to the provider as needed.
4. Performs independent double check of original orders with a second RN for accuracy of
   a. Protocol or regimen
   b. Agents
   c. Calculated body surface area
   d. Patient dose
   e. Schedule
   f. Route
5. Verifies that patient education, premedication, prehydration, and other preparations are completed.

ADMINISTRATION

1. Compares original order to dispensed drug label at the bedside with another RN.
2. Verifies patient identification.
3. Applies gloves and gown and uses safe handling precautions.
4. Verifies adequacy of venous access and appropriate IV site selection.
5. Checks patency of IV and flushes with 5 to 10 mL normal saline.
6. Demonstrates safe administration
   a. Pushes through side arm or at hub closest to the patient, checks patency every 2 to 5 mL.
   b. Verifies appropriate rate of administration.
7. Demonstrates appropriate monitoring/observation for specific acute drug effects.
8. Verbalizes appropriate action in the event of extravasation.
9. Verbalizes appropriate action in the event of hypersensitivity reaction.

AFTER ADMINISTRATION

1. Flushes line with enough fluid to clear IV tubing of drug.
2. Removes peripheral IV device or flushes/maintains vascular access device.
3. Disposes of chemotherapy waste according to policy.
4. Documents medications, education, and patient response.
5. Communicates posttreatment considerations to the patient, caregivers, and appropriate personnel.

IV, intravenous; ONS, Oncology Nursing Society; RN, registered nurse.

8. Use syringes and IV tubing with Luer locks (which have a locking device to hold needle firmly in place).
9. Label all syringes and IV tubing containing chemotherapeutic agents as hazardous material.
10. Place an absorbent pad directly under the injection site to absorb any accidental spillage.
11. Do not eat, drink, or chew gum while preparing or handling chemotherapy agents.
12. Keep all food and drink away from preparation area.
13. Avoid hand-to-mouth or hand-to-eye contact while handling chemotherapeutic agents or body fluids of the patient receiving chemotherapy.
14. If any contact with the skin occurs, immediately wash the area thoroughly with soap and water.
15. If contact is made with the eye, immediately flush the eye with water and seek medical attention.
16. Spill kits should be available in all areas where chemotherapy is stored, prepared, and administered.

Safe Disposal of Antineoplastic Agents, Body Fluids, and Excreta

1. Discard gloves and gown into a leak-proof container, which should be marked as contaminated or hazardous waste.
2. Use puncture- and leak-proof containers for needles and other sharp or breakable objects.
3. Linens contaminated with chemotherapy or excreta from patients who have received chemotherapy within 48 hours should be contained in specially marked hazardous waste bags.
4. Wear nonsterile nitrile gloves for disposing of body excreta and handling soiled linens within 48 hours of chemotherapy administration.
5. In the home, wear gloves when handling bed linens or clothing contaminated with chemotherapy or patient excreta within 48 hours of chemotherapy administration. Place linens in a separate, washable pillow case. Wash separately in hot water and regular detergent.

DRUG ALERT It is imperative that the nurse be alert for immediate complications that patients may experience during or shortly after cytotoxic therapy.

Extravasation

1. Occurs when the vesicant chemotherapy leaks out of the blood vessel and into the surrounding tissue resulting in:
   a. Blistering, begins within 3 to 5 days.
   b. Peeling and sloughing of skin, begins within 2 weeks.
   c. Tissue necrosis, usually in 2 to 3 weeks.
   d. Damage to tendons, nerves, and joints.
   e. Functional and sensory impairment of the area.
   f. Disfigurement.
   g. Loss of limb.
2. Steps to take if extravasation is suspected:
   a. STOP infusion of the vesicant.
   b. Disconnect the IV tubing from the IV device. DO NOT remove the IV device or port needle.
   c. Attempt to aspirate residual vesicant from the IV using a small syringe.
   d. Remove the IV or port needle.
   e. Assess the site of extravasation.
   f. Assess symptoms experienced by the patient.
   g. Notify the patient's provider.
   h. Initiate appropriate management measures in accordance with type of agent (see Table 4-4).

Chemotherapy Follow-up

1. Document drug dosage, site, and any occurrence of extravasation, including estimated amount of drug.

Table 4-4 Management of Chemotherapy Extravasation

CHEMOTHERAPEUTIC AGENT	ANTIDOTE	NURSING INTERVENTION
Anthracyclines (doxorubicin, epirubicin, daunorubicin)	Dexrazoxane	Apply ice, but remove at least 15 min before dexrazoxane. Dose of dexrazoxane is based on body surface area and should be administered intravenously in an area other than the extravasation site, opposite arm: Day 1: 1,000 mg/m^2 Day 2: 1,000 mg/m^2 Day 3: 500 mg/m^2
Alkylating agents (nitrogen mustard, cisplatin)	Sodium thiosulfate	Prepare ⅙ molar solution and inject 2 mL for each milligram of chemotherapy suspected to have extravasated. Inject solution subcutaneously in the site using a 25G needle (change the needle with each injection). Apply ice for 6–12 h following sodium thiosulfate injection.
Vinca alkaloids (vincristine, vinblastine, vinorelbine)	Hyaluronidase	Inject 1 mL of hyaluronidase locally as five separate injections subcutaneously into the extravasated area. Apply moderate heat for 15–20 min at least four times daily for the first 24–48 h to disperse drug and minimize pain.
Taxanes (paclitaxel, docetaxel)	No known antidote	Apply ice for 15–20 min at least four times daily for the first 24 h.
Antibiotics	None	Apply ice for 15–20 min at least four times daily for the first 24 h.

2. Observe regularly after administration for pain, erythema, induration, and necrosis, and notify the appropriate health care provider as indicated.
3. Monitor for other adverse effects of infusion.
   a. Patient may describe sensations of pain or pressure within the vessel, originating near the venipuncture site or extending 3 to 5 in (7.5 to 12.5 cm) along the vein.
   b. Discoloration or red streak following the line of the vein (called a flare reaction, common with doxorubicin) or darkening of the vein (with 5-fluorouracil).
   c. Itching, urticaria, muscle cramps, or pressure in the arm, caused by irritation of surrounding SC tissue.

Adverse Effects of Chemotherapy

All chemotherapy drugs have adverse effects. Adverse effects are exacerbated if the patient is an older adult, has comorbid conditions, or has impaired renal or hepatic function.

Adverse effects of chemotherapy are graded on a scale of 0 to 5, with 0 being no toxicity and 5 resulting in death. Scoring of adverse effects will determine if a delay in therapy is necessary, dose modification is necessary, or cessation of therapy must occur.

Alopecia

1. Most chemotherapeutic agents cause some degree of alopecia. This is dependent on the drug dose, half-life of drug, and duration of therapy.
2. Most commonly occurs on the scalp but can occur anywhere on the body.
3. Usually begins 1 to 3 weeks after administration of chemotherapy. Regrowth takes about 3 to 5 months.
4. Emotionally difficult for patients. Encourage patients to verbalize their feelings.
5. Scalp hypothermia may be utilized after careful consideration of side effects and efficacy. Scalp hypothermia is not recommended for pediatric patients, and contraindications exist for adults with some forms of cancer.

Anorexia

1. Chemotherapy changes the reproduction of taste buds.
2. Absent or altered taste can lead to a decreased food intake.
3. Concurrent renal or hepatic disease can increase anorexia.

Diarrhea

1. Defined as loose or watery stool. If left untreated, can lead to severe dehydration, electrolyte imbalances, hospitalizations, and treatment delays.
2. Cause is multifactorial, but up to 90% of all patients receiving chemotherapy can experience diarrhea.

Fatigue

The cause of fatigue is generally unknown but can be related to anemia, weight loss, altered sleep patterns, and emotional stress.

Nausea and Vomiting

1. Caused by the stimulation of the vagus nerve by serotonin released by cells in the upper GI tract.
2. Incidence depends on the particular chemotherapeutic agent and dosage.
3. Patterns of nausea and vomiting:
   a. Anticipatory—conditioned response from repeated association between therapy and vomiting; can be prevented with adequate antiemetic control.
   b. Acute—occurs 0 to 24 hours after chemotherapy administration.
   c. Delayed—can occur 1 to 6 days after chemotherapy administration; nausea is often worse than vomiting.

Mucositis

1. Caused by the destruction of the oral mucosa, causing an inflammatory response.
2. Initially presents as a burning sensation with no changes in the mucosa and progresses to significant breakdown, erythema, and pain of the oral mucosa.
3. Consistent oral hygiene is important to avoid infection.

Neutropenia

1. Defined as an absolute neutrophil count (ANC) of 1,500/mm^3 or less.
2. Primary dose-limiting toxicity of chemotherapy.
3. Risk of infection is greatest with an ANC less than 500/mm^3.
4. Caused by suppression of the stem cell.
5. Usually occurs 7 to 14 days after administration of chemotherapy but depends on the agent used.

6. Can be prolonged.
7. Patients should be taught to avoid infection through proper handwashing and hygiene and avoiding those with illness. Eliminating raw meats, seafood, eggs, or unwashed vegetables is also recommended.
8. Patients need to be monitored and treated promptly for fever or other signs of infection.
9. Can be prevented with the use of growth factors (e.g., granulocyte colony-stimulating factor [CSF], pegfilgrastim).

Anemia

1. Caused by suppression of the stem cell or interference with cell proliferation pathways.
2. May require red blood cell transfusion or injection of erythropoietin or darbepoetin.

Thrombocytopenia

1. Caused by suppression of megakaryocytes.
2. Incidence depends on the agent being used.
3. Risk of bleeding is present when platelet count falls below $50,000/mm^3$.
4. Risk is high when count falls below $20,000/mm^3$.
5. Risk is critical when count falls below $10,000/mm^3$.
6. Patient should be taught to avoid injury (e.g., no razors), vaginal douches, rectal suppositories, and dental floss during the period of thrombocytopenia.
7. May require platelet transfusions if count drops below $20,000/mm^3$.

Hypersensitivity Reactions

1. Nearly all of the available chemotherapeutic agents can produce hypersensitivity reactions (HSRs) in at least an occasional patient, and some cause reactions in 5% or more of patients receiving the drug. There are several agents (L-asparaginase, paclitaxel, docetaxel, teniposide, and carboplatin) for which HSRs are frequent enough to be a major form of treatment-limiting toxicity.
2. The mechanism is unknown for most of the chemotherapeutic agents.
3. Signs and symptoms include hives, pruritus, back pain, shortness of breath, hypotension, and anaphylaxis.
4. All unexpected drug reactions should be reported to the manufacturer.

Nursing Assessment

Skin and Mucous Membranes

1. Inspect for pain, swelling with inflammation or phlebitis, necrosis, or ulceration.
2. Inspect for skin rash and characteristics (e.g., whether pruritus is general or local).
3. Assess areas of erythema and associated tenderness or pruritus. Instruct the patient to avoid irritation to skin, sun exposure, or irritating soaps.
4. Assess changes in skin pigmentation.
5. Note reports of photosensitivity and tearing of the eyes.
6. Assess condition of gums, teeth, buccal mucosa, and tongue.
   a. Determine whether any taste changes have occurred.
   b. Check for evidence of stomatitis, erythematous areas, ulceration, infection, or pain on swallowing.
   c. Determine whether the patient has any complaints of pain or burning of the oral mucosa or on swallowing.

GI System

1. Assess for frequency, timing of onset, duration, and severity of nausea and vomiting episodes before and after chemotherapy.
   a. Usually occurs from 0 to 24 hours after chemotherapy but may be delayed. Anticipatory vomiting may occur after first course of therapy. Can be initiated by various cues, including thoughts, smell, or even sight of the medical personnel.
2. Observe for alterations in hydration and electrolyte balance.
3. Assess for diarrhea or constipation.
   a. Ascertain any changes in bowel patterns.
   b. Discuss the consistency of stools.
   c. Consider the frequency and duration of diarrhea (the number of stools each day for the number of days).
   d. Evaluate dietary changes or use of medications such as opioids or 5-HT3 blockers that have had an impact on diarrhea or constipation.
4. Assess for anorexia.
   a. Discuss taste changes and changes in food preferences.
   b. Ask about daily food intake and normal eating patterns.
5. Assess for jaundice, right upper quadrant abdominal pain, changes in the stool or urine, and elevated liver function tests that indicate hepatotoxicity.
6. Monitor liver function tests and total bilirubin.

Hematopoietic System

CLINICAL JUDGMENT Fever greater than 101°F (38.3°C) in a patient with an ANC less than $500/mm^3$ is an emergency requiring immediate administration of antibiotics.

1. Assess for neutropenia—ANC less than $500/mm^3$.
   a. Assess for any signs of infection (pulmonary, integumentary, central nervous system, GI, and urinary).
   b. Auscultate lungs for adventitious breath sounds.
   c. Assess for productive cough or shortness of breath.
   d. Assess for urinary frequency, urgency, pain, or odor.
   e. Monitor for elevation of temperature above 101°F (38.3°C) and chills.
2. Assess for thrombocytopenia—platelet count less than $50,000/mm^3$ (mild risk of bleeding); less than $20,000/mm^3$ (high risk of bleeding).
   a. Assess skin and oral mucous membranes for petechiae and bruises on extremities.
   b. Assess for signs of bleeding (including nose, urinary, rectal, or hemoptysis).
   c. Assess for blood in stools, urine, or emesis.
   d. Assess for signs and symptoms of intracranial bleeding if platelet count is less than $20,000/mm^3$; monitor for changes in level of responsiveness, vital signs, and pupillary reaction.
3. Assess for anemia.
   a. Assess skin color, turgor, and capillary refill.
   b. Ascertain whether patient has experienced dyspnea on exertion, fatigue, weakness, palpitations, or vertigo. Advise rest periods as needed.

Respiratory and Cardiovascular Systems

1. Assess lung sounds.
2. Assess for pulmonary fibrosis, evidenced by a dry, nonproductive cough with increasing dyspnea. Patients at risk include those over age 60, those who smoke, those receiving or having had pulmonary radiation, those receiving a cumulative dose of bleomycin, or those with any preexisting lung disease.

3. Assess for signs and symptoms of heart failure or irregular apical or radial pulses.
4. Verify baseline cardiac studies (e.g., electrocardiogram, multiple-gated acquisition scan/ejection fraction) before administering cardiotoxic chemotherapy such as doxorubicin.

Neuromuscular System

1. Determine whether the patient is having difficulty with fine motor activities, such as zipping pants, tying shoes, or buttoning a shirt.
2. Determine the presence of paresthesia (tingling, numbness) of fingers or toes.
3. Evaluate deep tendon reflexes.
4. Evaluate the patient for weakness, ataxia, or slapping gait.
5. Determine impact on activities of daily living and discuss changes.
6. Discuss symptoms of urinary retention or constipation.
7. Assess for ringing in ears or decreased hearing acuity.

Genitourinary System

1. Monitor urine output.
2. Assess for urinary frequency, urgency, or hesitancy.
3. Evaluate changes in odor, color, or clarity of urine sample.
4. Assess for hematuria, oliguria, or anuria.
5. Monitor blood urea nitrogen (BUN) and creatinine.

Nursing Interventions

Preventing Infection

1. Monitor vital signs every 4 hours; report occurrence of fever greater than 101°F (38.3°C) and chills.
2. Provide patient education.
   a. Instruct patient to report signs and symptoms of infection:
      i. Fever greater than 101°F (38.3°C) and/or chills.
      ii. Mouth lesions, swelling, or redness.
      iii. Redness, pain, or tenderness at rectum.
      iv. Change in bowel habits.
      v. Areas of redness, swelling, induration, or pain on skin surface.
      vi. Pain or burning when urinating or odor from urine.
      vii. Cough or shortness of breath.
   b. Reinforce good personal hygiene habits (routine bathing [preferably a shower], clean hair, nails, and mouth care).
   c. Avoid contact with people who have a transmittable illness.
   d. Encourage deep breathing and coughing to decrease pulmonary stasis.
3. Avoid performing invasive procedures—rectal temperatures, enemas, or insertion of indwelling urinary catheters.
4. Monitor white blood cell (WBC) count and differential.
5. Be aware that hematologic nadirs (lowest level) generally occur within 7 to 14 days after drug administration. Length of myelosuppression depends on specific drug. Institution of further therapy usually depends on an adequate WBC count and ANC.
6. Calculate ANC to determine the number of neutrophils capable of fighting an infection by:
7. Total WBC count × (% polys + % bands) = ANC. Example: 700 × (10% + 5%) = 105.
8. Interpretation: 105 of the 700 WBCs are neutrophils and capable of fighting an infection (indicates severe neutropenia).
9. Administer prophylactic antibiotics, as prescribed (if WBC count is less than 500).
10. Administer growth factors, as prescribed: SC filgrastim 5 µg/kg starting 24 hours after chemotherapy for 5 to 10 days for neutropenia prophylaxis or pegfilgrastim 6 mg SC for a single dose 24 hours after chemotherapy. Should also be administered with subsequent courses of chemotherapy to hasten neutrophil maturity.

Preventing Bleeding

1. Avoid invasive procedures when platelet count is less than 50,000/mm^3, including IM injections, suppositories, enemas, and insertion of indwelling urinary catheters.
2. Apply pressure on injection sites for 5 minutes.
3. Monitor platelet count; administer platelets as prescribed.
4. Monitor and test all urine, stools, and emesis for blood.
5. Provide patient education.
   a. Instruct patient to avoid straight-edge razors, nail clippers, and vaginal or rectal suppositories.
   b. Avoid intercourse when platelet count is less than 50,000/mm^3.
   c. Encourage patient to blow their nose gently.
   d. Avoid dental work or other invasive procedures while thrombocytopenic.
   e. Avoid the use of nonsteroidal anti-inflammatory drugs (NSAIDs), aspirin, and aspirin-containing products.

Minimizing Fatigue

1. Monitor blood counts (hemoglobin and hematocrit).
2. Administer blood products as prescribed.
3. Administer growth factors as prescribed, such as erythropoietin or darbepoetin.
4. Provide patient education and counseling.
   a. Information about fatigue.
   b. Reassurance that treatment-related fatigue does not mean your cancer is worse.
   c. Why fatigue and shortness of breath may occur.
   d. Suggestions for ways to cope with fatigue.
      i. Encourage aerobic and strength training exercise. Balance activity and rest.
      ii. Plan frequent rest periods between daily activities; take naps that do not interrupt nighttime sleep.
      iii. Set priorities and delegate tasks to others.
   e. Stress management.
   f. Explain that blood transfusions, if given, are a part of therapy and not necessarily an indication of a setback.
   g. Observe skin color.
   h. Monitor nutritional status.

Promoting Nutrition

EVIDENCE BASE National Comprehensive Cancer Network. (2024). *Evidence-based NCCN clinical practice guidelines: Version 1.2024.* www.nccn.org

1. Prevention of nausea/vomiting is the goal. Administer antiemetics before chemotherapy and on a routine schedule (not as needed).
2. Be aware that antiemetic combinations are more effective than single agents.
3. High emetogenic potential
   a. Day 1: Use the following combination:
      i. Olanzapine 5–10 mg PO once
      ii. NK1 receptor antagonist (RA) (choose one):
         - Aprepitant 125 mg PO once
         - Aprepitant injectable emulsion 130 mg intravenous (IV) once
         - Fosaprepitant 150 mg IV once
         - Netupitant 300 mg/palonosetron 0.5 mg PO once
         - Fosnetupitant 235 mg/palonosetron 0.25 mg (IV once)
         - Rolapitant 180 mg PO once

iii. 5-HT3 RA (choose one):
  - Dolasetron 100 mg PO once
  - Granisetron 10 mg subcutaneous (SQ) once, or 2 mg PO once, or 0.01 mg/kg (max 1 mg) IV once, or 3.1 mg/24-h transdermal patch applied 24–48 h prior to first dose of anticancer therapy
  - Ondansetron 16–24 mg PO once, or 8–16 mg IV once
  - Palonosetron 0.25 mg IV once

iv. Dexamethasone 12 mg PO/IV once

b. Day 2-4
  i. Olanzapine 5–10 mg PO daily on days 2, 3, 4
  ii. Aprepitant 80 mg PO daily on days 2, 3 (if aprepitant PO is used on day 1)
  iii. Dexamethasone 8 mg r,s PO/IV daily on days 2, 3

4. For moderate emetogenic risk
  a. Day 1
    i. 5-HT3 RA (choose one):
      - Dolasetron 100 mg PO once
      - Granisetron 10 mg SQ once (preferred), or 2 mg PO once, or 0.01 mg/kg (max 1 mg) IV once, or 3.1 mg/24-h transdermal patch applied 24–48 h prior to first dose of anticancer therapy
      - Ondansetron 16–24 mg PO once, or 8–16 mg IV once
      - Palonosetron 0.25 mg IV once (preferred)
    ii. Dexamethasone 12 mg PO/IV once r,s
  b. Day 2-4
    - Dexamethasone 8 mg r,s PO/IV daily on days 2, 3 or
    - 5-HT3 RA monotherapy:
      - Granisetron 1–2 mg (total dose) PO daily or 0.01 mg/kg (max 1 mg) IV daily on days 2, 3
      - Ondansetron 8 mg PO twice daily or 16 mg PO daily or 8–16 mg IV daily on days 2, 3
      - Dolasetron 100 mg PO daily on days 2, 3
5. Low emetogenic potential
  a. Start before anticancer therapy
  b. Repeat daily for multiday doses of anticancer therapy
    - Dexamethasone 8–12 mg PO/IV once, or
    - Metoclopramide 10–20 mg PO/IV once, or
    - Prochlorperazine 10 mg PO/IV once, or
    - 5-HT3 RA (select one):
      - Dolasetron 100 mg PO once
      - Granisetron 1–2 mg (total dose) PO once
      - Ondansetron 8–16 mg PO once
6. Extrapyramidal reactions occur frequently in patients under age 30 and over age 65. Treat dystonic reactions with diphenhydramine; treat restlessness with lorazepam.
7. Consider alternative measures for relief of anticipatory nausea, such as relaxation therapy, imagery, acupuncture, and distraction.
8. Encourage small, frequent meals appealing to patient preferences, but including high calories and proteins. Provide a high-protein supplement as needed.
9. Discourage smoking and alcoholic beverages, which may irritate mucous membranes.
10. Encourage fluid intake to prevent constipation.
11. Monitor intake and output, including emesis.
12. Consult dietitian about patient's food preferences, intolerances, and individual dietary interventions.
13. Recognize that the patient may have alterations in taste perception, such as a keener taste of bitterness and loss of ability to detect sweet tastes.

Minimizing Stomatitis

1. Report signs of infection—erythematous areas, white patches, ulcers.
2. Encourage good oral hygiene.
  a. Soft nylon-bristled toothbrush, brush two to three times daily, rinse frequently.
  b. Floss once daily.
3. Encourage the use of oral agents to promote cleansing, debridement, and comfort. Mouthwashes with more than 25% alcohol should be avoided.
4. Assess the need for antifungal, antibacterial, or antiviral therapy (each infection has a different appearance).
5. Administer local oral therapy, such as combinations with viscous lidocaine, for symptomatic control and maintenance of calorie intake.

Preventing and Managing HRs

1. Be alert for signs of allergic reactions such as pruritus, urticaria, and difficulty breathing as well as back pain. The situation may worsen suddenly to hypotension and anaphylaxis.
2. Stop the medication or infusion immediately, notify the health care provider, and monitor the patient closely. Treatment is supportive and dependent on type of reaction and its severity.
  a. Do not administer the agent again if there was a severe reaction resulting in significant hypotension.
  b. Premedicate the patient with antihistamine or corticosteroid, as directed, if there is a history of moderate reaction.

Strengthening Coping for Altered Body Image

1. Reassure patient that hair will grow back; however, it may grow back a different texture or different color.
2. Suggest wearing a turban, wig, or headscarf, preferably purchased before hair loss occurs. Many insurance companies will pay for a wig with a prescription.
3. Encourage patient to stay on therapeutic program.
4. Cold caps can minimize hair loss, but are presently only partially covered by insurance and can be cost prohibitive for some patients.

Patient Education and Health Maintenance

1. Make sure patient uses good hygiene, knows the symptoms of infection to report, and avoids crowds and people with infection while neutropenic.
2. Advise patient to avoid using a razor blade to shave, contact sports, manipulation of sharp articles, use of a hard-bristle toothbrush, and passage of hard stool to prevent bleeding while thrombocytopenic.
3. Advise females to report symptoms of vaginal infection because of opportunistic fungal or viral infection.
4. Encourage patient participation in plan for chemotherapy and to set realistic goals for work and activities.
5. Assure patient that changes in menses, libido, and sexual function are usually temporary during therapy.

Evaluation: Expected Outcomes

- Afebrile, no signs of infection.
- No bruising or bleeding noted; stool and urine heme test negative.
- Denies shortness of breath or severe fatigue.
- Tolerates small, frequent meals following antiemetic.
- No oral lesions or pain on swallowing.
- No urticaria, shortness of breath, or change in vital signs.
- Wears turban and expresses feelings about body image.

Radiation Therapy

Radiation therapy is the use of high-energy x-rays or other radiation particles to treat malignant diseases. Radiation with sufficient energy to disrupt atomic structures by ejecting orbital electrons is called ionizing radiation. The goal of radiation is to deliver a precisely measured dose of irradiation to a defined tumor volume with minimal damage to surrounding healthy tissue. This results in eradication of tumor, high quality of life, and prolongation of survival and allows for effective palliation or prevention of symptoms of cancer, with minimal morbidity. Because of advances in imaging and treatment delivery, radiation therapy offers improved targeting and increased sparing of normal tissues.

General Considerations

1. Different irradiation doses are required for tumor control, depending on tumor type and the number of cells present. Varying radiation doses can be delivered to specific portions of the tumor (periphery vs. central portion) or to the tumor bed in cases in which all gross tumor has been surgically removed.
2. Treatment portals must adequately cover all treatment volumes plus a margin.

Goals of Therapy

1. Curative—when there is a probability of long-term survival after adequate therapy, some adverse effects of therapy, although undesirable, may be acceptable.
2. Palliative—when there is no hope of survival for extended periods, radiation can be used to palliate symptoms, primarily pain. Lower doses of irradiation (75% to 80% of curative dose) can control the tumor and palliate symptoms without excessive toxicity.

Principles of Therapy

1. Radiosensitivity is the sensitivity of cells, tissues, or tumors to radiation. Rapidly dividing cells are most sensitive.
2. Radioresistance is the lack of tumor response to radiation because of tumor characteristics (slow growing, less responsive), tumor cell proliferation, and circulation. Radiation is most effective during the mitotic stage of the cell cycle.
3. Radioresistant tumors: Many tumors are resistant to radiation, such as squamous cell, ovarian, soft tissue sarcoma, and gliomas. Many other tumors can become resistant after a period of time. Normal radioresistant tissues include mature bone, cartilage, liver, thyroid, muscle, brain, and spinal cord.
4. Role of oxygen: The presence of oxygen enhances radiation. Without oxygen, chemical damage to DNA may be repaired. Giving multiple, daily doses allows reoxygenation and enhances radiosensitivity. The dose should allow for repair of normal tissues.
5. Tissue tolerance dose is the amount of radiation that a healthy cell can receive and still function. This is what limits the dose of radiation one can receive.
6. Tumor size is a major factor in response to radiation therapy. Smaller tumors are more responsive than larger tumors.

Types of Radiation Therapy

There are generally two types of ionizing radiation: external beam (teletherapy) and internal radiation (radioactive source in or near the cancer site) and several ways in which it is delivered.

1. External beam radiation is most commonly delivered through a linear accelerator machine. A number of techniques are used to administer external beam radiation:
   a. Proton therapy uses a beam of protons to deliver radiation directly to the tumor. A proton beam conforms to the shape and depth of a tumor while sparing healthy tissues and organs.
   b. Magnetic resonance imaging (MRI) linear accelerator is used to constantly obtain images of soft tissue–based tumors in real time during radiation. This allows for real-time control of the radiation beam during treatment.
   c. Stereotactic body radiation therapy (SBRT) has a narrower beam of radiation that is delivered precisely to the tumor itself sparing surrounding healthy brain tissue.
2. Internal Radiation Therapy
   a. Brachytherapy involves radioactive material that is implanted in the body. Small seeds containing radioactive iodine are placed at the tumor site with a needle or catheter. This is done as an outpatient procedure. Brachytherapy is commonly used to treat prostate, cervical, endometrial, vaginal, and breast cancers.
   b. Intraoperative radiation therapy (IORT) is used to treat an exposed tumor during cancer surgery. IORT delivers a high dose of radiation to a surgically exposed treatment area. Surrounding healthy organs and tissues are protected by lead shields.
   c. Stereotactic radiosurgery (SRS) uses dozens of tiny radiation beams to treat tumors in the head and neck with a single radiation dose.

Chemical and Thermal Modifiers of Radiation

1. Radiosensitization is the use of medications to enhance the sensitivity of the tumor cells.
2. Radioprotectors increase therapeutic ratio by promoting repair of normal tissues.
3. Hyperthermia is combined with radiation. Uses a variety of sources (ultrasound, microwaves) and produces a greater effect than radiation alone. It is usually applied locally or regionally immediately after radiation.

Units for Measuring Radiation Exposure or Absorption

1. Centigray (cGy) is a unit of radiation dose absorbed by the body equal to one hundredth of a gray; formerly called a rad (e.g., 1 cGy equals 1 rad). Gray (Gy) is the unit of absorbed radiation dose equal to 100 rad.
2. Hyperfractionated radiation therapy is the division of the total radiation dose into smaller daily doses. Administering fractions allows treatment of tumor cells while giving healthy cells time to repair themselves.

Nature and Indications for Use

Used alone or in combination with surgery or chemotherapy, depending on the stage of disease and goal of therapy.

1. Adjuvant radiation therapy—used in combination with other treatment modalities, such as chemotherapy or surgery, when a high risk of local recurrence or large primary tumor exists.
2. Curative radiation therapy—used in anatomically limited tumors (retina, optic nerve, certain brain tumors, skin, oral cavity). Course is usually longer and the dose higher.
3. Palliative—for treatment of symptoms:
   a. Provides excellent pain control for bone metastasis.
   b. Used to relieve obstruction.
   c. Relief of neurologic dysfunction for brain metastasis.
   d. Given in short, intensive courses.

Treatment Planning

1. Evaluation of tumor extent (staging), including diagnostic studies before treatment.

2. Define the goal of therapy (cure or palliation).
3. Select appropriate treatment modalities (irradiation alone or combined with surgery, chemotherapy, or both).
4. Treatment planning is known as simulation. This is the process of aiming and defining radiation beams to meet the goals of prescribed therapy.
   a. Simulation is used to accurately identify target volumes and sensitive structures. Computed tomography (CT) simulation allows for accurate three-dimensional treatment planning of target volume and anatomy of critical normal structures.
   b. Treatment aids (e.g., shielding blocks, molds, masks, immobilization devices, compensators) are extremely important in treatment planning and delivery of optimal dose distribution. Repositioning and immobilization devices are critical for accurate treatment.
   c. Lead blocks are made to shape the beam and protect normal tissues.
   d. Skin markings are applied to define the target and portal. These are generally replaced later by permanent tattoos.
5. Usual schedule is Monday through Friday.
6. Actual therapy lasts minutes. Most time is spent on positioning.
7. Determine optimal dose of irradiation and volume to be treated, according to anatomic location, histologic type, stage, potential regional nodal involvement (and other tumor characteristics), and normal structures in the region.

Complications

Complications depend on the site of radiation therapy, type of radiation therapy (external beam and internal radiation), total radiation dose, daily fractionated doses, and overall health of the patient. Adverse effects are predictable, depending on the normal organs and tissues involved in the field.

Acute Adverse Effects

1. Fatigue and malaise.
2. Skin: may develop a reaction as soon as 2 weeks into the course of treatment.
   a. Erythema—may range from mild to severe.
   b. Dry desquamation—shedding of the skin.
   c. Moist desquamation—shedding of the skin to reveal moist, edematous skin underneath. Areas having folds, such as the axilla, under the breasts, groin, and gluteal fold, are at an increased risk because of increased warmth and moisture.
   d. Folliculitis—infection of the hair follicles, which may result in pustule formation.
3. GI effects: nausea and vomiting, diarrhea, and esophagitis.
4. Oral effects: changes in taste, mucositis, dryness, and xerostomia (dryness of mouth from lack of normal secretions).
5. Pulmonary effects: dyspnea, productive cough, and radiation pneumonitis (usually occurs 1 to 3 months after radiation to the lung).
6. Renal and bladder effects: cystitis and urethritis.
7. Cardiovascular effects: damage to vasculature of organs and thrombosis (heart is relatively radioresistant).
8. Recall reactions: acute skin and mucosal reactions when concurrent or past chemotherapy (doxorubicin, dactinomycin).
9. Bone marrow suppression: more common with pelvic or large bone radiation.

Chronic Adverse Effects

After 6 months with variability in time of expression:

1. Skin effects: fibrosis, telangiectasia, permanent darkening of the skin, and atrophy.
2. GI effects: fibrosis, adhesions, obstruction, ulceration, and strictures.
3. Oral effects: permanent xerostomia, permanent taste alterations, and dental caries.
4. Pulmonary effects: fibrosis.
5. Renal and bladder effects: radiation nephritis and fibrosis.
6. Second primary cancer: patients who have received combined radiation and chemotherapy with alkylating agents have a rare risk of developing acute leukemia.

Nursing Assessment

1. Assess skin and mucous membranes for adverse effects of radiation.
2. Assess GI, respiratory, and renal function for signs of adverse effects.
3. Assess patient's understanding of treatment and emotional status.

Nursing Interventions

Maintaining Optimal Skin Care

1. Inform the patient that some skin reaction can be expected but that it varies from patient to patient. Examples include dry erythema, dry desquamation, wet desquamation, epilation, and tanning.
2. Do not apply lotions, ointments, or cosmetics to the site of radiation unless prescribed.
3. Discourage vigorous rubbing, friction, or scratching because this can destroy skin cells. Apply ointments as instructed by health professionals.
4. Avoid wearing tight-fitting clothing over the treatment field; prevent irritation by not using rough fabric such as wool and corduroy.
5. Take precautions against exposing the radiation field to sunlight and extremes in temperature.
6. Do not apply adhesive or other tape to the skin.
7. Avoid shaving the skin in the treatment field.
8. Use lukewarm water only and mild soap when bathing.

Ensuring Protection From Radiation

1. To avoid exposure to radiation while the patient is receiving therapy, consider the following:
   a. Time—exposure to radiation is directly proportional to the time spent within a specific distance to the source.
   b. Distance—amount of radiation reaching a given area decreases as resistance increases.
   c. Shield—sheet of absorbing material placed between the radiation source and the nurse decreases the amount of radiation exposure.
2. Individual monitoring devices should be worn by personnel exposed to radiation or radioactive material.
3. Take appropriate measures associated with sealed sources of radiation implanted within a patient (sealed internal radiation).
   a. Follow directives on precaution sheet that is placed on the charts of all patients receiving radiotherapy.
   b. Do not remain within 3 feet (1 m) of the patient any longer than required to give essential care.
4. Know that the casing material absorbs all alpha radiation and most beta radiation but that a hazard concerning gamma radiation may exist.
5. Do not linger longer than necessary in giving patient care, even though all precautions are followed.
6. Be alert for implants that may have become loosened (those inserted in cavities that have access to the exterior); for example, check the emesis basin following mouth care for a patient with an oral implant.
7. Notify the radiation therapist of any implant that has moved out of position.
8. Use long-handled forceps or tongs and hold at arm's length when picking up any dislodged radium needle, seeds, or tubes. Never pick up a radioactive source with your hands.

9. Do not discard dressings or linens unless you are sure that no radioactive source is present.
10. After the patient is discharged from the facility, it is a good policy for the radiologist to check the room with a radiograph or survey meter to be certain that all radioactive materials have been removed.
11. Continue radiation precautions when a patient has a permanent implant, until the radiologist declares precautions unnecessary.

Evaluation: Expected Outcomes

- Skin without breakdown or signs of infection.
- Radiation precautions maintained.

Immunotherapy

Immunotherapy is targeted cancer treatment. It has emerged as an important modality of cancer treatment and one where intensive research is actively being conducted. The goal is to produce antitumor effects through the action of natural host defense mechanisms. It is capable of altering the immune system with either stimulatory or suppressive effects. The underlying principle is that the primary function of the immune system is to detect and eliminate substances that are recognized as "nonself." This represents the most promising new cancer treatment approach since the development of chemotherapy.

Types of Immunotherapy

Cytokines

Cytokines are soluble proteins produced by mononuclear cells of the immune system (usually the lymphocytes and monocytes) that have regulatory actions on other cells in the immune system. Cytokines produced by lymphocytes are referred to as *lymphokines*, and cytokines produced by monocytes are referred to as *monokines*.

1. Examples of cytokines include interleukins, interferons, CSFs, and tumor necrosis factor.
2. Many other biologic agents are currently under investigation.

Monoclonal Antibody Therapy

Monoclonal antibodies work on cancer cells in the same way natural antibodies work, by identifying and binding to the target cells. They then alert other cells in the immune system to the presence of the cancer cells.

1. Some monoclonal antibodies target the cancer cell and others work through specific antibody–antigen response.
2. Monoclonal antibodies may be used alone or in combination with chemotherapy.
3. Examples of monoclonal antibodies include:
   a. Rituximab—a murine/human chimeric monoclonal antibody specific for the CD20 surface marker on B cells. It is approved for the treatment of relapsed or refractory low-grade/follicular non-Hodgkin lymphoma.
   b. Ibritumomab—combines the targeting power of monoclonal antibodies with the cell-damaging ability of localized radiation. It is developed to recognize and attach to substances on the surface of certain cells and deliver cytotoxic radiation directly to the cancerous cells.
   c. Trastuzumab—a recombinant DNA–derived humanized monoclonal antibody that selectively binds with high affinity in a cell-based assay to the extracellular domain of the human epidermal growth factor receptor (EGFR) 2 (HER2) protein. It is approved for the treatment of patients with early stage and advanced metastatic breast cancer whose tumors overexpress the HER2 protein.
   d. Cetuximab—binds to extracellular EGFR, resulting in inhibition of cell growth and induction of apoptosis.
   e. Bevacizumab—binds to and inhibits the activity of human vascular endothelial growth factor (VEGF) to its receptors blocking proliferation and formation of new blood vessels that supply tumor cells.
   f. Panitumumab—inhibits the binding of ligand to the EGFR receptor, resulting in inhibition of cell growth.
   g. Alemtuzumab—recognizes the CD52 antigen expressed on malignant and normal B lymphocytes. It has come to be used therapeutically in B-cell malignancies.
4. Potential adverse effects of monoclonal antibodies include dyspnea and mild wheezing, fever and chills, headache, rash, nausea and vomiting, tachycardia, bleeding, and allergic reactions.

Checkpoint Inhibitors

Immune checkpoint inhibitors—these drugs block tumor cells from inactivating T cells. This allows the T cell to remain active and fight the tumor cells. Examples include nivolumab, pembrolizumab, and ipilimumab.

Chimeric Antigen Receptor T-cell therapy

With this treatment, T cells are collected from the patient's bloodstream. These cells are then genetically engineered to recognize and target a specific protein on the cancer cells. They are then infused back into the patient via an IV. The goal is for the chimeric antigen receptor (CAR) T cells to then recognize and attack the cancer cells.

Nursing Assessment

1. Review patient's record or obtain history from the patient to determine site of cancer, previous cancer therapies, current medications, and other medical conditions.
2. Assess current cardiovascular and respiratory status.
3. Assess patient's understanding of immunotherapy and associated toxicities.
4. Assess for common side effects of immune system stimulation, including fever, chills, body aches, nausea, vomiting, and fatigue, as well as serious and potentially life-threatening adverse reactions, including dyspnea, wheezing, tachycardia, bleeding, hypotension, and anaphylaxis.

Nursing Interventions

Controlling Hyperthermia

1. Discuss the overall goal of immunotherapy, expected adverse effects, and the method of administration.
2. Instruct the patient to report fever, chills, diarrhea, nausea and vomiting, itching, or weight gain.
3. Administer or advise self-administration of antipyretics, such as acetaminophen, for fever.
4. Emphasize that adverse effects are temporary and will usually cease within 1 week after treatment ends.

Maintaining Tissue Perfusion

1. Monitor vital signs at least every 4 hours for hypotension, tachycardia, tachypnea, and fever.
   a. Instruct the patient to remain in bed if blood pressure is low.
   b. Monitor apical heart rate.
2. Assess respirations for rate and depth, and auscultate breath sounds for evidence of pulmonary edema.
3. Assess for signs of restlessness, apprehension, discomfort, or cyanosis, which may indicate respiratory distress.
4. Administer oxygen as prescribed.
5. Maintain patent IV line and administer serum albumin as prescribed.
6. Check extremities for warmth, color, and capillary refill.

Evaluation: Expected Outcomes

- Relief of fever after medication.
- Blood pressure stable and lungs clear.

SPECIAL CONSIDERATIONS IN CANCER CARE

Pain Management

Pain related to cancer may be caused by direct tumor infiltration of bones, nerves, viscera, or soft tissue, as well as by therapeutic measures (surgery, radiation). Pain is the most common symptom associated with cancer and has a negative impact on a patient's functional status and quality of life. Cancer pain can be controlled with medication in 80% to 95% of patients, and there is increasing evidence that survival is linked to pain management. See Appendix D, page 1505 for more information on pain management.

Oncologic Emergencies

Oncologic emergencies are a group of life-threatening metabolic syndromes or abnormalities associated with cancer and/or cancer treatment.

Septic Shock

Septic shock is a systemic disease associated with the presence and persistence of pathogenic microorganisms or their toxins in the blood. It is characterized by hemodynamic instability, abnormal coagulation, and altered metabolism.

Risk Factors

1. Neutropenia, absolute neutrophil count (ANC) less than 500.
2. Patients who are neutropenic longer than 7 days most susceptible.
3. Patients with HIV and concomitant neutropenia.
4. Prolonged hospitalization.
5. Older patients.
6. Patients with comorbid conditions, such as diabetes and pulmonary diseases.

Clinical Manifestations

1. Fever greater than 100.5°F (38.3°C).
2. Warm, flushed, dry skin.
3. Hypotension.
4. Tachycardia.
5. Tachypnea.
6. Decreased level of consciousness.
7. Patients will not have the usual symptoms of infection because of the lack of neutrophils. For example, skin infections may manifest as subtle rash or erythema. Urinary tract infections may be asymptomatic and patients with lung infections may be without pulmonary infiltrates.

Diagnostic Evaluation

1. Vital signs.
2. Culture—blood, urine, stool, sputum, central and peripheral intravenous (IV) lines, and any open wounds to determine source and type of infection.
3. Chest x-ray—to detect underlying pneumonia.
4. Computed tomography (CT) scans as necessary.
5. Arterial blood gas analysis—decreased pH reflects acidosis.
6. Blood urea nitrogen (BUN) and creatinine—elevated because of decreased circulating blood volume.
7. Complete blood count (CBC) with differential—elevated white blood cell (WBC) count with shift to left.

Management

1. Antibiotics are started immediately; broad-spectrum antibiotics are given until organism is identified.
2. IV fluids and plasma expanders are used to restore circulating volume.
3. Colony-stimulating factors (CSFs) are administered to increase ANC.
4. Vasopressors are administered to support blood pressure.
5. Oxygen is administered, as needed, to prevent tissue hypoxia.
6. Vital signs, respiratory status, urine output, and any signs of bleeding are monitored carefully.
7. Complications, such as renal failure, respiratory failure, cardiac failure, metabolic acidosis, and disseminated intravascular coagulation, are treated aggressively.

Spinal Cord Compression

Spinal cord compression (SCC) is the result of tumor compression on the dural sac. This can result in neurologic impairment or permanent loss of function if not treated immediately.

Incidence

1. Affects 5% of all patients with terminal cancer in the last 2 years of their lives with less than a 6-month median survival from diagnosis.
2. Lung, breast, and prostate cancer account for 15% to 20% of all cases.
3. Multiple myeloma, non-Hodgkin lymphoma, and renal carcinoma account for 5% to 10% of cases.

Clinical Manifestations

1. Cervical spine:
   a. Vertigo.
   b. Radicular pain in neck and back of head that is aggravated by neck flexion.
   c. Upper extremity weakness.
   d. Sensory loss in area of weakness (i.e., paresthesia, numbness).
   e. Abnormal deep tendon reflexes.
   f. Gastric hypersecretion and paralytic ileus.
2. Thoracic spine:
   a. Local or radicular pain (or both).
   b. Lower extremity weakness.
   c. Sensory loss below the level of the lesion.
   d. Band of hyperesthesia at dermatome of tumor site.
   e. Impaired bladder or bowel control.
3. Lumbar spine:
   a. Local or radicular pain (or both).
   b. Lower extremity weakness and paralysis.
   c. Atrophy of lower extremity muscles.
   d. Sensory loss below level of the lesion.
   e. Urinary symptoms (hesitancy, retention), constipation, or bowel incontinence.
4. Weakness and unsteadiness may be noted before changes in motor function. (Progression is usually rapid with foot drop and impaired ambulation. Urgent investigation and treatment are crucial to minimize the risk of paraplegia. The degree of weakness and ability to walk at presentation are important clinical predictors of outcome.)
5. Changes in sensation—paresthesia, numbness, tingling. (Severity usually mirrors the severity of motor weakness.)

CLINICAL JUDGMENT Any abnormal neurologic symptoms in a patient with cancer should be considered an SCC until proven otherwise.

Diagnostic Evaluation

1. Neurologic examination—early diagnosis is important.
2. X-ray of the painful site—may be abnormal; can be used as an initial screen for complaints of back pain.
3. Bone scan—more sensitive to bony metastasis than x-ray to detect abnormal vertebral bodies.
4. Magnetic resonance imaging (MRI)—most useful in detecting spinal cord lesions. The entire spine can be viewed. Immediately indicated if radiculopathy or myelopathy is present or x-rays are abnormal.

Management

1. Treatment is usually palliative because it is associated with metastatic disease.
2. Treatment goals are to relieve pain, minimize complications, and preserve or restore neurologic function.
3. Corticosteroids are the initial treatment until more definitive treatment can be instituted, reduce inflammation and swelling at site, increase neurologic function, and relieve pain.
   a. A loading dose of dexamethasone is usually given followed by tapering doses over a period of weeks.
   b. Steroids must be tapered and not abruptly discontinued.
   c. Monitor patient's glucose levels during dexamethasone treatment because it can cause hyperglycemia.
4. Radiation therapy to the tumor on spinal column is the most common treatment. Radiation is effective with 70% of patients having improvement in pain and function.
5. Surgery is considered when tumors are not radiosensitive or located in an area that has been previously radiated. It is also indicated for spinal instability.

Complications

1. Respiratory impairment, including pneumonia and atelectasis.
2. Mobility impairment, foot drop, skin impairment, and postural hypotension.
3. Sensory losses creating safety concerns.
4. Bladder or bowel dysfunction.

Patient Education

1. Facilitate referral to home care services for nursing assessment, nursing intervention, and rehabilitation for residual deficits.
2. Facilitate referral to appropriate outpatient services, including physical therapy, occupational therapy, and psychosocial support.
3. Provide instruction about safety issues for residual sensory deficits (e.g., test bath water temperature, careful use of extreme hot or cold).

Hypercalcemia

Hypercalcemia is an elevated serum calcium level above 11 mg/dL. It results when bone resorption exceeds both bone formation and the ability of the kidneys to excrete extracellular calcium released from the bones.

Incidence

1. The most common life-threatening disorder associated with malignancy; occurs in 20% to 30% of patients at some point in their illness.
2. Occurs most commonly in patients with carcinoma of the lung, breast, and renal cells; multiple myeloma; and adult lymphomas.
3. Can occur with or without skeletal metastasis, but more than 80% of patients do have bony disease.
4. Associated with a poor prognosis.

Clinical Manifestations

1. Signs and symptoms may vary, depending on the severity, and may be nonspecific and insidious.
   a. Early symptoms include anorexia, weakness, polyuria, polydipsia, and fatigue.
   b. Late symptoms include apathy, irritability, profound muscle weakness, nausea, vomiting, constipation, pruritus, lethargy, and confusion.
2. A rapid and life-threatening increase in calcium may cause dehydration, renal failure, coma, and death.

Diagnostic Evaluation

1. Serum calcium level greater than 11 mg/dL in adults, but ionized calcium of greater than 1.29 mmol/L is the most reliable test.
2. Electrolyte levels, BUN, and creatinine are obtained to determine hydration status and renal function.
3. Electrocardiogram (ECG) may show shortening of the QT interval and prolongation of the PR interval.

Management

1. Management includes treating the primary malignancy with chemotherapy, surgery, or radiation.
2. Acute, symptomatic hypercalcemia should be treated as an emergency.
3. Hydration and diuresis—IV normal saline (0.9% NaCl) is the initial treatment for patients with acute hypercalcemia and clinical symptoms to dilute the calcium and promote its renal excretion. Diuresis is induced with furosemide. (Thiazide diuretics aggravate hypercalcemia and should be avoided.)
4. Pharmacotherapy includes:
   a. Bisphosphonates—primary drug therapy, administered IV; pamidronate or zoledronic acid inhibits osteoclast resorption in the bone.
   b. Calcitonin—used in combination with glucocorticoids and inhibits bone resorption. It has a rapid onset but a short duration of action. Used most commonly in patients with multiple myeloma. It should not be used for longer than 72 hours.
   c. Denosumab—a monoclonal antibody that should be used in the setting of hypercalcemia at least 7 days after bisphosphonates.

Nursing Interventions

1. Prevent or detect hypercalcemia early.
   a. Recognize patients at risk and monitor for signs and symptoms, such as nausea and vomiting, constipation, lethargy, and anorexia.
   b. Emphasize importance of mobility to minimize bone demineralization and constipation.
   c. Instruct patient on the importance of adequate hydration.
2. Administer normal saline infusions as prescribed.
3. Administer medications as prescribed.
4. Maintain accurate intake and output; observe for oliguria or anuria.
5. Take vital signs every 4 hours, especially apical pulse and blood pressure.
6. Monitor electrolyte values and renal function.
7. Assess mental status.
8. Assess cardiorespiratory status for signs of fluid overload.

Superior Vena Cava Syndrome

Superior vena cava syndrome (SVCS) is obstruction and thrombosis of the superior vena cava caused by direct compression by a tumor or an enlarged lymph node, resulting in impaired venous drainage of the head, neck, arms, and thorax.

Incidence

1. Eighty percent to 95% of patients with SVCS are patients with cancer.
2. Eighty percent of cases arise from advanced lung cancer, specifically small cell lung cancers, and 15% from lymphoma.
3. Other malignancies associated with SVCS are thymoma and breast cancer.

Clinical Manifestations

1. Signs and symptoms may vary, depending on the degree of obstruction and how rapidly the obstruction occurs.
2. A rapid onset of SVCS is dramatic and potentially life threatening and requires immediate intervention.
3. Facial edema is found in 80% of cases and is the most common initial finding.
4. Early symptoms include progressive dyspnea, cough, feeling of fullness in the head, difficulty buttoning shirt collar (Stoke sign), dysphagia and hoarseness, and chest pain.
5. Cyanosis and edema of the head and upper extremities may be apparent. Collateral circulation with dilated chest wall veins may be visible.
6. Late symptoms include respiratory distress, headache, vision disturbances, dizziness and syncope, lethargy, irritability, and mental status changes.
7. Pleural effusion on chest x-ray may also be seen.

Diagnostic Evaluation

1. CT scan is the most common imaging technique used to diagnose SVCS.

Management

1. Radiation therapy and corticosteroids are the gold standard of treatment for SVCS to reduce tumor size and relieve pressure. Most patients experience a relief of symptoms within the first 4 days of therapy.
2. Chemotherapy may be used in conjunction with radiation. Specific chemotherapeutic agents depend on the tumor type.
3. Surgery is rarely used because of the associated high morbidity and mortality risks.
4. Percutaneous stent placement—an expandable stent may be placed inside the superior vena cava to keep it patent. Anticoagulants are also used in conjunction.
5. Thrombolytic and anticoagulant therapy may be used if a thrombus is suspected or to prevent the formation of a thrombus; must be used within the first 7 days to be effective.
6. Oxygen is given for relief of dyspnea and maintenance of tissue oxygenation.
7. Analgesics and tranquilizers are used for discomfort and anxiety.

Nursing Interventions

1. Administer oxygen, as prescribed, to relieve hypoxia.
2. Place patient in Fowler position—facilitates gravity drainage and reduces facial edema.
3. Limit patient's activity and provide a quiet environment.
4. Reassure patient that cyanotic color and facial edema will subside with treatment.

Psychosocial Components of Care

Nursing Assessment

1. Assess lifestyle before illness. How did patient solve other problems?
2. Assess for signs of anxiety and coexistence of depression: agitation and restlessness, sleep disturbances, excessive autonomic activity, weight gain or loss, mood changes.
3. What activities of daily living can patient perform?
4. What changes in lifestyle have resulted from cancer and its treatment?
5. Determine patient's perception of the disease and treatment.
6. Evaluate available social support; who is the most significant other?
7. Ask patient if any complementary or alternative medicine (CAM) modalities are being utilized for cancer treatment. Be aware that many patients seek herbal and other remedies despite lack of scientific evidence of any benefit. Encourage patient and family to discuss CAM use with health care provider to ensure safety.
8. Try to gain a sense of emotional strength and potential problem areas. Ask if patient and family have a plan for end-of-life care as appropriate.

Nursing Interventions

Reducing Anxiety

1. Establish and sustain an unhurried approach to give the patient time to organize fears, thoughts, and feelings.
2. Allow patient to share feelings about having cancer.
3. Reflect and amplify insights and judgments; try to reduce anxiety through reflection and reorientation.
4. Recognize feelings of losing control.
5. Discuss methods of stress reduction (imagery, relaxation).
6. Discuss the positive aspects of treatment.
7. Encourage expression of positive emotions—emphasis on living in the here and now, greater appreciation of life.
8. Reinforce effective coping behaviors.
9. Encourage patient to join a support group. Refer to local chapter of the American Cancer Society (ACS), call 1-800-ACS-2345 or visit www.cancer.org.
10. Remain available as problems arise. Give patient telephone numbers of people to call when needed.
11. Initiate referrals for additional rehabilitation and psychosocial services as appropriate.

Promoting Effective Coping

1. Encourage patient and family members to enroll in cancer education program.
2. Encourage patient to learn everything about treatment plan because this promotes a sense of control.
3. Provide expert physical care and teach patient about care.
4. Assist patient in strengthening support system (family, friends, visitors, health care staff and volunteers, support groups)—strengthens self-esteem through the experience of feeling accepted and valued.
5. Help patient readjust expectations and goals to promote ongoing adjustment.
6. Support patient in coping mechanisms chosen.

Allaying Fear of Death and Dying

1. Educate patient and family about prognosis and end-of-life choices, as outlined by patient's health care provider. Be direct, stating the statistics but stressing the positive aspects of the situation.

2. Assess and respect patient's beliefs.
3. Help patient and family agree on goals.
4. Facilitate emotional support for patient.
5. Provide bereavement support to survivors.

Evaluation: Expected Outcomes

- Discusses feelings; practices stress reduction.
- Patient and family attend cancer education program.
- Asks questions about prognosis and sets goals for care.

Survivorship

With earlier diagnosis and better treatment, more and more patients are surviving and living beyond cancer. Recent estimates show that as of 2022, the number of cancer survivors has surpassed 18 million. This expected continual increase in cancer survivors has put a strain on the health care delivery system. Primary care providers and oncologists have not been able to keep up with the growing number of patients who have completed their therapy.

The oversight of a health care provider is important as patients transition from active cancer care to survivorship. Sadly, many needs of cancer survivors are not being met. In 1986, the National Coalition for Cancer Survivors was created to address these issues. Accredited cancer centers are now required to have survivorship programs. Nurses are uniquely positioned to help transform survivorship care and improve the quality of care and patient outcomes.

Principles of Survivorship Care

1. Survivorship care is the process of learning how to live through cancer and beyond.
2. The goals of cancer survivorship programs as recommended by the American Society of Clinical Oncology (ASCO) include the following:
   a. Prevention of recurrent and new cancers.
   b. Surveillance for cancer spread or recurrence.
   c. Assessment of late medical and psychological effects of therapy.
   d. Adherence and interventions for consequences of cancer and its treatment.
   e. Coordination between specialist and other health care providers.
3. There are different models of survivorship programs. Most include a transition visit at the end of treatment. During this visit, current symptoms are addressed and patients are provided a survivorship care plan and education to include prevention of recurrent and new cancers, surveillance and late effects, health promotion, and a follow-up plan.
4. These visits are often conducted by providers and/or nurse practitioners. Nurses, however, have a pivotal role in survivorship programs. As patients often receive care from each of the treatment disciplines (medical oncology, surgical oncology, radiation oncology), nurses have the skills to integrate, coordinate care, and serve as the patient advocate. Nurses possess the skills and knowledge to educate and manage treatment-related side effects.

Management and Nursing Interventions

1. Realize that patients themselves have a difficult time adjusting to life after cancer treatment. They are often challenged with long-term side effects, both physical and psychological.
2. Provide education regarding the symptoms of recurrence, identification of late side effects, and an adoption of healthy lifestyle changes.
3. Ensure the patient has a knowledgeable provider that specifically addresses survivorship needs, and coordinate referrals to specialists as needed.
4. Encourage and set goals for healthy living, including physical activity, nutrition, and weight management.

Palliative Care

Palliative cancer care is the integration of therapies that address the multiple issues that cause patients with cancer and their families suffering. It is the care of the whole person along the illness trajectory, not just the end of life, to promote quality of life and relieve suffering. Palliative care comprises the management of pain, as well as other physical, psychological, and spiritual problems, and may be integrated into anticancer treatment and life-prolonging therapy. The hospice model of palliative care provides intensive end-of-life care, bereavement services, and support of the family after death of a loved one. Although palliative care is appropriate for many patients with cancer, it is not limited to cancer; many neurologic, cardiac, pulmonary, and other types of disorders call for palliative care in their more severe or advanced forms.

There are facility- and community-based programs as well as inpatient facilities and home care services (including hospice). Care of patients with advanced illness, such as cancer, and dealing with death and dying is an integral part of oncology nursing. Palliative care has been added to most medical and nursing schools across the country in recent years.

Principles of Palliative Care

1. Palliative care is an interdisciplinary team approach, including experts from medicine, nursing, social work, the clergy, and nutrition. This team approach is needed to make the necessary assessments and to institute appropriate interventions.
2. The essential components of palliative care are relief of symptom distress, improved quality of life, opening of communication on a regular basis with patients to provide appropriate care on their terms, and psychosocial support for patients and families.
3. The goal is to provide comfort and maintain the highest possible quality of life for as long as possible.
4. The traditional focus of palliative care is not on death but on a compassionate, specialized care for the living. It is based on a comprehensive understanding of patient suffering and focuses on providing effective pain and symptom management to seriously ill patients while improving quality of life.

End-of-Life Care

1. Hospice and palliative care provide care during progressive illness, but hospice eligibility begins only when a patient has a life expectancy of 6 months or less. In contrast, palliative care begins when the patient has been diagnosed with a life-limiting illness. It recognizes that the goals of care may change, but the focus is always on the quality of life.
2. Unfortunately, hospice is equated with care of the dying, causing it to be underutilized; thus, many patients only live a few days to a week after contacting hospice.

3. Only 14% of patients with cancer in the world are receiving palliative care, and most nurses lack the adequate knowledge and education to implement palliative care for those with cancer.
4. It has been shown that early referral to palliative care and hospice not only improves patient's symptoms and quality of life but also improves survival.
5. Hospice care and palliative care offer end-of-life care, which can be achieved by:
   a. Enhancing physical well-being through effective symptom management: pain, nausea, vomiting, constipation, sleeplessness.
   b. Enhancing psychological well-being through management of anxiety, depression, fear, denial, and hopelessness. Rather, happiness, enjoyment, and leisure are promoted.
   c. Enhancing social well-being by addressing financial burden, caregiver burden, roles and relationships, affection and sexual function, and concerns about appearance.
   d. Enhancing spiritual well-being through minimization of suffering and instead focusing on religious beliefs, hope, and meaning.

Management and Nursing Interventions

1. Provide pain relief, symptom control (dyspnea, nausea, constipation, anxiety, agitation), and prevention of complications.
2. Encourage patient and family to accept their current situation.
   a. Encourage patient and family to pursue enjoyable activities.
   b. Assist patient and family to focus on present and past joys.
   c. Share positive and hope-inspiring stories.
3. Facilitate participation in religious or spiritual activities.
4. Encourage families to minimize social isolation.
5. Provide private time for relationships.
6. Discuss end-of-life issues early in patient's treatment plan.
7. Encourage patients to express their preferences about end of life in the form of a legal document.
   a. Advance directives, such as medical orders for life-sustaining treatment or health care proxy and durable power of attorney, allow for the refusal of further treatment or authorize a family member or friend to make decisions for the patient (see p. 125).
   b. After discussion with the patient and family, the primary care provider in an inpatient setting can write orders based on the directives such as "do not resuscitate."
8. Make referrals for respite care, counseling, pastoral care, and bereavement services, as needed.
9. Assist patients and families with decisions for withholding or withdrawing life-sustaining therapies and transfer in and out of inpatient settings by explaining such therapies and clarifying how they fit with the goals of care.
10. Promote ethical practice by organizing interdisciplinary rounds on patients with end-of-life care issues, setting up a partnership in care with family members, collaborating with other nurses who have been through similar situations, and consulting with the ethics committee within your facility.
11. It is important for health care professionals to have open and frank discussions with patients about their preferences regarding end-of-life care. This discussion should not occur during a life-threatening event when patients and families are stressed and feel rushed to make a decision.

SELECTED READINGS

American Cancer Society. (2020). *Colorectal cancer early detection, diagnosis, and staging.* www.cancer.org/cancer/screening/american-cancer-society-guidelines-for-the-early-detection-of-cancer

American Cancer Society. (2022). *Cancer facts and figures for African American/Black people 2022–2024.* Author.

American Joint Committee on Cancer. (2017). *Cancer staging manual* (8th ed.). Springer International Publishing.

Cancer.Net. https://www.cancer.gov/about-cancer/treatment/clinical-trials

Centers for Disease Control and Prevention. (2023). *Vaccine schedules.* www.cdc.gov/vaccines/schedules/hcp/index.html

Devita, V. T., Lawrence, T. S., & Rosenberg, S. A. (2023). *Cancer: Principles and practice of oncology* (12th ed.). Wolters Kluwer.

Fontham, E., Wolf, A., Church, T., Etzioni, R., Flowers, C., Herzig, A., Guerra, C., Oeffinger, K., Shih, Y., Walter, L., Kim, J., Andrews, K., DeSantis, C., Fedewa, S., Manassaram-Baptiste, D., Saslow, D., Wender, R., & Smith, R. (2022). Cervical cancer screening guidelines for individuals at average risk: 2020 guideline update from the American cancer society. *CA: A Cancer Journal for Clinicians, 70*(5), 321–346. https://doi.org/10.3322/caac.21628

Giaquinto, A., Mille, K., Tossas, K., Winn, R., Jemel, A., & Siegel, R. (2022). Cancer statistics for African American/Black people 2022. *CA: A Cancer Journal for Clinicians, 72*(3), 202–229. https://doi.org/10.3322/caac.21628

Hassankhani, H., Rahmani, A., Taleghani, F., Sanaat, Z., & Dehghannezhad, J. (2020). Palliative care models for cancer patients: Learning for planning in nursing (review). *Journal of Cancer Education, 35*(1), 3–13. https://doi.org/10.1007/s13187-019-01532-3

Kamarudin, M. N. A., Sarker, M. M. R., Zhou, J. R., & Parhar, I. (2019). Metformin in colorectal cancer: Molecular mechanism, preclinical and clinical aspects. *Journal of Experimental & Clinical Cancer Research: CR, 38*(1), 491. https://doi.org/10.1186/s13046-019-1495-2

Love, M., Debay, M., Hudley, A. C., Sorsby, T., Lucero, L., Miller, S., Sampath, S., Amini, A., Raz, D., Kim, J., Pathak, R., Chen, Y. J., Kaiser, A., Melstrom, K., Fakih, M., & Sun, V. (2022). Cancer survivors, oncology, and primary care perspectives on survivorship care: An integrative review. *Journal of Primary Care & Community Health, 13*, 21501319221105248. https://doi.org/10.1177/21501319221105248

Miller, K. D., Nogueira, L., Devasia, T., Mariotto, A. B., Yabroff, K. R., Jemal, A., Kramer, J., & Siegel, R. L. (2022). Cancer treatment and survivorship statistics, 2022. *CA: A Cancer Journal for Clinicians, 72*(5), 409–436. https://doi.org/10.3322/caac.21731

Oncology Nursing Society. (2021). *Manual for radiation oncology nursing practice and education* (5th ed.). Author.

Oncology Nursing Society. (2024). *Core curriculum for oncology nursing* (7th ed.). Elsevier.

Rock, C. L., Thomson, C., Gansler, T., Gapstur, S. M., McCullough, M. L., Patel, A. V., Andrews, K. S., Bandera, E. V., Spees, C. K., Robien, K., Hartman, S., Sullivan, K., Grant, B. L., Hamilton, K. K., Kushi, L. H., Caan, B. J., Kibbe, D., Black, J. D., Wiedt, T. L., McMahon, C., … & Doyle, C. (2020). American Cancer Society guideline for diet and physical activity for cancer prevention. *CA: A Cancer Journal for Clinicians, 70*(4), 245–271. https://doi.org/10.3322/caac.21591

Gould Rothberg, B. E., Quest, T. E., Yeung, S. J., Pelosof, L. C., Gerber, D. E., Seltzer, J. A., Bischof, J. J., Thomas, C. R., Jr, Akhter, N., Mamtani, M., Stutman, R. E., Baugh, C. W., Anantharaman, V., Pettit, N. R., Klotz, A. D., Gibbs, M. A., & Kyriacou, D. N. (2022). Oncologic emergencies and urgencies: A comprehensive review. *CA: A Cancer Journal for Clinicians, 72*(6), 570–593. https://doi.org/10.3322/caac.21727

Rugo, H., & Van den Hurk, C. (2023). Alopecia related to systemic cancer therapy. *UpToDate.* Retrieved October 15, 2023, from https://www.uptodate.com/contents/alopecia-related-to-systemic-cancer-therapy

Siegel, R. L., Giaquinto, A. N., & Jemal, A. (2024, January–February). Cancer statistics, 2024. *CA: A Cancer Journal for Clinicians, 74*(1), 12–49. https://doi.org/10.3322/caac.21820. (Erratum in: *CA: A Cancer Journal for Clinicians* 2024, February 16.) PMID: 38230766.

Siegel, R. L., Miller, K. D., Wagle, N. S., & Jemal, A. (2023). Cancer statistics, 2023. *CA: A Cancer Journal for Clinicians, 73*(1), 17–48. https://doi.org/10.3322/caac.21763

Yarbro, C. H., Wujciki, D., & Gobel, B. H. (2018). *Cancer nursing: Principles and practice* (8th ed.). Jones & Bartlett.

5

Care of the Older Adult or the Person With a Disability*

OVERVIEW AND ASSESSMENT

The older adult and the person with a disability often present with similar health care and nursing care needs due to mobility challenges and altered functional ability. The effects of altered activity and function may cause particular problems among these groups, more commonly than in the general population. Be aware, however, that there is wide variation of health and ability among individuals in both populations. The older adult is generally considered as a person age 65 and older, according to the U.S. organizations of the National Institute on Aging (NIA), Centers for Disease Control and Prevention (CDC), Center for Medicare and Medicaid Services (CMS), and the United Kingdom organization of National Institute for Health and Clinical Excellence (NICE). The World Health Organization (WHO) and the United Nations (UN) define older adult as a person 60 years and older. The Americans with Disabilities Act (ADA) defines an individual with a disability as "a person who has a physical or mental impairment that substantially limits one or more major life activities, a person who has a history or record of such an impairment, or a person who is perceived by others as having such an impairment" (United States Department of Justice Civil Rights Division, 2020).

Normal Changes of Aging

There are a number of normal age-related changes that occur in all major systems of the body. These may present at different times for different people. It is important to be able to differentiate between normal and abnormal changes in older adults in order to provide appropriate care. A comprehensive geriatric evaluation (CGE) is essential to understand the holistic health needs of older adults. The CGE is performed by an interdisciplinary team, which typically includes a nurse, a physician or advanced practice provider, and a social worker. Other members of the team may include a pharmacist, a physical therapist, an occupational therapist, a recreational therapist, and a dietitian. The Hartford Institute for Geriatric Nursing provides many tools for the assessment of older adults on their website in their *Try This:* Series (https://hign.org/consultgeri-resources/try-this-series).

Vision

Characteristics

1. Decreased visual acuity.
2. Decreased visual fields, resulting in decreased peripheral vision.
3. Decreased dark adaptation.
4. Elevated minimal threshold of light perception.
5. Presbyopia (farsightedness) because of decreased visual accommodation from loss of lens elasticity.
6. Decreased color discrimination because of the yellowing of the lens; short wavelength colors, such as blues and greens, are more difficult to see.
7. Increased sensitivity to glare.
8. Decreased depth perception.
9. Decreased tear production.

Assessment Findings

1. Arcus senilis—deposits of lipid around the eye, seen as a white or gray circle around the iris; causes no vision impairments and does not require treatment.
2. Cataracts—clouding of the normally clear lens of the eye. (This results in lens thickening and decreased permeability;

*Please note that the term "male" in this chapter refers to a person assigned male at birth, and the term "female" in this chapter refers to a person assigned female at birth.

noted on examination with an ophthalmoscope; fuzziness of vision, like looking through wax paper. Cataracts cause blurring, sensitivity to light, or double vision.) Can be corrected surgically.
3. Macular degeneration—because of damage to macula that results in loss of central vision. (Objects seem blurred or distorted or are not seen); the leading cause of vision loss.
4. Glaucoma—increased intraocular pressure with tonometer testing. (Often is asymptomatic in early stages and later may result in blurring, colored "halos" around lights, pain or redness of eyes, and loss of peripheral vision.)
5. Smaller pupil size.
6. Complaints of decreased ability to read, discomfort from light, changes in depth perception, falls, motor vehicle accidents, difficulty handling small objects, difficulty with activities of daily living (ADLs), and tunnel vision.
7. Dry, red eyes.
8. Vitreous floaters, which are lightning flashes in the visual field.
9. Be aware that patients with vision loss may experience feelings of depression or anxiety.

Nursing Considerations and Teaching Points

1. Make sure objects are in the patient's visual field, and do not move objects around.
2. Use large lettering to label medications and any distributed written information.
3. Allow the person more time to focus and adjust to the environment.
4. Minimize glare—may help to wear sunglasses.
5. Use nightlights to help with dark adaptation problems.
6. Use adequate lighting and bright colors to enhance vision.
7. Mark the edges of stairs and curbs to help with depth perception problems.
8. Use microspiral telescopes or magnifying glasses and high-intensity lighting.
9. Encourage yearly eye examination and refer for examination if vision changes worsen (flashing lights in fields or "veil over the eye").
10. Encourage use of isotonic eyedrops as needed for dry eyes.
11. Encourage use of low vision aids, such as magnifying lens, light filtering lens, telescopic lenses, or electronic devices.
12. If patient reports depression or anxiety, refer patient for further evaluation of symptoms.
13. Refer patients to the following resources for vision impairments:
    - Prevent Blindness America: 800-331-2020; www.preventblindness.org
    - American Foundation for the Blind: 800-232-5463; www.afb.org
    - American Council of the Blind: www.acb.org
    - National Eye Institute: Low Vision: https://www.nei.nih.gov/learn-about-eye-health/eye-conditions-and-diseases/low-vision

Hearing

Characteristics

1. Hearing loss is common among older adults. Approximately 25% to 30% of people 60 to 69 years old have significant hearing loss, and the prevalence doubles every decade.
2. Two major types of hearing disorders are common in the older population.
    a. Sensorineural—progressive, irreversible bilateral loss of high-tone perception often associated with aging. This results in difficulty with discriminating sounds. Sound waves reach the inner ear but are not properly transmitted to the brain.
    b. Conduction deafness—results from blockage or impairment of the mechanical movement in the outer or middle ear (also a pathologic condition). Sound waves are not conducted to the inner ear, resulting in sounds that are muffled.
3. Hearing loss in older adults is usually a combined problem. The majority of the loss is due to auditory nerve changes or deterioration of the structures of the ear. There may also be nerve damage beyond the ear. Presbycusis and central deafness can result in permanent hearing loss; conduction deafness is reversible.
4. Usual progression from high-tone or high-frequency loss to a general loss of both high and low tones.
5. Consonants (higher-pitched sounds) are not heard well.
6. Hearing loss increases with age and is greater in males.
7. Increase in the sound threshold (i.e., greater sound needed to stimulate the older adult).
8. Decreased speech discrimination, especially with background noise.
9. Cerumen impaction, the most common cause of conductive hearing loss, is reversible.

Assessment Findings

1. Increased volume of patient's own speech.
2. Turning of head toward the speaker.
3. Requests of a speaker to repeat.
4. Inappropriate answers, but otherwise cognitively intact.
5. The person may withdraw; demonstrate a short attention span; and become frustrated, angry, and depressed.
6. Lack of response to a loud noise.

Nursing Considerations and Teaching Points

1. Be aware that hearing loss can impact the safety and quality of life of older adults in many ways. For example, the older adult may not hear instructions, alerting signals, telephones, or oncoming traffic. Hearing loss can contribute to social isolation and lower self-esteem.
2. Suggest hearing testing with an audiologist for further evaluation and consideration of an assistive device.
3. Face the person directly so they can lip-read.
4. Use gestures and objects to help with verbal communication.
5. Touch the person to get their attention before talking.
6. Speak into the patient's "good ear."
7. *Do not shout.* Shouting increases the tone of the voice, and older adults are unable to hear these high tones. Try speaking in a deeper or lower tone of voice.
8. Speak slowly and clearly.
9. Suggest amplifiers on telephones and alarms.
10. Allow the person more time to answer your questions.
11. Evaluate the person's ear canals regularly and assist with cerumen removal. Cerumen removal is facilitated by:
    a. Use of ceruminolytic agents, such as carbamide peroxide, 10 drops in the affected ear twice per day for 5 days, followed by flushing the ear with warm water via a 50-mL irrigation syringe or an electronic irrigation device.
    b. Careful use of an ear spoon to mechanically remove cerumen.
12. Refer patients to the following organizations:
    - American Speech–Language–Hearing Association: www.asha.org

- Hearing Loss Association of America: https://www.hearingloss.org
- National Institute on Deafness and Other Communication Disorders: www.nidcd.nih.gov/health/hearing/pages/older.aspx

Smell

Characteristics

1. Changes in smell (olfaction) are due to nasal sinus disease preventing odors from reaching smell receptors, a decrease in nerve fibers, chronic injury from infections, or bleeding.
2. Discrimination of fruity odors seems to persist the longest.
3. Generally, olfaction decreases in males more than in females.

Assessment Findings

1. Inability to notice unpleasant odors, such as fire, body odor, or excessive perfume.
2. Decreased appetite.

Nursing Considerations and Teaching Points

1. Age-related changes can impact safety and quality of life. For example, an older adult may not be able to recognize the smell of smoke or gas.
2. The inability to smell food may cause a decrease in the consumption of nutritious food.
   a. At mealtimes, name food items and give the person time to think of the smell/taste of the food.
   b. Suggest use of stronger spices and flavorings to stimulate the sense of smell.

Taste

Characteristics

1. Taste buds decrease with age, especially in males. People older than age 60 have lost half of their taste buds. By age 80, only one sixth of the taste buds remain.
2. Taste buds are lost from the front to the back (i.e., sweet and salty tastes are lost first, whereas bitter and sour tastes remain longer).

Assessment Findings

1. Complaints that food has no taste.
2. Excessive use of sugar and salt.
3. Inability to identify foods.
4. Decrease in appetite and weight loss.
5. Decreased pleasure from food.

Nursing Considerations and Teaching Points

1. Age-related changes can impact safety. For example, the older adult may not be able to detect spoiled food.
2. Serve food attractively, and separate different types of foods.
3. Vary the texture of foods.
4. Encourage good oral hygiene.
5. Season food.

Kinesthetic Sense

Characteristics

1. Awareness of body movement occurs through sensations from the receptors in the joints and muscles that tell us where we are in space; as we age, these receptors lose their ability to function. Therefore, there is a change in balance.
2. Walking with shorter step length, less leg lift, a wider base, and a tendency to lean forward.
3. With age, less ability to stop a fall from occurring.

Assessment Findings

1. Alterations in posture, ability to transfer, and gait.
2. Complaint of dizziness.

Nursing Considerations and Teaching Points

1. Position items within reach.
2. Give the person more time to move.
3. Take precautions to prevent falls.
4. Suggest physical therapy with balance training after periods of immobility.

Cardiovascular

Characteristics

1. With age, the valves of the heart become thick and rigid as a result of sclerosis and fibrosis, compounding any cardiac disease already present.
2. Blood vessels also become thick and rigid, resulting in elevated blood pressure (BP), which is present in half of the U.S. population older than age 65.
3. Maximum heart rate and aerobic capacity decrease with age.
4. Slower response to stress. Once the pulse rate is elevated, it takes longer to return to baseline.
5. Decline in maximum oxygen consumption.
6. About 50% of older adults have an abnormal resting electrocardiogram.
7. Subtle changes in artery walls result in a less flexible vasculature.
8. Decreased baroreceptor sensitivity.

Assessment Findings

1. According to the Eighth Joint National Committee (JNC-8) guidelines, high BP over age 60 requiring treatment is greater than or equal to 150/90 mm Hg and greater than or equal to 140/90 for adults with diabetes and kidney disease; however, the American Heart Association and American College of Cardiology (AHA/ACC) high BP guidelines recommend treatment for all ages if BP is greater than 130/80 mm Hg. The AHA/ACC guideline acknowledges that clinical judgment is required for older patients and that medical comorbidities, life expectancy, treatment preference, and the risk/benefit relationship of treatment need to be considered.
2. Prolonged tachycardia may occur following stress.

EVIDENCE BASE James, P. A., Oparil, S., Carter, B. L., Cushman, W. C., Dennison-Himmelfarb, C., Handler,J., Lackland, D. T., LeFevre, M. L., MacKenzie, T. D., Ogedegbe, O., Smith, S. C., Jr, Svetkey, L. P., Taler, S. J., Townsend, R. R., Wright, J. T., Jr, Narva, A. S., & Ortiz, E. (2014). Evidence-based guideline for the management of high blood pressure in adults. Report from the panel members appointed to the Eighth Joint National Committee (JNC 8). *Journal of the American Medical Association, 311*(5), 507–520. https://doi.org/10.1001/jama.2013.284427

EVIDENCE BASE Whelton, P., Carey, R., Aronow, W., Casey, D. E., Jr, Collins, K. J., Dennison-Himmelfarb, C., DePalma, S. M., Gidding, S., Jamerson, K. A., Jones, D. W., MacLaughlin, E. J., Muntner, P., Ovbiagele, B., Smith, S. C., Jr, Spencer, C. C., Stafford, R. S., Taler, S. J., Thomas, R. J., Williams, K. A., Sr, ... & Wright, J. T.. (2018). 2017 ACC/AHA/AAPA/ABC/ACPM/AGS/APhA/ASH/ASPC/NMA/PCNA guideline for the prevention, detection, evaluation, and management of high blood pressure in adults: A report of the American College of Cardiology/American Heart Association Task Force on Clinical Practice Guidelines. *Hypertension, 71*(6), e13–e115. https://doi.org/10.1161/HYP.0000000000000065

Nursing Considerations and Teaching Points

1. Encourage regular BP evaluation as well as lifestyle modifications and medication adherence, if indicated, for hypertension.
2. Check for postural BP changes to detect orthostatic hypotension and prevent falls. Instruct patients to rise slowly from lying to sitting to standing.
3. Encourage longer cooldown period after exercise to return to baseline cardiac function.
4. Encourage moderate physical activity: walking, biking, or swimming for 30 minutes five times per week (150 minutes/week), in addition to muscle-strengthening exercises two times a week, and balance training.

Pulmonary

Characteristics

1. With age, there is a weakening of the intercostal respiratory muscles, and the elastic recoil of the chest wall diminishes.
2. There is no change in total lung capacity; however, residual volume and functional residual capacity increase.
3. Partial pressure of oxygen decreases with age because of ventilation–perfusion mismatches. However, older adults are not hypoxic without coexistent disease.
4. There is a decrease in the mucus transport/ciliary system. Therefore, there is decreased clearance of mucus and foreign bodies, including bacteria.

Assessment Findings

1. Prolonged cough, inability to raise secretions.
2. Increased frequency of respiratory infections.

Nursing Considerations and Teaching Points

1. Older adults who are undergoing surgical treatment should engage in deep breathing exercises.
2. Teach measures to prevent pulmonary infections—avoid crowds or wear surgical masks or respirators in crowds during COVID-19 outbreaks and cold and flu season, wash hands frequently, and report early signs of infection.
3. Avoid smoking and exposure to secondhand smoke.
4. Encourage COVID-19, pneumococcal, and annual influenza immunizations as recommended by ongoing research.

Immunologic

Characteristics

1. The function of T-cell lymphocytes, such as cell-mediated immunity, declines with age because of involution and atrophy of the thymus gland.
2. Decreased T-cell helper activity; increased T-cell suppressor activity.
3. Declining B-cell function as a result of T-cell changes.

Assessment Findings

1. More frequent infections.
2. Increased incidence of many types of cancer.

Nursing Considerations and Teaching Points

1. Teach older adults that they are at increased risk of infection, cancer, and autoimmune disease; therefore, routine follow-up and screening are essential.
2. Encourage healthy lifestyle practices to maintain optimal health.

Neurologic

Characteristics

1. There is gradual loss in the number of neurons with age, but no major change in neurotransmitter levels.
2. Some brain tissue atrophy is normal and does not relate to cognitive impairment.
3. Decrease in muscle tone, motor speed, and nerve conduction velocity.
4. Decrease in gait speed of 1.6% per year after age 63; decreased step length, stride length, and arm swing.

Assessment Findings

1. Decreased position and vibration sense.
2. Diminished reflexes, possible absent ankle jerks.
3. Complaint of falls and impaired balance.
4. Wide-based gait with decreased arm swing.

Nursing Considerations and Teaching Points

1. Because of gait, strength, balance, and sensory changes in older adults, it is essential to teach them fall prevention techniques.
2. Decrease in gait speed is highly associated with increased disability and mortality. An older adult who takes longer than 12 seconds to walk 10 feet is at increased risk of falls and requires further evaluation and intervention.
3. Teach environmental safety techniques, including the use of proper footwear, nonslip surfaces, securely fastened handrails, sufficient light, glare-free lights, avoidance of low-lying objects, chairs of the proper height with armrests, skidproof strips or mats in the tub or shower, toilet and tub grab bars, and elevated toilet seats.
4. Refer for home safety evaluations, which may be available through state and local health departments. A home safety checklist can be obtained from the Consumer Product Safety Commission at https://www.cpsc.gov/s3fs-public/701.pdf.

Musculoskeletal

Characteristics

1. Declining muscle mass and endurance with age, although deconditioning may be an associated factor.
2. Decreased bone density, less so in males.
3. Decreased thickness and resiliency of cartilage, with a resulting increase in the stiffness of joints.
4. Bone resorption exceeds bone formation, resulting in a decline in bone density.
5. Injuries to the cartilage accumulate with age.

Assessment Findings

1. Muscle atrophy.
2. Increased incidence of fractures.
3. Complaint of joint stiffness in the absence of arthritis.
4. Decreased bone density (<2.5 standard deviations below normal).

Nursing Considerations and Teaching Points

1. Early intervention to encourage regular exercise (including weight-bearing exercise and resistance training) in older adults is important to prevent exacerbation of these normal changes.
2. Encourage increased dietary intake of calcium and vitamin D, consideration of oral calcium and vitamin D supplementation in conjunction with primary care provider, and decreased alcohol and nicotine use.

Community and Home Care Considerations

1. Encourage older adults to engage in 30 minutes of moderate physical activity, including walking, biking, or swimming, at least five times per week, in addition to muscle-strengthening exercises at least two times a week.
2. For older adults who will be exercising at less than 80% of the maximum heart rate (use the formula 220 − age), stress testing before starting an exercise program is not needed.
3. To help with adherence to the exercise program, older adults should be encouraged to exercise at a set time, include an accountability partner if feasible, relieve pain before exercising, and engage in an activity they enjoy. Provide positive reinforcement for those who do exercise, and continually reinforce the benefits of exercise (increased bone strength, cardiovascular fitness, decreased pain, decreased risks of falls, and overall sense of well-being).

Endocrine

Characteristics

1. Decreased secretion of trophic hormones from the pituitary gland.
2. Blunted growth hormone release during stress.
3. Elevated vasopressin (antidiuretic hormone); exaggerated response to osmotic challenge.
4. Elevated levels of follicle-stimulating hormone and luteinizing hormone because of reduced end-organ response.
5. Decreased insulin secretion after meals; this may be a function of weight or genetic factors.

Assessment Finding

Usually asymptomatic.

Nursing Considerations and Teaching Points

1. Encourage routine screening for elevated blood glucose—both fasting and postprandial.
2. Provide education about a well-balanced diet.

Reproductive

Characteristics

1. In females, menopause leads to decreases in the size of the ovaries and hormone production. This results in uterine involution, vaginal atrophy, and loss of breast mass.
2. With age, there is an increased risk in females of cystocele, rectocele, and uterine prolapse.
3. In males, testosterone production and secretion decrease with age. However, serum levels may be in the low-normal range through age 80.

Assessment Findings

1. Vaginal dryness, painful intercourse.
2. Atrophic vaginitis.
3. Urinary incontinence.

Nursing Considerations and Teaching Points

1. Suggest the use of additional lubrication during sexual intercourse.
2. Advise sexually active older males that spermatogenesis may continue into advanced age.
3. Address risks and benefits of time-limited hormone replacement therapy for symptomatic relief related to menopause.
4. Refer the patient for further evaluation for urinary incontinence.
5. For pelvic organ prolapse that negatively impacts quality of life, refer the patient for consideration of pessary placement or surgical intervention.

Renal and Body Composition

Characteristics

1. Increased body fat and decreased lean muscle mass, even when weight remains stable.
2. Decreased renal function, measured by the glomerular filtration rate, or creatinine clearance.
3. Despite reduced total body creatinine because of decreased muscle mass in the older adult, serum creatinine often remains within the normal range. This is because of decreased elimination of creatinine by the kidneys.
4. About 10% decline in creatinine clearance per decade after age 40; however, relatively unchanged serum creatinine.

Assessment Findings

1. Usually asymptomatic.
2. Increased incidence of anemia.

Nursing Considerations and Teaching Points

1. Be aware that although serum creatinine may be within normal range, creatinine clearance may be decreased. To obtain an estimated creatinine clearance in an older adult, the following formula may be used: (140 − age) (weight [kg])/(72)(serum creatinine [mg/dL]).
2. Drugs that are cleared through the kidneys may be given in decreased dosage. Adverse effects and toxicity must be closely monitored.
3. Consider the advantages and disadvantages of drug management for anemia associated with renal disease.

Skin

Characteristics

1. Thinning of all three layers of the skin—epidermis, dermis, and subcutaneous tissue—leads to greater fragility of the skin and decreased ability of the skin to function as a barrier to external factors.
2. Fewer melanocytes and decreased tanning.
3. Less efficient thermoregulation of heat because of fewer sweat glands.
4. Drier skin because the decreased number of sebaceous glands results in reduced oil production.
5. Other changes in aging skin include reduced sensory input, decreased elasticity, and impaired cell-related immune response.

Assessment Finding

1. Dry, irritated skin.

Nursing Considerations and Teaching Points

1. Excessive use of soap, which can be drying to the skin, should be avoided.
2. Careful skin evaluation and lubrication are necessary to prevent fissures and breakdown.
3. Heat regulation needs to be controlled by proper clothing and avoidance of extreme temperatures.
4. Avoid direct application of extreme heat or cold to the skin because damage may occur without feeling it.
5. Encourage use of sunscreen during all outdoor activities.

Community and Home Care Considerations

Xerosis (dry skin) is a common problem for older adults. Treatment should include:

1. Total body immersion in warm water (90°F to 105°F [32.2°C to 40.6°C]) for 10 minutes.
2. Use of nonperfumed soap without hexachlorophene.
3. Application of emollient, particularly those with alpha-hydroxy acids, after bathing and at bedtime.

Hematopoietic

Characteristics

1. Unchanged number of stem cells in all three cell lines; however, bone marrow cellularity is decreased by 33% during adult life.
2. Declining marrow activity, especially in response to stress, such as with blood loss or infection.

Assessment Finding

Asymptomatic.

Nursing Considerations and Teaching Points

1. Anemia and granulocytopenia are not normal consequences of aging and should be investigated.
2. Teach patients that there is no need to take oral iron unless there is an actual documented decrease in iron levels.
3. Encourage oral B_{12} and folate replacement to manage associated anemias.

Altered Presentation of Disease

Characteristics

1. In part because of the physiologic changes that occur with aging, the manifestations of illness in older patients are less dramatic than in younger patients.
2. Most older adults have at least one chronic condition. These coexisting conditions can complicate the evaluation of new symptoms.
3. Some risk factors make it more likely that older adults will present with an altered presentation of disease. For those older than age 85, risk factors include multiple comorbid conditions, taking over five medications, and having cognitive or functional impairment.

EVIDENCE BASE Blain, H., Rolland, Y., Benetos, A., Giacosa, N., Albrand, M., Miot, S., & Bousquet, J. (2020). Atypical clinical presentation of COVID-19 infection in residents of a long-term care facility. *European Geriatric Medicine, 11*(6), 1085–1088. https://doi.org/10.1007/s41999-020-00352-9

Assessment Findings

1. The classic indicators of disease are usually absent or disorders present atypically (see Table 5-1).
2. Older people are less likely to report new symptoms; rather, they attribute them to aging or existing conditions. Many older adults minimize symptoms because of fear of hospitalization or health care costs.
3. Older adults infected with SARS-CoV-2 are more likely to initially present with nonrespiratory symptoms such as diarrhea, fall, temperature fluctuations with hypothermia, and change in mental status.

Nursing Considerations and Teaching Points

1. Have a high index of suspicion for underlying illness if the older adult presents with an acute change in cognition, behavior, or function.

Functional Assessment

Functional assessment is the measurement of a person's ability to complete functional tasks and fulfill social roles, specifically addressing a patient's ability to complete tasks ranging from simple self-care to higher level activities. It is especially valuable in the care of an older adult or a person with a disability. It provides the nurse with objective data to help determine the person's needs and to plan interventions. Across the United States, there is an imperative to reduce hospital readmissions. Many programs have been successful. A common feature in most of the programs is the need to complete a functional assessment

Purpose

1. Functional assessment is essential because it:
   a. Offers a systematic approach to assessing patients for deficits that commonly go undetected.

Table 5-1 Atypical Presentation of Disorders in the Older Adult

DISORDER	ATYPICAL PRESENTATION
Acute intestinal infection	• Abdominal pain may be absent. • May present with acute confusional state, leukocytosis, and acidosis.
Appendicitis	• Pain may be diffuse, not localized in the right lower quadrant.
Biliary disease	• Confusion, declining function, and other nonspecific symptom. • Abnormal liver function tests may be the only sign.
Heart failure	• Initially, may have change in mental status and fatigue.
Hyperthyroidism	• Apathy, palpitations, weight loss, weakness.
Hypothyroidism	• Presents with weight loss.
Myocardial infarction	• Chest pain may be absent. • May present with syncope, dyspnea, vomiting, or confusion.
Perforated ulcer	• Rigidity may be absent until late.
Pneumonia	• May present with confusion. • Fever and cough may be absent.
Pulmonary embolism	• May present with change in mental status. • May not have fever, leukocytosis, or tachycardia.
Septicemia	• May be afebrile.
Systemic lupus erythematosus	• Pneumonitis, subcutaneous nodules, and discoid lesions are more common. • Malar rash, Raynaud phenomenon, and nephritis are less common.
Urinary tract infection	• Confusion.

b. Helps the nurse to identify problems and utilize appropriate resources.
c. Provides a way to assess progress and decline over time.
d. Helps the nurse evaluate the safety of the patient's ability to live alone.

2. Functional status includes the evaluation of sensory changes, ability to complete ADLs and instrumental ADLs, gait and balance problems, and elimination.

Instruments to Measure Functional Ability

1. Functional status may be assessed by several methods: self-report, direct observation, or family or caregiver report. Performance measures or direct observation are the best methods, when possible.
2. The instrument chosen should be based on the specific goal or purpose for the evaluation. For example, if the focus is on basic function, self-care, and mobility, the Barthel index should be used.
3. The Katz Index for Activities of Daily Living and Instrumental Activities of Daily Living is another rating scale for measuring functional ability and instrumental ADLs. Use this scale to determine level of independence of the older adult and repeat periodically to compare level of functioning over time.
4. Performance measures, such as the Tinetti Gait and Balance measure, Functional Reach Test, Get Up and Go, or the Chair Rise test, can be used to evaluate higher level functioning. Consider referral to rehabilitation (physical and occupational therapy) if screening identifies deficits.

Psychosocial Assessment

Altered Mental Status

1. Assessment of mental status to detect altered cognition involves examination of memory, perception, communication, orientation, calculation, comprehension, problem-solving, thought processes, language, executive function, visual–spatial abilities, abstraction, attention, aphasia, and apraxia.
2. Assessment can be facilitated by use of cognitive screening tools. A commonly utilized instrument is the Mini-Mental State Examination (MMSE), a 30-point cognitive screening instrument that assesses orientation to time and place, registration and recall, calculation, language skills, and visual–spatial abilities.
3. The total possible score is 30. A score of 24 to 30 suggests intact cognitive function; 20 to 23, mild cognitive impairment; 16 to 19, moderate cognitive impairment; and 15 or less, severe cognitive impairment. The MMSE can help to follow the patient's cognition over time and assess for acute and chronic changes.
4. Although success on scales such as this has been associated with language abilities, education, and socioeconomic status, this scale continues to be used as an appropriate screening tool for abnormal cognitive function.
5. Another cognitive screening instrument is the Mini-Cog examination, which is composed of a three-item recall and the clock drawing test (CDT). The Mini-Cog can be administered in less than 3 minutes, does not appear to be affected by the patient's education or language abilities, and has been successfully used to screen for dementia across a variety of clinical settings. The Mini-Cog can be administered as follows:
   a. Tell the patient to listen carefully and remember and repeat three unrelated words.
   b. Tell the patient to draw the face of a clock including numbers and hands to read a specific time. The CDT is considered normal if all numbers are present in the correct sequence and position and the hands display the requested time.
   c. Ask the patient to repeat the three previously stated words.
   d. Unsuccessful recall of all three items suggests dementia. Successful recall of all three items suggests intact cognition. An abnormal CDT with one to two errors on recall suggests dementia. A normal CDT with one error on recall suggests no dementia.
6. Assessment of altered mental status or behavior may elicit criteria that lead to a diagnosis of dementia. It is essential to differentiate dementia from delirium (which is treatable and reversible).
7. *Delirium* is a change in mental status that is abrupt in onset and is common because of an underlying medical condition, such as infection, electrolyte imbalance, medication intolerance or toxicity, cardiac decompensation, or hypoxia. The Confusion Assessment Method (CAM) can be utilized to screen for delirium.
   a. Occurs at any age with fairly sudden onset, and the behavior is variable hour to hour. May be superimposed upon dementia, mental health conditions, or intellectual disabilities, making identification difficult.
   b. Clouded, altered, or fluctuating level of consciousness (lethargic to hypervigilant), short attention span, and disturbed sleep–wake cycle. Hallucinations (sensory experiences without a stimulus) are common.
   c. Reversible with treatment of the underlying cause; however, individuals with an unrecognized and prolonged episode of delirium may not return to their previous cognitive baseline.
   d. Underrecognized and is associated with morbidity and mortality, especially among older adults.

EVIDENCE BASE Ho, M., Nealon, J., Igwe, E., Traynor, V., Chang, H. R., Chen, K. H., & Montayre, J. (2021). Postoperative delirium in older patients: A systematic review of assessment and incidence of postoperative delirium. *Worldviews on Evidence-Based Nursing, 18*(5), 290–301. https://doi.org/10.1111/wvn.12536

8. *Dementia* has an insidious, gradual onset with slow, progressive decline. Behavior may be consistent, and disorientation occurs late in the course. Consciousness is not clouded, attention span is generally not reduced, and day–night reversal of sleep–wake cycles can occur rather than hour-to-hour variation. Delusions (fixed false beliefs) are more common than hallucinations.

Social Activities and Support

1. Social support can be instrumental, informational, or emotional. The social environment is important with regard to recovery of acute medical problems and management of chronic illness.
2. Elicit information by asking such questions as:
   a. How often do you socialize with others?
   b. With whom do you socialize?
   c. What type of activities do you enjoy?

d. Do you enjoy socializing?
e. Who can you call for help?
f. Do you know of any place of worship or community groups you can call for help?

Emotional and Affective Status

Characteristics

1. Depression may occur in the older adult or person with a disability due to the many changes they are experiencing:
   a. Adjusting to new routines due to change in ability and function.
   b. The loss of roles, income, spouse, friends, family, home, pets, functional ability, health, and ability to participate in leisure activities.
   c. Ageist messages from society supporting and encouraging the value of youth.
   d. Prejudice and discrimination toward those with disabilities.
2. Depression may also be associated with underlying illnesses, such as Alzheimer disease (AD), Parkinson disease, and stroke; by substances such as alcohol; and by medications such as antihypertensives (beta-blockers), antiarthritics, and antianxiety agents.
3. Depression is usually difficult to identify in the older adult because the presentation is different than in younger people. Obtain the following information to assess for depression:
   a. Complaints of insomnia, weight loss, anorexia, and constipation (vegetative symptoms).
   b. Presence of anhedonia (lack of joy in usually pleasurable activities).
   c. Decrease in concentration, memory, and decision-making.
   d. Other somatic complaints, such as decreased appetite, musculoskeletal aches and pains, chest pain, and fatigue.
   e. History of chronic illness or other health problems.
   f. Impact of current medications.
4. Evaluate depression using one of the following tools:
   a. The Geriatric Depression Scale is a screening tool for older adults without or with mild cognitive impairment.
   b. The Cornell Scale for Depression in Dementia can be used as a screening tool for older adults with dementia.
   c. The Patient Health Questionnaire 9 (PHQ-9) has also been validated for use across the lifespan.
   d. The Depression Checklist or the Depression Scale for Severe Disability can be used for persons with intellectual disabilities.
5. Suicide is sometimes associated with depression, with suicides being especially high in older White males and adult males with disabilities. Assess for suicide risk.
6. Pain is underdetected and may be undertreated in older adults and can contribute to depressive symptoms and behavioral changes. Assess pain by asking and observing the patient, and provide appropriate measures to make the patient more comfortable.

Nursing and Patient Care Considerations

1. Older adults and persons with disabilities should be treated for depression; this may include medications, psychotherapy, bright light therapy, and, in some cases, electroconvulsive therapy.
2. Complement other therapeutic measures by providing opportunities to increase the patient's self-esteem.
   a. Encourage participation in meaningful activities.
   b. Encourage routine engagement in physical activity and exercise appropriate to ability.
   c. Promote the patient's positive self-image.
   d. Help the patient develop a sense of mastery.
   e. Encourage reminiscence of meaningful past events.
3. Help patient identify and use social supports.
4. For behavioral problems (agitation, combative behavior, or irritability), consider options such as aromatherapy, music therapy, pet therapy, relaxation techniques, massage, or physical activity.

Motivation in Older Adults and Persons With Disabilities

Characteristics

1. Motivation is an important variable in the patient's ability to recover from any health event and the ability to maintain the highest level of wellness.
2. Understanding individual motivational factors for engaging in health promotion activities like exercise is an approach that can improve adherence. It is possible to evaluate a patient's motivation to adhere to a given treatment plan and adopt interventions to help improve the patient's motivation.
3. Factors that influence motivation include:
   a. Needs such as hunger.
   b. Past experiences, specifically with health care providers.
   c. Negative attitudes toward aging.
   d. Self-efficacy expectations or the belief in one's ability to perform a specific activity.
   e. Outcome expectations or the belief that if a specific activity is performed there will be an expected outcome.
   f. The cost of performing a specific activity in terms of time, money, pain, fatigue, or fear.
   g. Internal factors, such as sensory changes, cognitive status, resilience, and adverse drug effects.
   h. External factors, such as social norms (particularly if those norms conflict with treatment) and the influence of social supports.
4. Problems in motivation because of age-related or functional ability differences:
   a. A shift from achievement motivation to conservative motivation.
   b. Establishment of meaningful rewards for people because of losses.
   c. Greater significance placed on the meaningful to the older person or the person with a disability.
   d. Evidence that older adults and individuals with a disability do not do well on tasks if they are asked to do them rapidly, under a time limit, or in a stressful situation.
   e. Increased importance placed on the cost of participating in an activity; fear of failing can be expressed either as increased anxiety or decreased willingness to take risks.
5. The Motivation Wheel (see Figure 5-1) can be used to evaluate motivation in the older adult or the person with a disability.
   a. Motivation is influenced by beliefs about physical and emotional benefits, mastery experiences, individualized care, social support, the environment, goals, physical sensations, and new activities.
   b. Motivation can be increased by strengthening beliefs about potential benefits, providing opportunities for mastery, identifying individualized care approaches and goals, using social supports, accessing supportive environments, decreasing unpleasant sensations, and trying new activities.

Nursing and Patient Care Considerations

1. Strategies to improve motivation include:
   a. Establish whose motives are being discussed. Involve the patient, family, and health care providers in setting patient-centered goals.

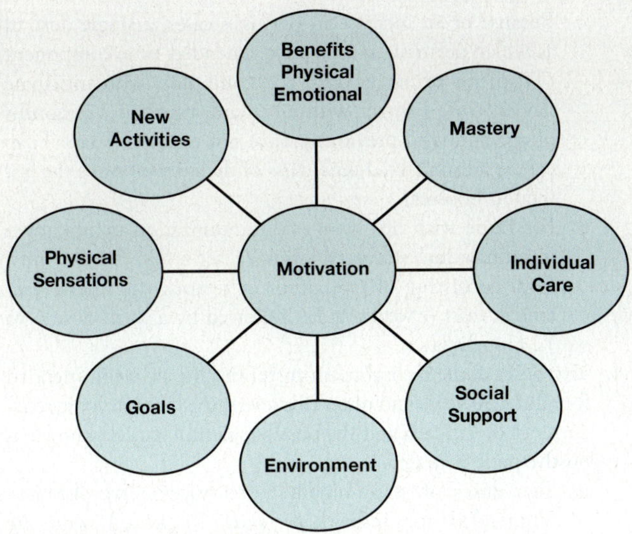

Figure 5-1. The wheel that moves.

   b. Explore with the patient any indication of fear or other unpleasant sensation associated with the activity, such as pain or fatigue, and implement interventions to decrease these unpleasant sensations.
   c. Evaluate the spokes of the wheel to consider the many factors that influence motivation and implement interventions as appropriate.
   d. Encourage patient to verbally express emotional factors associated with the activity.
   e. Examine the setting for the desired behavior to occur. Is the environment too stressful, too dark, or too noisy?
   f. Attempt to use role models. Older adult role models can change ageist attitudes and stimulate patients to perform the desired behavior.
   g. Set small goals to be met either daily or each shift. This provides frequent rewards.
   h. Do not be afraid to use yourself. Research has indicated that being nice, demonstrating caring, using humor, verbal encouragement, and support, can all help motivate the older adult.
2. Educate the older adult about the benefits of the activity, whether these are physical or psychological.

EVIDENCE BASE Lynch, K. A., Merdjanoff, A., Wilson, D., Chiarello, L., Hay, J., & Mao, J. J. (2022). "Moving forward": Older adult motivations for group-based physical activity after cancer treatment. *International Journal of Behavioral Medicine, 29*(3), 286–298. https://doi.org/10.1007/s12529-021-10018-w

HEALTH MAINTENANCE

EVIDENCE BASE United States Preventive Services Task Force. *The guide to clinical preventive services: Recommendations of the U.S. Preventive Services Task Force.* https://www.uspreventiveservicestaskforce.org/uspstf/

Health maintenance may easily be overlooked when caring for older adults and persons with disabilities due to other health concerns. However, health maintenance is imperative to prevent disease, promote wellness, and maximize quality of life.

Primary Prevention

There are three levels of health promotion and disease prevention. Primary prevention is the prevention of disease before it occurs. Primary prevention can be broken down into counseling, immunizations, and chemoprophylaxis.

Counseling

1. Encourage smoking cessation:
   a. According to the Centers for Disease Control and Prevention (CDC, 2023), approximately 8% of people in the United States age 65 and older smoke, and approximately 28% of adults with a disability smoke.
   b. Tobacco use has been linked to heart disease; peripheral vascular disease; cerebrovascular disease; chronic obstructive pulmonary disease; cancer such as lung, bladder, and esophageal malignancies; and numerous other health problems that decrease quality of life or cause premature death.
   c. Although much damage has been done to the lungs and blood vessels by years of smoking, all adults can benefit from smoking cessation by increasing quality of life.
   d. The U.S. Preventive Service Task Force recommends the "5-A" behavioral counseling framework as a useful strategy for engaging patients in smoking cessation discussions: (1) Ask about tobacco use; (2) Advise to quit through clear personalized messages; (3) Assess willingness to quit; (4) Assist to quit; and (5) Arrange follow-up and support.
2. Encourage physical activity:
   a. Approximately 75% of older Americans are inactive.
   b. The CDC (2021) recommends that all adults participate in regular physical activity for 30 minutes, 5 days a week, especially aerobic activities that promote cardiovascular fitness, such as walking, cycling, or swimming, but activity can be tailored to the individual's ability.
   c. Refer to a physical, occupational, or rehabilitation therapist. An individualized exercise prescription should be developed and cleared with the health care provider.
3. Identify patients with alcohol use disorder:
   a. The consequences of alcohol use disorder include liver disease, gastrointestinal (GI) bleeding, and motor vehicle accidents.
   b. Question patients about their use of substances or alcohol. Although current street drug use is less common, the patient may be misusing prescription drugs or may be using alcohol to combat pain.
   c. Recognize the signs and symptoms of alcohol use disorder in older adults (see Box 5-1).
   d. Refer for counseling.
4. Evaluate and counsel on dental health:
   a. Dental problems, especially in older adults, include missing teeth, ill-fitting dentures, periodontal disease, and tooth decay.
   b. Dental problems commonly lead to poor eating habits, apathy, and fatigue.
   c. Regular dental care should be encouraged to improve nutrition and the quality of life.

BOX 5-1 Signs of Alcohol Use Disorder in Older Adults

- Difficulty with gait and balance.
- Acute change in cognition.
- Frequent falls or accidents.
- Change in drinking patterns.
- Poor nutritional intake.
- Poor hygiene and self-care.
- Lack of physical exercise.

Immunizations

EVIDENCE BASE Centers for Disease Control and Prevention. (2022). *Advisory Committee for Immunization Practices (ACIP) recommendations*. Author. https://www.cdc.gov/vaccines/acip/recommendations.html

1. Pneumococcal pneumonia is a significant cause of mortality and morbidity in older adults and in those with a disability.
   a. There are two types of vaccines that prevent pneumococcal disease: pneumococcal conjugate vaccine (PCV13, PVC15, and PVC20) and pneumococcal polysaccharide vaccine (PPSV23). The CDC recommends that two pneumococcal vaccines be given to all people age 65 or older. For those individuals who have never received any pneumococcal vaccine, a dose of PCV15 should be given first, followed by a dose of PPSV23 at least 1 year later. Individuals who have been previously vaccinated with PPSV23 should receive a dose of PCV15 or PCV20 at least 1 year following their most recent dose of PPSV23. For individuals who have previously received PCV13, give PPSV23. If individuals received PCV13, but did not receive the recommended PPSV23, it is acceptable to give one dose of PCV20 if PPSV23 is not obtainable.
   b. The above vaccination schedule is also recommended for individuals aged 19 to 64 who smoke or who have chronic medical conditions or immunocompromising conditions.
2. Influenza may cause significant complications in older adults and those with a disability. Annual influenza vaccination is recommended for all people older than age 6 months without contraindications (e.g., severe allergic reaction to an influenza vaccine in the past or severe reaction to a vaccine ingredient such as gelatin; egg allergy is no longer a concern with current vaccines).
   a. Patients 65 years of age or older should receive an adjuvanted flu vaccine as they have been demonstrated to be more effective than the typical unadjuvanted flu vaccine.
   b. The intranasal live-attenuated influenza vaccine has not been approved for individuals 50 years of age or older.
   c. Several antiviral agents are effective against influenza. These agents can be effective in ameliorating symptoms if given within 48 hours of onset of illness.
3. Tetanus–diphtheria (Td) immunization is an important but frequently forgotten component of health maintenance, especially in older adults.
   a. The mortality rate of tetanus exceeds 50% in those older than age 65.
   b. Combined tetanus–diphtheria boosters should be given every 10 years; no age for discontinuation has been stated.
   c. Because of an increase in pertussis cases, a single dose of acellular pertussis is also recommended as a component (Tdap) for adults aged 65 years and older who anticipate having close contact with an infant less than 12 months of age and who previously have not received Tdap. Tdap can be administered regardless of the interval since the last tetanus booster.
   d. For those with no history of immunization or unknown immunization status, a primary series should be initiated, consisting of two doses of tetanus–diphtheria vaccine at least 4 weeks apart, followed by a third dose 6 to 12 months later.
4. Two doses of the recombinant zoster vaccine are recommended for adults 50 years and older to prevent the dermatologic reoccurrence of varicella and the possible painful sequela known as postherpetic neuralgia.
   a. Two doses of recombinant zoster vaccine are also recommended for individuals aged 19 to 64 who are immunocompromised.
   b. Recombinant zoster vaccine should be administered even for individuals who previously received zoster vaccine live, had shingles, or received a varicella vaccination. Recombinant zoster vaccine is highly effective in preventing shingles in comparison to zoster vaccine live (97% to 51%).
   c. Age is the most important factor in the development of herpes zoster, with a large increase beginning between age 50 and 60, and about 50% of people experience herpes zoster by age 85.

Chemoprophylaxis

1. The U.S. Preventive Services Task Force (USPSTF) recommends against starting low-dose aspirin use for the primary prevention of cardiovascular disease in individuals 60 years and older. Individuals who are 40 to 59 years old and have a 10% or greater risk of cardiovascular disease may consider the individual risks and benefits of aspirin use for primary prevention of cardiovascular disease.
2. Aspirin may be used for secondary prevention in individuals who have had a previous myocardial infarction, stroke, or coronary artery disease requiring a coronary artery stent or coronary artery bypass graft surgery.
3. Calcium, vitamin D, and other agents, such as selective estrogen receptor modulators or bisphosphonates, may be considered for those at risk for osteoporosis.

Secondary Prevention

Secondary prevention is the detection of disease in an early stage for best treatment outcomes, such as cancers, cardiovascular disease, osteoporosis, and tuberculosis.

Screening Recommendations

EVIDENCE BASE United States Preventive Services Task Force. *The guide to clinical preventive services: Recommendations of the U.S. Preventive Services Task Force*. https://www.uspreventiveservicestaskforce.org/uspstf/.

Age alone is not a criterion as to when to stop screening. Rather, the patient and health care provider should discuss values, expectations, functional status, and quality of life. A guide to shared decision-making for cancer screening is available at the USPSTF website at https://www.uspreventiveservicestaskforce.org/uspstf/recommendation-topics

The USPSTF has made the following recommendations for cancer screenings for adults:

1. Females between the ages of 40 to 74 who are at average risk of breast cancer should have a mammogram every other year. The precise age at which to discontinue screening mammography is uncertain. No clinical trials have been conducted on females older than age 74. Furthermore, although older females face a higher probability of developing breast cancer, they also have a greater chance of dying from other causes. Females with a disability are less likely to have regular mammogram screening due to difficulty with positioning for the equipment.
2. Regarding cervical cancer, it is appropriate for females to discontinue cervical cancer screening after age 65 only if they have had adequate recent screening with normal results and are not at high risk for cervical cancer.
3. Colorectal cancer screening is recommended for adults from ages 45 to 75. The age to discontinue colorectal cancer screening has not been determined; however, the USPSTF recommends selective screening for colorectal cancer in adults aged 76 to 85 if there are conditions to support screening for these individuals.
4. The USPSTF states that there is insufficient evidence to recommend for or against screening for prostate cancer. Older males and males with other significant medical conditions who have a life expectancy of fewer than 10 years are unlikely to benefit from the prostate-specific antigen test and digital rectal examination.

Tertiary Prevention

Tertiary prevention addresses the treatment of established disease to avoid complications and death. The major areas of focus for the older adult and the adult with a disability are preventing the complications of immobility and rehabilitation.

Preventing Complications of Immobility

Positioning

1. The goal of frequent position changes is to prevent contractures, stimulate circulation and prevent pressure injuries, prevent thrombophlebitis and pulmonary embolism, promote lung expansion and prevent pneumonia, and decrease edema of the extremities. Changing position from lying to sitting several times per day can help to prevent the negative changes in cardiovascular health from immobility which is known as *deconditioning*.
2. The recommendation is to change body position every 2 hours and, preferably, more frequently for patients who have no spontaneous movement. However, Yap and colleagues (2022) found that protocols for 2-hour repositioning of nursing home residents on high-density foam mattresses could be increased to 3- or 4-hour intervals without negatively impacting pressure injury prevention. Nursing home staff exhibited increased adherence for the 4-hour repositioning interval (95%) compared to 2-hour (80%) and 3-hour (90%) intervals.

EVIDENCE BASE Yap, T. L., Horn, S. D., Sharkey, P. D., Zheng, T., Bergstrom, N., Colon-Emeric, C., Sabol, V. K., Alderden, J., Yap, W., & Kennerly, S. M. (2022). Effect of varying repositioning frequency on pressure injury prevention in nursing home residents: Team-UP trial results. *Advances in Skin and Wound Care, 35*(6), 315–325. https://doi.org/10.1097/01.ASW.0000817840.68588.04

Proper Body Alignment

1. Dorsal or supine position
   a. The head is in line with the spine, both laterally and anteroposteriorly.
   b. The trunk is positioned, so flexion of the hips is minimized to prevent hip contracture.
   c. The arms are flexed at the elbow with the hands resting against the lateral abdomen.
   d. The legs are extended in a neutral position with the toes pointed toward the ceiling.
   e. The heels are suspended in a space between the mattress and the footboard to prevent heel pressure.
   f. Trochanter rolls are placed under the greater trochanters in the hip joint areas.
2. Sidelying or lateral position
   a. The head is in line with the spine.
   b. The body is in alignment and is not twisted.
   c. The uppermost hip joint is slightly forward and supported by a pillow in a position of slight abduction.
   d. A pillow supports the arm, which is flexed at both the elbow and shoulder joints.
3. Prone position
   a. The head is turned laterally and is in alignment with the rest of the body.
   b. The arms are abducted and externally rotated at the shoulder joint; the elbows are flexed.
   c. A small, flat support is placed under the pelvis, extending from the level of the umbilicus to the upper third of the thigh.
   d. The lower extremities remain in a neutral position.
   e. The toes are suspended over the edge of the mattress.

Therapeutic Exercise

1. It has been reported that there is a daily loss of 1% to 1.5% of initial strength in an immobilized older adult.
2. The goals of therapeutic exercise are to develop and retrain deficient muscles, to restore as much normal movement as possible to prevent deformity, to stimulate the functions of various organs and body systems, to build strength and endurance, and to promote relaxation.
3. Perform passive range-of-motion (ROM) exercise.
   a. Carried out without assistance from the patient.
   b. The purpose is to retain as much joint ROM as possible and to maintain circulation.
   c. Move the joint smoothly through its full ROM (see Box 5-2, pages 106 to 109). Do not push beyond the point of pain.
4. Perform active assistive ROM.
   a. Carried out by the patient with the encouragement and assistance of the nurse.
   b. The purpose is to encourage normal muscle function.
   c. Support the distal part and encourage the patient to take the joint actively through its ROM.
   d. Give only the amount of assistance necessary to accomplish the action.

BOX 5-2 Range of Motion

SHOULDER

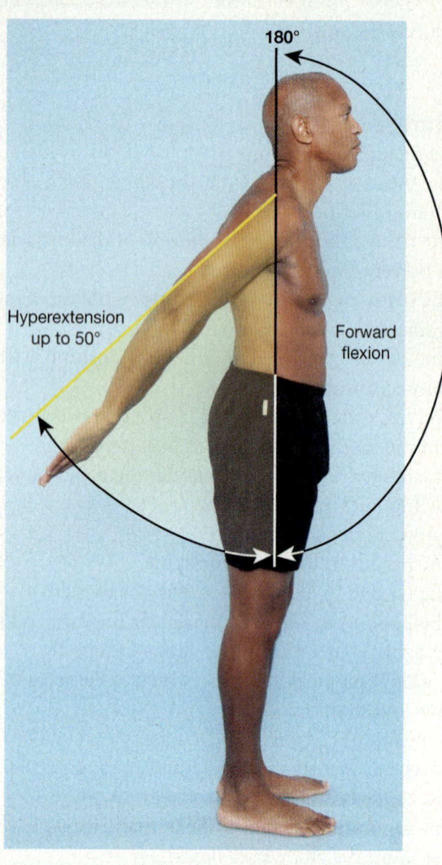

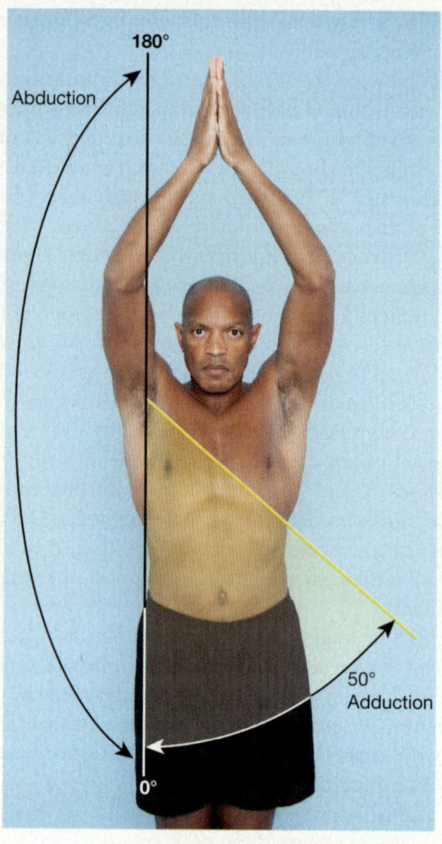

ELBOW

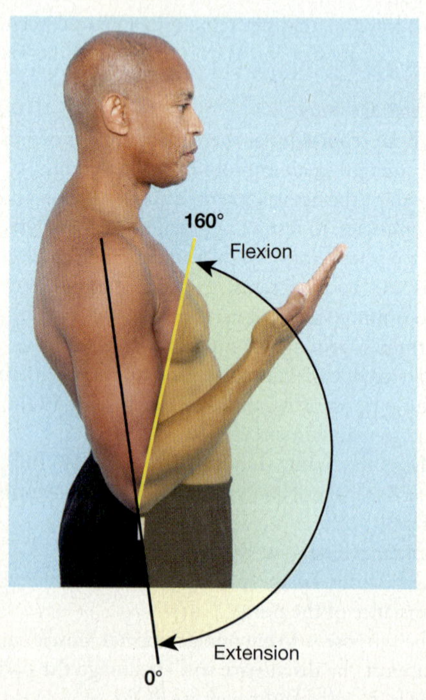

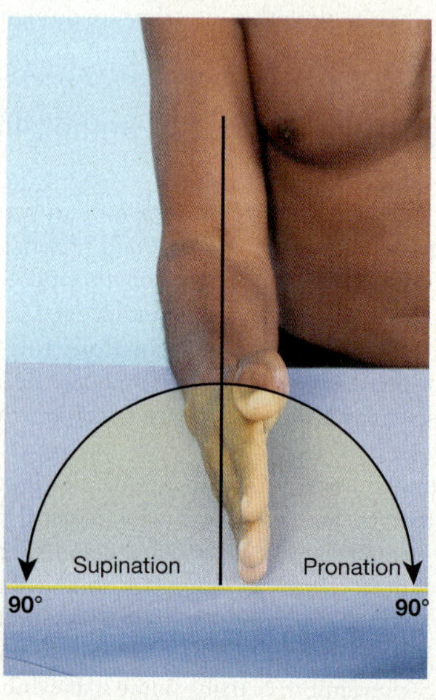

BOX 5-2 **Range of Motion (*continued*)**

WRIST

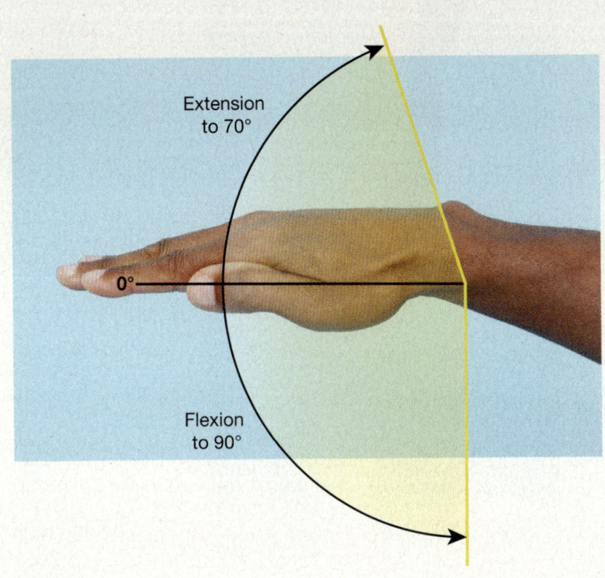

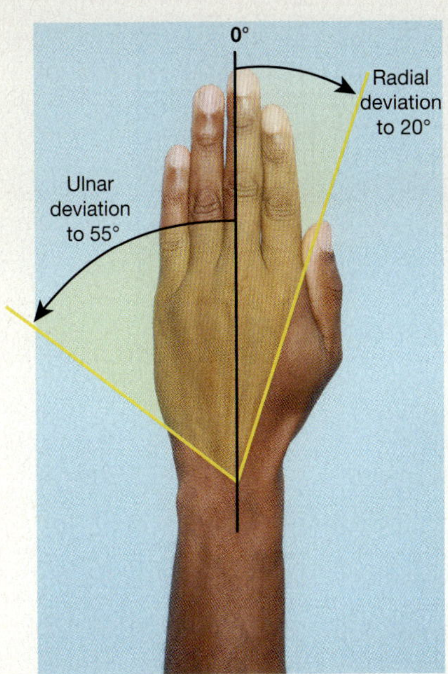

THUMB

Flexion

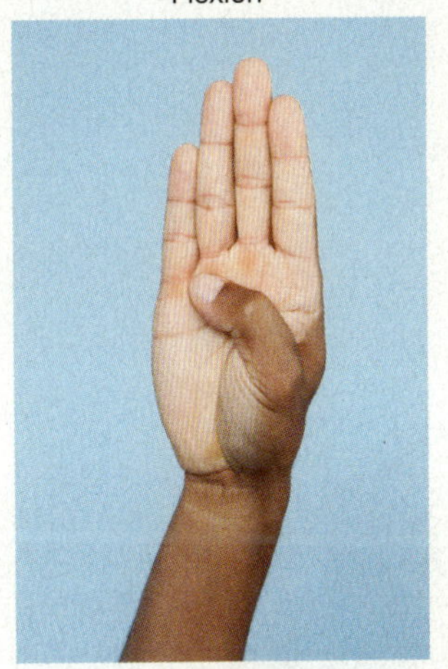

Extension

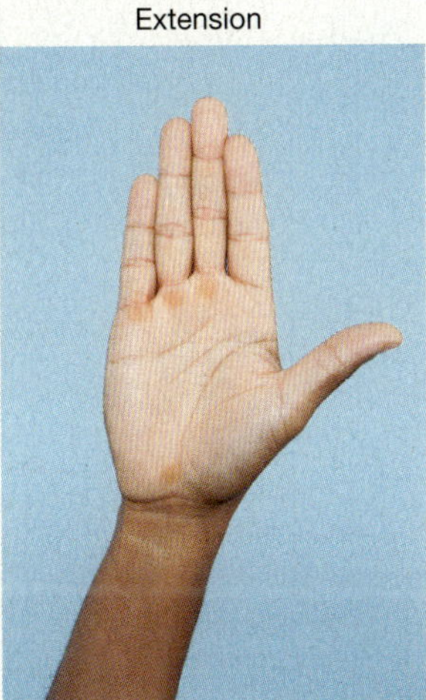

Opposition

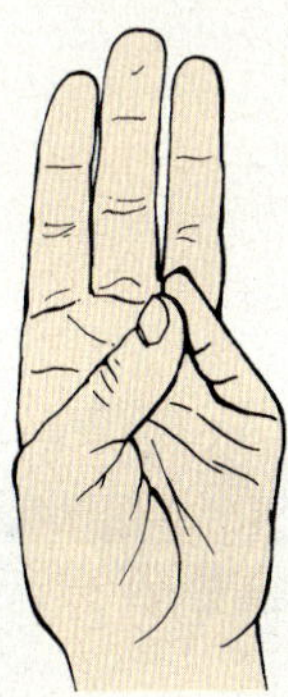

FINGERS

Adduction

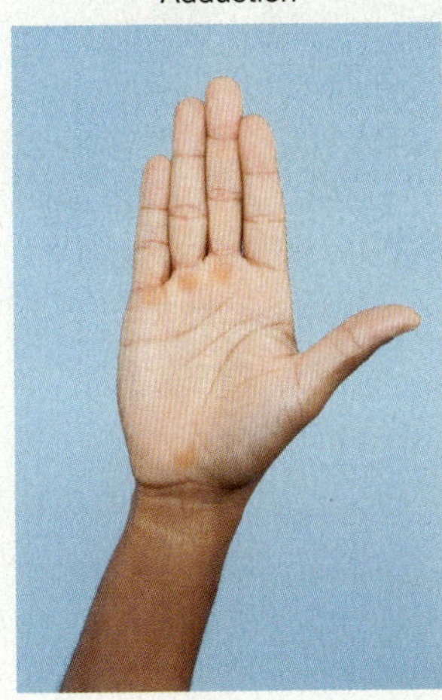

Abduction

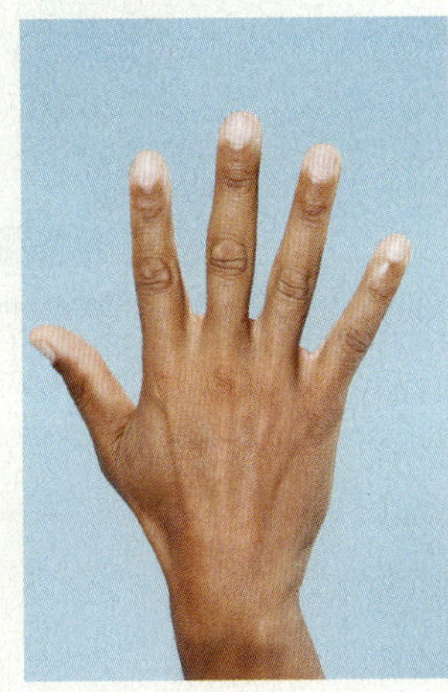

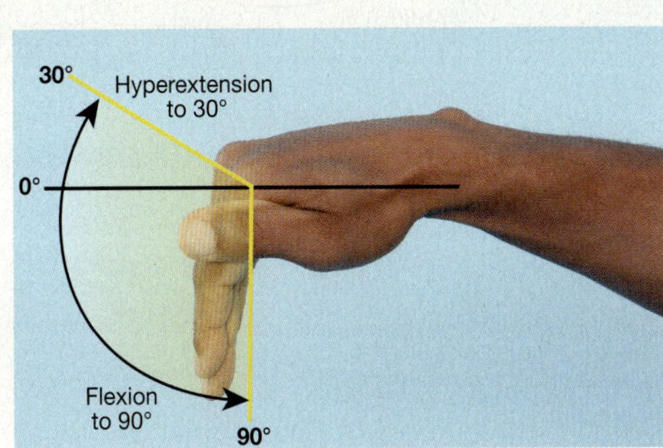

(*continued*)

BOX 5-2 Range of Motion (*continued*)

ANKLE

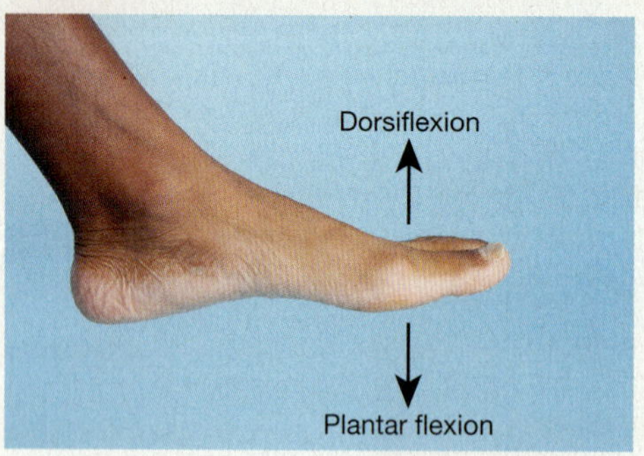

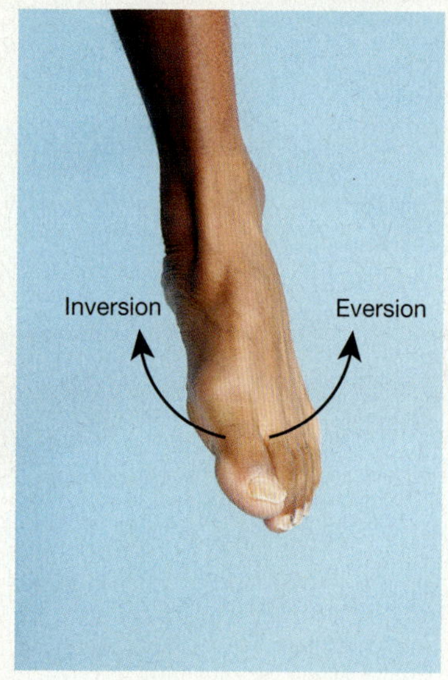

TOES

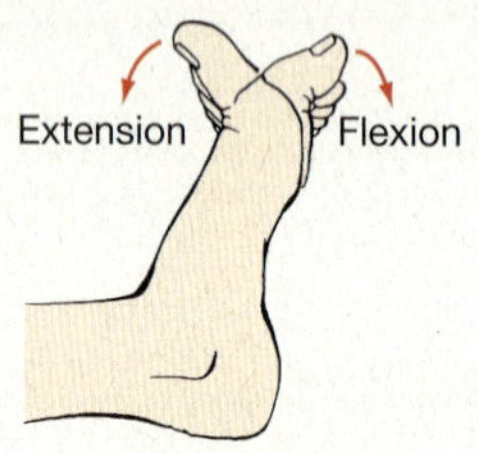

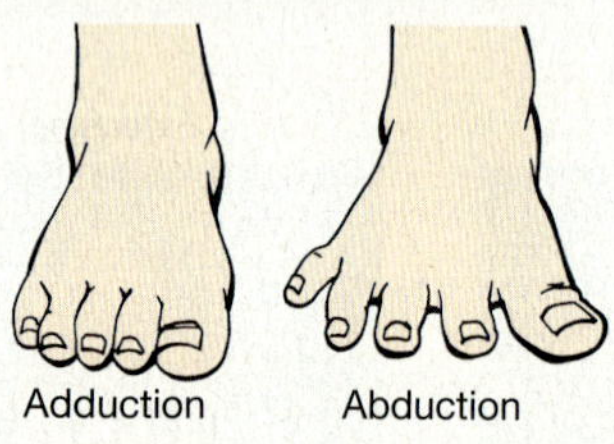

HIP

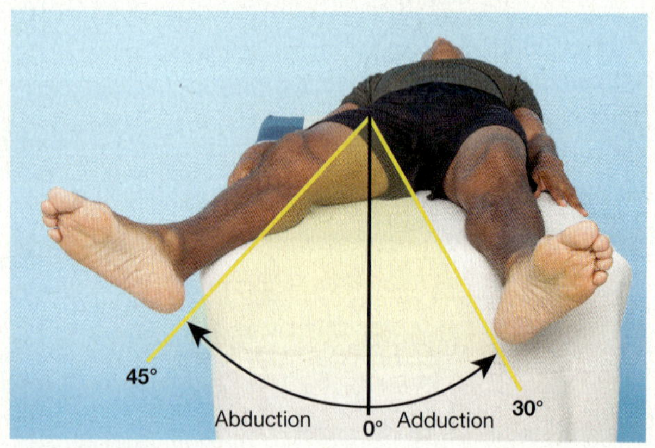

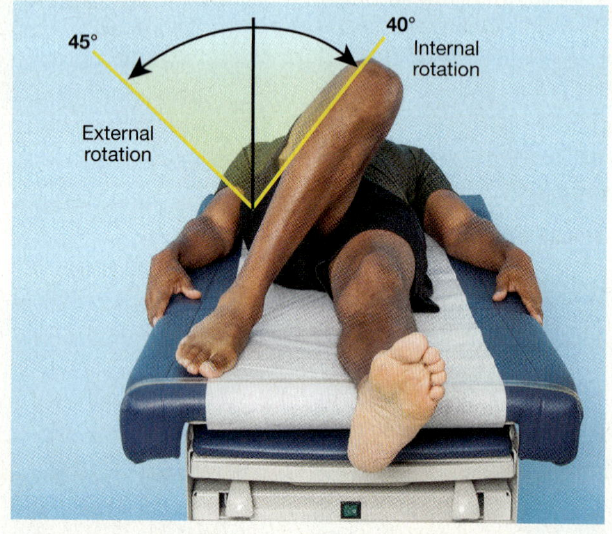

BOX 5-2 Range of Motion (*continued*)

KNEE

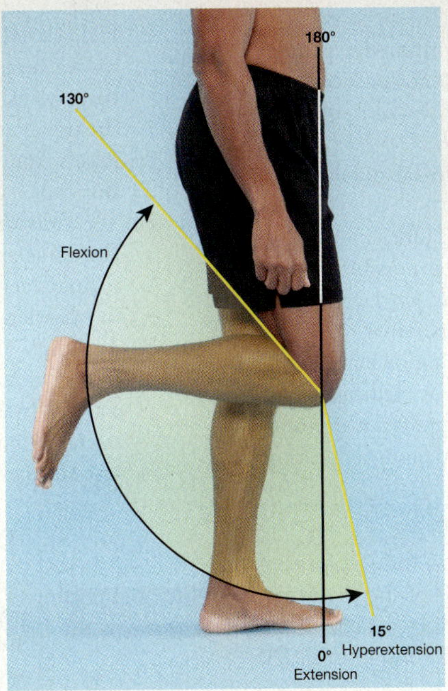

CERVICAL SPINE

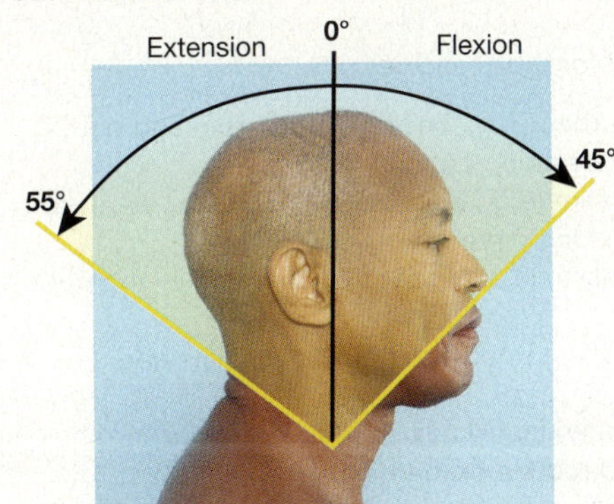

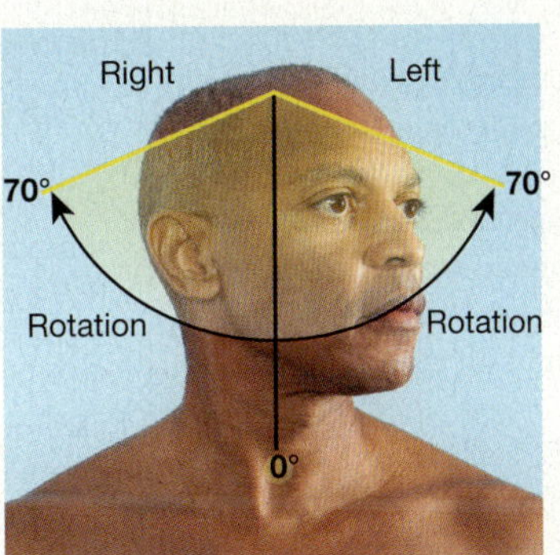

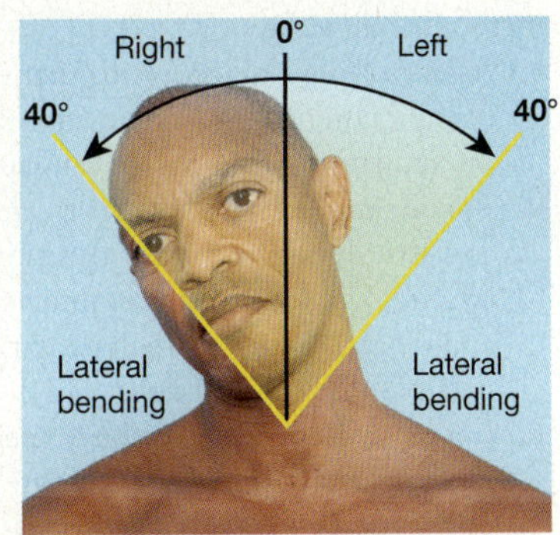

Most images in this box are reprinted with permission from Weber, J., & Kelley, J. (2022). Health assessment in nursing (7th ed., Figs. 24-6; 24-7; 24-8; 24-13; 24-14; 24-16A, B; 24-20A, B; 24-23A, C, D, E; 24-34A, B; 24-25C, D; 24-30). Wolters Kluwer; the exceptions are images for Thumb (Opposition) and Toes, which are from Weber, J., & Kelley, J. (2006). Health assessment in nursing (3rd ed.). Lippincott Williams & Wilkins (photographs by Barbara Proud).

5. Encourage active ROM.
   a. Accomplished by the patient without assistance.
   b. The purpose is to increase muscle strength.
   c. When possible, active exercise should be done against gravity.
   d. Encourage the patient to move the joint through the full ROM without assistance.
   e. Make sure that the patient does not substitute another joint movement for the one intended.
   f. Other active forms of exercise include turning from side to side, turning from back to abdomen, and moving up and down in bed.
6. Assist with resistive exercise.
   a. Carried out by the patient working against resistance produced by either manual or mechanical means.
   b. The purpose is to increase muscle strength.
   c. Encourage the patient to move the joint through its ROM while you or someone else provides slight resistance at first and then progressively increases resistance.
   d. Weights may be used and are attached at the distal point of the involved joint.
   e. The movements should be done smoothly.
7. Teach isometric or muscle-setting exercise.
   a. Involve alternately contracting and relaxing a muscle while keeping the part in a fixed position; performed by the patient.
   b. The purpose is to maintain strength when a joint is immobilized.
   c. Teach the patient to contract or tighten the muscle as much as possible without moving the joint.
   d. The patient holds the position for several seconds and then relaxes.

Rehabilitation and Restorative Care

Characteristics

1. The primary goal is restoring the patient to the maximum functional level.
2. Multidisciplinary service involving input from the primary care provider; nursing personnel; physical, occupational, speech, and recreational therapists; social worker; psychologist; and dietitian.
3. Rehabilitation and restorative nursing involve developing a rehabilitation philosophy of care.
   a. Patients are encouraged, and allowed sufficient time, to perform as much of their personal care as possible.
   b. Goals are set *with* the patient rather than *for* the patient.
   c. Prevention of further impairment is imperative.
   d. Focus on skin and wound care, regaining or maintaining bowel and bladder function, independent medication use, good nutritional status, psychosocial support, an appropriate activity–rest balance, and patient and family education.

EVIDENCE BASE Resnick, B., Boltz, M., Galik, E., Fix, S., Holmes, S., Zhu, S., & Barr, E. (2021). Testing the implementation of function-focused care in assisted living settings. *Journal of the American Medical Directors Association, 22*(8), 1706–1713.e1. https://doi.org/10.1016/j.jamda.2020.09.026

Nursing and Patient Care Considerations

1. Impaired cognitive function may have an impact on the quality of rehabilitation.
   a. Assess for physical problems that may exacerbate cognitive dysfunction (e.g., infection, adverse drug effects, metabolic or circulatory problems, or fatigue).
   b. Provide innovative measures to encourage ambulation, active ROM, and increased function; provide frequent verbal cues and large-print reminders; focus on basic self-care abilities and activities that are consistent with the individual's past life experiences.
   c. Implement appropriate safety measures, such as bed side rails, proper lighting, appropriate staffing, and avoidance of chemical and physical restraints.
2. Disability has a tremendous impact on a patient's body image and requires an adjustment by the patient. Be aware of the stages of psychological reaction the patient may undergo.
   a. Period of confusion, disorganization, and denial.
   b. Period of depression or anxiety and grief.
   c. Period of adaptation and adjustment.
3. Interventions in rehabilitation nursing include:
   a. Provide an atmosphere of acceptance.
   b. Identify and encourage positive coping patterns.
   c. Encourage socialization and participation in group activities.
   d. Give positive reinforcement and feedback about progress.
   e. Involve families as much as possible.
4. Use suggested interventions to motivate patients to engage in functional activities and exercise.

Community and Home Care Considerations

1. Family or significant other caring for the patient at home can have a major impact on the rehabilitation process.
   a. Assist family or significant other to face the reality of the patient's disability and to set appropriate and achievable goals.
   b. Involve family or significant other in the decision-making and in the patient's care for them to develop and practice the skills necessary for the patient to reach rehabilitation goals.
   c. Help extend and enlarge family's or significant other's skills by teaching problem-solving, treatment needs of the patient, ways to communicate to health care providers, and the use of community resources.
   d. Assess the level of caregiver fatigue or burnout (see Box 5-3).
2. For the individual living independently:
   a. Encourage adherence to a regular exercise program, which includes aerobic exercise, stretching, and strength training to maintain optimal function.
   b. The CDC (2021) recommends that all adults should accumulate at least 150 minutes of moderate-intensity physical activity (walking, biking, swimming, etc.) per week and strength training (heavy gardening, yoga, lifting weights, resistance exercises) at least 2 days a week.

BOX 5-3 Caregiver Strain Index

Instructions given to the caregiver: I am going to read a list of things that other people have found to be difficult in caring for patients after they come home from the hospital. Would you tell me whether any of these apply to you? (Give the examples.)

Score one point for "yes" and zero for "no"

1. Sleep is disturbed (e.g., because _____ is in and out of bed or wanders around at night).
2. It is inconvenient (e.g., because helping takes so much time or it is a long drive over to help).
3. It is a physical strain (e.g., because of lifting in and out of a chair).
4. It is confining (e.g., because helping restricts free time or cannot visit).
5. There have been family adjustments (e.g., because helping has disrupted routine or there has been no privacy).
6. There have been changes in personal plans (e.g., had to turn down a job or could not go on vacation).
7. There have been other demands on my time (e.g., from other family members).
8. There have been emotional adjustments (e.g., because of severe arguments).
9. Some behavior is upsetting (e.g., incontinence; _____ has trouble remembering things; _____ accuses others of taking things).
10. It is upsetting to find that _____ has changed so much from before (e.g., _____ is a different person from before).
11. There have been work adjustments (e.g., because of having to take time off).
12. It is a financial strain.
13. It has been completely overwhelming (e.g., because of worry about _____ or concerns about how to continue to manage).

Scoring: Total score of 7 or more suggests a greater level of stress.

Reprinted with permission from Robinson, B. C. (1983). Validation of a caregiver strain index. Journal of Gerontology, 38(3), 344–348. https://doi.org/10.1093/geronj/38.3.344. The Gerontological Society of America.

c. Based on individual functional ability, physical activity recommendations may be achieved with the following sample schedule:
   i. Aerobic exercise: Brisk walking 5 days per week for at least 30 minutes.
   ii. Flexibility: Stretch every day.
   iii. Strength training: Do strength-building activities 2 to 3 days per week that involve all major muscle groups.
d. For further information on exercise for older adults living independently, see www.cdc.gov/physicalactivity/everyone/guidelines/olderadults.html.

CARE OF SELECT HEALTH PROBLEMS

Some health problems are more common in older adults and persons with a disability due to mobility impairment and other altered functional ability. These include urinary and fecal incontinence, urinary retention, pressure injuries, osteoporosis, and altered nutrition. Older adults may also deal with altered response to medications and Alzheimer disease (AD).

Altered Nutritional Status

There is growing evidence that a balanced diet along with other health promotion behavior contributes to wellness and longevity. However, normal age-related changes, behavioral changes, and pathologic conditions may lead to malnutrition in the older adult or the person with a disability.

Pathophysiology and Etiology

1. Changes in the oral cavity, including loss of teeth, diminished saliva production, and difficulty with mastication, may cause decreased food intake.
2. A decrease in gastric secretion with reduced pepsin hinders protein digestion and iron, vitamin B_{12}, calcium, and folic acid absorption; there are no significant changes in the small or large bowel.
3. Sensory changes involving taste and smell cause anorexia.
4. Psychosocial factors including changes in living situation, depression, loneliness, decreased choice of food for institutionalized adults, need to adhere to special diets, socioeconomic status, and ability to obtain and prepare food all impact what is eaten.
5. Alcohol use interferes with the absorption of B-complex vitamins. Additionally, alcohol is high in calories and low in nutritional value.
6. Medications can alter nutrition by directly decreasing absorption and utilization of nutrients. Indirectly, medications can result in anorexia, xerostomia, dysgeusia, and early satiety.
7. Dysphagia, which commonly occurs after stroke, intubation, or head and neck surgery, or is related to developmental disability, chronic neuromuscular disorder, or dementia, may cause decreased food intake.
8. With age, there is a decrease in energy needs because of a decrease in muscle mass (total caloric need decreases by 30%).

Nursing Assessment

1. Be alert for patients who complain of difficulty swallowing and difficulty managing saliva. Watch for coughing after swallowing, sounding "wet" after eating, and pocketing food in the cheeks.
2. Assess for absent or diminished gag reflex.
3. Assess for a 10% weight loss over 6 months (marasmus) or weight loss along with low serum albumin levels (kwashiorkor), which are signs of protein–energy malnutrition.
4. Determine if the cholesterol level is below 130 mg/dL, which also may indicate malnourishment.

Nursing Interventions

1. Encourage good mouth care and promote oral health.
2. Encourage patients to avoid alcohol if possible; refer for counseling if necessary and compensate for the nutritional consequences of alcohol use disorder with liquid supplements and B vitamins.
3. Review all prescription and over-the-counter (OTC) medications with patients, and evaluate the influence of these on nutritional status.
4. If food procurement, preparation, and enjoyment are a problem, identify community resources to offer assistance in obtaining food and community meals.
5. In large facility settings, environmental factors may influence food enjoyment. Encourage socialization when eating, and try to minimize the negative effects of disruptive people or settings. Try to improve aesthetics.
6. To compensate for age-related changes in taste and smell, encourage the use of low-sodium food additives.
7. Encourage proper body position (e.g., sitting upright during mealtimes) and staying up for 30 minutes after eating to help with digestion.
8. If possible, encourage five to six small meals per day rather than three large meals.
9. If appropriate, encourage family to bring in favorite foods for patient.
10. Position food on the plate so that if there is visual neglect, or impairment, patient is best able to see the food served.
11. Identify patients with dysphagia and obtain a referral to a speech therapist.
    a. Work with the speech therapist and primary health care provider to determine what consistency of food is safe for patient to swallow.
    b. Use good compensatory techniques if indicated. These include sitting upright, tucking and turning the head, placing the food on the unaffected side of the tongue, swallowing twice to clear the pharyngeal tract, tucking the chin to the chest, and bringing the tongue up and back and holding the breath to swallow.
    c. Write out swallowing instructions for patient and family and educate family regarding the importance of maintaining these precautions.

Patient Education and Health Maintenances

1. Educate the patient and their family or significant other about basic nutritional requirements and on overcoming barriers that interfere with optimal nutrition.
   a. The Required Dietary Allowances for healthy adults are not age dependent, with three exceptions: decreased caloric intake and decreased protein intake (1 g/kg) for older adults, and decreased iron requirements for postmenopausal females.
2. Encourage the patient at home to eat a well-balanced diet to maintain an optimal nutritional state.
3. Suggest vitamin preparations with the fewest number of minerals and vitamins needed to prevent interactions and avoid megadoses.

4. Advise taking calcium carbonate, iron, and zinc at least 2 hours apart and taking vitamins at the same time daily.
5. Advise taking iron on an empty stomach and taking fat-soluble vitamins (A, D, E, and K) with food.
6. Educate about different types of calcium preparations:
   a. Calcium carbonate is more difficult to absorb on an empty stomach; it needs an acidic environment to enhance absorption. The percentage of calcium absorbed decreases as the calcium load increases; therefore, calcium carbonate absorption is greatest in doses of 500 mg or less, with food.
   b. Because calcium citrate is highly soluble in acid, it is better absorbed on an empty stomach. The citrate form does not need gastric acid for absorption.
   c. Calcium lactate can be absorbed at various pHs and does not need to be taken with food for absorption.

Urinary Incontinence

EVIDENCE BASE Batmani, S., Jalali, R., Mohammadi, M., & Bokaee, S. (2021). Prevalence and factors related to urinary incontinence in older adults women worldwide: A comprehensive systematic review and meta-analysis of observational studies. *BMC Geriatrics, 21*(1), 212. https://doi.org/10.1186/s12877-021-02135-8

Approximately 13 million Americans suffer from urinary incontinence. Approximately 35% of older adults admitted to an acute care hospital will develop urinary incontinence. The prevalence increases significantly for older adults living in nursing homes; it is estimated that 77% to 90% of residents in nursing homes are incontinent of urine. A person with a disability may have urinary incontinence for a variety of reasons, often due to mobility challenges.

Pathophysiology and Etiology

1. There are five basic types of urinary incontinence:
   a. Stress—an involuntary loss of urine with increases in intra-abdominal pressure. Usually caused from weakness and laxity of pelvic floor musculature or bladder outlet weakness.
   b. Urge—involves leakage of urine because of inability to delay voiding after sensation of bladder fullness is perceived. This is associated with detrusor hyperactivity, central nervous system (CNS) disorders, or local genitourinary conditions.
   c. Overflow—because of a leakage of urine resulting from mechanical forces on an overdistended bladder. This results from mechanical obstruction or hypomobility of the detrusor muscle.
   d. Mixed—symptoms of both stress and urge incontinence secondary to both an overactive detrusor and pelvic floor/urethral incompetence.
   e. Functional—involves urinary leakage associated with inability to get to the toilet because of cognitive or physical functioning.

Nursing Assessment

Because of the prevalence and increased incidence of incontinence in older adults and adults with a disability, it is imperative that nurses include urine function in their assessments.

1. Identify reversible causes of incontinence using the DRIP acronym:
   D—Delirium, especially new-onset delirium.
   R—Restricted mobility, retention.
   I—Infection (especially sudden-onset cystitis), inflammation (such as atrophic vaginitis or urethritis), impaction (fecal).
   P—Polyuria (from poorly controlled diabetes or diuretic treatment), pharmaceuticals (including psychotropics, anticholinergics, alpha-agonists, beta-agonists, calcium channel blockers, opioids, alpha-antagonists, and alcohol).
2. Evaluate lower urinary tract function.
   a. Stress maneuvers are evaluated by asking the patient, with a full bladder, to cough three times while standing. Observe for urine leakage.
   b. Check for postvoid residual by inserting a 12- or 14-Fr straight catheter a few minutes after the patient voids or use a portable ultrasound bladder scanner to measure postvoid urine residual.
   c. Evaluate bladder filling by leaving the straight catheter in place and using a 50-mL syringe to fill the bladder with sterile water. Hold the syringe about 6 inch (15 cm) above the pubic symphysis. Continue to fill the bladder in 25-mL increments until the patient feels the urge to void. Observe for involuntary bladder contractions. These contractions are detected by continuous upward movement of the column of fluid in the absence of abdominal straining.

Nursing Interventions

1. For stress or urge incontinence, teach Kegel (pelvic floor muscle) exercises.
   a. Teach the patient to first practice stopping the stream of urine while voiding to identify proper contraction of the pubococcygeal muscle; contraction will result in stopping flow, and relaxation allows flow.
   b. Once proper contraction is verified, advise patient to practice contraction of the muscle for 3 seconds and then relaxation of the muscle for 3 seconds in sets of 15 three times per day.
   c. The exercise can be practiced anywhere at any time because it involves contraction of an internal muscle; encourage patient to try them sitting, standing, and lying down. The abdomen should be relaxed, and no movement should be visible by doing Kegel exercises.
2. Assist with biofeedback that involves the use of bladder, rectal, or vaginal pressure recordings to train patients to contract pelvic floor muscles and relax the abdomen.
3. Institute a behavioral training program, using bladder records, biofeedback, and pelvic floor exercises for patients with stress or urge incontinence.
4. Institute other interventions such as:
   a. Bladder retraining—progressive lengthening or shortening of voiding intervals to restore the normal pattern of voiding; this is useful after period of immobility or catheterization.
   b. Scheduled toileting—using a fixed toileting schedule to prevent wetting episodes for patients with urge or functional incontinence.
   c. Habit training—involves using a variable toileting schedule based on patient's pattern of voiding; also incorporates positive reinforcement.
   d. Prompted voiding—includes regular prompts to void every 1 to 2 hours with positive reinforcement.
   e. Appropriate use of incontinence aids, such as pads or diapers.
   f. Judicious use of medications to help control urge incontinence. These include oxybutynin and tolterodine, among

others. Contraindicated in urinary or gastric retention, myasthenia gravis, and uncontrolled glaucoma. Monitor carefully for anticholinergic effects—dry mouth, heat intolerance, urine retention, constipation, drowsiness, dry eyes, and blurred vision.

Urine Retention

Urine retention is a common problem in the older adult and the person with a disability, frequently related to a neurologic or other underlying condition.

EVIDENCE BASE Fagard, K., Hermans, K., Deschodt, M., Van de Wouwer, S., Vander Aa, F., & Flamaing, J. (2021). Urinary retention on an acute geriatric hospitalisation unit: Prevalence, risk factors and the role of screening, an observational cohort study. *European Geriatric Medicine, 12*(5), 1011–1020. https://doi.org/10.1007/s41999-021-00495-3

DRUG ALERT Anticholinergic medications, such as antipsychotics, antidepressants, and antihistamines, also contribute to urinary retention. Additionally, opioids, anesthetics, alpha-agonists, beta-agonists, calcium channel blockers, urinary antispasmodics, and nonsteroidal anti-inflammatory agents are associated with urinary retention.

Pathophysiology and Etiology

1. Frequently encountered in the acute care setting, post catheterization, after stroke, in patients with diabetes because of atonic neuropathic bladder, because of fecal impaction, and in males with prostatic enlargement.
2. The patient with urine retention may void small amounts or may be incontinent continuously because of overflow of urine.
3. Patients with urine retention will usually have incontinence during the night.

POPULATION AWARENESS Urine retention may cause urinary tract infection, which can lead to poor outcomes for older adults.

Nursing Assessment

1. Take a complete history and perform a physical examination to rule out causes of urine retention.
2. Understand and identify the risk factors for urinary retention.
3. Monitor for a distended bladder and perform postvoid catheterization; there is no consensus of the upper or lower limits of a postvoid residual. However, residual of greater than 100 mL of urine is often used as a sign of urine retention.

Nursing Interventions

1. Remove fecal impaction to help patient regain bladder function.
2. If prostatic disease is suspected, appropriate referral is necessary.
3. Encourage male to use the standing position and female to use the sitting position to facilitate urinary flow; provide privacy.
4. Teach "double voiding." Finish voiding and then reposition oneself to void again. Also teach Credé method: have the patient massage the area of the abdomen directly over the bladder to "milk" the bladder to express any residual urine.
5. Evaluate medication regimen and discuss with health care provider the necessity or substitution of offending medication.
6. If no underlying condition is suspected, attempt intermittent catheterizations every 8 hours, in combination with regular voiding attempts by patient. If there is no response in 2 weeks (i.e., no decrease in postvoid residuals), referral to a urologist may be necessary for medical management of the urine retention.

Fecal Incontinence

Fecal incontinence is an inability to voluntarily control the passage of gas or feces. It occurs in an estimated 15% of females and 6% to 10% of males who live in the community and in an estimated 45% of older adults who live in nursing homes.

EVIDENCE BASE Pasricha, T., & Staller, K. (2021). Fecal incontinence in the elderly. *Clinics in Geriatric Medicine, 37*(1), 71–83. https://doi.org/10.1016/j.cger.2020.08.006

Pathophysiology and Etiology

1. Fecal continence depends on normal rectal and anal sensation, rectal reservoir capacity, and internal and external sphincter mechanisms.
2. In institutionalized older adults, fecal impaction is a primary cause of fecal incontinence because of stool leaking around a fecal mass.
3. In noninstitutionalized adults, fecal incontinence is commonly associated with dysfunction of one of the anorectal continence mechanisms, such as impaired contractile strength of the sphincters and lower rectal volume capacity. Stroke and spinal cord injuries cause loss of sensation in the rectal area.
4. Sometimes, functional or cognitive impairment and depression may inhibit motivation and the ability to remain continent.
5. Commonly, no cause can be determined for the fecal loss, and it is believed that the incontinence may be due to a degenerative injury to the pudendal nerve.

Nursing Assessment

1. Assess overall function, cognition, and affect.
2. Assess baseline bowel status through health history or observation.
3. Assess severity and frequency of symptoms, including quantity of fecal incontinence.
4. Perform a rectal examination to check for impaction or decreased rectal sphincter tone.
5. If the fecal incontinence is diarrheal in nature, stool evaluation for leukocytes, culture and sensitivity, ova and parasites, and *Clostridium difficile* may be indicated.

Nursing Interventions

1. Increase dietary fiber to add bulk to the stool to stimulate regular defecation, if there is no infection and no impaction present.
2. Try antidiarrheals such as loperamide, as directed, for managing diarrhea.
3. Try to set up a regular bowel evacuation pattern once an impaction is detected and removed. This includes regular

toileting times, set preferably after breakfast, and increased fluid and fiber intake. Use laxatives only as a last resort.
4. In patients who are bedbound, increased fiber in the diet is contraindicated. These patients may require a bisacodyl suppository or an enema to help with rectal evacuation two to three times per week.
5. Treat those with neurogenic fecal incontinence, such as patients with spinal cord injuries and poststroke, to induce fecal evacuation at regularly scheduled times.
6. Administer glycerin or bisacodyl suppository two to three times per week before breakfast (to use the normal gastrocolic reflex that starts after the first meal of the day) to help induce a complete rectal evacuation and decrease stool incontinence.

Patient Education and Health Maintenance

1. Explain to patient and family that it is not necessary to have bowel movements every day.
2. Advise avoidance of laxatives, which may induce diarrhea.
3. Encourage fibrous foods that stimulate the bowel to be eaten daily, preferably at breakfast, such as stewed prunes, citrus fruits, and bran cereals. Make sure that help is available to toilet patient when the urge to defecate is felt.
4. Recommend a home remedy to maintain regular bowel movements: 3 tbsp applesauce, 2 tbsp bran, and 1 tbsp prune juice mixed, refrigerated, and given at least 1 tbsp each morning.

Pressure Injuries

EVIDENCE BASE Cowan, L., Broderick, V., & Alderden, J. G. (2020). Pressure injury prevention considerations for older adults. *Critical Care Nursing Clinics of North America, 32*(4), 601–609. https://doi.org/10.1016/j.cnc.2020.08.009

National Pressure Injury Advisory Panel, European Pressure Ulcer Advisory Panel and Pan Pacific Pressure Injury Alliance. (2019). *Prevention and treatment of pressure ulcers/injuries: Quick reference guide 2019*. Cambridge Media.

Pressure injuries involve both deep tissue injuries that may include unbroken skin and localized broken or ulcerations of the skin or deeper structures. They most commonly result from prolonged periods of bed rest in acute- or long-term care facilities; however, they can develop within hours in the compromised individual (see Figure 5-2).

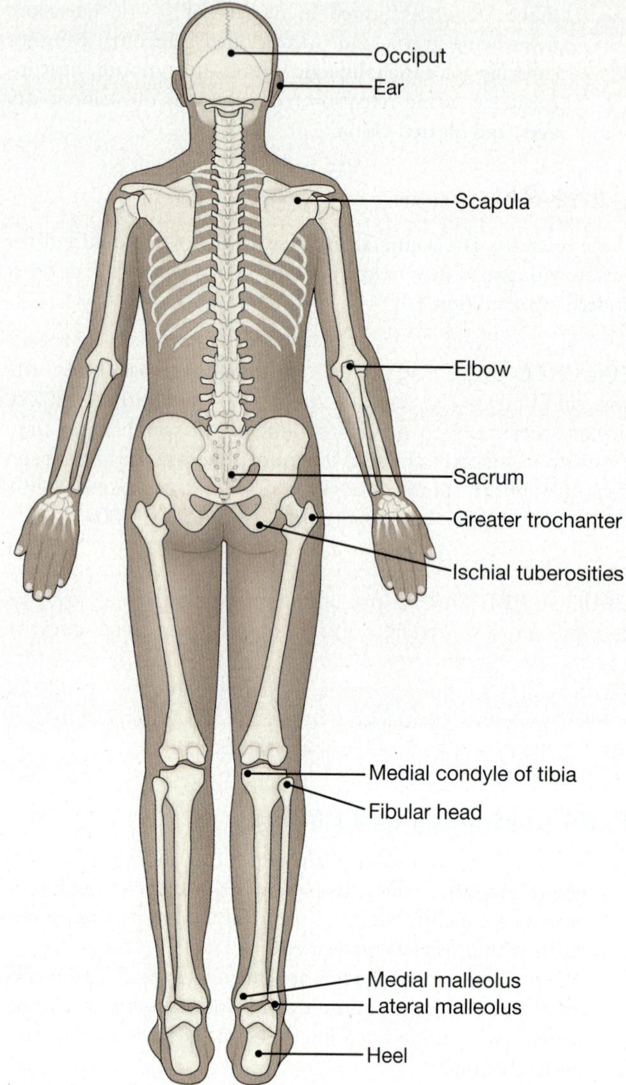

Figure 5-2. Areas susceptible to pressure injuries. (Reprinted with permission from Hinkle, J. L., Cheever, K. H., & Overbaugh, K. [2022]. *Brunner and Suddarth's textbook of medical-surgical nursing* [15th ed., Fig. 56-1]. Wolters Kluwer.)

Pathophysiology and Etiology

Factors in the Development of Pressure Injuries

1. Pressure of 70 mm Hg applied for longer than 2 hours can produce tissue destruction; healing cannot occur without relieving the pressure.
2. Friction contributes to pressure injury development by causing abrasion of the stratum corneum.
3. Shearing force, produced by sliding of adjacent surfaces, is particularly important in the partial sitting position. This force ruptures capillaries over the sacrum.
4. Moisture on the skin results in maceration of the epithelium.

Risk Factors for Pressure Injuries

1. Bowel or bladder incontinence.
2. Malnourishment or significant weight loss.
3. Edema, anemia, hypoxia, or hypotension.
4. Neurologic impairment or immobility.
5. Altered mental status, including delirium or dementia.

Nursing Assessment

1. Assess for risk factors for pressure injury development and alter those factors, if possible.
2. Assess skin of the older adult frequently for the development of pressure injuries. The Braden Scale for Predicting Pressure Sore Risk is one of the most commonly used instruments for predicting the development of pressure injuries. The Braden Scale assesses pressure injury risk in six areas: sensory perception, skin moisture, activity, mobility, nutrition, and friction/shear.
3. Stage the injury so appropriate treatment can be started. The National Pressure Injury Advisory Panel advocates the following staging system (see Figure 5-3):
   a. Stage 1A—intact skin with non-blanchable redness of a localized area, usually over a bony prominence.

A

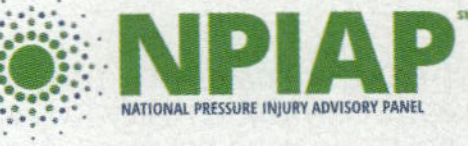

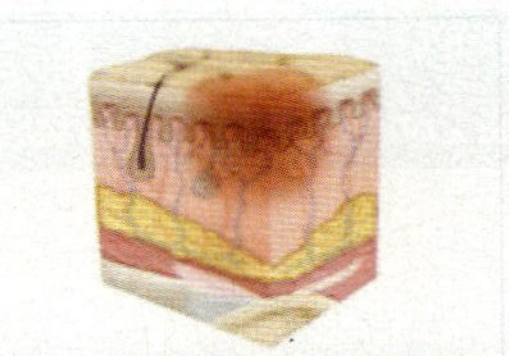
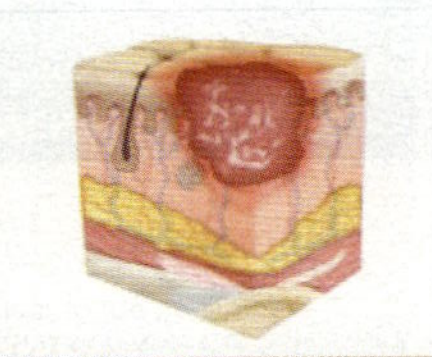
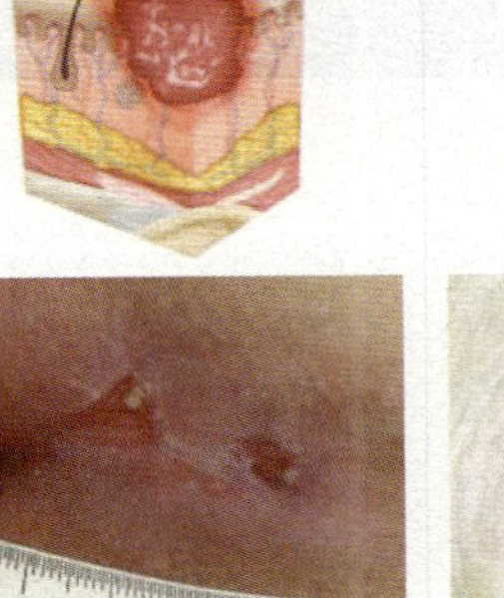
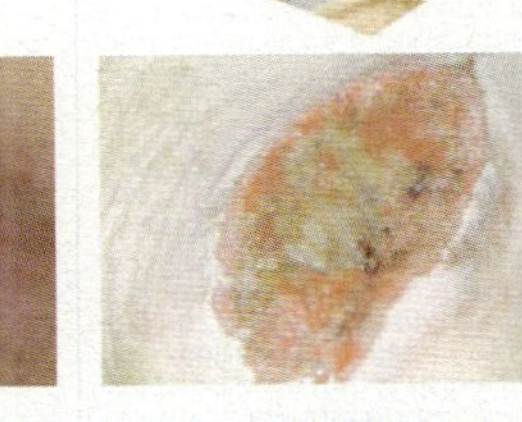
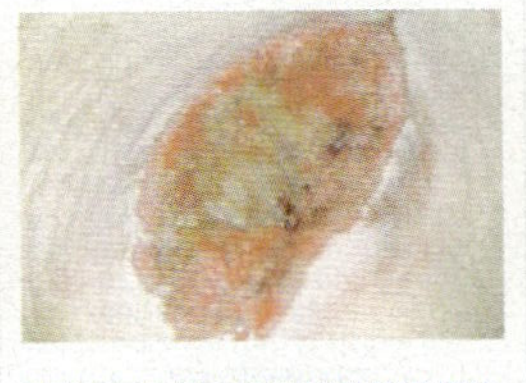
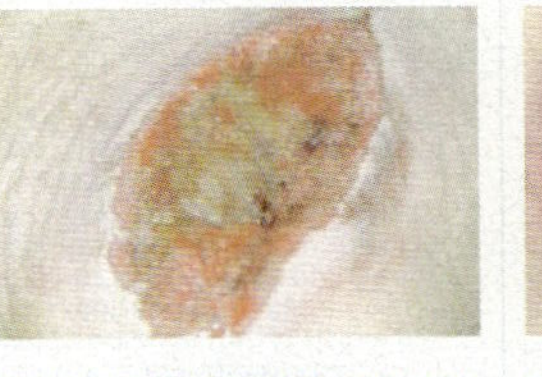
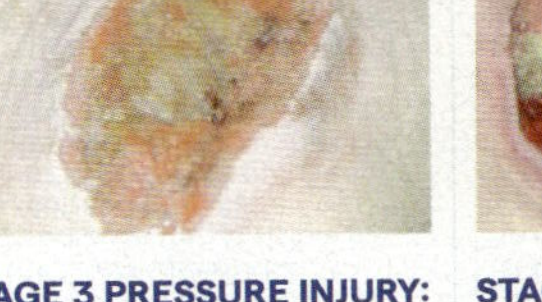
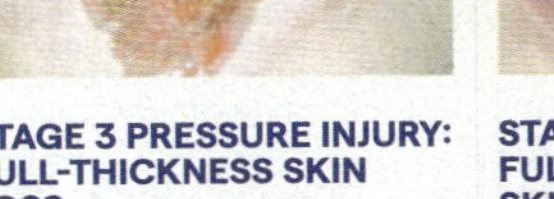
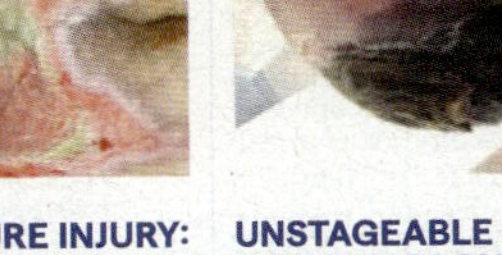

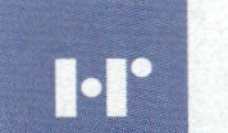

Figure 5-3. Stages of pressure injury. **(A)** For lightly pigmented skin and

B

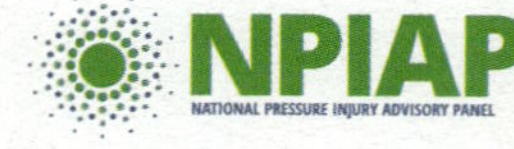

NPIAP STAGING FOR DARKLY PIGMENTED SKIN

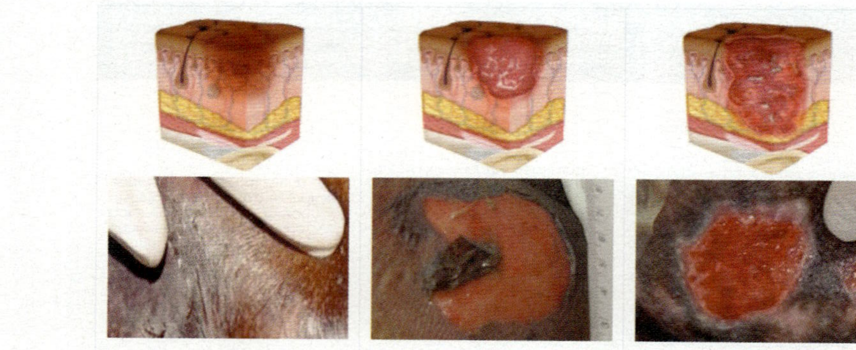

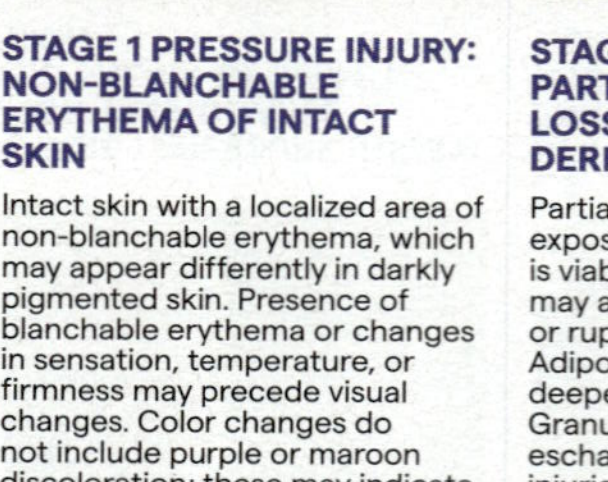

STAGE 1 PRESSURE INJURY: NON-BLANCHABLE ERYTHEMA OF INTACT SKIN

Intact skin with a localized area of non-blanchable erythema, which may appear differently in darkly pigmented skin. Presence of blanchable erythema or changes in sensation, temperature, or firmness may precede visual changes. Color changes do not include purple or maroon discoloration; these may indicate deep tissue pressure injury.

STAGE 2 PRESSURE INJURY: PARTIAL-THICKNESS SKIN LOSS WITH EXPOSED DERMIS

Partial-thickness skin loss with exposed dermis. The wound bed is viable, pink or red, moist, and may also present as an intact or ruptured serum-filled blister. Adipose (fat) is not visible and deeper tissues are not visible. Granulation tissue, slough and eschar are not present. These injuries commonly result from adverse microclimate and shear in the skin over the pelvis and shear in the heel.

STAGE 3 PRESSURE INJURY: FULL-THICKNESS SKIN LOSS

Full-thickness loss of skin, in which adipose (fat) is visible in the ulcer and granulation tissue and epibole (rolled wound edges) are often present. Slough and/or eschar may be visible. The depth of tissue damage varies by anatomical location; areas of significant adiposity can develop deep wounds. Undermining and tunneling may occur. Fascia, muscle, tendon, ligament, cartilage or bone is not exposed. If slough or eschar obscures the extent of tissue loss this is an Unstageable Pressure Injury.

STAGE 4 PRESSURE INJURY: FULL-THICKNESS LOSS OF SKIN AND TISSUE

Full-thickness skin and tissue loss with exposed or directly palpable fascia, muscle, tendon, ligament, cartilage or bone in the ulcer. Slough and/or eschar may be visible. Epibole (rolled edges), undermining and/or tunneling often occur. Depth varies by anatomical location. If slough or eschar obscures the extent of tissue loss this is an Unstageable Pressure Injury.

UNSTAGEABLE PRESSURE INJURY: OBSCURED FULL-THICKNESS SKIN AND TISSUE LOSS

Full-thickness skin and tissue loss in which the extent of tissue damage within the ulcer cannot be confirmed because it is obscured by slough or eschar. If slough or eschar is removed, a Stage 3 or Stage 4 pressure injury will be revealed. Stable eschar (i.e. dry, adherent, intact without erythema or fluctuance) on an ischemic limb or the heel(s) should not be softened or removed.

DEEP TISSUE PRESSURE INJURY: PERSISTENT NON-BLANCHABLE DEEP RED, MAROON OR PURPLE DISCOLORATION

Intact or non-intact skin with localized area of persistent non-blanchable deep red, maroon, purple discoloration or epidermal separation revealing a dark wound bed or blood-filled blister. Pain and temperature change often precede skin color changes. Discoloration may appear differently in darkly pigmented skin. This injury results from intense and/or prolonged pressure and shear forces at the bone-muscle interface.

TIPS FOR STAGING DARKLY PIGMENTED SKIN:

- Moisten the skin
- Inspect for changes in pigmentation
- Palpate for edema
- Ask about pain in the area
- Avoid direct light

Hillrom™

Educational materials produced by Hillrom in collaboration with NPIAP.

APR41801 REV 1 14-FEB-2020 ENG – US

Figure 5-3. (*continued*) **(B)** for darkly pigmented skin. (National Pressure Ulcer Advisory Panel, European Pressure Ulcer Advisory Panel, & Pan Pacific Pressure Injury Alliance. (2014). Prevention and treatment of pressure ulcers: Quick reference guide (E. Haesler, Ed.). Cambridge Media. Used with permission of the National Pressure Ulcer Advisory Panel (2024).)

b. Stage 2—partial thickness skin loss with exposed dermis presenting as a shallow open ulcer with a red–pink wound bed, without slough; may also present as an intact or open/ruptured serum-filled blister.
c. Stage 3—full-thickness skin loss, with subcutaneous fat that may be visible but bone, tendon, or muscle is not exposed; may include undermining and tunneling. Slough may be present but does not obscure the depth of tissue loss.
d. Stage 4—full-thickness skin and tissue loss with exposed bone, tendon, or muscle; slough or eschar may be present on some parts of the wound bed; often includes undermining and tunneling.
e. Unstageable—full-thickness tissue loss in which the base of the ulcer is covered by slough or eschar in the wound bed.
f. Suspected deep tissue injury—a localized area of intact skin or blood-filled blister, maroon or purple in color, caused by damage of the underlying soft tissue from shear or pressure.

Nursing Interventions

Prevent Pressure Injury Development

1. Provide meticulous care and positioning for immobile patients.
   a. Inspect skin several times daily.
   b. Wash skin with mild soap, rinse, and pat dry with a soft towel.
   c. Lubricate skin with a bland lotion to keep skin soft and pliable.
   d. Avoid poorly ventilated mattress that is covered with plastic or impermeable material.
   e. Employ bowel and bladder programs to prevent incontinence.
   f. Encourage ambulation and exercise.
   g. Promote nutritious diet with optimal protein, vitamins, and iron.
2. Teach patient and family or significant other the importance of good nutrition, hydration, activity, positioning, and avoidance of pressure, shearing, friction, and moisture.

Relieve the Pressure

1. Avoid elevation of the head of bed greater than 30 degrees.
2. Reposition every 2 hours.
3. Use special devices to cushion specific areas (especially bony areas), such as lamb's wool or fleece pads, convoluted foam mattresses, booties, or elbow pads. Lift heels off the bed in patients who are bedbound. Do not use donut devices or flotation rings because they cause increased pressure to the surrounding area.
4. Use an alternating-pressure mattress or air-fluidized bed for patients at high risk to prevent or treat pressure injuries.
5. Provide for activity and ambulation as much as possible.
6. Advise frequent shifting of weight and occasional raising of buttocks off chair while sitting.

Clean and Debride the Wound

1. Use normal saline for cleaning and disinfecting wounds.
2. Apply wet-to-dry dressings or enzyme ointments for debridement as directed or assist with surgical debridement.

Treat Local Infection

1. Avoid obtaining wound cultures because open wounds are always colonized with bacteria unless there is evidence of systemic infection or progressive local infection such as cellulitis.
2. Apply topical antibiotics to locally infected pressure injury as prescribed.

Cover the Wound

1. Cover the wound with a protective dressing as this minimizes disruption of migrating fibroblasts and epithelial cells and results in a moist, nutrient-rich environment for healing to occur.
   a. Polyurethane thin film dressings can be used for superficial low-exudate wounds. They are air and water permeable but do not absorb exudate.
   b. Hydrocolloids can provide padding to wounds but can lead to maceration; they are not oxygen permeable.
   c. Polyurethane foam/membrane dressings absorb exudate and are oxygen permeable.
   d. Hydrogel dressings are multilayered and include properties of both hydrocolloids and polyurethane (see Table 5-2 for a comparison of selected occlusive dressings).

Osteoporosis

Osteoporosis is a condition in which the bone matrix is lost, thereby weakening the bones and making them more susceptible to fracture. Bone mineral density is 2.5 standard deviations below the peak bone density for young adults (T score −2.5). Decrease in bone density of 1.5 to 2.5 below mean young adult bone density is termed *osteopenia* (T score −1.5 to −2.5). It is the most age-related metabolic bone disorder.

Pathophysiology and Etiology

1. The rate of bone resorption increases over the rate of bone formation, causing loss of bone mass.
2. Calcium and phosphate salts are lost, creating porous, brittle bones.
3. Occurs most commonly in postmenopausal females but may also occur in males.
4. Other factors include:
   a. Age.
   b. Inactivity.
   c. Chronic illness.
   d. Medications, such as corticosteroids, excessive thyroid replacement, and cyclosporine.
   e. Calcium and vitamin D deficiency.
   f. Family history.
   g. Smoking and alcohol use.
   h. Diet—caffeine has been linked as a risk factor.
   i. White and Asian individuals have higher risk incidence.
   j. Body type—small frame/short stature, low body fat.

Clinical Manifestations

1. Asymptomatic until later stages.
2. Fracture after minor trauma may be first indication. Most frequent fractures associated with osteoporosis include fractures of the distal radius, vertebral bodies (compression fractures), proximal humerus, pelvis, and proximal femur (hip).
3. May have vague complaints related to aging process (stiffness, pain, weakness).
4. Estrogen deficiency may be noted.

Diagnostic Evaluation

1. X-rays show changes only after 30% to 60% loss of bone.
2. Dual-energy x-ray absorptiometry (DEXA) scanning shows decreased bone mineral density (T score −2.5 or lower).
3. Serum and urine calcium levels are normal.

Table 5-2 Comparison of Selected Occlusive Dressing

DRESSING TYPE	EXAMPLES	APPROPRIATE USE	ADVANTAGES	DISADVANTAGES
Absorption	Debrisan Hydrophilic Beads	• Stage 2–4 pressure injuries with drainage	• Absorbs drainage and deodorizes wound	• Need to change dressing 1–2 times daily
Hydrocolloid	DuoDerm	• Stage 1–2 pressure injuries	• Provides padding • Easy to apply • Water impermeable • No skin excoriation	• Poor absorptive capacity • Poor oxygen exchange • Messy residue • Pressure areas possible
Polyurethane	OpSite, Tegaderm	• Nondraining wounds	• Transparent • Self-adhesive • Oxygen permeable	• No absorptive capacity • May cause excoriation • Difficult to apply
Polyurethane membrane	Mitraflex	• Skin tears • Tape burns • Blisters • Stage 2 pressure injuries • Low-moderate exudate wounds	• Good absorptive ability • Good oxygen exchange • Water impermeable • May debride	• May cause excoriation
Polyurethane foam	Epi-Lock Optifoam	• Skin tears • Tape burns • Blisters • Stage 2 pressure injuries • Low to moderate exudate wounds	• Good absorptive ability • Good oxygen exchange • Water impermeable • May debride • No skin excoriation	• Nonadhesive
Hydrogel	Vigilon, Biofilm	• Stage 1–3	• No skin excoriation • Transparent • Some ability to absorb drainage • Easy to apply	• Difficult to apply • Nonadherent
Debriding enzyme	Elase, Travase	• Stage 3–4	• Acts against devitalized tissue • Not appropriate for hard, dry eschar	• May damage healthy tissue

4. Serum bone matrix Gla protein (a marker for bone turnover) is elevated.
5. Bone biopsy shows thin, porous, otherwise normal bone.

Management

Management is primarily preventive.

1. Identify patients at risk for fractures.
2. Reduce modifiable risk factors through improved diet, smoking cessation, decreased alcohol consumption, and other healthy lifestyle choices.
3. Adequate intake of calcium—1.2 g/day—may be preventive.
4. Adequate intake of vitamin D.
   a. Vitamin D plays a major role in calcium absorption and bone health. With age, there is a decreased ability to take in vitamin D through the skin; therefore, replacement is recommended.
   b. Food sources are milk products, egg yolks, fish, and liver; however, dietary intake of vitamin D is limited.
   c. Vitamin D can be manufactured in the skin through sunlight exposure; however, this may be limited by cloud cover, latitude, season, and skin cancer prevention methods that limit exposure.
   d. Recommended daily allowance for adults age 70 and older is 800 international units.
5. Weight-bearing exercise (e.g., walking) throughout life.
6. Hormone replacement therapy is no longer recommended for osteoporosis prevention or treatment because the risks outweigh the benefits.
7. Raloxifene, an estrogen receptor agonist, is an alternative to estrogen. Not as effective as estrogen, but does show some benefits in preserving bone density. No increase in the risk of breast cancer.
8. Calcitonin administered by nasal spray may help prevent spinal fracture. Adverse effects are nasal burning and a runny nose.
9. Bisphosphonates, such as risedronate, alendronate, and ibandronate, bind to and inhibit osteoclast action, remain active on bone resorptive surfaces for 3 weeks, and do not impede normal bone formation. Bisphosphonates may cause gastrointestinal (GI) symptoms.
   a. Associated with improved bone density and decreased hip and spinal fracture rate.
   b. Bisphosphonates must be taken with fluid but not food, and the patient must remain upright for 30 minutes after taking the pill to prevent esophagitis.

c. Long-acting injectables, such as zoledronic acid, and teriparatide are protective for females at high risk for fractures and increase bone mass in males and females who are on long-term glucocorticoid therapy.
d. Long-term use of bisphosphonates typically requires drug holidays of 1 to 2 years to decrease the risk of femoral fractures.

10. Parathyroid hormones, teriparatide, and abaloparatide have limited utility because they require daily subcutaneous injections.
11. Denosumab, a monoclonal antibody treatment that is administered by subcutaneous injection every 2 months. Unlike bisphosphonates, denosumab is not contraindicated among individuals with renal disease.
12. Prevention of falls in older adults helps to prevent fractures.

EVIDENCE BASE Camacho, P. M., Petak, S. M., Binkley, N., Diab, D. L., Eldeiry, L. S., Farooki, A., Harris, S. T., Hurley, D. L., Kelly, J., Lewiecki, E. M., Pessah-Pollack, R., McClung, M., Wimalawansa, S. J., & Watts, N. B. (2020). American Association of Clinical Endocrinologists/American College of Endocrinology clinical practice guidelines for the diagnosis and treatment of postmenopausal osteoporosis-2020 update. *Endocrine Practice*, *26*(Suppl. 1), 1–46. https://doi.org/10.4158/GL-2020-0524SUPPL

Complications

1. Fractures.
2. Progressive kyphosis, loss of height (see Figure 5-4).
3. Chronic back pain from compression fracture.

Nursing Assessment

1. Obtain history of risk factors for osteoporosis, fractures, and other musculoskeletal disease.
2. Assess risk for falls and fractures—sensory or motor problems, improper footwear, lack of knowledge of safety precautions, and so forth. See Table 5-3 for assessment factors and interventions.
3. Assess pain level and efficacy of therapeutic interventions in patient with history of compression fractures.

Nursing Interventions

1. Administer non-opioid pain relievers, including topical analgesics, and educate patient on appropriate use.
2. Assist with putting on back brace and ensure proper fit, if ordered, while patient is ambulatory.
3. Encourage adherence to physical therapy appointments and practicing exercises at home to increase muscle strength surrounding bones and to relieve pain.
4. Encourage exercise for all age groups. Teach the value of walking daily throughout life to provide stress required for strong bone remodeling.
5. Provide dietary education in relation to adequate daily intake of calcium (1,200 mg) and vitamin D replacement. Calcium can be obtained through milk and dairy products, vegetables, and supplements. Anyone with a history of urinary tract calculi should consult with a health care provider before increasing calcium intake.
6. Suggest that perimenopausal females confer with their health care provider about the need for calcium supplements.

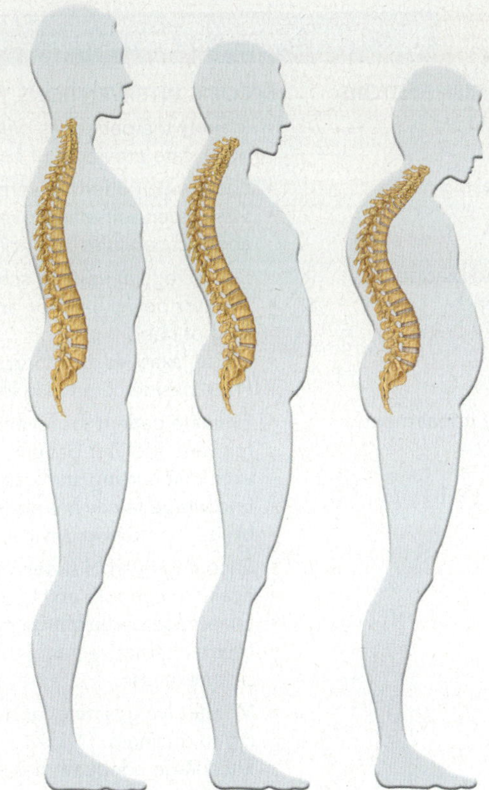

Figure 5-4. Progressive kyphosis in osteoporosis. (Reprinted with permission from Anatomical Chart Company.)

7. Alert patients to resources such as the National Osteoporosis Foundation. https://www.bonehealthandosteoporosis.org/

Patient Education and Health Maintenance

EVIDENCE BASE U.S. Preventive Services Task Force. (2018). *Osteoporosis to prevent fractures: Screening.* https://www.uspreventiveservicestaskforce.org/uspstf/recommendation/osteoporosis-screening

1. Encourage screening according to the U.S. Preventive Services Task Force (USPSTF) guidelines for all females older than age 65 and in postmenopausal women younger than 65 years who are at increased risk of osteoporosis.
2. According to the USPSTF, there is insufficient evidence to recommend osteoporosis screening in males.
3. Identify females at high risk for osteoporotic fractures in the community—frail, older White or Asian females with poor dietary intake of dairy products and little exposure to sun—and provide education and safety measures to prevent falls and fracture.
4. Make sure that diet contains optimal dietary calcium. Teach family and caregivers how to read labels, encourage dairy products, and add powdered milk to foods as possible. Use skim milk if cholesterol and fat intake is a consideration.
5. Make sure that supplements and other medications are being taken properly.
   a. Patient teaching is critical in dosing of bisphosphonates to prevent esophagitis. Patient must take this upon waking with 6 to 8 oz of water, at least 30 minutes before

Table 5-3 Assessment Factors and Interventions to Decrease Risk of Falls

KNOWN RISK FACTORS	SPECIFIC INTERVENTIONS TO DECREASE INDIVIDUAL RISK
History of falls	• Identify the patient as being at risk for falls: May use sticker on chart or door, inform families and other care providers of increased risk.
Fear of falling	• Encourage patient to verbalize feeling. • Strengthen self-efficacy related to transfers and ambulation by providing verbal encouragement about capabilities and ability to perform safely.
Bowel and bladder incontinence	• Set up regular voiding schedule (every 2 h or as appropriate based on patient need). • Monitor bowel function and encourage sufficient fluids and fiber (eight 8-oz glasses daily and 24 g of fiber). • Utilize laxatives as appropriate. • Place beside commode for night use.
Cognitive impairment	• Evaluate patient for reversible causes of cognitive impairment or delirium and eliminate causes as relevant. Monitor patient with cognitive impairment at least hourly with relocation of the patient such that nursing staff can observe and monitor regularly. • Encourage family member to hire staff or stay with patient continuously. • Utilize monitoring devices if available (i.e., bed/chair or exit alarms) rather than restraint.
Mood	• Encourage verbalization of feeling. • Evaluate patient's ability to concentrate and learn new information. • Encourage participation in daily activities. • Utilize alternative interventions, such as massage, aromatherapy, pet and plant therapy, and music or exercise.
Dizziness	• Monitor lying, sitting, and standing blood pressures and continually evaluate for factors contributing to dizziness. • Encourage adequate fluid intake (eight 8-oz glasses daily). • Set up environment to avoid movements that result in dizziness or vertigo. • Decrease or avoid alcohol use.
Functional impairment, immobility, impaired gait	• Encourage participation in personal care activities at the highest level (i.e., if possible encourage ambulation to bathroom rather than use of bedpan). • Refer to physical and occupational therapy as appropriate. • Facilitate adherence to exercise program when indicated. • Maintain safe and appropriate use of assistive device.
Medications	• Review medications with the primary health care provider and determine the need for each medication. • Make sure that medications are being used at the lowest possible dosages to obtain desired result.
Medical problems	• Work with primary health care provider to augment management of primary medical problem, such as Parkinson disease, heart failure, or anemia.
Environment	• Remove furniture if patient cannot be seated with feet reaching the floor. • Remove clutter. • Make sure furniture and any assistive devices used are in good condition. • Make sure lighting is adequate. • Make sure safety bars are available in the bathroom.

ingesting first food of the day, and must remain upright for 30 minutes after taking the medication. Weekly or monthly dosing increases adherence.

b. Calcitonin nasal spray dose is one spray in one nostril once per day; alternate nostrils each day.

6. Teach strategies to prevent falls. Assess home for hazards (e.g., scatter rugs, slippery floors, extension cords, inadequate lighting).
7. Obtain physical and occupational therapy consultations, as needed, to encourage use of walking aids when balance is poor and to improve muscle strength.

Altered Response to Medication

Adults older than age 65 consume 30% to 40% of all prescription drugs and OTC drugs. Age-related changes predispose older adults to problems with adverse drug effects.

Pathophysiology and Etiology

1. Drug absorption is affected by such age-related changes as:
   a. Decreased gastric acid.
   b. Decreased GI motility.
   c. Decreased gastric blood flow.
   d. Changes in GI villi.
   e. Decreased blood flow and body temperature in the rectum.
2. Drug distribution is affected by:
   a. Decreased body size.
   b. Decreased water content in the body.
   c. Increased total body fat.
   d. Drugs distributed in water have a higher concentration in older adults (e.g., gentamicin).
   e. Drugs distributed in fat have a wider distribution and less intense but prolonged effect (e.g., phenobarbital).

3. Drug metabolism in the older adult:
   a. Is altered by a decrease in liver size, blood flow, enzyme activity, and protein synthesis.
   b. Requires more time than in younger adults. Therefore, there is increased drug activity time in drugs that are metabolized in the liver (e.g., propranolol, theophylline).
4. Excretion of drugs is altered in older adults because of the following renal changes:
   a. Decreased renal tubular function and blood flow.
   b. This causes a decrease in renal filtration and an increase in blood levels of drugs that are excreted through the kidneys (e.g., cimetidine).

DRUG ALERT Drugs that may have severe adverse effects in older adults include anticholinergics (antihistamines, tricyclic antidepressants, drugs for treating urinary incontinence), nonsteroidal anti-inflammatory drugs (NSAIDs), any drug with a long half-life, and drugs with action on the central nervous system (CNS).

Nursing Assessment

1. Drug toxicities in older adults are different than they are in younger people.
2. Fewer symptoms may be identified, and they may develop slower; however, the reactions may be more pronounced and further advanced once they do present.
3. Behavioral and cognitive adverse effects are more common in older adults because the blood–brain barrier becomes less effective; the first reaction to a drug is confusion.
4. Many potential adverse drug effects are not identified because they are attributed to old age; fatigue, dementia, anorexia, or indigestion as adverse drug effects may not be reported.
5. Allergic reactions to drugs increase with age because of a greater likelihood of earlier exposure.

Nursing Interventions

1. Maintain awareness that the older adult is at greater risk for adverse drug reactions.
   a. This risk increases from 6% when two drugs are taken to 50% when five different drugs are taken and to 100% when eight or more drugs are taken.
2. Assess patient's ability to follow medication regimen by evaluation of:
   a. Cognition.
   b. Ability to read drug labels.
   c. Hand and muscle coordination.
   d. Swallowing difficulty.
   e. Lifestyle patterns, specifically smoking and alcohol use.
   f. Cultural beliefs toward medication.
   g. Ability to afford medication.
   h. Caregiver involvement in medication administration; assess caregiver if indicated.
3. Identify problems in the use of medications, such as:
   a. Lack of knowledge about drugs.
   b. Multiple medications and difficult administration techniques.
   c. Caregiver misunderstanding of medication use.
4. Appropriate interventions for safe drug use include:
   a. Obtain a complete drug history.
   b. Reinforce verbal instructions with written instructions using large-print and simple wording. If necessary, use color-coding rather than drug names.
   c. Write what the drug is used for and what the adverse effects can be.
   d. Make sure the patient or caregiver can open the medication container.
   e. Arrange medication schedules to coincide with regular activity, such as eating (if appropriate for that drug). Simplify the drug regimen as much as possible.
   f. If necessary, arrange a check-off system using a chart to ensure adherence or weekly pillbox.
   g. If possible, visibly evaluate all medications in the home, or ask patient to bring all medications for evaluation.
   h. Encourage patient to check expiration dates and discard all old or unneeded medications.
   i. Encourage patient to store medications in original containers in a dry, dark place.
   j. Encourage patient to avoid OTC medication without checking with the primary care provider before use.
   k. Encourage patient to report adverse drug effects.
   l. Work with prescribing caregiver and patient to maintain a medication regimen that follows the principles for geriatric drug use; start dosages low and go slow, use only necessary medications, titrate the dose to patient response, simplify the regimen, and have frequent reevaluations of the medication regimen.

POPULATION AWARENESS Physiologic changes with aging lead to increased blood alcohol level in older adults compared to younger individuals, especially in females. This may lead to falls, especially when alcohol is combined with other CNS agents.

Patient Education and Health Maintenance

1. Ask the patient or family to bring in all the patient's medications for clinic or office visits or whenever the patient goes to a facility to obtain an accurate medication history.
2. Ask the patient what vitamins, minerals, herbal supplements, and other OTC products are being used. Many patients do not consider these medications and will not readily supply the information unless specifically asked.
3. Alert patients and family members that many "natural" products sold over the counter still may cause adverse reactions and toxicity as well as interactions with other drugs.
4. Warn patients and families that many complementary and alternative medicine (CAM) therapies do not have proven effectiveness despite advertisements. CAM should be used as an adjunct to conventional therapy, and the patient should notify all health care providers of supplements and therapies being used.

Alzheimer Disease

The most common form of dementia is characterized by progressive impairment in memory, cognitive function, language, judgment, perception, and learned motor skills. Ultimately, patients cannot perform self-care activities and require total care.

Pathophysiology and Etiology

1. Gross pathophysiologic changes in the brain include cortical atrophy most prominent in the frontal and temporal lobes, enlarged ventricles, and atrophy of the hippocampus.

2. Microscopically, changes occur in the proteins of the nerve cells of the cerebral cortex and lead to accumulation of neurofibrillary tangles composed of the tau protein and neuritic plaques composed of the amyloid protein (deposits of protein and altered cell structures on the interneuronal junctions) and granulovascular degeneration. There is loss of cholinergic nerve cells, which are important in memory, function, and cognition.
3. Biochemically, neurotransmitter systems are impaired.
4. The cause is unknown, but risk factors include advanced age, female sex assigned at birth, family history of AD, and head trauma with a loss of consciousness. Indeed, research has identified four specific genes involved in predisposition to AD. Genes on chromosomes 1, 14, and 21 have been implicated in the causation of early-onset AD, whereas the #4 allele of the apolipoprotein gene on chromosome 19 appears to be associated with the development of AD after age 65.
5. Viruses, environmental toxins, cerebrovascular disease, and educational level may also play a role.

Clinical Manifestations

1. Disease onset is subtle and insidious. Initially, a gradual decline of cognitive function from a previously higher level may be noticed. Short-term memory impairment and problems with executive functioning (planning and organizing) is commonly the first characteristic in the earliest stages of the disease. Patients are forgetful and have difficulty learning and retaining new information. At least one of the following functional deficits is present:
   a. Memory impairment.
   b. Language disturbance (aphasia, may be receptive, expressive, or both).
   c. Visual processing and recognition difficulty (agnosia).
   d. Inability to perform skilled motor activities, such as dressing and walking (apraxia).
   e. Poor abstract reasoning, concentration, and impairment in executive functioning (planning and organizing).
2. Patients may have difficulty planning meals, managing finances, using a telephone, or driving without getting lost. Other classic signs include personality changes, such as irritability and suspiciousness, personal neglect of appearance, and disorientation to time and place.
3. The following clinical manifestations are typical in the middle stage of AD:
   a. Repetitive thoughts and actions (perseveration).
   b. Nocturnal restlessness.
   c. Apraxia (impaired ability to perform purposeful activity).
   d. Aphasia (impaired ability to speak).
   e. Agraphia (inability to write).
4. With disease progression, signs of frontal lobe dysfunction appear, including loss of social inhibitions and loss of spontaneity. Apathy, delusions, hallucinations, aggression, and wandering behavior often occur in the middle and late stages.
5. Patients in the advanced stage of AD require total care. Symptoms may include:
   a. Urinary and fecal incontinence.
   b. Emaciation.
   c. Resistiveness or rejection of care
   d. Inability to walk.
   e. Decreased responsiveness to verbal and physical stimulation.
   f. Difficulty swallowing (dysphagia).

Diagnostic Evaluation

1. Detailed patient history with corroboration by an informed source to determine cognitive and behavioral changes, their duration, and symptoms that may be indicative of other medical or psychiatric illnesses.
2. Noncontrast computed tomography (CT) scan to rule out other neurologic conditions, such as a stroke or tumor. Magnetic resonance imaging and single-photon emission CT may be used.
3. Neuropsychological evaluation, including some form of mental status assessment, to identify specific areas of impaired mental functioning in contrast to areas of intact functioning.
4. Laboratory tests include complete blood count, sedimentation rate, chemistry panel, thyroid-stimulating hormone, test for syphilis, urinalysis, serum B_{12}, folate level, and test for human immunodeficiency virus to rule out infectious or metabolic disorders.
5. Commercial assays for cerebrospinal fluid tau protein and beta-amyloid are available, but their use is limited. Genetic testing is available, but its use is controversial.

Management

DRUG ALERT Cholinesterase inhibitors were initially aimed at improving memory and cognition. These drugs, however, seem to have an important impact on the behavioral changes that occur in patients with cognitive impairment. Specifically, research studies have demonstrated that use of cholinesterase inhibitors improves the apathy, disinhibition, pacing, and hallucinations commonly noted in dementia. Be alert for drug interactions with NSAIDs, succinylcholine-type muscle relaxants, cholinergic and anticholinergic agents, drugs that slow the heart, and other drugs that are metabolized by the hepatic CYP2D6 or CYP3A4 pathways.

1. Primary goals of treatment for AD are to optimize functional abilities and improve quality of life by enhancing mood, cognition, and behavior. No curative treatment exists. Treatment includes pharmacologic and nonpharmacologic approaches.
2. Cholinesterase inhibitors were the first treatment for cognitive impairment of AD. These drugs improve cholinergic neurotransmission to help delay decline in cognition and function over time. There is also evidence that cholinesterase inhibitors may be helpful in decreasing agitated behaviors common in dementia.
   a. Donepezil is widely used in mild to moderate cases because it can be given once daily and is well tolerated; starting at 5 mg at bedtime and increased to 10 mg after 4 to 6 weeks. In patients with moderate to severe AD, the dose of donepezil may be increased to 23 mg daily; however, there is an increased risk of adverse GI side effects at this higher dose. Donepezil has also been shown to be beneficial in individuals with severe dementia.
   b. Galantamine is given with food in a dosage of 4 to 12 mg twice per day. Should be restarted at 4 mg bid if interrupted for several days. Dose should be reduced in cases of renal or hepatic impairment. Galantamine ER is an extended-release formula that can be given in once-daily dosing with dose ranges from 8 to 24 mg/day.
   c. Rivastigmine is given 1.5 mg twice per day with meals and increased up to 6 to 12 mg/day. Rivastigmine is also available in an oral solution and a patch form. Use of the

rivastigmine patch is associated with fewer GI side effects than oral use.

3. Memantine, an N-methyl D-aspartate-receptor antagonist, is approved for moderate to severe AD. Its mechanism of action involves regulation of the neurotransmitter glutamate. The immediate-release dosage is 10 mg bid, and the ER dosage begins at 7 mg once a day and is gradually increased to a maximum dose of memantine XR 28 mg once a day. The drug can be used concurrently with a cholinesterase inhibitor.
4. Studies indicate that other drugs, such as estrogen and NSAIDs, have not proven helpful in the treatment and prevention of AD.
5. Intravenous infusions of anti-amyloid beta monoclonal antibodies, such as aducanumab and lecanemab, have resulted in the reduction of beta-amyloid plaques in patients with mild cognitive impairment, but evidence of their clinical effectiveness has been mixed. Anti-amyloid beta monoclonal antibodies are associated with a significant risk of amyloid-related imaging abnormalities (ARIA) and brain bleeds.
6. Patients with depressive symptoms should be considered for antidepressant therapy.
7. Nonpharmacologic treatments used to optimize cognition and behavior include environmental manipulation that decreases stimulation, pet therapy, aromatherapy, massage, music therapy, and exercise.
8. If nonpharmacologic approaches have been applied consistently and have failed to adequately reduce the frequency and severity of behavioral symptoms that have the potential to cause harm to the patient or others, then the introduction of medications such as antipsychotics, benzodiazepines, anticonvulsants, antidepressants, and sedatives may be appropriate but will still need to be carefully and routinely monitored over time.
   a. The risk and potential benefits of any medication must be discussed with the patient (when appropriate) and the patient's family/decision maker.
   b. The minimum amount of a medication should be used for the shortest time possible.

DRUG ALERT Be aware that no medications are specifically approved by the U.S. Food and Drug Administration (FDA) to treat the neuropsychiatric and behavioral symptoms of individuals with dementia. Antipsychotics have been linked to a higher risk of death among older adults with dementia. This led the FDA to issue a boxed warning for antipsychotic use in dementia.

Complications

1. Increased incidence of functional decline.
2. Injuries such as falls due to lack of insight, hallucinations, and confusion.
3. Malnutrition because of inattention to mealtimes and hunger or lack of ability to prepare meals or feed self.

Nursing Assessment

1. Perform cognitive assessment for orientation, insight, abstract thinking, concentration, memory, and verbal ability.
2. Assess for changes in behavior and ability to perform ADLs.
3. Evaluate nutrition and hydration; check weight, skin turgor, and meal habits.
4. Assess motor ability, strength, muscle tone, and flexibility.

Nursing Interventions

Improving Cognitive Response

1. Simplify the environment: Reduce noise and social interaction to a level tolerable for the patient.
2. Maintain a predictable, structured routine, limit the number of choices available to the patient, use pictures to identify activities, and use structured group activities.
3. Encourage active participation in care as tolerated and provide positive feedback for tasks that are accomplished.
4. Provide opportunities for physical activity alternating with rest periods.
5. Avoid confrontations and arguments. Follow the patient's direction and individualize care as much as possible.
6. Maintain consistency in interactions and introduce new people slowly.

Preventing Injury

1. Avoid restraints, but maintain observation of the patient as necessary.
2. Provide for adequate lighting to avoid misinterpretation of the environment.
3. Remove unneeded furniture and equipment from the room.
4. Provide medical alert identification such as a bracelet.
5. Make sure patient has nonslip shoes or slippers that are easy to put on.
6. Encourage use of assistive safety devices, such as handrails and shower chairs.
7. Ensure physical activity as tolerated and range-of-motion (ROM) exercises to maintain mobility.

Ensuring Adequate Rest

1. Attempt to limit the use of medications that act on the CNS, such as anxiolytics and antipsychotics; however, if used, monitor for clinical response and potential adverse effects, including increased confusion, excess sedation, parkinsonism, extrapyramidal symptoms, and cardiovascular events.
2. Provide periods of physical exercise to expend energy.
3. Support normal sleep habits and bedtime rituals.
   a. Keep regular bedtime.
   b. Have patient change into pajamas at bedtime.
   c. Allow desired bedtime activity, such as snack, warm noncaffeinated beverage, listening to music, or prayer.
4. Maintain quiet, relaxing environment to avoid confusion and agitation.

Supporting Caregiver

1. Encourage caregiver to discuss feelings.
2. Encourage caregiver to maintain own health and emotional well-being.
3. Stress the need for relaxation time or respite care.
4. Assist the caregiver in finding resources, such as community or faith-based groups, social service programs, or facility-based support groups.
5. Assess caregiver's stress and refer for counseling.
6. Support decision to place patient in a long-term care facility.

Patient Education and Health Maintenance

1. Encourage regular medical checkups with attention to health maintenance every 3 to 6 months to provide ongoing medical surveillance of patient and stamina of caregivers. Include influenza vaccine and ensure that patient has had pneumococcal pneumonia vaccine.

2. Discuss advance directives for patients and discuss long-term placement options in anticipation of future needs to help family members adjust and plan arrangements.
3. Encourage patients to be involved in social and intellectual activities as long as possible, such as family events, exercise, and recreational activities and sharing the newspaper and other forms of media.
4. Assist caregivers to modify the home environment for safety, and advise families of safety hazards such as wandering and driving a car. Encourage use of door locks, electronic wander-alert guards, and registration with the "Safe Return" program through the Alzheimer's Association or local police department.
5. Remind family members of possible dangers around the house as patient becomes less responsible for behavior. Encourage caregivers to reduce the temperature of the hot water heater, remove dials from stove and other electrical appliances, remove matches and lighters, and safely store away tools and other potentially dangerous items.
6. Encourage activities that provide physical exercise and repetitive movement but that require little thought, such as dancing, painting, doing laundry, or vacuuming.
7. Teach patient and family to eliminate stimulants, such as caffeine, and maintain good nutrition.
8. Discuss with the family the need to organize finances and to make advanced directive decisions and guardianship arrangements before they are needed to allow the patient input into the process.
9. Advise about OTC products, such as ginkgo biloba, that have gained popularity; however, their clinical benefits have not been demonstrated to be better than placebo in well-designed randomized clinical trials. Although high doses of vitamin E (2,000 international units) have been shown to delay nursing home placement by a few months, there is no evidence of cognitive improvements, and doses higher than 400 international units have been associated with bleeding and cardiovascular events. Families should be encouraged to discuss their use with the health care provider and not abandon conventional treatment.
10. For additional information, refer families and caregivers to:
    Alzheimer's Association: www.alz.org
    National Institute on Aging: www.nia.nih.gov/Alzheimers
    Nursing Home Toolkit: Promoting Positive Behavioral Health: http://www.nursinghometoolkit.com/
    Function Focused Care: Optimizing Function with Physical Activity in Long Term Care Residents and Acute Care Patients: https://functionfocusedcare.wordpress.com/
    Dementia Care Caregiver Training Videos: https://www.uclahealth.org/medical-services/geriatrics/dementia/caregiver-education/caregiver-training-videos

LEGAL AND ETHICAL CONSIDERATIONS

All patients deserve to be treated with dignity. In addition, older adults and persons with a disability have special legal and ethical concerns. These populations deserve special attention to their rights when they cannot advocate or speak for themselves.

Restraint Use

Since the Nursing Home Reform Act took effect in October 1990, long-term care facilities throughout the United States have been required to follow guidelines emphasizing individualized, less restrictive care for residents.

The goal should be to minimize restraint use. And, although most nurses cite the rationale for placing a restraint on a patient is for patient safety, there is little evidence that patient safety or a reduction in injuries is achieved.

There are many alternative approaches to care as well as how to minimize risks associated with falls, as outlined at https://hign.org/consultgeri/resources/protocols/physical-restraints.

Guidelines

1. The following are the federal requirements for the use of restraints based on the 1987 Omnibus Budget Reconciliation Act and are consistent with the Centers for Medicare and Medicaid State Operations Manual: Appendix PP: Guidance to Surveyors for Long-Term Care Facilities: https://www.cms.gov/Regulations-and-Guidance/Guidance/Manuals/downloads/som107ap_pp_guidelines_ltcf.pdf.
2. These guidelines must be met in any long-term care facility that participates in Medicare or Medicaid. However, these guidelines are useful for health care providers working with older adults in all settings.
    a. The resident has the right to be free from any physical restraints imposed or psychoactive drug administered for purposes of discipline or convenience and not required to treat the resident's medical symptoms.
    b. Physical restraints are any manual method of physical or mechanical device, material, or equipment attached or adjacent to the resident's body that the person cannot remove easily, which restricts freedom of movement or access to one's body (includes leg and arm restraints, hand mitts, soft ties or vest, wheelchair safety bars, and geriatric chairs).
    c. There must be a trial of less restrictive measures unless the physical restraint is necessary to provide lifesaving treatment. If physical restraints are clinically indicated, the least restrictive intervention must be used for the least amount of time possible. Documentation must include frequent reevaluation of the need for restraints.
    d. The resident or legal representative must consent to the use of restraints.
    e. Residents who are restrained should be released, exercised, toileted, and checked for skin redness every 2 hours.
    f. The need for restraints should be reevaluated frequently.
    g. The specific facility will have to develop policies and procedures for the appropriate use of restraints and psychoactive drugs.
    h. Primary health care providers will have to write appropriate orders for restraints and psychoactive drugs.
3. The most frequently reported reason for nurses' use of restraints is to prevent patients from harming themselves or others. Specifically, they are used to prevent falls and prevent removal of catheters or IV lines.
4. Multiple studies have found that restraints actually increase incidence of falls, can result in patient strangulation, can increase patient confusion, can cause pressure injuries and nosocomial infections, can decrease functional ability, and can result in social isolation.
5. In regard to the patient's personal and social integrity, restraints have resulted in emotional responses of anger, fear, resistance, humiliation, demoralization, discomfort, resignation, and denial.

Alternative Interventions Instead of Restraints

1. Evaluate those patients who are considered to be in need of a restraint. Evaluation should include physical function and

cognitive status, elimination history, history of falls, vision impairment, BP (specifically evaluating for orthostatic hypotension), and medication use.
2. Attempt to correct any problems identified in the evaluation, such as vision impairment or unsafe gait.
3. Use the evaluation to determine patients at high risk of falling (e.g., those with confusion, orthostatic hypotension, multiple medication regimens, and altered gait).
4. Use interventions as alternatives to restraints as outlined in Box 5-4.

BOX 5-4 Techniques to Prevent Falls as Alternative to Restraints

FOR ALL PATIENTS

- Familiarize patient with the environment (i.e., identify call light or bell to ring, label the bathroom, kitchen, and closet).
- Have patient demonstrate ways to obtain help if needed.
- Place bed in low position with brakes locked if possible, or mattress on the floor.
- Make sure that footwear is fitted and nonslip and is used properly.
- Determine appropriate use of side rails based on cognitive and functional status.
- Utilize nightlight.
- Keep floor surfaces clean and dry.
- Keep room uncluttered and make sure that furniture is in optimal condition.
- Make sure patient knows where personal possessions are and can safely access them.
- Ensure adequate handrails in the bathroom (commode, shower, and tub), room, and hallway.
- Establish a care plan to maintain bowel and bladder function.
- Evaluate effects of medications that increase the patient's risk of falling.
- Encourage participation in functional activities and exercise at patient's highest possible level and refer to physical therapy as appropriate.
- Monitor patient regularly and encourage safe activities.

FOR PATIENTS AT HIGH RISK FOR FALLING WHEN WALKING INDEPENDENTLY

- Use specially designed chairs that make independent transfer difficult.
- Use a chair alarm and bed alarm when the patient cannot be visually supervised.
- Institute physical therapy and increased exercise activities to help strengthen muscles and improve function.
- For the patient who interferes with treatment, evaluate the need for invasive treatments. When such treatments are essential, use mittens or gloves rather than restraints.
- For the patient who wanders, provide an exercise program or establish a bounded environment in which the person can ambulate freely.
- For aggressive and agitated patients, be aware that restraints may only make the behavior worse. Provide a low-stimulus environment, consistent caregivers, and appropriate medications to help control the agitation. Music therapy has also been shown to decrease aggressive behavior.

Advance Directives

The 1990 Patient Self-Determination Act, which requires that patients be asked about the existence of advanced directives at the time of enrollment into a health care facility, has increased awareness of older adults' rights to determine their own care. Based on the ethical principle of autonomy (a person's privilege of self-rule), advance directives provide a clear and detailed expression of a person's wishes for care. Providing a patient with the opportunity to discuss their end-of-life plans is helpful. A four-step process includes initiating a discussion, facilitating the discussion, completing the document, and updating it.

Durable power of attorney for health care is also called medical power of attorney or *health care proxy*. It involves the designation of another person to make health care decisions for an incapacitated person. Many states have official documents that can be downloaded from their websites with detailed information about advanced directives and health care proxy.

EVIDENCE BASE Dinescu, A. (2021). Advance care planning. *Clinics in Geriatric Medicine*, *37*(4), 605–610. https://doi.org/10.1016/j.cger.2021.06.001

Types of Advance Directives

Living Wills

1. Living wills were the first and most widespread type of advance directive.
2. They were proposed as a mechanism for refusing "heroic" or unwanted medical intervention for the dying person.
3. They allow a person to state in writing that certain life-sustaining treatments should be withdrawn or withheld when that person is dying and unable to directly communicate their wishes.
4. Living wills only allow for the refusal of further treatment. They are not precise in terms of directives and focus only on the patient who is clearly terminally ill.

Health Care Proxy

1. This document appoints a proxy to act on behalf of another person, provides guidance for the proxy, and endures even when the maker is incapacitated.
2. This is always a written document.
3. The document states the preferences and perhaps even the values of its maker. It outlines the types of decisions the person would want to have made on their behalf.
4. Because no health care proxy document can cover all situations, the document should name a person who has the task of ensuring that the patient's wishes are honored. The proxy has the responsibility to interpret the document and extrapolate its contents to situations not specifically covered.

Medical Orders for Life-Sustaining Treatment (MOLST)

1. Many states have implemented a standard health care provider order form that indicates patient choices for a variety of life-sustaining treatment and is used across health care facilities.
2. MOLST is particularly important for patients with serious health conditions who:
   a. Want to avoid or receive any or all life-sustaining treatment.
   b. Are residents of long-term care facilities.
   c. Might die within a year.
3. Completion of the MOLST begins with a conversation or a series of conversations between the patient, patient's health

care agent or surrogate, primary care provider, and specialist care provider.
4. The health care provider should help delineate the patient's goals for care, review possible treatment options on the entire MOLST form, and facilitate informed medical decision-making.
5. The completed form can then also be used as a medical order across health care settings, from emergency personnel responding to the patient at home and to the staff of an intensive care unit.

Nursing and Patient Care Considerations

1. Under the Patient Self-Determination Act, all patients who enter a Medicare- or Medicaid-certified facility, nursing home, or home health agency must:
   a. Be provided with information about the state's laws and the facility's policies regarding advance directive.
   b. Be asked if they have advance directives.
   c. Have their advance directives placed in their medical record.
2. Education of patients and families is essential in helping them to understand the difference between living wills, MOLST, or health care proxy and determining which document best suits their needs.
3. Patients and families need to be educated about what is involved in undergoing various life-sustaining procedures, so they can make a decision regarding their future treatment.
4. Patients need to be informed that they can have more than one advance directive. That is, if a patient has a living will but is not terminally ill, encourage the patient to obtain a health care proxy to ensure that health care wishes will be met in any situation.
5. Information about completing advance directives can be obtained by contacting the National Palliative Care and Hospice Organization at *www.caringinfo.org*.

Advocacy for the Person With a Disability

There are an estimated 54 million Americans with a disability. Disability may strike any age group, ethnic or racial origin, and socioeconomic group. Nurses must not only provide skilled physical care to reduce complications and enhance the rehabilitation potential of persons with a disability, they must also act as advocates to help these individuals transcend their disabilities to be as independent, functional, and self-actualized as possible. The U.S. Surgeon General's Call to Action to Improve the Health and Wellness of Persons with Disability requests that all health care providers do the following:

- Give each patient the information necessary to live a long and healthy life.
- Listen and respond to the patient's health concerns.
- Communicate clearly and directly.
- Take the time needed to meet the patient's health care needs.

Definition of Disability

1. A disability can be viewed as any restriction or lack of ability to perform activities in a manner that is typical for most people.
2. The Americans with Disabilities Act (ADA) of 1990 defines a disability as a physical or mental impairment that substantially limits one or more major life activities. A person can also be considered disabled if there is a record of such an impairment or is regarded as having such an impairment.
3. Categories of disability include behavioral or emotional, sensory impaired disorder (hearing, vision, etc.), physical, and developmental.

Disability Laws

1. Many laws were enacted in the United States in the 20th century to provide funding for health care, education, and vocational rehabilitation.
   a. Initial laws were limited and focused on groups, such as wounded soldiers, injured workers, and veterans.
   b. The Social Security Act of 1935 broadened vocational rehabilitation to cover civilians and gave rehabilitation a permanent legislative basis.
   c. Medicare and Medicaid were created in 1965 as an amendment to the Social Security Act to provide health insurance and benefits to individuals based on age, presence of disability, and low income. Medical and nursing care are covered.
2. The Rehabilitation Act of 1973 was the first federal law in the United States to protect persons with a disability from discrimination.
   a. This law focused on access to public buildings and transportation, discrimination in the workplace, and independent living situations.
   b. However, this law applied only to facilities and programs supported by the federal government and did not affect the private sector.
3. The ADA amended previous legislation and made it illegal to discriminate against individuals with disabilities in the private sector as well as the public sector. Areas of focus are:
   a. Employers with 15 or more employees must provide qualified individuals with disabilities an equal opportunity to benefit from employment, including the hiring, training, promotion, and other privileges of employment. Employers are required to provide reasonable accommodations for the known physical or mental limitations of otherwise qualified individuals, so long as accommodations do not cause undue hardship to the employer.
   b. All state and local government institutions are required to provide equal opportunities for individuals with disabilities to take part in all programs, services, and activities, regardless of federal funding status.
   c. Public accommodations, which calls for the removal of barriers in public places that may be owned by private entities, such as restaurants, shops, hotels, and private schools. In addition, courses and examinations related to educational programs must be provided in a manner accessible to all despite obstacles such as hearing, vision, or speech limitations.
   d. Telecommunication relay services are required in all areas to allow those with hearing and speech limitations to communicate with others through a third party.

Challenges for Persons With Disabilities

1. Psychosocial adaptation to a disability is an ongoing process that progresses through stages: shock, denial, depression, ambivalence, and adaptation. It may become stalled at one or more stages and not reach adaptation.
2. Caregiver and family strain because of loss of income, hopelessness, and physical and mental exhaustion from taking over

roles and responsibilities from the person with a disability may impede successful rehabilitation.

3. Despite laws, persons with disabilities are still discriminated against when applying for jobs and educational programs. To get around the laws, employers and educational systems may list multiple physical requirements of a job or program that are meant to discourage persons with a disability from applying or that would prompt failure, even though these physical requirements may have nothing to do with the actual job.
4. In addition to physical barriers at workplaces and educational institutions, persons with disabilities must overcome tremendous attitude barriers. Once a disability is known, stereotyping and prejudice may overshadow a person's potential.

Nursing Interventions for Advocacy

1. Become familiar with Medicare and Medicaid regulations and coverage in the United States and assist patients with the medical forms.
   a. Medicare is available to individuals with a disability after 2 continuous years of disability with inability to work. Medicare is provided through the federal government and is not driven by income level.
   b. Medicare does cover health care provider visits, hospitalizations, and medications, but does not cover some durable medical equipment.
   c. Eligibility for Medicaid is based on income level and how many persons are in the household and is controlled by the state and local government. This may cover under-resourced individuals with disabilities.
2. Help individuals in the United States understand the eligibility for Social Security disability income if their medical condition lasts for 1 year or longer and they are unable to perform substantial employment. The individual must have worked within the last 5 years and have adequate employment credits.
3. Become aware of social services in your geographic area, both through government and charitable programs, such as public transportation that will transport individuals who use wheelchairs to medical appointments.
4. Assist patients in obtaining prescription drugs through discounted and free programs that may be available through pharmaceutical companies to those who do not have limited prescription coverage. Contact pharmaceutical companies directly or *www.ppaRx.com* (Partnership for Pharmaceutical Assistance) for eligibility requirements and applications.
5. If your facility is not fully accessible for persons with disabilities, advocate for structural changes that allow access.
6. When providing care for a person with a disability, always ask if you can assist and allow the individual to direct your assistance. Most individuals with disabilities know what works for them and what causes the least amount of discomfort.
7. Be aware that an individual with an acquired disability goes through an adjustment phase that can be compared with bereavement. Allow the individual time and respect for where they are in the process. Denial can last a year or more, and the individual must be supported, not pushed, to move on in the process.
8. Be aware of your own biases and attitudes toward individuals with a disability. Refrain from stereotyping. Also be aware that not all disabilities are visible (e.g., mental illness or impairment from a head injury). Treat all persons with respect and understanding.
9. Encourage sensitivity training in your facility for all employees to ensure compassionate care and polite interactions with all individuals with a disability.
10. Utilize the following resources for additional information and support:
    - Americans with Disabilities Act: *www.ada.gov*
    - Centers for Disease Control and Prevention; Disability and Health: *www.cdc.gov/ncbddd/disabilityandhealth/index.html*
    - Youreable (products, services, and information for persons with a disability): *www.youreable.com*
    - National Organization on Disability: *www.nod.org*
    - National Council on Disability: *www.ncd.gov*
    - Association of Rehabilitation Nurses: *www.rehabnurse.org*
    - ExceptionalNurse.com (resources for nurses with disabilities): *www.exceptionalnurse.com*

SELECTED READINGS

Aranda, M. P., Kremer, I. N., Hinton, L., Zissimopoulos, J., Whitmer, R. A., Hummel, C. H., Trejo, L., & Fabius, C. (2021). Impact of dementia: Health disparities, population trends, care interventions, and economic costs. *Journal of the American Geriatrics Society, 69*(7), 1774–1783. https://doi.org/10.1111/jgs.17345

Centers for Disease Control and Prevention, & Division of Nutrition, Physical Activity, and Obesity. (2021, July 29). *Physical activity for different groups.* https://www.cdc.gov/physicalactivity/basics/age-chart.html

Centers for Disease Control and Prevention, & Office on Smoking and Health. (2023, May 4). *Current cigarette smoking among adults in the United States.* https://www.cdc.gov/tobacco/data_statistics/fact_sheets/adult_data/cig_smoking/index.htm#:~:text=By%20Age&text=Current%20cigarette%20smoking%20was%20highest,people%20aged%2018%2D24%20years

Chen, S., Kent, B., & Cui, Y. (2021). Interventions to prevent aspiration in older adults with dysphagia living in nursing homes: A scoping review. *BMC Geriatrics, 21*(1), 429. https://doi.org/10.1186/s12877-021-02366-9

Cummings, J., Rabinovici, G. D., Atri, A., Aisen, P., Apostolova, L. G., Hendrix,S., Sabbagh, M., Selkoe, D., Weiner, M., & Salloway, S. (2022). Aducanumab: Appropriate use recommendations update. *The Journal of Prevention of Alzheimer's Disease, 9*(2), 221–230. https://doi.org/10.14283/jpad.2022.34

de Abreu, D. C. C., Porto, J. M., Tofani, P. S., Braghin, R. de M. B., & Freire Junior, R. C. (2022). Prediction of reduced gait speed using 5-time sit-to-stand test in healthy older adults. *Journal of the American Medical Directors Association, 23*(5), 889–892. https://doi.org/10.1016/j.jamda.2021.11.002

Galik, E. M., Resnick, B., Holmes, S. D., Vigne, E., Lynch, K., Ellis, J., Zhu, S., & Barr, E. (2021). A cluster randomized controlled trial testing the impact of function and behavior focused care for nursing home residents with dementia. *Journal of the American Medical Directors Association, 22*(7), 1421–1428.e4. https://doi.org/10.1016/j.jamda.2020.12.020

Izquierdo, M., Merchant, R. A., Morley, J. E., Anker, S. D., Aprahamian, I., Arai, H., Aubertin-Leheudre, M., Bernabei, R., Cadore, E. L., Cesari, M., Chen, L.-K., de Souto Barreto, P., Duque, G., Ferrucci, L., Fielding, R. A., García-Hermoso, A., Gutiérrez-Robledo, L. M., Harridge, S. D. R., Kirk, B., ... & Fiatarone Singh, M. (2021). International exercise recommendations in older adults (ICFSR): Expert consensus guidelines. *The Journal of Nutrition, Health & Aging, 25*(7), 824–853. https://doi.org/10.1007/s12603-021-1665-8

Juhn, Y. J., Wi, C.-I., Ryu, E., Sampathkumar, P., Takahashi, P. Y., Yao, J. D., Binnicker, M. J., Natoli, T. L., Evans, T. K., King, K. S., Volpe, S., Pirçon, J.-Y., Damaso, S., & Pignolo, R. J. (2021). Adherence to public health measures mitigates the risk of COVID-19 infection in older adults: A community-based study. *Mayo Clinic Proceedings, 96*(4), 912–920. https://doi.org/10.1016/j.mayocp.2020.12.016

Kennerly, S. M., Sharkey, P. D., Horn, S. D., Alderden, J., & Yap, T. L. (2022). Nursing assessment of pressure injury risk with the Braden scale validated against sensor-based measurement of movement. *Healthcare (Basel), 10*(11), 2330. https://doi.org/10.3390/healthcare10112330

Lichterfeld-Kottner, A., El Genedy, M., Lahmann, N., Blume-Peytavi, U., Büscher, A., & Kottner, J. (2020). Maintaining skin integrity in the aged: A systematic review. *International Journal of Nursing Studies, 103*, 103509. https://doi.org/10.1016/j.ijnurstu.2019.103509

Loretan, C. G., Cornelius, M. E., Jamal, A., Cheng, Y. J., & Homa, D. M. (2022). Cigarette smoking among US adults with selected chronic diseases associated with smoking, 2010-2019. *Preventing Chronic Disease, 19,* E62. https://doi.org/10.5888/pcd19.220086

Cantuaria, M. L., Pedersen, E. R., Waldorff, F. B., Wermuth, L., Pedersen, K. M., Poulsen, A. H., Raaschou-Nielsen, O., Sørensen, M., & Schmidt, J. H. (2024). Hearing Loss, Hearing Aid Use, and Risk of Dementia in Older Adults. *JAMA Otolaryngology–Head & Neck Surgery, 150*(2), 157-164. https://10.1001/jamaoto.2023.3509. PMID: 38175662; PMCID: PMC10767640.

Omaña, H., Bezaire, K., Brady, K., Davies, J., Louwagie, N., Power, S., Santin, S., & Hunter, S. W. (2021). Functional reach test, single-leg stance test, and Tinetti performance-oriented mobility assessment for the prediction of falls in older adults: A systematic review. *Physical Therapy, 101*(10), pzab173. https://doi.org/10.1093/ptj/pzab173

Patrizio, E., Calvani, R., Marzetti, E., & Cesari, M. (2021). Physical functional assessment in older adults. *The Journal of Frailty & Aging, 10*(2), 141–149. https://doi.org/10.14283/jfa.2020.61

Reid, I. R., & Billington, E. O. (2022). Drug therapy for osteoporosis in older adults. *Lancet (London, England), 399*(10329), 1080–1092. https://doi.org/10.1016/S0140-6736(21)02646-5

Resnick, B., Boltz, M., Galik, E., Holmes, S., Vigne, E., Fix, S., & Zhu, S. (2023). Assessing Pain in Older Adults. *Home Health Now. 41*(3), E3. https://10.1097/NHH.0000000000001181. PMID: 37144939

Rotenberg, S., Rodríguez Gatta, D., Wahedi, A., Loo, R., McFadden, E., & Ryan, S. (2022). Disability training for health workers: A global evidence synthesis. *Disability and Health Journal, 15*(2), 101260. https://doi.org/10.1016/j.dhjo.2021.101260

Sansone, S., Sze, C., Eidelberg, A., Stoddard, M., Cho, A., Asdjodi, S., Mao, J., Elterman, D. S., Zorn, K. C., & Chughtai, B. (2022). Role of pessaries in the treatment of pelvic organ prolapse: A systematic review and meta-analysis. *Obstetrics and Gynecology, 140*(4), 613–622. https://doi.org/10.1097/AOG.0000000000004931

United States Department of Justice Civil Rights Division. (2020, February 28). *Guide to disabilities rights laws.* Ada.gov/resources/disability-rights-guide

UNIT

II RESPIRATORY HEALTH

6 Respiratory Function and Therapy

OVERVIEW AND ASSESSMENT

See additional online content: Procedure Guidelines 6-1 and 6-2.

Respiratory Function

The major function of the pulmonary system (lungs and pulmonary circulation) is to deliver oxygen (O_2) to and remove carbon dioxide (CO_2) from the cells (gas exchange). The adequacy of oxygenation and ventilation is measured by partial pressure of arterial oxygen (PaO_2) and partial pressure of arterial carbon dioxide ($PaCO_2$). The pulmonary system also functions as a blood reservoir for the left ventricle when it is needed to boost cardiac output, as a protector for the systemic circulation by filtering debris/particles, and as a provider of metabolic functions such as surfactant production and endocrine functions.

Terminology

1. Alveolus—air sac where gas exchange takes place.
2. Apex—top portion of the upper lobes of the lungs.
3. Base—bottom portion of the lower lobes of the lungs, located just above the diaphragm.
4. Bronchoconstriction—constriction of smooth muscle surrounding bronchioles.
5. Bronchus—large airways; lung divides into right and left bronchi.
6. Carina—a ridge at the base of the trachea that separates the right and left mainstem bronchi.
7. Cilia—hairlike projections on the tracheobronchial epithelium, which aid in the movement of secretions and removal of debris.
8. Compliance—ability of the lungs to distend and change in volume relative to an applied change in pressure (e.g., emphysema—lungs very compliant; fibrosis—lungs noncompliant or stiff).
9. Dead space—the volume of ventilated air that does not participate in gas exchange; also known as wasted ventilation when there is adequate ventilation but no perfusion, as in pulmonary embolus or pulmonary vascular bed occlusion. Normal dead space is 150 mL.
10. Diaphragm—primary muscle used for respiration; located just below the lung bases; it separates the chest and abdominal cavities.
11. Diffusion (of gas)—movement of gas from area of higher to lower concentration.
12. Dyspnea—subjective sensation of breathlessness associated with discomfort, often caused by a dissociation between motor command and mechanical response of the respiratory system as in:
    a. Respiratory muscle abnormalities (hyperinflation and airflow limitation from chronic obstructive pulmonary disease [COPD]). Abnormal ventilatory impedance (narrowing airways and respiratory impedance from COPD or asthma).
    b. Abnormal breathing patterns (strenuous exercise, pulmonary congestion or edema, recurrent pulmonary emboli).
    c. Arterial blood gas (ABG) abnormalities (hypoxemia, hypercarbia).

13. Hemoptysis—the expectoration of blood or of blood-stained sputum from the larynx, trachea, bronchi, or lungs.
14. Hypoxemia—PaO_2 less than normal, which may or may not cause symptoms. (Normal PaO_2 is 80 to 100 mm Hg on room air.)
15. Hypoxia—insufficient oxygenation at the cellular level because of an imbalance in oxygen delivery and oxygen consumption. (Usually causes symptoms reflecting decreased oxygen reaching the brain and heart.)
16. Mediastinum—large anatomic area between lungs containing intrathoracic structures including the trachea, heart, great vessels, main stem bronchi, thymus, and venous and lymphatic structures.
17. Orthopnea—shortness of breath when in reclining position.
18. Paroxysmal nocturnal dyspnea—sudden shortness of breath associated with sleeping in recumbent position.
19. Perfusion—blood flow, carrying oxygen and cellular waste products that passes the alveoli.
20. Pleura—serous membrane enclosing the lung; composed of visceral pleura, covering all lung surfaces, and parietal pleura, covering chest wall and mediastinal structures, between which exists a potential space.
21. Pulmonary circulation—network of vessels that supply oxygenated blood to and remove CO_2-laden blood from the lungs.
22. Pulmonary hypertension—an increase in pressure in the pulmonary arteries, pulmonary vein, or pulmonary capillaries.
23. Respiration—inhalation and exhalation; at the cellular level, a process involving uptake of oxygen and removal of CO_2 and other products of oxidation.
24. Shunt—adequate perfusion without ventilation, with deoxygenated blood conducted into the systemic circulation, as in pulmonary edema, atelectasis, pneumonia, and COPD.
25. Surfactant—lipid–protein complex secreted by alveolar cells that reduces surface tension of pulmonary fluids and aids in elasticity of pulmonary tissue. Plays a role in the barrier against the entry of pathogens.
26. Ventilation—the process by which oxygen and CO_2 are transported to and from the lungs.
27. Ventilation–perfusion (V/Q) imbalance or mismatch—imbalance of ventilation and perfusion; a cause for hypoxemia. V/Q mismatch can be due to:
    a. Blood perfusing an area of the lung where ventilation is reduced or absent.
    b. Ventilation of parts of the lung that is not perfused.

Subjective Data

Assess symptoms obtained from the patient's description of an event through characterization and history taking to help anticipate needs and plan care. Encourages the patient to give a full description of the onset, the course, and the character of the problem and any factors that aggravate or relieve it.

Dyspnea

EVIDENCE BASE Chen, Y., Coxson, H., & Reid, W. D. (2016). Reliability and validity of the brief fatigue inventory and dyspnea inventory in people with chronic obstructive pulmonary disease. *Journal of Pain and Symptom Management*, *52*(2), 298–304. https://doi.org/10.1016/j.jpainsymman.2016.02.018

1. Characteristics—Is the dyspnea acute or chronic? Has it occurred suddenly or gradually? Is more than one pillow required to sleep? Is the dyspnea progressive, recurrent, or paroxysmal? Walking how far leads to shortness of breath? How does it compare with the patient's baseline level of dyspnea? Ask patient to rate dyspnea on a scale of 1 to 10, with 1 being no dyspnea and 10 being the worst imaginable. What relieves and what aggravates the dyspnea?
2. Associated factors—Is there a cough associated with the dyspnea and is it productive? What activities precipitate the shortness of breath? Does it seem to be worse when upset? Is it influenced by the time of day, seasons, or certain environments? Does it occur at rest or with exertion? Any fever, chills, night sweats, ankle/leg swelling? Any change in body weight?
3. History—Is there a patient or family history of chronic lung disease, cardiac or neuromuscular disease, cancer, problems with blood clotting, or immunocompromise? What is the smoking history?
4. Significance—Sudden dyspnea could indicate pulmonary embolus, pneumothorax, myocardial infarction (MI), acute heart failure, or acute respiratory failure. In a postsurgical or postpartum patient, dyspnea may indicate pulmonary embolus or edema. Orthopnea can be indicative of heart disease or COPD. If dyspnea is associated with a wheeze, consider asthma, COPD, heart failure, or upper airway obstruction. When dyspnea occurs in combination with fatigue, pulmonary hypertension may exist. Metabolic disorders, psychiatric conditions, and neuromuscular disorders may also contribute to dyspnea.

Chest Pain

1. Characteristics—Is the pain sharp, dull, stabbing, or aching? Is it intermittent or persistent? Is the pain localized or does it radiate? If it radiates, where? How intense is the pain? Are there factors that alleviate or aggravate the pain, such as position or activity?
2. Associated factors—What effect do inspiration and expiration have on the pain? What other symptoms accompany the chest pain? Is there diaphoresis, shortness of breath, or nausea?
3. History—Is there a smoking history or environmental exposure? Has the pain ever been experienced before? What was the cause? Is there a preexisting pulmonary or cardiac diagnosis? Has there been recent trauma?
4. Significance—Chest pain related to pulmonary causes is usually felt on the side where pathology arises, but it can be referred. Dull persistent pain may indicate carcinoma of the lung, whereas sharp, stabbing pain usually arises from the pleura. Dyspnea with pleuritic chest pain indicates clinically significant pulmonary embolism.

Cough

EVIDENCE BASE Weinberger, S. (2022). Evaluation and treatment of subacute and chronic cough in adults. *UpToDate*. Retrieved December 1, 2022, from https://www.uptodate.com/contents/evaluation-and-treatment-of-subacute-and-chronic-cough-in-adults

1. Characteristics—Is the cough dry, hacking, loose, barky, wheezy, or more like clearing the throat? Is it strong or weak? How frequent is it? Is it worse at night or at any time of day?

Does the intensity change on days off from work? Is there seasonal variation? Is it aggravated by food intake or exertion? Is it alleviated by any medication? How long has it been going on?
2. Associated factors—Is the cough productive? If so, what is the consistency, amount, color, and odor of the sputum? Is there hemoptysis? How does sputum compare with the patient's baseline? Is it associated with shortness of breath, pain, or nausea?
3. History—Is there a smoking/vaping history? Is the smoking/vaping current or in the past? Has there been any environmental or occupational exposure to dust, fumes, or gases that could lead to cough? Are there past pulmonary diagnoses, asthma, rhinitis, allergy, or exposure to allergens, such as pollen, house dust mites, animal dander, birds, mold or fungi, cockroach waste, and irritants (smoke, odors, perfumes, cleaning products, exhaust, pollution, cold air)? Has there been prolonged exposure to dampness, chemical sanitizers, cobalt or other hard metals, beryllium, asbestos, dusts from coal, wood, or grains? Does the patient have a history of acid reflux or postnasal drip or use an angiotensin-converting enzyme inhibitor with a common adverse effect of cough? Has there been a concurrent voice change? Has the patient recently traveled outside the country? Can the patient identify any specific triggers? Is the patient immunocompromised?
4. Significance—A dry, irritative cough may indicate viral respiratory tract infection. A cough at night should alert to potential left-sided heart failure, asthma, or postnasal drip worsening at night. A morning cough with sputum might be bronchitis. A cough that is less severe on days off from work may be related to occupational or environmental exposures. A patient with severe or changing cough should be evaluated for bronchogenic carcinoma. Consider bacterial pneumonia if sputum is rusty and lung tumor if it is pink tinged. A profuse, pink frothy sputum could be indicative of pulmonary edema. A cough associated with food intake could indicate problems with aspiration. A dry cough may be associated with pulmonary fibrosis. History of recent travel may be associated with infection from a source not commonly identified in the United States.

Hemoptysis

1. Characteristics—Is the blood from the lungs? It could be from the gastrointestinal (GI) system (hematemesis) or upper airway (epistaxis). Is it bright red or frothy? How much? Is onset associated with certain circumstances or activities? Was the onset sudden, and is it intermittent or continuous?
2. Associated factors—Was there an initial sensation of tickling in the throat? Was there a salty taste or burning or bubbling sensation in the chest? Has there been shortness of breath, chest pain, or difficulty with exertion?
3. History—Was there any recent chest trauma or respiratory treatment (chest percussion)? Does the patient have an upper respiratory infection, sinusitis, or recent epistaxis? Has the patient used cocaine or other illicit drugs?
4. Significance—Hemoptysis can be linked to pulmonary infection, pulmonary edema, COPD, lung carcinoma, abnormalities of the heart or blood vessels, pulmonary artery or vein abnormalities, or pulmonary emboli and infarction. Small amounts of blood-tinged sputum may be from the upper respiratory tract, and regurgitation of blood comes from a GI bleed.

Objective Data

The process in which data relating to the patient's problem are obtained through direct physical examination, including observation, palpation, percussion, and auscultation; laboratory analysis; or radiologic and other studies.

EVIDENCE BASE Heuer, A. (2022). *Wilkins clinical assessment in respiratory care* (9th ed.). Elsevier.

Key Observations

1. What is the respiratory rate, depth, and pattern? Are accessory muscles being used? Is the patient breathing through the mouth or pursing lips during exhalation? Is sputum being expectorated, and what is its appearance and odor?
2. Is there an increase in the anterior to posterior chest diameter, suggesting air trapping?
3. Is there obvious orthopnea or splinting?
4. Is there clubbing of the fingers, associated with bronchiectasis, lung abscess, empyema, cystic fibrosis, pulmonary neoplasms, and various other disorders?
5. Is there central cyanosis indicating possible hypoxemia or cardiac disease? Are mucous membranes and nail beds pink?
6. Are there signs of tracheal deviation, as seen with pneumothorax?
7. Are the jugular veins distended? Is there peripheral edema or other signs of cardiac dysfunction?
8. Does palpation of the chest cause pain? Is chest expansion symmetrical? Is there any change in tactile fremitus or egophony?
9. Is percussion of lung fields resonant bilaterally? Is diaphragmatic excursion equal bilaterally?
10. Are breath sounds present and equal bilaterally? Are the lung fields clear upon auscultation or are there rhonchi, wheezing, crackles, stridor, or pleural friction rub? Does auscultation reveal egophony, bronchophony, or whispered pectoriloquy?

Laboratory Studies

ABG Analysis

Description

1. An ABG is a laboratory test that measures (PaO_2) oxygen tension, ($PaCO_2$) carbon dioxide tension, acidity (pH), oxyhemoglobin saturation SaO_2, and bicarbonate (HCO_3). This provides a means of assessing the adequacy of ventilation.
2. ABG allows assessment of body's acid–base (pH) status, indicating if acidosis or alkalosis is present, whether acidosis or alkalosis is respiratory or metabolic in origin, and whether it is compensated or uncompensated.
3. ABG is used for diagnostic evaluation and evaluation of response to clinical interventions (oxygen therapy, mechanical ventilation, noninvasive ventilation, etc.).

Nursing and Patient Care Considerations

1. Blood can be obtained from any artery but is usually drawn from the radial, brachial, or femoral site. It can be drawn directly by percutaneous needle puncture or accessed by way of indwelling arterial catheter. Determine facility policy for qualifications for ABG sampling and site of arterial puncture.
2. If the radial artery is used, an Allen test must be performed before the puncture to determine whether collateral circulation is present.

3. Arterial puncture should not be performed through a lesion, through or distal to a surgical shunt, or in area where peripheral vascular disease or infection is present.
4. Absolute contraindications include an abnormal modified Allen test (absence of a radial arterial pulse), severe peripheral vascular disease of the artery being sampled, active Raynaud syndrome, and local infection at the arterial site.
5. Use caution with patients receiving anticoagulant therapy or thrombolytic medications.
6. Results may be affected by recent changes in oxygen therapy, suctioning, or positioning.
7. Interpret ABG values by reviewing patient trends as well as the following normal values:
   a. PaO_2—partial pressure of arterial oxygen (80 to 100 mm Hg).
   b. $PaCO_2$—partial pressure of arterial carbon dioxide (35 to 45 mm Hg).
   c. SaO_2—arterial oxygen saturation (>95%).
   d. pH—hydrogen ion concentration or degree of acid–base balance (7.35 to 7.45).
   e. (HCO_3^-)—bicarbonate primarily a metabolic buffer (22 to 26 mEq/L).

Sputum Examination

Description

1. Sputum may be obtained for evaluation of gross appearance, microscopic examination, Gram stain, culture and sensitivity, acid-fast bacillus, and cytology.
   a. The direct smear shows presence of white blood cells and intracellular (pathogenic) bacteria and extracellular (mostly nonpathogenic) bacteria.
   b. Gram stain shows whether bacteria is gram positive or gram negative and can be used to guide therapy until culture and sensitivity results are available.
   c. The sputum culture is used to identify presence of specific pathogens; sensitivity determines drug efficacy and serves as a guide for drug treatment (i.e., choice of antibiotic).
   d. Acid-fast smears detect presence of pathogens such as *Mycobacterium tuberculosis.*
   e. Cytology identifies abnormal and possibly malignant cells.

Nursing and Patient Care Considerations

1. Patients receiving antibiotics, steroids, and immunosuppressive agents for a prolonged time may have periodic sputum examinations because these agents may give rise to opportunistic pulmonary infections.
2. It is important that the sputum be collected correctly and that the specimen be sent to a laboratory immediately. Allowing it to stand in a warm room will result in overgrowth of organisms, making identification of pathogen difficult; this also alters cell morphology. A series of three early-morning specimens is needed for acid-fast bacillus examination. Cytology samples should be collected in container with fixative solution.
3. Sputum can be obtained by various methods:
   a. Deep breathing and coughing.
      i. An early-morning specimen obtained before eating or drinking yields best sample of deep pulmonary secretions from all lung fields.
      ii. Have patient clear nose and throat and rinse mouth with plain water—to decrease contamination by oral and upper respiratory flora.
      iii. Position patient upright or in high Fowler's unless contraindicated. Instruct patient to take several deep breaths, exhale, and perform a series of short coughs.
      iv. Have patient cough deeply and expectorate the sputum into a sterile container.
      v. If patient is unable to produce specimen, increasing oral fluid intake may be useful (unless oral intake is contraindicated/patient is on a fluid restriction).
   b. Induction through use of ultrasonic or hypertonic saline nebulization.
      i. Patient inhales mist through mouth slowly and deeply for 10 to 20 minutes.
      ii. Nebulization increases the moisture content of air going to lower tract; particles will condense on tracheobronchial tree and aid in expectoration.
   c. Suctioning—aspiration of secretions via mechanical means; must be used with caution because it may cause bleeding, cardiac dysrhythmias, and increased intracranial pressure (ICP).
      i. Tracheal, through endotracheal (ET) or tracheostomy tube.
      ii. Nasotracheal (NT), through nose and into back of throat or trachea.
   d. Bronchoscopy with bronchoalveolar lavage, in which 60 to 100 mL is instilled and aspirated from various lung segments. Sedation or anesthesia is required.
   e. Gastric aspiration (rarely necessary since advent of ultrasonic nebulizer).
      i. Nasogastric (NG) tube is inserted into the stomach, approximately 50 mL sterile water is instilled, and swallowed pulmonary secretions are siphoned out.
      ii. Useful only for culture of tubercle bacilli, not for direct examination.
      iii. Must be done as soon as patient wakes up in the morning.
   f. Transtracheal aspiration involves passing a needle and then a catheter through a percutaneous puncture of the cricothyroid membrane. Transtracheal aspiration bypasses the oropharynx and avoids specimen contamination by mouth flora.
4. Generally, a sputum sample of 15 mL is adequate for laboratory testing.

Pleural Fluid Analysis

Description

1. Pleural fluid is continuously produced and reabsorbed, with a thin layer normally in the pleural space. Abnormal pleural fluid accumulation (effusion) occurs in diseases of the pleura, heart, or lymphatics. The pleural fluid is studied, with other tests, to determine the underlying cause.
2. The fluid is obtained by aspiration (thoracentesis) or by tube thoracotomy (see Figure 6-1).
3. The fluid is examined for cancerous cells, cellular makeup, chemical content, and microorganisms.
4. Pleural cavity contains 10 to 20 mL clear yellow (serous) fluid that lubricates the surfaces of the pleura, the thin membrane that lines the chest cavity and surrounds the lungs. A pleural effusion is an abnormal collection of this fluid.
5. The test is performed to determine the cause of a pleural effusion and to relieve associated shortness of breath.

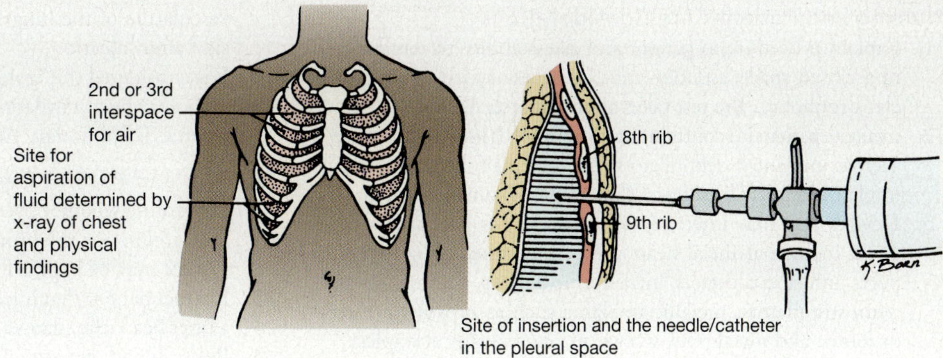

Figure 6-1. Thoracentesis for removal of pleural effusion and pleural fluid analysis.

Nursing and Patient Care Considerations

1. If done at bedside, prepare the patient by assisting to a supported upright position with lateral and posterior thorax of particular side exposed or in side-lying position with head of bed elevated 30 to 45 degrees and arm overhead. Support the patient through the process.
2. Observe and record total amount of fluid withdrawn, nature of fluid, color, and viscosity.
3. Prepare and label sample of fluid and ensure transport to the laboratory.
4. A chest x-ray may be done before or after the fluid is withdrawn.
5. Patient should not cough, breathe deeply, or move while fluid is being withdrawn.
6. Instruct patient to inform provider immediately if sharp chest pain or shortness of breath occurs.

Radiology and Imaging

Chest X-Ray

Description

1. Normal pulmonary tissue is radiolucent and appears black on film. Thus, densities produced by tumors, foreign bodies, and infiltrates can be detected as lighter or white images.
2. Commonly, two views—posterior–anterior and lateral—are obtained.
3. This test shows the position of normal structures, displacement, and presence of abnormal shadows. It may reveal pathology in the lungs in the absence of symptoms.

Nursing and Patient Care Considerations

1. X-ray should be taken upright if patient's condition permits. Assist technician at bedside in preparing patient for portable chest x-ray.
2. Encourage patient to take deep breath, hold breath, and remain still as x-ray is taken.
3. Make sure that all jewelry, electrocardiogram (ECG) or monitor leads, and metal objects (including metal-containing transdermal patches) in x-ray field are removed so as not to interfere with film.
4. Consider the contraindication of x-rays for pregnant patients.

Computed Tomography (CT) Scan

Description

1. Cross-sectional x-rays of the lungs are taken from many different angles and processed through a computer to create three-dimensional images. This three-dimensional imaging provides more complete diagnostic information than the two-dimensional x-ray.
2. It may be used to define pulmonary nodules and pulmonary abnormalities or to demonstrate mediastinal abnormalities and hilar adenopathy.

Nursing and Patient Care Considerations

1. Describe test to patient and family, including that table will slide into doughnut-shaped scanner and patient must lie still during test. The test usually takes about 30 minutes but may take longer.
2. Be alert to allergies to iodine or other radiographic contrast media that might be used during testing.
3. For scans performed with contrast, informed consent and intravenous (IV) access are required. Patient should take nothing by mouth (NPO) for 4 hours before scan. Blood urea nitrogen and creatinine should be evaluated 24 to 48 hours before the test or according to facility protocol.
4. Hydrate patient well to facilitate excretion of contrast, if used.
5. Check regarding weight limit of equipment before scanning patients with obesity.
6. Consider the contraindication of radiologic studies for the patient who are pregnant, especially CT scans with contrast media.

Magnetic Resonance Imaging

Description

1. Noninvasive procedure that uses a powerful magnetic field, radio waves, and a computer to produce detailed pictures of the organs, soft tissue, bone, and other internal structures.
2. Provides contrast between various soft tissues and is performed to:
   a. Assess abnormal growths, including cancer of the lungs or other tissues inadequately assessed with other imaging modalities.
   b. Determine stage of cancer, including tumor size, extent, and degree to which cancer has spread.
   c. Visualize lymph nodes and blood vessels.
   d. Assess disorders of the vertebrae, ribs, and sternum.
3. Traditional radiographic contrast media are not used but gadolinium injection or ingestion may be necessary, depending on patient's medical history and anatomy to be imaged.
4. It is helpful to synchronize the magnetic resonance imaging (MRI) picture to the ECG in thoracic studies.
5. The hazards of MRI during pregnancy are unknown, although ionizing radiation (x-ray) is not used during MRI.

Nursing and Patient Care Considerations

1. Explain procedure to patient and assess ability to remain still in a closed space; sedation may be necessary if the patient is claustrophobic. The test takes approximately 1 hour.
2. Evaluate patient for contraindications to MRI: implanted devices, such as implanted defibrillators that may malfunction; cochlear implants; or metallic surgical clips used on brain aneurysms.
3. Devices that may interfere with the exam or potentially pose a risk include artificial heart valves, implanted drug infusion ports, infusion catheters, intrauterine devices, pacemakers and neurostimulators, metallic implants such as prosthetic valves or joints, and metal pins, screws, plates, or surgical staples.
4. Make sure that all jewelry, ECG or monitor leads, hearing aids, pins/hairpins, removable dental work, and metal objects (including metal-containing transdermal patches) are removed.
5. Kidney disease and sickle cell anemia may contraindicate MRI with contrast material.
6. Check with MRI technician about the use of equipment, such as ventilator or mechanical IV pump, in MRI room.
7. Earplugs may be used to muffle loud thumping and humming noises during imaging.
8. Evaluate the patient for claustrophobia, and teach relaxation techniques to use during test or advocate for use of open MRI. Prepare to administer sedation, if necessary.
9. Check regarding size capacity of equipment before scanning patients with obesity.
10. It is recommended that nursing patients not breastfeed for 36 to 48 hours after MRI with contrast.

Positron Emission Tomography Scan

Description

1. Physiologic images are obtained on the basis of the detection of radiation from the emission of positrons. Positrons are tiny particles emitted from a radioactive isotope–administered IV to the patient. Radioactivity localizes in the area(s) being scanned and is detected by positron emission tomography (PET). Different colors or degrees of brightness on a PET image represent different levels of tissue or organ function.
2. Radioisotope is administered 30 to 90 minutes before scan via IV or inhalation.
3. Distinguishes between benign and malignant lung nodules.

Nursing and Patient Care Considerations

1. Describe test to patient and family, including that table will slide into doughnut-shaped scanner and patient must lie still during the test. The test usually takes 30 to 45 minutes.
2. Isotope has a short half-life and is not considered a radiologic hazard.
3. Encourage fluids to facilitate excretion of isotope.
4. Consider the contraindication of radiologic studies for the patient who is pregnant or breastfeeds.
5. Test results may be inaccurate for patients who have diabetes or for patients who have eaten within a few hours before the scan if blood glucose or insulin levels are not normal.

CT Pulmonary Angiography

Description

1. An imaging method used to study pulmonary vessels and pulmonary circulation.
2. For visualization, radiopaque medium is injected by way of a catheter in the main pulmonary artery rapidly into the vasculature of the lungs. Films are then taken in rapid succession after injection.
3. It is considered the "gold standard" for diagnosis of pulmonary embolus, but ventilation–perfusion V/Q scan may be used when CT Pulmonary Angiography is contraindicated.

Nursing and Patient Care Considerations

1. Determine whether patient is allergic to radiographic contrast media, describe the procedure, and obtain informed consent.
2. Patient may be kept NPO for 4 to 8 hours before procedure.
3. Instruct patient that injection of dye may cause flushing, cough, a brief headache, nausea, vomiting, and/or a warm sensation.
4. Pulse, blood pressure (BP), and respirations are monitored during the procedure.
5. After the procedure, make sure pressure is maintained over access site and monitor pulse rate, BP, and circulation distal to the injection site.
6. Patient may be advised to keep extremity straight for up to 12 hours after the procedure.
7. Necessity of test should be carefully evaluated in patients with bleeding disorders and pregnant people.

Ventilation–Perfusion Scan

Description

1. Ventilation–Perfusion Scan is a pair of nuclear scan tests using inhaled and injected radioisotopes to measure breathing (ventilation) and blood flow (perfusion) in all areas of the lungs. The two tests may be performed either separately or together.
2. Perfusion scan is done after injection of a radioactive isotope. It measures blood perfusion through the lungs and evaluates lung function on a regional basis.
3. Ventilation scan is done after inhalation of radioactive gas (e.g., xenon with O_2), which diffuses throughout the lungs. It indicates how well air reaches all parts of the lung.
4. Usually performed to detect pulmonary embolus. Also useful in evaluating advanced pulmonary disease (COPD), detecting abnormal circulation (shunts) in the pulmonary blood vessels, evaluating lung function, and identifying fibrosis.
5. It is also referred to as *V/Q scan* because the initials are used in mathematical equations that calculate air and blood flow.

Nursing and Patient Care Considerations

1. Determine if patient is allergic to radiographic dye before V/Q scan.
2. Determine if patient is pregnant or breastfeeding.
3. Explain the procedure to patient and encourage cooperation with inhalation and brief episodes of breath holding.
4. False positives may occur in patients with vasculitis, mitral stenosis, and pulmonary hypertension and when tumors obstruct a pulmonary artery with airway involvement, fatty tissues, and presence of parasites.
5. False negatives are associated with partially occluded vessels.

Other Diagnostic Tests

Bronchoscopy

EVIDENCE BASE Paradis, T., Dixon, J., & Tieu, B. (2016). The role of bronchoscopy in the diagnosis of airway/disease. *Journal of Thoracic Disease*, 8(12), 3826–3837. https://doi.org/10.21037/jtd.2016.12.68

Description

1. Bronchoscopy is the direct inspection and observation of the upper and lower respiratory tract through fiberoptic (flexible) or rigid bronchoscope as a means of diagnosing and managing inflammatory, infectious, and malignant diseases of the airway and lungs including airway injury and obstruction by a foreign body tumor or mass.
2. Flexible fiberoptic bronchoscopy allows for more patient comfort and better visualization of smaller airways, including nasal passages. It is usually performed using local anesthesia with or without moderate sedation. Fluoroscopy may be needed to facilitate specimen collection. It is used for therapeutic and diagnostic procedures such as:
   a. Bronchoalveolar lavage.
   b. Endobronchial or transbronchial biopsies.
   c. Cytologic wash or brush.
   d. Transbronchial needle aspiration.
   e. Endobronchial ultrasound.
   f. Autofluorescence bronchoscopy.
   g. Balloon dilation.
   h. Endobronchial laser ablation.
   i. Electrocautery.
   j. Photodynamic therapy.
   k. Brachytherapy.
   l. Tracheobronchial stents.
3. Rigid bronchoscopy, which often requires general anesthesia with adequate sedation and muscle relaxants, may be combined with flexible bronchoscopy for better access to distal airways. Diagnostic and therapeutic indications include:
   a. Control of massive hemoptysis.
   b. Foreign body extraction.
   c. Deeper biopsy specimen collection than can be obtained fiberoptically.
   d. Dilation of tracheal or bronchial strictures.
   e. Relief of airway obstruction.
   f. Insertion of stents.
   g. Tracheobronchial laser therapy or other mechanical tumor ablation.

Nursing and Patient Care Considerations

1. Check that an informed consent form has been signed and that risks and benefits have been explained to the patient.
2. Make sure that IV access is present and patent.
3. Absolute contraindications include uncorrectable coagulopathy, severe refractory hypoxemia, unstable hemodynamic status, facial trauma, and unstable cervical spine. Patients with increased risk are those with MI within past 6 weeks, head injuries susceptible to increased ICPs, and known or suspected pregnancy (because of possible radiation exposure).
4. Review and follow facility policy and procedure for anesthesia and sedation.
5. Administer prescribed medication to reduce secretions, block the vasovagal reflex and gag reflex, and relieve anxiety. Give encouragement and nursing support.
6. Restrict fluid and food, as ordered, before procedure to reduce risk of aspiration when reflexes are blocked. Patient may be kept NPO for 4 hours before flexible bronchoscopy with minimal sedation; if deeper sedation is used, patient's time on NPO is extended.
7. Remove dentures, contact lenses, and other prostheses.
8. After the procedure:
   a. Monitor cardiac rhythm and rate, BP, and level of consciousness (LOC).
   b. Monitor respiratory effort and rate.
   c. Monitor oximetry.
   d. Withhold ice chips and fluids until patient demonstrates gag reflex.
   e. Monitor patient's perceptions of pain, discomfort, and dyspnea.
   f. Assess for bleeding, noting that a minimal amount of blood streak in sputum may be expected.
9. Promptly report cyanosis, hypoventilation, hypotension, tachycardia or dysrhythmia, hemoptysis, dyspnea, and decreased breath sounds.
10. Provide outpatients with specific instructions regarding signs and symptoms of complications and what to do if they arise.

CLINICAL JUDGMENT After bronchoscopy, be alert for complications, such as pneumothorax, dysrhythmias, laryngospasm, and bronchospasm.

Lung Biopsy

Description

1. Procedures used for obtaining histologic material from the lung to aid in diagnosis include:
   a. Transbronchial biopsy—biopsy forceps inserted through bronchoscope and specimen of lung tissue obtained.
   b. Transthoracic needle aspiration biopsy—specimen obtained through needle aspiration under fluoroscopic guidance.
   c. Open lung biopsy—specimen obtained through small anterior thoracotomy; used in making a diagnosis when other biopsy methods have not been effective or are not possible.

Nursing and Patient Care Considerations

1. Obtain permission for consent, if required.
2. Observe for possible complications, including pneumothorax, hemorrhage (hemoptysis), and bacterial contamination of pleural space.
3. A chest x-ray should be done 1 hour after transbronchial biopsy to exclude pneumothorax.
4. See "Bronchoscopy" (page 134) or "Thoracic Surgeries" (page 151) for postprocedure care.

Pulmonary Function Tests (PFTs)

EVIDENCE BASE Graham, B. L., Steenbruggen, I., Miller, M. R., Barjaktarevic, I. Z., Cooper, B. G., Hall, G. L., Hallstrand, T. S., Kaminsky, D. A., McCarthy, K., McCormack, M. C., Oropez, C. E., Rosenfeld, M., Stanojevic, S., Swanney, M. P., & Thompson, B. R. (2019). Standardization of spirometry 2019 update: An official American Thoracic Society and European Respiratory Society technical statement. *American Journal of Respiratory and Critical Care Medicine*, *200*(8), e70–e88. https://doi.org/10.1164/rccm.201908-1590ST

Description

1. PFTs are used to detect and measure abnormalities in respiratory function and quantify severity of various lung diseases. Such tests include measurements of lung volumes, ventilatory function, diffusing capacity, gas exchange, lung compliance, airway resistance, and distribution of gases in the lung.
2. Ventilatory studies (spirometry) are the most common group of tests.
   a. Requires electronic spirometer, water spirometer, or wedge spirometer that plots volume against time (timed vital capacity).

Table 6-1 Pulmonary Function Tests

TERM	SYMBOL	DESCRIPTION	REMARKS
Vital capacity	VC	Maximum volume of air exhaled after a maximum inspiration.	• VC <10–15 mL/kg suggests need for mechanical ventilation. • VC >10–15 mL/kg suggests ability to wean.
Forced vital capacity	FVC	Total volume of air a patient is able to exhale for the total duration of the test during maximal effort.	• Reduced in obstructive disease (COPD) because of air trapping and restrictive disease. • Reflects airflow in large airways.
Forced expiratory volume in 1 sec	FEV_1	Volume of air exhaled in the first second of the performance of the FVC.	• Reduced in obstructive disease (COPD) because of air trapping. • Reflects airflow in large airways.
Ratio of FEV_1/FVC	FEV_1/FVC	FEV_1 expressed as a percentage of the FVC. The percentage of FVC expired in 1 sec.	• Decreased in obstructive disease. • Normal in restrictive disease.
Forced midexpiratory flow	$FEF_{25\%–75\%}$	Average flow during the middle half of the FVC.	• Reflects airflow in small airways. • Patients who smoke may have change in this test before other symptoms develop.
Peak expiratory flow rate	PEFR	Most rapid flow during a forced expiration after a maximum inspiration.	• Used to measure response to bronchodilators, airflow obstruction in patients with asthma.
Maximal voluntary volume	MVV	Volume of air expired in a specified period (12 sec) during repetitive maximal effort.	• An important factor in exercise tolerance. • Decreases in neuromuscular diseases.

b. Patient is asked to take as deep a breath as possible and then to exhale into spirometer as completely and either slowly or as forcefully as possible, depending on the type of test.
c. Results are compared with normal for patient's age, height, and sex assigned at birth (Table 6-1).
d. A reduction in the vital capacity, inspiratory capacity, and total lung capacity may indicate a restrictive form of lung disease (disease because of increased lung stiffness).
e. An increase in functional reserve capacity, total lung capacity, and reduction in flow rates usually indicate an obstructive flow because of bronchial obstruction or loss of lung elastic recoil.

3. Lung volumes are determined by body plethysmography (considered the gold standard). Additional methods include helium dilution, nitrogen washout, and chest measurements, which are based on chest images.
   a. Yields thoracic volume (total lung capacity, plus any unventilated blebs or bullae).
   b. An increased residual volume is found in air trapping because of obstructive lung disease.
   c. A reduction in several parameters usually indicates a restrictive form of lung disease or chest wall abnormality.
4. Diffusing capacity measures lung surface effective for the transfer of gas in the lung by having patient inhale gas containing known low concentration of carbon monoxide and measuring carbon monoxide concentration in exhaled air. Difference between inhaled and exhaled concentrations is related directly to uptake of carbon monoxide across alveolar–capillary membrane. Diffusing capacity is useful in evaluating restrictive and obstructive lung disease and pulmonary vascular disease.

Nursing and Patient Care Considerations

1. Instruct the patient in correct technique for completing PFTs; coach the patient through test, if needed. Appropriate interpretation requires adequate patient cooperation and effort and accurate equipment. Instruct patient not to use oral or inhaled bronchodilator (e.g., albuterol), caffeine, or tobacco at least 4 to 6 hours before the test (longer for long-acting bronchodilators).
2. Used with caution in patients with hemoptysis of unknown origin; pneumothorax; unstable cardiovascular status; recent MI or pulmonary embolus; thoracic, abdominal, or cerebral aneurysm; or recent eye, thoracic, or abdominal surgery.
3. Using a noseclip for all spirometric maneuvers is strongly recommended.
4. Although forced expiratory volume in the first second of a forced vital capacity is the "gold standard" for diagnosing airway obstruction, there is no single cutoff value separating normal from abnormal. This determination is based more on trending of individual results.

Pulse Oximetry

Description

1. Noninvasively provides an estimate of arterial oxyhemoglobin saturation by using selected wavelengths of light to determine the saturation of oxyhemoglobin. Oximeters function by passing a light beam through a vascular bed, such as the finger or earlobe, to determine the amount of light absorbed by oxygenated (red) and deoxygenated (blue) blood.
2. Calculates the amount of arterial blood that is saturated with oxygen (SaO_2) and displays this as a percentage.
3. Provides indication only of oxygenation, not ventilation.
4. Indications include:
   a. Monitor adequacy of oxygen saturation; quantify response to therapy.

b. Monitor unstable patient who may experience sudden changes in blood oxygen level.
c. Evaluation of need for home oxygen therapy.
d. Determine supplemental oxygen needs at rest, with exercise, and during sleep.
e. Need to follow the trend and need to decrease number of ABG sample drawn.

5. The oxyhemoglobin dissociation curve allows for correlation between SaO_2 and PaO_2 (see Figure 6-2).
   a. Increased body temperature, exercise, acidosis, and increased phosphates (2,3-DPG) cause a shift in the curve to the right, thus increasing the ability of hemoglobin to release oxygen to the tissues.
   b. Decreased temperature, decreased 2,3-DPG, and alkalosis cause a shift to the left, causing hemoglobin to hold on to the oxygen, reducing the amount of oxygen being released to the tissues.
6. Increased bilirubin, increased carboxyhemoglobin, low perfusion, or SaO_2 less than 80% may alter light absorption and interfere with results.

CLINICAL JUDGMENT There is a potential error in SaO_2 readings of ±2% that can increase to greater than 2% if the patient's SpO_2 drops below 80%. Oximeters rely on differences in light absorption to determine SaO_2. At lower saturations, oxygenated hemoglobin appears bluer in color and is less easily distinguished from deoxygenated hemoglobin. ABG analysis should be used in this situation.

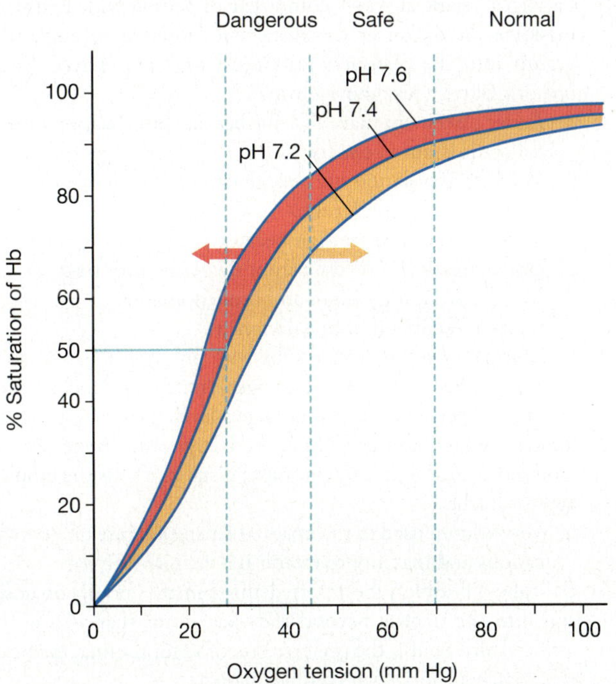

Figure 6-2. The oxyhemoglobin dissociation curve shows the relation between the partial pressure of oxygen and the oxygen saturation. At pressures greater than 60 mm Hg, the curve is essentially flat with blood oxygen content not changing with increases in the oxygen partial pressure. As oxygen partial pressures decrease in the slope of the curve, the oxygen is unloaded to peripheral tissue as the hemoglobin's affinity decreases. The curve is shifted to the right by an increase in temperature, 2,3-DPG, or $PaCO_2$, or a decrease in pH and to the left by the opposite of these conditions.

Nursing and Patient Care Considerations

1. Assess patient's hemoglobin. SaO_2 may not correlate well with PaO_2 if hemoglobin is not within normal limits.
2. Remove patient's nail polish because it can affect the ability of the sensor to correctly determine oxygen saturation, particularly polish with blue or dark colors.
3. Correlate oximetry with ABG values and then use for single reading or trending of oxygenation (does not monitor $PaCO_2$).
4. Display heart rate should correlate with patient's heart rate.
5. To improve quality of signal, hold finger dependent and motionless (motion may alter results) and cover finger sensor to occlude ambient light.
6. Assess site of oximetry monitoring for perfusion on a regular basis because pressure injury may occur from prolonged application of probe. Rotate probe every 2 hours.
7. Device limitations include motion artifact, abnormal hemoglobins (carboxyhemoglobin and methemoglobin), IV dye, exposure of probe to ambient light, low perfusion states, skin pigmentation, nail polish or nail coverings, and nail deformities such as severe clubbing.
8. Document inspired oxygen or supplemental oxygen and type of oxygen-delivery device.
9. Accuracy can be affected by decreased peripheral perfusion, ambient light, IV dyes, nail polish, deeply pigmented skin, cold extremities, hypothermia, patients in sickle cell crisis, jaundice, severe anemia, and use of antibiotics such as sulfas.
10. In patients with COPD, oxygen saturation levels may remain unchanged, even though CO_2 levels may be rising as the patient becomes acidotic. Pulse oximetry will not detect this deterioration.
11. Contraindicated for monitoring patients who have high levels of arterial carboxyhemoglobin, such as fire patients.

Capnometry/Capnography

Description

1. Used to noninvasively determine and monitor end-tidal carbon dioxide ($ETCO_2$)—the amount of CO_2 that is expired with each breath—via colorimetric indicator.
2. $ETCO_2$ is displayed as a capnogram (a waveform that may be time based or volume based and a numeric reading).
3. Normally, 2 to 5 mm Hg less than $PaCO_2$ in adults, with the difference being greater in the presence of lung disease, or increase in dead space, and can be used as an indirect estimate of V/Q mismatching for the lung.
4. Indicated for monitoring severity of pulmonary disease and monitoring response to therapy; evaluating efficacy of mechanical ventilatory support; monitoring adequacy of pulmonary, systemic, and coronary blood flow; and assessing metabolic rate and alveolar ventilation.
5. A standard in anesthesia care, it is being increasingly used in the critical care setting as well as in emergency care via pocket-sized models.

Nursing and Patient Care Considerations

1. Draw ABGs initially to correlate $ETCO_2$ with $PaCO_2$ and to establish the gradient between $PaCO_2$ and $ETCO_2$.
2. Accuracy of measurement can be affected by alterations in breathing pattern or tidal volume (V_T), breathing frequency, presence of freon from metered-dose inhalers, contamination of the system by secretions or condensate, low cardiac output, use of antacids or carbonated beverages, and leaks around tracheal tube cuffs or uncuffed tubes.

3. Does not evaluate pH or oxygenation.
4. Effective for confirming ET tube placement and for monitoring CO_2 in patients who tend to retain CO_2 (e.g., COPD).
5. Not a reliable method for determining inadvertent pulmonary placement of gastric tubes.
6. Clean and disinfect sensors and monitors per manufacturer's instructions.

Exhaled Breath Condensate

EVIDENCE BASE Konstaninidi, E., Lappa, A., Tzortzi, A., & Panagiotis, B. (2015). Exhaled breath condensate: Technical and diagnostic aspects. *The Scientific World Journal, 2015*, 435160. https://doi.org/10.1155/2015/435160

Description

1. Emerging as a source for determining biomarkers of lung disease mainly from the lower respiratory tract. Exhaled breath condensate (EBC) is a matrix of exhaled particles and droplets in which biomarkers may be identified, such as:
   a. Volatile (acetic acid, formic acid, ammonia) and nonvolatile compounds.
   b. Very-low- and low-molecular-weight compounds.
   c. Polypeptides.
   d. Proteins.
   e. Nucleic acids.
   f. Lipid mediators.
   g. Inorganic molecules.
   h. Organic molecules.
   i. Redox relevant molecules.
   j. pH-relevant molecules.
   k. Cytokines and chemokines.
2. Currently, there is no gold standard—either invasively or noninvasively—for determining absolute concentrations with which EBC can be easily compared.
3. The pH of EBC depends on disease state, ranging from 3.5 to 9.0, which can affect the reactivity and stability of other biomarkers being assayed.

Nursing and Patient Care Considerations

1. Collect condensate sample. Collection methods vary, depending on specific biomarkers to be analyzed. Ten minutes of tidal breathing yields 1 to 2 mm of sample; smaller sample sizes may be adequate for analysis of only one or two biomarkers.
2. Be aware that lower airway condensate may be contaminated by particles from oral and retropharyngeal mucosa.
3. Saliva trapping systems may be used with patients who drool, to reduce salivary contamination.

GENERAL PROCEDURES AND TREATMENT MODALITIES

See additional online content: Procedure Guidelines 6-3 to 6-24.

Artificial Airway Management

EVIDENCE BASE Burns, S., & Delgado, S. (2024). *AACN essentials of critical care nursing* (5th ed.). McGraw-Hill.

Airway management may be indicated in patients with loss of consciousness, facial or oral trauma, aspiration, tumor, infection, copious respiratory secretions, respiratory distress, and the need for mechanical ventilation (see Figure 6-3).

Types of Airways

1. Oropharyngeal airway—curved plastic device inserted through the mouth and positioned in the posterior pharynx to move tongue away from palate and open the airway.
   a. Usually for short-term use in the unconscious patient or may be used along with an oral endotracheal (ET) tube.
   b. Not used if recent oral trauma or surgery or if loose teeth are present.
   c. Does not protect against aspiration.
   d. Not recommended for use in alert patients because the device may trigger the gag reflex and induce vomiting, which may lead to aspiration.
2. Nasopharyngeal airway (nasal trumpet)—soft rubber or plastic tube hollow inserted through nose into posterior pharynx.
   a. Facilitates frequent nasopharyngeal suctioning.
   b. Useful in the semiconscious patient as an adjunct to help maintain airway patency.
   c. Use extreme caution with patients on anticoagulants or bleeding disorders.
   d. Select size that is slightly smaller than diameter of nostril and slightly longer than distance from tip of nose to earlobe.
   e. Check nasal mucosa for irritation or ulceration, and clean airway with hydrogen peroxide and water.
3. Laryngeal mask airway—composed of a tube with a cuffed masklike projection at the distal end; inserted through the mouth into the pharynx; seals the larynx and leaves distal opening of tube just above glottis.
   a. Easier placement than ET tube because visualization of vocal cords is not necessary.
   b. Provides ventilation and oxygenation comparable to that achieved with an ET tube.
   c. Cannot prevent aspiration because it does not separate the gastrointestinal (GI) tract from the respiratory tract.
   d. May cause laryngospasm and bronchospasm.
   e. Greater likelihood of misplacement.
4. Combitube—double-lumen tube with pharyngeal lumen and tracheoesophageal lumen; pharyngeal lumen has blocked distal end and perforations at pharyngeal level; tracheoesophageal lumen has open upper and lower end; large oropharyngeal balloon serves to seal mouth and nose; distal cuff seals the esophagus or trachea.
   a. Very seldom used in the hospital setting because of complications and inability to establish a definitive airway.
5. ET tube—flexible tube inserted through the mouth or nose and into the trachea beyond the vocal cords that acts as an artificial airway. It is the preferred method for trauma, medical emergencies, short-term complex patient.
   a. Maintains a patent airway.
   b. Allows for deep tracheal suction and removal of secretions.
   c. Permits mechanical ventilation.
   d. Inflated balloon seals off trachea, so aspiration from the GI tract cannot occur.
   e. Generally easy to insert in an emergency but maintaining placement is more difficult, so this is not for long-term use.

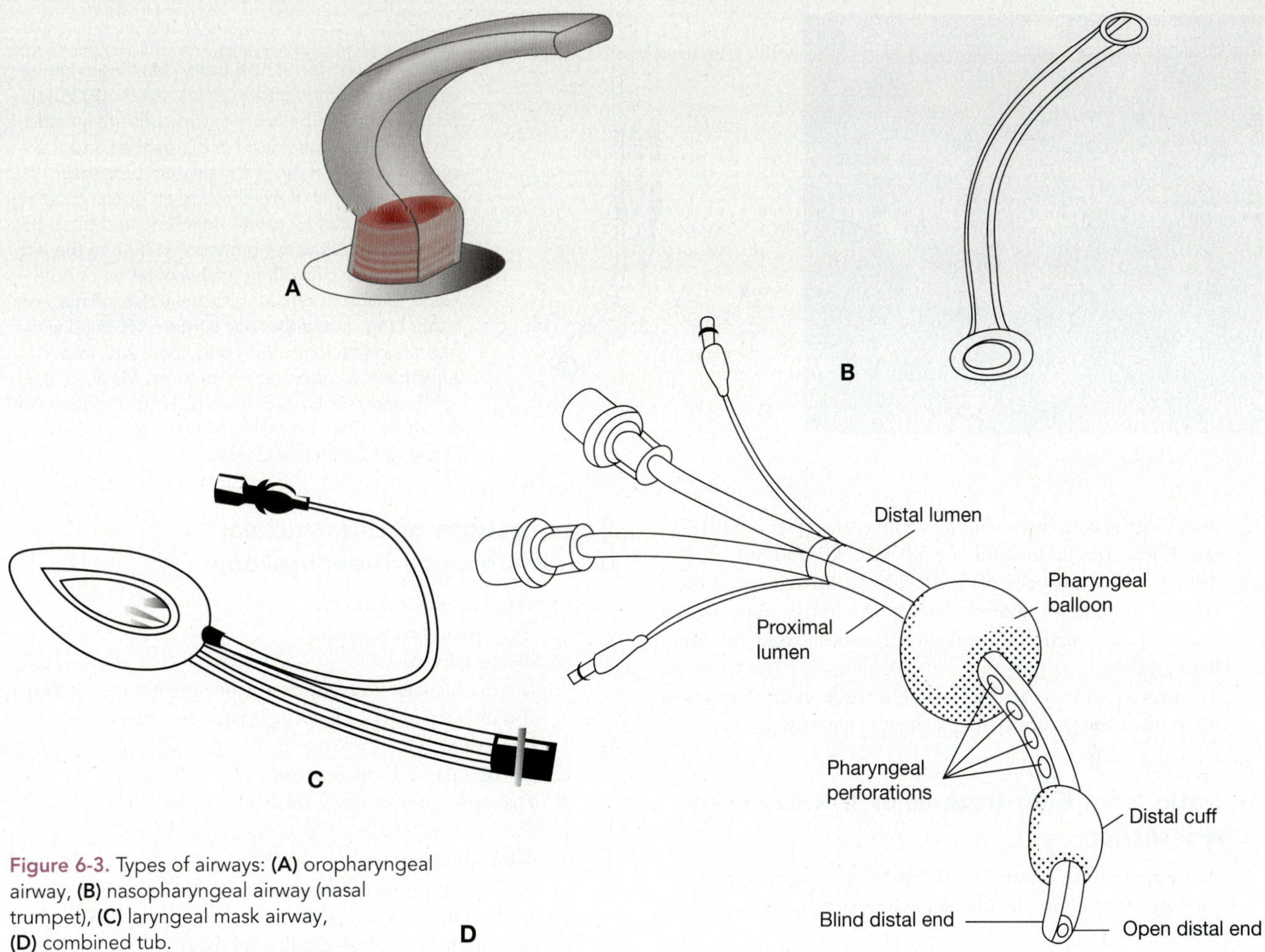

Figure 6-3. Types of airways: **(A)** oropharyngeal airway, **(B)** nasopharyngeal airway (nasal trumpet), **(C)** laryngeal mask airway, **(D)** combined tub.

6. Tracheostomy tube—firm, curved artificial airway inserted directly into the trachea at the level of the second or third tracheal ring through a surgically made incision.
   a. Permits mechanical ventilation and facilitates secretion removal.
   b. Can be for long-term use.
   c. Bypasses upper airway defenses, increasing susceptibility to infection.
   d. Allows the patient to eat and swallow.

CLINICAL JUDGMENT Position patient on side and suction oral cavity frequently to prevent aspiration of oral secretions or vomitus when an oral airway is in place.

CLINICAL JUDGMENT Nasopharyngeal airways may obstruct sinus drainage and produce acute sinusitis. Be alert to fever and facial pain.

Endotracheal Tube Insertion

1. Orotracheal insertion is technically easier because it is done under direct visualization with a laryngoscope. Disadvantages are increased oral secretions, decreased patient comfort, difficulty with tube stabilization, and inability of patient to use lip movement as a communication means.
2. Nasotracheal (NT) insertion may be more comfortable to the patient and is easier to stabilize. Disadvantages are that blind insertion is required and the possible development of pressure necrosis of the nasal airway, sinusitis, and otitis media.
3. Tube types vary according to length and inner diameter, type of cuff, and number of lumens.
   a. Usual sizes for adults are 6.0, 7.0, 8.0, and 9.0 mm.
   b. Most cuffs are high volume, low pressure, with self-sealing inflation valves, or the cuff may be of foam rubber.
   c. Most tubes have a single lumen; however, dual-lumen tubes may be used to ventilate each lung independently (see Figure 6-4).
4. May be contraindicated when glottis is obscured by vomitus, bleeding, foreign body, or trauma or cervical spine injury or deformity.

Tracheostomy Tube Insertion

1. Tube types vary according to presence of inner cannula and presence and type of cuff (see Figure 6-5).
   a. Tubes with high-volume, low-pressure cuffs with self-sealing inflation valves, with or without inner cannula.
   b. Fenestrated tube.
   c. Foam-filled cuffs.
   d. Speaking tracheostomy tube.
   e. Tracheal button or Passy-Muir valve.

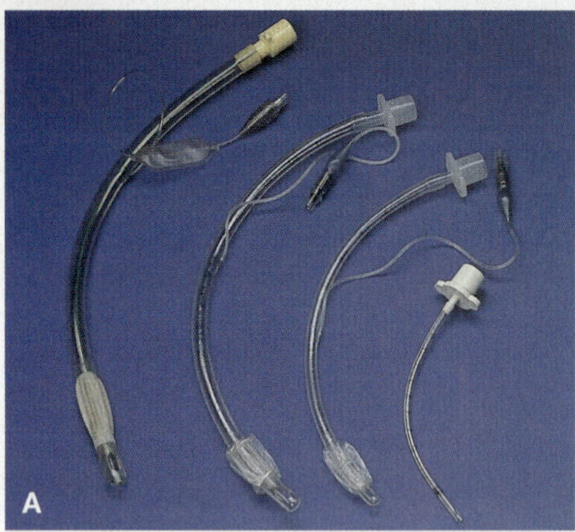

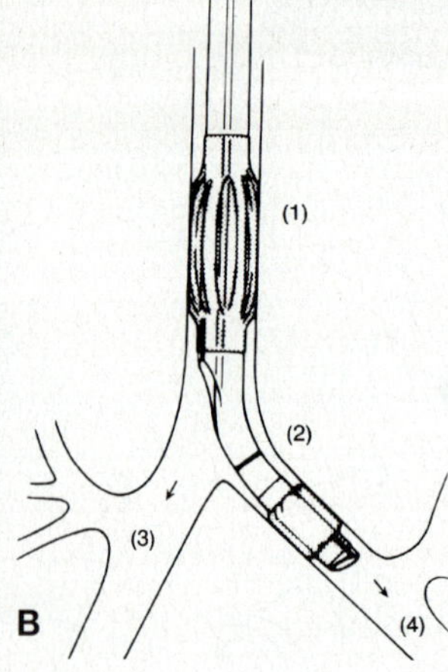

Figure 6-4. Endotracheal tubes. **(A)** Single-lumen and double-lumen endotracheal tubes. **(B)** When a double-lumen tube is used, two cuffs are inflated. One cuff (*1*) is positioned in the trachea and the second cuff (*2*) in the left mainstem bronchus. After inflation, air flows through an opening below the tracheal cuff (*3*) to the right lung and through an opening below the bronchial cuff (*4*) to the left lung. This permits differential ventilation of both lungs, lavage of one lung, or selective inflation of either lung during thoracic surgery. (*B*: Used with permission of John Wiley and Sons, Inc., from *Anesthesia for thoracic procedures*, *Marshall*, B. E., Longnecker, D. E., & Fairley, H. B. (Eds.), Blackwell Scientific, 1988; permission conveyed through Copyright Clearance Center, Inc.)

2. Tubes vary according to length and inner diameter in millimeters. Usual sizes for an adult are 5.0, 6.0, 7.0, and 8.0.
3. Tracheostomy is usually planned, either as an adjunct to therapy for respiratory dysfunction or for longer-term airway management when ET intubation has been used for more than 14 days.
4. The procedure may be done at the bedside in an emergency when other means of creating an airway have failed.

Indications for Endotracheal or Tracheostomy Tube Insertion

1. Acute respiratory failure, central nervous system (CNS) depression, neuromuscular disease, pulmonary disease, and chest wall injury.
2. Upper airway obstruction (tumor, inflammation, foreign body, or laryngeal spasm).
3. Anticipated upper airway obstruction from edema or soft tissue swelling because of head and neck trauma, some postoperative head and neck procedures involving the airway, facial or airway burns, or decreased level of consciousness (LOC).
4. Need for airway protection (vomiting, bleeding, or altered mental status).
5. Aspiration prophylaxis.
6. Fracture of cervical vertebrae with spinal cord injury; may require ventilatory assistance.

Complications of Endotracheal or Tracheostomy Tube Insertion

1. Laryngeal or tracheal injury.
   a. Sore throat, hoarse voice.
   b. Glottic edema.
   c. Trauma (damage to teeth or mucous membranes, perforation or laceration of pharynx, larynx, or trachea).
   d. Aspiration.
   e. Laryngospasm, bronchospasm.
   f. Ulceration or necrosis of tracheal mucosa.
   g. Vocal cord ulceration, granuloma, or polyps.
   h. Vocal cord paralysis.
   i. Postextubation tracheal stenosis.
   j. Tracheal dilation.
   k. Formation of tracheal–esophageal fistula.
   l. Formation of tracheal–arterial fistula.
   m. Innominate artery erosion.
2. Pulmonary infection and sepsis.
3. Dependence on artificial airway.

Nursing Care for Patients With Artificial Airways

General Care Measures

1. Handwashing and application of alcohol gel should be followed before and after all procedures.

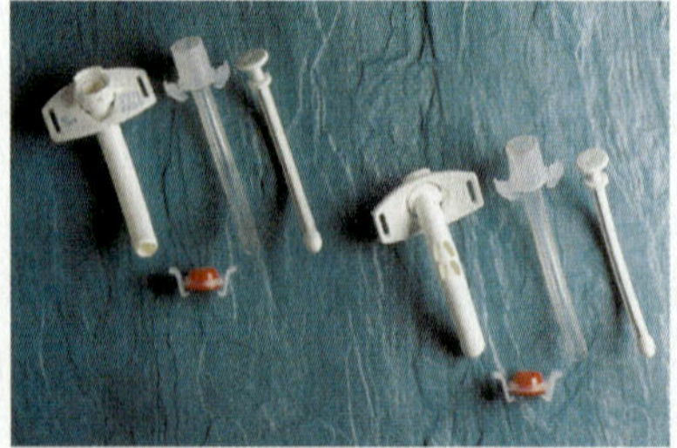

Cuffless: nonfenestrated (left) and fenestrated (right). Tracheostomy plug to allow breathing through upper airway is also shown.

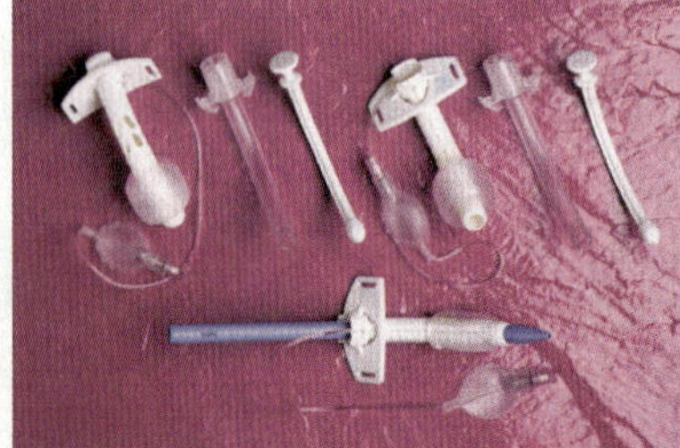

Cuffed: fenestrated (left) and nonfenestrated (right) with inner cannula and obturator for insertion. Percutaneous tracheostomy inducer (bottom).

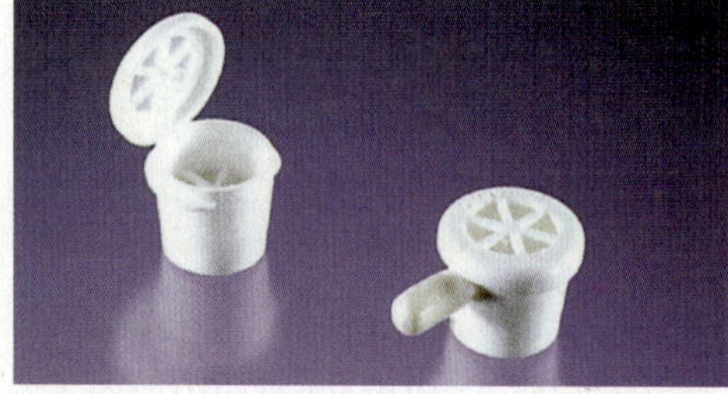

Speaking valve.

Figure 6-5. Types of tracheostomy tubes. (2018 Medtronic. All rights reserved. Used with the permission of Medtronic.)

2. Ensure adequate ventilation and oxygenation through the use of supplemental oxygen or mechanical ventilation as indicated.
3. Assess breath sounds every 2 hours. Note evidence of ineffective secretion clearance (rhonchi, crackles), which suggests need for suctioning.
4. Provide adequate humidity when the natural humidifying pathway of the oropharynx is bypassed.
5. Provide adequate suctioning of oral secretions to prevent aspiration and decrease oral microbial colonization.
6. Use clean technique when inserting an oral or nasopharyngeal airway, and take it out and clean it with hydrogen peroxide and rinse with water at least every 8 hours.
7. Perform oral care every 2 to 4 hours with soft toothbrush or swabs and prepackaged oral care kits. Frequent oral care will aid in prevention of ventilator-associated pneumonia. The patient's lips should be kept moisturized to prevent them from becoming sore and cracked.
8. Ensure that aseptic technique is maintained when inserting an ET or tracheostomy tube. The artificial airway bypasses the upper airway, and the lower airways are sterile below the level of the vocal cords.
9. Elevate the patient to a semi-Fowler's or sitting position, when possible; these positions result in improved lung compliance. The patient's position, however, should be changed at least every 2 hours to ensure ventilation of all lung segments and prevent secretion stagnation and atelectasis. Position changes are also necessary to avoid skin breakdown.
10. If an oral or nasopharyngeal airway is used, turn patient's head to the side to reduce the risk of aspiration (because there is no cuff to seal off the lower airway).

Nutritional Considerations

1. Consciousness is usually impaired in patient with an oropharyngeal airway, so oral feeding is contraindicated.
2. To enhance comfort, remove a nasopharyngeal airway in the conscious patient during mealtimes.
3. Recognize that an ET tube holds the epiglottis open. Therefore, only the inflated cuff prevents the aspiration of oropharyngeal contents into the lungs. The patient must not receive oral feeding. Administer enteral tube feedings or parenteral feedings, as ordered.
4. Administer oral feedings to a conscious patient with a tracheostomy, usually with the cuff inflated. The inflated cuff prevents aspiration of food contents into the lungs but causes the tracheal wall to bulge into the esophageal lumen and may make swallowing more difficult. Patients who are not on mechanical ventilation and are awake, alert, and able to protect the airway are candidates for eating with the cuff deflated. With the help of a speech therapist, evaluate the patient's ability to eat.
5. Patients should receive thickened rather than regular liquids; this will assist in effective swallowing.

CLINICAL JUDGMENT Consider the patient's nutritional needs early in the process of intubation so nutritional status does not decline further. It is difficult to wean patients who have compromised nutritional status.

Cuff Maintenance

1. ET tube cuffs should be inflated continuously and deflated only during intubation, extubation, and tube repositioning.
2. Tracheostomy tube cuffs also should be inflated continuously in patients on mechanical ventilation or continuous positive airway pressure (CPAP).
3. Patients who have undergone tracheostomy and who are breathing spontaneously may have the cuff inflated continuously (in the patient with decreased LOC without ability to fully protect airway), deflated continuously, or inflated only for feeding if the patient is at risk of aspiration.
4. Monitor cuff pressure every 4 hours.

External Tube Site Care

1. Secure an ET tube so it cannot be disrupted by the weight of ventilator or oxygen tubing or by patient movement.
   a. Use commercially available ET tube holder to secure tube. Check skin frequently to avoid pressure injury.
   b. Replace when soiled or insecure or when repositioning of tube is necessary.
   c. Position tubing so traction is not applied to ET tube.
2. Perform tracheostomy site care at least every 8 hours using 0.9% NS, and change tracheostomy ties when soiled and according to facility policy.
   a. Make sure ventilator or oxygen tubing is supported so traction is not applied to the tracheostomy tube.
3. Have available at all times at the patient's bedside a replacement ET tube in the same size as patient is using, resuscitation bag, oxygen source, and mask to ventilate the patient in the event of accidental tube removal. Anticipate your course of action in such an event.
   a. ET tube—know location and assembly of reintubation equipment including replacement ET tube. Know how to contact someone immediately for reintubation.
   b. Tracheostomy—have extra tracheostomy tube, obturator, and hemostats at bedside. Be aware of reinsertion technique, if facility policy permits, or know how to contact someone immediately for reinserting the tube.

CLINICAL JUDGMENT In the event of accidental ET or tracheostomy tube removal, use a bag/mask resuscitation device to ventilate the patient by mouth while covering tracheostomy stoma.

Psychologic Considerations

1. Assist patient to deal with psychological aspects related to artificial airway.
2. Recognize that patient is usually apprehensive, particularly about choking, inability to communicate verbally, inability to remove secretions, uncomfortable suctioning, difficulty in breathing, or mechanical failure.
3. Explain the function of the equipment carefully.
4. Inform patient and family that speaking will not be possible while the tube is in place, unless using a tracheostomy tube with a deflated cuff, a fenestrated tube, a Passy-Muir speaking valve, or a speaking tracheostomy tube.
   a. A Passy-Muir valve is a speaking valve that fits over the end of the tracheostomy tube. Air that is inhaled is exhaled through the vocal cords and out through the mouth, allowing speech.
5. Develop with patient the best method of communication (e.g., sign language; lip reading; alphabet, picture, or writing boards; digital communication tools).
   a. Patients with tracheostomy tubes or nasal ET tubes may effectively use orally operated electrolarynx devices.

b. Devise a means for patient to get the nurse's attention when someone is not immediately available at the bedside, such as call bell, soft-touch call bell, hand-operated bell, or rattle.

6. Anticipate some of patient's questions by discussing: "Is it permanent?" "Will it hurt to breathe?" or "Will someone be with me?"
7. If appropriate, advise patient that as condition improves, a tracheostomy button may be used to plug the tracheostomy site. A tracheostomy button is a rigid, closed cannula that is placed into the tracheostomy stoma after removal of a cuffed or uncuffed tracheostomy tube. When in proper position, the button does not extend into the tracheal lumen. The outer edge of the button is at the skin surface and the inner edge is at the anterior tracheal wall.

Community and Home Care Considerations

1. Teach patient and caregiver procedure. Patient will need to use stationary mirror to visualize tracheostomy and perform procedure.
2. Suctioning patient in the home: whenever possible, patient and caregiver should be taught to perform procedure. Patient should use controlled cough and other secretion-clearance techniques.
3. Preoxygenation and hyperinflation before suctioning may not be routinely indicated for all patients cared for in the home. Preoxygenation and hyperinflation are based on patient need and clinical status.
4. Normal saline should not be instilled unless clinically indicated (e.g., to stimulate cough).
5. Clean technique and clean examination gloves are used. At the end of suctioning, the catheter or tonsil tip should be flushed by suctioning recently boiled and cooled, or distilled, water to rinse away mucus, followed by suctioning air through the apparatus. The outer surface may be wiped with alcohol or hydrogen peroxide. The catheter and tonsil tip should be air-dried and stored in a clean, dry place. Generally, suction catheters should be discarded after 24 hours. Tonsil tips may be boiled and reused.
6. Care of tracheostomy stoma: clean with half-strength hydrogen peroxide (diluted with sterile water) and wipe with sterile water or sterile saline.

Mobilization of Secretions

The goal of airway clearance techniques is to improve clearance of airway secretions, thereby decreasing obstruction of the airways. This serves to improve ventilation and gas exchange. Patients with respiratory disorders, neuromuscular disorders, or CNS disorders, such as loss of consciousness that may impair respiratory function, typically require help with mobilization and removal of secretions. Increased amount and viscosity of secretions or inability to clear secretions through the normal cough mechanism may lead to pooling of secretions in lower airways. Pooling of secretions leads to infection and inadequate gas exchange. Secretions should be removed by coughing or, when necessary, by suctioning. However, routine suctioning should be avoided. Auscultation and visual inspection of the patient should be used to determine the need for suctioning. Secretions can be mobilized through the chest physical therapy measures of postural drainage, directed cough, positive expiratory pressure (PEP), high-frequency oscillation (oral devices such as Flutter or Acapella device, or chest devices such as the vest) mucus clearance devices, autogenic drainage, intrapulmonary vibration, percussion and vibration, and other secretion-clearance measures.

Nasotracheal Suctioning

1. Intended to remove accumulated secretions or other materials that cannot be moved by the patient's spontaneous cough or less-invasive procedures. Suctioning of the tracheobronchial tree in a patient without an artificial airway can be accomplished by inserting a sterile suction catheter lubricated with water-soluble jelly through the nares into the nasal passage, down through the oropharynx, past the glottis, and into the trachea.
2. NT suction is a blind, high-risk procedure with uncertain outcome. Complications include mechanical trauma, hypoxia, dysrhythmias, bradycardia, increased blood pressure (BP), vomiting, increased intracranial pressure (ICP), and misdirection of catheter.
3. Contraindications include:
   a. Bleeding disorders, such as disseminated intravascular coagulation, thrombocytopenia, leukemia.
   b. Laryngeal edema, laryngeal spasm.
   c. Esophageal varices.
   d. Tracheal surgery.
   e. Gastric surgery with high anastomosis.
   f. Myocardial infarction (MI).
   g. Occluded nasal passages or nasal bleeding.
   h. Epiglottitis.
   i. Head, facial, or neck injury.
4. May cause trauma to the nasal passages.
   a. Do not attempt to force the catheter if resistance is met.
   b. Report if significant bleeding occurs.
5. Insert a nasal airway if repeated suctioning is necessary to protect the nasal passages from trauma.
6. Be alert for signs of laryngeal edema because of irritation and trauma.
   a. Stop if suctioning becomes difficult or if the patient develops new upper airway noise or obstruction.
   b. Duration of the suctioning should be limited to less than 15 seconds.

CLINICAL JUDGMENT Suctioning should not be routinely performed. Only indicated when other methods to remove secretions from airway have failed.

Suctioning Through an Endotracheal or Tracheostomy Tube

1. Ineffective coughing may cause secretion collection in the artificial airway or tracheobronchial tree, resulting in narrowing of the airway, respiratory insufficiency, and stasis of secretions.
2. Assess the need for suctioning at least every 2 hours through auscultation of the chest.
3. Ventilation with a manual resuscitation bag will facilitate auscultation and may stimulate coughing, decreasing the need for suctioning.
4. Maintain sterile technique while suctioning.
5. Administer supplemental 100% oxygen through the mechanical ventilator or manual resuscitation bag before, after, and between suctioning passes to prevent hypoxemia.
6. Closed-system suctioning may be done with the suction catheter contained in the mechanical ventilator tubing. Ventilator disconnection is not necessary, so positive end–expiratory

pressure (PEEP) is maintained, sterility is maintained, risk of exposure to body fluids is eliminated, and time is saved. However, studies have not demonstrated that closed-system suctioning is more effective when compared with open suctioning in actually removing secretions.

Community and Home Care Considerations

1. Encourage patient to use directed cough or other airway clearance technique before suctioning. Auscultate the lungs to assess need for suctioning.
2. Teach caregivers to suction in the home situation using a clean technique rather than sterile. Wash hands well before suctioning.
3. Put on fresh examination gloves for suctioning, and reuse catheter after rinsing it in warm water.
4. Be aware that appropriate and aggressive airway clearance will assist in preventing pulmonary complications, thus lessening the need for hospitalization.
5. Hazards and complications are the same for the patient on home care as they are for a patient who is hospitalized.

Chest Physical Therapy

EVIDENCE BASE Wang, M. Y., Pan, L., & Hu, X. J. (2019). Chest physiotherapy for the prevention of ventilator associated pneumonia: A meta-analysis. *American Journal of Infection Control*, *47*(7), 755–760. https://doi.org/10.1016/j.ajic.2018.12.015

Strickland, S. L., Rubin, B. K., Drescher, G. S., Haas, C. F., O'Malley, C. A., Volsko, T. A., Branson, R. D., Hess, D. R., & American Association for Respiratory Care, Irving, Texas. (2013). AARC clinical practice guideline: Effectiveness of nonpharmacologic airway clearance therapies in hospitalized patients. *Respiratory Care*, *58*(12), 2187–2193. https://doi.org/10.4187/respcare.02925

Breathing Exercises

1. Techniques used to compensate for respiratory deficits and conserve energy by increasing efficiency of breathing. Have patient breathe in through the nose and out through the mouth at a ratio of 1:2.
2. The overall purposes for doing breathing exercises are:
   a. To relax muscles, relieve anxiety, and improve control of breathing.
   b. To eliminate useless, uncoordinated patterns of respiratory muscle activity.
   c. To slow the respiratory rate.
   d. To decrease the work of breathing.
   e. To improve efficiency and strength of respiratory muscles.
   f. To improve ventilation and oxygen saturation during exercise.
3. Diaphragmatic abdominal breathing is used primarily to strengthen the diaphragm, which is the main muscle of respiration. It also aids in decreasing the use of accessory muscles and allows for better control over the breathing pattern, especially during stressful situations and increased physical demands.
4. Pursed-lip breathing is used primarily to slow the respiratory rate and assist in emptying the lungs of retained CO_2. This technique is always helpful to patients, but especially when they feel extreme dyspnea because of exertion.
5. Breathing exercises are most helpful to patients when practiced and used on a regular basis.

CLINICAL JUDGMENT For patients with severe chronic obstructive pulmonary disease (COPD), evidence does not support the use of diaphragmatic breathing because this type of breathing may result in hyperinflation as a result of increased dyspnea and fatigue.

Percussion and Vibration

1. Postural drainage uses gravity and, possibly, external manipulation of the thorax to improve mobilization of bronchial secretions, to enhance matching of ventilation and perfusion, and to normalize functional residual capacity.
2. Indicated for difficulty with secretion clearance, evidence of retained secretions, and lung conditions that cause increased production of secretions such as bronchiectasis, cystic fibrosis, chronic bronchitis, and emphysema.
3. Contraindicated in undrained lung abscess, lung tumors, pneumothorax, diseases of the chest wall, lung hemorrhage, painful chest conditions, tuberculosis, severe osteoporosis, increased ICP, uncontrolled hypertension, and gross hemoptysis.
4. Percussion is movement done by "clapping" the chest wall in a rhythmic fashion with cupped hands or a mechanical device directly over the lung segments to be drained. The wrists are alternately flexed and extended so the chest is cupped or clapped in a painless manner. A mechanical percussor may be used to prevent repetitive motion injury. Research is mixed on the benefit of this technique.
5. Vibration is the technique of applying manual compression with oscillations or tremors to the chest wall during the exhalation phase of respiration. Research is mixed on the benefit of this technique.

Postural Drainage

1. Gravity-assisted positions, deep breathing, chest clapping, shaking, or vibration to assist in the removal of bronchial secretions from affected lung segments to central airways (see Figure 6-6).
2. The patient is positioned so the diseased areas are in a near-vertical position, and gravity is used to assist drainage of the specific segments.
3. The positions assumed are determined by the location, severity, and duration of mucus obstruction.
4. The exercises are usually performed two to four times daily, before meals and at bedtime. Each position is held for 3 to 15 minutes.
5. The procedure should be discontinued if tachycardia, palpitations, dyspnea, or chest pain occurs. These symptoms may indicate hypoxemia. Discontinue if hemoptysis occurs.
6. Contraindications include increased ICP, unstable head or neck injury, active hemorrhage with hemodynamic instability or gross hemoptysis, recent spinal surgery or injury, empyema, bronchopleural fistula, rib fracture, flail chest, and uncontrolled hypertension.
7. Bronchodilators, mucolytic agents, water, or saline may be nebulized and inhaled, or an inhaled bronchodilator may be used before postural drainage and chest percussion to reduce bronchospasm, decrease thickness of mucus and sputum, and combat edema of the bronchial walls, thereby enhancing secretion removal.
8. Perform secretion-clearance procedures before eating or a minimum of 1 hour after eating.

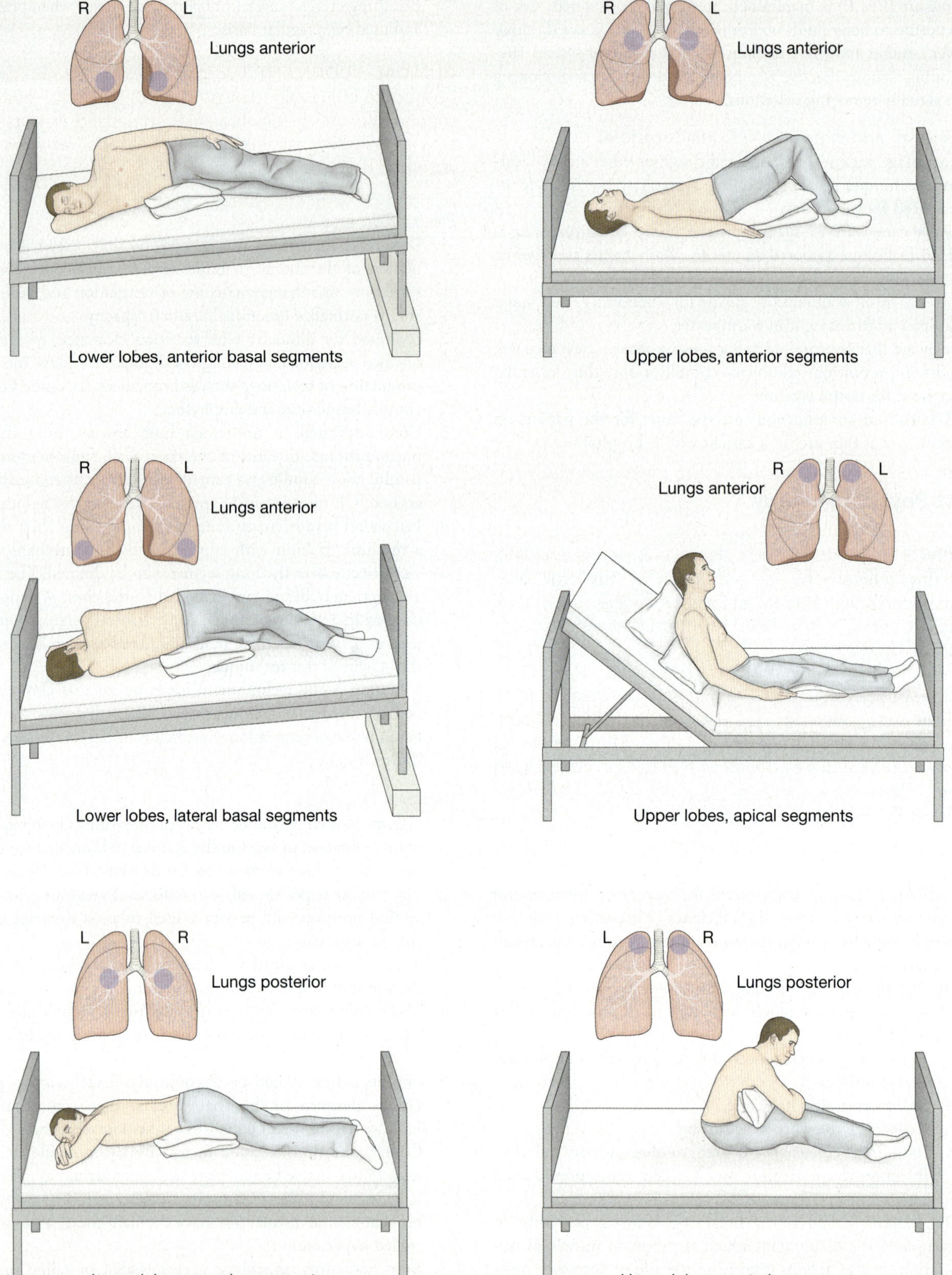

Figure 6-6. Postural drainage positions and the areas of lung drained by each position. (Reprinted with permission from Hinkle, J. L., Cheever, K. H., & Overbaugh, K. (2022). *Brunner and Suddarth's medical-surgical nursing* (15th ed., Fig. 20-6). Wolters Kluwer.)

9. Make sure patient is comfortable before the procedure starts and as comfortable as possible while assuming each position.
10. Auscultate the chest to determine the areas of needed drainage.
11. Encourage the patient to deep-breathe and cough after spending the allotted time in each position (normally 3 to 15 minutes).
12. Encourage diaphragmatic breathing throughout postural drainage; this helps widen airways so secretions can be drained.

CLINICAL JUDGMENT Postural drainage and chest percussion may result in hypoxia and should only be used if secretions are believed to be present.

Forced Expiratory Technique

1. Used to enhance effects of a spontaneous cough and compensate for physical limitations. Used for secretion clearance, atelectasis, prophylaxis against postoperative pulmonary complications, routine bronchial hygiene for cystic fibrosis, bronchiectasis, and chronic bronchitis and to obtain sputum specimen for diagnostic analysis.
2. Procedure includes a forced expiratory technique of two to three "huffs" (forced expirations), from mid- to low-lung volume, with glottis open, followed by a period of relaxed, controlled diaphragmatic breathing. Explain to the patient that to huff cough is the same maneuver that fogs eyeglasses. The forced expiration can be augmented by brisk adduction of the upper arms to self-compress the thorax.
3. Contraindications include increased ICP or known intracranial aneurysm, as well as acute or unstable head, neck, or spinal injury.

Manually Assisted Cough

This is the external application of mechanical pressure to the epigastric region coordinated with forced exhalation. This procedure may improve cough efficiency in those individuals with neuromuscular weakness or structural defects of the abdominal wall.

Positive Expiratory Pressure

1. Positive back pressure is created in the airways when the patient breathes in and out 5 to 20 times through a flow resistor or fixed orifice device.
2. During prolonged exhalation against positive pressure, peripheral airways are stabilized while air is pushed through collateral pathways (pores of Kohn and canals of Lambert) into distal lung units past retained secretions.
3. Expiratory airflow moves secretions to larger airways to be removed by coughing.
4. The pressure generated can be monitored and adjusted with a manometer (usually ranges from 10 to 20 cm H_2O).
5. Active exhalation with an inspiratory-to-expiratory (I:E) ratio of 1:3 or 1:4 is suggested.
6. The cycle is repeated until secretions are expelled, usually within 20 minutes or less if patient tires.

Autogenic Drainage

1. Controlled breathing used at three lung volumes, beginning at low-lung volume to unstick mucus, moving to midlung volume to collect mucus, and then to high-lung volume to expel mucus.
2. This method may be difficult for some patients to learn and to perform independently.
3. This can be performed in a seated position.

Flutter Mucus Clearance Device

1. Provides PEP and high-frequency oscillations at the airway opening; provides approximately 10 cm H_2O positive airway pressure.
2. The flutter valve is a pipe-shaped device with an inner cone and bowl loosely supporting a steel ball. The bowl containing the steel ball is covered by a perforated cap.
3. Indications include atelectasis, bronchitis, bronchiectasis, cystic fibrosis, and other conditions producing retained secretions.
4. Mucus clearance is based on:
   a. Vibration of the airways, which loosens mucus from airway walls.
   b. Intermittent increase in endobronchial pressure that keeps airways open.
   c. Acceleration of expiratory airflow to facilitate upward movement of mucus.
5. Contraindications include pneumothorax and right-sided heart failure.
6. Directions:
   a. Patient should be seated upright with chin tilted slightly upward to further open airway.
   b. Instruct patient to inhale slowly to three fourths of normal breath.
   c. Place flutter in mouth with lips firmly sealed around stem or mouthpiece.
   d. Position flutter at horizontal level or raise bulb end up to 30 degrees for greater force.
   e. Instruct patient to hold breath for 2 to 3 seconds.
   f. Exhale through flutter at moderately fast rate, keeping cheeks stiff. Urge to cough should be suppressed.
   g. Repeat for 5 to 10 more breaths.
7. Have patient perform same technique with one to two forced exhalations to generate mucus elimination and huff coughs as needed.
8. Generally used for 10 to 20 breaths with device followed by several directed coughs, repeating series four to six times or for 10 to 20 minutes up to four times daily.
9. Clean flutter device every other day by disassembling and using a liquid soap and tap water. Disinfect regularly by soaking cleaned disassembled parts in one part alcohol to three parts tap water for 1 minute; rinse, wipe, reassemble, and store.

Acapella Vibratory PEP Device

1. Enhances movement of secretions to larger airways, prevents collapse of airways, and facilitates filling of collapsed alveoli.
2. Airway vibration provides percussive effect, disengages mucus from airway walls, causes pulsation of mucus toward larger airways, and reduces viscoelasticity of mucus.
3. Select color-coded device: green for expiratory flow 15 L/min or greater, blue for less than 15 L/min.
4. Place mask tightly and comfortably over patient's mouth and nose (or seal lips tight around mouthpiece if mask is not used). Patient may sit, stand, or recline.
5. Instruct patient to perform diaphragmatic breathing, inhale to near-total lung volume, and exhale actively but not forcefully through device fully. Set resistance to achieve I:E ratio of 1:3 to 1:4. Use inline manometer to select expiratory pressure of 10 to 20 cm H_2O.
6. Use every 1 to 6 hours, according to response.
7. Assessment includes improving breath sounds, patient's report of improved dyspnea, improved chest x-ray, and improved oxygenation.

8. Acapella choice can be disassembled for cleaning in dishwasher, boiled, or autoclaved.

AeroPEP Valved Holding Chamber

1. Combines aerosol therapy from a metered-dose inhaler with a fixed orifice resister PEP therapy.
2. Place disposable mouthpiece over AeroPEP mouthpiece and attach manometer. Instruct patient to seal lips tightly around mouthpiece.
3. Although performing diaphragmatic breathing, inhale fully.
4. Exhale actively and fully to achieve PEP of 10 to 20 cm H_2O. Set AeroPEP between 0 and 6 at desired pressure on manometer.
5. Repeat for up to 20 minutes four times daily or as clinically indicated.

Intrapulmonary Percussive Ventilation or Percussionaire

1. Therapy is delivered by a percussionator, which delivers mini-bursts of air into the lungs at a rate of 100 to 300 per minute. Process includes delivery of a dense aerosol mist through a mouthpiece. The treatment lasts about 20 minutes.
2. Patient uses in sitting or recumbent position.
3. Instill nebulizer bowl with 20 mL of saline or aqueous water and prescribed bronchodilator.
4. Clinician or patient programs percussive cycle by holding down a button for 5 to 10 seconds for percussive inspiratory cycle and releasing to expectorate or pause during therapy.
5. Seal lips around mouthpiece with "pucker" to minimize cheek flapping.
6. Observe chest for percussive shaking.
7. Use twice daily for approximately 20 minutes with increased frequency as needed.

Mechanical Insufflation–Exsufflation

1. Assists in secretion clearance by applying positive pressure to the airway and then rapidly shifting to negative pressure by way of a face mask, mouthpiece, ET tube, or tracheostomy tube to increase cough effectiveness.
2. Used in patients with impaired cough who are unable to clear secretions.

Electrical Stimulation of the Expiratory Muscles

This procedure involves electrical stimulation of the abdominal muscles to increase cough effectiveness. An advantage is that presence of a caregiver is not required.

The Vest Airway Clearance System

1. Enhances secretion clearance through high-frequency chest wall oscillation. High-frequency compression pulses are applied to the chest wall by way of an air pulse delivery system and inflatable vest.
2. Variable-frequency large-volume air pulse delivery system attached to inflatable vest. Pressure pulses that fill the vest and vibrate the chest wall are controlled by a foot pedal. Pulse frequency ranges from 5 to 25 Hz and pressure in the vest ranges from 28 to 39 mm Hg.
3. A foot or hand control starts and stops pulsations.
4. Treatment length is usually 10 to 30 minutes. Therapy should include a break at least every 10 minutes for directed cough. Use twice daily, with increased frequency as needed.

Community and Home Care Considerations

1. Nebulizer tubing and mouthpiece can be reused at home repeatedly. Recommend thorough rinsing with warm water after each use, shake off excess water, and let air-dry.
2. Twice-weekly cleaning should include washing with liquid soap and hot water, followed by 30-minute soak in one part white vinegar and two parts tap water, and then rinsing with tap water, air-drying, and storing in a clean, dry place.

Administering Oxygen Therapy

EVIDENCE BASE Pirano, T., Madden, M., Roberts, K., Lamberti, J., Ginier, E., & Strickland, S. L. (2022). AARC clinical practice guideline: Management of adult patients with oxygen in the acute care setting. *Respiratory Care, 67*(1), 115–128. https://doi.org/10.4187/respcare.09294

Oxygen is an odorless, tasteless, colorless, transparent gas that is slightly heavier than air. It is used to treat or prevent symptoms and manifestations of hypoxia. Oxygen can be dispensed from a cylinder, piped-in system, liquid oxygen reservoir, or oxygen concentrator. It may be administered by nasal cannula, transtracheal catheter, nasal cannula with reservoir devices, or various types of face masks, including CPAP mask. It may also be applied directly to the ET or tracheal tube by way of a mechanical ventilator, T-piece, or manual resuscitation bag. The method selected depends on the required concentration of oxygen, desired variability in delivered oxygen concentration (none, minimal, moderate), and required ventilatory assistance (mechanical ventilator, spontaneous breathing).

Methods of Oxygen Administration

1. Nasal cannula—nasal prongs that deliver low or high flow of oxygen.
   a. Requires nose breathing.
   b. High flow devices can deliver up to 100% humidified, heated oxygen at a flow rate of 60 L/min
2. Simple face mask—mask that delivers moderate oxygen flow to nose and mouth. Delivers oxygen concentrations of 40% to 60%.
3. Venturi mask—mask with device that mixes air and oxygen to deliver constant oxygen concentration.
   a. Total gas flow at the patient's face must meet or exceed peak inspiratory flow rate. When other mask outputs do not meet inspiratory flow rate of patient, room air (drawn through mask side holes) mixes with the gas mixture provided by the face mask, lowering the inspired oxygen concentration.
   b. Venturi mask mixes a fixed flow of oxygen with a high but variable flow of air to produce a constant oxygen concentration. Oxygen enters by way of a jet (restricted opening) at a high velocity. Room air also enters and mixes with oxygen at this site. The higher the velocity (smaller the opening), the more room air is drawn into the mask.
   c. Mask output ranges from approximately 30% to 50% oxygen.
   d. It virtually eliminates rebreathing of CO_2. Excess gas leaves through openings in the mask, carrying with it the expired CO_2.
4. Partial rebreather mask—has an inflatable bag that stores 100% oxygen.
   a. On inspiration, the patient inhales from the mask and bag; on expiration, the bag refills with oxygen and expired gases exit through perforations on both sides of the mask and some enters bag (see Figure 6-7A).
   b. High concentrations of oxygen (50% to 75%) can be delivered.
   c. Often used to conserve oxygen supply during patient transport.

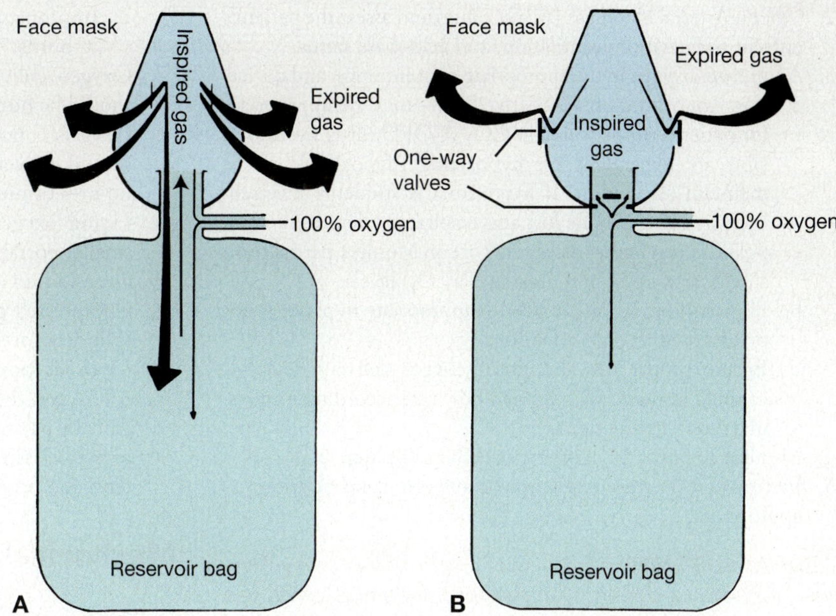

Figure 6-7. **(A)** Airflow diagram with partial rebreathing mask. **(B)** Airflow diagram with nonrebreathing mask. Arrows indicate direction of flow.

5. Nonrebreathing mask (see Figure 6-7B)—has an inflatable bag to store 100% oxygen and a one-way valve between the bag and mask to prevent exhaled air from entering the bag.
   a. Has one-way valves covering one or both of the exhalation ports to prevent entry of room air on inspiration.
   b. Has a flap or spring-loaded valves to permit entry of room air should the oxygen source fail or patient needs exceed the available oxygen flow.
   c. Optimally, all the patient's inspiratory volume will be provided by the mask/reservoir, allowing delivery of nearly 100% oxygen.
6. CPAP mask, a form of noninvasive positive pressure ventilation (NIPPV)—used to provide expiratory and inspiratory positive airway pressure in a manner similar to PEEP and does not require ET intubation.
   a. Has an inflatable cushion and head strap designed to tightly seal the mask against the face. See Figure 6-8.
   b. A PEEP valve is incorporated into the exhalation port to maintain positive pressure on exhalation.
   c. High inspiratory flow rates are needed to maintain positive pressure on inspiration.
7. Bilevel positive airway pressure (BiPAP) mask, a form of NIPPV—a combination of inspiratory and expiratory positive airway pressure often used to avoid intubation and mechanical ventilation.
   a. Preset pressure to be delivered during inspiration and preset pressure to be maintained during expiration.
   b. Mask with airtight seal is used, similar to CPAP.
8. T-piece (Briggs) adapter—used to administer oxygen to patient with ET or tracheostomy tube who is breathing spontaneously.
   a. High concentration of aerosol and oxygen delivered through wide-bore tubing.
   b. Expired gases exit through open reservoir tubing.
9. Manual resuscitation bag—delivers high concentration of oxygen to patient with insufficient inspiratory effort.
   a. With mask, uses upper airway by delivering oxygen to mouth and nose of patient.
   b. Without mask, adapter fits on ET or tracheostomy tube.
   c. Usually used in cardiopulmonary arrest, hyperinflation during suctioning, or transport of patients who are ventilator dependent.

Nursing Assessment and Interventions

1. Assess need for oxygen by observing for symptoms of hypoxia:
   a. Tachypnea.
   b. SaO_2 less than 88%.
   c. Tachycardia or dysrhythmias (premature ventricular contractions).
   d. A change in LOC (symptoms of decreased cerebral oxygenation are irritability, confusion, lethargy, and coma, if untreated).
   e. Cyanosis occurs as a late sign (PaO_2 ≤45 mm Hg).
   f. Labored respirations indicate severe respiratory distress.
   g. Myocardial stress—increase in heart rate and stroke volume (cardiac output) is the primary mechanism for compensation for hypoxemia or hypoxia; pupils dilate with hypoxia.

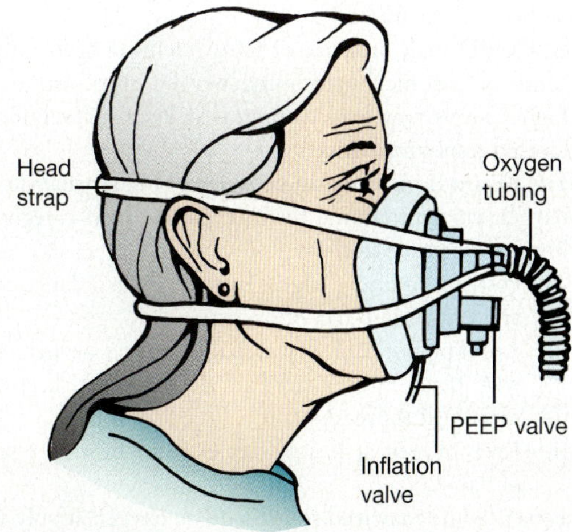

Figure 6-8. Continuous positive airway pressure mask with airtight seal. PEEP, positive end–expiratory pressure

2. Obtain Arterial blood gas (ABG) values and assess the patient's current oxygenation, ventilation, and acid–base status.
3. Administer oxygen in the appropriate concentration and device.
   a. Low concentration (24% to 28%)—may be appropriate for patients prone to retain CO_2 (COPD, drug overdose), who are dependent on hypoxemia (hypoxic drive) to maintain respiration. If hypoxemia is suddenly reversed, hypoxic drive may be lost and respiratory depression and, possibly, respiratory arrest may occur. Monitor partial pressure of arterial carbon dioxide ($PaCO_2$) levels.
   b. High concentration (≥30%)—appropriate in patients not predisposed to CO_2 retention.
   c. Ensure proper use and fit of oxygen-delivery device—cannula or mask, with oxygen flow rate according to manufacturer's instructions.
4. Monitor response by oximetry or ABG sampling.
5. Increase or decrease the inspired oxygen concentration, as appropriate.

CLINICAL JUDGMENT Success of any Positive Airway Pressure (PAP) device depends on patient adherence, which can be improved by proper education, proper mask fit, and frequent follow-up care.

CLINICAL JUDGMENT All accredited hospitals must be smoke free; however, other facilities and homes where oxygen is used may allow smoking. Make sure that no smoking is permitted where oxygen is used.

Community and Home Care Considerations

1. Indications for supplemental oxygen based on Medicare reimbursement guidelines:
   a. Documented hypoxemia: In adults: PaO_2 being 55 torr or SaO_2 being 88% or less when breathing room air, or PaO_2 being 56 to 59 torr or SaO_2 being 89% or less in association with cor pulmonale, heart failure, or polycythemia with hematocrit greater than 56%.
   b. Some patients may not qualify for oxygen therapy at rest but will qualify for oxygen during ambulation, exercise, or sleep. Oxygen therapy is indicated during these specific activities when SaO_2 is demonstrated to fall to 88% or less.
   c. Determine oxygen prescription for rest, exercise, and sleep, and instruct patient and caregiver to follow these flow rates.
2. Precautions in the home:
   a. In COPD with presence of CO_2 retention (generally because of chronic hypoxemia), oxygen administration at higher levels may lead to increased $PaCO_2$ level and decreased respiratory drive.
   b. Fire hazard is increased in presence of higher-than-normal oxygen concentrations. Instruct patient and caregiver of home oxygen precautions:
      i. Post "no smoking" signs. Instruct on avoidance of cigarettes within 6 feet of oxygen.
      ii. Avoid potential electrical sparks around oxygen (shave with blade razor instead of electric razor; keep away from heat sources).
      iii. Keep oxygen at least 6 feet (1.8 m) from any source of flame.
   c. Power failure may lead to inadequate oxygen supply when an oxygen concentrator is used without backup tank.
   d. Oxygen tanks must be secured in stand to prevent falling over.
   e. Improper use of liquid oxygen (touching liquid) may result in burns.
3. Oxygen delivered by way of tracheostomy collar or T tube should be humidified.
4. Oxygen concentrators extract oxygen from ambient air and should deliver oxygen at concentrations of 85% or greater at up to 4 L/min.
5. Liquid oxygen is provided in large reservoir canisters with smaller portable units that can be transfilled by patient or caregiver. Liquid oxygen evaporates from canister when not in use.
6. Compressed gas may be supplied in large cylinders (G or H cylinders) or smaller cylinders (D or E cylinders) with wheels for easier movement.
7. All oxygen-delivery equipment should be checked at least once daily by patient or caregiver, including function of equipment, prescribed flow rates, remaining liquid or compressed gas content, and backup supply.

Mechanical Ventilation

EVIDENCE BASE Meng, M., Zhang, J., Chen, L., & Wang, L. (2022). Prehospital, non-invasive ventilation for severe respiratory distress in adult patients: An updated meta-analysis. *Journal of Clinical Nursing, 31*(23/24), 3327–3337. https://doi.org/10.1111/jocn.16224

Burns, S., & Delgado, S. (2024). *AACN essentials of critical care nursing* (5th ed.). McGraw-Hill.

The mechanical ventilator device functions as a substitute for the bellows action of the thoracic cage and diaphragm. The mechanical ventilator can maintain ventilation automatically for prolonged periods. It is indicated when the patient is unable to maintain safe levels of oxygen or CO_2 by spontaneous breathing even with the assistance of other oxygen-delivery devices.

Clinical Indications

Mechanical Failure of Ventilation

1. Neuromuscular disease.
2. CNS disease.
3. CNS depression (drug intoxication, respiratory depressants, cardiac arrest).
4. Inefficiency of thoracic cage in generating pressure gradients necessary for ventilation (chest injury, thoracic malformation).
5. When ventilatory support is needed postoperatively.

Disorders of Pulmonary Gas Exchange

1. Acute respiratory failure.
2. Chronic respiratory failure.
3. Left-sided heart failure.
4. Pulmonary diseases resulting in diffusion abnormality.
5. Pulmonary diseases resulting in V/Q mismatch.
6. Acute lung injury.

Underlying Principles

1. Variables that control ventilation and oxygenation include:
   a. Ventilator rate—adjusted by rate setting, also known as frequency.
   b. Tidal volume V_T—volume of gas required for one breath (mL/kg), calculated based on predicted body weight.
   c. Fraction of inspired oxygen concentration (FiO_2)—set on ventilator and measured with an oxygen analyzer.

   d. Ventilator dead space—circuitry (tubing) common to inhalation and exhalation; tubing is calibrated.
   e. PEEP—set within the ventilator or with the use of external PEEP devices; measured at the proximal airway.
2. CO_2 elimination is controlled by V_T, rate, and dead space.
3. Oxygen tension is controlled by oxygen concentration and PEEP (also by rate and V_T).
4. In most cases, the duration of inspiration should not exceed exhalation.
5. The inspired gas must be warmed and humidified to prevent thickening of secretions and decrease in body temperature. Sterile or distilled water is warmed and humidified by way of a heated humidifier.

Types of Ventilators

Negative Pressure Ventilators

1. Applies negative pressure around the chest wall. This causes intra-airway pressure to become negative, thus drawing air into the lungs through the patient's nose and mouth.
2. No artificial airway is necessary; patient must be able to control and protect own airway.
3. Examples are the iron lung and cuirass (shell unit) ventilator.
4. Not widely used in clinical practice.

Positive Pressure Ventilators

During mechanical inspiration, air is actively delivered to the patient's lungs under positive pressure. Exhalation is passive and requires use of a cuffed artificial airway.

1. Pressure ventilation.
   a. Delivers selected gas pressure during inspiratory phase.
   b. Volume delivered depends on lung compliance and resistance.
   c. Use of volume-based alarms is recommended because any obstruction between the machine and lungs that allows a buildup of pressure in the ventilator circuitry will cause the ventilator to cycle, but the patient will receive no volume.
   d. Exhaled tidal volume is the variable to monitor closely.
2. Volume ventilation.
   a. Designated volume of air is delivered with each breath regardless of resistance and compliance. Usual starting volume is 6 to 8 mL/kg.
   b. Delivers the predetermined volume regardless of changing lung compliance (although airway pressures will increase as compliance decreases). Airway pressures vary from patient to patient and from breath to breath.
   c. Pressure-limiting valves, which prevent excessive pressure buildup within the patient-ventilator system, are used. Without this valve, pressure could increase indefinitely and pulmonary barotrauma could result. Usually equipped with a system that alarms when selected pressure limit is exceeded. Pressure-limited settings terminate inspiration when reached.

Modes of Operation

Controlled Mandatory Ventilation

1. Patient receives a predetermined set rate and tidal volume.
2. Provides a fixed level of ventilation, but will not cycle or have gas available in circuitry to respond to patient's own inspiratory efforts. This typically increases work of breathing for patients attempting to breathe spontaneously. Ventilator dyssynchrony may occur.
3. Generally used for patients who are unable to initiate spontaneous breaths.
4. Patient may require sedation/neuromuscular blockade while on this setting.

Assist/Control

1. Inspiratory cycle of ventilator is activated by the patient's voluntary inspiratory effort and delivers a preset tidal volume.
2. Ventilator also cycles at a rate predetermined by the operator. Should the patient not initiate a spontaneous breath, or breathe so weakly that the ventilator cannot function as an assistor, this mandatory baseline rate will provide a minimum respiratory rate.
3. Indicated for patients who are breathing spontaneously, but who have the potential to lose their respiratory drive or muscular control of ventilation. In this mode, the patient's work of breathing is greatly reduced.

Synchronized Intermittent Mandatory Ventilation (SIMV) or Intermittent Mandatory Ventilation (IMV)

1. Allows patient to breathe at their own rate and volume spontaneously through the ventilator circuitry.
2. Periodically, at a preselected time, a mandatory breath is delivered. The ventilator delivers the mandatory breath in synchrony with the patient's inspiratory effort.
3. If no inspiratory effort is delivered, the ventilator will deliver a mandatory breath at a scheduled time.
4. Gas provided for spontaneous breathing flows continuously through the ventilator.
5. Ensures that a predetermined number of breaths at a selected V_T are delivered each minute.
6. Indicated for patients who are breathing spontaneously, but at a V_T or rate less than adequate for their needs. Allows the patient to do some of the work of breathing.

Pressure Support

1. Augments inspiration to a patient who is breathing spontaneously.
2. Maintains a set positive pressure during spontaneous inspiration.
3. The patient ventilates spontaneously, establishing own rate, V_T, and inspiratory time.
4. Pressure support may be used independently as a ventilatory mode or used in conjunction with other modes of ventilation such as SIMV.

Positive Pressure Ventilation Techniques

Positive End–Expiratory Pressure

1. Maneuver by which pressure during mechanical ventilation is maintained above atmospheric at end of exhalation, resulting in an increased functional residual capacity. Airway pressure is therefore positive throughout the entire ventilatory cycle.
2. Purpose of PEEP is to increase functional residual capacity (or the amount of air left in the lungs at the end of expiration). This aids in:
   a. Increasing the surface area of gas exchange.
   b. Preventing collapse of alveolar units and development of atelectasis.
   c. Decreasing intrapulmonary shunt.
   d. Improving lung compliance.
   e. Improving oxygenation.
   f. Recruiting alveolar units that are totally or partially collapsed.

3. Benefits:
   a. Because a greater surface area for diffusion is available and shunting is reduced, it is often possible to use a lower FiO_2 than otherwise would be required to obtain adequate arterial oxygen levels. This reduces the risk of oxygen toxicity in conditions such as acute respiratory distress syndrome (ARDS).
   b. Positive intra-airway pressure may be helpful in reducing the transudation of fluid from the pulmonary capillaries in situations where capillary pressure is increased (i.e., left-sided heart failure).
   c. Increased lung compliance resulting in decreased work of breathing.
4. Hazards:
   a. Because the intrathoracic pressure is increased by PEEP, venous return is impeded. This may result in:
      i. Decreased cardiac output and decreased oxygen delivery to the tissues (especially noted in patients with hypovolemia).
      ii. Decreased renal perfusion.
      iii. Increased ICP.
      iv. Hepatic congestion.
   b. The decreased venous return may cause antidiuretic hormone formation to be stimulated, resulting in decreased urine output.
5. Precautions:
   a. Monitor frequently for signs and symptoms of respiratory distress (shortness of breath, dyspnea, tachycardia, chest pain).
   b. Monitor frequently for signs and symptoms of pneumothorax (increased PAP, increased size of hemothorax, uneven chest wall movement, hyperresonant percussion, distant or absent breath sounds).
   c. Monitor for signs of decreased venous return (decreased BP, decreased cardiac output, decreased urine output, peripheral edema).
   d. Abrupt discontinuance of PEEP is not recommended. The patient should not be without PEEP for longer than 15 seconds. The manual resuscitation bag used for ventilation during suction procedure or patient transport should be equipped with a PEEP device. Inline suctioning may also be used so that PEEP can be maintained.
   e. Intrapulmonary blood vessel pressure may increase with compression of the vessels by increased intra-airway pressure. Therefore, central venous pressure (CVP), PAP, and pulmonary capillary wedge pressure may be increased. The clinician must bear this in mind when determining the clinical significance of these pressures.

Continuous Positive Airway Pressure

1. Assists the patient who is breathing spontaneously to improve oxygenation by elevating the end-expiratory pressure in the lungs throughout the respiratory cycle.
2. May be delivered through ventilator circuitry when ventilator rate is at "0" or may be delivered through a separate CPAP circuitry that does not require the ventilator.
3. Indicated for patients who are capable of maintaining an adequate V_T, but who have pathology preventing maintenance of adequate levels of tissue oxygenation or for sleep apnea.
4. CPAP has the same benefits, hazards, and precautions noted with PEEP. Mean airway pressures may be lower because of lack of mechanical ventilation breaths. This results in less risk of barotrauma and impedance of venous return.

Newer Modes of Ventilation

Pressure-Regulated Volume Control (PRVC)

1. PRVC ventilator mode is a volume-targeted mode used in acute respiratory failure that combines the advantages of the decelerating inspiratory flow pattern of a pressure-control mode with the ease of use of a volume-control (VC) mode.
2. Ventilator uses feedback on a breath-by-breath basis to adjust the pressure delivered to achieve a target tidal volume.
3. A mandatory rate is set for the patient, and they may breathe above the set rate.

Airway Pressure Release Ventilation

1. Ventilator cycles between two different levels of CPAP.
2. The baseline airway pressure is the upper CPAP level and the pressure is intermittently released.
3. Uses a short expiratory time.
4. Used in severe ARDS/acute lung injury and other disorders with poor lung compliance.

Noninvasive Positive Pressure Ventilation

1. Uses a nasal or face mask or nasal pillows. Delivers air through a volume- or pressure-controlled ventilator.
2. Used primarily in the past for patients with chronic respiratory failure associated with neuromuscular disease. Now it is being used successfully during acute exacerbations. Some patients are able to avoid invasive intubation. Other indications include acute or chronic respiratory distress, acute pulmonary edema, pneumonia, COPD exacerbation, weaning, and postextubation respiratory decompensation.
3. Can be used in the home setting. Equipment is portable and relatively easy to use.
4. Eliminates the need for intubation; preserves normal swallowing, speech, and the cough mechanism.
5. May include BiPAP, which is essentially pressure support with CPAP. The system has a rate setting as well as inspiratory and expiratory pressure setting.

High-Frequency Ventilation

1. Uses very small V_T (dead space ventilation) and high frequency (rates >100/min).
2. Gas exchange occurs through various mechanisms, not the same as conventional ventilation (convection).
3. Types include:
   a. High-frequency oscillatory ventilation.
   b. High-frequency jet ventilation.
4. Theory is that there is decreased barotrauma by having small V_T and that oxygenation is improved by constant flow of gases.
5. Successful with infant respiratory distress syndrome; much less successful with adult pulmonary complications.

Nursing Assessment and Interventions

1. Monitor for complications:
   a. Airway aspiration, decreased clearance of secretions, ventilator-acquired pneumonia, tracheal damage, and laryngeal edema.
   b. Impaired gas exchange.
   c. Ineffective breathing pattern.
   d. ET tube kinking, cuff failure, mainstem intubation.
   e. Sinusitis.
   f. Pulmonary infection.
   g. Barotrauma (pneumothorax, tension pneumothorax, subcutaneous emphysema, pneumomediastinum).
   h. Decreased cardiac output.

i. Atelectasis.
j. Alteration in GI function (stress ulcers, gastric distension, paralytic ileus).
k. Alteration in renal function.
l. Alteration in cognitive–perceptual status.

2. Suction the patient as indicated.
   a. When secretions can be seen or sounds resulting from secretions are auscultated with or without the use of a stethoscope.
   b. After chest physiotherapy.
   c. After bronchodilator treatments.
   d. Increased peak airway pressure in patients who are mechanically ventilated that is not due to the artificial airway or ventilator tube kinking, the patient biting the tube, the patient coughing or struggling against the ventilator, or a pneumothorax.
3. Provide routine care for patient on mechanical ventilator, including good oral care and repositioning to prevent ventilator-associated pneumonia. Provide humidity to help mobilize secretions.
4. Assist with the weaning process, when indicated (patient gradually assumes responsibility for regulating and performing own ventilations).
   a. Patient must have acceptable ABG values, have no evidence of acute pulmonary pathology, and be hemodynamically stable.
   b. Obtain serial ABGs or oximetry readings, as indicated.
   c. Monitor very closely for change in pulse and BP, anxiety, and increased rate of respirations.
   d. The patient is awake and cooperative and displays optimal respiratory drive.
5. Once weaning is successful, extubate and provide alternate means of oxygen.
6. Extubation will be considered when the pulmonary function parameters of V_T, VC, and negative inspiratory pressure are adequate, indicating strong respiratory muscle function.

Community and Home Care Considerations

Patients may require mechanical ventilation at home to replace or assist normal breathing. Ventilator support in the home is used to keep patient clinically stable and to maintain life.

1. Candidates for home ventilation are those patients who are unable to wean from mechanical ventilation or have disease progression requiring ventilator support. Candidates for home mechanical ventilator support:
   a. Have a secure artificial airway (tracheostomy tube).
   b. Have FiO_2 requirement 40% or less.
   c. Are medically stable.
   d. Are able to maintain adequate ventilation on standard ventilator settings.
2. Patients may choose not to receive home ventilation. Examples of inappropriate candidates for home ventilation include patients who:
   a. Have an FiO_2 40% or greater.
   b. Use PEEP greater than 10 cm H_2O.
   c. Require continuous invasive monitoring.
   d. Lack a mature tracheostomy.
   e. Lack able, willing, appropriate caregivers, or caregiver respite.
   f. Lack adequate financial resources for care in home.
   g. Lack adequate physical facilities:
      i. Inadequate heat, electricity, sanitation.
      ii. Presence of fire, health, or safety hazards.
3. For patients on mechanical ventilation in the home, a contract and relationship with a home medical equipment company and home nursing agency must be developed to provide:
   a. Care of patient who is ventilator dependent.
   b. Provision and maintenance of equipment.
   c. Timely provision of disposable supplies.
   d. Ongoing monitoring of patient and equipment.
   e. Training of patient, caregivers, and clinical staff on proper management of patient on ventilator and use and troubleshooting of equipment.
4. Equipment required:
   a. Appropriate ventilator with alarms (disconnect and high pressure).
   b. Power source.
   c. Humidification system.
   d. Manual resuscitation bag with tracheostomy adapter.
   e. Suction equipment.
   f. Replacement tracheostomy tubes.
   g. Supplemental oxygen, as medically indicated.
   h. Communication method for patient.
   i. Backup charged battery/generator to run ventilator during power failures.
5. Lay caregiver training and return demonstration must include the following:
   a. Proper setup, use, troubleshooting, maintenance, and cleaning and infection control of equipment and supplies.
   b. Appropriate patient assessment and management of abnormalities, including cardiopulmonary resuscitation, response to emergencies, and power and equipment failure.
6. Potential complications include:
   a. Patient deterioration, decannulation, and need for emergency services.
   b. Equipment failure and malfunction.
   c. Psychosocial complications, including depression, anxiety, and loss of resources (caregiver, financial, detrimental change in family structure or coping capacity).
7. Communication is essential with local emergency medical services (fire, police, rescue) and utility (telephone, electric) companies from whom the patient would need immediate and additional assistance in event of emergency (e.g., power failure, fire).

Thoracic Surgeries

Thoracic surgeries (see Table 6-2) are operative procedures performed to aid in the diagnosis and treatment of certain pulmonary conditions and when performing surgery that compromises the integrity of the thoracic cavity. Procedures include thoracotomy, video-assisted thoracoscopy, decortication, lung volume reduction surgery, lobectomy (see Figure 6-9, page 152), pneumonectomy, segmental resection, and wedge resection. These procedures may or may not require chest drainage immediately after surgery.

CLINICAL JUDGMENT Meticulous attention must be given to the preoperative and postoperative care of patients undergoing thoracic surgery. These operations are wide in scope and represent a major stress on the cardiorespiratory system.

Table 6-2 Thoracic Surgery Types

TYPE	DESCRIPTION	INDICATIONS
Exploratory thoracotomy	*Internal view of lung* • Usually posterolateral parascapular but could be anterior incision. • Chest tubes after procedure.	May be used to confirm carcinoma or for chest trauma (to detect source of bleeding).
Lobectomy	*One-lobe removal* • Thoracotomy incision at site of lobe removal. • Chest tubes after procedure.	Used when pathology is limited to one area of lung: bronchogenic carcinoma, giant emphysematous blebs or bullae, benign tumors, metastatic malignant tumors, bronchiectasis, and fungal infections.
Pneumonectomy	*Removal of an entire lung* • Posterolateral or anterolateral thoracotomy incision. • Sometimes there is a rib resection. • Normally no chest drains or tubes because fluid accumulation in empty space is desirable.	Performed chiefly for carcinoma but may be used for lung abscesses, bronchiectasis, or extensive tuberculosis. *Note: Right lung is more vascular than left; may cause more physiologic problems if removed.*
Segmentectomy (segmental resection)	• *Removal of one or more lung segments.* Segments function as individual units.	Used when pathology is localized (such as in bronchiectasis) and when the patient has preexisting cardiopulmonary compromise.
Wedge resection	*Removal of small, localized lesion that occupies only part of a segment.* • Incision made without regard to segments. • Chest tubes after procedure.	Performed for random lung biopsy and small peripheral nodules. Considered when less-invasive tests have failed to establish a diagnosis. May be used as a therapeutic procedure.
Thoracoscopy	*Direct visualization of pleura with thoracoscope via an intercostal incision* • Medical thoracoscopy under sedation or local anesthesia; allows for visualization and biopsy. • Video-assisted thoracoscopic surgery (VATS) under general anesthesia; multiple puncture sites and video screen allow for visualization and manipulation of the pleura, mediastinum, and lung parenchyma.	VATS may be used for lung biopsy, lobectomy, resection of nodules, repair of fistulas.
Decortication	*Removal or stripping of thick fibrous membrane from visceral pleura* • Use of chest tube drainage system postoperatively.	Empyema unresponsive to conservative management.
Thoracotomy not involving lungs	• Incision into the thoracic cavity for surgical procedures on other structures.	Used for hiatal hernia repair, open-heart surgery, esophageal surgery, tracheal resection, aortic aneurysm repair.
Lung volume reduction surgery (LVRS)	• Involves reducing lung volume by multiple wedge excisions or VATS.	Performed in advanced bullous emphysema, alpha[1]-antitrypsin emphysema.

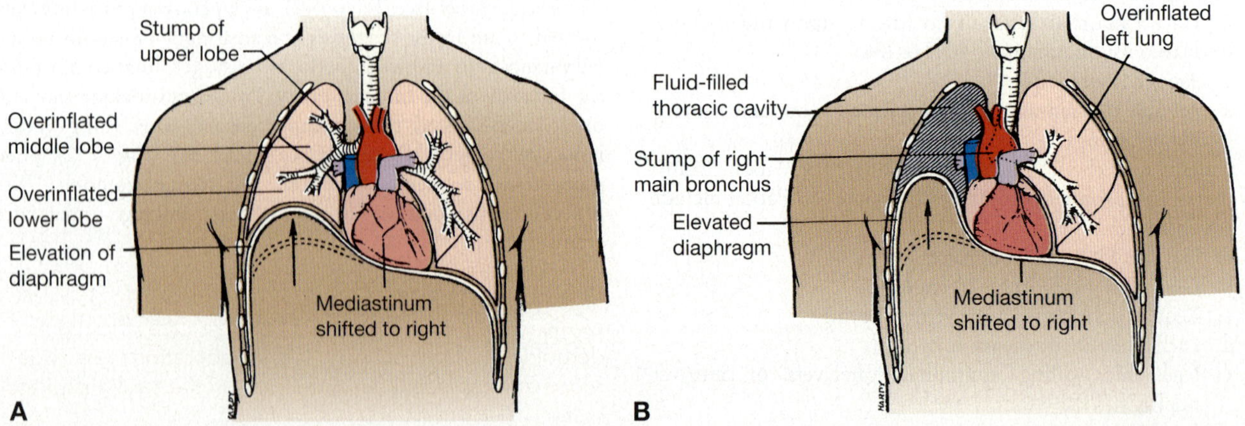

Figure 6-9. Operative procedures. **(A)** Lobectomy. **(B)** Pneumonectomy.

Preoperative Management

Goal is to maximize respiratory function to improve the outcome postoperatively and reduce risk of complications.

1. Encourage the patient to stop smoking to restore bronchial ciliary action and to reduce the amount of sputum, and likelihood of postoperative atelectasis, by decreasing secretions and increasing oxygen saturation.
2. Teach an effective coughing technique.
   a. Sit upright with knees flexed and body bending slightly forward (or lie on side with hips and knees flexed if unable to sit up).
   b. Splint the incision with hands or pillow.
   c. Take three short breaths, followed by a deep inspiration, inhaling slowly and evenly through the nose.
   d. Contract abdominal muscles and cough twice forcefully with mouth open and tongue out.
   e. Alternate technique—huffing and coughing—is less painful. Take a deep diaphragmatic breath and exhale forcefully against hand; exhale in a quick, distinct pant, or "huff."
3. Humidify the air to loosen secretions.
4. Administer bronchodilators to reduce bronchospasm.
5. Administer antimicrobials for infection.
6. Encourage deep breathing with the use of incentive spirometer to prevent atelectasis postoperatively.
7. Teach diaphragmatic breathing.
8. Carry out chest physical therapy and postural drainage to reduce pooling of lung secretions (see page 143).
9. Evaluate cardiopulmonary status for risk and prevention of complication.
10. Encourage activity to improve exercise tolerance.
11. Diagnostic studies may include pulmonary function test (PFT), chest x-ray, electrocardiogram (ECG), ABGs, serum electrolytes, CBC, and coagulation studies.
12. Administer medications and limit sodium and fluid to improve heart failure, if indicated.
13. Correct anemia, dehydration, and hypoproteinemia with intravenous (IV) infusions, tube feedings, and blood transfusions as indicated.
14. Give prophylactic anticoagulant, as prescribed, to reduce perioperative incidence of deep vein thrombosis and pulmonary embolism.
15. Provide teaching and counseling.
    a. Orient the patient to events that will occur in the postoperative period—coughing and deep breathing, suctioning, chest tube and drainage system, oxygen therapy, ventilator therapy, pain control, leg exercises, and range-of-motion (ROM) exercises for affected shoulder.
16. Make sure that patient fully understands surgery and is emotionally prepared for it; verify that informed consent has been obtained.

Postoperative Management

1. Use mechanical ventilator or supplemental oxygen until respiratory function and cardiovascular status stabilize. Assist with weaning and extubation.
2. Auscultate chest, monitor vital signs, monitor ECG, and assess respiratory rate and depth frequently. Arterial line, CVP, and pulmonary artery catheter are usually used.
3. Monitor ABG values or SaO_2 frequently.
4. Monitor and manage chest drainage system to drain fluid, blood, clots, and air from the pleura after surgery (see page 154). Chest drainage is usually not used after pneumonectomy because it is desirable that the pleural space fills with an effusion, which eventually obliterates the space.

Complications

1. Hypoxia—assess for restlessness, tachycardia, tachypnea, and elevated BP.
2. Postoperative bleeding—monitor for restlessness, anxiety, pallor, tachycardia, and hypotension.
3. Pneumonia; atelectasis—monitor for fever, chest pain, dyspnea, changes in lung sounds on auscultation.
4. Bronchopleural fistula from disruption of a bronchial suture or staple; bronchial stump leak.
   a. Observe for sudden onset of respiratory distress or cough productive of serosanguineous fluid.
   b. Position with the operative side down.
   c. Prepare for immediate chest tube insertion or surgical intervention.
5. Cardiac dysrhythmias (usually occurring third to fourth postoperative day); MI or heart failure.

Nursing Interventions

Maintaining Adequate Breathing Pattern

1. Monitor rate, rhythm, depth, and effort of respirations.
2. Auscultate chest for adequacy of air movement to detect bronchospasm, consolidation.
3. Monitor pulse oximetry and obtain ABG analysis and pulmonary function measurements as ordered.
4. Monitor LOC and inspiratory effort closely to begin weaning from ventilator as soon as possible.
5. Suction, as needed, using meticulous aseptic technique.
6. Elevate the head of the bed 30 to 40 degrees when patient is oriented and BP is stabilized to improve movement of diaphragm and alleviate dyspnea.
7. Encourage coughing and deep-breathing exercises and use of an incentive spirometer to prevent bronchospasm, retained secretions, atelectasis, and pneumonia.
8. Provide optimal pain relief to promote deep breathing, turning, and coughing.

CLINICAL JUDGMENT Tracheobronchial secretions are present in excessive amounts in patients after thoracotomy because of trauma to the tracheobronchial tree during operation, diminished lung ventilation, and diminished cough reflex.

CLINICAL JUDGMENT Look for changes in color and consistency of suctioned sputum. Colorless, fluid sputum is not unusual; opacification or coloring of sputum may mean dehydration or infection.

Stabilizing Hemodynamic Status

1. Evaluate BP, pulse, and respiration every 15 minutes or more frequently as indicated; extend the time intervals according to the patient's clinical status.
2. Monitor heart rate and rhythm by way of auscultation and continuous ECG because dysrhythmias are frequently seen following thoracic surgery.
3. Monitor CVP for prompt recognition of hypovolemia and for effectiveness of fluid replacement.

4. Monitor cardiac output and pulmonary artery systolic, diastolic, and wedge pressures. Watch for subtle changes, especially in the patient with underlying cardiovascular disease.
5. Assess chest tube drainage for amount and character of fluid.
   a. Chest drainage should progressively decrease after first 12 hours.
   b. Prepare for blood replacement and possible reoperation to achieve hemostasis if bleeding persists.
   c. Chest tube drainage in excess of 1,000 to 1,200 mL per 24-hour period should be reported to the health care provider for follow-up.
   d. Chest drainage greater than 200 mL in the first hour, development of subcutaneous emphysema, or any signs and symptoms of respiratory distress should be reported to the health care provider immediately.
6. Maintain intake and output record, including chest tube drainage.
7. Monitor infusions of blood and parenteral fluids closely because the patient is at risk for fluid overload if portion of pulmonary vascular system has been reduced.

Achieving Adequate Pain Control

1. Perform comprehensive pain assessment including onset, location, duration, characteristics, precipitating factors, and response to interventions.
2. Provide appropriate pain relief—pain limits chest excursions, thereby decreasing ventilation. Severity of pain varies with type of incision and with the patient's reaction to and ability to cope with pain. Usually, a posterolateral incision is the most painful.
3. Give opioids (usually by continuous IV infusion or by epidural catheter by way of patient-controlled analgesia pump) for pain relief, as prescribed, to permit patient to breathe more deeply and cough more effectively. To avoid respiratory and CNS depression, limit high doses of opioids; patient should be alert enough to cough.
4. Assist with intercostal nerve block or cryoanalgesia (intercostal nerve freezing) for pain control as ordered.
5. Position for comfort and optimal ventilation (head of bed elevated 15 to 30 degrees); this also helps residual air to rise in upper portion of pleural space where it can be removed by the chest tube.
   a. Patients with limited respiratory reserve may not be able to turn on unoperated side because this may limit ventilation of the operated side.
   b. Vary the position from horizontal to semierect to prevent retention of secretions in the dependent portion of the lungs.
6. Encourage splinting of incision with pillow or folded towel while turning, changing position, or coughing.
7. Teach relaxation (nonpharmacologic) techniques, such as progressive muscle relaxation and imagery, to help reduce pain.

CLINICAL JUDGMENT Evaluate for signs of hypoxia thoroughly when anxiety, restlessness, and agitation of new onset are noted before administering as-needed sedatives.

Increasing Mobility of Affected Shoulder

1. Begin ROM exercise of arm and shoulder on affected side immediately to prevent ankylosis of the shoulder ("frozen" shoulder).
2. Perform exercises at time of maximal pain relief.
3. Encourage patient to actively perform exercises three to four times per day, taking care not to disrupt chest tube or invasive lines (i.e., IV).

Patient Education and Health Maintenance

1. Advise that there will be some intercostal pain for several weeks, which can be relieved by local heat and oral analgesia. Many patients experience intercostal pain up to 1 year following surgery.
2. Advise that weakness and fatigability are common during the first 3 weeks after a thoracotomy, but exercise tolerance will improve with conditioning.
3. Suggest alternating walking and other activities with frequent, short rest periods. Walk at a moderate pace and gradually extend walking time and distance.
4. Encourage continuing deep-breathing exercises for several weeks after surgery to attain full expansion of residual lung tissue.
5. Instruct on maintaining good body alignment to ensure full lung expansion.
6. Advise that chest muscles may be weaker than normal for 3 to 6 months after surgery. Patient must avoid lifting more than 10 pound (4.5 kg) until complete healing has taken place.
7. Any activity that causes undue fatigue, increased shortness of breath, or chest pain should be stopped immediately.
8. Because all or part of one lung has been removed, warn patient to avoid respiratory irritants (smoke, fumes, and high level of air pollution).
   a. Avoid irritants that may cause coughing spasms.
   b. Sit in nonsmoking areas in public places.
9. Encourage patient to receive an annual influenza vaccine and obtain a pneumococcal pneumonia vaccine.
10. Encourage patient to keep follow-up visits.
11. Instruct patient to prevent respiratory infections by frequent handwashing and avoiding others with respiratory infections.

Evaluation: Expected Outcomes

- Respirations with normal range, adequate depth; lungs clear; ABG values and SaO_2 within normal limits.
- BP, CVP, and pulse within normal limits for individual.
- Coughs and turns independently; reports relief of pain.
- Performs active ROM of affected arm and shoulder; reports improved exercise tolerance.

Chest Drainage

Chest drainage is the insertion of a tube into the pleural space to evacuate air or fluid or help regain negative pressure. Whenever the chest is opened, there is loss of negative pressure in the pleural space, which can result in collapse of the lung. The collection of air, fluid, or other substances in the thoracic cavity can compromise cardiopulmonary function and cause collapse of the lung.

It is necessary to keep the pleural space evacuated postoperatively and to maintain negative pressure within this potential space. Therefore, during or immediately after thoracic surgery, chest tubes/catheters are positioned strategically in the pleural space, sutured to the skin, and connected to a drainage apparatus to remove the residual air and fluid from the pleural or mediastinal space. This assists in the reexpansion of remaining lung tissue.

Table 6-3 Indications for Chest Tube Use

INDICATION	ACCUMULATING SUBSTANCE
Pneumothorax	Air
Hemothorax	Blood
Pleural effusion	Fluid
Chylothorax	Lymphatic fluid
Empyema	Pus

Chest drainage can also be used to treat spontaneous pneumothorax or hemothorax/pneumothorax caused by trauma (see Table 6-3). Sites for chest tube placement are:

1. For pneumothorax (air)—second or third interspace along midclavicular or anterior axillary line.
2. For hemothorax (fluid)—sixth or seventh lateral interspace in the midaxillary line.

Principles of Chest Drainage

1. Many types of commercial chest drainage systems are in use, many of which use the water-seal principle. The chest tube/catheter and collecting tubing is attached to a chest drainage system using a one-way valve principle. Water acts as a seal and permits air and fluid to drain from the chest. However, air cannot reenter the chest cavity.
2. There are numerous types of chest drainage units available including water-seal/and dry-seal systems (see Figure 6-10).

Water-Seal System

1. Most commercially available units contain three chambers. Fluid or air from the pleural space is collected in the first compartment.
2. The water seal is the second chamber and typically contains 2 cm of water. This chamber functions as a one-way valve, which prevents backflow of air. Tidaling in the water-seal chamber (movement of water) is reflective of breathing and is considered a normal finding.
3. The suction control or third compartment is responsible for application of suction to the drainage unit. This chamber is filled with a prescribed amount of water, which determines the amount of suction. The unit is attached to a wall suction unit. Maximum recommended suction is −20 cm H_2O. Additional H_2O may need to be added to account for evaporation.

Dry Suction System

1. The unit does not contain water. The water chamber is replaced by a dial and valves to control suction at a prescribed level. Typical suction pressure is −20 cm H_2O. A bellow provides a visual confirmation of functioning suction.
2. Dry suction provides the following benefits: less opportunity for fluid spills, elimination of evaporation of water, quiet operation, and easier control of suction.

Nursing and Patient Care Considerations

1. Assist with chest tube insertion.
2. Assess patient's pain at insertion site and give medication appropriately. If patient is in pain, chest excursion and lung inflation will be hampered. Medicate for pain as needed. Assess for effectiveness and respiratory depression.
3. Maintain chest tubes to provide drainage and enhance lung reinflation. Ensure the tubing does not loop, kink, or restrict movements of the patient.
4. Maintain integrity of insertion site, observing for drainage, redness, impaired healing, and subcutaneous emphysema.

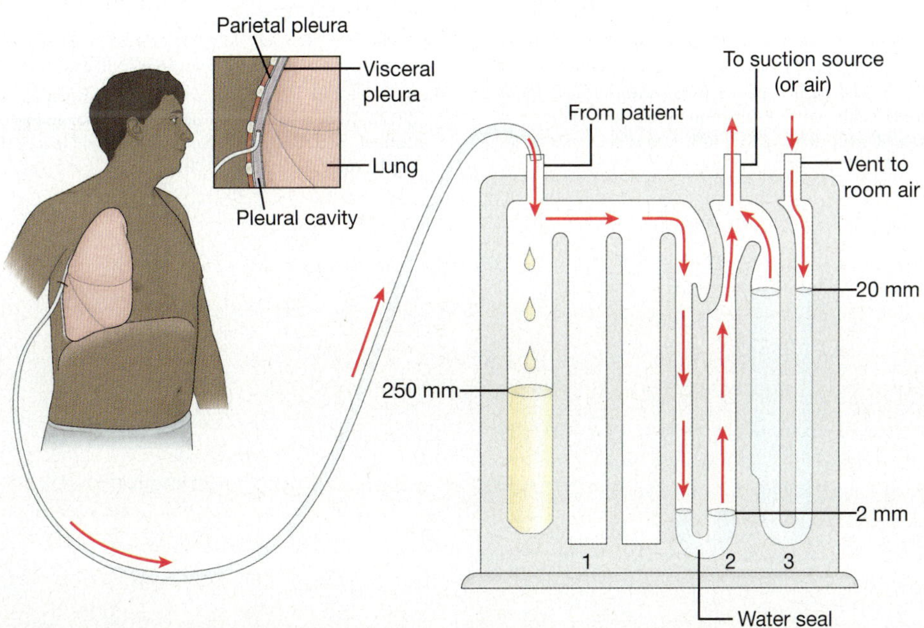

Figure 6-10. Chest drainage systems. Chest catheter placed in right pleural space and attached to Pleur-Evac system with three chambers. (Reprinted with permission from Timby, B. K., & Smith, N. E. (2022). *Introductory medical-surgical nursing* (13th ed., Fig. 21-14). Wolters Kluwer.)

5. Make sure there is fluctuation of the fluid level in the drainage container ("tidaling"). Fluctuation will stop if a dependent loop develops or the tubing is obstructed by blood clots or fibrin and when the lung is reexpanded.

CLINICAL JUDGMENT Clamping of chest tubes is not recommended because of the increased danger of tension pneumothorax from rapid accumulation of air in the pleural space. Follow facility policy regarding clamping of chest tubes. Check for leaks to assess the patient's tolerance for removal of the chest tube (perhaps up to 24 hours).

CLINICAL JUDGMENT Milking and stripping of chest tubes to maintain patency are not recommended. This practice has been found to cause significant increases in intrathoracic pressures and damage to the pleural tissue. New chest tubes contain a nonthrombogenic coating, thus decreasing the potential for clotting. If it is necessary to help the drainage move through the tubing, apply a gentle squeeze-and-release motion to small segments of the chest tube between your fingers.

SELECTED READINGS

American Association for Respiratory Care. (2021). Clinical practice guidelines: Management of adult patients with tracheostomy in the acute care setting. *Respiratory Care, 66*(1), 156–169. https://doi.org/10.4187/respcare.08206

American Association for Respiratory Care. (2022). Clinical practice guidelines: Artificial airway suctioning. *Respiratory Care, 67*(2), 258–271. https://doi.org/10.4187/respcare.09548

American Heart Association. (2020). *Highlights of the 2015 American Heart Association guidelines update for cardiopulmonary resuscitation and emergency cardiovascular care.* Author.

American Society of Anesthesiologists. (2022). Practice guidelines for management of the difficult airway: An updated report by the American Society of Anesthesiologists Task Force on Management of the Difficult Airway. *Anesthesiology, 136*, 31–81.

Cartuliares, M. B., Skjøt-Arkil, H., Rosenvinge, F. S., Mogensen, C. B., Skovsted, T. A., & Pedersen, A. K. (2021). Effectiveness of expiratory technique and induced sputum in obtaining good quality sputum from patients acutely hospitalized with suspected lower respiratory tract infection: A statistical analysis plan for a randomized controlled trial. *Trials, 22*(1), 675. https://doi.org/10.1186/s13063-021-05639-1

Gelzinis, T. (2022). Pulmonary hypertension in 2021: Part I—Definition, classification, pathology and presentation. *Journal of Cardiothoracic and Vascular Anesthesia, 36*(6), 1552–1564. https://doi.org/10.1053/j.jvca.2021.06.036

Golamari, R., & Gilchrist, I. (2021). Collateral circulation testing of the hand—Is it relevant now? A narrative review. *The American Journal of Medical Sciences, 361*(6), 702–710. https://doi.org/10.1016/j.amjms.2020.12.001

Harris, D. (2022). Essential critical care skills 6: Arterial blood gas analysis. *Nursing Times, 118*(4), 1–3.

Hyzy, R., & McSparron, J. (2022). Noninvasive ventilation in adults with acute respiratory failure: Practical aspects of initiation. *UpToDate.* Retrieved December 1, 2022, from https://www.uptodate.com/contents/noninvasive-ventilation-in-adults-with-acute-respiratory-failure-practical-aspects-of-initiation

Islam, S. (2022). *Flexible bronchoscopy in adults: Overview. UpToDate.* Retrieved December 3, 2022, from https://www.uptodate.com/contents/flexible-bronchoscopy-in-adults-overview

Johnson, K. (2024). *AACN procedure manual for critical care* (8th ed.). Elsevier Saunders.

Kaminsky, P. (2022). Overview of pulmonary function testing in adults. *UpToDate.* Retrieved December 7, 2022, from https://www.uptodate.com/contents/overview-of-pulmonary-function-testing-in-adults

Krauss, B., Falk, J., & Ladde, J. (2022). Carbon dioxide monitoring (capnography). *UpToDate.* Retrieved December 17, 2022, from https://www.uptodate.com/contents/carbon-dioxide-monitoring-capnography

Nagler, J. (2023). Continuous oxygen delivery systems for infants, children, and adults. *UpToDate.* Retrieved November 6, 2023, from https://www.uptodate.com/contents/continous-oxygen-delivery-systems-for-infants-adults-children

Pritchett, M. A., Oberg, C. L., Belanger, A., De Cardenas, J., Cheng, G., Cumbo Nacheli, G., Franco-Paredes, C., Singh, J., Toth, J., Zgoda, M., & Folch, E. (2020). Society for Advanced Bronchoscopy Consensus Statement and Guidelines for bronchoscopy and airway management amid the COVID-19 pandemic. *Journal of Thoracic Disorders, 12*(5), 1781–1798. http://dx.doi.org/10.21037/jtd.2020.04.32

Rauniyar, N., Pujari, S., & Shrestha, P. (2020). Study of oxygen saturation by pulse oximetry and arterial blood gas in ICU patients: A descriptive cross-sectional study. *JNMA: Journal of the Nepal Medical Association, 58*(230), 789–793. https://doi.org/10.31729/jnma.5536

Strohleit, D., Galetin, T., Kosse, N., Lopez-Pastorini, A., & Stoelben, E. (2021). Guidelines on analgosedation, monitoring, and recovery time for flexible bronchoscopy: A systematic review. *BMC Pulmonary Medicine, 21*(1), 198. https://doi.org/10.1186/s12890-021-01532-4

Toplis, E., & Mortimore, G. (2020). The diagnosis and management of pulmonary embolism. *British Journal of Nursing, 29*(1), 22–26. https://doi.org/10.12968/bjon.2020.29.1.22

Van Leeuwen, A., & Bladh, M (2021). *Davis's comprehensive manual of laboratory and diagnostic tests with nursing implications* (9th ed.). McGraw-Hill

Wang, C. H., Tsai, J. C., Chen, S. F., Su, C. L., Chen, L., Lin, C. C., & Tam, K. W. (2017). Normal saline instillation before suctioning: A meta-analysis of randomized controlled trials. *Australian Critical Care, 30*(5), 260–265. https://doi.org/10.1016/j.aucc.2016.11.001

7 Respiratory Disorders

ACUTE DISORDERS

See additional online content: Procedure Guidelines 7-1.

Respiratory Failure

Respiratory failure is a failure of one or both of the respiratory gas exchange systems: oxygenation (hypoxemia respiratory failure) and carbon dioxide elimination (hypercapnic respiratory failure).

Hypoxemic respiratory failure is characterized by arterial oxygen (PaO_2) level below 60 mm Hg (hypoxemia) with a normal (40 mm Hg) or low arterial carbon dioxide level ($PaCO_2$). It is the most common form of respiratory failure, usually associated with acute diseases of the lung generally involving fluid collection or collapse of alveolar units. Examples include cardiogenic or noncardiogenic pulmonary edema, pneumonia, and pulmonary hemorrhage.

Hypercapnic respiratory failure is characterized by an arterial carbon dioxide ($PaCO_2$) level of greater than 50 mm Hg. Hypoxemia is common while breathing room air. The pH depends on the bicarbonate level, which, in turn, is dependent on the duration and degree of hypercapnia.

Respiratory failure may be further classified as acute, chronic, or both. Acute respiratory failure is characterized by life-threatening abnormalities in arterial blood gases (ABGs) and acid–base levels, whereas chronic respiratory failure abnormalities may be less dramatic and more insidious.

Classification

Acute Respiratory Failure

1. Characterized by hypoxemia (PaO_2 <60 mm Hg) or hypercapnia ($PaCO_2$ >50 mm Hg) and acidosis (pH <7.35).
2. Occurs rapidly, usually in minutes to hours or days.

Chronic Respiratory Failure

1. Characterized by hypoxemia and/or hypercapnia with a normal pH (7.35 to 7.45).
2. Occurs over a period of days, months, or years, allowing activation of compensatory mechanisms, including renal bicarbonate retention (normal, ~22 to 26 mEq/L) with normalization of pH (or only slightly decreased, ~7.30 to 7.34).

Combined Acute and Chronic Respiratory Failure

1. Characterized by an abrupt increase in the degree of hypoxemia and/or hypercapnia in patients with preexisting chronic respiratory failure.
2. May occur during or following acute upper respiratory infection, pneumonia, exacerbation, or without obvious cause.
3. Extent of deterioration is best assessed by comparing the patient's present ABG levels with previous ABG levels (patient baseline).

Pathophysiology and Etiology

Hypoxemic Respiratory Failure

Characterized by a decrease in PaO_2 and normal or decreased $PaCO_2$.

1. The primary problem is the inability to adequately oxygenate blood, resulting in hypoxemia, because of an abnormality in one or more parts of the respiratory system, central nervous system (CNS), respiratory muscles, or chest wall.
2. Hypoxemia occurs because damage to the alveolar–capillary membrane causes leakage of fluid into the interstitial space or into the alveoli and slows or prevents movement of oxygen from the alveoli to the pulmonary capillary blood.
   a. Damage is either widespread (e.g., acute respiratory distress syndrome [ARDS]) or relatively localized (e.g., lobar pneumonia), resulting in decreased or absent ventilation in affected areas of the lung.
   b. Consequences are severe ventilation–perfusion mismatch and shunt (perfusion without ventilation).
3. Hypocapnia may result from hypoxemia and decreased pulmonary compliance or stiffness because of fluid within the lung.
   a. Change in compliance reflexively stimulates the increased ventilation.
   b. Ventilation is also increased as a response to hypoxemia.

4. Ultimately, if treatment is unsuccessful, $PaCO_2$ will increase and the patient will experience both an increase in $PaCO_2$ and a decrease in PaO_2.
5. Etiology includes the following:
   a. Cardiogenic or noncardiogenic pulmonary edema, pneumonia, and pulmonary hemorrhage.
   b. ARDS: The four main causes of ARDS are aspiration, pneumonia, sepsis, and trauma. However, there are numerous other causes of lung injury including pancreatitis, smoke inhalation, and near drowning.
   c. Hypercapnic respiratory failure: drug overdose, neuromuscular disease, chest wall abnormalities, asthma, and chronic obstructive pulmonary disease (COPD).

Ventilatory Failure Without Underlying Lung Disease

Characterized by a decrease in PaO_2 that is proportional to the increase in $PaCO_2$ and a decrease in pH.

1. The primary problem is insufficient respiratory center stimulation or insufficient chest wall movement, resulting in alveolar hypoventilation.
2. Hypercapnia occurs because impaired neuromuscular function or chest wall expansion limits the amount of carbon dioxide removed from the lungs.
   a. The primary problem is not the lungs. The patient's minute ventilation (tidal volume [V_T] × respiratory rate) is insufficient to allow normal alveolar gas exchange.
3. Carbon dioxide (CO_2) not excreted by the lungs combines with water (H_2O) to form carbonic acid (H_2CO_3). This predisposes to acidosis and a fall in pH.
4. Hypoxemia occurs as a consequence of inadequate ventilation and hypercapnia. When $PaCO_2$ rises, PaO_2 falls unless supplemental oxygen is used.
5. Etiology includes the following:
   a. Insufficient respiratory center activity (drug intoxication, e.g., opioid overdose, oversedation, general anesthesia; vascular disorders, such as cerebral vascular insufficiency, brain tumor; trauma, such as head injury, increased intracranial pressure).
   b. Insufficient chest wall function (neuromuscular disease, such as Guillain-Barré syndrome, myasthenia gravis, amyotrophic lateral sclerosis, poliomyelitis; chest wall trauma resulting in multiple fractures; spinal cord trauma; kyphoscoliosis).

Ventilatory Failure With Intrinsic Lung Disease

Characterized by a decrease in PaO_2, increase in $PaCO_2$, and decrease in pH.

1. The primary problem is acute exacerbation or chronic progression of previously existing lung disease, resulting in CO_2 retention.
2. Hypercapnia occurs because of damage to the lung parenchyma primarily caused by chronic airway obstruction (chronic bronchitis, emphysema, or severe asthma). This limits the amount of CO_2 removed by the lungs because the lungs are hyperinflated and poorly perfused.
3. The CO_2 not excreted by the lungs combines with H_2O to form H_2CO_3. This predisposes to acidosis with a fall in pH.
4. Hypoxemia occurs due to hypoventilation and hypercapnia. In addition, damage to the lung parenchyma and/or airway obstruction limits the amount of oxygen that enters the pulmonary capillary blood.
5. Etiology includes the following:
   a. COPD, chronic bronchitis, emphysema.
   b. Severe asthma.
   c. Cystic fibrosis.

Clinical Manifestations

1. Hypoxemia—restlessness, agitation, dyspnea, disorientation, confusion, delirium, loss of consciousness.
2. Hypercapnia—headache, somnolence, dizziness, confusion.
3. Tachypnea initially; when no longer able to compensate, bradypnea.
4. Accessory muscle use.
5. Asynchronous respirations.

CLINICAL JUDGMENT Obtain ABG levels whenever the history or signs and symptoms suggest that the patient is at risk for developing respiratory failure. Initial and subsequent values should be recorded, so comparisons can be made over time. The need for ABG analysis can be decreased by continuous oximetry monitoring of oxygen saturation (SpO_2). Correlate oximeter values with ABG values and then use oximeter for trending. Be aware that oximetry does not measure $PaCO_2$ and pH, important determinants of respiratory acidosis.

Diagnostic Evaluation

1. ABG analysis—shows changes in PaO_2, $PaCO_2$, pH, and possibly HCO_3 from the patient's normal levels or PaO_2 less than 60 mm Hg, $PaCO_2$ greater than 50 mm Hg, and pH less than 7.35.
2. Pulse oximetry—decreasing SpO_2 ($<90\%$).
3. End-tidal CO_2 monitoring—elevated (>40 mm Hg or >5 mm Hg above $PaCO_2$).
4. Complete blood count, serum electrolytes, chest x-ray, urinalysis, electrocardiogram (ECG), and blood and sputum cultures—to aid in determination of underlying cause and patient's condition.

Management

Hypoxemia is the major acute concern impacting organ function. Once corrected with stable ventilation and hemodynamics, identification and correction of underlying causes is essential and used to direct treatment.

1. Oxygen therapy to correct hypoxemia.
2. Turn the patient regularly and mobilize when clinically stable to improve ventilation and oxygenation. When appropriate, early ambulation of the patient.
3. Bronchodilators and possibly corticosteroids to reduce bronchospasm and inflammation.
4. Diuretics for pulmonary vascular congestion or pulmonary edema.
5. Ventilatory support using mechanical ventilation or noninvasive positive pressure ventilation using a facemask.

CLINICAL JUDGMENT Unless mechanically ventilated, high-flow oxygen in patients with COPD with CO_2 retention is contraindicated because it may cause depression of the respiratory center drive. In this population, the drive to breathe may be hypoxemia.

Complications

1. Oxygen toxicity if prolonged high FiO_2 required (≥ 0.80 for ≥ 3 days).
2. Barotrauma from mechanical ventilation intervention—damage to alveoli causing extra-alveolar air, primarily caused by the use of nonphysiologic tidal volumes (>8 mL/kg predicted body weight).

Nursing Assessment

See Standards of Care Guidelines 7-1.

1. Note objective signs suggesting increased work of breathing that include some combination of the following: tachypnea, pronounced use of sternocleidomastoid muscles, tracheal tugging, nasal flaring, sternal retractions (or intercostal muscle retraction) recruitment of abdominal muscles during exhalation, and diaphoresis. Patient may also complain of dyspnea ("can't catch my breath," "my breathing is hard," etc.).
2. Assess breath sounds.
   a. Diminished or absent sounds may suggest inability to ventilate the lungs sufficiently to prevent atelectasis. Decreased breath sounds may be common in moderate to severe COPD.
   b. Crackles may indicate ineffective airway clearance and fluid in the lungs.
   c. Wheezing indicates narrowed airways and bronchospasm.
   d. Rhonchi and crackles suggest ineffective secretion clearance.
3. Assess level of consciousness (LOC) and ability to tolerate increased work of breathing.
   a. Confusion and lethargy.
   b. Rapid shallow breathing, abdominal paradox (inward movement of the abdominal wall during inspiration), and accessory muscle retractions suggest inability to maintain adequate minute ventilation.
4. Assess for signs of hypoxemia and hypercapnia.
5. Analyze ABG and compare it with previous values.
   a. If the patient cannot maintain a minute ventilation sufficient to prevent CO_2 retention, pH will fall.
   b. Mechanical ventilation or noninvasive ventilation may be needed if pH falls to 7.30 or below.
6. Determine vital capacity (VC) and respiratory rate, and compare with values indicating the need for mechanical ventilation:
   a. VC less than 15 mL/kg.
   b. Respiratory rate greater than 30 breaths/min.
   c. Negative inspiratory force less than -30 cm H_2O.
   d. Refractory hypoxemia.
7. Determine hemodynamic status through assessment of blood pressure (BP), heart rate, pulmonary wedge pressure, cardiac output, and SvO_2, and compare with previous values. If the patient is on mechanical ventilation with positive end-expiratory pressure (PEEP), venous return may be limited, resulting in decreased cardiac output.

STANDARDS OF CARE GUIDELINES 7-1

Respiratory Compromise

When caring for patients at risk for respiratory compromise, consider the following assessments and interventions:

- Monitor closely and document complete assessments. Evaluate closely for any changes in clinical assessments.
- Perform thorough systematic assessment, including mental status, vital signs, respiratory status, and cardiovascular status.
- Evaluate for signs of hypoxia when anxiety, restlessness, confusion, or aggression of new onset are noted. Do not administer sedatives unless hypoxia has been ruled out by performing respiratory assessment.
- Notify appropriate health care provider of significant findings of hypoxia: SpO_2 less than 92%, cyanosis, circumoral pallor, rapid and shallow respirations, abnormal breath sounds, change in behavior or level of consciousness (LOC). Request assessment and intervention by health care provider, as indicated.
- Use extreme caution in administering sedatives and opioids to patients at risk for respiratory compromise.

This information should serve as a general guideline only. Each patient situation presents a unique set of clinical factors and requires nursing judgment to guide care, which may include additional or alternative measures and approaches.

Nursing Interventions

Improving Gas Exchange

1. Administer oxygen to maintain PaO_2 of 60 mm Hg or SaO_2 greater than 90% using devices that provide increased oxygen concentrations (aerosol mask, partial rebreathing mask, nonrebreathing mask, noninvasive positive pressure ventilation, or mechanical ventilation).
2. Administer diuretics and, as indicated, antibiotics and/or cardiac medications as ordered for an underlying disorder.
3. Monitor fluid balance by intake and output measurement, daily weight, and direct measurement of pulmonary capillary wedge pressure to detect hypovolemia or hypervolemia.
4. Provide measures to prevent hypoventilation and atelectasis, and promote chest expansion and secretion clearance, such as incentive spirometer, nebulization, head of bed elevated 30 degrees, turn frequently, and out of bed when clinically stable.
5. Monitor adequacy of alveolar ventilation by frequent measurement of SpO_2, ABG levels, respiratory rate, and forced vital capacity (FVC).
6. Compare monitored values with criteria indicating the need for mechanical ventilation (see "Nursing Assessment" section). Report and prepare to assist with noninvasive ventilation or intubation and initiation of mechanical ventilation, if indicated.

Maintaining Airway Clearance

1. Where indicated, administer medications to increase alveolar ventilation—bronchodilators to reduce bronchospasm and corticosteroids to reduce airway inflammation.
2. Teach slow, pursed lip breathing to reduce dyspnea and improve oxygen saturation. Secretion clearance techniques may be considered for retained secretions.
3. Promote effective cough with positioning, deep breathing, and bronchodilators if ordered. If cough effort is poor and/or ineffective for mucus clearance, suction the patient, if needed, to assist with removal of secretions.
4. If the patient becomes increasingly lethargic, cannot cough or expectorate secretions, and cannot cooperate with therapy, or if pH falls below 7.30, despite the use of the above therapy, report and prepare to assist with intubation and initiation of mechanical ventilation.

Patient Education and Health Maintenance

1. Instruct the patient with preexisting pulmonary disease to seek early intervention for infections to prevent acute respiratory failure, pneumonia, and exacerbations.
2. Teach the patient about medication regimen.
   a. Return demonstrate proper technique for inhaler use.
   b. Actions, dosage, and timing of medications.
   c. Monitoring for adverse effects of oral corticosteroids to report to health care provider: weight gain because of fluid retention and/or increased appetite, hyperglycemia, mood changes, insomnia, bruising, fragile skin, and vision changes because of cataracts or glaucoma.

Community and Home Care Considerations

1. Encourage patients at risk, especially older adults and those with preexisting lung disease, to get pneumococcal pneumonia and annual influenza vaccination.
2. All adults aged 65 years and older who have not received a prior pneumococcal conjugate vaccine (PCV) or with an unknown vaccination history should receive one dose of PCV (PCV 20 or PCV 15). When PCV 15 is used, it should be followed by a dose of PCV 23. When PCV 15 is used, the recommended interval between PCV 15 and PCV 23 is greater than or equal to 1 year.
3. Adults age 65 years and older with immunocompromising conditions should receive the PCV 23 greater than or equal to 8 weeks after PCV 13.
4. Encourage annual immunization for influenza in persons 6 months and older.
5. Intranasal live attenuated vaccine is an alternative for people ages 5 to 49 without chronic conditions, human immunodeficiency virus (HIV), or asthma.

EVIDENCE BASE Centers for Disease Control and Prevention. (2022). Prevention and control of seasonal influenza with vaccines: Recommendations of the Advisory Committee on Immunization Practices—United States, 2022–2023 influenza season. *MMWR, 71*(1), 1–28. www.cdc.gov/mmwr/volumes/71/rr/rr7101a1.htm

Kobayashi, M., Farra, J., Gierke, R., Britton, A., Childs, L., Leidner, A. J., Campos-Outcalt, D., Morgan, R. L., Long, S. S., Talbot, H. K., Poehling, K. A., & Pilishvili, T. (2022). Use of 15 valent pneumococcal conjugate vaccine and 20 valent pneumococcal conjugate vaccine among U.S. adults: Updated recommendations of the advisory committee on immunization practices—United States 2022. *MMWR, 71*(4), 109–117.

Evaluation: Expected Outcomes

- ABG values within the patient's normal limits.
- Decreased secretions; lungs clear.

Acute Respiratory Distress Syndrome

ARDS or acute *lung injury* results from acute insult at the level of the alveoli leading to severe hypoxemia and decreased pulmonary compliance. Hallmarks of ARDS include a risk factor for ARDS (e.g., sepsis, trauma, pancreatitis), severe hypoxemia with the need for high FiO_2, decreased lung compliance, bilateral pulmonary infiltrates, and absence of cardiogenic pulmonary edema. Mortality is 55% and improves with early intervention.

Pathophysiology and Etiology

1. Pulmonary and/or nonpulmonary insult to the alveolar–capillary membrane causing protein-rich fluid leakage into interstitial and alveolar spaces, resulting in edema.
   a. Inflammation in the interstitium and alveolar space promotes atelectasis and lung damage.
   b. This is associated with severe hypoxemia and reduced pulmonary compliance.
   c. Fibroproliferative state is often accompanied by capillary thrombosis, lung fibrosis, and neovascularization follows.
2. Diffuse alveolar damage with ventilation–perfusion (V/Q) mismatch caused by shunting of blood (see Figure 7-1).

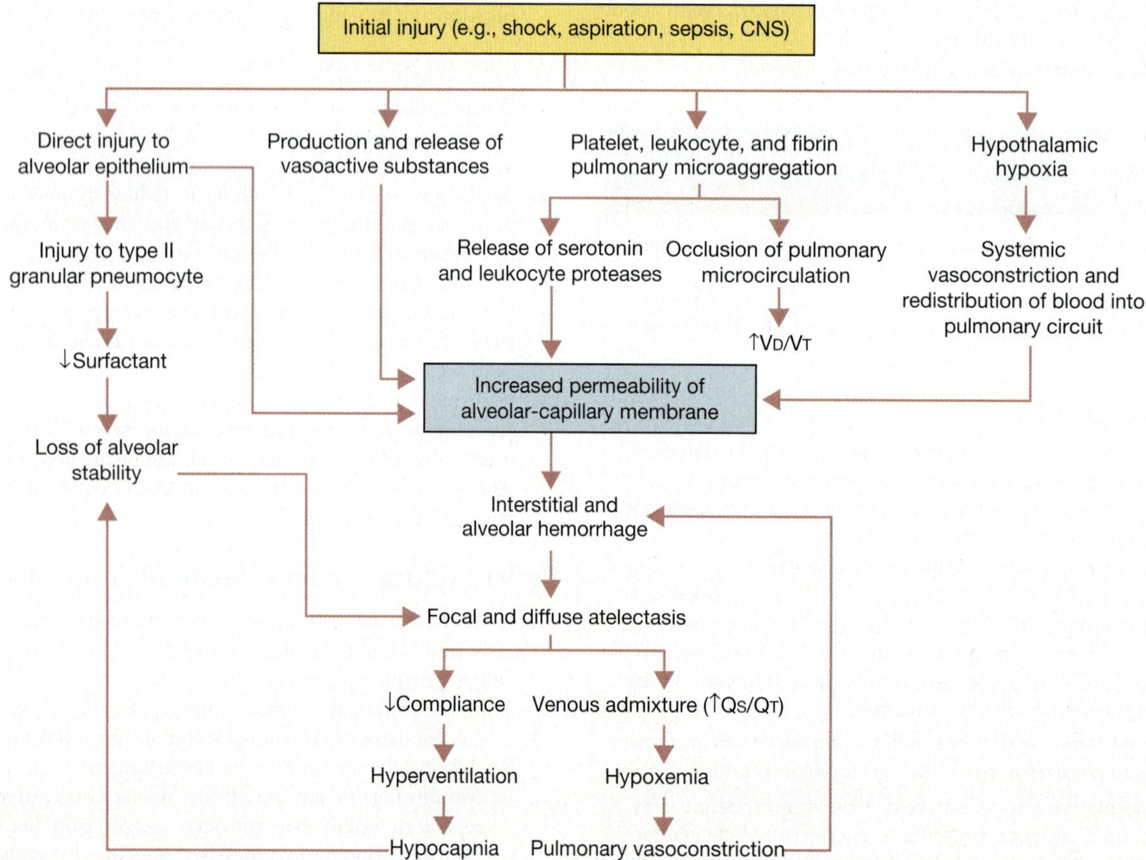

Figure 7-1. Pathogenesis of ARDS. ARDS, acute respiratory distress syndrome; CNS, central nervous system.

3. Mechanisms are unclear. Acute lung injury includes both pulmonary capillary endothelium and alveolar epithelium. Etiologies are numerous and can be pulmonary or nonpulmonary. Predisposing factors include (but are not limited to):
   a. Infections, including sepsis, COVID-19, pneumonia (usually bacterial or aspiration).
   b. Shock (any cause), trauma, pulmonary contusion, near drowning, direct or indirect lung injury, burns, pancreatitis.
   c. Inhaled agents—smoke, high concentration of oxygen, corrosive substances.
   d. Major surgery including coronary artery bypass graft, fat emboli, lung or bone marrow transplantation, transfusion of blood products, reperfusion pulmonary edema.

Clinical Manifestations

1. Acute onset of severe dyspnea, tachypnea, tachycardia, use of accessory muscles, cyanosis.
2. Increasing requirements of oxygen therapy. Hypoxemia refractory to supplemental oxygen therapy.
3. Scattered crackles and rhonchi heard on auscultation.
4. Decreased pulmonary compliance, evidenced by increasing pressure required to ventilate patient on mechanical ventilator.

Diagnostic Evaluation

1. Diagnosis is based on clinical, hemodynamic, and oxygen criteria. The hallmark signs for ARDS include acute-onset, severe hypoxemia, despite increasing oxygen therapy, and chest x-ray exhibiting bilateral infiltrates.
2. Pulmonary artery (PA) catheter readings show PA wedge pressure greater than 18 mm Hg, absence of left atrial hypertension, and no clinical signs of heart failure.

Management

1. Current ARDS treatment is primarily supportive. The underlying cause for ARDS should be determined so appropriate treatment can be initiated.
2. Mechanical ventilation is nearly always required to decrease the work of breathing and improve oxygenation.
   a. Low V_T by mechanical ventilation (6 mL/kg of predicted body weight) reduces mortality compared to high-volume ventilation.
   b. Protective ventilation (i.e., maximum inspiratory pressure of less than 35 cm) should be instituted.
   c. PEEP should be used to improve PaO_2 (keeps the alveoli open, thereby improving gas exchange). Therefore, a lower oxygen concentration (FiO_2) may be used to maintain satisfactory oxygenation.
3. Fluid management must be maintained. The patient may be hypovolemic because of the movement of fluid into the interstitium of the lung. PA catheter monitoring and inotropic medication can be helpful.
4. Medications are aimed at treating the underlying cause. Corticosteroids are used infrequently because of their controversial benefits.
5. Adequate nutrition should be initiated early and maintained.
6. Initiate prone positioning if indicated.

CLINICAL JUDGMENT The treatment for ARDS is aimed at maximizing clinical stability and managing symptoms, but the underlying cause must be treated or ARDS will not resolve. Supportive measures assist the patient while the underlying cause is being treated.

Complications

1. Infections, such as pneumonia, sepsis.
2. Respiratory complications, such as pulmonary emboli, barotrauma, oxygen toxicity, subcutaneous emphysema, or pulmonary fibrosis.
3. Gastrointestinal (GI) complications, such as stress ulcer, ileus, and pancreatitis.
4. Cardiac complications, such as decreased cardiac output and dysrhythmias.
5. Renal failure, disseminated intravascular coagulation.
6. Multisystem organ failure and sepsis, which may result in death.
7. Cognitive impairment.

Nursing Interventions

Care is similar to patients with respiratory failure (page 157) and pulmonary edema (page 276). Also see "Mechanical Ventilation" section, page 148.

Acute Bronchitis

Acute bronchitis is an inflammation of the airways resulting from infection (viral, bacterial) or an irritant (smoke, gastric acid). The inflammation causes airway narrowing and congestion, with an increase in secretions.

Pathophysiology and Etiology

1. Primarily viral etiology, such as rhinovirus, respiratory syncytial virus (RSV), and influenza.
2. Bacterial etiology more common in people with underlying pulmonary disease.
3. Exposure to irritants may be acute or chronic.
4. Airways become inflamed, narrowed, and congested with increased mucus production.

Clinical Manifestations

1. Dry cough, which may become productive with clear to purulent sputum.
2. Rhinorrhea, sore throat, and nasal congestion may precede and accompany lower respiratory tract symptoms.
3. Occasional pleuritic chest pain and fever.
4. Diffuse rhonchi and crackles and occasional wheezing heard on auscultation.

Diagnostic Evaluation

1. Chest x-ray—no evidence of infiltrates or consolidation.
2. Sputum Gram stain and culture have limited value.
3. Spirometry to determine FVC, forced expiratory volume in 1 second (FEV_1), and FEV_1/FVC ratio, which may indicate underlying airflow limitation as found in COPD (chronic bronchitis +/or emphysema).

Management

1. Antibiotic therapy is normally avoided due to predominantly viral cause of infection. If bacterial infection is present or strongly suspected, or for patients with underlying COPD, antibiotics are usually prescribed based on community resistance patterns and patient history and physical examination.
2. Hydration and humidification.
3. Secretion clearance interventions for retained or excess mucus (may include controlled cough, positive expiratory pressure [PEP] valve therapy, chest physical therapy) and mobilization.

4. Bronchodilators for bronchospasm, secretion clearance, and treatment of airflow obstruction if present.
5. Symptom management for cough and fever.
6. Management of irritants through acid reflux therapy, smoking cessation, and use of air filter.

Nursing Assessment

1. Obtain history of respiratory infection, course, and length of symptoms.
2. Assess severity of cough and characteristics of sputum production.
3. Auscultate chest for diffuse rhonchi and crackles as opposed to localized crackles usually heard with pneumonia.
4. Obtain medical history including COPD, gastroesophageal reflux disease (GERD), smoking history, and exposure to irritants.

Nursing Interventions

Establishing Effective Airway Clearance

1. Supportive care with symptom management is usually the first line in otherwise healthy patients. For those with bacterial infections and/or underlying COPD, administer or teach self-administration of antibiotics, as ordered.
2. Encourage mobilization of secretions through patient mobilization and, possibly, hydration, effective cough technique, and, if needed, the use of secretion clearance devices such as PEP and, possibly, chest physical therapy. Educate patient that beverages with caffeine or alcohol do not promote hydration.
3. If ordered, administer or teach self-administration of inhaled bronchodilators to reduce bronchospasm and enhance secretion clearance.
4. Caution patients on the use of over-the-counter cough suppressants, antihistamines, and decongestants that may cause drying and retention of secretions. Cough preparations containing the mucolytic guaifenesin may be appropriate.

Patient Education and Health Maintenance

1. Instruct patient about medication regimen, including the completion of the full course of antibiotics, if prescribed, and the effects of food or alcohol on the absorption of the selected medications. If patient is not being treated with antibiotics, reassure patient that full recovery without antibiotic treatment occurs in most cases, but to advise health care provider if symptoms do not improve.
2. Encourage patient to seek medical attention for shortness of breath, severe fatigue, and worsening condition.
3. Advise patient that a dry cough may persist after bronchitis because of irritation of the airways. A bedside humidifier and avoidance of dry environments may help. Humidifiers must be cleaned frequently to avoid growth of mold.
4. Encourage patient to discuss complementary and alternative therapies with health care provider. When questioned, some people use garlic as an antimicrobial. Other herbs that many believe to be helpful for asthma and bronchitis are echinacea, eucalyptus, and thyme; however, there are no definitive studies that show benefit. Because herbal products and supplements are not standardized, and may be mixed with other ingredients, safety and effectiveness cannot be ensured.

Evaluation: Expected Outcomes

- Coughs up clear secretions effectively.

Pneumonia

Pneumonia is an inflammatory process, involving the terminal airways and alveoli of the lung, caused by infectious agents (see Table 7-1, pages 163–165). It may be classified according to its causative agent.

Pathophysiology and Etiology

1. Community-acquired pneumonia (CAP) is a common infectious disease often caused by bacteria such as *Streptococcus pneumoniae*, *Haemophilus influenzae*, and *Moraxella catarrhalis*, as well as the viruses rhinovirus and influenza.
2. Development of CAP may be due to a defect in host defenses, exposure to a virulent microorganism, or an overwhelming exposure. An organism gains access to the lungs through aspiration of oropharyngeal contents, by inhalation of respiratory secretions from infected individuals, via the bloodstream, or from direct spread to the lungs as a result of surgery or trauma.
3. Risk factors include altered mental status, smoking, alcohol use, hypoxemia, toxic inhalations, pulmonary edema, uremia, malnutrition, bronchial obstruction, advanced age, immunosuppression, heart disease, underlying lung disease (cystic fibrosis, bronchiectasis, COPD, ciliary dysfunction, lung cancer), viral respiratory infection, and history of pneumonia.
   a. Patients who are immunocompromised include those receiving corticosteroids, immunosuppressants, chemotherapy, or radiotherapy; those with cancer, HIV infection, acquired immunodeficiency syndrome (AIDS), and alcohol use disorder; those who use intravenous (IV) drugs; and those undergoing organ transplantation.
   b. These people have an increased risk of developing overwhelming infection. Infectious agents include aerobic and anaerobic gram-negative bacilli, *Staphylococcus*, *Nocardia*, fungi, *Candida*, viruses such as cytomegalovirus, *Pneumocystis jiroveci*, reactivation of tuberculosis (TB), and others.
4. When bacterial pneumonia occurs in a healthy person, it may be preceded by a viral illness.
5. Other predisposing factors include conditions interfering with normal secretion clearance of the lung, such as tumor, general anesthesia, postoperative immobility; depression of the CNS from drugs, neurologic disorders, alcohol; and intubation.
6. Pneumonia may be divided into three groups:
   a. Community acquired, because of several organisms.
      i. "Typical" organisms include *S. pneumoniae* (most common organism), *H. influenzae*, *Staphylococcus aureus*, *M. catarrhalis*, anaerobes, and aerobic gram-negative bacteria, and rhinovirus and influenza virus.
      ii. Atypical pneumonia may be caused by *Legionella* species, *Mycobacterium pneumoniae*, and *Chlamydophila pneumoniae*.
   b. Nosocomial pneumonia is a term used to describe hospital-acquired pneumonia (HAP) and ventilator-acquired pneumonia (VAP). HAP is due primarily to gram-negative bacilli and staphylococci. HAP includes patients who have recently been hospitalized within 90 days of the infection; resided in a nursing home or long-term

Table 7-1 Commonly Encountered Pneumonias

TYPE	ORGANISM RESPONSIBLE	MANIFESTATIONS	CLINICAL FEATURES	TREATMENT[a]	COMPLICATIONS
Bacterial					
Streptococcal pneumonia (pneumococcal pneumonia)	• *Streptococcus pneumoniae*	• May be history of previous respiratory infection • Sudden onset, with shaking and chills • Rapidly rising fever; tachypnea • Cough, with expectoration of rusty or green (purulent) sputum • Pleuritic pain aggravated by cough • Chest dull to percussion; crackles, bronchial breath sounds **POPULATION AWARENESS** Confusion and/or increase in respiratory rate may be only presenting feature in older patient.	• Usually involves one or more lobes. • Chest x-ray shows consolidation of affected areas. • Common community-acquired pneumonia as well as seen in residents of nursing homes, those with alcohol use disorder, those who smoke, those with chronic obstructive pulmonary disease (COPD), those who use IV drugs, early human immunodeficiency virus (HIV), endobronchial obstruction.	*Nonhospitalized* • Amoxicillin, amoxicillin–clavulanate plus a macrolide (azithromycin, clarithromycin, or doxycycline). Alternatives include fluoroquinolones: levofloxacin. *Hospitalized* • Ceftriaxone, cefotaxime, ertapenem, or ampicillin–sulbactam plus a macrolide (azithromycin or clarithromycin) • Monotherapy with fluoroquinolone may also be used as an alternative to beta-lactams	• Shock • Pleural effusion • Superinfections • Pericarditis • Otitis media
Staphylococcal pneumonia	• *Staphylococcus aureus*	• Commonly, history of viral infection, especially influenza • Insidious development of cough, with expectoration of yellow, blood-streaked mucus • Onset may be sudden if patient is outpatient • Fever, pleuritic chest pain, progressive dyspnea • Pulse varies; may be slow in proportion to temperature	• Commonly seen in facility setting; during influenza epidemics; in IV drug use; and COPD, those who smoke, bronchiectasis. • These infections commonly lead to necrosis and destruction of lung tissue. • Treatment must be vigorous and prolonged owing to the disease's tendency to destroy the lungs. • Organism may develop rapid drug resistance. • Prolonged convalescence usual.	• Methicillin susceptible: nafcillin, oxacillin, or cefazolin • Methicillin resistant: vancomycin or linezolid	• Effusion/pneumothorax • Lung abscess • Empyema • Meningitis
Pneumonia because of gram-negative enteric bacilli	• *Klebsiella* species, *Pseudomonas* organisms, *Escherichia coli*, *Serratia*, *Proteus* species	• Sudden onset with fever, chills, dyspnea • Pleuritic chest pain and production of purulent sputum	• Infection usually occurs from aspiration of pharyngeal flora into bronchioles. • Seen in persons with severe illness; among the more common causes of hospital-acquired pneumonia.	• Enterobacteriaceae: third-generation cephalosporin, carbapenem (drug of choice if extended-spectrum beta-lactamase producer) beta-lactam/beta-lactamase inhibitor, fluoroquinolone • *Pseudomonas aeruginosa*:	• Early necrosis of lung tissue with rapid abscess formation • High mortality

(continued)

Table 7-1 Commonly Encountered Pneumonias (*continued*)

TYPE	ORGANISM RESPONSIBLE	MANIFESTATIONS	CLINICAL FEATURES	TREATMENT[a]	COMPLICATIONS
				• Empiric therapy: antipseudomonal quinolone or antipseudomonal beta-lactam plus an aminoglycoside, or antipseudomonal quinolone plus an aminoglycoside • Once susceptibilities are available: • Switch to single antibiotic therapy such as beta-lactam	
Legionella species	• *Legionella pneumophila*	• High fever, chills, cough, chest pain, tachypnea • Respiratory distress	• Peak incidence in people older than age 50 who smoke cigarette and have underlying diseases that increase susceptibility to infection or who have been on a cruise ship in the past 2 wk.	Levofloxacin and azithromycin	• Respiratory failure
Haemophilus influenza pneumonia, *Moraxella catarrhalis* pneumonia	• *H. influenzae* • *M. catarrhalis*	• Abrupt onset of coughing, fever, chills, tachypnea	• Common in patients who smoke and those who formerly smoked. • May affect healthy young adults. • X-ray may show consolidation. • Often seen in early HIV and may be the first indication of endobronchial tumor.	• Non-beta-lactam-producing organisms: amoxicillin, fluoroquinolones, doxycycline, azithromycin, clarithromycin • Beta-lactam–producing organisms: second- or third-generation cephalosporins, amoxicillin–clavulanate, fluoroquinolones, doxycycline, azithromycin, clarithromycin	• High mortality in patients with underlying disease (cancer, COPD) • Pleural effusion common
Atypical and Nonbacterial					
Mycoplasma or chlamydial pneumonia (*Legionella pneumoniae* may also be included in this category)	• *Mycoplasma pneumoniae, Chlamydia trachomatis*, or *L. pneumophila*	• Gradual onset; severe headache; irritating hacking cough producing scanty, mucoid sputum • Anorexia; malaise • Fever; nasal congestion; sore throat	• Occurs most commonly in children and young adults, as well as in older adults in community or hospital setting. • Rise in serum complement–fixing antibodies to the organism. • More common in patients with COPD and in those who smoke.	• For mycoplasma or *Chlamydophila pneumoniae*: macrolides, fluoroquinolones • For *Legionella*: fluoroquinolones, azithromycin	• Persisting cough, meningoencephalitis, polyneuritis, monoarticular arthritis, pericarditis, myocarditis • Chlamydial pneumonia has been implicated in cardiac atheromatous lesions in some patients

Viral pneumonia	• Influenza viruses • Parainfluenza viruses • Respiratory syncytial viruses • Rhinoviruses • Adenovirus • Varicella, rubella, rubeola, herpes simplex, cytomegalovirus, Epstein-Barr virus	• Cough • Constitutional symptoms may be pronounced (severe headache, anorexia, fever, and myalgia)	• In majority of patients, influenza begins as an acute coryza and myalgias; others have bronchitis and pleurisy, whereas still others develop GI symptoms. • Risk of developing influenza related to crowding and close contact with groups.	• Treat symptomatically • Prophylactic vaccination recommended for high-risk persons (older than age 65; chronic cardiac or pulmonary disease, diabetes, and other metabolic disorders) • For influenza virus: oseltamivir, zanamivir, peramivir • Follow yearly CDC guidelines for approved medication	• Persons with underlying disease have increased risk of complications, primary influenzal pneumonia, and secondary bacterial pneumonia • Bacterial superinfection • Pericarditis • Endocarditis
Pneumocystis jiroveci pneumonia (PCP)	• *P. jiroveci*	• Insidious onset • Increasing dyspnea and nonproductive cough • Tachypnea; progresses rapidly to intercostal retraction, nasal flaring, and cyanosis • Lowering of arterial oxygen tension • Chest x-ray will reveal diffuse, bilateral interstitial pneumonia	• Usually seen in a host whose resistance is compromised; most common opportunistic infection in AIDS in the United States. • Organism invades the lungs of patients who have suppressed immune system (from AIDS, cancer, leukemia) or after immunosuppressive therapy for cancer, organ transplant, or collagen disease. • Frequently associated with concurrent infection by viruses (cytomegalovirus), bacteria, and fungi.	• TMP-SMX; dapsone with trimethoprim, clindamycin with primaquine • Pentamidine	• Patients are critically ill • Prognosis guarded because it is usually a complication of a severe underlying disorder
Fungal pneumonia	• *Aspergillus fumigatus*	• Fever, productive cough, chest pain, hemoptysis • Chest x-ray reveals a broad range of abnormalities from infiltration to consolidation, cavitation, and empyema	• Individuals with neutropenia most susceptible. • May develop Aspergillus as a superinfection. • Often seen in late HIV disease.	• Antifungal therapy: voriconazole, amphotericin B	• High mortality rate • Invades blood vessels and destroys lung tissue by direct invasion and vascular infarction

CDC, Centers for Disease Control and Prevention; TMP-SMX, trimethoprim–sulfamethoxazole.
[a]Patients with community-acquired pneumonia (CAP) should be treated a minimum of 5 days and should be afebrile for 48 to 72 hours and clinically stable before discontinuing antibiotics.

care facility; or received parenteral antimicrobial therapy, chemotherapy, or wound care within 30 days of pneumonia. HAP is diagnosed greater than or equal to 48 hours after being admitted to the hospital. VAP is diagnosed after endotracheal (ET) intubation.
    c. Pneumonia in the person who is immunocompromised.
7. People older than age 65 have a high rate of mortality, even with appropriate antimicrobial therapy. Recurring pneumonia commonly indicates underlying disease, such as cancer of the lung, multiple myeloma, bronchiectasis, or COPD.

Clinical Manifestations

For the most common forms of bacterial pneumonia:

1. Typical bacterial CAP typically presents with fever, dyspnea, fatigue, and productive cough and often with pleuritic chest pain.
2. Pleuritic chest pain may be aggravated by respiration/coughing.
3. Dyspnea and tachypnea use of accessory muscles of respiration and fatigue.
4. Tachycardia may be present.

Diagnostic Evaluation

1. Chest x-ray shows a discernible infiltrate and presence/extent of pulmonary disease, typically consolidation.
2. Gram stain and culture and sensitivity of sputum are reliable and diagnostic if performed on a well-collected specimen without saliva contamination (excess squamous epithelial cells are present if saliva contamination) and if a predominant organism is present.
    a. Many patients, especially older adults, are not able to produce an adequate suitable sputum sample.
    b. Endobronchial specimens should be obtained from intubated patients.
    c. CAP is often diagnosed presumptively, without culture, but should be investigated for specific pathogens that would significantly alter standard management decisions, based on sputum culture (Gram stain typically shows few or no predominant organisms in atypical CAP).
3. Indications for sputum culture include:
    a. All patients requiring intubation and mechanical ventilation.
    b. Patients who do not require ventilation and who have risk factors for *Pseudomonas aeruginosa* or other multidrug-resistant gram-negative enteric pathogen infection, including severe COPD, use of chronic oral corticosteroids, and those with active alcohol misuse.
    c. Patients who do not require ventilation and who have risk factors for *S. aureus*, including end-stage renal disease, receiving hemodialysis, history of injection drug use, cavitary pulmonary infiltrates, and acute postinfluenza pneumonia.
4. Pretreatment blood samples for culture to detect bacteremia should be obtained from patients with admission to intensive care unit, cavitary lesion on chest x-ray, leukopenia, active alcohol misuse, chronic severe liver disease, asplenia, positive pneumococcal urinary antigen test, or pleural effusion.
5. Immunologic tests may be ordered to detect microbial antigens in serum, sputum, and urine.
6. Severity-of-illness scores, such as the CURB-65 criteria (confusion, uremia, respiratory rate, low BP, age 65 or greater), or pneumonia severity index can be used to identify patients with CAP who may be candidates for outpatient treatment.

Management

1. Antimicrobial therapy—depends on empiric recommendations and/or laboratory identification of causative organism and sensitivity to specific antimicrobials.
2. Oxygen therapy, if patient has inadequate gas exchange.
3. Patients with hypoxemia or respiratory distress who are refractory to oxygen should receive a cautious trial of noninvasive ventilation unless they require immediate intubation because of severe hypoxemia or acute respiratory failure.
4. Low V_T ventilation (6 mL/kg ideal body weight) for diffuse bilateral pneumonia or ARDS.
5. Early mobilization when clinically stable reduces the length of facility stay.
6. Assess influenza and pneumococcal vaccination status, and if not currently vaccinated or status uncertain, perform prior to hospital discharge.
7. Advise and assist with smoking cessation in patients who currently smoke.
8. Respiratory hygiene measures, including the use of hand hygiene and masks or tissues for patients with cough, should be used in outpatient settings and emergency departments (EDs) to reduce the spread of respiratory infections.

Complications

1. Pleural effusion.
2. Sustained hypotension and shock, especially in gram-negative bacterial disease, particularly in older patients.
3. Empyema.
4. Superinfection: pericarditis, bacteremia, and meningitis.
5. Delirium—considered a medical emergency.
6. Atelectasis—because of mucus plugs.
7. Delayed resolution.

Nursing Assessment

1. Take a careful history to help establish etiologic diagnosis. Local epidemiology and patient travel history, history of exposures, and local or national outbreaks may help in pneumonia identification.
    a. History of recent respiratory illness, complete medical history, and social history including risk factors for pneumonia.
    b. Presence of purulent sputum, increased amount of sputum, fever, chills, pleuritic pain, dyspnea, and tachypnea.
    c. Any pattern of family illness.
    d. Medications (including recent antibiotics) and allergies.
2. Observe for dyspnea, excess fatigue, change in mental status, anxiety, or respiratory distress.
3. Auscultate for crackles overlying the affected region and for bronchial breath sounds when consolidation (filling of airspaces with exudate) is present.

Nursing Interventions

Improving Gas Exchange

1. Observe for dyspnea, hypoxia, cyanosis, and confusion, indicating worsening condition.
2. Follow ABG levels/SpO_2 to determine oxygen need and response to oxygen therapy.
3. Administer oxygen at a concentration to maintain PaO_2/SpO_2 at an acceptable level. Hypoxemia may be due to abnormal V/Q mismatch with shunt in affected lung segments.

4. Use caution with high concentrations of oxygen in patients with COPD, particularly with evidence of CO_2 retention; use of high oxygen concentrations may worsen alveolar ventilation in some patients by depressing the patient's only remaining ventilatory drive. If high concentrations of oxygen are given, monitor alertness and PaO_2 and $PaCO_2$ levels for signs of CO_2 retention.
5. Place patient in an upright position as tolerated to obtain greater lung expansion and improve aeration. Frequent turning and increased activity (up in a chair, ambulate as tolerated) should be employed if clinically stable.

Enhancing Airway Clearance

1. If ordered, obtain freshly expectorated sputum for Gram stain and culture initially prior to antibiotic treatment. Early morning specimens are preferable for subsequent specimens. Instruct the patient as follows:
   a. Perform oral care and rinse mouth with water to minimize contamination by normal flora.
   b. Breathe deeply several times.
   c. Cough deeply and expectorate raised sputum into a sterile container.
2. Auscultate the chest for crackles and rhonchi. Encourage patient to deep breath and cough to reduce retained secretions that interfere with gas exchange. Suction as necessary.
3. Encourage increased fluid intake, unless contraindicated, to replace fluid losses caused by fever, diaphoresis, dehydration, and tachypnea.
4. Humidify oxygen over 4 L/min to reduce dryness of mucus membranes.
5. Employ PEP device use, huff cough, and possibly chest wall percussion and postural drainage, when appropriate, to loosen and mobilize secretions.
6. When clinically stable, mobilize patient to improve ventilation and secretion clearance and reduce the risk of atelectasis and worsening pneumonia.

Relieving Pleuritic Pain

1. Place patient in a comfortable position (semi-Fowler) for resting and breathing; encourage frequent change of position to prevent pooling of secretions in lungs and atelectasis.
2. Demonstrate how to splint the chest while coughing.
3. Avoid suppressing a productive cough.
4. Administer prescribed nonsedating analgesic agent to relieve pain.
5. Use comfort measures to improve symptom control.
6. Encourage modified bed rest during febrile period.
7. Watch for abdominal distention or ileus, which may be due to swallowing of air during intervals of severe dyspnea. Insert a nasogastric (NG) or rectal tube, as directed.

POPULATION AWARENESS Sedatives, opioids, and cough suppressants should be used cautiously in older patients because of their tendency to suppress cough and gag reflexes and respiratory drive. Also, provide or encourage frequent oral care for pneumonia prevention.

Monitoring for Complications

1. Be aware that fatal complications may develop during the early period of antimicrobial treatment.
2. Monitor temperature, pulse, respiration, BP, oximetry, mentation, and for evidence of dyspnea at regular intervals to assess the patient's response to therapy.
3. Auscultate lungs and heart. Heart murmurs or friction rub may indicate acute bacterial endocarditis, pericarditis, or myocarditis.
4. Employ special nursing surveillance for patients with:
   a. Alcohol use disorder, COPD, and immunosuppression—these people as well as older patients may have little or no fever.
   b. Chronic bronchitis—it may be difficult to detect subtle changes in condition because the patient may have seriously compromised pulmonary function and regular mucus production.
   c. Epilepsy—pneumonia may result from aspiration after a seizure.
   d. Delirium—may be caused by hypoxia, meningitis, and alcohol withdrawal.
5. Assess these patients for unusual behavior, alterations in mental status, stupor, and heart failure.
6. Assess for resistant fever or return of fever, potentially suggesting bacterial resistance to antibiotics.

CLINICAL JUDGMENT Delirium causes and treatment must be identified to control symptoms and prevent exhaustion and cardiac failure. Prepare for lumbar puncture, if indicated, to rule out meningitis, which may be lethal. Mild sedation should be considered with caution.

Patient Education and Health Maintenance

1. Advise patient to complete the entire course of antibiotics.
2. Advise patient that fatigue and weakness may persist after pneumonia.
3. Once clinically stable, encourage a gradual increase in activities to improve ventilation and reduce hazards of immobility.
4. Encourage breathing exercises to clear the lungs and promote full expansion and function.
5. Explain that a chest x-ray is usually taken 4 to 6 weeks after recovery to evaluate lungs for clearing and detect any tumor or underlying cause.
6. Advise smoking cessation. Cigarette smoke destroys tracheobronchial cilial action, which is the first line of defense of lungs, also irritates mucosa of bronchi, and inhibits function of alveolar scavenger cells (macrophages).
7. Advise the patient to keep up natural resistance with good nutrition, adequate rest, and physical activity, when tolerated. One episode of pneumonia may make the patient susceptible to recurring respiratory infections.
8. Instruct patient to avoid fatigue, sudden extremes in temperature, and excessive alcohol intake, which lower resistance to pneumonia.
9. Assess for and facilitate vaccination with pneumococcal and influenza vaccines (see page 104). Influenza vaccine is associated with reduced hospitalizations for pneumonia, influenza, and death in community-dwelling older adults.
10. Advise avoidance of contact with people with upper respiratory infections for several months after pneumonia resolves.
11. Respiratory and hand hygiene includes frequent handwashing, especially after contact with others.

Evaluation: Expected Outcomes

- Cyanosis and dyspnea reduced; ABG levels and SaO_2 improved.
- Coughs effectively; absence of crackles.
- Appears more comfortable; free of pain.
- Fever controlled; no signs of resistant infection.

Aspiration Pneumonia

Aspiration is the inhalation of oropharyngeal secretions and/or stomach contents into the lower airways. It may lead to acute pneumonia.

Pathophysiology and Etiology

1. Loss of protective airway reflexes (swallowing, cough) may be caused by an altered state of consciousness, alcohol or drug overdose, seizures, stroke, head trauma, general anesthesia, intercranial mass or lesion, during resuscitation procedures, seriously ill or debilitated patients, and abnormalities of gag and swallowing reflexes.
2. Other conditions and risk factors associated with aspiration include the following:
   a. Esophageal strictures and diverticula, head and neck neoplasms, tracheoesophageal fistula, and gastroesophageal reflux.
   b. Multiple sclerosis, dementia, Parkinson disease, myasthenia gravis, and pseudobulbar palsy.
   c. Intubation, tracheostomy, endoscopy, and bronchoscopy.
   d. Obstetric patients—from general anesthesia, lithotomy position, delayed emptying of the stomach from the enlarged uterus, and labor contractions.
   e. GI conditions—hiatal hernia, intestinal obstruction, abdominal distention, NG or feeding tube, and gastric or postpyloric tube feedings.
   f. Prolonged vomiting or recumbent position.
3. Effects of aspiration depend on the volume and character of aspirated material.
   a. Gastric acid causes chemical pneumonitis.
   b. Bacteria from the oropharynx cause aspiration pneumonia.
   c. Oil (mineral oil or vegetable oil) causes exogenous lipoid pneumonia.
   d. Foreign body may cause an acute respiratory emergency and may predispose the patient to bacterial pneumonia.
   e. Many cases of pneumonia result from aspiration of pathogens from the oral cavity or nasopharynx caused by *S. pneumoniae, H. influenza, S. aureus,* and gram-negative bacteria. These bacteria are relatively virulent, so that only a small inoculum is required to result in pneumonia. The aspiration episode may be subtle.

POPULATION AWARENESS Oropharyngeal dysphagia has been found in the majority of older adult patients (mean age, 84 years).

Clinical Manifestations

1. Tachycardia and fever.
2. Dyspnea, cough, and tachypnea.
3. Hypoxemia and cyanosis.
4. Decreased breath sounds, rales, pleural friction rub, and dullness to percussion overconsolidation.
5. Purulent sputum.

Diagnostic Evaluation

1. Chest x-ray may be normal initially; with time, shows consolidation and other abnormalities.

Management

1. Clearing the obstructed airway.
   a. If foreign body is visible, it may be removed manually.
   b. Suction trachea/ET tube—to remove particulate matter.
   c. Optimize secretion clearance and manage hypoxia with supplemental oxygen.
2. Antimicrobial therapy or specific therapy depending on the material aspirated.
3. Laryngoscopy/bronchoscopy may be performed for aspiration of solid material.
4. Oxygen therapy and assisted ventilation if adequate oxygenation cannot be maintained.
5. Fluid volume replacement and correction of acidosis for correction of hypotension and shock.

Complications

1. Lung abscess and empyema.
2. Necrotizing pneumonia.
3. ARDS.

Nursing Assessment

1. Assess for airway obstruction and hypoxemia.
2. Assess for development of fever, foul-smelling sputum, and congestion.
3. Assess LOC, gag reflex, swallowing ability, and other risk factors for aspiration.

Nursing Interventions

See pages 166 to 167 for nursing interventions.

Additional Nursing Interventions

1. Carefully monitor patients at risk for aspiration.
2. Elevate head of bed for debilitated patients, for those receiving tube feedings, and for those at risk for aspiration.
3. For patients with feeding tubes, make sure the tube is positioned properly and the tube is patent.
   a. Give tube feedings slowly, with the head of bed elevated. Check for residual volume if the facility requires.
   b. Check position of the tube in the stomach before feeding.
   c. Check seal of the cuff of the tracheostomy or ET tube before feeding.
4. Keep the patient in a fasting state before anesthesia (at least 8 hours).
5. Feed patients with impaired swallowing slowly, and make sure that no food is retained in the mouth after feeding.

CLINICAL JUDGMENT Morbidity and mortality rates of aspiration pneumonia remain high even with optimum treatment. Prevention is the key to the problem. Recent studies are uncertain about the effect of gastric residual volume on clinical outcomes including mortality, pneumonia, vomiting, and hospital length of stay.

Pulmonary Embolism

Pulmonary embolism (PE) refers to the obstruction of one or more pulmonary arteries by a thrombus (or thrombi) usually originating in the deep veins of the legs, the right side of the heart, or, rarely, an upper extremity, which becomes dislodged and is carried to the pulmonary vasculature.

Acute PE is a common form of venous thromboembolism (VTE), leading to V/Q mismatch, increase in pulmonary vascular resistance, pulmonary artery pressure (PAP), right heart workload and heart failure, decrease in cardiac output, and shock. Pulmonary infarction refers to necrosis of lung tissue because of reduction in blood supply.

Pathophysiology and Etiology

1. Obstruction, either partial or full, of pulmonary arteries, which causes decrease or absent blood flow; therefore, there is ventilation but no perfusion (V/Q mismatch).
2. Hemodynamic consequences:
   a. Increased pulmonary vascular resistance.
   b. Increased PAP.
   c. Increased right-sided heart workload to maintain pulmonary blood flow.
   d. Right-sided heart failure.
   e. Decreased cardiac output.
   f. Decreased BP.
   g. Shock.
   h. Risk of hypoxemia.
3. Pulmonary emboli can vary in size and seriousness of consequences.
4. Predisposing factors include the following:
   a. Stasis and prolonged immobilization.
   b. Concurrent phlebitis.
   c. Heart failure and stroke.
   d. Injury to the vessel wall.
   e. Coagulation disorders and hypercoagulable state.
   f. Malignancy.
   g. Advancing age, estrogen therapy, and oral contraceptives.
   h. Fracture of long bones.
   i. Obesity.

CLINICAL JUDGMENT Be aware of high-risk patients for PE—immobilization, trauma to the pelvis (especially surgical) and lower extremities (especially hip fracture), obesity, history of thromboembolic disease, varicose veins, pregnancy, heart failure, myocardial infarction (MI), malignant disease, postoperative patients, and older patients.

Clinical Manifestations

1. Rapid onset of dyspnea at rest, pleuritic chest pain, cough, syncope, delirium, apprehension, tachypnea, diaphoresis, and hemoptysis. Onset may be prolonged and presentation more subtle if obstruction is partial.
2. Chest pain with apprehension and a sense of impending doom occur when most of the PA is obstructed.
3. Tachycardia, rales, fever, hypotension, cyanosis, heart gallop, and loud pulmonic component of S_2 (split S_2).
4. Calf or thigh pain, edema, erythema, tenderness, or palpable cord (signs suggestive of deep vein thrombosis [DVT]).

CLINICAL JUDGMENT Have a high index of suspicion for pulmonary embolus if there is a subtle or significant deterioration in the patient's condition and unexplained cardiovascular and pulmonary findings.

Diagnostic Evaluation

1. Thoracic imaging: V/Q scan (possibly using single-photon emission computed tomography) or helical contrast-enhanced computed tomography (CT).
2. Pulmonary angiography if noninvasive testing is inconclusive or not a candidate for noninvasive testing. Contrast studies should be avoided in persons who are pregnant or have advanced renal failure.
3. D-Dimer assay for low to intermediate probability of PE.
4. ABG levels—decreased PaO_2 is usually found because of perfusion abnormality of the lung.
5. Chest x-ray—normal or possible wedge-shaped infiltrate.

Management

Emergency Management

For massive PE, the goal is to stabilize cardiorespiratory status.

CLINICAL JUDGMENT Massive PE is a medical emergency; the patient's condition tends to deteriorate rapidly. There may be a profound decrease in cardiac output, with an accompanying increase in right ventricular pressure.

1. Oxygen is administered to relieve hypoxemia, respiratory distress, and cyanosis and to dilate pulmonary vasculature.
2. An infusion is started to open an IV route for drugs and fluids.
3. Vasopressors, inotropic agents such as dopamine, and antiarrhythmic agents may be indicated to support circulation if the patient is unstable.
4. ECG is monitored continuously for findings suggestive of right-sided heart failure, which may have a rapid onset. Changes may include sinus tachycardia, Q waves, late T-wave inversion, S wave in lead I, right bundle-branch block, right axis deviation, atrial fibrillation, and T-wave changes.
5. Small doses of IV morphine may be given to relieve anxiety, alleviate chest discomfort (which improves ventilation), and ease adaptation to a mechanical ventilator, if this is necessary.
6. Pulmonary angiography, thoracic imaging, hemodynamic measurements, ABG analysis, and other studies are carried out.

Subsequent Management: Anticoagulation and Thrombolysis

1. Anticoagulant therapy includes subcutaneous low-molecular-weight heparin (LMWH), IV or subcutaneous unfractionated heparin (UFH) with monitoring, unmonitored weight-based subcutaneous UFH, or subcutaneous fondaparinux.
2. Anticoagulants prevent further thrombus formation and extend the clotting time of the blood; they do not dissolve clots.
   a. UFH is given as IV loading dose usually followed by continuous pump or drip infusion or given intermittently every 4 to 6 hours.
   b. Dosage adjusted to maintain the partial thromboplastin time (PTT) at 1½ to 2 times the pretreatment value (if the value was normal). Monitoring may also include antifactor Xa and activated clotting time.
   c. Protamine sulfate may be given to neutralize heparin in the event of severe bleeding.
3. Oral anticoagulation with warfarin is usually used for follow-up anticoagulant therapy after heparin therapy has been established and interrupts the coagulation mechanism by interfering with the vitamin K–dependent synthesis of prothrombin and factors VII, IX, and X.
   a. Dosage is controlled by monitoring serial tests of international normalized ratio (INR), achieving 2.0 to 3.0 as the norm.
   b. Fresh frozen plasma (FFP) should be given for emergent reversal of INR greater than 9 (two units FFP for patients with low to moderate risk of bleeding, four units for those with high risk).
   c. Vitamin K may be given orally when INR is greater than 5, in addition to holding doses of warfarin, or by slow IV infusion for significant bleeding.

d. Four-factor prothrombin complex concentrate can also be utilized for reversal of vitamin K antagonists.

4. Thrombolytic (fibrinolytic) agents, such as streptokinase, may be used in patients with massive PE.
   a. Effective in lysing recently formed thrombi.
   b. Improved circulatory and hemodynamic status.
   c. Administered IV in a loading dose followed by constant infusion.
5. Newer clot-specific thrombolytics (tissue plasminogen activator, streptokinase activator complex, single-chain urokinase) are preferred.
   a. Activate plasminogen only within the thrombus itself rather than systematically.
   b. Minimize occurrence of generalized fibrinolysis and subsequent bleeding.
6. Absolute contraindications to fibrinolytics include any prior intracranial hemorrhage, known structural intracranial cerebrovascular diseases such as arteriovenous malformation, known intracranial neoplasm, ischemic stroke within 3 months, suspected aortic dissection, bleeding, recent surgery of spinal canal or brain, and recently closed head or facial trauma. Caution should be used in patients greater than 75 years, current use of anticoagulation, pregnancy, non-compressible vascular punctures, traumatic or prolonged cardiopulmonary resuscitation, recent internal bleeding, history of severe hypertension, current systolic BP greater than 180 or diastolic BP greater than 110, dementia, remote ischemic stroke, and major surgery within 3 weeks.
7. Graduated compression stockings with 30 to 40 mm Hg compression, knee-high, and sized to fit help dilate deep veins and decrease swelling and venous ulcers that can develop due to postthrombosis syndrome and reduce the risk of recurrent DVT and PE.

POPULATION AWARENESS Consider the patient's age and INR level in the dosing of anticoagulation therapy. Older patients will usually need a decreased dosing regimen.

Surgical Intervention

1. When anticoagulation and thrombolysis are contraindicated or the patient has recurrent embolization or develops serious complications from drug therapy.
2. Placement of transvenously inserted intraluminal filter in inferior vena cava to prevent migration of emboli (see Figure 7-2); inserted through femoral or jugular vein by way of catheter.
3. Embolectomy (removal of pulmonary embolic obstruction), either by open surgical embolectomy or catheter embolectomy with fragmentation.

EVIDENCE BASE Goldberg, J. B., Spevack, D. M., Ahsan, S., Rochlani, Y., Dutta, T., Ohira, S., Kai, M., Spielvogel, D., Lansman, S., & Malekan, R. (2020). Survival and right ventricular function after surgical management of acute pulmonary embolism. *Journal of the American College of Cardiology*, *76*(8), 903–911. https://doi.org/10.1016/j.jacc.2020.06.065

Complications

1. Bleeding as a result of treatment.
2. Respiratory failure.
3. Chronic thromboembolic pulmonary hypertension (CTEPH) and cor pulmonale.

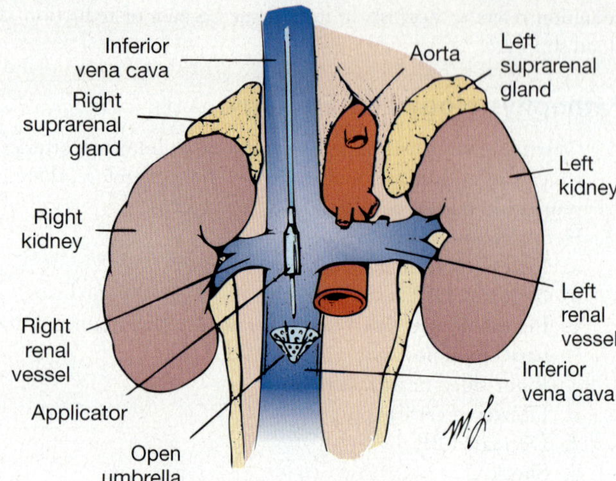

Figure 7-2. Insertion of umbrella filter in inferior vena cava to prevent pulmonary embolism. Filter (compressed within an applicator catheter) is inserted through an incision in the right internal jugular vein. The applicator is withdrawn when the filter fixes itself to the wall of the inferior vena cava after ejection from the applicator.

Nursing Assessment

1. Take nursing history with an emphasis on the onset and severity of dyspnea and nature of chest pain, as well as past medical history (PMH) for contraindications to thrombolytic therapy.
2. Examine the patient's legs carefully. Assess for swelling of the leg, duskiness, warmth, pain on pressure over gastrocnemius muscle, which may indicate thrombophlebitis as the source.
3. A positive Homans sign (pain on dorsiflexion of the foot) has low specificity and sensitivity for diagnosis of DVT.
4. Monitor respiratory rate—may be accelerated out of proportion to degree of fever and tachycardia.
   a. Observe rate of inspiration to expiration.
   b. Percuss for resonance or dullness.
   c. Auscultate for friction rub, crackles, rhonchi, and wheezing.
5. Auscultate heart; listen for splitting of second heart sound.
6. Evaluate results of laboratory data for patients on anticoagulants and report results that are outside of therapeutic range promptly; anticipate a dosage change.

Nursing Interventions

Correcting Breathing Pattern

1. Assess for hypoxia, dyspnea, headache, restlessness, apprehension, pallor, cyanosis, and behavioral changes.
2. Monitor vital signs, ECG, oximetry, and ABG levels for adequacy of oxygenation.
3. Monitor patient's response to IV fluids/vasopressors.
4. Monitor oxygen therapy—used to relieve hypoxemia.
5. Prepare patient for assisted ventilation when hypoxemia does not respond to supplemental oxygen. Hypoxemia is due to ventilation/perfusion mismatch.

Improving Tissue Perfusion

1. Closely monitor for shock—decreasing BP, tachycardia, and cool, clammy skin.
2. Monitor prescribed medications given to preserve right-sided heart filling pressure and increase BP.

3. Maintain patient on bed rest during acute phase to reduce oxygen demands and risk of bleeding.
4. Monitor urinary output hourly because there may be reduced renal perfusion and decreased glomerular filtration.
5. Provide antiembolism compression stockings with 30 to 40 mm Hg of compression.

Relieving Pain

1. Watch patient for signs of discomfort and pain.
2. Ascertain if pain worsens with deep breathing and coughing; auscultate for friction rub.
3. Give morphine, as prescribed, and monitor for pain relief and signs of respiratory depression.
4. Position with the head of bed slightly elevated (unless contraindicated by shock) and with chest splinted for deep breathing and coughing.
5. Evaluate patient thoroughly for signs of hypoxia when anxiety, restlessness, and agitation of new onset are noted, before administering as-needed sedatives. Consider calling a health care provider when these signs are present, especially if accompanied by cyanotic nail beds, circumoral pallor or cyanosis, and increased respiratory rate.

Reducing Anxiety

1. Correct dyspnea and relieve physical discomfort.
2. Explain diagnostic procedures and the patient's role; correct misconceptions.
3. Listen to the patient's concerns; attentive listening relieves anxiety and reduces emotional distress.
4. Speak calmly and slowly.
5. Do everything possible to enhance the patient's sense of control.

Intervening for Complications

1. Be alert for bleeding—related to anticoagulant or thrombolytic therapy. Major bleeding may occur from GI tract, brain, lungs, nose, and genitourinary (GU) tract.
2. Perform stool guaiac test to detect occult blood loss.
3. Monitor platelet count to detect heparin-induced thrombocytopenia.
4. Minimize risk of bleeding by performing essential ABG analysis on upper extremities; apply digital compression at puncture site for 30 minutes; apply pressure dressing to previously involved sites; check site for oozing.
5. Maintain patient on strict bed rest during thrombolytic therapy; avoid unnecessary handling.
6. Discontinue infusion in the event of uncontrolled bleeding.
7. Notify health care provider on call immediately for change in LOC or sensation or ability to follow commands, move limbs, or respond to questions with clear articulation. Intracranial bleed may necessitate discontinuation of anticoagulation promptly to avert a massive neurologic catastrophe.
8. Be alert for shock from low cardiac output secondary to resistance to right-sided heart outflow or to myocardial dysfunction because of ischemia.
   a. Assess for skin color changes, particularly nail beds, lips, earlobes, and mucous membranes.
   b. Monitor BP, pulse, and SpO_2.
   c. Measure urine output.
   d. Monitor IV infusion of vasopressor or other prescribed agents.

Patient Education and Health Maintenance

1. Advise patient of the possible need to continue taking anticoagulant therapy for 6 weeks up to an indefinite period as well as safety considerations and drug and food interactions with anticoagulants.
2. Teach regarding food and drug interactions if taking warfarin.
3. Teach about signs of bleeding, especially of the gums and nose, bruising, and blood in urine and stools.
4. For patients on anticoagulants, instruct to use soft toothbrush, avoid shaving with blade razor (use electric razor instead), and avoid aspirin-containing products. Notify health care provider of bleeding or increased bruising.
5. Warn against taking medications unless approved by health care provider because many drugs interact with anticoagulants.
6. Instruct patient to tell dentist about taking an anticoagulant.
7. Warn against inactivity for prolonged periods or sitting with legs crossed to prevent recurrence.
8. Warn against sports/activities that may cause trauma or injury to legs and predispose to a thrombus.
9. Encourage wearing a medical alert bracelet, identifying patient as a person who uses an anticoagulant.
10. Instruct patient to lose weight, if applicable; obesity is a risk factor.
11. Discuss contraceptive methods with patient, if applicable; people assigned female at birth with a history of pulmonary embolus are advised against taking hormonal contraceptives.

Evaluation: Expected Outcomes

- Verbalizes less shortness of breath.
- Vital signs stable; adequate urinary output.
- Reports freedom from pain.
- Appears more relaxed; sleeping at long intervals.
- Progresses without major bleeding or other complications.

Tuberculosis

Tuberculosis (*TB*) is an infectious disease caused by bacteria (*Mycobacterium tuberculosis*). It is usually spread from person to person through droplet aerosolization (droplet nuclei). It usually infects the lung but can occur at virtually any site in the body.

Pathophysiology and Etiology

Transmission

1. The term *Mycobacterium* is descriptive of a bacterium that resembles a fungus. The organisms multiply at varying rates and are characterized as acid-fast aerobic organisms that can be killed by heat, sunshine, and ultraviolet light.
2. TB is an airborne disease transmitted by droplet nuclei, usually from within the respiratory tract of an infected person who exhales them during coughing, talking, sneezing, or singing.
3. When a susceptible person inhales the droplet-containing air, the organism is carried into the lung to the pulmonary alveoli.
   a. About 2½ to 12 weeks after initial TB infection, TB testing (purified protein derivative [PPD] or quantiFERON blood test) is positive; however, most people who become infected do not develop clinical illness because the body's immune system brings the infection under control.
   b. Some bacilli remain viable in the body for years, such as with latent tuberculosis infection (LTBI). Persons with LTBI have no symptoms and are not infectious.

4. Persons at increased risk for TB include close contacts of persons with active TB; persons traveling from Africa, Asia, Eastern Europe, Latin America, and Russia; residents of high-risk congregate settings (correctional facilities, long-term care facilities, and homeless shelters); health care workers exposed to high-risk patients; and infants and children or adolescents exposed to high-risk adults.
5. Of concern in controlling TB in the United States is the prevalence of infection among persons born outside the country residing in the United States, delays in detecting and reporting pulmonary TB, and deficiencies in identifying and screening close contacts and persons with LTBI who are at risk for progression to active TB. The population at risk for progression include the following:
   a. Those who are HIV positive.
   b. Those who have acquired TB infection within the last 2 years.
   c. Children younger than age 4.
   d. Those with already immunocompromised conditions such as silicosis; diabetes mellitus; chronic renal failure; leukemia, lymphoma, and carcinoma of the head, neck, or lung; 10% or more below ideal body weight; prolonged corticosteroid use; use of tumor necrosis factor–alpha (TNF-α) antagonists; organ transplant; intestinal bypass or gastrectomy; and history of untreated or inadequately treated TB.

Pathology

1. The bacilli of TB infect the lung, forming a tubercle (lesion).
2. The tubercle:
   a. May heal, leaving scar tissue.
   b. May continue as a granuloma, then heal, or be reactivated.
   c. May eventually proceed to necrosis, liquefaction, sloughing, and cavitation.
3. The initial lesion may disseminate tubercle bacilli by extension to adjacent tissues, by way of the bloodstream, the lymphatic system, or through the bronchi.
4. Extrapulmonary TB occurs more commonly in children and immunocompromised individuals and can involve lymph nodes, bones, joints, pleural space, pericardium, CNS, GI tract, GU tissue, and the peritoneum.

Clinical Manifestations

Patient may be asymptomatic or may have insidious symptoms that may be ignored.

1. Constitutional symptoms.
   a. Fatigue, anorexia, weight loss, low-grade fever, and night sweats.
   b. Some patients have acute febrile illness, chills, and flulike symptoms.
2. Pulmonary signs and symptoms.
   a. Cough (insidious onset) progressing in frequency and producing mucoid or mucopurulent sputum and hemoptysis.
   b. Chest pain and dyspnea (suggest extensive involvement).
3. Extrapulmonary TB: pain, inflammation, and dysfunction in any of the tissues infected.

Diagnostic Evaluation

1. Testing for suspected TB infection includes sputum smear evaluated by microscopy for acid-fast bacilli (AFB) following Centers for Disease Control and Prevention guidelines. Three sputum specimens are collected 8 to 24 hours apart with one being an early morning specimen.
   a. Results of sputum sample are needed to drive decisions regarding the discontinuation of isolation precautions for patients with suspected TB in health care settings.
   b. For patients with a diagnosis of TB, decisions regarding discontinuation of precautions should be based on sputum smear (i.e., three consecutive negative smears) and other clinical criteria.
   c. In patients unable to produce sputum, induction with hypertonic saline should be attempted.
2. Sputum culture—a positive culture for *M. tuberculosis* confirms a diagnosis of active TB infection and can detect drug-resistant strains.
3. Chest x-ray to determine the presence and extent of disease.
4. Tuberculin skin test (PPD or Mantoux test)—inoculation of tuberculin-PPD into the intradermal layer of the inner aspect of the forearm. It is used to detect *M. tuberculosis* infection, past or present, active or inactive (latent).
   a. Skin reaction is observed 48 to 72 hours after injecting 0.1 mL of PPD intradermally. Inspect and palpate for induration and measure the maximum transverse diameter.
   b. An induration of 5 or more millimeters is considered positive in persons infected with HIV, recent contact of a person with TB disease, persons with chest x-ray changes consistent with prior TB, organ recipients, and persons immunosuppressed for other reasons.
   c. An induration of 10 or more millimeters is considered positive in recent immigrants (<5 years) from high-prevalence countries, people who use injection drugs, those exposed to high-risk congregate settings, mycobacteriology laboratory personnel, other clinical conditions considered high risk, children less than 4 years of age, infants, children, and adolescents exposed to adults in high-risk categories.
   d. An induration of 15 or more millimeters is considered positive in any person, including persons with no known risk factors for TB. However, targeted skin testing programs should only be conducted among high-risk groups.
5. Interferon-gamma release assay for *M. tuberculosis* may serve as an alternative to PPD, but it does not distinguish between active and latent TB.
   a. Unaffected by past exposure to bacille Calmette-Guérin (BCG) vaccine.
   b. Negative tests should be interpreted with caution in the immunocompromised, those at high risk for TB, and children.
   c. Is an alternative for those who may have a difficult time returning for a second appointment when receiving a PPD.

EVIDENCE BASE Centers for Disease Control and Prevention. (2022). *Testing for TB infection.* www.cdc.gov/tb/topic/testing/tbtesttypes.htm/

Management

See Table 7-2.

1. In patients with active TB, a combination of drugs to which the organisms are susceptible is given to destroy viable bacilli as rapidly as possible and to protect against the emergence of drug-resistant organisms.

Table 7-2 Recommended Drugs for the Initial Treatment of Tuberculosis in Adults

DRUG	DOSAGE FORMS	DAILY DOSE	TWICE-WEEKLY DOSE	THRICE-WEEKLY DOSE	MAJOR ADVERSE EFFECTS
Isoniazid	• Tablets: 50 mg, 100 mg, 300 mg • Syrup: 50 mg/5 mL • Vials: 1 g	5 mg/kg PO or IM (maximum 300 mg)	15 mg/kg (maximum 900 mg) (can also be given once per week)	15 mg/kg (maximum 900 mg)	Paresthesias, nausea, vomiting, elevated liver transaminases peripheral neuropathy, hepatitis, hypersensitivity, hepatotoxicity, seizures, irritability, lack of concentration, lupuslike syndrome
Rifampin	• Capsules: 150 mg, 300 mg • Syrup: formulated from capsules, 10 mg/mL	10 mg/kg PO (maximum 600 mg)	10 mg/kg (maximum 600 mg)	10 mg/kg (maximum 600 mg)	Red-orange discoloration of body fluids, nausea, vomiting, anorexia, hepatitis, elevated liver transaminases, febrile reaction, purpura (rare), pruritus and rash, caution regarding drug interactions
Pyrazinamide	Tablets: 500 mg	Dosages are variable by weight	Dosages are variable by weight	Dosages are variable by weight	Anorexia, rash, urticaria, nausea, vomiting, hepatotoxicity, hyperuricemia, arthralgias, acute gouty arthritis
Ethambutol	Tablets: 100 mg, 400 mg	15–20 mg/kg	240–250 mg/kg	25–35 mg/kg	Optic neuritis (decreased red-green color discrimination, decreased visual acuity), peripheral neuritis, joint pain, anorexia, nausea, vomiting, skin rash

IM, intramuscularly; PO, orally.

2. There are several currently recommended treatment options that may include a 4-month rifapentine–moxifloxacin TB treatment regimen or a 6- or 9-month RIPE TB treatment regimen which is described below. An initial phase of 2 months of bactericidal drugs, including isoniazid (INH), rifampin, pyrazinamide (PZA), and ethambutol (EMB). This regimen should be followed until the results of drug susceptibility studies are available unless there is little possibility of drug resistance.
   a. If drug susceptibility results are known and the organism is fully susceptible, EMB does not need to be included.
   b. For children whose visual acuity cannot be monitored, EMB is not normally recommended except with an increased likelihood of INH resistance or if the child has upper lobe infiltration and/or cavity formation.
   c. Because of increasing frequency of global streptomycin resistance, streptomycin is not considered interchangeable with EMB unless the organism is known to be susceptible to streptomycin.
   d. PZA may be withheld in patients with severe liver disease, gout, and, possibly, pregnancy.
   e. Adverse effects, including liver injury, have been noted with rifampin and pyrazinamide in a once-daily or twice-weekly combination; therefore, this combination is not recommended for the treatment of latent TB infection.
3. Follow up with 4 months of INH and rifampin. Six months of therapy is usually effective for killing the three populations of bacilli: those rapidly dividing, those slowly dividing, and those only intermittently dividing.
4. Sputum smears may be obtained every 2 weeks until they are negative; sputum cultures do not become negative for 3 to 5 months.
5. Rifabutin is used as a substitute for rifampin if the organism is susceptible to rifabutin and for patients taking medications that may interact with rifampin.
6. Second-line drugs—such as cycloserine, ethionamide, streptomycin, amikacin, kanamycin, capreomycin, para-aminosalicylic acid, and some fluoroquinolones—are used in patients with resistance, for retreatment, and in those with intolerance to other agents. Patients taking these drugs should be monitored by health care providers experienced in their use.
7. Extensively drug-resistant tuberculosis (XDR TB) is a relatively rare type of multidrug-resistant TB resistant to almost all oral drugs used to treat TB, including INH, rifampin, fluoroquinolones, and at least one of the three injectable drugs (i.e., amikacin, kanamycin, or capreomycin). XDR TB is of special concern for persons with HIV infection and/or immunocompromised persons because of the increased risk of infection and mortality.
8. For people with suspected LTBI, treatment should begin after active TB has been ruled out (see Table 7-3). Several treatment regimens are currently recommended for LTBI. Drug therapy may include INH, rifapentine, and rifampin. Shorter courses of therapy (3 to 4 months) with rifampin are recommended over longer courses (6 to 9 months) of monotherapy with INH. To prevent neurotoxicity, pyridoxine 25 to 50 mg daily is also recommended.

DRUG ALERT Adverse reactions to anti-TB drugs may be significant. Monitor liver function tests and instruct patients to seek immediate medical attention if signs or symptoms of hepatitis occur (nausea, emesis, anorexia, jaundice, dark urine, light gray or clay-colored stool, and/or abdominal pain).

EVIDENCE BASE Centers for Disease Control and Prevention. (2020). *Treatment regimens for latent tuberculosis infections (LTBI).* https://www.cdc.gov/tb/topic/treatment/tbdisease.htm

Table 7-3 Drug Therapy for Latent Tuberculosis Infection

DRUG	DURATION (MONTHS)	INTERVAL	TOTAL DOSES
Isoniazid and rifapentine	3	Once weekly	12
Isoniazid and rifampin	3	Daily	90
Isoniazid	9	Daily	270
		Twice weekly	76
Isoniazid	6	Daily	180
		Twice weekly	52
Rifampin	4	Daily	120

Adapted from Centers for Disease Control and Prevention. (2020). Treatment options for latent tuberculosis infection (LTBI). https://www.cdc.gov/tb/education/faqforproviders.htm

Complications

1. Pleural effusion.
2. TB pneumonia.
3. Other organ involvement with TB.
4. Serious reactions to drug therapy.

Nursing Assessment

1. Obtain a history of exposure to TB.
2. Assess for symptoms of active disease—productive cough, night sweats, afternoon temperature elevation, unintentional weight loss, and pleuritic chest pain.
3. Cavitation on chest x-ray, positive sputum AFB smear, and ongoing cough increase the risk of infection transmission.
4. Auscultate lungs for crackles.
5. During drug therapy, assess for liver dysfunction.
   a. Question the patient about loss of appetite, fatigue, joint pain, fever, tenderness in the liver region, clay-colored stools, dark urine, and vision changes.
   b. Monitor for fever, right upper quadrant abdominal tenderness, nausea, vomiting, rash, and persistent paresthesia of hands and feet.
   c. Monitor results of periodic liver function studies.

Nursing Interventions

Improving Breathing Pattern

1. Administer and teach self-administration of medications as ordered.
2. Encourage rest and avoidance of exertion if acutely ill.
3. Monitor breath sounds, respiratory rate, sputum production, dyspnea, and urine and stool color.
4. Provide supplemental oxygen as ordered.

Preventing Transmission of Infection

1. Be aware that TB is transmitted by respiratory droplets.
2. Provide care for hospitalized patient in a negative pressure room to prevent respiratory droplets from escaping when the door is opened.
3. Enforce rule that all staff and visitors use well-fitted standard N-95 particulate masks for contact with patient.
4. Use high-efficiency particulate masks, such as high-efficiency particulate air (HEPA) filter masks or positive air pressure respirators, for high-risk procedures, including suctioning, bronchoscopy, or pentamidine treatments.
5. Use standard precautions for additional protection: gowns and gloves for direct contact with the patient, linens or articles in room, and meticulous hand hygiene.
6. Educate the patient to control the spread of infection through secretions.
   a. Cover mouth and nose with double-ply tissue when coughing or sneezing. Do not sneeze into bare hands.
   b. Wash hands after coughing or sneezing.
   c. Dispose of tissues promptly into a closed plastic bag.
   d. Limit contact with others while infectious.

Improving Nutritional Status

1. Explain the importance of eating a nutritious diet to promote healing and improve defense against infection.
2. Provide small, frequent meals and liquid supplements during the symptomatic period.
3. Monitor weight.
4. Administer vitamin supplements, as ordered, particularly pyridoxine (vitamin B_6), to prevent peripheral neuropathy in patients taking INH.

Improving Adherence

1. Educate the patient about the etiology, transmission, and effects of TB. Stress the importance of continuing to take medicine for the prescribed time because bacilli multiply slowly and thus can only be eradicated over a long period.
2. Review adverse effects of the drug therapy (see pages 183–187). Question the patient specifically about common toxicities of drugs being used and emphasize immediate reporting should these occur.
3. Patient adherence remains a major problem in eradicating TB. Directly observed therapy (DOT) can be helpful (taking medication in an observed setting) and is especially critical for patients with drug-resistant TB, patients who are infected with HIV, those with a history of nonadherence to treatment, and those on intermittent treatment regimens (i.e., two or three times weekly). Coordinate with case manager, local health department, and home health agency to ensure needed follow-up.

Community and Home Care Considerations

1. Improve ventilation in the home by opening windows in the room of the affected person and keeping bedroom door closed as much as possible.
2. Instruct patient to cover mouth with fresh tissue when coughing or sneezing and to dispose of tissues promptly in plastic bags.
3. Discuss TB testing of people residing with patient.
4. Investigate living conditions, availability of transportation, financial status, alcohol and drug misuse, and motivation, which may affect adherence with follow-up and treatment. Initiate referrals to a social worker for interventions in these areas.
5. Report new cases of TB to local or state public health department for screening of close contacts and monitoring.

Patient Education and Health Maintenance

1. Review possible complications: hemorrhage, pleurisy, and symptoms of recurrence (persistent cough, fever, or hemoptysis).
2. Instruct patient on avoidance of job-related exposure to excessive amounts of silicone (working in foundry, rock quarry, sand blasting), which increases the risk of reactivation.
3. Encourage patient to report at specified intervals for bacteriologic (smear) examination of sputum to monitor therapeutic response and adherence.
4. Instruct patient in basic hygiene practices and investigate living conditions. Crowded, poorly ventilated conditions contribute to the development and spread of TB.
5. Encourage regular symptom screening. Follow-up chest x-ray is recommended if an individual with LTBI chooses not to be treated. A single posteroanterior chest x-ray annually for 2 years is sufficient. Any individual with a history of positive TB test who develops symptoms suggestive of TB (fever, night sweats, weight loss, productive cough, or hemoptysis) should be screened with a chest x-ray as part of the clinical evaluation for possible recurrent TB disease.
6. Provide instructions on prophylaxis with recommended medication regimens for people with LTBI or for children or patients infected with HIV who are close household contacts of patients with active TB because these individuals are at high risk of becoming infected.
7. Educate asymptomatic people about PPD testing and treatment of latent TB for positive results, based on risk grouping.

Evaluation: Expected Outcomes

- Afebrile; dyspnea relieved.
- Appropriate precautions observed; disposes of respiratory secretions properly.
- Maintains body weight.
- Takes medications as prescribed.

Pleurisy

Pleurisy or *pleuritis* is inflammation of the parietal and visceral pleura of the lung.

Pathophysiology and Etiology

1. Inflammation may occur in the course of pulmonary infectious, vascular, or neoplastic disorders:
   a. Pneumonia (bacterial, viral), TB, abscess, and some upper respiratory infections.
   b. PE or infarction.
   c. Lung cancer.
2. Inflammation of the pleura stimulates nerve endings, causing pain.
3. Additional fluid may develop in pleural space, causing pleural effusion.

Clinical Manifestations

1. Chest pain—becomes severe, sharp, and knifelike on inspiration (pleuritic pain).
   a. May become minimal or absent when breath is held.
   b. May be localized or radiate to the shoulder or abdomen.
2. Intercostal tenderness on palpation.
3. Pleural friction rub—grating or leathery sounds heard in both phases of respiration; heard low in the axilla or over the lung base posteriorly; may be heard for only a day or so.
4. Evidence of infection: fever, malaise, and increased white blood cell count.

Diagnostic Evaluation

1. Chest x-ray may show pleural thickening.
2. Sputum examination may indicate an infectious organism.
3. Examination of pleural fluid obtained by thoracentesis for smear and culture.
4. Pleural biopsy may be necessary to rule out other conditions.

Management

1. Treatment for the underlying primary disease (pneumonia, infarction); inflammation usually resolves when the primary disease subsides.
2. Pain relief, using pharmacologic and nonpharmacologic methods.
3. Intercostal nerve block may be necessary when pain causes hypoventilation.

Complications

1. Severe pleural effusion.
2. Atelectasis because of shallow breathing to avoid pain.

Nursing Assessment

1. Assess patient's level of pain.
2. Evaluate for pleural effusion (dyspnea, decreased breath sounds, and dullness to percussion on affected side).
3. Auscultate lungs for pleural friction rub.

Nursing Interventions

Easing Painful Respiration

1. Assist patient to find a comfortable position that will promote aeration; lying on the affected side decreases stretching of the pleura and, therefore, the pain decreases.
2. Instruct patient in splinting chest while taking a deep breath or coughing.
3. Administer or teach self-administration of pain medications, as ordered.
4. Employ nonpharmacologic interventions for pain relief, such as application of heat, muscle relaxation, and imagery.
5. Assist with intercostal nerve block if indicated.
6. Evaluate patient for signs of hypoxia (with SpO_2 or ABG) when anxiety, restlessness, and agitation of new onset are noted, before administering as-needed sedatives. Consider evaluation by a health care provider when these signs are present, especially if accompanied by cyanotic nail beds, circumoral pallor, and increased respiratory rate.

Patient Education and Health Maintenance

1. Instruct patient to seek early intervention for pulmonary diseases so pleurisy can be avoided.
2. Reassure and encourage patience because pain will subside.
3. Advise patient on reporting shortness of breath, which could indicate pleural effusion.

Evaluation: Expected Outcomes

- Respirations deep without pain.

Pleural Effusion

Pleural effusion refers to a collection of fluid in the pleural space. It is almost always secondary to other diseases.

Pathophysiology and Etiology

1. May be either transudative or exudative.
2. Transudative effusions occur primarily in noninflammatory conditions such as congestive heart failure (CHF); it is an accumulation of low-protein, low-cell-count fluid.
3. Exudative effusions occur in an area of inflammation caused by pneumonia, TB, or malignancy; it is an accumulation of high-protein fluid.
4. Occurs as a complication of:
   a. Disseminated cancer (particularly lung and breast) and lymphoma.
   b. Pleuropulmonary infections (pneumonia).
   c. Heart failure, cirrhosis, and nephrosis.
   d. Other conditions—sarcoidosis, lupus, and peritoneal dialysis.
   e. Medications such as procainamide, hydralazine, quinidine, nitrofurantoin, dantrolene, methysergide, procarbazine, and methotrexate.

Clinical Manifestations

1. Dyspnea, pleuritic chest pain, and cough.
2. Dullness or flatness to percussion (over areas of fluid) with decreased or absent breath sounds.

Diagnostic Evaluation

1. Chest x-ray or ultrasound detects the presence of fluid.
2. Thoracentesis—biochemical, bacteriologic, and cytologic studies of pleural fluid indicate cause.

Management

General

1. Transudative effusions are normally managed by treating the underlying cause (CHF, fluid overload) with diuretics and other medications; however, thoracentesis may be necessary for refractory effusion.
2. Thoracentesis is done to remove fluid that is impeding lung expansion and relieve dyspnea.
   a. Chest x-ray, ultrasound, or fluoroscopy may assist in localization.
   b. Repeated thoracentesis may be necessary until the underlying cause is resolved, as fluid redevelops.

For Malignant Effusions

1. Video-assisted thoracoscopy, chest tube drainage, radiation, and/or chemotherapy.
2. In malignant conditions, pleurodesis may be required. Thoracentesis may provide only transient benefits because effusion may reaccumulate within a few days.
3. Pleurodesis—production of adhesions between the parietal and visceral pleura accomplished by tube thoracostomy, pleural space drainage, and intrapleural instillation of a sclerosing agent (tetracycline, doxycycline, or minocycline).
   a. Drug introduced through tube into pleural space; tube clamped.
   b. Patient is assisted into various positions for 3 to 5 minutes each to allow the drug to spread to all pleural surfaces.
   c. Tube is unclamped, when directed, and chest drainage is facilitated for 24 hours or longer.
   d. Resulting pleural irritation, inflammation, and fibrosis cause adhesion of the visceral and parietal surfaces when they are brought together by the negative pressure caused by chest suction.

Complications

1. Large effusion could lead to respiratory failure.

Nursing Assessment

1. Obtain history of previous pulmonary condition.
2. Assess patient for dyspnea, tachypnea, and signs of fluid overload.
3. Auscultate and percuss the lungs for abnormalities.

Nursing Interventions

Maintaining Normal Breathing Pattern

1. Institute treatments to resolve the underlying cause, as ordered.
2. Assist with thoracentesis, if indicated (may be done at bedside or in interventional radiology suite).
3. Maintain chest drainage, as needed (see page 154).
4. Provide care after pleurodesis.
   a. Monitor for excessive pain from the sclerosing agent, which may cause hypoventilation.
   b. Administer prescribed analgesic.
   c. Report uncontrolled pain, which may necessitate intrapleural lidocaine instillation.
   d. Administer oxygen as indicated by dyspnea and hypoxemia.
   e. Observe patient's breathing pattern, oxygen saturation, and other vital signs for evidence of improvement or deterioration.

Patient Education and Health Maintenance

1. Instruct patient to seek early intervention for unusual shortness of breath, along with signs of worsening heart or lung disease.

Evaluation: Expected Outcomes

- Reports absence of shortness of breath.

Lung Abscess

A *lung abscess* is a localized, pus-containing, necrotic lesion in the lung characterized by cavity formation.

Pathophysiology and Etiology

1. Most commonly occurs due to aspiration of vomitus or infected material from the upper respiratory tract.
2. Secondary causes include:
   a. Aspiration of a foreign body into the lung.
   b. Pulmonary embolus.
   c. Trauma.
   d. TB and necrotizing pneumonia.
   e. Bronchial obstruction (usually a tumor) causes obstruction to bronchus, leading to infection distal to the growth.
3. The right lung is involved more frequently than the left because of dependent position of the right bronchus, the less

acute angle that the right main bronchus forms within the trachea, and its larger size.
4. In the initial stages, the cavity in the lung may communicate with the bronchus.
5. Eventually, the cavity becomes surrounded or encapsulated by a wall of fibrous tissue, except at one or two points where the necrotic process extends until it reaches the lumen of some bronchus or pleural space and establishes a communication with the respiratory tract, the pleural cavity (bronchopleural fistula), or both.
6. Lung abscesses are typically polymicrobial. Organisms typically seen are *Klebsiella pneumonia*, *S. aureus*, and *P. aeruginosa*.

Clinical Manifestations

1. Cough, fever, and malaise from segmental pneumonitis and atelectasis.
2. Headache, anemia, weight loss, dyspnea, and weakness.
3. Pleuritic chest pain from extension of suppurative pneumonitis to pleural surface.
4. Production of mucopurulent sputum, usually foul-smelling; blood streaking common; may become profuse after abscess ruptures into the bronchial tree.
5. The chest may be dull to percussion, with decreased or absent breath sounds and intermittent pleural friction rub.

Diagnostic Evaluation

1. Chest x-ray to help diagnose and locate the lesion.
2. Chest CT to locate and identify if lesion is singular or multiple areas of involvement.
3. Direct bronchoscopic visualization to exclude the possibility of tumor or foreign body; bronchial washings and brush biopsy may be done for cytopathologic study.
4. Sputum culture and sensitivity tests to determine causative organisms and antimicrobial sensitivity.

Management

1. Administration of appropriate antimicrobial agent, usually by IV route, until clinical condition improves, and then oral administration.
2. Percutaneous drainage by interventional radiology.
3. Bronchoscopy to drain abscess is controversial.
4. Surgical intervention only if the patient fails to respond to medical management, sustains a hemorrhage, or has a suspected tumor.
5. Nutritional management is usually a high-calorie, high-protein diet.

Complications

1. Hemoptysis from erosion of a vessel.
2. Empyema and bronchopleural fistula.
3. Entrapment of the lung.
4. Hemoptysis.
5. Further expansion of abscess.
6. Lung necrosis.

Nursing Assessment

1. Examine the oral cavity because poor condition of teeth and gums increases the number of anaerobes in the oral cavity and could be a source for infection. Promote frequent oral care.
2. Perform chest examination for abnormalities.
3. Monitor temperature to evaluate the effectiveness of therapy.

Nursing Interventions

Minimizing Respiratory Dysfunction

1. Monitor patient's response to antimicrobial therapy by vital signs, energy level, and appetite.
2. Evaluate patient thoroughly for signs of hypoxia, including SpO_2, when anxiety, restlessness, and agitation of new onset are noted before administering as-needed sedatives. Notify the health care provider for evaluation when these signs are present, especially if accompanied by cyanotic nail beds, circumoral pallor, and increased respiratory rate.
3. Perform postural drainage as directed (positions to be assumed depend on location of abscess) and encourage coughing and breathing exercises.
   a. Give adequate fluids to enhance liquefying of secretions.

Attaining Comfort

1. Use nursing measures to combat generalized discomfort: oral hygiene, positions of comfort, and relaxing massage.
2. Encourage rest and limitation of physical activity during febrile periods.
3. Monitor chest tube functioning.
4. Administer analgesics as directed. Use caution with opioids that might depress respirations.

Improving Nutritional Status

1. Provide a high-protein, high-calorie diet.
2. Offer liquid supplements for additional nutritional support when anorexia limits the patient's intake. Monitor weight weekly.
3. Obtain nutritional consult and consider medication side effects causing anorexia.

Patient Education and Health Maintenance

1. Teach the patient that an extended course of antimicrobial therapy (4 to 8 weeks) is usually necessary; mixed infections are common and may require multiple antibiotics.
2. Encourage patient to have periodontal care, especially in the presence of gingival lesions.
3. Stress importance of follow-up x-rays to monitor abscess cavity closure.
4. Remind the family that the patient may aspirate if weakness, confusion, alcohol misuse, seizures, and swallowing difficulties are present. Train in aspiration precautions.
5. Encourage patient to assume responsibility for attaining and maintaining an optimal state of health through a planned program of nutrition, rest, and exercise.

Evaluation: Expected Outcomes

- Respirations unlabored; temperature in normal range; less purulent sputum expectorated.
- Appears more comfortable; verbalizes less pain.
- Eats better; weight stable.

Cancer of the Lung (Bronchogenic Carcinoma)

Bronchogenic carcinoma is the most common cause of cancer deaths worldwide. It is classified according to cell type:

- Non–small cell lung cancer (NSCLC) (80%) includes epidermoid (squamous cell) carcinoma, adenocarcinoma, and bronchoalveolar carcinoma. This requires careful staging that will determine prognosis and treatment. Surgery may be an option for stage I-II and offers the best chance of survival but is only appropriate for approximately 20% to 25% of patients.

- Small cell lung cancer (about 20%) is almost always metastatic and is commonly treated with combination chemotherapy. The overall 5-year survival rate is low because of initial presentation with locally advanced or metastatic disease. Approximately 65% to 80% of patients present with unresectable disease.

Pathophysiology and Etiology

Predisposing Factors

1. Cigarette, pipe, cigar smoking, and secondhand smoke exposure—amount, frequency, and duration of smoking have a positive relationship to cancer of the lung.
2. Occupational exposure to radon, asbestos, air pollution, polycyclic aromatic hydrocarbons (from incomplete combustion of carbon-based fuels, such as wood, coal, diesel, fat, tobacco, incense, or tar), arsenic, chromium, nickel, iron, radioactive substances, isopropyl oil, and petroleum oil mists alone or in combination with tobacco smoke.
3. History of lung cancer.
4. Age greater than 65 years.

Staging and Classification

1. Staging refers to anatomic extent of tumor, lymph node involvement, atelectasis, bronchus involvement, and metastatic spread, including malignant pleural effusions. Classification refers to criteria that classify pathologic type of lung cancer.
2. Staging done by the tumor, node, and metastasis staging system for NSCLC is an internationally accepted system used to determine the disease stage and extent of disease and is used to guide management (particularly surgical) and determine prognosis.
   a. Imaging including chest CT and positron emission tomography (PET) scan.
   b. Pathology including biopsy (mediastinoscopy, tissue).
3. The International Association for the Study of Lung Cancer (IASLC) has developed a classification system using standardized criteria and terminology for the pathologic diagnosis of lung cancer in small biopsies and cytology. NSCLC can be further classified into a more specific type, such as adenocarcinoma or squamous cell carcinoma, based on this system. This classification system is important because 70% of patients with lung cancer present with advanced stages that are potentially unresectable.

EVIDENCE BASE Detterbeck, F. C., Boffa, D. J., Kim, A. W., & Tanoue, L. T. (2017). The eighth edition lung cancer stage classification. *Chest, 151*(1), 193–203. https://doi.org/10.1016/j.chest.2016.10.010

Clinical Manifestations

Symptoms are related to size and location of the tumor, extent of spread, and involvement of other structures.

1. Cough, especially a new type or changing cough, results from bronchial irritation.
2. Dyspnea and wheezing (suggests partial bronchial obstruction).
3. Chest pain (poorly localized and aching).
4. Excessive sputum production and repeated upper respiratory infections.
5. Hemoptysis.
6. Malaise, fever, weight loss, fatigue, and anorexia.
7. Paraneoplastic syndrome—metabolic or neurologic disturbances related to the secretion of substances by the neoplasm.
8. Symptoms of metastasis—bone pain; abdominal discomfort, nausea, and vomiting from liver involvement; pancytopenia from bone marrow involvement; and headache from CNS metastasis.
9. Usual sites of metastasis—lymph nodes, bones, liver, and CNS.

Diagnostic Evaluation

1. Abnormal findings seen on chest x-ray are typically followed with chest CT. If suggestive of possible cancer, a needle biopsy or bronchoscopy is typically performed to establish diagnosis, followed by a PET scan for staging and consideration of surgical options.
2. CT scan of the chest and abdomen and whole-body PET scan are indicated in most candidates for surgical resection.
3. Cytologic examination of sputum/chest fluids for malignant cells for pleural effusion.
4. Fiberoptic bronchoscopy for observation of location and extent of tumor and for biopsy or surgery.
5. PET scan—sensitive in detecting small nodules and metastatic lesions.
6. Lymph node biopsy; mediastinoscopy to establish lymphatic spread; to plan treatment.
7. Pulmonary function tests (PFTs)—to determine if the patient will have adequate pulmonary reserve to withstand surgical procedure.
8. Laboratory testing, including complete blood count, metabolic panel, calcium level, and liver function tests.

Management

Treatment depends on the cell type, the stage of disease, and the physiologic status of the patient. It includes a multidisciplinary approach that may be used separately or in combination, including surgical resection, radiation, chemotherapy, and biotherapy.

Complications

1. Hypercoagulable state.
2. Complications of treatment including pancytopenia, rash, and hair loss.
3. Superior vena cava syndrome—oncologic complication caused by obstruction of major blood vessels draining the head, neck, and upper torso.
4. Pleural effusion and pulmonary scarring.
5. Infectious complications, especially upper respiratory infections.
6. Brain metastasis.
7. With advanced lung cancer—massive hemoptysis, central airway obstruction, malignant pleural effusion, venous thrombosis, spinal cord compression, hypercalcemia, and syndrome of inappropriate antidiuretic hormone (SIADH).

Nursing Assessment

1. Determine onset and duration of coughing, sputum production (purulent vs. bloody), and degree of dyspnea. Auscultate breath sounds. Observe symmetry of the chest during respirations.

2. Take anthropometric measurements: weigh patient, review laboratory tests, and conduct appraisal of 24-hour food intake.
3. Ask about pain, including location, intensity, and factors influencing pain.
4. Monitor vital signs including oximetry.

Nursing Interventions

See also Chapter 4, page 77, for interventions related to cancer treatment.

Improving Breathing Patterns

1. Teach breathing retraining exercises to increase diaphragmatic excursion with resultant reduction in work of breathing.
2. Give prescribed treatment for productive cough (expectorant, antimicrobial agent) and mobilize patient, as tolerated, to potentially control thickened or retained secretions and subsequent dyspnea.
3. Augment the patient's ability to cough effectively.
   a. Splint chest manually with hands.
   b. Instruct patient to inspire fully and cough two to three times in one exhalation.
   c. Provide humidifier/vaporizer to provide moisture to loosen secretions.
4. Support patient undergoing removal of pleural fluid (by thoracentesis or tube thoracostomy) and instillation of sclerosing agent to obliterate pleural space and prevent fluid recurrence.
5. Administer oxygen by way of nasal cannula as prescribed.
6. Encourage energy conservation through pacing of activities and sitting for tasks.
7. Allow patient to sleep in a reclining chair or with head of bed elevated if severely dyspneic.
8. Recognize the anxiety associated with dyspnea; teach relaxation techniques.

Improving Nutritional Status

1. Emphasize that nutrition is an important part of the treatment of lung cancer.
   a. Encourage small amounts of high-calorie, high-protein foods frequently, rather than three daily meals.
   b. Ensure adequate protein intake—milk, eggs, chicken, fowl, fish, cheese, and oral nutritional supplements if the patient cannot tolerate meats or other protein sources.
2. Administer or encourage prescribed vitamin supplements to avoid deficiency states, glossitis, and cheilosis.
3. Change consistency of diet to soft or liquid if patient has esophagitis from radiation therapy.
4. Give enteral or total parenteral nutrition for the patient who is malnourished and unable or unwilling to eat.
5. Obtain nutritional consultation.

Controlling Pain

1. Take thorough history of pain; assess presence/absence of support system.
2. Administer prescribed drugs, usually starting with nonsteroidal anti-inflammatory drugs (NSAIDs) and progressing to adjuvant analgesic and short- and long-acting opioids.
   a. Administer regularly to control pain.
   b. Titrate to achieve pain control.
3. Consider alternative methods, such as cognitive and behavioral training, biofeedback, and relaxation, to increase patient's sense of control. Mind–body modalities (meditation, hypnosis, relaxation techniques, cognitive–behavioral therapy, biofeedback, and guided imagery) and massage therapy may be helpful for mood disorders and chronic pain. Acupuncture may improve pain control.
4. Evaluate problems of insomnia, depression, anxiety, and so forth, that may be contributing to patient's pain.
5. Initiate bowel training program because constipation is an adverse effect of some analgesic/opioid agents.
6. Facilitate referral to pain clinic/specialist if pain becomes refractory (unyielding) to usual methods of control.
7. Radiation therapy may be used to treat pain caused by bone metastasis.

Minimizing Anxiety

1. Realize that shock, disbelief, denial, anger, and depression are all normal reactions to the diagnosis of lung cancer.
2. Try to have the patient express concerns; share these concerns with health professionals. Link patient and family with cancer support groups.
3. Encourage the patient to communicate feelings to significant people in their life.
4. Prepare patient physically, emotionally, and intellectually for prescribed therapeutic program.
5. Expect some feelings of anxiety and depression to recur during illness.
6. Encourage the patient to keep active and remain in the mainstream. Continue with usual activities (work, recreation, sexual) as much as possible.
7. Administer antidepressants that may be used to treat depression; however, therapeutic effect is delayed 3 to 4 weeks.

Patient Education and Health Maintenance

1. Teach patient to use NSAIDs or other prescribed medication, as necessary, for pain without being overly concerned about developing dependence.
2. Help the patient realize that not every ache and pain is caused by lung cancer; some patients do not experience pain.
3. Radiation therapy may be used for pain control if the tumor has spread to the bone, control of hemoptysis, bronchial obstruction, or brain metastasis.
4. Advise the patient to report new or persistent pain; it may be due to some other cause such as arthritis.
5. Suggest talking to a social worker about financial assistance or other services that may be needed.
6. For additional information, contact the American Cancer Society, 1-800-ACS-2345, www.cancer.org; National Comprehensive Cancer Network, www.nccn.org.
7. Facilitate referral to cancer support group or mental health professional.
8. Support patient and family to make decisions regarding long-term care, possibly pulmonary rehabilitation.

Evaluation: Expected Outcomes

- Performs self-care without dyspnea.
- Eats small meals four to five times per day; weight stable.
- Reports decreased level of pain or a level that patient reports as tolerable for completing activities of daily living (ADLs) when treated with medication.
- Verbalizes emotions and concerns associated with cancer diagnosis; practices relaxation techniques.

CHRONIC DISORDERS

See additional online content: Patient Education Guidelines 7-1.

Bronchiectasis

Bronchiectasis is a chronic inflammation and dilatation of the bronchi caused by immune defects, cystic fibrosis, aspiration, and lung infections.

Pathophysiology and Etiology

1. May be a complication of respiratory infections including pneumonia, mycobacterium, and other organisms leading to damage to the bronchial wall, and buildup of thick sputum, causing obstruction.
2. Causes chronic coughing and excess mucus production, which is often purulent.
3. May involve a single lobe or segment or one or both lungs more diffusely.
4. As the condition progresses, there may be atelectasis and fibrosis, which lead to respiratory insufficiency.
5. Other causes include pulmonary infections; obstruction of bronchi; aspiration of foreign bodies, vomitus, chemicals, or material from the upper respiratory tract; cilial dysmotility syndrome; alpha$_1$-antitrypsin deficiency; and immunodeficiency.

Clinical Manifestations

1. Persistent cough with production of increased amounts of sputum that may be purulent.
2. Intermittent hemoptysis; dyspnea.
3. Recurrent fever and pulmonary infections.
4. Crackles and rhonchi heard over involved lobes.
5. Finger clubbing.

Diagnostic Evaluation

Early diagnosis is essential to prevent complications.

1. High-resolution CT is necessary for diagnosis of bronchiectasis.
2. Chest x-ray may reveal areas of atelectasis with widespread dilation of bronchi.
3. Sputum examination may detect offending pathogens.
4. Pulmonary function test (PFT) to evaluate airflow obstruction and impairment.

Management

The goal is to prevent progression of the disease, thereby improving symptoms, limiting exacerbations, decreasing complications, and reducing morbidity and mortality.

1. Infection controlled by:
    a. Smoking cessation.
    b. Prompt antimicrobial treatment of exacerbations of infection.
    c. Immunization against potential pulmonary pathogens (influenza and pneumococcal vaccine).
2. Secretion clearance techniques may be helpful, such as postural drainage, devices that provide positive expiratory pressure (PEP) and/or oscillations to lung walls including PEP valve, flutter valve, Acapella device, vest therapy, and, possibly, percussion and vibration or other methods.
3. Bronchodilators for bronchodilation and improved secretion clearance.
4. Mobilization and exercise such as in a pulmonary rehabilitation program.
5. Early management of acute exacerbations, including antibiotics, corticosteroids, and oxygen for hypoxemia. Severe exacerbation is normally managed with hospitalization, IV antibiotics, bronchodilators, and secretion clearance.
6. Surgical resection (segmental resection) when conservative management fails.

Complications

1. Progressive excess mucus production or suppuration.
2. Hemoptysis, major pulmonary hemorrhage.
3. COPD, emphysema, chronic respiratory failure, pulmonary hypertension, cor pulmonale.

Nursing Assessment

1. Obtain history regarding amount and characteristics of sputum produced, including hemoptysis.
2. Auscultate lungs for diffuse rhonchi and crackles.

Nursing Interventions

Maintaining Airway Clearance

1. Encourage use of secretion clearance therapy techniques to empty the bronchi of accumulated secretions (see page 142).
    a. Assist with postural drainage positioning for involved lung segments to drain the bronchiectatic areas by gravity, thus reducing the degree of infection and symptoms. Contraindicated with increased intracranial pressure, uncontrolled hypertension, and recent face or head surgery.
    b. Vibratory vest therapy and PEP devices (such as PEP valve, flutter valve, and Acapella device) for enhanced secretion clearance.
    c. Chest percussion and vibration may be used to assist in mobilizing secretions (use after bronchodilators and before meals). Contraindicated with osteoporosis, known rib or vertebral fractures.
    d. Encourage effective coughing to help clear secretions.
2. Encourage increased mobilization and intake of fluids to reduce viscosity of sputum and make expectoration easier.
3. Consider vaporizer to provide humidification and keep secretions thin.

Patient Education and Health Maintenance

1. Instruct the patient to avoid smoking, noxious fumes, dust, smoke, and other pulmonary irritants.
2. Teach the patient to monitor sputum. Report if untoward change in quantity or character occurs.
3. Instruct the patient and family about the importance of pulmonary drainage.
    a. Teach drainage exercises, use of secretion clearance device(s), and chest physical therapy techniques.
    b. Encourage morning postural drainage to address nocturnal accumulation of secretions.
    c. Encourage patient to engage in physical activity throughout the day to help mobilize mucus.
4. Encourage regular oral hygiene and dental care.

5. Emphasize the importance of influenza and pneumococcal immunizations and prompt evaluation of treatment of respiratory infections.

Evaluation: Expected Outcomes

- Decreased sputum and pulmonary infections; lungs clear after chest physical therapy.

Chronic Obstructive Pulmonary Disease

EVIDENCE BASE Global Strategy for the Diagnosis, Management and Prevention of COPD. (2023). *Global Initiative for Chronic Obstructive Lung Disease (GOLD)*. http://goldcopd.org

Chronic obstructive pulmonary disease (*COPD*) is a common, preventable, and treatable disease influenced by host factors and characterized by persistent respiratory symptoms and airflow limitation because of airway and/or alveolar abnormalities usually caused by significant exposure to noxious particles or gases, which cause an abnormal inflammatory response in the airways. Airflow limitation is not fully reversible. Emphysema or destruction of the gas-exchanging surfaces of the lungs describes one component of COPD. Chronic bronchitis is another component occurring in some patients. Asthma is not considered part of COPD because of reversibility seen on spirometry (see Chapter 24).

Pathophysiology and Etiology

1. Irritants from cigarette smoke and pollutants deposited in the lower respiratory tract cause inflammation and a cellular response that leads to alveolar wall destruction causing hyperinflation of the terminal bronchioles (emphysema) and increased size and number of mucus glands in bronchiole walls, which increases mucus production (chronic bronchitis) (see Figure 7-3).
   a. In chronic bronchitis, the diameter of the bronchiole lumen is reduced, cilia are damaged, and mucus obstructs the bronchioles.

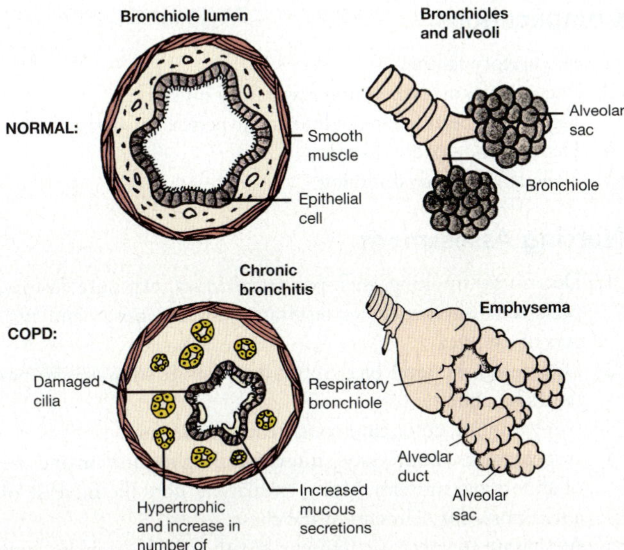

Figure 7-3. Airway changes in chronic obstructive pulmonary disease compared with normal.

   b. In emphysema, hyperinflation causes trapped air to remain in the terminal bronchioles and alveoli, reducing oxygenation.
2. Risk factors for COPD include the following:
   a. Cigarette smoking (primary risk factor).
   b. Environmental air pollution.
   c. Indoor air pollution from heating and cooking with biomass (energy sources from organic material).
   d. Host factors including genetic predisposition, abnormal lung development, and accelerated aging.
3. Alpha$_1$-antitrypsin deficiency is a genetically determined cause of emphysema and liver disease. Alpha$_1$-antitrypsin is the most common protease inhibitor in the blood and inhibits neutrophil elastase, an elastin and basement membrane–degrading protease released by neutrophils. When alveolar structures are left unprotected from exposure to elastase, progressive destruction of elastin tissues results in the development of emphysema.

Clinical Manifestations

Chronic Bronchitis and Emphysema

Usually insidious, gradual in onset, and steadily progressive.

1. Dyspnea (particularly with stairs or inclines) and decreased exercise tolerance occur in all cases. Skeletal muscle dysfunction is common.
2. Cough, which may be productive. Chronic bronchitis is characterized by cough and increased sputum production for at least 3 months during 2 consecutive years.
3. Increased anteroposterior diameter of the chest (barrel chest) because of air trapping, causing hyperinflation and diaphragmatic flattening in emphysema.
4. Wheezing, decreased breath sounds, and chest tightness may be present.

Exacerbation of COPD

Episodic and often recurrent, contributing to disease worsening because of increased inflammatory airway response.

1. Acute change in the patient's baseline dyspnea, cough, and sputum amount and color, which requires a change in treatment (typically oral steroids and/or antibiotics).
2. Triggers may include viral and/or bacterial infection or environmental pollutants or irritants. One third of exacerbations have no identifiable cause.
3. Exacerbations are associated with increased hyperinflation and air trapping with decreased expiratory flow contributing to worsening dyspnea as well as worsening ventilation/perfusion abnormalities, which may lead to hypoxemia.
4. Because exacerbations have increased risk of mortality and morbidity and decreased quality of life, prevention and early detection and management are important.

Diagnostic Evaluation

1. Spirometry or PFTs are necessary to accurately diagnose COPD. Airflow obstruction based on spirometry or pulmonary function including a postbronchodilator FEV_1/FVC of less than 70% of predicted for age, height, and sex assigned at birth. FEV_1 percent predicted is used to stage severity of COPD.
   a. Stage I (mild)—FEV_1/FVC less than 0.7; FEV_1 greater than or equal to 80% predicted.
   b. Stage II (moderate)—FEV_1/FVC less than 0.7; 50% less than or equal to FEV_1 50% to less than 80% predicted.

c. Stage III (severe)—FEV_1/FVC less than 0.7; 30% less than or equal to FEV_1 to less than 50% predicted.
d. Stage IV (very severe)—FEV_1/FVC less than 0.7; less than 30% FEV_1 predicted.
2. The Global Initiative for Chronic Obstructive Lung Disease (GOLD) COPD guidelines also emphasize exacerbation history and COPD Assessment Test (CAT) and modified Medical Research Council Dyspnea Scale (mMRC) scores to further characterize COPD.
3. Arterial blood gases (ABGs) or oximetry can be used to detect hypoxemia (SaO_2 or SpO_2 less than 92%). ABG can additionally detect respiratory failure ($PaO_2 < 60$ mm Hg with or without $PCO_2 > 50$ mm Hg on room air).
4. Chest x-ray—for differential diagnosis of pneumonia and pneumothorax.
5. Exercise testing and assessment of physical activity tolerance.
6. $Alpha_1$-antitrypsin assay is useful in identifying genetically determined deficiency in emphysema (helpful when COPD occurs at young age or in those who do not smoke).

Management

The goals of COPD management are to relieve symptoms, prevent disease progression, reduce mortality, improve exercise tolerance, improve health status/quality of life, and prevent and treat complications and exacerbations. The goal of acute care is to improve airflow obstruction. Treatment regimens are based on severity.

1. Smoking cessation is essential to reduce disease progression and improve survival.
2. Inhaled bronchodilators (see Table 7-4, pages 183–187) reduce dyspnea and bronchospasm and improve secretion clearance; these are delivered by metered-dose inhalers (MDIs), dry powder inhalers, or nebulizer devices. One or more long-acting agents are normally used for daily control, with short-acting "rescue" agents used as needed prior to exertion or when symptoms worsen.
   a. Anticholinergics such as tiotropium (a long-acting agent) and ipratropium (a short-acting agent).
   b. Short-acting beta-adrenergic agonists such as albuterol and levalbuterol.
   c. Long-acting beta-adrenergic agonists such as salmeterol, formoterol, and arformoterol.
3. Methylxanthines, such as theophylline, are oral bronchodilators but are not considered first-line treatment because of suboptimal effectiveness, side effects, and drug interactions.
4. Inhaled corticosteroids are recommended for patients with symptomatic COPD with FEV_1 that is less than 50% of the predicted value and repeated exacerbations and asthma COPD overlap syndrome (ACOS).
5. Oral corticosteroids are used in acute exacerbations for anti-inflammatory effect and may also be given an IV line in severe cases. Long-term treatment with systemic corticosteroids is not recommended due to significant adverse effects (see page 510).
6. For retained secretions, mobilizing the patient, bronchodilators, and for some, use of chest physical therapy, including postural drainage for secretion clearance, and breathing retraining, may be used for improved ventilation and control of dyspnea.
7. Supplemental oxygen therapy for patients with hypoxemia. Use caution in increasing oxygen flow rates in patients with CO_2 retention.
8. Noninvasive positive pressure ventilation (NIPPV) in patients with stable COPD.
9. Pulmonary rehabilitation to improve function, strength, symptom control, disease self-management techniques, independence, mood, and quality of life and reduce health care utilization.
10. Antimicrobial agents for pneumonia, exacerbations, or bronchitis suspected or known to be because of bacterial infections.
11. Lung volume reduction surgery is a potential option for the treatment of upper lobe emphysema in patients with poor exercise capacity.
12. Influenza (annual), pneumococcal, and COVID-19 vaccines are recommended.
13. Lung transplantation may be considered for people with advanced COPD.
14. Self-management strategies such as prevention and management of exacerbations. Disease self-management strategies include the use of action plans, frequent hand hygiene, physical activity, and regular medical follow-up.
15. Treatment for $alpha_1$-antitrypsin deficiency:
   a. Regular IV infusions (normally every week) of human $alpha_1$-antitrypsin as replacement therapy to correct the antiprotease imbalance in the lungs.
   b. Smoking cessation.
   c. Lung transplantation may be considered.

DRUG ALERT Long-acting inhaled bronchodilators are the gold standard of COPD management because of their effectiveness and safety.

DRUG ALERT High-dose or long-term prednisone therapy is associated with significant side effects including hypertension, edema, muscle weakness, increased risk of cataracts and glaucoma, weight gain, hyperglycemia, depression, insomnia, gastric and esophageal ulcer, osteoporosis, skin frailty, and bruising. Ensure that a plan is implemented for tapering steroid dose after an exacerbation, prescription is written, instructions are communicated to patient and family, and follow-up can be scheduled with health care provider.

Complications

1. Respiratory failure.
2. Pneumonia, overwhelming respiratory infection.
3. Right-sided heart failure, pulmonary hypertension, dysrhythmias.
4. Depression, anxiety disorder.
5. Skeletal muscle dysfunction.

Nursing Assessment

1. Determine smoking pack-per-year history, exposure history, positive family history of respiratory disease, onset, and triggers of dyspnea.
2. Determine the level of dyspnea and how it compares to patient's baseline.
3. Note amount, color, and consistency of sputum.
4. Inspect for use of accessory muscles during respiration and use of abdominal muscles during exhalation; note the increase of anteroposterior diameter of the chest.
5. Auscultate for decreased/absent breath sounds, crackles, and decreased heart sounds.
6. Determine oxygen saturation, pulse, and respiratory rate at rest and with activity.

Table 7-4 Commonly Used Pulmonary Drugs

DRUGS/ ADMINISTRATION	PHARMACOLOGIC EFFECTS	INDICATIONS	ADVERSE EFFECTS	NURSING CONSIDERATIONS
Bronchodilators				
Albuterol (metered-dose inhaler [MDI], nebulized solution, oral)	• Short-acting sympathomimetic (beta-2-adrenergic agonist) with highly selective beta-2 activity	• MDI, nebulized liquid: rapid relief of bronchospasm, acute exacerbation—works within 3–5 min • *Oral (rarely used)*: Maintenance therapy for bronchospasm, works within 30 min	• Throat irritation, URI symptoms, cough, tremor, dizziness, nervousness, tachycardia, headache, nausea, tremors, hypokalemia, tachyphylaxis. • Continuous nebulization may cause hypokalemia.	• Observe inhalation by patient to be certain that correct technique is used. • Caution patient not to exceed prescribed dose. Adverse effects may be associated with excessive use. Does not reduce inflammation. • HFA MDIs must be primed for four puffs before initial use and after not using for long periods.
Levalbuterol (HFA and nebulized solution)	• Short-acting sympathomimetic with selective beta-2 activity	• Treatment and prevention of bronchospasm	• Tachycardia, hypertension, nervousness.	• Administered every 4–6 h.
Salmeterol xinafoate (dry powder inhaler [DPI])	• Selectively stimulates beta-2 adrenergic receptors, relaxing airway smooth muscle; long-acting	• Maintenance therapy for asthma, COPD, exercise-induced bronchospasm; long-acting (12 h)	• Headache, throat irritation, nasal congestion, rhinitis, palpitations, tachycardia, tremor, hypertension, bronchospasm. • Possible increased risk of asthma-related deaths.	• Observe inhalation by patient to make sure that correct technique is used. • Instruct patient that it is not for immediate relief of bronchospasm and dyspnea. • Maximum dose two puffs every 12 h.
Formoterol (DPI)	• Selectively stimulates beta-2 adrenergic receptors, relaxing airway smooth muscle; long-acting	• Treatment and prevention of bronchospasm; long-acting	• URI, dyspepsia, chest pain, back pain, fever, diarrhea, nausea, vomiting, dry mouth, dizziness, insomnia, nervousness, tremor, palpitations, bronchospasm; possible increased risk of asthma-related deaths.	• Train patient for proper use of aerolizer. • Instruct patient that it is not for immediate relief of bronchospasm and dyspnea. • Administer twice daily or 15 min before exercise.
Indacaterol (DPI)	• Selectively stimulates beta-2 adrenergic receptors, relaxing airway smooth muscle; long-acting	• Treatment and prevention of bronchospasm; long-acting	• Cough, throat irritation, headache, tremor, palpitations.	• Once-daily dosing.
Arformoterol (nebulized solution)	• Selectively stimulates beta-2 adrenergic receptors, relaxing airway smooth muscle	• Maintenance therapy for COPD; long-acting	• Pain, chest pain, back pain, diarrhea, sinusitis, leg cramps, dyspnea, rash, flulike symptoms, bronchospasm. • Possible increased risk of asthma-related deaths.	• Not indicated for acute bronchospasm.

(continued)

Table 7-4 Commonly Used Pulmonary Drugs (*continued*)

DRUGS/ ADMINISTRATION	PHARMACOLOGIC EFFECTS	INDICATIONS	ADVERSE EFFECTS	NURSING CONSIDERATIONS
Ipratropium bromide (MDI, nebulized liquid)	• Anticholinergic	• Maintenance therapy for COPD, asthma, bronchospasm • Acts within 15 min	• Bronchitis, dyspnea, URI, cough, COPD exacerbation, nausea, dry mouth, flulike symptoms Rare: can cause blurring of vision if sprayed into the eyes (atropine derivative). • Voice hoarseness. • Urinary retention.	• Instruct patient to use spacer device with MDI or close lips around inhaler mouthpiece; close eyes during inhalation.
Tiotropium (DPI)	• Long-acting anticholinergic	• Maintenance therapy for COPD	• Dry mouth, pharyngitis, constipation, increased heart rate, blurred vision, urinary retention, URI symptoms, chest pain, UTI, dyspepsia, rhinitis, abdominal pain, angioedema.	• Not indicated for acute bronchospasm. • Eye discomfort and visual changes require prompt ophthalmology evaluation.
Aclidinium bromide (DPI)	• Long-acting anticholinergic	• Maintenance therapy for COPD	• Urinary retention. • Increased interocular pressures. • Headache, URI, cough.	• Acute dyspnea, avoid in severe allergies to milk proteins. • Rash, hives, facial swelling, itching.
Aminophylline (IV injection)	• Methylxanthine compound—relaxes smooth muscle by increasing the level of cyclic adenosine monophosphate	• Acute exacerbation of asthma or bronchitis	• CNS: irritability, restlessness, insomnia. • CV: palpitations, tachycardia, hypotension. • GI: nausea, vomiting, diarrhea.	• Too rapid administration can cause hypotension, extra systoles, and muscle tremors. Administer at prescribed rate with an IV infusion pump. • Requires monitoring of blood levels, associated with frequent drug interactions.
Theophylline preparations (oral)	• Methylxanthine compound—relaxes muscle by increasing cyclic adenosine monophosphate	• Mild bronchodilator, maintenance therapy for bronchospasm, asthma, COPD maintenance	• CNS: irritability, restlessness, insomnia, seizures in toxic ranges. • CV: palpitations, tachycardia, hypotension. • GI: nausea, vomiting, diarrhea.	• Teach patients to take at equal intervals throughout the day. • To decrease GI irritation, take with milk or crackers. • Monitor theophylline blood level periodically as directed to ensure therapeutic range and prevent toxicity. • Be alert for drug interactions.
Albuterol + ipratropium combination (MDI nebulized solution)	• Sympathomimetic with selective beta-2 and anticholinergic activity	• Fast-acting and maintenance therapy for bronchospasm; exacerbation of COPD	• See albuterol and ipratropium.	• See albuterol and ipratropium. • One puff of combivent equals one puff of albuterol and one puff of ipratropium.
Tiotropium bromide and olodaterol	• Long-acting selective beta-2 and anticholinergic activity	• Long-acting control of COPD	• See tiotropium and formoterol.	• See tiotropium and formoterol.

Umeclidinium	• Long-acting anticholinergic activity	• Long-acting control of COPD	• Nasal and throat irritation, URI, cough, muscle aches urinary retention.	• Bronchospasm. • Narrow-angle glaucoma closure.
Umeclidinium and vilanterol	• Long-acting selective beta-2 and anticholinergic activity	• Long-acting control of COPD	• Increase in heart rate, BP, ECG changes, hyperglycemia. • Nasal and throat irritation, URI, cough, muscle aches urinary retention.	• See salmeterol and umeclidinium.
Fluticasone furoate and vilanterol trifenatate	• See fluticasone and vilanterol	• See fluticasone and vilanterol	• See fluticasone and vilanterol.	• See fluticasone and vilanterol.
Corticosteroids				
Prednisone, prednisolone (IV injection, oral preparation)	• Potent anti-inflammatory activity	• Acute exacerbation of asthma or bronchitis (IV preparation) • Acute exacerbation (oral preparation) of asthma or COPD	• CNS: depression, euphoria, mood changes, insomnia. • GI: gastric irritation, peptic ulcer. • Metabolic: hypernatremia, hypokalemia, hyperglycemia, water retention, and weight gain. • Long-term, high-dose: adrenal insufficiency, osteoporosis, muscle weakness, cataracts, glaucoma, fragile and easily bruised skin, immunosuppression.	• Long-term use: do not stop abruptly because of adrenal suppression. • Take oral form with food. • Usually given as taper from higher dose to lowest possible dose that achieves desired effect. Alternatively, short course may be recommended. Long-term use should be avoided if possible. • Advise patient of possible increased appetite and weight gain risk; advise to eat small, frequent meals high in protein, fruits, and vegetables, and low in simple carbohydrates.
Beclomethasone (MDI)	• Synthetic corticosteroid with potent anti-inflammatory activity; effective only by inhalation • Not effective in acute attack; must be used for 2–4 wk to show effectiveness	• Asthma • Severe COPD with frequent exacerbations	• Oral candidiasis, dysphonia, cough, pharyngitis, bronchospasm, headache, sinusitis, URI, rhinitis, pain, back pain, bronchospasm. • May experience skin bruising in high doses.	• Bronchospasm, glaucoma, cataracts, osteoporosis. • Not used with status asthmaticus or acute asthma episodes. • Use a spacer device with MDI. • Gargle, rinse, and spit after use to prevent oral candidiasis.
Mometasone (DPI)	• Anti-inflammatory steroid; effective only by inhalation • Not effective in acute attack; must be used for up to 2–4 wk to show effectiveness	• Asthma maintenance • COPD (severe COPD with frequent exacerbations)	• Oral candidiasis, dysphonia. • Risk for systemic adverse effects associated with oral steroids is low. • May experience skin bruising in high doses. • Headache, rhinitis, URI, sinusitis, bronchospasm.	• Use water gargle, rinse, and spit after use to prevent oral yeast growth.

(continued)

Table 7-4 Commonly Used Pulmonary Drugs (*continued*)

DRUGS/ ADMINISTRATION	PHARMACOLOGIC EFFECTS	INDICATIONS	ADVERSE EFFECTS	NURSING CONSIDERATIONS
Ciclesonide (MDI)	• Anti-inflammatory steroid; effective only by inhalation • Not effective in acute attack; must be used for up to 2–4 wk to show effectiveness	• Asthma maintenance	• Oral candidiasis, dysphonia. • Risk for systemic adverse effects associated with oral steroids is low. • May experience skin bruising in high doses. • Headache, rhinitis, URI, sinusitis, bronchospasm.	• Use water gargle, rinse, and spit after use to prevent oral yeast growth; avoid eyes.
Fluticasone (MDI, DPI)	• Anti-inflammatory steroid; effective only by inhalation • Not effective in acute attack; must be used for 2–4 wk to show effectiveness	• Asthma • COPD (severe COPD with frequent exacerbations)	• Oral candidiasis, dysphonia. • Risk for systemic adverse effects associated with oral steroids is low. • May experience skin bruising in high doses. • URI, headache, sinusitis, bronchospasm.	• Longer acting. • Use a spacer device with MDI; use water gargle, rinse, and spit after use to prevent oral candidiasis.
Budesonide (DPI, nebulized liquid)	• Anti-inflammatory steroid; effective only by inhalation • Not effective in acute attack; must be used for 2–4 wk to show effectiveness	• Asthma • COPD (severe COPD with frequent exacerbations)	• Oral candidiasis. • Risk for systemic adverse effects associated with oral steroids is low. • May experience skin bruising in high doses. • Nasopharyngitis, rhinitis, nausea, bronchospasm.	• Longer acting. • Use water gargle, rinse, and spit after use to prevent oral candidiasis.
Fluticasone and salmeterol (MDI, DPI)	• Combination inhaled corticosteroid and long-acting beta-agonist bronchodilator	• Asthma maintenance • COPD maintenance • Maintenance therapy for controlled bronchospasm	• See fluticasone and salmeterol.	• See fluticasone and salmeterol.
Budesonide and formoterol (MDI)	• Combination inhaled corticosteroid and long-acting beta-agonist	• Asthma maintenance • COPD maintenance	• See budesonide and formoterol.	• See budesonide and formoterol.
Mometasone and formoterol (MDI)	• Combination inhaled corticosteroid and long-acting beta-agonist	• Asthma maintenance • COPD maintenance	• See mometasone and formoterol.	• See mometasone and formoterol.
Mast Cell Stabilizers				
Cromolyn (solution for inhalation, powder used with special inhaler)	• Inhibits activation of a variety of inflammatory cells associated with asthma, prevents bronchospasm • Not effective in acute attack; must be used for 2–4 wk to show effectiveness	• Maintenance therapy for asthma	• Cough, bronchospasm.	• Should not be used with status asthmaticus or acute asthma episodes. May be given in combination with bronchodilator if administration causes bronchospasm.

Leukotriene Receptor Antagonists				
Zafirlukast	• Blocks leukotriene receptors	• Prophylaxis and chronic treatment of mild to moderate asthma for persons older than age 4	• Potential drug interactions, particularly warfarin, cisapride. • Headache, infection, nausea, diarrhea.	• Will not reverse acute bronchospasm.
Zileuton	• Blocks leukotriene receptors	• Prophylaxis and chronic treatment of mild to moderate asthma for persons older than age 12	• Potential drug interactions. • Headache, sinusitis, nausea.	• Will not reverse acute bronchospasm.
Montelukast	• Blocks leukotriene receptors	• Prophylaxis and chronic treatment of mild to moderate asthma for persons older than age 5 • Exercise-induced bronchospasm	• Potential drug interactions, particularly phenobarbital, amiodarone. • Headache, flu, abdominal pain.	• Will not reverse acute bronchospasm.
Antifibrotics				
Nintedanib	• Treatment of idiopathic pulmonary fibrosis, binds to multiple tyrosine kinases, inhibiting intracellular signaling of fibroblasts	• Reduce progression of idiopathic pulmonary fibrosis	• Diarrhea, nausea, abdominal pain, vomiting, decreased appetite, headache, weight loss.	• Arterial thromboembolism, MI, hypertension, GI perforation, bleeding. • Monitor LFTs at baseline, monthly × 6 mo, and then every 3 mo thereafter.
Pirfenidone	• Treatment of idiopathic pulmonary fibrosis, mechanism unknown	• Reduce progression of idiopathic pulmonary fibrosis	• Nausea, rash, abdominal pain, URI, diarrhea, fatigue. • Photosensitivity: patient must wear sunscreen when outdoors.	• Angioedema. • Agranulocytosis. • Monitor LFTs at baseline, monthly × 6 mo, and then every 3 mo thereafter.
Other				
Roflumilast	• Inhibits phosphodiesterase type 4 leading to increased intracellular cyclic adenosine monophosphate	• Chronic bronchitis and frequent exacerbations	• Diarrhea, weight loss, nausea, headache, suicidality.	
Omalizumab	• Inhibits IgE binding to mast cells and basophils, decreasing mediator release	• Asthma prophylaxis, aeroallergen associated	• Injection site reaction, viral infection, URI, sinusitis, anaphylaxis.	

BP, blood pressure; CNS, central nervous system; ECG, electrocardiogram; GI, gastrointestinal; HFA, hydrofluoroalkane; IV, intravenous; LFT, liver function test; MDI, metered-dose inhaler; MI, myocardial infarction; URI, upper respiratory infection; UTI, urinary tract infection.

CLINICAL JUDGMENT If disease is moderately advanced, issues of an advance directive and resuscitation status need to be addressed. Although effective treatment and prevention and management of exacerbations and comorbidities often stabilize disease, COPD is progressive. It is better to have these discussions with the patient before a crisis situation.

Nursing Interventions

Improving Airway Clearance

1. Eliminate pulmonary irritants, particularly cigarette smoking.
   a. Cessation of smoking is a top priority, improving survival, slowing progression of COPD, and reducing pulmonary irritation, sputum production, and cough.
   b. Keep patient's room as free from pulmonary irritants as possible.
2. Administer bronchodilators to improve dyspnea, reduce hyperinflation at rest and with activity, control bronchospasm and dyspnea, and assist with raising sputum.
   a. Train, teach back, and monitor patient's inhaler technique.
   b. Assess for adverse effects—tremors, tachycardia, cardiac dysrhythmias, central nervous system (CNS) stimulation, hypertension.
   c. Auscultate the chest after administration of aerosol bronchodilators to assess for improvement of aeration and reduction of adventitious breath sounds.
   d. Observe if patient has reduction in dyspnea.
   e. Monitor serum theophylline level, as ordered, to ensure therapeutic level and prevent toxicity.
3. Use controlled coughing (see page 55).
4. Mobilize the patient when stable. Use pursed lip breathing, controlled cough, and possibly postural drainage positions to aid in clearance of secretions, particularly if secretions are tenacious, excessive, and/or mucopurulent (see page 143).
5. Keep secretions thin.
   a. Encourage fluid intake within the level of cardiac reserve.
   b. If appropriate, give continuous aerosolized sterile water or nebulized normal saline to humidify bronchial tree and liquefy sputum.

Improving Breathing Pattern

1. Teach and supervise breathing retraining exercises to improve dyspnea and decrease work of breathing (see page 143). Use pursed lip breathing at intervals and during periods of dyspnea especially associated with activity and/or panic to reduce hyperinflation, control rate and depth of respiration, and improve respiratory muscle coordination. Pursed lip breathing should be practiced for 10 breaths four times daily before meals and before sleep. Evidence for effectiveness of diaphragmatic breathing is less robust, particularly given flattened diaphragm in COPD.
2. Discuss and demonstrate relaxation exercises to reduce stress, tension, and anxiety.
3. Encourage patient to assume position of comfort to decrease dyspnea. Positions might include leaning the trunk forward with arms supported on a fixed object, sleeping with two or three pillows, or sitting upright.

Controlling Infection

1. Recognize early manifestations of respiratory infection—increased dyspnea; change in color, amount, and character of sputum including purulence; cough; wheeze; and possibly irritability and low-grade fever. Promptly report findings to provider for possible workup and treatment.
2. If ordered, obtain sputum for Gram stain and culture and sensitivity.
3. Administer prescribed antimicrobials to control bacterial infections in the bronchial tree, thus clearing the airways. Administer bronchodilators to improve ventilation.

Improving Gas Exchange

1. Monitor for hypoxemia with a typical goal of SaO_2 or SpO_2 of 92% to 93%. Watch for and report excessive somnolence, restlessness, anxiety, headaches, irritability or confusion, central cyanosis, and dyspnea at rest, which is caused by acute respiratory insufficiency and may signal respiratory failure.
2. Review ABG levels; document for evaluation and comparisons by clinical team.
3. Give supplemental oxygen, as ordered, to correct hypoxemia in a controlled manner. Monitor and minimize CO_2 retention. Patients that experience CO_2 retention may need lower oxygen flow rates.
4. Be prepared to assist with noninvasive ventilation *or* intubation and mechanical ventilation if acute respiratory failure and significant CO_2 retention occur.

CLINICAL JUDGMENT Normally, CO_2 levels in the blood provide a stimulus for respiration. However, in some patients with COPD, chronically elevated CO_2 may impair this mechanism and low oxygen levels may act as a stimulus for respiration. Giving a high flow rate or percentage of supplemental oxygen to people who retain CO_2 may suppress the hypoxic drive, leading to worsening hypoventilation, respiratory depression and decompensation, and the development of a worsening respiratory acidosis.

Improving Nutrition

1. Take nutritional history, weight, and height and calculate body mass index (BMI). Patients are at risk for cachexia (survival is decreased with BMI <21) and obesity because of poor nutritional intake, work of breathing, and inactivity.
2. Encourage frequent, small meals if patient is dyspneic and/or underweight; even a small increase in abdominal contents may press on the diaphragm and impede breathing and decrease interest in eating. Encourage snacking on nutritious, calorie-appropriate, and high-protein snacks, such as nuts, avocados, and dairy if tolerated.
3. Offer liquid nutritional supplements, if needed, to improve nutrient intake and provide appropriate calorie intake.
4. Encourage foods high in potassium (including bananas, dried fruits, dates, figs, orange juice, grape juice, milk, peaches, potatoes, and tomatoes), and monitor for low potassium, which may occur with COPD, corticosteroid use, and diuretic use.
5. Restrict sodium, as directed, if fluid retention is a problem or comorbidity of congestive heart failure (CHF), hypertension, or heart disease.
6. Avoid foods producing gas and abdominal distention and/or discomfort.
7. Employ good oral hygiene before meals to sharpen taste sensations.
8. Avoid hurrying and encourage pursed lip breathing between bites if patient is short of breath; rest after meals.

9. Give supplemental oxygen while patient is eating to relieve dyspnea if ordered.
10. Monitor body weight and evaluate BMI.

Increasing Activity Tolerance

1. Reemphasize the importance of exercise and physical conditioning programs (may reverse skeletal muscle dysfunction, improve dyspnea, improve muscle utilization of oxygen, and improve independence). This is part of pulmonary rehabilitation and may be included as part of physical therapy.
   a. Discuss walking, stationary bicycling, swimming, and "sit and be fit"–type videos.
   b. Encourage use of portable lightweight oxygen system for ambulation for patients with hypoxemia.
2. Encourage patient to carry out regular exercise program 3 to 7 days per week to increase physical endurance, but to discuss with provider before beginning the program.
3. Train patient in energy conservation techniques and pacing of activities.

Improving Sleep Patterns

1. Use nocturnal oxygen therapy, when ordered.
2. Avoid the use of high-dose sedatives and hypnotics that may cause respiratory depression.
3. Administer long- or short-acting inhaled anticholinergics, as directed (have been found to improve nocturnal respiratory symptoms in COPD).
4. Sleep with head of bed elevated based on patient's preference to improve pulmonary mechanics.

Enhancing Coping

1. Recognize signs of depression and anxiety disorders or use validated questionnaires to screen for mood disorders, which are common and often undiagnosed and untreated in COPD. Contributing factors include persistent dyspnea, fatigue, loss of independence, personal identity, social isolation, and quality of life that may make the patient irritable, apprehensive, anxious, and depressed, with feelings of helplessness and hopelessness.
2. Assess the patient for thoughts of suicide or self-harm and intentions. Communicate any positive findings promptly to the patient's provider, social worker, and appropriate resources, if needed.
3. Demonstrate a sincere, supportive, and open approach to the patient.
   a. Be a good listener and show that you care.
   b. Be sensitive to patient's fears, anxiety, and depression; provide emotional support.
   c. Provide patient with control of as many aspects of care as possible.
4. Administer antidepressants and antianxiety agents as directed, but avoid oversedation.
5. Support and encourage the patient to discuss concerns about disease, symptoms, and impact on the patient.
6. Be aware that dyspnea, fatigue, and altered self-image may lead to discomfort with sexuality and intimacy in patients with COPD. Encourage discussion of concerns and fears, and discuss adaptations and clarify misunderstandings. Encourage patient to use a bronchodilator and secretion clearance techniques before sexual activity, plan for sexual relations at the time of day when patient has the highest level of energy, use supplemental oxygen, if needed, and consider alternative displays of affection to loved one.
7. Support patient and spouse/family members. Refer to local or national support groups (American Lung Association: https://www.lung.org or 1-800-LUNGUSA).

Community and Home Care Considerations

1. Help to relax and pace activities. Obtain occupational therapy consult to help employ work simplification techniques, such as sitting for tasks, pacing activities, and using dressing aids (grabber, sock aid, long-handled shoe horn), shower bench, and handheld shower head.
2. Encourage enrollment in a pulmonary rehabilitation program where available and Better Breathers club or other support group found through the American Association for Cardiovascular and Pulmonary Rehabilitation at (312) 321-5146 or www.aacvpr.org. Components of pulmonary rehabilitation include supervised exercise training, breathing retraining techniques, proper use of medications and inhalers, secretion clearance techniques, prevention and management of respiratory infection, panic control, controlling dyspnea with ADLs and stair climbing, control of pulmonary irritants, monitored and supervised exercise, proper use of oxygen systems, and group support.
3. Suggest vocational counseling to help patient maintain gainful employment within physical limits for as long as possible.
4. Warn patient to avoid excessive fatigue, which is a factor in producing respiratory distress. Advise to adjust activities per individual fatigue patterns.
5. Advise in strategies and mechanisms to cope with emotional stress and mood disorders. Stress may trigger worsening dyspnea and panic. Teach coping strategies, such as pursed lip breathing, relaxation techniques, meditation, and guided imagery.
6. Stress that progression of worsening lung function may be slowed through smoking cessation and prevention of exacerbations. Long-term ongoing medical follow-up is a key aspect of disease self-management.
7. For patients who use oxygen or who are hypoxic, coordinate with oxygen supplier and patient to promote safe adherence to oxygen prescription and use of appropriate oxygen system so the patient can maintain activities and control hypoxemia.
8. Use community resources, such as Meals on Wheels or a home care aide, if energy level is low.

Patient Education and Health Maintenance

General Education

1. Give the patient a clear explanation of the disease, what to expect, and how to treat and live with it. Reinforce by frequent explanations, reading material, demonstrations, and question-and-answer sessions.
2. Review with the patient the objectives of treatment and nursing management.
3. Work with the patient to set goals (e.g., stair climbing, return to work).
4. Encourage patient involvement in disease self-management techniques, such as identification and prompt reporting of respiratory infection or respiratory deterioration and physical activity. Encourage patient to have open communication, partnership, and regular follow-up with primary care provider.

Avoid Exposure to Respiratory Irritants

1. Advise patient to stop smoking and avoid exposure to secondhand smoke. Offer strategies to promote long-term cessation including the use of medications, support groups, and counseling.
2. Advise patient to avoid exposure to indoor and outdoor pulmonary irritants and particulates, including dust, smog, and other respiratory irritants.
3. Advise patient to keep entire house well ventilated.
4. Warn patient to avoid extremely hot/cold weather if exposure causes bronchospasm and dyspnea. Use a scarf over the nose and mouth, and drink warm beverages in cold weather.
5. Stay indoors and exercise indoors with air conditioning when air pollution level is high.
6. Shower with warm (*not hot*) water to avoid excess exposure to steam.
7. If sensitive to dry air, instruct patient to humidify indoor air in winter; maintain 30% to 50% humidity for optimal mucociliary function. Clean and dry humidifier frequently to avoid mold and bacterial growth.
8. If the patient is sensitive to dust, pollen, and other particles, consider the use of a high-efficiency particulate air (HEPA) air cleaner to remove particles from air. Advise regular replacement.

Improve Airflow

1. Teach the proper technique for inhalation of medication to maximize aerosol deposition in the bronchial tree. See page 793 for patient education on inhaler use.
   a. Use spacer device if unable to use MDI effectively.
   b. If using a dried powder inhaler, instruct in proper use according to the manufacturer's instructions. Spacer devices are not necessary.
2. MDIs with hydrofluoroalkane (HFA) propellants require priming (spray four puffs of medication before first use and if not used for several days). Rinse plastic cartridge holder well daily and air-dry to prevent blockage.
3. Inhalers have built-in courter. Advise patient to refill inhaler well in advance of running out of medication.

DRUG ALERT To prevent oral candidiasis with use of inhaled corticosteroids, instruct patient on use of a spacer device and to rinse mouth after use.

Evaluation: Expected Outcomes

- Coughs up secretions easily; decreased wheezing and crackles.
- Reports less dyspnea; effectively using pursed lip breathing.
- No fever or change in sputum.
- ABG levels and/or SpO_2 improved.
- Tolerates small, frequent meals; weight stable.
- Reports walking longer distances without tiring.
- Sleeping in 4- to 6-hour intervals; uses low-flow oxygen at night as prescribed.
- Demonstrates more effective coping; expresses feelings; seeks support group.

Cor Pulmonale

Pulmonary heart disease (*cor pulmonale*) is typically due to right heart strain caused by excessively high pressures in pulmonary circulation. This alteration in the structure or function of the right ventricle results from disease of lung structure or function or its vasculature, such as pulmonary hypertension (except when this alteration results from disease of the left side of the heart or from congenital heart disease). It is heart disease caused by lung disease.

Pathophysiology and Etiology

1. Chronic lung disease or alteration of the pulmonary vasculature causes increased pressure in pulmonary circuit producing strain on the right ventricle, leading to right-sided heart failure.
2. Often chronic (associated with right ventricular hypertrophy), but may develop acutely because of pulmonary embolism and, less commonly, ARDS associated with right ventricular dilatation.
3. May develop due to pulmonary vasoconstriction because of alveolar hypoxia or acidosis and anatomic compromise of the pulmonary vascular bed.
4. Causes include:
   a. Pulmonary vascular disease (acute or chronic).
   b. Idiopathic pulmonary hypertension.
   c. Underlying lung disease such as COPD, cystic fibrosis, and interstitial lung disease.
   d. Polycythemia vera, sickle cell disease, macroglobulinemia.
   e. Significant kyphoscoliosis.
   f. Obstructive sleep apnea.

Clinical Manifestations

1. Fatigue, tachypnea, exertional dyspnea, and cough.
2. Anterior chest pain and hemoptysis.
3. Distended jugular veins, peripheral edema (often associated with hypercapnia), and possible cyanosis.
4. In advanced stages, right upper abdominal discomfort, jaundice, and syncope with exertion.
5. Split second heart sound on auscultation of the chest.

Diagnostic Evaluation

1. Chest x-ray shows right-sided heart enlargement and enlargement of central pulmonary arteries.
2. Electrocardiogram (ECG) changes are consistent with right-sided heart hypertrophy and/or right heart strain.
3. Echocardiogram shows right-sided heart enlargement.
4. Right heart catheter examination to confirm diagnosis and evaluate for pulmonary hypertension and underlying disease.
5. ABG levels—decreased PaO_2 and pH and increased $PaCO_2$.
6. PFTs to confirm underlying lung disease such as obstruction.
7. V/Q scanning or chest CT if history and physical examination suggest pulmonary thromboembolism as the cause or if other diagnostic tests do not suggest other etiologies. If interstitial lung disease is suspected, chest CT will aid in diagnosis.
8. Hematocrit for polycythemia, serum $alpha_1$-antitrypsin if deficiency is suspected, antinuclear antibody level for collagen vascular disease, such as scleroderma, coagulation studies to evaluate hypercoagulability states.

Management

The goal is the treatment of underlying lung disease and management of heart disease.

1. In cases of hypoxemia, supplemental oxygen to improve oxygen delivery to peripheral tissues, thus decreasing cardiac work and lessening sympathetic vasoconstriction. Liter flow individualized during activities, rest, and sleep.

2. Targeted therapy such as prostacyclin analogues and endothelin receptor antagonists may be used in primary pulmonary hypertension (PPH).
   a. Epoprostenol, treprostinil, and iloprost are prostacyclin (PGI2) analogues and have potent vasodilatory properties. Epoprostenol and treprostinil are administered via the IV route, and iloprost is inhaled.
   b. Bosentan is a mixed endothelin-A and endothelin-B receptor antagonist indicated for pulmonary arterial hypertension, including PPH. In clinical trials, bosentan improved exercise capacity, decreased rate of clinical deterioration, and improved hemodynamics.
   c. The PDE5 inhibitors sildenafil and tadalafil promote selective smooth muscle relaxation in lung vasculature. Their use in secondary pulmonary hypertension, such as in patients with COPD, is unclear.
3. The use of cardiac glycoside digoxin is somewhat controversial; it can improve right ventricular (RV) function but must be used with caution and should be avoided during acute hypoxia.
4. Oral anticoagulants in underlying thromboembolic event or primary PAH.
5. Diuretics are used if RV filling volume is markedly elevated and to manage peripheral edema.
   a. Used cautiously because of hemodynamic adverse effects with excessive volume depletion.
   b. Can lead to a decline in cardiac output as well as hypokalemic metabolic alkalosis.
6. Vasodilators including calcium channel blockers, particularly oral sustained-release nifedipine and diltiazem, can lower pulmonary pressures, although these agents appear more effective in primary rather than secondary pulmonary hypertension.
7. Bronchodilators to improve lung function.
8. Mechanical ventilation, if patient in respiratory failure.
9. Sodium restriction to reduce edema.

Complications

1. Respiratory failure.
2. Dysrhythmias.

Nursing Assessment

1. Determine if patient has a long-standing history of lung disease.
2. Assess the degree of dyspnea, fatigue, and hypoxemia.
3. Inspect for jugular vein distention and peripheral edema.

Nursing Interventions

Improving Gas Exchange

1. Monitor ABG values and/or oxygen saturation as a guide in assessing adequacy of ventilation.
2. Use continuous low-flow oxygen as directed to reduce pulmonary artery pressure.
3. Avoid CNS depressants (opioids, hypnotics). They have depressant action on respiratory centers and mask symptoms of hypercapnia.
4. Monitor for signs of respiratory infection because infection causes CO_2 retention and hypoxemia.

Attaining Fluid Balance

1. Watch alterations in electrolyte levels, especially potassium, which can lead to disturbances of cardiac rhythm.
2. Employ ECG monitoring when necessary and monitor closely for dysrhythmias.
3. Limit physical activity until improvement is seen.
4. Restrict sodium intake based on evidence of fluid retention.

Patient Education and Health Maintenance

1. Emphasize the importance of stopping cigarette smoking; cigarette smoking is a major cause of pulmonary heart disease.
   a. Ask patient about smoking habits.
   b. Inform patient of risks of smoking and benefits to be gained when smoking is stopped.
   c. Discuss the use of behavior modification techniques and smoking cessation aids.
2. Teach patient to recognize and treat infections immediately.
3. Advise patient to avoid environments with poor air quality, have good ventilation, but keep windows closed, and use air conditioning, if necessary.
4. Explain to patient and family that restlessness, depression, and poor sleeping as well as irritable and angry behavior may be characteristic; patient should improve with rise in oxygen and fall in CO_2 levels.
5. Explain the use of supplemental oxygen, which will reduce further workload on the right side of the heart.

Evaluation: Expected Outcomes

- Less dyspneic; ABG levels improved, oxygen saturation.
- Edema reduced; no dysrhythmias.

INTERSTITIAL LUNG DISEASE (PULMONARY FIBROSIS)

Interstitial lung disease (*ILD*) is a general term that refers to a variety of chronic lung disorders, such as *idiopathic pulmonary fibrosis (IPF)*, *sarcoidosis*, *asbestosis*, *silicosis*, *scleroderma*, *hypersensitivity pneumonitis*, and *coal worker's pneumoconiosis* (*CWP*). There are estimated to be 130 types of ILD; only about one third have known causes. Causes include abnormal immune response or abnormal healing in response to a variety of causes, including connective tissue diseases, occupational and environmental exposure, drugs and poisons, radiation, and infections. The most common ILD is IPF.

Overview

Unknown etiology such as IPF.

1. Connective tissue diseases including scleroderma, rheumatoid arthritis, Sjögren syndrome, systemic lupus erythematosus (SLE), polymyositis, dermatomyositis, and mixed connective tissue disease. Sarcoidosis is considered a multisystem disorder although it may resemble a connective tissue disorder.
2. Hypersensitivity pneumonitis (acute or chronic) may be due to repeated inhalation of certain fungal, bacterial, animal protein, or reactive antigens from occupational or environmental exposure. Susceptible persons develop immune reactions leading to pulmonary inflammation and possible scarring.
3. Occupational exposure may include asbestosis (increased risk for lung cancer), silicosis, and CWP.
4. Environmental exposure may include:
   a. Hard metal disease (cobalt, tungsten, carbide).
   b. Gas, fumes, vapors, and aerosols.
   c. Poison exposure.

d. Cancer drugs (nitrofurantoin, methotrexate, busulfan, bleomycin).
e. Anti-inflammatory drugs (aspirin, gold, penicillamine).
f. Cardiac drugs (amiodarone).
g. IV use of heroin, methadone, propoxyphene, and talc.
h. Exposure to radiation.
i. Infections.

5. Chronic changes include lung tissue damage, inflammation of alveoli with scarring, and fibrosis and stiffening of the interstitium tissue.
6. The damage limits oxygen transport through scarred alveolar–capillary membranes into the bloodstream.

Presentation

Additional information follows on IPF, ILD because of sarcoidosis and other connective tissue diseases, and occupational lung diseases. A generalized nursing process appears on page 194.

1. The most prevalent symptom is dyspnea, particularly with exercise, along with dry cough and fatigue.
2. Bibasilar crackles are heard on auscultation.
3. Connective tissue diseases may be associated with joint pain and swelling, rash, dry eyes, and dry mouth.
4. Symptoms may vary in severity, and the course of the disease may be unpredictable.

Idiopathic Pulmonary Fibrosis

EVIDENCE BASE Raghu, G., Remy-Jardin, M., Richeldi, L., Thomson, C. C., Inoue, Y., Johkoh, T., Kreuter, M., Lynch, D. A., Maher, T. M., Martinez, F. J., Molina-Molina, M., Myers, J. L., Nicholson, A. G., Ryerson, C. J., Strek, M. E., Troy, L. K., Wijsenbeek, M., Mammen, M. J., Hossain, T., Bissell, B. D., … Wilson, K. C. (2022). Idiopathic Pulmonary Fibrosis (an Update) and Progressive Pulmonary Fibrosis in Adults: An Official ATS/ERS/JRS/ALAT Clinical Practice Guideline. *American Journal of Respiratory and Citical Care Medicine, 205*(9), e18–e47. https://doi.org/10.1164/rccm.202202-0399ST

Pathophysiology and Etiology

1. *IPF* is a chronic, progressive fibrosing interstitial pneumonia of unknown cause, occurring primarily in older adults and limited to the lungs. It is characterized by progressive worsening of dyspnea and lung function and associated with a poor prognosis.
2. Lung function may worsen gradually or more rapidly, worsen due to acute exacerbation of IPF, or remain stable based on pulmonary function testing (PFT, usually measurement of forced vital capacity [FVC] and/or diffusion capacity of oxygen [DLCO]) or findings on chest COPD Assessment Test (CAT) scan.
3. Incidence is approximately 7 to 16 cases per 100,000 people, although this number is believed to be much higher than reported.
4. It is generally diagnosed between ages 50 and 70 with increased incidence with age.

Clinical Manifestations

1. Dyspnea and hypoxemia are common with exertion and may be present at rest.
2. Chronic, dry cough.
3. Breath sounds commonly include bibasilar inspiratory crackles.
4. Finger clubbing may be present.
5. Patients may have pulmonary hypertension and gastroesophageal reflux disorder.
6. History of smoking is common.

Diagnostic Evaluation

1. A multidisciplinary diagnosis that includes pulmonology, radiology, and pathology is recommended. Exclusion of other causes of ILD is important.
2. High-resolution chest CT shows usual interstitial pneumonia, basilar honeycombing, traction bronchiectasis with predominant subpleural reticular distribution, and absence of other features that would be inconsistent with IPF.
3. PFTs show decreased FVC with decreased diffusion capacity.
4. ABG may show low arterial oxygen level.
5. Exercise test shows hypoxemia.
6. Chest x-ray may demonstrate patchy, nonuniform infiltrates, ground-glass pattern, reticular nodular pattern, and small lung volume.
7. Right-sided heart catheterization may be performed if pulmonary hypertension is suspected or if elevated pulmonary artery (PA) pressures seen on echocardiogram.

Management

1. Two medications (pirfenidone and nintedanib) have been found to reduce loss of lung function.
2. Other agents such as prednisone, azathioprine, *N*-acetylcysteine, and warfarin do not provide clinical benefit when used specifically to treat IPF. They may be used for other non-IPF disorders or appropriate comorbidities.
3. Several promising clinical trials are developing. Patients should be informed of the National Institutes of Health registry of clinical trials at www.clinicaltrials.gov. The database includes information about a trial's purpose, who may participate, locations, and study contacts.
4. Supportive measures include oxygen for hypoxemia and pulmonary hypertension.
5. Options for cough include management of comorbidities (rhinitis, asthma), cough lozenges, and possibly prednisone (controversial).
6. Treatment of dyspnea includes pulmonary rehabilitation, which also works to improve endurance.
7. Lung transplantation may offer improved symptoms, function, and survival for some patients.

Sarcoidosis and Other Connective Tissue Diseases

For comprehensive management of connective tissue disorders, see Chapter 26.

General Considerations

1. *Sarcoidosis* is an inflammatory, multisystem disorder of unknown cause that affects the connective tissue and lungs.
   a. Granulomatous disease in which clumps of inflammatory epithelial cells (nodules) occur in many organs, primarily in the lungs.
   b. Nodules in the lungs can lead to narrowing of the airways, inflammation, and fibrosis of lung tissue.
   c. Other tissues including the skin, eyes, nose, muscles, heart, liver, spleen, bowel, kidney, testes, nerves, lymph nodes, and brain.

2. Rheumatoid arthritis is an inflammatory connective tissue disorder that causes ILD because of pleural inflammation in about 20% of cases, mostly people assigned female at birth between ages 50 and 60.
3. SLE is a multisystem autoimmune disease that causes pleural inflammation and pneumonitis.
4. Scleroderma is a connective tissue disorder that causes hardening of the skin and fibrotic changes, resulting in interstitial fibrosis.
5. Ankylosing spondylitis is a seronegative arthropathy causing back pain and possible pulmonary manifestations.

Occupational Lung Diseases

Pathophysiology and Etiology

1. *Asbestosis*: Asbestos fibers are inhaled and enter alveoli, which, in time, are obliterated by fibrous tissue that surrounds the asbestos particles.
   a. Fibrous pleural thickening and pleural plaque formation produce restrictive lung disease, decrease in lung volume, diminished gas transfer, and hypoxemia with subsequent development of cor pulmonale.
   b. Found in workers involved in the manufacture, cutting, and demolition of asbestos-containing materials; there are more than 4,000 known sources of asbestos fiber (asbestos mining and manufacturing, construction, roofing, demolition work, brake linings, floor tiles, paints, plastics, shipyards, and insulation).
   c. Asbestosis is strongly associated with bronchogenic cancer and mesotheliomas of the pleura and peritoneal surfaces. Smoking increases the risk of lung cancer 50 to 100 times.
2. *Silicosis*: When silica particles (which have fibrogenic properties) are inhaled, nodular lesions are produced throughout the lungs. These nodules undergo fibrosis, enlarge, and fuse.
   a. Dense masses form in the upper portion of the lungs; restrictive and obstructive lung disease results.
   b. Exposure to silica dust is encountered in almost any form of mining because the earth's crust is composed of silica and silicates (gold, coal, tin, copper mining); also stone cutting, quarrying, manufacture of abrasives, ceramics, pottery, and foundry work.
3. *CWP* ("black lung") is a variety of respiratory diseases found in coal workers in which there is an accumulation of coal dust in the lungs, causing a tissue reaction in its presence.
   a. Dusts (coal, kaolin, mica, silica) are inhaled and deposited in the alveoli and respiratory bronchioles.
   b. There is an increase of macrophages that engulf the particles and transport them to terminal bronchioles.
   c. When normal clearance mechanisms can no longer handle the excessive dust load, the respiratory bronchioles and alveoli become clogged with coal dust, dying macrophages, and fibroblasts, which lead to the formation of the coal macule, the primary lesion of CWP.
   d. As macules enlarge, there is dilation of the weakening bronchiole, with subsequent development of focal or centrilobular emphysema.
4. Hypersensitivity pneumonitis is considered a disease of exposure to various agents including mold and birds (feathers and related products such as down). Diagnosis can be difficult and requires good history taking about exposure to potential occupational and environmental antigens and detailed home and work history.
   a. Effects of inhaling organic dust (moldy hay, mushroom compost, malt, moldy maple bark, pigeon or parrot droppings, feathers, microwave popcorn fumes, hot tub exposure, or contaminated grain), noxious particles, gases, or fumes. Development of disease depends on composition of the inhaled substance, its antigenic (precipitating an immune response) or irritating properties, the dose inhaled, the length of time inhaled, and the host's response.
   b. Exposure to inorganic dust stimulates pulmonary interstitial fibroblasts, resulting in pulmonary interstitial fibrosis.
   c. Acute symptoms of fever, cough, and chills may occur 4 to 12 hours after exposure and recur with repeated exposure. Chronic disease develops years later.
   d. Noxious fumes may cause acute injury to alveolar wall with increasing capillary permeability and pulmonary edema.

Clinical Manifestations

Occupational lung diseases may develop slowly (over 20 to 30 years) and may be asymptomatic in the early stages.

1. Chronic cough; productive in silicosis and CWP.
2. Dyspnea on exertion; progressive and irreversible in asbestosis and CWP.
3. Susceptibility to lower respiratory tract infections.
4. Bibasilar crackles in asbestosis.
5. Expectoration of varying amounts of black fluid in CWP.

Diagnostic Evaluation

1. Chest x-ray—nodules of upper lobes in silicosis and CWP; diffuse parenchymal fibrosis, especially of lower lobes, in asbestosis.
2. High-resolution chest CT to evaluate and characterize fibrosis.
3. PFTs primarily show restrictive pattern.
4. Bronchoscopy with lavage to identify specific exposure.
5. Lung tissue biopsy may be needed to rule out other disorders.

Management

1. Pulmonary rehabilitation may be considered for patients with chronic, disabling symptoms.
2. For hypersensitivity pneumonitis, anti-inflammatory medications may be recommended if the condition is worsening, including prednisone and possibly azathioprine, mycophenolate, or cyclophosphamide.
3. For most other occupational lung diseases, there is no specific treatment; exposure is eliminated, and the patient is treated symptomatically.
4. Silicosis is associated with a high risk of tuberculosis (TB); patients should receive evaluation and appropriate treatment for TB.
5. Smoking cessation measures for people who have been exposed to asbestos to decrease the risk of lung cancer.
6. Keep asbestos worker under cancer surveillance; watch for changing cough, hemoptysis, weight loss, and melena.
7. Bronchodilators may be of some benefit if any degree of airway obstruction is present.

Complications

1. Respiratory failure.
2. Lung cancer in asbestosis.
3. Hypoxemia.

Nursing Care of the Patient With Interstitial Lung Disease

Nursing Assessment

1. Obtain occupational and environmental exposure history. Determine length and degree of exposure.
2. Obtain full medical history and family history for connective tissue disorders.
3. Obtain medication history and allergies.
4. Obtain history of smoking, respiratory infections, and other chronic lung disease.
5. Evaluate symptoms and functional capacity, and auscultate lungs for crackles.

Nursing Interventions

Improving Breathing Pattern

1. Administer oxygen therapy, as required.
2. If ordered, administer or teach self-administration of bronchodilators.
3. Encourage smoking cessation.

Promoting Gas Exchange

1. Encourage mobilization of secretions through hydration and breathing and coughing exercises.
2. Advise patient on pacing activities to prevent excess dyspnea or fatigue.

Patient Education and Health Maintenance

1. Provide information about the importance of smoking cessation as well as methods and resources for smoking cessation.
2. Instruct patient in health maintenance, such as adequate nutrition and exercise and immunizations, so additional medical problems can be avoided.
3. Encourage participation in pulmonary rehabilitation.
4. Advise patient that compensation may be obtained for impairment related to occupational lung disease through the Worker's Compensation Act.
5. Provide information to healthy workers on prevention of occupational lung disease.
    a. Enclose toxic substances to reduce their concentration in the air.
    b. Employ engineering controls to reduce exposure.
    c. Monitor air samples.
    d. Use standards established by the National Institute of Occupational Safety and Health (NIOSH) and the United States Public Health Service (USPHS) to eliminate exposure to asbestos and other pulmonary toxins. These may include the use of appropriate masks, respirators, and hoods depending on the toxin.

Evaluation: Expected Outcomes

- Reports less dyspnea.
- Reports improved quality of life.

TRAUMATIC DISORDERS

Pneumothorax

A *pneumothorax* is air in the pleural space occurring spontaneously or from trauma (see Figure 7-4). In patients with chest trauma, it is usually the result of a laceration to the lung parenchyma, tracheobronchial tree, or esophagus. The patient's clinical status depends on the rate of air leakage and size of wound. Pneumothorax is classified as:

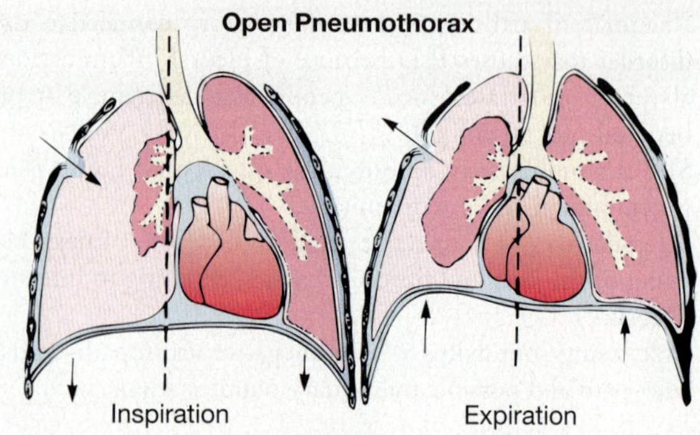

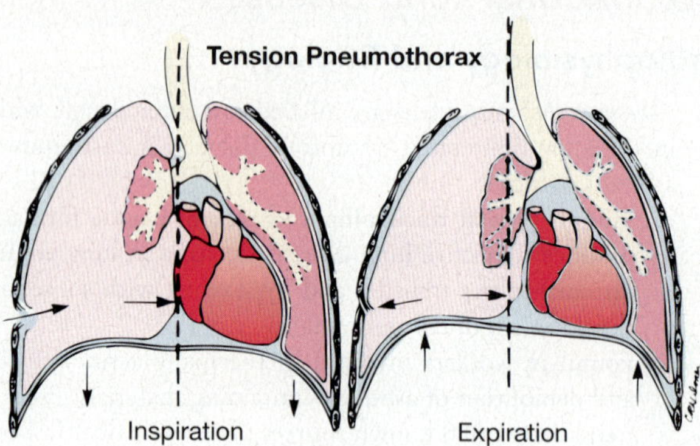

Figure 7-4. Open pneumothorax and tension pneumothorax. In open pneumothorax, air enters the chest during inspiration and exits during expiration. There may be slight inflation of the affected lung because of a decrease in pressure as air moves out of the chest. In tension pneumothorax, air can enter but not leave the chest. As the pressure in the chest increases, the heart and great vessels are compressed and the mediastinal structures are shifted toward the opposite side of the chest. The trachea is pushed from its normal midline position toward the opposite side of the chest, and the unaffected lung is compressed.

Spontaneous pneumothorax—sudden onset of air in the pleural space with deflation of the affected lung in the absence of trauma.

Tension pneumothorax—buildup of air under pressure in the pleural space resulting in interference with filling of both the heart and lungs.

Open pneumothorax (sucking wound of the chest)—implies an opening in the chest wall large enough to allow air to pass freely in and out of thoracic cavity with each attempted respiration.

Pathophysiology and Etiology

1. When there is a large, open hole in the chest wall, the patient will have a "steal" in ventilation of the other lung.
2. A portion of the V_T will move back and forth through the hole in the chest wall, rather than the trachea as it normally does.
3. Spontaneous pneumothorax is usually due to rupture of a subpleural bleb.
    a. May occur secondary to chronic respiratory diseases or idiopathically.
    b. May occur in healthy people, particularly in thin, White people assigned male at birth and those with a family history of pneumothorax.

Clinical Manifestations

1. Moderate to very severe dyspnea and often severe chest discomfort radiating to the back.
2. Hyperresonance and diminished breath sounds on the affected side.
3. Reduced mobility of the affected half of the thorax.
4. Tracheal deviation away from the affected side in tension pneumothorax.
5. Clinical picture of open or tension pneumothorax is one of air hunger, agitation, hypotension, and cyanosis.

Diagnostic Evaluation

- Chest x-ray confirms the presence of air in the pleural space.

Management

Spontaneous Pneumothorax

1. Observe and allow for spontaneous resolution for less than 50% pneumothorax in an otherwise healthy person.
2. Needle aspiration or chest tube if greater than 50% pneumothorax.
3. Pleurodesis may be done to prevent recurrence. Chemical pleurodesis uses various solutions inserted through the chest tube to irritate and thereby cause adhesion of parietal and visceral pleura. Surgical pleurodesis uses mechanical irritation to achieve adhesion, with possible removal of parietal pleura.
4. Thoracotomy to remove apical blebs in some cases.

Tension Pneumothorax

1. Immediate decompression to prevent cardiovascular collapse by chest tube insertion to let air escape.
2. Chest tube drainage with underwater seal suction to allow for full lung expansion and healing.

Open Pneumothorax

1. Close the chest wound immediately to restore adequate ventilation and respiration.
   a. Patient is instructed to inhale and exhale gently against a closed glottis (Valsalva maneuver) as a pressure dressing (petroleum gauze secured with elastic adhesive) is applied.
   b. This maneuver helps to expand collapsed lung.
2. Chest tube is inserted and water seal drainage is set up to permit evacuation of fluid/air and produce reexpansion of the lung.
3. Surgical intervention may be necessary to repair trauma.

Complications

1. Acute respiratory failure.
2. Cardiovascular collapse with tension pneumothorax.

Nursing Assessment

1. Obtain history for chronic respiratory disease, trauma, and onset of symptoms.
2. Inspect the chest for reduced mobility and tracheal deviation.
3. Auscultate the chest for diminished breath sounds and percuss for hyperresonance.

Nursing Interventions

Achieving Effective Breathing Pattern

1. Provide emergency care as indicated.
   a. Apply petroleum gauze to sucking chest wound (see "Management" section).
   b. Assist with emergency thoracentesis or thoracotomy.
   c. Be prepared to perform cardiopulmonary resuscitation or administer medications if cardiovascular collapse occurs.
2. Maintain patent airway; suction as needed.
3. Position patient upright if the condition permits to allow greater chest expansion.
4. Maintain patency of chest tubes.
5. Assist patient to splint chest while turning or coughing and administer pain medications, as needed.

Resolving Impaired Gas Exchange

1. Encourage patient to use the incentive spirometer.
2. Monitor oximetry and arterial blood gas (ABG) levels to determine oxygenation.
3. Provide oxygen as needed.

Patient Education and Health Maintenance

1. Instruct patient to continue use of the incentive spirometer at home.
2. For patients with spontaneous pneumothorax, there is an increased risk for recurrence; therefore, encourage these patients to report sudden dyspnea immediately.

Evaluation: Expected Outcomes

- Breath sounds equal bilaterally; less dyspneic.
- ABG levels improved.

Chest Injuries

Chest injuries are potentially life threatening because of immediate disturbances of cardiorespiratory physiology and hemorrhage and later developments of infection, damaged lung, and thoracic cage. Traumatic chest injuries include *rib fracture or contusion*, *hemothorax*, *flail chest*, *pulmonary contusion*, and *cardiac tamponade or contusion*. Patients with chest trauma may have injuries to multiple organ systems. The patient should be examined for intra-abdominal injuries, which must be treated aggressively.

Pathophysiology and Clinical Manifestations

Rib Fracture

1. Most common chest injury may be severe if several ribs are fractured, especially unstable fractures or in the presence of other morbidities.
2. May interfere with ventilation and may lacerate the underlying lung.
3. Causes pain at fracture site; painful, shallow respirations; and localized tenderness and crepitus (crackling) over fracture site.

Hemothorax

1. Blood in pleural space as a result of penetrating or blunt chest trauma.
2. Accompanies a high percentage of chest injuries.
3. Can result in hidden blood loss and increased risk of empyema.
4. Patient may be asymptomatic, dyspneic, hypoxemic, hypotensive, apprehensive, or in shock.
5. Diminished or absent breath sounds of the affected side, tracheal deviation to the unaffected side.

Flail Chest

1. Loss of stability of chest wall as a result of multiple rib fractures or combined rib and sternum fractures.
   a. When this occurs, one portion of the chest has lost its bony connection to the rest of the rib cage.

   b. During respiration, the detached part of the chest will be pulled in on inspiration and moved outward on expiration (paradoxical movement).
2. Normal mechanics of breathing are impaired to a degree that seriously jeopardizes ventilation, causing dyspnea, hypoxemia, cyanosis, and risk of acute respiratory failure.
3. Generally associated with other serious chest injuries: lung contusion, lung laceration, and diffuse alveolar damage. Also associated with tracheal damage, acute respiratory distress syndrome (ARDS), and pneumonia.

Pulmonary Contusion

1. Injury of the lung parenchyma that results in leakage of blood and edema fluid into the alveolar and interstitial spaces of the lung. May occur with rib fracture or chest trauma.
2. May not be fully developed for 24 to 72 hours.
3. Signs and symptoms include:
   a. Tachypnea, tachycardia, and hypoxemia.
   b. Crackles on auscultation.
   c. Pleuritic chest pain.
   d. Secretions may be copious.
   e. Cough—constant, loose, rattling.

Cardiac Tamponade

1. Compression of the heart as a result of accumulation of fluid within the pericardial space.
2. Caused by penetrating injuries, metastasis, cardiac rupture, cardiac surgery, pericarditis, and other disorders.
3. Signs and symptoms include:
   a. Tachycardia.
   b. Muffled heart sounds.
   c. Falling BP.
   d. Distended jugular veins, elevated central venous pressure (CVP).
   e. Pulsus paradoxus (audible BP fluctuation with respiration).
   f. Dyspnea, cyanosis, shock.

CLINICAL JUDGMENT A rapidly developing tamponade interferes with ventricular filling and causes impairment of circulation. Thus, there is a reduced cardiac output and poor venous return to the heart. Cardiac collapse can result. In the patient with hypovolemia caused by associated injuries, the CVP may not rise, thus masking the signs of cardiac tamponade.

Management and Nursing Interventions

The goal is to restore normal cardiorespiratory function as quickly as possible. This is accomplished by performing effective resuscitation if required while simultaneously assessing the patient, restoring chest wall integrity when possible, and reexpanding the lung. The order of priority is determined by the clinical status of the patient.

Rib Fracture

1. Give analgesics (usually nonopioid) to assist in effective coughing and deep breathing.
2. Encourage deep breathing with slow, full inspiration; give local support to injured area by splinting with pillow or hands.
3. Assist with intercostal nerve block to relieve pain so coughing and deep breathing may be accomplished. An intercostal nerve block is the injection of a local anesthetic into the area around the intercostal nerves to relieve pain temporarily after rib fractures, chest wall injury, or thoracotomy.
4. For multiple rib fractures, epidural anesthesia may be used.

Hemothorax

1. Assist with chest tube insertion and set up drainage system for complete and continuous removal of blood and air.
   a. Auscultate lungs and monitor for relief of dyspnea.
   b. Monitor amount of blood loss in drainage.
2. Assist with thoracentesis to aspirate blood from pleural space, if being done before a chest tube insertion.
3. Replace volume with IV fluids or blood products.
4. Trauma patients with pulmonary contusion and flail chest should receive adequate IV fluids to maintain adequate tissue perfusion. Once adequately resuscitated, unnecessary fluid administration should be meticulously avoided. A pulmonary artery catheter may be useful to avoid fluid overload.
5. The use of optimal analgesia and chest physiotherapy should be applied to minimize the likelihood of respiratory failure and ensuing ventilatory support.
6. Patients may require noninvasive positive pressure ventilation or mechanical ventilation with PEEP.
7. Steroids should not be used in therapy for pulmonary contusion.
8. Diuretics may be used in the setting of hydrostatic fluid overload as evidenced by elevated pulmonary capillary wedge pressures in hemodynamically stable patients or in the setting of known concurrent heart failure.

Flail Chest

1. Analgesia for pain management. Thoracic epidural analgesia may be used for some patients to relieve pain and improve ventilation.
2. Stabilize cardiopulmonary status. If respiratory compromise or failure is present, prepare for immediate endotracheal (ET) intubation and mechanical ventilation—treats underlying pulmonary contusion and serves to stabilize the thoracic cage for healing of fractures, improves alveolar ventilation, and restores thoracic cage stability and intrathoracic volume by decreasing work of breathing.
3. Prepare for operative stabilization of chest wall in select patients. Surgical fixation may be considered in severe unilateral flail chest or in patients requiring mechanical ventilation when thoracotomy is otherwise required.

Pulmonary Contusion

For moderate lung contusion:

1. Employ mechanical ventilation to keep lungs inflated.
2. Administer diuretics for pulmonary edema.
3. Use pulmonary artery pressure (PAP) monitoring.
4. Monitor for the development of pneumonia and ARDS.

Cardiac Tamponade

For penetrating injuries:

1. Assist with pericardiocentesis (see page 223) to provide emergency relief and improve hemodynamic function until surgery can be undertaken.
2. Prepare for emergency thoracotomy to control bleeding and to repair cardiac injury.

Additional Responsibilities

1. Secure and support the airway as indicated. ET intubation or tracheostomy may be needed.

2. Assist with noninvasive continuous positive airway pressure (CPAP) or mechanical ventilation to help to clear tracheobronchial tree, help the patient breathe with less effort, and reduce paradoxical motion.
3. Secure one or more IV lines for fluid replacement and obtain blood for baseline studies, such as hemoglobin level and hematocrit.
4. Monitor serial CVP readings to prevent hypovolemia and circulatory overload.
5. Monitor ABG/SpO_2 results to determine requirements for supplemental oxygen and mechanical ventilation.
6. Obtain urinary output hourly to evaluate tissue perfusion.
7. Continue to monitor thoracic drainage to provide information about the rate of blood loss, whether bleeding has stopped, and whether surgical intervention is necessary.
8. Institute electrocardiogram (ECG) monitoring for early detection and treatment of cardiac dysrhythmias (dysrhythmias are a frequent cause of death in chest trauma).
9. Maintain ongoing surveillance for complications:
   a. Aspiration.
   b. Atelectasis.
   c. Pneumonia.
   d. Mediastinal/subcutaneous emphysema.
   e. ARDS.
   f. Respiratory failure.

Patient Education and Health Maintenance

1. Instruct patient in splinting techniques.
2. Make sure patient is aware of the importance of seat belt use to reduce serious chest injuries caused by automobile accidents.
3. Teach patient to report signs of complications—increasing dyspnea, fever, and cough.

SELECTED READINGS

Ambesh, P., Obiagwu, C., & Shetty, V. (2017). Homan's sign for deep vein thrombosis: A grain of salt? *Indian Heart Journal, 69*(3), 418–419. https://doi.org/10.1016/j.ihj.2017.01.013

Bagai, J., & Beavers, C. J. (2020). *Anticoagulation monitoring during cardiac procedures: Considerations for anticoagulation safety.* Society for Cardiovascular Angiography and Interventions. https://scai.org/anticoagulation-monitoring-during-cardiac-procedures-considerations-anticoagulation-safety

Boka, K. (2021). *Pleural effusion treatment & management.* Medscape Drugs and Diseases. http://emedicine.medscape.com/article/299959-treatment

Centers for Disease Control and Prevention. (2020). *Treatment regimens for latent tuberculosis infection (LTBI).* www.cdc.gov/tb/topic/treatment/ltbi.htm

Clark, S. B., & Hicks, M. A. (2022). Staphylococcal pneumonia. In *StatPearls.* StatPearls Publishing. Retrieved January 30, from https://www.ncbi.nlm.nih.gov/books/NBK559152/

Dheda, K., Perumal, T., Moultrie, H., Perumal, R., Esmail, A., Scott, A. J., Udwadia, Z., Chang, K. C., Peter, J., Pooran, A., von Delft, A., von Delft, D., Martinson, N., Loveday, M., Charalambous, S., Kachingwe, E., Jassat, W., Cohen, C., Tempia, S., … Pai, M. (2022). The intersecting pandemics of tuberculosis and COVID-19: Population-level and patient-level impact, clinical presentation, and corrective interventions. *The Lancet. Respiratory Medicine, 10*(6), 603–622. https://doi.org/10.1016/S2213-2600(22)00092-3

Du, W., Liu, J., Zhou, J., Ye, D., OuYang, Y., & Deng, Q. (2018). Obstructive sleep apnea, COPD, the overlap syndrome, and mortality: Results from the 2005–2008 National Health and Nutrition Examination Survey. *International Journal of Chronic Obstructive Pulmonary Disease, 13,* 665–674. https://doi.org/10.2147/COPD.S148735

File, T. (2022). Treatment of community acquired pneumonia in adults in the outpatient setting. *UpToDate.* Retrieved January 25, 2022, from https://www.uptodate.com/contents/treatment-of-community-acquired-pneumonia-in-adults-in-the-outpatient setting

Grieco, D. L., Maggiore, S. M., Roca, O., Spinelli, E., Patel, B. K., Thille, A. W., Barbas, C. S. V., de Acilu, M. G., Cutuli, S. L., Bongiovanni, F., Amato, M., Frat, J. P., Mauri, T., Kress, J. P., Mancebo, J., & Antonelli, M. (2021). Non-invasive ventilatory support and high-flow nasal oxygen as first-line treatment of acute hypoxemic respiratory failure and ARDS. *Intensive Care Medicine, 47*(8), 851–866. https://doi.org/10.1007/s00134-021-06459-2

Jacobs, S., Lindell, K. O., Collins, E. G., Garvey, C. M., Hernandez, C., McLaughlin, S., Schneidman, A. M., & Meek, P. M. (2018). Patient perceptions of the adequacy of supplemental oxygen therapy. Results of the American Thoracic Society Nursing Assembly Oxygen Working Group Survey. *Annals of the American Thoracic Society, 15*(1): 24–32.

Kanj, S., & Sexton, D. (2021). *Pseudomonas aeruginosa pneumonia. UpToDate.* Retrieved February 1, 2022, from https://www.uptodate.com/contents/pseudomonas-aeruginosa-pneumonia

Kobayashi, M., Bennett, N. M., Gierke, R., Almendares, O., Moore, M. R., Whitney, C. G., & Pilishvili, T. (2015). Intervals between PCV13 and PPSV23 vaccines: Recommendations of the Advisory Committee on Immunization Practices (ACIP). *Morbidity and Mortality Weekly Report (MMWR), 64*(34), 944–947.

Li, X., & Ma, X. (2020) Acute respiratory failure in COVID-19: Is it "typical" ARDS? *Critical Care, 24*(198), 198. https://doi.org/10.1186/s13054-020-02911-9

Ramirez, J. (2022). *Overview of community-acquired pneumonia in adults. UpToDate.* https://www.uptodate.com/contents/overview-of-community-acquired-pneumonia-in-adults

Shin, D., Lebovic, G., & Lin, R. J. (2023). In-hospital mortality for aspiration pneumonia in a tertiary teaching hospital: A retrospective cohort review from 2008 to 2018. *Journal of Otolaryngology—Head & Neck Surgery, 52*(1), 23. https://doi.org/10.1186/s40463-022-00617-2

Tomaselli, G. F., Mahaffey, K. W., Cuker, A., Dobesh, P. P., Doherty, J. U., Eikelboom, J. W., Florido, R., Gluckman, T. J., Hucker, W. J., Mehran, R., Messé, S. R., Perino, A. C., Rodriguez, F., Sarode, R., Siegal, D. M., & Wiggins, B. S. (2020). 2020 ACC expert consensus decision pathway on management of bleeding in patients on oral anticoagulants: A report of the American College of Cardiology Solution Set Oversight Committee. *Journal of the American College of Cardiology, 76*(5), 594–622. https://doi.org/10.1016/j.jacc.2020.04.053

Yasuda, H., Kondo, N., Yamamoto, R., Asami, S., Abe, T., Tsujimoto, H., Tsujimoto, Y., & Kataoka, Y. (2021). Monitoring of gastric residual volume during enteral nutrition. *Cochrane Database of Systematic Reviews, 9,* 1–53. https://doi.org/10.1002/14651858.CD013335.pub2

Yates, G., & Saunders, K. (2019). Pulmonary hypertension: A review for nurses. *Canadian Journal of Cardiovascular Nursing, 29*(1), 7–14.

UNIT

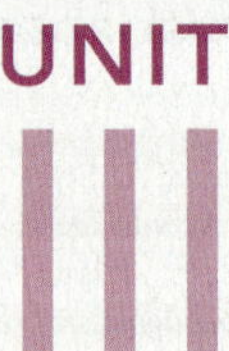

CARDIOVASCULAR HEALTH

8 Cardiovascular Function and Therapy*

OVERVIEW AND ASSESSMENT

Common Manifestations of Heart Disease

In patients with cardiac disease, chest pain is the most common manifestation and is the second most common chief complaint presenting to emergency departments. Chest pain remains a leading diagnostic challenge in the outpatient setting. Heart disease may also be characterized by shortness of breath, palpitations, weakness, fatigue, dizziness, altered mental status, syncope, diaphoresis, edema or swelling, or gastrointestinal (GI) complaints that may be caused by esophagitis or gastric reflux disease.

CLINICAL JUDGMENT Patients who are 65 and older, female, or who have diabetes may not present with typical symptoms of acute coronary syndrome (ACS). Consider the diagnosis of ACS in these patients when they present with other complaints, such as back pain, nausea, fatigue, dyspnea, presyncope or syncope, lightheadedness, vague abdominal discomfort, cold sweats, jaw pain, and right arm pain (without chest pain). Dyspnea is often the only complaint among older adult patients. Most patients who present to the emergency room with chest pain are females over the age of 65. Females in general tend to present with chest pain symptoms similar to males, but also with a greater prevalence of other symptoms such as palpitation and jaw, neck, and back pain. Males tend to report chest pain as their primary complaint.

Chest Pain

Characterization

1. How does the patient describe chest pain? Is it mild or severe, transient or constant? What activity or other factors make it worse, or better? When and where did the pain start? Was it substernal, back, chest wall, diffuse, or localized? Was the onset abrupt or gradual? Can it be characterized as tightness, discomfort, fullness, pressure-like, crushing, or searing? Does it radiate to the jaw, neck, back, or arm (particularly left)?
2. Assess chest pain systematically (see Box 8-1). Most pain management scales (visual analogues or numerical scales) are fast and easy to use but can only be used to measure the intensity of the pain; these scales do not measure the other essential elements for describing chest pain. In your assessment, ascertain the character and quality of the pain; location and radiation of the pain; factors that precipitate, aggravate, or relieve the pain; the duration of the pain; and any associated symptoms.

*Please note that the term "male" in this chapter refers to a person assigned male at birth, and the term "female" in this chapter refers to a person assigned female at birth.

BOX 8-1 Chest Pain Assessment Tips

Consider all chest pain and associated symptoms to be signs of myocardial ischemia (angina pectoris or MI) until it is ruled out.

The severity of the chest pain does not correlate with the cause of the pain. Indigestion and vague symptoms in a female patient, for example, may indicate myocardial ischemia or infarction. Older patients and patients with diabetes may present with noncardiac symptoms that, with further testing, are found to be related to ischemia.

The patient's perception of pain should also be considered, including such factors as sex assigned at birth, response to pain, cultural beliefs, and level of stress.

Location of perceived pain may be misleading. Referred pain occurs with many diseases—that is, pain is perceived by the patient to be in one area, but its source is actually located in another area.

The patient may present with one problem but have multiple coexisting problems. Older patients, for example, may have several health problems in addition to the reason for the present visit. Likewise, patients who delay seeking medical attention sometimes present with multisystem problems.

The patient may experience no symptoms at all.

MI, myocardial infarction.

3. Use one of two popular and similar assessment mnemonics—OLD CARTS or the PQRST assessment (see Chapter 1, page 3) to evaluate chest pain.

Significance

1. Ischemia caused by an increase in demand for coronary blood flow and oxygen delivery, which exceeds available blood supply, may result from coronary artery disease (CAD) or a decreased supply without an increased demand because of coronary artery spasm or thrombus.
2. Pain that is brought on by exertion and relieved by rest suggests angina pectoris or psychogenic pain. Psychogenic pain differs from angina in that it is usually associated with other symptoms, such as headache, back pain, stomach pain, and hyperventilation. Angina is usually caused by three Es: exercise, emotion, and eating.
3. Chest pain that worsens on deep inspiration or cough is suggestive of pleural, pericardial, or chest wall–type pain.
4. Chest wall tenderness and pain on inspiration are suggestive of costochondritis.
5. Chest pain that is relieved by leaning forward and aggravated by lying down suggests pericarditis.
6. Sudden onset of chest pain accompanied by dyspnea is suggestive of pulmonary emboli or pneumothorax.
7. Dissecting aortic aneurysm is likely in the patient with hypertension who complains of a sudden onset of tearing, ripping pain.
8. If the patient reports chest pain while eating, this suggests angina or esophageal spasm or biliary (cholecystitis), pancreatic (pancreatitis), or gastric disease (gastroesophageal reflux disease or ulcers).
9. A panic attack may imitate a heart attack but is more common in younger people and in females more than in males.
10. If the patient reports a sharp, well-localized pain reproduced with palpation of the chest wall or movement, the pain may be caused by musculoskeletal causes. Ask patient if they have a history of trauma or strenuous exercise prior to developing pain.

Shortness of Breath (Dyspnea)

Characterization

1. What precipitates or relieves dyspnea?
2. How many pillows does the patient sleep with at night?
3. How far can the patient walk or how many flights of stairs can the patient climb before becoming dyspneic?
4. Determine the type of dyspnea.
   a. Exertional—breathlessness on moderate exertion that is relieved by rest.
   b. Paroxysmal nocturnal—sudden dyspnea at night; awakens patient with feeling of suffocation; sitting up relieves breathlessness.
   c. Orthopnea—shortness of breath when lying down. Patient must keep their head elevated with more than one pillow to minimize dyspnea.

Significance

1. Exertional dyspnea occurs as a result of elevated pulmonary artery pressure (PAP) because of left ventricular dysfunction.
2. Paroxysmal (nocturnal) dyspnea, also known as cardiac asthma, is precipitated by stimuli that aggravate previously existing pulmonary congestion, resulting in shortness of breath that generally occurs at night and usually awakens the patient.
3. Orthopnea (dyspnea in the supine position) is caused by alterations in gravitational forces resulting in an elevation in pulmonary venous pressure and PAP. These, in turn, increase the pulmonary closing volume and reduce vital capacity. Orthopnea indicates advanced heart failure.
4. Patients with cardiac dyspnea tend to take short, shallow breaths, and patients with pulmonary dyspnea will likely breathe slower and deeper.

Palpitations

Characterization

1. Does the patient feel heart pounding, fluttering, beating too fast, or skipping beats?
2. Does the patient experience dizziness, pain, or dyspnea with palpitations?
3. What brings on this sensation?
4. How long does it last?
5. What does the patient do to relieve these sensations?

Significance

1. Pounding, jumping, and fluttering sensations occur in the chest because of a change in the patient's heart rate (HR) or rhythm or an increase in the force of its contraction.
2. Palpitations can occur as a result of cardiac arrhythmia as well as many other cardiac and noncardiac conditions.
3. Palpitations can be a manifestation of anxiety and panic disorders.
4. Palpitations can be intermittent, sustained and regular, or irregular.
5. Palpitations are most significant if dizziness and difficulty breathing occur simultaneously.
6. Palpitations that have a gradual onset and terminate in a pounding heartbeat may indicate sinus tachycardia.
7. Palpitations may be caused by noncardiac causes, such as thyrotoxicosis, hypoglycemia, pheochromocytoma, and fever.

8. Certain substances, such as tobacco, coffee, tea, unregulated synthetic cannabinoids, and alcohol, as well as certain drugs, including epinephrine, ephedrine, aminophylline, and atropine, may also precipitate arrhythmias and palpitations.

Weakness and Fatigue

Characterization

1. What activities can you perform without becoming tired?
2. What activities cause you to become tired, weak, or fatigued?
3. Is the fatigue relieved by rest?
4. Is leg weakness accompanied by pain or swelling?

Significance

1. Fatigue can be produced by low cardiac output (CO) because of right- or left-sided heart failure. The heart can't provide sufficient blood to meet the increased metabolic needs of cells.
2. As heart disease advances, fatigue is precipitated by less effort.
3. Weakness or tiring of the legs may be caused by peripheral arterial or venous disease.
4. Weakness and tiredness may be related to electrolyte imbalances, such as hypokalemia, hyperkalemia, hypercalcemia, hypernatremia, hyponatremia, hypophosphatemia, and hypermagnesemia.
5. Other disorders, such as chronic fatigue syndrome, multiple sclerosis, fibromyalgia, influenza, and Lyme disease, may also cause weakness and fatigue.

Dizziness and Syncope

Characterization

1. Is the dizziness characterized as lightheadedness, feeling faint, off balance, vertigo, or spinning?
   a. How long does the dizziness last and what relieves it?
2. How many episodes of syncope or near syncope have been experienced?
3. Did a hot room, hunger, sudden position change, defecation, or pressure on your neck precipitate the episode?

Significance

1. Patients who experience anxiety attacks and hyperventilation syndrome frequently experience faintness and dizziness.
2. Patients who suffer repeated bouts of unconsciousness may be experiencing seizures rather than syncope.
3. Syncope can be a result of hypoglycemia, anemia, or hemorrhage.
4. Vasovagal (vasodepressor or neurocardiogenic) syncope can be precipitated by a hot or crowded environment, alcohol, extreme fatigue, severe pain, hunger, prolonged standing, and emotional or stressful situations. Vasovagal syncope is caused by temporary slowing of the heart and reduction of brain perfusion.
5. Orthostatic or postural hypotension, another cause of dizziness, occurs when the patient stands up suddenly.
6. Cardiac syncope results from a sudden reduction in CO because of bradyarrhythmias or tachyarrhythmias.
7. Cerebrovascular diseases such as carotid stenosis can cause dizziness and syncope because of reduced cerebral blood flow.

Nursing History

History of Present Illness

1. The patient's history is the single most important aspect in evaluating chest discomfort. The quality, location, duration, and modifying (i.e., aggravating and relieving) factors are essential to making a correct diagnosis.
2. How long has the patient been ill? What has the course of the illness been, including current management? Obtain a characterization and review of systems (see Chapter 1).

Medical History

Medical and Surgical History

1. Assess childhood and adult illnesses, hospitalizations, accidents, and injuries.
   a. Does the patient have hypertension, diabetes mellitus, hyperlipidemia, chronic obstructive pulmonary disease (COPD), or other chronic illnesses (bleeding disorders or acquired immunodeficiency syndrome)? These may increase the risk of cardiac disease or aggravate disease.
   b. Review the patient's past illnesses and hospitalizations: trauma to the chest (possible myocardial contusion), sore throat and dental extractions (possible endocarditis), rheumatic fever (valvular dysfunction, endocarditis), and thromboembolism (myocardial infarction [MI], pulmonary embolism). Is the patient on dialysis or diagnosed with kidney disease? Kidney disease can increase the risk of cardiac disease and warrants further screening.

Review of Allergies

1. Ask if the patient is allergic to any drugs, foods, environmental agents, or animals and what reaction occurred.
   a. Allergies to penicillin or other commonly used emergency drugs, such as lidocaine or morphine, may influence the choice of drug treatments, if needed.
   b. Allergies to shellfish indicate iodine allergy; many contrast dyes used in radiologic procedures contain iodine.
   c. Does the patient have allergies to aspirin or nonsteroidal anti-inflammatory drugs, such as naproxen and ibuprofen? (An upset stomach or indigestion from aspirin is not an allergy—rather, it is sensitivity; the patient may still be able to take an enteric-coated aspirin.)

Medications

1. Assess the patient's prescription drugs, if any. Many cardiac drugs must be tapered to prevent a "rebound effect," whereas other drugs affect HR and may cause orthostatic hypotension. Estrogen preparations may lead to thromboembolism.
2. Assess the patient's use of over-the-counter medications, which may cause an increase in HR and blood pressure (BP).
3. Assess the patient's use of herbal preparations, vitamin and mineral supplements, and other alternative or complementary therapies. Herbal preparations can interact with other drugs and anesthesia and interfere with normal blood clotting.
4. Assess patient adherence to the prescribed medication regimen.
5. Assess financial ability to pay for medications.

Family History

1. Note the ages and health status of the patient's biological family members (biological parents, grandparents, siblings, and other blood relatives).
2. A family history of CAD, MI, sudden death, hypertension, hyperlipidemia, hypercholesterolemia, or diabetes could place the patient at an increased risk for heart disease.

Personal and Social History

1. Assess the patient's health habits, such as alcohol or illicit drug use (cocaine may cause MI), tobacco use, nutrition, obesity, pattern of recurrent weight gain after dieting, occupation,

stress, sleeping patterns, and physical activity (do they have a sedentary lifestyle?) (see Chapter 1 for additional information).
2. Many lifestyle choices increase the risk of acute and chronic cardiovascular disease.

Physical Examination

General Appearance

1. Is the patient awake, alert, and oriented, or are they lethargic, stuporous, or comatose?
2. Does the patient appear to be in acute distress, for example, clenching the chest (Levine sign)? Focus the physical assessment on what is essential when examining a patient in acute distress. Observe for diaphoresis, and assess skin temperature.
3. Observe the patient's general build (e.g., thin, emaciated, or obese) and skin color (e.g., pink, pale, ruddy, flushed, or cyanotic).
4. Assess the patient for shortness of breath and distention of jugular veins.

Vital Signs

1. Obtain temperature and note route.
2. Determine HR and rhythm.
   a. Assess pulse rate and rhythm using the radial artery.
   b. Time for one full minute; note regularity.
   c. Compare apical and radial HRs (pulse deficit).
   d. Rhythm should be noted as regular, regularly irregular, or irregularly irregular.
3. Monitor BP.
   a. BP can be measured indirectly using a sphygmomanometer, a stethoscope, and electronic devices, or directly by way of an arterial catheter. Be sure to use the right cuff size. Small cuff will result in overestimated BP.
   b. Avoid taking BP in an arm with an arteriovenous shunt or fistula, peripherally inserted central line, or on the same side as a mastectomy site or any type of lymphedema.
   c. If possible, take pressure in both arms and note differences (5 to 10 mm Hg difference is normal). Differences of more than 10 mm Hg may indicate subclavian steal syndrome or dissecting aortic aneurysm.
   d. Determine pulse pressure (systolic pressure minus diastolic pressure), which reflects stroke volume (SV), ejection velocity, and systemic resistance and is a noninvasive indicator of CO (30 to 40 mm Hg, normal; <30 mm Hg, decreased CO).
   e. Note the presence of pulsus alternans—loud sounds alternate with soft sounds with each auscultatory beat (hallmark of left-sided heart failure).
   f. Note the presence of pulsus paradoxus—abnormal fall in BP more than 10 mm Hg during inspirations (cardinal sign of cardiac tamponade).
   g. Vital signs are dependent on age, sex assigned at birth, weight, exercise tolerance, and medical conditions, so note patient's baseline for future comparison.
4. Assess for orthostatic hypotension.
   a. Orthostatic hypotension occurs when a patient's BP drops 15 to 20 mm Hg or more (with or without an increase in HR of at least 20 beats/min) when rising from a supine to a sitting or standing position.
   b. Autonomic compensatory factors for upright posture are inadequate because of volume depletion; bed rest; drugs, such as beta- or alpha-adrenergic blockers; or neurologic disease; prompt hypotension occurs with the assumption of the upright position.
   c. Note changes in HR and BP in at least two of three positions: lying, sitting, and standing; allow at least 3 minutes between position changes before obtaining rate and pressure.
5. Obtain oxygen saturation.

DRUG ALERT Note that patients taking beta-adrenergic blockers may not exhibit a compensatory increase in HR when changing to an upright position.

Head, Neck, and Skin

1. Examination of the head includes assessment of facial characteristics and facial expressions and color of skin and eyes, any of which can reveal underlying cardiac disease.
   a. Earlobe creases in a patient younger than age 45 may indicate a genetic tendency toward CAD.
   b. Facial color: look for a malar flush, cyanotic lips, or slightly jaundiced skin (rheumatic heart disease).
   c. de Musset sign (head bobbing with each heartbeat) may indicate severe aortic insufficiency.
   d. Facial edema may be noted with constrictive pericarditis and associated tricuspid valve disease.
2. Examine the neck for jugular venous pulse. Jugular vein distention is characteristic of heart failure and other cardiovascular disorders, such as constrictive pericarditis, tricuspid stenosis, and obstruction of the superior vena cava.
3. Examine the skin for temperature, diaphoresis, cyanosis, pallor, and jaundice.
   a. Warm, dry skin indicates adequate CO; cool, clammy skin indicates compensatory vasoconstriction because of low CO.
   b. Cyanosis may be central (noted on the tongue, buccal mucosa, and lips) because of bronchiectasis, COPD, heart failure, lung cancer, pneumothorax, polycythemia vera, pulmonary edema, pulmonary emboli, shock, and sleep apnea or peripheral (noted on distal aspects of extremities, tip of the nose, and earlobes) because of chronic arteriosclerotic occlusive disease, Buerger disease, deep vein thrombosis (DVT), heart failure, acute peripheral occlusions, and Raynaud disease and cold exposure.
   c. Jaundice may be a sign of right-sided heart failure or chronic hemolysis from prosthetic heart valve.
   d. Xanthelasmas are yellow plaque (fatty deposits) evident on the skin, commonly seen along the nasal side of one or both eyelids, palms, and tendons. Xanthelasmas are associated with hyperlipidemia and CAD and may occur normally in the absence of hyperlipidemia.
   e. Pallor indicates decreased peripheral oxyhemoglobin or decreased total oxyhemoglobin. Onset may be sudden or gradual and extent may be generalized (most apparent on the face, conjunctiva, oral mucosa, and nail beds) or local (seen only in the affected limb).

Chest

See page 16.

Extremities

1. Inspect nail beds for color, splinter hemorrhages, clubbing, and capillary refill.
   a. Color—pale nail beds may be indicative of anemia, whereas cyanosis may be indicative of decreased oxygenation.
   b. Splinter hemorrhages are thin brown lines in nail bed and are associated with endocarditis. Janeway lesions (non-tender, small erythematous, or hemorrhagic macular or nodular lesions on the palm and soles) are indicative of infective endocarditis.
   c. Clubbing (swollen nail base and loss of normal angle) is associated with chronic pulmonary or cardiovascular disease.
   d. Capillary refill indicates an estimate of the rate of peripheral blood low.
2. Inspect and palpate for edema—if pitting edema, describe the degree of edema in terms of depth of pitting that occurs with slight pressure: 1+ or mild, 0 to ¼ inch (0 to 0.6 cm); 2+ or moderate, ½ inch (1.3 cm); and 3+ to 4+ or severe, ¾ to 1 inch (2 to 2.5 cm).
3. Inspect hands and feet for tenderness. Tender nodes (Osler nodes) may be associated with infective endocarditis.
4. Palpate arterial pulses (see page 6).

Laboratory Studies

Cardiovascular function and disease are evaluated by blood tests that indirectly monitor heart function and structural damage.

Enzymes and Isoenzymes

The diagnostic utilization of cardiac markers has evolved dramatically over the past 50 years. When myocardial tissue is damaged (e.g., because of MI), cellular injury results in the release of intracellular enzymes and proteins (cardiac enzymes, isoenzymes, and biochemical markers) into the bloodstream, which, in turn, causes elevated peripheral blood enzyme levels (see Table 8-1).

1. The troponin complex is located on the thin filament of the contractile apparatus of striated and skeletal muscle and consists of three subunits: troponin C (TnC), troponin T (TnT), and troponin I (TnI). In the presence of myocardial damage, the troponin complex on the myofibril breaks down, and the subunits of troponin are slowly released into the bloodstream.
   a. TnC is not sensitive or specific for myocardial injury.
   b. TnT has a sensitivity of approximately 50% within 4 hours of the onset of chest pain, but increases to approximately 75% sensitivity after 6 hours of onset and approximately 100% sensitivity in 12 hours. However, its specificity for myocardial injury is lower.
   c. TnI has been found to be the most sensitive and specific for myocardial injury. It has little sensitivity within 4 hours of the onset of chest pain, but increases to 96% sensitivity after 6 hours of the onset of symptoms.
   d. Troponins are the preferred test for the diagnosis of acute myocardial infarction (AMI). Can be used for late diagnosis since elevation can persist for as long as 10 to 14 days.
2. High-sensitivity troponin (hs-cTnT and hs-cTnI) testing detects troponins at much lower levels, increasing sensitivity and reducing diagnostic time. Also detects circulating troponins in stable CAD in the absence of myocardial necrosis. Potentially can be used to monitor therapeutic response in patients with CAD.
3. Creatine kinase (CK) has a 98% sensitivity for AMI 72 hours after infarction. CK is a catalyst for energy production and is found in the brain, myocardium, and skeletal muscle. CK is sensitive but not specific for myocardial injury. CK isoenzymes are more specific than CK. Three CK isoenzymes have been identified: CK-MM, CK-MB, and CK-BB, with only CK-MB related to the heart. CK-MB is no longer recommended for most patients being evaluated for an ACS. Therefore, use has markedly diminished over time.

Other Biochemical Markers

1. Homocysteine is a toxic byproduct of the metabolism of the amino acid methionine into cysteine. Homocysteine exerts a direct cytotoxic effect on the endothelium of blood vessels by blocking the production of nitrous oxide, resulting in decreased pliability of vessels and the development of atherosclerotic plaque. Increased homocysteine levels ultimately result in atherosclerosis, CAD, MI, stroke, thromboembolism, and peripheral vascular disease.
   a. Hyperhomocysteinemia (increased homocysteine levels) is related to sex assigned at birth (male), advanced age, smoking, hypertension, elevated cholesterol, decreased folate, decreased levels of vitamin B_6 and B_{12}, and lack of exercise.
   b. Homocysteine can also be elevated in the presence of other diseases, substance use disorder, alcohol use disorder, and caffeine intake.
2. B-type natriuretic peptide (BNP) is synthesized in the ventricular myocardium and released as a response to increased wall stress. BNP is used for the diagnosis and prognosis of suspected heart failure. Plasma levels of BNP increase in the presence of left ventricular systolic and diastolic dysfunction, particularly in the presence of decompensating heart failure.

Table 8-1 Cardiac Markers—Normal Values, Rise, Peak, Advantages, and Disadvantages

ENZYME	RISE (HR)	PEAK (HR)	NORMALIZATION	ADVANTAGES	DISADVANTAGES
TnT	3–12	12–96	5–14 d	• Cardiac specific and sensitivity in late AMI	• Low sensitivity in early AMI • Inability to diagnose subsequent MI
TnI	3–12	12–24	5–10 d	• Cardiac specific and sensitivity in late AMI	• Low sensitivity in early AMI • Inability to diagnose subsequent MIs

AMI, acute myocardial infarction; MI, myocardial infarction; TnI, troponin I; TnT, troponin T.

a. Elevations in BNP are associated with increased mortality in patients with an ACS.
b. An increased BNP level identifies patients at the highest risk of developing sudden cardiac death and those who need a heart transplant. It is also associated with heart failure readmissions.
c. BNP is considered a useful marker of myocardial function and is used to guide therapy.
d. Pre- and postoperative elevations in BNP are associated with an increased risk of adverse cardiovascular events at 30 days.

3. C-reactive protein (CRP) is an inflammatory marker that may be an important risk factor for atherosclerosis and ischemic heart disease. CRP is produced by the liver in response to systemic cytokinesis. Elevated CRP is associated with AMI, stroke, and the progression of peripheral vascular disease. However, it can also be elevated with any inflammatory process. In addition to revealing events associated with CAD, CRP can be used to identify patients at risk for developing CAD. CRP appears to add the greatest predictive value in a subset of patients with intermediate coronary heart disease risk as determined by other measures such as the Framingham Risk Score.
4. Lipoprotein(a), also referred to as Lp(a), is a molecule that is similar to low-density lipoprotein cholesterol (LDL-C). It increases cholesterol deposits in the arterial wall, enhances oxidation of LDL-C, and inhibits fibrinolysis, resulting in the formation of atherosclerotic plaque and thrombosis. Treatment of elevated Lp(a) is suggested only for patients with a history of premature vascular disease without other risk factors. Measurement of Lp(a) concentrations has been challenging due to the complexity of composition of this lipoprotein, and different laboratories use different methods of measuring Lp(a) concentrations.
5. Factor I, or fibrinogen, is directly linked to increased cardiovascular risk. It is involved in the coagulation cascade (converting fibrinogen to fibrin by thrombin), stimulates smooth muscle cell migration and proliferation, and promotes platelet aggregation, which increases blood viscosity.
6. D-dimer may be done to evaluate for aortic dissection when chest pain is present. It is a degradation product of cross-linked fibrin and reflects activation of the extrinsic pathway of the coagulation cascade by tissue factor exposed in the aortic media by the intimal tear. It is also used to evaluate for the presence of thrombus or embolus (see page 309).

Nursing and Patient Care Considerations

1. A single set of negative cardiac biomarkers is not sufficient to rule out MI. Make sure that enzymes are drawn in a serial pattern, usually on admission and every 3 to 6 hours until three samples are obtained; enzyme activity is then correlated with the extent of heart muscle damage.
2. Maintain standard precautions while obtaining blood specimens and properly dispose of all equipment.
3. Advise patient that results of blood tests will be interpreted based on time and within the context of risk factors and other diagnostic tests. Greater peaks in enzyme activity and the length of time an enzyme remains at its peak level are correlated with serious damage to the heart muscle and, thus, a poorer prognosis.

Electrocardiogram

Basic Principles

1. Despite its limited sensitivity and specificity, the 12-lead electrocardiogram (ECG) is still the standard for the evaluation of myocardial ischemia. An ECG should be completed within 10 minutes of the development of chest pain to categorize the patient with a suspected MI into one of three ACS groups based on the pattern.
2. Electrical activity is generated by the cells of the heart as ions are exchanged across cell membranes.
3. Electrodes that are capable of conducting electrical activity from the heart to the ECG machine are placed at strategic positions on the extremities and chest precordium (see Figure 8-1).

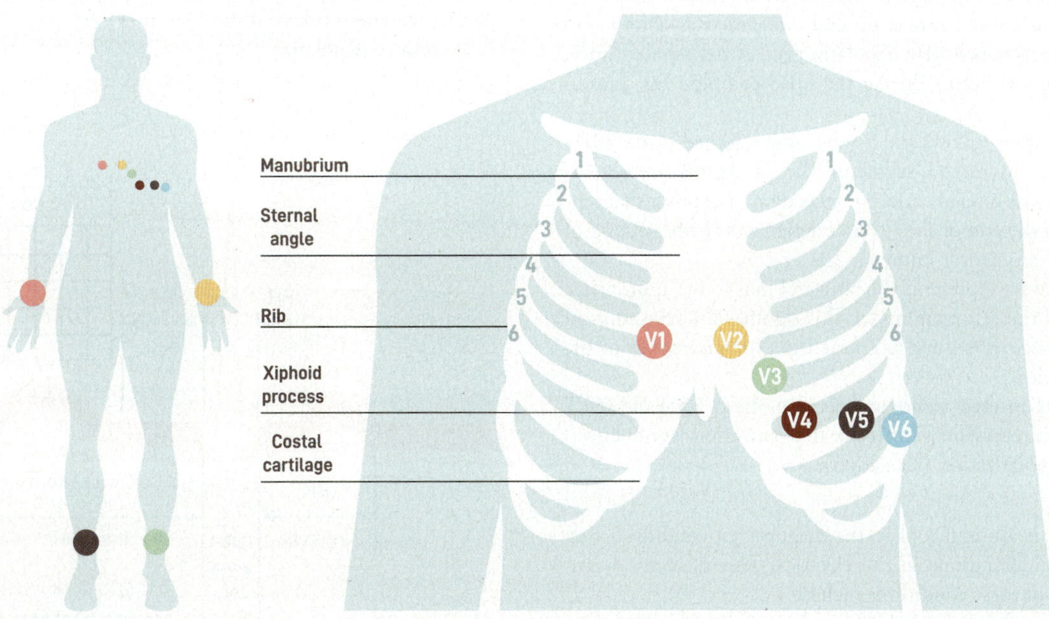

Figure 8-1. Electrodes that conduct electrical activity from the heart to the ECG machine are placed at strategic positions on the extremities and chest precordium. ECG, electrocardiogram (Shutterstock/inspiring.team).

4. The electrical energy sensed is then converted to a graphic display by the ECG machine. This display is referred to as the ECG. A normal ECG is composed of several different waveforms that represent electrical events during each cardiac cycle in various parts of the heart.
5. Each ECG lead consists of a positive and negative pole; each lead also has an axis that represents the direction in which the current flows.
6. The direction in which electrical current flows determines how the waveform will appear.
7. ECG leads are placed at each extremity right arm (RA), left arm (LA), right leg (RL), and left leg (LL), with the RL being the grounding lead.
8. ECG leads are divided into two groups: six extremity (limb) and six chest (precordial) leads.
   a. Standard limb or bipolar leads (I, II, III). These leads utilize three electrodes and form a triangle known as Einthoven triangle. Lead I records the difference between the right arm and left arm, lead II records the difference between the right arm and left leg, and lead III between the left arm and left leg.
   b. Augmented unipolar leads (aVR, aVL, aVF). The augmented leads use a limb electrode for one electrode and the average of the other two limb electrodes as the other electrode. The "a" indicates that these potentials are augmented by 50%.
   c. Precordial unipolar leads (V_1, V_2, V_3, V_4, V_5, and V_6). These leads measure the electrical field in a horizontal plan.
9. A heart contraction is represented on the ECG graph paper by the designated P wave, QRS complex, and T waves.
   a. The P wave is the first positive deflection and represents atrial depolarization or atrial contraction.
   b. The PR interval represents the time it takes for the electrical impulse to travel from the sinoatrial node to the atrioventricular (AV) node and down the bundle of His to the right and left bundle branches.
   c. The Q wave is the first negative deflection after the P wave; the R wave is the first positive deflection after the P wave.
   d. The S wave is the negative deflection after the R wave.
   e. The QRS waveform is generally regarded as a unit and represents ventricular depolarization. Atrial repolarization (relaxation) occurs during the QRS complex, but cannot be seen.
   f. The T wave follows the S wave and is joined to the QRS complex by the ST segment. The ST segment represents ventricular repolarization or relaxation. The point that represents the end of the QRS complex and the beginning of the ST segment is known as the J point.
   g. The T wave represents the return of ions to the appropriate side of the cell membrane. This signifies the relaxation of the muscle fibers and is referred to as *repolarization* of the ventricles.
   h. The QT interval is the time between the Q wave and the T wave; it represents ventricular depolarization (contraction) and repolarization (relaxation).

Indications

1. The ECG is a useful tool in the diagnosis of conditions that may cause aberrations in the electrical activity of the heart. Examples of these conditions include:
   a. MI and other types of CAD such as angina.
   b. Cardiac dysrhythmias.
   c. Cardiac enlargement.
   d. Heart valve disease.
   e. Cardiomyopathy.
   f. Hypertensive disorders.
   g. Electrolyte disturbances (calcium, potassium, magnesium, and phosphorous).
   h. Inflammatory diseases of the heart.
   i. Effects on the heart by drugs, such as beta-blockers, antiarrhythmics, and tricyclic antidepressants.
2. Despite its many advantages, however, the ECG also has several shortcomings:
   a. Fifty percent of all patients with AMI have no ECG changes.
   b. A patient may have a normal ECG, present pain free, and still have significant risk for myocardial ischemia.
   c. Several disease processes can mimic that of an AMI, including left bundle-branch blocks, ventricular paced rhythms, and left ventricular hypertrophy.

ECG Leads and Normal Waveform Interpretation

See Figure 8-2.

1. The normal amplitude of the P wave is 3 mm or less; the normal duration of the P wave is 0.04 to 0.11 second. P waves that exceed these measurements are considered to deviate from normal.
2. The PR interval is measured from the upstroke of the P wave to the QR junction and is normally between 0.12 and 0.20 second. There is a built-in delay in time at the AV node to allow for adequate ventricular filling to maintain normal SV.
3. The QRS complex contains separate waves and segments, which should be evaluated separately. Normal QRS complex should be between 0.06 and 0.10 second.
   a. The Q wave, or first downward stroke after the P wave, is usually less than 3 mm in depth. A Q wave of significant deflection is not normally present in the healthy heart. A pathologic Q wave usually indicates a completed MI.
   b. The R wave is the first positive deflection after the P wave, normally 5 to 10 mm in height. Increases and decreases in amplitude become significant in certain disease states. Ventricular hypertrophy produces very high R waves because the hypertrophied muscle requires a stronger electrical current to depolarize.

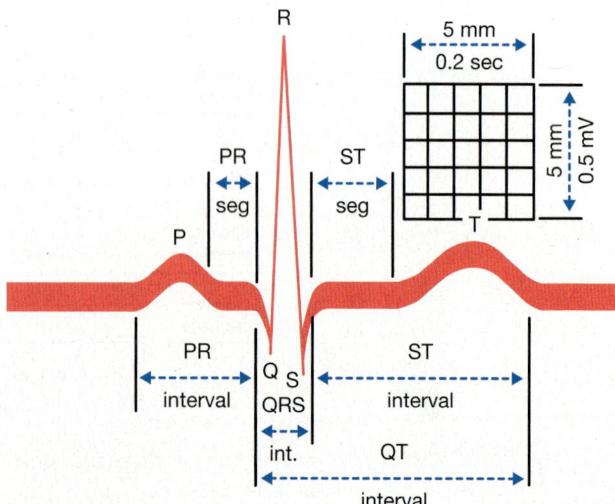

Figure 8-2. Waveform analysis.

4. The ST segment begins at the end of the S wave, the first negative deflection after the R wave, and terminates at the upstroke of the T wave.
5. The T wave represents the repolarization of myocardial fibers or provides the resting state of myocardial work; the T wave should always be present.
   a. Normally, the T wave should not exceed a 5-mm amplitude in all leads except the precordial (V_1 to V_6) leads, where it may be as high as 10 mm.
6. The P, Q, R, S, and T waves all appear differently depending on which lead you are viewing.

Nursing and Patient Care Considerations

1. Perform ECG or begin continuous ECG monitoring as indicated.
   a. Provide privacy and ask patient to undress, exposing the chest, wrists, and ankles. Assist with draping as appropriate. Remove large jewelry or metal from upper body to avoid interference.
   b. Place leads on the chest and extremities as labeled, using self-adhesive electrodes or water-soluble gel or other conductive material.
   c. Instruct patient to lie still, avoiding movement, coughing, or talking, while ECG is recording to avoid artifact.
   d. Make sure the ECG machine is plugged in and grounded and operate according to the manufacturer's directions.
   e. If continuous cardiac monitoring is being done, advise patient on the parameters of mobility as movement may trigger alarms and false readings. Advise the patient to notify someone if any leads come loose or fall off so they can be replaced in the correct location.
2. Interpret the rhythm strip (see Figure 8-3). Develop a systematic approach to assist in accurate interpretation.
   a. Determine the rhythm—is it regular, irregular, regularly irregular, or irregularly irregular? Use calipers, count blocks between QRS complexes, or measure the distance between R waves to determine regularity.
   b. Determine the rate—is it fast, slow, or normal?
      i. A gross determination of rate can be accomplished by counting the number of QRS complexes within a 6-second time interval (use the superior margin of ECG paper) and multiplying the complexes by a factor of 10.
      Note: This method is accurate only for rhythms that are occurring at normal intervals and should not be used for determining the rate in irregular rhythms. Irregular rhythms are always counted for 1 full minute for accuracy.
      ii. Another means of obtaining the rate is to divide the number of large five-square blocks between each two QRS complexes into 300. Five large five-square blocks represent 1 minute on the ECG paper. For example, in Figure 8-3, the number of large square blocks between complexes no. 5 and no. 6 equals 5, and 300 divided by 5 equals 60, or a rate of 60.
   c. Evaluate the P wave—are P waves present? Is there a P for every QRS complex? If there is not a P for every QRS, do the P waves have a normal configuration?
   d. Measure and evaluate the PR interval.
   e. Evaluate the QRS complex—measure the QRS complex and examine its configuration.
   f. Evaluate the ST segment—an elevated ST segment heralds a pattern of injury and usually occurs as an initial change in acute MI. ST depression occurs in ischemic states. Calcium and potassium changes also affect the ST segment.
   g. Evaluate the T wave—are T waves present? Do all T waves have a normal shape? Could a P wave be hidden in the T wave, indicating a junctional rhythm or third-degree heart block? Is it positively or negatively deflected (inverted T waves indicate ischemia) or peaked (indicative of hyperkalemia)?
   h. Evaluate the QT interval—should be less than one half the R-R interval. Prolonged QT interval can be congenital or acquired. Acquired usually results from drug therapy. Other causes include electrolyte abnormalities, eating disorders, CAD, and bradyarrhythmia.

See Chapter 9 for common cardiac dysrhythmias.

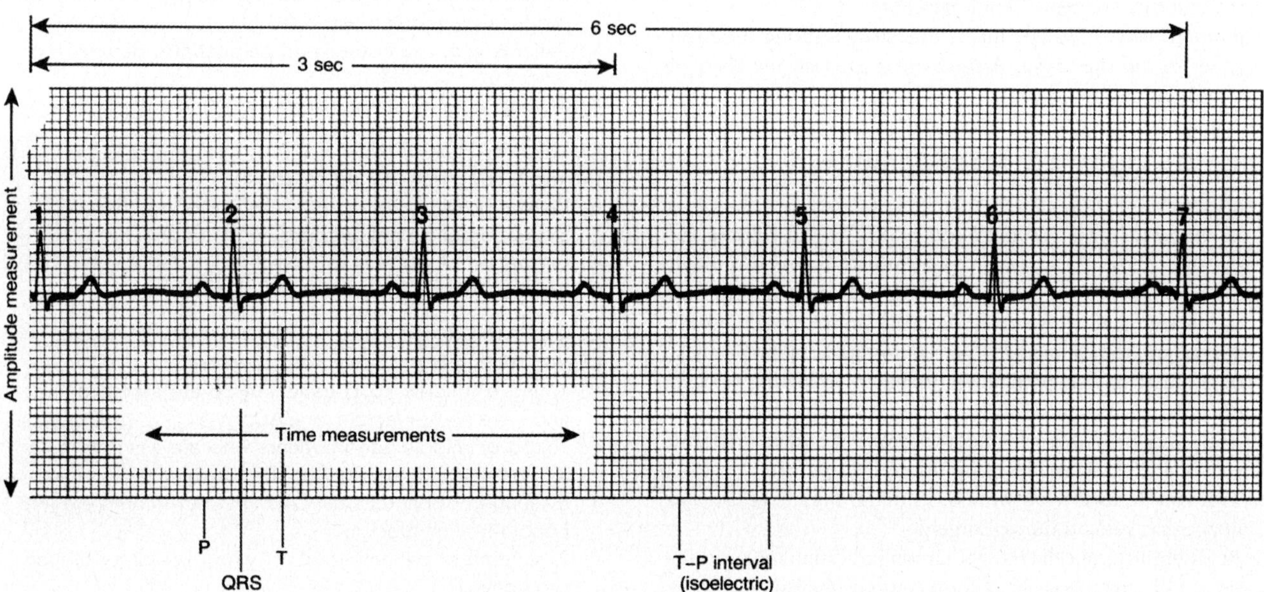

Figure 8-3. Lead II shows normal sinus rhythm on ECG paper. ECG, electrocardiogram.

Radiology and Imaging

Chest X-Ray

Chest x-rays can be used to assess heart size, contour, and position and may also reveal cardiac and pericardial calcification as well as physiologic alterations in pulmonary circulation. For further description and nursing considerations, see page 133.

Echocardiography (Ultrasound Cardiography)

Description

1. *Echocardiography* (ECHO) is used to visualize and assess cardiac function, structure, and hemodynamic abnormalities. It is the most commonly used noninvasive cardiac imaging tool.
2. It records high-frequency sound vibrations that are sent into the heart through the chest wall. The cardiac structures return the echoes derived from the ultrasound. The motions of the echoes are traced on an oscilloscope and recorded on film, CD, or DVD.
3. Clinical usefulness includes demonstration of valvular and other structural deformities; detection of pericardial effusion; evaluation of prosthetic valve function; diagnosis of cardiac tumors of asymmetric thickening of interventricular septum, cardiomegaly (heart enlargement), clots, vegetations on valves, wall motion abnormalities, and acute aortic dissection; and diagnosis of cardiomyopathies, such as stress cardiomyopathy or hypertrophic cardiomyopathy.
4. Types include two-dimensional (2-D), M-mode, and Doppler mode. The methods are complementary and are commonly used in conjunction.
   a. 2-D echocardiography—provides a wider view of the heart and its structures because it involves a planar ultrasound beam.
   b. M-mode—utilizes a single ultrasound beam and provides a narrow segmental view.
   c. Doppler mode—evaluates pressures and blood flow across the valves; also assesses for atrial and ventricular septal defects.

Nursing and Patient Care Considerations

1. Advise patient that traditional echocardiography is noninvasive and that no preparation is necessary.
2. Position patient on left side, if tolerated, to bring the heart closer to the chest wall. Assist patient to clean the chest of transducer gel after the test.

Transesophageal Echocardiography

Description

1. In *transesophageal echocardiography* (*TEE*), an ultrasound transmitter located at the end of a catheter is passed through the esophagus to the stomach, where flexion of the tip permits imaging of the heart through the stomach wall and the diaphragm, thus allowing clearer and more accurate diagnostic evaluation. It is particularly useful in evaluating valvular disease.
2. As the catheter is slowly withdrawn, views of cardiac structures are obtained at several levels in various 2-D planes.
3. TEE can be used for continuous monitoring of cardiac and noncardiac patients during surgery.
4. Atrial fibrillation is the most common indication for performing a TEE, used to evaluate for thromboembolism, especially prior to cardioversion.

Nursing and Patient Care Considerations

1. Explain procedure to patient and provide written information, if possible.
2. This is an invasive procedure; patient will require mild sedation and must be kept on nothing-by-mouth (NPO) status for a specified time—usually 4 to 6 hours—before the procedure.
3. The entire procedure takes less than 30 minutes.
4. Results of the study will be discussed with patient by the patient's health care provider after it is interpreted by the radiologist.

Treadmill Stress Testing

Description

1. In treadmill stress testing, the patient walks on a treadmill or rides a stationary bicycle until reaching a target HR, typically 70% to 80% of the maximum predicted HR. Treadmill stress testing has 70% sensitivity and specificity among the general population.
2. Indications for stress testing have been adapted from the American Heart Association (AHA) and the American College of Cardiology (see Box 8-2).
3. Contraindications for performing a stress test include:
   a. AMI within 2 to 3 days.
   b. Unstable coronary syndrome.
   c. Wolff-Parkinson-White syndrome.
   d. Uncontrolled arrhythmias.
   e. High-degree AV blocks.
   f. Acute myocarditis, pericarditis, or endocarditis.
   g. Symptomatic severe aortic stenosis.
   h. Uncontrolled hypertension.

BOX 8-2 Indications for Stress Test

CLASS I INDICATIONS
(Clear indications for stress testing)
- Suspected or proven coronary artery disease (CAD).
- Male patients who present with atypical chest pain.
- Evaluation of functional capacity and assessment of prognosis in patients with CAD.
- Patients with exercise-related palpitations, dizziness, or syncope.
- Evaluation of recurrent exercise-induced arrhythmias.

CLASS II INDICATIONS
(Stress testing may be indicated.)
- Evaluation of typical or atypical symptoms in females.
- Evaluation of variant angina.
- Evaluation of patients who are on digoxin preparations or who have a right bundle-branch block.

CLASS III INDICATIONS
(Stress testing is probably not necessary.)
- Young or middle-aged patients who are asymptomatic and have no risk factors for CAD.
- Young or middle-aged patients who are asymptomatic and present with noncardiac chest pain.
- Evaluation of patients for CAD who have complete left bundle-branch block.
- Evaluation of patients for CAD who have preexcitation syndrome.

i. Acute aortic dissection.
j. Acute pulmonary embolism or pulmonary infarct.
k. Severe pulmonary hypertension.

4. Reasons for terminating a stress test include:
   a. Absolute indications for termination of the test:
      i. A drop in systolic blood pressure (SBP) of greater than 10 mm Hg from baseline when accompanied by other indications of ischemia.
      ii. Moderate to severe angina.
      iii. Increasing neurologic symptoms, such as ataxia, dizziness, and near syncope.
      iv. Signs of impaired perfusion, such as cyanosis or pallor.
      v. Technical difficulties in monitoring ECG tracings or SBP.
      vi. Patient's desire to stop.
      vii. Sustained ventricular tachycardia.
      viii. ST elevation or more than 1 mm in leads without diagnostic Q waves, other than V or a VR.
   b. Relative indications for the termination of the test:
      i. A drop in SBP of 10 mm Hg or more from baseline in the absence of the evidence of ischemia.
      ii. ST or QRS changes (excessive horizontal or downsloping ST depression of >2 mm) or marked axis shift.
      iii. Arrhythmias, such as superficial vein thrombosis (SVT), multifocal premature ventricular contractions (PVCs), heart block, or bradyarrhythmia.
      iv. Fatigue, shortness of breath, leg cramps, wheezing, or claudication.
      v. Development of intraventricular conduction delay or bundle-branch block that cannot be differentiated from ventricular tachycardia (VT).
      vi. Increasing chest pain.
      vii. Hypertension response SBP of 250 mm Hg, diastolic blood pressure (DBP) higher than 115 mm Hg or both.
      viii. Complications of stress testing include hypotension during or immediately after exercise. Arrhythmias that occur during the test generally stop soon after the termination of the test and rarely cause an MI during the test.

Nursing and Patient Care Considerations

1. Explain the procedure to the patient and provide written information, if possible.
2. Explain to the patient that their HR and BP will be monitored throughout the test and during recovery.
3. Withhold caffeine-containing products for 24 hours before adenosine and dipyridamole stress testing.
4. Instruct the patient to avoid smoking on the day of the test because the presence of nicotine may interfere with the HR.
5. Discuss with the cardiologist which medications should be withheld before the test.
6. Maintain NPO status before testing for 2 hours or according to facility policy. If the patient has diabetes, discuss with the cardiologist about skipping a meal.
7. Establish a patent intravenous (IV) access.
8. Instruct patient to wear comfortable shoes such as walking or running shoes.
9. Patient may need to wear patient gown or loose-fitting clothes.
10. Results of the study will be discussed with the patient by the patient's health care provider after fully interpreted.

Stress Echocardiography

Description

1. *Stress (treadmill) echocardiography* has been found to have better sensitivity and specificity than treadmill stress testing alone.
2. Stress echocardiography is used to evaluate cardiac function at rest, during pharmacologic stress, and during or immediately following vigorous exercise.
3. Used primarily to detect the presence and extent of CAD by provoking regional ischemia with resulting wall motion abnormalities. This can define ischemic severity and risk stratification.
4. With the addition of Doppler, the evaluation of exercise-induced changes in valvular function, pulmonary artery systolic pressure, left ventricular outflow tract gradient, and global left ventricular systolic and diastolic function can be evaluated.
5. Stress echocardiography can be coupled with pharmacologic stress testing for patients who cannot exercise because of degenerative joint disease, physical deconditioning, neurologic disorders, COPD, or peripheral vascular disease. The most commonly administered drug is dobutamine with the addition of atropine to achieve the needed HR. The American Society of Echocardiography (ASE) guidelines recommend dobutamine as preferable to vasodilators (dipyridamole, adenosine, regadenoson).

Nursing and Patient Care Considerations

1. Explain procedure to the patient and provide written information, if possible.
2. Explain to the patient that their HR and BP will be monitored throughout the test and during recovery.
3. Withhold caffeine-containing products for 24 hours before adenosine and dipyridamole stress testing.
4. Instruct the patient to avoid smoking on the day of the test because the presence of nicotine may interfere with the HR.
5. Discuss with the cardiologist which medications should be withheld before test.
6. Maintain NPO status before testing for 2 hours or according to facility policy. If patient has diabetes, discuss with the cardiologist about skipping a meal.
7. Establish a patent IV access.
8. Instruct patient to wear comfortable shoes such as walking or running shoes.
9. Patient may need to wear patient gown or loose-fitting clothes.
10. Results of the study will be discussed with patient by the patient's health care provider after fully interpreted.

DRUG ALERT Theophylline-containing products should be discontinued 48 to 72 hours before an adenosine or dipyridamole stress test. Patients receiving oral dipyridamole should not be given IV adenosine because of potential for precipitating severe heart block. If possible, beta-adrenergic blockers should be withheld for 48 to 72 hours before a dobutamine stress test.

Myocardial Imaging

Positron-Emission Tomography

Description

1. Considered the most sensitive modality for detecting hibernating viable myocardium and predicting left ventricular recovery after coronary revascularization.

2. ^{18}F fluorodeoxyglucose (F-FDG), a glucose analogue that is transported into cells through a glucose membrane transporter, is injected. It does not undergo any further metabolism (unlike glucose) and essentially is trapped within the cell.
3. Trapped F-FDG accumulates and becomes an index of cellular glucose utilization signifying ongoing cellular metabolism. Reduced FDG uptake (reduced or absent glucose metabolism) signifies myocardial scar. Also see page 521.
4. Used to determine blood flow to the heart muscle and viability of areas with decreased function because of previous MI.
5. Allows for the differentiation of nonfunctioning heart muscle from heart muscle that would benefit from a procedure.
6. Additional cardiac positron-emission tomography (PET) evaluations with the use of radionuclides and scintillation cameras, and radionuclide angiograms can be used to assess left ventricular performance.
   a. Thallium 201 is a radionuclide (an unstable atom that produces a small amount of energy) that behaves like potassium in the body and is distributed throughout the myocardium in proportion to blood flow.
      i. Negative result of "cold spot" imaging with thallium 201 rules out MI.
      ii. A positive result, on the other hand, is inconclusive because it cannot differentiate between old and new infarction or areas of ischemia versus infarction.
   b. Technetium-99m-labeled sestamibi is a myocardial perfusion marker used to assess cell membrane and mitochondrial integrity and to reveal myocardial perfusion.
      i. Sestamibi is not taken up by acute or chronic infarct tissue, and the amount of uptake of the radionuclide by other tissue correlates with the size of the infarction, the amount of CK released in the blood, and the postinfarction left ventricular ejection fraction (LVEF).
      ii. "Hot spot" or positive imaging with technetium-99m is used when diagnosis of MI is unclear.
   c. Radionuclide ventriculogram with technetium-99m is used to evaluate valve structure and ventricular function.
      i. Contrast medium is injected through a catheter, opacifying the ventricular cavity to enable measuring of right and LVEF.
      ii. Also distinguishes regional from global ventricular wall motion and allows subjective analysis of cardiac anatomy to detect intracardiac shunts as well as valvular or congenital abnormalities.
      iii. Complications include arrhythmias, intramyocardial or pericardial injection of contrast medium, and, possibly, development of emboli because of injection of air or a thrombosis through the catheter.
   d. Dual single-photon emission computed tomography with simultaneous imaging using two isotopes improves the accuracy of assessing the infarcted area. The overlap of two isotopes may reflect the presence of salvaged myocardium adjacent to necrotic tissue.

Nursing and Patient Care Considerations

1. Advise patient that a radionuclide will be injected through a central venous or peripheral IV catheter.
2. Inform patient not to eat for 4 hours prior to the scan.
3. Check blood glucose prior to test for patients with diabetes; if greater than 200, may need to reschedule the test.
4. Encourage patient to drink water following the scan to assist excretion of contrast medium.
5. Reassure patient that the radionuclide will not cause radiation injury or affect heart function.
6. Explain to patient that hot flashes and nausea or vomiting may occur. A test dose will be administered before the dose required for contrast to assess patient's tolerance of radionuclide.
7. Results of the study will be discussed by the patient's health care provider after the study is interpreted by the radiologist.

Cardiac Magnetic Resonance Imaging

Magnetic Resonance Imaging (MRI) is used to evaluate diseased heart muscle. Currently, three techniques are being used. Resting MRI can assess end-diastolic wall thickness and contractile function. Dobutamine MRI is used to evaluate contractile reserve. Contrast-enhanced MRI allows for the visualization of the in vivo regions of microvascular obstruction. The extent of microvascular obstruction determines the magnitude of myocardial scarring. Once determined, the extent of microvascular obstruction is a strong predictor of myocardial remodeling and outcome after revascularization. It may eventually replace cardiac catheterization. Safety has been demonstrated in patients with permanent pacemakers and implantable cardioverter–defibrillators. For further description and nursing considerations, see page 134. Newer technologies combining MRI and PET use the strengths of each technology to produce integrated MRI and PET images.

Coronary Computed Tomography

Description

Cardiac computed tomography (CT) is most often performed as contrast-enhanced coronary CT angiography (CCTA) to evaluate the presence and extent of CAD. It has a high sensitivity and a corresponding low rate of false negatives. CCTA is a test best suited to identify patients at low risk for future major adverse cardiovascular events. It detects not only the presence and extent of stenosis but also coronary plaque.

The most common contraindication to CCTA is severe renal insufficiency or a history of allergy to iodinated contrast.

Nursing and Patient Care Considerations

1. Patient should be NPO for 4 to 6 hours before the test.
2. Instruct the patient to avoid any caffeinated drinks on the day before or the day of the test.
3. Instruct patient to avoid energy or diet pills on the day before or the day of the test.
4. Advise patient to drink plenty of water after the scan to flush out the contrast.

Phlebography (Venography)

Description

An x-ray visualization of the vascular tree after the injection of a contrast medium to detect venous occlusion.

Nursing and Patient Care Considerations

1. Inform patient that an intense burning sensation in the vessel where the solution is injected may be experienced. This will last for only a few seconds.
2. Note evidence of allergic reaction to the contrast medium; this may occur as soon as the contrast medium is injected, or it may occur after the test.
   a. Perspiring, dyspnea, nausea, and vomiting.
   b. Rapid HR and numbness of extremities.
   c. Hives.

3. Advise patient to notify health care provider of signs of allergic reaction.
4. Observe injection site for redness, swelling, bleeding, and thrombosis.

Other Diagnostic Tests

Angiography

Description

1. Invasive imaging procedure that enables visualization of blood vessels for their patency of blood flow versus blockage through the insertion of a catheter into an artery or vein followed by injection of contrast dye.
2. Various types include coronary, aortic, renal, peripheral, cerebral, and pulmonary angiography; lymphangiogram; ventriculography; and fluorescein angiography.
3. Provide information that may direct assessment and management of cardiovascular and cerebrovascular disease, peripheral blockage (arterial and venous), aneurysms, arterial and venous malformations, thrombosis (deep vein or pulmonary embolus), and fistulae, guide mapping prior to interventional procedures, and diagnose internal bleeding.

Nursing and Patient Care Considerations

Preprocedure

1. Question patient for known allergies, particularly to iodine (shellfish). If so, notify health care provider, who may want to prepare patient with oral corticosteroids and diphenhydramine before the study.
2. Make sure there is a signed consent and that patient/family questions have been answered.
3. Make sure fasting guidelines have been followed, varying from NPO to liquid or light diet. Follow facility policy; should be in accordance with American Society of Anesthesiologists guidelines (minimum fasting 6 hours from light meal, 2 hours from clear liquids) to minimize risk of pulmonary aspiration should emesis occur.
4. Make sure laboratory testing has been ordered and results have been reviewed, including blood urea nitrogen (BUN) and creatinine, to evaluate kidney function for ability to clear contrast dye; hemoglobin/hematocrit, platelet count, and coagulation values, to ensure clotting and anticoagulation baseline; white blood cell (WBC) count, to rule out infection that may be exacerbated by invasive procedure; electrolytes; pregnancy test (in female of childbearing age); and blood type and screen, in case blood transfusion is necessary.
5. Make sure baseline ECG is on file.
6. Ensure IV patency for medication administration.
7. Make sure patient has voided.
8. Administer premedication, if ordered.

Postprocedure

1. Record vital signs according to facility policy and stability of patient.
2. Check for bleeding or hematoma formation at insertion site.
3. Check distal extremity for normal color and intact pulses.
4. Patient may complain of discomfort in the groin or other site depending on the route by which contrast medium was administered. Check for bed rest/activity progression and special fluid instructions. Encourage fluids/hydration to ensure clearance of contrast dye.
5. Provide patient with discharge instructions, including follow-up care, medications, and driving and activity restrictions.

Diagnostic Electrophysiology Studies

Description

Electrophysiology studies (EPS) are a complex invasive procedure in which flexible catheters (with 2 to 10 electrodes) are placed percutaneously in the right or left femoral vein, the subclavian vein, the internal jugular vein, or the median cephalic veins. EPS assesses pacing thresholds and measures conduction intervals in the high RA, the right ventricular apex, the right ventricular outflow tract, the coronary sinuses, the bundle of His, and, occasionally, the left ventricle (LV). The test is followed by programmed stimulation protocols to evaluate the heart's conduction system.

Indications for EPS

1. Definite indications for EPS include:
   a. Sustained ventricular tachycardia.
   b. Cardiac arrest in the absence of AMI, antiarrhythmic drug toxicity, or electrolyte imbalance.
   c. Syncope of uncertain origin (for which noncardiac causes have been ruled out).
   d. Wide QRS tachycardia of uncertain etiology.
   e. To evaluate the effectiveness of a device for the detection and electrical termination of tachycardias (pacemakers or implanted defibrillators).
   f. Symptomatic Wolff-Parkinson-White syndrome.
   g. Frequent symptomatic regular supraventricular tachycardia unresponsive to medications.
2. Possible indications for EPS include:
   a. Asymptomatic Wolff-Parkinson-White syndrome.
   b. Post-MI.
   c. Nonsustained ventricular tachycardia.
   d. Cardiomyopathy.
   e. Frequent ventricular ectopy.
   f. Supraventricular tachycardia.
3. Contraindications for EPS include:
   a. Asymptomatic sinus bradycardia.
   b. Asymptomatic bundle-branch blocks.
   c. Palpitation.
   d. Atrial fibrillation or flutter.
   e. Third-degree AV blocks.
   f. Second-degree Mobitz type II AV blocks.

Nursing and Patient Care Considerations

1. Anticoagulants (warfarin) should be discontinued at least 3 days before EPS.
2. Discuss with health care provider which cardiac medications should be discontinued and when they should be discontinued.
3. Instruct patient to fast for at least 6 hours before the study.
4. Ensure laboratory tests are sent; may include BUN and creatinine, to evaluate kidney function for ability to clear contrast dye; hemoglobin/hematocrit, platelet count, and coagulation values to ensure clotting and anticoagulation baseline; WBC count, to rule out infection that may be exacerbated by invasive procedure; electrolytes; blood type and screen, in case blood transfusion is necessary; and pregnancy test in females of childbearing age.
5. Place electrodes for a 12-lead ECG, which will be recorded during the procedure.

6. Discuss with patient any feelings about the procedure and their physical condition. Patients frequently experience anxiety, fear of loss of control, denial, depression, and uncertainty.
7. Explain the procedure, its purpose, and the preparation involved.
8. Inform patient that pain medication and conscious sedation will be used during the procedure.
9. Postprocedure care includes:
   a. Keeping extremity used for IV straight, restraining if necessary.
   b. Monitoring patient's groin for bleeding or hematoma formation.
   c. Monitoring vital signs as ordered.
   d. Providing emotional support to patient and family.

Cardiac Catheterization

Description

1. *Cardiac catheterization* is a diagnostic procedure in which a catheter is introduced into the heart and blood vessels to provide physiologic data to guide treatment; measure cardiovascular hemodynamics; acquire radiographic images of coronary arteries, cardiac chambers, and aorta; collect blood from various chambers for analysis; and evaluate pulmonary blood flow and shunts.
2. The radial approach is becoming the preferred access site especially when there is peripheral vascular disease or morbid obesity. The femoral vein is another frequently used site. The catheter is directed up the aorta and into the coronary vasculature to visualize coronary anatomy (right or left) and measure hemodynamics. In rare instances of aortic disease, a transseptal approach may be used.
3. Right-sided heart catheterization—right side of the heart is accessed to evaluate pulmonary shunts, cardiac anomalies, and valvular disease. A radiopaque catheter is passed from the femoral vein and through the inferior vena cava or from the basilic vein and through the superior vena cava into the RA, RV, and pulmonary vasculature under direct visualization with a fluoroscope.
   a. RA and RV pressures are measured; blood samples are taken for hematocrit and oxygen saturation.
   b. After entering the RA, the catheter is then passed through the tricuspid valve and similar tests are performed on blood within the RV.
   c. Finally, the catheter is passed through the pulmonic valve, and as far as possible beyond that point, capillary samples are obtained, capillary wedge pressure is recorded, and CO can be determined.
   d. Complications include cardiac dysrhythmias, venous spasm, thrombophlebitis, infection at insertion site, cardiac perforation, and cardiac tamponade.
4. Left-sided heart catheterization—primarily done to diagnose CAD; usually done by retrograde approach by advancing the catheter up the aorta into the coronary anatomy.
   a. Retrograde approach—catheter may be introduced percutaneously by puncture of the femoral artery or by direct radial or brachial approach and advanced under fluoroscopic control into the ascending aorta and into the LV.
   b. Transseptal approach—catheter is passed from the right femoral vein (percutaneously or by saphenous vein cut down) upward into the RA. A long needle is passed up through the catheter and is used to puncture the septum separating the right and left atria; needle is withdrawn and the catheter is advanced under fluoroscopic control into the LV.
   c. The catheter tip is placed at the coronary sinus, and contrast medium is injected directly into one or both of the coronary arteries to evaluate patency.
   d. Gives hemodynamic data—permits flow and pressure measurements of left side of the heart.
   e. Usually performed to evaluate the patency of coronary arteries and function of the left ventricular muscle and mitral and aortic valves; may also be done to evaluate patients before surgery.
   f. Ventriculography—study of the LV; catheter is passed into the LV, and dye is injected with a rapid, uniform rate via an injector machine to measure ejection fraction or function of the LV.
   g. Complications of left-sided heart catheterization and implications for nursing assessment include dysrhythmias (ventricular fibrillation), syncope, vasospasm, pericardial tamponade, MI, pulmonary edema, allergic reaction to contrast medium, perforation of great vessels of the heart, systemic embolization (stroke, MI), loss of pulse distal to arteriotomy, and possible ischemia of the lower arm and hand.
5. Angiography is usually combined with heart catheterization for coronary artery visualization.
6. Contraindications for cardiac catheterization include uncontrolled ventricular irritability, electrolyte imbalance, medication toxicity (digitalis), uncontrolled heart failure, renal failure, recent stroke (within the past 3 months), active GI bleeding, active infection, uncontrolled hypertension, patient's refusal, and pregnancy. Some of these conditions can be reversed or improved prior to catheterization.

Nursing and Patient Care Considerations

Preprocedure

1. Question patient for known allergies, particularly iodine (shellfish), and make health care provider aware so that premedication with corticosteroid and antihistamine may be considered.
2. Make sure that there is a signed consent form and that patient and family questions have been answered.
3. Make sure that fasting guidelines have been followed, varying from NPO to liquid or light diet. Follow facility policy; should be in accordance with American Society of Anesthesiologists guidelines (minimum fasting 6 hours from light meal, 2 hours from clear liquids).
4. Make sure laboratory testing has been ordered and results reviewed (see pages 202–203). Make sure baseline ECG is on file.
5. Ensure IV patency for administration of medications.
6. Mark distal pulses.
7. Explain to patient that they will be lying on an examination table for a prolonged period and may experience certain sensations:
   a. Occasional thudding sensations in the chest—from extrasystoles, particularly when the catheter is manipulated in ventricular chambers.
   b. Strong desire to cough, which may occur during contrast medium injection into right side of heart during angiography.
   c. Transient feeling of hot flashes or nausea as the contrast medium is injected.

8. Evaluate patient's emotional status before catheterization, dispel myths, and provide factual information.
9. Have patient void before the procedure.
10. Allow for premedication (if any) to take effect prior to the procedure.

Postprocedure

1. Record vital signs according to facility protocol and patient's condition.
2. Check for bleeding or hematoma formation at insertion site.
3. Check distal extremity for normal color and intact pulses, and evaluate complaints of pain, numbness, or tingling sensation to determine signs of arterial insufficiency.
4. Assess for complaints of chest pain and respond immediately.
5. Follow activity restriction/progression directions, which are based on coagulation status and whether a vascular closure method was employed.
6. Evaluate complaints of back, thigh, or groin pain (may indicate retroperitoneal bleeding).
7. Obtain postprocedure ECG and labs according to facility protocol.
8. Be alert for signs and symptoms of vagal reaction (nausea, diaphoresis, hypotension, bradycardia); treat as directed with atropine and fluids.
9. Assess neurologic status if receiving IIB/IIIA platelet inhibitors or thrombolytics according to facility protocol.
10. Provide discharge instructions, including follow-up care, medications, driving and activity restrictions, and the need to report any pain or above-listed problems.

GENERAL PROCEDURES AND TREATMENT MODALITIES

See additional online content: Procedure Guidelines 8-1 to 8-2.

Hemodynamic Monitoring

Hemodynamic monitoring is the assessment of the patient's circulatory status; it includes measurements of heart rate (HR), precise measurements of intra-arterial pressure, cardiac output (CO), central venous pressure (CVP), pulmonary artery pressure (PAP), pulmonary artery (PA) wedge pressure, mixed venous oxygenation data, and blood volume. It describes the intravascular pressure and flow of blood that occurs when the heart muscle contracts and pumps blood throughout the body.

The primary purpose is the early detection, identification, and treatment of life-threatening conditions, such as acute myocardial infarction (AMI), heart failure, cardiac tamponade, and all types of shock (septic, cardiogenic, neurogenic, anaphylactic). It is also used to manage patients with suspected or known pulmonary hypertension. In addition, it is useful in determining fluid and vasoactive therapy during the acute phase of patient's care, especially for patients with multiorgan dysfunctions. It is also indicated for pre-, peri-, and postoperative surgery as well as for research studies.

CVP Monitoring

1. Refers to the measurement of right atrial pressure or the pressure of the great veins within the thorax (normal range: 5 to 10 cm H_2O or 2 to 8 mm Hg).
   a. Right-sided cardiac function is assessed through the evaluation of CVP.
   b. Left-sided heart function is less accurately reflected by the evaluation of CVP, but may be useful in assessing chronic right- and left-sided heart failure and differentiating right and left ventricular infarctions.
2. Requires the threading of a catheter into a large central vein (subclavian, internal, or external jugular, median basilic, or femoral). The catheter tip is then positioned in the right atrium (RA), upper portion of the superior vena cava, or the inferior vena cava (femoral approach only) (see Figure 8-4).
   a. To obtain venous access when peripheral vein sites are inadequate.
   b. To obtain central venous blood samples.
   c. To administer blood products, total parenteral nutrition, and some drug therapies contraindicated for peripheral infusion.
   d. To insert a temporary pacemaker.

Cardiac Output

CO is the amount (volume) of blood ejected by the left ventricle (LV) into the aorta in 1 minute. Normal CO is 4 to 8 L/min. CO measurements are used to evaluate the patient's responses to clinical interventions, mechanical assist devices, and vasoactive and inotropic medications.

Underlying Considerations

1. CO is determined by stroke volume (SV) and HR. Thus, CO = SV × HR. CO must be maintained to adequately oxygenate the body.
   a. HR = number of cardiac contractions per minute. The integrity of the conduction system and nervous system innervation of the heart influence functioning of this determinant.

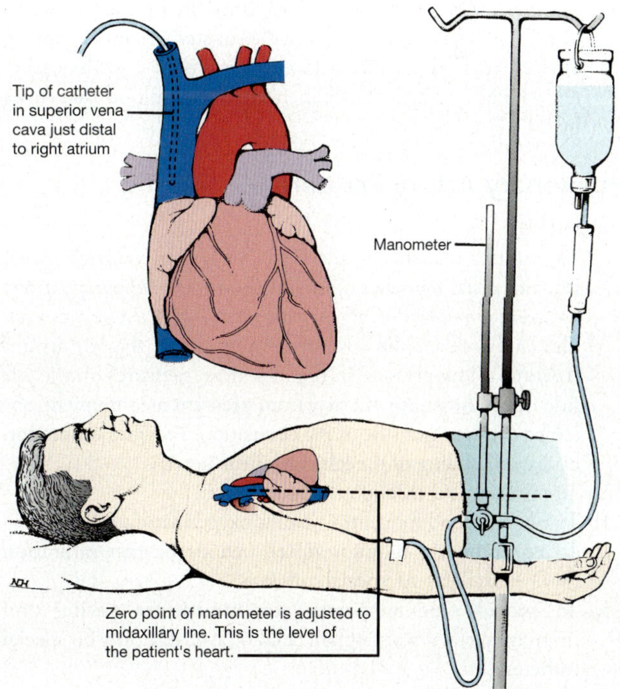

Figure 8-4. CVP monitoring. CVP, central venous pressure.

b. SV = amount of blood ejected from ventricle per beat (normal SV is 50 to 100 mL/beat). The amount of blood returning to the heart (preload), venous tone, resistance imposed on the ventricle before ejection (afterload), and the integrity of the cardiac muscle (contractility) influence the functioning of this determinant.

2. The body alters CO through increases or decreases in one or both of these parameters. CO is maintained if the HR falls by an increase in SV. Likewise, a decrease in SV produces a compensatory rise in HR to keep the CO normal.
3. CO will decrease if either of the determinants cannot inversely compensate for the other.
4. CO measurements are adjusted to patient size by calculating the cardiac index (CI). CI equals CO divided by body surface area (BSA); BSA is determined through standard charts based on individual height and weight. Normal CI is 2.5 to 4 $L/min/m^2$.

Assessment of CO

Signs of low CO include:

1. Changes in mental status.
2. An increase in HR.
3. Shortness of breath.
4. Cyanosis or duskiness of buccal mucosa, nail beds, and earlobes.
5. Falling blood pressure (BP).
6. Low urine output.
7. Cool, moist skin.
8. Decreased or no appetite.
9. Low oxygen saturation.

Methods

1. CO is measured by various techniques. In the clinical setting, it is usually measured by the thermodilution technique in conjunction with a flow-directed balloon-tipped PA catheter (commonly known as the Swan-Ganz catheter after the inventors).
2. The Swan-Ganz catheter is positioned in its final position in a branch of the PA; it has a thermistor (external sensing device) situated 1½ inches (4 cm) from the tip of the catheter, which measures the temperature of the blood that flows by it.

Pulmonary Artery Pressure Monitoring

Purposes

1. To monitor pressures in the RA (CVP), right ventricle (RV), PA, and distal branches of the PA (known as *pulmonary artery occlusion pressure* [PAOP] or *pulmonary artery wedge pressure*). The latter reflects the level of the pressure in the left atrium (LA) (or filling pressure in the LV); thus, pressures on the left side of the heart are inferred from pressure measurement obtained on the right side of the circulation. Provides estimation of diastolic filling of the left side of the heart.
2. To measure CO through thermodilution.
3. To obtain blood for central venous oxygen saturation.
4. To continuously monitor mixed venous oxygen saturation (SvO_2); available on special catheters.
5. To provide for temporary atrial/ventricular pacing and intra-atrial electrocardiogram (ECG) (available only on special catheters).
6. To evaluate the hemodynamic response to fluid therapy, medications, and other treatments.

Underlying Considerations

1. Left atrial pressure is closely related to left ventricular end-diastolic pressure (LVEDP—filling pressure of the LV) and is therefore an indicator of left ventricular function. Because there are no valves in the pulmonary arterial system when the Swan-Ganz catheter is wedged, it reflects an uninterrupted flow of blood to the LA.
2. The pulmonary artery diastolic pressure (PADP) reflects the LVEDP in patients with normal lungs and mitral valve. The PADP can be continuously monitored as an approximation of LVEDP (limits excessive balloon inflation to obtain a PAOP and subsequent risk of balloon rupture or damage to the PA.
3. SaO_2 is affected by four factors: CO, hemoglobin, arterial oxygen saturation (SaO_2), and tissue oxygen consumption.
4. Changes in SaO_2 alert the clinician to changes in these factors. More rapid detection of change facilitates interventions to correct problems before significant deterioration in patient's condition occurs.
5. If the amount of oxygen supplied to the tissues is inadequate to meet demands, more oxygen will be extracted from venous blood and SaO_2 will decrease. If oxygen supply exceeds demand, SaO_2 will increase.
6. PA catheters are associated with significant risk and disadvantages, including increased cost and mortality. Placement of a PA catheter is invasive and does not directly impact patient outcomes.

Methods

1. The Swan-Ganz catheter is a flow-directed (1.5 mL), balloon-tipped, 4- to 5-lumen catheter that is percutaneously inserted at the bedside and allows for continuous PAP monitoring as well as periodic measurement of PAOP and other parameters.
2. The catheter is 110 cm long, marked at increments of 10 cm, and is available in varying diameters (see Figure 8-5).
3. Most catheters in use incorporate thermodilution for the determination of CO.
4. If monitoring of SvO_2 is desired, a PA catheter incorporating fiberoptics is used.
5. If temporary cardiac pacing capability is desired, a catheter with a lumen for a pacing wire may be used.
6. Catheter may be inserted under fluoroscopy or at the bedside using the hemodynamic waveform as a guide to correct position.

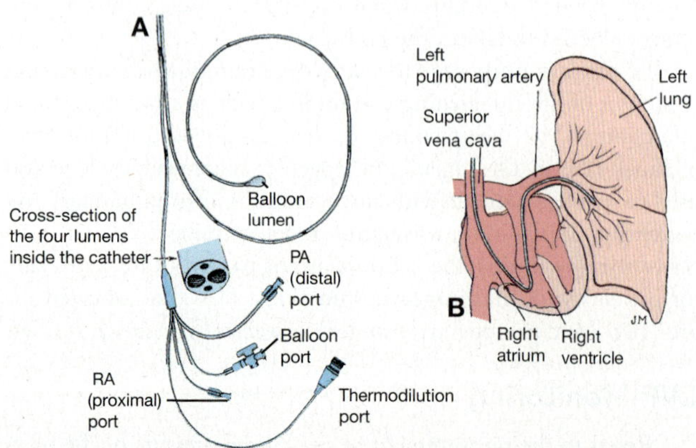

Figure 8-5. Swan–Ganz catheter showing (**A**) multiple lumens and (**B**) location within the heart. PA, pulmonary artery; RA, right atrium.

Newer Technology for Hemodynamic Monitoring

Complications associated with insertion of invasive PA catheters have led to the development of newer noninvasive or minimally invasive methods of hemodynamic monitoring.

1. Indirect Fick method—modification of the original Fick principle first developed in 1870.
2. Thoracic electrical bioimpedance (TEB)—noninvasive measurement of the electrical resistance of the thorax to a high-frequency, very-low-magnitude current. As thoracic fluid in the chest increases, TEB decreases; changes in CO correspond to changes in aortic blood flow.
3. Pulse contour devices—measure CO by assessing the contours of arterial pressure waveforms in relationship to the patient's SV.
4. Continuous SvO_2 monitoring—measures mixed venous oxygen by means of a modified PA catheter to assess oxygen-carrying hemoglobin (oxyhemoglobin) and non-oxygen-carrying hemoglobin (deoxyhemoglobin).
5. Continuous CO monitoring—utilizes a modified PA catheter.
6. Right ventricular ejection fraction measurement—assesses the amount of blood forced from the ventricle during systole; it is an indication of the strength or contractility of the heart as determined by a special type of arterial catheter.
7. Esophageal Doppler CO monitoring—utilizes sound waves to measure aortic blood flow and thereby determine SV.
8. Exhaled CO_2 monitoring—completely noninvasive technique based on the Fick equation that measures CO.
9. Lithium dilution CO is another thermodilution method that assesses CO through injection of lithium chloride into a central or peripheral venous catheter and measurement of the concentration of lithium chloride over time using lithium-sensitive electrodes.
10. Cardiac magnetic resonance imaging (MRI) measures CO by looking at blood flow generated by the picture from the magnetic current. It calculates SV, which is multiplied by HR.
11. Bioimpedance CO determination measures changes in the body's resistance to small electrical current. Blood volume in the chest changes during every ejection, which can be detected using eight electrical patches positioned on the neck and thorax. Based on these changes in impedance, a computer can calculate the CO.
12. Bioreactance is a novel noninvasive method for CO measurement that involves analysis of blood flow-dependent changes in phase shifts of electrical currents applied across the thorax.
13. Ultrasound indicator dilution (mostly used in pediatrics) works off in situ catheters and uses an unobjectionable indicator to allow for routine measurements of CO and blood volumes.
14. Point-of-care echocardiography using a pulse wave Doppler calculates CO by determining velocity time of the Doppler or tracing.

Cardiac Pacing

EVIDENCE BASE Johnson, K. (Ed.). (2024). *AACN procedure manual for progressive and critical care* (8th ed.). Elsevier.

A *cardiac pacemaker* is an electronic device that delivers direct electrical stimulation to stimulate the myocardium to depolarize, initiating a mechanical contraction. The pacemaker initiates and maintains the HR when the heart's natural pacemaker is unable to do so. It reestablishes effective circulation and normalizes hemodynamics that are compromised by a slow HR. Pacemakers can be used to correct bradycardias, tachycardias, sick sinus syndrome, and second- and third-degree heart blocks and for prophylaxis. Pacing may be accomplished through a permanent implantable system, a temporary system with an external pulse generator and percutaneously threaded leads, or a transcutaneous external system with electrode pads placed over the chest. A recent development is the leadless pacemaker.

Clinical Indications

1. Symptomatic bradydysrhythmias.
2. Symptomatic sinus bradycardia that results from required drug therapy.
3. Symptomatic heart block.
   a. Mobitz II second-degree heart block.
   b. Complete heart block.
   c. Bifascicular and trifascicular bundle-branch blocks.
4. Hypersensitive carotid sinus syndrome and neurocardiogenic syncope.
5. Prophylaxis.
   a. After AMI: dysrhythmia and conduction defects.
   b. Before or after cardiac surgery.
   c. During cardiac resynchronization therapy in patients with severe systolic heart failure.
   d. During diagnostic and therapeutic procedures such as cardiac catheterization, electrophysiology studies (EPS), percutaneous transluminal coronary angioplasty (PTCA), stress testing, before permanent pacing, and during transcatheter aortic valve replacement (TAVR).
6. Tachydysrhythmias (supraventricular tachycardia, ventricular tachycardia); to override rapid rhythm disturbances.

Types of Pacing

Permanent Pacemakers

There are three types of permanent pacemakers (PPMs); the standard pacer that paces one side of the heart causing uncoordinated contraction of the LV and RV, biventricular that coordinates the contraction of the LV and RV, and leadless.

Standard Pacemakers

1. Used to treat chronic heart conditions; surgically placed utilizing a local anesthetic, the leads are placed transvenously in the appropriate chamber of the heart and then anchored to the endocardium.
2. The pulse generator is placed in a surgically made pocket in subcutaneous tissue under the clavicle (most common) or in the abdomen. Choices for types of generators include single- or dual-chamber devices, biventricular devices, unipolar or bipolar pacing/sensing configuration, and various types of sensors for rate response.
3. Standard pacemaker consists of one to two leads, either one in the ventricle or one in the atrium and one in the ventricle.
4. Once placed, it can be programmed externally as needed.
5. Implantable cardioverter–defibrillators (ICDs) can also have standard pacing functionality.

Biventricular Pacemakers

1. Biventricular pacemakers are also referred to as cardiac resynchronization therapy.
2. Biventricular pacing is used to treat moderate to severe heart failure as a result of left ventricular dyssynchrony.

3. Intraventricular conduction defects result in an uncoordinated contraction of the LV and RV, which causes a wide QRS complex and is associated with worsening heart failure and increased mortality.
4. Biventricular pacemakers utilize three leads (one in the RA, one in the RV, and one in the LV via the coronary sinus) to coordinate ventricular contraction and improve CO.
5. Biventricular pacemakers can incorporate ICDs or be used alone.

Leadless Pacemakers

1. Self-contained, single chamber, implanted directly through femoral vein into RV. In select patients, these have been implanted via transjugular approach.
2. Fixated into the myocardium by a screw helix or nitinol tines.
3. Developed to eliminate complications of pocket or lead-related problems.
4. Ten-year estimated battery life; retrievable if necessary.
5. Leadless pacemakers only have the capacity to pace the ventricle.

Temporary Pacemakers

1. Temporary pacemakers are usually placed during an emergency, such as when a patient demonstrates signs of decreased CO due to bradycardia.
2. Indicated for patients with high-grade atrioventricular (AV) blocks, bradycardia, or low CO. They serve as a bridge until the patient becomes stable enough for placement of a PPM.
3. Indicated for patients in whom extrinsic causes of bradydysrhythmias are reversible, such as medication toxicity or metabolic and electrolyte disturbances.
4. Placement can be transcutaneous, transvenous, epicardial, or transthoracic.
   a. Transcutaneous pacing is noninvasive and the first step in the advanced cardiac life support (ACLS) bradycardia algorithm when the patient is unstable. With transcutaneous pacing, noninvasive multifunction electrode pads are placed either anterior-posteriorly (anterior chest wall under the left nipple, slightly midaxillary, and on the patient's back directly behind the anterior pad) or anterior-laterally (anterior chest wall under the left nipple, slightly midaxillary, and on patient's upper right chest wall below the clavicle). The multifunction electrode pads are connected to an external energy source (defibrillator with pacing capability). The electrical impulses flow through the multifunction electrode pads and subcutaneous skin to the heart, thereby pacing the heart. Note: Transcutaneous pacing should not be utilized continuously for more than 2 hours; transvenous pacing should then be initiated, along with a consult with the electrophysiology team for a PPM. American Heart Association (AHA) does not recommend transcutaneous pacing be used in patients who have a bradyasystolic cardiac arrest.
   b. Transvenous pacemakers are inserted transvenously (into a vein, usually the subclavian, internal jugular, antecubital, or femoral) into the right ventricle (or RA and RV for dual-chamber pacing) and then attached to an external pulse generator. This procedure may be done at the bedside or under fluoroscopy. If the pacemaker wires have a protective sheath covering to allow for adjustment of the wires sterilely, do not place tape over the sheath as it could rip the sheath when removing the tape. Keep hydrogen peroxide away from the sheath as it will cause the sheath to degrade.
   c. Epicardial pacemaker wires are attached to the endocardium, brought out through a surgical incision in the thorax. These wires are then connected to an external pulse generator. This is commonly seen after cardiac surgery.
   d. The transthoracic pacemaker is a type of temporary pacemaker that is placed only in an emergency via a long needle, using a subxiphoid approach. The pacer wire is then placed directly into the RV.
5. Monitor for evidence of lead migration and perforation of the heart.
   a. Observe for muscle twitching and/or cough or hiccup (may indicate chest wall or diaphragmatic pacing).
   b. Evaluate patient's complaints of chest pain (may indicate perforation of pericardial sac).
   c. Auscultate for pericardial friction rub.
   d. Observe for signs and symptoms of cardiac tamponade: distant heart sounds, distended jugular veins, pulsus paradoxus, and hypotension.
6. Provide an electrically safe environment for patient. Stray electrical current can enter the heart through temporary pacemaker lead system and induce dysrhythmias.
   a. Protect exposed parts of the electrode lead terminal in temporary pacing systems per the manufacturer's recommendations.
   b. Wear rubber gloves when touching temporary pacing leads. Static electricity from your hands can enter the patient's body through the lead system. To minimize static electricity, touch something metal (e.g., a light switch cover) before touching the patient.
   c. Make sure all equipment is grounded with three-prong plugs inserted into a proper outlet when using an external pacing system.
   d. Epicardial pacing wires should have the terminal needle protected by a plastic tube; place tube in rubber glove to protect it from fluids or electrical current when disconnected from generator.
7. When transcutaneous pacing a patient, use sedation if BP is stable. The milliamperes (mA) used to overcome the impedance to reach the heart through the skin is high and can be quite painful to the patient.
8. Monitor for infection by checking temperature every 4 hours; report elevations and assess central intravenous (IV) site (transvenous) and surgical incision site (epicardial or transthoracic) for signs and symptoms of infection, such as redness and drainage.
9. Prevent accidental pacemaker malfunctions.
   a. Use clear plastic covering over external temporary generators at all times (eliminates potential manipulation of programmed settings).
   b. Secure temporary pacemaker generator to patient's chest or waist; never hang it on an IV pole. Secure pacer wires to the patient with a safety loop.
   c. Transfer of patient from bed to stretcher should only be attempted with an adequate number of personnel so that patient can remain passive; caution personnel to avoid underarm lifts.
   d. Evaluate transcutaneous pacing electrode pads every 2 hours for secure contact to chest wall; change electrode pads every 24 hours or if pads do not have complete contact with the skin.
   e. Transport patient to other parts of facility with a nurse, portable ECG monitoring, and the direct current defibrillator

as it has the ability to transcutaneous pace the patient in the event of loss of capture. Patients with temporary pacemakers should never be placed in unmonitored areas.

CLINICAL JUDGMENT Do not use asynchronous (fixed rate) pacing if there is an intrinsic rhythm; this could lead to R on T syndrome and send the patient into lethal arrhythmia.

Pacemaker Design

Pulse Generator

Contains the circuitry and batteries to generate the electrical signal.

1. The pulse generator in a PPM is encapsulated in a metal box that is embedded under the skin. The box protects the generator from electromagnetic interferences and trauma.
2. In the leadless pacemaker, the pulse generator is self-contained in the device implanted in the RV.
3. A temporary pacing generator is an external system that either utilizes the defibrillator with pacing capability or is contained in a small box with dials for programming. It is an external system.
   a. Transcutaneous pacing systems utilize an external energy source such as a defibrillator with pacing ability. Dials for programming the unit are on the device.
   b. Electromechanical interference is more likely to occur with temporary systems.
   c. Temporary pacing systems use batteries, which need replacement based on the use of device. The transcutaneous system has rechargeable battery circuitry but should be plugged into an electrical outlet most of the time to ensure adequate battery life for transport.
4. Permanent pacing systems use reliable power sources such as lithium batteries. Lithium batteries have a projected life span of 8 to 12 years.

Pacemaker Lead

Transmits the electrical signal from the pulse generator to the heart. One, two, or three leads may be placed in the heart.

1. "Single-chamber" pacemaker.
   a. "Single-chamber" pacemakers have one lead in either the atrial or ventricular chamber.
   b. The sensing and pacing capabilities of the pacemaker are confined to the chamber where the lead is placed.
2. "Dual-chamber" pacemaker.
   a. A "dual-chamber" pacemaker has two leads.
   b. One lead is in the RA and the other lead is located in the RV.
   c. Pacing and sensing can occur in both heart chambers, closely "mimicking" normal heart function (physiologic pacing).
3. Biventricular pacemaker.
   a. One lead is in the RA, one is in the RV, and one is in the LV via the coronary sinus.
   b. In single RV (traditional) pacing, there is slight delay of the LV contracting as the electrical impulse begins in the RV and moves to the LV, giving the characteristic left bundle-branch block appearance. By pacing both RV and LV at the same time, the pacemaker can resynchronize a heart whose opposing walls do not contract in synchrony.
4. Pacemaker leads may be threaded through a vein into the RA or RV (endocardial/transvenous approach) or introduced by direct penetration of the chest wall and attached to the LV or RA (see Figure 8-6).
5. Fixation devices located at the end of the pacemaker lead allow for secure attachment of the lead to the heart, reducing the possibility of lead dislodgement.
6. Temporary leads protrude from the incision and are connected to the external pulse generator. Permanent leads are connected to the pulse generator implanted underneath the skin.

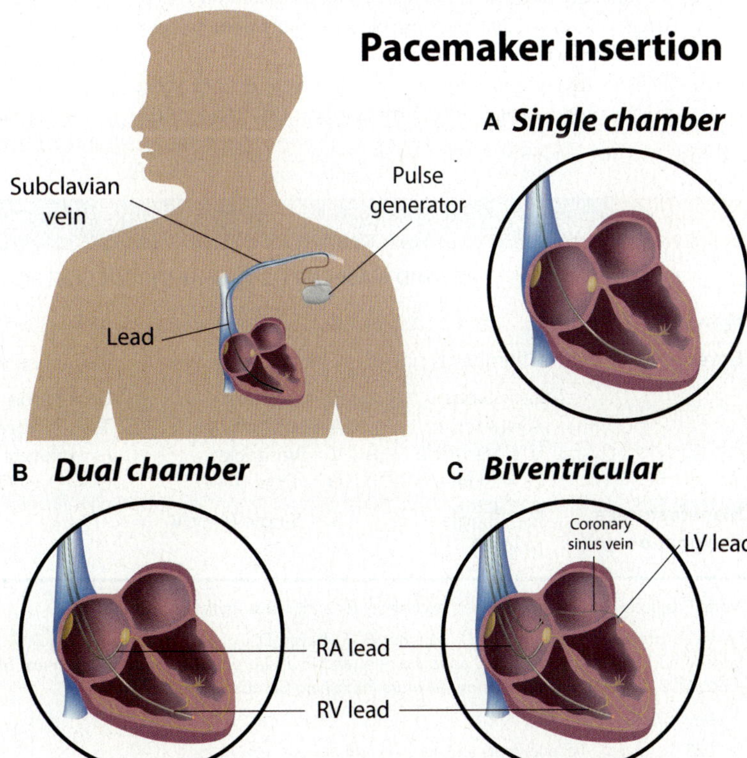

Figure 8-6. Permanent pacemaker insertion with (A) single-chamber lead (threaded through a central vein into the RV), (B) dual-chamber lead (one in the RA, one in the RV), and (C) biventricular pacemaker with one lead in the right ventricle, one lead in the LV and a third lead (not always present) guided into the RA. LV, left ventricle; RA, right atrium; RV, right ventricle (Shutterstock/Alila Medical Media).

Pacemaker Function

Cardiac pacing refers to the ability of the pacemaker to stimulate the atrium, the ventricle, or both heart chambers in sequence and initiate electrical depolarization and cardiac contraction. Cardiac pacing is evidenced on the ECG by the presence of a "spike" or "pacing artifact."

Pacing Functions

1. Atrial pacing—direct stimulation of the RA producing a "spike" on the ECG preceding a P wave.
2. Ventricular pacing—direct stimulation of the RV or LV producing a "spike" on the ECG preceding a QRS complex causing a widen QRS complex (bundle-branch block appearance).
3. AV pacing—direct stimulation of the RA and either ventricle in sequence; mimics normal cardiac conduction, allowing the atria to contract before the ventricles. ("Atrial kick" received by the ventricles allows for an increase in CO.)

Sensing Functions

Cardiac pacemakers have the ability to "see" intrinsic cardiac activity when it occurs (sensing).

1. Demand—ability to "sense" intrinsic cardiac activity and deliver a pacing stimulus only if the HR falls below a preset rate limit.
2. Fixed—no ability to "sense" intrinsic cardiac activity; the pacemaker can't "synchronize" with the heart's natural activity and consistently delivers a pacing stimulus at a preset rate.
3. Triggered—ability to deliver pacing stimuli in response to "sensing" a cardiac activity.
   a. "Sees" atrial activity (P waves) and delivers a pacing spike to the ventricle after an appropriate delay (usually 0.16 second, similar to PR interval).
   b. Maintains AV synchrony and increases HR based on increases in the body demands that occur with exercise or during stress.
   c. "Physiologic" sensors are being developed as alternatives to "trigger" a ventricular response because many patients have atrial dysfunction.
   d. "Sensor-driven" rate-responsive pacemakers do not sense atrial activity; a triggered ventricular beat occurs when the pacemaker senses either increases in muscle activity, temperature, and oxygen utilization or changes in blood pH.

Capture Functions

1. The pacemaker's ability to generate a response from the heart (contraction) after electrical stimulation is referred to as capture. Capture is determined by the strength of the electrical stimulus, measured in mA, the amount of time the stimulus is applied to the heart (pulse width), and by contact of the distal tip of the pacing lead to healthy myocardial tissue.
   a. "Electrical" capture is indicated by a pacer spike followed by a corresponding P wave or QRS complex.
   b. "Mechanical" capture of the ventricles is determined by a palpable pulse corresponding to the electrical event.
   c. During transcutaneous pacing, verify mechanical capture by palpating a femoral pulse, the preferred pulse check. This avoids interference while checking for a pulse from the jerking caused by the transcutaneous pacing.

Pacemaker Codes

The Intersociety Commission for Heart Disease (ICHD) has established a five-letter code to describe the normal functioning of today's sophisticated pacemakers. Each letter indicates the particular characteristic of the pacer (see Table 8-2).

Nursing Process for PPM Implantation

Nursing Assessment and Preprocedure Care

1. Assess patient's knowledge level of procedure.
2. Instruct patient that they may have nothing by mouth before the procedure.
3. Establish a peripheral IV.
4. Temporary transvenous pacemaker:
   a. Explain to the patient that there will be a central line placed either in the neck area or the groin area. Local anesthetic will be used to minimize discomfort during the insertion. Educate the patient on the prevention of central line–associated bloodstream infections.
   b. During the procedure, the patient will need to remain still and quiet.

Table 8-2 Five-Letter Code for Pacemakers

REVISED NASPE/BPEG Generic (NBG) CODE FOR PACING NOMENCLATURE

Position	I	II	III	IV	V
Category	Chamber(s) paced	Chamber(s) sensed	Response to sensing	Rate modulation	Multisite pacing
	O = None A = Atrium V = Ventricle D = Dual (A+V)	O = None A = Atrium V = Ventricle D = Dual (A+V)	O = None T = Triggered I = Inhibited D = Dual (T+I)	O = None R = Rate modulation	O = None A = Atrium V = Ventricle D = Dual (A+V)
Manufacturer's designation only	S = Single (A or V)	S = Single (A or V)			

Note: Positions I through III are used exclusively for antibradyarrhythmia function.

From Bernstein, A. D., Daubert, J. C., Fletcher, R. D., Hayes, D. L., Lüderitz, B., Reynolds, D. W., Schoenfeld, M. H., & Sutton, R. (2002), The revised NASPE/BPEG generic code for antibradycardia, adaptive-rate, and multisite pacing. *Pacing and Clinical Electrophysiology, 25*(2), 260–264. https://doi.org/10.1046/j.1460-9592.2002.00260.x, with permission.© Futura Publishing Company, Inc. 2002

Graphic 68327 Version 3.0.

c. Discuss with the patient the precautions and restrictions required with a temporary pacemaker in place.

5. PPM:
   a. Explain to patient that pacemaker insertion will be performed in an operating or special procedures room with fluoroscopically and continuous ECG monitoring.
   b. Describe local anesthetic that will be used to minimize discomfort; sedation.
   c. Explain to patient that the usual placement for a PPM is in the left upper chest.
   d. If the patient had a recent infection, ensure that blood cultures are taken and are negative according to hospital policy, before any implantable device procedure so that implant or leads do not become infected.
   e. Advise the patient that the incision will be closed with Steri-Strips (suture or staples may also be used). Instruction about keeping the area dry will be provided when the patient is discharged.

Nursing Interventions

Maintaining Adequate CO

1. Record the following information after insertion of the pacemaker:
   a. Pacemaker manufacturer, model, and lead type.
   b. Operating mode (based on ICHD code).
   c. Programmed settings: lower rate limit, upper rate limit, AV delay, and pacing thresholds.
   d. Patient's underlying rhythm.
   e. Patient's response to procedure.
2. Attach ECG electrodes for continuous monitoring of HR and rhythm. If the monitor has a pacer detection mode, turn it on to see the pacer spikes.
   a. Set alarm limits 5 beats below the lower rate limit and 5 to 10 beats above the upper rate limits (ensures immediate detection of pacemaker malfunction or failure).
   b. Keep alarms on at all times.
3. Analyze rhythm strips per facility protocol and as necessary.
   a. Identify the presence or absence of pacing artifact.
   b. Differentiate paced P waves and paced QRS complexes from spontaneous beats.
   c. Measure AV delay (if pacemaker has dual-chamber functions).
   d. Determine the paced rate.
   e. Analyze the paced rhythm for presence and consistency of capture (every pacing spike is followed by atrial or ventricular depolarization).
   f. Analyze the rhythm for presence and consistency of proper sensing. (After a spontaneous beat, the pacemaker should not fire unless the interval between the spontaneous beat and the paced beat equals the lower pacing rate or the paced beat follows the programmed AV delay.)
4. Monitor vital signs as per facility protocol and as necessary.
5. Monitor urine output and level of consciousness—ensures adequate CO achieved with paced rhythm.
6. Observe for dysrhythmias (ventricular ectopic activity can occur because of irritation of ventricular wall by lead wire).
   a. Monitor for competitive rhythms, such as runs of atrial fibrillation or flutter, accelerated junctional, or idioventricular or ventricular tachycardia.
   b. Report dysrhythmias.
   c. Administer antiarrhythmic therapy, as directed.
7. Obtain 12-lead ECG, as ordered.

Avoiding Injury

1. Note that a postpacemaker insertion chest x-ray has been taken to ensure correct lead wire position and that no fluid is in the lungs.
2. Ensure the pacemaker was interrogated prior to discharge.
3. Monitor for signs and symptoms of hemothorax—inadvertent punctures of the subclavian vein or artery, which can cause fatal hemorrhage; observe for diaphoresis, hypotension, shortness of breath, chest deviation, and restlessness; immediate surgical intervention may be necessary.
4. Monitor for signs and symptoms of pneumothorax—inadvertent puncture of the lung; observe for acute onset of dyspnea, cyanosis, chest pain, absent breath sounds over involved lung, acute anxiety, and hypotension. Prepare for chest tube insertion.
5. Evaluate continually for evidence of bleeding/hematoma.
   a. Check incision site frequently for bleeding/hematoma.
   b. Apply manual pressure carefully without pushing against pacemaker generator box.
   c. Palpate for pulses distal to the insertion site. (Swelling of tissues from bleeding may impede arterial flow.)
6. Be aware of hazards in the facility that can interfere with pacemaker function or cause pacemaker failure and PPM damage.
   a. Avoid use of electric razors.
   b. Avoid direct placement of defibrillator paddles over pacemaker generator; anterior placement of paddles should be 4 inches (10 cm) away from pacemaker; always evaluate pacemaker function after defibrillation.
   c. Electrocautery devices and transcutaneous electrical nerve stimulator (TENS) units pose a risk.
   d. Studies have shown that patients may safely have an MRI with a PPM. Check with the cardiologist.
   e. Caution must be used if patient will receive radiation therapy; the pacemaker should be repositioned if the unit lies directly in the radiation field.
7. Monitor for electrolyte imbalances, hypoxia, and myocardial ischemia. (The amount of energy the pacemaker needs to stimulate depolarization may need adjustment if any of these are present.)

Preventing Infection

1. Take temperature every 4 hours; report elevations. (Suspect PPM as infection source if temperature elevation occurs.)
2. Observe incision site for signs and symptoms of local infection: redness, purulent drainage, warmth, and soreness.
3. Be alert to manifestations of bacteremia. (Patients with endocardial leads are at risk for endocarditis; see page 258.)
4. Observe incision site for swelling as a hematoma may occur. Usually, any form of heparin is held for 24 to 48 hours post insertion.
5. Clean incision site, as directed, using sterile technique.
6. Instruct patient to keep incision site dry, which means no showers for 24 hours or as instructed.
7. Evaluate patient's complaints of increasing tenderness and discomfort at incision site.
8. Administer antibiotic therapy, as prescribed, after PPM insertion.

Relieving Anxiety

1. Offer careful explanations regarding anticipated procedures and treatments, and answer the patient's questions with concise explanations.
2. Encourage patient and family to use coping mechanisms to overcome anxieties—talking, crying, and walking.

3. Encourage patient to accept responsibility for care.
   a. Review care plan with patient and family.
   b. Encourage patient to make decisions regarding a daily schedule of self-care activities.
   c. Engage patient in goal setting. Establish with patient priorities of care and time frames to accomplish goals up until discharge.
4. Monitor for unwarranted fears expressed by patient and family (commonly, pacemaker failure) and provide explanations to alleviate fear. Explain to patient the life expectancy of batteries and the measures taken to check for failure (see "Patient Education").

Minimizing the Effects of Immobility

1. Encourage patient to take deep breaths frequently each hour (promotes pulmonary function); however, caution against vigorous coughing because this could cause lead dislodgement.
2. Instruct patient in dorsiflexion exercises of ankles and tightening of calf muscles. This promotes venous return and prevents venous stasis. Exercises should be done hourly.
3. Restrict movement of affected extremity (no restriction for leadless pacemaker).
   a. Place arm nearest to PPM implant in a sling as directed. Sling use can range from 6 to 24 hours, according to the prescribed order.
   b. Instruct patient to gradually resume range of motion (ROM) of extremity as directed (usually 24 hours for permanent implants). Instruct the patient not to raise their arm on the incision side above shoulder level or stretch their arm behind their back for as long as directed by the health care provider; this allows the leads a chance to secure themselves inside the heart.
   c. Evaluate patient's arm movements to ensure normal ROM progression; assist patient with passive ROM of extremity as necessary (prevents development of shoulder stiffness caused by prolonged joint immobility); consult physical therapy as directed if stiffness and pain occur.
4. Assist patient with activities of daily living (ADLs) as appropriate.

Relieving Pain

1. Prepare patient for the discomfort they may experience after pacemaker implant.
   a. Explain to patient that incisional pain will occur after procedure; pain will subside after the first week, but they may have some soreness for up to 4 weeks.
2. Administer analgesics as directed; attempt to coincide peak analgesic effect with performance of ROM exercises and ADLs.
3. Offer back rubs to promote relaxation.
4. Provide patient with diversional activities.
5. Evaluate effectiveness of pain-relieving modalities.
6. Explain to the patient about the potential for discomfort during transcutaneous pacing; however, assure patient that the lowest energy possible will be used and analgesics/anxiolytics will be given.

Maintaining a Positive Body Image

1. Encourage patient and family to express concerns regarding self-image and pacemaker implant.
2. Reassure patient and significant other that sexual activity and modes of dressing will not be altered by pacemaker implantation.
3. Offer pacemaker support group information to the patient.
4. Encourage spouse or significant other to discuss concerns of self-image with patient.

Patient Education and Health Maintenance

Anatomy and Physiology of the Heart

Use diagrams to identify heart structure, conduction system, area where pacemaker is inserted, and why the pacemaker is needed.

Pacemaker Function

1. Give patient the manufacturer's instructions (for particular pacemaker) and help familiarize patient with pacemaker.
2. If available, give patient a pacemaker to hold and identify unique features of patient's pacemaker, or show patient a picture of pacemaker.
3. Explain to patient the purpose and function of the component parts of the pacemaker: generator and lead system.

Activity

1. Reassure patient that normal activities will be able to be resumed.
2. Explain to patient that it takes about 2 months to develop full ROM of the arm (fibrosis occurs around the lead and stabilizes it in the heart).
3. Review driving restrictions.
4. Specific instructions include the following:
   a. Instruct patient not to lift items over 3 pounds (1.4 kg) or perform difficult arm maneuvers.
   b. Tell patient to avoid activities that involve rough contact around the pacemaker site.
   c. Caution patient not to fire a rifle with it resting over pacemaker implant.
   d. Sexual activity may be resumed when desired.
   e. Instruct patient not to rub or massage around pacemaker site.
5. Instruct patient to gauge activities according to sensations of moderate pain in the arm or site of implant and stretching sensation in and around implant site.

Pacemaker Failure

1. Teach patient to check own pulse rate daily for 1 full minute and to keep a chart for provider visit. This pulse check should be done at rest. (Patients may check pulse daily to ensure all is well and promote a sense of control.)
2. Teach patient to:
   a. Immediately report slowing of pulse lower than set rate or greater than 100.
   b. Report signs and symptoms of dizziness, fainting, palpitation, prolonged hiccups, and chest pain to health care provider immediately. These signs are indicative of pacemaker failure.
   c. Take pulse while these feelings are being experienced.
3. Instruct the patient to wear identification bracelet and carry pacemaker identification card that lists pacemaker type, rate, health care provider's name, and facility where the pacemaker was inserted; encourage the significant other to also keep a card with patient's pacemaker information.

Electromagnetic Interference

1. Advise patient that improvements in pacemaker design have reduced problems of electromagnetic interference (EMI).
2. Caution patient that EMI could interfere with pacemaker function.
   a. Inappropriate inhibition or triggering of pacemaker stimuli causing lightheadedness, syncope, or death.

b. Atrial oversensing may cause inappropriate pacemaker acceleration and can cause palpitations, hypotension, or angina in patients.
c. Rapid pacing can also result in ventricular fibrillation.
d. Reversion to a synchronous pacing mode. A common response to transient reversion is asynchrony pacing, which can cause irregular heartbeats or a decrease in CO, and that may stimulate ventricular tachyarrhythmias.
e. Reprogramming of the pacemaker or permanent damage to the pacemaker's circuitry or the electrode–tissue interface is less frequent in occurrence.
f. Teach patient to move 4 to 6 feet away from the source and to check pulse if dizziness or palpitations occur. Pulse should return to normal after moving away from interference.

3. Explain that high-energy radiation, linear power amplifiers, antennas, industrial arc welders, electrocautery equipment, TENS, unshielded motors (cars, boats), MRI equipment found in facilities, and junkyards may affect pacemaker function.
4. Tell patient that metal detectors or handheld wands may affect pacemaker function and that pacemakers will set off the alarm at metal detector gates. Therefore, patient should show pacemaker identification card and request a hand search.
5. Antitheft devices may interfere with pacemaker function if the patient remains stationary for an extended period of time near the device. Walking by the device should not interfere with pacemaker function.
6. Tell patient that household and kitchen appliances will not affect pacemaker function. Microwave ovens are no longer a threat to pacemaker operation (however, old warning signs may still be near microwave ovens). Cell phones are safe as long as they are 6 inches away from pacemaker site. Encourage patient to use the ear on the opposite side of the pacemaker site.

Care of Pacemaker Site

1. Advise patient to wear loose-fitting clothing around the area of pacemaker implantation until it has healed.
2. Watch for signs and symptoms of infection around generator and leads—fever, heat, pain, and skin breakdown at the implant site.
3. Advise patient to keep incision clean and dry. Encourage tub baths rather than showers for the first 10 days after pacemaker implantation.
   a. Instruct patient not to scrub incision site or clean site with bath water.
   b. Teach patient to clean the incision site with antiseptic, as directed.
4. Explain to patient that healing will take approximately 3 months.
   a. Instruct patient to maintain a well-balanced diet to promote healing.
5. Inform patient that there is no increased risk of endocarditis with dental cleaning or procedures, so antibiotic prophylaxis is not necessary.

POPULATION AWARENESS Older patients may experience delayed wound healing because of poor nutritional status. Evaluate nutritional intake carefully and offer a balanced diet including vitamin C to ensure proper healing.

Follow-Up

1. Make sure that the patient has a copy of ECG tracing (according to facility policy) for future comparisons. Encourage patient to have regular pacemaker checkups for monitoring function and integrity of the pacemaker. Encourage an appointment with the cardiologist in 7 to 10 days.
2. Inform patient that trans-telephonic evaluation of implanted cardiac pacemakers for battery and electrode failure is available.
3. Review medications with patient before discharge.
4. Inform patient that the pulse generator will have to be surgically removed to replace the battery and that it is a relatively simple procedure performed under local anesthesia.

Evaluation: Expected Outcomes

- Vital signs stable; pacing spikes rated on ECG tracing.
- Breath sounds noted throughout; respirations unlabored.
- Incision without drainage.
- Asks questions and participates in care.
- Affected arm and pacer site show decreased edema.
- Reports pain relief.
- Verbalizes acceptance of pacemaker.

Defibrillation and Cardioversion

Defibrillation is the use of electrical energy, delivered over a brief period, to temporarily depolarize the heart, so that when it repolarizes, it has a better chance of resuming normal electrical activity. It is used to treat ventricular fibrillation and ventricular tachycardia without a pulse, with the goal of converting to normal sinus rhythm.

Synchronized cardioversion is the use of electrical energy that is synchronized to the QRS complex so as not to hit the T wave during the cardiac cycle, which may cause ventricular fibrillation. It is used to treat atrial fibrillation, atrial flutter, supraventricular tachycardia, and ventricular tachycardia with a pulse.

Concepts

1. Types of defibrillators:
   a. Direct current defibrillators contain a transformer, an alternating current–direct current converter, a capacitor to store direct current, a charge switch, and a discharge switch to the electrodes to complete the circuit.
   b. Portable defibrillators have a battery as a power source and must be plugged in at all times when not in use.
   c. Automatic external defibrillator (AED) may be used inside the facility or in the community to deliver electric shock to the heart before trained personnel arrive with a manual defibrillator. AEDs are accurate to be used by less trained individuals because the device has a detection system that analyzes the person's rhythm, detects the presence of ventricular fibrillation or tachycardia, and instructs the operator to discharge a shock.
2. Steps in defibrillation:
   a. Immediately implement cardiopulmonary resuscitation (CPR) until the defibrillator is available.
   b. Expose the patient's bare chest and apply defibrillator paddles or pads according to manufacturer's instructions (see Figure 8-7).
   c. Turn the defibrillator to recommended setting, usually 200 joules, and charge paddles.
   d. Once the defibrillator is charged, give the "all-clear" warning, and ensure that no one is touching the patient. Shock the patient by doing the following:
      i. Paddles: push the discharge buttons (shock) on the paddles while exerting 25 pounds of pressure on the patient's chest.

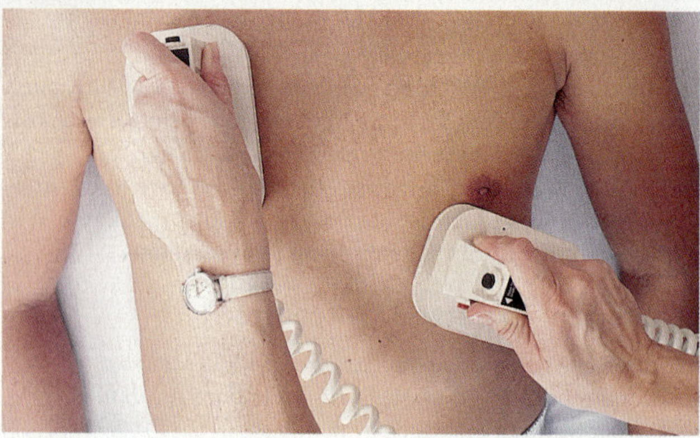

Figure 8-7. Paddle placement for ventricular fibrillation.

ii. Pads: push the discharge buttons (shock) on the defibrillator device.

e. Continue CPR for 2 minutes and repeat defibrillation process unless return of spontaneous circulation (ROSC) has occurred.

f. Once ROSC is restored, continue supportive care of the patient.

3. Steps in cardioversion:
   a. Ensure that laboratory results are available, serum potassium level is normal, digoxin has not been given, and oxygen is available. The procedure is usually elective; therefore, fasting may be ordered.
   b. Have emergency equipment available in the room, such as oxygen and suction.
   c. Apply paddles or multifunctional pads according to manufacturer's instructions; for cardioversion, pads are preferred.
   d. Turn defibrillator to synchronize setting and charge to the ordered level. Ensure that the synchronized marking is visible.
   e. Once the machine is charged, give the "all-clear" warning and ensure that no one is touching the patient. Shock the patient by doing the following:
      i. Paddles: push the discharge buttons (shock) on the paddles while exerting 25 pounds of pressure on the patient's chest.
      ii. Pads: Push the discharge buttons (shock) on the defibrillator device.
   f. Be aware that when the shock button is pressed, there may be a delay while synchronizing with the R wave until the shock is delivered.

CLINICAL JUDGMENT Synchronized cardioversion is generally contraindicated when a patient has been taking a significant amount of digoxin because more lethal dysrhythmias may occur after electric discharge.

Implantable Cardioverter–Defibrillator

The *ICD* is a device that delivers electric shocks directly to the heart muscle (defibrillation) to terminate lethal dysrhythmias: ventricular fibrillation and ventricular tachycardia. The ICD is surgically placed by one of four approaches: lateral thoracotomy, median sternotomy (in conjunction with cardiac surgery), subxiphoid, or subintercostal. All ICDs have a pacing function, if needed (see Figure 8-8).

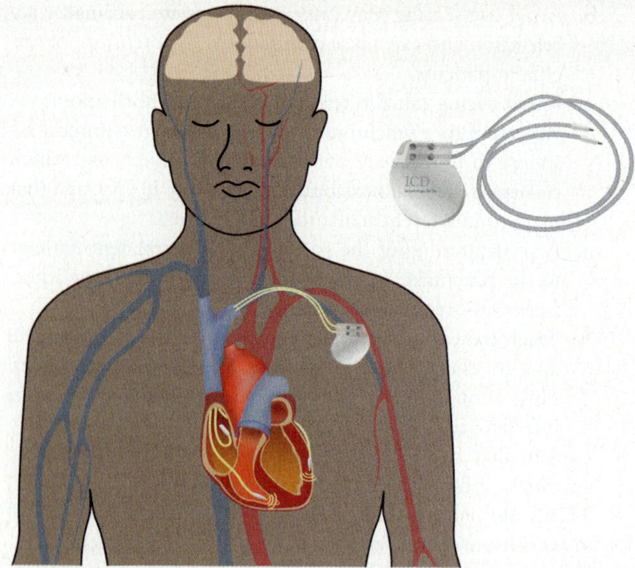

Figure 8-8. Implantable cardioverter–defibrillator (Shutterstock/Yoko Design).

Concepts

1. Sudden cardiac death as a result of ventricular tachycardia or fibrillation remains the leading cause of death in the United States.
2. ICDs terminate ventricular fibrillation and tachycardia automatically, thereby preventing sudden death.
3. Current ICDs have a variety of flexible programming and therapeutic options. For patients who also need pacemaker functions, the ICD serves this purpose. At the basic level, ICDs detect dysrhythmia based on duration and rate criteria. The ICD has the ability to distinguish dysrhythmias requiring ICD therapy from other cardiac dysrhythmias. ICDs can treat VT with antitachycardia pacing (ATP) or shock. This therapy allows the ICD to attempt to pace the patient out of VT for a preset amount of tries before shocking the patient. The ICD can be programmed with up to three zones to provide different therapies for tachyarrhythmias. ICDs have the ability to store information and transmit it to the interrogation device.

Indications

May be divided into two subgroups:

1. Secondary prevention of sudden cardiac death in patients with prior sustained VT/Ventricular fibrillation (VF):
   a. Episode of resuscitated VT/VF or sustained hemodynamically unstable VT in which reversible causes cannot be identified. This includes underlying heart diseases, idiopathic VT/VF, and congenital long QT syndrome.
   b. Patients with episodes of spontaneous sustained VT in the presence of heart disease.
   c. The key point is the prevention of total mortality.
2. Primary prevention of sudden cardiac death in patients at risk of life-threatening VT/VF:
   a. Patients who have received optimal medical management yet remain at high risk of sudden cardiac death.
3. Patients with prior myocardial infarction (MI) and left ventricular ejection fraction (LVEF) $\leq$30%.

4. Patients with cardiomyopathy New York Heart Association (NYHA) class II to III and LVEF ≤ 35%. Non-ischemic cardiomyopathy generally requires 3 months of optimal therapy and persistent LVEF ≤ 35%. If revascularized, also wait 3 months to be reevaluated for ICD.
5. Some patients with heart failure who also have intraventricular conduction delay are candidates for ICD.
6. Congenital long QT syndrome.
7. High-risk patients with Brugada syndrome, catecholaminergic polymorphic VT, or other channelopathies.

Design

The ICD is slightly larger than a pacemaker and consists of two parts:

1. Pulse generator—contains the circuitry and battery to detect dysrhythmias and generate the electric shock. The generator is usually placed in the left pectoral region and is commonly referred to as the active can or hot-can.
   a. Battery life depends on the amount of shocks and pacing and is usually 5 to 6 years.
   b. The direct current electric shock delivered is 25 to 35 joules. Depending on the device, it can be programmed up to 41 joules.
2. Lead system—consists of two components.
   a. Pace–sense component: monitors the heart rhythm and can deliver pacing output.
   b. Shocking coils: deliver the electrical shocks needed for defibrillation.
3. Most ICDs (but not all) can be noninvasively deactivated by a doughnut-shaped magnet. This will disable the ICD therapies of ATP and electrical cardioversion–defibrillation but will not turn off the pacemaker function. However, the magnet may initiate asynchronous pacing.

Function

Electric shocks are delivered in a programmed sequence:

1. The device detects a lethal dysrhythmia, charges and reconfirms that the lethal dysrhythmia is still present, and then "defibrillates" the heart. The lethal dysrhythmia must meet two programmed criteria (rate and amount of time spent from the isoelectric line) to trigger the device to emit an initial electric shock. The number of joules necessary to convert each patient is determined during insertion and testing of the device; it is usually 15 to 25 joules.
2. Nontermination of the lethal dysrhythmia by the initial shock triggers the device to continue the sequence (detect, charge, and defibrillate) until a total of four or five shocks have been delivered (the number of shocks depends on the device model implanted).
   a. Subsequent shocks are slightly higher, at 30 to 32 joules.
   b. The total sequence lasts approximately 2 minutes.
3. Termination of the lethal dysrhythmia after the shock sequence signals the device to revert to the "detection" mode of operation and not to reinitiate the shocking sequence. The device will reinitiate the shocking sequence only if a rhythm other than the lethal dysrhythmia is detected and maintained for at least 35 seconds. If this criterion is met and another lethal dysrhythmia is detected, the device will cycle through the shocking sequence again.
4. Termination of a lethal dysrhythmia at any time during the shocking sequence signals the device to interrupt the sequence, return to a detection mode, and reinitiate the shocking sequence if another lethal dysrhythmia is detected.

Complications

1. Many complications that occurred previously with ICDs have been decreased by the use of the transvenous technique for implantation that is similar to that of PPM insertion.
2. Complications associated with the implantation of the ICD include:
   a. Acceleration of arrhythmias.
   b. Air emboli.
   c. Bleeding.
   d. Perforation of the myocardium.
   e. Pneumothorax.
   f. Puncture of the subclavian vein.
   g. Thromboemboli.
   h. Venous occlusion.
3. Complications that can occur after placement of an ICD:
   a. Chronic nerve damage.
   b. Diaphragmatic stimulation.
   c. Erosion of pulse generator.
   d. Formation of pocket hematoma.
   e. Fluid accumulation/seroma.
   f. Infection of pocket/system.
   g. Keloid formation.
   h. Lead dislodgement.
   i. Lead fracture and insulation breaks.
   j. Venous thrombosis.

Nursing Interventions

Reducing Anxiety

1. Explain to patient and family the reason for implant, surgical procedure, and preprocedure and postprocedure management:
   a. Performed in the operating room or in an electrophysiology laboratory.
   b. Incision location.
   c. May need endotracheal (ET) intubation if unable to sedate.
   d. IV line; continuous ECG monitoring.
   e. Early mobilization after procedure.
   f. Coughing and deep breathing exercises.
   g. Management of incisional pain.
   h. Device turned on once implanted.
2. Provide emotional support to patient and family.
   a. Assess patient's and family's knowledge level, support systems, and usual coping mechanisms.
   b. Psychiatric counseling may be beneficial because patient is facing life-threatening issues.
   c. Encourage patient and family to verbalize fears or expectations of hospitalization, lifestyle adjustments, self-concept, body image, and device malfunction (misfiring or failure to fire).
   d. Reinforce to patient that daily activities will not increase the risk of the device misfiring.
   e. Explain the sensation that might be felt if the device fires and the patient is conscious. (Many patients will become unconscious before the device fires and

therefore feel no sensations.) Sensations experienced in conscious patients vary, but are commonly described as a severe chest blow.

3. Allow patient to participate in care as much as possible.
   a. Encourage patient to dress in street clothes during hospitalization. (Loose-fitting clothes are recommended to prevent chafing and irritation at the implant site.)
   b. Allow patient to look at the incision site.
   c. Give patient instructional booklets about the device.

Preventing Infection

1. Check temperature every 4 hours; report elevations. (Early postoperative fever may be due to atelectasis; defibrillator system as an infection source commonly occurs within 5 to 10 days of implantation.)
2. Evaluate incision site every 4 hours for signs of infection.
3. Culture drainage from the incision.
4. Evaluate incision for tissue erosion.
5. Monitor white blood cell (WBC) count and differential.
6. Clean incision and change dressing as directed, using aseptic technique.
7. Administer antibiotics, as ordered, before and after the procedure.

POPULATION AWARENESS Older patients may not demonstrate abnormal temperature elevations with infections and experience prolonged wound healing.

Maintaining Adequate CO

1. Monitor vital signs frequently until stable.
2. Evaluate incision site for evidence of bleeding or hematoma.
3. Evaluate urine output.
4. Be alert to risk for dysrhythmias postoperatively. (Manipulation of the heart and swelling may induce dysrhythmias 24 to 48 hours after implant.)
5. Monitor for changes in BP as a sudden drop may indicate cardiac tamponade.
6. Evaluate carefully all complaints of chest pain (noncardiac pain may be due to lead fracture or dislodgement; pain may be noted along wire pathways).
7. Auscultate heart sounds every 4 hours for the presence of friction rub or muffled heart sounds.
8. CPR should be started immediately on any patient with an implantable defibrillator who becomes unconscious and has no pulse. A slight "buzz" sensation will be felt if the implanted device delivers a shock, but it is not harmful. Gloves may be worn to minimize the sensation.

Promoting Effective Breathing Pattern

1. Ask patient to take several deep breaths every hour to expand lung fields.
2. Encourage coughing and deep breathing exercises frequently; medicate with analgesics before exercises and provide a pillow for splinting.
3. Monitor use of incentive spirometer.
4. Elevate head of bed to promote adequate ventilation.
5. Ausculate lung fields every 4 hours.
6. Assist with position changes every 2 hours while on bed rest.
7. Encourage early ambulation.
8. Administer analgesics, as ordered.

Patient Education and Health Maintenance

Introduction to Implantable Defibrillator

1. Review anatomy of the heart with emphasis on the conduction system, using a diagram of the heart.
2. Give accurate explanations, using correct medical terminology (allows patient to interact with the health care team more effectively), regarding reason for device implantation, components of system, and function of device.
   a. Use manufacturer's instructional booklet and video presentation about the device.
   b. Encourage family members to participate in the education process.

Living With the Implantable Defibrillator

1. Instruct patient and family on actions to be taken if the device fires.
   a. Explain signs and symptoms that may be experienced if a lethal dysrhythmia occurs: palpitations, dizziness, shortness of breath, and chest pain.
   b. If signs and symptoms occur, lie down and try to call 911 for help if alone.
   c. Family members should check for a pulse if patient becomes unconscious. CPR should be started immediately if no pulse is present and 911 has been called.
   d. Reinforce that shocks emitted from the device are not harmful, and CPR should never be delayed to wait for the device to complete the shocking sequence.
   e. If patient remains conscious or is unconscious with a pulse, family members should monitor patient during episode, continually assessing for a pulse during shocking sequence. After the episode, follow health care provider's instructions as directed.
   f. Notify health care provider immediately.
2. Explore with patient and family fears about failure of device, sensation associated with a shock, and injury to others if a shock occurs.
   a. Sensations experienced vary but are most commonly described as a severe blow to the chest.
   b. No injury will occur to others if in contact with patient during a shock; a slight shock may be felt by your partner if the device fires during sexual intercourse.
   c. Battery life depends on the frequency of use. The device is evaluated in 4 to 6 weeks after implantation and then every 3 months. Newer devices may allow for checks from home.
3. Review sources of EMI that should be avoided (see pages 218–219).
4. Advise patient that there is no increased risk of endocarditis, so antibiotic prophylaxis before dental work is not necessary.
5. Review with health care provider the resumption of activities, such as lifting, driving, sports, and sexual activity.

Other Instructions

1. Review care of incision site (see page 219).
2. Loose-fitting clothing should be worn until healing takes place.
3. Provide MedicAlert card; encourage carrying card at all times and obtaining a corresponding medical alert device.
4. Explain how to keep a diary of episodes and record dates of 4- to 6-month follow-up appointments.
5. Provide information to family members regarding CPR training courses.
6. Encourage use of support groups.

7. Always carry a list of current medications and name and number of provider and emergency contacts.

Evaluation: Expected Outcomes

- Verbalizes understanding of device and surgical procedure.
- Afebrile; incision without drainage.
- Vital signs stable; no dysrhythmias.
- Respirations unlabored; lungs clear.

Pericardiocentesis

Pericardiocentesis is an invasive procedure, which involves the puncture of the pericardial sac to aspirate fluid. The pericardium typically contains 10 to 50 mL of sterile fluid. Excessive fluid within the pericardial sac can cause compression of the heart chambers, resulting in an acute decrease in CO (cardiac tamponade). Fluid accumulation (pericardial effusion) can occur rapidly (acute) or slowly (subacute). The amount of excess fluid the pericardium is able to accommodate is individually based on the ability of the pericardium to stretch. Once the stretch has been maximized, intrapericardial pressure rises, possibly causing circulatory compromise.

Acute—a rapid increase of fluid into pericardial space (as little as 200 mL) causes a marked rise in intrapericardial pressure. Emergency intervention is required to prevent severe circulatory compromise.

Subacute—slow accumulation of fluid into pericardial sac over weeks or months, causing the pericardium to stretch and accommodate up to 2 L of fluid without severe increases in intrapericardial pressure.

Both of these situations require intervention to remove the pericardial fluid. Pericardiocentesis is frequently performed in the cardiac catheterization laboratory under fluoroscopy or assisted by echocardiographic imaging. In the case of severely decompensated cardiac tamponade, pericardiocentesis can be safely performed at the bedside with echocardiography.

Purposes

1. To remove fluid from the pericardial sac caused by:
   a. Infection.
   b. Malignant neoplasm or lymphoma.
   c. Trauma (blunt or penetrating wounds or from cardiac surgery or procedure).
   d. Drugs and toxins.
   e. Radiation.
   f. MI.
   g. Collagen vascular disease.
   h. Aortic dissection extending to the pericardium.
   i. Metabolic disorders, especially uremia, dialysis, and hypothyroidism.
   j. Cardiac diagnostic or interventional procedures.
   k. An idiopathic condition.
2. To obtain fluid for diagnosis.
3. To instill certain therapeutic drugs.

Sites for Pericardiocentesis

1. Subxiphoid—needle inserted in the angle between left costal margin and xiphoid.
2. Near cardiac apex, three-fourth inch (2 cm) inside left border of cardiac dullness.
3. To the left of the fifth or sixth interspace at the sternal margin.
4. Right side of fourth intercostal space just inside border of dullness.

Nursing Considerations

1. Administer sedation as prescribed to reduce anxiety.
2. If performed at bedside, ensure that patient is monitored and that emergency resuscitation equipment, defibrillator, and pacemaker are immediately available.
3. During and following the procedure, monitor for complications including dysrhythmias and bloody drainage (hemopericardium).
4. Following the procedure, report the presence of pericardial friction rub and distant heart sounds, indicating reaccumulation of fluid causing cardiac tamponade.

Percutaneous Coronary Intervention

EVIDENCE BASE Writing Committee Members, Lawton, J. S., Tamis-Holland, J. E., Bangalore, S., Bates, E. R., Beckie, T. M., Bischoff, J. M., Bittl, J. A., Cohen, M. G., DiMaio, J. M., Don, C. W., Fremes, S. E., Gaudino, M. F., Goldberger, Z. D., Grant, M. C., Jaswal, J. B., Kurlansky, P. A., Mehran, R., Metkus, T. S., Jr, … Zwischenberger, B. A. (2022). 2021 ACC/AHA/SCAI guideline for coronary artery revascularization: A report of the American College of Cardiology/American Heart Association Joint Committee on clinical practice guidelines. *Journal of the American College of Cardiology, 79*(2), e21–e129. https://doi.org/10.1016/j.jacc.2021.09.006

Percutaneous coronary intervention (PCI) is a broad term used to describe all invasive coronary interventions. Initially, PCI was limited to balloon angioplasty; however, it now includes intracoronary stenting and a wide spectrum of percutaneous procedures utilized to treat coronary disease. PCI has also replaced coronary artery bypass grafting (CABG) as the preferred treatment for coronary artery disease (CAD). Commonly performed PCIs include PTCA with intracoronary stenting, laser-assisted PTCA, and direct coronary atherectomy (DCA). Radial vascular access is recommended over femoral access for PCI, because of lower vascular complication rate and comparable efficacy and safety in relation to the primary outcome of death.

Types of Procedures

Percutaneous Transluminal Coronary Angioplasty

PTCA accesses the femoral, brachial, or radial artery, with the right femoral artery being the most common access site. The site is anesthetized and an arterial sheath is placed into the vessel. Under fluoroscopy, a catheter is advanced through the arterial sheath and directed to the coronary lesion. To visualize the coronary anatomy, specific radiographic projections are used with the fluoroscopy tube through the use of an injection of contrast dye. Once a coronary lesion or narrowing is identified, a balloon-tipped catheter is advanced through wire to the lesion. The balloon is then inflated to displace coronary plaque against the vessel wall (see Figure 8-9). Balloon inflation and deflation may be repeated until optimal flow is achieved in the affected vessel.

Intracoronary Stenting

Intracoronary stents are small meshed metal tubes that are mounted onto a balloon angioplasty catheter. Once initial angioplasty is performed, the angioplasty catheter is removed and replaced with a stent catheter. When the balloon is inflated, the stent is deployed and pressed into the intima of the artery where the occlusion existed. The balloon is deflated and the catheter is removed; however,

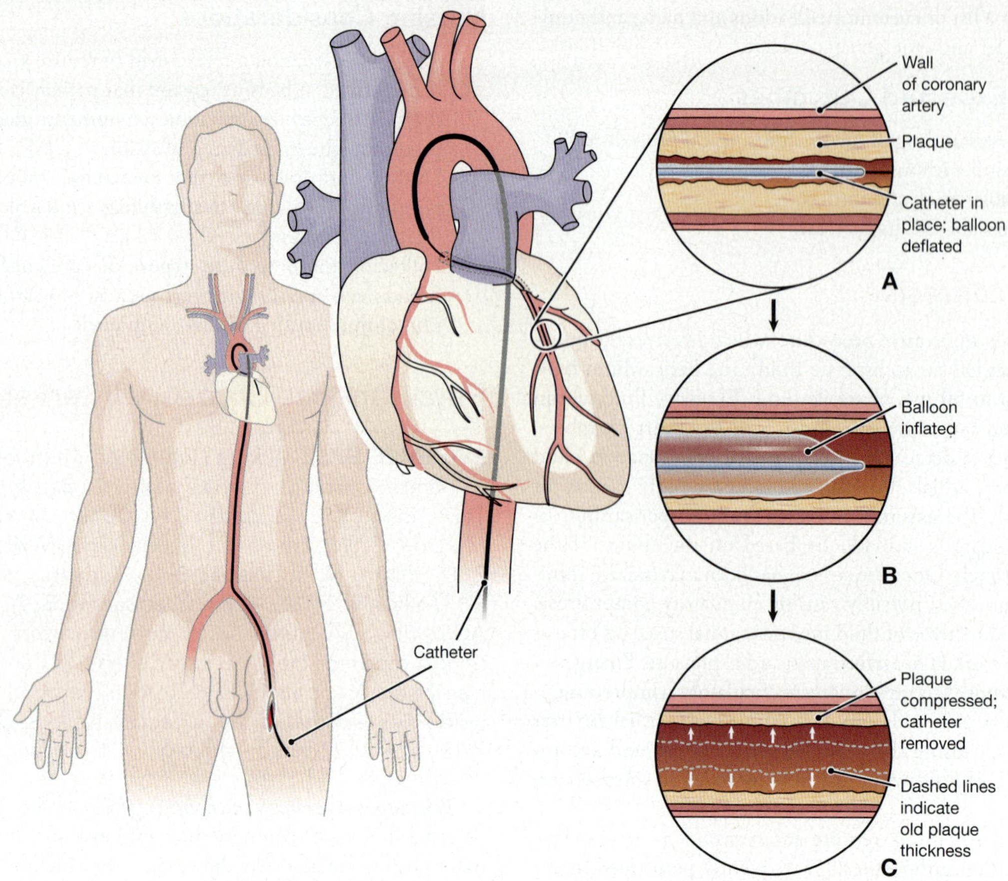

Figure 8-9. Percutaneous transluminal coronary angioplasty. (**A**) The balloon-tipped catheter is passed into the affected coronary artery. (**B**) The balloon is then rapidly inflated and deflated with controlled pressure. (**C**) The balloon disrupts the intima and causes changes in the atheroma, resulting in an increase in the diameter of the lumen of the vessel and improvement of blood flow. (Adapted from Purcell, J. A., & Giffin, P. A. [1981]. Percutaneous transluminal coronary angioplasty. *American Journal of Nursing, 9*, 1620–1626.)

the stent remains. The intracoronary stent acts as a scaffold helping to hold the artery open, thereby improving blood flow and relieving symptoms once caused by the blockage. Stents may be uncoated, called bare metal stents, or coated, called drug-eluting stents (DESs). DESs are intended and are preferred over bare metal stents to limit the overgrowth of normal tissue following implantation.

Laser-Assisted Balloon Angioplasty

A laser light is directed by a percutaneously inserted flexible fiberoptic catheter and can "vaporize" atheromatous lesions in the coronary vessels. Balloon angioplasty of the vessel may then be performed. This technique may minimize damage to the intimal lining, open diseased vessels more effectively, prevent early and long-term restenosis, and expand the use of angioplasty to calcified, unusual lesions and total occlusions. The most important complication of laser-assisted balloon angioplasty involves minor to major coronary dissection of the treated lesion.

Direct Coronary Atherectomy

DCA permits more controlled vascular injury and decreases the degree of arterial mural stretch that can occur with PTCA and balloon angioplasty. To remove plaque, DCA works by changing plaque into microscopic debris, thereby opening the diseased vessel more effectively, especially in patients who have coronary lesions not amenable to standard angioplasty. Complications associated with DCA include vascular spasm at the site of plaque removal or distal to the treated site; possible myocardial necrosis, evidenced by elevations of CK-MB; vessel perforation (infrequent but devastating); and groin complications and groin bleeding (more common with atherectomy procedures because of the size of the catheters involved).

Indications

Indications for PCI include the following (only after a comprehensive risk–benefit analysis has been reviewed): recurrent ischemia despite anti-ischemia therapy, elevated troponin levels, new ST-segment depression, symptoms of heart failure or new or worsening mitral insufficiency, depressed left ventricular systolic function, hemodynamic instability, sustained ventricular tachycardia, PCI within 6 months, prior CABG, and high-risk findings from noninvasive testing, including unprotected left main artery disease.

Contraindications

1. PCI is not indicated for patients who have no evidence of high-risk findings associated with single-vessel or multivessel CAD.
2. Procedure-related morbidity or mortality may be linked to the following relative contraindications, many of which may be avoided or reversed prior to PCI:
   a. Allergy (severe) to radiographic contrast dye.
   b. Anticoagulated state.

c. Decompensated heart failure (e.g., acute pulmonary edema).
d. Digoxin toxicity.
e. Febrile state.
f. Severe renal insufficiency.
g. Uncorrected hypertension.
h. Uncorrected hypokalemia.
i. Ventricular irritability, uncontrolled.

Complications

1. Major complications or adverse outcomes include death, post-procedure MI, or the need for emergent cardiac bypass surgery.
2. Other complications include:
   a. Anaphylaxis.
   b. Arrhythmias.
   c. Arterial dissection/coronary artery dissection.
   d. Bleeding.
   e. Cardiac perforation.
   f. Coronary occlusion, total.
   g. Hematoma at the access site.
   h. Renal failure.
   i. Restenosis—occurs in 30% to 50% of PTCA and 10% to 30% of intracoronary stenting procedures.
   j. Stroke.
   k. Tamponade.

DRUG ALERT Missed doses of anticoagulants following intracoronary stenting procedures are clearly linked to restenosis. The patient's ability to adhere to strict anticoagulation protocol will have an impact on the success of the procedure.

Nursing Interventions

Reducing Anxiety

1. Reinforce the reasons for the procedure.
   a. Describe the location of the coronary vessels using a diagram of the heart.
   b. Describe/draw the location of the patient's lesion using a heart diagram.
2. Explain the events that will occur before, during, and after the procedure. Preparation minimizes anxiety and increases adherence to the care regimen.
   a. Performed in the cardiac catheterization laboratory; similar to the cardiac catheterization procedure (see page 1196).
   b. Mild sedation given; patient remains awake throughout the procedure to report any chest pain (indicates myocardial ischemia).
   c. Assure patient that chest pain will be taken care of during the procedure.
3. Prepare patient for complications of procedure. Provide preoperative teaching to patient and family regarding procedure, potential complications, and risks associated with heart surgery (see page 1197).
4. Explain the necessity of the IV, ECG monitoring, frequent vital sign and groin checks, and remaining nothing by mouth (NPO) before the procedure.

Maintaining Adequate CO

1. Check vital signs according to facility policy, typically every 15 minutes for 1 hour, then every 30 minutes for 2 hours, and subsequently every 1 to 2 hours.
2. Continually evaluate for signs and symptoms of restenosis.
   a. Emphasize importance of reporting any chest discomfort or jaw, back, or arm pain and/or nausea and abdominal distress.
   b. Perform ECG for all complaints suspicious of possible myocardial ischemia.
   c. Administer oxygen and vasodilator therapy for pain, as directed.
   d. Obtain creatine kinase (CK) and isoenzymes as directed.
   e. Keep patient NPO if prolonged chest pain occurs (patient may return to catheterization laboratory).
3. Administer medications to maintain vessel patency.
   a. Antiplatelet or antithrombin agents may be given during and after procedure to prevent reocclusion (e.g., cangrelor, tirofiban, bivalirudin, eptifibatide, abciximab). Clopidogrel, or prasugrel, or ticagrelor may be given prior to PCI after ST-elevation myocardial infarction (STEMI).
   b. Low-dose heparin or low-molecular-weight heparin (enoxaparin) may also be used.
   c. Many patients are then maintained on medications such as clopidogrel, ticagrelor, or prasugrel. Aspirin and statins are also used. Reinforce adherence with drug therapy.
4. Evaluate fluid and electrolyte balance.
   a. Record intake and output.
   b. Encourage fluid intake or maintain IV fluids pre- and post-procedure to ensure adequate hydration to prevent contrast medium–induced nephropathy.
   c. Observe for dysrhythmias possibly related to potassium imbalance. Excessive diuresis causes potassium depletion.
   d. Administer potassium supplement, as prescribed.
5. Be alert to the risk of vasovagal reaction during removal of groin catheter if closure device is not employed.
   a. Observe for bradycardia, hypotension, diaphoresis, or nausea.
   b. Administer IV atropine, as directed.
   c. Place patient in Trendelenburg position to promote blood return to the heart and improve hypotension.
   d. Give fluid challenge as directed.

Preventing Bleeding

1. Refer to facility policy for activity progression regimen, usually gradual head elevation with ambulation within 4 to 6 hours after sheath removal. Maintain bed rest with affected extremity immobilized and head of bed elevated no more than 30 degrees (in the event the catheter remains) to prevent catheter dislodgement and bleeding.
2. Mark peripheral pulses before the procedure with indelible ink.
3. Check peripheral pulse of affected extremity and insertion site with each vital sign check.
4. Observe color, temperature, and sensation of affected extremity with each vital sign check.
5. Report if extremities become cool and pale and pulses become significantly diminished or absent.
6. Look for presence of hematoma and mark hematoma to note change in size. Report if hematoma continues to enlarge.
7. Note petechiae, hematuria, and complaints of flank pain (vessel patency is maintained by not reversing intraprocedure heparinization; chance of bleeding is increased).
8. Apply direct pressure over insertion site if bleeding is observed and report it immediately.
9. Check bed linen under patient frequently for blood.
10. Ask patient to report sensation of warmth in groin area.

Relieving Pain

1. Administer analgesics and anxiolytic medication, as directed.
2. Ensure a restful environment.
   a. Provide back rubs for muscle relaxation.
   b. Minimize noise and interruptions.
   c. Offer sleep medication, as indicated.
3. Progress patient's diet as tolerated (clear liquids/full liquid diet until catheters removed); assist patient with meals.

Patient Education and Health Maintenance

Instruct patient as follows:

1. Modification of cardiac risk factors as means of controlling progression of CAD.
2. Name of medications, action, dosage, and adverse effects.
   a. Common medications to prevent clot formation.
   b. Medications to slow HR and reduce chest pain.
   c. Medications to increase blood flow and prevent coronary artery spasm.
3. Dates and importance of any follow-up tests.
4. Symptoms for which patient should seek medical attention, such as adverse effects of medication and chest pain—especially chest pain unrelieved by nitroglycerin.
5. Restenosis (with or without stent) can occur; the patient typically presents with the previous same symptoms; however, the symptoms may vary if a different lesion is involved.

Evaluation: Expected Outcomes

- Verbalizes understanding of procedure.
- Vital signs stable; urine output adequate.
- No bleeding or hematoma at the insertion site.
- Verbalizes relief of pain.

Intra-Aortic Balloon Pump Counterpulsation

Counterpulsation is a method of assisting the failing heart and circulation by mechanical support when the myocardium is unable to generate adequate CO. The mechanism of counterpulsation therapy is opposite to the normal pumping action of the heart; counterpulsation devices pump while the heart muscle relaxes (diastole) and relax when the heart muscle contracts (systole).

Indications

1. Postcardiotomy support; low CO after cardiopulmonary bypass.
2. Severe unstable angina (UA) that is refractory to pharmacologic therapy.
3. Cardiogenic shock/left-sided heart failure after MI, myocarditis, cardiomyopathy, myocardial contusion, and refractory heart failure.
4. Postinfarction ventricular septal defects or mitral insufficiency resulting in shock.
5. Emergency support following PTCA or high-risk PCIs.
6. Hemodynamic deterioration in patients awaiting heart transplant.
7. Refractory ventricular arrhythmias.
8. Patients with severe left main coronary arterial stenosis for whom surgery is pending.
9. Adjunctive therapy after fibrinolysis in patients at high-risk restenosis.

Function

1. A balloon catheter is introduced into the femoral artery percutaneously or surgically, threaded to the proximal descending thoracic aorta, and positioned 1 to 2 cm distal to the origin of the left subclavian artery (see Figure 8-10).
2. In patients with severe peripheral arterial disease, axillary artery approach should be considered, especially if longer support is needed (see Figure 8-10). This allows for early mobilization and reduces the risk of infection.
3. The balloon catheter is attached to an external console, allowing for inflation and deflation of the balloon with gas such as He (helium). Helium has low viscosity that allows quick travel through the long connecting tubes, and it has low potential for gas embolization should the balloon rupture.

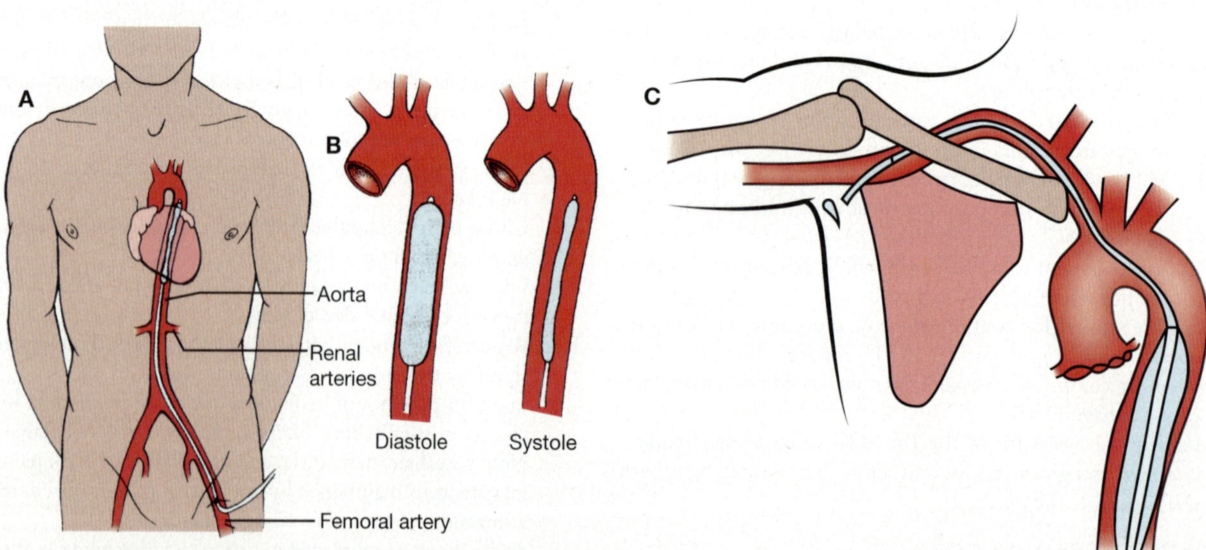

Figure 8-10. Counterpulsation. (A) Introduction of the intra-aortic balloon catheter via the femoral artery. (B) The intra-aortic balloon pump augments diastole, resulting in increased perfusion of the coronary arteries and myocardium and a decrease in the left ventricular workload. (C) Axillary approach.

4. The external console integrates the inflation and deflation sequence with the mechanical events of the cardiac cycle (systole–diastole) by "triggering" gas delivery in synchronization with the patient's ECG, the patient's arterial waveform, atrial/ventricular paced rhythm, or intrinsic pump rate.
   a. The most common method of "triggering" or signaling the intra-aortic balloon pump (IABP) is from the R wave of the patient's ECG signal.
   b. The balloon is automatically set to inflate in the middle of the T wave or at the dicrotic notch of the arterial waveform. This occurs immediately after aortic valve closure.
   c. V/AV trigger is only available in the semiautomatic mode. The ventricular spike of a ventricular or atrial-ventricular pacemaker is the trigger event. Patient must be 100% paced.
   d. Internal is used when there is no mechanical cardiac cycle (i.e., asystole or cardiopulmonary bypass). Rate can be set between 40 and 120 beats per minute (BPM).
5. The balloon is inflated at the onset of diastole; this results in an increase in diastolic aortic pressure (diastolic augmentation), which increases blood flow through the coronary arteries, thus easing the workload of a damaged heart by increasing coronary blood flow.
6. The balloon is deflated just before the onset of systole (just before aortic valve opening), facilitating the emptying of blood from the LV and decreasing pressure within the aorta as well as decreasing the resistance in the arterial tree against which the heart must pump (afterload reduction). This action results in less work for the LV.
7. This results in an increase in CO and a reduction in myocardial oxygen requirements.

CLINICAL JUDGMENT When the patient is in cardiac arrest, use the pressure trigger (semiautomatic mode) in order for the pump to identify the systolic upstroke during CPR for pump to trigger. The balloon will inflate and deflate in sync with compressions. Do not turn pump off or place on standby when needing to defibrillate the patient.

Contraindications

1. Aortic insufficiency—IABP will increase aortic insufficiency.
2. Aortic aneurysm or aortic dissection—IABP catheter may perforate a weakened vessel wall leading to thrombus formation, and inflation and deflation of the catheter may cause a thrombus to break off to become an embolus.
3. Peripheral vascular disease—femoral or iliac artery insertion may be impossible in a patient with severe vascular disease.
4. Terminal illness—outcome will not be affected, unless the patient meets the criteria for heart transplantation.
5. Prosthetic graft in thoracic aorta—may disrupt graft.
6. Coagulopathy—increases the risk of bleeding.
7. Uncontrolled sepsis.

Complications

1. Vascular injuries that may occur from IABP are:
   a. Plaque dislodging.
   b. Dissection of the aorta.
   c. Laceration of the aorta.
   d. Ischemia of the limb distal to the insertion site.
   e. Arterial perforation.
2. Peripheral nerve damage can occur from IABP if a cut down was used to insert the catheter.
3. Impairment of cerebral circulation because of balloon migration occluding the subclavian artery or by embolus and impairment of renal circulation because of balloon malposition or embolus. (Impaired circulation occurs more frequently in patients with peripheral vascular occlusive disease, in females with small vessels, and in patients with insulin-dependent diabetes.)
4. Infection at the insertion site and septicemia occur in 0.2% of patients with IABP.
5. Thrombocytopenia.
6. Hemorrhage because of anticoagulation.
7. Aortic dissection.

Nursing Interventions

Relieving Anxiety

1. Explain IABP therapy to patient and family geared to their level of understanding.
   a. Review purpose of therapy and how the IABP functions.
   b. Reinforce mobility restrictions: supine position with head of bed elevated 15 to 30 degrees and no movement or flexing of leg with IABP catheter.
   c. Explain the need for frequent monitoring of vital signs, rhythm, insertion site of affected extremity, and pulses.
   d. Discuss the sounds associated with functioning external console: balloon inflation and deflation and alarms.
2. Encourage family members to participate in patient's care.
   a. Allow family to visit patient frequently.
   b. Solicit family members' assistance in reinforcing mobility restrictions to patient and notifying nursing staff of patient comfort needs.
   c. Encourage family members to ask questions.
3. Allow patient to verbalize fears regarding therapy and illness.
4. Make sure that informed consent is obtained.
5. Administer anxiolytic medications as prescribed and indicated.
6. Keep the family informed of changes in the patient's condition.
7. Encourage realistic hope based on the patient's condition and discuss the patient's progress with the family.
8. Determine the family's previous coping mechanism to stressful situations.

Maintaining Adequate CO

1. Assist during insertion of IABP catheter.
   a. Offer patient reassurance and comfort measures (patient is only mildly sedated).
   b. Ensure strict aseptic environment during insertion.
   c. Establish ECG monitoring, choosing the lead with the largest R wave (external console senses R wave of ECG to trigger gas delivery) and without artifact (integration of the patient's cardiac cycle with the inflation and deflation balloon sequence depends on a continuous clear ECG tracing).
   d. Record date, time, and the patient's tolerance to procedure.
   e. Obtain chest x-ray to ensure placement of IABP catheter.
2. Start IABP counterpulsation immediately after insertion, as directed; review manufacturer's manual for IABP equipment in use. Updated manufacturer software allows the IABP to start up with one press of a button and automatically adjust balloon inflation or timing. Deflation can be manually adjusted. New software automatically chooses the best trigger and mode that best suits the patient's condition.
   a. Adjust the duration of balloon deflation by the arterial waveform because inflation is timed automatically;

inflation is "timed" to begin at the dicrotic notch of the arterial waveform, and deflation occurs before the next systole. Current IABPs can choose the best trigger for the patient (mostly ECG trigger and if in "auto" mode) independently from a user.

b. Set the augmentation alarm 10 mm Hg below the augmented diastolic pressure. The alarm should be on continuously and on maximum volume.
c. Compare the patient's arterial pressure waveform with and without balloon augmentation to evaluate the effectiveness of therapy. Note difference in patient's end-diastolic pressure and balloon-assisted end-diastolic pressure (the balloon-assisted end-diastolic pressure should be lower, indicating a reduction in afterload).
d. Monitor hemodynamic parameters with Swan-Ganz catheter (see page 212). Record mean arterial pressure (MAP), CVP, PAP, pulmonary capillary wedge pressure (PCWP), and CO to evaluate the overall effectiveness of therapy. Perform hemodynamic calculations to evaluate systemic vascular resistance and left ventricular stroke work. Use IABP MAP when titrating vasoactive medications.
e. Assess capillary refill, left radial pulses, and pedal and radial pulse on insertion site every 15 minutes for the first hour and then hourly or per facility policy. The balloon catheter or a thrombus can obstruct flow to the distal extremities. If the catheter migrates too high, it can obstruct flow of the left subclavian artery.

3. Monitor vital signs every 15 to 30 minutes for 4 to 6 hours and then hourly, if stable.
4. Monitor the IABP catheter site with vital signs and check for distal pulses to prevent limb ischemia.
5. Monitor neurologic status at least every 2 to 4 hours.
6. Monitor urine output from indwelling catheter every hour.
7. Maintain accurate intake and output and weigh patient daily (preferably at the same time every day).
8. Report chest pain immediately.
9. Treat dysrhythmias as directed.
10. Check for blood oozing around the IABP catheter hourly and then every 1 to 2 hours or per facility policy (anticoagulation therapy is used to prevent thrombus formation); apply direct pressure and report bleeding.
11. Axillary IABP: promote early mobilization in conjunction with physical therapy. Early mobilization may improve functional recovery, improve delirium, and provide optimization prior to transplant.
12. Blood draws are not recommended from the IABP arterial line; if needed, obtain a provider order. Place the pump in standby mode while blood is drawn and line is flushed. Povidone–iodine solution and hydrogen peroxide may degrade the catheter site and cause sheath disintegration.
13. Check facility policy for dressing changes. Refrain from placing tape on the sheath to avoid shearing and exposing the catheter to keep it sterile.

Maintaining Adequate Tissue Perfusion

1. Evaluate for ischemia of extremity with IABP catheter.
   a. Mark pulses with indelible ink to facilitate checks.
   b. Monitor peripheral pulses (dorsalis pedis, posterior tibial, popliteal, and left radial) for rhythm, character, and pulse quality every 15 minutes for 1 hour, then every 30 minutes for 1 hour, and then hourly.
   c. Use Doppler device for pulses difficult to palpate and to auscultate for bruits and hums.
   d. Observe skin temperature, color, sensation, and movement of the affected extremity. (Dusky, cool, mottled, painful, numb/tingling extremity indicates ischemia.)
2. Observe for possible indications of thromboemboli.
   a. Note decreases in urine output after initiation of therapy—may indicate renal artery emboli.
   b. Perform neurologic checks every hour to evaluate for cerebral emboli.
   c. Auscultate bowel sounds to detect evidence of ischemia.
3. Recognize early signs and symptoms of compartment syndrome. Increased pressure in tissue reduces blood flow.
   a. Note complaints of pain, pressure, and numbness of affected extremity induced by passive stretching.
   b. Palpate affected extremity for swelling and tension.
   c. Monitor CK values. Highly elevated CK may indicate compartment syndrome.
4. Ideally, keep head of bed elevated 30 degrees versus supine to avoid aspiration, but prevent upward migration of catheter.

Maintaining Skin Integrity

1. Assess skin frequently for signs of redness or breakdown.
2. Place patient on specialty mattress or bed designed to prevent pressure injuries (preferably before balloon insertion).
3. Pad bony prominences.
4. Implement passive ROM exercises with the exception of extremity with IABP catheter.
5. Turn patient from side to side as a unit every 2 hours. Patients are usually debilitated and prone to pressure injuries.
6. Follow facility guidelines for dressing change policy.

Evaluation: Expected Outcomes

1. States activity restrictions and rationale.
2. Blood pressure and CO readings improved.
3. Peripheral pulses strong; extremities warm and nail beds pink.
4. No skin redness or breakdown.

Percutaneous Left Ventricular Assist Device

Percutaneous left ventricular assist device (PLVAD) is a device placed either femorally or axillary to assist CO. PLVAD is considered a short-term device to provide hemodynamic support in patients with left ventricular failure. Device benefits include improved end-organ perfusion, reduced intracardiac filling pressures, reduced left ventricular volumes, reduced wall stress, and increased MAPs and myocardial oxygen consumption. Compared to IABP, the PLVAD provides greater improvement in hemodynamic parameters but is more costly, takes longer to insert, and has a higher rate of complications.

Indications

1. Temporary placement during high-risk PCIs.
2. Management of cardiogenic shock.
3. Acutely decompensated heart failure.
4. Cardiopulmonary arrest.

Function

The PLVAD works by creating a left ventricular bypass utilizing two different methods.

1. A cannula is placed through the aorta into the LV and sealed across the aortic valve.
   a. Placement is accomplished with the guidance of fluoroscopy or ECHO either in a procedural area or at the bedside.

b. The catheter contains a micro-axial flow pump composed of impeller blades/rotors that spin around a central shaft and move blood through the device. The pump pulls blood from the LV and ejects it into the ascending aorta.
c. The device is controlled by an automatic controller that displays flow rate performance level. The device has the capacity to deliver 2.5 or 5 L/min of flow depending on the catheter size.
d. The longer catheter requires surgical cut down and has the ability to be placed right axillary through a conduit. This placement allows for longer term use.
e. The device also contains a purge solution that runs through the cannula to prevent blood from compromising the pump and ensuring the pump stays cool.
f. The device is currently the only Food and Drug Administration (FDA)-approved treatment of cardiogenic shock that is refractory to medical management.
2. A device is placed percutaneously into the LA to the aorta.
a. A 21 Fr cannula is placed via the right femoral vein into the inferior vena cava and advanced through the RA to the LA through transseptal puncture.
b. The device uses a centrifugal pump that contains a spinning impeller.
c. The blood is pumped from the LA and ejected back into the arterial circulation through a percutaneously placed arterial cannula inserted into the iliofemoral arterial system.
d. The device runs through a console that manages rate per minute (RPM). A heparinized solution runs continuously to the pump head to promote lubrication, cooling, and decrease clot formation within the pump chamber.
e. The device has the capacity to deliver up to 5 L/min of flow.
f. The patient must have adequate right ventricular function, and the device can only be inserted through the femoral approach.
g. This device is indicated for those with poor left ventricular function.

Contraindications

1. Moderate to severe aortic insufficiency.
2. Contraindication to anticoagulation.
3. Severe peripheral vascular disease.
4. Irreversible neurologic disease.
5. LV thrombus (not for the second method as it bypasses the LV).
6. Mechanical aortic valves (not for the second method as it bypasses the LV).
7. Tortuous iliac artery or vessel.
8. Anatomic disorders precluding placement or correct positioning.
9. LV rupture or tamponade.

Complications

1. Air embolism during cannula insertion.
2. Limb ischemia.
3. Bleeding at insertion site.
4. Malposition of cannula.
5. Hemolysis.
6. Sacral pressure injury.

Nursing Interventions

Relieving Anxiety

1. Explain PLVAD therapy to patient and family.
a. Review purpose of therapy and how the PLVAD functions.
2. Reinforce mobility restrictions:
a. Femoral approach; supine position with head of bed elevated 15 to 30 degrees and no movement or flexing of leg with PLVAD cannula.
b. Femoral approach for the LA aortic approach: head of bed (HOB) flat and log rolling.
c. Axillary approach: limited ROM on affected upper limb. Out of bed with assistance.
3. Explain the need for frequent monitoring of vital signs, rhythm, insertion site of affected extremity, and pulses.
4. Discuss the sounds associated with functioning external console.
5. Encourage family members to participate in patient's care.
a. Allow family to visit patient frequently.
b. Solicit family members' assistance in reinforcing mobility restrictions to patient and notifying nursing staff of patient comfort needs.
c. Encourage family members to ask questions.
6. Allow patient to verbalize fears regarding therapy and illness.
7. Make sure that informed consent is obtained.
8. Administer anxiolytic medications as prescribed and indicated.
9. Keep the family informed of changes in the patient's condition.
10. Encourage realistic hope based on the patient's condition and discuss the patient's progress with the family.
11. Determine the family's previous coping mechanism to stressful situations.

Maintaining Adequate CO

1. Assist during insertion of PLVAD.
a. Ensure strict aseptic environment during insertion.
b. Record date, time, and the patient's tolerance to procedure.
c. Obtain bedside ECHO to ensure placement of PLVAD.
2. Monitor hemodynamic parameters with Swan-Ganz catheter (see page 212) if available. Record MAP, CVP, PAP, PCWP, and CO to evaluate overall effectiveness of therapy. Perform hemodynamic calculations to evaluate systemic vascular resistance and left ventricular stroke work.
3. Assess capillary refill, pedal, or radial pulses of the affected limb every 15 minutes for the first hour, every 30 minutes for the next hour, and then every 1 to 2 hours.
4. Monitor vital signs every 15 minutes for the first hour, every 30 mins for the next hour, and then every 1 to 2 hours.
5. Depending on the device, monitor with vital signs.
a. LV to aortic approach: monitor the performance level, motor current, liters per minute value, purge solution pressures, and purge rate.
b. RA to LA approach: monitor the RPM and liters per minute value.
6. Monitor for signs of cannula migration.
a. LV to aortic approach: placement signal alarms, motor current pulsatile or flattened.
b. LA to aortic approach placement signal alarms, motor current pulsatile or flattened.
7. Monitor for decreased blood oxygen saturation change in color of blood in pump.
8. Monitor the PLVAD cannula site for bleeding or migration with vital signs and check for distal pulses to prevent limb ischemia.
9. Monitor neurologic status at least every 2 to 4 hours.

10. Monitor urine output and weight of patient daily.
11. Report chest pain immediately.
12. Treat dysrhythmia as directed.
13. Monitor for chattering of tubing or suction down alarms. Both devices are preload dependent.

CLINICAL JUDGMENT Either PLVAD approach has heparin in the solution to keep the motors cool. This needs to be considered when calculating systemic heparin dosing.

Maintaining Adequate Tissue Perfusion

1. Evaluate for ischemia of extremity with PLVAD.
   a. Mark pulses with indelible ink to facilitate checks.
   b. Monitor peripheral pulses (dorsalis pedis, posterior tibial, popliteal, and left radial) for rhythm, character, and pulse quality every 15 minutes for 1 hour, then every 30 minutes for 1 hour, and then hourly.
   c. Use Doppler device for pulses difficult to palpate and to auscultate for bruits and hums.
   d. Observe skin temperature, color, sensation, and movement of the affected extremity. (Dusky, cool, mottled, painful, and numb/tingling extremity indicates ischemia.)
2. Observe for possible indications of thromboemboli.
   a. Note decreases in urine output after initiation of therapy—may indicate renal artery emboli.
   b. Perform neurologic checks every hour to evaluate for cerebral emboli.
   c. Auscultate bowel sounds to detect evidence of ischemia.
3. Recognize early signs and symptoms of compartment syndrome. Increased pressure in tissue reduces blood flow.
   a. Note complaints of pain, pressure, and numbness of affected extremity induced by passive stretching.
   b. Palpate affected extremity for swelling and tension.
   c. Monitor CK values. Highly elevated CK may indicate compartment syndrome.
4. Ideally, keep head of bed elevated 30 degrees versus supine to avoid aspiration, but prevent upward migration of catheter.

Maintaining Skin Integrity

1. Assess skin frequently for signs of redness or breakdown.
2. Place patient on specialty mattress or bed designed to prevent pressure injuries (preferably before balloon insertion).
3. Place protective pads over bony prominences to prevent pressure injury.
4. Implement passive ROM exercises with the exception of extremity with PLVAD.
5. Turn patient from side to side as a unit every 2 hours. Patients are usually debilitated and prone to pressure injuries.
6. For patients able to be out of bed, limit time in chair if unable to shift their weight.

Evaluation: Expected Outcomes

1. States activity restrictions and rationale.
2. Blood pressure and CO readings improved.
3. Peripheral pulses strong; extremities warm and nail beds pink.
4. Absence of skin redness or breakdown.

Heart Surgery

Open-heart surgery is most commonly performed for CAD, valvular dysfunction, and congenital heart defects. The procedure may require temporary cardiopulmonary bypass (blood is diverted from the heart and the lungs and mechanically oxygenated and circulated) to provide a bloodless field that leads to increased visibility of cardiac structures during the operation.

Newer and less invasive procedures include *minimally invasive direct coronary artery bypass (MIDCAB)* and *robotic-assisted coronary bypass and valve surgeries*. An estimated 405,000 coronary bypass graft surgeries occur yearly in the United States. Heart transplant will not be discussed.

Types of Procedures

Coronary Artery Bypass Graft

EVIDENCE BASE Writing Committee Members, Lawton, J. S., Tamis-Holland, J. E., Bangalore, S., Bates, E. R., Beckie, T. M., Bischoff, J. M., Bittl, J. A., Cohen, M. G., DiMaio, J. M., Don, C. W., Fremes, S. E., Gaudino, M. F., Goldberger, Z. D., Grant, M. C., Jaswal, J. B., Kurlansky, P. A., Mehran, R., Metkus, T. S., Jr, ... Zwischenberger, B. A. (2022). 2021 ACC/AHA/SCAI guideline for coronary artery revascularization: Executive summary: A report of the American College of Cardiology/American Heart Association Joint Committee on clinical practice guidelines. *Journal of the American College of Cardiology, 79*(2), 197–215. https://doi.org/10.1016/j.jacc.2021.09.005

Al-Maskari, A., Al-Noumani, H., & Al-Maskari, M. (2021). Patients' and nurses' demographics and perceived learning needs post-coronary artery bypass graft. *Clinical Nursing Research, 30*(8), 1263–1270. https://doi.org.pluma.sjfc.edu/10.1177/1054773821990266

AHC MEDIA. (2021). Management of the cardiac surgery patient. *Critical Care Alert, 28*(12), 1–6.

1. CABG surgery involves anastomosis of a graft (vein or artery) with distal portion bypassing the blocked coronary vessel restoring adequate blood supply to the heart muscle. The proximal end, in some cases, is anastomosed to the aorta (when the internal mammary artery is chosen as conduit, the proximal end remains attached in its normal circulation pattern). The choice of conduit is often multifactorial. Arterial conduit has been shown to have a longer patency rate. For this reason, the internal mammary artery is often chosen if time allows for its dissection from the chest wall and the length is adequate to bypass the blocked vessel. The saphenous vein remains the most commonly used because it is easily accessed and does not require extra prepping to prevent spasm (as is the case with a radial graft). Several studies suggest poor graft vein patency and increased revascularization rate for patients undergoing off-pump CABG compared to on-pump CABG.
   a. Multiple grafts can be placed to bypass multiple lesions.
   b. Traditional procedure is done through sternotomy, whereas newer procedures are less invasive.
2. The heart is stopped (in some cases) and the patient is placed on a cardiopulmonary bypass machine (on-pump CABG). In other situations, CABG is performed while the heart is beating using a stabilizer to decrease movement (off-pump CABG). Compared to CABG, PCI with DESs has been shown to increase the relative risk of death, risk of MI, and revascularization rates at 3.4 years after initial treatment. Primarily done to alleviate anginal symptoms and improve survival and quality of life.

3. Indications for CABG include:
   a. Left main coronary artery stenosis of 70% or greater.
   b. Proximal vessel disease greater than 50% to 70% stenosis of three main coronary arteries.
   c. Multivessel disease and decreased left ventricular function.
   d. UA.
   e. Chronic stable angina that is lifestyle limiting and unresponsive to medical therapies or PTCA and stenting cannot be achieved.
4. Relative contraindications for CABG include:
   a. Small coronary arteries distal to the stenosis.
   b. Severe aortic stenosis.
   c. Severe left ventricular failure with coexisting pulmonary, renal, carotid, and peripheral vascular disease.

Valvular Surgery

1. Prosthetic or biologic valves are placed in the heart as definitive therapy for incompetent heart valves. Mechanical valves are of man-made material and require a lifetime of anticoagulation therapy. Biologic valves are generally either porcine or bovine derivatives. The decision for mechanic or biologic valve is a shared decision between the patient and provider.
2. Valve repair or replacement can be done in conjunction with CABG surgery.
3. Usually done as an open-heart procedure through sternotomy incision or minithoracotomy. A selected group of patients may need a transcatheter valvular replacement (TAVR).
4. Postoperative care of a patient with either a mitral valve or an aortic valve is similar to that of a patient who has undergone post-CABG surgery. Patients who have mechanical valve need lifetime anticoagulation therapy regardless of the position of the valve replaced. Generally, MVR needs higher international normalized ratio (INR) goals (i.e., INR ≥3) than AVR (i.e., INR ≤2.5 in cases of increased risk of bleeding), which is partially influenced by the pressure gradient. In the immediate postoperative period, heparin infusion can be used as a bridge anticoagulation until warfarin can be instituted to the therapeutic INR goal. It is important to educate patients to not stop the anticoagulation and to always seek medical advice prior to doing so.

Congenital Heart Surgery

1. Defects of the heart can be surgically repaired and reconstructed.
2. Temporary cardiopulmonary bypass is not always required.

Minimally Invasive Direct Coronary Artery Bypass

1. Done through a left anterior small thoracotomy, a short parasternal incision, or a small incision using a port access and video-assisted technology.
2. Cardiopulmonary bypass machine is not needed because the heart remains beating.
3. The procedure is limited to proximal disease of the left anterior descending or right coronary artery.
4. With this procedure, there is less blood transfusion, less pain and discomfort, less infection, and less time under anesthesia; therefore, intensive care unit (ICU) length of stay is significantly shorter.

Off-Pump CABG (Beating-Heart Bypass Surgery)

1. CABG surgery is done using a median sternotomy without the use of cardiopulmonary bypass machine; preferred method in high-risk patients (e.g., patients with poor ventricular function or with severe aortic atherosclerosis).
2. Postaccess procedures are performed through a small anterior thoracotomy incision and a few 1-cm lateral port incisions that allow direct access to the heart and good visualization through a thoracoscope.
   a. Multiple vessel bypass can be performed as well as mitral valve surgery and repair of atrial septal defect.
   b. In emergency, if the heart stops, cardiopulmonary bypass can be used during surgery.
   c. Reduces postoperative length of stay to 1 to 3 days.
   d. Contraindicated in patients with occlusion in posterior and lateral arteries, severe atherosclerosis, and aortic aneurysms.
3. Transmyocardial laser revascularization (TMLR) provides relief to patients having refractory angina that is not amendable to conventional revascularization. Indications for TMLR include severe coronary heart disease, viable myocardium with reversible ischemia, LVEF of more than 20%, and target vessels that are too small for catheter revascularization.

Preoperative Management

1. Review of patient's condition to determine the status of vascular, pulmonary, renal, hepatic, hematologic, and metabolic systems.
   a. Cardiac history; circulatory studies.
   b. Pulmonary health—patients with chronic obstructive pulmonary disease (COPD) may require prolonged postoperative respiratory support. Chest computed tomography scans, baseline arterial blood gas (ABG), or pulmonary function tests should be ordered and used as reliable predictors of long-term pulmonary outcomes. (Vital capacity >2.5 L and forced expiratory volume in 1 second >1.5 L are ideal for favorable outcomes.)
   c. Depression—can produce a serious postoperative depressive state and can affect postoperative morbidity and mortality.
   d. Present alcohol intake; smoking history.
2. Preoperative laboratory studies.
   a. Complete blood count, serum electrolytes, lipid profile, and hemoglobin A1C, if patient has diabetes.
   b. Ensure active blood type and cross with the correct number of packed red blood cells (PRBCs) and other blood products on hold at the blood bank.
   c. Antibody screen, urine, and other cultures.
   d. Preoperative coagulation survey (platelet count, prothrombin time, partial thromboplastin time)—extracorporeal circulation will affect certain coagulation factors.
   e. Renal and hepatic function tests.
3. Evaluation of medication regimen. These patients are usually taking multiple drugs.
   a. Digoxin—may be receiving large doses to improve myocardial contractility; may be stopped several days before surgery to avoid digitoxic dysrhythmias from cardiopulmonary bypass.
   b. Diuretics—assess for potassium depletion and volume depletion; give potassium supplement to replenish body stores.
   c. Beta-adrenergic blockers such as metoprolol and propranolol—usually continued.
   d. Psychotropic drugs such as benzodiazepines (diazepam, alprazolam)—postoperative withdrawal may cause extreme agitation.

   e. Alcohol—sudden withdrawal may produce delirium.
   f. Anticoagulant/antiplatelet aggregate drugs, such as warfarin and clopidogrel—discontinued several days before operation to allow coagulation mechanism to return to normal.
   g. Corticosteroids—if taken within the year before surgery, may lead to adrenal crisis. It is essential that these patients be dosed adequately to prevent hypotension or death.
   h. Prophylactic antibiotics—may be given preoperatively.
   i. Drug sensitivities or allergies are noted.
   j. If patients are taking herbal supplements, they should be discontinued as far in advance as possible to prevent interactions with certain types of anesthesia.
4. If patient is taking any antihyperglycemic agents (i.e., insulin, metformin), discuss with the provider the need to reduce basal insulin doses and hold metformin before surgery. Ensure that basal insulin is not completely withheld, because this may result in diabetic ketoacidosis or hyperosmolar hyperglycemia state.
5. Improvement of underlying pulmonary disease and respiratory function to reduce the risk of complications.
   a. Encourage patient to stop smoking.
   b. Treat infection and pulmonary vascular congestion.
6. Preparation for events in the postoperative period.
   a. Take the patient and family on tour of ICU. This lessens anxiety about being in the ICU.
      i. Introduce the patient to staff personnel who will be caring for them.
      ii. Give family a schedule of visiting hours and times for phone contact.
   b. Teach chest physical therapy procedures to optimize pulmonary function.
      i. Have the patient practice with an incentive spirometer.
      ii. Show and practice diaphragmatic breathing techniques.
      iii. Have the patient practice effective coughing and leg exercises.
   c. Prepare patient for the presence of monitors, chest tubes, IV lines, blood transfusion, ET tube, nasogastric (NG) tube, pacing wires, arterial line, and indwelling catheter.
      i. Explain to the patient that chest tubes will be inserted below incision into the chest cavity for drainage and maintenance of negative pressure.
      ii. Explain to the patient that the ET tube will prevent speaking, but communication will be possible through writing until tube is removed (usually within 6 hours when the patient is awake and able to maintain own airway).
      iii. Explain to the patient that the diet will consist of liquids until 24 hours after surgery.
      iv. Explain that monitoring equipment and IV lines will restrict movement and nursing staff will position the patient comfortably every 2 hours and as necessary.
   d. Discuss with the patient the need to monitor vital signs frequently and the likelihood of frequent disturbances of the patient's rest.
   e. Discuss pain management with the patient; assure the patient that analgesics will be administered as necessary to control pain. Discuss the use of the patient control analgesia (PCA) machine.
   f. Tell the patient that both hands may be loosely restrained for a few hours after surgery to eliminate the possibility of pulling out tubes and IV lines inadvertently.
   g. Discuss with the patient the importance of physical and occupational therapy to increase mobility and decrease hospital stay. Patient will be assisted from the bed to chair by the morning of postoperative day 1.
7. Evaluation of emotional state to reduce anxieties.
   a. Patients undergoing heart surgery are more anxious and fearful than other surgical patients. (Moderate anxiety assists patient to cope with stresses of surgery. Low anxiety level may indicate that the patient is in denial. High anxiety may impair the patient's ability to learn and listen.)
   b. Offer support and help patient and family mobilize positive coping mechanisms.
   c. Answer questions and alleviate fears and misconceptions.
8. Surgical preparation.
   a. Shave anterior and lateral surfaces of the trunk and neck; shave entire body down to ankles (for coronary bypass).
   b. Shower or bathe per facility policy. Assist patient with antiseptic scrubs used on their chest prior to surgery.
   c. Give sedative or antibiotics before going to the operating room, as ordered.
   d. Ensure removable dental work, jewelry, and nail polish removed.

POPULATION AWARENESS Older patients with underlying respiratory problems (i.e., smoking, COPD, asthma) and patients who are debilitated are at greater risk for postoperative respiratory complications.

Complications

Complications following cardiac surgery can be divided into early complications (cardiovascular, pulmonary, renal, gastrointestinal [GI], and neuropsychologic) and late postoperative complications.

Early Complications

EVIDENCE BASE Bowden, T., Hurt, C. S., Sanders, J., & Aitken, L. M. (2022). Predictors of cognitive dysfunction after cardiac surgery: A systematic review. *European Journal of Cardiovascular Nursing, 21*(3), 192–204. https://doi-org.pluma.sjfc.edu/10.1093/eurjcn/zvab086

Charitos, E. I., Herrmann, F. E. M., & Ziegler, P. D. (2021). Atrial fibrillation recurrence and spontaneous conversion to sinus rhythm after cardiac surgery: Insights from 426 patients with continuous rhythm monitoring. *Journal of Cardiovascular Electrophysiology, 32*(8), 2171–2178. https://doi-org.pluma.sjfc.edu/10.1111/jce.15126

1. Cardiovascular dysfunction or low output syndrome can occur as a result of decreased preload (from bleeding or volume loss), increased afterload, arrhythmias, cardiac tamponade, or myocardial depression with or without myocardial necrosis.
2. Postoperative bleeding can occur secondary to coagulopathy, uncontrolled hypertension, or inadequate hemostasis.
3. Cardiac tamponade results from bleeding into the pericardial sac or accumulation of fluids in the sac, which compresses the heart and prevents adequate filling of the ventricles. Cardiac tamponade should be suspected when there is low CO, hypotension, tachycardia, increased CVP, narrow pulse pressure, or sharp drop in chest tube output postoperatively.
4. Myocardial depression (impaired myocardial contractility), which can be reversible, occurs secondary as a result of myocardial necrosis in 15% of all CABG surgeries.

5. Perioperative MI continues to be a serious problem that can occur in 5% of patients with stable angina and up to 10% of patients with UA postoperatively as a result of the surgical procedure.
6. Cardiac dysrhythmias commonly occur after heart surgery. Ischemia, hypoxia, electrolyte imbalances, alterations in the autonomic nervous system, hypertension, and increased catecholamine levels, among others, may attribute to dysrhythmia development.
   a. Atrial arrhythmias may occur after CABG or after valvular surgery; can occur anytime during the first 2 to 3 weeks postoperatively, but peak incidence is 3 to 5 days. Studies suggest perioperative beta-blockade is an effective therapy for prevention.
   b. Premature ventricular contractions (PVCs) occur in 8.9% to 24% of patients, most frequently after aortic valve replacement and CABG.
7. Hypotension may be caused by inadequate cardiac contractility and reduction in blood volume or by mechanical ventilation (when the patient "fights" the ventilator or positive end-expiratory pressure is used), all of which can produce a reduction in CO.
8. Pulmonary complications occur as a result of intubation and coronary pulmonary bypass.
   a. Continuous pulse oximetry, ABG studies, and chest x-ray are done frequently to monitor pulmonary function of a patient after heart surgery.
   b. Noncardiac pulmonary edema can occur immediately after surgery and can occur the first several days after surgery as a result of increased pulmonary capillary permeability.
   c. Pneumothorax can occur anytime postoperatively, especially when chest tubes are removed.
   d. Phrenic nerve damage can occur, resulting in diaphragmatic paralysis.
   e. Pulmonary emboli, although uncommon, can result from atrial fibrillation, heart failure, obesity, hypercoagulability, and immobilization.
   f. Older patients are at increased risk of developing pneumonia, atelectasis, and pulmonary effusions.
   g. Be vigilant and report copious amounts of secretion or any changes in patient's secretion.
9. Renal insufficiency or failure can occur as a result of deficient perfusion (can be due to heart–lung machine), hemolysis, low CO before and after open-heart surgery, hypotension, and by use of vasopressor agents to increase BP.
10. GI postoperative complications can include abdominal distention, ileus, gastroduodenal bleeding, cholecystitis, hepatic dysfunction, "shock liver syndrome," pancreatitis, mesenteric ischemia, diarrhea, or constipation.
11. Neuropsychologic complications postoperatively include ischemic stroke, neuropsychologic dysfunction, postcardiotomy delirium, and peripheral neurologic deficits.

POPULATION AWARENESS Older patients postoperatively are more sensitive to hypovolemia, excessive bleeding, and cardiac tamponade, which affect preload and result in a decrease in CO.

POPULATION AWARENESS Atrial fibrillation occurs in 35% of older patients postoperatively and may need to be treated with antiarrhythmics, cardioversion, and anticoagulants.

POPULATION AWARENESS Neurologic complications increase disproportionately to cardiac risk in older patients.

Late Complications

1. Late complications of cardiac surgery usually occur after the fourth day of surgery and include postpericardiotomy syndrome, cardiac tamponade, and incisional wound infections.
2. Postpericardiotomy syndrome is a group of symptoms occurring in 10% to 40% of patients several days after cardiac surgery.
   a. The cause of postpericardiotomy syndrome is not certain, but it may result from anticardiac antibodies, viral etiology (such as cytomegalovirus), or other causes.
   b. Postpericardiotomy syndrome occurs as the result of tissue trauma, which triggers an autoimmune response and inflammation of the pericardial cavity, resulting in pericardial and severe pleural pain.
   c. Manifestations—fever, malaise, arthralgias, dyspnea, pericardial effusion, pleural effusion and friction rub, and pleural/pericardial pain.
   d. Treatment regimen may include corticosteroids, aspirin, or colchicine. Pericardiocentesis or thoracentesis may be needed for persistent effusion.
3. Cardiac tamponade can occur in 1% to 2% of patients and is commonly associated with the administration of anticoagulants or antiplatelet therapy, usually occurring after 72 hours following surgery.
4. Wound infections, including sternal wound infections and mediastinitis, occur in 0.4% to 5% of all patients having cardiac surgery. Mortality rate associated with sternal wound infection and mediastinitis can vary between 8% and 45%.
   a. Wound infections usually appear 4 to 14 days postoperatively with symptoms of fever, leukocytosis, inflammation, and purulent drainage.
   b. *Staphylococcus epidermidis* and *Staphylococcus aureus* organisms are the most common causative organisms, but the infection can be caused by a number of pathogens ranging from gram-positives, gram-negatives, or even fungi.
5. MIs (postoperative) can occur at a rate of 1.34% because of bypass time greater than 100 minutes and the presence of UA.
6. Constrictive pericarditis has an incidence of 0.2% to 2.0%. Risk factors reveal normal left ventricular function, warfarin administration, and inadequate drainage of early postoperative pericardial effusion as the significant causes.
7. Respiratory complications—chest wall pain and prolonged ventilation—more than 14 days of ventilatory support (morbidity rate of 9.9%).
8. Renal dysfunction—up to 40% developed transient oliguria, with 2% progressing to renal failure requiring dialysis. Postoperative renal dysfunction results from postoperative hypovolemia, anemia, hypotension, low output syndrome, sepsis, and pericardial tamponade.

Other Complications

1. Postperfusion syndrome—diffuse syndrome characterized by systemic inflammatory response syndrome.
2. Febrile complications—probably from body's reaction to tissue trauma or accumulation of blood and serum in pleural and pericardial spaces.
3. In older patients, decreased kidney function can increase the risk of developing drug toxicities, adverse reactions, oliguria, and renal failure.

4. Failure to wean from the ventilator because of underlying pulmonary disease or postoperative pulmonary complications.

Postoperative Management

1. Adequate oxygenation is ensured; respiratory insufficiency is common after open-heart surgery.
   a. Patients require intubation during cardiac surgery, and the majority of them continued to require mechanical ventilation after being transported to the cardiac surgery ICU.
   b. Chest x-ray taken immediately after surgery and daily thereafter to evaluate state of lung expansion, to detect atelectasis or pneumothorax, and to demonstrate heart size and contour and confirm the placement of central line, ET tube, and chest drains.
2. Hemodynamic monitoring during the immediate postoperative period for cardiovascular and respiratory status and fluid and electrolyte balance to prevent or recognize complications.
3. Drainage of mediastinal and pleural chest tubes is monitored.
4. Fluid and electrolyte balance is monitored closely with daily weight.
5. Hypokalemia may be caused by inadequate intake, diuretics, vomiting, excessive NG drainage, and stress from surgery.
   a. Hyperkalemia may be caused by increased intake, red cell breakdown (from the pump, bleeding, or transfusion), acidosis, renal insufficiency, tissue necrosis, and adrenal cortical insufficiency.
   b. Hyponatremia may be due to a reduction of total body sodium or to an increased water intake, causing a dilution of body sodium.
   c. Hypocalcemia may be due to alkalosis (which reduces the amount of calcium in the extracellular fluid) because hydrogen ions dissociate from serum albumin and more calcium binds to albumin, reducing ionized calcium level in the blood, and multiple blood transfusions.
   d. Hypercalcemia may cause dysrhythmias imitating those caused by digoxin toxicity.
6. Postoperative medications include:
   a. Aspirin daily as MI prophylaxis.
   b. Analgesics.
   c. Antihypertensives or antiarrhythmics, if needed.
   d. Beta-blockers.
   e. Angiotensin-converting enzyme (ACE) inhibitors for patients with ejection fraction less than 30%.
   f. Antibiotics, if indicated.
7. Monitoring for complications.
8. Cardiac pacing, if indicated, by way of temporary pacing wires from the incision.

Nursing Interventions

Minimizing Anxiety

1. Orient to surroundings as soon as patient awakens from surgical procedure. Tell patient that the surgery is over and orient to location, time of day, and your name.
2. Allow family members to visit patient as soon as the condition stabilizes. Encourage family members to talk to and touch patient. (Family members may be overwhelmed by intensive care environment.)
3. As patient becomes more alert, explain purpose of all equipment in the environment. Continually orient patient to time and place. Make sure patient has glasses and hearing aids, if needed.
4. Administer anxiolytics, as directed.
5. Remove lines and tubing once medically appropriate.

Promoting Adequate Gas Exchange

1. Frequently check function of mechanical ventilator, patient's respiratory effort, and ABG levels.
2. Check ET tube placement (note location and measurement).
3. Auscultate chest for breath sounds. Crackles indicate pulmonary congestion; decreased or absent breath sounds indicate pneumothorax; rales may indicate pulmonary edema.
4. Sedate patient adequately to help tolerate ET tube and cope with ventilatory sensations. Implement ventilator care bundle (i.e., routine mouth care with chlorhexidine, keep HOB at 30 degrees) to prevent ventilator-associated pneumonia.
5. Use chest physiotherapy for patients with lung congestion to prevent retention of secretions and atelectasis.
6. Promote coughing, deep breathing, and turning to keep airway patent, prevent atelectasis, and facilitate lung expansion. Have patient sit at least 30 degrees unless medically contraindicated.
7. Suction tracheobronchial secretions carefully. Prolonged suctioning leads to hypoxia and possible cardiac arrest.
8. Administer diuretics, as prescribed.
9. Institute ventilatory weaning protocol when patient is awake and can initiate own breaths and assist with extubation (see page 151), when indicated.

Maintaining Adequate CO

1. Monitor cardiovascular status to determine the effectiveness of CO. Continuous monitoring of BP by way of intra-arterial line, HR, CVP, left atrial or PAP, and PCWP from monitor modules is observed, correlated with the patient's condition, and recorded.
2. Monitor and record urine output every hour (normal urinary output 0.5 to 1 mL/kg/h).
3. Observe buccal mucosa, nail beds, lips, earlobes, and extremities for duskiness, cyanosis—late signs of low CO.
4. Feel the skin; cool, moist skin or weak pulses reveal lowered CO. Note temperature and color of extremities.
5. Monitor neurologic status.
   a. Observe for symptoms of hypoxia—restlessness, headache, confusion, dyspnea, hypotension, and cyanosis. Obtain ABG values and core temperature.
   b. Note the patient's neurologic status hourly in terms of the level of responsiveness, response to verbal commands and painful stimuli, pupillary size and reaction to light, and movement of extremities, handgrasp ability.
   c. Monitor for and treat postoperative seizures.

Maintaining Adequate Fluid Volume

1. Administer IV fluids as ordered, but limit if signs of fluid overloading occur.
2. Keep intake and output flow sheets as a method of determining the positive or negative fluid balance and the patient's fluid requirements.
   a. IV fluids (including flush solutions through arterial and venous lines) are considered intake.
   b. Measure postoperative chest drainage—should not exceed 200 mL/h for the first 4 to 6 hours.
3. Be alert to changes in serum electrolyte levels.
   a. Hypokalemia may cause dysrhythmias, digoxin toxicity, metabolic alkalosis, weakened myocardium, and cardiac arrest.
      i. Watch for specific ECG changes.
      ii. Replace electrolytes, as needed.

b. Hyperkalemia may cause mental confusion, restlessness, nausea, weakness, and paresthesia of the extremities. Treatment may include administering an ion-exchange resin and sodium polystyrene sulfonate, which binds the potassium or hemodialysis. Temporary treatment includes sodium bicarbonate, insulin (with dextrose), albuterol, and calcium.
c. Hyponatremia may cause weakness, fatigue, confusion, seizures, and coma.
d. Hypocalcemia may cause numbness and tingling in the fingertips, toes, ears, and nose, carpopedal spasm, muscle cramps, and tetany. Give replacement therapy, as needed.
e. Hypercalcemia may cause digoxin toxicity.
   i. Treatment may include fluids, diuretics, calcitonin, or hemodialysis.
   ii. This condition may lead to asystole and death.
4. Monitor hematocrit and hemoglobin (frequency depends on hemodynamics and evidence of bleeding) and report any significant change in findings.
   a. Ensure that patient has current blood type and screen. Transfuse blood products, as ordered.
   b. Check coagulation tests, including prothrombin time, INR, and partial thromboplastin time, if patient is coagulopathic, bleeding, or anticoagulated for mechanical device.

Relieving Pain

1. Examine surgical incision sites.
2. Record nature, type, location, duration of pain, and contributing factors.
3. Differentiate between incisional pain and anginal pain. Obtain ECG and have the provider confirm if there are any changes.
4. Report restlessness and apprehension not corrected by analgesics—may be from hypoxia or a low output state.
5. Administer medications as prescribed, or monitor constant infusion to reduce the amount of pain and to aid the patient in performing deep breathing and coughing exercises more effectively.
6. Assist patient to position of comfort.
7. Encourage early mobilization.

Promoting Sleep and Recovery

1. Watch for symptoms of postcardiotomy delirium (may appear after a brief lucid period).
   a. Signs and symptoms include delirium (impairment of orientation, memory, intellectual function, judgment), transient perceptual distortions, visual and auditory hallucinations, disorientation, and paranoid delusions.
   b. Symptoms may be related to sleep deprivation, increased sensory output, disorientation to night and day, prolonged inability to speak because of ET intubation, age, and preoperative cardiac status.
2. Keep the patient oriented to time and place; notify the patient of procedures and expectations of cooperation.
3. Encourage family to visit at regular times—helps patient regain sense of reality.
4. Plan care to allow rest periods, day–night pattern, and uninterrupted sleep.
5. Encourage mobility as soon as possible.
   a. Keep environment as free as possible of excessive auditory and sensory input.
   b. Prevent bodily injury.
   c. Have physical therapy work with patient and provide analgesics prior to therapy.
6. Reassure patient and family that psychiatric disorders after cardiac surgery are usually transient.
7. Remove patient from the ICU as soon as possible. Allow patient to talk about psychotic episode—helps deal with and assimilate experience.

Avoiding Complications

1. Monitor ECG continuously for arrhythmias.
   a. Evaluate possible cause of dysrhythmias—inadequate oxygenation, electrolyte imbalance, MI, mechanical irritation (e.g., pacing wires, invasive lines, chest tubes), and any vasopressor or inotropic medications.
   b. Treat dysrhythmias immediately because they may lead to decreased CO. Atrial or AV pacing is used to treat sinus bradycardia or junctional rhythm with HRs less than 70 beats/min.
2. Assess for signs of cardiac tamponade—arterial hypotension; rising CVP; rising left atrial pressure; muffled heart sounds; weak, thready pulse; jugular vein distention; and falling urine output.
   a. Check for diminished amount of drainage in the chest collection bottle; may indicate that fluid is accumulating elsewhere, reposition as needed to facilitate fluid drainage.
   b. Prepare for pericardiocentesis.
   c. Assist with echocardiogram to evaluate tamponade.
3. Check cardiac enzyme levels daily. Elevations may indicate MI. (Symptoms may be masked by the usual postoperative discomfort.)
   a. Watch for decreased CO in the presence of normal circulating volume and filling pressure.
   b. Obtain serial ECGs and isoenzymes to determine the extent of myocardial injury.
   c. Assess pain to differentiate myocardial pain from incisional pain.
4. Monitor for hypertension or hypotension.
   a. Mild systolic hypertension occurs in 48% to 55% of all patients who have undergone CABG surgery within the first 6 hours postoperatively.
   b. Hypotension may be caused by bleeding, hypovolemia, decreased systemic vascular resistance (e.g., systemic inflammatory response syndrome), cardiogenic shock, tamponade, medications, or arrhythmias.
   c. Blood pressure goal following cardiac surgery is dependent on the patient's conditions (e.g., carotid disease, renal disease, bleeding).
5. Initiate measures to prevent embolization such as antiembolic stockings, not putting pressure on popliteal space (leg crossing, raising knee gatch), and starting passive and active exercises.
   a. Assess for signs of deep vein thrombosis (DVT) and pulmonary embolism.
   b. Maintain integrity of all invasive lines.
6. Monitor for bleeding.
   a. Watch for steady and continuous drainage of blood.
   b. Assess for arterial hypotension, low CVP, increasing pulse rate, low left atrial pressure, and PCWP.
   c. Prepare to administer blood products, IV solutions, protamine sulfate, antifibrinolytics, desmopressin [acetate] (DDAVP), or vitamin K.
   d. Prepare for potential return to surgery if bleeding persists (over 300 mL/h) for 2 hours.
   e. Monitor hemoglobin levels; if the patient's hemoglobin drops below 8 g/dL, transfusions of red blood cells or platelets may be necessary.

f. During the first 4 to 12 hours, blood recovered from mediastinal tubes can be autotransfused to the patient.

7. Be alert for fever and signs of infection. Check blood glucose levels as ordered.
   a. Administer prophylactic antibiotics, if ordered, for the first 48 hours.
   b. Control higher degrees of fever through use of a hypothermia mattress.
   c. Evaluate for atelectasis, pleural effusion, or pneumonia if fever persists. (The most common cause of early postoperative fever [within 24 hours] is atelectasis.)
   d. Evaluate for urinary tract infection and wound infection.
   e. Draw blood cultures to rule out infectious cause if fever persists.
8. Measure urine volume; less than 0.5 to 1 mL/kg/h can indicate decreased renal function.
   a. Monitor blood urea nitrogen (BUN) and serum creatinine levels as well as urine and serum electrolyte levels.
   b. Give rapid-acting diuretics or inotropic drugs (dopamine, dobutamine) to increase CO and renal blood flow.
   c. Prepare the patient for peritoneal dialysis or hemodialysis if indicated. (Renal insufficiency may produce serious cardiac dysrhythmias.)

Community and Home Care Considerations

Preparing the patient with cardiovascular disease or after cardiac surgery for the return home and optimizing the patient's health status in the home are important nursing functions. The key areas on which to focus include assessment, education, and evaluating responses.

1. Perform a thorough assessment of the patient's clinical condition, functional status, and home safety and support systems. Based on assessment, determine the patient's need for supportive services.
2. Coordinate services such as home health aides.
3. Refer patients to area meal delivery service as appropriate. These services provide special diets in most cases (e.g., low sodium or low cholesterol).
4. Coordinate outpatient cardiac rehabilitation services as appropriate.
5. Establish outpatient or home-based physical and occupational therapy as appropriate for graduated exercise and energy conservation techniques.
6. If therapist recommends inpatient rehabilitation, coordinate with facility social worker/discharge planner to find a rehabilitation facility suited for patient as well as their family.
7. Educate patient, family, and caregivers about potential complications and medication regimen. Medication management is a key issue when a cardiac surgery patient is leaving the hospital. Ensure that patient is discharged with an accurate medication list and clear instructions on what has changed compared to previous home medications. Ensure that prescriptions are given to the patient or transmitted to chosen pharmacy and that insurance coverage of medications and cost of all medications have been determined.

Patient Education and Health Maintenance

Note: Specific guidelines will vary slightly among facilities and health care providers. Check facility policy and orders.

1. Instruct about activities.
   a. Increase activities gradually within limits. (Avoid strenuous activities until after exercise stress testing.)
   b. Take short rest periods.
   c. Avoid lifting more than 20 pounds (9.1 kg).
   d. Participate in activities that do not cause pain or discomfort.
   e. Increase walking time and distance each day.
   f. Stairs (one to two times daily) the first week; increase as tolerated.
   g. Avoid large crowds at first.
   h. Avoid driving until after the first postoperative checkup.
   i. Resumption of sexual relations parallels the ability to participate in other activities.
      i. Usually may resume sexual activity 2 weeks after surgery.
      ii. Avoid sexual activity if tired or after a heavy meal.
      iii. Consult health care provider if chest discomfort, difficult breathing, or palpitations occur and last longer than 15 minutes after intercourse.
   j. Return to work after the first postoperative checkup, as advised by health care provider.
2. Expect some chest discomfort.
3. Advise about diet.
   a. Some patients are placed on minimum salt restriction (e.g., no salt added at table); cholesterol may be limited. Have a dietitian talk to the patient and family regarding diet.
   b. Weigh daily and report weight gain of more than 5 pounds (2.3 kg) per week.
   c. If the patient is taking warfarin, advise patient not to change normal dietary habits, but to maintain a similar intake pattern each day to prevent changes in INR.
4. Tight blood glucose control is recommended (keeping blood sugars 80 to 110 mg/dL) to prevent sternal wound infection.
5. Teach patient and family about wound care and how to avoid infections.
6. Teach about medications.
   a. Label all medications; give purposes and adverse effects.
   b. Patients with mechanical valves may continue warfarin regimen indefinitely. Explain bleeding precautions and the need for periodic laboratory studies.
7. Advise patients with prosthetic valves.
   a. Pregnancy is usually discouraged because of anticoagulation therapy.
   b. Need for antibiotic coverage before dental and surgical procedures.
   c. Patients taking anticoagulants should watch for bleeding and should avoid use of aspirin (and many other drugs)—interferes with action of warfarin.
8. Advise the patient to carry an identification card stating cardiac condition and medications being taken.
9. Encourage adherence to rehabilitation and exercise program after exercise stress testing.
10. Inform the patient whom to contact (and how) in case of an emergency.
11. See also section on patient education after MI, page 251, and patient education about infective endocarditis, page 261.
12. Explore community support groups such as AHA (*www.americanheart.org*).
13. Be diligent in providing older patients with education and discharge instructions that they will be able to follow because of sensory impairments, immobility, and transportation barriers.

POPULATION AWARENESS Older patients are extremely vulnerable to complications because of decreased functional ability and the normal process of aging.

Evaluation: Expected Outcomes

- Verbalizes understanding of surgical procedure, reduction of fear.
- Extubated 24 hours postoperative; spontaneous unlabored respirations 14 to 18 per minute.
- Blood pressure and HR stable; adequate urine output.
- Serum electrolytes within normal range.
- Verbalizes reduced pain.
- Sleeps for 2- to 3-hour intervals during night; oriented to time and place; no hallucinations.
- No bleeding noted; afebrile; ECG shows normal sinus rhythm.

SELECTED READINGS

Almarzooq, Z. I., & Mora, S. (2022). The curious case of synergy between lipoprotein (a), coronary calcification, and cardiovascular disease risk. *Clinical Chemistry, 68*(10), 1235–1237. https://doi.org/10.1093/clinchem/hvac094

Alvin, M. D., Jaffe, A. S., Ziegelstein, R. C., & Trost, J. C. (2017). Eliminating creatine kinase-myocardial band testing in suspected acute coronary syndrome: A value-based quality improvement. *JAMA Internal Medicine, 177*(10), 1508–1512. https://doi.org/10.1001/jamainternmed.2017.3597

Barrionuevo-Sánchez, M. I., Ariza-Solé, A., Ortiz-Berbel, D., González-Costello, J., Gómez-Hospital, J. A., Lorente, V., Alegre, O., Llaó, I., Sánchez-Salado, J. C., Gómez-Lara, J., Blasco-Lucas, A., & Comin-Colet, J. (2022). Usefulness of Impella support in different clinical settings in cardiogenic shock. *Journal of Geriatric Cardiology: JGC, 19*(2), 115–124. https://doi.org/10.11909/j.issn.1671-5411.2022.02.003

Bessman, E. S. (2019). Emergency cardiac pacing. In J. R. Roberts, C. B. Custalow, & T. W. Thomsen (Eds.), *Roberts and Hedges' clinical procedures in emergency medicine and acute care* (7th ed., pp. 288–308). Elsevier.

Bittner, V. A., Szarek, M., Aylward, P. E., Bhatt, D. L., Diaz, R., Edelberg, J. M., Fras, Z., Goodman, S. G., Halvorsen, S., Hanotin, C., Harrington, R. A., Jukema, J. W., Loizeau, V., Moriarty, P. M., Moryusef, A., Pordy, R., Roe, M. T., Sinnaeve, P., Tsimikas, S., ... ODYSSEY OUTCOMES Committees and Investigators. (2020). Effect of alirocumab on lipoprotein(a) and cardiovascular risk after acute coronary syndrome. *Journal of American College of Cardiology, 75*(2), 133–144. https://doi.org/10.1016/j.jacc.2019.10.057

Charitos, E. I., Herrmann, F. E. M., & Ziegler, P. D. (2021). Atrial fibrillation recurrence and spontaneous conversion to sinus rhythm after cardiac surgery: Insights from 426 patients with continuous rhythm monitoring. *Journal of Cardiovascular Electrophysiology, 32*(8), 2171–2178. https://doi-org.pluma.sjfc.edu/10.1111/jce.15126

Edvardsen, T., Asch, F. M., & Davidson, B. D. V. (2022). Guidelines and standards non-invasive imaging in coronary syndromes: Recommendations of the European Association of Cardiovascular Imaging and the American Society of Echocardiography, in collaboration with the American Society of Nuclear Cardiology, Society of Cardiovascular Computed Tomography, and Society for Cardiovascular Magnetic Resonance. *Journal of the American Society of Echocardiography*, (April), 329–354. https://doi.org/10.1093/ehjci/jeab244

Gorski, L. A., Hadaway, L., Hagle, M. E., Broadhurst, D., Clare, S., Kleidon, T., Meyer, B. M., Nickel, B., Rowley, S., Sharpe, E., & Alexander, M. (2021). Infusion therapy standards of practice, 8th Edition. *Journal of Infusion Nursing, 44*(1S), S1–S224. https://doi.org/10.1097/nan.0000000000000396

Gulati, M., Levy, P. D., Mukherjee, D., Amsterdam, E., Bhatt, D. L., Birtcher, K. K., Blankstein, R., Boyd, J., Bullock-Palmer, R. P., Conejo, T., Diercks, D. B., Gentile, F., Greenwood, J. P., Hess, E. P., Hollenberg, S. M., Jaber, W. A., Jneid, H., Joglar, J. A., Morrow, D. A., ... Shaw, L. J. (2021). 2021 AHA/ACC/ASE/CHEST/SAEM/SCCT/SCMR guideline for the evaluation and diagnosis of chest pain: Executive summary: A report of the American College of Cardiology/American Heart Association Joint Committee on clinical practice guidelines. *Circulation, 144*(22), e336–e367. https://doi.org/10.1161/CIR.0000000000001030

Hempel, T. T., & Wyatt, A. (2022). High sensitivity troponins. *Emergency Medicine Clinics of North America, 40*(4), 809–821. https://doi.org/10.1016/j.emc.2022.07.002

Jaffe, A. S., Lindahl, B., Giannitsis, E., Mueller, C., Cullen, L., Hammarsten, O., Mockel, M., Mair, J., Krychtiuk, K. A., Huber, K., Mills, N. L., & Thygesen, K. (2021). ESC study group on cardiac biomarkers of the association for acute cardiovascular care: A fond farewell at the retirement of CKMB. *European Heart Journal, 42*(23), 2260–2264. https://doi.org/10.1093/eurheartj/ehaa1079

Kontos, M. C., De Lemos, J. A., Deitelzweig, S. B., Diercks, D. B., Gore, M. O., Hess, E. P., McCarthy, C. P., McCord, J. K., Musey, P. I., Villines, T. C., & Wright, L. J. (2022). 2022 ACC expert consensus decision pathway on the evaluation and disposition of acute chest pain in the emergency department. *Journal of the American College of Cardiology, 80*(20), 1925–1960. https://doi.org/10.1016/j.jacc.2022.08.750

Kuang, R. J., Pirakalathanan, J., Lau, T., Koh, D., Kotschet, E., Ko, B., & Lau, K. K. (2021). An up-to-date review of cardiac pacemakers and implantable cardioverter defibrillators. *Journal of Medical Imaging and Radiation Oncology, 65*(7), 896–903. https://doi.org/10.1111/1754-9485.13319

Mierke, J., Loehn, T., Ende, G., Jahn, S., Quick, S., Speiser, U., Jellinghaus, S., Pfluecke, C., Linke, A., & Ibrahim, K. (2021). Percutaneous left ventricular assist device leads to heart rhythm stabilisation in cardiogenic shock: Results from the Dresden Impella Registry. *Heart, Lung & Circulation, 30*(4), 577–584. https://doi.org/10.1016/j.hlc.2020.08.005

Nyström, A., Strömberg, S., Jansson, K., Faresjö, Å. O., & Faresjö, T. (2022). Cardiovascular risks before myocardial infarction differences between men and women. *BMC Cardiovascular Disorders, 22*(1), 110. https://doi.org/10.1186/s12872-022-02555-3

O'Malley, P. G., Arnold, M. J., Kelley, C., Spacek, L., Buelt, A., Natarajan, S., Donahue, M. P., Vagichev, E., Ballard-Hernandez, J., Logan, A., Thomas, L., Ritter, J., Neubauer, B. E., & Downs, J. R. (2020). Management of dyslipidemia for cardiovascular disease risk reduction: Synopsis of the 2020 updated U.S. Department of Veterans Affairs and U.S. Department of Defense clinical practice guideline. *Annals of Internal Medicine, 173*(10), 822–829. https://doi.org/10.7326/M20-4648

Otto, C. M., Nishimura, R. A., Bonow, R. O., Carabello, B. A., Erwin, J. E., Gentile, F., Jneid, H., Krieger, E. V., Mack, M. J., McLeod, C. J., O'Gara, P. T., Rigolin, V. H., Sundt, T. M., Thompson, A., & Toly, C. (2021a). 2020 ACC/AHA guideline for the management of patients with valvular heart disease: Executive summary: A report of the American College of Cardiology/American Heart Association Joint Committee on clinical practice guidelines. *Circulation, 143*(5), e35–e71. https://doi.org/10.1161/cir.0000000000000932

Panchal, A. R., Bartos, J. A., Cabañas, J. G., Donnino, M. W., Drennan, I. R., Hirsch, K. G., Kudenchuk, P. J., Kurz, M. C., Lavonas, E. J., Morley, P. T., O'Neil, B. J., Peberdy, M. A., Rittenberger, J. C., Rodriguez, A. J., Sawyer, K. N., Berg, K. M., & Adult Basic and Advanced Life Support Writing Group. (2020). Part 3: Adult basic and advanced life support: 2020 American Heart Association guidelines for cardiopulmonary resuscitation and emergency cardiovascular care. *Circulation, 142*(16_Suppl_2), S366–S468. https://doi.org/10.1161/CIR.0000000000000916

Pieri, M., & Pappalardo, F. (2020). Bedside insertion of impella percutaneous ventricular assist device in patients with cardiogenic shock. *International Journal of Cardiology, 316*, 26–30. https://doi.org/10.1016/j.ijcard.2020.05.080

Puri, R., Nissen, S. E., Arsenault, B. J., St John, J., Riesmeyer, J. S., Ruotolo, G., McErlean, E., Menon, V., Cho, L., Wolski, K., Lincoff, A. M., & Nicholls, S. J. (2020). Effect of C-reactive protein on lipoprotein(a)-associated cardiovascular risk in optimally treated patients with high-risk vascular disease: A prespecified secondary analysis of the ACCELERATE trial. *JAMA Cardiology, 5*(10), 1136–1143. https://doi.org/10.1001/jamacardio.2020.2413

Rossignol, P., & Pitt, B. (2021). Heart failure and chronic kidney disease patients: First it is necessary to act. *Journal of the American College of Cardiology, 78*(4), 344–347. https://doi.org/10.1016/j.jacc.2021.05.027

Safirstein, J. G., Tehrani, D. M., Schussler, J. M., Reid, N., Mukerjee, K., Weber, L., Liu, H., Skenderian, S., Simeon, M., Yang, T., & Seto, A. H. (2022). Radial hemostasis is facilitated with a potassium ferrate hemostatic patch. *JACC: Cardiovascular Interventions, 15*(8), 810–819. https://doi.org/10.1016/j.jcin.2021.12.030

Steinwender, C., Khelae, S., Garweg, C., Chan, J. Y. S., Ritter, P., Johansen, J. B., Sagi, V., Epstein, L. M., Piccini, J. P., Pascual, M., Mont, L., Sheldon, T., Splett, V., Stromberg, K., Wood, N., & Chinitz, L. (2020). Atrioventricular synchronous pacing using a leadless ventricular pacemaker: Results from the MARVEL 2 study. *JACC Clinical Electrophysiology, 6*(1), 94–106. https://doi.org/10.1016/j.jacep.2019.10.017

Stiles, M. K., Fauchier, L., Morillo, C. A., & Wilkoff, B. L. (2020). 2019 HRS/EHRA/APHRS/LAHRS focused update to 2015 expert consensus statement on optimal implantable cardioverter-defibrillator programming and testing. *Heart Rhythm, 17*(1), e220–e228. https://doi.org/10.1016/j.hrthm.2019.02.034

Tachibana, M., Banba, K., Matsumoto, K., & Ohara, M. (2020). The feasibility of leadless pacemaker implantation for superelderly patients. *Pacing Clinical Electrophysiology, 43*(4), 374–381. https://doi.org/10.1111/pace.13894

Vilcant, V., & Zeltser, R. (2022). *Treadmill stress testing.* StatPearls Publishing.

Walter, J., du Fay de Lavallaz, J., Koechlin, L., Zimmermann, T., Boeddinghaus, J., Honegger, U., Strebel, I., Twerenbold, R., Amrein, M., Nestelberger, T., Wussler, D., Puelacher, C., Badertscher, P., Zellweger, M., Fahrni, G., Jeger, R., Kaiser, C., Reichlin, T., & Mueller, C. (2020). Using high-sensitivity cardiac troponin for the exclusion of inducible myocardial ischemia in symptomatic patients: A cohort study. *Annals of Internal Medicine, 172*(3), 175–185. https://doi.org/10.7326/M19-0080

Wiegand, D. L. (Ed.). (2017). *AACN procedure manual for critical care* (7th ed.). Saunders.

Zeppenfeld, K., Tfelt-Hansen, J., de Riva, M., Winkel, B. G., Behr, E. R., Blom, N. A., Charron, P., Corrado, D., Dagres, N., de Chillou, C., Eckardt, L., Friede, T., Haugaa, K. H., Hocini, M., Lambiase, P. D., Marijon, E., Merino, J. L., Peichl, P., Priori, S. G., ... ESC Scientific Document Group. (2022). 2022 ESC Guidelines for the management of patients with ventricular arrhythmias and the prevention of sudden cardiac death. *European Heart Journal, 43*(40), 3997–4126. https://doi.org/10.1093/eurheartj/ehac262

Zhang, W., Speiser, J. L., Ye, F., Tsai, M. Y., Cainzos-Achirica, M., Nasir, K., Herrington, D. M., & Shapiro, M. D. (2021). High-sensitivity C-reactive protein modifies the cardiovascular risk of lipoprotein(a): Multi-ethnic study of atherosclerosis. *Journal of American College of Cardiology, 78*(11), 1083–1094. https://doi.org/10.1016/j.jacc.2021.07.016

9 Cardiac Disorders*

CARDIAC DISORDERS

See additional online content: Nursing Care Plan 9-1

Coronary Artery Disease

EVIDENCE BASE Fihn, S. D., Blankenship, J. C., Alexander, K. P., Bittl, J. A., Byrne, J. G., Fletcher, B. J., Fonarow, G. C., Lange, R. A., Levine, G. N., Maddox, T. M., Naidu, S. S., Ohman, E. M., & Smith, P. K. (2014). 2014 ACC/AHA/AATS/PCNA/SCAI/STS focused update of the guideline for the diagnosis and management of patients with stable ischemic heart disease: A report of the American College of Cardiology/American Heart Association Task Force on Practice Cardiovascular Guidelines, and the American Association for Thoracic Surgery, Preventive Cardiovascular Nurses Association, Society for Cardiovascular Angiography and Interventions, and Society of Thoracic Surgeons. *Circulation*, *130*(19), 1749–1767. https://doi.org/10.1161/CIR.0000000000000095

Coronary artery disease (CAD) is the leading cause of death worldwide. CAD is characterized by the accumulation of plaque within the layers of the coronary arteries. The plaques progressively enlarge, thicken, and calcify, causing a critical narrowing (greater than 70% occlusion) of the coronary artery lumen, resulting in a decrease in coronary blood flow and an inadequate supply of oxygen to the heart muscle.

Acute coronary syndrome (ACS) is an umbrella term that is used to describe many of the complications associated with CAD. These include unstable angina (UA), non–ST-elevation myocardial infarction (NSTEMI), and ST-elevation myocardial infarction (STEMI).

Pathophysiology and Etiology

1. The most widely accepted cause of CAD is atherosclerosis (see Figure 9-1), which is the gradual accumulation of plaque within an artery forming an atheroma. Plaque consists of lipid-filled macrophages (foam cells), fibrin, cellular waste products, and plasma proteins, covered by a fibrous outer layer (smooth muscle cells and dense connective tissue).
   a. When the endothelium is injured by being exposed to low-density lipoproteins (LDLs), by-products of cigarette smoke, hypertension, hyperglycemia, infection, and increased homocysteine, hyperfibrinogenemia, and lipoprotein(a), an inflammatory response occurs, making the endothelium sticky and thereby attracting adhesion molecules.
   b. Over time, the plaque thickens, extends, and calcifies, causing narrowing of the lumen.
   c. Eventual hemorrhage and ulceration of the plaque may cause significant coronary obstruction.
2. Angina pectoris, caused by inadequate blood flow to the myocardium, is the most common manifestation of CAD.
   a. Angina is usually precipitated by physical exertion or emotional stress, which puts an increased demand on the heart to circulate more blood and oxygen.
   b. The ability of the coronary artery to deliver blood to the myocardium is impaired because of obstruction by a significant coronary lesion (greater than 70% narrowing of the vessel).
   c. Angina can also occur in other cardiac problems, such as arterial spasm, aortic stenosis, cardiomyopathy, or uncontrolled hypertension.
   d. Noncardiac causes include anemia, fever, thyrotoxicosis, and anxiety/panic attacks.

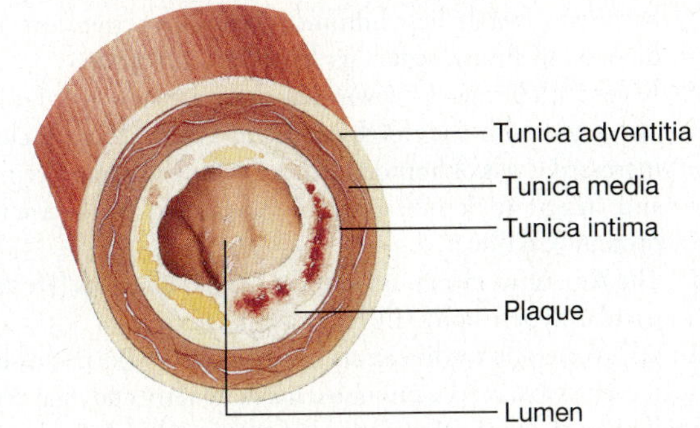

Figure 9-1. The pathogenesis of atherosclerosis.

*Please note that the term "male" in this chapter refers to a person assigned male at birth, and the term "female" in this chapter refers to a person assigned female at birth.

3. ACS is caused by a decrease in the oxygen available to the myocardium because of:
   a. Unstable or ruptured atherosclerotic plaque.
   b. Coronary vasospasm.
   c. Atherosclerotic obstruction without clot or vasospasm.
   d. Inflammation or infection.
   e. Stable angina that becomes unstable because of a noncardiac cause.
   f. Thrombus formation with subsequent coronary artery occlusion (the most common cause) (see "Myocardial Infarction," page 245).
4. Risk factors for the development of CAD include:
   a. Nonmodifiable: age (risk increases with age), sex (being a person assigned male at birth; females typically suffer from heart disease 10 years later than males because of the postmenopausal decrease in cardiac-protective estrogen), ethnicity (Black, Hispanic, Latino, and Southeast Asian populations have increased risk), and family history.
   b. Modifiable: elevated lipid levels, hypertension, obesity, tobacco use, metabolic syndrome (obesity, hypertension, and diabetes mellitus), sedentary lifestyle, and stress.
   c. Recent studies have shown that there are new risk factors associated with the development of CAD. These include increased levels of homocysteine, fibrin, and lipoprotein(a) and infection or inflammation (measured by C-reactive protein [CRP]).
   d. The American Heart Association (AHA) also lists left ventricular hypertrophy (LVH) as a risk factor.
5. An atherosclerotic cardiovascular disease (ASCVD) risk assessment every 4 to 6 years is promoted for short-term and long-term prediction of the development of cardiovascular disease based on age, sex assigned at birth, ethnicity, lipid panel, systolic blood pressure (BP), BP medication use, smoking status, and diabetes status. Additional risk markers are diastolic BP, chronic kidney disease, body mass index (BMI), and family history.

EVIDENCE BASE Wilson, P. (2024). Cardiovascular disease risk assessment for primary prevention. *Risk Calculators*. Retrieved from https://www.uptodate.com/contents/cardiovascular-disease-risk-assessment-for-primary-prevention-risk-calculators

Clinical Manifestations

See Standards of Care Guidelines 9-1

Chronic Stable Angina Pectoris

Chest pain or discomfort that is provoked by exertion or emotional stress and relieved by rest and nitroglycerin.

1. Character—substernal chest pain, pressure, heaviness (like something sitting on the chest), or discomfort. Other sensations include a squeezing, aching, burning, fullness, choking, strangling, and/or cramping pain.
   a. Pain may be mild or severe and typically presents with a gradual buildup of discomfort and subsequent gradual fading.
   b. May produce numbness or weakness in the arms, wrists, or hands.
   c. Associated symptoms include diaphoresis, nausea, indigestion, dyspnea, tachycardia, dizziness, feeling of profound fatigue, and increase in BP.
   d. Females may experience atypical symptoms of chest pain, such as jaw pain, shortness of breath, or indigestion. Patients with diabetes or history of heart transplant may not experience chest pain.

STANDARDS OF CARE GUIDELINES 9-1

Chest Pain

- Thoroughly evaluate any complaint of chest pain.
- Be alert to those at highest risk for myocardial infarction (MI)—those who smoke, those with hypertension, diabetes, or hyperlipidemia—but do not discount the possibility of MI occurring in those without risk factors.
- Be alert to common alternative presentation of coronary artery disease (CAD) and MI in females, patients with diabetes, and older patients (nausea, indigestion, fatigue).
- Notify health care provider, and obtain electrocardiogram for complaint of chest pain.
- For chest pain not relieved by rest or nitroglycerin, assist and advise patient to obtain emergency care immediately. Call 911 for emergency response team if pain is consistent with MI.

This information should serve as a general guideline only. Each patient situation presents a unique set of clinical factors and requires nursing judgment to guide care, which may include additional or alternative measures and approaches.

2. Location—behind middle or upper third of the sternum; the patient will generally make a fist over the site of the pain (positive Levine sign, indicating diffuse deep visceral pain) rather than point to it with their finger.
3. Radiation—usually radiates to the neck, jaw, shoulders, arms, hands, and posterior intrascapular area. Pain occurs more commonly on the left side than the right.
4. Duration—usually lasts 2 to 15 minutes after stopping activity; nitroglycerin relieves pain within 1 minute.
5. Other precipitating factors—exposure to weather extremes, eating a heavy meal, and sexual intercourse all increase the workload of the heart, thus increasing oxygen demand.

Unstable (Preinfarction) Angina Pectoris

Chest pain occurring at rest; no increase in oxygen demand is placed on the heart, but an acute lack of blood flow to the heart occurs because of coronary artery spasm or the presence of an enlarged plaque or hemorrhage/ulceration of a complicated lesion. Critical narrowing of the vessel lumen occurs abruptly in either instance.

1. A change in frequency, duration, and intensity of stable angina symptoms is indicative of progression to UA.
2. UA pain lasts longer than 10 minutes, is unrelieved by rest or sublingual nitroglycerin, and mimics signs and symptoms of impending MI.

CLINICAL JUDGMENT UA can cause sudden death or result in MI. Early recognition and treatment are imperative to prevent complications.

Silent Ischemia

The absence of chest pain with documented evidence of an imbalance between myocardial oxygen supply and demand (ST depression of 1 mm or more) as determined by electrocardiography (ECG), exercise stress test, or ambulatory (Holter) ECG monitoring.

1. Silent ischemia most commonly occurs during the first few hours after awakening (circadian event) because of an

increase in sympathetic nervous system activity, causing an increase in heart rate, BP, coronary vessel tone, and blood viscosity.
2. Populations at increased risk include people with diabetes and older people, particularly females.

Diagnostic Evaluation

1. Characteristic chest pain and clinical history.
2. Nitroglycerin test—relief of pain with nitroglycerin.
3. Blood tests.
   a. Cardiac markers, particularly troponin-I, to determine the presence and severity if acute cardiac insult is suspected; creatine kinase (CK) and its isoenzyme CK-MB are losing favor for diagnosing MI.
   b. HbA1C and fasting lipid panel to rule out modifiable risk factors for CAD.
   c. Coagulation studies, CRP, homocysteine, and lipoprotein(a) (increased levels are associated with a twofold risk in developing CAD).
   d. Hemoglobin to rule out anemia, which may reduce myocardial oxygen supply.
4. Twelve-lead ECG—may show LVH, ST- and T-wave changes (2 mm or greater ST elevation in contiguous leads for male and 1.5 mm or greater in female diagnostics for myocardial infarction), arrhythmias, and Q waves.
5. ECG stress testing—progressive increases in speed and elevation while walking on a treadmill increase the workload of the heart. ST- and T-wave changes occur if myocardial ischemia is induced.
6. Radionuclide imaging—a radioisotope, thallium-201, injected during exercise is imaged by camera. Low uptake of the isotope by heart muscle indicates regions of ischemia induced by exercise. Images taken during rest show a reversal of ischemia in those regions affected.
7. Radionuclide ventriculography (gated blood pool scanning)—red blood cells tagged with a radioisotope are imaged by camera during exercise and at rest. Wall motion abnormalities of the heart can be detected and ejection fraction estimated.
8. Cardiac catheterization—coronary angiography performed during the procedure determines the presence, location, and extent of coronary lesions.
9. Positron emission tomography (PET)—cardiac perfusion imaging with high resolution to detect very small perfusion differences caused by stenotic arteries. Not available in all settings.
10. Coronary computed tomography angiography (CTA)—scans the coronary arteries that supply blood to the heart and determines whether they are narrowed by plaques. Three-dimensional images can be created. Recommended for low- to intermediate-risk patients with chest pain.

Management

Drug Therapy

Antianginal medications (nitrates, beta-adrenergic blockers, calcium channel blockers, and angiotensin-converting enzyme [ACE] inhibitors) are used to maintain a balance between oxygen supply and demand. Coronary vessel relaxation promotes blood flow to the heart, thereby increasing oxygen supply. Reduction of the workload of the heart decreases oxygen demand and consumption. The goal of drug therapy is to maintain a balance between oxygen supply and demand.

1. Nitrates—caused by generalized vasodilation throughout the body. Nitrates can be administered via oral, sublingual, transdermal, intravenous (IV), or intracoronary (IC) route and may provide short- or long-acting effects.
   a. Short-acting nitrates (sublingual) provide immediate relief of acute anginal attacks or prophylaxis if taken before activity.
   b. Long-acting nitrates prevent anginal episodes and/or reduce severity and frequency of attacks.
2. Beta-adrenergic blockers—inhibit sympathetic stimulation of receptors that are located in the conduction system of the heart and in heart muscle.
   a. Some beta-adrenergic blockers (e.g., "nonselective" beta-adrenergic blockers) inhibit sympathetic stimulation of receptors in the lungs as well as the heart, causing vasoconstriction of the large airways of the lung.
   b. "Cardioselective" beta-adrenergic blockers (in recommended dose ranges) affect only the heart and can be used safely in patients with lung disease.

DRUG ALERT Beta-adrenergic blockers are generally contraindicated in people with COPD and asthma because of the risk of vasoconstriction of airways, causing shortness of breath and wheezing.

3. Calcium channel blockers—inhibit movement of calcium within the heart muscle and coronary vessels; promote vasodilation and prevent/control coronary artery spasm.
4. ACE inhibitors—have therapeutic effects by remodeling the vascular endothelium and have been shown to reduce the risk of worsening angina.
5. Antilipid agents—reduce total cholesterol (TC) and triglyceride (TG) levels and have been shown to assist in the stabilization of plaque.
6. Antiplatelet agents—decrease platelet aggregation to inhibit thrombus formation.
7. Folic acid and B complex vitamins—treat increased homocysteine levels.

Percutaneous Coronary Interventions

1. Percutaneous transluminal angioplasty.
   a. A balloon-tipped catheter is placed in a coronary vessel narrowed by plaque.
   b. The balloon is inflated and deflated to stretch the vessel wall and flatten the plaque (see page 280).
   c. Blood flows freely through the unclogged vessel to the heart.
2. IC atherectomy.
   a. A blade-tipped catheter is guided into a coronary vessel to the site of the plaque.
   b. Depending on the type of blade, the plaque is cut, shaved, or pulverized and then removed.
   c. Requires a larger catheter introduction sheath, so its use is limited to larger vessels.
3. IC stent.
   a. A diamond mesh tubular device (bare metal or drug-eluding) is placed in the coronary vessel.
   b. Prevents restenosis by providing a "skeletal" support.
   c. Drug-eluting stents contain an anti-inflammatory drug that is slowly released from the stent, decreasing the inflammatory response within the artery.

Other Interventional Strategies

1. Coronary artery bypass graft (CABG) surgery.
   a. A graft is surgically attached to the aorta, and the other end of the graft is attached to a distal portion of a coronary vessel.

   b. Bypasses obstructive lesions in the vessel and returns adequate blood flow to the heart muscle supplied by the artery (see page 230).
   c. Recommended for patients with diabetes mellitus, multivessel CAD, and acceptable surgical risk instead of percutaneous cardiac intervention (PCI).
2. Transmyocardial revascularization—by means of a laser beam, small channels are formed in the myocardium to encourage new blood flow.

Secondary Prevention

EVIDENCE BASE Eckel, R. H., Jakicic, J. M., Ard, J. D., de Jesus, J. M., Houston Miller, N., Hubbard, V. S., Lee, I. M., Lichtenstein, A. H., Loria, C. M., Millen, B. E., Nonas, C. A., Sacks, F. M., Smith, S. C., Jr., Svetkey, L. P., Wadden, T. A., Yanovski, S. Z., Kendall, K. A., Morgan, L. C., Trisolini, M. G., ... American College of Cardiology/American Heart Association Task Force on Practice Guidelines. (2014). 2013 AHA/ACC guideline on lifestyle management to reduce cardiovascular risk: A report of the American College of Cardiology/American Heart Association Task Force on Practice Guidelines. *Circulation, 129*(25 Suppl 2), S76–S99. https://doi.org/10.1161/01.cir.0000437740.48606.d1

1. Cessation of smoking.
2. Control of high BP (below 130/85 mm Hg in those with chronic kidney disease or heart failure; below 130/80 mm Hg in those with diabetes; below 140/90 mm Hg in all others).
3. Diet low in saturated fat (less than 7% of calories), cholesterol (less than 200 mg/day), trans fatty acids, sodium (less than 2 g/day), alcohol (2 or fewer drinks/day in males, 1 or fewer in females).
4. Low-dose aspirin daily for those at high risk.
5. Physical exercise (at least 30 to 60 minutes of moderate-intensity exercise most days).
6. Weight control (ideal BMI 18.5 to 24.9 kg/m^2); waist circumference less than 40 in for males and less than 35 in for females.
7. Control of diabetes mellitus (fasting glucose less than 110 mg/dL and HbA1C less than 7%).
8. Control of blood lipids with goal of LDL less than 100 mg/dL (less than 70 mg/dL in high-risk patients).

Complications

1. Sudden death because of lethal dysrhythmias.
2. Heart failure.
3. MI.

Nursing Assessment

1. Ask patient to describe anginal attacks.
   a. When do attacks tend to occur? After a meal? After engaging in certain activities? After physical activities in general? After visits of family/others?
   b. Where is the pain located? Does it radiate?
   c. What does the pain feel like? Is it equivalent to atypical chest pain?
   d. Was the onset of pain sudden? Gradual?
   e. How long did it last—Seconds? Minutes? Hours?
   f. Was the pain steady and unwavering in quality?
   g. Is the discomfort accompanied by other symptoms? Sweating? Light-headedness? Nausea? Palpitations? Shortness of breath?
   h. Is there anything that makes it worse (such as moving, deep breathing, food)?
   i. How is the pain relieved? How long does it take for pain relief?
2. Obtain a baseline 12-lead ECG.
3. Assess patient's and family's knowledge of disease.
4. Identify patient's and family's level of anxiety and use of appropriate coping mechanisms.
5. Gather information about the patient's cardiac risk factors. Use the patient's age, TC level, LDL and high-density lipoprotein (HDL) levels, systolic BP, and smoking status to determine the patient's 10-year risk for development of coronary heart disease (CHD). (https://static.heart.org/riskcalc/app/index.html#!/baseline-risk).
6. Evaluate patient's medical history for such conditions as diabetes, heart failure, previous MI, or obstructive lung disease that may influence choice of drug therapy.
7. Identify factors that may contribute to barriers or nonadherence to prescribed drug therapy.
8. Review renal and hepatic studies and complete blood count (CBC).
9. Discuss with patient current activity levels. (Effectiveness of antianginal drug therapy is evaluated by patient's ability to attain higher activity levels.)
10. Discuss patient's beliefs about modification of risk factors and willingness to change.

Nursing Interventions

Relieving Pain

1. Determine intensity of patient's angina.
   a. Ask patient to compare the pain with other pain experienced in the past and, on a scale of 0 (no pain) to 10 (worst pain), rate current pain.
   b. Observe for associated signs and symptoms, including diaphoresis, shortness of breath, protective body posture, dusky facial color, and/or changes in level of consciousness (LOC).
   c. If chest pain is equivalent to previously experienced pain, is this the usual pattern?
2. Position patient for comfort; Fowler position promotes ventilation.
3. Administer oxygen, if appropriate.
4. Obtain BP, apical heart rate, and respiratory rate.
5. Obtain a 12-lead ECG.
6. Administer antianginal drug(s), as prescribed.
7. Report findings to health care providers.
8. Monitor for relief of pain and note duration of anginal episode.
9. Take vital signs every 5 to 10 minutes until angina pain subsides.
10. Monitor for progression of stable angina to UA: increase in frequency and intensity of pain, pain occurring at rest or at low levels of exertion, pain lasting longer than 5 minutes.
11. Determine level of activity that precipitated anginal episode.
12. Identify specific activities patient may engage in that are below the level at which anginal pain occurs.
13. Reinforce the importance of notifying nursing staff when angina pain is experienced.

Maintaining Cardiac Output

1. Carefully monitor the patient's response to drug therapy.
   a. Take BP and heart rate in a sitting and a lying position on initiation of long-term therapy (provides baseline data to evaluate for orthostatic hypotension that may occur with drug therapy).

b. Recheck vital signs as indicated by onset of action of drug and at the time of drug's peak effect.
c. Note changes in BP of more than 10 mm Hg and changes in heart rate of more than 10 beats/min.
d. Instruct patient to rise slowly from lying to sitting position and sitting to standing position to reduce dizziness.
e. Note patient complaints of headache (especially with use of nitrates) and dizziness (more common with ACE inhibitors).
    i. Administer or teach self-administration of analgesics, as directed, for headache.
    ii. Encourage supine position to relieve dizziness (usually associated with a decrease in BP; preload is enhanced by lying supine, thereby providing a temporary increase in BP).
f. Institute continuous ECG monitoring, or obtain 12-lead ECG as directed.
    i. Interpret rhythm strip every 4 hours and as needed for patients on continuous monitoring (beta-adrenergic blockers and calcium channel blockers can cause significant bradycardia and varying degrees of heart block).
    ii. Assess for changes in ST segment (elevation or depression, worsening or improving).
g. Evaluate for development of heart failure (beta-adrenergic blockers and some calcium channel blockers have negative inotropic properties).
    i. Obtain daily weight and intake and output.
    ii. Auscultate lung fields for crackles, and assess for shortness of breath and decrease in oxygen saturation.
    iii. Monitor for the presence of edema.
    iv. Monitor central venous pressure (CVP), if applicable.
    v. Assess jugular vein distention.
    vi. Assess liver engorgement and check liver function studies.
h. Monitor laboratory tests as indicated (cardiac markers).

2. Monitor for poor perfusion.
    a. Decreasing BP.
    b. Weak pulses.
    c. Dizziness.
    d. Shortness of breath.
    e. Cool extremities.
    f. Pale.
    g. Diaphoretic.
3. Be sure to remove previous nitrate patch or paste before applying new paste or patch (prevents hypotension) and to reapply on different body site.
    i. To decrease nitrate tolerance, transdermal nitroglycerin may be worn only in the daytime hours and taken off at night when physical exertion is decreased.
    ii. Wear gloves to prevent accidentally getting paste on hands, which may cause lightheadedness.
4. Be alert to adverse reaction related to abrupt discontinuation of beta-adrenergic blocker and calcium channel blocker therapy. These drugs must be tapered to prevent a "rebound phenomenon": tachycardia, increase in chest pain, hypertension.
5. Discuss use of chromotherapeutic therapy with health care provider (tailoring of antianginal drug therapy to the timing of circadian events).
6. Report adverse drug effects to health care provider.

Decreasing Anxiety

1. Rule out physiologic etiologies for increasing or new-onset anxiety before administering as-needed sedatives. Physiologic causes must be identified and treated in a timely fashion to prevent irreversible adverse or even fatal outcomes; sedatives may mask symptoms delaying timely identification and diagnosis and treatment.
2. Assess patient for signs of hypoperfusion, auscultate heart and lung sounds, obtain a rhythm strip, and administer oxygen, as prescribed. Notify the health care provider immediately.
3. Document all assessment findings, health care provider notification and response, and interventions and response.
4. Explain to patient and family reasons for hospitalization, diagnostic tests, and therapies administered.
5. Encourage patient to verbalize fears and concerns about illness through frequent conversations—conveys to patient a willingness to listen.
6. Answer patient's questions with concise explanations.
7. Administer medications to relieve patient's anxiety as directed. Sedatives and tranquilizers may be used to prevent attacks precipitated by aggravation, excitement, or tension.
8. Explain to patient the importance of anxiety reduction to assist in control of angina. (Anxiety and fear put increased stress on the heart, requiring the heart to use more oxygen.) Teach relaxation techniques.
9. Discuss measures to be taken when an anginal episode occurs. (Preparing patient decreases anxiety and allows patient to describe angina accurately.)
    a. Review the questions that will be asked during anginal episodes.
    b. Review the interventions that will be employed to relieve anginal attacks.

Patient Education and Health Maintenance

Instruct Patient and Family About CAD

1. Assess readiness to learn (pain free, shows interest, and comfortable), learning style, cognition, and education level.
2. Review the chambers of the heart and the coronary artery system, using a diagram of the heart.
3. Show patient a diagram of a clogged artery; explain how the blockage occurs; point out on the diagram the location of patient's lesions.
4. Explain that angina is a warning sign from the heart that there is decreased oxygen and blood flow to arteries of the heart due to a blockage in the artery or spasm.
5. Review specific risk factors that affect CAD development and progression; highlight those risk factors that can be modified and controlled to reduce risk.
6. Discuss the signs and symptoms of angina, precipitating factors, and treatment for attacks. Stress to patient the importance of treating angina symptoms at once.
7. Distinguish for patient the different signs and symptoms associated with stable angina versus preinfarction angina.
8. Give patient and family handouts to review and encourage questions for a later teaching session.

Identify Suitable Activity Level to Prevent Angina

Advise the patient about the following:

1. Participate in a normal daily program of activities that do not produce chest discomfort, shortness of breath, and undue fatigue. Spread daily activities out over the course of the day; avoid doing everything at one time. Begin regular exercise regimen, as directed by health care provider.
2. Avoid activities known to cause anginal pain—sudden exertion, walking in extreme weather conditions, extremes of temperature, high altitude, and emotionally stressful situations,

which may accelerate heart rate, raise BP, and increase cardiac workload.

3. Refrain from engaging in physical activity for 2 hours after meals. Rest after each meal, if possible.
4. Do not perform activities requiring heavy effort (e.g., carrying heavy objects).
5. Try to avoid cold weather, if possible; dress warmly and walk more slowly. Wear scarf over the nose and mouth when in cold air.
6. Lose weight, if necessary, to reduce stress on the heart.
7. Instruct patient that sexual activity is not prohibited and should be discussed with health care provider; it is usually allowed if patient can climb two flights of stairs.

Instruct About Appropriate Use of Medications and Adverse Effects

1. Carry nitroglycerin at all times.
   a. Nitroglycerin is volatile and is inactivated by heat, moisture, air, light, and time; keep container tightly closed and away from moisture.
   b. Keep nitroglycerin in original dark glass container, tightly closed to prevent absorption of drug by other pills or pillbox.
   c. Nitroglycerin should cause a slight burning or stinging sensation under the tongue when it is potent.
2. Place nitroglycerin under the tongue at first sign of chest discomfort.
   a. Stop all effort or activity, sit, and take nitroglycerin tablet—relief should be obtained in a few minutes.
   b. Repeat dosage in 5 minutes for total of three tablets if relief is not obtained.
   c. Keep a record of the number of tablets taken to evaluate change in anginal pattern.
   d. Take nitroglycerin prophylactically to avoid pain known to occur with certain activities.
3. Demonstrate for patient how to administer nitroglycerin paste correctly.
   a. Place paste on calibrated strip.
   b. Remove previous paste on the skin by wiping gently with tissue. Be careful to avoid touching paste to fingertips as this will lead to increased dosing from absorption.
   c. Rotate site of administration to avoid skin irritation.
   d. Apply paste to the skin; use plastic wrap to protect clothing if not provided on strip.
   e. Have patient return demonstration.
4. Instruct patient on administration of transdermal nitroglycerin patches.
   a. Remove previous patch; fold in half so that medication does not touch fingertips and will not be accessible in trash. Wipe area with tissue to remove any residual medication.
   b. Apply patch to a clean, dry, nonhairy area of the body.
   c. Rotate administration sites.
   d. Instruct patient not to remove patch for swimming or bathing.
   e. If patch loosens and part of it becomes nonadherent, it should be folded in half and discarded. A new patch should be applied.
   f. Patch must be removed prior to magnetic resonance imaging (MRI) scan to prevent skin burn.
5. Teach patient about potential adverse effects of other medications. Instruct patient not to stop taking any of these without discussing with health care provider.
   a. Constipation—verapamil.
   b. Ankle edema—nifedipine.
   c. Heart failure (shortness of breath, weight gain, edema)—beta-adrenergic blockers or calcium channel blockers.
   d. Dizziness—vasodilators, antihypertensives.
   e. Impotence—decreased libido and sexual functioning—beta-adrenergic blockers.
6. Ensure that patient has enough medication until next follow-up appointment or trip to the pharmacy. Warn against abrupt withdrawal of beta-adrenergic blockers or calcium channel blockers to prevent rebound effect.

CLINICAL JUDGMENT Instruct patient to call 911 if chest pain persists or has worsened after the first sublingual nitroglycerin tablet was administered (5 minutes). Furthermore, instruct patient to continue to take other sublingual nitroglycerin tablets every 5 minutes until emergency medical services have arrived (instruct patient not drive self to the hospital).

Counsel on Risk Factors and Lifestyle Changes

EVIDENCE BASE US Preventive Services Task Force, Krist, A. H., Davidson, K. W., Mangione, C. M., Barry, M. J., Cabana, M., Caughey, A. B., Donahue, K., Doubeni, C. A., Epling, J. W., Jr., Kubik, M., Landefeld, S., Ogedegbe, G., Pbert, L., Silverstein, M., Simon, M. A., Tseng, C. W., & Wong, J. B. (2020). Behavioral counseling interventions to promote a healthy diet and physical activity for cardiovascular disease prevention in adults with cardiovascular risk factors: US Preventive Services Task Force recommendation statement. *JAMA, 324*(20), 2069–2075. https://doi.org/10.1001/jama.2020.21749

1. Inform patient of methods of stress reduction, such as biofeedback and relaxation techniques.
2. Review low-fat and low-cholesterol diet. Explain AHA guidelines (see www.heart.org), which recommend eating fish at least twice per week, especially fish high in omega-3 oils.
   a. Omega-3 oils have been shown to improve arterial health and decrease BP, TG, and the growth of atherosclerotic plaque.
   b. Omega-3 oils can be found in fatty fish, such as mackerel, salmon, sardines, herring, and albacore tuna.
   c. Suggest available cookbooks (AHA) that may assist in planning and preparing foods.
   d. Have patient meet with dietitian to design a menu plan.
3. Inform patient of available cardiac rehabilitation programs that offer structured classes on exercise, smoking cessation, and weight control.
4. Instruct patient to avoid excessive caffeine intake (coffee, cola drinks), which can increase the heart rate and produce angina.
5. Tell patient not to use "diet pills," nasal decongestants, or any over-the-counter (OTC) medications that can increase heart rate or stimulate high BP.
6. Encourage patient to avoid alcohol or drink only in moderation (alcohol can increase hypotensive adverse effects of drugs).
7. Encourage follow-up visits for control of diabetes, hypertension, and hyperlipidemia.
8. Have patient discuss supplement therapy (i.e., vitamins B_6, B_{12}, C, E, folic acid, and L-arginine) with health care provider.
9. For additional information, refer patient to the AHA (www.americanheart.org).
10. Refer patient to health care provider to discuss the use of phosphodiesterase inhibitors (PDE5) for erectile dysfunction.

DRUG ALERT Patient should not take PDE5, such as sildenafil, concurrently with nitrates or alpha-adrenergic blockers because severe hypotension and cardiac event may occur.

Evaluation: Expected Outcomes

- Verbalizes relief of pain.
- BP and heart rate stable.
- Verbalizes lessening anxiety, ability to cope.

Myocardial Infarction

Myocardial infarction (MI) is one of the manifestations of ACS and refers to a dynamic process by which one or more regions of the heart experience a prolonged decrease or cessation in oxygen supply because of insufficient coronary blood flow; subsequently, necrosis or "death" to the affected myocardial tissue occurs. The onset of the MI process may be sudden or gradual, and the progression of the event to cell death takes approximately 3 to 6 hours.

As described in the Fourth Universal Definition of MI, the term acute myocardial infarction (AMI) should be used when there is acute myocardial injury with clinical evidence of acute myocardial ischemia and with detection of a rise or fall of cardiac troponin values. In addition, the diagnosis is secured with supportive evidence in the form of typical symptoms, suggestive ECG changes, or imaging evidence of new loss of viable myocardium or new regional wall motion abnormality.

EVIDENCE BASE Thygesen, K., Alpert, J. S., Jaffe, A. S., Chaitman, B. R., Bax, J. J., Morrow, D. A., White, H. D., & Executive Group on behalf of the Joint European Society of Cardiology/American College of Cardiology/American Heart Association/World Heart Federation Task Force for the Universal Definition of Myocardial Infarction. (2018). Fourth universal definition of myocardial infarction. *Journal of the American College of Cardiology, 72*(18), 2231–2264. https://doi.org/10.1016/j.jacc.2018.08.1038

Pathophysiology and Etiology

1. Acute coronary thrombosis (partial or total)—associated with 90% of MIs.
   a. Severe atherosclerosis (greater than 70% narrowing of the artery) precipitates thrombus.
   b. Thrombus formation begins with plaque rupture and platelets' adhesion to the damaged area.
   c. Activation of the exposed platelets causes expression of glycoprotein IIb/IIIa receptors that bind fibrinogen.
   d. Further platelet aggregation and adhesion occurs, enlarging the thrombus and occluding blood supply.
2. Other etiologic factors include coronary artery spasm, coronary artery embolism, infectious diseases causing arterial inflammation, hypoxia, anemia, and severe exertion or stress on the heart in the presence of significant CAD (i.e., surgical procedures, shoveling snow).
3. Different degrees of damage occur to the heart muscle (see Figure 9-2):
   a. Zone of necrosis—death to the heart muscle caused by extensive and complete oxygen deprivation; irreversible damage.
   b. Zone of injury—region of the heart muscle surrounding the area of necrosis; inflamed and injured, but still viable if adequate oxygenation can be restored.

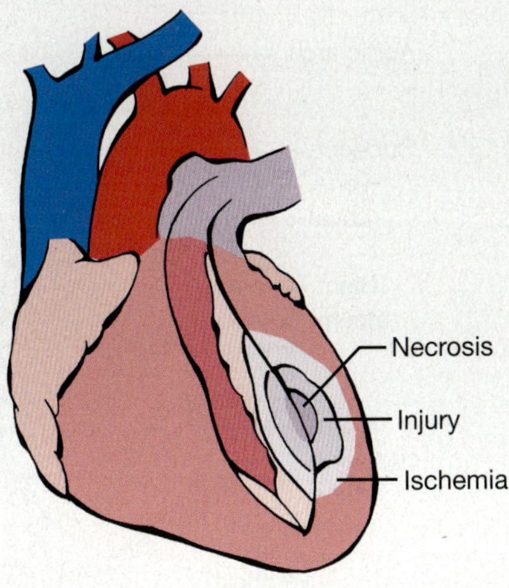

Figure 9-2. Different degrees of damage occur to the heart muscle after a myocardial infarction. This diagram shows zones of necrosis, injury, and ischemia.

   c. Zone of ischemia—region of the heart muscle surrounding the area of injury, which is ischemic and viable; not endangered unless extension of the infarction occurs.
4. The term acute coronary syndrome is applied to patients in whom there is a suspicion or confirmation of myocardial ischemia, which may be classified in the following ways:
   a. STEMI—whereby ST-segment elevations are seen on ECG. The area of necrosis may or may not occur through the entire wall of heart muscle.
   b. NSTEMI—no ST-segment elevations can be seen on ECG. ST depressions may be noted as well as positive cardiac markers, T-wave inversions, and clinical equivalents (chest pain). Area of necrosis may or may not occur through the entire myocardium.
   c. UA—considered to be present in patients with ischemic symptoms suggestive of an ACS without elevation in biomarkers with or without ECG changes indicative of ischemia. ST-segment and T wave changes on ECG are usually transient in UA.
5. Clinical classification of acute MI is based on the cause of myocardial ischemia; depending on clinical circumstances such as chest discomfort. Types 1 and 2 are the most common.
   a. Type 1: MI caused by acute atherothrombotic CAD and precipitated by atherosclerotic plaque rupture or erosion. There is an acute shortage of myocardial oxygen supply and demand; may be STEMI or NSTEMI.
   b. Type 2: when the event is secondary to ischemia due to either an increased oxygen demand or a decreased supply in the absence of an acute primary coronary thrombotic event.
   c. Type 3: cardiac death with symptoms suggestive of MI and new left bundle branch block, but death occurring before blood samples for biomarkers could be drawn.
   d. Type 4a: MI associated with percutaneous coronary intervention (PCI).
   e. Type 4b: MI related to stent/scaffold thrombosis.
   f. Type 5: MI related to CABG (either new graft occlusion or new native coronary artery occlusion).
6. The region(s) of the heart muscle that become(s) affected depends on which coronary artery(ies) is/are obstructed (see Figure 9-3).
   a. The left ventricle is a common and dangerous location for an MI because it is the main pumping chamber of

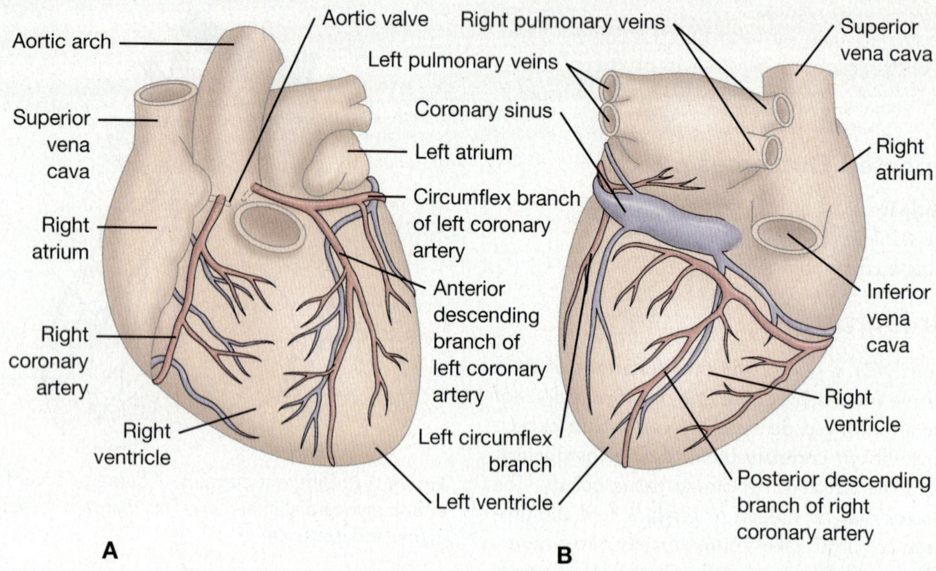

Figure 9-3. The coronary arteries supply the heart muscle with oxygenated blood, adjusting the flow according to metabolic needs. **(A)** Anterior view of the heart. **(B)** Posterior view of the heart. (Reprinted with permission from Hinkle, J. L., Cheever, K. H, & Overbaugh, K. [2022]. *Brunner and Suddarth's textbook of medical-surgical nursing* [15th ed., Fig. 23-2]. Lippincott Williams & Wilkins.)

the heart. The left anterior descending artery supplies oxygen to this part of the heart.
   b. Right ventricular infarctions commonly occur with damage to the inferior and/or posterior wall of the left ventricle. Occlusion in the right coronary or circumflex arteries can lead to this type of infarct.
7. The severity and location of the MI determine prognosis.

Clinical Manifestations

1. Chest pain.
   a. Severe, diffuse, steady substernal pain; may be described as crushing, squeezing, or dull.
   b. Not relieved by rest or sublingual vasodilator therapy such as nitroglycerine but requires opioids (i.e., morphine).
   c. May radiate to the arms (usually the left), shoulders, neck, back, and/or jaw.
   d. Continues for more than 15 minutes.
   e. May produce anxiety and fear, resulting in increased heart rate, BP, and respiratory rate.
   f. Some patients, especially older adults, females, and those with diabetes, may exhibit no complaints of pain (silent MI).
2. Diaphoresis; cool, clammy skin; facial pallor.
3. hypertension or hypotension.
4. Bradycardia or tachycardia.
5. Premature ventricular and/or atrial beats.
6. Palpitations, severe anxiety, dyspnea.
7. Disorientation, confusion, restlessness.
8. Fainting, marked weakness.
9. Nausea, vomiting, hiccups.
10. Atypical symptoms: epigastric or abdominal distress, dull aching or tingling sensations, shortness of breath, extreme fatigue.

POPULATION AWARENESS Females and patients with diabetes usually present with atypical and/or vague complaints (e.g., indigestion, fatigue). These patients are at higher risk of death during hospitalization. This is influenced by delay in seeking medical attention, and they are less likely to receive therapies that have been shown to be effective in MI treatment. Older adults may experience stroke-like symptoms, dizziness, or change in mental status.

11. Silent MI may go unrecognized until later. Three criteria qualify for a diagnosis of prior or silent MI:
    a. Abnormal Q waves with or without symptoms in the absence of nonischemic causes.
    b. Imaging evidence of loss of viable myocardium in a pattern consistent with ischemic etiology.
    c. Recent noncardiac surgery.

Diagnostic Evaluation

ECG Changes

1. Generally occurs within 2 to 12 hours, but may take 72 to 96 hours.
2. Necrotic, injured, and ischemic tissues alter ventricular depolarization and repolarization.
   a. ST-segment depression and T-wave inversion indicate a pattern of ischemia.
   b. ST elevation indicates an injury pattern.
   c. Q waves (see Figure 9-4) indicate tissue necrosis and are permanent. A pathologic Q wave is one that is greater than 3 mm in depth or greater than one third the height of the R wave.
3. Location of the infarction (anterior, anteroseptal, inferior, posterior, lateral) is determined by the leads in which the ST changes (elevation vs. depression) are seen. Of note, the changes must be in two contiguous or related leads to be diagnostic (see Figure 9-5)
4. Size or the amount of myocardium affected is another factor that influences ECG findings.
5. Early ECG is essential to allow initial categorization of suspected MI as STEMI, NSTEMI, or undifferentiated chest pain syndrome.

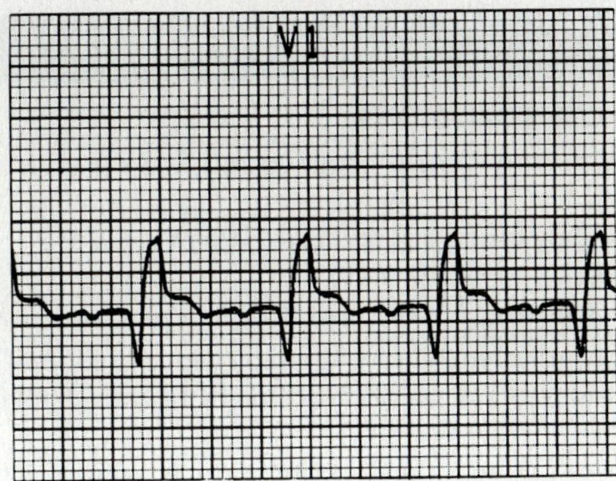

Figure 9-4. Abnormal Q wave.

CLINICAL JUDGMENT A normal ECG does not rule out the possibility of infarction, because ECG changes can be subtle and obscured by underlying conditions (bundle-branch blocks, electrolyte disturbances). Be aware that left bundle branch block is often present in patients with pacemakers and in acute MI. This is why clinical history and cardiac enzymes are important when suspecting or diagnosing MI.

Cardiac Markers

1. Cardiac enzymes (biochemical markers) are not diagnostic of an acute MI with a single elevation; serial markers are drawn (see page 202).
   a. Marker elevation is then correlated with the extent of heart muscle damage.
   b. Characteristic elevation over several hours confirms an MI.
   c. Cardiac troponin I and T are specific and sensitive biomarkers of myocardial injury. They are the preferred serologic tests for the evaluation of patients with suspected acute MI. Measurement of cardiac troponin I and T can be performed using sensitive or highly sensitive (preferred) tests.

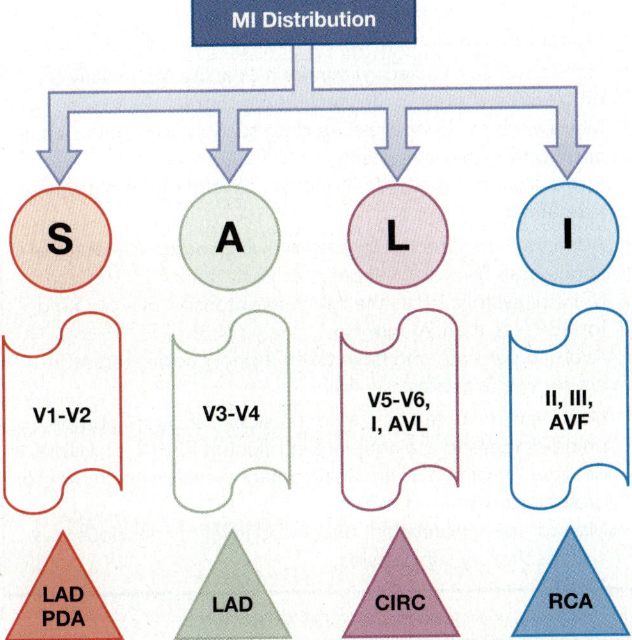

Figure 9-5. SALI pneumonic for MI distribution by ECG lead changes. ECG, electrocardiography; MI, myocardial infarction; S, septal; A, anterior; L, lateral; I, inferior; LAD, left anterior descending; PDA, posterior descending artery; CIRC, circumflex; RCA, right coronary artery.

   d. CK-MB is used in some institutions if troponin test is unavailable. This is relatively specific to myocardial injury, when skeletal muscle damage is not present. It typically begins to rise between 4 and 6 hours after the onset of infarction, but an elevation may not be seen until about 12 hours. This test is valuable when it shows an increased CK-MB level after the level has begun to decline, which is an important indicator of MI extension.

EVIDENCE BASE Thygesen, K., Alpert, J. S., Jaffe, A. S., Chaitman, B. R., Bax, J. J., Morrow, D. A., White, H. D., & Executive Group on behalf of the Joint European Society of Cardiology/American College of Cardiology/American Heart Association/World Heart Federation Task Force for the Universal Definition of Myocardial Infarction. (2018). Fourth universal definition of myocardial infarction. *Journal of the American College of Cardiology, 72*(18), 2231–2264. https://doi.org/10.1016/j.jacc.2018.08.1038

Other Findings

1. Elevated CRP and lipoprotein(s) because of inflammation in the coronary arteries.
2. Abnormal coagulation studies (prothrombin time [PT], partial thromboplastin time [PTT]).
3. Elevated white blood cell (WBC) count and sedimentation rate because of the inflammatory process involved in heart muscle cell damage.
4. Radionuclide imaging allows recognition of areas of decreased perfusion.
5. PET scan determines the presence of reversible heart muscle injury and irreversible or necrotic tissue; extent to which the injured heart muscle has responded to treatment can also be determined.
6. Cardiac MRI provides an accurate assessment of myocardial structure and function.
7. Echocardiography can detect regional wall motion abnormalities induced by ischemia when greater than 20% transmural myocardial thickness is affected.

Management

The goals of therapy are immediate relief of ischemia and prevention of severe outcomes. To achieve this requires administration of anti-ischemic therapy (i.e., rest, supplemental oxygen, nitroglycerin, beta-blockers, ACE inhibitors) and antithrombotic therapy (i.e., aspirin, clopidogrel, ticlopidine, ticagrelor); ongoing risk stratification; and use of invasive procedure (i.e., cardiac catheterization) to provide early restoration of coronary blood flow. See Table 9-1.

Growing evidence suggests that the use of supplemental oxygen in the absence of hypoxia may lead to increase in infarct size. Caution should be exercised when administering oxygen to patients experiencing STEMI. Supplemental oxygen is indicated in patients with hypoxemia (SaO_2 <90% or PaO_2 <60 mm Hg).

EVIDENCE BASE Ibanez, B., James, S., Agewall, S., Antunes, M. J., Bucciarelli-Ducci, C., Bueno, H., Caforio, A. L. P., Crea, F., Goudevenos, J. A., Halvorsen, S., Hindricks, G., Kastrati, A., Lenzen, M. J., Prescott, E., Roffi, M., Valgimigli, M., Varenhorst, C., Vranckx, P., Widimský, P., ... Gale, C. P. (2017). 2017 ESC guidelines for the management of acute myocardial infarction in patients presenting with ST-segment elevation. *European Heart Journal, 39*(2), 119–177. https://doi.org/10.1093/eurheartj/ehx393

Table 9-1 Medications Used in the Treatment of Myocardial Infarction

DRUGS AND MECHANISM OF ACTION	NURSING CONSIDERATIONS
Aspirin Potent inhibitor of prostaglandin synthesis and platelet aggregation	• Administer immediately; continue 160–325 mg daily as directed. • If not already taking aspirin, have patient chew the first dose. • Monitor for bleeding, tinnitus, renal compromise.
Clopidogrel, ticagrelor A selective P2Y(12) receptor antagonist, inhibits platelet aggregation	• Research indicates that dual therapy with clopidogrel and aspirin reduces the risk of myocardial infarction, stroke, and death. • Lower levels of active metabolite occur in patients with the CYP2C19 gene and those taking omeprazole. • Obtain full medication history because many drug interactions may occur.
Unfractionated heparin, lower molecular weight heparin (dalteparin, enoxaparin) Inactivates thrombin, prevents the conversion of fibrinogen to fibrin	**Unfractionated heparin** • Obtain weight to calculate dose to achieve therapeutic partial thromboplastin time (PTT) and activated clotting time (ACT). • Administer IV or subcutaneously. • Reversal agent: Protamine Sulfate • Monitor patient for thrombocytopenia. **Low molecular weight heparin** • PTT is not monitored. • Protamine may be used as a reversal agent, only reduces 65%–70% of enoxaparin. • Subcutaneous route only.
Glycoprotein (GP) IIb/IIIa inhibitors (eptifibatide) Reduces thrombus burden and increases myocardial perfusion	• Indicated for intermediate or high-risk ACS, percutaneous coronary intervention. • There are multiple agents in this category. Follow package insert for administration guidelines.
Fibrinolytics (alteplase, streptokinase) Insoluble fibrin molecules are broken down to soluble fragments by plasmin. Disruption of fibrin meshwork in clots	• Indicated in ST segment elevation ACS only. • Obtain weight and follow package insert for administration guidelines. • Monitor for active bleeding.
β-Adrenergic blockers (metoprolol, atenolol) Decreases contractility, decreases heart rate, increases relaxation, and decreases cardiac conduction times.	• Administer as directed, within 24 h to all patients with ACS without contraindications. • Titrate dosage to meet therapeutic goals. • Monitor for hypotension and HR <60.
Angiotensin-converting enzyme inhibitors (captopril, enalapril) Decrease endothelial dysfunction and prevent conversion of angiotensin I to angiotensin II. Decrease blood pressure and have cardioprotective properties.	• Administer as directed, within 24 h of acute MI, usually a drug with a short half-life, such as captopril. • May switch to a longer acting drug such as lisinopril or enalapril, with once daily dosing. • Instruct patient that a dry nonproductive cough is a common side effect.
Nitroglycerin Relaxation of smooth muscle resulting in a vasodilatory effect; reduction in preload.	• Administer as directed by the following routes: SL tablet or spray; oral; IV; or topical patch or paste for long-term use. • Monitor systolic BP as the risk of hypotension is high; hold for SBP less than 90 mm Hg. • Avoid in patients who have taken a phosphodiesterase inhibitor within the last 24–48 h.
Morphine Acts as an analgesic and sedative. May modulate sympathetic response, thus decreasing myocardial oxygen demand.	• Despite widespread use, recent research shows that morphine decreased the antiplatelet effect of P2Y12 inhibitors. • Reserve for patients with unacceptable levels of pain, not for prolonged use. • Monitor for hypotension, decreased level of consciousness, and respiratory suppression.

ACS, acute coronary syndrome; BP, blood pressure; HR, heart rate; IV, intravenous; MI, myocardial infarction; SBP, systolic blood pressure.

EVIDENCE BASE Nehme, Z., Stub, D., Bernard, S., Stephenson, M., Bray, J. E., Cameron, P., Meredith, I. T., Barger, B., Ellims, A. H., Taylor, A. J., Kaye, D. M., Smith, K., & AVOID Investigators. (2016). Effect of supplemental oxygen exposure on myocardial injury in ST-elevation myocardial infarction. *Heart (British Cardiac Society), 102*(6), 444–451. https://doi.org/10.1136/heartjnl-2015-308636

Immediate Interventions

EVIDENCE BASE Collet, J. P., Thiele, H., Barbato, E., Barthélémy, O., Bauersachs, J., Bhatt, D. L., Dendale, P., Dorobantu, M., Edvardsen, T., Folliguet, T., Gale, C. P., Gilard, M., Jobs, A., Jüni, P., Lambrinou, E., Lewis, B. S., Mehilli, J., Meliga, E., Merkely, B., ... ESC Scientific Document Group. (2020). 2020 ESC guidelines for the management of acute coronary syndromes in patients presenting without persistent ST-segment elevation. *European Heart Journal, 42*(14), 1289–1367. https://doi.org/10.1093/eurheartj/ehaa575

Use the MONA acronym to outline immediate pharmacologic interventions.

1. M (morphine)—IV rather than intramuscular (IM) is used to treat chest pain. Endogenous catecholamine release during pain imposes an increase in the workload on the heart, thus causing an increase in oxygen demand. Morphine's analgesic effects decrease the pain, relieve anxiety, and improve cardiac output (CO) by reducing preload and afterload.
2. O (oxygen)—given via nasal cannula or face mask. Increases oxygenation to ischemic heart muscle.
3. N (nitrates)—given sublingually via spray or through IV administration. Vasodilator therapy reduces preload by decreasing blood return to the heart and decreasing oxygen demand. IV nitrates are more effective than sublingual with regard to symptom relief and regression of ST depression (NSTEMI). Caution: Nitrate side effects are headache and hypotension.
4. A (aspirin)—immediate dosing by mouth (chewed) is recommended to halt platelet aggregation.

Additional Pharmacologic Therapy

1. Beta-blockers should be considered to reduce myocardial oxygen consumption by lowering heart rate, BP, and myocardial contractility. For long-term management of MI, beta-blockers are recommended in patients with left ventricular ejection fraction (LVEF) less than 40% if no other contraindications are present.
2. Platelet inhibitors (P2Y12 inhibitors) such as clopidogrel, prasugrel, and ticagrelor help inhibit adenosine triphosphate (ATP)-induced platelet aggregation.

DRUG ALERT Patients undergoing PCI should be treated with dual antiplatelet therapy: such as aspirin plus clopidogrel.

DRUG ALERT Beta blockers should not be used when coronary vasospasm is suspected.

3. Fibrinolytic agents such as tissue plasma activator, streptokinase, and reteplase are given IV to reestablish blood flow in coronary vessels by dissolving thrombus. Preferred procedure if catheterization laboratory unavailable for other interventions.
   a. Contraindicated in the management of UA or NSTEMI or posterior wall MI. Studies have shown no clinical benefits in the absence of ST elevation MI or bundle-branch block.
   b. No effect on the underlying stenosis that precipitated the thrombus to form.
4. Antiarrhythmics, such as amiodarone, to decrease the ventricular irritability that occurs after MI.
   a. Bolus of amiodarone is given via IV line over 10 minutes; then, an infusion is given in varying doses over 24 hours (1 mg/min for 6 hours, then 0.5 mg/min for 18 hours).
   b. Correction of electrolyte imbalances, such as hypo/hyperkalemia and hypomagnesemia, that also cause ventricular irritability.

Percutaneous Coronary Interventions

EVIDENCE BASE Ibanez, B., James, S., Agewall, S., Antunes, M. J., Bucciarelli-Ducci, C., Bueno, H., Caforio, A. L. P., Crea, F., Goudevenos, J. A., Halvorsen, S., Hindricks, G., Kastrati, A., Lenzen, M. J., Prescott, E., Roffi, M., Valgimigli, M., Varenhorst, C., Vranckx, P., Widimský, P., ... Gale, C. P. (2017). 2017 ESC guidelines for the management of acute myocardial infarction in patients presenting with ST-segment elevation. *European Heart Journal, 39*(2), 119–177. https://doi.org/10.1093/eurheartj/ehx393

1. PCI is a group of procedures that create mechanical opening of the coronary vessel(s).
2. Procedures include percutaneous transluminal coronary angioplasty, coronary stenting, and atherectomy.
3. PCI can be performed during an evolving infarction and can be used instead of, or as an adjunct to, fibrinolytic therapy (see page 223).
4. If PCI cannot be performed within 90 minutes for patients with STEMI, fibrinolytic therapy is considered. The guidelines suggest that patients presenting to non–PCI capacity facilities should be transferred to PCI-capable facility within 120 minutes of presentation for immediate PCI. However, if delays are anticipated (i.e., transfer delay by greater than 120 minutes), then fibrinolytic therapy should be considered within 30 minutes of presentation to facility.

Surgical Revascularization

1. Cardiac surgery (i.e., CABG) following STEMI is associated with high mortality in the first 3 to 7 days; thus, the benefit of revascularization must be weighed against the risk of cardiac surgery. In most cases, PCI or fibrinolysis can usually restore flow to the ischemic myocardium more quickly than CABG surgery, largely owing to delay in getting patient to the operating room and the time it takes to complete the surgical procedure. However, newer surgical approaches such as off-pump CABG have mitigated this risk for some patients.
2. Bypass surgery is uncommonly used as the reperfusion strategy of choice in STEMI. It is considered after unsuccessful or complicated PCI, patient in cardiogenic shock, mechanical complications, or early recurrent ischemia.
3. Benefits of this therapy include definitive treatment of the stenosis and less scar formation on the heart.

Complications

1. Dysrhythmias.
2. Sudden cardiac death because of ventricular arrhythmias.
3. Infarct expansion (thinning and dilation of the necrotic zone).

4. Infarct extension (additional heart muscle necrosis occurring after 24 hours of acute infarction).
5. Heart failure (with 20% to 35% left ventricle damage).
6. Cardiogenic shock.
7. Reinfarction.
8. Ischemic cardiomyopathy.
9. Cardiac rupture.
10. Papillary muscle rupture.
11. Ventricular mural thrombus.
12. Ischemic stroke.
13. Thromboemboli (deep vein thrombosis and pulmonary embolism [PE]).
14. Ventricular aneurysm.
15. Cardiac tamponade.
16. Pericarditis (2 to 3 days after MI).
17. Dissection of coronary arteries during angioplasty.
18. Psychiatric problems—depression, personality changes.

Nursing Assessment

1. Gather information regarding the patient's chest pain:
   a. Nature and intensity—describe the pain in patient's own words, and compare it with pain previously experienced.
   b. Onset and duration—exact time pain occurred as well as the time pain relieved or diminished (if applicable).
   c. Location and radiation—point to the area where the pain is located and to other areas where the pain seems to travel.
   d. Precipitating and aggravating factors—describe the activity performed just before the onset of pain and if any maneuvers and/or medications alleviated the pain.
2. Question patient about other symptoms experienced associated with the pain. Observe patient for diaphoresis, facial pallor, dyspnea, guarding behaviors, rigid body posture, extreme weakness, and confusion.
3. Evaluate cognitive, behavioral, and emotional status.
4. Question patient about prior health status with emphasis on current medications, allergies (opiate analgesics, iodine, shellfish), recent trauma or surgery, nonsteroidal anti-inflammatory drug (NSAID) ingestion, peptic ulcers, fainting spells, drug and alcohol use.
5. Gather information about presence or absence of cardiac risk factors.

Nursing Interventions

Alleviating Anxiety

1. Rule out physiologic etiologies for increasing or new-onset anxiety before administering as-needed sedatives. Physiologic causes must be identified and treated in a timely fashion to prevent irreversible adverse or even fatal outcomes; sedatives may mask symptoms, delaying timely identification, diagnosis, and treatment.
   a. Autonomic signs of anxiety are increases in heart rate, BP, respiratory rate, and tremulousness, but they may also be signs of physiologic complications.
   b. Anxiety with dyspnea, tachypnea, and tachycardia may indicate PE; frothy pink sputum and orthopnea indicate pulmonary edema.
   c. Appearance of heart murmurs or friction rub indicates valvular dysfunction, possible intraventricular septal rupture, and pericarditis.
2. Whenever anxiety increases, assess patient for signs of hypoperfusion, auscultate heart and lung sounds, obtain a rhythm strip, and administer oxygen, as prescribed. Notify the health care provider immediately.
3. Assess and document emotional status frequently. Document all assessment findings, health care provider notification and response, and interventions and response.
4. Explain to patient and family reasons for hospitalization, diagnostic tests, and therapies administered.
5. Explain equipment, procedures, and need for frequent assessment to patient and significant others.
6. Discuss with patient and family the anticipated nursing and medical regimen.
   a. Explain visiting hours and need to limit number of visitors per facility policy.
   b. Offer family preferred times to phone unit to check on patient's status.
7. Administer antianxiety agents, as prescribed.
   a. Explain to patient the reason for sedation: undue anxiety can make the heart more irritable and require more oxygen.
   b. Assure patient that the goal of sedation is to promote comfort and, therefore, should be requested if anxious, excitable, or "jittery" feelings occur.
   c. Observe for adverse effects of sedation, such as lethargy, confusion, and/or increased agitation.
8. Maintain consistency of care, with one or two nurses regularly assisting patient, especially if severe anxiety is present.
9. Offer massage, imagery, and progressive muscle relaxation to promote relaxation, reduce muscle tension, and reduce workload on the heart.

Increasing Activity Tolerance

1. Promote activity tolerance with early gradual increase in mobilization—prevents deconditioning, which occurs with bed rest.
   a. Minimize environmental noise.
   b. Provide a comfortable environmental temperature.
   c. Avoid unnecessary interruptions and procedures.
   d. Structure routine care measures to include rest periods after activity.
   e. Discuss with patient and family the purpose of limited activity and visitors—to help the heart heal by lowering heart rate and BP, maintaining cardiac workload at lowest level, and decreasing oxygen consumption.
   f. Promote restful diversional activities for patient (reading, listening to music, coloring, crossword puzzles, crafts).
   g. Encourage frequent position changes while in bed.
2. Assist patient with prescribed activities.
   a. Assist patient to rise slowly from a supine position to minimize orthostatic hypotension related to medications.
   b. Encourage passive and active range-of-motion (ROM) exercise as directed while on bedrest.
   c. Measure the length of hallway so patients can gradually increase their activity levels with specific guidelines (walk one width [150 feet] of the unit).
   d. Elevate patient's feet when out of bed in chair to promote venous return.
   e. Implement a step-by-step program for progressive activity, as directed. Typically, can progress to the next step if free from chest pain and ECG changes during the activity.

Preventing Bleeding

1. Take vital signs every 15 minutes during infusion of fibrinolytic agent and then hourly.
2. Observe for hematomas or skin breakdown, especially in potential pressure areas such as the sacrum, back, elbows, ankles.

3. Be alert to verbal complaints of back pain indicative of possible retroperitoneal bleeding.
4. Observe all puncture sites every 15 minutes during infusion of fibrinolytic therapy and then hourly for bleeding.
5. Apply manual pressure to venous or arterial sites if bleeding occurs. Use pressure dressings for coverage of all access sites.
6. Observe for blood in stool, emesis, urine, and sputum.
7. Minimize venipunctures and arterial punctures; use heparin lock for blood sampling and medication administration.
8. Avoid IM injections.
9. Caution patient about vigorous toothbrushing or shaving.
10. Avoid trauma to patient by minimizing frequent handling of patient.
11. Monitor laboratory values: PT, international normalized ratio, PTT, hematocrit (HCT), and hemoglobin.
12. Check for current blood type and cross-match.
13. Administer proton pump inhibitor or other medication for gastrointestinal (GI) protection, as directed, to prevent stress ulcers.
14. Implement emergency interventions, as directed, in the event of bleeding: fluid, volume expanders, blood products.
15. Monitor for changes in mental status and headache.
16. Avoid vigorous oral suctioning.
17. Avoid use of automatic BP device above puncture sites or hematoma. Use care in taking BP; use arm not being used for fibrinolytic therapy.

Maintaining Cardiac Tissue Perfusion

1. Observe for persistence and/or recurrence of signs and symptoms of ischemia, including chest pain, diaphoresis, hypotension—may indicate extension of MI and/or reocclusion of coronary vessel.
2. Report immediately.
3. Administer oxygen, as directed.
4. Record a 12-lead ECG.
5. Prepare patient for possible emergency procedures: cardiac catheterization, bypass surgery, PCI, fibrinolytic therapy, intra-aortic balloon pump (IABP).

Strengthening Coping Abilities

1. Listen carefully to patient and family to ascertain their cognitive appraisals of stressors and threats. Encourage patient and family to ask questions.
2. Assist patient to establish a positive attitude toward illness and progress adaptively through the grieving process.
3. Manipulate environment to promote restful sleep by maintaining patient's usual sleep patterns.
4. Be alert to signs and symptoms of sleep deprivation—irritability, disorientation, hallucinations, diminished pain tolerance, aggressiveness.
5. Provide extra support on transfer from the intensive care unit to the intermediate care unit by familiarizing the patient with the new staff, layout of the unit, and nursing routine.

Patient Education and Health Maintenance

Goals are to restore patient to optimal physiologic, psychological, social, and work level; to aid in restoring confidence and self-esteem; to develop patient's self-monitoring skills; to assist in managing cardiac problems; and to modify risk factors.

1. Inform the patient and family about what has happened to patient's heart.
   a. Explain basic cardiac anatomy and physiology.
   b. Identify the difference between angina and MI.
   c. Describe how the heart heals and that healing will not be complete for 6 to 8 weeks after infarction.
   d. Discuss what the patient can do to assist in the recovery process, and reduce the chance of future heart attacks.
2. Instruct patient on how to judge the body's response to activity.
   a. Introduce the concept that different activities require varying expenditures of oxygen.
   b. Emphasize the importance of rest and relaxation alternating with activity.
   c. Instruct patient how to take pulse before and after activity as well as guidelines for the acceptable increases in heart rate that should occur.
   d. Review signs and symptoms indicative of a poor response to increased activity levels: chest pain, extreme fatigue, shortness of breath.
3. Design an individualized activity progression program for patient as directed.
   a. Determine activity levels appropriate for patient, as prescribed, and by predischarge low-level exercise stress test.
   b. Encourage patient to list activities they enjoy and would like to resume.
   c. Establish the energy expenditure of each activity (i.e., which are most demanding on the heart), and rank activities from lowest to highest.
   d. Instruct patient to move from one activity to another after the heart has been able to manage the previous workload as determined by signs and symptoms and pulse rate.
4. Give patient specific activity guidelines, and explain that activity guidelines will be reevaluated after the heart heals.
   a. Walk daily, gradually increasing distance and time, as prescribed.
   b. Avoid activities that tense muscles, such as weight lifting, lifting heavy objects, isometric exercises, pushing and/or pulling heavy loads, all of which can cause vagal stimulation.
   c. Avoid working with arms overhead.
   d. Gradually return to work.
   e. Avoid extremes in temperature.
   f. Do not rush; avoid tension.
   g. Advise getting at least 7 hours of sleep each night and taking 20- to 30-minute rest periods twice per day.
   h. Advise limiting visitors to three to four daily for 15 to 30 minutes, and shorten phone conversations.
5. Tell patient that sexual relations may be resumed on advice of health care provider, usually after exercise tolerance is assessed.
   a. If patient can walk briskly or climb two flights of stairs, they can usually resume sexual activity; resumption of sexual activity parallels resumption of usual activities.
   b. Sexual activity should be avoided after eating a heavy meal, after drinking alcohol, or when tired.
   c. Discuss erectile dysfunction as an adverse effect of drug therapy and phosphodiesterase contraindications.
6. Advise eating three to four small meals per day rather than large, heavy meals. Rest for 1 hour after meals.
7. Advise limiting caffeine and alcohol intake.
8. Driving a car must be cleared with health care provider at a follow-up visit.
9. Teach patient about medication regimen and adverse effects.
10. Instruct the patient to call 911 when chest pressure or pain not relieved in 5 minutes by nitroglycerin or rest.

11. Instruct the patient to notify health care provider when the following symptoms appear:
    a. Shortness of breath.
    b. Unusual fatigue.
    c. Swelling of feet and ankles.
    d. Fainting, dizziness.
    e. Very slow or rapid heartbeat.
12. Assist patient to reduce risk of another MI by risk factor modification.
    a. Explain to patient the major risk factors that can increase chances of having another MI.
    b. Instruct patient in strategies to modify risk factors.
13. For additional information and support, refer patient to AHA (www.americanheart.org) and the ACC (www.acc.org).

Evaluation: Expected Outcomes

- No signs of anxiety or agitation.
- Activity slowly progressing and tolerated well.
- No signs of bleeding.
- No recurrent chest pain.
- Sleeps well; emotionally stable.

Hyperlipidemia

Hyperlipidemia is a group of metabolic abnormalities resulting in combinations of elevated serum cholesterol. TC and TG are two of the major lipids in the body. The liver serves as the key organ for cholesterol metabolism and regulation. Lipids are transported through the bloodstream by lipoproteins. Lipoproteins are made up of a phospholipid and specific proteins called *apoproteins* or *apolipoproteins*. There are five main classes of lipoproteins:

- Chylomicrons.
- Very-low-density lipoproteins (VLDLs).
- Intermediate-density lipoproteins (IDLs).
- Low-density lipoproteins (LDLs).
- High-density lipoproteins (HDLs).

Pathophysiology and Etiology

Primary Hyperlipidemias

1. Genetic metabolic abnormalities resulting in the overproduction or underproduction of specific lipoproteins or enzymes. They tend to be familial, autosomal codominant genetic disorders characterized by raised serum LDL-cholesterol (LDL-C) levels resulting from defects in hepatic uptake.
2. Primary hyperlipidemias include hypercholesterolemia, defective apolipoproteinemia, hypertriglyceridemia, combined hyperlipidemia, dysbetalipoproteinemia, polygenic hypercholesterolemia, lipoprotein lipase deficiency, apoprotein C-II deficiency, and lecithin cholesterol acetyltransferase deficiency.

Secondary Hyperlipidemias

1. Very common and are multifactorial.
2. Etiologic factors include chronic diseases, such as diabetes, hypothyroidism, nephrotic syndrome, and liver disease.
3. Other etiologic factors are obesity, dietary intake, pregnancy, alcohol dependency.
4. Medications include beta-adrenergic blockers, alpha-adrenergic blockers, diuretics, glucocorticoid and anabolic steroids, and estrogen preparations.

Consequences

1. Atherosclerotic plaque formation in blood vessels.
2. Causes narrowing and possible ischemia and may lead to thromboembolus formation.
3. Result in cardiovascular, cerebrovascular, and peripheral vascular disease.
4. Familial genetic hyperlipidemia increases the risk of early onset of cardiovascular disease.

Clinical Manifestations

1. Usually asymptomatic until significant target organ damage is done.
2. May be metabolic signs, such as corneal arcus, xanthoma, xanthelasma, pancreatitis.
3. Chest pain, MI.
4. Carotid bruit, transient ischemic attacks, stroke.
5. Intermittent claudication, arterial occlusion of lower extremities, loss of pulses.

Diagnostic Evaluation and Management

Diagnosis and management of hyperlipidemia begin with serum lipoprotein evaluation and assessment of ASCVD. Risk reduction has been a major focus since the first guidelines were introduced in 2013. Medical history and review of risk factors are used to determine which of four statin benefit groups the individual falls within. Statin therapy is tailored in those most likely to benefit in terms of primary and secondary risk reduction. Therapeutic lifestyle changes (TLC), also known as heart-healthy lifestyle habits, should be encouraged for all individuals (Table 9-2 and Box 9-1).

EVIDENCE BASE Grundy, S. M., Stone, N. J., Bailey, A. L., Beam, C., Birtcher, K. K., Blumenthal, R. S., Braun, L. T., de Ferranti, S., Faiella-Tommasino, J., Forman, D. E., Goldberg, R., Heidenreich, P. A., Hlatky, M. A., Jones, D. W., Lloyd-Jones, D., Lopez-Pajares, N., Ndumele, C. E., Orringer, C. E., Peralta, C. A., ... Yeboah, J. (2019). 2018 AHA/ACC/AACVPR/AAPA/ABC/ACPM/ADA/AGS/APhA/ASPC/NLA/PCNA guideline on the management of blood cholesterol: A report of the American College of Cardiology/American Heart Association Task Force on Clinical Practice Guidelines. *Circulation*, *139*(25), e1082–e1143. https://doi.org/10.1161/CIR.0000000000000625

Table 9-2 Categorizing Serum Lipids

TOTAL CHOLESTEROL (TC) mg/dL (mmol/L)	CATEGORY
<200 (<5.2)	Normal
200–239 (5.2–6.1)	Borderline high
≥240 (≥6.2)	High
LDL-Cholesterol mg/dL (mmol/L)	
<100 (<2.6)	Normal
100–129 (2.6–3.3)	Above, near optimal
130–159 (3.4–4.0)	Borderline high
160–189 (4.1–4.8)	High
≥190 (≥4.9)	Very high
HDL-Cholesterol mg/dL (mmol/L)	
<40 (<1.0)	Low
≥60 (≥1.6)	High
Triglycerides (TG) mg/dL (mmol/L)	
<150 (<1.7)	Normal
150–499 (1.7–5.6)	Moderate hypertriglyceridemia
500–999 (5.6–11.3)	Moderate to severe hypertriglyceridemia
>1,000 (>11.3)	Severe hypertriglyceridemia

HDL, high-density lipoprotein; LDL, low-density lipoprotein.

BOX 9-1 LDL Goal-Directed Hyperlipidemia Treatment

LDL goal <70 mg/dL: Considered an optional goal for high-risk patients with CHD or a risk equivalent (peripheral artery disease, carotid artery disease, diabetes, aortic aneurysm). Treatment recommendation: therapeutic lifestyle changes; optional drug therapy if LDL <100 mg/dL.

LDL goal <100 mg/dL: Goal for high-risk patients who have CHD or a risk equivalent and 10-year risk >20%. Treatment recommendations: therapeutic lifestyle changes and drug therapy if LDL ≥100 mg/dL; optional drug therapy if LDL <100 mg/dL.

LDL goal <130 mg/dL: Goal for moderately high-risk patients with two or more risk factors and 10-year risk 10% to 20%. Treatment recommendations: therapeutic lifestyle changes initiated if LDL ≥130 mg/dL; drug therapy if LDL ≥130 mg/dL; optional drug therapy if LDL is 100 to 129 mg/dL.

LDL goal <130 mg/dL: Goal for moderate-risk patients with two or more risk factors and 10-year risk <10%. Treatment recommendation: therapeutic lifestyle changes initiated if LDL ≥130 mg/dL; drug therapy initiated if LDL ≥160 mg/dL.

LDL goal <160 mg/dL: Goal for lower-risk patients with 0 to 1 risk factors. Treatment recommendations: therapeutic lifestyle changes initiated if LDL ≥160 mg/dL; drug therapy initiated if LDL ≥190 mg/dL; optional drug therapy if LDL is 160 to 189 mg/dL.

CHD, coronary heart disease; LDL, low-density lipoprotein.

1. The appropriate intensity of statin therapy should be initiated or continued:
   a. Clinical ASCVD (history of MI, unstable or stable angina, coronary artery procedures or evidence of clinically significant MI or other revascularization, stroke, transient ischemic attack (TIA), and peripheral arterial disease presumed to be of atherosclerotic origin)
      i. Age ≤75 years and no safety concerns: high-intensity statin.
      ii. Age greater than 75 years or safety concerns: moderate-intensity statin.
   b. Primary prevention—primary LDL-C ≥190 mg/dL.
      i. Rule out secondary causes of hyperlipidemia.
      ii. Age ≥21 years: high-intensity statin.
      iii. Achieve at least a 50% reduction in LDL-C.
      iv. LDL-C–lowering nonstatin therapy may be considered to further reduce LDL-C.
   c. Primary prevention—diabetes 40 to 75 years of age and LDL-C 70 to 189 mg/dL.
      i. Moderate-intensity statin.
      ii. Consider high-intensity statin when ≥7.5% 10-year ASCVD risk using the Pooled Cohort Equations (defined as nonfatal MI, coronary heart disease [CHD] death, or nonfatal and fatal stroke).
   d. Primary prevention—no diabetes 40 to 75 years of age and LDL-C 70 to 189 mg/dL.
      i. Estimate 10-year ASCVD risk using the Risk Calculator based on the Pooled Cohort Equations in those NOT receiving a statin; estimate risk every 4 to 6 years.
      ii. To determine whether to initiate a statin, engage in a clinician–patient discussion of the potential ASCVD risk reduction, adverse effects, drug–drug interaction, and patient preferences.
      iii. Reemphasize heart-healthy lifestyle habits, and address other risk factors.
      iv. ≥7.5% 10-year ASCVD risk: consider moderate- or high-intensity statin.
      v. 5 to less than 7.5% 10-year ASCVD risk: consider moderate-intensity statin.
      vi. Other factors may be considered: LDL-C ≥160 mg/dL, family history of premature ASCVD, hs-CRP ≥2.0 mg/L, CAC score ≥300 Agatston units, ABI less than 0.9, or lifetime ASCVD risk.
   e. Primary prevention when LDL-C less than 190 mg/dL and age less than 40 or greater than 75 years or less than 5% 10-year ASCVD risk.
      i. Statin therapy may be considered in selected individuals.
   f. Statin therapy is not routinely recommended for individuals with New York Heart Association (NYHA) class II to IV heart failure or who are receiving maintenance hemodialysis.
2. Regularly monitor adherence to lifestyle and drug therapy with lipid and safety assessments, and assess adherence, response to therapy, and adverse effects with 4 to 12 weeks following statin initiation or change in therapy.
   a. Measure a fasting lipid panel.
   b. Do not routinely monitor alanine transaminase (ALT) or CK unless symptomatic.
   c. Screen and treat type 2 diabetes according to current practice guidelines. Heart-healthy lifestyle habits should be encouraged to prevent progression to diabetes.
   d. Anticipate therapeutic response: approximately ≥50% reduction in LDL-C from baseline for high-intensity statin and 30% to less than 50% for moderate-intensity statin.
      i. Insufficient evidence for LDL-C or non–HDL-C treatment targets from randomized-controlled trials (RCTs).
      ii. For those with unknown baseline LDL-C, and LDL-C, 100 mg/dL was observed in RCTs of high-intensity statin therapy.
   e. Less than anticipated therapeutic response:
      i. Reinforce improved adherence to lifestyle and drug therapy.
      ii. Evaluate for secondary causes of hyperlipidemia if indicated.
      iii. Increase statin intensity, or, if on maximally tolerated statin, consider addition of nonstatin therapy in selected high-risk individuals.
   f. Regularly monitor adherence to lifestyle and drug therapy every 3 to 12 months once adherence has been established. Continue assessment of adherence for optimal ASCVD risk reduction and safety.
3. In individuals intolerant of the recommended intensity of statin therapy, use the maximally tolerated intensity of statin. If there are muscle or other symptoms, establish that they are related to the statin.

Hypertriglyceridemia

1. Hypertriglyceridemia is associated with pancreatitis and ASCVD. The goals of management are to lower the risk of both conditions; however, in regard to ASCVD, efficacy of lowering TG is not well established compared to lowering LDL. Levels of LDL may underrepresent the cardiovascular risk in patients with hypertriglyceridemia.
   a. High TG levels are associated with small, dense cholesterol-depleted LDL particles that falsely decrease the LDL value.

b. Since TG levels are not directly involved in the development of atherosclerosis, the efficacy of targeting lower TG levels is problematic. Treatment to lower TC may not be effective if elevated TC is due to elevated TG where LDL is normal.
c. TG-rich lipoproteins may contribute to atherosclerotic events by increasing endothelial activation, facilitating monocyte infiltration into the arterial wall, and increasing activation of pro-inflammatory genes. Factors affecting the development of hypertriglyceridemia include insulin resistance conditions, renal disease, hypothyroidism, multiple myeloma, systemic lupus erythematosus, alcohol consumption, and diet with excessive calories.

2. Patients with hypertriglyceridemia should still undergo an assessment of their atherosclerotic cardiovascular risk and LDL levels. Most LDL lowering drugs also reduce fasting TG levels. TLC may also be of some benefit.

Drug Classifications

See Table 9-3.

1. HMG-CoA reductase inhibitors (statins) are the most effective way to lower elevated LDL and TC, as a result of lower intrahepatic cholesterol and an uptake of hepatic cell surface LDL receptors. They also raise levels of HDL, lower levels of CRP, and may lower TGs. They can be used alone or in combination with other lipid-lowering drugs.
   a. Require periodic liver function monitoring.
   b. Should not be taken with large volume of grapefruit juice; can increase risk of myopathy.
   c. Should not be taken by patients who are pregnant, lactating, or who plan to get pregnant.
   d. Musculoskeletal side effects include myalgia, rhabdomyolysis, elevated CK.

DRUG ALERT Currently, statins are contraindicated during pregnancy. Patients of childbearing age should be counselled on the risk of becoming pregnant while on these medications.

2. Cholesterol absorption inhibitors—the newest class of lipid-lowering drugs; inhibit intestinal absorption of phytosterols and cholesterol and reduce LDL. Do not require liver function testing if given as monotherapy.
3. Bile acid sequestrants bind to cholesterol in the gut, decreasing absorption. Contraindicated in those with history of bile obstruction and phenylketonuria (aspartame-containing agent only).
4. Nicotinic acid (vitamin B_3)—works by inhibiting VLDL secretion, thus decreasing production of LDL. The main adverse effect is severe flushing; however, taking 81 to 325 mg of aspirin beforehand may help. Newer sustained-release forms have fewer adverse effects. Niacin should be avoided in patients with severe peptic disease.
5. Fibric acid derivatives—inhibit synthesis of VLDL, decrease TG, increase HDL. Contraindicated in liver, biliary, or kidney disease.
6. PCSK9 inhibitors are monoclonal antibodies. They target and inactivate a specific protein in the liver called proprotein convertase subtilisin/kexin 9. This protein binds to the LDL receptor and acts as an enzyme to break down the receptor so it can no longer remove LDL from the bloodstream. By inhibiting this protein, a dramatic reduction of LDL is seen in the bloodstream.

Other Treatment Considerations

1. TLC should be considered immediately for all patients with hyperlipidemia and is an important adjunct therapy for patients who receive medications. Diet should be low-fat, balanced, and healthy.
2. Children and adolescents should be considered for screening and treatment of hyperlipidemia if they have positive family history and a family history of obesity. Other indications for screening (in these populations) include being overweight and exhibiting features of metabolic syndrome (hypertension, type 2 diabetes, central adiposity).
3. Drug therapy is recommended for males age 10 or older and after the onset of menses in females following a 6- to 12-month dietary trial. HMG-CoA reductase inhibitors are the drug class of choice.
4. Some dietary products may serve as adjunct therapy, such as omega-3 fatty acids, soy protein, plant stanols, and fiber.

Complications

1. Disability from MI, stroke, and lower extremity ischemia.

Nursing Interventions and Patient Education

1. Teach diet basics and obtain nutritional consult.
2. Teach patient to engage in exercise.
3. Engage patient in smoking cessation program.
4. Tell patients that for every 1% increase in HDL, there is a 2% to 3% decrease in risk for CHD.
5. Explain the goal of recommended cholesterol levels. Encourage patients to keep a log of lipid results.
6. Encourage follow-up laboratory work—repeat lipoprotein analysis and liver function test monitoring every 3 months for those on HMG-CoA reductase inhibitors.
7. Teach patient taking bile acid sequestrants not to take other medications for 1 hour before or 2 hours after because it prevents absorption of many medications.
8. For more information on hyperlipidemia and TLC, refer patient to AHA (www.heart.org) or the National Heart, Lung, and Blood Institute diseases and conditions index (www.nhlbi.nih.gov/health/dci).

Cardiogenic Shock

Cardiogenic shock is the failure of the heart to pump blood adequately to meet the oxygenation needs of the body. It occurs when the heart muscle loses its contractile power. It most commonly occurs as a result of AMI, and left ventricular pump failure is the primary insult. It is the most common cause of death in the post-AMI patient (about 5% to 10% of patients with AMI develop cardiogenic shock), with a resulting mortality of 50% to 80%. Mortality rate in cardiogenic shock after 6 to 12 months is about 50%, unchanged in the past two decades. See Figure 9-6.

Pathophysiology and Etiology

1. Persistent hypotension with a marked systolic of less than 80 to 90 mm Hg or mean arterial pressure (MAP) 30 mm Hg lower than baseline because of left ventricular failure.
2. Compensatory peripheral vasoconstriction may initially improve coronary and peripheral perfusion; however, it increases cardiac afterload that overwhelms damaged myocardium. The result is diminished oxygenated blood flow to peripheral tissue and the heart.

Table 9-3 Drugs Affecting Lipoprotein Metabolism

DRUG CLASS	AGENTS AND DAILY DOSES	LIPID/LIPOPROTEIN EFFECTS		ADVERSE EFFECTS	CONTRAINDICATIONS
HMG-CoA reductase inhibitors (statins)	• Lovastatin (20–80 mg) • Pravastatin (20–40 mg) • Simvastatin (20–80 mg) • Fluvastatin (20–80 mg) • Atorvastatin (10–80 mg) • Rosuvastatin (5–40 mg) • Pitavastatin (1–4 mg)	LDL HDL TG	↓ 18%–55% ↑ 5%–15% ↓ 7%–30%	• Myopathy • Increased liver enzymes	*Absolute*: • Active or chronic liver disease *Relative:* • Concomitant use of certain drugs[a]
Bile acid sequestrants	• Cholestyramine (4–16 g) • Colestipol (5–20 g) • Colesevelam (2.6–3.8 g)	LDL HDL TG	↓ 15%–30% ↑ 3%–5% No change or increase	• GI distress • Constipation	*Absolute*: • Bowel obstruction • Biliary obstruction
Nicotinic acid	• Immediate-release (crystalline) nicotinic acid (1.5–3 g) • Extended-release nicotinic acid (Niaspan[a]) (1–2 g); sustained-release nicotinic acid (1–2 g)	LDL HDL TG	↓ 5%–25% ↑ 15%–35% ↓ 20%–50%	• Flushing (may be reduced by taking with aspirin and food) • Hyperglycemia • Hyperuricemia, gout • Upper GI distress • Hepatotoxicity • New onset of atrial fibrillation • Weight loss	*Absolute*: • Hepatic dysfunction • Active peptic ulcer disease *Relative:* • Diabetes • Hyperphosphatemia • Gout • Unstable angina, MI
Fibric acids	• Gemfibrozil (600 mg BID) • Fenofibrate (200 mg) • Clofibrate (1,000 mg BID)	LDL (*may be increased in patients with high TG*) HDL TG	↓ 5%–20% ↑ 10%–20% ↓ 20%–50%	• Dyspepsia • Gallstones • Myopathy • Pancreatitis • Rhabdomyolysis in conjunction with statin use • Muscle symptoms	*Absolute*: • Severe renal disease • Severe hepatic disease
Cholesterol absorption inhibitors	• Ezetimibe (10 mg)	LDL Apoprotein B	↓ (additional 25% over a statin when used in combination; also a TG reduction) ↓	• Back pain • Arthralgia • Diarrhea • Abdominal pain • Sinusitis	• Contraindicated in active liver disease if combined with a statin
PCSK9 inhibitors	• Alirocumab (75–150 mg SQ every 2 wk) • Evolocumab (140 mg SQ every 2 wk or 420 mg SQ monthly in the abdomen, thigh, or upper arm)	LDL-C	↓29.9%–67%	• Nasopharyngitis • Injection site reaction • Influenza-like symptoms • Bruising	

[a]*Cyclosporine, macrolide antibiotics, various antifungal agents, and cytochrome P-450 inhibitors (fibrates and niacin) should be used with appropriate caution.*

Adapted from National Cholesterol Education Program. (n.d.). ATP III guidelines at-a-glance quick desk reference. *https://www.nhlbi.nih.gov/files/docs/guidelines/atglance.pdf*

BID, two times a day; GI, gastrointestinal; HDL, high-density lipoprotein; LDL, low-density lipoprotein; LDL-C, LDL-cholesterol; MI, myocardial infarction; SQ, subcutaneously; TG, triglyceride.

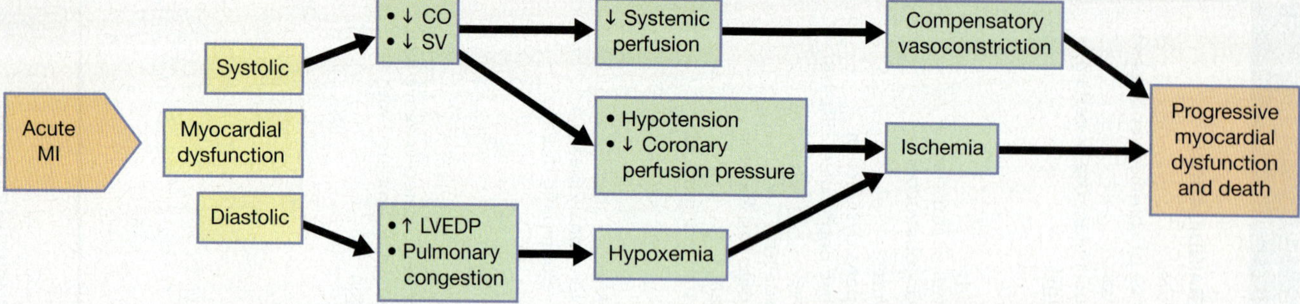

Figure 9-6. How cardiogenic shock can lead to death following MI. CO, cardiac output; LVEDP, left ventricular end-diastolic pressure; MI, myocardial infarction; SV, stroke volume.

3. Impaired contractility causes a marked reduction in CO and ejection fraction.
4. Decreased CO results in a lack of blood and oxygen to the heart as well as other vital organs (brain and kidneys).
5. Lack of blood and oxygen to the heart muscle results in continued damage to the muscle, a further decline in contractile power, and a continued inability of the heart to provide blood and oxygen to vital organs.
6. MI causing extensive damage (40% or greater) to the left ventricular myocardium is the most common cause.

DRUG ALERT Be aware that the standard treatment of acute MI with beta-adrenergic blockers, ACE inhibitors, analgesics, and nitrates does not prevent cardiogenic shock and may exacerbate systolic hypotension.

7. Mechanical complications such as ventricular septal rupture, contained free wall rupture, and papillary muscle rupture are strongly suspected in patients with shock, particularly a first MI.
8. In addition to MI with or without complications, common causes of cardiogenic shock include:
   a. Aortic dissection—complicated by acute severe aortic insufficiency or MI.
   b. Acute decompensation of heart failure.
   c. Acute myocarditis.
   d. Takotsubo stress-induced cardiomyopathy.
   e. Postcardiotomy.
   f. Cardiac tamponade.
   g. Peripartum cardiomyopathy.
   h. Hypertrophic cardiomyopathy with severe outflow obstruction.
   i. Massive PE.

Clinical Manifestations

1. Confusion, restlessness, mental lethargy (because of poor perfusion of the brain or metabolic encephalopathy).
2. Low systolic BP (90 or 30 mm Hg less than previous levels) or MAP <65 mm Hg.
3. Oliguria—urine output less than 30 mL/h for at least 2 hours (because of decreased perfusion of kidneys).
4. Cold, clammy skin (blood is shunted from the peripheral circulation to perfuse vital organs); profoundly diaphoretic with mottled extremities.
5. Weak, thready, diminished peripheral pulses, fatigue, hypotension (because of inadequate CO).
6. Dyspnea, tachypnea, cyanosis, respiratory distress (increased left ventricular pressures result in elevation of left atrial and pulmonary pressures, causing pulmonary congestion).
7. Dysrhythmias (because of lack of oxygen to heart muscle) and sinus tachycardia (as a compensatory mechanism for a decreased CO).
8. Chest pain (because of lack of oxygen and blood to heart muscle).
9. Decreased bowel sounds, nausea, or abdominal pain (because of paralytic ileus from decreased perfusion to GI tract).
10. Metabolic acidosis because of increased lactate production and reduced clearance (caused by anaerobic metabolism and liver dysfunction).
11. Hypoperfusion causes release of catecholamines, which increase contractility and peripheral blood flow but may also increase myocardial oxygen demand and have proarrhythmic effects.

Diagnostic Evaluation

1. Altered hemodynamic parameters (pulmonary artery wedge pressure 15 mm Hg or greater, cardiac index [CI] less than 2.0, elevated systemic vascular resistance [SVR], high right ventricular end-diastolic pressure [RVEDP] greater than 20 mm Hg and decreased mixed venous oxygen saturation).
2. Chest x-ray—pulmonary vascular congestion.
3. Abnormal laboratory values—elevated blood urea nitrogen (BUN) and creatinine, elevated liver enzymes, increased PTT and PT, elevated serum lactate, elevated brain natriuretic peptide (BNP). BNP may be useful as an indicator of heart failure and as an independent prognostic indicator of survival. Abnormally elevated cardiac enzymes. Higher levels of lactic acid can be associated with increased mortality.
4. ECG—acute injury pattern consistent with an AMI.
5. Doppler echocardiogram—reveals any ventricular wall motion or surgically correctable cause, such as valvular dysfunction and tamponade.
6. Pulmonary artery catheterization for severely hypotensive patient.

Management

Studies have suggested that treatment for cardiogenic shock resulting from an AMI should focus on revascularization and thrombolytics. Reduction in mortality related to early revascularization in patients with STEMI is supported by research. Augmenting CO with devices (IABP is a method of choice) is crucial until revascularization is established. Mechanical ventilation is supportive, and left ventricular assist device (LVAD) and extracorporeal membrane oxygenation (ECMO) may be used.

Pharmacologic Therapy

Pharmacologic therapy may need to be discontinued or its use decreased when a patient has gone into cardiogenic shock. Standard therapy for a failing heart includes:

1. Positive inotropic drugs (epinephrine, dopamine, dobutamine, amrinone, milrinone) stimulate cardiac contractility.

Dobutamine, amrinone, and milrinone may lower BP because of vasodilatory effect.
2. Vasodilator therapy.
   a. Decreases the workload of the heart by reducing venous return and lessening the resistance against which the heart pumps (preload and afterload reduction).
   b. CO improves, left ventricular pressures and pulmonary congestion decrease, and myocardial oxygen consumption is reduced.
3. Vasopressor therapy may be needed to maintain adequate perfusion pressure (MAP 70 mm Hg or greater). These medications are norepinephrine, epinephrine, vasopressin, and phenylephrine. These should be used in the lowest possible dose. Higher vasopressor doses are associated with poor survival.
4. Diuretic therapy is used to reduce plasma volume and peripheral edema. The reduction in extracellular fluid and plasma volume associated with diuresis may initially decrease CO and, consequently, BP, with a compensatory increase in peripheral vascular resistance. Continuous renal replacement therapy (CRRT) has been considered for patients in cardiogenic shock if unable to diurese because of low renal perfusion. CRRT should be considered with stage 2 kidney injury or when life-threatening changes in fluid, electrolyte, and acid–base balance precipitate the need for dialysis.

DRUG ALERT Use vasoactive drugs with extreme caution in the presence of cardiogenic shock. They require constant vigilance and astute observation to maintain an adequate perfusion pressure while achieving afterload reduction.

Reperfusion Therapy

Revascularization in cardiogenic shock patient may increase the patient's survival rate. See page 249.

1. PCI—prompt restoration of blood flow can lead to improved left ventricular function and thus salvaged ischemic myocardium. Timing of revascularization less than 90 minutes of door-to-door angioplasty after onset of symptoms provides better survival rates of patients with cardiogenic shock. Antithrombotic therapy with antiplatelet agents and anticoagulants during PCI has shown reduced mortality owing to cardiogenic shock following acute MI.
2. Thrombolytics—use of fibrinolytic drugs leads to improved left ventricular systolic function and survival in patients with MI associated with either ST-segment elevation or left bundle-branch block. Use may be limited owing to allergy or bleeding concerns such as recent hemorrhagic stroke.

Counterpulsation Therapy

See page 226.

1. Improves blood flow to the heart muscle and reduces myocardial oxygen needs.
2. Helps increase diastolic BP, which increases coronary blood flow to territory perfused by a vessel with a critical stenosis.
3. Results in improved CO (1.5 L/min increase) and preservation of viable heart tissue.
4. Should be instituted as quickly as possible to increase survival because of its overall benefits.

Total Circulatory and Mechanical Support

1. LVAD or right ventricular assist device may be used as bridge to recovery in some patients. See page 228. Percutaneous axial heart pump helps unload the left ventricle and reduces diastolic volume. It is a miniaturized, percutaneously inserted vascular access device that can be placed via a retrograde approach across the aortic valve using a femoral arterial access.
2. Extracorporeal life support (ECMO)—circulates blood using a membrane oxygenator, which relieves both left and right heart and the lungs of part of their workload.

Emergency Cardiac Surgery

1. CABG (see page 230).
2. Heart transplantation.

Complications

1. Neurologic impairment/stroke.
2. Acute respiratory distress syndrome.
3. Renal failure.
4. Cardiopulmonary arrest.
5. Dysrhythmia.
6. Ventricular aneurysm.
7. Multiorgan dysfunction syndrome.
8. Bowel ischemia.
9. Limb ischemia.
10. Death.

Nursing Assessment

Clinical assessment begins with attention to the airway/breathing/circulation and vital signs.

1. Identify patients at risk for development of cardiogenic shock.
2. Assess for early signs and symptoms indicative of shock:
   a. Restlessness, confusion, or change in mental status.
   b. Increasing heart rate and decreasing BP.
   c. Decreasing pulse pressure (indicates impaired CO).
   d. Presence of pulsus alternans (indicates left-sided heart failure).
   e. Decreasing urine output, weakness, fatigue.
3. Observe for presence of central and peripheral cyanosis.
4. Observe for development of edema and cool extremities.
5. Identify signs and symptoms indicative of extension of MI—recurrence of chest pain, diaphoresis.
6. Identify patient's and significant other's reaction to crisis situation.

CLINICAL JUDGMENT Monitor closely for any signs of respiratory compromise, and act immediately to prevent death. Use continuous pulse oximetry, and report oxygen saturation 90% or less.

Nursing Interventions

Improving Cardiac Output

1. Monitor and record BP, pulse, and respiratory rate every 1 to 5 minutes until the patient stabilizes.
2. Establish continuous ECG monitoring to detect dysrhythmias, which increase myocardial oxygen consumption.
3. Monitor hemodynamic parameters continually with pulmonary artery catheter (see page 212) to evaluate effectiveness of implemented therapy.
   a. Obtain pulmonary artery pressure (PAP), pulmonary artery wedge pressure, and CO readings, as indicated.
   b. Calculate the CI (CO relative to body size) and SVR (estimation of afterload).
   c. Cautiously titrate vasoactive drug therapy according to hemodynamic parameters.

4. Administer vasoactive drug therapy through central venous access if possible (peripheral tissue necrosis can occur if peripheral IV access infiltrates and peripheral drug distribution may be lessened from vasoconstriction).
5. Be alert to adverse responses to drug therapy.
   a. Dopamine may cause an increase in heart rate, which may result in ischemia.
   b. Vasodilators, such as nitroglycerin and nitroprusside, may worsen hypotension.
   c. Dobutamine may result in dysrhythmias.
   d. Diuretics may cause hyponatremia, hypokalemia, and hypovolemia.
6. Monitor BP and MAP with intra-arterial line continuously during active titration of vasoactive drug therapy.
7. Maintain MAP greater than 65 mm Hg (blood flow through coronary vessels is inadequate with MAP less than 65 mm Hg).
8. Measure urine output every hour from indwelling catheter, and document hourly intake and output.
9. Obtain daily weight.
10. Evaluate serum electrolytes for hyponatremia, hypomagnesemia, and hypokalemia.

CLINICAL JUDGMENT Be aware that chest pain indicates myocardial ischemia and may further heart damage. Report immediately; obtain a 12-lead ECG; check cardiac enzymes; and anticipate use of counterpulsation therapy and additional interventions.

Improving Oxygenation

1. Monitor rate and rhythm of respirations every hour.
2. Auscultate lung fields for abnormal sounds (coarse crackles indicate severe pulmonary congestion) every hour; notify health care provider.
3. Evaluate arterial blood gas (ABG) levels and correlate with oxygen saturation.
4. Administer oxygen therapy to increase oxygen tension and improve hypoxia.
5. Elevate head of bed 20 to 30 degrees, as tolerated (may worsen hypotension), to facilitate lung expansion.
6. Reposition patient frequently to promote ventilation and maintain skin integrity.
7. Observe for frothy pink sputum and cough (may indicate pulmonary edema); report immediately.

Maintaining Tissue Perfusion

1. Perform a neurologic check every hour using the Glasgow Coma Scale. Report change in mental status immediately.
2. Obtain BUN and creatinine blood levels, and monitor urine output to evaluate renal function.

DRUG ALERT If diuretic is ordered in an attempt to increase renal blood flow and urine output, administer with caution, because worsening hypotension may occur.

3. Auscultate for bowel sounds every 2 to 4 hours. Report absent bowel sounds and abdominal distention, indicating ileus and need for gastric decompression. Evaluate peripheral arterial pulses and assess skin color and temperature every 2 hours and note changes. Cold and clammy skin may be a sign of continuing peripheral vascular constriction, indicating progressive shock.
4. Protect skin from pressure injury.
5. Obtain serum lactate to evaluate tissue perfusion and acidosis. Report rising lactate, which may be an ominous sign.

Relieving Anxiety

1. Evaluate increasing anxiety or new-onset anxiety for a physiologic cause before treating with anxiolytics.
2. Explain equipment and rationale for therapy to patient and family. Increasing knowledge assists in alleviating fear and anxiety.
3. Encourage patient to verbalize fears about diagnosis and prognosis.
4. Explain sensations patient will experience before procedures and routine care measures.
5. Offer reassurance and encouragement.
6. Utilize social worker or pastoral care for support.
7. Provide for periods of uninterrupted rest and sleep to ease emotional stress.
8. Assist patient to maintain as much control as possible over environment and care.
   a. Develop a schedule for routine care measures and rest periods with patient.
   b. Make sure that a calendar and clock are in view of patient.

Patient Education and Health Maintenance

1. Provide education after patient is stabilized, rested, and ready to learn.
2. Teach patient about medications, including their indications, monitoring parameters, therapeutic effects, and adverse reactions.
3. Teach signs of impending heart failure—increasing edema, shortness of breath, decreasing urine output, decreasing BP, increasing pulse—and tell patient to notify health care provider immediately.
4. See specific measures for MI (see page 245), cardiomyopathy (see page 268), and valvular disease (see page 279).
5. Teach patient importance of keeping follow-up appointments with primary care physician and cardiologist.
6. Have dietitian teach patient and family about a low-sodium, low-fat diet, and reiterate the importance of adhering to this diet.
7. Explain to the patient the need to work with a physical and occupational therapist—especially if the patient has low ejection fraction—for energy conservation.

Evaluation: Expected Outcomes

- CO greater than 4 L/min; CI greater than 2.2; pulmonary capillary wedge pressure (PCWP) less than 18 mm Hg.
- Respirations unlabored and regular; normal breath sounds throughout lung fields.
- Normal sensorium; urine output adequate; skin warm and dry.
- Verbalizes lessened anxiety and fear.

Infective Endocarditis

Infective endocarditis (IE; bacterial endocarditis) is an infection of the inner lining of the heart caused by direct invasion of bacteria or other organisms that could potentially result in myocardial abscess or heart failure and other complications.

Pathophysiology and Etiology

1. When the inner lining of the heart (endocardium) becomes inflamed, a fibrin clot (vegetation) forms.
2. The fibrin clot may become colonized by pathogens during transient episodes of bacteremia resulting from invasive procedures (venous and arterial cannulation, dental work causing

gingival bleeding, GI tract surgery, liver biopsy, sigmoidoscopy), indwelling catheters, urinary tract infections, and wound and skin infections.

3. Platelets and fibrin surround the invading microorganisms, forming a protective covering and causing the infected vegetation to enlarge.
   a. The enlarged vegetation (the basic lesion of endocarditis) can deform, thicken, stiffen, and scar the free margins of valve leaflets as well as the fibrous ring (annulus) supporting the valve.
   b. The vegetations may also travel to various organs and tissues (spleen, kidney, coronary artery, brain, and lungs) and obstruct blood flow.
   c. The "protective covering" surrounding the vegetation makes it difficult for WBCs and antimicrobial agents to infiltrate and destroy the infected lesion.
4. Some of the bacterial causes include:
   a. *Streptococcus viridans*—bacteremia occurs after dental work or upper respiratory infection. This group is a part of normal human flora in the upper respiratory tract and oral cavity. It also affects some older populations and can be community acquired.
   b. *Staphylococcus aureus*—most common cause of IE; bacteremia occurs after cardiac surgery, increasing health care exposures (intravascular catheters, hemodialysis, surgical wounds, indwelling prosthetic devices), or parenteral drug misuse.
   c. *Staphylococcus epidermidis*—bacteremia occurs owing to prosthetic heart valves and IV access procedures.
   d. Enterococci (penicillin-resistant group *D. streptococci*)—bacteremia usually occurs in older patients (over age 60) with genitourinary tract infection.
   e. Gram-negative bacteria such as *Pseudomonas aeruginosa*, *Actinobacter*, and HACEK group bacteria. The HACEK group consists of *Haemophilus* species, *Aggregatibacter* species, *Cardiobacterium hominis*, *Eikenella corrodens*, and *Kingella* group species.
   f. Facultative intracellular parasites such as *Bartonella* and other opportunistic pathogens such as *Salmonella* and *Brucella* can cause IE.
5. Fungi (*Candida albicans*, *Aspergillus*) and rickettsiae are additional causes.
6. IE may develop on a heart valve already injured by rheumatic fever, congenital defects, on abnormally vascularized valves, normal heart valves, and mechanical and biologic heart valves.
7. IE may be acute or subacute, depending on the microorganisms involved. Acute IE manifests rapidly with danger of intractable heart failure and occurs more commonly on normal heart valves.
8. Subacute IE manifests as a prolonged chronic course with a lesser risk of complications and occurs more commonly on damaged or defective valves.
9. IE may follow cardiac surgery, especially when prosthetic heart valves are used. Foreign bodies, such as pacemakers, patches, grafts, and dialysis shunts, predispose to infection.
10. High incidence among those with substance use disorder, in whom the disease mainly affects normal valves, usually the tricuspid.
11. Patients who are hospitalized, with indwelling catheters, those on prolonged IV therapy or prolonged antibiotic therapy, those with burns, and those on immunosuppressive drugs or steroids may develop fungal endocarditis.
12. Relapse because of metastatic infection is possible, usually within the first 2 months after completion of antibiotic regimen.
13. Genitourinary disorders, infection, and manipulations, which include pregnancy, delivery, and abortion, may predispose to infection as well.
14. A prior history of IE is another risk factor.

CLINICAL JUDGMENT Be alert for patients who are hospitalized and at increased risk for IE due to nosocomial bacteremia associated with intravascular lines and wound care.

Clinical Manifestations

Severity of manifestations depends on invading microorganism.

General Manifestations

1. Fever, chills, sweats (fever may be absent in older patients or those with uremia).
2. Anorexia, weight loss, weakness.
3. Cough and back and joint pain (especially in patients over age 60).
4. Splenomegaly.
5. Subacute IE is characterized by nonspecific symptoms such as dyspnea, tiredness, weight loss, joint pain, slight fever, chills, and sweats, making it difficult to diagnose.

Skin and Nail Manifestations

1. Janeway lesions—light pink macules on palms or soles, nontender, may change to light tan within several days or fade in 1 to 2 weeks; usually an early sign of endocardial infection.
2. Petechiae—conjunctiva and mucous membranes.
3. Splinter hemorrhages in nail beds.
4. Osler nodes—painful red nodes on pads of fingers and toes; usually late sign of infection and found with a subacute infection.
5. Clubbing of fingers and toes—occurs primarily in patients who have an extended course of untreated IE.

Heart Manifestations

1. New pathologic or changing murmur—new onset heart murmur is a hallmark of acute IE when accompanied by fever, stroke, heart failure, and septic or pulmonary embolization. No murmur with other signs and symptoms may indicate right-sided heart infection.
2. Tachycardia—related to decreased CO.
3. Pericardial friction rub, and symptoms consistent with heart failure.
4. New heart block or dysrhythmia.
5. Perivalvular abscess—manifests as conduction abnormalities on ECG, persistent bacteremia, and fever despite antimicrobial therapy.
6. Pericarditis—may cause chest pain and signs of cardiac tamponade.

EVIDENCE BASE Rajani, R., & Klein, J. L. (2020). Infective endocarditis: A contemporary update. *Clinical Medicine (London, England)*, *20*(1), 31–35. https://doi.org/10.7861/clinmed.cme.20.1.1

Central Nervous System Manifestations

1. Localized headaches, stiff neck.
2. Transient cerebral ischemia or other neurologic symptoms.
3. Altered mental status, aphasia.
4. Hemiplegia.
5. Cortical sensory loss.
6. Roth spots on fundi (retinal hemorrhages).

Pulmonary Manifestations

1. Pneumonitis, pleuritis, pulmonary edema, infiltrates, effusions (causing friction rub)—occur with right heart involvement.

Embolic Phenomena

Septic embolization—can occur prior to presentation or after initiation of antimicrobial therapy. Embolization can cause stroke, paralysis, PE, ischemia of the extremities, splenic or renal infarction, and AMI. Symptoms vary by embolic location.

1. Lung—hemoptysis, chest pain, shortness of breath.
2. Kidney—hematuria, abnormal urine color.
3. Spleen—pain in the left upper quadrant of the abdomen radiating to left shoulder.
4. Heart—MI, aortic insufficiency, heart failure, valvular abscess.
5. Brain—sudden blindness, paralysis, brain abscess, meningitis, cerebrovascular accident (CVA).
6. Blood vessels—mycotic aneurysms.
7. Abdomen—melena, acute pain.

Diagnostic Evaluation

Varied clinical manifestations and similarities to other diseases make early diagnosis of IE difficult. Accurate diagnosis is essential to guide therapy. A definitive clinical diagnosis can be made based on the finding of two major criteria, five minor criteria, or one major and three minor criteria.

Major Criteria (Based on Modified Duke Criteria)

1. Blood cultures—at least two positive serial blood cultures (90% of patients with IE have positive blood cultures).
2. Endocardial involvement (diagnosed with transesophageal echocardiogram)—identification of vegetations and assessment of location and size of lesions.
3. New valvular insufficiency/regurgitation.
4. Development of abscess or new partial dehiscence of prosthetic valve or new valvular regurgitation.

Minor Criteria

1. Predisposing cardiac condition or IV drug use.
2. Fever higher than 100.4°F (38°C).
3. Vascular factors—pulmonary complication, arterial emboli, Janeway lesions, mycotic aneurysm, intracranial hemorrhage, conjunctival hemorrhages.
4. Immunologic factors—Osler nodes, Roth spots, rheumatoid factor, glomerulonephritis.
5. Microbiology—positive bacterial or fungal cultures but not meeting major criteria; or serologic evidence of active infection with organism consistent with IE.

Management

1. IV antimicrobial therapy, based on sensitivity of causative agent. Six weeks of therapy is recommended for most patients except uncomplicated right-sided IE, in whom 2 weeks of combination therapy is recommended.
2. Combination antibiotic therapy is highly effective and can be given for 2 weeks, depending on the group of pathogens identified. Bactericidal serum levels of selected antibiotics are monitored by serial titers; if serum lacks adequate bactericidal activity, higher dosage or a different antibiotic is needed.
3. Supplemental nutrition.
4. Surgical intervention for specific complications, but surgery should be delayed for at least a month in patients who suffered a hemorrhagic CVA. Surgery should not be delayed in patients following silent embolic event or TIA, associated heart failure, abscess, or high embolic risk patients.
   a. Acute destructive valvular lesion—excision of infected valves or removal of prosthetic valve.
   b. Hemodynamic impairment, severe heart failure.
   c. Recurrent emboli.
   d. Resistant infection.
   e. Drainage of abscess or empyema.
   f. Repair of peripheral or cerebral mycotic aneurysm.

DRUG ALERT Antimicrobial therapy for IE should be targeted at the organism from the blood cultures; however, it is highly recommended to initiate empiric antibiotic therapy while waiting for blood culture results. Empiric therapy is for patients who manifest hemodynamic instability, have clinical presentation suggestive of acute endocarditis (e.g., new murmur and fever, especially with history of IE or congenital heart disease, IV drug use, immunosuppression, or recent surgery). Two sets of blood cultures should be obtained, ideally from two separate venipunctures

Complications

1. Severe heart failure because of valvular insufficiency.
2. Uncontrolled/refractory infection due to perivalvular abscess. This causes conduction abnormalities as the abscess extends into adjacent conduction tissues, leading to heart blocks.
3. Embolic episodes (brain ischemia or necrosis of extremities and organs). Septic embolization.
4. Organ dysfunction resulting from immunologic process (kidneys, eyes, skin).
5. Tissue destruction by microorganism, valvular damage, mycotic aneurysms, hemorrhage, and abscess formation.

Nursing Assessment

1. Identify factors that may predispose to IE, such as rheumatic heart disease, congenital heart defects, idiopathic hypertrophic subaortic stenosis, IV drug misuse, prosthetic heart valves, aortic or mitral stenosis, previous history of endocarditis, recent genitourinary surgery or other interventions that may have precipitated transient bacteremia, as well as homelessness or squalid living conditions.
2. Determine onset of signs and symptoms of endocarditis (early treatment of infection improves prognosis).
3. Obtain thorough history of allergies, with special emphasis on adverse reactions to antibiotic therapy. Note if patient is currently on antibiotic therapy (may affect blood culture results).
4. Perform thorough physical examination and document findings, particularly cardiac murmur, presence of skin lesions, and signs of heart failure, and assess for changes day to day.
5. Identify patient's and family's level of anxiety and use of appropriate coping mechanisms. Drug misuse, living conditions, and other social determinants may complicate treatment and recovery from illness.
6. Obtain blood cultures, CBC, sedimentation rate, CRP, renal and hepatic studies, and a baseline 12-lead ECG.

Nursing Interventions

Maintaining Adequate Fluid Balance and Cardiac Output

1. Auscultate heart, and report any new murmur or change in existing murmur; presence of gallop.

2. Monitor BP and pulse.
   a. Note presence of pulsus alternans (indicative of left-sided heart failure).
   b. Evaluate pulse pressure (30 to 40 mm Hg indicates adequate CO).
3. Evaluate for jugular vein distention, indicating heart failure.
4. Record intake and output.
5. Record daily weight.
6. Auscultate lung fields for evidence of crackles (rales).
7. Monitor liver function studies (elevated with liver engorgement related to right heart failure).
8. Assess skin turgor for dehydration and edema for heart failure.
9. Administer diuretics and other medications as ordered, oxygen via nasal cannula as needed.
10. Maintain bedrest and provide assistance with activities.

Maintaining Tissue Perfusion

1. Observe patient and promptly report altered mentation, aphasia, loss of muscle strength, and any sensory deficits.
2. Monitor respiratory rate and effort and oxygen saturation, and evaluate for dyspnea on exertion. Be alert for chest pain, dyspnea, hemoptysis, tachycardia, and hypoxemia, indicating pulmonary embolus or infarction. Elevate head of bed and position for maximum chest expansion.
3. Monitor renal function and color of urine (oliguria, hematuria, concentrated urine, indicating renal infarction caused by septic emboli).
4. Assess skin color and temperature for peripheral occlusion. Protect skin from pressure injury.

Maintaining Normothermia

1. Observe basic principles of asepsis, good handwashing techniques, and continuity of care by excellent documentation and communication.
2. Employ meticulous IV care for long-term antibiotic therapy.
   a. Note the date of needle or cannula insertion on nursing care plan.
   b. If a peripheral site is used, rotate the site every 72 hours or if site becomes tender, reddened, infiltrated, or has purulent drainage.
   c. Change gauze dressing every 48 hours or transparent dressing every 5 to 7 days (for midline and central venous access) and as needed to prevent infection.
   d. If a continuous venous access device is used, follow facility policy for site care, IV tubing and dressing changes, and flushing procedures.
3. For IM antibiotic therapy, develop chart for rotation of sites.
4. Note that missed doses of antibiotic may have irreversible deleterious consequences, so scheduling is essential to prevent the patient from being off the unit when antibiotic is due.
5. Observe for allergic reaction to antibiotic therapy (severe respiratory distress, rash, itching, fever), stop the antibiotic, and notify health care provider promptly so a substitute can be ordered.
6. Obtain audiogram before potentially ototoxic antibiotic is started, and observe for adverse effects such as ototoxicity and renal failure.
7. Assess effectiveness of therapy by obtaining urine culture after 48 hours of drug therapy and blood cultures after 24 to 48 hours of therapy.
8. Monitor temperature every 4 hours.
   a. Document results on a graph.
   b. Note increases in heart rate and/or respirations with elevated temperatures.
   c. Provide blankets and temperature-controlled comfortable environment if patient has shaking chills; change bed linens, as necessary.
   d. Administer antipyretic or analgesic medications, as directed.
9. Observe patient for a general "sense of well-being" within 5 to 7 days after initiation of therapy.
10. Promote adequate hydration because diaphoresis and increased metabolic rate may cause dehydration.
11. Encourage oral fluid intake.
12. Administer IV fluids as directed.
13. Observe skin turgor and mucous membranes.

DRUG ALERT Rapid infusion of vancomycin (less than 1 hour) may cause red neck syndrome (intense red rash over the upper half of the body) because of histamine release. Slow the rate of infusion and the rash will clear. Vancomycin and gentamicin dosages and intervals should be adjusted in patients with impaired renal function.

Patients with unknown history of penicillin allergy or history of any hypersensitivity reaction should be evaluated by infectious disease specialist with possible challenge test, versus choosing alternative to penicillin.

Improving Nutritional Status

1. Assess patient's daily caloric intake and monitor weight.
2. Discuss food preferences and ability to chew with patient.
3. Consult with a dietitian about nutritional needs and appropriate diet for patient.
4. Encourage small meals and snacks throughout the day.
5. Educate family about the patient's caloric needs.
6. Encourage family to assist the patient with meals, and bring in patient's favorite foods as needed.

Reducing Anxiety

1. Rule out physiologic etiologies for increasing or new-onset anxiety before administering as-needed sedatives. Physiologic causes must be identified and treated in a timely fashion to prevent irreversible adverse or even fatal outcomes; sedatives may mask symptoms, delaying timely identification, diagnosis, and treatment.
2. Assess patient for signs of hypoperfusion, auscultate heart and lung sounds, obtain a rhythm strip, and administer oxygen, as prescribed. Notify the health care provider immediately.
3. Document assessment findings, health care provider notification and response, and interventions and response.
4. Explain to patient and family reasons for hospitalization, diagnostic tests, and therapies administered.
5. Encourage patient to verbalize fears about illness and hospitalization. Use motivational interviewing and active listening to encourage patient to open up about substance misuse and other life problems.
6. Explain procedures to patient before initiation.
7. Encourage diversional activities for patient, such as television, reading, and interaction with other patients.

Patient Education and Health Maintenance

For Patients at Risk for IE

1. Discuss anatomy of the heart and changes that occur during endocarditis, using diagrams of the heart.
2. Give patient written literature on early signs and symptoms of disease; review these with patient.

3. Discuss with patient the mode of entry of infection.
4. Indicate that antibiotic prophylaxis is recommended prior to dental procedures that manipulate the gingival and some respiratory procedures (see Table 9-4), for patients with the following conditions:
   a. Congenital heart disease (particularly unrepaired cyanotic defects) repaired with prosthetic material (for 6 months following repair) or repaired with residual defect.
   b. Prosthetic cardiac valve.
   c. Previous IE.
   d. Heart transplantation recipient with cardiac valvular disease.
5. Identify individual steps necessary to prevent infection.
   a. Practice good oral hygiene, regular toothbrushing, and flossing. See dentist regularly.
   b. Notify health care personnel of any history of congenital heart disease or valvular disease.
   c. Discuss importance of carrying emergency identification with information of medical history at all times.
   d. Take temperature if infection is suspected, and notify health care provider of elevation.
   e. Educate patients at risk to look for and treat signs and symptoms of illness indicating bacteremia—injuries, sore throats, furuncles, and so forth.
6. Encourage at-risk individuals to receive pneumococcal and influenza vaccines.

For Individuals Who Have Had Endocarditis Regarding Possible Relapse

1. Discuss importance of keeping follow-up appointments after discharge (infection can recur in 1 to 2 months).
2. Review the tests that will be performed after discharge—blood cultures, physical examination, echocardiography.
3. Teach patient to inspect soles for Janeway lesions (indicative of possible relapse).
4. Contact social worker or case manager to assist patient with financial planning and home discharge arrangements, if applicable.

Evaluation: Expected Outcomes

- BP stable; no change in murmur; no gallop noted.
- No change in LOC, strength, or neurologic function.
- Normal temperature; negative blood cultures; no hearing impairment.
- Tolerates increased daily caloric intake well.
- Verbalizes decrease in anxiety.

Rheumatic Endocarditis (Rheumatic Heart Disease)

Rheumatic endocarditis is an acute, recurrent inflammatory disease that causes damage to the heart as a sequela to group A beta-hemolytic streptococcal infection, particularly the valves, resulting in valve leakage (insufficiency) and/or obstruction (narrowing or stenosis). There are associated compensatory changes in the size of the heart's chambers and the thickness of chamber walls. Acute rheumatic fever occurs around 2 to 3 weeks after streptococcal infection occurs. After multiple episodes of rheumatic fever, progressive fibrosis of heart valves ensue, which then leads to rheumatic valvular heart disease. If this remains untreated, heart failure or death may occur.

Rheumatic endocarditis is a major burden in developing countries, where it causes most of the cardiovascular morbidity and mortality in young people, leading to about 250,000 deaths per year worldwide. Since 1990, the prevalence of rheumatic heart disease world-wide has been steadily rising, reaching 40 million in 2019.

EVIDENCE BASE Roth, G. A., Mensah, G. A., Johnson, C. O., Addolorato, G., Ammirati, E., Baddour, L. M., Barengo, N. C., Beaton, A. Z., Benjamin, E. J., Benziger, C. P., Bonny, A., Brauer, M., Brodmann, M., Cahill, T. J., Carapetis, J., Catapano, A. L., Chugh, S. S., Cooper, L. T., Coresh, J., ... GBD-NHLBI-JACC Global Burden of Cardiovascular Diseases Writing Group. (2020). Global burden of cardiovascular diseases and risk factors, 1990–2019: Update from the GBD 2019 Study. *Journal of the American College of Cardiology, 76*(25), 2982–3021. https://doi.org/10.1016/j.jacc.2020.11.010

Table 9-4 Preventing Endocarditis: Regimens for a Dental Procedure

		REGIMEN: SINGLE DOSE 30–60 MIN PROCEDURE	
Situation	**Agent**	**Adults**	**Children**
Oral	Amoxicillin	2 g	50 mg/kg
Unable to take oral medication	Ampicillin OR	2 g IM or IV	50 mg/kg IM or IV
	Cefazolin or ceftriaxone	1 g IM or IV	50 mg/kg IM or IV
Allergic to penicillins or ampicillin—oral	Cephalexin[a,b] OR	2 g	50 mg/kg
	Clindamycin OR	600 mg	20 mg/kg
	Azithromycin or clarithromycin	500 mg	15 mg/kg IM or IV
Allergic to penicillins or ampicillin and unable to take oral medication	Cefazolin or ceftriaxone[b] OR	1 g IM or IV	50 mg/kg IM or IV
	Clindamycin	600 mg IM or IV	20 mg/kg IM or IV

IM, intramuscular; IV, intravenous.
[a]*Or other first- or second-generation oral cephalosporin in equivalent adult or pediatric dosage.*
[b]*Cephalosporins should not be used in individuals with a history of anaphylaxis, angioedema, or urticaria with penicillins or ampicillin.*

See discussion of rheumatic fever in children in Chapter 41, page 1215.

Pathophysiology and Etiology

1. Rheumatic fever is a sequela to group A beta-hemolytic streptococcal infection that occurs in about 3% of untreated infections. It is a preventable disease through detection and adequate treatment of streptococcal pharyngitis.
2. Connective tissue of the heart, blood vessels, joints, and subcutaneous tissues can be affected.
3. Lesions in connective tissue are known as Aschoff bodies, which are localized areas of tissue necrosis surrounded by immune cells.
4. Heart valves, mainly the mitral valve, are most commonly affected, resulting in valve leakage and narrowing. Combined lesions of both aortic and mitral valves occur in 20% of cases, while tricuspid valve involvement occurs in about 10% in association with mitral and aortic disease and when current infections have occurred. Pulmonary valve is rarely affected.
5. Compensatory changes in the chamber sizes (enlargement, bulging) and thickness of chamber walls occur.
6. Heart involvement also includes pericarditis, myocarditis, epicarditis, and endocarditis, known as pancarditis.

Clinical Manifestations

1. Symptoms of streptococcal pharyngitis may precede rheumatic symptoms.
   a. Sudden onset of sore throat; throat reddened with exudates.
   b. Swollen, tender lymph nodes at angle of the jaw.
   c. Headache and fever 101°F to 104°F (38.3°C to 40°C).
   d. Abdominal pain (children).
   e. Some cases of streptococcal throat infection relatively asymptomatic.
2. Warm and swollen joints (polyarthritis), beginning in the lower extremities (knees and ankles) and may include the large joints in the upper extremities (elbows, wrists). Pain in joints.
3. Sydenham chorea (irregular, jerky, involuntary, unpredictable muscular movements).
4. Erythema marginatum (transient mesh-like macular rash on the trunk and extremities, never on the face, in about 5% to 13% of patients).
5. Subcutaneous nodules (hard, painless nodules over extensor surfaces of extremities; rare).
6. Fever.
7. Prolonged PR interval, as shown on ECG.
8. Heart murmurs; pleural and pericardial friction rubs.
9. History of previous rheumatic fever or rheumatic heart disease.
10. If there is heart valve damage, symptoms may include chest pain or discomfort, shortness of breath, fatigue, swelling of hands/feet, and rapid or irregular heartbeat.

Diagnostic Evaluation

Major Diagnostic Criteria

1. Carditis—caused by regurgitation of the valves.
2. Arthritis—earliest symptom of infection; presents around 21 years of age. It is more common and severe in teenagers and young adults. Joint pain is typical and can be severe, limiting movement.
3. Subcutaneous nodules—small, painless bumps or nodules beneath the skin.
4. Chorea—Sydenham chorea, also known as chorea minor, is a neurologic disorder consisting of abrupt, involuntary movement, muscular weakness (often in hands, feet, and face), and emotional disturbance. Common in prepubescent and young adult females.
5. Erythema marginatum—flat, slightly raised, painless rash with ragged edge.

Minor Manifestation

1. Fever >38.5°C (101.3°F) orally. Painful and tender.
2. Arthralgia—painful and tender joints—often in wrist, elbows, ankles, and knees.
3. Prolonged PR interval on ECG—prolonged PR interval for age on ECG.
4. Elevated acute phase reactants—elevated peak erythrocyte sedimentation rate or CRP during acute illness.

Diagnostic Findings

1. Throat culture—streptococcal organisms.
2. Sedimentation rate, WBC count and differential, and CRP—increased during acute phase of infection.
3. Elevated antistreptolysin-O (ASO)/streptococcal antibody titer.
4. ECG—prolonged PR interval or heart block.
5. Echocardiography and Doppler study.
6. Cardiac catheterization to evaluate valvular damage and left ventricular function in those with severe cardiac dysfunction.
7. Chest x-ray to help evaluate cardiomegaly or pulmonary vascular congestion, which can be a sign of congestive heart failure.
8. Rapid detection test—immunofluorescence technique that can identify 90% of patients with rheumatic fever and those at risk for developing one.
9. Rapid antigen detection test—detects group A streptococci antigen that allows the diagnosis of streptococcal pharyngitis to be made and initiate antibiotics.

CLINICAL JUDGMENT Throat culture on family members should also be considered to treat them and prevent reinfection of patient

Management

Primary prevention of rheumatic heart disease centers on quick recognition and treatment of streptococcal infection to prevent the development of acute rheumatic fever.

1. Antimicrobial therapy—penicillin, erythromycin, or cephalosporin. Early treatment is key to survival.
2. Rest—to maintain optimal cardiac function.
3. Salicylates or NSAIDs to treat fever and pain.

DRUG ALERT Recommend and administer NSAIDs with caution in patients with reduced renal function, age >65, and those with history of or risk factors for GI bleeding.

4. Corticosteroids—during acute inflammatory phase.
5. Prevention of recurrent episodes through long-term penicillin therapy for 5 years or until 21 years old, whichever is longer, if patient does not have carditis, or 10 years if with carditis; periodic prophylaxis throughout life.
6. Beta-blockers, ACE inhibitors, digoxin, other afterload reduction medications, diuretics, supplemental oxygen, rest, sodium and fluid restrictions—to manage heart failure.
7. Although chorea is self-limiting, corticosteroids, phenobarbital, and diazepam may relieve the symptom.

8. Percutaneous mitral balloon valvuloplasty (PMBV) is recommended for patients with rheumatic mitral stenosis.
9. Meticulous dental hygiene and thorough dental evaluation is required if dental infection was the factor that contributed to rheumatic heart disease (more common in IE).

Complications

1. Valvular heart disease.
2. Cardiomyopathy.
3. Heart failure.
4. Atrial arrhythmias.
5. Pulmonary and systemic embolism.

Nursing Assessment

1. Obtain history of recent symptoms of fever, sore throat, or joint pain; recurrent episodes of pharyngitis, fever, and arthralgias; and possible exposure to streptococcus infections through family, school, or community.
2. Ask patient about chest pain, dyspnea, fatigue.
3. Observe for skin lesions or rash on the trunk and extremities.
4. Palpate for firm, nontender movable nodules near tendons or joints.
5. Auscultate heart sounds for murmurs and/or rubs.

Nursing Interventions

Reducing Fever

1. Administer penicillin therapy, as prescribed, to eradicate hemolytic streptococcus; an alternative drug may be prescribed if patient is allergic to penicillin, or sensitivity testing and desensitization may be done.
   a. Coordinate schedule to prevent missed or delayed dose of antibiotic because of patient being off unit to prevent deleterious effects.
2. Give salicylates or NSAIDs, as prescribed, to suppress rheumatic activity by controlling toxic manifestations, to reduce fever, and to relieve joint pain.
3. Assess for effectiveness of drug therapy.
   a. Take and record temperature every 3 hours.
   b. Evaluate patient's comfort level every 3 hours.

Maintaining Adequate Cardiac Output

1. Assess for signs and symptoms of acute rheumatic carditis.
   a. Be alert to patient's complaints of chest pain, palpitations, and/or precordial "tightness."
   b. Monitor for tachycardia (usually persistent when patient sleeps) or bradycardia.
   c. Monitor cardiac rhythm and be alert to development of second-degree heart block or Wenckebach disease (acute rheumatic carditis causes PR-interval prolongation).
2. Auscultate heart sounds every 4 hours.
   a. Document presence of murmur or pericardial friction rub.
   b. Document extra heart sounds (S_3 gallop, S_4 gallop).
3. Monitor for development of chronic rheumatic endocarditis, which may include valvular disease and heart failure.

Maintaining Activity

1. Maintain bedrest for duration of fever or if signs of active carditis are present.
2. Provide ROM exercise program.
3. Provide diversional activities that prevent exertion.
4. Discuss the need for tutorial services with caregivers to help child keep up with schoolwork.

Patient Education and Health Maintenance

1. Counsel patient to maintain good nutrition.
2. Counsel patient on hygienic practices.
   a. Discuss proper handwashing, disposal of tissues, covering mouth when coughing, and maintaining distance to reduce transmission of respiratory infections.
   b. Discuss importance of using patient's own toothbrush, soap, and washcloths when living in group situations.
3. Counsel patient on importance of receiving adequate rest.
4. Instruct patient to seek treatment immediately should sore throat or fever occur.
5. Support patients in long-term antibiotic therapy to prevent relapse (5 years for most adults).
6. Instruct patient with valvular disease to use prophylactic antibiotic therapy an hour before certain procedures and surgery (see page 50).
7. Discuss patient's ability to pay for medical treatment. If appropriate, contact social services for patient. (Financial difficulties may inhibit patient from seeking early treatment of symptoms.)

Evaluation: Expected Outcomes

- Afebrile.
- Denies chest pain; normal sinus rhythm.
- Maintains bedrest while febrile.

Myocarditis

Myocarditis is an inflammatory process involving the myocardium, thus damaging the heart muscle. Although the exact cause of myocarditis is still unknown, it is thought to attack otherwise healthy individuals. It is believed to be the cause of sudden death among young adults and the cause of acute or chronic dilated cardiomyopathy.

Pathophysiology and Etiology

1. Focal or diffuse inflammation of the myocardium; may be acute or chronic.
2. May follow infectious process—viral or "idiopathic" (particularly coxsackie group B and may develop after influenza A or B, herpes simplex, parvovirus, cytomegalovirus, adenovirus, enterovirus, Epstein-Barr, rubella, and human immunodeficiency virus [HIV]), bacterial, parasitic, protozoal, rickettsial, spirochetal, and fungal (*Candida*, *Aspergillus*, and *Histoplasma*).
3. Lyme disease, an infection caused by the spirochete *Borrelia burgdorferi*, has been associated with myocarditis; seen in patients with history of travel to endemic regions or history of a tick bite.
4. *Trypanosoma cruzi*, a parasitic infection seen in areas of Central and South America, can present as myocarditis.
5. Hepatitis C virus has been associated with myocarditis by identification of HCV antibodies.
6. May be associated with chemotherapy (especially doxorubicin), immunosuppressive therapy, or vaccinia virus inoculation for protection against smallpox infection.
7. Systemic disorders such as sarcoidosis and celiac disease, autoimmune conditions such as systemic lupus, and other collagen diseases may cause myocarditis.
8. May be associated with exposures to certain chemicals (arsenic and hydrocarbons); allergic or toxic reactions to penicillin or

sulfonamides; insect/snakebites; cocaine use. Other medications, including anticonvulsants and antipsychotics, have been implicated in hypersensitivity myocarditis.

9. Radiation exposure—most cases are the result of therapy for Hodgkin lymphoma or breast or lung cancer. Less common is exposure to a nuclear reactor or after detonation of a nuclear device.
10. SARS-CoV-2, the virus that causes COVID-19, and vaccines—case reports described findings consistent with a diagnosis of "clinically suspected myocarditis." More studies and case evaluations are needed to confirm their association with myocarditis.

Clinical Manifestations

1. Symptoms depend on type of infection, degree of myocardial damage, capacity of the myocardium to recover, and host resistance. Can be acute or chronic and can occur at any age. Symptoms may be minor and go unnoticed.
   a. Fatigue and dyspnea.
   b. Palpitations.
   c. Occasional precordial discomfort/vague chest pain.
2. Cardiac enlargement.
3. Abnormal heart sounds: murmur, S_3 or S_4, or friction rubs.
4. Signs of heart failure (e.g., pulsus alternans, dyspnea, crackles, lower extremity edema, low urine output) or unexplained cardiogenic shock.
5. Fever with tachycardia or other signs of viral infection, such as headache, joint pain, and sore throat.

Diagnostic Evaluation

1. Transient ECG changes—ST segment flattened, T-wave inversion, conduction defects, extrasystoles, supraventricular and ventricular ectopic beats, brady- or tachyarrhythmias.
2. Elevated WBC count, CRP, and sedimentation rate.
3. Measurement of serum cardiac biomarkers such as creatinine phosphokinase (CPK) and troponin (T or I)—may be elevated.
4. Chest x-ray—may show heart enlargement and lung congestion.
5. Elevated antibody titers (ASO titer as in rheumatic fever).
6. Stool and throat cultures isolating bacteria or a virus.
7. Endomyocardial biopsy for definitive diagnosis. This is the gold standard for establishing the diagnosis.
8. Echocardiogram—defines size, structure, and function of the heart.
9. Cardiovascular MRI—may be helpful to determine structural alterations; can provide accurate tissue characterization.
10. Nuclear imaging using *gallium* (detects the extent of myocardial inflammation) or *indium* (antimyosin antibodies—shows the extent of myocyte necrosis)

Management

Treatment objectives are targeted toward management of complications. Supportive care is the first line of treatment.

1. Elevated ventricular filling pressures should be treated with IV diuretics and vasodilators (when feasible) such as nitroprusside.
2. Antidysrhythmic therapy (usually amiodarone) and, possibly, an implantable cardioverter defibrillator (ICD) for symptomatic or sustained ventricular arrythmias, even if active inflammation is still present.
3. Strict bedrest to promote healing of damaged myocardium.
4. Antimicrobial therapy if causative bacteria are isolated.
5. Anticoagulation therapy.
6. ACE inhibitor or beta-adrenergic blocker (should be used with caution; may cause hypotension)—to strengthen the heart's pumping ability and to reduce its workload, thus improving left ventricular systolic dysfunction. Diuretics should be considered with caution.
7. In severe cases, aggressive therapy may be necessary: inotropes, such as dobutamine, milrinone, and dopamine (at a lower dose); IABP counterpulsation therapy.
8. In acute cases, temporary pacemakers may be required for patients with symptomatic bradycardia or complete heart block.
9. A ventricular assist device or extracorporeal membrane oxygenation may rarely be required to sustain patients with refractory cardiogenic shock as well as consideration of urgent heart transplantation.
10. IV immunoglobulin has antiviral effects; interferon-alpha and interferon-beta; immunosuppressive regimen of steroids and cyclosporine or azathioprine improves systolic function.

Complications

1. Heart failure, pericarditis.
2. Cardiomyopathy.
3. Arrhythmias.
4. Sudden cardiac death.

Nursing Assessment

1. Assess for fatigue, palpitations, fever, dyspnea, and chest pain.
2. Auscultate heart sounds.
3. Assess limbs for swelling, discoloration of the skin, and temperature of the skin.
4. Evaluate history for precipitating factors.
5. Pay special attention to variation in BP, irregular or rapid heart rate, and tachypnea.

Nursing Interventions

Reducing Fever

1. Administer antipyretics and antibiotics as directed.
2. Check temperature every 4 hours.
3. Provide comfort measures such as cool compresses, ice chips, change of clothing and sheets, and comfortable environmental temperature.

Maintaining Fluid Balance and Adequate Cardiac Output

1. Evaluate for clinical evidence that disease is subsiding—monitor pulse, auscultate for abnormal heart sounds (murmur or change in existing murmur), check temperature, auscultate lung fields, monitor respirations.
2. Record and monitor hemodynamic pressures as indicated—CVP, pulmonary arterial pressure, pulmonary wedge pressure, cardiac output/index, and mixed venous gas saturation—to detect worsening hemodynamic compromise.
3. Record intake and output.
4. Record daily weight.
5. Check for peripheral edema and elevate extremities as indicated.
6. Elevate head of bed, if necessary, to enhance respiration. Encourage use of incentive spirometry.

7. Treat the symptoms of heart failure as indicated (see page 270).
8. Evaluate patient's pulse and apical rate for signs of tachycardia and gallop rhythm—indications that heart failure is recurring.
9. Evaluate for evidence of dysrhythmias—patients with myocarditis are prone to develop dysrhythmias.
   a. Institute continuous cardiac monitoring if evidence of a dysrhythmia develops.
   b. Have equipment for resuscitation, defibrillation, and cardiac pacing available in case of life-threatening dysrhythmia.

DRUG ALERT Digoxin should not be considered for patients with myocarditis. High doses of digoxin may increase production of proinflammatory cytokines and may worsen myocardial injury. If digoxin was given, assess for toxic signs and symptoms, such as anorexia, nausea, fatigue, weakness, yellow-green halos around visual images, or prolonged PR interval.

Reducing Fatigue

1. Ensure bedrest to reduce heart rate, stroke volume, BP, and heart contractility; also helps to decrease residual damage and complications of myocarditis and promotes healing. Prolonged bedrest may be required until there is reduction in heart size and improvement of function.
2. Provide diversional activities for patient.
3. Allow patient to use bedside commode rather than bed pan (reduces cardiovascular workload).
4. Discuss with patient activities that can be continued after discharge.
   a. Discuss the need to modify activities in the immediate future.
   b. Explore patient's feelings and concerns about role fulfillment.

Reducing Chest Pain

1. Assess for chest pain; provide pain medication if not contraindicated.
2. Provide a quiet environment and comfort measures such as change in position, back rub, emotional support.
3. Provide supplemental oxygen as indicated.

Patient Education and Health Maintenance

Instruct patient as follows:

1. There is usually some residual heart enlargement; physical activity may be slowly increased; begin with chair rest for increasing periods; follow with walking in the room and then outdoors.
2. Report any symptom involving rapid heartbeat.
3. Avoid competitive sports, cigarettes, illicit drugs, and alcohol. Myocardial toxic medications such as doxorubicin cannot be used.
4. Pregnancy is not advisable for patients with cardiomyopathies associated with myocarditis.
5. Prevent infectious diseases with appropriate immunizations (pneumococcal and influenza vaccines).
6. Refer patient to cardiac phase II rehabilitation—a safe, monitored environment to increase patient's exercise work capacity.

Evaluation: Expected Outcomes

- Afebrile.
- BP and heart rate stable; no dysrhythmias noted.
- Maintains bedrest.
- Pain reported at 2 on a scale of 0 to 10.

Pericarditis

Pericarditis is an inflammation of the pericardium, the membranous sac enveloping the heart. It is usually a manifestation of a more generalized disease. In healthy individuals, the pericardial cavity contains about 15 to 50 mL of an ultrafiltrate of plasma. Diseases of the pericardium present clinically in four ways:

Acute and recurrent pericarditis. Pericardial effusion is an abnormal accumulation of fluid in the pericardial cavity.

Cardiac tamponade is an acute type of pericardial effusion in which the heart is compressed, either by blood or by a penetrating injury so that its normal function is impeded.

Constrictive pericarditis is a condition in which a chronic inflammatory thickening of the pericardium compresses the heart so it is unable to fill normally during diastole.

Pathophysiology and Etiology

1. Acute idiopathic pericarditis is the most common and typical form; etiology unknown.
2. Infection.
   a. Viral—Coxsackievirus, Herpes viruses, adenovirus, parvovirus B19, HIV, influenza, and echovirus.
   b. Bacterial—*Staphylococcus*, meningococcus, *Streptococcus*, pneumococcus, gonococcus, *Mycobacterium tuberculosis*.
   c. Fungal (rare)—Histoplasma, Aspergillus, Blastomyces, and Candida species.
   d. Parasitic (rare)—Echinococcus and Toxoplasma.
3. Connective tissue disorders (lupus erythematosus, periarteritis nodosa) and GI diseases (ulcerative colitis, Crohn and Whipple disease).
4. MI; early, 24 to 72 hours; or late, 1 week to 2 years after MI (Dressler syndrome).
5. Malignant disease; thoracic irradiation (primary or metastatic pericardial tumors).
6. Chest trauma, heart surgery, pacemaker insertion, coronary percutaneous interventions, and radiofrequency ablation.
7. Drug-induced—procainamide, phenytoin, hydralazine, methyldopa, and isoniazid.
8. Asbestosis (may induce pericardial as well as lung lesions).
9. Metabolic disorders such as uremia; hypothyroidism may cause pericardial effusion, not necessarily pericarditis.

Clinical Manifestations

1. Pain in anterior chest, aggravated by thoracic motion—may vary from mild to sharp and severe; located in precordial area (may be felt beneath the clavicle, neck, scapular region); may be relieved by leaning forward.
2. Pericardial friction rub—scratchy, raspy, grating, or creaking sound occurring due to friction of the pericardial layers during systole.
3. Edema, ascites, and dyspnea—from pericardial effusion and cardiac tamponade.
4. Fever, sweating, chills—because of inflammation of the pericardium.
5. Dysrhythmias.

Diagnostic Evaluation

1. Echocardiogram—most sensitive method for detecting pericardial effusion.
2. Chest x-ray—may show enlarged cardiac silhouette with clear lung fields.

3. ECG—to evaluate for MI (acute stage of pericarditis, ST elevation is found in several or all leads).
4. WBC count and differential indicating infection.
5. Antinuclear antibody and serologic tests elevated in lupus erythematosus.
6. Purified protein derivative test positive in tuberculosis.
7. ASO titers—elevated if rheumatic fever is present.
8. BUN—to evaluate for uremia.
9. Elevated erythrocyte sedimentation rate and serum CRP levels.
10. Elevated cardiac biomarkers—troponin and MB fraction of creatinine kinase.
11. Pericardiocentesis—for examination of pericardial fluid for etiologic diagnosis and relief from cardiac tamponade.
12. Cardiac MRI or CT.

Management

The objectives of treatment are targeted toward determining the etiology of the problem; administering pharmacologic therapy for specified etiology, when known; and being alert to the possible complication of cardiac tamponade.

1. Penicillin or other antibiotics for bacterial pericarditis; penicillin G is preferred for rheumatic fever (see page 1215).
2. Antitubercular drugs such as rifampin and isoniazid for confirmed tuberculosis (see page 171).
3. Amphotericin B and fluconazole for fungal pericarditis.
4. Corticosteroids for lupus; high-dose prednisolone may be used to reduce constrictive pericarditis but may increase the risk of HIV-associated malignancies.
5. Dialysis is necessary to control pericarditis in patients with end-stage renal disease.
6. Intrapericardial instillation of chemotherapy and radiotherapy are necessary to control neoplastic pericarditis.
7. Bedrest, aspirin, and prednisone are used to treat post-MI syndrome.
8. Postpericardiotomy syndrome (after open heart surgery) is treated symptomatically.
9. Emergency pericardiocentesis is necessary if cardiac tamponade develops.
10. Partial pericardiectomy (pericardial "window") or total pericardiectomy for recurrent constrictive pericarditis.
11. NSAIDs are recommended for symptom relief of acute pericarditis; colchicine and steroid regimen are used as adjunct to NSAID therapy.

DRUG ALERT Aspirin should be substituted for other NSAIDs in patients following MI and those on antiplatelet therapy. It is the first-line therapy in the first trimester of pregnancy but should not be used past 20 weeks; acetaminophen may be used at 20 weeks and later.

12. Steroid-sparing immunosuppressive agent such as IVIG may be used for corticosteroid-dependent recurrent pericarditis.

Complications

1. Cardiac tamponade.
2. Heart failure.
3. Hemopericardium (especially patients receiving anticoagulants after MI).

DRUG ALERT Anticoagulants should be used with caution since some forms of acute pericarditis, such as uremic and iatrogenic pericarditis, have been associated with increased risk of hemorrhagic pericardial effusion and cardiac tamponade.

Nursing Assessment

1. Assess chest pain.
   a. Ask the patient if pain is aggravated by breathing, turning in bed, twisting body, coughing, yawning, or swallowing.
   b. Assess for relief with sitting up and/or leaning forward.
   c. Be alert to the patient's medical diagnoses when assessing pain. Post-MI patients may experience a dull, crushing pain radiating to the neck, arm, and shoulders, mimicking an extension of infarction. Report change in character of chest pain or worsening pain.
2. Auscultate heart sounds.
   a. Listen for pericardial friction rub by asking patient to hold breath briefly.
   b. Listen to the heart with patient in different positions.
   c. Assess for pulsus paradoxus.
3. Evaluate history for precipitating factors.

Nursing Interventions

Reducing Discomfort

1. Administer prescribed drug regimen for pain and symptomatic relief.
2. Relieve anxiety of patient and family by explaining the difference between pain of pericarditis and pain of recurrent MI. (Patients may fear extension of myocardial tissue damage.)
3. Explain to patient and family that pericarditis does not indicate further heart damage.
4. Encourage patient to remain on bedrest when chest pain, fever, and friction rub occur.
5. Assist patient to position of comfort.

Maintaining Cardiac Output

CLINICAL JUDGMENT Normal pericardial sac contains less than 30 mL of fluid; pericardial fluid may accumulate slowly without noticeable symptoms. However, a rapidly developing effusion can produce serious hemodynamic alterations. Be alert for chest pain with hypotension, tachycardia, and narrow pulse pressure.

1. Assess heart rate, rhythm, BP, respirations at least hourly in the acute phase; continuously if hemodynamically unstable.
2. Assess for signs of cardiac tamponade—increased heart rate, decreased BP, presence of paradoxical pulse, distended jugular veins, restlessness, muffled heart sounds.
3. Prepare for emergency pericardiocentesis or surgery. Keep pericardiocentesis tray at bedside (see page 223).
4. Assess for signs of heart failure (see page 270).
5. Monitor closely for the development of dysrhythmias.

Patient Education and Health Maintenance

1. Advise restriction of activity until biomarkers are normal.
2. Instruct patient about signs and symptoms of pericarditis and the need for long-term medication therapy to help relieve symptoms.
3. Review all medications with the patient—purpose, adverse effects, dosage, and special precautions.

Evaluation: Expected Outcomes

- Verbalizes relief of pain.
- Pulse and heart rate stable, no dysrhythmias, no friction rub.

Cardiomyopathy

Cardiomyopathy refers to disease of the heart muscle. Currently, it is considered a disorder in which heart muscle is structurally and functionally abnormal in the absence of CAD, hypertension, valvular disease, and congenital heart disease. Causes of cardiomyopathy are classified as primary or secondary. Primary cardiomyopathies have genetic, mixed, or acquired etiologies, whereas secondary cardiomyopathies have infiltrative, toxic, or inflammatory causes. The four main types are dilated (DCM), hypertrophic (HCM), restrictive (RCM, less common), and arrhythmogenic right ventricular cardiomyopathy (ARVCM). There are additional types of less common cardiomyopathies.

Pathophysiology and Etiology

Dilated Cardiomyopathy

Dilated cardiomyopathy (DCM), the most common form of cardiomyopathy, is characterized by dilation and impaired contraction of one or both ventricles. Affected patients have impaired systolic function and present with features of heart failure. DCM can be divided into ischemic and nonischemic cardiomyopathy.

1. Ischemic cardiomyopathy.
   a. It is caused by inadequate oxygen supply because of obstruction in coronary arteries.
   b. The lack of oxygen interrupts both mechanical and electrical functions of the cells, decreases contractility, and causes dysrhythmia.
   c. The scar formed from MI leads to systolic dysfunction.
2. Nonischemic cardiomyopathy.
   a. Cause is primarily idiopathic (unknown).
   b. 10% to 50% of cases are identified by genetic mutation.
   c. Viruses may play a role.
3. Both the right and the left ventricles dilate (enlarge) significantly, causing a decrease in the ability of the heart to pump blood efficiently to the body.
4. Blood remaining in the ventricles after contraction causes increases in ventricular, atrial, and pulmonary pressures.
5. Increased pressures continue to diminish the ability of the heart to pump blood to the body, and heart failure symptoms occur after all compensatory mechanisms are exhausted.
6. Alcohol misuse, chemotherapy, chemical agents, myocarditis, pregnancy (third trimester, postpartum), valve disease, endocrine disorders such as thyroid disease, and infections, such as HIV, can cause dilated cardiomyopathy.

Hypertrophic Cardiomyopathy

1. Hypertrophic cardiomyopathy (HCM) is primarily due to the abnormal thickening of the ventricular septum of the heart.
2. The thickening of the heart muscle commonly occurs asymmetrically (septum is proportionately thicker than the other ventricular walls) but may also occur symmetrically (septum and the ventricular free wall both become equally thickened).
3. The ultrastructure of the heart is also disrupted by patches of myocardial fibrosis, disorganization of myocardial fibers, and abnormalities of the coronary microvasculature.
4. The thickened heart muscle and ultrastructure disruption change the shape, size, and distensibility of the ventricular cavity and alter the normal thickness and functioning of the mitral valve; as a result, the heart's ability to relax and contract normally is impaired.
   a. Muscle stiffness impairs the filling of the ventricle with blood during relaxation.
   b. Forceful contractions eject blood from the heart too rapidly, causing abnormal pressure gradients; mechanical narrowing of the passage by which the blood leaves the heart may also occur, acutely obstructing blood flow to the body.
   c. The LV volume is normal or reduced in HCM, and diastolic dysfunction is usually present.
5. Some forms of HCM have familial presentation suggestive of genetic mutations.

Restrictive Cardiomyopathy

1. Restrictive cardiomyopathy (RCM) is characterized by nondilated ventricles with impaired ventricular filling.
2. The heart muscle becomes infiltrated by various substances, resulting in severe fibrosis.
3. The heart muscle becomes stiff and nondistensible, impairing the ability of the ventricle to fill with blood adequately.
4. Amyloidosis and hemochromatosis (excess iron deposition) may cause RCM.
5. Can be classified as familial noninfiltrative, infiltrative, storage diseases, and other disorders (diabetic CM, scleroderma, endomyocardial fibrosis).
6. Endomyocardial fibrosis occurs mainly in children and adolescents in the tropics. Cause is unknown.

Arrhythmogenic Right Ventricular Cardiomyopathy

1. Prevalence in the general adult population is 1 in 2,000 to 5,000; more common among males.
2. ARVCM is an inherited CM that affects the first-degree relative of the family member that has the genetic disorder.
3. Pathophysiology is characterized by placement of the right ventricular myocytes by fibrofatty tissue, right ventricular dysfunction, and ventricular dysrhythmias.
4. Sudden death may occur in young adults (11% of sudden cardiac death is due to ARVCM). May be due to atrial or ventricle septal defects, pulmonary valve stenosis, tricuspid valve regurgitation, tetralogy of Fallot.

Unclassified CMs

1. The term was introduced in the 2008 ESC classification system.
2. LV noncompaction: a rare CM with an altered myocardial wall due to intrauterine arrest of compaction of the loose interwoven meshwork.
3. Stress-induced CM: also called apical ballooning syndrome, broken heart syndrome, and takotsubo CM. Characterized by transient systolic dysfunction of the apical and/or mid-segments of the LV.
4. Cirrhotic CM: cirrhosis is associated with myocardial dysfunction independent of alcohol exposure.
5. Endocardial fibroelastosis: Characterized by diffuse thickening of the LV endocardium secondary to proliferation of fibrous and elastic tissue. Occurs primarily in infants during the first year of life.

Clinical Manifestations

1. Exertional dyspnea.
2. Chest pain.
3. Signs of heart failure (see page 270).
4. Pulmonary edema (see page 276).
5. Dysrhythmias (frequent atrial/ventricular ectopic beats; sinus, atrial, and ventricular tachycardia [VT]).
6. Pericardial effusions (with RCM).
7. Cardiac murmur.
8. Syncope.
9. Sudden cardiac death may be the first sign with ARVCM.

Diagnostic Evaluation

1. Chest x-ray (cardiomegaly).
2. ECG—may show dysrhythmia, LV hypertrophy.
3. Echocardiogram to detect abnormalities of heart wall movements, thickness or thinness, ventricle cavity size, and impaired valve function.
4. Twenty-four–hour Holter monitoring to detect dysrhythmias.
5. Radionuclide imaging to assess ventricular function.
6. Cardiac catheterization to help determine cause (ischemic or nonischemic).
7. Pulmonary artery catheter for hemodynamic monitoring.

Management

The goal of therapy is to maximize ventricular function and prevent complications. Guidelines for the management of cardiomyopathy and heart failure, in general, center around the measurement of ejection fraction.

Dilated Cardiomyopathy

1. Effective management of heart failure by conventional therapy (see page 270).
2. Oral anticoagulants may be instituted to prevent thrombus and pulmonary embolus.
3. Heart transplantation may be considered in eligible patients.
4. Mechanical circulatory support device (i.e., LVAD or biventricular assist devices [BiVAD]) may also be considered.

DRUG ALERT Patients with dilated cardiomyopathy and other forms of heart failure are susceptible to digoxin toxicity, especially with the concomitant use of amiodarone, furosemide, or verapamil, and so are patients with renal impairment. Monitor patient carefully for evidence of nausea, vomiting, yellow vision, and dysrhythmias.

Hypertrophic Cardiomyopathy

1. Guidelines for the management of cardiomyopathy and heart failure, in general, center around the measurement of ejection fraction. Patients with EF greater than 50 are considered to have heart failure with preserved ejection fraction (HF*p*EF). Those with EF less than or equal to 40 are considered to have heart failure with reduced ejection fraction (HF*r*EF). Beta-adrenergic blockers reduce the force of the heart muscle's contraction, diminish obstructive pressure gradients, and decrease oxygen requirements. Three different beta-blockers have been shown to be effective in reducing mortality in patients with chronic HF*r*EF; these include metoprolol sustained release, bisoprolol, and carvedilol.
2. Antidysrhythmic therapy—digoxin is most commonly used to slow ventricular response and increase myocardial contractility in patients with heart failure, although beta-blockers have been shown to be more effective than digoxin during exercise. Combination of beta-blockers and digoxin is more effective than either drug alone. If contraindicated, amiodarone may be an alternative.
3. Myotomy and myectomy—surgical resection of a portion of the septum to reduce muscle thickness and provide symptom relief.
4. Alcohol septal ablation when performed by experienced HCM teams at dedicated centers have improved outcomes.
5. Device implantation—pacemakers and automatic internal defibrillators may be implanted to prevent sudden death.

DRUG ALERT Verapamil and diltiazem should be avoided in heart failure treatment because they depress myocardial function with increasing heart failure. Agents that increase contractility of the heart muscle (dopamine, dobutamine) should also be avoided or used with extreme caution.

CLINICAL JUDGMENT Be aware that nitroglycerin may worsen chest pain by decreasing venous return to the heart and further increasing obstruction of blood flow from the heart. Chest pain experienced by patients with HCM should be managed by rest and elevation of the feet (improves venous return to the heart).

Restrictive Cardiomyopathy

1. Therapy is palliative unless specific underlying process is established.
2. Heart failure can be controlled with fluid restriction and diuretic therapy.
3. Digoxin is beneficial for controlling atrial fibrillation.
4. Oral anticoagulants are instituted to prevent thromboemboli.
5. Heart transplant if patient is considered to have a long-term survival. Unfortunately, patients have the highest waitlist mortality due to other end organ damage.

Arrhythmogenic Right Ventricular Cardiomyopathy

1. Antidysrhythmic agents such as carvedilol, sotalol, amiodarone.
2. ICD.
3. Myocardial ablation or transplantation.
4. Beta-blockers for patients with definite ARVCM and a prior history of sudden cardiac arrest or documented VT.
5. Refractory ventricular arrhythmias may require radiofrequency catheter ablation (RFA).
6. Bilateral cardiac sympathetic denervation (BCSD) has been shown to reduce ICD shocks in patients with structural heart disease and refractory VT.
7. Patients should avoid any endurance and competitive sports.
8. Heart transplant if eligible.

Complications

1. Mural/apical thrombus (because of blood stasis in ventricles with dilated cardiomyopathy).
2. Severe heart failure.
3. Sudden cardiac death.
4. PE.

Nursing Assessment

1. Evaluate patient's chief complaint, which may include fever, syncope, general aches, fatigue, palpitations, dyspnea.
2. Evaluate etiologic factors, such as alcohol misuse, pregnancy, recent viral infection, or history of endocrine disorders.
3. Assess for positive family history.
4. Auscultate lung sounds for crackles (pulmonary edema) or decreased breath sounds (pleural effusion).
5. Assess heart size through palpation of the chest for point of maximal impulse (PMI) and auscultate for abnormal sounds.
6. Evaluate cardiac rhythm and ECG for evidence of atrial or ventricular enlargement and infarction.
7. Evaluate JVD for fluid overload.

Nursing Interventions

Improving Cardiac Output

1. Monitor heart rate, rhythm, temperature, and respiratory rate at least every 4 hours.
2. Evaluate CVP, PAP, and PCWP by pulmonary artery catheter to assess progress and effect of drug therapy.
3. Calculate CO, CI, SV, and SVR.
4. Observe for changes in CO, such as decreased BP, change in mental status, decreased urine output.
5. Monitor mixed venous oxygenation saturation or central oxygenation saturation.
6. Administer pharmacologic support, as directed, and observe for changes in hemodynamic and clinical status.
7. Administer medications to control or eradicate dysrhythmias, as directed.
8. Administer anticoagulants as directed, especially for patients in atrial fibrillation or reduced EF.
   a. Monitor coagulation studies.
   b. Observe for evidence of bleeding.

Relieving Anxiety

1. Always evaluate increasing and/or new-onset anxiety for a physiologic cause and report to the health care provider before administration of anxiolytics.
2. Explain all procedures and treatments.
3. Inform patient and visitors of visiting hours and policy and whom to contact for information.
4. Orient patient to unit, purpose of equipment, and care plan.
5. Encourage questions and voicing of fears and concerns.

Reducing Fatigue

1. Make sure that patient and visitors understand the importance of rest.
2. Assist patient in identifying stressors and reducing their effect (important for patients with HCM because stress worsens the outflow obstruction).
3. Provide uninterrupted periods and assist with ambulation, as ordered.
4. Teach the use of diversional activities and relaxation techniques to relieve tension.
5. Obtain a physical therapy consult to maintain and increase patient functioning.

Patient Education and Health Maintenance

1. Medication education includes the following:
   a. Dosing schedule of each medication.
   b. Signs and symptoms of adverse reactions and when to notify health care provider.
   c. How to take pulse before certain medications such as digoxin and beta-blockers.
   d. Fluid intake, urine output, and daily weight monitoring if taking diuretic.
   e. Need for follow-up for periodic blood levels.
   f. Importance of reading the information sheet that comes with each medication and consulting pharmacist or health care provider with any questions.
   g. Instruction to not stop any medication before consulting health care provider.
2. Advise low-sodium diet (less than 1,500 g daily). Teach how to read labels.
3. Advise reporting signs of heart failure—weight gain, edema, shortness of breath, increased fatigue.
4. Encourage discussion with health care provider about recreational exercise, especially with HCM, before starting any type of exercise or sports.
5. Make sure that family members know cardiopulmonary resuscitation (CPR), because sudden cardiac arrest is possible.

Evaluation: Expected Outcomes

- BP and hemodynamic parameters stable; urine output adequate; baseline mental status.
- Asks questions and cooperates with care.
- Rests at intervals.

Heart Failure

EVIDENCE BASE Heidenreich, P. A., Bozkurt, B., Aguilar, D., Allen, L. A., Byun, J. J., Colvin, M. M., Deswal, A., Drazner, M. H., Dunlay, S. M., Evers, L. R., Fang, J. C., Fedson, S. E., Fonarow, G. C., Hayek, S. S., Hernandez, A. F., Khazanie, P., Kittleson, M. M., Lee, C. S., Link, M. S., ... Yancy, C. W. (2022). 2022 AHA/ACC/HFSA guideline for the management of heart failure: A report of the American College of Cardiology/American Heart Association Joint Committee on Clinical Practice Guidelines. *Journal of the American College of Cardiology, 79*(17), e263–e421. https://doi.org/10.1016/j.jacc.2021.12.012

Heart failure is a clinical syndrome that results from the progressive process of remodeling, in which mechanical and biochemical forces alter the size, shape, and function of the ventricle's ability to fill with or pump enough oxygenated blood to meet the metabolic demands of the body. Heart failure is a growing health and economic burden in the United States.

Pathophysiology and Etiology

1. Cardiac compensatory mechanisms (increased heart rate, vasoconstriction, heart enlargement) initially occur to assist the struggling heart.
   a. These mechanisms are able to "compensate" for the heart's inability to pump effectively and maintain sufficient blood flow to organs and tissue at rest.
   b. Physiologic stressors that increase the workload of the heart (exercise, infection) may cause these mechanisms to fail and precipitate the "clinical syndrome" associated with a failing heart (elevated ventricular/atrial pressures, sodium and water retention, decreased CO, circulatory and pulmonary congestion).
   c. The compensatory mechanisms may hasten the onset of failure because they increase afterload and cardiac work.
2. Caused by disorders of heart muscle, resulting in decreased contractile properties of the heart, such as CAD, hypertension, dilated cardiomyopathy, and valvular heart disease.
3. Risk factors include:
   a. hypertension.
   b. Hyperlipidemia.
   c. Diabetes.
   d. CAD.
   e. Family history.
   f. Smoking.
   g. Alcohol consumption.
   h. Use of cardiotoxic drugs.

i. Ventricular dysrhythmias.
j. Atrial dysrhythmias.
k. Metabolic disorders.
l. Arteriosclerotic disease (coronary, cerebral, peripheral).
m. Obesity.

Systolic Versus Diastolic Failure

Heart failure is classified as either HFpEF or HFrEF. Systolic and/or diastolic dysfunction may exist in either heart failure type (see Figure 9-7).

1. Systolic failure—poor contractility of the myocardium results in decreased CO and an elevated SVR.
2. Diastolic failure—stiff myocardium, which impairs the ability of the left ventricle to fill up with blood. This causes an increase in pressure in the left atrium and pulmonary vasculature, causing the pulmonary signs of heart failure.

Acute Versus Chronic Heart Failure

1. Acute failure—sudden onset of symptoms such as acute pulmonary edema and decreased CO; requires intervention and medical attention.
2. Chronic failure—long-term process with accompanying compensatory mechanism; can progress to acute phase in the setting of dysrhythmias, ischemia, or sudden illness.
3. Acute or chronic heart failure—patients with established history of heart failure who present with exacerbation.

Neurohormonal Compensatory Mechanisms in Heart Failure

1. Sympathetic nervous system changes
   a. Increased catecholamines to compensate for low CO.
   b. Shunting of blood from nonvital to vital organs.
   c. Increased oxygen demand, decreased coronary artery perfusion, and decreased diastolic filling.
2. Renin–Angiotensin–Aldosterone System Changes
   a. Increased fluid retention in response to decreased CO.
   b. Increased vasoconstriction (action of angiotensin II).
   c. Increased SVR.
   d. Increased workload of the heart.
   e. Further decreased CO over time.

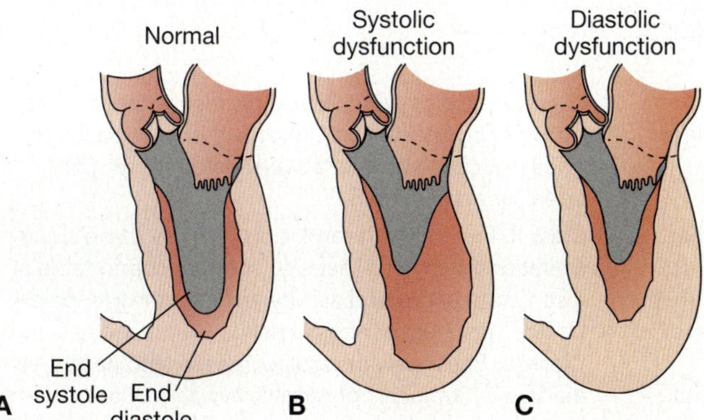

Figure 9-7. Heart failure because of systolic and diastolic dysfunction. The ejection fraction represents the difference between end-diastolic function and end-systolic volume. **(A)** Normal systolic and diastolic function with normal ejection fraction; **(B)** systolic dysfunction with decreased ejection fraction because of impaired systolic function; **(C)** diastolic dysfunction with decreased ejection fraction because of decreased diastolic filling. (Reprinted with permission from Porth, C. M. [2005]. *Pathophysiology: Concepts of altered health states* [7th ed.]. Lippincott Williams & Wilkins.)

3. Ventricular hypertrophy occurs to overcome the increased afterload.
4. Ventricular remodeling—change in size, shape, structure, and function of the heart.

Clinical Manifestations

Initially, there may be isolated left-sided heart failure, but, eventually, the right ventricle fails because of the additional workload. Combined left- and right-sided heart failure is common. Heart failure may be classified according to physical activity (NYHA Functional Classification) or disease progression (American College of Cardiology/American Heart Association [ACC/AHA] Guidelines); see page 271.

Signs of Left-Sided Heart Failure (Forward Failure)

Altering the filling and pumping function of left ventricle, congestion occurs mainly in the lungs from blood backing up into pulmonary veins and capillaries.

1. Shortness of breath, dyspnea on exertion, tachypnea, paroxysmal nocturnal dyspnea (because of reabsorption of dependent edema that has developed during the day), orthopnea, cyanosis, pulmonary edema, and hemoptysis.
2. Cough—may be dry, unproductive; usually occurs at night.
3. Fatigability—from low CO, nocturia, insomnia, dyspnea, catabolic effect of chronic failure.
4. Insomnia, restlessness.
5. Tachycardia—ventricular gallop (S_3 and S_4).

Signs of Right-Sided Heart Failure (Backward Failure)

Altering the pumping function of right ventricle, there are signs and symptoms of elevated pressures and congestion in systemic veins and capillaries.

1. Edema of ankles; unexplained weight gain (pitting edema is obvious only after retention of at least 10 pound [4.5 kg] of fluid).
2. Liver congestion—may produce upper abdominal pain.
3. Distended jugular veins, increased CVP, pulmonary hypertension (increased PCWP).
4. Abnormal fluid in body cavities (pleural space, abdominal cavity), splenomegaly.
5. Anorexia and nausea—from hepatic and visceral engorgement.
6. Nocturia—diuresis occurs at night with supine position and improved CO.
7. Weakness.

Cardiovascular Findings in Both Types

1. Cardiomegaly (enlargement of the heart)—detected by physical examination and chest x-ray.
2. Ventricular gallop—evident on auscultation.
3. Rapid heart rate.
4. Development of pulsus alternans (alternation in strength of beat).

Diagnostic Evaluation

Heart failure is largely a clinical diagnosis based on a careful history, physical examination, and laboratory and imaging data.

1. Echocardiography—two-dimensional with Doppler flow studies—may show ventricular hypertrophy, dilation of chambers, and abnormal wall motion; most common test used to measure ejection fraction.
2. ECG (resting and exercise)—may show ventricular hypertrophy and ischemia.

3. Chest x-ray may show cardiomegaly, pleural effusion, and vascular congestion.
4. Cardiac catheterization—
   a. Left heart catheterization to evaluate for CAD.
   b. Right heart catheterization—to measure pulmonary pressure and left ventricular function.
5. ABG studies may show hypoxemia because of pulmonary vascular congestion.
6. Mixed venous blood gas saturation measures the oxygen content of the blood that returns to the heart after meeting the tissue needs.
7. General bloodwork: CBC, electrolytes, Ca, Mg, renal function, glycohemoglobin, lipid profile, thyroid function, and liver function studies to fully assess patient condition that may impact heart failure.
8. Heart failure specific bloodwork: Human B-type natriuretic peptide (BNP, triage BNP, N-terminal prohormone brain NP, or proBNP).
   a. As volume and pressure in the cardiac chambers rise, cardiac cells produce and release more BNP. This test aids in the differentiation of heart failure from other pulmonary diseases (i.e., chronic obstructive pulmonary disease) and establishes acute exacerbation of heart failure.
   b. A level less than 100 pg/mL is normal. BNP level 100 to 300 pg/mL indicates that heart failure is present in some form. Levels greater than 300 indicate mild heart failure is currently happening. Levels above 600, moderate heart failure; levels greater than 900, severe heart failure. BNP has inverse relationship with BMI, so severity or degree of volume retention cannot be determined by the BNP values in patients with obesity.
   c. BNP is used in emergency departments to quickly diagnose and start treatment.
9. Radionuclide ventriculogram.
10. Thallium scan to rule out underlying causes.

Management

Management is based on stage. There are two classification systems that stage heart failure: the NYHA Functional Classification and the ACC/AHA Stages. The most common classification system is the NYHA Functional Classification that has four categories (Class I to Class IV), which differentiate patients based on limitations during physical activity. The ACC/AHA staging system defines four stages and correlates to treatment plans. The stages range from a high risk of developing heart failure to advanced heart failure. There is no reversal through the stages. The objective is to delay progression through the stages.

Overview Based on ACC/AHA Stage

See Table 9-5.

1. Stage A—focuses on eliminating risk factors by initiating TLC, such as smoking cessation, increasing physical activity, and decreasing alcohol consumption. This stage also focuses on controlling chronic diseases, such as hypertension, high cholesterol, and diabetes. Beta-adrenergic blockers, ACE inhibitors, and diuretics are useful in treating this stage.
2. Stage B—treatment similar to stage A, with emphasis on use of ACE inhibitors and beta-adrenergic blockers.
3. Stage C—same as A and B but with closer surveillance and follow-up.
   a. Digoxin is typically added to the treatment plan in this stage.
   b. Use of diuretic, hydralazine, nitrate, aldosterone antagonist, as indicated.
   c. Drug classes to be avoided due to worsening of heart failure symptoms include antiarrhythmic agents, calcium channel blockers, and NSAIDs.
   d. Patients post-MI (i.e., 40 days post MI) with EF 35 or less who have New York State Heart Association class II or III

Table 9-5 Heart Failure Staging and Guidelines

AMERICAN COLLEGE OF CARDIOLOGY/ AMERICAN HEART ASSOCIATION STAGE	MANAGEMENT GUIDELINES	NEW YORK STATE HEART ASSOCIATION CLASSIFICATION
Stage A. People at high risk of developing heart failure but without structural heart disease or symptoms of heart failure.	Initiate therapeutic lifestyle changes and, possibly, ACE inhibitor.	
Stage B. People who have structural heart disease but no symptoms of heart failure.	Add ACE inhibitor and β-adrenergic blocker unless contraindicated.	**Class I.** Patients with cardiac disease without limitations of physical activity. Ordinary physical activity does not cause undue fatigue, palpitations, dyspnea, or anginal pain.
Stage C. People who have structural heart disease with current or prior symptoms of heart failure.	Add sodium-restricted diet, diuretics, digoxin. Avoid or withdraw antiarrhythmics, most calcium channel blockers, NSAIDs. Consider aldosterone antagonists, ARBs, hydralazine, nitrates.	**Class II.** Patients with cardiac disease who have slight limitations of physical activity. They are comfortable at rest. Ordinary physical activity results in fatigue, palpitations, dyspnea, or anginal pain. **Class III.** Patients with cardiac disease who have marked limitation of physical activity. They are comfortable at rest. Less than ordinary physical activity causes fatigue, palpitations, dyspnea, or anginal pain.
Stage D. People with refractory heart failure who require specialized interventions.	Add mechanical assist device, continuous inotropic therapy. Consider hospice care.	**Class IV.** Patients with cardiac disease who cannot carry out any physical activity without discomfort. Symptoms of cardiac insufficiency or of anginal syndrome may be present even at rest. Any physical activity increases discomfort.

ACE, angiotensin-converting enzyme; ARB, angiotensin receptor blocker; NSAID, nonsteroidal anti-inflammatory drug.

symptoms and on guideline-supported medical therapies are recommended for ICD placement.

4. Stage D—may need mechanical circulatory support, continuous inotropic therapy, cardiac transplantation, or palliative care.
   a. Treatment aimed at decreasing excess body fluid.
   b. May not tolerate other classes of drugs used in previous stages.
5. Unlike NYHA functional class, once a patient progresses to stage C, for example, they cannot go back to stage B.

Drug Classes

1. Diuretics (preload reduction) to eliminate excess body fluid and decrease ventricular pressures.
   a. Loop diuretics are the preferred diuretic for use in most patients with heart failure.
   b. Thiazide diuretics may be considered for patients with hypertension and heart failure where fluid retention is mild. There is no evidence to support the common misconception that patients who are allergic to sulfa drugs are also allergic to thiazide diuretics.
   c. Metolazone or chlorothiazide may be added to loop diuretics with refractory edema that is unresponsive to loop diuretics alone.
   d. The infusion of hypertonic saline prior to diuretics could temporarily reduce neurohormonal sodium retention, leading to increase in diuresis.
   e. A low-sodium diet and fluid restriction complement this therapy.
2. Positive inotropic agents—increase the heart's ability to pump more effectively by improving the contractile force of the muscle.
   a. Digoxin strengthens the force of heart muscle contractions. It may be initiated at any time to reduce symptoms of heart failure prevent hospitalizations, control rhythm, and improve exercise tolerance.
   b. Dopamine improves BP in advanced heart failure and increases blood flow to the kidneys and increases urine output.
   c. Dobutamine improves CO, decreases PCWP, and decreases SVR with little effect on heart rate or systemic arterial pressure.
   d. Milrinone and amrinone are potent vasodilators and increase contractility.
3. Vasodilator therapy—decreases the workload of the heart by dilating peripheral vessels. By relaxing capacitance vessels (veins and venules), vasodilators reduce ventricular filling pressures (preload) and volumes. By relaxing resistance vessels (arterioles), vasodilators can reduce impedance to left ventricular ejection and improve stroke volume.
   a. Nitrates (nitroglycerin, isosorbide, nitroglycerin ointment)—predominantly dilate systemic veins and work by decreasing left ventricular filling pressure and SVR.
   b. Hydralazine—predominantly affects arterioles; reduces arteriolar tone.
   c. Prazosin—balanced effects on both arterial and venous circulation.
   d. Sodium nitroprusside—potent afterload reducer; predominantly affects arterioles.
   e. Morphine—analgesic of choice because it enhances peripheral dilation, decreases venous return, and decreases anxiety, thus decreasing workload of the heart.
4. ACE inhibitors—inhibit the formation of angiotensin II, thereby producing vasodilation. This decreases left ventricular dilation and can prevent ventricular remodeling with chronic use.
   a. Studies have shown ACE inhibitors can alleviate heart failure symptoms and improve clinical status as well as overall sense of well-being among patients with heart failure.
   b. The following ACE inhibitors have been shown to reduce morbidity and mortality: captopril, enalapril, lisinopril, perindopril, ramipril, and trandolapril.
   c. Renal function must be monitored with ACE inhibitor use.
5. Beta-adrenergic blockers—negative inotropes that decrease myocardial workload and protect against fatal dysrhythmias by blocking norepinephrine effects of the sympathetic nervous system.
   a. Metoprolol or metoprolol sustained release is commonly used.
   b. Carvedilol is a nonselective beta- and alpha-adrenergic blocker. Patients may actually experience increase in general malaise for a 2- to 3-week period while they adjust to the medication. To reduce the risk of orthostatic hypotension, instruct patient to take medicine with food.
   c. Bisoprolol works by relaxing blood vessels and slowing heart rate to decrease BP and increase left ventricular function.
6. Angiotensin II-receptor blockers—similar effects as ACE inhibitors, although mechanism of action is different. Used in patients who cannot tolerate ACE inhibitors because of cough or angioedema.
7. Aldosterone antagonists or antimineralocorticoids—decrease sodium retention, sympathetic nervous system activation, and cardiac remodeling.
   a. Spironolactone is most commonly used; eplerenone is also used.
   b. May cause hyperkalemia, especially in those with impaired renal function, in those taking high doses of ACE inhibitors, or in those who use potassium supplements.
   c. Angiotensin receptor/neprilysin inhibitor (ARNI) is a newer agent, consisting of combination of sacubitril and valsartan. Valsartan is the angiotensin receptor blocker (ARB) that lowers BP by keeping blood vessels from constricting. Sacubitril is the NI that allows the body to get rid of more sodium, dilates the blood vessels, and increases urine output.

DRUG ALERT When switching from an ACE to an ARNI, there must be a washout period for the ACE (usually 48 hours) before starting the ARNI to prevent severe hypotension.

8. Calcium channel blockers may be used in acute heart failure due to high BP when other BP medications are not effective.
9. Nesiritide is a natriuretic peptide used in patients with decompensated heart failure. It decreases PAP by causing smooth muscle cell relaxation and diuresis, resulting in afterload reduction and less dyspnea.
10. Amiodarone—to treat arrhythmias.
11. Sodium-glucose cotransporter-2 inhibitors (SGLT2i), such as canagliflozin, dapagliflozin, and empagliflozin promote osmotic diuresis and natriuresis in patients with and without diabetes and reduce preload. May have vascular effects that promote vasodilation and reduce afterload.

Mechanical Circulatory Support

May be used in stage D heart failure and acute exacerbation of heart failure.

1. IABP; see page 226, helps decrease afterload.
2. Percutaneous LVAD to improve CO, see page 228.
3. Cardiac resynchronization therapy or biventricular pacing—helps to restore synchronous ventricular contractions, improves ventricular left ventricle filling, and improves CO.
4. Total artificial heart or left, right, or biventricular assist device.
5. Partial left ventriculectomy (reduction ventriculoplasty or Batista procedure)—a triangular section of the weakened heart muscle is removed to reduce ventricular wall tension. This procedure is not commonly used.
6. Endoventricular circular patch plasty or the Dor procedure—removal of diseased portion of septum or left ventricle with a synthetic or autologous tissue patch, thus providing a more normal shape and size of the heart, which improves hemodynamics.
7. Acorn cardiac support device—a polyester mesh, custom-fitted jacket is surgically placed on the epicardial surface, providing diastolic support. Over time, it decreases or halts remodeling.
8. Intubation—for pulmonary edema or respiratory distress.
9. ICD—for patients with previous cardiac arrest, sustained ventricular arrhythmias, and in those post MI with ejection fraction less than 30%.
10. Heart transplant.

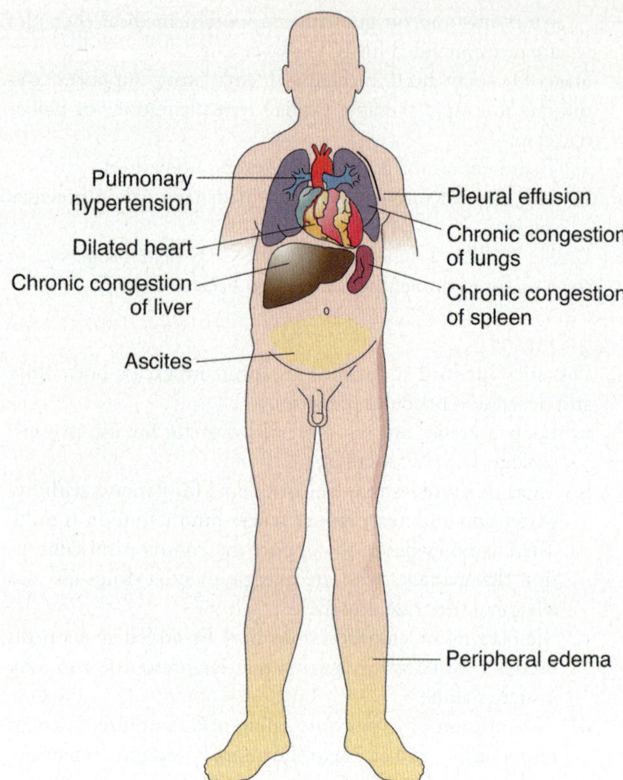

Figure 9-8. Consequences of heart failure.

Complications

1. Intractable or refractory heart failure unresponsive to treatment, leading to death.
2. Cardiac arrhythmias.
3. Myocardial failure and cardiac arrest.
4. Digoxin toxicity—from decreased renal function and potassium depletion.
5. Pulmonary infarction, pneumonia, and emboli.

Nursing Assessment

1. Obtain history of symptoms, onset and duration of the symptoms, limits of activity, response to rest, and history of response to drug therapy. Determine neurologic status during the history.
2. Assess heart sounds, rhythm, PMI, and BP. Assess peripheral vascular system, particularly for edema (see Figure 9-8). Assess respiratory effort, auscultate chest for breath sounds and presence of wheezes and crackles, and percuss for possible pleural effusion.
3. Inspect for jugular vein distention and obtain hemodynamic measurements, as indicated, and note change from baseline.
4. Assess abdomen for ascites, and determine weight and change from baseline weight.
5. Note results of serum electrolyte levels and other laboratory tests.
6. Identify sleep problems and signs of depression that are often present in patients with heart failure.

Nursing Interventions

Maintaining Adequate Cardiac Output

1. Place patient at physical and emotional rest to reduce work of the heart.
   a. Provide rest in semirecumbent position or in armchair in climate-controlled environment—reduces work of the heart, increases heart reserve, reduces BP, decreases work of respiratory muscles and oxygen utilization, and improves efficiency of heart contraction; recumbency promotes diuresis by improving renal perfusion.
   b. Provide bedside commode—to reduce work of getting to bathroom and the stress of defecation.
   c. Provide for psychological rest—emotional stress produces vasoconstriction, elevates arterial pressure, and increases heart rate.
      i. Promote physical comfort with measures such as medication, pillows, reassuring presence.
      ii. Avoid loud noises, bright lights, and chaotic care environment that tend to promote anxiety and agitation.
      iii. Offer careful explanations and answers to the patient's questions.
2. Evaluate frequently for progression of left-sided heart failure. Take frequent BP readings.
   a. Watch for decreasing mean arterial pressure.
   b. Note narrowing of pulse pressure.
   c. Note alternating strong and weak pulsations (pulsus alternans).
3. Auscultate heart sounds frequently and monitor cardiac rhythm.
   a. Note presence of S_3 or S_4 gallop (S_3 gallop is a significant indicator of heart failure).
   b. Monitor for premature ventricular beats.
   c. Assess chest pain.
   d. Measure CVP or jugular venous pressure (JVP).
4. Observe for signs and symptoms of reduced peripheral tissue perfusion: cool temperature of the skin, facial pallor, poor capillary refill of nail beds.
5. Administer pharmacotherapy as directed.
   a. Monitor for adverse effects and therapeutic effect of drug therapy.

6. Monitor clinical response of patient with respect to relief of symptoms (lessening dyspnea and orthopnea, decrease in crackles, relief of peripheral edema).

CLINICAL JUDGMENT Watch for sudden unexpected hypotension, which can cause myocardial ischemia and decrease perfusion to vital organs. Take immediate measures to increase blood pressure—elevate legs and notify health care provider.

Improving Oxygenation

1. Raise head of bed 8 to 10 in (20 to 25 cm)—reduces venous return to heart and lungs; alleviates pulmonary congestion.
   a. Support lower arms with pillows—eliminates pull of patient's weight on shoulder muscles.
   b. Sit orthopneic patient on side of bed with feet supported, head and arms resting on an over-the-bed table, and lumbosacral area supported with pillows.
2. Auscultate lung fields at least every 4 hours for crackles and wheezes in dependent lung fields (fluid accumulates in areas affected by gravity).
3. Observe for increased rate of respirations (could be indicative of falling arterial pH).
4. Observe for Cheyne-Stokes respirations (may occur in older patients because of a decrease in cerebral perfusion, stimulating a neurogenic response).
5. Reposition the patient (or encourage the patient to change position) frequently—to help prevent atelectasis and pneumonia. Encourage ambulation as tolerated.
6. Encourage deep breathing exercises every 1 to 2 hours—to avoid atelectasis. The use of incentive spirometry can be beneficial.
7. Offer small, frequent feedings—to avoid excessive gastric filling and abdominal distention with subsequent elevation of diaphragm that causes decrease in lung capacity.
8. Administer oxygen, as directed.

Restoring Fluid Balance

1. Administer prescribed diuretic, as ordered.
2. Give diuretic early in the morning—nighttime diuresis disturbs sleep if patient is not catheterized. If evening dose is ordered, give by 6 pm to prevent disrupted sleep from getting up to go to the bathroom.
3. Keep input and output record—patient may lose large volume of fluid after a single dose of diuretic. Watch fluid intake. Monitor urinary output; it should be 0.5 to 1 mL/kg/h.
4. Weigh patient daily—to determine if edema is being controlled; weight loss should not exceed 1 to 2 pound (0.5 to 1 kg/day).
5. Assess for signs of hypovolemia caused by diuretic therapy—thirst; decreased urine output; orthostatic hypotension; weak, thready pulse; increased serum osmolality; and increased urine specific gravity.
6. Be alert for signs of hypokalemia, which may cause weakening of cardiac contractions and dysrhythmias. Watch for signs and symptoms of anorexia, nausea, vomiting, abdominal distention, and loss of bowel sounds due to paralytic ileus, paresthesias, muscle weakness and cramps, and confusion.
7. Monitor electrolytes frequently, and give potassium replacement therapy orally or IV, as prescribed.
8. Monitor renal function. Creatinine may rise with overdiuresis or as an indicator that more advance therapies are needed.
9. Be aware of conditions that may be worsened by diuretic therapy, including hyperuricemia, gout, volume depletion, hyponatremia, magnesium depletion, hyperglycemia, and diabetes mellitus.
10. Watch for signs of bladder distention in older male patients with prostatic hyperplasia.
11. Administer IV fluids carefully and monitor intake, including all medications being infused, to prevent fluid overload.
12. Monitor for pitting edema of lower extremities and sacral area (dependent areas based on positioning).
13. Observe for pressure injury (especially in patients with edema on bedrest). These patients may need frequent repositioning, lower extremities elevated, and possible special support surfaces (gel cushion, air-loss, or alternating pressure mattresses).
14. Administer deep venous thrombosis (DVT) prophylaxis, and maintain mechanical lower extremity compression device to prevent phlebothrombosis and PE, as directed.
15. Be alert to complaints of right upper quadrant abdominal pain, poor appetite, nausea, and abdominal distention (may indicate hepatic and visceral engorgement or paralytic ileus).
16. Monitor patient's diet. Diet may be limited in sodium—to prevent, control, or eliminate edema. Watch for outside snacks and favorite foods being brought in.
17. Monitor fluid intake closely if fluid restriction is prescribed. Less than 2 liters daily may be difficult to maintain when IV fluids are included, leading to patient nonadherence.
18. Prepare patient for short-term CRRT to remove fluid if resistant to diuresis and BP/MAP is low.

Improving Activity Tolerance

1. Assist patient to increase activities gradually. Alter or modify activities to keep within the limits of cardiac reserve.
   a. Assist patient with self-care activities early in the day (fatigue sets in as day progresses).
   b. Be alert to complaints of chest pain or discomfort during or after activities.
   c. Obtain occupational therapy consult as indicated for safe activities of daily living and energy conservation techniques.
2. Observe for symptoms and behavioral response to increased activity.
3. Monitor patient's heart rate during self-care activities. Allow heart rate to decrease to preactivity level before initiating a new activity.
   a. Note time lapse between cessation of activity and decrease in heart rate (decreased stroke volume causes immediate rise in heart rate).
   b. Document time lapse and revise patient care plan as appropriate (progressive increase in time lapse may be indicative of increased left-sided heart failure).
4. Relieve nighttime anxiety and provide for rest and sleep—patients with heart failure have a tendency to be restless at night because of cerebral hypoxia with superimposed nitrogen retention. Provide oxygen via nasal cannula as needed, and administer medications for insomnia and restlessness, as ordered.

Improving Knowledge

1. Explain the disease process; note that the term "failure" may be terrifying.
   a. Explain that the pumping action of the heart is impaired; treatment is necessary to move blood through the body to provide nutrients and oxygen and aid in the removal of waste.
   b. Explain the difference between heart failure and heart attack.

2. Provide teaching about the signs and symptoms of worsening condition or recurrence.
   a. Weigh daily (at the same time) and report a weight gain or loss of more than 2 to 3 pound (1 to 1.4 kg) in a few days.
   b. Watch for other signs of fluid retention: swelling of ankles, feet, sacrum, buttocks, abdomen; persistent cough; tiredness; loss of appetite; frequent urination at night.
3. Review medication regimen.
   a. A combination of medications are used based on ejection fraction to reduce preload and afterload, control heart rate, and prevent blood clots.
   b. IV medications will be transitioned to oral medications, which may be reduced and discontinued as condition improves, but follow-up is important to maintain control for life.

Patient Education and Health Maintenance

1. Advise patient of symptoms that need to be reported to health care provider.
   a. Weight gain of greater than 2 pounds in a day or 5 pounds in a week; weigh daily at the same time with same amount of clothing.
   b. Increased shortness of breath, inability to lie down, wheezing, increased cough.
   c. Increased swelling of feet, legs, abdomen.
2. Help patient understand all medications.
   a. Give medication information sheets, and review the indication/therapeutic benefit of each medication.
   b. Make sure the patient has a pill organizer or check-off system to show that medications have been taken at the proper time each day.
   c. Inform the patient of adverse drug effects, and point to information on how to reduce them.
   d. If the patient is taking oral potassium, advise that solution may be diluted with juice and taken after a meal to avoid stomach upset; tablets should not be crushed or chewed to prevent disruption of slow-release mechanism.
   e. Obtain history of supplement use, such as coenzyme Q10, and advise patient to discuss with health care provider to identify interactions.

CLINICAL JUDGMENT To reduce readmission for heart failure, ensure that the patient and caregiver understand how each medication works to optimize heart function and that they will be able to obtain all prescriptions; that they understand whom to notify for increase in daily weight or worsening symptoms; that salt and fluid restriction are clear; and that follow-up for lab work and office visit is arranged. Identify patients who may benefit from home health care, televisits, and other resources such as remote monitoring.

3. Review activity program instructions:
   a. Increase walking and other activities gradually, provided they do not cause fatigue and dyspnea.
   b. In general, continue at whatever activity level can be maintained without the appearance of symptoms.
   c. Avoid excesses in eating and drinking.
   d. Undertake a balanced weight reduction program until optimal weight is reached.
   e. Avoid extremes in heat and cold, which increase the work of the heart; air conditioning may be essential in a hot, humid environment.
   f. Keep *regular* appointment with health care provider or clinic.
   g. Suggest cardiac rehabilitation program if available in the area.
4. Restrict sodium as directed.
   a. Teach restricted sodium diet (less than 1,500 mg/day) and the DASH diet; see page 323.
   b. Give patient a written diet plan with lists of permitted and restricted foods.
   c. Advise patient to look at all labels for sodium/salt content per serving size. Many packaged foods may seem like 1 serving but actually contain multiple servings.
   d. Teach the patient to rinse the mouth well after using tooth cleansers and mouthwashes—some of these contain large amounts of sodium. When water softeners are used, water should be checked for salt content.
   e. Teach the patient that sodium may be contained in medications such as antacids, cough remedies, pain relievers, estrogens, and other drugs.
   f. Encourage use of salt-free flavorings, spices, herbs, and lemon juice rather than salt.
   g. Advise patients with renal disease to use salt substitutes cautiously and discuss with health care provider.
   h. Instruct patient to check for hidden sodium in foods that do not taste salty, such as bread, frozen foods, and, especially, canned foods.
5. Make sure patient sets up follow-up appointments.
6. Advise patient to stop smoking, and provide resources to help with smoking cessation.

Evaluation: Expected Outcomes

- Normal BP and heart rate.
- Respiratory rate, 16 to 20 breaths/min; oxygen saturation within normal range; ABG levels within normal limits.
- Weight decrease of 2.2 pound (1 kg) every 2 days; no pitting edema of lower extremities and sacral area.
- Completes activities of daily living with minimal shortness of breath; rests between activities.
- States recurrent symptoms to watch for and knows medications and doses.

Acute Pulmonary Edema

Acute pulmonary edema refers to the movement of excess fluid into the alveoli or interstitial spaces of the lung. "Flash" pulmonary edema is a term used to describe sudden cardiogenic alveolar pulmonary edema.

Pathophysiology and Etiology

1. The presence of fluid in the alveoli impedes gas exchange, especially oxygen movement into pulmonary capillaries (see Figure 9-9).
2. May be caused by:
   a. Heart disease—acute increase in left arterial filling pressure occurs as a result of left-sided heart failure due to conditions such as MI, aortic stenosis, severe mitral valve disease, hypertension, heart failure.
   b. Circulatory overload—transfusions and infusions.
   c. Drug hypersensitivity, allergy, poisoning.
   d. Lung injuries—smoke inhalation, shock lung, PE, or infarct.

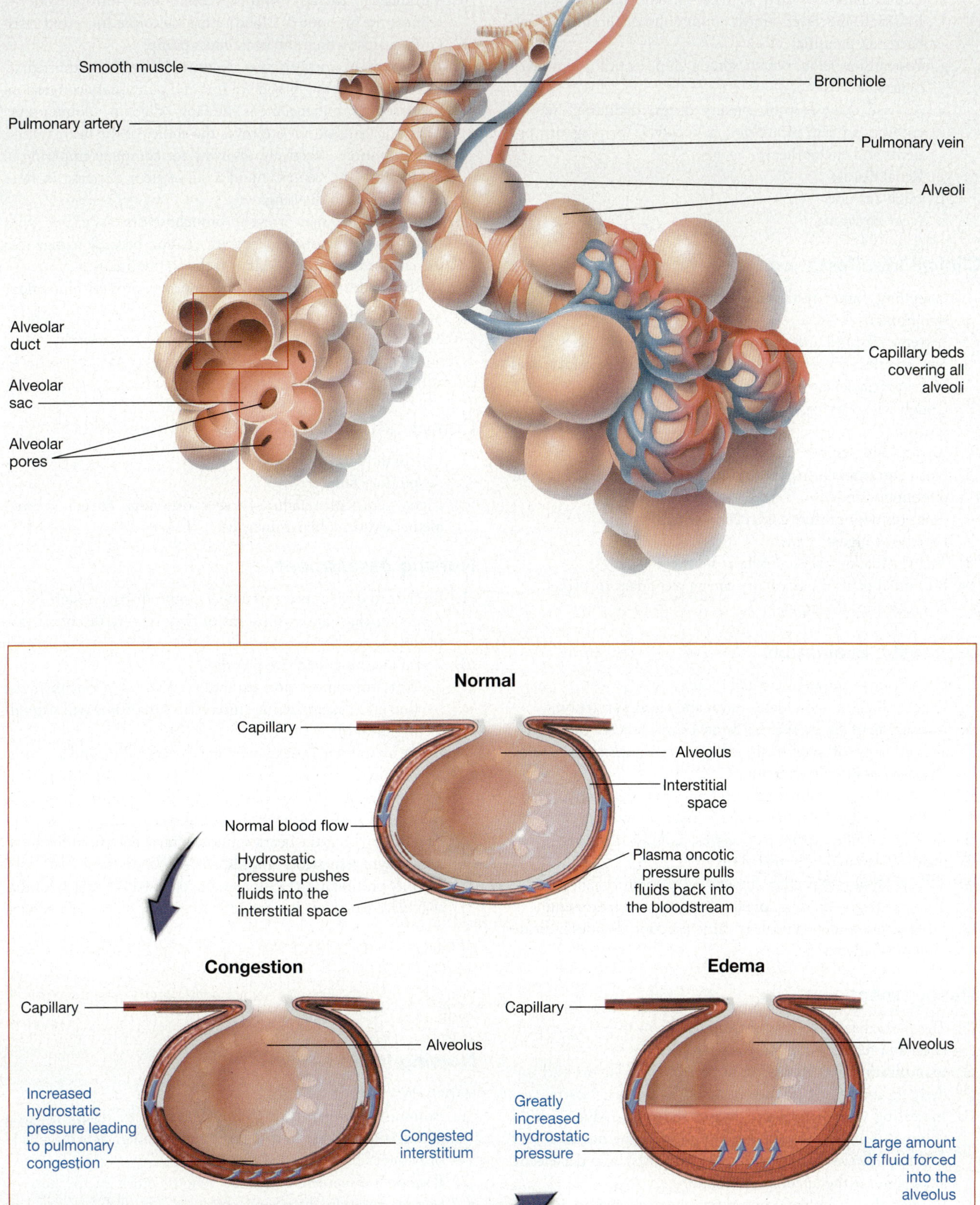

Figure 9-9. Normal alveoli and how pulmonary edema develops.

e. Central nervous system injuries—stroke, head trauma.
f. Infection and fever—most commonly, pneumonia (viral, bacterial, parasitic).
g. Postcardioversion, postanesthesia, or postcardiopulmonary bypass.
h. Adverse drug reaction—many drugs, including heroin, cocaine, aspirin, nicardipine as tocolytic for pregnant patients and chemotherapy agents.
i. Renal disease.
j. High altitude.
k. Near drowning.

Clinical Manifestations

1. Coughing and restlessness during sleep (premonitory symptoms).
2. Extreme dyspnea and orthopnea—patient usually uses accessory muscles of respiration with retraction of intercostal spaces and supraclavicular areas.
3. Cough with varying amounts of white- or pink-tinged frothy sputum.
4. Anxiety and panic.
5. Noisy breathing—inspiratory and expiratory wheezing and bubbling sounds.
6. Cyanosis with profuse cold, clammy perspiration.
7. Distended jugular veins.
8. Tachycardia, new S3 or S4 heart sound.
9. Precordial pain (if pulmonary edema secondary to MI).
10. Decreased urine output.

Diagnostic Evaluation

1. Chest x-ray—shows interstitial edema.
2. Echocardiogram—evaluates valves and ejection fraction.
3. Measurement of PCWP by Swan-Ganz catheter (differentiates etiology of pulmonary edema—cardiogenic or altered alveolar–capillary membrane).
4. Blood cultures in suspected infection—may be positive.
5. Cardiac markers in suspected MI—may be elevated.
6. BUN, creatinine, serum electrolytes, and blood counts.
7. proBNP elevated in heart failure.
8. ABG analysis—may show impending respiratory failure.
9. Thoracentesis—fluid sample for diagnosis and treatment.
10. Lung ultrasound—valuable in early detection; B-lines indicate interstitial edema.

Management

1. The immediate objective of treatment is to improve oxygenation and reduce pulmonary congestion.
2. Identification and correction of precipitating factors and underlying conditions are then necessary to prevent recurrence.
3. Increasing oxygen tension (oxygen therapy), reducing fluid volume (diuretics, vasodilators), improving the heart's ability to pump effectively (glycosides, beta agonists), and decreasing anxiety guide therapeutic interventions.
4. Oxygen therapy—high concentrations of oxygen are used to combat hypoxemia. Intubation and/or ventilatory support may be necessary to improve hypoxemia and prevent hypercarbia. Noninvasive ventilation (NIV) is the first line of intervention.
5. Morphine—reduces anxiety, promotes venous pooling of blood in the periphery, and reduces resistance against which the heart must pump.
6. Vasodilator therapy (nitroglycerin and nitroprusside)—reduces the amount of blood returning to the heart and resistance against which the heart must pump.
7. Reduction of intravascular volume (diuresis or immediate dialysis)—decreases blood volume and pulmonary congestion.
8. Contractility enhancement therapy (digoxin, dobutamine, nesiritide, milrinone) improves the ability of the heart muscle to pump more effectively, allowing for complete emptying of blood from the ventricle and a subsequent decrease in fluid backing up into the lungs.
9. Aminophylline may prevent bronchospasm associated with pulmonary congestion. Use with caution because it may also increase heart rate and induce tachydysrhythmias.
10. IABP—to decrease afterload and improve coronary blood flow.

DRUG ALERT Use extreme caution in administering nitroglycerin to patients with aortic stenosis who are preload dependent. May cause drop in blood pressure.

Complications

1. Dysrhythmias.
2. Respiratory failure.
3. Right ventricular failure—lower extremity edema, ascites, pleural effusion, hepatomegaly.

Nursing Assessment

1. Be alert to development of a new nonproductive cough.
2. Assess for signs and symptoms of hypoxia—restlessness, confusion, headache.
3. Auscultate lung fields frequently.
   a. Note inspiratory and expiratory wheezes, rhonchi, moist fine crackles appearing initially in lung bases and extending upward.
   b. Be aware that patients who have heart failure and are compensated may not present with crackles. In this patient population, this is a late sign. Their symptoms may be shortness of breath without crackles.
4. Auscultate for extra heart sounds, which may be difficult to hear due to respiratory sounds.
5. Identify precipitating factors, such as elevated BP or tachycardia, that place patient at risk for development of pulmonary edema.

CLINICAL JUDGMENT Acute pulmonary edema is a true medical emergency; it is a life-threatening condition. Act promptly to assess patient and notify health care provider of findings.

Nursing Interventions

Improving Oxygenation

1. Administer oxygen in high concentration to relieve hypoxia and dyspnea and to keep oxygen saturation greater than 94% or patient's baseline.
2. Position the patient to reduce venous return to the heart—upright position, head and shoulders up, and feet and legs hanging down to favor pooling of blood in dependent portions of body by gravitational forces and to decrease venous return.
3. Give morphine in small, titrated intermittent doses (IV) as directed.
   a. Morphine is usually not given if pulmonary edema is caused by stroke or occurs with chronic pulmonary disease or cardiogenic shock.

b. Watch for excessive respiratory depression.
c. Monitor BP because morphine may intensify hypotension.
d. Have morphine antagonist available—naloxone.

4. Give diuretics IV, or monitor diuresis during dialysis.
   a. Monitor urine output closely; some patients have a strong response to diuretics.
   b. Watch for falling BP, increasing heart rate, and decreasing urinary output—indications that the total circulation is not tolerating diuresis and that hypovolemia may develop.
   c. Check electrolyte levels because potassium loss may be significant.
   d. Watch for signs of urinary obstruction in males with prostatic hyperplasia.
5. Administer vasodilator if patient fails to respond to therapy, and monitor BP, PAP, and CO as indicated.
6. Assist with insertion of IABP, if needed, and monitor patient according to facility's protocol.
7. Administer aminophylline, if ordered.
   a. Monitor blood levels of drug.
   b. Evaluate for adverse effects of drug—ventricular dysrhythmias, hypotension, headache.
8. Administer cardiac glycosides as ordered.
9. Assist with cardioversion, if indicated (pulmonary edema may precipitate tachycardias).
10. Give appropriate drugs for severe, sustained hypertension.
11. Continually evaluate the patient's response to therapy. Reevaluate lung fields and cardiac assessment, and monitor urine output and laboratory values.

Decreasing Anxiety

1. Stay with patient and display a confident attitude—the presence of another person is therapeutic because the acute anxiety of the patient may tend to intensify the severity of patient's condition. (Arterial vasoconstriction diminishes as anxiety is relieved.)
2. Explain to patient in a calm manner all therapies administered and the reason for their use. Explain to patient the importance of wearing oxygen mask. Assure patient that mask will not increase sensation of suffocation.
3. Inform patient and family of progress toward resolution of pulmonary edema.
4. Allow time for patient and family to voice concerns and fears.

Patient Education and Health Maintenance

During convalescence, instruct patient as follows to prevent recurrence of pulmonary edema:

1. Remind patient of early symptoms before onset of acute pulmonary edema; these should be reported promptly.
2. If coughing develops (a wet cough), sit with legs dangling over side of bed.
3. See "Patient Education, Heart Failure," page 276.

Evaluation: Expected Outcomes

- Unlabored respirations at 12 to 20 breaths/min, lungs clear on auscultation, pulse oximetry greater than 94%.
- Appears calm and rests comfortably.

Acquired Valvular Disease of the Heart

EVIDENCE BASE Nishimura, R. A., Otto, C. M., Bonow, R. O., Carabello, B. A., Erwin, J. P., 3rd, Fleisher, L. A., Jneid, H., Mack, M. J., McLeod, C. J., O'Gara, P. T., Rigolin, V. H., Sundt, T. M., 3rd, & Thompson, A. (2017). 2017 AHA/ACC focused update of the 2014 AHA/ACC guideline for the management of patients with valvular heart disease: Executive summary: A report of the American College of Cardiology/American Heart Association Task Force on Practice Guidelines. *Circulation, 135*(25), e1159–e1195. https://doi.org/10.1161/CIR.0000000000000503

The function of normal heart valves is to maintain the forward flow of blood from the atria to the ventricles and from the ventricles to the great vessels.

Valvular damage may interfere with valvular function by stenosis (obstruction) or by impaired closure that allows backward leakage of blood (valvular insufficiency, regurgitation, or incompetence).

Pathophysiology and Etiology

Mitral Stenosis

1. Mitral stenosis is the progressive thickening and contracture of valve cusps with narrowing of the orifice and progressive obstruction to blood flow. Rheumatic fever is the most common cause of mitral stenosis in adults. Calcium deposit around the valves is rare with mitral stenosis. In children, the cause may be congenital.
2. Acute rheumatic valvulitis has "glued" the mitral valve flaps (commissures) together, thus shortening the chordae tendineae, so that the flap edges are pulled down, greatly narrowing the mitral orifice.
3. The left atrium has difficulty emptying itself through the narrow orifice into the left ventricle; therefore, it dilates and hypertrophies. Pulmonary circulation becomes congested.
4. As a result of the abnormally high PAP that must be maintained, the right ventricle is subjected to a pressure overload and may eventually fail.

Mitral Insufficiency

1. Mitral insufficiency (regurgitation or incompetence) is incomplete closure of the mitral valve during systole, allowing blood to flow back into the left atrium.
2. Left atrial pressures increase, reflected by increases in PAP and PCWP.
3. LVH may develop due to inefficient emptying.
4. May be due to myxomatous (connective tissue) degeneration, which causes stretching of leaflets and chordae tendineae; chronic rheumatic heart disease, ischemic heart disease, CAD, and IE; may also result due to medications and penetrating and nonpenetrating trauma.

Aortic Stenosis

1. Aortic stenosis is a narrowing of the orifice between the left ventricle and the aorta.
2. The obstruction to the aortic outflow places a pressure load on the left ventricle that results in hypertrophy and failure.
3. Left atrial pressure increases.
4. Pulmonary vascular pressure increases, which may eventually lead to right-sided heart failure.
5. May be caused by congenital anomalies (bicuspid aortic valve), calcification, or acute rheumatic fever.
6. Aortic valve sclerosis (thickening) is an important finding because it can lead to aortic stenosis and increased cardiovascular risk.

Aortic Insufficiency

1. Abnormalities of aortic valve or aortic root prevent valve flaps from completely sealing the aortic orifice during diastole and thus permit backflow of blood from the aorta into the left ventricle.

2. The left ventricle increases the force of contraction to maintain an adequate CO, usually resulting in hypertrophy.
3. The low aortic diastolic pressures result in decreased coronary artery perfusion.
4. May be caused by rheumatic or IE, congenital malformation, aortic root dilation, Marfan syndrome, Ehlers-Danlos syndrome, Reiter syndrome, hypertension, systemic lupus erythematosus, or diseases that cause dilation or tearing of the ascending aorta (syphilitic disease, rheumatoid spondylitis, dissecting aneurysm).

Tricuspid Stenosis

1. Tricuspid stenosis is restriction or narrowing of the tricuspid valve orifice because of commissural fusion and fibrosis.
2. Usually follows rheumatic fever and is commonly associated with diseases of the mitral valve. Could be congenital in origin.

Tricuspid Insufficiency

1. Tricuspid insufficiency (regurgitation) allows the regurgitation of blood from the right ventricle into the right atrium during ventricular systole.
2. Common causes include dilation of right ventricle, rheumatic fever, congenital anomalies, left-sided heart disease, and pulmonary hypertension.

Clinical Manifestations

1. Fatigue, weakness.
2. Dyspnea, cough, orthopnea, nocturnal dyspnea.
3. Characteristic murmur (see "Nursing Assessment").
4. Dysrhythmias, palpitations.
5. Hemoptysis (from pulmonary hypertension) and hoarseness (from compression of left recurrent laryngeal nerve by dilated left atrium) in mitral stenosis.
6. Low BP, dizziness, syncope, angina, and symptoms of heart failure in aortic stenosis.
7. Arterial pulsations visible and palpable over the precordium and visible in the neck, widened pulse pressure, and water-hammer (Corrigan) pulse (pulse strikes palpating finger with a quick, sharp stroke and then suddenly collapses) in aortic insufficiency.
8. Symptoms of right-sided heart failure—edema, ascites, hepatomegaly—in tricuspid stenosis and insufficiency.

Diagnostic Evaluation

1. ECG may show dysrhythmias.
2. Echocardiography (including 3D) may show abnormalities of valve structure and function and chamber size and thickness.
3. Chest x-ray may show cardiomegaly and pulmonary vascular congestion.
4. Cardiac catheterization and angiocardiography confirm diagnosis and determine severity.
5. Cardiac MRI provides more information and confirms diagnosis.
6. Exercise testing for patients with severe valvular disease to determine prognosis.

Management

Medical Therapy

1. Antibiotic prophylaxis for endocarditis before invasive procedures—indicated in most cases; see page 258.
2. Treatment of heart failure—diuretics, sodium restriction, vasodilators, cardiac glycosides, as indicated.

Surgical Intervention

See page 230 for care of the patient undergoing heart surgery.

1. For mitral stenosis:
   a. Closed mitral valvotomy—introduction of a dilator through the mitral valve to split its commissures.
   b. Open mitral valvotomy—direct incision of the commissures.
   c. Mitral valve replacement.
   d. Balloon valvuloplasty—a balloon-tipped catheter is percutaneously inserted, threaded to the affected valve, and positioned across the narrowed orifice. The balloon is inflated and deflated, causing a "cracking" of the calcified commissures and enlargement of the valve orifice.
2. For mitral insufficiency—mitral valve replacement or annuloplasty (retailoring of the valve ring). Various percutaneous mitral valve repair techniques are currently being evaluated.
   a. MitraClip—a small implanted clip is introduced through the femoral artery catheter and attached to the mitral valve to help it close more completely.
   b. Transcatheter mitral valve in valve replacement (TMVR)—compressed prosthetic valve is introduced through femoral artery via catheter and placed inside diseased mitral valve.
3. For aortic stenosis or insufficiency:
   a. Replacement of aortic valve with prosthetic (mechanical) or tissue (bioprosthetic) valves.
   b. Complications include risk of thromboembolism with mechanical valve, requiring long-term anticoagulation with risk of bleeding; and degeneration of bioprosthetic valve, limiting its durability.
   c. Balloon valvuloplasty may be done for aortic stenosis (see previously).
   d. Transcatheter aortic valve implantation or replacement (TAVR)—a less invasive procedure, where a bioprosthetic valve is used. Mostly for patients with severe symptomatic AS aged 75 years or older with surgical risk but expected to survive.
4. For tricuspid stenosis or insufficiency—valvuloplasty or replacement may be done at the time of surgical intervention for associated rheumatic mitral or aortic disease.
5. Percutaneous pulmonary valve implantation (PPVI)—for patients with pulmonic valve and right ventricular outflow tract defects.

Complications

1. Left-sided heart failure.
2. Possible, right-sided heart failure.
3. Dysrhythmias.
4. Pulmonary edema.

Nursing Assessment

Mitral Stenosis

1. Auscultate for accentuated first heart sound, usually accompanied by an "opening snap" (because of sudden tensing of valve leaflets) at the apex with diaphragm of stethoscope.
2. Place the patient in left lateral recumbent position. With bell of stethoscope at the apex, auscultate for a low-pitched diastolic murmur (rumbling murmur). Note duration of murmur (long duration is indicative of significant stenosis).

Mitral Insufficiency

1. Auscultate for diminished first heart sound.

2. Auscultate for systolic murmur (prominent finding), commencing immediately after first heart sound at apex, and note radiation of sound to the axilla and left intrascapular area.
3. Mild insufficiency may produce a pansystolic murmur (little connection between severity of mitral insufficiency and intensity of murmur auscultated).

Aortic Stenosis

1. Auscultate for prominent fourth heart sound and possible paradoxical splitting of second heart sound (suggestive of associated left ventricular dysfunction). First heart sound is normal.
2. Auscultate for a midsystolic murmur at the base of the heart (right upper sternal border) and at the apex of the heart. Note harsh and rasping quality at the base of the heart and a higher pitch at the apex of the heart.
3. There may be a palpable thrill.

Aortic Insufficiency

1. Auscultate for soft first heart sound.
2. Place the patient in sitting position, leaning forward.
3. Place diaphragm of stethoscope along left sternal border at the third and fourth intercostal space and then along the right sternal border. Auscultate for a high-pitched decrescendo diastolic murmur. To increase audibility of murmur, ask the patient to hold breath at end of deep expiration. Reauscultate for murmur.

Tricuspid Stenosis

1. Auscultate for a rumbling or blowing middiastolic murmur at the left sternal border (increases with inspiration).

Tricuspid Insufficiency

1. Auscultate for a third heart sound (may be accentuated by inspiration).
2. Auscultate for a pansystolic murmur in the parasternal region at the fourth intercostal space. Murmur is usually high-pitched.

Nursing Interventions

Maintaining Adequate Cardiac Output

1. Assess vital signs frequently and for change in existing murmur or new murmur.
2. Assess for signs of left- or right-sided heart failure; see page 271.
3. Assess for pulmonary edema.
4. Monitor and treat dysrhythmias, as ordered.
5. Prepare the patient for surgical intervention (see page 231).

Improving Tolerance

1. Maintain bedrest while symptoms of heart failure are present.
2. Allow patient to rest between interventions.
3. Begin activities gradually (e.g., chair sitting for brief periods).
4. Assist with activities of daily living for patient to reserve strength for ambulation.

Strengthening Coping Abilities

1. Instruct the patient about specific valvular dysfunction, possible etiology, and therapies implemented to relieve symptoms.
   a. Include family members in discussions with the patient.
   b. Stress the importance of adapting lifestyle to cope with illness.
2. Discuss with patient their questions and fears about surgical intervention, if applicable.
3. Assess the patient's use of appropriate coping mechanisms.
4. Refer the patient to appropriate counseling services, if indicated (vocational, social work, cardiac rehabilitation, substance use disorder).

Patient Education and Health Maintenance

1. Review activity restriction and schedule with patient and family.
2. Instruct patient to report signs of impending or worsening heart failure—dyspnea, cough, increased fatigue, ankle swelling.
3. Review sodium and fluid restrictions.
4. Review medications—purpose, action, schedule, and adverse effects.
5. See "Patient Education, Heart Failure," page 276; "Infective Endocarditis," page 258; and "Rheumatic Endocarditis," page 262.

Evaluation: Expected Outcomes

- BP and heart rate within normal limits.
- Tolerates chair sitting for 15 minutes every 2 hours.
- Discusses ways to cope with lifestyle and activity changes.

Cardiac Dysrhythmias

Cardiac dysrhythmias are disturbances in regular heart rate and/or rhythm because of change in electrical conduction or automaticity. Dysrhythmias may arise from the sinoatrial (SA) node (sinus bradycardia or tachycardia) or anywhere within the atria or ventricles (known as ectopy or ectopic beats). Some may be benign and asymptomatic, whereas other dysrhythmias are life-threatening.

Dysrhythmias may be detected by change in pulse, abnormality on auscultation of heart rate, or ECG abnormality. Continuous cardiac monitoring is indicated for potentially life-threatening dysrhythmias.

Sinus Tachycardia

See Figure 9-10.

Etiology

1. Sympathetic nerve fibers, which act to speed up excitation of the SA node, are stimulated by underlying causes, such as anxiety, exercise, fever, shock, drugs, altered metabolic states (such as hyperthyroidism), or electrolyte disturbances.
2. There is recent increased prevalence associated with long COVID-19 infection.
3. The wave of impulse is transmitted through the normal conduction pathways; the rate of sinus stimulation is simply greater than normal (rate exceeds 100 beats/min).

Analysis

Rate: 100 to 150 beats/min.
Rhythm: R–R intervals are regular.
P wave: present for each QRS complex, normal configuration, and each P wave is identical or may be buried in previous T wave.
PR interval: falls between 0.12 and 0.20, or 0.16 second. P wave may be hidden in preceding T wave in rapid rates.
QRS complex: normal in appearance; one follows each P wave.
QRS interval: less than 0.11 seconds.
T wave: follows each QRS complex and is positively conducted.
QT interval: less than 0.48 seconds. This is usually corrected for heart rate and sex assigned at birth.

Management

1. Treatment is directed toward elimination of the cause rather than the dysrhythmia. Sometimes, this is a compensatory mechanism for decreased CO; thus, correction is not needed.

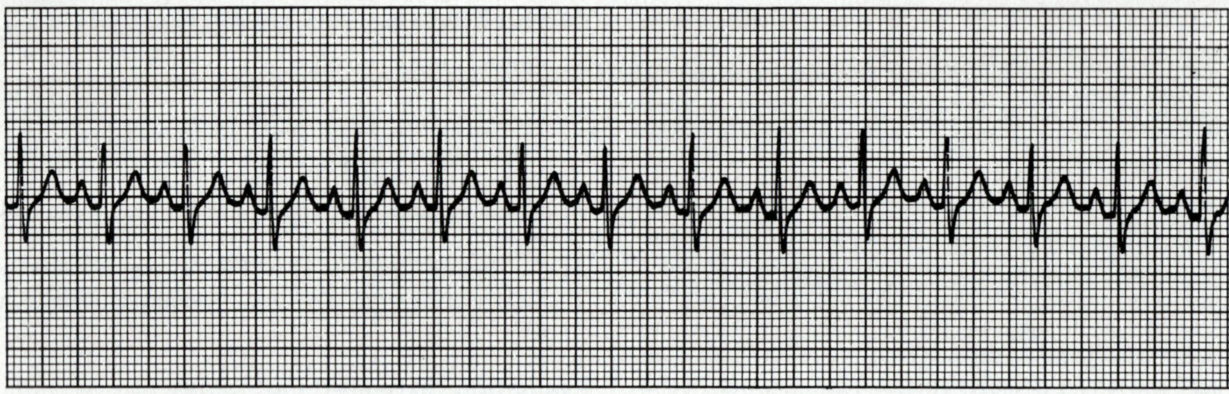

Figure 9-10. Sinus tachycardia.

2. Urgency is dependent on the effect of rapid heart rate on coronary artery filling time to prevent cardiac ischemia.
3. Administration of oxygen and normal saline solution should be considered as initial treatment.

Sinus Bradycardia

See Figure 9-11.

Etiology

1. The parasympathetic fibers (vagal tone) are stimulated and cause the sinus node to slow.
2. Underlying causes:
   a. Many drugs, including anesthesia.
   b. Altered metabolic states such as hypothyroidism.
   c. The process of aging, which causes increasing fibrotic tissue and scarring of the SA node.
   d. Certain cardiac diseases such as acute MI (especially inferior wall MI).
   e. Genetic mutations related to SA node dysfunction, such as Brugada syndrome.
3. The wave of impulse is transmitted through the normal conduction pathways; the rate of sinus stimulation is simply less than normal (less than 60 beats/min).

Analysis

Rate: less than 60 beats/min.
Rhythm: R–R interval is regular.
P wave: present for each QRS complex, normal configuration, and each P wave is identical.
PR interval: falls between 0.12 and 0.18 second.
QRS complex: normal in appearance; one follows each P wave.
QRS interval: 0.04 to 0.11 second.
T wave: follows each QRS and is positively conducted.

Management

1. The urgency of treatment depends on the effect of the slow rate on maintenance of CO.
2. Atropine 0.5 mg IV push blocks vagal stimulation to the SA node and therefore accelerates heart rate. Dopamine and epinephrine are alternatives if atropine is ineffective.
3. If bradycardia persists, a pacemaker may be required.
4. Sinus bradycardia is common in athletic individuals. Asymptomatic and hemodynamically stable SB needs no treatment.

Premature Atrial Contraction

See Figure 9-12.

Etiology

1. May occur in the healthy heart, where they are idiopathic and benign.
2. In the diseased heart, premature atrial contractions (PACs) may represent ischemia and a resultant irritability in the atria. They may increase in frequency and be the precursor of more serious dysrhythmias.
3. May be caused by electrolyte abnormalities, hypoxia, MI, heart failure, and acid–base disturbances.
4. The wave of impulse of the PAC originates within the atria and outside the sinus node. Because the impulse originates within the atria, the P wave will be present, but it will be different in appearance as compared with those beats originating within the sinus node. The impulse traverses the remainder of the conduction system in a normal pattern; thus, the QRS complex is identical in configuration to the normal sinus beats.

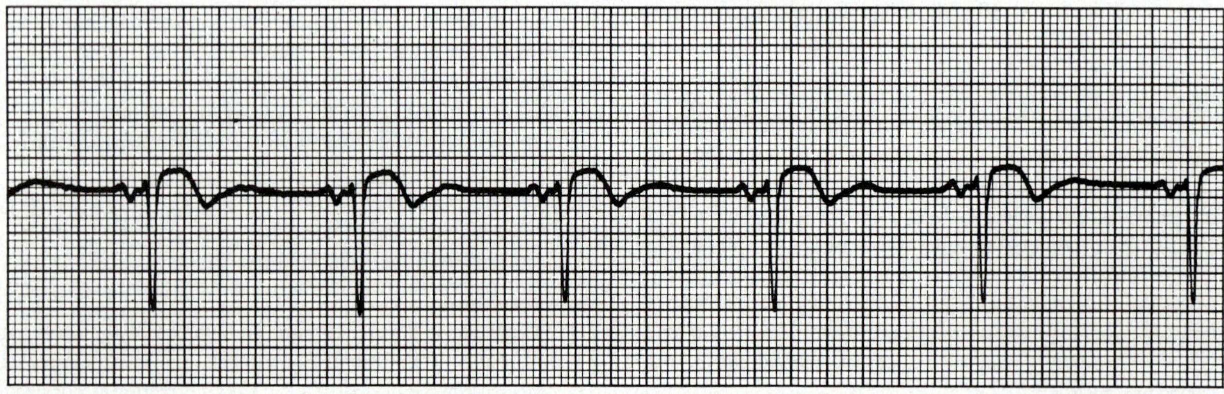

Figure 9-11. Sinus bradycardia.

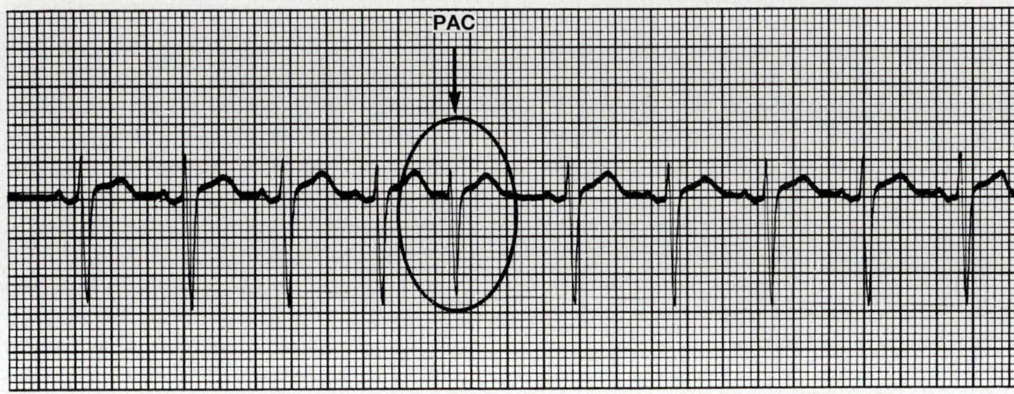

Figure 9-12. Normal sinus rhythm with premature atrial contraction.

Analysis

Rate: may be slow or fast.

Rhythm: will be irregular; caused by the early occurrence of the PAC.

P wave: will be present for each normal QRS complex; the P wave of the premature contraction will be distorted in shape.

PR interval: may be normal but can also be shortened, depending on where in the atria the impulse originated. (The closer the site of atrial impulse formation to the atrioventricular [AV] node, the shorter the PR interval will be.)

QRS complex: within normal limits because all conduction below the atria is normal.

T wave: normally conducted.

Management

1. Generally requires no treatment if laboratory values are normal.
2. PACs should be monitored for increasing frequency.

Paroxysmal Atrial Tachycardia

See Figure 9-13.

Etiology

1. Causes include:
   a. Syndromes of accelerated pathways (e.g., Wolff-Parkinson-White syndrome).
   b. Syndrome of mitral valve prolapse.
   c. Ischemic CAD.
   d. Excessive use of alcohol, cigarettes, caffeine.
   e. Drugs—digoxin is a frequent cause.
2. An ectopic atrial focus generates the rhythm of the heart and is stimulated at a very rapid rate; the impulse is conducted normally through the conduction system, so the QRS complex usually appears within normal limits.
3. The rate is often so rapid that P waves are not obvious but may be "buried" in the preceding T wave.

Analysis

Rate: between 150 and 250 beats/min.

Rhythm: regular.

P wave: present before each QRS complex; however, the faster the rate, the more difficult it becomes to visualize P waves. (The P waves can frequently be measured with calipers by observing the varying configuration of the preceding T waves.)

PR interval: usually not measurable.

QRS complex: will appear normal in configuration and within 0.06 to 0.10 second.

T wave: will be distorted in appearance as a result of P waves being buried in them.

Management

1. Treatment is directed first to slowing the rate and, second, to reverting the dysrhythmia to a normal sinus rhythm.
2. Reducing the rate may be accomplished by having the patient perform a Valsalva maneuver. This stimulates the vagus nerve to slow the heart.
   a. A Valsalva maneuver may be done by having the patient gag or "bear down" as though attempting to have a bowel movement.
   b. The health care provider may choose to perform carotid massage.

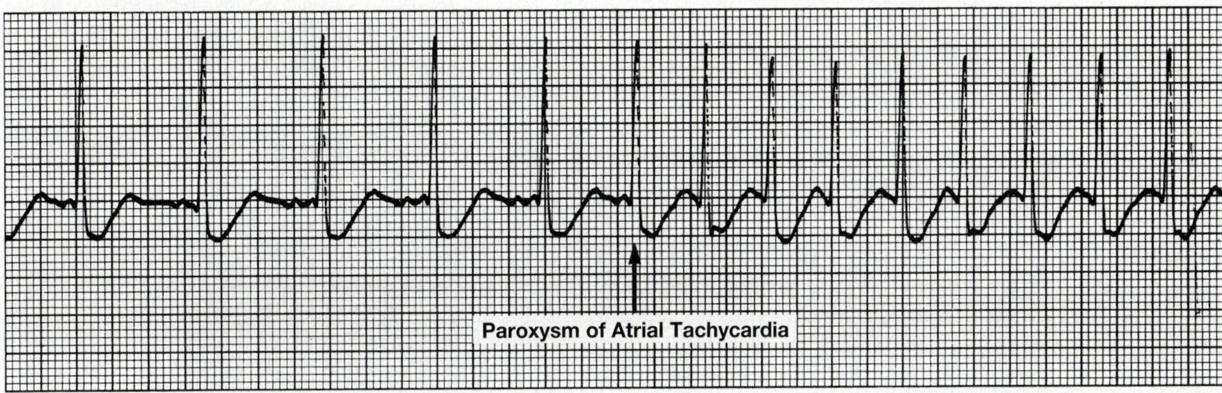

Figure 9-13. Paroxysmal atrial tachycardia.

3. Adenosine is the drug of choice for paroxysmal atrial tachycardia associated with hypotension, chest pain, or shortness of breath.
   a. The initial dose is 6 mg rapid IV push, followed by a fast normal saline flush. If there is no response in 1 to 2 minutes, a second and third bolus of 12 mg may be given, each followed by fast normal saline flushes.
   b. Has a very short half-life and is therefore eliminated quickly.
4. IV beta-adrenergic blockers, such as esmolol, may be used.
5. Calcium channel blockers (e.g., verapamil) are effective in reverting this dysrhythmia. Beware of hypotension, however, especially in the volume-depleted patient.
6. If drug therapy is ineffective, elective cardioversion can be used.

Atrial Flutter

See Figure 9-14.

Etiology

1. Occurs with atrial stretching or enlargement (as in AV valvular disease), MI, and heart failure.
2. An ectopic atrial focus captures the rhythm in atrial flutter and fires at an extremely rapid rate (200 to 400 beats/min) with regularity.
3. Conduction of the impulse through the conduction system is normal; thus, the QRS complex is unaffected.
4. An important feature of this dysrhythmia is that the AV node sets up a therapeutic block, which disallows some impulse transmission.
   a. This can produce a varying block or a fixed block (i.e., sometimes, the AV node will transmit every second flutter wave, producing a 2:1 block, or the rhythm can be 3:1 or 4:1).
   b. If the AV node conducted 1:1, then the outcome would be a ventricular rate of about 300 beats/min. The patient would rapidly deteriorate.

Analysis

Rate: atrial rate between 250 and 400 beats/min; ventricular rate will depend on degree of block.

Rhythm: regular or irregular, depending on kind of block (e.g., 2:1, 3:1, or a combination).

P wave: not present; instead, it is replaced by a saw-toothed pattern that is produced by the rapid. firing of the atrial focus. These waves are also referred to as "F" waves.

PR interval: not measurable.

QRS complex: normal configuration and normal conduction time.

T wave: present but may be obscured by flutter waves.

Management

1. The urgency of treatment depends on the ventricular response rate and resultant symptoms. Too rapid or too slow a rate will decrease CO.
2. A calcium channel blocker, such as diltiazem, may be used to slow AV nodal conduction. Use with caution in the patient with heart failure, hypotension, or concomitant beta-adrenergic blocker therapy.
3. Digoxin may be used.
4. An IV beta-adrenergic blocker, such as esmolol, may also be used.
5. If drug therapy is unsuccessful, atrial flutter will typically respond to cardioversion. Small doses of biphasic electrical current (50 to 100 joules) are usually successful.
6. Electrophysiologic studies and subsequent ablation therapy are highly effective because the ectopic focus is usually readily identified.

Atrial Fibrillation

See Figure 9-15.

Etiology

1. Fibrotic changes associated with the aging process, acute MI, valvular diseases, and digoxin preparations may cause atrial fibrillation.
2. Fluid shifts in the body (i.e., after hemodialysis or surgery).
3. Multiple atrial foci fire impulses at rapid and disorganized rates.
4. The atria are not depolarized effectively; thus, there are no well-formed P waves.
5. Instead, the baseline between QRS complexes is filled with a "wiggly" line that is described as fine or coarse.
6. If the atrial rate is rapid enough, the line will appear almost flat. The atria are said to be firing at rates of between 300 and 500 times per minute.
7. The conduction of a QRS complex is so random that the rhythm is extremely irregular.
8. Atrial fibrillation may be described as controlled if the ventricular response is 100 beats/min or less; the dysrhythmia is uncontrolled if the rate is above 100 beats/min.

Analysis

Rate: atrial fibrillation is usually immeasurable because fibrillatory waves replace P waves; ventricular rate may vary from bradycardia to tachycardia.

Rhythm: classically described as an "irregular irregularity."

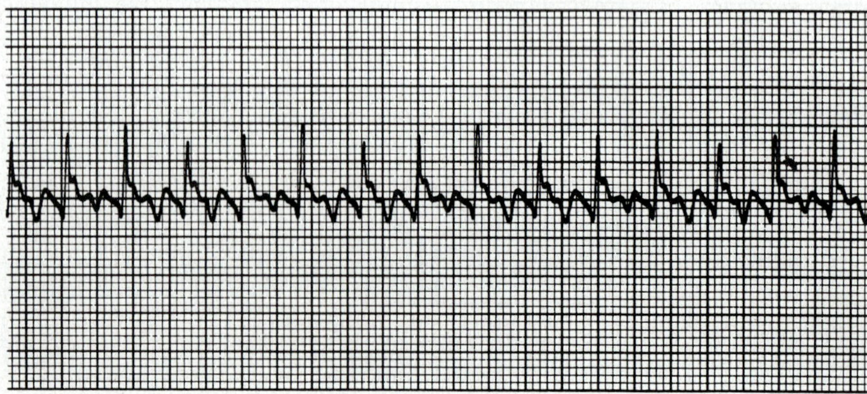

Figure 9-14. Atrial flutter.

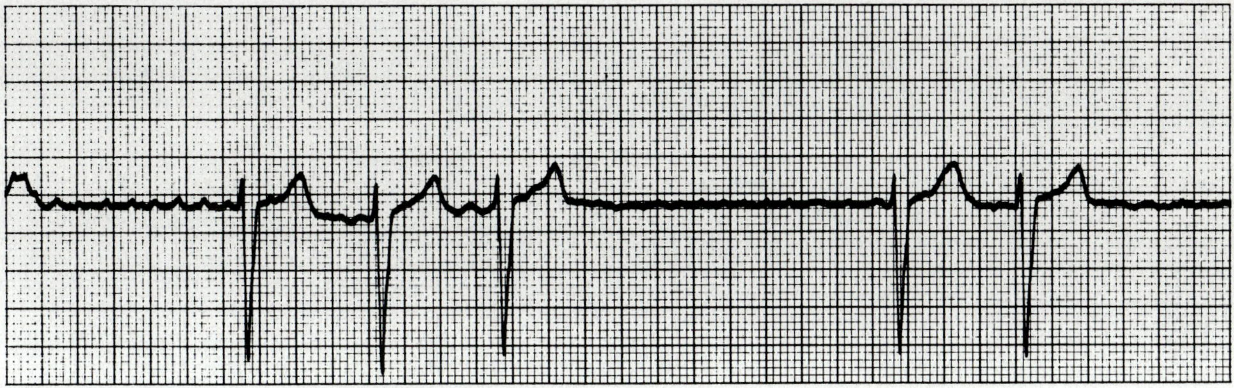

Figure 9-15. Atrial fibrillation with slow ventricular response (controlled).

P wave: replaced by fibrillatory waves, sometimes called "little f" waves.
PR interval: not measurable.
QRS complex: a normally conducted complex.
T wave: normally conducted.

Management

1. Controlled atrial fibrillation of long-standing duration requires no treatment as long as the patient is experiencing no untoward effects. Most cardiologists agree that reversion of long-standing atrial fibrillation is hazardous because of the potential for a thrombus to be dislodged from the atria at the time of reversion.
2. Goal is rate control. Uncontrolled atrial fibrillation (ventricular responses of 100 beats/min or greater) is treated with beta-adrenergic blocker or calcium channel blockers to control rate at rest and activity. Amiodarone may be added as antiarrhythmic. If the atrial fibrillation is of recent onset, the cardiologist may choose to revert the rhythm to a sinus rhythm.
3. Catheter ablation aims to isolate the signals from the pulmonary vein.
4. Cardioversion (electrical) for recent-onset atrial fibrillation may be required, starting with low amounts of biphasic electrical current (100 to 200 joules). Chemical cardioversion is accomplished with the drugs tikosyn or ibutilide.
5. Chronic anticoagulation therapy may be warranted to prevent microemboli. If anticoagulation cannot be tolerated, left atrial appendage (LAA) closure device may be implanted.

DRUG ALERT Digoxin is a second-line drug for rate because it only controls rate at rest.

Premature Ventricular Contraction

See Figure 9-16.

Etiology

1. May be caused by acute MI, other forms of heart disease, pulmonary diseases, electrolyte disturbances, metabolic instability, and substance use disorder.
2. The wave of impulse originates from an ectopic focus (foci) within the ventricles at a rate faster than the next normally occurring beat.
3. Because the normal conduction pathway is bypassed, the configuration of the premature ventricular contraction (PVC) is wider than normal and is distorted in appearance. PVCs may occur in regular sequence with normal rhythm—every other beat (bigeminy), every third beat (trigeminy), and so forth (see Figure 9-17).

Analysis

Rate: may be slow or fast.
Rhythm: will be irregular because of the premature firing of the ventricular ectopic focus.
P wave: will be absent because the impulse originates in the ventricle, bypassing the atria and AV node.
PR interval: not measurable.
QRS complex: will be widened greater than 0.12 second, bizarre in appearance when compared with normal QRS complex.

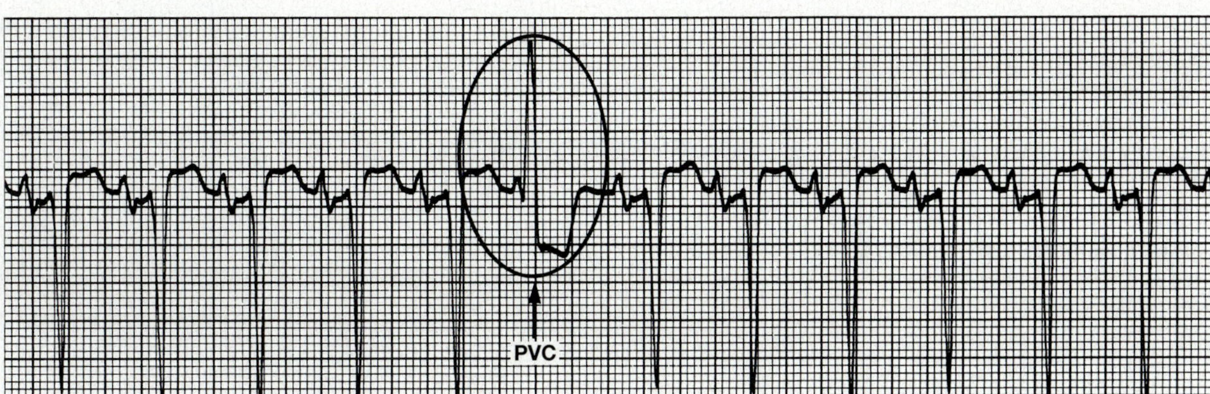

Figure 9-16. Normal sinus rhythm with premature ventricular contraction.

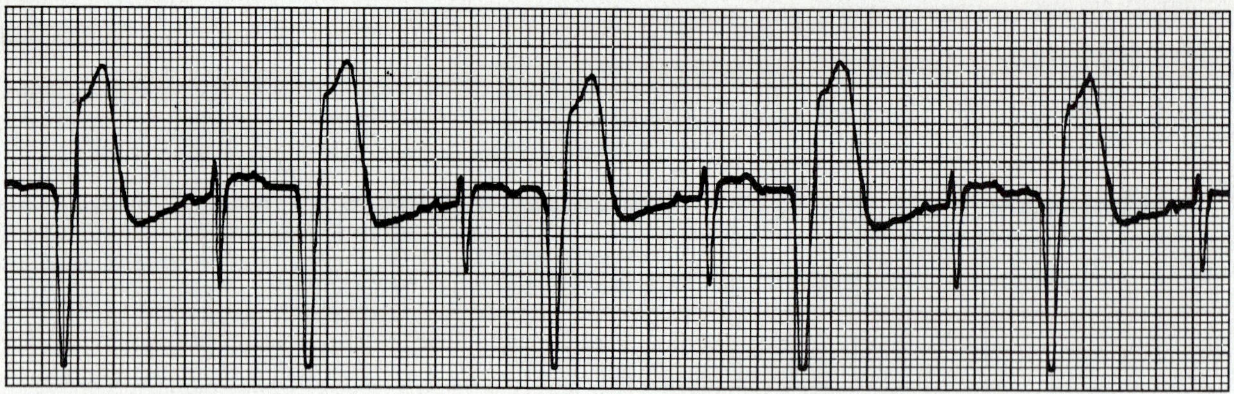

Figure 9-17. Ventricular bigeminy.

(The QRS of a PVC is commonly referred to as having a "sore thumb" appearance.)

T wave: the T wave of the PVC is usually deflected opposite to the QRS.

Management

1. PVCs are usually the precursors of more serious ventricular dysrhythmias. The following conditions involving PVCs require prompt and vigorous treatment, especially if the patient is symptomatic or unstable:
   a. PVCs occurring at a rate exceeding six per minute.
   b. Occurring as two or more consecutively.
   c. PVCs falling on the peak or down slope of the T wave (period of vulnerability, Ron T phenomenon).
   d. Are of varying configurations, indicating a multiplicity of foci.
2. Historically, the standard treatment for PVCs has been lidocaine. Today, however, amiodarone IV is the preferred method because of lidocaine's risk for toxicity.
   a. Can be given by bolus of 150 mg IV over 10 minutes.
   b. IV infusion consists of a loading dose of 1 mg/min for 6 hours, followed by a maintenance rate of 0.5 mg/min for 18 hours.
   c. After IV load, patient may require oral dosing.
3. Lidocaine toxicities include confusion and slurred speech. It should be used with caution in older adults and in those with liver disease.
4. Amiodarone toxicities include pulmonary fibrotic changes, hypothyroidism, and liver dysfunction.
5. If ventricular premature beats occur in conjunction with a bradydysrhythmia, atropine may be chosen to accelerate the heart rate and eliminate ectopic beats.
6. Atropine should be used with caution with acute MI. The injured myocardium may not be able to tolerate the accelerated rate.
7. Electrolyte infusions may also be needed to treat PVCs. Magnesium sulfate may be used, especially in patients with acute MI. It may be given as 1 g IV over 1 hour or according to facility policy. Potassium infusions can be given at 10 mmol/h and should be diluted accordingly to route of IV administration.

DRUG ALERT Be alert to the development of confusion, slurring of speech, and diminished mentation because lidocaine toxicity affects the central nervous system. Should these symptoms appear, slowing the lidocaine may cause them to abate.

8. Electrophysiology studies aim to isolate and eliminate the foci of PVCs.

Ventricular Tachycardia

See Figure 9-18.

Etiology

1. Occurs with:
   a. Acute MI, cardiomyopathy.
   b. Syndromes of accelerated rhythm that deteriorate (e.g., Wolff-Parkinson-White syndrome).
   c. Metabolic acidosis, especially lactic acidosis.
   d. Electrolyte disturbance.
   e. Toxicity to certain drugs, such as digoxin or isoproterenol.
2. A life-threatening dysrhythmia that originates from an irritable focus within the ventricle (due to lack of perfusion) at a

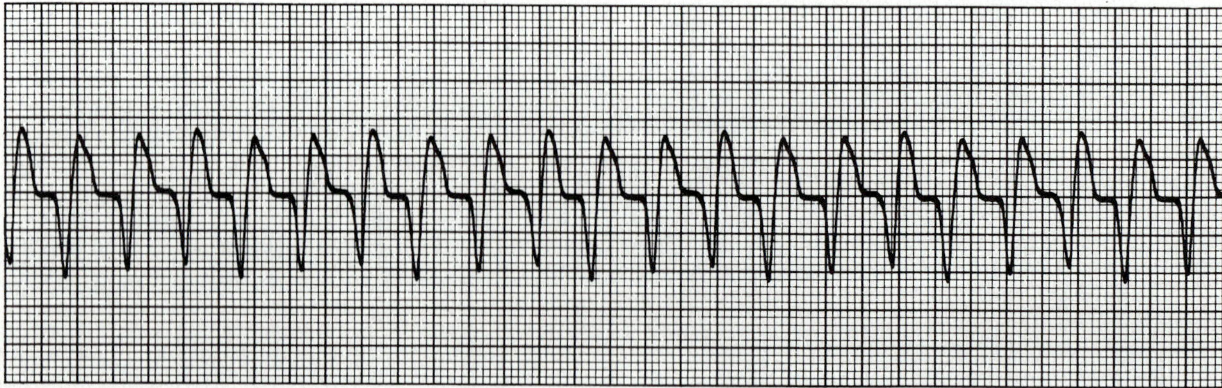

Figure 9-18. Ventricular tachycardia.

rapid rate. Because the ventricles are capable of an inherent rate of 40 beats/min or less, a ventricular rhythm at a rate of 100 beats/min may be considered tachycardia.

Analysis

Rate: usually between 100 and 220 beats/min.
Rhythm: usually regular but may be irregular.
P wave: not present.
PR interval: not measurable.
QRS complex: broad, bizarre in configuration, widened greater than 0.12 second.
T wave: usually deflected opposite to the QRS complex.

Management

1. VT less than 30 seconds is called nonsustained VT. VT more than 30 seconds is sustained VT and requires immediate treatment.
2. If the patient has a pulse and is hemodynamically stable, medications are the initial treatments. Amiodarone IV bolus can be given to halt the dysrhythmia. Other potential medications that may be used (if amiodarone fails) include lidocaine and procainamide. If patient becomes hemodynamically unstable, prepare for synchronized cardioversion with 200 joules of biphasic electrical current.
3. If the patient is pulseless, defibrillation is recommended with 200 joules of biphasic electrical current.
4. The purpose of cardioversion–defibrillation is to abolish all abnormal electrical activity and allow the intrinsic cardiac rhythm the opportunity to restart.
5. In some cases, VT may be refractory to drug therapy. Nonpharmacologic treatments, such as endocardial resection, aneurysmectomy, antitachycardia pacemakers, automatic internal defibrillators, and catheter ablation, are alternative treatment modalities.
6. An atypical form of VT, referred to as polymorphous VT or *torsades de pointes* (twisting of the points), can result as a consequence of drug therapy (e.g., quinidine therapy) or electrolyte imbalance such as hypomagnesemia. It is important to diagnose polymorphous VT as the treatment differs from monomorphic VT.
   a. *Torsades de pointes* is characterized by a QT interval prolonged to greater than 0.60 second, varying R–R intervals, and polymorphous QRS complexes.
   b. The treatment of choice is administration of magnesium sulfate 1 g IV over 5 to 60 minutes.
   c. If the patient loses consciousness and pulse, defibrillate with 120 to 200 joules of biphasic electrical current.
   d. Ventricular pacing to override the ventricular rate and thus capture the rhythm is also an acceptable treatment.
   e. Procainamide should be avoided because its effect is to prolong the QT interval.

CLINICAL JUDGMENT VT is life-threatening, and its presentation calls for immediate identification and intervention by the nurse.

Ventricular Fibrillation

See Figure 9-19.

Etiology

1. Occurs in acute MI, acidosis, electrolyte disturbances, and other deteriorating ventricular rhythms.
2. The ventricles are firing chaotically at rates that exceed 300 beats/min, resulting in ineffective impulse conduction. CO ceases, and the patient loses pulse, BP, and consciousness.
3. Must be reversed immediately or the patient will die.

Analysis

Rate: not measurable because of absence of well-formed QRS complexes.
Rhythm: chaotic.
P wave: not present.
QRS complex: bizarre, chaotic, no definite contour.
T wave: not apparent.

Management

1. The only treatment for ventricular fibrillation is immediate defibrillation. Defibrillate at 120 to 200 joules with a biphasic defibrillator. Current advanced cardiac life support guidelines no longer recommend three stacked shocks before initiating CPR and medication administration. Epinephrine and vasopressin are first-line drugs after defibrillation because these drugs may make the fibrillation more vulnerable to defibrillation.
2. Unsuccessful defibrillation may be a result of lactic acidosis (treatable with sodium bicarbonate).
3. Check adequacy of the high-quality CPR being performed: 100 compressions/min at a 2 to 2½-in depth.

Atrioventricular Block

Etiology

1. May be caused by ischemia or inferior wall MI, digoxin toxicity, hypothyroidism, or Stokes-Adams syndrome.
2. Impaired tissue at the level of the AV node prevents the timely passage of the wave of impulse through the conduction system.

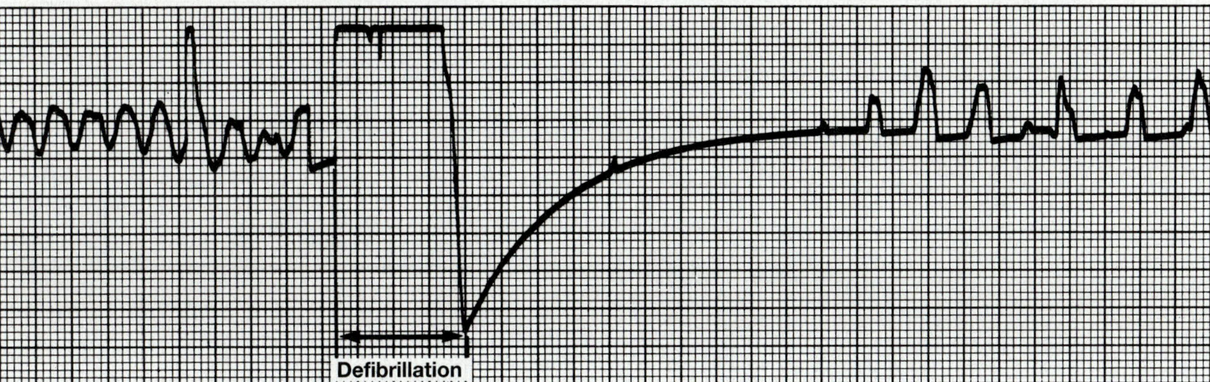

Figure 9-19. Ventricular fibrillation with defibrillation.

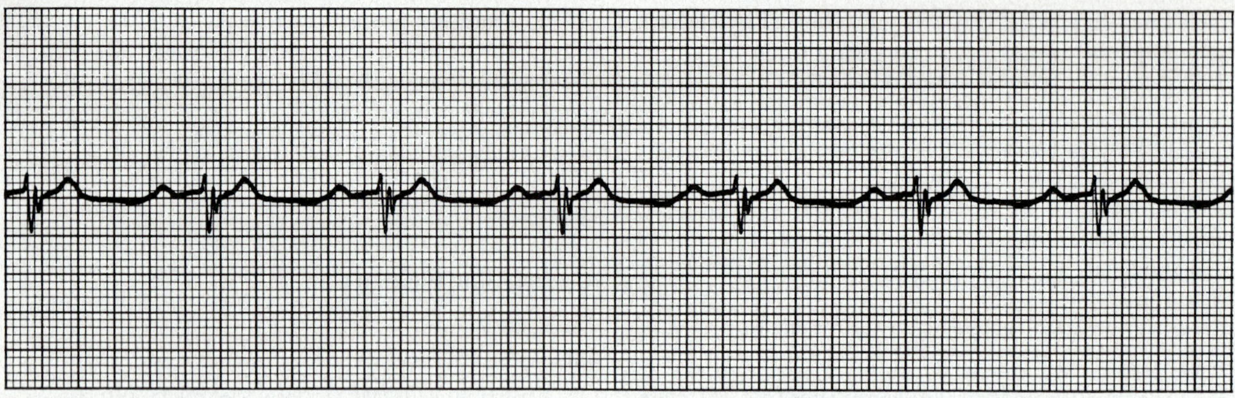

Figure 9-20. First-degree atrioventricular (AV) block.

3. In first-degree AV block, the impulse is transmitted normally, but it is delayed at the level of the AV node. The PR interval exceeds 0.20 second.
4. In second-degree AV block, two or more atrial impulses occur before the ventricles are stimulated.
   a. Second-degree type 1 (Mobitz 1 Wenckebach)—block occurs above the AV node. There is an increase in delay of electrical impulse (increasing PR interval) with every beat until one P wave fails to conduct and is not followed by a QRS complex (beat is dropped). Mobitz type 1 is usually a temporary and benign dysrhythmia and seldom requires intervention (pacing) unless ventricular rate is slow and the patient is unstable.
   b. Second-degree type 2 (Mobitz 2)—block occurs below the AV node in the bundle of His or bundle-branch system. The atria and ventricles are discharging impulses, but the activity bears no relationship to each other. There is a sudden failure to conduct an atrial impulse to the ventricles without a delay of the PR interval.
5. In third-degree AV block, or complete heart block, the electrical impulse is completely blocked from the SA node to the AV node. An independent pacemaker in the ventricles takes over at a much slower rate than the atria and are firing independently of each other.

Analysis

1. First-degree AV block (see Figure 9-20).

Rate: usually normal but may be slow.
Rhythm: regular.
P wave: present for each QRS complex, identical in configuration.
PR interval: prolonged to greater than 0.20 second.
QRS complex: normal in appearance and between 0.06 and 0.10 second.
T wave: normally conducted.

2. Second-degree AV block (see Figure 9-21).

Rate: usually normal.
Rhythm: may be regular or irregular.
P wave: present, but some may not be followed by a QRS complex. A ratio of two, three, or four P waves to one QRS complex may exist.
PR interval: varies in Mobitz I (Wenckebach), usually lengthens until one is not conducted; constant in Mobitz II, but not all P waves conducted.
T wave: normally conducted.

3. Third-degree AV block (complete heart block) (see Figure 9-22).

Rate: atrial rate is measured independently of the ventricular rate; the ventricular rate is usually very slow.
Rhythm: each independent rhythm will be regular, but they will bear no relationship to each other.
P wave: present but no consistent relationship with the QRS.
PR interval: not really measurable.
QRS complex: depends on the escape mechanism (i.e., AV node will have normal QRS, ventricular will be wide, and the rate will be slower).
T wave: normally conducted.

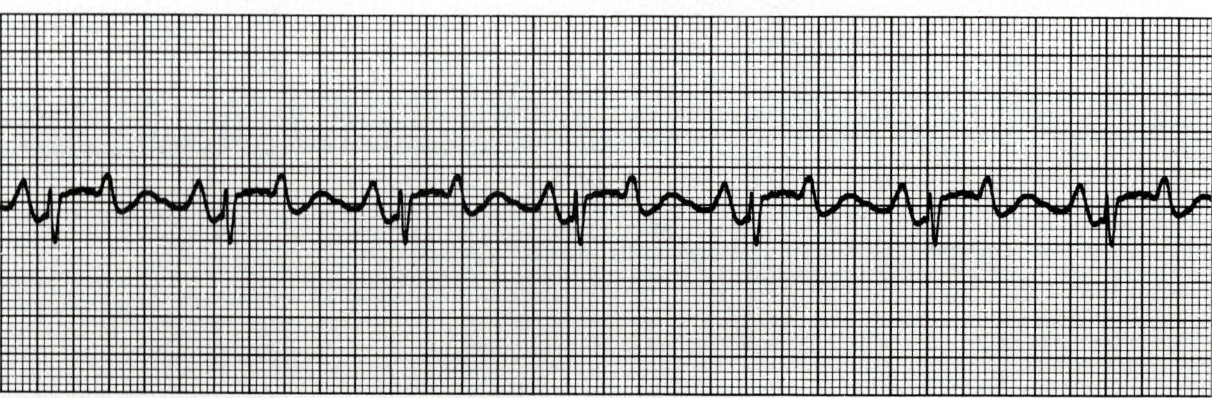

Figure 9-21. Second-degree atrioventricular (AV) block (Mobitz I).

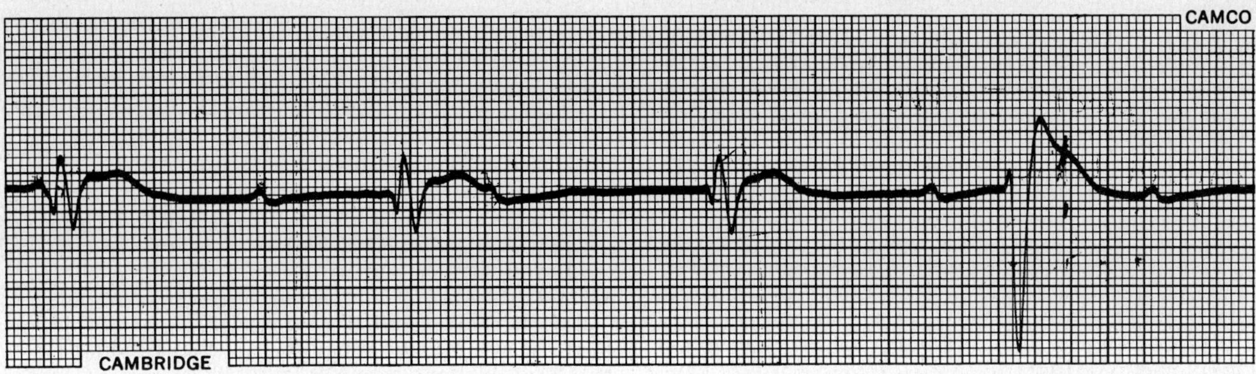

Figure 9-22. Third-degree atrioventricular (AV) block.

Management

Like that of other dysrhythmias, the treatment of heart blocks depends on the effect the rate is having on CO.

1. First-degree AV block usually requires no treatment.
2. Second-degree AV block, type 1 and type 2, may require treatment if the ventricular rate falls too low to maintain effective CO. Mobitz type 2 is more serious than Mobitz type 1.
3. Third-degree AV block usually requires intervention. Some patients may be able to tolerate third-degree block for a length of time; however, it is not sustainable long-term.
4. Transcutaneous pacing should be employed in the emergent situation while transvenous pacing is being set up. Permanent pacemaker may be necessary (see page 213).
5. Atropine may be given while awaiting the pacemaker, but it must be remembered that the effect of atropine is to block vagal tone and the vagus acts on the sinus node. Because the AV node is the culprit in heart block, atropine may not be helpful.

SELECTED READINGS

Abdul-Rahmi, A., Shhen, L., Rush, C., Jhund, P. S., Lees, K. R., McMurray, J. J. V., & VICCTA-Heart Failure Collaborators. (2018). Effect of digoxin in patients with heart failure and mid-range (borderline) left ventricular ejection fraction. *European Journal of Heart Failure, 20*(7), 1139–1145. https://doi.org/10.1002/ejhf.1160

Ai, S., Liu, J., Ma, G., Ye, W., Hu, R., Zhang, S., Fan, X., Liu, B., Miao, Q., Qin, Y., & Li, X. (2022). Endocarditis-associated rapidly progressive glomerulonephritis mimicking vasculitis: A diagnostic and treatment challenge. *Annals of Medicine, 54*(1), 754–763. https://doi.org/10.1080/07853890.2022.2046288

Al-Khatib, S. M., Stevenson, W. G., Ackerman, M. J., Bryant, W. J., Callans, D. J., Curtis, A. B., Deal, B. J., Dickfeld, T., Field, M. E., Fonarow, G. C., Gillis, A. M., Granger, C. B., Hammill, S. C., Hlatky, M. A., Joglar, J. A., Kay, G. N., Matlock, D. D., Myerburg, R. J., & Page, R. L. (2018). 2017 AHA/ACC/HRS guideline for management of patients with ventricular arrhythmias and the prevention of sudden cardiac death: Executive summary: A report of the American College of Cardiology/American Heart Association Task Force on Clinical Practice Guidelines and the Heart Rhythm Society. *Heart Rhythm, 15*(10), e190–e252. https://doi.org/10.1016/j.hrthm.2017.10.035

Arnett, D. K., Blumenthal, R. S., Albert, M. A., Buroker, A. B., Goldberger, Z. D., Hahn, E. J., Himmelfarb, C. D., Khera, A., Lloyd-Jones, D., McEvoy, J. W., Michos, E. D., Miedema, M. D., Muñoz, D., Smith, S. C., Jr, Virani, S. S., Williams, K. A., Sr, Yeboah, J., & Ziaeian, B. (2019). 2019 ACC/AHA Guideline on the Primary Prevention of Cardiovascular Disease: A Report of the American College of Cardiology/American Heart Association Task Force on Clinical Practice Guidelines. *Circulation, 140*(11), e596–e646. https://doi.org/10.1161/CIR.0000000000000678

Asber, S. R., Shanahan, K. P., Lussier, L., Didomenico, D., Davis, M., Eaton, J., Esposito, M., & Kapur, N. K. (2020). Nursing management of patients requiring acute mechanical circulatory support devices. *Critical Care Nurse, 40*(1), e1–e11. https://doi.org/10.4037/ccn2020764

Assis, F. R., Krishnan, A., Zhou, X., James, C. A., Murray, B., Tichnell, C., Berger, R., Calkins, H., Tandri, H., & Mandal, K. (2019). Cardiac sympathectomy for refractory ventricular tachycardia in arrhythmogenic right ventricular cardiomyopathy. *Heart Rhythm, 16*(7), 1003–1010. https://doi.org/10.1016/j.hrthm.2019.01.019

Atwood, J. (2022). Management of acute coronary syndrome. *Emergency Medicine Clinics of North America, 40*(4), 693–706. https://doi.org/10.1016/j.emc.2022.06.008

Authors/Task Force Members; ESC Committee for Practice Guidelines; & ESC National Cardiac Societies. (2019). 2019 ESC/EAS guidelines for the management of dyslipidaemias: Lipid modification to reduce cardiovascular risk. *Atherosclerosis, 290*, 140–205. https://doi.org/10.1016/j.atherosclerosis.2019.08.014

Baddour, L. M., Wilson, W. R., Bayer, A. S., Fowler, V. G., Tleyjeh, I. M., Rybak, M. J., Barsic, B., Lockhart, P. B., Gewitz, M. H., Levison, M. E., Bolger, A. F., Steckelberg, J. M., Baltimore, R. S., Fink, A. M., O'Gara, P., & Taubert, K. A. (2015). Infective endocarditis in adults: diagnosis, antimicrobial therapy, and management of complications. *Circulation, 132*(15), 1435–1486. https://doi.org/10.1161/cir.0000000000000296

Bainey, K. R., Bates, E. R., & Armstrong, P. W. (2020). ST-segment–elevation myocardial infarction care and COVID-19. *Circulation: Cardiovascular Quality and Outcomes, 13*(6). https://doi.org/10.1161/circoutcomes.120.006834

Barnes, G. (2020). Combining antiplatelet and anticoagulant therapy in cardiovascular disease. *Hematology American Society of Hematology Education Program, 2020*(1), 642–648. https://doi.org/10.1182/hematology.2020000151

Brown, R. M. (2022). Acute coronary syndrome in women. *Emergency Medicine Clinics of North America, 40*(4), 629–636. https://doi.org/10.1016/j.emc.2022.06.003

Brown, J. C., Gerhardt, T. E., & Kwon, E. (2023, updated). Risk factors for coronary artery disease. In *StatPearls* [Internet]. StatPearls Publishing. https://www.ncbi.nlm.nih.gov/books/NBK554410/

Brugada, J., Katritsis, D. G., Arbelo, E., Arribas, F., Bax, J. J., Blomström-Lundqvist, C., Calkins, H., Corrado, D., Deftereos, S. G., Diller, G. P., & Gomez-Doblas, J. J. (2020). 2019 ESC guidelines for the management of patients with supraventricular tachycardia. The Task Force for the management of patients with supraventricular tachycardia of the European Society of Cardiology (ESC): Developed in collaboration with the Association for European Paediatric and Congenital Cardiology (AEPC). *European Heart Journal, 41*(5), 655–720. https://doi.org/10.1093/eurheartj/ehz467

Chapman, A. R., Shah, A. S., Lee, K. K., Anand, A., Francis, O., Adamson, P., McAllister, D. A., Strachan, F. E., Newby, D. E., & Mills, N. L. (2018). Long-term outcomes in patients with type 2 myocardial infarction and myocardial injury. *Circulation, 137*(12), 1236–1245. https://doi.org/10.1161/circulationaha.117.031806

Cholesterol Treatment Trialists' Collaboration. (2019). Efficacy and safety of statin therapy in older people: A meta-analysis of individual participant data from 28 randomised controlled trials. *Lancet (London, England), 393*(10170), 407–415. https://doi.org/10.1016/S0140-6736(18)31942-1

Claessen, B. E., Guedeney, P., Gibson, C. M., Angiolillo, D. J., Cao, D., Lepor, N., & Mehran, R. (2020). Lipid management in patients presenting with acute coronary syndromes: A review. *Journal of the American Heart Association, 9*(24), e018897. https://doi.org/10.1161/JAHA.120.018897

Cleland, J., Bunting, K., Flater, M., Altman, D. G., Holmes, J., Coats, A. J. S., Manzano, L., McMurray, J. J. V., Ruschitzka, F., van Veldhuisen, D. J., von Lueder,

T. G., Böhm, M., Andersson, B., Kjekshus, J., Packer, M., Rigby, A. S., Rosano, G., Wedel, H., Hjalmarson, Å., ... Beta-blockers in Heart Failure Collaborative Group. (2018). Beta-blocker for heart failure with reduced, mid-range, and preserved ejection fraction: An individual patient-level analysis of double-blind randomized trails. *European Heart Journal, 39*(1), 26–35. https://doi.org/10.1093/eurheartj/ehx564

Costello, B. T., & Younis, G. A. (2020). Acute coronary syndrome in women: An overview. *Texas Heart Institute Journal, 47*(2), 128–129. https://doi.org/10.14503/THIJ-19-7077

Crowley, J., Cronin, B., Essandoh, M., D'Alessandro, D., Shelton, K., & Dalia, A. A. (2019). Transesophageal echocardiography for impella placement and management. *Journal of Cardiothoracic and Vascular Anesthesia, 33*(10), 2663–2668. https://doi.org/10.1053/j.jvca.2019.01.048

Dass, C., & Kanmanthareddy, A. (2022). Rheumatic heart disease. *In: StatPearls [Internet]*. StatPearls Publishing.

Dembowski, E., Freedman, I., Grundy, S., & Stone, N. (2022). Guidelines for the management of hyperlipidemia: How can clinicians effectively implement them? *Progress in Cardiovascular Diseases, 75*, 4–11. https://doi.org/10.1016/j.pcad.2022.11.009

Dron, J. S., Wang, J., Cao, H., McIntyre, A. D., Iacocca, M. A., Menard, J. R., Movsesyan, I., Malloy, M. J., Pullinger, C. R., Kane, J. P., & Hegele, R. A. (2019). Severe hypertriglyceridemia is primarily polygenic. *Journal of Clinical Lipidology, 13*(1), 80–88. https://doi.org/10.1016/j.jacl.2018.10.006

Duarte, G. S., Nunes-Ferreira, A., Rodrigues, F. B., Pinto, F. J., Ferreira, J. J., Costa, J., & Caldeira, D. (2019). Morphine in acute coronary syndrome: Systematic review and meta-analysis. *BMJ Open, 9*(3), e025232. https://doi.org/10.1136/bmjopen-2018-025232

Dunlay, S. M., Roger, V. L., & Redfield, M. M. (2017). Epidemiology of heart failure with preserved ejection fraction. *Nature Reviews Cardiology, 14*(10), 591–602. https://doi.org/10.1038/nrcardio.2017.65

Ergle, K., Parto, P., & Krim, S. R. (2016). Percutaneous ventricular assist devices: A novel approach in the management of patients with acute cardiogenic shock. *Ochsner Journal, 16*(3), 243–249.

Fan, W., Philip, S., Granowitz, C., Toth, P. P., & Wong, N. D. (2019). Hypertriglyceridemia in statin-treated US adults: The National Health and Nutrition Examination Survey. *Journal of Clinical Lipidology, 13*(1), 100–108. https://doi.org/10.1016/j.jacl.2018.11.008

Fiedler, A., Dalia, A., Axetell, A. L., Ortoleva, J., Thomas, S. M., Roy, N., Villavicencio, M. A., D'Alessandro, D. A., & Cudemus, G. (2018). Impella placement guided by echocardiography can be used as a strategy to unload the left ventricle during peripheral venoarterial extracorporeal membrane oxygenation. *Journal of Cardiothoracic and Vascular Anesthesia, 32*(6), 2585–2591. https://doi.org/10.1053/j.jvca.2018.05.019

Frankline, B., Thompson, P., Al-Zaiti, S., Albert, C. M., Hivert, M. F., Levine, B. D., Lobelo, F., Madan, K., Sharrief, A. Z., Eijsvogels, T. M. H; American Heart Association Physical Activity Committee of the Council on Lifestyle and Cardiometabolic Health; Council on Cardiovascular and Stroke Nursing; Council on Clinical Cardiology; & Stroke Council. (2020). Exercise-related acute cardiovascular events and potential deleterious adaptations following long-term exercise training: Placing the risks into perspective—An update: A scientific statement from the American Heart Association. *Circulation, 141*(13), e705–e736. https://doi.org/10.1161/CIR.0000000000000749

Garrote-Coloma, C., & Fernandez-Vazques, F. (2020). To clip, or not to clip, in patients with functional mitral regurgitation. *Cardiovascular Revascularization Medicine, 21*(2), 249–250. https://doi.org/10.1016/j.carrev.2019.12.013

Haas, P., Felton, A., & Felton, S. (2019). *Understanding EP: A comprehensive guide: Part 1 of 2* (1st ed.). KDP.

Hedayati, T., Yadav, N., & Khanagavi, J. (2018). Non-ST-segment acute coronary syndromes. *Cardiology Clinics, 36*(1), 37–52. https://doi.org/10.1016/j.ccl.2017.08.003

Heidenreich, P. A., Bozkurt, B., Aguilar, D., Allen, L. A., Byun, J. J., Colvin, M. M., Deswal, A., Drazner, M. H., Dunlay, S. M., Evers, L. R., Fang, J. C., Fedson, S. E., Fonarow, G. C., Hayek, S. S., Hernandez, A. F., Khazanie, P., Kittleson, M. M., Lee, C. S., Link, M. S., Milano, C. A., ... Yancy, C. W. (2022). 2022 AHA/ACC/HFSA Guideline for the Management of Heart Failure: A Report of the American College of Cardiology/American Heart Association Joint Committee on Clinical Practice Guidelines. *Circulation, 145*(18), e895–e1032. https://doi.org/10.1161/CIR.0000000000001063

Hensey, M., Brown, R., Lal, S., Sathananthan, J., Ye, J., Cheung, A., Blanke, P., Leipsic, J., Moss, R., Boone, R., & Webb, J. G. (2021). Transcatheter mitral valve replacement: An update on current techniques, technologies, and future directions. *JACC: Cardiovascular Interventions, 14*(5), 489–500. https://doi.org/10.1016/j.jcin.2020.12.038

Hershberger, R. E., Givertz, M. M., Ho, C. Y., Judge, D. P., Kantor, P. F., McBride, K. L., Morales, A., Taylor, M. R. G., Vatta, M., & Ware, S. M. (2018). Genetic evaluation of cardiomyopathy—A Heart Failure Society of America practice guideline. *Journal of Cardiology Failure, 24*(5), 281–302. https://doi.org/10.1016/j.cardfail.2018.03.004

Hiemstra, Y. L., Debonnaire, P., van Zwet, E. W., Bootsma, M., Schalij, M. J., Bax, J. J., Delgado, V., & Marsan, N. A. (2018). Development of and progression of overt heart failure in nonobstructive hypertrophic cardiomyopathy. *American Journal of Cardiology, 122*(4), 656–662. https://doi.org/10.1016/j.amjcard.2018.04.038

Katsiki, N., & Doumas, M. (2021). Emerging cardiovascular risk factors and specific patient populations at increased cardiovascular risk. *Current Vascular Pharmacology, 19*(3), 241–242. https://doi.org/10.2174/157016111903201231115755

Khan, S. S., Coresh, J., Pencina, M. J., Ndumele, C. E., Rangaswami, J., Chow, S. L., Palaniappan, L. P., Sperling, L. S., Virani, S. S., Ho, J. E., Neeland, I. J., Tuttle, K. R., Rajgopal Singh, R., Elkind, M. S. V., Lloyd-Jones, D. M., & American Heart Association (2023). Novel prediction equations for absolute risk assessment of total cardiovascular disease incorporating cardiovascular-kidney-metabolic health: A scientific statement from the American Heart Association. *Circulation, 148*(24), 1982–2004. https://doi.org/10.1161/CIR.0000000000001191

Kirresh, A., Candilio, L., & Stone, G. W. (2021). Intralesional delivery of glycoprotein IIb/IIIa inhibitors in acute myocardial infarction: Review and recommendations. *Catheterization and Cardiovascular Interventions, 99*(3), 641–649. https://doi.org/10.1002/ccd.30008

Kociol, R. D., Cooper, L. T., Fang, J. C., Moslehi, J. J., Pang, P. S., Sabe, M. A., Shah, R. V., Sims, D. B., Thiene, G., & Vardeny, O. (2020). Recognition and initial management of fulminant myocarditis. *Circulation, 141*(6), e69–e92. https://doi.org/10.1161/cir.0000000000000745

Kusumoto, F. M., Schoenfeld, M. H., Barrett, C., Edgerton, J. R., Ellenbogen, K. A., Gold, M. R., Goldschlager, N. F., Hamilton, R. M., Joglar, J. A., Kim, R. J., Lee, R., Marine, J. E., McLeod, C. J., Oken, K. R., Patton, K. K., Pellegrini, C. N., Selzman, K. A., Thompson, A, & Varosy, P. D. (2019). 2018 ACC/AHA/HRS guideline on the evaluation and management of patients with bradycardia and cardiac conduction delay: A report of the American College of Cardiology/American Heart Association Task Force on Clinical Practice Guidelines and the Heart Rhythm Society. *Circulation, 140*(8), e382–e482. https://doi.org/10.1161/CIR.0000000000000628

Lawton, J. S., Tamis-Holland, J. E., Bangalore, S., Bates, E. R., Beckie, T. M., Bischoff, J. M., Bittl, J. A., Cohen, M. G., DiMaio, J. M., Don, C. W., Fremes, S. E., Gaudino, M. F., Goldberger, Z. D., Grant, M. C., Jaswal, J. B., Kurlansky, P. A., Mehran, R., Metkus, T. S., Nnacheta, L. C., ... Zwischenberger, B. A. (2022). 2021 ACC/AHA/SCAI guideline for coronary artery revascularization. *Journal of the American College of Cardiology, 79*(2), e21–e129. https://doi.org/10.1016/j.jacc.2021.09.006

Markatis, E., Afthinos, A., Antonakis, E., & Papanikolaou, I. C. (2020). Cardiac sarcoidosis: Diagnosis and management. *Reviews in Cardiac Medicine, 21*(3), 321–338. https://doi.org/10.31083/j.rcm.2020.03.102

McCarthy, C., Murphy, S., Cohen, J. A., Rehman, S., Jones-O'Connor, M., Olshan, D. S., Singh, A., Vaduganathan, M., Januzzi, J. L., & Wasfy, J. H. (2019). Misclassification of myocardial injury as myocardial infarction. *JAMA Cardiology, 4*(5), 460–464. https://doi.org/10.1001/jamacardio.2019.0716

McKenna, W., Maron, B., & Thiene, G. (2017). Classification, epidemiology, and global burden of cardiomyopathies. *Circulation Research, 121*(7), 722–730. https://doi.org/10.1161/CIRCRESAHA.117.309711

O'Gara, P. T., Kushner, F. G., Ascheim, D. D., Casey, D. E., Jr., Chung, M. K., de Lemos, J. A., Ettinger, S. M., Fang, J. C., Fesmire, F. M., Franklin, B. A., Granger, C. B., Krumholz, H. M., Linderbaum, J. A., Morrow, D. A., Newby, L. K., Ornato, J. P., Ou, N., Radford, M. J., Tamis-Holland, J. E., ... Zhao, D. X. (2013). 2013 ACCF/AHA guideline for the management of ST-elevation myocardial infarction: A report of the American College of Cardiology Foundation/American Heart Association Task Force on Practice Guidelines. *Journal of the American College of Cardiology, 61*(4), e78–e140. https://doi.org/10.1016/j.jacc.2012.11.019

Ojha, N., & Dhamoon, A. S. (2022). Myocardial infarction. In: *StatPearls* [Internet]. StatPearls Publishing.

Ommen, S., Mital, S., Burke, M., Day, S. M., Deswal, A., Elliott, P., Evanovich, L. L., Hung, J., Joglar, J. A., Kantor, P., Kimmelstiel, C., Kittleson, M., Link, M. S., Maron, M. S., Martinez, M. W., Miyake, C. Y., Schaff, H. V., Semsarian, C., & Sorajja, P. (2020). 2020 AHA/ACC guidelines for the diagnosis and treatment of patients with hypertrophic cardiomyopathy: A report of the American College of Cardiology/American Heart Association Joint Committee on Clinical

Practice Guidelines. *Circulation, 142*(25), e533–e631. https://doi.org/10.1161/CIR.0000000000000937

Otto, C. M., Nishimura, R. A., Bonow, R. O., Carabello, B. A., Erwin, J. P., Gentile, F., Jneid, H., Krieger, E. V., Mack, M., McLeod, C., O'Gara, P. T., Rigolin, V. H., Sundt, T. M., Thompson, A., & Toly, C. (2021). 2020 ACC/AHA guideline for the management of patients with valvular heart disease: Executive summary: A report of the American College of Cardiology/American Heart Association Joint Committee on Clinical Practice Guidelines. *Circulation, 143*(5), e35–e71. https://doi.org/10.1161/cir.0000000000000932

Park, J., Choi, K. H., Lee, J. M., Kim, H. K., Hwang, D., Rhee, T., Kim, J., Park, T. K., Yang, J. H., Song, Y. B., Choi, J., Hahn, J., Choi, S., Koo, B., Chae, S. C., Cho, M. C., Kim, C. J., Kim, J. H., Jeong, M. H., ... Kim, H. (2019). Prognostic implications of door-to-balloon time and onset-to-door time on mortality in patients with ST-segment–elevation myocardial infarction treated with primary percutaneous coronary intervention. *Journal of the American Heart Association, 8*(9). https://doi.org/10.1161/jaha.119.012188

Pelliccia, A., Solberg, E. E., Papadakis, M., Adami, P. E., Biffi, A., Caselli, S., La Gerche, A., Niebauer, J., Pressler, A., Schmied, C. M., Serratosa, L., Halle, M., Van Buuren, F., Borjesson, M., Carrè, F., Panhuyzen-Goedkoop, N. M., Heidbuchel, H., Olivotto, I., Corrado, D., ... Sharma, S. (2019). Recommendations for participation in competitive and leisure time sport in athletes with cardiomyopathies, myocarditis, and pericarditis: Position statement of the Sport Cardiology Section of the European Association of Preventive Cardiology (EAPC). *European Heart Journal, 40*(1), 19–33. https://doi.org/10.1093/eurheartj/ehy730

Pieri, M., & Pappalardo, F. (2020). Bedside insertion of impella percutaneous ventricular assist device in patients with cardiogenic shock. *International Journal of Cardiology, 316*, 26–30. https://doi.org/10.1016/j.ijcard.2020.05.080

Redfors, B., Mohebi, R., Giustino, G., Chen, S., Selker, H. P., Thiele, H., Patel, M. R., Udelson, J. E., Ohman, E. M., Eitel, I., Granger, C. B., Maehara, A., Ali, Z. A., Ben-Yehuda, O., & Stone, G. W. (2021). Time delay, infarct size, and microvascular obstruction after primary percutaneous coronary intervention for ST-segment–elevation myocardial infarction. *Circulation: Cardiovascular Interventions, 14*(2). https://doi.org/10.1161/circinterventions.120.009879

Rogers, E., Torres, C., Rao, S. V., Donatelle, M., & Beohar, N. (2022). Clinical characteristics, outcomes, and epidemiological trends of patients admitted with type 2 myocardial infarction. *Journal of the Society for Cardiovascular Angiography & Interventions, 1*(5), 100395. https://doi.org/10.1016/j.jscai.2022.100395

Roth, G. A., Mensah, G. A., & Fuster, V. (2020). The global burden of cardiovascular diseases and risks. *Journal of the American College of Cardiology, 76*(25), 2980–2981. https://doi.org/10.1016/j.jacc.2020.11.021

Simko, L. C. (2022). Cardiogenic Shock and the Use of Percutaneous Mechanical Assist Devices. *Critical care nurse, 42*(1), 56–67. https://doi.org/10.4037/ccn2022140

Tisdale, J. E., Chung, M. K., Campbell, K. B., Hammadah, M., Joglar, J. A., Leclerc, J., Rajagopalan, B., & American Heart Association Clinical Pharmacology Committee of the Council on Clinical Cardiology and Council on Cardiovascular and Stroke Nursing. (2020). Drug-induced arrhythmias: A scientific statement from the American Heart Association. *Circulation, 142*(15), e214–e233. https://doi.org/10.1161/CIR.0000000000000905

Toth, P. P., Fazio, S., Wong, N. D., Hull, M., & Nichols, G. A. (2020). Risk of cardiovascular events in patients with hypertriglyceridaemia: A review of real-world evidence. *Diabetes Obesity Metabolism, 22*(3), 279–289. https://doi.org/10.1111/dom.13921

Tschöpe, C., Ammirati, E., Bozkurt, B., Caforio, A. L., Cooper, L. T., Felix S. B., Hare, J. M., Heidecker, B., Heymans, S., Hubner, N., Kelle, S., Klingel, K., Maatz, H., Parwani, A. S., Spillman, F., Starling, R. C., Tsutsui, H., Seferovic, P. M., & Van Linthout, S. (2021). Myocarditis and inflammatory cardiomyopathy: Current evidence and future directions. *Nature Reviews Cardiology, 18*(3), 169–193. https://doi.org/10.1038/s41569-020-00435-x

US Preventive Services Task Force, Mangione, C. M., Barry, M. J., Nicholson, W. K., Cabana, M., Chelmow, D., Coker, T. R., Davis, E. M., Donahue, K. E., Jaén, C. R., Kubik, M., Li, L., Ogedegbe, G., Pbert, L., Ruiz, J. M., Stevermer, J., & Wong, J. B. (2022). Statin use for the primary prevention of cardiovascular disease in adults: US Preventive Services Task Force recommendation statement. *JAMA, 328*(8), 746–753. https://doi.org/10.1001/jama.2022.13044

Vahanian, A., Beyersdorf, F., Praz, F., Milojevic, M., Baldus, S., Bauersachs, J., Capodanno, D., Conradi, L., De Bonis, M., De Paulis, R., Delgado, V., Freemantle, N., Gilard, M., Haugaa, K. H., Jeppsson, A., Jüni, P., Pierard, L., Prendergast, B. D., Sádaba, J. R., ... ESC/EACTS Scientific Document Group. (2022). 2021 ESC/EACTS guidelines for the management of valvular heart disease. *European Heart Journal, 43*(7), 561–632. https://doi.org/10.1093/eurheartj/ehab395

Vasan, R., Enserro, D., Beiser, A., & Xanthakis, V. (2022). Lifetime risk of heart failure among participants in the Framingham study. *Journal of American College of Cardiology, 79*(3), 250–263. https://doi.org/10.1016/j.jacc.2021.10.043

Virani, S. S., Morris, P. B., Agarwala, A., Ballantyne, C. M., Birtcher, K. K., Kris-Etherton, P. M., Ladden-Stirling, A. B., Miller, M., Orringer, C. E., & Stone, N. J. (2021). 2021 ACC expert consensus decision pathway on the management of ASCVD risk reduction in patients with persistent hypertriglyceridemia: A report of the American College of Cardiology Solution Set Oversight Committee. *Journal of the American College of Cardiology, 78*(9), 960–993. https://doi.org/10.1016/j.jacc.2021.06.011

Watkins, D. A., Beaton, A. Z., Carapetis, J. R., Karthikeyan, G., Mayosi, B. M., Wyber, R., Yacoub, M. H., & Zühlke, L. J. (2018). Rheumatic heart disease worldwide: JACC Scientific Expert Panel. *Journal of the American College of Cardiology, 72*(12), 1397–1416. https://doi.org/10.1016/j.jacc.2018.06.063

Wilson, W. R., Gewitz, M., Lockhart, P. B., Bolger, A. F., DeSimone, D. C., Kazi, D. S., Couper, D. J., Beaton, A., Kilmartin, C., Miro, J. M., Sable, C., Jackson, M. A., & Baddour, L. M. (2021). Prevention of viridans group streptococcal infective endocarditis: A scientific statement from the American Heart Association. *Circulation, 143*(20), e963–e978. https://doi.org/10.1161/cir.0000000000000969

10 Vascular Disorders*

GENERAL PROCEDURES AND TREATMENT MODALITIES

See additional online content: Procedure Guidelines 10-1

Anticoagulant Therapy

EVIDENCE BASE Ortel, T. L., Neumann, I., Ageno, W., Beyth, R., Clark, N. P., Cuker, A., Hutten, B. A., Jaff, M. R., Manja, V., Schulman, S., Thurston, C., Vedantham, S., Verhamme, P., Witt, D. M., Florez, I. D., Izcovich, A., Nieuwlaat, R., Ross, S., Schünemann, H. J., ... Zhang, Y. (2020). American Society of Hematology 2020 guidelines for management of venous thromboembolism: Treatment of deep vein thrombosis and pulmonary embolism. *Blood Advances*, 4(19), 4693–4738. https://doi.org/10.1182/bloodadvances.2020001830

Anticoagulant therapy is the administration of medications to achieve the following:

- Disrupt the blood's natural clotting cascade when there is a risk of pathologic clotting.
- Prevent formation of a thrombus in immobile and/or postoperative patients.
- Interrupt the extension of a thrombus once it has formed.
- Agents are used in the acute treatment of thromboembolic disorders, for long-term treatment and prevention of recurrent thromboembolism, or for short-term prevention of thromboembolism following certain surgeries.

Types of anticoagulants include heparins (unfractionated [UFH] and low-molecular-weight [LMW] heparin), indirect thrombin inhibitors, vitamin K antagonist (VKA), direct thrombin inhibitors, and direct factor Xa inhibitors.

CLINICAL JUDGMENT Anticoagulants may be contraindicated or used with extreme caution in patients who are at risk for bleeding due to difficult follow-up, fall risk, and age, and in patients with hepatic and renal insufficiency.

Anticoagulant Indications

1. UFH and LMW heparin (enoxaparin, tinzaparin, nadroparin) are used extensively as anticoagulants. Heparins act indirectly by binding to antithrombin (AT) rather than binding directly to coagulation factors that efficiently inactivate factor Xa via AT. UFH is a more efficient inactivator of thrombin due to a ternary complex formed between heparin, AT, and thrombin.
   a. Indications for use include COVID-19 hypercoagulability state, venous thromboembolism (VTE) prophylaxis, deep vein thrombosis (DVT), pulmonary embolism (PE), myocardial infarction (MI), acute coronary syndrome (ACS), stroke or transient ischemic attack (TIA), pre- and postoperatively for high-risk procedures or orthopedic surgical procedures.
   b. Advantages to UFH compared to LMW heparin include:
      i. Rapid onset and offset of action.
      ii. Ability to monitor using activated partial thromboplastin time (aPTT), anti-factor Xa activity, or activated clotting time (ACT).
      iii. Ability to fully and rapidly reverse activity using protamine sulfate.
   c. Disadvantages to UFH include:
      i. No oral form is available; prophylactic dose is generally administered as a subcutaneous injection.
      ii. Acute treatment dose must be given by intravenous (IV) infusion to maintain therapeutic level, due to short half-life.
      iii. Variable bioavailability occurs due in part to competitive occupation of binding sites by proteins other than AT and coagulation factors.

*Please note that the term "male" in this chapter refers to a person assigned male at birth, and the term "female" in this chapter refers to a person assigned female at birth.

iv. Potential development of heparin-induced thrombocytopenia (HIT).
v. Potential increased risk of hemorrhagic complications.

d. Advantages of LMW heparin compared to UFH include:
   i. Greater bioavailability.
   ii. Longer duration of the anticoagulant effect.
   iii. Better correlation between dose and anticoagulation response.
   iv. Lower risk of HIT.
e. Disadvantages of LMW heparin include:
   i. Slightly delayed onset of action than UFH.
   ii. Longer duration of therapy, more difficult to stop suddenly.
   iii. Not as easy to inactivate with protamine sulfate as UFH.
   iv. Prolonged half-life in renal failure.
f. Life-threatening HIT may occur as an immune-mediated reaction to either form of heparin but is most common with UFH use (see Box 10-1).

POPULATION AWARENESS UFH and LMW heparins can be safely used in pregnancy because they do not cross the placenta. Multidose vials contain benzyl alcohol that does cross the placenta and may cause fetal harm. Preservative-free preparations should be used during pregnancy. They are also considered safe in breastfeeding.

BOX 10-1 Heparin-Induced Thrombocytopenia

Heparin-induced thrombocytopenia (HIT), also known as type 2 HIT and heparin-induced thrombocytopenia and thrombosis (HITT), is an immune-mediated disorder occurring 4–10 days after exposure to heparin due to the emergence of antibodies that bind to heparin and platelet factor 4 (PF4), activating the platelets and causing a prothrombotic state. Rather than causing significant bleeding as in other forms of thrombocytopenia, venous thromboembolism (deep vein thrombosis [DVT], pulmonary embolism) and occasionally arterial thrombosis (myocardial infraction, stroke, and arterial occlusion of limb) may occur due to platelet activation. Type 1 HIT is a nonimmune drop in platelet count occurring within 2 days of initiation of heparin. Platelet count normalizes with continued therapy.

Clinical presentation includes platelet reduction of 50% or greater below patient's baseline. Skin lesions at the injection site may also occur, as well as acute systemic reaction after intravenous (IV) bolus, causing chills, fever, dyspnea, chest pain, and flushing. Diagnostic testing includes immunoassay to identify antibodies and functional assays to measure platelet activity of PF4–heparin antibody complexes.

Management involves discontinuation of all heparin products (including flushes) whenever HIT is suspected. Imaging for thrombosis should be considered even if asymptomatic. Alternate anticoagulation should be initiated, usually with a direct thrombin inhibitor. There is a high degree of morbidity (such as amputation) and mortality of 20% with this condition, so prompt attention to platelet counts and potential thromboembolic events is essential to save life and limb.

2. Fondaparinux is a synthetic anticoagulant based on the pentasaccharide sequence that makes up the minimal AT-binding region of heparin. It is an indirect inhibitor of factor Xa, but it does not inhibit thrombin. It has a higher affinity than UFH or LMW heparin to bind to AT. This causes a conformational change in AT that leads to the inactivation of factor Xa.
   a. Indications for use are DVT, superficial vein thrombosis, thromboprophylaxis, ACS, and HIT.
   b. Major advantages are once-daily dosing due to longer half-life and no need to monitor for therapeutic level. Also, lack of platelet interaction reduces the risk of HIT. It is given subcutaneously.
   c. A disadvantage is that there is no approved antidote or reversal agent if severe bleeding should occur.
3. VKAs such as warfarin are extremely effective in reducing the risk of venous or arterial thromboembolic events. The therapeutic range is narrow, and dosing is affected by many factors including drug interactions and diet. Patients who are supratherapeutic are at risk for bleeding, whereas patients who are subtherapeutic are at risk for developing thromboembolism.
   a. Indications are atrial fibrillation (AF), ACS, heart failure (HF), prosthetic heart valve, stroke, DVT, PE, and antiphospholipid syndrome.
   b. Advantages include the following:
      i. Large body of clinical experience.
      ii. Greater efficacy than other oral anticoagulants in patients with prosthetic heart valve.
      iii. Low cost and wide availability.
      iv. Reversal treatments with vitamin K and/or fresh frozen plasma (FFP), or prothrombin complex concentrates (contain four vitamin K–dependent clotting factors II, VII, IX, and X).
   c. Disadvantages include the following:
      i. Requires frequent monitoring of international normalized ratio (INR), with associated cost and burden.
      ii. Dosing is affected by illness, changes in diet, and interactions with numerous different medications.
      iii. Higher rates of thromboembolic and bleeding complications in patients with AF.
4. Direct thrombin inhibitors bind directly to prevent thrombin from cleaving fibrinogen to fibrin. Parenteral forms are bivalirudin and argatroban.
   a. Bivalirudin and argatroban are indicated for patients undergoing a percutaneous coronary intervention (PCI) and management of patients who are HIT+. Monitored by either aPTT or ACT.
   b. The oral formulation, dabigatran, is indicated to reduce the risk of systemic embolism and stroke in patients with nonvalvular AF. It is also indicated in the treatment of DVT and PE in patients who have been treated with a parental anticoagulant for 5 to 10 days.
5. Direct Xa inhibitors bind directly to prevent factor Xa from cleaving prothrombin to thrombin. There is no parenteral formulation available. The oral formulation includes rivaroxaban, apixaban, and edoxaban.
   a. Indications for direct Xa inhibitors include VTE prophylaxis (nonorthopedic and orthopedic, individuals with or without cancer), AF, ACS, and HIT. Not for use in patients with mechanical prosthetic heart valves, severe kidney disease, severe hepatic impairment, pregnancy, or antiphospholipid syndrome.

6. The oral preparations of either direct thrombin inhibitors or direct Xa inhibitors are known as direct oral anticoagulants (DOACs).
   a. Advantages of DOACs include:
      i. Lower risk of bleeding than VKAs.
      ii. Possible lower risk of fracture than VKA has been identified in several retrospective studies
      iii. Less laboratory monitoring.
   b. Disadvantages of DOACs include:
      i. Not recommended for mechanical prosthetic heart valves, in pregnancy, severe hepatic disease, or antiphospholipid syndrome.
      ii. More expensive than VKAs. No generic equivalents.
      iii. Not titratable for patients with an aggressive hypercoagulable state who would need a higher level of therapeutic dosing.

DRUG ALERT Oral anticoagulants should be discontinued preoperatively according to manufacturer guidelines (based on half-life) and according to discussion between the primary health care team and surgeon or proceduralist to reduce the risk of thrombus in the preoperative phase and hemorrhage in the intraoperative phase.

Nursing and Patient Care Considerations

Administering UFH and LMW Heparin

Obtain baseline coagulation studies, including prothrombin time (PT) and aPTT to ensure the patient does not have an underlying coagulopathy, as well as complete blood count to evaluate for anemia or platelet abnormality.

1. Obtain creatinine level prior to LMW heparin therapy to ensure kidney function.
2. In some patients, checking liver function test (specifically transaminases) may be appropriate.
3. Weigh the patient before initiating therapy. Dosing may be calculated based on the patient's weight.
4. For continuous IV UFH administration:
   a. Nomograms may be based on the aPTT or anti-factor Xa activity and are either weight based or non-weight based. Low-, standard-, or high-goal therapies may be used based on the indication for therapy and the patient's risk for bleeding.
   b. Use a continuous infusion pump.
   c. Verify the concentration and dose of heparin programmed against the chosen nomogram. This may involve an independent double check by another nurse with initiation, dose change, and a new bag.
   d. Monitor aPTT and/or anti-Xa levels and adjust dosing according to the nomogram.
5. LMW heparin is administered in fixed or weight-based doses, adjusted for renal function.
6. When transitioning UFH to a VKA, it is important to overlap heparin with warfarin generally 4 to 5 days and at least 24 hours of a therapeutic INR before discontinuing heparin.
7. When transitioning UFH to a DOAC, IV heparin can be stopped when the first dose of DOAC is given. When transitioning from LMW heparin, the DOAC is given right before the next dose of LMW heparin is scheduled.

Administering Other Anticoagulants

1. Administer fondaparinux daily as ordered, from preloaded syringe, subcutaneously into the abdomen, alternating sides.
2. Administer warfarin daily at the same time, usually in the late afternoon or evening, in case INR monitoring done earlier indicates the need for modification in dose. Monitor INR routinely, and with change in other medication or dietary intake that may affect therapeutic level, as directed.
3. Administer DOACs according to order, based on indication and patient characteristics. Edoxaban can be administered daily and apixaban is usually twice daily. Rivaroxaban and dabigatran may be ordered as either once or twice daily. Apixaban dosage may be reduced in patients age 80 or older, in those weighing less than or equal to 60 kg, and with creatine greater than or equal to 1.5 mg/dL.

DRUG ALERT Be aware that dabigatran needs to stay in original container and has a 60-day shelf life.

Monitoring Clotting Profiles

1. aPTT is the coagulation test used to monitor the anticoagulation effects of UFH.
   a. Therapeutic aPTT is 2 to 2½ times the control.
   b. Obtain aPTT levels per nomogram or order and adjust dosage accordingly.
2. PT and INR are the coagulation tests used to monitor the anticoagulation effects of VKAs.
   a. Therapeutic INR is 2 to 3, or 2.5 to 3.5 for higher intensity therapeutic range.
   b. Obtain PT/INR levels daily or as ordered. Warfarin dose will be adjusted to achieve the desired level of anticoagulation.
   c. Possible drug–drug or food–drug interactions may require more frequent monitoring.
3. Other laboratory studies to monitor as ordered:
   a. Platelet count—to monitor for occurrence of HIT, indicated by a 50% decrease in platelet count or steady down trending results.
   b. Hemoglobin and hematocrit—baseline and periodically to monitor for anemia due to occult or overt bleeding.
   c. Fibrinogen—if abnormal bleeding occurs on UFH.
4. No monitoring of aPTT or other coagulation tests are required for LMW heparin, factor Xa inhibitors, or direct thrombin inhibitors; however, aPTT may be monitored for LMW heparin therapy in patients with renal disease and in patients weighing less than 50 kg or more than 80 kg.

Preventing Bleeding

1. Follow precautions to prevent bleeding.
   a. Handle patient carefully while turning and positioning.
   b. Maintain pressure on IV and venipuncture sites for at least 5 minutes after removal. Apply ice if patient is prone to bleeding.
   c. Assist with ambulation and implement fall precautions.
2. Observe carefully for any possible signs of bleeding and report immediately so that anticoagulant dosage may be reviewed and altered, if necessary:
   a. Hematuria—frank blood in urine or microhematuria as detected on the test strip.
   b. Melena—dark/tarry stools; use test cards for occult blood.
   c. Hemoptysis—frank blood in emesis; use test cards for occult blood.
   d. Bleeding gums—note any pink saliva or frank bleeding with dental hygiene.
   e. Epistaxis—frequent/persistent nosebleeds.
   f. Bruising/hematomas—inspect skin carefully.

3. Have on hand the antidotes to reverse anticoagulants being used (see Table 10-1, page 296).
   a. Heparin—protamine sulfate, by IV injection.
   b. Warfarin—phytonadione (vitamin K_1, AquaMEPHYTON); oral or IV and dose is dependent on the INR level and the degree or risk of patient bleeding.
   c. Dabigatran—idarucizumab by IV injection.

CLINICAL JUDGMENT When epidural anesthesia or spinal puncture is employed, anticoagulants increase the risk of epidural or spinal hematoma, which may result in paralysis. Anticoagulants may be held before procedures, but even slight risk of bleeding should be taken seriously. Monitor these patients closely for sensory and motor dysfunction.

POPULATION AWARENESS There is a risk of bleeding in any patient receiving anticoagulants; however, advanced age and hypertension increase the risk of intracerebral hemorrhage. Any fall in an older adult that may involve the head, or a fall with head injury at any age, may require computed tomography (CT) imaging.

Patient Education and Health Maintenance

1. Instruct patient about taking anticoagulants.
   a. Follow instructions carefully and take medications exactly as prescribed. Know the strength and the look of the pill (color, shape). If you miss a dose or accidentally take more than you were supposed to, refer to your medication instructions or call your provider.
   b. Notify all health care providers, including dentist, that you are taking anticoagulants.
   c. Avoid foods that may alter the effects of anticoagulants or, if used, should be used regularly (every day, if possible): green, leafy vegetables, fish, liver, green tea, and tomatoes.
   d. Take medications at the same time each day and do not stop taking them unless directed by health care provider, even if symptoms of thrombus/embolus are not present.
   e. Use a pill minder to stay organized. One exception is that dabigatran should remain in the original bottle or package it came in.
   f. Wear a medical identification bracelet or carry a card indicating the name of the anticoagulants and dose and include name, address, and telephone number of your health care provider.
2. Advise the patient to notify the health care providers of the following:
   a. All medications, both prescribed and over-the-counter (OTC) (including vitamins and herbal supplements), that patient is currently taking.
   b. Accidents, infections, excessive diarrhea, and other significant illnesses that may affect the patient's ability to take the anticoagulant and/or the risk for developing a thrombosis.
   c. When scheduling invasive procedures by other health care providers, including routine dental examinations and other dental procedures, cardiac catheterizations, or surgical procedures, inform the team that you are taking anticoagulants. Have the surgical/procedure team consult with your primary health care provider about what is an acceptable time to stop your anticoagulant for the procedure and when to restart the medication after the procedure.
   d. Discuss with your health team if you plan to get pregnant. Some anticoagulants are not recommended during pregnancy.
3. Advise the patient to avoid:
   a. Taking any other medications without first checking with health care provider, particularly:
      i. Vitamins, especially if they contain vitamin K.
      ii. Herbal supplements.
      iii. Aspirin or nonsteroidal anti-inflammatory drugs (NSAIDs).
      iv. Mineral oil (can decrease absorption of vitamin K).
      v. Cold medicines and antibiotics.
      vi. Oral contraceptives and hormones.
      vii. Anti-reflux medicines.
      viii. Oral antifungals.
   b. Excessive use of alcohol; may affect your ability to clot; check on acceptable limits for social drinking.
   c. Participation in activities in which there is a high risk of injury (e.g., contact sports).
   d. Foods that may cause diarrhea or upset stomach or sudden changes in your diet.
   e. Shaving with a sharp razor.
4. Instruct the patient to be alert for these warning signs:
   a. Excessive bleeding that does not stop quickly (such as following shaving, a small cut, bleeding gums, nosebleed).
   b. Excessive menstrual bleeding.
   c. Skin discoloration or bruises that appear suddenly—particularly on the fingers and toes or deep purple spots anywhere on the body ("blue toe syndrome").
   d. Black or bloody stools; for questionable stool discoloration, test for occult blood.
   e. Vomit that is bloody or looks like coffee grounds.
   f. Blood in urine.
   g. Faintness, dizziness, or unusual weakness.
   h. Severe headache.
5. Stress the importance of close follow-up and adherence with periodic laboratory work for blood clotting profiles, need to notify health care provider if unable to keep scheduled appointments, and contact provider with questions about dosage.

Thrombolytic Therapy

Thrombolytic agents activate plasminogen to form plasmin, which accelerates lysis of thromboemboli. Most commonly used agents include recombinant tissue plasminogen activator (tPA), streptokinase, and recombinant human urokinase. These agents are only available in parenteral formulation. Currently, the most commonly used agent in the United States is tPA (alteplase). It is administered either systemically or by catheter-directed therapy depending on the indication.

Clinical Indications

1. Acute PE (see page 168)—limited to patients with pulmonary and hemodynamic compromise. Many centers have PE response teams for rapid diagnosis and management, including to determine if patient is a candidate for thrombolytic therapy.

EVIDENCE BASE Zuo, Z., Yue, J., Dong, B. R., Wu, T., Liu, G. J., & Hao, Q. (2021). Thrombolytic therapy for pulmonary embolism. *Cochrane Database of Systematic Reviews, 4*(4), CD004437. https://doi.org/10.1002/14651858.CD004437.pub6

Table 10-1 Guide to Anticoagulants

DRUG	CONTRAINDICATIONS AND PRECAUTIONS	MONITORING	ANTIDOTE	OTHER CONSIDERATIONS
Unfractionated heparin (UFH)	• Allergy • Acute major bleeding • Thrombolytic therapy given within past 24 h in patient with stroke • Be aware that HIT most frequently develops 1–2 wk after starting therapy	• Get baseline complete blood count, platelet count, prothrombin time/INR, and creatinine before starting therapy; liver function tests and albumin with suspected liver disease. • Daily aPTT or heparin assay. • Monitor platelet count every other day (for HIT).	• Protamine sulfate IV over 10 min. • Risk for anaphylaxis is 1%.	• Generally safe in pregnancy unless patient has mechanical heart valve. • Safe in the patient who breastfeeds. • Monitor for HIT: reaction at injection site, systemic reaction after bolus injection, 50% decrease in platelets.
Low-molecular-weight heparins (LMWH)	• Allergy • Acute major bleeding • Thrombolytic therapy given within past 24 h in patient with stroke • HIT • Renal failure	• Same baseline as UFH. • Monitor platelet count every 2–3 d if also receiving UFH.	• No agent for complete reversal. • Protamine sulfate provides for 60%–75% reversal.	• Generally safe in pregnancy unless patient has mechanical heart valve. • Generally safe in the patient who breastfeeds. • Monitor for HIT.
Factor Xa inhibitors	• Allergy • Acute major bleeding • Thrombolytic therapy given within past 24 h in patient with stroke • Renal failure	• Same baseline as UFH. • No routine monitoring of PTT or INR. • Fondaparinux: monitor heparin assay regularly in those with renal insufficiency, body weight <50 kg, or those with obesity.	• No antidote for apixaban, edoxaban. • Idarucizumab is the reversal agent for dabigatran; 5-g dose (2–50 mL vials of 2.5 g) given IV. • Fondaparinux: possible partial reversal with recombinant factor VIIa. • Rivaroxaban: activated charcoal to reduce absorption in overdose.	• Safety not known in pregnancy or breastfeeding. • Use cautiously in bacterial endocarditis, uncontrolled hypertension, and other conditions. • Increased risk of bleeding in renal or hepatic impairment. • Risk of spinal or epidural hematoma with spinal procedures.
Warfarin sodium	• Allergy • Hemorrhage • Pregnancy	• Same baseline as UFH. • Monitor INR daily to every few days until stable and then monthly (best time is at least 16 h after last dose). • If starting medication that can affect warfarin, check INR in 3–4 d.	• Vitamin K orally or IV over 60 min. • May lead to warfarin resistance and thromboembolism. • Transfusion of fresh frozen plasma may be given.	• Only small amount secreted in breast milk. • Hold for 4 d prior to surgery. • Increased risk of thromboembolism if INR <1.7; increased risk of bleeding if INR >4.0. • Purple toe syndrome may occur 3–10 wk after starting therapy. • Numerous drug and food interactions.
Direct thrombin inhibitors	• Allergy • Active bleeding	• Assess baseline renal function, and annually if creatinine clearance <50 mL/min or age >75 yr.	• No known antidote. • About 60% of drug may be cleared with dialysis over 3–4 h. • Transfusion of fresh frozen plasma or packed red cells may be given.	• Safety not known in pregnancy or breastfeeding. • Risk of bleeding increases with age. • Consult medication reference for drug interactions.

HIT, heparin-induced thrombocytopenia; INR, international normalized ratio; IV, intravenous; PTT, partial thromboplastin time.

2. Acute occlusion of peripheral arteries/prosthetic grafts.
3. DVT (popliteal, femoral, or iliofemoral)—limited to severe symptomatic swelling or limb-threatening ischemia. Catheter-directed therapy is preferred due to the reduced risk of major bleeding.
4. Acute ST elevation MI when PCI is not readily available (see page 245).
5. Stroke (see page 345).

Contraindications

Absolute Contraindications

1. Intracranial neoplasm.
2. Recent (<2 months) intracranial or spinal surgery or trauma.
3. History of hemorrhagic stroke.
4. Active bleeding or bleeding diathesis or nonhemorrhagic stroke within the previous 3 months.

Relative Contraindications

1. Severe uncontrolled hypertension.
2. Nonhemorrhagic stroke more than 3 months prior.
3. Surgery within the previous 10 days.
4. Pregnancy.

Nursing and Patient Care Considerations

1. Obtain complete blood count (CBC) and coagulation studies prior to initiation and during therapy.
2. Monitor for allergic reactions presenting as new rash, fever, and/or chills.
3. Be aware that minor bleeding during thrombolytic therapy is common and is not generally an indication to stop therapy. This usually occurs at site of invasive procedures such as IV puncture sites.
4. During the infusion, monitor the patient closely for stability, development of neurologic deficits, obvious bleeding, and hemodynamic changes indicative of bleeding. Notify the provider immediately and be prepared to stop the thrombolytic therapy.
5. Ensure that blood type and screening are current and that cross-matched blood is on hold in the blood bank for immediate access. If refractory bleeding persists after therapy stops, FFP and/or cryoprecipitate may be given.
6. If given for acute ST elevation MI, monitor the electrocardiogram (ECG) for dysrhythmias, return of ST changes, and/or chest pain.
7. If given for arterial or venous thrombosis of an extremity, monitor the extremity for color, temperature, sensation, a reduction in swelling, and pain level. Assess pulses by manual palpation or by Doppler to ensure that arterial flow is intact. A venogram is generally performed 12 to 24 hours after initiating therapy to decide whether therapy needs to continue or stop.
8. Minimize invasive procedures during therapy.

POPULATION AWARENESS Risk of major bleeding from thrombolytic therapy increases with age greater than or equal to 65. Use of catheter-directed therapy reduces that risk.

Care of the Patient Undergoing Vascular Surgery

Vascular surgery may involve operations of the arteries, veins, or lymphatic system. Surgery may be performed on an urgent basis, as in *thoracoabdominal or abdominal aortic repair* for aortic dissection or *embolectomy* for acute arterial embolism. Surgery can also be elective for *vein ligation and stripping* for varicose veins after conservative management fails. Other vascular procedures include *thrombectomy* and *vena cava filter insertion* for venous problems and *arterial bypass grafting* (aortoiliac, aortofemoral, femoral–femoral, femoropopliteal, and femoral–distal), *endarterectomy, endovascular grafting,* and *percutaneous transluminal angioplasty (PTA)* for arterial problems with or without placement of an intraluminal stent.

Preoperative Management

1. Additional health conditions, such as heart disease, hypertension, hypercholesterolemia, diabetes mellitus, and chronic lung disease, are fully evaluated, and management is adjusted to decrease intraoperative risks and postoperative complications.
2. Skin alterations are assessed preoperatively, and impairment is minimized through protection of the affected parts, treatment with antibiotics, and proper positioning to enhance circulation (elevated for venous and lymphatic problems, level or slightly dependent for arterial problems).
3. Nutritional status is assessed and improved preoperatively to aid in wound healing postoperatively.
4. Risk factors for vascular disease, such as smoking, obesity, and sedentary lifestyle, are reviewed, and patient teaching is initiated to prevent the recurrence or progression of vascular disorder.
5. The patient is prepared emotionally and physically for surgery, with teaching focusing on postoperative care including frequent circulation and wound checks, and prevention of complications, such as bleeding, infection, and neurovascular compromise. Discharge education will cover follow-up appointments, risk factor modification, and medication changes.

Postoperative Management

1. After revascularization, peripheral pulses are assessed distal to the operative site to ensure adequate tissue perfusion using Doppler. Sensation, range of motion, color, temperature, and pulses should be assessed on the affected extremity after surgery.
2. If revascularization was obtained with the use of bypass graft, the graft site is protected and assessed for patency as well.
3. Endovascular and PTA procedures are less invasive but require careful monitoring of the catheter incision site for bleeding, in addition to peripheral circulation.
4. Surgical incisions are assessed for redness, drainage, and approximation and may be covered with dry dressings, and possible incisional wound vacuum devices.
5. Patients are positioned to promote circulation, reduce swelling, and maintain skin integrity.
6. Anticoagulation may be continued but increases the chance of bleeding following surgery.
7. Hydration, nutrition, and oxygenation are promoted to ensure wound healing.
8. Breathing exercises using an incentive spirometer are performed every 2 hours while patient is awake to prevent postoperative pulmonary complications.

CLINICAL JUDGMENT Be alert for postoperative complications, which may be generalized or specific to the type of surgery. Postoperative MI; neurologic, pulmonary, or renal complications; thromboembolism; hemorrhage;

compartment syndrome; and hyperperfusion syndrome may result in the patient who has undergone vascular surgery.

CLINICAL JUDGMENT If severe headache on the operative side occurs after a carotid procedure, report immediately. Cerebral hyperperfusion syndrome is a rare but life-threatening complication that may result up to 1 month after surgery when increased carotid blood flow leads to cerebral edema and bleeding. Permanent disability and death may result. Close monitoring of blood pressure and treatment of hypertension are also important.

Nursing Interventions

Promoting Tissue Perfusion

1. Maintain dressing or compression bandages, as directed.
2. Monitor for bleeding through dressing—reinforce and notify the surgeon, as indicated.
3. Monitor for hematoma formation beneath the skin—increased pain and swelling. Apply pressure and notify the surgeon.
4. Measure vital signs frequently for tachycardia and hypotension, which may indicate hemorrhage.
5. Perform frequent neurovascular checks on involved extremity. Check warmth, color, capillary refill, sensation, movement, and pulses; compare with the other side.
6. Position as directed—usually legs elevated and fully supported.

Preventing Infection

1. Maintain IV infusion or heparin lock for antibiotic administration, as ordered, and assess daily for signs of infiltration and infection.
2. Check incision site for drainage, warmth, and erythema, which indicate infection.
3. Change incision dressing, as ordered and as needed, for drainage or soiling.
4. Monitor temperature for elevation.
5. Monitor hematologic profiles for elevation in white blood cell (WBC) count.

Relieving Pain

1. Assess pain level and administer analgesic as ordered.
2. If patient-controlled anesthesia is being used, instruct patient on use and make sure the pump is functioning properly.
3. Position for comfort, using pillows for support.
4. Watch for adverse effects of opioids, such as hypotension, respiratory depression, nausea and vomiting, and constipation.
5. Time pain medication before activity or treatments, if possible.
6. Instruct patient in alternative coping methods such as visualization and muscle relaxation.

Minimizing Immobility

1. Encourage isometric and range-of-motion (ROM) exercises while on bed rest.
   a. Exercise affected extremity by pushing the foot into footboard, making a fist, or simply contracting muscles without movement if approved by the surgeon.
   b. Perform full ROM of other extremities.
2. Encourage ambulation as soon as allowed.
   a. Avoid dangling legs because of possible compression against the back of the bed or chair.
   b. Avoid long periods of sitting or standing.
   c. Encourage multiple short periods of walking throughout the day.

Patient Education and Health Maintenance

1. Discuss individualized risk factors with the patient and caregiver. Advise the patient to reduce weight, eat a healthy diet, increase activity, stop smoking, and take prescribed medicines for hypertension, hypercholesterolemia, and diabetes.
2. Refer patient to vascular rehabilitation (if available), physical therapy, and occupational therapy as indicated.
3. Instruct patient and caregiver in care of incision and wound at home. Make sure that patient has supplies and resources for additional help available.
4. Instruct patient and caregiver on signs of infection, graft failure, or worsening circulatory compromise that should be reported.
5. For venous or lymphatic surgeries, instruct patient about wearing compression stockings or garments, or applying elastic wrap bandages, if ordered. Have patient perform return demonstration.
6. For arterial surgeries, instruct patient to avoid restrictive clothing (including socks, hose, and shoes), especially over areas of revascularization.
7. Instruct patient to inspect feet (using a mirror, if necessary), including plantar aspect and between toes, daily and to inspect shoes for foreign objects, such as small stones, before putting them on.
8. Instruct patient to wear thick socks and well-fitting shoes with wide toe box to avoid the development of breakdown/ulceration on pressure points. Instruct patient not to wear sandals or walk barefoot.
9. Review any medications, especially anticoagulants.
10. Make sure that the patient knows when and where to follow up.

Evaluation: Expected Outcomes

- Affected extremity with good color, capillary refill, and pulses; warm and sensitive to touch; moving adequately.
- Incision site is well approximated and without signs and symptoms of infection.
- Reports adequate pain control on current regimen.
- Mobility, including ambulation, returning to baseline, without difficulty or shows signs of progressing independence with the assistance of physical or occupational therapy.

CONDITIONS OF THE ARTERIES

See additional online content, Patient Education Guidelines 10-1, 10-2, and 10-3.

Arteriosclerosis and Atherosclerosis

Arteriosclerosis is an arterial disease manifested by a loss of elasticity and a hardening of the vessel wall. This "hardening of the arteries" causes a restriction in blood flow. The damage can be caused by hypercholesterolemia, hypertension, and diabetes, or can be a result of heredity factors.

Atherosclerosis is the most common type of arteriosclerosis, manifested by the formation of atheromas (patchy lipoidal degeneration of the intima). Lesions, or plaques, form throughout the arterial wall, reducing the size of the vessel and limiting the flow of blood. The process begins in early childhood; over time, atherosclerotic lesions can completely occlude the lumen by buildup of the plaque material and may contribute to thrombus formation. Atherosclerosis commonly affects the heart and brain leading to ischemic heart disease (IHD) and ischemic stroke, the world's first and fifth causes of death, respectively. Approximately 5 million people in the United States have atherosclerosis.

Pathophysiology and Etiology

1. Multiple factors that are interrelated are thought to contribute to atherosclerosis including:
   a. Endothelial dysfunction—vasodilator dysfunction caused by the loss of endothelial-derived nitric oxide is an initial step in atherosclerosis; occurs as a result of risk factors including hypercholesterolemia, oxidized low-density lipoprotein (LDL), diabetes, hypertension, and smoking.
   b. Dyslipidemia.
      i. High levels of LDL cholesterol accumulate in the macrophages (foam cells) and in the lipid core of the plaque.
      ii. Cholesterol accumulation in foam cells leads to mitochondrial dysfunction, apoptosis, and necrosis, which results in the release of cellular proteases, inflammatory cytokines, and prothrombotic molecules.
   c. Inflammatory and immunologic factors:
      i. Inflammation is seen in the earliest histologic studies. Macrophages that have ingested oxidized LDL release a variety of inflammatory substances, cytokines, and growth factors.
      ii. These inflammatory substances, cytokines, and growth factors disrupt the endothelium-dependent vasodilation potentially through a decrease in available nitric oxide.
   d. Plaque rupture—acute coronary and cerebrovascular syndromes are typically due to rupture or erosion of plaques leading to thrombosis.
   e. Smoking:
      i. Cigarette smoking decreases endothelium-dependent vasodilation and availability of platelet-derived nitric oxide.
      ii. There is also an increase in multiple inflammatory markers including C-reactive protein, interleukin-6, and tumor necrosis factor-alpha, an increase in fibrinogen levels, and a decreased in fibrinolysis.
      iii. Finally, cigarette smoking increases the oxidation of LDL and decreases the activity of paraoxonase that protects against LDL oxidation.
2. The pathologic process may affect the coronary, cerebral, peripheral, or aortic arterial systems. There are two types of atherosclerotic lesions: fatty streaks and fibrous plaques (see Figure 10-1).
3. Risk factors include age, diabetes, high blood pressure (BP), high levels of cholesterol and triglycerides, smoking, diet high in saturated fats and trans-fatty acids, heredity conditions such as hypercholesterolemia, obesity, physical inactivity, and a family history of atherosclerosis in a male under 55 or a female under 65.

Clinical Manifestations

1. Symptoms and signs are based on the area affected (the entire vascular system or one segment may be affected).
   a. Brain (cerebral and carotid arteries)—transient ischemic attacks (TIAs); stroke; vision disturbances, such as amaurosis fugax (one type of TIA), which is described by patients as a shade over a portion of eye (see Chapter 11).
   b. Heart (coronary artery disease [CAD])—angina, myocardial infarction (MI), and heart failure (see Chapter 9).
   c. Gastrointestinal (GI) tract (aortic occlusive disease, aortic aneurysm, and mesenteric ischemia)—abdominal pain, unintentional weight loss, and lower back pain.
   d. Kidneys (renal artery stenosis)—renal insufficiency and poorly controlled hypertension.
   e. Extremities (peripheral arterial disease [PAD])—intermittent claudication (pain in a muscle associated with exercise caused by lack of oxygen to the muscle), pain at rest, tissue loss (with or without the presence of infection or gangrene), and embolic events.
2. Decreased or absent pulses; bruits of major vessels.

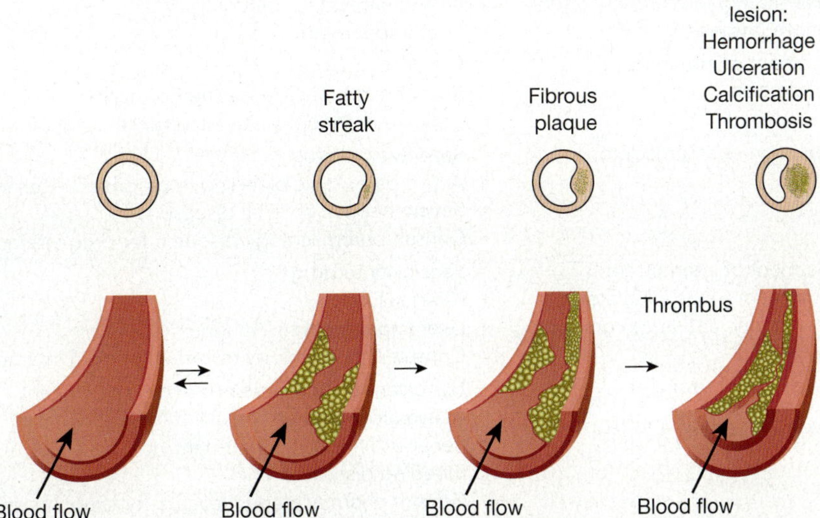

Figure 10-1. Atherosclerosis is a progressive process that occurs over decades. The earliest lesion is a fatty streak, which may regress or progress to a fibrous plaque. Irreversible fibrous plaques may eventually develop into atheroma, which may be complicated by hemorrhage, ulceration, calcification, and thrombus. Target organ disease includes myocardial infarction, stroke, and peripheral arterial occlusion.

Diagnostic Evaluation

Specific to body system affected:

1. Arteriography of the involved area may show stenosis and increased collateral circulation.
2. Computed tomography (CT) scan.
3. Magnetic resonance imaging (MRI)/magnetic resonance angiography (MRA).
4. Noninvasive testing of the vascular system: duplex studies, sequential Doppler studies, pulse volume resistance, and ankle–brachial index (ABI).
   a. For ABI, systolic pressure of the posterior tibial and dorsalis pedis arteries is determined by Doppler for each side as measures of ankle pressure.
   b. The greater ankle systolic pressure for each side is divided by the brachial systolic pressure of the same side. Normally, the systolic pressures are equal. In the presence of atherosclerotic disease, the pressure below an occluded area is less than the arm pressure.
   c. Normal ABI is 1.00 to 1.40.
   d. Result below 0.90 indicates obstruction of the lower extremity arteries.
   e. Result greater than 1.40 indicates noncompressible vessels because of calcification, so ABI cannot be interpreted.
5. Electrocardiogram (ECG), Holter monitoring, exercise stress testing, echocardiogram, cardiac CT, cardiac MRI, and cardiac catheterization may be done to evaluate CAD.

Management

Medical Management

1. Modification of risk factors—stress reduction, improvement in sleep, weight loss, moderate- to high-intensity exercise, dietary changes, and monitoring for type 2 diabetes.
2. Prescriptive management—anticoagulants, antiplatelet therapy (see Table 10-2), lipid-lowering agents, and antihypertensives.
3. Specific treatment for end-organ dysfunction—see cerebrovascular insufficiency (page 345), CAD (page 239), and peripheral arterial occlusive disease (page 301).
4. Vascular rehabilitation/exercise.

Surgical Management

1. Endovascular procedures:
   a. Percutaneous transluminal angioplasty (PTA) with or without placement of intraluminal stent—to relieve arterial stenosis when lesions are accessible, as in superficial femoral and iliac arteries, through the use of special inflatable balloon catheters and metal stents.

Table 10-2 Antiplatelet Therapy

Antiplatelet therapy is used to prevent platelet aggregation and thrombus formation. It is used in the treatment of cerebrovascular disease, coronary artery disease, and intermittent claudication. This table lists some common antiplatelet medications, their indications, and potential contraindications/precautions.

MEDICATION	USE	CONTRAINDICATIONS/PRECAUTIONS
Aspirin	Prevention of MI, TIA, stroke	• Allergy to ASA • Active gastric ulcers
Ticlopidine	Prevention of stroke	• Sensitivity to drug • Neutropenia, thrombocytopenia, history of TTP, active bleeding disorders[a] • Liver and renal impairment • Consult pharmacology resource for drug interactions
Ticagrelor	Decreased platelet aggregation Prevention of MI/coronary artery stent thrombosis	• Sensitivity to drug • GI and intracranial bleeding • Liver impairment
Pentoxifylline	Treatment of intermittent claudication	• Sensitivity to drug • Recent cerebral or retinal hemorrhage • Caffeine or theophylline intolerance
Clopidogrel	Reduction of atherosclerotic events	• Sensitivity to drug • Active pathologic bleeding (e.g., peptic ulcer, intracranial hemorrhage) • Severe hepatic or renal disease • Consult pharmacology resource for drug interactions
Cilostazol	Treatment of intermittent claudication—has antiplatelet, vasodilatory, and antithrombotic effects	• Sensitivity to drug • Heart failure • Liver impairment • Consult pharmacology resource for drug interactions
Dipyridamole, 200 mg; aspirin, 25 mg	Prevention of stroke	• Hypersensitivity reaction to either component • Active ulcer disease • Renal and hepatic impairment • Bleeding disorders • Consult pharmacology resource for drug interactions

ASA, acetylsalicylic acid; GI, gastrointestinal; MI, myocardial infarction; TIA, transient ischemic attack; TTP, thrombotic thrombocytopenia.

[a]Monitor complete blood count and platelet count every 2 weeks.

b. Endovascular grafting—placement of prosthetic graft via a transluminal approach. Graft material covers a metallic stent, which may or may not be impregnated with medication to decrease failure. The stent is placed via femoral artery or radial artery and is deployed. This is commonly used for abdominal aortic aneurysms, renal arteries, and mesenteric and iliac arteries.
c. Rotational atherectomy—high-speed rotary cutter that removes lesions by abrading plaque. Benefits of this therapy are minimal damage to the normal endothelium and low incidence of complications.
d. Laser angioplasty—amplified light waves are transmitted by fiberoptic catheters. Laser beam heats the tip of a percutaneous catheter and vaporizes the atherosclerotic plaque.

2. Surgical revascularization of the affected vessels, including:
   a. Embolectomy—removal of blood clot from the artery.
   b. Thrombectomy—removal of thrombus from the artery.
   c. Endarterectomy—removal of atherosclerotic plaque from the artery.
   d. Bypass—use of a graft, either vein graft or prosthetic material, to route blood flow around the blocked area.

Complications

Long-term complications of atherosclerosis are related to the specific body system affected:

1. Brain—long- and short-term disabilities associated with stroke.
2. Heart—stable or unstable angina, MI, and heart failure.
3. Aorta—aneurysms (thoracoabdominal, abdominal), ischemic bowel, impotence, renal failure, and loss of kidney.
4. Lower extremities—intermittent claudication, nonhealing ulcers, infections or gangrene, and amputation.

Nursing Interventions and Patient Education

See "Care of the Patient Undergoing Vascular Surgery," page 297. In addition, attention is directed at reducing risk factors to halt the process, through smoking cessation, stress reduction, weight reduction, optimal control of hypertension (see page 318) and diabetes (see Chapter 21), diet modification to reduce cholesterol, and lipid-lowering therapy (see page 254).

Peripheral Arterial Disease

PAD is a form of arteriosclerosis in which the peripheral arteries become blocked. Chronic occlusive arterial disease occurs much more frequently than does acute occlusion (which is the sudden and complete blocking of a vessel by a thrombus or embolus). Patients at increased risk for PAD include those with the following risk factors: aged 50 or older; being African American; having a personal or family history of coronary or peripheral artery disease; having diabetes, hypertension, hyperlipidemia, abdominal obesity, a blood clotting disorder, or kidney disease; and having a history of smoking or tobacco use.

PAD and coronary artery disease are related diseases. Not only do they share risk factors but a patient who has PAD has a higher risk of CAD, MI, and a TIA or stroke than a patient without PAD. A patient with heart disease has a one in three chance of having PAD in their lower extremities.

EVIDENCE BASE Abramson, B. L., Al-Omran, M., Anand, S. S., Albalawi, Z., Coutinho, T., de Mestral, C., Dubois, L., Gill, H. L., Greco, E., Guzman, R., Herman, C., Hussain, M. A., Huckell, V. F., Jetty, P., Kaplovitch, E., Karlstedt, E., Kayssi, A., Lindsay, T., Mancini, G. B. J., ... Virani, S. (2022). Canadian Cardiovascular Society 2022 Guidelines for peripheral arterial disease. *Canadian Journal of Cardiology, 38*(5), 560–587. https://doi.org/10.1016/j.cjca.2022.02.029

Pathophysiology and Etiology

1. Most commonly caused by atherosclerosis with contributing risk factors as discussed in the previous section.
2. May involve the following vessels in isolation or combination:
   a. Aortoiliac system—from the renal arteries to iliac arteries.
   b. Femoral arteries—superficial femoral, profunda femoris.
   c. Popliteal artery.
   d. Trifurcating vessels—anterior tibial, posterior tibial, and peroneal arteries.
   e. Dorsalis pedis artery.
   f. Pedal arch.
3. Lesions tend to form at areas of bifurcation of the vessels.
4. Pattern of disease differs in those without diabetes and those with diabetes:
   a. Without diabetes—disease usually involves macrocirculation (larger vessels [e.g., aorta, iliac, femoral arteries]) and is more common in isolated segments.
   b. With diabetes—disease usually involves microcirculation (smaller vessels [e.g., popliteal, tibial, peroneal, and small vessels in the foot/digits]) and occurs in more diffuse segments.

POPULATION AWARENESS Diabetes is considered a major risk factor for PAD. Patients with diabetes are three times more likely to develop PAD than patients without diabetes. Diabetes also increases the risk of critical limb ischemia, lower extremity amputation, restenosis rates, cardiovascular event rates, longer hospital stays, impaired daily physical activity, and mortality.

5. PAD can be categorized based on the level of symptoms that a patient reports. The Fontaine Stages are:
   a. Asymptomatic.
   b. IIa: Mild claudication (leg pain during exercise).
   c. IIb: Moderate to severe claudication.
   d. III: Ischemic rest pain.
   e. IV: Ulcers or gangrene.
6. Thromboangiitis obliterans (Buerger disease) is a nonatherosclerotic type of PAD that is caused by an inflammatory process of small- to medium-sized arteries and veins in the extremities.
   a. The thrombus is a highly cellular and inflammatory plaque, and the blood vessel wall is spared from the damage seen with an atherosclerotic plaque.
   b. This disease is associated with heavy cigarette smoking and is seen most commonly in young patients under the age of 45 years.
   c. Patients present with distal extremity ischemia, ischemic digit ulcers, or gangrene.

Clinical Manifestations

Symptoms appear gradually and are specific to the area affected.

Aortoiliac

1. Mesenteric ischemia, pain after eating that increases as the disease progresses.
2. Unintentional weight loss.

3. Renal insufficiency.
4. Poorly controlled hypertension.
5. Impotence.
6. Intermittent claudication (including gluteal claudication).

Femoral, Popliteal, and Distal Arteries

1. Intermittent claudication (calf, thigh, and foot).
2. Pain at rest—associated with severe arterial ischemia. Severe pain in feet aggravated by elevation of lower extremity. Pain is relieved by placing foot in a dependent position.
3. Dependent rubor—dusky purple color of extremity when in dependent position; changes to pallor when elevated.
4. Numbness or tingling of feet or toes.
5. Trophic changes associated with tissue malnutrition:
   a. Hair loss.
   b. Thick toenails.
   c. Thin, shiny skin.
   d. Cool temperature of extremity.
6. Tissue loss or nonhealing ulcers, which may develop wet or dry gangrene (see Figure 10-2). Arterial ulcers are usually painful, pale, and have well-demarcated (punched-out) edges.

Diagnostic Evaluation

Noninvasive

1. Vascular physical examination.
2. ABI—see page 300; may be done before and after exercise.
   a. A toe brachial index (TBI) should be measured in patients who have suspected PAD when the resting ABI is greater than 1.40.
   b. This is particularly useful in patients with diabetes as the associated increased calcification of the distal arteries may artificially elevate the ABI result.
3. Doppler ultrasound—decreased velocity of flow through a stenotic vessel or no flow with total occlusion.
4. Segmental plethysmography/pulse volume recordings (PVR)—decreased pressure distal to the region of occlusion.

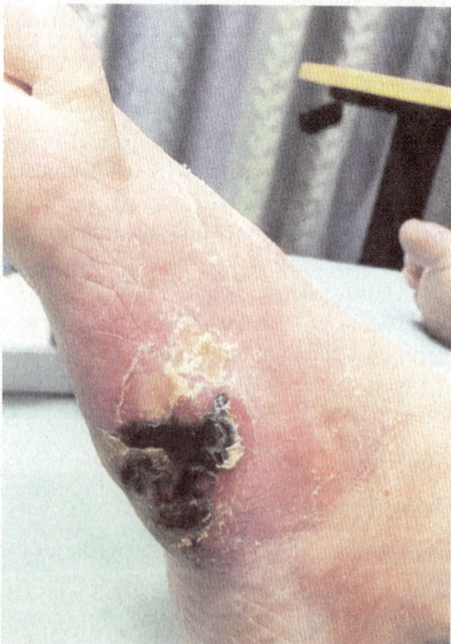

Figure 10-2. Arterial ulcer.

Invasive

1. Computed tomography angiography (CTA) to obtain a three-dimensional view of artery and occlusion.
2. MRA to confirm occlusion.
3. Angiography to confirm occlusion.

Management

Management Goals for Patient With PAD

1. Reestablish blood flow to areas of critical ischemia.
2. Preserve the extremity.
3. Relieve pain associated with intermittent claudication or pain at rest.
4. Provide sufficient blood flow for wound healing.

Lifestyle Management

1. Tobacco cessation.
2. Dietary modification—high fiber, low cholesterol/fat and sodium.
3. Exercise—including a structured walking plan to improve endurance.
4. Weight management.
5. Manage other health conditions such as hypertension, diabetes, and hypercholesterolemia/hyperlipidemia.
6. Manage stress levels.
7. Practice good foot and skin care.

Pharmacologic Management

1. Antiplatelet therapy—medications like aspirin or clopidogrel can be used to decrease the risk of thromboembolic events (see page 300).
2. Antihypertensive therapy (see page 320).
3. Cholesterol reduction—statins are the first line for treatment. Statins lower serum lipids but also slow the progression of carotid atherosclerosis (see page 75).
4. Antidiabetic agents—patients can be prescribed oral antidiabetic agents or insulin based on hemoglobin A1C and fasting and postprandial glucose levels.
5. Treatment of other underlying risk factors (i.e., smoking cessation products).
6. Medication, such as cilostazol, for relief of intermittent claudication.

Surgical Management

1. Minimally invasive procedures—endovascular procedures, such as atherectomy or angioplasty with or without stenting, may be used alone or with revascularization surgery for dilatation of localized noncalcified segments of narrowed arteries.
2. Peripheral artery bypass surgery may be required. There are many different options for bypass grafting depending on the level of disease.
3. Amputation (see page 858) is usually the last option for patients when the affected extremity has severe infection and gangrene, failed attempts at revascularization, or when revascularization is not considered a viable option.

Hyperbaric Management

1. Hyperbaric oxygen therapy may be used for nonhealing wounds and gas gangrene. This is limited to centers that have a hyperbaric oxygen chamber (most commonly used for diving accidents).
2. Increased atmospheric pressure inside the chamber combined with 100% oxygen delivery allows for greater concentration of oxygen to be delivered to all parts of the body.

3. Typical treatment programs last 2 hours, five or six times per week for 4 weeks or more.
4. Adverse effects include pressure or popping in ears, slight lightheadedness at the end of treatment sessions, and possible temporary change in vision.

Complications

1. Swelling, bleeding, or pain around the incision or at the puncture site if a percutaneous procedure was performed.
2. Peripheral edema.
3. Ulceration with slow healing.
4. Gangrene, sepsis.
5. Severe occlusion may necessitate limb or partial limb amputation.

Nursing Assessment

1. Auscultate the abdomen and listen for the presence of bruits.
2. Observe lower extremities for capillary refill, color, sensation, and temperature. Compare bilaterally for differences.
3. Palpate pulses (see Figure 10-3) and record. If pulses are nonpalpable, attempt to locate the pulse with a handheld Doppler. About 10% of people have absent dorsalis pedis artery from birth.
4. Inspect nails for thickening and opacity; inspect skin for shiny, atrophic, hairless, and dry appearance—reflect chronic changes.

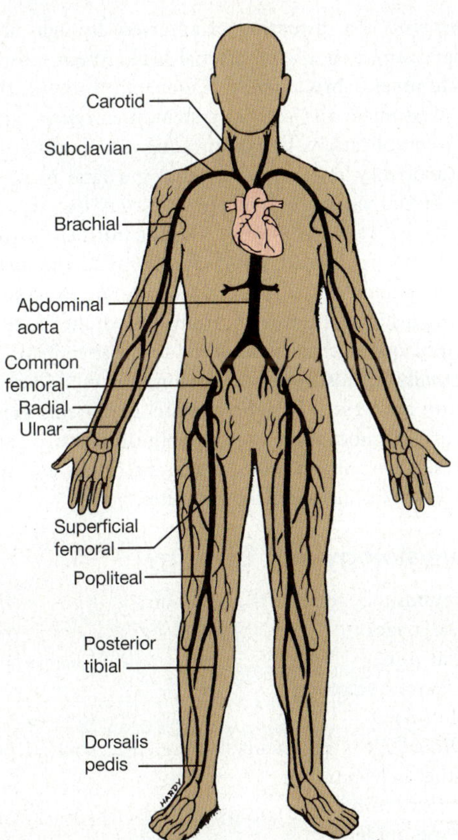

Figure 10-3. Salient points in evaluating peripheral arterial insufficiency. Reduced or absent femoral pulses indicate aortoiliac disease. Absent popliteal pulses indicate superficial femoral occlusion. Pulse deficits in one extremity, with normal pulses in the contralateral extremity, may suggest acute arterial embolus. Absent pedal pulses indicate tibioperoneal artery involvement.

5. Assess for pain:
   a. Severe abdominal pain after eating.
   b. Pain in legs with exercise.
   c. Pain in feet at rest.
6. Assess for ulcers of toes and feet.

CLINICAL JUDGMENT Have a high index of suspicion for PAD in patients with a history of smoking. Current or previous tobacco use is the most important risk factor for PAD and the complications associated with PAD. Tobacco use increases the risk for PAD by 400%.

Nursing Interventions

Promoting Tissue Perfusion

1. Perform frequent neurovascular checks of the affected extremity.
2. Inspect lower extremity and feet for new areas of ulceration or extension of existing ulceration.
3. Provide and encourage a well-balanced diet to enhance wound healing.
4. Encourage walking or performance of range-of-motion (ROM) exercises to increase blood flow, which will increase collateral circulation.
5. Administer or teach self-administration of pain medication to achieve a comfort level conducive to ambulation.

Protecting Lower Extremities

1. Encourage patient to wear protective footwear, such as rubber-soled slippers or shoes with closed, wide toe box when out of bed.
2. Instruct patient and family to keep hallways and walkways free of clutter to avoid injury.
3. Avoid tight-fitting socks and shoes.
4. Instruct patient to avoid sitting with legs crossed.
5. Avoid using adhesive tape and harsh soaps on the affected skin.
6. Instruct patient to check temperature of bath water with thermometer or forearm before entering the tub.
7. Perform and teach foot care, including washing, carefully drying, and inspecting feet daily.

Preventing Infection

1. Apply moisturizing lotion to intact skin of lower extremities to prevent drying and cracking of the skin.
2. Encourage patient to wear clean hose or socks daily: woolen socks for winter and cotton for summer.
3. Teach patient to:
   a. Trim toenails straight across after soaking the feet in warm water.
   b. Place wisps of cotton under the corner of great toenail if there is a tendency toward ingrown toenails.
   c. Have a podiatrist treat corns and calluses; do not use corn pads or strong medications.
4. Teach patient signs to report:
   a. Redness, swelling, irritation, blistering, and foul odor.
   b. Itching, burning, and rashes.
   c. Bruises, cuts, and unusual appearance of the skin.
   d. New areas of ulceration.
5. Instruct patient to check with health care provider before using any over-the-counter (OTC) or topical lotions or creams on the wound.
6. Administer antibiotics postoperatively to prevent infection around prosthetic graft material.

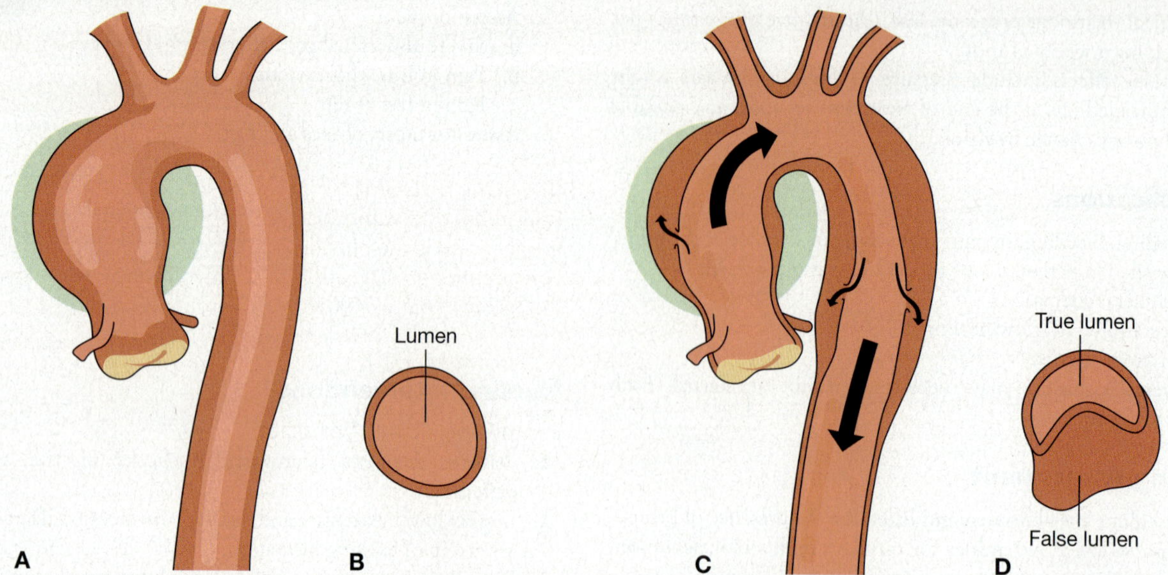

Figure 10-4. Aortic aneurysm and dissection: **(A)** ascending thoracic aortic aneurysm, **(B)** enlarged lumen, **(C)** dissection through intima and media, **(D)** expanding false lumen. (A: Shutterstock/logika600)

Patient Education and Health Maintenance

1. Instruct patient on the importance of walking to improve circulation; set up a plan for incremental increase in distance.
2. Instruct patient not to sit or stand in one position for long periods.
3. Instruct patient, when sitting, to keep knees below the level of the hips to avoid hip flexion.
4. Instruct patient to avoid tight-fitting clothing (e.g., elastic-topped socks or clothing made out of Lycra/Spandex), especially over area of graft placement.
5. Instruct patient not to cross legs when sitting or lying down.
6. Instruct patient on methods to promote vasodilation by keeping extremity warm and stopping use of other vasoconstricting substances such as caffeine.
7. Instruct patient on the importance of daily foot care.
8. Encourage patient to stop smoking.
9. Encourage follow-up for control of chronic conditions and ongoing risk factor management.

Evaluation: Expected Outcomes

- No new ulcer formation.
- Verbalizes the importance of wearing protective shoes and washing and inspecting feet daily.
- No signs of infection of lower extremities.

Aneurysm

EVIDENCE BASE Isselbacher, E. M., Preventza, O., Hamilton Black, J., Augoustides, J. G., Beck, A. W., Bolen, M. A., Braverman, A. C., Bray, B. E., Brown-Zimmerman, M. M., Chen, E. P., Collins, T. J., DeAnda, A., Fanola, C. L., Girardi, L. N., Hicks, C. W., Hui, D. S., Schuyler Jones, W., Kalahasti, V., Kim, K. M., ... Woo, Y. J. (2022). 2022 ACC/AHA guideline for the diagnosis and management of aortic disease: A report of the American Heart Association/American College of Cardiology Joint Committee on Clinical Practice Guidelines. *Circulation, 146*(24), e334–e482. https://doi.org/10.1161/cir.0000000000001106

An *aneurysm* is a distention of an artery brought about by a weakening/destruction of the arterial wall. Aneurysms are lined with intraluminal debris, such as plaque and thrombi. Because of the high pressure in the arterial system, aneurysms can enlarge, producing complications by compressing surrounding structures; left untreated, they may rupture, causing a fatal hemorrhage. A dissection occurs when the layers of the artery become separated. Blood flows between the layers, causing further disruption of the arterial wall (see Figure 10-4). Additionally, the intraluminal thrombus may totally occlude the artery, leading to acute ischemia to all arteries distal to the area of thrombosis, or they may embolize clot and/or plaque to the arteries distal to the aneurysm.

The *aorta* is the most common site for aneurysms; however, they may form in any vessel. Peripheral vessel aneurysms may involve the renal artery, subclavian artery, popliteal artery, or any major artery. These aneurysms produce a pulsating mass and may cause pain or pressure on surrounding structures.

Pathophysiology and Etiology

1. Aneurysms may form as the result of:
   a. Older age.
   b. Male sex.
   c. Cigarette smoking.
   d. Heredity.
   e. Other large artery aneurysms (e.g., iliac, femoral, popliteal).
   f. Atherosclerosis.
   g. Hypertension.
   h. Hyperlipidemia.
   i. Diabetes.
   j. Trauma.
   k. Immunologic conditions.
   l. Obesity.
2. False aneurysms (pseudoaneurysm) are associated with trauma to the arterial wall, as in blunt trauma or trauma

associated with arterial punctures for angiography and/or cardiac catheterization.

3. The ascending aorta and the aortic arch are the sites of greatest hemodynamic stress and are the most common sites of arterial dissection.
4. Morphologically, aneurysms may be classified as follows:
   a. Saccular—distention of a vessel projecting from one side.
   b. Fusiform—distention of the whole artery (i.e., entire circumference is involved).
   c. Dissecting—hemorrhagic or intramural hematoma, separating the medial layers of the aortic wall.
5. Aneurysms of the thoracic aorta are classified as:
   a. Ascending aortic aneurysms—aortic valve to brachiocephalic trunk (innominate artery).
   b. Aortic arch aneurysms—thoracic aneurysm involving the brachiocephalic vessels.
   c. Descending aortic aneurysms—distal to left subclavian artery.
   d. Thoracoabdominal aneurysms.
6. Abdominal aortic aneurysms are described based on the involvement of the renal or visceral arteries:
   a. Suprarenal aneurysm—involves the origins of one or more visceral arteries but does not extend into the thoracic region.
   b. Pararenal aneurysm—renal arteries arise from the aneurysmal aorta, but the aneurysm does not extend to the level of the mesenteric arteries.
   c. Juxtarenal aneurysm—the aneurysm begins just after the renal arteries.
   d. Infrarenal aneurysm—the aneurysm begins distal to the renal arteries.

Clinical Manifestations

Aneurysm of the Thoracoabdominal Aorta

For some people, chest pain is the first and only sign of a thoracic aortic aneurysm.

1. Pulse and BP difference in upper extremities if aneurysm interferes with circulation in the left subclavian artery.
2. Pain and pressure symptoms.
3. Constant, boring pain because of pressure.
4. Intermittent and neuralgic pain because of impingement on nerves.
5. Dyspnea, causing pressure against trachea.
6. Cough, often paroxysmal and brassy in sound.
7. Hoarseness, voice weakness, or complete aphonia, resulting from pressure against recurrent laryngeal nerve.
8. Dysphagia because of impingement on esophagus.
9. Edema of chest wall—infrequent.
10. Dilated superficial veins on the chest.
11. Cyanosis because of vein compression of chest vessels.
12. Ipsilateral dilation of pupil because of pressure against cervical sympathetic chain.
13. Abnormal pulsation apparent on chest wall because of erosion of aneurysm through rib cage—in syphilis.

Abdominal Aneurysm

1. Many of these patients are asymptomatic.
2. Abdominal pain most common, either persistent or intermittent—often localized in middle or lower abdomen to the left of midline.
3. Lower back and flank pain caused by pressure on the spine from enlarging aneurysm.
4. Feeling of an abdominal pulsating mass, palpated as a thrill, auscultated as a bruit.
5. Hypertension.
6. Distal variability of BP; pressure in arm greater than the thigh.
7. Upon rupture, will present with hypotension and/or hypovolemic shock.

Diagnostic Evaluation

1. Abdominal or chest x-ray may identify asymptomatic aneurysms.
2. CT scanning and ultrasonography are used to detect and monitor the size of aneurysm.
3. MRI/MRA can determine diameter, define anatomy, and identify rupture or dissection.
4. Spiral CT gives a three-dimensional view of the aneurysm and any atherosclerosis of arteries.
5. Contrast arteriography allows visualization of aneurysm and vessel. However, this should be used with caution in patients with connective tissue disorders due to the risk of injury or dissection.
6. Evaluation for genetic syndrome if thoracic aortic aneurysm/dissection presents at a young age, including Marfan syndrome (most common), Ehlers–Danlos syndrome, Loeys–Dietz syndrome, and Turner syndrome. If one or more first-degree relatives are found to have thoracic aortic dilatation, aneurysm, dissection, an abdominal aortic aneurysm, or brain aneurysm, then referral to a geneticist is recommended. Family members (biological siblings, biological children) may also require genetic screening. Family members with the genetic mutation should undergo aortic imaging.

Management

Surveillance

1. For thoracoabdominal aortic aneurysms:
   a. In patients with a dilated thoracic aorta, monitor by transthoracic echocardiogram, CT scan, or MRI in 6 to 12 months.
   b. If aneurysm is stable, surveillance imaging can be performed every 6 to 24 months depending on diameter.
2. For abdominal aortic aneurysms:
   a. For small aneurysms (3.0 to 3.9 cm) monitor by CT imaging every 3 years.
   b. For aneurysms 4.0 to 4.9 cm in males and 4.0 to 4.4 cm in females, monitor by CT imaging every 12 months.
   c. For aneurysms greater than or equal to 5.0 cm in males or greater than or equal to 4.5 cm in females, monitor by CT imaging every 6 months.
3. An aortic aneurysm diameter of greater than or equal to 5.5 cm meets the criteria for elective surgical repair. The risk for aortic dissection or rupture increases with increasing aneurysm diameter and with increasing rate of growth.

Surgery

1. Open repair of aneurysm—method of choice in patients requiring aortic root replacement and/or aortic valve replacement. This will require cardiopulmonary bypass.
2. Endovascular repair of aneurysm—this is called a TEVAR (for thoracic endovascular aortic repair) or EVAR (for endovascular aortic repair) using a stent graft, which is deployed via the iliac or femoral artery. It attaches above and below the aneurysm, and it redirects the flow of blood away from the aneurysm.

3. Thoracic aneurysms are the most difficult to treat, but endovascular grafting is possible. One concern during any thoracic aneurysm repair is blood flow to the brachiocephalic (innominate) artery. Its vertebral branch supplies the spinal cord, and interruption in flow can cause permanent paralysis.

Other Interventions

1. Smoking cessation.
2. Aggressive BP control with medications including beta-blockers, angiotensin-converting enzyme (ACE) inhibitors, and angiotensin receptor blockers (ARBs).
3. Activity restrictions—patients with aneurysms often are restricted from participating in contact sports or heavy weight lifting.

Complications

1. Fatal hemorrhage.
2. Myocardial ischemia.
3. Stroke.
4. Paraplegia (decreased perfusion of spine as complication of repair because of interruption of anterior spinal artery).
5. Abdominal ischemia.
6. Ileus.
7. Graft occlusion.
8. Graft infections.
9. Acute renal failure.
10. Impotence.
11. Lower extremity ischemia.

Nursing Assessment

1. In patients with thoracoabdominal aortic aneurysm, be alert for sudden onset of sharp, ripping, or tearing pain located in the anterior chest, epigastric area, shoulders, or back, indicating acute dissection or rupture.
2. In patients with abdominal aortic aneurysm, assess for abdominal (particularly left lower quadrant) pain and intense lower back pain caused by rapid expansion. Be alert for syncope, tachycardia, and hypotension, which may be followed by fatal hemorrhage because of rupture.

Nursing Interventions

Maintaining Perfusion of Vital Organs

Preoperatively:

1. Assess for chest pain and abdominal pain.
2. Prepare patient for diagnostic studies or surgery, as indicated.
3. Monitor for signs and symptoms of hypovolemic shock.
4. Perform mental status and neurologic assessment regularly.

Postoperatively:

1. Monitor vital signs frequently.
2. Assess for signs and symptoms of bleeding:
   a. Hypotension.
   b. Tachycardia.
   c. Tachypnea.
   d. Diaphoresis.
3. Monitor laboratory values, as ordered.
4. Monitor urine output hourly.
5. Assess abdomen for bowel sounds and distention. Observe for diarrhea, which occurs sooner than one would expect return of bowel function.
6. Perform regular neurovascular checks on distal extremities.
7. Assess feet for signs and symptoms of embolization:
   a. Cold feet.
   b. Cyanotic toes or patchy blue areas on the plantar surface of feet.
   c. Pain in feet.
8. Maintain intravenous (IV) infusion to administer medications to control BP and provide fluids postoperatively.
9. Position patient to avoid hip flexion, keeping knees below the level of the hips when sitting in a chair.
10. If thoracoabdominal aneurysm repair has been performed, monitor for signs and symptoms of spinal cord ischemia:
    a. Pain.
    b. Numbness.
    c. Paresthesia.
    d. Weakness.

Preventing Infection

1. Monitor temperature.
2. Monitor changes in white blood cell (WBC) count.
3. Monitor incision for signs of infection.
4. Administer antibiotics, if ordered, to prevent bacterial seeding of the graft.

Relieving Pain

1. Administer pain medication, as ordered, or monitor patient-controlled analgesia.
2. Keep head of bed elevated no more than 45 degrees for the first 3 days postoperatively to prevent pressure on the incision site.
3. Rarely—administer nasogastric decompression for ileus following surgery, until bowel sounds return.
4. Assess abdomen for bowel sounds and distention.

Patient Education and Health Maintenance

1. Instruct patient about medications to control BP and the importance of taking them.
2. Discuss disease process and signs and symptoms of expanding aneurysm or impending rupture, or rupture, to be reported.
3. For postsurgical patients, discuss warning signs of postoperative complications (fever, inflammation of operative site, bleeding, and swelling).
4. Encourage adequate balanced intake for wound healing.
5. Encourage patient to maintain an exercise schedule postoperatively.
6. Instruct patient that due to use of a prosthetic graft to repair the aneurysm, prophylactic antibiotics will be used for invasive procedures, including routine dental examinations and dental cleaning for 6 to 12 months after aneurysm repair.
7. Make all patients aware that a one-time screening for abdominal aortic aneurysm by ultrasound has been recommended for males ages 65 to 75 who ever smoked. If the patient has an aortic aneurysm, members of the family over age 55 of any gender should be screened with ultrasound to rule out abdominal aortic aneurysm.
8. Encourage genetic counseling and testing if there is suspicion of a genetic/familial component.

Evaluation: Expected Outcomes

- No change in mental status, bowel sounds, vital signs, or urine output.
- Afebrile and no signs of infection.
- Reports control of pain with medication.

Acute Arterial Occlusion

Acute arterial occlusion is the sudden interruption of blood flow, which may cause complete or partial obstruction of the artery. There is no time for the development of collateral circulation. Critical ischemia of the extremity develops and may result in loss of affected extremity and/or death.

Pathophysiology and Etiology

1. Embolization is the most common cause of acute arterial occlusion.
2. Emboli may consist of thrombus, atheromatous debris, or tumor.
3. Emboli most commonly originate in the heart as a result of atrial fibrillation, MI, or heart failure (~85%) but can also occur after invasive procedures, such as cardiac catheterization, angiography, and surgery.
4. Arteriosclerosis may cause roughening or ulceration of atheromatous plaques, which can lead to emboli.
5. May also be associated with immobility, anemia, and dehydration.
6. Emboli tend to lodge at bifurcations and areas of atherosclerotic narrowing.
7. Other causes of acute occlusion include:
   a. Trauma.
   b. Thrombus.
   c. Venous outflow obstruction, which includes compartment syndrome.

Clinical Manifestations

1. Acute pain due to associated vasomotor spasm.
2. Paralysis of part.
3. Anesthesia of part.
4. Pallor and coldness.
5. Edema.
6. Rigidity of extremity.
7. Pulselessness.

Diagnostic Evaluation

1. Neurovascular assessment of the affected area.
2. Doppler ultrasonography, segmental limb pressure, and pulse volume recordings may indicate decreased flow.
3. Arteriography confirms diagnosis.
4. MRA or spiral CT confirms diagnosis and gives a three-dimensional view of the area.
5. Digital subtraction angiography, MRA, and MRI may be done for cerebral embolization.

Management

1. Drug therapy—anticoagulants (see page 292) and thrombolytics (see page 295).
2. Surgery:
   a. Intra-arterial thrombolysis—percutaneous catheter delivers thrombolytic directly into an artery to break down the thrombus.
   b. Embolectomy (see Figure 10-5) must be performed within 6 to 10 hours to prevent muscle necrosis and loss of extremity.
   c. Transcatheter embolectomy—percutaneous catheter that will directly aspirate the embolus. This is often done in conjunction with thrombolysis or angioplasty and stenting.

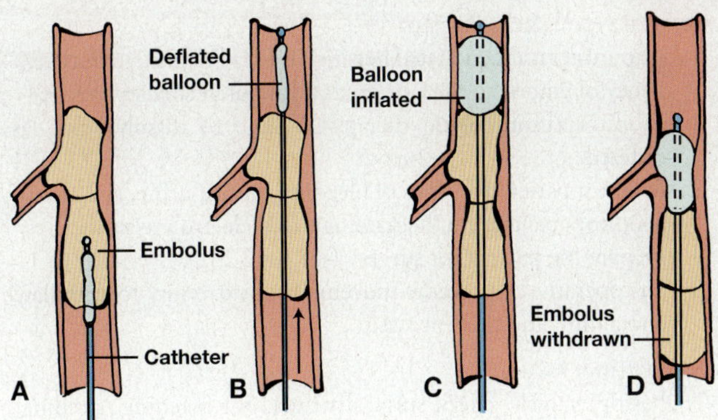

Figure 10-5. Extracting an embolus from a vessel can be done with the use of a Fogarty embolectomy catheter. The catheter, with a soft, deflated balloon near the tip, is threaded through the artery via an arteriotomy. **(A, B)** It is passed through the embolus and its thrombus; **(C)** it is then inflated. **(D)** A steady pull downward withdraws the embolus along with the catheter.

   d. Fasciotomy—incisions made over leg compartments to aid the expansion of edematous tissue and relief of pressure on the arterial system.
   e. Amputation of the affected limb if revascularization is inappropriate due to metabolic complications.
3. Support of BP.

Complications

1. Irreversible ischemia and loss of extremity.
2. Metabolic complications:
   a. Acidosis.
   b. Hyperkalemia.
   c. Renal failure.
3. Shock.

Nursing Assessment

1. Assess for acute, severe pain.
2. Assess for gradual or acute loss of sensory and motor function.
3. Check for aggravation of pain by movement of and pressure on the extremity.
4. Palpate for loss of distal pulses.
5. Inspect for pale, mottled, and numb extremity.
6. Inspect for collapse of superficial veins because of decreased blood flow to the extremity.
7. Inspect for sharp line of color and temperature demarcation. This may occur distal to the site of occlusion as a result of ischemia.
8. Assess for edema.

Nursing Interventions

Protecting the Extremity

1. Protect extremity by keeping it at or below the body's horizontal plane.
2. Protect leg from hard surfaces, tight or heavy surfaces, and tight or heavy overlying bed linens.
3. Handle extremity gently and prevent pressure or friction while repositioning.
4. Administer pain medications, as ordered.

Promoting Tissue Perfusion

1. Administer unfractionated heparin (UFH) IV line to reduce tendency of emboli to form or expand (useful in smaller arteries).
2. Monitor thrombolytic therapy IV line to dissolve clot, as ordered.
3. Monitor patient for signs of bleeding (gums, urine, and stool).
4. Monitor coagulation, hematology, and electrolyte studies.
5. Prepare the patient for surgery (see page 231).
6. Postoperatively, promote movement of extremity to stimulate circulation and prevent stasis.

Preventing Infection

1. Postoperatively, check surgical wound for bleeding, swelling, erythema, and discharge.
2. Maintain IV infusion or venous access device to administer IV antibiotics, if indicated.
3. Continue to monitor the patient for tachycardia, fever, pain, erythema, warmth, swelling, and drainage at the incision site.

Patient Education and Health Maintenance

1. Teach prevention techniques, such as daily aerobic activity, observation for skin breakdown, and prevention of injury.
2. Teach patient the medical regimen and importance of taking prescribed medications, such as oral anticoagulants, to prevent reembolization.
3. Encourage patient to report symptoms of arterial occlusion: paralysis, numbness, tingling, pallor, and coldness of the extremity.

Evaluation: Expected Outcomes

- Patient reports no pain; no injury noted.
- Limb has normal color, sensation, movement, and temperature.
- No signs of infection.

Vasospastic Disorder (Raynaud Phenomenon)

Raynaud phenomenon is a vasospastic disorder that is brought on by an unusual sensitivity to cold, emotional stress, or autoimmune disorders. It is termed primary Raynaud disease when it is idiopathic and unaccompanied by other systemic manifestations. It is termed secondary Raynaud syndrome when it is associated with autoimmune disorders.

Pathophysiology and Etiology

1. The condition is a form of intermittent arteriolar vasoconstriction that results in coldness, pallor, and numbness of fingertips, toes, or tip of the nose with sharply demarcated color changes and a rebound circulation with redness and pain.
2. The cause is unknown, although it may be secondary to connective tissue and other immunologic disorders such as scleroderma, systemic lupus, polymyositis, and Sjögren syndrome.
3. Episodes may be triggered by emotional factors or by unusual sensitivity to cold.
4. Most common in females between ages 16 and 40 and seen much more commonly in cold climates and during the winter months.

Clinical Manifestations

1. Intermittent arteriolar vasoconstriction resulting in coldness, numbness, paresthesias, pallor, and pain when blood flow resumes.
2. Involvement of the fingers appears to be asymmetric; thumbs are less often involved.
3. Characteristic color changes: white–blue–red (see Figure 10-6).
   a. White—blanching, dead-white appearance if spasm is severe.
   b. Blue—cyanotic, relatively stagnant blood flow.
   c. Red—a reactive hyperemia on rewarming.
4. Episodes may last several minutes to several hours.
5. Occasionally, there is ulceration of the fingertips (most common in autoimmune disorders).

Diagnostic Evaluation

1. There are no simple office tests that can be used to diagnose Raynaud phenomenon.
2. Patients are asked three questions:
   a. Are your fingers unusually sensitive to cold?
   b. Do your fingers change color when exposed to cold?
   c. If the fingers change color, do they turn white, blue/purple, or both?
3. Tests may be done to rule out secondary disease processes, such as chronic arterial occlusive or connective tissue disease.
4. Noninvasive blood flow tests for finger pressures and arterial waveforms may be done.

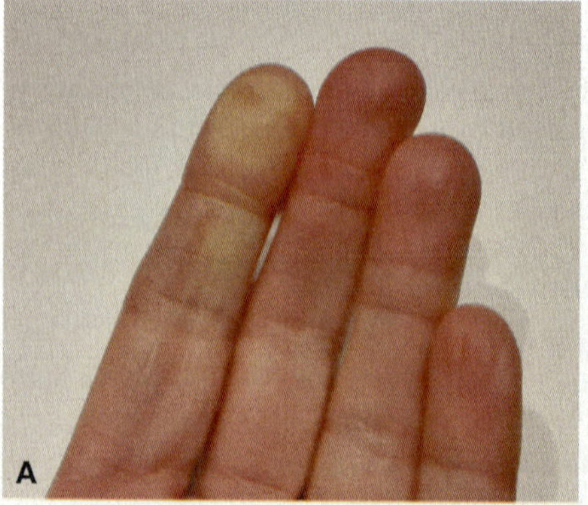

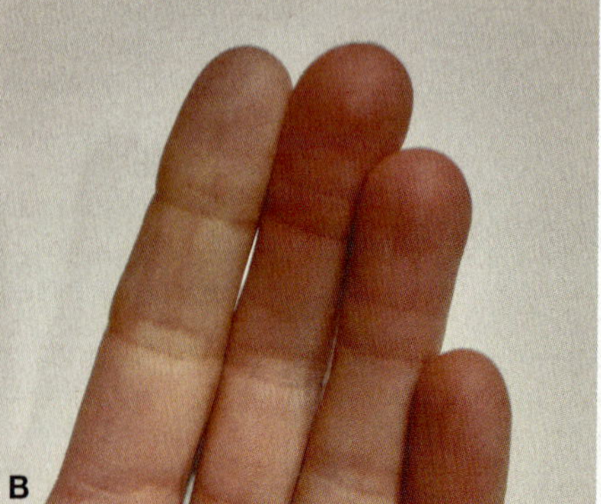

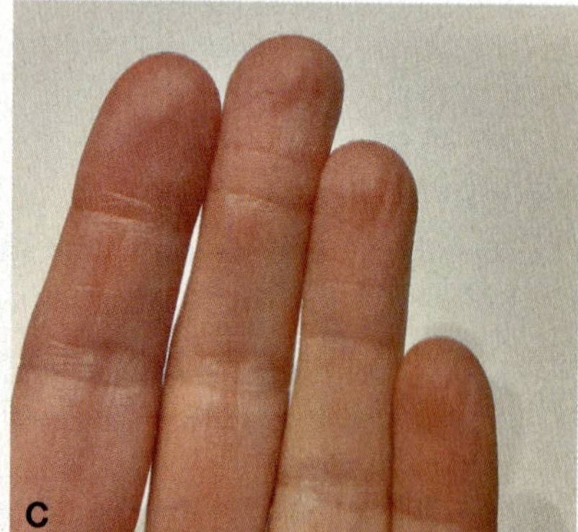

Figure 10-6. Raynaud phenomenon shows color changes through progression of episodes (note the tip of the index finger): **(A)** white (pallor due to spasm), **(B)** blue (cyanosis), **(C)** red (hyperemia). Middle finger also shows color change from earlier spasm: resolving cyanosis **(A)**, hyperemia **(B)**, return to normal color **(C)**.

Management

1. Avoidance of trigger and aggravating factors.
2. Protection of the fingers and toes with warm mittens (not gloves) and warm boots in cold weather.
3. Control or limitation of emotional stress.
4. Avoidance of vasoconstricting medications such as OTC nasal decongestants, medications for attention deficit hyperactivity disorder (ADHD), and medications used for migraine headaches.
5. Smoking cessation.
6. Longer acting calcium channel blockers (e.g., amlodipine or nifedipine) are frequently used to prevent or reduce vasospasm.
7. Phosphodiesterase type 5 inhibitors (e.g., sildenafil) cause vasodilatation.
8. Nitroglycerin, angiotensin II receptor blockers (e.g., losartan), or selective serotonin reuptake inhibitors (e.g., fluoxetine) may be helpful for some. Adverse effects, such as headache, dizziness, and orthostatic hypotension, may be prohibitive.

Complications

1. Chronic disease may cause atrophy of the skin and muscles.
2. Ulceration and gangrene (rare).

Nursing Assessment

1. Perform thorough history and review of systems for clues to underlying disorder.
2. Assess for blanching of digits when exposed to cold. Color turns cyanotic and then red with normal temperature.
3. Note whether warmth brings about symptom relief.

Nursing Interventions

Minimizing Vasospasm

1. Assist patient in avoiding skin exposure to cold; for example, use mittens to handle cold items (water pitcher, refrigerated items). Always dress warmly with insulated, water- and wind-resistant garments for outside in the cold, including warm hat, mittens, coat, socks, and boots. Battery-operated gloves and handwarmers are available.
2. Encourage patient to stop smoking.
3. Help patient to understand the need to avoid stressful situations and offer options for stress management.
4. Teach rewarming techniques—warm water, holding fingers in axillary or groin areas.
5. Administer and teach patient about drug therapy.
6. Instruct patient about the need to take drugs every day to prevent or minimize symptoms.
7. Monitor for orthostatic hypotension when initiating drug therapy.
8. Advise patient that episode may be terminated by placing hands (or feet) in warm water.

Relieving Pain

1. Explain to patient that pain may be experienced when spasm is relieved—hyperemic phase.
2. Administer or teach self-administration of analgesics.
3. Reassure patient that pain is temporary; persistent pain, ulceration, or signs of infection should be reported.

Patient Education and Health Maintenance

1. Avoid whatever provokes vasoconstriction of vessels of hands.
2. Prevent injury to hands, which can aggravate vasoconstriction and lead to ulceration.
3. Minimize exposure to cold because this precipitates a reaction. Avoid wet and windy environments.
4. Advise wearing warm clothing—boots, mittens, and hooded jackets—when going out in cold weather and waterproof clothing when raining or snowing.
5. Avoid placing hands in cold water, the freezer, or the refrigerator unless protective mittens are worn.
6. Use extra precautions to avoid injuries to fingers and hands from needlesticks and knife cuts.

Evaluation: Expected Outcomes

- Follows medication regimen, avoiding triggers.
- Reports decreased length of painful phase with episodes.

CONDITIONS OF VEINS

See additional online content: Procedure Guidelines 10-2 and 10-3.

Venous Thrombus

EVIDENCE BASE National Institute for Health and Care Excellence. (2020). *Venous thromboembolic disease diagnosis, management, and thrombophilia testing.* https://www.nice.org.uk/guidance/ng158

See Table 10-3.

There are several types of venous thrombosis:

Phlebitis is an inflammation in the wall of a vein. The term is used clinically to indicate a superficial and localized condition that can be treated with application of heat.

Superficial phlebitis is an inflammation in the wall of a vein in the presence of pain but in the absence of a thrombus (or clot).

Superficial thrombophlebitis is a condition in which a clot forms in a vein secondary to phlebitis. Although superficial thrombophlebitis can be found in any vein, when found in the lower extremities, the term superficial vein thrombosis (SVT) is used to describe

Table 10-3 Comparison of Arterial and Venous Obstruction

FACTOR	ARTERIAL OBSTRUCTION	VENOUS OBSTRUCTION
Onset	May be sudden	Gradual
Color	Pale later—mottled, cyanotic	Slightly cyanotic rubescent
Skin temperature	Cold	Warm
Leg size	May be reduced	Enlarged
Leg hair and nails	Decreased hair; thick, brittle nails	No change
Edema	None to mild	Typically calf to foot
Sensation	Sensory changes	Normal sensation
Arterial pulses	Pulse deficit	Normal
Effect of elevating leg	Condition worsens	Slight improvement

inflammation and thrombus in the great saphenous, accessory saphenous, and small saphenous veins.

Deep vein thrombosis (DVT) is thrombosis of deep rather than superficial veins. Two serious complications are pulmonary embolism (PE) and postthrombotic syndrome.

Pathophysiology and Etiology

General Points

1. Three antecedent factors are believed to play a significant role in the development of venous thromboses: (1) stasis of blood, (2) injury to the vessel wall, and (3) altered blood coagulation (Virchow triad). Thrombosis does not occur with stasis alone.
2. Usually, two of the three factors occur before thrombosis develops.

Thrombosis-Related Situations

1. Venous stasis—following operations, childbirth, or bed rest for any prolonged illness.
2. Prolonged sitting or as a complication of varicose veins.
3. Injury (bruise) to a vein; may result from direct trauma or internal trauma such as from intravenous (IV) catheters, infusion of medications, and/or infiltration of medications.
4. Extension of an infection of tissues surrounding the vessel.
5. Continuous pressure of a tumor, aneurysm, or excessive weight gain in pregnancy.
6. Unusual activity in a person who has been sedentary (particularly heavy lifting or prolonged holding of heavy objects) increases the risk of upper extremity thromboses.
7. Hypercoagulability associated with malignant disease and blood dyscrasias.

High-Risk Factors

1. Malignancy/hypercoagulable states.
2. Previous venous insufficiency.
3. Conditions causing prolonged bed rest—myocardial infarction (MI), heart failure, sepsis, traction, end-stage cancer, and human immunodeficiency virus/acquired immunodeficiency syndrome.
4. Leg trauma—fractures, cast, joint replacements.
5. General surgery—over age 40.
6. Obesity, smoking.
7. Inherited coagulopathy (e.g., antithrombin III deficiency, protein C&S deficiency, factor V Leiden thrombophilia).

Clinical Manifestations

Clinical features vary with site and length of affected vein.

1. DVT may occur asymptomatically or may produce severe pain, fevers, chills, malaise, and swelling and cyanosis of the affected arm or leg. The chief symptom is unilateral limb edema in which the onset is sudden.
2. Superficial thrombophlebitis produces visible and palpable signs, such as heat, pain, swelling, erythema, tenderness, and induration, along the length of the affected vein.
3. Extensive vein involvement may cause lymphadenitis or arterial compromise if the swelling is extensive enough.

Diagnostic Evaluation

1. Venous duplex/color duplex ultrasound—this commonly done, noninvasive test allows for visualization of the thrombus, including any free-floating or unstable thrombi that may cause emboli. It is to detect thrombi of the upper and lower extremities.
2. Compression ultrasound is a quick, simple method using only transducer pressure to survey proximal leg veins. Doppler ultrasound may be added to determine if thrombus is occlusive.
3. Impedance plethysmography—a noninvasive measurement of changes in calf volume corresponding to changes in blood volume brought about by temporary venous occlusion with a high-pneumatic cuff. Electrodes measure electrical impedance as the cuff is deflated. Slow decrease in impedance indicates diminished blood flow associated with thrombus.
4. Venography—IV injection of a radiocontrast agent. The vascular tree is visualized and obstruction is identified.
5. Intravascular ultrasound (IVUS)—a catheter-based intervention for venous thromboembolism (VTE), 360-degree ultrasound imaging of a vein.
6. Coagulation profiles—partial thromboplastin time (PTT), prothrombin time/international normalized ratio (PT/INR), circulating fibrin, monomer complexes, fibrinopeptide A, serum fibrin, high-sensitivity D-dimer, proteins C and S, antithrombin III levels, factor V Leiden, and prothrombin gene mutation. Detect intravascular coagulation or coagulopathies.

Management

Goals of management are to prevent the propagation of the thrombus, prevent recurrent thrombus formation, prevent pulmonary emboli, and limit venous valvular damage.

Anticoagulation

For documented cases of DVT, oral or IV anticoagulation may be used to prevent embolization.

Oral and subcutaneous anticoagulants may be used to prevent DVT related to hip and knee replacement surgery and immobility (see page 63).

Thrombolytic Therapy

May be used in life- or limb-threatening situations (see page 295).

Nonpharmacologic Therapies

For patients with phlebitis and SVT, elevation of the extremity, warm or cool compresses, compression stockings, and pain management are the focus of care.

For patients with an acute DVT of the lower extremity:

1. Ambulation is encouraged in patients who are therapeutically anticoagulated.
   a. Elevation of effected extremity: at least 10 to 20 degrees above the level of the heart to enhance venous return and decrease swelling. The popliteal space should be supported but not constricted.
   b. If the upper extremity is affected, a sling or stockinette attached to an IV pole may be used.
2. Graduated compression stockings: promote venous return and reduce swelling.
   a. Electrically or pneumatically controlled stockings, boots, or sleeve.
   b. Graduated compression can be started after anticoagulation therapy, within 2 weeks of diagnosis, to prevent postthrombotic syndrome and/or to treat the symptoms of postthrombotic syndrome.
   c. Should supply 30 to 40 mm Hg of ankle pressure (see Table 10-4).

Table 10-4 Compression Level for Venous Disorders

LEVEL OF SUPPORT	PRESSURE	INDICATIONS
Mild	15–20 mm Hg	Minor varicose veins; tired, aching legs; minor edema
Moderate	20–30 mm Hg	Moderate to severe varicose veins, phlebitis, moderate edema, post vein ablation
Firm	30–40 mm Hg	Severe varicose veins, active venous ulcer, severe edema, following DVT, post venous surgery
Extra firm	>40 mm Hg	Lymphedema

DVT, deep vein thrombosis.

d. Stockings should be continued for 2 years after diagnosis, be replaced every 6 months, and should be refitted as necessary to ensure the appropriate amount of compression on the limb.

Surgery

1. Placement of a filter into the inferior vena cava to prevent fatal pulmonary embolism in a patient who cannot tolerate prolonged anticoagulant therapy or who has recurrent emboli in the presence of adequate anticoagulation.
2. Thrombectomy may be necessary for severely compromised venous drainage of the extremity.
3. Endovascular thrombolysis with direct catheter-infused lytic therapy to the affected limb.

Complications

1. Pulmonary embolism.
2. Postthrombotic syndrome.

Nursing Assessment

1. Obtain history of risk factors for thrombophlebitis.
2. Note symmetry or asymmetry of legs. Measure and record leg circumferences daily. Acute, unilateral edema may be the first sign of a DVT.
3. Observe for evidence of venous distention or edema, puffiness, stretched skin, and hardness to touch.
4. Examine for signs of obstruction because of occluding thrombus—swelling, particularly in loose connective tissue or popliteal space, ankle, or suprapubic area.
5. Monitor for signs of pulmonary embolus, including shortness of breath, chest pain, and tachycardia.
6. Hand-test extremities for temperature variations—use dorsum (back) of the same hand; first compare ankles, then move to the calf and up to the knee to detect increased inflammation of the vessel.
7. Assess for calf pain, which may be aggravated when the foot is dorsiflexed with the knee flexed. Unfortunately, this sign is nonspecific and has a low sensitivity for detecting thrombophlebitis.
8. Assess all IV catheter insertion sites for signs and symptoms of infection and infiltration.

Nursing Interventions

1. Elevate extremity to promote venous drainage and reduce swelling.
2. Apply warm or cool compresses for patients experiencing phlebitis or SVT.
3. Initiate anticoagulation for patients experiencing DVT, and for patients with SVT at risk of developing DVT, as directed.
4. Administer pain medication as needed.
5. Apply compression stockings after anticoagulation therapy has started and 2 weeks after the identification of a DVT.

Preventing Bleeding

See page 294 for nursing interventions for patients on anticoagulant therapy.

Preventing Other Hazards of Immobility

1. Prevent venous stasis by proper positioning in bed.
   a. Support full length of legs when they are to be elevated.
   b. Prevent pressure injuries that may occur over bony prominences, such as sacrum, hips, knees, and heels. Be aware of bony prominence of one leg pressing on soft tissue of other leg (in side-lying position, place a soft pillow between the legs).
   c. Avoid hyperflexion at knee as in jackknife position (head up, knees up, pelvis, and legs down); this promotes stasis in pelvis and extremities.
2. Encourage mobility to the highest level tolerated by patient and state of anticoagulation.
   a. Encourage ambulation, if able, for patient therapeutically anticoagulated.
   b. If patient is restricted to bed rest, encourage the patient to move as much as possible (based on restrictions).
   c. Patients can perform toe raises or ankle pumps using the foot board, can simulate walking, or if available, use a pedal system. Passive range of motion can be used to assist patients that are unable to move against gravity.
3. Encourage adequate fluid intake, frequent changes of position, and effective coughing and deep-breathing exercises.

CLINICAL JUDGMENT Be alert for signs of pulmonary embolism—chest pain, dyspnea, anxiety, and apprehension—and report immediately.

4. Discourage crossing of legs and long periods of sitting because compression of vessels can restrict blood flow.

Patient Education and Health Maintenance

1. Teach patient the signs of recurrent venous thrombus and pulmonary embolism to report immediately.
2. Provide thorough instructions about anticoagulant therapy (see page 292).
3. Teach patient to promote circulation and prevent stasis by applying compression stockings at home.
4. Advise against straining or any maneuver that increases venous pressure in the leg. Eliminate the necessity to strain at bowel movement by increasing fiber and fluids in the diet.
5. Encourage lifestyle modification—educate the patient on the benefits of smoking cessation, weight reduction, and increasing activity.
6. Advise patient to avoid prolonged periods of sitting or standing. If necessary, perform exercises to encourage venous return.

Evaluation: Expected Outcomes

- Patient verbalizes reduced pain.
- No bleeding is observed.
- Normal respiratory status is maintained.

Chronic Venous Insufficiency

Various terms are used to describe chronic venous conditions.

Chronic venous disease—this is used when abnormalities (venous valvular incompetence and/or venous obstruction) have been present for a long time but now symptoms and/or signs indicating the need for treatment and/or further investigation are present.

Chronic venous insufficiency—this is used when patients have chronic venous disease displaying more advanced clinical signs such as severe edema, skin changes, or ulceration.

Pathophysiology and Etiology

1. Following venous thrombosis, smaller vessels dilate because the main channel for returning blood from the leg to the heart is blocked by a thrombus.
2. Valves of diseased connecting veins (perforators) that serve to keep blood flowing from the superficial system into the deep system can no longer prevent backflow. The result is chronic venous stasis, resulting in swelling and edema, as well as superficial varicose veins.
3. Most commonly involved deep veins are the iliac and femoral veins. The saphenous vein is the most common superficial vein affected.
4. Risk factors for chronic venous disease include:
   a. History of venous thrombosis.
   b. Varicose veins or a family history of varicose veins.
   c. Obesity and/or not getting enough physical activity.
   d. Pregnancy.
   e. Smoking/tobacco use.
   f. Sitting or standing for long periods of time.
   g. Sleeping in a chair or recliner.
   h. May-Turner syndrome.
   i. Being female.
   j. Being over age 50.

Clinical Manifestations

1. Symptoms include pain, leg heaviness, aching, swelling, dryness and tightness of skin, itching, irritation, and muscle cramps.
2. Telangiectasias (spider veins), reticular veins, small varicose veins.
3. Varicose veins are dilated, elongated, tortuous, subcutaneous veins.
4. Dependent edema at the ankle, which may progress over time to include the calf region. Edema may be present only at the end of the day in the early stages but will become persistent throughout the day with progression of disease (intractable induration).
5. Skin changes occur with severe disease and include pigmentation (hemosiderin buildup in the skin resulting in a brownish discoloration), dermatitis (itchy, dry skin), and lipodermatosclerosis (hardening of the skin).
6. Ulceration (especially surrounding medial malleolus) may be seen in advanced disease.

Diagnostic Evaluation

1. Physical examination to identify symptoms of chronic venous disease.
2. Air plethysmography, photoplethysmography, or ambulatory venous pressure measurements.
3. Lower extremity duplex, computed tomography (CT), magnetic resonance imaging (MRI), catheter-based contrast venography, or IVUS may also be done.

Management

1. Skin care, leg elevation, exercise, and weight management.
2. Compression therapy which includes compression stockings, wraps, or in more advanced stages intermittent pneumatic compression devices.
3. Nonsurgical treatment:
   a. Sclerotherapy or endovenous thermal ablation (surface laser or high-frequency radio wave therapy) to treat telangiectasias and reticular veins.
4. Surgical treatment:
   a. Ligation and stripping.
   b. Microincision/ambulatory phlebectomy—used to treat superficial varicose veins by removing the damaged portion of the vein.
   c. Subfascial endoscopic perforator surgery—damaged veins are clipped to block blood flow through those veins. This will help heal and prevent reoccurrence of venous ulcers.
   d. Vein bypass—in severe disease, a healthy vein will be used to bypass the damaged vein.

CLINICAL JUDGMENT Be aware that in the hospital setting, the use of pneumatic compression devices consistently has been proven to prevent venous thrombus in patients at risk. However, for these devices to prevent venous stasis leading to thrombus, they must be active. Once the device is removed or turned off, risk increases.

Complications

1. Venous ulcers.
2. Cellulitis.
3. Recurrent thrombosis.

Nursing Interventions and Patient Education

Instruct the patient as follows:

1. Exercise regularly.
2. Manage your weight.
3. Wear 30- to 40-mm compression stockings, as prescribed by provider.
4. Avoid sitting or standing for long periods or sitting with legs crossed.
5. When sitting or lying down, elevate legs.
6. Check your skin daily. Keep skin moisturized to prevent scaling and dryness.
7. Avoid constricting bandages.
8. Prevent injury, bruising, scratching, or other trauma to the skin of the leg and foot.
9. Be alert for signs of ulceration, drainage, warmth, erythema, and pain, indicating infection.
10. Stop using tobacco products.

Venous Ulcers

Venous ulcer is an excavation of the skin surface produced by sloughing of inflammatory necrotic tissue, usually caused by chronic venous insufficiency in the lower extremity.

Pathophysiology and Etiology

1. Venous ulcers result from a complex process involving cellular, molecular, and hemodynamic changes in the microcirculation. These changes lead to a cascade of events resulting in venous structural changes that exacerbate venous hypertension.
1. Secondary bacterial infection occurs because of decreased microcirculation that limits the body's response to infection.
2. Postthrombotic syndrome and stasis with uncontrolled edema are responsible for most leg ulcers.
3. Risk factors associated with venous ulcer formation include:
   a. Age.
   b. Obesity and inactivity.
   c. Arterial hypertension.
   d. Lipodermatosclerosis.
   e. Family history of venous ulceration.

Clinical Manifestations

Severity of symptoms depends on the extent and duration of venous insufficiency. Venous ulcers may be characterized as healed, active (nonhealed), or recurrent. If left without treatment, venous ulcers can extend circumferentially around the leg.

1. Open lesions that are commonly found from midcalf to approximately 1 inch below the malleolus.
2. Venous ulcers tend to be shallow, have a base of red granulation tissue, with irregular wound edges (see Figure 10-7).
3. Exudate and odor may be present depending on the extent of leg edema and bacterial growth. Severe infection can lead to osteomyelitis.
4. The area may be covered by a dark crust or there may be crusting of skin around the ulcer.
5. Edema and pigmentation around the ulcer may be present.
6. Patient may complain of swelling, heaviness, aching, and fatigue.

Diagnostic Evaluation

1. Noninvasive tests, such as plethysmography and venous Doppler, may show impeded blood flow and incompetent valves.
2. Wound cultures will identify microorganisms, if infected.

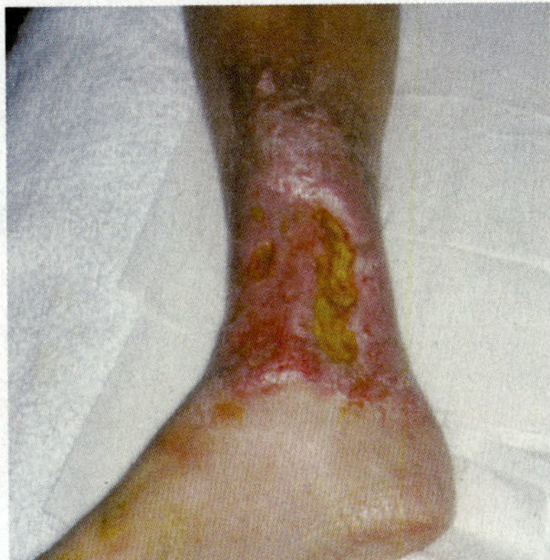

Figure 10-7. Venous ulcer.

Management

General Wound Management

1. Odor—minimizing microbial bioburden through interval mechanical débridement and/or the use of odor-absorbing dressings can help to reduce odor.
2. Bleeding—use of nonadherent and alginate dressings can minimize bleeding.
3. Pruritus—maintain a proper moisture balance. If needed, apply topical corticosteroid creams.
4. Exudate—use of an absorptive dressing over the nonadherent dressing will help to control drainage. Negative pressure wound therapy can be helpful in this situation.
5. Pain—patient should be asked about pain related to dressing changes and treated as appropriate.

Surgical Management

1. Wound cultures—ideally should be collected from the wound base to minimize false-positive results from a chronic wound environment.
   a. Prior to surgery, wound cultures should be collected if there are signs/symptoms of infection, so that antimicrobial therapy can be started.
   b. During surgical débridement, wound cultures should also be obtained to aid detection of infectious organism and to direct antimicrobial therapy.
2. Débridement—removal of nonviable tissue, biofilm, contaminants, and other foreign material is important to assist with healing. Surgical débridement allows for aggressive débridement of the chronic wound in a controlled environment that provides adequate pain management and the ability to control bleeding. This also allows for débridement of wounds that extend to the soft tissue or bone.

Stimulating Formation of Granulation Tissue

1. Dressing of choice:
   a. Nonadherent so that removal is painless and does not damage newly forming tissue.
   b. Highly absorbent.
   c. Safe, nontoxic.
   d. Sterile, accessible, and inexpensive.
2. Application of compression over dressings, generally through the use of bandages or elastic stockings.
   a. Unna's boot or other layered compression bandage, an effective treatment of choice, is an example of a combined dressing and compression bandage.
   b. In some circumstances, inflatable pneumatic leggings may be appropriate.
3. The use of human growth factor ointment to the ulcer may be appropriate to stimulate tissue growth.
4. Bed rest with leg elevation.
5. Diuretic therapy for edema reduction may improve capillary circulation.
6. Negative pressure wound therapy can be used in vascularized wounds. This therapy also allows for irrigation with saline or antibiotic solution.

Wound Closure

1. Application of skin grafts for ulcers that have not healed within 12 months of medical therapy.
2. Skin grafts are not recommended for first-line treatment.
3. Skin-equivalent grafts may be used, particularly if skin grafts fail.

Preventing Recurrence

1. Ligation of the saphenofemoral or saphenopopliteal vessels with stripping.
2. Laser or radiofrequency ablation of the saphenofemoral or greater saphenous vein and saphenofemoral junction.
3. Ligation of the lower leg communicating veins (usually endoscopic).
4. Deep vein bypass or reconstruction.
5. Injection compression sclerotherapy.

Complications

1. Infection.
2. Sepsis.

Nursing Assessment

1. Observe appearance and temperature of the skin.
2. Note location and appearance of ulcer.
3. Determine the presence and quality of all peripheral pulses. Use Doppler, if needed.
4. Observe for drainage and signs of infection.

Nursing Interventions

Restoring Skin Integrity

1. Elevate affected extremity to decrease edema.
2. Place lamb's wool between toes to prevent pressure on a toe.
3. Provide overbed cradle to protect leg from pressure of bed linens.
4. Consider an air-fluidized bed to provide pressure relief.
5. Administer prescribed antibiotics.
6. Apply wet-to-moist dressings, chemical beads or ointments, and topical antibiotics, as ordered. Wounds should not be allowed to completely dry out. Slight moisture aids the healing process.
7. Apply Unna boot or other compression system to lower extremity, as ordered.
8. Ensure adequate nutritional intake to enhance wound healing.

Reducing Pain

1. Administer prescribed analgesics, such as nonsteroidal anti-inflammatory drugs (NSAIDs), to reduce pain and inflammation.
2. Medicate 30 to 45 minutes before a dressing change.
3. Encourage short periods of ambulation when pain relief is achieved.

Ensuring Adherence to Treatment Plan at Home

1. Make sure that all supplies are obtained for home care. Utilize community nursing and social work support for additional resources and to help with financial arrangements, as needed.
2. Assess the patient's and caregiver's ability to perform dressing changes at home. Include additional significant others in teaching to assist patient.
3. Arrange for home visits one to several times per week to assess healing of ulcer, assess for infection, and assist family in carrying out dressing changes and other measures.

Patient Education and Health Maintenance

1. Stress the importance of following explicitly the recommendations of the health care provider.
2. Explain the hazards of trying other remedies without professional advice.
3. Indicate that the treatment may be long but that patience is an important aspect.
4. Encourage maintenance of healthy tissue when the ulcer has healed by continuing with the safeguards practiced before because breakdown of healed tissue frequently occurs.
5. Encourage participation in physical therapy and a regular exercise program.
6. Encourage weight control and proper dietary intake to ensure adequate amounts of protein, vitamins (A, C, E), zinc, and a reduced sodium intake.
7. Teach patient the correct method of dressing changes.
8. Instruct patient on injury prevention, including keeping hallways and walkways clear of obstacles and using a nightlight to avoid injury if awakened at night.
9. Encourage use of compression stockings when ordered.

Evaluation: Expected Outcomes

- Skin is of normal color and temperature, nontender and nonswollen, and demonstrates new epithelium.
- Verbalizes only minimal discomfort with dressing changes.

Varicose Veins

Varicose veins are the tortuous, twisted, dilated veins commonly involving the great saphenous vein and the small saphenous vein or their superficial tributaries. As venous insufficiency progresses through increased hydrostatic pressure and vein weakness, the vein walls become asymmetrically distended and some of the valves become incompetent. The process is irreversible. *Secondary varicose veins* result from obstruction of deep veins.

Telangiectasias (spider veins) are dilated superficial capillaries, arterioles, and venules. They may be cosmetically unattractive but do not pose a threat to circulation.

Pathophysiology and Etiology

1. Valvular reflux caused by incompetent valves (failure of valve leaflets), weakened vascular walls (loss of elasticity), and increased IV pressure (with bidirectional flow of blood) produces the varicosity (see Figure 10-8).

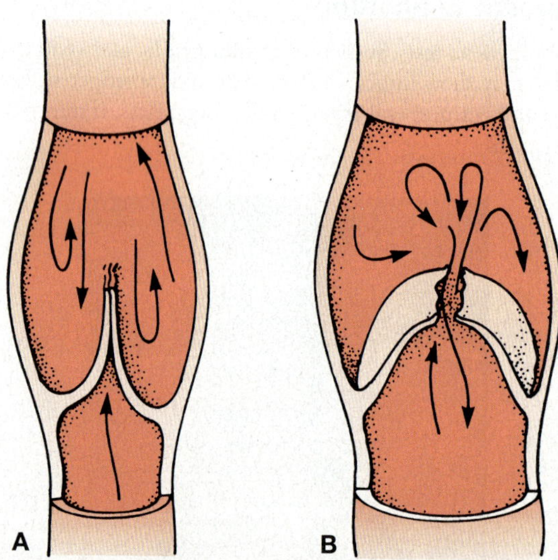

Figure 10-8. Valve incompetence develops as dilation of a vessel prevents effective approximation of valve cusps. **(A)** Closed venous valve. **(B)** Incompetent venous valve.

2. Varicosities may occur elsewhere in the body (esophageal and hemorrhoidal veins) when flow or pressure is abnormally high.
3. Predisposing factors:
   a. Female.
   b. Hereditary weakness of vein wall or valves.
   c. Long-standing distention of veins brought about by pregnancy, obesity, or prolonged standing.
   d. Advanced age—loss of tissue elasticity.

Clinical Manifestations

1. Disfigurement because of large, discolored, tortuous leg veins.
2. Easy leg fatigue, cramps in leg, heavy feeling, increased pain during menstruation, and nocturnal muscle cramps.

Diagnostic Evaluation

1. Doppler ultrasound and duplex imaging—can detect accurately and rapidly the presence or absence of venous reflux in deep or superficial vessels.
2. Other diagnostic tests are used if the Doppler ultrasound is inconclusive or for more complex situations:
   a. CT.
   b. MRI.
   c. Photoplethysmography—a noninvasive technique to observe venous flow hemodynamics by noting changes in the blood content of the skin; used to detect incompetence in valves located inside the vein.
   d. Venous outflow and reflux plethysmography—able to detect deep venous occlusion.
   e. Ascending and descending venography—an invasive technique that can also demonstrate venous occlusion and patterns of collateral flow. This test is expensive and may not be required if a careful history, physical examination, and laboratory testing are done.

Management

1. Conservative therapies, such as encouraging weight loss if appropriate and avoiding activities that cause venous stasis by obstructing venous flow.
2. Surgery may be considered for ulceration, bleeding, and cosmetic purposes in selected patients if patency of deep veins is ensured. The goal of procedures is to eliminate diseased veins and shunt blood to deeper veins with competent valves.
3. Surgical procedures—a single method or combination of methods is tailored to meet the needs of the individual:
   a. Sclerosing injection—may be combined with ligation or limited to treatment of isolated varicosities. The affected vessel may be sclerosed by injecting sodium tetradecyl sulfate or similar sclerosing agent. Compression bandage is then applied without interruption for 2 to 6 weeks; inflamed endothelial surfaces adhere by direct contact.
   b. Multiple vein ligation—either by multiple incisions or ambulatory phlebectomy (veins are removed using tiny incisions and hooks to grasp the veins).
   c. Ligation and stripping of the greater and lesser saphenous systems.
   d. Laser or radiotherapy treatment—small catheter is inserted via the groin and the veins ablated.
   e. Laser therapy—eliminates small veins under the skin.

Complications

1. Hemorrhage because of weakening of and pressure on the vein wall.
2. Skin infection and breakdown, producing ulcers (rare in primary varices).
3. Skin discoloration over the veins injected.

Nursing Assessment

1. Inspect for dilated, tortuous vessel.
2. Perforating veins that are incompetent may be felt as bulging circles at intervals beneath the skin. New varices are palpated along the surface of the muscle or bone. Chronic varices create deep pockets and may feel "boggy" with deep palpation.
3. Assess for any ulceration, chronic venous insufficiency, or signs of infection.

Nursing Interventions

Promoting Tissue Integrity Postoperatively

1. Maintain compression bandages from toes to groin. Monitor neurovascular status of feet (color, warmth, capillary refill, sensation, and pulses) to prevent compromise from swelling.
2. Elevate legs about 30 degrees, providing support for the entire leg. Make sure that knee gatch of the bed is positioned for straight incline. Encourage early ambulation.
3. Monitor for signs of bleeding, especially during the first 24 hours.
   a. Blood soaked through bandages.
   b. Increased pain, hematoma formation.
   c. Hypotension and tachycardia.

CLINICAL JUDGMENT If incisional bleeding occurs, elevate the leg above the level of the heart, apply pressure over the site, and notify the surgeon.

4. Be alert for complaints of pain over bony prominences of the foot and ankle; if the elastic bandage is too tight, loosen it.
5. Maintain IV for fluids and antibiotics, as ordered.
6. After removal of compression bandages (about 7 days postoperatively), observe or teach patient to observe for signs of cellulitis or incisional infection.
7. Encourage use of prescription compression stockings for several weeks to months following surgery.

Relieving Pain

1. Administer analgesics or teach self-administration, as prescribed.
2. Encourage early and frequent ambulation with legs elevated when not walking.
3. When ambulatory, advise patient to avoid prolonged standing, sitting, or crossing or dangling legs to prevent obstruction.

Patient Education and Health Maintenance

Postoperative Instructions

Instruct the patient to:

1. Wear pressure bandages or compression stockings as prescribed—usually for 3 to 4 weeks after surgery.
2. Elevate legs about 30 degrees and provide adequate support for entire leg.

3. Take prescribed or recommended analgesics for pain, as needed.
4. Report such signs as sensory loss, calf pain, or fever to the health care provider.
5. Avoid dangling of legs.
6. Walk frequently.
7. Be aware that patchy numbness can be expected but should disappear in less than 1 year.
8. Follow conservative management instructions (below) to prevent recurrence.

Conservative Management

Instruct the patient to:

1. Avoid activities that cause venous stasis by obstructing venous flow:
   a. Wearing tight garters, tight spandex, or compression around the popliteal area.
   b. Sitting or standing for prolonged periods of time.
   c. Crossing the legs at knees for prolonged periods while sitting (reduces circulation by 15%).
2. Control excessive weight gain.
3. Wear firm elastic support, as prescribed, from toe to knee when in upright position.
   a. Put compression stockings on in bed before getting up.
   b. If thigh-high compression is ordered, this may be difficult but adherence is important. Do not discontinue without notifying the surgeon.
4. Elevate foot of bed 6 to 8 inches (15 to 20 cm) or use a wedge for night sleeping.
5. Avoid injuring legs.

Evaluation: Expected Outcomes

- Skin is of normal color and temperature, nontender and nonswollen, and intact.
- Actively moves extremity; verbalizes reduced pain.

LYMPHATIC DISORDERS

The lymphatic system is a network of vessels and nodes that are interrelated with the circulatory system. It removes tissue fluid from intercellular spaces and protects the body from bacterial invasion. Lymph nodes are located along the course of the lymphatic vessels and filter lymph before it is returned to the bloodstream.

Lymphedema and Lymphangitis

Lymphedema is a swelling of the tissues (particularly in the dependent position) produced by an obstruction to the lymph flow in an extremity. This results in excessive accumulation of fluid in the interstitial space, which is composed of high molecular weight proteins. Lymphedema can result from injury, infection, obstruction, or congenital abnormalities.

Lymphangitis is an acute inflammation of lymphatic channels, which most commonly arises from a focus of infection in an extremity.

Pathophysiology and Etiology

Lymphedema

1. Classified as primary (congenital malformations) or secondary (acquired obstruction).
2. Swelling in the extremities occurs due to an increased quantity of lymph fluid that results from an obstruction of lymphatics.
3. Obstruction may be in both the lymph nodes and the lymphatic vessels. Eventually, subcutaneous tissue becomes fibrotic, impairing vascular flow and oxygen transfer to tissues.
4. It may be caused or aggravated by radiation therapy, trauma, cancer, morbid obesity, or surgery involving the lymph tissue (particularly radical mastectomy). It may be associated with varicose veins and chronic phlebitis.

Lymphangitis

1. Most commonly caused by infection in an extremity. The pooled protein-rich lymph fluid creates a good medium for the growth of bacteria and fungi.
2. The characteristic red streak extending up an arm or leg from the infected wound outlines the course of the lymphatics as they drain.
3. Recurrent lymphangitis is typically associated with lymphedema.
4. Can occur in:
   a. Normal lymphatic channels with acute infection.
   b. Damaged lymphatic channels (e.g., after saphenous vein harvesting for coronary artery bypass).
   c. Anatomic abnormalities.

Clinical Manifestations

Lymphedema

1. The majority of cases are unilateral; however, the etiology of lymphedema will determine if the lymphedema is unilateral or bilateral.
2. Initially, there will be pitting edema.
3. With worsening lymphedema, dermal thickening occurs and the skin becomes dry and firm with less pitting due to cutaneous fibrosis and adipose disposition.
4. A positive Stemmer sign indicates lymphedema. This occurs when there is inability to lift a skin fold at the base of the second toe or finger, compared to the unaffected extremity.

Lymphangitis

1. Acute lymphangitis—occurs as an infection at a distal site, leading to lymphangitis with red, tender streaks extending proximately, with involvement of regional lymph nodes. The patient often presents with fever.
2. Nodular lymphangitis—presents with nodular subcutaneous swellings along the course of the lymphatic channels. The patient may or may not report pain. The lesions may ulcerate leading to regional lymphadenopathy. Diagnosis normally requires aspiration or biopsy of a nodule.
3. Filarial lymphangitis—the presence of a parasite leads to inflammation, dilatation, and thickening and tortuosity of the lymphatic channels with eventual valvular incompetence. Unlike the other presentations, filarial lymphangitis presents with the distal spread away from the parasite-containing lymph node.

Diagnostic Evaluation

1. Limb circumference measurements, comparing sides.
2. Optoelectronic volume—infrared measurement of limb volume.
3. Lymphangiography (dye injection into lymphatic channels) and/or lymphoscintigraphy (intradermal technetium injection

at distal site of affected limb) to identify anatomic abnormalities or obstruction.
4. Computed tomography (CT) to visualize causes such as obstructing mass.
5. MR imaging/MR lymphography.
6. Indocyanine green (ICG) lymphangiography.
7. Histology, microscopy, and culturing of samples to identify infectious cause in suspected lymphangitis.

Management

Lymphedema

1. Lymphedema therapy.
   a. Compression garments to help squeeze the fluid out of tissues. This may be in the form of medical-grade stockings or garments or pneumatic compression, which provides intermittent pumping to squeeze fluid from the extremity. These may be used in the upper or lower extremities.
   b. Manual lymphatic drainage, massage to help move fluid, and myofascial release to break up fibrotic tissue.
   c. Complete decongestive therapy (see Table 10-5).
2. Diuretics are usually not effective and can worsen edema and promote volume depletion.
3. Low-level laser therapy for breast cancer–related upper extremity lymphedema.
4. Surgery:
   a. Lymphatic bypass procedures.
   b. Excision of affected subcutaneous tissue and fascia with skin grafting.
   c. Transfer of superficial lymphatics to deep lymphatic system by buried dermal flap.
   d. Liposuction of lower extremity lymphedema—limited; more common for upper extremity.
5. Adjunct lifestyle changes include leg elevation, diet, and exercise to promote ideal body weight, and self-monitoring of condition by serial measurement of limb circumference.

Lymphangitis

1. Administer empiric antibiotics, until diagnostic studies are completed.
2. Incise and drain if necrosis and abscess formation occur.
3. Surgical débridement in some cases.

Table 10-5 Complete Decongestive Therapy

PHASE/TIME FRAME Goals	COMPONENTS
Phase 1: Intensive treatment	Manual lymphatic drainage
Five times weekly for 2–4 weeks, or more	Compression dressings or garments
Mobilization of fluid	Therapeutic exercises
Initiation of connective tissue reduction	Meticulous skin and nail care to prevent infection
Phase 2: Maintenance	Elastic compression garments during awake hours
Daily, months to years	
Maintenance of swelling reduction	Self-compression bandaging at night
Optimization of connective tissue reduction	Skin care and continue therapeutic exercises
	Self-manual lymphatic drainage 20 min daily

Complications

1. Abscess formation (rare, with lymphangitis).
2. Septicemia.
3. Complications of surgery include flap necrosis, hematoma, abscess under flap, and cellulitis.
4. Reduced function of extremity.

Nursing Assessment

1. Assess patient for any areas of compromised skin integrity.
2. Assess extremity for edema and inflammation.
   a. Palpate edema to evaluate its quality: soft and pitting (venous) or firm and nonpitting (lymph).
   b. Note any areas of abscess formation (suppurative lymphadenitis).
3. Monitor for signs of fever and chills.

Nursing Interventions

Maintaining Skin Integrity

1. Apply elastic bandages or prescription compression stockings or garments daily (after acute attack with lymphangitis).
2. Advise the patient to rest frequently with affected part elevated—each joint higher than the preceding one.
3. Make sure the patient washes and dries thoroughly the crevices of the skin if edema has caused skin folds.
4. Administer or teach self-administration of antibiotics and other antimicrobials, as prescribed.
5. Recommend isometric exercises with extremity elevated to use muscle contraction to help mobilize fluid.
6. Suggest moderate sodium restriction in diet.
7. Observe postoperatively for signs of infection.

Relieving Pain From Inflammation and Postoperatively

1. Provide for comfortable positioning using soft pillows and bedding; ensure that patient can move the affected area easily.
2. Administer or teach patient to administer analgesics, as prescribed; monitor for adverse effects.
3. Ensure that clothing and bedding are not causing pressure on the affected extremity; use a bed cradle if available.

Patient Education and Health Maintenance

1. Instruct patient on proper application of compression garments.
2. Encourage adherence to therapy, which often involves frequent rewrapping of compression bandages, exercise, and massage for several months.
3. Advise patient to avoid trauma to extremity.
4. Instruct patient to use lotions that are free of perfumes, which may irritate skin.
5. Advise patient to practice good hygiene to avoid superimposed infections.
6. Instruct patient about the signs and symptoms of infection to report to health care providers.
7. Instruct patient to inspect feet and legs daily for evidence of skin breakdown, particularly between toes, and to report itching or rash that may indicate superimposed tinea infection.

Evaluation: Expected Outcomes

- Skin is normal color and temperature, nontender, and intact.
- Verbalizes no pain on actively moving extremity.

HYPERTENSIVE DISORDERS

Hypertension

EVIDENCE BASE Whelton, P. K., Carey, R. M., Aronow, W. S., Casey, D. E., Jr., Collins, K. J., Dennison Himmelfarb, C., DePalma, S. M., Gidding, S., Jamerson, K. A., Jones, D. W., MacLaughlin, E. J., Muntner, P., Ovbiagele, B., Smith, S. C., Jr., Spencer, C. C., Stafford, R. S., Taler, S. J., Thomas, R. J., Williams, K. A., Sr, ... Wright, J. T., Jr. (2018). 2017 ACC/AHA/AAPA/ABC/ACPM/AGS/APhA/ASH/ASPC/NMA/PCNA guideline for the prevention, detection, evaluation, and management of high blood pressure in adults: A report of the American College of Cardiology/American Heart Association Task Force on Clinical Practice Guidelines. *Hypertension, 71*(6), e13–e115. https://doi.org/10.1161/HYP.0000000000000065

The American Heart Association defines *blood pressure* (BP) as the force of blood pushing against the arterial wall as it relates to blood viscosity (thickness) and resistance of blood vessel. Systolic blood pressure (SBP) is the highest arterial pressure when the heart contracts and empties. Diastolic blood pressure (DBP) is the lowest arterial pressure when the heart relaxes to fill with blood. *Hypertension* (high BP) is a disease of vascular regulation in which the mechanisms that control arterial pressure within the normal range are altered. The predominant mechanisms of BP control are the central nervous system (CNS), the renin–angiotensin–aldosterone system, and extracellular fluid volume. Why these mechanisms fail is not known.

Pathophysiology and Etiology

Elevated diastolic pressure leads to strain on the arterial wall, which over time causes thickening and calcification of the arterial media (a condition called sclerosis) and eventually narrowing of the blood vessel lumen. Elevated BP is seen when there is increased cardiac output and increased peripheral resistance.

Primary or Essential Hypertension

(Approximately 95% of patients with hypertension.)

1. When the diastolic pressure is 90 mm Hg and/or the systolic pressure is 140 mm Hg or higher and other causes of hypertension are absent, the condition is said to be primary hypertension. More specifically, an individual is considered hypertensive when the average of two or more properly measured, seated BP readings taken at rest on each of two or more office visits exceeds the upper limits of normal (see Box 10-2).
2. Cause of essential hypertension is unknown; however, there are several areas of investigation:
   a. Hyperactivity of sympathetic vasoconstricting nerves.
   b. Presence of vasoactive substance released from the arterial endothelial cells, which acts on smooth muscle, sensitizing it to vasoconstriction.
   c. Increased cardiac output, followed by arteriole constriction.
   d. Excessive dietary sodium intake, sodium retention, insulin resistance, and hyperinsulinemia play roles that are not clear. There is a growing body of evidence implicating excess sodium intake in the pathogenesis of elevated BP.
   e. Familial (genetic) tendency.
3. SBP elevation in the absence of elevated DBP is termed isolated systolic hypertension and is treated in the same manner.

BOX 10-2 Hypertension Classification for Adults

- Normal: <120 systolic and <80 diastolic
- Elevated: 120–129 systolic and >80 diastolic
- Stage 1: 130–139 systolic or 80–89 diastolic
- Stage 2: 140 or greater systolic or 90 or greater diastolic
- Hypertensive crisis[a]: >180 systolic and/or diastolic >120

[a]*A prompt change in medication is required in patients with no other indications of problems; immediate hospitalization is required if there are signs of organ damage.*

Secondary Hypertension

1. Occurs in approximately 5% of patients with hypertension secondary to other pathology.
2. Renal pathology:
   a. Chronic kidney disease, congenital anomalies, pyelonephritis, renal artery stenosis, acute and chronic glomerulonephritis, and obstructive uropathy (hydronephrosis).
   b. Reduced blood flow to kidney causes release of renin. Renin reacts with a serum protein to form angiotensin I, which is converted to angiotensin II through the action of angiotensin-converting enzyme in the lungs, leading to vasoconstriction and increased salt and water retention.
3. Coarctation of the aorta (stenosis of the aorta)—blood flow to upper extremities is greater than flow to the kidneys. The kidneys release renin when they sense hypotension.
4. Endocrine disturbances:
   a. Pheochromocytoma—a tumor of the adrenal gland that causes release of epinephrine and norepinephrine and a rise in BP (extremely rare).
   b. Adrenal cortex tumors lead to an increase in aldosterone secretion (hyperaldosteronism) and an elevated BP (rare).
   c. Cushing syndrome leads to an increase in adrenocortical steroids (causing sodium and fluid retention) and hypertension.
   d. Hyperthyroidism causes increased cardiac output.
5. Obstructive sleep apnea causes nocturnal hypertension, which leads to sustained daytime hypertension.
6. Prescription medications such as estrogens and steroids (cause fluid retention), sympathomimetics (cause vasoconstriction and tachycardia), antidepressants (prevent the breakdown of epinephrine), appetite suppressants (cause tachycardia and vasoconstriction), and nonsteroidal anti-inflammatory drugs (NSAIDs; cause fluid retention and can lead to renal insufficiency).
7. Nonprescription drugs and substances such as methamphetamines and cocaine (cause vasoconstriction and tachycardia); NSAIDs; herbal agents such as St. John's wort, ginseng, ephedra (unclear etiology of hypertension); antihistamines (cause vasoconstriction and tachycardia); some weight loss medications and nicotine (causes vasoconstriction).
8. Food substrates such as sodium chloride, ethanol, licorice, and glucose, all of which can cause increased fluid retention.

Consequences of Hypertension

1. Hypertension can cause intimal wall injury in the arteries, which can lead to arteriosclerosis in which smooth muscle cell proliferation, lipid infiltration, and calcium accumulation occur in the vascular endothelium.
2. Over time, the constant pressure of blood moving through a weakened artery can cause a section of the wall to enlarge

and form a bulge that could potentially rupture leading to a life-threatening bleed.
3. Prolonged hypertension damages small blood vessels in the brain, eyes, heart, and kidneys.
4. The major objective in patients with high BP is to prevent target organ damage of the heart (left ventricular hypertrophy, angina, myocardial infarction [MI], heart failure), brain (stroke, transient ischemic attack [TIA], dementia), kidneys (chronic kidney disease), eyes (retinopathy, blindness), or vasculature (aneurysm, peripheral arterial disease [PAD]).
5. Hypertension is either the strongest or one of the strongest risk factors for almost all different types of cardiovascular diseases acquired during the life span.

Prevalence and Risk Factors

EVIDENCE BASE World Health Organization. (2023). *Hypertension.* https://www.who.int/news-room/fact-sheets/detail/hypertension

Tsao, C. W., Aday, A. W., Almarzooq, Z. I., Alonso, A., Beaton, A. Z., Bittencourt, M. S., Boehme, A. K., Buxton, A. E., Carson, A. P., Commodore-Mensah, Y., Elkind, M. S. V., Evenson, K. R., Eze-Nliam, C., Ferguson, J. F., Generoso, G., Ho, J. E., Kalani, R., Khan, S. S., Kissela, B. M., ... Martin, S. S. (2022). Heart disease and stroke statistics—2022 update: A report from the American Heart Association. *Circulation, 145*(8), e153–e639. https://doi.org/10.1161/CIR.0000000000001052

1. According to the World Health Organization, hypertension affects approximately 1.28 billion people worldwide and is the most common modifiable risk factor for arteriosclerosis. An estimated 46% of adults with hypertension are unaware that they have the condition, and only one in five people have hypertension under control.
2. According to the AHA 2022 Heart Disease and Stroke Statistics, using data from 2015 to 2018, 121.5 million (47.3%) of Americans have hypertension, and this number is expected to increase due to the aging of the population. Only a fraction of these people are aware of their hypertension and are treated for it, and even fewer have gained adequate control of their BP. In 2019, 102,072 U.S. deaths were attributable to hypertension.
3. Risk factors:
   a. Nonmodifiable—age, family history, ethnicity.
   b. Modifiable—obesity, high-sodium diet, excessive alcohol consumption, physical inactivity, insufficient sleep, smoking, diabetes, metabolic syndrome.
4. Social determinants such as low socioeconomic status, lack of health insurance, food and housing insecurity, and lack of safe space to exercise contribute to the risk factors.

POPULATION AWARENESS There is a higher incidence of hypertension in the African American population, along with a higher mortality rate and risk for complications such as stroke, left ventricular hypertrophy, heart failure, and kidney disease.

Clinical Manifestations

1. Usually asymptomatic; known as the silent killer.
2. May cause headache, dizziness, blurred vision, chest pain, and shortness of breath when greatly elevated.
3. Elevated BP readings taken in a seated position on at least two occasions.

Diagnostic Evaluation

1. Electrocardiogram (ECG)—to determine the effects of hypertension on the heart (left ventricular hypertrophy, ischemia) or the presence of underlying heart disease.
2. Chest x-ray—may show cardiomegaly or aortic dilation by the presence of a widened mediastinum.
3. Proteinuria, elevated serum blood urea nitrogen (BUN), and elevated creatinine levels—indicate kidney disease as a cause or effect of hypertension; first voided urine microalbumin or spot urine for albumin–creatinine ratio are early indicators.
4. Serum potassium—decreased in primary hyperaldosteronism; elevated in Cushing syndrome; both are causes of secondary hypertension.
5. Urine (24-hour) for catecholamines—increased in pheochromocytoma.
6. Renal ultrasound to detect renal vascular diseases.
7. Renal artery duplex imaging to identify renal artery stenosis.
8. Outpatient ambulatory BP measurements.
9. Tests for causes of secondary hypertension are done if hypertension is resistant to treatment or specific signs and symptoms of secondary hypertension are present.

Management

BP Target Goals

1. BP goals are based on research and published guidelines and/or consensus statements. Clinicians must be aware of their patients' target BP goals.
2. Guidelines from the Eighth Report of the Joint National Commission (JNC-8):
   a. BP goals for patients aged 60 and older are less than 150/90 mm Hg.
   b. BP goals for patients younger than aged 60 are less than 140/90 mm Hg.
   c. BP goals for patients with diabetes and chronic kidney disease are less than 140/90 mm Hg.
3. Guidelines from the American Heart Association:
   a. Individuals with or without ischemic heart disease, coronary artery disease (CAD) equivalents, and high risk for CAD have a target BP goal of less than 130/80 mm Hg.
   b. If the patient has left ventricular (LV) dysfunction, the target BP is less than 120/80 mm Hg.
4. Guidelines from the American Diabetes Association indicate that individuals with diabetes should have a target BP of less than 140/90 mm Hg.

Lifestyle Modifications

1. Lifestyle modifications reduce BP, prevent or delay the incidence of hypertension, enhance antihypertensive drug therapy, and decrease cardiovascular risk (see Box 10-3).
2. If, despite lifestyle changes, BP remains at or above 140/90 mm Hg (or is not at optimal level in the presence of other cardiovascular risk factors) over 3 to 6 months, drug therapy should be initiated.
3. If BP is extremely elevated or in the presence of cardiovascular risk factors, single-drug therapy may be initiated right away.

BOX 10-3 Lifestyle Therapy for Blood Pressure (BP) Control

- Weight control—may reduce BP 1 mm Hg for every 1 kg (2.2 lb) weight loss; goal is ideal body weight.
- DASH eating plan—may reduce systolic BP 11 mm Hg; diet is rich in fruits, vegetables, and low-fat dairy products; reduced intake of saturated and total fats.
- Reduced sodium intake—may reduce systolic BP 5 mm Hg; optimal goal is no more than 1,500 mg sodium per day.
- Physical activity—may reduce systolic BP 5 mm Hg; regular aerobic physical activity (such as brisk walking) should occur at least 90–150 minutes per week.
- Moderate alcohol intake—may reduce systolic BP 4 mm Hg; alcohol intake is limited to no more than two drinks per day for most males and no more than one drink per day for females and lighter weight persons. One drink is equivalent to 12-ounce beer, 5-ounce wine, or 1-ounce 80-proof whiskey.

Table 10-6 Evidence-Based Dosing for Antihypertensive Drugs

ANTIHYPERTENSIVE MEDICATION	INITIAL DAILY DOSE/NO. OF DOSES PER DAY	TARGET DOSE IN RCTs REVIEWED (mg)
ACE inhibitor		
Captopril	50 (2)	150–200
Enalapril	5 (1–2)	20
Lisinopril	10 (1)	40
Angiotensin receptor blockers		
Eprosartan	400 (1–2)	600–800
Candesartan	4 (1)	12–32
Losartan	50 (1–2)	100
Valsartan	40–80 (1)	160–320
Irbesartan	75 (1)	300
Beta-blockers		
Atenolol	25–50 (1)	100
Metoprolol	50 (1–2)	100–200
Calcium channel blockers		
Amlodipine	2.5 (1)	10
Diltiazem extended release	120–180 (1)	360
Nitrendipine	10 (1–2)	20
Thiazide-type diuretics		
Bendroflumethiazide	5 (1)	10
Chlorthalidone	12.5 (1)	12.5–25
Hydrochlorothiazide	12.5–25 (1–2)	25–100
Indapamide	1.25 (1)	1.25–2.5

ACE, angiotensin-converting enzyme; RCT, randomized controlled trial.

These dosages may vary from those listed in the Physicians' Desk Reference. Please review current medication reference materials for most current dosing. Many antihypertensive agents are combination medications.

Drug Therapy

See Table 10-6.

1. Considerations in selecting therapy include:
   a. Ethnicity—African American individuals respond well to calcium channel blockers and thiazide diuretics, if compelling conditions are not noted. A renin–angiotensin system (RAS) blocker is the first line for African American individuals with kidney disease, diabetes, or heart failure. White individuals respond well to angiotensin-converting enzyme (ACE) inhibitors.
   b. Age—diuretics are typically the first drug prescribed, but some adverse effects such as fatigue and lightheadedness may not be tolerated by older adults.
   c. Concomitant diseases and therapies—some agents also treat migraines, benign prostatic hyperplasia, heart failure; have beneficial effects on conditions such as renal insufficiency; or have adverse effects on such conditions as diabetes or asthma.
   d. Quality-of-life impact—tolerance of adverse effects.
   e. Cost considerations—newer and brand name agents usually more expensive.
   f. Dosing—multiple doses may reduce adherence.
2. Most guidelines and recommendations, including the 2017 American College of Cardiology/American Heart Association (ACC/AHA) guidelines, recommend that initial therapy be chosen among the following four classes of medications:
   a. Thiazide-like or thiazide-type diuretics—lower BP by promoting urinary excretion of water and sodium to lower blood volume.
   b. Long-acting calcium channel blockers—prevent calcium from entering cells of the heart and blood vessel walls, resulting in lower BP by relaxing and vasodilating blood vessels. May work better at lowering BP in Black individuals and older adults.
   c. ACE inhibitors—lower BP by blocking the enzyme that converts angiotensin I to the potent vasoconstrictor angiotensin II and reducing sympathetic nervous system activity; also raise the level of bradykinin, a potent vasodilator, and lower aldosterone levels. Some patients may not tolerate ACE inhibitors due to the dry cough side effect from the buildup of bradykinin.
   d. Angiotensin receptor blockers (ARBs)—similar in action to ACE inhibitors but act by blocking the effect of angiotensin II. Because there is no buildup of bradykinin, patient may tolerate ARBs better than ACE inhibitors.
   e. Both ACE inhibitors and ARBs in patients with chronic kidney disease with increased albuminemia reduce the risk of progression to end-stage kidney disease.
3. Other medications:
   a. Beta-adrenergic blockers—lower BP by slowing the heart and reducing cardiac output by blocking beta-adrenergic receptors that produce epinephrine. Not recommended as initial monotherapy or part of a combination therapy unless started as a treatment for MI.
   b. Alpha-receptor blockers—lower BP by dilating peripheral blood vessels and lowering peripheral vascular resistance. Research has indicated these medications provide little

protection against heart failure but are effective in improving benign prosthetic hypertrophy.

c. Central alpha agonists—lower BP by diminishing sympathetic outflow from the CNS, thereby lowering peripheral resistance.

d. Peripheral adrenergic agents/blockers—inhibit peripheral adrenergic release of vasoconstricting catecholamines such as norepinephrine.

e. Combined alpha- and beta-adrenergic blockers—work through alpha- and beta-receptors.

f. Direct vasodilators—act directly on the blood vessel walls, relaxing muscles to allow blood to flow more easily.

g. Aldosterone inhibitors—antagonize aldosterone receptors and inhibit sodium reabsorption in the collecting duct of the nephron in the kidneys.

h. Direct renin inhibitors—block the RAS pathway at the point of activation; prevent potent vasoconstriction.

4. If hypertension is not controlled with the first drug within 1 to 3 months, three options can be considered:
   a. If the patient has faithfully taken the drug and not developed adverse effects, the dose of the drug may be increased.
   b. If the patient has had adverse effects, another class of drugs can be substituted.
   c. A second drug from another class could be added. If adding the second agent lowers the pressure, the first agent can be slowly withdrawn or, if necessary, combination therapy can be continued.
   d. Some patients require two medications at the time of diagnosis. This should be considered for patients who are 20 mm Hg above their systolic goal or 10 mm Hg above their diastolic goal.
5. The best management of hypertension is to use the fewest drugs at the lowest doses while encouraging the patient to maintain lifestyle changes. After BP has been under control for at least 1 year, a slow, progressive decline in drug therapy can be attempted. However, most patients need to resume medication within 1 year.
6. If the desired BP is still not achieved with the addition of a second drug, a third agent or a diuretic or both (if not already prescribed) could be added. Seventy-five percent of individuals with hypertension require two or more antihypertensive agents to reach their BP goal.
7. Resistant hypertension is defined as an individual that requires three or more antihypertensive agents to control BP.

DRUG ALERT ACE inhibitors are a drug of choice for patients with diabetes as they delay progression to end-stage renal disease. However, they may worsen renal function in the presence of renal artery stenosis. Evaluation of renal function following their initiation is indicated.

Complications

See Figure 10-9.

1. Angina pectoris or MI because of decreased coronary perfusion.
2. Left ventricular hypertrophy and heart failure because of consistently elevated aortic pressure.
3. Renal failure because of diminished perfusion to the glomerulus.
4. TIAs, stroke, or cerebral hemorrhage because of cerebral ischemia and arteriosclerosis.
5. Retinopathy.
6. Accelerated hypertension (see page 323).

Nursing Assessment

Nursing History

Query the patient about the following:

1. Family history of high BP.
2. Previous episodes of high BP.
3. Dietary habits and salt intake.
4. Target organ disease or other disease processes that may place the patient in a high-risk group—diabetes, CAD, kidney disease.

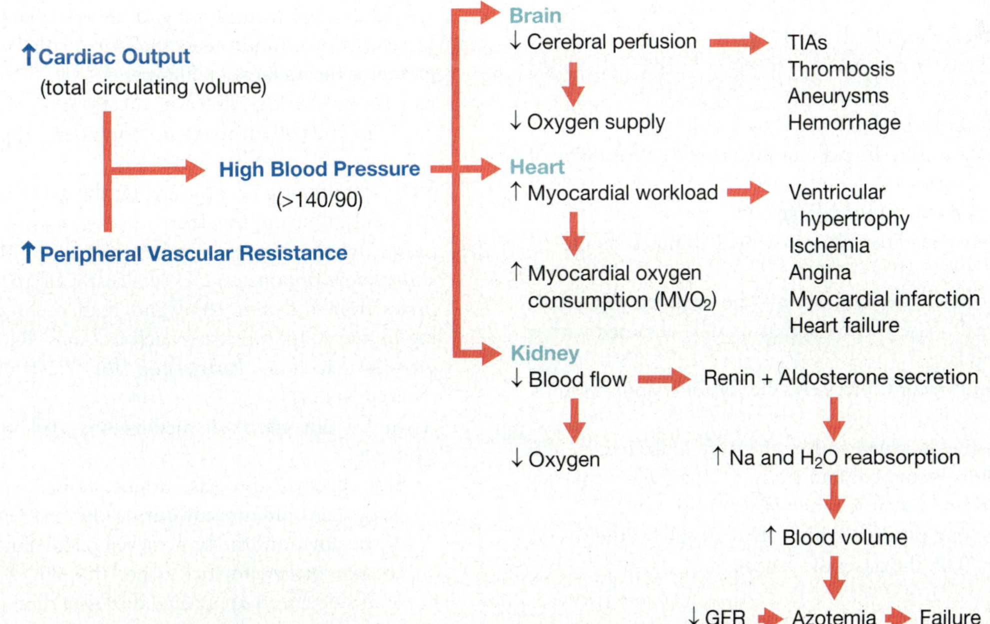

Figure 10-9. Determinants and clinical effects of high blood pressure. GFR, glomerular filtration rate; TIA, transient ischemic attack.

5. Tobacco use.
6. Episodes of headache, weakness, muscle cramps, tingling, palpitations, sweating, and vision disturbances.
7. Medication that could elevate BP (refer to "Secondary Hypertension," above):
   a. Hormonal contraceptives, corticosteroids.
   b. NSAIDs.
   c. Nasal decongestants, appetite suppressants, and tricyclic antidepressants.
8. Other disease processes, such as gout, migraines, asthma, heart failure, and benign prostatic hyperplasia, which may be helped or worsened by particular antihypertensive drugs.

Physical Examination

1. Auscultate heart rate and heart sounds for the presence of an S4, indicating stiffening of the walls of the left ventricle, which may occur in hypertension.
2. Palpate the chest wall for a shift of the point of maximal impulse to the left, which occurs in heart enlargement. Palpate peripheral pulses for possible PAD.
3. Auscultate for bruit over the aorta, renal arteries, and peripheral arteries to determine the presence of atherosclerosis.
4. Determine mental status by asking patient about memory, ability to concentrate, and ability to perform simple mathematical calculations.

BP Determination

1. Measure BP in both arms to determine whether there is a difference. If the SBP is greater than 15 mm Hg in one arm than the other, this may indicate the presence of subclavian stenosis in the arm with the lower SBP. If this BP differential is found, BP should be monitored in the arm with the highest SBP.
2. Avoid taking BP readings immediately after stressful or taxing situations. Wait 30 minutes after patient has smoked.
3. Have the patient assume position of comfort and remain silent. Make sure feet are on the floor or otherwise supported. The patient should be seated and relaxed for at least 5 minutes, and the BP should be taken around the same time each day it is taken to observe for trends in BP.
4. Support the bared arm; avoid constriction of arm by a rolled sleeve.
5. Use a BP cuff of the correct size.
   a. The bladder within the cuff should encircle at least 80% of the patient's arm.
   b. Many adults will require a large cuff.
   c. Two or more readings separated by 2 minutes should be averaged.
6. Be aware that falsely elevated BPs may be obtained with a cuff that is too small; falsely low readings may be obtained with a cuff that is too large.
7. Auscultate and record precisely the systolic and diastolic pressures.
   a. Systolic—the pressure within the cuff indicated by the level of the mercury column at the moment when the first clear, rhythmic pulsatile sound is heard (Phase 1).
   b. Diastolic—the pressure within the cuff just as the sound disappears (i.e., the onset of silence).

CLINICAL JUDGMENT The finding of an isolated elevated BP does not necessarily indicate hypertension. However, the patient should be regarded as at risk for high BP until further assessment—through history taking, repeat BP measurements, and diagnostic testing—either confirms or refutes the diagnosis.

POPULATION AWARENESS Older adult patients are more likely to have hypertension and isolated systolic hypertension because of age-related changes of decreased arterial compliance and arterial stenosis. Another age-related change, autonomic dysregulation, may cause orthostatic hypotension—a risk factor for syncope and falls. In such cases, an elevated BP may be acceptable.

Nursing Interventions/Patient Education

Increasing Knowledge for Better Outcomes

1. Explain the meaning of high BP and the term hypertension and risk factors.
2. Explain how high BP/hypertension affects the cardiovascular, cerebral, and renal systems.
3. Stress to the patient that they may not have any symptoms of elevated BP. There is no correlation between how they feel and whether BP is normal or high.
4. Explain that high BP/hypertension is a chronic disease and that it is important to keep regular follow-up appointments to monitor their BP and prevent any complications related to high BP. It is also important to keep BP controlled and in the range prescribed by the health care provider.
5. Instruct the patient to monitor their BP at home, including the proper method to take a BP and how to record the readings. Instruct the patient to contact the health care provider when BP is higher than the health care provider's goal BP.
6. Explain to the patient what factors can affect BP (e.g., dehydration, diarrhea, and other illnesses).
7. Provide written materials or online resources for enhanced learning.

Enhancing Adherence to Treatment

1. Assist the patient in developing an individualized plan to manage BP through medication and lifestyle changes.
2. Develop a medication schedule that is convenient and appropriate for the medication and patient.
   a. Provide a written list of medications.
   b. Assist the patient to set up reminders (e.g., phone alarms, use of pill minder containers).
3. Stress the importance of knowing the generic/brand name of the medication and the dose.
4. Assess the ability of the patient to pay for their medication and explore options such as less costly alternatives, obtaining prices from different retail and mail order pharmacies, using online coupon services such as Good Rx, and subsidized programs such as Partnership for Prescription Assistance (www.pparx.org).
5. Assess for side effects of medications and how they may be managed.
   a. Side effects of anorexia, fatigue, nausea, diarrhea, or lightheadedness often occur during the first few days or weeks of therapy until the body develops tolerance to them. Encourage patient to stick it out through the initial period, or, if side effects are severe, discuss a dose titration plan to get used to the medication gradually.
   b. If constipation occurs, encourage a high-fiber diet.
   c. Warn patients about orthostatic hypotension. Instruct patient to get up slowly from a lying/sitting position to

standing, to maintain hydration, and to be cautious during warm, humid weather.
   d. Instruct the patient to notify the health care provider of a persistent dry cough as the dosage or medication may need to be changed.
6. Advise the patient not to stop taking any medication without discussing it with their health care provider.
7. Discuss with the patient what lifestyle changes they can make.
   a. Acknowledge the difficulty when making changes and provide support.
   b. Find out patient's usual diet and diet preferences, and educate about modifications within that framework that will improve BP.
   c. Explain that sodium is another word for salt; reducing sodium can reduce BP by 20 mm Hg according to research.
   d. Provide website and written information on the Dietary Approaches to Stop Hypertension (DASH) Eating Plan as a guide, if patient is receptive to a structured eating plan (https://www.nhlbi.nih.gov/education/dash-eating-plan).
   e. Teach the patient and family how to read food labels to monitor sodium/salt intake and calories.
   f. Refer the patient to a dietitian for a thorough dietary education and meal planning.
   g. Find out what patient sees as barriers to physical activity and explore ways to increase activity within patient's schedule and environment.
   h. Encourage and discuss with patient how to form a plan to cut down or quit smoking. Advise patient that the longer the interval between cigarettes increases the time BP will not be as elevated, lowering mean arterial pressure (MAP).
8. Assist patient to make follow-up appointment and ensure they have transportation available.

POPULATION AWARENESS Polypharmacy, cognitive changes, and sensory deficits in older adults may make dosage adjustment and control of BP difficult. Work with the patient, family, and home health team to devise a simple method for the patient to take the proper medications. Older patients are also more sensitive to therapeutic levels of drugs and may demonstrate adverse effects while on an otherwise average dosage. Monitor closely for safety and efficacy of therapy.

Evaluation: Expected Outcomes

- Patient is able to name medications and dosages.
- Patient has all prescriptions, has not missed doses, and has follow-up appointment scheduled.

Malignant Hypertension

Malignant hypertension, also called *accelerated hypertension*, occurs when the BP rapidly elevates to an extreme level, threatening one or more of the target organs: brain, kidneys, or heart. Malignant hypertension is defined as BP greater than or equal to 180/120 mm Hg or isolated diastolic BP greater than 130 mm Hg and is a medical emergency.

Pathophysiology and Etiology

1. When rapid hypertension occurs, the normal autoregulation of the artery eventually fails.
2. The rise in pressure in the arterioles and capillaries leads to damage to the vascular wall, which disrupts the endothelium and allows fibrinous material to enter the vascular wall, thereby narrowing or obliterating the vascular lumen.
3. For example, within the brain, the breakthrough vasodilation from failure of autoregulation leads to the development of cerebral edema and symptoms of hypertensive encephalopathy.
4. Etiology includes collagen vascular disorders, aortic dissection, renal failure, renal artery stenosis, and toxemia of pregnancy.

Clinical Manifestations

1. Brain effects:
   a. Encephalopathy.
   b. Stroke.
   c. Progressive headache, stupor, and seizures.
2. Kidney effects:
   a. Decreased blood flow and vasoconstriction.
   b. Elevated BUN.
   c. Increased plasma renin activity.
   d. Lowered urine-specific gravity.
   e. Proteinuria.
   f. Renal failure.
3. Cardiac effects:
   a. Acute MI.
   b. Left-sided heart failure.
   c. Right-sided heart failure.

Diagnostic Evaluation

Tests are done to evaluate the presence of end-organ damage.
1. ECG.
2. Chest x-ray.
3. Urinalysis if pregnant.
4. Serum electrolytes and serum creatinine.
5. CT or MRI of the brain.
6. CT or MRI of chest if aortic dissection is suspected.

Management

Goal is to lower BP to reduce the probability of permanent damage to target organs. This should be done gradually as not to cause more damage. General rule is to decrease MAP by 10% to 20% in the first hour and then 5% to 15% over the next 23 hours.
1. If DBP exceeds 115 to 130 mm Hg, clinical condition is assessed very carefully.
2. Immediate hospitalization and treatment if the following are present:
   a. Seizures.
   b. Abnormal neurologic signs.
   c. Severe occipital headache.
   d. Pulmonary edema.
3. The patient is hemodynamically monitored in the ICU.
4. Antihypertensive agents are administered parenterally. Agents include:
   a. Nitroprusside—a rapidly acting arteriolar and venous dilator, given as an intravenous (IV) infusion. Initial dose: 0.25 to 0.5 µg/kg/min; maximum dose: 8 to 10 µg/kg/min. Avoid in neurologic emergencies or in pregnancy. Preferred in perioperative hypertension.
   b. Nitroglycerin—produces a greater venodilator effect than arteriolar dilation effect, given as an IV infusion. Initial dose: 5 µg/min; maximum dose: 200 µg/min. Preferred perioperative.

c. Labetalol—an alpha- and beta-adrenergic blocker, given as an IV bolus or infusion. Bolus: 20 mg initially, followed by 20 to 80 mg every 10 minutes to a total dose of 300 mg. Infusion: 0.5 to 2 mg/min. Preferred in acute ischemic stroke. Should be avoided in patients with asthma, chronic obstructive pulmonary disease (COPD), heart failure, and bradycardia.
d. Esmolol—antagonizes beta-1 adrenergic receptors, given as bolus 1,000 μg/kg IV, then 150 μg/kg/min IV prn, max 300 μg/kg/min, may continue 50 μg/kg/min IV q4min prn, titrate to taper off.
e. Nicardipine—a dihydropyridine calcium channel blocker, given as an IV infusion. Initial dose: 5 mg/h; maximum dose: 15 mg/h. Preferred in acute ischemic stroke. Major limitations are a longer onset of action.
f. Clevidipine—an ultra-short-acting dihydropyridine calcium channel blocker. Initial dose: 1 to 2 mg/h; maximum dose: 21 mg/h.
g. Fenoldopam—a peripheral dopamine-1 receptor agonist, maintains or increases kidney perfusion while it lowers BP. Given as an IV infusion. Initial dose: 0.01 μg/kg/min; the dose is titrated at 15-minute intervals, depending on the BP response normal dosing: 0.01 to 1.6 μg/kg/min.
h. Hydralazine—an arteriolar dilator, given as an IV bolus. Initial dose: 10 mg given every 20 to 30 minutes; maximum dose: 20 mg. Avoid in neurologic emergencies.
i. Propranolol—a beta-adrenergic blocker, given as an IV infusion and then followed by oral therapy. Dose: 1 to 10 mg load, followed by 3 mg/h.
j. Phentolamine—an alpha-adrenergic blocker, given as an IV bolus. Dose: 5 to 10 mg every 5 to 15 minutes.
k. Enalaprilat—an ACE inhibitor, given as an IV bolus. Dose: 1.25 to 5 mg every 6 hours. Used cautiously because hypotensive response is unpredictable.

5. Diuretics may be administered to maintain a sodium diuresis when the arterial pressure falls.
6. Vasopressor agents should be available if the BP responds too vigorously to antihypertensive agents.

CLINICAL JUDGMENT BP should be reduced gradually and wide pressure variations avoided because lowered BP may not be adequate to perfuse vital organs.

Nursing Interventions

1. Record BP frequently or monitor BP via an intra-arterial line or electronically controlled cuff. Some drugs necessitate the taking of BP readings every 5 minutes or more frequently while titrating drug therapies.
2. Monitor for adverse effects of medications—headache, tachycardia, and orthostatic hypotension.
3. Measure urine output accurately.
4. Observe for hypokalemia, especially if diuretic therapy is initiated. Monitor for ventricular dysrhythmias.
5. Observe for CNS complications.
   a. Note signs of confusion, irritability, lethargy, and disorientation.
   b. Listen for complaints of headache, difficulty with vision.
   c. Check for evidence of nausea or vomiting.
   d. Be alert for signs of seizure activity. Provide a safe environment—padded side rails. Keep bed in lowest position.
6. Reduce activity and provide a quiet environment.
7. Monitor ECG continuously.
8. Maintain constant vigilance until BP is decreased and stable and then begin a hypertension teaching program.

SELECTED READINGS

Chaikof, E. L., Dalman, R. L., Eskandari, M. K., Jackson, B. M., Lee, W. A., Mansour, M. A., Mastracci, T. M., Mell, M., Murad, M. H., Nguyen, L. L., Oderich, G. S., Patel, M. S., Schermerhorn, M. L., & Starnes, B. W. (2018). The Society for Vascular Surgery practice guidelines on the care of patients with an abdominal aortic aneurysm. *Journal of Vascular Surgery, 67*(1), 2–77.e2. https://doi.org/10.1016/j.jvs.2017.10.044

Cheung, C. Y. S., Parikh, J., Farrell, A., Lefebvre, M., Summa-Sorgini, C., & Battistella, M. (2021). Direct oral anticoagulant use in chronic kidney disease and dialysis patients with venous thromboembolism: A systematic review of thrombosis and bleeding outcomes. *Annals of Pharmacotherapy, 55*(6), 711–722. https://doi.org/10.1177/1060028020967635

Chopard, R., Albertsen, I. E., & Piazza, G. (2020). Diagnosis and treatment of lower extremity venous thromboembolism. *JAMA, 324*(17), 1765–1776. https://doi.org/10.1001/jama.2020.17272

Correia, M. A., Ritti-Dias, R. M., Cucato, G. G., Wolosker, N., Puech-Leão, P., Consolim-Colombo, F., Trombetta, I. C., Longano, P., & Silva, G. O. (2021). In peripheral artery disease, diabetes is associated with reduced physical activity level and physical function and impaired cardiac autonomic control: A cross-sectional study. *Annals of Physical and Rehabilitation Medicine, 64(2)*, 101365. https://doi.org/10.1016/j.rehab.2020.01.006

Criqui, M. H., Matsushita, K., Aboyans, V., Hess, C. N., Hicks, C. W., Kwan, T. W., McDermott, M. M., Misra, S., & Ujueta, F. (2021). Lower extremity peripheral artery disease: Contemporary epidemiology, management gaps, and future directions: A scientific statement from the American Heart Association. *Circulation, 144*(9), e171–e191. https://doi.org/10.1161/cir.0000000000001005

Crouch, A., Ng, T. H., Kelley, D., Knight, T., Edwin, S., ASCEND-HIGHER, & Giuliano, C. (2022). Multi-center retrospective study evaluating the efficacy and safety of apixaban versus warfarin for treatment of venous thromboembolism in patients with severe obesity. *Pharmacotherapy, 42*(2), 119–133. https://doi.org/10.1002/phar.2655

Dawwas, G. K., Leonard, C. E., Lewis, J. D., & Cuker, A. (2022). Risk for recurrent venous thromboembolism and bleeding with apixaban compared with rivaroxaban: An analysis of real-world data. *Annals of Internal Medicine, 175*(1), 20–28. https://doi.org/10.7326/M21-0717

Executive Committee of the International Society of Lymphology. (2020). The diagnosis and treatment of peripheral lymphedema: 2020 Consensus Document of the International Society of Lymphology. *Lymphology, 53*(1), 3–19. PMID: 32521126.

Gerhard-Herman, M. D., Gornik, H. L., Barrett, C., Barshes, N. R., Corriere, M. A., Drachman, D. E., Fleisher, L. A., Fowkes, F. G., Hamburg, N. M., Kinlay, S., Lookstein, R., Misra, S., Mureebe, L., Olin, J. W., Patel, R. A., Regensteiner, J. G., Schanzer, A., Shishehbor, M. H., Stewart, K. J., … Walsh, M. E. (2017). 2016 AHA/ACC guideline on the management of patients with lower extremity peripheral artery disease: A report of the American College of Cardiology/American Heart Association Task Force on Clinical Practice Guidelines. *Circulation, 135*(12), e726–e779. https://doi.org/10.1161/CIR.0000000000000471

Hennemeyer, C., Khan, A., McGregor, H., Moffett, C., & Woodhead, G. (2019). Outcomes of catheter-directed therapy plus anticoagulation versus anticoagulation alone for submassive and massive pulmonary embolism. *American Journal of Medicine, 132*(2), 240–246. https://doi.org/10.1016/j.amjmed.2018.10.015

Holt, A., Strange, J. E., Rasmussen, P. V., Blanche, P., Nouhravesh, N., Jensen, M. H., Schjerning, A. M., Schou, M., Torp-Pedersen, C., Gislason, G. H., Hansen, M. L., McGettigan, P., & Lamberts, M. (2022). Bleeding risk following systemic fluconazole or topical azoles in patients with atrial fibrillation on apixaban, rivaroxaban, or dabigatran. *American Journal of Medicine, 135*(5), 595–602. e5. https://doi.org/10.1016/j.amjmed.2021.11.008

Jones, N. R., & Round, T. (2021). Venous thromboembolism management and the new NICE guidance: What the busy GP needs to know. *British Journal of General Practice, 71*(709), 379–380. https://doi.org/10.3399/bjgp21X716765

Martin, K. A., Beyer-Westendorf, J., Davidson, B. L., Huisman, M. V., Sandset, P. M., & Moll, S. (2021). Use of direct oral anticoagulants in patients with obesity for treatment and prevention of venous thromboembolism: Updated communication from the ISTH SSC Subcommittee on Control of Anticoagulation. *Journal of Thrombosis Haemostasis, 19*(8), 1874–1882. https://doi.org/10.1111/jth.15358

O'Kane, C. P., Avalon, J. C. O., Lacoste, J. L., Fang, W., Bianco, C. M., Davisson, L., & Piechowski, K. L. (2022). Apixaban and rivaroxaban use for atrial fibrillation in patients with obesity and BMI ≥50 kg/m^2. *Pharmacotherapy, 42*(2), 112–118. https://doi.org/10.1002/phar.2651

Ozemek, C., Tiwari, S., Sabbahi, A., Carbone, S., & Lavie, C. J. (2020). Impact of therapeutic lifestyle changes in resistant hypertension. *Progress in Cardiovascular Diseases, 63*(1), 4–9. https://doi.org/10.1016/j.pcad.2019.11.012

Pahwa, R., & Jialal, I. (2023). *Atherosclerosis.* [Updated August 8, 2023]. In: *StatPearls* [Internet]. StatPearls Publishing. https://www.ncbi.nlm.nih.gov/books/NBK507799/

Pei, D. T., Liu, J., Yaqoob, M., Ahmad, W., Bandeali, S. S., Hamzeh, I. R., Virani, S. S., Hira, R. S., Lakkis, N. M., & Alam, M. (2019). Meta-analysis of catheter directed ultrasound-assisted thrombolysis in pulmonary embolism. *American Journal of Cardiology, 124*(9), 1470–1477. https://doi.org/10.1016/j.amjcard.2019.07.040

Qin, Y., Chen, Z., Gao, S., Shen, Y., & Ye, Y. (2024, Feb). Development and validation of a risk prediction model for linezolid-induced thrombocytopenia in elderly patients. *European Journal of Hospital Pharmacy, 31*(2), 94-100. https://doi.org/10.1136/ejhpharm-2022-003258. PMID: 35477677; PMCID: PMC10895188.

Raetz, J., Wilson, M., & Collins, K. (2019). Varicose veins: Diagnosis and treatment. *American Family Physician, 99*(11), 682–688. PMID: 31150188.

Raffetto, J. D., Ligi, D., Maniscalco, R., Khalil, R. A., & Mannello, F. (2020). Why venous leg ulcers have difficulty healing: Overview on pathophysiology, clinical consequences, and treatment. *Journal of Clinical Medicine, 10*(1), 29. https://doi.org/10.3390/jcm10010029

Roerecke, M., Kaczorowski, J., & Myers, M. G. (2019). Comparing automated office blood pressure readings with other methods of blood pressure measurement for identifying patients with possible hypertension: A systematic review and meta-analysis. *JAMA Internal Medicine, 179*(3), 351–362. https://doi.org/10.1001/jamainternmed.2018.6551

Stergiou, G. S., Palatini, P., Parati, G., O'Brien, E., Januszewicz, A., Lurbe, E., Persu, A., Mancia, G., & Kreutz, R. (2021). European Society of Hypertension Council and the European Society of Hypertension Working Group on Blood Pressure Monitoring and Cardiovascular Variability. 2021 European Society of Hypertension practice guidelines for office and out-of-office blood pressure measurement. *Journal of Hypertension, 39*(7), 1293–1302. https://doi.org/10.1097/HJH.0000000000002843

Stevens, S. M., Woller, S. C., Kreuziger, L. B., Bounameaux, H., Doerschug, K., Geersing, G. J., Huisman, M. V., Kearon, C., King, C. S., Knighton, A. J., Lake, E., Murin, S., Vintch, J. R. E., Wells, P. S., & Moores, L. K. (2021). Antithrombotic therapy for VTE disease: Second update of the CHEST guideline and expert panel report. *Chest, 160*(6), e545–e608. https://doi.org/10.1016/j.chest.2021.07.055

Tang, T., Chen, L., Chen, J., Mei, T., & Lu, Y. (2019). Pharmacomechanical thrombectomy versus catheter-directed thrombolysis for iliofemoral deep vein thrombosis: A meta-analysis of clinical trials. *Clinical and Applied Thrombosis/Hemostasis, 25*, 1076029618821190. https://doi.org/10.1177/1076029618821190

Zasadzka, E., Trzmiel, T., Kleczewska, M., & Pawlaczyk, M. (2018). Comparison of the effectiveness of complex decongestive therapy and compression bandaging as a method of treatment of lymphedema in the elderly. *Clinical Interventions in Aging, 13*, 929–934. https://doi.org/10.2147/CIA.S159380

UNIT IV NEUROLOGIC AND SENSORY HEALTH

11 Neurologic Disorders*

OVERVIEW AND ASSESSMENT

See additional online content: Procedure Guidelines 11-1

A baseline neurologic assessment is needed to detect changes in neurologic function and includes a patient history, general physical examination, and thorough neurologic examination. An important goal of the neurologic assessment is to identify the minimum amount of stimulation required to elicit maximum response. Common manifestations of neurologic dysfunction include motor, sensory, autonomic, and cognitive deficits. By exploring these symptoms, obtaining a pertinent history, and performing a thorough neurologic examination, the reader will gain an understanding of the underlying disorder and become skilled in planning care for patients with neurologic disorders (see Standards of Care Guidelines 11-1, page 327). See Chapter 1, page 98, for neurologic examination techniques. Documentation using appropriate terminology and comparison of right to left for asymmetrical findings are important. See Box 11-1, page 327, for definitions of findings.

Radiology and Imaging

Structural and functional imaging techniques have evolved to facilitate the rapid diagnosis and treatment of neurologic disorders. Brain mapping describes the process of translating the brain into a functionally useful group of dynamic maps or patterns. The diagnosis and evaluation of neurologic disorders are increasingly guided by functional brain mapping techniques that detect changes in brain patterns associated with neuropathology. Structural or anatomic imaging reveals information about the structure of the nervous system, including the brain and spinal cord. Functional or physiologic imaging focuses on the function of the brain and biochemical and metabolic processes in brain cells.

Computed Tomography

Description

1. Computed tomography (CT) is a structural imaging study that uses a computer-based x-ray to provide a cross-sectional image of the brain. A computer calculates differences in tissue absorption of the x-ray beams. The CT scan produces a three-dimensional (3D) view of structures in the brain and

*Please note that the term "male" in this chapter refers to a person assigned male at birth, and the term "female" in this chapter refers to a person assigned female at birth.

STANDARDS OF CARE GUIDELINES 11-1

Neurologic Disorders

When caring for patients with neurologic disorders, consider the following assessments and interventions:

- Use age-appropriate assessment and examination techniques.
- Be aware of the status of the patient when assuming care so comparison can be made with subsequent assessments.
- Perform a thorough systematic assessment, including mental status, vital signs, and cardiovascular status.
- Document the patient's condition to provide a record for continuity of care.
- Provide translation services for patients who have difficulty understanding or speaking English because this may impact the interpretation of the neurologic examination.
- Evaluate for signs of worsening neurologic condition through a systematic examination. Follow the institutional guidelines and clinician's orders regarding the frequency of assessments. If the patient shows signs of neurologic deterioration, more frequent assessment and/or interventions may be necessary.
- Be cautious in the administration of sedatives, opiates, or other medications that affect neurologic functioning because these may mask signs of neurologic deterioration.
- Notify appropriate health care provider of new or worsening neurologic symptoms, such as a change in behavior or level of consciousness; a change in functioning of the cranial nerves; motor, sensory, or neurovascular deficits; or alterations in the pattern of breathing or vital signs. Implement appropriate interventions for acute changes in neurologic status.
- Institute safety precautions for patients with neurologic deficits because they may be especially prone to falls. Follow institutional guidelines for patients with seizure disorder.
- Assess the patient's level of functioning in their activities of daily living. For those with cranial nerve or motor deficits, assess for difficulty swallowing prior to eating. For patients with difficulty swallowing, implement appropriate institutional protocols to prevent aspiration. This may include contacting the primary clinician to obtain an evaluation from a speech therapist or changing the diet.
- Use a multidisciplinary approach to care when indicated, including medical and surgical specialists, pharmacists, dietitian/nutritional therapist, physical/occupational/speech therapists, and rehabilitation specialists.
- Be aware that families or caregivers of patients with cognitive impairment or who are nonverbal may be able to provide assistance in the interpretation of behavioral cues.
- Assess family support and coping throughout the trajectory of the disease. Social issues (such as financial, community support systems) may require the expertise of a social worker or other clinical resource support personnel.

BOX 11-1 Definitions of Neurologic Findings

Acalculia—inability to do mathematical calculations.
Agnosia—inability to recognize sensory input.
Amaurosis fugax—sudden, temporary, or fleeting blindness, not caused by disease of the eye.
Anisocoria—inequality in size of the pupils.
Apraxia—inability to perform coordinated movements.
Confabulation—fluent, nonsensical speech.
Decerebrate rigidity (extensor posturing)—dysfunction of vestibulospinal tract and the reticular activating system (RAS) of the upper brainstem; jaw clenched, neck extended, elbows extended, forearms pronated, wrists flexed, knees extended, and feet plantar flexed.
Decorticate rigidity (flexor posturing)—dysfunction of corticospinal tract above the brainstem; arms adducted, elbows and wrists flexed, legs extended and internally rotated, and feet plantar flexed.
Dyslexia—visual aphasia.
Dysarthria—difficulty speaking.
Dyspraxia—partial loss of ability to perform coordinated movements.
Fluent aphasia (Wernicke, sensory)—comprehension is poor, but speech is fluent and nonsensical.
Homonymous hemianopsia—corresponding visual field deficits in half of the visual field bilaterally.
Micrographia—change in handwriting with the script becoming smaller and more cramped.
Nonfluent aphasia (Broca, motor)—comprehension intact but has poor expression through speech.
Nystagmus—involuntary oscillation of the eyeball, vertical, horizontal, or rotary.
Paratonia—progressively increasing and irregular resistance to passive movements.

distinguishes between soft tissues and water. Intravenous (IV) contrast dye may be used to examine the integrity of the blood–brain barrier. Multidetector scanners allow for rapid imaging.

2. CT of the head is primarily used to detect cerebral hemorrhage, whereas CT of the head with contrast is used to detect tumors and inflammatory disorders.
3. Spinal CT may be used to evaluate lower back pain due to bony lesions or degenerative changes. CT myelography is typically reserved for those who have had previous spinal surgery or a questionable diagnosis.
4. May be used when magnetic resonance imaging (MRI) is contraindicated (metallic or electronic implants) or not tolerated (claustrophobia).
5. *Advantages of CT*: widespread availability, short imaging time, excellent images of bone, and 100% sensitivity for detection of cerebral hemorrhage.
6. *Disadvantages of CT*: does not provide information about function of tissues; exposes the patient to ionizing radiation at higher doses than traditional x-rays; imposes a weight restriction of 300 pounds; if contrast is used, there is the risk of contrast-induced nephropathy.

Nursing and Patient Care Considerations

1. Instruct the patient to remove metal items, such as earrings, eyeglasses, and hair clips.
2. Ask whether the patient has an allergy to iodine or shellfish, or history of previous allergy to IV dye to determine whether the patient needs to be premedicated.
3. Evaluate for adequate renal function if contrast will be used; creatinine level is usually checked.
4. Tell the patient to expect a sensation of feeling flushed if contrast dye is injected through the IV catheter.

5. Inform the patient that the procedure usually takes less than 5 minutes.
6. Request that the patient remain as immobile as possible during the examination.
7. Tell the patient to resume usual activities after the procedure.
8. Encourage increased fluid intake for the rest of the day to assist in expelling the contrast dye.

Magnetic Resonance Imaging

Description

1. Conventional MRI is a noninvasive structural imaging procedure that uses powerful magnetic field and radiofrequency waves to create an image. When tissue is placed in a strong magnetic field, hydrogen atoms in the tissue line up within the field. In MRI, pulsating radiofrequency waves are applied to the magnetic field to alter the tissue magnetization, creating a clear image of the tissue.
2. MRI is the imaging procedure of choice for most neurologic diseases (e.g., detection of demyelinating diseases, nonacute hemorrhage, and cerebral tumors; evaluation of spinal cord injury [SCI], acute herniated disks, cerebral infarction, spinal cord tumors) and has largely replaced myelography, a more invasive procedure. See Table 11-1 for comparison to CT.
3. Specific protocols have been developed for trauma, stroke, brain tumors, and epilepsy.
4. MRI may be ordered with or without contrast. The contrast (gadolinium) alters the magnetic properties of tissue to differentiate tissue types. Contrast may be administered via IV line, by mouth, or through insertion into the rectum.
5. Closed MRI uses scanning equipment that resembles a tunnel-like chamber. Open MRI uses more sophisticated equipment that does not involve a closed chamber. During open MRI, the patient can comfortably see the surroundings from all views while the scan is in progress. This is ideal for patients who are claustrophobic or anxious, children, older adults, and those with class 3 obesity.
6. Two magnet strengths, 1.5 and 3.0 T. The letter "T" stands for "tesla." Three Tesla refers to the highest imaging strength, able to produce highly detailed images.
7. Imaging orientation:
   a. Axial—slice dividing the head into the upper and lower halves.
   b. Coronal—slice dividing the head into the front and back halves.
   c. Sagittal—slice dividing the head into the left and right halves.
8. Imaging sequences:
   a. T1—excellent tissue discrimination that provides anatomic images.
   b. T2—sensitive to the presence of increased water and visualization of edema for differentiation of normal tissue and pathologic changes.
   c. MRI with gadolinium—improves the specificity of normal/abnormal tissue. With blood–brain barrier disruption, there is leakage of contrast medium. The pattern of contrast uptake into brain tissue helps differentiate conditions such as central nervous system (CNS) infections, neoplasms, meningeal diseases, and noninfectious inflammatory processes.
   d. Fluid-attenuated inversion recovery—evaluates edema within white matter; also used to identify subarachnoid disease.
   e. Diffusion-weighted imaging (DWI)—helps to evaluate the extent of a stroke and demyelinating disease and differentiates tumors from abscesses; shows increased enhancement with cytotoxic edema.
   f. Apparent diffusion coefficient (ADC)—shows decreased attenuation associated with acute stroke.
   g. DWI/ADC mismatch—increased enhancement on DWI in conjunction with decreased enhancement on ADC indicates acute stroke.
   h. Perfusion-weighted imaging (PWI)—evaluates cerebral blood flow, transit time, and blood volume. Useful in the evaluation of the extent of the ischemia stroke and determination of whether there is salvageable tissue or a penumbra.
   i. DWI/PWI mismatch—increased enhancement on DWI with flow deficit on PWI indicates acute stroke.
   j. MRI single-photon emission computed tomography (SPECT)—provides assessment of neurochemicals (choline, lactate, *N*-acetylaspartate, glutamine/glutamate) for differentiation of brain tumors, abscess, demyelinating disease, and postradiation necrosis.
   k. Swan—useful in the evaluation microscopic bleeds and small blood vessels.
   l. Gradient recalled echo (GRE)—useful in the evaluation of small lesions and hemorrhage.
9. *Advantages of MRI*: no ionizing radiation, sensitivity to blood flow, imaging in several planes, and superior visualization of soft tissues. An important advantage is its ability to distinguish water, iron, fat, and blood. Sensitive to detection of white matter changes and valuable in detecting changes associated with Alzheimer disease and multiple sclerosis.
10. *Disadvantages of MRI*: contraindicated for patients with pacemakers (however, some pacemakers are MRI compatible), cochlear implants, nontitanium aneurysm clips, or other implanted objects that could be dislodged by the magnetic

Table 11-1 Comparison of CT and MRI

CONSIDERATIONS	CT	MRI
Radiation exposure	• Minimal	• None
Imaging planes	• Axial, coronal, and sagittal	• Axial, coronal, and sagittal
Cost	• Several hundred dollars	• Several thousand dollars, but dependent on protocol being used
Advantages	• Rapid evaluation for intracranial hemorrhage and subarachnoid hemorrhage	• Detection of stroke, multiple sclerosis, epilepsy, tumors
Disadvantages	• Poor visualization of anatomic structures; radiation exposure	• May result in claustrophobia • May need prior x-rays if metallic fragments are suspected—if identified, cannot complete study

CT, computed tomography; MRI, magnetic resonance imaging.

BOX 11-2 Contrast-Induced Nephropathy

When intravenous (IV) contrast medium is to be used in any radiologic study, renal function must be adequate to clear the substance. Check for risk factors for contrast-induced nephropathy:

- Renal insufficiency (creatinine level greater than 1.5 or a glomerular filtration rate of less than 60 mL/min).
- Diabetic nephropathy and other conditions that cause reduced renal perfusion.
- High total dose of contrast (less than 5 mL/kg or greater than 100 mL).

If risk factors are present, hydration with normal saline starting 1 hour prior to the procedure and for 6 hours following the procedure is recommended.

Metformin should be held for 24 hours before any procedure and for 48 hours after the procedure if IV contrast is utilized.

field. Dental amalgam, gold, and stainless steel are generally considered safe but may distort the image. If contrast is used, there is the risk of contrast-induced nephropathy. MRI scanner has the appearance of a tunnel-like chamber, and its constricted opening prevents its use for people with extreme obesity. Because of its narrow dimensions, MRI may induce claustrophobic and anxiety reactions, so antianxiety medication may be necessary before the procedure or an open MRI may be used.

Nursing and Patient Care Considerations

1. Encourage the patient to use the bathroom before the procedure because it may take from 20 to 60 minutes, though the scan time is dependent on the protocol requested and number of scans performed.
2. Instruct the patient to remove metal items, including eyeglasses, jewelry, hair clips, hearing aids, dentures, and clothing with zippers, buckles, or metal buttons.
3. Evaluate for adequate renal function if contrast will be used (see Box 11-2).
4. Encourage the patient to remain as still as possible during the procedure.
5. Describe the tunnel-like narrow chamber of the closed MRI scanner and inform the patient that it sometimes causes feelings of anxiety or claustrophobia. Evaluate the need for sedation.
6. Inform the patient the scanner will make a dull, thumping noise throughout the procedure.
7. Tell the patient to resume usual activities after the procedure.

Functional Magnetic Resonance Imaging

Description

1. Functional MRI (fMRI) is an imaging study that aids in identifying regions of the brain activated by particular stimuli and tasks. Imaging is performed during presentation of a stimulus or performance of a specific task and during rest periods. A statistical comparison is performed with images obtained during the stimulus/task periods compared with those performed during the rest periods by evaluating the conversion of oxyhemoglobin to deoxyhemoglobin and utilization of glucose, which occurs during normal brain activity. Involves IV administration of contrast material that lowers signal intensity on MRI in relation to blood flow as the material passes through the brain.
2. *Advantages of fMRI*: does not use ionizing radiation and can be applied repeatedly in the same patient without risk. Offers potential in early detection of patients with prodromal dementia. It is also useful in preoperative evaluation of patients with lesions (tumors, seizure foci) adjacent to eloquent areas of the brain (speech center, premotor and motor cortex, and memory centers).
3. *Disadvantages of fMRI*: same as MRI.

Nursing and Patient Care Considerations

1. Instruct the patient for MRI. Full cooperation of the patient is vital for head motion and task performance reasons. Global cognitive impairment, aphasia, neglect, substantial sensory disturbances, and severe depression are usually exclusion criteria. The performance of motor tasks during imaging should be monitored.
2. Medications that may interfere with the performance of tasks during the procedure should be avoided, if possible, including benzodiazepines, sedatives, and opioids.

Positron Emission Tomography

Description

1. Positron emission tomography (PET) is a computer-based imaging technique that permits the study of the brain's function by evaluating the metabolism, blood flow, and chemical processes within the brain. PET measures emissions of particles of injected radioisotopes—called *positrons*—and converts them to an image of the brain.
2. PET scanners are not frequently used or widely available because of their high cost, and PET requires sophisticated equipment to produce its radioisotopes, or positron emitter.
3. A glucose-like solution and mildly radioactive tracers are combined for injection or inhalation. After injection into the arterial bloodstream or inhalation of this radioactive compound, pairs of gamma rays are emitted into adjacent tissue during radioactive decay. The PET scanner measures the gamma rays to determine how quickly the tissues absorb the radioactive isotopes. A computer processes the data into an image that shows where the radioactive material is located, corresponding to cellular metabolism.
4. *Advantages of PET*: provides information on patterns of glucose and oxygen metabolism. Areas of decreased metabolism indicate dysfunction. PET is useful for the early detection of Alzheimer disease and other dementias, Parkinson disease, amyotrophic lateral sclerosis (ALS), Huntington disease, multiple sclerosis, and psychiatric disorders, such as depression or schizophrenia. PET can also help locate/identify abnormal brain activity, such as seizure foci, and assess brain function after stroke.
5. *Disadvantages of PET*: ionizing radiation, high initial cost.

Nursing and Patient Care Considerations

1. Inform the patient that this procedure requires injection or inhalation of a radioactive substance that emits positively charged particles. Explain that the image is created when the negative particles found in the body combine with the positive particles of the imaging substance.
2. Explain that, after injection of the radioisotope, the patient will be asked to rest quietly on a stretcher for about 45 minutes to allow the substance to circulate.

3. Reassure the patient that radiation exposure is minimal.
4. Encourage the patient to void before the test because the scan and associated procedures may take several hours.
5. Advise the patient to increase fluid intake after the procedure to flush out the radioisotope and to resume meals.
6. Tell the patient that it may take a few days to get the results of the PET scan because it requires processing before it is available for interpretation.

Single-Photon Emission Computed Tomography

Description

1. SPECT is a widely available noninvasive functional imaging technique that evaluates cerebral vascular supply. A radioactive tracer is administered by inhalation or injection into the bloodstream; the tracer then decays to emit only a single photon. It uses a rotating camera to track the single photons emitted from radioactive decay and collects information from multiple views. Evaluation of the radioactive tracers creates images that show cerebral blood flow in various regions of the brain.
2. The radioactive tracer compounds used are commercially prepared and do not require the specialized equipment used in PET scanning.
3. SPECT is typically used to evaluate cerebral blood flow in patients with ischemic stroke, subarachnoid hemorrhage (SAH), migraine, dementia (including Alzheimer disease), epilepsy, and other degenerative diseases.
4. *Advantages of SPECT*: can perform hemodynamic, chemical, and functional imaging; widely available.
5. *Disadvantages of SPECT*: ionizing radiation; provides only relative measurements.

Nursing and Patient Care Considerations

1. Inform the patient that this is a noninvasive procedure that should cause minimal discomfort.
2. Tell the patient that results of the scan are typically available for interpretation by a specialist immediately after the procedure.

Transcranial Doppler Studies

Description

1. Transcranial Doppler (TCD) ultrasonography involves noninvasive testing to measure flow changes in the form of velocities of the cerebral arteries. It helps evaluate vasospasm post-SAH, occlusion, or flow abnormalities as with stroke.
2. Bone windows (temporal, transorbital, or foramen magnum) are accessed using a fiberoptic probe after the application of ultrasound gel. The fiberoptic probe is directed at a specific artery, and the velocities are then recorded.
3. Specific criteria are utilized for the identification of each cerebral vessel prior to assessment of the vessel (specific bone window, depth, flow direction, and waveform).
4. *Advantages of TCD studies*: low cost; can be performed at bedside and repeated as needed (useful in monitoring trends).
5. *Disadvantages of TCD studies*: Results are operator dependent; inability to obtain signal; limited data on sensitivity and specificity.

Nursing and Patient Care Considerations

1. Explain that the study will be done with the patient in a reclining position.
2. Inform the patient that the test normally takes less than 1 hour, depending on the number of arteries that are to be studied.

Computed Tomography Perfusion

Description

1. CT perfusion involves rapid injection (5 to 10 mL/second) of 40 mL of iodine contrast during continuous scanning. Computer analysis of "washin" and "washout" of the contrast generates a single-slice acquisition blood flow map.
2. The test requires a 20-gauge catheter or larger for injection of the contrast. Contrast is cleared through the kidneys; therefore, renal function should be evaluated prior to study to reduce the risk of contrast-induced nephropathy.
3. CT scan is programmed to analyze specific area of concern. Three 1-cm thick computer-generated images are produced that reflect relative cerebral blood flow, relative blood volume, and mean transit time.
4. *Advantages of CT perfusion*: 90% sensitivity and 100% specificity for cerebral ischemia; can be performed in conjunction with CT angiogram. Can be used in evaluating cerebral vasospasm in aneurysmal SAH, though the sensitivity and specificity are unknown.
5. *Disadvantages of CT perfusion*: limited anatomic assessment; radiation exposure; if contrast is used, there is the risk of contrast-induced nephropathy; requires large-bore catheter.

Nursing and Patient Care Considerations

1. Instruct the patient about the rationale for placement of large-bore catheter.
2. Assess the patient for contrast allergy and premedicate, if indicated.
3. Inform the patient that radiation exposure, although present, is minimal.

Cerebral Angiography

Description

1. Following local anesthesia, a radiopaque dye is injected through a catheter in the femoral artery (or brachial artery if femoral is inaccessible) and passed through one of the major cervical blood vessels to assess cerebral circulation. Serial x-rays are taken after contrast dye illuminates the cerebral arterial and venous systems. The structure and patency of cerebral arteries are examined. Contrast is cleared through the kidneys. The test is frequently performed on an outpatient basis, unless the patient is already hospitalized.
2. 3D imaging is available for more thorough evaluation of vascular abnormalities.
3. *Advantages of cerebral angiography*: useful in detection of stenosis or occlusion, aneurysms, and vessel displacement due to pathologic processes (e.g., tumor, abscess, hematoma).
4. *Disadvantages of cerebral angiography*: involves considerable exposure to radiation. Contraindicated in patients with a stroke in evolution. Potential complications: temporary or permanent neurologic deficit, including stroke, anaphylaxis, bleeding or hematoma at the IV site, and impaired circulation in the extremity distal to the injection site, usually the femoral artery. There is a risk of contrast-induced nephropathy.

Nursing and Patient Care Considerations

1. Omit the meal before the test, although clear liquids may be taken.

2. Evaluate for adequate renal function; should have recent normal serum creatinine.
3. Ask the patient about allergies and specifically rule out the presence of iodine allergy, which requires pretest preparation. Commonly, patients with allergy to iodine also have allergies to radiopaque contrast media that may cause severe reaction.
4. Options for pretest allergy prevention include the following:
   a. Elective procedure: Give prednisone 50 mg orally 13, 7, and 1 hour prior to contrast and diphenhydramine 50 mg orally 1 hour prior to contrast.
   b. Urgent procedure: Give methylprednisolone IV and diphenhydramine 50 mg orally, intramuscularly (IM), or IV 1 hour prior to contrast.
5. Mark pedal peripheral pulses.
6. Explain that a local anesthetic will be used to insert a catheter into the femoral artery (brachial artery may be used) and threaded into the required cerebral vessel.
7. Tell the patient to expect some discomfort when the catheter is inserted into the artery. In addition, the sensation of a warm, flushed feeling and metallic taste should be expected when the dye is injected.
8. Caution the patient that they will need to lie still during the procedure and that they will be asked to hold breath intermittently during scanning.
9. After angiography:
   a. Maintain bed rest and do not flex lower extremities, as ordered, and monitor vital signs. Instruct the patient to maintain bed rest for up to 6 hours. If a closing device is utilized, the time can be reduced to 2 to 3 hours.
   b. Check the patient frequently for neurologic symptoms, such as motor or sensory alterations, reduced level of consciousness (LOC), speech disturbances, dysrhythmias, or blood pressure (BP) fluctuations.
   c. Monitor puncture site for bleeding, hematoma, and pulses, as ordered. Apply pressure if bleeding or hematoma is noted and inform provider.
   d. Evaluate renal function and monitor for adverse reaction to contrast medium (e.g., restlessness, respiratory distress, tachycardia, facial flushing, nausea, and vomiting).
   e. Assess skin color, temperature, and peripheral pulses of the extremity distal to the IV site—change may indicate impaired circulation due to occlusion. Inform provider if noted.

Computed Tomographic Angiography

Description

1. CT angiography is a minimally invasive 3D imaging technique that uses multisectional spiral CT imaging in conjunction with rapid power injection of contrast (50 mL) into a large antecubital vein. Multiple, thin slices are reconstructed to provide 3D imaging of cerebral vasculature.
2. Proper timing of contrast injection with initialization of CT scans is essential to optimize intravascular enhancement.
3. The test requires a 20-gauge catheter or larger for injection of the contrast. Contrast is cleared through the kidneys; therefore, renal function should be evaluated prior to the study to reduce the risk of contrast-induced nephropathy (see page 329).
4. *Advantages of CT angiography*: Speed of scanning allows for unstable patients to be evaluated; increasing in availability.
5. *Disadvantages of CT angiography*: exposure to radiation; need for large-bore (18 to 20 gauge) catheter; potential for anaphylaxis; contraindicated for patients with acute/chronic renal failure.

Nursing and Patient Care Considerations

1. Restrict food for 4 to 6 hours before the procedure.
2. Assess for contrast allergy and premedicate, if indicated.
3. Evaluate renal function as contrast is cleared through the kidneys. Elevated creatinine may preclude the individual from obtaining the study.

Magnetic Resonance Angiography/Venography of the Brain

1. Magnetic resonance angiography/venography (MRA/MRV) is a 3D phase contrast technique. The test focuses on high signal or blood flow while suppressing background nonactive tissue.
2. Two flow-opposing acquisitions are obtained, and the computer subtracts the background signal to construct the cerebral vasculature.
3. *Advantages of MRA/MRV*: no exposure to radiation.
4. *Disadvantages of MRA/MRV*: less sensitivity than CT angiography (sensitivity increases in aneurysms larger than 5 mm).

Nursing and Patient Care Considerations

1. Same as those for MRI, page 328.

Dynamic Volume Computed Tomography

Description

1. This scanning technique can include entire organs, such as the heart or brain, in a single rotation and enables dynamic processes, such as blood volume and time to peak, to be observed.
2. The scanning process takes less time and requires a smaller dose of iodinated contrast and less radiation than does conventional CT, making it an ideal diagnostic test in emergency situations (heart attack or stroke) or for those who cannot tolerate large doses of iodine contrast (renal disease).

Nursing and Patient Care Considerations

1. The general considerations for conventional CT are the same.
2. Inform the patient about lying flat on the table while the tube revolves around the area to be scanned.
3. If contrast will be used, the patient will most likely have an IV catheter placed for the injection of dye. A sensation of warmth or metallic taste in the mouth may be experienced after the dye injection.

Other Diagnostic Tests

Other diagnostic tests include lumbar puncture, which provides information about the CNS through direct contact with the cerebrospinal fluid (CSF); a variety of tests that measure electrical impulses in portions of the nervous system; and neuropsychological evaluation.

Lumbar Puncture

Description

1. A needle is inserted into the lumbar subarachnoid space, usually between the third and fourth lumbar vertebrae, and CSF is withdrawn for diagnostic and therapeutic purposes.
2. Purposes include the following:
   a. Obtaining CSF for examination (microbiologic, serologic, cytologic, or chemical analysis).

b. Measuring cerebrospinal pressure and assisting in the detection of obstruction of CSF circulation.
c. Determining the presence or absence of blood in the spinal fluid.
d. Aiding in the diagnosis of viral or bacterial meningitis, SAH or intracranial hemorrhage, tumors, and brain abscesses.
e. Administering antibiotics and cancer chemotherapy intrathecally in certain cases.
f. Determining levels of tau protein and beta-amyloid in the CSF—a test that may be used to assist in the diagnosis of Alzheimer disease. Elevated levels of tau protein and decreased levels of beta-amyloid are associated with Alzheimer disease.

Nursing and Patient Care Considerations

1. Assist the patient to side-lying position with a small pillow under the head and a pillow between legs with back arched and knees drawn up toward the abdomen. Alternately, a sitting position, leaning forward, may be used, particularly for persons with obesity.
2. Assist in sending CSF sample tubes for evaluation.
3. After the procedure, support the patient in lying flat for 2 hours, ensuring hydration, and monitor for a spinal headache and CSF leak.

Electroencephalography

Description

1. Electroencephalography (EEG) measures electrical activity of the brain cells. Electrodes are attached to multiple sites on the scalp to provide a recording of electrical activity that is generated in the cerebral cortex. Electrical impulses are transmitted to an EEG, which magnifies and records these impulses as brain waves on a strip of paper. Devices allow for continuous EEG monitoring of selective areas of the brain; thus, limited data are collected. It is useful in the intensive care unit (ICU) or epilepsy monitoring unit (EMU) setting for continuous monitoring to evaluate for seizure activation.
2. Provides physiologic assessment of cerebral activity for diagnosis of epilepsy, alterations in brain activity in coma, and organic brain syndrome and sleep disorders. Particularly helpful in the investigation of patients with seizures.
3. Usually performed in a room designed to eliminate electrical interference; however, in the case of a comatose patient, it may be performed at bedside using a portable unit.
4. Restlessness and fatigue can alter brain wave patterns.
5. For a baseline recording, the patient is instructed to lie still and relax with eyes closed. After a baseline recording in a resting phase, the patient may be tested in various stress situations (e.g., asked to hyperventilate for 3 minutes, look at a flashing strobe light) to elicit abnormal electrical patterns.
6. In patients with epilepsy, continuous monitoring is performed with video monitoring. This is useful for interpretation and correlation of physiologic seizure activity and clinical seizures.
   a. Grids, strips, or intracranial electrodes are placed intraoperatively for more accurate assessment of seizure foci.
   b. Mapping of seizure activity is performed to determine the precise location of seizure foci.
   c. Once foci are located, the site is evaluated for possible surgical resection.

Nursing and Patient Care Considerations

1. For routine EEG, tranquilizers, anticonvulsants, sedatives, and stimulants should be held for 24 to 48 hours before the study.
2. Thoroughly wash and dry the patient's hair to remove hair sprays, creams, or oils.
3. Explain that the electrodes will be attached to the patient's skull with a special paste.
4. Assure the patient that the electrodes will not cause shock, and encourage the patient to relax during the procedure because anxiety can affect brain wave patterns.
5. Meals should be taken as usual to avoid sudden changes in blood glucose levels.

Evoked Potential Studies

Description

1. These tests measure the brain's electrical responses to visual, somatosensory, or auditory stimuli.
   a. Visual evoked potentials—produced by asking the patient to look at rapidly reversing checkerboard patterns. These assist in evaluating multiple sclerosis and traumatic injury. EEG electrodes are placed over the occiput and record the transmission time from the retina to the occiput.
   b. Somatosensory evoked potentials—generated by stimulating a peripheral sensory nerve and useful in diagnosing peripheral nerve disease and injury. These measure transmission time up the spinal cord to the sensory cortex.
   c. Auditory evoked potentials—produced by applying sound, such as clicks, to help locate auditory lesions and evaluate integrity of the brainstem. The transmission time up the brainstem into the cortex is measured.
2. Can be performed intraoperatively or during interventional procedures in which the patient is under general anesthesia. Acute changes may indicate potential for deficits.

Nursing and Patient Care Considerations

1. Explain that the electrodes will be attached to the patient's scalp to measure the electrical activity of the nervous system. Placement of the electrodes will depend on the type of evoked potentials being measured.
2. Ask the patient to remove all jewelry.
3. Assure the patient that the procedure is not painful and does not cause any electric shock.
4. Inform the patient that the test usually takes 45 to 60 minutes.

Needle Electromyography

Description

1. In combination with nerve conduction studies, needle electromyography (EMG) is the gold standard for assessing the neurophysiologic characteristics of neuromuscular diseases. Because it is invasive and painful, its use is limited when activity from several muscles needs to be monitored simultaneously. It is the recording of a muscle's electrical impulses at rest and during contraction. A needle is attached to an electrode and inserted into a muscle. A mild electrical charge is delivered to stimulate the muscle at rest and during voluntary contraction. The response of the muscle is measured on an oscilloscope screen.
2. Useful in distinguishing lower motor neuron (LMN) disorders from muscle disorders (e.g., ALS from muscular dystrophy).
3. Nerve conduction time, another diagnostic test, is often measured simultaneously.

Nursing and Patient Care Considerations

1. Explain that this test measures the electrical activity of muscles.
2. Advise the patient to avoid caffeine and tobacco products for 3 hours before the test, as these substances can affect test results.

3. Inform the patient that the procedure normally takes at least 1 hour.
4. Tell the patient a needle will be inserted through the skin into select muscles and to expect some degree of discomfort when the needle is inserted.
5. Inform the patient that, after the test, a mild analgesic or warm compresses may be needed to relieve muscle soreness.
6. Inform the patient to observe the needle insertion sites for bleeding, hematoma, redness, or other signs of infection and to notify the health care provider if any of these are observed.

Nerve Conduction Studies (Electroneurography)

Description

1. A peripheral nerve is stimulated electrically through the skin and underlying tissues. A recording electrode detects the response from the stimulated nerve. The time between the stimulation of the nerve and the response is measured on an oscilloscope, and speed of conduction along the nerve is calculated.
2. Used to determine LMN dysfunction, differentiating disease or injury in peripheral nerves, spinal nerve roots, or the anterior horn of the spinal cord by measuring nerve conduction velocity.

Nursing and Patient Care Considerations

1. Explain that surface-stimulating electrodes with a special paste are applied and taped to the nerve site (leg, arm, or face).
2. Advise the patient that an electric current is passed through the electrode and that a mild sensation or slight discomfort may be experienced while the current is applied.

Neuropsychological Testing

Description

1. A series of tests that evaluate the effects of neurologic disorders on cognitive functioning and behavior.
2. A neuropsychologist selects appropriate tests to determine the extent and type of functional deficits.
3. Paper-and-pencil tests, puzzles, and word-and-recall games are commonly used. Testing may assess the following:
   a. Intelligence, attention span, memory, judgment.
   b. Motor, speech, and sensory function.
   c. Affect, coping, and adaptation.
   d. Language quality, abstraction, distractibility.
   e. Ability to sequence learned behaviors.
   f. Used in diagnosis of organic brain dysfunction and dementia.
   g. Valuable in determining vocational rehabilitation training needs.
4. Utilized in some facilities to determine competency of a patient with regard to instituting durable power of attorney or need for guardianship.

Nursing and Patient Care Considerations

1. Assure the patient that these tests are not intended to evaluate mental illness.
2. Explain that testing evaluates the ability to remember, calculate numbers, and perform abstract reasoning.
3. The patient should be well rested because testing is mentally tiring and lengthy. A complete examination is a 4- to 6-hour process, depending on the patient's ability to concentrate.
4. Anticipate fatigue and frustration after the examination.

Polysomnography

Description

1. Polysomnography is a noninvasive, all-night sleep study that measures character of sleep, simultaneously monitoring EEG, cardiac and respiratory function, and movements during sleep. It is used to confirm fragmented sleep patterns in narcolepsy and sleep-related epilepsy.
2. Testing is time-consuming and labor-intensive. Procedures typically include multiple physiologic measures, such as EEG, EMG, electrocardiogram [ECG]), heart rate, respiratory effort, airflow, and oxygen saturation.

Nursing and Patient Care Considerations

1. Explain that the electrodes placed on the scalp, chest, extremities, and face will be uncomfortable but do not deliver electrical current.
2. Reassure the patient that a technician will be in the next room.
3. Testing can also be performed on an outpatient basis.
4. Advise the patient to wear comfortable nightwear.

Multisleep Latency Test

Description

1. Multisleep latency test (MSLT) is a sleep study performed during the day. It is the most widely objective assessment of daytime sleepiness and is commonly used to confirm a diagnosis of narcolepsy.
2. Testing consists of four "napping" periods of 20 to 35 minutes, during which time the patient lies down on a bed in a darkened room and is allowed to fall asleep. The multiple short sleep periods during the MSLT increase the observation of rapid eye movement (REM) periods.

Nursing and Patient Care Considerations

1. Explain the time and duration of the naps.
2. Reassure the patient of freedom to move about between naps.
3. Tell the patient to wear comfortable clothing and to bring reading or other materials for use between naps.

GENERAL PROCEDURES AND TREATMENT MODALITIES

See additional online content: Procedure Guidelines 11-2

Nursing Management of the Patient With an Altered State of Consciousness

Unconsciousness is a condition in which there is a depression of cerebral function ranging from stupor to coma. Coma results from impairment in both the arousal and awareness of consciousness. The arousal of consciousness is mediated by the reticular activating system (RAS) in the brainstem, whereas the awareness component is mediated by cortical activity within the cerebral hemispheres.

Both arousal and awareness are assessed when using the Glasgow Coma Scale (GCS) as a measure of level of consciousness (LOC) (see Table 11-2).

When using the GCS, *coma* may be defined as no eye opening on stimulation, absence of comprehensible speech, and failure to obey commands. The GCS is designed to provide a rapid assessment of LOC and does not provide a means to monitor or localize

Table 11-2 Glasgow Coma Scale

PARAMETER	FINDING	SCORE
Eye opening	Spontaneously	4
	To speech	3
	To pain	2
	Do not open	1
Best verbal response	Oriented	5
	Confused	4
	Inappropriate speech	3
	Incomprehensible sounds	2
	No verbalization	1
Best motor response	Obeys command	6
	Localizes pain	5
	Withdraws from pain	4
	Abnormal flexion	3
	Abnormal extension	2
	No motor response	1

Interpretation: Best score = 15; worst score = 3; 7 or less generally indicates coma; changes from baseline are most important.

neurologic dysfunction. Facility-generated neurologic assessment tools may be used in combination with the GCS to assess, monitor, and trend neurologic function.

An altered state of consciousness may be caused by many factors, including hypoxemia; trauma; neoplasms; vascular, degenerative, and infectious disorders; as well as a variety of metabolic disorders and structural neurologic lesions. Diagnostic evaluation and management depend on the underlying cause, overall intracranial dynamics, age, comorbidities, and general state of health.

Nursing Assessment

1. Assess eye opening (level of responsiveness).
   Eye opening = arousal
   Tracking = awareness
2. Assess neurologic function using the GCS. The GCS addresses eye opening, verbal responses, and motor responses. If the patient's eyes do not open spontaneously or to your voice, then assess responses using painful stimuli by applying pressure against trapezius/axillary pinch or sternum. Use the least amount of pain for the best response.
3. Assess cognitive function.
   a. Orientation.
      i. Person, place, and time.
      ii. Where are you, why are you here.
      iii. General information—national and local current events.
   b. Speech—aphasia and other problems (see Table 11-3).
      i. Expressive aphasia (motor/Broca)—inability to express self.
      ii. Receptive aphasia (sensory/Wernicke)—inability to understand the spoken language.
      iii. Global aphasia—inability to speak or understand spoken language.
      iv. Other aphasia syndromes—amnesia, conduction.
   c. Other alterations include the following:
      i. Confabulation—fluent, nonsensical speech.
      ii. Perseveration—continuation of thought process with an inability to change train of thought without direction or repetition.
4. Assess motor function—voluntary versus reflexive:
   a. Voluntary movement.
      i. Normal complex movement—strength and symmetry in the upper extremities (UE), pronator drift proximally and grip strength distally; in the lower extremities (LE), leg lifts proximally and dorsi/plantar flexion distally.
      ii. Localization—ability to determine the location of stimuli; patient localizes area of painful stimuli.
      iii. Withdrawal—abduction of the UE; moving away from the stimuli.
   b. Reflexive movement.
      i. Abnormal flexor posturing (decorticate)—dysfunction of corticospinal tracts above the brainstem. Abnormal flexion of the UE with adduction of the UE, internal

Table 11-3 Differentiating Aphasia

APHASIA	FLUENCY	RATE	COMPREHENSION	GRAMMAR	REPETITION
Fluent (Wernicke/receptive aphasia)	Intact, although speech is nonsensical	Normal	Absent to poor	Intact	Intact
Nonfluent (Broca/expressive aphasia)	Poor	Slow, halting	Intact	Absent	Poor
Global	Poor	Slow	Absent	Absent	Poor
Conduction	Intact, although there is functional transposition of sounds with phonetic paraphrases	Normal	Intact	Intact	Poor
Anomic or amnesiac aphasia	Difficulty naming and finding words	Halting	Intact	Intact	Intact

rotation of the UE, wrist and extension, and internal rotation and plantar flexion of the LE.

ii. Abnormal extension posturing (decerebrate)—dysfunction of vestibulospinal tract and the RAS of the upper brainstem. Abnormal extension, hyperpronation, and adduction of the UE and wrist flexion; abnormal extension and internal rotation of the LE with plantar flexion of the feet and toes.

iii. Mixed posturing—varied extensor and flexor tone in UE.

iv. Flaccid—medullary compression with complete loss of motor tone.

5. Test cranial nerve (CN) reflexes to assess for brainstem dysfunction.
   a. Assess pupil size, symmetry, and reaction to light.
   b. Assess extraocular movements (CN III, CN IV, CN VI) and reflex eye movements elicited by head turning (oculocephalic response). This should not be performed on patients with suspected cervical spine injury, patients in a cervical collar, or patients known to have cervical spine injuries.
   c. The oculovestibular (caloric) response (CN III, CN IV, CN VI, CN VIII) is tested by medical staff when the patient is comatose, as part of the brain death examination.
   d. Assess CN V and CN VII together to evaluate facial pain, blink, eye closure, and grimace.
   e. Assess CN IX, CN X, and CN XII to evaluate gag, swallowing reflex, tongue protrusion, and patient's ability to handle own secretions.
6. Assess respiratory rate and pattern (normal, Kussmaul, Cheyne-Stokes, apneic).
7. Assess deep tendon reflexes; evaluate tone for spasticity, rigidity, and paratonia (abnormal resistance increasing throughout flexion and extension, indicating frontal lobe dysfunction).
8. Examine head for signs of trauma, and mouth, nose, and ears for evidence of edema, blood, and cerebrospinal fluid (CSF) (may indicate basilar skull fracture).
9. Monitor any change in neurologic status over time and report changes to health care provider, as indicated.

KEY DECISION POINT A critical indicator of neurologic function is the LOC. A change in GCS of 2 or more points may be significant. If patient demonstrates deterioration, as evidenced by a change in neurologic examination, notify the health care provider without delay and reevaluate the neurologic status more often than required by orders based on nursing judgment.

Nursing Interventions

Minimizing Secondary Brain Injury

1. Monitor for change in neurologic status, decreased LOC, onset of CN deficits.
2. Identify trends in neurologic function and communicate findings to medical staff.
3. Monitor response to pharmacologic therapy, including drug levels, as indicated.
4. Monitor laboratory data, CSF cultures, and Gram stain, if applicable, and communicate findings to medical staff.
5. Assess neurologic drains and dressings for patency and characteristics of drainage.
6. Institute measures to minimize risk for increased intracranial pressure (ICP), cerebral edema, seizures, or neurovascular compromise.
7. Adjust care to reduce risk of increasing ICP: body positioning in a neutral position (head aligned with shoulders) without flexing head, reduce hip flexion, distribute care throughout 24-hour period sufficiently for ICP to return to baseline.
8. Monitor temperature status; maintain normothermia. Institute cooling procedure as ordered.

Maintaining an Effective Airway

1. Position the patient to prevent the tongue from obstructing the airway, encourage drainage of respiratory secretions, and promote adequate exchange of oxygen and carbon dioxide.
2. Keep the airway free from secretions with suctioning. In the absence of cough and swallowing reflexes, secretions rapidly accumulate in the posterior pharynx and upper trachea and can lead to respiratory complications (e.g., aspiration).
   a. Insert oral airway if the tongue is paralyzed or is obstructing the airway. An obstructed airway increases ICP. This is considered a short-term measure.
   b. Prepare for insertion of a cuffed endotracheal (ET) tube to protect the airway from aspiration and to allow efficient removal of tracheobronchial secretions.
   c. See Chapter 6 for technique of tracheal suctioning.
   d. Use oxygen therapy as prescribed to deliver oxygenated blood to the central nervous system (CNS).
   e. Before suctioning, pretreat with sedative, opioid, or ET lidocaine, if indicated.

Attaining and Maintaining Fluid and Electrolyte Balance

1. Monitor prescribed intravenous (IV) fluids carefully, maintaining euvolemia and minimizing large volumes of "free water," which may aggravate cerebral edema.
2. Maintain hydration and enhance nutritional status with the use of enteral or parenteral fluids.
3. Measure urine output.
4. Evaluate pulses (radial, carotid, apical, and pedal) and measure blood pressure (BP); these parameters are a measure of circulatory adequacy/inadequacy.
5. Maintain circulation; support the BP and treat life-threatening cardiac dysrhythmias.

Maintaining Healthy Oral Mucous Membranes

1. Remove dentures. Inspect the patient's mouth for dryness, inflammation, and the presence of crusting.
2. Provide mouth care by brushing teeth and cleansing the mouth with an appropriate solution every 2 to 4 hours to prevent parotitis (inflammation of parotid gland).
3. Apply lip emollient to maintain hydration and prevent dryness.

Skin Integrity

1. Keep the skin clean, dry, well lubricated, and free from pressure because comatose patients are susceptible to the formation of pressure injuries.
2. Turn the patient from side to side on a regular schedule to relieve pressure areas and help clear lungs by mobilizing secretions; turning also provides kinesthetic (sensation of movement), proprioceptive (awareness of position), and vestibular (equilibrium) stimulation.
3. Reposition carefully after turning to prevent ischemia and shearing over pressure areas.
4. Position extremities in functional position, and monitor the skin underneath splints/orthosis to prevent skin breakdown and pressure neuropathies.
5. Perform range of motion (ROM) exercises of extremities at least four times daily; contracture deformities develop early in unconscious patients.

Maintaining Corneal Integrity

1. Protect the eyes from corneal irritation as the cornea functions as a shield. If the eyes remain open for long periods, corneal drying, irritation, and ulceration are likely to result.
2. Make sure the patient's eye is not rubbing against bedding if blinking and corneal reflexes are absent.
3. Inspect the condition of the eyes with a penlight.
4. Ensure that contact lenses have been removed.
5. Irrigate eyes with sterile saline or prescribed solution to remove discharge and debris.
6. Instill prescribed ophthalmic ointment in each eye to prevent glazing and corneal ulceration.
7. Apply eye patches, when indicated, ensuring that eyes remain closed under patch.

Reducing Fever

1. Look for possible sites of infections (respiratory, CNS, urinary tract, wound) when fever is present in an unconscious patient.
2. Monitor temperature frequently or continuously.
3. Control persistent elevations of temperature. Fever increases metabolic demands of the brain, decreases circulation and oxygenation, and results in cerebral deterioration.
   a. Monitor core temperature continuously and treat hyperthermia promptly. Hyperthermia increases the brain's metabolic rate and the risk of secondary injury. A body core temperature is 4°C to 5°C lower than brain temperature.
   b. Maintain a cool ambient temperature. Anticipate potential for overcooling and make environmental adjustments accordingly (e.g., operating room environment).
   c. Minimize excess covering on bed.
   d. Administer prescribed antipyretics.
   e. Use cool water sponging and an electric fan blowing over the patient to increase surface cooling for hyperthermia resistant to antipyretics.
   f. Use an external cooling device to maintain normothermia, but avoid rapid overcooling. Intravascular cooling devices may also be used.

Promoting Urinary Elimination

1. An indwelling or external urethral catheter may be used for short-term management.
2. Use intermittent bladder catheterization for distention as soon as possible to minimize the risk of infection. Palpate over the patient's bladder at intervals or use a bladder scan to detect urine retention and an overdistended bladder.
3. Monitor for fever and cloudy, foul-smelling urine.
4. Initiate a bladder training program as soon as consciousness is regained.

Promoting Bowel Function

1. Auscultate for bowel sounds; palpate the lower abdomen for distention.
2. Observe for constipation due to immobility and lack of dietary fiber. Stool softener or laxative, scheduled or as needed, may be prescribed to promote bowel elimination. The goal is bowel movement every other day.
3. Monitor for diarrhea resulting from infection, antibiotics, enteric feedings, hyperosmolar fluids, and fecal impaction.
   a. Perform a rectal examination if fecal impaction is suspected.
   b. Use fecal collection bags and provide meticulous skin care if the patient has fecal incontinence.

Family Education and Support

1. Develop a supportive and trusting relationship with the family or significant other.
2. Provide information and frequent updates on the patient's condition and progress.
3. Involve them in routine care and teach procedures that they can perform at home.
4. Demonstrate and teach methods of sensory stimulation to be used frequently.
   a. Use physical touch and reassuring voice.
   b. Talk to the patient in a meaningful way even when the patient does not seem to respond. Assume the patient is able to hear even if unresponsive.
   c. Orient the patient periodically to person, time, and place.
5. Demonstrate and teach methods frequently used to manage restlessness/agitation.
   a. Eliminate distractions.
   b. Reduce environmental stimuli (turn off television and radio, close door).
   c. Use one-to-one communication.
   d. Talk slowly and simplify information without talking down to the person.
6. Teach the family to recognize and report unusual restlessness, which could indicate cerebral hypoxia, metabolic imbalance, or pain.
7. Enlist the help of the social worker, home health agency, or other resources to assist family with issues such as financial concerns, guardianship, need for additional follow-up care (rehabilitation, long-term care facility), need for medical equipment in home, and/or respite care.

Evaluation: Expected Outcomes

- Neurologic status remains at baseline or improved.
- Maintains clear airway; coughs up secretions.
- Absence of signs of dehydration.
- Intact, pink mucous membranes.
- No skin breakdown or erythema.
- Absence of trauma to cornea.
- Core temperature within normal limits.
- Absence of urinary tract infection (UTI); maintenance of normal bladder emptying.
- Bowel movement on regular basis in response to bowel regimen.

Nursing Management of the Patient With Increased Intracranial Pressure

ICP is the pressure exerted by the contents inside the cranial vault—the brain tissue (gray and white matter), CSF, and the blood volume. A pressure reading at or greater than 20 mm Hg is defined as increased ICP.

EVIDENCE BASE American Association of Neuroscience Nurses. (2022). *AANN core curriculum for neuroscience nursing* (7th ed.). Author.

Pathophysiology and Etiology

1. ICP is composed of the following components and volume ratio: brain tissue, 80%; CSF, 10%; blood volume, 10%.
2. The Monro-Kellie doctrine states that the intracranial vault is a closed structure with a fixed intracranial volume. The intracranial contents must be kept in equilibrium, and the ratio

between volume and pressure must remain constant. Any increase in the volume of one component must be accompanied by a reciprocal decrease in one of the other components. When this volume–pressure relationship becomes unbalanced, ICP increases.

3. The brain attempts to compensate for rises in ICP by:
   a. Displacement/shunting of CSF from the intracranial compartment to the lumbar subarachnoid space (SAS). Normally, about 500 mL of CSF are produced and absorbed in 24 hours. About 125 to 150 mL circulates throughout the ventricular system and the SAS in the following ratio: 25 mL in the ventricles, 90 mL in the lumbar SAS, and 35 mL in the cisterns and surrounding SAS.
   b. Increased CSF absorption.
   c. Decreased cerebral blood volume by displacement of cerebral venous blood into the venous sinuses. Compensatory measures are finite. Increased ICP will ultimately occur if the volume of the intracranial mass exceeds the volume compensated.
4. Intracranial compliance is "tightness" of the brain. Compliance is the relationship between intracranial volume and ICP. It is a nonlinear relationship; as ICP increases, compliance decreases. With functional compensatory mechanisms, an increase in volume causes a small, transient increase in ICP. As compliance decreases, small increases in volume result in moderate increases in pressure. When compensatory mechanisms are exhausted, very slight increases in volume will produce large increases in pressure. The patient's response to changes in ICP will depend on where the patient is on the volume–pressure curve.
5. Factors that influence the ability of the body to achieve this steady state include the following:
   a. Systemic BP.
   b. Ventilation and oxygenation.
   c. Metabolic rate and oxygen consumption (fever, shivering, physical activity).
   d. Regional cerebral vasospasm.
   e. Oxygen saturation and hematocrit.
6. Inability to maintain a steady state results in increased ICP. Traumatic brain injury (TBI), cerebral edema, intracerebral hemorrhage, ischemic stroke, abscess and infection, lesions, intracranial surgery, and radiation therapy can be potential etiologies of increased ICP.
7. Increased ICP constitutes an emergency and requires prompt treatment. ICP can be monitored by means of an intraventricular catheter, a subarachnoid screw or bolt, or an epidural pressure recording device.
8. Alterations or compromise in cerebral blood flow can be measured noninvasively by a transcranial Doppler (TCD) study. Increased velocities indicate vasospasm, diminished velocities indicate low blood flow, and absent velocities are consistent with no flow or brain death.

Nursing Assessment

Change in LOC

Caused by increased ICP. Assess for the following:

1. Change in LOC (awareness): drowsiness, lethargy.
2. Early behavioral changes: restlessness, irritability, confusion, and apathy.
3. Falling score on the GCS (see page 334).
   a. Change in orientation: disorientation to time, place, or person.
   b. Difficulty or inability to follow commands.
   c. Difficulty or inability in verbalization or in responsiveness to auditory stimuli.
   d. Change in response to painful stimuli (e.g., purposeful to inappropriate or absent responses).
   e. Posturing (abnormal flexion or extension).

Changes in Vital Signs

Caused by pressure on brainstem. Assess for the following:

1. Rising BP or widening pulse pressure (the difference between systolic [SBP] and diastolic BP). This may be followed by hypotension and labile vital signs, indicating further brainstem compromise.
2. Pulse changes with bradycardia changing to tachycardia as ICP rises.
3. Respiratory irregularities: tachypnea (early sign of increased ICP); slowing of rate with lengthening periods of apnea; Cheyne-Stokes (rhythmic pattern of increasing and decreasing depth of respirations with periods of apnea) or Kussmaul (paroxysms of difficult breathing) breathing; central neurogenic hyperventilation (prolonged, deep breathing); apneustic (sustained inspiratory effort) breathing; and ataxic (incoordinated and spasmodic) breathing. Respiratory irregularities may not be apparent if the patient is mechanically ventilated.
4. Hyperthermia followed by hypothermia.

KEY DECISION POINT Watch for Cushing triad—bradycardia, hypertension (with widening pulse pressure), and irregular respirations; this is classic symptomatology related to uncompensated increased ICP and is considered a neurologic medical emergency. Alert health care provider and prepare for therapeutic intervention.

Pupillary Changes

1. Caused by increased pressure on optic and oculomotor nerves. Fundoscopic examination may reveal changes.
2. Inspect the pupils with a penlight to evaluate size, configuration, and reaction to light.
3. Compare both eyes for similarities or differences, particularly pupillary changes related to location and progression of brainstem herniation.
   a. Midbrain involvement—fixed and dilated.
   b. Pontine involvement—pinpoint pupils.
   c. Uncal herniation.
      i. Unilaterally dilating pupil ipsilateral to lesion.
      ii. Anisocoria (unequal) with sluggish light reaction in dilated pupil.
      iii. If treatment is delayed or unsuccessful, contralateral pupil becomes dilated and fixed to light.
      iv. When herniation of the brainstem occurs, both pupils assume midposition and remain fixed to light.
   d. Central transtentorial herniation.
      i. Pupils are small bilaterally (1 to 3 mm).
      ii. Reaction to light is brisk but with small range of constriction.
      iii. If treatment is delayed or unsuccessful, small pupils dilate moderately (3 to 5 mm) and fix irregularly at midposition.
      iv. When herniation of the brainstem occurs, both pupils dilate widely and remain fixed to light.
4. Pupillometer can be used to measure pupillary size and reactivity, detecting subtle change by utilizing infrared light.

Extraocular Movements

1. Evaluate gaze to determine whether it is conjugate (paired, working together) or dysconjugate (eye deviates or movement is asymmetric).
2. Evaluate movement of eyes.
   a. Inability to abduct or adduct: deviation of one or both eyes.
   b. Alteration in vision (e.g., blurred vision, diplopia, field cut).
   c. Spontaneous roving, random eye movements.
   d. Nystagmus on horizontal/vertical gaze.
3. Oculocephalic reflex (doll's eyes): brisk turning of the head left, right, up, or down with observation of eye movements in response to the stimulus. Tests brainstem pathways between CN III, CN IV, CN VI, and CN VIII. This should not be performed on patients with suspected cervical spine injury, patients in a cervical collar, or patients with known cervical spine injuries unless part of the brain death examination.
4. Oculovestibular reflex (cold calorics): 30 to 60 mL of ice water instilled into the ear with the head of the bed elevated to 30 degrees. Tests brainstem pathways between CN III, CN IV, CN VI, and CN VIII. Response preserved longer than the doll's eyes maneuver. Performed by health care provider as part of brain death examination.

Other Changes

Be alert for the following:

1. Headache increasing in intensity and aggravated by movement and straining.
2. Vomiting recurrent with little or no nausea, especially in early morning; may be projectile.
3. Papilledema from optic nerve compression.
4. Subtle changes, such as restlessness, headache, forced breathing, purposeless movements, and mental cloudiness.
5. Motor and sensory dysfunctions (proximal muscle weakness, presence of pronator drift).
6. Contralateral hemiparesis progressing to complete hemiplegia.
7. Speech impairment (expressive, receptive, or global aphasia) when dominant hemisphere involved.
8. Seizure activity: focal or generalized.
9. Decreased brainstem function (CN deficits, such as loss of corneal reflex, gag reflex, and ability to swallow).
10. Pathologic reflexes: Babinski, grasp, chewing, sucking.

Nursing Interventions

Decreasing Intracranial Pressure

CLINICAL JUDGMENT Increased ICP is a true life-threatening medical emergency that requires immediate recognition and prompt therapeutic intervention.

1. Establish and maintain airway, breathing, and circulation.
2. Promote normal PCO_2. Hyperventilation is not recommended for prophylactic treatment of increased ICP as cerebral circulation is reduced by 50% the first 24 hours after injury. Hyperventilation causes cerebral vasoconstriction and decreases cerebral blood flow to decrease ICP; this can potentiate secondary injury to the brain. Hyperventilation should be used only after all other treatment options have been exhausted or in an acute crisis.
3. Avoid hypoxia. Decreased PO_2 (less than 60 mm Hg) causes cerebral vasodilation, thus increasing ICP.
4. Maintain cerebral perfusion pressure (CPP) greater than 50 mm Hg. CPP is determined by subtracting the ICP from the mean arterial pressure (MAP): CPP = MAP − ICP.
5. Administer mannitol (0.25 to 1 g/kg), an osmotic diuretic, if ordered. Osmotic diuretics act by establishing an osmotic gradient across the blood–brain barrier that depletes the intracellular and extracellular fluid volume within the brain and throughout the body. Mannitol will be ineffective if the blood–brain barrier is not intact.
6. Administer hypertonic saline (2% or 3%), if ordered. It creates an osmotic gradient that pulls extra fluid from the brain with an intact blood–brain barrier, lowers ICP, improves cerebral blood flow by reducing viscosity, and improves oxygen-carrying capacity. Saline (23.4%) is used as a bolus to treat acute increases in ICP in conjunction with or in place of mannitol; requires central access for administration and should be given over 5 minutes.
7. Insert an indwelling urinary catheter for the management of diuresis.
8. Administer corticosteroids, such as dexamethasone, as ordered, to reduce vasogenic edema associated with brain tumors. Corticosteroids are not recommended in the treatment of cytotoxic (intracellular) cerebral edema related to trauma or stroke.
9. Maintain balanced fluids and electrolytes. Watch for increased or decreased serum sodium due to the following conditions that may occur with increased ICP.
   a. Diabetes insipidus (DI) results from the absence of antidiuretic hormone (ADH); this is reflected by increased urine output with elevation of serum osmolarity and sodium.
   b. The syndrome of inappropriate antidiuretic hormone (SIADH) results from the secretion of ADH in the absence of changes in serum osmolality. This is a hypervolemic state reflected by decreased urine output with decreased serum sodium and increased free water.
   c. Cerebral salt wasting is associated with abnormal release of aldosterone, resulting in increased elimination of sodium and decreased interstitial volume (hypovolemic state) (see Table 11-4).

Table 11-4 Differentiating Etiology of Hyponatremia

	CEREBRAL SALT WASTING	SIADH
Volume		
Plasma	Decreased CVP <6	Increased
Urine output	Marked increase	Normal or decreased
Sodium		
Serum	Decreased	<135 mEq/L
Urine	Marked increase	>20 mEq/L
Osmolality		
Serum	Increased or no change	Decreased (<280 mmol/L)
Urine	Increased or no change	Increased (>100 mmol/kg)
Serum K^+	Increased	Decreased or no change
Hematocrit	Increased	Decreased or no change
Treatment	Fludrocortisone	Fluid restriction Oral: Salt replacement IV: 3% saline

CVP, central venous pressure; IV, intravenous; SIADH, syndrome of inappropriate antidiuretic hormone.

10. Monitor the effects of anesthetic agents, such as propofol, and sedatives, such as midazolam or dexmedetomidine hydrochloride, which may be given to prevent sudden changes in ICP due to coughing, straining, or "fighting" the ventilator. Short-acting medications are preferred to allow for intermittent neurologic assessment.
11. High-dose barbiturates, such as pentobarbital, may be used in patients with refractory increased ICP. (*Note*: Prophylactic use is not recommended. It is utilized when all other treatments have failed.) Dosing: 10 mg/kg over 30 minutes; then 5 mg/kg every hour for 3 hours followed by a maintenance dose of 1 mg/kg/h. (Goal serum barbiturate level of 3 to 4 mg/dL.)
    a. High-dose barbiturates induce a comatose state and suppress brain metabolism, which, in turn, reduces cerebral blood flow and ICP. Only pupillary response is assessed.
    b. Be alert to the high level of nursing support required. All responses to environmental and noxious stimuli (suctioning, turning) are abolished as well as all protective reflexes.
    c. Cough or gag reflex will be absent, and the patient will be unable to protect the airway, increasing susceptibility to pneumonia.
    d. Monitor ICP, arterial pressure, and serum barbiturate levels, as indicated. Perform continuous electroencephalography (EEG) monitoring to document burst suppression (suppression of cortical activity) and ensure adequate dosing of barbiturates, if used.
    e. Monitor temperature because barbiturate coma causes hypothermia.
    f. Diminished gastrointestinal (GI) motility and high risk for ileus.
12. Maintain normothermia and treat fever aggressively. Fever increases cerebral blood flow and cerebral blood volume; acute increases in ICP occur with fever spikes. Cerebral temperature is 4°C to 5°C higher than body core temperature; therefore, small increases in body core temperature can create drastic increases in the core temperature of the brain. Infection is a common complication of ICP, and in the presence of fever, an infectious workup should be completed.
13. Avoid positions or activities that may increase ICP. Keep head in alignment with shoulders; neck flexion or rotation increases ICP by impeding venous return. Keep the head of the bed elevated 30 degrees to reduce jugular venous pressure and decrease ICP.
    a. Minimize suctioning, keep procedure less than 15 seconds, and, if ordered, instill lidocaine via ET tube before suctioning. Coughing and suctioning are associated with increased intrathoracic pressure, which is associated with ICP spikes. Inject 5 to 10 mL of lidocaine into ET tube before suctioning to dampen the cough response.
    b. Minimize other stimuli, such as alarms, television, radio, and bedside conversations, which may precipitously increase ICP (stimuli that create elevation in ICP are patient dependent).
14. Maintain normal blood sugar levels. Treat with sliding scale insulin or insulin drip as ordered.
15. Initiate treatment modalities, as ordered, for increased ICP (above 20 mm Hg or if there is a significant shift in pressure).
16. Pretreat prior to known activities that raise ICP and avoid taking pressure readings immediately after a procedure. Allow patient to rest for approximately 5 minutes.
17. Record ICP readings every hour and correlate with significant clinical events or treatments (suctioning, turning).

Evaluation: Expected Outcomes

- ICP and vital signs stable; alert and responsive.

Intracranial Monitoring

EVIDENCE BASE Nag, D. S., Sahu, S., Swain, A., & Kant, S. (2019). Intracranial pressure monitoring: Gold standard and recent innovations. *World Journal of Clinical Cases, 7*(13), 1535–1553. https://doi.org/10.12998/wjcc.v7.i13.1535

Intracranial monitoring, including ICP monitoring, is a technology that helps the nurse assess, plan, intervene, and evaluate patient responses to care. ICP monitoring is widely used (see Figure 11-1).

1. External ventricular drain (EVD): Catheter is inserted into lateral ventricle (right is preferred) through a drilled burr hole opening; connected to fluid-filled transducer, which converts mechanical pressure to electrical impulses and waveform; allows ventricular drainage. EVD is the most accurate method to measure ICP.
2. Subarachnoid (bolt) hollow screw inserted into SAS beneath the skull and dura through drill hole; also connected to pressure transducer system.
3. Epidural sensor inserted beneath skull but not through dura, so does not measure pressure directly; fiberoptic cable is connected directly to monitor.
4. Parenchymal device is inserted directly into brain tissue.

Intracranial Pressure Waveforms

ICP pulse waveforms are generated from a pressure wave transmitted through the cardiovascular system into the tissues within the intracranial cavity (see Figure 11-2).

1. The normal pulse waveform consists of three identifiable components: P-1, P-2, and P-3.

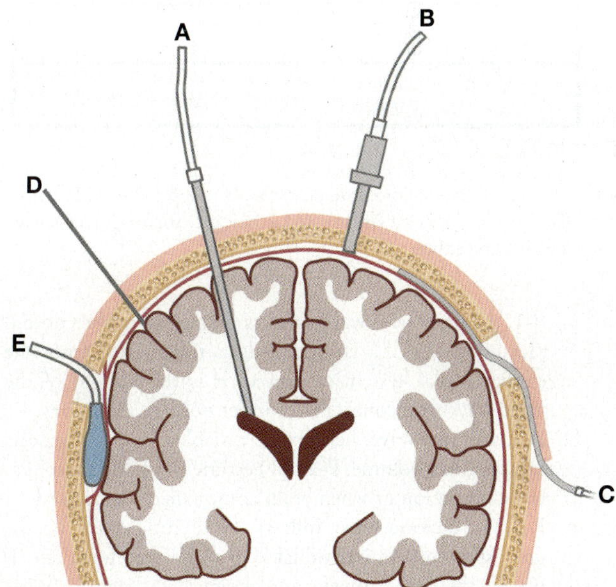

Figure 11-1. Intracranial pressure monitoring system. **(A)** Intraventricular; **(B)** subarachnoid; **(C)** subdural; **(D)** parenchymal; **(E)** epidural. (Adapted with permission from Diepenbrock, N. H. [2015]. *Quick reference to critical care* [5th ed., Fig. 1.28]. Lippincott Williams & Wilkins.)

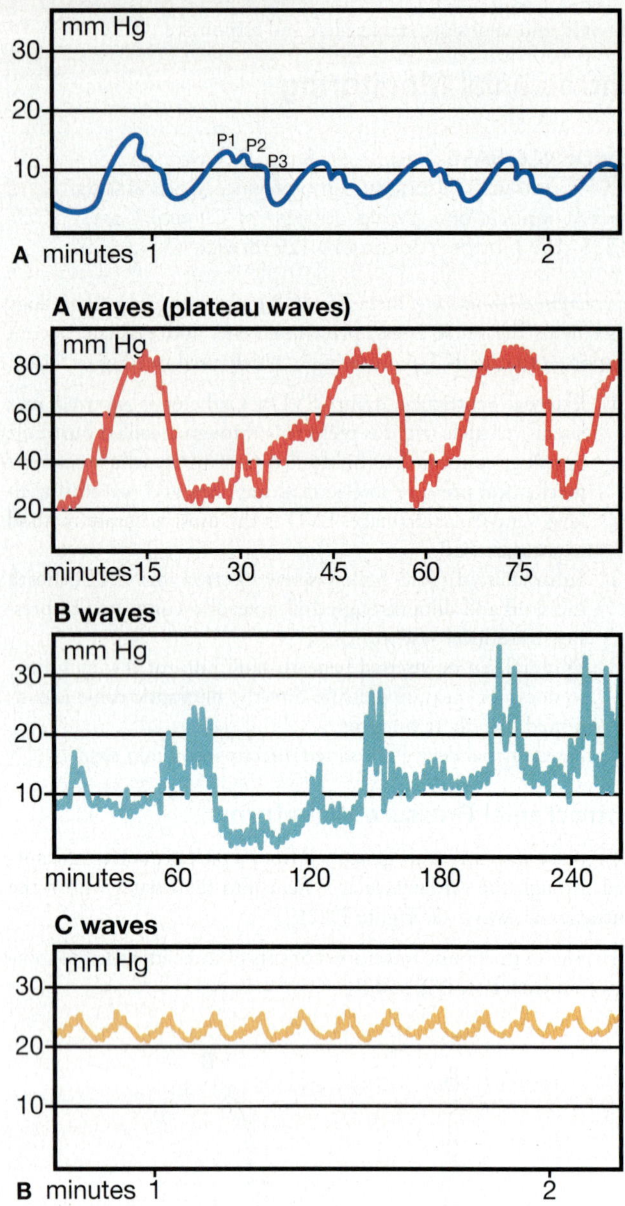

Figure 11-2. Intracranial pressure (ICP) waves. **(A)** Normal ICP waveform. **(B)** *A waves* (plateau waves) are pathologic. *B and C waves* have little clinical significance.

a. P-1, the percussive wave, reflects pulsations of the choroid plexus, where CSF is produced, as transmitted from the cardiovascular system at systole. It is the highest of the three waveform components under normal conditions.

b. P-2, the tidal wave, has a more variable shape and reflects relative brain volume. P-2 can become elevated in response to a mass lesion or when brain compliance is decreased.

c. P-3, the dicrotic wave, follows the dicrotic notch on the downslope of the individual ICP pulse waveform and is usually the lowest waveform segment.

2. Plateau or A-wave patterns are pathologic, reflecting a rapid rise in ICP up to 50 to 100 mm Hg, and may be followed by a variable period during which the ICP remains elevated and then falls to baseline. Truncated patterns that do not exceed an elevation of 50 mm Hg are early indicators of neurologic deterioration. Waves are clinically significant as elevation in ICP is related to compromise in autoregulation secondary to increased cerebral blood volume and decreased cerebral blood flow.

3. B- and C-wave patterns are related to respiration and are of little clinical significance. B-wave patterns are of shorter duration and smaller amplitude than A-wave patterns and may precede A-wave patterns. C-wave patterns are small, rhythmic oscillations that fluctuate with changes in respiration and BP.

Other Monitoring Systems

1. Licox brain oxygen monitoring system—placed in the brain tissue through a burr hole and monitors brain tissue partial pressure of oxygen ($PbrO_2$), cerebral temperature, and indirect ICP. Continual monitoring of the cerebral temperature and oxygenation levels provides direct information on the acute changes in the intracranial tissue that can potentiate secondary brain injury.
2. Microdialysis—catheter is placed into the brain tissue through a burr hole for monitoring of cerebral oxygen, glucose, lactate, lactate–pyruvate, glutamate, and glycerol. The catheter is connected to a 2.5-mL syringe and into a microinfusion pump. The pump is perfused with Ringer solution. Samples are obtained periodically for analysis.
3. Jugular venous oximetry—a fiberoptic oximetry catheter is placed into the jugular bulb of the internal jugular vein for measurement of jugular venous oxygen saturation ($SjvO_2$). $SjvO_2$ is helpful in evaluating arterial saturation, cerebral metabolic rate for oxygen, and cerebral blood flow. The normal range is between 54% and 75%. A low $SjvO_2$ is suggestive of increased brain extraction of oxygen related to systemic arterial hypoxia, decreased cerebral blood flow from hypotension or vasospasm, or an elevated ICP with a low CPP. Desaturation is thought to be associated with ischemic events and directly related to increased morbidity.

Nursing Interventions

1. Note the pattern of waveforms and any sustained elevation of pressure above 20 mm Hg.
2. Avoid overstimulation of the patient.
   a. Note the stimuli that cause increased pressure, such as bathing, suctioning, repositioning, or visitors. Adjust care, as indicated.
   b. Premedicate, as indicated.
   c. Provide rest periods between periods of care.
   d. Limit visitors as status indicates.
   e. Limit unnecessary conversation at patient's bedside.
   f. Eliminate external environmental stimuli. Close doors, turn off suction equipment when not in use, limit television or radio as status indicates.
3. Watch for developing or increasing P-2 waves and frequency of A (plateau) waves. Report these, and begin measures to lower increased ICP.

CLINICAL JUDGMENT Sustained elevation in ICP greater than 20 mm Hg and CPP less than 50 mm Hg correlates with worsening outcomes following TBI. Measures to reduce increased ICP should be performed immediately and the health care provider notified when the ICP remains elevated for more than 5 minutes.

Nursing Management of the Patient Undergoing Intracranial Surgery

Craniotomy is the surgical opening of the skull to gain access to intracranial structures to perform a biopsy, remove a tumor, relieve increased ICP, evacuate a blood clot, evaluate and treat the cause of intracranial hemorrhage, or remove epileptogenic tissue. Surgical approach is based on the location of the lesion and may be supratentorial (above the tentorium or dural covering that divides the cerebrum from cerebellum) or infratentorial (below the tentorium, including the brainstem). Craniotomy may be performed by means of burr holes (made with a drill or hand tools) or by making a bony flap. *Craniectomy* is excision and removal of a portion of the skull. *Cranioplasty* is repair of a cranial defect by means of a plastic or metal plate. *Transsphenoidal surgery* is an approach that gains access to the pituitary gland through the nasal cavity and sphenoidal sinus (see Chapter 204).

Preoperative Management

1. Diagnostic findings, surgical procedure, and expectations are reviewed with the patient.
2. Presurgical shampoo with an antimicrobial agent may be ordered. Skull preparation is performed in the operating room.
3. Depending on primary diagnosis, corticosteroids may be ordered preoperatively to reduce vasogenic cerebral edema.
4. Depending on the type and location of lesion, anticonvulsants may be ordered to reduce the risk of seizures.
5. The patient is prepared for the use of intraoperative antibiotics to reduce the risk of infection.
6. Urinary catheterization is performed to assess urinary volume during operative period.
7. If cerebral edema develops, intraoperative or postoperative osmotic diuretic (mannitol) or corticosteroids may be ordered for its treatment.
8. Neurologic assessment is performed to evaluate and record the patient's neurologic baseline and vital signs for postoperative comparison.
9. Family and patient are made aware of the immediate postoperative care and where the provider will contact the family after surgery.
10. Supportive care is given, as needed, for neurologic deficits.

Postoperative Management

1. Respiratory status is assessed by monitoring rate, depth, and pattern of respirations. A patent airway is maintained.
2. Vital signs and neurologic status are monitored using a facility-based neurologic assessment tool; findings are documented. Arterial line may be used for blood pressure monitoring.
3. Pharmacologic agents may be prescribed to control increased ICP.
4. Incisional and headache pain may be controlled with analgesic such as an opioid or acetaminophen, as prescribed. Monitor response to medications.
5. Position head of bed at 15 to 30 degrees, or per clinical status of the patient, to promote venous drainage. Determining appropriate position of head of bed is patient dependent and should be adjusted based on observed changes in the patient's clinical response and ICP to positioning.
6. Turn side to side every 2 hours; positioning restrictions will be ordered by the health care provider (craniectomy patients should not be turned on the side of the cranial defect).
7. Computed tomography (CT) scan of the brain is performed if the patient's status deteriorates.
8. Oral fluids are provided when the patient is alert and swallow reflex has returned. Intake and output are monitored. Speech therapy may be ordered for bedside swallow study or radiographic swallow study.
9. Signs of infection are monitored by checking craniotomy site, ventricular drainage, nuchal rigidity, or presence of CSF (fluid collection at surgical site).
10. Periorbital edema is controlled by measures such as elevation of head of bed and cold compresses. Removal of surgical dressing and increase in activity will assist in the resolution of periorbital edema.

Potential Complications

1. Intracranial hemorrhage/hematoma.
2. Cerebral edema.
3. Infections (e.g., postoperative meningitis, pulmonary, wound).
4. Seizures.
5. CN dysfunction.
6. Decreased CPP causing cerebral ischemia.

Nursing Interventions

Maintaining Intracranial Pressure Within Normal Range

1. Closely monitor LOC, vital signs, pupillary response, and ICP, if indicated. Notify health care provider if ICP is greater than 20 mm Hg or CPP is less than 50 mm Hg.
2. Teach the patient to avoid activities that can raise ICP, such as excessive flexion or rotation of the head and Valsalva maneuver (coughing, straining with defecation).
3. Administer medications, as prescribed, to reduce ICP.
4. Check ICP waveform before nursing interventions that create noxious tactile stimuli, such as suctioning, prolonged physical assessment, turning, and ROM exercises and delay interventions based on patient response.

Preventing Aspiration

1. Offer fluids only when the patient is alert and swallow reflexes have returned; the patient may require speech language pathology assessment for ability to swallow.
2. Have suction equipment available at bedside. Suction only if indicated. Pretreat with sedation or ET lidocaine to prevent elevation of ICP.
3. Elevate head of bed to maximum of order, or per clinical status, and patient comfort.

Preventing Nosocomial Infections

1. Use sterile technique for dressing changes, catheter care, and ventricular drain management.
2. Be aware of patients at higher risk of infection—those undergoing lengthy operations, those with ventricular drains left in longer than 72 hours, and those with operations of the third ventricle.
3. Assess surgical site for redness, tenderness, and drainage.
4. Watch for leakage of CSF, which increases the danger of meningitis.
   a. Watch for sudden discharge of fluid from wound; a large leak usually requires surgical repair.
   b. Warn against coughing, sneezing, or nose blowing, which may aggravate CSF leakage.
   c. Assess for elevation of temperature and neck rigidity.
   d. Note patency of ventricular catheter system.

5. Early removal of urinary catheter.
6. Institute measures to prevent respiratory or UTI postoperatively.

Relieving Pain

1. Medicate patient as prescribed and according to assessment findings.
2. Elevate head of bed per protocol to relieve headache.
3. Provide distractive measures for pain management.
4. Darken room if patient is photophobic.

Avoiding Constipation

1. Encourage fluids when the patient is able to manage liquids.
2. Ambulate as soon as possible.
3. Change to nonopioid agents for pain control as soon as possible.
4. Avoid Valsalva-like maneuvers.
5. Use stool softeners and laxatives, as ordered.

Family Education and Support

1. Keep the patient and family aware of progress and plans to transfer to step-down unit, general nursing unit, subacute care, or rehabilitation facility.
2. Encourage frequent visiting and interaction of family for stimulation of patient as care allows.
3. Begin discharge planning early, and obtain referral for home care nursing, social work, or physical and occupational therapy, as needed.

Evaluation: Expected Outcomes

- Normal ICP and CPP maintained between 50 and 70 mm Hg.
- Gag reflex present; breath sounds clear.
- Afebrile without signs of infection.
- Verbalizes decreased pain.
- Passed soft stool.

CRANIAL NERVE DISORDERS

Bell Palsy

Idiopathic *Bell palsy* is an acute peripheral facial paralysis of the infratemporal portion of cranial nerve (CN) VII (facial nerve) that most often occurs unilaterally. The annual incidence of Bell palsy is approximately 15 to 20 cases per 100,000 persons. It is typically a self-limiting process that improves in 3 to 6 months.

Pathophysiology and Etiology

1. Cause is unknown. Possible etiologies include sensory ganglionitis of the central nervous system (CNS) with secondary muscle palsy, caused by inflammation, vascular ischemia, and autoimmune demyelination.
2. Most patients experience a viral prodrome (e.g., upper respiratory infection, herpes simplex virus) 1 to 3 weeks before the onset of symptoms.
3. Can affect anyone at any age; however, it disproportionately affects those who are pregnant and those who have diabetes, hypertension, or influenza.
4. Generally self-limiting. With or without treatment, most patients improve significantly within 2 weeks and about 80% recover completely within 3 months. In rare cases, the symptoms may never completely resolve or may recur. Risk factors thought to be associated with a poor outcome include (1) over age 60 years, (2) complete paralysis, and (3) decreased taste or salivary flow on the side of paralysis.

Clinical Manifestations

1. Acute onset of unilateral upper and lower facial paralysis (over a 48-hour period and reaches its peak within 72 hours). Paralysis of the ipsilateral side of the face from vertex of scalp to chin; facial muscles weak throughout the forehead, cheek, and chin; can affect speech and taste, distort face, decrease tearing, and cause posterior auricular pain.
2. Involvement of all branches of facial nerve: facial weakness, diminished taste from anterior two thirds of the tongue, decreased blink reflex, decreased lacrimation, inability to close eye, painful eye sensations, photophobia, drooling.
3. Patients may experience neck, mastoid, or ear pain or hyperacusis on the affected side.

Diagnostic Evaluation

1. History to determine previous illness, onset of paralysis, and associated symptoms.
2. Exclusion of lesions that mimic Bell palsy, such as tumor, infection (Lyme disease, meningitis), trauma, stroke, or other conditions (sarcoidosis, multiple sclerosis, Guillain-Barré syndrome) through thorough neurologic examination and computed tomography (CT) scan or brain magnetic resonance imaging (MRI) with contrast media.
3. Electrophysiologic testing, specifically action potentials, electromyographies (EMGs), and nerve conduction velocities, to evaluate nerve function.
4. Lyme disease serologic testing a history of tick bite or bilateral weakness. About 5% to 10% of untreated Lyme disease patients may develop Bell palsy.

CLINICAL JUDGMENT A rapid neurologic examination should be performed to differentiate Bell palsy from other conditions that could be causing facial droop. The patient with Bell palsy should have normal level of consciousness (LOC), motor strength (except in the area of facial nerve), sensation, and reflexes. Depending on the clinical concern, a head CT scan or brain MRI may be indicated for abnormal neurologic findings beyond the facial nerve.

Management

1. Corticosteroid therapy should be initiated within 72 hours of onset to decrease inflammation (e.g., prednisone 50 to 60 mg for the first 5 days, followed by a tapering dose). Acyclovir combined with prednisone may improve facial function. When using corticosteroids for the treatment of Bell palsy, caution should be used in patients with tuberculosis, peptic ulcer disease, diabetes mellitus, renal or hepatic dysfunction, or malignant hypertension. For patients who have a contraindication to steroid therapy, acyclovir alone may be given.
2. Eye care to maintain lubrication and moisture if unable to close. May need to be patched during sleep.
3. Physical therapy, electrical stimulation to maintain muscle tone.
4. Biofeedback as adjunct therapy.
5. Surgical treatment of Bell palsy may include to anastomose facial nerve to other CN (CN VII to CN XI or CN VII to CN XII), surgical closure of eyelid to protect cornea (tarsorrhaphy), facial nerve decompression, placement of gold weights into the eyelid and facial lifts. Bell palsy is usually self-limiting and, therefore, generally does not require surgical treatment.

Complications

1. Corneal ulceration.
2. Impairment of vision.
3. Synkinesis (an abnormal, involuntary facial muscle contraction during normal facial muscle movements).
4. Psychosocial adjustment to prolonged paralysis.

Nursing Assessment

1. Test motor components of facial nerve (VII) by assessing patient's smile and ability to whistle, purse lips, wrinkle forehead, and close eyes. Observe for facial asymmetry.
2. Observe patient's ability to handle secretions, food, and fluids; observe for drooling.
3. Assess patient's ability to blink and speak clearly.
4. Assess effect of altered appearance on body image.

Nursing Interventions

Preventing Eye Dryness and Maintaining Corneal Integrity

1. Administer and teach the patient to administer artificial tears and ophthalmic ointment as prescribed.
2. Patch eye to keep shut at night, as directed.
3. Inspect eye for redness or discharge.
4. Advise the patient to report eye pain immediately.
5. Protect the cornea if the eye does not close. Keratitis (inflammation of the cornea), ulceration, and vision loss are major threats to a patient with Bell palsy.

Enhancing Body Image

1. Encourage the patient to express feelings related to body image disturbance.
2. Encourage the patient to use mirror as means to obtain feedback about actual versus perceived appearance.
3. Perform and teach the patient to perform facial massage to alleviate feelings of stiffness and enhance recovery.

Patient Education and Health Maintenance

1. Instruct the patient to wear wraparound sunglasses to decrease normal evaporation from the eye from sun and wind, to avoid eye irritants, and to increase environmental humidity.
2. Instruct the patient in use of ophthalmic drops and ointment, proper methods of lid closure, and patching of the eye.
3. Demonstrate facial exercises (e.g., raise eyebrows, squeeze eyes shut, purse lips) and stress their importance to prevent muscle atrophy.

Evaluation: Expected Outcomes

- Cornea without redness, pain, or discharge.
- Verbalizes adjustment to body image disturbance.

Trigeminal Neuralgia (Tic Douloureux)

Trigeminal neuralgia (TN) (tic douloureux) is an intensely painful neurologic condition that affects one or more branches of the fifth cranial (trigeminal) nerve. Patients experience sudden paroxysms of "lancinating" or electric shock–like facial pain localized to one or more branches of the nerve (see Figure 11-3). The pain is often precipitated by trigger points that "fire" when the patient talks, shaves, eats, touches the face, brushes the teeth, or is exposed to cold wind. Approximately 15,000 patients in the United States are diagnosed with TN annually. Patients who present with the disease between ages 20 and 40 are more likely to suffer from a demyelinating lesion in the pons secondary to multiple sclerosis (MS).

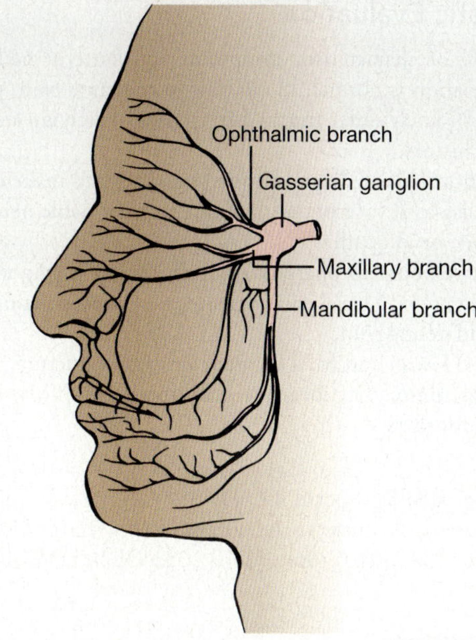

Figure 11-3. The main divisions of the trigeminal nerve are the ophthalmic, maxillary, and mandibular. Sensory root fibers arise in the Gasserian ganglion.

Pathophysiology and Etiology

1. Unknown cause, but degenerative or viral origin suspected.
2. Any of the three trigeminal nerve branches can be affected:
   a. V_1: ophthalmic branch; pain involves the eye and forehead.
   b. V_2: maxillary branch; pain involves the cheek, upper teeth, upper gums, and nose.
   c. V_3: mandibular branch; pain involves the lower jaw, side of the tongue, lower teeth, and lower gum and extends to the ear.
3. Compression from artery adjacent to the nerve strips myelin from the nerve when it pulsates. Loss of myelin acts like an uninsulated wire that "fires" abnormally in response to stimuli.

POPULATION AWARENESS TN is commonly seen in older adults. Pain typically appears to be localized to one or more teeth. Patients may seek dental care for pain relief, resulting in one or more tooth extractions without alleviation of pain.

Clinical Manifestations

1. Sudden, severe episodes of intense facial pain localized to one or more of the branches of the nerve, lasting less than 30 to 60 seconds and ending abruptly.
2. Pain may occur spontaneously or be precipitated by activation of trigger points, such as touching the face, talking, chewing, yawning, and brushing the teeth, that place pressure on the terminal end of the branch affected.
3. Pain is always unilateral and does not cross the midline. Bilateral pain is sometimes seen in patients with MS and should result in a high index of suspicion for this condition. MS and hypertension are the two risk factors found in epidemiologic studies.
4. Some patients experience numbness, particularly around the mouth.

Diagnostic Evaluation

1. History of characteristic symptoms and pattern; neurologic examination is normal. In contrast to migraine pain, persons with TN rarely suffer attacks during sleep, which is a key point in the history.
2. Classification and diagnostic grading system to make diagnosis of classic TN, secondary TN due to identifiable neurologic disorder, or idiopathic TN.
3. Quick response to pharmacologic treatment is important to rule out atypical facial pain, vasomotor or postherpetic neuralgia, and dental pain.
4. Head CT scan and MRI of the brain show structural lesions, such as tumor, arteriovenous malformation (AVM), MS, or other disorders.

EVIDENCE BASE Cruccu, G., Di Stefano, G., & Truini, A. (2020). Trigeminal neuralgia. *New England Journal of Medicine, 383*(8), 754–762. https://doi.org/10.1056/NEJMra1914484

Management

Pharmacologic

1. Carbamazepine and oxcarbazepine are the first-line and most effective medications used to treat this condition. Other drugs such as levetiracetam, phenytoin, baclofen, pregabalin, and gabapentin may be substituted.
2. Although pain generally responds to pharmacologic intervention, it gradually becomes refractory over time, or patients suffer undesirable adverse effects.

Surgical

Operative procedure selected is one that will provide the greatest chance of long-term pain relief with the fewest complications.

1. Alcohol, phenol block, or glycerol injection for pain may last several months after injection.
2. Percutaneous radiofrequency trigeminal gangliolysis directs low-voltage stimulation of nerve by electrode inserted through foramen ovale; sensory function is destroyed with goal to preserve motor function; may cause decreased corneal sensation if V1 affected; paresthesias, jaw weakness, or undesirable, painful numbness (anesthesia dolorosa). Pain may recur as nerve regenerates, necessitating repeat procedure.
3. Rhizotomy (transection of nerve root at Gasserian ganglion) causes complete loss of sensation; other complications include burning, stinging, discomfort in and around eye, herpetic lesions of face, keratitis, and corneal ulceration. Pain may recur as nerve regenerates.
4. Percutaneous balloon microcompression for selective destruction of nerve fibers that mediate light touch and trigger pain. Relieves pain in ophthalmic branch while sparing corneal sensation.
5. Microvascular decompression of trigeminal nerve. Most effective form of therapy, with 75% to 80% of patients pain free without need for long-term medication after the procedure. Treatment of choice for younger patients who are at low anesthesia risk, do not want facial numbness, and are willing to accept craniotomy.
6. Gamma knife surgery is less invasive than the percutaneous procedures. It is about as effective as the percutaneous procedures; however, relief may not come for weeks to months, and it is a bit more expensive.

Complications

1. Anorexia and weight loss.
2. Dehydration.
3. Anxiety, fear.
4. Depression, social isolation, and suicidal ideations in extreme cases.

Nursing Assessment

1. Take history of the pain, including duration, severity, and aggravating factors.
2. Assess nutritional status and hydration.
3. Assess for anxiety and depression, including problems with sleep, social interaction, and coping ability/skills.

Nursing Interventions

Relieving Pain

1. To minimize painful episodes, review with patient potential trigger factors, and develop individualized methods of coping with identified triggers.
2. Encourage the patient to take medication regularly, including "rescue" medication for breakthrough periods.
3. Help the patient maintain a method of communication without causing pain from talking.

Maintaining Adequate Nutrition

1. To maximize nutritional intake, instruct the patient to take foods and fluids at room temperature and to chew on the unaffected side.
2. Have the patient consult with the dietitian for appropriate meal texture and composition.
3. Encourage small, frequent meals to avoid fatigue and pain.
4. Advise about the use of nutritional supplements, if indicated.

Increasing Control

1. Support the patient through treatment trials.
2. Teach relaxation exercises, such as relaxation breathing, progressive muscle relaxation, and guided imagery, to relieve tension.
3. Encourage participation in support groups (e.g., Facial Pain Association) and facilitate a therapeutic relationship with the health care provider.

Patient Education and Health Maintenance

1. Educate the surgical patient regarding self-care after denervation procedures.
   a. Instruct the patient to inspect the eye for redness and foreign bodies three to four times per day if corneal sensation is impaired.
   b. Instruct the patient to instill lubricating eye drops every 4 hours if corneal sensation is impaired.
   c. Instruct the patient to avoid drinking hot or very cold liquids.
   d. Instruct the patient to chew on the unaffected side to avoid biting tongue, lips, and inside of mouth.
   e. Instruct the patient who wears dentures that jaw muscle will regenerate over time; avoid having dentures refitted, but maintain regular dental checkups because pain will not be felt.
   f. Instruct the patient to report any change in sensation.
2. Refer patient to the Facial Pain Association for education and support network (www.fpa-support.org) or the National Institute of Neurological Disorders and Stroke (www.ninds.nih.gov).

Evaluation: Expected Outcomes

- Verbalizes reduced pain.
- Maintains weight.
- Verbalizes decreased anxiety and depression.

CEREBROVASCULAR DISEASE

Cerebrovascular Insufficiency

EVIDENCE BASE Kleindorfer, D. O., Towfighi, A., Chaturvedi, S., Cockroft, K. M., Gutierrez, J., Lombardi-Hill, D., Kamel, H., Kernan, W. N., Kittner, S. J., Leira, E. C., Lennon, O., Meschia, J. F., Nguyen, T. N., Pollak, P. M., Santangeli, P., Sharrief, A. Z., Smith, S. C., Jr., Turan, T. N., & Williams, L. S. (2021). 2021 guideline for the prevention of stroke in patients with stroke and transient ischemic attack: A guideline from the American Heart Association/American Stroke Association. *Stroke*, *52*(7), e364–e467. https://doi.org/10.1161/STR.0000000000000375

Greenberg, S. M., Ziai, W. C., Cordonnier, C., Dowlatshahi, D., Francis, B., Goldstein, J. N., Hemphill, J. C., III, Johnson, R., Keigher, K. M., Mack, W. J., Mocco, J., Newton, E. J., Ruff, I. M., Sansing, L. H., Schulman, S., Selim, M. H., Sheth, K. N., Sprigg, N., Sunnerhagen, K. S., & American Heart Association /American Stroke Association. (2022). 2022 guideline for the management of patients with spontaneous intracerebral hemorrhage: A guideline from the American Heart Association/ American Stroke Association. *Stroke*, *53*, e282–e361. https://doi.org/10.1161/STR.0000000000000407

Rodgers, M. L. (2021). Care of the patient with acute ischemic stroke (endovascular/intensive care unit-postinterventional therapy): Update to 2009 comprehensive nursing care scientific statement: A scientific statement from the American Heart Association. *Stroke*, *52*, e198–e210. https://doi.org/10.1161/STR.0000000000000358

Cerebrovascular insufficiency is an interruption or inadequate blood flow to a focal area of the brain, resulting in transient or permanent neurologic dysfunction. *Transient ischemic attack* (TIA) lasts less than 24 hours. *Ischemic stroke* is similar to myocardial infarction, in that the pathogenesis is loss of blood supply to the tissue, which can result in irreversible damage if blood flow is not restored quickly.

Pathophysiology and Etiology

1. Cerebrovascular insufficiency can be caused by atherosclerotic plaque or thrombosis, resulting in increased PCO_2, decreased PO_2, decreased blood viscosity, hyperthermia/hypothermia, and increased intracranial pressure (ICP).
2. Carotid arteries, vertebral arteries, major intracranial vessels, or microcirculation may be affected.
3. Cardiac causes of emboli include atrial fibrillation, mitral valve prolapse, infectious endocarditis, and prosthetic heart valve.
4. Event may be classified as TIA—transient episode of cerebral dysfunction with associated clinical manifestations lasting usually minutes to an hour, possibly up to 24 hours.
5. Symptoms persisting longer than 24 hours are classified as stroke (also known as *brain attack*).

Risk Factors for Stroke

Medical Conditions

1. Diabetes mellitus: Of the patients presenting with acute ischemic stroke, new cases of type 2 DM have been detected in about 11.5%, and prediabetes has been detected in about 36.2%.
2. Hypertension.
3. Hyperlipidemia.
4. Coronary artery disease and cardiac disorders, such as congenital heart disease, valvular conditions, endocarditis, and atrial fibrillation.
5. History of TIA or stroke: Approximately 23% of strokes each year are recurrent. Risk of recurrent stroke or TIA is high (5% at 1 year), but risks can be reduced with prevention strategies.
6. Hypercoagulable disorders, such as protein C deficiency: Protein C deficiency is an autosomal dominant disorder and a well-established cause for stroke development, especially in young adults.
7. Rare: endothelial damage (inflammation or infection, drug-induced, fibromuscular dysplasia, carotid or vertebral artery dissections).

Behaviors

1. Cigarette smoking approximately doubles the risk of stroke.
2. Alcohol misuse.
3. Physical inactivity.
4. Cocaine use (hemorrhagic stroke).

Nonmodifiable Factors

1. Increasing age—risk doubles for each decade over age 50.
2. Sex assigned at birth—females have more stokes than males, and stroke kills more females than males.
3. Heredity—increased risk with family history of stroke, especially before the age of 65.
4. Ethnic background—African Americans are 50% more likely to have a stroke than their White adult counterparts.

Other

Factors that may increase stroke risk for females include pregnancy, history of preeclampsia/eclampsia or gestational diabetes, oral contraceptive use, and postmenopausal hormone therapy. There have been reports in the literature of increased risk in individuals with migraine headaches. Chiropractic manipulation has been associated with ischemic stroke related to dissection.

DRUG ALERT Increased stroke risk has been associated with individuals who smoke cigarettes and take oral contraceptives.

Clinical Manifestations of Transient Ischemic Attacks

1. Temporary, focal brain ischemia that is sudden in onset and that results in a neurologic deficit that resolves within 24 hours. Diagnostic imaging demonstrates no permanent ischemic changes.
2. Carotid system involvement: (anterior circulation): amaurosis fugax (temporary blindness in one eye), vision change (temporary blurring of vision, graying or fogginess of vision), unilateral weakness, unilateral numbness or paresthesias.
3. Vertebrobasilar system involvement: (posterior circulation) vertigo, ataxia, dizziness, diplopia, dysarthria, dysphagia, weakness, and sensory changes that are bilateral or unilateral.

Diagnostic Evaluation

1. Facilities will have a stroke protocol for ordering of diagnostic studies for patients suspected of a TIA or stroke. These include computed tomography (CT) scan, CT perfusion, CT angiography, digital subtraction angiography, magnetic resonance angiogram (MRA), magnetic resonance imaging (MRI), and transcranial Doppler (TCD) ultrasound.

2. MRI stroke protocol—consists of a standard MRI with specific sequences to identify ischemia (refer to page 328 for descriptions of these sequences).
3. Transthoracic echocardiography (TTE) with a bubble study—can provide information when searching for the etiology of the ischemic event. Specifically, cardioembolic sources.
4. Transesophageal echocardiography (TEE)—may be ordered in place of a TTE or to follow-up findings noted on the TTE.
5. Heart recording device:
   a. Implantable loop recorder (ILR)—monitors heart rhythm continually. Monthly data are sent remotely for rhythm analysis.
   b. Ambulatory cardiac monitor.
6. Laboratory studies—determined on an individual basis and may include:
   a. Prothrombotic states—protein C, protein S, antithrombin II, thrombin time, hemoglobin, anticardiolipin antibody, lupus anticoagulant, syphilis antibody.
   b. Anticoagulation monitoring—heparin (activated partial thromboplastin time [aPTT]), warfarin (prothrombin time/international normalized ratio [PT/INR]), antiplatelets (clopidogrel), prasugrel, ticagrelor monitored with P_2Y_{12} assay. Aspirin—aspirin platelet assay.

Management

1. Management decisions (medical and surgical) will depend on the results of the diagnostic workup and can include the following:
   a. Medications—antiplatelet medications, anticoagulation.
   b. Surgical or endovascular interventions to improve blood flow to the brain. These include carotid endarterectomy, placement of a carotid stent, carotid angioplasty, and extracranial–intracranial anastomosis (EC-IC bypass).
   c. Treatment of dysrhythmias.
   d. Risk factor reduction—control of hypertension, diabetes, hyperlipidemia, and smoking cessation.

Complications

1. Complete ischemic stroke.
2. Hemorrhagic conversion of ischemic stroke.
3. Cerebral edema.

Nursing Assessment

1. Obtain a history of presenting complaints, medical history addressing known risk factors. Hypertensive and diabetic control; hyperlipidemia; cardiovascular disease or dysrhythmias, such as atrial fibrillation; smoking. Complete medication history with attention to any antiplatelet, anticoagulants, and over-the-counter (OTC) medications.
2. Perform physical examination, including neurologic, cardiac, and circulatory systems; be sure to listen for carotid bruit.
3. Assess the patient for a history of headache and, if positive, for duration of headache.

Nursing Interventions

Improving Cerebral Perfusion

1. Teach the patient signs and symptoms of TIA and need to notify health care provider immediately. Use the acronym FAST to know what to look for: F, face weakness; A, arm weakness; S, speech difficulties; T, time—immediately seek medical assistance.
2. Administer or teach self-administration of anticoagulants, antiplatelet agents, antihypertensives, and other medication; also teach about monitoring for adverse effects and therapeutic effect.
3. Prepare the patient for surgical or endovascular intervention as indicated (see page 355).

Providing Care and Preventing Complications After Surgical Procedure

Also see "Nursing Management of the Patient Undergoing Intracranial Surgery" section, page 341, and "Cerebral Angiography" section, page 330.

1. After surgical procedure, monitor vital signs as ordered and administer prescribed medications to avoid hypotension (which can cause cerebral ischemia) or hypertension (which can precipitate cerebral hemorrhage).
2. Perform frequent neurologic checks as ordered. Including level of consciousness (LOC), speech, pupil size, equality, and reaction; motor strength and sensation. Notify the health care provider of any deficits immediately.
3. Observe operative area/puncture site closely for development of hematoma. Mild swelling is expected, but if hematoma formation is suspected, notify provider and prepare the patient for possible intervention.
4. Medicate for pain and avoid agitation or sudden changes in position, which could affect blood pressure (BP).
5. Elevate head of bed when vital signs are stable.
6. Following carotid endarterectomy:
   a. Monitor BP closely as patients after surgery may experience BP instability for 12 to 24 hours.
   b. Monitor for hoarseness, impaired gag reflex, or difficulty swallowing and facial weakness, which indicate cranial nerve (CN) injury.
   c. Keep head in neutral position to relieve stress on surgical site; monitor drainage.
   d. Keep tracheostomy tube at bedside and assess for stridor; hematoma formation can cause airway obstruction.
7. Following EC-IC bypass, avoid pressure over the anastomosis of the superior temporal artery (EC) and the middle cerebral artery (MCA) (IC) to prevent rupture or ischemia of the site. If the patient wears glasses, remove the eyeglass arm on the operative side to avoid this possible pressure point.
8. Following carotid stenting, administer medications, as directed. Following placement of a carotid stent, the patient will be on dual-antiplatelet therapy (DAPT) for a designated period of time.
   a. Heparin—bolus given intraprocedure, then possible continuous intravenous (IV) drip postprocedure to maintain partial thromboplastin time (PTT) within ordered range; monitor PTT every 6 hours or according to institution protocol. In the event of an acute neurologic deficit, the heparin drip should be stopped until an acute intracerebral bleed has been ruled out.
   b. Clopidogrel before procedure, as ordered. Can be given as a loading dose of 150 mg the evening before procedure, 300-mg loading dose before procedure, 75 mg daily 48 hours before procedure, or 75 mg daily 1 week before procedure. Dosing is according to surgeon preference.
   c. Daily dosing of 75 mg clopidogrel for 30 to 90 days (specific duration varies), as directed.
   d. Aspirin 81 mg daily, as directed.
9. Monitor puncture site for bleeding, hematoma, and pulse, as ordered. Apply pressure if bleeding or hematoma is noted and inform provider.

DRUG ALERT Loading dose of clopidogrel, intraprocedural heparin bolus, postprocedural heparin drip, and postprocedural clopidogrel and aspirin daily dosing minimize the risk of thromboembolic complications following carotid stenting while increasing the risk of hemorrhagic complications. Close monitoring of neurologic status and PTT is warranted. Inform health care provider of any changes in neurologic status, PTT levels out of ordered range, and signs of bleeding.

Encouraging Lifestyle Changes to Reduce Risk

1. Help the patient begin to formulate a plan for smoking cessation.
2. Teach the patient and family members the basics of nutrition, how to read labels, and how to follow a low-fat diet (particularly one low in saturated fats).
3. Obtain a referral to a nutritionist for help with weight management and low-fat, low-sodium diet, as indicated.
4. Encourage physical activity if possible. The American Heart Association (AHA) recommends adults get at least 150 minutes per week of moderate-intensity aerobic exercise, 75 minutes per week of vigorous aerobic exercise, or a combination of both. Obtain a physical therapy referral for endurance training and monitoring, as indicated.
5. Monitor INR if warfarin is prescribed, and educate the patient about the risk of bleeding.

Patient Education and Health Maintenance

1. Encourage the patient receiving long-term oral anticoagulants requiring laboratory monitoring to adhere to follow-up monitoring and to report any signs of bleeding.
2. Encourage patients receiving antiplatelet agents to report any signs of bleeding.
3. Encourage the use of electric razors and toothbrushes to prevent bleeding.
4. Reinforce with patient and family the importance of accessing the medical system, by calling 911, when symptoms first occur.
5. Recommend a medical alert device if patient is on antiplatelets or anticoagulation. There are multiple styles of devices, including one that can be attached to the band of a smart watch.
6. Recommend the patient keep a list of their medications on their person so it will be available in an emergency.
7. Refer the patient to the American Stroke Association (ASA) (www.strokeassociation.org) or the National Institute of Neurologic Disorders and Stroke (www.ninds.nih.gov) for additional information and support.

Evaluation: Expected Outcomes

- Alert without neurologic deficits.
- Respirations unlabored, vital signs stable, no swelling of neck; reports relief of pain.
- Expresses readiness to quit smoking and adhere to recommended dietary changes.

Cerebrovascular Accident (Stroke, Brain Attack)

Stroke, cerebrovascular accident (CVA), or *brain attack* is the onset and persistence of neurologic dysfunction resulting from disruption of blood supply to the brain and indicates infarction rather than ischemia. Every year in the United States, more than 795,000 people have a stroke. Stroke is the leading cause of long-term disability and the fourth leading cause of death in the United States, with 162,890 deaths in 2021.

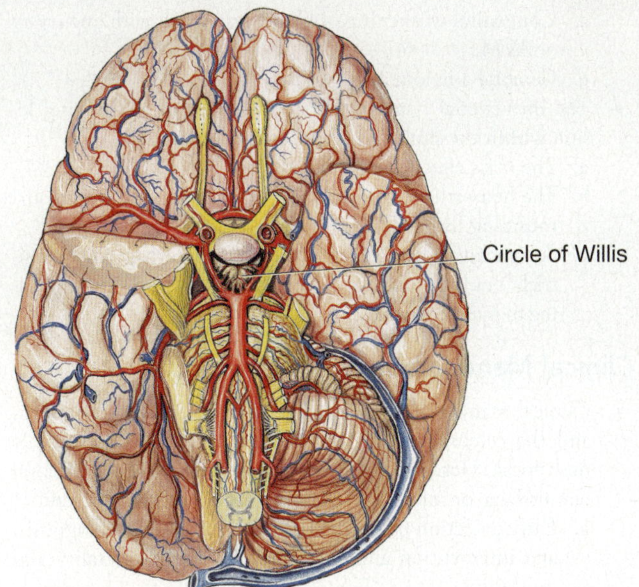

Figure 11-4. The circle of Willis as seen at the base of a brain removed from the skull. (Reprinted with permission from Anatomical Chart Company.)

Strokes are classified as ischemic (87% of strokes) or hemorrhagic (13%). About 60% of hemorrhagic strokes are the result of hypertension.

Pathophysiology and Etiology

Ischemic Stroke

1. Partial or complete occlusion of a cerebral blood flow to an area of the brain due to the following:
   a. Thrombus (most common)—due to arteriosclerotic plaque in a cerebral artery, usually at bifurcation of larger arteries; occurs over several days.
   b. Embolus—a moving clot of cardiac origin (frequently due to atrial fibrillation) or from a carotid artery that travels quickly to the brain and lodges in a small artery; occurs suddenly with immediate maximum deficits.
2. Area of brain affected is related to the vascular territory that was occluded. Subtle decrease in blood flow may allow brain cells to maintain minimal function, but as blood flow decreases, focal areas of ischemia occur, followed by infarction to the vascular territory (see Figure 11-4 for cerebral circulation).
3. An area of injury includes edema, tissue breakdown, and small arterial vessel damage. The small arterial vessel damage poses a risk of hemorrhage. The larger the area of infarction, the greater the risk of hemorrhagic conversion.
4. Ischemic strokes are not activity dependent; may occur at rest.

Hemorrhagic Stroke

1. Leakage of blood from a blood vessel and subsequent hemorrhage into brain tissue, causing edema, compression of brain tissue, and spasm of adjacent blood vessels.
2. May occur outside the dura (extradural), beneath the dura mater (subdural), in the subarachnoid space (SAS), or within the brain tissue (intracerebral).
3. Causal mechanisms include the following:
   a. Increased pressure due to hypertension.
   b. Head trauma causing dissection or rupture of vessel.
   c. Deterioration of vessel wall from chronic hypertension, diabetes mellitus, or cocaine use.

d. Congenital weakening of blood vessel wall with aneurysm or AVM.
e. Cerebral amyloid angiopathy.
4. The intracranial hemorrhage becomes a space-occupying lesion within the skull and compromises brain function.
a. The mass effect causes pressure on brain tissue.
b. The hemorrhage irritates local brain tissue, leading to surrounding focal edema.
c. Subarachnoid hemorrhage (SAH) or hemorrhage into a ventricle can block normal cerebrospinal fluid (CSF) flow, leading to hydrocephalus.

Clinical Manifestations

1. Clinical manifestations vary depending on the vessel affected and the cerebral territories perfused. Symptoms are usually multifocal. Headache may be a sign of impending cerebral hemorrhage or infarction; however, it is not always present.
a. Early detection of warning signs promotes early diagnosis, and intervention aimed at lessening stroke mortality and morbidity.
2. Common clinical manifestations related to vascular territory (see Table 11-5).
a. Numbness (paresthesia), weakness (paresis), or loss of motor ability (plegia) on one side of the body.
b. Difficulty in swallowing (dysphagia).
c. Aphasia (expressive, receptive, and global).
d. Visual difficulties of inattention or neglect (lack of acknowledgment of one side of the sensory field), loss of half of a visual field (hemianopsia), double vision, photophobia.
e. Altered cognitive abilities and psychological affect.
f. Self-care deficits.

Diagnostic Evaluation

1. Facilities will have a stroke protocol for ordering of diagnostic studies for patients suspected of a TIA or stroke. These include CT scan of head, CT perfusion scan (provides evaluation of cerebral blood flow, cerebral blood volume, and mean transient time to determine the extent of ischemic changes, CT angiography (head and neck), digital subtraction angiography, MRA, MRI, and TCD ultrasound.
2. MRI stroke protocol—consists of a standard MRI with specific sequences to identify ischemia (refer to page 328 for descriptions of these sequences).
3. TTE with a bubble study—can provide information when searching for the etiology of the ischemic event. Specifically, cardioembolic sources.
4. TEE—may be ordered in place of a TTE or to follow-up findings noted on the TTE.
5. Heart recording device:
a. ILR—monitors heart rhythm continually. Monthly data are sent remotely for rhythm analysis.
b. Ambulatory cardiac monitor.
6. Laboratory studies—determined on an individual basis and may include:
a. Prothrombotic states—protein C, protein S, antithrombin II, thrombin time, hemoglobin, anticardiolipin antibody, lupus anticoagulant, syphilis antibody.
b. Anticoagulation monitoring—heparin (aPTT), warfarin (PT/INR), antiplatelets (clopidogrel, prasugrel, ticagrelor) monitored with P_2Y_{12} assay. Aspirin—aspirin platelet assay.
7. TCD—noninvasive method used to evaluate cerebral perfusion. Useful in bedside evaluation and to provide a means for ongoing monitoring of cerebral blood flow to document changes and trends.

Management

Acute Treatment: Ischemic Stroke

1. Support of vital functions—maintain adequate airway and oxygenation. Monitor for cardiac dysrhythmias, control fever.

Table 11-5 Stroke Deficits Related to Vascular Territory

CEREBRAL ARTERY	BRAIN AREA INVOLVED	SIGNS AND SYMPTOMS[a]
Anterior cerebral	Infarction of the medial aspect of one frontal lobe if lesion is distal to communicating artery; bilateral frontal infarction if flow in other anterior cerebral artery is inadequate	Paralysis of contralateral foot or leg; impaired gait; paresis of contralateral arm; contralateral sensory loss over toes, foot, and leg; problems making decisions or performing acts voluntarily; lack of spontaneity, easily distracted; slowness of thought; urinary incontinence; cognitive and affective disorders
Middle cerebral	Massive infarction of most of lateral hemisphere and deeper structures of the frontal, parietal, and temporal lobes; internal capsule; basal ganglia	Contralateral hemiplegia (face and arm); contralateral sensory impairment; aphasia; homonymous hemiplegia; altered consciousness (confusion to coma); inability to turn eyes toward paralyzed side; denial of paralyzed side or limb (hemiattention); possible acalculia, alexia (visual aphasia), finger agnosia, and left right confusion; vasomotor paresis and instability
Posterior cerebral	Occipital lobe; anterior and medial portion of temporal lobe	Homonymous hemianopia and other visual defects, such as color blindness, loss of central vision, and visual hallucinations; memory deficits; perseveration (repeated performance of same verbal or motor response)
	Thalamus involvement	Loss of all sensory modalities; spontaneous pain; intentional tremor; mild hemiparesis; aphasia
	Cerebral peduncle involvement	Oculomotor nerve palsy with contralateral hemiplegia
Basilar and vertebral	Cerebellum and brainstem	Visual disturbance such as diplopia, dystaxia, vertigo, dysphagia, dysphonia

[a]Dependent on hemisphere involved and adequacy of collaterals.

2. Neurologic assessments utilizing the National Institutes of Health (NIH) Stroke Scale (https://www.stroke.nih.gov/documents/NIH_Stroke_Scale_508C.pdf) and management of increased ICP.
3. IV fluids (normal saline) at maintenance until able to tolerate oral diet. Colloids may be used for reperfusion and hemodilution.
4. Maintain BP within prescribed parameters. The AHA and ASA recommend treatment of hypertension in the early poststroke period if BP >220/120 mm Hg. If the patient is a candidate for thrombolysis, treatment is initiated with BP >185/110.
   a. Management of systemic hypertension with labetalol, nicardipine, or clevidipine.
   b. Goal is to promote adequate cerebral perfusion to prevent further ischemia. Avoid lowering BP greater than 15% within the first 24 hours as stroke progression can occur.
   c. Management of hypotension—systolic BP (SBP) goal greater than 100. Vasopressor agents to maintain SBP within prescribed range. Sustained hypotensive episodes are associated with poor outcome.
5. Hyperglycemia and BP fluctuations or rapid increases in BP increase the risk of hemorrhagic conversion.
6. Pretreatment with tissue plasminogen activator (tPA)—unable to receive tPA if SBP greater than 185 mm Hg or diastolic BP greater than 110 mm Hg.
7. Post-tPA—maintain SBP less than 180 mm Hg or diastolic BP less than 105 mm Hg for the first 24 hours post-tPA.
8. Thrombolytic therapy (see Box 11-3).
   a. Recombinant tPA administered IV is the only Food and Drug Administration (FDA)-approved medical treatment for acute ischemic stroke. Dosing: IV 0.9 mg/kg within 3 hours of the onset of symptoms.
   b. Intra-arterial (IA) tPA within 6 hours of the onset of symptoms. Benefits have been demonstrated in acute ischemic stroke related to occlusion of MCA. Advantages include the following:
      i. Higher concentration delivered to clot.
      ii. Can be performed in conjunction with mechanical disruption of clot.
      iii. Provides precise imaging of pathology and evaluation of collateral circulation.
      iv. Defines extent of injury and recanalization.
   c. Disadvantages include the following:
      i. Risk of hemorrhage related to catheter manipulation.
      ii. Dislodgement of clot.
      iii. Delay in thrombolytic therapy due to access delays.
      iv. Limited facility-based accessibility
   d. Following tPA administration:
      i. Monitor for signs of neurologic deterioration.
      ii. Monitor for reperfusion injury.
      iii. Monitor for signs of bleeding (catheter sites, urine, stool, gastric).
9. Endovascular procedures.
   a. Mechanical thrombectomy (MT):
      i. Mechanical intervention procedure where a blood clot/thrombus is removed using endovascular devices.
      ii. The AHA/ASA guidelines for the performance of MT.
         a. May be performed up to 24 hours after symptoms began.
         b. Utilized for large vessel occlusion (MCA).
   b. IA thrombolysis:
      i. Abciximab—antiplatelet agent delivered IA.
      ii. Verapamil—potent vasodilator injected into intracranial vessel to treat acute spasm.
   c. Other—angioplasty and stenting have been utilized in acute dissection.
10. Maintain normal glucose levels as hypoglycemia and hyperglycemia have been associated with a poor outcome.
11. Maintain normothermia because hyperthermia is associated with a poor neurologic outcome.
12. Deep vein thrombosis (DVT) prophylaxis—sequential stockings and low-dose heparin or low-molecular-weight heparin (LMWH) should be utilized. Data do not suggest any increased risk of hemorrhage in this population.
13. Focus on early rehabilitation.

BOX 11-3 Inclusion and Exclusion Criteria for Tissue Plasminogen Activator Therapy

INCLUSION

- Onset of symptoms.
  - Within 4.5 hours intravenous (IV) tPA.
  - Within 6 hours intra-arterial (IA) tPA.
- Ischemic stroke with measurable deficits using the National Institutes of Health Stroke Scale (see page 349).
- No hemorrhage noted on computed tomography (CT) scan of the brain.
- Clearly defined time of symptom onset.

EXCLUSION

- Head CT demonstrates early signs of infarction or hemorrhage.
- Uncontrolled hypertensive nonresponsive to IV or oral agent (systolic greater than 185 or diastolic greater than 110 mm Hg).
- Glucose level greater than 400 mg/dL.
  - Heparin within past 48 hours.
  - Patient on warfarin.
  - Elevated partial thromboplastin time (PTT) or prothrombin time.
  - Platelet count less than 100,000.
- History of previous intracranial hemorrhage, head trauma, or stroke within past 3 months.
- Gastrointestinal (GI) or genitourinary tract hemorrhage in the past 3 weeks.
- History of major surgery in the past 2 weeks.

Acute Treatment: Hemorrhagic Stroke

1. Support of vital functions—maintain adequate airway and oxygenation. Monitor for cardiac dysrhythmias, control fever.
2. Neurologic assessment—facility-based neurologic assessment tool should be used. Notify the health care provider of changes in examination. Deterioration can be related to rebleed or development of cerebral edema.
3. Reversal of coagulopathies:
   a. Obtain patient's medication history. Medications to be concerned about include antiplatelet agents (aspirin, clopidogrel, ticagrelor, prasugrel, ticlopidine, dipyridamole/aspirin) and anticoagulants (warfarin, apixaban, dabigatran, rivaroxaban).
   b. Laboratory studies:
      i. For warfarin, a PT/INR will be ordered.
      ii. Antiplatelet agents:

a. If patient is on aspirin, an aspirin platelet function will be ordered to determine whether the platelets have been inhibited and to what degree.
b. If on clopidogrel, ticagrelor or prasugrel, a test (P_2Y_{12} assay) will be obtained to determine the degree of platelet inhibition.
c. Reversal agents.

iii. For warfarin, vitamin K and prothrombin complex may be used. Platelets may also be ordered. The 2022 AHA/ASA guidelines for intracerebral hemorrhage (ICH) recommend four-factor prothrombin complex concentrate to fresh frozen plasma for quick INR correction and limiting expansion of hematoma.
iv. Reversal agent for dabigatran is idarucizumab.
v. Reversal agent for apixaban and rivaroxaban is Andexxa.
vi. Currently, there is no specific agent to reverse antiplatelet effects. Guidelines from the Neurocritical Care Society suggest a single dose of desmopressin (DDAVP). Platelets may also be ordered.

4. Management of BP within prescribed parameters—2022 AHA/ASA guidelines recommend for patients with ICH of mild-to-moderate severity and SBP between 150 and 220 mm Hg at the time of arrival to hospital that a reduction of SBP to a target of 140 mm Hg is safe and may improve outcomes. Goal is to prevent rebleeding while promoting adequate cerebral perfusion. Labetalol, hydralazine, nicardipine, or alternative IV antihypertensive agents may be used.
5. Neurosurgical consultation for possible evacuation of ICH may be ordered.
6. Treatment of clinical seizures with phenytoin or levetiracetam. Seizures commonly occur within the first 24 hours of ICH. Prophylactic antiepileptic drugs (AEDs) are not recommended.
7. Maintain normal glucose level because hypoglycemia/hyperglycemia is associated with a poor outcome. Sliding scale insulin or insulin drip should be given to maintain normoglycemia.
8. Maintain normothermia because hyperthermia is associated with a poor neurologic outcome.
9. DVT prophylaxis—sequential stockings and low-dose heparin or LMWH should be utilized. Data do not suggest any increased risk of hemorrhage in this population.
10. Focus on early rehabilitation.

Subsequent Treatment

1. Ischemic stroke and TIA—aspirin is recommended within 24 hours poststroke. (In tPA patients, aspirin should not be given until 24 hours post-tPA.) Alternative antiplatelet agents include clopidogrel, ticagrelor, prasugrel, ticlopidine, and dipyridamole/aspirin.
   a. DAPT is recommended after high-risk TIA or minor stroke for 21 to 90 days for the reduction of recurrent ischemic stroke. This plays a role in secondary prevention. After the designated time period, the patient will remain on one antiplatelet (generally aspirin unless contraindicated). During this period, the patient is at a higher risk for bleeding.
2. Antispasmodic agents can be used for spastic paralysis.
3. Early initiation of a rehabilitation program, including physical therapy, occupational therapy, and speech therapy, and counseling, as needed.
4. Depression is common; therefore, early initiation of antidepressants can be beneficial, such as selective serotonin reuptake inhibitors.

Complications

1. Aspiration pneumonia.
2. Dysphagia.
3. Spasticity, contractures.
4. DVT, pulmonary embolism.
5. Brainstem herniation.
6. Poststroke depression.

Nursing Assessment

1. Maintain neurologic flow sheet (NIH Stroke Scale for ischemic stroke and facility-based neurologic assessment tool for hemorrhagic stroke).
2. Assess for voluntary or involuntary movements, tone of muscles, presence of deep tendon reflexes (reflex return signals end of flaccid period and return of muscle tone).
3. Also assess mental status, CN function, sensation/proprioception.
4. Monitor bowel and bladder function/control.
5. Monitor effectiveness of anticoagulation therapy.
6. Frequently assess level of function and psychosocial response to condition.
7. Assess for skin breakdown, contractures, and other complications of immobility.

DRUG ALERT Warfarin is adjusted to maintain an INR at 2 to 3 (goal of 2.5) to prevent stroke associated with atrial fibrillation. Monitor for potential complications of ICH and subdural hemorrhage. Report INRs that are elevated to reduce the risk of bleeding or decreased levels to adjust therapy to be more effective.

CLINICAL JUDGMENT Use of clinical pathways maximizes patient with stroke outcomes across the care continuum. Case management models of care foster interdisciplinary utilization, timeliness of referrals, patient education, patient satisfaction, and efficient use of health care resources. The specific role of the nurse in stroke recovery integrates therapeutic aspects of coordinating, maintaining, and training.

Nursing Interventions

Preventing Falls and Other Injuries

1. Maintain bed rest during acute phase (24 to 48 hours after the onset of stroke) with head of bed slightly elevated and side rails in place.
2. Administer oxygen, as ordered, during acute phase to maximize cerebral oxygenation.
3. Frequently assess respiratory status, vital signs, heart rate and rhythm, and urine output to maintain and support vital functions.
4. When patient becomes more alert after acute phase, maintain frequent vigilance and interactions aimed at orienting, assessing, and meeting the needs of the patient.
5. Try to allay confusion and agitation with calm reassurance and presence.
6. Assess the patient for risk for fall status.

Preventing Complications of Immobility

Interventions to improve functional recovery require active participation of the patient and repetitive training. Functional demand and intensive training are believed to trigger central nervous system (CNS) reorganization—responsible for late functional recovery after stroke. Collaborate with physical and occupational therapy to support exercise and mobility.

1. Maintain functional position of all extremities.
   a. Apply a trochanter roll from the crest of the ilium to the midthigh to prevent external rotation of the hip.
   b. Place a pillow in the axilla of the affected side when there is limited external rotation to keep arm away from chest and prevent adduction of the affected shoulder.
   c. Place the affected upper extremity slightly flexed on pillow supports, with each joint positioned higher than the preceding one to prevent edema and resultant fibrosis; alternate elbow extension.
   d. Place the hand in slight supination with fingers slightly in flexion.
   e. Avoid excessive pressure on ball of foot after spasticity develops.
   f. Do not allow top bedding to pull affected foot into plantar flexion; may use tennis shoes in bed.
   g. Encourage neutral positioning of affected limbs to promote relaxation and to limit abnormal increases in muscular tone to enhance functional recovery (reflex-inhibiting positioning).
2. Apply splints and braces, as indicated, to support flaccid extremities or on spastic extremities to decrease stretch stimulation and reduce spasticity. Collaborate with therapists for recommendations on slings, braces.
   a. Volar splint to support functional position of wrist.
   b. Sling to prevent shoulder subluxation of flaccid arm.
   c. High-top sneaker for ankle and foot support. Ankle–foot orthosis for patient with footdrop.
3. Exercise the affected extremities passively through range of motion (ROM) four to five times daily to maintain joint mobility and enhance circulation; encourage active ROM exercise as able (see page 105). Educate family members/significant others on how to perform ROM.
4. Teach the patient to use the unaffected extremity to move the affected one.
5. Assist with ambulation, as needed, with the help of physical therapy, as indicated.
   a. Check for orthostatic hypotension when dangling and standing.
   b. Gradually position the patient from a reclining position to head elevated, and dangle legs at the bedside before transferring out of bed or ambulating; assess sitting balance in bed.
   c. Assess the patient for excessive exertion.
   d. Have the patient wear walking shoes or tennis shoes.
   e. Assess standing balance and have the patient practice standing.
   f. Help the patient begin ambulating as soon as standing balance is achieved; ensure safety with a patient waist belt.
   g. Provide rest periods as patient will tire easily.

Optimizing Orientation and Awareness

1. Be aware of the patient's cognitive alterations and adjust interaction and environment accordingly.
2. Participate in cognitive retraining program—reality orientation, visual imagery, cueing procedures—as outlined by rehabilitation nurse or therapist.
3. In patients with increased awareness, use pictures of family members, clock, calendar; postschedule of daily activities where patient can see it.
4. Focus on the patient's strengths and give positive feedback.
5. Be aware that depression is common and therapy should include psychotherapy and early initiation of antidepressants.

Facilitating Communication

1. Speak slowly, using visual cues and gestures; be consistent and repeat as necessary.
2. Speak directly to the patient while facing them.
3. Give plenty of time for response and reinforce attempts as well as correct responses.
4. Minimize distractions.
5. Use alternative methods of communication other than verbal, such as written words, gestures, pictures, message boards, tablets, phones.

Fostering Independence

1. Teach the patient to use nonaffected side for activities of daily living (ADLs), but not to neglect affected side.
2. Adjust the environment (e.g., call light, tray) to the side of awareness if spatial neglect or visual field cuts are present; approach the patient from the uninvolved side.
3. Teach the patient to scan environment if visual deficits are present.
4. Encourage the family to provide clothing a size larger than patient wears, with front closures, Velcro, and stretch fabric; teach the patient to dress while sitting to maintain balance.
5. Make sure personal care items, urinal, and commode are nearby and that patient obtains assistance with transfers and other activities, as needed.
6. Be aware that ADLs require anticipatory (automatic coordination of multiple muscle groups in anticipation of a specific movement) and reactive (adjustment of posture to stimuli) postural adjustments.
7. Be aware that patients usually have clear goals in relation to functional abilities, against which all success and forward progress will be measured; help them set realistic short- and long-term goals.

Promoting Adequate Oral Intake

1. Perform a bedside swallow screen before ANY oral intake (including medication) is provided. Follow institutional protocol. If any coughing or difficulties are noted, contact speech therapy for official consult.
2. Initiate referral for a speech therapist for individuals with compromised LOC, dyspraxia speech, or speech difficulties, which do not allow for evaluation of swallowing function at bedside. A radiographic swallow study may be required to evaluate swallowing (often called a *barium swallow*) performed in radiology with a speech therapist.
3. Note that speech therapist will evaluate and provide dietary recommendations for consistency of liquids and solids.
4. Help the patient relearn swallowing sequence using compensatory techniques (see page 111).
5. Encourage small, frequent meals and allow plenty of time to chew and swallow. Dietary consults can be helpful for selection of food preferences.
6. Remind the patient to chew on the unaffected side.
7. Encourage the patient to drink small sips from a straw with chin tucked to the chest, strengthening effort to swallow while chin is tucked down.
8. Inspect mouth for food collection and pocketing before entry of each new bolus of food.
9. Inspect oral mucosa for injury from biting tongue or cheek.
10. Encourage frequent oral hygiene.
11. Teach the family how to assist the patient with meals to facilitate chewing and swallowing.

a. Reduce environmental distractions to improve patient concentration.
b. Provide oral care before eating to improve aesthetics and afterward to remove food debris.
c. Position the patient so they are sitting with 90 degrees of flexion at the hips and 45 degrees of flexion at the neck. Use pillows to achieve correct position.
d. Maintain position for 30 to 45 minutes after meals to prevent regurgitation and aspiration.

Attaining Bladder Control

1. Insert indwelling bladder catheterization during acute stage for accurate fluid management; remove as soon as status stabilizes.
2. Establish regular voiding schedule—every 2 to 3 hours, correlated with fluid intake—when bladder tone returns. If the patient is unable to void, intermittent catheterization can be used to empty bladder and prevent overstretching of bladder. The bladder scan device is useful in monitoring bladder capacity and identifying individuals at risk.
3. Assist with standing or sitting to void (especially males).
4. See page 112 for bladder retraining program details.

Strengthening Family Coping

1. Consult a social worker for assistance with patient/family support, to obtain copy of durable power of attorney, address guardianship, and long-term care decisions, as needed.
2. Encourage the family to maintain outside interests.
3. Teach stress management techniques, such as relaxation exercises, use of community and faith-based support networks.
4. Encourage participation in support group for family respite program for caregivers or other available resources in area.
5. Involve as many family and friends in care as possible.
6. Provide information about stroke and expected outcome.
7. Teach the family that stroke survivors may show depression in the first 3 months of recovery.

Community and Home Care Considerations

1. Hemiplegic complications resulting from stroke commonly include "frozen" shoulder; adduction and internal rotation of arm with flexion of elbow, wrist, and fingers; external rotation of the hip with flexion of the knee and plantar flexion of the ankle.
2. Perform ROM exercises and instruct the patient and family on these as well as on proper positioning.
3. Reinforce that these muscle and ligament deformities resulting from stroke can be prevented with daily stretching and strengthening exercises.
4. Depression after stroke is a major problem because it can increase morbidity. Monitor for signs of depression, such as difficulty sleeping, frequent crying, anorexia, feelings of guilt, or sadness. Notify the health care provider for possible medication therapy.
5. Continue to support family who may be caring for a person with hemiplegia or aphasia at home or in long-term care for a long time.

Patient Education and Health Maintenance

1. Teach the patient and family to adapt home environment for safety and ease of use. Physical therapy evaluation will also include the home environment and make recommendations as indicated.
2. Instruct the patient of the need for rest periods throughout day.
3. Reassure the family that it is common for poststroke patients to experience emotional lability and depression; treatment can be given.
4. Encourage consistency in the environment without distraction.
5. Assist the family to obtain self-help aids for the patient.
6. Instruct the family in the management of aphasia (see Box 11-4).
7. Educate those at risk for stroke about lifestyle modifications and medication therapy that can lower risk.

BOX 11-4 Management of Aphasia

Aphasia is an acquired disorder of communication resulting from brain damage due to stroke, head injury, brain tumors, or brain cysts. It may involve impairment of the ability to speak, to understand speech of others, and to read, write, calculate, and understand gestures. Most individuals with aphasia have difficulty with expression and comprehension to varying degrees. Fatigue has adverse effect on speech.

To enhance your communication with the patient with aphasia, keep the environment simple and relaxed, minimize distractions, and use multiple sensory channels.

Refer the family to:
American Speech-Language-Hearing Association
10801 Rockville Pike
Rockville, MD 20852
301-897-5700
www.asha.org

APHASIA SYNDROMES

- Fluent aphasia (Wernicke or receptive aphasia): Patient retains verbal fluency but may have difficulty in understanding speech. Speech is effortless and lacks clear content, information, and direction (nonsensical).
- Nonfluent aphasia (Broca or expressive aphasia): Varied degrees of difficulty in initiation of speech, difficulty in formation of words with poor articulation, and difficulty in finding appropriate words. Speech is slow and laborious. Auditory comprehension is preserved.
- Anomic or amnesiac aphasia: Characteristic feature is difficulty naming and finding words. However, grammar, comprehension, and repetition remain intact.
- Conduction aphasia: Major difficulty is with sequencing phonemes resulting in literal paraphasic errors. Auditory comprehension remains intact; however, patient has difficulty repeating spoken language.
- Global aphasia: Severe disruption of communication (verbal speech, written, reading, and auditory comprehension).

NURSING INTERVENTIONS

- Speak at your normal rate and volume: The patient is not hard of hearing.
- Allow plenty of time to answer.
- Do not ask questions that require complex answers.
- Be aware that patient use of rote phrases may be spontaneous.
- Provide pad and pen if the patient prefers and is able to write.
- Avoid forcing speech.
- Watch the patient for clues and gestures if their speech is jargon; make neutral statements.
- Allow plenty of time for response.
- Ask for minimal word response.
- Encourage the patient to speak slowly.
- Expect frustration and anger at inability to communicate.
- Keep environment simple.
- Use gestures as well as language.
- Allow the patient to manipulate objects for additional sensory input.

8. Refer the patient and family for more information and support to agencies such as the National Stroke Association (*www.stroke.org*).

Evaluation: Expected Outcomes

- No falls, vital signs stable.
- Maintains body alignment, no contractures.
- Intact skin integrity.
- Oriented to person, place, and time.
- Communicates appropriately.
- Brushes teeth, puts on shirt and pants independently (if condition permits).
- Feeds self two thirds of meal.
- Voids on commode at 2-hour intervals.
- Family seeks help and assistance from others.

Rupture of Intracranial Aneurysm

EVIDENCE BASE Torregrossa, F., & Grasso, G. (2022). Therapeutic approaches for cerebrovascular dysfunction after aneurysmal subarachnoid hemorrhage: An update and future perspectives. *World Neurosurgery, 159*, 276–287. https://doi.org/10.1016/j.wneu.2021.11.096

An *intracranial aneurysm* is an abnormal localized dilation of the wall of a cerebral artery due to congenital absence of the muscle layer of the vessel. Constant blood flow against the weakened area results in growth of the aneurysm and thinning of the vessel wall. Aneurysms usually occur at a bifurcation of an artery or major branches of the circle of Willis. They may be of congenital, traumatic, arteriosclerotic, or infectious origin. Most are saccular and asymptomatic until rupture; other types are fusiform and berry (see Figure 11-5). When an aneurysm ruptures, sudden bleeding occurs in the SAS between the arachnoid and the pia, causing SAH, which produces symptoms related to meningeal irritation. Hemorrhage can extend into the ventricular system, causing obstruction of CSF flow (hydrocephalus) or into the brain tissue (intracerebral bleed), causing further neurologic compromise. Depending on the extent of SAH, cerebral vasospasm (transient thickening of intralumen of a vessel) can occur, producing decreased cerebral blood flow, ischemia, and potential infarction or delayed cerebral ischemia (DCI). Transient thickening of the vessel is believed to be in response to the circulating blood and/or its breakdown products in the CSF. Vasospasm commonly occurs 3 to 14 days after SAH and peaks on day 5.

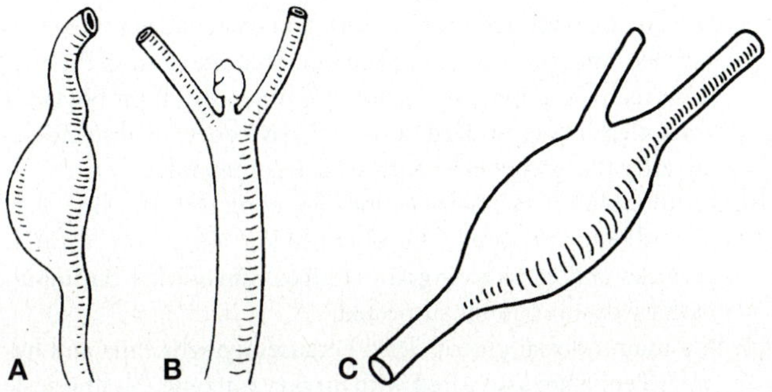

Figure 11-5. Types of aneurysms. **(A)** Saccular aneurysm; **(B)** berry aneurysm; **(C)** fusiform aneurysm.

Grading of Aneurysms

Hunt-Hess Scale is the most commonly used scale. It is a numeric grading scale that correlates to the patient's presentation and neurologic examination. It is used to describe the severity of the hemorrhage and to help predict outcome.

0, Unruptured; asymptomatic discovery.
I, Asymptomatic or minimal headache with slight nuchal rigidity.
II, Moderate-to-severe headache, nuchal rigidity; no neurologic deficit other than CN deficit.
III, Drowsiness, confusion, or mild focal deficit (e.g., hemiparesis), or combination of these findings.
IV, Stupor, moderate-to-severe deficit, possibly early decerebrate rigidity and vegetative disturbances.
V, Deep coma, decerebrate rigidity, moribund appearance.

Pathophysiology and Etiology

1. Etiology is believed to be multifactorial and includes structural abnormality of the cerebral vessel wall, atherosclerotic changes, hypertension, and environment. It is believed that inflammation has a role in the growth of the aneurysm.
2. Associated conditions: polycystic disease, Ehlers-Danlos syndrome, Marfan, Osler-Weber-Rendu syndrome, fibromuscular dysplasia, moyamoya syndrome, sickle cell anemia, collagen type III disorder, bacterial endocarditis (mycotic aneurysms), trauma (dissecting aneurysms).
3. Risk factors for rupture:
   a. Modifiable: hypertension, smoking, alcohol misuse, illicit drug use (e.g., cocaine).
   b. Nonmodifiable: sex assigned at birth (female), ethnicity (incidence is higher and has increased in Black patients), first-degree relative with history of aneurysm, history of previous aneurysm rupture, and having more than one aneurysm.
4. May become symptomatic because of pressure of enlarging aneurysm on nearby CNs or brain tissue.
5. Rupture and hemorrhage into SAS may cause increased ICP, hydrocephalus, and ischemia.
6. Vasospasm may occur within 3 to 14 days, peak 5 to 7 days after rupture, causing ischemia and infarction.
7. Rebleeding may occur because of lysis of clot with greatest risk for rebleeding in the first 6 to 72 hours after initial bleed. Securing the aneurysm as soon as possible reduces this risk. Higher mortality rate (70%) after rebleed.

Incidence

1. In the general population, aneurysms are found in about 3% to 5% of the individuals in the United States and are more common in older adults. In females, aneurysms are more common in those over 50 years of age.
2. About 20% of those with an aneurysm will have more than one aneurysm.
3. Incidence of SAH is 10 to 14 per 100,000 persons in the United States.
   a. In children, aneurysms are more common in prepubescent males than prepubescent females and more common in posterior than anterior circulation.

Clinical Manifestations

1. Sudden onset of severe headache, often accompanied by nausea and vomiting, but no neurologic deficits; leaking of aneurysm or AVM may cause a warning bleed.

2. Sudden, severe headache (commonly described as the "worst headache of my life"), meningeal signs (nuchal rigidity, photophobia, irritability), and neurologic dysfunction (related to vascular territory) are commonly related to SAH secondary to ruptured intracranial aneurysm, which can be catastrophic.
3. Neurologic deficit related to vascular territory (see page 348); progressive CN III, CN IV, CN VI deficits due to mass effect.
4. Sentinel bleeds—10% to 20% of patients with SAH experience an acute, sudden headache that appears days or weeks before admission for SAH. Etiology of sentinel bleed is unclear.

Diagnostic Evaluation

1. History and physical examination.
2. CT scan—to determine presence of blood in SAS, rule out other lesions, and evaluate mass effect. Modified Fischer grade—estimates blood volume and location on CT. Assists in predicting risk for vasospasm. The Modified Fisher scale was adapted from the Fisher scale and adjusted based on clinical analysis of the occurrence of vasospasm.
   a. Grade 0: no SAH; no intraventricular hemorrhage (IVH), 0% risk of vasospasm.
   b. Grade 1: focal or diffuse, thin SAH, no IVH; 24% risk of vasospasm.
   c. Grade 2: thin focal (less than 1 mm) or diffuse SAH, IVH present; 33% risk of vasospasm.
   d. Grade 3: thick focal (greater than 1 mm) or diffuse SAH, no IVH; 33% risk of vasospasm.
   e. Grade 4: thick focal (greater than 1 mm) or diffuse SAH; 40% risk of vasospasm.
3. Lumbar puncture (if no mass effect on CT)—may be performed if initial imaging is negative for SAH but clinical picture is concerning for hemorrhage. Spinal fluid evaluated for blood or xanthochromia.
4. MRA or CT angiogram—noninvasive evaluation of cerebral vascular structures. Can be useful in the workup of suspected aneurysms (individuals with persistent headaches or unexplained neurologic deficits such as CN palsies). CT angiogram is the preferred study, though renal function must be assessed secondary to use of contrast dye.
5. Cerebral angiogram—gold standard test; provides definitive evaluation of aneurysm etiology, presence, location, and configuration. Useful in determining the presence of vasospasm, extent of vasospasm, and collateral circulation.
6. TCD—noninvasive method to evaluate cerebral perfusion. Useful in the bedside evaluation and to provide a means for ongoing monitoring of cerebral blood flow to document changes and trends. Results are operator dependent.
7. Laboratory studies—complete blood count, metabolic panel, coagulation parameters, toxicology.

Management

Unruptured

1. Evaluation of diagnostic studies is key to determine need for intervention, scheduling of elective surgical clipping, or endovascular embolization, if indicated.
2. Normalize BP if hypertensive (SBP goal 120 to 140).
3. Smoking cessation.
4. Cessation of illicit drug use (if applicable).

After Rupture

1. Neurologic assessments hourly and as clinically indicated.
2. Intracranial aneurysm precautions to minimize the risk of rebleeding and control BP—bed rest with the head elevated 30 degrees, avoidance of Valsalva maneuver and neck flexion, physical care as condition indicates.
3. Rapid repair of aneurysm should be performed by surgical clipping or endovascular embolization.
4. Management of systemic hypertension with labetalol, nicardipine, hydralazine, or alternative IV antihypertensive agent can be used to maintain SBP within ordered parameters. Close BP monitoring should be maintained to prevent fluctuations in BP.
5. Fluid goal is euvolemia. Prophylactic or therapeutic hypervolemia is avoided. Strict monitoring of intake and output (I&O), including running total I&O, and daily weights should be obtained to accurately assess fluid status. Routine use of central venous access for central venous pressure (CVP) monitoring is not recommended.
6. Neuroprotective agents.
   a. Nimodipine, a calcium channel blocker, has demonstrated reduced incidence of delayed neurologic deficits and is felt to be neuroprotective during SAH and vasospasm. The medication is administered on admission and continues for 21 consecutive days. Dosing: 60 mg orally/via nasogastric tube every 4 hours. Close monitoring for potential drop in BP after administration. If noted drop in BP, inform provider for dosing modification. Often changed to 30 mg every 2 hours and BP reassessed for impact on BP.
      i. Nimodipine has cerebral specificity to block the influx of calcium at the intracellular space. It is the only drug approved by the FDA for the treatment of vasospasm. For optimal effect, nimodipine should be started within 96 hours of SAH.
7. Hypertensive therapy—used with symptomatic vasospasm. Increasing the BP is believed to improve cerebral blood flow. Colloids should be used initially with the use of vasopressors as a secondary measure. Common vasopressor agents utilized are phenylephrine and norepinephrine. Neurologic examination should be utilized to determine specific SBP or mean arterial pressure (MAP) goal.
8. Management of acute obstructive hydrocephalus related to IVH by placement of ventriculostomy or external ventricular drain (EVD).
   a. Adjustment of drain to promote drainage of CSF.
   b. Intraventricular tPA clot lysis may be used to promote CSF drainage. Current studies indicate low risk for intracranial bleeding with reduced risk for vasospasm.
   c. Surgical placement of permanent shunt (e.g., ventricular-peritoneal shunt) may be necessary.
9. Witnessed seizures: Phenytoin, fosphenytoin, and levetiracetam are the preferred medications. Duration of drug therapy is variable, and levels are monitored for accurate dosing. Prophylactic use of antiepileptics is not recommended. If prophylactic antiepileptics are utilized, a 3- to 7-day course or discontinuing after the aneurysm is secured is recommended.
10. Cardiopulmonary complications are common. Baseline electrocardiography should be obtained on admission. Cardiac enzymes and echocardiogram are recommended if cardiopulmonary dysfunction is suspected.
11. Maintain normal glucose level because hypoglycemia and hyperglycemia are associated with a poor outcome. Sliding scale insulin or insulin drip should be utilized to maintain blood sugar at 80 to 180. Glucose level less than 80 and greater than 200 should be avoided.

12. Monitor electrolytes, especially serum sodium, as hyponatremia is often seen after an SAH. Serum magnesium is to be maintained at or above 2.0 mg/dL.
13. Maintain normothermia. Hyperthermia is associated with a poor neurologic outcome. Antipyretic agents are first-line treatment for the management of fever. External surface cooling devices or intravascular cooling devices should be employed when antipyretics are ineffective. Fever workup should be performed to evaluate for potential infectious etiology of fever.
14. DVT prophylaxis—sequential stockings and low-dose heparin or LMWH should be utilized. Data do not suggest any increased risk of hemorrhage in this population. Low-dose heparin or LMWH should be held prior to and after any intracranial procedure for 24 hours.

Surgical Intervention

1. Surgical obliteration of aneurysm by clipping, ligation, or endovascular technique.
2. Assessment of Hunt-Hess grade and medical stability assist in determining the timing of intervention, usually within 24 to 72 hours.
3. Method of treatment is determined by evaluating aneurysm size, location, neck width, condition of the patient, and associated medical conditions.
4. Surgical methods:
   a. Craniotomy is performed to access the aneurysm. Placement of titanium clips across the neck of the aneurysm or wrapping of fusiform aneurysm. Multiple size titanium clips are available to secure aneurysm.
   b. *Advantages*: removal of ICH/subarachnoid blood; low rate of aneurysm recurrence.
   c. *Disadvantage*: open procedure.
5. Endovascular techniques:
   a. Cerebral angiography with placement of titanium coils into the aneurysm.
   b. Obliteration of the aneurysm.
      i. Multiple types of coils are available. Type and length of coil utilized are dependent on configuration of aneurysm. Coils fill the aneurysm and are detached using electronic heating. Multiple coils are placed until there is no blood flow noted on angiography to the aneurysm.
      ii. Coil embolization with aid of a stent. When the base of the aneurysm is broad, a stent is used to form a bridge across the neck of the aneurysm, allowing for placement of coils within the aneurysm.
      iii. Flow-diverting stent—stents that do not use coils; used in treatment of internal carotid artery aneurysm.
      iv. *Advantages*: minimally invasive treatment; shorter duration of anesthesia.
      v. *Disadvantage*: potential for recurrence if aneurysm not completely occluded. Aneurysms treated with a stent require DAPT.
   c. Interventional treatment of vasospasm. Often treatment will combine both angioplasty and an IA injection.
      i. Balloon angioplasty—dilation of vessel by expansion of a transarterial balloon to treat vasospasm.
      ii. IA injection—verapamil, nicardipine, or papaverine for temporary local vasodilation.

DRUG ALERT Heparin can be used intraprocedurally and postprocedurally, as directed, to minimize the risk of thromboembolic events. Risks include thromboembolic complications and rupture of aneurysm with extension of SAH.

Complications

1. Aneurysm rebleed—risk is 4% on day 1, then 1.5% per day on days 2 to 13, 20% within 14 days, and 50% within 6 months; highest risk within first 6 hours. Seventy percent mortality in rebleed.
2. Delayed ischemic neurologic deficit occurs secondary to diminished cerebral blood flow. Cerebral vasospasm and DCI are the most common cause. Greatest risk: 3 to 14 days after SAH. Current theory is that cerebral vasospasm is a reversible thickening of medial wall and smooth muscle proliferation, causing narrowing of the vessel lumen. Seventy percent to 80% of patients have radiographic vasospasm, with 30% being symptomatic or demonstrating the effects of DCI.
3. Obstructive hydrocephalus—20% to 30% of patients develop obstructive hydrocephalus. EVD placement allows for temporary CSF drainage; 18% to 26% will require placement of a ventricular-peritoneal shunt.
4. Seizures after SAH occur in 3% to 28% of the patients, with 1% to 7% at presentation. Witnessed seizures are treated with AEDs, although specific duration of treatment remains controversial. Prophylactic use of AEDs is not recommended, although it may be considered. If prophylactic AEDs are used, a 3- to 7-day course or discontinuing after the aneurysm is secured is recommended.
5. Hyponatremia—occurs in up to 35% of patients; thought to be caused by syndrome of inappropriate antidiuretic hormone (SIADH) or cerebral salt wasting. It is essential to differentiate between SIADH and cerebral salt wasting to ensure appropriate treatment (see Chapter 20).
6. Hyperglycemia—believed to be a result of the body's stress response. Associated with poorer outcomes and must be avoided.
7. Cardiopulmonary complications (related to abnormal catecholamine release).
   a. Cardiovascular changes ranging from atrial fibrillation, bradycardia, and T-wave abnormalities to left ventricular dysfunction with or without myocardial failure and myocardial injury in severe cases.
   b. Neurogenic pulmonary edema.
8. Median mortality rate in the United States is approximately 32%. Moderate-to-severe disability is found in about 30% of those who survive an SAH. Rebleed and DCI secondary to vasospasm is directly related to mortality and morbidity.

Nursing Assessment

1. Perform and document neurologic assessment with vital signs and as patient condition warrants.
2. Monitor for changes in or decreasing LOC, CN dysfunction, pupillary abnormality, and motor deficit, which signify increased ICP, cerebral vasospasm, DCI, or expanding lesion.
3. Assess for increasing headache, which could signal rebleeding.
4. Monitor for focal neurologic deficits, which may indicate vasospasm.
5. Review laboratory results for electrolyte abnormalities. Notify provider and/or treat according to institution protocols.
6. Review results of TCD. Inform provider if velocities have increased.

Nursing Interventions

Modifying Activity to Prevent Complications

1. Prior to treatment, reduce environmental stimuli, limit stress, and decrease the risk of rebleed and/or increased ICP.

a. Maintain complete bed rest with head elevated 30 degrees to reduce cerebral edema.
b. Maintain quiet environment with low lighting, noise control, and limit activity to prevent photophobia, agitation, and pain.
c. Encourage the awake patient to avoid activities that increase BP or ICP: straining, sneezing, acute flexion/rotation of the neck; assist the patient with position changes.
d. Avoid Valsalva maneuver, which may increase ICP, by administering stool softeners to prevent straining; avoiding rectal temperatures, enemas, and suppositories; and teaching the awake patient to exhale through mouth during defecation.
e. Avoid caffeinated beverages and extremes of temperatures.
f. Provide physical care, such as bathing and feeding, as needed.

2. Implement nursing interventions to minimize ICP and cerebral swelling (e.g., elevate head of bed 30 degrees, maintain proper head and neck alignment to avoid jugular vein compression, avoid prolonged suctioning procedures, keep procedure less than 15 seconds, collaborate with provider to use lidocaine before suctioning if intubated).
3. Medicate the patient, as ordered, during periods of extreme agitation.
4. Perform and document neurologic assessment with vital signs and as patient condition warrants, which includes monitoring LOC, CN function, pupillary function, and motor function. Insidious onset of confusion, disorientation, and decreased LOC or focal deficit associated with vascular territory associated with aneurysm bleed may indicate vasospasm (peak occurrence is 5 days after bleed, up 14 days after bleed). Speech slurring or onset of pronator drift may be the first sign of deterioration.
5. Assess for signs of increased ICP, including agitation, change in LOC, bradycardia, and widening pulse pressure, and changes in respiratory pattern (Cheyne-Stokes pattern, apneustic, ataxic).
6. Monitor arterial blood gas (ABG) values for hypoxia and hypercapnia, which aggravate ICP.
7. Monitor ventriculostomy, if present, for patency, amount, and character of drainage, and correct height level every hour.
8. Recognize need for maintenance of BP parameters based on status of treated versus untreated aneurysm.
9. Evaluate effectiveness of antihypertensive or vasopressor therapy.
10. Perform ongoing physical assessment, including respiratory, cardiac, gastrointestinal (GI), and genitourinary (GU) function to detect potential complications.

CLINICAL JUDGMENT There are no evidence-based data to support daily sampling of CSF. If CSF is cloudy or purulent, notify the provider. CSF will be sent for culture and Gram stains, white blood cell (WBC) count, red blood cell (RBC) count, glucose, and protein analysis. Institutional policy and procedure will determine who is permitted to obtain CSF samples.

Maintaining Safety

1. Monitor neurologic status based on condition, including LOC, pupillary reaction, motor and sensory function, CN function, speech, and presence of headache.
2. Administer crystalloid to maintain euvolemia.
3. Monitor BP, hemodynamic monitoring, neurologic status, and input and output status at least every hour, or as status indicates, while in the intensive care unit (ICU).
4. Maintain safety factors based on neurologic deficits; prevent physical injury related to vision, hearing, and body awareness deficits.
5. Monitor for seizure activity and administer AEDs as directed.
6. See "Nursing Management of the Patient With an Altered State of Consciousness" section, page 333.

Reducing Pain

1. Assess level of pain and pain relief; report any increase in headache.
2. Administer analgesics, as prescribed.
3. Administer dexamethasone, as prescribed, for headache control. May be useful for headaches as a result of inflammatory changes secondary to coils.
4. Encourage distraction and relaxation techniques to promote calming effect.
5. Explain to the patient/significant other the limited use of opioids secondary to need to assess the patient's LOC at all times.
6. Encourage elevated head of bed to minimize cerebral swelling.
7. Provide cool compresses to head.
8. Assess the patient for experiences of unrelieved or increased pain; assess for any changes in neurologic signs, nuchal rigidity, photophobia, and/or changes in vision, which could signal hemorrhage, hydrocephalus, or meningeal irritation.

Reducing Anxiety

1. Provide ongoing assessment of psychosocial issues (sexuality, anxiety, fear, depression, frustration, emotional lability).
2. Be attuned to verbal and nonverbal cues from the patient/family that signal problems with coping.
3. Inform the patient regarding all treatment modalities.
4. Encourage discussion of risks/benefits with the surgeon/interventional neuroradiologist.
5. Use reassurance and therapeutic conversation to relieve fear and anxiety.
6. Provide support to the patient/family in dealing with the stress and uncertainty of hospitalization.
7. Consult social services for assistance with patient/family support to obtain copy of advance directives, including durable power of attorney, address guardianship, and long-term care decisions, as needed.
8. Prepare the patient and family for surgery or endovascular treatment.

Community and Home Care Considerations

1. Assess the level of knowledge and ability of the patient/significant other to retain information.
2. Assess ongoing home care needs.
3. Assess the need for skilled nursing or rehabilitation center placement and obtain social service referral to help with planning.
4. Provide teaching to the family and caregivers and act as liaison between health care team and family.

Patient Education and Health Maintenance

1. Instruct the patient/family on purpose and frequency of neurologic radiologic procedures.
2. Explain what an aneurysm is, signs/symptoms of rupture, and possible threats of rupture.
3. Educate the patient about activities to avoid to prevent sudden increased pressure, such as heavy lifting and straining prior to definitive treatment.
4. Encourage lifelong medical follow-up and immediate attention if severe headache develops.

5. Instruct the patient/family on need for and use of invasive monitoring and drainage systems.
6. Reinforce the need for head of bed not to be adjusted.
7. Provide educational material for procedures.
8. Set mutual goals for discharge and communicate discharge preparations with other disciplines (registered nurse, provider physical therapist, discharge coordinator).
9. Explain medications to the patient/significant other and potential adverse effects. Explain the importance of continued nimodipine therapy and correct usage.
10. Have the patient verbalize discharge instructions regarding wound care, activity restrictions, medications, and reportable signs/symptoms.

Evaluation: Expected Outcomes

- No signs of rebleeding, increased ICP, vasospasm; vital signs and neurologic signs stable.
- Safety maintained; no seizure activity.
- Verbalizes decreased pain or control of pain to an intensity that is acceptable.
- The patient and family able to state reason for surgery/endovascular intervention, possible risks; openly discuss fears and uncertainties.

Rupture of Intracranial Arteriovenous Malformation

EVIDENCE BASE Chen, C.-J., Ding, D., Derdeyn, C. P., Lanzino, G., Friedlander, R. M., Southerland, A. M., Lawton, M. T., & Sheehan, J. P. (2020). Brain arteriovenous malformations: A review of natural history, pathobiology, and interventions. *Neurology, 95*(20), 917–927. https://doi.org/10.1212/WNL.0000000000010968

Sugiyama, T., Grasso, G., Torregrossa, F., & Fujimura, M. (2022). Current concepts and perspectives on brain arteriovenous malformations: A review of pathogenesis and multidisciplinary treatment. *World Neurosurgery, 159*, 314–326. https://doi.org/10.1016/j.wneu.2021.07.106

An *arteriovenous malformation* (AVM) is a system of dilated arteries and veins with dysplastic vessels. The normal capillary beds are absent, and the arterial blood flows directly into the draining veins (fistula). AVMs are congenital lesions that can enlarge over the patient's lifespan; these lesions are often asymptomatic until rupture. The lifetime risk of bleed in an unruptured AVM is 2% to 4% per year throughout the patient's lifespan, depending on size and structural configuration of the lesion.

Pathophysiology and Etiology

1. AVMs generally contain a nidus (central core) and "red" engorged veins (oxygenated veins) and have been described as a tangled mass of discolored vessels that have the appearance of a cluster of grapes.
2. The artery to venous connection, or fistula, creates increased pressure within the venous system, resulting in vascular dilation, congestion, and hypoperfusion.
3. AVMs are generally low-pressure abnormalities at birth and can progress to a high-flow, high-pressure abnormality in adulthood.
4. Parenchymal AVMs can be located in the pia matter, subcortical tissue, paraventricular region, or a combination of these regions.

Table 11-6 Spetzler-Martin Grading System

	POINTS
Size of Nidus	
Small	1
Medium	2
Large	3
Eloquence of Brain Tissue	
No	0
Yes	1
Deep Vascular Component	
No	0
Yes	1

Grading scale of 1 to 5: 1 = lowest risk, 5 = greatest risk for treatment.

5. Approximately 50% of patients with AVMs present with hemorrhage. Other signs of AVM rupture include seizures and signs of mass effect.
6. Intracerebral bleeding in a ruptured AVM tends to be superficial; cerebral vasospasm rarely occurs. The Spetzler-Martin grading system is used as a prognostic indicator as well as a tool to define risks associated with treating AVMs. Grading scale of 1 to 5: 1 = lowest risk, 5 = greatest risk for treatment (see Table 11-6).

Clinical Manifestations

1. Sudden onset of severe headache, often accompanied by nausea and vomiting, but without neurologic deficits, may be an early sign of a ruptured AVM.
2. Progressively worsening headache, as well as new onset of seizure activity due to spontaneous superficial ICH, are commonly related to a ruptured AVM.
3. May present with LOC and severe deficits if massive bleed. Focal signs or deficits are dependent on the location of the bleed and compression of adjacent brain structures (visual disturbances, CN deficits, hemiparesis, etc.).

Diagnostic Evaluation

1. History and physical examination.
2. CT scan—to determine presence of blood, rule out other lesions; increased density if blood present, may also show increased ICP or mass effect.
3. MRI and MRA or CT angiogram—noninvasive evaluation of cerebral vascular structures. Useful in the diagnosis of AVM, but does not define vascular changes and flow patterns.
4. Cerebral angiogram—gold standard test and the only diagnostic tool that provides definitive evaluation of AVM presence, location, and vascular structure. Will also evaluate flow patterns, pressure gradients, and collateral circulation and identify intranidal aneurysms and feeding vessels.

Management

Unruptured

1. Aimed at diagnostic evaluation of AVM to determine appropriate intervention. Interventions include observation, single or combination of modalities of surgery, endovascular therapy, or radiosurgery.

2. Surgical resection—dependent on location, eloquence of brain tissue, and size.
3. Endovascular management—infrequently used as sole treatment since AVMs may reestablish flow and few are able to be completely resolved with embolization. Materials used are classified as solid or liquid agents. Solids include *N*-butyl cyanoacrylate liquid polymer, polyvinyl alcohol particles, detachable coils, and balloon occlusion. Liquid agents include glue, onyx, and alcohol.
   a. Staged embolization is generally performed on larger AVMs to reduce flow patterns gradually.
   b. Initial embolization is aimed at protecting area at risk for rupture, reducing the nidus, or controlling the area at highest risk for bleeding.
4. Stereotactic radiosurgery (SRS)—lesions less than or equal to 2.5 to 3 cm in size. Radiation creates vessel wall injury, initiating clot formation that leads to eventual blockage of vessel (this can take 1 to 3 years to occur). During this time, the AVM remains at risk for rupture.
5. AEDs for seizures as presenting symptom—fosphenytoin, phenytoin, or levetiracetam may be given initially via IV for rapid loading. Levels should be monitored for accurate dosing.
6. Normalize BP if hypertensive.
7. Smoking cessation.

After Rupture

1. Maintenance and close monitoring of SBP within prescribed limits to prevent rebleed from hypertension and ischemia from decreased cerebral perfusion with nicardipine, labetalol, apresoline, or alternative IV antihypertensive agents.
2. Vasopressor agents may be needed to maintain SBP within prescribed range.
3. Antiepileptics for seizures as presenting symptom—phenytoin, fosphenytoin, and levetiracetam; duration based on provider preference and the location and extent of bleed.
4. Surgical intervention—after a bleed, surgery is not performed immediately unless to evacuate a hematoma. Partial embolization of the AVM, specifically area of suspected rupture, may be performed and then followed by surgery several weeks later.

Complications

1. Bleed or rebleed.
2. Hydrocephalus; obstructive initially requiring ventriculostomy, nonobstructive long term, may require shunt.
3. Seizures.
4. Permanent deficit or deterioration and death.

Nursing Assessment

1. Perform and document neurologic assessment with vital signs and as patient condition warrants.
2. Monitor for changes in or decreasing LOC, CN function, pupillary function, and motor function, including drift (inability to maintain unsupported position).
3. Assess for increasing headache or focal neurologic deficits, which could signal rebleeding.
4. Assess vital signs and pupillary changes frequently for the development of increased ICP.

Nursing Interventions

Maintaining Cerebral Perfusion and Preventing Complications

1. Medicate the patient as ordered during periods of extreme agitation.
2. Institute seizure precautions by providing padded side rails, suction equipment, and oral airway at the bedside.
3. Perform and document neurologic assessment with vital signs and as patient condition warrants, which includes monitoring LOC, CN function, pupillary function, and motor function.
   a. Assess for signs of increased ICP, including bradycardia and widening pulse pressure, changes in respiratory pattern (Cheyne-Stokes pattern, apneustic, ataxic).
   b. Assess for subjective neurologic complaints specific to decreased perfusion (e.g., diplopia, headache, blurred vision).
   c. Assess for signs and symptoms of rebleed: insidious onset of confusion, disorientation, and decreased LOC, or focal deficit associated with area of bleed.
   d. Document findings and report any changes such as drowsiness and speech slurring or onset of pronator drift, which may be first sign of deterioration.
4. Implement nursing interventions to minimize ICP and cerebral swelling (e.g., elevate head of bed 30 degrees, maintain proper head and neck alignment to avoid jugular vein compression), avoid prolonged suctioning procedures, keep procedure less than 15 seconds, collaborate with providers to use lidocaine presuctioning if intubated).
5. Monitor ABG values for hypoxia and hypercapnia, which aggravate ICP.
6. Monitor ventriculostomy, if present, to manage acute hydrocephalus, for patency, amount, and character of drainage, and correct height level every 1 hour.
   a. If CSF is cloudy or purulent or other signs of potential infection are present, contact the health care provider.
   b. CSF will be sent for culture and Gram stains, WBC count, RBC count, glucose, and protein analysis. Institutional policy and procedure will determine who is permitted to obtain CSF samples.
7. Recognize need for maintenance of BP parameters and evaluate effectiveness of antihypertensive or vasopressor therapy.
8. Maintain fluid volume status, evaluate electrolytes, evaluate hemoglobin and hematocrit, and monitor input and output status at least every hour, or as status indicates
9. Maintain safety factors for neurologic deficits (e.g., prevent sensory overload, physical injury related to vision, or hearing, body awareness deficits).
10. Also see "Nursing Management of the Patient With an Altered State of Consciousness" section, page 333.

Reducing Pain

1. Assess level of pain and pain relief; report any increase in headache.
2. Administer analgesics as prescribed.
3. Encourage distraction and relaxation techniques to promote calming effect.
4. Explain to the patient/significant other the limited use of opioids secondary to need to assess patient's LOC at all times.
5. Encourage elevated head of bed to minimize cerebral swelling.
6. Provide cool compresses to head.
7. Assess the patient for experiences of unrelieved or increased pain; assess for any changes in neurologic signs, which could signal hemorrhage, hydrocephalus, or meningeal irritation.

Reducing Anxiety

1. Provide ongoing assessment of psychosocial issues (anxiety, fear, depression, frustration, emotional lability).
2. Be attuned to verbal and nonverbal cues from the patient/family that signal problems with coping.

3. Inform the patient regarding all treatment modalities.
4. Encourage discussion of risks/benefits with the surgeon/interventional neuroradiologist.
5. Use reassurance and therapeutic conversation to relieve fear and anxiety.
6. Provide support to the patient/family in dealing with the stress and uncertainty of hospitalization.
7. Consult social services for assistance with the patient/family support and long-term care decisions, as needed.
8. Prepare the patient and family for surgery or endovascular treatment.

Community and Home Care Considerations

1. Assess level of knowledge and ability of the patient/significant other to retain information.
2. Assess ongoing home care needs.
3. Assess need for nursing home or rehabilitation center placement and obtain social service referral to help with planning.
4. Provide teaching to family and caregivers and act as liaison between health care team and family.

Patient Education and Health Maintenance

1. Instruct the patient/family on purpose and frequency of neurologic/radiologic procedures.
2. Explain what an AVM is, signs/symptoms of rupture, and possible threats of rupture.
3. Educate the patient to the risk of rebleed, which is 50% within 6 months if untreated, and remains for rest of life if not definitively treated.
4. Encourage lifelong medical follow-up and immediate attention if severe headache develops.
5. Explain the need for follow-up angiograms to verify complete eradication of AVM or to define extent of eradication to facilitate treatment planning.
6. Provide educational material for procedures.
7. Set mutual goals for discharge, and communicate discharge preparations with other disciplines (registered nurse, provider, physical therapist, discharge coordinator).
8. Explain medications to the patient/significant other and potential adverse effects.
9. Have patient verbalize discharge instructions regarding wound care, activity restrictions, medications, and reportable signs/symptoms.

Evaluation: Expected Outcomes

- No signs of rebleeding, increased ICP, decreased cerebral perfusion, or seizures; vital signs stable; neurologic parameters stable.
- Verbalizes decreased pain or control of pain to an intensity that is acceptable.
- Decrease in anxiety sufficient to allow the completion of necessary procedures and to promote recovery.

INFECTIOUS DISORDERS

Meningitis

Meningitis is an inflammation of the pia mater and arachnoid membranes that surround the brain and the spinal cord. The subarachnoid space between these two meninges contains cerebrospinal fluid (CSF) that may reflect the signs and symptoms of meningitis.

EVIDENCE BASE Wall, E. C., Chan, J. M., Gil, E., & Heyderman, R. S. (2021). Acute bacterial meningitis. *Current Opinion in Neurology, 34*(3), 386–395. https://doi.org/10.1097/WCO.0000000000000934

Carter, E., & McGill, F. (2022). The management of acute meningitis: An update. *Clinical Medicine, 22*(5), 396–400. http://doi.org/10.7861/clinmed.2022-cme-meningitis

Pathophysiology and Etiology

1. Viral meningitis (aseptic nonbacterial) is the most common form. More than 75,000 cases occur in the United States yearly. Viral meningitis is usually self-limiting; management is supportive. It is usually caused by a nonpolio enterovirus (e.g., coxsackie, echovirus) accounting for 85% to 95% of cases. The incidence of viral meningitis drops with age. As a general rule, the younger the patient, the greater the risk of viral meningitis. This organism is spread by the fecal–oral route and through sewage.
2. In the United States, the incidence of acute, bacterial meningitis is 0.7 to 0.9 per 100,000 population. The mortality is 10% to 30%, and many who recover are left with long-term problems (e.g., hearing deficit).
3. Bacterial meningitis may cause damage to the central nervous system (CNS) from the inflammatory process rather than the pathogen. The organisms causing these infections seem to vary depending on the age and immune status of the patient. *Streptococcus pneumoniae* (pneumococcal meningitis) is the leading cause of bacterial meningitis accounting for 50% to 70% of cases. It also has the highest mortality rate (50% in developing countries and 20% to 37% in developed countries). *Neisseria meningitidis* (meningococcal meningitis), which is a gram-negative diplococcus, is the second most common pathogen in children and adults.
   a. Most bacteria that cause meningitis begin by colonizing the nasopharynx and then invade the circulation and CSF, causing an inflammatory response mediated by cytokines.
   b. Bacterial meningitis can result in brain damage due to chemicals released by bacteria that kill or damage neurons, purulent exudates that may result in vasculitis and vasospasm, and increased intracranial pressure (IICP) that causes cerebral edema.
4. Fungal meningitis, particularly *Cryptococcus neoformans*, affects patients who are immunosuppressed (e.g., those with human immunodeficiency virus [HIV]), through soil contaminated with excrement from pigeons and chickens. Cryptococcal antigen, or culture, is found in the CSF, but meningeal signs may be minimal. In patients who are HIV positive, tuberculous meningitis, tuberculomas, and atypical mycobacterial infections of the brain may be noted.
5. Parasitic meningitis is usually cause by flukes, worms, or amoeba.
6. Other avenues of infection include:
   a. Spread of nearby infection (e.g., acute and chronic sinusitis [with *S. pneumoniae* and *Streptococcus aureus* most common], mastoiditis, otitis media, osteomyelitis of skull or vertebrae, or pneumonia).
   b. Access via blood-borne route (e.g., neoplastic meningitis)—malignant cells infiltrate the leptomeninges as a complication of breast cancer, lung cancer, malignant melanoma, non-Hodgkin lymphoma, and acute leukemia.

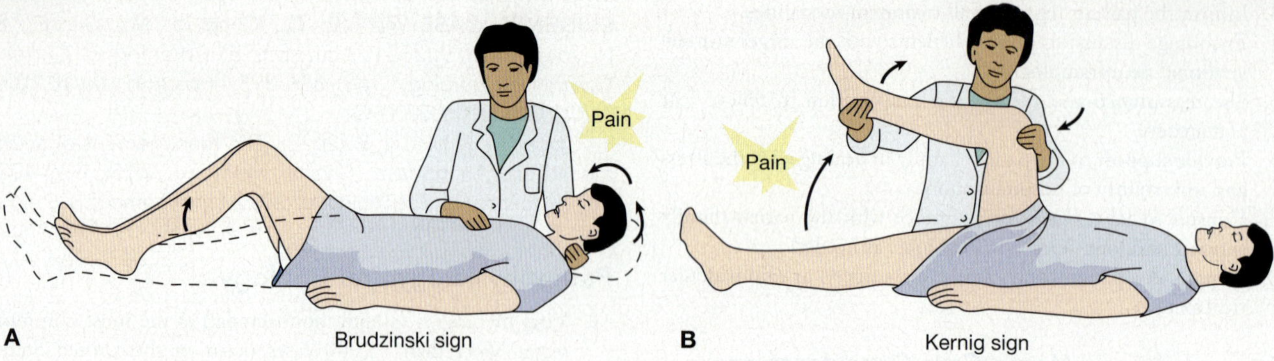

Figure 11-6. Signs of meningeal irritation include nuchal rigidity and positive Brudzinski and Kernig signs. **(A)** To elicit Brudzinski sign, place the patient supine and flex the head upward. Resulting flexion of both hips, knees, and ankles with neck flexion indicates meningeal irritation. **(B)** To test for Kernig sign, once again place the patient supine. Keeping the bottom leg straight, flex the other hip and knee to form a 90-degree angle. Slowly extend the upper leg. This places a stretch on the meninges, resulting in pain and spasm of the hamstring muscle. Resistance to further extension can be felt.

   c. CSF contamination—post-op craniotomy, contamination of external ventricular drain (EVD), open penetrating wounds.
   d. *Listeria monocytogenes*, a gram-positive bacilli, may cause meningitis through contaminated hot dogs, cold meats, and unpasteurized dairy products.
7. The incidence of *Haemophilus influenzae* meningitis has decreased because of the *Haemophilus* b conjugate vaccine.

Clinical Manifestations

1. Classic symptoms are fever, headache, and nuchal rigidity. Constitutional symptoms of vomiting, diarrhea, cough, and myalgias appear in more than 50% of patients. History of temperature elevation occurs in 76% to 100% of patients who seek medical attention. A common pattern is low-grade fever in the prodromal stage and higher temperature elevations at the onset of neurologic signs.
2. Altered mental status; confusion in older patients.
3. Petechial (appears like "rug" burn) or purpuric rash from coagulopathy, especially with *N. meningitidis.*
4. Photophobia.
5. Neck tenderness or a bulging anterior fontanel in infants.
6. Children may exhibit behavioral changes, arching of the back and neck, a blank stare, refusal to feed, and seizures. Viral meningitis can cause a red, maculopapular rash in children.
7. Positive Brudzinski and Kernig signs (see Figure 11-6).
8. Neonates may exhibit poor feeding, altered breathing patterns, or listlessness.
9. Onset may be over several hours or several days depending on the infectious agent, the patient's age, immune status, comorbidities, and other variables. Some viruses cause rapid onset of symptoms, whereas others may involve prodromal nonspecific flulike symptoms, such as malaise, myalgia, and upper respiratory symptoms. In many cases, symptoms have a biphasic pattern; the nonspecific flulike symptoms and low-grade fever precede neurologic symptoms by approximately 48 hours. With the onset of neck stiffness and headache, the fever usually returns.

KEY DECISION POINT If the patient presents with meningitis-like symptoms and appears very ill, evaluation and treatment for bacterial meningitis must be urgently initiated. Patients with bacterial meningitis are typically sicker than patients with a viral etiology, with high fever, severe headache with or without photophobia, and mental status changes. Blood and CSF cultures should be taken as soon as possible as the goal of treatment is to administer appropriate intravenous (IV) antibiotics within 30 minutes of presentation.

Diagnostic Evaluation

1. Complete blood count (CBC) with differential is indicated to detect an elevated leukocyte count in bacterial and viral meningitis, with a greater percentage of polymorphonuclear leukocytes (90%) in bacterial and (less than 50%) in viral meningitis (normal 0% to 15%).
2. Blood cultures are obtained to indicate the organism.
3. CSF evaluation for pressure, leukocytes, protein, glucose—CSF normally has five or fewer lymphocytes or mononuclear cells/mm^3.
   a. In acute bacterial meningitis, the CSF looks turbid or cloudy, opening pressure on lumbar puncture (LP) may be elevated, elevated leukocytes (several thousand with predominance of polymorphonuclear neutrophils), elevated protein, and low glucose. A Gram stain will identify if the organism is gram positive or gram negative, culture will identify the organism, and sensitivity will provide antibiotic choice selection for treatment. White blood cell (WBC) differential should be done by a stained smear of sediment.
   b. In viral encephalitis, the CSF may indicate normal/moderately elevated pressure, few/elevated leukocytes (fewer than 1,000), normal or slightly elevated protein, and normal glucose.

KEY DECISION POINT Prior to an LP being performed, the patient is assessed for signs of elevated ICP. A computed tomography (CT) scan may also be needed, as performing an LP with IICP can result in cerebral herniation.

4. New developments in laboratory techniques allow detection of bacterial antigens in the CSF in 1 to 2 hours. This is especially important in patients who received antibiotics prior to obtaining CSF, as the sensitivity of the Gram stain is reduced 20% when antibiotics have been administered.

5. Magnetic resonance imaging (MRI)/CT with and without contrast rules out other disorders. A CT scan with contrast must be obtained to detect abscesses.

Management

1. The assessment and management of meningitis should be approached through a team effort with nursing, infectious disease and otolaryngology specialists, neurology, internal medicine, and laboratory and diagnostic staff. Droplet precautions are warranted for suspected *N. meningitidis* and *H. influenzae* meningitis.
2. The Infectious Disease Society of America (IDSA) guidelines are utilized. Most patients are given IV antibiotics as soon as possible until the laboratory findings determine the type of meningitis (e.g., viral, bacterial). Broad-spectrum antibiotics are given until organism has been identified and sensitivities have been received. Once sensitivities are known, the antibiotics can be modified. However, cultures should be taken before initiating antibiotics.
   a. The use of corticosteroids (e.g., dexamethasone) as an adjunctive therapy varies among providers. Rationale for use is the anti-inflammatory effect and reduction in edema. The IDSA recommends corticosteroids be given before or at the same time the first dose of antibiotics is administered. IV dose is 0.6 mg/kg/day in four divided doses for the first 4 days of antibiotics and should be confined to patients older than age 6 weeks.

DRUG ALERT In patients with diabetes mellitus or prediabetes, the glucose level will be impacted with the use of corticosteroids. These patients must have blood glucose checks and glycemic management.

3. Antifungal agents, such as amphotericin B and the triazoles, fluconazole, and itraconazole, are indicated for cryptococcal meningitis. Relapse is common if the patient does not have chronic suppressive therapy with fluconazole or another antifungal agent.
4. Empiric antituberculosis drugs must be initiated if infection by *Mycobacterium tuberculosis* is suspected.
5. Be aware that bacterial resistance to antibiotics has been increasing, making meningitis very difficult to treat in some instances. Infectious disease practitioners will be consulted for antibiotic treatment and course.

Complications

1. Bacterial meningitis, particularly in children, may result in deafness, learning difficulties, spasticity, paresis, or cranial nerve (CN) disorders.
2. Seizures.
3. Possible blindness, optic atrophy, optic neuritis with meningeal fibrosis around the optic nerve.
4. IICP may result in cerebral edema, decreased perfusion, infarction.
5. Paresis or paralysis.
6. Bilateral adrenal hemorrhage (Waterhouse-Friderichsen syndrome).
7. Purpura may be associated with disseminated intravascular coagulation.

Nursing Assessment

1. Obtain a history of recent infections such as upper respiratory infection and exposure to causative agents. Meticulous history-taking is essential and must include evaluation of exposure to ill contacts, mosquitoes, ticks, and outdoor activities in areas of endemic Lyme disease; travel history with possible exposure to tuberculosis; as well as history of medication use, IV drug use, and sexually transmitted infection risk. Another important part of history is prior antibiotic use, which may alter the clinical picture of bacterial meningitis.
2. Assess neurologic status and vital signs.
3. Evaluate for signs of meningeal irritation.
4. Assess sensorineural hearing loss (vision and hearing), CN damage (e.g., facial nerve palsy), and diminished cognitive function.

Nursing Interventions

Reducing Fever

1. Administer antimicrobial agents on time to maintain optimal blood levels.
2. Monitor temperature frequently or continuously and administer antipyretics, as ordered.
3. Institute other cooling measures, such as a hypothermia blanket, as indicated.

Maintaining Fluid Balance

1. Prevent IV fluid overload, which may worsen cerebral edema.
2. Monitor intake and output closely.

Enhancing Cerebral Perfusion

1. Assess level of consciousness (LOC), vital signs, and neurologic parameters frequently. Observe for signs and symptoms of IICP (e.g., decreased LOC, dilated pupils, widening pulse pressure).
2. Maintain a quiet, calm environment to prevent agitation, which may cause an IICP.
3. Prepare the patient who will be undergoing an LP for CSF evaluation and/or repeat spinal tap, if indicated. Evaluate the patient for ICP prior to LP.
4. Notify the health care provider of signs of deterioration: increasing temperature, decreasing LOC, seizure activity, or altered respirations.

Reducing Pain

1. Administer analgesics, as ordered; monitor for response and adverse reactions. Avoid opioids, which may mask a decrease in LOC.
2. Darken the room if photophobia is present.
3. Assist with position of comfort for neck stiffness, and turn the patient slowly and carefully with head and neck in alignment.
4. Elevate the head of the bed to decrease ICP and reduce pain.

Promoting Mobility

1. Frequently turn and reposition the patient to prevent skin breakdown.
2. Progress from passive to active exercises based on the patient's neurologic status.
3. Suggest early physical and occupational therapy referrals to promote return to optimal level of functioning.

DRUG ALERT Note and report to the provider if any doses of antibiotics, osmotic diuretics, and steroids are missed.

Community and Home Care Considerations

1. Prevent bacterial meningitis by eliminating colonization and infection with the offending organism.
   a. Administer vaccines against *H. influenzae* type b for children; *N. meningitidis* serogroups A, C, Y, and W135 for

patients at high risk (especially college students, those without spleens, those who are immunodeficient); and *S. pneumoniae* for patients with chronic illnesses and older adults.

   b. Administer vaccines for travelers to countries with a high incidence of meningococcal disease and household contacts of someone who has had meningitis.
   c. Chemoprophylaxis for meningococcal disease, most commonly with rifampin, may be necessary for health care workers, household contacts in the community, day care centers, and other highly susceptible populations.
2. If maintenance antifungal prophylaxis is initiated for patients with low CD4$^+$ counts, as seen in some patients with acquired immune deficiency syndrome (AIDS), the patient must understand the importance of long-term pharmacologic therapy.

Patient Education and Health Maintenance

1. Advise close contacts of the patient with meningitis that prophylactic treatment may be indicated; they should check with their health care providers or the local public health department.
2. Encourage the patient to follow medication regimen as directed to eradicate the infectious agent completely.
3. Encourage follow-up and prompt attention to infections in future.
4. Direct the patient and family to the Centers for Disease Control and Prevention (www.cdc.gov/meningitis/index.html) for support and additional information.

Evaluation: Expected Outcomes

- Afebrile.
- Adequate urine output; central venous pressure (CVP) in normal range.
- Alert LOC; normal vital signs.
- Pain controlled.
- Optimal level of functioning after resolution.

Encephalitis

Encephalitis is an inflammation of cerebral tissue, typically accompanied by meningeal inflammation resulting in neurologic dysfunction. Encephalitis is most commonly caused by a viral infection. Like meningitis, encephalitis can be infectious or noninfectious and acute, subacute, or chronic.

Pathophysiology and Etiology

1. Approximately 12.6 per 100,000 individuals are diagnosed with encephalitis each year. Viral encephalitis accounts for 60% of the cases. In the United States, this is approximately 20,000 cases per year.
2. Once the pathogen enters the body (portal of entry varies among viruses) and reaches the CNS, neurons are attacked, which results in dysfunction and injury.
3. Many viruses can cause encephalitis; major ones include:
   a. Arboviruses (arthropod borne) (e.g., Eastern equine encephalitis, Western equine encephalitis, St. Louis encephalitis, California virus encephalitis, West Nile virus [WNV], and Japanese B encephalitis).
   b. Postviral, which results in CNS infection (e.g., measles, mumps, chickenpox).
   c. Postvaccination encephalitis.
   d. Other (e.g., polio, rabies, herpes simplex, herpes zoster, infectious mononucleosis).

Clinical Manifestations

1. Signs and symptoms may develop hours or weeks after exposure.
2. Classic symptoms include fever, headache, and changes in LOC.
3. Symptoms demonstrated are related to the area of the brain experiencing inflammation.
4. Symptoms can include seizures, aphasia, hemiparesis, myoclonic movements, ataxia, nystagmus, ocular paralysis, facial weakness. May also have behavioral changes.
5. Involvement of the temporal lobe—the patient may experience temporal lobe seizures.
6. Clinical criteria utilized to diagnose encephalitis (International Encephalitis Consortium).
   a. Altered LOC.
   b. At least two of the following:
      i. Fever ≥38.5°C within 72 hours.
      ii. Seizures.
      iii. New focal neurologic deficit.
      iv. CSF WBC count ≥5/mm^3.
      v. Electroencephalography (EEG) abnormalities.

Diagnostic Evaluation

1. Diagnosis is based on the clinical presentation, serologic assays, and CSF analysis.
2. A comprehensive history is obtained and must include if the patient has any risk factors for a CNS infection, including recent travel, recent animal/insect bites, immunosuppressed state (e.g., receiving chemotherapy), occupational exposure.
3. Physical examination.
4. CT scan of the brain without contrast may be performed prior to an LP if there is a concern for IICP. an LP is contraindicated with IICP.
5. LP, with evaluation of CSF, is performed to detect leukocytosis, increased mononuclear cell pleocytosis, increased proteins, and normal or slightly lowered glucose.
6. Polymerase chain reaction (PCR) analysis of the virus DNA and antigen is recommended. Detection of antigens is essential in diagnosing the specific virus (e.g., herpes simplex virus, cytomegalovirus).
7. Specific antibody titers (immunoglobulin M [IgM], IgG) are also obtained.
8. EEG may demonstrate slow brain wave complexes in encephalitis.
9. MRI of the brain with contrast is performed unless contraindicated. If contraindicated, a brain CT scan with contrast is obtained. MRI is recommended as specific patterns can be identified to aid in identification of the etiology.

Management

1. Differentiate acute viral encephalitis from noninfectious diseases, such as sarcoidosis, vasculitis, systemic lupus erythematosus, and others.
2. In patients who are immunosuppressed, the provider must differentiate acute viral encephalitis from cytomegalovirus encephalitis, toxoplasmic encephalitis, and fungal infections.
3. Medical management includes empiric therapy with IV broad-spectrum antibiotics and acyclovir. Once agent has been identified, the therapy can be narrowed.
4. Acyclovir is administered IV for 14 to 22 days. Dosed at 10 mg/kg every 8 hours.
5. Monitor neurologic examination and vital signs, maintain fluid and electrolyte balance, and manage IICP (if develops) and seizures (if develop).

DRUG ALERT Acyclovir dose must be adjusted for impaired renal function.

Complications

1. IICP and cerebral edema—can result in neurologic deficits depending on area of brain affected.
   a. Herpes simplex encephalitis (HSE) has a propensity for the temporal lobes, which results in edema and areas of necrosis. IICP places the patient at risk for temporal lobe herniation. The patient may also experience olfactory and gustatory hallucinations, anosmia, temporal lobe seizures, and aphasia.
2. Seizures.
3. Headache.
4. Fever.
5. Mortality and morbidity depend on the infectious agent, host status, prompt start of antiviral medication, and other considerations.

Nursing Assessment

1. Obtain patient history of recent infection, animal exposure, tick or mosquito bite, recent travel, and exposure to ill contacts.
2. Perform a complete physical assessment.
3. Assess vital signs and neurologic status as indicated.
4. Assess for signs of meningeal irritation.
5. Assess respiratory function.

CLINICAL JUDGMENT Although most cases of viral encephalitis only require universal precautions to prevent infection, patients who present with open lesions to the skin, as occurs in herpes simplex or herpes zoster, should have contact isolation procedures implemented.

Nursing Interventions

Preventing Injury

1. Maintain a quiet environment and provide care gently, avoiding overactivity and agitation, which may cause IICP.
2. Maintain seizure precautions with side rails padded, airway, and suction equipment at bedside.
3. Administer medications, as ordered; monitor response and adverse reactions.

Promoting Cerebral Perfusion

1. Monitor neurologic status closely. Observe for subtle changes, such as behavior or personality changes, weakness, or CN involvement, and notify the health care provider.
2. Elevate head of bed 30 degrees.
3. Maintain neck in neutral position.
4. Monitor blood gas levels.

Relieving Fever

1. Monitor temperature and vital signs frequently.
2. Administer antipyretic medications.
3. Provide tepid baths.
4. Use cooling blanket if indicated.
5. Reduce room temperature to provide a cool environment.
6. Monitor fluid intake and output and provide fluid replacement through IV lines as needed.

Managing Safe Behavior in the Environment

1. Frequently orient to person, place, time, and purpose.
2. Provide simple instructions and frequent cues to perform required activities.
3. Maintain consistency in care and avoid overstimulation.
4. Maintain constant surveillance and safety precautions.

Community and Home Care Considerations

1. Promote vaccination of patient, family, and significant others for measles, mumps, and rubella.
2. Pregnant people who have a history of genital herpes simplex, or their partners, should inform their provider of this history.
3. Contacts of rabies-infected patients should be offered rabies prophylaxis.
4. Direct the patient and family to the Encephalitis Society (www.encephalitis.info) for support and additional information.

Patient Education and Health Maintenance

1. Explain the effects of the disease process and the rationale for care.
2. Reassure significant others based on patient's prognosis.
3. Encourage follow-up for evaluation of deficits and rehabilitation progress.
4. Educate others about the signs and symptoms of encephalitis if epidemic is suspected.
5. Educate on measures for the prevention of WNV, advise the use of repellants when outdoors and removal of standing water that acts as a breeding ground for mosquitoes.

Evaluation: Expected Outcomes

- No seizures or signs of IICP.
- Alert with no neurologic deficits.
- Afebrile.
- Participating safely in ADLs.

Brain and Spinal Abscesses

EVIDENCE BASE Michali, M. C., Kastanioudakis, I. G., Basiari, L. V., Alexiou, G., & Komnos, I. D. (2021). Parenchymal brain abscess as an intracranial complication after sinusitis. *Cureus, 13*(8), e17365. https://doi.org/10.7759/cureus.17365

1. A brain abscess is an area of encapsulated pus within the brain parenchyma. Annual incidence is estimated from 0.2 to 1.3 per 100,000 people.
2. An empyema is a collection of pus in the subdural and/or epidural spaces. Subdural empyema is more common than epidural empyema. These account for 15% to 25% of all intracranial infections. Paranasal sinus disease accounts for over two-thirds of infections in older children and adults.
3. Spinal abscesses typically occur in the epidural space. A spinal epidural abscess (SEA) is localized between the thecal sac of the spinal cord and the spinal ligaments and vertebrae.

Pathophysiology and Etiology

1. Brain (intraparenchymal) abscess.
   a. Infection may come from a contiguous spread (e.g., otitis media or mastoiditis, sinusitis, penetrating trauma, or neurosurgery) or hematogenous (e.g., dental infections, lung abscess, empyema, bacterial endocarditis, congenital heart disease).

   b. Infectious agents will vary depending on the predisposing condition (e.g., otitis media, mastoiditis, or sinusitis is polymicrobial, mainly streptococci, Enterobacteriaceae, *S. pneumoniae*, anaerobes, *S. aureus* sinusitis).
2. Empyema.
   a. Epidural empyema is a result of direct spread of infection from the sinuses, mastoids, or calvarium or spread of infection following surgery.
   b. Subdural empyema may result from hematogenous or direct spread. The falx cerebri prevents it from crossing the midline.
3. SEAs.
   a. Infection from a hematogenous source is believed to occur through the arterial route. Infection from a contiguous spread may occur from infected skin, pressure injury, or contamination from spinal surgery or spinal instrumentation (e.g., LP).

Clinical Manifestations

1. Brain abscess and empyema.
   a. The clinical presentation varies depending on the location and size of abscess, virulence of the pathogen, immune status of the individual, and any preexisting conditions.
   b. Classic symptoms: Headache, fever, and a focal neurologic deficit occur in only about 20% of patients.
   c. Headache is the most frequent symptom (60%), followed by fever (53%) and neurologic deficit (48%).
   d. Abnormal mental status and focal deficits are most frequently reported findings on examination. Seizures may occur.
   e. Potential for IICP with nausea, vomiting, and decreased LOC.
2. SEAs.
   a. Most common symptom is pain located at the level of the infection. Radicular pain may also be experienced.
   b. Other symptoms may include fever, motor weakness, and changes in sensation.

Diagnostic Evaluation

1. For suspected abscess or empyema, a CT scan with contrast is often the initial study as this can be obtained quickly in the emergency setting. An MRI with contrast is obtained after the initial CT. CT scan and MRI with contrast will provide information on the location(s) of the abscess. Follow-up imaging will be obtained once treatment has been instituted to evaluate resolution of the infection.
   a. There are four stages of abscess development (early and late cerebritis, early and late capsule). These stages can be identified based on the changes seen on the imaging. In the inflammatory stages of cerebritis on a contrast CT, an irregular peripheral rim of enhancement surrounding the abscess is seen. As the abscess transitions into the capsule stage(s), a thin, distinct capsule is seen with a low-density center. On a contrast MRI, the T1- and T2-weighted images will provide information for staging.
   b. On imaging, there are distinct differences seen for epidural and subdural empyema. On CT scan, an epidural empyema appears as a lens shaped collection, while a subdural appears as a crescent shape. An epidural empyema often crosses the midline, while a subdural is confined by the falx. T1- and T2-weighted images are viewed in contrast MRI.
2. For suspected SEA, an MRI with contrast is the recommended study. If unable to obtain an MRI, a CT with contrast will be obtained.
   a. There will be enhancement in the areas of inflammation (vertebral end plates and abscesses).
   b. A hyperintense T2 signal on MRI demonstrates edema in the area of bone and disk involved.
   c. Destruction of the vertebral end plates, collapse of vertebra, and kyphotic deformities reflect late findings.
3. Laboratory studies.
   a. CBC with differential, erythrocyte sedimentation rate (ESR), and C-reactive protein (CRP).
   b. Blood cultures.

CLINICAL JUDGMENT LP is contraindicated in patients suspected of having a brain abscess because such patients are at risk for herniation if the abscess is acting as a space-occupying lesion.

4. Other diagnostic tests may be obtained based upon patient presentation.
   a. CT Panorex—poor dental hygiene or dentition is a source of infection.
   b. CT of the temporal bones—history of otitis media and an abscess in the temporal lobe.
   c. EEG—concern for seizure activity.

Management

1. Brain abscess.
   a. Surgical intervention will be based on several factors (size, number, location, and stage of abscess).
      i. Options include:
2. Stereotactic aspiration by neuronavigation.
3. Craniotomy to remove the abscess. This is performed when the abscess is large, multiloculated, and the patient is experiencing intracranial hypertension.
   a. The aspirated or resected material will be sent for culture and sensitivity (C&S) and stat Gram stain.
   b. An EVD may be required if the patient has IICP and/or the abscess had ruptured into the ventricle.
   c. Broad-spectrum IV antibiotics will be initiated (aerobic, anaerobic, fungal coverage). Once C&S results received, treatment will be adjusted.
   d. Infectious disease consult for antibiotic selection and duration.
   e. Follow-up imaging will be obtained at specific time frames during treatment course.
4. Cerebral empyema.
   a. Surgical intervention:
      i. Epidural empyema—patient will undergo a craniectomy and washout of the epidural space. The craniectomy is required because the skull has been in contact with the pathogen. This will be replaced at a later time (cranioplasty) once the infection has been cleared. Time frame is at the neurosurgeon's discretion (generally 3 to 6 months).
      ii. Subdural empyema—the procedure is determined by the neurosurgeon and based upon factors such as location and if adequate drainage can be achieved via a burr hole.

5. Burr hole drainage.
6. Craniotomy.
   a. Broad-spectrum IV antibiotics will be initiated (aerobic, anaerobic, fungal coverage). Once C&S results received, treatment will be adjusted.
   b. Infectious disease consults for antibiotic selection and duration.
   c. Follow-up imaging will be obtained at specific time frames during treatment course.
   d. Protective helmet if craniectomy performed.
7. SEA.
   a. For patients presenting with a neurologic deficit, surgical decompression is performed. A laminectomy and drainage of the abscess are performed. Aspirated material is sent for C&S.
   b. For patients presenting without a neurologic deficit, a referral to interventional radiology may be made. The abscess is drained under image guidance and sent for C&S.
   c. Broad-spectrum IV antibiotics will be initiated (e.g., aerobic, anaerobic, fungal coverage). Once C&S results received, treatment will be adjusted.
   d. Infectious disease consults for antibiotic selection and duration.
   e. Follow-up imaging will be obtained at specific time frames during treatment course.
8. Adjunctive therapy for abscess and empyema may include corticosteroids and osmotic diuretics to reduce cerebral edema and anticonvulsants to manage seizures.
9. If a subdural drain is used to provide continuous drainage of the abscess, the patient should be placed in a supine position to prevent rapid fluid shifts into the drainage device.

Complications

1. IICP and cerebral edema.
2. Headache.
3. Seizures.
4. Permanent neurologic deficits.

Nursing Assessment

1. Obtain a history of previous infections, immunosuppression, headache, and related symptoms.
2. Obtain medication list (prescribed and over the counter [OTC]).
3. Assess vital signs and neurologic status as ordered and, if noted, change in condition.
4. If EVD present—monitor ICP, CSF drainage, color, clarity, ICP wave form.
5. If surgical drain present—record output.
6. Assess surgical dressing for drainage.
7. Assess surgical site for erythema, drainage, integrity of sutures/staples.

Nursing Interventions

Relieving Pain

1. Administer pain medications, as ordered.
2. Provide comfort measures, such as quiet environment, positioning with head slightly elevated, and assistance with hygiene needs.
3. Provide passive relaxation techniques, such as soft music and back rubs.

Promoting Cerebral Perfusion

1. Monitor neurologic status closely. Observe for subtle changes, such as behavior or personality changes, weakness, or CN involvement, and notify the health care provider.
2. Elevate head of bed 30 degrees.
3. Maintain neck in neutral position.
4. Monitor blood gas levels.

Minimizing Neurologic Deficits

1. Maintain a safe environment with side rails up, call light within reach, and frequent observation.
2. Evaluate other CN function and report changes.
3. Refer to occupational therapist, speech therapist, or other rehabilitation specialist to provide adjunct to nursing rehabilitation.

Reducing Anxiety

1. Prepare the patient and family for surgery when indicated. Encourage discussion with surgeon to understand risks and benefits of the procedure.
2. Explain postoperative progression and nursing care (see page 341).

Reducing Fever

1. Administer antipyretic agents as indicated.
2. Administer antimicrobial agents on time to maintain optimal blood levels.
3. Monitor temperature frequently or continuously and administer antipyretics, as ordered.
4. Institute other cooling measures, such as a hypothermia blanket, as indicated.

Community and Home Care Considerations

1. Patient follow-up is essential for sinusitis, otitis media, respiratory infections, and other infectious processes that may have been the etiology for brain abscess or empyema.
2. Ensure follow-up appointments with required providers have been made prior to discharge.
3. Ensure referrals for home care have been made and set up prior to discharge. This will include home health registered nurse (RN) for medication management and possible physical therapy/occupational therapy if recommended by inpatient therapists.

Patient Education and Health Maintenance

1. Instruct patient and significant other on medication regimen. This may include administration of IV antibiotics via peripherally inserted central catheter (PICC) line.
2. Instruct on wound care (if applicable) and signs/symptoms to report to provider.
3. If protective helmet prescribed—understands importance of wearing helmet.
4. Follow-up after discharge with primary care provider.
5. Dental follow-up for patients with dental caries/dentition as etiology of infection.

Evaluation: Expected Outcomes

- Verbalizes discharge medications' purpose, administration, and signs/symptoms to report to provider.
- Verbalizes wound care instructions.
- Verbalizes reduced pain.

- Oriented to person, place, and time; follows simple commands.
- No injury related to neurologic deficits.
- Reduced anxiety regarding disease process and procedures.

DEGENERATIVE DISORDERS

Parkinson Disease

Parkinson disease (PD) is a chronic, progressive neurologic disease affecting the brain centers responsible for control and regulation of movement. It is characterized by tremor, bradykinesia, rigidity, and postural abnormalities. Parkinson can complicate the diagnosis, clinical course, and recovery from other illness. Approximately 1% of the total U.S. population older than age 60 years is affected by idiopathic PD, and it less commonly affects people of younger ages. It is the second most common neurodegenerative disease.

Pathophysiology and Etiology

1. A deficiency of dopamine, due to degenerative changes in the substantia nigra of the brain, is thought to be responsible for the symptoms of PD.
2. Underlying etiology may be related to a virus; genetic susceptibility; toxicity from pesticides, herbicides, methyl-phenyltetrahydropyridine, or welding fumes; repeated head injuries; or other unknown cause.
3. The clinical diagnosis of PD may be difficult because older patients may have other causes of rigidity, bradykinesia, and tremor.

Clinical Manifestations

1. Bradykinesia (slowness of movement), loss of spontaneous movement, and delay in initiating movements.
2. Resting ("pill-rolling") tremor of 4 to 5 Hz. The tremor may be worse on one side of the body, affecting the limbs and sometimes involving the head, neck, face, and jaw.
3. Rigidity in performance of all movements. Rigidity is always present but increases during movement. May lead to sensations of pain, especially in the arms and shoulders.
4. Poor balance when moving abruptly or suddenly changing body position. May lead to falls.
5. Autonomic disorders—sleeplessness, salivation, sweating, orthostatic hypotension, dizziness.
6. Depression, dementia.
7. Masklike facies secondary to rigidity.
8. Gait difficulties characterized by a decreased or nonexistent arm swing; short, shuffling steps (festination); difficulty in negotiating turns; and sudden freezing spells (inability to take the next step).
9. Verbal fluency may be impaired.
10. Finger-tapping responses are slowed.
11. Micrographia (change in handwriting, with the script becoming smaller).
12. Problems with speech, breathing, swallowing, and sexual function.

Diagnostic Evaluation

1. Observation of clinical symptoms; may perform imaging studies to rule out other disorders.
2. Physical examination of upper extremity elbow flexion/extension reveals rigidity on extension.
3. Sensorimotor assessment of grip reveals abnormally high grip forces and longer than normal to complete object lift, particularly with lighter loads.
4. Favorable response to a single dose of levodopa or apomorphine helps confirm the diagnosis.

Management

Pharmacologic

1. Anticholinergics, including trihexyphenidyl, benztropine, and procyclidine, to reduce transmission of cholinergic pathways, which are thought to be overactive when dopamine is deficient. These medications are most effective in controlling tremor but are known to cause confusion and hallucinations.
2. Amantadine, originally an antiflu medication, blocks the reuptake of dopamine or increases the release of dopamine by neurons in the brain, thereby increasing the supply of dopamine in the synapses. Widely used as an early monotherapy, its effect may be augmented by drug-free days.
3. Levodopa, a dopamine precursor, combined with carbidopa, a decarboxylase inhibitor, to inhibit destruction of L-dopa in the bloodstream, making more available to the brain. The addition of carbidopa prevents levodopa from being metabolized in the gut, liver, and other tissues and allows more to get to the brain. Therefore, a smaller dose of levodopa is required to treat symptoms, and the unpleasant adverse effects are greatly reduced.
4. Bromocriptine, pramipexole, and ropinirole are dopaminergic agonists that activate dopamine receptors in the brain. Can be taken either alone or in combination with levodopa–carbidopa.
5. Use of the monoamine oxidase inhibitor selegiline or deprenyl boosts the effect of levodopa–carbidopa when levodopa becomes less effective.
6. Tolcapone and entacapone are catechol-*O*-methyltransferase inhibitors for adjunct treatment. They prolong the duration of symptom relief by blocking the action of an enzyme that breaks down levodopa before it reaches the brain. Must be taken with levodopa.
7. Other medications that include levodopa include:
   a. Combination formula of carbidopa/levodopa with entacapone (Stalevo), which is useful in patients stable on both medications.
   b. An enteral suspension of carbidopa/levodopa infused directly into the small intestine, for those with advanced PD who experience unpredictable gastric emptying (requires jejunostomy tube).
   c. An extended-release capsule (Rytary) used as a secondary drug in those patients who experience early wearing off levodopa therapy.
8. Apomorphine is an injectable, long-acting dopamine agonist, beneficial in patients experiencing early wearing off of levodopa therapy.
9. Inhalation with levodopa 50 can also be prescribed in patients who experience early wearing off.
10. Both injectable and inhalation therapies can be used up to 5 times a day.

DRUG ALERT History of melanoma and angleclosure glaucoma are contraindications to levodopa therapy; patients should have suspicious skin lesions removed before initiating therapy, as it may activate a malignant melanoma.

POPULATION AWARENESS Older patients may have reduced tolerance to anti-Parkinson drugs and may require smaller doses. Watch for and report psychiatric reactions, such as anxiety, confusion, and hallucinations; cardiac effects, such as dizziness, orthostatic hypotension, and pulse irregularity; and blepharospasm (twitching of the eyelid), an early sign of toxicity. Other adverse effects may include dry mouth, nausea, drowsiness, and insomnia.

Surgery

1. Surgical treatments for PD and essential tremor are promising.
2. Medial pallidotomy (electrode destroys cells in the globus pallidus) often improves long-standing symptoms, such as dyskinesia, akinesia, rigidity, and tremor, and for patients who have developed dyskinetic movements in reaction to their medications.
3. Deep brain stimulation (DBS) of the thalamus decreases tremor and uncontrollable movements unresponsive to medication. Electrodes are implanted in the thalamus or globus pallidus and connected to a pacemaker-like device, which are programmed by a provider trained in DBS programming. Patients are provided the ability to adjust programs if deemed appropriate by the provider.
4. Gamma knife surgery provides concentrated gamma rays and destroys cells within the thalamus; beneficial in patients with essential tremor and who are unable to tolerate surgery.
5. Brain tissue transplants are still in the experimental stages but have produced encouraging results using stem cells and genetically engineered animal cells that can be made to produce dopamine.

Complications

1. Dementia.
2. Aspiration.
3. Injury from falls.

Nursing Assessment

1. Obtain a history of symptoms and their effect on functioning. Mobility, feeding, communication, and self-care difficulties will have many nursing implications (see Figure 11-7).
2. Assess cranial nerves (CNs), cerebellar function (coordination), motor function.
3. Observe gait and performance of activities.
4. Assess speech for clarity and pace.
5. Assess for signs of depression.
6. Assess family dynamics, support systems, and access to social services.

Nursing Interventions

Improving Mobility and Reducing Risk of Falls

1. Encourage the patient to participate in daily exercise, such as walking, riding a stationary bike, swimming, or gardening.
2. Advise the patient to do stretching and postural exercises as outlined by a physical therapist.
3. Encourage the patient to take warm baths and receive massages to help relax muscles.
4. Instruct the patient to take frequent rest periods to overcome fatigue and frustration.
5. Teach postural exercises and walking techniques to offset shuffling gait and tendency to lean forward.
   a. Instruct the patient to use a broad-based gait.
   b. Have the patient make a conscious effort to swing arms, raise the feet while walking, use a heel–toe gait, and increase the width of stride.
   c. Tell the patient to practice walking to marching music or sound of ticking metronome to provide sensory reinforcement.
6. Assess for proper supportive footwear and safe use of mobility aid such as walker or cane.

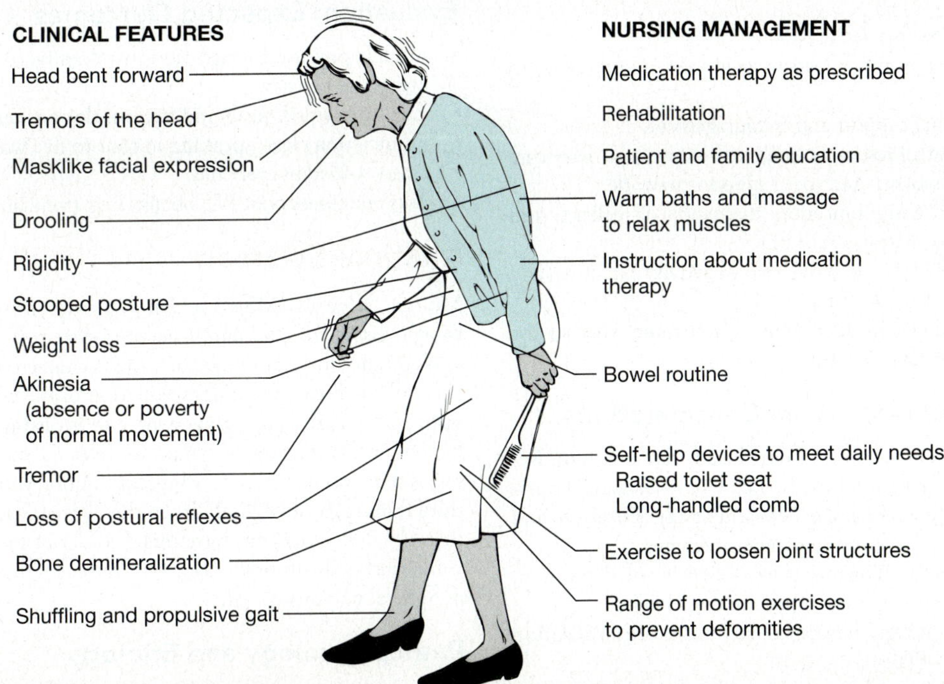

Figure 11-7. Appearance of person with Parkinson disease. (LifeART image copyright (c) 2024. Lippincott Williams & Wilkins. All rights reserved.)

Optimizing Nutritional Status

1. Teach the patient to think through the sequence of swallowing—close lips with teeth together lift tongue up with food on it; then move tongue back and swallow while tilting head forward.
2. Instruct the patient to chew deliberately and slowly, using both sides of mouth.
3. Tell the patient to make conscious effort to control accumulation of saliva by holding head upright and swallowing periodically.
4. Have the patient use secure, stabilized dishes and eating utensils.
5. Suggest smaller meals and additional snacks.
6. Monitor weight.
7. Suggest nutritionist and speech therapist referrals to improve oral intake and nutritional status.

Maximizing Communication Ability

1. Encourage adherence with medication regimen.
2. Suggest referral to speech therapist.
3. Teach the patient facial exercises and breathing methods to obtain appropriate pronunciation, volume, and intonation.
   a. Take a deep breath before speaking to increase the volume of sound and number of words spoken with each breath.
   b. Exaggerate pronunciation and speak in short sentences; read aloud in front of a mirror or into a tape recorder to monitor progress.
   c. Exercise facial muscles by smiling, frowning, grimacing, and puckering.

Preventing Constipation

1. Encourage foods with moderate fiber content—whole grains, fruits, and vegetables.
2. Increase water intake.
3. Obtain a raised toilet seat to encourage normal position.
4. Encourage the patient to follow regular bowel regimen that may include stool softener and other mild medications for constipation.

Strengthening Coping Ability

1. Help the patient establish realistic goals and outline ways to achieve goals.
2. Provide emotional support and encouragement.
3. Encourage use of all resources, such as therapists, primary care provider, social worker, and social support network.
4. Encourage open communication, discussion of feelings, and exchange of information about PD.
5. Have the patient take an active role in activity planning and evaluation of treatment plan.
6. Observe for changes in depression to determine whether the patient is responding to antidepressants.

Community and Home Care Considerations

1. Recommend interdisciplinary home health care program. Requires skilled assessment of needs of patient, professional nursing and therapeutic services, patient and family education, and case management to optimize patient outcomes.
2. Encourage use of soothing music to reduce pain and depression.
3. Assess safety in environment to reduce risk of falls.
4. Utilize physical therapy services to encourage safe ambulation and reduce fear of falls.
5. Encourage use of social services, respite care and health visitors, mental health counselors, and support groups to prevent caregiver strain.
6. Use occupational therapy aids to ensure mobility and safety, such as grab rails in the tub or shower, raised toilet seat, hand rails on both sides of the stairway, rope secured to foot of bed to achieve sitting position, and straight-backed wooden chairs with armrests.
7. Bowel and bladder management is an extremely important factor in the decision to keep the patient at home. Techniques to reduce incontinence episodes, such as having frequently scheduled toileting time, and to handle episodes of incontinence, such as having cleaning supplies and a change of clothes/briefs in the bathroom, should be taught to decrease caregiver burden.

Patient Education and Health Maintenance

1. Instruct the patient to avoid sedatives, unless specifically prescribed, which have additive effect with other medications.
2. Instruct the patient in medication regimen, signs of toxicity, and adverse reactions, such as orthostatic hypotension, dry mouth, dystonia, muscle twitching, urine retention, impaired glucose tolerance, anemia, and elevated liver function tests.
3. Encourage follow-up and monitoring for diabetes, glaucoma, hepatotoxicity, and anemia while undergoing drug therapy. Increasing episodes of freezing should be reported.
4. Teach the patient ambulation cues to avoid "freezing" in place and possibly avoid falls by doing one of the following:
   a. Raise head, raise toes, and then rock from one foot to another while bending knees slightly.
   b. Raise arms in a sudden short motion.
   c. Take a small step backward and then start forward.
   d. Step sideways and then start forward.
5. Instruct the family not to pull patient during episodes of "freezing," which increases the problem and may cause falling.
6. Refer the patient/family for more information and support to agencies such as National Parkinson's Foundation (www.parkinson.org) and National Institute of Neurologic Disorders and Stroke (www.ninds.nih.gov).

Evaluation: Expected Outcomes

- Attends physical therapy sessions; does facial exercises 10 minutes twice per day.
- Eats three small meals and two snacks; no weight loss.
- Enunciation clear; speaking in four to five words per breath.
- Passes soft stool every day.
- Asks questions about PD; obtains help from family and/or friends.

Multiple Sclerosis

Multiple sclerosis (MS) is a chronic, frequently progressive neurologic disease of the central nervous system (CNS) of unknown etiology and uncertain trajectory. MS is characterized by the occurrence of small patches of demyelination of the white matter of the optic nerve, brain, and spinal cord. MS is distinguished by exacerbations and remissions of symptoms over the course of the illness. MS is the most common CNS disease among young adults and the third leading cause of disability in the United States. It is estimated that 400,000 Americans have this disorder of the brain and spinal cord, causing disruption of electrical messages from the brain to the peripheral nervous system.

Pathophysiology and Etiology

1. *Demyelination* refers to the destruction of the myelin, the fatty and protein material that covers certain nerve fibers in the brain and spinal cord (see Figure 11-8).

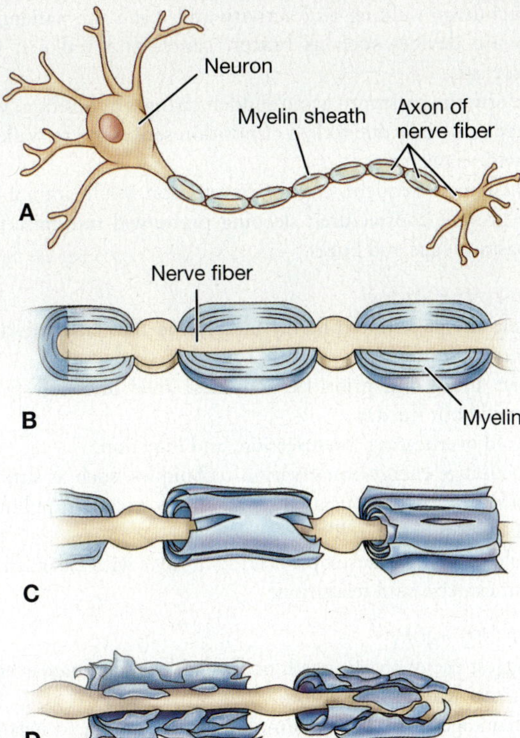

Figure 11-8. The process of demyelination. (**A** and **B**) A normal nerve cell and axon with myelin. (**C** and **D**) The slow disintegration of myelin, resulting in a disruption in axon function. (Reprinted with permission from Hinkle, J. L., Cheever, K. H., & Overbaugh, K. [2022]. *Brunner & Suddarth's textbook of medical-surgical nursing* [15th ed., Fig. 64-3.]. Wolters Kluwer.)

2. Demyelination results in disordered transmission of nerve impulses.
3. Inflammatory changes lead to scarring of the affected nerve fibers.
4. Cause is unknown but may possibly be related to autoimmune dysfunction, genetic susceptibility, or an infectious process.
5. More prevalent in the northern latitudes and among White populations.

Classification

The National Multiple Sclerosis Advisory Committee recognizes four clinical forms of MS:

1. Relapsing remitting (RR)—clearly defined acute attacks evolve over days to weeks. Partial recovery of function occurs over weeks to months. Average frequency of attacks is once every 2 years, and neurologic stability remains between attacks without disease progression. (At the time of onset, 90% of cases of MS are diagnosed as RR.)
2. Secondary progressive (SP)—always begins as RR, but clinical course changes with increasing relapse rate, with a steady deterioration in neurologic function unrelated to the original attack. (Fifty percent of those with RR will progress to SP within 10 years; 90% will progress within 25 years.)
3. Primary progressive (PP)—characterized by steady progression of disability from onset without exacerbations and remissions. More prevalent among males and older individuals. Worst prognosis for neurologic disability. (Ten percent of cases of MS are diagnosed as PP.)
4. Progressive relapsing (PR)—the same as PP, except that patients experience acute exacerbations along with a steadily progressive course (rarest form).

Clinical Manifestations

Lesions can occur anywhere within the white matter of the CNS. Symptoms reflect the location of the area of demyelination.

1. Fatigue and weakness.
2. Abnormal reflexes—absent or exaggerated.
3. Vision disturbances—impaired and double vision, nystagmus.
4. Motor dysfunction—weakness, tremor, incoordination.
5. Sensory disturbances—paresthesias, impaired deep sensation, impaired vibratory and position sense.
6. Impaired speech—slurring, scanning (dysarthria).
7. Urinary dysfunction—hesitancy, frequency, urgency, retention, incontinence; upper urinary tract infection (UTI). Urinary dysfunction affects about 90% of patients with MS and may exacerbate relapse of MS.
8. Neurobehavioral syndromes—depression, cognitive impairment, emotional lability.
9. Symptoms of MS are often unpredictable, varying from person to person and from time to time in the same person.

Diagnostic Evaluation

1. Establishing a definitive diagnosis is often difficult, with much uncertainty concerning prognosis once the diagnosis is made.
2. Serial brain magnetic resonance imaging (MRI) studies have proved to be useful for diagnosing and monitoring patients with MS—show small plaques scattered throughout white matter of CNS.
3. Magnetic resonance spectroscopy is now being studied to monitor specific pathophysiology of evolving MS plaques.
4. Electrophoresis study of cerebrospinal fluid (CSF) shows abnormal immunoglobulin G (IgG) antibody.
5. Visual, auditory, and somatosensory evoked potentials—slowed conduction is evidence of demyelination.

Management

MS treatment is dynamic and rapidly evolving, covering two main areas: direct treatment of MS and treatment of the effects or symptoms resulting from MS. Treatment is aimed at relieving symptoms and helping the patient function. However, a therapeutic relationship between the patient and nurse creates a critical and strong bond that is essential across the long trajectory of the illness.

Current Disease-Modifying Drugs

1. Corticosteroids or adrenocorticotropic hormones are used to decrease inflammation and shorten duration of relapse or exacerbation.
2. Immunosuppressive agents may stabilize the course.
3. Interferon beta-1a and interferon beta-1b are being used for the treatment of rapidly progressing symptoms in some patients.
4. Glatiramer acetate, fingolimod, and natalizumab are immunomodulators used in RR disease.
5. Mitoxantrone, a chemotherapeutic agent used for the treatment of SP (chronic), PR, or worsening RR MS not responding to other disease-modifying drugs.

Treating Exacerbations

1. A true exacerbation of MS is caused by an area of inflammation in the CNS.
2. The treatment most commonly used to control exacerbations is intravenous (IV), high-dose corticosteroids. Methylprednisolone is one of the most commonly used corticosteroids in MS.
3. Plasmapheresis (plasma exchange) is only considered for the 10% who do not respond well to standard corticosteroid treatment.

Chronic Symptom Management

1. Treatment of spasticity with agents such as baclofen, dantrolene, diazepam; physical therapy; nerve blocks and surgical intervention.
2. Control of fatigue with amantadine and lifestyle changes.
3. Treatment of depression with antidepressant drugs and counseling.
4. Bladder management with anticholinergics, intermittent catheterization for drainage, prophylactic antibiotics.
5. Bowel management with stool softeners, bulk laxative, suppositories.
6. Multidisciplinary rehabilitation management with physical therapy, occupational therapy, speech therapy, cognitive therapy, vocational rehabilitation, and complementary and alternative medicine, as indicated, to restore or maintain functions essential to daily living in individuals who have lost these capacities through the disease process.
7. Control of dystonia with carbamazepine.
8. Management of pain syndromes with carbamazepine, phenytoin, perphenazine/amitriptyline, and nonpharmacologic modalities.

Complications

1. Dysphagia and respiratory dysfunction.
2. Infections: bladder, respiratory, sepsis.
3. Complications from immobility.
4. Speech, voice, and language disorders such as dysarthria.

Nursing Assessment

1. Observe motor strength, coordination, and gait.
2. Perform CN assessment.
3. Evaluate elimination function.
4. Explore coping, effect on activity and sexual function, emotional adjustment.
5. Assess patient and family coping, support systems, and available resources.
6. Assess for anxiety, depression, sleep disturbances, cognitive impairment, and pain, which commonly occur in patients with MS.

Nursing Interventions

Promoting Motor Function

1. Perform muscle-stretching and muscle-strengthening exercises daily, or teach the patient or family to perform, using a stretch–hold–relax routine to minimize spasticity and prevent contractures.
2. Apply ice packs before stretching to reduce spasticity.
3. Tell the patient to avoid muscle fatigue by stopping activity just short of fatigue and to take frequent rest periods.
4. Encourage walking and activity and teach the patient how to use devices such as braces, canes, and walkers, when necessary.
5. Inform the patient to avoid sudden changes in position, which may cause falls due to loss of position sense, and to walk with a wide-based gait.
6. Encourage frequent change in position while immobilized to prevent contractures; sleeping prone will minimize flexor spasm of hips and knees.

Minimizing Fatigue

1. Help the patient and family understand that fatigue is an integral part of MS.
2. Plan ahead and prioritize activities. Take brief rest periods throughout the day.
3. Avoid overheating, overexertion, and infection.
4. Encourage energy-conservation techniques, such as sitting to perform activity, limiting trips up and down stairs, pulling, or pushing rather than lifting.
5. Help the patient develop a healthy lifestyle with balanced diet, rest, exercise, and relaxation.

Preventing Injury

1. Suggest use of an eye patch or frosted lens (alternate eyes) for patients with double vision.
2. Encourage regular ophthalmologic consultation to maximize vision and be aware of potential for hearing changes and assess as needed.
3. Provide a safe environment for patient with any sensory alteration.
   a. Orient the patient to the environment and keep arrangement of furniture and personal articles constant.
   b. Make sure floor is free from obstacles, loose rugs, or slippery areas.
   c. Teach the use of all senses to maintain awareness of environment.

Managing Dysphagia

1. Initiate referrals to speech/language pathologist and dietician for evaluation and treatment of swallowing problems.
2. Ensure that the patient is alert and distractions are minimized at mealtimes: provide supervision, as indicated.
3. Use safe swallowing practices, including proper positioning, double swallow, and chin tuck.
4. Monitor the patient for signs and symptoms of choking or aspiration; use suctioning as indicated.
5. Educate and counsel patients and care partners about feeding options as disease progresses.

Maintaining Urinary Elimination

1. Ensure adequate fluid intake to help prevent infection and stone formation.
2. Assess for urine retention and catheterize for residual urine, as indicated.
3. Teach the patient to report signs of UTI immediately.
4. Set up bladder training program to reduce incontinence.
   a. Encourage fluids every 2 hours.
   b. Follow regular schedule of voiding, every 1 to 2 hours, lengthening as tolerated.
   c. Restrict fluid volume and salty foods 1 to 2 hours before bedtime.
5. See Chapter 17 for more information on urine retention and incontinence.

Normalizing Family Processes

1. Encourage verbalization of feelings of each family member.
2. Encourage counseling and use of church or community resources.
3. Suggest dividing up household duties and childcare responsibilities to prevent strain on one person.
4. Explore adaptation of some roles so the patient can still function in family unit.
5. Expand treatment efforts to include the whole family.
6. Support mothers with MS who often face fatigue and episodic exacerbations during their childrearing years.

Promoting Sexual Function

1. Encourage open communication between partners.
2. Discuss birth control options, if appropriate.
3. Suggest sexual activity when the patient is most rested.
4. Suggest consultation with sexual therapist to help obtain greater sexual satisfaction.

Community and Home Care Considerations

1. The nurse case manager functions as care provider, facilitator, advocate, educator, counselor, and innovator aimed at intervening in a wide variety of settings to improve patient function and mobility.
2. Teach the patient receiving interferon beta-1a and interferon beta-1b to expect adverse effects of flulike symptoms, fever, asthenia, chills, myalgias, sweating, and local reaction at the injection site. Liver function test elevation and neutropenia may also occur. Adverse effects may persist for up to 6 months of treatment before subsiding.
3. Instruct the patient receiving interferon beta-1a and interferon beta-1b in self-injection technique.
4. Teach the patient and family to use their own judgment, knowledge, and ingenuity to control MS symptoms.
5. Teach the patient and family how to conduct periodic self-assessment of daily functioning so that home care team can continue to make modifications in treatment plan.

DRUG ALERT Ensure rotation of subcutaneous injection site of disease-modifying drugs to prevent skin reactions. Avoid injections into an area of skin that is sore, reddened, infected, or damaged. Injection sites include the inner thigh, outer surface of the upper arm, stomach, or buttocks. If the patient is thin, thigh and arm sites are preferred. Use a diagram or log of the date and site location for each injection.

Patient Education and Health Maintenance

1. Encourage the patient to maintain previous activities, although at a lowered level of intensity, and reinforce appropriate and safe use of adaptive equipment and aides.
2. Teach the patient to respect fatigue and avoid physical overexertion and emotional stress; remind the patient that activity tolerance may vary from day to day.
3. Advise the patient to avoid exposure to heat and cold or infectious agents.
4. Encourage a nutritious diet that is high in fiber to promote health and good bowel elimination.
5. Advise the patient that some medications may accentuate weakness, such as some antibiotics, muscle relaxants, antiarrhythmics and antihypertensives, antipsychotics, oral contraceptives, and antihistamines; check with health care provider or pharmacist before taking any new medications.
6. Try to include children in the education of MS and the relationship of fatigue and functional status.
7. Refer the patient/family for more information and support to agencies such as the National Multiple Sclerosis Society (www.nmss.org).

Evaluation: Expected Outcomes

- Performs exercises correctly without spasm.
- Rests at intervals; tolerates activity well.
- Moves about in environment without injury.
- No episodes of aspiration.
- Voids every 2 hours with no incontinent episodes.
- Family sharing care, discussing feelings.
- Reports satisfaction with sexual activity.

Amyotrophic Lateral Sclerosis

Amyotrophic lateral sclerosis (ALS), also known as *Lou Gehrig disease*, is an incapacitating, fatal neuromuscular disease that affects as many as 1.75 to 3 in 100,000 persons each year. ALS results in progressive muscle weakness and progressive muscle wasting and paralysis. ALS can affect both upper motor neurons (UMNs) and lower motor neurons (LMNs). It is accompanied by other LMN signs, such as atrophy or fasciculations and bulbar symptoms. Average age of onset for patients with ALS is 58 to 63 years and 40 to 60 years for those with familial ALS.

Pathophysiology and Etiology

1. Degeneration of UMNs (nerves leading from the brain to medulla or spinal cord) and LMNs (nerves leading from the spinal cord to the muscles of the body).
2. Results in progressive loss of voluntary muscle contraction and functional capacity, involving the legs, feet, arms, and hands, and those that control swallowing and breathing. Patients develop variable hyperreflexia, clonus, spasticity, extensor plantar responses, and limb or tongue fasciculations. Extraocular muscles and bladder and anal sphincter muscles are typically spared. ALS rarely affects cognitive functions.
3. Cause is unknown. Usually affects males in the fifth or sixth decade of life.
4. Nearly 10% of ALS cases are familial; the disease is transmitted in an autosomal dominant manner. The copper/zinc *SOD1* gene is mutated in 10% to 20% of these familial cases. Although the primary mechanism of SOD1-mediated neural injury is currently unknown, apoptosis, excitotoxicity, and oxidative stress are thought to play major roles in pathogenesis. Sporadic ALS shares clinical features with familial ALS. However, no SOD1 mutations or polymorphisms have been identified in these patients. Common pathways of disease pathogenesis may play a role, with different molecular abnormalities that lead to similar phenotypes.
5. Several studies have shown an inflammatory component to the affected spinal cord regions, with the presence of activated microglia, reactive astrocytes, and IgG deposition. Whether this reaction precedes or accompanies the molecular events that promote neuronal cell death is unknown.

Clinical Manifestations

1. Progressive weakness and wasting of muscles of arms, trunk, and legs.
2. Fasciculations and signs of spasticity.

3. Progressive difficulty swallowing with drooling (sialorrhea) and regurgitation of liquids through the nose, speaking (nasal and unintelligible sounds), and, ultimately, breathing.
4. CN deficits (bulbar symptoms) are present in 20% of cases (prevalence increases with age), along with dysarthria, voice deterioration, and dysphagia. (Patients with bulbar presentation have poorer prognosis; these symptoms also have a profound impact on quality of life because of nutritional risk factors, aspiration, and respiratory complications.)

Diagnostic Evaluation

1. ALS is a clinical diagnosis.
2. Electromyography to evaluate denervation and muscle atrophy.
3. Nerve conduction study to evaluate nerve pathways.
4. Pulmonary function tests to evaluate respiratory function.
5. Barium swallow to evaluate ability to achieve various phases of swallowing mechanisms.
6. MRI, computed tomography (CT) to rule out other disorders.
7. Laboratory tests: creatine kinase, heavy metal screen, thyroid function tests, CSF evaluation to rule out other causes of muscle weakness.
8. Interdisciplinary approach to care; will require assessments including physical rehabilitation and medicine, speech language pathologist, registered dietician, social worker, case manager.

Management

1. There is no cure for ALS, nor is there a proven therapy that will prevent or reverse the course of the disorder.
2. Riluzole has been shown to prolong the survival of patients with ALS by 2 to 3 months. There are currently multiple clinical trials examining others agents to treat ALS.
3. Most treatment is palliative and symptomatic.
4. Botulinum toxin B injections into the parotid and submandibular glands, amitriptyline therapy, or low-dose radiation therapy to the salivary glands may be used to treat drooling.
5. There are insufficient data to support or refute any specific intervention for the treatment of cramps, spasticity, depression, anxiety, insomnia, pain, dyspnea, or cognitive/behavioral impairments in ALS.
6. Neuropsychological screening may be conducted to assess for cognitive and behavioral impairments.
7. Feeding gastrostomy.
8. Tracheostomy and mechanical ventilation eventually become necessary and should be discussed prior to need to ascertain the patient's wishes regarding these measures.
9. Although no formal research has been conducted addressing the best time to discuss care preferences and end-of-life care in ALS, it is important to elicit this information to guide the selection of various therapeutics, such as intubation, tube feeding, treatment of infection, and management of changes in level of consciousness (LOC). Having the family or significant other present when these discussions occur can help alleviate miscommunication or disagreements in the plan of care.

EVIDENCE BASE Masrori, P., & Van Damme, P. (2020). Amyotrophic lateral sclerosis: A clinical review. *European Journal of Neurology, 27*(10), 1918–1929. https://doi.org/10.1111/ene.14393

Complications

1. Respiratory failure.
2. Aspiration pneumonia.
3. Cardiopulmonary arrest.
4. Locked-in syndrome—fully conscious but unable to respond in any way.

Nursing Assessment

1. Evaluate respiratory function: rate, depth, tidal volume.
2. Perform CN assessment, particularly gag reflex and swallowing.
3. Assess voluntary motor function and strength.

Nursing Interventions

Maintaining Respiration

1. Monitor vital capacity frequently. Document pattern and report any decrease below patient's baseline.
2. Position patient upright, suction upper airway, and perform chest physical therapy to enhance respiratory function.
3. Encourage use of incentive spirometer to exercise respiratory muscles.
4. Assess for signs of hypoxia, such as tachypnea, hypopnea, restlessness, poor sleep, and excessive fatigue.
5. Obtain arterial blood gas (ABG) values as ordered.
6. Establish the wishes of the patient in terms of life support measures; obtain copy of advance directive for chart, if applicable.
7. Assist with intubation, tracheostomy, and mechanical ventilation when indicated (see Chapter 6).
8. Provide suctioning and routine care of a patient with artificial airway and mechanical ventilation.

Optimizing Mobility

1. Encourage the patient to continue usual activities as long as possible but modify exertion to avoid fatigue.
2. Encourage physical therapy exercises to strengthen unaffected muscles and perform range of motion (ROM) exercises to prevent contractures.
3. Encourage energy-conservation techniques.
4. Obtain assistive devices, as needed, to help the patient maintain independence, such as special feeding devices, remote controls, and a motorized wheelchair.

Meeting Nutritional Requirements

1. Provide high-calorie, small, frequent feedings.
2. Provide meals that are of a texture the patient can handle; semisolid food is usually easiest to swallow.
   a. Avoid easily aspirated, pureed, and mucus-producing foods (e.g., milk).
   b. Try warm or cold foods that stimulate temperature receptors in mouth and may help in swallowing.
   c. Do not wash down solids with fluids—may cause choking and aspiration.
3. Allow the patient to make their own food selection.
4. Provide assistive devices for self-feeding when possible.
5. Make mealtimes a pleasant experience in a bright room, with quiet company so the patient may concentrate on eating and avoid undue embarrassment.
6. Examine oral cavity for food debris before and after meals, and assess swallowing function and buildup of saliva.
7. Encourage rest periods before meals to alleviate muscle fatigue.
8. Place the patient upright for meals with neck flexed to partially protect the airway.
9. Instruct the patient to take a breath before swallowing, hold breath to swallow, exhale or cough after swallow, and swallow again.
10. Tell the patient to avoid talking while eating.
11. Prepare the patient for gastrostomy or other alternate feeding methods when appropriate and desired by patient.

Minimizing Fatigue

1. Encourage activity alternating with frequent naps.
2. Encourage the patient to accomplish most important activities early in day.
3. Consult with occupational therapist about energy-conservation techniques in performing activities of daily living (ADLs).

Maintaining Social Interaction

1. Use mechanical speech aids or communication board.
2. Use an environmental control board.
3. Eye movements/blinks may be the last voluntary movement; develop a code system to serve as a communication method.
4. Because standard call lights cannot be activated by the severely debilitated patient with ALS, provide adaptive call light (environmental control unit) and/or some type of constant monitoring and surveillance to meet patient's needs.
5. Allow the patient to select which social activities are meaningful.
6. Refer to counselor or psychologist for coping with communication barriers and inevitability of losses.

Preventing Aspiration and Infection

1. Consult with a speech therapist for techniques and devices to assist swallowing.
2. Discourage bed rest to prevent pulmonary stasis.
3. Perform chest physiotherapy, as tolerated.
4. Monitor for fever and tachycardia and obtain sputum, urine, and other cultures, as indicated.

Community and Home Care Considerations

1. Teach caregivers how to perform suctioning, tracheostomy care, and ventilator care in the home, as indicated. Clean technique will be used rather than sterile.
2. Teach caregivers how to perform gastrostomy feedings and care of tube.
3. Assess for adequate supplies for care and ability of caregivers to carry out procedures.
4. Encourage cleanliness in home environment and avoidance of contact with anyone with respiratory infection. Give influenza and pneumonia vaccines, as indicated.

Patient Education and Health Maintenance

1. Stress the importance of maintaining physical exercise.
2. Review with the patient and family proper eating mechanics to avoid fatigue and aspiration.
3. Inform the patient of right to make decisions early in the disease process regarding an advance directive and life-sustaining treatment.
4. Encourage the family to seek support and respite care.
5. Remind the family that the patient with ALS maintains full alertness, sensory function, and intelligence. Encourage them to maintain interaction, socialization, and stimulation and to seek out technology such as mind-activated computer-driven communication devices.
6. Refer the patient/family for more information and support to agencies such as the ALS Association (www.alsa.org).

Evaluation: Expected Outcomes

- Normal respiratory rate and rhythm, shallow, unlabored at rest.
- Does active ROM exercises for 15 minutes twice per day; uses assistive utensils to feed self.
- Tolerates small, frequent feedings without aspiration.
- Naps twice per day for 1 to 2 hours.
- Communicates needs effectively to staff and family.
- No signs of respiratory or urinary infection.

NEUROMUSCULAR DISORDERS

Guillain-Barré Syndrome (Polyradiculoneuritis)

Guillain-Barré syndrome (GBS) is an acute, rapidly progressing, ascending inflammatory demyelinating polyneuropathy of the peripheral sensory and motor nerves and nerve roots. GBS is most often, but not always, characterized by muscular weakness and distal sensory loss or dysesthesias. GBS is the most frequently acquired demyelinating neuropathy. It affects 0.2 to 2 in 100,000 people and must be identified quickly to initiate treatment and decrease life-threatening complications. Usually, GBS occurs a few days or weeks following symptoms of a respiratory or gastrointestinal (GI) viral infection. Occasionally, surgery or vaccinations will trigger the syndrome. The disorder can develop over the course of hours, days, or weeks. Maximum weakness usually occurs within the first 2 weeks after symptoms appear, and by the third week of the illness, 90% of all patients are at their weakest. About 30% of those with GBS have residual weakness after 3 years, and the recurrence rate is approximately 3%.

Mortality results from respiratory failure, autonomic disturbances, sepsis, and complications of immobility and occurs at a rate of about 5% despite intensive medical care.

Pathophysiology and Etiology

1. Believed to be an autoimmune disorder that causes acute neuromuscular paralysis due to destruction of the myelin sheath surrounding peripheral nerve axons and subsequent slowing of transmission.
2. Viral infection, immunization, or other event may trigger the autoimmune response.
3. About 30% to 40% of cases are preceded by *Campylobacter* infection, an acute infectious diarrheal illness.
4. There are current case reports that relate the coronavirus disease 2019 (COVID-19) virus to the occurrence of GBS.
5. Cell-mediated immune reaction is aimed at peripheral nerves, causing demyelination and, possibly, axonal degeneration.

Clinical Manifestations

1. Paresthesias and, possibly, dysesthesias.
2. Acute onset of symmetric progressive muscle weakness, most often beginning in the legs and ascending to involve the trunk, upper extremities, and facial muscles; paralysis may develop.
3. Difficulty with swallowing, speech, and chewing due to cranial nerve (CN) involvement.
4. Decreased or absent deep tendon reflexes, position, and vibratory perception.
5. Autonomic dysfunction (increased heart rate and postural hypotension).
6. Decreased vital capacity, depth of respirations, and breath sounds.
7. Occasionally spasm and fasciculations of muscles.

Diagnostic Evaluation

1. History and neurologic examination. Progressive weakness, decreased sensation, decreased deep tendon reflexes.

2. Lumbar puncture for cerebrospinal fluid (CSF) examination—reveals low blood cell count, high protein.
3. Electrophysiologic studies—nerve conduction velocity shows decreased conduction velocity of peripheral nerves.

Management

1. Plasmapheresis produces temporary reduction of circulating antibodies to reduce the severity and duration of the GBS episode.
2. High-dose immunoglobulin (Ig) therapy and corticosteroids are used to reduce the severity of the episode.
3. Electrocardiogram (ECG) monitoring and treatment of cardiac dysrhythmias.
4. Analgesics and muscle relaxants, as needed.
5. Intubation and mechanical ventilation if respiratory paralysis develops.

Complications

1. Respiratory failure.
2. Cardiac dysrhythmias.
3. Complications of immobility and paralysis.
4. Anxiety and depression.

Nursing Assessment

1. Assess pain level due to muscle spasms and dysesthesias.
2. Assess cardiovascular function including orthostatic blood pressures (BPs).
3. Assess respiratory status closely to determine hypoventilation due to weakness.
4. Perform CN assessment, especially CN IX for gag reflex.
5. Assess motor strength.

Nursing Interventions

Maintaining Respiration

1. Monitor respiratory status through vital capacity measurements, rate and depth of respirations, breath sounds.
2. Monitor level of weakness as it ascends toward respiratory muscles.
3. Watch for breathlessness while talking, a sign of respiratory fatigue.
4. Maintain calm environment and position the patient with head of bed elevated to provide for maximum chest excursion.
5. As much as possible, avoid opioids and sedatives that may depress respirations.
6. Monitor the patient for signs of impending respiratory failure; heart rate above 120 or below 70 beats/min; respiratory rate above 30 breaths/min; prepare to intubate.
7. Long-term respiratory management may be necessary with placement of a tracheostomy.

Avoiding Complications of Immobility

1. Position the patient correctly and provide range of motion (ROM) exercises.
2. Encourage physical and occupational therapy exercises to regain strength during the rehabilitative period.
3. Assess for complications, such as contractures, pressure injuries, edema of lower extremities, and constipation.
4. Provide assistive devices, as needed, such as cane or wheelchair, for patient to take home.
5. Recommend referral to rehabilitation services or physical therapy for evaluation and treatment.

Promoting Adequate Nutrition

1. Assess chewing and swallowing ability by testing CN V, CN IX, and CN X; if function is inadequate, provide alternate nutrition through enteral or parenteral methods.
2. During rehabilitation period, encourage a well-balanced, nutritious diet in small, frequent feedings with vitamin supplement, if indicated.
3. Recommend referral to dietitian for evaluation and proper diet therapy.

Maintaining Communication

1. Develop a communication system with the patient who cannot speak.
2. Have frequent contact with the patient and provide explanation and reassurance, remembering that the patient is fully conscious.
3. Provide some type of patient call system. Because standard call lights cannot be activated by the severely weak patient, provide adaptive call light and/or some type of constant monitoring and surveillance to meet the patient's needs.
4. Recommend referral to speech therapy for evaluation and treatment.
5. Refer to counselor, social worker, or psychologist to develop/enhance coping skills and regain sense of control.

Relieving Pain

1. Administer analgesics, as required; monitor for adverse reactions, such as hypotension, nausea and vomiting, and respiratory depression.
2. Provide adjunct pain management therapies, such as therapeutic touch, massage, diversion, and guided imagery.
3. Provide explanations to relieve anxiety, which augments pain.
4. Turn the patient frequently to relieve painful pressure areas.

Reducing Anxiety

1. Get to know the patient and build a trusting relationship.
2. Discuss fears and concerns while verbal communication is possible.
3. Reassure the patient that recovery is probable.
4. Use relaxation techniques such as listening to soft music.
5. Provide choices in care and give the patient a sense of control.
6. Enlist the support of significant others.

Community and Home Care Considerations

1. Be aware that GBS is a significant cause of new long-term disability for at least 1,000 people per year in the United States, necessitating long-term rehabilitation and community reintegration. Outcome can range from mild paresthesias to death. The chance of recovery is significantly affected by age, antecedent gastroenteritis, disability, electrophysiologic signs of axonal degeneration, latency to nadir, and duration of active disease.
2. Given the young age at which GBS sometimes occurs, the patient and family must be treated as an integral unit, assessing family communication, knowledge, adjustment, and use of support systems.
3. Include in caregiver training strategies the need for exercise, positioning, and activity to prevent secondary complications, such as contractures, deep vein thrombosis (DVT), hypercalcemia, and pressure injuries.

Patient Education and Health Maintenance

1. Advise the patient and family that acute phase lasts 1 to 4 weeks, then the patient stabilizes and rehabilitation can begin; however, convalescence may be lengthy, from 3 months to 2 years.

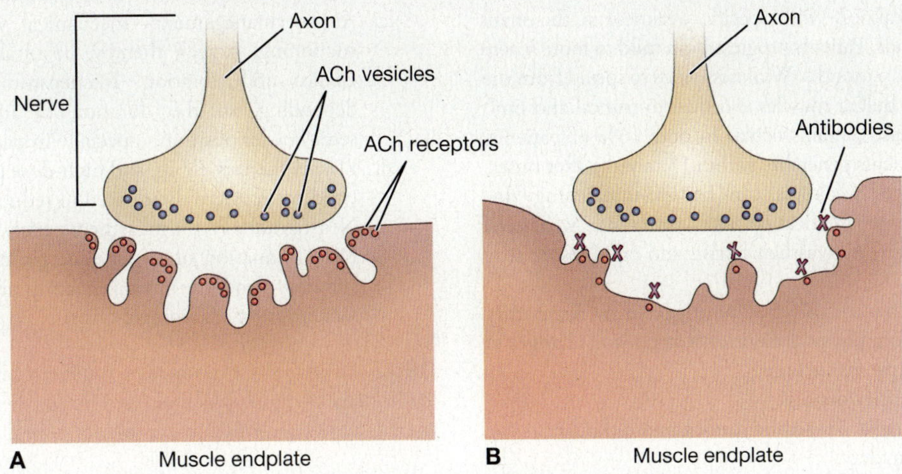

Figure 11-9. Myasthenia gravis. **(A)** Usual acetylcholine (ACh) receptor site. **(B)** ACh receptor site in myasthenia gravis. (Reprinted with permission from Hinkle, J. L., Cheever, K. H., & Overbaugh, K. [2022]. *Brunner & Suddarth's textbook of medical-surgical nursing* [15th ed., Fig. 64-4.]. Wolters Kluwer.)

2. Instruct the patient in breathing exercises or use of incentive spirometer to reestablish normal patterns.
3. Teach the patient to wear good supportive and protective shoes while out of bed to prevent injuries due to weakness and paresthesia.
4. Instruct the patient to check feet routinely for injuries because trauma may go unnoticed because of sensory changes.
5. Reinforce maintenance of optimal weight; additional weight will further stress motor abilities.
6. Encourage the use of scheduled rest periods to avoid overfatigue.
7. Refer the patient/family for more information and support to agencies such as Guillain-Barré Syndrome Foundation International (www.gbsfi.com).

Evaluation: Expected Outcomes

- Normal respiratory rate and rhythm, shallow, unlabored.
- Performs assistive ROM exercises every 2 hours; no pressure injuries or edema present.
- Gag reflex present; eating small meals without aspiration.
- Uses short phrases and head nodding to communicate effectively.
- Verbalizes decreased pain.
- Verbalizes reduced anxiety.

Myasthenia Gravis

Myasthenia gravis (MG) is a chronic autoimmune disorder affecting the neuromuscular transmission of impulses in the voluntary muscles of the body. MG is characterized by fluctuating weakness increased by exertion. Weakness increases during the day and improves with rest. Presentation and progression vary because of an antibody-mediated attack against acetylcholine receptors at the neuromuscular junction. Loss of acetylcholine receptors leads to a defect in neuromuscular transmission. Cardinal features are muscle weakness and fatigue. Evidence suggests that the frequency and recognition of MG is increasing.

Pathophysiology and Etiology

1. MG is idiopathic in most patients. Penicillamine is known to induce various autoimmune disorders, including MG.
2. Depletion of acetylcholine receptors at neuromuscular junctions brought about by an autoimmune attack (see Figure 11-9). In about 90% of patients, no specific cause can be identified, but genetic makeup is a predisposing factor, suggesting environmental factors may be involved in the development of this disorder.
3. The reduced number of acetylcholine receptors results in diminished amplitude of end-plate potentials. Failed transmission of nerve impulses to skeletal muscle at the myoneural junction results in decreased muscle power, clinically manifested as extreme fatigue and weakness. The pattern of muscle involvement varies among individuals.
4. About 80% to 90% of patients with MG have serum antibodies to acetylcholine.
5. Thyroid gland abnormalities are present in 80% of patients. Thymic tumor is the most important known cause; 10% of patients with MG have a thymoma.
6. *Cholinergic crisis* can result from overmedication with anticholinergic drugs, which release too much acetylcholine at the neuromuscular junction.
7. *Brittle crisis* occurs when the receptors at the neuromuscular junction become insensitive to anticholinesterase medication.
8. Females are three times more susceptible to developing MG than males.
9. Spontaneous remissions are rare. Long and complete remissions are even less common. Most remissions (with treatment) occur during the first 3 years of disease.

Clinical Manifestations

1. Extreme muscular weakness and easy fatigability.
2. Vision disturbances—diplopia and ptosis from ocular weakness. Extraocular muscle weakness or ptosis is present initially in 50% of patients and occurs during the course of illness in 90%. Bulbar muscle weakness is also common, along with weakness of head extension and flexion.
3. Facial muscle weakness causes a masklike facial expression. Patients may present a snarling appearance when attempting to smile.
4. Dysarthria and dysphagia from weakness of laryngeal and pharyngeal muscles.

5. Proximal limb weakness, with specific weakness in the small muscles of the hands. Patients progress from mild to more severe disease over weeks to months. Weakness tends to spread from the ocular to facial to bulbar muscles and then to truncal and limb muscles. The disease remains ocular in only 16% of patients. About 87% of patients generalize within 13 months after onset.
6. Respiratory muscle weakness can be life-threatening. Intercurrent illness or medication can exacerbate weakness, quickly precipitating a myasthenic crisis and rapid respiratory compromise.
7. Impending myasthenic crisis may be triggered by respiratory infection, aspiration, physical/emotional stress, and changes in medications. Symptoms include:
   a. Sudden respiratory distress.
   b. Signs of dysphagia, dysarthria, ptosis, and diplopia.
   c. Tachycardia, anxiety.
   d. Rapidly increasing weakness of extremities and trunk.

Diagnostic Evaluation

1. Serum test for acetylcholine receptor antibodies—positive in up to 90% of patients.
2. Electrophysiologic testing, such as electromyography (EMG), shows decreased response to repetitive nerve stimulation.
3. Edrophonium (Tensilon) test—intravenous (IV) injection of this short-acting anticholinesterase relieves symptoms temporarily. After injection, a marked but temporary improvement in muscle strength identified by performance of repetitive movements or EMG testing suggests MG. It also differentiates myasthenic crisis from cholinergic crisis.
4. Thyroid function tests should be done to evaluate for coexistent thyroid disease and computed tomography (CT) scan to assess enlargement of thymus gland. Chest CT scan is mandatory to identify thymoma in all cases of MG. This is especially true in older individuals.

Management

1. With treatment, most patients can lead productive and fulfilling live.
2. Oral anticholinesterase drugs, such as neostigmine and pyridostigmine, are first-line treatments for mild MG, enhancing neuromuscular transmission.
3. Immunosuppressive drugs, such as prednisone, are the mainstay of treatment when weakness is not adequately controlled by anticholinergic medication. Azathioprine may be added as a steroid-sparing agent. Immunosuppressant treatment is often permanent.
4. Newer agents including eculizumab have been approved by the Food and Drug Administration (FDA) for the treatment of patients with MG.
5. Plasmapheresis removes antibodies from the blood and is used for patients in myasthenic crisis or for short-term treatment of patients undergoing thymectomy. IV Ig is also an option and has less side effects.
6. Thymectomy is indicated for patients with tumor or hyperplasia of the thymus gland (thymectomy is not usually beneficial in late-onset patients).
7. Interventions for myasthenic crisis:
   a. Immediate hospitalization and may require intensive care.
   b. Edrophonium to differentiate crisis and treat myasthenic crisis; temporarily worsens cholinergic crisis; unpredictable results with brittle crisis.
   c. Airway management—mechanical ventilation, vigorous suctioning, oxygen therapy, postural drainage with percussion and vibration. Tracheostomy may be required, depending on the duration of intubation. Maintain semi-Fowler position, especially in patients with obesity.
   d. Plasmapheresis, IV Ig, and high-dose parenterally administered corticosteroids are used to reduce symptoms.
   e. Neostigmine IV for myasthenic crisis.
   f. Discontinuation of anticholinergic medications until respiratory function improves; atropine to reduce excessive secretions for cholinergic crisis.

DRUG ALERT Plasmapheresis must be carried out before IV Ig therapy because plasmapheresis will remove the IV Ig proteins that are effective in symptom reduction.

Complications

1. Aspiration.
2. Complications of decreased physical mobility.
3. Respiratory failure.

Nursing Assessment

1. Expect the patient to complain of extreme muscle weakness and fatigue.
2. Assess CN function, motor fatigability with repetitive activity, and speech. Observe eye muscles (usually affected first) for ptosis, ocular palsy, and diplopia.
3. Assess respiratory status—breathlessness, respiratory weakness, tidal volume, and vital capacity measurements.
4. Assess complications secondary to drug treatment—long-term immunomodulating therapies may predispose patients with MG to various complications.
   a. Long-term steroid use may lead to or aggravate many conditions, such as osteoporosis, cataracts, hyperglycemia, weight gain, avascular necrosis of hip, hypertension, and gastritis or peptic ulcer disease. To decrease the risk of ulcer, patients should take an H_2-blocker or antacid.
   b. Increased risk for infection from immunomodulating therapy, especially if the patient is on more than one agent. Such infections include tuberculosis, systemic fungal infections, and *Pneumocystis carinii* pneumonia.
   c. Risk of lymphoproliferative malignancies may be increased with chronic immunosuppression.
   d. Immunosuppressive drugs may have teratogenic effects. In addition, risk of congenital deformity (arthrogryposis multiplex) is increased in offspring of females with severe MG.

DRUG ALERT Neonates born to females with MG need to be monitored for respiratory failure for 1 to 2 weeks after birth. Discuss these aspects with females in reproductive years prior to beginning therapy with these drugs.

Nursing Interventions

Minimizing Fatigue

1. Plan exercise, meals, and other activities of daily living (ADLs) during energy peaks. Time administration of medications 30 minutes before meals to facilitate chewing and swallowing.
2. Assist the patient in developing realistic activity schedule.
3. Provide an eye patch and alternate eyes for the patient with diplopia to allow safe participation in activity.

4. Allow for rest periods throughout the day.
5. Obtain assistive devices to help the patient perform ADLs.

DRUG ALERT Many medications can accentuate the weakness experienced by the patient with MG, including some antibiotics (such as ciprofloxacin, aminoglycosides, chloroquine, and procaine penicillin), antiarrhythmics (such as procainamide, beta-adrenergic blockers, and quinidine), local and general anesthetics, muscle relaxants, and analgesics such as nonsteroidal anti-inflammatory drugs (NSAIDs). Assess function after administering any new drug, and report deterioration in condition.

Preventing Aspiration

1. Assess the patient's oral motor strength before each meal.
2. Teach the patient to position their head in a slightly flexed position to protect airway during eating.
3. Modify diet, as needed, to minimize the risk of aspiration; for instance, soft, solid foods instead of liquids. Teach the patient that eating warm foods (not hot foods) can ease swallowing difficulties.
4. Have suction available that the patient can operate.
5. Administer IV fluids and nasogastric tube feedings to the patient in crisis or with impaired swallowing; elevate head of bed after feeding.
6. Suction the patient frequently if on a mechanical ventilator; assess breath sounds and check chest x-ray reports because aspiration is a common problem.

Maintaining Social Interactions

1. Encourage the patient to use an alternate communication method, such as flash cards or a letter board, if speech is affected.
2. Instruct the patient to speak in a slow manner to avoid voice strain; refer to speech therapy, as needed.
3. Show the patient how to cup chin in hands during speech to support lower jaw and assist with speech.
4. Teach the patient to tilt head and to carry a handkerchief to manage secretions in public.
5. Encourage family participation in care.
6. Refer the patient to the Myasthenia Gravis Foundation of America (www.myasthenia.org) to meet other patients with the disease who lead productive lives.

Community and Home Care Considerations

1. Assess the home environment for physical and emotional stressors, such as uncomfortable temperature, draft, or loud noises.
2. Emphasize continued follow-up and adherence with treatment regimen.
3. Identify the need for additional home care services such as respiratory therapy, physical therapy, and nutritional services.
4. Assess the patient frequently for fluctuation in condition and inform caregivers that this is common.
5. Teach the patient and family how to use home suction in case of aspiration. Make sure everyone in household knows the Heimlich maneuver.

Patient Education and Health Maintenance

1. Instruct the patient and family regarding the symptoms of crisis. Intercurrent infection or treatment with certain drugs may worsen symptoms of MG temporarily. Mild exacerbation of weakness is possible in hot weather.
2. Review the peak times of medications and how to schedule activity for best results. For patients on anticholinesterase therapy:
   a. Stress accurate dosage and times; take anticholinesterase drugs 30 to 45 minutes before meals.
   b. Tell the patient not to skip medication.
   c. Instruct the patient to avoid taking medication with fruit, coffee, tomato juice, or other medications.
   d. Inform the patient of adverse effects such as GI distress.
3. Stress the importance of activity with scheduled rest periods before fatigue develops.
4. Teach the patient ways to prevent crisis and aggravation of symptoms.
   a. Avoid exposure to colds and other infections.
   b. Avoid excessive heat and cold.
   c. Inform the dentist of condition because the use of procaine is not well tolerated.
   d. Avoid emotional upset; plan ahead to minimize stress.
5. Encourage the patient to wear a medical alert device.
6. Stress the importance of adequate nutrition; instruct to chew food thoroughly and eat slowly.
7. Advise the patient to avoid alcohol, tonic water.
8. Refer the patient/family for more information to the Myasthenia Gravis Foundation of America (www.myasthenia.org).

Evaluation: Expected Outcomes

- Demonstrates optimal self-care in bathing, eating, toileting, and dressing without fatigue.
- Breathes effectively; cough is effective; suctioning own secretions; lungs clear.
- Visits with friends, participates in social activities, uses alternative method of communications.

TRAUMA

Traumatic Brain Injury

EVIDENCE BASE Zrelak, P. A., Eigsti, J., Fetzick, A., Gebhardt, A., Moran, C., Moyer, M., & Yahya, G. (2020). *Evidence-based review: Nursing care of adults with severe traumatic brain injury—Literature review.* American Association of Neuroscience Nursing.

Godoy, D. A., Seifi, A., Chi, G., Paredes Saravia, L., & Rabinstein, A. A. (2022). Intracranial pressure monitoring in moderate traumatic brain injury: A systematic review and meta-analysis. *Neurocritical Care, 37*(2), 514–522. https://doi.org/10.1007/s12028-022-01533-z

Traumatic brain injury (TBI) is the disruption of normal brain function due to a trauma-related injury. TBI produces compromised neurologic function, resulting in focal or diffuse symptoms. Falls are the most common etiology of TBI-related hospitalizations (52%), followed by motor vehicle accidents (20%). The goal of treatment is to prevent secondary brain injury by providing supportive care (see Chapter 31 for emergency management of TBI).

Pathophysiology and Etiology

Types of Traumatic Brain Injury

1. Concussion—diffuse brain injury that occurs from a traumatic event resulting in a rapid onset of impaired neurologic function(s); resolves spontaneously. Imaging shows no structural abnormalities. May range from mild to severe.

2. Contusion—bruising of the brain parenchyma with associated swelling. May occur from blunt force trauma, a depressed skull fracture with penetration of tissue by bone, or an acceleration–deceleration injury. In an acceleration–deceleration injury, the initial point of contact is coup, and contrecoup is the opposite point.
3. Intracerebral hematoma—bleeding directly into the brain tissue commonly associated with edema.
4. Epidural hematoma (EDH)—blood between the inner table of the skull and dura. Frequently associated with injury or laceration of the middle meningeal artery secondary to a temporal bone fracture. EDH is commonly associated with a lucid interval, followed by unresponsiveness.
5. Subdural hematoma—blood between the dura and the arachnoid caused by venous bleeding; commonly associated with additional cerebral injuries: contusion or intracerebral hematoma.
6. Diffuse axonal injury (DAI) or shear injury—axonal tears within the white matter of the brain. Frequently occurs within the corpus callosum or brainstem and at the junction of the frontal/temporal poles. Associated with prolonged coma and poor prognosis.

Mechanism of Injury and Effects

1. Mechanism of injury is related to acceleration and deceleration of the brain (soft gelatin matter) within the skull (hard external surface with sharply edged internal surface). May be caused by blunt or penetrating injury.
2. The initial insult is the primary injury, and the injury related to the sequela is the secondary injury. Cellular changes (release of oxygen-free radicals and neurotransmitters, calcium loss, and increase in lactate acid) and systemic instability (hypotension, anemia, hypoxia, hypercarbia, hypovolemia) potentiate secondary injury.
3. Neurologic deficits result from primary brain injury (contusion, hematoma, DAI, or shearing of white matter) or secondary injury (ischemia and mass effect from hemorrhage and cerebral edema of surrounding brain tissue).
4. Second impact syndrome (SIS) occurs in repetitive concussion when there is insufficient time for the brain to recover from the previous injury. SIS is common in sports-related injuries and is associated with cerebral injury and cerebral edema, which can be severe.
5. Coagulopathy may result from increased release of intracranial thromboplastin, causing elevation in partial thromboplastin time (PTT) and fibrinogen levels, which, in turn, results in clotting dysfunction, from mild bleeding to disseminated intravascular coagulation.
6. Paroxysmal sympathetic hyperactivity (PSH) or sympathetic storming may result from uncontrolled release of sympathetic hormones spontaneously or in response to some stressor. PSH results in tachycardia, tachypnea, hyperthermia, diaphoresis, agitation, and dystonia.
7. Diabetes insipidus (DI)—reduced secretion of antidiuretic hormone (ADH) with excessive fluid and electrolyte loss through the kidneys due to edema or compression of the pituitary/hypothalamic region; may cause severe dehydration.
8. Syndrome of inappropriate antidiuretic hormone (SIADH)—oversecretion of ADH with normal to increased intravascular volume (hypervolemic state) and dilutional hyponatremia (see Chapter 20).
9. Cerebral salt wasting (CSW)—increase in urinary secretion of sodium accompanied by volume depletion (hypovolemic state).

Classification

See page 334 for Glasgow Coma Scale (GCS).

1. Mild (GCS 13 to 15).
2. Moderate (GCS 9 to 12).
3. Severe (GCS 3 to 8).

Associated Injuries: Extracranial Trauma

1. Facial trauma and skull fractures—occur in 20% of major TBI. Temporal bone is the thinnest; frontal and occipital bones are thickest.
   a. Linear fracture—fracture through entire thickness of bone that runs in linear pattern.
   b. Basilar skull fracture.
      i. Occurs at the base of the skull and characterized by location.
      ii. Anterior fossa results in contusions around the eyes (raccoon eyes) and risk of rhinorrhea.
      iii. Posterior fossa results in contusions around the ears (Battle sign) and risk of otorrhea.
   c. Depressed fracture—displaced by more than half the width of the bone. There is a risk of dural tear, cerebrospinal fluid (CSF) leak, and intracranial injury; may be closed or open. Open fracture high risk of infection.
   d. Facial fractures—orbital (LeFort I to II), mandible, zygoma, maxillary, nasal fractures.
2. Vascular injuries—vertebral or carotid artery dissection.
3. Spine fracture with or without spinal cord injury (SCI).
4. Soft tissue injuries.

Clinical Manifestations

Clinical presentation will vary depending on the severity of injury, location, and any associated injuries.

1. Change in level of consciousness (LOC).
2. Pupillary abnormalities.
3. Changes in motor strength or sensation.
4. Changes in pattern of respiration.
5. Cardiac dysrhythmias.
6. Hemodynamic instability—often systolic hypertension.
7. Cognitive deficits (confusion, aphasia, reading difficulties, writing difficulties, acalculia [inability to perform simple arithmetic], concentration difficulties, and memory deficits such as retrograde and antegrade amnesia and difficulty learning new information).
8. Nausea, vomiting.
9. Headache, vertigo.
10. Agitation, restlessness.
11. Otorrhea may indicate leakage of CSF from ear (otorrhea) due to posterior fossa skull fracture; rhinorrhea may indicate leakage of CSF from nares (rhinorrhea) due to anterior fossa skull fracture.
12. Episodes of altered LOC, tachycardia, tachypnea, hyperthermia, agitation due to sympathetic storming (aggravated stress response).
13. Abnormal bleeding due to coagulopathy.

Diagnostic Evaluation

1. Computed tomography (CT) scan of the brain without contrast to identify intraparenchymal injury, subdural hematoma or EDH, basilar skull fractures.
2. Skull and cervical spine films to identify fracture, displacement. Lumbar and thoracic films may be required.

3. Computed tomographic angiogram (CTA) of the neck if concern for vertebral dissection.
4. CTA of the head if concern for intracranial vascular injury.
5. Magnetic resonance imaging (MRI) may be obtained later to help identify and diagnose DAI.
6. Laboratory studies: complete blood count (CBC), chemistry, prothrombin time/international normalized ratio (PT/INR), activated partial thromboplastin time aPTT), serum osmolarity, serum alcohol level, drug screen, urinalysis (U/A), pregnancy (if applicable).
7. Additional studies—chest x-ray, pelvic x-rays. Depending on presentation may require abdominal x-rays, abdominal/pelvic CT scan, and focused abdominal sonography in the trauma bay to evaluate for abdominal trauma.
8. Neuropsychological tests during rehabilitation phase to determine the extent of cognitive deficits.

Management

1. Airway—assess and maintain patent airway.
   a. Anticipate that patients with a GCS of 8 or less, facial fractures, or other injuries that will impact oxygenation will be intubated and ventilated.
2. Breathing.
   a. Oxygen with goal of PaO_2 greater than 100 mm Hg.
   b. Maintain $PaCO_2$ 35 to 45 mm Hg.
   c. Avoid use of hyperventilation.
   d. Early tracheostomy if anticipate intubation greater than 2 weeks.
3. Circulation—prevent hypotension. Absolutely critical.
   a. Maintain mean arterial pressure (MAP) 90 mm Hg.
   b. Maintain systolic blood pressure (SBP) 140 to 160 mm Hg.
   c. Normovolemia.
4. Management of increased intracranial pressure (ICP) and cerebral edema.
5. Management of paroxysmal sympathetic storming or PSH. Medications utilized include opiates, beta-adrenergic blockers, alpha-agonists, neuromodulators, and benzodiazepines. Response to medications varies. This has been associated with poorer functional outcomes.
6. Maintenance of normoglycemia.
7. Supportive care—rehabilitation services, skin care.
8. Nutritional support. Consult dietician for caloric needs and supplement recommendations. Recommended that patients be fed by at least day 5. Studies have shown patients who are not fed within 5 days of injury have a twofold increase in mortality, which increases to fourfold by day 7.
9. Antibiotics, as ordered, to prevent infection with open skull fractures or penetrating wounds.
10. Surgery to evacuate intracranial hematomas, debridement of penetrating wounds, elevation of skull fractures, or repair of CSF leaks.
11. Treatment of hypernatremia (due to DI, dehydration, diaphoresis) with fluid replacement, vasopressin therapy.
12. Treatment of hyponatremia.
    a. CSW and SIADH are the two etiologies for the development of hyponatremia.
    b. See Chapter 17, page 586 for discussion of hyponatremia and volume changes.
13. Seizure prophylaxis is not recommended to prevent posttraumatic seizures. Antiepileptic drugs (AEDs) will be given if the patients experience a seizure. Refer to Chapter 11, Table 11-8, for information of antiepileptic medications.

Complications

1. Infections: systemic (respiratory, urinary), neurologic (meningitis, ventriculitis).
2. Increased ICP, hydrocephalus, brain herniation.
3. Posttraumatic seizures and seizure disorder.
4. Permanent neurologic deficits: cognitive, motor, sensory, speech.
5. Neurobehavioral alterations: impulsivity, uninhibited aggression, emotional lability.
6. Persistent PSH.
7. Disseminated intravascular coagulation.
8. DI, SIADH, CSW.
9. Death.

Nursing Assessment

1. Monitor for signs of increased ICP—altered LOC, abnormal pupil responses, vomiting, increased pulse pressure, bradycardia, hyperthermia.
2. Monitor for signs of PSH—altered LOC, diaphoresis, tachycardia, tachypnea, hypertension, hyperthermia, agitation, and dystonia. PSH is generally seen in patients with severe TBI.
3. Monitor cardiac status for hypotension and arrhythmias (bradycardia, elevated T waves, premature ventricular contractions, premature atrial contractions, and sinus arrhythmias)—common and frequently asymptomatic. Tachycardia with hypotension is indicative of hypovolemia; patient should be evaluated for additional source of blood loss.
4. Be alert for DI—excessive urine output, dilute urine (specific gravity less than 1.005), hypernatremia.
5. Be alert for hyponatremia and assess etiology (SIADH or CSW); see page 338.
6. Monitor laboratory findings and report abnormal values:
   a. Abnormal PTT, PT, and fibrinogen levels indicating coagulopathy.
   b. Electrolyte imbalance—alterations in serum potassium (hypokalemia) and sodium (hypernatremia/hyponatremia) levels are common.
   c. Anemia—related to additional trauma or may be dilutional.
   d. Elevated white blood cell (WBC) count—indicating infection related to trauma or invasive procedures.
   e. Hypoxia or hypercarbia.
7. Perform CN, motor, sensory, and reflex assessment.
8. Assess for behavior that warrants potential for injury to self or others.

CLINICAL JUDGMENT Regard every patient who is unresponsive with a brain injury as having a potential SCI. Cervical collar and spine precautions should be maintained until spinal fracture has been ruled out. A significant number of patients are under the influence of alcohol at the time of injury, which may mask the nature and severity of the injury.

Nursing Interventions

Maintaining Adequate Cerebral Perfusion

1. Maintain a patent airway.
2. Monitor ICP, as ordered (see page 339).
3. Monitor cerebral oxygenation, temperature, or neurochemicals, as ordered. Provide oxygen therapy to maintain PaO_2 above 100 and carbon dioxide within normal range.
4. Monitor BP and maintain within ordered parameters. Alert provider if BP not within desired range.

5. Assess neurologic status—monitor LOC, CN function, and motor and sensory function; identify emerging trends in neurologic function; and communicate findings to provider.
6. If the patient has severe TBI, monitor for signs of PSH (abnormal stress response) and identify triggers and effective treatment modalities. Institute nursing measures that have been found to be helpful, such as maintaining normothermia, pretreating before known trigger, applying cool compress to forehead, and providing relaxing music.
7. Monitor response to pharmacologic therapy, including antiepileptic levels, as directed.
8. Monitor laboratory data, CSF cultures, and Gram stains, if applicable, and institute prompt antibiotic therapy, as directed.
9. Administer prescribed treatments for hypernatremia or hyponatremia (if applicable).
10. Assess dressings and drainage tubes after surgery for patency, security, and characteristics of drainage.
11. Institute measures to minimize increased ICP, ischemic changes, cerebral edema, seizures, or neurovascular compromise, such as careful positioning, to avoid flexing head, reducing hip flexion (can reduce venous drainage, causing congestion), and spreading out care evenly over 24-hour period.

CLINICAL JUDGMENT PSH places the patient at high risk for secondary brain injury, cardiac abnormalities, weight loss, skin breakdown, and infection. Be alert to triggers (suctioning, turning, hyperthermia, infection, auditory stimuli) and treat promptly to control symptoms.

CLINICAL JUDGMENT Severe states of hypernatremia and hyponatremia can cause further neurologic compromise (seizures, nausea, confusion, irritability/agitation, coma). Close monitoring of laboratory values is indicated to evaluate trends and maintain normal range. Hypernatremia and hyponatremia should not be reversed quickly because the rapid change can create rebound cerebral edema and be detrimental to the patient. Rapid increase in serum sodium level can cause central pontine myelinolysis and results in severe damage of myelin sheath of white matter in pons.

Maintaining Respiration

1. Auscultate breath sounds; note any change or development of adventitious sounds.
2. Monitor respiratory rate, depth, and pattern of respirations; report any abnormal patterns.
3. Administer or monitor impact of respiratory treatments.
4. Assist with intubation and ventilatory assistance, if needed.
5. Monitor arterial blood gas (ABG) results for PaO_2 and levels.
6. Ensure continuous pulse oximetry.
7. Maintain head of bed at 30 degrees.
8. Alternate patient position every 2 hours.
9. Suction the patient, as needed.

Meeting Nutritional Needs

1. Nutritional support should be initiated by day 5. Determination of caloric needs and formula selection and quantity will be evaluated by dietitian.
   a. Continuous enteric feedings.
      i. Elevate the head of the bed during feedings.
      ii. Check residuals to prevent aspiration. Follow institution's policy for enteral feeding.
      iii. Monitor for diarrhea.
      iv. Transgastric jejunal feedings reduce the risk of aspiration pneumonia.
   b. Consider IV hyperalimentation—for patients unable to tolerate or initiate enteral feedings.
2. Oral feeding—bedside swallow screen before any oral food/fluids begun. Consult speech therapist for bedside or radiographic swallow study if patient fails swallow screen or appears at risk for dysphagia. Assessment of swallowing function decreases risk of aspiration. Speech therapy is essential for retraining and developing adaptive techniques. Caloric needs of a patient with a head injury increase by 100% to 200%. Consult your dietitian to institute nutritional support within the first 5 days after injury to support the recovery process. Weight loss is generally in the form of muscle loss and can be as much as 25 to 30 pounds (11.3 to 13.6 kg).
3. Administer H_2-blocking agents to prevent gastric ulceration and hemorrhage from gastric acid hypersecretion.
4. Normoglycemia—monitor glucose levels utilizing fingerstick samples and glucose monitor. Insulin (IV drip/sliding scale) may be required to regulate serum glucose levels within a normal range to avoid hypoglycemia and hyperglycemia, which worsens the effects of secondary brain injury.

Promoting Cognitive Function

1. Assess the patient's LOC and compare to baseline.
2. Be aware of the patient's cognitive alteration and adjust interaction and environment accordingly.
3. Provide meaningful stimulation using all senses—visual, olfactory, gustatory, acoustic, and tactile.
4. Observe the patient for fatigue or restlessness from overstimulation.
5. Involve the family in sensory stimulation program to maximize its effectiveness.
6. Decrease environmental stimuli when the patient is in agitated state.
7. Reorient to surroundings using repetition, verbal and visual cues, and memory aids; routinely orient the patient after awakening.
8. Use pictures of family members, clock, and calendar as outlined by occupational and speech therapist.
9. Encourage the family to provide items from home to increase sense of identity and security.
10. Anticipate the need for additional help with toileting, eating, and performing activities of daily living (ADLs) due to cognitive impairment.
11. Break down ADLs into simple steps that patient can progressively take part in.
12. Structure the environment and care activities to minimize distraction and provide consistency.
13. Identify and maintain usual patterns of behavior—sleep, medication use, elimination, food intake, and self-care routine.
14. Refer the patient for cognitive retraining, if appropriate.

Preventing Injury

1. Instruct the family regarding the behavioral phases of recovery from brain injury, such as restlessness and combativeness.
2. Investigate for physical sources of restlessness, such as uncomfortable position, signs of urinary tract infection (UTI), or pressure injury development.
3. Reassure the patient and family during periods of agitation and irrational behavior.
4. Pad side rails and wrap hands in mitts if patient is agitated. Maintain constant vigilance and avoid restraints, if possible.

5. Keep environmental stimuli to a minimum to avoid confusion and agitation. Veil beds can be useful in reducing injury in the agitated patient.
6. Provide adequate light if the patient is hallucinating.
7. Avoid sedatives to avoid medication-induced confusion and altered states of cognition.

Strengthening Family Coping

1. Refer the family to community support services, such as respite care, faith-based groups, city and state social services, and resources on the internet. Suggest the Brain Injury Association of America (www.biausa.org) for further information.
2. Assist the family members to establish stress management techniques that can be integrated into their lifestyle, such as ventilation of feelings, use of respite care, relaxation techniques.
3. Consult with social worker or psychologist to assist the family in adjusting to patient's permanent neurologic deficits.
4. Help the family assist the patient to recognize current progress and not focus on limitations.

Community and Home Care Considerations

1. Observe for signs of postconcussion syndrome (PCS), which include headache, decreased concentration, irritability, dizziness, insomnia, restlessness, diminished memory, anxiety, easy fatigability, and alcohol intolerance.
2. Be aware that persistence of these symptoms can interfere with relationships and employability of the patient.
3. Encourage the patient and family to report these symptoms and obtain additional support and counseling, as needed. PCS may persist as long as 2 years.
4. Act as liaison to coordinate all home care services the patient will need while keeping in touch with the patient's primary care provider, neurologist, and neurosurgeon.
5. Provide the necessary education to caregivers in tube feedings, positioning, range of motion (ROM) exercises, and medications.
6. Make sure that coaches and caregivers from community recreation programs and schools are familiar with and follow guidelines for sports-related concussion. Many states have specific recommendations.
   a. The American Academy of Pediatrics (AAP) and the Centers for Disease Control and Prevention (CDC) have published guidelines for the individuals returning to play sports. There is a six-step return to play progression. Each step increases the individual's exertion level.
      i. Symptoms and cognitive function are monitored at each level.
      ii. Progression to the next level only occurs when the individual is experiencing symptoms at current level.
      iii. If symptoms return at any step, activities are stopped. After a minimum of 24 hours without symptoms, the individual may start again at the step where symptoms were experienced.
   b. HEADS UP is a free online training for health care professions developed by the CDC and AAP. It provides an overview of the evidence-based recommendations in the CDC guideline.

Patient Education and Health Maintenance

1. Review the signs of increased ICP with the family.
2. Reinforce the lability of cognitive, language, and physical functioning of the person with brain injury and the lengthy recovery period.
3. Teach the family techniques to calm the agitated patient.
   a. Therapeutic use of touch, massage, and music.
   b. Elimination of distractions (television, radio, alarms, crowds).
   c. Provide one-on-one communication.

Evaluation: Expected Outcomes

- No signs of increased ICP.
- Stable vital signs.
- Nutrition meeting caloric needs.
- Improving neurologic status.
- Less agitated; side rails maintained.

Spinal Cord Injury

EVIDENCE BASE Thomas, A. X., Riviello, J. J., Jr., Davila-Williams, D., Thomas, S. P., Erklauer, J. C., Bauer, D. F., & Cokley, J. A. (2022). Pharmacologic and acute management of spinal cord injury in adults and children. *Current Treatment Options in Neurology, 24*(7), 285–304. https://doi.org/10.1007/s11940-022-00720-9

Krysa, J. A., Gregorio, M. P., Pohar Manhas, K., MacIsaac, R., Papathanassoglou, E., & Ho, C. H. (2022). Empowerment, communication, and navigating care: The experience of persons with spinal cord injury from acute hospitalization to inpatient rehabilitation. *Frontiers in Rehabilitation Sciences, 3,* 904716. https://doi.org/10.3389/fresc.2022.904716

SCI is a traumatic injury to the spinal cord that may vary from a mild cord concussion with transient numbness to immediate and complete tetraplegia. The most common sites are the cervical areas C5, C6, and C7, and the junction of the thoracic and lumbar vertebrae, T12 and L1. Injury to the spinal cord may result in loss of function below the level of cord injury (see Figure 11-10). SCI requires comprehensive and specialized care. The Model Spinal Cord Injury System is a network of comprehensive, federally funded, regional SCI centers in the United States. The Department of Veterans Affairs operates 23 SCI centers. (Also see Chapter 31 for emergency management of SCI.)

Pathophysiology and Etiology

1. The estimated annual incidence of SCI is about 17,500. The average age has increased and is now 42, with an increase in fall-related injuries in older adults. The most common cause of SCI is motor vehicle crashes, followed by falls, violence, and sports-related injuries.

   The level most often injured is C2 (32%), resulting in quadriplegia.
2. The life expectancy for an individual with SCI is lower than that of a person without SCI. The leading causes of death are pneumonia, emboli, and septicemia.
3. SCI may result from trauma, vascular disorders, infectious conditions, tumor, and other insults.
4. SCI can affect upper motor neurons (UMNs) or lower motor neurons (LMNs). UMNs extend from the motor strip in the cerebral cortex of the brain through the corticospinal tract in the spinal cord, where they synapse with interneurons in the ventral horn. LMNs originate in the ventral horn, exit the spinal cord at each segment, and extend to the neuromuscular junction. Each LMN innervates 10 to 2,000 muscle fibers.

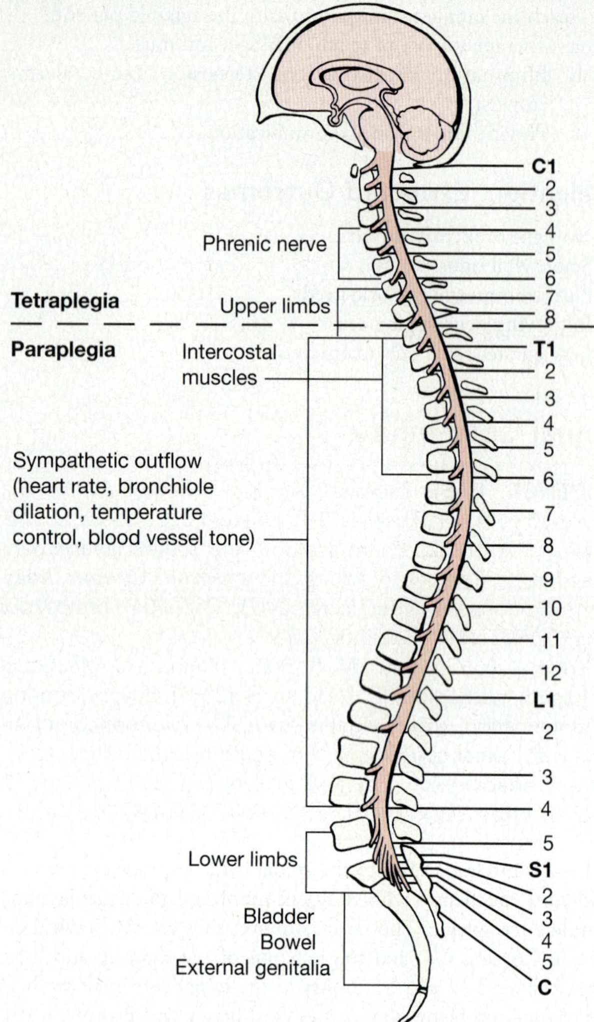

Figure 11-10. Levels of spinal cord innervation.

a. Spasticity results from injury above T12 or a UMN lesion (intact reflex arch below level of injury [LOI]).
b. Flaccidity/reflex loss results from injury at L1 or an LMN injury.

POPULATION AWARENESS Older patients are at greater risk for altered glucose metabolism, loss of bone minerals leading to fractures, musculoskeletal pain and weakness, and greater loss of function with SCI.

Clinical Manifestations

1. Patients with tetraplegia have damage to the cervical segments of nerves (C1–C8) in the spinal canal. Function may be impaired in the upper extremities, trunk, pelvic organs, and lower extremities.
2. Patients with paraplegia have damage to the thoracic, lumbar, or sacral segments of nerves in the spinal cord. The arms are unaffected, but function may be impaired in the trunk, pelvic organs, and lower extremities.
3. The International Standards for Neurological Classification of Spinal Cord Injury (ISNCSCI), promoted by the American Spinal Injury Association (ASIA), are used (available: http://asia-spinalinjury.org). The ASIA Impairment Scale (AIS) is based on completeness of injury and motor/sensory function.
   a. ASIA A = complete. No sensory and motor function in the sacral segments S4–S5.
   b. ASIA B = incomplete; intact sensory but absent motor function below the neurologic LOI and includes levels S4–S5.
   c. ASIA C = motor incomplete. Motor function is preserved below the LOI, and more than half of key muscle functions distal to LOI have muscle grade less than 3.
   d. ASIA D = motor incomplete. Motor function is preserved below the LOI, and at least half of key muscles distal to LOI have muscle grade greater than or equal to 3.
   e. ASIA E = normal if the individual was graded with the ISNCSCI and graded as normal in all segments, AND THE PATIENT HAD PRIOR DEFICITS, graded as ASIA E. A patient without an initial SCI does not receive an ASIA grade.
4. Sacral sensation is intact if there is deep sensation and sensation at the anal mucocutaneous junction; sacral motor is intact if the patient has voluntary contraction of the external anal sphincter with digital stimulation.
5. The zone of partial preservation (ZPP) indicates areas of partial sensory/motor innervation below the LOI; the ZPP is applicable only to complete injuries.
6. The neurologic LOI is the lowest neural level with normal sensory and motor function on both sides of the body. When describing the LOI, the neurologic level is noted unless stated specifically that the skeletal LOI, which is the level of greatest vertebral damage, is being discussed.
7. Various syndromes (incomplete injuries) may characterize the clinical presentation (see Table 11-7).
8. Sensation function (e.g., sensitivity of pinprick/light touch) is tested on each of the 28 dermatomes on both sides of the body. The following grading is suggested: 0 = absent; 1 = impaired; 2 = normal. The external anal sphincter should also be tested (sensory incomplete if sensate).
9. Motor function is tested on each of the 10 paired myotomes on both sides of the body. The following grading is suggested: 0 = total paralysis; 1 = contraction visible or palpable; 2 = active movements and full ROM without gravity; 3 = active movement and full ROM against gravity; 4 = active movement and full ROM with moderate resistance; 5 = normal motor with active movement and full ROM against full resistance. The external anal sphincter tone should also be tested (motor incomplete if contraction).
10. Most recovery occurs within 6 months of injury; patients with incomplete injuries have greater recovery than patients with complete injuries.
11. Instability exists when ligamentous structures and vertebra cannot protect the vulnerable spinal cord and movement can further damage the injured spinal cord; stability exists when ligamentous structures and vertebra can protect the spinal cord from further neurologic injury.
12. Vertebral fractures may be simple, compressed or wedge, dislocated (vertebra overrides another vertebra), subluxed (vertebra partially dislocated over another vertebrae), comminuted (vertebrae shattered), or teardrop (vertebrae chipped). Jefferson fractures, which may occur with head injuries, involve the C1 level.

Diagnostic Evaluation

1. CT of the spine—to detect bony fracture.
2. MRI of the spine—to detect soft tissue injury, hemorrhage, edema, bony injury; syringomyelia (cystic degeneration in

Table 11-7 Incomplete Spinal Cord Clinical Syndromes

SYNDROME	AFFECTED SITE	DEFICIT	PRESERVATION
Central cord	Central cervical spinal cord	More motor deficit in upper extremities than lower extremities caused by medial damage of corticospinal tract	Sacral sensory; lower extremities have better motor function than upper extremities because of lateral sparing of corticospinal tract
Brown-Sequard	Hemisection of spinal cord	Ipsilateral motor function and fine touch, vibration, and proprioception (posterior tract); contralateral sensory function pain and temperature (spinothalamic tract)	Ipsilateral sensory function of pain and temperature (spinothalamic tract); contralateral motor function, fine touch, vibration, and proprioception (posterior tract)
Anterior cord	Main anterior spinal artery of anterior spinal cord affecting anterior two-thirds of spinal cord	Variable motor deficit; variable sensory deficit of pain and temperature (spinothalamic tract)	Posterior one-third of spinal cord (posterior spinal artery); sensory function of proprioception, light touch, vibration (posterior tract)
Conus medullaris	Conus and lumbar nerve roots in spinal cord	Variable motor deficit; bowel, bladder, and lower extremity reflexes (flaccid)	Lesions of proximal conus may be reflexic (e.g., butocavernosa, micturition).
	Lumbosacral nerve roots in spinal cord (distal from conus medullaris)	Variable motor deficit; bowel, bladder, and lower extremity reflexes (flaccid)	Lesions proximal to level of injury may be reflexic (e.g., bulbocavernosus, micturition).

spinal cord) may present as cord compression, syrinx (cavity) at the fracture site, and kyphosis at fracture site. Performed prior to application of cervical traction (if indicated) and surgical intervention.

3. Electrophysiologic monitoring to determine function of neural pathways.
4. Urodynamic studies may include urine flow to detect bladder outlet obstruction and/or impaired bladder contractility; cystometrogram to determine bladder sensation, compliance, and capacity; and sphincter EMG and other studies. The gold standard in urodynamics is to measure bladder and urethral pressure under fluoroscopy monitoring.
5. If deep vein thrombosis (DVT) or pulmonary emboli (PE) are suspected, an ultrasound of the lower extremity to check for thrombosis can be performed, and a spiral CT or ventilation/perfusion scan can be performed to check for PE.
6. Heterotopic ossification may be diagnosed in the inflammatory stages using ultrasound. Alkaline phosphatase and erythrocyte sedimentation rate (ESR) are typically elevated.
7. Nutritional status should be assessed using nutritional history, anthropometric measurements, prealbumin (half-life 12 to 36 hours), and transferrin (half-life 6 to 10 days).
8. Total lymphocyte count and creatinine height index are also used to establish nutritional risk.

Management

Requires a multidisciplinary approach because of multiple system involvement and the psychosocial aspects of catastrophic injuries.

Immediately After Trauma (Less Than 1 Hour)

1. Immobilization with hard cervical collar (HCC), sandbags, and rigid spine board to transport from the field to acute care facility. Monitor for respiratory failure, hypotension, and/or bradycardia and treat appropriately.

CLINICAL JUDGMENT C1 to C4 innervate the diaphragm. Injury at these levels results in respiratory compromise, necessitating intubation and ventilation. Edema of the spinal cord occurs with injury and can quickly ascend the spinal cord. Patients must be monitored closely for respiratory compromise.

Acute Phase

1. Maintenance of pulmonary and cardiovascular stability.
   a. Intubation and mechanical ventilation, if needed.
   b. Vasopressors to maintain adequate perfusion to sustain MAP greater than 85 mm Hg.
   c. Medical stabilization before spinal stabilization and decompression.
2. Spinal cord immobilization.
   a. Cervical collars:
      i. Used in initial stabilization.
      ii. May be utilized following surgical stabilization and to immobilize ligaments when a ligamentous injury has also occurred.
   b. Cervical traction:
      i. With early surgery, the use of traction has decreased. It may be used in situations where surgery is delayed or in certain types of fractures.
         a. Types of tongs include:
            1. Gardner Wells tongs—applied at the bedside.
            2. Crutchfield and Vinke tongs require predrilled holes in the skull under local anesthesia.
      ii. Weight is added to traction gradually to reduce the vertebral fracture; weight maintained at a level to ensure vertebral alignment. Lateral spine films are taken after the addition of weight to assess spinal alignment. Motor and sensory assessment is performed before and after weight application.
3. Rigid kinetic turning bed can be used to immobilize patients with thoracic and lumbar injuries.

4. Surgical interventions are considered when the patient has vertebral instability that may result in further neurologic damage; an injury that is incomplete at onset may become complete if instability exists. The objectives are to remove all of the bony and soft tissues that are compressing the spinal cord, thereby minimizing the possibility of deteriorating neurologic status, and stabilize the vertebra surrounding the spinal cord so that rehabilitation may begin as soon as possible. Goals of treatment of the spinal fractures are aimed at protecting the neural elements and preventing deformity and instability.
   a. Surgical timing: Current practice is early surgical intervention (less than 24 hours), though there is no class I evidence that clearly defines the timing of surgery. STASCIS (Surgical Treatment of Acute Spinal Cord Injury Study), a prospective, nonrandomized clinical trial, revealed that early surgical decompression (within 24 hours) is safe, with 19.8% demonstrating neurologic improvement (greater than 2 grade improvement AIS) compared with 8.8% in the late decompressive group (2012).
   b. Procedures:
      i. An unstable injury or one that has the possibility to become unstable in the cervical region will require surgery. The surgeon takes into consideration the type of fracture, location, body habitus, and comorbidities when determining the type of surgery (fusion, screws, levels involved) and approach (anterior, posterior).
      ii. Thoracic thoracolumbar/lumbar procedures are performed when the spinal canal has been compromised and a neurologic deficit exists. If there is ligamentous injury without deficit, surgery is also required. A three-column injury usually requires surgery. Stabilization, typically done using the posterior approach, involves the use of wires, bone grafts, plates, screws, and other fixation devices to prevent movement at the damaged bony site.
5. Methylprednisolone sodium (Solu-Medrol) is not recommended (class I evidence) in SCI related to high rate of significant complications
   a. Higher rate of hyperglycemia, gastrointestinal (GI) hemorrhage, wound infections, and higher mortality in concomitant TBI (class I evidence).
   b. Higher rate of pneumonia, steroid-induced myelopathy (class II evidence).
6. Management of neurogenic bladder—indwelling urinary catheter initially, then a straight catheterization schedule.
7. Pressure injury prevention—assessment of skin integrity, provide skin care and turn patient every 2 hours. May use special bed. Pressure relief cushions when out of bed and weight shifts every 2 hours.
8. Prevention of DVT and its sequelae is an important aspect of the treatment of patients who have sustained SCI because of the high risk of thromboembolic complications.
   a. Class I, II, and III evidence supports the utilization of external device in conjunction with low-molecular-weight heparin (LMWH)/adjusted-dose heparin within 1 to 2 days postinjury.
9. Autonomic dysreflexia—can occur in patients with an injury at T6 or above. A syndrome where there is excessive sympathetic stimulation caused by spinal reflexes, which are still intact. Precipitated by a noxious stimulus (most often, it is seen when there is a full bladder but can also be from many other stimuli, e.g., impaction/constipation). This is a medical emergency. Treatment is identification of the cause. If unable to resolve, may require antihypertensive agent.

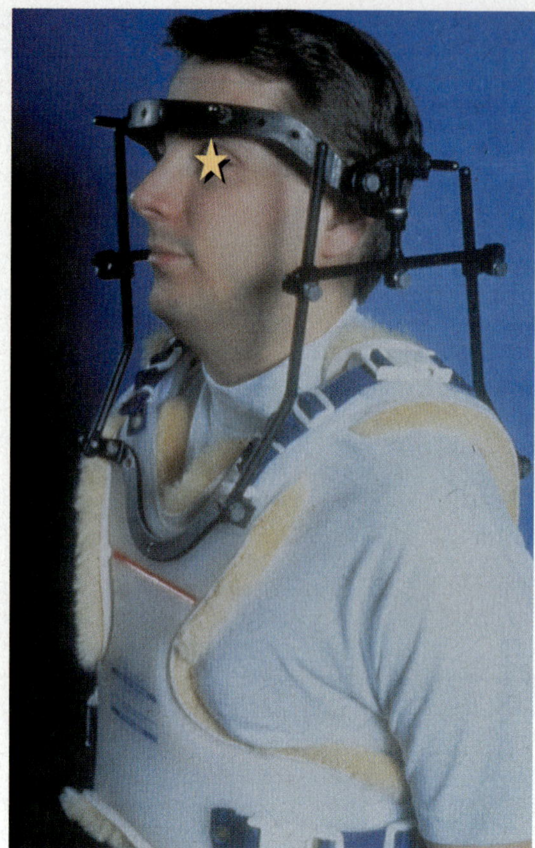

Figure 11-11. Halo brace. (Reprinted with permission from Hinkle, J. L., Cheever, K. H., & Overbaugh, K. [2022]. *Brunner & Suddarth's textbook of medical-surgical nursing* [15th ed., Fig. 63-6.]. Wolters Kluwer; Adapted from Schwartz, E. D., Adam, E., & Flander, S. [2007]. *Spinal trauma: Imaging, diagnosis, and management.* Lippincott Williams & Wilkins.)

Subacute Phase

1. Stiff orthosis is utilized for external stabilization of cervical fractures. Devices include the halo brace (see Figure 11-11) and HCCs. Device is selected based on the type of fracture and extent of instability. Average length of time in a halo brace is 12 weeks; x-rays are used to evaluate bony healing. Once vest is removed, patient will be transitioned to a cervical collar (CCC) for a period of time followed by a Philadelphia collar for 4 weeks.
   a. Halo vest.
      i. The materials used in the halo ring and vest are now made with MRI-compatible materials. However, the nurse must always confirm this prior to having the patient go to MRI.
      ii. The ring is attached to stainless steel pins (two anterior pins, two posterior pins) and attached to a vest by four connecting rods.
      iii. Torque wrenches connect the rods to the ring and vest; pressures are typically 8 in/pound for pins (2 to 5 in/pound in children), and locking bolts are 28 in/pound. Torque wrenches are kept with the patient at all times, often taped directly onto the vest, in case of an emergency.

   iv. Pins and locking bolts must be retightened (by provider) approximately 24 to 48 hours after placement and periodically thereafter.
   v. Pin sites should be cleaned once or twice daily as prescribed.
2. Thoracic and lumbar orthotic devices—these may be used to maintain alignment or as part of the postoperative management, or as the nonoperative management for the injury.
   a. The clamshell brace used for thoracolumbar fractures is an example of a brace in this category.
3. H_2-receptor blockers to prevent gastric irritation and hemorrhage.
4. Early mobilization and passive exercise as soon as the patient is surgically and medically stable. Referrals to physical and occupational therapy.
5. Providing adequate nutrition for caloric needs is essential. Referral to dietitian for recommendations. Depending on condition, may require enteral feedings.
6. Interventions to help prevent thromboembolism include compression hose, compression boots, ROM, adjusted-dose heparin, or LMWH.
   a. Prior to applying mechanical compression, tests to exclude the presence of lower extremity DVT should be performed if thromboprophylaxis has been delayed for more than 72 hours after injury.
   b. Vena cava filters are not recommended, though may be utilized in patients who have not achieved success with anticoagulant prophylaxis or who have a contraindication to anticoagulation. They are not a substitute for thromboprophylaxis due to morbidity related to DVT (e.g., postphlebitic syndrome) and propagation of vena cava embolism.
   c. Recommend a minimum of 8 weeks from time of injury for those with limited mobility.

Chronic Phase

This phase begins with the transition from the acute care setting into a subacute or rehabilitation setting.

1. DVT prophylaxis is recommended a minimum of 8 weeks from time of injury for those with limited mobility.
2. Spasticity—may develop 1 to 3 days postinjury or up to several weeks later. It negatively impacts the patient's ability to carry out ADLs and rehabilitation.
   a. Identify patient triggers that precipitate spasticity and work to avoid as much as possible (known potential triggers include UTI, constipation, pressure injury, ingrown toenail).
   b. Provide passive ROM at least four times daily. Teach family or significant others how to perform ROM for the patient.
   c. Turn and reposition every 2 hours.
   d. Prevent contractures.
   e. Treatment begins with conservative therapies and then progress to pharmacologic therapy, muscle relaxants (baclofen—orally or via intrathecal pump), botulism toxin injections.
3. Autonomic dysreflexia.
4. Neurogenic bowel and bladder.
5. Sexual dysfunction.
6. Rehabilitation includes medical and psychosocial support, physical therapy, urologic evaluation, occupational therapy, and multiple other interventions to facilitate an increased level of function and community participation.

Complications

1. Spinal shock lasting a few hours to a few weeks noted by loss of all reflex, motor, sensory, and autonomic activity below the level of the lesion.
2. Respiratory arrest, pneumonia, atelectasis requiring mechanical ventilation with cervical injury.
3. Cardiac arrest may result from initial trauma, worsening of initial injury from edema, concomitant injuries, and other illnesses.
4. Thromboembolic complications.
5. Infections—respiratory, urinary, pressure injuries, sepsis.
6. Autonomic dysreflexia—exaggerated autonomic response to stimuli below the level of the lesion in patients with lesions at or above T6 is a medical emergency and can result in dangerous elevation of BP.
7. Autonomic dysfunction resulting in orthostatic hypotension, thermodysregulation, and vasomotor abnormalities.
8. Urologic—bladder storage pressure greater than 35 to 40 cm due to neurogenic bladder may result in renal injury.
9. Paralytic ileus—common in subacute and acute stages.
10. Heterotopic ossification—bony overgrowth that occurs below the LOI any time after SCI.
11. Syringomyelia—cystic formation in the spinal cord may occur any time after SCI.
12. Depression.
13. Pressure injuries.
14. Neuropathic pain occurs in 34% to 94% of patients with SCI.
15. Complications can arise from the halo apparatus in persons with cervical injuries.
   a. Pin/ring loosening—can result from bone reabsorption. Signs and symptoms include increased pain, altered pin position, and drainage.
   b. Infection—can result from bacterial infections. Signs and symptoms include drainage and erythema.
   c. Skull/dural penetration—can result from inner table penetration, usually due to a fall. Signs and symptoms include a headache, visual disturbances, and CSF leak from the pin site.
   d. Dysphagia and respiratory problems—can result from halo or vest positioning. Signs and symptoms include difficulty swallowing and respiratory distress.

Nursing Assessment

1. Assess cardiopulmonary status and vital signs to help determine the degree of autonomic dysfunction, especially in patients with tetraplegia.
2. Determine LOC and cognitive function indicating TBI or other pathology.
3. Perform frequent motor and sensory assessment of trunk and extremities—extent of deficits may increase because of edema and hemorrhage. Later, increasing neurologic deficits and pain may indicate development of syringomyelia.
4. Note signs and symptoms of spinal shock, such as flaccid paralysis, urine retention, absent reflexes.
5. Assess bowel and bladder function.
6. Assess quality, location, and severity of pain.
7. Perform psychosocial assessment to evaluate motivation, support network, financial, or other problems.
8. Assess for indicators of powerlessness, including verbal expression of no control over situation, depression, nonparticipation, dependence on others, passivity.

Nursing Interventions

Attaining an Adequate Breathing Pattern

1. For patients with high-level lesions, continuously monitor respirations and maintain a patent airway. Be prepared to intubate if respiratory fatigue or arrest occurs.
2. Frequently assess cough and vital capacity. Teach effective coughing, if patient is able (see Box 11-5).
3. Provide adequate fluids and humidification of inspired air to loosen secretions.
4. Suction, as needed; observe vagal response (bradycardia—should be temporary).
5. When appropriate, implement chest physiotherapy regimen to assist pulmonary drainage and prevent infection.
6. Monitor results of ABG values, chest x-ray, and sputum cultures.
7. Tape halo wrench to body jacket or halo traction in the event the jacket must be removed for basic or advanced life support or respiratory distress.

Promoting Mobility

1. Place the patient on firm surface until spinal cord stabilization. After stabilization, turn every 2 hours on a pressure reduction surface, ensuring good alignment. Specialized beds, such as a kinetic turning bed, may be used.
2. Logroll the patient with unstable SCI.
3. Perform ROM exercises to prevent contractures and maintain rehabilitation potential.
4. Monitor BP with position change in the patient with lesions above midthoracic area to prevent orthostatic hypotension.
5. Encourage physical therapy and practicing of exercises as tolerated. Functional electrical stimulation may facilitate independent standing and walking.
6. Encourage weight-bearing activity to prevent osteoporosis and risk of kidney stones.

CLINICAL JUDGMENT Never attempt to reposition the patient by grasping a halo or any other stabilization device. This may result in severe damage to the brain, head, or vertebra.

BOX 11-5 Assisted Coughing

Many patients with tetraplegia have an impairment of the diaphragmatic and intercostal muscles. The result is a weak or ineffective cough. To increase the mechanical effectiveness of the patient's cough, perform or teach the assisted cough technique.

1. Place the patient in supine, low semi-Fowler position.
2. Place the heels of your hands on the costophrenic angle of the patient's rib cage.
3. With the patient's head turned away, ask the patient to hyperventilate and exhale once or twice. Allow your hands to move with the patient.
4. During the next breath, ask the patient to take a deep breath and cough while exhaling.
5. As the patient coughs, thrust your hands down and in (inferiorly and medially) to add power to the diaphragm during exhalation.
6. Allow one or two normal breaths and repeat the procedure.

CLINICAL JUDGMENT Incorrect hand placement may cause injury to the internal organs, ribs, and xiphoid process.

Protecting Skin Integrity

1. Pay special attention to pressure points when repositioning patient. Seating and mobility requirements must be determined.
2. Obtain pressure relief mattress and appropriate wheelchair and cushion.
3. Inspect for pressure injury development daily over bony prominences, including the back of the head, ears, trunk, heels, and elbows. Observe under stabilization devices for pressure areas, particularly on the scapulae. Use a risk assessment tool to determine the risk of developing pressure injury.
4. Keep the skin clean, dry, and well lubricated.
5. Turn the patient a minimum of every 2 hours and instruct patient to perform wheelchair weight shifts every 15 minutes. Place the patient in prone position at intervals, unless contraindicated.
6. Institute treatment for pressure injuries immediately and relieve pressure to promote healing.

Promoting Urinary Elimination

1. Remove indwelling catheter when medically appropriate. Intermittent catheterization, typically beginning every 4 hours, utilizes bladder scanner in monitoring frequency needs.
2. Encourage fluid intake with goal of 3,000 mL of fluid per day to prevent infection and urinary calculi.

Promoting Bowel Elimination

1. Assess bowel sounds and note abdominal distention. Paralytic ileus is common immediately after injury.
2. Encourage intake of high-calorie, high-protein, and high-fiber (15 g) diet when food is tolerated.
3. Assess for loose stool oozing from rectum and perform rectal examination to check for fecal impaction; remove fecal matter, if necessary.
4. Institute a bowel program as early as possible. Bowel plans are individualized for each patient.
   a. Schedule bowel care at the same time of day to develop a predictable outcome.
   b. Stimulate the gastrocolic reflex 30 minutes before bowel care with food or liquid intake.
   c. Perform bowel care with the patient in a bowel chair or in left side-lying position; the procedure should not take more than 2 hours.
5. Medications utilized include stool softeners, bowel stimulants. A glycerin suppository is utilized to stimulate the defecation reflex and promote bowel emptying. Alternatively, digital stimulation with gloved, lubricated finger can be used.

Preventing Autonomic Dysfunction and Orthostatic Hypotension

1. Be alert to signs of autonomic dysreflexia (see Box 11-6), try to avoid triggers, assess for causes, and treat, as directed.
2. Be alert for, prevent, and manage orthostatic hypotension, especially in patients with cervical SCI.
3. Other conservative strategies consist of use of embolic hose, abdominal binder, and high-salt diet.
4. Administer a sympathomimetic, such as ephedrine or pseudoephedrine, as ordered, before the patient is transferred to wheelchair.

DRUG ALERT Caution should be exercised for patients with SCI who are taking tricyclic antidepressants because of autonomic dysfunction. Patients with SCI are more vulnerable to anticholinergic adverse effects and orthostatic hypotension. In addition, numerous potential drug reactions are associated with monoamine oxidase inhibitors and SCI.

BOX 11-6 Autonomic Dysreflexia

Be aware of and try to prevent common causes of autonomic dysreflexia whenever possible:

- Bladder distention, urinary tract infection (UTI), bladder or kidney stones.
- Urinary abnormalities or procedures.
- Bowel distention, bowel impaction.
- Constrictive clothing, shoes, or apparatus.
- Noxious stimuli such as pain, strong smells, pressure.

Be alert for signs and symptoms of autonomic dysreflexia:

- Sudden and significant increase in systolic blood pressure (SBP) and diastolic BP 20 to 40 mm Hg above the patient's baseline. (Normal SBP for a person with tetraplegia is 90 to 110 mm Hg.) In children and adolescents, a systolic increase of greater than 15 to 20 mm Hg above baseline is significant.
- Pounding headache.
- Bradycardia and/or cardiac arrhythmias.
- Profuse sweating, piloerection, and flushing above the level of injury (LOI).
- Blurred vision and spots in visual field.
- Nasal congestion.
- Apprehension and anxiety.

Take the following actions if autonomic dysreflexia occurs:

- Check BP; if elevated, call health care provider immediately.
- Immediately sit the patient up.
- Loosen clothing and other constrictive apparatus.
- Monitor BP every 2 to 5 minutes.
- Check the urinary system—catheterize patient (use 2% lidocaine jelly and wait 2 minutes); if catheter in place, check for kinks in tubing obstructing drainage; if catheter blockage suspected, gently irrigate with 10–15 mL normal saline (use 5 to 10 mL in children younger than age 2); replace catheter if not draining adequately.
- If BP remains greater than 150 mm Hg systolic, check for impaction (use 2% lidocaine jelly and wait 2 minutes). Remove stool.
- If BP remains greater than 150 mm Hg systolic, administer immediate-release nifedipine 10 mg (bite and swallow), nitroglycerin ointment 2% 1 in (2.5 cm) above the LOI, or another antihypertensive agent.
- If autonomic dysreflexia is still unresolved, check for additional causes (e.g., pressure injury, ingrown toenail).

After the episode of autonomic dysreflexia, document the following:

- Monitor BP for at least 2 hours for recurrent hypertension or symptomatic hypotension. Notify the health care provider as indicated.
- Provide patient teaching for prevention and treatment of complication.
- Make sure all caregivers understand autonomic dysreflexia and that the patient carries an identification card indicating LOI and emergency information.

Empowering the Patient

1. Explain all procedures to the patient. Answer questions.
2. Make sure that the patient plays an integral part in decision-making about care plan. Allow the patient to make modifications to treatment plan when possible.
3. Schedule procedures and planning sessions when the patient is rested and experiencing decreased anxiety.
4. Recognize incremental gains in function or participation.
5. Discuss stress management techniques, such as relaxation therapy, counseling, and problem-solving.
6. Refer to vocational training program if the patient expresses an interest.
7. Use peer counseling for patient to gain support from others with SCI.
8. Be alert for signs of depression (problems with sleep, loss of interest, guilt, loss of energy, lack of concentration, change in appetite, feeling sad) or risk for suicide and refer to mental health counselor. Administer antidepressant medications, as directed.
9. Explore the use of hands-free environmental control units to control environment (e.g., turn on television).

Minimizing Alteration in Sexuality and Fertility

1. Encourage the patient to discuss alternate expression of feelings with partner.
2. Advise bowel care and urinary elimination before intercourse.
3. Advise females that 90% regain regular menstrual cycles by 1 year. Pregnancy can occur, and delivery occurs in 40% before 37 weeks of gestation. Autonomic dysreflexia may occur as a complication of delivery.
4. Refer the patient to a urologist or other health care provider to explore sexuality options.
   a. Females with SCI experience little sensation during sexual intercourse, but fertility and ability to bear children are usually not affected.
   b. Males with SCI may consider implantation of a penile prosthesis or an assistive device to obtain an erection. Sildenafil has been used to manage erectile dysfunction in males with SCI. Ejaculation is more common with lower motor neuron or incomplete injuries; males with injuries at T10 and above may ejaculate with vibrostimulation.

Reducing Pain

1. Assess pain using consistent pain scale. Report changes from baseline or new location or type of pain.
2. Manage neurogenic pain with pharmacologic agents, as directed.
3. Help the patient assess the effects of nonpharmacologic treatment, such as acupuncture.

Community and Home Care Considerations

Promoting Optimal Function

1. Determine short- and long-term functional goals. Expected outcomes should relate to motor recovery, level of functional independence, social integration, and quality of life.
2. Monitor neurologic status, including functional outcomes, periodically throughout the patient's lifespan. Functional outcomes may relate to:
   a. Respiratory, bowel, bladder, and skin.
   b. Bed/wheelchair mobility, transfers, positioning.
   c. Standing and ambulation.
   d. Independent ADLs, such as eating, grooming, bathing, and dressing.

e. Communication, including speech, computer skills, handwriting, telephone.
f. Transportation, including driving, adapted vehicle use, public transportation.
g. Homemaking, including meal planning and preparation and chores.
3. Periodically evaluate the need for an increased level of assistance and equipment as the patient with an SCI ages.
4. Assist the patient in arranging modifications necessary to their home and in obtaining financial assistance for modifications to the environment.
5. Coordinate continued rehabilitation efforts to ensure social support, ongoing pharmacologic treatment, and monitoring for long-term complications, such as depression; vocational training; and adaptation to home and work environments. Use functional independence measure or other instrument to set and achieve goals with the patient in ADLs, transferring, locomotion, and other functional aspects.
6. Teach bowel care and urinary elimination procedures to the patient and all caregivers to ensure continuity.
7. Teach care of traction and immobilization devices.
8. Enlist help of occupational therapist, physical therapist, vocational therapist, recreational therapist, and other specialists, as needed.
9. Alert caregivers that autonomic dysreflexia is a complication that may occur up to several years after SCI involving T6 and above. Teach the patient and caregivers preventive and emergency treatment measures.

Patient Education and Health Maintenance

1. Teach the patient and family about the physiology of nerve transmission and how the SCI has affected normal function, including mobility, sensation, and bowel and bladder function.
2. Reinforce that rehabilitation is lengthy and involves adherence with therapy to increase function.
3. Explain that spasticity may develop 2 weeks to 3 months after injury and may interfere with routine care and ADLs.
4. Teach the patient to protect skin from pressure injury development by frequent repositioning while in bed, weight shifting and liftoffs every 15 minutes while in a wheelchair, and avoiding shear forces and friction.
5. Teach inspection of skin daily for development of pressure injuries, using a mirror, if necessary.
6. Encourage sexual counseling, if indicated, to promote satisfaction in personal relationships.
7. Teach importance of seat belts.

Evaluation: Expected Outcomes

- Respirations adequate, ABG values within normal limits.
- Repositioning hourly, no orthostatic changes.
- No evidence of pressure injuries or DVT.
- Reflex (or areflexic) voiding without retention.
- Bowel evacuation controlled.
- No episodes of autonomic dysreflexia.
- Verbalizes feeling of control over condition.
- Patient and partner exploring sexuality and sexual options.
- Reports pain at or lower than 2 to 3 levels on a scale of 1 to 10.

Vertebral Compression Fractures

Vertebral fractures commonly occur with trauma but can also be associated with osteoporosis or cancer.

Pathophysiology and Etiology

1. The vertebral body is made up of cancellous (soft) and outer cortical (hard) bone. The fracture creates an area of weakness within the vertebral column.
2. This weakness is further stressed and compressed with normal biomechanical stresses (weight-bearing activities from standing, sitting, and lifting). Over time, the fracture loses height, compressing the vertebral body.
3. The periosteum layer of the bone contains many pain receptors and, with weight-bearing activities that apply pressure on the fractured bone, stimulates the nerve endings, thereby producing pain.
4. Risk factors include:
   a. Osteoporosis—females over age 50; males over age 70; prolonged use of steroids.
   b. Metastatic cancer—breast, lung, renal, prostate, melanoma, multiple myeloma.
5. Other risk factors include the following:
   a. Smoking.
   b. Inactivity.
   c. Poor nutrition.

Clinical Manifestations

General Considerations

1. A vertebral body may fracture without causing debilitating pain.
2. Symptoms depend on the location and extent of fracture, progression of fracture, and effect on surrounding structures.
3. Most symptomatic fractures result in pain, although the development of instability can result in sensory changes, loss of reflex, and muscle weakness from canal compromise.

Cervical

1. Pain and stiffness in the neck, top of shoulders, and region of the scapula.
2. Pain with rotation, flexion, and extension.
3. Paresthesias and numbness of upper extremities.
4. Weakness of upper extremities.

Thoracic/Lumbar

1. Middle to lower back pain at site of fracture.
2. Pain aggravated with activity and relieved with rest and flexion.
3. Progressive kyphosis or postural deformity of the lumbar spine. Progressive thoracic kyphosis decreases lung capacity and can compromise pulmonary function.
4. Point tenderness to palpation on clinical examination.

Diagnostic Evaluation

1. Plain x-rays (anteroposterior and lateral views)—evaluate vertebral structure, height loss, and alignment.
2. CT scan—evaluation of the extent of fracture and canal involvement.
3. MRI—differential diagnosis includes infectious process or metastatic lesion. MRI has greater sensitivity for soft tissue abnormalities.
4. Bone scan—evaluation of microscopic changes within the bone. Identification of additional metastatic lesions, infectious process, microscopic fractures.

Management

Conservative Treatment

1. Orthosis/brace; heat or ice to affected area.
2. Physical therapy.

3. Anti-inflammatory drugs.
4. Analgesics, opioids may be necessary during acute phase.
5. Treatment and prevention of osteoporosis.

Surgical/Invasive Intervention

1. Surgical intervention—spinal instrumentation is not considered an option in patients with advanced osteoporosis secondary to the risk of nonunion and hardware failure.
2. Vertebroplasty—injection of methyl methacrylate (bone cement) with barium (radiopaque) into vertebral body aimed at providing stabilization of vertebral body.
3. Kyphoplasty—partial restoration of vertebral height using percutaneous placement of a balloon into vertebral body, inflation of the balloon with radiopaque solution (creates a cavity), and deflation and removal of the balloon followed by insertion of methyl methacrylate with barium. May be done under moderate sedation or general anesthesia. Reduced risk of glue leakage secondary to creation of the cavity.

Complications

1. PE due to leakage of cement into venous system following vertebroplasty or kyphoplasty.
2. Spinal cord or nerve root compromise due to leakage of cement following vertebroplasty or kyphoplasty.
3. Muscular spasms related to preprocedural deconditioning and postprocedural change in posture.

Nursing Assessment

1. Perform repeated assessments of motor function and sensation.
2. Assess for localized tenderness.
3. Assess pain level on scale of 1 to 10.

Nursing Interventions

Minimizing Pain

1. Administer or teach self-administration of analgesics as prescribed; inform patient about potential adverse effects (sedation, constipation, GI upset). Advise use of over-the-counter stool softeners.
2. Administer or teach self-administration of anti-inflammatories, as prescribed; advise taking with food or antacid to prevent GI upset.
3. Teach self-administration of muscle relaxants, as prescribed; inform patient about potential adverse effects of sedation.
4. Instruct in proper application and use of orthosis, if ordered.
5. Apply moist ice or heat to affected area of back, per patient-defined relief of pain.
6. Inspect skin several times a day, especially under stabilization devices, for redness and evidence of pressure injury development. Pressure injuries can cause severe pain.
7. Educate the patient about vertebroplasty or kyphoplasty, as indicated.
   a. One to two small punctures with a large-bore needle will be made at site of vertebral body to be treated. Level will be verified using fluoroscopy before insertion of bone cement.
   b. Routine postprocedural care will include assessment of vital signs and neurologic function, pain control, and ambulation, as ordered. Assess movement and sensation of extremities. Report any new deficit. CT of the spine may be ordered if encroachment on spinal cord or nerve root is suspected.
8. Encourage adherence with physical therapy treatments, as ordered.

Preventing Respiratory Complications Postoperatively

1. Monitor vital signs and assess respiratory status and report any breathing difficulties. Chest x-ray or CT of the chest (PE protocol) may be ordered if PE is suspected.
2. Administer analgesics and nonsteroidal anti-inflammatory drugs (NSAIDs) to control pain from incision and muscular inflammation due to procedure. Differentiate increased respiratory rate due to pain and anxiety rather than hypoxemia.
3. Enforce bed rest for 2 to 3 hours; patient may turn side to side, as directed; gradually increase activity, as tolerated.
4. Position for comfort. May apply heat or ice to affected muscles if spasm occurs and administer muscle relaxant, as indicated.
5. Report any increasing pain, weakness, or breathing difficulties. Auscultate lungs and report abnormalities.

Patient Education and Health Maintenance

1. Advise the patient of 10- to 25-pound lifting restriction for 1 week after vertebroplasty/kyphoplasty, as ordered, and to avoid strenuous activities; level of activity may be increased gradually as status indicates.
2. Demonstrate proper body mechanics to be used for bending, reaching, and lifting in all activities.
3. Alternate ice and heat for 20-minute intervals five to six times per day, as needed.
4. No soaking baths for 1 week to enhance wound healing of puncture sites.
5. Encourage the patient to do stretching and strengthening exercises for back and aerobic exercise for endurance on a daily basis.
6. Physical therapy may be indicated for reconditioning, heat therapy, and massage.
7. Instruct the patient to report any changes in neurologic function or recurrence of pain.

Evaluation: Expected Outcomes

- Verbalizes reduced pain.
- Vital signs stable, respirations unlabored, out of bed without difficulty.

Peripheral Nerve Injury

Peripheral nerve injury (PNI) is an injury to nerves in the upper extremity (e.g., radial, ulnar, median) or lower extremity (e.g., peroneal, sciatic, femoral, tibial). PNI may include damage to major nerves, the nerve root, the plexus (e.g., brachial or lumbar), and other peripheral sites.

Pathophysiology and Etiology

1. The incidence of PNI is approximately 2% to 3% in populations with multiple injuries. Males have higher incidence than females.
2. PNI damage may occur by congenital, traumatic, chemical, pathologic, thermal, or mechanical means. Focal trauma is the most common of all PNI. Injuries can be direct (e.g., gunshot) or indirect (e.g., casting).
3. The most frequently injured site is the upper extremity, specifically the upper arm. Childhood PNIs occur predominantly in the lower extremities.
4. Injury to the nerve causes impairment in axonal function and, possibly, disruption of myelination. Approximately 50% of

motor nerves and 75% of cutaneous nerves are myelinated. Schwann cells contain multiple axons. Myelinated axons enhance conduction between nodes, accelerating transmission compared with nonmyelinated axons. Fibers are classified according to diameter, conduction speed, myelination, and target.

5. Sensory regeneration, as opposed to motor regeneration, may take years following a PNI.
6. Nerve injuries are classified according to the Sunderland system, which establishes grades of nerve function on which to base recovery and need for surgery.
   a. First-degree PNI (neuropraxia)—there is a conduction impairment, but the anatomy is intact. Complete recovery is anticipated in 3 months.
   b. Second-degree PNI (axonotmesis)—Wallerian degeneration occurs distal to the PNI site, and axons disintegrate. Complete recovery is anticipated.
   c. Third-degree PNI—scarring occurs in the endoneural tube. Axons recover 1 in (2.5 cm) per month. Incomplete recovery is anticipated.
   d. Fourth-degree PNI (e.g., crush injury)—axonal regeneration is blocked by scar tissue. Surgical repair is typically required.
   e. Fifth-degree PNI (e.g., penetrating trauma)—the peripheral nerve is severed. Surgical intervention is required.
7. Compression neuropathy depends on the amount and extent of compression force. Edema, connective tissue thickening, and segmental demyelization of large fibers occur.
8. Useful function can be achieved when up to 75% of axons are damaged.

Clinical Manifestations

1. Flaccid paralysis.
2. Absent deep tendon reflexes.
3. Atonic/hypotonic muscles.
4. Progressive muscle atrophy.
5. Fasciculations peak 2 to 3 weeks after injury.
6. Trophic changes: Skin is warm and dry 3 weeks after injury and then becomes cold and cyanotic with loss of hair, brittle fingernails, and ulceration.
7. Causalgia (chronic pain syndrome): Neuropathic pain may be crawling, electric, tingling, or burning. (It typically follows the cutaneous sensory nerve distribution of the PNI.)
8. Specifics to area affected:
   a. Radial nerve injury—weakness in extension, possible wrist drop, inability to grasp objects/make a fist, impaired sensation over posterior forearm and dorsum of the hand.
   b. Brachial plexus—difficulty in abduction of shoulder, weakness with supination and flexion of the forearm (upper trunk) or extension of the forearm (middle trunk), or paralysis and atrophy of small muscles of the hand (lower trunk).
   c. Median and ulnar nerve injuries—sensory (median nerve) and motor (ulnar) loss of function in the hand (pronation, opposition of thumb, paralysis of finer flexor muscles).
   d. Femoral—weakness of knee and hip extension, atrophy of quadriceps, absence of knee jerk, loss of sensation of anterior aspect of the thigh.
   e. Common peroneal—footdrop, sensory loss on dorsum of foot, difficulty with eversion.
   f. Sciatic—footdrop, pain across gluteus and thigh, loss of knee flexion, weakness/paralysis of muscles below knee.
9. Chronic nerve compression may begin with intermittent signs and symptoms; these may only occur in specific maneuvers, such as digital pressure or position. For example, damage to the brachial plexus, entrapped at the supra/infraclavicular junction, may elicit symptoms following arm elevation for 1 minute. In carpal tunnel syndrome (compression of the median nerve), wrist flexion or external pressure applied proximally to the carpal tunnel may evoke symptoms.

Diagnostic Evaluation

1. The electrodiagnostic examination consists of nerve conduction studies (sensory, motor, mixed) and needle electrode examination.
   a. The electrodiagnostic examination tests only large myelinated axons; it does not assess pain, temperature, or paresthesia.
   b. It can confirm PNI occurrence and determine the type of axon, pathophysiology, severity, location, and injury prognosis.
2. Muscle ultrasonography evaluates the extent of muscle involvement and assesses acute nerve injuries.
3. MRI and electrophysiologic studies such as electroneurography and EMG detect the site and degree of nerve injury.
4. Muscle imaging may detect atrophy and mesenchymal alteration of skeletal muscles.
5. Tinel sign (tapping the axons of the regenerating nerve produces a paresthesia in the normal distribution of the nerve) reveals the rate of axonal regeneration.

Management

1. Microsurgery reapproximates the severed peripheral nerve endings. The sooner the repair is performed, the better the chance of recovery. Microsurgical repair can be done with tension-free coaptation using technology, such as carbon dioxide laser welding, fibrin gluing, and ring coupling. Autogenous nerve grafts are the gold standard.
2. Primary nerve repair (neurorrhaphy) may be done within 1 week of injury (e.g., open wounds—except gunshots). Secondary nerve repair is performed after 1 week (e.g., crush injury with soft tissue damage). In partially transected nerves, surgery may be delayed 2 to 3 months to determine whether regeneration will take place.
   a. Nerve grafting—two neurorrhaphy sites are used. Thin, cutaneous nerve grafts with large fascicles and minimal connective tissue are optimal. Common donor sites include the sacral nerve (lateral aspect of the foot), lateral antebrachial cutaneous nerve (lateral forearm), and the median antebrachial cutaneous nerve (medial arm and elbow). Small segments of nerve grafts may be placed to create a bridge to facilitate axonal and Schwann cell growth. Nerve "conduits," connectors of nerve sites, may be composed of bone, vein, artery, silicone, or other material.
   b. End-to-side neurorrhaphy—the severed nerve's distal end is attached to the side of a healthy nerve.
   c. Nerve transfer—ideally, the donor nerve fascicles are in close proximity to the target muscle motor end plate or target sensory nerve. If the patient has multiple nerve injuries, such as a complete brachial plexus injury, nerve transfer priority is given to promoting elbow flexion, shoulder abduction, and external rotation. Sensory nerve priorities are given to the ulnar thumb and radial index finger.
3. Tissue expansion is used to compensate for tissue deficit.

4. Insulin-like growth factor and acidic fibroblast growth factor have enhanced regeneration when administered systemically or topically and other factors are being investigated.
5. Corticosteroids may be used to decrease edema.
6. Occupational therapy may be consulted to splint or cast the patient. Splinting (e.g., hands) or casting may be indicated to reduce tension on the PNI site and facilitate healing. Day splints are typically functional splints; night splints are positioning splints. Splint material depends on the amount of resistance to be exerted by the orthosis, the splint size, and the patient's compensatory movements.
   a. Radial nerve splint—volar or dorsal cock-up splints are indicated if wrist extension is impaired.
   b. Median nerve splint—a thumb opposition splint preserves the function of the hand grip.
   c. Ulnar nerve splint—this functional and positioning splint prevents "claw hand" deformity and contractures of fingers four and five.
7. Flexibility is primarily due to connective tissues stretching as opposed to muscle contraction. Passive and active ROM exercises are essential to provide stretch and prevent contractions. Ultrasound diathermy may be used on deep muscles, and topical heat may be used for superficial muscles to promote stretching. Progressive resistance and strengthening, including isometric activities, are used to restore function. Functional electrical stimulation may also be used.
8. Fibrosis, caused by edema, may be minimized by elevating the affected limb. Using static graduated compression devices (e.g., sleeves, gloves, hose) or sequential compression devices, distal to proximal wrapping, may also minimize edema. Likewise, massage may reduce edema.
9. Desensitization techniques (e.g., scheduled exposure to irritating textures, vibration) may be used to manage hyperesthesia. Sensory reeducation may be protective (compensatory). Sensory restoration is progressive, with temperature and pain returning first, followed by transient light touch and vibration.
10. Neuropathic pain may be managed by traditional analgesics, antidepressants (e.g., tricyclic), anticonvulsants (e.g., gabapentin), topical and transdermal agents (e.g., capsaicin), NSAIDs, alpha-adrenergic agonists (e.g., clonidine), calcium channel blockers (e.g., nicardipine), or transcutaneous electrical stimulation.
11. Carpal tunnel syndrome management may include activity modification, NSAIDs, serial steroid injections, vitamin B_6, diuretics, and a wrist splint for 6 months. Endoscopic surgical release of the ligament may also be an option.
12. Complex peripheral injuries, such as injury to the brachial plexus, may require multimodal treatment, including surgery, pain management, and functional rehabilitation. A multidisciplinary team approach is most effective in maximizing outcomes.

Complications

1. Infection, if injury is penetrating and site becomes contaminated.
2. Compartment syndrome due to edema or positioning.
3. Muscle atrophy/flaccid paralysis; disuse syndrome.
4. Sensory deficit.
5. Contractures.
6. Chronic pain.
7. Nerve damage resulting from surgical repair.

Nursing Assessment

1. Perform frequent neurovascular checks of the affected extremity (pressure, vibration, and two-point discrimination sensation; motor function, strength; pulses; temperature; capillary refill; degree of swelling).
2. Assess degree of pain on a scale of 0 to 10.
3. Test reflexes of affected extremity.
4. Observe for signs of infection if there is an open wound.
5. Assess for concomitant injuries such as head or skeletal trauma.

Nursing Interventions

Protecting Neurovascular Function

1. Administer corticosteroids and diuretics, as ordered, to decrease swelling and development of compartment syndrome.
2. Keep extremity elevated to promote venous drainage.
3. Perform neurovascular check to evaluate status of injury.
   a. Incorporate Tinel sign into assessment.
   b. Report any changes in condition.
4. Postoperatively assist rehabilitation team in reeducating nerves and muscles to achieve function.
5. Observe for paresthesias, pain, or altered skin integrity in areas of splinting and casting.

Promoting Comfort

1. Administer and teach self-administration of analgesics, as ordered.
2. Elevate extremity.
3. Avoid exposing denervated areas to temperature extremes.
4. Apply devices such as splints and slings, as ordered.
5. Maintain mobility with ROM exercises. Perform gently, following administration of analgesics.

Preventing Infection

1. Assess wound and dressing frequently for erythema, warmth, swelling, odor, and drainage.
2. Monitor temperature with vital signs for hyperthermia and tachycardia, indicating infection.
3. Encourage deep breathing exercises and ambulation to prevent pulmonary complications.

Patient Education and Health Maintenance

1. Teach management of wound and dressing and casts or splints.
2. Review analgesia schedule and need for elevation of injured area.
3. Teach exercises for involved area.
4. Suggest assistive devices to promote independence.
5. Stress the importance of adhering with long-term rehabilitation, physical therapy, and follow-up evaluations.
6. Support a community accident prevention program, including the use of seat belts, industrial regulations, and sports and recreational safety measures.

Evaluation: Expected Outcomes

- Stable neurovascular status; functional use of extremity.
- Patient reports adequate relief of pain.
- Wound/surgical site free of erythema, drainage, odor.

CENTRAL NERVOUS SYSTEM TUMORS

Brain Tumors

EVIDENCE BASE Miller, K. D., Ostrom, Q. T., Kruchko, C., Patil, N., Tihan, T., Cioffi, G., Fuchs, H. E., Waite, K. A., Jemal, A., Siegel, R. L., & Barnholtz-Sloan, J. S. (2021). Brain and other central nervous system tumor statistics, 2021. *CA: A Cancer Journal for Clinicians*, *71*(5), 381–406. https://doi.org/10.3322/caac.21693

Louis, D. N., Perry, A., Wesseling, P., Brat, D. J., Cree, I. A., Figarella-Branger, D., Hawkins, C., Ng, H. K., Pfister, S. M., Reifenberger, G., Soffietti, R., von Deimling, A., & Ellison, D. W. (2021). The 2021 WHO classification of tumors of the central nervous system: A summary. *Neuro-oncology*, *23*(8), 1231–1251. https://doi.org/10.1093/neuonc/noab106

Intracranial neoplasms are the result of abnormal proliferation of cells within the central nervous system (CNS). A *tumor* is a mass of cancerous cells within the brain. It is believed that there is a 2- to 3-cm surrounding area of cancer cells with the potential to develop into a tumor. Tumors require blood to grow and recruit a vascular supply to support the metabolic needs of the tumor. Intracranial tumors are primary or metastatic tumors, and malignancy depends on cell type and location. Primary tumors include tumors of the brain itself, the skull or meninges, the pituitary gland, and the blood vessels. Metastatic tumors spread from the primary site of cancer (breast, lung, prostate, kidney) through the vascular supply and lymphatic systems. Defining primary cancer cell type determines the treatment modality and influences the overall prognosis.

Primary CNS tumor etiology remains unknown. Glioma research has identified a genetic mutation of p53 on chromosome 17 occurs in 50% of all cancers. Loss of heterozygosity of chromosome arm 10q also has been reported in gliomas, although research continues into potential genetic mutation and growth factors, as well as attempting to identify a tumor marker. No known environmental risks have been identified. Primary CNS tumors rarely metastasize outside the CNS.

Pathophysiology and Etiology

Tumors may originate in the CNS or metastasize from elsewhere in the body (50% of all brain tumors) and may be benign or malignant; all tumors produce effects of space-occupying lesion (edema, increased intracranial pressure [ICP]). Malignancy may be related not only to cell type and invasiveness but also to location and operative accessibility (i.e., the tumor is located in an area of the brain that will not tolerate compression of the brain structures or is not surgically accessible). The World Health Organization grading scale is currently used to classify gliomas, although other grading scales are available. The grading system evaluates the probability of tumor recurrence and malignancy from low (grades I to II) to high (grades III to IV). Tumors arise from any tissue of the CNS (see Figure 11-12).

1. Gliomas—tumors of the neuroepithelial/glial cells (supportive tissue of the brain; account for 40% to 50% of intracranial neoplasms):
   a. Astrocytoma—overgrowth of the astrocyte cells (connective tissue) of the brain. Tumors are graded on a scale from

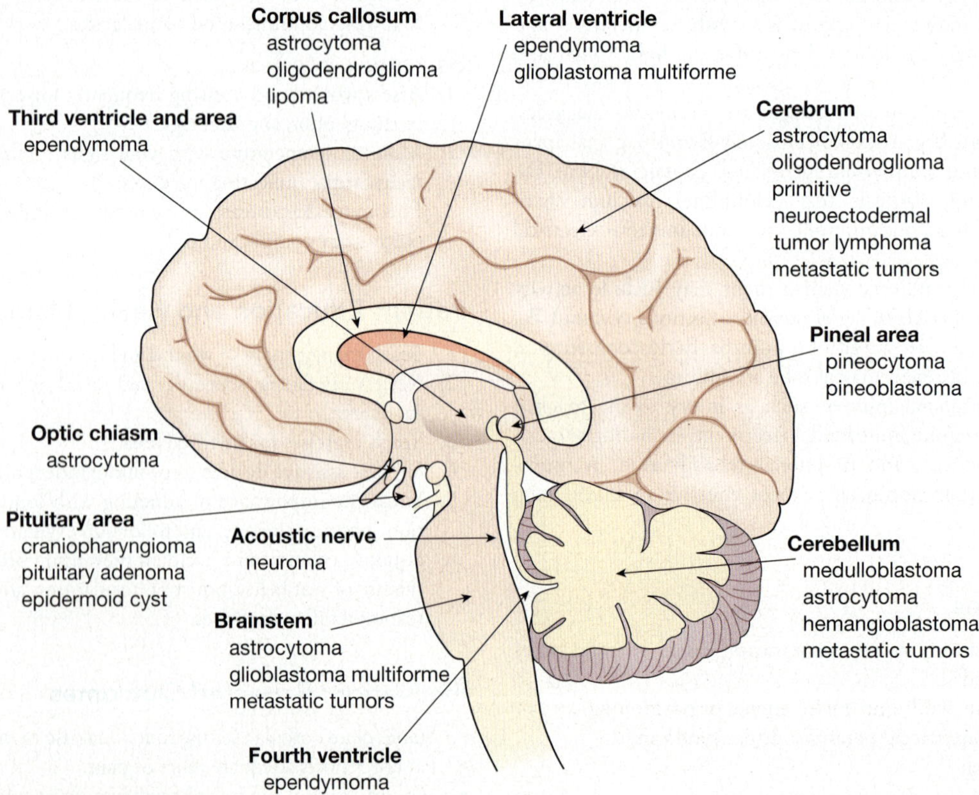

Figure 11-12. Common brain tumor sites.

I to IV that defines growth pattern, invasiveness, infiltration, cell differentiation, margination, and necrosis.
   i. Grade I (astrocytoma)—slow-growing tumor with well-defined cells and minimal infiltration.
   ii. Grade II (astrocytoma)—some atypical cells with higher rate of recurrence and risk of advancing to grade III or IV with recurrence.
   iii. Grade III (anaplastic astrocytoma) that is highly invasive and infiltrative, with poorly marginated borders and a rapid growth pattern and risk of advancing to grade IV with recurrence.
   iv. Grade IV (glioblastoma multiforme)—a malignant tumor that is highly invasive, infiltrative, and poorly marginated, with necrosis and a very rapid growth pattern (accounts for 55% of gliomas).
  b. Oligodendroglioma—overgrowth of oligodendroglial cells with calcification. Begins as a less invasive tumor but demonstrates malignancy as it progresses. The frontal and temporal lobes of the cerebrum are common locations. Rare in children.
  c. Ependymoma (5% to 6% of intracranial gliomas)—overgrowth of the ependymal cells of the brain. Slow growing; commonly occurs in the floor of the fourth ventricle; presents with signs and symptoms of increased ICP and hydrocephalus; 69% of cases occur in children.
  d. Mixed gliomas—two or more cell types within a tumor.
  e. Medulloblastoma—most common pediatric malignant tumor. Commonly located in the fourth ventricle/cerebellar vermis; rapid growth pattern, highly invasive; high risk for metastasis within cerebrospinal fluid (CSF).
  f. Hemangioblastoma—rare, benign tumor commonly located in the posterior fossa; von Hippel-Lindau disease is multiple hemangiomas within CNS.
  g. Colloid cyst—a rare cyst that contains neuroepithelial cells; occurs in the third ventricle.
2. Meningioma—arises from meningeal lining of the brain. Can involve the skull; accounts for 20% of primary brain tumors (90% are benign; 10% are atypical or anaplastic). Higher incidence in females aged 40 to 70 years. Rare in children.
  a. Grade I meningiomas are benign, slow-growing, encapsulated lesions without brain tissue infiltration—but may have a dural tail.
  b. Grade II (atypical meningiomas), rapid-growing tumors with increased miotic activity and higher risk of recurrence after resection; risk of advancing to anaplastic tumor.
  c. Grade III (anaplastic meningioma), which has malignant features and invasion of brain tissue.
3. Peripheral nerve tumors—generally benign tumors that occur secondary to nerve sheath overgrowth.
  a. Acoustic neuroma/schwannoma, located on cranial nerve (CN) VIII.
  b. Neurofibromatosis type 1 (von Recklinghausen).
  c. Neurofibromatosis type 2.
4. Pituitary tumors.
  a. Pituitary adenoma, occurs primarily in the anterior of the pituitary and can be:
   i. Secreting tumor—prolactin (causes amenorrhea/galactorrhea in females, impotence in males, and infertility in all genders), adrenocorticotrophic hormone (causes Cushing syndrome), or growth hormone (causes acromegaly).
   ii. Nonsecreting tumor.
  b. Craniopharyngioma (considered a developmental tumor)—a benign cystic lesion with calcification, occurring in the anterior pituitary margin. Fifty percent occur in children.
5. Germ cell tumors and tumor-like cysts.
  a. Dermoid cysts—occur in the ectodermal layer and contain hair and sebaceous glands.
  b. Epidermoid cysts containing cell debris and keratin.
  c. Pineal tumor—overgrowth of germ cells, pineal cells, or mixed germ types (includes teratomas) within the pineal region (more common in children and males).
  d. Chordoma—rare neoplasm that contains embryonic remnant occurring along the neuraxis.
6. Hematopoietic tumors—include primary malignant lymphoma (rare, diffusely infiltrating tumor of the brain, occurs in adults, high rate of recurrence) and secondary lymphoma associated with acquired immune deficiency syndrome (AIDS).
7. Secondary CNS tumors/metastatic lesions—commonly from lung cancer (40% to 50%), breast cancer (14% to 20%), melanoma (10%), renal (5%), and undetermined primary sites (10% to 15%). Single lesions common with lung and breast cancer can have multiple lesions that are unresectable. Indicate systemic spread of primary cancer.

Clinical Manifestations

Manifestations depend on the location and biologic nature of the tumor. If the tumor is in a noneloquent area of the brain or is slow growing, specific symptoms may not develop until the late stages of the process. Instead, the tumor may produce generalized symptoms related to the increasing size of the tumor and the expanding area of cerebral edema surrounding the margins of the tumor. This is referred to as the "mass" effect of the tumor.

1. Generalized symptoms (due to increased ICP)—headache (especially in the morning), vomiting, papilledema, malaise, altered cognition, and consciousness.
2. Focal neurologic deficits (related to region of tumor):
  a. Parietal area—sensory alterations, speech and memory disturbances, neglect, visuospatial deficits, right–left confusion, depression.
  b. Frontal lobe—personality, behavior, and memory changes; contralateral motor weakness; expressive aphasia.
  c. Temporal area—memory disturbances, auditory hallucinations, receptive aphasia, complex partial seizures, visual field deficits.
  d. Occipital area—visual agnosia and visual field deficits.
  e. Cerebellar area—coordination, gait, and balance disturbances, dysarthria.
  f. Brainstem—dysphagia, incontinence, cardiovascular instability, respiratory depression, coma, CN dysfunction.
  g. Hypothalamus—loss of temperature control, diabetes insipidus, syndrome of inappropriate antidiuretic hormone (SIADH).
  h. Pituitary/sella turcica—visual field deficits, amenorrhea, galactorrhea, impotence, cushingoid symptoms, elevated growth hormone, panhypopituitarism.
3. Referred symptoms (related to the vasogenic [extracellular] edema surrounding the tumor).
4. Seizures.

Diagnostic Evaluation

1. Computed tomography (CT)—with and without contrast to visualize tumor, hemorrhage, shift of midline, cerebral edema.

2. Magnetic resonance imaging (MRI)—to visualize tumor; more useful than CT and gold standard for diagnostic evaluation.
3. Electroencephalography (EEG)—to detect locus of irritability, if seizures are present.
4. Angiography—to detect and evaluate the vascular supply of the tumor.
5. MR spectroscopy—evaluates the neurochemicals located within a core segment of the lesion; useful in differentiating tumors from infectious lesions.
6. Functional MRI—evaluates the functional eloquence of the brain tissue affected by the tumor, and the tissue at risk, for mass effect.
7. Skull radiography—to determine bone involvement, identify pineal shift, helpful in children.
8. Stealth-guided surgery or stereotactic biopsy surgery—needed for definitive diagnosis, cell type.

Management

Effectiveness of treatment depends on tumor type and location, capsulation, or infiltrative status. Tumors in vital areas, such as the brainstem, or nonencapsulated and infiltrating tumors, may not be surgically accessible, and treatment may produce severe neurologic deficits (blindness, paralysis, mental impairment). Treatment is usually multimodal. Treatment of high-grade gliomas is palliative. There is no current treatment modality that provides a definitive cure. Treatment is aimed at improving duration of survival.

1. Surgery—removal/debulking by way of craniotomy, stealth guidance, laser resection, or ultrasonic aspiration.
   a. Craniotomy: Goal is gross total resection of the tumor for maximum removal of tumor cells. Biopsy may be performed on tumors in eloquent locations; whereas surgery may not be an option for some tumors secondary to location. Gross total resection is associated with longer survival compared with subtotal resection in glioblastoma multiforme; 10% are inoperable based on location of the tumor.
   b. Awake craniotomy—allows intraoperative brain mapping.
   c. Image-guided surgery—computer-generated intraoperative localization of lesion.
   d. Laser resection or ultrasonic aspiration—may augment surgical resection.
   e. Endovascular treatment—useful in embolization of the arterial feeders to the meningiomas to reduce surgical risk related to blood loss.
2. Radiation therapy—external radiation to tumor bed with 2- to 3-cm border.
   a. Conventional therapy daily for 6 weeks; shorter to brainstem.
   b. Prophylactic radiation to brainstem for other brain tumors with high risk of metastasis.
3. Radiosurgery—stereotactic radiosurgery by way of linear accelerator scalpel, proton beam, or gamma knife delivers a single, high dose of radiation to a precisely targeted tumor area. Destroys only targeted abnormal tissue, limiting damage to surrounding brain tissue.
4. Chemotherapy (the blood–brain barrier limits the effectiveness of chemotherapy agents).
   a. Metastatic tumors—single or combination drug therapy; may require autologous bone marrow transplantation (aspirated before chemotherapy and reinfused afterward to treat bone marrow depression).
   b. Primary glioma:
      i. Maximal surgical resection of tumor, when possible, improves overall outcome survival.
      ii. External beam radiation therapy with concurrent chemotherapy with temozolomide for 6 weeks in patients with high-grade glioma. Followed by adjuvant temozolomide 5 days every 28 days for 12 cycles.
      iii. Carmustine (BCNU) wafers are biodegradable chemotherapy wafers that are surgically placed into the tumor bed during tumor debulking. Up to eight wafers are placed in the space where the tumor was located, and they slowly break down over time.
      iv. Bevacizumab is Food and Drug Administration (FDA) approved for the treatment of recurrent glioblastoma multiforme. Studies demonstrate a reduction in cerebral edema, though there is no change in length of survival.
      v. Lomustine (CCNU) alternative oral chemotherapy can be used as monotherapy or in conjunction with other agents including bevacizumab.
      vi. Immunotherapy (epidermal growth factor receptor variant III) remains investigational, though has shown promising results in phase II studies.
      vii. Tumor treating fields with NovoTTF destroys glioblastoma cells through electromagnetic fields. FDA approved for adjuvant therapy with current investigations examining outcome survival in patients treated concurrently with radiation therapy and temozolomide.
5. Shunting procedure—to manage hydrocephalus, which may be obstructive or nonobstructive depending on the location, tumor type, degree of necrosis, and associated edema and inflammation.
6. Supportive therapy and medications.
   a. Antiepileptics for treatment of seizure activity; may be utilized for prophylaxis.
   b. Dexamethasone to reduce swelling and reduce radiation edema; also given during end stage to enhance quality of life.
   c. The presence of tumors creates a hypercoagulable state. Prophylactic use of anticoagulant may or may not be ordered, though may be required in the presence of deep vein thrombosis (DVT) or pulmonary embolism (PE).
7. Investigational therapies currently in progress:
   a. Multiple trials examining targeted treatments based on molecular and genetic properties of brain tumors.
   b. Use of combination therapies including bevacizumab and lomustine is currently in phase III of evaluation.

Complications

1. Increased ICP and brain herniation; death.
2. Neurologic deficits from expanding tumor or treatment.

Nursing Assessment

1. Assess vital signs and signs of increased ICP (see page 337).
2. Assess CN function, level of consciousness (LOC), mental status, affect, and behavior.
3. Monitor for seizures.
4. Assess level of pain using visual analogue scale (0 to 10) or face scale, as indicated.
5. Assess level of anxiety.
6. Assess patient and family patterns of coping, support systems, and resources.
7. If treated with chemotherapy, assess bone marrow function by monitoring neutrophil and platelet counts.

Nursing Interventions

Also see care of the patient undergoing chemotherapy (Chapter 4), and craniotomy (page 341)

Relieving Pain

1. Provide analgesics around the clock at regular intervals that will not mask neurologic changes.
2. Maintain the head of the bed at 15 to 30 degrees to reduce cerebral venous congestion.
3. Provide a darkened room or sunglasses if the patient is photophobic.
4. Maintain a quiet environment to increase patient's pain tolerance.
5. Provide scheduled rest periods to help the patient recuperate from stress of pain.
6. Instruct the patient to lie with the operative side up.
7. Alter diet, as tolerated, if the patient has pain on chewing.
8. Collaborate with the patient on alternative ways to reduce pain such as use of music therapy.

Preventing Injury

1. Report any signs of increased ICP or worsening neurologic condition to health care provider immediately.
2. Adjust care to reduce the risk of increased ICP; body positioning without flexion of head, reduce hip flexion, distribute care throughout the 24-hour period to allow ICP to return to baseline.
3. Monitor laboratory data, CSF cultures, and Gram stains, and communicate results to medical staff.
4. Monitor intake and output, osmolality studies, and electrolytes; prevent overhydration, which can worsen cerebral edema.
5. Monitor response to pharmacologic therapy, including drug levels.
6. Initiate seizure precautions; pad the side rails of the bed to prevent injury if seizures occur; have suction equipment available.
7. Maintain availability of medications for the management of status epilepticus (see page 403).
8. Initiate fall precautions; side rails up at all times, call light within reach at bedside, assist with toileting on a regular basis.
9. Gradually progress patient to ambulation with assistance as tolerated, enlist help from physical therapist, occupational therapist early, as indicated, to prevent falls.
10. If the patient is dysphagic or unconscious, initiate aspiration precautions: Elevate head of the bed 30 degrees and position the patient's head to the side to prevent aspiration.
11. If dysphagic, position the patient upright and instruct in sequenced swallowing to maintain feeding function.
12. Maintain oxygen and suction at the bedside in case of aspiration.
13. For the patient with visual field deficits, place materials in visual field.

Minimizing Anxiety

1. Provide a safe environment in which the patient may verbalize anxieties.
2. Help the patient to express feelings related to fear and anxiety.
3. Answer questions and provide written information.
4. Include the patient/family in all treatment options and scheduling.
5. Introduce stress management techniques.
6. Provide consistency in care and continually provide emotional support.
7. Assess the patient's usual coping behaviors and provide support in these areas.
8. Consult with social worker for community resources.
9. Be aware that anxiety and depression prior to and following surgery are associated with shorter postsurgical survival in patients with glioblastoma multiforme. Screening assessments can be performed with standard instruments, and levels indicating a high risk of anxiety or depression should be reported to the health care provider.

Optimizing Nutrition

1. Medicate for nausea before position changes, radiation, or chemotherapy, and as needed.
2. Maintain adequate hydration within guidelines for cerebral edema.
3. Offer small, frequent meals as tolerated.
4. Consult with dietitian to evaluate food choices and provide adequate caloric needs through enteral or parenteral nourishment if unable to take oral nutrition.
5. Alter consistency of diet, as necessary, to enhance intake.

Strengthening Family Coping

1. Recognize stages of grief.
2. Foster a trusting relationship.
3. Provide clear, consistent explanations of procedures and treatments.
4. Encourage family involvement in care from the beginning.
5. Establish a means of communication for family with patient when verbal responses are not possible.
6. Consult with social worker and mental health provider if the family needs assistance in adjusting to neurologic deficits.
7. Assist the family to use stress management techniques and community resources such as respite care.
8. Encourage discussion with health care provider about prognosis and functional outcome.
9. Discuss development of advance directive and durable power of attorney (DPA). Maintain positive attitude and define that rationale as a way to allow for patient-defined extent of care in the advent of deterioration.

Patient Education and Health Maintenance

1. Explain the adverse effects of treatment.
2. Encourage close follow-up after diagnosis and treatment.
3. Explain the importance of continuing corticosteroids and how to manage adverse effects, such as weight gain and hyperglycemia.
4. Encourage the use of community resources for physical and psychological support, such as transportation to medical appointments, financial assistance, and respite care.
5. Refer the patient/family for more information and support to agencies such as the National Institute of Neurologic Disorders and Stroke (www.ninds.nih.gov) and the National Brain Tumor Foundation (www.braintumor.org).

Evaluation: Expected Outcomes

- Reports satisfactory comfort level.
- No new neurologic deficits, seizures, falls, or other complications.
- Expresses decreased anxiety.
- Nutritional intake meeting metabolic demands.
- Patient and family verbalize understanding of treatment and available resources.

Tumors of the Spinal Cord and Canal

Tumors of the spinal cord and canal may be extradural (existing outside the dural membranes), including chordoma and osteoblastoma; intradural–extramedullary (within the lumbar subarachnoid space [SAS]), including meningiomas, neurofibromas, and schwannomas; or intramedullary (within the spinal cord), including astrocytomas, ependymomas, and neurofibromatosis "dumbbell tumors." Vascular tumors can affect any part of the spinal cord or canal.

Pathophysiology and Etiology

1. Astrocytomas, characterized by asymmetrical expansion in the spinal cord, are more common in children than adults. Ependymomas, usually with a cyst, are the most common intramedullary tumor in the adult but are rare in children. These tumors are central in the spinal cord.
2. Vascular tumors can affect the spinal cord in various ways. Hemangioblastomas often cause edema and syrinx (fluid-filled cavity) formation. Cavernomas are located on the dorsal surface of the spinal cord.
3. Approximately 85% of all patients with cancer develop bony metastasis, with the spinal column as the primary site. Spinal cord compression due to cancer typically presents with incomplete paraplegia involving the thoracic spine.
4. Cause for abnormal cell growth is unknown.
5. Extradural tumors spread to the vertebral bodies.
6. Spinal cord and/or nerve compression can result.

Clinical Manifestations

Depends on the location and type of tumor and extent of spinal cord compression.

1. Back pain that is localized or radiates; may be absent in more than 50% of patients.
2. Weakness of extremity with abnormal reflexes.
3. Sensory changes.
4. Bladder, bowel, or sexual dysfunction.

Diagnostic Evaluation

1. A plain x-ray or CT scan can detect a pathologic fracture, collapse, or destruction resulting from a mass.
2. MRI is sensitive to tumor detection.

Management

1. Two surgical approaches may be used to manage spinal cord tumors:
   a. Anterior decompression is typically indicated because most spinal cord tumors are anterior.
   b. The posterolateral approach may be used for excision of thoracic tumors. Endoscopy, or other surgical techniques using instrumentation, can be used to visualize the anterior part of the cord. In thoracic tumors above T_5, posterolateral decompression negates the need for an anterior thoracotomy or sternotomy.
2. Intraoperative somatosensory evoked potentials and motor evoked potentials can be used to "map" the optimal spinal cord site for incision and identify sensory and motor tracts within the spinal cord. This mapping reduces the neurologic deficits that are frequently associated with tumor incisions.
3. Various techniques are used to remove spinal cord tumors, including the following:
   a. Intramedullary tumors are totally resected. Corticosteroids are administered before and after surgery. MRI verifies tumor characteristics preoperatively (e.g., exact level). Microsurgical laser techniques, ultrasound, and x-rays may be used intraoperatively. In surgery, every effort must be made to keep the anterior spinal artery intact.
   b. Vascular tumors may be managed in different ways. Hemangioblastomas are usually removed from the outside inward by exterior coagulation and progressive tumor shrinkage before removal. Cavernomas are usually removed by exterior coagulation and progressive tumor shrinkage before removal but from the inside outward.
   c. Neoplastic tumors may be treated with radiation or surgically excised using an anterior approach because these tumors typically cause anterior cord compression.
4. Radiation therapy may be used over 2 to 4 weeks; dosing protocols vary. Spinal radiation before surgical decompression may adversely affect wound healing. In patients who have a good functional status, radiotherapy to a malignant spinal cord tumor can significantly improve survival time.
5. Corticosteroids, such as dexamethasone and prednisone in moderate to high doses, are indicated for use before radiation therapy to improve the ambulation rate in the paretic patient.
   a. Corticosteroids are not typically used in patients who are nonparetic and ambulatory.
   b. They are tapered over 2 weeks before discontinuing.
6. Chemotherapy is considered experimental.
7. When compared with patients with traumatic spinal cord injury (SCI), the rehabilitation of patients with spinal cord tumors is shorter; however, patients with cancer have more limited functional improvement than patients with SCI.

Complications

1. Spinal cord infarction secondary to compression.
2. Nerve or spinal compression from tumor expansion.
3. Tetraplegia or paraplegia due to spinal cord compression.

Nursing Assessment

1. Perform motor and sensory components of the neurologic examination.
2. Assess pain using scale of 0 to 10, as indicated.
3. Assess autonomic nervous system relative to level of lesion—pupillary responses, vital signs, bowel and bladder function.
4. Assess for spinal or nerve compression—progressive increase in pain, paralysis or paresis, sensory loss, loss of rectal sphincter tone, and sexual dysfunction.

Nursing Interventions

Relieving Anxiety

1. Provide an accepting environment for patient to verbalize anxieties.
2. Provide explanations regarding all procedures. Answer questions or refer the patient to someone who can answer questions.
3. Refer to cancer and SCI support groups, as needed.
4. Provide the patient/family with written information regarding disease process and medical interventions.
5. Reduce environmental stimulation.
6. Promote periods of rest to enhance coping skills.
7. Involve the family in distraction techniques.
8. Provide options in care when possible.

Relieving Pain

1. Administer analgesics, as indicated, and evaluate for pain control.
2. Instruct the patient in the use of patient-controlled analgesia, if available.
3. Instruct the patient in relaxation techniques, such as deep breathing, distraction, and imagery.
4. Position patient off surgical site postoperatively.

Compensating for Sensory Alterations

1. Reassure the patient that the degree of sensory/motor impairment may decrease during the postoperative recovery period as the amount of surgical edema decreases.
2. Instruct the patient with sensory loss to visually scan the extremity during use to avoid injury related to lack of tactile input.
3. Instruct the patient with painful paresthesias in appropriate use of ice, exercise, and rest.
4. Assess the patient with sensory and motor alterations and refer to physical therapy for assistance with activities of daily living (ADLs), ambulation.

Achieving Urinary Continence

1. Assess the urinary elimination pattern of the patient.
2. Instruct the patient in the therapeutic intake of fluid volume and relationship to elimination.
3. Instruct the patient in an appropriate means of urinary elimination and bowel management (see Chapter 17).

Preventing Postoperative Complications

1. Provide routine postoperative care to prevent complications.
2. Monitor surgical site for bleeding, CSF drainage, signs of infection.
3. Keep surgical dressing clean and dry.
4. Clean surgical site, as ordered.
5. Pad the bed rails and chair if the patient experiences numbness or paresthesias to prevent injury.
6. Support the weak/paralytic extremity in a functional position.

Patient Education and Health Maintenance

1. Encourage the patient with motor impairment to use adaptive devices.
2. Demonstrate proper positioning and transfer techniques.
3. Instruct the patient with sensory losses about dangers of extreme temperatures and the need for adequate foot protection at all times.
4. If the patient has suspected or confirmed neurofibromatosis, suggest referral to genetic counselor. Also, encourage follow-up for MRI every 12 months to monitor disease progression.
5. Refer to cancer and SCI support groups, as needed.

Evaluation: Expected Outcomes

- Asks questions and discusses care options.
- Reports that pain is relieved.
- Reports decreased paresthesias; ambulatory postoperatively.
- Voids at intervals without residual urine.
- Incision healing, skin intact.

OTHER DISORDERS

Seizure Disorders

Seizures (also known as *epileptic seizures* and, if recurrent, *epilepsy*) are defined as a sudden alteration in normal brain activity that causes distinct changes in behavior and body function. Seizures are thought to result from disturbances in the cells of the brain that cause cells to give off abnormal, recurrent, uncontrolled electrical discharges.

Pathophysiology and Etiology

Altered Physiology

1. The pathophysiology of seizures is unknown. It is known, however, that the brain has certain metabolic needs for oxygen and glucose. Neurons also have certain permeability gradients and voltage gradients that are affected by changes in the chemical and humoral environment.
2. Factors that change the permeability of the cell population (ischemia, hemorrhage) and ion concentration (Na+, K+) can produce neurons that are hyperexcitable and demonstrate hypersynchrony, producing an abnormal discharge.
3. A seizure may manifest itself as an altered behavior, motor, or sensory function relating to any anatomic location in the brain.

Classification

The International League Against Epilepsy developed an international classification of epileptic seizures that divides seizures into two major classes: partial-onset seizures and generalized-onset seizures. Partial-onset seizures begin in one focal area of the cerebral cortex, whereas generalized-onset seizures have an onset recorded simultaneously in both cerebral hemispheres.

1. Partial-onset seizures indicate that seizure focus is emanating from a specific area in the brain, either in a hemisphere or in particular lobe. Can be subdivided into two subtypes: focal aware, which indicates patient is able to respond to their environment; and focal with impaired awareness, which indicates patient is unaware of their environment.
2. Generalized-onset seizures indicate that seizure activity may originate in one area of the brain but rapidly progresses to involve both hemispheres of the brain. Consciousness is impaired with generalized seizures.

Etiology

The etiology may be unknown or due to one of the following:

1. Trauma to head or brain resulting in scar tissue or cerebral atrophy.
2. Tumors.
3. Cranial surgery.
4. Metabolic disorders (hypocalcemia, hypoglycemia/hyperglycemia, hyponatremia, anoxia).
5. Central nervous system (CNS) infection.
6. Circulatory disorders.
7. Drug withdrawal states (alcohol, barbiturates).
8. Congenital neurodegenerative disorders.
9. Nonepileptogenic behaviors, which can emulate seizures but have a psychogenic, rather than an organic, origin.

Clinical Manifestations

Manifestations are related to the area of the brain involved in the seizure activity and may range from single abnormal sensations, aberrant motor activity, altered consciousness or personality to loss of consciousness, and convulsive movements.

1. Impaired consciousness.
2. Disturbed muscle tone or movement.
3. Disturbances of behavior, mood, sensation, or perception.
4. Disturbances of autonomic functions.

Table 11-8 Antiepileptic Drugs

GENERIC NAME	DOSAGE FORMS	USUAL DOSES	HALF-LIFE	USUAL TARGET RANGE
Carbamazepine				
	• Suspension 100 mg/5 mL • Tablet 200 mg • Chew tab 100 mg • Extended-release tablets 100, 200, 400 mg • Extended-release sprinkle capsules 200, 300 mg	• 10–40 mg/kg/d divided bid for extended release; tid to qid for immediate release	Initial 20–50, then 5–14 h; induces own metabolism over the first 2 wk	4–12 μg/mL
Clonazepam				
	• Tablets 0.5, 1, 2 mg	• 0.01–0.3 mg/kg/d divided tid or given QHS • 0.5 mg PO tid—adults maximum 20 mg/d	20–40 h	20–70 μg/mL
Diazepam (rectal)				
	• Pediatric rectal gel 2.5, 5, 10 mg • Adult rectal gel 10, 15, 20 mg	• 2–5 y/o—0.5 mg/kg • 6–11 y/o—0.3 mg/kg • >12 y/o—0.2 mg/kg	30–60 h	Not applicable
Ethosuximide				
	• Capsule 250 mg • Solution 250 mg/5 mL	• 15–40 mg/kg/d divided bid	30–60 h	40–100 μg/mL
Felbamate				
	• Tablets 400, 600 mg • Suspension 600 mg/5 mL	• 15–45 mg/kg/d (or 1,200–3,600 mg) divided tid to qid; usual maximum 60 mg/kg/d	14–23 h	30–100 μg/mL
Gabapentin				
	• Capsule 100, 300, 400 mg • Tablets 600, 800 mg • Solution 250 mg/5 mL	• Initially 10–20 mg/kg/d divided tid to qid; titrate up to 40–60 mg/kg/d; usual maximum 90 mg/kg/d	5–9 h	4–20 μg/mL
Lamotrigine				
	• Tablets 25, 100, 150, 200 mg • Chew tablets 2, 5, 25 mg	• 200–500 mg/d divided bid • 2–15 mg/kg/d; start dose slowly	12–50 h up to 70 h with VPA	3–20 μg/mL
Lacosamide				
	• 50, 100, 150, 200 mg tablets. Oral solution 10 mg/mL; injection solution 10 mg/mL	• 200–400 mg/d in two divided doses	12–16 h	10–20 μg/mL
Levetiracetam				
	• Tablets 250, 500, 750 mg	• Initially 10 mg/kg PO divided bid or 500 mg PO bid; increase every 2 wk to 40–60 mg/kg/d	Adults 7 h	5–50 μg/mL
Lorazepam				
	• Tablets 0.5, 1, 2 mg • Solution 2 mg/mL • Injection 2, 4 mg/mL	• 0.05–0.1 mg/kg/dose; 4 mg/dose maximum may repeat in 10–15 min	10–20 h	50–240 μg/mL
Oxcarbazepine				
	• Tablets 150, 300, 600 mg	• Adult initially 300 mg PO bid, increase weekly to a usual maintenance dose of 1,200–2,400 mg/d • Child initially 10 mg/kg/d; titrate to a dose of 30–60 mg/kg/d	Parent 1–2.5 h; metabolite 8–15 h	10–35 μg/mL for the monohydroxy derivative

MECHANISM OF ACTION	INDICATIONS	DOSE-RELATED ADVERSE EFFECTS
Modulates sodium channels	• Simple-partial • Complex partial • Generalized tonic/clonic seizures	Double or blurred vision, lethargy (reduced by slow-dose titration)
Enhances GABA	• Myoclonic • Lennox-Gastaut syndrome • Atonic • Absence	Drowsiness (50%), ataxia (30%), behavioral disturbances (25%), movement disorders, slurred speech, hypersecretion
Enhances GABA	• Acute repetitive seizures	Sedation
Reduces current in the T-type calcium channel	• Absence	GI distress, drowsiness, hiccups, sedation
Blocks glycine binding to the NMDA receptors, modulates sodium channel, enhances GABA	• Lennox–Gastaut syndrome • Complex partial seizures	Anorexia, weight loss, vomiting, insomnia, headache, somnolence; rare cases of aplastic anemia (25 cases per 100,000) and liver failure (8 cases per 100,000) have also been seen.
Not known	• Partial seizures with or without secondary generalized tonic/clonic seizures	Somnolence, dizziness, ataxia, nystagmus, weight gain, nausea, vomiting, blurred vision, tremor, slurred speech, peripheral edema, dyspepsia, hiccups
Blocks sodium channels and blocks release of glutamate	• Simple partial seizures • Complex partial seizures • Generalized tonic/clonic seizures • Lennox-Gastaut syndrome • Absence	Fatigue, drowsiness, ataxia, dizziness, headache, nausea, vomiting, double or blurred vision, nystagmus
Modulates Na^+ channels	• Adjunctive treatment focal seizures with or without secondary generalization in patients aged 16 y and older in age	Dizziness, ataxia, fatigue, headache. Tremor, somnolence, balance disorder, memory impairment, vertigo, asthenia, gait disturbance, depression and bradycardia. Blurred vision, diplopia, nystagmus. Nausea, vomiting, and diarrhea
Inhibits propagation of seizure by unknown mechanism	• Partial-onset seizures	Somnolence (14.8%), asthenia (14.7%), coordination difficulties (3.4%), dizziness, nervousness, behavioral problems, decreased blood counts
Enhances GABA	• Status epilepticus	Sedation with risk of respiratory depression, amnesia, abnormal behavior, withdrawal reactions
Modulates sodium channels	• Partial-onset seizures	Headache, drowsiness, fatigue, nausea, dizziness, hyponatremia (hematologic toxicity not observed to date); dermatologic reactions (rash)

(continued)

Table 11-8 Antiepileptic Drugs *(continued)*

GENERIC NAME	DOSAGE FORMS	USUAL DOSES	HALF-LIFE	USUAL TARGET RANGE
Phenobarbital C-IV				
	• Capsule 16 mg • Elixir 15 mg/5 mL, 20 mg/5 mL • Tablet 8, 15, 16, 30, 32, 60, 65, 100 mg • Injection 30, 60, 65, 130 mg/mL	• 2–6 mg/kg/d divided qid to bid (high end of range for infants/young children)	40–140 h	15–40 µg/mL
Phenytoin, fosphenytoin				
	• Injection 50 mg/mL (fosphenytoin is 50 mg/mL phenytoin equivalent) • Suspension 125 mg/5 mL, 30 mg/5 mL • Chew tablets 50 mg • Capsules 30, 100 mg	• 4–12 mg/kg/d divided bid to tid for children getting PO; qid to bid for adults getting PO; divided q6h for IV dosing	5–34 h	10–20 µg/mL total 1–2 µg/mL free (for patients with protein binding)
Primidone				
	• Suspension 250 mg/5 mL • Tablets 50, 250 mg	• 10–25 mg/kg/d divided bid to tid; maximum 2 mg/d	4–20 h (PEMA ½ 30–36 h)	5–20 µg/mL
Rufinamide				
	200 and 400 mg film-coated tablets Oral suspension: 40 mg/mL	1,800–3,200 mg bid Children: 45 mg/kg/d.	6–10 h	10–25 µg/mL
Tiagabine				
	• Tablets 2, 4, 12, 16, 20 mg	• Adult 32–56 mg/d divided bid to qid (start with a 4 mg PO qid, adjust weekly) • Child 0.1 mg/kg/d divide tid, increase to 0.6 mg/kg/d (1 mg/kg/d with enzyme inducers)	2–9 h	5–70 µg/mL
Topiramate				
	• Tablets 25, 100, 200 mg • Sprinkle capsules 15, 25 mg	• Children initiate at 0.5–1 mg/kg/d divided bid; usual dose is 6–12 mg/kg/d divided bid to tid • Adult: 200–800 mg/d divided bid; initiate slowly with 25 mg qh, increase weekly	12–30 h	2–25 µg/mL
VPA/divalproex sodium				
	• Solution 250 mg/5 mL • Capsule 250 mg • Sprinkle 125 mg • Extended release 500 mg • Tablet 125, 200, 500 mg	• 15–60 mg/kg/d divided bid to tid	7–20 h	50–150 µg/mL
Vigabatrin				
	• Tablet 500 mg scored	• Adult: 2–4 mg/d divided bid • Children: 1–2 mg/d or 40–100 mg/kg/d	5–7 h	Not known
Zonisamide				
	• Capsule 100 mg	• Adult 200–400 mg/d PO bid (max 600 mg), initially 100 mg PO qid and adjust every 2 wk • Children initially 1 mg/kg/d, adjust every 2 wk (maximum 15 mg/kg/d)	27–60 h	15–40 µg/mL

bid, twice daily; GABA, gamma-aminobutyric acid; GI, gastrointestinal; IV, intravenous; NMDA, N-methyl-D-aspartate; PEMA, phenylethylmalonamide; PO, orally; q, every; tid, three times daily; VPA, valproic acid.

MECHANISM OF ACTION	INDICATIONS	DOSE-RELATED ADVERSE EFFECTS
Enhances GABA	• Generalized tonic/clonic seizures • Simple partial seizures • Complex partial seizures	Sedation, mental dullness, cognitive impairment, hyperactivity, ataxia
Modulates sodium channels	• Generalized tonic/clonic seizures • Complex partial seizures • Simple partial seizures	Nystagmus, ataxia, lethargy, propylene glycol in IV preparation can cause myocardial depression, bradycardias, other electrocardiogram changes, hypotension, rash.
Enhances GABA	• Generalized tonic/clonic seizures • Simple partial seizures • Complex partial seizures	Same as phenobarbital
Modulates Na^+ channel	Adjunctive treatment focal seizures with or without secondary generalization. In children >4 yr used as adjunctive treatment of seizures associated with Lennox-Gastaut syndrome	Somnolence, coordination abnormalities. Dizziness, gait disturbances, and ataxia. Vomiting, rash, headache, increased risk of suicide thoughts or behavior. Contraindicated in patients with familial short QT syndrome
Inhibits neuronal and glial uptake of GABA	• Partial-onset seizures	Sedation, dizziness, memory impairment, inattention, emotional lability, headache, abdominal pain, anorexia, tremor
Modulates sodium channels, enhances GABA activity, and modulates NMDA receptor	• Partial-onset seizures • Lennox-Gastaut syndrome • Generalized tonic/clonic • Juvenile myoclonic epilepsy	Speech and language problems, difficulty with concentration and attention, confusion, fatigue, paresthesias, weight loss
Unknown (may modulate sodium channel, enhance GABA)	• Generalized tonic/clonic seizures • Absence • Myoclonic • Partial-onset seizures • Lennox-Gastaut syndrome	GI upset, lethargy, changes in menstrual cycle, thrombocytopenia
Inhibits GABA transaminase (preventing GABA metabolism)	• Infantile spasms due to tuberous sclerosis	Drowsiness, fatigue, ataxia, behavioral changes, weight gain, psychosis (in predisposed patients and upon abrupt withdrawal), hematologic, visual field problems
Modulates sodium and T-type calcium channels	• Partial-onset seizures • Generalized seizures • Absence • Myoclonic • Lennox-Gastaut • Infantile spasms	Drowsiness, psychosis (2%)

Diagnostic Evaluation

1. Electroencephalography (EEG) with or without video monitoring—locates epileptic focus, spread, intensity, and duration; helps classify seizure type.
2. Magnetic resonance imaging (MRI), computed tomography (CT) scan—to identify lesion that may be cause of seizure.
3. Single-photon emission computed tomography (SPECT) or positron emission tomography (PET) scan—additional tests to identify seizure foci.
4. Neuropsychological studies—to evaluate for behavioral disturbances.
5. Serum laboratory studies or lumbar puncture—to evaluate for infectious, hormonal, or metabolic etiology.

Management

1. Pharmacotherapy—antiepileptic drugs (AEDs) selected according to seizure type (see Table 11-8, pages 398-401).
2. Biofeedback—useful in the patient with reliable auras.
3. Surgery considered in patients who are refractory to antiepileptic medications or require the use of more than two AEDs. Standardized surgical procedures include anteromesial temporal resection, corpus callosotomy, hemispherectomy.
4. Modulation therapy—in those who are refractory to medication and not candidates for traditional surgery.
   a. Vagal nerve stimulation—sends regular electrical impulses to the brain via the vagus nerve to reduce seizures.
   b. Intracranial neurostimulator—new procedure that monitors electrical activity of the brain and is programmed to deliver impulses at a certain rate and pulse width to reduce seizures.
   c. Deep brain stimulation—electrodes placed within deeper structures of the brain and connected to a stimulator placed in the anterior upper chest wall. Delivers chronic stimulation, thus preventing seizure activity.

Complications

1. Status epilepticus (see Box 11-7).
2. Injuries due to falls, especially head injuries.
3. SUDEP (sudden unexplained death in epilepsy).

Nursing Assessment

1. Obtain seizure history, including prodromal signs and symptoms, seizure behavior, postictal state, history of status epilepticus.
2. Document the following about seizure activity:
   a. Circumstances before attack, such as visual, auditory, olfactory, or tactile stimuli; emotional or psychological disturbances; sleep; hyperventilation.
   b. Description of movement, including where movement or stiffness started; type of movement and parts involved; progression of movement; whether beginning of seizure was witnessed.
   c. Position of the eyes and head; size of pupils.
   d. Presence of automatisms, such as lip smacking or repeated swallowing.
   e. Incontinence of urine or feces.
   f. Duration of each phase of the attack.
   g. Presence of unconsciousness and its duration.
   h. Behavior after attack, including inability to speak, any weakness or paralysis (Todd paralysis), sleep.
3. Investigate the psychosocial effect of seizures.
4. Obtain history of drug or alcohol misuse.
5. Assess adherence and medication-taking strategies. Nonadherence to medication regimen as well as toxicity of antiepileptic medications can increase seizure frequency. Obtain drug levels before implementing medication changes.

Nursing Interventions

Maintaining Cerebral Tissue Perfusion

1. Maintain a patent airway until the patient is fully awake after a seizure.
2. Provide oxygen during the seizure if color change occurs.
3. Stress the importance of taking medications regularly.
4. Monitor serum levels for therapeutic range of medications.
5. Monitor the patient for toxic adverse effects of medications.
6. Monitor platelet and liver functions for toxicity due to medications.

Preventing Injury

1. Provide a safe environment by padding side rails and removing clutter.
2. Place the bed in a low position.
3. Do not restrain the patient during a seizure.
4. Do not put anything in the patient's mouth during a seizure.
5. Place the patient on their side during a seizure to prevent aspiration.
6. Protect the patient's head during a seizure. If seizure occurs while ambulating or from chair, cradle head or provide cushion/support for protection against head injury.
7. Stay with the patient who is ambulating or who is in a confused state during seizure.
8. Provide a helmet to the patient who falls during seizure.
9. Manage the patient in status epilepticus.

Strengthening Coping

1. Consult with social worker for community resources for vocational rehabilitation, counselors, support groups.
2. Teach stress reduction techniques that will fit into the patient's lifestyle.
3. Initiate appropriate consultation for the management of behaviors related to personality disorders, brain damage secondary to chronic epilepsy.
4. Answer questions related to the use of computerized video EEG monitoring and surgery for epilepsy management.

Community and Home Care Considerations

1. Counsel patients with uncontrolled seizures about driving or operating dangerous equipment. Be familiar with state laws regarding driving while on or tapering AEDs.
2. Assess home environment for safety hazards in case the patient falls, such as crowded furniture arrangement, sharp edges on tables, and glass. Soft flooring and furniture and padded surfaces may be necessary.
3. Provide instructions on safety precautions while performing activities alone to prevent injury, drowning, or choking.
4. Support the patient in discussion about seizures with employer, school, and so forth.
5. SUDEP can be reduced by decreasing the number of seizures that a patient experiences and by taking medications, as prescribed. Although multiple medications may be required to reduce seizure frequency, it should be considered within the context of quality of life and risk reduction.

BOX 11-7 Emergency Management of Status Epilepticus

Status epilepticus (acute, prolonged, repetitive seizure activity) is a series of generalized seizures without return to consciousness between attacks. The term has been broadened to include continuous clinical and/or electrical seizures lasting at least 5 minutes, even without impairment of consciousness. Status epilepticus is considered a serious neurologic emergency. It has high mortality and morbidity (permanent brain damage, severe neurologic deficits). Factors that precipitate status epilepticus in patients with preexisting seizure disorder include medication withdrawal, fever, metabolic or environmental stresses, alcohol or drug withdrawal, and sleep deprivation.

NURSING INTERVENTIONS

- Establish airway and maintain blood pressure (BP).
- Obtain blood studies for glucose blood urea nitrogen, electrolytes, and anticonvulsant drug levels to determine metabolic abnormalities and serve as a guide for maintenance of biochemical homeostasis.
- Administer oxygen—there is some respiratory depression associated with each seizure, which may produce venous congestion and hypoxia of the brain.
- Establish intravenous (IV) lines and keep open for blood sampling, drug administration, and infusion of fluids.
- Administer IV anticonvulsant (lorazepam, phenytoin, diazepam) *slowly* to ensure effective brain tissue and serum concentrations.
  - Give additional anticonvulsants, as directed—effects of lorazepam are of short duration.
  - Monitor anticonvulsant drug levels regularly.
- Monitor the patient continuously; depression of respiration and BP induced by drug therapy may be delayed.
- Use mechanical ventilation, as needed.
- If initial treatment is unsuccessful, general anesthesia may be required.
- Assist with search for precipitating factors.
  - Monitor vital and neurologic signs on a continuous basis.
  - Use electroencephalographic monitoring to determine nature and abolition (after diazepam administration) of epileptic activity.
  - Determine (from family member) whether there is a history of epilepsy, alcohol/drug use, trauma, recent infection.

Patient Education and Health Maintenance

1. Encourage the patient to determine existence of trigger factors for seizures (e.g., skipped meals, lack of sleep, emotional stress, menstrual cycle).
2. Remind the patient of the importance of following medication regimen.
3. Tell the patient to avoid alcohol because it interferes with metabolism of antiepileptic medications.
4. Encourage the patient and family to discuss feelings and attitudes about epilepsy.
5. Encourage the patient to carry or wear a medical alert device.
6. Encourage a moderate lifestyle that includes exercise, mental activity, and nutritional diet.
7. For the surgical candidate, reinforce instructions related to surgical outcome of the specific surgical approach (temporal lobectomy, corpus callosotomy, hemispherectomy, and extratemporal resection).
8. Refer the patient/family for more information and support to agencies such as the Epilepsy Foundation of America (www.efa.org).

Evaluation: Expected Outcomes

- Takes medication as ordered, drug level within normal range.
- No injuries observed.
- Reports using support services and stress management techniques.

Narcolepsy

Narcolepsy is a neurologic disorder characterized by abnormalities of rapid eye movement (REM) sleep, some abnormalities of non-REM sleep, and excessive daytime sleepiness.

Pathophysiology and Etiology

1. Recent advances suggest that this common sleep disorder may be a neurodegenerative or autoimmune disorder resulting in the loss of hypothalamic neurons that contain a peptide, hypocretin (orexin). Hypocretin plays a central role in the timing of sleep and wakefulness and inhibits REM sleep. The deficiency in hypocretin contributes to the abnormalities of sleep and wakefulness in narcolepsy.
2. Genetic susceptibility—associated with class II human leukocyte antigens.
3. Although considered a hypersomnia disorder, the person does not experience excessive amounts of sleep in a 24-hour period. Typically, patients with narcolepsy have an optimal amount of sleep over 24 hours. They have abnormal REM sleep that intrudes into wakefulness.
4. Onset is usually between ages 15 and 25 years.

Clinical Manifestations

1. Four classic symptoms (all symptoms not present in all patients):
   a. Excessive daytime sleepiness is usually the first symptom.
   b. Cataplexy (abrupt loss of muscle tone after emotional stimulation such as laughter, anger).
   c. Sleep paralysis (powerless to move limbs, speak, open eyes, or breathe deeply while fully aware of condition).
   d. Hypnagogic hallucinations (drowsiness before sleep, usually visual or auditory).
2. Symptoms enhanced by high temperature, indoor activity, and idleness.
3. Clinical manifestations may abate, but never phase out completely.
4. Patient may complain of inability to focus vision or thought process rather than have a feeling of sleepiness.
5. Nocturnal sleep disturbance—occurs 2.5 to 3 hours after falling asleep.
   a. After being awake for 45 to 60 minutes, the patient will fall back to sleep for another 2.5 to 3 hours and then awaken again.
   b. This is believed to be the source of the daytime somnolence.

Diagnostic Evaluation

1. An overnight polysomnogram in a sleep disorders lab is included in the evaluation to assess nighttime sleep—indicates the underlying cause for the complaint of sleepiness. The polysomnogram helps evaluate sleep quality and excludes other disorders, such as sleep apnea.
2. The polysomnogram is followed the next day by a multiple sleep latency test to assess daytime sleepiness—indicates severity of the problem. Patients are given four or five opportunities to nap every 2 hours. Patients with narcolepsy typically fall asleep more rapidly than the norm of 10 to 15 minutes.

Management

1. Long-term treatment is required. Mutual goal setting is imperative because not everyone derives benefit from treatment. Even with medication, patients may never attain normal levels of alertness.
2. Nonpharmacologic therapy includes support groups, short naps (10 to 20 minutes, three times daily), caffeinated beverages, exercise, sleep hygiene techniques, and avoidance of heavy meals.
3. Stimulants prescribed may include pemoline, methylphenidate, dextroamphetamine, and methamphetamine.
4. Antidepressants for cataplexy; protriptyline, desipramine, fluoxetine.
5. Other medications for cataplexy can include modafinil (Provigil), sodium oxybate (XYWAV), pitolisant (SUNOSI), and methylphenidate (Ritalin).

Complications

1. Injury related to falling asleep.
2. Psychosocial problems, such as disturbed relationships, loss of employment, and depression.

Nursing Assessment

1. Obtain history of sleep and activity pattern.
2. Assess emotional status and social interactions.
3. Assess response to medication and lifestyle treatment.

Nursing Interventions

Promoting Normal Sleep–Wake Cycle

1. Review daily schedule to determine periods of sleep and cataplexy. Advise to wake at the same time daily.
2. Help the patient establish nondrug therapies (exercise, diet) that will fit into lifestyle.
3. Make sure that the bedroom is dark, cool, and quiet to facilitate sleep.
4. Administer or teach self-administration of prescribed medications.
   a. Advise of adverse effects of amphetamines, such as nervousness, irritability, tremors, and gastrointestinal (GI) upset.
   b. Warn the patient to take only as prescribed and not to increase dosage because of tolerance and drug dependence.

Reducing Fatigue

1. Schedule 10- to 20-minute rest periods two or three times per day. Help the patient incorporate naps into lifestyle.
2. Encourage the patient to incorporate small amounts of caffeinated beverages at intervals and smaller, more frequent meals rather than large, heavy meals during the day to maintain energy.
3. Plan diversional activities and relaxation during fatigued periods.

Strengthening Coping

1. Encourage active participation in selection of treatment modalities.
2. Assist the patient in identifying trigger factors of worsening symptoms.
3. Teach problem-solving strategy to promote sense of control over activities and symptoms during the day.
4. Review patient coping mechanisms and reinforce positive ones.
5. Assist the patient to discuss information about narcolepsy with friends, family, school, and employers to help reduce anxiety and/or embarrassment about their condition.
6. Encourage the use of support groups and community resources, such as the American Sleep Association (www.sleepassociation.org).

Patient Education and Health Maintenance

1. Review the normal sleep cycle and the pathophysiology of narcolepsy.
2. Stress the importance of nonpharmacologic measures as an adjunct to treatment.
3. Inform the patient of rights of employment conditions under the Americans with Disabilities Act.
4. Advise caution with using alcohol, working with machinery, or using dangerous equipment to prevent injury to self or others during sleepiness or cataplexy.
5. If the patient drives, advise using caution and avoiding lengthy trips.
6. Encourage the patient to wear a medical alert device.
7. Encourage follow-up with health care provider, specialist, and mental health counselor, as needed.

Evaluation: Expected Outcomes

- Complies with medication regimen.
- Reports working without undue fatigue.
- Identifies trigger factors.

Headache Syndromes

Headaches are one of the most common complaints of people seeking health care. Pain in the head is a symptom of underlying pathology. The International Headache Society instituted a classification system that is the standard for defining various types of headaches. It divides headaches into two categories: primary headache disorders, which include migraine, tension-type headache, and cluster headache, and secondary headache disorders. Identifying the etiology of headaches requires an understanding of the characteristics of each type of headache.

EVIDENCE BASE Eigenbrodt, A. K., Ashina, H., Khan, S., Diener, H. C., Mitsikostas, D. D., Sinclair, A. J., Pozo-Rosich, P., Martelletti, P., Ducros, A., Lantéri-Minet, M., Braschinsky, M., Del Rio, M. S., Daniel, O., Özge, A., Mammadbayli, A., Arons, M., Skorobogatykh, K., Romanenko, V., Terwindt, G. M., & Ashina, M. (2021). Diagnosis and management of migraine in ten steps. *Nature Reviews Neurology*, *17*(8), 501–514. https://doi.org/10.1038/s41582-021-00509-5

Pathophysiology and Etiology

Primary Headaches

Diagnosis is generally based on the characteristic clinical history and elimination of other pathology, such as stroke, intracranial bleed, arteriovenous malformation (AVM), or brain tumor.

1. Migraine headache—consists of initial vasospasm followed by dilation of intracranial and extracranial arteries; occurs in about 10% of the population.
   a. Caused by hyperactivity to the neurotransmitter serotonin; familial predisposition.
   b. Attack may consist of any of four phases: premonitory phase, aura phase, headache phase, and postdrome phase.
   c. Classified with or without aura (usually visual); aura is due to reduced cortical neuronal activity.
2. Tension headache—due to irritation of sensitive nerve endings in the head, jaw, and neck from prolonged muscle contraction in the face, head, and neck; mild or moderate intensity that does not prohibit activity.
   a. Precipitating factors include fatigue, stress, and poor posture.
   b. Characterized by hatband distribution.
3. Cluster headache—release of increased histamine results in vasodilation.
   a. Usually unilateral, recurring.
   b. Occurs more often in males.

Secondary Headaches

Headache due to a neurologic or systemic disease.

1. Mass lesion (tumor, abscess, AVM, subdural or epidural hematoma [EDH]).
2. Intracranial infection (bacterial/viral/fungal meningitis or encephalitis).
3. Inflammation (giant cell arteritis, vasculitis).
4. Cerebrovascular disease (subarachnoid hemorrhage [SAH], intracranial hemorrhage, occlusive vascular disease).
5. Increased ICP.
6. Low-pressure headache (post–lumbar puncture, trauma induced).
7. Sinus infection, viral infection such as influenza, systemic illness.

Clinical Manifestations

1. Migraine: Sensory, motor, or mood alterations precede headache; gradual onset of severe unilateral, throbbing headache; may become bilateral.
   a. Migraine with aura (classic migraine), characteristic aura may include scintillating scotoma (area of decreased vision surrounded by area of less abnormal or normal vision with zigzag appearance), hemianopsia (loss of half of field of vision), and paresthesias; headache follows aura in less than 1 hour; usually lasts less than a day.
   b. Migraine without aura (common migraine), nausea, vomiting, and photophobia may accompany moderate-to-severe headache; worsened by activity; may last 4 to 72 hours and greatly impair activities.
   c. Either type of migraine may be triggered in females by hormonal fluctuations (menses, pregnancy), excess or lack of sleep, change in eating habits, and certain food additives.
2. Tension/muscle contraction: dull, bandlike, constricting, persistent pain and pressure in the back of the head and neck, across forehead, bitemporal areas; may be tender points of head or neck.
   a. Not aggravated by activity, but may be worsened by noise and light.
   b. No nausea and vomiting, but may be associated with anorexia.
3. Cluster headache: sudden, sharp, burning, excruciating, unilateral pain; always involving facial area from neck to temple and often occurs during the evening or night; more frequent in males.
   a. Occurs in clusters of 2 to 8 weeks, followed by headache-free periods.
   b. Associated with unilateral excessive tearing, redness of the eye, stuffiness of nostril on affected side, facial swelling, flushing, and sweating.
   c. Attacks last several minutes to several days. Multiple attacks may occur in 1 day.

Diagnostic Evaluation

1. Skull/sinus films to rule out lesions, sinusitis.
2. CT scan/MRI to rule out lesions, hemorrhage, chronic sinusitis.
3. Erythrocyte sedimentation rate (ESR) and other blood studies to help determine inflammatory process with temporal arteritis.

CLINICAL JUDGMENT "Red flags" for possible serious cause of headache (hemorrhage, stroke, tumor, infection) include altered LOC; neurologic findings such as weakness, facial droop, dysarthria, or aphasia; nausea and vomiting; new onset of or change in characteristic headaches; and patient reporting that it is "the worst headache of my life." These patients should be evaluated with a brain CT scan.

Management

Pharmacologic Treatment

Medications are intended to reduce the frequency, severity, and duration of the headache. Effectiveness of medication is individualized. Some persons may need a combination of medications.

1. Management includes combination of diet, sleep hygiene, consistent caffeine intake, regular exercise, and avoidance of triggers.
2. Management of migraine headaches includes abortive and preventive medications.
3. Abortive agents include methysergide, a serotonin antagonist; ergotamine, a vasoconstrictor; or 5-hydroxytryptamine (5HT)-agonists such as sumatriptan. Newer agents include lasmiditan (Reyvow), a 5HT-receptor agonist (does not affect the 5HT receptor that mediates vasoconstriction); ubrogepant and rimegepant, which target to lock calcitonin gene–related peptide (CGRP). Other oral 5HT-agonists include zolmitriptan, naratriptan, and rizatriptan.
4. Preventive medications commonly used in the treatment of migraine headaches include antiseizure medications, antidepressants, beta-blockers, and calcium channel blockers.
5. Aspirin, acetaminophen, and nonsteroidal anti-inflammatory drugs (NSAIDs) may be used for mild-to-moderate pain of tension, sinus, or mild vascular headaches.
6. Inhalation of 100% oxygen may abort a cluster headache.
7. Antihistamines and decongestants may be effective for sinus headaches.
8. Corticosteroids may be used for temporal arteritis.
9. Occasionally, opioid analgesics, muscle relaxants, and antianxiety agents may be needed for severe pain.
10. Vitamin supplements including magnesium and vitamin B_2 may be beneficial in preventing headache episodes.

DRUG ALERT Vasoconstrictors and 5HT-agonists used to abort vascular headaches are contraindicated in patients with uncontrolled hypertension, coronary artery disease, and peripheral vascular disease.

Nonpharmacologic Management

1. Relaxation techniques, guided imagery, paced breathing.
2. Biofeedback, cognitive therapy.
3. Trigger identification and control of factors such as intake of alcohol (red wine), skipped meals, oversleeping, or undersleeping. Anticipatory guidance in proper sleep hygiene.
4. To prevent migraine: avoidance of monosodium glutamate, mixed spices such as "seasoned salt," nitrates and nitrites commonly contained in bacon, hot dogs, or deli meats.
5. Rest in a quiet, dark room at the onset of headache.
6. If a person who uses caffeine, spread caffeine intake evenly over the day.
7. Routine exercise program.

Complications

1. Usually none from primary headaches.

Nursing Assessment

1. Obtain a history of related symptoms, triggering factors, degree of pain, and medications used.
2. Perform a complete neurologic examination to detect any focal deficits or signs of increased intracranial pressure (ICP) that indicate tumor or hemorrhage.
3. Assess coping mechanisms and emotional status.

Nursing Interventions

Controlling Pain

1. Reduce environmental stimuli: light, noise, and movement to decrease the severity of pain.
2. Suggest light massage for tight muscles in neck, scalp, or back for tension headaches.
3. Apply warm, moist heat to areas of muscle tension.
4. Encourage patient to lie down and attempt to sleep.
5. Teach progressive muscle relaxation to treat and prevent tension headaches.
   a. Alternately tense and relax each group of muscles for a count of five, starting with the forehead and working downward to the feet.
   b. Try to maintain a state of relaxation of each muscle group until the whole body feels relaxed.
   c. Relaxation of just head and neck may also be helpful if time is limited.
6. Teach patient the cause of headache and proper use of medication.
7. Encourage adequate rest once headache is relieved to recover from fatigue of the pain.

Promoting Positive Coping

1. Encourage patient to become aware of triggering factors and early symptoms of headache so it can be prevented or promptly treated. Hunger, lack of exercise, and erratic sleep schedules may trigger headaches.
2. Encourage adequate nutrition, rest and relaxation, and avoidance of stress and overexertion to better cope with headaches.
3. Implement problem-solving to help patient manage problems that arise in social or work situations related to headaches.
4. Review coping mechanisms and strengthen positive ones.
5. Promote use of headache diary.

Patient Education and Health Maintenance

1. Teach proper administration of medication.
   a. Self-injection of sumatriptan given subcutaneously with autoinjector.
   b. Oral inhalation technique of ergotamine through metered-dose inhaler.
   c. Nasal spray dosing of sumatriptan.
2. Teach about adverse effects of medications.
   a. GI upset, gastritis, and possible ulcer formation with NSAIDs—take with food.
   b. Numbness, coldness, paresthesias, and pain of extremities with ergot derivatives—report to health care provider.
   c. Chest pain, wheezing, flushing with sumatriptan—report to health care provider.
   d. Hypotension with beta-adrenergic blockers and calcium channel blockers—arise slowly, do not exceed prescribed dosage, do not discontinue beta-adrenergic blockers abruptly.
3. Advise avoidance of alcohol, which can worsen headaches.
4. Teach about foods that are high in tyramine, which may trigger migraines—aged cheese, red wine, some processed meats. Some food additives such as nitrates may also trigger migraines, and many people identify their own individual triggers.
5. Teach patient how to perform relaxation techniques to reduce stress and promote inner well-being.
6. Refer patient for more information to the International Headache Society (http://www.ihs-headache.org/).

Evaluation: Expected Outcomes

- Reports fewer, less severe headaches.
- Describes use of positive coping mechanisms.

Herniated Intervertebral Disk

Herniation of the intervertebral disk (ruptured disk) is a protrusion of the nucleus of the disk into the annulus (fibrous ring around the disk) with subsequent nerve compression. The herniation may occur in any portion of the vertebral column (see Figure 11-13). The pressure on spinal nerve roots or the spinal cord causes severe, chronic, or recurrent back and leg pain.

Pathophysiology and Etiology

1. The intervertebral disk is a cartilaginous plate made up of gelatinous material in the center, known as the *nucleus pulposus*, and is encapsulated in the fibrous annulus.
2. About 90% of herniated disks involve the lumbar and lumbosacral spine. The most common site is the L4–L5 disk space. The cause of a herniated lumbar disk is usually a flexion injury, but many patients do not recall experiencing a traumatic event. Cervical herniation is less common; but when it does occur, it is usually in individuals aged 45 years or older.
3. Risk factors for herniation include:
   a. Degeneration (aging), trauma, and congenital predisposition.
   b. Biomechanical factors, such as twisting and repetitive motions in occupational settings.
   c. Sedentary occupations.
   d. Obesity.
   e. Smoking.

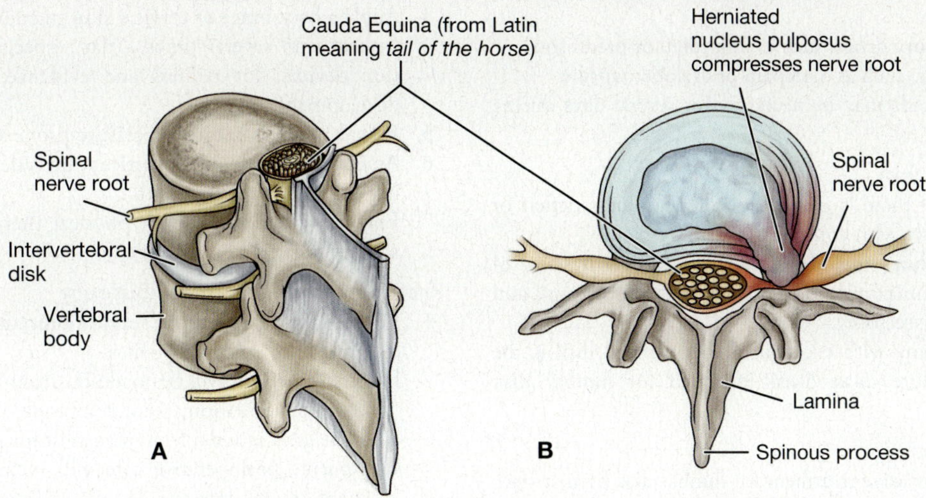

Figure 11-13. **(A)** Normal lumbar spine vertebrae, intervertebral disks, and spinal nerve root. **(B)** Ruptured vertebral disk. (Reprinted with permission from Hinkle, J. L., Cheever, K. H., & Overbaugh, K. [2022]. *Brunner & Suddarth's textbook of medical-surgical nursing* [15th ed., Fig. 65-6.]. Wolters Kluwer.)

4. The herniation compresses the spinal nerve root, usually restricted to one side and, with further degeneration of the disk, may eventually produce pressure on the spinal cord.
5. This sequence may take months to years, producing acute and chronic symptoms.

Clinical Manifestations

General Considerations

1. An intervertebral disk may herniate without causing symptoms.
2. Symptoms depend on the location, size, rate of development, and effect on surrounding structures.
3. Most symptomatic disk herniations result in pain, sensory changes, loss of reflex, and muscle weakness that resolve without surgery.

Cervical

1. Pain and stiffness in the neck, top of shoulders, and region of the scapula.
2. Pain in upper extremities and head.
3. Paresthesias and numbness of upper extremities.
4. Weakness of upper extremities.

Lumbar

1. Lower back pain with varying degrees of sensory and motor dysfunction.
2. Pain radiating from the lower back into the buttocks and down the leg, referred to as *sciatica*.
3. A stiff or unnatural posture.
4. Some combination of paresthesias, weakness, and reflex impairment.
5. Positive straight-leg raise test: Pain occurs in leg below the knee when leg is raised from a supine position.

CLINICAL JUDGMENT Cauda equina syndrome is an urgent condition caused by an acute compression of the cauda equina area of the spinal cord by massive disk extrusion. Symptoms include progressive sensory and motor loss of lower extremities, saddle anesthesia (loss of sensation around perineum), bowel and/or bladder incontinence, or sexual dysfunction. It must be recognized early, and compression must be relieved to prevent permanent loss of these functions. If patients report such symptoms, emergent assessment and intervention is indicated.

Diagnostic Evaluation

1. CT scan or MRI—demonstrates herniation; MRI has greater sensitivity.
2. Electromyography—localizes specific spinal nerve involvement.
3. Myelogram—rarely done, but demonstrates herniation and pressure on spinal cord or nerve roots.

Management

Nonpharmacologic Measures

1. Bed rest on a firm mattress (2 days usually sufficient) usually results in improvement in 80% of patients.
2. Heat or ice massage to affected area.
3. Cervical collar or possibly cervical traction is widely used, although efficacy is not proven.
4. Physical therapy may be prescribed to maximize function and assist the patient in recovery.
5. Epidural steroid injection may be administered by interventional radiologist, particularly with the presence of radiculopathy, radiating/shooting pain down the extremity, to relieve symptoms.
6. Nonpharmacologic and pharmacologic measures may be used together for 4 to 6 weeks as conservative management if there is no progressive neurologic deficit.
   a. More than 90% of low back pain episodes resolve completely by 4 to 6 weeks, and those with herniated disk may experience spontaneous remission of pain.
   b. Surgical intervention is reserved for those with neurologic deficits or persistent symptoms over 6 weeks and is designed to relieve radicular (sciatic) pain.

Pharmacotherapy

1. Anti-inflammatory drugs, such as ibuprofen or prednisone.
2. Muscle relaxants, such as diazepam or cyclobenzaprine.
3. Analgesics; opioids may be necessary for several days during acute phase.

Surgical Intervention

1. May be done if there is progression of neurologic deficit or failure to improve with conservative management.
2. Surgical procedures include discectomy (decompression of nerve root), laminectomy, spinal fusion, microdiscectomy, and percutaneous discectomy.
3. Hemilaminectomy with excision of the involved disk is the surgical procedure most often indicated for lumbar disk disease.

Chemonucleolysis

1. Less common invasive treatment for lumbar disk herniation.
2. Injection of chymopapain into herniated disk that produces loss of water and proteoglycans from the disk, reducing the size of the disk and subsequent pressure on the nerve root.
3. May cause severe complications, such as transverse myelitis, allergic reactions, and persistent muscle spasm.

Alternative and Complementary Measures

1. Acupuncture.
2. Manipulative therapy.
3. Massage therapy for adjunct pain relief.
4. Homeopathic remedies.
5. Various nutritional supplements.

Complications

1. Permanent neurologic dysfunction (weakness, numbness).
2. Chronic pain with associated psychosocial issues.
3. Cauda equina syndrome.

Nursing Assessment

1. Perform repeated assessments of motor function, sensation, and reflexes to determine progression of condition.
2. Assess level at which straight-leg raise test is positive; generally, radiation of pain below knee at 45 degrees of elevation is considered positive for nerve root involvement; positive at lesser elevation may indicate worsening condition.
3. Assess pain level on scale of 0 to 10.

Nursing Interventions

Minimizing Pain

1. Administer or teach self-administration of anti-inflammatory drugs, as prescribed, and with food or antacid to prevent GI upset.
2. Administer or teach self-administration of prescribed muscle relaxant; observe safety because drowsiness may result.
3. Administer or teach self-administration of analgesics, as prescribed; be prepared for sedation.
4. Encourage regular activity with limits of pain.
5. Apply dry or moist heat to affected area of back, as desired.
6. Encourage relaxation techniques, such as imagery and progressive muscle relaxation.

Maintaining Mobility

1. Encourage range of motion (ROM) exercises while in bed.
2. Properly fit and use a cervical collar (if appropriate to level of injury).
3. Apply a back brace or cervical skin traction, if ordered.
4. Inspect skin several times a day, especially under stabilization devices, for redness and evidence of pressure injury development.
5. Provide good skin care to pressure-prone areas.
6. Assist the patient with activities at bedside and discourage lifting or straining of any kind.
7. Encourage adherence with physical therapy treatments and activity restrictions, as ordered.

Preparing the Patient for Surgery

1. Educate the patient about surgical procedure.
   a. Procedure is generally short.
   b. Small incision will be made on front or back of neck for cervical herniation; second incision may be on hip if a bone graft is taken from iliac crest for spinal fusion.
   c. Routine postoperative care will include frequent assessment of vital signs and neurologic function, frequent turning and deep breathing, pain control, and ambulation on the first postoperative day.
2. Document baseline neurologic assessment to compare with after surgery.
3. Explain your actions to the patient as you prepare the operative area, administer preoperative medications, and perform any other preoperative order.

Preventing Complications Postoperatively

1. Monitor vital signs and surgical dressing frequently because hemorrhage is a possible complication.
2. If the patient has a wound drainage system, check tubing frequently for patency and secure vacuum seal.
3. Assess movement and sensation of extremities regularly, report new deficit.
4. Administer analgesics and steroid medications to control pain from incision and swelling around nerve roots and spinal cord due to surgery.
5. Maintain cervical collar, if ordered.
6. Logroll the patient to reposition frequently and encourage coughing and deep breathing.
7. Position the patient for comfort with a small pillow under their head (but avoid extreme neck flexion) and pillow under knees to take pressure off lower back.
8. Provide fluids as soon as gag reflex and bowel sounds are noted.
9. Assess for hoarseness, which suggests that cervical surgery resulted in a recurrent laryngeal nerve injury; this injury may cause an ineffective cough.
10. Watch for dysphagia due to edema of the esophagus and provide dietary modifications, as necessary.
11. Make sure that the patient voids after surgery; report urine retention.
12. Encourage ambulation as soon as possible by having the patient lie on the side close to the edge of the bed and push up with arms while swinging legs toward floor in one motion; alternate walking with bed rest, discourage sitting.
13. Report any sudden reappearance of radicular pain (may indicate nerve root compression from slipping of bone graft or collapsing of disk space) or burning back pain radiating to buttocks (may indicate arachnoiditis).

Community and Home Care Considerations

1. Demonstrate and encourage back strengthening, aerobic exercise (walking, biking, swimming), and endurance exercises.

2. Make sure that the patient avoids heavy lifting and bending/twisting from the waist and uses proper body mechanics in all activities.
3. Discourage prolonged bed rest and inactivity.
4. Refer for vocational counseling, if indicated.
5. If cervical skin traction is ordered for home use, teach the patient how to apply the chinstrap and head halter. The weight should hang freely over the back of a chair or doorknob near the head of the bed. Make sure the patient maintains proper alignment of the neck and removes traction before moving the head.

Patient Education and Health Maintenance

1. Educate the patient regarding lifestyle changes—smoking cessation, increased activity, weight loss.
2. Provide instructions regarding back anatomy and back care to reduce symptoms.
3. Teach the patient the importance of cervical collar use and other conservative measures to try to reduce inflammation and heal disk herniation.
4. Tell the patient who has had a cervical disk herniation to avoid extreme flexion, extension, or rotation of the neck and to keep the head in neutral position during sleep.
5. Encourage the patient with a lumbar disk herniation to maintain ADLs within pain limits, but lifting and sitting for prolonged periods are discouraged.
6. Encourage the patient to do stretching and strengthening exercises of the extremities and abdomen after acute symptoms have subsided. The back can be gently stretched by lying on the back and bringing the knees up toward the chest.
7. Teach the patient about proper body mechanics and the use of leg and abdominal muscles rather than the back. Knees should be bent on lifting and load should be carried close to midtrunk.
8. Encourage follow-up with physical therapy, as indicated, for reconditioning and work hardening.
9. Tell the patient to avoid the prone position, long car rides, and sitting in a soft chair.
10. Instruct the patient to report any changes in neurologic function or recurrence of radicular pain.
11. Encourage good nutrition, avoidance of obesity, and proper rest to reduce the risk of recurrence.

Evaluation: Expected Outcomes

- Verbalizes reduced pain.
- Maintains mobility with active lifestyle.
- Expresses understanding of preoperative preparation and postoperative care.
- Incision healing without signs of infection; patient ambulating with minimal pain.

SELECTED READINGS

American Headache Society. (2019). The American Headache Society position statement on integrating new migraine treatments into clinical practice. *Headache: The Journal of Head and Face Pain, 59*(1), 1–18. https://doi.org/10.1111/head.13456

Armstrong, M. J., & Okun, M. S. (2020). Diagnosis and treatment of Parkinson disease: A review. *JAMA, 323*(6), 548–560. https://doi.org/10.1001/jama.2019.22360

Bassetti, C. L., Adamantidis, A., Burdakov, D., Han, F., Gay, S., Kallweit, U., Khatami, R., Koning, F., Kornum, B. R., Lammers, G. J., Liblau, R. S., Luppi, P. H., Mayer, G., Pollmächer, T., Sakurai, T., Sallusto, F., Scammell, T. E., Tafti, M., & Dauvilliers, Y. (2019). Narcolepsy—Clinical spectrum, aetiopathophysiology, diagnosis and treatment. *Nature Reviews Neurology, 15*(9), 519–539. https://doi.org/10.1038/s41582-019-0226-9

Cooper, A. S. (2021). Carotid endarterectomy for symptomatic carotid stenosis. *Critical Care Nurse, 41*(6), 76– 78. https://doi.org/10.4037/ccn2021863

Corsini, C., Castillo Almeida, N. E., O'Horo, J. C., Esquer Garrigos, Z., Wilson, W. R., Cano, E., DeSimone, D. C., Baddour, L. M., Van Gompel, J. J., & Sohail, M. R. (2021). Bacterial brain abscess: An outline for diagnosis and management. *The American Journal of Medicine, 134*(10), 1210–1217.e2. https://doi.org/10.1016/j.amjmed.2021.05.027

Dresser, L., Wlodarski, R., Rezania, K., & Soliven, B. (2021). Myasthenia gravis: Epidemiology, pathophysiology and clinical manifestations. *Journal of Clinical Medicine, 10*(11), 2235. https://doi.org/10.3390/jcm10112235

Goadsby, P. J. (2019). Primary headache disorders: Five new things. *Neurology: Clinical Practice, 9*(3), 233–240. https://doi.org/10.1212/CPJ.0000000000000654

Green, T. L., McNair, N. D., Hinkle, J. L., Middleton, S., Miller, E. T., Perrin, S., Power, M., Southerland, A. M., Summers, D. V., & on behalf of the American Heart Association Stroke Nursing Committee of the Council on Cardiovascular and Stroke Nursing and the Stroke Council. (2021). Care of the patient with acute ischemic stroke (posthyperacute and prehospital discharge): Update to 2009 comprehensive nursing care scientific statement: A scientific statement from the American Heart Association. *Stroke*, 52(5), e179–e198. https://doi.org/10.1161/STR.0000000000000357

Harmison, L. E., Beckham, J. W., & Adelman, D. S. (2023). Autonomic dysreflexia in patients with spinal cord injury. *Nursing, 53*(1), 21–26. https://doi.org/10.1097/01.NURSE.0000902944.16062.1f

Hauser, S. L., & Cree, B. A. (2020). Treatment of multiple sclerosis: A review. *The American Journal of Medicine, 133*(12), 1380–1390.e2. https://doi.org/10.1016/j.amjmed.2020.05.049

Helliesen, E. A., & Scheffel, K. (2022). *Spine disorders* (7th ed.). American Association of Neuroscience Nurses.

Hickey, J. V., & Strayer, A. L. (Eds.). (2020). *The clinical practice of neurological and neurosurgical nursing* (8th ed.). Wolters Kluwer.

Littlejohns, L., McNett, M., & Olson, D. (Eds.). (2022). *AANN core curriculum for neuroscience nursing* (7th ed.). AANN.

Menon, D., Barnett, C., & Bril, V. (2020). Novel treatments in myasthenia gravis. *Frontiers in Neurology, 11*, 538. https://doi.org/10.3389/fneur.2020.00538

Miller, T. R., Wessell, A., Jindal, G., Malhotra, J., Simard, J., & Gandi, D. (2022). The utility of platelet inhibition testing in patients undergoing Pipeline embolization of intracranial aneurysms. *Journal of Neurointerventional Surgery, 14*(1), 34–40. https://doi.org/10.1136/neurintsurg-2021-017681

Nevin, S., & Melby, V. (2022). Talking about post-injury sexual functioning: The views of people with spinal cord injuries—A qualitative interview study. *International Journal of Nursing Practice, 28*(3), e12977. https://doi.org/10.1111/ijn.12977

Nguyen, T. P., & Taylor, R. S. (2022). Guillain Barre syndrome. In *StatPearls* [Internet]. StatPearls Publishing.

Portelli Tremont, J. N., Cook, N., Murray, L. H., Udekwu, P. O., & Motameni, A. T. (2022). Acute traumatic spinal cord injury: Implementation of a multidisciplinary care pathway. *Journal of Trauma Nursing: The Official Journal of the Society of Trauma Nurses, 29*(4), 218–224. https://doi.org/10.1097/JTN.0000000000000664

Pressler, R. M., Cilio, M. R., Mizrahi, E. M., Moshé, S. L., Nunes, M. L., Plouin, P., Vanhatalo, S., Yozawitz, E., de Vries, L. S., Puthenveettil Vinayan, K., Triki, C. C., Wilmshurst, J. M., Yamamoto, H., & Zuberi, S. M. (2021). The ILAE classification of seizures and the epilepsies: Modification for seizures in the neonate. Position paper by the ILAE Task Force on Neonatal Seizures. *Epilepsia, 62*(3), 615–628. https://doi.org/10.1111/epi.16815

Pryor, J., Haylen, D., & Fisher, M. J. (2022). The usual bowel care regimes of people living in the community with spinal cord injury and factors important for integrating bowel care into everyday life. *Disability and Rehabilitation, 44*(21), 6401–6407. https://doi.org/10.1080/09638288.2021.1966678

Sexton, G. P., Nae, A., Cleere, E. F., O'Riordan, I., O'Neill, J. P., Lacy, P. D., Amin, M., Colreavy, M., Caird, J., & Crimmins, D. (2022). Concurrent management of suppurative intracranial complications of sinusitis and acute otitis media in children. *International Journal of Pediatric Otorhinolaryngology, 156*, 111093. https://doi.org/10.1016/j.ijporl.2022.111093

Toscano, G., Palmerini, F., Ravaglia, S., Ruiz, L., Invernizzi, P., Cuzzoni, M. G., Franciotta, D., Baldanti, F., Daturi, R., Postorino, P., Cavallini, A., & Micieli, G. (2020). Guillain-Barré syndrome associated with SARS-CoV-2. *New England Journal of Medicine, 382*(26), 2574–2576. https://doi.org/10.1056/NEJMc2009191

Tschoepe, R., Benfield, A., Posey, R., & Mercer, V. (2022). A systematic review of the effects of community transition programs on quality of life and hospital readmissions for adults with traumatic spinal cord injury. *Archives of Physical Medicine and Rehabilitation, 103*(5), 1013–1022.e12. https://doi.org/10.1016/j.apmr.2021.08.002

Venkatesan, A. (2021). Encephalitis and brain abscess. *Continuum (Minneapolis, Minn.), 27*(4), 855–886. https://doi.org/10.1212/CON.0000000000001006

Xiang, L., Li, H., Xie, Q. Q., Siau, C. S., Xie, Z., Zhu, M. T., Zhou, B., Li, Z. P., & Wang, S. B. (2023). Rehabilitation care of patients with neurogenic bladder after spinal cord injury: A literature review. *World Journal of Clinical Cases, 11*(1), 57–64. https://doi.org/10.12998/wjcc.v11.i1.57

Zangiabadi, N., Ladino, L. D., Sina, F., Orozco-Hernández, J. P., Carter, A., & Téllez-Zenteno, J. F. (2019). Deep brain stimulation and drug-resistant epilepsy: A review of the literature. *Frontiers in Neurology, 10*, 601. https://doi.org/10.3389/fneur.2019.00601

Zhang, W., Xu, L., Luo, T., Wu, F., Zhao, B., & Li, X. (2020). The etiology of Bell's palsy: A review. *Journal of Neurology, 267*, 1896–1905. https://doi.org/10.1007/s00415-019-09282-4

12 Eye Disorders

INTRODUCTION

Terms and Abbreviations

Definitions of Terms

1. *Accommodation:* Focusing apparatus of the eye that adjusts to objects at different distances by means of increasing the convexity of the lens (brought about by contraction of the ciliary muscles).
2. *Ametropia:* Abnormal vision.
   a. *Myopia:* Nearsightedness: rays of light coming from an object at a distance of 20 feet or more are brought to a focus in front of the retina.
   b. *Hyperopia:* Farsightedness: rays of light coming from an object at a distance of 20 feet or more are brought to a focus in the back of the retina.
3. *Astigmatism:* Uneven curvature of the cornea causing the patient to be unable to focus horizontal and vertical rays of light on the retina at the same time.
4. *Emmetropia:* Normal vision: rays of light coming from an object at a distance of 20 feet (6 m) or more are brought to focus on the retina by the lens (see Figure 12-1).
5. *Presbyopia:* The elasticity of the lens decreases with increasing age; an emmetropic person with presbyopia will read the paper at arm's length and will require prescription lenses to correct the problem.
6. *Strabismus:* Deviation of the eye so that the visual axes are not physiologically coordinated.
7. *Vision:* Passage of rays of light from an object through the cornea, aqueous humor, lens, and vitreous humor to the retina and its appreciation in the cerebral cortex.
8. *Visual acuity:* Measurement of a person's ability to see at a distance or near (reading distance) and is measured against a standard of a normal person's visual ability.

Eye Care Specialists

1. **Ophthalmologist:** Physician specializing in diagnosis, surgery, and treatment of the eye; may specialize in a specific part of the eye or disorder, such as a cornea specialist or glaucoma specialist.
2. **Optometrist:** Doctor of optometry who can examine, diagnose, and manage visual problems and diseases of the eye but does not perform surgery.
3. **Optician:** Technician who fits, adjusts, and gives eyeglasses or other devices on the written prescription of an ophthalmologist or optometrist.
4. **Ocularist:** Technician who makes ophthalmic prostheses.

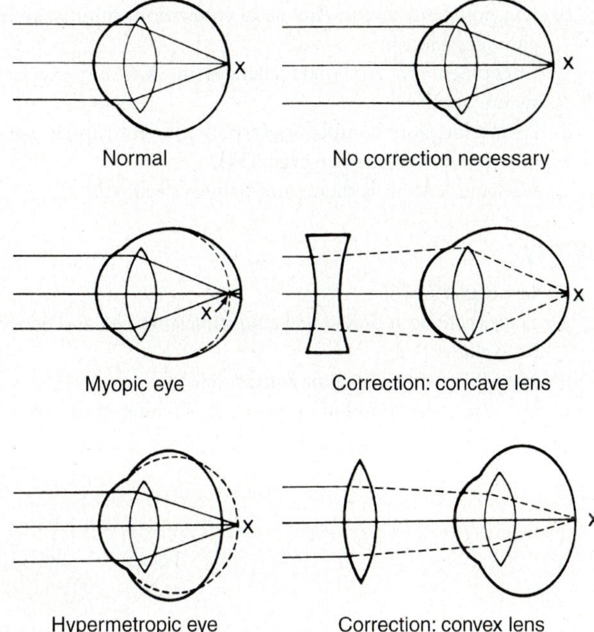

Figure 12-1. Normal vision and refractory errors.

Subjective Data

EVIDENCE BASE Dean, E. C., Gomez, J. L., & Welch, R. M. (2022). *Essentials of ophthalmic nursing. Book 1* (2nd ed., rev., pp. 39–45). American Society of Ophthalmologic Registered Nurses.

Subjective data for eye assessment include complaints of altered vision or other symptoms, associated lifestyle and other factors, and recent and past health history.

Presenting Symptoms

1. Explore the chief complaint from the patient by asking the following questions:
   a. Is there pain, foreign body sensation (scratchy, something in the eye), photophobia, dryness, redness, itchiness, lacrimation, or drainage?
   b. Is there blurred vision, double vision, loss of vision, or change in vision in a portion of the visual field?
   c. Are there other visual symptoms such as glare, halos, floaters?
   d. Is there difficulty in functioning, such as driving or reading, because of visual problems?
2. Review related systems.
   a. Neurologic: Are there scintillations, scotomas, transient ischemic attacks, headache, sensory or motor dysfunction?
   b. Ear, nose, and throat: Any nasal congestion, rhinitis, sinus pain, dry mouth?
   c. Integumentary: Are there changes in skin and mucous membranes?
   d. Endocrine: Any complaints of polyuria, polydipsia; signs of hyperthyroidism (see page 634)?
   e. Musculoskeletal: Is there joint pain or swelling?

History

1. Review ocular history.
   a. Have there been previous eye injuries, surgeries, and ocular procedures?
   b. Is patient using glasses or contact lenses?
   c. Was there childhood poor vision or patching of the eye?
   d. Are there current visual problems such as glaucoma, cataracts, macular degeneration, or diabetic retinopathy?
2. Obtain medication history, including nonprescription, herbal, topical, and inhalant products.
3. Determine allergies to medications; note type of reaction.
4. Determine history of systemic conditions such as diabetes, cardiovascular disease, arthritis, Marfan syndrome, albinism, sickle cell anemia.
5. Obtain family history of ocular conditions such as glaucoma, cataracts, macular degeneration, color blindness, retinitis pigmentosa, retinoblastoma, nystagmus, keratoconus, choroideremia, corneal dystrophies, and other chronic diseases.
6. Perform functional assessment.
   a. Depending on the patient's circumstance, administer the National Eye Institute Visual Function Questionnaire (VFQ-25) available at *www.rand.org/health/surveys_tools/vfq.html*, or other valid visual functioning questionnaires such as the VF-14.
   b. This helps determine the need for surgery based on the extent to which the eye disorder interferes with the patient's ability to carry out a visually dependent activity of daily living such as driving or reading.

POPULATION AWARENESS Question older patients about driving. Change in driving pattern, such as avoidance of night driving and less rush-hour driving, may indicate visual dysfunction as well as impaired reflexes and ability to concentrate in complex situations. A common complaint is not being able to read road signs in time to respond to them.

Ocular Examination

See Figure 12-2. Also see "Adult Physical Assessment," pages 6 to 32.

CLINICAL JUDGMENT Every patient who seeks medical attention for an eye complaint should have visual acuity tested.

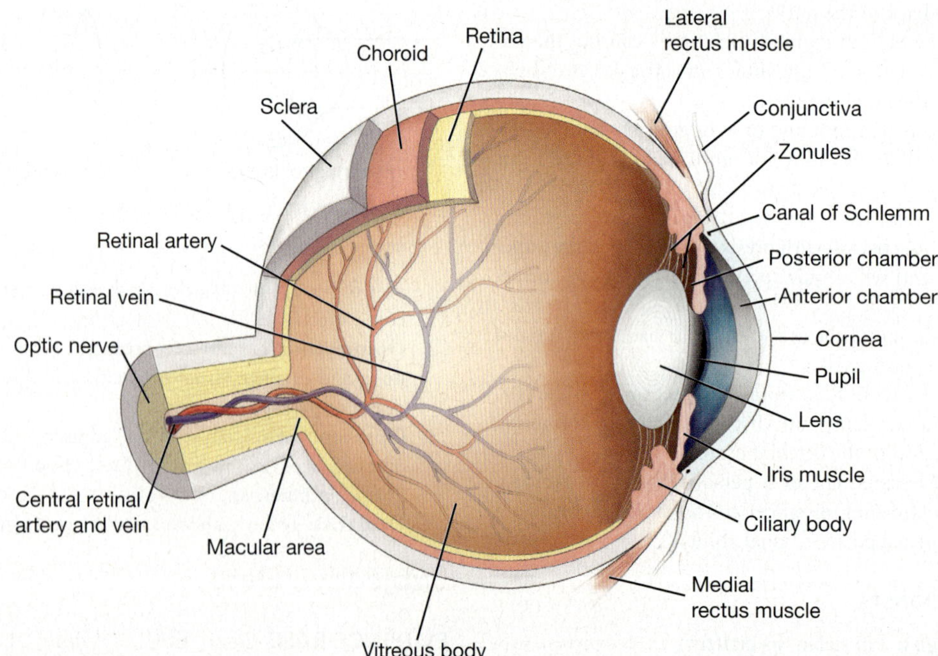

Figure 12-2. Three-dimensional cross-section of the eye. (Reprinted with permission from Hinkle, J. L., Cheever, K. H., & Overbaugh, K. J. [2022]. *Brunner and Suddarth's textbook of medical-surgical nursing* [15th ed., Fig. 58-3]. Lippincott Williams & Wilkins.)

External Examination

Includes examination of the eye and accessory organs without the aid of special apparatus.

Visual Acuity at Distance (Snellen Chart and Other Methods)

1. Letters and objects are of different sizes that can be seen by the normal eye at a distance of 20 feet (6 m) from the chart.
2. Letters appear in rows and are arranged, so the normal eye can see them at distances of 30, 40, and 50 feet (9, 12, and 15 m), and so forth.
3. Each eye is tested separately, with and without correction (glasses or contact lenses), whereas the nontesting eye is completely occluded.
4. Test the right eye (oculus dexter [OD]) first and then the left eye (oculus sinister [OS]).
5. A person who can identify letters of size 20 at 20 feet (6 at 6 m) is said to have 20/20 (6/6) vision.
6. If vision is less than 20/200 (6/60), additional tests may be recorded as:
   a. Counting fingers (CF)—at feet (meters).
   b. Hand motion (HM)—ability to detect hand movement at a certain distance.
   c. Light perception and projection (LP).
   d. Light perception only.
   e. No light perception.

Visual Acuity at Near (Jaeger Chart and Other Methods)

1. Letters and objects are of different sizes that can be seen by the normal eye at a reading distance of 14 in (36 cm) from the chart.
2. Letters appear in rows and are arranged, so the normal eye can read them at different levels on the Jaeger chart.
3. Each eye is tested separately, with and without correction (glasses or contact lenses), whereas the nontesting eye is completely occluded.
4. Test the right eye (OD) first and then the left eye (OS).
5. The vision is documented in Jaeger or Snellen notation where J1+ is equivalent to 20/20, J2 is equivalent to 20/30, and so forth.

Visual Fields

Determines function of optic pathways and identifies loss of visual field and functional capacity.

1. Equipment—light source and test objects. May be performed manually or as automated visual fields.
2. Peripheral field—useful in detecting decreased peripheral vision in one or both eyes.
   a. Patient is seated 18 to 24 in (45.5 to 61 cm) in front of the examiner.
   b. The left eye is covered, whereas the patient focuses with the right eye on a spot about 12 in (30.5 cm) from the eye.
   c. A test object is brought in from the side at 15-degree intervals through a complete 360 degrees.
   d. The patient signals when they see the test object and again when the object disappears through the 360 degrees.

Color Vision Tests

These tests are done to determine the person's ability to perceive primary colors and shades of colors. It is particularly significant for people whose occupation requires discerning colors, such as artists, interior decorators, transportation workers, surgeons, and nurses. (Useful in diagnosing diffuse retinal dysfunction and various types of optic neuropathies.)

1. Equipment:
   a. Polychromatic plates—dots of primary colors printed on a background of similar dots in a confusion of colors.
   b. Individual colored discs—each disc is matched to its next closest color.
2. Procedure:
   a. Various polychromatic plates are presented to the patient under specified illumination.
   b. The patterns may be letters or numbers that the normal eye can perceive instantly, but that are confusing to the person with a perception defect.
3. Outcome:
   a. Color blindness—person cannot perceive the figures.
   b. Red-green blindness—8% of people assigned male at birth, 0.4% of people assigned female at birth.
   c. Blue-yellow blindness—rare.

Refraction

Refraction is a clinical measurement of the error of focus in an eye.

1. Refraction and internal examination may be accomplished by instilling a medication with cycloplegic and mydriatic properties into the conjunctiva of the eye. Tropicamide and cyclopentolate are two such medicines that cause ciliary muscle relaxation, pupil dilation (mydriasis), and lowered accommodative power (cycloplegia).
2. In older children and adults, refraction without the use of drugs is preferred.
3. Visual screening through a multiple pinhole card can help differentiate refractive causes of decreased vision versus decreased vision secondary to organic disease.
4. The refractive state of the eye can be determined in two ways:
   a. Objectively—through retinoscopy or by automatic refraction (special instrument that measures, computes, and prints out refraction errors of each eye).
   b. Subjectively—trial of lenses to arrive at the best visual image.

Internal Examination

Ophthalmoscopic Examination

1. Direct ophthalmoscopy—uses a strong light reflected into the interior of the eye through an instrument called an ophthalmoscope.
2. Indirect ophthalmoscopy—allows the examiner to obtain a stereoscopic view of the retina. Light source is from a head-mounted light. The examiner views the retina through a convex lens held in front of the eye and a viewing device on the head mount. The image appears inverted. This method of examination allows the examiner to use binocular vision with depth perception and a wider viewing field.
3. Clinical significance:
   a. Detection of cataracts, vitreous opacities, corneal scars.
   b. Close examination for the pathologic changes in retinal blood vessels that may occur with diabetes or hypertension.
   c. Examination of the choroid for tumors or inflammation.
   d. Examination of the retina for retinal detachment, scars, or exudates and hemorrhages.

Slit-Lamp Examination

1. Special equipment that magnifies the cornea, sclera, and anterior chamber and provides oblique views into the trabeculum for examination by the ophthalmologist.
2. Helps detect disorders of the anterior portion of the eye.

3. The room is generally darkened and the pupils are dilated.
4. The patient sits with chin and forehead resting against equipment supports.

Tonometry

1. Measures intraocular pressure (IOP), which depends on the amount of aqueous humor secreted into the eye and ease by which it leaves.
2. Tonometry is indicated as one of the measurements to screen for glaucoma, assess the development of glaucoma if suspected, evaluate glaucoma therapy, and diagnose phthisis and diagnose drug-induced IOP increase or phthisis bulbi (end-stage eye disease).
3. Normal tension is considered less than or equal to 20 mm Hg.
4. Tonometry techniques:
   a. Goldmann applanation tonometry (see Figure 12-3):
      i. This is the most effective measuring method for determining IOP; however, it requires a biomicroscope and a trained interpreter. May be part of the slit-lamp examination or done by handheld device.
      ii. After instillation of topical anesthesia, the cornea is flattened by a known amount (3.14 mm).
      iii. The pressure necessary to produce this flattening is equal to the IOP, counterbalancing the tonometer.
   b. Schiotz tonometry (rarely used at present).
   c. Electronic tonometer that provides a digital reading of IOP, such as the Tono-Pen.
   d. Pneumatonometer or air applanation tonometry—requires no topical anesthesia and measures tension by sensing deformation of the cornea in reaction to a puff of pressurized air.
   e. Perkins handheld tonometer.
   f. Finger tension—pressure determined by use of digital pressure.

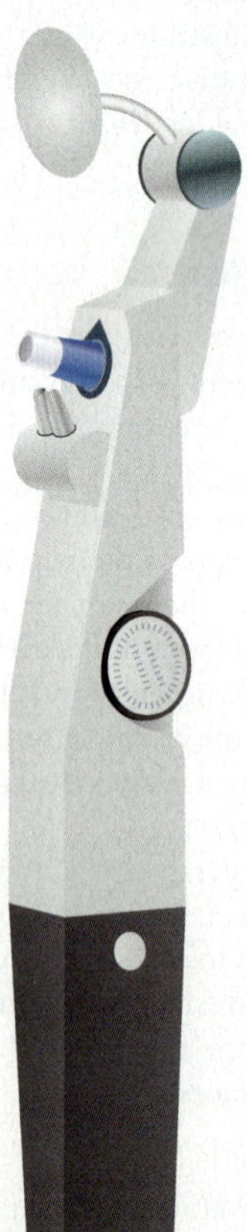

Figure 12-3. Example of an applanation tonometer.

Radiology and Imaging

Several imaging studies beyond the basic eye examination may be done to further evaluate eye disease.

Fluorescein Angiography

Description

1. Provides information concerning vascular obstructions, microaneurysms, abnormal capillary permeability, and defects in retinal pigment permeability.
2. Introduction of sodium fluorescein intravenous (IV) administration over several minutes, usually through a brachial vein.
3. Indirect ophthalmoscopy using a blue filter may be done and photographs of the ocular fundus are obtained.

Nursing and Patient Care Considerations

1. Advise the patient that a series of eye drops will be given to dilate the pupil for better visualization of the retina. The patient will be positioned in a special chair with head immobilized.
2. Dye will be injected into the arm over several minutes. Photographs will be taken during injection and up to 1 hour after injection.
3. Adverse effects include nausea because of dye injection, burning in eye from eye drop instillation, blurred vision and photophobia for 4 to 8 hours because of pupil dilation, and possible yellow skin and urine discoloration for up to 48 hours after dye injection.

DRUG ALERT Serious reactions, such as hoarseness, respiratory obstruction, tachycardia, and anaphylactic reaction leading to death, may result from sodium fluorescein IV administration.

Eye and Orbit Sonography

Description

1. Sound waves are used in the diagnosis of intraocular and orbital lesions. Three types of ultrasonography are used in ophthalmoscopy:
   a. A-scan—uses stationary transducers to measure the distance between changes in acoustic density. This is used to differentiate between benign and malignant tumors and to measure the length of the eye to determine the power of an intraocular lens (IOL).
   b. B-scan—moves linearly across the eye; increases in acoustic density are shown as an intensification on the line of the scan that presents a picture of the eye and the orbit.
   c. IOL Master technology—evaluates the length of the eye, surface curvature, and IOL power; has increased the accuracy of biometry by fivefold. It is also less technician-dependent for accuracy.
2. Abnormal patterns are seen in alkali burns, detached retina, keratoprosthesis, thyroid ophthalmopathy, foreign bodies, vascular malformations, benign and malignant tumors, and a variety of other conditions.

Nursing and Patient Care Considerations

1. Advise the patient that topical anesthetic drops are applied to the eye before the procedure so the patient will not feel the transducer contacting the eye.

2. The procedure may take as little as 8 to 10 minutes or 30 minutes or longer, if a lesion is detected, to locate the lesion.
3. Warn patient not to rub eyes until the anesthetic has worn off to avoid trauma to the eye.

Electroretinography

Description

Used to evaluate hereditary and acquired disorders of the retina; an electrode is placed over the eye to evaluate the electrical response to light.

Nursing and Patient Care Considerations

1. Advise the patient that the eyes are propped open and the patient will be positioned lying or sitting down.
2. Topical anesthetic drops are instilled.
3. A cotton wick electrode saturated in saline is applied to the cornea.
4. Various intensities of light are produced and the electrical potential is measured.
5. Caution the patient not to rub eyes for up to 1 hour after procedure to avoid trauma while eyes are anesthetized.

GENERAL PROCEDURES AND TREATMENT MODALITIES

See additional online content: Procedure Guidelines 12-1–12-5.

Common Eye Procedures

Instillation of Medications

1. Ophthalmic medications may be used for diagnostic and therapeutic purposes:
   a. To dilate or contract the pupil.
   b. To relieve pain, discomfort, itching, and inflammation.

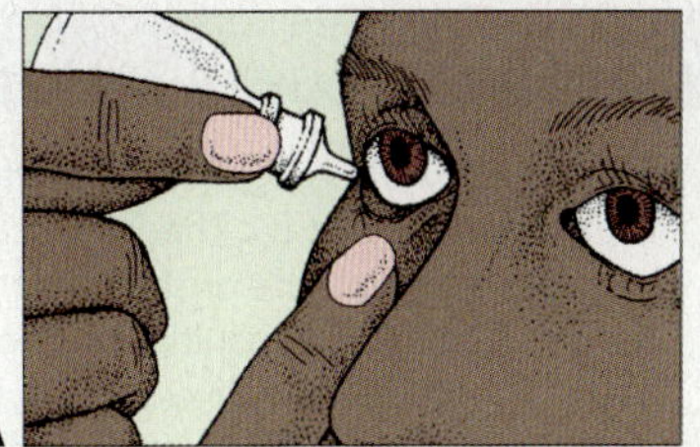

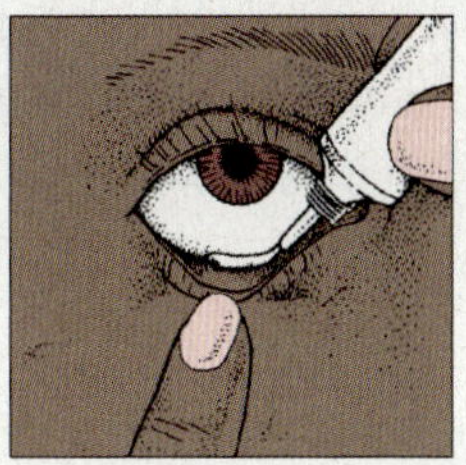

Figure 12-4. Instilling eye medication: (A) Solution (drops). (B) Ointment.

   c. To act as an antiseptic in cleansing the eye.
   d. To combat infection.
2. Solution or ointment is administered using clean technique:
   a. Use one finger to pull downward on skin of lower lid.
   b. Drop solution or squeeze out 1/8-in ribbon of ointment into center of conjunctival sac.
   c. Instruct the patient to close eye slowly but do not squeeze lids tightly or rub them.

See Figure 12-4 and Table 12-1.

Irrigation of the Eye

1. Ocular irrigation is often necessary for the following:
   a. To irrigate chemicals or foreign bodies from the eyes.
   b. To remove secretions from the conjunctival sac.
   c. To treat infections or relieve itching.
   d. To provide moisture on the surface of the eyes of an unconscious patient.
2. Use prescribed solution or 1,000 mL of normal saline solution with intravenous (IV) tubing.
3. Test pH with litmus paper before flushing if chemical injury is suspected and after irrigation until pH is 7.
4. Evert the lower conjunctival sac and have the patient look up, and then direct the irrigating solution from the inner canthus toward the outer canthus along the lower conjunctival sac.

Table 12-1 Ophthalmic Pharmacologic Agents

PHARMACOLOGY	ACTION	PRODUCTS
Sympathomimetics	Given topically for the treatment of glaucoma. Immediate effect is decrease in production of aqueous humor. Long-term effect is an increase in outflow of aqueous humor. May be used in combination with miotics, beta-adrenergic blockers, carbonic anhydrase inhibitors, or hyperosmotic agents.	• Epinephrine • Dipivefrin • Phenylephrine
Miotics, direct acting	Cholinergic agents given topically that affect the muscarinic receptors of the eye; results include miosis and contraction of the ciliary muscle. In narrow-angle glaucoma, miosis opens the angle to improve aqueous outflow. Contraction of the ciliary muscle enhances the outflow of aqueous humor by indirect action of the trabecular network—the exact mechanism is unknown. Primary use of miotics is in glaucoma but can be used to counter the effects of cycloplegics/mydriatics.	• Acetylcholine • Carbachol • Pilocarpine
Miotics, cholinesterase inhibitors	Topical agents that inhibit the enzyme cholinesterase, causing an increase in the activity of the acetylcholine already present in the body. Causes intense miosis and contraction of the ciliary muscle. Decrease in IOP that is seen as a result of increased outflow of aqueous humor. Used for treatment of open-angle glaucoma, conditions where the outflow of aqueous is obstructed; post-iridectomy problems; and accommodative esotropia (inward deviation of one eye).	• Demecarium bromide • Isoflurophate • Physostigmine

(continued)

Table 12-1 Ophthalmic Pharmacologic Agents (*continued*)

Beta-adrenergic blockers	Act on the beta receptors of the adrenergic nervous system. Two types of beta sites: B_1 and B_2. The B_1 site is primarily the myocardium resulting in decreased heart rate and cardiac output. B_2 primarily bronchial and vascular smooth muscle resulting in bronchoconstriction, decreased blood pressure. The cardioselective blocker (betaxolol) acts only on B_1 sites and may on rare occasions cause cardiac effects if absorbed systemically. All other nonselective blockers act on B_1 and B_2 sites and cause significant cardiac and pulmonary effects if absorbed systemically. Used for treatment of increased IOP by decreasing the formation of aqueous humor and causing a slight increase in the outflow facility.	• Betaxolol • Levobunolol • Timolol • Carteolol
Carbonic anhydrase inhibitors	Oral agents that act to inhibit the action of carbonic anhydrase. Suppression of this enzyme results in a decreased production of aqueous humor. Used in combination regimen to treat glaucoma and postoperative rise in IOP.	• Acetazolamide • Methazolamide
Osmotic diuretics	Osmotic agents given intravenously used for reduction of IOP in acute attack of glaucoma or before ocular surgery where preoperative reduction of IOP is indicated.	• Mannitol • Glycerin
Prostaglandin analogs	Reduce IOP presumably by increasing uveoscleral flow or filtration of aqueous. Used in open-angle glaucoma resistant to other agents.	• Latanoprost • Travoprost • Bimatoprost • Unoprostone
Mydriatics	Topical agents that result in dilation of the pupil, vasoconstriction, and an increase in the outflow of aqueous humor. Used for pupillary dilation for surgery and examination.	• Phenylephrine
Cycloplegic mydriatics	Topical agents that block the reaction of the sphincter muscle of the iris and the muscle of the ciliary body to cholinergic stimulation, resulting in dilation of the pupil (mydriasis) and paralysis of accommodation (cycloplegia). Used in conditions requiring pupil to be dilated and kept from accommodation.	• Atropine • Homatropine • Scopolamine • Cyclopentolate • Tropicamide
Ophthalmic anti-infectives	Topical agents used for treatment of ophthalmic infections. Commercial products are intended for treatment of superficial ocular problems, such as conjunctivitis and blepharitis. Extemporaneous (compounded) drops are used for more serious topical infections (i.e., corneal ulcer, endophthalmitis [intraocular infection]).	*Antibiotics* • Bacitracin • Chloramphenicol • Ciprofloxacin • Erythromycin • Gentamicin • Gatifloxacin • Levofloxacin • Moxifloxacin • Neomycin/polymyxin/bacitracin • Norfloxacin • Sulfacetamide • Tobramycin *Antifungal* • Amphotericin B • Fluconazole • Natamycin *Antiviral* • Trifluridine • Vidarabine
Local anesthetics	Block the transmission of nerve impulses. Used topically to provide local anesthetic for tests, such as tonometry, and for procedures of short duration. Injections used in ophthalmology for retrobulbar blocks.	• Proparacaine • Tetracaine injection • Lidocaine
Ophthalmic steroid anti-inflammatories	Mostly corticosteroids. Used topically to relieve pain and photophobia as well as suppress other inflammatory processes of the conjunctiva, cornea, lid, and interior segment of the globe.	• Dexamethasone • Fluorometholone • Loteprednol • Prednisolone acetate

Table 12-1 Ophthalmic Pharmacologic Agents (*continued*)

Nonsteroidal anti-inflammatory drugs (NSAIDs)	Act by inhibiting an enzyme involved in the synthesis of prostaglandins, which are key in the body's response to inflammation. These drugs, given topically, are analgesics and anti-inflammatories.	• Diclofenac sodium • Flurbiprofen • Ketorolac • Suprofen
Anti-allergy medications	There are a number of different types of drugs, given topically, in this category, including antihistamine, mast cell stabilizers, NSAID anesthetics, and astringents (some in combination).	*Antihistamines* • Emedastine • Levocabastine • Olopatadine • Pheniramine *Mast cell stabilizers* • Cromolyn • Lodoxamide *Astringent* • Zinc sulfate
Vasoconstrictors	Topical agents that contract local blood vessels, resulting in less redness and irritation.	• Naphazoline
Alpha-selective adrenergic agonist agents	Topical agents that mimic the effects of endogenous adrenergic compounds by selectively binding to alpha-2 receptors used for lowering elevated IOP by reducing aqueous production and increasing uveoscleral outflow.	• Apraclonidine hydrochloride • Brimonidine tartrate
Anti-VEGF agents	Slow growth of abnormal blood vessels under the retina by blocking the effects of VEGF to slow vision loss and possibly improve vision in wet age-related macular degeneration.	• Bevacizumab • Pegaptanib • Ranibizumab

IOP, intraocular pressure; VEGF, vascular endothelial growth factor.
All pharmacologic agents should be reviewed from manufacturer's information or drug reference source before administration for contraindications, adverse reactions, and cautions.

Application of Dressing or Patch

1. One or both eyes may need shielding for the following:
   a. To keep an eye at rest, thereby promoting healing.
   b. To prevent the patient from touching eye.
   c. To absorb secretions.
   d. To protect the eye.
   e. To control or lessen edema.
2. Instill ointment if directed and make sure that eye is closed before securing gauze patch or eye shield with tape strips placed diagonally from midforehead to outer cheek.

Removing a Particle From the Eye

1. Typically, removing a foreign body from the eye is an uncomplicated first-aid measure.
   a. As the patient looks upward, place your finger below the lower lid and pull downward to expose the conjunctival sac.
   b. Inspect for particles using a light and magnifying lens.
   c. Remove particle with cotton-tipped applicator moistened in saline by gently wiping across the conjunctival sac.
2. If no offending particle is found, proceed to the upper lid.
   a. As the patient looks downward, place the cotton applicator horizontally on the upper lid and gently pull the lid outward and upward (see Figure 12-5) over the applicator.
   b. Remove particle if found and return eyelid to neutral position.
3. If a particle appears to be embedded, medical intervention is required, that is, local anesthetic, antibiotic therapy, and clinical expertise, in using other instruments.
4. The cornea should be evaluated for abrasion from the foreign body by use of fluorescein staining, even if a foreign body cannot be found.

Removing Contact Lenses

1. Because contact lenses need regular cleaning and changing, if a person is injured and incapacitated because of an accident, sickness, or other cause, the lenses should be removed.
2. Determine the type of lens from the patient or family.
   a. Soft corneal lenses are widely used. The diameter covers the cornea plus a portion of the sclera of the eye. Extended- and daily-wear soft lenses are available.
   b. Rigid or gas-permeable lenses are usually smaller than the cornea of the eye, although some are made to extend beyond the cornea onto the sclera of the eye. These lenses need to be removed promptly.
3. Do not remove lenses if the iris is not visible on opening the eyelids; await the arrival of an ophthalmologist. If patient is to be transported, note that contacts are in the eyes. (Write out the message and tape it to the patient or send with transporter.)
4. To remove soft lenses, retract the lower lid and attempt to slide the lens off the cornea using your index finger, and then pinch the lens between two fingers and gently remove it.

Ocular Surgery

Common types of ocular surgery are described, followed by a nursing process overview for any patient having ocular surgery. Also see the following entries for specific surgical care: conditions of

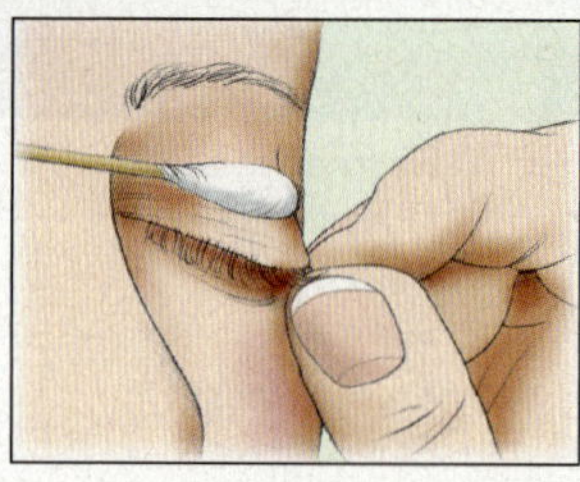
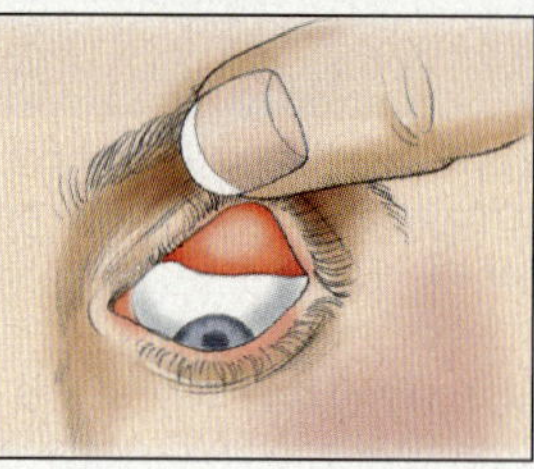

Figure 12-5. Removing a particle from the eye.

the eyelids, page 420; cataract, page 422; retinal detachment, page 427; and acute glaucoma and chronic glaucoma, page 426.

Corneal Transplantation (Keratoplasty)

Description

1. The transplantation of a donor cornea, usually obtained at autopsy, to repair a corneal scar, burn, deformity, or dystrophy.
2. Types of grafts:
   a. Full thickness (6.5 to 8 mm)—most common.
   b. Partial-thickness lamellar.
3. Fresh cornea is the preferred tissue; it is removed from the donor within 12 hours after death and used within 24 hours.
4. Special solutions for storage of fresh cornea are available, which may extend storage up to 3 days.
5. *Cryopreservation* is the care and handling of a corneal graft by freezing to retain its transparency.

Complications

1. Hemorrhage.
2. Graft dislocation.
3. Infection.
4. Postoperative glaucoma.
5. Graft rejection—may occur 10 to 14 days postoperatively; signs and symptoms include decreased vision, ocular irritation, corneal edema, and red sclera.

Refractive Surgery

Description

1. A variety of procedures used to correct nearsightedness, farsightedness, and astigmatism; may eliminate need for glasses or contact lenses, especially with aging.
2. May not be appropriate with corneal disease, retinal disease, glaucoma, severe diabetes, uncontrolled vascular disease, autoimmune disease, or pregnancy.
3. There is no guarantee on desired effect, but complication rate is extremely low.
4. Procedures are quick, performed in physician's office or clinic, and most people are back to full activity in 1 to 3 days.
5. Specific procedures are used to correct nearsightedness, farsightedness, or astigmatism.
6. May eliminate need for glasses, especially with aging.

Types of Procedures

1. Radial keratotomy:
   a. Procedure designed to provide correction of myopia (nearsightedness).
   b. The cornea is anesthetized topically, and under a microscope, the surgeon marks the visual axis.
   c. Eight to 16 radial incisions are made into the corneal surface to flatten it. This permits images to fall on the retina instead of in front of it.
   d. Time to optimal correction is about 3 months. (Procedure is being performed much less frequently now with the development of laser surgery for refraction.)
2. Excimer photorefractive keratectomy.
   a. Limited to correcting myopia and some astigmatism.
   b. The front surface of the corneal epithelium is removed (by laser, manual scraping, or both).
   c. The laser is then used to change the corneal curvature by vaporizing the tissue (reshaping or sculpting the cornea).
   d. Optimal visual recovery about 6 months.
3. Laser-assisted in situ keratomileusis (LASIK).
   a. Procedure is designed to treat a wider range of prescriptions than the other refractive procedures.
   b. Microsurgical instrument (microkeratome) is used to create a corneal flap.
   c. A cool laser beam (using an excimer laser) reshapes the cornea and the flap is then closed.
   d. The excimer laser can remove corneal tissue with an accuracy of up to 0.25 μm.
   e. Only about 50 μm of tissue is removed to achieve the desired correction.
   f. Refractive recovery about 3 months.
4. Holmium laser thermokeratoplasty (holmium LTK).
   a. Tissue is heated, not vaporized.
   b. Cornea is marked to pinpoint where to aim the laser.
   c. The laser heats only selected portions of the cornea to shrink collagen fibers around the cornea edges.

Vitrectomy

1. This procedure is performed for conditions such as unresolved hemorrhage with diabetic retinopathy, intraocular foreign body, and vitreoretinal adhesions.
2. It involves the removal of all or part of the vitreous humor, the transparent, gelatinlike substance behind the lens.
3. As the vitreous is removed, saline is infused to replace the vitreous. At the end of the procedure, gas, air, or silicone oil may be introduced into the eye to act as a tamponade to keep the retina in place.
   a. If gas is used, the patient may be restricted to prone position (for at least 50 minutes of each hour) for 1 to 6 weeks until the SF6 gas is absorbed.
   b. If air or oil is used, a semi-Fowler position is allowed.
4. Precautions should be taken to prevent increased intraocular pressure (IOP), which would disrupt healing.
   a. Avoid straining to have bowel movement or bend over.
   b. Avoid coughing or sneezing or sudden movements of the head.
   c. Monitor for headache, which may be a sign of increased IOP.

Enucleation

1. Complete removal of the eyeball, usually performed due to trauma, infection, tumor such as melanoma, or prevention of sympathetic ophthalmia.
2. At surgery, the eye is removed by opening the conjunctiva and extraocular muscles, severing the optic nerve, and removing the eyeball.
3. A ball implant is then covered by the muscles and maintains the contour of the eye. The conjunctiva is then closed and a plastic conformer is placed to maintain the integrity of the eyelid.
4. An individualized prosthesis can be fitted 4 to 6 weeks later and a second procedure may be done to improve ocular motility.

5. Care considerations include acceptance of body image, adjustment to mononuclear vision, and care of the enucleated socket and prosthesis, including the following:
   a. Inspecting eye and lid.
   b. Instilling medication.
   c. Irrigating site to remove mucus.
   d. Removing the prosthesis.
   e. Using aseptic technique when performing care.
6. Complications include hemorrhage, infection, and implant extrusion.

Nursing Assessment

1. Collect subjective and objective data about patient's general state of health.
2. Ascertain what symptoms the patient has been having (eye pain, visual loss, drainage, history of trauma) and how that has impacted usual activity.
3. Assess the patient's mobility and self-care ability.
4. Assess visual as well as other sensory impairments, which may impact safety and independence.
5. Gather data regarding usual support systems used by the patient. Is family nearby? Do friends visit regularly? Is increased supervision required after surgery because of visual impairment?
6. Review patient's medications and determine if anticoagulants have been taken. They are usually stopped just prior to retinal surgery; however, they are usually continued for patients undergoing cataract surgery.

Nursing Interventions

Preparing for Surgery

1. Explain to the patient preoperative orders as well as postoperative expectations. (These will be specific for each type of surgery and particular health care provider.)
   a. Eye surgery is usually performed under local anesthesia and that they will be awake but sedated and must remain still during procedure.
   b. Postoperatively, a specific position in bed may be maintained for a few hours.
      i. The patient may be required to lie on the unoperated side.
      ii. Following vitrectomy, the patient may be required to lie prone for at least 50 minutes of every hour. Advise the patient they can stand up to use bathroom and shower but must keep nose pointing to the ground. Although this is a difficult restriction to follow, it's the only way to improve visual outcome with this procedure.
      iii. Following some surgeries, supine position may be required with only a small pillow.
2. Instruct the patient to wash hair the evening before surgery; long hair of patients should be arranged so it is off the face. There may be restrictions on using makeup to prevent makeup flakes from entering the operative site, thereby increasing the risk for infection and inflammation.
3. Check agency surgical policy regarding skin preparation. Patients may be requested to shower with antibacterial soap the evening before or morning of surgery.
4. Check that operative permit is correct and signed with specified eye having surgery noted. Ask patient which eye (do not suggest an eye). Verification can prevent two thirds of wrong site incidents.
5. Remove dentures, contact lenses, or eye prosthesis and metal objects before patient goes to the operating room based on facility policy and type of anesthesia. (Wedding band can usually be taped in place.)
6. Inform the patient if eye bandages are necessary postoperatively.
   a. Eye patch used following keratoplasty.
   b. Pressure patch used after vitrectomy. Drainage is expected for 2 days postoperatively.
   c. Pressure dressing and ice used after enucleation.
7. Administer preoperative medications, including eye drops, as prescribed.
8. Put bed side rails up after administering medications and place the call bell next to the patient.
9. Be available to answer questions the patient may have relating to the surgery or postoperative period.

CLINICAL JUDGMENT For patients requiring bed rest (i.e., after keratoplasty, eye injury, retinal detachment surgery), take measures to prevent pulmonary and/or circulatory complications, including range-of-motion exercises, antiembolism stockings, and pneumatic compression devices.

Preventing Injury Postoperatively

1. Position the patient, as permitted, for specific surgery.
   a. Prone if vitrectomy was done with gas to hold retina in place.
   b. Semi-Fowler for vitrectomy when air or oil was used.
2. Position side rails (up) to offer the patient a sense of security.
3. Place the call bell next to the patient; have the patient call the nurse rather than risk increased IOP from the stress and strain of attempting to be self-sufficient.
4. Advise the patient to avoid bending over, quick movements of the head, or straining that may cause increase in IOP. Medicate, if indicated, for excessive coughing or sneezing. (May not be a concern for current, small-incision cataract surgery.)
5. Monitor for headache, which may be a sign of IOP.
6. Instruct caregivers to tell the patient when they enter and leave the room.
7. Avoid activities such as combing hair that may cause tension on sutures or operative site.
8. Apply cold compresses to control edema and associated discomfort following vitrectomy.

POPULATION AWARENESS Be aware that older people may have additional sensory/perceptual alterations, such as hearing loss and decreased position sense, which increases their risk of falls and feeling of isolation.

Reducing Fear

1. Be aware that dependence on sight is recognized when one faces diminishment or loss of sight.
2. Recognize that patients' concern of surgical outcome may be manifested differently, for example, fear, depression, tension, resentment, anger, or rejection.
3. Encourage the patient to express feelings.
4. Demonstrate interest, empathy, and understanding.
5. Reassure the patient that rehabilitative programs and personnel are available.
6. Refer patient to the local blind or low-vision association for training and adaptive equipment (see page 1455).

Increasing Self-care Activities

1. Orient patient to the environment and assist with activities as needed.
2. Provide diversional and occupational therapy to keep the patient occupied mentally within the limits of decreased vision.
3. Encourage self-care as much as able, with rest periods as necessary.
4. Provide adequate diet and fluids to promote proper elimination and decreased straining.
5. Discourage the patient from smoking, shaving with a straight edge, and use of pointed objects near eyes for safety reasons.
6. Caution the patient against rubbing eyes or wiping them with soiled tissues.
7. Instruct the patient to wear dark glasses if eyes are light sensitive.
8. Maintain safe environment—doors should be completely open or closed, floors kept clear of articles.

Patient Education and Health Maintenance

1. Advise the patient to consult ophthalmologist before undertaking diversional or recreational therapy that may be fatiguing to the eyes—such as reading, working on computer, and craft work.
2. Emphasize that lights should not be too bright or glaring.
3. Before the patient leaves the hospital, provide discharge instructions about medications, including topical antibiotics, corticosteroids, and pain medications.
4. Instruct the patient and family on instillation of eye medications, proper cleansing of the eyelids and lashes, and application of an eye shield or patch.
5. Provide instructions on massaging the eyelid in the postoperative period following eyelid surgery.
6. Assure patient of temporary bruising and swelling of eyelids.
7. Ensure that patient has follow-up information about eyeglasses, prosthesis fitting, and follow-up visits. Advise patient that improved vision may not occur quickly following keratoplasty.
8. Advise watching for signs of graft rejection 10 to 14 days following keratoplasty: decreased vision, irritation, corneal edema, and redness of sclera.
9. Educate the patient about talking books, records, tapes, and audio machines available from most public libraries without charge.
10. Encourage the use of smartphone-based assistive technology, such as apps designed for low vision, which may improve independent functioning.
11. Confirm the following points with the patient and family before discharge:
    a. Is a return appointment date with health care provider confirmed?
    b. Are prescriptions for patient's medications in hand or have been sent to pharmacy?
    c. Do the patient and family member know how to use the prescribed medications?
    d. Does the patient understand the restrictions placed on them (e.g., positioning, straining, return to usual activities) and the reasons for the restrictions?
    e. Does the patient understand visual limitation and expected outcome?
    f. Do the patient and family know what signs and symptoms to report to health care provider between appointments (i.e., pain, temperature above 101°F [38.3°C], bleeding or discharge from operative site)?

EVIDENCE BASE Senjam, S. S., Manna, S., & Bascaran, C. (2021). Smartphones-based assistive technology: Accessibility features and apps for people with visual impairment, and its usage, challenges, and usability testing. *Clinical Optometry, 13*, 311–322. https://doi.org/10.2147/OPTO.S336361

Evaluation: Expected Outcomes

- Adheres to preoperative routine; asks appropriate questions.
- Adheres to measures to prevent increased IOP and falls.
- Appears relaxed and positive concerning outcome of surgery.
- Manages self-care with minimal assistance.

COMMON EYE DISORDERS

Conditions of the Conjunctiva and Eyelids

The *eyelids* are the outermost defense mechanisms of the eyes, functioning as a physical barrier as well as to maintain moisture and disperse tears. The *palpebral conjunctiva* lines the upper and lower lids and the bulbar conjunctiva forms a protective coating over the sclera. The conjunctiva responds to infections, inflammatory disorders, and environmental irritants. Blood vessels in the conjunctiva dilate readily, causing redness, and pain receptors respond to inflammatory changes. Inflammatory disorders are outlined in Table 12-2. Structural disorders that may be amenable to surgery include:

- Entropion—inward turning of the eyelid margin.
- Ectropion—outward turning of the eyelid margin.
- Ptosis (blepharoptosis)—drooping of the upper eyelid.
- Lagophthalmos—inadequate closure of the eyelids.
- Pinguecula—overgrowth of tissue on the conjunctiva.
- Pterygium—overgrowth of tissue on the cornea.

Pathophysiology and Etiology

1. Entropion and ectropion are classified as congenital, involutional, paralytic (cranial nerve [CN] VII palsy), cicatricial, or mechanic. Caused by severe eye disease, trauma, surgery, chemical burn.
2. Ptosis is classified according to the underlying cause and timing of onset described as acquired or congenital. General causes include neurologic, muscular, and autoimmune disorders; eye socket tumors may also cause ptosis.
3. Pinguecula is a degenerative lesion and pterygium is a fibrovascular lesion; both typically result from ultraviolet light exposure.

Clinical Manifestations

1. Sagging and/or irritation of eyelid.
2. Redness, tearing, burning of the eye.
3. Superficial punctate keratitis (inflammation of cornea).
4. Yellowish nodules in bulbar conjunctiva (pinguecula); wing-shaped folds of tissue across limbus of the cornea (pterygium).
5. Loss of superior field of vision with ptosis or reduced visual acuity may be seen with pterygium.
6. Lashes roll back against the ocular surface after eyelid is released—positive digital inversion test (entropion).

Table 12-2 Conditions of the Eyelids and Conjunctiva

CONDITION	TREATMENT AND NURSING CONSIDERATIONS
Blepharitis	
An inflammatory reaction of the eyelid margin caused by bacteria (usually *Staphylococcus aureus*) or seborrheic skin condition, resulting in flaking, redness, irritation, and possibly recurrent styes of the upper or lower lid, or both.	Diagnostic culture usually not necessary. Mild cases treated with eyelid margin scrub at least once daily (baby shampoo may be used). If *S. aureus* is likely, antibiotic ointment is prescribed one to four times per day to eyelid margin. Teach patient to scrub eyelid margin with cotton swab to remove flaking and then apply ointment with cotton swab, as directed.
Hordeolum (stye)/chalazion	
The term "stye" refers to an inflammation or infection of the glands and follicles of the eyelid margin. External hordeolum involves the hair follicles of the eyelashes; chalazion is a granulomatous (chronic) infection of the meibomian glands. Bacteria, usually *Staphylococcus*, and seborrhea are the causes. Pain, redness, foreign body sensation, and a pustule may be present.	Treatment usually consists of warm soaks to help promote drainage, good handwashing and eyelid hygiene, and possible application of antibiotic ointment. In some cases, incision and drainage in the office with local anesthetic may be necessary. Teach patient how to clean eyelid margins and not to squeeze the stye.
Conjunctivitis	
Inflammation or infection of the bulbar (covering the sclera and cornea) or palpebral (covering inside lids) conjunctiva. May be allergic; bacterial (*S. aureus, Streptococcus pneumoniae, Haemophilus influenzae*, and others); gonococcal; viral (adenovirus, herpes simplex, coxsackievirus, and others); or irritative (topical medication, chemicals, wind, smoke, contact lenses, ultraviolet light) causes. Trachoma is caused by *Chlamydia trachomatis* and is a major cause of blindness worldwide, but is rare in North America. Symptoms of conjunctivitis vary from mild pruritus and tearing to severe drainage, burning, hyperemia, and chemosis (edema). The term "pink eye" usually refers to infectious conjunctivitis.	Fluorescein staining may be done to rule out ulceration or keratitis (involvement of cornea). Culture if purulent exudate; special culture for *Neisseria gonorrhoeae*. Warm soaks (10 min four times per day) used when crusting and drainage present; cold compresses helpful for allergic and irritative causes. If topical antibiotic ordered, teach patient instillation technique. Urge good handwashing to prevent spread. Allergic conjunctivitis treated with topical or oral antihistamines, vasoconstrictors, and mast cell stabilizers.

Diagnostic Evaluation

1. External examination detecting appearance and function of eyelids.
2. Inspection of the conjunctiva, sclera, and cornea, followed by slit-lamp examination.
3. Lid position measurements—margin-reflex distance (MRD), palpebral fissure, levator function, and distance between upper lid crease to lid margin.
4. CN testing for extraocular movements (3rd, 4th, 6th CN) and visual fields (2nd CN).
5. Pharmacologic testing—phenylephrine or cocaine test to rule out Horner syndrome and edrophonium (Tensilon) test to rule out myasthenia gravis as causes of ptosis.

Management

1. Lubricating agents to treat inflammation of the cornea.
2. Massaging of eyelid, especially with cicatricial ectropion to help stretch scarring and improve anatomic position.
3. Manual inversion of eyelid margin for entropion.
4. Treatment of trichiasis by removing lashes with fine forceps.
5. Taping upper eyelid in ptosis.
6. Surgical management for ectropion and entropion.
   a. Ectropion and entropion repair—involves a horizontal tightening technique of the lower lid.
   b. Lateral canthoplasty (elongation of the eye opening).
   c. Lower lid retractor insertion.
7. Surgical management for ptosis.
   a. Approach depends on the cause and degree of ptosis and considers the object of the surgery, which is to balance the lid position in primary gaze.
   b. Complications of surgery include overcorrection and undercorrection of the eyelids, corneal or conjunctival irritation, abnormal contour of the eyelids, lagophthalmos.
8. Surgical excision of pterygium may be necessary due to large size. Other options include strontium 90 beta-irradiation or mitomycin C administration.
9. Surgery for pinguecula is indicated when tissue growth passes the limbus and invades the Bowman layer of the cornea.

For nursing management see page 51.

Disorders of the Cornea and Uveal Tract

The *cornea* is the outermost tissue that functions in vision. It must remain clear and smooth to admit light to the retina. Blood vessels are contained in the *limbus* (periphery). Epithelial layers of the cornea repair rapidly, but if they are penetrated, infection can rapidly spread inward and vision may be lost.

The *uveal tract* is made up of the iris, which controls pupil size; ciliary body, which secretes aqueous humor and controls accommodation; and choroid layer, which provides vasculature to the anterior uveal tract. Disorders of the uveal tract may cause pupil changes, problems with accommodation, clouding of the anterior chamber or vitreous, and more serious problems because of adhesions (see Table 12-3).

Table 12-3 Conditions of the Cornea and Uveal Tract

CONDITION	TREATMENT AND NURSING CONSIDERATIONS
Corneal abrasion and ulceration (keratitis)	
Loss of epithelial layers of cornea because of some type of trauma—contact with fingernail, tree branch, spark or other projectile, or overwearing contact lens. May lead to corneal ulceration and secondary infection into cornea (keratitis), which may lead to blindness. Symptoms are pain, redness, foreign body sensation, photophobia, increased tearing, and difficulty opening eye.	Treatment is urgent. Fluorescein staining and examination with wood lamp or slit lamp to identify the abrasion or ulceration. Antibiotic ointment may be instilled and eye patched for 24 h. No benefit to patching has been found for simple abrasions, however. Cycloplegic drops may also be used in large abrasions or ulcers. Abrasion heals in 24–48 h. Ulceration should be followed by an ophthalmologist. Make sure that patch is secure enough so patient cannot open eyelid, but not so tight that patient "sees stars." Teach patient to use topical antibiotic (or antiviral in cases of herpes simplex dendritic keratitis) after patch is removed, and follow up as directed. Review safety practices, such as wearing protective eye shields, not rubbing eyes, using contact lenses properly, and washing hands frequently.
Iritis/uveitis	
Uveitis is an inflammation of the intraocular structures. It is classified by involved structures: (1) anterior uveitis—iris (iritis) or iris and ciliary body (iridocyclitis), (2) intermediate uveitis—structures posterior to the lens (pars planitis or peripheral uveitis), and (3) posterior uveitis—choroid (choroiditis), retina (retinitis), or vitreous near the optic nerve and macula. Anterior uveitis is most common and is usually unilateral. Posterior uveitis is usually bilateral. Causes of uveitis are infections; immune-mediated disorders, such as ankylosing spondylitis, Crohn disease, Reiter syndrome, and lupus; and trauma, or it may be idiopathic. Onset is acute with deep eye pain, photophobia, conjunctival redness, small pupil that does not react briskly, ciliary flush (redness around limbus), and decreased visual acuity.	Urgent ophthalmology evaluation is needed. Inflammation is treated with a topical corticosteroid and a cycloplegic agent. Teach patient how to instill medications and adhere to dosing schedule to prevent permanent eye damage. Suggest sunglasses to decrease pain from photophobia. Encourage follow-up for IOP measurements because corticosteroids can increase IOP.

IOP, intraocular pressure.

Cataract

Clouding or opacity of the crystalline lens that impairs vision.

Pathophysiology and Etiology

1. Senile cataract—commonly occurs with aging.
2. Congenital cataract—occurs at birth.
3. Traumatic cataract—occurs after injury.
4. Aphakia—absence of crystalline lens.
5. Additional risk factors for cataract formation include diabetes; ultraviolet light exposure; high-dose radiation; and drugs such as corticosteroids, phenothiazines, and some chemotherapy agents.

Clinical Manifestations

1. Blurred or distorted vision.
2. Glare from bright lights.
3. Gradual and painless loss of vision.
4. Previously dark pupil may appear milky or white.

Diagnostic Evaluation

1. Slit-lamp examination—to provide magnification and visualize opacity of lens.
2. Tonometry—to determine intraocular pressure (IOP) and rule out other conditions.
3. Direct and indirect ophthalmoscopy to rule out retinal disease.
4. Perimetry—to determine the scope of the visual field (normal with cataract).

Management

General

1. Surgical removal of the lens is indicated:
   a. When a cataract interferes with activities, the patient is a candidate for cataract surgery.
   b. Because cataract often occurs in both eyes, surgery is recommended when vision in the better eye causes problems in daily activities. Surgery is done on only one eye at a time.
2. Cataract surgery is usually done under either regional block or topical anesthesia, with or without intravenous (IV) sedation, and on an outpatient basis.
3. Oral medications may be given to reduce IOP.
4. Intraocular lens (IOL) implants are usually implanted at the time of cataract extraction, replacing thick glasses that may provide suboptimal refraction.
5. In the rare instance that IOL implant is not used, the patient will be fitted with appropriate eyeglasses or a contact lens to correct refraction after the healing process.

Surgical Procedures

1. There are two types of extractions:
   a. Intracapsular extraction—the lens as well as the capsule are removed through a small incision. (This technique is rarely used in the United States.)

   b. Extracapsular extraction—the lens capsule is incised and the nucleus, cortex, and anterior capsule are extracted.
      i. The posterior capsule is left in place and is usually the base to which an IOL is implanted.
      ii. A conservative procedure of choice, simple to perform, is usually done under local anesthesia.
2. Phacoemulsification is usually used to remove the lens.
   a. A hollow needle vibrating at ultrasonic speed is used to emulsify the lens.
   b. Then the emulsified particles are irrigated and aspirated from the anterior chamber.
3. Cryosurgery is rarely used to remove the lens. A pencil-like instrument with a metal tip is supercooled (−35°C [−31°F]) and then touched to the exposed lens, freezing it so the lens is easily lifted out.

IOL Implantation

1. The implantation of a synthetic lens (IOL) is designed for distance vision; the patient may wear prescription glasses for reading and near vision. IOL implant restores binocular vision.
2. Previously, most IOLs were spherical with the front surface curved. Aspheric IOLs increase contrast sensitivity.
   a. The multifocal IOL incorporates more than one optical power to permit focusing at different distances.
   b. The aspheric IOL can reduce postoperative spherical aberrations and, therefore, improve the ability to see in varying light conditions, such as rain, snow, fog, twilight, and nighttime darkness.
   c. The toric IOL is designed to correct astigmatism.
      i. Sophisticated calculations are required to determine the prescription for the lens.
      ii. Numerous types of IOLs are available. Designs and materials change as new developments occur.
3. Advantages of the IOL include:
   a. Provides an alternative for the person who cannot wear contact lenses.
   b. Cannot be lost or misplaced like conventional glasses.
   c. Provides superior vision correction and better depth perception than glasses.
4. Complications (specific to implantation):
   a. Pain from inflammation of various eye structures—usually controlled by nonsteroidal anti-inflammatories, but systemic antibiotics and immunosuppression may be required.
   b. Rosy vision (glare) because of keeping pupil from full constriction; excessive light enters pupil, causing a dazzling of macula (minute corneal opacity).
   c. Degeneration of the cornea.
   d. Malposition or dislocation of lens.
5. Implants may not be advisable for patients with severe myopia, history of chronic iritis, retinal detachment, diabetic retinopathy, glaucoma, and complications during surgery.

Contact Lens

Extended-wear contact lens is an option for those who do not receive IOL implants. They restore binocular vision and result in magnification of images in the range of 7% to 10%.

The patient will need to take the lens out for cleaning periodically or, if the patient is an older adult or debilitated, will need to follow up at intervals for cleaning at the ophthalmologist's office.

Complications

1. Blindness.

Nursing Assessment

Preoperative

1. Assess knowledge level regarding procedure.
2. Determine visual limitations and effect on daily living.
3. Assess anxiety and fears about loss of vision and surgery.

Postoperative

1. Assess pain level.
   a. Sudden onset—may be due to ruptured vessel or suture and may lead to hemorrhage.
   b. Severe pain—accompanied by nausea and vomiting; may be caused by increased IOP and may require immediate treatment.
2. Assess visual acuity in unoperated eye.
3. Assess for signs of infection—fever, inflammation, pain, drainage.
4. Assess the patient's functional level and ability to be independent.

Nursing Interventions

Preparing the Patient for Surgery

1. Orient the patient and explain procedures and plan of care to decrease anxiety.
2. Instruct the patient not to touch eyes to decrease contamination.
3. Obtain conjunctival cultures, if requested, using aseptic technique.
4. Administer preoperative eye drops—antibiotic, mydriatic–cycloplegic, and other medications—mannitol solution IV, sedative, antiemetic, and opioid, as directed. Explain medication actions to patient.

Preventing Complications Postoperatively

1. Medicate for pain, as prescribed, to promote comfort.
2. Administer medication to prevent nausea and vomiting, as needed.
3. Notify the health care provider of sudden pain associated with restlessness and increased pulse, which may indicate increased IOP, or fever, which may indicate infection.
4. Caution the patient against coughing or sneezing and medicate, as needed, to prevent increased IOP.
5. Advise the patient against rapid movement or bending from the waist to minimize IOP. The patient may be more comfortable with head elevated 30 degrees and lying on the unaffected side.
6. Allow the patient to ambulate as soon as possible and to resume independent activities.
7. Assist the patient in maneuvering through environment with the use of one eye while eye patch is on (1 to 2 days).
8. Encourage the patient to wear eye shield at night to protect operated eye from injury while sleeping.

Patient Education and Health Maintenance

Promoting Independence

1. Advice the patient to increase activities, as tolerated, unless given restrictions by the surgeon.
2. Caution against activities that cause patient to strain (e.g., lifting heavy objects, straining at defecation, and strenuous activity) for up to 6 weeks, as directed.
3. Instruct the patient and family about proper eye drop or ointment instillation.
4. Advise the patient to bring all medications to follow-up visits to permit dosage adjustments by ophthalmologist. Discontinued medications can then be discarded to prevent confusion.

Adjusting to Visual Change

1. Inform the patient receiving corrective lenses that fitting for temporary corrective lenses for the first 6 weeks will occur several days after surgery.
   a. Prescription for permanent lenses will be determined 6 to 12 weeks after surgery.
   b. Prescription for a permanent contact lens will be determined about 3 to 6 weeks after surgery.
2. Encourage the patient to wear dark glasses after eye dressings are removed to provide comfort from photophobia because of lack of pupil constriction from mydriatic–cycloplegic drops.

Adjusting to the Eyeglasses

1. Stress the importance of patience in the coming weeks of adjustment—it is easy to become frustrated.
2. Tell the patient that if glasses are to be worn, they will cause the perceived image to be about one third larger than normal. Glasses cannot restore binocular vision as an IOL implant or contact lens will because of the discrepancy of image size between the treated eye and untreated eye.
3. If glass is used in the prescription, it is heavier and thicker than the more expensive plastic cataract eyeglass lenses.
4. Instruct the patient to look through the center of corrective glasses and to turn head when looking to the side because peripheral vision is markedly distorted.
5. It is necessary to relearn space judgment—walking, using stairs, reaching for articles on the table (such as a cup of coffee), and pouring liquids—because of loss of binocular vision and peripheral distortion.
6. Advise patients to use handrails while walking and doing steps and to reach out slowly for objects to be picked up.

Becoming Familiar With Contact Lenses

Teach the patient that:

1. With contact lenses, magnification is only about 7% to 10%; peripheral vision is not distorted so binocular vision is achieved and spatial distortion is usually not an issue.
2. Patients do need to learn how to remove daily-wear and extended-wear lenses or return to the ophthalmologist's office for replacement of extended-wear lens periodically.

Becoming Familiar With Intraocular Lens

1. Teach the patient that with an intraocular lens, magnification problems are negligible. Both the operated eye and the unoperated eye can work together after cataract surgery with lens implantation, and the preoperative glasses can usually be worn in the recuperative period.
2. Advise the patient that eyeglasses may not be required for distance but may be needed for reading and writing.
3. Caution the patient against straining of any type. Bend knees only if necessary to reach for something on the floor.
4. Recommend sponge bathing. Avoid getting soap in the eyes.
5. Advice avoidance of tilting head forward when washing hair; tilt head slightly backward. Vigorous shaking of the head is to be avoided.

Evaluation: Expected Outcomes

- Vision maximized and distortions or limitations in vision described by patient.
- Independent activities demonstrated, denies discomfort.

Acute (Angle-Closure) Glaucoma

A condition in which an obstruction occurs at the access to the trabecular meshwork and the canal of Schlemm. IOP is normal when the anterior chamber angle is open, and glaucoma occurs when a significant portion of that angle is closed. Glaucoma is associated with progressive visual field loss and eventual blindness if allowed to progress. This is most commonly an acute painful condition (about 10% of glaucoma cases), not to be confused with chronic open-angle glaucoma (about 90% of cases).

Pathophysiology and Etiology

1. Mechanical blockage of anterior chamber angle results in accumulation of aqueous humor (fluid). See Figure 12-6.
2. Anterior chamber is anatomically shallow in most cases.
3. The shallow chamber with narrow anterior angles is more prone to physiologic events that result in closure.
4. Angle closure occurs because of pupillary dilation or forward displacement of the iris.
5. Angle closure can occur in subacute, acute, or chronic forms.
6. Episodes of subacute closure may precede an acute attack and cause transient blurred vision and pain but no increased IOP.
7. Acute angle closure causes a dramatic response with sudden elevation of IOP and permanent eye damage within several hours if not treated.
8. Within several days, scar tissue forms between the iris and cornea, closing the angle. The iris and ciliary body begin to

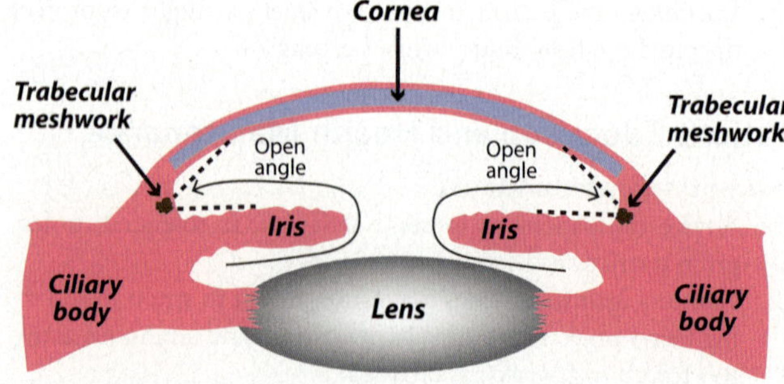

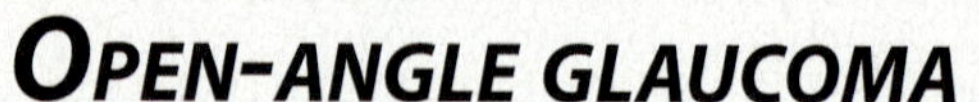

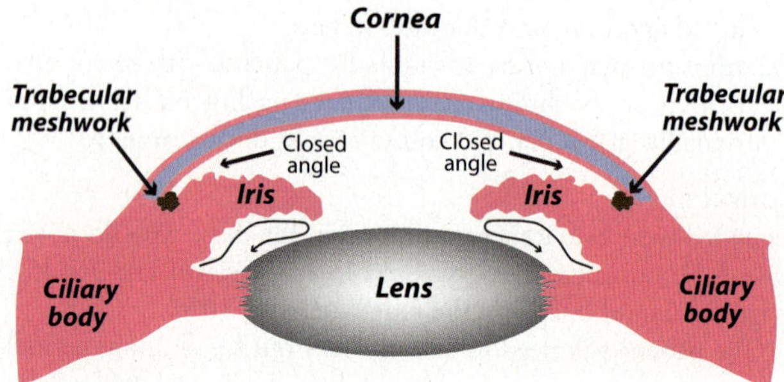

Figure 12-6. Angle-closure glaucoma compared with open-angle glaucoma (Shutterstock/Timonina).

atrophy, the cornea degenerates because of edema, and the optic nerve begins to atrophy.

Clinical Manifestations

1. Pain in and around eyes because of increased ocular pressure; may be transitory attacks.
2. Rainbow of color (halos) around lights.
3. Vision becomes cloudy and blurred.
4. Pupil mid-dilated and fixed.
5. Nausea and vomiting may occur.
6. Hazy-appearing cornea because of corneal edema.
7. Although onset may have initial subclinical symptoms, severity of symptoms may progress to cause acute symptoms of increased IOP—nausea and vomiting, sudden onset of blurred vision, severe pain, profuse lacrimation, and ciliary injection.

CLINICAL JUDGMENT Acute angle-closure glaucoma is a medical emergency. If nausea and vomiting occur with visual impairment, contact health care provider for immediate evaluation and treatment. Untreated, blindness can result in less than 1 week.

Diagnostic Evaluation

1. Tonometry—elevated IOP, usually greater than 50 mm Hg.
2. Ocular examination may reveal a pale optic disc.
3. Gonioscopy (using special instrument called gonioscope) to study the angle of the anterior chamber of the eye.

DRUG ALERT Dilating drops are avoided if the anterior chamber is shallow. This is determined by oblique illumination of the anterior segment of the eye. A flashlight is shined across the iris from the temporal side. If the iris is bulging (with a shallow anterior chamber), a crescent shadow appears on the nasal side of the iris.

Management

Pharmacologic

1. Emergency pharmacotherapy is initiated to decrease eye pressure before surgery.
2. Medications are based on the patient's condition but may include:
   a. Parasympathomimetic drugs used as miotic drugs—pupil contracts; iris is drawn away from cornea; aqueous humor may drain through lymph spaces (meshwork) into canal of Schlemm.
   b. Carbonic anhydrase inhibitor—restricts action of enzyme that is necessary to produce aqueous humor.
   c. Beta-adrenergic blockers—nonselective—may reduce production of aqucous humor or may facilitate outflow of aqueous humor.
   d. Hyperosmotic agents—to reduce IOP by promoting diuresis.

Surgery

1. Surgery is indicated if:
   a. IOP is not maintained within normal limits by medical regimen.
   b. There is progressive visual field loss with optic nerve damage.
2. Types of surgery include:
   a. Peripheral iridectomy—excision of a small portion of the iris whereby aqueous humor can bypass pupil. Treatment of choice is typically a laser procedure.
   b. Trabeculectomy—partial-thickness scleral resection with small part of trabecular meshwork removed and iridectomy. Necessary if peripheral anterior adhesions (synechiae) have developed due to repeated glaucoma attacks.
   c. Laser iridotomy—multiple tiny laser incisions to iris to create openings for aqueous flow; may be repeated.
3. Other eye is usually operated on eventually as a preventive measure.

Complications

Uncontrolled IOP that can lead to optic atrophy and total blindness.

Nursing Assessment

1. Evaluate the patient for severe pain, nausea, and vomiting and signs of increased IOP.
2. Assess visual symptoms and effect on daily activity.
3. Establish history of onset of attack and previous attacks.
4. Assess the patient's level of anxiety and knowledge base of glaucoma and treatment.

Nursing Interventions

Relieving Pain

1. Notify the health care provider immediately of the patient's condition.
2. Administer opioids and other medications, as directed. Medications that may cause nausea and vomiting are avoided. The patient may be medicated with antiemetic if nausea occurs.
3. Explain to the patient that the goal of treatment is to reduce IOP as quickly as possible.
4. Explain procedures to the patient.
5. Reassure the patient that, with reduction in IOP, pain and other signs and symptoms should subside.
6. Explain adverse effects of medications:
   a. Mannitol (IV)—transient blurred vision, rhinitis, thirst, nausea, transient circulatory overload, and headache.
   b. Acetazolamide or methazolamide (oral)—drowsiness, anorexia, paresthesia, stomach upset, tinnitus, fluid and electrolyte imbalance, rare kidney or liver dysfunction.
   c. Pilocarpine (topical)—burning and redness of eye, headache, constricted pupil, poor vision in dim light, retinal detachment, and rare lens opacity.

Relieving Fear

1. Provide reassurance and calm presence to reduce anxiety and fear.
2. Prepare the patient for surgery, if necessary.
3. Describe procedure to the patient; surgery will likely be done on an outpatient basis.
   a. Patch will be worn for several hours and sunglasses may help with photophobia.
   b. Vision will be blurred for first few days after the procedure.
   c. Frequent initial follow-up will be necessary for tonometry to make sure there is control of IOP.

Patient Education and Health Maintenance

1. Instruct the patient in use of medications. Stress the importance of long-term medication use to control this chronic

Table 12-4 Drugs That Affect Intraocular Pressure

MEDICATION	ROUTE	EFFECT
Corticosteroids	Oral, inhalant, intravenous, intravitreal, periocular topical solutions (creams and drops)	Elevates IOP
Alpha-chymotrypsin	Intraocular	Transient elevation of IOP
Topiramate (anticonvulsant)	Oral	Elevates IOP
Anticholinergics	Topical	Causes angle-closure glaucoma
Sulfonamides	Oral	Causes angle-closure glaucoma
Tricyclic antidepressants	Oral	Causes acute angle-closure glaucoma
Monoamine oxidase inhibitors	Oral	Causes acute angle-closure glaucoma
Antihistamines	Oral	Causes acute angle-closure glaucoma
Antiparkinsonian	Oral	Causes acute angle-closure glaucoma
Antipsychotics	Oral	Causes acute angle-closure glaucoma
Anti-spasmolytics	Oral	Causes acute angle-closure glaucoma
Cycloplegic agents	Topical	Contraindicated in narrow-angle glaucoma
Mydriatic agents	Topical	Contraindicated in narrow-angle glaucoma
Sympathomimetic agents	Topical	Contraindicated in narrow-angle glaucoma

IOP, intraocular pressure.

disease. Patients commonly forget that eye drops are medications and that glaucoma is a chronic illness.
2. Remind the patient to keep follow-up appointments.
3. Instruct the patient to seek immediate medical attention if signs and symptoms of increased IOP return—severe eye pain, photophobia, and excessive lacrimation.
4. Advise the patient to notify all health care providers of condition and medications and to avoid use of medications that may increase IOP, such as corticosteroids and anticholinergics (such as antihistamines), unless the benefit outweighs the risk (see Table 12-4).

Evaluation: Expected Outcomes

- Pain is decreased.
- Describes treatment regimen and verbalizes reduced fear.

Chronic (Open-Angle) Glaucoma

Glaucoma is characterized as a disorder of increased IOP, degeneration of the optic nerve, and visual field loss. Incidence increases with age: 2% at age 40, 7% at age 70, and 8% at age 80.

Pathophysiology and Etiology

1. Degenerative changes occur in the trabecular meshwork and canal of Schlemm, causing microscopic obstruction. See Figure 12-6 (page 14).
2. Aqueous fluid cannot be emptied from the anterior chamber, increasing IOP.
3. IOP varies with activity and some people tolerate elevated IOP without optic damage (ocular hypertension), whereas others exhibit visual field defects and optic damage with minimal or transient IOP elevation.
4. The risk of eye damage increases with age, family history of glaucoma, diabetes, and hypertension.

Clinical Manifestations

1. Mild, bilateral discomfort (tired feeling in eyes, foggy vision).
2. Slowly developing impairment of peripheral vision—central vision unimpaired.
3. Progressive loss of visual field.
4. Halos may be present around lights with increased ocular pressure.
5. May be asymptomatic but detected during routine eye exam.

Diagnostic Evaluation

1. Tonometry—IOP usually greater than 24 mm Hg but may be within normal limits.
2. Ocular examination—to check for clipping and atrophy of the optic disc.
3. Visual fields testing for deficits.

Management

1. Commonly treated with a combination of topical miotic agents (increase the outflow of aqueous humor by enlarging the area around trabecular meshwork) and oral carbonic anhydrase inhibitors and beta-adrenergic blockers (decrease aqueous production).
2. Remission may occur; however, there is no cure. The patient should continue to see health care provider at 3- to 6-month intervals for control of IOP.
3. If medical treatment is not successful, surgery may be required, but is delayed as long as possible.
4. Types of surgery include:
   a. Laser trabeculoplasty.
      i. An outpatient procedure, treatment of choice if increased ocular pressure unresponsive to medical regimen only.
      ii. As many as 100 superficial surface burns are placed evenly at junction of pigmented and nonpigmented

trabeculum meshwork for 360 degrees in anesthetized eye, which allows increased outflow of aqueous humor.

iii. Maximum decrease in IOP is achieved in 2 to 3 months, but IOP may rise again in 1 to 2 years.

b. Iridencleisis—an opening is created between anterior chamber and space beneath the conjunctiva; this bypasses the blocked meshwork and aqueous humor is absorbed into conjunctival tissues.

c. Cyclodiathermy or cyclocryotherapy—the ciliary body's function of secreting aqueous humor is decreased by damaging the body with high-frequency electrical current or supercooled probe applied to the surface of the eye over the ciliary body.

d. Corneoscleral trephine (rarely done)—a permanent opening at the junction of the cornea and sclera is made through the anterior chamber so aqueous humor can drain.

DRUG ALERT Using beta-adrenergic blocker eye drops in the treatment of glaucoma can cause an adverse reaction in patients taking oral beta-adrenergic blockers for cardiovascular disease. Monitor vital signs due to the risk for bradycardia.

Nursing Assessment

1. Assess frequency, duration, and severity of visual symptoms.
2. Assess the patient's knowledge of disease process and anxiety about the diagnosis.
3. Assess the patient's motivation to participate in long-term treatment.

Nursing Interventions

Providing Information About Glaucoma

1. Review the normal anatomy and physiology of the eye as well as the changes that occur in the drainage of aqueous humor with glaucoma.
2. Make sure the patient understands that, although asymptomatic, IOP could still be elevated and damage to the eye could be occurring. Therefore, ongoing use of medication and follow-up are essential.
3. Teach the patient the action, dosage, and adverse effects of all medications. Make sure of adequate administration of eye drops by watching the patient give return demonstration.
   a. Timolol and betaxolol—adverse effects include headache, eye irritation, decreased corneal sensitivity, blurred vision, bradycardia, palpitations, bronchospasm, hypotension, and heart failure.
   b. Pilocarpine—adverse effects include eye irritation, blurring, and redness; headache; pupil constriction; poor vision in dim light; possible hypertension and tachycardia; and rare retinal detachment and lens opacity.
   c. Acetazolamide and methazolamide—adverse effects include drowsiness, anorexia, paresthesia, stomach upset, tinnitus, fluid and electrolyte imbalance, and rare kidney and liver dysfunction.
4. Discuss visual defects with the patient and ways to compensate. Vision loss is permanent and treatment is aimed at stopping the process.
5. Inform the patient that surgery is done on an outpatient basis and recovery is quick. Prolonged restrictions are not required.
   a. After surgery, elevation of head 30 degrees will promote aqueous humor drainage after a trabeculectomy.
   b. Additional medications after surgery include topical steroids and cycloplegics to decrease inflammation and to dilate the pupil.

Patient Education and Health Maintenance

1. Patient must remember that glaucoma cannot be cured, but it can be controlled.
2. Remind the patient that periodic eye checkups are essential because pressure changes may occur.
3. Alert the patient to avoid, if possible, circumstances that may increase IOP:
   a. Upper respiratory infections.
   b. Emotional upsets—worry, fear, anger.
   c. Exertion, such as snow shoveling, pushing, and heavy lifting.
4. Recommend the following:
   a. Continuous daily use of eye medications as prescribed.
   b. Moderate use of the eyes.
   c. Exercise in moderation to maintain general well-being.
   d. Unrestricted fluid intake: alcohol and coffee may be permitted unless they are noted to cause increased IOP in the particular patient.
   e. Maintenance of regular bowel habits to decrease straining.
   f. Wearing a medical identification tag indicating the patient has glaucoma.

Evaluation: Expected Outcomes

- Verbalizes understanding of glaucoma as a chronic disease; demonstrates proper instillation of ophthalmic medications.

Retinal Detachment

Retinal detachment is defined as detachment of the sensory area of the retina (rods and cones) from the pigmented epithelium of the retina. A break in the continuity of the retina may first occur from small degenerative holes and tears, which may lead to detachment.

Pathophysiology and Etiology

1. Spontaneous detachment may occur due to degenerative changes in the retina or vitreous.
2. Trauma, inflammation, or tumor causes detachment by forming a mass that mechanically separates the retinal layers.
3. Diabetic retinopathy commonly leads to retinal degeneration and tears, disrupting the integrity of the retina.
4. Myopia and loss of a lens from a cataract (aphakia) also predispose to retinal tears and detachment because the posterior chamber is enlarged, leading to vitreous pull.
5. After detachment occurs, that portion of the retina cannot perceive light because the blood and oxygen supply is cut off; hence, part of the visual field is lost.
6. Detachment occurs most commonly in patients over age 40.

Clinical Manifestations

1. Retinal detachment may occur slowly or rapidly, but without pain.
2. The patient complains of flashes of light or blurred, "sooty" vision because of stimulation of the retina by vitreous pull.
3. The patient notes sensation of particles moving in line of vision (more so than usual—"floaters" that a person can see floating across field of vision when looking at a light background).

4. Delineated areas of vision may be blank.
5. A sensation of a veil-like coating coming down, coming up, or coming sideways in front of the eye may be present if detachment develops rapidly.
   a. This veil-like coating, or shadow, is commonly misinterpreted as a drooping eyelid or elevated cheek.
   b. Straight-ahead vision may remain good in early stages.
6. Unless the retinal holes are sealed, the retina will progressively detach; ultimately, there will be a loss of central vision as well as peripheral vision, leading to legal blindness.

Diagnostic Evaluation

Indirect ophthalmoscopy shows gray or opaque retina. The retina is normally transparent. Slit-lamp examination and three-mirror gonioscopy magnify the lesion.

Management

General

1. Sedation, bed rest, and eye patch may be used to restrict eye movements.
2. Surgical intervention may be indicated.
3. Return of visual acuity with a reattached retina depends on:
   a. Amount of retina detached before surgery.
   b. Whether the macula (area of central vision) was detached.
   c. Length of time the retina was detached.
   d. Amount of external distortion caused by the scleral buckle.
   e. Possible macular damage as a result of diathermy of cryocoagulation.
4. Surgical reattachment is successful approximately 90% to 95% of the time. If the retina remains attached 2 months postoperatively, the condition is likely to be corrected and is unlikely to recur.

Surgical Procedures

1. Photocoagulation—a light beam (either laser or xenon arc) is passed through the pupil, causing a small burn and producing an exudate between the pigment epithelium and retina.
2. Electrodiathermy—an electrode needle is passed through the sclera to allow subretinal fluid to escape. An exudate forms from the pigment epithelium and adheres to the retina.
3. Cryosurgery or retinal cryopexy—a supercooled probe is touched to the sclera, causing minimal damage; as a result of scarring, the pigment epithelium adheres to the retina.
4. Scleral buckling—a technique whereby the sclera is shortened to allow buckling to occur, which forces the pigment epithelium closer to the retina (often accompanied by vitrectomy).

Complications

1. Glaucoma.
2. Infection.

Nursing Assessment

Preoperative

1. Assess for history of trauma or other risk factors.
2. Assess level of anxiety and knowledge level regarding procedures.
3. Determine visual limitations and obtain visual description from patient to determine assistance needed.

Postoperative

1. Assess pain level.
2. Assess visual acuity if unoperated eye not patched.
3. Determine the patient's ability to ambulate and assume independent activities, as tolerated.

Nursing Interventions

Reducing Anxiety Before Surgery

1. Instruct the patient to remain quiet in prescribed position. (Detached area of retina remains in dependent position.) Assist with all activities and offer frequent reassurance.
2. Patch both eyes. Make sure that the patient is oriented to surroundings and can call for assistance.
3. Describe preoperative procedures before carrying them out.
4. Wash the patient's face with antibacterial solution.
5. Administer preoperative medications, as ordered.
6. Instruct the patient not to touch eyes.

Preventing Postoperative Complications

1. Caution the patient to avoid bumping head.
2. Advise the patient to try to avoid coughing or sneezing and medicate if needed to prevent increased IOP.
3. Encourage ambulation and independence, but assist with activities as needed.
4. Administer medications for pain, nausea, and vomiting, as prescribed.
5. Provide safe diversional activities such as radio, audio books.
6. If the patient's anticoagulation therapy has been stopped, provide preventive measures such as compression stockings, leg exercises, and carefully monitor for signs and symptoms of thrombosis and embolism.

Patient Education and Health Maintenance

1. Encourage self-care at discharge, if done in an unhurried manner. (Avoid falls, jerks, bumps, or accidental injury.)
2. Instruct the patient about the following:
   a. Rapid eye movements should be avoided for several weeks.
   b. Driving is restricted.
   c. Within 3 weeks, light activities may be pursued.
   d. Within 6 weeks, heavier activities and athletics are possible. Define such activities for the patient.
   e. Avoid straining and bending head below the waist.
   f. Use meticulous cleanliness when instilling eye medications.
   g. Apply a clean, warm, moist washcloth to eyes and eyelids several times a day for 10 minutes to provide soothing and relaxing comfort.
   h. Symptoms that indicate a recurrence of the detachment: floating spots, flashing light, and progressive shadows. Recommend that the patient contact health care provider if they occur.
3. Advise on follow-up. The first follow-up visit to the ophthalmologist should occur in 2 weeks, with other visits scheduled thereafter.

Evaluation: Expected Outcomes

- Verbalizes understanding of treatment.
- Follows activity restrictions.

Other Problems of the Retina and Vitreous

The retina is a multilayered structure that receives images and transmits them to the brain. It is nourished by retinal arteries and veins. Problems result from inflammation, trauma, vascular changes, congenital defects, and aging. Central lesions affect the macula, impairing central vision, near vision, and color discrimination. Peripheral lesions impair peripheral vision, causing blind spots, night blindness, and eventual tunnel vision. See Table 12-5 for treatment of individual disorders.

CLINICAL JUDGMENT Central retinal artery occlusion is a medical emergency. Vision may be salvaged if treated within 24 hours of onset.

Nursing Assessment

1. Take history of eye problems, general health, and family history of eye disease.
2. Obtain functional history of how eye problem may be impairing work, recreation, and other activities.
3. Assess bilateral visual acuity, peripheral vision, and color discrimination.
4. Assist with pupil dilation and ophthalmoscopy, as directed.

Table 12-5 Other Conditions of the Retina and Vitreous

CONDITION	TREATMENT AND NURSING CONSIDERATIONS
Vitreous hemorrhage Bleeding into the vitreous may occur due to trauma, sickle cell disease, hypertension, diabetic retinopathy, retinal tear or detachment, intraocular lens displacement, and clotting abnormalities. It causes decrease or loss of vision in affected eye.	The underlying cause is treated and surgery to repair the retina may include photocoagulation, cryotherapy, scleral buckle, or vitrectomy. (See "Retinal Detachment," page 17.) Assist the patient with visual deficit and activity and position restrictions before surgery. Maintain eye patches, activity restriction, and medication administration after surgery.
Central retinal artery occlusion Sudden occlusion of the central retinal artery causes painless loss of vision in one eye with loss of light perception. It may have been preceded by episodes of transient blindness (amaurosis fugax) for 10–15 min. It is caused by an embolus, usually from the ipsilateral carotid artery.	Treatment consists of massaging the globe in an attempt to break up the embolus or move it distally, inhalation of a mixture of 95% oxygen and 5% CO_2 to get the retinal vessels to dilate, and IV infusion of acetazolamide to lower IOP. Place the patient in Trendelenburg position and monitor vital signs, as directed. Offer reassurance and assist with additional testing and treatment, as indicated.
Central retinal vein occlusion Occlusion of the central retinal vein or a branch causes sudden (over several hours), painless decrease in visual acuity. Usually occurs in people with hypertension or other vascular disorders.	Urgent ophthalmologic evaluation is needed. Photocoagulation may be used to prevent local hemorrhage and promote neovascularization. Corticosteroids are used to treat retinal edema and an aspirin or anticoagulant may be used to prevent further occlusive disease. Encourage regular screening for glaucoma in follow-up as a complication from scar tissue formation after photocoagulation.
Macular degeneration Age-related changes in the choroid deprive the fovea centralis of blood supply, causing a dry (atrophic) form (onset over several years) or wet (exudative) form (onset over several days to weeks with neovascularization and hemorrhaging). Central and near vision are affected, but some peripheral vision remains bilateral.	Support patient and family. Be realistic about prognosis—there is no cure but treatment may include laser, anti-VEGF therapy, diet, and vitamins (AREDS formulation) to slow the progression of the disease. Anti-VEGF therapy involves intraocular injection of medication every few weeks; can be painful and may raise the risk of infection. Refer patient to the local chapter of The Lions Club or other agencies for vision rehabilitation in order to assist with adaptive devices for low vision.
Retinitis Inflammation of the retina, usually caused by cytomegalovirus as a complication of human immunodeficiency virus disease. Symptoms include blurred vision, floaters and/or flashes in the eye, and loss of peripheral vision and eventually blindness. Determination of the progression of the disease is made by direct and indirect ophthalmoscopy and intravenous fluorescein angiography.	Antiviral medications can help control the symptoms and slow the progression of retinitis. Other treatment modalities include vitrectomy, silicone oil injection, and retinal detachment repair. Nursing interventions focus on patient education of drug side effects, care of central venous lines for intravenous medication, and monitoring blood count and for signs of kidney damage. Patient may be referred to community resources for low-vision assistance.
Diabetic retinopathy A vascular disorder of the retina that leads to diminished vision as a complication of diabetes mellitus. Classified as nonproliferative or proliferative and typically occurs in four stages.	See page 427. Untreated diabetic retinopathy may cause complications such as retinal detachment, vitreous hemorrhage, clinically significant macular edema, glaucoma, and blindness.

AREDS, age-related eye disease study; IOP, intraocular pressure; IV, intravenous; VEGF, vascular endothelial growth factor.

Nursing Interventions

Ensuring Safety Following Sudden Loss of Vision

1. Orient the patient to the layout of the facility and explain procedures.
2. Assist with self-care activities and educate patient on how to call for assistance.
3. Have personal articles placed nearby and take care not to move things without alerting the patient.
4. Ensure clear path for patient to move and ambulate; remove obstacles; provide ambulation aids as needed.
5. Help the patient understand visual weaknesses, such as where blind spots are and how to compensate by turning head to scan environment, using magnifying glass, having environment brightly lit.
6. Use side rails and direct visual supervision, if needed.
7. Assist the patient on stairs, make sure good footwear is worn, and obtain occupational therapy referral if needed.

Relieving Anxiety

1. Keep the patient informed during the diagnostic process.
2. Encourage patient to discuss feelings and frustrations.
3. Refer patients with vision less than 20/70 for telerehabilitation, or other resource for education and assistive devices (see page 430).
4. Advise patient to memorize environment while some vision is intact and to subsequently avoid changing the environment.
5. Encourage participation in support groups.

EVIDENCE BASE Bittner, A. K., Yoshinaga, P. D., Rittiphairoj, T., & Li, T. (2023). Telerehabilitation for people with low vision. *Cochrane Database of Systematic Reviews*, (1). Art. No.: CD011019. https://doi.org/10.1002/14651858.CD011019.pub4

Patient Education and Health Maintenance

1. Encourage frequent follow-up with ophthalmologist.
2. Advise the patient to use corrective lenses as directed and keep lens prescription up to date and to have a spare pair of glasses available.
3. Warn the patient against straining eyes by excessive exposure to the sun, reading, or computer work.
4. Rest eyes, as needed.
5. Report sudden deterioration in vision or other changes: sudden loss of vision, increase in floaters, flashes of light, sharp pain.

Evaluation: Expected Outcomes

- Performs daily activities without injury.
- Discusses feelings and participates in support group.

Eye Trauma

Trauma to the eye may be caused by blunt or sharp injury or chemical or thermal burns. The eyelids, protective layers, surrounding soft tissue, or the globe itself may be injured. Vision may be impaired by direct injury or latent scarring. See Table 12-6 for specific conditions.

Nursing Assessment

1. Obtain history of mechanism of injury as well as extent of other injuries.
2. Assess level of pain and visual symptoms.
3. Perform neurologic assessment and assess vital signs.
4. Assess visual acuity.

Nursing Interventions

Relieving Pain

1. Medicate for pain, as directed.
2. Provide ice and cool compresses to relieve swelling and pain.
3. Provide additional comfort measures, such as positioning, dimmed lights, and quiet environment.
4. Irrigate and patch eye, as directed.
5. Monitor vital signs and neurologic status, as indicated.
6. Watch for and report signs of infection, such as fever, drainage, increased pain, warmth, and redness.

CLINICAL JUDGMENT Monitor for respiratory depression, hypotension, and decreased level of consciousness if opioid analgesic is used. Medications that depress the central nervous system may be contraindicated if head injury is suspected.

Strengthening Coping

1. Provide psychological support and assist with self-care activities, as needed.
2. Describe procedures and treatments to the patient and family.
3. Maintain safe environment.
4. Assist patient with coping measures such as relaxation breathing, imagery, and distraction.
5. Prepare the patient for surgery, as indicated (see page 56).

Patient Education and Health Maintenance

1. Teach the patient how to administer medications such as topical antibiotics.
2. Instruct on use of patch or shield.
3. Advise the patient to report increase in pain, decrease in vision, redness, and fever.
4. Teach safety measures with decreased visual acuity.
5. Advise the use of corrective lenses, as prescribed.
6. Stress follow-up care.
7. Attempt to prevent future trauma with protective eyewear.

Evaluation: Expected Outcomes

- Rests comfortably, reports less pain.
- Cooperates with procedures; uses coping mechanisms.

Resources

For further information regarding eye disorders and resources, contact:

- American Academy of Ophthalmology (*www.eyecareamerica.org*).
- American Council of the Blind (*www.acb.org*).
- American Foundation for the Blind (*www.afb.or*).
- American Macular Degeneration Foundation (*www.macular.org*).
- Lions Club International (www.lionsclub.org).
- National Eye Institute, Eye Health Information (*www.nei.nih.gov/health*).
- Royal National Institute of Blind People (*www.rnib.org.uk*).

Table 12-6 Eye Trauma

CONDITION	CLINICAL MANIFESTATIONS	MEDICAL MANAGEMENT
Blunt contusion		
Bruising of periorbital soft tissue	• Swelling and discoloration of the tissue • Bleeding into the tissue and structures of the eye • Pain • Diagnosis: Tests must determine if injury to parts of eye and systemic trauma	• Treatment to reduce swelling • Pain management dependent on structures involved *Note:* If there is any possibility of a ruptured globe, a loose patch and shield should be placed and ocular manipulation discouraged until ophthalmologist assessment completed.
Hyphema		
Presence of blood in the anterior chamber	• Pain • Blood in anterior chamber • Increased intraocular pressure	• Usually spontaneous recovery • If severe, bed rest or chair rest with bathroom privileges, eye shield, interior chamber paracentesis, topical steroids, and cycloplegics
Orbital fracture		
Fracture and dislocation of walls of the orbit, orbital margins, or both	• May be accompanied by other signs of head injury • Rhinorrhea • Contusion • Diplopia • Diagnosis: x-ray, computed tomography	• May heal on own if no displacement or impingement on other structures • Surgery (repair the orbital floor with plate freeing entrapped orbital tissue)
Foreign body		
On cornea (25% all ocular injuries), conjunctiva Intraocular particles penetrate sclera, cornea, globe	• Severe pain • Lacrimation • Foreign body sensation • Photophobia • Redness • Swelling *Note:* Wood and plant foreign body may cause severe infection within hours.	• Medical emergency • Removal of foreign body through irrigation, cotton-tipped applicator, or magnet • Treatment of intraocular foreign body depends on size, magnetic properties, tissue reaction, location • Surgical removal
Laceration/perforation		
Cutting or penetration of soft tissue or globe	• Pain • Bleeding • Lacrimation • Photophobia	• Medical emergency • Surgical repair—method of repair depends on severity of injury • Antibiotics—topically and systemically
Ruptured globe		
Concussive injury to globe with tears in the ocular coats, usually the sclera	• Pain • Altered intraocular pressure • Limitation of gaze in field of rupture • Hyphema • Hemorrhage (poor prognostic sign) • Diagnosis: computed tomography, ultrasound	• Medical emergency • Surgical repair • Vitrectomy • Scleral buckle • Antibiotics • Steroids • Enucleation may be necessary
Burns		
Chemical—caused by alkali or acid agent	• Pain • Burning • Lacrimation • Photophobia	• Medical emergency • Copious irrigation until pH is 7 • Severe scarring may require keratoplasty • Antibiotics
Thermal—usually burn to eyelids—may be first-, second-, or third-degree burn	• Pain • Burned skin • Blisters	• First aid—apply sterile dressings • Pain control • Leave fluid blebs intact • Suture eyelids together to protect eye—if perforation a possibility • Skin grafting with severe second- and third-degree burns
Ultraviolet—excessive exposure to sunlight, sunlamp, snow blindness, welding	• Pain—delayed several hours after exposure • Foreign body sensation • Lacrimation • Photophobia *Note:* Symptoms occur sometime after exposure.	• Pain relief • Condition self-limiting • Bilateral patching with antibiotic ointment and cycloplegics

SELECTED READINGS

Agarwal, S., Srinivasan, B., Harwani, A. A., Fogla, R., & Iyer, G. (2022). Perioperative nuances of cataract surgery in ocular surface disorders. *Indian Journal of Ophthalmology, 70*(10), 3455–3464. https://doi.org/10.4103/ijo.IJO_624_22

Chauhan, M. Z., Rather, P. A., Samarah, S. M., Elhusseiny, A. M., & Sallam, A. B. (2022). Current and novel therapeutic approaches for treatment of diabetic macular edema. *Cells, 11*(12), 1950. https://doi.org/10.3390/cells11121950

Clapp, C. M., Pepper, J. V., Schmidt, R., & Stern, S. (2020). Overview of vocational rehabilitation data about people with visual impairments: Demographics, services, and long-run labor market trends. *Journal of Visual Impairment & Blindness, 114*(1), 43–56. https://doi.org/10.1177/0145482X20901380

Dean, E. C., & Welch, R.M. (Eds.). (2017). *Ophthalmic procedures in the office and clinic* (4th ed.). American Society of Ophthalmologic Registered Nurses.

Ferguson, T. J., & Randleman, J. B. (2024). Cataract surgery following refractive surgery: Principles to achieve optical success and patient satisfaction. *Survey of Ophthalmology, 69*(1), 140–159. https://doi.org/10.1016/j.survophthal.2023.08.002

Fleckenstein, M., Schmitz-Valckenberg, S., & Chakravarthy, U. (2024). Age-related macular degeneration: A review. *JAMA, 331*(2), 147–157. https://doi.org/10.1001/jama.2023.26074

Guo, H., Hosseini-Moghaddam, S. M., & Hodge, W. (2019). Corneal biomechanical properties after SMILE versus FLEX, LASIK, LASEK, or PRK: A systematic review and meta-analysis. *BMC Ophthalmology, 19*(1), 167. https://doi.org/10.1186/s12886-019-1165-3

Joseph, S., Selvaraj, J., Mani, I., Kumaragurupari, T., Shang, X., Mudgil, P., Ravilla, T., & He, M. (2024). Diagnostic accuracy of artificial intelligence based automated diabetic retinopathy screening in real-world settings: A systematic review and meta-analysis. *American Journal of Ophthalmology, S0002-9394*(24), 00066-7. Advance online publication. https://doi.org/10.1016/j.ajo.2024.02.012

Keskinbora, K., & Güven, F. (2020). Artificial intelligence and ophthalmology. *Turkish Journal of Ophthalmology, 50*(1), 37–43. https://doi.org/10.4274/tjo.galenos.2020.78989

Linaburg, T., Choi, D., Bunya, V. Y., Massaro-Giordano, M., & Briceño, C. A. (2021). Systematic review: Effects of pterygium and pingueculum on the ocular surface and efficacy of surgical excision. *Cornea, 40*(2), 258–267. https://doi.org/10.1097/ICO.0000000000002575

Lorenzini, M. C., & Wittich, W. (2021). Head-mounted visual assistive technology-related quality of life changes after telerehabilitation. *Optometry and Vision Science: Official Publication of the American Academy of Optometry, 98*(6), 582–591. https://doi.org/10.1097/OPX.0000000000001705

Mangione, C. M., Lee, P. P., Gutierrez, P. R., Spritzer, K., Berry, S., Hays, R. D., & the National Eye Institute Visual Function Questionnaire Field Test Investigators. (2001). Development of the 25-item National Eye Institute Visual Function Questionnaire (VFQ-25). *Archives of Ophthalmology, 119*, 1050–1058. https://doi.org/10.1001/archopt.119.7.1050

Milde, N., Schmidt, D. C., Larsen, A., & Kessel, L. (2024). Which rehabilitation initiatives can effectively improve participation in an educational setting for visually impaired and blind adolescents? A systematic review. *BMC Ophthalmology, 24*(1), 10. https://doi.org/10.1186/s12886-023-03267-8

Muir, K. W., Rosdahl, J. A., Hein, A. M., Woolson, S., Olsen, M. K., Kirshner, M., Sexton, M., & Bosworth, H. B. (2022). Improved glaucoma medication adherence in a randomized controlled trial. *Ophthalmol Glaucoma, 5*(1), 40–46. https://doi.org/10.1016/j.ogla.2021.04

Pacheco, L. (Ed.). (2017). *Care and handling of ophthalmic microsurgical instruments* (4th ed.). American Society of Ophthalmologic Registered Nurses.

Papadopoulos Z. (2020). Recent developments in the treatment of wet age-related macular degeneration. *Current Medical Science, 40*(5), 851–857. https://doi.org/10.1007/s11596-020-2253-6

Pelusi, L., Mandatori, D., Mastropasqua, L., Agnifili, L., Allegretti, M., Nubile, M., & Pandolfi, A. (2023). Innovation in the development of synthetic and natural ocular drug delivery systems for eye diseases treatment: Focusing on Drug-loaded ocular inserts, contacts, and intraocular lenses. *Pharmaceutics, 15*(2), 625. https://doi.org/10.3390/pharmaceutics15020625

Smith, L., & Vasile, E. (2021). A pathway to independent living: A collaborative approach between families, education and rehabilitation professionals. *Journal of Visual Impairment & Blindness, 115*(6), 568–573. https://doi.org/10.1177/0145482X211062255

Soekamto, C., Rosignoli, L., Zhu, C., Johnson, D. A., Sohn, J. H., & Bahadorani, S. (2022). Visual outcomes of acute bacterial endophthalmitis treated with adjuvant intravitreal dexamethasone: A meta-analysis and systematic review. *Indian Journal of Ophthalmology, 70*(8), 2835–2841. https://doi.org/10.4103/ijo.IJO_955_

Sultan, Z. N., Agorogiannis, E. I., Iannetta, D., Steel, D., & Sandinha, T. (2020). Rhegmatogenous retinal detachment: A review of current practice in diagnosis and management. *BMJ Open Ophthalmology, 5*(1), e000474. https://doi.org/10.1136/bmjophth-2020-000474

Welch, R. M., Waldo, M. N., Gomez, J. L., & Dean, E. C. (2022). *Essentials of ophthalmic nursing. Book 2.* American Society of Ophthalmologic Registered Nurses.

Welch, R. M., Waldo, M. N., Gomez, J. L., & Dean, E. C. (2022). *Essentials of ophthalmic nursing. Book 3.* American Society of Ophthalmologic Registered Nurses.

Welch, R. M., Waldo, M. N., Gomez, J. L., & Dean, E. C. (2022). *Essentials of ophthalmic nursing. Book 4.* American Society of Ophthalmologic Registered Nurses.

13 Ear, Nose, and Throat Disorders

OVERVIEW AND ASSESSMENT

History

Obtaining a history, including the patient's signs and symptoms, current health patterns, and previous past medical history, will help in identifying ear, nose, and throat (ENT) problems and developing an individualized plan of care.

Key Signs and Symptoms

1. Epistaxis.
   a. When did the bleeding first begin? Did it occur spontaneously or occur after facial or nasal trauma, nose blowing, digital manipulation, or recent nasal or sinus surgery? In many cases, anterior bleeding commonly flows from the nasal vestibule and, in the reclining position, will drip into the throat. Posterior bleeding commonly causes dripping into the oropharynx when upright or supine. Nasal endoscopy or examination via anterior rhinoscopy is performed to confirm the site of bleeding.
   b. Unilateral or bilateral? What side of the nose is the bleeding coming from, and, if bilateral, on what side did it begin? Ask the patient about measures employed to control the bleeding thus far.
   c. Assess current medication history: Is the patient taking acetylsalicylic acid (ASA/aspirin), nonsteroidal anti-inflammatory drugs (NSAIDs), antiplatelet agents, or anticoagulants? When was the last dose taken?
   d. Is there a history of current oxygen therapy? Is there a history of chronic bleeding disorders? Obtain results of recent blood work: complete blood count (CBC), prothrombin time (PT), international normalized ratio (INR), or partial prothrombin time (PTT).
2. Headache.
   a. Exactly what parts of the head or face hurt? Is it pain or a pressure sensation? Use the mnemonic OLD CARTS or PQRST (see page 3) to assess pain, with emphasis on location, duration, and symptom onset.
   b. Assess for associated neck, dental, or jaw pain; nausea; vomiting; visual changes; and/or sensitivity to light or sound. Assess for associated nasal congestion, postnasal drip, or clear or purulent rhinorrhea. Assess for a history of migraine disease.
3. Sore throat—assess onset and duration of symptoms, previous medical treatment, and symptom response.
   a. Is it accompanied by swollen glands, high fever, nasal congestion, and postnasal drip? Assess for associated weight loss; head, neck, or ear pain; voice changes; neck mass; trismus; or difficulty breathing. Has the patient been able to eat or drink?
   b. Is it acute or chronic? Was there any exposure to others with throat infection?
4. Nasal congestion.
   a. Is it acute or chronic? Accompanied by fever and purulent drainage? Assess the severity and duration of symptoms, associated purulent or clear rhinorrhea, fever, facial pain or sinus tenderness, itchy eyes, sneezing, or postnasal drip. If symptoms are chronic, assess if worsened with changes in barometric pressure, vary with seasons, or brought on by odors or allergen exposure.
   b. Assess for current/chronic history of use of nasal sprays containing oxymetazoline or if the patient is experiencing anosmia/hyposmia (complete or partial loss

of smell). Ask if the patient has a previous history of nasal polyps, previous nasal or sinus surgery, or nasal fracture.

5. Hoarseness.
   a. Assess history of recent surgical procedures involving the head or neck, recent endotracheal intubation, radiation treatment to the head/neck, history of tobacco/alcohol use, occupation as vocal performer, or history of lung disease with the use of inhaled steroids, chronic or recent antibiotic therapy, and symptoms of gastroesophageal reflux.
   b. Is it acute (less than 2 weeks), recurrent, or chronic (more than 2 weeks)? Assess onset and duration of symptoms, subjective impairment in communication, or voice-related quality.
   c. Assess for recent upper respiratory infection (URI) symptoms, associated dysphagia, odynophagia (pain with swallowing), globus sensation (sensation of something in the throat), throat pain, weight loss, ear pain, neck mass or enlarged lymph nodes in neck, hemoptysis, or shortness of breath.
6. Earache (otalgia).
   a. Is it worsened by manipulation of the auricle or is it a deep, throbbing pain? Is there otorrhea? Assess the onset and duration of pain using the PQRST mnemonic. Assess for associated erythema or edema of the external ear canal or external auricle, pruritus, hearing loss, or otorrhea. Is the pain intermittent or constant?
   b. Were there preceding URI symptoms? Is the pain associated with hearing loss, aural fullness, vertigo, headache, or fluctuation of hearing? Have there been any recent dental procedures?
   c. Assess history for nighttime bruxism (grinding teeth), clenching of the jaw or teeth, malocclusion, or pain worsened with movement of the jaw, dental pain, or swelling of the muscles of mastication.
   d. Assess for ear pain that occurs with swallowing and associated symptoms of head and neck cancer.
7. Hearing loss.
   a. Was it sudden or gradual in onset? Assess subjective onset of hearing loss. Did the patient experience sudden or gradual onset of the hearing loss? Is there associated tinnitus, vertigo, aural fullness, or ear pain?
   b. Unilateral or bilateral? Assess for a history of noise exposure; recreational shooting; occupational, acoustic trauma; or history of chronic otitis media. Assess for a history of familial/hereditary hearing loss. Assess for ototoxic medication use.
8. Dizziness.
   a. Is the patient light-headed or experiencing vertigo (as if the room or self is spinning)? Assess for subjective lightheadedness, room spinning, or imbalance. Are symptoms acute or chronic and associated with symptoms of fluctuation of hearing, aural fullness, or tinnitus (symptoms of Ménière disease)?
   b. Is the dizziness associated with a change in head or body position? Do symptoms occur with rolling over in bed, looking up or bending over, or when going from sitting to standing? Are there feelings of presyncope or a history of syncopal episode when rising from sitting to standing? Are there changes in blood pressure associated with lying, sitting, and standing?
   c. Assess for duration of symptoms and associated nausea, vomiting, headache, or focal neurologic symptoms.

CLINICAL JUDGMENT Hoarseness for longer than 4 weeks, or earlier if accompanied by hemoptysis and weight loss, is an indication for ENT evaluation and laryngoscopy.

Current Health Patterns

1. Inquire about nutrition, dental care, normal mouth care habits, dental caries, use of partial or full dentures, and stress-related grinding, clenching, or clamping of teeth.
2. Ask about the history of alcohol, smoking, use of a pipe, and smokeless tobacco. Is there a personal history of human immunodeficiency virus (HIV), sexually transmitted infection, recreational drug use, or human papillomavirus (HPV)?
3. Determine personal hygiene about ears. Are cotton swabs or other objects used for cleaning or to relieve itching? Does the patient wear hearing aids or earplugs?
4. Is there any loud noise exposure? Is there a history of noise exposure via recreational shooting or in the patient's occupation? Ask about the use of noise protection when exposed to prolonged and loud noise. Is there family history of hearing loss?
5. Does the patient frequently strain voice through talking, singing, or shouting? Is the patient a singer?
6. What medications is the patient taking? Have antibiotics been used? For how long?

Medical History

1. Is there a history of allergic rhinitis, other allergy symptoms, immunotherapy, chronic or recurrent sinusitis, previous nasal surgery, chronic otitis media, chronic pharyngitis, history of snoring, or obstructive sleep apnea?
2. Is there any immunosuppressive illness, such as diabetes mellitus, cancer, HIV infection, autoimmune disease, recent radiation, or chemotherapy?
3. Is there a history of previous thyroid, carotid artery, or other surgery involving the laryngeal nerve?
4. Any history of previous or recent head, facial, or nasal trauma?

See Chapter 1, pages 9 to 10, for physical assessment of the ears, nose, throat, and neck.

Diagnostic Tests

Audiometry

Description

1. Audiometry is the most basic and accurate testing to determine and measure hearing ability. The results are plotted on a graph known as an audiogram. Testing is performed by an audiologist. The following points describe aspects of audiometry:
   a. Pure tone threshold audiometry is the lowest level at which sound is heard across various sound frequencies. This is compared to normative data to measure hearing loss and used to monitor hearing sensitivity over time.
   b. Speech audiometry provides information about the patient's communication ability. Speech reception threshold is defined as the softest level at which the patient can repeat a word. Speech recognition or speech discrimination is the percentage of words that a patient can repeat accurately at the comfortable listening level. This helps to determine the ability to understand conversational speech.
   c. Pure tone testing is performed by presenting pure tones via air and bone conduction. Air conduction testing is done by

presenting pure tones at various octave levels from 250 to 8,000 Hz through a transducer, such as insert earphone or cushion headphone. The patient sits in a soundproof booth, and the audiologist presents tones and the patient is asked to indicate when the sound is heard. Testing by bone conduction is done with the use of a bone oscillator, which is placed on the mastoid of the test ear, and pure tones are presented at 500, 1,000, 2,000, and 4,000 Hz.

d. Immittance testing includes tympanometry and acoustic reflex testing.
   i. Acoustic reflex testing measures the response of the stapedius muscle in response to auditory signals. It provides information about the acoustic and the facial nerves as well as about a conductive or sensorineural hearing loss.
   ii. Tympanometry measures the changes that occur to the tympanic membrane and middle ear when changes in air pressure are introduced into the ear canal. It can provide information about eustachian tube dysfunction, middle ear fluid, tympanic membrane perforation, patency of pressure-equalizing tubes, and middle ear disease, such as otosclerosis.

Nursing and Patient Care Considerations

1. The patient wears earphones and signals upon hearing a tone.
2. A soundproof room is used to increase accuracy.
3. No special patient preparation or participation is necessary for tympanometry.

Cineradiography

Description

1. This motion study is performed to study the functional dynamics of the pharynx and esophagus.
2. It provides a more physiologic examination than esophagram (barium swallow). Mucosal detail is seen better with cineradiography, whereas video capture allows more dynamic evaluation with less radiation.
3. "Modified barium swallow" evaluates laryngotracheal aspiration while a speech pathologist provides various consistencies of food and swallowing techniques. An esophagram evaluates the pharyngeal and esophageal mucosa.

Nursing and Patient Care Considerations

1. The patient is usually kept nothing by mouth (NPO) the night before surgery.
2. The patient will be given radioprotective gear to prevent radiation from reaching other parts of the body.

Electronystagmography

Description

1. *Electronystagmography* (ENG) is the recording of eye movements, specifically nystagmus, during various oculomotor and vestibular testing. Videonystagmography is the recording of eye movements using infrared video image analysis in three dimensions. The pattern of nystagmus, in conjunction with the patient's neurotologic examination and clinical history, may provide information about the underlying etiology of the patient's symptoms.
2. Used to establish the diagnosis of Ménière disease, vestibular neuronitis or labyrinthitis, benign paroxysmal positional vertigo (BPPV), or migraine-associated vertigo and to assist in ruling out vestibular pathology in a patient with symptoms of dizziness.
3. The test takes place in a dimly lit room, with the patient on an examination table, and lasts for 60 to 90 minutes.
4. Electrodes are placed on the forehead and lateral to each eye in ENG testing. Video goggles are used in videonystagmography. Eye movements are recorded in response to various position changes and visual stimuli, with eyes open and eyes closed.
5. Caloric testing is the evaluation of nystagmus induced by warm or cold water irrigation into the external ear canals. Caloric testing can also be obtained by instilling cool and warm air into the ear canal. Caloric testing is used to measure the degree of vestibular dysfunction. Testing of patients with a normally functioning vestibular system will induce vertigo.
6. The audiologist may perform the vertebral artery test with older adults, patients who have a history of neck trauma, or patients in whom vertebral artery disease is suspected. Patients who elicit symptoms when the head is hyperextended may not be able to have portions of the positional testing completed.

Nursing and Patient Care Considerations

1. Patient preparation includes avoiding a heavy meal before the procedure and avoiding caffeine and alcohol for 48 hours before the procedure.
2. Medications that may affect the vestibular system, such as sedatives, antianxiety agents, narcotics, and medications ordered for dizziness, may be held for several days before the procedure.
3. The patient will receive instructions from the facility/provider who will be administering the test for specific medications that will need to be held and for how long before testing is performed. The patient should be counseled on the importance of following these preprocedural instructions, as they may affect the accuracy of the testing.

GENERAL PROCEDURES AND TREATMENT MODALITIES

Nasal Surgery

Types of Surgery and Indications

Facial Trauma and Nasal Fractures

1. Nasal bone fractures are common after blows to the nose during sports activities, interpersonal altercations, motor vehicle accidents, or falls. These can be diagnosed via physical examination or nasal/facial images, including high-resolution computed tomographic (CT) scans (three-dimensional reconstruction can be generated).
2. Nasal fractures are treated with observation, closed reduction, closed reduction with septoplasty, or open reduction with or without internal stabilization, based on the severity of the injury. The best time to perform surgery is within the first few hours after injury or after 7 to 10 days when acute edema begins to resolve. Closed reduction should be performed before fibrosis of fracture lines, usually within 2 weeks after injury but up to 3 weeks after diagnosed.
   a. Observation should be performed 7 to 10 days after the injury, especially when the swelling has subsided, to ensure noticing any deformity.
   b. Closed reduction is effective for noncomminuted and mild nasal fractures with or without dorsal septal disruption.
3. Repair and stabilization of other maxillofacial fractures usually require an operating room procedure for wiring or plating.

Nasal Septal Surgery

1. Septoplasty is an intranasal procedure performed under general anesthesia to remove portions of, straighten, or trim the septal bone and/or cartilage. Silastic splints are sutured on either side of the septum to stabilize the repositioned septum. The splints are removed within 1 week postoperatively. This surgery is performed to treat chronic nasal obstruction and may be done in conjunction with sinus surgery to promote a clear nasal airway.
2. Submucosal turbinate reduction or excision of middle turbinate concha bullosa is an intranasal procedure performed under local or general anesthesia in the operating room to surgically trim, excise, or reduce tissue in the nasal cavity that contributes to nasal obstruction. May be done in conjunction with septoplasty.

Rhinoplasty

1. Involves changing the nose's external appearance. Grafted cartilage or bone harvested from other parts of the body may be used. Use of local anesthesia with sedation or general anesthesia. Full cosmetic results will not be seen until swelling is completely gone (about 1 year).
2. A septorhinoplasty may be done when there are external and internal nasal deformities.

Sinus Surgery

1. Functional endoscopic sinus surgery (FESS) is corrective sinus surgery performed under general anesthesia in the operating room using direct visualization via a rigid nasal endoscope or, more recently, with the assistance of image-guided systems. Image-guided systems utilize CT scans to provide the surgeon with intraoperative landmarks and map.
2. Diseased mucosa is removed, and the natural sinus ostia are widened to facilitate the normal sinus drainage patterns.
3. In addition to nasal and sinus conditions, surgery may also be used to treat traumatic optic neuropathy, cerebrospinal fluid (CSF) leaks, nasolacrimal duct obstruction, dysthyroid orbitopathy (also known as Graves ophthalmopathy and thyroid eye disease), posterior orbital lesions, and choanal atresia.
4. Packing may be placed intraoperatively depending on the surgeon's preference and amount of bleeding. Packing is usually very small, filling only the area adjacent to the sinus ostia, so that it is not visible, except for a retrieval string extending outside the nasal ala.
5. Balloon catheter sinuplasty: The procedure uses a small balloon catheter to open blocked sinus passageways. The procedure is done to widen and restructure the blocked passageways without surgical removal of bone and tissue. Usually used to treat chronic sinusitis (see Figure 13-1).
6. Other approaches to the sinuses, such as the Caldwell–Luc procedure (opening under the lip to enter the maxillary sinus and strip out diseased mucosa), may be performed. A naso-antral window (creating an opening between the maxillary sinus and the anterior inferior nose) and anterior/posterior ethmoidectomies may be performed, as well as opening and draining the frontal or sphenoid sinuses. Newer procedures are favored over the Caldwell–Luc procedure, which is now used only in selected complicated cases.

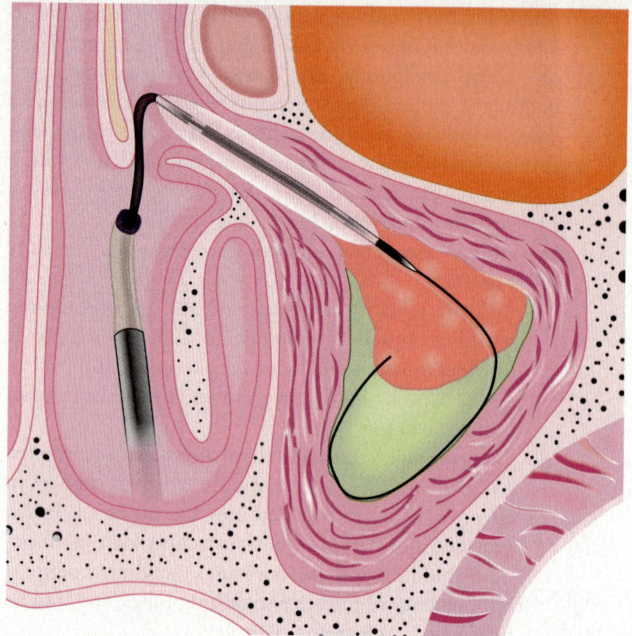

Figure 13-1. Balloon catheter sinus surgery. A catheter is introduced through the nose and into the sinus ostia, where the balloon is inflated to enlarge the sinus opening and promote drainage.

Preoperative Management

1. The head of the bed should be raised to promote drainage, lessen edema, and make the patient more comfortable.
2. Intermittent cold compresses, oral steroids, and pain medications should be utilized, as ordered, for pain and swelling.
3. Antibiotics may be used preoperatively to reduce bacterial colonization of the nose and sinuses.
4. The patient should be advised that a sensation of pressure may be felt in the nasal area during surgery performed under local anesthetic.
5. The patient should be counseled about the possible use of packing with some surgeries, which may be removed several days postoperatively, and the need to breath through mouth.
6. Instructions for stopping aspirin, nonsteroidal anti-inflammatory drugs (NSAIDs), and antiplatelet and anticoagulant medications will be provided by the surgeon and individualized after collaboration with the patient's cardiologist or primary care provider.
7. The patient should abstain from smoking 3 weeks prior to the surgery and 4 weeks after the surgery.

DRUG ALERT In most cases, the patient should avoid the use of aspirin, NSAIDs, anticoagulants, antiplatelet agents, vitamin E, and herbal medications such as *Ginkgo biloba*, *St. John wort*, *ginseng*, garlic, green tea, and any other drugs that may affect platelet function 14 days before surgery. If the patient has taken these medications within a week of surgery, make sure the surgeon is notified.

Complications

1. Hematoma/hemorrhage: septal hematoma or postoperative bleeding. A septal hematoma will need to be drained by the surgeon immediately if this should occur.
2. Local infection—contaminated nasal packing is an excellent culture medium for pathogens. Most patients are treated postoperatively with antibiotics, but this is surgeon specific.
3. Aspiration.

4. Pressure necrosis (from packing) may occur, but the current trend is toward less packing.
5. Blindness from orbital hematoma or unintended orbital involvement in endoscopic sinus surgery.
6. CSF rhinorrhea from unintended or traumatic violation of the cribriform plate. This is commonly referred to as a CSF leak.
7. Pulmonary decompensation.
8. Alteration in taste and smell and change in voice.

POPULATION AWARENESS Due to increased age, comorbidities, and physiologic changes associated with aging, older adults are at an increased risk for postoperative complications. Monitor urine output, signs of confusion, electrolytes, and hematocrit and hemoglobin. Implement coughing and deep breathing, incentive spirometry, and early mobilization.

Nursing Interventions

Facilitating Breathing and Comfort

1. Keep the head elevated (three to four pillows) day and night to minimize swelling. This also promotes comfort.
2. Apply cold compresses or ice packs intermittently for 24 hours to lessen edema and discoloration and to promote comfort. (Use great caution and only with the approval of surgeon after rhinoplasty.)
3. Advise the patient that packing will be removed within 1 week of placement.
4. Encourage the use of a humidifier to relieve crusting of the nasal mucosa and prevent irritation from dryness in the nose and throat.
5. Encourage relaxation techniques and deep breathing exercises for anxiety associated with nasal passages being blocked.
6. Be alert for worsening pulmonary conditions, such as asthma, chronic obstructive pulmonary disease (COPD), and sleep apnea, when the nose is congested or packed.
7. Encourage the use of nonnarcotic analgesics, and caution the use of opioids, which may cause respiratory depression. Medicate with analgesics as prescribed. Topical decongestants may be prescribed to relieve nasal congestion in the first few days postoperatively. Pain after nasal surgery is usually mild to moderate.

Preventing Bleeding and Aspiration

1. Monitor closely for bleeding; check for increased swallowing, blood dripping down back of the throat (use flashlight and tongue blade), and expectoration of large amounts of clots and blood.
2. Change the 4 × 4 gauze pad under the nose as it becomes soaked with blood; bleeding should gradually decrease. Teach family and patient that blood will be bright red at first and will gradually lessen over the next several days.
3. Notify the surgeon if bleeding increases. Expect a temporary minor increase in bleeding with vomiting, sneezing, ambulation, or crying in the first 48 hours.
4. Teach the patient that mild nausea is normal postoperatively and may be from anesthesia, pain medications, or swallowing of blood; however, be alert for continuous trickle of blood postnasally.
5. Instruct the patient not to blow the nose but to blot secretions with tissue and spit out any secretions collecting in the oropharynx.

PATIENT EDUCATION GUIDELINES 13-1

Nasal Saline Irrigation

This procedure will help clear nasal passages of crusted drainage that may be blocking the sinus opening. Perform this once or twice a day, following clearance by the surgeon, to feel less nasal congestion and to help sinuses drain.

1. Wash hands.
2. Prepare saline solution right before irrigation. *Commercially prepared sinus irrigation kits are readily available that contain packets and sinus rinse bottle.*
3. Mix ½ tsp noniodized salt and ¼ tsp baking soda with 8 ounce warm distilled or sterilized water until well dissolved. Do not use tap water.
4. Lean forward from the waist over a sink.
5. Fill a bulb syringe (1 ounce infant ear or nasal bulb) or rinse bottle with the saline solution by squeezing it in the solution and letting it fill by suction. If using sinus rinse kit, follow instructions.
6. Insert the tip of the filled syringe into one nostril, aimed toward the eye away from the nasal septum.
7. Squeeze the syringe gently and feel the solution run backward in the nose and out the other nostril and possibly down the back of the throat and out of the mouth.
8. When comfortable with this procedure, you may be able to rotate head forward, backward, and from side to side to irrigate the sinuses as well as the nose.

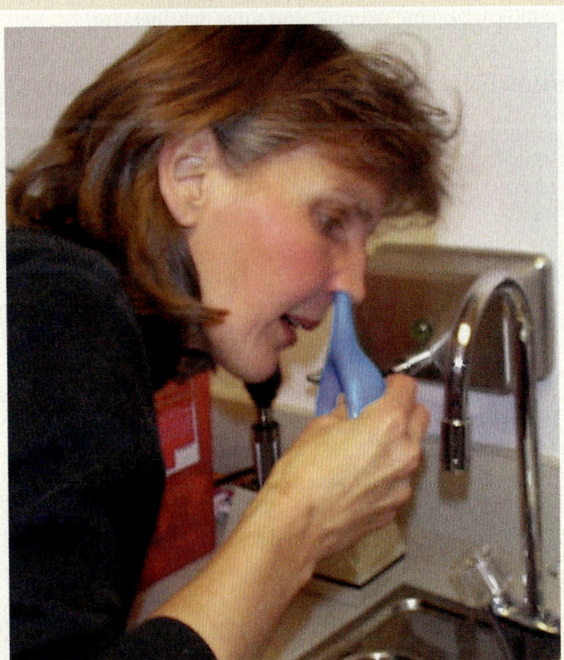

Nose irrigation with bulb syringe or sinus irrigation kit.

6. Regularly observe and document visible packing-retrieval strings external to nose, taped to cheek, if present. Postoperative instructions should be given upon discharge with appointments for postoperative splint removal or sinus debridement, if indicated. The surgeon will discuss activity and work restrictions specific to the patient.

Ensuring Proper Nasal Hygiene

1. Encourage the patient to use a vaporizer to help relieve crusting of nasal mucosa from dryness.
2. Remind the patient that sneezing, straining, and nose blowing increase venous pressure and can result in bleeding/hematoma.
3. Advise the patient to keep the mouth open while sneezing if unable to control sneezing.
4. Teach the patient an appropriate method of nasal hygiene as approved by the surgeon. After FESS, the patient will need regular appointments for sinus debridement by the surgeon. Advise the patient that sinus irrigation will need to be done to control nasal crusting and to facilitate healing (Patient Education 13-1)
5. In general, the patient may gently clean the nasal ala area with saline and/or peroxide for comfort, but large crusts should be removed by the surgeon or allowed to work themselves free.
6. Instruct the patient to avoid environmental irritants, especially smoke.

Protecting Oral Mucous Membranes

1. Administer frequent mouth care because the patient is forced to breathe through the mouth.
2. Use a flexible straw to sip mouthwash for rinsing purposes.
3. Encourage fluid intake and use of lip protectant.

Preventing Infection

1. Be alert for uncontrolled postoperative pain, fever, foul odor or taste in the mouth, or unusual drainage.
2. Administer or teach self-administration of prophylactic antibiotics at regularly scheduled times, if ordered.
3. Advise the patient to keep follow-up appointment for splint removal, packing removal, and sinus debridement.

Patient Education and Health Maintenance

1. Tell the patient to notify the surgeon immediately for uncontrolled postoperative pain, any visual changes postoperatively, fever, unilateral clear nasal discharge with leaning the head forward, uncontrolled excessive nasal bleeding, dyspnea, or blanching or necrosis of the external nasal tissues or the palate while packing is in place.
2. After Caldwell–Luc procedure or rhinoplasty, advise the patient that numbness in the operative area may be present for several weeks to months.
3. Instruct the patient to avoid strenuous activity, lifting, bending, straining, and trauma to the nose.
4. After splint removal, avoid trauma to the nose and sleep in the supine position. The operating surgeon will provide more specific postoperative instructions.
5. Excessive sun exposure should also be avoided after rhinoplasty for 6 months to 1 year because of a tendency for hyperpigmentation.
6. If a nasal splint is present, tell the patient to avoid getting it wet; do not attempt to remove it.
7. Advise the patient that postoperative follow-up may need to continue for several weeks to months to monitor for excess scar formation or cosmetic deformity.

Evaluation: Expected Outcomes

- Mouth breathing without difficulty.
- No excessive bleeding; protects airway without aspiration.
- Nasal and palatal tissues free from blanching or darkening.
- Oral mucous membranes dry, but pink and intact.
- Afebrile; no signs of infection.

Ear Surgery

Ear surgery may involve the tympanic membrane, the middle ear cavity, the mastoid, or the inner ear. It may be done for perforation of the eardrum to facilitate drainage and remove diseased tissue in cases of infection or cholesteatoma, to relieve vertigo, or to treat hearing loss.

Types of Surgery

1. Myringotomy—creating a surgical opening into the tympanic membrane (with knife or laser) for possible drainage tube insertion.
2. Tympanoplasty—reconstruction of diseased or deformed middle ear components (see Table 13-1).
   a. Type I (myringoplasty)—purpose is to close perforation by placing a graft over it to create a closed middle ear to improve hearing and decrease the risk of infection and cholesteatoma. Perforation is closed using one of the following:
      i. Fascia from temporalis muscle (this is the most commonly used material).
      ii. Other materials: vein grafts from hand or forearm, epithelium from auditory canal, fat, synthetic materials such as gel foam, platelet-rich plasma.
   b. Types II to V—suitable replacement (polyethylene, Teflon or titanium prosthesis, bone, cartilage) is used to maintain continuity of conduction sound pathway. A two-stage procedure is usually performed for a tympanoplasty and mastoidectomy.
3. Mastoidectomy—removal of mastoid process of the temporal bone.
   a. Simple or cortical mastoidectomy is done via a postauricular approach, but the bony ear canal is left intact.
   b. Modified radical mastoidectomy or canal wall down mastoidectomy is done with a meatoplasty for the best results. A wide excision of the mastoid and diseased middle ear contents through a postauricular incision is performed with the bony canal being drilled out. A new larger ear canal is created that gives better access to the areas where cholesteatoma usually occurs (the attic and antrum).
4. Stapedectomy—removal of the footplate of stapes and insertion of a graft or prosthesis.
5. Stapedotomy—removal of the stapes suprastructure, allowing a hole to be created with a laser in the stapes footplate. The base of the prosthesis will be inserted into the opening, and the other end will be crimped around the incus.
6. Labyrinthectomy—destruction of the labyrinth (inner ear) through the middle ear and aspiration of the endolabyrinth to treat intractable Ménière disease, which leads to total hearing loss.
7. Endolymphatic decompression and shunt—release of pressure on the endolymphatic system in the labyrinth and creation of a shunt for fluid to the subarachnoid space or the mastoid to treat vertigo associated with Ménière disease. Preserves hearing and vestibular function.

Table 13-1 Types of Tympanoplasty

	MIDDLE EAR DAMAGE		REPAIR PROCESS
Type	**Tympanic Membrane**	**Ossicles**	
I	Perforated	Normal	• Close perforation—myringoplasty
II	Perforated	Erosion of malleus and/or incus	• Close perforation; graft against incus or whatever remains of malleus
III	Tympanic membrane destroyed or widely perforated	Rest of ossicular chain destroyed but stapes are intact and mobile.	• Grafts implanted to contact the normal stapes • Tympanostapedopexy
IV	Tympanic membrane destroyed or widely perforated	Ossicular chain destroyed. Head, neck, and crura of stapes destroyed. Stapes footplate mobile.	• Expose mobile stapes footplate—graft implanted. Air pocket between graft and round window provides protection. • The cavum minor operation
V	Tympanic membrane destroyed or widely perforated	Ossicular chain destroyed. Head, neck, and crura of stapes destroyed. Stapes footplate fixed.	• Make opening in horizontal semicircular canal; graft seals off middle ear to give sound protection for round window. • Tympanoplasty and fenestration of lateral semicircular canal

8. Cochlear implant—implantation of electronic device that bypasses the damaged cochlea and stimulates the auditory nerve (cochlear branch of cranial nerve VIII).
9. Osseointegrated bone conduction prosthesis is a hearing implant placed in the temporal bone for single-sided deafness or for conductive hearing loss. Takes the place of a conventional hearing aid. Provides sound amplification via bone conduction.

Preoperative Management

1. Hearing function is fully evaluated along with a baseline assessment of the facial nerve.
2. Antibiotics are given to treat infection.
3. The patient is prepared emotionally for the effects of surgery.
4. Careful assessment for signs of acute infection is performed, which may delay surgery.
5. Avoid aspirin, ibuprofen, vitamin E, herbal supplements, and smoking 2 weeks prior to surgery.

Postoperative Management

1. Antibiotics may be continued to prevent local and central nervous system (CNS) infection.
2. Patients are advised to have limited activity for the first 24 hours to decrease symptoms of nausea and vertigo (if the inner ear was disturbed) or to prevent disruption of prosthesis.
3. Analgesics, antiemetics, and antihistamines are given, as needed.
4. The patient is positioned to promote drainage but maintain some immobility. Using two extra pillows for 2 weeks to elevate the head, thereby preventing edema, is advised.
5. The patient is often seen 7 to 10 days after surgery to remove any metal stent placed. Additional packing may be removed up to 6 weeks postoperatively if prosthesis or graft procedure was performed. Often, an eardrop will be used to slowly dissolve the remaining packing over a period of 6 to 8 weeks to give some weight to the grafted tympanic membrane.
6. Hearing will be reevaluated after edema has subsided and healing has occurred. The time frame for this varies by procedure but may be as long as 3 to 4 months after surgery to allow for healing.
7. With an osseointegrated implant, a fitting of the outer processor is usually delayed by 2 to 3 months to allow the bone to osseointegrate around the implant. In children, or in radiated bone, this may be done in two stages separated by 6 months to allow for a slower rate of bone growth.
8. Cochlear implant activation and placement of the outer speech processor and external transmitter occur approximately 3 to 4 weeks after surgery to allow for healing.

Complications

1. Infection: local, CNS (meningitis, brain abscess).
2. Hearing loss.
3. Facial nerve paralysis—rare.
4. Dizziness—usually temporary.

Nursing Interventions

Relieving Pain

1. Administer or teach self-administration of analgesic, as indicated, postoperatively.
2. Tell the patient to expect pain to subside within the first few hours with simple procedures or within the first day or 2 with major procedures.
3. Position the patient for comfort following the instructions from the surgeon.
   a. On the side with surgical ear upward to maintain graft position and immobility.
   b. Lying on the side with surgical ear down to promote drainage from the ear canal.
   c. Position of patient preference.
4. Elevate the head of the bed to reduce swelling and pressure.
5. Advise the patient to avoid sudden movement. Use pillows for support.

Preventing Infection

1. Reinforce external dressings, as needed, until after first changed by the surgeon, then change when saturated to prevent bacterial growth in damp dressings.
2. Loosely pack cotton or gauze in the ear canal, as indicated, without causing increased pressure.

3. Do not probe or insert anything into the ear canal.
4. Administer or teach self-administration of antibiotics, as prescribed. Do not use eardrops unless specifically ordered postoperatively.
5. Wash hands before ear care, and instruct the patient not to touch the ear.
6. Take care not to get the dressing or ear wet.
7. Advise the patient not to blow the nose, which could cause nasopharyngeal secretions to be forced up the eustachian tube into the middle ear.
8. Instruct the patient to report any increased pain, fever, ear inflammation, or drainage, indicating local infection.
9. Be alert for headache, fever, stiff neck, or altered level of consciousness, which may indicate CNS infection.

Ensuring Safety

1. Be aware that dizziness or vertigo may occur for the first several days postoperatively.
2. Maintain side rails up while the patient is in bed.
3. Assist the patient with ambulation for the first time after surgery and as needed thereafter.
4. Encourage the patient to move slowly because sudden movements may exacerbate vertigo.
5. Administer or teach self-administration of antiemetics and antihistamines, as ordered and as needed; watch for sedation.
6. Instruct the patient not to blow nose, cough, lean forward, or perform the Valsalva maneuver to avoid disrupting the graft or prosthesis, aggravating vertigo, or forcing bacteria up the eustachian tube. If coughing or blowing nose is necessary, do so with an open mouth to relieve pressure.

Patient Education and Health Maintenance

1. Advise the patient that there may be a temporary hearing loss for a few weeks after surgery because of tissue edema, packing, and so forth. The effects of a hearing restoration operation will not be known for several weeks, and additional rehabilitation may be necessary to optimize results.
2. Advise the patient to protect the ear, perform dressing changes, or place loose cotton in the outer ear, as indicated. Replace cotton twice daily or sooner if saturated by drainage.
3. Encourage follow-up for packing removal, as directed.
4. Instruct the patient to avoid sudden pressure changes in the ear.
   a. Do not blow the nose.
   b. Do not fly in a small plane. The date for which a patient may fly is individualized by their surgery and surgeon's preference.
   c. Do not dive under water.
   d. Avoid lifting, straining, bending.
5. Advise against smoking.
6. Tell the patient to protect their ears when going outdoors for the first week. A cotton ball is all that is needed.
7. Tell the patient to avoid getting the ear wet until completely healed.
8. Tell the patient to avoid crowds or exposure to colds so upper respiratory infection is prevented.
9. Instruct the patient about signs and symptoms of complications to report.
   a. Return of tinnitus.
   b. Vertigo.
   c. Fluctuations of hearing ability.
   d. Fever, headache, ear inflammation, increased pain, stiff neck.
   e. Facial drooping or numbness.
10. Advise the patient that facial nerve paralysis may be temporary and to increase fluid intake through a straw during this time.

Evaluation: Expected Outcomes

- Verbalizes relief of pain.
- No signs of infection.
- Ambulates without difficulty.

CONDITIONS OF THE MOUTH AND JAW

Candidiasis

EVIDENCE BASE Talapko, J., Juzbasic, M., Pustijanac, E., Bekic, S., & Kotris, I. (2021). *Candida albicans*—The virulence factors in clinical manifestations of infection. *Journal of Fungi, 7*(2), 1–19. https://doi.org/10.3390/jof7020079

Candidiasis is an opportunistic fungal infection commonly caused by *Candida albicans*. It may be localized in the mouth and pharynx but may also occur in the esophagus. Candidiasis can become a source of systemic dissemination, particularly in high-risk persons.

Pathophysiology and Etiology

1. Commonly seen in individuals with immunosuppression from disease states or treatment regimens such as diabetes, cancer, or human immunodeficiency virus (HIV) and those receiving radiation therapy and/or chemotherapy.
2. May be caused by altered oral environment from xerostomia (dry mouth), use of inhaled steroids for asthma and chronic obstructive pulmonary disease (COPD), chronic antibiotic therapy, preexisting infections, poor oral hygiene or nutritional status, smoking, or wearing dentures.

Clinical Manifestations

1. Oral examination reveals diffuse, white, painless plaques. Underlying mucosa may be erythematous.
2. May be asymptomatic but may result in mild oral discomfort, burning, or alterations in taste.
3. Patients with disease spread beyond the oral cavity may present with chest pain, pain and difficulty with swallowing, or hoarseness.

Diagnostic Evaluation

1. Microscopic smear of plaques shows characteristic hyphae.
2. Oral fungal culture positive for *C. albicans*.
3. Occasionally, a biopsy of lesions may be necessary to rule out leukoplakia (premalignant plaques).
4. Blood culture for invasive *C. albicans*.
5. T2 Candida Panel—non–culture-based diagnostic test for the rapid identification of the five most common strains of *Candida* from whole blood. Can identify candidemia when a patient presents with sepsis.

Management

1. Topical antifungal medications such as nystatin suspension or clotrimazole troches are most often used.

2. Systemic treatment is indicated if topical agents fail or for esophageal cases with fluconazole, ketoconazole (used cautiously in immunosuppressed patients), or amphotericin B.
3. Topical oral rinses or preparations containing combinations of hydrocortisone, diphenhydramine, antifungals, or antibiotics may be used to enhance healing and lessen discomfort.
4. Viscous lidocaine may be used topically to coat the oral mucosa before meals to lessen pain and enhance oral intake.
5. Oral prostheses may also be treated to avoid harboring and reintroducing infection.

Complications

1. Candidal infection throughout the gastrointestinal (GI) tract.
2. Candidal sepsis in patients who are immunocompromised.

Nursing Assessment

1. Carefully examine the oral cavity daily to monitor lesions as well as response to prescribed antifungal therapy.
2. Assess the level of pain; administer analgesics, as prescribed; and monitor response to analgesics.
3. Assess nutritional status and the effect of pain on oral intake. Monitor oral intake, nutritional and hydration status, weight loss/gain, and signs of dehydration.
4. Teach patients who are prescribed inhaled steroid therapy for asthma/COPD to rinse their mouth after each use to prevent oropharyngeal candidiasis.

Nursing Interventions

Attaining Adequate Nutrition

1. Administer analgesics, as prescribed, 30 to 60 minutes before meals.
2. Provide soft foods, soothing liquids; avoid temperature extremes.
3. Provide gentle suctioning if the pain becomes so severe that the patient cannot handle secretions.
4. Administer intravenous (IV) fluids as directed.

Ensuring Adequate Therapy

1. Administer antifungal agents, as prescribed. Observe the patient for proper use of topical preparation.
   a. Make sure that the mouth is clean and free of food debris before administering the drug.
   b. For swish-and-swallow preparations, tell the patient to swish and hold in the mouth for at least 10 minutes before swallowing.
   c. For troches, have the patient suck until dissolved.
2. Observe for signs and symptoms of systemic drug adverse effects: nausea, vomiting, diarrhea. Renal, bone marrow, cardiovascular, hepatic, or neurologic toxicities may occur in patients receiving systemic antifungals with underlying chronic disease states. Monitor chemistry profile and complete blood count as directed.
3. Explain the importance of continuing therapy for duration prescribed, which may be up to 21 days.

Patient Education and Health Maintenance

1. Instruct high-risk patients about daily oral examination and signs and symptoms to observe.
2. Teach the patient to avoid highly seasoned foods, extremes in temperature, alcoholic beverages, and smoking, all of which irritate the oral mucosa.
3. Encourage good oral hygiene.
4. May need to refrain from wearing dentures because of oral discomfort.
5. Encourage the patient on long-term systemic antifungal therapy to follow up for liver function test monitoring, as directed.
6. Use of probiotics could be beneficial for the maintenance of oral health.

Evaluation: Expected Outcomes

- Adequate intake of liquids and soft foods as evidenced by stable body weight and signs of dehydration.
- Swishes oral suspension for 10 minutes before spitting or swallowing.

Herpes Simplex Infection (Type 1)

Also known as *cold sores* or *fever blisters*, herpes simplex virus (HSV; usually type 1) is commonly associated with lip and oral lesions 80% of the time. HSV-1 causes genital outbreaks in 20% of the cases. This virus is very contagious. HSV-1 is declining in Western countries due to improvement in hygiene and living conditions.

Pathophysiology and Etiology

1. After a primary infection and the patient produces antibodies, the virus remains latent in the sensory ganglia.
2. Recurrent herpes labialis may be precipitated by sun exposure, fever, oral trauma, fatigue, emotional upset, hormonal changes, and other factors.
3. The spread of HSV-1 is through respiratory droplets or exposure to infected saliva via a break in the skin or mucous membranes.
4. HSV-2 (and rarely HSV-1) is associated with genital lesions and is sexually transmitted.

Clinical Manifestations

Symptoms occur 2 to 12 days after exposure.

1. Prodromal period—tingling, soreness, and burning in area where the lesion will develop.
2. Small vesicles appear on erythematous, edematous base, frequently near the mucocutaneous junction of the lips and oral mucosa. Lesions may be spread to genitalia during oral sex.
3. Lesions may be quite severe in the immunosuppressed.
4. Vesicles rupture, causing painful ulcerations.
5. Lesions heal spontaneously in 7 to 14 days, but reoccur.

Diagnosis and Management

1. No diagnostic tests are necessary, but serologic testing may be done. The diagnosis of herpes simplex is made from viral culture from skin vesicles, serology, or monoclonal antibody testing. HSV-1 serology–antibody detection via Western blot is the gold standard for diagnosis.
2. Treatment may not be necessary if cases are mild and are usually short lived.
3. Comfort measures, such as mild oral or topical analgesics.
4. Good hygiene (washing hands) and avoiding close contact prevent the spread to self and others.
5. Antiviral agents, including acyclovir, famciclovir, and valacyclovir, are available to decrease the duration of symptoms. Best to start antivirals within 24 hours of symptoms.

6. Penciclovir 1% cream—Food and Drug Administration (FDA) approved; applied every 2 hours while awake at the earliest sign. If used within 1 hour of an outbreak, will decrease the duration of viral shedding.
7. Acyclovir 5% cream may be used on topical lesions. Oral or IV antivirals may also be used if clinically indicated.

Nursing Interventions and Patient Education

1. Advise adequate rest and nutrition and avoidance of identified triggers.
2. Advise that the virus is transmitted through close contact, such as kissing and sharing food and cups, so avoid these from prodromal period until well healed.
3. Recommend good handwashing and hygiene.
4. Aphthous ulcers or canker sores are not caused by HSV-1.

Temporomandibular Disorders

Temporomandibular disorders (TMDs) are conditions affecting the jaw joint that consist of one or more of the following:

1. Myofascial pain—pain in the muscles serving the jaw (temporalis, masseter, medial and lateral pterygoids), neck, and shoulder.
2. Internal derangement of the jaw joint (dislocated or displaced joint disk or injured condyle).
3. Degenerative joint disease (e.g., arthritis).

Pathophysiology and Etiology

1. Causes include rheumatoid or osteoarthritis, scleroderma, ankylosing spondylitis, trauma, teeth clenching or bruxism (teeth grinding). Neoplasms and acute infections such as parotitis, dental infections, and peritonsillar abscesses cause referred ear pain and should be differentiated from TMDs.
2. Any mental and physical stresses can induce or exacerbate symptoms.
3. Abovementioned factors result in inflammation and muscle spasm of the temporomandibular joint (TMJ).

Clinical Manifestations

1. Pain at the joint, temples, mandible, or masticatory muscles may worsen with jaw movement. Referred muscle spasm of the neck, trapezius, and sternocleidomastoid muscle causes discomfort.
2. Clicking or crepitus from opening and closing of the jaw or popping of the joint.
3. Limitation of movement, dislocation, or jaw locking.
4. May be associated with headaches, earaches, or tinnitus.
5. Change in the bite where the upper and lower teeth do not match in the normal comfortable way.
6. May experience deteriorating oral hygiene or halitosis from limited oral opening (trismus), making dental hygiene difficult.
7. May experience difficulty chewing because of limited jaw excursion, resulting in altered diet and weight loss.
8. Jaw clicking alone is common and requires no workup or intervention if asymptomatic.

Diagnostic Evaluation

1. Diagnosis can usually be achieved by history and physical examination without extensive testing. Provocative maneuvers performed on physical examination that reproduce pain with opening and closing of the jaw are generally suggestive of TMJ arthralgia.
2. Dental and TMJ x-rays may or may not be helpful.
3. Occlusal analysis evaluates for malocclusion of the jaw and teeth in a bite position.
4. Computed tomography (CT) scan and magnetic resonance imaging (MRI) are usually normal unless there are underlying degenerative changes, fracture, or neoplasm of the jaw or cervical spine.
5. Arthrography (joint x-rays using dye).
6. Arthroscopy (endoscopic invasive joint examination).

Management

1. Initial management employs jaw rest (soft, no-chew diet for 2 weeks, plus avoiding extreme jaw movements, such as wide yawning and gum chewing).
2. Anti-inflammatory/analgesic medications such as ibuprofen, corticosteroid intra-articular injections, and anticonvulsants (gabapentin).
3. Application of warm, moist heat or ice packs.
4. Muscle relaxants may be prescribed.
5. Therapeutic night guard or splint—to realign malocclusion or joint disk and to optimize muscle relaxation.
6. Massage and physical therapy for gentle stretching and relaxing exercises with or without ultrasound (deep heat) therapy—to enhance analgesia and muscle relaxation and to promote local tissue metabolism.
7. Transcutaneous electrical nerve stimulation (TENS) reduces muscle spasm of the head, neck, and back and reduces pain.
8. In general, conservative reversible measures mentioned earlier are employed as long as possible before progressing to invasive/surgical management.
    a. Arthroscopy—investigational procedure to visualize the joint, reposition disk, lyse adhesions, or debride joint.
        i. Reserved for conditions not improved by medical management.
        ii. Complications include cranial nerve (CN) VII damage with facial paralysis and paresis, perforation of the external auditory canal, and piercing of the middle cranial fossa.
    b. Surgery—to remove the disk or reshape bony prominences.
9. Complications include malocclusion, CN VII damage, and infection.

Nursing Interventions and Patient Education

1. Assess the character, frequency, location, and duration of pain. Evaluate what triggers and relieves the pain. Determine how effective previous treatments have been.
2. Explore the effect of the disorder on the patient's lifestyle, especially eating habits. Assist the patient to alter methods of oral hygiene and eating if severe trismus is present.
3. Instruct the patient on the indications, dosages, and adverse effects of analgesics and anti-inflammatory medications.
4. Teach the patient proper use of heat therapies. Cold applications may be preferred by some patients to reduce pain and spasm.
5. Encourage the patient to perform active mouth opening, protrusion, and lateral movement exercises of the jaw for 5 minutes, four to five times per day, as prescribed, to stretch muscles and reduce spasm.
6. Encourage the use of soft food and liquid supplements during times of acute pain exacerbated by eating. Advise reduction of

foods that require excessive chewing, such as raw vegetables, tough meat, and nuts. Discourage gum chewing.
7. Explore tension-reducing modalities with the patient, especially progressive muscle relaxation to reduce muscle tension and spasm.
8. Encourage follow-up with dentist; oral surgeon; ear, nose, and throat (ENT) specialist; or other caregiver, as indicated.
9. Encourage proper use of the night guard or dental splint, including periodic appointments to assess fit.
10. May need medical alert device bracelet and preoperative anesthesia consultation for elective surgeries if maximum jaw opening is less than 30 mm, limiting access for airway intubation.

Maxillofacial and Mandibular Fractures

Fractures of the maxillofacial bones or mandible may occur as the result of industrial, athletic, and motor vehicle accidents; violent acts; and falls.

Pathophysiology and Etiology

1. Maxillofacial fractures usually occur due to blow to the cheek or face.
2. Mandibular fractures frequently occur due to blow to the chin (most common fracture).
3. May be nondisplaced or displaced, usually closed, and includes soft tissue injury.
4. May also occur as part of planned surgical reconstruction for jaw problems.
5. Injuries sustained in altercations or motor vehicle accidents may be associated with alcohol intoxication or recreational drug use.

Clinical Manifestations

1. Malocclusion, asymmetry, abnormal mobility, crepitus (grating sound with movement), pain, or tenderness; difficulty opening mouth (trismus).
2. Tissue injury: swelling, ecchymosis, bleeding, and pain.

Diagnostic Evaluation

1. CT is the gold standard for evaluating the extent of injuries.
2. Panorex can also be used if CT is not available.

Management

Goal is to restore facial aesthetics and function.

1. Maintenance of adequate respiratory functioning—may include oxygen support, endotracheal intubation, or tracheostomy. See Chapter 31, page 939.
2. Control of bleeding—usually accomplished with direct pressure.
3. Reduction of the fracture—usually closed reduction.
4. Immobilization—depends on the location, type, and severity of the fracture.
   a. Barton bandage with a Kling or stockinette bandage.
   b. Interdental fixation with rubber bands or wiring.
   c. Intermaxillary fixation with rubber bands or wiring.
   d. Interosseous fixation with open reduction.
5. Maintenance of adequate nutritional intake with liquid or soft diet—to maintain immobilization of fracture site.
6. Pain control—to promote comfort.
7. Control of infection with antibiotics in the presence of positive cultures.

Complications

1. Airway obstruction, aspiration.
2. Hemorrhage, infection.
3. Disfigurement.
4. Extraocular muscle entrapment/orbital globe displacement with resultant visual disturbance.
5. Acute drug or alcohol withdrawal.
6. Hardware failure.
7. Malunion or malocclusion.

Nursing Assessment

1. Obtain description of injury and review chart and diagnostic tests for the extent of injury.
2. Continually assess respiratory status.
3. Assess the level of pain.
4. Assess visual acuity and extraocular movement.
5. Assess for tremors, delirium or hallucinations, anxiety, and seizure activity related to alcohol or drug withdrawal.

Nursing Interventions

Preventing Aspiration

1. Maintain effective airway.
   a. Elevate the head of the bed 30 to 45 degrees or position leaning over a bedside stand to reduce edema and improve handling of secretions.
   b. Make sure suctioning equipment is readily accessible; teach patient oral and nasal suctioning; position on side or upright during suctioning.
   c. Administer antiemetic, as prescribed, for nausea and vomiting to prevent aspiration.
   d. Make sure wire cutters or scissors are present for immediate removal of the wires or rubber bands if the airway becomes obstructed. (Vertical rubber bands or wires should be cut.)
   e. Make sure that a method for calling the nurse (call bell) is within easy access for the patient at all times in case of emergency.
2. Monitor blood pressure, pulse, respirations, and temperature to note the early onset of infection or aspiration.

Maintaining Nutritional Status

1. Administer liquid diet, as prescribed; place a straw against the teeth or through any gaps in the teeth. Teeth may initially be sensitive to hot and cold.
2. Position in upright position before, during, and for 45 to 60 minutes after all feedings.
3. Evaluate ongoing nutritional and hydration status; weight; intake, output, and specific gravity; laboratory values—24-hour urea nitrogen, transferrin level, electrolytes, and albumin.
4. Advance to puree diet, as tolerated.
5. Make the environment as pleasant as possible to enhance appetite—remove all sources of odor, decrease interruptions, position comfortably.

Increasing Comfort

1. Administer IV or oral liquid analgesics, as prescribed—avoid opioids on an empty stomach, which may cause nausea and vomiting.
2. Administer diazepam as prescribed to reduce anxiety and control reflex muscle spasm.
3. Apply paraffin wax to the ends of wire fixation devices to decrease irritation to the gums and oral mucosa.

4. Apply petroleum jelly to the lips to decrease dryness and prevent cracking.

Strengthening Body Image

1. Provide firm reassurance regarding progress to reduce anxiety and allay fears.
2. Avoid unrealistic promises in relation to scars or disfigurement.
3. Allow the patient to choose the first time for looking in the mirror.
4. Provide privacy, as requested. The patient may be sensitive to appearance.
5. Provide alternative form of communication, such as magic slate or picture board, because maxillomandibular fixation limits articulating ability, making speech difficult to understand.

Preventing Infection

1. Provide mouth care every 2 hours while awake for the first several days, then four to six times per day.
2. Initially, provide mouth care with warm normal saline mouth swishes.
3. As the diet is progressed, remove collected debris with a pressurized water stream cleaner and encourage the patient to brush their teeth with a soft, child-size toothbrush.
4. Observe facial injuries for swelling, erythema, pain, or warmth to detect the onset of infection.
5. Change facial dressings as needed to prevent soiling with secretions, food, or drainage, which may promote bacterial growth.

Patient Education and Health Maintenance

1. Encourage adequate nutrition—inform the patient and family that foods can be blenderized and thinned with juices or broths to a consistency that can be taken through a straw.
2. Explore with the patient options for maintaining proper oral care; encourage the patient to practice the options of choice.
3. Discuss the use of antiemetic medications to prevent nausea and vomiting, stressing the complications this could cause.
4. Make sure the patient has wire cutters or scissors at all times and knows how to use them should airway obstruction occur.
5. Encourage follow-up health care visits, including counseling for alcohol or substance use disorder.

Evaluation: Expected Outcomes

- No evidence of aspiration.
- Tolerates fluids through straw; maintains adequate body weight.
- Expresses relief of pain.
- Views self in mirror; notices improvement in appearance.
- No signs of infection; oral hygiene maintained.

PROBLEMS OF THE NOSE, THROAT, AND SINUSES

Rhinopathies

Rhinopathies are disorders of the nose that interrupt its normal functions of olfaction and warming, filtering, and humidifying inspired air. These include allergic, nonallergic, and infectious conditions.

Pathophysiology and Etiology

Three groups: allergic, nonallergic, infectious rhinitis.

1. Allergic rhinitis—immunoglobulin E (IgE)–mediated response causing release of vasoactive substances from mast cells (see page 781).
2. Nonallergic, noninfectious rhinitis—eight subgroups
   a. Drug induced (rebound rhinitis; rhinitis medicamentosa)—caused by excessive use of topical nasal decongestants. These products include oxymetazoline and phenylephrine. Many systemic medications may induce nasal congestion and stuffiness and include specific beta-blockers, antihypertensives, and antidepressants.
   b. Idiopathic/vasomotor rhinitis—consists of symptoms caused by autonomic instability with disruption of the normal balance of sympathetic and parasympathetic innervation. This produces nasal congestion, rhinorrhea, and postnasal drip. Symptoms may be manifested on exposure to cold weather.
   c. Hormone induced/rhinitis of pregnancy—nasal congestion resulting from estrogen-mediated mucosal engorgement, especially in the last trimesters of pregnancy; may also occur with oral contraceptive use, postmenopausal estrogen therapy, and during the last portion of the menstrual cycle. Edema of the nasal mucosa and turbinate congestion occur.
   d. Senile rhinitis related to nasal changes due to aging.
   e. Gustatory rhinitis caused by eating of spicy, hot, or cold foods.
   f. Occupational rhinitis associated with nasal congestion and rhinorrhea from agents in the workplace.
   g. Atrophic rhinitis is associated with nasal dryness and lack of mucosal secretions.
   h. Nonallergic rhinitis with eosinophilia syndrome (NARES)—patients have symptoms of rhinitis, negative allergy testing, but a large number of eosinophils in nasal secretions.
3. Infectious rhinitis is either viral (common cold) or bacterial (purulent rhinitis).

Clinical Manifestations

1. Rhinorrhea—wet, running/dripping nose or postnasal drip.
2. Eyes—edema of the conjunctivae, tearing and itching of the eyes, increase in vascularity; characteristic allergic shiners (dark staining under eyes) with allergic rhinitis.
3. Nasal cavity—congestion, pressure, or stuffiness (see Figure 13-2). Chronic nasal crusting and erythema around outer nares and turbinates are often swollen, edematous with pale or bluish hue. Characteristic allergic salute often seen in children caused by upward lifting of the tip of the nose with the hand.
4. Oral cavity—chronic mouth breathing, enlarged lymph tissue in the oropharynx, prominent vascularity, or cobblestoning in the posterior pharynx.
5. Headache.

Management

1. Treatment of underlying cause.
   a. Allergy—antihistamines (see Chapter 24).
   b. Nonallergic rhinitis—treatment modalities can include avoidance if caused by chemical, food, or other irritants.
   c. Infectious—no specific treatment.
   d. Vasomotor rhinitis—treated with ipratropium, which blocks vagally mediated reflexes that cause congestion.
2. Symptom control.
   a. Decongestants—short-term usage of topical or systemic decongestants, no more than 2 to 3 days.
   b. Intranasal corticosteroids—used for their anti-inflammatory effects.

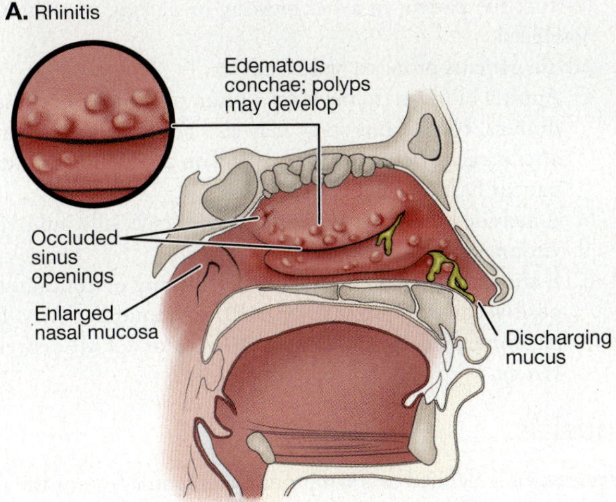

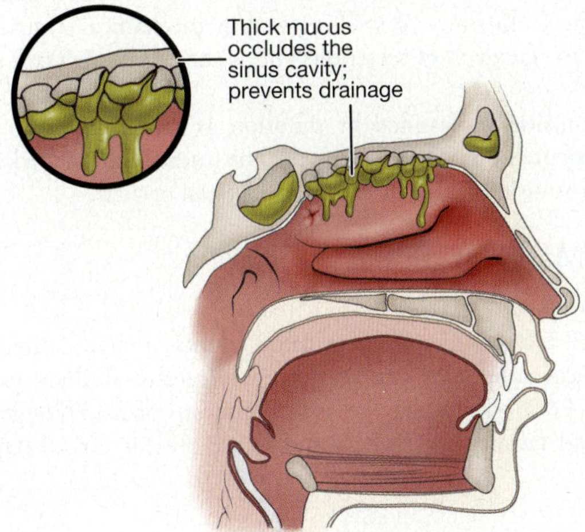

Figure 13-2. Pathophysiologic processes in rhinitis and rhinosinusitis. Although pathophysiologic processes are similar in rhinitis and rhinosinusitis, they affect different structures. **(A)** In rhinitis, the mucous membranes lining the nasal passages become inflamed, congested, and edematous. The swollen nasal conchae block the sinus openings, and mucus is discharged from the nostrils. **(B)** Rhinosinusitis is also marked by inflammation and congestion, with thickened mucous secretions filling the sinus cavities and occluding the openings. (Reprinted with permission from Hinkle, J. L., Cheever, K. H., & Overbaugh, K. J. [2022]. Brunner and Suddarth's textbook of medical-surgical nursing [15th ed., Fig. 18-1]. Lippincott Williams & Wilkins.)

DRUG ALERT Severe rebound nasal obstruction may occur with the overuse of topical decongestants. Stress the importance of only using for 2 to 3 days, as directed.

Nursing Interventions and Patient Education

1. Educate patients about avoidance measures for known or suspected allergens or irritants such as smoke.
2. Do not overuse topical nasal sprays and drops.
3. Advise about the adverse effect of systemic decongestants is stimulation of sympathetic nervous system—insomnia, nervousness, palpitations.
4. Be aware that intranasal corticosteroids do not cause significant systemic absorption in usual doses but, occasionally, may cause nasal fungal infections and, in rare cases, nasal septal perforation and epistaxis.
5. Educate patients about correct administration technique for nasal sprays, particularly to direct the tip of the spray bottle away from the septum, toward the outward corner of the eye or toward the ear.

Epistaxis

Epistaxis refers to nosebleed or hemorrhage from the nose. It most commonly originates in the anterior portion of the nasal cavity. Most nosebleeds are anterior; posterior bleeds are more difficult to control.

Pathophysiology and Etiology

1. Local causes:
   a. Dryness leading to crust formation—bleeding occurs with removal of crusts by nose picking, rubbing, or blowing.
   b. Trauma—direct blows.
   c. Deviated septum.
   d. Chronic nasal cannula use.
2. Systemic causes are less common—hypertension, arteriosclerosis, renal disease, bleeding disorders. Episodic epistaxis is most commonly seen in patients on antiplatelet, anticoagulant, and antithrombolytic agents. Osler–Weber–Rendu syndrome or hereditary hemorrhagic telangiectasia, hemophilia, von Willebrand disease, and liver disease are examples of bleeding disorders that can predispose patients to frequent episodes of epistaxis.
3. Environmental causes such as allergies, dryness during winter months.
4. Medication causes: nonsteroidal anti-inflammatory drugs (NSAIDs), anticoagulants, platelet aggregation inhibitors, topical nasal steroid sprays, some herbal supplements, drug use (cocaine).

Diagnostic Evaluation

1. Inspection with nasal speculum to determine the site of bleeding or nasal endoscopy by otolaryngologist. Important to determine which side bled first.
2. Laboratory evaluation to exclude blood dyscrasias and coagulopathy.

Management

Depends on the severity and source of bleeding in the nasal cavity.

1. The patient is placed in an upright posture, leaning forward to reduce venous pressure, and instructed to breathe gently through the mouth to prevent swallowing of blood. The patient is asked to sit at a 90-degree angle, while the nasal ala, or the soft part of the anterior nose, is pinched and pressure is applied for 10 to 15 minutes, or as needed to control the bleeding.
2. With anterior bleeds, the patient is instructed to compress the soft part of the nose with the index finger and thumb for 5 to 10 minutes to maintain pressure on the nasal septum.
3. A cotton pledget soaked with a vasoconstricting agent may be inserted into each nostril, and pressure is applied if bleeding is not controlled. After 5 to 10 minutes, the cotton is removed and the site of bleeding is identified. Oxymetazoline, in

combination with a topical anesthetic agent such as lidocaine, may be sprayed directly into the nasal cavity or applied on pledgets or cotton balls. Suction may be used to evacuate the bloody contents of the nasal cavity to visualize the source of bleeding.
4. The blood vessel may be cauterized with the use of silver nitrate sticks or with electrocautery.
5. If bleeding continues despite the use of pressure or cautery, anterior or posterior packing may be placed into the nasal cavity or nasopharynx. Packing is usually kept in for 72 hours or more. Balloon tamponade may be required to apply pressure over a larger area.
6. Surgical ligation of vessels may be required if bleeding is unable to be controlled with the abovementioned measures.

CLINICAL JUDGMENT Monitor the patient for a vasovagal episode during insertion and with removal of nasal packing. This is best prevented with reclining the patient back when symptoms first occur.

Complications

1. Rhinitis, maxillary and frontal sinusitis.
2. Orthostatic hypotension from sudden blood loss.
3. Rebleeding with packing removal.
4. Aspiration.
5. Pressure necrosis of nasal mucosa from packing.
6. Airway obstruction from packing dislodgement.

Nursing Interventions and Patient Education

1. Monitor vital signs and assist with control of bleeding. Assess for changes in blood pressure and pulse indicative of hypovolemia.
2. Be aware that packing is uncomfortable and painful and may be in place for 48 to 72 hours. Antibiotics may be prescribed to prevent secondary infection from packing.
3. Nosebleed precautions and postprocedural instructions should be given to the patient. Instructions for holding specific antiplatelet and anticoagulant medications will be coordinated in conjunction with the patients' clinical history. The patient should be advised to avoid sneezing with mouth closed, blowing nose, removing the packing, avoiding any strenuous activity, and avoiding straining with bowel movement.
4. Monitor the patient with posterior packing for hypoxia (from aspiration of blood, sedation, and preexisting pulmonary dysfunction). Patients who require posterior balloon packing are admitted for observation and monitoring. These patients are at risk for soft palate necrosis and airway obstruction. If coagulopathies are found on blood work, these are corrected while the patient is hospitalized. Monitor prothrombin time (PT), international normalized ratio (INR), and partial prothrombin time (PTT), if ordered.
5. Instruct the patient as follows for self-management of minor bleeding episodes:
   a. Sit up and lean forward while compressing the soft part (lower half) of the nose between the index finger and the thumb.
   b. If bleeding continues, moisten a small piece of cotton with vasoconstricting nose drops (phenylephrine or oxymetazoline) and place inside the nose.
   c. Apply pressure to the bleeding site for 5 to 10 minutes.
6. Instruct the patient to avoid blowing or picking nose after a nosebleed.
7. Advise patients prone to nosebleeds to:
   a. Apply a lubricant to the nasal septum twice daily to reduce dryness. Nasal saline spray may also be advised a few days after nasal cautery is performed and on a regular basis if the patient has recurrent episodes.
   b. A bedside humidifier is recommended, especially if the environmental air is dry.
   c. If the patient uses chronic oxygen therapy or continuous positive airway pressure (CPAP), a humidifier may be recommended on the oxygen delivery or CPAP delivery system.

Sinusitis

Rhinosinusitis is defined as a symptomatic inflammation of the sinuses and nasal cavity. It may be precipitated by congestion from viral upper respiratory infection and/or nasal allergy. A patient with chronic allergic disease may be prone to recurrent episodes of sinusitis or chronic rhinosinusitis. Obstruction of the sinus ostia (resulting from mucosal swelling and/or mechanical obstruction) leads to retention of secretions and is the usual precursor to sinusitis.

Rhinosinusitis is classified by duration as acute (less than 4 weeks), subacute (4 to 12 weeks), or chronic (more than 12 weeks). Acute rhinosinusitis can be classified as bacterial or viral.

Clinical Manifestations

Acute Sinusitis

1. Defined as up to 4 weeks of purulent, nonclear nasal drainage with nasal congestion and/or facial pain/pressure/fullness (see Figure 13-3). There may be both symptoms of nasal congestion and facial pain, and symptoms are present for 10 days

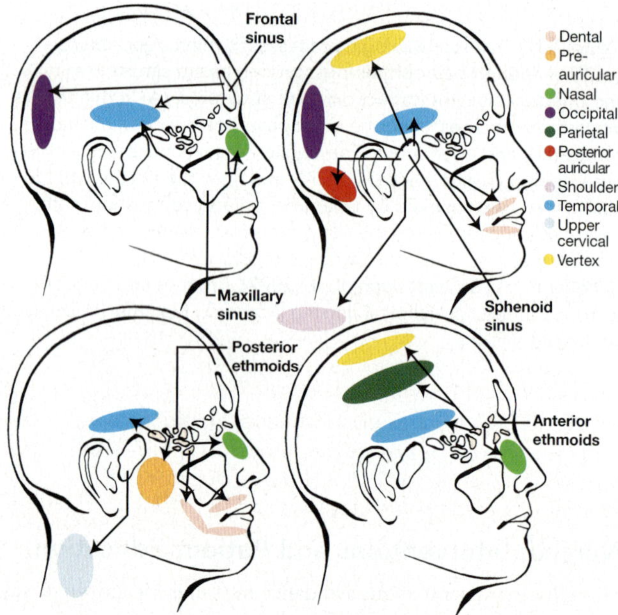

Figure 13-3. Referred pain from the paranasal sinuses. (Adapted with permission from Galen, B. [1997]. Chronic recurrent sinusitis: Recognition and treatment. *Lippincott's Primary Care Practice, 1*[2], 183–197.)

or more. There may be chronic exacerbations of symptoms within 4 weeks.

2. Nasal congestion or obstruction is defined as subjective symptoms of difficulty breathing through the nose and/or red and edematous nasal mucosa visualized on physical examination.
3. Anosmia (lack of smell) may be reported.
4. Other symptoms that may be present include fever, cough, ear pressure, maxillary dental pain, and fatigue.
5. Viral rhinosinusitis is differentiated from bacterial by duration—symptoms for 10 days or less without worsening symptoms. Bacterial rhinosinusitis manifests for 10 days with worsening symptoms.

Chronic Rhinosinusitis

1. Mucopurulent nasal drainage, nasal obstruction, facial pain/pressure/fullness, and/or decreased sense of smell. May also have malaise and ear pain or pressure and cough. Patients may have recurrent episodes or continued symptoms for 12 weeks or more.
2. Symptoms may or may not be present but are nondiagnostic of chronic rhinosinusitis.

Diagnostic Evaluation

1. Sinus plain film consisting of Caldwell, Waters, and lateral views may be obtained but not routinely recommended for acute, isolated, or noncomplicated cases. X-rays may reveal air–fluid level, mucosal thickening, or opacification of one or more sinus cavities.
2. Computed tomographic (CT) scanning is recommended when complication is suspected or in patients with chronic sinus disease.
3. Nasal endoscopy, performed by an ear, nose, and throat (ENT) specialist, is considered the gold standard to evaluate the nasal and sinus cavity and to obtain cultures of material for the purpose of directing appropriate antibiotic therapy.
4. CT with contrast or magnetic resonance imaging (MRI) with gadolinium may be obtained if cranial extension suspected.

Management

1. Topical decongestant spray or drops or systemic decongestants may be used to treat the nasal congestion associated with rhinosinusitis. Topical therapy should be limited to no more than 3 successive days of use as increased use beyond 3 days may cause rebound nasal congestion (rhinitis medicamentosa).
2. Topical nasal corticosteroids are frequently used in chronic sinusitis and may be used in acute cases. Nasal corticosteroids have been shown to decrease the severity of symptoms when used with appropriate antibiotic therapy.
3. Antibiotics—amoxicillin is the initial drug of choice in adults with acute rhinosinusitis. For penicillin-allergic patients, sulfamethoxazole–trimethoprim or macrolide antibiotics may also be used as first-line therapy. The most common organisms identified in patients with acute bacterial rhinosinusitis are *Streptococcus pneumoniae*, *Haemophilus influenzae*, and *Moraxella catarrhalis*. Other less common organisms include *Staphylococcus aureus* and anaerobes.
4. Usually 10- to 14-day course for acute sinusitis; azithromycin or fluoroquinolones may be prescribed for 3 to 5 days.
5. Prolonged therapy for chronic sinusitis (up to several months).
6. Analgesics—pain may be significant.
7. Warm compresses; cool vapor humidity for comfort and to promote drainage; nasal saline irrigation.
8. Surgical interventions (for chronic sinusitis when conservative treatment is unsuccessful).
   a. Functional endoscopic sinus surgery (FESS)—endoscopic removal of diseased tissue from affected sinus; used to treat chronic sinusitis of maxillary, ethmoid, and frontal sinuses.
   b. Nasal antrostomy (nasal–antral window)—surgical placement of an opening under inferior turbinate to provide aeration of the antrum and to permit exit for purulent materials.
   c. Balloon sinuplasty is a minimally invasive procedure where a balloon is inflated to increase the diameter of passageways in the sinuses and promote drainage.
   d. For nursing care, see page 436.

Complications

1. Extension of infection to the orbital contents and eyelids.
2. Bone infection (osteomyelitis) may spread by direct extension or through blood vessels. Frontal bone commonly affected.
3. Central nervous system (CNS) complications include meningitis, subdural and epidural purulent drainage, brain abscess, and cavernous sinus thrombosis (acute thrombophlebitis originating from an infection in an area having venous drainage to cavernous sinus).

CLINICAL JUDGMENT Watch for lid edema, edema of ocular conjunctiva, drooping lid, limitation of extraocular motion, vision loss; may indicate orbital cellulitis, which necessitates immediate treatment.

Nursing Interventions and Patient Education

1. Teach the patient signs and symptoms of acute, bacterial rhinosinusitis versus signs and symptoms of rhinitis. Educate the patient in regard to symptoms that prompt medical attention.
2. Advise the patients about adverse reactions of antibiotic therapy, including side effects, drug interactions, and symptoms that prompt medical attention.
3. Stress the importance of adhering to antibiotic therapy for complete duration and following up for recurrence.
4. Teach the patient with recurrent sinusitis how to irrigate nasal passages with saline to remove crusted mucus near the sinus openings and enhance drainage (page 437).
5. Instruct the patient not to smoke.
6. Encourage the patient to receive influenza vaccine yearly.

Pharyngitis

Pharyngitis is a rapid onset of inflammation of the pharynx, including palate, tonsils, and posterior wall of the pharynx, most commonly caused by acute infection, usually transmitted through respiratory secretions. Streptococcal pharyngitis (*strep throat*) and rhinoviruses (the common cold) are frequent causes. Pharyngitis is diagnosed in 11 million emergency departments and outpatient office visits per year.

Pathophysiology and Etiology

1. Acute bacterial pharyngitis is usually caused by group A beta-hemolytic streptococci.
2. Other bacterial causes include *H. influenzae*, *M. catarrhalis*, *Corynebacterium diphtheriae* (diphtheria), *Neisseria gonorrhoeae* (gonorrhea), and other groups of streptococcus. Transmission

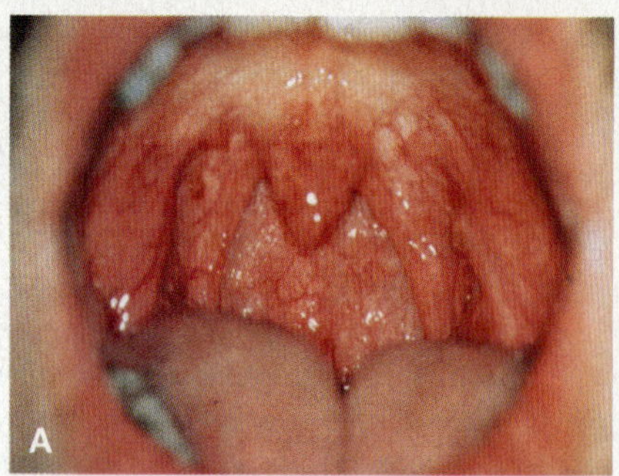

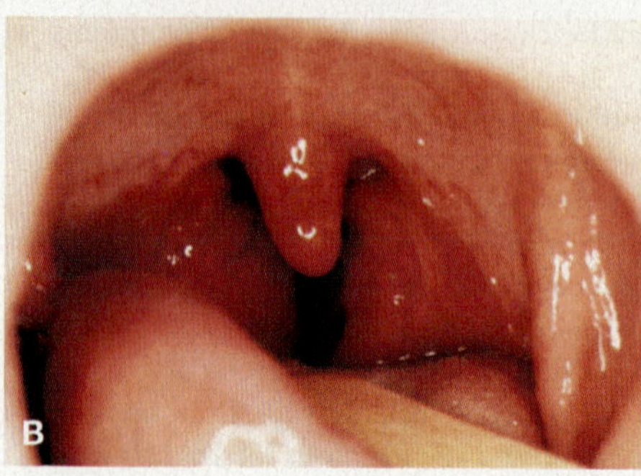

Figure 13-4. Pharyngitis—inflammation without exudate. **(A)** Redness and vascularity of the pillars and uvula are mild to moderate. **(B)** Redness is diffuse and intense. Each patient would probably complain of a sore throat. (**A:** Reprinted with permission from Hinkle, J. L., Cheever, K. H., & Overbaugh, K. J. [2022]. Brunner and Suddarth's textbook of medical-surgical nursing [15th ed., Fig. 18-2]. Lippincott Williams & Wilkins; **B:** Reprinted with permission from the Wellcome Trust, National Medical Slide Bank, London, UK.)

of *N. gonorrhoeae* is through oral contact with genital secretions; it is a sexually transmitted disease.

3. Viral pharyngitis is common and causes include rhinovirus, adenovirus, parainfluenza virus, coxsackievirus, coronavirus, and others.
4. More chronic causes are irritation from postnasal drip of allergic rhinitis and chronic sinusitis, chemical irritation, and systemic diseases.

Clinical Manifestations

1. For acute bacterial infections, abrupt onset of sore throat and fever, usually above 100.4°F (38.0°C), and exposure to *Streptococcus* within the preceding 2 weeks are suggestive of streptococcal pharyngitis.
   a. Throat pain is aggravated by swallowing.
   b. Pharynx appears reddened with edema of uvula; tonsils enlarged and reddened; pharynx and tonsils may be covered with exudate (see Figure 13-4).
   c. Palatal petechiae and a scarlatiniform rash are highly specific but uncommonly seen.
2. Varying degrees of sore throat, nasal congestion, fatigue, and fever with other bacterial and viral causes.
3. Cough, conjunctivitis, and diarrhea are common with viral causes.
4. Swollen, palpable, and tender cervical lymph nodes in most cases. Anterior cervical lymph node swelling and enlargement are common.

Diagnostic Evaluation

1. Throat culture or streptococcal rapid antigen detection test (RADT) to rule out streptococci. Rapid strep tests provide results within 5 minutes; false-negative rate is higher than with culture method.
2. Gonococcal antigen detection test to rule out gonococcal pharyngitis, if genital gonococcal infection or positive sexual contact is suspected.
3. Mono Spot test to rule out mononucleosis.
4. Viral testing is not practical, and viral causes are self-limiting.

Management

1. For group A streptococcal pharyngitis, penicillin V 250 mg four times a day orally for 10 days or penicillin G benzathine in a single intramuscular (IM) dose of 2.4 million units appears to shorten the duration of symptoms and prevents rheumatic fever (see page 263).
2. Amoxicillin, amoxicillin–clavulanate, clindamycin, macrolides, erythromycin, and cephalosporins are used for bacterial pharyngitis.

Complications

1. Acute rheumatic fever.
2. Peritonsillar abscess/cellulitis.
3. Acute glomerulonephritis.
4. Scarlet fever.
5. Sinusitis, otitis media, and mastoiditis.

DRUG ALERT Acute rheumatic fever, a complication of streptococcal pharyngitis, can be prevented if the patient is treated adequately with penicillin and, possibly, another antibiotic. Unfortunately, there is no evidence that antibiotic therapy will prevent acute glomerulonephritis.

Nursing Interventions and Patient Education

1. Advise the patient to have any sore throat with fever evaluated, especially in the absence of cold symptoms.
2. Encourage adherence to full course of antibiotic therapy, despite feeling better in several days, to prevent complications.
3. Advise lukewarm saline gargles and use of antipyretic/analgesics, as directed, to promote comfort.
4. Encourage bed rest with increased fluid intake during episodes of fever.
5. Promote good hand hygiene to prevent spread.

DRUG ALERT Reye Syndrome Warning—aspirin should not be used in children or teenagers who have a viral infection, whether they have a fever, due to association with Reye syndrome (see page 1126).

EAR DISORDERS

See additional online content: Procedure Guidelines 13-1

Hearing Loss

Hearing loss ranks high as a health disability. There are multiple causes, and the range of hearing loss varies from mild hearing loss to profound hearing loss with complete inability to understand the spoken word. Two major types of hearing loss are conductive and sensorineural. There are 48 million Americans (14%) with hearing loss.

Classification of Hearing Loss

1. Conductive loss—any condition interfering with sound transmission through the external auditory canal or transmission of tympanic membrane vibrations through the middle ear ossicles to the inner ear.
2. Sensorineural (perceptive) loss—hearing loss due to disease of the inner ear or nerve pathways; sensitivity to and discrimination of sounds are impaired. Hearing aids usually are helpful.
3. Combined or mixed hearing loss—combination of the above-mentioned conditions; commonly occurs with trauma to the ear.
4. Sudden sensorineural hearing loss—30-dB hearing loss in one or both ears in three contiguous frequencies that occurs within 3 days or less. It can be caused by an acute viral infection, vascular event, or head trauma.

See Table 13-2 for tuning fork tests that assist in differentiating conductive from sensorineural hearing loss.

Presbycusis

A progressive, bilaterally perceptive hearing loss of older adults, usually involving high frequencies, that occurs with the aging process.

1. An audiogram should be obtained by a professional audiologist to evaluate the degree of hearing loss, word discrimination ability, and identification of any hearing loss suggestive of a retrocochlear etiology.
2. The patient should be counseled by an otolaryngologist in collaboration with an audiologist, who can make recommendations for hearing amplification.
3. Helpful aids should be considered, such as a telephone amplifier, radio and television earphone attachments, and a buzzer instead of a doorbell.
4. Understanding and help from family members are important.

Table 13-2 Tuning Fork Tests

EAR CONDITION	WEBER TEST	RINNE TEST
Normal, no hearing loss	No shifting of sounds laterally/equal Sound in both ears	Sound perceived two times longer by *air* conduction
Conductive loss	Shifting of sounds to poorer ear	Sound perceived as long or longer by *bone* conduction
Sensorineural loss	Shifting of sounds to better ear	Sound perceived longer by *air* conduction

Otosclerosis

Otosclerosis is defined as an abnormal growth of bone of the middle ear that prevents the ossicles, or middle ear bones, from working properly and impeding movement of the stapes. Causes progressive hearing loss in one or both ears, vertigo, and tinnitus.

The cause is unknown, but there is a familial tendency, and people assigned female at birth are affected more often than people assigned male at birth.

Clinical Manifestations

1. Young adults present with a history of slow, progressive hearing loss of soft-spoken tones, with no signs of middle ear infection. In people of childbearing age, often progresses during pregnancy.
2. Audiometry findings substantiate conductive or mixed hearing loss.

Management

1. No known medical treatment exists for this form of deafness, but amplification with a hearing aid may be helpful.
2. Surgery—stapedotomy or stapedectomy.
   a. The removal of otosclerotic lesions at the footplate of stapes or complete removal of the stapes and the creation of a tissue implant with prosthesis to maintain suitable conduction.
   b. To perform such delicate surgery, an otologic binocular microscope is used.

Cochlear Implant

A *cochlear implant* (CI) is a device that emits auditory signals for profoundly deaf people (see Figure 13-5). The single-electrode system bypasses the damaged cochlear system and stimulates the remaining auditory nerve fibers. This results in the perception of sound.

Description

1. Purpose is for the patient to detect louder environmental sounds but will not restore normal hearing. Many recipients continue to rely on speech reading (formerly called lip reading) to make sense of the sound input being received. Some patients are able to rely entirely on hearing with their CI device and may even be able to use the telephone.
2. The microphone and sound processor are positioned externally; the electrode array is implanted internally and inserted into the cochlea. The receiver–stimulator is inserted into a bony well created in the mastoid behind the ear.
3. Electrical stimuli converted from the sound processor are sent inside the body to the implanted electrode. These electrical signals stimulate the auditory nerve fibers, which are interpreted by the brain.
4. Success rate is highly variable and depends on several different parameters. According to the Acoustical Society of America, as of 2022, over one million registered devices have been implanted worldwide.

Patient Criteria

According to the American Academy of Audiology, the use of a team approach and updated guidelines for screening will lead to more candidates for CIs who will benefit from improved hearing and quality of life. Some of the recommendations for identification of candidates include the following:

1. Any patient who gains limited benefit from current hearing aids and is interested in improvement in hearing.
2. Unilateral or bilateral hearing loss.

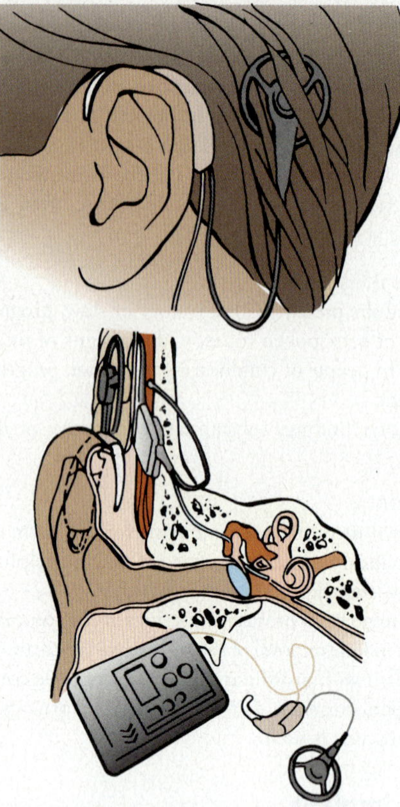

Figure 13-5. Nucleus 24 cochlear implant system. Sounds are picked up by the small, directional microphone located in the headset at the ear. A thin cord carries the sound from the microphone to the speech processor, a powerful miniaturized computer. The speech processor filters, analyzes, and digitizes the sound into coded signals that are sent from the speech processor to the transmitting coil. The transmitting coil sends the coded signals as FM radio signals to the cochlear implant under the skin. The cochlear implant delivers the appropriate electrical energy to the array of electrodes, which have been inserted into the cochlea. The electrodes along the array stimulate the remaining auditory nerve fibers in the cochlea. The resulting electrical sound information is sent through the auditory system to the brain for interpretation. The entire process takes microseconds.

3. Hearing loss cause and duration, and history of hearing aid use.
4. Physical, mental, emotional health and support systems.
5. Monosyllabic word testing and sentence recognition testing scores.

Nursing Interventions

1. Encourage the prospective patient to visit with someone who is currently using an implant to learn its positive and negative results.
2. Explain the rehabilitation process; usually begins 2 to 4 weeks after surgery to activate the CI, including:
   a. Adjustment of controls.
   b. Operation and maintenance of stimulator unit.
   c. Listening critically and learning speech reading.
   d. Learning discrimination of sounds through CI. Understanding speech through CI is not possible with this device alone.
   e. Many people trained with such an implant can speech-read more easily and can distinguish voices and environmental sounds.
3. Pneumococcal vaccination is important for all CI candidates and recipients. This should be given at least 2 weeks prior to surgery.
4. For care after surgery, see page 451.

Other Implantable Devices

1. Osseointegrated devices transmit sound from an external device, worn above the ear, through the skin and into the skull to the inner ear. This device is indicated in those with conductive hearing loss when a hearing aid is contraindicated such as chronic ear infection, those with aural atresia or microtia without the normal ear canal needed to carry sound to the middle ear, and those with single-sided deafness.
2. Implantable middle ear hearing devices (IMEHDs) to increase the transmission of sound to the inner ear. Attaches to one of the ossicles in the middle ear.
3. Bone-anchored hearing aid (BAHA) is like a CI for individuals with middle ear problems, mixed hearing problems, or unilateral hearing loss.

Maximizing Communication With the Person Who Is Hard of Hearing

When hearing loss is permanent or not amenable to medical or surgical intervention, aural rehabilitation is necessary for the patient to maintain communication and prevent isolation. Aural rehabilitation is a multifaceted process that includes auditory training (listening skills), speech reading, and the use of hearing aids. Nurses strive to maintain effective communication with patients. These suggestions promote better communication.

Strategies for Communicating With the Person Who Is Hard of Hearing and Able to Speech-Read

1. Face the person as directly as possible when speaking.
2. Place yourself in good light so the person can see your mouth.
3. Do not chew, smoke, or have anything in your mouth when speaking.
4. Speak slowly and enunciate distinctly.
5. Provide contextual clues that will assist the person in following your speech. For example, point to a tray if you are talking about the food on it.
6. To verify that the patient understands your message, write it for them to read (i.e., if you doubt that the patient is understanding you).

Strategies for Communicating With the Person Who Is Hard of Hearing and Has Difficulty Being Understood

1. Pay attention when the person speaks; facial and physical gestures may help you understand what person is saying.
2. Exchange conversation with person when it is possible to anticipate replies. This is particularly helpful in your initial contact with person and may help you become familiar with speech peculiarities.
3. Anticipate context of speech to assist in interpreting what the person is saying.
4. If unable to understand the person, resort to writing or include in your conversation someone who does understand; request that the person repeat that which is not understood.

Organizations That Help the Hard of Hearing

- Alexander Graham Bell Association for the Deaf (*www.agbell.org*)
- American Speech-Language-Hearing Association (*www.asha.org*)

- National Association of the Deaf (*www.nad.org*)
- The National Institute on Deafness and other Communication Disorders has a directory of organizations for individuals with communication disorders (*www.nidcd.nih.gov*).

Community and Home Care Considerations

1. Prevention of hearing loss should be discussed in the community—in schools, the workplace, and community gatherings.
2. Preventable hearing loss includes
   a. Noise-induced hearing loss—long periods of exposure to loud noise from machinery or engines.
   b. Acoustic trauma—single exposure to intense noise, such as an explosion or amplified music.
3. Prevention involves avoidance of both types of noise, generally noise above 85 or 90 dB.
4. Teach people to be aware of their surroundings and avoid noisy places or turn off sources of noise in the environment whenever possible.
5. Teach proper use of ear protection including earplugs and headsets both in the workplace and elsewhere.
6. Advise people that the Occupational Safety and Health Administration requires ear protection when noise exposure is above the legal limits, so workers have a right to protective equipment.

Otitis Externa

Otitis externa is an inflammation/infection of the external ear, pinna, and/or ear canal.

Pathophysiology and Etiology

1. Bacterial causes: Most common causes are *Pseudomonas aeruginosa*, *Proteus mirabilis*, and *Staphylococcus aureus*.
2. May be caused by fungal source: *Aspergillus niger*, *C. albicans*.
3. Commonly caused by chronic dermatologic conditions, such as seborrhea, psoriasis, eczema, or contact dermatitis. Allergic reaction to topical otic such as neomycin/polymyxin preparations may also occur in some patients.
4. Trauma to the ear canal, usually from cleaning the canal.
5. Stagnant water in ear canal after swimming or from water irrigation for cerumen removal is a common etiology.
6. Necrotizing malignant otitis externa is a serious infection into deeper tissue adjacent to the ear canal, including cellulitis and osteomyelitis. It is usually caused by *Pseudomonas* and may be seen in patients with diabetes, patients aged 60 years and above, patients who are debilitated, or patients with compromised immune systems.
7. Methicillin-resistant *S. aureus* otorrhea has been a common cause of chronic ear drainage. Treatment is based on culture and sensitivity of the ear drainage.

Clinical Manifestations

1. Otalgia or ear pain, increased by manipulation of auricle or tragus; hearing loss and aural fullness. Itching may also be present.
2. Periauricular lymphadenopathy.
3. Foul-smelling white to purulent drainage otorrhea. Drainage may be thick and purulent or thin and white, depending on the causative organism.
4. Red, swollen ear canal with discharge on otoscopic examination; ear canal can be swollen shut.

Management

1. Instillation of isopropyl alcohol drops (dries moisture), acetic acid solution (restores acidity), or topical antibiotics (curbs infection). A combination of these treatments may be used depending on the cause. Antifungal agents, in ointment, powder, or drop form, may be used.
   a. Prophylactic use of alcohol drops or acetic acid solution by swimmers or those prone to otitis externa may be indicated.
   b. Antibiotic drops include combination products containing polymyxin, neomycin, and hydrocortisone; ciprofloxacin; and ofloxacin. Tobramycin preparations may be used with methicillin-resistant infections (confirmed by culture and sensitivity).
   c. A 10-day course of treatment is usually indicated.
   d. Parenteral antibiotics will be used for necrotizing otitis externa.
2. If canal is swollen and tender, an antibiotic solution containing a corticosteroid is chosen to reduce inflammation and swelling. If acute inflammation and closure of the ear canal prevent drops from saturating canal, a wick may need to be inserted by an ear, nose, and throat (ENT) specialist so drops will gain access to walls of entire ear canal.
3. Burow solution (aluminum acetate solution) or topical corticosteroid cream or lotion may be used in otitis externa caused by dermatitis.
4. Fungal infections may be treated with a topical antifungal, such as nystatin or ketoconazole.
5. In chronic otitis externa, debris from the ear canal may need to be removed through suction after pain and swelling have subsided. Avoid water irrigation, as this promotes bacterial and fungal growth from stagnant moisture.
6. Warm compresses and analgesics may be needed.

Nursing Interventions and Patient Education

1. Demonstrate proper application of eardrops. See Patient Education Guidelines 13-2.
2. Advise the patient that otitis externa can be prevented or minimized by thoroughly drying the ear canal after coming into contact with water or moist environment.
3. Teach the patient to use prophylactic eardrops after swimming to assist in preventing swimmer's ear, as directed by health care provider.
4. Advise the use of properly fitting earplugs for recurrent cases.
5. Teach proper ear hygiene: Clean auricle and outer canal with washcloth only; do not insert anything smaller than a finger wrapped in washcloth in the ear canal. Avoid inserting cotton swabs or sharp objects into the ear canal because:
   a. Cerumen may be forced against the tympanic membrane, causing impaction.
   b. The canal lining may be abraded, making it more susceptible to infection.
   c. The tympanic membrane may be injured.

Impacted Cerumen and Foreign Bodies

Cerumen impaction is defined as accumulation of cerumen, or "ear wax," that causes symptoms of ear pain, fullness, or hearing loss and/or prevents visualization of the tympanic membrane.

Etiology and Clinical Manifestations

1. Cerumen is a mixture of glandular secretions from the ear canal mixed with squamous epithelium. Cerumen builds up

over a period of time, causing a decrease in hearing acuity and a feeling that the ear is plugged.
   a. May be underlying seborrhea or other dermatologic condition that causes flaking of skin that mixes with cerumen and becomes obstructive.
   b. Cerumen may be pushed back into external canal and cover the tympanic membrane by action of cotton swab.
2. Insect may fly or crawl into the ear, causing initial low rumbling sound; later, feeling that ear is plugged and decreased hearing acuity. Foreign bodies may be placed into the ear canal, especially by children, and include food particles, small objects, or tips of cotton swabs.
3. The patient often seeks treatment for symptoms related to the foreign body or impacted cerumen.

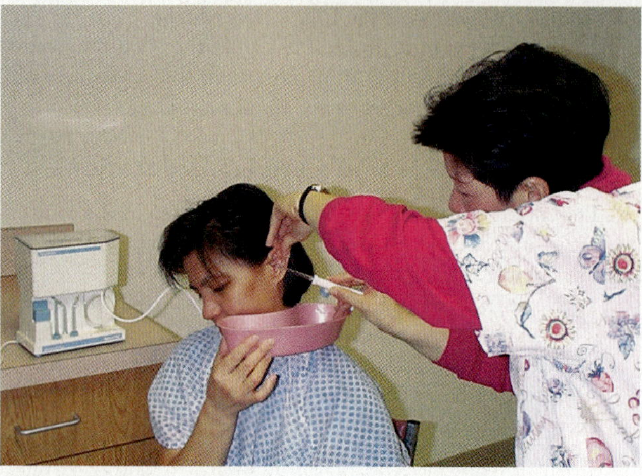

Figure 13-6. Using an electronic irrigation device to irrigate the external auditory cavity.

Management

1. Accumulated cerumen does not have to be removed unless it causes symptoms, interferes with examination of the ear drum, or interferes with hearing. May be removed by curette or by irrigation with a syringe or electronic irrigation device (see Figure 13-6).
   a. Avoid directing irrigation stream directly at the tympanic membrane, rather direct stream at the wall of canal.
   b. Use warm water at approximately body temperature.
2. Foreign bodies may be removed by instrumentation or irrigation by health care provider.
   a. Insects—treat by instilling oil drops to smother insect, which then can be removed with ear spatula or irrigation.
   b. Vegetable foreign bodies (e.g., peas)—irrigation is contraindicated because vegetable matter absorbs water, which would further wedge it in the canal.
   c. Only a skilled person should attempt to remove foreign body to prevent tympanic membrane perforation and trauma to canal.
   d. General anesthesia may be required to remove foreign bodies from young children, if they are unable to cooperate.

CLINICAL JUDGMENT Do not attempt to irrigate the ear or instill anything into the external canal if the eardrum may be perforated; otoscopic examination should be done to rule out tympanic membrane rupture or acute infection. If the tympanic membrane is unable to be visualized and perforation is suspected, or acute infection is suspected, do not irrigate and refer to ENT specialist. Some antibiotic eardrops are contraindicated if the tympanic membrane is not intact.

Nursing Interventions and Patient Education

1. Teach proper ear hygiene, especially not putting anything in ears.
2. Explain the normal protective function of cerumen.
3. If patient has a problem with cerumen buildup and has been advised by health care provider to use a ceruminolytic periodically, make sure that the patient is getting cerumen out of the ear before more medication is instilled. A bulb syringe may be used by the patient at home to help remove softened cerumen.
4. Advise the patient to report persistent fever, pain, drainage, or hearing impairment.

Acute Otitis Media

Acute otitis media or *acute suppurative otitis* is a rapid onset of inflammation and infection of the middle ear caused by contamination from bacteria from the middle ear fluid through the eustachian tube. Prevalent in children due to the anatomically shorter eustachian tube, but also occurs in adults.

Pathophysiology and Etiology

1. Pathogenic organisms gain entry into the normally sterile middle ear, usually through a dysfunctional eustachian tube.
2. Organisms include *Streptococcus pneumoniae, Haemophilus influenzae, Moraxella catarrhalis*, and *S. aureus*.

PATIENT EDUCATION GUIDELINES 13-2

Instilling Ear Drops

1. Wash hands.
2. Hold the medication bottle between your hands for 1 to 2 minutes to warm drops before administering.
3. Lie on the side with affected ear facing upward. Shake drops. Pull ear up and back and then instill drops by squeezing the bulb the ordered number of times.
4. Pump tragus by pushing on the flap of skin protecting the ear canal five to six times to ensure drops reach eardrum.
5. Remain on the side for 1 to 2 minutes. Repeat, if necessary, on opposite ear.

3. In serous (secretory) otitis media, no purulent infection occurs, but blockage of the eustachian tube causes negative pressure and transudation of fluid from blood vessels and development of effusion in the middle ear.

Clinical Manifestations

1. Pain is usually the first symptom. Child will tug, rub, or hold the ear.
2. Fever may rise to 104°F to 105°F (40°C to 40.6°C).
3. Purulent drainage (otorrhea) is present if the tympanic membrane is perforated.
4. Irritability may be noted in the young person.
5. Headache, hearing loss, anorexia, nausea, and vomiting may be present.
6. Purulent effusion may be visible behind the tympanic membrane, or tympanic membrane may be reddened and bulging on otoscopic examination.
7. History may reveal previous upper respiratory infection (URI), allergic rhinitis, eustachian tube dysfunction, history of reflux, adenoid hypertrophy, history of cleft palate, smoking in household, sibling otitis media in children, or child in daycare. Patients who have received radiation therapy of the head and neck or experienced barotrauma or those with nasopharyngeal tumor may develop middle ear effusions.

Diagnostic Evaluation

1. Pneumatic otoscopy shows a tympanic membrane that is full, bulging, and opaque with impaired mobility (or retracted with impaired mobility).
2. Cultures of discharge through ruptured tympanic membrane may suggest causative organism.

Management

1. Antibiotic treatment—amoxicillin is first-line treatment; cephalosporins, macrolides, or trimethoprim–sulfamethoxazole may be used in patients with penicillin allergy.
2. Amoxicillin/clavulanate and cephalosporins are used for treatment failure due to increasing rate of beta-lactamase–producing bacteria that inactivate penicillin and other antibiotics.
3. Usual treatment course is 10 days.
4. Follow-up is indicated to determine the effectiveness of therapy.
5. Nasal or topical decongestants and antihistamines have a limited role in promoting eustachian tube drainage.
6. Surgery—myringotomy with placement of pressure-equalizing tubes.
   a. An incision is made into the posterior inferior aspect of the tympanic membrane for relief of persistent effusion. A pressure-equalizing tube may be inserted to prevent recurrent episodes.
   b. Performed in selected patients to prevent recurrent episodes or in patients with middle ear effusion for 3 months or more.
   c. May be done because of failure of patient to respond to antimicrobial therapy; for severe, persistent pain; and for persistent conductive hearing loss.
   d. Full recovery in 4 weeks. Tubes fall out in 6 to 12 months.

Complications

1. Perforation of tympanic membrane.
2. Chronic otitis media and mastoiditis.
3. Conductive hearing loss.
4. Meningitis and brain abscess.

Nursing Assessment

1. Obtain history of URI, previous ear infections, allergies, and progression of symptoms.
2. Assess fever and level of pain.
3. Obtain baseline hearing evaluation, if indicated.

Nursing Interventions

Relieving Pain

1. Administer or teach self-administration of anti-inflammatories and other analgesics, as prescribed.
2. Administer or teach self-administration of antibiotics, as prescribed. Oral corticosteroids may be prescribed, as well as nasal steroids.
3. Encourage the use of local warm compresses or heating pad to promote comfort and help resolve infectious process.
4. Be alert for symptoms such as headache, slow pulse, vomiting, and vertigo, which may be significant for sequelae that involve the mastoid or the brain.

Patient Education and Health Maintenance

1. Encourage follow-up after treatment to ensure resolution.
2. Advise the patient that sudden relief of pain may indicate tympanic membrane rupture. Do not instill anything in ear and call health care provider.
3. Instruct the patient to follow up for recurrence of symptoms, such as pain, fever, ear congestion, or hearing loss.

Evaluation: Expected Outcomes

- Verbalizes relief of pain at follow-up visit.

Chronic Suppurative Otitis Media and Mastoiditis

Chronic suppurative otitis media is a chronic inflammation of the middle ear with tissue damage, usually caused by repeated episodes of acute otitis media. It may be caused by an antibiotic-resistant organism or a particularly virulent strain of organism. It may be associated with tympanic membrane perforation. *Mastoiditis* is inflammation of the mastoid air cells of the temporal bone adjacent to the ear and is a common complication of acute otitis media.

Pathophysiology and Etiology

1. The accumulation of purulent inflammatory exudate under pressure in the middle ear cavity may result in necrosis of tissue, with damage to the tympanic membrane and, possibly, the ossicles.
   a. The most common organisms are *S. pneumoniae*, *H. influenzae*, and *M. catarrhalis*.
   b. Other organisms may be present, such as *Pseudomonas*, *Proteus*, and *Bacteroides* species.
2. Persistent rupture of the tympanic membrane and damage to the ossicles lead to conductive hearing loss.
3. Extension of infection may occur into the mastoid cells (mastoiditis), facial nerve, labyrinth, lateral sinus, and the meninges of the brain.
4. Cholesteatoma may form (mass of squamous epithelium and desquamated debris in the middle ear), which may cause erosion of the ossicles or inner ear.

Clinical Manifestations

1. Painless or dull ache, decreased hearing, tenderness of mastoid.
2. Otorrhea may be odorless or foul smelling.
3. Vertigo and pain may be present if central nervous system (CNS) complications have occurred.
4. History will indicate several episodes of acute otitis media with recent antibiotic treatment and possible rupture of tympanic membrane.
5. Fever and postauricular erythema and edema.

Diagnostic Evaluation

1. Conductive hearing loss is present through audiometric tests.
2. Computed tomography (CT) of the temporal bone may show mastoid pathology, for example, cholesteatoma or opacification of mastoid cells.
3. Culture of exudate from the middle ear (through ruptured tympanic membrane or at the time of surgery).
4. Pneumatic otoscope to evaluate mobility of the tympanic membrane and assess the presence of fluid in the middle ear.

Management

Note: If advanced chronic ear disease is left untreated, inner ear and life-threatening CNS complications may develop because of erosion of surrounding structures.

Medical Therapy

1. Antibiotic and steroid eardrops may control middle ear infection and inflammation, but when mastoiditis develops, parenteral antibiotic therapy is necessary.
2. Eardrops containing neomycin, gentamicin, tobramycin, and quinolones, such as ciprofloxacin, are instilled into the middle ear when the tympanic membrane is ruptured. Otic drops containing antibiotics or antibiotic powder preparations may be used for infection and otorrhea.
3. Local cleaning using microscope and instrumentation is the mainstay of treatment and done by ENT specialist.
4. Intravenous (IV) antibiotics must cover beta-lactamase–producing organisms—ampicillin–sulbactam, cefuroxime—based on culture results.

DRUG ALERT Quinolones are the preferred treatment. Use extreme caution with ototoxic antibiotics, such as aminoglycosides, which may cause hearing loss.

Surgical Interventions

1. Indicated when cholesteatoma is present.
2. Indicated when there is pain, profound deafness, dizziness, sudden facial paralysis, or stiff neck (may lead to meningitis or brain abscess).
3. Types of procedures:
   a. Simple mastoidectomy—removal of diseased bone and insertion of a drain; indicated when there is persistent infection and signs of intracranial complications.
   b. Radical mastoidectomy (canal wall down)—removal of complete mastoid as well as posterior wall of ear canal, remnants of the tympanic membrane, and the malleolus and incus.
   c. Posteroanterior mastoidectomy (canal wall up)—combines simple mastoidectomy with tympanoplasty (reconstruction of middle ear structures). Leaves ear canal intact.

Complications

1. Acute and chronic mastoiditis.
2. Labyrinthitis.
3. Cholesteatoma.
4. CNS infection (meningitis, intracranial abscess).
5. Postoperatively—facial nerve paralysis, bleeding, vertigo.

Nursing Assessment

1. Assess for a history of ear infection and treatment adherence. Identify social determinants that may prevent adherence to treatment in the future—lack of finances/prescription coverage, lack of transportation, language and cultural barriers, education and intellectual challenges, and so forth.
2. Assess for ear drainage and patency of tympanic membrane.
3. Assess for hearing loss.
4. Palpate for mastoid tenderness.

For nursing process related to patients undergoing surgical treatment, see "Care Related to Ear Surgery," page 438.

Patient Education and Health Maintenance

1. Teach the patient to keep the ear dry—use ENT-approved or molded earplugs during showering, washing hair, and swimming—to prevent any water from gaining access to the middle ear.
2. Encourage the patient to follow up for frequent ear cleaning.
3. Stress the importance of adhering to antibiotic schedule and to notify the home care nurse or health care provider if there is any problem with venous access or a dose is missed for any reason.
4. Advise of complications and to report headache, change in mental status or arousal, or increased ear pain.
5. Stress the importance of follow-up hearing evaluations and early intervention for any signs of ear infection in the future.

Ménière Disease

Ménière disease (or *endolymphatic hydrops*) is a chronic inner ear disease characterized by spontaneous episodes of vertigo, fluctuating hearing loss, aural fullness, and tinnitus.

Pathophysiology and Etiology

1. There is no cure, cause is unknown, and it is not fatal.
2. Fluid distention of the endolymphatic spaces of the labyrinth destroys cochlear hair cells. Pathology of the disease is endolymphatic hydrops, which is thought to be caused by overaccumulation of endolymphatic fluid and distention of the endolymphatic-containing areas in the cochlea and vestibular organs.
3. Usually unilateral, later may become bilateral. Diagnoses primarily based on clinical symptoms, but audiometry and electronystagmography (ENG) are traditionally obtained.
4. Occurs most frequently between ages 40 and 60 years.
5. Severity of attacks may diminish over the years, but hearing loss increases.

Clinical Manifestations

1. Sudden attacks occur, in which the patient feels that the room is spinning (vertigo); may last 30 minutes to several hours or days.

2. Aural fullness, tinnitus, and reduced hearing or fluctuating hearing loss occur on involved side.
3. Headache, nausea, vomiting, and disequilibrium may be present.
4. After multiple attacks, tinnitus and impaired hearing may be continuous.

Diagnostic Evaluation

1. ENG or electrocochleography (ECoG) (see page 435), along with the patients' history (two or more episodes of vertigo lasting at least 20 minutes each), and neurotologic examination, is used to establish the diagnosis of Ménière disease.
2. Audiogram may reveal low-frequency sensorineural hearing loss in affected ear.
3. CT scan and magnetic resonance imaging (MRI) to rule out acoustic neuroma. Only MRI of the internal auditory canal with gadolinium can differentiate Ménière disease symptoms from the symptoms of an intracranial lesion.

Management

Medical

Focuses on treatment of the symptoms.

1. Administration of a vestibular suppressant to control symptoms.
   a. Meclizine up to 25 mg four times a day.
   b. Diphenhydramine 25 to 50 mg three or four times a day.
   c. Diazepam or lorazepam may be helpful as vestibular suppressant.
2. Intratympanic injections of aminoglycosides and corticosteroids can improve vertigo control.
3. Streptomycin (intramuscular [IM]) or gentamicin (transtympanic injection) may be given to selectively destroy vestibular apparatus if vertigo is uncontrollable.
4. An antiemetic, such as promethazine, may be needed to reduce nausea, vomiting, and resistant vertigo.
5. Diuretics.
6. Positive pressure device used to reduce the severity of vertigo. Produces intermittent air pressure pulses to the middle ear from a device placed in the external ear canal and transmitted through a tube placed in the tympanic membrane. However, research is very uncertain on the effectiveness.

EVIDENCE BASE Webster, K. E., George, B., Galbraith, K., Harrington-Benton, N. A., Judd, O., Kaski, D., Maarsingh, O. R., MacKeith, S., Ray, J., Van Vugt, V. A., & Burton, M. J. (2023). Positive pressure therapy for Ménière's disease. *Cochrane Database of Systematic Reviews*, (2), CD015248. https://doi.org/10.1002/14651858.CD015248.pub2

DRUG ALERT In general, meclizine is not recommended on a long-term basis, as it prevents CNS compensation. Meclizine may be used for symptomatic relief on a short-term basis.

Surgical

1. Conservative—endolymphatic subarachnoid or mastoid shunt to relieve symptoms without destroying function.
2. Destructive surgery.
   a. Labyrinthectomy—recommended if the patient experiences progressive hearing loss and severe vertigo attacks so normal tasks cannot be performed; results in total deafness of affected ear.
   b. Vestibular nerve section—neurosurgical suboccipital approach to the cerebellopontine angle for intracranial vestibular nerve neurectomy.

Complications

1. Irreversible hearing loss.
2. Disability and social isolation due to vertigo and hearing loss.
3. Injury due to falls.

Nursing Assessment

1. Assess for frequency and severity of attacks.
2. Provide screening hearing tests.
3. Evaluate effect on the patient's activities and potential for fall or injury.

Nursing Interventions

For care related to labyrinth surgery, see page 439.

Ensuring Safety

1. Help the patient recognize an aura so that they have time to prepare for an attack.
2. Encourage the patient to lie down during attack, in safe place, and lie still.
3. Put side rails up on bed if in hospital.
4. Have the patient close eyes if this lessens symptoms.
5. Inform the patient that the dizziness may last for varying lengths of time. Maintain safety precautions until attack is complete.

Minimizing Feelings of Isolation

1. Provide encouragement and understanding. Show the patient that you understand the seriousness of this disorder, even though there is little that can be done to ease the discomfort.
2. Assist the patient to identify specific triggers to control attacks.
   a. Remind the patient to move slowly because jerking or making sudden movements may precipitate an attack.
   b. Avoid noises and glaring, bright lights, which may initiate an attack.
   c. Control environmental factors and personal habits that may cause stress or fatigue.
   d. If there is a tendency to allergic reactions to foods, eliminate those foods from the diet.
3. Avoid oversedation of the patient through polypharmacy with sedatives, anticholinergics, and opioids that may increase the risk of falling if attack occurs.
4. Teach the patient to be aware of other sensory cues from the environment, visual, olfactory, and tactile, if hearing is affected.

Patient Education and Health Maintenance

1. Teach about medication therapy, including adverse effects of vestibular suppressants—drowsiness, dry mouth.
2. Advise sodium restriction as adjunct to vestibular suppressant therapy.
3. Advise the patient to keep a diary or log of attacks, triggers, and severity of symptoms.
4. Encourage follow-up hearing evaluations and provide information about surgical care if planned.
5. Teach the patient hearing conservation methods—avoid loud noises, wear earplugs if necessary, avoid smoking, and avoid use of ototoxic drugs, such as aspirin, quinine, and some antibiotics. Limit caffeine, chocolate, and alcohol consumption.

Evaluation: Expected Outcomes

- Lays down with side rails up and eyes closed during attack; resolves without injury.
- Identifies dietary triggers and follows treatment plan.

Vestibular Labyrinthitis

Labyrinthitis is an inflammation of the inner ear caused by a viral or bacterial infection. It is characterized by hearing loss, vertigo, and, usually, nausea and vomiting.

See Box 13-1, for other causes of vertigo, including benign paroxysmal positional vertigo (BPPV).

BOX 13-1 Vertigo

Vertigo is a type of dizziness characterized by the illusion of movement: a perception either that the surroundings are moving while the body remains still or that one's body is moving while the surroundings remain still. It is caused by vestibular dysfunction—in either the peripheral vestibular system (inner ear) or the central vestibular system (brainstem and cerebellum).

- Common causes of vertigo of peripheral origin include Ménière disease, labyrinthitis, acoustic neuroma, and benign paroxysmal positional vertigo (BPPV).
- Causes of central vertigo include multiple sclerosis, basilar migraine, transient ischemic attack or stroke of the basilar artery, brain tumor, trauma, and cerebral hemorrhage.
- Other causes of dizziness are vasovagal syncope, hypovolemia, autonomic neuropathy of diabetes, severe anemia, aortic stenosis, hypoglycemia, hypoxia, hypocarbia, multiple sensory deficits, adverse drug effects, and emotional illness.

BPPV is the most common cause of vertigo. Its onset is sudden, it can be severe in intensity, and it is always related to change in position of the head. It can be diagnosed by thorough history and physical examination, including some provocative maneuvers such as the Dix–Hallpike maneuver. Diagnostic tests are required only to rule out central vestibular dysfunction and dizziness caused by other disorders. Patients with BPPV may be very concerned about their symptoms and are at risk for injury due to imbalance.

NURSING CONSIDERATIONS

- Ensure safety by creating an uncluttered environment, using side rails and handrails as necessary, using proper footwear, and encouraging the patient to call for help.
- Teach patient to avoid sudden position changes, including simple head movements, such as looking up or turning over in bed.
- Discourage the use of alcohol and sedating drugs, which may further impair safe ambulation.
- Most episodes of BPPV last seconds to minutes and completely resolve within 3 months; however, if severe or prolonged, suggest referral to a physical therapist for vestibular rehabilitation.

Pathophysiology and Etiology

1. Bacterial labyrinthitis is usually associated with acute otitis media or cholesteatoma. Infectious organisms may enter the inner ear through the oval or round window. Bacterial meningitis can cause labyrinthitis by spread of the bacterial infection via the cochlear aqueduct and internal auditory canal. Diagnostic imaging may include CT of the temporal bone, MRI of the internal auditory canal with gadolinium, and lumbar puncture, if bacterial meningitis is suspected.
2. The most common cause of viral labyrinthitis is a viral illness of the respiratory tract system and may include measles, mumps, rubella, or herpetic infections of the facial or acoustic nerve. This may be seen in Ramsey–Hunt syndrome.
3. Vestibular neuronitis or neuritis is a disorder of the vestibular nerve (cranial nerve [CN] XII) characterized by severe, sudden onset of vertigo with normal hearing. Etiology most commonly from viral illness but may be attributed to other causes. The course is usually self-limiting. The patient may have an unsteady gait but is able to walk. (This is differentiated by cerebellar disease, in which the patient has vertigo and nystagmus and is usually unable to walk.) Treatment is supportive with meclizine, benzodiazepines, antiemetics, or vestibular rehabilitation.

Clinical Manifestations

1. Sudden onset of incapacitating vertigo, with varying degrees of nausea and vomiting, hearing loss, and tinnitus.
2. Issues with balance and gait.
3. Persists; does not occur in episodic attacks like Ménière disease.

Management

1. The rare cases of bacterial labyrinthitis are treated with antibiotics, as with the suspected predisposing infection.
   a. Bacterial labyrinthitis is treated by antibiotics, antiemetics, vestibular suppressants, and vestibular rehabilitation.
2. Viral labyrinthitis is treated with symptomatic support. Management may include antiviral therapy, antiemetics, vestibular suppressants, and, later in illness, vestibular rehabilitation.
3. A vestibular suppressant and antiemetic medication such as meclizine, diazepam, or promethazine may be needed, as with Ménière disease.
4. Surgical intervention—pressure equalization with a myringotomy.
5. Audiometric evaluation should be obtained with all patients with vertigo to differentiate between vestibular labyrinthitis and vestibular neuronitis. MRI of the brain and internal auditory canal is obtained when asymmetrical hearing loss is present to rule out acoustic neuroma.

Complications

1. Permanent hearing loss.
2. Injury from fall.
3. Visual impairment and impaired spatial awareness.

Nursing Assessment

1. Assess past history of previous attacks, including frequency and severity of attacks and how patient handles them.
2. Assess for fever related to bacterial infection.
3. Assess for additional neurologic symptoms—visual changes, change in mental status, sensory and motor deficits—that may indicate CNS pathology.

4. Assess for effectiveness of vestibular stimulants and antiemetics.
5. If fall occurs, assess for injury.

Nursing Interventions

Preventing Injury

1. At the onset of attack, have the patient lie still in darkened room with eyes closed or fixed on stationary object until the vertigo passes.
2. Make sure that the patient can obtain help at all times through the use of call system, close proximity to staff, or companion.
3. Remove obstacles in the patient's environment.
4. Make sure that sensory aids are available—glasses, hearing aid, proper lighting.
5. Use side rails while the patient is in bed.
6. Administer medications, as directed; assess for and avoid oversedation.
7. Recommend physical and occupational therapy evaluations if deficits are severe.

Minimizing Anxiety

1. Explain the physiology behind vertigo and the possible triggers.
2. Support patient and family through the diagnostic process.
3. Assist the patient to adjust activities to minimize the impact.
4. Teach stress reduction techniques, such as deep breathing, talking and asking questions, and distraction.

Ensuring Adequate Fluid

1. Keep diet light while vertigo is present.
2. Administer antiemetics, as directed.
3. Assess intake and output, as indicated.
4. Encourage fluids and small feedings while patient is feeling better.

Encouraging Safe Self-care

1. Encourage activity while vertigo is minimal; rest during attacks.
2. Set up environment for the patient's safety and convenience—chair near sink, walker to hold on to while walking, if necessary, and so forth.
3. Assist the patient with hygiene and other care, as needed.
4. Advise caregiver assistance if needed.

Patient Education and Health Maintenance

1. Teach patients with viral labyrinthitis that attacks are self-limiting, will become less severe, and should leave no permanent disability.
2. Teach safety measures during vertigo attacks.
3. Tell the patient that vertigo is best tolerated while lying flat in bed in a darkened room, with eyes closed or looking at stable object.
4. Teach patients how to take medications and to avoid other CNS depressants, such as alcohol.
5. Encourage follow-up and prompt diagnosis and treatment of otitis media.

Evaluation: Expected Outcomes

- Verbalizes need to rest in bed during attack with side rails up.
- Verbalizes feelings and questions about treatment.
- Takes fluids, light diet every 4 hours, after medication administration.
- Performs appropriate hygiene and dressing by oneself at bedside.

MALIGNANT DISORDERS

See additional online content: Procedure Guidelines 13-2

Cancer of the Oral Cavity, Oropharynx, Nasopharynx, and Paranasal Sinuses

Cancer of the oral cavity may arise from the lips, buccal mucosa, gums, retromolar trigone, hard palate, floor of the mouth, salivary glands, and anterior two thirds of the tongue. Cancer of the oropharynx may arise from the tonsillar fossa, pharyngeal wall, and palatal arch (soft palate, uvula, and anterior border of the anterior tonsillar pillar). Cancer of the nasopharynx may arise from the fossa of Rosenmüller (projection of nasopharynx just below base of skull). Cancer of the paranasal sinuses may arise from the maxillary sinuses (80%) or, less commonly, in the ethmoid, frontal, and sphenoid sinuses.

Pathophysiology and Etiology

EVIDENCE BASE NIH National Cancer Institute. (2021). *Head and neck cancer fact sheet.* https://www.cancer.gov/types/head-and-neck/head-neck-fact-sheet

1. Oral and oropharyngeal cancer accounts for approximately 4% of all cancers diagnosed annually in the United States. About 54,000 people will be diagnosed with oral cavity and pharynx cancer, and about 11,200 will have died from this disease in 2022. Prevalence is greater in people assigned male at birth and people between the ages of 55 to 64 years. Approximately 90% are squamous cell carcinoma.
   a. High-risk factors include use of tobacco and excessive use of alcohol (particularly in combination), use of smokeless tobacco (snuff), pipe smoking, marijuana use, exposure to human papillomavirus (HPV) (causes greater than 60% of all oropharyngeal cancers in the United States), poor oral hygiene, and genetic factors.
   b. Overall survival rate depends on the primary location of the tumor and the stage of the disease at diagnosis. On average, 68% of those with this disease will survive more than 5 years.
2. Nasopharyngeal carcinoma is most prevalent in persons with Chinese or Asian ancestry because of a diet high in preservation (e.g., salted fish, paan-betel quid). These types of cancers have a high genetic predisposition.
   a. Strong association with the Epstein–Barr virus and drinking large amounts of alcohol.
   b. The most common presentation is neck mass. Blood-stained saliva or sputum is the second most common presentation.
   c. Occurs 75% of the time in people assigned male at birth, usually between ages 30 and 60 years. Overall survival rate is 50% to 90%, depending on the stage of disease at diagnosis.
3. Malignant paranasal sinus tumors are rare and have relatively poor survival outcomes. They are usually squamous cell in origin.
   a. The majority of cancer occurs in the maxillary sinus (50% to 70%), in the nasal cavity (15% to 30%), and ethmoid sinus (10% to 20%).

b. Pathology is classified into epithelial and nonepithelial categories, with many subsets being attributable to environmental or occupational toxins.
c. Overall survival rate is 27% to 94%, with the higher stage of cancer contributing to poorer prognosis.

Clinical Manifestations

1. Commonly asymptomatic in early stages.
2. Oral cancer—nonhealing, nonpainful crusting and ulcerated leukoplakic and erythemic lesions.
3. Cancer of the lip—presence of a lesion that fails to heal.
4. Cancer of the tongue—swelling, ulceration, areas of tenderness or pain, bleeding, abnormal texture, or limited movement of the tongue.
5. Floor of the mouth cancer—red, slightly elevated, mucosal lesion with ill-defined borders, leukoplakia, indurated, ulceration, or wartlike growth.
6. Cancer of the tonsil—swelling, neck mass, wartlike growth, odynophagia, otalgia.
7. Cancer of the retromolar trigone area—trismus, otalgia, dysphagia, odynophagia.
8. Cancer of the pharyngeal wall—dysphagia, odynophagia, otalgia, neck mass.
9. Cancer of the nasopharynx—epistaxis, unilateral serous otitis, unilateral nasal blockage, loss of sense of smell (cranial nerve [CN] I), eye movement abnormalities (CN III, CN IV, and CN V), and tongue movement impairment and dysphagia (CN IX, CN X, and CN XII).
10. More advanced stages characterized by ulceration, bleeding, pain, induration, CN impairments, dysphagia, odynophagia, weight loss, and/or cervical lymphadenopathy (neck mass).

POPULATION AWARENESS Of all new cancer diagnoses, 44% involve people greater than 70 years of age. Older adults may experience cancer-related or cancer therapy–related cognitive changes, sometimes referred to as "chemo brain." Difficulty in concentration, diminished multitasking ability, and short-term memory loss may occur.

Diagnostic Evaluation

1. Careful inspection of the oral cavity with indirect mirror examination of pharynx.
2. Flexible or rigid nasopharyngoscopy to directly examine the nasopharynx and pharynx.
3. Excisional biopsy of suspected tissue is the gold standard.
4. Radiologic studies: computed tomography (CT), with or without contrast as clinically indicated; magnetic resonance imaging (MRI); and, possibly, fluorodeoxyglucose-positron emission tomography (FDG-PET)/CT for stages III to IV disease.

Management

EVIDENCE BASE Caudell, J. J., Gillison, M. L., Maghami, E., Spencer, S., Pfister, D. G., Adkins, D., Birkeland, A. C., Brizel, D. M., Busse, P. M., Cmelak, A. J., Colevas, A. D., Eisele, D. W., Galloway, T., Geiger, J. L., Haddad, R. I., Hicks, W. L., Hitchcock, Y. J., Jimeno, A., Leizman, D., Mell, L. K., Mittal, B. B., Pinto, H. A., Rocco, J. W., Rodriguez, C. P., Savvides, P. S., Schwartz, D., Shah, J. P., Sher, D., St John, M., Weber, R. S., Weinstein, G., Worden, F., Yang Bruce, J., Yom, S. S., Zhen, W., Burns, J. L., & Darlow, S. D. (2022). NCCN Guidelines® Insights: Head and Neck Cancers, Version 1.2022. *Journal of the National Comprehensive Cancer Network, 20*(3), 224-234. https://doi.org/10.6004/jnccn.2022.0016

Selection of treatment depends on the size and site of lesion and how extensively surrounding tissues are involved. Also see Chapter 4, page 76.

1. Oral cavity cancer treatment consists of the following:
   a. Surgery to remove the primary disease plus any neck lymph nodes, or definitive radiotherapy.
   b. For more advanced cancer, surgery followed by chemoradiation or multimodal clinical trials is recommended.
2. Surgical resection of nasopharyngeal cancer may be difficult because of the location and the relationship to many important structures.
   a. Radiation therapy is the treatment of choice in early-stage cancers of these areas.
   b. For more advanced nasopharyngeal cancer, the recommendation is to perform multimodal clinical trials, or concurrent chemoradiation, or induction chemotherapy followed by chemoradiation.
   c. If metastasis is present, clinical trials are recommended, or concurrent platinum-based combination chemotherapy, or concurrent chemoradiation.
3. Oropharynx cancer (base of tongue cancer, tonsil, posterior pharyngeal wall and soft palate) should be tested for HPV status to determine prognosis; however, this does not affect the treatment recommendations.
   a. For low-grade cancer, the treatment choice is definitive radiation, or transoral or open resection of the primary tumor with neck dissection followed by chemoradiation, or multimodal clinical trials.
   b. For high-grade cancers, the treatment choices remain the same as earlier, except for the addition of induction chemotherapy with radiation or systemic chemotherapy and radiation therapy.
4. Paranasal sinus cancer treatment usually consists of minimally invasive or open surgery followed by radiation; chemotherapy may also be utilized.

Complications

1. Second primary cancers of the larynx, hypopharynx, esophagus, and lungs.
2. Secondary to treatment:
   a. Surgery—transient salivary outflow obstruction, infection, voice changes, fistula formation, loss of swallowing, cosmetic defects.
   b. Radiation (early effects)—taste alterations, mucositis, xerostomia, dysphagia, odynophagia, anorexia, dermatitis, fatigue, pain.
   c. Radiation (late effects)—thyroid dysfunction, radiation caries, osteoradionecrosis, xerostomia, trismus, nasopharyngeal stenosis, cerebrospinal fluid (CSF) leak and other neurologic complications, tissue fibrosis, trismus, laryngeal edema, vascular complications.
   d. Chemotherapy—nausea, vomiting, dehydration, skin reaction, mucositis, hyperuremia, liver abnormalities, weight loss, anorexia, myelosuppression, peripheral neuropathy, hypomagnesemia, ototoxicity, nephrotoxicity, alopecia, and cognitive effects.

CLINICAL JUDGMENT Chemotherapy-induced complications, including anemia, neutropenia, and thrombocytopenia, require early intervention and precautions to prevent debilitating anemia, infection, and hemorrhage. Severe blood count values: hemoglobin (≤8 g/dL), neutrophils (<1,500 μL; severe <500 μL), and platelets (<60,000 μL; severe <20,000 μL). Monitor and implement preventative measures when needed.

DRUG ALERT Erythropoietin-stimulating medications may be given as supportive therapy to boost erythrocyte proliferation to patients receiving chemotherapy. Due to the effect of increasing blood viscosity, caution should be exercised in patients with a history of seizures, stroke, cardiovascular disease, deep venous thrombosis (DVT), and pulmonary emboli.

Nursing Assessment

1. Obtain complete history, noting risk factors such as smoking and alcohol use, exposure to Epstein–Barr virus, diet, high-risk sexual behavior, and exposure to environmental toxins.
2. Question the patient regarding changes in swallowing, smell or taste, salivation, discomfort when eating, sore throat, foul breath odor, weight loss, epistaxis, unilateral nasal obstruction, changes in hearing, neck mass, changes in tongue movement, and changes in vision.
3. Note the quality of voice patterns and odor of breath.
4. Inspect the oral cavity: erythema, red velvety areas; white patches; crusting, bleeding; swelling; record the size, location, and description.
5. Use nasal speculum to inspect the nares for obstruction.
6. Palpate cervical lymph nodes for size, firmness, tenderness.

Nursing Interventions

Also see page 460 if radical neck dissection has been performed.

Achieving an Acceptable Level of Comfort

1. Provide regular assessments of pain and administer oral analgesics or topical analgesic gargles, as prescribed.
2. If cleared by the provider, assist with mouth care with soft toothbrush and flossing between teeth.
3. If the patient cannot tolerate brushing and flossing:
   a. Gently lavage oral cavity with a catheter inserted between the patient's cheek and gums with warm water or salt water rinses.
4. Provide management of excessive salivation and mouth odors.
   a. Insert a gauze wick in corner of mouth; place basin conveniently to catch drooling; replace frequently to absorb and direct excess saliva.
   b. Suction secretions with a soft rubber catheter, if not allergic to latex, as needed; instruct the patient on suctioning methods.
5. Provide management of decreased salivation, if necessary.
   a. Encourage intake of fluids, particularly water, if not contraindicated.
   b. Instruct the patient to avoid dry, bulky, and irritating foods.
   c. Offer lemon lozenges or chewing gum to stimulate salivation.
   d. Encourage use of humidifier.
   e. Suggest foods with sauces and gravies to make them moist and easier to swallow.
6. Maintain a clean and odor-free environment by removing soiled dressings, tissues, and gauzes and providing room deodorants.

EVIDENCE BASE Lalla, R. V. (2020). Evidence-based management of oral mucositis. *JCO Oncology Practice, 16*(3), 111–112. https://doi.org/10.1200/JOP.19.00766

Improving Nutritional Status

1. Handle feeding problems in one or a combination of the following ways, as ordered:
   a. Intravenous (IV) fluid to prevent dehydration.
   b. Nasogastric (NG) tube feedings or prophylactic placement of gastrostomy tube for feedings.
   c. Orally—small frequent meals high in protein and vitamin content and low in acidity and salt.
2. Provide mouth care before and after eating.
3. Allow the patient to have meals in privacy, if desired.
4. Offer easily chewed foods; mash or puree, if necessary.
5. Add herbs or sweeteners to enhance flavor.
6. Provide methods to compensate for decreased salvation by offering the following:
   a. Sip fluids, especially water, and carry water bottle throughout day.
   b. Avoid dry, bulky, and irritating foods.
   c. Use lemon lozenges or chewing gum to stimulate salvation.
   d. Use cholinergic stimulants or saliva substitutes as prescribed.
   e. Use a humidifier.
   f. Add gravy and sauces to food.
7. Encourage daily fluoride treatment as prescribed while undergoing radiation.
8. Have patient remove dentures if mucositis is present.
9. If swallowing difficulties persist, consult the speech–language pathologist.
10. Monitor weight, intake and output, and laboratory tests, such as 24-hour urine for urea nitrogen, C-reactive protein, albumin, prealbumin, transferrin level, and electrolytes.
11. Maintain a clean and odor-free environment by removing soiled material and using room deodorizer.

Strengthening Body Image

1. Assess the patient's reaction to condition.
   a. Evaluate the patient's apprehension and offer emotional support.
   b. Correct misinformation.
   c. Determine therapeutic care plan for the patient's rehabilitation.
2. Recognize that face and neck surgery can be disfiguring and the patient is often embarrassed, withdrawn, and depressed.
3. Assist the patient in caring for personal appearance.
4. Observe closely for indications of the patient's needs, which may be communicated in other ways, such as acting out or withdrawn behavior.
5. Allow verbalization of fears, anger, and distaste with body changes in a nondefensive manner.
6. Communicate acceptance of appearance in an honest manner.
7. Encourage the patient's family and friends to visit so the patient is aware that others care about them.
8. Provide diversional activities.

Community and Home Care Considerations

1. Teach mouth care procedure and dressing care to maintain cleanliness and prevent odor.
2. Emphasize adequate nutrition—proper consistency, proper seasoning, and right temperature. Show the family how to prepare food in blender or food processor, as necessary. Teach tube feeding procedure, if applicable.
3. If suctioning is required, instruct as to method, use, and care of equipment and obtain supplies for family.

4. Provide detailed instructions and demonstration to the patient and caregiver on incisional care.
5. Assess for signs of obstruction, hemorrhage, infection, and depression, and teach caregivers what to do about them if they occur.
6. If the patient is undergoing radiation therapy, encourage them to perform appropriate skin care, avoid exposure to potential chemical irritants, limit direct sun exposure, and avoid application of lotions, ointments, or fragrances to the head and neck region, which might alter the depth at which the maximum radiation dose is delivered.
7. Encourage the radiated patient to use sialogogues such as hard candy to stimulate saliva flow. Pilocarpine may be prescribed to prevent xerostomia for patients who have completed radiation therapy.

Patient Education and Health Maintenance

1. Encourage cessation of high-risk behaviors, such as smoking, alcohol consumption, use of smokeless tobacco, pipe smoking.
2. Emphasize the need for routine follow-up examinations with specialists, dentist (for the use of fluoride trays during radiation), and speech pathologist, if indicated.
3. Stress the importance of using lip balm with sunscreen.

Evaluation: Expected Outcome

- Reports adequate comfort levels, is pain free, and handles secretions adequately.
- Achieves adequate nutritional status, able to eat prescribed diet, and maintains weight.
- Verbalizes acceptance of body image, demonstrates behaviors that reflect positive self-esteem (e.g., shaves, dresses, applies makeup).

Neck Dissection for Head and Neck Malignancy

Systematic removal of lymph nodes with their surrounding fibrofatty tissue from the various compartments of the neck. The goal of neck dissection is to eradicate metastases involving the cervical lymph nodes. Metastases originate from primary lesions involving the oral cavity, pharynx, and larynx. The cervical lymph nodes are grouped into six major levels (I to VI) with additional division into two sublevels (A and B) of levels I, II, and V.

Surgical Procedures

1. Resection of lesion is the primary intervention.
2. Radical neck dissection—removal of lymph nodes in levels I through V and internal jugular (IJ) vein, sternocleidomastoid muscle (SCM), and the spinal accessory nerve (CN XI).
3. Modified radical neck dissection—removal of lymph nodes in levels I through V, and preservation of one or more of IJ, SCM, CN XI.
4. Selective neck dissection—removal of one or more lymph node groups that are at greatest risk for harboring metastasis.
5. Minimally invasive neck dissection (MIND), via endoscopic or robotic approach, has been shown to have comparable efficacy to conventional neck dissection procedures, with shorter length of stay, fewer postoperative complications, and better cosmetic outcomes; however, the procedure is longer.

EVIDENCE BASE Nayak, S. P., Sreekanth Reddy, V., Gangadhara, B., & Sadhoo, A. (2022). Efficacy and safety of novel minimally invasive neck dissection techniques in oral/head and neck cancer: A systematic review and meta-analysis. *Indian Journal of Otolaryngology and Head & Neck Surgery, 74*(Suppl. 2), s2166–s2176. https://doi.org/10.1007/s12070-020-02066-7

6. Commonly followed by postoperative radiation therapy. In some instances where resection is impossible, radiation therapy is the sole treatment for head and neck malignancy.
7. Based on cancer's location, extent, and treatment, surgical reconstruction may be performed with a rotational flap, skin graft, or free flap to promote healing and improve aesthetics.

Preoperative Management

1. Interventions to improve nutritional status preoperatively include nutritional supplements, hyperalimentation, alcohol withdrawal, and counseling.
2. The patient's general health status is evaluated, and underlying conditions, such as cirrhosis, diabetes mellitus, pulmonary, and cardiovascular disease, are identified and treated, if possible.
3. The patient is evaluated for level of understanding of disease process, treatment regimen, and follow-up care.
4. Emotional preparation for major surgery, long rehabilitation, and change in body image is provided.

Postoperative Management

1. A major goal of postoperative management is protection of the airway. After the patient has fully recovered from anesthesia, the endotracheal tube is removed (unless respiratory compromise occurs).
2. The patient is closely monitored for hemorrhage. Wound drainage is facilitated with a negative pressure drain. The drain is removed when output is less than 25 mL in a 24-hour period.
3. Prophylactic antibiotics are given to prevent infection because of extensive incision, lymph node resection, and close proximity to oral secretions.
4. Oral nutritional supplements, enteral feedings, or hyperalimentation is provided until oral intake is adequate and nutritional status is improved.
5. Provide adequate pain control with analgesics, in addition to narcotics as needed. When the patient is taking narcotics, provide stool softeners and/or laxatives to prevent narcotic-induced constipation.
6. Shoulder range of motion assessment is performed to determine if CN XI (spinal accessory) has been weakened during surgery. Physical therapy will provide strengthening exercises.

Complications

1. Surgery—air leaks, infection, wound dehiscence, bleeding, hematoma, chylous fistula, facial or cerebral edema, blindness, carotid artery rupture, and damage to nerves, such as the phrenic, vagus, brachial plexus, spinal accessory, and cutaneous nerves and the mandibular branch of the facial, hypoglossal, or lingual nerves.
2. Radiation.
   a. Early—radiation mucositis, xerostomia erythema, desquamation, dysphagia, secondary infection, oral pain.

b. Long term—atrophy, fibrosis, salivary dryness, hoarseness, difficulty swallowing, bone pain, osteonecrosis, pathologic fractures, limitation of movement, poor wound healing.

Nursing Interventions

Maintaining Effective Breathing Pattern

1. Place the patient in Fowler position.
2. Observe for signs of respiratory embarrassment, such as dyspnea, cyanosis, edema, hoarseness, or dysphagia.
3. Provide supplemental oxygen by face mask, if necessary; if tracheostomy is present, provide humidified air or oxygen by tracheostomy collar or adequate ambient humidification.
4. Auscultate for decreased breath sounds, crackles, or wheezes; auscultate over the trachea in the immediate postoperative period to assess for stridor indicative of edema.
5. Encourage deep breathing and coughing.
6. Assist the patient in assuming a sitting position to bring up secretions.
7. Suction secretions orally or aseptically through a tracheostomy if patient is unable to cough them up.

Preventing Infection

1. Assess vital signs for indication of infection—increased heart rate, elevation of temperature.
2. Inspect wound for hemorrhage, drainage, or tracheal constriction; reinforce dressings, as needed.
3. Inspect incision for signs of infection—increased pain and tenderness, redness, warmth, swelling, drainage.
4. If a drain is used, expect approximately 80 to 120 mL of serosanguineous secretions to be drawn off during the first postoperative day; this diminishes with each day. Ensure that the drain is milked at the insertion site at least three times per day to prevent clotting. Assess for color and amount of drainage.
   a. The initial output will be serosanguineous and eventually will turn serous. If the fluid appears milky, the surgeon should be notified right away as this may be indicative of a chyle leak.
   b. A high output of several hundred milliliters or more per day may also indicate chyle leak. If the output is less than 600 mL of chyle per day, the leak is initially managed conservatively with closed wound drainage, pressure dressings, and zero-fat nutritional support. Parenteral alimentation through a central line may also be utilized to further reduce chylous output.
5. Aseptically clean skin area around drain exit, using saline or prescribed solution.
6. Make sure that the incision site remains clean and dry; remove secretions immediately.

Improving Nutritional Status

1. Postoperatively provide IV fluids and hyperalimentation, tube feedings through NG tube or gastrostomy tube, or oral feedings as soon as swallowing is established.
2. Provide mouth care before and after meals.
3. Assess for excessive or decreased salivation, which may impair swallowing.
4. Make sure that emergency suctioning and airway equipment is available at the bedside during meals in the event of choking or aspiration. Utilize speech–language therapist to evaluate dysphagia.
5. Position the patient in an upright position, supporting shoulders and neck with pillows, if necessary.
6. Ask whether the patient would prefer privacy during meals.
7. Provide an environment that is clean and free from interruptions and odor.
8. Assist with oral intake, providing easily chewed foods. Mash or puree meals, if necessary.

Strengthening Body Image

1. Respect the patient's desire for privacy during treatments, dressing changes, and feedings.
2. Prepare visitors for the patient's change in appearance.
3. If the patient has difficulty speaking, assist with alternate communication methods and allow adequate time for communication.
4. Observe for lower facial paralysis; this may indicate facial nerve injury.
5. Watch for shoulder dysfunction, which may follow resection of spinal accessory nerves.
   a. Use muscle exercises provided by the physical therapist and muscle reeducation postoperatively.
   b. Work with the patient to obtain good functional range of motion.
6. Encourage the patient to verbalize concerns and feelings.
   a. Consult the health care provider to determine the nature and extent of explanation and prognosis that has been given to the patient.
   b. Encourage the patient to seek confirmation of personal philosophy and religious beliefs because this may provide answers.
   c. Accentuate the positive.
   d. Encourage the patient to participate in the plan of care.
   e. Recognize that a great effort has to be made in behavior modification to change a lifestyle that included alcohol consumption and cigarette smoking. Provide educational material and support.

Community and Home Care Considerations

1. Determine if the patient requires home care for drain care and/or home physical therapy.
2. If the patient has a permanent tracheostomy, instruct the patient and caregivers about the following:
   a. Need for increased humidification in the home environment.
   b. Avoiding activities that may cause aspiration (e.g., swimming).
3. Referral for speech–language pathologist to meet ongoing communication needs.

Patient Education and Health Maintenance

Exercises

1. Instruct the patient and family regarding exercises to prevent limited range of shoulder motion and discomfort (see Figure 13-7).
2. Perform exercises morning and evening. Initially, exercises are done only once; the number is increased by one each day until each exercise is done 10 times.
3. After each exercise, the patient is instructed to relax.

Follow-Up Visits

1. Emphasize the need for frequent follow-up visits and completion of radiation therapy, if prescribed.
2. Recommend a dental follow-up to ensure good oral hygiene and dental rehabilitation, if indicated.

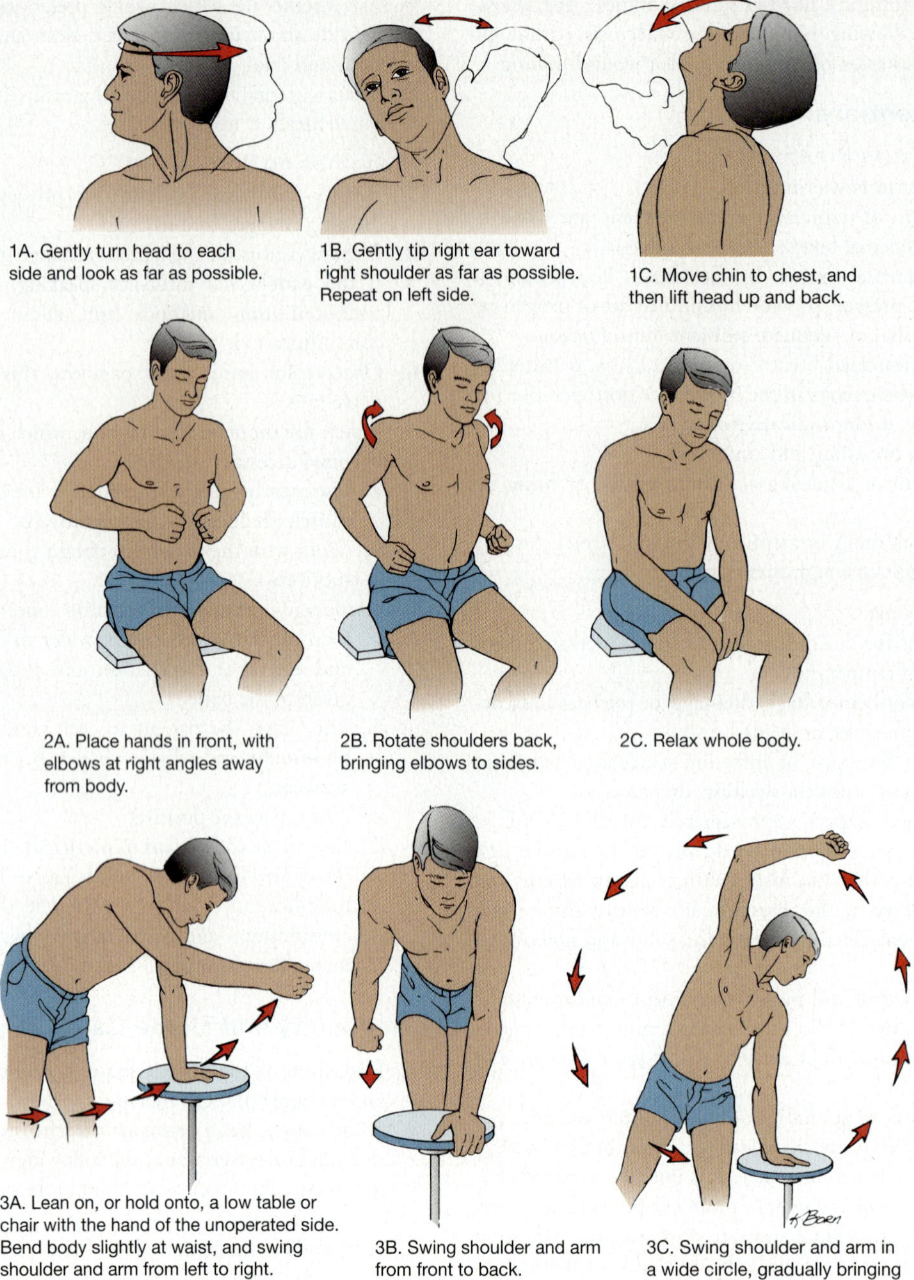

Figure 13-7. Rehabilitation exercises after head and neck surgery to regain maximum shoulder function and neck motion.

Evaluation: Expected Outcomes

- Maintains adequate breathing pattern; absence of dyspnea, shortness of breath; is able to handle secretions.
- Is free from signs and symptoms of infection; vital signs stable; incision is clean, dry, without redness or drainage.
- Is adequately hydrated; maintains stable nutrition and weight; can tolerate diet without choking or aspiration.
- Discusses concerns about condition; verbalizes positive aspects of self.

Cancer of the Larynx

Cancer of the larynx is a malignant growth of the vocal cords. It accounts for 0.7% of all cancers. The supraglottic larynx refers to the area above the vocal cords, including the epiglottis. The subglottic larynx refers to the area below the vocal cords to about the first tracheal ring. When treated early, the likelihood of cure is great. The National Cancer Institute at the National Institutes of Health estimated that in 2022, there were approximately 12,470 new cases diagnosed in the United States and 3,820 persons were estimated to die from the disease. The 5-year survival rate (2012 to 2018) is estimated to be 61%.

Pathophysiology and Etiology

1. Occurs predominantly in people assigned male at birth older than age 60.
2. Most patients have a history of smoking and heavy alcohol intake. Other risk factors include laryngopharyngeal reflux;

industrial exposure to diesel exhaust, asbestos, organic solvents, sulfuric acid, mustard gas, certain mineral oils, metal dust, asphalt, wood dust, stone dust, mineral wool, and cement dust; genetic susceptibility; and diet.
3. In North America, about 60% of carcinomas of the larynx arise in the glottis, almost 35% arise in the supraglottic region, and about 5% arise in the subglottic region of the larynx.
4. When limited to the vocal cords, spread is slow because of lessened blood supply; 5-year survival is 83%.
5. When cancer involves the supraglottis, cancer spreads more rapidly to the lymph nodes of the neck than does glottis cancer; 5-year survival is 46%.

EVIDENCE BASE American Cancer Society. (2023). *Key statistics for laryngeal and hypopharyngeal cancers.* https://www.cancer.org/cancer/types/laryngeal-and-hypopharyngeal-cancer/about/key-statistics.html

Clinical Manifestations

Depend on tumor location; sequence in appearance related to pattern and extent of tumor growth.

Supraglottic Cancer (Above the Vocal Cords)

1. Tickling sensation in throat.
2. Dryness and fullness (lump) in throat.
3. Painful swallowing (odynophagia) associated with invasion of extralaryngeal musculature.
4. Coughing on swallowing.
5. Pain radiating to ear (otalgia; late symptom).

Glottic Cancer (Cancer of the Vocal Cord)

1. Most common cancer of the larynx.
2. Hoarseness or aphonia (loss of voice for more than 4 to 6 weeks).
3. Aspiration.
4. Dyspnea.
5. Hemoptysis.
6. Ear ache.
7. Pain (in later stages).

Subglottic Cancer (Uncommon)

1. Coughing.
2. Short periods of difficulty in breathing.
3. Hemoptysis; fetid odor, which results from ulceration and disintegration of tumor.
4. Acute airway compromise; stridor (late stages).

Diagnostic Evaluation

1. Indirect mirror examination or indirect laryngoscopy of larynx may indicate lesion.
2. Direct laryngoscopy and biopsy to identify lesion.
3. CT scan and other special radiologic tests to detect tumor.
4. The T, N, M classification system is used for staging (see page 77). In larynx cancer, prognosis can be predicted by the tumor size and nodal involvement. If lymph nodes are involved, the prognosis is usually poorer than when none are involved.

Management

General Considerations

1. Depends on sites and stages of cancer. Early malignancy may be removed endoscopically.
2. Laryngeal cancers, stage I or stage II, may be treated with either radiation therapy or surgery. The goal of surgical treatment, at this stage, is to preserve the larynx.
3. Today due to treatment progress for laryngeal cancer, stage III and stage IV cancers may be treated with chemotherapy, radiation, and laryngeal preservation surgery.
4. Surgery is still considered the primary treatment for patients with large tumors and advanced laryngeal cancer.

EVIDENCE BASE Johnson, J. T. (2021). *Malignant tumors of the larynx treatment and management.* Medscape. https://urldefense.com/v3/__https://emedicine.medscape.com/article/848592-treatment*d9__;Iw!!I1GahPdV!a5DH2huaU5ebpUyuMCTkbpjOgIp7Ju_Xms2mhoHIQT_yIPH7mv7lCSKmupo3MR7piKqZ5rzeiP9y1wfBVWb6s7INjw$

Surgery

1. Laser excision for early-stage disease via endoscopic transoral resection.
2. Partial laryngectomy—removal of small lesion on true cord, along with a substantial margin of healthy tissue. Preserves the patient's ability to talk.
3. Supraglottic laryngectomy—removal of all laryngeal structures superior to the floor of the ventricle, maintaining both true vocal cords, both arytenoids, the base of the tongue, and the hyoid bone. Is performed for T1, T2, or selected T3 supraglottic tumors. An acceptable alternative to supraglottic laryngectomy is transoral laser microsurgery for T1 to T2 and selected T3 tumors. Able to speak but limited.
4. Hemilaryngectomy—removal of one true vocal cord, false cord, one half of thyroid cartilage, arytenoid cartilage. Preserves ability to talk; no stoma; increased risk for aspiration.
5. Total laryngectomy—removal of entire larynx (epiglottis, false or true cords, cricoid cartilage, hyoid bone; two or three tracheal rings are usually removed when there is extrinsic cancer of the larynx [extension beyond the vocal cords]). A radical neck dissection may also be performed because of metastasis to cervical lymph nodes. Creation of permanent stoma.
6. Total laryngectomy with tracheoesophageal puncture (TEP). During surgery, a puncture is made in the posterior wall of the trachea, which is also the anterior wall of the esophagus. A voice prosthesis or a red rubber catheter is inserted into the puncture. The red rubber catheter serves two purposes: to mature the track until a voice prosthesis is inserted and to provide enteral feedings until the patient is allowed to swallow. If a voice prosthesis is inserted at the time of surgery, the patient is fed through either an NG or gastrostomy tube.

Complications

1. Pharyngocutaneous fistula may develop after any surgical procedure that involves entering the pharynx or esophagus.
   a. Monitor for saliva collecting beneath the skin flaps or leaking through suture line into neck drains.
   b. Management—NG tube or gastrostomy feeding, meticulous local wound care with frequent dressing changes, promotion of drainage.
2. Hemorrhage (carotid artery rupture) or hematoma formation.
   a. A major postoperative complication (e.g., skin necrosis or salivary fistula) usually precedes carotid artery rupture.

   b. Management—immediate wound exploration in operating room.
3. Drain failure.
4. Infection.
5. Wound dehiscence—patients who have been radiated prior to surgery and/or who are malnourished are more at risk for wound dehiscence.
6. Complications of radiation—edema of the larynx, soft tissue and cartilage necrosis, skin reaction, chondritis.
7. Long-term complications:
   a. Stomal stenosis.
   b. Pharyngoesophageal stenosis and stricture.
   c. Hypothyroidism.

Nursing Assessment

1. Ask about alcohol intake, smoking and drug history, and chronic illnesses.
2. Take a nutrition history and 24-hour food intake recall. Review results of laboratory test. Weigh the patient.
3. Observe ability to swallow.
4. Review recommendations of speech–language pathologist for communication.
5. Assess for independence, self-assuredness, and willingness to try new things; these are strengths on which to build.
6. Assess reality of the patient's expectations.
7. Assess patient's ability to care for self, particularly concerning stomal care.
8. Assess the patient's social support system. Who will be home with the patient after discharge?

Nursing Interventions

Preparing for Total Laryngectomy

1. Collaborate with the surgeon in preparing the patient; interpret and reiterate what surgeon and speech–language pathologist have explained.
   a. Inform the patient that breathing will occur through an opening (tracheostoma) in the neck.
   b. Advise the patient that speech will be altered by surgery.
2. Expect reactions of anxiety and depression because the psychosocial effects of voice loss are substantial.
3. Practice a means of communication (pad and pencil, sign language, pictures, word cards, artificial larynx) that can be used until speech therapy begins.
4. Arrange for the patient to be visited by laryngectomee (one who has had larynx removed) for support.
5. Provide portable battery-operated suction machine, suction catheter kits, and other supplies from a home care company, and educate patient on suctioning procedure prior to the patient's discharge. Initiate referral for home care nursing and other community services.
6. Provide information about other community support services such as the International Association of Laryngectomees or Supporting Patients with Oral Head and Neck Cancer.
7. Reinforce information about alternative modes of communication.
   a. Artificial larynx, using either neck or intraoral placement: Electrolarynx provides communication assistance in early postoperative period or later to those unable to learn alternative method.

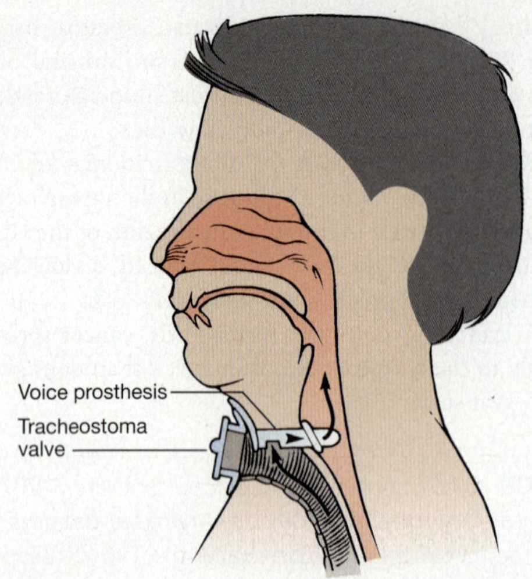

Figure 13-8. Schematic representation of tracheoesophageal puncture speech. When the patient plugs the stomal opening, air is forced from the lungs through a one-way valve voice prosthesis. Air travels into the esophagus and out the mouth, creating speech.

   b. TEP with voice prosthesis: A one-way valve voice prosthesis is inserted through TEP to allow the patient to shunt pulmonary air into esophagus for voice production (see Figure 13-8).
   c. Esophageal speech is accomplished by training the patient to force air down the esophagus and release it in a controlled manner.

Improving Breathing Pattern

1. Elevate the head of the bed and monitor for signs of difficulty breathing—suprasternal and intercostal retractions, tachypnea, dyspnea, tachycardia, and changes in sensorium.
2. Auscultate trachea/chest for evidence of stridor or wheezing and for the absence of breath sounds.
3. Make sure the patient uses a specific signal to indicate need for suctioning; enter on nursing care plan.
4. Suction secretions according to the prescriber's orders to prevent accumulation of mucus, which may lead to mucus plugging.
   a. Also suction nasal secretions because the patient is unable to blow nose.
   b. Remove crusts from stoma at least three times daily to prevent webbing of mucus across the stoma.
5. Use chest physical therapy, as necessary, to remove secretions.
6. Assist the patient in secretion removal.
   a. Teach the patient to bend forward until stoma is below lung level and to exhale rapidly. This aids in secretion removal from lungs.
   b. Teach the patient to wipe resultant secretions away from tracheostoma with a handkerchief.
7. Encourage breathing exercises because most patients smoke heavily.
8. Supply constant humidification to moisten tracheostoma and avoid viscous secretions; tracheal air will require additional warmth and moisture.
9. Keep calm and maintain sense of security.
   a. Reassure the patient that someone is always near to assist.
   b. Have call bell within reach.

10. Remind patient that they are now a neck breather and can no longer breathe out of their nose or mouth.
11. In the event of airway obstruction, clear the stoma and ventilate through stoma.

Facilitating Adequate Nutrition

1. Monitor IV fluids during the first few postoperative days.
2. Administer fluids and nutrients by NG or gastrostomy tube.
   a. Tube feedings may be started after bowel sounds are heard and continued until sufficient healing of pharynx has occurred (approximately 7 to 14 days) and patient is ready to resume oral feedings.
   b. Avoid manipulating NG tube as it is resting on or near suture line.
   c. Clean nostrils and lubricate with water-soluble lubricant.
   d. Clean crust on the outside of tube.
   e. Pay attention to oral hygiene, with regular toothbrushing and prescribed antiseptic mouthwashes.
3. Assure the patient that swallowing is safe and may feel differently than before surgery. Some structures and muscles removed during surgery may cause the patient to "work harder" to swallow.
   a. Patients may need more liquids to wash down foods.
   b. It may be easier to eat smaller, more frequent meals.
   c. A modified barium swallow may be ordered several days after surgery to be sure adequate healing has occurred and that there are no leaks or fistulas opening into the airway.
   d. After a total laryngectomy, there is a separation of the airway (trachea) from the esophagus; and theoretically, there is no risk for aspiration. However, if a TEP is present and occupied by either a voice prosthesis or red rubber catheter, leakage around the TEP site could occur.
4. The speech–language pathologist will educate the patient and family about the presence, care, and maintenance of the TEP and any potential problems.

Providing Alternative Communication

1. Advise the patient to communicate by writing or with artificial larynx until voice work can begin with speech–language pathologist.
2. Discourage forced whispering, which increases pharyngeal tension.
3. Encourage the patient to join local (Lost Chord Club) or web-based (Web Whispers, webwhispers.org) laryngectomy support group that offer information, support, and services for patients and caregivers adjusting to laryngectomee.
4. Inform the patient of the various communication methods:
   a. An electrolarynx, which is placed against the neck, cheek, or in the mouth for a monotone, mechanical sound, can be used immediately after surgery. The speech–language pathologist will provide instruction on the use of the device.
   b. Esophageal speech is the act of air charging, which is achieved by thrusting the tongue back and forcing a bolus through the cricopharyngeus. The air bolus then is regurgitated through the pharyngoesophageal segment, which vibrates to produce sound.
   c. Tracheoesophageal speech, which is the most common voice restoration option, involves placing a one-way valve voice prosthesis into the TEP. The patient takes a breath and occludes the stoma with either a finger or stoma button. This air is forced through the voice prosthesis into the pharynx, which vibrates and produces sound.

EVIDENCE BASE Nair, N. P., Sharma, V., Dixit, A., Kaushal, D., Soni, K., Choudhury, B., & Goyal, A. (2022). Future solutions for voice rehabilitation in laryngectomees: A review of technologies based on electrophysiological signals. *Indian Journal of Otolaryngology and Head & Neck Surgery, 74*(Suppl.), s5082–s5090. https://doi.org/10.1007/s12070-021-02765-9

Providing Information About Laryngectomy

1. Inform the patient that it is very important to keep the stoma clear of mucus. This is accomplished through regular tracheal suctioning and by cleaning mucus from the stoma several times per day.
2. A laryngectomy or tracheostomy tube may be worn if there is neck edema and narrowing of the stoma. The tube is not always permanent. The type of tube used is determined by the provider or speech–language pathologist.
3. Demonstrate procedure for cleaning and changing tube.
   a. See page 140 for tracheostomy tube care. A laryngectomy tube is cleaned the same way as an inner cannula.
   b. Place gauze dressing under tube to absorb secretions, as prescribed. Change when it becomes soiled to prevent skin irritation and odor.
   c. Encourage the patient to change the laryngectomy or tracheostomy fastener when soiled.
4. Tracheostoma care—teach the patient to:
   a. Wash hands before touching stoma to prevent infection.
   b. Wet washcloth with warm water; wring dry and gently wipe stoma. Do not use soap, tissues, or cotton balls because these may enter airway.
   c. Apply petroleum around exterior of stoma to prevent skin irritation.
   d. Report excessive redness, swelling, purulent secretions, or bleeding.
5. Stoma cover.
   a. Stoma cover is necessary to filter air and increase humidity of air; also necessary for hygienic purposes.
   b. Stoma cover can be crocheted, made of cotton cloth, or commercially available as foam filters.
   c. Clothing and accessories:
      i. Ascot or turtleneck sweaters may be worn. When a regular shirt is worn, the second button from the top can be sewed over the buttonhole as though it were fastened. This leaves a wide opening through which a handkerchief can be inserted when coughing.
      ii. A variety of fashionable scarves, jewelry, and high-neck outfits can be worn.
6. Bowel care: Discuss high-fiber diet and use of stool softener because patient with tracheostoma is usually not able to hold breath to "bear down" for bowel movement.
7. If the patient snored before surgery, they will no longer snore after laryngectomy because air no longer passes through the nose and mouth. For the same reason, the patient may have difficulty sniffing and blowing their nose. The speech–language pathologist can provide techniques for briefly sniffing through the nose.
8. Swallowing after laryngectomy will resume no sooner than 5 days after surgery. A barium swallow may be ordered to detect a leak in the internal incision line. Swallowing may be a little slower and/or more difficult. The speech–language pathologist will provide swallowing therapy.

Community and Home Care Considerations

1. Provide humidification in the home; use heat moisture exchanger, a humidifier, or cool mist vaporizer, especially in bedroom and when dry heat is used.
2. Tell the patient to avoid cold air; cover tracheostoma with a thin layer of foam or other cover to warm and humidify air.
3. Encourage the patient to drink fluids liberally (2 to 3 quarts [2 to 3 L]) to help liquefy secretions.
4. Have the patient always keep stoma covered for hygienic management of secretions and to keep dust and foreign matter from entering trachea.
5. Place a protective shield over stoma before bathing, showering, or shampooing hair and while getting a haircut or shaving. Use an electric razor instead of blade because shaving cream can irritate.
6. Swimming is to be avoided as there is no way to prevent water from entering the stoma.
7. Ensure working smoke detectors are available in the home as the sense of smell is decreased.

Patient Education and Health Maintenance

1. Tell the patient to expect some loss of smell and taste sensation.
2. Advise the patient to check with health care provider before taking over-the-counter medication because many drugs (such as antihistamines and cold products) tend to dry the mucous membranes of the stoma.
3. Warn the patient to seek immediate attention for pain, difficulty breathing or swallowing, appearance of pus or blood-streaked sputum.

Evaluation: Expected Outcomes

- Verbalizes understanding of tracheostoma and communication options.
- Breathes quietly; no evidence of noisy secretions.
- Swallows soft foods; maintains weight.
- Makes needs known; speech therapy has started.
- Manages tracheostomal care; has made provisions for home humidification and tracheostomal supplies.

SELECTED READINGS

Alam, M., Suttan, A., & Chandra, K. (2022). Microbiological assessment of chronic otitis media: Aerobic culture isolates and their antimicrobial susceptibility patterns. *Indian Journal of Otolaryngology and Head & Neck Surgery, 74*(Suppl. 3), s3706–s3712. https://doi.org/10.1007/s12070-021-02496-x

Barkwill, D., & Arora, R. (2023). *Labyrinthitis*. In *StatPearls*. StatPearls Publishing. https://www.ncbi.nlm.nih.gov/books/NBK560506/

Beckman, S., & Anschuetz, L. (2021). Minimally invasive tympanoplasty: Review of the outcomes and technical refinements. *Operative Techniques in Otolaryngology—Head and Neck Surgery, 32*(2), 143–149. https://doi.org/10.1016/j.otot.2021.05.014

Centers for Disease Control and Prevention. (2022, January 27). *Cochlear implants and vaccination recommendations.* https://www.cdc/gov/vaccines/vpd/mening/public/dis-cochlear-faq-gen.html

Crotty, T. A., Cleere, E. F., & Keogh, I. J. (2023). Endoscopic versus microscopic type-1 tympanoplasty: A meta-analysis of randomized trials. *The Laryngoscope, 133*(7), 1550–1557. https://doi.org/10.1002/lary.30479

Davy, C., & Heathcote, S. (2021). A systematic review of interventions to mitigate radiotherapy-induced oral mucositis in head and neck cancer patients. *Supportive Care in Cancer, 29*(4), 2187–2202. https://doi.org/10.1007/s00520-020-05548-0

DeBoer, D. L., & Kwon, E. (2023). Acute sinusitis. In *StatPearls*. StatPearls Publishing. https://ncbi.nlm.nih.gov/books/NBK547701/

Dong, Y. L., Hou, W. F., Chang, C., Cao, X. Z., & Li, Z. Y. (2023). Effectiveness of honey on radiation-induced oral mucositis among patients with head and neck malignancies: A systematic review and meta-analysis. *Current Topics in Nutraceutical Research, 21*(1), 53–59. https://doi.org/10.37290/ctnr2641-452x.21:53-59

Espada-Sanchez, M., deSanta Maria, R. S., Martin-Astorga, M. D. C., Lebron-Martin, C., Delgado, M. J., Eguiluz-Garcia, I. Rondon, C., Mayorga, C., Torres, M. J., Aranda, C. J., & Canas, J. A. (2023). Diagnosis and treatment in asthma and allergic rhinitis: Past, present, and future. *Applied Sciences, 13*, 1–26. https://doi.org/10.3390/app13031273

Garstka, A. A., Kozowska, A., Kijak, K., Brzozka, M., Gronwald, H., Skomro, P., & Lietz-Kijak, D. (2023). Accurate diagnosis and treatment of painful temporomandibular disorders: A literature review supplemented by own clinical experience. *Pain Research and Management, 1002235.* https://doi.org/10.1155/2023/1002235

Houssein, F.A., Phillips, K.M., & Sedaghat, A.R. (2024). When its not allergic rhinitis: Clinical signs to raise a patient's suspicion for chronic rhinosinusitis. *Otolaryngology-Head and Neck Surgery.* https://doi.org/10.1002/ohn.646

Khademi, S., Kazemi, A., Divanbeigi, R., & Afzalzadeh, M. (2022). A review of the revisions and complications management procedure in sinus surgery. *Journal of Family Medicine and Primary Care, 11*(3), 887–895. https://doi.org/10.4103/jfmpc.jfmpc_897_21

Leadon, M. & Hohman, M. H. (2023). *Posterior epistaxis nasal pack*. In *StatPearls*. StatPearls Publishing. https://www.ncbi.nlm.nih.gov/books/NBK576436/

Li, M. L. (2022). Rhinoplasty. *JAMA Otolaryngology—Head & Neck Surgery, 148*(12), 1188. https://doi.org/10.1001/jamaoto.2022.2626

Li, X., Wang, Q., Hu, X., & Liu, W. (2022). Current status of probiotics as supplements in the prevention and treatment of infectious diseases. *Frontiers in Cellular and Infection Microbiology, 12.* https://doi.org/10.3389/fcimb.2022.789063

Liao, Z., Guo, J., Mi, J., Liao, W., Chen, S., Huang, Y., Xu, Y., Zhang, J., Yang, Q., & Hong, H. (2021). Analysis of bleeding site to identify associated risk factors of intractable epistaxis. *Therapeutics and Clinical Risk Management, 17*, 817-822. https://doi.org/10.2147/TCRM.S301706

Lindeborg, M. M., Jung, D. H., Chan, D. K., & Mitnick, C.D. (2022). Prevention and management of hearing loss in patients receiving ototoxic medications. *Bulletin of the World Health Organization, 100*(12), 789–796. https://doi.org/10.2471/BLT.21.286823

Liva, G. A., Karatzanis, A. D., & Prokopakis, E. P. (2021). Review of rhinitis: Classification, types, pathophysiology. *Journal of Clinical Medicine, 10*(14), 3183. https://doi.org/10.3390/jcm10143183

Monday, L. M., Acosta, T. P., & Alangaden, G. (2021). T2Candida for the diagnosis and management of invasive *Candida* infections. *Journal of Fungi, 7*(3), 178. https://doi.org/10.3390/jof7030178

Panesar, K., & Susarla, S. M. (2021). Mandibular fractures: Diagnosis and management. *Seminars in Plastic Surgery, 35*(4), 238–249. https://doi.org/10.1055/s-0041-1735818

PDQ® Screening and Prevention Editorial Board. (2022). *PDQ oral cavity, oropharyngeal, hypopharyngeal, and laryngeal cancers prevention*. National Cancer Institute. https://www.cancer.gov/types/head-and-neck/hp/oral-prevention-pdq

Peker, S., Korkmaz, F. D., & Cukurova, I. (2021). Perioperative nursing care of the patient undergoing a cochlear implant procedure. *AORN Journal—The Official Voice of Perioperative Nursing, 113*(6), 595–608. https://doi.org/10.1002/aorn.13401

Risk, H. G., Mehta, N. K., Qureshi, V., Yuen, E., Zhang, K., Nkrumah, Y., Lambert, P. R., Lui, Y. F., McRackon, T. R., Nguyen, S. A., & Meyer, T. A. (2022). Pathogenesis and etiology of Ménière disease: A scoping review of a century of evidence. *JAMA Otolaryngology Head and Neck Surgery, 148*(4), 360–368. https://doi.org/10.1001/jamaoto.2021.4282

Sanchez-Perez, J. & March, A. R. (2023). *Osseointegrated bone-conducting hearing protheses*. In *StatPearls*. StatPearls Publishing. https://www.ncbi.nlm.nih.gov/books/NBK564385/

Shetty, N., Anchan, S. V., Jalisatgi, R. R., Naik, A. S., Pandurangi, A. S., Siddappa, R., & Yadrami, P. G. (2022). Topical use of autologous platelet rich fibrin in tympanoplasty: A prospective interventional study. *Journal of Clinical and Diagnostic Research, 16*(6), 1–4. https://doi.org/10.7860/JCDR/2022/56206.16465

Tabassom, A., & Cho, J. J. (2022). Epistaxis. In *StatPearls*. StatPearls Publishing. https://www.ncbi.nlm.nih.gov/books/NBK435997/

Wolford, R. W., Goyal, A., Belgam Syed, S. Y., & Schaefer, T. J. (2023). Pharyngitis. In *StatPearls*. StatPearls Publishing. https://www.ncbi.nlm.nih.gov/books/NBK519550/

Zeitler, D.M, Prentiss, S.M, Sydlowski, S.A, Dunn, C.C. (2023). American Cochlear Implant Alliance Task Force: Recommendations for determining cochlear implant candidacy in adults. *Laryngoscope, 134*(53), S1–S14. https://doi.org/10.1002/lary.30879

Zeng, F. (2022). Celebrating the one millionth cochlear implant. *JASA Express Letters, 2*, 077201. https://doi.org/10.1121/10.0012825

UNIT

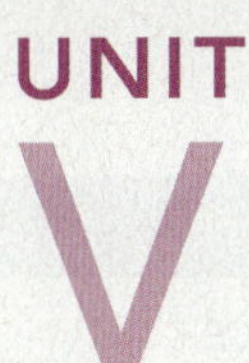

GASTROINTESTINAL AND NUTRITIONAL HEALTH

14 Gastrointestinal Disorders*

OVERVIEW AND ASSESSMENT

The gastrointestinal (GI) system is composed of the alimentary canal and its accessory organs. The alimentary canal begins at the mouth and extends through the pharynx, esophagus, stomach, small intestine, colon, and rectum and ends at the anus. The accessory organs include the tongue, salivary glands, liver, gallbladder, and pancreas.

The functions of the GI system include ingestion and propulsion of food; mechanical and chemical digestion of food; synthesis of nutrients, such as vitamin K; absorption of nutrients into the bloodstream; and the storage and elimination of nondigestible waste products from the body through feces.

Subjective Data

A comprehensive health history should be obtained to elicit subjective data related to major manifestations of GI problems. Common manifestations include nutritional problems, abdominal pain, indigestion, nausea, vomiting, diarrhea, constipation, bloody bowel movements, change in bowel habits, weight loss, and dysphagia (see Standards of Care Guidelines 14-1, page 468).

Nutritional Problems

1. Characteristics: What is your typical 24-hour food intake? What is your usual weight? Has there been a recent weight gain or loss? If a recent weight change, how many pounds and over what time period? How is your appetite?
2. Associated factors: Explore other factors that may influence weight changes—food preferences; family/individual routines associated with eating; cultural and religious values; psychological factors, such as depression, anxiety, stress; physical factors, such as activity level, health status, dental problems, allergies; access/transportation to grocery stores; limited finances; eating habits, self-imposed dietary restrictions or supplements; body image; nutritional knowledge; and alternative therapy such as use of essential oils.
3. History: Any history of eating disorders? Any family history of ulcer, GI cancer, inflammatory bowel disease, obesity?

Abdominal Pain

1. Characteristics: Can you describe the pain (sharp, dull, superficial, or deep)? Is the pain intermittent or continuous? Was the onset sudden or gradual? Can you point to where the pain is located? What makes the pain better, worse?

*Please note that the term "male" in this chapter refers to a person assigned male at birth, and the term "female" in this chapter refers to a person assigned female at birth.

STANDARDS OF CARE GUIDELINES 14-1

Gastrointestinal Dysfunction

When caring for a patient after abdominal surgery or with any type of gastrointestinal (GI) disorder:

- Make sure that adequate bowel sounds are present before allowing anything by mouth. Periodically reassess for bowel sounds, bloating, nausea, vomiting, and abdominal distension or tenderness.
- Monitor food/fluid intake and output as indicated.
- Periodically monitor weight, and watch for trend in weight loss or weight gain.
- Assess stools for frequency, consistency, color, and amount.
- Report increase in pain, fever, nausea, vomiting, bloating, change in stools, or signs of wound infection to health care provider promptly.
- Monitor complete blood count, electrolytes, albumin, and protein as directed.

This information should serve as a general guideline only. Each patient situation presents a unique set of clinical factors and requires nursing judgment to guide care, which may include additional or alternative measures and approaches.

2. Associated factors: Are there other symptoms associated with the pain—fever, chills, night sweats, nausea, vomiting, diarrhea, constipation, anorexia, weight loss, dyspepsia, black tarry stools or blood in the stool?
3. History: Any family history of GI cancer, ulcer disease, inflammatory bowel disease? Any previous history of tumors, malignancy, ulcers?

Indigestion (Dyspepsia)

1. Characteristics: Have you experienced any of the following symptoms—a feeling of fullness, heartburn, excessive belching, flatus, nausea, a bad taste, mild or severe pain? How is your appetite? If pain or tenderness, where is it located? Does the pain radiate to any other areas? What precipitating factors are associated with the pain? What makes the symptoms better, worse? Are the symptoms associated with food intake? If associated with food, the amount and type?
2. Associated factors: Is there nausea, vomiting, dysphagia, blood in bowel movements, or diarrhea? Is there a history of alcohol, nonsteroidal anti-inflammatory drug (NSAID), bisphosphonate, or aspirin use?
3. History: Any family history of cancer or inflammatory bowel disease? Any history of bowel obstruction? Any previous abdominal surgeries?

Nausea and Vomiting

1. Characteristics: Is the nausea or vomiting associated with certain stimuli, such as specific foods, odors, activity, or a certain time of day? Does it occur before or after food intake? How many times per day does vomiting occur? What specific fluids/foods can be tolerated when vomiting occurs? What is the amount, color, odor, and consistency of the vomitus (see Table 14-1)?
2. Associated factors: Is there fever, headache, dizziness, weakness, or diarrhea? Missed menstrual period? Any weight loss? Any new medications? Any psychological stress, depression, or emotional problems?
3. History: Any history of gallbladder disease? Ulcer disease? GI cancer? Unprotected intercourse?

Table 14-1 Nature of Vomitus

COLOR/TASTE/CONSISTENCY	POSSIBLE SOURCE
Yellowish or greenish	• May contain bile • Medication—senna
Bright red (arterial)	• Hemorrhage, peptic ulcer
Dark red (venous)	• Hemorrhage, esophageal or gastric varices
"Coffee grounds"	• Digested blood from slowly bleeding gastric or duodenal ulcer
Undigested food	• Gastric tumor • Ulcer, obstruction • Gastric paresis
"Bitter" taste	• Bile
"Sour" or "acid"	• Gastric contents
Fecal components	• Intestinal obstruction

Dysphagia

1. Characteristics: Is the onset acute or gradual? Is the problem with swallowing intermittent or continuous? Is this associated with solid foods, liquids, or both? Has there been any nasal regurgitation? Where does the food stick: neck (cricopharyngeal), midesophagus, or sternal xiphoid process?
2. Associated factors: Is there any regurgitation, heartburn, chest or back pain, weight loss? Any hoarseness, voice change, or sore throat? Have there been any fevers, chills, night sweats, or weight loss?
3. History: Is there a family history of esophageal cancer? Is there a history of stroke, palsy, or any other neurologic conditions? Is there a history of alcohol or tobacco intake?

Diarrhea

1. Characteristics: How long has the diarrhea been present? Determine the frequency, consistency, color, quantity, and odor of stools. Are there blood, mucus, pus, or food particles in the stools? Does this represent a change in bowel habits? Any nocturnal diarrhea? What makes the diarrhea worse, better? Any associated weight loss? (see Box 14-1, page 469).
2. Associated factors: Any fever, nausea, vomiting, abdominal pain, abdominal distention, flatus, cramping, urgency with straining? Is the patient taking antibiotics? Has there been any recent travel to foreign countries? (Mexico, South America, Africa, and Asia are areas with the highest risk of traveler's diarrhea.) Is the patient experiencing emotional stress or anxiety? Are there any recently prescribed medications?
3. History: Is there a history of celiac disease, colon cancer, ulcerative colitis, Crohn disease, malabsorption syndrome? Has the patient undergone surgery recently (e.g., bariatric surgery)?

DRUG ALERT Obtain a history of over-the-counter (OTC), herbal, or "natural" products the patient may be taking. Ginger is commonly used as an antiemetic, and although generally safe, it can cause heartburn. Licorice root is used for upset stomach and to soothe ulcers but can cause sodium and fluid retention and loss of potassium. Goldenseal is used as an antidiarrheal but can cause a number of adverse reactions, including skin and mucous membrane irritation, interference with anticoagulation, and cardiac and nervous system excitability. Peppermint oils, which are often used to treat irritable bowel syndrome (IBS), can interact with drugs that reduce stomach acid (e.g., antacids and histamine-2 [H_2] blockers). Also, many herbs can impair absorption of other medicines. Remind patients that herbal products are not found naturally in the body or in significant amounts in the daily diet, so should be treated like drugs.

Constipation

1. Characteristics: What is the frequency, consistency, color of the stools? Is there a change in bowel habits? If a change, has this been gradual or sudden? What is the size of the stools? Have there been dietary changes? Is there blood or mucus in the stools? Any laxative use?
2. Associated factors: Are there periods of diarrhea? Is there abdominal pain or distention? Is the patient experiencing stress? Is there a change in activity level? Does the patient have a regular time for defecation? Does the patient use antacids containing calcium or an anticholinergic? Have there been any fevers, chills, night sweats, or weight loss?
3. History: Any family history of colorectal cancer? Any history of depression or metabolic disorders, such as hypothyroidism or hypercalcemia?

Physical Examination

When performing a physical examination of the abdomen, include the following: inspection of the abdomen, auscultation of all four abdominal quadrants, percussion for tympany or dullness, light and deep palpation.

CLINICAL JUDGMENT Auscultation should be performed before percussion and palpation, which may stimulate bowel sounds. Deep palpation in noted areas of tenderness or pain should be performed last.

BOX 14-1 Causes of Diarrhea and Constipation

CAUSES OF DIARRHEA

- Infectious agents (*Escherichia coli, Salmonella, Shigella, Campylobacter, Giardia, Amoeba, Clostridium difficile, Yersinia, Cyclospora, Cryptosporidium, Rotavirus*).
- Drugs (antibiotics, magnesium) and some foods.
- Fecal impaction.
- Bowel disease (irritable bowel syndrome [IBS], ulcerative colitis, Crohn disease).
- Malabsorption syndromes (lactose intolerance, celiac sprue, fat malabsorption).
- Short bowel syndrome.
- Malignant syndromes (Zollinger–Ellison syndrome, carcinoid syndrome).

CAUSES OF CONSTIPATION

- Inadequate fluid intake.
- Psychological factors.
- Electrolyte imbalances.
- Hormonal abnormalities, such as hypothyroidism.
- Mechanical bowel obstruction, such as ileus.
- Drugs (laxative misuse, anticholinergic agents, calcium channel blockers, opiates) and some foods.
- Loss of innervation (Hirschsprung disease).
- Neuromuscular (paralysis, spinal cord injury or sacral lesion, multiple sclerosis).
- Anorectal disorders (hemorrhoids, fecal impaction, cancer, abscess, fissures).
- Sedentary lifestyle.

Key Findings

1. Mouth lesions, missing teeth, and swollen or bleeding gums may contribute to weight loss and nutritional deficiencies.
2. Body weight may indicate obesity or problems such as anorexia nervosa or malignancy.
3. Palpable mass may indicate an enlarged organ, inflammation, malignancy, hernia.
4. Rebound tenderness, guarding, and rigidity may indicate appendicitis, cholecystitis, peritonitis, pancreatitis, duodenal ulcer.
5. Protuberant or bulging abdomen or flanks can indicate ascites. Two physical assessment skills that may help confirm the presence of ascites are testing for shifting dullness and testing for a fluid wave.
6. Distention and absence of bowel sounds may indicate intestinal obstruction.
7. Tenting of the skin when the skin is rolled between the thumb and the index finger. Tenting may indicate dehydration.

Characteristics of Stool

1. The appearance of blood in the stool may be characteristic of its source.
   a. Upper GI bleeding—tarry black (melena).
   b. Lower GI bleeding—bright red blood.
   c. Lower rectal or anal bleeding—blood streaking on the surface of stool or on toilet paper.
2. Other characteristics of stool may indicate a particular GI problem.
   a. Bulky, greasy, foamy, foul smelling, gray with silvery sheen—steatorrhea (fatty stool).
   b. Light gray "clay colored" (because of the absence of bile pigments, acholic)—biliary obstruction.
   c. Mucus or pus visible—chronic ulcerative colitis, shigellosis.
   d. Small, dry, rocky-hard masses—constipation, obstruction.
   e. Marble-size stool pellets—IBS.

Laboratory Tests

Laboratory tests for GI disorders include a variety of stool studies and blood tests.

EVIDENCE BASE Engel-Nitz, N. M., Miller-Wilson, L.-A., Le, L., Limburg, P., & Fisher, D. A. (2023). Colorectal screening among average risk individuals in the United States, 2015–2018. *Preventive Medicine Reports, 31*, 102082. https://doi.org/10.1016/j.pmedr.2022.102082

Fecal Immunochemical Test for Occult Blood Detection

Description

An immunochemical test card has antibodies that detect human hemoglobin in stool. This test is used to screen for colon cancer when colonoscopy is not an option. Fecal immunochemical test (FIT) is preferred to the stool guaiac tests because of higher sensitivity and ease of use (e.g., no dietary restrictions).

Nursing and Patient Care Considerations

1. Advise patient not to collect specimen during menstruation or if hemorrhoidal bleeding is present. Usually, at least two stool specimens need to be collected, on separate occasions.
2. Collect specimen or advise patient regarding proper collection of specimen.
   a. Check expiration date of collection kit.

   b. Sit on toilet and proceed with bowel movement so that stool will be on top of collection paper. Do not put toilet paper in specimen.
   c. Use the sample probe and brush across the stool sample so that the groove of probe is filled with stool (obtain sample from several different locations within the stool).
   d. Insert probe back into the sample container and tighten the lid of the container, or place stool on the card depending on the type of collection kit being used.
   e. Write the date on sample container label.
3. Follow the manufacturer's instructions for processing.

Stool Guaiac Tests for Occult Blood

Description

Commercially available guaiac-impregnated slides or wipes test feces for blood. May be used as another option for colon cancer screening.

Nursing and Patient Care Considerations

1. Advise patient about the test preparation procedure. Common practices are listed here. For 3 days before the test and during the stool collection period:
   a. Diet should have a high-fiber content.
   b. Avoid red meat in the diet.
   c. Avoid foods with a high peroxidase content, such as turnips, cauliflower, broccoli, horseradish, and melon.
   d. Avoid iron preparations, iodides, bromides, aspirin, NSAIDs, or vitamin C supplements greater than 250 mg/day.
   e. Avoid enemas or laxatives before stool specimen collection.
2. Collect sample or advise patient on collection procedure.
   a. A wooden applicator is used to apply a stool specimen to the slide or a special wipe is used and placed in the packet.
   b. Avoid urine or toilet tissue contamination.
3. When hydrogen peroxide (denatured alcohol–stabilizing mixture) is added to samples, any blood cells present liberate their hemoglobin, and a bluish ring appears on the electrophoretic paper. Read precisely at 30 seconds.
4. Three stool samples are taken because of the possibility of intermittent bleeding and false-negative results.
   a. A single positive test is an indication for further diagnostic evaluation for GI lesions.
   b. False-positive results occur in about 10% of tests.
   c. Test may become false negative in 10% of specimens tested 4 or more days after streaking on paper.

Stool DNA Test

Description

This test detects DNA associated with colon cancer. Cells are shed from the tumor into the intestinal lumen as stool passes through. The procedure is similar to guaiac tests. The specificity of this type of testing is inferior to the FIT and colonoscopy so is not used as commonly.

Other Common Stool Studies

Description

There are multiple types of stool analyses that are helpful in detecting conditions affecting the GI tract, liver, and pancreas. Basic stool examination is for amount, consistency, and color. Normal color varies from light to dark brown, but various foods and medications may affect stool color. Additional testing may include tests for ova and parasites; stool cultures that can identify viruses and bacteria; fecal leukocytes; fecal fat, which can help in the diagnosis of malabsorption syndromes; testing for *Clostridioides difficile* (*Clostridium difficile, C. difficile*) colitis due to disruption of normal intestinal flora, typically after antibiotic therapy; and stool for *Helicobacter pylori*, which is performed at least 4 weeks after treatment to confirm eradication.

Nursing and Patient Care Considerations

1. Use a tongue blade to place a small amount of fresh stool in a container. The container may be sterile or may have a preservative depending on which test has been ordered. Remind patient not to mix urine or toilet paper in the specimen.
2. Save a sample of fecal material if unusual in appearance; contains worms or blood, blood streaked, unusual in color; or has excess mucus; show to health care provider.
3. For accurate specimen results, the vials must be sent to the laboratory as soon as possible. Certain stool studies allow for refrigeration of the sample, but this is test dependent.
4. Send specimens to be examined for parasites to the laboratory immediately so the parasites may be observed under a microscope while viable, fresh, and warm.
5. Consider that barium, bismuth, mineral oil, and antibiotics may alter the results.
6. *C. difficile* testing is indicated if watery diarrhea occurs at least three times in a 24-hour period; the sample must be liquid stool, because dormant spores often remain in solid stool.

Hydrogen Breath Test

Description

1. The hydrogen breath test is used to evaluate carbohydrate malabsorption and maldigestion, to detect the presence of excess bacteria in the small intestine, and to estimate small bowel transit time.
2. A substance, such as lactulose, lactose, or another carbohydrate, is ingested and, after a certain time period, exhaled gases are measured.
3. The test measures the amount of hydrogen, methane, and carbon dioxide produced in the colon, absorbed in the blood, and then exhaled in the breath. The levels of hydrogen and methane are indicators of bacterial metabolism in the small intestine.
4. This test is diagnostic for lactose intolerance, other carbohydrate malabsorption syndromes, and small intestine bacterial overgrowth (SIBO).

Nursing and Patient Care Considerations

1. Patient should have nothing by mouth (NPO) for 12 hours before the procedure.
2. Patient should not smoke after midnight before the test.
3. Antibiotics should not be used for 4 weeks, and laxatives/enemas should not be used for 1 week before the test. These products may alter the laboratory results.
4. Appropriate diet instructions should be given before discharge if the test is positive.

Helicobacter pylori Testing

Description

1. Diagnostic tests for *H. pylori* include a serum antibody test, urea breath test, and fecal antigen test. Alternatively, if an endoscopy is being performed, then biopsies of the gastric mucosa can be evaluated for *H. pylori* with rapid urea testing; histology review by a pathologist, or culture; or polymerase chain reaction testing.
2. A positive serum antibody test may not differentiate between current and past disease.

3. The urea breath test and fecal antigen test are useful in detecting active *H. pylori* prior to treatment with antibiotics. Both of these tests can be used to confirm eradication after antibiotic therapy has been completed.

Nursing and Patient Care Considerations

1. Patients with symptoms and those with an active or past history of ulcer disease or with gastric mucosa-associated lmphoid tissue (MALT) lymphoma should be tested for *H. pylori*. Endoscopy may be necessary for patients with symptoms of weight loss, anemia, or occult blood loss and for patients older than 45 years.
2. It is recommended that negative *H. pylori* test results in a patient with ulcer-related complications be confirmed by a second test.
3. Describe the procedure for urea breath testing to the patient.
   a. Antibiotics, proton pump inhibitors, and bismuth preparations must be held for 2 weeks prior to testing.
   b. Foods and fluids should be held for at least 1 hour prior to testing.
   c. A baseline breath sample will be taken by having the patient breathe into a container, then patient will ingest a carbon-labeled urea substance, and a final breath sample will be taken shortly after ingestion.
   d. The whole process takes about 40 minutes.
4. When confirming eradication of *H. pylori*, testing should not be done earlier than 4 weeks post-treatment.
5. False-positive results from *H. pylori* breath testing may be caused by achlorhydria or urease production associated with other GI disorders.

EVIDENCE BASE Cardos, I. A., Zaha, D. C., Sindhu, R. K., & Cavalu, S. (2021). Revisiting therapeutic strategies for *H. pylori* treatment in the context of antibiotic resistance: Focus on alternative and complementary therapies. *Molecules (Basel, Switzerland)*, *26*(19), 6078. https://doi.org/10.3390/molecules26196078

Radiology and Imaging Studies

Upper Gastrointestinal Series and Small Bowel Series

Description

1. Upper GI series and small bowel series are fluoroscopic x-ray examinations of the esophagus, stomach, and small intestine after the patient ingests barium sulfate.
2. As the barium passes through the GI tract, fluoroscopy outlines the GI mucosa and organs.
3. Spot films record significant findings.
4. Double-contrast studies administer barium first, followed by a radiolucent substance, such as air, to produce a thin layer of barium to coat the mucosa. This allows for better visualization of any type of lesion.

Nursing and Patient Care Considerations

1. Explain the procedure to patient.
2. Instruct patient to maintain low-residue diet for 2 to 3 days before test and a clear liquid dinner the night before the procedure.
3. Emphasize NPO after midnight before the test.
4. Encourage patient to avoid smoking before the test.
5. Explain that the health care provider may prescribe all opioids and anticholinergics to be withheld 24 hours before the test because they interfere with small intestine motility. Other medications may be taken with sips of water, if ordered.
6. Explain that the patient will be instructed at various times throughout the procedure to drink the barium (480 to 600 mL).
7. Explain that a cathartic will be prescribed after the procedure to facilitate expulsion of barium.
8. Instruct patient that stool will be light in color for the next 2 to 3 days from the barium.
9. Instruct patient to notify health care provider if they have not passed the barium in 2 to 3 days because retention of the barium may cause obstruction or fecal impaction.
10. Note that a water-soluble iodinated contrast agent (e.g., Gastrografin) may be used for a patient with a suspected perforation or colonic obstruction. Barium is toxic to the body if it leaks into the peritoneum with perforation. It can also worsen an obstruction; thus, it is not used if an obstruction is suspected.

Barium Enema

Description

1. Fluoroscopic x-ray examination visualizing the entire large intestine is administered after the patient is given an enema of barium sulfate.
2. Can visualize structural changes, such as tumors, polyps, diverticula, fistulas, obstructions, and ulcerative colitis.
3. Air may be introduced after the barium to provide a double-contrast study.

Nursing and Patient Care Considerations

1. Explain to patient:
   a. What the x-ray procedure involves.
   b. That proper preparation provides a more accurate view of the tract and that preparations may vary.
   c. That it is important to retain the barium so all surfaces of the tract are coated with opaque solution.
2. Instruct patient on the objective of having the large intestine as clear of fecal material as possible:
   a. Patient may be given a low-fiber, low-fat diet 1 to 3 days before the examination.
   b. The day before the examination, intake may be limited to clear liquids (no drinks with red dye).
   c. The day before the examination, an oral laxative, suppository, and/or cleansing enema may be prescribed.
3. Patient will be NPO after midnight the day of the procedure.
4. An enema or cathartic may be ordered after the barium enema to cleanse bowel of barium and prevent impaction.
5. Inform patient that barium may cause light-colored stools for several days after the procedure.
6. If barium enema and upper GI series are both ordered, the upper GI series is done last so that barium traveling down the digestive tract does not interfere with the results of the barium enema.

Ultrasonography (Ultrasound)

Description

1. A noninvasive test that focuses high-frequency sound waves over an abdominal organ to obtain an image of the structure.
2. Ultrasound can detect small abdominal masses, fluid-filled cysts, gallstones, dilated bile ducts, ascites, and vascular abnormalities.
3. Doppler ultrasonography may be ordered for vascular assessment.

Nursing and Patient Care Considerations

1. An ultrasound should be done prior to barium studies or at least 24 hours after barium administration because it may interfere with the images.
2. Abdominal ultrasound usually requires patient to be NPO for at least 6 hours before the procedure.
3. Change position of patient, as indicated, for better visualization of certain organs.

Computed Tomography

Description

1. Computed tomography (CT) is an x-ray technique that provides excellent anatomic definition and is used to detect tumors, cysts, and abscesses.
2. The CT scan can also reveal masses, dilated bile ducts, pancreatic inflammation, and some gallstones.
3. It identifies changes in intestinal wall thickness and mesenteric abnormalities.
4. Ultrasound and CT can be used to perform guided needle aspiration of fluid or cells from lesions anywhere in the abdomen. The fluid or cells are then sent for laboratory tests (e.g., cytology or culture).
5. CT colonography is a procedure that can take the place of colonoscopy. After a thin, flexible rectal tube is inserted to distend the colon with air or carbon dioxide, CT imaging captures a large volume of data about the colon through the abdomen in prone and supine positions.

EVIDENCE BASE Kim, D. H. (2023). CT colonography is the perfect colorectal screening test that unfortunately few people use yet. *Korean Journal of Radiology, 24*(2), 79–82. https://doi.org/10.3348/kjr.2022.0969

Nursing and Patient Care Considerations

1. Instruct patient to fast for 4 hours before the procedure. Patient can take usual medications with a sip of water, but should hold medications for diabetes.
2. A pregnancy test should be obtained on females of childbearing potential. If the patient is pregnant, do not proceed with scan, and notify health care provider.
3. Ask if there are known allergies to iodine or contrast media. Intravenous (IV) administration of contrast medium may be performed to provide better visualization of body parts. If allergic, notify the technician and health care provider immediately.
4. Instruct patient to report symptoms of itching or shortness of breath if receiving contrast media, and observe patient closely.
5. Preparation for CT colonography is the same as for endoscopy of the colon; to eliminate any stool that might obscure any polyps or lesions of the mucosal lining (see page 473). If ordered, administer smooth muscle relaxant before the procedure to help reduce peristalsis.

Endoscopic Procedures

Endoscopy is the use of a flexible tube (the fiberoptic endoscope) to visualize the GI tract and to perform certain diagnostic and therapeutic procedures. Images are produced through a video screen or telescopic eyepiece. The tip of the endoscope moves in four directions, allowing for wide-angle visualization. The endoscope can be inserted through the rectum or mouth, depending on which portion of the GI tract is to be viewed. Capsule endoscopy utilizes an ingestible camera device rather than an endoscope.

Endoscopes contain multipurpose channels that allow for air insufflation, irrigation, fluid aspiration, and the passage of special instruments. These instruments include biopsy forceps, cytology brushes, needles, wire baskets, laser probes, and electrocautery snares.

Endoscopic functions other than visualization include biopsy or cytology of lesions, removal of foreign objects or polyps, control of internal bleeding, and opening of strictures.

Capsule Endoscopy

Description

1. Adjunctive diagnostic tool used to detect abnormalities of the small bowel (angiodysplasias, areas of active bleeding, polyps, ulcerations, tumors or causes of diarrhea, and nutritional malabsorption).
2. The procedure involves swallowing a capsule (camera device), which passes through the digestive system while taking pictures of the intestine.
3. Images are transmitted to sensor array abdominal leads, which are attached to a Walkman-like recording device belted to the patient's waist.
4. After approximately 8 hours, the recording device is removed and is connected to a computer to download the images for review. The capsule will be excreted naturally through the digestive tract.

CLINICAL JUDGMENT Capsule endoscopy is contraindicated for patients with small bowel obstruction, dysphagia, fistulas, severe delayed gastric emptying, gastrectomy with gastrojejunostomy, or GI stricture. There is a risk of trapping the capsule, delayed passage, or impaired peristalsis. Pacemakers or implanted defibrillators may alter the quality and quantity of study information.

Nursing and Patient Care Considerations

1. Give patient instructions on bowel prep. Inform patient that a good bowel prep allows for better pictures. Patient will be NPO for about 12 hours before swallowing the camera.
2. Oral medications are discontinued 2 hours before the study. Antispasmodics, bismuth preparations, and antidiarrheal medications should be held for 24 hours before the study. Iron preparations and Carafate should be held 5 days before the study to prevent mucosal staining.
3. Instruct patient not to smoke 24 hours before the procedure to prevent mucosal staining.
4. Instruct patient to avoid strenuous activity, heavy lifting, bending or stooping, or immersion in water while wearing the leads and recorder. This is to prevent detachment of the leads or damage of the recorder.
5. After ingesting the capsule, patient is instructed not to eat or drink for at least 2 hours and then can advance to clear liquids. After 4 hours, patient can have a light snack and medications. When the procedure is completed, patient can resume a normal diet.
6. During the capsule endoscopy procedure, instruct the patient to check the blinking light on the top of the data recorder every 15 minutes. Avoid radio equipment (ham radio or broadcasting towers), which may interfere with the capsule's signal.

7. The capsule is naturally excreted within 1 to 3 days. Patient should be instructed to call the provider for the following symptoms: abdominal bloating or pain, chest pain, vomiting, or fever. These symptoms may indicate that the capsule has obstructed the GI tract.
   a. The patient should verify excretion of the capsule before undergoing magnetic resonance imaging (MRI).

Esophagogastroduodenoscopy

Description

1. Allows for visualization of the esophagus, stomach, and duodenum.
2. Esophagogastroduodenoscopy (EGD) can be used to diagnose acute or chronic upper GI bleeding, esophageal or gastric varices, polyps, malignancy, ulcers, gastritis, esophagitis, esophageal stenosis, and gastroesophageal reflux.
3. Instruments passed through the scope can be used to perform a biopsy or cytologic study, remove polyps or foreign bodies, control bleeding, or open strictures.

Nursing and Patient Care Considerations

1. Ensure that patient is NPO for 6 to 12 hours before the procedure to prevent aspiration and allow for complete visualization of the stomach.
2. Remove dentures and partial plates to facilitate passing the scope and preventing injury.
3. As an outpatient, advise that someone must accompany the patient to drive home because of the patient being sedated.
4. Inform the health care provider of any known allergies and current medications. Medications may be held until after the test is completed.
5. Obtain prior x-rays, and send with patient.
6. Describe what will occur during and after the procedure:
   a. The throat will be anesthetized with a spray or gargle.
   b. An IV sedative will be administered.
   c. Patient will be positioned on the left side with a towel or basin at the mouth to catch secretions.
   d. A plastic mouthpiece will be used to help relax the jaw and protect the endoscope. Emphasize that this will not interfere with breathing.
   e. Patient may be asked to swallow once while the endoscope is being advanced. Then, the patient should not swallow, talk, or move the tongue. Secretions should drain from the side of the mouth, and the mouth may be suctioned.
   f. Air is inserted during the procedure to permit better visualization of the GI tract. Most of the air is removed at the end of the procedure. Patient may feel bloated, burp, or pass flatus from remaining air.
   g. Keep patient NPO according to protocol until patient is alert and gag reflex has returned.
   h. May resume regular diet after gag reflex returns and fluids are tolerated.
   i. May experience a sore throat for 24 to 36 hours after the procedure. When the gag reflex has returned, throat lozenges or warm saline gargles may be prescribed for comfort.
7. Monitor vital signs every 30 minutes for 3 to 4 hours, and keep the side rails up until patient is fully alert.
8. Monitor patient for abdominal or chest pain, cervical pain, dyspnea, fever, hematemesis, melena, dysphagia, lightheadedness, or a firm distended abdomen. These may indicate complications.
9. Instruct patient on the above-listed signs and symptoms and advise to report immediately should any occur, even after discharge.
10. Possible complications include perforation of the esophagus or stomach, pulmonary aspiration, hemorrhage, respiratory depression or arrest, infection, cardiac arrhythmias or arrest.

CLINICAL JUDGMENT Perforation of the GI tract is a complication of endoscopy. Assess for abdominal or chest pain, dyspnea, fever, tachycardia, lightheadedness, and distended abdomen. Report immediately.

Flexible Sigmoidoscopy and Colonoscopy

1. Sigmoidoscopy is the visualization of the anal canal, rectum, sigmoid colon, and proximal colon through a fiberoptic sigmoidoscope.
2. Colonoscopy is the visualization of the entire large intestine, sigmoid colon, rectum, and anal canal. It is used as a screening test for colon cancer because it can be used to identify and remove potentially precancerous and cancerous polyps.
3. Sigmoidoscopy or colonoscopy can be used to diagnose malignancy, polyps, inflammation, or strictures.
4. Colonoscopy is used for surveillance in patients with a history of chronic ulcerative colitis, previous colon cancer, or colon polyps.
5. Lower GI endoscopy can be used to perform biopsy, remove foreign objects, or obtain diagnostic specimens.
6. Colonoscopy requires bowel preparation for 1 to 2 days before the procedure and use of conscious sedation during the procedure. The bowel preparation usually includes an oral laxative regime or approximately 1 gallon of an iso-osmolar electrolyte solution (Colyte, GoLYTELY, or NuLYTELY) to consume over a 3- to 4-hour period the day before the procedure, a clear liquid diet the day before, and an oral laxative the night before (protocols vary). Alternate prep may also be used.
7. CT colonography, also known as *virtual colonoscopy*, is evolving as a noninvasive screening method, see page 472.

DRUG ALERT Sodium phosphate preps should be avoided in people with congestive heart failure, renal impairment, and in others who may be more sensitive to fluid retention and electrolyte imbalances.

Endoscopic Ultrasound

Description

1. This procedure is a combination of endoscopy and ultrasonography to visualize the GI tract and can be used to evaluate the upper GI tract or the lower GI tract.
2. An ultrasonic transducer is built into the distal end of the endoscope.
3. This procedure allows for high-quality resolution and imaging of the walls of the esophagus, stomach, duodenum, small intestines, and colon. Adjacent abdominal structures can also be studied.
4. Endoscopic ultrasound (EUS) is also indicated to evaluate and stage lesions of the GI tract.

Nursing and Patient Care Considerations

1. Verify patient's adherence with the pretest bowel preparation the day before the procedure, usually an oral laxative (such as magnesium citrate) and a clear liquid diet.

2. Patient must be NPO after midnight.
3. Explain to patient that a feeling of fullness will occur when water is introduced into the GI tract. This eliminates airspace and provides for high resolution.
4. If an upper EUS is performed, maintain the NPO status until the gag reflex returns. A lower EUS can be performed using a rectal approach.
5. Observe patient for a change in vital signs, bleeding, pain, vomiting, and abdominal distention or rigidity.
6. Make sure that patients who have had endoscopic procedures requiring sedation have a caregiver to drive them home after the procedure.

GENERAL PROCEDURES AND TREATMENT MODALITIES

See additional online content: Procedure Guidelines 14-1 to 14-5

Relieving Constipation and Fecal Impaction

One method of evacuating the lower bowel is an enema, the installation of a solution into the rectum and sigmoid colon. If fecal impaction is discovered on examination, manual disimpaction may be performed to remove stool and promote bowel elimination (see Figure 14-1). However, it is best to try to prevent constipation by using fiber, laxatives, or stool softeners so that enemas and manual disimpaction are not needed.

Purposes of Enema Administration

1. Bowel preparation for diagnostic tests or surgery to empty the bowel of fecal content.
2. Delivery of medication into the colon (such as enemas containing steroids to treat ulcerative proctitis or a sodium polystyrene sulfonate enema to decrease the serum potassium level).
3. To soften the stool (oil retention enemas).
4. To relieve gas (tidal, milk and molasses, or Fleet enemas).
5. To promote defecation and evacuate feces from the colon for patients with constipation or an impaction (not a first-line therapy).

Nursing and Patient Care Considerations

1. Encourage exercise and early mobilization to promote bowel elimination.
2. Consider manual removal of fecal impaction in the following patients at risk:
   a. Older adults with chronic constipation or insufficient hydration or who are inactive.
   b. Patients with orthopedic disorders who have been in traction or in body casts.
   c. When barium has not been adequately removed after radiologic examination.
   d. Patients with neurologic disorders.
3. Fecal impaction can occur with a descending/sigmoid colostomy. The fingers may be used to break up feces through the stoma, followed by cleansing irrigation.
4. Contraindications of manual removal of fecal impaction include:
   a. Pregnancy.
   b. After genitourinary, rectal, perineal, abdominal, or gynecologic surgery.
   c. Myocardial infarction, coronary insufficiency, pulmonary embolus, heart failure, heart block.
   d. Gastrointestinal (GI) or vaginal bleeding.
   e. Blood dyscrasias, bleeding disorders.
   f. Hemorrhoids, fissures, and rectal polyps.
5. Prepare for enema administration by helping the patient to lying position on the left side with knees bent. Lubricate 3 to 4 in (7.5 to 10 cm) of the tip of enema tubing with water-soluble lubricant, even if prelubricated.
6. Insert enema tip 3 to 4 in into the rectum and instill slowly, to avoid cramping and rectal spasm. When completely instilled, ask the patient to hold the enema solution as long as possible, before gently withdrawing the tubing.
7. Ensure that patient can safely transfer to bathroom, commode, or bed pan when the overwhelming urge to defecate is felt.

CLINICAL JUDGMENT Be aware that manual removal of fecal impaction may cause syncope because of stimulation of the vagus nerve.

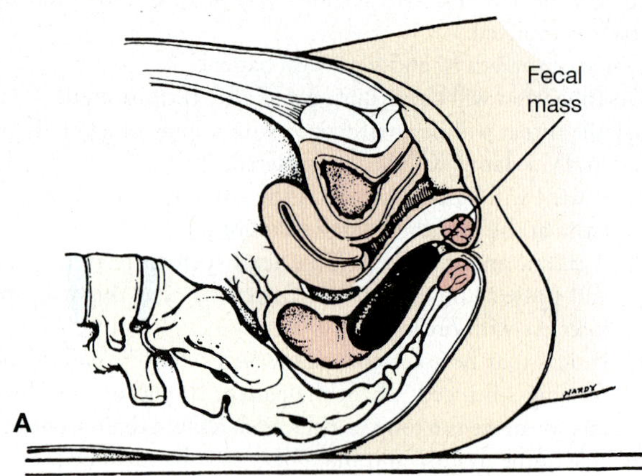

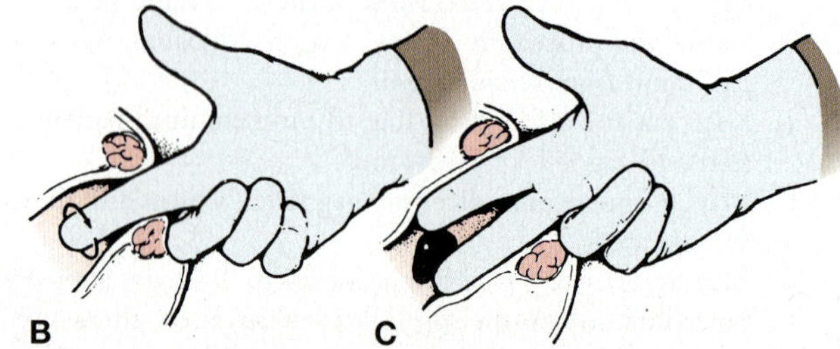

Figure 14-1. Fecal impaction. **(A)** Note the shaded area inside the rectal sphincter, which indicates fecal impaction. **(B)** By gently stimulating the rectal wall with a gloved index finger and using a circular motion, it is possible to loosen fecal material. **(C)** It may be necessary to gently insert two fingers in an attempt to crush the fecal mass. A scissor-like motion is used.

Nasogastric and Nasointestinal Intubation

EVIDENCE BASE Bloom, L., & Seckel, M. A. (2022). Placement of nasogastric feeding tube and postinsertion care review. *AACN Advanced Critical Care*, *33*(1), 68–84. https://doi.org/10.4037/aacnacc2022306

Nasogastric (NG) intubation refers to the insertion of a tube through the nasopharynx into the stomach. NG intubation has multiple purposes, including stomach decompression, stomach lavage (irrigation because of active bleeding or poisoning), medication administration, and short-term feeding. Extended-use NG tubes are made of a flexible, soft plastic material with manufacturer's recommendations that may include leaving the tube in place for up to 30 days before changing the tube.

Nasointestinal (NI) intubation is performed by a health care provider and may be assisted by a nurse. A small-bore tube is inserted into the duodenum or jejunum for the purpose of feeding and maintaining nutrition. It can be done manually, endoscopically, or fluoroscopically. Using fluoroscopy is considered the "gold standard" or preferred method of insertion. Intestinal feeding tubes are soft, flexible, small-diameter (8 or 12 Fr) tubes with a longer length than gastric feeding tubes (measuring up to 47 in [120 cm] as compared with approximately 30 in [76 cm] for a gastric feeding tube). Some tubes are weighted at the distal end of the tube, so they will be carried by peristalsis. All tubes should be routinely pretested for patency and function before passage, and radiologic confirmation of appropriate placement before use is standard.

Nursing and Patient Care Considerations

1. Before inserting the tube, ensure unobstructed nasal passage, then approximate the distance to the stomach by measuring from the tip of the patient's nose to the earlobe and down to the xiphoid process, and then mark this point on the tube with tape (see Figure 14-2). Lubricate the first 2 to 3 in of the tube with water-soluble lubricant.
2. With the patient's head in neutral position, insert the tube into the nostril and slowly direct the tube backward and downward. The patient may gag as the tube passes the pharynx, allow the patient to rest, tilt the head slightly forward, and take a sip of water. Turn the tube 180 degrees and continue to advance the tube slowly to the predetermined mark.

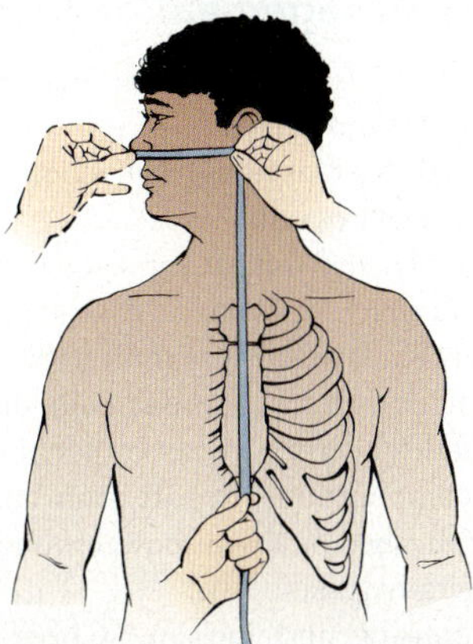

Figure 14-2. Measuring nasogastric tube length.

3. If patient is unconscious, advance the tube between respirations to make sure it does not enter the trachea.
   a. You will need to stroke the unconscious patient's neck to facilitate passage of the tube down the esophagus.
   b. Watch for cyanosis while passing the tube in an unconscious patient. Cyanosis indicates the tube has entered the trachea.
4. If patient has a nasal condition that prevents insertion through the nose, the tube is passed through the mouth.
   a. Remove dentures, slide the distal end of the tube over the tongue, and proceed the same way as a nasal intubation.
   b. Make sure to coil the end of the tube and direct it downward at the pharynx.
5. Be aware that pain or vomiting after the tube is inserted indicates tube obstruction or incorrect placement; may need to be pulled back or removed.
6. If the NG tube is not draining, reposition tube by advancing or withdrawing it slightly (with a provider's order). After repositioning, always check for placement.
7. Recognize the complications when the tube is in for prolonged periods: nasal erosion, sinusitis, esophagitis, esophagotracheal fistula, gastric ulceration, and pulmonary and oral infections.
8. Assess the color, consistency, and odor of gastric contents. Coffee ground–like contents may indicate GI bleeding. Report findings immediately.
9. The tube should be confirmed for placement prior to irrigation and before and after medication administration through the tube.
   a. Medications should be given in liquid form, if possible.
   b. Clamp the tube for 30 to 45 minutes to ensure medication absorption before reconnecting to suction, if ordered.
10. Check GI function by auscultating for bowel sounds on a regular basis after the tube has been clamped for 30 minutes.
11. When discontinuing an NG tube, remove all tape and have the patient take a deep breath, hold it, and pull steady and slowly (covering it with a towel as it emerges) and then more quickly when it reaches the pharynx.

CLINICAL JUDGMENT Be aware that NG tubes are contraindicated with basilar skull fractures or facial fractures. Oral gastric tube may be inserted instead.

Caring for the Patient Undergoing Gastrointestinal Surgery

Types of Procedures

Gastric Surgeries

1. Total gastrectomy—complete excision of the stomach with esophageal–jejunal anastomosis.
2. Subtotal or partial gastrectomy—a portion of the stomach excised:
   a. Billroth I procedure—gastric remnant anastomosed to the duodenum.
   b. Billroth II procedure—gastric remnant anastomosed to the jejunum.
3. Gastrostomy (Janeway or Spivak)—rectangular stomach flap created into abdominal stoma, used for intermittent tube feedings.

Hernia Surgeries

1. Herniorrhaphy—surgical repair of a hernia with suturing of the abdominal wall.
2. Hernioplasty—reconstructive hernia repair with mesh sewn over the defect for reinforcement.

Bowel Surgeries

1. Appendectomy—excision of the vermiform appendix.
2. Bowel resection—segmental excision of small and/or large bowels with varied approaches:
   a. Anastomosis of proximal and distal ends of the bowel.
   b. Anastomosis of proximal and distal ends of the bowel with temporary diverting loop ostomy.
   c. Both ends of bowel exteriorized to the abdominal wall with proximal ostomy and distal mucous fistula.
   d. Hartmann procedure—proximal large bowel as ostomy; distal end of large bowel oversewn inside the abdomen as Hartmann pouch.
3. Low anterior resection—subtotal resection of the rectum with colorectal or coloanal anastomosis.
4. Abdominoperineal resection—a combined abdominal and perineal approach for removal of the rectum and anus with permanent colostomy.
5. Subtotal colectomy—partial removal of the large bowel or colon.
6. Total colectomy—complete removal of the large bowel or colon with varied approaches:
   a. Ileorectal anastomosis—colon removal with the ileum anastomosed to the rectum.
   b. Proctocolectomy—colon removal including the rectum and anus with permanent ileostomy.
   c. Ileal reservoir—anal anastomosis. (Colon removal, subtotal proctectomy, possible distal rectal mucosectomy, creation of pelvic reservoir from two, three, or four loops of the ileum with anastomosis at anal canal. Usually, a temporary loop ileostomy is performed as fecal diversion to protect the reservoir and the ileal–anal anastomosis. After takedown of temporary loop ileostomy [2 to 3 months postoperatively], the reservoir stores feces and patient eliminates under voluntary control through the anus [see page 505].)
   d. Kock or Barnett continent internal reservoir (BCIR) procedures—proctocolectomy, creation of a continent small bowel reservoir with nipple valve abdominal stoma used for stool removal through routine intubation. (Continence is provided through the nipple valve.)
7. Roux-en-Y jejunostomy—the jejunum severed with distal end exteriorized as permanent stoma for intermittent tube feedings; proximal end reanastomosed to GI tract distal to stoma to reestablish pathway.

Laparoscopic Surgery

1. GI surgical procedures are increasingly being assisted by the use of a laparoscope, either partially or totally. The laparoscope is usually inserted through a 1-cm umbilical incision with additional trocars used for visualization and assistance. Dissection is performed with endocautery, scissors, or laser.
2. Advantages may include reduction in postoperative pain, shorter hospital and recuperative periods, decreased risk of infection, and improved cosmetic outcome. The direct cost of a laparoscopic procedure may be greater than an open procedure; however, the overall cost of the procedure and recuperative period may be lower due to a more rapid recovery.
3. Contraindications may include obesity, internal adhesions, and bowel obstruction with distention.
4. Cholecystectomies and appendectomies are routinely done through laparoscopy; hernia repairs can be done using the laparoscope. Other GI surgeries, including ostomies and bowel resections (may include select patients with cancer), are increasingly being done through this surgical approach.

Preoperative Management

1. The patient is assessed for symptoms, such as pain, dysphagia, cough, hoarseness, nausea/vomiting, diarrhea, and constipation. Nutritional status, dietary changes, and weight loss are considered.
2. Support system and personal coping mechanisms are evaluated.
3. All diagnostic tests and procedures are explained to promote cooperation and relaxation.
4. The patient is prepared for the type of surgical procedure as well as postoperative care (intravenous [IV], patient-controlled analgesia pump, NG tube, surgical drains, incision care, possibility of ostomy).
5. Measures to prevent postoperative complications are taught, including coughing, turning/early mobilization, and deep breathing; using the incentive spirometer (obtain baseline volume); and splinting the incision.
6. IV fluids or total parenteral nutrition (TPN) before surgery may be ordered to improve fluid and electrolyte balance and nutritional status.
7. Intake and output is monitored.
8. Preoperative laboratory studies are obtained.
9. Bowel cleansing will be initiated 1 to 2 days before surgery for better visualization. Preparation may include diet modifications, such as liquid or low residue, oral laxatives, suppositories, enemas, or polyethylene glycoelectrolyte solution (Colyte, GoLYTELY).
10. Antibiotics are ordered to decrease the bacterial growth in the colon.
11. An ostomy specialty nurse is consulted if patient is scheduled for an ostomy to initiate early understanding and management of postoperative care.
12. Patient may not have anything by mouth (NPO) after midnight the night before surgery. Medications may be withheld, if ordered. This will keep the GI tract clear.

Postoperative Management and Nursing Care

1. Physical assessment is completed at least once per shift, or more frequently, as indicated.
   a. Monitor vital signs for signs of infection and shock—fever, hypotension, tachycardia.
   b. Monitor intake and output for signs of imbalance, dehydration, and shock. Include all drains in evaluating intake and output. Replace fluids as indicated.
   c. Assess the abdomen for increased pain, distention, rigidity, and rebound tenderness because these may indicate postoperative complications. Report abnormal findings.
   d. Expect diminished or absent bowel sounds in the immediate postoperative phase.
   e. Evaluate dressing and incision. Check for purulent or bloody drainage, odor, and unusual tenderness or redness at incision site, which may indicate bleeding or infection.
   f. Evaluate for passing of flatus or feces.

g. Monitor for nausea and vomiting. Note the presence of fecal smell or material in vomitus because it may indicate an obstruction.
h. Check NG aspirate, vomitus, and stools for signs of bleeding. Record and report findings if present.

2. Laboratory values are monitored, and patient is evaluated for signs and symptoms of electrolyte imbalance and shock.
3. Wound drains, IV lines, and all other catheters are monitored and evaluated for signs of infection or infiltration.
4. To maintain patency of NG tube, the tube may be irrigated with 30 mL of normal saline solution every 2 hours and as needed. If there are large amounts of NG output, IV replacement may be necessary.
5. Deep vein thrombosis (DVT) prophylaxis treatment should be initiated (i.e., subcutaneous heparin or antiembolism stockings may be used).
6. Turning, coughing, deep breathing, and incentive spirometry are performed every 2 hours. Dangling at bedside or out of bed to a chair is encouraged the night of surgery, and an attempt at ambulation the first postoperative day is made, unless ordered otherwise.
7. Patient-controlled analgesia for pain control or other analgesics, as ordered, are administered to promote comfort.
8. Wound dressing is changed daily or as ordered, maintaining aseptic technique. Expect the use of wound drainage device.
9. Diet is advanced, as ordered, after the presence of bowel sounds indicates GI tract has regained motility. After 1 to 2 days of NPO postoperatively, the usual diet progression is ice chips, sips of water, clear liquids, full liquids, soft or regular diet.
10. Dietary education includes fiber, avoiding gas-producing foods, and maintaining adequate fluid intake.
11. Reinforcement of teaching and assistance with ostomy care, if indicated.
12. Administration of medications, as ordered, which may include a stool softener or laxative when bowel function has returned.

CLINICAL JUDGMENT Because of the type of abdominal surgery and location of the suture line, the health care provider may order not to irrigate or manipulate the NG tube.

Complications

1. Paralytic ileus or obstruction.
2. Adhesion formation.
3. Would dehiscence.
4. Dumping syndrome.
5. Nutrition deficiencies.
6. Peritonitis or sepsis.
7. Anastomotic leakage, which may result in peritonitis.

Nursing Interventions

Maintaining Fluid Volume and Hemodynamic Stability

1. Monitor intake and output every 8 hours, or more frequently, as needed, to assess changing status. Include amount of wound drainage from dressing changes and drains that may be in place. Watch for bleeding.
2. Be on the alert for shock and hemorrhage. In addition to increased pulse and respirations and decreased blood pressure (BP), observe for changes in mental status, pallor, clammy skin, and dizziness.
3. Assess the patient for signs of dehydration—flushed, dry skin; tenting of the skin; oliguria; tachycardia, hypotension, and rapid respirations; increase in hematocrit, blood urea nitrogen (BUN), and change in electrolytes; fever; weight loss.
4. Monitor laboratory results for electrolytes, creatinine, hemoglobin, and hematocrit, and report abnormal findings.
5. Assess the patient for signs of electrolyte imbalance—nausea or vomiting, cardiac dysrhythmia, tremor, seizures, anorexia, malaise, weakness, irregular pulse; changes in behavior, mental status.
6. Weigh the patient daily to gauge fluid volume status.
7. Administer parenteral fluids, enteral feedings, and blood products, as ordered, to maintain volume during period of decreased oral intake and blood loss.
8. Encourage early ambulation to stimulate circulation and prevent thromboembolism.
9. Prevent venous stasis by use of compression stockings, if indicated.
10. Check for tight dressings or binder that might restrict circulation.

Preventing Infection

1. Review signs and symptoms of wound infection with patient so early intervention may be instituted.
2. Monitor temperature every 8 hours, or as needed, and review previous readings to recognize early increases.
3. Change surgical dressings every 24 hours, or more frequently, as indicated. Maintain aseptic technique to avoid contamination.
4. Monitor wound for signs and symptoms of infection, such as redness, swelling, purulent drainage, odor, and pain.
5. Obtain a wound culture, as ordered.
6. Monitor the patient with an indwelling catheter for signs and symptoms of urinary tract infection (UTI), such as concentrated, cloudy urine; hematuria; fever. If catheter is discontinued, monitor for the abovementioned plus complaints of burning and frequency.
7. Assist the patient in washing perineum daily, and as needed if incontinence is present, for increased comfort and hygiene.
8. Assess breath sounds and monitor for crackles.
9. Instruct and encourage the patient to turn, cough, deep breathe, and use incentive spirometer every 2 hours to prevent atelectasis and pneumonia.
10. Encourage early ambulation to initiate bowel function and reduce the risk of embolus.
11. Administer antibiotics, as ordered, to maintain constant blood level.

Promoting Comfort

1. Assess pain location, intensity, and characteristics, and make sure they are appropriate for postoperative stage.
2. Administer prescribed pain medications, and provide instructions if using a patient-controlled analgesia pump, to keep patient comfortable.
3. Assess the effectiveness of the pain medications. If ordered, promethazine can potentiate the effectiveness of pain medication.
4. Encourage the patient to change positions frequently, get out of bed to chair/ambulate, and to splint incision when turning, coughing, or deep breathing to prevent vascular and pulmonary complications and promote comfort.
5. Be alert for respiratory depression, excessive drowsiness, and hypotension indicating adverse reaction or opiate overdose. Have naloxone on hand for reversal, if necessary.

Improving Nutritional Status

1. Monitor intake and output each shift, or more frequently if indicated, to maintain fluid balance.
2. Administer parenteral nutrition, if ordered.
3. Give fluids NPO when audible bowel signs are present.
4. Advance diet as tolerated, following prescribed diet progression. Increase fluids according to the patient's tolerance.
5. Offer a diet with vitamin supplements when the patient's condition permits.
   a. Usually high in protein and calories to promote wound healing.
6. Educate patient about dumping syndrome—a complex reaction that may occur because of excessively rapid emptying of gastric contents. Manifestations include nausea, weakness, perspiration, palpitation, some syncope, and, possibly, diarrhea. Instruct the patient as follows:
   a. Eat small, frequent meals rather than three large meals.
   b. Suggest a diet high in protein and fat and low in carbohydrates, and avoid meals high in sugars, milk, chocolate, and salt.
   c. Reduce fluids with meals, but take them between meals.
   d. Take anticholinergic medication before meals (if prescribed) to lessen GI activity.
   e. Relax when eating; eat slowly and regularly.
   f. Take a rest after meals.
7. Weigh the patient regularly to ensure adequate calorie intake.
8. Provide snacks or high-protein, high-calorie supplements and assist in menu selection, if needed.
9. Instruct the patient to avoid gas-producing foods, and encourage ambulation.
10. Educate the patient who has undergone a total gastrectomy that lifelong parenteral administration of vitamin B_{12} is necessary to prevent pernicious anemia. This may also apply to people with the terminal ileum removed and sometimes for those with ileostomies.

Improving Skin Integrity

1. Assess wound for signs of erythema, swelling, and purulent drainage, which may indicate infection.
2. Change surgical dressing as ordered, and as needed, to protect the skin from drainage and decrease the risk of infection.
3. Apply dressings around drains and tubes to protect the skin from leakage, if indicated.
4. Turn the patient frequently and encourage getting out of bed to chair/ambulate or position changes to prevent skin breakdown over bony prominences.
5. Obtain special support surfaces for patients at risk for pressure injuries.
6. Teach the patient about wound and/or ostomy care, if applicable, to promote independence and self-confidence.

Promoting Bowel Elimination

1. Instruct the patient to report promptly blood in the stool or coughing up blood, which may indicate GI bleeding. Explain signs and symptoms of postoperative complications to report: nausea or vomiting, abdominal distention, changes in bowel function and stool consistency or color.
2. Assess for the presence of bowel sounds to evaluate return of bowel function.
3. Ask the patient if passing flatus rectally or through an ostomy—also indicative of return of bowel function.
4. Evaluate for abdominal distention, nausea, or vomiting, which may indicate obstruction.
5. Monitor stool for frequency, amount, and consistency.
6. Administer stool softener or laxative, as ordered, to promote comfort with elimination.
7. Encourage diet with adequate fiber and fluid content for natural laxative effect.
8. Encourage and assist with ambulation to promote peristalsis.

Patient Education and Health Maintenance

1. Advise the patient that home health care may be ordered and initiate appropriate referrals, if indicated.
2. Reinforce discharge instructions and the importance of postoperative regimen to include health provider follow-up appointments and laboratory and other scheduled tests or therapies.
3. Change dressing and reinforce ostomy care as directed by health care provider. Report any signs of infection—unusual drainage, redness, warmth, increased pain, swelling.
4. Instruct the patient to gradually increase activities of daily living (ADLs). No heavy lifting (more than 10 pounds), pushing, pulling, or driving for 6 to 8 weeks postoperatively.
5. Educate patient about late complications and signs and symptoms to report to health care provider, particularly abdominal pain, which may be of gradual or sudden onset.
6. Provide referral to additional community resources if applicable (support groups, meal programs, social services).

CLINICAL JUDGMENT Phytobezoar formation (retained gastric concretion composed of vegetable matter) can be seen with partial gastrectomy and vagotomy. After a gastric resection, the remaining gastric tissue is not able to disintegrate and digest certain fibrous foods. This undigested fiber congeals to form masses that become coated by mucus secretions of the stomach. Be alert for gradual worsening of abdominal pain, distension, loss of appetite, change in bowel habits, and possible vomiting. Computed tomography (CT) or ultrasound of the abdomen may be ordered, and endoscopy may be necessary for treatment.

Evaluation: Expected Outcomes

- Vital signs stable; fluid and electrolytes in balance.
- No signs and symptoms of infection; incision healing well.
- Verbalizes increased comfort (using a 0 to 10 pain scale) with pain rating 0 to 3/10.
- Consumes 50% to 75% of each meal; no weight loss.
- Incisional flaps approximated and healing ridge present.
- Passing flatus and stool.

Caring for the Patient Undergoing Ostomy Surgery

See Standards of Care Guidelines 14-2.

Types of Fecal Ostomies

Colostomy

See Figure 14-3.

1. A surgically created opening between the colon and the abdominal wall to allow fecal elimination. It may be a temporary or permanent diversion.
2. A colostomy may be placed in any segment of the large intestine (colon), which will influence the nature of fecal discharge.

STANDARDS OF CARE GUIDELINES 14-2

Care of the Patient With an Ostomy

- Prepare patient and family preoperatively by explaining the surgical procedure, stoma characteristics, and ostomy management with a pouching system.
- Have ostomy specialty nurse mark an optimal stoma site.
- Postoperatively, monitor the stoma color and amount and color of stomal output every shift; document and report any abnormalities.
- Periodically change a properly fitting pouching system over the ostomy to avoid leakage and protect the peristomal skin. Use this time as an opportunity for teaching.
- Assess peristomal skin with each pouching system change, document findings, and treat any abnormalities (skin breakdown because of leakage, allergy, or infection) as indicated.
- Teach patient and/or caregiver self-care skills of routine pouch emptying, cleansing skin and stoma, and changing of the pouching system until independence is achieved.
- Instruct patient and family in lifestyle adjustments regarding gas and odor control, procurement of ostomy supplies, and bathing, clothing, and travel tips.
- Encourage patient to verbalize feelings regarding the ostomy, body image changes, and sexual issues.
- Inform patient of community resources, such as the United Ostomy Association, local and mail-order ostomy supply dealers, ostomy specialty nurses, the American Cancer Society, and the Crohn's & Colitis Foundation.

This information should serve as a general guideline only. Each patient situation presents a unique set of clinical factors and requires nursing judgment to guide care, which may include additional or alternative measures and approaches.

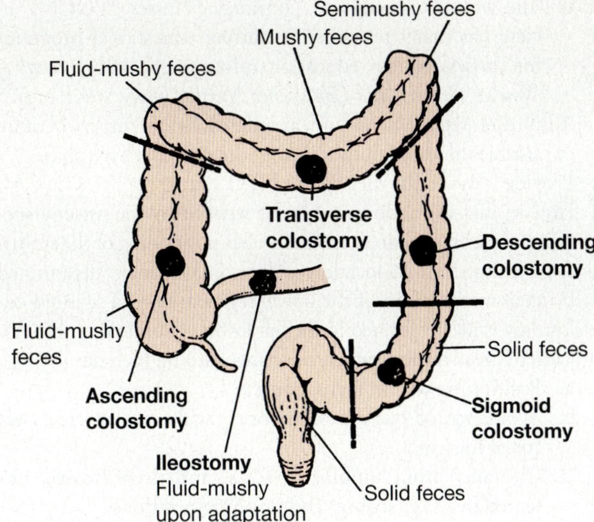

Figure 14-3. A diagrammatic representation of the placement of fecal ostomies and nature of discharge at these sites.

The more right sided the colostomy, the looser the stool. Transverse and descending/sigmoid colostomies are the most common types.

3. A colostomy may be performed as part of an abdominoperineal resection for rectal cancer, a fecal diversion for unresectable cancer, a temporary measure to protect an anastomosis, or a surgical treatment for inflammatory bowel diseases, trauma, perforated diverticulitis, ischemic bowel, cancer, and congenital conditions.

Ileostomy

1. A surgically created opening between the ileum of the small intestine and the abdominal wall to allow elimination of small bowel effluent.
2. An ileostomy is usually formed at the terminal ileum of the small bowel and is usually placed in the right lower quadrant of the abdomen. Stool from an ileostomy drains frequently (average four to five times per day) and contains proteolytic enzymes, which can be harmful to the skin.
3. Diagnoses that may require a temporary or permanent ileostomy include ulcerative colitis, Crohn disease, familial polyposis, cancer, congenital defects, and trauma.

Characteristics of Stomas

1. A stoma is the part of the intestine (small or large) that is brought above the abdominal wall to become the outlet for discharge of intestinal waste. Stoma is often used interchangeably with "ostomy."
2. Normal stomal characteristics: pink red, moist, bleeds slightly when rubbed, no feeling to touch, stool functions involuntary, and postoperative swelling gradually decreases over several months.
3. Stoma classifications:
   a. End stoma: After the bowel is divided, the proximal bowel is exteriorized to abdominal wall, everted (which exposes mucosal lining), and sutured to the dermis or subcutaneous tissue. There is only one opening that drains stool. The distal bowel is either surgically removed or sutured closed within the abdominal cavity.
   b. Double-barrel stoma: After the bowel is divided, the proximal and distal ends of the bowel are exteriorized to the abdominal wall, everted, and sutured to the dermis or subcutaneous tissue. If the stomas are brought up next to each other requiring them to be pouched together, they are referred to as a *double-barrel stoma*; if the stomas are apart to be pouched separately, they may be referred to as an *end stoma* (proximal), which drains stool, and a *mucous fistula* (distal), which drains mucus. This type of stoma is usually temporary.
   c. Loop stoma: A bowel loop is brought to the abdominal wall through an incision and stabilized temporarily with a rod, catheter, or a skin or fascial bridge. The anterior wall of the bowel is opened surgically or by electrocautery to expose the proximal and distal openings. The posterior wall of the bowel remains intact and separates the functioning proximal opening and the nonfunctioning distal opening. This type of stoma is usually temporary.

Preoperative Management and Nursing Care

1. Prepare the patient for general abdominal surgery (see page 691). Have the patient see an ostomy specialty nurse.
   a. An ostomy specialty nurse has the title of certified ostomy care nurse or certified wound, ostomy, and continence nurse (CWOCN, previously known as a *certified enterostomal therapy nurse*). These nurses play a vital role in the rehabilitation of patients with ostomies and related problems.

   b. The Wound Ostomy and Continence Nurses (WOCN) Society has many resources, including educational programs for nurses, patient education information, and *Journal of Wound, Ostomy, and Continence Nursing* (www.wocn.org).
2. Administer replacement fluid, as ordered, before surgery because of possible increased output during the postoperative phase.
3. Provide low-residue diet before NPO status.
4. Explain that the abdomen may be marked by the ostomy specialty nurse or surgeon to ensure proper positioning of the stoma. *Note:* The abdominal location of the stoma is usually determined by anatomic location of the bowel segment (e.g., a sigmoid colostomy is ideally located in the left lower abdominal quadrant).
5. Other considerations when selecting a stoma include:
   a. Positioning within rectus muscle.
   b. Avoidance of bony prominences, such as iliac crest and costal margin.
   c. Clearance from umbilicus, scars, and deep creases, observed in lying, sitting, and standing positions.
   d. Positioning on a flat pouching surface.
   e. Avoidance of beltline when possible.
   f. Positioning within patient's visibility to optimize independent ostomy care.
6. Support the patient and family with the many psychosocial considerations of ostomy surgery.

Postoperative Management and Nursing Care

1. Administer general abdominal surgery care (see page 468).
2. Assess stoma every shift for color and record findings:
   a. Normal color: pink red.
   b. Dusky: dark red; purplish hue (ischemic sign).
   c. Necrotic: brown or black; may be dry (notify health care provider to determine the extent of necrosis).
3. Apply pouching system as close to stoma as possible without it being rubbed. It is acceptable to have a 1/16- to 1/8-in clearance to prevent constriction, which can contribute to edema (see Figure 14-4).
4. Check for abdominal distention, which reduces blood flow to stoma through mesenteric tension.
5. Evaluate and empty drains and ostomy pouch frequently to promote patency and maintain seal.
6. Monitor intake and output with extreme accuracy because output may remain high during early postoperative period.
7. Suction and irrigate NG tube frequently, as ordered, to relieve pressure and decrease gastric contents.
8. Offer continued support to patient and family.

Complications

1. Mucocutaneous separation (between the skin and stoma).
2. Stomal ischemia.
3. Stomal stricture or stenosis (usually a long-term complication).
4. Stomal prolapse.
5. Peristomal hernia.
6. Stomal laceration.
7. Stomal retraction.
8. Peristomal skin breakdown from exposure to fecal output, allergic reaction to products, or infection, such as candidiasis.

Nursing Interventions

Educating the Patient

1. Review the surgical procedure with the patient and discuss the information that the surgeon and other providers have given. Clarify any misunderstandings.
2. Avoid overwhelming the patient with information.
3. Include family in discussions, when appropriate.
4. Use available educational materials, including pictures and drawings, if the patient is receptive.
5. Involve the WOCN in ostomy teaching and reinforce information, including lifestyle modifications.
6. Use a team approach; the need for information may come from many disciplines.
7. Assess the patient's response to teaching. If the patient is not interested, provide alternative times for teaching and review.

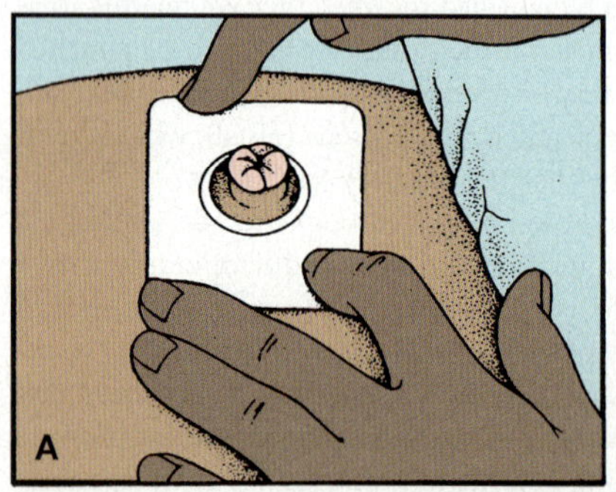

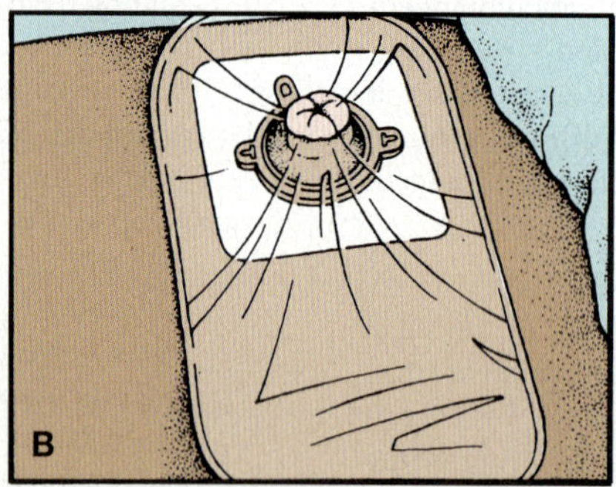

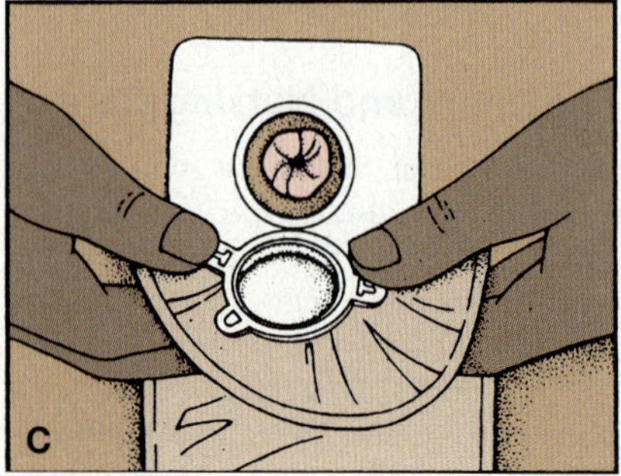

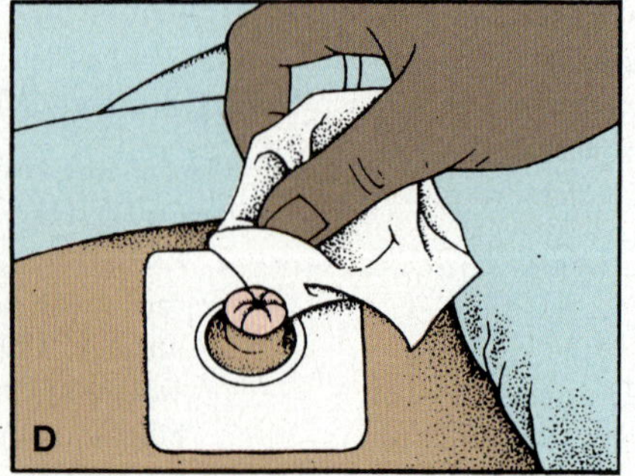

Figure 14-4. Changing a two-piece pouching system. Pouching systems are varied by manufacturer and chosen according to patient needs. Systems are one piece or two piece and disposable or reusable. A disposable, one-piece pouch is commonly used with backing as adhesive tape, skin barrier, or both. A disposable two-piece system consists of a skin barrier wafer with or without a tape border and a pouch. Reusable systems consist of double-backed adhesive disks, cement, or belt to provide a seal and can be used for weeks to months. **(A)** A wafer with flange (1.5 to 4 in) is applied after cleaning and drying of peristomal skin. **(B)** A transparent or opaque drainable pouch is positioned over stoma at desired angle. **(C)** Pouch may be removed without removal of wafer. **(D)** Stoma may be assessed without removing wafer.

8. Introduce gradual steps toward achieving independent ostomy management. The patient may progress through the following steps:
   a. Observe stoma, pouch change, and emptying procedure.
   b. Learn tail closure application and removal.
   c. Empty and rinse pouch.
   d. Assist with pouching system change until independent.
9. Consider the psychosocial issues of the patient and their effect on learning.

Maintaining Skin Integrity

1. Select pouching system based on the type of ostomy and condition of stoma and skin (see Figure 14-3).
2. Empty pouch when one-third to one-half full to avoid overfilling, which interferes with pouch seal.
   a. Remove tail closure from pouch tail.
   b. Cuff the bottom of pouch tail.
   c. Drain stool from pouch.
   d. Clean pouch tail with toilet tissue or wipe (may rinse pouch if desired).
   e. Uncuff pouch and reapply tail closure.
3. Treat peristomal skin breakdown as needed.
   a. Dust skin breakdown with skin barrier powder (e.g., Stomahesive powder).
   b. Seal powder with water or skin sealant (e.g., Skin-Prep). May be applied one to three times per day, depending on the severity of the skin breakdown.
   c. Allow skin to dry before applying pouching system.

CLINICAL JUDGMENT When peristomal skin is exposed to excess moisture, candidiasis can occur. It presents as an erythematous rash, which may include papules, pustules, or white patches. Patients may complain of pruritus. The treatment procedure is the same as for skin breakdown, using a prescribed antifungal powder (nystatin) in place of the skin barrier powder. The antifungal powder should be used at each pouching system change and continued 2 weeks after the condition has cleared. Positive identification of *Candida albicans* can be done through a culture or microscopic visualization. Treatment is usually initiated without culture or scraping if the signs and symptoms are classic.

Maximizing Nutritional Intake

1. Review dietary habits with the patient to determine patterns, preferences, and bowel irritants.
2. Advise the patient to avoid foods that stimulate elimination, such as nuts, seeds, and certain fruits.
3. Recommend consistency in dietary habits as well as moderation.
4. Coordinate consult with nutritionist, as needed.
5. Weigh daily; monitor vital signs and electrolytes to determine patient's nutritional status.

Promoting a Positive Self-Image

1. Encourage the patient to verbalize feelings about the surgical outcome. Acknowledge that it is normal to have negative feelings toward ostomy surgery; empathize with the patient.
2. Describe behaviors to attain a sense of control, such as resuming ADLs.
3. Provide support during initial viewing of the stoma and encourage the patient to touch the area.
4. Encourage spouse or significant other to view the stoma.
5. Arrange a visit by a United Ostomy Association ostomy visitor if the patient desires. This is preferably done preoperatively.
6. Suggest counseling, as necessary, and encourage the patient to use normal support systems, such as family, faith-based groups, and community groups.
7. Assess if patient has questions about sexual function, intimacy, and childbearing. Encourage the patient and significant other to express feelings about the ostomy and provide information to clear up misconceptions.
8. Discuss ways to conceal pouch during intimacy, if desired: pouch covers, special ostomy underwear. May briefly use small capacity pouch (minipouch or cap).
9. Advise that different positions for sexual activity can be tried to decrease stoma friction and skin irritation.
10. Review, when appropriate, that an ostomy in a female does not prevent a successful pregnancy and does not affect fertility for males or females.

Patient Education and Health Maintenance

Skin Care

1. Instruct the patient to inspect peristomal skin with each pouching system change.
2. Review techniques for treating peristomal skin problems.
3. Recommend alternative products if patient develops allergic reaction to an ostomy product.
4. Teach the patient to notify health care provider when skin care problems are not resolved by usual methods.

Colostomy Irrigation

1. Teach colostomy irrigation procedure, to patients with a descending or sigmoid colostomy. Reinforce its purposes of cleansing the colon and stimulating the colon to move at a desired time regularly to regain control of fecal elimination.
   a. Irrigation may occur every day or every other day depending on bowel pattern.
   b. It usually takes 1 to 2 months to establish control.
   c. Patients with a preoperative history of regular, formed bowel movements are more likely to realize success.
2. Set up patient in front of commode with irrigation sleeve directed into the commode, and lubricate tip of the enema before gently inserting no more than 3 in into stoma.
3. Allow solution to flow in slowly, over 5 to 10 minutes, and slower if cramping occurs.
4. Remove tubing and allow fecal matter to drain for 10 to 15 minutes before closing sleeve, which should be left in place for 20 more minutes before cleansing stoma and applying usual colostomy bag.

Odor Control

1. Encourage pouch hygiene through rinsing, keeping pouch tail free of stool, airing of reusable pouches, discarding odor-impregnated pouches.
2. Recommend the use of pouch deodorants, room deodorizers, and oral deodorizers, such as bismuth subgallate or parsley.
3. Avoid the use of pinholes in pouch.

Gas Control

1. Suggest avoidance of straws, excessive talking while eating, chewing gum, and smoking to reduce swallowed air.
2. Instruct about gas-forming foods, such as beans and cabbage, and eliminate when appropriate. It takes about 6 hours for gas to travel from the mouth to colostomy.
3. Recommend using the arm over stoma to muffle gas sounds when appropriate.

Activities of Daily Living

Educate the patient about the following:

1. Resumption of normal bathing habits (tub or shower) with or without pouching system.
2. Picture framing the edges of the pouching system with waterproof tape, if needed, for bathing or swimming.
3. Clothing modifications are usually minimal. Girdles without stays and pantyhose are acceptable.
4. Carrying an ostomy supply kit during work or travel in case of an emergency.
5. Participating in sports as desired. Caution must be exercised with contact sports. During vigorous activities, a belt or binder may provide extra security.
6. For additional information and support, refer to the United Ostomy Association, a self-help group for ostomates and other interested people, at www.uoa.org. The official membership publication is the *Ostomy Quarterly*. Encourage patients with an ostomy to participate in a local chapter. Chapters usually publish a local newsletter, conduct monthly meetings, and provide trained ostomy visitors on request by health care providers.
7. Ostomy manufacturers offer literature covering a wide variety of ostomy-related topics.
8. Encourage the patient to maintain contact with health care providers.

Evaluation: Expected Outcomes

- Verbalizes knowledge regarding ostomy surgery and general care of ostomy.
- No skin breakdown around ostomy.
- Plans menus with nutritionist; weight stable.
- Discusses ostomy appearance and intimacy concerns with partner.

ESOPHAGEAL DISORDERS

Esophageal varices are covered in Chapter 15, page 529.

Gastroesophageal Reflux Disease and Esophagitis

Gastric contents flow back into the esophagus, and sometimes further back into the mouth and lungs, in gastroesophageal reflux disease (GERD) because of incompetent lower esophageal sphincter (LES). Esophagitis, or inflammation of the esophageal mucosa, may result.

Pathophysiology and Etiology

1. Gastroesophageal (GE) reflux associated with an incompetent LES—gastric contents reflux (flow backward) through the LES into the esophagus.
2. Can be the result of impaired gastric emptying from gastroparesis or partial gastric outlet obstruction.
3. The acidity of gastric content and the amount of time in contact with esophageal mucosa are related to the degree of mucosal damage.
4. Inflammation and ulceration of the esophagus may result, causing esophagitis.
5. May be caused by motility disorders (scleroderma, esophageal spasm).
6. Eosinophilic esophagitis is a Th-2 antigen-mediated condition, which causes an influx of eosinophils into all layers of the esophagus, which sets off an inflammatory response. Chronic inflammation leads to esophageal remodeling, resulting in dysphagia.

Clinical Manifestations

Gastroesophageal Reflux Disease

1. The most common symptom is heartburn (pyrosis), typically occurring 30 to 60 minutes after meals and in reclining positions. May have complaints of spontaneous reflux (regurgitation) of sour or bitter gastric contents into the mouth.
2. Other typical symptoms include globus (sensation of something in the throat), mild epigastric pain, dyspepsia, and nausea and/or vomiting.
3. Dysphagia is a less common symptom.
4. Atypical symptoms include chest pain, hoarseness, recurrent sore throat, frequent throat clearing, chronic cough, dental enamel loss, bronchospasm (asthma/wheezing), and odynophagia (sharp substernal pain on swallowing).
5. Symptoms that may suggest other disease etiologies need further evaluation: atypical chest pain (rule out possible cardiac causes), dysphagia, odynophagia, gastrointestinal (GI) bleeding, shortness of breath, or weight loss (rule out cancer or esophageal stricture).

Esophagitis

1. Esophagitis is an acute or chronic inflammation of the esophagus. Severity of symptoms may be unrelated to the degree of esophageal tissue damage.
2. Symptoms vary according to etiology of esophagitis. Symptoms include dysphagia, odynophagia, severe burning, chest pain.
3. Causes of esophagitis other than GERD:
   a. Infectious—*Candida*, herpes, human immunodeficiency virus, cytomegalovirus.
   b. Chemical (alkali or acid) or radiation therapy.
   c. Medication induced—may include doxycycline, ascorbic acid, quinidine, potassium chloride, bisphosphonates, tetracycline.
   d. Immune-mediated eosinophilic esophagitis.

Diagnostic Evaluation

1. Uncomplicated GERD may be diagnosed on patient history of typical symptoms.
2. Endoscopy can visualize inflammation, lesions, or erosions. Biopsy can confirm diagnosis.
3. Esophageal manometry measures LES pressure and determines whether esophageal peristalsis is adequate. This study should be used before patients undergo surgical treatment for reflux. This test is also done before a pH probe for determination of correct catheter placement.
4. Acid perfusion (Bernstein test)—onset of symptoms after ingestion of dilute hydrochloric acid and saline is considered positive. This test differentiates between cardiac and noncardiac chest pain.
5. Ambulatory 24-hour pH monitoring is performed when GERD is suspected but not responding to standard therapies, prior to antireflux surgery, or when the patient's symptoms may not be typical. It determines the amount of GE acid reflux and has a 70% to 90% specificity rate.

6. The Bravo pH capsule system is a catheter-free system in which a capsule containing a radiotelemetry pH sensor is inserted into the esophagus. This sensor transmits signals to an external pager-size receiver, allowing the patient to be catheter free during the 24 hours of pH testing.
    a. The Bravo pH capsule system is contraindicated for patients with pacemakers, implantable defibrillators, or neurostimulators. It is also contraindicated for patients with a history of severe esophagitis, varices, obstructions, bleeding diatheses, or strictures.
    b. The patient should not undergo magnetic resonance imaging (MRI) within 30 days of Bravo capsule pH monitoring.
7. Barium esophagography—use of barium with radiographic studies to diagnose mechanical and motility disorders. This test is not recommended in diagnosing GERD.

Management

Treatment goals include eliminating symptoms, healing esophageal damage (if present), and preventing complications and relapse.

Lifestyle Modifications

1. Head of bed raised 6 to 8 in (15 to 20 cm).
2. Do not lie down for 2 to 3 hours after eating—time frame for greatest reflux.
3. Bland diet—avoid garlic, onion, peppermint, fatty foods, chocolate, coffee (including decaffeinated), citrus juices, colas, and tomato products.
4. Avoid overeating—causes LES relaxation.
5. No tight-fitting clothes.
6. Weight loss.
7. Smoking cessation.
8. Reduce alcohol intake.

Pharmacologic Treatment

1. Antacids—reduce gastric acidity. Use on an as-needed basis. Provide symptomatic relief, but are short acting and do not heal esophageal lesions.
2. Histamine-2 (H_2)-receptor antagonists, such as ranitidine, cimetidine, famotidine, nizatidine—decrease gastric acid secretions. Provide symptomatic relief. May require lifelong therapy.
3. If symptoms do not respond to H_2-receptor antagonist, change to a once-daily proton pump inhibitor (PPI), such as omeprazole, esomeprazole, pantoprazole, rabeprazole, or lansoprazole, to block gastric acid secretion.
4. PPIs have been shown to be more effective than H_2-receptor antagonists in achieving faster healing rates for erosive esophagitis.
5. Swallowed corticosteroid therapy, which is administered topically to the esophagus, such as fluticasone propionate and budesonide, helps decrease inflammatory response by reducing eosinophil infiltration.

EVIDENCE BASE Nennstiel, S., & Schlag, C. (2020). Treatment of eosinophilic esophagitis with swallowed topical corticosteroids. *World Journal of Gastroenterology, 26*(36), 5395–5407. https://doi.org/10.3748/wjg.v26.i36.5395

6. Drug maintenance therapy may be needed depending on the severity of disease and recurrence of symptoms after initial drug therapy is stopped.
7. Use the lowest effective drug dose of H_2-receptor blocker or PPI.

DRUG ALERT PPIs should be taken 30 minutes before a meal for optimal control of gastric acidity. Impaired absorption of calcium may occur with PPI use, leading to fracture risk. Calcium citrate is recommended because it is not dependent on an acid environment for absorption.

DRUG ALERT Swallowed corticosteroid therapy is accomplished by using the inhaler to spray into the mouth and then swallow. This medication is not inhaled, and patients should not eat or drink anything for 30 minutes after administration.

Endoscopic and Surgical Treatment

1. Nissen fundoplication and bariatric surgery (for the patient with obesity) are the most common surgical therapies for long-term management of GERD. Surgery is not recommended for those who do not respond to PPI therapy.
    a. Upper portion of the stomach is wrapped around the distal esophagus and sutured, creating a tight LES.
    b. This procedure can be performed laparoscopically.
    c. Combined with vagotomy–pyloroplasty if associated with gastroduodenal ulcer.
    d. Antireflux surgery may not eliminate the need for future pharmacologic treatment.
2. Many endoscopic therapies for the treatment of GERD have not been efficacious and are no longer used. In the United States, there are only two endoscopic therapies being used, and these are only used if patient has risks of Barrett esophagus or if symptom resolution did not occur with pharmacologic treatment:
    a. The Stretta procedure is a radiofrequency energy delivery system used to provide a thermal burn to the GE junction.
    b. Transoral incisionless fundoplication (TIF) is done using the EsophyX device on an endoscope to tighten the GE valve, thereby reducing reflux.

Complications

1. Esophageal stricture formation.
2. Ulceration of the esophagus, with or without fistula formation.
3. Aspiration may be complicated by pneumonia.
4. Development of Barrett esophagus—presence of columnar epithelium above the GE junction associated with adenocarcinoma of the esophagus.

Nursing Interventions and Patient Education

1. Teach the patient about prescribed medications, adverse effects, and when to notify the health care provider. PPIs may interact with carbamazepine, cyclosporine, diazepam, diclofenac, digoxin, iron, ketoconazole, lidocaine, methotrexate, metoprolol, nifedipine, phenytoin, propranolol, quinidine, theophylline, and warfarin.
2. Inform the patient about medications that may exacerbate symptoms. Anticholinergics may further impair functioning of the LES, allowing reflux; antihistamines, antidepressants, antihypertensives, antispasmodics, and some neuroleptics and antiparkinsonian drugs decrease saliva production, which may decrease acid clearance from the esophagus.
3. Advise the patient to sit or stand when taking any solid medication (pills, capsules): Emphasize the need to follow the drug with at least 100 mL of liquid.

4. Familiarize the patient and family with foods and activities to avoid, such as fatty foods, garlic, onions, alcohol, coffee, chocolate, and peppermint.
5. Caution the patient against straining, bending over, tight-fitting clothes, and smoking.
6. Encourage the patient to sleep with the head of the bed elevated (not pillow elevation).
7. Encourage a weight reduction program, if the patient is overweight, to decrease intra-abdominal pressure.

Hiatal Hernia

A hiatal hernia is a protrusion of a portion of the stomach through the hiatus of the diaphragm and into the thoracic cavity.

Pathophysiology and Etiology

1. There are two types of hiatal hernias (see Figure 14-5):
   a. Sliding hernia: The stomach and GE junction slip up into the chest (most common).
   b. Paraesophageal hernia (rolling hernia): Part of the greater curvature of the stomach rolls through the diaphragmatic defect.
2. Caused by muscle weakening because of aging or other conditions, such as esophageal carcinoma or trauma, or following certain surgical procedures.

Clinical Manifestations

1. May be asymptomatic.
2. Heartburn (with or without regurgitation of gastric contents into the mouth).
3. Dysphagia, chest pain.

Diagnostic Evaluation

1. Barium study of the esophagus outlines hernia.
2. Endoscopic examination visualizes defect.

Management

1. Elevation of the head of the bed (6 to 8 in [15 to 20 cm]) to reduce nighttime reflux.
2. Antacid therapy to neutralize gastric acid.
3. H_2-receptor antagonist (cimetidine, ranitidine) to reduce acid secretion.
4. Swallowed topical corticosteroid therapy (fluticasone propionate) if patient has esophagitis.
5. Surgical repair of hernia if symptoms are severe.

Complications

1. Aspiration of reflux contents.
2. Ulceration, hemorrhage.
3. Gastritis.
4. Stricture.
5. Incarceration of the portion of the stomach in the chest.

Nursing Interventions and Patient Education

1. Instruct the patient on the prevention of reflux of gastric contents into the esophagus by:
   a. Eating smaller meals.
   b. Avoiding stimulation of gastric secretions by omitting caffeine and alcohol.
   c. Refraining from smoking.
   d. Avoiding fatty foods: promote reflux and delay gastric emptying.
   e. Refraining from lying down for at least 1 hour after meals.
   f. Losing weight, if patient has obesity.
   g. Avoiding bending from the waist and/or wearing tight-fitting clothes.
2. Advise the patient to report to health care facility immediately for the onset of acute chest pain, which may indicate incarceration of a large paraesophageal hernia.

Esophageal Trauma and Perforations

Esophageal trauma or perforations are injuries to the esophagus caused by external or internal insult.

Pathophysiology and Etiology

1. External: stab or bullet wounds, crush injuries, blunt trauma.
2. Internal:
   a. Swallowed foreign objects (coins, pins, bones, dental appliances, caustic poisons).
   b. Spontaneous or postemetic rupture—usually in the presence of underlying esophageal disease (reflux, hiatal hernia).
   c. Mallory–Weiss syndrome—nonpenetrating mucosal tear at the GE junction. Caused by an increase in transabdominal pressure from lifting, vomiting, or retching. Substance use disorder is a predisposing condition.

Clinical Manifestations

1. Pain at the site of injury or impaction, aggravated by swallowing—chest pain, may be severe.

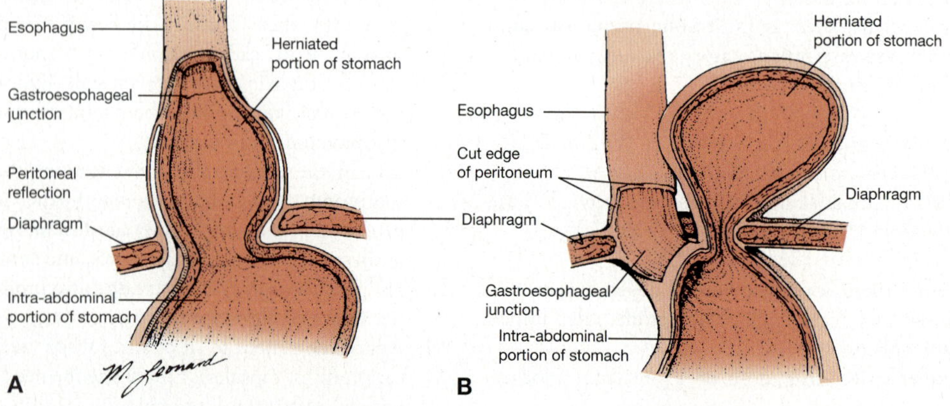

Figure 14-5. Hiatal hernia. **(A)** Sliding hernia. **(B)** Paraesophageal hernia.

2. Dysphagia or odynophagia.
3. Persistent foreign object sensation.
4. Subcutaneous emphysema and crepitus of the face, neck, or upper thorax—noted in esophageal perforation in the cervical or thoracic regions.
5. Temperature elevation occurring within 24 hours of trauma.
6. Blood-stained saliva or excessive salivation.
7. Hematemesis; previous history of vomiting or retching—Mallory–Weiss syndrome.
8. Respiratory difficulty if there is pressure on the tracheobronchial tree from injury or edema.

Diagnostic Evaluation

1. History of recent esophageal trauma.
2. Chest x-ray to look for foreign body.
3. Esophagogram to outline trauma.
4. Endoscopy to directly visualize trauma.

Management

1. Maintenance of adequate respiratory functioning; may require oxygen support or endotracheal intubation—to ensure an open airway in the presence of edema of the neck.
2. Replacement of fluids. May need blood transfusion. Bleeding may stop spontaneously; if not, endoscopic hemostatic therapy or surgery is indicated.
3. Restoration of the continuity of the esophagus by removing the cause.
4. For external wound injury, emergency first aid wound care and surgical repair may be indicated.
5. For swallowed foreign bodies:
   a. Barium swallow determines the location of foreign body; usually removed through endoscopy.
   b. Some patients with a history of food impaction may be treated with a spasmolytic, such as intravenous (IV) glucagon.
6. For chemical ingestion:
   a. If lye or other caustic or organic solvent was swallowed, do not try to induce vomiting.
   b. Treat with IV fluids, active charcoal, and analgesics, and notify poison control.
   c. A gastrostomy may be performed, either as a temporary or as a permanent means of feeding the patient.
   d. Resulting strictures may be relieved by dilating the narrow esophagus.
   e. Reconstructive surgery may be necessary to create a new passageway for food between the pharynx and the stomach.

Complications

1. Airway occlusion.
2. Shock.
3. Perforation with mediastinitis or pleural effusion.
4. Stricture formation.
5. Abscess or fistula formation.

Nursing Assessment

1. Assess the following to determine the status of patient:
   a. Airway—patency of airway, ability to swallow, any choking or gagging.
   b. Breathing—respiratory effort, movement of air in lungs.
   c. Circulation—pulses, any bleeding vital signs.
2. Monitor vital signs for hypovolemic shock.

Nursing Interventions

Maintaining Respiratory Function

1. Assess respiratory rate, depth, use of accessory muscles, and skin color.
2. Auscultate trachea and lung fields for stridor, crackles, or wheezes.
3. Position the patient in semi-Fowler position to facilitate breathing and reduce neck edema.
4. Administer oxygen as prescribed.
5. Have emergency airway equipment at bedside.

Maintaining Fluid Volume

1. Monitor vital signs frequently for signs of shock and report acute change or unfavorable trend.
2. Administer IV fluids and blood transfusion for volume replacement, as indicated.
3. Monitor intake and output. Urine output should be greater than 30 mL/h.
4. Monitor laboratory results (electrolytes, hemoglobin, hematocrit, lactic acid) and report abnormal findings.

Reducing Pain

1. Administer analgesics as prescribed—IV analgesia may be required to control pain and allow for rest.
2. Assess for pain relief and record patient's response to medication.
3. Instruct the patient to report increase in the severity or nature of pain.
4. Provide reassurance and support.

CLINICAL JUDGMENT Sudden onset of acute retrosternal chest pain may indicate acute inflammation of the mediastinum, due to chemical irritation from esophageal rupture. Report immediately.

Maintaining Nutritional Status

1. Monitor daily weights and skin turgor.
2. Administer parenteral hyperalimentation as prescribed—to prevent gastric reflux into the esophagus, which may occur with enteral feedings.
3. Encourage progression of diet through nasogastric (NG), esophagostomy, or oral feedings when esophagoscopy or esophagogram reveals adequate healing of the esophagus.
4. Continue to monitor intake and output.
5. Inform the patient about signs and symptoms of possible complications to report: difficulty breathing or swallowing.
6. Teach patient with dysphagia how to swallow (see Box 14-2). This assists the patient who has difficulty swallowing after injury or surgical correction of the oropharynx or upper esophagus (also helpful with neurologic deficit or stroke).

Evaluation: Expected Outcomes

- Respirations unlabored, breath sounds clear.
- Urine output greater than 30 mL/h; blood pressure (BP) and pulse stable.
- States pain decreased to level of 2 or 3 on 0 to 10 scale.
- Weight stable, tolerating parenteral feedings well.

Motility Disorders of the Esophagus

Primary motility disorders include achalasia, diffuse esophageal spasm, and those of nonspecific origin. Secondary motility disorders may be caused by neuromuscular, GI, endocrine, or connective tissue disorders.

BOX 14-2 Teaching a Patient With Dysphagia How to Swallow

1. Sit the patient upright and the head in midline and forward position, chin pointed toward the chest.
2. Instruct the patient to smell the food before each bite; hold each bite for a few seconds; hold lips together firmly; concentrate on swallowing; then, swallow.
3. If the patient has an increase in saliva during the meal, instruct the patient to collect the saliva with the tongue and consciously swallow it between bites throughout the meal.
4. If the patient complains of a dry mouth during meals, instruct them to move tongue in a circular manner against the insides of the cheeks to stimulate salivation.
5. Caution the patient against talking during the meal or with the mouth full of food.
6. Advise the following tips about food and fluid intake:
   a. Try foods that hold some shape and are moist enough to prevent crumbling but dry enough to hold a bolus shape—casseroles, custards, scrambled eggs.
   b. Use mugs and glasses with spouts or use a straw.
   c. Avoid sticky foods—peanut butter, chocolate, milk, ice cream.
   d. Moisten dry foods with margarine, gravy, or broths.
   e. Liquids such as juices can be thickened with sherbet.
   f. Safely try warm and cold foods and fluids, which are thought to maximally stimulate receptors that activate swallowing mechanism.

Pathophysiology and Etiology

Primary Motility Disorders

1. *Achalasia* refers to excessive resting tone of the LES, incomplete relaxation of the LES with swallowing, and failure of normal peristalsis in the lower two thirds of the esophagus. The pathology is related to defective innervation of the myenteric plexus innervating the involuntary muscles of the esophagus.
2. Diffuse esophageal spasm is a motor disorder in which high-amplitude, nonpropulsive, nonperistaltic tertiary contractions (a form of aperistalsis) are present. LES functioning is frequently normal.

Secondary Motility Disorders

1. Neuromuscular dysfunction includes myasthenia gravis, Parkinson disease, muscular dystrophy, amyotrophic lateral sclerosis, and cerebral palsy.
2. Connective tissue disorders include scleroderma.
3. GI causes include GERD.
4. Other secondary causes include the autonomic neuropathy of diabetes mellitus.

Clinical Manifestations

Achalasia

1. Gradual onset of dysphagia with solids and liquids.
2. Substernal discomfort or a feeling of fullness.
3. Regurgitation of undigested food during a meal or within several hours after a meal.
4. Weight loss.

Diffuse Esophageal Spasm

1. Intermittent dysphagia for solids or liquids—does not progress to continuous dysphagia.
2. Aggravation of symptoms (large volume of food and hot or cold liquids).
3. Anterior chest pain.

Secondary Motility Disorders

Symptoms of esophagitis from GE reflux.

Diagnostic Evaluation

Achalasia

1. Chest x-ray, which may show an enlarged, fluid-filled esophagus.
2. Barium esophagography showing dilation, decreased or absence of peristalsis, decreased emptying, and a "bird beak" narrowing of the distal esophagus.
3. Esophageal manometry to confirm the diagnoses suspected.
4. Endoscopic ultrasound (EUS) or a chest CT for suspected tumor.

Diffuse Esophageal Spasm

1. Barium esophagography showing simultaneous contractions of the esophagus having a "corkscrew" or "rosary bead" appearance.
2. Esophageal manometry showing intermittent contractions with episodes of normal peristalsis.

Secondary Motility Disorders

1. Diagnostic workup may include barium esophagography or manometry.
2. Additional testing for suspected or confirmed neurologic disorders, scleroderma, or diabetes.

Management

Achalasia

1. Drug therapy using calcium channel blockers such as nifedipine to reduce LES pressure. This type of treatment is usually best for patients presenting with mild symptoms and a nondilated esophagus or patients who are medically unstable to undergo invasive therapies.
2. Esophageal dilation using a balloon-tipped catheter is the preferred treatment for most patients.
3. Surgical therapy (Heller myotomy of the LES) may be used on patients who do not respond to balloon dilation. This surgery requires a laparotomy or thoracotomy or may be done through a thoracoscope.

Diffuse Esophageal Spasm

1. Drug therapy using nitrates and calcium channel blockers is the primary treatment.
2. Dilation may provide some symptom relief.
3. Surgical myotomy is used rarely for patients with a debilitating disorder who are able to withstand a surgical procedure.

Other Motility Disorders

1. Treatment of the GE reflux.
2. Dilation may be required for peptic stricture.

Complications

1. Malnutrition.
2. Pneumonia, lung abscess, bronchiectasis from nocturnal regurgitation causing aspiration.
3. Esophagitis and esophageal diverticula.
4. Perforation from dilation procedure.
5. Peptic stricture or Barrett esophagus from severe erosive esophagitis.

Nursing Assessment

1. Assess for difficulty with swallowing, vomiting, weight loss, chest pain associated with eating.
2. Inquire as to what facilitates passage of food, such as position changes, use of liquids.

Nursing Interventions

Improving Nutritional Status

1. Direct the patient to eat sitting in an upright position; eat slowly and chew food thoroughly.
2. Avoid food and beverages that precipitate symptoms.
3. Suggest that the patient sleep with head elevated to avoid reflux or aspiration.
4. Provide a bland diet and tell the patient to avoid alcohol as well as spicy, very hot, and very cold foods, to minimize symptoms.
5. Eliminate sources of tension as a precipitating factor producing stress during mealtimes.
6. Administer pharmacologic agents as prescribed.

Promoting Comfort

1. Assess the patient for discomfort, chest pain, regurgitation, and cough. If a surgical procedure was performed, assess for incisional pain.
2. Provide appropriate postoperative care. Incisional approach determines the nature of postoperative care (e.g., an incision through the chest implies nursing care similar to that given to a patient with a thoracotomy [see page 151]).
3. Administer analgesics as ordered.
4. Assess for effectiveness of pain medication.

Patient Education and Health Maintenance

1. Encourage lifestyle activity changes similar to those for patients with reflux (see page 482).
2. See Box 14-2 on page 486 to help the patient with dysphasia with swallowing.
3. Provide information on all diagnostic procedures or surgery performed. Clarify any misunderstandings.

Evaluation: Expected Outcomes

- Demonstrates proper positioning for eating; describes dietary habits that minimize symptoms; adherent to medications regimen.
- States pain decreased to 2 or 3 on 0 to 10 scale.

Esophageal Diverticulum

An esophageal diverticulum is an outpouching of the esophageal wall, usually in the cervical posterior region of the esophagus, secondary to an obstructive or inflammatory process.

Pathophysiology and Etiology

1. *Zenker diverticulum*—protrusion of pharyngeal mucosa at the pharyngoesophageal junction between the interior pharyngeal constrictor and the cricopharyngeal muscle (see Figure 14-6).
2. Often due to tightening of the cricopharyngeal muscle over time.
3. Mid- or distal esophageal diverticula may develop above strictures or may be secondary to motility disorders.

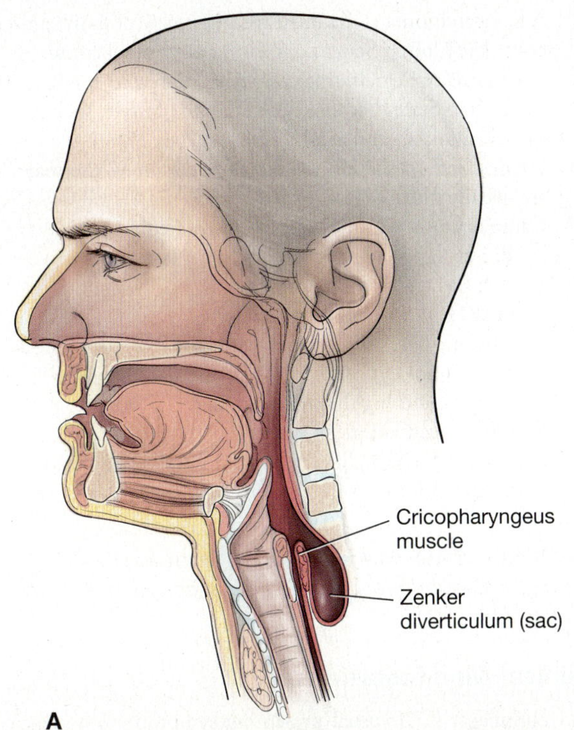

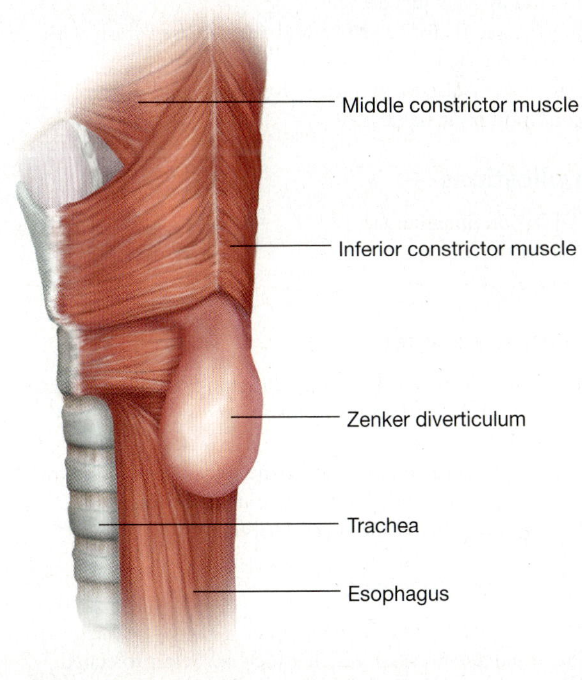

Figure 14-6. Zenker diverticulum. **(A)** Cross section. **(B)** Posterior view. (**A:** Reprinted with permission from LoCicero, J. [2018]. *Shields' general thoracic surgery* [8th ed., part of Fig. 125-14]. Wolters Kluwer. **B:** Reprinted with permission from Hawn, M. [2015]. *Operative techniques in thoracic and esophageal surgery* [Fig. 13-2]. Wolters Kluwer.)

Clinical Manifestations

Zenker Diverticulum

1. Difficulty in swallowing, fullness in the neck, throat discomfort, a feeling that food stops before it reaches the stomach, and regurgitation of undigested food.
2. Belching, gurgling, or nocturnal coughing brought about by diverticulum becoming filled with food or liquid, which is regurgitated and may irritate the trachea.
3. Halitosis and foul taste in the mouth caused by food decomposing in a pouch (diverticulum).
4. Weight loss because of nutritional depletion.

POPULATION AWARENESS Hoarseness, asthma, and pneumonitis may be the only signs of esophageal diverticula in older adults.

Mid- or Distal Esophageal Diverticula

Generally no symptoms.

Diagnostic Evaluation

1. Barium esophagogram outlines diverticulum.
2. Endoscopy is not indicated and may be dangerous because of the possibility of rupture.

Management

Zenker Diverticulum

1. Small Zenker diverticula may not be treated, but the underlying cause is treated with dilation or myotomy.
2. For larger Zenker diverticula, transverse cervical diverticulectomy or diverticulopexy with suspension and cricopharyngeal myotomy may be done.
   a. Caution is taken to avoid injury to common carotid artery and internal jugular vein.
   b. The sac is dissected free and then excised flush with the esophageal wall.
3. For mid- or distal esophageal diverticula, underlying primary condition must be treated.

Complications

1. Aspiration pneumonia.
2. Malnutrition.
3. Lung abscess.

Nursing Assessment

1. Obtain a history of dysphagia, coughing, throat discomfort, choking, and regurgitation of food.
2. Evaluate for halitosis.
3. Determine what measures assist the patient with food intake and what foods and fluids the patient can tolerate.
4. Evaluate weight loss and dietary habits.

Nursing Interventions

Improving Nutritional Status

1. Provide frequent, small meals, which are better tolerated.
2. Elevate the head of bed for 2 hours after eating.
3. Monitor intake and output.
4. Weigh daily.

Maintaining Comfort and Preventing Complications

1. Preoperatively, or if the condition is nonoperative, implement nursing interventions similar to those for esophagitis.
2. Postoperatively, wound care is similar to that of other surgical incisions of the same anatomic position (e.g., thoracotomy [see page 151]).
3. Administer appropriate pain medications and assess effectiveness.
4. Patient may need oral suctioning to control drooling.
5. Maintain NG tube if in place.
   a. Irrigate the tube as ordered.
   b. Do not manipulate NG tube because of the location of the tube and suture line.

Patient Education and Health Maintenance

1. Instruct patient regarding treatment of esophagitis caused by GE reflux (see page 482).
2. Advise patient that small diverticulum may not require surgery and can be managed by eating small bites of food that are easy to swallow; drinking a lot of water after eating; and avoiding nuts, skins, or seeds that could get stuck in diverticulum.
3. Instruct patient on the importance of good oral hygiene.

Evaluation: Expected Outcomes

- Tolerates oral feedings; maintains weight.
- States pain decreased to 2 or 3 on 0 to 10 scale.

Cancer of the Esophagus

Malignant lesions of the esophagus occur in two main types that are defined histologically: squamous cell and adenocarcinoma.

Pathophysiology and Etiology

1. Adenocarcinoma is the most common type of esophageal cancer in the United States comprising 60% of all cases.
2. Squamous cell carcinoma cases have decreased significantly in the United States because of changes in lifestyle, such as reduction of smoking and alcohol use.
3. Highest rate in the United States occurs in White males who are usually older than age 60.
4. Cause is unknown but has been associated with:
   a. Barrett esophagus.
   b. Achalasia.
   c. GERD.
   d. Chronic use of alcohol and tobacco (squamous cell carcinoma).
   e. Obesity and highly processed diet.
   f. Other head and neck cancers.
5. Represents 1.1% of all cancers, and 2.6% of all cancer deaths; 5-year survival rate is 21.7%.

EVIDENCE BASE National Cancer Institute. (2023). *Cancer stat facts: Esophageal cancer.* seer.cancer.gov/statfacts/html/esoph.html

Clinical Manifestations

1. Dysphagia is the usual presenting symptom, although it is a late sign, by which time there is often regional or systemic involvement.

2. Mild, atypical chest pain associated with eating precedes dysphagia but is rarely significant enough for the patient to seek health care.
3. Pain on swallowing (odynophagia).
4. Progressive weight loss.
5. Hoarseness (if laryngeal involvement).
6. Lymphadenopathy (supraclavicular or cervical) or hepatomegaly with metastatic involvement.
7. Later symptoms—hiccups, respiratory difficulty, foul breath, and regurgitation of food and saliva.

Diagnostic Evaluation

1. Chest x-ray may show adenopathy, mediastinal widening, metastasis, or a tracheoesophageal fistula.
2. Endoscopy with cytology and biopsy.
3. Surveillance endoscopy of Barrett esophagus is beneficial for early detection of malignant changes.
4. Barium esophagogram may show polypoid, infiltrative, or ulcerative lesion requiring biopsy.
5. CT scanning may be helpful in delineating the extent of the tumor as well as in identifying the presence of adjacent tissue invasion and metastases.

Management

1. The goal of treatment may be cure or palliation, depending on the staging of the tumor and the patient's overall condition in relation to nutritional, cardiovascular, pulmonary, and functional status.
2. The wide variability in treatment reflects the overall poor results from any one approach.
3. Surgery.
   a. Lesions of the middle and lower esophagus are excised with the use of the thoracotomy approach with esophagogastrectomy or colon interposition (section of the colon is used to replace the excised portion of the esophagus).
   b. Lesions of the cervical esophagus are excised with a bilateral neck dissection and esophagogastrectomy; laryngectomy and thyroidectomy may be necessary.
   c. A two-step approach may be selected when resection with a cervical esophagostomy and feeding gastrostomy is performed initially; subsequent reconstructive surgery is performed.
   d. Anemia is common with esophageal cancer and is associated with poorer outcomes following surgery; thus, treatment should be pursued aggressively, including perioperative transfusions.
4. Radiation, chemotherapy, or their combination; combination therapy appears to have better results.
5. Palliative treatment of dysphagia through dilation done by endoscopy or laser therapy.
6. The goal of palliative treatment is to reduce the complications of the tumor to improve quality of life. Any one or a combination of the aforementioned therapies can be used for palliative treatment.

EVIDENCE BASE Connor, J. P., Destrampe, E., Robbins, D., Hess, A. S., McCarthy, D., & Maloney, J. (2023). Pre-operative anemia and peri-operative transfusion are associated with poor oncologic outcomes in cancers of the esophagus: Potential impact of patient blood management on cancer outcomes. *BMC Cancer, 23*, 99. https://doi.org/10.1186/s12885-023-10579-x

Complications

1. Preoperatively: malnutrition, aspiration pneumonitis, hemorrhage, anemia, sepsis, and tracheoesophageal fistula.
2. Postoperatively: pneumonia, dumping syndrome, nutritional deficiencies, reflux esophagitis, and anastomosis leakage.

Nursing Assessment

1. Obtain a history of symptoms, such as dysphagia, pain, cough, and hoarseness.
2. Evaluate for dietary changes and weight loss.
3. Assess support system and personal coping mechanisms.

Nursing Interventions

Also see "Caring for the Patient Undergoing Gastrointestinal Surgery" section, page 475.

Improving Nutritional and Fluid Status

1. Provide the preoperative patient with a high-protein, high-calorie diet as tolerated. Nutritional supplements may be indicated. Total parenteral nutrition (TPN) may be ordered if unable to take food or fluids orally.
2. Monitor blood counts perioperatively and administer blood transfusions for hemoglobin <7 g/dL, as directed.
3. Postoperatively, administer IV fluids as prescribed. Initially, the patient may require large volumes if extensive excision of lymph nodes was performed.
4. Assess for bowel sounds; administer fluids per NG tube and liquid feedings through jejunostomy, as prescribed.
5. Encourage patient in advancing diet from liquids to soft foods.
6. Remind patient to remain in upright position for approximately 2 hours after eating to avoid reflux.
7. Provide mouth care for patient comfort and hygiene.

Preventing Infection and Other Complications

1. Monitor BP, pulse, respiration, and temperature to note early onset of hemorrhage, infection, dysrhythmias, aspiration, or anastomosis leakage.
2. Observe drainage from incision and/or chest tube for bleeding or purulence.
3. Monitor arterial blood gas (ABG) levels, manage pain, suction, provide chest physiotherapy, and provide oxygen as indicated.

Strengthening Individual Coping

1. Encourage patient to utilize support system during treatment and recovery process.
2. Provide information about laryngectomy, gastrostomy, and other procedures related to surgery, as indicated.
3. Provide training in relaxation techniques and diversional therapy for anxiety and pain control after surgery.
4. Refer to the American Cancer Society (www.acs.org) for additional information and sources of support.

Patient Education and Health Maintenance

1. Encourage the patient to avoid overeating, take small bites, chew food well, and avoid chunks of meat and stringy raw vegetables and fruit.
2. Depending on type of surgery, small, frequent meals may be better tolerated.
3. Encourage rest postoperatively and advancing activities as tolerated.

4. Instruct the patient regarding signs and symptoms of complications to report: nausea, vomiting, elevated temperature, cough, and difficulty swallowing.

Evaluation: Expected Outcomes

- Good skin turgor; eating small, frequent meals; gaining weight.
- Vital signs stable; incision without drainage.
- Performing self-care with the help of support people.

GASTRODUODENAL DISORDERS

Gastrointestinal Bleeding

Gastrointestinal (GI) bleeding is not just a gastroduodenal disorder but may occur anywhere along the alimentary tract. Bleeding is a symptom of an upper or lower GI disorder. It may be obvious in emesis or stool, or it may be occult (hidden).

Pathophysiology and Etiology

1. Trauma anywhere along the GI tract.
2. Erosion of ulcers and fistulas.
3. Rupture of an enlarged vein, such as a varicosity (esophageal or gastric varices).
4. Inflammation, such as esophagitis (caused by acid or bile), gastritis, inflammatory bowel disease (chronic ulcerative colitis [UC], Crohn disease), and bacterial infection.
5. Alcohol and drugs (aspirin-containing compounds, nonsteroidal anti-inflammatory drugs [NSAIDs], anticoagulants, corticosteroids).
6. Diverticular disease.
7. Cancers.
8. Vascular lesions or disorders, such as bowel ischemia, aortoenteric fistula, and arteriovenous malformations.
9. Mallory–Weiss tear.
10. Anal disorders, such as hemorrhoids or fissures.

Clinical Manifestations

Characteristics of Blood

1. Bright red: vomited from high in the esophagus (hematemesis); passed from the rectum or distal colon (coating stool).
2. Dark red: higher up in the colon and small intestine; mixed with stool.
3. Shades of black ("coffee ground"): vomited from the esophagus, stomach, and duodenum.
4. Tarry stool (melena): occurs in patient who accumulates excessive blood in the stomach.

Signs and Symptoms of Bleeding

1. Massive bleeding.
   a. Acute, bright red hematemesis or large amount of melena with clots in the stool.
   b. Rapid pulse, drop in blood pressure (BP), hypovolemia, and shock.
2. Subacute bleeding.
   a. Intermittent melena or coffee-ground emesis.
   b. Hypotension.
   c. Weakness and dizziness.
3. Chronic bleeding.
   a. Intermittent appearance of blood.
   b. Increased weakness, paleness, or shortness of breath.
   c. Occult blood.
   d. Iron deficiency anemia.

Diagnostic Evaluation

1. It is not difficult to diagnose bleeding, but it may be difficult to locate the source of bleeding.
2. History: change in bowel pattern, presence of pain or tenderness, recent intake of food and what kind (e.g., red beets), alcohol consumption, and drugs (e.g., aspirin or steroids).
3. Complete blood count (CBC) (hemoglobin, hematocrit, platelets) and coagulation studies (partial thromboplastin time, prothrombin time with international normalized ratio) may show abnormalities.
4. A nasogastric (NG) tube may be used before endoscopy in some cases if there is uncertainty that bleeding is occurring in the upper GI tract; however, there is not good evidence to support this practice.
5. Endoscopy: identifies source of bleeding, determines risk of rebleeding, and provides endoscopic therapy, if needed.
6. Colonoscopy: identifies source of lower GI bleeding and allows for therapy if needed.
7. Imaging may detect the cause of bleeding.
8. Test of stool for occult blood.

Management

Based on Etiology

1. If aspirin or NSAIDs are the cause, discontinue medication and treat bleeding.
2. If ulcer is the cause, assess medications, dietary and lifestyle modifications, and tests for *Helicobacter pylori*.
3. Therapeutic endoscopic procedure (cautery, injection).
4. Surgery may be indicated for cancers, inflammatory diseases, and vascular disorders.

Emergency Intervention

1. Initiate nothing by mouth (NPO) status.
2. Intravenous (IV) lines and oxygen therapy initiated.
3. If life-threatening bleeding occurs, treat shock; administer blood replacement, intra-arterial vasopressin or embolization.
4. Surgical therapy, if indicated.

Other Measures

1. Electrocoagulation using a heater probe.
2. Injection of sclerosant or epinephrine.
3. Banding or clips.
4. IV proton pump inhibitors (PPIs) are sometimes used to reduce the risk of rebleeding.
5. IV antibiotics may be given to reduce the risk for secondary infections, which can occur after GI bleeding, and thereby reduce the risk for mortality.
6. Beta-blockers may be given to reduce rebleeding risk in those with esophageal/gastric varices.
7. Surgery is indicated when more conservative measures fail.

Complications

1. Hemorrhage.
2. Shock.
3. Death.
4. Infection.

Nursing Assessment

1. Obtain history regarding:
   a. Change in bowel patterns or hemorrhoids.
   b. Change in color of stools (dark black, red, or streaked with blood).

c. Alcohol consumption.
d. Medications, such as aspirin, NSAIDs, antibiotics, anticoagulants, and corticosteroids.
e. Hematemesis.
f. Other medical conditions.
2. Evaluate for the presence of abdominal pain or tenderness.
3. Monitor vital signs and laboratory tests for changes that indicate bleeding (hemoglobin, hematocrit, platelet count, coagulation studies).
4. Test for occult blood, if indicated.
5. Assess urine output as renal perfusion may be affected.

Nursing Interventions

Preventing Hypotension and Shock and Maintaining Fluid Volume

1. Monitor vital signs frequently.
2. Observe for changes indicating shock, such as tachycardia, hypotension, increased respirations, decreased urine output, and change in mental status.
3. Administer IV fluids and blood products, as ordered, to maintain volume.
4. Monitor intake and output, as ordered, to evaluate renal perfusion and fluid status.
5. Maintain NG tube and NPO status to rest GI tract, as ordered.

Attaining Balanced Nutritional Status

1. Weigh daily to monitor caloric status.
2. Administer total parenteral nutrition (TPN), if ordered, to promote nutrition while on oral restrictions.
3. Begin oral liquids when NPO restriction is discontinued. Advance diet as tolerated. Diet should be high calorie and high protein. Small, frequent feedings may be indicated.
4. Offer snacks as tolerated; include high-protein liquid supplements.

Patient Education and Health Maintenance

1. Discuss the cause and treatment of GI bleeding with patient.
2. Instruct patient on reporting signs and symptoms of GI bleeding: melena, emesis that is bright red or "coffee-ground" color, rectal bleeding, weakness, fatigue, and shortness of breath.
3. Instruct patient on how to test stool or emesis for occult blood, if applicable.
4. Encourage follow-up with gastroenterologist and for screening tests as indicated.

Evaluation: Expected Outcomes

- Intake and output equal; vital signs stable.
- Tolerates small feedings; weight stable.

Peptic Ulcer Disease

Peptic ulcer disease refers to ulcerations in the mucosa of the lower esophagus, stomach, or duodenum (see Figure 14-7).

Pathophysiology and Etiology

1. Etiology of peptic ulcer disease is multifactorial.
a. *H. pylori* infection—present in most patients with peptic ulcer disease.
b. NSAID-induced injury—presents as a chemical gastropathy.
c. Acid secretory abnormalities (especially in duodenal ulcers).
d. Zollinger–Ellison syndrome (hypersecretory syndrome) should be considered in refractory ulcers.

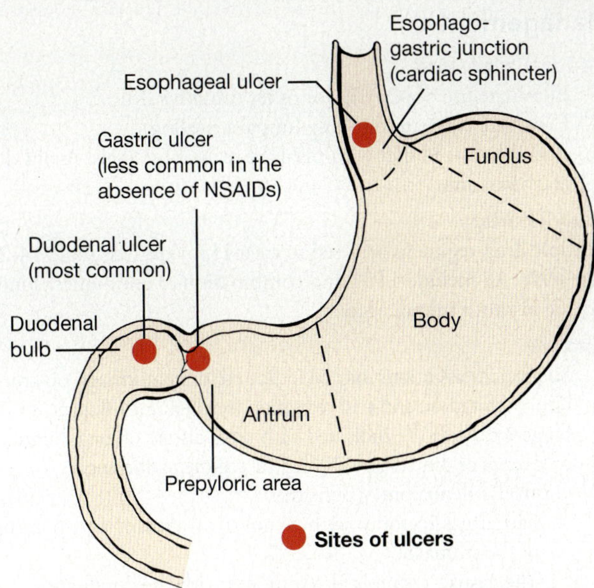

Figure 14-7. Esophageal, gastric, and duodenal ulcer sites. NSAIDs, nonsteroidal anti-inflammatory drugs.

2. Risk factors may include drugs (NSAIDs, prolonged high-dose corticosteroids), family history, Zollinger–Ellison syndrome, cigarettes, stress, O blood type, and lower socioeconomic status.
3. Studies are inconclusive in determining an association between ulcer formation and diet or the intake of alcohol and caffeine.

Clinical Manifestations

1. Gnawing or burning epigastric pain occurring 1.5 to 3 hours after a meal.
2. Nocturnal epigastric, abdominal pain or burning; may awaken patient at night, usually around midnight to 3 a.m.
3. Epigastric tenderness on examination.
4. Early satiety, anorexia, weight loss, heartburn, and belching (may indicate reflux disease).
5. Dizziness, syncope, hematemesis, or melena (may indicate hemorrhage).
6. Anemia.

CLINICAL JUDGMENT Sudden, intense midepigastric pain radiating to the right shoulder may indicate ulcer perforation. Report immediately.

Diagnostic Evaluation

1. Upper GI endoscopy with possible tissue biopsy and cytology.
a. PyloriTek, a biopsy urea test, is up to 97% specific and 96% sensitive for detection of *H. pylori*.
b. Point-of-service test with results within 1 hour.
2. Upper GI radiographic examination (barium study).
3. Serial stool specimens to detect occult blood.
4. Gastric secretory studies (gastric acid secretion test and fasting serum gastrin level)—elevated in Zollinger–Ellison syndrome.
5. Serology to test for *H. pylori* antibodies or stool test to assess for *H. pylori* antigen.
6. C-urea breath test to detect *H. pylori*.

DRUG ALERT Stop antisecretory PPI at least 2 weeks before the C-urea breath test. It can cause false-negative test result.

Management

General Measures

1. Eliminate use of NSAIDs or other causative drugs.
2. Eliminate cigarette smoking (impairs healing).
3. A well-balanced diet with meals at regular intervals. Avoid dietary irritants.

Drug Therapy

Multiple drug-regimens are used to treat H. pylori (see Table 14-2, page 492). All include a PPI and combination of antibiotics; some include bismuth subsalicylate.

Surgery

1. Surgical interventions may be indicated for hemorrhage, obstruction, perforation, and acid reduction (see Figure 14-8, page 493). Surgery may also be indicated with ulcer disease of long duration or severity or difficulty with medical regimen adherence.
2. Gastroduodenostomy (Billroth I).
   a. Partial gastrectomy with removal of antrum and pylorus of the stomach.
   b. The gastric stump is anastomosed with the duodenum.
3. Gastrojejunostomy (Billroth II).
   a. Partial gastrectomy with removal of antrum and pylorus of the stomach.
   b. The gastric stump is anastomosed with the jejunum.
4. Antrectomy.
   a. Gastric resection includes a small cuff of duodenum, the pylorus, and the antrum (lower half of the stomach).
   b. The duodenal stump is closed, and the jejunum is anastomosed to the stomach.
5. Total gastrectomy.
   a. Also called an *esophagojejunostomy*.
   b. Removal of the stomach with attachment of the esophagus to the jejunum or duodenum.
6. Pyloroplasty.
   a. A longitudinal incision is made in the pylorus, and it is closed transversely to permit the muscle to relax and to establish an enlarged outlet.
   b. Often, a vagotomy is performed at the same time.
7. Vagotomy.
   a. The surgical division of the vagus nerve to eliminate the impulses that stimulate HCl secretion.
   b. There are three types: *selective vagotomy*, which severs only the branches that interrupt acid secretion; *truncal vagotomy*, which severs the anterior and posterior trunks to decrease acid secretion and gastric motility; and *parietal vagotomy*, which severs only the part of vagus that innervates the parietal acid–secreting cells.
   c. Traditionally performed by laparotomy, the vagotomy procedure can also be done using a laparoscope.

Complications

1. GI hemorrhage.
2. Ulcer perforation.
3. Gastric outlet obstruction.

Nursing Assessment

1. Determine location, character, and radiation of pain, factors aggravating or relieving pain, how long it lasts, and when it occurs.
2. Ask about eating patterns, regularity, types of food, and eating circumstances.
3. Ask about medications (especially aspirin, NSAIDs, anticoagulants, and antiplatelet agents).
4. Inquire about a history of illnesses, including previous GI bleeds.
5. Obtain psychosocial history.
6. Perform physical assessment with documentation of positive abdominal findings.
7. Take vital signs, including lying, standing, and sitting BPs and pulses, to determine whether orthostasis is present due to bleeding.

Nursing Interventions

Avoiding Hypotension and Fluid Volume Deficit

1. Monitor vital signs frequently and observe for an increase in pulse and a decrease in BP (signs of shock).

Table 14-2 Medication Considerations for *Helicobacter pylori* Therapy

DRUG	DOSING	NURSING CONSIDERATIONS
Triple therapy: • PPI (omeprazole, lansoprazole, esomeprazole, pantoprazole, etc; standard dose) • Amoxicillin 1000mg • Clarithromycin 500mg or Metronidazole 500mg *(Antibiotics may be dosed sequentially each for 5 days, and PPI for total of 10 days).* **DRUG ALERT** Avoid treatment if patient may be pregnant.	bid × 14 days bid × 14 days bid × 14 days	• Antibiotics: Metronidazole and clarithromycin may cause unpleasant metallic taste, nausea, and vomiting; it may help to eat small, frequent meals, suck on sugar-free candy, take with food. Avoid alcohol within 72 h of taking metronidazole; can cause severe reaction. Clarithromycin may interact with lovastatin, salmeterol, phenytoin, and other medications; do not drink grapefruit juice during therapy. Report inability to take antibiotic or vomiting doses. Report watery or bloody diarrhea, which may indicate pseudomembranous colitis. • PPIs: may cause dizziness, headache, and stomach upset Best taken before meals Do not take with certain drugs, such as antiepileptics and warfarin.
Bismuth-based quadruple therapy: • PPI or H2 receptor blocker (famotidine; standard dose) • Bismuth subsalicylate 525mg • Metronidazole 250mg or Levofloxacin 500mg • Tetracycline 500mg	bid 10-14 days qid 10-14 days qid 10-14 days Daily 10-14 days qid 10-14 days	• Bismuth subsalicylate: interacts with many drugs, such as antiepileptics, salicylates, corticosteroids; may turn stool black; may interfere with radiologic testing of the GI tract. Report ringing in the ears, may indicate salicylate toxicity. • Tetracycline may increase sensitivity to sun; food and dairy products decrease absorption.

bid, two times a day; GI, gastrointestinal; H2, histamine 2; PPI, proton pump inhibitor; qid, four times a day.

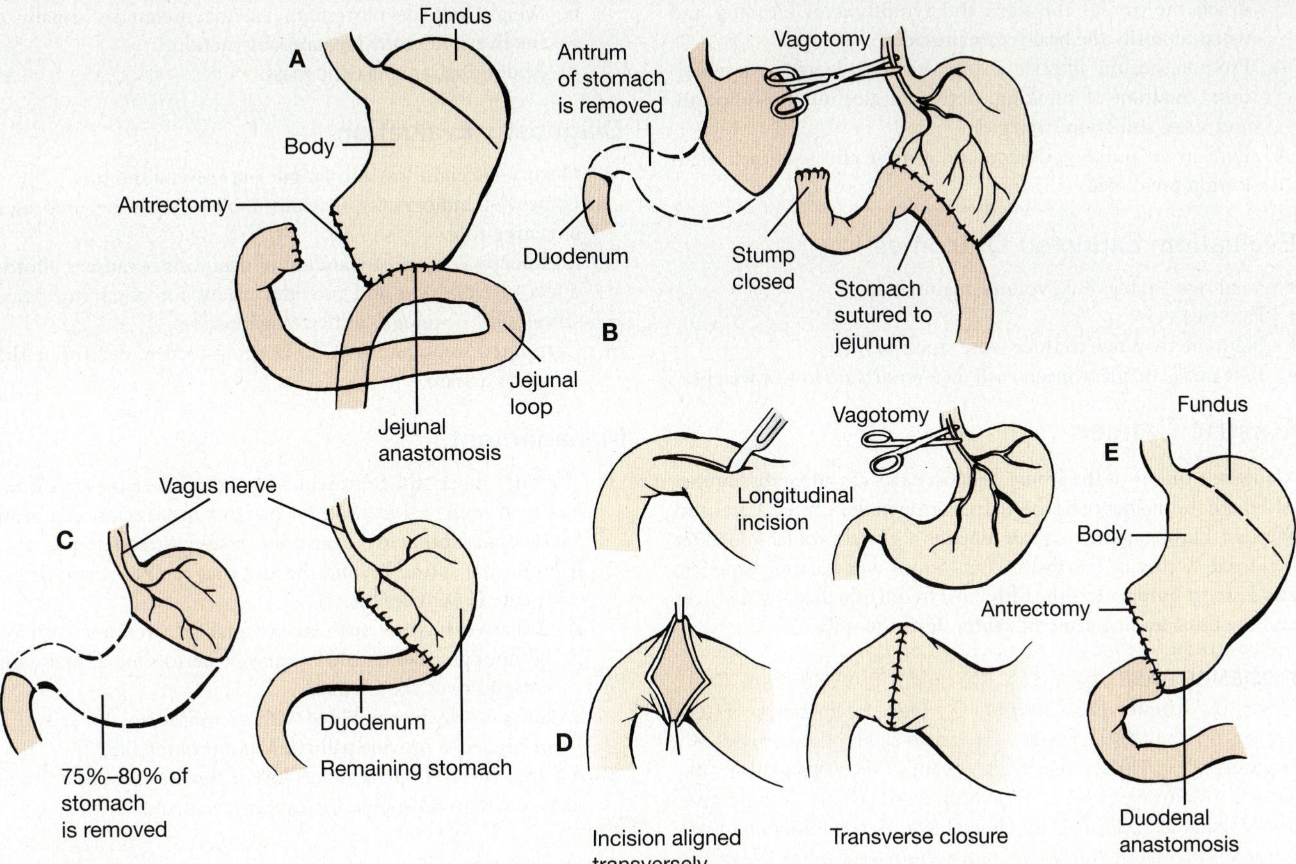

Figure 14-8. Surgical procedures for peptic ulcer. **(A)** Gastrojejunostomy (Billroth II). The jejunum is anastomosed to the gastric stump after a partial gastrectomy (removal of antrum and pylorus). **(B)** Antrectomy and vagotomy. The resected portion includes a small cuff of the duodenum, the pylorus, and the antrum (about one half of the stomach). The stump of the duodenum is closed by suture, and the side of the jejunum is anastomosed to the cut end of the stomach. **(C)** Subtotal gastrectomy. The resected portion includes a small cuff of the duodenum, the pylorus, and from two thirds to three quarters of the stomach. The duodenum or side of the jejunum is anastomosed to the remaining portion of the stomach. **(D)** Vagotomy and pyloroplasty. A longitudinal incision is made in the pylorus, and it is closed transversely to permit the muscle to relax and to establish an enlarged outlet. This compensates for the impaired gastric emptying produced by vagotomy. **(E)** Gastroduodenostomy (Billroth I). The duodenum is anastomosed to the gastric stump after removal of the antrum and pylorus (partial gastrectomy).

2. Monitor intake and output continuously to determine fluid volume status.
3. Monitor stools and emesis for blood.
4. Monitor hemoglobin and hematocrit and electrolytes.
5. Administer prescribed IV fluids and blood replacement, as prescribed.
6. Insert NG tube as prescribed, to remove clots and prepare patient for endoscopy.
7. Administer medications through the NG tube to neutralize acidity, as prescribed.
8. Prepare the patient for diagnostic procedure or surgery to determine or stop the source of bleeding.

Achieving Pain Relief

1. Administer prescribed medication.
2. Provide small, frequent meals to prevent gastric distention when NPO restriction is discontinued.
3. Advise the patient about the irritating effects of certain drugs and foods.

Decreasing Diarrhea

1. Monitor the patient's elimination patterns to determine the effects of medications.
2. Monitor intake and output, considering volume lost through the rectum and risk for dehydration.
3. Administer antidiarrheal medication as prescribed.
4. Watch for signs and symptoms of impaired skin integrity (erythema, discomfort, pruritus) around the anus and initiate protective measures, such as skin barrier to promote comfort and prevent breakdown.

Achieving Adequate Nutrition

1. Eliminate foods that cause pain or distress; otherwise, the diet is usually not restricted once NPO status is discontinued.
2. Provide small, frequent meals that neutralize gastric secretions and may be better tolerated.
3. Provide high-calorie, high-protein diet with nutritional supplements, as ordered.
4. Administer parenteral nutrition, as ordered, if bleeding is prolonged and patient is malnourished.

Patient Education and Health Maintenance

1. Explain all tests and procedures to increase knowledge and cooperation and minimize anxiety.
2. Review the health care provider's recommendations for diet, activity, medication, and treatment. Allow time for questions and clarify any misunderstandings.
3. Give the patient a chart listing medications, dosages, times of administration, and desired effects to promote adherence.

Teach the patient the signs and symptoms of bleeding and when to notify the health care provider.
4. Promote healthy lifestyle changes to include adequate nutrition, cessation of smoking, decreased alcohol consumption, and stress reduction strategies.
5. Explain the purpose, dosage, and adverse effects of each medication prescribed.

Evaluation: Expected Outcomes

- Vital signs stable; fluid volume maintained.
- Pain free.
- No more than two to three loose stools per day.
- Eats small, frequent meals each day; reports no loss of weight.

Gastric Cancer

Malignant tumor of the stomach; most cases are adenocarcinoma. Although the incidence has been decreasing in the United States and Western Europe, gastric cancer remains a global problem. Greater incidence occurs in Northeast Asia, South and Central America, and Eastern Europe. It is the fifth most frequently diagnosed cancer and the third leading cause of cancer deaths worldwide.

EVIDENCE BASE Ajani, J. A., D'Amico, T. A., Bentrem, D. J., Chao, J., Cooke, D., Corvera, C., Das, P., Enzinger, P. C., Enzler, T., Fanta, P., Farjah, F., Gerdes, H., Gibson, M. K., Hochwald, S., Hofstetter, W. L., Ilson, D. H., Keswani, R. N., Kim, S., Kleinber, L. R., … Pluchino, L. A. (2022). Gastric cancer, Version 2.2022, NCCN clinical practice guidelines in oncology. *Journal of National Comprehensive Cancer Network, 20*(2), 167–192. https://doi.org/10.6004/jnccn.2022.0008

Pathophysiology and Etiology

1. Gastric cancer occurs due to an imbalance between the normal process of cell proliferation and apoptosis (cell death). It is a slow process, with etiologic determinants being chemical carcinogen exposure and/or infection with *H. pylori*.
2. Major risk factors include *H. pylori* infection, smoking, older age, dietary factors such as high processed foods and high salt content, obesity, and heavy alcohol consumption. Other risk factors include a history of adenomatous gastric polyp, pernicious anemia, atrophic gastritis; family history of gastric cancer; and lower socioeconomic status.
3. Gastric adenocarcinoma arises from a single cell. Proximal tumors (in the cardia of the stomach) are becoming more common than distal tumors and have a worse prognosis.
4. Tumor growth may follow a polypoid, fungating, ulcerating, or diffusely infiltrative pattern.

Clinical Manifestations

1. Typically, patient presents with same symptoms as gastric ulcer; later, on evaluation, the lesion is found to be malignant.
2. Progressive loss of appetite, noticeable change in or appearance of common GI symptoms—gastric fullness (early satiety) and dyspepsia lasting longer than 4 weeks.
3. Blood (usually occult) in the stools.
4. Vomiting—may indicate pyloric obstruction or cardiac–orifice obstruction. Occasionally, vomiting has a coffee-ground appearance because of slow leaks of blood from ulceration of the cancer.
5. Later manifestations include the following:
   a. Pain, usually induced by eating and relieved by vomiting.
   b. Weight loss, loss of strength, anemia, metastasis (usually to the liver), hemorrhage, and obstruction.
   c. Abdominal or epigastric mass.

Diagnostic Evaluation

1. History—weight loss and fatigue over several months.
2. Upper GI radiography (barium swallow) may be used as a screening tool.
3. Endoscopy is the gold standard of diagnosis because it affords direct visualization and provides means for obtaining tissue samples for histologic and cytologic review.
4. Computed tomography (CT) imaging used to determine the extent of disease.

Management

1. The only successful treatment of gastric cancer is surgical removal. A preferred method for patients meeting criteria is an endoscopic submucosal dissection versus gastrectomy.
2. If tumor has spread beyond the area that can be excised surgically, cure is not possible.
   a. Palliative surgery, such as subtotal gastrectomy with or without gastroenterostomy, may be performed to maintain continuity of the GI tract.
   b. Surgery may be combined with chemotherapy for stage T2 or higher to provide palliation and prolong life.
3. A 5-year survival rate is about 70% if treated early, but plummets to 6% to 33% if gastric cancer has spread.

EVIDENCE BASE American Cancer Society. (2023). *Stomach cancer survival rates.* https://www.cancer.org/cancer/stomach-cancer/detection-diagnosis-staging/survival-rates.html

Complications

1. If surgery is performed, possible risk of hemorrhage or infection.
2. Dumping syndrome following gastrectomy.
3. Metastasis and death.

Nursing Assessment

1. Assess for anorexia, weight loss, and GI symptoms (gastric fullness, dyspepsia, vomiting).
2. Evaluate for pain, noting characteristics/location.
3. Check stool for occult blood, as directed.
4. Monitor CBC to assess for anemia.

Nursing Interventions

See "Caring for the Patient Undergoing Gastrointestinal Surgery" section, page 475.

Intestinal Conditions

Abdominal Hernias

An abdominal hernia occurs when the contents of the abdomen, usually the small intestine, push through a weak point in the muscular wall of the abdomen. The weakness of the abdominal wall can be congenital in nature, because of acquired weakness (e.g., aging or trauma) or because of increased intra-abdominal pressure (e.g., because of heavy lifting, obesity, pregnancy, straining, coughing, ascites, or proximity to tumor).

Pathophysiology and Etiology

Classification by Site

1. Inguinal—a hernia into the inguinal canal that is more common in males (see Figure 14-9). This type of hernia is further differentiated based on the causative factor.
   a. Indirect inguinal—congenital hernia that occurs when the entrance of the inguinal canal does not close after birth, causing a weakness in the abdominal wall. Through this weakened area, the hernia extends down the inguinal canal and often into the scrotum or labia.
   b. Direct inguinal—caused by degeneration of the abdominal muscles, allowing the small intestine to pass through the posterior inguinal wall into the groin.
2. Femoral—hernia follows the tract below the inguinal ligament through the femoral canal.
3. Umbilical—intestinal protrusion at the umbilicus because of failure of umbilical orifice to close. Occurs most often in females with obesity, in children, and in patients with increased intra-abdominal pressure from cirrhosis and ascites.
4. Ventral or incisional—intestinal protrusion because of weakness at the abdominal wall; may occur after impaired incisional healing because of infection or drainage.
5. Peristomal—hernia through the fascial defect around a stoma and into the subcutaneous tissue.

Classification by Severity

1. Reducible—the protruding mass can be placed back into the abdominal cavity.
2. Irreducible—the protruding mass cannot be moved back into the abdomen.
3. Incarcerated—an irreducible hernia in which the intestinal flow is completely obstructed.
4. Strangulated—an irreducible hernia in which the blood and intestinal flow are completely obstructed; develops when the loop of the intestine in the sac becomes twisted or swollen and a constriction is produced at the neck of the sac.

Clinical Manifestations

1. Bulging over herniated area appears when the patient stands or strains and disappears when supine.
2. Hernia tends to increase in size and recurs with intra-abdominal pressure.
3. Strangulated hernia presents with pain, vomiting, swelling of hernial sac, lower abdominal signs of peritoneal irritation, and fever.

Diagnostic Evaluation

1. Usually diagnosed by clinical manifestations:
2. Abdominal x-rays—reveal abnormally high levels of gas in the bowel.
3. Laboratory studies (CBC, electrolytes)—may show hemoconcentration (increased hematocrit), dehydration (increased or decreased sodium), and elevated white blood cell (WBC) count, if strangulated.

Management

1. Mechanical (reducible hernia only).
   a. A truss is an appliance with a pad and belt that is held snugly over a hernia to prevent abdominal contents from entering the hernial sac. A truss provides external compression over the defect and should be removed at night and reapplied in the morning before patient arises. This nonsurgical approach may be used only when a patient is not a surgical candidate.
   b. Peristomal hernia is often managed with a hernia support belt with Velcro, which is placed around an ostomy pouching system (similar to a truss).
   c. Conservative measures—no heavy lifting, straining at stool, or other measures that would increase intra-abdominal pressure.
2. Surgical—recommended to correct hernia before strangulation occurs, which then becomes an emergency situation.
   a. Herniorrhaphy—removal of hernial sac; contents replaced into the abdomen; layers of muscle and fascia sutured. Laparoscopic herniorrhaphy is a possibility and often performed as outpatient procedure.
   b. Hernioplasty involves reinforcement of suturing (often with mesh) for extensive hernia repair.
   c. Strangulated hernia requires resection of ischemic bowel in addition to repair of hernia.

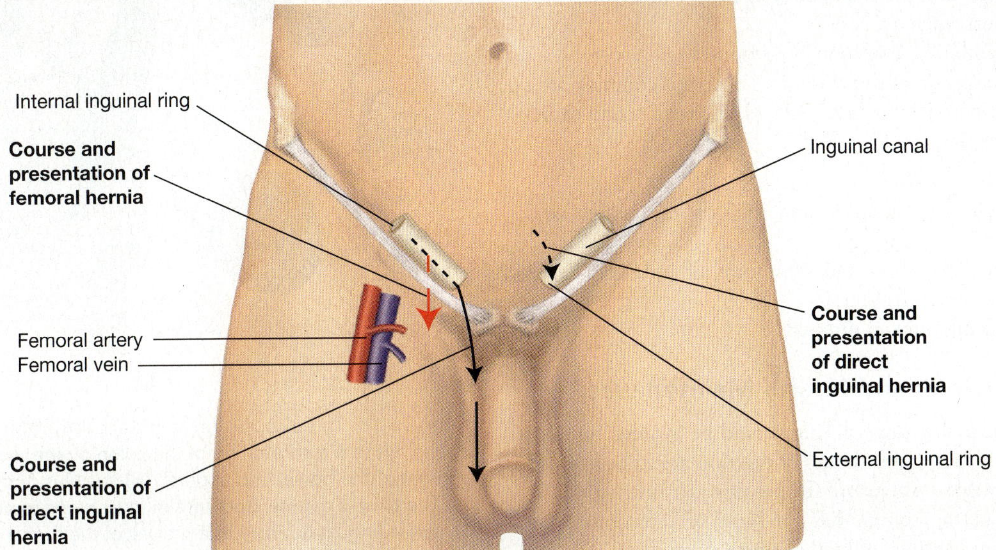

Figure 14-9. Direct and indirect inguinal hernia. (Reprinted with permission from Bickley, L. [2021]. *Bates' guide to physical examination and history taking* [13th ed., first figure in Table 20-5]. Lippincott Williams & Wilkins.)

Complications

1. Bowel obstruction.
2. Recurrence of hernia.

Nursing Assessment

1. Ask the patient if hernia is enlarging and uncomfortable, reducible or irreducible; determine relationship to exertion and activities.
2. Assess bowel sounds and determine bowel pattern.
3. Determine whether the patient is exhibiting signs and symptoms of strangulation, such as distention, fever, nausea, and vomiting.

Nursing Interventions

Achieving Comfort

1. Fit the patient with truss or belt when hernia is reduced, if ordered.
2. Trendelenburg position may reduce pressure on hernia, when appropriate.
3. Emphasize to the patient to wear truss under clothing and to apply before getting out of bed when hernia is reduced.
4. Advise that pain and scrotal swelling may be present for 24 to 48 hours after repair of an inguinal hernia.
   a. Apply ice intermittently.
   b. Elevate scrotum and use scrotal support.
   c. Take medication prescribed to relieve discomfort.
5. Give stool softeners, as directed.
6. Evaluate for signs and symptoms of hernial incarceration or strangulation.
7. Insert NG tube for incarcerated hernia, if ordered, to relieve intra-abdominal pressure on herniated sac.

Relieving Pain Postoperatively

1. Have the patient splint the incision site with hand or pillow when coughing to lessen pain and protect site from increased intra-abdominal pressure.
2. Advise the patient that scrotal swelling and pain may be present for 24 to 48 hours after repair of hernia.
   a. Administer analgesics and teach self-administration, as ordered.
   b. Apply ice intermittently.
   c. Elevate scrotum on small pillow or towel roll and use scrotal support when up.
3. Encourage ambulation as soon as permitted.
4. Advise the patient that difficulty in urinating is common after surgery; promote elimination to avoid discomfort, and catheterize if necessary.

Preventing Infection

1. Check dressing for drainage and incision for redness and swelling.
2. Monitor for other signs and symptoms of infection: fever, chills, malaise, and diaphoresis.
3. Administer antibiotics, as directed.

Patient Education and Health Maintenance

1. Inform patient that heavy lifting should be avoided for 4 to 6 weeks. Athletics and extremes of exertion are to be avoided for 8 to 12 weeks postoperatively, per provider instructions.
2. Teach patient to monitor self for signs of infection: pain, drainage from incision, and temperature elevation.
3. Advise patient to report continued difficulty in voiding or new urinary symptoms.

Evaluation: Expected Outcomes

- Hernia effectively reduced with truss or belt; patient comfortable.
- Verbalizes pain decreased to 2 or 3 on 0 to 10 scale.
- No swelling present; afebrile and no drainage from incision.

Intestinal Obstruction

Intestinal obstruction is an interruption in the normal flow of intestinal contents along the intestinal tract. The block may occur in the small or large intestine, may be complete or incomplete, may be mechanical or paralytic, and may or may not compromise the vascular supply. Obstruction most frequently occurs in the young and the old.

Pathophysiology and Etiology

Types and Causes

1. Mechanical obstruction—a physical block to passage of intestinal contents without disturbing blood supply of the bowel. High small bowel (jejunal) or low small bowel (ileal) obstruction occurs four times more frequently than colonic obstruction (see Figure 14-10). Causes include:
   a. Extrinsic—adhesions from surgery, hernia, wound dehiscence, masses, volvulus (twisted loop of the intestine). Up to 70% of small bowel obstructions are caused by adhesions.
   b. Intrinsic—hematoma, tumor, intussusception (telescoping of intestinal wall into itself), stricture or stenosis, congenital conditions (atresia, imperforate anus), trauma, inflammatory diseases (Crohn, diverticulitis, UC).
   c. Intraluminal—foreign body, fecal or barium impaction, polyp, gallstones, meconium in infants.
   d. In postoperative patients, approximately 90% of mechanical obstructions are due to adhesions. In nonsurgical patients, hernia (most often inguinal) is the most common cause of mechanical obstruction.

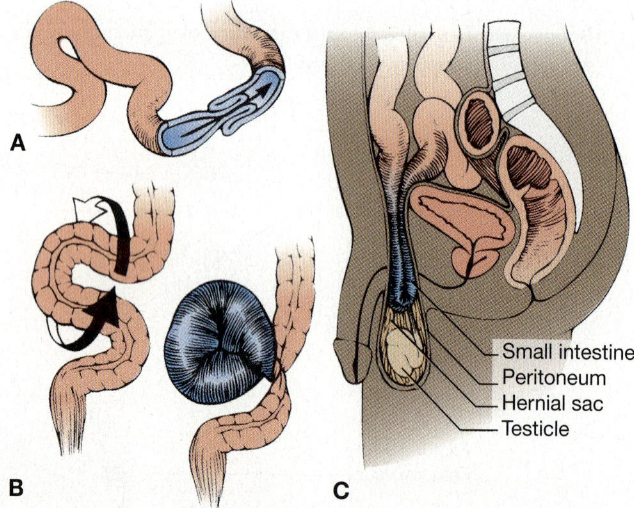

Figure 14-10. Three causes of intestinal obstruction. **(A)** Intussusception. Note the shortening of the colon by the movement of one segment of the bowel into another. **(B)** Volvulus of the sigmoid colon. The twist is counterclockwise in most cases of sigmoid volvulus. **(C)** Hernia (inguinal). Note that the sac of the hernia is a continuation of the peritoneum of the abdomen and that the hernial contents are the intestine, omentum, or other abdominal contents that pass through the hernial opening into the hernial sac.

2. Paralytic (adynamic, neurogenic) ileus.
   a. Peristalsis is ineffective (diminished motor activity perhaps because of toxic or traumatic disturbance of the autonomic nervous system).
   b. There is no physical obstruction and no interrupted blood supply.
   c. Disappears spontaneously after 2 to 3 days.
   d. Causes include:
      i. Spinal cord injuries; vertebral fractures.
      ii. Postoperatively after any abdominal surgery.
      iii. Peritonitis, pneumonia.
      iv. Wound dehiscence (breakdown).
      v. GI tract surgery.
3. Strangulation—obstruction compromises blood supply, leading to gangrene of the intestinal wall. Caused by prolonged mechanical obstruction.

Altered Physiology

1. Increased peristalsis, distention by fluid and gas, and increased bacterial growth proximal to obstruction. The intestine empties distally.
2. Increased secretions into the intestine are associated with diminution in the bowel's absorptive capacity.
3. The accumulation of gases, secretions, and oral intake above the obstruction causes increasing intraluminal pressure.
4. Venous pressure in the affected area increases, and circulatory stasis and edema result.
5. Bowel necrosis may occur because of anoxia and compression of the terminal branches of the mesenteric artery.
6. Bacteria and toxins pass across the intestinal membranes into the abdominal cavity, thereby leading to peritonitis.
7. "Closed-loop" obstruction is a condition in which the intestinal segment is occluded at both ends, preventing either the downward passage or the regurgitation of intestinal contents.

Clinical Manifestations

Fever, peritoneal irritation, increased WBC count, toxicity, and shock may develop with all types of intestinal obstruction.

1. Simple mechanical—high small bowel: colic (cramps); mid to upper abdomen, some distention, early bilious vomiting, increased bowel sounds (high-pitched tinkling heard at brief intervals), minimal diffuse tenderness.
2. Simple mechanical—low small bowel: significant colic (cramps), midabdominal, considerable distention, vomiting slight or absent, later feculent, increased bowel sounds and "hush" sounds, minimal diffuse tenderness.
3. Simple mechanical—colon: cramps (mid to lower abdomen), later-appearing distention, and then vomiting may develop (feculent); increase in bowel sounds; minimal diffuse tenderness.
4. Partial chronic mechanical—may occur with granulomatous bowel in Crohn disease. Symptoms are cramping, abdominal pain, mild distention, and diarrhea.
5. Strangulation symptoms are initially those of mechanical obstruction, but progress rapidly—pain is severe, continuous, and localized. There is moderate distention, persistent vomiting, usually decreased bowel sounds, and marked localized tenderness. Stools or vomitus becomes bloody or contains occult blood.

Diagnostic Evaluation

1. Fecal material aspiration from NG tube.
2. Abdominal and chest x-rays.
   a. May show presence and location of small or large intestinal distention, gas, or fluid.
   b. "Bird beak" lesion in colonic volvulus.
   c. Foreign body visualization.
3. Contrast studies—small bowel follow-through with water-soluble contrast (e.g., Gastrografin) can be both diagnostic and therapeutic.
4. Laboratory tests.
   a. Electrolytes, blood urea nitrogen (BUN), and creatinine may be abnormal because of hypovolemia and vomiting.
   b. Elevated WBC counts because of inflammation; marked increase with necrosis, strangulation, or peritonitis.
   c. Lactate level may be increased if ischemia of small bowel is present.
5. Flexible sigmoidoscopy or colonoscopy may identify the source of the obstruction, such as tumor or stricture.

Management

Nonsurgical Management

1. Correction of fluid and electrolyte imbalances with normal saline or Ringer's solution with potassium as required.
2. NG suction to decompress bowel and decrease risk of perforation. Small bowel follow-through with water-soluble contrast (e.g., Gastrografin).
3. Treatment of shock and peritonitis.
4. TPN may be necessary to correct protein deficiency from chronic obstruction, paralytic ileus, or infection.
5. Analgesics and sedatives, avoiding opiates because of GI motility inhibition.
6. Antibiotics to prevent or treat infection.
7. Ambulation for patients with paralytic ileus to encourage return of peristalsis.

Surgery

Consists of relieving obstruction. Options include:

1. Closed bowel procedures: lysis of adhesions, reduction of volvulus, intussusception, or incarcerated hernia.
2. Enterotomy for removal of foreign bodies or bezoars.
3. Resection of the bowel for obstructing lesions or strangulated bowel with end-to-end anastomosis.
4. Intestinal bypass around obstruction.
5. Temporary ostomy may be indicated (see "Caring for the Patient Undergoing Ostomy Surgery" section, page 478).

Complications

1. Dehydration because of loss of water, sodium, and chloride.
2. Peritonitis.
3. Shock because of loss of electrolytes and dehydration.
4. Death because of shock.

Nursing Assessment

1. Assess the nature and location of the patient's pain and the presence or absence of distention, flatus, defecation, emesis, and obstipation.
2. Listen for high-pitched bowel sounds, peristaltic rushes, or the absence of bowel sounds.
3. Assess vital signs.

POPULATION AWARENESS Watch for air–fluid lock syndrome in older patients, who typically remain in the recumbent position for extended periods. Fluid collects in dependent bowel loops, and peristalsis is too weak to push fluid "uphill." Conduct frequent checks of the patient's level of responsiveness; decreasing responsiveness may offer a clue to a worsening electrolyte imbalance or impending shock.

Nursing Interventions

Maintaining Adequate Lung Ventilation

1. Keep the patient in Fowler position to promote ventilation and relieve abdominal distention.
2. Maintain NG tube as prescribed to decompress bowel.
3. Monitor respiratory rate, breath sounds, and oxygen saturation, or arterial blood gas (ABG) levels, as indicated.

Maintaining Electrolyte and Fluid Balance

1. Measure and record all intake and output, including NG drainage and liquidy stool output.
2. Administer IV fluids and parenteral nutrition as prescribed.
3. Monitor electrolytes, urinalysis, hemoglobin, and blood cell counts, and report any abnormalities. Collect stool samples to test for occult blood, if ordered.
4. Explain the rationale for NG suction, NPO status, and IV fluids initially, to rest bowel and try to relieve obstruction, or prepare for surgery.
5. Maintain urinary catheter if there is urine retention because of bladder compressions by the distended intestine.
6. Monitor vital signs; a drop in BP or increased pulse may indicate decreased circulatory volume because of blood loss from strangulated hernia.

Achieving Pain Relief

1. Administer prescribed analgesics.
2. Provide supportive care during NG intubation to assist with discomfort.
3. To relieve air–fluid lock syndrome, turn the patient from supine to prone position every 10 minutes until enough flatus is passed to decompress the abdomen. A rectal tube may be indicated.
4. To reduce fear and anxiety associated with pain, recognize the patient's concerns and initiate measures to provide emotional support. Encourage presence of support person.

Ensuring GI Perfusion to Prevent Complications

1. Prevent infarction by carefully assessing the patient's status; pain that increases in intensity or becomes localized or continuous may herald strangulation.
2. Detect early signs of peritonitis, such as rigidity and tenderness, in an effort to minimize this complication.
3. Avoid enemas, which may distort an x-ray or make a partial obstruction worse.
4. Observe for signs of shock—pallor, tachycardia, hypotension.
5. Watch for signs of:
   a. Metabolic alkalosis (slow, shallow respirations; changes in sensorium; tetany).
   b. Metabolic acidosis (disorientation; deep, rapid breathing; weakness; and shortness of breath on exertion).

Patient Education and Health Maintenance

1. Advise plenty of rest and slow progression of activity as directed by surgeon or other health care provider.
2. Teach wound care, if indicated.
3. Advise slow progression of diet, as tolerated, once home.
4. Encourage the patient to follow up as directed and to call surgeon or health care provider if increasing abdominal pain, vomiting, or fever occurs prior to follow-up.

Evaluation: Expected Outcomes

- Respirations 20/min and unlabored with head of bed elevated 45 degrees.
- Urine output greater than 30 mL/h; vital signs stable.
- Maintains position of comfort; states pain decreased to 3 or 4 on 0 to 10 scale.
- Alert and oriented, vital signs stable, abdomen firm, not rigid.

Appendicitis

Appendicitis is inflammation of the vermiform appendix caused by an obstruction of the intestinal lumen from infection, stricture, fecal mass, foreign body, or tumor.

Pathophysiology and Etiology

1. Obstruction is followed by edema, infection, and ischemia.
2. As intraluminal tension develops, necrosis and perforation usually occur.
3. Appendicitis can affect any age group; most common in adolescents/young adults, especially males.

Clinical Manifestations

1. Generalized or localized abdominal pain in the epigastric or periumbilical areas and upper right abdomen. Within 2 to 12 hours, the pain localizes in the right lower quadrant and intensity increases.
2. Anorexia, moderate malaise, mild fever, nausea, and vomiting.
3. Usually, constipation occurs, occasionally diarrhea.
4. Rebound tenderness, involuntary guarding, generalized abdominal rigidity.

Diagnostic Evaluation

1. Physical examination consistent with clinical manifestations.
2. WBC count reveals moderate leukocytosis (10,000 to 16,000/mm^3) with shift to the left (increased immature neutrophils).
3. Urinalysis to rule out urinary disorders.
4. Abdominal x-ray may visualize shadow consistent with fecalith in the appendix; perforation will reveal free air.
5. Abdominal ultrasound or CT scan can visualize the appendix and rule out other conditions, such as diverticulitis and Crohn disease. Focused appendiceal CT can quickly evaluate for appendicitis.

POPULATION AWARENESS In older adults, be aware of vague symptoms: milder pain, less pronounced fever, and leukocytosis with shift to the left on differential.

Management

EVIDENCE BASE Podda, M., Poillucci, G., Pacella, D., Mortola, L., Canfora, A., Aresu, S., Pisano, M., Erdas, E., Pisanu, A., & Cillara, N. (2021). Appendectomy versus conservative treatment with antibiotics for patients with uncomplicated acute appendicitis: A propensity score-matched analysis of patient-centered outcomes (the ACTUAA prospective multicenter trial). *International Journal of Colorectal Disease, 36*(3), 589–598. https://doi.org/10.1007/s00384-021-03843-8

1. Antibiotics and careful monitoring for uncomplicated/unperforated appendicitis.
2. Surgery (appendectomy) is the preferred treatment when indicated.

a. Simple appendectomy or laparoscopic appendectomy in the absence of rupture or peritonitis.
b. An incisional drain may be placed if an abscess or rupture occurs.
3. Preoperatively maintain bed rest, NPO status, IV hydration, possible antibiotic prophylaxis, and analgesia.

Complications

1. Perforation (in 95% of cases).
2. Abscess.
3. Peritonitis.

Nursing Assessment

1. Obtain a history for location and extent of pain.
2. Auscultate for the presence of bowel sounds; peristalsis may be absent or diminished.
3. On palpation of the abdomen, assess for tenderness anywhere in the right lower quadrant, but usually localized over McBurney point (point just below midpoint of line between the umbilicus and iliac crest on the right side). Assess for rebound tenderness in the right lower quadrant as well as referred rebound when palpating the left lower quadrant.
4. Assess for positive psoas sign by having the patient attempt to raise the right thigh against the pressure of your hand placed over the right knee. Inflammation of the psoas muscle in acute appendicitis will increase abdominal pain with this maneuver.
5. Assess for positive obturator sign by flexing the patient's right hip and knee and rotating the leg internally. Hypogastric pain with this maneuver indicates inflammation of the obturator muscle.

DRUG ALERT Do not give antipyretics, which may mask fever, and do not administer laxatives/cathartics because they may cause rupture.

Nursing Interventions and Patient Education

See page 475, Caring for the Patient Undergoing Gastrointestinal Surgery.

Diverticular Disease

EVIDENCE BASE Bailey, J., Dattani, S., & Jennings, A. (2022). Diverticular disease: Rapid evidence review. *American Family Physician, 106*(2), 150–156. PMID: 35977135

Diverticular disease encompasses the intestinal problems that can be caused by diverticula. A *diverticulum* is a pouch or saccular dilation of the colon wall. *Diverticulosis* is a condition exhibiting multiple diverticula without inflammation. *Diverticulitis* is inflammation and infection of one or more diverticula. Diverticular disease is usually categorized into complicated or uncomplicated disease. Incidence of diverticular disease has been increasing.

Pathophysiology and Etiology

Diverticulosis

1. Marks the formation of diverticula, which are herniations of the mucosal and submucosal layers of the colon developing at weak points where nutrient blood vessels penetrate the colon wall (see Figure 14-11).
2. Causes for diverticular disease are unclear, but data suggest excessive intraluminal pressure plays a key role. A contributing factor may be a low-residue diet, which reduces fecal residue, narrows the bowel lumen, and leads to higher pressure intra-abdominally during defecation.
3. The prevalence of diverticulosis increases with age, to about 80% by age 85.

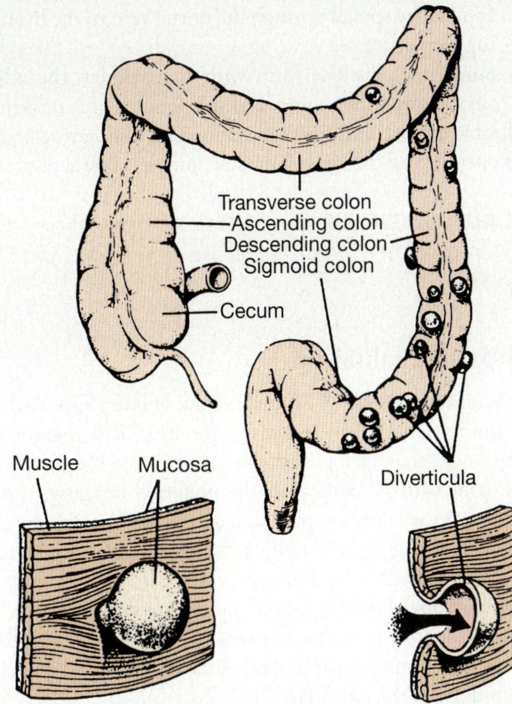

Figure 14-11. Diverticula are most common in the sigmoid colon; they diminish in number and size as the colon approaches the cecum. Diverticula are rarely found in the rectum.

Diverticulitis

1. Results when one or more diverticula become inflamed and usually perforate the thin diverticular wall, which consists of mucosal and serosal layers. The exact cause is unknown but postulated to be caused by stasis or obstruction of the diverticula, leading to bacterial overgrowth, inflammation, and ischemia.
2. *Complicated diverticulitis* refers to diverticular disease that has led to abscess, perforation, fistula, stricture, or obstruction.
3. Uninflamed or minimally inflamed diverticula may erode adjacent arterial branches, causing acute massive rectal bleeding.
4. It is estimated that only 1% to 4% of people with diverticulosis will develop diverticulitis in their lifetime.

Clinical Manifestations

Diverticulosis

1. May be asymptomatic.
2. Crampy abdominal pain.
3. Bowel irregularity—constipation or diarrhea.
4. Periodic abdominal distention.
5. Sudden massive hemorrhage may be the first symptom.

Diverticulitis

1. Left lower quadrant pain.
2. Low-grade fever, chills, leukocytosis.
3. Abdominal distension and rigidity may be present.
4. Urinary frequency and dysuria are associated with bladder involvement in the inflammatory process.
5. Complicated diverticulitis occurs when ruptured diverticula produce abscesses or peritonitis with abdominal rigidity; signs of shock and sepsis (hypotension, chills, high fever). Near a blood vessel, a rupture may cause massive hemorrhage.

a. Sepsis may spread through the portal vein to the liver, causing liver abscesses.
b. Sometimes, fistulae form with the bladder, the adjacent small bowel, the vagina, and the perianal area or skin.

6. Chronic diverticulitis may cause adhesions that narrow the bowel's opening and can cause partial or complete bowel obstruction.

CLINICAL JUDGMENT Tenderness on palpation of the left lower quadrant alone is the most specific finding for diverticulitis.

Diagnostic Evaluation

1. Laboratory studies: WBC may show leukocytosis with shift to the left; elevated C-reactive protein (CRP); hemoglobin/hematocrit may be low with chronic or acute bleeding.
2. CT scan with IV contrast is the preferred imaging study because it is the most accurate in correctly identifying diverticulitis and in staging its severity. CT guidance can also be used if an abscess needs to be drained.
3. Colonoscopy should not be done during an acute attack but should be done 6 weeks after resolution of symptoms, for patients with complicated diverticulitis, if a colonoscopy has not been done in the past year.
4. Barium enema (after infection subsides)—may visualize diverticular sacs, narrowing of colonic lumen, partial or complete obstruction, or fistulae. In patients with acute diverticulitis, a barium enema may rupture the bowel.

Management

Diverticulosis

EVIDENCE BASE Aune, D., Sen, A., Norat, T., & Riboli, E. (2020). Dietary fibre intake and the risk of diverticular disease: A systematic review and meta-analysis of prospective studies. *European Journal of Nutrition, 59*(2), 421–432. https://doi.org/10.1007/s00394-019-01967-w

1. Vegetarian or high-quality diet (rich in fruit, vegetables, whole grains, and legumes); limited red meat and sweets have been shown to reduce the incidence of diverticulitis. There is no compelling evidence that a high-fiber diet will prevent recurrence of diverticulitis.
2. Normal body mass index, physical activity, and avoidance of tobacco are also recommended for prevention.
3. Avoidance of long-term use of NSAIDs may also be preventative (except low-dose aspirin for cardiovascular secondary prevention).

Uncomplicated Diverticulitis

1. Medical management.
   a. Research has shown that antibiotic treatment may not be necessary but can be used selectively in those with mild acute symptoms. It is strongly recommended for patients who are immunocompromised.
   b. For more severe symptoms, patient may be treated with modified diet, bowel rest, and oral or IV broad-spectrum antibiotic.
2. Surgical management.
   a. Elective partial colectomy is not routinely recommended but may be considered on an individual basis depending on disease severity, comorbidities, and complications.

Complicated Diverticulitis

Treatment is dependent upon the associated complication that has occurred.

1. Abscess—may be managed with bowel rest and antibiotics while under close observation; however, percutaneous drainage may be needed if patient becomes septic. Sigmoid resection may also be considered for multiple abscesses.
2. Perforation—surgical resection of the diseased area with possible colostomy (Hartmann procedure) may be necessary.
3. Fistulae—may require surgical repair depending on the type of fistula and its associated symptoms.
4. Stricture/obstruction—if the obstruction is complete, surgery is required. If a partial obstruction has occurred, bowel rest, IV hydration, and possible antibiotics may successfully treat symptoms.
5. Hemorrhage—NPO, IV fluids, blood transfusion as necessary, and NG tube placement. Colonoscopy to identify source of bleeding.
   a. If colonoscopy is not successful in identifying source of bleeding, a technetium 99–labeled red blood cell scan will be done.
   b. Mesenteric angiography is an alternative study that may be used and has potential to be therapeutic, because the bleeding source can be thrombosed if identified.
   c. Surgical resection is not typical, because this type of hemorrhage is usually self-limited.

Complications

1. Hemorrhage from colonic diverticula, usually in the right colon.
2. Bowel obstruction.
3. Fistula formation (colovesical fistula is the most common).
4. Septicemia.
5. Perforation.

Nursing Assessment

1. Have the patient describe the amount of fiber and fluid intake per day and past and present bowel patterns. Any constipation, diarrhea, or alternating of both?
2. Ask if experiencing abdominal cramping or pain, bloody stools, or stool/gas passage from the vagina or in urine.
3. Watch for signs and symptoms of peritonitis: increasing abdominal pain, guarding, rebound tenderness, abdominal distention, and nausea/vomiting.
4. Monitor vital signs: Temperature may be elevated; tachycardia and hypotension may indicate peritonitis/massive bleeding.

Nursing Interventions

Maintaining Fluid Balance

1. Maintain NPO status and NG suction until bowel sounds return.
2. Provide IV fluid as directed and prepare for blood transfusion if indicated.
3. Monitor intake and output, including NG aspirate.
4. Report any occult or frank blood in stool, tachycardia, drop in BP, fever, or increased pain.

Achieving Pain Relief

1. Observe for signs and location of pain, type, and severity, and intervene when appropriate.
   a. Administer nonopiate analgesics as prescribed (opiates may mask signs of perforation).
   b. Administer anticholinergics, as prescribed, to decrease colon spasm.
2. Auscultate bowel sounds to monitor bowel motility.
3. Advise the patient to report left lower quadrant pain, generalized abdominal tenderness, and fever, which may signal complication.
4. Palpate abdomen to determine rigidity or tenderness caused by perforation or peritonitis.

Promoting Normal Bowel Elimination

1. Follow prescribed diet that is low residue and low in sugar to promote bowel rest during acute phase.
2. Review patient's dietary pattern and recommend diet that is high in fruits, vegetables, whole grains, and legumes; and low in red meat and sugar once acute episode has resolved.
3. Monitor weight and determine patient's nutritional needs to attain ideal body mass index.
4. Observe and record color, consistency, and frequency of stools.
5. Encourage oral fluids to promote bowel stimulation.

Patient Education and Health Maintenance

1. Explain the disease process to the patient and its relationship to diet and healthy lifestyle.
2. Encourage medical and surgical follow-up and reporting any worsening symptoms, especially left lower quadrant abdominal pain.
3. Emphasize the importance of establishing regular bowel habits through diet, physical activity, fluid intake, and regular schedule of elimination.
4. Refer to nutritionist, as needed.

Evaluation: Expected Outcomes

- No change in vital signs; stool negative for occult blood.
- Expresses relief of pain and has a decrease in symptoms.
- Reports daily bowel movements (BMs).

Peritonitis

Peritonitis occurs when bacteria or other microorganisms cause a generalized or localized inflammation of the peritoneum, the membrane lining the abdominal cavity and abdominal organs (see Figure 14-12).

Pathophysiology and Etiology

1. Primary peritonitis, also known as *spontaneous bacterial peritonitis* (SBP), occurs when bacteria cross through the intestinal wall into the peritoneum, causing infection. SBP can occur in patients with cirrhosis, nephrotic syndrome, and ovarian diseases (e.g., cancer).
2. Secondary peritonitis is due to perforation, rupture of an organ, trauma, or peritoneal dialysis.

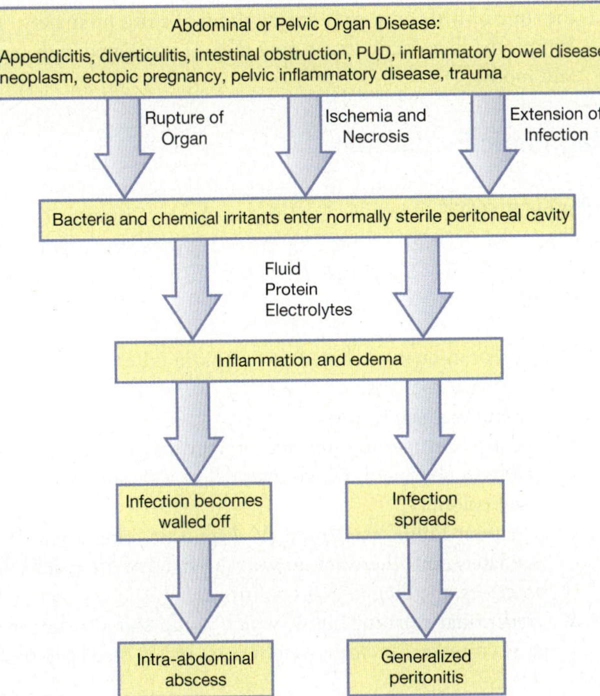

Figure 14-12. Pathophysiology of peritonitis. PUD, peptic ulcer disease.

Clinical Manifestations

1. Initially, local type of abdominal pain tends to become constant, diffuse, and more intense.
2. The abdomen becomes extremely tender, and muscles become rigid; rebound tenderness and ileus may be present; the patient lies very still, usually with legs drawn up.
3. Percussion: resonance and tympany because of paralytic ileus; loss of liver dullness may indicate free air in the abdomen.
4. Auscultation: decreased bowel sounds.
5. Nausea and vomiting often occur; peristalsis diminishes; anorexia is present.
6. Elevation of temperature and pulse as well as leukocytosis.
7. Fever; thirst; oliguria; dry, swollen tongue; signs of dehydration.
8. Weakness, pallor, diaphoresis, and cold skin are the results of the loss of fluid, electrolytes, and protein into the abdomen.
9. Hypotension, tachycardia, and hypokalemia may occur.
10. With generalized peritonitis, large volumes of fluid may be lost into abdominal cavity (ascites). Shallow respirations may result from abdominal distention and upward displacement of the diaphragm.

Diagnostic Evaluation

1. WBC count to determine whether leukocytosis is present (leukopenia if severe).
2. ABG levels may show hypoxemia or metabolic acidosis with respiratory compensation.
3. Urinalysis may indicate urinary tract problems as primary source.
4. Peritoneal aspiration (paracentesis) to demonstrate blood, pus, bile, bacteria (Gram stain), amylase.
5. Abdominal x-rays may show free air in the peritoneal cavity, gas and fluid collection in small and large intestines, generalized bowel dilation, intestinal wall edema.
6. CT scan of the abdomen or sonography may reveal intra-abdominal mass, abscess, ascites.
7. Radionuclide scans (gallium, hepatobiliary iminodiacetic acid, and liver/spleen scan) may identify an intra-abdominal abscess.
8. Chest x-ray may show elevated diaphragm.
9. Exploratory laparotomy may be performed to identify the underlying cause.

Management

1. Treatment of inflammatory conditions preoperatively and postoperatively with antibiotic therapy may prevent peritonitis. Broad-spectrum antibiotic therapy to cover aerobic and anaerobic organisms is the initial treatment, followed by specific antibiotic therapy after culture and sensitivity results.
2. Bed rest, NPO status, and respiratory support, if needed.
3. IV fluids and electrolytes, possibly TPN.
4. Analgesics for pain; antiemetics for nausea and vomiting.
5. NG intubation to decompress the bowel.
6. Possibly rectal tube to facilitate passage of gas.
7. Operative procedures to close perforations, remove infection source (i.e., inflamed organ, necrotic tissue), drain abscesses, and lavage peritoneal cavity.
8. Abdominal paracentesis may be done to remove accumulating fluid.

9. Blood transfusions, if appropriate.
10. Oral feedings after return of bowel sounds and passage of gas and/or feces.

Complications

1. Intra-abdominal abscess formation (i.e., pelvic subphrenic space).
2. Septicemia.
3. Hypovolemic problems.
4. Renal or liver failure.
5. Respiratory insufficiency.

Nursing Assessment

1. Assess for abdominal distention and tenderness, guarding, rebound, hypoactive or absent bowel sounds to determine bowel function.
2. Observe for signs of shock—tachycardia and hypotension.
3. Monitor vital signs, ABG levels, CBC, electrolytes, and central venous pressure to monitor hemodynamic status and assess for complications.

Nursing Interventions

Maintaining Fluid and Electrolyte Volume

1. Keep the patient NPO to reduce peristalsis.
2. Provide IV fluids to establish adequate fluid intake and to promote adequate urine output, as prescribed.
3. Record accurately intake and output, including the measurement of vomitus and NG drainage.
4. Minimize nausea, vomiting, and distention by use of NG suction, antiemetics.
5. Monitor for signs of hypovolemia: dry mucous membranes, oliguria, postural hypotension, tachycardia, diminished skin turgor. Report to health care provider.

Achieving Pain Relief

1. Maintain semi-Fowler position to enhance comfort and breathing pattern.
2. Provide analgesics as prescribed, monitor for adverse reactions, assess effectiveness, and advocate for dosage change as needed.

Achieving Adequate Nutrition

1. Administer TPN, as ordered, to maintain positive nitrogen balance until patient can resume oral diet.
2. Reduce parenteral fluids and give oral food and fluids per order when the following occur:
   a. Temperature and pulse return to normal.
   b. Abdomen becomes soft.
   c. Peristaltic sounds return (determined by abdominal auscultation).
   d. Flatus is passed, and patient has BMs.

Patient Education and Health Maintenance

1. Teach the patient and family how to care for open wounds and drain sites, if appropriate.
2. Assess the need for home care nursing to assist with wound care and assess healing; refer as necessary.
3. Encourage follow-up as directed and reporting of increased pain, fever, and anorexia.

Evaluation: Expected Outcomes

- Balanced intake and output; no evidence of dehydration.
- States pain reduced to 3 or less on 0 to 10 scale.
- Bowel sounds present; tolerating soft diet.

Irritable Bowel Syndrome

Irritable bowel syndrome (IBS) is a functional bowel disorder characterized by abdominal pain and altered bowel function. It is the most common functional GI disorder and is estimated to affect 10% of people worldwide.

EVIDENCE BASE Lacy, B. E., Pimentel, M., Brenner, D. M., Chey, W. D., Keefer, L. A., Long, M. D., & Moshiree, B. (2021). ACG clinical guideline: Management of irritable bowel syndrome. *American Journal of Gastroenterology, 116*(1), 17–44. https://doi.org/10.14309/ajg.0000000000001036

Pathophysiology and Etiology

The exact etiology of IBS is unknown. Pathophysiology involves disordered communication between the gut and the brain, leading to motility disturbance, visceral hypersensitivity, and altered central nervous system processing. IBS is not a life-threatening disorder, and surgery is not necessary. It does not transform into inflammatory bowel disease and does not increase the risk for colorectal cancer. It is most common in young adult to middle-aged females.

Clinical Manifestations

1. Functional abnormalities vary and may come and go, leading to a chronic problem.
2. Symptoms may include:
   a. Lower abdominal pain.
   b. Diarrhea, constipation, or alternating of both.
   c. Bloating, distention.
   d. Mucous drainage.
   e. Fecal urgency, feeling of incomplete evacuation.
3. Patients usually have a characteristic pain pattern ranging from pain in the postprandial period, occurring before or at the time of BM, or arising during times of stress or anxiety.
4. Symptoms that occur after eating may be associated with certain foods.

Diagnostic Evaluation

EVIDENCE BASE Ford, A. C., Serber, A. D., Corsetti, M., & Camilleri, M. (2020). Irritable bowel syndrome. *Lancet, 396*(10263), 1675–1688. https://doi.org/10.1016/S0140-6736(20)31548-8

1. Diagnosis can be made based on symptom criteria, in the absence of warning signs.
   a. Careful medical history.
   b. Rectal examination—normal or tenderness at left lower quadrant abdomen, which may reflect a spasm in the sigmoid colon.
   c. If patient fulfills the Rome IV diagnostic criteria for IBS (see later), and there are no warning signs of other disease processes, the diagnosis is confirmed.
   d. Traditional warning signs, which could signal other organic diseases, include weight loss, rectal bleeding, and

family history of inflammatory bowel disease or celiac disease.

2. Rome IV diagnostic criteria include recurrent abdominal pain or discomfort at least 3 days per month in the past 3 months associated with two or more of the following:
   a. Improvement in abdominal pain or discomfort with defecation.
   b. Onset associated with a change in frequency of stool.
   c. Onset associated with a change in form or appearance of stool.
3. Tests to rule out other disease processes include:
   a. Serology testing for celiac disease, in cases with diarrhea.
   b. Fecal calprotectin to rule out inflammatory bowel disease, in cases of diarrhea.
   c. Other testing such as CBC, CT imaging, and colonoscopy may be considered if other symptoms are present.

Management

1. Treatment should focus on management of symptoms through education, dietary awareness, addition of soluble fiber, and use of antispasmodic agents and other medications for severe symptoms, according to bowel habit. Keeping a diary of symptoms and possible triggers for several weeks may help provide information on how to individually manage IBS.
   a. Emotional stress, anticipation of stressful interactions, depression, or mood changes can exacerbate symptoms of IBS.
   b. Stress-relieving activities such as yoga, journaling, and deep breathing exercises may be helpful; or professional gut-directed psychotherapy, using techniques such as cognitive behavioral therapy, may be needed.
   c. Foods that exacerbate symptoms may be identified and eliminated from the diet. A trial of the FODMAP diet (fermentable oligosaccharides, disaccharides, monosaccharides, and polyols) may be helpful in identifying individual triggers.
   d. It is recommended that the diet contain soluble fiber, but research is inconclusive about its association with reduced symptoms.
2. Antispasmodic medications are used for painful contractions and spasms.
   a. Anticholinergic drugs: Dicyclomine or hyoscyamine may be taken daily or 30 to 60 minutes before meals as needed; reduce pain but do not change bowel habit or other symptoms.
   b. Direct smooth muscle relaxants such as cimetropium, mebeverine, and others; not available in the United States.
   c. Peppermint oil helps with symptoms of pain and bloating through a variety of mechanisms; side effects include nausea and heartburn.
3. Antidepressants act as neuromodulators to impact nerve signaling in the gut, reducing global symptoms.
   a. Tricyclic antidepressants (TCAs).
   b. Selective serotonin reuptake inhibitors (SSRIs).
4. Secretagogues to treat irritable bowel syndrome with constipation (IBS-C).
   a. Lubiprostone activates chloride channels in the bowel to increase BM frequency and reduce pain through unknown mechanism.
   b. Linaclotide increases fluid secretion and gut motility to relieve constipation; also reduces pain by decreasing activity of sensory nerves in the gut.
5. Direct serotonin (5-hydroxytryptamine or 5-HT) agonist/antagonists—target serotonin receptors in the GI tract.
   a. Tegaserod is approved for IBS-C; improves pain and bloating as well as constipation; may be associated with increased cardiovascular events, such as myocardial infarction, stroke, and transient ischemic attacks.

DRUG ALERT Tegaserod should only be prescribed for females <65 years of age with IBS-C who do not have a history of cardiovascular disease or more than one risk factor.

   b. Alosetron delays gut motility and improves pain; approved for irritable bowel syndrome with diarrhea (IBS-D) but is associated with adverse effects of constipation and rare ischemic colitis. Therefore, it is approved for females whose IBS symptoms limit quality of life.
6. Retainagogues are a newer class of medications that block the absorption of sodium in the GI tract, causing more water to be retained. This speeds up intestinal transit time, causing softer BMs; also reduces pain and other symptoms. Tenapanor is the first approved drug in this class.
7. Osmotic laxatives—polyethylene glycol 3350 powder is the only laxative that has been studied in IBS-C; it improves stool texture and frequency, but does not help with pain or global symptoms.
8. Antidiarrheal loperamide solidifies stool but has no effect on pain or other symptoms.
9. Nonabsorbable antibiotic—rifaximin helps reduce diarrhea and improve global symptoms, although mechanism is not fully understood; it is approved for IBS-D as a 2-week treatment that can be repeated if needed.

DRUG ALERT Opioids are inappropriate as treatment for IBS because it is a chronic condition and opioids have a tendency to worsen constipation.

Complications

1. This disorder is associated with:
   a. Psychological distress.
   b. Sexual dysfunction.
   c. Interference with work and sleep.
   d. Decreased quality of life.
2. Unnecessary surgery because of misdiagnosis (such as cholecystectomy, appendectomy, or partial colectomy).

Nursing Assessment

1. Assess the patient for contributing factors that may affect symptoms, such as diet and lifestyle habits, emotional stress, past trauma, relationships, and other concerns.
2. Record BM characteristics to understand pattern to determine best treatment options.
3. Explore pain, discomfort, bloating, and other symptoms and their characteristics: frequency, duration, location, timing, and intensity.

Nursing Interventions

Minimizing Pain or Discomfort

1. Assess and evaluate abdominal pain using a pain scale.
2. Review patient's medication regimen for proper usage and effect on pain and other symptoms.

3. Identify adverse effects that may be limiting use and overall benefit, such as drowsiness, dry mouth, nausea, bloating, diarrhea, or constipation.

Decreasing Diarrhea or Constipation

1. Monitor amount, consistency, and frequency of stool.
2. Encourage regular exercise and adequate fluid and soluble fiber intake to promote regular movements.
3. Discourage the use of laxatives or antidiarrheal medications without consulting health care provider; always follow package instructions for over-the-counter (OTC) medications.

Improving Self-Management and Coping

1. Educate the patient on the diagnosis and the natural course of IBS.
2. Validate the patient's feelings and frustrations about symptoms.
3. Encourage a strong, trusting relationship between patient and health care provider.
4. Encourage patient to try positive coping mechanisms to relieve stress, such as yoga, progressive muscle relaxation, relaxation breathing, journaling, music therapy.
5. Refer the patient for psychological counseling if indicated.

Patient Education and Health Maintenance

1. Instruct the patient about all prescribed medications, including purpose, dosage, and adverse effects.
2. Encourage healthy eating pattern, including eating at regular times, eating slowly, avoiding eating beyond feeling full, avoiding gas-forming foods, drinking 8 cups of fluid daily, and limiting intake of coffee, tea, alcohol, and carbonated and sugary drinks.
3. Assist patient in identifying trigger foods and situations by keeping and analyzing journal. Look at the timing of events in relation to eating and symptoms.
4. For trial of low FODMAP diet, support the patient, but ensure that the patient is receiving guidance from a registered dietician. FODMAP foods will be restricted for 6 to 8 weeks and then are gradually introduced based on the patient's response to restriction.
   a. Fermentable—gas producing.
   b. Oligosaccharides—simple sugars linked together.
   c. Disaccharides—double sugar (lactose).
   d. Monosaccharides—single sugar (fructose).
   e. Pylols—sugar alcohol (sorbitol, xylitol, mannitol, glycerol).

EVIDENCE BASE Wilson, B., Cox, S. R., & Whelan, K. (2021). Challenges of the low FODMAP diet for managing irritable bowel syndrome and approaches to their minimisation and mitigation. *Proceedings of the Nutrition Society, 80*(1), 19–28. https://doi.org/10.1017/S0029665120006990

Evaluation: Expected Outcomes

- Expresses pain reduced to level of 2 on a 0 to 10 scale after eating.
- Reports regular, formed BMs daily.
- Verbalizes strategies successful in coping with symptoms.

Ulcerative Colitis

Ulcerative colitis (UC) is a chronic idiopathic, diffuse inflammatory disease of the mucosa and, less frequently, the submucosa of the colon and rectum. If only the rectum is involved, it may be called *ulcerative proctitis*.

Pathophysiology and Etiology

1. The exact cause of UC is unknown. Possible theories include:
   a. Genetic predisposition.
   b. Environmental factors (viral or bacterial pathogens, dietary).
   c. Immunologic imbalance or disturbances.
   d. Defect in intestinal barrier causing hypersensitive mucosa and increased permeability.
   e. Defect in repair of mucosal injury, which may develop into a chronic condition.
2. Multiple crypt abscesses develop in intestinal mucosa that may become necrotic and lead to ulceration and perforation.
3. May manifest as a systemic disease with inflammatory changes of connective tissue (see Figure 14-13). Most common in young adulthood and middle age, with peak incidence at ages 20 to 40.
4. Incidence greatest in White people of Jewish descent.

Clinical Manifestations

1. Bloody diarrhea is a key symptom.
2. Tenesmus (painful straining), sense of urgency, and frequency.
3. Increased bowel sounds; the abdomen may appear flat, but, as condition continues, the abdomen may appear distended.
4. There is often weight loss, fever, dehydration, hypokalemia, anorexia, nausea and vomiting, iron deficiency anemia, and cachexia (general lack of nutrition and wasting with chronic disease).

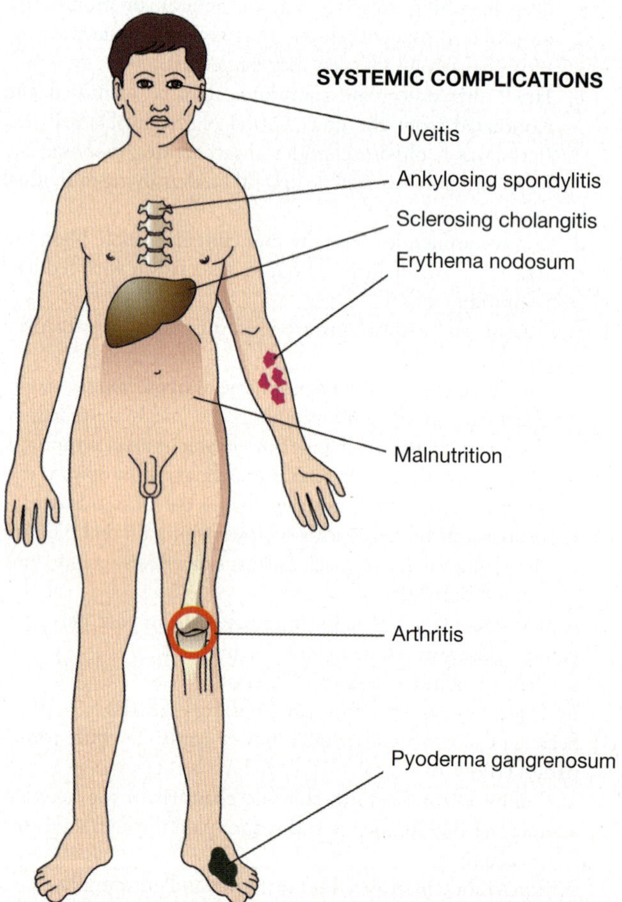

Figure 14-13. Gastrointestinal and systemic complications of ulcerative colitis. (Reprinted with permission from Rubin, R., & Strayer, D. S. [2011]. *Rubin's pathology: Clinicopathologic foundations of medicine* [6th ed., part of Fig. 13-54]. Lippincott Williams & Wilkins.)

5. Crampy abdominal pain.
6. The disease usually begins in the rectum and sigmoid and spreads proximally, at times, involving the entire colon. Anal area may be irritated and reddened; left lower abdomen may be tender on palpation.
7. There is a tendency for the patient to experience remissions and exacerbations.
8. Increased risk of developing colorectal cancer.
9. May exhibit extracolonic manifestations of eye (iritis, uveitis), joint (polyarthritis), and skin complaints (erythema nodosum, pyoderma gangrenosum).

Diagnostic Evaluation

Diagnosis is based on a combination of laboratory, radiologic, endoscopic, and histologic findings.

Laboratory Tests

1. Stool examination to rule out enteral pathogens; fecal analysis positive for blood during active disease.
2. CBC—hemoglobin and hematocrit may be low because of bleeding; WBC may be increased.
3. Elevated markers of inflammation such as erythrocyte sedimentation rate (ESR), CRP.
4. Serology for perinuclear antineutrophil cytoplasmic antibodies (P-ANCAs) will be elevated in most patients.
5. Fecal calprotectin is nonspecific but usually elevated; it correlates to neutrophils in the intestine.
6. Decreased serum levels of potassium, magnesium, and albumin may be present due to loss through diarrhea.

Other Diagnostic Tests

1. Barium enema to assess the extent of disease and detect pseudopolyps, carcinoma, and strictures. May show absence of haustral markings; narrow, lead-pipe appearance; superficial ulcerations.
2. Flexible proctosigmoidoscopy/colonoscopy findings reveal mucosal erythema and edema, ulcers, and inflammation that begins distally in the rectum and spreads proximally for variable distances. Pseudopolyps and friable tissue may be present.
3. Histologic findings from biopsies of the colon include changes in crypt height, loss of crypts, and neutrophil infiltrates in the crypts.
4. CT scan can identify complications such as toxic megacolon.
5. Rectal biopsy—differentiates from other inflammatory diseases or cancer.

Management

EVIDENCE BASE Yuan, W., Marwaha, J. S., Rakowsky, S. T., Palmer, N. P., Kohane, I. S., Rubin, D. T., Brat, G. A., & Feuerstein, J. D. (2022). Trends in medical management of moderately to severely active ulcerative colitis: A nationwide retrospective analysis. *Inflammatory Bowel Diseases, 29*(5), 695–704. https://doi.org/10.1093/ibd/izac134

General Measures

1. Activity as tolerated, IV fluid replacement, clear liquid diet or diet as tolerated.
2. For patients with severe dehydration and excessive diarrhea, TPN may be recommended to rest the intestinal tract and restore nitrogen balance. However, bowel rest does not affect underlying disease activity.
3. Treatment of anemia—iron supplements for chronic bleeding and blood replacement for massive bleeding.

Drug Therapy

1. Sulfasalazine and 5-aminosalicylates (5-ASA) oral and rectal formulations are available for initial and maintenance therapy. Dose-related adverse effects include vomiting, anorexia, headache, fever, rash, dyspepsia, and lowered sperm count (sulfasalazine).
2. Corticosteroids—may be used initially for moderate-to-severe UC and dose increased as needed; however, not for maintenance therapy due to potential long-term side effects. Enema available for proctitis and left-sided colitis.
3. Immunosuppressive drugs—purine analogs, azathioprine, and 6-mercaptopurine may be indicated when the patient is refractory or dependent on corticosteroids.
4. Biologic agents include anti–tumor necrosis factor (TNF) therapy (e.g., infliximab, adalimumab) and antiadhesion molecule inhibitors (vedolizumab), which can be used to target proteins made by immune system and maintain remission of symptoms. Side effects can include opportunistic infections, headache, rash, and arthralgias.
5. Anticoagulation therapy to prevent venous thrombosis embolisms.

DRUG ALERT Avoid antimotility agents, opioids, and anticholinergics in patients with UC due to increased risk of ileus and megacolon.

Surgical Measures

1. Surgery is recommended when patients fail to respond to medical therapy, if clinical status is worsening, for uncontrollable adverse effects of medications, severe hemorrhage, perforation, toxic megacolon, dysplasia, or cancer.
2. Noncurative approaches (possible curative, reconstructive procedure at later date):
   a. Temporary loop colostomy for decompression if toxic megacolon present without perforation.
   b. Subtotal colectomy, ileostomy, and Hartmann pouch.
   c. Colectomy with ileorectal anastomosis.
3. Reconstructive procedures—curative:
   a. Total proctocolectomy with permanent end ileostomy.
   b. Total proctocolectomy with continent ileostomy (Kock or Barnett continent internal reservoir [BCIR]).
   c. Total colectomy with ileal reservoir—anal (or ileal reservoir–distal rectal) anastomosis—procedure of choice. Multiple reservoir shapes can be surgically created; however, the J-shaped pouch (reservoir) is the easiest to construct (see Figure 14-14).
   d. The ultimate surgical goal is to remove the entire colon and rectum to cure patient with UC.

Complications

1. Perforation, hemorrhage.
2. Toxic megacolon (life-threatening)—fever, tachycardia, abdominal distention, peritonitis, leukocytosis, dilated colon on abdominal x-ray.
3. Abscess formation, stricture, anal fistula.
4. Malnutrition, anemia, electrolyte imbalance.
5. Skin lesions (erythema nodosum, pyoderma gangrenosum).
6. Arthritis, ankylosing spondylitis.
7. Colon malignancy.
8. Liver disease (sclerosing cholangitis).
9. Eye lesions (uveitis, conjunctivitis).
10. Growth retardation in prepubertal children.
11. Possible infertility in females.

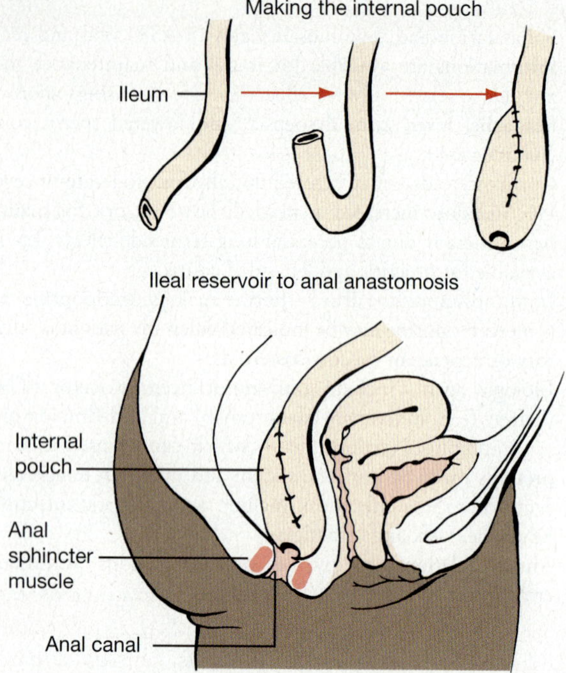

Figure 14-14. Ileal reservoir–anal anastomosis. This reservoir is constructed of two loops of the small intestine, forming a J configuration (J pouch).

Nursing Assessment

1. Review symptoms such as fatigue, shortness of breath, and palpitations due to anemia.
2. Assess food habits and use of any dietary or herbal supplements as alternative therapies that may have a bearing on triggering symptoms (milk intake may be a problem). Many patients use vitamins, herbs, and homeopathic remedies without realizing the effect on bowel function.
3. Determine the number and consistency of BMs, any rectal bleeding, and if patient is having episodes of urgency and incontinence that are impacting lifestyle.
4. Listen for hyperactive bowel sounds; assess weight.

Nursing Interventions

Promoting Comfort

1. Follow prescribed treatment of reducing or eliminating food and fluid and instituting parenteral feeding or low-residue diets to rest the intestinal tract as directed.
2. Give sedatives and tranquilizers, as prescribed, not only to provide general rest but also to slow peristalsis.
3. Be aware of skin breakdown around the anus, which causes discomfort.
   a. Cleanse the skin gently after each BM.
   b. Apply a protective emollient, such as petroleum jelly, skin sealant, or moisture barrier ointment.
4. Relieve painful rectal spasms (produced by frequent diarrheal stools) with anodyne suppositories, as prescribed.
5. Report any evidence of sudden abdominal distention—may indicate toxic megacolon.
6. Reduce physical activity to a minimum, or provide frequent rest periods.
7. Provide commode or bathroom next to bed because urgency of movements may be a problem.

Achieving Nutritional Requirements

1. Maintain an acutely ill patient on parenteral replacement of vitamins, fluids, and electrolytes (potassium), as prescribed.
2. When resuming oral fluids and foods, select those that are nonirritating to the mucosa (mechanically, thermally, and chemically). If this fails, an elemental diet may be prescribed to provide low residue to rest the lower intestinal tract.
3. Avoid dairy products if the patient is lactose intolerant.
4. Provide a well-balanced, low-residue, high-protein diet to correct malnutrition.
5. Determine which foods the patient can tolerate and modify diet plan accordingly.
6. Bolster with supplemental vitamin therapy, including vitamins C, B complex, and K, as prescribed.
7. Possibly avoid cold fluids, which may increase intestinal motility.
8. Administer prescribed medications for symptomatic relief of diarrhea.

Maintaining Fluid Balance

1. Maintain accurate intake and output records, including urine, stool, and any other fluid output.
2. Weigh daily; rapid increase or decrease may relate to fluid imbalance.
3. Monitor serum electrolytes and report abnormalities.
4. Observe for decreased skin turgor, dry skin, oliguria, decreased temperature, weakness, and increased hemoglobin, hematocrit, BUN, and specific gravity, all of which are signs of fluid loss leading to dehydration.

Minimizing Infection and Complications

1. Give antibacterial drugs as prescribed.
2. Administer corticosteroids as prescribed.
3. Provide conscientious skin care after severe diarrhea.
4. Alert the patient to possible postoperative problems with skin care, aesthetic difficulties, and surgical revisions.
5. For severe proctitis, instill rectal steroids, as prescribed, to produce a remission of symptoms.
6. Administer prescribed therapy to correct existing anemia.
7. Observe for signs of colonic perforation and hemorrhage—abdominal rigidity, distention, hypotension, and tachycardia. Inform patients that early indications of relapse, such as bleeding or increased diarrhea, should be reported immediately so treatment may be initiated.

Enhancing Positive Coping

1. Teach the patient about chronic aspects of UC and each component of care prescribed.
2. Encourage self-care in monitoring symptoms, seeking medical checkups, and maintaining health (e.g., immunizations).
3. Acknowledge the patient's complaints; do not minimize symptoms.
4. Encourage the patient to talk; actively listen and offer support.
5. Arrange for the patient to share experiences with others undergoing similar procedures.
6. Answer questions about the permanent or temporary ostomy, if appropriate.
7. Initiate patient education about living with chronic disease.
8. Include the patient as part of the health care team to provide continuity of care, communication, and periodic evaluation.
9. Offer educational and emotional support to family members.
10. Refer for psychological counseling, as needed.

Patient Education and Health Maintenance

1. For further information and support, refer to the Crohn and Colitis Foundation of America at www.ccfa.org. If the patient has an ileostomy, provide information about the local chapter of the United Ostomy Association (www.uoa.org).
2. Teach patients who have undergone one of the continent restorative procedures (Kock, BCIR, or ileal reservoir–anal anastomosis) to be alert for a common late postoperative complication called *pouchitis*.
   a. The symptoms include increased stool output, cramps, and malaise.
   b. It is thought to be related to stasis within the pouch/reservoir and usually responds to metronidazole.
   c. Advise patient to notify health care provider.
3. Teach patients with a temporary or permanent ileostomy how to prevent a food blockage by limiting certain foods the first few months after surgery—Chinese vegetables (such as bok choy and bamboo shoots), skins and seeds, fatty meats, bean hulls, popcorn, and other foods that do not digest well. Also chew foods well and drink plenty of fluid with meals.
4. Teach patients with temporary or permanent ileostomy to be alert for signs and symptoms of a food blockage.
   a. This is a mechanical blockage of undigested foodstuffs at the level of the fascia.
   b. It is most likely to occur in the first 6 weeks postoperatively when the bowel is edematous; however, patients with an ileostomy must be aware that it can occur at any time if precautions are not taken.
   c. Symptoms may include spurty, watery stool with strong odor, decreased or no stool output, abdominal discomfort, cramping or bloating, and stomal swelling. Nausea and vomiting are late symptoms and require immediate attention.
   d. Treatment includes avoiding solid foods and drinking clear liquids as soon as symptoms occur, gently massaging the abdomen around the stoma, pulling the knees to the chest and rocking the body back and forth, taking a warm shower or bath to help with relaxation.

CLINICAL JUDGMENT If food blockage lasts for more than 2 to 3 hours or if nausea/vomiting occur, advise the patient to seek medical attention immediately. Usually, an ileostomy lavage is done by a health care provider or ostomy specialty nurse to relieve the blockage. Advise a patient with ileostomy never to take laxatives.

   e. Applying a pouching system with a larger opening to allow for stomal swelling may prevent this from recurring.

Evaluation: Expected Outcomes

- Reports lessening of pain; functions well with minimal analgesics.
- Demonstrates improved food and fluid intake; avoids roughage intake.
- Controls diarrhea; vital signs stable.
- Afebrile, no skin breakdown, vital signs stable, no abdominal rigidity.
- Shows improved mood, caring for self, talking about change in lifestyle.

Crohn Disease

Crohn disease is a chronic, idiopathic inflammatory disease that can affect any part of the GI tract. It is predominantly a transmural disease of the bowel wall. Other names for this disease include *regional enteritis*, *granulomatous colitis*, *transmural colitis*, *ileitis*, and *ileocolitis*.

EVIDENCE BASE Ranasinghe, I. R., & Hsu, R. (2023). Crohn disease. In *StatPearls* [Internet]. StatPearls Publishing. https://www.ncbi.nlm.nih.gov/books/NBK436021/

Pathophysiology and Etiology

1. The exact etiology is unknown for this disease. It is thought to be multifactorial with the following theories:
   a. Genetic predisposition.
   b. Environmental agents, such as infections (viral or bacterial overload) or dietary factors, may trigger the disease.
   c. Immunologic imbalance or disturbances.
   d. Defect in the intestinal barrier that increases the permeability of the bowel.
   e. Defect in the repair of mucosal injury, leading to chronic condition.
   f. Cigarette smoking is a risk factor in developing disease and increases exacerbations. In contrast, cigarette smoking seems to have a protective effect with UC.
2. Intestinal tissue is thickened and edematous; ulcers enlarge, deepen, and form transverse and longitudinal linear ulcers that intersect, resembling a cobblestone appearance. The deep penetration of these ulcers may form fissures, abscesses, and fistulae. The healing and fibrosis of these lesions may lead to stricture (see Figure 14-15).
3. The rectum is typically spared from disease, and "skip lesions" are discontinuous areas of diseased bowel.
4. Transmural inflammation is a characteristic finding of this disease as well as granulomas.
5. Involvement of the upper GI tract (mouth, esophagus, stomach, and duodenum) is rare, and if present, there is usually disease elsewhere.
6. May occur at any age; however, peak incidence is in the third decade, with a smaller peak in the fifth decade.
7. Most common in White people and those of Jewish descent.
8. The clinical presentation can be divided into three patterns:
   a. Inflammatory.
   b. Fibrostenotic (stricturing).
   c. Perforating (fistulizing).
9. Recurrences tend to fall into the same pattern for each individual patient and may provide an approach to treatment.

Clinical Manifestations

These are characterized by exacerbations and remissions—may be abrupt or insidious.

1. Crampy intermittent pain, anorexia, weight loss, malaise, nausea.
2. Chronic diarrhea—usual consistency is soft or semiliquid. Bloody stools or steatorrhea (because of malabsorption) may occur.
3. Fever may indicate infectious complication, such as abscess.
4. Fecal urgency and tenesmus.
5. Extraintestinal symptoms include erythema nodosum, uveitis, stomatitis, liver and gallbladder disease, arthritis, and nephrolithiasis.

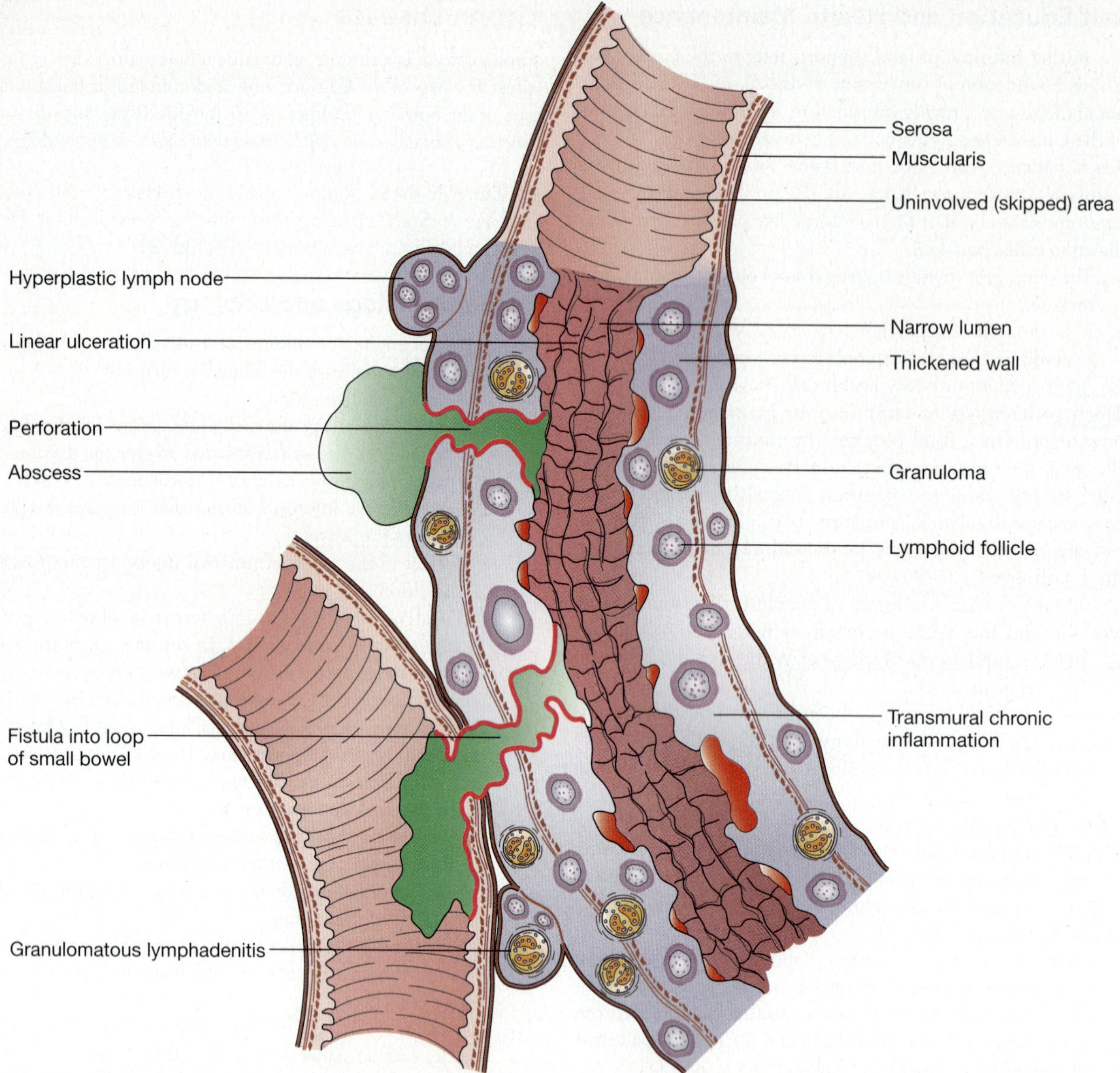

Figure 14-15. Transmural intestinal changes in Crohn disease. (Reprinted with permission from Strayer, D. S., Saffitz, J. E., & Rubin, E. [2020]. *Rubin's pathology: Mechanisms of human disease* [8th ed., Fig. 19-60]. Lippincott Williams & Wilkins.)

6. Rectal examination may reveal a perirectal abscess, fistula, fissure, or skin tags (which represent healed perianal lesions).
7. Characteristics by pattern:
   a. *Inflammatory pattern* may display malabsorption, weight loss, and less abdominal pain.
   b. *Fibrostenotic pattern* may display a partial small bowel obstruction, diffuse abdominal pain, nausea, vomiting, and bloating.
   c. *Perforating pattern* may display a sudden profuse diarrhea because of enteroenteric fistula, fever, and localized tenderness because of abscess, or other fistulizing symptoms, such as pneumaturia and recurrent urinary tract infections (UTIs).

Diagnostic Evaluation

1. The diagnosis is based on a combination of laboratory, radiologic, endoscopic, and histologic findings.
2. CBC may show mild leukocytosis, thrombocytosis, anemia.
3. Elevated ESR and CRP, hypoalbuminemia, reduced serum B_{12} and iron.
4. Stool analysis may reveal leukocytes but no enteric pathogens; guaiac-positive stool. Fecal calprotectin to assess amount of inflammation (disease activity).
5. Special serology such as normal ANCAs and raised antisaccharomyces cerevisiae antibodies (ASCAs) can distinguish Crohn disease from UC.
6. Upper GI and small bowel follow-through barium studies may show the classic "string sign" at the terminal ileum, which suggests a constriction of an intestinal segment.
7. A barium enema may permit visualization of lesions in the large intestine and terminal ileum.
8. CT of the abdomen and pelvis is helpful with diagnosis but is more often used to evaluate complications, such as abscesses or fistulae.
9. Colonoscopy is the procedure of choice. Typical findings include the presence of skip lesions, cobblestoning, ulcerations, and rectal sparing.

10. Biopsy may reveal granulomas, infiltration of lymphocytes, and monocytes.
11. Thiopurine methyltransferase level may be checked before starting drug therapy; low level is associated with more side effects, very high level is associated with reduced effectiveness.

Management

Medical Management

1. The goals of medical management include managing symptoms, reducing complications, inducing remissions, improving nutrition, and avoiding surgical interventions when possible. Management is also based on the location and severity of disease and extraintestinal complications.
2. Weight loss, water and electrolyte imbalances, and iron, vitamin, mineral, and protein deficiencies occur in 80% of patients.
3. During acute episodes, bowel rest is usually required.
4. Nutritional replacements may include an elemental diet (Vivonex) administered orally or through an NG tube.
5. TPN may be ordered.
6. For milder cases, a low-residue diet may be indicated and avoidance of untolerated foods. Nutritional supplements may be ordered to provide additional nutrients and calories.

Drug Therapy

1. There is no known cure for this disease; it is primarily treated with medications. The disease severity and the area of the GI tract influence drug therapy (see Table 14-3, page 510).
2. Sulfasalazine may be used for mild disease.
3. Corticosteroids—to reduce inflammation; given orally, by IV line, or by suppository, retention enema, or foam, depending on the severity of disease. Steroids should be tapered off whenever possible.
4. Immunomodulators (6-mercaptopurine, azathioprine, methotrexate, cyclosporine, and tacrolimus)—used in patients who are steroid dependent or steroid refractory. Assists with fistula improvement or healing.
5. Biologic agents used either in combination with immunomodulators or alone.
   a. TNF agents such as infliximab and adalimumab—monoclonal antibodies that block the activity of the inflammatory agent and TNF. They are indicated for moderate-to-severe disease not responding to traditional therapies and for patients with draining fistulae.
   b. Adhesion molecule inhibitors such as vedolizumab, which has lower systemic side-effect profile.
6. Antibiotics to treat fistulas and abscesses.
7. Patients with inflammation of intestines are at increased risk of venous thromboembolism, and prophylactic treatment should be used during the acute stage.
8. Antidiarrheals (loperamide, cholestyramine, or codeine [but try to avoid])—decrease stool frequency in mild-to-moderate disease; use with caution.
9. Miscellaneous drugs—antispasmodics (dicyclomine), bulking agents (psyllium), or TCAs (amitriptyline) for treatment of abdominal pain. Vitamins and supplements may be needed long term.

Surgery

Indicated only for the complications of Crohn disease. Approximately 70% of patients with Crohn disease will eventually require one or more operations to relieve obstruction, close fistulae, drain abscesses, repair perforations, manage hemorrhage, or widen strictures. Depending on the patient, surgical options include:

1. Segmental bowel resection with anastomosis.
2. Subtotal colectomy with ileorectal anastomosis.
3. Total colectomy with ileostomy for severe disease in the colon and rectum (see page 478 for care of the patient with ostomy).
4. Kock pouch and ileal reservoir–anal anastomosis are contraindicated in patients with Crohn disease. These procedures require the use of the small intestine in which Crohn disease may develop.

Complications

1. Abscess (occurs in 20%) and fistulae (occur in 40%).
2. Strictures—may result from inflammation, edema, abscess, and adhesions, but usually from fibrostenosis.
3. Hemorrhage, bowel perforation, intestinal obstruction.
4. Nutritional deficiencies: poor caloric intake because of food avoidance, malabsorption of bile salts and fat, vitamin B_{12} deficiency with ileal disease, short-gut syndrome after extensive surgical resections.
5. Dehydration and electrolyte disturbances.
6. Peritonitis and sepsis.

Nursing Assessment

1. Assess frequency and consistency of stools to evaluate volume losses and effectiveness of therapy.
2. Have the patient describe the location, severity, and onset of abdominal cramping or pain.
3. Ask the patient about weight loss and anorexia; weigh daily to monitor changes.
4. Have the patient describe foods eaten to understand dietary exacerbations.
5. Determine whether the patient smokes, including duration and amount.
6. Ask about family history of GI diseases.

Nursing Interventions

Achieving Adequate Nutritional Balance

1. Provide comprehensive education about anatomy and physiology of the GI system, the chronic disease process, drug therapy, potential complications, and potential surgery.
2. Encourage a diet that is low in residue, fiber, and fat and high in calories, protein, and carbohydrates, with vitamin and mineral supplements.
3. Explain the importance of adequate hydration and nutrition (based on individual tolerance) and daily weight monitoring.
4. Provide small, frequent feedings to prevent distention.
5. Have the patient participate in meal planning to encourage adherence and increase knowledge.
6. Prepare the patient for elemental diet or TPN if the patient is debilitated.

Maintaining Fluid and Electrolyte Balance

1. Monitor intake and output.
2. Provide fluids, as prescribed, to maintain hydration (1,000 mL/24 hours is minimum intake to meet body fluid needs).
3. Monitor stool frequency and consistency.
4. Monitor electrolytes (especially potassium) and acid–base balance because diarrhea can lead to metabolic acidosis.

Table 14-3 Drugs Used to Treat Inflammatory Bowel Disease

CATEGORY	ROUTE	DRUG	ADVERSE EFFECTS	CONSIDERATIONS
Corticosteroids	Oral	Budesonide, prednisone, and methylprednisolone	Cushingoid appearance, hypertension, acne, water retention, weight gain, hair loss, increased appetite, hypokalemia, gastric irritation, ulcer formation, adrenal suppression, decreased resistance to infection. Complications associated with prolonged use include osteoporosis, cataract development, growth retardation, peptic ulceration, hyperglycemia, hypertension, aseptic joint necrosis, and glaucoma.	• May be administered in IV form when the gastrointestinal tract is not able to absorb drugs properly • Budesonide is approved for treating mild to moderately active Crohn disease of the terminal ileum. Because of budesonide's first-pass metabolism, systemic adverse effects are less common than those that occur with conventional steroids. Corticosteroids are not indicated for maintenance therapy in treating IBD secondary to associated long-term adverse effects.
	IV	Hydrocortisone and methylprednisolone		
	Rectal	Hydrocortisone/pramoxine and hydrocortisone		
Immune-modulating agents	Oral	6-Mercaptopurine and azathioprine	Bone marrow suppression, increased vulnerability to infection, rash, fever, malaise, arthralgias, hepatic dysfunction, nausea, vomiting, diarrhea, pancreatitis, hair loss, and neoplasm development	• Monitor for bone marrow suppression. • Pregnancy category D • Testing available that evaluates the patient's ability to metabolize the drug, determines therapeutic levels, and monitors for hepatotoxicity.
	SQ	Methotrexate		
Biologic agents	IV	Infliximab	Infusion-related reactions: pruritus, rash, chest pain, hypotension, hypertension, dyspnea, headache, nausea, vomiting, fatigue, and fever	• Infusion reactions usually resolve with decreasing the rate of infusion.
	IV	Vedolizumab, ustekinumab, and risankizumab	Other potential adverse effects (rare): autoantibody development (lupus-like syndrome) and increased susceptibility to infection	• Perform tuberculosis (TB) skin test prior to the first dose because of the drug's ability to allow latent TB to become active; a positive skin test (>5-mm induration) indicates the need for treatment for latent TB, before initiation of infliximab therapy. • Do not administer to patients with an active infection.
	SQ	Adalimumab, vedolizumab, ustekinumab, and risankizumab		
5-ASA drugs	Oral	Mesalamine and balsalazide	Headache, diarrhea, abdominal pain, abdominal cramping, malaise, rash, arthralgias, and nephrotoxicity	• Use mesalamine with caution in patients with renal insufficiency. Researchers have yet to determine the safety of balsalazide in patients with renal impairment. • Mesalamine (Asacol bran tablets) may be excreted whole in stool. Ask patients to report frequent passage of whole tablets.
	Oral	Sulfasalazine	Headache, diarrhea, abdominal pain, abdominal cramping, malaise, hair loss, rash, orange discoloration of urine, bone marrow suppression, photosensitivity, and decreased sperm motility in males	• Monitor CBC for signs of bone marrow suppression. • Recommend daily sunscreen use. • Decreased sperm motility is reversible upon drug discontinuation. • Urine discoloration is harmless.

CBC, complete blood count; IBD, inflammatory bowel disease; IV, intravenous; SQ, subcutaneous; 5-ASA, 5-aminosalicylic acid.

5. Watch for cardiac dysrhythmias and muscle weakness because of loss of electrolytes.
6. Encourage regular follow-up and report signs of complications: increasing abdominal distention, cramping pain, diarrhea, malaise, anorexia, fever, and passing stool through the urethra or vagina.

Controlling Pain

1. Administer medications for control of inflammatory process, as prescribed.
2. Observe and record changes in pain—frequency, location, characteristics, precipitating events, and duration.
3. Monitor for distention, increased temperature, hypotension, and rectal bleeding—all signs of obstruction because of the inflammation.
4. Clean rectal area and apply ointments, as necessary, to decrease discomfort from skin breakdown.
5. Prepare the patient for surgery if response to medical and drug therapy is unsatisfactory.
6. Surgery is determined specifically for each patient.
7. Recurrence of the disease is possible after surgery.

Providing Psychosocial Support

1. Offer understanding, concern, and encouragement—this person is often embarrassed about frequent and malodorous stools and often is fearful of eating.
2. Facilitate supportive psychological counseling, if appropriate.
3. Encourage the patient's usual support people to be involved in management of the disease and seek additional support groups as needed.
4. Encourage health-promoting behavior.
5. Encourage the patient to participate in stress-reducing activities, such as exercise, relaxation techniques, music therapy.

Patient Education and Health Maintenance

1. Instruct patient about all prescribed medications, including the purpose, dosage, and adverse effects as well as to discuss the use of any OTC drugs with health care provider.
2. Encourage healthy lifestyle including smoking cessation and avoidance of NSAIDs, which may exacerbate disease.
3. Encourage follow-up with gastroenterologist and surgeon as indicated, as well as routine health checkups with primary care provider.
4. Encourage routine screening tests and preventative practices, such as immunizations.
   a. Tuberculosis testing should be done before starting immunomodulator or biologic therapy, which affects immune system.
   b. Obtain immunization history or titers prior to starting medication, particularly measles, mumps, and rubella (MMR), to ensure immunity.
5. For further information and support, refer to Crohn's & Colitis Foundation at www.ccfa.org.

Evaluation: Expected Outcomes

- Improved nutritional intake; weight stable.
- Adequate fluid intake; no evidence of dehydration; electrolyte levels within normal limits.
- Demonstrates relief of pain and manageable symptoms.
- Verbalizes improved attitude toward ways to live with the disease.

Colorectal Cancer

EVIDENCE BASE American Cancer Society. (2023). *Colorectal cancer facts & figures.* https://www.cancer.org/research/cancer-facts-statistics/colorectal-cancer-facts-figures.html

Colorectal cancer refers to malignancies of the colon and rectum. This type is the second leading cause of cancer death in the United States, for men and women combined. Colorectal tumors are nearly all adenocarcinomas. Lymphoma, carcinoid, melanoma, and sarcomas account for only 5% of colorectal lesions.

Pathophysiology and Etiology

1. Risk factors include:
   a. Age: Risk increases sharply after age 45. African Americans can present earlier.
   b. Previous history of resected colorectal cancer or adenomatous polyps.
   c. Family history of colorectal cancer or adenomatous polyps, especially if one first-degree relative diagnosed before age 60 or two first-degree relatives diagnosed at any age.
   d. Familial adenomatous polyposis (FAP; also a variant called *Gardner syndrome*) is an inherited condition characterized by multiple adenomatous polyps of the colon, in which cancer will inevitably develop in all affected individuals.
   e. Hereditary nonpolyposis colorectal cancer (HNPCC)—hereditary condition with a markedly increased risk of developing colorectal cancer as well as other cancers, such as endometrial, ovarian, renal, pancreatic, gastric, and small intestinal. There are few or no adenomatous polyps, and the bowel may undergo rapid change from normal tissue to polyp to cancer.
   f. Chronic UC—increasing risk after 10-year history.
   g. Incidence is higher in industrialized countries and lower in underdeveloped countries. Reason unclear but may be related to diet. The Western diet, which is high in refined grains, processed and red meats, high-fat dairy products, desserts, and fried foods, has been shown to increase the risk of colorectal cancer.
   h. Immunodeficiency disease.
2. Colorectal lesions occur most frequently in the rectum and sigmoid areas; however, it appears there is a trend toward increasing frequency of right-sided lesions.
3. Most adenocarcinomas are ulcerative in appearance. A left-sided lesion tends to be annular and scar-like; a right-sided lesion tends to be a cauliflower-like mass that protrudes into the bowel lumen.
4. A lesion starts in the mucosal layers of the colonic wall and eventually penetrates the wall and invades surrounding structures and organs (bladder, prostate, ureters, vagina). Cancer spreads by direct invasion, lymphatic spread, and through the bloodstream. The liver and lungs are the most common metastatic sites.

EVIDENCE BASE Engel-Nitz, N. M., Miller-Wilson, L.-A., Le, L., Limburg, P., & Fisher, D. A. (2023). Colorectal screening among average risk individuals in the United States, 2015–2018. *Preventive Medicine Reports, 31*, 102082. https://doi.org/10.1016/j.pmedr.2022.102082

Clinical Manifestations

Colorectal cancer is often asymptomatic. If present, symptomatology varies according to the location of the lesion and the extent of involvement.

1. Right-sided lesions—change in bowel habits, usually diarrhea; vague abdominal discomfort; black, tarry stools; anemia; weakness; weight loss; palpable mass in right lower quadrant.
2. Left-sided lesions—change in bowel habits, often increasing constipation with bouts of diarrhea because of partial obstruction; bright, streaked red blood in stool; cramping pain; weight loss; anemia; palpable mass.
3. Rectal lesions—change in bowel habits with possible urgent need to defecate, alternating constipation and diarrhea, and narrowed caliber of stool; bright red blood in stool; feeling of incomplete evacuation; rectal fullness progressing to dull constant ache.

Diagnostic Evaluation

1. Fecal immunochemical test (FIT)—replaces the older guaiac-based tests.
2. Flexible sigmoidoscopy—can be used if colonoscopy is declined.
3. Colonoscopy with biopsy—diagnostic procedure of choice after strong suspicious clinical history or abnormal barium enema. CT colonography (CTC), also known as *virtual colonoscopy*, may be used for screening.
4. Pelvic MRI and endorectal ultrasonography—provide information about cancer penetration and pararectal lymph nodes.
5. Carcinoembryonic antigen (CEA)—70% of patients have elevated CEA levels. The CEA level monitors possible recurrence or metastasis.
6. CT scan of the abdomen, liver, lungs, and brain—may reveal metastatic disease.

Management

Surgical Resection

Treatment of choice for those with resectable lesions. Regional lymph node dissection determines staging and guides decisions regarding adjuvant therapy. Surgical options include:

1. Laparotomy with wide segmental bowel resection of tumor, including regional lymph nodes and blood vessels (right hemicolectomy, transverse colectomy, left hemicolectomy, or sigmoid resection).
2. Transanal excision—select people with tumors less than 1¼ in (3 cm) and well differentiated less than 3 in (7.5 cm) from the anal verge and localized to the rectal wall may avoid laparotomy.
3. Low anterior resection for upper rectal lesions—may include temporary loop colostomy to protect anastomosis with second procedure for takedown of colostomy.
4. Colonic J pouch—may be offered as a new surgical technique for rectal cancer (see page 506).
5. Select patients may be offered laparoscopic cancer surgery, although this remains controversial.
6. Abdominoperineal resection with permanent end colostomy for lower rectal lesions when adequate margins cannot be obtained, or there is involvement of anal sphincters. Because of improved stapling devices used deep in the pelvis, abdominoperineal resection accounts for fewer than 5% of colorectal resections.
7. Temporary loop colostomy to decompress bowel and divert fecal stream, followed by later bowel resection, anastomosis, and takedown of colostomy.
8. More extensive surgery involving the removal of other organs if cancer has spread, such as liver wedge, bladder, uterus, and/or small intestine, may be performed.
9. Unresectable colorectal cancer—diverting colostomy or ileostomy as palliation for obstructing tumor, laser fulguration, or the placement of an expandable wire stent.
10. Total proctocolectomy or ileal reservoir–anal anastomosis procedure for patients with FAP and chronic UC before colorectal cancer develops.

Other Therapy

1. Radiation therapy may be used preoperatively to improve resectability of the tumor and may be used postoperatively as adjuvant therapy to treat residual disease.
2. Chemotherapy may be used as adjuvant therapy to improve survival time.
   a. Used for residual disease, recurrence of disease, unresectable tumors, and metastatic disease.
   b. Drug combinations may include 5-fluorouracil plus levamisole or 5-fluorouracil plus leucovorin.
   c. A newer drug, irinotecan, is being used in protocols for advanced colorectal cancer.
3. Blood replacement of whole blood or packed red blood cells if severe anemia exists.

Complications

1. Obstruction.
2. Hemorrhage.
3. Anemia.
4. Metastasis.

Nursing Assessment

1. Interview patient regarding dietary habits and family and medical history to identify risk factors.
2. Question the patient regarding symptomatology of colorectal cancer, changes in bowel habits, rectal bleeding, tarry stools, abdominal discomfort, weight loss, weakness, and anemia.
3. Palpate the abdomen for tenderness (usually not tender), presence of mass.
4. Monitor stool for blood and other changes.

Nursing Interventions

Achieving Adequate Nutrition

1. Meet the patient's nutritional needs by serving a high-calorie, low-residue diet for several days before surgery, if condition permits.
2. Observe and record fluid losses, such as may be sustained by vomiting and diarrhea.
3. Maintain hydration through IV therapy and record urine output. Metabolic tissue needs are increased, and more fluids are needed to eliminate waste products.
4. Serve smaller meals spaced throughout the day to maintain adequate calorie and protein intake if not restricted to NPO status.
5. Encourage the patient to participate in meal planning to promote adherence.

6. Adjust diet before and after treatments, such as chemotherapy or radiation. Serve clear liquids, bland diet, or follow restrictions as prescribed.
7. Instruct the patient to take prescribed antiemetic, as needed, especially if receiving chemotherapy.

Relieving Constipation or Diarrhea

1. Monitor amount, consistency, frequency, and color of stool.
2. For constipation, use laxatives or enemas, as needed, and encourage exercise and adequate fluid/fiber intake to promote bowel motility.
3. For diarrhea, encourage adequate fluid intake to prevent fluid volume deficit and electrolyte imbalance.
4. For diarrhea related to radiation or chemotherapy, administer antidiarrheal medications and discuss foods that may slow transit time of bowel, such as bananas, rice, peanut butter, and pasta.

CLINICAL JUDGMENT Antidiarrheal medications and foods to control diarrhea are contraindicated for the patient with an obstructing lesion. Use these measures only postoperatively after lesion resection for control of diarrhea related to cancer therapy.

Relieving Pain

1. Assess type and severity of pain and administer analgesics, as needed.
2. Evaluate effectiveness of analgesic regimen.
3. Investigate different approaches, such as relaxation techniques, repositioning, imaging, laughter, music, reading, and touch, for control or relief of pain.

Maintaining Energy Level

1. Institute an individualized activity plan after assessing the patient's activity level and tolerance, noting shortness of breath or tachycardia.
2. Allow for frequent rest periods to regain energy.
3. Administer blood products or recombinant human erythropoietin, as ordered, if fatigue is related to severe anemia.
4. Facilitate physical and occupational therapy referrals as indicated.

Minimizing Fears and Enhancing Coping

1. Encourage the patient and family to express feelings and fears together and separately.
2. Acknowledge that it is normal to have negative feelings toward cancer, surgery, colostomy, and treatment options.
3. Stress the positive aspects of treatment and future outcomes.
4. Provide detailed information and answer questions to increase sense of control. Review disease process, treatment modalities of radiation and chemotherapy, and complications. Offer educational materials suited to the patient, such as brochures and interactive internet programs.
5. Teach and demonstrate to the patient and/or family the skills necessary for colostomy management, which may include colostomy irrigation. The ostomy specialty nurse can provide formal education in this area.
6. Suggest counseling, if needed, due to overwhelming fear, inability to cope with daily activities, and unresolved trauma impacting emotions.

Patient Education and Health Maintenance

1. Initiate a home care nursing referral to assist with wound care, to manage treatment adverse effects, and to continue teaching colostomy care.
2. Discuss genetic testing with patient and family; can confirm a hereditary diagnosis such as FAP or HNPCC.
3. Become an advocate for colon cancer prevention by educating the public about screening. Beginning at age 45 or sooner for African Americans, males and females should follow one of the following American Cancer Society guidelines for early detection of colon cancer.
   a. Flexible sigmoidoscopy every 5 years.
   b. Colonoscopy every 10 years.
   c. Double-contrast barium enema every 5 years.
   d. CTC every 5 years.
   e. Alternately, stool-based testing can be done annually, but if positive, a colonoscopy must follow. Tests include guaiac-based fecal occult blood test (gFOBT) with high sensitivity for cancer, FIT with high sensitivity for cancer, and stool DNA (sDNA) with high sensitivity for cancer (interval uncertain pending further research).
4. For additional information and support, refer to the American Cancer Society at www.cancer.org.

Evaluation: Expected Outcomes

- Exhibits weight gain and improves nutritional status by adequate dietary intake.
- Has regular soft BMs.
- Minimal pain, controlled with analgesics or other techniques.
- Able to perform activities of daily living (ADLs) with adequate amounts of energy; no shortness of breath on exertion.
- Sleeping well; able to discuss feelings and fears related to surgery, prognosis, and treatment options.

ANORECTAL CONDITIONS

Hemorrhoids

Hemorrhoids are vascular masses in the lower rectum or anus. External hemorrhoids appear outside the external sphincter, whereas internal hemorrhoids appear above the internal sphincter (see Figure 14-16). When blood within the hemorrhoids becomes clotted because of obstruction, the hemorrhoids are referred to as *thrombosed*.

Pathophysiology and Etiology

1. The exact pathogenesis remains controversial. Theories include:
   a. Abnormal dilation of veins of internal hemorrhoidal venous plexus.
   b. Abnormal distention of the arteriovenous anastomoses.
   c. Downward displacement or prolapse of anal cushions.
   d. Destruction of the anchoring connective tissue system.
2. Predisposing factors include:
   a. Pregnancy, prolonged sitting/standing.
   b. Straining at stool, chronic constipation/diarrhea.
   c. Anal infection, rectal surgery, or episiotomy.
   d. Hereditary factor.
   e. Exercise.
   f. Coughing, sneezing, vomiting.
   g. Loss of muscle tone because of age.
   h. Anal intercourse.
3. Increased intra-abdominal pressure causes engorgement in the vascular tissue lining the anal canal.
4. Loosening of vessels from surrounding connective tissue occurs with protrusion or prolapse into anal canal.

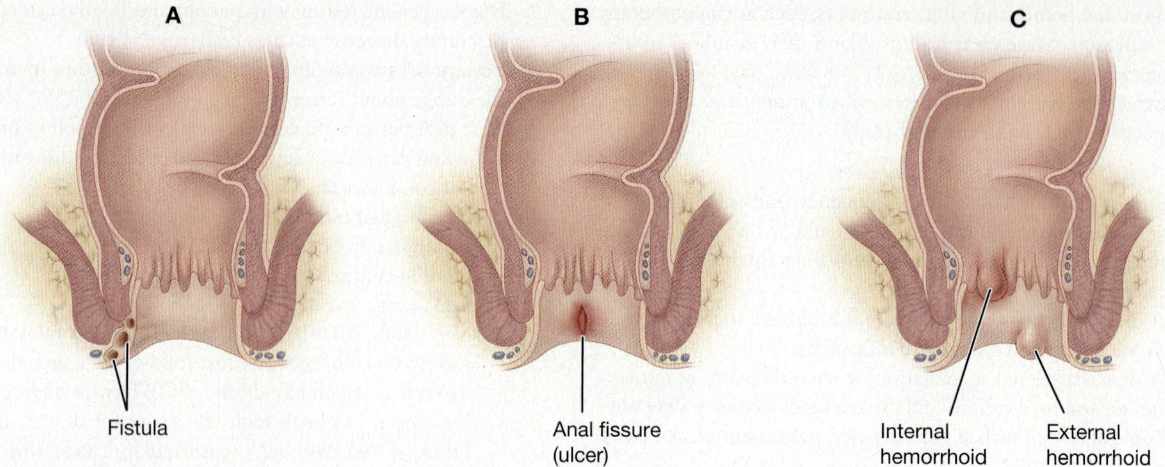

Figure 14-16. Various types of anal lesions. (A) Fistula. (B) Fissure. (C) External and internal hemorrhoids. (Reprinted with permission from Hinkle, J. L., Cheever, K. H., & Overbaugh, K. [2022]. *Brunner and Suddarth's textbook of medical-surgical nursing* [15th ed., Fig. 41-12]. Lippincott Williams & Wilkins.)

Clinical Manifestations

1. Bleeding during or after defecation, bright red blood on stool because of injury of mucosa covering hemorrhoid (most common).
2. Visible (if external) and palpable mass.
3. Constipation and anal itching.
4. Sensation of incomplete fecal evacuation.
5. Infection or ulceration, mucus discharge.
6. Pain noted more in external hemorrhoids.
7. Sudden rectal pain because of thrombosis in external hemorrhoids.

Diagnostic Evaluation

1. History and visualization by external examination through anoscopy or proctosigmoidoscopy.
2. Barium enema or colonoscopy to rule out more serious colonic lesions causing rectal bleeding.

Management

Asymptomatic hemorrhoids require no treatment.

Medical

1. Bowel habits should be regulated with nonirritating stool softeners and high-fiber diet to keep stools soft.
2. Frequent, warm sitz baths to ease pain and combat swelling.
3. Control of itching by improved anal hygiene measures and control of moisture.
4. Analgesics as needed.
5. Topical creams, lotions, pads, and suppositories containing active ingredients, such as witch hazel, zinc monohydrate, pramoxine hydrochloride, glycerol stearate, phenylephrine, and hydrocortisone, to reduce swelling and provide comfort.
6. Avoid prolonged use of topical anesthetics on hemorrhoids or fissures because they often produce hypersensitive (allergic) perianal skin rashes with severe itching.

DRUG ALERT Avoid prolonged use of over-the-counter or prescription hemorrhoidal products without medical evaluation. Skin irritation and other adverse effects, or masking of more serious conditions may occur

7. Manual reduction of external hemorrhoids if prolapsed.
8. Injection of sclerosing solutions (phenol 5%) to produce scar tissue and decrease prolapse.
9. Cryodestruction (cryosurgery)—freezing of hemorrhoids.
   a. Causes profuse drainage and swelling.
   b. Foul-smelling discharge may last for 7 to 10 days after cryosurgery.
10. Other procedures include infrared coagulation (infrared radiation) and bipolar diathermy (heat).

Surgical

1. Surgery may be indicated when the following conditions exist:
   a. Prolonged bleeding.
   b. Disabling pain.
   c. Intolerable itching.
   d. Prolapse.
2. Rubber ring ligation is the treatment of choice.
   a. During anoscopy, the apex of the hemorrhoid is grasped and drawn through a drum.
   b. A trigger device expels two rubber bands, which encircle the base of the hemorrhoid.
   c. After a period of time, the hemorrhoid sloughs away.
3. Dilation of the anal canal and lower rectum under general anesthesia is another treatment.
   a. This procedure is not advocated for patients whose main complaints are prolapse or incontinence.
   b. It is also not recommended for older patients with weak sphincters.
4. Incision and removal of clot from acutely thrombosed hemorrhoid.
5. Hemorrhoidectomy—excision of internal/external hemorrhoids.

Complications

1. Hemorrhage, anemia.
2. Incontinence.
3. Prolapse and strangulation.

Nursing Interventions and Patient Education

1. After thrombosis or surgery, assist with frequent positioning, using pillow support for comfort.

2. Provide analgesics, warm sitz baths, or warm compresses to reduce pain and inflammation.
3. Apply anal pads, creams, or suppositories, as ordered, to relieve discomfort.
4. Observe anal area postoperatively for drainage and bleeding; report if excessive.
5. Administer stool softener/laxative to assist with bowel movements soon after surgery to reduce the risk of stricture.
6. Encourage regular exercise, high-fiber diet, and adequate fluid intake (8 to 10 glasses/day) to avoid straining and constipation.
7. Discourage regular use of laxatives—firm, soft stools dilate the anal canal, decreasing stricture formation.
8. Determine the patient's normal bowel habits, and identify predisposing factors to educate patient about changes necessary to prevent recurrence of symptoms.

Other Conditions of the Anorectum

See Table 14-4, pages 515 to 516.

Table 14-4 Anorectal Disorders

CONDITION	ETIOLOGY	CLINICAL MANIFESTATIONS	MANAGEMENT	NURSING CONSIDERATIONS
Fissure				
Linear laceration of anal epithelium; typically located in the posterior midline	• Constipated stools may tear anal lining. • Perineum strain during childbirth. • Tuberculosis, syphilis, and Crohn disease are less common causes.	• Tearing acute pain during and after bowel movement; discomfort may continue several hours after bowel movement. • Spotting of bright red blood with stool; spasm of anal canal; burning	• Promotion of regular, soft bowel movements through stool softeners, suppositories, high-fiber diet, bulking agents • Topical creams • Fissurectomy; sphincterotomy	• Assist with warm sitz baths and local application of anesthetic ointment to reduce pain. • Instruct to eat high-fiber foods and drink fluids to prevent constipation.
Abscess				
Localized area of pus from inflammation of anorectal tissue	• Infection develops from abrasion from foreign object, such as enema tip or fishbone. • Acute phase of anal fistula, suspect Crohn disease • Tuberculosis or actinomycosis	• Painful, reddened bulge or swelling near the anus; pain increases with sitting; moderate-to-severe pain. • Purulent drainage	• Incision and drainage of purulent exudate • Placement of drainage catheter for 7–10 d; possible packing dressing • Warm sitz baths; pulsed lavage	• Wound assessment • Pain medications as needed • Alert for passage of bowel movements, postoperatively.
Fistula				
Abnormal tubelike passage from the skin near the anus into anal canal	• Often preceded by anal abscess • May be associated with inflammatory bowel disease, cancer, or foreign body • Hidradenitis suppurativa	• Purulent drainage from opening • Itching and pain	• Fistulotomy • Fistulectomy • Bowel rest to allow fistula to heal; possible fecal diversion temporarily	• Wound assessment • Pain medications as needed • Alert for passage of bowel movements, postoperatively.
Anal Condylomas; Venereal Warts				
	• Infectious cauliflower-like papillomas; probably sexually transmitted papillomavirus • Differentiate from syphilitic warts, hemorrhoids, and anal/skin cancers	• Thrive in moist, macerated surfaces, as with purulent drainage • Often recur • Rarely invade the urethra, bladder, or rectum	• Application of podophyllum resin (may be painful) • Electrofulguration • α-Interferon injections/synergistic with podophyllum resin • Fluorouracil	• Encourage good anal hygiene and frequent use of talc dusting powder. • Schedule follow-up visits to assess area periodically for recurrence.
Proctitis				
Acute or chronic inflammation of rectal mucosa	• Common infecting organisms: *Neisseria gonorrhoeae*, *Chlamydia*, herpes simplex virus, *Treponema pallidum* (syphilis) • Radiation	• Anorectal pain; purulent, mucoid, or bloody discharge; pruritus; tenesmus • Diarrhea and/or constipation	• Treatment specific to isolated organism—antibiotics, antivirals • Bulking agents, antispasmodics	• Review medications. • Assist with examination and treatment.

(continued)

Table 14-4 Anorectal Disorders (*continued*)

CONDITION	ETIOLOGY	CLINICAL MANIFESTATIONS	MANAGEMENT	NURSING CONSIDERATIONS
Stricture				
Narrowing of the anorectal lumen, preventing dilation of sphincter	• Usually results from scarring after anorectal surgery (hemorrhoidectomy) or inflammation • Congenital anomalies	• Constipation, ribbon stools, may not completely evacuate stools • Pain with bowel movement; itching	• Treatment of inflammatory cause • Dilation by digital, instrumentation, or balloon methods • If stenosis severe, may need plastic surgery to anal canal	• Prevention of stenosis after anal surgery facilitated by anal hygiene, warm sitz baths, and dilation • Postoperative care includes stool softeners, warm sitz baths, and wound care.
Rectal Prolapse				
Mucosal membrane protrudes through the anus.	• The support structures are weakened (sphincters and muscles), leading to rectal intussusception. • Conditions may include neurologic disorders, chronic diseases, aging.	• Associated with constipation and straining; rectal fullness • Bloody diarrhea; rectal ulcer secondary to intussusception	• Treatment depends on underlying cause. • Sclerosing agent injection may fix the rectum in place. • Surgery may include sphincter repair or resection of prolapsed tissue.	• Diet/fluid instructions to avoid constipation. • Teach perineum-strengthening exercises.

SELECTED READINGS

Aspiras, O., Lucas, T., Thompson, H. S., Manning, M. A., Blessman, J., Dawadi, A., Hirko, K. A., & Penner, L. A. (2023). Culturally targeted message framing and colorectal cancer screening preferences among African Americans. *Health Psychology, 42*(1), 1–4. https://doi.org/10.1037/hea0001246

Balk, E. M., Adam, G. P., Cao, W., Danko, K., Buhma, M. R., Mehta, S., & Saldahna, S. (2020). *Management of colonic diverticulitis* (Comparative Effectiveness Review No. 233. AHRQ Publication No. 20(21)-EHC025). Agency for Healthcare Research and Quality. https://effectivehealthcare.ahrq.gov/sites/default/files/pdf/cer-233-diverticulitis-final-report.pdf

Bergemalm, D., Andersson, E., Hultdin, J., Eriksson, C., Rush, S. T., Kalla, R., Adams, A. T., Keita, Å. V., D'Amato, M., Gomollon, F., Jahnsen, J., IBD Character Consortium, Ricanek, P., Satsangi, J., Repsilber, D., Karling, P., & Halfvarson, J. (2021). Systemic inflammation in preclinical ulcerative colitis. *Gastroenterology, 161*(5), 1526–1539.e9. https://doi.org/10.1053/j.gastro.2021.07.026

Buensalid, J. A., Valencia, J. C., & Chandrasekar, P. H. (2023) Helicobacter pylori infection treatment. *Medscape Drugs and Diseases.* https://emedicine.medscape.com/article/2172395-overview

Castaneda, D., Franco Azar, F., Hussain, I., Lara, L. F., Pimentel, R. R., Alemar, G., Hrelec, C., Ponsky, J., & Erim, T. (2022). A cooperative approach for treatment of Zenker's diverticulum. *Surgical Endoscopy, 36*(6), 4129–4135. https://doi.org/10.1007/s00464-021-08736-z

Cholin, L., Ashour, T., Mehdi, A., Taliercio, J. J., Daou, R., Arrigain, S., Schold, J. D., Thomas, G., Nally, J., Nakhoul, N. L., & Nakhoul, G. N. (2021). Proton-pump inhibitor vs. H2-receptor blocker use and overall risk of CKD progression. *BMC Nephrology, 22*(1), 264. https://doi.org/10.1186/s12882-021-02449-0

Hall, J., Hardiman, K., Lee, S., Lightner, A., Stocchi, L., Paquette, I. M., Steele, S. R., & Feingold, D. L.; Prepared on behalf of the Clinical Practice Guidelines Committee of the American Society of Colon and Rectal Surgeons. (2020). The American Society of Colon and Rectal Surgeons clinical practice guidelines for the treatment of left-sided colonic diverticulitis. *Diseases of the Colon & Rectum, 63*(6), 728–747. https://doi.org/10.1097/DCR.0000000000001679

Hibi, T., Ishibashi, T., Ikenoue, Y., Yoshihara, R., Nihei, A., & Kobayashi, T. (2020). Ulcerative colitis: Disease burden, impact on daily life, and reluctance to consult medical professionals: Results from a Japanese internet survey. *Inflammatory Intestinal Diseases, 5*(1), 27–35. https://doi.org/10.1159/000505092

Hoegberg, L. C. G., Shepherd, G., Wood, D. M., Johnson, J., Hoffman, R. S., Caravati, E. M., Chan, W. L., Smith, S. W., Olson, K. R., & Gosselin, S. (2021). Systematic review on the use of activated charcoal for gastrointestinal decontamination following acute oral overdose. *Clinical Toxicology (Philadelphia, PA), 59*(12), 1196–1227. https://doi.org/10.1080/15563650.2021.1961144

Hosseini, S. M., Dadgar Moghaddam, M., Yazdan Panah, S., & Vafaeimanesh, J. (2020). Effect of gastric lavage with hemostasis powder® on upper gastrointestinal bleeding (Conversion of emergency endoscopy to elective endoscopy). *Caspian Journal of Internal Medicine, 11*(3), 304–309. https://doi.org/10.22088/cjim.11.3.304

Kao, C., & Lin, C. (2024). Catastrophic Gastrointestinal Bleeding Caused by Aorto-gastric Fistula. *Journal of Radiological Science,* Publish Ahead of Print. https://doi.org/10.4103/jradiolsci.JRADIOLSCI-D-23-00028

Killian, R. E., Gillespie, P. G. J. A., Bishop-Royse, J., Wolf, D. L. A., & Gates, L. (2019). Clinical practice guideline: Gastric tube placement verification. *Journal of Emergency Nursing, 45*(3), 306.e1–306.e19. https://doi.org/10.1016/j.jen.2019.03.011

Kittscha, J., Fairbrother, G., Bliokas, V., & Wilson, V. (2022). Adjustment to an ostomy. *Journal of Wound, Ostomy and Continence Nursing, 49*(5), 439-448. https://doi.org/10.1097/WON.0000000000000895

Lynch, W. D., & Hsu, R. (2022). Ulcerative colitis. In *StatPearls* [Internet]. StatPearls Publishing. https://www.ncbi.nlm.nih.gov/books/NBK459282/

Mak, M. Y., & Tam, G. (2020). Ultrasonography for nasogastric tube placement verification: An additional reference. *British Journal of Community Nursing, 25*(7), 328–334. https://doi.org/10.12968/bjcn.2020.25.7.328

Ngamruengphong, S., Ferri, L., Aihara, H., Draganov, P. V., Yang, D. J., Perbtani, Y. B., Jue, T. L., Munroe, C. A., Boparai, E. S., Mehta, N. A., Bhatt, A., Kumta, N. A., Othman, M. O., Mercado, M., Javaid, H., Aadam, A. A., Siegel, A., James, T. W., Grimm, I. S., … Kalloo, A. N. (2021). Efficacy of endoscopic submucosal dissection for superficial gastric neoplasia in a large cohort in North America. *Clinical Gastroenterology and Hepatology, 19*(8), 1611–1619. https://doi.org/10.1016/j.cgh.2020.06.023

Patel, C. K., Kahrilas, P. J., Hodge, N. B., Tsikretsis, L. E., Carlson, D. A., Pandolfino, J. E., & Tétreault, M.-P. (2022). RNA-sequencing reveals molecular and regional differences in the esophageal mucosa of achalasia patients. *Scientific Reports, 12*(1), 1–13. https://doi.org/10.1038/s41598-022-25103-7

Peery, A. F., Shaukat, A., & Strate, L. L. (2021). AGA clinical practice update on medical management of colonic diverticulitis: Expert review. *Gastroenterology, 160*(3), 906–911.e1. https://doi.org/10.1053/j.gastro.2020.09.059

Taylor, S., & Manara, A. R. (2021). X-ray checks of NG tube position: A case for guided tube placement. *The British Journal of Radiology, 94*(1124), 20210432. https://doi.org/10.1259/bjr.20210432

Zhang, Y., Zhang, Y., Peng, L., & Zhang, L. (2023). Research progress on the predicting factors and coping strategies for postoperative recurrence of esophageal cancer. *Cells, 12*(1), 114. https://doi.org/10.3390/cells12010114

Zondervan, N., Snelgrove, R., & Bradley, N. (2022). Management of acute diverticulitis. *CMAJ: Canadian Medical Association Journal = Journal de l'Association Medicale Canadienne, 194*(34), E1171. https://doi.org/10.1503/cmaj.220139

15 Hepatic, Biliary, and Pancreatic Disorders*

OVERVIEW AND ASSESSMENT

Assessment of Accessory Organ Dysfunction

The liver and its bile ducts, the gallbladder, and the pancreas are called accessory glands in the gastrointestinal (GI) system. Their function is to aid digestion through the delivery of bile and enzymes to the small intestine. The liver plays additional roles in detoxification of chemicals and synthesis and storage of important nutrients. The pancreas also functions as an endocrine gland, as discussed in Chapter 15.

Effects of Aging on Liver and Gallbladder

Liver laboratory tests generally remain within normal range, but a number of other physiologic changes occur within the hepatic and biliary systems with aging:

1. Decline in liver volume and size.
2. Decrease in blood flow.
3. Reduced drug metabolism.
4. Decline in capability of drug clearance.
5. Slower repair of damaged liver cells after injury.
6. Decreased production and flow of bile with decline in gallbladder contraction after meals.
7. Atypical clinical presentation of gallbladder and bile duct disorders.
8. Increased cholesterol secretion in bile leading to increased occurrence of gallstones.
9. Slower clearance of hepatitis B surface antigen, if infected.
10. Rapid progression of hepatitis C infection with lower response rate to therapy.

POPULATION AWARENESS Use caution with administering potentially hepatotoxic drugs, such as acetaminophen, to older adults.

History

1. Was the patient born between the years 1945 and 1965?
2. Have there been blood transfusions (before 1992)? Are there known blood disorders? GI bleeding?
3. Has there been contact with a person who has an infection such as hepatitis? Any unprotected sexual activity or ingestion of potentially contaminated food?
4. Has there been drug or chemical toxicity, such as carbon tetrachloride, chloroform, phosphorus, arsenicals, ethanol, halothane, isoniazid, or acetaminophen? Have amanita mushrooms been ingested recently? Are certain medications being taken, such as phenothiazine derivatives, sulfonamides, antidiabetic drugs, propylthiouracil, monoamine oxidase inhibitors, methyldopa, azathioprine, corticosteroids, thiazide diuretics, estrogens, and valproic acid? Have any antiviral medications been taken for HIV, including protease inhibitors or antineoplastic agents (note that many of these drugs can cause hepatic, biliary, and pancreatic GI symptoms)?
5. Is there a history of nonsterile needle puncture, as in subcutaneous ("skin popping"), intramuscular ("muscling"), or intravenous (IV) drug use? Tattoos?
6. Does medical history include gallstones, hepatitis, pancreatitis, Wilson disease, Budd–Chiari syndrome, biliary cirrhosis, liver surgery, or transplantation?
7. Any family history of gallstones, pancreatitis, gallbladder, or pancreatic cancer or related cancers such as breast or ovarian cancer?
8. Is there a history of organ transplantation (before 1992)?

*Please note that the term "male" in this chapter refers to a person assigned male at birth, and the term "female" in this chapter refers to a person assigned female at birth.

9. Assess alcohol consumption: "How many times in the past year have you had five or more drinks in a day (for males) or four or more drinks in a day (for females)?"

Common Manifestations

1. Any jaundice/icterus—yellow color of sclera and skin, pruritus, dark tea-colored urine, light gray or clay-colored (acholic) stool?
2. Any dyspepsia, anorexia, nausea, vomiting, right upper quadrant or epigastric pain, or pain radiating to the back or shoulder blade? What is the relationship of pain to eating or to position?
3. Has there been fatigue, malaise, loss of vigor and strength, easy bruising, or weight loss?
4. Any fever, chills, headache, myalgias, arthralgias, photophobia?
5. Any steatorrhea—stools that are loose, greasy, foamy, orange in color, and foul smelling and that float?

Physical Examination Findings

1. Skin—yellow sclera or skin? Rashes or scratches on body from severe scratching because of pruritus? Any signs of bruising or petechiae on body, palmar erythema, or overt bleeding?
2. Neurologic—what is the level of consciousness (LOC)? Any asterixis (flapping tremor elicited when the arms are extended and wrists dorsiflexed)?
3. Abdomen—any tenderness or liver enlargement in the right upper quadrant? Any ascites? Any palpable masses in the abdomen? Any fluid wave?
4. Peripheral vascular—any edema, anasarca, or telangiectasia?

Laboratory Tests

See Table 15-1, pages 518 to 519.

Table 15-1 Liver Diagnostic Studies

TEST AND PURPOSE	NORMAL	NURSING CONSIDERATIONS
Bile Formation and Secretion		
Serum Bilirubin		
Measures bilirubin in the blood; this determines the ability of the liver to take up, conjugate, and excrete bilirubin. Bilirubin is a product of the breakdown of hemoglobin.		
Direct (conjugated)—soluble in water	0–0.3 mg/dL	• Abnormal in biliary and liver disease, causing jaundice clinically.
Indirect (unconjugated)—insoluble in water	0–1 mg/dL	• Abnormal in hemolysis and in functional disorders of uptake or conjugation.
Total serum bilirubin	0.1–1.2 mg/dL	• Used as screening test for liver or biliary dysfunction.
Urine Bilirubin		
Not normally found in urine, but if direct serum bilirubin is elevated, some spills into urine.	None (0)	• Tea-colored urine; when specimen is shaken, yellow-green tinted foam can be observed. • If the patient is receiving phenazopyridine, mark the laboratory slip to this effect because there may be a false-positive bilirubin result.
Urobilinogen		
Formed in the small intestine by action of bacteria on bilirubin. Related to amount of bilirubin excreted into bile.	Urine urobilinogen <1 mg in 2-h specimen or 0.5–4 mg/dL in 24-h specimen. Fecal urobilinogen 50–300 mg/24 h	• Random urine specimen is collected over 2 h after lunch, or a total level is collected over a 24-h period. • Place specimen in dark brown container and send it to laboratory immediately or refrigerate to prevent decomposition. • If the patient is receiving antimicrobials, mark laboratory slip to this effect because production of urobilinogen can be falsely reduced.
Protein Studies		
Albumin and Globulin Measurement		
Is of greater significance than total protein measurement.		• As one increases, the other decreases.
Albumin—produced by liver cells	3.5–5.5 g/dL	• Albumin ↓ (decrease) in cirrhosis, chronic hepatitis
Globulin—produced in lymph nodes, spleen, bone marrow, and Kupffer cells of liver	2.5–5.9 g/dL	• Globulin ↑ (increase) in cirrhosis, chronic obstructive jaundice, viral hepatitis

Table 15-1 Liver Diagnostic Studies (*continued*)

Coagulation		
PT		
Prothrombin and other clotting factors are manufactured in the liver; its rate is influenced by the supply of vitamin K.	9.6–12.5 sec	• PT may be prolonged in liver disease, in which case it will not return to normal with vitamin K. It may also be prolonged in malabsorption of fat and fat-soluble vitamins, in which case it will return to normal with vitamin K.
Calculated from PT		
INR	0.8–1.2	Used to monitor warfarin therapy.
Fat Metabolism		
Cholesterol		
Measures lipid metabolism by determining serum cholesterol levels.	140–200 mg/dL	• Serum cholesterol level is decreased in parenchymal liver disease. • Serum lipid level is increased in biliary obstruction.
Liver Detoxification		
Serum Alkaline Phosphatase		
Because bile disposes this enzyme, any impairment of liver cell excretory function will cause an elevation. In cholestasis or obstruction, increased synthesis of enzyme causes very high levels in blood.	30–120 IU/L	• Elevated to more than three times normal in extrahepatic obstructive jaundice, intrahepatic cholestasis, liver metastasis, or granulomas. Also elevated in osteoblastic diseases, Paget disease, and hyperparathyroidism.
Enzyme Production		
These enzymes are found in high concentration in the liver as well as some other tissues. Liver injury results in enzyme release into blood.		
AST	0–37 IU/L	• An elevation in these enzymes indicates liver cell damage.
ALT	0–40 IU/L	• Some drugs such as opioids may also cause a rise in AST and ALT.
LDH	105–333 IU/L	• LDH is found in liver, heart, kidney, muscle, and blood cells.
GGT	0–51 IU/L	• GGT is also found in the kidneys, pancreas, and bile ducts but is most sensitive to alcohol-induced liver damage.
Ammonia (NH_3), serum	0–32 mmol/L	• Ammonia levels rise when the liver is unable to convert ammonia to urea.

ALT, alanine aminotransferase; AST, aspartate aminotransferase; GGT, gamma glutamyl transpeptidase, INR, international normalized ratio; LDH, lactate dehydrogenase; PT, prothrombin time

Carbohydrate Antigen 19-9

Description

A tumor antigen found in serum; used as a marker to assess the efficacy of treatment, surgical outcomes, and survival for pancreatic, biliary, and hepatocellular cancers. Also known as cancer-associated antigen 19-9.

Nursing and Patient Care Considerations

1. Tell patient a blood test will be taken and the results will be ready in 1 to 2 days.
2. Not a screening test for pancreatic cancer, this is an adjunct with other tests to provide support for a diagnosis of pancreatic cancer and to better measure the recurrence of pancreatic cancer after treatment.
3. Level may be elevated with benign conditions including acute cholangitis, cirrhosis, and gallstones.

Serum Alpha-Fetoprotein Concentration

Description

A glycoprotein normally produced during gestation by the fetal liver and yolk sac. It reappears in the serum when a tumor returns to a more primitive state. Alpha-fetoprotein (AFP) is elevated in up to 95% of hepatocellular carcinomas (primary liver cancer).

Nursing and Patient Care Considerations

1. Tell patient a blood test will be taken and the results will be ready in 1 to 3 days.
2. Not a screening test for primary liver cancer, this is an adjunct with other tests to provide support for a diagnosis of primary liver cancer and to detect/predict liver metastasis.
3. AFP may also be elevated in the setting of nonmalignant liver diseases, pregnancy, certain tumors of the gonads (testes and ovaries), and gastric cancer.

Radiology and Imaging Studies

Ultrasonography

Description

1. A noninvasive test that focuses high-frequency sound waves over an area in the abdomen to generate an image of the structure.
2. Ultrasound of the abdomen can detect gallstones, dilated bile duct, fluid-filled cysts, ascites, and small abdominal masses.
3. This test is the preferred diagnostic procedure. It is rapid and accurate, and does not expose the patient to radiation. It can be used safely in patients with liver dysfunction and jaundice.
4. It is reported to be able to detect gallstones with 95% accuracy.
5. Ultrasound with Doppler can assess the patency of the portal vein, hepatic artery, hepatic vein, and direction of blood flow. It can be used to diagnose patients with Budd–Chiari syndrome or vessel thrombosis after major liver surgery or liver transplant.

Nursing and Patient Care Considerations

1. The patient should have nothing to eat or drink for 4 to 8 hours prior to the exam, and a fat-free meal is preferred the evening before the test, in order to minimize air in the stomach and bowel, which would obscure images of the gallbladder, liver, pancreas, and spleen. Medications may be taken with small sips of water.
2. Explain to the patient that a gel is applied to the skin over the selected area and a wandlike transducer is swept across the area of interest.
3. Images of organs will be obtained.

Cholescintigraphy (Hepatobiliary Iminodiacetic Acid [HIDA] Scan)

Description

1. A noninvasive nuclear medicine study using radioactive isotopes to evaluate gallbladder function and aid in the diagnosis of hepatobiliary disorders, such as common bile duct obstruction, acute and chronic cholecystitis, bile leaks, bile reflux, and hepatocellular dysfunction after liver transplantation.
2. A radioactive agent is administered in an IV line. It is taken up by the hepatocytes and excreted rapidly through the biliary tract.
3. The biliary tract is scanned with a gamma camera as the radiotracer moves through the body, and images of the gallbladder and biliary tract are obtained.

Nursing and Patient Care Considerations

1. Patient should have nothing by mouth (NPO) for at least 4 hours before the procedure to optimize emptying of gallbladder.
2. If possible, no opiates should be administered for at least 6 hours before the procedure because of opiate effects on smooth muscle motility of biliary tree and gallbladder.
3. Inform the patient that the scan takes approximately 2 to 4 hours and additional images may need to be taken up to 24 hours later.

Endoscopic Retrograde Cholangiopancreatography

Description

1. Involves visualization of the common bile, pancreatic, and hepatic ducts with a flexible fiber-optic endoscope inserted into the esophagus, passed through the stomach, and into the duodenum.
2. The common bile duct and the pancreatic duct are cannulated, and contrast medium is injected into the ducts, permitting visualization and radiographic evaluation.
3. Done to detect extrahepatic biliary obstruction, such as calculi, tumors of the bile duct, strictures or injuries to the bile duct; intrahepatic biliary obstruction caused by stones or tumor; and pancreatic disease, such as chronic pancreatitis, pseudocyst, pancreatic duct anomalies, or tumor.
4. May be combined with a therapeutic biliary or pancreatic procedure, such as endoscopic sphincterotomy, placement of biliary or pancreatic stents, tissue biopsy, removal of fluid for cytology, or retrieval of retained gallstones from the common bile duct.

Nursing and Patient Care Considerations

Preprocedure

1. Assess for allergies to iodine, seafood, or contrast media to determine the need for premedication with antihistamines or steroids (per facility protocol) to prevent a reaction.
2. Patient must be NPO for at least 6 hours before the procedure. Withhold medications according to provider order.
3. Any patient receiving heparin should have the infusion stopped for 4 to 6 hours before the procedure and a partial thromboplastin time (PTT) assessed. If patient is receiving warfarin, a recent international normalized ratio (INR) must be available.
4. Make sure that dentures are removed; instruct the patient to gargle and swallow topical anesthetic to decrease gag reflex, as ordered.
5. Verify that the patient has a signed consent form before sedation is given.
6. Establish baseline vital signs.
7. Establish IV access.
8. Administer antibiotic prophylaxis, as ordered.
9. Assist in placing patient in the prone position.
10. If outpatient procedure, the patient must have a responsible adult to drive them home as patient is not allowed to drive or operate machinery for 24 hours because of the effects of mild sedation.

Postprocedure

1. Monitor and document vital signs.
2. Observe for and report abdominal distention and signs of perforation, GI bleeding, or pancreatitis, including chills, fever, abdominal pain, vomiting, hypotension, and tachycardia. Notify the health care provider immediately.
3. Maintain NPO status until the patient is alert and gag reflex returns, at which time clear liquid diet is initiated and advanced as tolerated.

Endoscopic Ultrasound

Description

1. In endoscopic ultrasound (EUS), a high-frequency ultrasound probe is placed at the tip of an endoscope to assess the pancreas through the GI lumen and provide images of the pancreas and adjacent organs.
2. It is useful in staging pancreatic tumors and establishing the size of the tumor, its extension into adjacent structures, local and regional nodal involvement, and any blood vessels that may be involved.
3. Tissue may also be obtained by fine needle aspiration biopsy through EUS guidance to confirm the diagnosis of a pancreatic malignancy.

Nursing and Patient Care Considerations

1. Instruct the patient that tissue may be obtained for analysis.
2. Verify that the patient has a signed consent form for the procedure and tissue aspiration before sedation is given.
3. Preprocedure and postprocedure care is the same as for endoscopic retrograde cholangiopancreatography (ERCP).

Magnetic Resonance Cholangiopancreatography

Description

1. A noninvasive, nonradiation radiologic technique that produces images of the pancreatic ducts and biliary tree similar in appearance to those obtained from an ERCP with the advantage of providing images of the surrounding parenchyma.
2. Able to detect the level and presence of biliary obstruction, but cannot offer therapeutic intervention.
3. Magnetic resonance cholangiopancreatography (MRCP) does not require the administration of contrast material and provides ideal imaging for patients with allergies to iodine-based contrast materials or kidney disease. Noniodine contrast agent may be given to enhance the picture of the biliary anatomy or secretin may be given as it stimulates exocrine secretion of the pancreas and improves visualization of the pancreatic duct by increasing its caliber.

Nursing and Patient Care Considerations

Preprocedure

1. Confirm that the patient does not have a pacemaker or internal defibrillator because the magnetic field could cause malfunction.
2. Confirm that the patient does not have any metal hardware in or on the body, such as intracranial aneurysm clips, intraocular metal fragments, cochlear ear devices, metal joint replacements, retained bullets or shrapnel, or steel sutures, because this may cause artifact and a distorted picture from the magnetic pull by the metal.
3. Remove all metal attachments from the patient, such as watch, jewelry, piercings, cell phone, IV poles, and infusion devices.
4. Confirm that the patient does not have a fear of enclosed spaces (claustrophobia) or anxiety as the patient may not be able to undergo the procedure or may require a sedative.
5. The patient must be NPO for at least 4 hours before the procedure.
6. Inform the patient that the test takes about 10 to 30 minutes and is quite loud. They may choose to use ear plugs for comfort.

Postprocedure

1. The patient may resume usual activities.
2. The health care provider will notify the patient of the results when available, usually in 1 to 3 days.

Positron Emission Tomographic Scan

Description

1. Positron emission tomography (PET) is an imaging technique that uses positively charged radioactive particles to detect subtle changes in the body's metabolism and chemical activities.
2. Fluorodeoxyglucose 18F (^{18}F-FDG) is injected via IV line as a radiotracer and has a short half-life of 110 minutes and is cleared rapidly from the body.
3. The radiotracer used most often for PET scan has a glucose component; because malignant tumors use glucose and grow at a faster rate than normal tissue, PET scans are able to locate areas of high tracer uptake, which represents tumor growth.
4. A PET scan provides a black-and-white or color-coded image of the function of a particular area of the body, rather than its structure. Functional change precedes structural change in tissues and organs; therefore, PET scans can detect abnormalities earlier than a computed tomography (CT) scan or magnetic resonance imaging (MRI).
5. PET scan application in hepatic, biliary, and pancreatic disease includes the detection of cancer—particularly when other conventional imaging findings are negative—and response to cancer treatment. PET scan can also be used to evaluate the physiology of the heart and brain at baseline or following an event to determine remaining function.

Nursing and Patient Care Considerations

Preprocedure

1. The patient should begin a limited carbohydrate diet 24 hours prior to the procedure. The test provides images showing where certain molecules are in the body, including where glucose is located. This is greatly affected by the level of sugar in the blood; therefore, the diet the day before the scan impacts the quality of pictures.
2. The patient must be NPO, except for plain water, for at least 6 hours before the procedure.
3. Patients with diabetes or patients with glucose intolerance may require adjustments in diet and diabetes medications or insulin dosage on the day of the test as blood glucose levels must be no higher than 200 mg/dL. Adjustments should be made on an individual basis.
4. Patients are not to do exercise of any sort for the 48 hours prior to the exam. This includes even nominal activity such as golf and gardening.
5. Advise the patient to remove jewelry or other items containing metal.
6. Inform the patient that scanning time varies from 15 minutes to 2 hours, depending on the areas to be scanned, but the total time in the imaging center is longer (2 to 3 hours).
7. Caution the patient that it is essential to arrive on time for this test because the FDG tracer is radioactive only for a short time. Some centers order the tracer on a per case basis, scheduling delivery of the radiotracer to coincide with the patient's time of arrival.
8. Inform the patient that an IV line will be used to inject the radiotracer. To allow the radiotracer to disperse throughout the body, the scan will be performed 30 to 60 minutes after the injection.
9. Make sure that a bowel preparation has been carried out, if ordered. Ask the patient to void prior to the scan.
10. Inform the patient that the radiotracer is rapidly cleared from the body and that the test has no adverse effects.

Postprocedure

1. The patient may resume usual activities.
2. The patient may be encouraged to increase fluid intake to assist in flushing out the radiotracer.

Percutaneous Transhepatic Cholangiography

Description

1. Percutaneous transhepatic cholangiography (PTC) is a fluoroscopic examination of the intrahepatic and extrahepatic biliary ducts after injection of contrast medium into the biliary tree through percutaneous needle injection.

2. Distinguishes obstructive jaundice caused by liver disease from jaundice caused by biliary obstruction, such as from a tumor, injury to the common bile duct, stones within the bile ducts, or sclerosing cholangitis.
3. A biliary catheter may be placed during the procedure to drain the biliary tree, called percutaneous transhepatic biliary drainage (PTBD). This relieves jaundice, decreases pruritus, improves nutritional status, allows easy access into the biliary tree for further procedures, and can be used as an anatomic landmark and stent of a surgical anastomosis to allow for healing.

Nursing and Patient Care Considerations

Preprocedure

1. Assess for allergies to iodine, seafood, or contrast media to determine need to be premedicated with antihistamines or steroids (per facility protocol) to prevent reaction.
2. The patient must be NPO for at least 6 hours before the procedure.
3. Verify that the patient has had all questions answered and has a signed consent form before sedatives are given.
4. Inform the patient that the procedure takes 30 to 60 minutes.
5. Establish baseline hemoglobin, hematocrit, and platelet count.
6. Inquire if the patient is taking any blood thinners. Make sure prothrombin time (PT) and INR are within normal limits.
7. Establish baseline vital signs.
8. Establish an IV line.
9. Administer antibiotic prophylaxis, as ordered.

Postprocedure

1. Monitor and document vital signs and assess puncture site for bleeding, hematoma, or bile leakage.
2. Assess for and report signs of peritonitis from bile leaking into the abdomen (fever, chills, diffuse abdominal pain, tenderness, distention) or cholangitis (infection in the biliary tree) from bacteria in the bile being released into the GI tract and then into the bloodstream.
3. Continue antibiotic prophylaxis per facility protocol.
4. If the patient has PTBD, monitor the catheter exit site for bleeding or bile drainage and monitor drainage in bile bag for color, amount, and consistency. The drainage initially may have some blood mixed with bile but should clear within a few hours. The liver makes 700 to 1,000 mL of bile in 24 hours, and there should be adequate drainage when bile is draining into a bile bag (called external drainage).
   a. Report frank blood and blood clots that appear in the bile bag.
   b. Large amounts of bile drainage may require fluid replacement.
   c. Maintain patency and security of biliary catheter; perform routine care and dressing at catheter exit site.
   d. Perform routine flushing of biliary catheter per order. Cap off the end of the biliary catheter to allow internal drainage of bile, if indicated. Teach the patient the care and flushing of biliary catheter and signs of complications, if indicated.
   e. Do not aspirate from a PTBD catheter because this draws bacteria from the bowel back through the liver and may cause cholangitis. Gently push solution into the PTBD catheter to prevent increased pressure within the biliary tree.
5. Signs of complications include fever, chills, persistent jaundice, abdominal bloating, exquisite abdominal tenderness, inability to flush the catheter, bleeding from the catheter, redness or discharge from the catheter site, leakage around the exit site of the catheter, and dislodgment of the catheter.

Other Diagnostic Tests

Transient Elastography

Description

1. Noninvasive measure to evaluate the liver. The probe measures the velocity as this wave passes through the liver.
2. Superior to ultrasound and can replace biopsy to evaluate fibrosis and cirrhosis.
3. Used for initial assessment of liver scarring, as well as follow-up for progression of disease.

Nursing and Patient Care Considerations

1. Technical limitations of the test preclude its use in patients who have ascites, individuals with morbid obesity, and/or patients who have large amounts of chest wall fat.
2. Ensure that the patient has maintained NPO status for at least 2 hours before the procedure, with no eating or drinking of high sugar items on the day of the test.
3. Inform the patient that the test takes about 10 minutes and causes no discomfort.
4. Following the procedure, the patient may resume normal activity and diet.

Liver Biopsy

EVIDENCE BASE Chowdhury, A. B., & Mehta, K. J. (2022). Liver biopsy for assessment of chronic liver diseases: A synopsis. *Clinical and Experimental Medicine, 23*, 273–285. https://doi.org/10.1007/s10238-022-00799-z

Description

Liver biopsy is the gold standard for the diagnosis of cirrhosis or cancer. Sampling of liver tissue through needle aspiration establishes a diagnosis of liver disease through histologic review. The sample may be taken from the liver directly (percutaneous) or through the internal jugular vein (transjugular). Both forms of biopsy include the risks of an invasive procedure: pain, risk for bleeding, and close monitoring and observation. The transjugular liver biopsy utilizes fluoroscopy and is a safer option for patients with diffuse liver disease and severe alteration in coagulation or massive ascites.

Nursing and Patient Care Considerations

Preprocedure

1. Establish baseline hemoglobin level, hematocrit, and platelet count.
2. Any patient receiving heparin should have the infusion stopped for 4 to 6 hours before the procedure. If the patient is receiving warfarin, aspirin, clopidogrel, or other platelet-inhibiting or blood-thinning medication, a recent INR, PTT, and PT must be available and within normal limits.
3. Verify informed consent.
4. Establish baseline vital signs.
5. Inform the patient that cooperation in holding breath for about 10 seconds during the procedure is important to obtain biopsy without damaging the diaphragm.
6. An IV may be inserted for sedation, as needed.

Postprocedure

1. Position the patient on their right side with pillow supporting lower rib cage for several hours following transcutaneous biopsy to prevent bleeding.
2. Neck discomfort is common following transjugular liver biopsy. Utilize positioning and nonpharmacologic methods to promote comfort.

3. Check vital signs and observe biopsy site frequently for bleeding or drainage.
4. Complications include bleeding, pneumothorax, infection, dysrhythmia, and from sedation.

Fine Needle Aspiration

Description

1. The removal of cells or fluid from a mass to establish a diagnosis through histologic review.
2. A fine needle is inserted into the suspicious area, and a small sample is withdrawn.
3. The needle is guided by fluoroscopy, CT scan, or ultrasound and can usually reach most internal organs with minimal risk to the patient.

Nursing and Patient Care Considerations

Preprocedure

1. Establish baseline hemoglobin, hematocrit, and platelet count.
2. Verify informed consent.
3. Establish baseline vital signs.
4. Tell the patient that a mild sedative may be given and a pain block may be performed in the area where the needle will be placed.
5. Encourage the patient to cooperate with body position to obtain the necessary cells.
6. An IV may be inserted for sedation, as needed.

Postprocedure

1. Monitor vital signs per facility protocol.
2. Assess the patient for any signs of complications, including pain, hypotension, tachycardia, and abdominal distention or hematoma at the biopsy site.
3. Inform the patient that bruising or some discomfort may be experienced at the biopsy site.
4. Instruct the patient on resuming anticoagulants based on health care provider directions.
5. If performed as an outpatient procedure, the patient must have a responsible adult to drive them home as the patient is not allowed to drive or operate machinery for 24 hours after the procedure because of the effects of sedation.

HEPATIC DISORDERS

See additional online content: Procedure Guidelines 15-1, 15-2

Hepatic disorders may disrupt normal liver function, which include the following:

- Storage of vitamins A, B, D; iron; and copper.
- Synthesis of plasma proteins, including albumin and globulins.
- Synthesis of the clotting factors vitamin K and prothrombin.
- Storage of glycogen and synthesis of glucose from other nutrients (gluconeogenesis).
- Breakdown of fatty acids for energy.
- Production of bile.
- Detoxification and excretion of waste products.

Hepatitis

EVIDENCE BASE Yang, W., Tian, X., & Liang, J. (2022). A comprehensive nursing model combined with high-quality nursing intervention for antiviral therapy in patients with chronic hepatitis B. *Evidence-Based Complementary and Alternative Medicine, 2022*, 6244637. https://doi.org/10.1155/2022/6244637

Di Marco, L., La Mantia, C., & Di Marco, V. (2022). Hepatitis C: Standard of treatment and what to do for global elimination. *Viruses, 14*(3), 505. https://doi.org/10.3390/v14030505

Hepatitis is defined as inflammation of the liver. Viral infection is a common cause associated with a broad spectrum of clinical manifestations from nonsymptom-producing infection, through icteric hepatitis, to hepatic necrosis. Five types of viral hepatitis have been identified.

Pathophysiology and Etiology

Type A Hepatitis

1. Hepatitis A virus (HAV) is caused by an RNA virus of the enterovirus family.
   a. Mode of transmission is usually via the fecal–oral route, either via person-to-person contact or through consumption of contaminated food or water. Prevalent in underdeveloped countries or in instances of overcrowding and poor sanitation.
   b. Commonly spread by person-to-person contact and, rarely, by blood transfusion or illicit drug use.
   c. Vaccines are available.
2. Incubation period is 15 to 50 days, with the average being 28 days.
3. Occurrence is worldwide, usually among children and young adults.
4. Nearly all recover within 6 months. Mortality is less than 1%.

Type B Hepatitis

1. Hepatitis B virus (HBV) is a double-stranded DNA virus from the family of hepadnaviruses that contains an outer envelope and inner core.
   a. HBcAg—hepatitis B core antigen (antigenic material in an inner core).
   b. HBsAg—hepatitis B surface antigen (antigenic material in an outer coat).
   c. HBeAg—hepatitis B envelop antigen (an independent protein circulating in the blood).
2. Each antigen stimulates a specific antibody:
   a. Anti-HBc—hepatitis B core antibodies (persists during the acute phase of illness; may indicate continuing HBV in the liver).
   b. Anti-HBs—hepatitis B surface antibodies (detected during late convalescence; usually indicates recovery and development of immunity).
   c. Anti-HBe—hepatitis B envelop antibodies (usually signifies reduced infectivity).
3. Significance:
   a. HBsAg—usually detected transiently in blood of 80% to 90% of infected people; may be noted in blood for months or years, indicating that the patient has acute or chronic hepatitis B infection or is a viral carrier.
   b. HBeAg—if absent, the patient is an asymptomatic carrier. If present, it indicates highly infectious period of acute, active hepatitis. If it persists, it indicates progression to chronic state.

4. Mode of transmission is primarily through blood (percutaneous and mucosal route).
   a. Oral route through saliva or through breastfeeding.
   b. Sexual activity through blood, semen, saliva, or vaginal secretions. Hepatitis B is recognized as a sexually transmitted infection.
   c. Gay males and those with HIV are at high risk.
5. Incubation period is 60 to 150 days (average of 90 days).
6. Occurrence is for all ages, but it mostly affects young adults worldwide. Vaccines are available.
7. Fifteen percent to 25% of chronically infected persons develop chronic liver disease, including cirrhosis, liver failure, or liver cancer. It causes 1,800 deaths per year in the United States and is the main cause of cirrhosis and hepatocellular carcinoma (HCC) worldwide.

Type C Hepatitis

1. Hepatitis C virus (HCV) is an RNA virus of the enterovirus family.
2. Mode of transmission is through direct exposure to blood and body fluids, primarily through: sharing contaminated needles, syringes, or other equipment to inject drugs.
   a. Less commonly through: transmission from birthing parent who is infected to fetus, sexual contact with a person who is infected, unregulated tattooing, and needlestick or other sharp instrument injuries.
3. Incubation period varies from 14 to 182 days (average range 14 to 84 days).
4. Occurs in all age groups.
   a. May occur sporadically or in epidemic proportions.
   b. Increasing number of cases diagnosed in baby boomer generation, born between the years of 1945 and 1965; 70% of newly infected persons develop chronic hepatitis C infection.
   c. There is currently no vaccine available.
   d. As many as 30% of those infected with HCV will develop cirrhosis or liver cancer within 20 years.

Type D Hepatitis (Delta Hepatitis)

EVIDENCE BASE Wasuwanich, P., Striley, C. W., Kamili, S., Teshale, E. H., Seaberg, E. C., & Karnsakul, W. (2022). Hepatitis D–associated hospitalizations in the United States: 2010–2018. *Journal of Viral Hepatitis, 29*(3), 218–226. https://doi.org/10.1111/jvh.13645

1. Hepatitis Delta virus (HDV) is a defective RNA agent that appears to replicate only with HBV. It requires HBsAg to replicate.
   a. Occurs along with HBV or may superinfect a chronic HBV carrier.
   b. Cannot outlast a hepatitis B infection.
   c. May be acute or chronic.
2. Mode of transmission and incubation are the same as for HBV.
3. Rarely seen in the United States because of high rates of hepatitis B vaccination beginning in infancy. Occurrence in the United States is primarily in individuals who inject intravenous (IV) drugs, veterans who have served in high-infection areas, or patients requiring multiple transfusions.
4. The highest incidence exists in the Mediterranean, the Middle East, and South America. Prevalence is low in North America and Northern Europe, South Africa, and Eastern Asia.
5. Chronic infection can be treated with interferon alfa, but response rate is low.

Type E Hepatitis

1. Nonenveloped, single-strand RNA virus.
2. Mode of transmission is fecal–oral.
3. Incubation is 15 to 60 days (mean 40 days).
4. Occurrence is primarily in India, Africa, Asia, and Central America, but may be found in recent travelers to these areas and is more common in young adults. More severe cases occur in pregnant people (third trimester) and those with preexisting chronic liver disease.
5. Most people recover completely. In those with severe cases, mortality rates can be as high as 30%.

Autoimmune Hepatitis

1. In addition to viral hepatitis, autoimmune hepatitis (AIH) has also been identified. It is a chronic form of hepatitis that is progressive and fluctuates with degree of liver damage.
2. Although the cause of AIH is unknown, it is thought to be self-antigen mediated.
3. Treatment usually consists of anti-inflammatory or immunosuppressive agents, which may need to be taken throughout the patient's life.
4. AIH may lead to abrupt and severe or chronic (fulminant) liver failure and need for transplantation.

Clinical Manifestations

Type A Hepatitis

1. May have no symptoms.
2. Prodromal symptoms: fatigue, anorexia, malaise, headache, low-grade fever, nausea, and vomiting.
3. Highly contagious during this period, usually 2 weeks before the onset of jaundice.
4. Icteric phase: jaundice, tea-colored urine, clay-colored stool, and right upper quadrant tenderness.
5. Symptoms may be mild in children; adults are more likely to have severe symptoms and a prolonged course of disease.

Type B Hepatitis

1. An estimated 30% of the world's population shows serologic evidence of current or past HBV infection. Symptom onset usually more insidious and prolonged compared with HAV but may be asymptomatic.
2. Prodromal symptoms: fatigue, anorexia, transient fever, abdominal discomfort, nausea and vomiting, headache; can last 1 week to 2 months.
3. Extrahepatic manifestations may include myalgias, photophobia, arthritis, angioedema, urticaria, maculopapular eruptions, skin rashes, and vasculitis.
4. Icteric phase: jaundice.
5. May become chronic active or chronic persistent (asymptomatic) hepatitis.
6. In rare cases, it may progress to fulminant hepatitis.

Type C Hepatitis

1. Similar to those associated with HBV but usually less severe.
2. Symptoms usually occur 6 to 7 weeks after exposure but may be attributed to another viral infection and not diagnosed as hepatitis.
3. Genotype 1 HCV is the most common infection, accounting for approximately 70% to 75% of all hepatitis C infections.
4. Approximately 60% to 85% of people infected with HCV go on to develop a chronic infection. Complications of

chronic HCV include cirrhosis, decompensated liver disease, and HCC.
5. Patients not treated for chronic HCV are at increased risk of developing HCC.
6. It is recommended that high-risk individuals be tested for HCV because many may remain asymptomatic for approximately 20 years.

Type D Hepatitis

1. Similar to HBV but more severe.
2. With superinfection of chronic HBV carriers, causes sudden worsening of condition and rapid progression of cirrhosis.

Diagnostic Evaluation

1. Elevated serum transferase levels (aspartate transaminase [AST], alanine transaminase [ALT]) for all forms of hepatitis.
2. Radioimmunoassays that reveal immunoglobulin (Ig)M antibodies to hepatitis virus in the acute phase of HAV.
3. Radioimmunoassays to include HBsAg, anti-HBc, and anti-HBsAg detected in various stages of HBV (see Figure 15-1).
4. Hepatitis C antibody—may not be detected for 6 weeks after exposure; antibody test used for screening purposes for past exposure of current infection. Positive results should be confirmed by nucleic acid testing for HCV RNA, which indicates active infection.
5. Anti-delta antibodies of HBsAg for HDV or the detection of IgM in acute disease and IgG in chronic disease.
6. Hepatitis E IgM.
7. Liver biopsy to detect chronic active disease, progression, and response to therapy.

Management

All Types of Hepatitis

1. Rest according to the patient's level of fatigue.
2. Therapeutic measures to control dyspeptic symptoms and malaise.

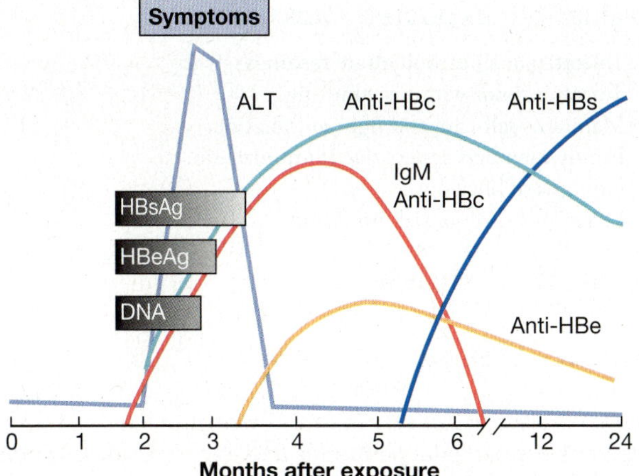

Figure 15-1. Time course for clinical, laboratory, and virologic features of acute hepatitis B infection. ALT, alanine aminotransferase; HBeAg, hepatitis B envelop antigen; HBsAg, hepatitis B surface antigen; anti-HBc, antibody to hepatitis B core antigen; anti-HBe, antibody to hepatitis B envelop antigen; anti-HBs, antibody to hepatitis B surface antigen; IgM, immunoglobulin M. (Reprinted with permission from Betts, R. F., Chapman, S. W., & Penn, R. L. [2003]. Reese and Betts' a practical approach to infectious diseases [5th ed.]. Lippincott Williams & Wilkins.)

3. Small, frequent feedings of high-calorie, low-fat foods.
4. Administration of antiemetic for nausea.
5. Hospitalization for protracted nausea and vomiting or life-threatening complications; enteral feedings may be necessary.
6. IV fluid and electrolyte replacement, as indicated.
7. Vitamin K is administered if international normalized ratio (INR)/prothrombin time (PT) is prolonged.
8. After jaundice has cleared, gradual increase in physical activity. This may require many months.

Patients With HBV

1. Decision to initiate treatment is primarily based upon the presence or absence of cirrhosis, the ALT level, and the HBV DNA level. Pregnancy and presence of malignancy are also considered.
2. Treatment strategies for chronic HBV typically include pegylated interferon or nucleoside analogs (NA), such as entecavir, or tenofovir.
3. All patients should be vaccinated for hepatitis A.

Patients With HCV

EVIDENCE BASE Bhattacharya, D., Aronsohn, A., Price, J., Lo Re, V., & AASLD-IDSA HCV Guidance Panel. (2023). Hepatitis C guidance 2023 update: AASLD-IDSA recommendations for testing, managing, and treating hepatitis C virus infection. *Clinical Infectious Diseases*, ciad319. Advance online publication. https://doi.org/10.1093/cid/ciad319

1. HCV infection will clear spontaneously in 30% of patients within 6 months of the estimated time of infection.
2. Antiviral treatment should be considered for all patients with chronic infection of HCV lasting at least 6 months.
3. Treatment of the virus is guided by genotype and presence or absence of cirrhosis. An 8-week course of multiple direct-acting antivirals such as glecaprevir–pibrentasvir or a 12-week course of elbasvir–grazoprevir, ledipasvir–sofosbuvir, or sofosbuvir–velpatasvir. Ninety percent of all patients who complete treatment achieve sustained virologic response (SVR).
4. Close monitoring includes treatment adherence and identification of adverse drug reactions. Laboratory monitoring includes complete blood count, kidney function, liver enzymes, and bilirubin levels.
5. Patients should be vaccinated against hepatitis A and B if they do not have immunity. Patients who complete treatment can recontract the disease, making education on prevention imperative.

Complications

1. Dehydration, hypokalemia.
2. Chronic "carrier" hepatitis or chronic active hepatitis.
3. Cholestatic hepatitis.
4. Fulminant hepatitis (liver transplantation may be necessary).
5. HBV and HCV chronic infections have a higher risk of developing HCC.

Nursing Assessment

1. Assess for systemic and liver-related symptoms.
2. Obtain history on risk factors, such as IV drug use, sexual activity, travel to endemic countries, and ingestion of possible contaminated food or water to assess for any mode of transmission of the virus.

3. Assess size and texture of liver to detect enlargement or characteristics of cirrhosis.
4. Obtain vital signs, including temperature.

Nursing Interventions

Maintaining Adequate Nutrition

1. Encourage frequent small feedings of high-calorie, low-fat/low-cholesterol diet. Avoid large quantities of protein during acute phase of illness as the body is unable to metabolize protein by-products.
2. Vitamin D deficiency is common in patients with chronic liver disease and may require dietary or nutritional supplementation.
3. Encourage eating meals in an upright sitting position to decrease pressure on the liver.
4. Encourage taking pleasing meals in an environment with minimal noxious stimuli (i.e., odors, noise, interruptions).
5. Administer or teach self-administration of antiemetics, as prescribed.

DRUG ALERT In patients with liver dysfunction, avoid the use of phenothiazines as an antiemetic, as drugs such as prochlorperazine have a cholestatic effect and may cause or worsen jaundice. Granisetron or haloperidol is preferred.

Maintaining Adequate Fluid Intake

1. Provide frequent oral fluids, as tolerated.
2. Administer IV fluids for patients with inability to maintain oral fluids, as prescribed.
3. Monitor intake and output.

Maintaining Adequate Rest and Activity

1. Promote periods of rest during symptom-producing phase, according to level of fatigue.
2. Promote comfort by administering or teaching self-administration of analgesics as prescribed.
3. Provide emotional support and diversional activities when recovery and convalescence are prolonged.
4. Encourage gradual resumption of activities and mild exercise during convalescent period.

Ensuring Prevention of Disease Transmission

1. Educate the patient about disease and disease transmission.
2. Emphasize the self-limiting nature of most forms of hepatitis and the need for follow-up of liver function tests and viral studies.
3. Stress importance of proper public and home sanitation and of proper preparation and dispensation of foods.
4. Encourage specific protection for close contacts.
   a. Immunoglobulin or vaccine should be administered within 2 weeks to household contacts of patients with HAV.
   b. Hepatitis B immune globulin as soon as possible to blood or body fluid contacts of patients with HBV, followed by HBV vaccine series.
5. Explain precautions to the patient and family about transmission and prevention of transmission to others.
   a. Good handwashing and hygiene after using the bathroom.
   b. Avoidance of sexual activity (especially for HBV) until free of HBsAg.
   c. Avoidance of sharing needles, drug paraphernalia, eating utensils, and toothbrushes to prevent blood or body fluid contact (especially for HBV and HCV).
6. Report all cases of hepatitis to public health officials.

Preventing and Controlling Bleeding

1. Monitor and teach the patient to monitor and report signs of bleeding.
2. Monitor PT/INR and administer vitamin K, as ordered.
3. Avoid trauma that may cause bruising, limit invasive procedures, if possible, and maintain adequate pressure on needlestick sites.

Monitoring Thought Processes

1. Monitor for signs of encephalopathy—lethargy and somnolence with mild confusion and personality changes, such as excessive sexual or aggressive activity and loss of usual inhibitions. Lethargy may alternate with excitability, euphoria, or unruly behavior.
2. Monitor for worsening of condition, from stupor to coma; assess for asterixis.
3. Maintain calm, quiet environment and reorient the patient, as needed.

Patient Education and Health Maintenance

1. Identify persons at high risk for each type of hepatitis and advise prevention and screening.
2. Educate adolescents about the risk of piercing and tattooing in transmission of HCV.
3. Encourage vaccination for HBV with series of three injections for high-risk patients, such as health care workers or persons living in institutions, as well as vaccination of all children.
4. Instruct all patients who have received a blood transfusion to refrain from donating blood for 12 months. Anyone testing positive for hepatitis B or C is ineligible to donate blood.
5. Stress the need to follow precautions with blood and secretions until the patient is deemed free of HBsAg.
6. Explain to patients who are carriers of HBV that their blood and secretions will remain infectious.
7. For additional information, refer to the local public health department, American Red Cross, or the Centers for Disease Control and Prevention (*www.cdc.gov*).

Evaluation: Expected Outcomes

- Tolerates small carbohydrate feedings.
- Tolerates fluids without vomiting.
- Maintains self-care and light ambulation.
- Family members seek active immunization.
- No signs of bleeding.
- Lethargic but oriented, no tremor.

Hepatic Cirrhosis

EVIDENCE BASE Biggins, S. W., Angeli, P., Garcia-Tsao, G., Ginès, P., Ling, S. C., Nadim, M. K., Wong, F., & Kim, W. R. (2021). Diagnosis, evaluation, and management of ascites, spontaneous bacterial peritonitis and hepatorenal syndrome: 2021 practice guidance by the American Association for the Study of Liver Diseases. *Hepatology, 74*, 1014–1048. https://doi.org/10.1002/hep.31884

It is a chronic disease with diffuse destruction and fibrotic regeneration of hepatic cells (see Figure 15-2). As necrotic tissue is replaced by fibrotic tissue, normal liver structure and vasculature are altered, impairing blood and lymph flow, resulting in hepatic insufficiency and portal hypertension.

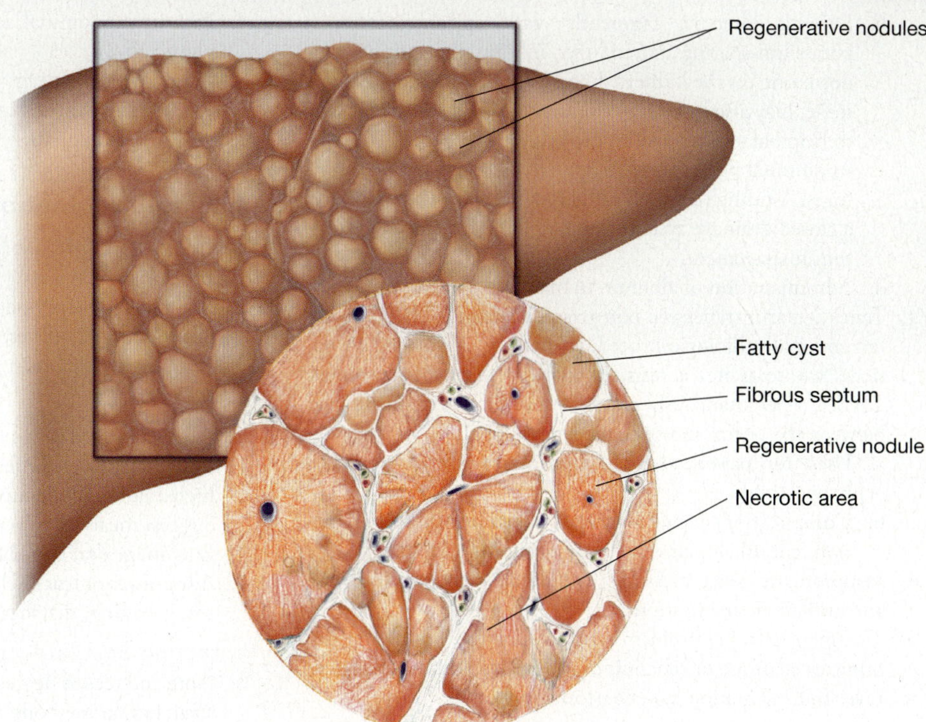

Figure 15-2. Fibrotic changes to liver tissue in cirrhosis. (Reprinted with permission from Anatomical Chart Company.)

Pathophysiology and Etiology

1. Laënnec cirrhosis (macronodular), also known as alcoholic cirrhosis.
   a. Fibrosis—mainly around central veins and portal areas.
   b. Usually due to chronic alcohol toxicity and malnutrition.
2. Postnecrotic cirrhosis (micronodular).
   a. Broad bands of scar tissue.
   b. Because of previous acute viral hepatitis or drug-induced massive hepatic necrosis.
3. Biliary cirrhosis.
   a. Scarring around bile ducts and lobes of the liver.
   b. Results from chronic biliary injury and obstruction of the intrahepatic or extrahepatic biliary system.
   c. Partial or total obstruction of the bile ducts can lead to infectious cholangitis and cirrhosis, which is much rarer with Laënnec or postnecrotic cirrhosis.

Clinical Manifestations

1. Onset is insidious; may take years to develop.
2. Early symptoms include fatigue, anorexia, ankle edema in the evening, epistaxis and bleeding gums, and weight loss.
3. Later signs and symptoms because of chronic failure of the liver and obstruction of portal circulation.
   a. Chronic dyspepsia, constipation, or diarrhea.
   b. Esophageal varices, dilated cutaneous veins around the umbilicus (caput medusa), internal hemorrhoids, ascites, splenomegaly, and pancytopenia.
   c. Plasma albumin is reduced, leading to edema and contributing to ascites.
   d. Anemia and poor nutrition lead to fatigue and weakness, wasting, and depression.
   e. Deterioration of mental function from lethargy to delirium to coma and eventual death.
   f. Estrogen–androgen imbalance causes spider angioma and palmar erythema; menstrual irregularities in females; and, in males, testicular and prostatic atrophy, gynecomastia, loss of libido, and impotence.
4. Bleeding tendencies, such as nosebleeds, easy bruising, hematemesis, occult blood in stool, or profuse hemorrhage from stomach and esophageal varices.

Diagnostic Evaluation

1. Computed tomography (CT) scan is helpful to determine the size of the liver and its irregularities and in detection of a mass.
2. Transient elastography to diagnose cirrhosis.
3. Liver biopsy detects degree of destruction and fibrosis of hepatic tissue in those who are not candidates for transient elastography.
4. Gastrointestinal (GI) endoscopy to determine esophageal varices.
5. Paracentesis to examine ascitic fluid for cell, protein, and bacterial counts.
6. Percutaneous transhepatic cholangiography (PTC) differentiates extrahepatic from intrahepatic obstructive jaundice.
7. Laparoscopy allows direct visualization of the liver.
8. Serum liver function test results may be elevated, but normal enzymes do not rule out cirrhosis.

Management

1. Minimize further deterioration of liver function through the withdrawal of toxic substances, alcohol, and medications.
2. Correction of nutritional deficiencies with vitamins and nutritional supplements and a high-calorie and moderate- to high-protein diet.
3. Treatment of ascites and fluid and electrolyte imbalances.
   a. Restrict sodium and water intake, depending on amount of fluid retention.

b. Diuretic therapy, frequently with spironolactone, a potassium-sparing diuretic that inhibits the action of aldosterone on the kidneys. Loop diuretics, including torsemide, may also be used in conjunction with spironolactone to help balance potassium depletion.
c. Abdominal paracentesis to remove fluid and relieve symptoms. A tunneled cuffed catheter with a one-way valve and a closed drainage system may be placed for chronic symptom management.
d. Administration of albumin to maintain osmotic pressure.

4. Transjugular intrahepatic portosystemic shunt (TIPS), an interventional radiologic procedure, may be performed in patients whose ascites is resistant to other forms of treatment. TIPS is a percutaneously created connection within the liver between the portal and systemic circulations.
   a. Used for patients with complications related to portal hypertension.
   b. Complications include bacterial infections, shunt obstruction, encephalopathy, and worsening coagulopathies.
5. Symptomatic relief measures include analgesic, antipruritic, and antiemetic medications.
6. Treatment of other problems associated with liver failure. Administer lactulose or rifaximin, for hepatic encephalopathy.
7. Liver transplantation may be necessary.

Complications

1. Hyponatremia and water retention.
2. Bleeding esophageal varices.
3. Coagulopathies.
4. Spontaneous bacterial peritonitis (SBP).
5. Hepatic encephalopathy, which may be precipitated by the use of sedatives, sepsis, or electrolyte imbalance.

Nursing Assessment

1. Obtain history of precipitating factors, such as alcohol use, viral hepatitis, or biliary disease.
2. Establish present pattern of alcohol intake.
3. Assess mental status through interview and interaction with the patient.
4. Perform abdominal examination, assessing for ascites (see Figure 15-3).
5. Observe for bleeding.
6. Assess daily weight first thing in the morning and abdominal girth measurements.

Nursing Interventions

Promoting Activity Tolerance

1. Encourage alternating periods of rest and ambulation.
2. Maintain some periods of bed rest with legs elevated to mobilize edema and ascites.
3. Encourage and assist with gradually increasing periods of activity.

Improving Nutritional Status

1. Encourage the patient to eat multiple, small, frequent high-calorie, moderate-protein meals.
2. Suggest meals in an aesthetically pleasing environment.
3. Encourage oral hygiene before meals.
4. Administer or teach self-administration of medication for nausea, vomiting, diarrhea, or constipation.

Protecting Skin Integrity

1. Note and record degree of jaundice of skin and sclera as well as scratches on the body.
2. Encourage frequent skin care, bathing without soap, and massage with emollient lotions.
3. Advise the patient to keep fingernails short.
4. Administer antipruritic medications as ordered.

Preventing Bleeding

1. Observe stools and emesis for color, consistency, and amount; test for occult blood.
2. Be alert for symptoms of anxiety, epigastric fullness, weakness, and restlessness, which may indicate GI bleeding.
3. Observe for external bleeding: ecchymosis, leaking needlestick sites, epistaxis, petechiae, and bleeding gums.
4. Keep the patient quiet and limit activity if signs of bleeding are exhibited.
5. Administer vitamin K or other reversal agents, as prescribed.
6. Stay in constant attendance during episodes of bleeding.

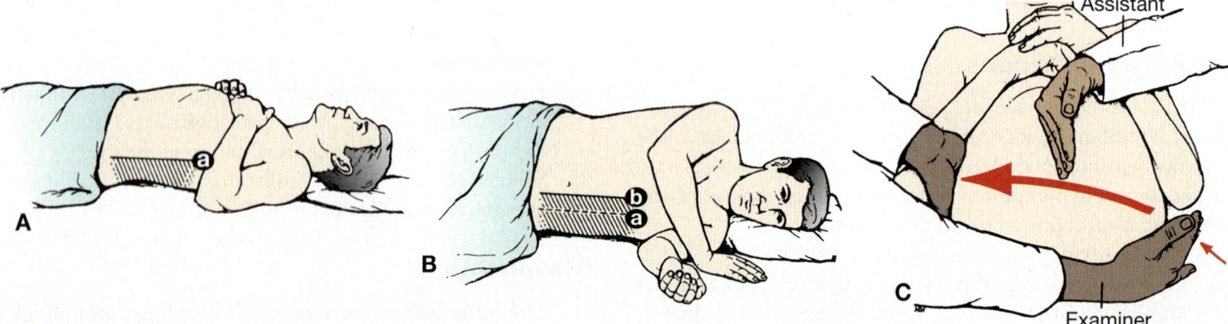

Figure 15-3. Assessing for ascites. **(A)** To percuss for shifting dullness, each flank is percussed with the patient in a supine position. If fluid is present, dullness is noted at each flank. The most medial limits of the dullness should be marked as indicated in *a*. The patient should then be shifted to the side. **(B)** Note what happens to the area of dullness if fluid is present; the area of dullness begins at *b*. **(C)** To detect the presence of a fluid wave, the examiner places one hand alongside each flank. A second person then places a hand, ulnar side down, along the patient's midline and applies light pressure. The examiner then strikes one flank sharply with one hand, while the other hand remains in place to detect any signs of a fluid impulse. The assistant's hand should dampen any wave impulses traveling through the abdominal wall, unless fluid is present.

7. Institute and teach measures to prevent trauma:
   a. Maintain safe environment.
   b. Gentle blowing of nose.
   c. Use of soft toothbrush.
8. Use small-gauge needles for injections and maintain pressure over site until bleeding stops.
9. Management of bleeding from esophageal varices can include endoscopic variceal ligation (banding) or injection sclerotherapy.

Promoting Improved Thought Processes

1. Limit sedatives and promote sleep/wake cycles to prevent delirium.
2. Protect from sepsis through good handwashing and prompt recognition and management of infection.
3. Monitor fluid intake and output and serum electrolyte levels to prevent dehydration and hypokalemia (may occur with the use of loop diuretics), which may precipitate hepatic coma.
4. Keep environment warm.
5. Pad the side rails of the bed, keep the bed in the lowest position, and provide careful nursing surveillance to ensure the patient's safety.
6. Assess level of consciousness (LOC) and frequently reorient, as needed.
7. Administer lactulose through a retention enema or nasogastric (NG) tube, as ordered, for elevated ammonia levels and decreasing LOC.

DRUG ALERT Opioids, sedatives, and barbiturates are used cautiously in the patient with cirrhosis who is restless to prevent precipitation of hepatic coma.

Patient Education and Health Maintenance

1. Advise the patient to avoid substances (over-the-counter medications, herbals, illicit drugs, toxins) that may affect liver function.
2. Stress the necessity of giving up alcohol completely.
3. Urge acceptance of assistance from a substance use program.
4. Involve the person closest to the patient because recovery usually is not easy and relapses are common.
5. Provide written dietary instructions.
6. Encourage daily weighing for self-monitoring of fluid retention or depletion.
7. Discuss adverse effects of diuretic therapy.
8. Emphasize the importance of rest, a sensible lifestyle, and an adequate, well-balanced diet.
9. Stress the importance of continued follow-up for laboratory tests and evaluation by a health care provider.

Evaluation: Expected Outcomes

- Ambulates three times daily.
- Tolerates small, frequent meals.
- Skin without breakdown or scratches.
- No bleeding or bruising; results of occult blood stool tests are negative.
- Drowsy but easily aroused and oriented.

Bleeding Esophageal Varices

Esophageal varices are dilated tortuous veins usually found in the submucosa of the lower esophagus; however, they may develop higher in the esophagus or extend into the stomach.

Pathophysiology and Etiology

1. Nearly always because of portal hypertension, which may result from obstruction of the portal venous circulation and cirrhosis of the liver.
   a. Because of increased obstruction of the portal vein, venous blood from the intestinal tract and spleen seeks an outlet through collateral circulation, which creates new pathways of return to the right atrium and causes an increased strain on the vessels in the submucosal layer of the lower esophagus and upper part of the stomach.
   b. These collateral vessels are tortuous, fragile, and bleed easily.
2. Other causes of varices are abnormalities of the circulation in the splenic vein or superior vena cava and hepatic vein thrombosis.
3. Mortality is high because of further deterioration of liver function to hepatic coma and complications, such as aspiration pneumonia, sepsis, and renal failure.

Clinical Manifestations

1. Hematemesis—vomiting of bright red blood.
2. Melena—passage of black, tarry stools, which indicates that blood has been in the GI tract for at least 14 hours.
3. Bright red rectal bleeding from hypermotility of the bowel or rectal varices.
4. Blood loss may be sudden and massive, causing shock.

Diagnostic Evaluation

1. Upper GI endoscopy for patients with a suspected upper GI source of bleeding.
2. Hemoglobin and hematocrit may be decreasing, and liver function tests can be abnormal.

Management

EVIDENCE BASE Zia, H. A., Aby, E. S., & Rabiee, A. (2021). An update on the management of esophageal variceal hemorrhage. *Clinical Liver Disease, 18*(4), 179–183. https://doi.org/10.1002/cld.1108

1. Restoration of circulating blood volume with blood transfusions and IV fluids.
2. Use of IV vasoconstrictors, such as octreotide or vasopressin, to control bleeding. These medications may be used to reduce portal pressure by decreasing splanchnic blood flow and to increase clotting and hemostasis. Vasopressin has a significant vasoconstrictive effect on other organs, such as the heart and intestine.
3. Gastric lavage to remove blood from the GI tract and to enhance visualization for endoscopic examination.
4. Endoscopic esophageal ligation (variceal banding) may be urgent or nonurgent and is usually the first-line treatment to control acute bleeding. The procedure may need to be repeated until all varices are obliterated. The goal is to achieve rapid hemostasis and prevent early rebleeding.
5. Esophageal balloon tamponade, whereby balloons are inflated in the distal esophagus and the proximal stomach to collapse the varices and induce hemostasis. This procedure should be reserved for patients who are known, without a doubt, to be bleeding from esophageal varices and in whom all forms of conservative therapy have failed.
   a. Complications include esophageal necrosis, perforation, aspiration, asphyxiation, and stricture.

   b. If hemostasis is not achieved within 2 hours, another treatment should be immediately considered. Tamponade should not be used for more than 24 hours.
   c. Patients must be continuously monitored in the intensive care setting.
   d. Precaution must be taken during balloon tamponade therapy to ensure that the patient does not pull or inadvertently displace the tube. Keep scissors taped to the head of the bed. In the event of *acute respiratory distress*, use the scissors to cut across tubing (to deflate both balloons) and remove tubing.
6. Endoscopic sclerotherapy—during endoscopy, a sclerosing agent is injected directly into the varix to promote thrombosis and sclerosis of bleeding sites.
   a. To control bleeding and reduce the frequency of subsequent variceal hemorrhages, but repeated treatments may be required.
   b. Complications include esophageal ulceration, stricture, and perforation.
7. Portal systemic shunt (portocaval or portorenal) done through TIPS procedure or surgically, to treat portal hypertension and bleeding.
8. Evaluation for liver transplantation if TIPS or surgical shunt does not control portal hypertension.
9. Nonselective beta-adrenergic blocker therapy, such as nadolol, to lower the portal pressure by reducing portal blood flow.
10. High-dose proton pump inhibitor (PPI) therapy for long-term management of erosive gastropathy.
11. Antibiotics, as patients with variceal hemorrhage are at high risk for SBP.

Complications

1. Exsanguination or recurrent hemorrhage.
2. Portal systemic encephalopathy.
3. SBP.

Nursing Assessment

1. Monitor vital signs and respiratory status.
2. Assess LOC and impending signs of liver failure.

Nursing Interventions

Maintaining Adequate Tissue Perfusion

1. Assess blood pressure (BP), heart rate, skin condition, and urine output for signs of hypovolemia and shock.
2. Monitor frequently the patient receiving vasopressin infusion for complications: hypertension, bradycardia, abdominal cramps, chest pain, or water intoxication.
3. Observe the patient for straining, gagging, or vomiting; these increase pressure in the portal system and increase the risk of further bleeding.
4. Check all GI secretions and stool for occult and frank blood.
5. Administer infusion of blood products including packed red blood cells (PRBCs) and fresh frozen plasma (FFP), as prescribed.
6. Administer vitamin K and four-factor prothrombin complex concentrate, as prescribed.

Preventing Aspiration

1. Assess respirations and monitor oxygen saturation of blood.
2. Note and report occurrence of signs of obstructed airway or ruptured esophagus from the esophageal balloon: changes in skin color, respirations, breath sounds, LOC, or vital signs; chest pain.
3. Check location and inflation of esophageal balloon; maintain traction on tubes, if applicable.
4. Have scissors readily available. Cut tubing and remove esophageal balloon immediately if the patient develops acute respiratory distress.
5. Keep head of bed elevated to avoid gastric regurgitation and aspiration of gastric contents.
6. When using the Sengstaken–Blakemore esophageal balloon tube, ensure removal of secretions above the esophageal balloon: position NG tube in the esophagus for suctioning purposes; provide intermittent oropharyngeal suctioning.
7. Inspect nares for skin irritation; clean and lubricate frequently to prevent bleeding.

Reducing Anxiety and Fear

1. Explain all procedures to the patient.
2. Provide care in a supportive, nonjudgmental manner.
3. Remain with the patient or maintain close observation and place call bell within the patient's reach.
4. Work swiftly and confidently, not hurriedly and anxiously.
5. Provide alternate means of communication if tubes or other equipment interferes with the patient's ability to talk.
6. Use touch and other tactile stimuli to provide reassurance to the patient.
7. Use protective restraints to prevent dislodging of tubes in a confused, combative patient.

Patient Education and Health Maintenance

1. Discuss signs and symptoms of recurrent bleeding and the need to seek emergency medical treatment if these occur.
2. Instruct the patient to avoid behaviors that increase portal system pressure: straining, gagging, and Valsalva maneuver.
3. Explain to the patient that alcohol consumption can cause further complications.
4. Encourage the patient to abstain from alcohol consumption; discuss support organizations such as Alcoholics Anonymous.

Evaluation: Expected Outcomes

- Airway maintained without aspiration.
- BP stable; urine output adequate.
- Cooperates and indicates understanding of treatment.

Liver Cancer

EVIDENCE BASE Falette Puisieux, M., Pellat, A., Assaf, A., Ginestet, C., Brezault, C., Dhooge, M., Soyer, P., & Coriat, R. (2022). Therapeutic management of advanced hepatocellular carcinoma: An updated review. *Cancers, 14*(10), 2357. https://doi.org/10.3390/cancers14102357

Cancer of the liver, or HCC, is a primary cancer of the liver and is the most rapidly growing cause of cancer deaths in the United States. It is the fourth leading cause of cancer-associated death around the world.

Cholangiocarcinoma is a primary malignant tumor of the bile ducts, which can be intrahepatic or extrahepatic. This type of cancer is uncommon in the United States but is more commonly seen in Asia.

Liver metastasis may occur from a primary site, which is found in about one half of all late cancer cases. Neoadjuvant therapy is given to shrink metastatic liver tumor(s) to make them more amenable to resection.

Pathophysiology and Etiology

1. Incidence of primary cancer of the liver is increasing in the United States.
2. Alcoholic cirrhosis, chronic HBV or HCV infections, nonalcohol-associated steatohepatitis, and chronic liver disease have been implicated in its etiology.
3. Rarer associated causes are metabolic syndrome; hemochromatosis; alpha$_1$-antitrypsin deficiency; aflatoxins; chemical toxins, such as vinyl chloride and Thorotrast; carcinogens in herbal medicines; nitrosamines; and ingestion of hormones, as in oral contraceptives.
4. Arises in normal tissue as a discrete tumor or in end-stage cirrhosis in a multinodular pattern.
5. Liver metastasis reaches the liver by way of the portal system, lymphatic channels, or direct extension from an abdominal tumor.

Clinical Manifestations

1. Depends on the state of the liver in which it arises; without cirrhosis and with good liver function, carcinoma of the liver may grow to huge proportions before becoming symptomatic, but in a cirrhotic patient, the lack of hepatic reserve usually leads to a more rapid course.
2. The most common presenting symptom is right upper quadrant abdominal pain, usually dull or aching, and may radiate to the right shoulder.
3. A right upper quadrant mass, weight loss, abdominal distention with ascites, fatigue, anorexia, malaise, and unexplained fever.
4. Jaundice is present only in a minority of patients at diagnosis in primary cancer of the liver. In cholangiocarcinoma, the presenting symptom is usually painless obstructive jaundice.
5. With portal vein obstruction, ascites and esophageal varices occur.

Diagnostic Evaluation

1. Increased levels of serum bilirubin, alkaline phosphatase, and liver enzymes.
2. Alpha-fetoprotein (AFP) is the principal tumor marker for HCC and is elevated in 70% to 95% of patients with the disease.
3. Ultrasonography, CT, and magnetic resonance imaging (MRI) are the most useful noninvasive tests to detect liver cancer and assess if the tumor can be surgically resected.
4. Positron emission tomography (PET) scan to look for recurrent or metastatic disease.
5. Percutaneous needle biopsy assisted by ultrasonography or CT scan.
6. Laparoscopy with liver biopsy may be performed.

Management

EVIDENCE BASE National Comprehensive Cancer Network. (2023). *Clinical practice guidelines in oncology: Hepatobiliary cancers.* Version 1.2023. www.nccn.org/professionals/physician_gls/f_guidelines.asp

Nonsurgical Treatment

Varying degrees of success with nonsurgical management. These therapies may prolong survival and improve the patient's quality of life by reducing pain, but the overall effect is palliative.

1. Indicated in patients who are not surgical candidates because of inadequate hepatic reserve or tumor location. Regional therapies are used to reduce the size of the tumor and make surgical excision possible.
2. Local thermal ablation (radiofrequency ablation [RFA], microwave ablation [MWA]) is a preferred approach for those with one or a few relatively small tumors. Hepatic arterial embolization for large unresectable or multifocal tumors.
3. Radiation therapy can help reduce pain and discomfort of large unresectable tumors.
4. Systemic treatment with a multikinase inhibitor, sorafenib, or immune checkpoint inhibitor immunotherapy, lenvatinib, is reserved for those with advanced unresectable HCC who are unsuitable for locoregional therapy and whose liver function is adequate to tolerate therapy.
5. Clinical trials on chemotherapy administered systemically or intra-arterially, to the site of the tumor, continue to show low efficacy in liver cancer.
6. Percutaneous transhepatic biliary drainage (PTBD) is used to drain obstructed biliary ducts in patients with inoperable tumors or in patients considered poor surgical risks.
7. Percutaneous or endoscopic placement of internal stents may also palliate a patient with obstructed bile ducts with a terminal diagnosis.

Surgical Treatment

EVIDENCE BASE Banama, M. (2022). Factors affecting the survival and long-term outcomes in patients undergoing hepatic resection for hepatocellular carcinoma: A narrative review. *Journal of Health Informatics in Developing Countries, 16*(1). https://jhidc.org/index.php/jhidc/article/view/372

1. Partial hepatectomy is the best treatment for patients who meet the following criteria: tumor size is less than 5 cm, lack of macrovascular involvement, and confined to the liver with no extrahepatic disease.
   a. The 5-year survival rate is less than 65%; recurrence and metastasis are frequent.
   b. Surgery is an option only after the extent of the tumor and hepatic reserve have been considered.
2. Surgical resection may be along anatomic divisions of the liver or nonanatomic resections.
3. Percutaneous portal vein embolization may be performed prior to surgery of large liver tumors. Cutting off blood supply to the diseased portion of the liver allows enlargement of the nondiseased portion of the liver. An adequate amount of reserved liver is needed to sustain a patient and prevent postoperative complications.
4. Liver transplantation is an accepted treatment for liver cancer, especially if hepatic reserve is low and the patient meets the surgical criteria.
   a. The Model for End-stage Liver Disease-Na (MELD-Na) is a severity scoring system for chronic liver disease that uses a patient's laboratory values for serum bilirubin, serum sodium, serum creatinine, and the INR to predict 3-month survival.

b. MELD-Na is used by the United Network for Organ Sharing (UNOS) for prioritization of patients awaiting liver transplantation in the United States.
c. Patients may be treated with nonsurgical therapies including embolization or radiation while waiting for a liver transplant.

Complications

1. Malnutrition, biliary obstruction with jaundice.
2. Sepsis, liver abscesses.
3. Acute blood loss.
4. Cancer metastasis.
5. Fulminant liver failure.

Nursing Assessment

1. Obtain history of viral hepatitis, alcoholic liver disease, cirrhosis, exposure to toxins, or other potential causes.
2. Assess for signs and symptoms of malnutrition, including recent weight loss, loss of strength, anorexia, and anemia.
3. Assess for abdominal pain, right shoulder pain, and enlargement of the liver.
4. Assess for fever, jaundice, ascites, or bleeding.
5. Note any change in mental status as a sign of hepatic encephalopathy.

Nursing Interventions

Care of the patient after liver surgery is similar to general abdominal surgery (see page 468).

Controlling Pain

1. Administer pharmacologic agents, as ordered, to control pain, considering metabolism through a liver with decreased function.
   a. Titrate drugs carefully, using lowest dose that is effective.
   b. Monitor for signs of drug toxicity, particularly respiratory depression and decreased LOC.
2. Provide nonpharmacologic methods of pain relief, such as massage, heat/cold, and guided imagery.
3. Position the patient for comfort, usually in semi-Fowler position.
4. Assess the patient's response to pain control measures.

Improving Nutritional Status

1. Encourage the patient to eat small meals and take liquid supplements.
2. Assess and report changes in factors affecting nutritional needs: increased body temperature, pain, signs of infection, stress level. Encourage additional calories, as tolerated.
3. Monitor daily weight.

Relieving Excess Fluid Volume

1. Monitor vital signs and record accurate fluid intake and output.
2. Restrict sodium and fluid intake, as prescribed.
3. Administer diuretics and replacement potassium and phosphate, as prescribed.
4. Administer albumin and protein supplements, as prescribed, to draw fluid from interstitial to intravascular space.
5. Measure and record abdominal girth daily at the level of the umbilicus.
6. Weigh daily, watching for increases that indicate increased fluid retention such as abdominal and lower-extremity edema.
7. Monitor laboratory tests as directed and report abnormal values.

Improving Mental Status

1. Assess the patient's LOC and changes in behavior.
2. Limit noise and environmental stimuli.
3. Frequently reorient to person, place, and time.
4. Speak slowly and clearly while allowing the patient to respond.
5. Provide for precautions to prevent falls and promote safety.

Patient Education and Health Maintenance

1. Instruct the patient and family on preparation for surgery, reinforce and clarify surgical procedure proposed, and review postoperative instructions.
2. Instruct the patient and family on nonsurgical treatment, if appropriate.
3. Explore pain management options.
4. Inform the patient of signs and symptoms of complications.
5. Instruct the patient in continued surveillance for recurrence.
6. Instruct the patient and family in care of tubes or drains.

Evaluation: Expected Outcomes

- Verbalizes reduced pain.
- Tolerates small feedings; no weight loss.
- Abdominal girth decreased; urine output greater than intake.
- Patient safety maintained.

Acute Liver Failure

Acute liver failure is acute injury of the liver cells without preexisting liver disease, resulting in the inability of the liver to perform its many functions.

Pathophysiology and Etiology

1. Several viruses have been associated with acute liver failure, including viral hepatitis A, B, C, D, and E, herpes simplex virus (HSV), varicella zoster virus, Epstein–Barr virus, adenovirus, and cytomegalovirus.
2. Drug-related hepatotoxicity accounts for more than 50% of acute liver failure cases, including acetaminophen overdose and idiosyncratic drug reactions, such as reactions to antibiotics, nonsteroidal anti-inflammatory drugs (NSAIDs), and anticonvulsants. Herbal medications and dietary supplements have also been associated with acute liver failure.
3. Hypoperfusion may result from systemic hypotension due to causes such as cardiac dysfunction, sepsis, or drugs. May also be seen with Budd–Chiari syndrome (hepatic vein thrombosis), veno-occlusive disease, or the use of vasoconstricting drugs such as cocaine and methamphetamine.
4. Miscellaneous causes include acute fatty liver of pregnancy, AIH, partial hepatectomy, complication of liver transplantation.
5. Progression of acute liver failure is rapid, with development of mental status changes, jaundice, or right upper quadrant pain within 6 weeks of onset of disease.
6. Overall, survival rates are greater than 60%. Approximately 55% of patients will survive without needing a liver transplantation.

Clinical Manifestations

1. Right upper quadrant tenderness.
2. Malaise, anorexia, nausea, vomiting, fatigue.
3. Jaundice.

4. Tea-colored urine that is frothy when shaken.
5. Pruritus caused by bile salts deposited on skin.
6. Steatorrhea and diarrhea because of decreased fat absorption.
7. Peripheral edema or ascites as the fluid moves from the intravascular to the interstitial spaces, secondary to hypoproteinemia or portal hypertension.
8. Easy bruising, petechiae, melena, or hematemesis caused by clotting deficiency.
9. Hypotension, tachycardia due to reduced systemic vascular resistance.
10. Altered LOC, ranging from irritability and confusion to stupor, somnolence, and coma.
11. Change in deep tendon reflexes—initially hyperactive, become flaccid, asterixis.
12. Fetor hepaticus—breath odor of acetone.
13. Portal systemic encephalopathy, also known as hepatic coma or hepatic encephalopathy, can occur in conjunction with cerebral edema.
14. Cerebral edema may lead to signs of increased intracranial pressure (ICP) (e.g., papilledema, hypertension, and bradycardia). This is commonly the cause of death because of brain stem herniation and/or respiratory arrest.

Diagnostic Evaluation

1. Prolonged PT/INR; sensitive markers of hepatic failure.
2. Decreased platelet count.
3. Elevated AST and ALT result from hepatocellular necrosis.
4. Elevated ammonia and bilirubin levels.
5. Hypoglycemia due to impaired glycogen production and gluconeogenesis.
6. Dilutional hyponatremia or hypernatremia, hypokalemia, hypocalcemia, and hypomagnesemia.

Management

EVIDENCE BASE Vasques, F., Cavazza, A., & Bernal, W. (2022). Acute liver failure. *Current Opinion in Critical Care, 28*(2), 198–207. https://doi.org/10.1097/MCC.0000000000000923

1. Acetaminophen overdose treated with *N*-acetylcysteine (NAC).
2. Airway protection as encephalopathy worsens and coma ensues. May require intubation and mechanical ventilation.
3. Oral or rectal administration of lactulose to minimize formation of ammonia and other nitrogenous by-products in the bowel.
4. Rectal administration of neomycin to suppress urea-splitting enteric bacteria in the bowel and decrease ammonia formation.
5. Cerebral edema management may include head of bed elevated to 30 degrees, ICP monitoring, administration of an osmotic diuretic such as mannitol, or barbiturates.
6. Careful hemodynamic monitoring and administration of vasopressors as ordered.
7. Low-molecular-weight dextran or albumin followed by a potassium-sparing diuretic (spironolactone) to enhance fluid shift from interstitial back to intravascular spaces.
8. Pancreatic enzymes, if diarrhea and steatorrhea are present, to permit better tolerance of fats in the diet.
9. Cholestyramine to promote fecal excretion of bile salts to decrease itching.
10. Antacids, PPIs, and histamine-2 (H_2) antagonists to reduce the risk of bleeding from stress ulcers.
11. Restriction of sodium while maintaining adequate caloric intake with hypertonic IV dextrose solution, enteral tube feedings, or total parenteral nutrition.
12. Supplemental vitamins (A, B complex, C, and K) and folate.
13. Infusion of FFP to maintain PT/INR; cryoprecipitate, as needed, to manage coagulopathy.
14. Additional medical interventions, depending on the patient's condition, may include hemodialysis, hemofiltration, hemoperfusion, or plasmapheresis.
15. Liver transplantation has become the treatment of choice.
16. Current research underway regarding use of liver support dialysis.

Complications

1. Acute respiratory failure.
2. Infections and sepsis.
3. Cardiac dysfunction, hypotension.
4. Hepatorenal failure.
5. Hemorrhage.

Nursing Assessment

1. Obtain history of exposure to medications, chemicals, or toxins; exposure to infectious hepatitis; and course of illness.
2. Assess respiratory status, LOC, and vital signs.
3. Assess for ascites, edema, jaundice, bleeding, asterixis, and presence or absence of reflexes.
4. Assess results of arterial blood gas (ABG) tests, electrolytes, INR, hemoglobin level, and hematocrit.

Nursing Interventions

Maintaining Adequate Fluid Volume

1. Monitor vital signs frequently.
2. Weigh the patient daily and keep an accurate intake and output record; record frequency and characteristics of stool.
3. Measure and record abdominal girth at the level of the umbilicus daily.
4. Assess and record peripheral edema.
5. Restrict sodium and fluids; replace electrolytes, as directed.
6. Administer colloid plasma expanders, such as dextran, or albumin and diuretics, as prescribed.
7. Assess for signs and symptoms of hemorrhage or bleeding.

Improving Respiratory Status

1. Monitor respiratory rate, depth, use of accessory muscles, nasal flaring, and breath sounds.
2. Monitor ABG values, hemoglobin level, and hematocrit; report abnormalities.
3. Elevate head of the bed to lower diaphragm and decrease respiratory effort.
4. Turn the patient frequently to prevent stasis of secretions.
5. Administer oxygen therapy, as directed.

Improving Nutritional Status

1. Enlist a nutrition specialist to evaluate nutritional status and needs.
2. Encourage the patient to eat in an upright sitting position to decrease abdominal tenderness and feeling of fullness.
3. Provide small, frequent meals or dietary supplements.
4. Provide mouth care if the patient has bleeding gums or fetor hepaticus.

5. Restrict intake of sodium, as directed.
6. Provide enteral and parenteral feedings, as needed.

Maintaining Skin Integrity

1. Inspect skin for alteration in integrity.
2. Provide good skin care.
3. Bathe with mild soap and apply soothing lotions.
4. Keep the patient's fingernails short to prevent scratching from pruritus.
5. Administer medications, as prescribed, for pruritus.
6. Assess for signs of bleeding from broken areas on the skin.
7. Turn and position the patient frequently to prevent pressure injury.
8. Avoid trauma and friction to the skin.

Preventing Infection

1. Be alert for signs of infection, such as fever, cloudy urine, abnormal breath sounds.
2. Use good handwashing and aseptic technique when caring for a break in the skin or mucous membranes.
3. Restrict visits with anyone who may have an infection.
4. Encourage the patient not to scratch the skin.

Preventing Injury

1. Maintain close observation, bed side rails up, and nurse call system within reach.
2. Assist with ambulation, as needed, and avoid obstructions to prevent falls.
3. Have a well-lit room and frequently reorient the patient.
4. Observe for subtle changes in behavior or change in sleeping pattern to detect worsening encephalopathy.

Patient Education and Health Maintenance

1. Teach the patient and family to notify health care provider of increased abdominal discomfort, bleeding, increased edema or ascites, hallucinations, or changes in consciousness.
2. Instruct the patient to avoid activities that increase the risk of bleeding: scratching, falling, forceful nose blowing, aggressive toothbrushing, and use of straight-edged razor.
3. Advise limiting activities when fatigued and encourage use of frequent rest periods.
4. Maintain close follow-up for laboratory testing and evaluation by health care provider.

Evaluation: Expected Outcomes

- BP stable, urine output adequate.
- Respirations unlabored.
- Tolerates multiple small feedings per day.
- Skin intact without abrasions.
- No fever or signs of infection.
- No falls.

BILIARY DISORDERS

The gallbladder and bile ducts constitute the biliary system. The gallbladder stores and concentrates bile produced by the liver. The hormone cholecystokinin, secreted by the small intestine, stimulates contraction of the gallbladder and relaxation of the sphincter of Oddi for delivery of bile into the small intestine.

Bile assists in the breakdown of fat; absorption of fatty acids, cholesterol, and other lipids from the small intestine; and excretion of conjugated bilirubin from the liver.

Common terms related to the gallbladder and bile ducts are as follows:

Cholecyst—gallbladder.
Cholecystitis—inflammation of the gallbladder.
Cholelithiasis—presence or formation of gallstones in the gallbladder.
Cholecystectomy—removal of the gallbladder.
Cholecystostomy—drainage of the gallbladder through a tube.
Choledocho—common bile duct.
Choledochotomy—incision into the common bile duct.
Choledocholithiasis—presence of stones in the common bile duct.
Choledocholithotomy—incision of the common bile duct for the extraction of an impacted gallstone.
Choledochoduodenostomy—surgical formation of a communication between the common bile duct and the duodenum.
Choledochojejunostomy—surgical formation of a communication between the common bile duct and the jejunum.

Cholelithiasis, Cholecystitis, Choledocholithiasis

These conditions refer to stones or inflammation of the biliary system (see Figure 15-4). Cholecystitis may be acute or chronic.

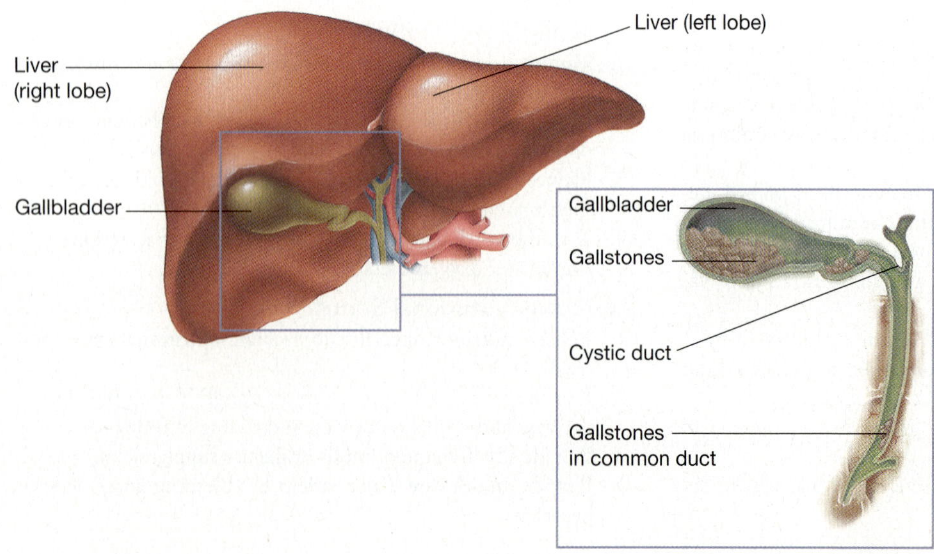

Figure 15-4. Cholelithiasis and choledocholithiasis. (Reprinted with permission from Anatomical Chart Company.)

Pathophysiology and Etiology

Cholelithiasis

1. Cholesterol stones occur when cholesterol supersaturates the bile in the gallbladder and precipitates out of the bile. The cholesterol-saturated bile predisposes to the formation of gallstones and acts as an irritant, producing inflammatory changes in the gallbladder.
   a. Cholesterol stones make up 80% of gallstones in the United States.
   b. Females develop cholesterol stones at four times the rate that males do.
   c. Females are usually older than age 40 and have obesity.
   d. Stone formation increases in those who use contraceptives, estrogens, and cholesterol-lowering drugs, which are known to increase biliary cholesterol saturation.
   e. Gallstones are associated with high-calorie diets, type 2 diabetes mellitus, dyslipidemia, hyperinsulinism, obesity, and metabolic syndrome.
   f. Bile acid malabsorption, genetic predisposition, and rapid weight loss are also risk factors for cholesterol gallstones.
2. Pigment stones occur when free bilirubin combines with calcium.
   a. Found in patients with cirrhosis, hemolysis, and infections in the biliary tree.
   b. These stones cannot be dissolved.
3. In the United States, approximately 6% of males and 9% of females have gallstones.
   a. Incidence of stone formation increases with age because of increased hepatic secretion of cholesterol and decreased bile acid synthesis.
   b. Increased risk in patients with malabsorption of bile salts with gastrointestinal (GI) disease, post gastric bypass, with bile fistula, with gallstone ileus, with carcinoma of the gallbladder, or in those who have had ileal resection or ileal bypass.

Cholecystitis

1. Acute cholecystitis, an acute inflammation of the gallbladder, is most commonly caused by gallstone obstruction.
   a. Secondary bacterial infection may occur and progress to empyema (purulent effusion of the gallbladder).
2. Acalculous cholecystitis is acute gallbladder inflammation without obstruction by gallstones.
   a. Occurs after major surgical procedures, severe trauma, or severe burns.
3. Chronic cholecystitis occurs when the gallbladder becomes thickened, rigid, and fibrotic and functions poorly. Results from repeated attacks of cholecystitis, calculi, or chronic irritation.

Choledocholithiasis

1. Small gallstones can pass from the gallbladder into the common bile duct and travel to the duodenum. More commonly, they remain in the common bile duct and can cause obstruction, resulting in jaundice and pruritus.
2. Common bile duct stones are frequently associated with infected bile and can lead to cholangitis (inflammation/infection in the biliary system).
3. Patients experience biliary pain in the upper abdomen, jaundice, chills and fever, mild hepatomegaly, abdominal tenderness, and, occasionally, rebound tenderness.

Clinical Manifestations

1. Gallstones that remain in the gallbladder are usually asymptomatic.
2. Biliary colic can be caused by gallstones.
   a. Steady, severe, aching pain or sensation of pressure in the epigastrium or right upper quadrant, which may radiate to the right scapular area or right shoulder.
   b. Begins suddenly and persists for 1 to 3 hours until the stone falls back into the gallbladder or passes through the cystic duct.
3. Acute cholecystitis causes biliary colic pain that persists for more than 4 hours and increases with movement, including respirations.
   a. Also causes nausea and vomiting, low-grade fever, and jaundice (with stones or inflammation in the common bile duct).
   b. Right upper quadrant guarding and Murphy sign (inability to take a deep inspiration when examiner's fingers are pressed below the hepatic margin) are present.
4. Chronic cholecystitis causes heartburn, flatulence, and indigestion. Repeated attacks of symptoms may occur resembling acute cholecystitis.

Diagnostic Evaluation

1. Ultrasonography, computed tomography (CT) scan, and hepatobiliary iminodiacetic acid (HIDA) scan may show stones or inflammation.
2. Magnetic resonance cholangiopancreatography (MRCP) is a noninvasive exam that can identify gallstones anywhere in the biliary tract.
3. Endoscopic retrograde cholangiopancreatography (ERCP) or percutaneous transhepatic cholangiography (PTC) to visualize location of stones and extent of obstruction.
4. Elevated conjugated bilirubin and alkaline phosphatase result from obstruction.
5. Elevated amylase and lipase levels, with gallstone pancreatitis.
6. Elevated white blood cell (WBC) count and positive blood cultures if sepsis.

Management

1. Supportive management may include intravenous (IV) fluids, nasogastric (NG) tube to suction, antibiotics, and pain management with NSAIDs or oral antispasmodics.
2. A cholecystostomy tube may be placed percutaneously into the gallbladder to decompress the organ in preparation for future surgery. This may be placed by interventional radiology.
3. Oral therapy with ursodeoxycholic acid to dissolve the stone, inhibit and reduce intestinal absorption of cholesterol, and improve gallbladder emptying.
   a. Indicated for patients at high risk for surgery because of comorbid conditions.
   b. Major adverse effects include diarrhea, abnormal liver function tests, and increases in serum cholesterol.
   c. Ultrasound is repeated every 6 to 12 months to assess response to therapy, may eventually result in dissolution of small gallstones, but with a recurrence rate of more than 50%.
4. Surgical management:
   a. Cholecystectomy, open or laparoscopic.
   b. Intraoperative cholangiography and choledochoscopy for common bile duct exploration.
   c. Placement of a T tube in the common bile duct to decompress the biliary tree and allow access into the biliary tree postoperatively.

5. After cholecystectomy, intracorporeal lithotripsy may be used to fragment retained stones in the common bile duct by pulsed laser or hydraulic lithotripsy applied through an endoscope directly to the stones. The stone fragments are removed by irrigation or aspiration. Retained stones may also be removed by basket retrieval through the endoscopic or percutaneous transhepatic biliary approach.

Complications

1. Cholangitis.
2. Gangrene, empyema, or perforation of the gallbladder.
3. Biliary fistula through the duodenum or jejunum.
4. Gallstone ileus.

Nursing Assessment

1. Obtain history and demographic data that may indicate risk factors for biliary disease.
2. Assess the patient's pain for location, quality, intensity, and relieving and exacerbating factors.
3. Assess for signs of dehydration: dry mucous membranes, poor skin turgor, and low urine output with elevated specific gravity.
4. Assess sclera and skin for jaundice.
5. Monitor temperature and WBC count for indications of infection.

Nursing Interventions

Also see "Care of the Patient Undergoing Cholecystectomy" section.

Relieving Pain

1. Assess pain location, severity, and characteristics.
2. Administer medications or monitor patient-controlled analgesia (PCA) to control pain, as prescribed.
3. Assist in attaining position of comfort.

Restoring Normal Fluid Volume

1. Administer IV fluids and electrolytes, as prescribed.
2. Administer antiemetics, as prescribed, to decrease nausea and vomiting.
3. Maintain NG decompression, if needed.
4. Begin food and fluids, as tolerated, after acute symptoms subside or postoperatively.
5. Observe and record amount of biliary tube drainage, if applicable.

Patient Education and Health Maintenance

1. Instruct the patient in care of tubes or catheters that may be in place at discharge.
   a. Observe for bleeding or drainage around insertion site.
   b. Replace dressing per facility protocol.
   c. Report change or decrease in drainage.
2. Review discharge instructions for activity, diet, medications, and follow-up.
3. Emphasize symptoms of complications to be reported, such as increased or persistent pain, fever, abdominal distention, nausea, anorexia, jaundice, unusual drainage.
4. Encourage follow-up, as indicated.

Evaluation: Expected Outcomes

- Verbalizes reduced pain level.
- Tolerates oral fluids and solid food; adequate urine output.

Care of the Patient Undergoing Cholecystectomy

EVIDENCE BASE Melly, C., McGeehan, G., O'Connor, N., Johnston, A., Bass, G., Mohseni, S., Donohoe, C., Bucholc, M., & Sugrue, M. (2022). Patient-reported outcome measures (PROMs) after laparoscopic cholecystectomy: Systematic review. *BJS Open*, 6(3), zrac062. https://doi.org/10.1093/bjsopen/zrac062

Cholecystectomy is surgical removal of the gallbladder for acute and chronic cholecystitis. Cholecystectomy is one of the most commonly performed abdominal surgical procedures. Laparoscopic cholecystectomy is considered the "gold standard" for the surgical treatment of gallstone disease.

Procedure

1. Open laparotomy—gallbladder removed after making an abdominal incision.
2. Laparoscopy—gallbladder removed from a small opening just above the umbilicus through the use of a laparoscope for viewing (see Figure 15-5).
   a. Three other small punctures are made in the abdomen to place other special instruments used to assist in the manipulation and removal of the gallbladder.
   b. The organs in the abdomen can be viewed through the laparoscope and via a television monitor through a camera attached to the laparoscope.
3. If the patient is scheduled for a laparoscopic cholecystectomy, consent is also obtained for a traditional open cholecystectomy

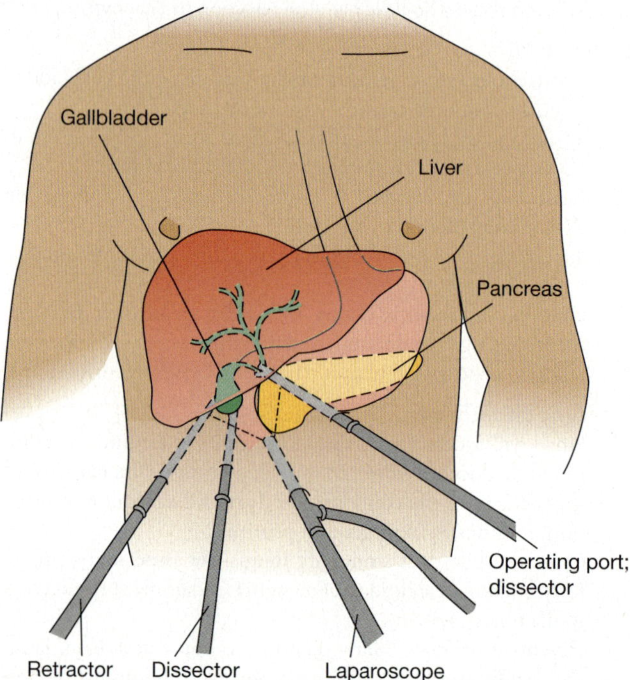

Figure 15-5. Laparoscopic cholecystectomy. The surgeon makes four small incisions (less than ½ inch each) in the abdomen and inserts a laparoscope with a miniature camera into the opening. The camera apparatus displays the gallbladder and adjacent tissues on a screen, allowing the surgeon to visualize the organ for removal.

in case the gallbladder is not accessible through the laparoscopic technique.
4. After cholecystectomy, bile ducts will eventually dilate to accommodate the volume of bile once held by the gallbladder to aid in the digestion of fats.

Preoperative Management

1. The patient must have nothing by mouth (NPO) from midnight the night before surgery.
2. IV fluids are given before surgery to improve hydration status if the patient has been vomiting.
3. Antibiotics are ordered for acute cholecystitis.
4. Educate the patient about the procedure and what to expect postoperatively.

Postoperative Management

1. Postoperatively, the patient is evaluated for the following:
   a. Vital signs, LOC.
   b. Level of pain.
   c. Appearance of surgical sites: wound drain or T-tube patency (if common bile duct exploration also performed), security and drainage (if present).
   d. Intake and output.
   e. Postoperative nausea and vomiting.
2. Early ambulation is encouraged.
3. Monitor for complications including: incisional infection, hemorrhage, and bile duct injury (persistent pain, fever, abdominal distention, nausea, anorexia, or jaundice).

Potential Complications

1. Infection, hemorrhage, or bile duct injury.
2. Pneumonia or atelectasis.
3. Deep vein thrombosis or pulmonary embolism.
4. Impaired wound healing.

Nursing Interventions

Relieving Pain

1. Assess pain location, level, and characteristics.
2. Administer pain medications or monitor PCA, as prescribed.
3. Encourage splinting of incision when moving.
4. Encourage ambulation as soon as prescribed to prevent thromboembolism, to facilitate voiding, and to stimulate peristalsis.
5. Instruct the patient that usual activities can normally be resumed within 5 to 7 days after laparoscopic cholecystectomy or within 4 to 6 weeks of open cholecystectomy.
   a. Sexual activity may be resumed when pain has abated.
   b. Obtain specific instructions for incision care; activity, such as heavy lifting; strenuous activity; showers and tub baths; and driving per surgeon's protocol.

Preventing Infection

1. Assess dressings for any increased or purulent drainage.
2. Assess wound drain or T-tube site for drainage, and note amount, color, and odor.
3. Assess bile drainage from T tube into bile bag:
   a. Maintain T-tube patency and security.
   b. Report decrease in drainage.
4. Report right upper quadrant pain, abdominal distention, fever, chills, or jaundice, as these may indicate a bile duct injury.
5. Administer antibiotics, as prescribed.
6. Encourage use of incentive spirometer, coughing and deep breathing, and ambulation to decrease risk of pulmonary infection.

Maintaining Skin Integrity

1. Assess incisions for healing.
2. Perform incisional care as prescribed.
3. Assess for adequate hydration.
4. Assess and report any signs of redness, swelling, pain, or drainage from the wounds.

Providing Adequate Nutrition

1. Assess for nausea and vomiting and administer antiemetics, as prescribed.
2. Encourage fluid intake and advance to regular diet, as tolerated.
3. Administer replacement fluids for bile drainage from T tube, if indicated.
4. Clamp T tube, when indicated, and assess tolerance of food and color of stools.

Patient Education and Health Maintenance

1. Teach the patient and family that rapid postoperative recovery should be expected.
2. Advise the patient and family to notify the surgeon immediately of any subtle change in the patient's postoperative course or persistent symptoms. A bile duct injury should be suspected after a laparoscopic cholecystectomy in patients who do not show the expected recovery during the early postoperative period.
3. Advise the patient to advance diet, as tolerated. Fats can be taken *as tolerated* because the bile ducts dilate to accommodate storage of bile, as needed.

Evaluation: Expected Outcomes

- Verbalizes decreased pain.
- No fever or signs of infection.
- Incision healing without drainage.
- Tolerates fluids and small solid feedings.

PANCREATIC DISORDERS

The pancreas secretes enzymes, including amylase and lipase, through the pancreatic duct when stimulated by cholecystokinin and secretin to aid in digestion of carbohydrates and fat in the small intestine. The pancreas also secretes hormones, such as insulin and glucagon, which help to regulate and maintain normal serum glucose.

Acute Pancreatitis

Acute pancreatitis is an inflammation of the pancreas, ranging from mild edema to extensive hemorrhage, resulting from various insults to the pancreas. It is defined by a discrete episode of abdominal pain and serum pancreatic enzyme elevations. The structure and function of the pancreas usually return to normal after an acute attack. Chronic pancreatitis occurs when there is persistent cellular damage to the pancreas (see Table 15-2 for comparison).

Pathophysiology and Etiology

1. Excessive alcohol consumption is the most common cause in the United States.
2. Also commonly caused by biliary tract disease, such as cholelithiasis and cholecystitis.

Table 15-2 Acute Versus Chronic Pancreatitis: Comparing Findings

	ACUTE PANCREATITIS	CHRONIC PANCREATITIS
Definition	• Inflammation that leads to swelling of the pancreas • Autodigestion—enzymes normally secreted by the pancreas become activated inside the pancreas and start to digest the pancreatic tissue	• Associated with widespread scarring and destruction of pancreatic tissue • Affects more males than females
Etiology	• Gallstones passing through the common bile duct • Alcohol misuse • Viral infection, hereditary conditions, traumatic injury, certain medications (especially estrogens, corticosteroids, thiazide diuretics, and azathioprine), pancreatic or common bile duct surgical procedures, or ERCP • Underlying pancreatic tumor • Hypercalcemia • Hypertriglyceridemia • Idiopathic	• Alcohol misuse • Cigarette smoking • Hereditary pancreatitis • Ductal destruction (from trauma, stones, tumors) • Systemic diseases (cystic fibrosis, systemic lupus erythematosus, hyperparathyroidism) • Congenital conditions such as pancreas divisum • Hypercalcemia • Hypertriglyceridemia • Idiopathic
Symptoms	• Sudden attack of constant, severe upper abdominal pain that may radiate to the back • Pain that is sudden and steady • Pain that may be aggravated by walking or lying down supine, and relieved by positioning on one side with knees flexed, sitting up, and leaning forward (pancreatic position) • Other possible symptoms: nausea, vomiting, diarrhea, bloating, fever, diaphoresis, and jaundice	• Constant, dull mid- to upper abdominal pain; may also have back pain • Pain that worsens with eating food or drinking alcohol; relieved by positioning on one side with knees flexed, sitting up, and leaning forward (pancreatic position) • As disease progresses, attacks of pain that last longer and occur more frequently • May have nausea, vomiting • Weight loss
Course	• Mild disease in 85% of patients with rapid recovery within a few days of onset of illness	• Destruction of pancreatic tissue that slowly progresses from chronic inflammatory damage
Diagnosis	• Medical history • Social history • Serum amylase and lipase • Serum triglycerides • Ultrasound, CT scan, MRI	• Medical history • Social history • Liver function tests • Fecal elastase test • Abdominal x-ray that may reveal calcium deposits in the pancreas • Imaging studies, such as ultrasound, CT scan, ERCP, EUS, MRI/MRCP • CEA and CA 19-9 to assess for pancreatic cancer
Treatment	• Depends on severity as acute pancreatitis may be mild, moderate, or severe • IV fluids • Pain medication • Diet advancement based on pain and nausea • Surgery for such complications as necrosis, infection, bleeding	• Pain management • Nutritional support and diet modification with smaller, frequent, low-fat meals • Pancreatic enzymes • Diabetes control • Pancreatic duct drainage procedures or excision of damage of all or part of the pancreas • Alcohol abstinence

Complications	• Severe acute pancreatitis may lead to:
	  • Multiple organ system failure, such as lung, liver, kidney, and heart
	  • Infected pancreatic necrosis
	  • Pancreatic abscess
	  • Pancreatic pseudocysts
	  • Pancreatic fistula
	  • Pancreatic ascites
	  • Damage to surrounding organs, such as small bowel, colon, and duodenum (due to inflammation)
		• Malnutrition from poor absorption of nutrients, especially fats
		• Frequent bowel movements that are loose, greasy, foul smelling (steatorrhea)
		• Insulin-dependent diabetes
		• Increased risk of pancreatic cancer
		• Pseudocyst
		• Bleeding from the stomach
		• Increased risk of venous thromboembolism
		• Possible bouts of acute pancreatitis

Prognosis	• Can usually fully recover without recurrence if cause is removed	• Can maintain quality of life with supportive care and adherence to medical regimen

CA, carbohydrate antigen; CEA, carcinoembryonic antigen; CT, computed tomography; ERCP, endoscopic retrograde cholangiopancreatography; EUS, endoscopic ultrasound; IV, intravenous; MRCP, magnetic resonance cholangiopancreatography; MRI, magnetic resonance imaging.

3. Less common causes are bacterial or viral infection, blunt abdominal trauma, peptic ulcer disease, ischemic vascular disease, hypertriglyceridemia (greater than 1,000 mg/dL), hypercalcemia; the use of corticosteroids, thiazide diuretics, and oral contraceptives; surgery on or near the pancreas or after instrumentation of the pancreatic duct by endoscopic retrograde cholangiopancreatography (ERCP); tumors of the pancreas or ampulla; and (rarely) hereditary pancreatitis.
4. The overall mortality in acute pancreatitis is under 5%, and as high as 17% with necrotizing pancreatitis because of shock, anoxia, hypotension, or multiple-organ dysfunction.
5. Attacks may resolve with complete recovery, may recur without permanent damage, or may progress to chronic pancreatitis.
6. Autodigestion of all or part of the pancreas is involved, but the exact mechanism is not completely understood.

Clinical Manifestations

(Depends on severity of pancreatic damage.)

1. Abdominal pain, usually constant, midepigastric or periumbilical, radiating to the back or flank. The patient assumes a fetal position on one side with knees flexed, or sits up and leans forward while sitting (known as "pancreatic position") to relieve pressure of the inflamed pancreas on celiac plexus nerves. Pain can be mild to incapacitating.
2. Nausea and vomiting.
3. Fever.
4. Involuntary abdominal guarding, epigastric tenderness to deep palpation, and reduced or absent bowel sounds.
5. Dry mucous membranes; hypotension; cold, clammy skin; cyanosis; and tachycardia, which may reflect mild-to-moderate dehydration from vomiting or capillary leak syndrome (third space loss).
6. Shock may be the presenting manifestation in severe episodes, with respiratory distress and acute renal failure.
7. Purplish discoloration of the flanks (Turner sign) or of the periumbilical area (Cullen sign) occurs in extensive hemorrhagic necrosis of the pancreas.

Diagnostic Evaluation

1. A minimum of two out of three criteria must be met to diagnose acute pancreatitis: abdominal pain; elevated serum lipase (or amylase) at least three times greater than the upper limit of normal; characteristic findings of acute pancreatitis on imaging studies.
2. Serum glucose, bilirubin, alkaline phosphatase, lactate dehydrogenase, aspartate transaminase (AST), alanine transaminase (ALT), white blood cell (WBC) count, hematocrit/hemoglobin, potassium, and cholesterol may be elevated.
3. Serum albumin, calcium, sodium, magnesium, and, possibly, potassium may be low from dehydration, vomiting, and the binding of calcium in areas of fat necrosis.
4. Elevated C-reactive protein (CRP) level in the first 48 hours is suggestive of severe pancreatitis and is predictive of a worse clinical course.
5. Abdominal x-ray to detect an ileus or isolated loop of small bowel overlying pancreas. Pancreatic calcifications or gallstones may suggest an alcohol or biliary etiology.
6. Abdominal ultrasound to determine if the patient has gallstones or obstruction in the common bile duct. Can also detect peripancreatic fluid indicative of pancreatic necrosis.
7. Computed tomography (CT) scan to assess for acute interstitial edematous pancreatitis, pancreatic enlargement, and necrosis of pancreas.
8. Magnetic resonance imaging (MRI) has a higher sensitivity for the diagnosis of early acute pancreatitis and can better characterize the pancreatic and bile ducts and complications of acute pancreatitis than CT scan.
9. Chest x-ray for detection of pulmonary complications. Pleural effusions are common, especially on the left, but may be bilateral.

Management

EVIDENCE BASE de-Madaria, E., Buxbaum, J. L., Maisonneuve, P., de Paredes, A. G. G., Zapater, P., Guilabert, L., Vaillo-Rocamora, A., Rodríguez-Gandía, M. A., Donate-Ortega, J., Lozada-Hernández, E. E., Collazo Moreno, A. J. R., Lira-Aguilar, A., Llovet, L. P., Mehta, R., Fernández-Cabrera, I., Casals-Seoane, F., Deza, D. C., Lauret-Braña, E., Martí-Marqués, E., ... Bolado, F.; ERICA Consortium. (2022). Aggressive or moderate fluid resuscitation in acute pancreatitis. *The New England Journal of Medicine, 387*, 989–1000.

Depending on severity of the episode, management focuses on alleviation of symptoms and support of the patient to prevent complications.

1. Intravenous hydration with lactated Ringer should be provided to all patients for the first 24 to 48 hours, with attention to volume status.
2. Adequate oxygenation, which is often reduced by pain, anxiety, acidosis, abdominal pressure, or pleural effusions.
3. Pain control to alleviate pain and anxiety, which increases pancreatic secretions.
4. Nasogastric (NG) intubation and suction to relieve gastric stasis, distention, and ileus, if needed. Maintenance of alkaline gastric pH with proton pump inhibitors (PPIs) or histamine-2 (H_2)-receptor antagonists and antacids to suppress acid drive of pancreatic secretions and to prevent stress ulcers.
5. Begin oral nutrition within 24 hours, for mild cases if the pain is improved. This may help to protect the gut mucosal barrier and limit bacterial movement, reducing the risk for complications of acute pancreatitis.
6. For more severe cases, feeding may be delayed due to symptoms of pain, nausea, or vomiting. If nothing by mouth by Day 5, nasojejunal enteral feeds may be initiated.
7. Supportive pharmacotherapy:
   a. Electrolyte replacements, as needed.
   b. Sodium bicarbonate to treat metabolic acidosis.
   c. Insulin to treat hyperglycemia.
   d. Antibiotic therapy for documented infection or sepsis.
8. Cholecystectomy is indicated during the hospital admission for acute gallstone pancreatitis.
9. Surgical intervention if complications occur.
   a. Incision and drainage of abscess and infected pseudocysts.
   b. Debridement or pancreatectomy to remove necrotic pancreatic tissue.

Complications

1. Pancreatic ascites, abscess, or pseudocyst.
2. Acute necrotic collections or walled-off pancreatic necrosis.

3. Pulmonary infiltrates, pleural effusion, acute respiratory distress syndrome.
4. Hemorrhage with hypovolemic shock.
5. Acute renal failure.
6. Sepsis and multiple-organ dysfunction syndrome.

Nursing Assessment

1. Obtain history of gallbladder disease, alcohol use, hypertriglyceridemia, or precipitating factors.
2. Assess gastrointestinal (GI) symptoms, including nausea and vomiting, diarrhea, and passage of stools containing fat.
3. Assess characteristics of abdominal pain.
4. Assess nutritional and fluid status.
5. Assess respiratory rate and pattern and breath sounds.

POPULATION AWARENESS The incidence of severe, systemic complications of pancreatitis increases with age. Assess for any changes in mental status in an older person with pancreatitis as an indicator of an underlying complication. Acute pancreatitis in an older person without other precipitating factors may indicate an underlying pancreatic tumor obstructing the pancreatic duct.

Nursing Interventions

Controlling Pain

1. Administer opioid analgesics, as ordered.
2. Assist the patient to a comfortable position.
3. Maintain patency of NG suction to remove gastric secretions and to relieve abdominal distention, if indicated.
4. Provide frequent oral hygiene and care.
5. Administer antacids, PPIs, or H_2-receptor antagonists, as prescribed.
6. Report increase in severity of pain, which may indicate hemorrhage of the pancreas, rupture of a pseudocyst, or inadequate dosage of the analgesic.

Restoring Adequate Fluid Balance

1. Monitor and record vital signs, skin color, and temperature.
2. Monitor intake and output and weigh daily.
3. Evaluate laboratory data for hemoglobin, hematocrit, albumin, calcium, potassium, sodium, and magnesium levels and administer replacements, as prescribed.
4. Observe and measure abdominal girth if pancreatic ascites is suspected.
5. Report trends in falling blood pressure (BP) or urine output or rising pulse because this may indicate hypovolemia and shock or renal failure.

Improving Respiratory Function

1. Assess respiratory rate and rhythm, effort, oxygen saturation, and breath sounds frequently.
2. Position in upright or semi-Fowler position to enhance diaphragmatic excursion.
3. Administer oxygen supplementation, as prescribed, to maintain adequate oxygen levels.
4. Report signs of respiratory distress immediately.
5. Instruct the patient in coughing and deep breathing to improve respiratory function.

Nutrition

1. Assess nutritional status, history of weight loss, and dietary habits, including alcohol intake.
2. Administer antacids or H_2-receptor antagonists to prevent neutralization of enzyme supplements, as indicated.
3. Monitor intake and output and daily weight.
4. Assess for GI discomfort with meals and character of stools.
5. Monitor blood glucose levels and teach balanced, low-concentrated carbohydrate diet and insulin therapy as indicated.
6. Identify foods that aggravate symptoms, and teach low-fat diet.

Patient Education and Health Maintenance

1. Instruct the patient to gradually resume a low-fat diet.
2. Instruct the patient to increase activity gradually, providing for rest periods as needed.
3. Reinforce information about the disease process and precipitating factors. Stress that subsequent bouts of acute pancreatitis may destroy the pancreas, cause additional complications, and lead to chronic pancreatitis.
4. If pancreatitis is a result of alcohol use, the patient needs to be reminded of the importance of eliminating all alcohol; advise about Alcoholics Anonymous or other substance use counseling.

Evaluation: Expected Outcomes

- Verbalizes reduced pain level.
- BP stable; urine output adequate.
- Respirations unlabored; breath sounds clear.

Chronic Pancreatitis

Chronic pancreatitis is a syndrome involving inflammation, fibrosis, and loss of pancreatic cells, resulting in chronic abdominal pain, fatty stools, exocrine and endocrine insufficiency, and visible pancreatic damage on imaging studies. Prevalence of chronic pancreatitis is 50 per 100,000 people.

Pathophysiology and Etiology

1. Chronic pancreatitis often develops in patients between the ages of 30 and 40, and is more common in males.
2. Alcohol use and smoking are the most common causes; less common causes are hyperparathyroidism, hereditary pancreatitis, autoimmune pancreatitis, malnutrition, and trauma to the pancreas.
3. With chronic inflammation, destruction of the secreting cells of the pancreas causes maldigestion and malabsorption of protein and fat and possibly diabetes mellitus if islet cells of the pancreas have been affected.
4. As cells are replaced by fibrous tissue, obstruction of the pancreatic and common bile ducts and duodenum may result.

Clinical Manifestations

1. Pain is usually located in the epigastrium or left upper quadrant, frequently radiating to the back, similar to that observed in acute pancreatitis, but more constant and occurring at unpredictable intervals. As the disease progresses, recurring attacks of pain will be more severe, more frequent, and of longer duration.
2. Weight loss, nausea, vomiting, and anorexia.
3. Malabsorption and steatorrhea occur late in the course of the disease.
4. Glucose intolerance.

Diagnostic Evaluation

1. Serum amylase and lipase may be normal to low because of decreased pancreatic exocrine function.
2. Fecal fat analysis determines need for pancreatic enzyme replacement.
3. Fasting triglyceride level to assess for severe elevation.
4. Genetic testing including serine protease 1 gene, to assess for cause.
5. Serum immunoglobulin 4 (IgG4) to assess for autoimmune etiology.
6. Plain abdominal x-ray to determine diffuse calcification of the pancreas.
7. CT scan identifies pancreatic structural changes, such as calcifications, masses, ductal irregularities, enlargement, and pseudocysts.
8. ERCP defines ductal anatomy and localizes complications, such as pancreatic pseudocysts and ductal disruptions.

Management

1. Alcohol abstinence and tobacco cessation.
2. Pain management, including supportive behavioral therapy.
3. Small meals and hydration with correction of nutritional deficiencies.
4. Pancreatic enzyme replacement.
5. Treatment of diabetes mellitus.
6. Endoscopic placement of pancreatic stent allowing free flow of pancreatic juices through distorted and irregular/narrowed pancreatic duct.
7. Surgical interventions to reduce pain, restore drainage of pancreatic secretions, correct structural abnormalities, and manage complications.
   a. Pancreatojejunostomy—side-to-side anastomosis of pancreatic duct to jejunum to drain pancreatic secretions into jejunum.
   b. Revision of sphincter of ampulla of Vater by a sphincteroplasty, in which the sphincter is sewn open to allow free flow of pancreatic juices.
   c. Drainage of pancreatic pseudocyst into nearby structures or by external drain.
   d. Resection of part of pancreas (pancreatoduodenectomy [Whipple operation]) or removal of entire pancreas (total pancreatectomy) with autotransplantation of islet cells.

Complications

1. Pancreatic pseudocyst formation.
2. Pancreatic ascites and pleural effusions.
3. GI hemorrhage.
4. Biliary tract obstruction.
5. Pancreatic fistula.
6. Splenic vein thrombosis.
7. Diabetes mellitus.

Nursing Assessment

1. Assess level of abdominal pain.
2. Assess nutritional status.
3. Assess for steatorrhea and malabsorption.
4. Assess for signs and symptoms of diabetes mellitus.
5. Assess current level of alcohol intake and motivation and resources available to abstain from drinking such as Alcoholics Anonymous.

Nursing Interventions

Controlling Pain

1. Assess and record the character, location, frequency, and duration of pain.
2. Determine precipitating and alleviating factors of the patient's pain.
3. Explore the effect of pain on the patient's lifestyle and eating habits.
4. Administer or teach self-administration of analgesics, as ordered.
5. Use nonpharmacologic methods to promote relaxation, such as distraction, imagery, and progressive muscle relaxation.
6. Assess response to pain control measures and refer to pain management clinic, if indicated.

Improving Nutritional Status

1. Assess nutritional status, history of weight loss, and dietary habits, including alcohol intake.
2. Administer pancreatic enzyme replacement with meals, as prescribed.
3. Administer antacids, PPIs, or H_2-receptor antagonists to prevent neutralization of enzyme supplements, as indicated.
4. Monitor intake and output and daily weight.
5. Assess for GI discomfort with meals and character of stools.
6. Monitor blood glucose levels and teach balanced, low-concentrated carbohydrate diet and insulin therapy, as indicated.
7. Identify foods that aggravate symptoms and teach low-fat diet.

DRUG ALERT Warn the patient that dangerous hypoglycemic reaction may result from use of insulin while drinking alcohol and skipping meals.

Relieving Anxiety About Surgical Intervention

1. Describe planned surgical intervention and the expected results, including improved pain and improved ability to eat.
2. Prepare the patient for adverse effects and complications of surgery.
   a. Total pancreatectomy will cause permanent diabetes mellitus, dependence on insulin, severe malabsorption, and the need for lifelong pancreatic enzyme replacement. Consultation and close monitoring by endocrinologist and diabetes educator.
   b. Malnutrition and debility increase the patient's risk for poor healing and complications of surgery.
3. Assist the patient to prepare for surgery by encouraging intake of nutritional and vitamin supplements and alcohol abstinence.
4. Encourage the patient to enlist the help of support network and strengthen appropriate coping mechanisms.
5. After surgery, provide meticulous care to prevent infection, promote incision healing, and prevent routine complications of surgery.

Patient Education and Health Maintenance

1. Instruct the patient regarding correct use of analgesics.
2. Instruct in proper administration of pancreatic enzyme replacement.
   a. Take just before or during meals.
   b. May be enteric coated. Do not crush or chew tablets; powder may be sprinkled on food if swallowing tablets is difficult.

c. Take with antacid, PPI, or H_2-receptor antagonist, as directed, to prevent pancreatic enzyme from being destroyed by gastric acid secretions.
3. Advise the patient to monitor number and characteristics of stools; report increased stools or food intolerance.
4. Teaching about diabetes with follow-up to monitor progression of condition, if applicable.
5. Stress that treatment will be ineffective if alcohol consumption is continued.

Evaluation: Expected Outcomes

- Verbalizes reduced pain level.
- Weight stabilized or weight gain noted.
- Verbalizes understanding of effects of surgical procedure.

Pancreatic Cancer

Cancer of the pancreas is a highly lethal malignancy that may arise in the head (about 70% of cases) or body and tail of the pancreas. Adenocarcinoma of the cells that line the ducts of the pancreas is the most common (85%) type. Pancreatic cancer is the fourth leading cause of cancer deaths in the United States because 90% of tumors are not resectable at the time of diagnosis.

Pathophysiology and Etiology

1. Incidence is increasing, with 64,000 cases diagnosed each year in the United States.
2. Pancreatic cancer is the seventh leading cause of cancer deaths worldwide.
3. Occurs more commonly in males than in females, and in Black Americans than in White Americans.
4. Rarely before the age of 45 years, usually occurs between ages 60 and 80 years.
5. Cigarette smoking, prolonged exposure to industrial chemicals, high-fat diet, diabetes mellitus, obesity, physical inactivity, and chronic pancreatitis are considered risk factors. A small percentage of pancreatic cancer is inherited.
6. Obstruction of bile flow may occur with tumors in the head of the pancreas because of compression of the distal common bile duct.
7. Obstruction of pancreatic duct produces pain and exocrine dysfunction.

Clinical Manifestations

1. Symptoms are commonly vague and nonspecific, preventing early detection.
2. Weakness, weight loss, anorexia, nausea, vomiting, and abdominal pain may occur.
3. Pain usually occurs in the upper abdomen and is gnawing or boring and may radiate around the flank to the back.
   a. Pain is usually worse at night, and patients tend to lie on one side with knees to chest position or may sit up and lean forward when seated to relieve pain (pancreatic position).
   b. Pain may become more localized, severe, and unremitting as the disease progresses.
4. Early satiety and a feeling of bloating after eating may occur.
5. Hepatomegaly.
6. Biliary obstruction produces jaundice, dark tea-colored urine, clay-colored stools, and pruritus.
7. Depression and lethargy may be present.

Diagnostic Evaluation

1. Liver function tests and pancreatic enzymes elevated; coagulation studies may be prolonged.
2. Carcinoembryonic antigen (CEA) and carbohydrate antigen (CA) 19-9 may be elevated.
3. Transabdominal ultrasonography detects tumors larger than 3 cm.
4. ERCP defines anatomy and allows placement of biliary stent for unobstructed flow of bile by tumor in the head of the pancreas prior to surgery or as palliation in patients not deemed surgical candidates.
5. Magnetic resonance cholangiopancreatography (MRCP)—defines anatomy without contrast dye.
6. Abdominal CT scan to assess resectability and presence of metastatic disease.
7. Positron emission tomography (PET) scan to differentiate cancer from cyst as well as to assess for recurrence or metastatic disease.
8. Biopsy through percutaneous fine needle aspiration or endoscopic ultrasound (EUS) for cytology and to confirm malignancy.

Management

The goal of treatment may be cure or palliation, depending on the staging of the tumor. Despite advances in treatment, the 5-year survival rate is 5%; for those with localized disease, the 5-year survival rate is somewhat improved and is around 12%.

Surgery

Surgical resection is the only potentially curative treatment. Unfortunately, because of the late presentation of the disease, only 15% to 20% of patients are candidates for pancreatectomy.

1. Whipple procedure (pancreaticoduodenectomy) is the removal of the head of the pancreas and distal portion of the common bile duct including the gallbladder, duodenum, and the distal stomach with anastomosis of the remaining pancreas, stomach, and common bile duct to the jejunum (see Figure 15-6). If the gallbladder is present, it is also removed. Modifications of the conventional pancreaticoduodenectomy procedure have been developed in an attempt to improve outcomes or minimize the morbidity associated with the operation.
   a. Stomach and pylorus may be preserved—pylorus-preserving pancreaticoduodenectomy. This procedure may decrease the incidence of postoperative dumping, marginal ulceration, and bile reflux gastritis.
   b. Subtotal stomach-preserving pancreaticoduodenectomy—preserve as much stomach as possible while minimizing problems related to delayed gastric emptying.
2. Total pancreatectomy, including a splenectomy, may be performed for diffuse tumor throughout the pancreas.
3. Distal pancreatectomy is the removal of the distal pancreas and spleen for tumors localized in the body and tail.
4. Palliative bypass for nonresectable tumors: choledochojejunostomy or cholecystojejunostomy for obstructive jaundice or gastrojejunostomy for gastric outlet obstruction.

Other Measures

1. Chemotherapy alone or in combination with radiation therapy may be given before surgery to shrink tumors that involve major blood vessels.
2. Chemotherapy combined with radiation therapy may be given for resectable tumors after surgery for microscopic or undetectable disease left behind.

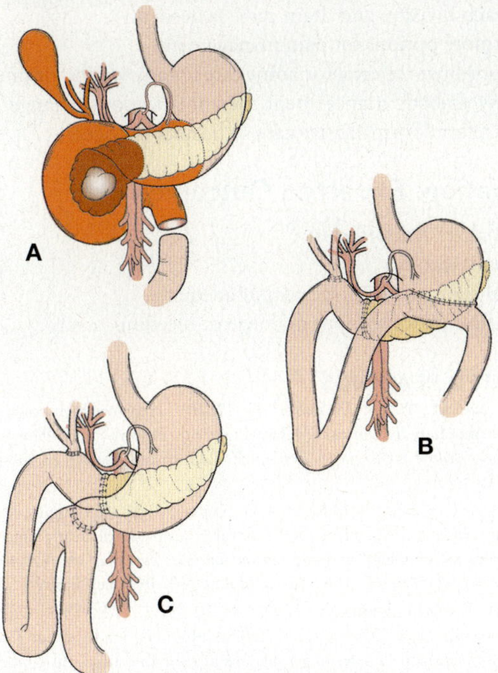

Figure 15-6. Pancreaticoduodenectomy. **(A)** The standard pancreaticoduodenectomy (Whipple procedure) involves a wide area of resection around the tumor, including the gallbladder, distal stomach including the pyloric region, duodenum, and head of the pancreas, as indicated. **(B)** Anastomoses of the common bile duct, fundus of the stomach, and body and tail of the pancreas to the jejunum. **(C)** Pylorus-preserving variant involves conservation of the stomach, including the pyloric valve anastomosed to the jejunum.

3. Chemotherapy and radiation therapy may be given for tumors deemed unresectable at the time of surgery and after palliative bowel bypass surgery.
4. Chemotherapy may be given alone for treatment of unresectable or metastatic disease.
5. Radiation therapy may be used alone.
   a. External beam irradiation for local control, to reduce pain, and to palliate obstruction.
   b. Intraoperative radiation therapy given after the pancreas resection has also been used in some centers.
6. Endoscopic or percutaneous stent placement for relief of biliary or duodenal obstruction.
7. Chemical splanchnicectomy, injection of alcohol into the celiac plexus, numbs the nerves in the area of the pancreas to provide temporary pain relief.
   a. May be performed intraoperatively by the surgeon or percutaneously under CT guidance as an outpatient procedure by an anesthesia pain service.
8. Immunotherapies under investigation that show promising results include immune modulators, therapeutic vaccines, monoclonal antibodies, oncolytic viruses, adjuvant immunotherapies, and cytokines.

EVIDENCE BASE Robatel, S., & Schenk, M. (2022). Current limitations and novel perspectives in pancreatic cancer treatment. *Cancers, 14*, 985. https://doi.org/10.3390/cancers14040985

Complications

1. Biliary, gastric, and duodenal obstruction.
2. Metastasis and liver failure/ascites secondary to metastasis.
3. Portal hypertension and pain because of encasement of major blood vessels and celiac nerve plexus in the area of the pancreas.
4. Venous thromboembolism (VTE): incidence of VTE is four- to sevenfold higher in pancreatic cancer as in other common adenocarcinomas.
5. Malnutrition, weight loss, anorexia, and cachexia.

Nursing Assessment

1. Obtain history for risk factors, pain, and symptoms of pancreatic dysfunction.
2. Assess nutritional status and hydration, including diet history, anorexia, weight loss, nausea and vomiting, steatorrhea, skin turgor.
3. Evaluate laboratory results for alterations in glucose, pancreatic enzymes, liver function, and coagulation studies.
4. Assess psychosocial status to determine depression, usual coping strategies, support systems, and experience with past serious illness.
5. Assess use of alternative therapies or over-the-counter medications.

DRUG ALERT The efficacy of herbal medications to treat or cure pancreatic cancer has not been proven. Little is known about the interaction of herbal medications with conventional medications or treatments. Herbal medications may interact with chemotherapy drugs and compromise treatment. If a patient is using alternative treatments or herbal medications, this must be known to all health care providers.

Nursing Interventions

For surgical care, see "Care of the Patient Undergoing Gastrointestinal Surgery" (page 475).

Controlling Pain

1. Administer opioids, as ordered, or monitor person-controlled analgesia (PCA).
2. Teach relaxation techniques, such as relaxation breathing, progressive muscle relaxation, and imagery, as adjuncts for pain relief.
3. Assist with frequent turning and comfortable positioning.
4. Administer adjuvant medications, such as antidepressants and anxiolytics, as prescribed.
5. Assess the patient's response to pain and symptom control measures.
6. Consider palliative care or hospice services for symptom management if the patient no longer benefits from therapy.

Improving Nutritional Status

1. Administer enteral or parenteral nutrition, as prescribed, preoperatively and postoperatively.
2. Monitor serum glucose level for hyperglycemia or hypoglycemia.
3. Progress diet slowly when oral intake is tolerated; observe for nausea, vomiting, and gastric distention.
4. Administer high-protein, high-carbohydrate diet with vitamin supplements and pancreatic enzymes, as prescribed.

5. Encourage use of spices to stimulate taste buds, provide cool foods to decrease odor, use plastic utensils if the patient complains of metallic taste from treatments, and offer small, frequent meals.
6. Provide appetite stimulant, such as megestrol, as needed.
7. Monitor serum albumin.
8. Weekly weights.
9. Assess for fat and protein malabsorption: stools that float, have greasy appearance, are orange in color, and are foul smelling.

Attaining Adequate Fluid Volume

1. Monitor vital signs and record accurate intake and output.
2. Monitor wound drain output.
3. Evaluate laboratory values for hypoalbuminemia, hyponatremia, hypochloremia, and metabolic alkalosis; replace electrolytes, as prescribed.
4. Administer fluid replacement, as indicated.
5. Report change in vital signs or increased pain: may indicate hemorrhage, leak from anastomosis, or tumor progression.

Maintaining Tissue Integrity

1. Observe skin for jaundice, breakdown, irritation, or excoriation.
2. Administer antipruritic medication, provide frequent skin care with mild soap and with thorough rinsing, apply emollient lotions, trim fingernails short to prevent scratching.
3. Maintain aseptic technique in handling wound dressings and drainage of all secretions.
4. Inspect skin around drains for irritation and protect skin from leakage of fluids from drains or tubes.
5. Inspect surgical dressings and incision for bleeding, drainage, or signs of infection.
6. Prevent tension on anastomoses by monitoring for abdominal distention and maintaining patency of surgically placed tubes and drains.

Community and Home Care Considerations

1. Educate the patient and family about course of disease and support them through the process.
2. Provide assistive devices and direct care to help with energy conservation. Patients who die of pancreatic cancer may have progressive weight loss from anorexia leading to severe cachexia, fatigue, and muscle wasting, which is refractory to any intervention.
3. Assess for bowel obstruction, which may also deplete energy and lower nutritional status. Notify health care provider of reduced bowel activity, increased pain, or abdominal distention.
4. Emphasize to the patient and family that pain can always be managed and patients need not die in pain. The plan for pain management should be aggressive and should provide the patient an optimal quality of life.
5. Encourage the family to take advantage of palliative care or hospice services.

Patient Education and Health Maintenance

1. Instruct the patient and family on self-care measures for pancreatic insufficiency.
   a. Glucose monitoring, insulin administration, signs and symptoms of hypoglycemia and hyperglycemia.
   b. Pancreatic enzyme replacement; high-protein, high-carbohydrate diet.
2. Teach incision and drain care, as needed.
3. Explore options for pain management.
4. Coordinate referral for home care for any wound or drain care, new diabetic management, new medications, change in diet, or referral for palliative care or hospice services.

Evaluation: Expected Outcomes

- Verbalizes reduced pain.
- Weight stable.
- Vital signs stable; urine output adequate.
- Incision intact without drainage or bleeding.

SELECTED READINGS

Berkan-Kawińska, A., & Piekarska, A. (2020). Hepatocellular carcinoma in non-alcohol fatty liver disease—Changing trends and specific challenges. *Current Medical Research and Opinion, 36*(2), 235–243. https://doi.org/10.1080/03007995.2019.1683817

Blackford, A. L., Canto, M. I., Klein, A. P., Hruban, R. H., & Goggins, M. (2020). Recent trends in the incidence and survival of stage 1A pancreatic cancer: A surveillance, epidemiology, and end results analysis. *Journal of the National Cancer Institute, 112*(11), 1162–1169. https://doi.org/10.1093/jnci/djaa004

Butaru, A. E., Mămuleanu, M., Streba, C. T., Doica, I. P., Diculescu, M. M., Gheonea, D. I., & Oancea, C. N. (2022). Resource management through artificial intelligence in screening programs-key for the successful elimination of hepatitis C. *Diagnostics (Basel, Switzerland), 12*(2), 346. https://doi.org/10.3390/diagnostics12020346

Chaouch, M. A., Leon, P., Cassese, G., Aguilhon, C., Khayat, S., & Panaro, F. (2022). Total pancreatectomy with intraportal islet autotransplantation for pancreatic malignancies: A literature overview. *Expert Opinion on Biological Therapy, 22*(4), 491–497. https://doi.org/10.1080/14712598.2022.1990261

Cohen, C., Moraras, K., Jackson, M., Kamischke, M., Gish, R. G., Brosgart, C. L., Toy, M., Hutton, D., Block, T. M., Wang, S., & So, S. (2022). Letter to the editor: Importance of universal screening for chronic hepatitis B infection in adults in the United States. *Hepatology (Baltimore, Md.), 75*(4), 1062–1063. https://doi.org/10.1002/hep.32304

Conners, E. E., Panagiotakopoulos, L., Hofmeister, M. G., Spradling, P. R., Hagan, L. M., Harris, A. M., Rogers-Brown, J. S., Wester, C., & Nelson, N. P. (2023). Screening and testing for hepatitis B virus infection: CDC recommendations—United States, 2023. *Morbidity and Mortality Weekly Report (MMWR), 72*(1), 1–25. https://doi.org/10.15585/mmwr.rr7201a1

Crosignani, A., Spina, S., Marrazzo, F., Cimbanassi, S., Malbrain, M. L. N. G., Van Regenmortel, N., Fumagalli, R., & Langer, T. (2022). Intravenous fluid therapy in patients with severe acute pancreatitis admitted to the intensive care unit: A narrative review. *Annals of Intensive Care, 12, 98.* https://doi.org/10.1186/s13613-022-01072-y

Dahmarde, H., Parooie, F., & Salarzaei, M. (2020). Is ^{18}F-FDG PET/CT an accurate way to detect lymph node metastasis in colorectal cancer: A systematic review and meta-analysis. *Contrast Media & Molecular Imaging, 2020*, 5439378. https://doi.org/10.1155/2020/5439378

Fraquelli, M., Nadarevic, T., Colli, A., Manzotti, C., Giljaca, V., Miletic, D., Štimac, D., & Casazza, G. (2022). Contrast-enhanced ultrasound for the diagnosis of hepatocellular carcinoma in adults with chronic liver disease. *The Cochrane Database of Systematic Reviews, 9*(9), CD013483. https://doi.org/10.1002/14651858.CD013483.pub2

Jaber, S., Garnier, M., Asehnoune, K., Bounes, F., Buscail, L., Chevaux, J. Dahyot-Fizelier, C., Darrivere, L., Jabaudon, M., Joannes-Boyau, O., Launey, Y., Levesque, E., Levy, P., Montravers, P., Muller, L., Rimmelé, T., Roger, C., Savoye-Collet, C., Seguin, P., … De Jong, A. (2022). Guidelines for the management of patients with severe acute pancreatitis, 2021. *Anaesthesia Critical Care & Pain Medicine, 41*(3), 101060. https://doi.org/10.1016/j.accpm.2022.101060

James, T. W., & Baron, T. H. (2021). Endoscopic and radiologic treatment of biliary disease. In: M. Feldman, L. S. Friedman, & L. J. Brandt (Eds.), *Sleisenger and Fordtran's gastrointestinal and liver disease* (11th ed., chap 70). Elsevier.

Jayaprakasam, V. S., Paroder, V., & Schöder, H. (2021). Variants and pitfalls in PET/CT imaging of gastrointestinal cancers. *Seminars in Nuclear Medicine, 51*(5), 485–501. https://doi.org/10.1053/j.semnuclmed.2021.04.001

Kaufman, C. S., & Cretcher, M. R. (2021). Transjugular liver biopsy. *Techniques in Vascular and Interventional Radiology, 24*(4), 100795. https://doi.org/10.1016/j.tvir.2021.100795

Llovet, J. M., Villanueva, A., Marrero, J. A., Schwartz, M., Meyer, T., Galle, P. R., Lencioni, R., Greten, T. F., Kudo, M., Mandrekar, S. J., Zhu, A. X., Finn, R. S., & Roberts, L. R.; AASLD Panel of Experts on Trial Design in HCC. (2021). Trial design and endpoints in hepatocellular carcinoma: AASLD consensus conference. *Hepatology (Baltimore, Md.)*, *73*(Suppl. 1), 158–191. https://doi.org/10.1002/hep.31327

Mahmud, N., Fricker, Z., Hubbard, R. A., Ioannou, G. N., Lewis, J. D., Taddei, T. H., Rothstein, K. D., Serper, M., Goldberg, D. S., & Kaplan, D. E. (2021). Risk prediction models for post-operative mortality in patients with cirrhosis. *Hepatology (Baltimore, Md.)*, *73*(1), 204–218. https://doi.org/10.1002/hep.31558

Majumder, S., Taylor, W. R., Foote, P. H., Berger, C. K., Wu, C. W., Mahoney, D. W., Bamlet, W. R., Burger, K. N., Postier, N., de la Fuente, J., Doering, K. A., Lidgard, G. P., Allawi, H. T., Petersen, G. M., Chari, S. T., Ahlquist, D. A., & Kisiel, J. B. (2021). High detection rates of pancreatic cancer across stages by plasma assay of novel methylated DNA markers and CA19-9. *Clinical Cancer Research*, *27*(9), 2523–2532. https://doi.org/10.1158/1078-0432.CCR-20-0235

Meshram, R. J., Kathwate, G. H., & Gacche, R. N. (2022). Progress, evolving therapeutic/diagnostic approaches, and challenges in the management of hepatitis C virus infections. *Archives of Virology*, *167*, 717–736. https://doi.org/10.1007/s00705-022-05375-0

Nadig, V., Herrmann, K., Mottaghy, F. M., & Schulz, V. (2022). Hybrid total-body pet scanners-current status and future perspectives. *European Journal of Nuclear Medicine and Molecular Imaging*, *49*(2), 445–459. https://doi.org/10.1007/s00259-021-05536-4

Nam, H., Hong, S. S., Jung, K. H., Kang, S., Park, M. S., Kang, S., Kim, H. S., Mai, V. H., Kim, J., Lee, H., Lee, W., Suh, Y. J., Lim, J. H., Kim, S. Y., Kim, S. C., Kim, S. H., & Park, S. (2022). A serum marker for early pancreatic cancer with a possible link to diabetes. *Journal of the National Cancer Institute*, *114*(2), 228–234. https://doi.org/10.1093/jnci/djab191

Olakowski, M., & Bułdak, Ł. (2022). Current status of inherited pancreatic cancer. *Hereditary Cancer in Clinical Practice*, *20*(1), 26. https://doi.org/10.1186/s13053-022-00224-2

Paisi, M., Crombag, N., Burns, L., Bogaerts, A., Withers, L., Bates, L., Crowley, D., Witton, R., & Shawe, J. (2022). Barriers and facilitators to hepatitis C screening and treatment for people with lived experience of homelessness: A mixed-methods systematic review. *Health Expectations*, *25*(1), 48–60. https://doi.org/10.1111/hex.13400

Pobłocki, J., Jasińska, A., Syrenicz, A., Andrysiak-Mamos, E., & Szczuko, M. (2020). The neuroendocrine neoplasms of the digestive tract: Diagnosis, treatment and nutrition. *Nutrients*, *12*(5), 1437. https://doi.org/10.3390/nu12051437

Radkani, P., Hawksworth, J., & Fishbein, T. (2022). Biliary system. In: C. M. Townsend Jr, R. D. Beauchamp, B. M. Evers, & K. L. Mattox (Eds.), *Sabiston textbook of surgery* (21st ed., chap 55). Elsevier.

Ramzan, A., & Tafti, D. (2022). *Nuclear medicine PET/CT gastrointestinal assessment, protocols, and interpretation* [Updated October 1, 2022]. *StatPearls*. https://www.ncbi.nlm.nih.gov/books/NBK580532/

Szatmary, P., Grammatikopoulos, T., Cai, W., Huang, W., Mukherjee, R., Halloran, C., Beyer, G., & Sutton, R. (2022). Acute pancreatitis: Diagnosis and treatment. *Drugs*, *82*, 1251–1276. https://doi.org/10.1007/s40265-022-01766-4

Wolf, E., Rich, N. E., Marrero, J. A., Parikh, N. D., & Singal, A. G. (2021). Use of hepatocellular carcinoma surveillance in patients with cirrhosis: A systematic review and meta-analysis. *Hepatology (Baltimore, Md.)*, *73*(2), 713–725. https://doi.org/10.1002/hep.31309

Wood, L. D., Canto, M. I., Jaffee, E. M., & Simeone, D. M. (2022). Pancreatic cancer: Pathogenesis, screening, diagnosis, and treatment. *Gastroenterology*, *163*(2), 386.e1–402.e1. https://doi.org/10.1053/j.gastro.2022.03.056

Yang, F., Xu, Y., Dong, Y., Huang, Y., Fu, Y., Li, T., Sun, C., Pandanaboyana, S., Windsor, J. A., & Fu, D. (2022). Prevalence and prognosis of increased pancreatic enzymes in patients with COVID-19: A systematic review and meta-analysis. *Pancreatology*, *22*(4), 539–546. https://doi.org/10.1016/j.pan.2022.03.014

Yoo, J. E., Han, K., Shin, D. W., Kim, D., Kim, B. S., Chun, S., Jeon, K. H., Jung, W., Park, J., Park, J. H., Choi, K. S., & Kim, J. S. (2022). Association between changes in alcohol consumption and cancer risk. *JAMA Network Open*, *5*(8), e2228544. https://doi.org/10.1001/jamanetworkopen.2022.28544

16 Nutritional Problems*

OVERVIEW AND ASSESSMENT

See additional online content: Procedure Guidelines 16-1–16-3.

Nutrition Overview

Knowledge of nutrients and the basic principles of nutrition is important in the role of patient education for disease prevention and health promotion. The principles also help to provide an understanding and background to diseases affected by a person's nutritional status. The basic food groups and their placement on a plate help to serve as a guide to basic, healthy nutrition.

Key Principles

1. Nutrients, including carbohydrates, fats, proteins, vitamins, and minerals, have specific functions within the body. They work together to provide energy, regulate metabolic processes, and synthesize tissues.
2. Nutritional influences all body systems favorably and unfavorably. Examples of unfavorable effects include the link between cholesterol and heart disease or salt intake and high blood pressure (BP). Favorable effects are many, such as the association of fiber intake with improved gastrointestinal (GI) function and the role of folic acid in preventing neural tube defects.
3. Nutritional needs vary in response to metabolic changes, age, sex assigned at birth, growth periods, stress (trauma, disease, pregnancy, lactation), and physical condition.
4. Nutritional supplements may be needed depending on disease states, dietary intake, and other factors.
5. The types of foods eaten and eating patterns are developed during a lifetime and are determined by psychosocial, cultural, religious, and economic influences.
6. The nurse works with the registered dietitian to promote optimum nutrition for each patient.

MyPlate and the Dietary Guidelines for Americans

1. Dietary guidelines were first developed in 1958 and were based on four basic food groups: grains, vegetables and fruits, meat, and milk. In 2010, the Department of Health and Human Services and U.S. Department of Agriculture (USDA) Dietary Guidelines for Americans were restructured and divided the four basic food groups into five food groups, which now consist of grains, fruits, vegetables, protein, and dairy. Although the guidelines have been reformatted, it still holds true that a well-balanced diet consists of foods from each of these groups and is composed of foods low in fat, cholesterol, and sodium and high in fiber (*https://www.dietaryguidelines.gov*).
2. In response to growing scientific knowledge regarding the linkage between diet and disease, the USDA developed the MyPlate Plan (see Figure 16-1). It reflects making food choices for a healthy lifestyle and includes basic information on how to build a healthy plate by cutting back on foods high in solid fats, added sugars, and salt; eating the right amount of calories; and being physically active. Additionally, the 2020 to 2025 *Dietary Guidelines* endorse four overarching Guidelines to encourage healthy eating patterns such that people can enjoy foods that meet their personal, cultural, and traditional preferences and fit within their budget:
   a. Follow a healthy dietary pattern at every stage of life.
   b. Customize and enjoy nutrient-dense food and beverage choices to reflect personal preferences, cultural traditions, and budgetary considerations.
   c. Focus on meeting food group needs with nutrient-dense foods and beverages and stay within calorie limits.
   d. Limit food and beverages higher in added sugars, saturated fats, and sodium, and limit alcoholic beverages.

Nutritional Assessment

Nutritional assessment is an ongoing process designed to identify a person's nutritional status and the significance on the

*Please note that the term "male" in this chapter refers to a person assigned male at birth, and the term "female" in this chapter refers to a person assigned female at birth.

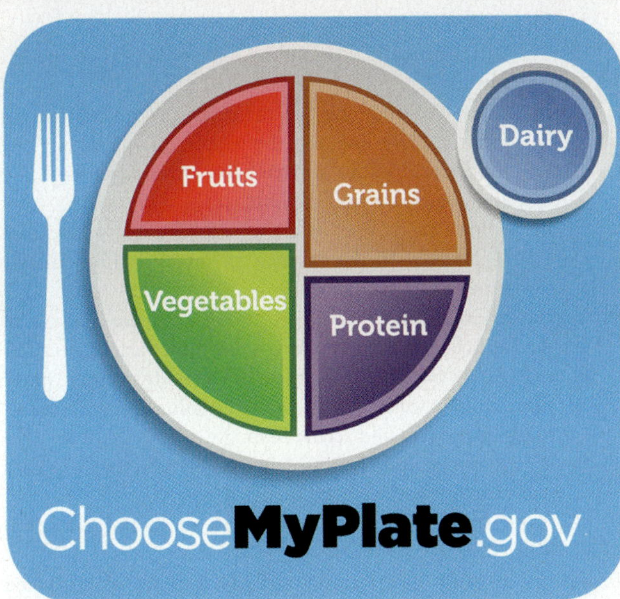

Figure 16-1. MyPlate illustrates healthy eating. (U.S. Department of Agriculture.)

person's well-being. Although there are many methods and tools for assessing nutritional status, there is no universal method or "gold standard." Weight loss is perhaps the most validated parameter of nutritional status. However, multiple factors must be evaluated and considered to determine the risk for or degree of malnutrition.

There are many methods to assess the nutritional status including the type and amount of food consumed. Assessing nutritional intake is one method to assist in identification of malnutrition caused by an imbalance in nutrition. Techniques to capture nutritional intake may include a 24-hour recall of foods eaten, a food diary kept by the patient for several days, or a food frequency questionnaire that reflects food intake patterns. In addition to these specific tools, the following information is useful to determine nutritional patterns and status.

Key Clinical History Points

1. General background information—name, age, sex, family composition, socioeconomic status, occupation.
2. General health status and any chronic conditions, including diabetes and associated dietary restrictions as well as any hospitalizations.
3. Cultural and religious factors influencing dietary patterns.
4. Family history of diseases, including diabetes and obesity.
5. Current medications, over-the-counter products, and herbal supplements.
6. Food habits.
   a. Typical daily intake, including meal frequency, meal timing, and meal location.
   b. Snacking patterns.
   c. Food intolerance or dislikes.
   d. Nutritional supplements, including vitamins, minerals, fortified beverages, and foods.
   e. Alcohol consumption.
   f. Use of specific diets or dietary restrictions.
7. Food purchase and preparation.
   a. Who purchases and prepares food and where food is purchased.
   b. Facilities for food storage and preparation.
   c. Factors influencing the types of food purchased.
8. Nutritionally related problems.
   a. General well-being, energy level.
   b. Changes in appetite.
   c. Weight change during the past 6 months.
   d. Difficulty chewing or swallowing, use of dentures.
   e. Change in sense of taste or smell.
   f. Eructation, flatulence, nausea, vomiting, diarrhea, constipation, or abdominal pain or swelling in relation to food intake.
   g. Bowel habits.
9. Physical activity and exercise.

Physical Examination and Anthropometrics

1. Perform a systematic physical examination, including vital signs, observing for a wide variety of physical findings associated with nutritional status.
   a. Listlessness, apathy.
   b. Cognitive and sensory deficits.
   c. Poor muscle tone or wasting of muscle.
   d. Dull, brittle hair; hair may be thin or sparse, easily plucked.
   e. Rough, dry, and scaly skin or dermatitis.
   f. Ecchymosis.
   g. Premature whitening of hair.
   h. Cheilosis (fissures at angles of mouth).
   i. Stomatitis (inflammation of mouth).
   j. Inflammation and easy bleeding of gums.
   k. Glossitis (inflammation of tongue).
   l. Dental caries and poor dentition.
   m. Spoon-shaped, brittle, ridged nails.
   n. Skeletal deformities such as bowlegs.
2. Perform anthropometry, as indicated. (Anthropometry comes from the word *anthropology* and is the science that studies the size, weight, and proportions of the human body to determine body fat mass, lean mass, and nutritional status.) Types of anthropometric measurements include height and weight, skin-fold thickness, and circumferential tests.
3. Height and weight are determined on patient admission and are later used as a baseline for comparisons in nutritional status.
   a. Height should be measured with a stadiometer.
   b. Weight should be measured using a consistent and reliable scale and at a consistent time, standing with shoes and overgarments removed.
   c. Unintended weight loss of more than 10% of body weight during 6 months is considered clinically significant and may be associated with physiologic abnormalities and increased morbidity and mortality.
4. Body mass index (BMI) is weight in kilograms divided by height in meters squared (see Table 16-1).
   a. BMI of less than 18.5 is classified as underweight.
   b. BMI of 18.5 to 24.9 is classified as normal weight.
   c. BMI of 25 to 29.9 is classified as overweight.
   d. BMI of 30 to 39.9 is classified as obese.
   e. BMI greater than 40 is classified as extremely obese.
5. Metabolism is generally faster in younger people, and for this reason, babies and children have higher energy requirement needs than do adults. Requirement needs are based on many factors including age, sex assigned at birth, activity level, and disease state. Exact measurements of caloric requirements for infants can be obtained by using charts; these estimate the

Table 16-1 Body Mass Index (BMI)[a]

Weight	5'	5'3"	5'6"	5'9"	6'	6'3"
140	27	25	23	21	19	18
150	29	27	24	22	20	19
160	31	28	26	24	22	20
170	33	30	28	25	23	21
180	35	32	29	27	25	23
190	37	34	31	28	26	24
200	39	36	32	30	27	25
210	41	37	34	31	29	26
220	43	39	36	33	30	28
230	45	41	37	34	31	29
240	47	43	39	36	33	30
250	49	44	40	37	34	31

[a]*Body mass index = weight (kg)/height (m²).*

body surface area by height and weight and the standard basal metabolic rate for a given weight (see Appendix B, page 1499).

6. Functional assessment including gait and strength of extremities.
7. Skin-fold thickness provides an estimate of body fat based on the amount of fat in subcutaneous tissue using calibrated calipers to measure the thickness of the skin at designated sites (see Figure 16-2).
   a. Grasp skin and subcutaneous fat, pulling it away from the underlying muscle, and place the caliper jaws over the skin-fold flap.
   b. Take the reading within 2 to 3 seconds and without using excessive pressure.
   c. Repeat the reading twice and take an average of the three readings to increase accuracy.
8. Skin-fold sites include the following:
   a. Vertical measurements:
      i. Triceps: on the posterior midline of the upper arm, midpoint between the acromion and olecranon processes.
      ii. Abdomen: two cm to the right of the umbilicus.
      iii. Thigh: on the anterior midline of the thigh, midway between the proximal border of the patella the inguinal crease (hip).
   b. Diagonal measurements:
      i. Subscapular: just below the inferior border of the left scapula.
      ii. Chest/Pectoral: one half the distance between the anterior axillary line and the nipple (in males); or one third the distance between the anterior axillary line and the nipple (in females).
      iii. Suprailiac: in line with the natural angle of the iliac crest taken in the anterior axillary line immediately superior to the iliac crest.
9. Circumferential tests provide information on the amount of skeletal muscle and adipose tissue. Mid-upper arm circumference (MAC)—an indirect estimate of the body's muscle mass:
   a. Place a tape measure around the midpoint of the nondominant upper arm and secure it snugly.
   b. To calculate, multiply the triceps skin fold by 3.14 and subtract the product from the MAC.
   c. Adult standards are 16.5 mm for females and 12.5 mm for males.
10. Advanced body composition analysis is a set of advanced techniques that provide various measurements including total-body fat, muscle mass percentages, bone weight, and visceral adipose tissue (VAT) score among other measurements of body composition. Methods may include the following:
    a. Dual-energy x-ray absorptiometry (DEXA).
    b. Underwater (hydrostatic) weighing.
    c. Air displacement plethysmography (ADP).
    d. Bioelectrical impedance analysis (BIA).

Laboratory Tests

1. Serum albumin, prealbumin and transferrin levels measure visceral proteins that inversely correlate with metabolic stress, such as inadequate nutrition, but not directly measure nutritional status.
   a. Albumin is a protein made by the liver and is responsible for maintaining blood volume and serum electrolyte balance. The half-life of albumin is about 21 days. A decrease in nutritional status may result in a drop in albumin synthesis. However, in chronic malnutrition, serum albumin levels are typically normal or high.
   b. Prealbumin is also made by the liver and is a more sensitive but expensive test that measures more recent nutritional status. Its half-life is 2 to 3 days.
   c. Transferrin is another transport protein made by the liver and is responsible for binding iron to plasma and

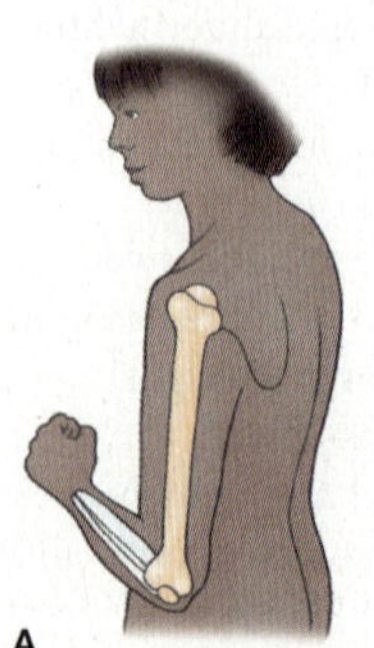

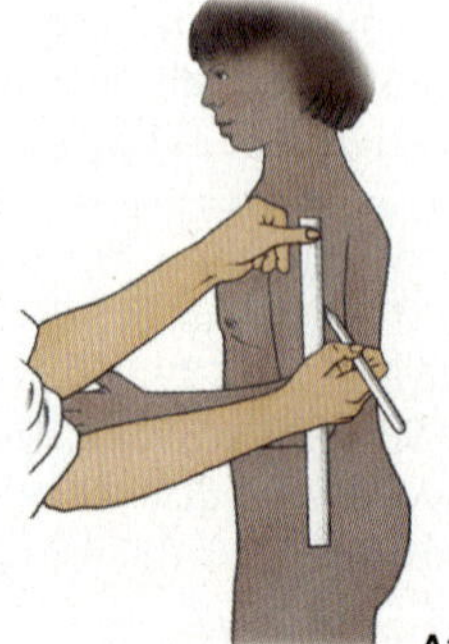

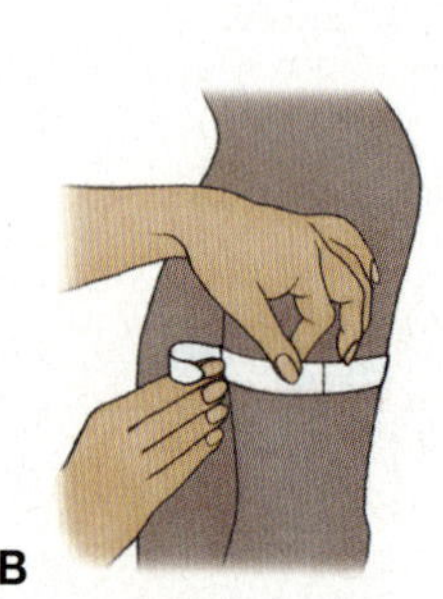

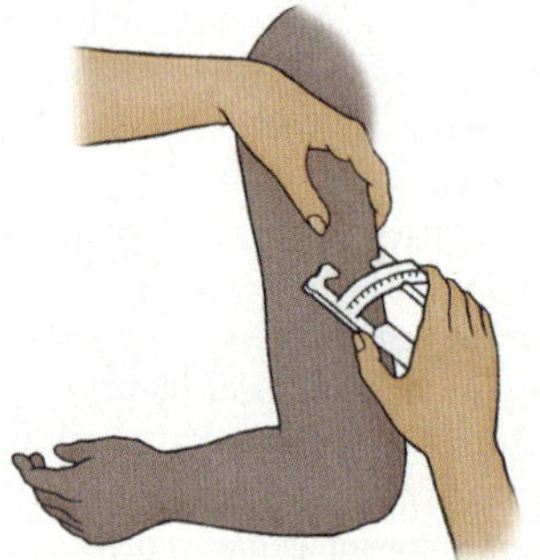

Figure 16-2. Anthropometric measurements. **(A and A1)** Marking the midpoint of the upper arm. **(B)** Obtaining the mid-upper arm circumference. **(C)** Measuring triceps skin-fold thickness.

transporting it to the bone marrow. Reduced levels are found in catabolic states and some chronic diseases.
2. Hemoglobin—made by the liver; decreased amounts are related to iron-deficiency anemia or other defect in hemoglobin synthesis or dilution of the blood such as during pregnancy.
3. Twenty-four-hour urine creatinine—an increase in this measure indicates increased tissue breakdown.
4. Twenty-four-hour urine urea nitrogen or total urinary nitrogen—this test can be used to determine nitrogen balance.
5. Electrolytes, blood urea nitrogen, and creatinine may help to assess hydration status.
6. Micronutrient levels to help identify nutritional deficiencies.

General Procedures and Treatment Modalities

The inability to take nutrients through the oral route either totally or in part may require alternative means to enhance and maintain nutritional status. Alternative methods of nutritional support include enteral feeding and parenteral nutrition. The decision as to which method is used will depend on many factors including the patient's acuity and nutritional status.

Enteral Feeding

Administration of nutrients directly into the stomach, duodenum, or jejunum through a tube is more physiologically beneficial and cost-effective than parenteral feeding. Enteral feeding carries less risk of infection than parenteral feeding and maintains a functional GI tract by preventing mucosal atrophy and biliary and hepatic dysfunction. Enteral therapy is appropriate for patients with at least a minimally functional GI tract who cannot take adequate nutrition by mouth.

Enteral therapy has become utilized more frequently as more commercially available enteral formulas have been developed and long-term enteral feeding tubes have become safer and more easily inserted.

Clinical Indications

1. Increased metabolic needs and inability to take adequate oral diet—trauma, burns, cancer, sepsis.
2. Coma or mechanical ventilation.
3. Head/neck surgery.
4. Malabsorption.
5. Obstruction of esophagus or oropharynx.
6. Severe anorexia nervosa.
7. Dysphagia.

Sites of Tube Insertion

Short-Term Nutritional Support (<30 Days)

1. Nasogastric (NG) feeding—tubes are passed through the nose or mouth (orogastric) into the stomach and secured in place.
   a. Tube placement must be verified by x-ray before use. Aspiration of contents for pH or auscultation of air injected through a tube has been shown to be of limited value. New techniques that are available include colorimetric carbon dioxide detectors and electronic capnographics, both of which measure end-tidal carbon dioxide to determine if the tube has gone into the trachea.
   b. If there is a question about tube placement in the respiratory tract, the tube should be removed.
2. Nasoenteric feeding (i.e., nasoduodenal or nasojejunal)—tube is passed through the nose into the duodenum or jejunum and secured in place. X-ray is usually needed to verify correct tube placement.

Long-Term Nutritional Support (>30 Days)

1. Gastrostomy—insertion of a tube surgically, radiologically, or by a percutaneous endoscopic procedure into the stomach.
2. Gastrostomy button—small device inserted through gastrostomy stoma to allow for long-term feeding with minimal effect on body image.
3. Jejunostomy—insertion of a tube directly into the jejunum either surgically or by a percutaneous endoscopic procedure. Jejunostomy feedings are generally done by continuous infusion using a feeding pump.
4. Gastrojejunostomy—a tube inserted endoscopically, less likely to be dislocated.

Types of Tubes

1. Large-bore NG polyurethane tube—size 12 to 18F, used very short term (e.g., Salem Sump).
2. Small-bore NG tube—made of polyurethane, silicone, or polyvinyl chloride with a tungsten-weighted tip or nonweighted tip, size 8 to 12F and 30 to 36 in (76 to 91.5 cm) long.
3. Nasointestinal tube—made of silicone, polyurethane, or polyvinyl chloride with a tungsten-weighted tip or nonweighted tip, size 8 to 12F and 40 to 60 in (101.5 to 152.5 cm) long.
4. Gastrostomy tube—catheter made of silicone, polyurethane, polyvinyl chloride, or latex; a balloon on the distal end to stabilize the tube may be used and ranges from 5 to 30 mL capacity, size 14 to 28F. Adults usually have 20F tubes, and children usually start with 14F.
5. Gastrostomy button—silicone; ranging from 18 to 28F and 1 in (2.5 cm) long; useful for the person wanting minimal alteration in body image.
6. Jejunostomy tube—size ranging from 5 to 14F with or without a balloon (a balloon may obstruct lumen of the jejunum). A plain red rubber catheter is occasionally used as a short-term jejunostomy tube, and some gastrostomy tubes may be used for jejunostomy.

Delivery Systems for Feeding Solution

1. Intermittent or continuous infusion of feeding solution by gravity is accomplished by hanging a container of feeding solution from an intravenous (IV) pole and adjusting the delivery rate by a flow regulator.
2. Continuous feeding by controller feeding pump allows uniform flow, particularly of viscous solutions.
3. Bolus feeding involves enteral formula poured into a barrel of a large (60 mL) syringe attached to a feeding tube and allowed to infuse by gravity.

CLINICAL JUDGMENT Bolus feeding may precipitate dumping syndrome, particularly if given into the small intestine. Dumping syndrome occurs when hyperosmolar substances enter the intestine quickly, causing an influx of water into the GI tract that can result in nausea, vomiting, bloating, cramping, and diarrhea. Dumping syndrome may also cause dizziness, nervousness, and nausea.

Community and Home Care Considerations

Teach patient and family:

1. Technique for administration of tube feeding (intermittent, continuous, bolus).
2. Signs and symptoms of potential complications.
3. Need to assess tube placement and residual before each feeding (for gastric feedings only).
4. Principles of medical asepsis, including careful handwashing, refrigeration of formula, cleaning of equipment with soap and water, and thorough drying between feedings.
5. When the gastrostomy or jejunostomy tube insertion site is well healed, the surrounding skin can be cleaned with soap and water.
6. Gauze dressing can be applied, as needed.
7. Leakage around the tube or signs of peristomal skin irritation should be reported.

Complications

See Table 16-2.

Parenteral Nutrition

Parenteral nutrition is the introduction of nutrients, including amino acids, lipids, dextrose, vitamins, minerals, electrolytes, trace elements, and water, through a venous access device (VAD) directly into the intravascular fluid to provide nutrients required for metabolic functioning of the body.

Table 16-2 Complications of Enteral Feeding and Treatment

COMPLICATIONS	CAUSES	INTERVENTIONS
Tube displacement	Tube migration into the esophagus	• Observe for eructation of air when injecting air to test for tube placement in the stomach. • Aspirate gastric contents; if none is obtained, suspect esophageal placement.
	Tube placement into the respiratory tract	• Observe for gagging, dyspnea, inability to speak, coughing when tube insertion attempted. • Obtain chest x-ray.[a] • Withdraw tube and attempt reinsertion with the patient's head flexed forward.[a]
Tube obstruction	Tube kinking	• Obtain chest x-ray to confirm and withdraw and reinsert the new tube.[a]
	Tube clogging	• Flush tube every 4 h with 30 mL of water and after administration of intermittent feeding and medication administration. • Administer medications in liquid form if possible. Crush medications finely (if crushable). • Attempt to declog by administering water first. If unsuccessful, then administer pancreatic enzyme/bicarbonate mixture.
Aspiration	Patient lying flat	• Elevate HOB 30°–45° during continuous feedings or for 30–60 min after bolus feeds.
	Absent or depressed gag reflex	• Elevate HOB 30°–45° during continuous feedings or for 30–60 min after bolus feeds.
	Reflux	• Elevate HOB 30°–45° during continuous feedings or for 30–60 min after bolus feeds. • Administer proton pump inhibitor per provider orders.
	Improper tube placement	• Confirm proper placement with x-ray imaging. • Tape tube in place.
Vomiting	Tube migration into the esophagus	• See interventions for tube displacement above.
	Decreased absorption	• Auscultate for decreased bowel sounds, observe for abdominal distention. • Consider decreasing the amount of tube feeding.[a] • Consider administration on a continuous basis.[a] • Consider placement of a small-bore, weighted-tip nasointestinal tube.[a]
	Rapid rate of infusion	• Administer no faster than 200–300 mL during 10–20 min. • Consider administration on a continuous basis.[a]
	Excessive infusion of air	• If giving a bolus feeding, pinch tubing off when refilling the syringe with formula. • If giving continuous feeding, make certain the bag does not empty before closing off tubing.
	Patient position	• Maintain the patient at 30°–45° angle of head elevation during and 30–60 min after feeding. If administering continuous feeding, maintain head elevation at all times.
	Nausea	• Antiemetics.
	Obstruction	• Assess for distention and decreased bowel sounds; obtain x-ray.
	Constipation	• Assess for impaction and review the frequency of bowel movements.

Table 16-2 Complications of Enteral Feeding and Treatment (*continued*)

COMPLICATIONS	CAUSES	INTERVENTIONS
Diarrhea	Drug therapy	• Evaluate drug regimen for possible causes of drug-induced diarrhea from antibiotics, elixirs with high osmolarity, elixirs with sorbitol, and magnesium-containing antacids.
	High osmolarity of formula	• Begin administration of formula at a slow rate.[a] • Consider continuous feeding rather than intermittent.[a]
	Lactose intolerance	• Administer lactose-free formula. (Few commercial formulas contain lactose.)
	Bacterial contamination of formula	• Change administration set daily or per facility protocol. • Maintain strict medical asepsis, including careful handwashing before administration of formula. • Allow formula to hang no longer than 8 h (unless it is a "ready-to-hang" container that can hang for 24–48 h).
	Rapid infusion rate	• Administer slowly; consider continuous rather than intermittent infusion.[a]
	Fecal impaction	• Manually clear the impaction.
	Clostridium difficile	• Administer antibiotics.
Constipation	Lack of fiber	• Ensure that the patient is not impacted and administer formula with fiber.[a]
	Decreased fluid intake	• Increase intake of water.[a]
	Drug therapy	• Evaluate drug regimen for possible cause, including aluminum-containing antacids or lack of stool softener.
Hyperglycemia	Diabetes, impaired metabolism	• Monitor serum glucose, assess for dehydration caused by hyperosmotic diuresis; observe for symptoms of hyperglycemia, including polyuria, polydipsia. • Administer insulin.[a] • Observe for hypercapnia (increased respirations, elevated PCO_2).
Hypernatremia	Dehydration	• Assess for signs and symptoms of dehydration (I&O, daily weight, skin turgor, blood urea nitrogen, CVP, tachycardia, hypotension). • Rehydrate with extra water via the feeding tube or, if the patient is severely hypernatremic, use the IV route. • Rehydrate with D_5W or hypotonic saline solutions.[a]
Hyponatremia	Overhydration, excessive sodium loss (diaphoresis, nasogastric suction)	• Observe for signs and symptoms of hypervolemia (shortness of breath, rales, I&O, daily weight, peripheral edema, elevated CVP). • Observe for signs and symptoms of hyponatremia (lethargy, headaches, mental status change, nausea, vomiting, abdominal cramping). • Replace sodium, administer diuretics, or, depending on the cause of hypernatremia, restrict fluids.[a]
Hyperkalemia	Metabolic acidosis/ renal insufficiency	• Observe for signs and symptoms of hyperkalemia (dysrhythmias, nausea, diarrhea, muscle weakness). • Treat underlying cause. • Administer exchange resin, glucose, and insulin.[a] • Choose a lower potassium formula.
Hypokalemia	Diarrhea, refeeding syndrome	• See interventions for diarrhea. • If severe, replace potassium.[a]
Hypophosphatemia	Refeeding	• Replace phosphorus.

CVP, central venous pressure; H_2, histamine; HOB, head of bed; I&O, intake and output.

[a]Obtain orders from the health care provider.

Clinical Indications

1. Patient cannot tolerate enteral nutrition because of:
   a. Paralytic ileus.
   b. Intestinal obstruction.
   c. Acute pancreatitis and enteral feedings not possible.
   d. Severe malabsorption.
   e. Persistent vomiting and jejunal route not possible.
   f. Enterocutaneous fistula and enteric feeding not possible.
   g. Inflammatory bowel disease.
   h. Short-bowel syndrome.
2. Hypermetabolic states for which enteral therapy is either not possible or inadequate, such as burns, trauma, or sepsis.
3. In these situations, additional components are added to the enteral therapy or individualized solutions are developed to meet the nutritional needs of the patient.

Methods of Parenteral Nutrition

Total Nutrient Admixture

1. Given through a central vein, commonly into the superior vena cava, total nutrient admixture (TNA) is a parenteral

formula that combines carbohydrates in the form of a concentrated (most commonly 40%, 50%, or 70%) dextrose solution; proteins in the form of essential and nonessential (except arginine and glutamine) amino acids (0.8 to 1.5 g of protein/kg/day); lipids in the form of an emulsion (25% to 30% of total calories); and vitamins, minerals, trace elements, and fluids individualized to meet the patient's needs.
2. Central TNA is indicated for patients requiring parenteral feeding for 7 or more days.

Peripheral Parenteral Nutrition

1. Given through a peripheral vein, this parenteral formula combines a less concentrated dextrose solution with amino acids, vitamins, minerals, and lipids.
2. Unlike TNA given centrally, peripheral parenteral nutrition provides fewer calories and, occasionally, a larger percentage of calories is supplied by lipids rather than by carbohydrates.
3. Indicated for patients requiring parenteral nutrition for fewer than 7 days who do not already have enteral access.

Total Parenteral Nutrition

1. Total parenteral nutrition (TPN) combines dextrose, amino acids, vitamins, and minerals and is given through a central IV line.
2. If lipids are needed, they are given intermittently or mixed with the TPN solution through a central IV line.

Fat Emulsion (Lipids)

1. About 10%, 20%, or 30% emulsion composed of triglycerides, egg phospholipids, glycerol, and water. It also contains vitamin K.
2. May be given centrally or peripherally.

Complications

See Table 16-3 on page 552.

Table 16-3 Complications of Total Parenteral Nutrition and Treatment

COMPLICATIONS	CAUSES	INTERVENTIONS
Sepsis	• High glucose content of fluid • Venous access device contamination	• Monitor temperature, white blood cell count, insertion site for signs and symptoms of infection. • Maintain strict surgical asepsis when changing dressing and tubing. • Consider removal of venous access device with replacement in alternate site.[a] • If blood cultures positive, consider institution of antibiotic therapy.[a]
Electrolyte imbalance	• Iatrogenic • Effect of underlying diseases (i.e., fistula, diarrhea, vomiting) • Blood sample contaminated by parenteral nutrition	• Monitor electrolyte levels at least daily initially. • Monitor signs and symptoms of electrolyte imbalance. • Treat underlying cause.[a] • Change the concentration of electrolytes in TPN as necessary to address blood levels.[a]
Hyperglycemia	• Insufficient insulin secretion • High glucose content of fluid • Blood sample contaminated by parenteral nutrition	• Monitor blood glucose frequently. • Administer exogenous insulin per addition to TPN, subcutaneously or through a separate IV drip.[a] • Decrease glucose content of fluid if warranted.[a]
Hypoglycemia	• Abrupt discontinuation of parenteral nutrition administered through a central vessel	• Reduce the rate of parenteral nutrition by 50% × 2 h, then discontinue. • If TPN/peripheral parenteral nutrition must be stopped abruptly, hang a separate dextrose solution if insulin has been administered.
Hypervolemia	• Iatrogenic • Underlying disease (i.e., heart failure, renal failure)	• Monitor intake and output, daily weights, CVP, breath sounds, peripheral edema. • Consider administering a more concentrated solution.[a]
Hyperosmolar diuresis	• High osmolarity of parenteral nutrition	• Monitor intake and output, daily weights, CVP. • Consider decreasing the concentration or increasing the amount of fluid administered.[a]
Hepatic dysfunction	• IV nutrition	• Monitor liver function tests, triglyceride levels, presence of jaundice. • Consider alteration in macronutrients.[a]
Hypercapnia	• Excessive calorie delivery	• Consider reducing total calories.[a]
Lipid intolerance	• Low birth weight or premature neonate • History of liver disease • History of elevated triglycerides	• Monitor for bleeding (check stools for occult blood, coagulation studies, platelet levels). • Monitor oxygen levels for impaired oxygenation. • Monitor for fat overload syndrome: monitor triglyceride levels and liver function tests, hepatosplenomegaly, decreased coagulation, cyanosis, dyspnea. • Monitor allergic reaction: nausea, vomiting, headache, chest pain, back pain, fever. • Administer lipid-containing solutions slowly initially, while observing for symptoms.
Lipid particulate aggregation	• Unstable mixture of dextrose solution with lipid emulsion	• Observe for cracking or creaming of fluid and discontinue use of fluid with these characteristics.

CVP, central venous pressure; IV, intravenous; TPN, total parenteral nutrition.
[a]Obtain orders from the health care provider.

Delivery Systems for Parenteral Nutrition

1. Central VADs:
   a. Insertion of long-term VADs, such as Hickman, Broviac, or Groshong catheters.
   b. Peripherally inserted central catheters (peripherally inserted central catheter lines) may be used.
   c. Multilumen, central VADs can allow concomitant administration of TNA and other solutions, including medications or blood, each running through a separate lumen.
2. Peripheral IV access:
   a. Insertion of an angiocatheter into a vein in the arm or leg.
   b. Midline catheters of longer length and with the ability to remain in place for more than 3 days.
3. Delivery of parenteral nutrition should be controlled by a volume control infuser.
4. Filters should be used whenever possible.
   a. A 0.22-µm filter may be used for TPN (without added fat emulsion).
   b. A 1.2-µm filter may be used for TNA or fat emulsion.

Nursing Interventions and Patient Education

1. Use strict sterile technique to attach IV tubing (with filter) to parenteral nutrition bag, purge air, make sure all clamps are closed, and then close the clamp on VAD before attaching IV tubing to VAD. If central VAD is being used, have the patient bear down and hold their breath to perform the Valsalva maneuver, which prevents air from being sucked into the tubing.
2. Regulate flow and monitor administration hourly for patient tolerance and development of complications.
3. Change central VAD dressing according to facility protocol, maintaining sterility.
   a. The patient should be in a supine position with head turned away from dressing.
   b. Clean the skin first with alcohol, then povidone–iodine, starting at the insertion site and moving outward in a circular pattern.
   c. Apply a transparent dressing over the insertion site when the skin is thoroughly dry.
   d. Loop and tape tubing outside of dressing.
4. Monitor for signs and symptoms of pneumothorax, air embolism, bleeding, venous thrombosis, and insertion site infection including but not limited to tachycardia, hypotension, fever, shortness of breath, chest pain, or lightheadedness.

NUTRITIONAL DISORDERS

Nutritional disorders can have a negative impact on the health and well-being of a person. In addition, some nutritional disorders may in turn lead to the development of other diseases or health issues. If not identified and treated in a timely fashion, these disorders can have a devastating effect.

Obesity

1. *Obesity* is an overabundance of body fat that impacts people of all ages, ethnicities, socioeconomic classes, and genders. Obesity is typically measured by a person's body mass index (BMI) (weight in kilograms divided by height in meters squared). A BMI greater than 30 is classified as obese. Obesity has become a global health issue affecting both rich and poor countries. Current global estimates find that more than 1 billion people worldwide—which includes 650 million adults, 340 million adolescents, and 39 million children—are affected by obesity. According to the Centers for Disease Control and Prevention, the prevalence of obesity among U.S. adults was 41.9% during the time period 2017 to 2020. During the same time period, the prevalence of severe obesity increased from 4.7% to 9.2%.
2. Obesity is limited not only to the adult population; it impacts children and adolescent populations as well. In 2023, the American Academy of Pediatrics identified essential components for treatment of children and adolescents with obesity to include:
   a. Providing intensive, longitudinal treatment in the medical home.
   b. Evaluating and monitoring child or adolescent for obesity-related medical and psychological comorbidities.
   c. Identifying and addressing social drivers of health.
   d. Using nonstigmatizing approaches to clinical treatment that honor the unique individual qualities of each child and family.

EVIDENCE BASE Centers for Disease Control and Prevention. (2023). http://www.cdc.gov/obesity/data/adult_html

Pathophysiology and Etiology

Increasing evidence reveals that obesity is a multifactorial disease and may be the result of several different factors. Such factors may include the following:

1. Heredity and genetic factors:
   a. Identical twins raised separately are more likely to have similar amounts of body fat than are fraternal twins raised separately.
   b. Genetic defects in certain disorders such as Bardet-Biedl syndrome and Prader-Willi syndrome can directly cause obesity.
2. Environmental factors:
   a. Some evidence shows that children reared by parental caregivers with obesity have an increased tendency toward obesity.
   b. Increased availability of high-fat, high-calorie foods.
   c. Reduction in physical activity.
   d. Modern-day conveniences (i.e., riding lawnmowers, escalators, elevators, etc.).
3. Psychological factors:
   a. Depression.
   b. Anxiety.
   c. Anger.
   d. Posttraumatic stress.
   e. Boredom.
4. Physiologic factors:
   a. Endocrine abnormalities (rare causes of obesity)—Cushing syndrome, polycystic ovary syndrome, hypothyroidism, hypogonadism, or hypothalamic lesions.
   b. Age—advancing age may be associated with obesity, usually due to changes in activity level and metabolic rate, or in females because of hormonal changes; early childhood and the start of puberty may also be associated with obesity.
5. Pharmacologic factors:
   a. Corticosteroids.
   b. Antidepressants.
   c. Hormones and other medications.

Clinical Manifestations

1. BMI greater than 30, depending on body composition.
2. Increased weight is correlated with an increased incidence of comorbid conditions.
   a. Cardiovascular disease.
   b. Type 2 diabetes mellitus.
   c. Hypertension.
   d. Obstructive sleep apnea.
   e. Osteoarthritis.
   f. Gastroesophageal reflux disease.
   g. Gallbladder disease.
   h. Cancer of the breast, endometrium, prostate, and colon.
   i. Stroke.
   j. Dyslipidemia.
   k. Stress urinary incontinence.
   l. Infertility.
   m. Depression (may be a cause of obesity as well as caused by obesity).
   n. COVID-19.
3. Metabolic syndrome (insulin resistance syndrome)—a group of characteristics that when co-occurring increase the risk of coronary artery disease, stroke, and type 2 diabetes.
   a. Obesity.
   b. Hypertension.
   c. Insulin resistance.
   d. High triglycerides.

Diagnostic Evaluation

1. Nutritional assessment—a systematic method for obtaining, verifying, and interpreting data needed to identify nutrition-related problems and their causes and significance.
2. Anthropometric and physical assessment—to evaluate increased body fat and effects of obesity on the body.
3. Selected hormonal studies (thyroid, cortisol levels)—to assess for potential underlying cause.

Management

Conservative Measures

1. Diet therapy—has been controversial, but a well-balanced diet containing all the major food groups is still advised and recommended as a first-step therapy.
   a. A 1,000-calorie deficit per day is required to lose 2.2 pounds (1 kg) of body weight per week.
   b. Diet therapy should be individualized to the patient; however, the overall goal is to create a calorie deficit through reduced calorie intake or increased calorie expenditure.
   c. A balance of food groups is essential to maintain vitamin and nutrient balance. Nutrient supplementation may be necessary (calcium, vitamin D, iron, B_{12}, zinc, and folate).
   d. Food preparation should include seasoning with herbs, onion, garlic, and pepper, and foods should be baked, broiled, steamed, sautéed using minimal oil or cooked in an air fryer.
   e. Food attractively arranged on smaller plates, using whole rather than processed foods and eaten slowly, will assist the overall process.
   f. Eliminating entire food groups from the diet, such as carbohydrates (in many popular protein- and fat-based diets), will eventually result in craving for those foods eliminated, disruption of normal metabolic processes, and quick weight gain when the food is added to the diet.
2. Exercise—regular physical activity is an important component in weight loss and weight maintenance along with reduced caloric intake. The most recent recommendations from the World Health Organization are for adults 18 to 64 years of age to incorporate at least 150 to 300 minutes per week of physical activity. Physical activity may also add other health benefits if done on a regular basis, such as improved cardiovascular status and emotional well-being.
3. Behavior modification is a cornerstone of any successful diet.
   a. Identify and eliminate situations or cues leading to overeating or high-calorie foods with the use of a food diary.
   b. Provide positive reinforcement of proper dietary habits.
   c. Should a lapse in diet habits occur, focus on a prompt and positive return to appropriate dietary habits.
   d. Stress reduction techniques, such as visual imagery or progressive muscle relaxation; peer support may be helpful.

EVIDENCE BASE Physical Activity. (2022). World Health Organization. Retrieved April 2023, from https://www.who.int/news-room/fact-sheets/detail/physica-activity

Pharmacotherapy

1. Anorexia medications include amphetamines, sympathomimetics, and norepinephrine-releasing agents or reuptake inhibitors; reduce appetite and stimulate weight loss initially.
   a. However, tolerance may develop and weight may be regained when the drugs are discontinued.
   b. Numerous long-term studies have failed to show long-term success with these agents.
2. Phentermine products are available in prescription form and primarily act on chemicals in the brain to decrease appetite. Phentermine products also have a stimulant component and should not be used in uncontrolled hypertension, advanced heart disease, history of drug use, or with monoamine oxidase (MAO) inhibitors.
3. Phentermine–topiramate extended release is a U.S. Food and Drug Administration (FDA)-approved drug available in prescription form. This drug combines the effects of phentermine with the weight loss effects of topiramate (a medication used to treat seizures).
4. Naltrexone hydrochloride and bupropion hydrochloride, branded as Contrave, is a combination of two medications, naltrexone (used to treat narcotic and alcohol dependency) and bupropion (an antidepressant), to help decrease appetite and control eating.
5. Liraglutide, semaglutide, and tirzepatide are all injectable medications used for the management of diabetes and FDA approved for weight loss and management. These medications decrease the production of glucagon, which in turn slows down the emptying of the stomach. It also works in the brain to reduce the amount of food consumed.
6. Orlistat, a pancreatic lipase inhibitor, blocks the breakdown of fat in the gastrointestinal (GI) system; about 30% of dietary fat is eliminated.
   a. Adverse effects include oily or fatty stool, flatulence, and GI distress.
   b. Long-term safety of the drug has not been determined, but addition of a fat-soluble vitamin supplement (vitamins A, D, E, and K and beta carotene) taken 1 hour before or 2 hours after orlistat will prevent a theoretical vitamin deficiency.
   c. Should not be used in cases of cholestasis or malabsorption.

d. Orlistat is available over the counter in a lower dosage than originally prescribed.
e. These medications are only adjunct to diet and exercise therapy.

7. Gelesis 100, also considered a medical device, is a capsule that is considered a medical device. The capsule contains super-absorbent hydrogel particles that expand in the stomach and increase fullness.
8. Setmelanotide is a melanocortin-4 receptor agonist that helps to decrease appetite.
9. Several other medications used to treat depression, seizures, and/or diabetes have been prescribed off-label to help promote weight loss. These medications have not been approved by the FDA for the treatment of obesity:
   a. Bupropion—an antidepressant medication.
   b. Topiramate—an anticonvulsant medication.
   c. Zonisamide—an anticonvulsant medication.
   d. Metformin—an oral medication used to treat diabetes.
10. Medications are only an adjunct to diet and exercise therapy.

Metabolic and Bariatric Surgery

Many surgical procedures have been used over the years to help treat obesity and metabolic disorders. For many years, the Roux-en-Y gastric bypass has been considered the gold standard. However, many new surgical treatment options have emerged, leading to a greater availability of treatment options (see Figure 16-3). These surgical therapies are generally reserved for patients with severe obesity (i.e., BMI > 35 with comorbid conditions or BMI > 40) who cannot lose weight and maintain weight loss through nonsurgical therapies. Metabolic and bariatric surgery has proven to be a safe and effective means for weight loss when performed by an experienced surgeon within a multidisciplinary center. In addition to the anatomic and mechanical changes created by the various procedures, there is increasing evidence of metabolic or hormonal changes that lead to weight loss. Metabolic/hormonal changes associated with these surgeries include a decrease in the hormone ghrelin, which produces a decrease in hunger and an increase in Peptide Tyrosine Tyrosine (PYY) and Glucagon-Like Peptide (GLP-1) creating an increase in satiety.

1. Roux-en-Y gastric bypass—a restrictive and malabsorptive procedure in which a small 1- to 2-ounce pouch/stomach (normal size = 30 to 50 ounces) is created by stapling and completely separating the smaller proximal stomach pouch from the larger distal stomach pouch. To this proximal pouch, a portion of the jejunum or Roux limb is attached, thus bypassing the distal stomach pouch and allowing the new pouch to empty food contents into the bowel. The biliopancreatic limb is then anastomosed to the Roux limb, thus creating a "Y" configuration and a method of elimination of digestive juices from the distal stomach and duodenum.
2. One-anastomosis gastric bypass (OAGB or mini gastric bypass)—combines restriction and malabsorption, but differs from the Roux-en-Y gastric bypass. The OAGB creates a long and narrow gastric pouch and connects a loop of bowel (jejunum) to the new gastric pouch with a single anastomosis.
3. Adjustable gastric banding—a silicone band or "belt" is placed at the gastroesophageal junction, creating a small upper segment of the stomach. An access port or reservoir, which is connected to the band by tubing, is placed midabdomen just under the skin, which allows for band adjustments to create a narrower passage into the larger remaining stomach. This in turn slows the emptying process from the upper segment into the lower segment of the stomach, thus causing satiety with a smaller amount of food. Hormonal changes with this surgery initially increase ghrelin production, which increases hunger.
4. Sleeve gastrectomy—a restrictive procedure in which a "sleeve" is created by stapling the stomach into a long tube from the esophagus to the duodenum. The remnant stomach is removed, whereas the pylorus remains intact and allows for normal emptying of stomach contents.
5. Biliopancreatic diversion with duodenal switch (BPD/DS)—a primarily malabsorptive procedure with some restrictive qualities. The BPD/DS is a complex surgical procedure in which a partial gastrectomy is performed along with the division and rerouting of the small intestine (i.e., duodenum—hence duodenal switch). This inhibits the absorption of calories and some nutrients, but allows for normal absorption of other key nutrients such as protein, calcium, iron, and vitamin B_{12}. In contrast to the gastric bypass, the BPD/DS maintains the pyloric valve, which prevents complications such as dumping syndrome, marginal ulcers, and/or stomal stenosis from occurring.
6. Single anastomosis duodenal–ileal bypass (SADI)—a modified version of the duodenal switch eliminating a second anastomosis by creating an end to side duodenal-ileal diversion. The SADI maintains the pyloric valve and may be a primary procedure or conversion.
7. Revisions and conversions—surgical procedures to either revise or convert (to another procedure) a primary metabolic and bariatric surgery typically for complications or weight recurrence.
8. Other—there are several investigational procedures for severe obesity on the horizon that may add viable options for weight loss in the future but are not endorsed as of yet.

Medical Devices

1. Intragastric balloons are available as single or double balloons that are inserted endoscopically into the stomach for no longer than 6 months. The balloon(s) mimic a sleeve gastrectomy by filling a portion of the stomach to reinforce proper portion control and a sensation of fullness. Both single (Orbera) and double (ReShape Dual Balloon) balloons are FDA approved but are not typically covered by insurance. Intragastric balloons are indicated for a maximum of 6 months duration. Prior history of metabolic and bariatric surgery may be a contraindication for these products.
2. Transpyloric bulb is an endoscopically inserted spherical bulb that delays emptying of the stomach. Indications for use include BMI 35.0 to 40.0 kg/m^2 or 30.0 to 34.9 kg/m^2 with an associated comorbidity. The device may be left in place for a duration of 1 year.
3. Endoscopic sleeve gastroplasty creates a smaller stomach with endoscopic suturing of the stomach, similar to a sleeve gastrectomy, but without the removal of the greater curvature of the stomach.
4. Transoral outlet reduction (TORe) involves endoscopic suturing to reduce the gastrojejunostomy of the gastric bypass for weight recurrence.

Complications

1. Obesity is a risk factor for many comorbid conditions including diabetes, gallbladder disease, osteoarthritis of weight-bearing joints, hypertension, coronary artery disease (CAD),

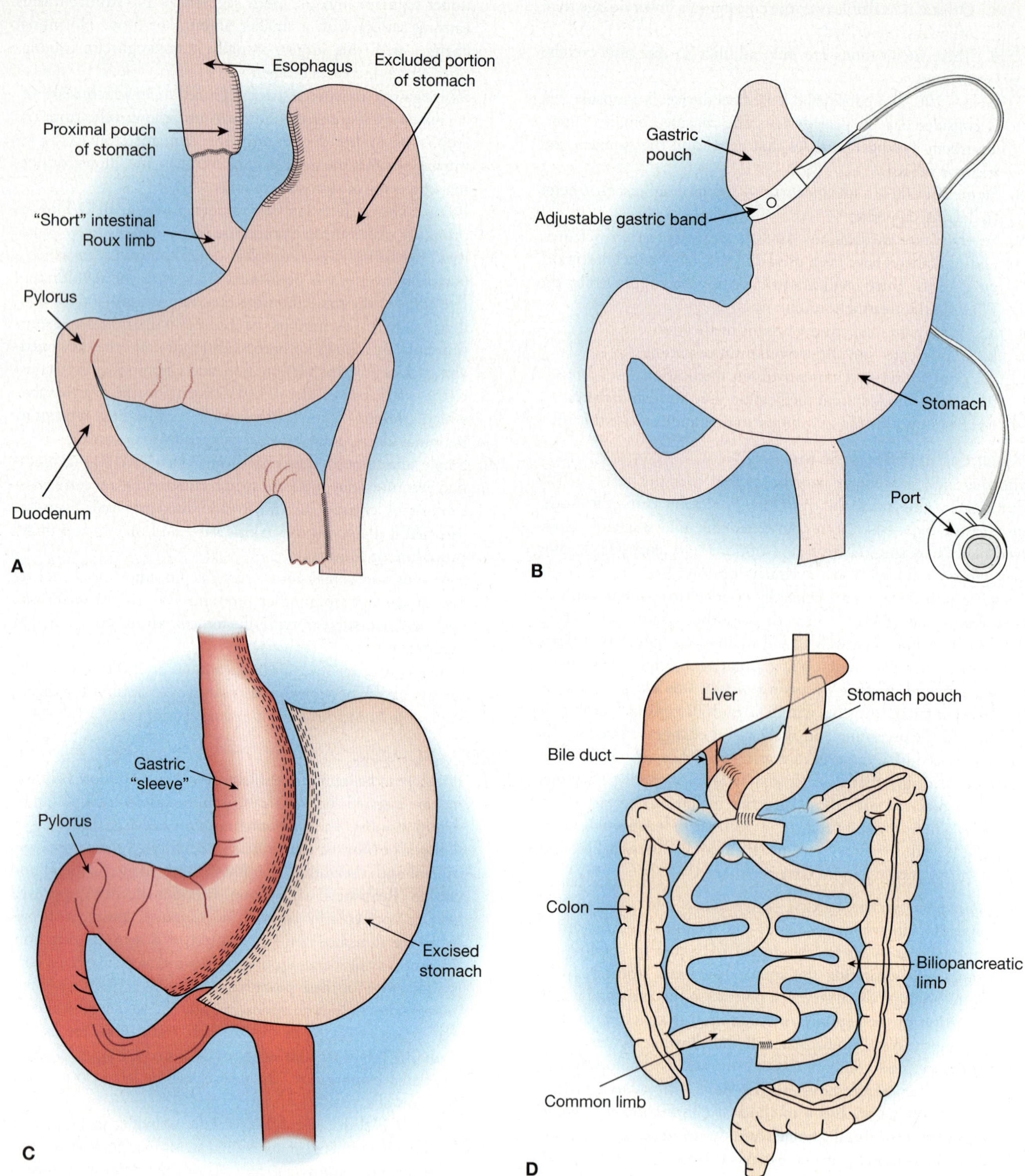

Figure 16-3. Selected bariatric procedures. **(A)** Adjustable gastric band. **(B)** Gastric bypass with Roux-en-Y anastomosis. **(C)** Sleeve gastrectomy. **(D)** Biliopancreatic diversion with duodenal switch.

obstructive sleep apnea, metabolic syndrome, dyslipidemia, COVID-19, as well as several other conditions.

2. Vitamin and mineral deficiencies because of surgical intervention, severely restricted diet, or nonadherence to recommended supplementation.
   a. A moderate, well-balanced weight reduction diet will generally not cause deficiencies, except with surgical intervention, although vitamin/mineral supplementation may be used and is strongly recommended post metabolic and bariatric surgery.
   b. A low-calorie diet (<800 to 1,000 calories per day) will require careful monitoring and vitamin/mineral supplementation.
   c. Complications of metabolic and bariatric surgery may include marginal ulcers, anastomotic or staple line leaks or bleeding, fistulas, infection, pulmonary emboli, chronic nausea and vomiting, vitamin D and B_{12} deficiency, thiamine, copper, and iron deficiency as well as other nutritional deficiencies. Daily vitamin and mineral supplementation is necessary.

Nursing Assessment

1. Assess vital signs including height, weight, BMI, blood pressure, heart and respiratory rate and tempa.
2. Obtain a complete nutritional assessment (may be in collaboration with a registered dietitian).
3. Assess behavioral and emotional components of eating, coping mechanisms, and past successes and failures with dieting.

Nursing Interventions

Modifying Nutritional Intake

1. Assist the patient in assessing current dietary habits and identifying poor dietary habits.
2. Assist the patient in developing an appropriate diet plan based on likes and dislikes, activity level, and lifestyle.
3. Suggest behavior modification strategies, such as exercise (i.e., walking) during lunch break, preventing access to quick snacks, and eating only at mealtimes at the table.
4. Provide emotional support to the patient during weight reduction efforts through positive reinforcement and creative problem-solving.
5. Provide the patient with alternative coping mechanisms, including stress reduction techniques such as progressive relaxation and guided imagery.
6. Assess the patient's ability to tolerate exercise through measurement of vital signs before, during, and after exercise and ask about symptoms of shortness of breath and chest pain.
7. Discourage fad dieting.

Preventing Complications Postoperatively

1. Provide initial postoperative care as for GI surgery (see page 475).
2. Administer IV fluids, as directed. Record intake and output.
3. Start oral fluids per surgeon's protocol (this will vary from facility to facility and surgeon to surgeon). General progression for most patients will be to start with small sips and gradually advance to larger sips of clear liquids.
4. Advance diet as per surgeon's protocol. Confirmation of the bariatric diet stages with the facility's bariatric program and/or surgeon is crucial, as this will vary from facility to facility and surgeon to surgeon.
5. Observe for and report increased abdominal pain, distention, or alteration in abdominal drain output (if utilized), which may indicate leakage or bleeding at anastomosis or staple sites or obstruction.
6. Monitor vital signs, breath sounds, and wounds for signs of infection, pneumonia, or other potential complications.
7. Watch for and report signs of dehydration (thirst, oliguria, dry mucous membranes) and hypokalemia (muscle weakness, anorexia, nausea, decreased bowel sounds, and dysrhythmias).
8. Educate the patient on the importance of physical activity to prevent venothrombosis.
9. Warn the patient that overeating may cause vomiting or painful esophageal distention. Dumping syndrome may occur especially in the postoperative Roux-en-Y gastric bypass patient with food products that are high in fat or high in sugar.
10. Stress the importance of good dietary habits and behavior modification to lose weight because metabolic and bariatric surgery is only an adjunct to treatment.
11. Encourage close, long-term follow-up for monitoring of weight loss and nutritional status. Additional long-term complications may include marginal ulcers, hernias, strictures, bowel obstruction, gallstones, and/or malnutrition.
12. Following metabolic and bariatric surgery, educate the patient on the importance of strict adherence to diet protocol and to avoid premature advancement to another stage without discussing with the surgeon, dietitian, or other staff member. Encourage the patient to meet fluid (48 to 64 oz fluid/day) and protein (individualized) goals. Advise the patient to notify the surgeon for fever (>101°F); tachycardia (heart rate >100); severe abdominal pain; nausea or vomiting; difficulty breathing or ability to catch breath; or any redness, drainage, or swelling from incisions. Prevention and prompt attention to signs of complications can prevent readmission and adverse outcomes.

Strengthening Self-Concept

1. Direct patient education and conversation in a nonjudgmental manner.
2. Get to know the patient and point out the positive aspects of patient's health and well-being.
3. Encourage the patient to make a change in weight for the positive health aspects, not just for cosmetic reasons.
4. Make referral to behavioral health professional and support groups as needed.
5. Be a good role model—show a healthy attitude toward sensible eating, exercise, and other healthy practices.
6. Be sensitive to discrimination, behaviors, and attitudes toward people with obesity.

Patient Education and Health Maintenance

1. Discuss fat, carbohydrate, and protein, their inclusion in common foods, and their calories per gram.
2. Describe the five basic food groups and their placement in the MyPlate Plan.
3. Explain the purpose of a balanced diet and the need for vitamins and minerals from food sources; supplement needed following bariatric surgery.
4. Review the health hazards of obesity.
5. Advise the patient of the plateau period that may occur without weight loss for some time, but advise the patient not to get discouraged.
6. Tell the patient to keep a food diary to show to nutritionist and to weigh self no more than once per week.
7. If the patient is interested in liquid diets or herbal supplements to lose weight, encourage discussion with the health care provider. Some preparations may contain ephedra, a powerful

stimulant that may cause increased BP, significant adverse effects, and many drug interactions.

8. Refer to such organizations as Obesity Action Coalition (*www.obesityaction.org*) and the National Institutes of Diabetes and Digestive and Kidney Disease: Weight-control Information Network (https://www.niddk.nih.gov/health-information/weight-management) for further information on weight loss options.

Evaluation: Expected Outcomes

- Loses 10% to 15% excess body weight during the first month.
- No abdominal distention, nausea or vomiting, or wound infection.
- Verbalizes feeling good about self, secondary to change in diet and exercise habits.

Eating Disorders

Disordered eating can run the full gamut from starvation as noted in anorexia nervosa, to overeating behaviors such as binge-eating disorder—or may include a combination of both as seen in bulimia nervosa. Eating disorders can affect all people but are generally more prevalent among females than among males. Lifetime prevalence is estimated at 0.3% for anorexia, 0.9% for bulimia, and 1.6% for binge-eating disorder. The disordered eating may develop during childhood or later in life, but is more common during teens or young adulthood, and may be chronic or intermittent during many years. There are multiple causes that may be attributable to the eating disorder including genetic, biologic, hormonal, environmental, behavioral, psychological, and social etiologies. See Table 16-4 on pages 558 to 559 for a comparison of the three most common eating disorders.

Although this section focuses on anorexia nervosa, bulimia nervosa, binge-eating disorder, and avoidant restrictive food intake disorder, there are other disordered or maladaptive eating behaviors, including pica, orthorexia, and Prader-Willi syndrome. Pica is a disorder of eating objects with no nutritional value, such as dirt, paper, or ice. Orthorexia is the unhealthy obsession with consuming healthy foods. Prader-Willi syndrome is a genetic disorder that produces hormonal symptoms such as constant hunger, leading to obesity. Another category of eating disorders on the rise is other specified feeding or eating disorder (OSFED) or other specified feeding or eating disorders and includes subtypes such as atypical anorexia nervosa, purging disorder, and night eating syndrome.

Diagnostic Evaluation

1. Serum chemistry for electrolytes, blood urea nitrogen (BUN), and creatinine and bicarbonate—may be abnormal, indicating fluid and electrolyte imbalances.
2. Hormonal tests may include thyroid function tests, luteinizing hormone (LH), follicle-stimulating hormone (FSH), estrogen, and testosterone.
3. Serum glucose and lipid testing to determine the body's response to dietary intake.
4. Electrocardiogram to determine arrhythmias caused by electrolyte imbalance.

Table 16-4 Comparison of Eating Disorders

DISORDER/DESCRIPTION	PATHOPHYSIOLOGY/ETIOLOGY	CLINICAL MANIFESTATIONS
Anorexia nervosa: characterized by self-induced weight loss >15% of normal weight for age and height and is associated with high morbidity and mortality. There are two subtypes of anorexia nervosa: • Restrictive subtype characterized by periods of starvation. • Binge-purge subtype in which periods of starvation are mixed with episodes of binging and purging and may include the use of laxatives and diuretics.	• Semistarvation state with glucose and protein sparing, fat utilization, endocrine changes, and fluid and electrolyte disturbances. Results in: • Loss of fat stores. • Decreased protein synthesis. • Decrease in thyroid hormone. • Hypothalamic or pituitary dysfunction—decrease in FSH, LH, and estrogen.	• Extremely restricted eating. • Extreme thinness (emaciation). • Relentless pursuit of thinness and unwillingness to maintain a normal or health weight. • Intense fear of gaining weight. • Distorted body image, a self-esteem that is heavily influenced by perceptions of body weight and shape, or a denial of the seriousness of low body weight. • Amenorrhea, bradycardia, hypotension, cold intolerance. • Multisystem organ failure.
Bulimia nervosa: characterized by recurrent episodes of binge eating and feeling of loss of control over eating behavior during these episodes. The binging episodes lead to self-disgust and are typically followed by inappropriate methods to prevent weight gain, including self-induced vomiting, excessive use of laxatives, diuretics, fasting, or excessive exercise.	• Onset of illness typically occurs in late adolescence or early 20s. • Ten times more common in young females than in young males. • May be associated with a personal or family history of obesity, substance use, depression, anxiety, or mood disorders. • Self-induced vomiting. • Starvation may be as evident as in anorexia nervosa. • Eating binges may occur as often as several times per day and be present for many months.	• Physical signs may include calluses or skin changes on hand and fingers, loss of dental enamel, swollen lymph nodes, and bad breath or mouthwash smell on breath because of self-induced vomiting. • Endocrine changes, such as amenorrhea, may be present. • Electrolyte imbalances. • Acid reflux. • Severe dehydration.

Table 16-4 Comparison of Eating Disorders (*continued*)

DISORDER/DESCRIPTION	PATHOPHYSIOLOGY/ETIOLOGY	CLINICAL MANIFESTATIONS
BED: disordered eating that results in a loss-of-control eating episode(s). BED is not associated with inappropriate compensatory behaviors; however, it is often associated with some type of psychopathology.	• Presence of comorbid psychopathology: specific phobia, social phobia, unipolar major depression, posttraumatic stress disorder, alcohol misuse, or dependence. • Increased risk for developing chronic pain, diabetes mellitus, and hypertension. • More likely to have obesity. • Binge episodes at least once a week for 3 mo.	• Eating unusually large amounts of food in a specific amount of time. • Eating even when full or not hungry. • Eating fast during binge episodes. • Eating until uncomfortably full. • Eating alone or in secret to avoid embarrassment. • Feeling distressed, ashamed, or guilty about eating. • Frequently dieting, possibly without weight loss.
Avoidant restrictive food intake disorder.	• Most commonly seen in middle childhood. • Eating is limited by the amount or type of food eaten. • Child-caloric limitation is insufficient to support growth and development. • Adult-caloric intake is insufficient to maintain basic body functions.	• Restriction of types or amounts of food eaten. • Lack of appetite. • Dramatic weight loss. • Upset stomach or abdominal pain.

BED, binge-eating disorder; FSH, follicle-stimulating hormone; LH, luteinizing hormone.

Management

Although pathophysiology, etiology, and symptoms may differ somewhat between each eating disorder, the assessment, diagnosis, and treatment and therapies are very similar. Paramount to the entire process, however, is the multidisciplinary clinical approach that should include nurses, nutritionists, behavioral health providers, advanced practice providers, primary providers, and other health care providers who specialize in treating patients with eating disorders.

1. Dietary modification and nutritional counseling to achieve gradual weight gain and/or normal eating habits.
   a. Balanced diet with incremental inclusion of foods previously perceived as restricted by the patient.
   b. Increased activity, exercise gradually.
2. Enteral or parenteral feeding as needed if the prescribed diet cannot be maintained by the patient and physical status warrants. Enteral feeding is preferred and is used more frequently.
3. Individual counseling focuses on the patient's need to control weight, alteration in body image, and associated diagnoses, including depression and suicidal ideation.
4. Psychological counseling and support, such as talk therapy or behavioral therapy.
   a. Assist the patient to develop insight into behavior and a more realistic body image.
   b. Assist the patient to develop effective coping strategies and problem-solving mechanisms.
5. Antidepressants, antianxiety, and other pharmacologic agents for associated psychiatric problems may be tried.
   a. Selective serotonin uptake inhibitor (SSRI) such as fluoxetine to treat bulimia nervosa.
   b. Stimulant such as lisdexamfetamine (Vyvanse) to treat binge-eating disorder.
6. Inpatient treatment (preferably on a specialized eating disorder unit) is recommended if weight is less than 75% ideal; marked orthostatic hypotension; bradycardia less than 40; sustained tachycardia greater than 100; inability to maintain a core body temperature of 98.6°F (37°C); suicidal or no response to outpatient therapy.

Complications

1. Fluid and electrolyte imbalance.
   a. Hypokalemia, hyponatremia, hypochloremia.
   b. Hyperkalemia.
   c. Metabolic alkalosis.
   d. Dehydration.
2. Cardiac disturbances.
   a. Dysrhythmias, bradycardia, tachycardia.
   b. Hypotension.
   c. Cardiac arrest.
3. Nutritional imbalance.
   a. Obesity.
   b. Cachexia.
4. Seizures due to hyponatremia.
5. Increased risk of infection related to a decrease in white blood cells.
6. Endocrine dysfunction.
   a. Amenorrhea, decreased estrogen in females.
   b. Decreased testosterone in males, decreased libido.
   c. Decreased thyroid hormone.
7. Esophageal tear or gastric rupture.
8. Dental erosion.
9. Comorbid psychiatric conditions.
   a. Depression.
   b. Anxiety disorders.
   c. High risk for suicide.

Nursing Assessment

1. Perform a complete nutritional assessment. Obtain a detailed dietary history and complete review of systems, including psychological, gynecologic, endocrine, GI systems, activities of daily living, and exercise history.

2. Perform physical examination, including vital signs, height and weight, heart rate and rhythm, bowel sounds, and observation for hematemesis and dental caries (which may indicate self-induced vomiting).
3. Evaluate fluid and electrolyte status and manifestations of associated problems.
4. Assess for signs and symptoms of depression, anxiety, personality disorder, associated eating behaviors, and history of family dysfunction.

Nursing Interventions

Attaining Appropriate Weight

1. Assist the patient to select well-balanced diet and maintain appropriate eating habits.
2. Encourage small, frequent meals or snacks of high-calorie foods and beverages. Liquid nutritional supplements may be best tolerated.
3. Monitor and assess daily intake and output, weight (before breakfast), urine for ketones, and serum electrolytes to determine physical response to nutritional interventions.
4. Provide positive reinforcement for appropriate eating behaviors.
5. Provide positive reinforcement for improved intake and weight gain or stabilization of weight.
6. Assess bowel function. Promote fluids and activity to prevent constipation if the patient cannot tolerate food high in fiber.
7. Teach the patient the risks associated with abnormal eating behavior and the benefits of maintaining healthful nutritional and exercise habits.

Fostering a Healthy Body Image

1. Establish a trusting relationship and provide for patient's safety and security needs.
2. Encourage the patient to verbalize feelings about body image, self-concept, fears, and frustrations.
3. Emphasize the importance of counseling, stress management, assertiveness training, and other therapies over the long term to strengthen body image and acceptance.

Improving Coping

1. Encourage the patient to set realistic goals for weight and appearance. Involve the patient in the treatment plan, offering choices to increase sense of control.
2. Assist the patient to identify and implement alternative coping strategies in times of stress, including expression and exploration of feelings, problem-solving, appropriate use of exercise, and relaxation techniques.
3. Set limits so that the patient will feel in control of self. Be alert for lying and manipulation that the patient may display to preserve control.
4. Include family in counseling and teaching sessions, as appropriate.

Preventing Suicide

1. Assess the level of risk by obtaining the history of past suicide attempts, recent suicidal thoughts, and current ideation, plan, and possible method.
2. Maintain the level of observance called for by situation.
3. Make sure that access to sharp objects is prohibited.
4. Make sure that a crisis intervention team is on call, if needed.

Patient Education and Health Maintenance

1. Teach principles of nutrition and healthful diet and eating habits. Discuss food matter-of-factly to avoid reinforcing patient's preoccupation with food.
2. Teach the effect of starvation on both physiologic and psychological functioning.
3. Involve patient's family and significant others in the treatment plan, as appropriate.
4. Describe the dangers of using laxatives and diuretics in weight control, such as electrolyte imbalances, dehydration, and bowel atony.
5. Stress the importance of maintaining follow-up visits and counseling.
6. Refer to such agencies as the American Anorexia-Bulimia Association (*www.aaba.org*), Eating Disorder Information Center (*www.nedic.ca*), National Association of Anorexia Nervosa and Associated Disorders (*www.anad.org*), and National Eating Disorder Association (*www.nationaleatingdisorders.org*).

Evaluation: Expected Outcomes

- Well-balanced dietary intake without evidence of vomiting. Gain of 1 pound (0.5 kg) during first week (anorexia nervosa).
- Verbalizes satisfaction with body image and weight.
- Verbalizes appropriate problem-solving approach.
- Denies suicidal ideation and thoughts.

Malabsorption Syndrome

Malabsorption syndrome is a group of symptoms and physical signs that occur because of poor nutrient absorption in the small intestine, particularly fat absorption, with a resultant decrease in absorption of fat-soluble vitamins A, D, E, and K. Poor absorption of other nutrients, including carbohydrates, minerals, and other vitamins and proteins, may also occur. *Celiac sprue* and *lactose intolerance* are common types of malabsorption syndromes.

Pathophysiology and Etiology

Malabsorption has multiple etiologies, including gallbladder, liver, or pancreatic disease, lymphatic obstruction, vascular impairment, and bowel resection. Two common causes:

1. Celiac sprue—malabsorption of nutrients resulting from atrophy of villi and microvilli of the small intestine because of an intolerance to gluten found in common grains, such as wheat, rye, oats, and barley (see Chapter 48).
2. Lactose intolerance—typically of genetic origin, this digestive enzyme deficiency prevents the digestion of lactose found in milk, causing osmosis of water into the lumen of the intestine.

Clinical Manifestations

1. Steatorrhea.
2. Abdominal distention and pain.
3. Flatulence.
4. Anorexia, weight loss, edema.
5. Vitamin deficiency—fat soluble (A, D, E, K).
6. Protein deficiency and negative nitrogen balance.
7. Anemia, weakness, and fatigue due to poor absorption of iron, folic acid, and vitamin B_{12}.

Diagnostic Evaluation

1. Fecal fat analysis—72-hour stool collection; fecal fat may be increased.
2. M2A Imaging System—a device that provides images via a receiver and recorder tracing the transit of a capsule that is swallowed by the patient. Used to evaluate and diagnose malabsorption syndromes as well as other GI diseases.

3. Lower GI series (barium enema)—may be used to evaluate the colon.
4. Serum measurement of vitamin levels, total protein, and albumin may be decreased.
5. Prothrombin time may be prolonged because of vitamin K deficiency.

Management

1. Treatment of the underlying cause, if possible, by eliminating causative agents, such as grains or milk.
2. Promotion of adequate nutritional intake through a carefully designed diet that substitutes alternatives to the offending agent and that ensures replacement of deficient nutrients through oral, enteral, or parenteral therapy.
3. Medications such as pancreatic enzymes.

Complications

1. Dehydration.
2. Electrolyte imbalance with possible cardiac dysrhythmias.
3. Protein deficiency with muscle atrophy and edema.
4. Vitamin deficiency with tetany, bleeding, anemia, and osteoporosis.
5. Skin breakdown.

Nursing Assessment

1. Assess fluid and electrolyte status through careful monitoring of intake and output, daily weight, serum electrolytes, vital signs, and other signs and symptoms of dehydration and electrolyte imbalance.
2. Assess GI function through observation of frequency and characteristics of stool, bowel sounds, distention, pain, and other associated symptoms.
3. Assess nutritional status.

Nursing Interventions

Improving Nutritional Status

1. Ensure that the diet is free from causative agents, such as dairy or wheat products.
2. Provide diet high in missing nutrients, including proteins, carbohydrates, fats, vitamins, and minerals.
3. Teach the patient to use substitute products for causative agents, such as gluten-free flour, corn, soybean, and lactose-free milk substitutes.
4. Monitor weight and characteristics of stool closely.

Restoring Fluid Balance

1. Monitor intake and output and urine-specific gravity.
   a. Include watery stool in output.
   b. Be aware that edema is caused by low serum proteins, not fluid overload.
2. Monitor vital signs frequently, based on condition.
3. Be alert for dehydration—orthostatic hypotension, tachycardia, decreased skin turgor, dry mucous membranes, thirst, oliguria.
4. Observe for signs and symptoms of potential electrolyte disturbances—nausea, vomiting, dysrhythmias, tremors, seizures, anorexia, weakness—and report abnormal results of serum electrolytes.
5. Administer IV fluids or parenteral or enteral nutrition, as ordered.

Relieving Pain

1. Assess timing, frequency, and character of pain and its relationship to food.
2. Encourage Fowler position and frequent change in position for comfort.
3. Administer analgesics, antidiarrheals, and antiflatulents, as ordered.

Maintaining Tissue Integrity

1. Provide meticulous perineal care after each stool with application of hydrophobic ointments, if necessary, to prevent skin breakdown.
2. Give careful attention to general skin condition, assessing for redness, breakdown, and poor turgor, and maintain general skin integrity through cleanliness, lubrication, padding of bony prominences, frequent turning, and adequate hydration and nutrition.

Patient Education and Health Maintenance

1. Provide nutritional counseling for the patient and family, particularly if symptoms are secondary to food intolerance; stress which foods to avoid and the importance of carefully reading all food labels, recommend appropriate food substitutions, and necessary nutritional supplements.
2. Advice regarding signs and symptoms that indicate worsening of disease—increased frequency of stool, diarrhea or steatorrhea, increased pain.
3. Suggest such support groups as the Celiac Sprue Association (*https://www.csaceliacs.org*) and the Crohn's and Colitis Foundation of America (*www.ccfa.org*).

Evaluation: Expected Outcomes

- Maintains weight and energy level.
- Vital signs stable; urinary output adequate.
- Verbalizes decreased pain after meals.
- No skin breakdown noted.

Vitamin and Mineral Deficiencies

Vitamins are organic compounds found in food needed for growth, reproduction, good health, and resistance to infection. Minerals are inorganic compounds found in nature and serve a variety of physiologic functions. Specific requirements depend on age, activity, metabolic rate (increased fever), and special processes, such as pregnancy, lactation, and disease processes.

See Table 16-5 on pages 562 to 566 for vitamin and mineral needs for healthy adults age 19 or older. Needs are different for children and pregnant or lactating people.

Dietary reference intake tables have been developed by the Food and Nutrition Board at the Institute of Medicine of the National Academies and include the following:

Recommended dietary allowance—the average daily dietary intake level sufficient to meet the nutrient requirements of nearly all (97% to 98%) healthy people in a group.

Adequate intake—amount believed to cover the needs of all healthy people in the groups, but lack of data or uncertainty in the data prevents being able to specify with confidence the percentage of people covered by this intake.

Estimated average requirement—average daily nutrient intake level estimated to meet the requirements of half of the healthy people in a group.

Table 16-5 Vitamin and Mineral Requirements and Imbalances

VITAMIN, RDA, AND EAR	FUNCTION	CLINICAL MANIFESTATIONS OF IMBALANCE	DIAGNOSTIC EVALUATION	MANAGEMENT
Vitamin A (Retinol) RDA: 700–900 mcg EAR: 500–625 mcg fat soluble	• Tissue maintenance via antioxidant ability • Helps regulate the immune system • Skeletal and soft tissue growth and development • Visual adaptation to light and dark • Supports reproductive function	*Deficiency:* Night blindness, xerophthalmia, keratinization, generalized mucosa dryness/damage, vomiting, diarrhea, weight loss, urinary and vaginal infections, tooth decay, follicular hyperkeratosis, fatigue *Toxicity:* Hair loss, joint pain, dry skin, mouth soreness, anorexia, vomiting, liver damage	*Deficiency:* • History and physical findings are helpful in the diagnosis of most vitamin imbalances. • Serum level <35 mg/dL suggests vitamin deficiency.	*Deficiency:* • Replacement therapy of 30,000 international units to treat night blindness. • Good dietary sources of vitamin A are green and yellow fruits and vegetables and liver. • In patients with malabsorption of fat-soluble vitamins and patients with low dietary intake of vitamin A, IV supplements are required.
Vitamin B_1 (Thiamine) RDA: 1.1–1.2 mg EAR: 0.9–1.0 mg water soluble	• Carbohydrate metabolism • Necessary for neurologic, gastric, cardiac, and musculoskeletal function	*Deficiency:* Appetite loss, constipation, dyspnea, fatigue, irritability, nervousness, memory loss, paresthesias, muscle pain, beriberi, blurred or double vision, difficulty swallowing, nausea, vomiting *Toxicity:* Large doses may be given generally without difficulty, although anaphylaxis has been reported	*Deficiency:* • Erythrocyte transketolase activity <15%–20%.	*Deficiency:* • Treat underlying cause. • High-protein diet with supplemental B complex vitamins. • Food sources rich in thiamine are brewer's yeast, meat, wheat germ, enriched grains and beans. • Parenteral therapy with 50–100 mg/day followed by 5–10 mg/day PO.
Vitamin B_2 (Riboflavin) RDA: 1.1–1.3 mg EAR: 0.9–1.1 mg water soluble	• Carbohydrate metabolism • Promotes growth, red blood cell formation, and healthy eyes and skin	*Deficiency:* Sore throat, cheilosis, dermatitis, burning and itching of eyes, tearing and vascularization of corneas; late-stage symptoms include neuropathy and growth retardation *Toxicity:* None known	*Deficiency:* • Erythrocyte glutathione activity >1.2–1.3. • Decreased urinary riboflavin levels.	*Deficiency:* • Good dietary sources of B_2 are dairy products, vegetables, enriched grains, eggs, nuts, liver. • Oral supplements of 5–15 mg/day.
Vitamin B_6 (Pyridoxine) RDA: 1.3–1.7 mg EAR: 1.1–1.4 mg water soluble	• Required for protein metabolism • Maintains neurologic function and RBC production	*Deficiency:* Anemia, weakness, glossitis, cheilosis, irritability, seizures *Toxicity:* Neuromuscular damage, peripheral neuropathy	*Deficiency:* • Pyridoxal phosphate levels <50 ng/mL.	*Deficiency:* • Oral supplementation: 10–20 mg. • Good dietary sources of B_6 are bananas, brewer's yeast, fish, meat, whole grains, liver. • People taking oral contraceptives or isoniazid may need to supplement their diets with pyridoxine. • Pregnancy also increases the need.
Vitamin B_{12} (Cobalamin) RDA: 2.4 mcg EAR: 2.0 mcg water soluble	• Maintains neurologic function and RBC development via hemoglobin synthesis	*Deficiency:* Megaloblastic anemia, memory impairment, confusion, depression, fatigue, nervousness, decreased reflex response, balance impairment, speech difficulties, demyelination of the large fibers of the spinal cord, anorexia, vomiting, weight loss, yellowing of skin, abdominal pain, dyspnea, diarrhea, glossitis, burning of lips or mouth, palpitations, tachycardia, sore tongue, weakness *Toxicity:* None	*Deficiency:* • Serum levels of <100 pg/mL. • Decreased hematocrit with elevation of MCV. • Schilling test also measures the absorption of radioactive B_{12}.	*Deficiency:* • B_{12} 200 mcg/day IM for 1 wk, then every month for life if deficiency is due to pernicious anemia. • Oral vitamin B_{12} may be necessary for strict vegetarians. • Good dietary sources of B_{12} are eggs, fish, organ meats, lean meat, dairy products.

Biotin RDA: 30 mcg EAR: Not established water soluble	• Metabolism of proteins, fats, and carbohydrates	*Deficiency:* Dry skin, fatigue, grayish skin discoloration, muscle pain, depression, insomnia, anorexia *Toxicity:* None	—	*Deficiency:* • Good sources of biotin are egg yolks, vegetables, yeast, milk, grains.
Folate (Folic Acid) RDA: 400 mcg EAR: 320 mcg water soluble	• RBC formation • DNA and RNA synthesis and support of cell growth and reproduction • Prevention of birth defects	*Deficiency:* Glossitis, diarrhea, megaloblastic anemia, digestive problems, fatigue, palpitations, restless leg syndrome *Toxicity:* Inactivation of anticonvulsants, masking of vitamin B_{12} deficiency	*Deficiency:* • Serum level <3 ng/mL.	*Deficiency:* • Nutritional supplementation: 1 mg/day PO. • Avoid alcohol. • Good sources of folate are citrus fruits, eggs, milk, green leafy vegetables, dairy products, organ meats, seafood, whole grains, yeast.
Niacin RDA: 14–16 mg EAR: 11–12 mg water soluble	• Metabolism of carbohydrates, fats, and proteins • Works with thiamine and riboflavin for the production of cellular energy • Promotes skin, neurologic, and GI function	*Deficiency:* Apathy, fatigue, appetite loss, headaches, indigestion, muscle weakness, nausea, insomnia, dermatitis, diarrhea, confusion, disorientation, memory impairment, glossitis, stomatitis, pellagra *Toxicity:* Liver damage, flushing	*Deficiency:* • Serum levels <30 mcg/100 mL. • Diminished or absent metabolites in urine.	*Deficiency:* • Good sources of niacin are eggs, lean meats, organ meats, poultry, seafood, fish, dairy products, nuts, whole and enriched grains, brewer's yeast. • Nutritional supplementation: 10–150 mg. • Supplemental niacin may also be necessary when taking oral contraceptives.
Pantothenic Acid RDA: 5 mg EAR: Not established water soluble	• Vital for overall metabolism • Aids in formation of carbohydrates, proteins, and fats • Aids in cortisone production, ATP production, stress tolerance, vitamin utilization, hemoglobin synthesis	*Deficiency:* Diarrhea, hair loss, respiratory infections, nervousness, muscle cramps, premature aging, intestinal disorders, eczema, kidney disorders *Toxicity:* None	—	*Deficiency:* • This vitamin is widely available in foods, especially organ meats, legumes, vegetables, fruits.
Vitamin C RDA: 75–90 mg EAR: 60–75 mg water soluble	• Antioxidant action decreases cellular dysfunction • Promotes wound healing • Aids in connective tissue, bone, tooth, and cartilage formation • Promotes capillary integrity • Promotes nonheme iron absorption	*Deficiency:* Bleeding gums, tooth decay, nosebleeds, low infection resistance, bruising, anemia, delayed wound healing, anorexia, joint pain, lethargy, perifollicular hemorrhage *Toxicity:* GI distress	*Deficiency:* • Serum levels <0.2 mg/100 dL.	*Deficiency:* • Nutritional supplementation: 100–1,000 mg/day of vitamin C. • Good sources of vitamin C are citrus fruits, green leafy vegetables, broccoli, tomatoes, peppers, potatoes, strawberries. • Avoid smoking.
Vitamin D RDA: 15 mcg EAR: 10 mcg fat soluble	• Regulates calcium and phosphate absorption and metabolism and bone formation	*Deficiency:* Rickets, osteomalacia, weakness, spasm/twitching of eyes, burning in mouth, sweating	*Deficiency:* • Low levels of vitamin D (serum 25 [OH] D).	*Deficiency:* • Nutritional supplementation: ergocalciferol, 25 mcg/day PO.

(continued)

Table 16-5 Vitamin and Mineral Requirements and Imbalances (*continued*)

VITAMIN, RDA, AND EAR	FUNCTION	CLINICAL MANIFESTATIONS OF IMBALANCE	DIAGNOSTIC EVALUATION	MANAGEMENT
	• Aids in renal phosphate clearance, myocardial function, nervous system maintenance, and normal blood clotting	*Toxicity:* Hypercalcemia, bone pain, nausea, vomiting, itching, thirst, agitation, weakness. Calcifications in soft tissue can be fatal	• Radiographic bone deformities. • Abnormal bone densitometry.	• Good sources of vitamin D are egg yolks, yeast, enriched milk, fish liver oils. • Exposure to sunlight.
Vitamin E (Tocopherol) RDA: 15 mg EAR: 12 mg fat soluble	• Antioxidant action decreases cellular dysfunction • Aids in RBC formation	*Deficiency:* Neuromuscular disturbances, including decreased reflexes, vibratory and position sense, ataxia, night blindness, fatigue, leg weakness or cramps, dry skin *Toxicity:* Interference with vitamin K	*Deficiency:* • Serum levels <0.5 mg/dL.	*Deficiency:* • Nutritional supplementation: 100–400 international units/day PO. • Parenteral therapy may be necessary to treat neurologic symptoms. • Good sources of vitamin E are vegetable oils, milk, eggs, meat, fish, green leafy vegetables.
Vitamin K RDA: 90–120 mcg EAR: Not established fat soluble	• Promotes coagulation through the formation of prothrombin and other clotting factors	*Deficiency:* Abnormal bleeding times, hemorrhage, epistaxis, hematemesis, and bleeding at any orifice or puncture site are possible *Toxicity:* No tolerable upper limit has been established	*Deficiency:* • Prothrombin time extended longer than PTT.	*Deficiency:* • Administration of vitamin K 15 mg subcutaneously. • Good sources of vitamin K are green leafy vegetables, liver, wheat germ, cheeses, egg yolks, soybean oil.
Minerals				
Calcium AI: 1,000–1,200 mg EAR: 800–1,000 mg	• Aids in bone and tooth formation, muscle contraction, blood coagulation, nerve impulse transmission, cardiac function, cell membrane permeability, enzyme activation	*Deficiency:* Tooth decay, muscle cramps, tetany, nervousness and delusion, cardiac palpitations, heart failure, and paresthesias *Toxicity:* Constipation, loss of appetite, nausea, vomiting, dry mouth, renal calculi	*Deficiency:* • Dual-energy x-ray absorptiometry (DEXA) for bone mineral density. *Toxicity:* • Serum level >10.5 mg/dL.	*Deficiency:* • Oral supplements of 1–2 g/day of elemental calcium. • In severe hypocalcemia, 10 mL of 10% calcium gluconate IV administered no faster than 2 mL/min. • Good sources of calcium are milk products, green leafy vegetables, legumes, tofu processed with calcium. *Toxicity:* • Force fluids, diuretics, and limit dietary intake; administration of phosphate salts and glucocorticoids may also be necessary.
Chloride AI: 2,000–2,300 mg	• Helps keep the body's acid–base balance • Helps with metabolism	*Deficiency:* Extremely rare but can cause loss of appetite, weakness, and lethargy *Toxicity:* May result in fluid retention	*Deficiency:* • Serum levels <98. *Toxicity:* • Serum levels >108.	• No specific treatment.
Chromium AI: 20–35 mcg EAR: Not established	• Maintains serum glucose levels • Maintains fat metabolism	*Deficiency:* Glucose intolerance, vertigo, abdominal pain, shock, convulsions, anuria, dermatitis *Toxicity:* Unknown	*Deficiency:* • Serum levels <0.3 mg/mL.	*Deficiency:* • Nutritional supplementation: 50–200 mg/day. • Good sources of chromium are brewer's yeast, whole grains, cereals.

Copper RDA: 900 mcg EAR: 700 mcg	• Hemoglobin synthesis • Maintenance of hemostasis • Energy production	*Deficiency:* Hypochromic anemia, bone disease, weakness, skin lesions, altered respiratory status *Toxicity:* Nausea, vomiting, diarrhea, abdominal pain, malaise	*Deficiency:* • In addition to diminished serum levels, 24-h urine samples showing levels of urinary excretion of copper below 15–60 mcg/24 h.	*Deficiency:* • Nutritional supplementation: 0.1 mg/kg/day PO. • IV supplementation: 1–2 mg/day. • Good sources of copper are nuts, seeds, organ meats, seafood.
Iodine RDA: 150 mcg EAR: 95 mcg	• Thyroid hormone synthesis	*Deficiency:* Hypothyroidism or goiter, nervousness, irritability, obesity, cold hands and feet, chills, brittle hair, fatigue, bradycardia, decreased cardiac output, thick tongue, hoarseness, poor memory, hearing loss, anorexia *Toxicity:* Goiter	*Deficiency:* • Low T_3 and T_4 levels. • Thyroid scan.	*Deficiency:* • Nutritional supplementation: 50–100 mg daily PO. • Good sources of iodine are iodized salt, seafood.
Iron RDA: 8–18 mg EAR: 5–8.1 mg	• Hemoglobin synthesis • Cellular oxidation • Transportation of oxygen	*Deficiency:* Iron-deficiency anemia, fatigue, tachycardia, palpitations, dyspnea, susceptibility to infection, brittle nails *Toxicity:* Iron poisoning; nausea, vomiting, gastrointestinal irritation, constipation, diarrhea	*Deficiency:* • Decreased hemoglobin, hematocrit, iron, and ferritin levels and increased total iron-binding capacity.	*Deficiency:* • Nutritional supplementation: ferrous sulfate 325 mg PO tid; Imferon 250 mg/day IM for each gram of hemoglobin below normal. • IV supplementation: 1.5–2 g over 4–6 h. • Good sources of iron are egg yolks, fish, organ meats, wheat germ, beef, peas, chicken, turkey, legumes, spinach.
Magnesium RDA: 310–420 mg EAR: 265–350 mg	• Parathyroid hormone regulation • Acid–base balance • Enzyme activation • Smooth muscle regulation • Metabolism of carbohydrates and protein • Cell growth and reproduction	*Deficiency:* Tetany, tremors, confusion, depression, tachycardia, dysrhythmias, seizures *Toxicity:* Nausea, vomiting, drowsiness, muscle weakness, decreased deep tendon reflexes, hypotension, respiratory depression	*Deficiency:* • Serum levels <1.3 mEq/L. *Toxicity:* • Serum levels >2.1 mEq/L.	*Deficiency:* • Nutritional supplementation: 1–2 g IV during 15 min. • Good sources of magnesium are nuts, meat, whole grains, green vegetables, seafood, dairy products. *Toxicity:* • Supportive measures.
Phosphorus RDA: 700 mg EAR: 580 mg	• Nerve and muscle activity • Vitamin utilization • Kidney function • Metabolism of carbohydrates, proteins, and fats • Cell growth and repair • Myocardial contraction • Energy production • Bone and tooth formation	*Deficiency:* Anorexia, weakness, tremor, paresthesias, anemia, mental status change, hypoxia, osteomalacia *Toxicity:* Tetany, soft tissue calcification, seizures, renal damage	*Deficiency:* • Serum levels <2.5 mg/dL. *Toxicity:* • Serum levels >4.5 mg/dL.	*Deficiency:* • Nutritional supplementation: PO or IV phosphate. • Good sources of phosphate are dairy products, eggs, fish, grains, meat, poultry, cheeses, beans, cocoa, chocolate, liver, milk, peas, nuts.

(continued)

Table 16-5 Vitamin and Mineral Requirements and Imbalances (*Continued*)

VITAMIN, RDA, AND EAR	FUNCTION	CLINICAL MANIFESTATIONS OF IMBALANCE	DIAGNOSTIC EVALUATION	MANAGEMENT
	• Acid–base balance • Red blood cell function			*Toxicity:* • Administration of phosphate-binding agents. • Hemodialysis or peritoneal dialysis.
Potassium AI: 4,700 mg	• Muscle contraction • Cardiac function • Protein synthesis • Nerve impulse transmission • Carbohydrate metabolism • Acid–base balance • Major intracellular cation	*Deficiency:* Muscle weakness, fatigue, malaise, flaccidity, mental confusion, irritability, depression, dysrhythmias, hypotension, nausea, vomiting, anorexia, decreased GI motility, muscle cramps, paresthesias, hyperglycemia, polyuria, metabolic alkalosis *Toxicity:* Muscle weakness, paralysis, paresthesias, nausea, vomiting, diarrhea, metabolic acidosis, prolonged cardiac conduction, ventricular dysrhythmias	*Deficiency:* • Serum levels <3.5 mEq/L. *Toxicity:* • Serum levels >5 mEq/L.	*Deficiency:* • Nutritional supplementation: PO or IV, IV replacement generally at a rate of 10 mEq/h with careful cardiac monitoring and frequent measurements of serum potassium levels. • Good sources of potassium are bananas, oranges, beef, prunes, beans, seafood, raisins. *Toxicity:* • Infuse calcium gluconate 10% (10 mL). • Sodium bicarbonate infusion. • Insulin and glucose infusion. • Oral or rectal exchange resins. • Hemodialysis or peritoneal dialysis.
Sodium AI: 1,300–1,500 mg	• Maintains fluid balance • Cell membrane permeability and absorption of glucose • Bioelectric potential of tissues • Cardiac function • Acid–base balance • Regulation of neuromuscular function	*Deficiency:* Muscle weakness, irritability, headache, seizures, nausea, vomiting, malaise, abdominal cramping, hypotension, tachycardia *Toxicity:* Flushed skin, oliguria, agitation, thirst, dry mucous membranes, seizures	*Deficiency:* • Serum levels <135 mEq/L. *Toxicity:* • Serum levels >145 mEq/L.	*Deficiency:* • Restrict free water intake. • Infuse 0.9% saline solution if the patient is hypovolemic. • Infuse 3% saline and administer diuretic if sodium levels significantly low. • Demeclocycline may be used to block ADH in the renal tubules to promote water excretion. *Toxicity:* • Administer salt-free solutions such as D_5W followed by 0.45% saline solution. • Low-sodium diet. • Administer vasopressin if diminished ADH is the cause.
Zinc RDA: 8–11 mg EAR: 6.8–9.4 mg	• Cellular metabolism • Maintenance of taste and smell • Burn and wound healing • Gonadal function • Maintenance of serum vitamin A concentration • Acid–base balance • Protein digestion • Promotion of growth	*Deficiency:* Fatigue, hair loss, poor wound healing, impaired growth, bone deformities, loss of taste, anorexia, iron-deficiency anemia, hypogonadism, hyperpigmentation *Toxicity:* Diminished deep tendon reflexes, malaise, decreased level of consciousness, diarrhea, leukopenia	*Deficiency:* • Serum levels <75 mcg/dL.	*Deficiency:* • Nutritional supplementation: zinc sulfate 200 mg PO tid. • Good sources of zinc are liver, seafood, beans, lentils, oatmeal, wheat bran, egg yolks, peas, chicken, and milk. *Toxicity:* • Supportive measures.

ADH, antidiuretic hormone; AI, adequate intake; ATP, adenosine triphosphate; DRI, dietary reference intake; EAR, estimated average requirement; IM, intramuscular; IV, intravenous; MCV, mean corpuscular volume; PO, by mouth; PTT, partial thromboplastin time; RBC, red blood cell; RDA, recommended daily allowance; tid, three times per day.

SELECTED READINGS

Adeyinka, A., Rouster, A. S., & Menogh, V. (2023, January). *Enteric feedings*. StatPearls Publishing. https://www.ncbi.nlm.nih.gov/books/NBK532876/

American Academy of Pediatrics. (2023). Clinical practice guideline for the evaluation and treatment of children and adolescents with obesity. *American Academy of Pediatrics, 151*(2). https://publications.aap.org/pediatrics/article/151/2/e2022060640/190443/Clinical-Practice-Guideline-for-the-Evaluation-and?autologincheck=redirected

American Society for Parental and Enteral Nutrition. (2019). *Appropriate dosing for parenteral nutrition: ASPEN recommendations*. https://www.nutritioncare.org/uploadedFiles/Documents/Guidelines_and_Clinical_Resources/PN%20Dosing%201-Sheet-Nov%202020-FINAL.pdf

Dhindsa, B. S., Saghir, S. M., Naga, Y., Dhaliwal, A., Ramai, D., Cross, C., Singh, S., Bhat, I., & Adler, D. G. (2020). Efficacy of transoral outlet reduction in Roux-en-Y gastric bypass patients to promote weight loss: A systematic review and meta-analysis. *Endoscopy International Open, 8*(10), E1332–E1340. https://www.ncbi.nlm.nih.gov/pmc/articles/PMC7511267/

Eisenberg, D., Shikora, S. A., Aarts E., Aminian, A., Angrisani, L., Cohen, R. V., De Luca, M., Faria, S. L., Goodpaster, K. P. S., Haddad, A., Himpens, J. M., Kow, L., Kurian, M., Loi, K., Mahawar, K., Nimeri, A., O'Kane, M., Papasavas, P. K., Ponce, J., … Kothari, S. N. (2022). 2022 American Society for Metabolic and Bariatric Surgery (ASMBS) and International Federation for the Surgery of Obesity and Metabolic Disorders: Indications for metabolic and bariatric surgery. *Surgery for Obesity and Related Diseases, 18*(12), 1345–1356. https://doi.org/10.1007/s11695-022-06332-1

Hamdan, M., & Puckett, Y. (2023, January). *Total parenteral nutrition*. StatPearls Publishing. https://www.ncbi.nlm.nih.gov/books/NBK559036/

Harris, B., & Szoka, N. (2019). *Transpyloric shuttle*. SAGES. https://www.sages.org/publications/tavac/transpyloric-shuttle/#:~:text=The%20TransPyloric%20Shuttle%20(TPS)%20is,locked%20into%20the%20correct%20shape

Harvard T.H. Chan School of Public Health. (2023). *The nutrition source. Vitamins and minerals*. https://www.hsph.harvard.edu/nutritionsource/vitamins/

Kesari, A., & Noel, J. Y. (2023, January). *Nutritional assessment*. StatPearls Publishing. https://www.ncbi.nlm.nih.gov/books/NBK580496/

Mechanick, J. I., Apovian, C., Brethauer, S., Garvey, W. T., Joffe, A. M., Kim, J., Kushner, R. F., Lindquist, R., Pessah-Pollack, R., Seger, J., Urman, R. D., Adams, S., Cleek, J. B., Correa, R., Kathleen Figaro, M., Flanders, K., Grams, J., Hurley, D. L., Kothari, S., … Still, C. D. (2020). Clinical practice guidelines for the perioperative nutrition, metabolic, and nonsurgical support of patients undergoing bariatric procedures—2019 update: Cosponsored by American Association of Clinical Endocrinologists/American College of Endocrinology, The Obesity Society, American Society for Metabolic & Bariatric Surgery, Obesity Medicine Association, and American Society of Anesthesiologists. *Surgery for Obesity and Related Diseases, 16*, 175–247. https://doi.org/10.1002/oby.22719

National Institute of Mental Health. (2023). *Eating disorders*. https://www.nimh.nih.gov/health/topics/eating-disorders

National Institutes of Mental Health, National Institutes of Health, and Health and Human Services. (2023, January). *Eating disorders*. https://www.nimh.nih.gov/health/topics/eating-disorders

Public Education Committee, American Society for Metabolic and Bariatric Surgery. (2021, May). *Bariatric surgery procedures*. https://asmbs.org/patients/bariatric-surgery-procedures

U.S. Department of Health and Human Services. (2022, May 17). *Adult obesity facts*. https://www.cdc.gov/obesity/data/adult.html

U.S. Department of Health and Human Services and U.S. Department of Agriculture. (2020). *Dietary guidelines for Americans: 2020–2025 make every bite count with the dietary guidelines* (9th ed.). https://www.dietaryguidelines.gov/resources/2020-2025-dietary-guidelines-online-materials

U.S. Food and Drug Administration. (2022). *Weight-loss and weight-management devices*. https://www.fda.gov/medical-devices/products-and-medical-procedures/weight-loss-and-weight-management-devices

World Health Organization. (2021). *Obesity and overweight*. https://www.who.int/news-room/fact-sheets/detail/obesity-and-overweight

World Health Organization. (2022). *World Obesity Day 2022—Accelerating action to stop obesity*. https://www.who.int/news/item/04-03-2022-world-obesity-day-2022-accelerating-action-to-stop-obesity#:~:text=More%20than%201%20billion%20people,adolescents%20and%2039%20million%20children

UNIT

VI RENAL, GENITOURINARY, AND REPRODUCTIVE HEALTH

17 Renal and Urinary Disorders*

OVERVIEW AND ASSESSMENT

See additional online content: Procedure Guidelines 17-1

Subjective Data

Subjective data include characterization of symptoms, history of present illness, past medical and surgical history, demographic data, and lifestyle factors. Signs and symptoms involving the urinary tract may be due to disorders of the kidneys, ureters, or bladder; surrounding structures; or disorders of other body systems (see Standards of Care Guidelines 17-1).

Changes in Micturition (Voiding)

Changes in the Amount or Color of Urine

1. Hematuria—blood in the urine, may be gross (visible by color change) or microscopic.
   a. Considered a serious sign and requires evaluation.
   b. Color of bloody urine depends on several factors, including the amount of blood present and the anatomic source of the bleeding.
   c. Microscopic hematuria is the presence of red blood cells (RBCs) in urine, which can be seen only under a microscope; urine appears normal.
   d. Hematuria may be due to a systemic cause, such as blood dyscrasias, anticoagulant therapy, or extreme exercise.
   e. Painless hematuria may indicate neoplasm in the urinary tract.
   f. Hematuria is common in patients with urinary tract stone disease, malignancy, acute infection, glomerulonephritis, trauma to the kidneys or urinary tract, thrombosis and embolism involving renal artery or vein, and polycystic kidney disease.
2. Polyuria—large volume of urine voided in a given time.
   a. Volume is out of proportion to the usual voiding pattern and fluid intake.
   b. Normally urine output exceeding 3 L/24 hours.
   c. Demonstrated in diabetes mellitus, diabetes insipidus, chronic renal disease, use of diuretics.

*Please note that the term "male" in this chapter refers to a person assigned male at birth, and the term "female" in this chapter refers to a person assigned female at birth..

STANDARDS OF CARE GUIDELINES 17-1

Renal Impairment

- Be aware that systemic factors, urologic status, and renal function affect urine output. Notify health care provider of decreased urine output.
- Patients at risk for renal impairment include those with cardiovascular disease, diabetes, and hypertension; patients who are postoperative or hypotensive; and those with prostate and other diseases of the urinary tract.
- Thorough assessment of the urinary tract includes:
  - Hourly intake and output measurement.
  - Assessment of color, clarity, and specific gravity of the urine.
  - Palpation of the abdomen for suprapubic tenderness.
  - Percussion of the flanks for costovertebral angle tenderness.
  - Prostate examination.
  - Subjective assessment for symptoms, such as urgency, frequency, nocturia, hesitancy, dribbling, decreased force of stream, hematuria, and incontinence.
- Be alert to drugs or agents that may impair urinary and renal function, such as nonsteroidal anti-inflammatory drugs, anticholinergics, sympathomimetics, aminoglycoside antibiotics, antifungals, calcineurin inhibitors, angiotensin-converting enzyme inhibitors, angiotensin receptor blockers, chemotherapeutic agents, and contrast media.
- Report abnormal urinalysis, urine culture, and renal function test results to health care provider promptly.

This information should serve as a general guideline only. Each patient situation presents a unique set of clinical factors and requires nursing judgment to guide care, which may include additional or alternative measures and approaches.

3. Oliguria—small volume of urine.
   a. Output between 50 and 500 mL/24 hours.
   b. May result from acute renal failure, chronic kidney disease (CKD) stage V, shock, dehydration, fluid and electrolyte imbalance, or obstruction.
4. Anuria—absence of urine output.
   a. Output less than 50 mL/24 hours.
   b. Indicates serious renal dysfunction requiring immediate medical or surgical intervention, or CKD stage V.

Symptoms Related to Irritation of the Lower Urinary Tract

1. Dysuria—painful or uncomfortable urination.
   a. Burning sensation seen in a wide variety of inflammatory and infectious urinary tract conditions.
2. Frequency—voiding occurs more frequently than usual when compared with patient's usual pattern or with a generally accepted norm of once every 3 to 6 hours.
   a. Determine whether patient's normal fluid intake has been altered—it is essential to know the normal voiding pattern to evaluate frequency.
   b. Increasing frequency can result from a variety of conditions, such as infection and diseases of the urinary tract, metabolic disease, hypertension, medications (diuretics).
3. Urgency—strong desire to urinate that is difficult to postpone.
   a. Because of inflammatory conditions of the bladder, prostate, or urethra; acute or chronic bacterial infections; neurogenic voiding dysfunctions; chronic prostatitis or bladder outlet obstruction in males; overactive bladder; and urogenital atrophy in postmenopausal females.
4. Nocturia—urination at night that interrupts sleep.
   a. Causes include urologic conditions affecting bladder function, poor bladder emptying, bladder outlet obstruction, or overactive bladder.
   b. Metabolic causes include decreased renal concentrating ability or heart failure, hyperglycemia, and remobilization of dependent edema.
   c. Increases in older age as kidneys lose circadian rhythm and physiologic regulation.
5. Strangury—slow and painful urination; only small amounts of urine voided. Wrenching sensation at the end of urination produced by spasmodic muscular contraction of the urethra and bladder.
   a. Blood staining may be noted.
   b. Seen in numerous urologic conditions, including severe cystitis, interstitial cystitis, urinary calculus, and bladder cancer.

Symptoms Related to Obstruction of the Lower Urinary Tract

1. Weak stream—decreased force of stream when compared to the usual stream of urine when voiding.
2. Hesitancy—undue delay and difficulty in initiating voiding.
   a. May indicate compression of the urethra, outlet obstruction, neurogenic bladder.
3. Terminal dribbling—prolonged dribbling or urine from the meatus after urination is complete. May be caused by bladder outlet obstruction.
4. Incomplete emptying—feeling that the bladder is still full even after urination. Indicates urinary retention, overactive bladder, small void volumes, or a condition that prevents the bladder from emptying well; may lead to infection.
5. Urinary retention—inability to void.

Involuntary Voiding

1. Urinary incontinence—involuntary loss of urine; may be due to pathologic, anatomic, or physiologic factors affecting the urinary tract (see page 112).
2. Nocturnal enuresis—involuntary voiding during sleep. May be physiologic during early childhood; thereafter, may be functional or symptomatic of obstructive or neurogenic disease (usually of the lower urinary tract) or dysfunctional voiding.

Urinary Tract Pain

1. Kidney pain—may be felt as a dull ache in costovertebral angle or may be a sharp, colicky pain felt in the flank area that radiates to the groin or testicle. Because of distention of the renal capsule; severity related to how quickly it develops.
2. Ureteral pain—felt in the back and/or abdomen and can radiate to the groin, urethra, penis, scrotum, or testicle.
3. Bladder pain (lower abdominal pain or pain over suprapubic area)—may be due to bladder infection, overdistended bladder, or bladder spasms.
4. Urethral pain—from irritation of the bladder neck, from foreign body in canal, or from urethritis because of infection or trauma; pain increases when voiding.
5. Pain in scrotal area—because of inflammatory swelling of the epididymis or testicle, torsion of the testicle, testicular mass, or

scrotal infection. May also be referred pain from neurologic, renal, or gastrointestinal (GI) source.

6. Testicular pain—because of injury, mumps, orchitis, torsion of the spermatic cord, testes, or testes appendix.
7. Perineal or rectal discomfort—because of acute or chronic prostatitis, prostatic abscess, or trauma.
8. Pain in glans penis—usually from prostatitis; penile shaft pain results from urethral problems; may also be referred pain from ureteral calculus.

Related Symptoms

1. GI symptoms related to urologic conditions include nausea, vomiting, diarrhea, abdominal discomfort, paralytic ileus.
2. Occur with urologic conditions because the GI and urinary tracts have common autonomic and sensory innervation and because of renointestinal reflexes.
3. Fever and chills may also occur with infectious processes.

History

Seek the following historical data related to urinary and renal function:

1. What are patient's present and past occupations? Look for occupational hazards related to the urinary tract—contact with chemicals, plastics, tar, rubber; also truck or school bus drivers, dry cleaners, farmers.
2. What is patient's smoking history?
3. What is the past medical and surgical history, especially in relation to urinary problem?
4. Is there any family history of renal disease?
5. What childhood diseases did patient have?
6. Is there a history of urinary tract infections (UTIs)? Did any occur before age 12? Risk factors for UTIs?
7. Did enuresis continue beyond the age when most children gain control?
8. Any history of genital lesions or sexually transmitted infections (STIs)?
9. For the female patient: number of children? Vaginal or cesarean delivery? Any forceps deliveries? When? Any signs of vaginal discharge? Vaginal/vulvar itch or irritation? Family history of pelvic organ prolapse ("dropped" bladder or uterus) or urinary incontinence? Age of menopause?
10. For the male patient: any history of benign prostatic hyperplasia (BPH)? Any issues starting the stream of urine, continuing the stream of urine, or feeling the bladder is full after urination? Any surgical or medical treatment of BPH? Any dry ejaculation, or orgasm without ejaculate (retrograde ejaculation)?
11. Does patient have diabetes mellitus? Hypertension? Allergies? Neurologic disease or dysfunction? Vascular disease?
12. Has patient ever been hospitalized for a UTI? What diagnostic tests were performed? Cystoscopy? Urodynamics? Kidney x-ray procedures? Was patient catheterized for a time? Were antibiotics administered via intravenous (IV) or oral route?
13. Has patient ever had surgery for bladder or traumatic injuries involving the pelvis?
14. Is patient taking any prescription or over-the-counter (OTC) drugs or herbal preparations that may affect renal or urinary function? Have any drugs been prescribed for renal or urinary problems?

Objective Data

Objective data should focus on physical examination of the abdomen, the genitalia, and rectal examination in some cases. Complete body system assessment may be indicated in some conditions, such as renal failure (see Chapter 1).

Laboratory Tests

Common laboratory studies pertaining to renal and urologic disorders include blood and urinary excretion tests for renal function, prostate-specific antigen (PSA), and urinalysis.

Tests of Renal Function

Description

1. Renal function tests are used to determine the effectiveness of the kidneys' excretory functioning, to evaluate the severity of kidney disease, and to follow patient's progress.
2. There is no single test of renal function; rather, optimal results are obtained by combining a number of clinical tests.

Nursing and Patient Care Considerations

Renal function may be within normal limits until about 50% of renal function has been lost (see Table 17-1).

Prostate-Specific Antigen

Description

1. PSA is an amino acid glycoprotein that is measured in the serum by a simple blood test.
2. An elevated PSA indicates the presence of prostate disease but is not exclusive to prostate cancer. Amide proton transfer (APT) magnetic resonance imaging (MRI) in combination with PSA testing differentiates malignant prostate lesions from benign prostate lesions. Prostate cancer is the most common cancer of the genitourinary (GU) tract in males.
3. Level rises continuously with the growth of prostate cancer.
4. No normal serum PSA level, previously less than 4 ng/mL, was considered normal. In general, higher levels of PSA are more likely to indicate prostate cancer.
5. Patients who have undergone surgical treatment for prostate cancer are monitored every 6 to 12 months with PSA levels for recurrence. Cancer recurrence is suspected with a trend of increasing PSA levels.

Nursing and Patient Care Considerations

1. No patient preparation is necessary.
2. Current or recent UTI, prostatitis, digital rectal examination, ejaculation or vigorous exercise, or urethral instrumentation can cause an artificial elevation of PSA.
3. Finasteride, dutasteride, or other medications used to treat BPH can cause low PSA levels.
4. Clinical laboratories may differ slightly in methods used for determining PSA; patients having serial PSA should be sent to the same laboratory.

Urinalysis

Description

Involves examination of the urine for overall characteristics, including appearance, pH, specific gravity (SG), and osmolality as well as microscopic evaluation for the presence of normal and abnormal cells.

1. Appearance—normal urine is clear. Foamy urine can be seen with proteinuria. Cloudy urine may or may not be pathologic.
   a. Nonpathologic causes: Normal urine may develop cloudiness on refrigeration, from standing at room temperature, or from precipitation of phosphates in alkaline urine (phosphaturia).

Table 17-1 Tests of Renal Function

TEST	PURPOSE/RATIONALE	TEST PROTOCOL
There is no single test of renal function because this function is subject to variation. The rate of change of renal function is more important than the result of a single test.		
Renal concentration test • Specific gravity • Osmolality of urine	• Both tests evaluate the ability of the kidney to dilute or concentrate urine. • Values are elevated in prerenal states, including dehydration. Concentration ability is lost (resulting in low values) in CKD and some types of AKI despite changes in volume status.	• Fluids may be withheld 12–24 h to evaluate the concentrating ability of the tubules under controlled conditions. Specific gravity measurements of urine are taken at specific times to determine urine concentration.
Creatinine clearance	• Provides a reasonable approximation of rate of glomerular filtration • Measures volume of blood in mL cleared of creatinine in 1 min • Most sensitive indication of early renal disease	• Collect all urine over 24-h period. • Draw one sample of blood within the period.
Serum creatinine	• A test of renal function reflecting the balance between production and filtration by renal glomerulus • Most sensitive test of renal function	• Obtain sample of blood serum.
Serum urea nitrogen (BUN)	• Serves as an index of renal excretory capacity • Serum urea nitrogen depends on the body's urea production and urine flow. (Urea is the nitrogenous end product of protein metabolism.) • Affected by protein intake, hydration status, and catabolism	• Obtain sample of blood serum.
Protein	• Random specimen may be affected by dietary protein intake. Proteinuria >300 mg/24 h may indicate renal disease.	• Collect all urine over 24-h period.
Microalbumin/creatinine ratio	• Sensitive test for the subsequent development of proteinuria; >25 mg/g for females and >17 mg/g for males predicts early nephropathy	• Collect random urine specimen.
Urine casts	• Mucoproteins and other substances present in renal inflammation; help to identify type of renal disease (e.g., red cell casts present in glomerulonephritis, fatty casts in nephrotic syndrome, white cell casts in pyelonephritis).	• Collect random urine specimen.

AKI, acute kidney injury; BUN, blood urea nitrogen; CKD, chronic kidney disease.

b. Pathologic causes: because of pus (pyuria), blood, epithelial cells, bacteria, fat, colloidal particles, phosphate, or lymph fluid (chyluria).
2. Odor—normal urine has a faint aromatic odor.
   a. Characteristic odors produced by ingestion of asparagus.
   b. Cloudy urine with ammonia odor: urea-splitting bacteria such as *Proteus*, causing UTIs.
   c. Offensive odor: may be due to bacterial action in the presence of pus.
   d. Acetone scent can be detected in diabetic ketoacidosis.
3. Color—varies with urine concentration and is affected by metabolites, medications, and certain foods.
   a. Normal urine is clear yellow or amber because of the pigment urochrome.
   b. Dilute urine is pale yellow or clear.
   c. Concentrated urine is tea colored and may be a sign of insufficient fluid intake.
   d. Blue, blue green: medication, namely, amitriptyline, propofol, indomethacin, and methenamine; pseudomonas infection.
   e. Red or red brown: because of blood pigments, porphyria, bleeding lesions in urogenital tract, some drugs such as phenazopyridine and foods (beets).
   f. Yellow brown, green brown, or tea colored: may reveal obstructive lesion of bile duct system, obstructive jaundice, or hepatitis.
   g. Dark brown or black: because of malignant melanoma, leukemia, methemoglobin or medications, namely, methyldopa, levodopa.
4. pH of urine—reflects the ability of the kidney to maintain normal hydrogen ion concentration in plasma and extracellular fluid; indicates *acidity* or *alkalinity* of urine.
   a. pH should be measured in fresh urine because the breakdown of urine to ammonia causes urine to become alkaline.
   b. Normal pH is 4.5 to 8.0.
   c. Urine acidity (pH less than 4.5) or alkalinity (pH greater than 8.0) has relatively little clinical significance unless the patient is being treated for renal calculus disease or being evaluated for renal tubular acidosis.

5. SG—reflects the kidney's ability to concentrate or dilute urine; may reflect the degree of hydration or dehydration.
   a. Normal SG ranges from 1.005 to 1.030.
   b. SG is low and matches the SG of plasma at 1.010 (isosthenuria) in the late stages of CKD.
   c. Volume depletion will cause the SG to be elevated, and volume overload will result in a low SG.
6. Osmolality—indication of the amount of osmotically active particles in urine (number of particles per unit volume of water). It is similar to SG but is considered a more precise test, and only 1 to 2 mL of urine is required. Osmolality can range from 50 to 1,200 mOsm/kg.

Nursing and Patient Care Considerations

1. Freshly voided urine provides the best results for routine urinalysis; some tests may require a first morning specimen.
2. The urine should be refrigerated to ensure accurate results if urine sample cannot be delivered to laboratory immediately.
3. Obtain sample of about 30 mL.
4. Urine culture and sensitivity tests are typically performed using the same specimen obtained for urinalysis; therefore, use clean-catch or catheterization technique.
5. Patients with urinary diversions, especially ileal conduit diversions, require catheterized urine specimen. The urinalysis will normally demonstrate bacteria if the specimen is collected from intestinal diversion.

Radiology and Imaging Studies

These tests include simple x-rays, x-rays with the use of contrast media, ultrasound, nuclear scans, and imaging via computed tomography (CT) and MRI. Patient age and pregnancy status help dictate imaging choice.

EVIDENCE BASE Kaul, I., Moore, S., Barry, E., & Pareek, G. (2023). Renal imaging in stone disease: Which modality to choose? *Rhode Island Medical Journal (2013)*, *106*(11), 31–35.

X-ray of Kidneys, Ureters, and Bladder

Description

1. Consists of plain film of the abdomen.
2. Delineates size, shape, and position of the kidneys.
3. Reveals deviations, such as radiopaque calcifications (stones), tumors, or kidney displacement.
4. Not reliable as sole imaging modality to diagnose stones as it will not show radiolucent stones.

Nursing and Patient Care Considerations

1. No preparation is needed.
2. Usually done before other testing.
3. Patient will be asked to wear a gown and remove all metal from the x-ray field.

Pyelogram

Description

1. Antegrade pyelogram: injection of small amount of radiopaque contrast directly into the renal pelvis, usually via an existing nephrostomy tube.
2. Retrograde pyelogram: injection of radiopaque contrast material through ureteral catheters, which have been passed into ureters by means of cystoscopic manipulation.
3. The radiopaque solution is introduced by syringe injection. May require sedation.
4. Mostly used to determine the location and severity of an obstruction in the urinary system.
5. Used in place of previously used intravenous pyelogram (IVP) for visualization of the collecting system.

Nursing and Patient Care Considerations

1. Contraindicated in patients with UTI.
2. May require sedation.
3. Allergic reactions are rare as only a small amount of dye is absorbed into the body.

Cystourethrogram

Description

1. Visualization of the urethra and bladder by x-ray after retrograde instillation of contrast material through a catheter. An examination of only the bladder is a *cystogram* and of only the urethra is a *urethrogram*.
2. Used to identify injuries, vesicoureteral reflux, tumors, or structural abnormalities of the urethra or bladder or to evaluate emptying problems or incontinence (voiding cystourethrogram).

Nursing and Patient Care Considerations

1. Carries risk of infection because of instrumentation.
2. Allergy to contrast material is a contraindication.
3. Additional x-rays may be taken after the catheter is removed and patient voids (voiding cystourethrogram).
4. Provide reassurance to allay patient's embarrassment.

Renal Angiography

Description

1. IV catheter is threaded through the femoral and iliac arteries into the aorta or renal artery.
2. Contrast material is injected to visualize the renal arterial supply.
3. Evaluates blood flow dynamics, demonstrates abnormal vasculature, and differentiates renal cysts from renal tumors.
4. May be done prior to renal transplant or to embolize a kidney before nephrectomy for renal tumor.

Nursing and Patient Care Considerations

1. NPO after midnight before the examination; clear liquids permitted up to 2 hours before the examination. Adequate hydration is essential.
2. Continue oral medications (special orders needed for patients with diabetes).
3. IV access required.
4. May not be done on the same day as other studies requiring barium or contrast material.
5. Maintain bed rest for approximately 4 hours after the examination, with the leg kept straight on the side used for groin access.
6. Observe frequently for hematoma or bleeding at the access site. Keep sandbag at bedside for use if bleeding occurs.

Renal Scan

Description

1. Radiopharmaceuticals (also called *radiotracers* or *isotopes*) are injected IV.
   a. Tc-DTPA, Tc^{99m}-DMSA is used for anatomic or MAG3 visualization and evaluation of glomerular filtration.
   b. Other radiopharmaceuticals may also be used depending on the purpose of the scan.

2. Assesses renal function and not used to assess for renal anatomy, mass, or stones.
3. Studies are obtained with a scintillation camera placed posterior to the kidney with patient in a supine, prone, or sitting position.

Nursing and Patient Care Considerations

1. Patient should be well hydrated. Give several glasses of water or IV fluids, as ordered, before scan.
2. Furosemide or captopril may be administered in conjunction with the scan to determine their effects.

Ultrasound

Description

1. Uses high-frequency sound waves passed into the body and reflected back in varying frequencies based on the composition of soft tissues. Organs in the urinary system create characteristic ultrasonic images that are electronically processed and displayed as an image.
2. Abnormalities, such as masses, malformations, stones, or obstructions, can be identified; useful in differentiating between solid and fluid-filled masses.
3. A noninvasive technique without the use of radiation.

Nursing and Patient Care Considerations

1. Ultrasound examination of the prostate is performed using a rectal probe. A laxative or enema may be ordered to be given several hours prior to the examination.
2. Ultrasound examination of the bladder requires that the bladder be full.
3. Patient should not have had any studies using barium for 2 days before ultrasound of the kidney or bladder.

Computed Tomography and Magnetic Resonance Imaging

CT urogram has replaced IVP and is now the radiographic modality of choice to visualize the kidneys, ureter, and bladder. Noncontrast CT known as "stone survey" is the preferred method for evaluating urolithiasis. MRI may be ordered to evaluate for tumors.

See descriptions on page 843.

Other Tests

Other tests that may be done to evaluate disorders of the renal and urologic systems include cystoscopy, urodynamic testing, and needle biopsy of the kidney.

Cystoscopy

Description

1. *Cystoscopy* is a method of direct visualization of the urethra and bladder by means of a cystoscope that is inserted through the urethra into the bladder. It has a self-contained optical lens system that provides a magnified, illuminated view of the bladder.
2. Uses include:
   a. To inspect the bladder wall directly for tumor, stone, or ulcer and to inspect the urethra for abnormalities or to assess the degree of prostatic obstruction.
   b. To allow insertion of ureteral catheters for radiographic studies or before abdominal or GU surgery.
   c. To see configuration and position of ureteral orifices.
   d. To remove calculi from the urethra, bladder, and ureter.
   e. To diagnose and treat lesions of the bladder, urethra, and prostate.
   f. To perform endoscopic prostate surgeries, including transurethral resection of the prostate (TURP) (see page 582).

Nursing and Patient Care Considerations

1. Simple cystoscopy is usually performed in an office setting. More complicated cystoscopies, involving resections or ureteral catheter insertions, are done in the operating room suite, where IV sedation or spinal or general anesthesia may be used.
2. Patient's genitalia are cleaned with an antiseptic solution just before the examination. A local topical anesthetic (lidocaine gel) is instilled into the urethra before insertion of cystoscope. Lidocaine gel may also be administered post-cystoscopy; however, it has not been shown to reduce urinary symptoms.
3. Because fluid flows continuously through the cystoscope, patient may feel an urge to urinate during the examination.
4. Contraindicated in patients with known UTI.
5. Nursing interventions after cystoscopic examination:
   a. Monitor for complications: urinary retention, urinary tract hemorrhage, infection within the prostate or bladder.
   b. Expect patient to have some burning on voiding, blood-tinged urine, and urinary frequency from trauma to mucous membrane of the urethra.
   c. Administer or teach self-administration of antibiotics prophylactically, as ordered, to prevent UTI.
   d. Advise warm sitz baths or analgesics, such as ibuprofen or acetaminophen, to relieve discomfort after cystoscopy. Increase hydration.
   e. Provide routine catheter care if urine retention persists and an indwelling catheter is ordered.

Urodynamics

Description

Urodynamics is a term that refers to any of the following tests that provide physiologic and functional information about the lower urinary tract. They measure the ability of the bladder to store and empty urine. Most urodynamic equipment uses computer technology with results visible in real time on a monitor.

1. Uroflowmetry (flow rate)—a record of the volume of urine passing through the urethra per unit of time (mL/s). It is shown on graph paper and gives information about the rate and flow pattern of urination. It is used to evaluate obstructive voiding. Minimum volume of urine needed for an accurate test is 150 mL.
2. Cystometrography—recording of the pressures exerted during filling and emptying of the urinary bladder to assess its function. Data about the ability of the bladder to store urine at low pressure and the ability of the bladder to contract appropriately to empty urine are obtained.
   a. A small catheter is placed through the urethra (or suprapubic area) into the bladder. The residual volume is measured if patient recently voided and the catheter is left in place.
   b. The catheters are connected to urodynamic equipment designed to measure pressure at the distal end of the catheter.
   c. Water, saline, or contrast material is infused at a slow rate into the bladder.
   d. When the bladder feels full, patient is asked to "void." A normal detrusor contraction of the bladder appears as a sharp rise in bladder pressure on the graph. If the patient is unable to void, the test may be considered normal because it is difficult to void normally with catheters in place.

3. Sphincter electromyography (EMG)—measures the activity of the pelvic floor muscles during bladder filling and emptying. EMG activity may be measured using surface (patch) electrodes placed around the anus or with percutaneous wire or needle electrodes.
4. Pressure flow studies—involve all of the abovementioned components, along with the simultaneous measurement of intra-abdominal pressure by way of a small tube with a fluid-filled balloon that is placed in the rectum. This permits better interpretation of actual bladder pressures without the influence of intra-abdominal pressure.
5. Video urodynamics—use all of the abovementioned components. The fluid used to fill the bladder is contrast material, and the entire study is performed under fluoroscopy, providing radiographic pictures in combination with the recording of bladder and intra-abdominal pressures. Video urodynamics are reserved for patients with complicated voiding dysfunction.

Nursing and Patient Care Considerations

1. Contraindicated in patients with UTI.
2. Frequently performed by nurses; essential to provide information and support throughout the test to ensure clinically significant results.
3. Patients may have burning on urination afterward (because of instrumentation); encourage fluids.
4. Short-term antibiotics are commonly given to prevent infection.

Needle Biopsy of the Kidney

Description

Performed by percutaneous needle biopsy through renal tissue with ultrasound guidance or by open biopsy through a small flank incision; useful in securing specimens for electron and immunofluorescent microscopy to determine diagnosis, treatment, and prognosis of renal disease.

Nursing and Patient Care Considerations

1. Prebiopsy nursing management.
   a. Ensure that coagulation studies, platelet count, and hematocrit results are reported to provide baseline values and to identify patients at risk for postbiopsy bleeding.
   b. Establish an IV line, as ordered.
   c. Ensure that patient is NPO for several hours before the procedure, as ordered.
   d. Describe the procedure to patient, including holding breath (to prevent movement of the thorax) during insertion of the biopsy needle.
   e. Instruct patient to urinate before the procedure.
2. Postbiopsy nursing management.
   a. Place patient in a supine position immediately after biopsy and on bed rest for 8 to 24 hours to minimize bleeding.
   b. Take vital signs every 5 to 15 minutes for the first hour and then with decreasing frequency if stable to assess for hemorrhage, which is a major complication.
   c. Watch for rise or fall in blood pressure (BP), anorexia, vomiting, or development of dull, aching discomfort in the abdomen.
   d. Assess for flank pain (usually represents bleeding into the muscle) or colicky pain (clot in the ureter).
   e. Assess for backache, shoulder pain, or dysuria.
   f. Persistent bleeding may be suspected when an enlarging hematoma is palpable through the abdomen.
   g. If perirenal bleeding develops, avoid palpating or manipulating the abdomen after the first examination has determined that a hematoma exists.
   h. Collect serial urine specimens to evaluate for hematuria.
   i. Assess for any patient complaints, especially frequency and urgency on urination.
   j. Keep fluid intake at 3,000 mL daily, if tolerated, unless patient has renal insufficiency.
   k. Hematocrit and hemoglobin may be ordered to assess for anemia prior to discharge.
3. Instruct patient on the following after biopsy:
   a. Avoid strenuous activity, strenuous sports, and heavy lifting for at least 2 weeks.
   b. Notify health care provider if any of the following occur: flank pain, hematuria, lightheadedness and fainting, rapid pulse, or any other signs and symptoms of bleeding.
   c. Report for follow-up 1 to 2 months after biopsy; will be checked for hypertension and the biopsy area is auscultated for a bruit.

GENERAL PROCEDURES AND TREATMENT MODALITIES

See additional online content: Procedure Guidelines 17-2 to 17-4

Catheterization

Catheterization may be done to relieve acute or chronic urinary retention, to drain urine preoperatively and postoperatively, to determine the amount of residual urine after voiding, or to determine an accurate measurement of urinary drainage in patients who are critically ill.

Catheterization of Female

1. Assess for latex allergy and utilize silicone catheter if allergic to latex.
2. Acquire assistance if needed for positioning patient with knees bent and legs (dorsal recumbent position) spread with light directed onto the vulva. Maintain strict sterile technique using prepackaged indwelling catheter tray, or sterile straight catheter, sterile gloves, lubricant, and cleansing components set up on sterile field as indicated. Nondominant hand usually used for spreading labia, and dominant hand remains sterile (see Figure 17-1).
3. Cleanse urethral meatus with povidone–iodine or other cleansing solution via cotton balls manipulated with sterile forceps or betadine swab sticks.
4. Introduce well-lubricated catheter 2 to 3 in (5 to 7.5 cm) into the urethral meatus using sterile gloved hand, watching for flow of urine. Once the flow of urine begins, advance additional 1 to 2 in.
5. Obtain specimen and secure the catheter and drainage bag as indicated. Note the amount of urine drained.

Catheterization of Male

1. Assess for latex allergy and utilize silicone catheter if allergic to latex.
2. Grasp the shaft of the penis with nondominant hand; elevate it, retracting the foreskin, if present.

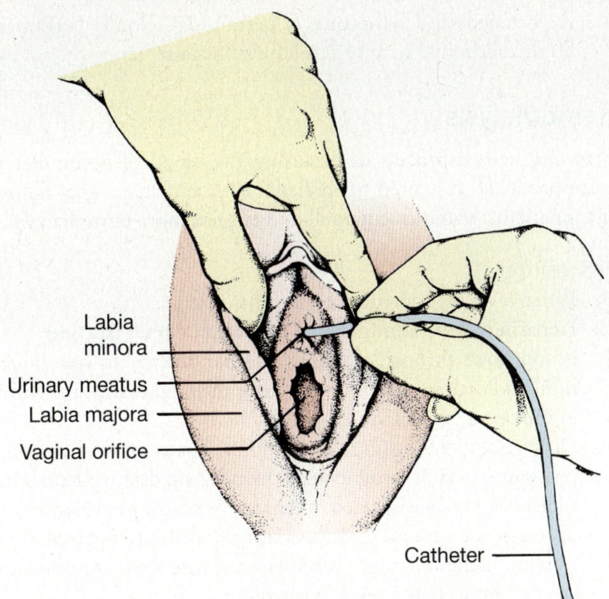

Figure 17-1. Urethral catheterization of the female patient.

3. Cleanse with spiral downward motion from urethral meatus, using a new sterile cotton ball with each stroke.
4. Apply gentle traction as you insert the well-lubricated catheter 6 to 10 in (15 to 25 cm) with your sterile hand. Watch for urine flow and advance the catheter another 1 in (2.5 cm).
5. Obtain specimen and secure the catheter and drainage bag as indicated. Note the amount of urine drained.

Suprapubic Catheterization

1. Establishes drainage from the bladder by introducing a catheter percutaneously through the anterior abdominal wall into the bladder.
2. May be done for acute urinary retention when urethral catheterization is not possible; for urethral trauma, stricture, or fistula to divert the flow of urine from the urethra; or for obtaining an uncontaminated urine specimen for culture.
3. Once the surgical tract is healed, the catheter may be changed by the nurse monthly.

Dialysis

Dialysis refers to the diffusion of solute molecules through a semipermeable membrane, passing from the side of higher concentration to that of lower concentration. The purpose of dialysis is to maintain fluid, electrolyte, and acid–base balance and to remove endogenous and exogenous toxins. It is a substitute for some kidney excretory functions but does not replace the kidneys' endocrine functions. Methods of dialysis include:

1. Peritoneal dialysis (PD).
   a. Continuous ambulatory peritoneal dialysis (CAPD).
   b. Automated peritoneal dialysis (APD)/continuous cycling PD—uses APD machine to do multiple exchanges overnight, with or without a prolonged dwell time during the day.
2. Hemodialysis (see page 576).
3. Continuous renal replacement therapy (CRRT)—this includes slow continuous ultrafiltration, continuous venovenous hemofiltration, continuous venovenous hemodialysis, and continuous venovenous hemodiafiltration. These use extracorporeal blood circulation through a small-volume, low-resistance filter to provide continuous removal of solutes and fluid in the intensive care setting.
   a. CRRT is indicated for patients who are hemodynamically unstable and cannot tolerate the rapid fluid shifts that occur with intermittent dialysis. It is also indicated for patients with oliguria who require large amounts of hourly intravenous (IV) fluids or parenteral nutrition. CRRT is often better tolerated by patients who are critically ill because it is a slower and less aggressive process for the removal of fluid and solutes than hemodialysis.
   b. CRRT is accomplished by insertion of a large-gauge double-lumen catheter into the internal jugular, subclavian, or femoral vein. A roller-type pump is used to propel blood through the system, and anticoagulation may be used to prevent clotting. This is the current standard of care because of consistent blood flow rates.
   c. Care for the patient on CRRT is provided in an intensive care setting, with special attention given to assessing and calculating fluid and electrolyte balance, aggressively managing hypotension, preventing and monitoring for hemorrhage, monitoring for heat loss through the extracorporeal circulation, assessing for infection, and preventing clotting.

Continuous Ambulatory Peritoneal Dialysis

CAPD is a form of intracorporeal dialysis that uses the peritoneum as the semipermeable membrane (see Figure 17-2).

Procedure

1. A permanent indwelling catheter is implanted into the peritoneum; the internal cuff of the catheter becomes embedded by fibrous ingrowth, which stabilizes it and minimizes leakage.
2. A tube for connecting the catheter to an administration set is attached via a locking mechanism to the distal end of the peritoneal catheter, called the *transfer set*. It remains with the

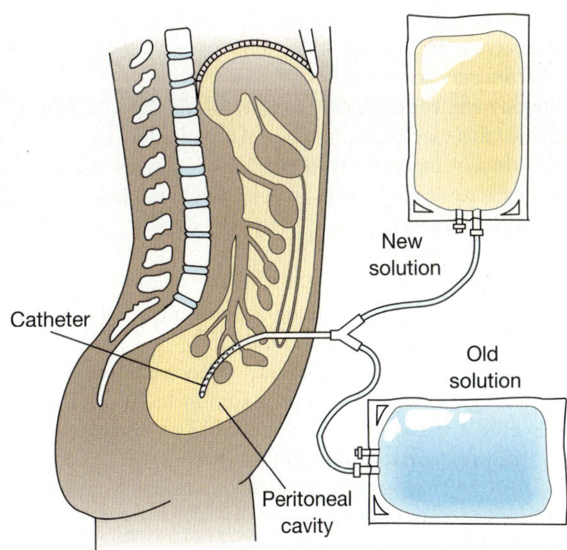

Figure 17-2. Continuous ambulatory peritoneal dialysis. The peritoneal catheter is implanted through the abdominal wall. Fluid infuses into the peritoneal cavity and drains after a prescribed time. (Adapted with permission from Norris, T. L. [2025]. *Porth's pathophysiology: Concepts of altered health states* [11th ed., Fig. 34-6]. Wolters Kluwer.)

patient (attached to the catheter tubing) and must be changed at regular intervals per the manufacturer's recommendations without contamination. Specific transfer sets may only fit administration tubing from the same manufacturer, but there are devices available to make the transfer set compatible with other PD systems.
3. There are many types of administration sets, the most common being the double bag system. The double bag system has a preattached bag of dialysate solution and drainage, which has been shown to reduce peritonitis rates.
4. In CAPD, a patient is prescribed a set number of exchanges (fill, drain, and dwell) throughout the day.
5. During the fill, the dialysate bag is raised to shoulder level and infused by gravity into the peritoneal cavity (approximately 10 minutes for a 2-L volume).
6. During the dwell time, diffusion and osmosis occur. The typical dwell time is 4 to 6 hours.
7. At the end of the dwell time, the dialysate fluid is drained from the peritoneal cavity by gravity. Drainage of 2 L plus ultrafiltration take about 10 to 20 minutes if the catheter is functioning optimally.
8. After the dialysate is drained, a fresh bag of dialysate solution is infused using aseptic technique, and the procedure is repeated.
9. Patient performs four to five exchanges daily, 7 days per week, with an overnight dwell time allowing uninterrupted sleep; most patients become unaware of fluid in the peritoneal cavity.

Advantages Over Hemodialysis

1. Physical and psychological freedom and independence.
2. More liberal diet and fluid intake.
3. Relatively simple and easy to use.
4. Satisfactory biochemical control of uremia.

Complications

1. Infectious peritonitis, exit site and tunnel infections.
2. Noninfectious catheter malfunction, obstruction, dialysate leak.
3. Peritoneal–pleural communication; hernia formation.
4. Gastrointestinal (GI) bloating, distention, nausea.
5. Hypervolemia, hypovolemia.
6. Bleeding at catheter site.
7. Bloody effluent secondary to internal bleeding. In female patients, this may occur during menstruation.
8. Obstruction may occur if the omentum becomes wrapped around the catheter or the catheter becomes caught in a loop of bowel.
9. Poor sleep quality.

Patient Education

1. The use of CAPD as a long-term treatment depends on the prevention of recurring peritonitis.
   a. Use strict aseptic technique when performing bag exchanges. All persons in the room, including patient, must wear a mask any time connecting or disconnecting the transfer set to or from another system.
   b. Perform bag exchanges in clean, closed-off area without pets and other activities.
   c. Wash hands before touching bag.
   d. Inspect bag and tubing for defects and leaks.
2. Do not omit bag changes—this will cause inadequate control of renal failure.
3. Some weight gain may accompany CAPD—the dialysate fluid contains a significant amount of dextrose, which adds calories to daily intake.
4. Report signs and symptoms of peritonitis—cloudy peritoneal fluid, abdominal pain or tenderness, malaise, fever.

Hemodialysis

Hemodialysis is a process of cleansing the blood of accumulated waste products. It is used for patients with end-stage renal failure or for patients who are acutely ill and require short-term dialysis.

Procedure

1. Patient's access is prepared and cannulated.
2. Heparin may be administered to prevent circuit clotting.
3. Blood flows through a semipermeable dialyzer in one direction, and dialysis solution surrounds the membranes and flows in the opposite direction.
4. Dialysis solution consists of highly purified water to which sodium, potassium, calcium, magnesium, chloride, and dextrose have been added. Bicarbonate is added to achieve the proper pH balance.
5. Through the process of diffusion, solutes in the form of electrolytes, metabolic waste products, and acid–base components can be removed or added to the blood.
6. Excess water is removed from the blood (ultrafiltration).
7. The blood is then returned to the body through patient's access.

Requirements for Hemodialysis

1. Access to patient's circulation.
2. Dialysis machine and dialyzer with semipermeable membrane.
3. Appropriate dialysate bath.
4. Time—approximately 4 hours, three times weekly.
5. Place—dialysis center or home (if feasible).

Methods of Circulatory Access

1. Arteriovenous fistula (AVF)—creation of a vascular communication by suturing a vein directly to an artery (see Figure 17-3).

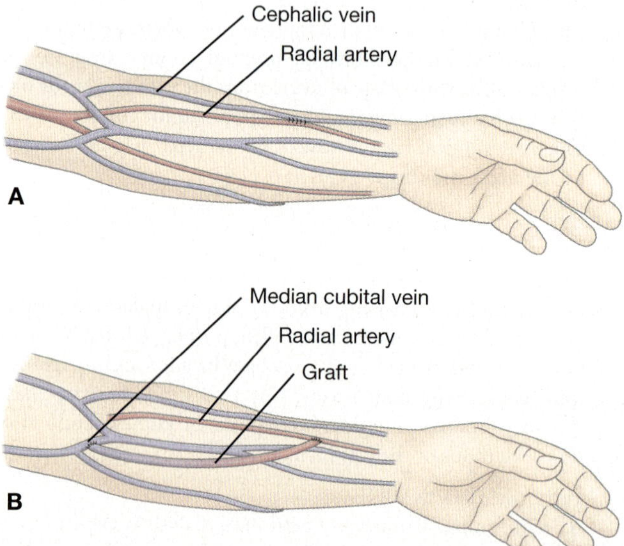

Figure 17-3. **(A)** Arteriovenous fistulas are created by anastomosing a patient's vein to an artery. This illustrates a side-to-side anastomosis. **(B)** Arteriovenous grafts are established by connecting the artery and vein using synthetic tubing. (Reprinted with permission from Hinkle, J. L., Cheever, K. H., & Overbaugh, K. [2022]. *Brunner and Suddarth's textbook of medical-surgical nursing* [15th ed., Fig. 48-5]. Lippincott Williams & Wilkins.)

a. Usually, radial artery and cephalic vein are anastomosed in nondominant arm; vessels in the upper arm may also be used. Leg vessels are used if unable to place in the upper extremity (UE).
b. Over time, the venous limb of the fistula system dilates. By means of two large-bore needles inserted into the dilated venous limb, blood may be obtained and passed through the dialyzer. The arterial end is used for arterial flow and the distal end for reinfusion of dialyzed blood.
c. Maturation of AVF requires at least 6 to 8 weeks; a central vein catheter (CVC) is used in the interim.

2. Arteriovenous graft (AVG)—arteriovenous connection consisting of a tube graft usually made from an autologous saphenous vein or from polytetrafluoroethylene. Ready to use in 3 to 4 weeks.
3. CVC—direct cannulation of veins (subclavian, internal jugular, or femoral) is used for temporary dialysis access. Tunneled catheters may be placed for permanent dialysis access in patients who refuse or are not candidates for AVF/AVG placement. CVC access is the least preferred permanent access because of increased risk of clotting and infection.

Complications of Vascular Access

1. Infection.
2. Clotting.
3. Central vein thrombosis or stenosis.
4. Stenosis or thrombosis of AVF/AVG.
5. Ischemia distal to the vascular access (steal syndrome).
6. Aneurysm or pseudoaneurysm.
7. Hemorrhage.

Monitoring During Hemodialysis

1. Involves constant monitoring of dialysis access, hemodynamic status, electrolyte, and acid–base balance as well as maintenance of sterility and a closed system.
2. Performed by specially trained nurses and dialysis technicians who are familiar with the protocol and equipment being used.

Chronic Hemodialysis Management

1. Dietary management involves restriction or adjustment of protein, sodium, potassium, phosphorous, or fluid intake. Ongoing consultation with a dietician is standard.
2. Careful adjustment of medications that are normally excreted by the kidney or are dialyzable. Certain medications are contraindicated.
3. Surveillance for complications:
   a. Arteriosclerotic cardiovascular disease, heart failure, disturbance of lipid metabolism (hypertriglyceridemia), coronary heart disease, stroke.
   b. Infections, systemic, or localized.
   c. Anemia.
   d. GI complications: gastric ulcers, GI bleeding, constipation, and diarrhea.
   e. Bone problems (renal osteodystrophy)—from alterations in mineral metabolism.
   f. Electrolyte imbalances.
   g. Hypertension.
   h. Hypervolemia/pulmonary edema.
   i. Psychosocial problems: depression, anxiety, suicide, alteration in body image, and sexual dysfunction.
4. Hepatitis B and hepatitis C surveillance. All patients are encouraged to be vaccinated against hepatitis B.
5. Support agencies are the American Association of Kidney Patients (*www.aakp.org*), National Kidney Foundation (www.kidney.org), National Kidney and Urologic Diseases Information Clearing House (www.niddk.nih.gov).

Kidney Surgery

Kidney surgery may include partial or total nephrectomy (removal of the kidney), kidney transplantation for end-stage renal disease (ESRD), procedures to remove stones or tumors, and procedures to insert drainage tubes (nephrostomy). Incisional approaches vary but may involve the flank, thoracic, and abdominal regions. Nephrectomy is most commonly performed for malignant tumors of the kidney but may also be indicated for trauma and kidneys that no longer function because of obstructive disorders and other renal disease. Nephrectomy is also the procedure of choice to remove a healthy kidney for donation to a transplant recipient. The absence of one kidney does not result in impaired renal function when the remaining kidney is normal and healthy.

Many surgical procedures were previously performed as "open" procedures but are now being done with laparoscopic "keyhole" surgeries. An endoscope is introduced, and the abdomen is inflated with carbon dioxide. Instruments are passed through other sites or a sleeve may be used, which allows a hand to be introduced at the operative site. Advantages are decreased postoperative pain, decreased blood loss, and, in some cases, decreased length of hospital stay.

Preoperative Management

1. Patient is prepared for surgery, and consent is witnessed. Preoperative antibiotics and bowel cleansing regimen may be prescribed.
2. Risk factors for thromboembolism are identified (smoking, oral contraceptive use, varicosities of lower extremities), and antiembolism stockings may be applied. Leg exercises are taught, and the patient is prepared for pneumatic/sequential compression stockings that will be used postoperatively.
3. Pulmonary status is assessed (presence of dyspnea, productive cough, other related cardiac symptoms), and deep breathing exercises, effective coughing, and use of incentive spirometer are taught.
4. If embolization of the renal artery is being done preoperatively for patients with renal cell carcinoma, the following symptoms of postinfarction syndrome are observed for (may last up to 3 days):
   a. Flank pain.
   b. Fever.
   c. Leukocytosis.
   d. Hypertension.

Postoperative Management

1. Vital signs are monitored, and incisional area is assessed for evidence of bleeding or hemorrhage.
2. Possible pulmonary complications of atelectasis, pneumonia, and pneumothorax are observed. Pulmonary clearance through deep breathing, percussion, and vibration is maintained. Chest tube drainage may be used in patients who have an open procedure (the proximity of the thoracic cavity to the operative area may result in the need for chest tube drainage postoperatively).
3. Patency of urinary drainage tubes is maintained (nephrostomy, suprapubic, or urethral catheter). Ureteral stents may be used.
4. Respiratory status and lower extremities are assessed for thromboembolic complications.

5. Bowel sounds, abdominal distention, and pain are monitored, which may indicate paralytic ileus and need for nasogastric decompression.
6. For patients who have undergone kidney transplantation, immunosuppressant drugs are ordered.
   a. A combination of medications is used, including a corticosteroid; calcineurin inhibitor, such as tacrolimus or cyclosporine; and mycophenolate mofetil.
   b. Early signs of rejection include temperature greater than 100.4°F (38°C), decreased urine output, weight gain of 3 pound (1.5 kg) or more overnight, pain or tenderness over the graft site, hypertension, increased serum creatinine.

CLINICAL JUDGMENT Use frequent and close observation of blood pressure (BP), pulse, and respiration to recognize hemorrhage (and shock)—chief danger after renal surgery. Watch for pain, sanguineous drainage from drain sites, or expanding pulsatile flank mass. Prepare for rapid blood and fluid replacement and reoperation.

Nursing Interventions

Relieving Pain

1. Assess pain location, level, and characteristics. Transient renal colic-like pain may be caused by passage of blood clots down the ureter; however, report any persistent increasing or unrelievable pain, which may indicate obstruction of urinary drainage or hemorrhage.
2. Administer pain medications; evaluate effectiveness of patient-controlled analgesia (PCA).
3. Encourage patient to ambulate; splint incision to move or cough.

Promoting Urinary Elimination

1. Maintain patency of urinary drainage tubes and catheters while in place. Prevent kinking or pulling.
2. Use handwashing and asepsis when providing care and handling urinary drainage system (especially important for patient taking immunosuppressants).
3. Make sure indwelling catheter is dependent and draining.
   a. Report decrease in output or excessive clots.
   b. Be alert for signs of urinary infection, such as cloudy urine, fever, or bladder or flank ache.
4. Intervene to encourage removal of catheter when patient becomes ambulatory.
5. Maintain adequate fluid intake, IV or oral, when allowed.

Preventing Infection

1. Monitor for fever, elevated leukocyte count, abnormal breath sounds.
2. Administer antibiotics, as prescribed.
3. Assist patient with use of incentive spirometer, coughing and deep breathing, and ambulation to decrease the risk of pulmonary infection. Provide meticulous care to chest tube sites.
4. Change dressings promptly if drainage is present—drainage is an excellent culture medium for bacteria.
5. Obtain specimens for bacteriologic testing of urine, wounds, sputum, and discontinued catheters, drains, and IV lines as indicated. Before removing catheters or urinary drains, disinfect skin around entry site, then remove. Using aseptic technique, cut off tip of catheter or drain and place in sterile container for laboratory culture.
6. Monitor vascular access to hemodialysis to ensure patency and watch for evidence of infection.
7. For patients who have undergone kidney transplantation, provide antimicrobial therapy.
   a. Oral antifungals to prevent mucosal candidiasis, which commonly occurs due to immunosuppression.
   b. Antiviral medications are routinely used to prevent cytomegalovirus infection.
8. Provide regular skin care and assist with hygiene.

Maintaining Fluid Balance

1. Closely monitor intake and output, especially after kidney transplantation.
   a. Expect normal urine output to be 0.5 to 1.5 mL/kg/h.
2. Report oliguria with less than 0.5mL/kg/h or polyuria of greater than 1.5mL/kg/h.
3. Monitor serum electrolyte results and electrocardiogram (EKG) for changes associated with electrolyte imbalance.
   a. T-wave inversion and U waves with hypokalemia; tall peaked T waves with hyperkalemia.
   b. Report arrhythmias or other cardiac symptoms immediately.
4. Monitor BP (goal is systolic greater than 110) and heart rate, central venous pressure (CVP), and pulmonary artery pressure (if indicated) to anticipate adjustment of fluid replacement.
5. Avoid using dialysis access extremity for IV lines, intra-arterial monitoring, or restraints.
6. Although rare, hemodialysis may be required in the postoperative period if the transplanted kidney does not function immediately.

Patient Education and Health Maintenance

After Nephrectomy

1. Provide information about continued recovery from surgery, including engaging in regular exercise, refraining from heavy lifting or strenuous activities, and resuming normal dietary intake.
2. Promote wearing a medical alert device and inform all health care providers of solitary kidney status.
3. Encourage close follow-up and need to seek medical attention for any signs of urinary infection, urinary obstruction, or urinary tract disease if there is only one kidney present to prevent damage to that kidney.

After Kidney Transplantation

1. Explain and reinforce symptoms of rejection—fever, chills, sweating, lassitude, hypertension, weight gain, peripheral edema, decrease in urine output.
   a. Hyperacute rejection—occurs within minutes or hours of transplantation and is rarely treatable.
   b. Accelerated rejection—occurs 24 hours to 5 days after transplantation and is treated by plasmapheresis and IV immunoglobulin G.
   c. Acute T-cell–mediated rejection (90% of all rejection episodes)—occurs days to weeks after transplantation and is treated by IV steroids or additional immunosuppression.
   d. Chronic rejection—occurs months to years after transplantation and results in slowly declining function of the allograft.
2. Observe for symptoms of urine leak, such as sudden loss of kidney function, pain over transplant site, and copious drainage of yellow fluid from the wound.
3. Explain continued protection of vascular access graft, which may still be enlarged, tender to palpation, and associated with edema of overlying tissues.

4. Encourage adherence with laboratory tests (blood urea nitrogen [BUN], creatinine, serum chemistry, hematology, bacteriology, cyclosporine, tacrolimus levels, neutrophil gelatinase-associated lipocalin, and other indicators of kidney damage or rejection), to monitor patient's immune status and detect early signs of rejection.
5. Instruct patient and family about prescribed immunosuppressant and complications of therapy—infection or incomplete control of rejection.
   a. Review immunosuppressive medications in detail, including color identification of pills, dose schedules, adverse effects, and the necessity for taking the medication.
   b. Review other medications, such as histamine-2 (H_2) blockers or proton pump inhibitors (PPIs), to prevent stress ulcers and prophylaxis for *Candida* and community-acquired infections.
6. Review in detail postoperative self-care regimen (may be inpatient or outpatient), including adequate fluid intake, daily weight, measurement of urine, stool test for occult blood, prevention of infection, exercise.
7. Instruct to report immediately:
   a. Decrease in urinary output.
   b. Weight gain, edema.
   c. Malaise, fever.
   d. Graft swelling and tenderness (visible and palpable below the skin).
   e. Changes in BP readings.
   f. Respiratory distress.
   g. Anxiety, depression, change in appetite or sleep.
8. Discuss with health care provider the feasibility of participating in contact sports because of the risk of trauma to the transplanted kidney.
9. Stress that follow-up care after transplantation is a lifelong necessity.
10. For additional support and information, refer to the American Association of Kidney Patients (www.aakp.org) and the United Network for Organ Sharing (https://unos.org).

Evaluation: Expected Outcomes

- Verbalizes relief of pain.
- Urinary drainage clear without clots.
- Absence of fever or signs of infection.
- Vital signs stable; urine output 50 mL/h.

Urinary Diversion

EVIDENCE BASE Partin, A., Dmochowski, R., Karoussi, L., Oetersm, C., & Wein, A. (Eds.). (2020). *Campbell-Walsh-Wein urology* (12th ed., Vols. 1–3). Elsevier.

Urinary diversion refers to diverting the urinary stream from the bladder so that it exits by way of a new avenue. A number of operative procedures may be performed to achieve this (see Figure 17-4). Methods of urinary diversion include:

1. Ileal conduit (or "Bricker loop")—most common; transplants the ureters into an isolated section of the terminal ileum, bringing one end through the abdominal wall to create a stoma. Urine flows from the kidney into the ureters, then through the ileal conduit, and exits through urinary stoma. The ureters may also be transplanted into a segment of the transverse colon (colon conduit).
2. Nephrostomy—insertion of a catheter into the renal pelvis by way of an incision into the flank or by percutaneous catheter placement into the kidney. They are rarely placed for long periods of time; they are a short-term method of diverting urine away from an obstruction or lesion below the level of the renal pelvis.
3. Continent urinary diversion procedures—create a urinary reservoir from an intestinal segment that is either brought to the skin using a valve mechanism that permits catheterization or anastomosed directly to the proximal urethra.
   a. Continent urinary reservoir (Kock pouch, Indiana pouch, Mainz pouch, and others)—transplants the ureters into a pouch created from small bowel or large and small bowel. Mechanisms to discourage ureteral reflux are used to implant the ureters into the pouch, including an intussuscepted nipple valve or tunneling the ureters through the teniae of the bowel. The existing ileocecal valve, or a surgically created intussuscepted nipple valve, provides the continence mechanism. Patient does not have to wear an external appliance, but the procedure does require intermittent self-catheterization of the pouch.
   b. Orthotopic bladder replacement (hemi-Kock pouch, neobladder, and others)—pouch created from small or large and small bowel is anastomosed to urethral stump; voiding is through the urethra. Patient usually has nocturnal incontinence; not all patients are candidates for this procedure.

Preoperative Management

1. Functional assessment should be performed, including the degree of manual dexterity and visual acuity along with cognitive function—essential for stoma care or self-catheterization postoperatively.
2. Patient's psychosocial resources are evaluated, including available support persons, education, occupation, and economic resources (including insurance coverage of ostomy supplies, if needed), coping strengths, attitudes toward urinary diversion.
3. Bowel preparation is performed to prevent fecal contamination during surgery and the potential complication of infection.
   a. Clear liquids only and prescribed laxatives for mechanical cleansing of the bowel.
   b. Antibiotics, as prescribed (nonabsorbable; active against enteric organisms), to reduce bacterial count in the bowel lumen.
4. Adequate hydration is ensured, including IV infusions, to ensure urine flow during surgery and to prevent hypovolemia.
5. The procedure is explained by the surgeon and the WOCN (wound, ostomy, continence nurse) before surgery.
   a. For ileal or colon conduit, the stoma site is planned preoperatively with patient standing, sitting, and lying—to place the stoma away from bony prominences, skin creases, and scars and where the patient can see it.
   b. Stoma site may also be marked, even though continent urinary diversion procedure is planned, in case findings during surgery prevent continent procedure and standard ileal or colon conduit is necessary.

Postoperative Management

1. Patient is assessed for immediate postoperative complications: wound or urinary tract infection (UTI), urinary or fecal anastomotic leakage, small bowel obstruction, paralytic ileus, deep vein thrombosis, pulmonary embolism, and necrosis of stoma.

Types of cutaneous diversions

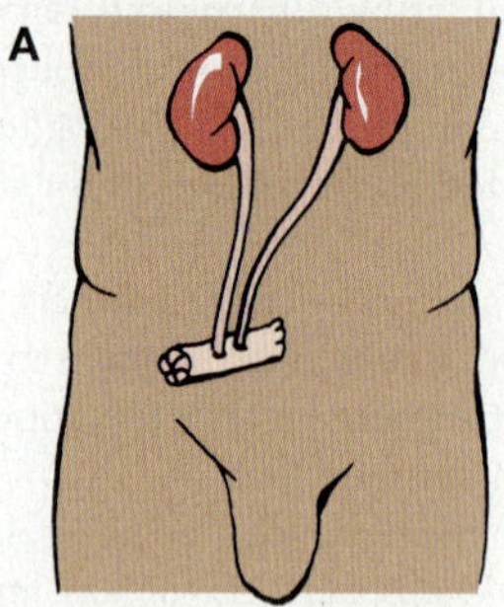

Conventional ileal conduit. The surgeon transplants the ureters to an isolated section of the terminal ileum (ileal conduit), bringing one end to the abdominal wall. The ureter may also be transplanted into the transverse sigmoid colon (colon conduit) or proximal jejunum (jejunal conduit).

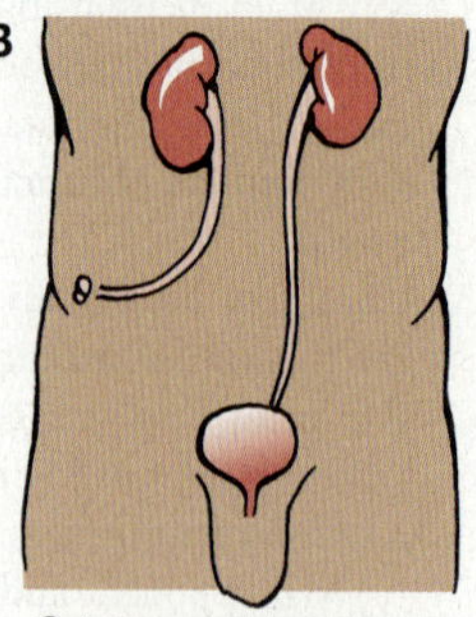

Cutaneous ureterostomy. The surgeon brings the detached ureter through the abdominal wall and attaches it to an opening in the skin.

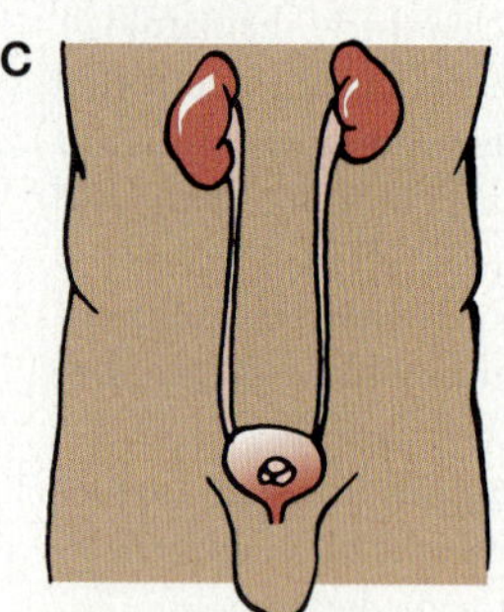

Vesicostomy. The surgeon sutures the bladder to the abdominal wall and creates an opening (stoma) through the abdominal and bladder walls for urinary drainage.

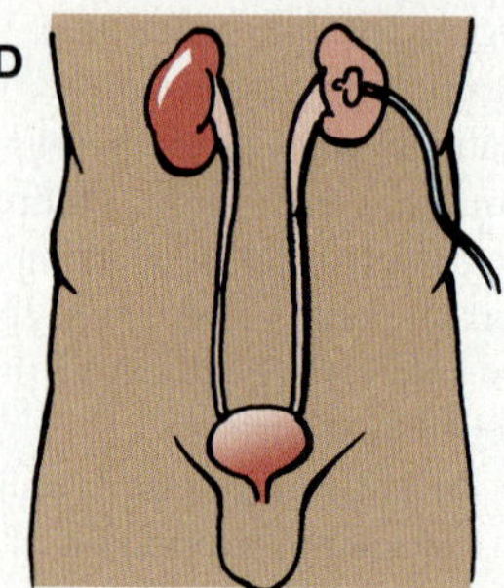

Nephrostomy. The surgeon inserts a catheter into the renal pelvis via an incision into the flank or by percutaneous catheter placement, into the kidney.

Types of continent urinary diversions

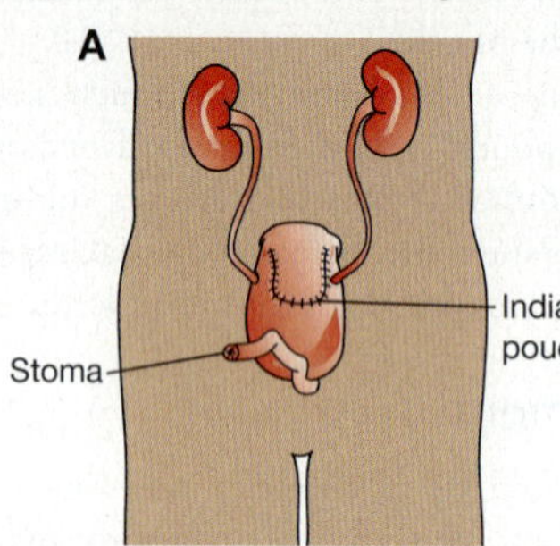

Indiana pouch. The surgeon introduces the ureters into a segment of ileum and cecum. Urine is drained periodically by inserting a catheter into the stoma.

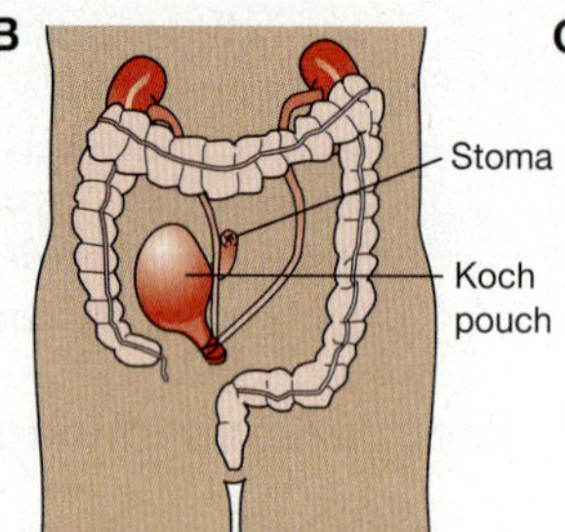

Continent ileal urinary diversions (Koch pouch). The surgeon transplants the ureters to an isolated segment of small bowel, ascending colon, or ileocolonic segment and develops an effective continence mechanism or valve. Urine is drained by inserting a catheter into the stoma.

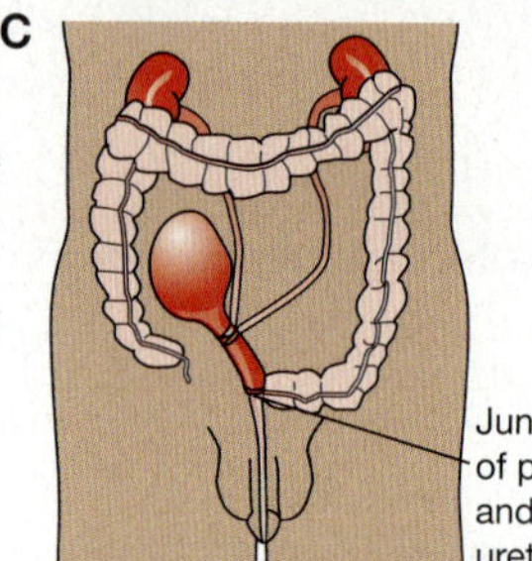

In male patients, the Koch pouch can be modified by attaching one end of the pouch to the urethra, allowing more normal voiding. The female urethra is too short for this modification.

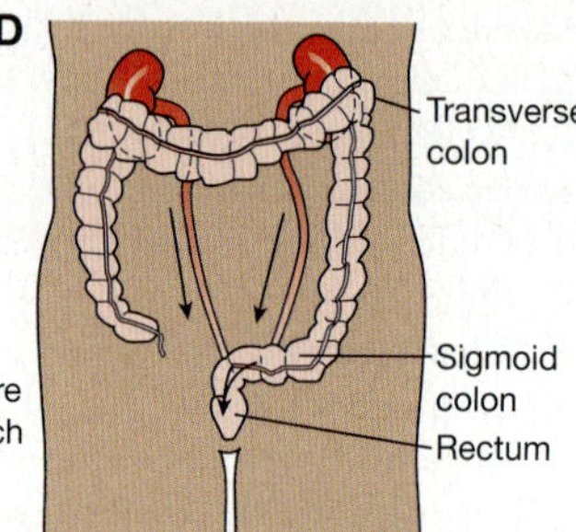

Ureterosigmoidostomy. The surgeon introduces the ureters into the sigmoid, thereby allowing urine to flow through the colon and out of the rectum.

Figure 17-4. Methods of urinary diversion. (Reprinted with permission from Smeltzer, S., & Bare, B. [2000]. *Brunner and Suddarth's textbook of medical-surgical nursing* [9th ed.]. Lippincott Williams & Wilkins.)

2. Intake and output are monitored, including the amount of urinary output, patency of drainage catheters, and degree of hematuria.
3. Pelvic gravity or suction drains are evaluated—sudden increase in drainage suggests an anastomotic leak; send specimen of drainage for creatinine, if ordered. (Presence of measurable creatinine in the drainage indicates urine in drainage, confirming a urine leak.)
4. Ureteral stents are used to protect ureterointestinal anastomoses; stents will emerge from stoma or through separate wound (stents are not visible in patients who have undergone orthotopic bladder replacement). They are removed in 3 weeks.

Nursing Interventions

Achieving Urinary Elimination

For patients with ileal or colon conduit:

1. Maintain a transparent urostomy pouch over the stoma postoperatively to allow for easy assessment.
2. Inspect the stoma for color and size; whether it is flush, nippled, or retracted; and the condition of the skin around the stoma. Document baseline information for subsequent comparison.
   a. Stoma should be red, wet with mucus, soft, and slightly rubbery to the touch (stoma lacks nerve ending, so feeling in stoma is absent).
   b. Cyanotic stoma indicates poor circulation.
   c. Necrotic stoma is blue black or tan brown.
3. Report bleeding, necrosis, sloughing, suture separation.
4. Check patency of ureteral stents.
5. Keep the pouch on at all times, and observe normal urine (but not fecal) drainage at all times.
   a. Connect pouches to drainage bag when patient is in bed and record urine volume hourly.
   b. Initial urostomy pouch remains in place for several days postoperatively; it is changed every 3 to 4 days when patient teaching begins.

For patients with continent urinary diversion:

1. Maintain patency of drainage catheters placed into internal urinary pouch during surgery; irrigate with 30-mL saline every 2 to 4 hours to prevent obstruction from mucous accumulation.

2. Assess stoma—should be very small and flush.
3. Record urine output and character of urine.
4. Monitor output of pelvic drain (on gentle suction or gravity drainage) every 8 hours.
5. Advise patient that approximately 3 weeks after surgery, the drainage catheter is removed from the pouch after a radiographic study ("pouchogram") confirms healing of all anastomoses.

Controlling Pain

1. Administer analgesic medications or teach use of and monitor PCA (IV or epidural).
2. Assess response to pain control.
3. Provide positioning for comfort, alternating with ambulation, as able.

Resolving Body Image Issues

1. Assess patient's reaction to looking at new urinary stoma, if applicable; provide reassurance and support.
2. Be on the alert for difficulty coping, which may be manifested in irritability or lack of motivation to learn.
   a. Give extra support until patient can cope.
   b. Reinforce the concept that the stoma will be manageable.
   c. Acknowledge feelings of fear and anxiety as normal.
3. Encourage patient to participate gradually in care of stoma or catheters.
4. Encourage verbalization of feelings and concerns related to urinary diversion.
5. If possible, arrange for patient to speak with another patient who has undergone the same surgery; this provides realistic expectations and support for a positive outcome.
6. Help patient and family to gain independence through learning to manage the ostomy. Provide for demonstrations, supervised practice, written instructions, and return demonstrations until patient is independent in self-care.

Coping With Sexual Dysfunction

1. Be aware that many males experience impotence as a result of surgery; provide information or referrals about options, including medications, pharmacologic erection programs, and penile prostheses.
2. Allow patient to express feelings related to loss of sexual function and encourage discussion with partner.
3. Tell females that they may usually resume sexual activity after healing is complete.

Patient Education and Health Maintenance

For Patients With Ileal or Colon Conduit

1. Obtain and familiarize patient with the appropriate equipment. Most urostomy pouching systems are disposable. The choice of pouch is determined by location of stoma, patient activity, body build, and economic status.
   a. Two-piece pouches consist of a skin barrier (or wafer) that fits around the stoma and adheres to the skin and a pouch that snaps onto the skin barrier.
   b. One-piece pouches may be precut for the correct stoma size and include the adhesive; the pouch is applied directly to the peristomal skin.
2. Assist patient to determine stoma size (for ordering correct appliance). The stoma will shrink considerably as edema subsides, and the size is recalibrated several times during the first 3 to 6 weeks postoperatively.
   a. Measuring guides are included with most urostomy pouches.
   b. The inside diameter of the skin barrier should not be more than 1/16 in larger than the diameter of the stoma.
3. Teach how to change the pouch.
   a. Change pouch early in the morning before taking fluids or before evening meal—urine output is lower at these times.
   b. Prepare the new pouching system according to manufacturer's directions.
   c. Wash the peristomal skin with non–cream-based soap and water. Rinse and pat dry. *The skin must be dry, or appliance will not adhere.*
   d. A gauze or tissue wick may be applied over the stoma to absorb urine while the appliance is being changed. Keep the skin free from direct contact with urine. Suggest the use of tampons to soak up urine from stoma while changing pouch at home, if desired; however, do not insert into stoma.
   e. Center the skin barrier directly over the stoma and apply it carefully. Apply gentle pressure around appliance for secure adherence.
   f. Apply a belt to keep pouch in place, if desired; it is especially useful in patients with soft abdomens.
4. Advise that additional adhesives, such as pastes or cements, are not usually necessary with a well-fitting pouch.
5. Tell patient that frequency of pouch changes depends on the type of pouch used—generally, pouches should be changed every 3 to 4 days.
6. Advise emptying the pouch when it is one third to one-half full to prevent weight of urine from loosening adhesive seal—open drain valve (spigot) for periodic emptying.
7. Teach how to attach outlet on pouch to a bedside urinary drainage container with plastic tubing (at least 5 feet to allow turning) and how to secure tubing to the leg to prevent twisting or kinking.
   a. Position the drainage bottle lower than the level of the bed to enhance flow by gravity.
   b. Clean nighttime drainage equipment with vinegar and water. Rinse well.
8. Advise patient to drink liberal amounts of fluids to flush the conduit free of mucus and reduce possibility of urinary infection.
9. Teach that the stoma may bleed if it is bumped or rubbed; report bleeding that continues for several hours.
10. Advise carrying spare pouches in handbag or pocket and bringing an extra pouch to every visit with health care provider.
11. Advise wearing cotton (rather than nylon) underwear or the use of specially made underwear for patients with an ostomy that prevents contact between plastic pouch and skin. Heavy girdles are not allowed because they may cause chafing of the stoma and prevent free flow of urine.
12. Advise reporting problems with peristomal skin or with leakage from the pouch or the development of fever, chills, pain, change in color of urine (cloudy, bloody), and diminishing urine output.
13. For additional information and support, refer to the United Ostomy Associations of America (www.ostomy.org).

For Patients With Continent Ileal Urinary Reservoir

1. Teach irrigation of catheter; this must be done every 4 to 6 hours at home.
2. Teach how to change stoma dressing.
3. Instruct in use of leg bag or bedside urinary drainage bag while catheter remains in place.

4. Teach how to catheterize continent urinary diversion when healing is verified:
   a. Red rubber or plastic, straight, or coudé catheters are used.
   b. Apply a small amount of water-soluble lubricant to the tip of the catheter.
   c. Use clean technique; wash hands before each catheterization.
   d. Maintain schedule of catheterizations during initial "training" period to allow the pouch to adapt gradually to holding larger amounts of urine (every 2 hours during day and every 3 hours at night; increase by 1 hour each week for 5 weeks).
   e. After training period, catheterize four to five times per day; pouch should not hold more than 400 to 500 mL.
   f. Irrigate pouch with saline through catheter once per day to clear it of accumulated mucus.
5. Teach patient to report problems such as leakage of urine from stoma between catheterizations.
6. Tell patient to shower or bathe normally, wear normal clothing; only a small dressing or an adhesive bandage needs to be worn over the stoma.
7. Advise patient to drink 8 to 10 glasses of water daily.

For Orthotopic Bladder Replacement

1. Teach patient to irrigate Foley catheter that will stay in place for 3 weeks after surgery; irrigate with 30-mL saline every 4 to 6 hours.
2. Instruct in use of leg bag or bedside drainage bag while catheter remains in place.
3. Instruct on how to change dressing.
4. After healing of pouch is confirmed and catheter is removed, teach patient to "void."
   a. Voiding is accomplished by abdominal straining; mucus is expected in voided urine.
   b. Voiding schedule must be maintained for the first 5 to 6 weeks (every 2 hours during day and every 3 hours at night; increase by 1 hour each week).
   c. Incontinence is anticipated after catheter is removed; usually more pronounced when patient is asleep and muscles are relaxed.
5. Teach patient to perform pelvic floor exercises, which must be done faithfully for the rest of their life; as pelvic floor sphincter muscles strengthen, incontinence subsides. Most patients continue to have small amounts of nocturnal incontinence.
   a. Contract pelvic floor muscles (as if stopping stream of urine or flatus) for 5 seconds; then relax for 5 to 10 seconds.
   b. Repeat approximately 15 to 20 times for one set, and do three sets per day.
   c. May require referral to physical therapist to assist in the process.
6. Provide information about absorbent products that may be used temporarily; also, teach about preventive skin care.
7. Instruct in clean self-catheterization, which may be needed if the urethra becomes obstructed with mucus; pouch should be irrigated with saline if catheterization is necessary.
8. Reassure patient that time, patience, and continued adherence to voiding and exercise schedule will result in continence.

Evaluation: Expected Outcomes

- Urine draining by way of urinary diversion.
- Verbalizes good pain control.
- Discusses feelings about change in body image; seeks support through family.
- Verbalizes reasonable expectations about sexual function.

Prostatic Surgery

Prostatic surgery may be done for benign prostatic hyperplasia (BPH) or prostate cancer. Surgical approach depends on the size of the gland, severity of obstruction, age, underlying health, and prostatic disease.

Surgical Procedures

EVIDENCE BASE Partin, A., Dmochowski, R., Kavoussi, L., Oetersm, C., & Wein, A. (Eds.). (2020). *Campbell-Walsh-Wein urology* (12th ed., Vols. 1–3). Elsevier.

1. Transurethral resection of the prostate (TURP; formerly the most common procedure) is done without an incision by means of endoscopic instrument.
2. Photovaporization of the prostate (PVP) is starting to replace TURP; it is done through a cystoscope, using a laser to vaporize diseased prostatic tissue.
3. Transurethral microwave thermotherapy (TUMT) of the prostate and transurethral needle ablation (TUNA) of the prostate are both office-based procedures that use heat to destroy diseased prostatic tissue.
4. Indigo interstitial laser therapy of the prostate is another procedure that is done on an outpatient basis.
5. Open prostatectomy.
   a. Suprapubic—incision into suprapubic area and through bladder wall; commonly done for BPH.
   b. Perineal—incision between the scrotum and the rectal area; may be done for patients with poor surgical risk but causes highest incidence of urinary incontinence and impotence.
   c. Radical retropubic—incision at the level of symphysis pubis; may preserve nerves responsible for sexual function; done for prostate cancer.
6. Robotic radical prostatectomy uses a laparoscopic approach for removal of cancerous prostate.

Preoperative Management

1. Information about the procedure and the expected postoperative care, including catheter drainage, irrigation, and monitoring of hematuria, is discussed.
2. Complications of surgery are discussed.
   a. For radical and laparoscopic prostatectomy, incontinence or dribbling of urine may occur for up to 1 year after surgery; pelvic floor (Kegel) exercises help regain urinary control.
   b. For TURP and PVP, retrograde ejaculation—seminal fluid released into the bladder and eliminated in the urine rather than through the urethra during intercourse occurs in 75% or patients; impotence is usually not a complication but occurs in 5% to 10% of patients with TURP and PVP and can be as high as 75% in those undergoing radical prostatectomy.
3. Bowel preparation is given, or patient is instructed in home administration and fasting after midnight.
4. Optimal cardiac, respiratory, and circulatory status should be achieved to decrease the risk of complications.
5. Prophylactic antibiotics are ordered.

Postoperative Management

1. Urinary drainage is maintained and observed for signs of hemorrhage.
2. Wound care is provided to prevent infection.
3. Pain is controlled, and early ambulation is promoted.
4. Surveillance is maintained for complications.
   a. Wound infection and dehiscence.
   b. Urinary obstruction or infection.
   c. Hemorrhage.
   d. Thrombophlebitis, deep vein thrombosis, and pulmonary embolism.
   e. Urinary incontinence, sexual dysfunction.

Nursing Interventions

Facilitating Urinary Drainage

1. Maintain patency of urethral catheter placed after surgery.
   a. For TURP and open prostatectomy for BPH, monitor flow of three-way closed irrigation and drainage system (see Figure 17-5) if used. Continuous irrigation helps prevent clot formation, which can obstruct catheter, cause painful bladder spasms, and lead to infection.
   b. If Foley is obstructed and with a health care provider order, manually irrigate with 50- to 60-mL irrigating fluid using aseptic technique.
   c. Avoid overdistention of the bladder, which could lead to hemorrhage.
   d. Administer anticholinergic medications to reduce bladder spasms, as ordered.
2. Assess the degree of hematuria and any clot formation; drainage should become light pink within 24 hours.
   a. Report bright red bleeding with increased viscosity (arterial)—may require surgical intervention.
   b. Report increase in dark red bleeding (venous)—may require traction of the catheter so the inflated balloon applies pressure to prostatic fossa.
   c. Prepare for blood transfusion if bleeding persists.
3. Administer IV fluids, as ordered, and encourage oral fluids when tolerated to ensure hydration and urine output.

DRUG ALERT Anticholinergic medications are contraindicated in patients with narrow angle-closure glaucoma.

Preventing Infection

1. After open prostatectomy, provide frequent monitoring of vital signs, intake and output, and observation of incisional dressing, if present.
2. Encourage ambulation to prevent venous thrombosis, pulmonary embolism, and pneumonia.
3. Observe urine for cloudiness or odor and obtain urine for evaluation of infection, as ordered.
4. Administer antibiotics, as prescribed.
5. Report testicular pain, swelling, and tenderness, which could indicate epididymitis from spreading infection.
6. Assist with perineal care if perineal incision is present to prevent contamination by feces.
7. Avoid rectal temperatures, enemas, or rectal tubes postoperatively to prevent hemorrhage or disruption of healing.

Relieving Pain

1. Administer pain medication or monitor PCA, as directed.
2. Position patient for comfort and tell them to avoid straining, which will increase pelvic venous congestion and may cause hemorrhage.

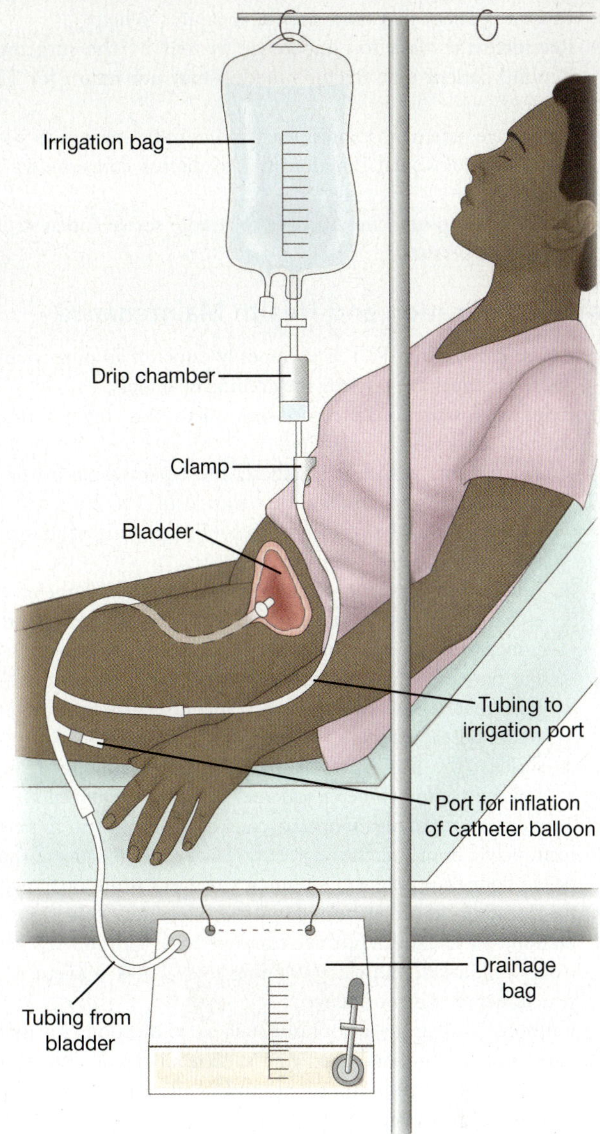

Figure 17-5. A three-way system for bladder irrigation. (Adapted with permission from Taylor, C. R., Lynn, P., & Bartlett, J. [2023]. *Fundamentals of nursing: The art and science of person-centered care* [10th ed., Fig. 38-14]. Wolters Kluwer.)

3. Administer stool softeners to prevent discomfort from constipation.
4. Make sure catheter is secured to patient's thigh and tubing is not creating traction on catheter, which will cause pain and potential hemorrhage.

Reducing Anxiety

1. Provide realistic expectations about postoperative discomfort and overall progress.
   a. Tell patient to avoid sexual intercourse, straining at stool, heavy lifting, and long periods of sitting for 6 to 8 weeks after surgery.
   b. Advise follow-up visits after treatment because urethral stricture or bladder neck contracture may occur.
2. Reassure patient that urinary incontinence and frequency, urgency, and dysuria are expected after removal of catheter and should gradually subside.

3. Reassure patient that there may be measures to help.
4. Reinforce the risks for impotence as told by the surgeon. Remind patient that erectile function may not return for 12 months.
5. Encourage patient to express fears and anxieties related to potential loss of sexual function and to discuss concerns with partner.
6. Advise that options are available to restore sexual function if impotence persists.

Patient Education and Health Maintenance

1. Advise patient that PVP is commonly done on an outpatient basis; patient may go home the evening of surgery.
2. Reinforce instructions provided on catheter care, maintaining patency, and catheter irrigation.
   a. For patients with open, radical, and laparoscopic prostatectomy, the catheter will be removed in 2 to 3 weeks. A cystogram may be performed to confirm healing of anastomosis prior to removing catheter.
   b. Advise that stress incontinence may occur after catheter is removed and is more pronounced when abdominal pressure is increased, such as with coughing, laughing, straining.
   c. For patients who experience urgency before surgery, caution that they may have urge incontinence for several weeks postoperatively.
   d. Discuss the use of absorbent products to contain urine leakage around catheter and after catheter is removed.
3. Teach measures to regain urinary control. Teach patient to perform pelvic floor exercises correctly. Have patient squeeze the pelvic floor muscles (as if stopping stream of urine or flatus) for 5 seconds and then relax for 5 to 10 seconds. This should be done 15 to 20 times, three times per day. Caution against using abdominal muscles (straining or Valsalva maneuver), which increases incontinence.
4. Reinforce availability of options such as medications for urinary urgency and oral medicine such as sildenafil, vacuum erectile device, penile injections, and penile prosthesis to restore sexual function.
5. Encourage patients with prostate cancer to have a PSA blood test 3 months after surgery and yearly thereafter.

Evaluation: Expected Outcomes

- Clear yellow drainage by way of catheter.
- Incision without drainage; afebrile.
- Verbalizes good pain relief.
- Verbalizes realistic expectations for urinary and sexual functioning.

RENAL AND UROLOGIC DISORDERS

Acute Kidney Injury

Acute kidney injury (AKI) is a clinical syndrome in which there is a sudden decline in renal function. This results in disturbances in fluid and electrolyte balance, acid–base homeostasis, blood pressure (BP) regulation, erythropoiesis, and mineral metabolism. It is frequently associated with an increase in blood urea nitrogen (BUN) and creatinine, decrease in glomerular filtration rate (GFR), oliguria, hyperkalemia, and sodium and fluid retention.

Pathophysiology and Etiology

Causes

See Figure 17-6.

1. Prerenal causes—result from conditions that decrease renal blood flow (hypovolemia, shock, hemorrhage, burns, impaired cardiac output, diuretic therapy, and renal artery disorders).
2. Intrarenal causes—result from injury to renal tissue and are usually associated with intrarenal ischemia, toxins, immunologic processes, systemic disorders, trauma, and vascular disorders.
3. Postrenal causes—arise from obstruction or disruption to urine flow anywhere along the urinary tract.

Clinical Course

1. Onset: begins when the kidney is injured and lasts from hours to days.
2. Oliguric–anuric phase: urine volume less than 400 to 500 mL/24 hours.
   a. Accompanied by rise in serum concentration of elements usually excreted by the kidney (urea, creatinine, organic acids, and the intracellular cations—potassium and magnesium).
   b. In approximately 50% patients with AKI, urine output remains greater than 500 mL/day. This is called *nonoliguric* AKI. These patients often have less complications and better prognosis for recovery than patient with oliguria.
3. Diuretic phase.
   a. Characterized by high urine output because of the kidney's inability to concentrate urine.
   b. Close monitoring of fluid volume and electrolytes is essential.
4. Recovery phase.
   a. Usually lasts several months to 1 year.
   b. Complete recovery of renal function may occur, or they may be some residual deficits because of scarring of kidney tissue.
   c. Avoiding secondary insults to the kidney, such as nephrotoxic drugs, contrast dye, hypotension, and infection, is important to minimize permanent kidney damage.

Clinical Manifestations

1. Prerenal—signs and symptoms consistent with hypovolemia may be present, such as decreased tissue turgor, dryness of mucous membranes, weight loss, hypotension, oliguria or anuria, reduced jugular venous distention, and tachycardia. However, if the prerenal cause is related to vasodilation, third spacing of fluid, or cardiovascular disease, signs/symptoms of increased extracellular fluid may be present.
2. Intrarenal—presentation based on the cause; edema usually present.
3. Postrenal—findings may include a distended bladder, an abdominal mass, and an enlarged prostate. Renal colic may be present with nephrolithiasis.

Diagnostic Evaluation

1. Urinalysis—reveals proteinuria, hematuria, casts, increased white blood cell (WBC) and nitrate (possible infection), glycosuria, and pH. Also, can give clues of hydration status (specific gravity).
2. Rising serum creatinine and BUN levels.

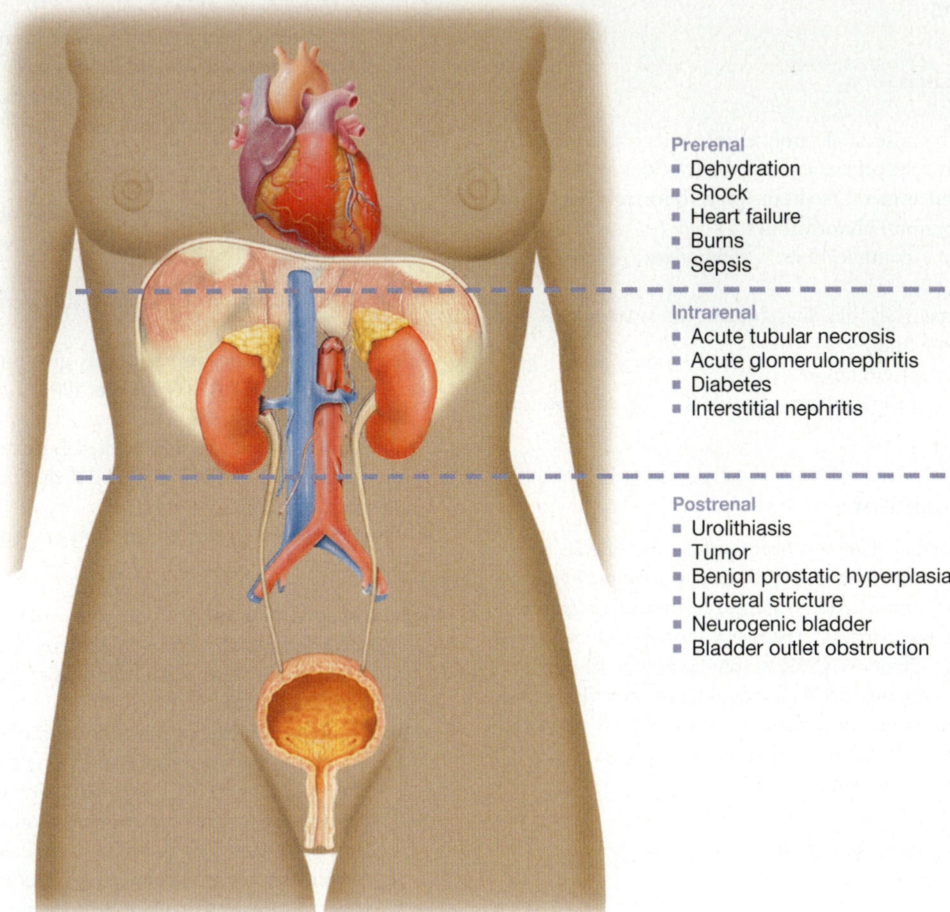

Figure 17-6. Causes of acute renal failure.

3. Urine chemistry examinations to help distinguish various forms of acute renal failure.
4. Renal ultrasonography—for estimate of renal size, to evaluate for masses, and to exclude a treatable obstructive uropathy.
5. Computed tomography/magnetic resonance imaging (CT/MRI) to evaluate for masses or vascular disorders and renal angiography to evaluate for renal artery stenosis.
6. Renal biopsy in selected cases of unexplained proteinuria.

Management

Preventive Measures

1. Identify patients with preexisting renal disease.
2. Initiate adequate hydration before, during, and after any procedure requiring NPO status.
3. Identify and stop nephrotoxic medications when possible. Prevent and treat shock with blood, fluid replacement, or vasopressors. Prevent prolonged periods of hypotension.
4. Close monitoring of urinary output and hydration status (central venous pressure [CVP], edema, pulmonary examination) in patients who are critically ill.
5. Ensure adequate hydration if contrast dye studies are indicated and attempt to avoid scheduling consecutive dye studies. Patients at most risk for contrast-induced nephropathy (CIN) are those with baseline renal impairment, diabetes, older adult patients, and patients with heart failure.
6. Avoid infections; give meticulous care to patients with indwelling catheters and intravenous (IV) lines.
7. Take every precaution to make sure that the right person receives the right blood to avoid severe transfusion reactions, which can precipitate renal complications.

DRUG ALERT Nonsteroidal anti-inflammatory drugs (NSAIDs) may reduce GFR in people at risk for renal insufficiency, causing renal failure.

Corrective and Supportive Measures

1. Correct reversible cause of acute renal failure (e.g., improve renal perfusion, maximize cardiac output, surgical relief of obstruction).
2. Be alert for and correct underlying fluid excesses or deficits.
3. Correct and control acid/base and electrolyte imbalances: hyperkalemia, hypocalcemia, hyperphosphatemia, and metabolic acidosis.
4. Restore and maintain mean arterial pressure (MAP) greater than 65.
5. Support nutrition.
6. Adjust renally excreted medication dosages/frequency. Timing of medications may also be adjusted in patient receiving intermittent hemodialysis.
7. Initiate hemodialysis, peritoneal dialysis, or continuous renal replacement therapy (CRRT) if indicated.

Complications

1. Infection.
2. Metabolic acidosis.
3. Anemia.
4. Arrhythmias because of electrolyte imbalances, including hyperkalemia, hypocalcemia, and metabolic acidosis.
5. Electrolyte and mineral (sodium, potassium, calcium, phosphorus, magnesium) abnormalities.
6. Hypervolemic complications: pulmonary edema and hypertension.
7. Gastrointestinal (GI) bleeding because of stress ulcers and platelet abnormalities.
8. Multiple organ system failure.
9. Progression to chronic kidney disease (CKD) or worsening of CKD.

Nursing Assessment

1. Determine whether there is a history of cardiac disease, hypovolemia, trauma, malignancy, sepsis, benign prostatic hypertrophy, abdominal tumors, kidney stones, or intercurrent illness.
2. Determine whether patient has been exposed to potentially nephrotoxic drugs (antibiotics, NSAIDs, contrast agents, solvents).
3. Conduct an ongoing physical examination for tissue turgor, pallor, alterations in mucous membranes, BP, heart rate changes, pulmonary edema, and peripheral edema.
4. Monitor intake and output.

Nursing Interventions

Monitoring and Maintaining Fluid Balance

See Table 17-2.

1. Monitor for signs and symptoms of hypervolemia.
   a. Crackles on auscultation of lungs, engorged neck veins (jugular venous distention), periorbital edema, ascites, edema of extremities/sacrum.
   b. Elevated BP.
   c. Elevated CVP.
2. Assess for evidence of hypovolemia.
   a. Dry mucous membranes, poor skin turgor.
   b. Hypotension, orthostatic BP changes.
3. Monitor urinary output and urine specific gravity, as ordered; measure and record intake and output including urine, gastric suction, stool, and wound drainage.
4. Monitor serum and urine electrolyte concentrations.
5. Weigh patient daily to provide an index of fluid balance.
6. Adjust fluid intake to avoid volume overload and volume depletion.
   a. Fluid restriction is usually initiated in patients with oliguria.
   b. During oliguric–anuric phase, give only enough fluids to replace losses (usually 400 to 500 mL/24 hours plus measured fluid losses).
   c. Fluid allowance should be distributed throughout the day.
   d. Restrict salt and water intake if there is evidence of extracellular excess.
7. Provide patient education on fluid and sodium restriction, if indicated.

Maintaining Electrolyte and Acid–Base Balance

1. Monitor and replace serum electrolytes ordered.
   a. Evaluate for signs and symptoms of hyperkalemia (see table 17-2 below).
   b. Notify health care provider of value above 5.5 mg/L.
   c. Watch for electrocardiogram (EKG) changes—tall, tented T waves; depressed ST segment; wide QRS complex.
   d. Administer sodium bicarbonate or glucose and insulin to shift potassium into the cells, as ordered.
   e. Administer cation exchange resin (sodium polystyrene sulfonate) orally or rectally to provide more prolonged correction of elevated potassium, as ordered.
   f. Instruct patient about the importance of following prescribed diet, avoiding foods high in potassium.
   g. Prepare for dialysis when rapid lowering of potassium is needed.
   h. Administer blood transfusions *during* dialysis to prevent hyperkalemia from stored blood.

Table 17-2 Signs and Symptoms of Fluid and Electrolyte Imbalances

	DEFICIT	EXCESS
Volume	Acute weight loss (>5%), drop in body temperature, dry skin and mucous membranes, postural hypotension, longitudinal wrinkles or furrows of tongue, oliguria or anuria	Acute weight gain (>5%), edema, hypertension, distended neck veins, dyspnea, rales
Sodium	Abdominal cramps, muscle weakness, apprehension, convulsions, hypotension and tachycardia, oliguria or anuria	Agitation, muscle irritability, dry, sticky mucous membranes, hypertension, tachycardia, edema, dyspnea, thirst, rough and dry tongue, increased viscosity of saliva
Potassium	Anorexia, abdominal distention, intestinal ileus, muscle weakness, tenderness, and cramps; dizziness, hypotension, cardiac arrhythmias	Diarrhea, intestinal colic, irritability, nausea, muscle weakness, flaccid paralysis, cardiac dysrhythmias and arrest
Calcium	Irritability, laryngospasm, positive Chvostek and Trousseau signs, tingling of extremities, tetany	Lethargy, mental confusion, anorexia, nausea, vomiting, abdominal pain and distention, constipation, bone pain
Bicarbonate	Deep, rapid breathing (Kussmaul), shortness of breath on exertion, stupor, weakness (metabolic acidosis)	Depressed respirations, muscle hypertonicity, tetany (metabolic alkalosis)
Magnesium	Positive Chvostek sign, seizures, disorientation, seizures, hyperactive deep tendon reflexes, dysrhythmias	Hypotension, bradycardia, lethargy, hypoactive deep tendon reflexes, respiratory depression

2. Monitor acid–base status as directed.
   a. Arterial blood gas (ABG) or venous blood gas.
   b. CO_2 on chemistry panel approximates ABG bicarbonate level.
3. Prepare for ventilator therapy if severe acidosis is present.
4. Administer oral alkalizing medications or IV sodium bicarbonate as ordered.
5. Be prepared to implement dialysis for uncontrolled acidosis.

Preventing and Monitoring for Infection

1. Monitor for signs of infection.
2. Remove bladder catheter as soon as possible, monitor for UTI.
3. Use intensive pulmonary hygiene—high incidence of lung edema and infection.
4. Carry out meticulous wound care.
5. If antibiotics are administered, care must be taken to adjust the dosage for renal impairment.

Maintaining Adequate Nutrition

1. Work collaboratively with dietitian to direct nutritional support.
2. Protein sources should be of high biologic value—rich in essential amino acids (fish, eggs, meat)—so that the patient does not rely on tissue catabolism for essential amino acids.
3. Encourage small frequent meals if the patient is experiencing nausea or reflux symptoms.
4. Weigh patient daily.
5. Monitor BUN, creatinine, electrolytes, serum albumin, prealbumin, total protein, and transferrin.
6. Be aware that food and fluids containing large amounts of sodium, potassium, and phosphorus may need to be restricted.

Monitoring for and Preventing Gastrointestinal Bleeding

1. Examine all stools and emesis for gross and occult blood.
2. Administer histamine-2 (H_2)-receptor antagonist or proton pump inhibitors (PPIs), as directed as prophylaxis for gastric stress ulcers. If an H_2-receptor antagonist is used, care must be taken to adjust the dose for the degree of renal impairment.
3. Prepare for endoscopy when GI bleeding occurs.

Monitoring Cognition and Orientation

1. Speak to the patient in simple orienting statements, using repetition when necessary.
2. Monitor for and report mental status changes—somnolence, lassitude, lethargy, and fatigue progressing to irritability, disorientation, twitching, seizures.
3. Use seizure precautions—padded side rails and airway and suction equipment at bedside, if indicated.
4. Prepare for dialysis, which may help prevent confusion related to uremia.

Patient Education and Health Maintenance

1. Explain to patient that they may have residual defects in kidney function and that AKI puts them at increased risk for CKD.
2. Educate patient on importance of follow-up with their provider for ongoing monitoring of renal function.
3. Advise avoidance of any medications unless specifically prescribed.
4. Provide education on means to slow the progression of kidney disease in patient with residual deficits in kidney function.
   a. Avoid or minimize exposure to nephrotoxins such as NSAIDs, radiocontrast dye, some antibiotics, some chemotherapeutic agents, and some anticonvulsants.
   b. Maintain good blood glucose control (target HgbA1C of 7).
   c. Monitor for and aggressively treat UTIs.
   d. Avoid intravascular volume depletion.
   e. Smoking cessation.
   f. Low-sodium diet.
   g. Maintain healthy body mass index (BMI) (20 to 25 kg/m^2).

Evaluation: Expected Outcomes

- BP stable; no edema or shortness of breath.
- Serum electrolytes and ABG values within normal range.
- No signs of infection.
- Adequate caloric intake, stable weight, and normal total protein and albumin level.
- Stool negative for occult; hemoglobin (Hgb) level stable.
- Alert and oriented 4×.

Chronic Kidney Disease

CKD is a progressive deterioration of renal function, which, if left untreated, eventually results in death from uremia (an excess of urea and other nitrogenous wastes in the blood) and its complications. The treatment for end-stage renal disease (ESRD) is dialysis or kidney transplantation. According to the National Kidney Foundation, approximately 30 million Americans have some type of CKD. Most cases are asymptomatic until later stages and most people die from other comorbidities (i.e., cardiac disease, diabetes mellitus [DM]) before reaching ESRD.

Pathophysiology and Etiology

Causes

1. Hypertension.
2. DM.
3. Glomerulopathies (from lupus or other disorders).
4. Interstitial nephritis.
5. Hereditary renal disease, polycystic disease.
6. Obstructive uropathy.
7. Developmental or congenital disorder.

Clinical Course and Consequences of Decreasing Renal Function

1. Rate of progression varies based on the underlying cause and severity of that condition.
2. Stages 1 to 5 based on GFR; stage 5 is most severe: ESRD.
3. Retention of sodium and water causes volume overload, which can lead to edema, heart failure, and hypertension.
4. Metabolic acidosis results from the kidney's inability to excrete hydrogen ions, produce ammonia, and conserve bicarbonate.
5. Decreased GFR causes increase in serum phosphate with reciprocal decrease in serum calcium, which can lead to bone demineralization.
6. Erythropoietin production by the kidney decreases, causing anemia.
7. Uremia affects the central nervous system (CNS), which, if left untreated, can cause altered cognitive function, personality changes, seizures, and coma.

Clinical Manifestations

1. GI—anorexia, metallic taste in the mouth, nausea, vomiting, diarrhea, constipation, ulceration of GI tract, and hemorrhage.
2. Cardiovascular—hyperkalemic EKG changes, hypertension, pericarditis, pericardial effusion, pericardial tamponade.
3. Respiratory—pulmonary edema, pleural effusions, pleural rub.
4. Neuromuscular—fatigue, sleep disorders, headache, lethargy, muscular irritability, peripheral neuropathy, seizures, coma.

5. Metabolic and endocrine—changes in insulin metabolism, decreased vitamin D_3 levels (resulting in decreased calcium absorption), secondary hyperparathyroidism (high parathyroid hormone levels), hyperlipidemia, sex hormone disturbances causing decreased libido, impotence, amenorrhea.
6. Electrolyte and acid–base disturbances—metabolic acidosis, hyperkalemia, hypermagnesemia, hypocalcemia (see page 586).
7. Dermatologic—pallor, hyperpigmentation, pruritus, ecchymosis, uremic frost (deposits of urate crystals on the skin from untreated ESRD).
8. Skeletal abnormalities—bone demineralization from metabolic acidosis and renal osteodystrophy.
9. Hematologic—anemia, impaired platelet function causing increased bleeding tendencies, and WBC dysfunction, resulting in a state of immunosuppression.
10. Psychosocial functions—personality and behavior changes, alteration in cognitive processes.

Diagnostic Evaluation

1. Complete blood count (CBC) for anemia.
2. Elevated serum creatinine, BUN, phosphorus, potassium.
3. Decreased serum calcium, bicarbonate, and proteins, especially albumin.
4. ABG levels—metabolic acidosis: low blood pH, low carbon dioxide, low bicarbonate.
5. Spot urine for protein/creatinine ratio. Findings can be validated with 24-hour urine collection.

Management

The goal is to conserve renal function as long as possible and prevent complications.

1. Detection and treatment of underlying causes of renal failure (e.g., glycemic control, optimal BP management).
2. Dietary regulation—protein restriction may be beneficial prior to initiation of dialysis to minimize uremic symptoms. Other dietary restrictions include sodium, potassium, and phosphorus restrictions and possible fluid restriction (ESRD).
3. Treatment of associated conditions:
   a. Anemia—erythropoiesis-stimulating agents, such as epoetin alfa and darbepoetin; oral or IV iron administration.
   b. Acidosis—replacement of bicarbonate stores by oral administration of sodium bicarbonate.
   c. Hyperkalemia—restriction of dietary potassium; administration of cation exchange resin.
   d. Phosphate retention and hypocalcemia—dietary PO_4 restriction, administration of phosphate-binding agents; IV or PO vitamin D_3 or vitamin D_3 analogs.
   e. Inability to activate vitamin D, administration of cholecalciferol.
4. Prevent fluid overload through sodium and fluid restriction. May give diuretics pre-ESRD.
5. Maintenance dialysis or kidney transplantation when symptoms can no longer be controlled with conservative management.
6. Provide patient education on lifestyle measures to help slow progression of CKD (see Acute Kidney Injury, page 584).

Complications

1. Cardiovascular events (i.e., myocardial infarction, heart failure, cerebral vascular accident)—leading cause of death in patients with CKD.
2. Bleeding: GI bleeding, vascular access bleeding in ESRD.
3. Infection: pulmonary, urinary, and systemic; access related.

Nursing Assessment

1. Obtain a history of chronic disorders and underlying health status.
2. Assess the degree of renal impairment and involvement of other body systems by obtaining a review of systems and reviewing laboratory results.
3. Perform a thorough physical examination, including vital signs, cardiovascular, pulmonary, GI, neurologic, dermatologic, and musculoskeletal systems.
4. Assess psychosocial response to disease process, including availability of resources and support network.

Nursing Interventions

Maintaining Fluid and Electrolyte Balance

See interventions related to AKI, page 586.

Maintaining Adequate Nutritional Status

See interventions related to AKI, page 586.

Maintaining Skin Integrity

1. Keep skin clean while relieving itching and dryness.
   a. Soap for sensitive skin.
   b. Oatmeal baths.
   c. Bath oil added to bathwater.
2. Apply ointments or creams for comfort and to relieve itching.
3. Keep nails short and trimmed to prevent excoriation.
4. Keep hair clean and moisturized.
5. Administer antihistamines for relief of itching, if indicated, but discourage patient from taking any over-the-counter (OTC) drugs without discussing with health care provider.

Preventing Constipation

1. Encourage high-fiber diet, bearing in mind the potassium content of some fruits and vegetables, such as apricots, dried fruit, and potato skins.
2. Medications.
   a. Commercial fiber supplements may be prescribed.
   b. Use stool softeners, as prescribed.
   c. Avoid laxatives and cathartics that cause electrolyte toxicities (compounds containing magnesium or phosphorus).
3. Increase activity as tolerated.

Prevent Injury

1. Inspect patient's gait, range of motion, and muscle strength.
2. Administer analgesics, as ordered, and provide massage/heat/IV fluid for severe muscle cramps.
3. Increase activity as tolerated—avoid immobilization because it increases bone demineralization.
4. Check orthostatic BPs. Alert provider to orthostatic BP changes and tachycardia.
5. Monitor for signs and symptoms of bleeding.

Increasing Understanding of and Adherence With Treatment Regimen

1. Prepare patient for dialysis or kidney transplantation.
2. Offer hope while providing realistic expectations.
3. Assess patient's understanding of treatment regimen as well as concerns and fears.
4. Explore alternatives that may reduce or eliminate adverse effects of treatment.
   a. Adjust schedule so rest can be achieved after dialysis.
   b. Offer smaller, more frequent meals to reduce nausea and facilitate taking medication.

5. Encourage strengthening of social support system and coping mechanisms to lessen the impact of the stress of CKD.
6. Provide social work and nutritionist referral.
7. Contract with patient for behavioral changes if nonadherent with therapy.
8. Discuss option of supportive psychotherapy for depression or anxiety.
9. Promote decision-making by patient.
10. Refer patients and family members to renal support agencies.

Patient Education and Health Maintenance

1. To promote adherence to the therapeutic program, teach the following:
   a. Weigh self every morning after voiding and defecating, if needed, to monitor for fluid overload.
   b. Fluid restriction requirements.
   c. Methods to adhere to fluid restrictions: Measure allotted fluids and save some for ice cubes. Thirst-quenching strategies: sucking on ice; sugarless candy or gum; citrus fruits like frozen orange wedges or ice cubes with lemon juice; frozen grapes; rinsing mouth with water; avoiding high-sodium intake.
2. For further information and support, refer to the National Kidney Foundation (www.kidney.org).
3. Encourage all people in the following at-risk patient groups to obtain screening for CKD: older adults, Native Americans, African Americans, Latinos, people with diabetes, people with hypertension, those with autoimmune disease, and those with a family history of kidney disease. More information on the National Kidney Foundation's Clinical Practice Guidelines for Chronic Kidney Disease can be obtained from www.kidney.org/professionals/kdoqi/index.cfm.

Evaluation: Expected Outcomes

- BP stable (less than 130/80); no excessive weight gain.
- Tolerates small meals and adheres to protein restriction.
- No skin excoriation; reports relief of itching.
- Regular soft bowel movements.
- Ambulates without falls.
- Asks questions and reads education materials about CKD and its treatment.

Acute Glomerulonephritis

Acute *glomerulonephritis* (GN) refers to a group of kidney diseases in which there is an inflammatory reaction in the glomeruli because of an immunologic mechanism.

Pathophysiology and Etiology

1. Occurs after an infection elsewhere in the body or may develop secondary to systemic disorders.
2. An antigen–antibody reaction produces immune complexes that lodge in the glomeruli, producing thickening of and damage to the glomerular basement membrane; the renal vasculature, interstitium, and tubular epithelium may also be affected.
3. Immune complexes activate a variety of secondary mediators, such as complement pathways, neutrophils, macrophages, prostaglandins, and leukotrienes. These affect vascular tone and permeability, resulting in tissue injury.
4. Eventual scarring and loss of filtering surface may lead to renal failure.

Clinical Manifestations

1. Mild disease is frequently discovered accidentally through a routine urinalysis.
2. Pharyngitis or impetigo from group A *Streptococcus* (if postinfectious GN).
3. Tea-colored urine, oliguria.
4. Periorbital edema, edema of extremities.
5. Fatigue and anorexia.
6. Hypertension, headache.

Diagnostic Evaluation

1. Urinalysis for hematuria (microscopic or gross), proteinuria, cellular elements, and various casts.
2. A 24-hour urine for protein (increased) and creatinine clearance (may be reduced) outline the degree of renal function.
3. Elevated BUN and serum creatinine levels, low albumin level, increased antistreptolysin titer (increased in postinfectious GN from reaction to streptococcal organism), and, in some cases, decreased serum complement.
4. Needle biopsy of the kidney reveals obstruction of glomerular capillaries from proliferation of endothelial cells.

Management

1. Management is symptomatic and includes antihypertensives, diuretics, drugs for the management of hyperkalemia, H_2 blockers, and phosphate-binding agents.
2. Antibiotic therapy is initiated to eliminate infection (if still present).
3. Fluid intake is restricted.
4. Potassium and sodium intake is restricted in the presence of hyperkalemia, edema, or signs of heart failure.

Complications

1. Hypertension and heart failure.
2. Endocarditis can occur in postinfectious GN.
3. Fluid and electrolyte imbalances: hyperkalemia, hyperphosphatemia, hypocalcemia, hypervolemia.
4. Malnutrition.
5. Hypertensive encephalopathy and seizures.
6. ESRD.

Nursing Assessment

1. Obtain medical history; focus on recent infections or symptoms of chronic immunologic disorders (systemic lupus erythematosus, scleroderma).
2. Assess urine specimen for blood, protein, color, and amount.
3. Perform physical examination, specifically looking for signs of edema, hypertension, and hypervolemia (engorged neck veins, elevated jugular venous pressure, adventitious lung sounds, gallop rhythm).
4. Evaluate EKG and serum laboratory values for electrolyte imbalance.

Nursing Interventions

Maintaining Adequate Nutritional Status

See interventions related to AKI, page 586.

Improving Fluid Balance

1. Carefully monitor fluid balance: strict intake and output and replace fluids according to patient's fluid losses (urine, feces, other drainage, and take into account insensible loss if rapid breathing or sweating) and record daily body weight, as prescribed.

2. Monitor pulmonary artery pressure and CVP during acute hospitalizations.
3. Monitor for signs and symptoms of heart failure: distended neck veins, tachycardia, gallop rhythm, enlarged and tender liver, crackles at the bases of lungs.
4. Monitor for hypertension; observe for hypertensive encephalopathy and any evidence of seizure activity. Hypertensive encephalopathy is a medical emergency, and treatment is aimed at reducing BP without impairing renal function.

Patient Education and Health Maintenance

1. Explain that patient must have follow-up evaluations of BP, urinary protein, and creatinine and serum electrolyte concentrations to determine whether there is exacerbation of disease activity.
2. Encourage patient to treat any infection promptly.
3. Tell patient to notify health care provider of signs of fluid accumulation or uremia (nausea, vomiting, decreased appetite, difficulty concentrating, pruritus).

Evaluation: Expected Outcomes

- Urine output adequate; vital signs stable.
- No edema, shortness of breath, or adventitious heart or lung sounds.

Nephrotic Syndrome

Nephrotic syndrome is a clinical disorder characterized by marked increase in protein in the urine (proteinuria), decrease in albumin in the blood (hypoalbuminemia), edema, and excess lipids in the blood (hyperlipidemia). These occur as a consequence of excessive leakage of plasma proteins into the urine because of increased permeability of the glomerular capillary membrane.

Pathophysiology and Etiology

1. Seen in any condition that seriously damages the glomerular capillary membrane.
   a. Chronic glomerulonephritis.
   b. DM with intercapillary glomerulosclerosis.
   c. Amyloidosis of the kidney.
   d. Systemic lupus erythematosus.
   e. Preeclampsia.
   f. Viral infections (hepatitis B, hepatitis C, or human immunodeficiency).
2. Hypoalbuminemia results in decreased oncotic pressure, causing generalized edema as fluid moves out of the vascular space (see Figure 17-7).
3. Decreased circulating volume then activates the renin–angiotensin system, causing retention of sodium and further edema.
4. Decreased plasma oncotic pressure stimulates synthesis of proteins (including lipoproteins), resulting in hypercholesterolemia. Impaired metabolism and clearance of lipids may also play a role in nephrotic syndrome hyperlipidemia.

Clinical Manifestations

1. Insidious onset of pitting-dependent edema, periorbital edema, and ascites; weight gain.
2. Fatigue, headache, malaise, irritability.
3. Marked proteinuria—leading to depletion of body proteins.
4. Hyperlipidemia (increased cholesterol and triglycerides)—may lead to accelerated atherosclerosis.

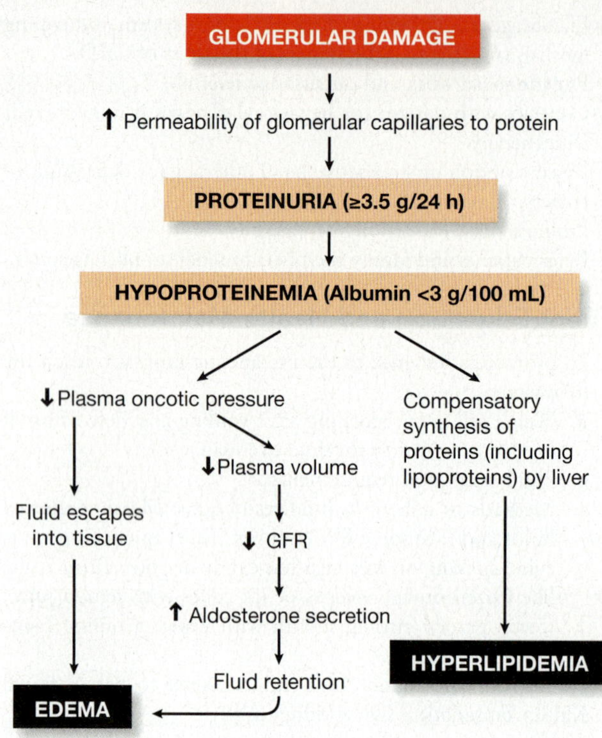

Figure 17-7. Pathophysiology of the nephrotic syndrome. GFR, glomerular filtration rate. (Reprinted with permission from Strayer, D. S., Saffitz, J. E., & Rubin, E. [2020]. *Rubin's pathology* [8th ed., Fig. 22-13]. Wolters Kluwer.)

Diagnostic Evaluation

1. Urinalysis—marked proteinuria, microscopic hematuria, urinary casts, appears "foamy."
2. A 24-hour urine for protein (increased) and creatinine clearance (may be decreased).
3. Protein electrophoresis and immunoelectrophoresis of the urine to categorize the proteinuria.
4. Needle biopsy of the kidney—for histologic examination of renal tissue to confirm diagnosis.
5. Serum chemistry—decreased total protein and albumin, normal or increased creatinine, increased triglycerides, and altered lipid profile.

Management

1. Treatment of causative glomerular disease.
2. Diuretics (used cautiously) and angiotensin-converting enzyme inhibitors (ACEIs) to control proteinuria (ACEI used only in chronic disease).
3. Corticosteroids or immunosuppressive agents to decrease proteinuria.
4. General management of edema.
   a. Sodium and fluid restriction.
   b. Infusion of salt-poor albumin.
   c. Dietary protein supplements if indicated.
5. Diet low in saturated fats.
6. Lipid-lowering agents.

Complications

1. Hypovolemia.
2. Thromboembolic complications—renal vein thrombosis, venous and arterial thrombosis in extremities, pulmonary

embolism, coronary artery thrombosis, and cerebral artery thrombosis secondary to loss of hemostasis control proteins, such as antithrombin III, protein S, and protein C.
3. Altered drug metabolism because of decrease in plasma proteins.
4. Progression to CKD and possibly ESRD.

Nursing Assessment

1. Obtain a history of onset of symptoms, including changes in characteristics of urine and onset of edema.
2. Perform physical examination looking for evidence of edema and hypovolemia.
3. Assess vital signs, daily weights, intake and output, and laboratory values.

Nursing Interventions

Increasing Circulating Volume and Decreasing Edema

1. Monitor daily weight, intake and output, and urine specific gravity.
2. Monitor CVP (if indicated), vital signs, orthostatic BP, and heart rate to detect hypovolemia.
3. Monitor serum BUN and creatinine to assess renal function.
4. Administer diuretics or immunosuppressive agents, as prescribed, and evaluate patient's response.
5. Infuse IV albumin, as ordered.
6. Enforce mild-to-moderate sodium and fluid restriction if edema is severe.

Preventing Infection

1. Monitor for signs and symptoms of infection.
2. Monitor temperature routinely.
3. Monitor CBC with diff as ordered.
4. Use aseptic technique for all invasive procedures and educate patient on the importance of strict handwashing.

Patient Education and Health Maintenance

1. Teach patient signs and symptoms of nephrotic syndrome; also, review causes, the purpose of prescribed treatments, and the importance of long-term therapy to prevent ESRD.
2. Instruct patient in adverse effects of prescribed medications and methods of preventing infection if taking immunosuppressive agents.
3. Carefully review with patient and family dietary and fluid restrictions; consult a dietitian for assistance in meal planning.
4. Discuss the importance of maintaining exercise, decreasing cholesterol and fat intake, and changing other risk factors, such as smoking, obesity, and stress, to reduce the risk of severe thromboembolic complications.
5. In patients with severe disease, prepare for dialysis and possible transplantation.

Evaluation: Expected Outcomes

- Vital signs remain stable, edema decreased.
- No signs of infection.

URINARY DISORDERS

Lower Urinary Tract Infections

EVIDENCE BASE Mayo Clinic. (2022, September 14). *Urinary tract infection (UTI)*. https://www.mayoclinic.org/diseases-conditions/urinary-tract-infection/symptoms-causes/syc-20353447

A *urinary tract infection* (UTI) is caused by the presence of pathogenic microorganisms in the urinary tract with or without signs and symptoms. Lower UTIs may predominate at the bladder (cystitis) or urethra (urethritis).

Bacteriuria refers to the presence of bacteria in the urine (10^3 bacteria/mL of urine or greater generally indicates infection).

In *asymptomatic bacteriuria*, organisms are found in urine, but patient has no symptoms.

Recurrent UTIs may indicate the following:

Unresolved—bacteria fails to respond to antimicrobial therapy.
Recurrent—reinfection after eradication of pathogens.

Pathophysiology and Etiology

1. Ascending infection after entry by way of the urinary meatus.
   a. Females are more susceptible to developing acute cystitis because of shorter length of urethra; anatomic proximity to the vagina, periurethral glands, and rectum (fecal contamination); and the mechanical effect of coitus.
   b. Females with recurrent UTIs typically have gram-negative organisms at the vaginal introitus; there may be some defect of the mucosa of the urethra, vagina, or external genitalia of these patients that allows enteric organisms to invade the bladder.
   c. Poor voiding habits may result in incomplete bladder emptying, increasing the risk of recurrent infection.
   d. Acute infection in females most commonly arises from organisms of the patient's own intestinal flora (*Escherichia coli*).
2. Although *E. coli* causes 86% of UTIs, other pathogens, such as *Klebsiella* species, *Proteus* species, and *Staphylococcus saprophyticus*, may also cause these infections.
3. In males, obstructive abnormalities (strictures, prostatic hyperplasia) are the most frequent cause.
4. UTI is a considerable source of nosocomial infection and sepsis in older adults.
5. Upper urinary tract disease may occasionally cause recurrent bladder infection.

Clinical Manifestations

1. Dysuria, frequency, urgency, and nocturia.
2. Suprapubic pain and discomfort.
3. Microscopic or gross hematuria.

POPULATION AWARENESS The only sign of UTI in the older patient may be mental status changes.

Diagnostic Evaluation

1. Urine dipstick may react positively for blood, white blood cells (WBCs), and nitrates, indicating infection.
2. Urine microscopy shows red blood cells (RBCs) and many WBCs per field without epithelial cells that indicate urogenital contamination.
3. Urine culture is used to detect the presence of bacteria and for antimicrobial sensitivity testing; however, it is not necessary in all cases.
4. Patients with indwelling catheters may have asymptomatic bacterial colonization of the urine without UTI. In these patients, UTI is diagnosed and treated only when symptoms are present.

CLINICAL JUDGMENT Urinalysis showing many epithelial cells is likely contaminated by vaginal secretions in females and is, therefore, inaccurate in indicating infection. Urine culture may be reported as contaminated as well. Obtaining a clean-catch, midstream specimen is essential for accurate results, and catheterization may be necessary in some patients.

Management

1. Antibiotic therapy according to sensitivity results.
    a. A wide variety of antimicrobial drugs are available.
    b. Urinary infections usually respond to drugs that are excreted in urine in high concentrations; a potentially effective drug should rapidly sterilize the urine and thus relieve the patient's symptoms.
2. For uncomplicated infection:
    a. First-line therapy for females with uncomplicated cystitis includes a 5-day course of nitrofurantoin or a 3-day course of co-trimoxazole or a fluoroquinolone such as ciprofloxacin, although fluoroquinolones are often reserved for serious infections. A single dose of fosfomycin has also shown effectiveness in females.
    b. For females over age 65, 7 to 10 days of antibiotic therapy is recommended.
    c. Males are treated with 7 to 10 days of antibiotic therapy.
    d. Follow-up culture to prove treatment effectiveness may be indicated.
    e. Adverse effects include nausea, diarrhea, drug-related rash, and vaginal candidiasis.
3. Pregnant females are usually treated for 7 to 10 days.
4. Females with recurrent infections may be treated longer, undergo diagnostic testing to rule out a structural abnormality, or be maintained on a daily dose of antibiotic as prophylaxis.
5. For complicated infection, see treatment of pyelonephritis (see page 594).
6. For severe discomfort with voiding, phenazopyridine may be ordered to reduce bladder irritation three times per day for 2 days.

Complications

1. Pyelonephritis.
2. Hematogenous spread resulting in sepsis.

Nursing Assessment

1. Determine whether patient has a history of UTIs in childhood or during pregnancy or has had recurrent infections.
2. Question about voiding habits, personal hygiene practices, and methods of contraception (use of diaphragm or spermicides is associated with the development of cystitis).
3. Ask if patient has any associated symptoms of vaginal discharge, itching, or irritation—dysuria may be a prominent symptom of vaginitis or infection from sexually transmitted pathogens, rather than UTI.
4. Examine for suprapubic tenderness, as well as abdominal tenderness, guarding, rebound, or masses that may indicate more serious process.

Nursing Interventions

Relieving Pain

1. Administer or teach self-administration of antibiotic—eradication of infection is usually accompanied by rapid resolution of symptoms.
2. Encourage patient to take prescribed analgesics and antispasmodics, if ordered.
3. Encourage rest during the acute phase if symptoms are severe.
4. Encourage plenty of fluids to promote urinary output and to flush out bacteria from urinary tract.

Increasing Understanding and Practice of Preventive Measures

1. For females with recurrent UTIs, give the following instructions:
    a. Reduce vaginal introital concentration of pathogens by hygienic measures.
    b. Wash genitalia in shower or while standing in bathtub—bacteria in bath water may gain entrance into the urethra.
    c. Cleanse around the perineum and urethral meatus after each bowel movement, with front-to-back cleansing to minimize fecal contamination of periurethral area.
2. Drink liberal amounts of water to lower bacterial concentrations in the urine.
3. Avoid bladder irritants—coffee, tea, alcohol, cola drinks, and aspartame.
4. Decrease the entry of microorganisms into the bladder during intercourse.
    a. Void immediately after sexual intercourse.
    b. A single dose of an oral antimicrobial agent may be prescribed after sexual intercourse.
5. Avoid external irritants such as bubble baths, talcum powders, perfumed vaginal cleansers, douches, or deodorants.
6. Patients with persistent bacteria may require long-term antimicrobial therapy to prevent colonization of periurethral area and recurrence of UTI.
    a. Take antibiotic at bedtime after emptying the bladder to ensure adequate concentration of drug overnight because low rates of urine flow and infrequent bladder emptying predispose to multiplication of bacteria.
    b. Use self-monitoring tests (dipsticks) at home to monitor for UTI.

Patient Education and Health Maintenance

1. Advise females with simple, uncomplicated cystitis that they do not require follow-up as long as symptoms are completely resolved with antibiotic therapy. Males usually need follow-up cultures and possibly additional testing if more than one episode of infection.
2. Instruct patient to void frequently (every 2 to 3 hours) and to empty bladder completely because this enhances bacterial clearance, reduces urine stasis, and prevents reinfection. Infrequent voiding distends the bladder wall, leading to hypoxia of bladder mucosa, which is then more susceptible to bacterial invasion.
3. Instruct patients who have had UTIs during pregnancy to have follow-up studies.
4. Female patients with uncomplicated but recurrent cystitis may self-administer a 2- or 3-day course of antibiotics when symptoms begin, if prescribed.
5. Cranberry juice or capsules may help prevent cystitis by altering the bladder mucosa so that the bacteria cannot attach. Acidophilus and cranberry capsules are available in health food and vitamin stores.

Evaluation: Expected Outcomes

- Verbalizes relief of symptoms.
- Verbalizes self-care measures to prevent recurrence.

Interstitial Cystitis/Bladder Pain Syndrome

EVIDENCE BASE Clemens, J. Q., Erickson, D. R., Varela, N. P., & Lai, H. H. (2022). Diagnosis and treatment of interstitial cystitis/bladder pain syndrome. *The Journal of Urology, 208*(1), 34–42. https://doi.org/10.1097/JU.0000000000002756

Interstitial cystitis (also called *painful bladder syndrome*) is a syndrome of chronic, cystitis-like symptoms in the absence of bacterial infection. It is a diagnosis of exclusion.

Pathophysiology and Etiology

1. The etiology of interstitial cystitis is unknown. However, theories include an inflammatory or autoimmune process that alters the normal configuration of cells in the bladder epithelium, although infectious, neurologic, psychological, and vascular origins are also considered possible.
   a. One plausible theory is a neurogenic origin, in which an initial peripheral inflammatory response later activates the sacral nerves to continue to respond without evidence of continued inflammation.
   b. Mast cell involvement in the inflammatory response also seems a plausible etiology, with many patients having a concomitant history of allergies.
2. The bladder is normally lined with a gel-like substance composed of glycosaminoglycans (heparin, hyaluronic acid, and chondroitin) that act as an impermeable barrier to irritating solutes such as potassium.
3. Disruption to the bladder epithelium leads to irritant seepage, which produces the symptoms.
4. The bladder wall is chronically inflamed with no evidence of bacterial infection.
5. Occurs far more frequently in females than in males.

Clinical Manifestations

1. History of slow, progressive increase in urinary frequency and urgency. Urgency may be extreme; frequency (as many as 16 times per day) and nocturia increase with duration of symptoms.
2. Symptoms of suprapubic pain and pressure occurring for at least 3 to 6 months.
   a. Bladder pain may be continuous, may increase prior to voiding when the bladder is full, or may present as diffuse perineal, vaginal, suprapubic, or lower back pain.
   b. Pain is usually relieved by voiding.
3. Symptoms are exacerbated by sexual intercourse and at the time of menstruation.
4. Symptoms may be present for 5 to 7 years before diagnosis is made.

Diagnostic Evaluation

1. Tender bladder base during pelvic examination, assessed by palpation of the anterior vaginal wall.
2. Urinalysis and urine culture to rule out infection.
3. Cystoscopy under anesthesia with bladder biopsies and bladder distention; presence of bleeding or ulcerations on bladder distention is characteristic of some cases of interstitial cystitis.
4. Urodynamic tests commonly reveal a small bladder capacity with early sensation of urgency and, in some cases, poor detrusor function with incomplete bladder emptying.
5. In potassium sensitivity testing, symptoms are produced when potassium is placed in the bladder; however, the use of this test is controversial as inflammation also produces a positive test.
6. Diagnosis is usually made by ruling out other potential causes of symptoms, including radiation or chemical cystitis, gynecologic or urologic malignancies, sexually transmitted infection (STI), and urolithiasis.

Management

1. Treatment is individualized and focused on symptom control.
2. Dietary modification to identify foods that act as triggers can be accomplished through an elimination diet. Possible triggers are citrus fruits, tomatoes, caffeinated beverages, carbonated beverages, chocolate, and spicy foods.
3. Bladder retraining (increasing intervals between voiding) is commonly necessary to increase bladder capacity that has been diminished by frequent voiding; pelvic floor strengthening with Kegel exercises can help with urgency and frequency.
4. Oral administration of pentosan polysulfate relieves symptoms in some patients, with maximal effect seen after 3 to 6 months; many continue this therapy for years. If no improvement after 3 to 6 months, the drug is discontinued.
5. Antihistamines may be beneficial for patients who have allergies. Hydroxyzine has been beneficial in patients.
6. Tricyclic antidepressants such as amitriptyline may be helpful for their analgesic, anticholinergic, and antihistaminic effects. Gabapentin is also used for chronic pain.
7. Bladder distention during cystoscopy under general anesthesia relieves symptoms in 30% to 50% of patients, especially those with small bladder capacity. Relapse commonly occurs 3 months post-treatment, however, and the effectiveness of this treatment diminishes with repeated use.
8. Intravesical therapy with various substances, including silver nitrate and dimethyl sulfoxide, may be used.
9. Transcutaneous electrical nerve stimulation has demonstrated some relief for the pain syndrome associated with interstitial cystitis.
10. Stress management techniques such as yoga and meditation.

DRUG ALERT Pentosan polysulfate has anticoagulant properties; therefore, it should not be used by patients taking other anticoagulant drugs or in conditions associated with increased risk for bleeding. Reversible alopecia may occur as well but resolves once the drug is discontinued.

Complications

1. Psychosocial problems related to pain, urgency, and frequency.
2. Secondary bacteriuria.

Nursing Assessment

1. Assess voiding patterns, including frequency, nocturia, and urgency (a voiding diary is helpful). Determine whether symptoms increase in relation to certain foods, menstrual cycle, or sexual intercourse.
2. Assess level of pain using a scale of 1 to 10; determine whether pain increases during or after voiding and if bladder spasms occur. Some practitioners may use a symptom questionnaire such as the O'Leary-Sant Interstitial Cystitis Symptom and Problem Index or the Pelvic Pain and Urgency/Frequency questionnaire.

3. Perform abdominal examination and assist with pelvic examination, if indicated, to rule out gynecologic causes and to identify the location of pain on palpation.
4. Assess impact on relationships and quality of life.

Nursing Interventions

Controlling Pain

1. Administer pharmacologic agents, as ordered, to relieve pain and other symptoms. Counsel patient on adverse effects, such as drowsiness, with antihistamines and tricyclic antidepressants.
2. Instruct patient in comfort and preventive measures, such as application of heating pad, avoidance of bladder irritants (caffeine, alcohol, chocolate, and acidic or spicy foods), and avoidance of known allergens.
3. If prescribed, teach patient self-catheterization and the self-administration of intravesical medications.

Improving Urinary Elimination

1. Encourage patient to use a voiding diary as well as a dietary record to make associations between intake of certain foods or fluids and increase in symptoms.
2. Set up bladder retraining program to increase bladder capacity and reduce symptoms.
   a. Have patient start with every 10- to 15-minute voiding intervals during the day.
   b. Instruct patient to gradually (every week or 2) increase intervals by 15 minutes.
   c. The ultimate goal (over a period of about 3 months) should be voiding intervals of 3.5 hours during the day.
   d. Teach Kegel exercises to help strengthen supporting muscles. Warm baths and perineal massage may help with relaxation before exercises.
   e. Make a referral for biofeedback training, if needed, to enhance Kegel exercises.
3. Advise patient to restrict fluids only when necessary because of impending limited access to toilet facilities; normal fluid intake should be encouraged otherwise.
4. Assess patient's response to pharmacologic therapy.

Strengthening Coping

1. Inquire about patient's ability to work and carry on roles as spouse, caregiver, based on frequency and discomfort.
2. Explore with patient positive coping strategies for self and family in dealing with chronic illness.
3. Encourage counseling, as needed.

Patient Education and Health Maintenance

1. Teach patient mechanism of action and adverse effects of pharmacologic therapies.
2. Teach self-catheterization using clean technique, if needed, to self-administer medications or accomplish complete bladder emptying.
3. Provide information about food and fluids known to be bladder irritants.
4. Refer for additional information and support to agencies such as the Interstitial Cystitis Association (www.ichelp.org).

Evaluation: Expected Outcomes

- Verbalizes some relief of pain.
- Verbalizes less urgency, frequency, and nocturia.
- Identifies coping strategies.

Acute Bacterial Pyelonephritis

Bacterial pyelonephritis is an acute infection and inflammatory disease of the kidney and renal pelvis involving one or both kidneys.

Pathophysiology and Etiology

1. Enteric bacteria, such as *E. coli*, are the most common pathogen; other gram-negative pathogens include *Proteus* species, *Klebsiella*, and *Pseudomonas*. Gram-positive bacteria are less common but include *Enterococcus* and *Staphylococcus aureus*.
2. Bacterial infection usually ascends from the lower urinary tract; however, hematogenous migration is possible (particularly with *S. aureus*).
3. Pyelonephritis can result from urinary obstruction, such as vesicoureteral reflux (incompetence of ureterovesical valve, which allows urine to regurgitate into ureters, usually at the time of voiding), other renal disease, trauma, or pregnancy.
4. Low-grade inflammation with interstitial infiltrations of inflammatory cells may lead to tubular destruction and abscess formation.
5. Chronic pyelonephritis may result in scarred, atrophic, and nonfunctioning kidneys.

Clinical Manifestations

1. Fever, chills.
2. Flank pain (with or without radiation to the groin).
3. Nausea, vomiting, anorexia, abdominal pain, diarrhea.
4. Costovertebral angle tenderness (unilateral or bilateral).
5. Urgency, frequency, and dysuria may be present.

POPULATION AWARENESS Older patients may not exhibit the usual febrile response to pyelonephritis but have nonspecific gastrointestinal (GI) or pulmonary symptoms instead.

Diagnostic Evaluation

1. Urinalysis (dipstick or microscopic) to identify leukocytes, bacteria, nitrites, and RBCs and WBCs in urine; white cell casts may also be seen.
2. Urine culture to identify causative bacteria.
3. Complete blood count (CBC) shows elevated WBC count consisting of neutrophils and bands.
4. Computed tomography (CT) scan of the abdomen—with contrast—is the imaging study of choice. Other studies include intravenous urography (IVU) or renal ultrasound to evaluate for urinary tract obstruction; other radiologic or urinary tests may be conducted, as necessary.
5. Blood cultures may be drawn, if indicated.

Management

1. For severe infections (dehydrated, cannot tolerate oral intake) or complicating factors (suspected obstruction, pregnancy, advanced age, immunocompromised), inpatient antibiotic therapy is recommended.
   a. Usually, immediate treatment is started with an intravenous (IV) fluoroquinolone, aminoglycoside, or extended-spectrum cephalosporin to cover the prevalent gram-negative pathogens; may be subsequently adjusted according to culture results.
   b. An oral antibiotic may be started 24 hours after fever has resolved, and oral therapy continued for 2 weeks.

2. Oral antibiotic therapy is acceptable for outpatient treatment.
   a. A fluoroquinolone or co-trimoxazole is used—10 to 14 days is the usual length of treatment.
3. Repeat urine cultures should be performed after the completion of therapy.
4. Supportive therapy is given for fever and pain control and hydration.

Complications

1. Bacteremia with sepsis.
2. Papillary necrosis leading to renal failure.
3. Renal abscess requiring treatment by percutaneous drainage or prolonged antibiotic therapy.
4. Perinephric abscess.
5. Paralytic ileus.

Nursing Assessment

1. Monitor symptoms and assess ability to tolerate oral fluids and food.
2. Obtain urologic history that could suggest recurrent infections or urinary tract obstruction.
3. Obtain vital signs; monitor for impending sepsis.
4. Assess bowel sounds for possible paralytic ileus.

Nursing Interventions

Reducing Body Temperature

1. Administer or teach self-administration of antibiotics, as prescribed, and monitor for effectiveness and adverse effects.
2. Assess vital signs frequently and monitor intake and output; administer antiemetic medications to control nausea and vomiting.
3. Administer antipyretic medications, as prescribed and according to temperature.
4. Report fever that persists beyond 72 hours after initiating antibiotic therapy; further testing for complicating factors will be ordered.
5. Use measures to decrease body temperature, if indicated: cooling blanket, application of ice to armpits and groins.
6. Correct dehydration by replacing fluids, orally if possible, or via IV administration.
7. Monitor CBC, blood cultures, and urine studies for resolving infection.

Relieving Pain

1. Administer or teach self-administration of analgesics and monitor their effectiveness.
2. Use comfort measures, such as positioning, for local relief of flank pain.
3. Assess patient's response to pain control measures.

Patient Education and Health Maintenance

1. Explain to patient possible causes of pyelonephritis and its signs and symptoms; also, review signs and symptoms of lower UTI.
2. Review antibiotic therapy and importance of completing prescribed course of treatment and having follow-up urine cultures.
3. Explain preventive measures, including good fluid intake, personal hygiene measures (wipe front to back), and healthy voiding habits.

Evaluation: Expected Outcomes

- Afebrile within 48 hours.
- Verbalizes reduced pain.

Nephrolithiasis and Urolithiasis

Nephrolithiasis refers to renal stone disease; *urolithiasis* refers to the presence of stones in the urinary system. Stones, or calculi, are formed in the urinary tract from the kidney to bladder by the crystallization of substances excreted in the urine.

EVIDENCE BASE Zeng, G., Zhu, W., Robertson, W. G., Penniston, K. L., Smith, D., Pozdzik, A., Tefik, T., Prezioso, D., Pearle, M. S., Chew, B. H., Veser, J., Fiori, C., Deng, Y., Straub, M., Türk, C., Semins, M. J., Wang, K., Marangella, M., Jia, Z., … Sarica, K. (2022). International Alliance of Urolithiasis (IAU) guidelines on the metabolic evaluation and medical management of urolithiasis. *Urolithiasis, 51*(1), 4. https://doi.org/10.1007/s00240-022-01387-2

Pathophysiology and Etiology

1. Most stones (75%) are composed mainly of calcium oxalate crystals; the rest are composed of calcium phosphate salts, uric acid, struvite (magnesium, ammonium, and phosphate), or the amino acid cysteine.
2. Causes and predisposing factors:
   a. Hypercalcemia and hypercalciuria caused by hyperparathyroidism, renal tubular acidosis, multiple myeloma, and excessive intake of vitamin D, milk, and alkali.
   b. Chronic dehydration, poor fluid intake, and immobility.
   c. Diet high in purines and abnormal purine metabolism (hyperuricemia and gout).
   d. Genetic predisposition for urolithiasis or genetic disorders (cystinuria).
   e. Chronic infection with urea-splitting bacteria (*Proteus vulgaris* and *Proteus mirabilis*).
   f. Chronic obstruction with stasis of urine and foreign bodies within the urinary tract.
   g. Excessive oxalate absorption in inflammatory bowel disease and bowel resection or ileostomy.
   h. Living in mountainous, desert, or tropical areas.
3. Stones may be found anywhere in the urinary system and vary in size from mere granular deposits (called *sand* or *gravel*) to bladder stones the size of an orange.
4. One of three patients with stones are males; in both sexes, the peak age of onset is 40 to 60 years.
5. Most stones migrate downward (causing severe colicky pain when the stone obstructs the ureter) and are discovered in the lower ureter. Spontaneous stone passage can be anticipated in 80% to 90% of patients with calculus less than 5 mm in size.
6. Some stones may lodge in the renal pelvis, ureters, or bladder neck, causing obstruction, edema, secondary infection, and, in some cases, nephron damage.
7. Those with stones for the first time have a 50% risk of recurrence within the next 7 to 10 years.

Clinical Manifestations

1. Pain pattern depends on site of obstruction (see Figure 17-8).
   a. Renal stones produce an increase in hydrostatic pressure and distention of the renal pelvis and proximal ureter causing renal colic. Pain relief is immediate after stone passage.

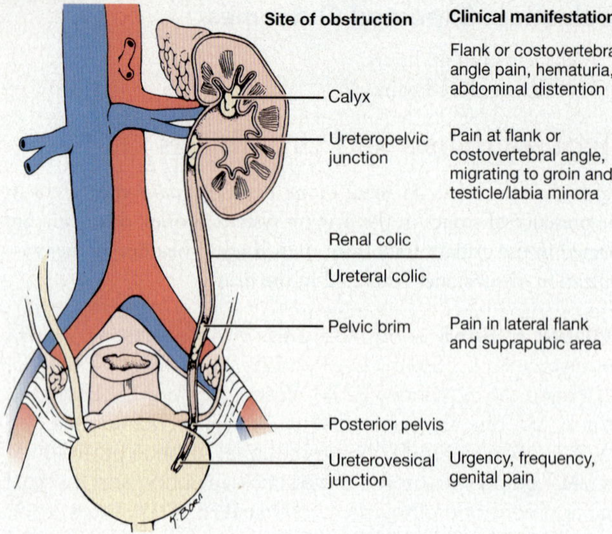

Figure 17-8. Areas where calculi may obstruct the urinary system. The ensuing clinical manifestations depend on the site of obstruction. Stones that have broken loose may obstruct the flow of urine, cause severe pain, and injure the kidney. (Reprinted with permission from Creason, C. [2010]. *Stedman's medical terminology: Steps to success in medical language*. Lippincott Williams & Wilkins.)

   b. Ureteral stones produce symptoms because of obstruction as they pass down the ureter (ureteral colic).
   c. Bladder stones may be asymptomatic or produce symptoms similar to cystitis.
2. Obstruction—stones blocking the flow of urine will produce symptoms of colic, chills, and fever.
3. GI symptoms include nausea, vomiting, diarrhea, and abdominal discomfort—because of renointestinal reflexes and shared nerve supply (celiac ganglion) between the ureters and the intestine.

Diagnostic Evaluation

1. Kidney, ureters, and bladder radiography may show stone.
2. IVU—to determine site and evaluate the degree of obstruction.
3. Regular ultrasound may be as sensitive with good technique; however, it will not show radiolucent stones.
4. Spiral CT scan stone study—special noncontrast CT technique to assess for stone in the ureter; it is the study of choice and will show all stones.
   a. Requires no preparation and is noninvasive.
   b. Takes only 10 minutes.
5. Analysis of available stone material—crystals can be identified by polarization microscopy, x-ray diffraction, and infrared spectroscopy.
6. Urinalysis—hematuria and pyuria; pH less than 5.5 may indicate uric acid stone; more than 7.5 may indicate struvite stone; urine culture and drug sensitivity studies to detect infection.
7. Serum kidney function tests; electrolytes, calcium, phosphorus, uric acid, and magnesium levels; serum parathyroid hormone may also be evaluated.

Management

General Principles

1. If it is a small stone (less than 5 mm) and able to treat as outpatient, 80% to 90% of patients will pass stone spontaneously with hydration, pain control, and reassurance.
2. Patient may be hospitalized for intractable pain, persistent vomiting, high-grade fever, obstruction with infection, bilateral ureteral calculi, and solitary kidney with obstruction.

Extracorporeal Shock Wave Lithotripsy

1. Noninvasive procedure used for both renal and ureteral radiopaque stones less than 2 cm and greater than 4 mm.
2. High-energy shock waves are directed at the kidney stone, disintegrating it into minute particles that pass in the urine. (A shock wave is a large, condensed wave of energy produced by high-speed motion.)
3. Patient is placed on specially designed table and immersed in a water bath or placed on an adjustable stretcher positioned over a cushion of water.
   a. In water bath model, shock waves travel through water surrounding the patient.
   b. In cushion model, a layer of gel lies between the stretcher and water; shock waves move through the cushion and gel.
4. Position of the kidney stone is located by fluoroscopy, and the shock waves are targeted directly at the stone. The shock waves do not affect soft tissue.
5. Eliminates need for surgery in majority of patients and can be repeated for recurrent stones with no apparent risk to kidney structure or function. Long-term adverse effects may include increased risk of hypertension or diabetes.
6. Complications include pain from both the procedure and passing stone fragments, urinary infection, and perirenal hematoma (bleeding around the kidney).
7. Contraindications to extracorporeal shock wave lithotripsy (ESWL) include pregnancy and uncorrected bleeding disorders.

Percutaneous Nephrolithotomy

For stones in renal collecting system or upper portion of ureter and larger than 2 cm in diameter (see Figure 17-9).

1. Under fluoroscopic guidance, a needle is advanced into collecting system; guide wire is advanced into renal pelvis or ureter.
2. Tract is dilated with mechanical dilators or high-pressure balloon dilator until nephroscope can be inserted up against stone.
3. Stones can be broken apart with hydraulic shock waves or a laser beam administered by way of nephroscope; fragments are removed using forceps, graspers, or basket.
4. May be combined with ESWL.
5. Complications include hemorrhage, infection, and extravasation of urine.

Ureteroscopy

1. Used for distal ureteral calculi; may be used for midureteral calculi.
2. Flexible or rigid ureteroscopes are used in conjunction with baskets or graspers.
3. Electrohydraulic, ultrasonic, or laser equipment may also be used to fragment stone.
4. A stent may be inserted and left in place after surgery to maintain patency of the ureter.

Open Surgical Procedures

Indicated for only 1% to 2% of all stones; rarely performed, most likely to be done percutaneously or laparoscopically, if indicated.

1. Pyelolithotomy—removal of stones from kidney pelvis.
2. Nephrolithotomy—incision into the kidney for removal of stone.

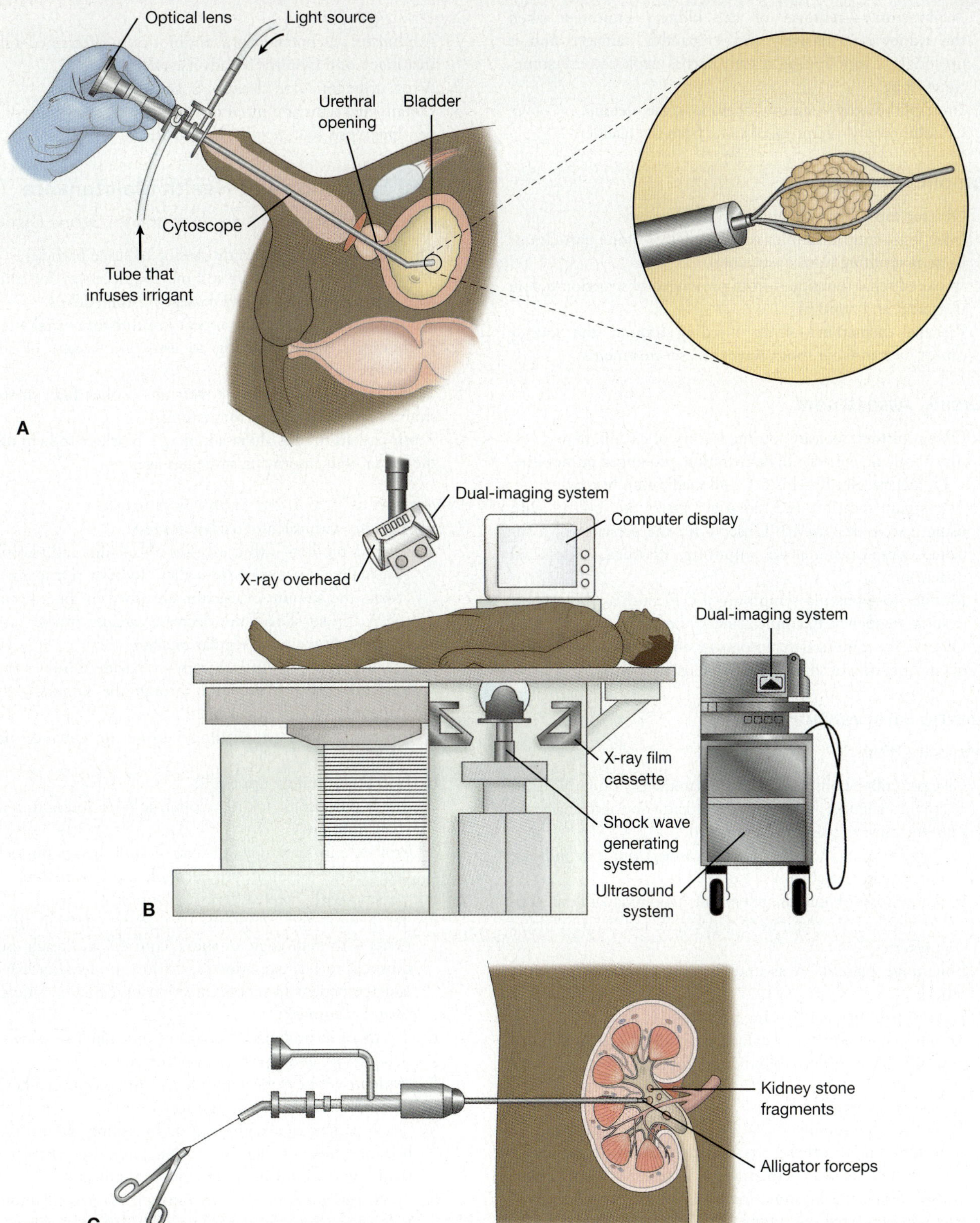

Figure 17-9. Methods of treating renal calculi. **(A)** During ureteroscopy, which is used for removing small stones located in the ureter close to the bladder, a ureteroscope is inserted into the ureter to visualize the stone. The stone is then fragmented or captured and removed. **(B)** Extracorporeal shock water lithotripsy is used for most symptomatic, nonpassable upper urinary stones. Electromagnetically generated shock waves are focused over the area of the renal calculus. The high-energy dry shock waves pass through the skin and fragment the stone. **(C)** Percutaneous nephrolithotomy is used to treat larger stones. A percutaneous tract is formed, and a nephroscope is inserted through it. Then, the stone is extracted or pulverized. (Reprinted with permission from Hinkle, J. L., Cheever, K. H., & Overbaugh, K. [2022]. *Brunner and Suddarth's textbook of medical-surgical nursing* [15th ed., Fig. 49-6]. Lippincott Williams & Wilkins.)

3. Nephrectomy—removal of the kidney; indicated when the kidney is extensively and irreparably damaged and is no longer a functioning organ; partial nephrectomy sometimes done.
4. Ureterolithotomy—removal of stone in the ureter.
5. Cystolithotomy—removal of stone from the bladder.

Complications

1. Obstruction—from remaining stone fragments.
2. Infection—from dissemination of infected stone particles or bacteria resulting from obstruction.
3. Impaired renal function—from prolonged obstruction before treatment and removal.
4. Perirenal hematoma—from bleeding around the kidney caused by trauma of shock waves or laser treatments.

Nursing Assessment

1. Obtain history, focusing on the history of calculi, family history of calculi, episodes of dehydration, prolonged immobility, UTI, dietary, bleeding history, and medication history.
2. Assess pain location and radiation; assess the level of pain using a scale of 1 to 10. Observe for the presence of associated symptoms: nausea, vomiting, diarrhea, abdominal distention.
3. Monitor for signs and symptoms of UTI, such as chills, fever, dysuria, frequency. Examine urine for hematuria.
4. Observe for signs and symptoms of obstruction, such as frequent urination of small amounts, oliguria, anuria.

Nursing Interventions

Controlling Pain

1. Give prescribed nonsteroidal anti-inflammatory drug (NSAID) or opioid analgesic (orally or via IV patient-controlled analgesia) until the cause of pain can be removed.
   a. Monitor patient closely for increasing pain; may indicate inadequate analgesia.
   b. Large doses of opioids are typically required to relieve pain; so monitor for respiratory depression and drop in blood pressure (BP).
2. Encourage patient to assume position that brings some relief.
3. Reassess pain frequently using pain scale.
4. Administer antiemetics (usually given orally IV, but rectal suppository may be given), as indicated, for nausea.

Maintaining Urine Flow

1. Administer fluids orally or via IV line (if vomiting) to reduce concentration of urinary crystalloids and ensure adequate urine output. Avoid overhydration, which may result in increased distention at stone location, causing an increase in pain and associated symptoms.
2. Monitor total urine output and patterns of voiding. Report oliguria or anuria.
3. Strain all urine through strainer or gauze to harvest the stone; uric acid stones may crumble. Crush clots and inspect sides of urinal/bed pan for clinging stones or fragments.
4. For outpatient treatment, patient may use a coffee filter to strain urine.
5. Help patient to walk, if possible, because ambulation may help move the stone through the urinary tract.

Controlling Infection

1. Administer parenteral or oral antibiotics, as prescribed during treatment, and monitor for adverse effects.
2. Assess urine for color, cloudiness, and odor.
3. Obtain vital signs and monitor for fever and symptoms of impending sepsis (tachycardia, hypotension).

Patient Education and Health Maintenance

Recovery From Surgical Interventions for Stone Disease

1. Encourage fluids to accelerate passing of stone particles.
2. Teach about analgesics that still may be necessary for colicky pain, which may accompany passage of stone debris.
3. Warn that some blood may appear in urine for several weeks.
4. Encourage frequent walking to assist in passage of stone fragments.
5. Teach patient to strain urine through a coffee filter or stone strainer and to save stone for analysis.
6. Teach patient to take alpha-adrenergic blockers to help dilate the ureter, thus improving stone passage.

Prevention of Recurrent Stone Formation

1. For patients with calcium oxalate stones:
   a. Instruct on diet—avoid excesses of calcium and phosphorus; maintain a low-sodium diet (sodium restriction decreases the amount of calcium absorbed in the intestine). (*Note:* Patient should not decrease calcium intake; rather, they should maintain regular intake.)
   b. Teach purpose of drug therapy—thiazide diuretics to reduce urine calcium excretion through the kidneys.
2. For patients with uric acid stones:
   a. Teach methods to alkalinize urine to enhance urate solubility.
   b. Instruct on testing urine pH.
   c. Teach purpose of taking allopurinol—to lower uric acid concentration.
   d. Provide information about reduction of dietary purine intake (reduce red meat, fish, alcohol, and fowl intake).
3. For patients with infected (struvite) stones:
   a. Teach signs and symptoms of urinary infection (in patients with neurologic or spinal cord disease, teach use of dipsticks to evaluate urine for nitrites and leukocytes); encourage patient to report infection immediately; must be treated vigorously.
   b. Try to avoid prolonged periods of recumbency—slows renal drainage and alters calcium metabolism.
4. For patients with cystine stones (occur in *cystinuria*, a hereditary disorder of amino acid transport):
   a. Teach patient to alkalinize urine by taking sodium bicarbonate tablets to increase cystine solubility; instruct patient how to test urine pH with a pH indicator.
   b. Teach patient about drug therapy with D-penicillamine—to lower cystine concentration or dissolution by direct irrigation with thiol derivatives.
   c. Explain the importance of maintaining drug therapy consistently.
5. For all patients with stone disease:
   a. Explain the need for consistently increased fluid intake (24-hour urinary output greater than 2 L)—lowers the concentration of substances involved in stone formation.
      i. Drink enough fluids to achieve a urinary volume of 2,000 to 3,000 mL or more every 24 hours.

ii. Drink larger amounts during periods of strenuous exercise and in hot, humid weather because of perspiration.

b. Encourage a diet low in sugar and animal proteins—refined carbohydrates appear to lead to hypercalciuria and urolithiasis; animal proteins increase urine excretion of calcium, uric acid, and oxalate.
c. Increase consumption of fiber—inhibits calcium and oxalate absorption.
d. Save any stone passed for analysis. (Only patients with more than one episode of urolithiasis are advised to have a metabolic evaluation.)
e. Can discontinue urine straining once stone is passed.

Evaluation: Expected Outcomes

- Verbalizes reduced pain level.
- Urine output adequate with low specific gravity.
- Afebrile; urine clear.

Renal Cell Carcinoma

Renal cell carcinoma accounts for 85% of primary malignant renal tumors, occurring twice as more frequently in males than in females. Most renal cell tumors are found in the renal parenchyma and develop with few (if any) symptoms.

Pathophysiology and Etiology

1. Unknown etiology; tobacco exposure, through the use of cigarettes or chew, causes a twofold increase in risk. Obesity and hypertension are additional risk factors for developing renal cell cancer. Exposure to asbestos, solvents, and cadmium also increases risk.
2. Occurs most frequently in persons between ages 50 and 70 years.
3. Early-stage renal cancer usually diagnosed incidentally during CT scan or sonogram for an unrelated health problem.
4. Incidence is 10% to 20% higher in African American males.

Clinical Manifestations

1. Many renal tumors produce no symptoms.
2. Weight loss, fever, and night sweats—from systemic effects of renal cancer.
3. Classic triad (late symptoms, occurs in only 7% to 10% of patients):
   a. Hematuria—intermittent or continuous, microscopic or gross.
   b. Flank pain—from distention of renal capsule, invasion of surrounding structures.
   c. Palpable mass in the flank or abdomen.
4. Hematuria, dyspnea, cough, and bone pain with advanced disease.

Diagnostic Evaluation

1. Ultrasonography—helpful in differentiating renal cyst from renal tumor.
2. Three-phase CT scan with and without IV contrast—primary technique for detecting, diagnosing, categorizing, and staging a renal mass.
3. Intravenous pyelogram (IVP)—used as a screening procedure and rarely performed, IVP alone may fail to detect some renal tumors.
4. Magnetic resonance imaging (MRI)—determines whether thrombosis is in renal vein and evaluates for vascular extension.

Management

The goal is to eradicate the tumor and prevent metastasis.

Radical Nephrectomy

Removal of the kidney and associated tumor, adrenal gland, surrounding perirenal fat, Gerota fascia, and, possibly, regional lymph nodes—provides maximum opportunity for disease control.

1. Performed through a vertical midline, subcostal, thoracoabdominal, or flank incision.
2. See page 577 for care of patient after renal surgery.
3. Increasingly done laparoscopically.
4. Partial nephrectomy is done for localized tumors as nephron sparing.

Renal Artery Embolization

Preoperative occlusion of renal artery followed by nephrectomy—limited to patient with large vascular tumor in which the renal artery may be difficult to reach early in procedure.

1. Catheter is advanced into renal artery.
2. Embolizing material (Gelfoam, steel coils) is injected into artery and carried with arterial blood flow to occlude the tumor vessels.
3. Monitor for postinfarction syndrome (lasts 2 to 3 days)—severe abdominal pain, nausea, vomiting, diarrhea, fever.
4. Complications—arterial obstruction, bleeding, diminution of renal function.

Chemotherapy and Immunotherapy

Renal cell carcinomas are generally refractory to chemotherapeutic agents, radiation, and hormonal manipulation.

1. Interleukin-2—lymphokine that stimulates the growth of T lymphocytes—may offer some benefit to patients with metastatic renal cancer, although toxicity is severe.
2. Sunitinib and sorafenib inhibit vascular endothelial growth factor and platelet-derived growth factors.
   a. Main adverse effects include rash, diarrhea, and hand–foot skin rash.
   b. Possible 3- to 5-month increase in survival.

Cryoablation

1. Freezing of tumor with liquid nitrogen or argon gas through percutaneous needles placed into tumors, using ultrasound guidance.
2. Appropriate for tumors 3.5 cm or less in size.

Thermal Ablation

1. Use of heat through percutaneous needles to cause tissue necrosis, thus killing tumor cells.
2. Appropriate for tumors 3.5 cm or less in size.

Complications

Metastasis to the lung, bone, liver, brain, and other areas.

Nursing Assessment

1. Assess for clinical manifestations of systemic disease—fatigue, anorexia, weight loss, pallor, fever, and bone pain—as well as evidence of metastasis.
2. Assess cardiopulmonary and nutritional status before surgery.

3. Monitor for adverse effects and complications of diagnostic tests and treatment.
4. Assess pain control and coping ability.

Nursing Interventions

Reducing Anxiety

1. Explain each diagnostic test, its purpose, and possible adverse reactions. Ensure that informed consent has been obtained, as indicated.
2. Assess patient's understanding about diagnosis and treatment options. Answer questions, and encourage a more thorough discussion with health care provider, as needed.
3. Encourage patient to discuss fears and feelings; involve family and significant others in teaching.

Controlling Symptoms of Postinfarction Syndrome

1. Administer analgesics, as prescribed, to control flank and abdominal pain.
2. Encourage rest and assist with positioning for 2 to 3 days until syndrome subsides.
3. Obtain temperature every 4 hours and administer antipyretics, as indicated.
4. Restrict oral intake and provide IV fluids while patient is nauseated.
5. Administer antiemetics, as ordered.

Patient Education and Health Maintenance

1. Ensure that patient understands where and when to go for follow-up (surgeon, primary care provider, oncologist, and radiologist for metastatic workup and treatment).
2. Explain the importance of follow-up for hypertension and renal function, even if patient feels well.
3. Advise patient with one kidney to wear a medical alert device and notify all health care providers because potentially nephrotoxic medications and procedures must be avoided.

Evaluation: Expected Outcomes

- Asks questions and verbalizes fears.
- Afebrile; states reduced pain.

Injuries to the Kidney

Trauma to the abdomen, flank, or back may produce renal injury. Suspicion is high in a patient with multiple injuries.

Pathophysiology and Etiology

1. *Blunt trauma* (falls, sporting accidents, motor vehicle accidents) can suddenly move the kidney out of position and in contact with a rib or lumbar vertebral transverse process, resulting in injury. This is the most common injury to the kidney, accounting for 80% to 85% of all renal injuries.
2. *Penetrating trauma* (gunshot and stab wounds) can injure the kidney if it lies in the path of the wound.
3. Renal trauma is classified according to the severity of injury (see Figure 17-10):
   a. Grade I (most common): renal contusion or bruising and subcapsular hematoma with normal radiographic imaging.
   b. Grade II: perirenal hematoma or laceration that extends into renal cortex less than or equal to 1 cm.
   c. Grade III: laceration that extends into renal cortex and renal medulla greater than 1 cm.

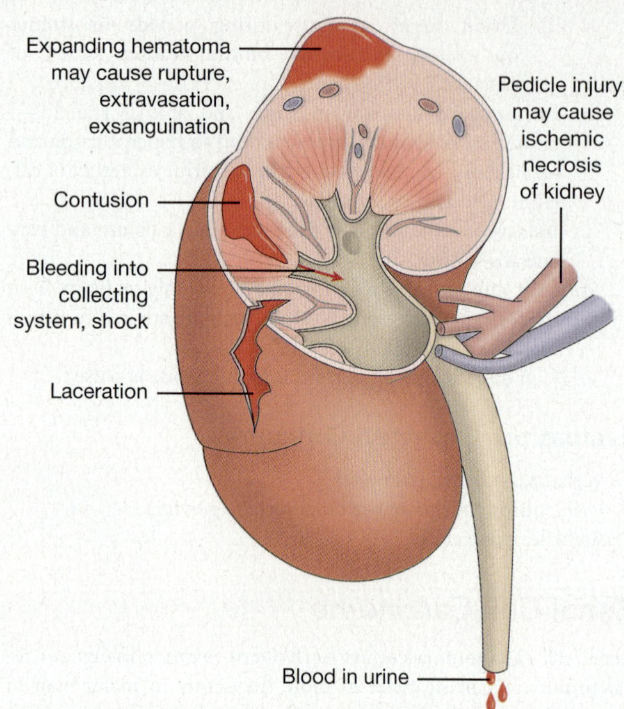

Figure 17-10. Types and pathophysiologic effects of kidney injuries: contusions, lacerations, rupture, and pedicle injury. (Reprinted from Hinkle, J. L., Cheever, K. H., & Hinkle, J. L. (2018). *Brunner & Suddarth's textbook of medical-surgical nursing* (14th ed.). Wolters Kluwer, with permission.)

   d. Grade IV: laceration that extends into collecting system, urine extravasation; requires surgical management.
   e. Grade V: shattered kidney or avulsion of renal artery or renal vein/artery injury; requires surgical management.
4. Eighty percent of patients with renal trauma will have injuries to other organ systems also necessitating treatment.

Clinical Manifestations

1. Hematuria is common but not indicative of severity of injury.
2. Flank pain; perirenal hematoma.
3. Nausea, vomiting, abdominal rigidity—from ileus (seen when there is retroperitoneal bleeding).
4. Shock—from severe or multiple injuries.

Diagnostic Evaluation

1. History of injury—determine whether injury was caused by blunt or penetrating trauma.
2. IVU with nephrotomograms—to define the extent of injury to the involved kidney and the function of contralateral kidney.
3. CT scan with IV contrast—differentiates between major and minor injuries.
4. Arteriography—to evaluate the renal artery, if necessary.

Management

1. Contusions and minor lacerations are managed conservatively with bed rest, IV fluids, and monitoring of serial urines for clearing of hematuria.

2. Major lacerations (grades IV and V) are surgically repaired.
3. Ruptures are surgically repaired, usually by partial nephrectomy.
4. Renal pedicle injury is a hemorrhagic emergency and requires immediate surgical repair and possible nephrectomy.

CLINICAL JUDGMENT If there is a history consistent with renal injury and patient presents in shock, suspect a renal pedicle injury. This is a hemorrhagic emergency, requiring immediate treatment of shock and preparation for surgery.

Complications

1. Hemorrhage, shock with cardiovascular collapse.
2. Hematoma or urinoma formation, abscess formation.
3. Hypertension.
4. Pyelonephritis.
5. Nephrolithiasis.
6. Hydronephrosis.
7. Arteriovenous fistula.

Nursing Assessment

1. Obtain a history of traumatic event and any history of renal disease.
2. Inspect for any abrasions, lacerations, or entrance and exit wounds to upper abdomen or lower thorax.
3. Monitor BP and pulse to assess for bleeding and impending shock; perirenal hemorrhage may cause rapid exsanguination.
4. Assess for the presence and degree of hematuria.

CLINICAL JUDGMENT Watch for any *sudden* change in patient's condition—drop in BP, increasing flank or abdominal pain and tenderness, or palpable mass in the flank. May indicate hemorrhage, which requires surgical intervention.

Nursing Interventions

Restoring and Maintaining Renal Perfusion

1. Assess vital signs frequently, including BP, heart rate, and central venous pressure (CVP) to monitor for hemorrhage and impending shock.
2. Assess abdomen and back for local tenderness and palpable mass, swelling, and ecchymosis, indicating hemorrhage or urine extravasation.
3. Outline original mass with marking pen for future comparison of size.
4. Establish IV access for support of BP with fluids or vasopressors, replacement of blood, and perfusion of kidneys.
5. Monitor serial hematocrit determinations to be sure that bleeding has stopped.

Preserving Urinary Elimination

1. Save, inspect, and compare each urine specimen—to follow the course and degree of hematuria.
   a. Label each specimen with date and time.
   b. If specimen is not grossly bloody, dipstick for blood or send to laboratory for microscopic examination.
2. Monitor intake and output carefully.
3. Give antibiotics, as directed, to discourage infection from perirenal hematoma or urinoma or severely contaminated wounds.
4. Monitor for paralytic ileus (lack of bowel sounds) caused by retroperitoneal bleeding.
   a. Keep patient NPO until bowel sounds return.
   b. Administer IV fluids to maintain urine output.

Controlling Pain

1. Administer analgesic medication, as prescribed; exercise caution with drugs that may aggravate hypotension or mask complications of hemorrhage.
2. Encourage bed rest and positioning of comfort until hematuria clears to facilitate healing of minor injuries.
3. Expect a low-grade fever with retroperitoneal hematomas as absorption of the clot occurs; administer antipyretics, as ordered, for comfort.

Patient Education and Health Maintenance

1. Instruct patient not to engage in strenuous activity for at least 1 month after blunt trauma to minimize incidence of delayed or secondary bleeding.
2. Teach patient signs and symptoms of late complications—infection and nephrolithiasis.
3. Advise patient to have BP measured frequently and consistently to monitor for hypertension.
4. Review safety precautions to prevent future injuries.

Evaluation: Expected Outcomes

- Vital signs stable.
- Serial urines clearing.
- Reports decreased pain.

Injuries to the Bladder and Urethra

Injuries to the bladder and urethra commonly occur along with pelvic fracture or may be due to surgical interventions.

Pathophysiology and Etiology

1. Bladder injuries are classified as follows:
   a. Contusion of the bladder.
   b. Intraperitoneal rupture.
   c. Extraperitoneal rupture.
   d. Combination of intraperitoneal and extraperitoneal bladder rupture.
2. Urethral injuries (occurring almost exclusively in men) are classified as follows:
   a. Partial or complete rupture.
   b. Anterior or posterior urethral rupture.
3. Injuries to the bladder and urethra are commonly associated with pelvic fractures and multiple trauma.
4. Certain surgical procedures (endoscopic urologic procedures, gynecologic surgery, surgery of the lower colon and rectum) also carry a risk of trauma to the bladder and urethra.
5. Intraperitoneal bladder rupture occurs when the bladder is full of urine and the lower abdomen sustains blunt trauma. The bladder ruptures at its weakest point, the dome. Urine and blood extravasate into the peritoneal cavity.
6. Extraperitoneal bladder rupture occurs when the lower bladder is perforated by a bony fragment during pelvic fracture or with a sharp instrument during surgery. Urine and blood extravasate into the pelvic cavity.
7. Urethral rupture occurs during pelvic fracture (posterior) or when the urethra or penis is manipulated accidentally during surgery or injury (anterior).

Clinical Manifestations

1. Inability to void.
2. Gross hematuria; presence of blood at urinary meatus may indicate ruptured urethra.
3. Shock and hemorrhage—pallor, rapid and increasing pulse rate.
4. Suprapubic pain and tenderness.
5. Rigid abdomen—indicates intraperitoneal rupture.
6. Absence of prostate on rectal examination in posterior urethral rupture.
7. Swelling or discoloration of the penis, scrotum, and anterior perineum in anterior urethral rupture.

Diagnostic Evaluation

1. Retrograde urethrogram—to detect rupture of the urethra.
2. Cystogram—to detect and localize perforation/rupture of the bladder.
3. Plain film of the abdomen—may show associated pelvic fracture.
4. Abdominal CT with contrast—best study to evaluate the extent of kidney injury.
5. Excretory urogram—to survey the kidneys and ureters for injury.

Management

Bladder Injury

1. Treatment instituted for shock and hemorrhage.
2. Surgical intervention carried out for intraperitoneal bladder rupture. Extravasated blood and urine will first be drained and urine diverted with suprapubic cystostomy or indwelling catheter.
3. Small extraperitoneal bladder ruptures will heal spontaneously with indwelling suprapubic or urethral catheter drainage. If ruptured urethra is suspected and/or blood at meatus observed, do not catheterize because doing so may complete a partial urethral rupture. A urethrogram must be obtained first to determine patency of the urethra.
4. Large extraperitoneal bladder ruptures are repaired surgically.

Urethral Injury Management—Controversial

1. Immediate repair—the urethra is manipulated into its correct anatomic position with reanastomosis after evacuation of hematoma.
2. Delayed repair—suprapubic cystostomy drainage for 6 to 12 weeks allows the urethra to realign itself while hematoma and edema resolve; then, surgical reanastomosis.
3. Two-stage urethroplasty—reconstruction of the urethra occurs in two separate surgeries with urinary elimination diverted until final procedure.

Complications

1. Shock, hemorrhage, peritonitis.
2. UTI.
3. Urethral stricture disease.
4. Impotence.
5. Incontinence.

Nursing Assessment

1. Obtain vital signs; assess for evidence of shock.
2. Obtain detailed history of injury, if possible.
3. Inspect urinary meatus for evidence of bleeding. If present, do not insert Foley until retrograde urethrogram verifies patent urethra.
4. Perform physical examination for symptoms of bladder rupture, dullness to palpation, and rebound tenderness or rigidity.

Nursing Interventions

Stabilizing Circulatory Volume

1. Monitor vital signs and CVP frequently, as indicated by condition.
2. Establish IV access and replace blood and fluids, as ordered.

Facilitating Urinary Elimination

1. Inspect urethral meatus for blood and, if present, do not catheterize but prepare for diagnostic evaluation and suprapubic cystostomy.
2. Obtain urine specimen, if possible, and assess for the degree of hematuria and presence of infection.
3. Prepare patient for surgical repair by assisting with preoperative workup and describing postoperative experiences.
4. Postoperatively, maintain patency and flow of indwelling urinary catheters.
5. Inspect suprapubic incision and Penrose drains from perivesical areas for bleeding, extravasation of urine, or signs of infection.

Controlling Pain

1. Administer analgesics, as ordered (when patient's vital signs are stable).
2. Assess patient's response to pain control medications.
3. Position for comfort (usually semi-Fowler position), if not contraindicated by other injuries, and prevent pulling of catheter tubing.

Relieving Fear

1. Provide information to the conscious patient throughout the stabilization and evaluation phase; prepare for surgery, if impending.
2. Keep patient's family or significant others informed of condition and progress.
3. Provide information on long-term outcome of treatment.

Patient Education and Health Maintenance

1. Teach patient to care for indwelling catheters that will remain in place during healing or after surgery.
   a. Empty catheter frequently.
   b. Clean catheter and insertion area with soap and water.
   c. Inspect urine for blood, cloudiness, or concentration.
   d. Drink plenty of fluids to keep urine flowing.
2. Teach patient to report signs and symptoms of UTI.
3. Instruct patient (after surgical repair of bladder rupture) that bladder capacity may be temporarily decreased, causing frequency and nocturia; this resolves over time.
4. Explain possibility of recurrent urethral stricture disease to patients with urethral injury; instruct in daily self-catheterization to dilate the urethra, if prescribed.
5. Support patient (after severe urethral injury) if there is a chance of impotence or incontinence.

Evaluation: Expected Outcomes

- Vital signs stable.
- Adequate urine output by way of catheter.
- Verbalizes relief of pain.
- Verbalizes reduction in fear.

Cancer of the Bladder

Cancer of the bladder is the second most common urologic malignancy. Approximately 90% of all bladder cancers are transitional cell carcinomas, which arise from the epithelial lining of the urinary tract; transitional cell tumors can also occur in the ureters, renal pelvis, and urethra. The remaining 10% of bladder cancers are adenocarcinoma, squamous cell carcinoma, or sarcoma.

Pathophysiology and Etiology

1. Many bladder tumors are diagnosed when the lesions are superficial; papillary tumors are easily resected.
2. One fourth of patients with bladder cancer present with nonpapillary, muscle invasive disease.
3. Bladder tumors tend to be either low-grade superficial tumors or high-grade invasive cancers.
4. Metastasis occurs in the bladder wall and pelvis, para-aortic or supraclavicular nodes, liver, lungs, and bone.
5. Although the specific etiology is unknown, it appears that multiple agents are linked to the development of cancer of the bladder, including:
   a. Cigarette smoking—the risk of developing bladder cancer is up to four times higher in those who smoke.
   b. Prolonged exposure to aromatic amines or their metabolites—generally dyes manufactured by the chemical industry and used by other industries.
   c. Exposure to cyclophosphamide, radiation therapy to the pelvis, chronic irritation of the bladder (as in long-term indwelling catheterization), and excessive use of the analgesic drug phenacetin, which has been taken off the market.
6. Bladder cancer is the fourth most common cancer in men; it occurs four times more frequently in males than in females; peak incidence occurs in the sixth to eighth decades.

Clinical Manifestations

1. Painless hematuria, either gross or microscopic—most characteristic sign.
2. Dysuria, frequency, urgency—bladder irritability.
3. Pelvic or flank pain—obstruction or distant metastases.
4. Leg edema—from invasion of pelvic lymph nodes.

Diagnostic Evaluation

1. Cystoscopy for visualization of number, location, and appearance of tumors; for biopsy.
2. Urine and bladder washing for cytologic study.
3. Urine for flow cytometry—uses a computer-controlled fluorescence microscope to scan and image the nucleus of each cell on a slide; based on the fact that cancer cells contain abnormally large amounts of DNA.
4. IVU—may reveal filling defect indicative of bladder tumor; also determines status of upper tracts.
5. CT urography (three-phase CT scan)—replacing IVU or IVP as the test of choice to evaluate kidneys, ureter, and bladder.
6. To evaluate for metastatic disease:
   a. CT scan or MRI—to evaluate the extent of disease and tumor responsiveness.
   b. Chest x-ray—to evaluate for pulmonary metastases.
   c. Pelvic lymphadenectomy (during cystectomy)—most accurate for staging.

Management

Surgery

1. Transurethral resection and fulguration—endoscopic resection for superficial tumors.
   a. May be followed by intravesical chemotherapy to prevent tumor recurrence.
   b. Complications include hemorrhage, infection, bladder perforation, and temporary irritative voiding.
   c. Laser irradiation of bladder tumors is also used to destroy tumors; however, it does not allow for tumor specimen collection for pathologic analysis.
2. Partial cystectomy when lesions are located only in the dome of the bladder, away from the ureteral orifices.
3. Radical cystectomy (removal of the bladder) for invasive or poorly differentiated tumors.
   a. Requires diversion of the urinary stream (see page 579).
   b. In males, includes removal of the bladder, prostate and seminal vesicles, proximal vas deferens, and part of proximal urethra.
   c. Males may be impotent.
   d. In females, consists of anterior exenteration with removal of the bladder, urethra, uterus, fallopian tubes, ovaries, and segment of anterior wall of the vagina.
   e. May be combined with chemotherapy and radiation.

Intravesical (Within the Bladder) Chemotherapy and Immunotherapy

1. Instillation of immunotherapeutic agent bacillus Calmette-Guérin (BCG) stimulates immune response to prevent recurrence of transitional cell bladder tumors. BCG is attenuated mycobacterium initially developed as a vaccine for tuberculosis and has demonstrated antitumor activity in selected cancers.
2. Instillation of antineoplastic agents, such as thiotepa, mitomycin-C, and doxorubicin, allows a high concentration of drug to come in contact with the tumor and urothelium with minimal systemic toxicity.
3. Patient is instructed as follows:
   a. Minimize fluid intake and avoid taking diuretic medications for several hours before the instillation period to maximize concentration of drug treatment period.
   b. Change position, as directed during instillation, in an effort to have drug contact as much of urothelial surface as possible.
   c. Wash hands and perineal area after voiding the medication to prevent contact dermatitis.
   d. Do not void for 2 hours after instillation; then, increase fluid intake and void frequently.
   e. When using BCG, place two cups of bleach into toilet with each void for 6 hours after starting voiding to neutralize the chemotherapeutic agent and prevent possible contamination to others.
   f. Course of treatment involves weekly instillations for 6 weeks followed by monthly instillations.
4. Complications from intravesical chemotherapy and immunotherapy include UTI, irritative voiding symptoms, allergic reaction, bone marrow suppression, or systemic BCG reaction. A systemic BCG reaction occurs when fever higher than 100°F (37.8°C) persists for more than 24 hours; it is treated with antituberculosis agents.

Systemic Chemotherapy

Metastatic bladder cancer is a chemotherapeutically responsive disease; gemcitabine and cisplatin have lower toxicity, improved tolerability, and similar overall survival to the MVDC combination (methotrexate, vinblastine, doxorubicin, and cisplatin), which had been in wide use.

Radiation Therapy

External beam radiation therapy is commonly used in combination with chemotherapy.

Complications

Regional metastasis through the pelvis as well as metastasis to the lung, liver, and bone.

Nursing Assessment

1. Assess for hematuria, irritative voiding symptoms, risk factors (especially smoking history), weight loss, fatigue, and signs of metastasis.
2. Assess coping ability and knowledge of the disease and explore feelings about impotence.

Nursing Interventions

Maintaining Urinary Elimination After Transurethral Surgery

1. Maintain patency of indwelling urinary drainage catheter; manual irrigation is not recommended due to dangers of bladder perforation; continuous bladder irrigation may be used, if necessary.
2. Ensure adequate hydration either orally or via IV line.
3. Monitor intake and output, including irrigation solution.
4. Monitor urine output for clearing of hematuria.

Controlling Pain

1. Administer analgesic medication for pelvic discomfort.
2. Administer anticholinergic medications or belladonna and opium suppositories to relieve bladder spasms.
3. Ensure patency of catheter drainage; do not irrigate unless specifically ordered.
4. Remove indwelling catheter as soon as possible after procedure.

Relieving Anxiety

1. Allow patient to verbalize fears and concerns about altered sexuality.
2. Provide realistic information about diagnostic studies, surgery, and treatments.

Patient Education and Health Maintenance

1. Advise patient that irritative voiding symptoms and intermittent hematuria are possible for several weeks after transurethral resection of bladder tumors.
2. Teach patient with superficial bladder cancer importance of vigilant adherence to follow-up schedule: After initial 6-week induction course of BCG, they need cystoscopy and 3 weekly instillations of BCG at 3 and 6 months and then every 6 months thereafter for 3 years. Yearly cystoscopy is required as 70% of superficial tumors will recur.
3. Review purpose and adverse effects of intravesical chemotherapy treatments (usually not given until after recurrence).

Evaluation: Expected Outcomes

- Urine output adequate and clear.
- Verbalizes relief of pain and bladder spasms.
- Verbalizes lessened anxiety.

CONDITIONS OF THE MALE REPRODUCTIVE TRACT

Urethritis

EVIDENCE BASE Centers for Disease Control and Prevention. (2021). Sexually transmitted infections treatment guidelines, 2021. *Morbidity and Mortality Weekly Report, 70*(4), 1–187. https://doi.org/10.15585/mmwr.rr7004a1

Urethritis is inflammation of the urethra. It is usually an ascending infection in males. In females, it is usually associated with cystitis (see page 656) or vaginitis (see page 637).

Pathophysiology and Etiology

1. Nongonococcal urethritis—urethritis not caused by *Gonococcus*; may be sexually transmitted:
   a. *Chlamydia trachomatis*—most clinically significant of the pathogens, three cases of chlamydia diagnosed for every one case of gonorrhea. Usually asymptomatic.
   b. *Ureaplasma urealyticum* and *Mycoplasma genitalium*—responsible for up to one third of cases.
   c. *Trichomonas vaginalis* and herpes simplex virus are other sexually transmitted organisms causing urethritis.
   d. Incubation period of 1 to 5 weeks depending on the organism; in some cases, infection may be subclinical for a period of time, particularly in males.
2. Gonococcal urethritis—caused by *Neisseria gonorrhoeae*, sexually transmitted; usually most virulent and destructive.
   a. Incubation period usually 3 to 10 days.
   b. Urethritis in gay males is more commonly gonococcal than nongonococcal.
3. Gonococcal and nongonococcal urethritis can both be present.
4. Nonsexually transmitted.
   a. Bacterial urethritis—may be associated with urinary tract infection (UTI).
   b. From trauma—secondary to passage of urethral sounds, repeated cystoscopy, indwelling catheter.

Clinical Manifestations

1. Can be asymptomatic.
2. Itching and burning around area of the urethra.
3. Urethral discharge: may be scant or profuse; thin, clear, or mucoid; or thick and purulent (gonococcal).
4. Dysuria and frequency.
5. Penile discomfort.

Diagnostic Evaluation

1. Gram stain—*N. gonorrhoeae* is detected as gram-positive diplococci on microscopic examination of urethral discharge or urine.
2. Culture of urethral discharge on selective medium.

3. DNA amplification tests on urethral voided specimen or other DNA/antibody tests of urethral discharge (currently, primary test)—to detect *C. trachomatis* and *N. gonorrhoeae*.
4. Wet mount microscopic examination of fresh urethral discharge—trichomonads may be visible and motile.
5. First voided urine for screening—either positive leukocyte esterase test by dipstick or greater than 10 white blood cell (WBC) per high-power field by microscopy indicates urethritis.
6. In rare cases, urethroscopy may be necessary to isolate a lesion such as warts caused by human papillomavirus (HPV).

Management

1. Gonococcal urethritis: one dose oral antibiotic of cefixime 400 mg or one dose intramuscular (IM) treatment with ceftriaxone 125 mg.
2. Chlamydial urethritis: single dose of oral antibiotic azithromycin 1 g or doxycycline 100 mg orally twice per day for 7 days.
3. Unless proven otherwise by negative testing, treatment for chlamydia is given along with treatment for gonorrhea.
4. Recurrent urethritis despite appropriate treatment for nongonococcal urethritis or confirmed presence of *T. vaginalis* treatment is one dose oral metronidazole 2 g.

DRUG ALERT Fluoroquinolones are now avoided in the treatment of gonococcal infections because of drug resistance.

Complications

Depends on cause, but may include:

1. Prostatitis, epididymitis, urethral stricture, sterility because of vas epididymal duct obstruction.
2. Rectal infection, pharyngitis, conjunctivitis, skin lesions, arthritis with gonococcal infection.
3. Long-term complications of these infections in females include pelvic inflammatory disease and infertility.

Nursing Assessment

1. Obtain a history of unprotected sexual contact and assess patient's understanding of risk.
2. Assess for signs and symptoms involving urinary and reproductive tracts.
3. Perform genital and abdominal examination to assess for the extent of infection.

Nursing Interventions

Resolving Infection and Preventing Complications

1. Collect urethral swab of discharge, urine, and blood, as ordered, for laboratory examination.
2. Use standard precautions when handling specimens.
3. Administer antibiotics, as prescribed.
   a. Usually ordered based on presumptive diagnosis before test results are obtained.
   b. Monitor for and advise patient of adverse effects or allergic reactions.

Preventing Spread of Infection

1. Encourage adherence with antimicrobial regimen for the prescribed time period.
2. Advise abstinence from sexual activity until treatment is complete and cure is established (usually 7 to 10 days).
3. Instruct the patient to avoid sexual activity with previous sexual partner until that person has been tested and treated for infection as well.
4. The use of condoms may prevent transmission but depends on technique.

Patient Education and Health Maintenance

1. Advise safer sex practices, such as abstinence, mutual monogamy, and use of male or female condom to prevent transmission of sexually transmitted organisms as well as unintended pregnancy.
2. Emphasize the need for follow-up care if symptoms persist or return.
3. Advise patient that reporting of gonorrhea to the public health department is required by law in all of the United States and Canada.
4. Tell patient that they will be called on to name all sexual partners within the past 60 days and that the process will be confidential.
5. Provide written information about all sexually transmitted infections (STIs) and ensure that patient understands the dangers of high-risk sexual behavior.

Evaluation: Expected Outcomes

- Signs of infection resolved.
- Reports sexual contacts have been treated.

Benign Prostatic Hyperplasia

Benign prostatic hyperplasia (BPH) is enlargement of the prostate that constricts the urethra, causing urinary symptoms. One in four males who reach age 80 will require treatment for BPH.

Pathophysiology and Etiology

1. The process of aging and the presence of circulating androgens are required for the development of BPH.
2. The prostatic tissue forms nodules as enlargement occurs.
3. The normally thin and fibrous outer capsule of the prostate becomes spongy and thick as enlargement progresses.
4. The prostatic urethra becomes compressed and narrowed, requiring the bladder musculature to work harder to empty urine.
5. Effects of prolonged obstruction cause trabeculation (formation of cords) of the bladder wall, decreasing its elasticity.

Clinical Manifestations

1. In early or gradual prostatic enlargement, there may be no symptoms because the bladder musculature can initially compensate for increased urethral resistance.
2. Obstructive symptoms—hesitancy, diminution in size and force of urinary stream, terminal dribbling, sensation of incomplete emptying of the bladder, urinary retention.
3. Irritative voiding symptoms—urgency, frequency, nocturia.

Diagnostic Evaluation

1. American Urologic Association Symptom Index score greater than 7 (uses rating of questions about the obstructive and irritative symptoms): 0 to 7, mild; 8 to 19, moderate; and 20 to 35, severe.
2. Rectal examination—smooth, firm, symmetric, or asymmetric enlargement of the prostate.

3. Urinalysis—to rule out hematuria and infection.
4. Serum creatinine and blood urea nitrogen (BUN)—to evaluate renal function.
5. Serum prostate-specific antigen (PSA)—may be elevated in patients with BPH.
6. Optional diagnostic studies for further evaluation:
   a. Urodynamics—measures peak urine flow rate, voiding time and volume, and status of the bladder's ability to effectively contract.
   b. Measurement of postvoid residual urine; by ultrasound or catheterization.
   c. Cystourethroscopy—to inspect the urethra and bladder and evaluate prostatic size.
   d. Uroflow—graphically demonstrates voiding pattern and can help characterize the severity of obstruction.

Management

1. Patients with mild symptoms (in the absence of significant bladder or renal impairment) are followed annually; BPH does not necessarily worsen in all males.
2. Pharmacologic management.
   a. Alpha-adrenergic blockers, such as doxazosin, tamsulosin, terazosin, and alfuzosin—relax smooth muscle of bladder neck and prostate to facilitate voiding.
   b. 5-Alpha-reductase inhibitors such as finasteride and dutasteride—exert antiandrogen effect on prostatic cells and can reverse or prevent hyperplasia. These drugs decrease the size of the prostate and improve urinary symptoms. Effect of drug may take up to 6 months. Females should not handle drug because it can be absorbed through the skin and is not recommended for use with pregnancy. In addition, patients taking dutasteride cannot donate blood.
3. Surgery (also see page 582)—options include transurethral resection of the prostate (TURP; formerly most common procedure), transurethral incision of the prostate, or open prostatectomy for very large prostates, usually by suprapubic approach.
4. Photovaporization of the prostate (PVP) is starting to replace TURP; it is done through a cystoscope, using a laser to vaporize diseased prostatic tissue.
5. Transurethral microwave thermotherapy (TUMT) and transurethral needle ablation (TUNA) are both office-based procedures that use heat to destroy diseased prostatic tissue.
6. Indigo interstitial laser therapy of the prostate is another procedure that is done on an outpatient basis.

DRUG ALERT Although prescribed for their effect on prostatic smooth muscle, alpha-adrenergic blockers (except for tamsulosin and alfuzosin) also have an antihypertensive effect. Dosage is usually titrated up from an initial small dose. It is commonly recommended that the first dose, or all once per day doses, be taken at bedtime.

DRUG ALERT Finasteride is present in semen and may have deleterious fetal effects.

Complications

1. Acute urinary retention, involuntary bladder contractions, bladder diverticula, and cystolithiasis.
2. Vesicoureteral reflux, hydroureter, hydronephrosis.
3. Gross hematuria, UTI.

Nursing Assessment

1. Obtain a history of voiding symptoms, including onset, frequency of day and nighttime urination, presence of urgency, dysuria, sensation of incomplete bladder emptying, and decreased force of stream. Determine impact on quality of life.
2. Perform rectal (palpate size, shape, and consistency) and abdominal examination to detect distended bladder, degree of prostatic enlargement.
3. Perform simple urodynamic measures—uroflowmetry and measurement of postvoid residual, if indicated.

Also see page 582 for care of the patient undergoing prostatic surgery.

Nursing Interventions

Facilitating Urinary Elimination

1. Provide privacy and time for patient to void.
2. Assist with catheter introduction with guide wire or by way of suprapubic cystotomy, as indicated.
   a. Monitor intake and output.
   b. Maintain patency of catheter.
3. Administer medications, as ordered, and monitor for and teach patient about adverse effects.
   a. Alpha-adrenergic blockers—hypotension, orthostatic hypotension, syncope (especially after the first dose), potential impotence, potential retrograde ejaculation, blurred vision, rebound hypertension if discontinued abruptly.
   b. Finasteride and dutasteride—hepatic dysfunction, potential impotence, interference with PSA testing, presence in semen with potential adverse effect on fetus of pregnant patient.
4. Assess for and teach patient to report hematuria and signs of infection.

DRUG ALERT Treatment with finasteride and dutasteride decreases the PSA by half, so this should be taken into account when obtaining PSA to monitor for prostate cancer.

Patient Education and Health Maintenance

1. Explain to patient the symptoms and complications of BPH—urinary retention, hydronephrosis, cystitis, increase in irritative voiding symptoms. Encourage reporting these problems and maintaining close follow-up.
2. Advise patients with BPH to avoid certain drugs that may impair voiding (see Table 17-3), particularly over-the-counter (OTC) cold medicines containing sympathomimetics, such as phenylpropanolamine.
3. Advise patient that irritative voiding symptoms do not immediately resolve after relief of obstruction; symptoms diminish over time.
4. Tell patient postoperatively to avoid sexual intercourse, straining at stool, heavy lifting, and long periods of sitting for 6 to 8 weeks after surgery, until prostatic fossa is healed.
5. Advise follow-up visits after treatment because urethral stricture may occur and regrowth of prostate is possible after TURP.
6. Be aware of herbal or "natural" products marketed for "prostate health."

Table 17-3 Bladder Function and Drug Actions

FUNCTION	DRUG GROUPS	EXAMPLES
Detrusor Muscle		
Increased tone and contraction	Cholinergic drugs (stimulate parasympathetic receptors that cause detrusor muscle contraction)	• Bethanechol • Neostigmine
Decreased tone, possible retention	Anticholinergic drugs (block parasympathetic receptors that cause detrusor muscle contraction)	• Methantheline • Propantheline • Oxybutynin • Darifenacin • Solifenacin • Trospium
Relaxes bladder tone	Calcium channel–blocking drugs (may interfere with influx of calcium to support detrusor muscle tone)	• Nifedipine • Verapamil • Diltiazem • Tolterodine tartrate
Internal Sphincter		
Increased tone, possible retention	α_1-adrenergic agonists (activate α receptors that cause contraction of muscles of the internal sphincter)	• Phenylephrine • Ephedrine • Phenylpropanolamine
Decreased tone	α_1-adrenergic blockers	• Alfuzosin • Prazosin • Doxazosin • Terazosin • Tamsulosin
External Sphincter		
Decreased tone, possible retention	Skeletal muscle relaxants	• Baclofen • Dantrolene • Diazepam

a. Advise patients that saw palmetto has shown some efficacy in reducing symptoms of BPH in a number of clinical trials.
b. The active ingredient in commercial preparations is lipidosterolic extract of *Serenoa repens*; dosage is 160 mg twice per day.
c. It should be taken with breakfast and an evening meal to minimize gastrointestinal (GI) adverse effects.
d. Although it appears safe and there are no known drug interactions, tell patients they must discuss use of saw palmetto with their health care providers.

7. Advise patient to notify all health care providers of medications. If cataract surgery is being planned, the ophthalmologist should be aware of tamsulosin use, which may increase the risk of floppy iris syndrome.

Evaluation: Expected Outcomes

- Voiding adequate without residual urine.

Prostatitis

Prostatitis is an inflammation of the prostate gland. It is classified as bacterial prostatitis (acute or chronic) or chronic pelvic pain syndrome (without the presence of bacterial invasion).

Pathophysiology and Etiology

Acute and Chronic Bacterial Invasion of the Prostate

1. From reflux of infected urine into ejaculatory and prostatic ducts.
2. From hematogenous (bloodstream) origin, lymphogenous spread, or direct extension from the rectum.
3. Secondary to urethritis—from ascent of bacteria from the urethra.
4. May be stimulated by urethral instrumentation or rectal examination of the prostate when bacteria are present.
5. May be caused by gram-negative enteric bacteria, such as *Pseudomonas aeruginosa*, *Escherichia coli*, and *Klebsiella pneumonia*, and gram-positive cocci, such as *Streptococcus* and *Staphylococcus*; may also be caused by *C. trachomatis*.

Chronic Pelvic Pain Syndrome

Pain or discomfort without other signs of infection and no known etiologic cause; difficult to diagnose and manage.

Clinical Manifestations

1. Sudden chills and fever (moderate-to-high fever) and body aches with acute prostatitis.
2. Symptoms are more subtle with chronic prostatitis and chronic pelvic pain syndrome.
3. Bladder irritability—frequency, dysuria, nocturia, urgency, hematuria to varying degrees.
4. Pain in the perineum, rectum, lower back, lower abdomen, and tip of the penis.
5. Pain after ejaculation, symptoms of urethral obstruction.

Diagnostic Evaluation

1. Urinalysis.
2. Urine culture and sensitivity tests.
   a. Prostate massage is inadvisable because it can precipitate frank sepsis or bacteremia.

   b. In acute bacterial prostatitis, there are numerous WBCs and a positive culture; in chronic bacterial prostatitis, there is a lower bacterial colony count; in chronic pelvic pain syndrome, there may be WBCs but a negative culture.
3. Rectal examination commonly reveals exquisitely tender, painful, swollen (boggy) prostate that is warm to the touch (with acute bacterial prostatitis).
4. Serum WBC count is elevated in acute bacterial prostatitis.
5. Bladder scan for postvoid residual evaluates bladder emptying.
6. Transrectal ultrasound detects prostate abscess.

Management

Acute Bacterial Prostatitis

1. Antimicrobial therapy generally for 2 to 4 weeks based on drug sensitivity; commonly a fluoroquinolone or sulfamethoxazole–trimethoprim.
2. IV therapy with ampicillin or an aminoglycoside in the hospitalized patient. Patients are hospitalized if there is suspected abscess, urosepsis, or immunocompromise.
3. Urinary retention is managed with suprapubic cystostomy; urethral catheterization is usually avoided.
4. Antipyretics, analgesics, hydration, stool softeners, and sitz baths for symptom relief.

Chronic Bacterial Prostatitis

1. Usually 4 to 6 weeks of oral antibiotic therapy with ability to diffuse into prostate.
   a. Quinolones such as ciprofloxacin, levofloxacin, ofloxacin, or norfloxacin.
   b. Sulfonamide such as sulfamethoxazole–trimethoprim.
2. Oral antispasmodic agents may provide relief from urinary frequency and urgency.
3. Alpha-adrenergic blockers may help with urination.

Chronic Pelvic Pain Syndrome

1. Usually requires multiple modalities.
2. Alpha-adrenergic blockers and skeletal muscle relaxants may provide some relief of symptoms.
3. Aggressive diagnostic intervention should take place to rule out other conditions, such as cancer of the prostate or interstitial cystitis.
4. Anti-inflammatory medications such as nonsteroidal anti-inflammatory drugs (NSAIDs) are helpful.
5. Tricyclic antidepressants may be helpful for pain control.
6. Pentosan may be helpful to relieve discomfort.
7. Quinoline antibiotics may be taken for 4 to 6 weeks.
8. Pelvic floor massage and biofeedback may help relieve perineal muscle spasms.

Complications

1. Bacteriuria, urethritis, epididymitis, prostatic abscess, bacteremia, septicemia.
2. Acute urinary retention.
3. Constipation.

Nursing Assessment

1. Obtain a history of previous lower UTIs or STIs and recent voiding patterns.
2. Perform examination of genitalia for urethral discharge; rectal examination (except in acute bacterial prostatitis because of tenderness and possibility of disseminating infection) to assess tenderness of the prostate.
3. Collect specimens: urine for culture and expressed prostatic secretions. To help distinguish urethral, bladder, and prostate infections, have the patient collect the first 10 mL of urine and label this voided bladder-1. This will be a urethral specimen. Next, have the patient collect a midstream urine specimen and label this voided bladder-2. This is a bladder specimen. Have the patient urinate after a prostatic massage and label this voided bladder-3. This is a prostatic specimen.

Nursing Interventions

Reducing Fever

1. Start antibiotic therapy as soon as specimens are obtained for culture.
2. Administer antipyretic medications; use cooling measures, if necessary.
3. Keep patient well hydrated, via IV administration or orally, because of fluid loss through fever; however, avoid overhydration, which increases urine volume and reduces antibiotic concentration in urine.

Relieving Pain

1. Administer analgesic or anti-inflammatory medication, as ordered.
2. Maintain bed rest in acute prostatitis to relieve perineal and suprapubic pain.
3. Maintain high-fiber diet and give stool softeners, as needed, to prevent constipation, which increases pain.

Controlling Chronic Pain

1. Administer or teach self-administration of analgesics, anti-inflammatory agents, alpha-adrenergic blockers, or skeletal muscle relaxants as ordered.
2. Advise warm sitz baths to relieve pain and promote muscular relaxation of pelvic floor and reduce potential for urinary retention.
3. Assess patient's response to supportive measures and coping with chronic pain.

Patient Education and Health Maintenance

1. Instruct patient to take antibiotic, as prescribed; emphasize the importance of completing long course of therapy to prevent recurrence and resistance of organisms.
2. Teach patient the symptoms of recurrence and of disseminated spread of infection.
3. Instruct patient in comfort measures: sitz baths (10 to 20 minutes) several times daily, continued use of stool softeners, and not sitting for long periods.
4. Advise patient to avoid sexual arousal and intercourse during period of acute inflammation; sexual intercourse may be beneficial in the treatment of chronic prostatitis to stimulate the secretion of prostatic fluid and relieve prostate congestion; chronic prostatic infection is not sexually transmittable.
5. Encourage prescribed follow-up because recurrence is possible.

Evaluation: Expected Outcomes

- Afebrile.
- Verbalizes relief of pain after analgesic.
- Verbalizes reduction of chronic pain.

Cancer of the Prostate

Cancer of the prostate is the leading cause of cancer and second leading cause of cancer death among American males and is the most common carcinoma in males older than 65.

Pathophysiology and Etiology

1. The incidence of prostate cancer is 30% higher in African American males.
2. The majority of prostate cancers arise from the peripheral zone of the gland.
3. Prostate cancer can spread by local extension, by lymphatics, or by way of the bloodstream.
4. The etiology of prostate cancer is unknown; however, there is an increased risk for persons with a family history of the disease.
5. The influences of dietary fat intake, serum testosterone levels, and industrial exposure to carcinogens are under investigation.

Clinical Manifestations

1. Most early-stage prostate cancers are asymptomatic.
2. Symptoms because of obstruction of urinary flow:
   a. Hesitancy and straining on voiding, frequency, and nocturia.
   b. Diminution in size and force of urinary stream.
3. Symptoms because of metastasis:
   a. Pain in lumbosacral area radiating to hips and down legs (from bone metastases).
   b. Perineal and rectal discomfort.
   c. Anemia, weight loss, weakness, nausea, oliguria (from uremia).
   d. Hematuria (from urethral or bladder invasion, or both).
   e. Lower extremity edema—occurs when pelvic node metastases compromise venous return.

Diagnostic Evaluation

1. Digital rectal examination—the prostate can be felt through the wall of the rectum; hard nodule may be felt (see Figure 17-11).
2. Transrectal ultrasound–guided needle biopsy (through anterior rectal wall or through the perineum) for histologic study of biopsied tissue includes Gleason tumor grade if carcinoma is present.
3. Transrectal ultrasonography—sonar probe placed in the rectum.

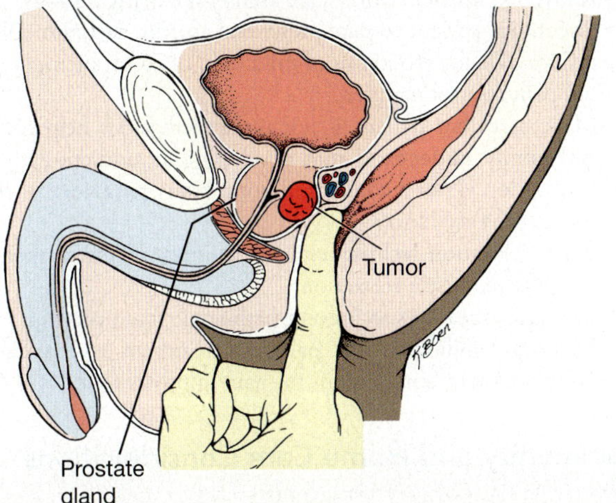

Figure 17-11. The prostate gland can be felt through the wall of the rectum. The size of the gland, overall consistency, and the presence of any firm areas and nodules are noted.

4. PSA—a protease produced by both benign and malignant prostate tissues. An elevated PSA may be due to BPH, prostatitis, or prostate cancer.
   a. Prostate cancer is suspected if PSA is above 4; however, prostate cancer may also occur at levels under 4.0.
   b. A free PSA level can be used to help stratify the risk of an elevated PSA. The lower the free PSA level, the higher the risk for prostate cancer.
   c. PSA velocity: PSA increases of 0.75 ng in 1 year could indicate prostate cancer.
   d. Age-specific PSA can help stratify risk for prostate cancer as well.
5. Guidelines among various cancer, urologic, and prevention organizations such as U.S. Preventive Services Task Force (USPSTF) and the American Urological Association (AUA) regarding prostate cancer screening vary. The USPSTF states that there is insufficient evidence to recommend screening. The American Cancer Society (2023) recommends screening at age 50 for males of average risk, age 45 for those at high risk, and age 40 for those at highest risk. All recommend informed discussion with patients.
6. Staging evaluation—skeletal x-rays, CT scan, MRI, bone scan, analysis of pelvic lymph nodes provide accurate staging information.
7. ProstaScint imaging study scan uses an IV infusion of monoclonal antibody to prostate-specific membrane antigen.
   a. Immediate and delayed images at 48 and 72 hours may identify soft tissue and bone metastasis for staging.
   b. Radiation is excreted through urine and feces and body fluids but is very low and not a risk to others.
   c. Patient is monitored for signs of allergic reactions following test.
8. Research is being conducted on numerous genetic and chromosomal abnormalities. Overexpression of the *AMACR* gene was found in 90% of patients with prostate cancer. Testing for this gene could result in identifying prostate cancer at an earlier stage.

Management

Conservative Measures

1. Watchful waiting/active surveillance may be indicated in males with Gleason 6 or lower stage prostate cancer or life expectancy of 10 years or less because prostate cancer may be slow growing and it is expected that many males will die from other causes. It is commonly recommended that these patients be followed closely with periodic PSA determinations and examination for evidence of metastases.
2. Symptom control for advanced prostatic cancer in which treatment is not effective:
   a. Analgesics and opioids to relieve pain.
   b. Short course of radiotherapy for specific sites of bone pain.
   c. IV administration of beta-emitter agent (strontium chloride 89) delivers radiotherapy directly to sites of metastasis.
   d. TURP to remove obstructing tissue if bladder outlet obstruction occurs.
   e. Suprapubic catheter placement.
   f. Zoledronic acid is given IV for bone metastasis pain.

Surgical Interventions

1. Radical prostatectomy—removal of entire prostate gland, prostatic capsule, and seminal vesicles; may include pelvic lymphadenectomy.

a. Procedure is used to treat stage T_1 and T_2 prostate cancers.
b. Complications may include urinary incontinence and impotence and possible rectal injury.
c. Nerve-sparing techniques may preserve sexual potency and continence.

2. Cryosurgery of the prostate freezes prostate tissue, killing tumor cells without removing the gland.

Radiation

1. External beam radiation or intensity-modulated radiotherapy focused on the prostate—to deliver maximum radiation dose to tumor and minimal dose to surrounding tissues.
2. Brachytherapy—interstitial implantation of radioactive substances into the prostate, which delivers doses of radiation directly to tumor while sparing uninvolved tissue.
3. Used to treat stages T_1, T_2, and T_3, especially if patient is not a good surgical candidate. Both forms of radiation are used in some patients; external beam followed by brachytherapy.
4. Complications include radiation cystitis (urinary frequency, urgency, nocturia), urethral injury (stricture), radiation enteritis (diarrhea, anorexia, nausea), radiation proctitis (diarrhea, rectal bleeding), impotence, skin reaction, and fatigue.

Hormone Manipulation (Palliative)

1. Prostate cancer is a hormone-sensitive cancer. The aim of hormonal treatment is to deprive tumor cells of androgens or their by-products and thereby alleviate symptoms and retard progress of disease.
2. Bilateral orchiectomy (removal of testes) results in reduction of the major circulating androgen, testosterone. A small amount of androgen is still produced by adrenal glands.
3. Pharmacologic methods of achieving androgen deprivation—also used to reduce tumor volume before surgery or radiation therapy.
   a. Luteinizing hormone–releasing hormone (LHRH) agonists (such as leuprolide and goserelin acetate) reduce testosterone levels as effectively as orchiectomy.
   b. Antiandrogen drugs (flutamide, bicalutamide, nilutamide) block androgen action directly at the target tissues (testes and adrenals) and block androgen synthesis within the prostate gland and adrenal glands.
   c. Combination therapy with LHRH agonist and an antiandrogen blocks the action of all circulating androgen.
4. Complications of hormonal manipulation include hot flashes, nausea and vomiting, gynecomastia, sexual dysfunction, and osteoporosis.

Complications

1. Bone metastasis—vertebral collapse and spinal cord compression, pathologic fractures.
2. Complications of treatment.

Nursing Assessment

1. Obtain a history of current symptoms; assess for family history of prostate cancer.
2. Palpate lymph nodes, especially in supraclavicular and inguinal regions (may be the first sign of metastatic spread); assess for flank pain and distended bladder.
3. Assess comorbidities, nutritional status, and coping before treatment.

Nursing Interventions

Reducing Anxiety

1. Help patient assess the impact of the disease and treatment options on quality of life.
2. Give repeated explanations of diagnostic tests and treatment options; help patient gain some feeling of control over disease and decisions.
3. Help patient and family set achievable goals.
4. Convey a sense of caring and reassurance in your physical care.

Achieving Optimal Sexual Function

1. Although patient may be ill while experiencing the effects of therapy, they may wonder about sexual function. Provide the opportunity to communicate concerns and sexual needs.
2. Let patient know that decreased libido is expected after hormonal manipulation therapy and that impotence may result from some surgical procedures and radiation.
3. Expect patient's behavior to reflect depression, anxiety, anger, and regression. Encourage expression of feelings and communication with partner.
4. Suggest options such as sexual counseling, learning other methods of sexual expression, and consideration of implant, pharmacologic agents, and other options for treatment of erectile dysfunction.
5. Have patient ask urologist about penile rehabilitation after radical open or laparoscopic prostatectomy. The early incorporation of phosphodiesterase-5 (PDE5) inhibitors, vacuum erectile device, or intracavernosal injections may increase the return of postprostatectomy erections.

DRUG ALERT Yohimbine is an herbal preparation sold OTC as an aphrodisiac and treatment for male erectile dysfunction. Caution patients that it is considered an unsafe herb by the U.S. Department of Agriculture because of its many drug and food interactions and adverse effects, including hypertension, tachycardia, and tremor.

Controlling Pain

1. Administer and teach self-administration of opioid analgesics, as ordered; oral sustained-release opioids, sustained-release transdermal patches, and subcutaneous or epidural patient–controlled infusion pumps are among the many options.
2. Encourage patient to take prescribed aspirin, acetaminophen, or NSAIDs for reduction of mild pain or to supplement opioid pain control regimen.
3. Make sure that patient is not undermedicated; help patient and family understand that developing an addiction to the medication is not a concern in hormonally refractory or metastatic prostate cancer.
4. Teach relaxation techniques, such as imagery, music therapy, progressive muscle relaxation.
5. Use safety measures to prevent pathologic fractures from falls.
6. Encourage follow-up and palliative treatment such as radiation therapy to bony lesions for pain improvement.

Community and Home Care Considerations

EVIDENCE BASE American Cancer Society. (2023, February 24). *American Cancer Society recommendations for prostate cancer early detection*. Author.

Encourage awareness of prostate cancer in the community.

1. Risks include being African American, over age 50, and having a first-degree relative with prostate cancer. High-fat diet has also been linked to prostate cancer.
2. Males who are asymptomatic with at least a 10-year life expectancy should have the opportunity to make an informed decision about screening.
3. If screening is desired after a detailed discussion between patient and health care provider, digital rectal examination and PSA blood testing begin at age 50 for males at average risk, at age 45 for African American males and those with a first-degree relative with history of prostate cancer, or at age 40 if a man has multiple relatives diagnosed with prostate cancer before age 65.
4. There is insufficient and conflicting evidence whether prostate cancer screening saves lives.
5. PSA less than 2.5 ng/mL indicates low risk for prostate cancer; therefore, recommendation is to repeat in 2 years.
6. If any urinary obstructions symptoms develop, patient should seek evaluation.

Patient Education and Health Maintenance

1. Teach patient importance of follow-up for check of PSA levels (every 6 to 12 months depending on pathology and recommendation of urologist) and evaluation for disease progression through periodic bone scan or CT scan. Cancer recurrence is suspected with PSA greater than 0.2 on two occasions.
2. Teach IM or subcutaneous administration of hormonal agents, as indicated.
3. If bone metastasis has occurred, encourage safety measures around the home to prevent pathologic fractures such as removal of throw rugs, use of handrail on stairs, use of night-lights.
4. Advise reporting symptoms of worsening urethral obstruction, such as increased frequency, urgency, hesitancy, and urinary retention.
5. Advise patient to monitor for signs of metastasis, such as fatigue, weight loss, weakness, pain, and bowel and bladder dysfunction.
6. For additional information and support, refer to agencies such as the Us TOO International (www.ustoo.com); Man to Man, a program of the American Cancer Society (www.cancer.org); and American Urological Association Foundation (www.urologyhealth.org).

Evaluation: Expected Outcomes

- Discusses treatment options; asks questions.
- Verbalizes understanding of sexual dysfunction and interest in seeking sexual counseling.
- Reports pain relief after opioid administration.

Testicular Cancer

Testicular cancer is a disease that occurs in younger males between ages 15 and 35 years. It is relatively uncommon, affecting 9 of 100,000 males annually. It is the most treatable form of urologic cancer.

Pathophysiology and Etiology

1. The majority of testicular cancers are of germ cell origin; the most common germinal tumors in adults are seminoma, embryonal carcinoma, teratoma, and choriocarcinoma (the latter three are also called *nonseminomas*).
2. The etiology of testicular tumors is unknown, but there is a relationship between cryptorchidism (failure of the testes to descend into the scrotum) and tumor occurrence.
3. Testicular tumors metastasize in a stepwise manner to the retroperitoneal lymph nodes with subsequent involvement of the mediastinal lymph nodes, lungs, and liver.
4. Testicular germ cell tumors are considered potentially curable; seminomas are extremely responsive to radiation therapy; nonseminomas are sensitive to platinum-based chemotherapy.

Clinical Manifestations

1. Painless swelling or enlargement of the testis; accompanied by sensation of heaviness in the scrotum.
2. Pain in the testis (if patient has epididymitis or bleeding into tumor).
3. Symptoms of metastatic disease: cough or dyspnea, lymphadenopathy, back pain, GI symptoms, lower extremity edema, or bone pain.

Diagnostic Evaluation

1. Elevated serum markers of human chorionic gonadotropin, lactic acid dehydrogenate, and alpha-fetoprotein; assay of tumor markers also used for diagnosis, detection of early recurrence, staging, and monitoring response to therapy.
2. Scrotal ultrasonography—to identify the location of lesion and differentiate between solid and cystic lesions.
3. Chest x-ray—to seek pulmonary or mediastinal metastasis.
4. CT scanning of the chest, abdomen, and pelvis—to evaluate retroperitoneal lymph nodes and to follow progress of therapy.

Management

Choice of treatment depends on tumor histology and stage of disease.

Surgery

1. Inguinal orchiectomy—removal of the testis and its tunica and spermatic cord.
2. Retroperitoneal lymph node dissection (RPLND) may be performed after orchiectomy in nonseminomas for staging and therapeutic purposes.
3. Complications of surgery:
    a. RPLND causes infertility because of ejaculatory dysfunction.
    b. Modified nerve-sparing unilateral lymphadenectomy can be done on selected patients, thus preserving ejaculation.
    c. Unilateral orchiectomy eliminates half of germinal cells, thus reducing sperm count.
    d. Libido and ability to attain an erection are preserved.

Radiation Therapy

1. Radiation therapy to lymphatic drainage pathways (after orchiectomy in seminomas); cure rate is close to 99%.
2. Other testicle is shielded, usually preserving fertility.

Chemotherapy

1. Cisplatin combination therapy is used in the treatment of nonseminomatous primary tumor and regional lymphatic metastases and in managing distant metastatic disease.
2. Discomforts of chemotherapy include significant nausea and vomiting, alopecia, myalgia, GI cramping, and mucositis.

Complications

1. Infertility; loss of testicle.
2. Retrograde ejaculation after retroperitoneal lymphadenectomy.
3. Death from metastatic disease.

Nursing Assessment

1. Examine testicular mass; ascertain when it was discovered and if it has changed or enlarged since initial discovery.
2. Examine supraclavicular and inguinal lymph nodes for enlargement.
3. Assess for symptoms of metastatic disease.

Nursing Interventions

Reducing Anxiety

1. Provide realistic information about impending surgery or treatment; dispel myths associated with testicular disease; emphasize positive cure rates.
2. Refer patient to educational and support services through the American Cancer Society and local cancer support groups.

Preserving Body Image

1. Reassure patient that orchiectomy will not diminish virility and RPLND will alter fertility and ejaculation, but not libido, erection, and sensation.
2. Advise patient that testicular prosthesis can preserve look and feel of the scrotum.
3. Refer the patient for counseling, as needed, for problems and concerns with relationships, peers, or work life.
4. Discuss possible donation of sperm because of infertility issues.

Preventing Complications of Treatment

1. Provide routine postoperative care, including early ambulation, respiratory care, and administration of pain medication.
2. After RPLND, monitor for paralytic ileus, which is common after extensive resection.
   a. Auscultate bowel sounds frequently and observe for abdominal distention.
   b. Withhold oral fluids until bowel sounds have returned.
   c. Report complaints of nausea and vomiting.
   d. Begin nasogastric decompression, if indicated.
3. For nursing care involving radiation and chemotherapy, see pages 86 and 77.

Patient Education and Health Maintenance

1. Teach all young males to perform monthly testicular self-examination (see Patient Education Guidelines 17-1); after orchiectomy, patient should examine remaining testicle monthly, preferably during or after a shower or bath.
2. Review schedule for radiation treatments or chemotherapy; teach patient and family possible adverse effects; discuss expectations for treatment period.
3. Provide information about retrograde ejaculation after RPLND and alternatives for fertility.

Evaluation: Expected Outcomes

- Verbalizes understanding of treatment and complications.
- No abdominal distention noted.
- Discusses concerns about sexual function with staff and partner.

Epididymitis

Epididymitis is an infection of the epididymis that usually spreads from the urethra or bladder to the epididymis by way of the ejaculatory duct and vas deferens.

Pathophysiology and Etiology

1. Occurs as a complication of UTI, urethral stricture disease, bacterial prostatitis, gonococcal or nongonococcal bacterial urethritis.

PATIENT EDUCATION GUIDELINES 17-1

Testicular Self-Examination

1. Examine for testicular tumor once per month, at a convenient time such as the first of the month or your birth date every month, preferably during or after showering or bathing.
2. Use both hands to feel the testes through the scrotal tissue.
3. Locate the epididymis; this is, the irregular cordlike structure on the top and at the back of the testicle that stores and transports sperm. The spermatic cord (and vas) extends upward from the epididymis.
4. Feel each testis between the thumb and the first two fingers of each hand. The testes lie freely in the scrotum, are oval shaped, and measure 4 to 5 cm in length, 3 cm in width, and about 2 cm in thickness.
5. Note size, shape, and abnormal tenderness. An abnormality may be felt as a firm area on the front or side of the testicle.
6. Stand in front of mirror and look for changes in size/shape of the scrotum. It is normal to find one testis larger than the other.
7. Report any evidence of a small, pea-sized lump or other abnormality.

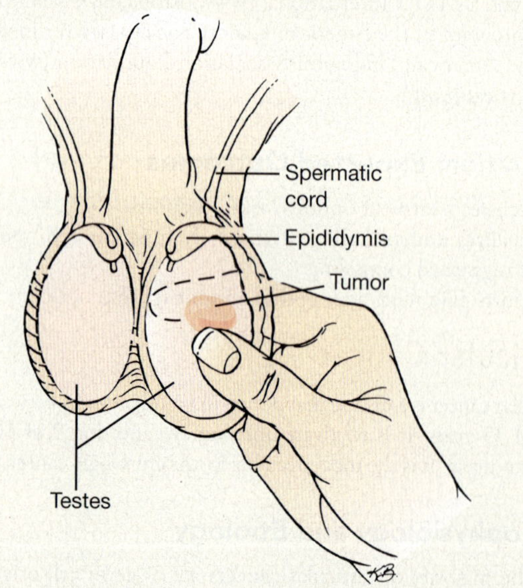

Using the fingertips and thumb, the epididymis, testes, and spermatic cord are located bilaterally.

2. In males under age 35, sexually transmitted organisms are the main etiologic agents, usually *C. trachomatis* and *N. gonorrhoeae*.
3. In gay males, *E. coli* is a common cause.
4. In older males, the main causes are bladder outlet obstruction and urinary bacteria (*E. coli, P. aeruginosa*).

Clinical Manifestations

1. Unilateral scrotal pain and tenderness.
2. Edema, redness, and tenderness of the scrotum.
3. Dysuria, frequency.
4. Fever, nausea, vomiting.
5. Pyuria, bacteriuria, leukocytosis.

Diagnostic Evaluation

1. Urine culture and sensitivity.
2. Examination (Gram stain, culture, gonorrhea, and *Chlamydia* testing) of urethral discharge and expressed prostatic secretions to establish causative organism.
3. Ultrasound with Doppler to rule out testicular torsion.

Management

1. Antimicrobial therapy after collection of specimens.
   a. Treatment of choice for presumed STIs is combination of ceftriaxone 250 mg IM in a single dose with doxycycline 100 mg orally twice per day for 10 days.
   b. For presumed *E. coli* and other infections, a quinolone, such as ciprofloxacin 500 mg orally twice a day for 10 days or co-trimoxazole for 10 days, is recommended.
2. Analgesics for pain relief.
3. Bed rest with the scrotum elevated on a towel to allow for lymphatic drainage.
4. In some cases, the spermatic cord is injected with a local anesthetic to relieve pain.

Complications

1. Spread of infection to testicle—epididymo-orchitis.
2. Infertility; risk is greater when infection is bilateral.

Nursing Assessment

1. Obtain a history of STIs (or symptoms), UTI, or prostatitis; recent urologic instrumentation or surgery.
2. Assess for elevated temperature, pain level, and swollen and tender scrotum.
3. Assess for sexual behavior risk—multiple partners, nonuse of condoms, history of STIs.

Nursing Interventions

Relieving Pain

1. Administer or teach self-administration of analgesics, as ordered—commonly NSAIDs or acetaminophen. Assess patient's response.
2. Encourage bed rest during the acute phase.
3. Apply scrotal support to relieve edema and discomfort, to improve lymphatic drainage, and to take tension off the spermatic cord.
   a. Use rolled towel under the scrotum or scrotal bridge.
   b. Suggest a cotton-lined athletic supporter for ambulation.

Patient Education and Health Maintenance

Instruct the patient as follows:

1. Avoid straining (lifting, straining at stool, and sexual activity) until infection is under control.
2. Sexual partners within the past 60 days of patients with chlamydial or gonorrheal urethritis or epididymitis should be examined and treated.
3. Follow-up with health care provider, as directed—it may take 2 to 4 weeks or longer for epididymitis to resolve completely.
4. Report signs of infection in the reproductive tract immediately to obtain treatment and prevent spread.
5. Obtain follow-up care to ensure complete resolution of infection; uncontrolled infection may impair fertility.
6. Use safer sex practices, such as abstinence, mutual monogamy, and condoms, to prevent further infection associated with sexual activity.

Evaluation: Expected Outcomes

- Verbalizes relief of pain.

Genital Lesions Caused by Sexually Transmitted Infections

EVIDENCE BASE Centers for Disease Control and Prevention. (2021). Sexually transmitted infections treatment guidelines, 2021. *Morbidity and Mortality Weekly Report, 70*(4), 1–187. https://doi.org/10.15585/mmwr.rr7004a1

Genital lesions are ulcerations or other skin or mucous membrane lesions that indicate infection with an STI and may actively shed the infecting organism.

Pathophysiology and Etiology

Causes include:

1. Syphilis—*Treponema pallidum*.
2. Chancroid—*Haemophilus ducreyi*.
3. Lymphogranuloma venereum—specific subtypes of *C. trachomatis*.
4. Genital herpes—herpes simplex virus.
5. Condylomataacuminata (genital warts)—specific subtypes of HPV.

Clinical Manifestations

See Table 17-4, for clinical manifestations, diagnosis, and treatment of genital lesions.

Nursing Considerations and Patient Education

1. Explain transmission of STIs and preventive measures, such as male or female condoms, abstinence, and mutual monogamy.
2. Encourage adherence with treatment regimen and follow-up to ensure cure before resuming sexual activity.
3. Explain that some shedding of herpes virus may occur even while asymptomatic, so patient must discuss this with partner; consider use of condoms at all times; reduce risk of transmission by abstaining at the first sign of an outbreak (tingling sensation) until 1 to 2 weeks after resolution of symptoms.
4. For additional information and support, refer to STI National Hotline at (800) 227-8922.

Table 17-4 Characteristics and Management of Genital Lesions Caused by STIs

DISORDER AND INCUBATION	CLINICAL MANIFESTATIONS	DIAGNOSIS AND TREATMENT
Herpes Genitalis		
2–20 d	Clustered vesicles on erythematous, edematous base that rupture, leaving shallow, painful ulcer that eventually crusts; mild regional lymphadenopathy; recurrent and may be brought on by stress, infection, pregnancy, sunburn.	• Diagnostic tests include Tzanck smear, viral culture, antigen test of tissue or exudate from lesion, or serum antibody tests. • No cure, but symptomatic period is diminished by acyclovir, valacyclovir, or famciclovir started with each recurrence; or recurrences greatly reduced or prevented by continuous treatment, decreases the risk of spread to partners. • Analgesics and sitz baths promote comfort.
Syphilis		
10–90 d for primary; up to 6 mo following lesion (chancre) for secondary	*Primary:* nontender, shallow, indurated, clean ulcer; mild regional lymphadenopathy *Secondary:* maculopapular rash including palms and soles, mucous patches, and condylomatous lesions; fever, generalized lymphadenopathy	• VDRL test or RPR blood test with confirmation by specific treponemal antibody tests • Preferred treatment is benzathine penicillin G 2.4 million units IM in a single dose; doxycycline, tetracycline, or ceftriaxone may be used in penicillin allergy.
Chancroid		
3–14 d	Bacterial disease caused by *Haemophilus ducreyi*. Vesiculopustule that erodes, leaving a tender, painful, shallow or deep, well-circumscribed ulcer with ragged, undermined borders and a friable base covered by purulent exudate; unilateral or bilateral large, tender inguinal lymph nodes (buboes) in 50% of patients	• Identification of *H. ducreyi* on special culture media • Treated with azithromycin, ciprofloxacin, erythromycin, or ceftriaxone IM. Single-dose regimens are available. • Apply warm soaks to buboes.
Lymphogranuloma Venereum		
3–30 d	Small, transient, nontender papule or superficial ulcer precedes firm, adherent unilateral inguinal and femoral lymph nodes (buboes) with characteristic groove in between (groove sign); may suppurate	• Microimmunofluorescence testing of bubo aspirate, if possible. Clinical diagnosis after ruling out other causes for genital lesions and lymphadenopathy. • Treatment of choice is doxycycline, but erythromycin may be effective. • Incision and excision of buboes should be avoided: aspiration may be helpful.
Condyloma Acuminatum		
3 wk to 3 mo, possibly years before grossly visible	Single or multiple, soft, fleshy, flat or vegetating growths may occur on the penis, anal area, urethra; no lymphadenopathy.	• Diagnosed by inspection or biopsy • Topical therapy with podofilox 0.5% for external warts, podophyllin 10%–25% solution, or trichloroacetic acid 80%–90% imiquimod. May require multiple applications. • Cryotherapy, electrodissection, electrocautery, carbon dioxide laser, and surgical excision may also be done. • Recurrence is common.

IM, intramuscular; RPR, rapid plasma reagin; STIs, sexually transmitted infections; VDRL, Venereal Disease Research Laboratory.

Carcinoma of the Penis

Carcinoma of the penis occurs primarily on the glans of the penis. Risk factors include uncircumcised, phimosis, HPV, lichen sclerosus, balanitis xerotica obliterans, increasing age, smoking, poor personal hygiene, and the accumulation of smegma under the skin of an uncircumcised penis. It primarily occurs in males older than age 50 and represents 0.5% of malignancies in males in the United States.

Pathophysiology and Etiology

1. Several types of penile lesions are potentially premalignant.
   a. Condylomataacuminata.
   b. Giant condylomataacuminata (Buschke–Löwensteintumor).
   c. Kaposi sarcoma.
   d. Leukoplakia.
2. Erythroplasia of the glans (erythroplasia of Queyrat) is a carcinoma in situ of the penis and may involve the glans, prepuce, or penile shaft or may spread to the remainder of the genitalia

and perineal region. It appears as a red, velvety lesion with ulcerations.
3. Bowen disease is a squamous cell carcinoma in situ resembling a red plague. Commonly involving the shaft of the penis.
4. Malignant lesions that ulcerate metastasize quickly to the regional femoral and iliac lymph nodes.
5. Distant metastasis occurs in the inguinal lymph nodes; in rare cases, to lungs, liver, bone, or brain.

Clinical Manifestations

1. Can present as a painless, wartlike growth or ulcer on the glans or prepuce or with painful, bleeding, or exudative lesion.
2. Phimosis (constriction of foreskin with inability to retract over glans) may obscure a lesion, preventing detection until advanced stages.
3. Lymphadenopathy; secondary infection of lesions or metastatic disease.
4. Malodorous and persistent discharge from the penis is a late symptom.

Diagnostic Evaluation

1. Biopsy of penile lesion and lymph nodes.
2. Ultrasonography and MRI of the inguinal lymph nodes.
3. Chest x-ray, CT or MRI scan, bone scan to assess for distant nodal metastases.
4. Positron emission tomography (PET) scans assist in primary staging or to assess for lymph node metastases.
5. Sentinel node biopsy to determine whether nonenlarged inguinal lymph nodes contain cancer.

Management

1. Localized lesions are surgically removed by partial penectomy, laser or cryotherapy, or Mohs micrographic surgery; total penectomy with perineal urethrostomy is necessary for more involved tumors.
2. Because inguinal lymphadenopathy may be due to inflammation and not malignancy, patients are prescribed a 4- to 6-week course of antibiotics after partial or total penectomy and are reassessed. If lymphadenopathy remains, then a bilateral lymphadenectomy is performed for cancer control.
3. Radiation therapy to small superficial tumors and lymph nodes may control the disease.

Complications

1. Disfigurement because of ulceration or treatment.
2. Complications of lymphadenectomy—necrosis and infection of skin flap, chronic edema of lower extremities.

Nursing Assessment

1. Obtain a history of current lesion, history of STIs, and hygiene.
2. Perform genital examination for characteristics of lesion, phimosis, inguinal lymph node enlargement.
3. Assess support system and personal coping mechanisms.

Nursing Interventions

Resolving Fears

1. Provide patient with opportunity to acquire information about causes and prognosis of disease.
2. Interpret diagnostic and staging results to patient.
3. Encourage realistic expectations regarding outcome of treatment.

Enhancing Coping With Body Image Changes

1. Maintain a nonjudgmental approach; allow patient to ventilate feelings about loss of part or all of the penis.
2. Provide routine postoperative care confidently, watching for bleeding, monitoring urination, and anticipating pain.
3. Provide opportunity for patient to discuss alternative methods of sexual expression with knowledgeable professional.
   a. About 40% of patients are able to participate in sexual activity and stand erect to void after partial penectomy.
4. Monitor patient for symptoms of depression requiring intervention.

Patient Education and Health Maintenance

1. Instruct the uncircumcised patient about proper hygiene—importance of daily removal of all retained smegma.
2. Explain expected postoperative function of the penis in patient undergoing partial penectomy.
3. Describe how voiding will occur to patient undergoing perineal urethroplasty.
4. Provide information about follow-up and monitoring for recurrences or radiation and chemotherapy, as appropriate.

Evaluation: Expected Outcomes

- Verbalizes understanding and acceptance of diagnosis and treatment plan.
- Discusses feelings and interest in seeking counseling.

SELECTED READINGS

Abufaraj, M., Shariat, S., Moschini, M., Rohrer, F., Papantoniou, K., Devore, E., McGrath, M., Zhang, X., Markt, S., & Schernhammer, E. (2020). The impact of hormones and reproductive factors on the risk of bladder cancer in women: Results from the Nurses' Health Study and Nurses' Health Study II. *International Journal of Epidemiology, 49*(2), 599–607. https://doi.org/10.1093/ije/dyz264

Anwar, M., Khadim, M. T., Asif, M., ud Din, H., Jamal, S., & Chaudary, M. (2022). Malignant male genital tract and urinary system tumors: Tumour registry data analysis at Armed Forces Institute of Pathology, Pakistan (2009-2018). *Pakistan Armed Forces Medical Journal, 72*(6), 1–4. https://doi.org/10.51253/pafmj.v72i6.2992

Atia, J., Evison, F., Gallier, S., Hewins, P., Ball, S., Gavin, J., Coleman, J., Garrick, M., & Pankhurst, T. (2023). Does acute kidney injury alerting improve patient outcomes? *BMC Nephrology, 24*(14), 1–10. https://doi.org/10.1186/s12882-022-03031-y

Borurbonnais, F. F., Slivar, S., & Malone-Tucker, S. (2020). Caring for patients on CRRT—Key safety concerns identified by nurses. *Canadian Journal of Critical Care Nursing, 31*(2), 13–19. https://cjccn.ca/wp-content/uploads/2020/09/CJCCN-31-3-2020Rev.pdf

Chow, E., Merchant, A. A., Molnar, F., & Frank, C. (2023). Approach to chronic kidney disease in the elderly. *Canadian Family Physician Medecin de Famille Canadien, 69*(1), 25–27. https://doi.org/10.46747/cfp.690125

Flagg, L. R., Julien, D. M., Lajiness, M. J., & Thompson, D. L. (2021). Urinary catheterization of the adult female. *Urologic Nursing, 41*(2), 65–69. https://www.suna.org/sites/default/files/download/resources/SUNA_catheterizationFemaleCCP.pdf

Flagg, L. R., Julien, D. M., Lajiness, M. J., & Thompson, D. L. (2021). Urinary catheterization of the adult male. *Urologic Nursing, 41*(2), 70–75.

Goyal, A., Daneshpajouhnejad, P., Hashmi, M. F., & Bashir, K. (2022). Acute kidney injury. In *StatPearls* [Internet]. StatPearls Publishing. https://www.ncbi.nlm.nih.gov/books/NBK441896/

Hosein, M., Paskar, D., Kodama, R., & Ditkofsky, N. (2019). Coming together: A review of the American Association for the Surgery of Trauma's updated kidney injury scale to facilitate multidisciplinary management. *American Journal of Roentgenology, 213*(5), 1091–1099. https://doi.org/10.2214/AJR.19.21486

Keane, K. G., Redmond, R. J., McIntyre, C., O'Connor, E., Madden, A., O'Connell, C., Inder, S. M., Smyth, L. G., Thomas, A. Z., Flynn, R. J., & Manecksha, R. P. (2021). Does instillation of lidocaine gel following flexible cystoscopy decrease the severity of post procedure symptoms? A randomized controlled trial assessing the efficacy of lidocaine gel post flexible cystoscopy. *Irish Journal of Medical Science, 190*, 1553–1559. https://doi.org/10.1007/s11845-020-02458-2

Koren, G., & Koren, D. (2020). Retrograde ejaculation—A commonly unspoken aspect of prostatectomy for benign prostatic hypertrophy. *American Journal of Men's Health, 14*(2). https://doi.org/10.1177/1557988320910870

Lee, K. S., & Koo, C. (2020). Clinical factors associated with the feeling of incomplete bladder emptying in women with little postvoided residue. *International Neurourology Journal, 24*(2), 172–179. https://doi.org/10.5213/inj.1938256.128

Manzoor, H., & Bhatt, H. (2022). Prerenal kidney failure. In *StatPearls* [Internet]. StatPearls Publishing. https://www.ncbi.nlm.nih.gov/books/NBK560678/

Mayo Clinic. (2022, February 26). *Glomerulonephritis.* https://www.mayoclinic.org/diseasesconditions/glomerulonephritis/diagnosis-treatment/drc-20355710

Mayo Clinic. (2023, March 1). *Belladonna and opium (rectal route).* https://www.mayoclinic.org/drugs-supplements/belladonna-and-opium-rectal-route/description/drg-20075097

Monaghan, T. F., Bliwise, D. L., Denys, M.-A., Goessaet, A.-S., Decalf, V., Kumps, C., Vande Walle, J., Weiss, J. P., Epstein, M. R., Weedon, J., Lazar, J. M., & Everaert, K. (2020). Phenotyping nocturnal polyuria: Circadian and age-related variations in diuresis rate, free water clearance and sodium clearance. *Age and Ageing, 49*(3), 439–445. https://doi.org/10.1093/ageing/afz200

National Cancer Institute. (2022, March 11). *Prostate-specific antigen (PSA) test.* https://www.cancer.gov/types/prostate/psa-fact-sheet

Oliveira, M. C., Flores, F. D. S., Barbosa, F. M., Fujii, C. D. C., Rabelo-Silva, E. R., & de Fátima Lucena, A. (2021). Evaluation of percutaneous renal biopsy complications based on outcomes and indicators of the nursing outcomes classification. *Revista Latino-Americana de Enfermagem, 29*(e3415). https://doi.org/10.1590/1518-8345.3759.3415

Pedreira-Robles, G., Garcimartín, P., Bach-Pascual, A., Giró-Formatger, D., Redondo-Pachón, D., & Morín-Fraile, V. (2023). Creating the nursing care map in the evaluation of kidney transplant candidates: A scoping review and narrative synthesis. *Nursing Open, 10*(10), 6668–6689. https://doi.org/10.1002/nop2.1937

Rahman, S., & Marathi, R. (2022). Sodium polystyrene sulfonate. In *StatPearls* [Internet]. StatPearls Publishing. https://www.ncbi.nlm.nih.gov/books/NBK559206/

Rogulska, K., Wojciechowska-Koszko, I., Dolegowska, B., Kwiatkowska, E., Roszkowska, P., Kapczuk, P., & Kosik-Bogacka, D. (2022). The most promising biomarkers of allogenic kidney transplant rejection. *Journal of Immunology Research, 2022*, Article 6572338. https://doi.org/10.1155/2022/6572338

Yan, C., Zeng, C., Ma, Y., Zhan, X., & Min, Y. (2022). Prevalence and risk factors of poor sleep quality in continuous ambulatory peritoneal dialysis patients in Nanchang, Southeast China. *Renal Failure, 44*(1), 1145–1150. https://doi.org/10.1080/0886022x.2022.2097406

Yang, L., Wang, L., Tan, Y., Dan, H., Xian, P., Zhang, Y., Tan, Y., Lin, M., & Zhang, J. (2023). Amide proton transfer-weighted MRI combined with serum prostate-specific antigen levels for differentiating malignant prostate lesions from benign prostate lesions: A retrospective cohort study. *Cancer Imaging, 23*(3), 1–8. https://doi.org/10.1186/s40644-022-00515-w

18 Gynecologic Disorders*

OVERVIEW AND ASSESSMENT

The Menstrual Cycle

The *menstrual cycle* is the cyclical pattern of ovarian hormone secretion (estrogen and progesterone) under the control of pituitary hormones (luteinizing hormone [LH] and follicle-stimulating hormone [FSH]) that results in thickening of the uterine endometrium, ovulation, and menstruation. Cycle length varies among individuals.

Phases of the Menstrual Cycle

The menstrual cycle is generally divided into two phases: follicular (or proliferative) and luteal (or secretory). See Figure 18-1. Further subdivisions of the cycle are:

1. Menstrual or bleeding phase (or early follicular phase): starts day 1 of the cycle and lasts approximately 5 days; endometrial sloughing and discharge occur because of low levels of estrogen and progesterone.
2. Postmenstrual phase (or early follicular phase); approximately days 5 to 8—thin endometrium. Ovarian follicles grow.
3. Proliferative phase (or mid- to late follicular phase): approximately days 8 to 15; estrogen starts to increase the thickness of the endometrium. A selected ovarian follicle continues to grow. A surge in LH occurs. Transition from proliferative phase to secretory phase occurs with ovulation, the expulsion of a mature follicle (or ovum) from the ovary.
4. Secretory phase (or luteal phase, which usually lasts 14 days after LH surge): approximately days 16 to 23; endometrium thickens because of increased progesterone; after ovulation, a corpus luteum forms and then regresses unless fertilization occurs.
5. Premenstrual phase (or late luteal phase): days 24 to 28; levels of estrogen and progesterone begin to fall.

Characteristics of Menstruation

See Table 18-1.

Subjective Data

Explore patient's gynecologic history, current symptoms, and general history to elicit important data. Provide a private and comfortable setting for history taking before the patient undresses. Reassure the patient about confidentiality and rationale for history taking (see Chapter 1).

Gynecologic Review of Systems

1. Menstrual history: date of start of last menstrual period (LMP) or age at last menses. Documented in this manner: age at menarche × cycle length × number of days of bleeding

*Please note that the term "male" in this chapter refers to a person assigned male at birth, and the term "female" in this chapter refers to a person assigned female at birth.

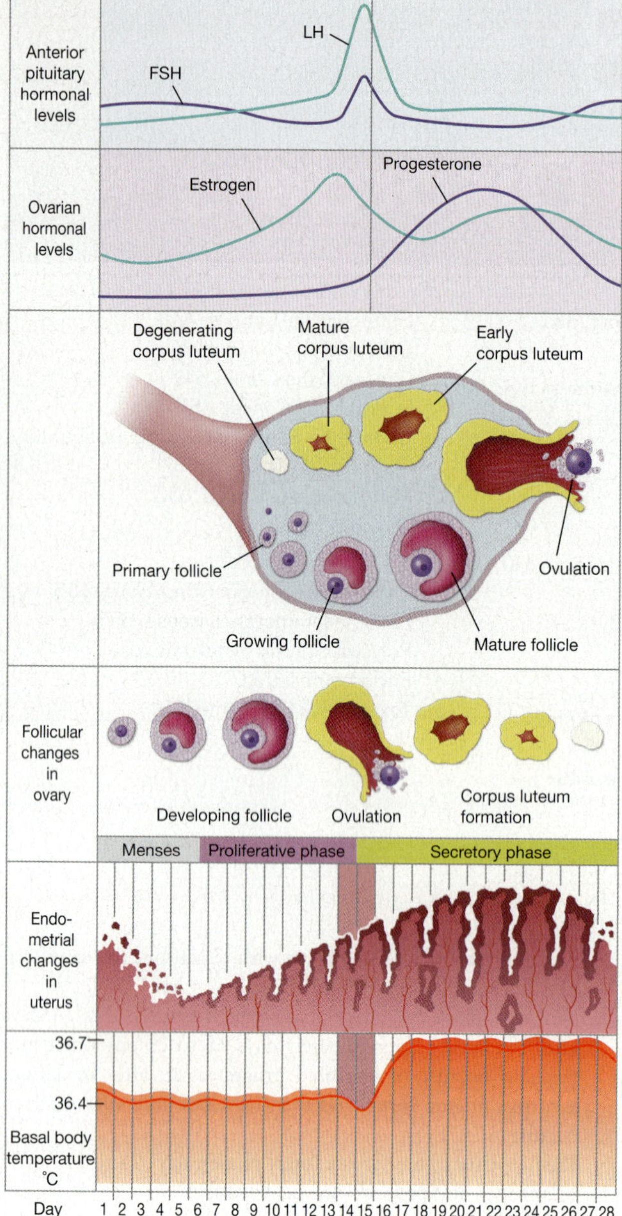

Figure 18-1. The menstrual cycle. FSH, follicle-stimulating hormone; LH, luteinizing hormone. (Adapted with permission from Premkumar, K. [2012]. *Anatomy & physiology: The massage connection* [3rd ed., Fig. 7-9]. Lippincott Williams & Wilkins.)

(e.g., 13 × 28 × 4). Symptoms of dysmenorrhea? Symptoms of premenstrual syndrome? Intermenstrual spotting/bleeding, postcoital bleeding, or postmenopausal bleeding?

2. Obstetric history: gravida (number of pregnancies) and para (number of term births, preterm births, miscarriages/abortions, living children) (e.g., G2P1102). Difficulty conceiving or assisted reproduction? For each pregnancy, list date; gestational age at delivery; mode of delivery; maternal complications (gestational diabetes, hypertension); and fetal, delivery, or neonatal complications.
3. Cervical cytology/Papanicolaou (Pap) test history: date and result of most recent test? Diagnosis and follow-up of abnormal Pap or human papillomavirus (HPV) tests? History of HPV vaccination (as age appropriate)?

Table 18-1 Characteristics of Menstruation

CHARACTERISTIC	RANGE	AVERAGE
Menarche (age at onset)	9–17 yr	12.5 yr
Cycle length	21–35 d	28 d
Flow—duration	2–8 d	3–5 d
Flow—amount	10–80 mL	35 mL
Menopause (age at onset)	45–55 yr	51 yr

4. Sexual history: age of first sexual activity? What is the preference for gender of sexual partner? Activity type? Satisfaction? Frequency? Number of partners in past year and during lifetime?
5. Methods of contraception and sexually transmitted infection (STI) prevention: desire for pregnancy testing or STI screening? Desire for other methods? Desire for preconceptual counseling? Use of condoms?
6. Screening for intimate partner violence and previous emotional, physical, or sexual abuse or assault.

Abnormal Bleeding

1. Characteristics: date of LMP? Frequency, duration, and amount of flow for most recent several cycles? Previous menstrual pattern and change? What is the color and consistency of blood? What are the sizes of the clots? Significant change in quantity or quality of menstrual flow? Bleeding or spotting between periods, postcoital bleeding, or postmenopausal bleeding? Pain with bleeding? Age at menarche? Age at menopause?
2. Associated factors: pregnancy and childbirth history? Is the patient sexually active? What method of contraception is used? Is the patient taking hormone replacement or hormonal contraceptives? Any other medications? Does the patient have obesity, or is the patient underweight? Does the patient have acne and hirsutism? History of amenorrhea? Coagulation disorders?
3. Significance: may indicate infection of the vagina or cervix; malignancy of the vulva, vagina, cervix, or uterus; benign tumor of the uterus; ovarian cyst; polyps; fibroids; adenomyosis; pregnancy; endometriosis; polycystic ovary syndrome; thyroid, hypothalamic, or pituitary disorder; coagulopathy; endometrial hyperplasia; or perimenopausal phase.

Vaginal Discharge

1. Characteristics: color, amount, and duration of the discharge? Any odor, itching, burning, urinary symptoms, or pain? Fever? Dyspareunia (painful intercourse—vulvar, vaginal, or internal pain with intercourse)? Onset related to menses or to intercourse?
2. Associated factors: LMP? What is the sexual history, such as number of partners or new partner within the past 6 months, type of sexual activity, and symptoms in partner? Is barrier method of contraception used? Is the patient menopausal or postmenopausal? Environmental factor changes? Vaginal dryness? Does the patient take estrogen replacement? Recent use of antibiotics? Recent douching? Recent over-the-counter product use or herbal/natural remedies? History of STIs?
3. Significance: may indicate normal or pathologic discharge, bacterial vaginosis, candidal vaginitis, cervicitis, gonorrhea, chlamydia, trichomoniasis, pelvic inflammatory disease (PID), or genital malignancy.

Pelvic Pain

1. Characteristics: frequency, duration, severity, and location of pain? Does the pain radiate? Was the onset sudden or gradual? What aggravates and what relieves it? Relationship to menstrual cycle, eating, physical exercise, bowel, or bladder function? Any dyspareunia? Does it feel like heaviness in the pelvis? Intensity and effect on daily activities?
2. Associated factors: LMP? Fever, nausea, vomiting, dizziness, abnormal bleeding? Urinary symptoms? Back pain? Recent significant weight loss or gain? Use of estrogen preparations? Difficulty conceiving? Did the patient perform a home pregnancy test? Use of an intrauterine system (IUS)? Any change in bowel habits or diarrhea? History of sexual abuse? Use of pain medications and home remedies?
3. Significance: may indicate condition arising from relaxed pelvic muscles, PID, endometriosis, interstitial cystitis, urinary tract infection, irritable bowel syndrome, history of sexual abuse (posttraumatic stress disorder), ectopic pregnancy, miscarriage, uterine fibroids, or cervical or uterine cancer.

Physical Examination

Physical examination for a patient with a gynecologic disorder should focus on the abdomen, pelvis, and genitalia. Palpate the abdomen for masses or tenderness. Request verbal permission before starting the pelvic examination. Consider using a chaperone during the examination. If the patient has presented as a survivor of sexual assault, then do not ask the patient to undress or examine the patient but ensure immediate transfer to a local emergency department with sexual assault nurse examiners or other professionals with expertise in forensic evidence collection and supportive services after assault. See Chapter 31, page 951.

The nurse in a gynecologic or obstetric setting may perform a vaginal examination to obtain specimens for diagnostic studies and assess the patient's condition.

Laboratory Tests

Cervical Cytology

Description

A Pap test of the cervix is obtained during pelvic examination to screen for cervical dysplasia or cancer. May also help to detect HPV, endometrial cancer, or infections. Classification by Bethesda system indicates any cellular abnormalities.

Bethesda System 2014

1. Specimen type—indicates conventional smear (slide) versus liquid based.
2. Specimen adequacy.
   a. Satisfactory for evaluation—result is given but presence of other factors, such as absence of transformation zone, is also listed.
   b. Unsatisfactory for evaluation—result may not be given; lists reason, such as inadequate number of cells or obscured by blood or inflammation, repeat cytology in 2 to 4 months
3. Interpretation of results—only a screening tool, not diagnostic.
   a. Negative for intraepithelial lesion or malignancy: no cell abnormalities.
      i. Presence of an organism (*Trichomonas*, fungal elements, shift in flora) and cellular changes consistent with herpes simplex virus (HSV) and cytomegalovirus may also be listed.
      ii. Other nonneoplastic findings (reactive reparative changes, glandular cells, atrophy) may be described.
   b. Epithelial cell abnormalities—atypical squamous cells are common.
      i. Atypical squamous cells of undetermined significance—management options based on population and can include HPV testing, repeat Pap test in 1-year intervals, and/or colposcopy.
      ii. Atypical squamous cells, cannot exclude high-grade intraepithelial lesion—potentially more serious; do immediate colposcopy and endocervical sampling for further evaluation.
      iii. Low-grade squamous intraepithelial lesion—management options based on population and can include repeat Pap test in 6-month intervals, HPV testing, and/or colposcopy.
      iv. High-grade squamous intraepithelial lesion—management options based on population and can include colposcopy with biopsy and endocervical curettage.
      v. Squamous cell carcinoma—colposcopy and biopsy.
   c. Glandular cell abnormalities—atypical, not otherwise specified (NOS) or atypical, favor neoplastic (require further evaluation); colposcopy, and HPV testing. Endometrial biopsy is performed if over 35 years of age and on younger females with risk factors for endometrial neoplasia such as unexplained uterine bleeding, chronic anovulation, or in females with obesity.
   d. Endocervical adenocarcinoma in situ; colposcopy, cervical biopsy, conization, and possible referral to oncologist. Hysterectomy may be performed for females who do not desire to preserve fertility.
   e. Adenocarcinoma—endocervical, endometrial, extrauterine, and NOS—biopsy and conization; consider referral to gynecologic oncologist.

Nursing and Patient Care Considerations

EVIDENCE BASE American College of Obstetricians and Gynecologists. (2021, April). *Updated cervical cancer screening guidelines.* Practice Advisory. https://www.acog.org/clinical/clinical-guidance/practice-advisory/articles/2021/04/updated-cervical-cancer-screening-guidelines

1. Pap test should not be performed during menses, unless the liquid-based system is used.
2. Instruct the patient not to use douche, medication, tampon, or cream in the vagina and to avoid sexual intercourse for 48 hours before the examination.
3. Recommend regular screening based on established guidelines set forth by the American Cancer Society, U.S. Preventive Services Task Force, and American College of Obstetricians and Gynecologists (ACOG). The same screening guidelines apply to all females whether vaccinated against HPV or not. More frequent testing is recommended if the female has human immunodeficiency virus (HIV), is immunosuppressed, was exposed to diethylstilbestrol (DES) in utero, or has been treated for cervical intraepithelial neoplasia (CIN) 2, CIN 3, or cervical cancer.
   a. Recommend starting Pap testing at age 21.
   b. Recommend testing every 3 years from ages 21 to 30 for females without risk factors such as DES exposure.
   c. For those ages 30 to 65, there are three options: continue cytology screening every 3 years; extend the screening interval to 5 years by doing HPV testing approved by the

U.S. Food and Drug Administration (FDA); or extend the screening interval to 5 years by continuing with HPV test and cytology.
   d. Discontinue screening after age 65 if adequate negative prior screening.
   e. Discontinue after total hysterectomy with removal of cervix if no history of dysplasia or cancer.
4. Make sure that the patient obtains results. If the patient has an abnormal cytology result, explain that this is not always conclusive but requires further testing based on age, such as repeat Pap test, HPV testing, colposcopy, biopsy, or conization. Encourage the patient to return for further testing.
5. Yearly examination for breast cancer screening; detection of other genital cancers, infections, and reproductive problems; and contraception management may be indicated.

Tests for Gonorrhea and Chlamydia

EVIDENCE BASE Workowski, K. A., Bachmann, L. H., Chan, P. A., Johnston, C. M., Muzny, C. A., Park, I., Reno, H., Zenilman, J. M., & Bolan, G. A. (2021). Sexually transmitted infections treatment guidelines, 2021. *MMWR Recommendations and Reports*, *70*(4), 1–187. https://doi.org/10.15585/mmwr.rr7004a1

Description

1. Commonly known as deoxyribonucleic acid (DNA) probe or antigen detection tests, a single specimen can detect both STI-causing organisms. Will detect even subclinical infection; can be used as a screening test.
2. Can also be done by culture method, but takes longer and requires separate specimens and special processing for each.
3. Screening for chlamydia and gonorrhea can also be done on urine specimen using amplified DNA technology. This method is more expensive, but saves time in specimen collection (especially for females) in screening centers.

Nursing and Patient Care Considerations

1. Explain the procedure to the patient before taking the specimen.
2. Specimens should be taken from the cervix without douching for 24 hours or from the male urethra before urinating.
3. Obtain specimen with cotton-tipped swab inserted and rotated in the cervical os for 10 seconds or urethral meatus in a male patient. Small-tipped swabs are available for the urethra. Send swab to laboratory in provided container with preservative.
4. For urine testing, ask the patient to provide the first 10 to 20 mL of voided urine in a specimen container (this represents a urethral specimen, i.e., more likely to contain the organism, if present, without being diluted by a larger amount of urine from the bladder).
5. May also use ThinPrep as a testing vehicle.
6. Retesting for reinfection is advised at 3 months posttreatment.

CLINICAL JUDGMENT Retesting for chlamydia is advised whether or not the patient believes that partner has been treated, so follow-up visit for 3 months should be scheduled at the time of treatment. If follow-up does not occur at that time, retesting at the next clinical visit within the next 12 months should occur.

Radiology and Imaging Studies

Hysterosalpingography

Description

1. This fluoroscopic x-ray study of the uterus and fallopian tubes is used to determine tubal patency, detect pathology in the uterine cavity, identify peritoneal adhesions, and treat unexplained fertility.
2. A bivalve speculum is introduced while the patient is in the lithotomy position and contrast medium is injected into the uterine cavity; the medium will enter the peritoneum in 10 to 15 minutes if tubes are patent.

Nursing and Patient Care Considerations

1. Determine the date of LMP; the test is done a few days after menses ends, before ovulation. Obtain pregnancy test if patient is within childbearing years, as indicated.
2. Verify that the patient does not have a history of allergy to contrast media or iodine.
3. Administer prescribed antibiotic and analgesic.
4. After procedure, apply a perineal pad for drainage of excess contrast medium or blood, and instruct the patient to notify the health care provider if bloody drainage continues after 3 days or if signs of infection are present.
5. Inform the patient that pain medication may be necessary for shoulder discomfort because of dye irritation of the phrenic nerve.

Pelvic Ultrasonography

EVIDENCE BASE AIUM practice parameter for the performance of an ultrasound examination of the female pelvis. (2020). *Journal of Ultrasound in Medicine*, *39*(5), E17–E23. https://doi.org/10.1002/jum.15205

Description

A noninvasive test that uses high-frequency sound waves to form images of the interior pelvic cavity; used to detect uterine, tubal, ovarian, and pelvic cavity pathology, to measure organ size, and to evaluate pregnancy.

Nursing and Patient Care Considerations

1. Inform patient that a full bladder may be necessary to make the uterus easier to visualize.
2. Instruct patient to drink 16 to 32 ounces of water (may differ among facilities) before the procedure and not to void. If transvaginal ultrasound will be performed, inform patient that a vaginal probe will be inserted to obtain more accurate measurements from internal organs. Have the patient empty the bladder prior to insertion of probe. (Probe is not used if patient is virginal.)
3. After the procedure, help the patient wipe off ultrasound gel from abdomen and allow them to empty the bladder.
4. Abnormalities are represented as different densities that differentiate solid from cystic masses and can help make a diagnosis; however, explain to the patient that further testing may be necessary.

Other Diagnostic Procedures

See Standards of Care Guidelines 18-1, page 5.

STANDARDS OF CARE GUIDELINES 18-1

Caring for a Patient Undergoing Gynecologic Surgery

When caring for a patient undergoing gynecologic surgery, the following are essential to prevent complications and to promote healthy adaptation:

- Discuss procedure with patient before surgery—Does patient know why surgery is being done? Does patient know which organs will be removed or altered? Does patent understand the implications for childbearing, sexuality, menopause? Answer questions and contact surgeon, if necessary.
- After the procedure, assess vital signs as frequently as indicated for signs of shock, infection, fluid overload, and atelectasis.
- Assess incision for drainage and signs of infection (redness, oozing, warmth, increased pain).
- Assess vaginal area for excessive bleeding or foul-smelling drainage.
- Monitor intake and output.
- If patient has an indwelling catheter, ensure that it is draining clear urine greater than 30 to 50 mL/h.
- After catheter has been removed, ensure that patient voids in adequate amounts and monitor for urinary retention or signs of infection.
- Ensure adequate intravenous (IV) and then oral fluids, but monitor for edema and shortness of breath, signs of fluid overload.
- Monitor level of pain and relief with analgesics, but watch for oversedation, hypotension, and decreased bowel sounds as adverse effects of opioids.
- Provide comfort measures, such as positioning, splinting incision during position changing, or coughing, applying ice pack to the perineum.
- Auscultate bowel sounds for return, signaling progression of diet. Report nausea, vomiting, and loss of or decrease in bowel sounds immediately; intervention for bowel obstruction may be needed.
- Institute thromboembolism prevention, as ordered, and monitor for calf tenderness.
- Encourage ambulation as early as possible, but encourage gradual resumption of activities, according to surgeon instructions.
- Notify surgeon of fever, shortness of breath, increased pain, excessive bleeding or drainage, foul odor, change in vital signs, urinary retention, decreased urine output, nausea and vomiting, or tender, swollen calf.

This information should serve as a general guideline only. Each patient situation presents a unique set of clinical factors and requires nursing judgment to guide care, which may include additional or alternative measures and approaches.

Colposcopy

Description

Examination of the cervix with a bright light and magnification of 10 to 40 times; done to determine distribution of abnormal squamous epithelium and to pinpoint areas from which biopsy tissue can be taken; may be done with cervicography (photographing the cervix).

Nursing and Patient Care Considerations

1. The procedure is preferably done when the cervix is least vascular (usually 1 week after the end of the menstrual flow). Obtain pregnancy test if the patient is within childbearing years, as indicated.
2. Explain that a vaginal speculum will be inserted and that a biopsy may be taken, causing only slight discomfort.
3. Help the patient into lithotomy position, drape appropriately, and provide emotional support throughout the procedure. Provide distraction techniques, such as music and posters (hung on the ceiling), as appropriate.
4. After the cervix and vagina are swabbed with acetic acid solution and inspected through the colposcope, biopsies may be taken. Biopsy tissue is preserved in 10% formalin, labeled, and sent to the laboratory. Saline may be used to rinse the area, and bleeding may be stopped with silver nitrate or ferric subsulfate (Monsel solution).
5. After the procedure, assist the patient to rise slowly and give the following discharge instructions:
   a. Avoid heavy lifting for 24 hours.
   b. There may be some bleeding and cramping; however, more than that of a normal period must be reported to the health care provider.
   c. Obtain the health care provider's instructions regarding douching and sexual intercourse.

Conization

Description

Excision of a cone-shaped piece of tissue from the cervix, including the area where the squamous and columnar epithelial tissue meet (transformation zone) for diagnostic and therapeutic purposes. The transformation zone is the area of most cervical cancers. The procedure can be done via scalpel, laser, or electrosurgery techniques.

Nursing and Patient Care Considerations

1. Explain to the patient that this test can be a minor surgical procedure that requires local or general anesthesia. Obtain pregnancy test if patient is within childbearing years, as indicated.
2. After excision, bleeding is controlled by cauterization or suturing and packing.
3. The patient should be observed for several hours after the procedure for excessive bleeding.
4. Instruct the patient to avoid tampons, douching, and intercourse as well as not to immerse self in water (no swimming, hot tub, tub bath) for 2 weeks, or as directed by the health care provider, to allow healing.

Hysteroscopy

Description

Endoscopic visualization of the uterine cavity used to evaluate endometrial cancer, check tubal patency, determine the cause of uterine bleeding, remove polyps or fibroids, and observe the placement and appearance of intrauterine conception (IUC).

Nursing and Patient Care Considerations

1. Obtain pregnancy test prior to the procedure if the patient is within childbearing years, as indicated.
2. Administer prescribed sedative before the procedure, and explain that a local anesthetic will also be injected into the cervix in the operating room.

3. The patient will be assisted into the lithotomy position, and the perineum and vagina will be cleaned immediately before sterile draping.
4. Explain that instruments called sounds are inserted into the cervical canal for dilation before insertion of the hysteroscope. With the scope in place, normal saline or CO_2 gas is slowly infused into the endometrial cavity to distend it and allow for viewing.
5. Observe patient for several hours and give discharge instructions.
   a. Over-the-counter analgesics may be needed for minor discomfort if analgesic has not been prescribed.
   b. Notify the health care provider of severe cramping or bleeding, fever, or unusual discharge.

Endometrial Biopsy

Description

1. The procedure is done with or without local anesthesia to obtain cells from the uterine lining to assist in the diagnosis of endometrial cancer, menstrual disorders, and infertility.
2. During speculum examination, a uterine sound is placed, followed by a curette or Pipelle suction device to withdraw specimen (may be done several times).

Nursing and Patient Care Considerations

1. Obtain pregnancy test if patient is within childbearing years, as indicated.
2. Administer prostaglandin inhibitor to decrease postoperative uterine cramping.
3. Assist patient into the dorsal lithotomy position and explain procedure.
4. Label the specimen, place in formalin, and send to the laboratory.
5. Inform the patient that light bleeding and occasional cramping may be experienced for a few days.
6. Instruct the patient to report fever, chills, and increased bleeding; no tampons, douching, or intercourse for 2 to 3 days.

GENERAL PROCEDURES AND TREATMENT MODALITIES

Fertility Control

Nurses who work in the gynecologic or any setting may be involved in contraceptive counseling.

Basic Principles

1. *Contraception* is the prevention of fertility on a temporary basis.
2. *Sterilization* is the permanent prevention of fertility. Female and male sterilization procedures can be performed. Some procedures can be reversed but with possible complications and variable success rates.
3. Contraception effectiveness depends on motivation, which is a result of education, culture, religious beliefs, and personal situation. It is best to include both partners in any contraception decision.
4. Nurses should be familiar with contraceptive methods and educate patients without moral judgment.
5. Failure rate (pregnancy) is determined by experience of 100 females for 1 year and is expressed as pregnancies per 100 female-years.

Contraceptive Methods

See Table 18-2.

Table 18-2 Contraceptive Methods

METHODS	DEFINITION	PROCEDURE	ADVANTAGES	DISADVANTAGES
Natural Methods				
Periodic abstinence	• Abstain from intercourse during fertile period of each cycle.	• Determine fertile period by: • Calendar method—ovulation occurs 14 d before the next menstrual period. • Cervical mucus method—increase in mucus at the time of ovulation; clear and stringy. • Basal body temperature—drops immediately before ovulation and rises 24–72 h after ovulation. • Symptothermal method—combines mucus and temperature.	• No health hazards. • Inexpensive. • May be religiously acceptable. • Increased knowledge of cycles.	• 20% failure rate. • Requires consistent record-keeping. • Decrease in spontaneity.
Coitus interruptus (withdrawal method)	• Withdrawal of the penis from the vagina when ejaculation is imminent.	• Must withdraw before ejaculation so that ejaculation occurs away from female genitalia.	• No cost. • No health hazards. • Always available.	• Failure rate of 20%; pre-ejaculatory fluid may contain sperm. • Interruption of sexual act.

Table 18-2 Contraceptive Methods (*continued*)

METHODS	DEFINITION	PROCEDURE	ADVANTAGES	DISADVANTAGES
Lactation amenorrhea method	• Breastfeeding has a contraceptive effect due to prolactin's inhibition of luteinizing hormone, which maintains menstrual cycle.	• Three requirements: Baby is <6 mo old and is breastfed on demand, around the clock, without formula or food supplementation, and the female has not had menses.	• No health hazards. • No cost.	• Need to use other methods such as spermicide or barrier, which has no effect on breast milk if the three conditions are not met.
Barrier Methods				
CLINICAL JUDGMENT Inform patients who use condoms, diaphragms, and the cervical cap that latex sensitivity may be a problem; they should watch for itching, swelling, and generalized reactions.				
Condom—male and female	• Latex or polyurethane or processed collagenous tissue sheaths, placed over an erect penis to prevent semen from entering the vagina. • Female condom is placed in the vagina.	• Place condom over an erect penis. • Leave dead space at the tip of condom (from which air has been expelled) to allow room for ejaculate. • Use spermicide on exterior for added protection. • Grasp ring around condom at withdrawal to avoid leaving condom in the vagina.	• Failure rate is low with proper use (2%–3%). • Prevention of STI. • Inexpensive. • No health hazard. • May help premature ejaculation by decreasing sensitivity. • Increases male involvement in contraception.	• Decreased sensitivity. • Interruption of sexual act. • Sensitivity to latex may be a problem. • Failure rate with typical use is 13%. • Female condoms are more expensive and made of polyurethane. • Failure rate with perfect use is 5% and 12% with typical use.
Diaphragm	• Rubber cap shaped like a dome with a flexible rim.	• Check for holes. • Place spermicide inside dome. • Place diaphragm against and covering cervical opening, behind lower edge of pubic bone. • Leave in place for 6–8 h after intercourse. • Requires fitting by a provider.	• Failure rate with perfect use is 6% and 12% with typical use. • May reduce the risk of developing cervical cancer. • May place in the vagina several hours before intercourse. • Can use while breastfeeding.	• Occasional toxic shock or allergic reactions. • May experience pelvic discomfort. • Possible increase in UTIs • Must be properly cleaned with soap and water, dried and stored to preserve integrity of rubber.
Cervical cap	• Rubber cap, shaped like a cup with a tall dome and flexible rim.	• Place spermicide inside cap and place cap over cervical opening prior to intercourse.	• Failure rate 14%–29%. • Can be left in place for up to 48 h. • Can use while breastfeeding.	• Must be properly cleaned with soap and water, dried, and stored. • Can be difficult to insert and remove.
Spermicides				
Nonoxynol-9 or octoxynol-9	• Available in a variety of forms: foam, jelly, cream, suppository, tablet.	• Place next to the cervix before intercourse; better if used with a barrier method.	• Available in a variety of forms. • Sold over the counter.	• Less effective if not used with barrier method; generally, 28% failure rate. • Some patients are allergic. • Increases risk of UTI. • Frequent use may cause genital lesions, increasing risk of HIV transmission.

(*continued*)

Table 18-2 Contraceptive Methods (*continued*)

METHODS	DEFINITION	PROCEDURE	ADVANTAGES	DISADVANTAGES
Intrauterine Contraception				
	• Small device made of plastic with exposed copper or progesterone release system; acts to inhibit implantation.	• Health care provider inserts device, usually at the time of menses. • Check intrauterine device string regularly—at least once per month—or after each intercourse when it is first inserted.	• Failure rate low, 1% or less. • Convenient; permits spontaneous intercourse. • Replace every 3–12 yr, depending on the type.	• Risk of PID for the first month and resultant tubal damage and infertility. • May cause spotting, bleeding, or pain. • Risk of spontaneous abortion. • Risk of uterine rupture (rare).
Hormones				
Combination oral contraceptive	• Tablets containing estrogen to inhibit ovulation and progestin to make cervical mucus impenetrable to sperm; lowest effective doses are used.	• Take daily in a cyclical or continuous manner.	• <1% failure rate in the first year with correct use. • Decreased pelvic pain due to endometriosis, decreased risk of ovarian and endometrial cancer, decreased bleeding due to uterine fibroids. • Aids in menstrual disorders. • Improves acne.	• Serious adverse reactions include thromboembolism, stroke, myocardial infarction, and cerebral embolism, especially for those who smoke cigarettes or are overweight. • Questionable risk of breast, cervical cancer. • May experience nausea, vomiting, headache, bloating. • Must remember to take at same time daily.
Progestin-only oral contraceptive (minipill)	• Smaller doses of progestins than in combined oral contraceptives.	• Take daily.	• As low as <1% failure rate during the first year with correct use. • Avoids estrogen-related adverse effects and possibly cardiovascular risks. • The thickened cervical mucus may reduce the risk of ascending infection with development of PID. • Safe in breastfeeding.	• May cause irregular menses, spotting, amenorrhea. • Must be taken at the same time daily (no more than 3 h late) or protection is lost.
Combination transdermal contraceptive patch	• Estrogen and progesterone are absorbed systemically, as efficacious as oral hormones.	• Apply weekly to buttocks, inner aspect of upper arms, or abdomen for 3 wk and then off for 1 wk for menses.	• Same as oral hormones but administered weekly. • Avoids first-pass metabolism through the liver.	• Same as oral hormones. • May become loose or cause minor skin reaction. • Increased risk of DVT compared to oral method. • Females >190 lb should not use.
Hormonal vaginal contraceptive	• Vaginal ring containing estrogen and progesterone, as effective as oral contraceptive.	• Insert ring into the vagina; remove after 3 wk for 1 wk for menses.	• Same as oral contraceptives except it is administered monthly. • Avoids first-pass metabolism through the liver, thereby increasing bioavailability, reducing drug interactions, and limiting adverse effects.	• Same as oral contraceptives. • Requires vaginal insertion and retrieval. • May cause vaginitis, leukorrhea.

Table 18-2 Contraceptive Methods *(continued)*

METHODS	DEFINITION	PROCEDURE	ADVANTAGES	DISADVANTAGES
Postcoital contraception (morning-after pill)	• May be combined estrogen and progestin, high-dose estrogen, or progestin.	• More effective if started within 24–72 h after intercourse, may be used up to 5 d after intercourse.	• Very effective.	• May be religiously opposed. • Can cause nausea.
Progesterone implant	• Progesterone release system made up of silastic rod.	• Implanted in subcutaneous fat of the upper arm.	• Long term (up to 3 yr). • Convenient. • Only 0.4% failure rate.	• May cause irregular bleeding, spotting, amenorrhea, acne, headaches. • May be difficult to remove. • High initial expense.
Progesterone injection	• IM injection of long-acting progesterone.	• Injections should be every 11–13 wk.	• Convenient. • <1% failure rate with correct use.	• Requires every 3-mo follow-up. • May cause irregular bleeding, spotting, amenorrhea, weight gain. • Long-term effects still unknown. • High discontinuation rate in adolescents due to adverse effects and missed appointments. • Need calcium supplementation.
Progesterone Antagonist				
RU-486; mifepristone	• Drug that prevents implantation and leads to menses (medical abortion).	• Given orally within 10 d of a missed period; may be combined with prostaglandin suppository.	• Causes abortion in 95% of users up to 5 wk after conception.	• Is an abortifacient; not a contraceptive in most cases. • May cause nausea, bleeding, incomplete abortion.

DVT, deep vein thrombosis; HIV, human immunodeficiency virus; IM, intramuscular; PID, pelvic inflammatory disease; STI, sexually transmitted infection; UTI, urinary tract infection.

Sterilization Procedures

Tubal sterilization is frequently performed for birth control. Hysterectomy and oophorectomy, performed for other reasons, also result in sterility. Male sterilization by vasectomy is another option.

General Considerations

1. Approaches.
   a. Abdominal is most frequently used: may be postpartum laparotomy, minilaparotomy, or laparoscopy. Laparoscopy with electrocoagulation is frequently performed. It is a safe and effective procedure.
   b. Uterine approach utilizing hysteroscopy to visualize the tubal ostia and insert coils or plugs.
2. Techniques vary by surgeon preference.
   a. Electrocoagulation: burn section of tube with or without excision; low reversal rate.
   b. Pomeroy: the tube is tied in midsection and section removed; may be reversed.
   c. Fimbriectomy: the fimbriated end removed and end tied; irreversible.
   d. Cornual resection: removal of the section of the tube nearest to the uterus and suture cornual opening closed.
   e. Silastic bands: plastic or metal clips to occlude tube; may be reversed, although rare.
   f. Coils or plugs inserted in the tubal ostia through hysteroscopy.

Complications

1. Failure to successfully block the tubes—pregnancy or tubal pregnancy.
2. Hemorrhage, infection, uterine perforation, and damage to the bowel, bladder, or aorta.

Nursing and Patient Care Considerations

1. Assess motivation for sterilization and level of knowledge about the procedure. Informed consent is needed. The couple should be thoroughly counseled about the permanence of the procedure.
   a. Teach the patient that there is no effect on hormones and menstruation will continue.
   b. Teach patient there should not be any adverse effect on sexual response.

2. Birth control should be used prior to sterilization unless performed during the menstrual period, during a cesarean section, immediately postpartum, or after an abortion procedure.
3. Prepare the patient to expect some abdominal soreness for several days; instruct patient to report any bleeding, increasing pain, or fever.
4. Sexual intercourse and strenuous activity should be avoided for 2 weeks.

Dilation and Curettage

Dilation and curettage is a common gynecologic surgery for diagnostic and therapeutic purposes, which consists of widening the cervical canal with a dilator and scraping the uterine cavity with a curette. Performed to control uterine bleeding, secure endometrial and endocervical tissue for cytologic examination, and treat missed, incomplete, or induced abortion.

Nursing and Patient Care Considerations

1. Prepare patient for the procedure—answer questions; request that patient void; administer an enema, if ordered; and administer nonsteroidal anti-inflammatory drug (NSAID) or a sedative, as directed.
2. Immediately postoperatively, monitor vital signs at frequent intervals; potential for hemorrhage exists.
3. Monitor perineal pads and the bed for amount of bleeding; report excessive amounts.
4. Offer prescribed analgesics for lower back and pelvic pain; cramping may occur for 2 to 3 days because of dilation of the cervix.
5. Instruct patient to maintain decreased activity for remainder of day to decrease cramping and bleeding.
6. Instruct patient to use perineal pads at home and to report fever (more than 100.4°F [38°C]), heavy bleeding (saturating a pad within 1 hour more than once), cramps lasting longer than 48 hours, increasing pain, and prolonged or a foul-smelling vaginal discharge.
7. Instruct patient to avoid strenuous activity until bleeding stops.
8. Inform patient that the procedure does not affect sexual functioning, but that sexual intercourse, douching, and tampons should be avoided for at least 2 weeks, according to preference of health care provider.

Laparoscopy

Laparoscopy is the endoscopic visualization of the pelvic and abdominal cavities through a small incision below the umbilicus. It is used to diagnose pelvic pain and infertility; differentiate between ovarian, tubal, and uterine masses; evaluate genital anomalies; treat endometriosis, ectopic pregnancy, and adhesions; perform tubal sterilizations; and as a major surgical tool to treat a multitude of gynecologic indications including laparoscopically assisted hysterectomy.

Nursing and Patient Care Considerations

1. Obtain pregnancy test if the patient is within childbearing years, as indicated.
2. Prepare patient by ensuring that nothing has been taken by mouth (NPO), answering questions about the procedure, and administering a sedative and enema, if ordered.
3. Inform the patient that shoulder or abdominal discomfort is common after the procedure from the infusion of carbon dioxide given to separate the intestines from pelvic organs. Elevation of feet higher than shoulders after the procedure helps relieve this.
4. The patient will receive local, general, or regional anesthesia and will be placed in Trendelenburg position to displace the intestines for better visualization.
5. After the procedure, monitor bleeding and vital signs and administer analgesics, as indicated.
6. Inform patient that passing gas and bowel movements may be difficult initially because of the manipulation of the intestines; ambulation and fluids will be helpful.
7. Advise patient to report bleeding, cramping, or fever; avoid strenuous activity for 2 to 3 days; and not to have intercourse for 1 week. Additional restrictions may be advised for complex procedures.

Hysterectomy

Hysterectomy is the surgical removal of the uterus. It is the second most common operation in the United States among reproductive-age females.

Types of Hysterectomy

1. Abdominal:
   a. Subtotal/supracervical hysterectomy—corpus of the uterus is removed, but cervical stump remains.
   b. Total hysterectomy—entire uterus is removed, including the cervix; tubes and ovaries remain.
   c. Total hysterectomy with bilateral salpingo-oophorectomy—entire uterus, tubes, and ovaries are removed.
2. Vaginal—removal of the uterus and cervix through the vagina.
3. Laparoscopically assisted vaginal hysterectomy—allows for the removal of pelvic adhesions that would otherwise prevent vaginal hysterectomy.
4. Laparoscopic supracervical hysterectomy—laparoscopic removal of the uterus that spares the cervix.
5. Laparoscopic total hysterectomy—laparoscopic removal of the entire uterus and cervix.

Indications

1. Uterine fibroids, endometriosis and adenomyosis, and dysfunctional uterine bleeding—most common.
2. Uterine prolapse and chronic pelvic pain.
3. Cancer of the vagina, cervix, uterus, ovaries, or fallopian tubes.
4. Obstetric complications—rare.

Preoperative Management

1. Procedure and reason for hysterectomy, what the procedure involves, and what to expect postoperatively are explained.
2. Patient must remain NPO from midnight the night before surgery and must void before surgery.
3. An enema may be administered before surgery to evacuate the bowel and prevent contamination and trauma during surgery.
4. Vaginal irrigation is performed before surgery and skin preparation is done, if ordered.
5. Implement the Universal Protocol for Preventing Wrong Site, Wrong Procedure, and Wrong Person Surgery (see https://www.jointcommission.org/standards/universal-protocol/).
6. Preoperative medication is given to help the patient relax.

Postoperative Management

1. Postoperatively, the following assessments are made:
   a. Wound appearance and drainage.
   b. Vital signs and level of consciousness.
   c. Level of pain and comfort to include nausea and vomiting.
   d. Vaginal drainage (serous, bloody).
   e. Intake and output.
   f. Urge to void, bladder distention, and residual urine (if appropriate).
   g. Clarity, color, and sediment of urine.
   h. Homans sign or impaired circulation.
   i. Return of bowel sounds, passage of flatus, and first bowel movement.
2. Exercise and ambulation are encouraged to prevent thromboembolism, facilitate voiding, and stimulate peristalsis.

Complications

1. Incisional/pelvic infection.
2. Hemorrhage.
3. Urinary tract injury.
4. Bowel obstruction.
5. Thrombophlebitis/venous thromboemboli.

Nursing Interventions

Relieving Pain

1. Assess pain location, level, and characteristics.
2. Administer prescribed pain medications. Ensure that patient knows how to use patient-controlled analgesia pump and is using it properly.
3. Encourage patient to splint incision when moving.
4. Encourage patient to ambulate as soon as possible to decrease flatus and abdominal distention.
5. Institute sitz baths or ice packs, as prescribed, to alleviate perineal discomfort.
6. Monitor level of sedation related to opioid administration—may interfere with ambulation and elimination.

Promoting Urinary Elimination

1. Monitor intake and output, bladder distention, and signs and symptoms of bladder infection.
2. Maintain patency of indwelling catheter if one is in place.
3. Catheterize patient intermittently if uncomfortable or if patient has not voided in 8 hours.
4. Catheterize to check for residual urine after patient voids; should be less than 100 mL. Continue to check if more than 100 mL of urine is retained (increases risk of bladder infection).
5. Encourage patient to empty bladder around the clock, not only when feeling the urge, because of loss of sensation of bladder fullness.
6. Encourage fluid intake to decrease risk of urinary infection.

Preventing Infection

1. Assess vaginal drainage amount, color, and odor; incision site; and temperature.
2. Administer antibiotics, as prescribed.
3. Assist use of incentive spirometer, coughing and deep breathing, and ambulation to decrease risk of pulmonary infection. Monitor respirations and breath sounds for compromise.

Strengthening Body Image

1. Allow the patient to discuss feelings about body image.
2. Encourage the patient to discuss feelings with spouse or significant other.
3. Reassure the patient that premature menopause will not occur if ovaries were not removed, but total hysterectomy with bilateral salpingo-oophorectomy will promote surgical menopause.
4. Discuss changes regarding sexual functioning, such as shortened vagina and possible dyspareunia because of dryness.
5. Offer suggestions to improve sexual functioning.
   a. Use of water-soluble lubricants.
   b. Change position—female-dominant position offers more control of depth of penetration.

Patient Education and Health Maintenance

1. Advise patient that surgical menopause may cause hot flashes, vaginal dryness, and mood swings unless short-term hormonal replacement therapy is instituted.
2. Advise patient against sitting too long at one time, as in driving long distances, because of the possibility of blood pooling in the lower extremities, which increases the risk of thromboembolism.
3. Suggest that patient delay driving a car until the third postoperative week because even pressing the brake pedal puts stress on the lower abdomen. Avoid hazardous activities when taking opioid analgesics.
4. Tell patient to expect a tired feeling for the first few days at home and not to plan too many activities for the first week. Patient can perform most usual daily activities within 4 to 6 weeks or per provider instruction. Teach patient that the recovery period differs for each individual and is dependent on medical history and any complications that may have occurred. Inform patients that it may be 2 to 3 months or even a year "to feel like themselves again."
5. Tell patient not to feel discouraged if, at times during convalescence, periods of depression, crying, and nervousness occur. This is common but will not last. Tell patient to call provider if the feelings persist.
6. Ensure that patient understands instructions on strenuous or lifting activities, which are usually restricted for 4 to 6 weeks.
7. Reinforce instructions given by the surgeon on intercourse, douching, and use of tampons, which are usually discouraged for 6 to 8 weeks. Sexual intercourse should be resumed cautiously to prevent injury and discomfort. Showers are permitted, but tub baths are deferred until healing is sufficient.
8. Instruct patient to report fever higher than 100.4 °F (38°C), heavy vaginal bleeding, drainage, increased pain or cramping, foul odor of discharge, and bleeding or increased drainage from incision site.
9. Emphasize the importance of follow-up visits and routine physical and gynecologic examinations.

Evaluation: Expected Outcomes

- Verbalizes decreased pain.
- Voids every 4 to 6 hours with no residual urine.
- No fever or signs of infection.
- Verbalizes positive statements about self and positive outlook on recovery.

MENSTRUAL CONDITIONS

Dysmenorrhea

Dysmenorrhea is painful menstruation; most common of gynecologic dysfunctions.

Pathophysiology and Etiology

Primary Dysmenorrhea

1. No pelvic lesion; usually intrinsic to the uterus.
2. Current research supports increased prostaglandin production by the endometrium as the chief cause.
3. May also be because of hormonal, obstructive, and psychological factors.

Secondary Dysmenorrhea

1. Caused by lesion, such as endometriosis, pelvic infection, congenital abnormality, uterine fibroids, or ovarian cyst.
2. May also be caused by passage of a clot through undilated cervix.

Clinical Manifestations

1. Pain may be caused by increased uterine contractility and uterine hypoxia.
2. Characteristics of pain—recurrent, crampy, colicky or dull, usually in lower midabdominal region, and spasmodic or constant.
3. Nausea, vomiting, diarrhea, headache, chills, tiredness, nervousness, and lower backache may be experienced.
4. Usually self-limiting without complications.

Diagnostic Evaluation

Tests to rule out underlying cause:

1. Chlamydia and gonorrhea tests—may show infection.
2. Pelvic ultrasound—may detect tumor, endometriosis, and cysts.
3. Serum or urine pregnancy test—to rule out ectopic pregnancy.
4. Possibly, hysteroscopy and laparoscopy—primarily to detect endometriosis.

Management

The following measures are for primary dysmenorrhea; treatment of secondary dysmenorrhea is aimed at underlying pathology.

1. Nonsteroidal anti-inflammatory agents, such as ibuprofen or naproxen sodium for their anti-prostaglandin action. Most effective with loading dose 1 to 2 days before onset of menses and taken on a regular schedule for 2 to 3 days.
2. Local heat, such as heating pad, to increase blood flow and decrease spasms, for 20-minute intervals with increased effectiveness with other therapies.
3. Hormonal contraceptives to decrease contractility and menstrual flow. Evidence supports decreased dysmenorrhea symptoms with monthly oral contraceptives, extended-cycle oral contraceptives, intravaginal hormonal devices, and intrauterine hormonal systems.
4. Exercise to increase endorphin release, which decreases pain perception, and to suppress prostaglandin release.

Nursing Assessment

1. Obtain menstrual and gynecologic history that could suggest underlying pathology.
2. Assess level of pain using scale of 1 to 10; assess the patient's emotional response to pain, coping mechanisms, and ability to carry out activities.
3. Obtain vital signs, including temperature, to rule out infection.
4. Perform abdominal and pelvic examination (if indicated) to obtain specimens.

Nursing Interventions

Controlling Pain

1. Administer pharmacologic agents, as ordered, or teach self-administration to control pain and menstrual flow.
2. Apply heating pad to lower back or abdomen, as indicated, for 20-minute intervals.
3. Assess the patient's response to pain control measures.
4. Encourage verbalization of feelings and reassure patient through the evaluation process.
5. Encourage activity and exercise, as tolerated.

Enhancing Coping Skills

Instruct the patient in stress reduction techniques, breathing techniques, and lifestyle changes that may improve symptoms such as exercise, healthy eating habits, adequate sleep, and smoking cessation.

Patient Education and Health Maintenance

1. Explain to the patient possible causes of dysmenorrhea.
2. Teach the patient nonpharmacologic methods to reduce pain.
   a. Apply a heating pad to the lower midabdomen or back or take warm tub baths for 20-minute intervals.
   b. Exercise regularly (30 minutes, five or more times per week).
   c. Healthy eating habits; see *www.myplate.gov*.
   d. Smoking cessation.
3. Teach the patient to use prescribed medications effectively by taking medication at the beginning of discomfort and repeating as necessary, especially on the first day of menses.
4. Teach the patient adverse effects of medications.
5. Encourage patient to reduce stress through adequate sleep, good nutrition, exercise, smoking cessation, and coping with stressors.
6. Discuss patient's feelings toward menstruation (hygienic issues, inconvenience, female identity).

Evaluation: Expected Outcomes

- Verbalizes reduced pain level.
- Demonstrates healthy coping skills.

Premenstrual Syndrome and Premenstrual Dysphoric Disorder

EVIDENCE BASE Tiranini, L., & Nappi, R. E. (2022). Recent advances in understanding/management of premenstrual dysphoric disorder/premenstrual syndrome. *Faculty Reviews, 11*, 11. https://doi.org/10.12703/r/11-11

Premenstrual syndrome (PMS) is a group of behavioral, psychological, and physical symptoms that include headache, irritability, depressed mood, breast tenderness, and abdominal bloating that are clearly related to onset of menstruation.

Premenstrual dysphoric disorder (PMDD) is a severe form of PMS.

Pathophysiology and Etiology

1. Etiologic theories include hormonal imbalances, such as ovarian steroid interaction; dysfunction of neurotransmitters (such as serotonin), prostaglandins, or endorphins; psychological factors, such as attitudes and beliefs related to menstruation; and environmental factors, such as nutrition and pollution.
2. Affects patients of childbearing age.
3. May occur in 20% to 32% of menstruating patients; up to 80% experience one or more of the symptoms during the luteal phase of their menstrual cycle.

Clinical Manifestations

1. Symptoms may begin 7 to 14 days before onset of menstrual flow; may diminish 1 to 2 days after menses begins.
2. Physical—edema of extremities, abdominal fullness, breast swelling and tenderness, headache, vertigo, palpitations, acne, backache, constipation, thirst, and weight gain.
3. Psychological and behavioral—labile mood, irritability, fatigue, lethargy, depressed mood, anxiety, crying spells, changes in appetite, and decreased concentration.
4. Diagnosis based on clinical manifestations; usually neither diagnostic laboratory nor radiologic evaluation is necessary.
5. Usually self-limiting without complications.

Management

1. First-line treatment is lifestyle changes. Stress management; dietary modifications including reduced caffeine, salt, and alcohol intake; regular aerobic exercise; adequate sleep; and relaxation can be effective for symptoms management.
2. Pharmacologic therapy includes nonsteroidal anti-inflammatory drugs (NSAIDs) such as ibuprofen and naproxen to reduce dysmenorrhea-related symptoms.
3. For severe PMS or PMDD, treatment includes selective serotonin reuptake inhibitors (SSRIs) such as citalopram, escitalopram, fluoxetine, and sertraline and serotonin–norepinephrine reuptake inhibitors such as venlafaxine.
4. Oral contraceptives may help relieve symptoms. Some studies have shown combined contraceptives using the progesterone drospirenone and extended-cycle regimens to be most effective.
5. Ulipristal acetate (UPA), a selective progesterone receptor modulator, has been shown in studies to be particularly effective for depression and irritability.
6. The gonadotropin-releasing hormone (GnRH) agonist leuprolide may be effective for some patients by suppressing the ovaries.
7. A variety of vitamins and herbal supplements have been promoted with limited evidence of effective treatment.

DRUG ALERT The SSRI paroxetine should be avoided in patients of childbearing age because of increased risk of congenital abnormalities.

Nursing Assessment

1. Ask the patient to describe symptoms, their onset, and means of relief.
2. Assess the patient's diet, activity, and rest habits.
3. Assess the patient's emotional response to symptoms and methods of coping.

Nursing Interventions

Increasing Control Through Healthy Coping

1. Encourage patient to keep a diary for several consecutive months, which includes dates, cycle days, stressors, symptoms, and their severity, to understand cyclical nature of the condition and determine if therapy is effective.
2. Use patient education with written materials and resources as a tool to help patient increase control over symptoms.
3. Administer or teach self-administration of medications, as ordered; teach patient about side effects such as changes in menstrual cycle and possible drowsiness or difficulty sleeping with antidepressants.
4. Provide emotional support for patient and significant others.
5. Teach stress management and relaxation measures such as imagery and progressive muscle relaxation.
6. Suggest counseling, as indicated.

Patient Education and Health Maintenance

1. Teach patient possible causes of the syndrome and the importance of healthy lifestyle in helping to control symptoms, particularly healthy diet and physical activity. Help patient identify any vitamins or nutrients that may be lacking in diet, such as calcium and vitamin D, for long-term health.
2. Refer for further resources and support to such groups as the National Association for Premenstrual Syndrome (UK) (http://pms.org.uk) or the U.S. Department of Health and Human Services Office on Women's Health (www.womenshealth.gov).

Evaluation: Expected Outcomes

- Verbalizes increased knowledge and sense of control over condition.

Amenorrhea

Amenorrhea is the absence of menstrual flow.

Pathophysiology and Etiology

Primary Amenorrhea

1. Menarche does not occur by age 15 with pubertal development or by age 14 with absence of secondary sex characteristics.
2. May be caused by chromosomal disorders, such as Turner syndrome, agenesis of the uterus, or constitutional delay of growth and puberty.
3. Transverse vaginal septum or imperforate hymen.

Secondary Amenorrhea

1. Menstruation stops for 3 months in people with previously established regular menstrual cycles or 9 months in a person with previously established oligomenorrhea (infrequent or longer menstrual cycles).
2. May be caused by pregnancy, lactation, menopause, or corpus luteal ovarian cysts.
3. Excessive exercise, inadequate nutrition with decreased body fat stores, and excessive weight loss may cause amenorrhea in young athletes (included in the female athlete triad: an eating disorder, amenorrhea, and osteoporosis).
4. Amenorrhea and anovulation secondary to polycystic ovary syndrome (PCOS) commonly occur in females with obesity but may be seen in those with normal body mass index (BMI). See page 547.
5. Ovarian, adrenal, or pituitary tumors and thyroid disorders are hormonal causes.

6. Some medications, such as antipsychotics (phenothiazines), antidepressants, antihypertensives, histamine H2 blockers, opiates, chemotherapy, and hormonal contraceptives, may also induce amenorrhea.
7. It may be a result of severe depression, severe psychological trauma, physical trauma, or radiation.

Diagnostic Evaluation

1. Pregnancy test.
2. Prolactin level (elevated) with pituitary tumor.
3. Thyroid-stimulating hormone (TSH).
4. Progesterone challenge test in secondary amenorrhea if both prolactin and TSH are normal and pregnancy test is negative.
   a. Positive result—bleeding occurs; chronic anovulation is most likely.
   b. Negative result—no bleeding occurs; may indicate ovarian insufficiency; other tests are needed.
5. Hormonal levels—luteinizing hormone (LH) and follicle-stimulating hormone (FSH)—to determine type of hypogonadism in primary amenorrhea or to detect ovarian insufficiency in secondary amenorrhea.
6. Dehydroepiandrosterone sulfate (DHEAS) level and serum testosterone are measured if there is evidence of hyperandrogenism.
7. Genetic karyotyping to detect chromosome abnormalities in primary amenorrhea.
8. Ultrasound to identify presence of the uterus and/or outflow obstruction.

Management

Treatment is based on causative factor.

1. Discontinue causative medications if benefit of discontinuance outweighs risk.
2. Nutritional, exercise, or psychological counseling, as indicated.
   a. Recommend decreased exercise in athletes to increase body fat stores and restore normal BMI.
   b. Recommend weight reduction if patient has obesity.
3. Low-dose hormonal contraceptives to regulate cycle after underlying cause has been determined.
4. In PCOS:
   a. Insulin-sensitizing agents decrease androgen levels, improve ovulation rate, and improve glucose tolerance.
   b. Clomiphene citrate is first-line treatment for ovulation induction.
   c. Laser treatment plus eflornithine is indicated for hirsutism in PCOS.
5. Treatment of tumor or other underlying cause, surgery, as indicated.

Complications

1. Amenorrhea increases risk for osteoporosis and endometrial hyperplasia, which may lead to atypia and cancer of the endometrium.
2. PCOS conveys risk of metabolic syndrome, type 2 diabetes, and cardiovascular disease. Improvement in ovulation rate increases the risk of pregnancy.

Nursing Assessment

1. Assess for signs of chromosomal disorders, such as abnormal genitalia, masculinization, short stature, and characteristic facies.
2. Assess for signs of pituitary tumor, such as headache, vision disturbances, dizziness, and galactorrhea.
3. Assess weight and body build, BMI, change in weight, and nutritional and exercise habits that may indicate anorexia or loss of body fat because of exercise.
4. Assess for signs of PCOS: elevated blood pressure, elevated BMI, waist circumference, stigmata of insulin resistance, and hirsutism.
5. Assess emotional status, areas of stress, and coping ability.

Nursing Interventions

Meeting Nutritional Requirements and Improving Body Image

1. Explore knowledge of the food groups, behavior regarding meals, and exercise routine; point out misconceptions, dangerous behavior, and how weight may be affecting menses.
2. Monitor weight and BMI and return of menstrual cycles.
3. Point out ineffective coping mechanisms and teach more positive coping mechanisms such as assertiveness. Instruct in relaxation techniques.
4. Refer for individual or group nutritional and psychological counseling as needed.

Patient Education and Health Maintenance

1. Teach patient the physiology of the normal menstrual cycle and possible causes in diagnostic workup for amenorrhea.
2. Teach proper use and adverse effects of prescribed medications.
3. Teach the patient to chart menstrual periods on a calendar and maintain regular gynecologic and medical follow-up visits.
4. Teach patients with PCOS that they should be screened for type 2 diabetes and cardiovascular risk factors such as fasting lipid levels and BMI.

Evaluation: Expected Outcomes

- Achieves normal BMI with restoration of menses.

Abnormal Uterine Bleeding

EVIDENCE BASE Khafaga, A., & Goldstein, S. R. (2019). Abnormal uterine bleeding. *Obstetrics and Gynecology Clinics of North America*, 46(4), 595–605. https://doi.org/10.1016/j.ogc.2019.07.001

Abnormal uterine bleeding (AUB) is irregular or excessively heavy menstrual bleeding. It may be acute or chronic and is abnormal in regularity, volume, frequency, or duration, and it occurs in the absence of pregnancy.

Pathophysiology and Etiology

Causes of AUB are subdivided into anovulatory and ovulatory patterns.

Anovulatory AUB

1. Common causes of anovulatory AUB include polycystic ovary syndrome (PCOS), uncontrolled diabetes mellitus, thyroid disorders (hypo- and hyperthyroidism), hyperprolactinemia, or medications (such as antipsychotics and antiepileptics).
2. In adolescents, AUB is frequently caused by immature hypothalamic–pituitary–ovarian axis.

3. Ovarian insufficiency in perimenopausal patients frequently causes dysfunctional uterine bleeding (DUB). Recurrent irregular menstrual cycles are considered abnormal if they occur 8 years before menopause.
4. Anovulation may be related to hypothalamic or pituitary dysfunction, impaired follicular formation or rupture, or corpus luteum dysfunction.
5. Temporary estrogen withdrawal at ovulation may cause midcycle ovulatory bleeding.

Ovulatory AUB

1. Excessive bleeding or duration may be related to hypothyroidism, late-stage liver disease, or bleeding disorders (such as von Willebrand disease).
2. Structural abnormalities, such as submucosal fibroids or endometrial fibroids, may cause AUB.
3. Approximately one half of people with ovulatory AUB have no identifiable cause.

Clinical Manifestations

Anovulatory AUB Patterns/Dysfunctional Bleeding

1. Amenorrhea—no bleeding for three cycles or more.
2. Oligomenorrhea—significantly diminished menstrual flow; infrequent intervals (greater than 35 days) or irregular intervals.
3. Metrorrhagia—bleeding from the uterus between regular menstrual periods; significant because it is usually a symptom of disease.
4. Menometrorrhagia—excessive bleeding at the usual time of menstruation and at other irregular intervals.

Ovulatory Patterns

1. Menorrhagia—excessive bleeding during regular menstruation cycles; can be increased in duration or amount.
2. Polymenorrhea—frequent menstruation occurring at intervals of less than 21 days.
3. Menometrorrhagia—excessive bleeding at the usual time of menstruation and at other irregular intervals.

Diagnostic Evaluation

Tests to rule out pathologic causes of abnormal bleeding include:

1. Pregnancy test.
2. Complete blood count (CBC) to detect anemia and platelet count.
3. TSH to rule out thyroid disorder; prolactin to rule out pituitary adenoma.
4. Thorough history and examination to look for anovulatory medical conditions (such as obesity and hirsutism—signs of PCOS) and to rule out enlarged uterus, trauma, or foreign body.
5. Other tests that may be done during physical exam include a Pap smear to rule out cervical dysplasia or malignancy; chlamydia and gonorrhea tests to rule out PID.
6. Endometrial biopsy to determine hormonal effect on the uterus and rule out malignancy.
7. Transvaginal ultrasound to rule out ovarian or uterine pathology or structural abnormality. Saline infusion sonohysterography is more sensitive and specific than transvaginal ultrasound.
8. Coagulation screen to rule out blood dyscrasias in adolescents with menorrhagia. Iron studies are not first-line, but are recommended if hematocrit and hemoglobin are low.
9. If cause is still undetermined, then hysteroscopy is recommended to detect uterine fibroids, polyps, and other lesions.

Management

Treatment is based on the underlying cause.

1. Hormonal contraceptives (birth control pills or hormone-releasing intrauterine conception [IUC]) to control chronic bleeding or induce regular withdrawal bleeding. Endometrial biopsy should be repeated after 3 to 6 months of treatment to monitor endometrial hyperplasia. Combination estrogen–progesterone oral contraceptives, although commonly prescribed first-line, lack adequate evidence for the treatment of AUB.
2. In females who cannot take estrogen because of an increased thrombotic risk, progesterone-only administration can be effective. Cyclical oral progesterone for 21 days significantly reduces menorrhagia. For patients with menorrhagia, levonorgestrel-releasing intrauterine system is superior to oral contraceptives. Long-acting progestin injections may reduce bleeding but cause irregular spotting.
3. In emergencies, parenteral conjugated estrogen may be used to stop acute bleeding. Because of increased risk of thromboembolism, concomitant use of low-molecular-weight heparin may be considered.
4. Treat underlying anemia with iron, possible transfusions.
5. NSAIDs are useful to decrease menstrual flow volume in menorrhagia.
6. Tranexamic acid, an antifibrinolytic agent, has demonstrated efficacy in decreasing menorrhagia. In an underlying bleeding disorder (such as von Willebrand disease), intranasal desmopressin may be indicated.
7. Androgen therapy with a gonadotropin-releasing hormone, such as leuprolide acetate, to reduce menstrual blood loss in perimenopausal females or to reduce the size of uterine fibroids before surgery.
8. Surgical procedures, such as hysteroscopic polypectomy or resection of uterine submucosal fibroids.
9. Hysteroscopic endometrial resection (removal of diseased or abnormal tissue) or endometrial ablation (application of heat to endometrium to induce scarring) when abovementioned methods are not helpful.
   a. By 5 years postablation, one third of patients require another surgery.
   b. The uterus is preserved, but it results in infertility.
10. Hysterectomy in refractory cases.

Complications

1. Recurrent anovulation in anovulatory AUB increases the risk of endometrial cancer because of the impact of unopposed estrogen on the endometrium. Individuals with regular ovulation and AUB have no greater risk of endometrial cancer because the endometrium regularly sloughs.
2. Severe anemia may result from menorrhagia or menometrorrhagia.

Nursing Assessment

1. Ask patient for menstrual and gynecologic history, sexual activity, and possibility of pregnancy.
2. Assess frequency, duration, and amount of menstrual flow.

3. Assess for other symptoms of underlying pathology, such as systemic hormonal conditions, pelvic pain, fever, and abdominal masses or tenderness.
4. Assess for signs and symptoms of anemia—fatigue, shortness of breath, pallor, and tachycardia.

Nursing Interventions

Reducing Fatigue and Signs of Anemia

1. Administer medications, as ordered. Teach patient indications and side effects.
2. Encourage good dietary intake with increased sources of iron-fortified cereals and breads, meat (especially red meat), and green, leafy vegetables.
3. Administer oral iron preparations with meals to prevent nausea and with vitamin C–rich foods or drinks to enhance absorption. Treat constipation, as necessary.
4. Monitor hemoglobin and infuse packed red blood cells, as ordered.
5. Encourage activity, as tolerated.

Patient Education and Health Maintenance

1. Teach patient the causes of AUB and about the diagnostic process to rule out pathologic causes of abnormal bleeding.
2. Teach about hormonal therapy, related adverse effects, and what bleeding patterns to expect. Bleeding should stop within the first week of hormonal contraceptives but should start again in the fourth week as regular menstrual period would with cyclical contraceptives.
3. Advise the patient to keep a calendar or log of menses. Help patient manage heavy flow and prevent accidents by wearing double pads, changing frequently, and expecting gushes when changing position from reclining to sitting or standing.

Evaluation: Expected Outcomes

- Verbalizes reduced fatigue and better ability to perform routine activities.

Menopause

EVIDENCE BASE Voedisch, A. J., Dunsmoor-Su, R., & Kasirsky, J. (2021). Menopause: A global perspective and clinical guide for practice. *Clinical Obstetrics and Gynecology*, *64*(3), 528–554. https://doi.org/10.1097/GRF.0000000000000639

Menopause is described as the physiologic cessation of menses. Climacteric or perimenopause is the period during which there is decline in ovarian function and the female experiences symptoms of estrogen deficiency and, possibly, irregular cycles. Menopause has occurred if menses has not occurred for 12 months.

Pathophysiology and Etiology

1. Menopause is caused by the cessation of ovarian function and decreased estrogen production by the ovary; average age range is 45 to 55, with the average age of 51.
2. Anovulation may occur during perimenopause, disrupting menstrual cycles.
3. Artificial or surgical menopause may occur secondary to surgery or radiation involving the ovaries. Some chemotherapeutic agents also cause a chemical menopause.
4. Hysterectomy without ovary removal may result in earlier menopause because of disruption of the blood supply to the ovaries.

Clinical Manifestations

1. Genitalia—atrophy of the vulva, vagina, and urethra results in dryness, bleeding, itching, burning, dysuria, thinning of pubic hair, loss of labia minora, and decreased secretions during intercourse.
2. Sexual function—vaginal dryness, discomfort, dyspareunia, and decreased intensity and duration of sexual response, but can still have active and satisfactory function.
3. Vasomotor—60% to 75% of females experience "hot flashes," which may be preceded by an anxious feeling and accompanied by sweating. These may occur at night, causing "night sweats."
   a. Psychological—insomnia, irritability, anxiety, memory loss, fear, and depression may be experienced.
   b. Some females experience palpitations.
   c. Symptoms, severity, and personal/cultural meanings vary with each individual.

Diagnostic Evaluation

1. Levels of LH and FSH will increase, and estradiol will decrease; however, levels may fluctuate often during perimenopause, so diagnosis is based on symptoms.
2. FSH greater than 30 to 40 IU/L indicates menopause; greater than 100 IU/L indicates complete ovarian insufficiency.
3. Laboratory studies of FSH are not necessary to diagnose the perimenopausal phase or menopause itself.

Management

Menopausal Hormone Therapy/Estrogen Replacement Therapy

1. Indicated at the smallest possible dose for the shortest time period (less than 5 years) to reduce vasomotor symptoms (with the added benefit to prevent osteoporosis). Common systemic routes of administration include oral and transdermal.
2. Progesterone cotherapy preparations (oral, transdermal; or in combination products with estrogen) are required in a cyclical dosage pattern if the uterus is intact to prevent endometrial hyperplasia and possible cancer. Continuous progesterone therapy is no longer recommended because of association with adverse breast outcomes.
3. Vaginal preparations are most effective for atrophic vaginitis. Concomitant progesterone is not indicated with vaginal estrogen because of minimal systemic absorption of estrogen.
4. Available as synthetic, animal-based, and natural (plant source) products.
5. Menopausal hormone therapy is contraindicated with the following conditions:
   a. Increased risk of thromboembolic disease, previous or current idiopathic deep vein thrombosis, or pulmonary embolism.
   b. Past, current, or suspected breast cancer.
   c. Estrogen-sensitive cancers (uterine, ovarian), untreated endometrial hyperplasia, and undiagnosed genital bleeding.
   d. Active or recent angina or myocardial infarction.
   e. Untreated hypertension.
   f. Active liver disease.
   g. Hypersensitivity to active substances in menopausal hormone therapy.
   h. Porphyria cutanea tarda (absolute contraindication).
6. Data are lacking to support progesterone or progestin alone for the treatment of hot flashes.

Other Measures

1. Vaginal lubricants to decrease vaginal dryness and dyspareunia.
2. Calcium and vitamin D supplements to prevent bone loss.
3. Nonhormonal treatment of menopausal symptoms that may be considered includes SSRIs for depressive symptoms, clonidine (central alpha-blocker) or gabapentin for vasomotor symptoms. These therapies are supported by evidence.
4. Dietary supplements (considered natural products by consumers)—limited data are available on efficacy and safety. The patient should discuss potential benefits and risks with a health care provider.
   a. Soy products contain varying amounts of isoflavones which act as phytoestrogens to reduce hot flashes. Most dietary soy products do not contain enough isoflavones to cause significant effects, but adverse effects may include headaches, nausea, and other gastrointestinal symptoms.
   b. Red clover isoflavones have been shown through meta-analysis to reduce hot flashes. Common adverse reactions are headaches, nausea, and vaginal spotting.
   c. Black cohosh has very limited evidence of reducing hot flashes. Adverse reactions include gastrointestinal upset, rash, and in rare cases, liver damage.
   d. Vitamin E supplementation shows some benefit in reducing hot flashes and atrophic vaginitis according to a recent systematic review of 16 studies.

DRUG ALERT Phytoestrogens may be contraindicated in females with strong risk for hormone-dependent conditions such as breast, uterine, and ovarian cancer.

   e. Multiple randomized clinical trials have shown evening primrose oil to reduce menopausal symptoms such as anxiety and irritability, hot flashes and night sweats, and improve quality of life. Mild gastrointestinal effects and headache may occur.
   f. A systematic review of randomized clinical trials of ginseng showed varying results, with several studies showing ginseng to reduce hot flashes and menopausal symptoms, and improve quality of life. Gastrointestinal effects, insomnia, hypertension, and bleeding may occur with excessive use.

DRUG ALERT Clinical trial data on the following commonly used herbal supplements have demonstrated improved symptom relief over placebo: evening primrose, ginseng, and red clover.

Complications

1. Osteoporosis has been clearly linked to estrogen depletion in menopause.
2. Coronary artery disease (CAD) rarely develops in females before menopause and may be associated with the effects of estrogen depletion on blood vessels.
3. Vaginal atrophy related to a dry, estrogen-depleted epithelium increases the risk for dyspareunia, recurrent vulvovaginitis, and urinary tract infections (UTIs). More research is required related to the etiology and treatment of postmenopausal stress and urge urinary incontinence.
4. Psychosocial issues of menopause: risk of depression increases.

Nursing Assessment

1. Obtain history of the patient's current symptoms and menstrual cycle.
2. Obtain history for other risk factors for CAD, osteoporosis, stroke, depression, breast cancer, and uterine cancer.
3. Assess genitalia for atrophy, dryness, and elasticity.
4. Assess the patient's emotional response to menopause.

Nursing Interventions

Maintaining Normal Activity and Sexuality Patterns

1. Explore with patient feelings about menopause, clear up misconceptions about sexual functioning, and encourage patient to discuss feelings with partner.
2. Tell the patient that sexual functioning may decrease during menopause but may even increase because of loss of fear of pregnancy and increased time if children are grown.
3. Instruct the patient how to use a water-based lubricant for intercourse to decrease dryness or discuss vaginal estrogen replacement therapy.

Increasing Knowledge and Self-Management

1. Provide patient with information related to estrogen replacement therapy, including dosage schedule, route, adverse effects, and what to expect of menstrual bleeding.
   a. Patients who still have a uterus can expect a period at the end of every month if they take hormones cyclically. Progesterone cyclical cotherapy is indicated to prevent endometrial hyperplasia.
   b. Systemic preparations (oral, transdermal) are indicated for systemic symptoms, such as hot flashes and mood swings.
   c. Vaginal preparations are indicated for vaginal atrophy and may help to reduce recurrent UTIs.
2. Help patient to understand the risks versus benefits of menopausal hormone therapy, formulate questions, and initiate discussion with health care provider about treatment options for vasomotor symptoms. Refer patient to clinical trial results from the Women's Health Initiative (www.nhlbi.nih.gov/whi).

Patient Education and Health Maintenance

1. Teach the patient about foods that are high in calcium and vitamin D—dairy products, dark green vegetables, salmon, and fortified foods. Encourage patient to maintain weight-bearing activities several times weekly to prevent osteoporosis.
2. Counsel patient on reducing risk factors for CAD, including smoking cessation.
3. Encourage patient to keep regular medical and gynecologic follow-up visits, including all age-appropriate screenings, such as mammography, pelvic exam, dual-energy x-ray absorptiometry (DEXA) scan for osteoporosis, lipid panel, and colonoscopy.
4. Advise patient that vulvovaginal infection and trauma are possible because of the dryness of the tissue and to seek prompt evaluation if pain and discharge occur or increases.
5. Encourage patient to talk to health care providers about concerns such as breast cancer with hormonal therapy. Also, refer the patient for information on postmenopausal hormone therapy to https://www.nih.gov/health-information/menopausal-hormone-therapy-information.
6. Encourage patients to report all use of supplements to their health care providers so they can use these preparations appropriately and safely.

POPULATION AWARENESS In postmenopausal patients, if vaginal bleeding occurs and is not associated with hormone replacement, report to health care provider immediately because endometrial cancer may be suspected.

Evaluation: Expected Outcomes

- Verbalizes confidence in sexual function and usual activities.
- Verbalizes satisfactory management of menopausal symptoms.

INFECTIONS AND INFLAMMATION OF THE VULVA, VAGINA, AND CERVIX

Some conditions are considered sexually transmitted, others are caused by inflammation or non–sexually transmitted infections (STIs). For syphilis, see page 645.

EVIDENCE BASE Workowski, K. A., Bachmann, L. H., Chan, P. A., Johnston, C. M., Muzny, C. A., Park, I., Reno, H., Zenilman, J. M., & Bolan, G. A. (2021). Sexually transmitted infections treatment guidelines, 2021. *MMWR Recommendations and Reports, 70*(4), 1–187. https://doi.org/10.15585/mmwr.rr7004a1. www.cdc.gov/std/treatment-guidlines/default.htm

Vulvitis

Vulvitis is inflammation of the vulva.

Pathophysiology and Etiology

Causative Factors

1. Infections—*Trichomonas*, molluscum contagiosum, bacteria, fungi, herpes simplex virus (HSV), and human papillomavirus (HPV; genital warts). Also, see pages 640–645.
2. Irritants.
   a. Urine, feces, and vaginal discharge.
   b. Close-fitting, synthetic fabrics.
   c. Chemicals, such as laundry detergents, vaginal sprays, deodorants, perfumes, some soaps, chlorine, dryer sheets, and bubble bath.
3. Carcinoma.
4. Chronic dermatologic conditions, such as psoriasis or eczema.

Predisposing Factors

1. Illnesses, such as diabetes mellitus and dermatologic disorders.
2. Atrophy due to menopause.

Clinical Manifestations

1. Pruritus—more acute at night, aggravated by warmth, often associated with candidal infections.
2. Reddened, edematous tissue, possible ulceration.
3. Pain, burning, and dyspareunia.
4. Exudate—possibly profuse and purulent—involving vaginitis.
5. Lesions of molluscum contagiosum are multiple, from 1 mm to 1 cm in size, and filled with white caseous material.
6. Lesions of HSV are vesicles with an erythematous base, clustered in a somewhat linear pattern.
7. Lesions of HPV are flesh-colored, irregular, raised, soft warty-like growths.

Diagnostic Evaluation

1. Vulvar smears and cultures—may show infectious organism.
2. Biopsy of vulvar tissue—may be necessary to rule out malignancy and chronic dermatologic conditions.

Management

1. Oral or topical anti-infectives (antibiotics, antifungals, antivirals) to treat infectious agents.
2. Extremely low-dose topical steroids to treat inflammation in some cases.
3. Vaginal estrogen to treat vaginal atrophy associated with menopause.
4. Treatment of underlying disorder.
5. Molluscum contagiosum may be treated by scalpel excision, silver nitrate, electrical cautery, or curette or may be left untreated, allowing spontaneous resolution.

Complications

1. Scarring and chronic discomfort.
2. Transmission of STI to partner.

Nursing Assessment

1. Question the patient about medical history, symptoms, and sexual activity.
2. Determine use of chemical-containing products on undergarments or directly on the vulva.
3. Examine the genitalia and lymph nodes.

Nursing Interventions

Relieving Pain

1. Administer prescribed medications and instruct the patient on their use, method of application, and adverse effects.
2. Instruct on use of sitz baths, or sitting in warm water for 15 to 20 minutes, three to four times daily. May also use cool compresses to soothe and clean vulva.
3. Instruct the patient about the nature of the condition (e.g., chronic recurrent or curable) and expectations for symptoms after treatment.

Patient Education and Health Maintenance

1. Teach the patient hygienic principles.
   a. Wipe from front to back after voiding.
   b. Use cotton with warm water and bland soap for cleansing, rinse, and pat dry. May also use fragrance-free hypoallergenic wet wipes.
2. Teach the patient to avoid chemical irritants, such as sprays, perfumed and deodorant soaps, new laundry detergents, static-control dryer sheets, and bubble bath.
3. Teach the patient to avoid mechanical irritants, such as tight clothing, synthetic fabrics, and undergarments; replace these with loose-fitting cotton undergarments. Avoid chronic moisture; change bathing suit after swimming.
4. Teach the patient how to use sitz bath and cool compresses at home and to avoid scratching.
5. Teach the patient that some infections, such as *Trichomonas*, molluscum contagiosum, and HSV, are sexually transmitted; so the partner needs to seek treatment before intercourse is resumed. Assist the patient with health communication techniques to inform partner.
6. Educate about STI prevention and encourage screening (see Box 18-1).

Evaluation: Expected Outcomes

- Verbalizes increased comfort level and control of symptoms.

BOX 18-1 Sexually Transmitted Infection Prevention Counseling

Sexually transmitted infections (STIs) can be prevented through interactive, patient-centered counseling approaches that address personal risk. Key techniques to facilitate rapport include use of open-ended questions and understandable language. Most effective strategies are performed in nonjudgmental and empathetic ways, incorporating the patient's culture, language, gender, sexual orientation, age, and developmental level. Motivational interviewing techniques and assessing for readiness to change are also helpful.

The first step in counseling is taking a sexual history, including:

- Type and number of partners.
- Methods for prevention of pregnancy.
- Methods for prevention of STIs.
- Past history of STIs.
- Exposure to intravenous drug use or sex workers.

An individualized prevention plan may incorporate one or more of the following specific methods of prevention:

- Abstinence from oral, vaginal, and anal sex. Encourage abstinence until beginning a mutually monogamous lifetime relationship.
- Monogamy: to be in a long-term, mutually monogamous relationship with an uninfected person. Before starting a mutually monogamous sexual relationship, individuals may consider screening for STIs.
- Reduce the number of lifetime sexual partners.
- Preexposure vaccination:
  - Human papillomavirus (HPV) vaccine (ages 9 to 26).
  - Hepatitis B vaccine (plus hepatitis A vaccine for males who have sex with males and people who use intravenous [IV] drugs).
- Proper use of male condoms (latex or polyurethane; not "natural" or "lambskin" condoms, which do not protect against viral transmission) with correct use:
  - A new condom with each new sex act.
  - Carefully handle the condom so as not to puncture it.
  - Put condom on after penis is erect.
  - Ensure adequate lubrication.
  - Use only water-based lubricants; oil-based lubricants (petroleum jelly, massage oil, cooking oils) will weaken condom.
  - Hold condom firmly at base during withdrawal to avoid it slipping off.
  - Condoms with spermicidal lubricants are not recommended to prevent STIs.
- Proper use of female condoms (lubricated polyurethane or nitrile sheath with a ring on each end, i.e., inserted into the vagina): Use as a protective barrier before intimate contact.
- Adolescents and adults who use nonbarrier methods of contraception (hormones, intrauterine conception [IUC] surgery) should be counseled about barrier methods to prevent STIs because they may incorrectly perceive that they are not at risk for STIs.
- Spermicides do not prevent STI/human immunodeficiency virus (HIV) transmission; they may increase it by disrupting normal epithelium.

EVIDENCE BASE Centers for Disease Control and Prevention. (2021). *Sexually transmitted infections treatment guidelines, 2021*. Author. www.cdc.gov/std/treatment-guidelines/STI-Guidelines-2021.pdf

Bartholin Cyst or Abscess

Bartholin cyst or *abscess*, also called *bartholinitis*, is an infection of the greater vestibular gland, causing cyst or abscess formation.

Pathophysiology and Etiology

1. These glands lie on both sides of the vagina at the base of the labia minora; they lubricate the vagina.
2. If they become obstructed secondary to infection, abscess or cyst formation may occur (see Figure 18-2).
3. Abscess or cyst may spontaneously rupture or enlarge and become painful.
4. Most are sterile or abscess/cellulitis caused by mixed vaginal flora.
5. May also be caused by sexual transmission of infection (gonorrhea or chlamydia).

Clinical Manifestations

1. Asymptomatic cyst.
2. Pain, erythema, tenderness, swelling.
3. Edema, cellulitis, possible abscess formation.

Diagnostic Evaluation

1. Culture, if draining or upon excision, to identify infectious organisms.
2. If older than age 40, or recurrent, carcinoma must be ruled out by biopsy.

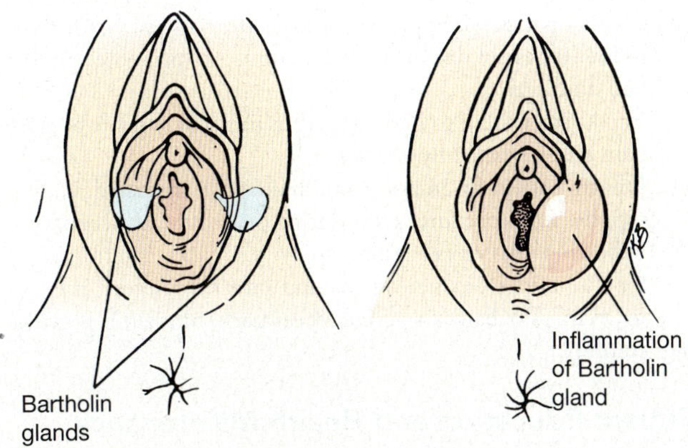

Figure 18-2. Site and infection of vestibular gland.

Management

1. May be treated conservatively with warm soaks or sitz baths if small or asymptomatic; antibiotics used if cellulitis is present.
2. May need incision and drainage; provides immediate relief, but may recur. Procedures are generally done under local anesthesia and take about 20 minutes in an outpatient office.
   a. Contents are opened and drained; culture sent. Then, sutures are closed.
      i. As an alternative, a Word catheter, Foley catheter, or Jacobi ring is inserted to keep cavity open (called fistulization).
      ii. Healing occurs around catheter and it is removed 2 to 4 weeks later to provide a new opening to the gland.
3. Marsupialization, for recurrent abscesses.
   a. Cyst is incised and sutured open to incision edges.
   b. Healing occurs from within the area of the abscess.
4. Other acceptable methods of treatment include silver nitrate gland ablation, cyst or abscess ablation or excision with a carbon dioxide laser, and needle aspiration with or without alcohol sclerotherapy.
5. Complete excision under general anesthesia if carcinoma is suspected.
6. All treatment methods heal within 2 weeks or less. Recurrence may occur in up to 20% of patients with all treatment methods. No method has been demonstrated to be superior in healing rate or recurrence rate.

Complications

Scarring from recurrent infection and rupture.

Nursing Assessment

1. Obtain history of sexual activity, including new partners and history of STIs. Risk for Bartholin gland cyst or abscess is similar to risk for STIs.
2. Inspect the labia minora for warmth, erythema, and swelling.
3. Assess for signs of other STIs—rash, genital ulcers, and vaginal discharge.

Nursing Interventions

Relieving Pain

1. Administer pain medications and antibiotics, or teach self-administration, as ordered; explain adverse effects to patient.
2. Instruct patient to apply warm soaks or to use sitz bath three to four times per day for 15 to 20 minutes to promote comfort and drainage.
3. Encourage patient to limit activity as much as possible because pain is exacerbated by activity.
4. Prepare patient for incision and drainage, if indicated. Gather supplies for procedure; assist during procedure, as necessary.
5. Following marsupialization: apply ice packs intermittently for 24 hours to reduce edema and provide comfort; thereafter, warm sitz baths, a perineal heat pack, or a lamp provides comfort.

Patient Education and Health Maintenance

1. If STI is the suspected cause of infection, advise patient to instruct partner to be tested and treated prophylactically.
2. Advise patient to abstain from intercourse until cyst or abscess has resolved, partner has been examined and treated, and patient has completed all antibiotics (approximately 2 weeks).
3. Review principles of perineal hygiene with patient.
4. Discuss STIs and methods of prevention—abstinence, monogamy, and proper use of female or male condoms. See page 613.
5. Encourage patient to follow-up for recurrent abscess to rule out malignant lesions. Surgical treatment is commonly necessary for recurrences.

Evaluation: Expected Outcomes

- Verbalizes relief of pain.

Vaginal Fistula

A *vaginal fistula* is an abnormal, tortuous opening between the vagina and another hollow organ (see Figure 18-3).

Pathophysiology and Etiology

Causes

1. Obstetric injury, especially in long labors and in countries with inadequate obstetric care (rarely occurs in developed nations).
2. Pelvic surgery (rare)—hysterectomy or vaginal reconstructive procedures.
3. Carcinoma (rare)—extensive disease or complication of treatment such as radiation therapy.

Types

1. *Vesicovaginal* fistula is an opening between the bladder and vagina.
2. *Rectovaginal* fistula is an opening between the rectum and vagina.
3. *Ureterovaginal* fistula is an opening between the ureter and vagina.
4. *Urethrovaginal* fistula is an opening between the urethra and vagina.
5. *Vaginoperineal* fistula is an opening between the vagina and perineum.

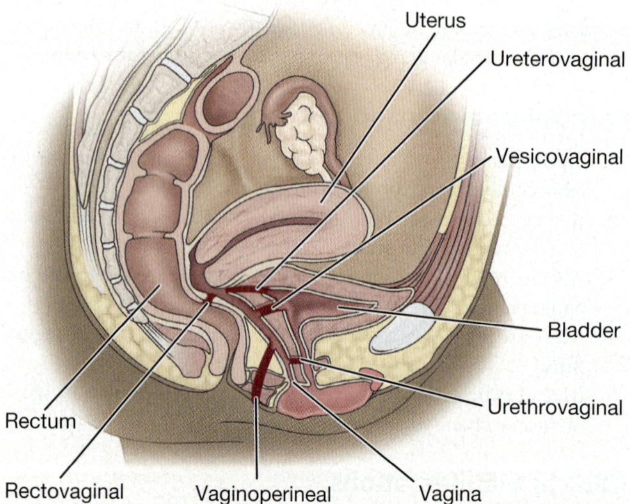

Figure 18-3. Sites of vaginal fistulas. (Adapted with permission from Hinkle, J. L., Cheever, K. H., & Overbaugh, K. [2022]. *Brunner and Suddarth's textbook of medical-surgical nursing* [15th ed., Fig. 51-2]. Wolters Kluwer.)

Clinical Manifestations

1. Vesicovaginal—the most common type of fistula.
   a. Constant trickling of urine into the vagina.
   b. Loss of urge to void because the bladder is continuously emptying.
   c. May cause excoriation and inflammation of the vulva.
2. Rectovaginal.
   a. Fecal incontinence and flatus through the vagina; malodorous.
   b. May present as vulvar cancer.
3. Ureterovaginal fistula—rare.
   a. Urine in the vagina but the patient still voids regularly.
   b. May cause severe UTIs.
4. Urethrovaginal fistula.
   a. Dysuria.
   b. Urine in the vagina on voiding.
5. Vaginoperineal fistula—pain and inflammation of the perineum.

Diagnostic Evaluation

1. Methylene blue test—after instillation of this dye in the bladder via catheter, place tampon in the vagina. Remove after the female has ambulated.
   a. Methylene blue appears in the vagina in vesicovaginal fistula.
   b. Methylene blue does not appear in the vagina in ureterovaginal fistula.
2. Indigo carmine test—after a methylene blue test shows negative results, indigo carmine is injected intravenously (IV). If dye appears in the vagina, this indicates ureterovaginal fistula.
3. Cystoscopy with retrograde pyelography.
4. Intravenous pyelography (IVP)—helps to detect ureteral fistulas.

Management

1. Fistulas recognized at the time of delivery should be corrected immediately.
2. Historically, surgeries were delayed for 8 to 12 weeks to allow recovery from infection or inflammation. However, early excision and repair within 1 to 2 weeks of urine leakage have become common.
3. Surgical closure of opening via vaginal route is most common in developing nations. In developed nations, laparoscopic, vaginal, or abdominal or robot-assisted routes may be used.
4. Fecal or urinary diversion procedure may be required for large fistulas.
5. Rarely, a fistula may heal without surgical intervention.
6. Medical approach.
   a. Prosthesis to prevent incontinence and allow tissue to heal; done for patients who are not surgical candidates.
   b. Prosthesis is inserted into the vagina; it is connected to drainage tubing leading to a leg bag.

Complications

1. Hydronephrosis, pyelonephritis, and possible renal failure with ureterovaginal fistula.
2. Vaginal infection and pelvic organ infection from rectovaginal fistula.

Nursing Assessment

1. Obtain obstetric, gynecologic, and surgical history.
2. Monitor intake and output and voiding pattern.
3. Assess drainage on perineal pads.
4. Watch for signs of infection (fever, chills, flank pain).

Nursing Interventions

Preventing Infection

1. Before repair surgery, encourage frequent sitz baths and recommend the use of incontinence products with frequent changing.
2. Perform vaginal irrigation, as ordered, and teach patient the procedure.
3. Administer prescribed antibiotics to reduce pathogenic flora in the intestinal tract. A single injectable dose of gentamicin before surgery is as effective as extended use of amoxicillin, chloramphenicol, or cotrimoxazole.
4. After rectovaginal repair:
   a. Maintain clear liquid diet, as prescribed, to limit bowel activity for several days.
   b. Encourage rest.
   c. Administer warm perineal irrigations to decrease healing time and increase comfort.
5. After vesicovaginal repair:
   a. Maintain proper drainage from indwelling catheter (intermittent flushing with sterile normal saline) to prevent pressure on newly sutured tissue (usually for about 7 days postoperatively).
   b. Administer vaginal or bladder irrigations gently because of tenderness at operative site.
   c. Maintain strict intake and output records. IV fluids or copious oral fluid intake may be recommended to maintain good urinary flow.
   d. Prophylactic antibiotics to prevent infection may be recommended.
6. If medical management is indicated, teach patient the use of prosthetic device.
7. Encourage patient to express feelings about self-esteem and sexual function.

Patient Education and Health Maintenance

1. Teach patient to report signs of infection early.
2. Teach the patient to clean the perineum gently and to follow surgeon's instructions on when to resume sexual intercourse and strenuous activity.
3. Advise patient to keep regular follow-up appointments.

Evaluation: Expected Outcomes

- No signs of infection—afebrile and no complaints of flank pain or difficulty voiding.

Vaginitis

Vaginitis is inflammation of the vagina caused by infectious pathogens.

Pathophysiology and Etiology

1. May be caused by sexually transmitted organisms or overgrowth of vaginal flora.
2. Normal vaginal secretions because of estrogen secretion and acidity inhibit the growth of pathogens.
3. Such conditions as diabetes, pregnancy, stress, coitus, and menopause alter normal vaginal environment.
4. Types of vaginitis (see Table 18-3).
   a. Simple (contact).
   b. Bacterial vaginosis (most often caused by *Gardnerella*).
   c. *Trichomonas*.
   d. *Candida albicans*.
   e. Atrophic.

Table 18-3 Types of Vaginitis

DESCRIPTION	MANIFESTATIONS	MANAGEMENT
Simple Vaginitis (Contact Vaginitis)		
• An inflammation of the vagina, with discharge; due to mechanical, chemical, allergic, or other noninfectious irritation, poor hygiene, imbalance in vaginal flora. • Urethritis commonly accompanies vaginitis because of the proximity of the urethra to the vagina. • Predisposing factors: contact allergens, excessive perspiration, synthetic underclothing, poor hygiene, foreign bodies (tampons, condoms, spermicides, condoms with spermicides, diaphragms that have been left in too long).	• Increased (yet minimal) vaginal discharge with itching, redness, burning, and edema. • Voiding and defecation aggravate the above symptoms.	• Stimulate the growth of lactobacilli (Doderlein bacilli) through consumption of yogurt with live active cultures. • Current evidence does not support douching. • Foster cleanliness by meticulous care after voiding and defecation. • Discontinue use of causative agent.
Bacterial Vaginosis		
• An inflammation of the vagina commonly referred to as nonspecific vaginitis because it is *not* caused by *Trichomonas*, *Candida*, or gonorrhea. It is not considered an STI. • Increased levels of *Gardnerella vaginalis* are usually responsible for symptoms.	• Vaginal discharge with odor. • Itching and burning may suggest concomitant organisms present. • It is benign in that when the discharge is wiped away, underlying tissue is healthy and pink. • Vaginal pH is >4.5. • May be asymptomatic. • Presence of "clue" cells on microscopic examination of saline slide • Positive KOH "whiff" test (fishy odor).	• Treatment only recommended for symptomatic patients. • Metronidazole taken orally for 7 d or topical clindamycin or metronidazole. • Alcohol intake should be avoided during metronidazole treatment and for 24 h after completion to avoid nausea and vertigo. Studies have demonstrated that metronidazole is not teratogenic. • Treating partners is not recommended. • Clindamycin cream weakens latex condoms. • Data do not support douching.
Trichomonas vaginalis		
• STI. A condition produced by a protozoan (pear-shaped and motile) that thrives in an alkaline environment. Recurrence may occur because of low levels of antimicrobial resistance.	• Copious malodorous discharge; may be frothy and yellow-green in color. • May have pruritus, dyspareunia, and spotting. • Red, speckled (strawberry) punctate hemorrhages on the cervix. • May also have vulvar edema, dysuria, and hyperemia secondary to irritation of discharge. • Motile organisms visible on saline microscopy. • Point-of-care rapid test and cultures are available.	• Destroy infective protozoa by taking oral metronidazole 2 g or tinidazole 2 g. • *Note:* Treatment during pregnancy is acceptable after the first trimester for tinidazole and throughout pregnancy for metronidazole. • Prevent reinfection by treating partner concurrently, even though male may be asymptomatic. • Avoid alcohol during treatment. • Rescreen after 3 mo because of possibility of low-level antimicrobial resistance.
Candida albicans		

• A fungal infection caused by *Candida albicans*. Associated factors include:
  • Steroid therapy
  • Obesity
  • Pregnancy
  • Antibiotic therapy
  • Diabetes mellitus
  • Oral contraceptives
  • Frequent douching
  • Chronic debilitative diseases
	• Vaginal discharge is thick and irritating; white or yellow patchy, cheeselike particles adhere to vaginal walls.
	• Itching is the most common complaint.
	• May also experience burning, soreness, vulvar edema, excoriations, fissures, dyspareunia, frequency, and dysuria.
	• Microscopic examination will reveal hyphae, buds, and pseudohyphae.
	• Vaginal pH is normal (<4.5).
		• Eradicate the fungus by applying antifungal vaginal cream (clotrimazole, miconazole, or ketoconazole), suppository, or tablet for 1–14 nights, as ordered; or take oral fluconazole in single dose.
		• Oral fluconazole is contraindicated in pregnancy; topical creams may be used.
		• Side effects of topical vaginal creams include burning and irritation. Systemic fluconazole is associated with GI intolerance, headaches, and rare and transitory elevations in liver function tests.
		• Azole antifungals have clinically important interactions with many medications.

Table 18-3 Types of Vaginitis (*continued*)

DESCRIPTION	MANIFESTATIONS	MANAGEMENT
• Characteristics • *C. albicans* is a normal inhabitant of the intestinal tract and therefore a frequent contaminant of the vagina. • Because this fungus thrives in an environment rich in carbohydrates, it is seen commonly in patients with poorly controlled diabetes. • This infection is observed in patients who have been on antibiotic or steroid therapy for a while (reduces natural protective organisms in the vagina).		• Incorporate live culture yogurt into diet to enhance lactobacillus colonization and improve microorganism balance in the vagina. • Treat the symptomatic or uncircumcised partner with balanitis by applying antifungal cream under the foreskin nightly for 7 nights. • For severe or recurrent cases, use systemic antifungal, such as weekly fluconazole for suppression therapy.
Atrophic Vaginitis		
• A common postmenopausal occurrence due to atrophy of the vaginal mucosa secondary to decreased estrogen levels; more susceptible to infection.	• Vaginal itching, dryness, burning, dyspareunia, and vulvar irritation. • May also have vaginal bleeding. • Vaginal mucosa appears dry and slightly paler. **CLINICAL JUDGMENT** In the postmenopausal female, if vaginal bleeding occurs, encourage patient to see health care provider immediately because bleeding is a warning sign of cancer.	• Vaginal estrogen treatment is most effective. • The condition reverses itself under treatment, which must be maintained. • If infection is also present, this is treated. • If the uterus is intact and systemic estrogen therapy is used to treat additional menopausal symptoms, progesterone must be added to prevent endometrial hyperplasia due to unopposed estrogen.

GI, gastrointestinal; STI, sexually transmitted infection.

Clinical Manifestations

Signs and symptoms vary with etiology or causative organism.

1. Vaginal itching, irritation, burning.
2. Odor and increased or unusual vaginal discharge.
3. Dyspareunia, pelvic pain, dysuria.
4. Asymptomatic.

Diagnostic Evaluation

1. History and physical examination.
2. Wet smear for microscopic examination.
   a. Saline slide: discharge mixed with saline; useful in detecting *Gardnerella* and *Trichomonas* organisms.
   b. Potassium hydroxide (KOH): useful in detecting *C. albicans* and *Gardnerella* by whiff test (if fishy odor is noted when KOH is applied, suspect *Gardnerella* organisms causing bacterial vaginosis).
3. Vaginal pH (not diagnostic, but may indicate infection)—use nitrazine paper.
   a. Normal pH: 4.0 to 4.5.
   b. Bacterial vaginosis: greater than 4.5.
   c. *Trichomonas*: greater than 4.5.
4. Chlamydia and gonorrhea cultures or DNA probe—to rule out chlamydia or gonorrhea cervicitis.
5. Pap smear—not considered a diagnostic tool for vaginitis: it has low sensitivity and specificity to detect bacterial vaginosis and *Trichomonas*.

Management

1. Anti-infectives (oral or vaginal preparations).
2. Estrogen replacement (systemic or vaginal preparation) for atrophic vaginitis.
3. Evaluation and treatment of sexual partners for STIs, such as *Trichomonas*.
4. Vaginal recolonization with lactobacilli through ingestion of yogurt with active cultures.

Nursing Assessment

1. Obtain a health history including questions specific to the condition.
   a. Nature of discharge: cheeselike, frothy, puslike, thick or thin, or scant? Onset? Color? Odor? Other symptoms: dysuria, itching, and dyspareunia?
   b. Menstrual history.
   c. Disease history: diabetes mellitus and its control? Previous vaginal infections? STIs?
   d. Obstetric history.
   e. Sexual history: age of onset of sexual activity? New partner? Numbers of current and lifetime partners? Frequency of sexual activity? Its nature? Urogenital symptoms or infections in partner? Current barrier use?
   f. Medications and allergies. Current contraceptive use?
   g. Vaginal hygiene: use of douches, deodorants, sprays, and ointments; types of tampons, bubble bath, shower/bath soap, and nature of clothing (tight-fitting)?

2. Perform or assist with a physical examination, including a vaginal examination, and obtain vaginal and/or cervical discharge specimens, as indicated.

Nursing Interventions

Improving Comfort

1. Instruct patient to discontinue use of irritating agents, such as bubble baths and vaginal douches.
2. Suggest that the patient take cool baths or sitz baths and pat dry or dry with hair dryer on low setting.
3. Encourage the patient to wear loose cotton undergarments.
4. Encourage the patient to take analgesics.
5. Provide emotional support.

Promoting Tissue Integrity

1. Teach the patient to clean the perineum and pat dry before applying medication.
2. Demonstrate application of prescribed medication.
3. Emphasize importance of taking prescribed medication for full length of therapy and as directed; teach patient adverse effects.
4. Stress importance of follow-up visits.

Reducing STI Transmission Risk

1. Emphasize importance of sexual abstinence and vaginal rest (nothing in the vagina) until therapy is complete and sexual partner has been treated, if indicated.
2. Tell patient use of condoms may be protective but may produce irritation.
3. Instruct the patient in the use of water-soluble lubricant if the vagina is dry and atrophic.
4. Instruct the patient that some oil-based vaginal medications may decrease the efficacy of condoms to protect against STIs and pregnancy.

Patient Education and Health Maintenance

1. Teach causes of vaginitis and its symptoms so patient can seek treatment promptly.
2. Discuss STIs and methods of prevention—abstinence, monogamy, and proper use of female or male condoms. See page 613.
3. Teach measures to prevent vaginitis.
   a. Wipe from front to back after toilet use.
   b. Keep area clean and dry.
   c. Wear loose cotton clothing to absorb moisture and provide good circulation.
   d. Change sanitary pads and tampons frequently so they do not become saturated.
   e. Avoid bubble baths, vaginal deodorants, sprays, and douches.
   f. If the patient insists on using douches (not recommended), use a mild vinegar solution (2 teaspoons white vinegar to 1 quart water) at the end of a menstrual cycle. Teach proper technique: to infuse gently to lightly bathe tissues and to avoid using a forceful stream that could push bacteria higher inside the pelvis.
4. For recurrent *Candida* infections, encourage good control if the patient has diabetes or encourage the patient to be tested for diabetes. Teach all patients to eliminate concentrated carbohydrates from diet to prevent recurrence.

Evaluation: Expected Outcomes

- Verbalizes relief of discomfort.
- Vaginal mucosa pink, with normal amount and color of secretions.
- Reports practice of prevention methods.

Human Papillomavirus Infection

HPV infection may be asymptomatic but frequently causes *condyloma acuminatum* or genital warts.

Pathophysiology and Etiology

1. Sexually transmitted; highly contagious.
2. More than 40 types of HPV can infect the genital tract, many are asymptomatic, and multiple types may coexist.
3. Ninety percent of visible genital warts are caused by HPV types 6 and 11. Up to 70% of cervical cancer and precancerous lesions are caused by types 16 and 18. Types 31, 33, 45, 52, 58, and others have been strongly associated with cervical dysplasia.
4. Incubation period of up to 8 months.

Clinical Manifestations

1. Single or multiple soft, fleshy painless growths of the vulva, vagina, cervix, urethra, or anal area that may be irritating or uncomfortable (see Figure 18-4).
2. May be subclinical infection and still contagious.
3. Occasional vaginal bleeding, discharge, odor, and dyspareunia.

Diagnostic Evaluation

1. Pap smear—shows characteristic cellular changes (koilocytosis).
2. Acetic acid swabbing on vaginal examination will whiten lesions and make them more identifiable in genital mucosa. However, this test is not specific to HPV and is not recommended for screening.
3. Cervical sampling for viral DNA tests to detect subclinical HPV; however, the significance of positive and negative results has not been determined. Liquid Pap smear done for cervical cancer screening for females older than 30 years—if the Pap smear is abnormal, DNA testing is done to confirm the presence of HPV causing cellular changes (known as reflex testing). DNA HPV testing is not recommended for genital wart diagnosis.
4. Colposcopy is also used to diagnose subclinical HPV infection.
5. Anoscopy or urethroscopy may be necessary to identify anal and urethral lesions.
6. Genital warts are usually diagnosed on physical exam through visual inspection.

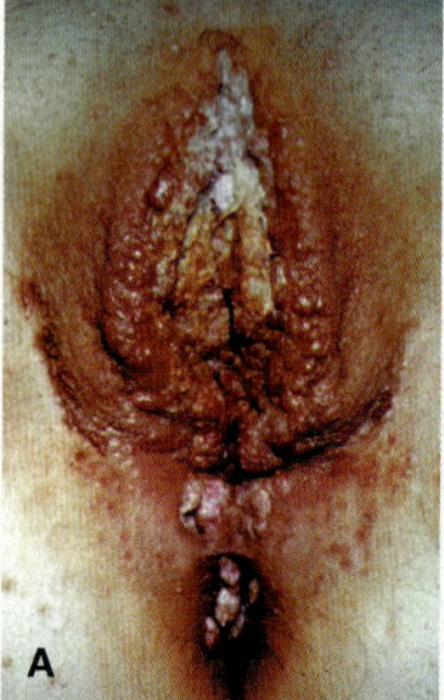

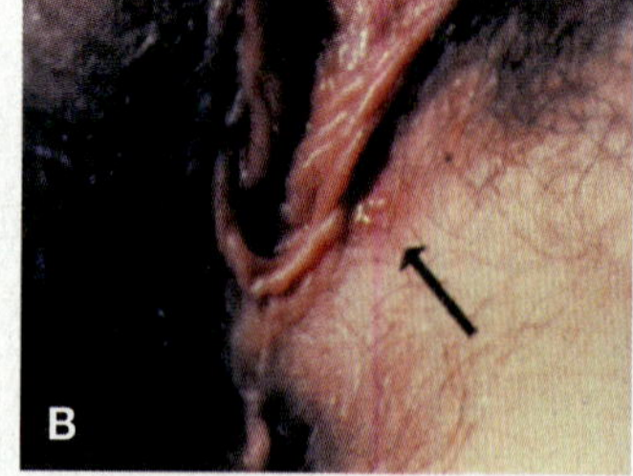

Figure 18-4. Genital lesions. **(A)** Condyloma acuminatum. **(B)** Genital herpes. Arrow indicates vesicular lesion.

Management

Therapies are likely to reduce HPV infectivity but do not eradicate HPV. Treatment method is guided by provider and patient preferences.

1. External lesions may be treated by the patient with multiple applications of a topical preparation. Perform hand hygiene before and after, or wear gloves for application.
   a. Podofilox—applied with cotton swab or finger to visible warts twice per day for 3 days and then no treatment for 4 days; may be repeated for up to four cycles of therapy.
   b. Imiquimod—applied by finger three times per week for up to 16 weeks; may be washed off 6 to 10 hours after application.
   c. Sinecatechins ointment—applied by finger three times daily for up to 16 weeks; not washed off after use.
   d. Safety of these products during pregnancy is unknown and therefore is not recommended.
2. Noncervical lesions may be treated by health care provider with topical preparations, such as podophyllin resin, trichloroacetic acid, or bichloroacetic acid.
   a. Requires multiple visits for repeat treatments.
   b. May require washing off several hours later.
3. Cryotherapy with liquid nitrogen or cryoprobe, electrocautery, laser treatment, or local excision of large warts or cervical lesions.
4. Highly recurrent, particularly in first 3 months—may require retreatment.
5. Subclinical genital HPV infection typically clears spontaneously and treatment is not recommended.
6. Three vaccines for HPV are available in the United States.
   a. Bivalent HPV vaccine types 16 and 18; recombinant.
   b. Quadrivalent HPV vaccine types 6, 11, 16, and 18; recombinant.
   c. 9-valent vaccine types 6, 11, 16, 18, 31, 33, 45, 52, and 58.
7. Vaccine schedule: Advisory Committee on Immunization Practices (ACIP) recommends anyone starting the series before age 15 receives two doses of vaccine at least 6 months apart. If the two doses are received less than 5 months apart, a third dose of vaccine is recommended.
   a. The Centers for Disease Control and Prevention (CDC) recommends all vaccines for females aged 11 or 12 to 26 (licensed for ages 9 to 26).
   b. The quadrivalent vaccine is recommended for males aged 11 or 12 to 26 (licensed for ages 9 to 26).
   c. They are most effective when all doses are administered before the onset of sexual activity.

Complications

1. Implicated in cervical intraepithelial neoplasia.
2. May cause neonatal laryngeal papillomatosis if infant born through infected birth canal.
3. Obstruction of anal canal and vagina by enlarging lesions.
4. Scarring and pigment changes if treatment not employed properly.

Nursing Assessment

1. Obtain history of STIs, Pap test results, and sexual partners.
2. Inspect external genitalia for lesions; assist with vaginal examination.

Nursing Interventions

Improving Understanding of HPV Treatment

1. Explain to the patient that the goal of therapy is to remove visible lesions; however, HPV will not be cured or eliminated. Genital warts are not life-threatening.
2. Encourage the patient to adhere with treatment schedule and inspect areas for resolution of lesions or redevelopment of new lesions.
3. Advise the patient of high recurrence rate; 3-month follow-up visit is advisable; if lesions redevelop, the patient should follow-up for retreatment.
4. Advise patient about proper use of male or female condoms to reduce the risk of transmission, although not fully because HPV can infect areas not covered by the condom. Condom use, abstinence, and monogamy will protect against other STIs.
5. Encourage female patients to follow up regularly for Pap tests because HPV has been associated with cervical neoplasia.
6. Advise patient of risk to neonate during delivery; patient should receive close prenatal care if pregnant.

Patient Education and Health Maintenance

1. Advise patient to discuss HPV with partner. Partner should receive treatment for visible lesions. Screening for other STIs in both patient and partner is recommended.
2. Make sure patient realizes that even though lesions may be gone, HPV may still be transmitted to new sexual partners. Abstinence, monogamy, and condoms are advisable to prevent transmission of all STIs. See page 613.

Evaluation: Expected Outcomes

- Presents with no visible lesions at follow-up visit.

Herpes Genitalis

Herpes genitalis is a viral infection that causes lesions of the cervix, vagina, and external genitalia.

Pathophysiology and Etiology

1. Caused by HSV, usually type 2, but may be type 1, which usually causes oral or skin lesions (see page 880).
2. Sexually transmitted.
3. About 12% of the U.S. population ages 14 to 49 is infected with HSV-2.
4. HSV-1 infection is more prevalent but less often associated with sexually transmitted genital infections.
5. Infection is chronic and often presents with recurrent exacerbations. The virus lies dormant in dorsal root ganglia of spinal nerves between outbreaks.

Clinical Manifestations

1. Lesions occur 2 to 30 days after initial exposure, sometimes with fever, malaise, lymphadenopathy, and headache for primary infection (see Figure 18-4, page 640).
2. Lesions are preceded by sensation of tingling; proceed from vesicles on erythematous, edematous base to painful ulcers that crust and heal without scars.
3. Internal lesions may cause watery discharge and dyspareunia.
4. Recurrent lesions may be stimulated by fever, stress, illness, local trauma, menses, and sunburn.
5. Infection can be asymptomatic.

Diagnostic Evaluation

1. Virologic tests—detect virus.
   a. Polymerase chain reaction (PCR) assay is a type of nucleic acid amplification test (NAAT) for HSV DNA (genetic material) used to diagnose genital herpes infection as long as type 1 or type 2. PCR assays are very sensitive and highly specific. A swab is used to collect a sample from lesions.
   b. Viral cultures also can detect HSV by type but are less sensitive than PCR. A swab of active lesions is preserved in viral medium and transported to the laboratory. Failure to detect HSV by PCR or culture does not rule out HSV infection because viral shedding is intermittent.
2. Serologic (blood) tests—detect antibodies to HSV; are available as type specific or type common.
   a. May be false negative during early infection but persist well after active lesions have resolved. Type-specific tests based on glycoprotein G1 or glycoprotein G2 are variable in sensitivity and specificity, so confirmation tests (western blot) may be done.
   b. Test often used when there is clinical diagnosis of genital herpes but without other laboratory confirmation or for person with partner who has genital herpes.
3. Screening in the general population for HSV-1 and HSV-2 is not recommended.

Management

1. Systemic antivirals, such as acyclovir, famciclovir, and valacyclovir, suppress virus and decrease length, severity, and shedding of infection.
   a. Oral therapy may be episodic—started as soon as the first episode is diagnosed and whenever the first signs of a recurrence are recognized (within 24 hours of onset of prodromal symptoms or lesion onset).
      i. Acyclovir 400 mg po TID for 7 to 10 days for first episode; 800 mg BID for 5 days for recurrent episodes.
      ii. Famciclovir 250 mg po TID for 7 to 10 days for first episode; 1 g BID for 1 day for recurrent episodes.
      iii. Valacyclovir 1 g po BID for 7 to 10 days for first episode; 1 g qd × 5 days for recurrent episodes.
   b. Oral therapy may be given continuously to suppress recurrences and viral shedding, which reduces transmission, especially within the first 12 months of disease onset.
      i. Acyclovir 400 mg orally twice daily.
      ii. Valacyclovir 500 mg orally once a day (if infrequent recurrences); valacyclovir 1 g orally once a day (more effective if 10 or more recurrences yearly).
      iii. Famciclovir 250 mg orally twice daily.
   c. IV administration (acyclovir) may be necessary for severe infections (disseminated infections, pneumonitis, hepatitis, meningoencephalitis) or for immunocompromised patients.
   d. Topical treatment (acyclovir) is the least effective and not recommended.
2. Pain medication—ranges from acetaminophen and nonsteroidal anti-inflammatory drugs (NSAIDs) to oral opioids.
3. Local comfort measures, such as lidocaine gel, sitz baths, compresses, and use of a hair dryer, to area on cool setting.
4. Immunization has been under investigation. See *www.clinicaltrials.gov.*

Complications

1. Disseminated infection, meningitis, pneumonitis, and hepatitis.
2. Neonatal infection if neonate born through infected canal.

Nursing Assessment

1. Question the patient about frequency and type of sexual activity and discomfort noted.
2. Question the patient about pruritus, burning, tenderness, urinary symptoms, and unusual discharge.
3. Assess the patient's view of herpes, transmission, stigmas, misconceptions, and fears.
4. Inspect genitalia for lesions, erythema, and edema. Use a speculum to examine the vagina and cervix, as indicated.

Nursing Interventions

Relieving Pain

1. Demonstrate and encourage the use of warm sitz baths to increase blood supply to the areas and facilitate healing.
2. Instruct patient to keep the area clean and dry. Pat dry with a clean towel or use blow dryer on cool setting. Wear loose cotton undergarments and loose clothing.
3. Encourage bed rest if case is severe.
4. Administer pain medications, as prescribed.
5. Encourage the patient to void in a warm sitz bath if urination is painful.
6. Insert indwelling catheter if urination is extremely painful or if retention occurs.
7. Encourage fluid intake.

Restoring Skin Integrity

1. Administer an antiviral agent and teach the patient proper use and adverse effects.
2. Keep lesions clean and dry.
3. Teach the patient not to rub or to scratch lesions.

Enhancing Coping

1. Explore with the patient feelings about herpes and its effects on relationships.
2. Teach and reinforce healthy coping mechanisms such as relaxation breathing, imagery, and mindfulness. Encourage the patient to discuss antiviral suppressive therapy to reduce the risk of transmission and to reduce frequency and duration of recurrent outbreaks.
3. Discuss effects of stress on future outbreaks. Assist the patient to identify life stressors and how to cope with them.
4. Encourage the patient to discuss feelings with family and significant others.

Eliminating Health Behavior Risks

1. Teach the patient to avoid intercourse from first sign of active outbreak (often a tingling sensation) to resolution of lesions (at least 2 weeks after primary infection, approximately 1 week after recurrent outbreaks).
2. Teach the patient that shedding of virus through genital secretions is possible even during asymptomatic period, so the partner must be notified.
3. Inform the patient that condoms should be used for intercourse, but condoms may not be fully protective. Encourage the patient to discuss suppressive antiviral therapy with health care provider.
4. Explore possibility of noncoital aspects of sexual relationship.
5. Teach patient that virus may be spread through the genital–oral route.

Patient Education and Health Maintenance

1. Inform the patient that initial outbreak is usually more painful than recurrent outbreaks and that outbreaks vary from monthly to only a few times per year.
2. Teach the patient to recognize precipitating factors and change lifestyle to prevent potential triggers, if possible.
3. Remind the patient of the effects on a neonate and the importance of notifying health care provider if pregnancy occurs.
4. Instruct the patient in methods to decrease risk of sexual transmission: abstinence, monogamy, male or female condom use, and antiviral suppressive therapy. See page 613. The patient must inform partner of the risk of transmission to a potential sexual partner before any intimate contact. Viral shedding is highest during the prodromal and active lesion stages.
5. Tell the patient that oral lesions can occur with HSV-2 because of transmission by oral intercourse, but that most oral cold sores are caused by HSV-1 infection.
6. Refer the patient to support groups, such as the American Sexual Health Association (www.ashasexualhealth.org/herpes-support-groups/ or 919-364-8400).

Evaluation: Expected Outcomes

- Verbalizes decreased pain.
- Skin intact, without signs of secondary infection and scarring.
- Verbalizes reduced anxiety and more confidence.
- Reports safer sexual behavior.

Chlamydial Infection

Chlamydia infection is the most common STI, particularly in adolescents and young adults. Females are asymptomatic or present with cervicitis; males are commonly asymptomatic but may present with urethritis.

Pathophysiology and Etiology

1. Chlamydia infection in females is the result of sexual intercourse, with infection entering the vagina, infecting the cervix, and, possibly, spreading up through the endometrium and fallopian tubes.
2. Young females ages 15 to 24 are at highest risk for infection, possibly because of susceptibility of cervical tissue to the organism and higher-risk sexual behaviors in this age group.
3. *Chlamydia trachomatis* is the most common sexually transmitted pathogen in males and females in the United States, with an incidence of more than 481.3 cases per 100,000 people.

Clinical Manifestations

1. May be asymptomatic or have vaginal discharge—may be clear mucoid to creamy discharge.
2. May have dysuria and mild pelvic discomfort.
3. May have intermenstrual spotting.
4. The cervix may be covered by thick mucopurulent discharge and be tender, erythematous, edematous, and friable.

Diagnostic Evaluation

1. DNA testing (or nucleic acid amplification tests [NAATs]) of sample from cervical swab, vaginal swab, urine, or male urethral swab—most sensitive and specific; can be done simultaneously for gonorrhea.
2. Chlamydia culture from cervical exudate and cervical mucosa.
3. The CDC recommends annual screening for all sexually active females younger than age 25 and for older females at high risk (multiple sex partners or new partner).

Management

1. Antibiotic regimens include:
   a. Azithromycin 1 g orally in a single dose.
   b. Doxycycline 100 mg orally twice per day for 7 days.
   c. Alternatives include erythromycin, levofloxacin, or ofloxacin.
2. Current and/or most recent sexual partners (during 60 days or more preceding onset) should be tested and treated despite test results.

DRUG ALERT Because chlamydia infection and gonorrhea frequently coexist, especially in adolescents and young adults, treatment of both STIs is recommended.

Complications

1. Pelvic inflammatory disease (PID).
2. Ectopic pregnancy or infertility secondary to untreated or recurrent PID.
3. Transmission to neonate born through infected birth canal.

Nursing Assessment

1. Obtain history of sexual activity and symptoms or infections in partner.
2. Perform abdominal and pelvic examination for tenderness caused by possible spread to pelvic organs.

Nursing Interventions

Preventing Infection Transmission

1. Advise abstinence from sexual intercourse until 7 days after treatment has been completed.
2. Ensure that partner is treated at the same time; recent partners should receive treatment despite lack of symptoms and negative chlamydia test result. Abstinence should continue until 7 days after partners have completed treatment.
3. Report case to local public health department (chlamydia is a reportable infectious disease in most of the United States).
4. Ensure that patient begins treatment and will have access to prescription and transportation for follow-up. Single-dose azithromycin as directly observed therapy is often a good choice for patients with limited access to health care resources.
5. Retesting for chlamydia is recommended 3 months after treatment to detect reinfection, particularly in adolescents and young adults.

Patient Education and Health Maintenance

1. Teach about all STIs, mode of transmission, symptoms, and complications. Clarify misconceptions.
2. Explain the treatment regimen to the patient, and advise of adverse effects and the importance of informing partner about the need for treatment.
3. Discuss STIs and methods of prevention—abstinence, monogamy, and proper use of female or male condoms. See page 613.

4. Stress the importance of follow-up examination and retesting. Recurrence rates are highest in younger patients.
5. Encourage screening periodically for at-risk patients.
6. For further information on STIs, refer patients to such agencies as the American Social Health Association (www.ashastd.org or 919-361-8400).

Evaluation: Expected Outcomes

- Returns for follow-up; states complied with abstinence during treatment of self and partner; verbalizes use of measures to prevent STI transmission.

Gonorrhea

Gonorrhea is a common STI that causes cervicitis or urethritis. From the cervix, it can easily ascend to the uterus and fallopian tubes, if untreated.

Pathophysiology and Etiology

1. Gonorrhea is caused by the gram-positive diplococci *Neisseria gonorrhoeae.*
2. Infection occurs through sexual transmission, causing cervicitis in females and possible conjunctivitis, pharyngitis, and proctitis.
3. Untreated infection may lead to PID, generalized dissemination, or gonococcal arthritis.
4. In 2020, 677,769 cases of gonorrhea were reported to the CDC. Gonorrhea is the second most common reportable sexually transmitted infection in the United States.
5. Teens and young adults are most commonly affected.

Clinical Manifestations

1. Frequently asymptomatic in females.
2. May cause mucopurulent vaginal discharge or a painful burning sensation when urinating.
3. Vaginal speculum examination may reveal cervical discharge and inflammation.
4. Cervical motion tenderness and tender pelvic organs on bimanual examination if infection has begun to ascend.

Diagnostic Evaluation

1. DNA testing (or NAATs) of sample obtained by cervical swab, vaginal swab, urine, or male urethral swab (most sensitive and specific; can be done simultaneously for chlamydia).
2. Endocervical culture should be performed to provide antimicrobial susceptibility results.
3. Pharyngeal or conjunctival secretions can be tested if pharyngitis or conjunctivitis is suspected. Follow laboratory specifications for these tests.
4. Joint aspiration and blood cultures may be necessary if disseminated infection is suspected.

Management

1. Uncomplicated gonococcal infection of the cervix, urethra (in males), or rectum (in males or females) can be treated with a single-dose antibiotic, such as the following (plus treatment for coinfection with chlamydia):
   a. Cefixime 400 mg orally.
   b. Ceftriaxone 500 mg intramuscular (IM).
   c. Alternative regimens involving other cephalosporins are also approved.
2. Pharyngeal infections should be treated for coinfection with chlamydia with the following:
   a. Ceftriaxone 500 mg IM single dose *plus*.
   b. Azithromycin 1 g orally single dose or doxycycline 100 mg orally twice daily × 7 days.
3. Gonococcal conjunctivitis should be treated with ceftriaxone 1 g IM single dose plus concomitant chlamydial treatment.
4. Disseminated infections require IV or IM therapy, such as:
   a. Ceftriaxone 1 g IM or IV every 24 hours.
   b. Cefotaxime 1 g IV every 8 hours.
   c. Ceftizoxime 1 g IV every 8 hours.
5. For IV or IM therapy, patient is switched to oral therapy 24 to 48 hours after improvement and then takes cefixime 400 mg orally twice daily to complete 7 days of antimicrobial therapy.
6. In all cases of suspected gonorrhea, concomitant treatment of chlamydia is recommended with appropriate second antibiotic agent.

DRUG ALERT Fluoroquinolone therapy is no longer recommended for the treatment of gonorrhea in the United States because of resistance.

Complications

1. PID, ectopic pregnancy, and infertility.
2. Disseminated infection.
3. Ophthalmia neonatorum and sepsis (rare) caused by infant born through infected birth canal.

Nursing Assessment

1. Question the patient on history of STIs, STI protection, sexual activity, and usual self-care practices.
2. Obtain history of symptoms in patient and partner—incubation period is usually 3 to 7 days in males, but symptoms are typically overlooked in females.
3. Assess for ability to change lifestyle practices that may have led to STI.

Nursing Interventions

Stopping Transmission of STIs

1. Administer antibiotics, as prescribed, explaining adverse effects to patient.
2. Make sure that patient can obtain prescription medication at discharge.
3. Monitor for relief of pain, discharge, and other symptoms.
4. Explain importance of sexual abstinence until symptoms are resolved completely and until 7 days after therapy is complete in patient and partner.
5. Report to public health department and tell patient that information will be obtained to ensure testing of sexual contacts.

Patient Education and Health Maintenance

1. Teach patient about all possible STIs, their prevalence, and their mode of transmission. Clarify misconceptions.
2. Advise patient of complications of gonorrhea and chlamydia.
3. Discuss STIs and methods of prevention—abstinence, monogamy, and proper use of female or male condoms. See page 613.
4. Stress the importance of follow-up examination and testing to ensure eradication of infection. Encourage follow-up for routine female health care and periodic STI screening.

5. For additional information, refer to the American Sexual Health Association (www.ashasexualhealth.org) or Centers for Disease Control and Prevention (www.cdc.gov/std/default.htm).

Evaluation: Expected Outcomes

- Reports resolution of symptoms and use of condoms, abstinence, or other prevention measures at follow-up visit.

Syphilis

Syphilis is an STI that initially causes a genital lesion but can spread systemically to body organs such as the brain, bones, and the heart. It is caused by the bacteria *Treponema pallidum*.

Pathophysiology and Etiology

1. Transmission is through sexual intercourse as well as from a pregnant patient who is infected to the fetus.
2. Symptoms can occur 10 to 90 days after contact; the average is 21 days.
3. In 2022, 207,000 cases were reported in the United States. Since 2000, the rate has steadily increased each year.

Clinical Manifestations

1. Primary syphilis: The first sign is a painless chancre at the site of infection, an average of 3 weeks after exposure. The chancre lasts 3 to 6 weeks and will go away even if not treated. If left untreated, it will progress to secondary syphilis.
2. Secondary syphilis: Usually within 2 weeks to 6 months of the chancre, a rash will appear even on the palms of the hands and soles of the feet. Lymphadenopathy, low-grade fever, sore throat, headache, fatigue, loss of appetite, hair loss, and sore joints may also occur. Symptoms typically last about 6 weeks and will go away. If left untreated, it will progress to latent syphilis.
3. Latent syphilis: At this stage, there will be no symptoms but the patient is infectious to other sexual partners.
   a. Early latent syphilis occurs within 1 year of infection or symptoms of primary or secondary syphilis.
   b. Late latent syphilis occurs after more than 1 year duration of infection.
4. Tertiary syphilis: One third of people infected with syphilis who are not treated will progress to the tertiary stage. The bones, skin, heart, and nervous symptom can be affected.
5. Congenital syphilis is transmitted during pregnancy, causing congenital syphilis and permanent damage in the baby.

Diagnostic Evaluation

1. Treponemal blood tests will detect antibodies specific for syphilis. These tests include *Treponema pallidum* particle agglutination (TP-PA), various enzyme immunoassays (EIAs), chemiluminescence immunoassays, immunoblots, and rapid treponemal assays.
2. Samples of cerebrospinal fluid can be used if nervous system complications are suspected.

Management

1. Treatment for adults (including pregnant patients) and adolescents with primary, secondary, or early latent syphilis: benzathine penicillin G 2.4 million units IM in a single dose.
2. Treatment recommendation for adults and adolescents with late latent syphilis or latent syphilis of unknown duration: benzathine penicillin G 7.2 million units total, administered as three doses of 2.4 million units IM each at weekly intervals.
3. Neonates should be immediately screened and treated if postpartum patient had syphilis during pregnancy.

Complications

1. Progression of the disease to tertiary stage, systemic disease (uveitis, meningitis, hearing loss, paresis), and death.
2. Transmission to a fetus causing stillbirth, liver damage, anemia, bone deformity, jaundice, deafness, blindness, and meningitis.

Nursing Assessment

1. Question patient about sexual history and the possibility of missed symptoms/stages of the disease.
2. Perform thorough neurologic assessment in cases of latent syphilis of undetermined duration.
3. Obtain history of any symptoms in the partner.

Nursing Interventions

Understanding Treatment Process

1. Administer treatment as prescribed. Penicillin desensitization may be necessary before treatment because alternative antibiotics may not be as effective.
2. Advise patient of possible Jarisch–Herxheimer reaction (fever, myalgias, headache), which is a reaction to treatment, not an allergic reaction. It may occur up to 24 hours after treatment and is managed symptomatically.
3. Perform HIV and other STI testing as directed, due to increased risk of coinfection.
4. Report cases to the local public health department and advise that patient will be contacted for names of sexual contacts.

Patient Education and Health Maintenance

1. Prevent STIs by modifying sexual activity, see page 613.
2. Question partner(s) about history and be alert for partner's signs and symptoms (chancre, rash, fever, swollen glands) before intercourse.
3. Return for testing after treatment for primary and secondary syphilis at 6 and 12 months; for latent syphilis, return at 6, 12, and 24 months.

PROBLEMS RESULTING FROM RELAXED PELVIC MUSCLES

Cystocele is a downward displacement (protrusion) of the bladder into the vagina (see Figure 18-5). *Urethrocele* is downward displacement of the urethra into the vagina.

Pathophysiology and Etiology

1. Associated with obstetric trauma to fascia, muscle, and ligaments during childbirth (results in poor support).
2. Typically becomes apparent years later, when genital atrophy associated with aging occurs.
3. May also be caused by congenital defect or may appear after hysterectomy.

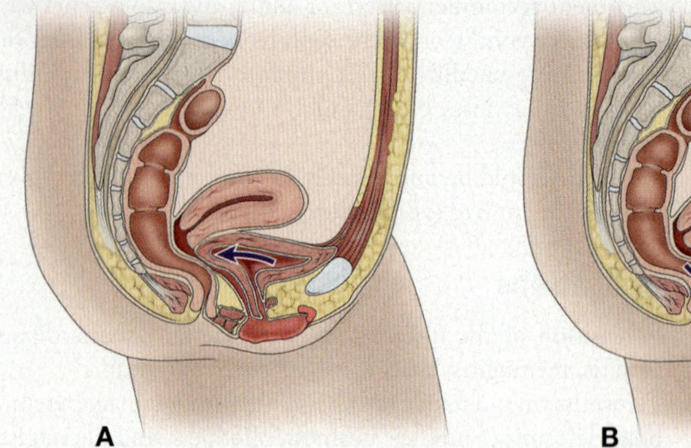

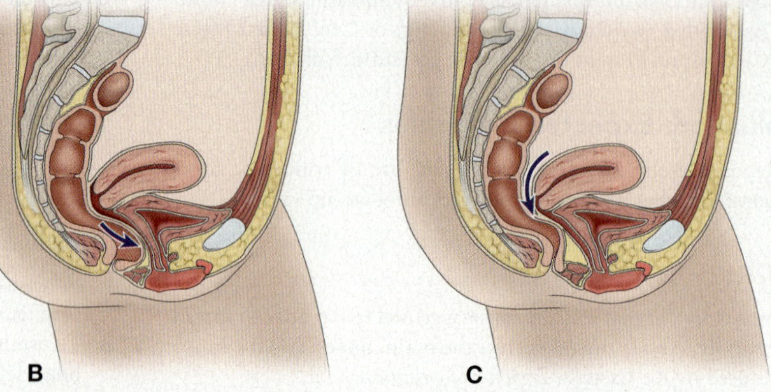

Figure 18-5. Pelvic support disorders. **(A)** Cystocele. **(B)** Rectocele. **(C)** Enterocele. (Reprinted with permission from Hinkle, J. L., Cheever, K. H., & Overbaugh, K. [2022]. *Brunner and Suddarth's textbook of medical-surgical nursing* [15th ed., Fig. 51-3]. Wolters Kluwer.)

Clinical Manifestations

1. May be asymptomatic in early stages.
2. Pelvic pressure or heaviness, backache, nervousness, and fatigue.
3. Urinary symptoms—urgency, frequency, incontinence, and incomplete emptying.
4. Aggravated by coughing, sneezing, standing for long periods, and obesity, which increase intra-abdominal pressure.
5. Relieved by resting or by lying down.

Diagnostic Evaluation

1. Pelvic examination identifies condition.
2. Urinalysis and culture are done to rule out infection.

Management

1. Vaginal pessary—silicone (can be latex or polycarbonate) device inserted into the vagina as temporary treatment to support pelvic organs.
   a. Prolonged use may lead to necrosis and ulceration.
   b. Should be removed and cleaned at least once weekly.
2. Estrogen therapy after menopause to decrease genital atrophy.
3. Pelvic floor muscle exercises to improve symptoms.
4. Surgery—if cystocele is large and interferes with bladder functioning.
   a. May do anterior vaginal colporrhaphy (repair of anterior vaginal wall).
   b. Complications of surgery include urinary retention and bleeding (requires vaginal packing).

Complications

Urinary incontinence and infection.

Nursing Assessment

1. Obtain history of obstetric trauma, abdominal surgery, menopause, and use of estrogen.
2. Ask about urinary symptoms and pain.
3. Observe the perineum while the patient bears down or is in upright position for bulge from the vagina.

Nursing Interventions

Relieving Pain

1. Encourage periods of rest with legs elevated to relieve strain on the pelvis.
2. Advise use of mild analgesics, as necessary.
3. Provide postoperative care.
   a. Encourage voiding every 4 to 8 hours to reduce pressure so that no more than 150 mL will accumulate in the bladder—intermittent catheterization or use of an indwelling catheter may be required.
   b. Administer perineal care to patient after each voiding and defecation.
   c. Use available sprays for anesthetic and antiseptic effects.
   d. Apply an ice pack locally to relieve congestion and discomfort.
   e. Administer analgesics, as prescribed, for relief of pain.

Optimizing Urine Elimination

1. Teach the patient Kegel pelvic floor exercises to regain muscle tone.
   a. Practice while voiding by stopping the flow of urine for 3 to 5 seconds and then releasing for 5 seconds.
   b. Patient can tighten pelvic floor muscle at any time, repeat 10 times, three times per day, and increase as able.
2. Encourage the patient to void frequently and respond to the urge to void promptly.
3. Warn the patient to avoid straining to prevent incontinence.
4. Encourage fluids to decrease bacterial flora in the bladder.
5. Catheterize patient if retention is suspected.
6. Obtain urine specimen for culture and sensitivity if infection is suspected.

Patient Education and Health Maintenance

1. Teach patients to avoid straining, remain active, avoid obesity, and perform Kegel exercises to minimize pelvic relaxation in their older years.
2. Encourage prompt attention to symptoms of urinary tract infection (UTI)—dysuria, urgency, frequency, and foul-smelling urine.

Evaluation: Expected Outcomes

- Verbalizes reduced pain.
- Reports decreased frequency of incontinence.
- Voids regularly without symptoms of infection.

Rectocele and Enterocele

Rectocele is displacement (protrusion) of the rectum into the vagina. *Enterocele* is displacement of the intestine into the vagina (see Figure 18-5).

Pathophysiology and Etiology

1. Posterior vaginal wall becomes weakened, allowing displacement.
2. Weakening caused by obstetric trauma, childbirth, pelvic surgery, and aging.

Clinical Manifestations

1. Pelvic pressure or heaviness, backache, and perineal burning.
2. Constipation—may have difficulty in fecal evacuation; the patient may use fingers in the vagina to push feces up so defecation may occur.
3. Incontinence of feces and flatus—if tear between the rectum and vagina.
4. Visible protrusion into the vagina.
5. Symptoms are aggravated by standing for long periods.

Diagnostic Evaluation

1. Vaginal examination reveals condition.
2. May use Sims speculum to uplift the cervix and fully evaluate condition.

Management

1. Pessary—plastic device inserted into the vagina to aid pelvic support.
2. Estrogen replacement vaginally to prevent atrophy.
3. Pelvic floor muscle exercises to improve symptoms.
4. Surgery, if rectocele is large enough to interfere with bowel functioning: posterior colpoplasty (perineorrhaphy)—repair of posterior vaginal wall.

Complications

Total fecal incontinence.

Nursing Assessment

1. Obtain history of childbirth, pelvic surgery, and symptoms of bowel function.
2. Observe for bulge into the vagina while the patient bears down or is in upright position.
3. Monitor bowel movements.

Nursing Interventions

Relieving Pain

1. Encourage periods of rest with legs elevated to relieve pelvic strain.
2. Encourage use of mild analgesics, as needed; avoid opioids, which may worsen constipation.
3. Postoperative care:
   a. Suggest low Fowler position to reduce edema and discomfort.
   b. Administer perineal care to patient after each voiding and defecation.
   c. Heat may enhance the healing process, but use cautiously to avoid burns.
   d. Use ice packs locally to relieve congestion and discomfort.
   e. Administer analgesics and stool softeners, as ordered.

Relieving Constipation

1. Teach the patient to increase fluid and fiber in diet.
2. Encourage use of stool softeners preventatively, or mild laxatives to make passage of stool easier.

Patient Education and Health Maintenance

1. Advise the patient to follow surgeon's instructions for resuming activity and to avoid heavy lifting, straining, and intercourse until cleared.
2. Educate the patient to avoid straining and obesity in future, which may cause return of rectocele or enterocele.

Evaluation: Expected Outcomes

- Verbalizes reduced pain.
- Passes soft stool daily.

Uterine Prolapse

Uterine prolapse is an abnormal position of the uterus in which the uterus protrudes downward.

Pathophysiology and Etiology

1. The uterus herniates through the pelvic floor and protrudes into the vagina (prolapse) and possibly beyond the introitus (procidentia).
2. Usually caused by obstetric trauma and overstretching of musculofascial supports.
3. Degrees (see Figure 18-6).
   a. First degree—the cervix prolapses into the vaginal canal.
   b. Second degree—the cervix is at the introitus.
   c. Third degree—the cervix extends over the perineum.
   d. Marked procidentia—the entire uterus protrudes outside the vaginal cavity.

Clinical Manifestations

1. Low backache or dyspareunia.
2. Pressure and heaviness in pelvic region.
3. Bloody discharge because of the cervix rubbing against clothing or inner thighs.
4. Urinary frequency, urgency, or repeated bladder infections.
5. Symptoms are aggravated by obesity, standing, straining, coughing, or lifting a heavy object because of increased intra-abdominal pressure.

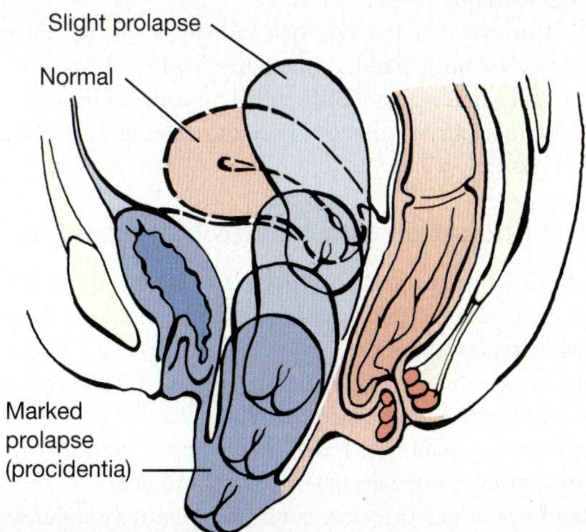

Figure 18-6. Degrees of uterine prolapse. (Reprinted with permission from Reeder, S., Martin, L., & Koniak-Griffin, D. [1997]. *Maternity nursing: Family, newborn, and women's health care* [18th ed.]. Lippincott-Raven Publishers.)

Diagnostic Evaluation

Pelvic examination identifies condition.

Management

1. Hysterectomy or surgical correction.
2. Vaginal pessary—plastic device inserted into the vagina as temporary or palliative measure if surgery cannot be done.
3. Pelvic floor muscle exercises to improve symptoms.
4. Estrogen cream—decrease genital atrophy.

Complications

1. Necrosis of the cervix and uterus.
2. Infection.

Nursing Assessment

1. Obtain history of childbirth and surgery.
2. Ask about symptoms and aggravating factors.
3. Examine patient in lying or standing position; if the cervix is not readily visible, spread labia gently; do not attempt to insert speculum.

Nursing Interventions

Relieving Discomfort

1. Administer sitz baths for comfort and cleansing and explain procedure to patient.
2. Provide heating pad for lower back or lower abdomen as needed for comfort.
3. Administer pain medications or teach self-administration, as ordered.
4. Check for proper placement of pessary.
5. Advise increased fluid intake and frequent voiding to prevent bladder infection; report urinary retention, dysuria, urgency, or hematuria.

Maintaining Cervical and Uterine Mucosal Integrity

1. For second- and third-degree prolapse, apply saline compresses frequently.
2. Provide postoperative care.
   a. Administer perineal care to patient after each voiding and defecation.
   b. If urinary retention occurs, catheterize or use indwelling catheter until bladder tone is regained.
   c. Apply an ice pack locally to relieve congestion.
   d. Promote ambulation but prevent straining to reduce pelvic pressure.

Patient Education and Health Maintenance

1. Encourage the patient with pessary to follow up, as directed, for removal and cleaning of pessary and evaluation of any vaginal irritation or trauma.
2. Encourage all patients to report vaginal discharge, pain, or bleeding before or after treatment.
3. Explain to patient that sexual intercourse is possible with pessary; however, vaginal canal may be shortened.
4. Reinforce surgeon's instructions postoperatively about waiting to have vaginal penetration.
5. Encourage the patient to explore with partner ways to engage in sexual activity without strain and with greatest comfort.

Evaluation: Expected Outcomes

- Verbalizes improved comfort.
- Cervix and uterus without ulceration.

GYNECOLOGIC TUMORS

Cancer of the Vulva

Cancer of the vulva is most commonly squamous cell carcinoma of the labia majora, labia minora, or clitoris; it may also originate as a urethral tumor.

Pathophysiology and Etiology

1. Most common in postmenopausal patients, although it may also occur in younger patients related to human papillomavirus (HPV) infection.
2. Represents 4% of gynecologic cancers.
3. Like many cancers, the cause is unknown, but HPV, vulvar intraepithelial neoplasia (VIN), older age, smoking, and human immunodeficiency virus (HIV) are risk factors.
4. Spreads primarily through local, direct extension and lymphatic system; distant metastasis can occur late in the disease process.

Clinical Manifestations

1. Early changes of external genitalia may include itching, color changes (white plaque or redness), tenderness, burning, ulceration, a lump or mass.
2. Discharge or bleeding; may be foul-smelling because of secondary infection.
3. Edema of tissues and lymphadenopathy.
4. Pain or dyspareunia.

Diagnostic Evaluation

1. Biopsy of lesion and lymph nodes. If small, lesion may be excised at the time of biopsy.
2. Additional imaging such as magnetic resonance imaging (MRI), computed tomography (CT), positron emission tomography (PET) for staging.

Management

EVIDENCE BASE PDQ® Adult Treatment Editorial Board. (n.d.). *Vulvar cancer treatment (PDQ®)–Health professional version*. National Cancer Institute. Updated 15 March, 2023. https://www.cancer.gov/types/vulvar/hp/vulvar-treatment-pdq

1. Surgery is generally the treatment of choice.
   a. For early stages, excision alone with at least 1 cm margins is performed.
   b. Unilateral lymph node dissection may be performed.
   c. Radiation may be added, or considered alone, if patient is not a good candidate for surgery.
2. VIN may be treated with surgery or the topical antineoplastic imiquimod.
3. Later stages of vulvar cancer are treated with surgery and systemic chemotherapy.
4. Recurrent vulvar cancer is treated with radical vulvectomy and pelvic exenteration.

Complications

1. Lymphatic spread.
2. Complications after surgery may occur—wound infection, wound breakdown, lymphedema, leg cellulitis, and introital stenosis.

Nursing Assessment

1. Obtain history of lesion, including when the patient first noticed it and any change in appearance.
2. Obtain gynecologic history, especially about past infections.
3. Assess overall health for tolerance of treatment.
4. Assess support systems and personal coping skills.

Nursing Interventions

Relieving Fear Preoperatively

1. Have patient describe understanding of the problem; answer questions and clear up misconceptions.
2. Emphasize the positive outcomes of the prescribed treatment plan; reinforce what the surgeon has already described.
3. Prepare the patient for surgery and describe the postoperative appearance of the wound and use of drains and urinary catheter (see Figure 18-7).
   a. Provide skin preparation as directed and cleanse the vulva via a chlorhexidine shower the night before surgery; 2% chlorhexidine gluconate antiseptic solution may also be ordered.
   b. Administer bowel preparation, as ordered, to evacuate intestinal tract before surgery; there will be no bowel movement for 2 to 3 days postoperatively.

Promoting Tissue Healing Postoperatively

1. Maintain drainage and compression of tissues to remove fluid that could cause edema and prevent wound healing. Empty drains, as needed (at least every 8 hours).
2. Keep wound clean and dry.
   a. Perform sterile dressing changes, as prescribed.
   b. Perform perineal care or sitz baths after each bowel movement or voiding (after catheter is removed).
   c. Maintain patency of urinary catheter, as ordered, to prevent wound contamination with urine.
   d. Encourage low Fowler position to promote comfort and reduce tension on sutures.
   e. Prevent straining with defecation by providing a low-residue diet initially and stool softeners later, as ordered.

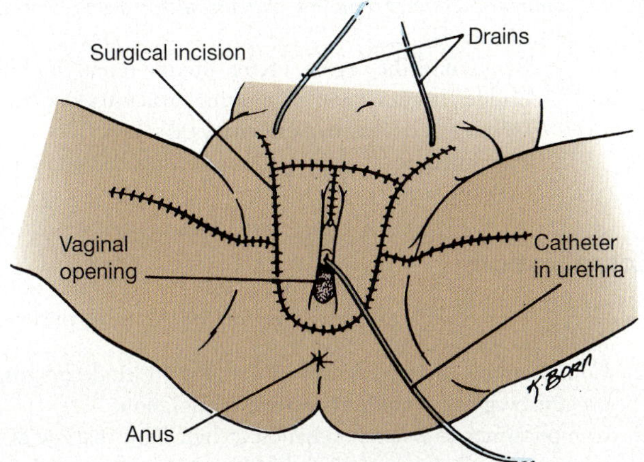

Figure 18-7. Postoperative appearance after radical vulvectomy.

   f. Provide deep vein thrombosis prophylaxis (anticoagulant or sequential compression device), as prescribed, and encourage leg exercises to prevent thrombus/embolus formation. Encourage careful ambulation when allowed while preventing perineal tension.

Restoring Sexual Function

1. Encourage the patient to ventilate feelings about sexual mutilation and altered functioning.
2. Tell the patient that if the vagina is still intact, vaginal intercourse is still possible.
3. Inform the patient of changes that may occur because of surgery—loss of sexual arousal if the clitoris is removed, shortening of the vagina, and decreased lubrication.
4. Help the patient explore alternative methods of sexual intimacy and encourage discussion of feelings with partner.

Patient Education and Health Maintenance

1. Encourage follow-up visits for additional therapy, if required.
2. Encourage regular health checkups and screening for cancer and other age-related illnesses.
3. Encourage early evaluation of any suspicious lesions, bleeding, or discharge.

Evaluation: Expected Outcomes

- Verbalizes reduced fear.
- Perineum healed without complications.
- Verbalizes understanding of anatomic changes and sexual function.

Cancer of the Cervix

Cancer of the cervix is the fourth most common gynecologic malignancy. There are about 11,500 new cases and 4000 deaths each year in the United States. There were 660,000 new cases estimated worldwide in 2022, and 350,000 deaths. Highest rates of incidence and mortality occur in low- and middle-income countries.

EVIDENCE BASE Center for Disease Control and Prevention. (2023). *Cervical cancer statistics.* US Department of Health and Human Services. https://www.cdc.gov/cancer/cervical/statistics/index.htm

Centers for Disease Control and Prevention. (n.d.). *Cervical cancer statistics.* Updated August 10, 2022. https://www.cdc.gov/cancer/cervical/statistics/index.htm

Sung, H., Ferlay, J., Siegel, R. L., Laversanne, M., Soerjomataram, I., Jemal, A., & Bray, F. (2021). Global cancer statistics 2020: GLOBOCAN estimates of incidence and mortality worldwide for 36 cancers in 185 countries. *CA: A Cancer Journal for Clinicians, 71*(3), 209–249. https://doi.org/10.3322/caac.21660

World Health Organization. (2024). Cervical cancer. WHO. https://www.who.int/news-room/fact-sheets/detail/cervical-cancer#:~:text=Cervical%20cancer%20is%20the%20fourth,%2D%20and%20middle%2Dincome%20countries

Pathophysiology and Etiology

1. Early sexual activity, multiple sexual partners, a high-risk sexual partner, history of HIV and other sexually transmitted infections (STIs)—especially HPV—and a history of vulvar

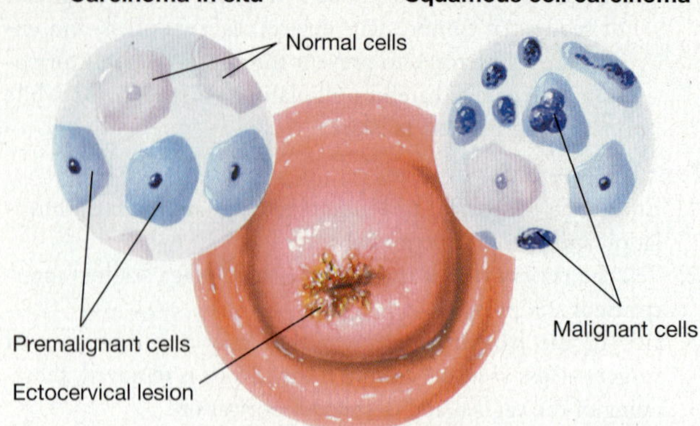

Figure 18-8. Cervical cancer. (Reprinted with permission from Anatomical Chart Company.)

or vaginal squamous intraepithelial neoplasia or cancer, and immunosuppression are major risk factors. There also appears to be an increased risk of cervical cancer associated with the use of oral contraceptives.
2. Incidence is higher in lower socioeconomic status and in Hispanics, African Americans, American Indians, and Alaska Natives—presumably related to decreased access to health care and screening.
3. Types (see Figure 18-8):
   a. Dysplasia (precancer)—atypical cells with some degree of surface maturation.
   b. Carcinoma in situ—cytology similar to invasive carcinoma but confined to the epithelium.
   c. Invasive carcinoma—stroma is involved; 69% are of the squamous cell type. Spreads by local invasion and lymphatics to the vagina and beyond.

Clinical Manifestations

1. Early disease is usually asymptomatic, although patient may notice watery, vaginal discharge.
2. Initial symptoms include postcoital bleeding, irregular vaginal bleeding or spotting between periods or after menopause, and malodorous discharge.
3. As disease progresses, bleeding becomes more constant and is accompanied by pain that radiates to buttocks and legs as well as urinary and rectal symptoms that may be due to invasion of these organs.
4. Weight loss, anemia, edema of lower extremities, and fever signal advanced disease.

Diagnostic Evaluation

1. Pap smear—routine screening measure; abnormal results warrant further diagnostic tests, such as colposcopy and biopsy or conization.
2. Staging is done clinically rather than surgically as with other cancers. Based on physical findings on abdominal and pelvic examination.
3. Supplemental imaging can include chest x-ray, intravenous pyelography (IVP), urography, colposcopy, cystoscopy, proctosigmoidoscopy, CT scan with intravenous (IV) contrast, and barium studies of the lower colon and rectum.

Management

EVIDENCE BASE National Cancer Institute. (2022). *Cervical cancer treatment (PDQ®)–Health professional version.* Author. https://www.cancer.gov/types/cervical/hp/cervical-treatment-pdq#_93

Treatment by Stage

1. Dysplasia to Carcinoma In Situ
   a. Techniques to destroy abnormal cells in the cervical transformation zone.
   b. Cryosurgery, laser therapy, electrocautery (loop electrosurgical excision procedure [LEEP]), or conization may be performed on outpatient basis.
   c. Vaginal discharge, bleeding, pain, and cramping result from these procedures in various degrees, but postoperative convalescence is minimal.
2. Microinvasive Stage
   a. Surgical conization—large excision of cervical tissue, may be done under local or general anesthesia.
   b. LEEP—using heated wire to excise portion of the cervical tissue.
3. Invasive Cervical Cancer
   a. Extent is staged and treated with hysterectomy, radiotherapy, or chemotherapy.

Management Modalities

1. Radiotherapy.
   a. Intracavitary (localized for earlier stage) or external (more generalized dosage to the pelvis for stages IIB through IVB).
   b. Cisplatin, a radiation sensitizer, is used to improve survival.
2. Chemotherapy—cisplatin may be used in combination with radiation for locally advanced disease or for metastatic disease in which recurrence is common. Other agents that may be used include ifosfamide, carboplatin, and topotecan.
3. Surgery.
   a. Total hysterectomy, conization, modified radical hysterectomy, and intracavitary radiation therapy may be performed for stage IA with or without oophorectomy and/or lymph node dissection.
   b. Radical hysterectomy and bilateral lymph node resections for stages IB and IIA. Radiation and chemotherapy may also be considered for these stages after hysterectomy.
   c. Pelvic exenteration for advanced cases if the patient is a candidate. Usually done for patients with isolated central recurrence.
      i. Removal of the vagina, uterus, uterine tubes, ovaries, bladder, rectum, and supporting structures and the creation of an ileal conduit and fecal stoma.
      ii. Performed for pelvic recurrence after radiation or chemotherapy.

Complications

1. Spread to the bladder and rectum; metastasis to lungs, mediastinum, bones, and liver.
2. Complications of intracavitary radiotherapy include cystitis, proctitis, vaginal stenosis, and uterine perforation.
3. Complications of external radiation include bone marrow depression, bowel obstruction, and fistula.

Nursing Assessment

1. Obtain history of Pap tests, sexual activity, and past STIs.
2. Obtain history of symptoms.
3. Assess understanding of disease and responses, such as guilt, fear, denial, and anxiety.

Nursing Interventions

Relieving Anxiety

1. Assist the patient to seek information on stage of cancer and treatment options.
2. Prepare the patient for hysterectomy or other surgery (see page 626 for nursing interventions for hysterectomy).
3. Prepare the patient for radiation therapy to the uterus (see page 620 for nursing interventions for radiation therapy).
4. Provide emotional support during diagnostic and treatment phases.
5. Encourage activity and socialization as patient is able.

Patient Education and Health Maintenance

1. Explain the importance of lifelong follow-up, regardless of treatments, to determine the response to treatment and detect spread of cancer.
2. Refer to cancer support group in community.
3. Encourage all patients to discuss cervical cancer screening guidelines with their health care providers (see page 663).

Evaluation: Expected Outcomes

- Reports decreased anxiety and increased participation in treatment process.

Endometrial Cancer

Cancer of the uterus is usually adenocarcinoma of the endometrium of the fundus or body of the uterus. Most common gynecologic cancer in the United States.

Pathophysiology and Etiology

1. Most patients are postmenopausal with an average age of early 60s at the time of diagnosis.
2. Cause is unknown but associated with increased estrogen exposure as in tamoxifen use and unopposed estrogen replacement, obesity, anovulation, or estrogen-secreting tumors.
3. Hypertension and diabetes mellitus are also risk factors.

Clinical Manifestations

1. Irregular bleeding before menopause or postmenopausal bleeding is the most common complaint.
2. Watery, usually malodorous vaginal discharge.
3. Pain, fever, and bowel and bladder dysfunctions are late signs.
4. Anemia secondary to bleeding.

Diagnostic Evaluation

1. Pelvic and rectovaginal examination—enlarged uterus may be palpated.
2. Endometrial biopsy is preferred as the initial diagnostic test; however, if less than 50% of the endometrium is affected, malignancy can be missed.
3. Transvaginal ultrasound to measure endometrial thickness.
4. Dilation and curettage—if endometrial sampling cannot be performed in office, hysteroscopy may also be helpful.
5. Hormone receptor status (especially progesterone and estrogen) is assessed as prognostic indicator.
6. Atypical glandular cells may be found on cervical cytology; however, cervical screening is not a reliable method for detecting endometrial cancer.
7. Metastatic workup—involves evaluation of lymph node involvement and imaging studies of the lungs, liver, bones, and brain, as indicated.

Management

EVIDENCE BASE National Cancer Institute. (2022). *Endometrial cancer treatment (PDQ®)–Health professional version.* Author. https://www.cancer.gov/types/uterine/hp/endometrial-treatment-pdq

1. Staging for endometrial cancer is based on surgical aspects versus clinical staging.
   a. Emphasis is placed on histologic grade, depth of myometrial invasion, and cervical involvement.
   b. These parameters assist in prediction of lymph node involvement and help determine need for lymph node dissection.
2. Early stage I requires total abdominal hysterectomy with bilateral salpingo-oophorectomy (TAH/BSO).
3. Advanced stage I and stage II require TAH/BSO and selective lymph node dissection.
4. Radiation therapy (intracavitary or external) may be added after surgery or chosen instead of surgery for more advanced stages or for patients who are high-risk surgical candidates.
   a. Acute complications include hemorrhagic cystitis, vaginitis, enteritis, and proctitis.
   b. Chronic complications include vaginal dryness, vaginal stenosis, cystitis, bladder dysfunction, proctitis, small bowel obstruction, fistulas, strictures, and leg edema.
5. Hormonal therapy—progestational agents may alter receptor sites in the endometrium for estrogen and thus decrease growth (for metastatic disease); may provide stabilization of disease.
6. Chemotherapy—for metastatic and recurrent disease; using cisplatin, doxorubicin, and possibly paclitaxel.

Complications

Spread throughout the pelvis; metastasis to lungs, liver, bone, and brain.

Nursing Assessment

1. Obtain history of menses, pregnancy, and estrogen replacement.
2. Ask about irregular or postmenopausal bleeding and other symptoms.
3. Assess the patient's response to possible diagnosis of cancer—fear, guilt, and denial.

Nursing Interventions

Relieving Fear

1. Support patient through the diagnostic process, and reinforce information given by health care provider about treatment options.

2. Prepare patient for radiation therapy, if indicated (see below).
3. Prepare patient for hysterectomy, if indicated (see page 626).
4. Provide complete and concise explanations for all care you provide; emphasize the positive aspects of patient's recovery.

Patient Education and Health Maintenance

1. Explain importance of reporting postmenopausal bleeding.
2. Encourage keeping follow-up visits.
3. Explain that surgery or radiation treatment does not prevent satisfying sexual activity.
4. Refer to local cancer support group or American Cancer Society (www.acs.org).

Evaluation: Expected Outcomes

- Verbalizes understanding of diagnosis and treatment chosen.

Care of the Patient Receiving Intracavitary Radiation Therapy

Procedural Considerations

1. An applicator (tandems and ovoids are most common) is positioned in the endocervical canal and vagina in the operating room with the patient under anesthesia. (High-dose remote brachytherapy is also used. This is an outpatient procedure and the treatment takes just minutes. The radioactive source is removed between treatments.)
2. After recovery from anesthesia, x-rays are taken to check correct placement.
3. Radiologist inserts radioactive material (radium or cesium) into applicator, which remains in place 24 to 72 hours. Therapy is individualized according to the stage of disease and patient's response to and tolerance of radiation.
4. External radiation over the pelvis may be supplemented to eliminate cancer spread via lymphatic system.

Nursing Interventions

Patient Preparation

1. Patients require a thorough medical evaluation before treatment to evaluate risks and precautions related to preexisting medical problems or special needs.
2. An indwelling catheter is placed in the operating room.
3. Encourage patient to bring diversional activities because patient will remain on bed rest during radiation treatment.
4. Instruct patient on radiation safety measures:
   a. Neither patient nor secretions are radioactive, but the applicator is.
   b. Do not touch source of radiation.
   c. Notify someone immediately if source is dislodged.
   d. When applicators are removed, no radioactivity remains.
   e. Radioactivity is monitored by specially trained personnel.
   f. No people who are pregnant or children younger than age 18 are allowed to visit.
   g. Lead shields may be used to decrease radiation that emanates from the patient.
5. Reinforce that help is readily available.

During Radiation Treatment

1. Maintain patient on strict bed rest on the back with head of bed elevated 15 to 30 degrees. Patient may be logrolled three or four times per day. Use convoluted foam mattress.
2. Have patient bathe upper body. Perineal care and linen changes are done by the nursing staff.
3. Maintain the patient on a low-residue diet to prevent bowel movements, which could dislodge the apparatus. Encourage the patient to eat several small portions rather than few large servings. Medication to induce constipation is given.
4. Inspect indwelling catheter frequently to ensure proper drainage. A distended bladder may cause severe radiation burns.
5. Encourage fluids to prevent bladder infection.
6. Observe for signs and symptoms of radiation sickness—nausea, vomiting, fever, diarrhea, and abdominal cramping.
7. Check applicator position every 8 hours and monitor amount of bleeding and drainage (a small amount is normal).
8. Check the patient frequently to minimize anxiety, but minimize time spent at bedside to reduce radiation exposure.
9. Mild sedatives or pain medication may be given for patient comfort.
10. Ensure that rules and regulations regarding radiation safety are strictly followed by all health care workers for the protection of everyone.

CLINICAL JUDGMENT Maintain cardinal rules of time, distance, and shielding when caring for the patient with intracavitary radiation. Long-handled forceps and a lead-lined container are left in the room after loading in the event the radioactive sources are dislodged.

During Radiation Removal

1. Before removal of the applicator, the patient is medicated with appropriate analgesic.
2. The radioactive sources are removed by radiation personnel and safely stored for transport.
3. The indwelling catheter is removed, and then the applicator is removed.
4. The patient is given an enema or suppository to reverse the induced constipation.
5. The patient should be evaluated for safe ambulation because of prolonged bed rest before discharge.

Myomas of the Uterus

Myomas (fibroids, leiomyomas, fibromyomas) are benign tumors of the uterine myometrium (smooth muscle).

Pathophysiology and Etiology

1. The most common pelvic tumor in females. Approximately 80% of females have fibroids, but many are not symptomatic.
2. May spontaneously regress after menopause.
3. Unknown cause; increased incidence in Black females.

Clinical Manifestations

1. Small myomas do not cause symptoms.
2. First indication may be palpable mass.
3. Irregular bleeding—usually menorrhagia.
4. Pain may come from pressure on adjacent organs—possible heavy feeling in the pelvis or degeneration associated with vascular occlusion.
5. Secondary symptoms include fatigue because of anemia, urinary disturbances, and constipation.

Diagnostic Evaluation

1. Transvaginal ultrasound or hysteroscopy—to identify size and location of myomas.
2. MRI may be helpful in clarifying anatomy and myoma location; however, it is expensive and best reserved for surgical planning of difficult procedures.

Management

1. Myomectomy may be done for small or accessible tumor and may be done through hysteroscopy, laparoscopy, or laparotomy. If fertility preservation is desired, abdominal myomectomy is preferred for symptomatic patients.
2. Hysterectomy for large or numerous tumors.
3. Medical therapies for the management of symptoms include gonadotropin-releasing hormone antagonist therapy to create hypoestrogenic environment and to try to shrink tumors. Hormonal birth control, nonsteroidal anti-inflammatory drugs (NSAIDs), or antifibrinolytic agents are used for heavy menstrual bleeding.
4. Frequently resolve on their own postmenopausally.
5. Uterine artery embolization—transvenous procedure in which the blood supply to the myoma is obstructed and the myoma degenerates.

Complications

1. Infertility with hysterectomy.
2. Habitual abortion.

Nursing Assessment

1. Ask about pain, menstrual irregularity, possible urinary symptoms, and constipation.
2. Assess the patient's understanding of condition as benign.

Nursing Interventions

Relieving Pain

1. Teach patient proper use and adverse effects of analgesics and use of heating pad, as desired.
2. Encourage the patient to avoid long periods of standing; rest with the pelvis in dependent position periodically to achieve comfort.
3. Encourage patient to void frequently to avoid increased pressure from distended bladder.
4. Advise a high-fiber diet to prevent constipation.
5. Prepare the patient for surgery, if indicated.

Patient Education and Health Maintenance

1. Tell the patient to report increased symptoms and worsening bleeding because myomas may be enlarging and treatment may be indicated.
2. Reassure the patient that myomas do not become malignant, but to keep regular follow-up visits for cancer screening.

Evaluation: Expected Outcomes

- Verbalizes control of pain.

Ovarian Cysts

Ovarian cysts are growths arising from ovarian components, usually benign.

Pathophysiology and Etiology

1. Commonly arise from functional changes in the ovary—from graafian follicle or from persistent corpus luteum.
2. Dermoid cysts may develop from abnormal embryonic epithelium.
3. Frequently found during childbearing years.

Clinical Manifestations

1. May be asymptomatic or cause minor pelvic pain.
2. Possible menstrual irregularity.
3. Tender, palpable mass.
4. Rupture causes acute unilateral lower abdominal pain and tenderness; may mimic usual pain at ovulation (mittelschmerz), pelvic inflammatory disease (PID), appendicitis, or ectopic pregnancy.
5. Discomfort during bowel movement or pressure on the bowel.

Diagnostic Evaluation

1. Pelvic sonogram to determine size and characteristics.
2. Pregnancy test to rule out ectopic pregnancy.
3. Biopsy (at the time of surgery) is done for suspicious cysts.
4. Additional testing may include hemoglobin and hematocrit if acute bleeding is suspected, endocervical swabs if pelvic infection is part of the differential diagnosis, and CA-125 if malignancy is identified.

Management

1. Cysts without malignant characteristics and that measure less than 10 cm in diameter can be observed with repeat ultrasound in 2 to 3 months.
2. Surgery for large, complex, or leaking cyst by laparoscopy or laparotomy.

Complications

Rupture may cause peritoneal inflammation.

Nursing Assessment

1. Obtain history of sexual activity, use of contraception, and past episodes of PID to rule out ectopic pregnancy.
2. Obtain history of recent menses—irregular bleeding and spotting commonly signal follicular cyst; delayed menses and prolonged bleeding signal corpus luteal cyst.
3. Perform vital signs and abdominal examination for tenderness, guarding, and rebound, which may indicate rupture.

Nursing Interventions

Relieving Pain

1. Administer or teach self-administration of analgesics, as prescribed, and provide heating pad, if desired.
2. Teach the patient the proper use of hormonal contraceptives, if prescribed, with adverse effects; encourage monthly follow-up visits to determine if cyst is resolving.
3. Tell the patient that heavy lifting, strenuous exercise, and sexual intercourse may increase pain.

Maintaining Fluid Volume

1. Monitor for nausea, vomiting, rigid abdomen, and change in vital signs related to rupture of cyst. Administer IV fluids, as

directed, and maintain nothing by mouth (NPO) status until abdominal rigidity resolves.
2. Reassure the patient that symptoms will resolve with supportive care.
3. Prepare the patient with large or nonresponsive cyst for surgery, as indicated.
4. Postoperatively monitor vital signs frequently and maintain IV infusion while restricted to NPO status.
5. Assess frequently for abdominal distention because of fluid and gas pooling in the abdominal cavity.
6. Place the patient in semi-Fowler position for greatest comfort, and encourage early ambulation to reduce distention (help patient arise slowly to prevent orthostatic hypotension).
7. Administer antiemetics and insert a nasogastric tube, as ordered, to prevent vomiting.
8. As distention resolves, assess bowel sounds and advance oral intake slowly.

Patient Education and Health Maintenance

1. Reassure patient that in most cases ovarian function and fertility remain.
2. Reassure patient about low malignancy rate of cysts.
3. Encourage the patient to report recurrent symptoms or worsening of pain if cyst is being treated medically.

Evaluation: Expected Outcomes

- Verbalizes reduced pain.
- Vital signs stable; no orthostasis.

Ovarian Cancer

Ovarian cancer is a gynecologic malignancy with high mortality because of advanced disease by the time of diagnosis. It is the leading cause of morbidity of gynecologic cancers.

Pathophysiology and Etiology

1. Median age is 63 years. One of 70 females will develop ovarian cancer.
2. Cause is unknown, but about 10% of cases are associated with family history of breast, endometrial, colon, or ovarian cancer.
3. Smoking and personal history of breast, colon, or endometrial cancer are also risk factors.
4. There is also higher incidence in nulliparous females.

Clinical Manifestations

1. No early manifestations.
2. First manifestations—(vague) bloating, increased abdominal size, urinary urgency or frequency, difficulty eating or feeling full, and abdominal or pelvic pain, which may occur with other symptoms, almost daily, and are more severe than expected.
3. Late manifestations—abdominal pain, ascites, pleural effusion, and intestinal obstruction.

Diagnostic Evaluation

1. Pelvic examination to detect enlargement, nodularity, and fixed position of the ovaries.
2. Pelvic sonography (transabdominal and transvaginal) is the most useful diagnostic test and CT scan is done to determine metastatic spread.
3. Color Doppler imaging may be used to detect vascular changes within the ovaries.
4. Paracentesis or thoracentesis if ascites or pleural effusion is present.
5. Laparotomy to stage the disease and determine effectiveness of treatment.
6. Increase of CA-125 signifies progression, but not as useful as diagnostic or screening tool because level can be elevated because of inflammation and other causes.

Management

1. TAH/BSO and omentectomy are usual treatment because of delayed diagnosis. Optimal debulking to less than 1 cm is the goal.
2. Chemotherapy is more effective if tumor is optimally debulked (less than 1-cm residual disease); usually follows surgery because of frequency of advanced disease; may be given IV or intraperitoneal.
3. Radiation therapy is not usually valuable.
4. Second-look laparotomy may be done after adjunct therapies to take multiple biopsies and determine effectiveness of therapy; however, this has not proven to affect survival.
5. Immunotherapy is being investigated in clinical trials as stand-alone treatment or in conjunction with other modalities.

Complications

Direct intra-abdominal or lymphatic spread and peritoneal seeding.

Nursing Assessment

1. Obtain history of irregular menses, pain, and postmenopausal bleeding.
2. Ask about vague gastrointestinal (GI)-related complaints.
3. Ask about history of other malignancy and family history of breast or ovarian cancer.
4. Assess the patient's general health status in terms of tolerating surgical and adjuvant therapy.

CLINICAL JUDGMENT A combination of a long history of ovarian dysfunction and persistent undiagnosed GI complaints raises suspicion for ovarian cancer. A palpable ovary in a postmenopausal female is abnormal and should be evaluated as soon as possible.

Nursing Interventions

Strengthening Coping

1. Provide emotional support through diagnostic process; allow patient to express feelings and encourage positive coping mechanisms.
2. Administer anxiolytic and analgesic medications, as prescribed, and teach patient and caregivers the potential adverse effects.
3. Refer patient to cancer support group locally or American Cancer Society (www.acs.org) or National Cancer Institute (www.cancer.org).

Maintaining Adequate Nutrition

1. Administer or teach the patient or caregiver to administer antiemetics, as needed, for nausea and vomiting.
2. Encourage small, frequent, bland meals or liquid nutritional supplements as able.
3. Assess the need for IV fluids if the patient is vomiting.

4. Monitor for passage of gas and bowel movements after surgery. Bowel dysfunction related to surgery may cause nausea and anorexia.

Maintaining Body Image

1. Prepare the patient for body image changes with chemotherapy (i.e., hair loss).
2. Encourage the patient to prepare ahead of time with turbans, wigs, and hats.
3. Encourage the patient to enhance appearance with makeup, clothing, and jewelry.
4. Stress the positive effects of the patient's treatment plan.

Relieving Pain

1. Prepare the patient for surgery, as indicated; explain the extent of incision, IV, catheter, packing, and drain tubes expected (see page 626 for a discussion of hysterectomy).
2. Postoperatively, administer analgesics, as needed, and explain that patient may be drowsy.
3. Reposition frequently and encourage early ambulation to promote comfort and prevent adverse effects.

Patient Education and Health Maintenance

1. Explain to the patient the onset of menopausal symptoms with ovary removal.
2. Tell the patient that disease progression will be monitored closely by laboratory tests and second-look laparoscopy may be necessary.
3. Female relatives of patient should notify their health care providers; biannual pelvic examinations may be necessary.

Evaluation: Expected Outcomes

- Openly discusses prognosis, asks appropriate questions, and makes plans for short-term future.
- Maintains weight.
- Verbalizes satisfaction in appearance with wig.
- Verbalizes good control over pain.

OTHER GYNECOLOGIC CONDITIONS

See additional online content: Nursing Care Plan 18-1

Pelvic Inflammatory Disease

EVIDENCE BASE Workowski, K. A., Bachmann, L. H., Chan, P. A., Johnston, C. M., Muzny, C. A., Park, I., Reno, H., Zenilman, J. M., & Bolan, G. A. (2021). Sexually transmitted infections treatment guidelines, 2021. *MMWR Recommendations and Reports*, *70*(4), 1–187. https://doi.org/10.15585/mmwr.rr7004a1. www.cdc.gov/std/treatment-guidlines/default.htm

Pelvic inflammatory disease (PID) includes several inflammatory disorders of the upper female genital tract, often with infection that may involve the fallopian tubes, ovaries, uterus, or peritoneum.

Pathophysiology and Etiology

1. Incidence has been increasing; high recurrence rate because of reinfections.
2. Commonly polymicrobial; causative agents include *Neisseria gonorrhoeae*, *Chlamydia trachomatis*, anaerobes (*Gardnerella vaginalis*), gram-negative bacteria, and *streptococci*. Cervical infection ascends through the endometrium, into the fallopian tubes, and possibly into the peritoneal cavity.
3. Predisposing factors include multiple sexual partners, early onset of sexual activity, use of intrauterine system (IUS; the wick promotes ascension of bacteria), and procedures such as therapeutic abortion, cesarean sections, and hysterosalpingograms.

Clinical Manifestations

1. Pelvic pain—most common presenting symptom; usually dull and bilateral.
2. Fever greater than 101°F (38.33°C)—especially with gonococcal infections.
3. Cervical discharge—mucopurulent.
4. Irregular bleeding.
5. Gastrointestinal (GI) symptoms—nausea, vomiting, and acute abdomen usually signify abscess.
6. Urinary symptoms—dysuria and frequency.
7. Presentation with chlamydia may be mild.

CLINICAL JUDGMENT Localized right or left lower quadrant tenderness with guarding, rebound, or palpable mass signifies tubo-ovarian abscess with peritoneal inflammation. Immediate evaluation and surgical intervention are necessary to prevent rupture and widespread peritonitis.

Diagnostic Evaluation

1. Clinical diagnosis can be made if any of the following minimum criteria are present in patients at risk for sexually transmitted infection (STI):
   a. Cervical motion tenderness.
   b. Uterine tenderness.
   c. Adnexal tenderness.
2. In addition to the presence of the minimum criteria, signs/symptoms of lower genital tract infection (such as cervical exudate, a friable cervix, and white blood cells on microscopic examination of cervical secretions) improve the specificity of the diagnosis.
3. Endocervical DNA testing or culture to identify organisms (*Gonorrhea* or *Chlamydia*).
4. Complete blood count (CBC) may show elevated leukocytes.
5. Elevated C-reactive protein or elevated erythrocyte sedimentation rate shows inflammation.
6. Some cases may warrant endometrial biopsy, hysterosalpingectomy, transvaginal ultrasound, magnetic resonance imaging (MRI), or laparoscopic visualization of the fallopian tubes.

Management

1. Patients with mild to moderate symptoms can be treated on an outpatient basis with oral antimicrobial regimens and timely follow-up 48 to 72 hours after initiation of antibiotic and at completion of 2-week antibiotic course.
2. Inpatient treatment is required for surgical emergencies; abscess; pregnancy; severe infection with nausea, vomiting, and high fever; cannot take oral fluids; immunodeficient patient; or more aggressive antibiotics required to preserve fertility.

3. Parenteral antimicrobial regimens recommended by the Centers for Disease Control and Prevention (CDC) during hospitalization include the following:
   a. Cefotetan 2 g intravenously (IV) every 12 hours or cefoxitin 2 g IV every 6 hours *plus* doxycycline 100 mg IV or orally every 12 hours. *Note:* Doxycycline is contraindicated during pregnancy and IV infusion is painful; oral administration is preferred when possible.
   b. Clindamycin 900 mg IV every 8 hours *plus* gentamicin 2 mg/kg of body weight IV or intramuscular (IM) as loading dose, followed by 1.5 mg/kg every 8 hours as maintenance dosage. (A single daily dose [3 to 5 mg/kg] of gentamicin may be substituted.)
4. Outpatient, oral antimicrobial regimens recommended by the CDC include:
   a. Ceftriaxone 500 mg IM single dose *plus* doxycycline 100 mg orally twice per day for 14 days, with or without metronidazole 500 mg orally twice per day for 14 days.
   b. Cefoxitin 2 g IM single dose *and* probenecid 1 g orally administered concurrently as a single dose *plus* doxycycline 100 mg orally twice daily for 14 days, with or without metronidazole 500 mg orally twice daily for 14 days.
   c. Other IM third-generation cephalosporin (ceftizoxime or cefotaxime) *plus* doxycycline 100 mg orally twice a day for 14 days, with or without metronidazole 500 mg twice a day for 14 days.
5. Parenteral therapy can be switched to oral therapy 24 to 48 hours after improvement is shown (reduced fever, decreased pain, resolution of nausea and vomiting). Ongoing oral therapy after parenteral therapy may be one of the following regimens:
   a. Doxycycline 100 mg orally twice per day to complete a total of 14 days.
   b. Clindamycin 450 mg orally four times per day to complete a total of 14 days.
   c. With or without addition of metronidazole 500 mg orally twice per day to complete 14 days.
6. Surgical treatment or interventional drain placement may be necessary to drain abscess or later to treat adhesions or tubal damage.

Complications

1. Abscess rupture and sepsis.
2. Infertility because of adhesions to fallopian tubes and ovaries.
3. Ectopic pregnancy caused by inability of fertilized egg to pass stricture.
4. Dyspareunia because of adhesions.

Nursing Assessment

1. Obtain history of menstruation, contraception, sexual activity (including number of partners and new partner), STI history, and symptoms in sexual partner.
2. Assess level of pain and fever; evaluate vital signs for hypotension and increased pulse, indicating hypovolemia.
3. Perform abdominal and pelvic examinations, if indicated; be alert for abdominal tenderness, rebound, guarding, or a mass.
4. Assess the patient's feelings about having an STI.

Nursing Interventions

Relieving Pain

1. Administer or teach the patient to self-administer analgesics as prescribed; monitor for adverse effect of drowsiness and constipation.
2. Assist to comfortable position of pelvic dependence, with upper body and legs slightly elevated. Suggest heating pad to lower abdomen or low back.
3. Administer IV antibiotics at scheduled time to maintain therapeutic blood levels.

Restoring Fluid Balance

1. Administer antiemetics as needed for nausea and vomiting impairing fluid intake.
2. Administer IV fluids as directed, and monitor intake and output.
3. Monitor vital signs as indicated; report decreased blood pressure (BP) and increased heart rate, which may indicate fluid volume deficit.
4. Restart oral intake with ice chips and sips of water when vomiting has ceased for 2 hours.

Patient Education and Health Maintenance

1. Encourage adherence with antibiotic therapy for full length of prescription.
2. Stress the need for sexual abstinence and pelvic rest (nothing in the vagina, including no douching or tampons) until completion of the patient's and partner's antimicrobial regimens, resolution of the patient's and partner's symptoms, and follow-up visit.
3. Advise testing and empiric treatment of gonorrhea and chlamydia for all sexual partners (within past 60 days or more). Tell patient that diagnosis of chlamydia or gonorrhea necessitates reporting to public health department and partners will be traced.
4. Repeat patient and partner testing for gonorrhea and chlamydia is recommended 3 months after treatment completion.
5. Discuss STIs and methods of prevention—abstinence, monogamy, and proper use of female or male condoms. See page 613.

Evaluation: Expected Outcomes

- Verbalizes relief of pain.
- Vital signs stable; intake equals output.

Polycystic Ovary Syndrome

Polycystic ovary syndrome (PCOS) is a complex endocrinologic condition characterized by at least two out of the following three conditions: anovulation, hyperandrogenism, and polycystic ovary morphology. There are various clinical presentations, which often makes diagnosis challenging.

Pathophysiology and Etiology

1. PCOS develops during the early pubertal years.
2. Genetic and environmental factors are believed to play a role in the development of PCOS.
3. Continuous oversecretion of androgens impairs the hypothalamic–pituitary–ovary feedback loop, leading to luteinizing hormone hypersecretion and follicles that do not mature. The cysts in PCOS are not true cysts but rather the follicles that stop developing.
4. Obesity and sedentary lifestyle are associated with metabolic dysfunction, which contributes to hyperinsulinemia and the resulting metabolic syndrome and type 2 diabetes mellitus.

Clinical Manifestations

1. Anovulatory cycles.
2. Amenorrhea/oligomenorrhea.

3. History of infertility.
4. Signs of hyperandrogenism including acne, hirsutism, and alopecia; acanthosis nigricans may also occur, appearing as hyperpigmented, leathery skin of the back of the neck.
5. Obesity and increased waist circumference are often present.
6. Mood disturbances such as depression and anxiety.

Diagnostic Evaluation

1. Thorough history and examination including pelvic exam to assess for masses.
2. Evaluation of ovarian failure—follicle-stimulating hormone (FSH), luteinizing hormone (LH), LH/FSH ratio.
3. Prolactin to rule out pituitary adenoma.
4. Glucose (fasting), insulin (fasting) to determine impaired glucose and diabetes.
5. Comprehensive metabolic panel for possible liver disease.
6. Lipid profile for hyperlipidemia.
7. Human chorionic gonadotropin (hCG) to rule out pregnancy.
8. Thyroid-stimulating hormone (TSH) to rule out thyroid disorder.
9. Testosterone (total and free), androstenedione may be elevated in PCOS.
10. Dehydroepiandrosterone sulfate (DHEAS), 17-ketosteroids, and other tests to evaluate hyperandrogenism.
11. Transvaginal ultrasound to assess ovaries and presence of cysts and endometrial hyperplasia.

Management

1. Weight loss and exercise program. Weight loss of as little as 5% to 10% has been shown to improve oligoanovulation and fertility.
2. Low-dose, low androgenic combination oral contraceptives to restore menstrual cycles and relieve hyperandrogen symptoms.
3. Anti-androgen medications such as spironolactone for acne and hirsutism.
4. Insulin-sensitizing agents such as metformin for those seeking pregnancy or those with a history of gestational diabetes; also improves menstrual cycles.

Complications

1. Insulin resistance and development of type 2 diabetes, metabolic syndrome.
2. Infertility.
3. Spontaneous abortion.
4. Endometrial hyperplasia and endometrial cancer.
5. Cardiovascular disease (atherosclerosis, hypertension, increased triglycerides, stroke).
6. Nonalcoholic fatty liver disease.

Nursing Assessment

1. Review menstrual cycle with patient; cycle of 35 days or longer points to anovulation.
2. Assess weight, body mass index (BMI), and waist and hip circumference; obesity and waist to hip ratio >0.87 is associated with PCOS.
3. Assess for hair and skin changes, which may not be obvious if the patient has been trying to conceal these.
4. Review risk factors for thromboemboli for patients starting hormonal contraceptives: smoking, hypertension, peripheral vascular disease, history of blood clot, obesity, sedentary lifestyle.

Nursing Interventions

Improving Body Image and Self-Care

1. Educate patient about the importance of weight loss to improve disease process and decrease complications, as well as to reduce hyperandrogen symptoms. Calorie restriction and exercise together are most effective.
2. Assist the patient with safe and effective methods for facial hair removal until treatment of hyperandrogenism with oral contraceptives or other medication takes effect (may take 6 months or more). Options include electrolysis and laser treatment, which can be time consuming and expensive; bleaching creams, which may or may not be effective; topical eflornithine, which works directly in the hair follicle to slow hair growth, is by prescription.
3. Provide emotional support for the patient and partner dealing with infertility. Educate about the menstrual cycle and medications that may be used to stimulate ovulation.

Patient Education and Health Maintenance

1. Encourage regular follow-up visits with endocrinologist, gynecologist, and fertility specialist, as indicated.
2. Encourage close surveillance for diabetes and hyperlipidemia to guide additional treatment and prevent complications.
3. Advise on overall healthy lifestyle to reduce cardiovascular risk, including avoidance of smoking; increase intake of fruits, vegetables, and fiber; reduce intake of saturated fats, sugars, and salt; limit alcohol intake; increase physical activity; and reduce stress.

Evaluation: Expected Outcomes

Patient verbalizes understanding of lifestyle changes and medications with hope for control of symptoms.

Endometriosis

EVIDENCE BASE Horne, A. W., & Missmer, S. A. (2022). Pathophysiology, diagnosis, and management of endometriosis. *BMJ (Clinical Research Ed.)*, *379*, e070750. https://doi.org/10.1136/bmj-2022-070750

Endometriosis is the abnormal proliferation of uterine endometrial tissue outside the uterus.

Pathophysiology and Etiology

1. May also be found outside the pelvic cavity; an intact uterus is not needed to have endometriosis (see Figure 18-9).
2. Peaks in females ages 25 to 45; may occur at any age. Increased risk in siblings, females with shorter menstrual cycles, and longer duration of flow. More common in White females than in Black females, in females who do not exercise, and in females with obesity.
3. Responds to ovarian hormonal stimulation—estrogen increases it; progestins decrease it.
   a. Bleeds during uterine menstruation, resulting in accumulated blood and inflammation and subsequent adhesions and pain.
   b. Regresses during amenorrhea (i.e., pregnancy and menopause) and hormonal contraceptive and androgen use.
4. Theories of origin:
   a. May be embryonic tissue remnants that differentiate as a result of hormonal stimulation and spread via lymphatic or venous channels.

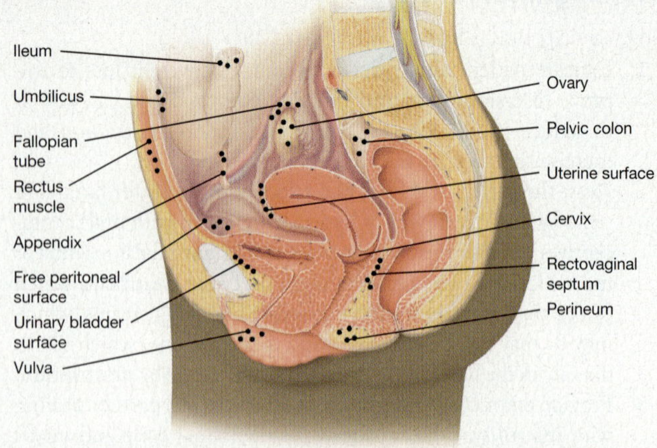

Figure 18-9. Common sites of endometriosis. Ectopic endometrial tissue can implant almost anywhere in the pelvic peritoneum. It can even invade distant sites such as the lungs. (Adapted with permission from Anatomical Chart Company.)

b. May be transferred via surgical instruments.
c. May be caused by retrograde menstruation through fallopian tubes into peritoneal cavity (but this theory does not account for some types of endometriosis).
d. Genetic predisposition may increase the likelihood in females with a first-degree relative with endometriosis.
e. Lymphatic or vascular distribution of endometrial tissue.

Clinical Manifestations

1. Depends on sites of implantation; may be asymptomatic.
2. Pelvic pain—especially during or before menstruation.
3. Dyspareunia.
4. Painful defecation—if implants are on the sigmoid colon or rectum.
5. Abnormal uterine bleeding.
6. Persistent infertility (in 30% to 40% of females with endometriosis).
7. Hematuria, dysuria, and flank pain—if bladder involved.

Diagnostic Evaluation

1. Pelvic and rectal examinations—tender, fixed nodules or ovarian mass or uterine retrodisplacement; nodules may not be palpable.
2. Transvaginal ultrasound—diagnostic tool of choice to first assess for endometriosis. MRI and computed tomography (CT) are reserved for inconclusive ultrasound results.
3. Laparoscopy—for definitive diagnosis to view implants, obtain tissue for histologic analysis, and determine extent of disease.

Management

Medical

The goal of medical suppressive therapy is to decrease pain. However, if therapy is stopped, pain recurs. Medical therapies are ineffective for infertility associated with endometriosis.

1. Hormonal contraceptives—such as combination oral contraceptives (OCs); use small amount of estrogen and maximum amount of progestin and androgen effect to decrease implant size. OC use for more than 24 months effectively decreases endometrioma recurrence and decreases the frequency and intensity of dysmenorrhea.
2. Progestins—such as depot medroxyprogesterone acetate; create a hypoestrogenic environment. Efficacy is equivalent to OCs.
3. Nonsteroidal anti-inflammatory drugs (NSAIDs)—such as ibuprofen and naproxen sodium—decrease dysmenorrhea with anti-prostaglandin action.
4. If after 3 months of OC and NSAID treatment has not provided adequate pain relief, then gonadotropin-releasing hormone (GnRH) agonist (leuprolide) injections may be administered during a 6-month period—create hypoestrogenic environment. Menopausal-like side effects, such as hot flashes and vaginal dryness, may not be tolerable to some patients. If GnRH therapy will continue later, then norethindrone acetate add-back therapy will be added to prevent bone mineral loss and alleviate some symptoms. Calcium, vitamin D, and bisphosphonates may also be added.
5. Aromatase inhibitors, such as letrozole—inhibit the action of aromatase, which converts androgens to estrogen, thereby reducing estrogen levels in all tissues including endometriosis.
6. Danazol—synthetic androgen suppresses endometrial growth. Use is limited secondary to adverse effects (increased facial hair, acne, weight gain, vasomotor symptoms) and other drugs are available with better side-effect profiles. Contraindicated in pregnancy.

Surgical

1. Laparoscopic surgery—preferred procedure to remove implants and lyse adhesions by excision; not curative; high recurrence rate.
2. Carbon dioxide laser laparoscopy—for minimal to moderate disease; vaporizes tissue; may be done at same time as diagnosis; good pregnancy rate.
3. Laparotomy—rarely performed; involves a larger abdominal incision than laparoscopy; for severe endometriosis or persistent symptoms.
4. Presacral neurectomy—rarely performed; to decrease central pelvic pain; preserves fertility; limited efficacy in relieving pain; severe constipation results.
5. Hysterectomy—if fertility is not desired and symptoms are severe; greater pain relief is achieved when ovaries are also removed.

Complications

1. Infertility.
2. Rupture of cyst—mimics ruptured appendix.
3. Chronic pelvic pain.
4. Dyspareunia.
5. Bowel or ureter obstruction.

Nursing Assessment

1. Obtain history of symptoms to determine spread and severity of disease.
2. Assess pain—level, location, frequency, duration, characteristics, and impact on functioning.
3. Perform abdominal examination to assess for areas of tenderness and nodules.
4. Assess for impact of endometriosis and/or infertility on patient and significant other.

Nursing Interventions

Reducing Pain

1. Teach use of analgesics and other prescribed medication, including adverse effects that may occur.
   a. Common adverse effects with medications include weight gain, depression, bloating, hot flashes (also known as hot flushes), menstrual irregularity, headaches, lethargy, and joint and muscle aches. Danazol may cause acne, abnormal hair growth, and reduced breast size, which can be distressing.
   b. Help the patient explore ways to minimize adverse effects such as adding exercise and reducing calories to counteract weight gain, dressing in layers and having a fan available if hot flashes occur, trying over-the-counter (OTC) products as needed for headache and nausea, seeking treatment if depression persists.
   c. Encourage patient to talk to health care provider about persistent or intolerable symptoms.
   d. Monitor the patient's weight, BP, and routine blood work including liver function tests regularly, as these may be affected by medications.
2. Encourage use of heating pad to painful areas, as needed.
3. Teach patient relaxation techniques to control pain, such as deep breathing, imagery, and progressive muscle relaxation.
4. Encourage patient to try position changes for sexual intercourse if experiencing dyspareunia.

Strengthening Personal Coping

1. Include patient in treatment planning; answer questions about drug and surgical treatment to enhance informed decision-making.
2. Encourage adequate rest and nutrition.
3. Provide emotional support and encourage patient to discuss treatment of infertility with significant other.
4. Encourage exploration and use of positive coping mechanisms such as journaling and positive self-talk.
5. Prepare the patient for surgery, as indicated (see page 56).

Patient Education and Health Maintenance

1. Encourage adherence to medication schedule and keeping follow-up appointments.
2. Refer patient to support groups such as Endometriosis Association (endometriosisassn.org) and reliable resources for information such as https://www.nichd.nih.gov/health/topics/endometriosis or https://www.nhs.uk/conditions/endometriosis/.

Evaluation: Expected Outcomes

- Verbalizes reduced pain and tolerates adverse effects of medications.
- Verbalizes increased coping ability.

Toxic Shock Syndrome

Toxic shock syndrome (TSS) is a rare condition caused by a bacterial toxin from *Staphylococcus aureus* or sometimes by group A *Streptococcus pyogenes* in the bloodstream; it can be life-threatening.

Pathophysiology and Etiology

1. Cause is uncertain, but 70% of cases historically were associated with menstruation and superabsorbent tampon use. Menstrual cases have declined since the withdrawal of superabsorbent tampons from the market around 1986. Now, half of TSS cases are not menstrually related.
2. TSS does occur in nonmenstruating or postmenopausal females, males, and children with conditions such as cellulitis, surgical wound infections, subcutaneous abscesses, vaginal infections, after childbirth, and with the use of contraceptive sponge or diaphragm.
3. See Figure 18-10 for pathophysiology.

Clinical Manifestations

1. Patients may initially present with fever, hypotension, and diffuse rash.
2. May have sudden onset of fever greater than 102°F (38.9°C), often with flulike symptoms (myalgias, headache, sore throat).
3. Hypotension and rapid progression to shock within 72 hours of onset.
4. Rash (similar to sunburn) that is diffuse, red, and macular; followed by desquamation, particularly of the palms and soles, 1 to 2 weeks after illness onset.
5. Mucous membrane hyperemia.
6. Vomiting and profuse watery diarrhea.
7. Rapid progression to multisystem involvement.

Diagnostic Evaluation

1. Blood, urine, throat, and vaginal or cervical cultures; possibly cerebrospinal fluid culture to detect or rule out infectious organism.

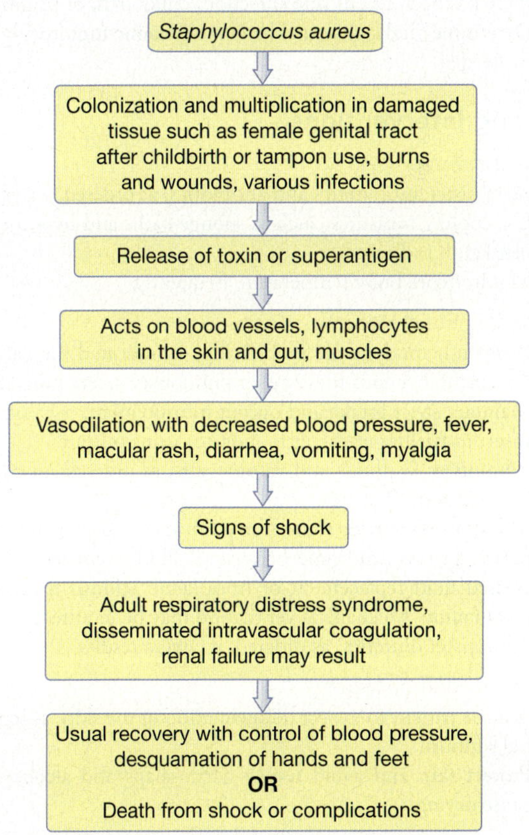

Figure 18-10. Pathophysiology of toxic shock syndrome.

2. Tests to rule out other febrile illnesses—Rocky Mountain spotted fever, Lyme disease, meningitis, and Epstein–Barr or coxsackie virus.
3. CBC, electrolytes, blood urea nitrogen, creatinine, coagulation studies, and other tests to monitor condition.

Management

Management will be achieved in an intensive care unit because of the nature of the rapidly progressing shock, circulatory compromise, impending potential acute renal failure, and multisystem organ failure.

1. Fluid and electrolyte replacement to increase BP and prevent renal failure.
2. Inotropes and vasopressor medications (i.e., dopamine), as needed.
3. IV antibiotics (i.e., penicillins, cephalosporins, vancomycin); methicillin-resistant *Staphylococcus aureus* has been reported in some cases of TSS.
4. Mechanical ventilation in acute respiratory distress and lactic acidosis.
5. The use of steroids and immunoglobulins is controversial and under investigation.
6. Surgery may be employed to remove causative infectious site or to debride skin and soft tissue.

Complications

Cardiovascular collapse and renal failure because of shock.

Nursing Assessment

1. Determine menstrual history, use of tampons, or whether there has been recent skin infection, childbirth, or surgery.
2. Determine vital signs quickly; hemodynamic monitoring may be needed.

Nursing Interventions

Reducing Fever

1. Administer antipyretics and antibiotics, as ordered.
2. Use cooling measures, such as sponge baths and hypothermia blanket, if indicated.
3. Monitor core body temperature frequently.

Restoring Fluid Volume

1. Perform hemodynamic monitoring, as indicated (i.e., arterial line, central venous pressure, or pulmonary artery pressure).
2. Maintain strict intake and output measurement.
3. Insert indwelling catheter to monitor urine output.
4. Administer IV fluids and vasopressors, as ordered, to control hypotension.
5. Monitor respiratory status for pulmonary edema and respiratory distress syndrome because of fluid overload from increased fluid replacement or from lactic acidosis from acute renal failure. Mechanical ventilation may be required.
6. Administer diuretics, as ordered, if edema results.

Restoring Skin Integrity

1. Tell the patient to expect desquamation of the skin, as in peeling sunburn.
2. Protect skin and avoid use of harsh soaps and alcohol that cause drying.
3. Tell the patient to apply mild moisturizer and avoid direct sunlight until healed.
4. Advise the patient that reversible hair loss may occur 1 to 2 months after TSS.

Patient Education and Health Maintenance

1. Tell the patient to expect fatigue for weeks to months after TSS.
2. Tell the patient not to use tampons in future to reduce risk of recurrence.
3. Encourage follow-up examination and cultures.
4. Teach prevention of TSS related to menstruation.
   a. Avoid use of tampons if menstrual flow is light. Use pads whenever possible.
   b. Alternate use of pads with tampons.
   c. Change tampons frequently and do not wear one longer than 8 hours—4 hours maximum in heavy discharge time.
   d. Be careful of vaginal abrasions that can be caused by some applicators.
   e. Be alert to symptoms of TSS.

Evaluation: Expected Outcomes

- Afebrile.
- Normotensive and good urine output.
- Skin heals without scar.

SELECTED READINGS

ACOG Committee Opinion, Number 800. (2020). The use of hysteroscopy for the diagnosis and treatment of intrauterine pathology. *Obstetrics and Gynecology, 135*(3), e138–e148. https://doi.org/10.1097/AOG.0000000000003712

Britton, L. E., Alspaugh, A., Greene, M. Z., & McLemore, M. R. (2020). CE: An evidence-based update on contraception. *The American Journal of Nursing, 120*(2), 22–33. https://doi.org/10.1097/01.NAJ.0000654304.29632.a7

Burness, J. V., Schroeder, J. M., & Warren, J. B. (2020). Cervical colposcopy: Indications and risk assessment. *American Family Physician, 102*(1), 39–48. PMID: 32603071

Center for Disease Control and Surveillance. (2024). *Sexually transmitted infections surveillance, 2022.* US Department of Health and Human Services. https://www.cdc.gov/std/statistics/2022/default.htm

Cooper, D. B., & Menefee, G. W. (2022). Dilation and curettage. In *StatPearls* [Internet]. StatPearls Publishing. Updated March 9, 2022. https://www.ncbi.nlm.nih.gov/books/NBK568791/

Crosbie, E. J., Kitson, S. J., McAlpine, J. N., Mukhopadhyay, A., Powell, M. E., & Singh, N. (2022). Endometrial cancer. *Lancet (London, England), 399*(10333), 1412–1428. https://doi.org/10.1016/S0140-6736(22)00323-3

Ebrahimi, A., Tayebi, N., Fatemeh, A., & Akbarzadeh, M. (2020). Investigation of the role of herbal medicine, acupressure, and acupuncture in the menopausal symptoms: An evidence-based systematic review study. *Journal of Family Medicine and Primary Care, 9*(6), 2638–2649. https://doi.org/10.4103/jfmpc.jfmpc_1094_19

Ethirajulu, A., Alkasabera, A., Onyali, C. B., Anim-Koranteng, C., Shah, H. E., Bhawnani, N., & Mostafa, J. A. (2021). Insulin resistance, hyperandrogenism, and its associated symptoms are the precipitating factors for depression in women with polycystic ovarian syndrome. *Cureus, 13*(9), e18013. https://doi.org/10.7759/cureus.18013

Fantasia, H. C., Harris, A. L., & Fontenot, H. B. (2020). *Guidelines for nurse practitioners in gynecologic settings.* Springer Publishing Company.

Farkas, A. H., Abumusa, H., & Rossiter, B. (2023). Structural gynecological disease: Fibroids, endometriosis, ovarian cysts. *The Medical Clinics of North America, 107*(2), 317–328. https://doi.org/10.1016/j.mcna.2022.10.010

Faubion, S. S., Crandall, C. J., Davis, L., El Khoudary, S. R., Hodis, H. N., Lobo, R. A., Maki, P. M., Manson, J. E., Pinkerton, J. V., Santoro, N. F., Shifren, J. L., Shufelt, C. L., Thurston, R. C., & Wolfman, W. (2022). The 2022 hormone therapy position statement of the North American Menopause Society. *Menopause, 29*(7), 767–794. https://doi.org/10.1097/GME.0000000000002028

Feduniw, S., Korczyńska, L., Górski, K., Zgliczyńska, M., Bączkowska, M., Byrczak, M., Kociuba, J., Ali, M., & Ciebiera, M. (2022). The effect of vitamin E supplementation in postmenopausal women—A systematic review. *Nutrients, 15*(1), 160. https://doi.org/10.3390/nu15010160

Ferries-Rowe, E., Corey, E., & Archer, J. S. (2020). Primary dysmenorrhea: Diagnosis and therapy. *Obstetrics and Gynecology, 136*(5), 1047–1058. https://doi.org/10.1097/AOG.0000000000004096

Font, M. D., Thyagarajan, B., & Khanna, A. K. (2020). Sepsis and septic shock—Basics of diagnosis, pathophysiology and clinical decision making. *The Medical Clinics of North America, 104*(4), 573–585. https://doi.org/10.1016/j.mcna.2020.02.011

Fontham, E. T. H., Wolf, A. M. D., Church, T. R., Etzioni, R., Flowers, C. R., Herzig, A., Guerra, C. E., Oeffinger, K. C., Shih, Y. T., Walter, L. C., Kim, J. J., Andrews, K. S., DeSantis, C. E., Fedewa, S. A., Manassaram-Baptiste, D., Saslow, D., Wender, R. C., & Smith, R. A. (2020). Cervical cancer screening for individuals at average risk: 2020 guideline update from the American Cancer Society. *CA: A Cancer Journal for Clinicians, 70*(5), 321–346. https://doi.org/10.3322/caac.21628

Huang, Y. C., & Chang, K. V. (2022). Kegel exercises. In *StatPearls*. StatPearls Publishing.

Hye Won Lee, Lin Ang, & Myeong Soo Lee. (2022). Using ginseng for menopausal women's health care: A systematic review of randomized placebo-controlled trials. *Complementary Therapies in Clinical Practice, 48*, 101615. https://doi.org/10.1016/j.ctcp.2022.101615

Jewson, M., Purohit, P., & Lumsden, M. A. (2020). Progesterone and abnormal uterine bleeding/menstrual disorders. *Best Practice & Research. Clinical Obstetrics & Gynaecology, 69*, 62–73. https://doi.org/10.1016/j.bpobgyn.2020.05.004

Kanadys, W., Barańska, A., Błaszczuk, A., Polz-Dacewicz, M., Drop, B., Kanecki, K., & Malm, M. (2021). Evaluation of clinical meaningfulness of red clover (*Trifolium pratense L.*) extract to relieve hot flushes and menopausal symptoms in peri- and post-menopausal women: A systematic review and meta-analysis of randomized controlled trials. *Nutrients, 13*(4), 1258. https://doi.org/10.3390/nu13041258

Kazemi, F., Masoumi, S. Z., Shayan A, Oshvandi K. (2021). The effect of evening primrose oil capsule on hot flashes and night sweats in ostmenopausal omen: A single-blind randomized controlled trial. *Journal of Menopausal Medicine, 27*(1), 8-14. https://doi-org/10.6118/jmm.20033

Kerns, J., Itriyeva, K., & Fisher, M. (2022). Etiology and management of amenorrhea in adolescent and young adult women. *Current Problems in Pediatric and Adolescent Health Care, 52*(5), 101184. https://doi.org/10.1016/j.cppeds.2022.101184

Kornstein, S. G., Pinkerton, J. V., Pace, D. T., Singer, A. J., Kingsberg, S. A., Ellis, L. E., Ashley, P., & Klein, W. (2022). Multidisciplinary Management of Menopause: Symposium Proceedings. *Journal of Women's Health (15409996), 31*(8), 1071–1078. https://doi-org.pluma.sjfc.edu/10.1089/jwh.2022.0175

Ladd, M., & Tuma, F. (2022). Rectocele. In *StatPearls*. StatPearls Publishing.

Long, S. (2021). Endometrial biopsy: Indications and technique. *Primary Care, 48*(4), 555–567. https://doi.org/10.1016/j.pop.2021.07.003

Makajeva, J., Watters, C., & Safioleas, P. (2022). Cystocele. In *StatPearls*. StatPearls Publishing.

McNeil, M., & Merriam, S. (2021). Menopause. *Annals of Internal Medicine, 174*(7), ITC97–ITC112. https://doi.org/10.7326/AITC202107200

Muldoon J. (2022). Uterine prolapse: Impact of the condition and practical advice. *British Journal of Nursing (Mark Allen Publishing), 31*(18), S8–S14. https://doi.org/10.12968/bjon.2022.31.18.S8

Olawaiye, A. B., Cuello, M. A., & Rogers, L. J. (2021). Cancer of the vulva: 2021 update. *International Journal of Gynecology and Obstetrics, 155*(1), 7–18. https://doi.org/10.1002/ijgo.13881

Perry, S. E., Hockenberry, M. J., Lowdermilk, D. L., Cashion, K., Alden, K. R., Olanshansky, E. F., & Rodgers, C.C. (2023). *Maternal child nursing care* (7th ed.). Elsevier.

Preti, M., Joura, E., Vieira-Baptista, P., Van Beurden, M., Bevilacqua, F., Bleeker, M. C. G., Bornstein, J., Carcopino, X., Chargari, C., Cruickshank, M. E., Erzeneoglu, B. E., Gallio, N., Heller, D., Kesic, V., Reich, O., Stockdale, C. K., Temiz, B. E., Woelber, L., Planchamp, F., … Gultekin, M. (2022). The European Society of Gynaecological Oncology (ESGO), the International Society for the Study of Vulvovaginal Disease (ISSVD), the European College for the Study of Vulval Disease (ECSVD) and the European Federation for Colposcopy (EFC) consensus statements on pre-invasive vulvar lesions. *Journal of Lower Genital Tract Disease, 26*(3), 229–244. https://doi.org/10.1097/LGT.0000000000000683

Safdari, F., Motaghi Dastenaei, B., Kheiri, S., & Karimiankakolaki, Z. (2021). Effect of evening primrose oil on postmenopausal psychological symptoms: A triple-blind randomized clinical trial. *Journal of Menopausal Medicine. 27*(2), 58-65. http://doi.org/10.6118/jmm.21010

Tan, A., Bieber, A. K., Stein, J. A., & Pomeranz, M. K. (2019). Diagnosis and management of vulvar cancer: A review. *Journal of the American Academy of Dermatology, 81*(6), 1387–1396. https://doi.org/10.1016/j.jaad.2019.07.055

Taylor, H. S., Kotlyar, A. M., & Flores, V. A. (2021). Endometriosis is a chronic systemic disease: Clinical challenges and novel innovations. *Lancet (London, England), 397*(10276), 839–852. https://doi.org/10.1016/S0140-6736(21)00389-5

US Preventive Services Task Force. (2018). Screening for cervical cancer: US Preventive Services Task Force recommendation statement. *JAMA, 320*(7), 674–686. https://doi.org/10.1001/jama.2018.10897

Watson, L. A. (2020). Cervical conization. In G. C. Fowler (Ed.), *Pfenninger and Fowler's procedures for primary care* (4th ed., Chap. 128). Elsevier.

Zhang, M., Cheng, S., Jin, Y., Zhao, Y., & Wang, Y. (2021). Roles of CA125 in diagnosis, prediction, and oncogenesis of ovarian cancer. *Biochimica et Biophysica Acta. Reviews on Cancer, 1875*(2), 188503. https://doi.org/10.1016/j.bbcan.2021.188503

19
Breast Conditions*

OVERVIEW AND ASSESSMENT

See additional online content: Procedure Guidelines 19-1.

Subjective Data

Obtain a nursing history about specific breast complaints and general health information from the patient to plan care and appropriate patient teaching.

Breast Manifestations

1. Palpable lumps—date noted; affected by menstruation; changes noted since detection.
2. Nipple discharge—date of onset, color, unilateral or bilateral, spontaneous or provoked.
3. Pain or tenderness—localized or diffuse, cyclic or constant, unilateral or bilateral.
4. Date of last breast imaging and result.
5. Patient's practice of breast self-examination (BSE).

History

General Information

1. Age.
2. Past medical–surgical history; injuries; bleeding tendencies.
3. Medications, including current or prior use of hormonal contraceptives and hormones, over-the-counter (OTC) products, vitamins, and herbal supplements.

Gynecologic and Obstetric History

1. Menarche.
2. Date of last menses.
3. Pregnancies, miscarriages, abortions, deliveries.
4. Lactation history.
5. Prior history of interventions affecting breast, including previous history of irradiation involving breast region.
6. Family history of breast cancer.

Examination and Screening

Perform a breast examination for any breast complaint and, if the patient desires, teach patient how to examine breasts. Although research has not shown that physical exams of the breast by a health professional are effective in reducing mortality, examination should be done for any breast complaint. Research has also not shown that BSE is effective in reducing mortality; however, BSE may allow females to become more comfortable and familiar with their own bodies. Mammography is the primary breast cancer screening method.

1. Breast exam is best done just after the menstrual period, because breasts are less engorged and a lump is easier to detect, and at regular monthly intervals after the cessation of menses.
2. Compare inspection and palpation findings with the opposite breast.
3. Remind patient that 90% of breast lumps are not cancerous.
4. Do not neglect males when there is a breast complaint—1% of breast cancers occur in males.
5. It is acceptable for the patient to choose not to do BSE or to do BSE irregularly.

POPULATION AWARENESS Normal breast changes in older patients include drooping, flaccid breasts caused by decreased subcutaneous tissue from decreased estrogen levels. Nipple size and erection are also reduced.

*Please note that the term "male" in this chapter refers to a person assigned male at birth, and the term "female" in this chapter refers to a person assigned female at birth

Guidelines for Early Detection

EVIDENCE BASE Qaseem, A., Lin, J. S., Mustafa, R. A., Horwitch, C. A., Wilt, T. J., Clinical Guidelines Committee of the American College of Physicians, Forciea, M. A., Fitterman, N., Iorio, A., Kansagara, D., Maroto, M., McLean, R. M., Tufte, J. E., & Vijan, S. (2019). Screening for breast cancer in average-risk women: A guidance statement from the American College of Physicians. *Annals of Internal Medicine, 170*(8), 547–560. https://doi.org/10.7326/M18-2147

Females at Average Risk

1. Recommendations vary by organization.
2. American Cancer Society recommends females begin annual mammography at age 45, biennial at age 55, but should be available to females at age 40, and continue as long as life expectancy is projected to be 10 years or longer. Because of lack of evidence, clinical breast exam and BSE are no longer recommended.
3. National Comprehensive Cancer Network (NCCN) and the American College of Radiology recommend females should have annual mammographic screening beginning at age 40.
4. U.S. Preventive Services recommends females aged 50 to 74 undergo biennial screening mammography and end screening at age 75. Clinical breast exam is not recommended after age 40.

POPULATION AWARENESS Long-term effects of endocrine treatment in transgender women have not been sufficiently studied. As a result, there are currently no established cancer screening guidelines for transgender patients at any point in their transition process. Breast cancer screening may be recommended based on shared decision-making and initiated sooner if there is a known family history of breast cancer.

Older Females

1. Screening decisions in females 75 years and older should be individualized by considering the potential benefits and risks of mammography in the context of current health status and estimated life expectancy.
2. As long as a patient is in reasonably good health and would be a candidate for treatment, mammography screenings should be continued.

POPULATION AWARENESS Many older females may not be aware of newer treatments for breast cancer and may fear radical mastectomy; therefore, they may avoid breast cancer screening. Provide information about incidence, screening, and treatment, and encourage discussion with a health care provider.

Females at Increased Risk

EVIDENCE BASE Nelson, H. D., Pappas, M., Cantor, A., Haney, E., & Holmes, R. (2019). Risk assessment, genetic counseling, and genetic testing for BRCA-related cancer in women: Updated evidence report and systematic review for the US Preventive Services Task Force. *Journal of the American Medical Association, 322*(7), 666–685. https://doi.org/10.1001/jama.2019.8430

1. Females at increased risk for breast cancer (see page 666) might benefit from additional screening strategies beyond those offered to those of average risk, such as earlier initiation of screening, shorter screening intervals, or the addition of screening modalities other than mammography and physical examination, such as ultrasound or magnetic resonance imaging (MRI).
2. Screening MRI, in addition to yearly screening mammogram, is recommended for females with an approximately 20% to 25% or greater lifetime risk of developing breast cancer, including those with a strong family history of breast or ovarian cancer, those who were treated for Hodgkin disease, those with a history of lobular carcinoma in situ (LCIS) or atypical hyperplasia, and those with a prior history of breast cancer. Annual MRI should be considered in these females. Several models exist that attempt to calculate lifetime risk of breast cancer for females with identifiable factors associated with the disease. The Gail model is the most commonly used. It is available on the National Cancer Institute website at www.bcrisktool.cancer.gov. The Tyrer-Cuzick model and the Claus model are examples of risk prevention models that estimate risk of breast cancer based on family history and other characteristics.

Laboratory Tests

Nipple Discharge Cytology

Description

Secretions are smeared on a slide, fixed, and submitted for cytologic examination. There is a high rate of false-negative test results with this method.

Nursing and Patient Care Considerations

1. Wash nipple area with water and pat dry before obtaining specimen if crusting of drainage is present.
2. Gently milk the breast or ask the patient to express fluid to obtain a large drop on nipple.
3. Carefully touch the slide to drop and draw slide across nipple to obtain a smear. Spray with fixative or drop into a container with fixative.
4. Inform patient of results promptly to reduce anxiety and explain that other tests may be needed.

Ductal Lavage

Description

A procedure that targets females without symptoms at increased risk for breast cancer. Breast duct epithelial cells are collected from the nipple for cytologic analysis.

Nursing and Patient Care Considerations

Advise patient to discuss questions with a health care provider. This test is not widely used, and there are insufficient data at this time to recommend its use for screening.

Tumor-Specific Tests

Tests to evaluate the characteristics of a tumor and/or its potential to regrow.

1. Presence of estrogen and progesterone receptors identifies patients as most likely to benefit from hormonal forms of therapy. Approximately 75% of breast cancers are estrogen receptor positive. A negative result is associated with a less favorable prognosis.

2. HER2—human epidermal growth factor receptor that has been demonstrated in 15% to 30% of breast cancers. Found by many investigators to be associated with poorer survival, regardless of clinical stage. May affect treatment decisions.
3. Histologic grade is reported using an Elston–Ellis modification of the Scarff–Bloom–Richardson Scale. It is a combination of nuclear grade, mitotic rate, and tubule formation with scores given for each. A low score equates to a low grade (grade I) and a higher score to a higher grade (grade III). In general, high-grade tumors are considered to be more aggressive and are more likely to recur when compared to low-grade tumors.
4. Multiparameter gene assays quantify the likelihood of distant breast cancer recurrence and measure how chemotherapy may assist with planning treatment. A mathematic formula that includes 16 genes was established to help estimate the likelihood of recurrent breast cancer despite tamoxifen therapy.
   a. The Oncotype DX assay is included in NCCN guideline treatment decision pathway. Breast cancer diagnostic and treatment guidelines are available at www.nccn.org.
   b. Another gene assay, MammaPrint (also known as The Amsterdam 70-gene prognostic profile) could be helpful in predicting the benefits of chemotherapy for patients with high clinical risk cancer and involved lymph nodes.
5. Cancer subtyping—as determined by gene expression profiling—is currently under investigation.
6. Pathologists may use other special stains to aid in diagnosis.

Tests to Detect Metastasis

1. Increased values on liver function tests may indicate possible liver metastasis.
2. Increased calcium and alkaline phosphatase levels may indicate possible bony metastasis.
3. Additional metastatic workup may include chest x-ray, bone scan, computed tomography (CT) scan, and positron emission tomography (PET) scan.
4. Biologic markers (i.e., CA15.3 and CA27.29) may be used for monitoring patients with metastatic disease in conjunction with diagnostic imaging, history, and physical examination. Present data are insufficient to recommend their use alone for screening, diagnosis, or staging. However, monitoring trends in values in metastatic breast cancer setting could indicate response to therapy or treatment failure.

Radiology and Imaging

Mammography

Description

1. Low-dose x-ray of breast is used to screen for breast abnormalities or may be used when a lump is found on physical examination. Can detect patients with clustered microcalcifications.
2. Compression of the breast is used to reduce the amount of radiation absorbed by the breast tissue and separate overlapping tissue.
3. Two views are taken routinely: craniocaudal and mediolateral; other views are done as necessary.
4. Best performed at a facility that is accredited by the American College of Radiology. The machines and staff at these facilities have met specific criteria. Computer-aided detection has been developed to aid radiologists in detecting abnormalities. Assessment categories have been developed to describe the results and provide follow-up recommendations. A category 0 is incomplete and needs additional images.
   a. Category 1 is a negative result (normal mammogram) with nothing on which to comment.
   b. Category 2 is a normal mammogram, but there is a benign finding on which to comment.
   c. Category 3 is probably benign, but short-interval follow-up may be recommended to determine the stability of the finding.
   d. Category 4 describes a suspicious abnormality, and biopsy should be considered.
   e. Category 5 is highly suggestive of malignancy; appropriate action should be taken.
   f. Category 6 describes a known, biopsy-proven malignancy requiring appropriate action.
5. Mammography is not routinely done during pregnancy.
6. The breasts of young females tend to be extremely dense and are poorly suited to mammography.
7. False-negative results occur even in the best facilities; figure may reach 10%.
8. Both screen film and digital mammography use x-rays to obtain images. With digital mammography, a film image is replaced with an electronic image similar to digital photography. For females younger than age 50, females with radiographically dense breasts, and premenopausal and perimenopausal females, digital mammography is more accurate than film mammography and thus has supplanted film mammography as the technology of choice. Digital tomosynthesis creates a three-dimensional picture of the breasts that may make breast cancers easier to see, and adding tomosynthesis has increased breast cancer detection and decreased false-positive results.
9. Interpretation of mammography using artificial intelligence (AI) has the potential to improve breast screening outcomes. Several products are approved by the U.S. Food and Drug Administration (FDA) and are available to assist radiologists with mammography interpretations. Further evaluation is required to determine the role of AI in primary and assistive interpretation of screening mammography.

EVIDENCE BASE Nielsen, S., & Narayan, A. K. (2023). Breast cancer screening modalities, recommendations, and novel imaging techniques. *Surgical Clinics of North America, 103*(1), 63–82. https://doi.org/10.1016/j.suc.2022.08.004

Nursing and Patient Care Considerations

1. Recommend regular screening based on established guidelines (see page 619). Tell patients that routine screening mammography has been shown to reduce mortality from breast cancer. Procedure takes approximately 15 minutes.
2. Remind patients not to apply deodorant, cream, or powder to breast, nipple, or underarm areas on examination day.
3. Advise that some discomfort may be felt from compressing the breast.
4. Patients should have an opportunity to become informed about the benefits, limitations, and potential harms associated with regular screening. Overdiagnosis of clinically insignificant disease is possible. Benefits are thought to outweigh the exposure to low doses of radiation.
5. Alert patient that extra views do not imply that the patient has breast cancer.
6. Advise patient of COVID-19 consideration. An increased rate of axillary adenopathy on the side of the injection following

COVID-19 mRNA vaccination has been reported. Although some recommendations suggest delaying breast imaging by 4 to 6 weeks after vaccination to avoid false-positive results, most recent studies recommend to avoid delays but to inform the radiologist of the vaccination to allow correct interpretation of the results.

CLINICAL JUDGMENT Because health teaching is an important nursing role, nurses should educate females about the importance of routine screening. Because of differences in screening guidelines, females may also need advice regarding the timing of mammograms.

Community Health Education

Implement patient teaching of importance of screening on a community level by:

1. Reinforcing that early detection is associated with decreased mortality.
2. Helping patients and families establish and maintain support networks.
3. Tailoring patient education messages to patients of different cultures.
4. Knowing the resources available and making people aware of them.
   a. National Cancer Institute—answers questions and provides booklets about cancer. Call 800-4-CANCER or go to www.cancer.gov
   b. American Cancer Society—offers many services to patients and their families. Call 800-ACS-2345 for local chapter or go to www.cancer.org.
   c. Susan G. Komen Foundation at www.komen.org.

Ultrasonography

Description

1. Uses high-frequency sound waves to get an image of the breast.
2. Helps determine if a lump is a cyst or a solid mass.
3. May be used if patient is pregnant or is younger than age 35.

Nursing and Patient Care Considerations

1. Advise that this test is painless and noninvasive.
2. No preparation is necessary.

Galactography/Ductogram

1. A contrast mammogram is obtained by injection of water-soluble contrast medium into a duct for patient with persistent bloody nipple discharge. It is a time-consuming procedure that is not routinely used.
2. It may outline an intraductal papilloma.
3. Its ability to differentiate benign from malignant lesions is limited.

Magnetic Resonance Imaging

1. Produces images from the combination of a magnetic field, radio waves, and computer processing.
2. May be used in patients newly diagnosed with breast cancer for presurgical planning. May help in determining the extent of disease, multifocality, and unsuspected disease in the contralateral breast, and after neoadjuvant chemotherapy, may help to downstage a patient and possibly decrease the magnitude of the planned procedure.
3. Useful in high-risk females, those with dense breasts, and in those with silicone implants.
4. Because MRI is less accessible and more expensive than mammography, it is not useful for generalized screening. There may be increased false-positive results.
5. See pages 665 to 666 for a description of MRI.

Other Tests

In addition to laboratory tests and imaging studies, biopsy methods are commonly used to evaluate breast conditions. A biopsy is the only certain way to learn whether a breast lump or suspicious area seen on a mammogram is cancerous.

Fine-Needle Aspiration

Description

1. Uses a thin needle and syringe to collect tissue or to drain lump after using a local anesthetic. If it is a cyst, removing the fluid will collapse it; no other treatment may be needed. Ultrasound may be used to locate a nonpalpable cyst.
2. Normal cyst fluid appears straw colored or greenish. Fluid should be sent for cytology if it appears suspicious (clear or bloody); otherwise, it is discarded.
3. This office procedure uses local anesthetic with results usually within 24 hours.
4. It has limited sensitivity, possibly because of insufficient acquisition of cytologic material.

Nursing and Patient Care Considerations

1. Inform patient of small risk of hematoma and infection.
2. Adhesive bandage applied after procedure; usually no discomfort.
3. Solid lesions may warrant an excisional biopsy.

Needle Biopsy

Description

1. Office procedure uses local anesthetic and removes a small piece of breast tissue using a needle with a special cutting edge.
2. For palpable lesions with a high suspicion of malignancy. May provide a tissue diagnosis quickly—usually approximately 24 hours—without doing an excisional biopsy to plan definitive surgery.
3. Ultrasound guidance may be used for nonpalpable lesions.

Nursing and Patient Care Considerations

1. Inform patient of small risk of hematoma and infection.
2. Tell patient that several passes may be necessary to obtain specimen, with minor discomfort.
3. Pressure dressing applied after procedure.
4. Recommend use of acetaminophen or ibuprofen for postprocedure discomfort—usually minimal, if any.

Stereotactic Core Needle Biopsy

Description

1. An x-ray–guided method for localizing and sampling nonpalpable lesions detected on mammography with 90% to 95% sensitivity in detecting breast cancer.
2. Performed as an outpatient procedure with the patient lying prone on a special table using an automated biopsy gun with

a vacuum system to draw tissue into a sampling chamber and rotate the cutter to excise tissue. There may be a weight limit for this table.
3. After local anesthetic is administered, a needle is placed in the lesion with confirmation of its position on stereotactic x-ray views. Multiple samples are taken from different portions of the lesion. Allows harvesting of larger quantities of tissue with a single needle insertion. A tiny clip may be left in place at the end of the procedure to mark the area.
4. The procedure is quicker and less expensive than mammographically guided needle localization followed by surgical excisional biopsy and is an alternative to surgical excisional biopsy to make a diagnosis.

Nursing and Patient Care Considerations

1. Inform patient that it is a 1-hour outpatient procedure that requires no special preparation.
2. The patient should dress comfortably and will need to remain still during the procedure.
3. Complications may include minor bleeding, hematoma, and infection.
4. Explain that nonspecific, suspicious, or atypical findings may result in proceeding to excisional biopsy.
5. Remind patient that the area in question will not be removed, only sampled.

Note: Many nonpalpable abnormalities that require breast biopsy are being identified because of increased use of screening mammography.

Excisional Biopsy

Description

1. Surgical removal of a palpable or nonpalpable lesion. A frozen section may be done for immediate tissue diagnosis.
2. Excisional biopsy or lumpectomy entails entire removal of a mass; incisional biopsy entails partial removal of a mass.
3. This outpatient procedure may be performed under local or general anesthesia.
4. Curvilinear incision is usually made directly over the mass, which is excised en bloc including a 1-cm grossly free margin of tissue.
5. Tumor ablation with insertion of a probe percutaneously that destroys cancer cells by freezing, heating, or with radiofrequency has been attempted; however, existing evidence is inadequate to recommend ablation as an alternative to surgical excision.

Nursing and Patient Care Considerations

1. Pressure dressing is placed, which can be removed in 24 to 48 hours.
2. Inform patient to watch for bleeding, hematoma, and signs of infection.
3. Recommend analgesics for discomfort and a support bra for comfort.
4. May take several days to get results, a stressful time for patients.

Needle Localization With Biopsy

Description

1. Performed when there is a nonpalpable mammographic finding.
2. Mammogram is used as a guide for placing a needle at the site of the breast change after injecting some local anesthetic.
3. A wire may be left in place for the surgeon, and dye may be injected to mark the site.
4. Excisional biopsy is then done by removing the area around the tip of the wire.

Nursing and Patient Care Considerations

Inform patient that this may be a tedious procedure because patient must remain immobile as the breast is compressed in the mammogram machine or stereotactic table and views are obtained.

Sentinel Lymph Node Biopsy

Description

1. A diagnostic surgical procedure utilizing selective lymph node sampling.
2. Pathologic study of the first (sentinel) axillary lymph node to receive drainage from a tumor; predicts the status of the remainder of the lymph nodes in the axilla.
3. Localization accomplished by injection of a blue dye and/or radioactive particles around a tumor to identify lymph nodes with afferent drainage.
4. The excised sentinel lymph nodes are subjected to routine pathologic examination and, possibly, immunohistochemical staining to detect micrometastasis.
5. The status of the sentinel lymph node is used to determine whether to proceed with full axillary dissection and/or determine treatment modalities.
6. If the sentinel lymph node tests negative, no further axillary surgery is indicated.
7. If the test result is positive, further axillary dissection may be needed. However, in patients undergoing breast-conserving surgery and having fewer than three involved lymph nodes, completion axillary lymph node dissection may be omitted per American Society of Clinical Oncology guidelines with no difference in overall survival.

EVIDENCE BASE Laws, A., Kantor, O., & King, T. A. (2023). Surgical management of the axilla for breast cancer. *Hematology/Oncology Clinics of North America, 37*(1), 51–77. https://doi.org/10.1016/j.hoc.2022.08.005

Nursing and Patient Care Considerations

1. This is a reliable procedure, which is usually performed at the same time as definitive surgery—in conjunction with a breast-preserving procedure or mastectomy.
2. There is less morbidity and cost than with axillary dissection.

GENERAL PROCEDURES AND TREATMENT MODALITIES

Surgery for Breast Cancer

Surgery for breast cancer may involve *mastectomy* or a *breast-preserving procedure*. The objective of breast-preserving procedures is a cosmetically acceptable breast after complete excision of the tumor. Research studies that compare breast conservation with mastectomy have demonstrated equivalent patient survival. Contraindications to breast conservation include multifocal disease; diffuse, extensive ductal carcinoma in situ (DCIS); inability to tolerate radiation therapy; and persistent positive margins. The evolving field of oncoplastic surgery uses

Table 19-1 Types of Surgery for Breast Cancer

PROCEDURE	DESCRIPTION	INDICATIONS
Lumpectomy (excisional biopsy)	Removal of tumor and surrounding tissue	For diagnosis of an abnormal mammographic finding or palpable breast lump if needle biopsy not performed. Further surgery may be needed.
Quadrantectomy (partial mastectomy)	Removal of a breast quadrant that includes the tumor area and possibly overlying skin	Normal- to large-sized breasts. Usually done at the same time as axillary surgery.
Sentinel lymph node biopsy	Removal of only a few gatekeeper lymph nodes	Performed to predict status of lymph nodes—if negative for tumor, axillary dissection is not performed. May be done in conjunction with quadrantectomy or mastectomy.
Axillary dissection	Surgical removal of the axillary lymph nodes	Performed when lymph node is positive for tumor, mainly for prognosis, staging, and locoregional disease control.
Simple mastectomy[a]	Surgical removal of the entire breast	Large or multifocal tumors; females with very small breasts in whom local excision of tumor will be cosmetically unacceptable; ineligibility for radiation therapy; patient preference; prophylaxis.
Modified radical mastectomy[a]	Surgical removal of the entire breast and the axillary lymph nodes (simple mastectomy plus axillary dissection)	Positive lymph nodes; advanced disease.
Radical mastectomy[a]	Removal of entire breast, pectoral muscles, axillary nodes	Rarely done today—may be performed for advanced disease.

[a]*Mastectomy may be followed by immediate or delayed reconstruction.*

techniques to allow the removal of large volumes of breast tissue while avoiding deformity. Although mastectomy rates have remained stable, risk-reducing contralateral prophylactic mastectomy has risen. See Table 19-1 for the surgical approach options that are available. The following discussion covers mastectomy and axillary node dissection.

Preoperative Management

See Chapter 3 for routine preoperative care. In addition:

1. The nature of the procedure is explained, along with expected postoperative care that includes drain care, location of the incision, and mobility of the arm.
2. Information is clarified about diagnosis and possibility of further therapy.
3. Measures are taken to recognize the extreme anxiety and fear that the patient, family, and significant others experience.
   a. Discuss patient's concerns and usual coping mechanisms.
   b. Explore support systems with the patient.
   c. Discuss concerns regarding body image changes.
4. Evaluate the patient's overall medical condition to guide preoperative care, help determine how well the patient will tolerate surgery, and help prepare for complications that may occur postoperatively.

POPULATION AWARENESS Assessment of preoperative mental status of the older patient will help determine if a cognitive change occurs postoperatively.

Potential Complications

1. Infection.
2. Hematoma, seroma.
3. Lymphedema.
4. Paresthesia, pain of axilla and arm.
5. Impaired mobility of arm.

Postoperative Management and Nursing Care

See Chapter 3 for routine postoperative care. In addition:

1. Dressing is removed and the wound is assessed for erythema, hematoma or seroma (fluid under incision), edema, tenderness, odor, and drainage. Report suspected hematoma promptly.
   a. Initial dressing may consist of gauze held in place by elastic, tape, or clear occlusive dressing wrap.
   b. Usually removed within 24 hours.
   c. Incision may remain open to air or elastic wrap may be replaced if patient prefers.
2. Suction drain from wound is maintained.
   a. May have 100 to 200 mL serous to serosanguineous drainage in the first 24 hours.
   b. Report if grossly bloody or excessive in amount.
3. Arm on the affected side is observed for edema, erythema, and pain.
4. Patient teaching about drain care, exercises, and surgical outcome occurs.
5. Breast cancer surveillance of female relatives, especially biological sisters, biological daughters, and biological mother, is discussed.

CLINICAL JUDGMENT Patients who have undergone mastectomy may have an elastic wrap bandage that should fit snugly but not so tightly that it hinders respiration. Assess to make sure the bandage fits comfortably and supports the unaffected breast, and report a bandage that may inhibit deep breaths.

Nursing Interventions

In addition to routine postoperative interventions, provide the following care.

Mobilizing Affected Arm

1. Assess patient's ability to perform self-care and factors impeding performance.
2. Encourage wrist and elbow flexion and extension initially. Encourage use of arm for washing face, combing hair, applying lipstick, and brushing teeth. Encourage patient to gradually increase use of arm.
3. Encourage patient to avoid abduction initially to help prevent seroma formation.
4. Support arm in a sling, if prescribed, to prevent abduction of the arm.
5. Instruct and provide patient with exercises to do when permitted (see Table 19-2).

Increasing Knowledge

1. Explain how wound will gradually change and that the newly healed wound may have less sensation because of severed nerves.
2. Instruct patient on signs of infection, hematoma, or seroma formation to be reported.
3. Teach patient to bathe incision gently and to blot carefully to dry, and later, with approval, massage the healed incision gently with cocoa butter to encourage circulation and increase skin elasticity.
4. Teach care of drains, if appropriate; empty contents, measure, and record.
5. Teach the importance of breast self-examination (BSE), mammograms, and regular follow-up visits.
6. Encourage discussion with health care provider about pregnancy after breast cancer, if indicated.

POPULATION AWARENESS Signs and symptoms of infection may not be obvious in older patients. Assess patients for mental status changes or loss of appetite.

Promoting Lymphatic Drainage

1. Instruct patient on potential problem of lymphedema of the arm, when lymph fluid collects in the arm. At particular risk are patients who undergo axillary node dissection in combination with radiation therapy to axilla. There is a decreased risk when sentinel lymph node biopsy only is performed. Explain that lymphedema may occur years postoperatively. May present as arm heaviness, decreased flexibility, aching, or swelling.
2. Do not take blood pressure, draw blood, inject medications, or start intravenous lines in affected arm. Post sign over the bed.
3. Elevate affected arm on pillows, above the level of heart, and hand above elbow to promote gravity drainage of fluid.
4. Teach patient to massage the affected arm, if prescribed, which will increase circulation and decrease edema. Treatment for severe lymphedema may also include the application of elastic bandages and/or intermittent pneumatic compression. Compressive sleeves and exercises may be recommended to prevent lymphedema.
5. Teach patient care of the affected arm to prevent lymphedema (see Patient Education Guidelines 19-1) and infection.

Table 19-2 Exercises for the Rehabilitation of the Patient Following Mastectomy

EXERCISE	EQUIVALENT DAILY ACTIVITIES
1. Stand. • Lean forward at waist. • Allow arms to hang. • Swing arms from side to side together, then in opposite direction. • Next, swing arms from front to back together, then in opposite direction.	• Broom sweeping • Vacuum cleaning • Mopping floor • Pulling out and pushing in drawers • Weaving • Playing golf
2. Stand facing wall with palms flat against wall, arms extended. • Relax arms and shoulders and allow upper part of body to lean forward against hands. • Push away to original position; repeat.	• Pushing self out of bath tub • Kneading bread • Breaststroke—swimming • Sawing or cutting types of crafts
3. Stand facing wall with palms flat against wall. • Climb the wall with the fingers; descend, repeat.	• Raising windows • Washing windows • Hanging clothes on line • Reaching to an upper shelf
4. Stand and clasp hands at small of back; raise hands; lower; repeat. • Clasp hands back of neck; reach downward; upward; repeat.	• Fastening brassiere • Buttoning blouse or dress • Pulling up a dress zipper • Fastening beads • Washing the back
5. Toss a rope over a sturdy shower or curtain rod. • Hold the ends of the rope (knotted) in each hand and alternately pull on each end. • Using a seesaw motion and with arms outstretched, slide the rope up and down over the rod.	• Drying the back with a bath towel • Raising and lowering a window blind • Closing and opening window drapes
6. Flex and extend each finger in turn.	• Sewing, knitting, crocheting • Typing, painting, playing piano or other musical instrument

PATIENT EDUCATION GUIDELINES 19-1

Prevention of Lymphedema

To reduce the risk of lymphedema of your arm after the removal of lymph nodes, follow these general guidelines to prevent infection and obstruction of blood and lymph fluid.

- Take care of your skin to prevent dryness, cracking, and irritation that may lead to infection.
- Keep your arm clean and cover any open areas.
- Take care of your fingernails to avoid ripped cuticles and nails.
- Avoid using a razor for underarm hair removal.
- Protect hands and fingers from injury while gardening, sewing, cooking, and other chores.
- Avoid constricting clothing around arms.
- Avoid having blood drawn or needles inserted into the affected arm.
- Avoid having blood pressure taken on the affected arm.
- Prevent insect bites and stings through use of repellent and protective clothing.

For more information, refer to American Cancer Society (www.cancer.org).

EVIDENCE BASE Executive Committee of the International Society of Lymphology. (2020). The diagnosis and treatment of peripheral lymphedema: 2020 Consensus Document of the International Society of Lymphology. *Lymphology, 53*(1), 3–19.

Enhancing Body Image

1. Assess mastectomy patient's knowledge of prosthesis and reconstruction options and provide information, as needed.
2. Discuss patient's views on their altered body image and sexuality.
3. Suggest clothing adjustments to camouflage loss of breast.
4. Assist patient to obtain a temporary prosthesis (may be provided by Reach to Recovery [see below]). First prosthesis should be light and soft to allow incision to heal. A heavier type usually may be worn 4 to 8 weeks after surgeon's approval has been secured. Provide information regarding where to obtain permanent prosthesis and bras.
5. Encourage patient to discuss feelings with their partner and explore alternate means of sexual expression.
6. Encourage patient to allow themselves to experience the grief process over the loss of their breast and to learn to cope with these feelings.
7. Assist patient and partner to view the incision when ready.

Reducing Anxiety

1. Familiarize patient with Reach to Recovery (www.cancer.org, then click on Support Programs), an American Cancer Society program that consists of volunteers who have had mastectomies or breast-preserving procedures and who make postoperative hospital visits to provide support and information. Clear first with patient's care provider.
2. Discuss patient's usual coping mechanisms.
3. Encourage and assist family to support patient.
4. Assist patient to maintain control by planning care with them and incorporating their usual routines.
5. Refer patient to postmastectomy support group, as needed and desired.
6. Offer a list of community resources.
7. Remind patient that stress related to breast cancer and mastectomy may persist for a year or more and to seek help.
8. Include family in supportive interventions and measures to increase coping skills.

Facilitating Individual and Family Coping

1. Allow patient and family members to acknowledge their feelings.
2. Approach family with warmth, respect, and support.
3. Acknowledge family strengths.
4. Involve family in care of patient.
5. Discuss stresses on the patient and family.
6. Direct family to community agencies, as indicated.

Community and Home Care Considerations

Because of short stays (1 to 2 days) after mastectomy, many patients can achieve the following benefits from home care:

1. Assess incision and drain tubes for proper healing and no signs of infection.
2. Teach patient drain tube and dressing care.
3. Support patient with adjustment back into home and community.
4. Monitor for lymphedema and reinforce teaching about arm care and exercises.
5. Goals of home care for these patients are to provide assessment of cardiovascular status and to ensure return of energy and proper healing.

CLINICAL JUDGMENT Help identify those patients who may require longer hospitalizations and, possibly, a short stay in a subacute unit for rehabilitation to avoid readmission to the hospital. Factors that may be related to a delay in recovery include increased age, comorbid conditions, reduced nutritional status, infection, limited mobility, and limited support system or lack of presence of a caregiver.

Patient Education and Health Maintenance

1. Advise patient to call surgeon for signs of infection, increased pain, or arm edema.
2. Make sure that patient knows schedule for follow-up with the surgeon.
3. Provide resources for patient for ongoing information and support: The American Cancer Society (800-ACS-2345 or www.cancer.org) has numerous pages of information about surgery, nutrition and cancer, lymphedema, psychosocial issues, and other concerns.
4. Stress the importance of continued yearly mammogram of the unaffected breast.

Evaluation: Expected Outcomes

- Moves affected arm within prescribed limits.
- States care of incision, drains, and follow-up guidelines.
- No infection or swelling in the affected arm.

- Expresses positive body image.
- Exhibits minimal anxiety.
- Maintains a functional support system.

Breast Reconstruction After Mastectomy

Breast reconstruction (mammoplasty) may be performed at the same time as mastectomy (immediate) or as long after surgery as desired (delayed). Benefits include improved psychological coping because of improved body image and self-esteem. Cost is usually covered by insurance. Reconstruction selection is based on an assessment of cancer treatment, patient body type, smoking history, comorbidities, and patient concerns. An advantage of immediate reconstruction is a smaller scar through the use of a skin-sparing mastectomy. Nipple-sparing mastectomy may be an option for some females as well, especially those undergoing prophylactic mastectomy or those with a low nipple involvement rate. It appears to be a safe procedure for properly selected patients. Trials are warranted to determine the best incision and reconstruction methods. Reconstruction does not interfere with the future detection of tumors.

CLINICAL JUDGMENT Because breast reconstruction does not affect disease recurrence or survival, the expectations and desires of the patient are paramount in the decision-making process. Identify patients with questions and fears about the procedure and facilitate open discussion with members of the breast cancer team.

Implants

Indicated for patients with inadequate breast tissue and skin of good quality.

Description

1. Uses prosthetic implants placed in pocket under the skin or pectoralis muscle. A variety of implants are available that contain saline, silicone gel, or a combination of both.
2. If opposite breast is ptotic (protruding downward), mastopexy may be necessary to achieve symmetry.
3. A dermal matrix may be used at surgery to help provide a foundation for the tissue expander and/or implant.
4. Complications include capsular contracture resulting in firmness; may be painful and cause infection.
5. Tissue expanders may be necessary before implants are inserted.
   a. Inflatable envelope is placed under muscle or skin and is filled with saline when incision is healed (about 4 weeks).
   b. Saline is instilled every 1 to 3 weeks until the expander is beyond desired size.
   c. Later, expander is removed and a permanent implant is placed.
   d. Some types of expanders may be left in permanently.
6. Advantages of implant reconstruction over other methods: surgical simplicity, faster postoperative recovery, and lack of complications related to donor site.
7. Disadvantages: difficulties obtaining symmetry to the normal breast; very small risk of anaplastic large cell lymphoma associated with textured implants.

Nursing and Patient Care Considerations

1. Identify patients who smoke and make them aware of increased rates of wound infections and healing complications for all types of reconstruction. Teach signs and symptoms of infection, hematoma, migration, and deflation.
2. Teach patient to massage breast to decrease capsule formation around implant.
3. Teach patient that discomfort may be felt with expanders, if used.

Flap Grafts

Description

1. Transfer of skin, muscle, and subcutaneous tissue from another part of the body to the mastectomy site.
2. Types:
   a. Latissimus dorsi—skin, fat, and muscles of back between shoulder blades—are tunneled under the skin to front of chest. Usually, an implant is also needed.
   b. Transverse rectus abdominis myocutaneous flap—muscle, fat, skin, and blood supply are tunneled to breast area.
   c. Perforator flap reconstruction, that is, deep inferior epigastric perforator (DIEP) or superior gluteal artery perforator (SGAP), uses tissue as above without using muscle. Because of its complexity, offered by few breast centers.
3. Disadvantages include cost, slow process (done in stages), and increased morbidity.
4. Complications include flap loss, hematoma, infection, seroma, and abdominal hernia.

Nursing and Patient Care Considerations

1. Assess flap and donor site for color, temperature, and wound drainage.
2. Control pain.
3. Provide support with a bra or abdominal binder to maintain position of prosthesis.
4. Teach patient to perform BSE monthly and that some asymmetry may be present.

Nipple–Areolar Reconstruction

1. Usually done at a separate time from breast reconstruction.
2. Uses skin and fat from reconstructed breast for nipple and upper thigh for areola; tanning or tattoo done to obtain appropriate color.

Other Surgeries of the Breast

Reduction mammoplasty may be done for cosmetic purposes or to relieve uncomfortable symptoms. Augmentation mammoplasty is considered a cosmetic procedure.

Reduction Mammoplasty

Description

1. Removal of excess breast tissue, which also involves a reduction in skin and possible transposition of nipple–areolar complex.
2. Used for alleviation of symptoms that may include back and neck pain, muscle spasm, and grooving at the shoulders secondary to bra straps.
3. Complications include hematoma, infection, necrosis of skin flap, and nipple inversion.

Nursing and Patient Care Considerations

1. Explore reasons patient may desire surgery.
2. Discuss postoperative expectations with patient.
3. Nursing interventions are similar to those in patient undergoing reconstruction.

Augmentation Mammoplasty

Description

1. Enlarging of the breasts with the use of implants.
2. Implants may be made of silicone or saline. In most cases, this is a self-pay procedure if for cosmetic purpose.

3. Complications include hematoma, wound infection, diminished sensation of the nipple, and capsular contracture, resulting in firmness of the breast.
4. Breast implants are not associated with an increased incidence of breast cancer.

Nursing and Patient Care Considerations

1. Discuss patient's expectations preoperatively.
2. Nursing interventions are similar to those in the patient undergoing reconstruction with implants.

DISORDERS OF THE BREAST

See additional online content: Patient Education Guidelines 19-2.

See Standard of Care Guidelines 19-1, page 671.

STANDARD OF CARE GUIDELINES 19-1

Problems of the Breast

When caring for any patient undergoing evaluation, diagnostic testing, treatment, or counseling for a breast-related problem, ensure optimal outcome by adhering to the following guidelines:

- Explain the mammogram procedure or other diagnostic test and make sure patient knows when and how results will be obtained.
- Perform breast examination according to American Cancer Society guidelines.
- Inform health care provider and patient of any suspicious findings on breast examination—asymmetry of breasts, dimpling, skin changes, nipple discharge, fixed or hard mass.
- Inform health care provider and patient of abnormal mammogram or other test result and make sure that follow-up is arranged.

AFTER SURGERY FOR BREAST CANCER

- Assess for evidence of bleeding from the incision or flaps, including increase in pain, and notify surgeon promptly for increased pain or bleeding.
- Assess drainage from suction drain for amount, color, and odor. Report if grossly bloody, purulent, or excessive in amount (may have 100 to 200 mL in the first 24 hours).
- Assess newly reconstructed breast flaps for viability by color, warmth, and wound drainage. Notify surgeon promptly for increased warmth, change in color, purulent or excessive drainage.
- Maintain proper protective positioning (avoid abduction to prevent edema) of arm and follow precautions for lymphedema.
- Assess patient's emotional response and provide support throughout the diagnostic and treatment process.

This information should serve as a general guideline only. Each patient situation presents a unique set of clinical factors and requires nursing judgment to guide care, which may include additional or alternative measures and approaches.

Fissure of the Nipple

A *fissure* is a type of ulcer that develops in the nipple of a nursing person.

Etiology and Clinical Manifestations

1. May be caused by lack of preparation of nipples in the prenatal period.
2. Condition aggravated by sucking infant.
3. Nipple appears sore and irritated.
4. Nipple bleeds.
5. Infection may result.

Management and Nursing Interventions

1. Wash nipples with sterile saline solution.
2. Use artificial nipple for nursing.
3. If above does not initiate healing process, stop nursing and use breast pump.
4. Teach proper breastfeeding techniques to prevent fissures.
   a. Wash, dry, and lubricate nipples in prenatal period in preparation for nursing.
   b. Make sure infant's mouth covers areola.
   c. Keep nipple clean by washing and drying after each nursing period.
   d. Use lanolin cream to prevent cracking; must remove before breastfeeding.

Nipple Discharge

Nipple discharge may be serous, serosanguineous, bloody, purulent, or multicolored. It is commonly associated with benign conditions; rarely, malignancy is responsible. It may be spontaneous or nonspontaneous (occurs only when breast is compressed), and it is important to differentiate between the two.

Etiology and Clinical Manifestations

1. Galactorrhea—bilateral, nonspontaneous, multiple ducts, milky gray or green discharge usually seen in patients in child-bearing years.
   a. Commonly seen after pregnancy and can last for 1 to 2 years.
   b. May also be secondary to excessive breast manipulation, increased production of prolactin, medication, an endocrine anovulatory syndrome, or pituitary adenoma.
2. Mastitis—usually unilateral, purulent (see below).
3. Discharge containing blood—usually caused by intraductal papilloma (wart) or other benign lesion but, in rare cases, may be malignant.

Diagnostic Evaluation

1. Evaluate a spontaneous nipple discharge with clinical examination, test for occult blood, mammography, and/or ultrasonography. MRI is not usually helpful.
   a. Use of a Hemoccult card gently pressed against the nipple when expressing discharge will help determine if the discharge is bloody, which warrants further workup.
   b. May get prolactin level; if elevated, may indicate pituitary adenoma.
2. Nonspontaneous milky gray or green discharge generally is not of pathologic significance and may not require workup.

Management and Nursing Interventions

1. Nursing interventions are aimed at alleviating anxiety and providing support to patient undergoing diagnostic testing. Reassure patient that nipple discharge rarely indicates cancer.
2. Bromocriptine may be given to suppress galactorrhea.
3. Treat for mastitis if purulent (see below).
4. Surgery may be indicated to treat cause of bloody and some other discharges caused by breast lesions.
   a. Most commonly because of wartlike intraductal papilloma in one of larger collecting ducts at edge of areola. May be secondary to fibrocystic changes or duct ectasia.
   b. Excisional biopsy and histologic examination may be done to rule out cancer.
   c. Ductoscopy, an image-guided excision using direct visualization of the ductal system and an intraductal biopsy, is being investigated at some larger centers.
5. Pituitary surgery for excision of adenoma (see page 709).

Acute Mastitis

Acute mastitis is inflammation of the breast secondary to infection. Breast infections may be lactational or nonlactational.

Pathophysiology and Etiology

1. Lactational infections usually occur at beginning of lactation in first-time, breastfeeding parent. May also occur later in chronic lactation mastitis and central duct abscesses.
2. Milk stasis may lead to obstruction, followed by noninfectious inflammation, then infectious mastitis.
3. Source of infection may be from hands of patient, personnel caring for patient, baby's nose or throat, or blood-borne.
4. Nonlactational infections usually present with central subareolar inflammation.
5. Most common pathogens: *Staphylococcus aureus*, *Escherichia coli*, and *Streptococcus*.

Clinical Manifestations

1. Redness, warmth, edema; breast may feel doughy and tough. Fever may be present.
2. Patient may complain of dull pain in affected area and may have nipple discharge.
3. Complication is mammary abscess (see below).

Management and Nursing Interventions

1. Diagnosis is usually made by characteristic manifestations.
2. Oral antibiotics are given—10- to 14-day course.
   a. Cephalexin—250 to 500 mg every 6 hours.
   b. Clindamycin—150 to 300 mg every 6 hours.
   c. Amoxicillin clavulanate—500 mg/125 mg three times daily or 875 mg/125 mg twice daily.
   d. Sulfamethoxazole/trimethoprim—800 mg/160 mg two times daily or doxycycline 100 mg two times daily recommended if penicillin resistance suspected.
3. May have patient stop breastfeeding (controversial).
4. Apply heat to resolve tissue reaction; may cause increased milk production and worsen symptoms.
5. May apply cold to decrease tissue metabolism and milk production.
6. Have the patient wear firm breast support.
7. Encourage the breastfeeding patient to practice meticulous personal hygiene to prevent mastitis.
8. Consider lactation consult.

Mammary Abscess

Mammary abscess is a localized collection of pus in a cavity of breast tissue. About 3% of patients with mastitis may develop a breast abscess.

Etiology and Clinical Manifestations

1. May follow acute mastitis if untreated. Some patients may develop a chronic subareolar abscess thought to be caused by a plugging of major mammary ducts in the nipple with infection of obstructed secretions. This usually occurs in patients who smoke.
2. Patient may have fever, chills, and malaise.
3. Affected area is sensitive and erythematous; may have palpable mass.
4. Pus may be expressed from nipple.

Management and Nursing Interventions

1. May perform needle aspiration if superficial mass.
2. Incision and drainage may be done, if deep.
3. A biopsy of the cavity wall may be done at time of incision and drainage to rule out breast carcinoma associated with abscess.
4. Administer antibiotics and analgesics, if ordered.
5. Apply hot, wet dressings to increase drainage and hasten resolution. Pack wound, as directed.
6. A diagnostic mammogram and sonogram may be ordered after resolution of the abscess to rule out cancer.

Fibrocystic Change/Breast Pain

Fibrocystic change is a general term that includes various changes in the breast, namely, fibrosis and cystic dilation of the ducts. May be present in up to 50% of females.

Pathophysiology and Etiology

1. Pathogenesis is not known but is related to the cyclic stimulation of the breast by estrogen and represents a change from the normal stimulation and regression pattern of this process.
2. Occurs usually in females between ages 35 and 50 and is a source of considerable discomfort in a sizable percentage of those affected.
3. Hormone replacement therapy (HRT) may be associated with fibrocystic changes in a female who has never experienced this previously.

Clinical Manifestations

1. Increased generalized breast lumpiness or excessive nodularity with tenderness, pain, and breast swelling. Symptoms may decrease after menses.
2. Lumps or cysts—soft or firm; single or multiple; smooth, round, and movable. Cysts may enlarge and become tender and painful. There may be many cysts of different sizes; some may be palpable.
3. Possible nipple discharge—may be milky, yellow, or greenish.

Diagnostic Evaluation

1. Physical examination detects changes.
2. Mammography or ultrasound.

3. Aspiration—if a palpable, symptomatic mass exists or the cyst is complex.
4. Cytology of cyst fluid is not cost-effective and rarely of clinical value in fibrocystic breast changes.

Management

There is no satisfactory treatment, and management is usually geared toward relief of symptoms.

Surgical Management

1. Needle aspiration and conservative medical follow-up if:
   a. The aspirate appears like normal cyst fluid and is not blood stained.
   b. Cyst completely resolves after aspiration.
   c. No indication of an underlying neoplasm.
2. Surgical excision—indicated if a cyst keeps recurring after several aspirations or if a single solid discrete lump is present.

Medical Management

1. Sporadic discomfort may be relieved by over-the-counter (OTC) analgesics, including topical nonsteroidal anti-inflammatory drugs such as diclofenac topical gel.
2. Evening primrose oil seems to be helpful in mastalgia management.
3. Supportive garments (e.g., support bra) tend to reduce mastalgia.
4. Warm compresses or ice packs could offer some relief.
5. Contraceptives or supplemental progestins during the secretory phase of the menstrual cycle may help with pain control.
   a. Mastalgia that begins after initiating hormonal contraceptive pills may resolve after a few cycles.
   b. Switching to a lower estrogen/higher progesterone ratio may help.

Other Measures

1. Diet modifications.
   a. Eliminating caffeine (coffee, tea, cola drinks, and chocolate) from the diet may help reduce symptoms.
   b. Decreasing fat intake may improve swelling, tenderness, and nodularity.
2. Stopping tobacco use has been suggested to relieve symptoms.
3. Prophylactic lumpectomy—rarely indicated for intractable pain not relieved with medical therapy in females with multiple previous biopsies or biopsy evidence of a precancerous lesion.

Nursing Interventions and Patient Teaching

1. Suggest monthly BSE if the patient is interested—cysts may mask underlying cancer.
2. Reinforce patient's confidence in breast self-examination (BSE) by rechecking their findings.
3. Offer suggestions for alternative methods if BSE is difficult to do (i.e., tender breasts).
4. Encourage patient to see health care provider regularly for examinations.
5. Recommend that patient wear a well-fitted support bra.
6. Offer emotional support for their anxiety and fear of cancer.
7. Reassure that discomfort is common and that it is rarely the only presenting sign of cancer.

Benign Tumors of the Breast

Benign tumors of the breast are characterized clinically as benign lesions that are distinct and persistent over time. Approximately 90% of breast lumps are benign.

Pathophysiology and Etiology

1. Fibrocystic changes—solid lumps may be fatty or fibrous tissue or fluid-filled cysts (see above).
2. Galactocele—a milk-filled cyst.
3. Fibroadenoma—a benign breast tumor composed of epithelial and stromal components.
   a. Common in young females.
   b. A slight increase in the risk of breast cancer among females with fibroadenomas.
4. Other benign tumors include adenosis, intraductal papillomas, lipomas, and neurofibromatosis that may produce a palpable mass.

Clinical Manifestations

1. Gross cysts—may be tender or nontender. Consistency depends on pressure of fluid within cyst and breast tissue around them; may be soft and fluctuant or may feel like a solid tumor if dense.
2. Galactocele—firm, nontender mass.
3. Fibroadenoma—may be a firm, smooth, movable lump that is usually painless. Size does not usually fluctuate with menstrual cycle changes but tends to enlarge over time.

Diagnostic Evaluation

1. Physical examination, mammography, and ultrasound identify and characterize lesion.
2. Cyst aspiration—diagnostic aspiration is usually curative in a galactocele or breast cyst.
3. If a lump does not respond to cyst aspiration, excisional biopsy remains the "gold standard" to rule out cancer.

Management and Nursing Interventions

1. Nonsuspicious or indeterminate masses in young females may be observed through one or two menstrual cycles for resolution of the mass.
2. In general, any distinct and persistent solid lump should have biopsy and possibly excision.
3. Nursing care is directed toward support as patient goes through diagnostic process.

Disorders of the Male Breast

Disorders of the male breast include gynecomastia (benign) and malignant breast cancer.

Clinical Features

Gynecomastia

1. Overdevelopment of breast tissue, usually bilateral.
2. Common in infants, adolescents, and males older than age 50.
3. Usually results from hormonal alterations—idiopathic systemic disorders, such as endocrine disorders, disease of the liver, pituitary adenoma, and chronic renal failure; such drugs as cimetidine, thiazides, spironolactone, omeprazole, phenytoin, reserpine, nifedipine, and theophylline; such neoplasms as testicular tumors and in association with lung and prostate cancer (may be related to therapy).
4. Pubertal gynecomastia has an onset in males ages 10 to 12 and generally regresses within 18 months. Need to rule out illicit

drugs in teens. Marijuana, alcohol, amphetamines, heroin, LSD, and methadone can cause gynecomastia.
5. Asymptomatic and pubertal gynecomastia does not require further tests but should be reevaluated in 6 months. There is no evidence that links gynecomastia with male breast cancer.
6. Investigation is warranted if the drugs used by the patient do not explain the gynecomastia and the breast is tender or the diameter of the breast tissue is more than 4 cm.
7. Reduction subcutaneous nipple-sparring mammoplasty is considered for patients with long-standing gynecomastia for cosmetic and accompanying psychosocial reasons.

POPULATION AWARENESS Ask teenagers and young adults with gynecomastia if they use alcohol and/or illicit drugs.

Breast Cancer

1. Resembles cancer of the breast in females.
2. Less than 1% of all breast cancers—incidence greatest in males in their 60s.
3. Carries poor prognosis because males may delay seeking treatment until disease is advanced.
4. Risk factors: family history (20% of males with breast cancer have a first-degree relative with the disease), estrogen exposure, occupation, and some genetic syndromes, such as Cowden and Klinefelter. Males chronically exposed to hot environments, such as steel mills, have been shown to be at increased risk as well those employed in the soap and perfume industry and those exposed to petroleum and exhaust fumes.
5. There are no specific screening recommendations for males.
6. Nursing care and treatment is essentially the same as for postmenopausal female breast cancer, including tamoxifen, chemotherapy, and/or radiation therapy.

Cancer of the Breast

Breast cancer is the most commonly diagnosed cancer among females in the United States, excluding nonmelanoma of the skin. It is the second leading cause of cancer death among females overall, after lung cancer, but it is the leading cause of cancer death among Black and Hispanic females.

EVIDENCE BASE Siegel, R. L., Miller, K. D., Wagle, N. S., & Jemal, A. (2023). Cancer statistics, 2023. *CA: A Cancer Journal for Clinicians, 73*(1), 17–48. https://doi.org/10.3322/caac.21763

Pathophysiology and Etiology

1. Most breast cancer (85% to 90%) begins in the lining of the milk ducts, sometimes in the lobule. Eventually, it grows through the wall of the duct and into the fatty tissue (see Table 19-3 for types of breast cancer).
2. Family history accounts for approximately 7% of all breast cancers.
   a. Current genetic models attribute 5% to 10% of all breast cancers to dominantly inherited breast cancer susceptibility genes. Several breast/ovarian susceptibility genes have been identified: presence of mutations in *BRCA1* and *BRCA2* as well as, less often, in *PALPB2* gene could increase patient's risk of developing breast or ovarian cancer. Females of Ashkenazi Jewish descent have an increased likelihood of *BRCA* mutations.
   b. Some hereditary breast cancers are due to other rare hereditary syndromes, such as Li-Fraumeni (associated pathogenic variants in the tumor protein p53 [TP53]) and

Table 19-3 Types of Breast Cancer

CELL TYPE	DESCRIPTION	INCIDENCE[a]	COMMENTS
In situ			
DCIS	Abnormal cells in duct	28% frequently found in combination with invasive cancer	A noninvasive breast cancer; the majority found by mammogram
Invasive			
Ductal	Classified on basis of microscopic appearance as ductal or lobular	85%–90%	Characterized by stony hardness on palpation
Lobular	As above	5%–10%	Relatively uncommon; tends to be more infiltrative
Others			
Tubular medullary mucinous papillary sarcoma	Types frequently associated with above; cell type must dominate to be assigned	<10% of all breast cancers	Axillary metastasis uncommon in tubular; medullary associated with fast growth rate and favorable prognosis
Inflammatory	Applies to distinctive inflamed appearance of skin; no consistent histologic type	1%–4%	Presents with erythema, warmth, tenderness, and edema; may be treated with chemotherapy or radiation therapy first
Paget disease of nipple	Usually associated with underlying intraductal or invasive carcinoma	2%	Presents as scaly, erythematous, periareolar eruption

DCIS, ductal carcinoma in situ.
[a]Percentage greater than 100—infiltrating carcinoma frequently includes small areas containing other special types or a combination of in situ and infiltrating carcinoma is seen.

Cowden syndromes (associated with pathogenic mutation in tumor suppressor [PTEN]).

c. Genetic testing may be performed on those patients with an increased likelihood of breast and ovarian cancer based on personal and family history. The National Comprehensive Cancer Network (NCCN) has outlined criteria for this testing. See their guidelines at nccn.org/guidelines/category_2.

3. Knowledge of a mutation can help patients make informed decisions to manage their risk for future breast cancers. It is important to have genetic counseling before the test because of its implications. Screening is not warranted for general population.
4. Present knowledge does not indicate that carcinogens play an important role in the development of breast cancer.

Epidemiology of Breast Cancer

EVIDENCE BASE Giaquinto, A. N., Sung, H., Miller, K. D., Kramer, J. L., Newman, L. A., Minihan, A., Jemal, A., & Siegel, R. L. (2022). Breast cancer statistic, 2022. *CA: A Cancer Journal for Clinicians, 72*(6), 524–541. https://doi.org/10.3322/caac.21754

Incidence

Each year in the United States, about 264,000 cases of breast cancer are diagnosed in females and about 2,400 in males. About 42,000 females and 500 males in the United States die each year from breast cancer. Black females have a higher rate of death from breast cancer than White females. In 2022, it was estimated that approximately 287,850 new cases of invasive breast cancer would be diagnosed.

Survival Rates

1. Five-year overall survival rates:
   Localized: 97%.
   Regional: 78.7%.
   Distant: 23.3%.
2. In the general population, the relative survival rate is lower among Black females than White females. Black females are more likely than White females to be diagnosed with large tumors and distant-stage disease. Similarly, Black males are more likely than White males to be diagnosed with large tumors and distant-stage disease.
3. Lymph node status is the most important prognostic indicator of disease-free survival.
4. Age, comorbidity, staging (tumor size, lymph node status, and distant metastasis), nuclear grade, histologic differentiation, possibly HER2 status, and treatment are important prognostic factors for survival (see Table 19-4). These factors can be used to estimate overall 10-year survival.
5. There has been a decline in the death rate in the United States from breast cancer. This may be related to:
   a. Change in lifestyle such as diet.
   b. Early diagnosis—increased use and improvement in screening mammography.
   c. Improved treatment.

Risk Factors

A female's lifetime risk of developing breast cancer is 12.5% based on a life span of 80 years.

1. Major—being a person assigned female at birth, increasing age, having a diagnosis of lobular carcinoma in situ, having a prior history of breast or ovarian cancer, and having a family history (especially biological mother, sisters). Approximately a twofold risk in females with affected biological sister or biological mother; this increases if more relatives were affected or if affected close relatives developed breast cancer before menopause.
2. Probable—nulliparity, older age at first live childbirth, late menopause, early menarche, benign proliferative breast disease, diagnosis of atypical ductal or lobular hyperplasia on biopsy, long-term use of estrogen replacement therapy that increases with duration of use, and previous exposure to chest wall irradiation.
3. Controversial—hormonal contraceptive use (estrogen and progestin may stimulate tumor growth with long-term use), multiple breast biopsies, decreased physical activity, alcohol use, obesity, and increased dietary fat intake.
4. Results of breast cancer prevention trials have shown a reduction in incidence of breast cancer in high-risk females treated with tamoxifen, exemestane, or raloxifene.

Table 19-4 Staging of Breast Cancer

STAGE	DESCRIPTION
0	Carcinoma in situ.
I	Tumor ≤2 cm in greatest dimension; no axillary lymph node metastasis other than micrometastasis; no evidence of distant metastasis.
II	Tumor <2 cm in greatest dimension but with one to three positive lymph nodes, a tumor 2–5 cm with or without axillary lymph node metastasis, or a tumor >5 cm without spread to lymph nodes; no evidence of distant metastasis.
III	Any size tumor with four or more positive axillary lymph nodes or with direct extension to the chest wall or skin; inflammatory breast cancer; no evidence of distant metastasis.
IV	Any of the above plus distant metastasis (i.e., liver, lungs, bone, brain).

POPULATION AWARENESS Age is the greatest single risk factor for the development of cancer. Cancer warning signals may be unheeded in older females, so thorough history-taking and physical examination are essential.

Clinical Manifestations

See Figure 19-1.

1. A firm lump or thickening in breast, usually painless; 50% located in upper outer quadrant of breast. Enlargement of axillary or supraclavicular lymph nodes may indicate metastasis.
2. Nipple discharge—spontaneous, may be bloody, clear, or serous.
3. Breast asymmetry—a change in the size or shape of the breast or abnormal contours. As female changes positions, compare one breast to other.
4. Nipple retraction or scaliness, especially in Paget disease.
5. Late signs—pain, ulceration, edema, orange-peel skin (peau d'orange) from interference of lymphatic drainage.
6. Inflammatory breast cancer may present with erythema.

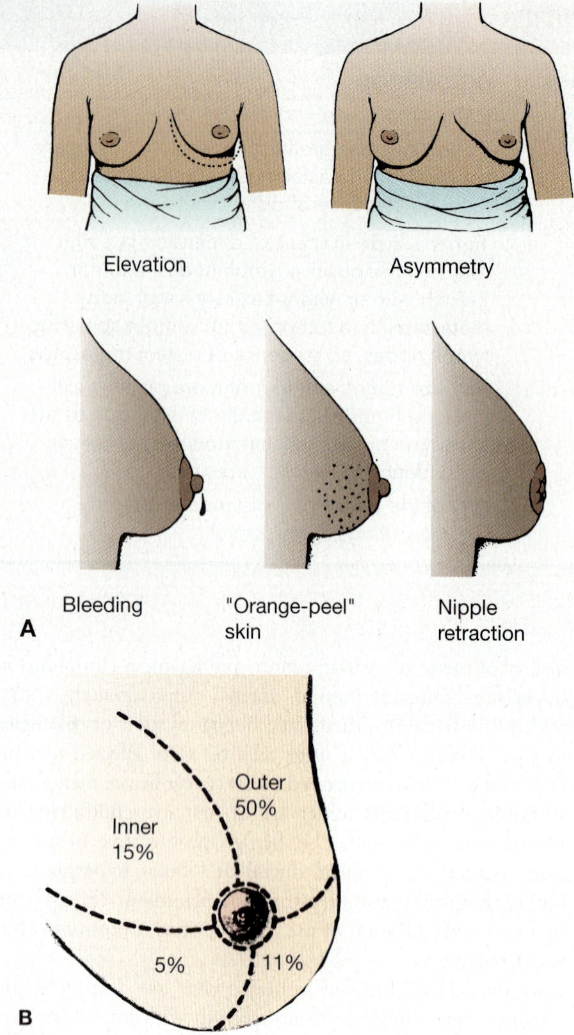

Figure 19-1. (A) Signs of cancer of the breast. (B) Distribution of carcinomas in different areas of the breast.

7. Many small invasive breast cancers as well as noninvasive breast cancer (ductal carcinoma in situ [DCIS]) do not present with a palpable mass but are found on mammography.

CLINICAL JUDGMENT Be aware that pain is not usually an early warning sign of breast cancer. Remain alert for other signs, such as those listed earlier.

Diagnostic Evaluation

See page 671.

Management

Based on type and stage of breast cancer, receptors, and menopausal status. For females with localized invasive breast cancer, information from clinical trials indicates that treatment with a breast-preserving procedure has similar survival rates as mastectomy. Surgery for DCIS (noninvasive breast cancer) may involve only a lumpectomy, but mastectomy may be necessary for extensive disease. Treatment for DCIS is becoming more and more controversial with concern by some that this entity is being overtreated.

Surgery

See page 666 for a discussion of surgery for breast cancer.

Radiation Therapy

1. In conjunction with breast-preserving procedure as adjuvant (additional) therapy to decrease incidence of local recurrence for invasive breast cancer and DCIS. In the patient with DCIS, if it is thought that the individual risk is low, some patients may be treated by excision alone. May be used preoperatively to shrink a large tumor to operable size.
2. May be used after a mastectomy in patients with large tumors that involve the chest wall and/or many positive axillary lymph nodes; may delay reconstruction.
3. Absolute contraindications to a breast-preserving procedure include widespread disease, diffuse malignant-appearing microcalcifications on mammography, radiation therapy during pregnancy, and positive margins. Relative contraindications include active connective tissue disease, tumors greater than 5 cm in size, positive genetic mutation linked to increased risk of breast cancer, and history of previous radiation therapy to the breast or chest wall.
4. Treatment may be individualized in pregnancy—that is, appropriate surgery followed by chemotherapy in the second or third trimester and delayed irradiation to preserve the breast.
5. May also be used to alleviate bone pain in metastatic breast cancer.
6. Radiation directed to breast, chest wall, and remaining lymph nodes.
   a. Usually five treatments per week for 6 or 7 weeks.
   b. A booster or second phase of treatment may be given.
   c. May include implants of radioactive material after external treatment completed.
   d. Proton beam radiation reduces the dose of radiation to normal tissues by allowing for more precise dose delivery. This therapy could be recommended in some cases, especially if left breast irradiation is planned, in order to minimize cardiac muscle exposure to radiation. Adverse effects include mild fatigue, sore throat, dry cough, nausea, and anorexia; later, skin will look and feel sunburned. Eventually, the breast may become firmer. Complications include increased arm edema, decreased arm mobility, pneumonitis, and brachial nerve damage. See page 669 for care of patient undergoing radiation therapy.
7. Partial breast irradiation may be performed only as part of a prospective trial. (Whole breast radiotherapy remains the gold standard).
   a. Accelerated partial breast irradiation through a balloon temporarily surgically implanted in the breast treats only the lumpectomy bed. Treatment is twice per day for 5 days. Early data suggest acceptable locoregional disease control with this approach; however, long-term follow-up studies are needed.
   b. A one-time dose of radiation intraoperatively is also under investigation and shows promise.

Chemotherapy

1. Major use is in adjuvant systemic treatment postoperatively; usually begins 6 to 8 weeks after surgery (stressful for patient who just finished major surgery).
2. In some cases, presurgical (neoadjuvant) chemotherapy could be indicated. For those patients, breast surgery generally is scheduled 4 to 6 weeks after final chemotherapy treatment.

3. Treatments are given every 2 to 4 weeks for 5 to 6 months. Because the drugs differ in their mechanisms of action, combinations of agents are used to treat cancer.
4. Main chemotherapy agents used for breast cancer include doxorubicin, cyclophosphamide, paclitaxel, docetaxel, and carboplatin. For advanced cancer, docetaxel, vinorelbine, capecitabine, gemcitabine, eribulin, and sacituzumab are used (also see Table 4-3 on page 79).
5. Indications for chemotherapy include:
   a. Large tumors, positive lymph nodes, premenopausal females, and poor prognostic factors. Currently, adjuvant chemotherapy and/or hormonal therapy are recommended for all patients with invasive breast cancers 1 cm wide or larger although the benefit in some patients may be relatively small.
   b. Patients who score high on gene assay as well as those tumors that are shown to be "triple negative"—ER/PR as well as HER2 negative.
   c. Data are insufficient to make definitive recommendations for patients older than 80 years.
6. Other agents that may be used include:
   a. Trastuzumab—a member of the epithelial growth receptor family; increased survival when added to chemotherapy in early-stage and well as metastatic breast cancer in patients whose cancer expresses the gene HER2.
   b. Pertuzumab—another monoclonal antibody used always in conjunction with trastuzumab. It could be used prior to surgery (neoadjuvant) in patients with early-stage, locally advanced, or metastatic HER2-positive breast cancer.
   c. Trastuzumab emtansine–antibody drug conjugate consisting of trastuzumab linked with cytotoxic agent. Used as an adjuvant treatment in patients who received trastuzumab-based neoadjuvant therapy and were found to have residual disease at the time of the surgery. It is also used in patients with metastatic HER2-positive breast cancer.
   d. Fam-trastuzumab-deruxtecan-nxki—another antibody drug conjugate containing trastuzumab linked to topoisomerase I inhibitor. It is used in the treatment of patients with metastatic HER2-positive as well as low HER2-positive breast cancers.
   e. Pamidronate zoledronic acid or denosumab may be added if bone metastasis is present to help reduce pain. Patients should undergo dental exam prior to initiation of this therapy for preventive maintenance and to correct dental problems, as osteonecrosis of the jaw is more common in those who have undergone invasive dental procedures. Use of these agents could be associated with hypocalcemia. Calcium and vitamin D supplementation is recommended for the patient undergoing therapy with those agents.
   f. Poly ADP ribose polymerase inhibitors, such as olaparib, are targetive agents that help repair DNA and may be helpful in triple-negative, BRCA-positive cancers.
7. Adverse effects include bone marrow suppression, cardiotoxicity, nausea and vomiting, diarrhea, alopecia, weight gain or loss, fatigue, stomatitis, anxiety, depression, and premature menopause (see page 78 for nursing care of patient undergoing chemotherapy). Risk of cardiomyopathy could be associated with anti-HER2 agents.
8. Chemotherapy may also be used as primary treatment in inflammatory breast cancer and occasionally in large tumors.
9. Hope for the future is the development of specific targeted biologic therapies and more individualized treatment.

Endocrine Therapy

1. Selective estrogen receptor modulators, such as tamoxifen and raloxifene, bind estrogen receptors, thereby blocking effects of estrogen.
   a. Adjuvant systemic therapy after surgery.
   b. Benefits patients who are estrogen receptor (ER)–positive, regardless of menopausal status.
   c. Given for at least 5 years; oral administration once or twice per day. Extended use, up to 10 years, may be recommended in some patients.
   d. Adverse effects include hot flashes, irregular periods, vaginal irritation, nausea and vomiting, headaches, increased risk of endometrial cancer, and thromboembolic events.
   e. Females on tamoxifen should have an annual gynecologic assessment if uterus present.
2. Aromatase inhibitors, such as anastrozole, exemestane, and letrozole, block conversion of androgen, which is secreted by the adrenal glands, into estrogen. Large clinical trials report more favorable outcomes with aromatase inhibitors, and treatment has shifted from 5 years of tamoxifen therapy to initial treatment with an aromatase inhibitor in postmenopausal females.
   a. Aromatase inhibitors as well as fulvestrant, an estrogen receptor agonist, may be used as a second-line therapy after tamoxifen in patients whose cancer has returned or progressed.
   b. Aromatase inhibitors are ineffective in premenopausal females and should be administered in conjunction with ovarian suppression.
   c. Adverse effects include hot flashes, vaginal dryness, musculoskeletal symptoms, osteoporosis, and increased rate of bone fracture. Therefore, females on aromatase inhibitors should have monitoring of bone health.

DRUG ALERT Traditionally, breast cancer survivors have not been considered candidates for vaginal estrogen. However, debates and studies continue to be conducted regarding the safety of vaginal estrogen in this population.

Bone Marrow Transplant

1. Autologous method after high-dose chemotherapy.
2. Clinical trials have shown it to be ineffective for breast cancer.

Oophorectomy

Removal of ovaries.

1. Treatment for recurrent or metastatic disease in estrogen receptor–positive premenopausal females.
2. Deprives tumor of primary estrogen source—remissions of 3 months to several years.
3. Pharmacologic ablation with goserelin or leuprolide has been compared to surgical oophorectomy in estrogen receptor–positive postmenopausal females, and response rates are similar.
4. Surgical ablation is now considered second choice because of its increased risks.

Complications

1. Metastasis—most common sites: lymph nodes, lung, bone, liver, and brain.
2. Signs and symptoms of metastasis may include bone pain, neurologic changes, weight loss, anemia, cough, shortness of breath, pleuritic pain, and vague chest discomfort.

Nursing Assessment

1. Assess general health status and underlying chronic illnesses that may have an impact on patient's response to treatment.
2. Identify what the patient and family need to know regarding breast cancer and its treatment, and take measures to decrease their impact. Base education on patient and family needs.
3. Determine the level of anxiety, fears, and concerns.
4. Identify coping ability and availability of support systems.

Nursing Interventions

Reducing Anxiety

1. Realize that diagnosis of breast cancer is a devastating emotional shock to patient. Support patient through the diagnostic process. Many females must make challenging decisions in a brief period of time. Some communities have developed nursing navigators as a way of assisting and supporting individuals through the process. Check if there is a nurse navigator in your community.
2. Provide the results of each test in language patient can understand.
3. Stress the advances made in earlier diagnosis and treatment options.
4. Facilitate referral for psychological evaluation or counseling if the patient experiences prolonged anxiety or depression.

Providing Information about Treatment

1. Involve patient in treatment planning.
2. Describe surgical procedures.
3. Prepare patient for the effects of chemotherapy; encourage patient to plan ahead for the common adverse effects of chemotherapy.
4. Educate patient about the effects of radiation therapy.
5. Teach patient about hormonal therapy. Patient may develop hot flashes with the start of hormonal therapy or with the discontinuation of HRT at the time of diagnosis of breast cancer (see Chapter 18 for information on menopausal symptoms). Measures that may help with symptoms of hot flashes include:
   a. Mediations such as gabapentin, antidepressants such as venlafaxine, and oxybutynin.
   b. Nutritional supplements and herbs have been used but have not been rigorously tested.
   c. Studies suggest that exercise routine may help to reduce hot flashes.

Strengthening Coping

1. Repeat information and speak in calm, clear manner.
2. Display empathy and acceptance of patient's emotions.
3. Explore coping mechanisms.
4. Evaluate where patient is in stages of acceptance.
5. Help patient identify and use support persons.
6. Arrange visit from support group member.
7. Refer for counseling, financial aid, and so forth.
8. Resources include American Cancer Society (800-ACS-2345 or www.cancer.org), National Cancer Institute (www.cancer.gov), National Alliance of Breast Cancer Organizations (www.nabco.org), and the Susan G. Komen Breast Cancer Foundation (www.komen.org).

Patient Education and Health Maintenance

1. Encourage patient to continue close follow-up and to report any new symptoms. Most females will be seen every 3 months for the first 2 years, every 6 months for the next 3 years, and once per year after 5 years.
2. Stress importance of continued yearly mammogram.
3. Inform patient that yearly laboratory work, bone scan, and chest x-ray may be performed when clinically indicated.
4. Encourage healthy lifestyle and ideal body weight (20 to 25 body mass index). Evidence suggests that this may lead to optimal breast cancer outcomes. There are no specific recommendations on the type of physical activity advisable for patients with a history of breast cancer; however, data from observational studies demonstrated that those who participated in a moderate amount of physical activity after breast cancer diagnosis have improved outcomes as compared with those who were less active.
5. Assist patient in assessing integrative and complementary therapies. A number of studies looked at benefits of complementary therapies, including acupressure and acupuncture, yoga, and mindfulness for patients with history of breast cancer. Although there is no evidence that any specific intervention decreases recurrences, the results suggest that they may improve quality of life and mood.

Evaluation: Expected Outcomes

- Verbalizes less anxiety.
- Verbalizes understanding of all treatment options and their adverse effects.
- Identifies appropriate coping mechanisms and support systems.

SELECTED READINGS

Bakker, M. F., de Lange, S. V., Pijnappel, R. M., Mann, R. M., Peeters, P. H. M., Monninkhof, E. M., Emaus, M. J., Loo, C. E., Bisschops, R. H. C., Lobbes, M. B. I., de Jong, M. D. F., Duvivier, K. M., Veltman, J., Karssemeijer, N., de Koning, H. J., van Diest, P. J., Mali, W. P. T. M., van den Bosch M. A. A. J., Veldhuis, W. B., & van Gils, C. H.; DENSE Trial Study Group. (2019). Supplemental MRI screening for women with extremely dense breast tissue. *New England Journal of Medicine, 381*, 2091–2102. https://doi.org/10.1056/NEJMoa1903986

Balci, F. L., Uras, C., & Feldman, S. (2020). Clinical factors affecting the therapeutic efficacy of evening primrose oil on mastalgia. *Annals of Surgical Oncology, 27*(12), 4844–4852.

Campbell, K. L., Winters-Stone, K. M., Wiskemann, J., May, A. M., Schwartz, A. L., Courneya, K. S., Zucker, D. S., Matthews, C. E., Ligibel, J. A., Gerber, L. H., Morris, G. S., Patel, A. V., Hue, T. F., Perna, F. M., & Schmitz, K. H. (2019). Exercise guidelines for cancer survivors: Consensus statement from international multidisciplinary roundtable. *Medicine and Science in Sport and Exercise, 51*(11), 2375–2390. https://doi.org/10.1249/MSS.0000000000002116.0

Eden, K. B., Ivlev, I., Bensching, K. L., Franta, G., Hersh, A. R., Case, J., Fu, R., & Nelson, H. D. (2020). Use of an online breast cancer risk assessment and patient decision aid in primary care practices. *Journal of Women's Health, 29*(6), 763–769. https://doi.org/10.1089/jwh.2019.8143

Fairchild, B., Ellsworth, W., Selber, J. C., Bogue, D. P., Zavlin, D., Nemir, S., Checka, C. M., & Clemens, M. W. (2020). Safety and efficacy of smooth surface tissue expander breast reconstruction. *Aesthetic Surgery Journal, 40*(1), 53–62. https://doi.org/10.1093/asj/sjy199

Franzoi, M. A., Agostinetto, E., Perachino, M., Del Mastro, L., de Azambuja, E., Vaz-Luis, I., Partridge, A. H., & Lambertini, M. (2021). Evidence-based approaches for the management of side-effects of adjuvant endocrine therapy in patients with breast cancer. *The Lancet Oncology, 22*(7), e303–e313. https://doi.org/10.1016/S1470-2045(20)30666-5

Goetz, M. P., Gradishar, W. J., Anderson, B. O., Abraham, J., Aft, R., Allison, K. H., Blair, S. L., Burstein, H. J., Dang, C., Elias, A. D., Farrar, W. B., Giordano, S. H., Goldstein, L. J., Isakoff, S. J., Lyons, J., Marcom, P. K., Mayer, I. A., Moran, M. S., Mortimer, J., ... Kumar, R. (2019). NCCN guidelines insights: Breast cancer, version 3.2018. *Journal of National Comprehensive Cancer Network, 17*(2), 118–126. https://doi.org/10.6004/jnccn.2019.0009

Houssami, N., Kirkpatrick-Jones, G., Noguchi, N., & Lee, C. I. (2019). Artificial Intelligence (AI) for the early detection of breast cancer: A scoping review to assess AI's potential in breast screening practice. *Expert Review of Medical Devices, 16*(5), 351–362. https://doi.org/10.1080/17434440.2019.1610387

Kowalchuk R. O., Corbin, K. S., & Jimenez, R. B. (2022). Particle therapy for breast cancer. *Cancers, 14*(4), 1066. https://doi.org/10.3390/cancers14041066

Lehman, C. D., Lamb, L. R., & Alessandro, H. A. (2021). Mitigating the impact of coronavirus disease (COVID-19) vaccinations on patients undergoing breast imaging examinations: A pragmatic approach. *American Journal of Roentgenoly, 3*, 584–586. https://doi.org/10.2214/AJR.21.25688

Narayan, P., Osgood, C. L., Singh, H., Chiu, H. J., Ricks, T. K., Chiu Yuen Chow, E., Qiu, J., Song, P., Yu, J., Namuswe, F., Guiterrez-Lugo, M., Hou, S., Pierce, W. F., Goldberg, K. B., Tang, S., Amiri-Kordestani, L., Theoret, M. R., Pazdur, R., & Beaver, J. A. (2021). FDA approval summary: Fam-trastuzumab deruxtecan-nxki for the treatment of unresectable or metastatic HER2-positive breast cancer. *Clinical Cancer Research, 27*(16), 4478–4485. https://doi.org/10.1158/1078-0432.CCR-20-4557

National Cancer Institute. (n.d.). *Breast cancer risk assessment tool.* National Cancer Institute and National Surgical Adjuvant Breast and Bowel Project. www.cancer.gov/bcrisktool/

National Cancer Institute. (2020). *Breast cancer risk in American Women.* https://www.cancer.gov/types/breast/risk-fact-sheet

Nuciforo, P., Townend, J., Piccart, M. J., Fielding, S., Gkolfi, P., El-Abed, S., de Azambuja, E., Werutsky, G., Bliss, J., Moebus, V., Colleoni, M., Aspitia, A. M., Gomez, H., Gombos, A., Coccia-Portugal, M. A., Tseng, L. M., Kunz, G., Lerzo, G., Sohn, J., … Di Cosimo, S. (2023). Ten-year survival of neoadjuvant dual HER2 blockade in patients with HER2-positive breast cancer. *European Journal of Cancer, 181*, 92–101. https://doi.org/10.1016/j.ejca.2022.12.020

Obeagu, E. I., & Obeagu, G. U. (2024). Breast cancer: A review of risk factors and diagnosis. *Medicine (Baltimore), 103*(3), e36905. https://doi.org/10.1097/MD.0000000000036905. PMID: 38241592; PMCID: PMC10798762

Ocaña, A., Amir, E., & Pandiella, A. (2018). Dual targeting of HER2-positive breast cancer with trastuzumab emtansine and pertuzumab: Understanding clinical trial results. *Oncotarget, 9*(61), 31915–31919. https://doi.org/10.18632/oncotarget.25739

Okines, A., & Turner, N. (2024). Developing therapies for triple-negative breast cancer subtypes. *Lancet Oncology, 25*(2), 149-151. https://doi.org/10.1016/S1470-2045(23)00639-3

Tischkowitz, M., Balmaña, J., Foulkes, W. D., James, P., Ngeow, J., Schmutzler, R., Voian, N., Wick, M. J., Stewart, D. R., & Pal, T.; ACMG Professional Practice and Guidelines Committee. (2021). Management of individuals with germline variants in PALB2: A clinical practice resource of the American College of Medical Genetics and Genomics (ACMG). *Genetics in Medicine, 23*(8), 1416–1423. https://doi.org/10.1038/s41436-021-01151-8

US Food and Drug Administration. (2021). *FDA strengthens safety requirements and updates study results on breast implants.* https://www.fda.gov/news-events/press-announcements/fda-strengthens-safety-requirements-and-updates-study-results-breast-implants

Whisenant, M. S., Alexander, A., Woodward, W. A., Teshome, M., Ueno, N. T., & Williams, L. A. (2024). Inflammatory breast cancer: Understanding the patient experience. *Cancer Nursing, 47*(1), E65-E72. https://doi.org/10.1097/NCC.0000000000001165

Wolfson, S., Kim, E., Plaunova, A., Bukhman, R., Sarmiento, R. D., Samreen, N., Awal, D., Sheth, M. M., Toth, H. B., Moy, L., & Reig, B. (2022). Axillary adenopathy after COVID-19 vaccine: No reason to delay screening mammogram. *Radiology, 303*(2), 297–299. https://doi.org/10.1148/radiol.213227

Yao, K., Tong, C., & Chao Cheng, C. (2022). A framework to predict the applicability of Oncotype DX, MammaPrint, and E2F4 gene signatures for improving breast cancer prognostic prediction. *Scientific Reports, 12*(1), 2211. https://doi.org/10.1038/s41598-022-06230-7

Zeng, C., Bastarache, L. A., Tao, R. Venner, E., Hebbring, S., Andujar, J. D., Bland, S. T., Crosslin, D. R., Pratap, S., Cooley, A., Pacheco, J. A., Christensen, K. D., Perez, E., Zawatsky, C. L. B., Witkowski, L., Zouk, H., Weng, C., Leppig, K. A., Sleiman, P. M. A., … Denny, J. C. (2022). Association of pathogenic variants in hereditary cancer genes with multiple diseases. *JAMA Oncology, 8*(6), 835–844. https://doi.org/10.1001/jamaoncol.2022.0373

Zirpoli, G. R., Pfeiffer, R. M., Bertrand, K. A., Huo, D., Lunetta, K. L., & Palmer, J. R. (2024). Addition of polygenic risk score to a risk calculator for prediction of breast cancer in US Black women. *Breast Cancer Research, 26*(1), 2. https://doi.org/10.1186/s13058-023-01748-8

UNIT VII METABOLIC AND ENDOCRINE HEALTH

20 Endocrine Disorders*

OVERVIEW AND ASSESSMENT

The Function of Hormones

The endocrine system and the nervous system maintain homeostasis. The endocrine glands produce hormones, chemical substances that are secreted into the bloodstream and that exert a stimulatory or inhibitory effect on target tissues or on glands. Hormones achieve their effect by binding with specific receptors located on the membrane on the target cell (e.g., catecholamines) or by penetrating the cell membrane and forming a complex that influences cellular metabolism (e.g., steroids). The target cell response may be reflected through the production and secretion of a second hormone or through a change in cell metabolism that alters the concentration of electrolytes or other substances in the bloodstream.

General Effects of Hormone Action

1. Regulate the overall metabolic rate and the storage, conversion, and release of energy.
2. Regulate fluid and electrolyte balance.
3. Initiate coping responses to stressors.
4. Regulate growth and development.
5. Regulate reproductive processes.

Regulation of Hormones

1. Hormone secretion is typically controlled through a negative feedback loop
   a. Reductions in blood concentration of hormone lead to activation of the regulator endocrine gland and to release of its stimulator hormones.
   b. Elevations in blood concentration of target cell hormones or changes in blood composition resulting from target cell activity can cause inhibition of hormone secretion.
2. Endocrine disorders are manifested as states of hormone deficiency or hormone excess. The underlying pathophysiology may be expressed as:
   a. *Primary*—the secreting gland releases inappropriate hormone because of disease of the gland itself.
   b. *Secondary*—the secreting gland releases abnormal amounts of hormone because of disease in a regulator gland (e.g., pituitary).

*Please note that the term "male" in this chapter refers to a person assigned male at birth and that the term "female" in this chapter refers to a person assigned female at birth.

c. *Tertiary*—the secreting gland releases inappropriate hormone because of hypothalamic dysfunction, resulting in abnormal stimulation by the pituitary.

3. Abnormal hormone concentrations may also be caused by hormone-producing tumors (adenomas) located at a remote site.

History

Patients with diseases of the endocrine system commonly report nonspecific complaints. Commonly, symptoms may reflect changes in general well-being, such as fatigue, weakness, weight change, appetite, sleep patterns, or emotional status. A thorough review of systems is necessary to detect changes in various body systems caused by an endocrine disorder (see Table 20-1).

Physical Examination

Objective findings may be obvious and related to the patient's complaints or may be "silent signs," of which the patient is completely unaware. Thorough physical examination of all body systems, particularly the integumentary, cardiovascular, and neurologic systems, may reveal key findings for endocrine dysfunction.

Tests of Thyroid Function

Total Thyroxine

Description

1. This is a direct measurement of the concentration of total thyroxine (T_4) in the blood, using a radioimmunoassay technique.
2. It is an accurate index of thyroid function when T_4-binding globulin (TBG) is normal.
3. Low plasma-binding protein states (malnutrition, liver disease) may give low values.
4. High plasma-binding protein values (pregnancy, estrogen therapy) may give high values.
5. It can be used to diagnose hypofunction and hyperfunction of the thyroid and to guide and evaluate thyroid hormone replacement therapy (HRT).

Nursing and Patient Care Considerations

1. The test to monitor thyroid hormone therapy may be performed 6 to 8 weeks after dosage adjustment because of the time required for thyroid-stimulating hormone (TSH) to reflect the body's response to the new dose.
2. Interpretation of test results:
   a. Hypothyroidism—below normal.
   b. Hyperthyroidism—above normal.

Free Thyroxine

Description

1. Direct measurement of free T_4 concentration in the blood using a two-step radioimmunoassay method.
2. Accurate measure of thyroid function independent of the variable influence of thyroid-binding globulin levels.
3. Used to aid in the diagnosis of hyperthyroidism and hypothyroidism.
4. Used to monitor and guide thyroid (HRT).

Nursing and Patient Care Considerations

1. Interpretation of test results:
   a. Hyperthyroidism—above normal.
   b. Hypothyroidism—below normal.
2. Results best interpreted in conjunction with TSH levels for diagnostic purposes.
3. Often used to monitor thyroid, levels meaningful only after 6 to 8 weeks of therapy to evaluate adequacy of dosage because of long half-life of T_4.

Thyroid-Binding Globulin

Description

1. This measures the concentration of the carrier protein for T_4 in the blood.
2. Because most T_4 is protein bound, changes in TBG will influence values of T_4.
3. Helpful in distinguishing between true thyroid disease and T_4 test abnormalities caused by TBG excess or deficit.

Nursing and Patient Care Considerations

Determine if patient is taking estrogen or is pregnant, both of which can elevate TBG; results may be depressed by malnutrition or by liver disease.

Triiodothyronine

Description

1. Directly measures concentration of triiodothyronine (T_3) in the blood using a radioimmunoassay technique.
2. T_3 is less influenced by alterations in thyroid-binding proteins; it binds to albumin.
3. T_3 has a shorter half-life than T_4 and occurs in minute quantities in the active form.
4. Useful to rule out T_3 thyrotoxicosis, hyperthyroidism when T_4 is normal and to evaluate effects of thyroid replacement therapy.

Nursing and Patient Care Considerations

1. T_3 can be transiently depressed in the acutely ill patient.
2. Interpretation of test results:
   a. Hypothyroidism—below normal.
   b. Hyperthyroidism—above normal.

T_3 Resin Uptake

Description

1. This is an indirect measure of thyroid function, based on the available protein-binding sites in a serum sample that can bind to radioactive T_3.
2. The radioactive T_3 is added to the serum sample in the test tube and will bind with available protein-binding sites. The unbound T_3 binds to resin for T_3 uptake, reflecting the amount of T_3 left over because of lack of binding sites.
3. Estrogen and pregnancy produce an increase in binding sites, thus causing a lowered T_3 resin uptake.

Nursing and Patient Care Considerations

1. Results may be altered if patient has been taking estrogens, androgens, salicylates, or phenytoin.
2. Interpretation of test results:
   a. Hypothyroidism—below normal.
   b. Hyperthyroidism—above normal.

Free Thyroid Index

Description

The free thyroid index is a laboratory estimate of free T_4 concentration with calculated adjustment for variations in patient's TBG concentration.

Table 20-1 Clinical Manifestations of Endocrine Dysfunction

SIGN OR SYMPTOM	POSSIBLE CAUSES
Cardiovascular	
Tachycardia or tachyarrhythmia	• Hyperthyroidism • Pheochromocytoma • Adrenal insufficiency
Bradycardia	• Hypothyroidism
Orthostatic hypotension	• Adrenal insufficiency
Hypertension	• Pheochromocytoma • Hyperaldosteronism • Cushing syndrome • Hyperparathyroidism • Hypothyroidism
Heart failure	• Hyperthyroidism • Hypothyroidism • Cushing syndrome
Neurologic	
Fatigue	• Adrenal insufficiency • Hypothyroidism • Hyperparathyroidism
Nervousness, tremor	• Pheochromocytoma • Hyperthyroidism
Confusion, lethargy, or coma	• Diabetic ketoacidosis • Hypothyroidism • Syndrome of inappropriate antidiuretic hormone
Paresthesia	• Hypothyroidism • Hypoparathyroidism • Diabetes mellitus
Headache	• Acromegaly • Pituitary tumor • Pheochromocytoma
Psychosis	• Hyperaldosteronism • Hypothyroidism • Hyperthyroidism • Cushing syndrome • Adrenal insufficiency • Hyperparathyroidism
Chvostek sign, Trousseau sign	• Hypoparathyroidism
Increased reflexes	• Hyperthyroidism
Decreased reflexes	• Hypothyroidism
Peptic ulcer	• Cushing syndrome
Diarrhea	• Adrenal insufficiency
Constipation	• Hypothyroidism • Hyperparathyroidism • Pheochromocytoma
Weight loss	• Hyperthyroidism • Hyperparathyroidism • Pheochromocytoma
Hyperdefecation	• Hyperthyroidism
Abdominal pain	• Addisonian crisis • Hyperparathyroidism
Musculoskeletal	
Weakness	• Hyperthyroidism • Hypothyroidism • Cushing syndrome • Adrenal insufficiency • Hyperparathyroidism • Hypoparathyroidism • Hyperaldosteronism
Pathologic fractures	• Hyperparathyroidism
Joint pain	• Hypothyroidism • Acromegaly
Bone pain	• Hyperparathyroidism
Bone thickening	• Acromegaly
Urologic	
Polyuria	• Diabetes insipidus • Diabetes mellitus
Kidney stones	• Hyperparathyroidism • Acromegaly • Cushing syndrome
Integumentary	
Hirsutism	• Adrenal hyperfunction • Acromegaly
Hair loss	• Hypoparathyroidism • Hypothyroidism • Cushing syndrome
Sparse body hair	• Pituitary insufficiency • Adrenal insufficiency • Hypogonadism
Hyperpigmentation	• Addison disease • Hyperthyroidism • Ectopic corticotropin production
Profuse diaphoresis	• Hyperthyroidism • Pheochromocytoma
Thin skin	• Cushing syndrome
Coarse hair	• Hypothyroidism
Fine hair	• Hyperthyroidism
Edema	• Cushing syndrome
Reproductive	
Amenorrhea	• Hyperthyroidism • Hypogonadism • Cushing syndrome • Acromegaly • Pituitary tumor
Gynecomastia	• Hypogonadism • Pituitary tumor
Loss of libido, impotence	• Hypogonadism • Hypothyroidism • Adrenal insufficiency • Diabetes mellitus
Ophthalmic/Visual	
Exophthalmos	• Graves disease
Diplopia	• Graves disease • Pituitary tumor
Visual field deficit	• Pituitary tumor
Periorbital swelling	• Hypothyroidism • Graves disease
Body Habitus	
Round face, "buffalo hump"	• Cushing syndrome
Abnormally tall stature	• Prepubertal growth • Acromegaly

Nursing and Patient Care Considerations

Interpretation of test results:

1. Below normal—hypothyroidism.
2. Above normal—hyperthyroidism.

Thyrotropin, Thyroid-Stimulating Hormone

Description

1. Direct measure of TSH, the hormone secreted by the anterior pituitary gland that regulates the production and secretion of T_4 by the thyroid gland.
2. Third-generation TSH chemiluminometric assays are most commonly utilized.
3. Preferred test differentiates between thyroid disorders caused by disease of the thyroid gland itself and disorders caused by disease of the pituitary or hypothalamus. Also useful to detect early stages of hypothyroidism (subclinical hypothyroidism) and to monitor HRT. Patient must be on a stable dose of thyroxine for 6 to 8 weeks for TSH levels to accurately reflect adequacy of treatment.
4. Morning samples are preferred.

Nursing and Patient Care Considerations

1. Interpretation:
   a. In primary hypothyroidism, TSH levels are elevated.
   b. In secondary hypothyroidism (failure of the pituitary gland), TSH levels are low.
   c. In hyperthyroidism, TSH levels are low.

Thyrotropin-Releasing Hormone Stimulation Test

Description

1. The thyrotropin-releasing hormone (TRH) stimulation test evaluates the patency of the pituitary–hypothalamic axis. Once used primarily to distinguish between primary and central hypothyroidism (secondary or tertiary), this test is rarely used for that purpose with the advent of more sensitive TSH assays. Now, its primary use is to distinguish between secondary and tertiary hypothyroidism and evaluate acromegaly.
2. A baseline sample is drawn, then TRH is administered via intravenous (IV) injection, and blood samples are drawn to determine TSH levels at 30, 90, and 120 minutes.

Nursing and Patient Care Considerations

1. Interpretation:
   a. Increased TSH should be seen within 30 minutes.
   b. No rise in secondary hypothyroidism.
   c. Blunted rise in hyperthyroidism.
   d. Delayed rise (90-minute sample) associated with tertiary hypothyroidism.
   e. Elevated growth hormone (GH) levels associated with acromegaly.
2. A subnormal response can occur in patients taking L-dopa or cortisol.

Thyroid Autoantibodies

Description

Used to detect selected autoantibodies associated with some thyroid diseases and the levels of those autoantibodies.

1. Thyroid-stimulating immunoglobulin (TSI)—autoantibodies that stimulate the TSH receptor on the thyroid gland, causing hyperfunction of the thyroid. Helpful in the diagnosis of Graves disease.
2. Thyroid peroxidase (TPO) antibodies—associated with Hashimoto thyroiditis and Graves disease.
3. Thyroglobulin antibodies—elevated with Hashimoto thyroiditis and Graves disease.

Tests of Parathyroid Function

Parathyroid Hormone

Description

1. Test is either an intact parathyroid hormone (PTH) (second-generation assay) or PTH 1-84 assay (third generation), which should be measured concurrently with serum calcium level.
2. Range of normal values may vary by laboratory and method.

Nursing and Patient Care Considerations

Elevated PTH in hyperparathyroidism; decreased PTH in hypoparathyroidism.

Serum Calcium, Total

Description

1. This is a direct measurement of protein-bound and "free" ionized calcium.
2. Ionized calcium fraction is the best indicator of changes in calcium metabolism.
3. Results can be affected by changes in serum albumin, the primary protein carrier.
4. Used to detect alterations in calcium metabolism caused by parathyroid disease or malignancy.

Nursing and Patient Care Considerations

1. Sample may be obtained from fasting patient and should be collected in tube with heparin as anticoagulant.
2. Test should be repeated to confirm parathyroid disease.
3. Elevations in serum calcium can be caused by dehydration, vitamin D intoxication, thiazide diuretics, immobilization, hyperthyroidism, or lithium therapy.
4. Low values may be seen in renal failure, chronic disease states, malabsorption syndrome, and vitamin D deficiency.
5. Interpretation of test results:
   a. Hyperparathyroidism, malignancy—elevated.
   b. Hypoparathyroidism—below normal.

Serum Calcium, Ionized

Description

1. Approximately 45% to 50% of total serum calcium is in biologically active ionized form.
2. This is the preferred method of testing changes in calcium metabolism caused by parathyroid disease, malignancy, or thyroid surgery.

Nursing and Patient Care Considerations

1. Sample should be collected in tube with heparin as anticoagulant.
2. Test should be repeated on three different occasions to confirm parathyroid disease.
   a. Hyperparathyroidism, malignancy—elevated.
   b. Hypoparathyroidism—below normal.
3. Tourniquet use during blood sample collection for calcium studies should be kept to a minimum. Prolonged constriction will cause migration of plasma proteins into the bloodstream locally; this results in spuriously high serum calcium values and pseudohypercalcemia.

Serum Phosphate

Description

1. Test measures the level of inorganic phosphorus in the blood.
2. Alteration in parathyroid function tends to have opposite effects on calcium and phosphorus metabolism.
3. Used to confirm metabolic abnormalities that affect calcium metabolism.

Nursing and Patient Care Considerations

Elevated in hypoparathyroidism; low values in hyperparathyroidism.

Tests of Adrenal Function

Plasma Cortisol

Description

1. This is a direct measure of the primary secretory product of the adrenal cortex by radioimmunoassay technique.
2. Serum concentration varies with circadian cycle, so normal values vary with time of day and stress level of patient (8:00 a.m. levels are typically double those of 8:00 p.m. levels).
3. Useful as an initial step to assess adrenal dysfunction, but further workup is usually necessary.

Nursing and Patient Care Considerations

1. A fasting sample is preferred.
2. Blood samples should coincide with circadian rhythm with draw time indicated on a laboratory slip.
3. Interpretation of test results:
   a. Decreased values seen in Addison disease, anterior pituitary hyposecretion, and secondary hypothyroidism.
   b. Increased values seen in hyperthyroidism, stress (e.g., trauma, surgery), carcinoma, Cushing syndrome, hypersecretion of corticotropin by tumors (oat cell cancer), adrenal adenoma, and obesity.

Salivary Cortisol

Description

1. Because cortisol-binding globulin (CBG) is normally absent from saliva, it does not interfere with cortisol levels. Therefore, salivary cortisol can be more reliably measured without variation because of fluctuating CBG levels.

Nursing and Patient Care Considerations

1. A mouth swab is collected from patient in the evening and can be done at home after rinsing the mouth before brushing teeth.

Twenty-Four–Hour Urinary Free Cortisol Test

Description

1. Test measures cortisol production during a 24-hour period.
2. Useful to establish diagnosis of hypercortisolism.
3. Less influenced by diurnal variations in cortisol.

Nursing and Patient Care Considerations

1. Instruct patient in appropriate collection technique.
2. Collection jug should be kept on ice and sent to laboratory promptly when collection completed.
3. Interfering factors:
   a. Elevated values—pregnancy, hormonal contraceptives, spironolactone, and stress.
   b. Recent radioisotope scans can interfere with test results.

Dexamethasone Suppression Tests

Description

1. The dexamethasone suppression test (DST) is a valuable method to evaluate adrenal hyperfunction.
2. Adrenal production and secretion of cortisol is stimulated by adrenocorticotropic hormone (ACTH; corticotropin) from the pituitary gland.
3. Dexamethasone is a synthetic steroid effective in suppressing corticotropin secretion.
4. In a healthy patient, the administration of dexamethasone will inhibit corticotropin secretion and will cause cortisol levels to fall below normal.
5. Certain drugs (rifampin, phenytoin) increase metabolic clearance of dexamethasone and may contribute to false-positive test results.
6. Those on estrogen-containing drugs should stop 6 weeks prior to test, and this test is not reliable in pregnancy.

Nursing and Patient Care Considerations

Explain the procedure to patient.

1. Overnight low-dose (1 mg) DST (used primarily to differentiate between those with endogenous Cushing syndrome and those without Cushing syndrome).
   a. Administer dexamethasone 1 mg orally at 11:00 p.m.
   b. Draw cortisol level at 8:00 a.m. before patient rises.
   c. Expect suppressed cortisol levels (less than 5 μg/dL). Test is highly sensitive when a 2-mg cutoff is used for diagnosis.
2. Forty-eight–hour low-dose (2 mg) DST.
   a. Patient is instructed to take 0.5 mg of dexamethasone every 6 hours for a 2-day period.
   b. Plasma cortisol sample is collected 2 or 6 hours after the last dose.
   c. It is essential that patient have clearly written instructions for adherence with dosing and blood sampling schedule for test to be valid.
3. High-dose overnight DST (helpful to distinguish Cushing disease from other forms of Cushing syndrome).
   a. Give patient dexamethasone 8 mg orally at 11:00 p.m.
   b. Draw cortisol level at 8:00 a.m. before patient rises.
   c. Suppressed cortisol levels (less than 50% of baseline value) indicative of patient with corticotropin-secreting pituitary adenoma (Cushing disease).
   d. Unsuppressed cortisol levels are associated with ectopic corticotropin secretion (malignancy) or adrenal tumors.
4. Encourage patient to take dexamethasone with milk because it may cause gastric irritation.

Adrenocorticotropic Stimulation Test

Description

1. ACTH stimulates the production and secretion of cortisol by the adrenal cortex.
2. Demonstrates the ability of the adrenal cortex to respond appropriately to ACTH.
3. This is an important test to evaluate adrenal insufficiency but may not distinguish primary insufficiency from secondary insufficiency.

Nursing and Patient Care Considerations

1. Obtain baseline cortisol level.
2. Administer 250 μg ACTH (cosyntropin IV or intramuscularly [IM]).
3. Collect cortisol levels at times ordered (usually at 30 and 60 minutes).

4. Interpretation of test results:
   a. Range of normal responses may vary; however, typically, a rise in cortisol of double baseline value is considered normal.
   b. Diminished response—adrenal insufficiency with low cortisol values.

DRUG ALERT Infusion of cosyntropin can cause flushing or slight reduction in blood pressure (BP). Warn patients about these effects, monitor BP, and ensure safety.

Corticotropin-Releasing Hormone Stimulation Test

Description

1. Test measures responsiveness of the pituitary gland to corticotropin-releasing hormone (CRH)—a hypothalamic hormone that regulates pituitary secretion of ACTH.
2. Useful to differentiate the cause of excess cortisol secretion when ectopic source of ACTH is suspected.
3. In general, CRH will stimulate ACTH secretion in the pituitary but not in nonpituitary corticotropin-secreting tissues.

Nursing and Patient Care Considerations

1. Describe procedure to patient.
   a. Fasting patient is given CRH (1 μg/kg or 100 μg) via IV line.
   b. Catheters are advanced through the femoral veins to areas near the adrenal glands, so sampling can take place near ACTH secretion.
   c. Blood samples for ACTH test are collected at 5, 10, 15, 30, 45, 60, 90, and 120 minutes.
2. Normal response is a rise in ACTH to at least double the baseline value.
3. Interpretation of test results:
   a. Brisk rise in ACTH double baseline value—Cushing disease.
   b. No response in ACTH—corticotropin-independent Cushing syndrome (adrenal tumor) or ectopic source of corticotropin secretion (ectopic tumor).
   c. Test can produce false-negative response; 15% of patients are misdiagnosed by the test.

Urine Vanillylmandelic Acid and Metanephrine

Description

1. Direct measure of metabolites of catecholamines secreted by the adrenal medulla.
2. Metanephrine is a more reliable measure of catecholamine secretion.
3. Preferred method to diagnose pheochromocytoma, neuroblastoma, and other neural crest tumors.

Nursing and Patient Care Considerations

1. Obtain proper urine collection jug with hydrochloride preservative, and explain 24-hour urine collection to patient.
2. A wide range of medications and foods may alter test performed by some laboratories. Verify with the laboratory and health care provider the need to hold some medications, such as sympathomimetics and methyldopa, and such foods as coffee, tea, vanilla extract, and bananas before and during urine collection.
3. Interpretation—pheochromocytoma: vanillylmandelic acid greater than 10 μg/mg of creatinine or greater than 10 mg/24 hours; metanephrine greater than 0.7 μg/mg of creatinine or greater than 0.7 mg/24 hours.

Plasma Catecholamines

Description

Direct measure of circulating catecholamines using radioimmunoassay technique; more sensitive test than urine test but more prone to false-positive results.

Nursing and Patient Care Considerations

1. Collect sample from IV catheter 20 to 30 minutes after venipuncture, if possible, to reduce the rise in catecholamine levels from pain and anxiety.
2. Collect the sample in a heparinized tube.
3. Interpretation—levels higher than 2,000 ng/L diagnostic for pheochromocytoma.

Clonidine Suppression Test

Description

1. Based on the principle that catecholamine production by pheochromocytomas is autonomous, as opposed to other causes of excess catecholamines, which are regulated by the sympathetic nervous system.
2. Clonidine, as a central alpha-adrenergic agonist, suppresses production of catecholamines.
3. Useful to differentiate pheochromocytoma from essential hypertension when test results are inconclusive.
4. Corticosteroids should be avoided prior to testing.

Nursing and Patient Care Considerations

1. Collect baseline catecholamine sample from IV catheter 20 to 30 minutes after venipuncture, if possible, to reduce the rise in catecholamine levels from pain and anxiety.
2. Give clonidine 0.3 mg orally.
3. After 3 hours, collect second catecholamine sample.
4. Interpretation—in patients without pheochromocytoma, a significant drop in catecholamines should be seen at 3 hours (less than 500 pg/mL or reduction of total catecholamines by 50%), whereas in patients with pheochromocytoma, no drop in catecholamines will be evident.

DRUG ALERT Warn patients not to rise quickly and monitor for orthostatic hypotension after clonidine administration.

Aldosterone (Urine or Blood)

Description

1. Direct measure, using radioimmunoassay technique, of aldosterone, a hormone secreted by the adrenal cortex that regulates renal control of sodium and potassium.
2. May be measured in the blood or in 24-hour urine collection specimen.
3. Urine test is more reliable because it is less influenced by short-term fluctuations in the bloodstream.
4. Useful to diagnose primary aldosteronism.

Nursing and Patient Care Considerations

1. Test results can be elevated by stress, strenuous exercise, upright posture, and medications such as diazoxide, hydralazine, and nitroprusside.
2. Test results may be decreased by excessive licorice ingestion and the medications, fludrocortisone and propranolol.

Tests of Pituitary Function

Serum Growth Hormone

Description

1. Direct radioimmunoassay measurement of human GH, secreted by the anterior pituitary gland; useful to diagnose acromegaly, gigantism, pituitary tumors, pituitary-related growth failure in children, or GH deficiency in adults.
2. Because GH secretion is episodic, single fasting samples may not be reliable to detect GH excess or deficiency.
3. These conditions are best evaluated by using a stimulation test (for deficiency states) or a suppression test (for hormone excess conditions).

Nursing and Patient Care Considerations

1. Blood sample is taken after an overnight fast (caloric intake will lower GH blood levels).
2. Patient should be restful and calm before blood sample collection.
3. Normal range: males—less than 5 ng/mL; females—less than 8 ng/mL.
4. May be elevated by the following substances and medications: alcohol, L-dopa, hormonal contraceptives, alpha-antagonists, and beta-adrenergic blockers.

Serum Prolactin

Description

Direct radioimmunoassay measurement of prolactin, secreted by the anterior pituitary gland; helps diagnose pituitary tumors.

Nursing and Patient Care Considerations

1. Blood sample is taken after an overnight fast.
2. Normal values: males—1 to 20 ng/mL; females—1 to 25 ng/mL.
3. Values above 300 ng/mL highly suggestive of pituitary tumor.
4. Elevated values may be caused by exercise or by breast stimulation, such as from friction.
5. Medications that will elevate test results include phenothiazines, reserpine, estrogens, tricyclic antidepressants, methyldopa, antihypertensive medications, and selective serotonin reuptake inhibitors.

Adrenocorticotropic Hormone

Description

1. Direct measurement of ACTH concentration in the bloodstream by radioimmunoassay technique.
2. One measure of pituitary gland function useful to provide important information regarding adrenal gland dysfunction.
3. Useful to identify cause of adrenal abnormalities when compared with serum cortisol levels.

Nursing and Patient Care Considerations

1. Because ACTH is rapidly degraded, blood samples should be centrifuged and frozen promptly to avoid falsely low results.
2. High stress levels in patient can invalidate results.
3. Interpretation of test results:
   a. Elevated levels with elevated cortisol—Cushing disease or ectopic production of ACTH.
   b. Elevated levels with low cortisol—Addison disease.
   c. Low levels with elevated cortisol—adrenal tumor.
   d. Low levels with low cortisol—hypopituitarism.

Insulin Tolerance Test

Description

1. Dynamic test measures pituitary response to induced hypoglycemia, particularly GH secretion and ACTH-stimulated cortisol production by the adrenal gland.
2. Useful to diagnose functional hypopituitarism that is caused by pituitary disease or that appears after pituitary surgery.
3. Considered the "gold standard" for diagnosis of GH deficiency.

Nursing and Patient Care Considerations

1. After overnight fast, insulin 0.15 unit/kg (usual dose but may vary) body weight is given via IV line.
2. Blood samples are collected, usually at baseline, every 15 minutes after insulin dose.
3. The test is considered valid if blood glucose falls to half of baseline or less than 35 mg/dL.
4. Peak response is seen at 60 to 100 minutes.
5. For adrenal response, a rise in cortisol by a factor of at least 1.5 is necessary to show normal response.
6. GH deficiency is present if GH levels fail to rise above 3 μg/L.
7. This test is contraindicated in people with epilepsy or heart disease. In people with suspected adrenal insufficiency, ACTH stimulation test should be done first.
8. For people in whom the insulin tolerance test is contraindicated, other agents may be used, such as clonidine, arginine, glucagon, L-dopa, or GH-releasing hormone, to stimulate GH secretion.
9. Test should be performed with health care provider present. Dextrose 50% solution should be available at bedside to treat hypoglycemia, and test stopped if blood sugar falls below 35 mg/dL.

Glucose Suppression Test

Description

Postprandial elevations of glucose inhibit the secretion of GH by the pituitary gland. Failure to suppress GH levels after ingestion of glucose suggests a GH-secreting tumor.

Nursing and Patient Care Considerations

1. Patient should fast for this test.
2. Seventy-five to hundred grams of concentrated glucose is administered by mouth.
3. Blood samples are collected at baseline, 30, and 60 minutes.
4. Interpretation of test results:
   a. GH levels less than 2 μg/L are considered normal.
   b. GH levels that are not suppressed are suggestive of acromegaly.
5. Failure of GH suppression may also be caused by starvation or protein calorie restriction.
6. Patients may complain of nausea after ingesting Glucola.

Water Deprivation Test

Description

1. Functional test of the adequacy of posterior pituitary secretion of antidiuretic hormone (ADH) and its ability to concentrate urine and to maintain serum osmolality in the face of water deprivation.
2. Useful to determine the diagnosis and etiology of diabetes insipidus (DI).

Nursing and Patient Care Considerations

1. The test is begun by obtaining patient's weight, BP, heart rate, serum, and urine osmolality at time 0.
2. Patient weight, BP, heart rate, urine output volume, and osmolality are determined hourly.
3. Deprivation is continued until urine osmolality "plateaus," as evidenced by a change of less than 10% in urine osmolality between consecutive measurements and a 2% reduction in patient's body weight. At this time, samples are collected for serum sodium, osmolality, and vasopressin.
4. The test may be stopped if patient loses more than 5% of their body weight or if cardiac instability occurs.
5. If urine osmolality remains below that of serum (usually 300 mOsm/kg), the diagnosis of DI is confirmed, and the second stage of the test, which distinguishes central and nephrogenic DI, is begun.
6. Artificial ADH (desmopressin acetate [DDAVP]) 2 µg is given SubQ or IM to determine changes in urine osmolality at 30, 60, and 120 minutes in response to the injected hormone.
7. If the highest urine osmolality value obtained after injection is more than 50% higher than the preinjection value, DI is caused by pituitary failure. If the osmolality value is less than 50% of preinjection value, then DI is caused by renal disease.
8. Patients with suspected DI who undergo the water deprivation test must be monitored closely because dehydration may occur rapidly in people with severe disease.

Radiology and Imaging

Radioactive ^{131}I Uptake

Description

1. Measures thyroid uptake patterns of iodine as a whole or within specified areas of the gland. A radioactive tracer of sodium iodide-131(^{131}I) or sodium iodide-123 (^{123}I) isotopes is administered orally or intravenously to fasting patient.
2. I-131 has a longer half-life than I-123; due to this, I-123 is the agent used more frequently to decrease radiation exposure.
3. After a prescribed interval, usually 24 hours after oral tracers and 30 minutes after IV tracers, measurements of radioactive counts per minute are taken with a scintillator.
4. Normal thyroid will remove 15% to 50% of the iodine from the bloodstream.
5. Hyperthyroidism may result in the removal of as much as 90% of the iodine from the bloodstream (e.g., Graves disease); it may also cause a low uptake with some forms of thyroiditis.
6. Hypothyroidism is reflected in low uptake.

Nursing and Patient Care Considerations

After the test, radioactive iodine is eliminated through urine. The following measures are recommended from 1 to 21 days (depending on dose given, most average 3 days):

1. Monitor for pain at the injection site.
2. Assess for hypersensitivity, anaphylactic reactions to the radioisotope.
3. Drink lots of fluids.
4. Flush toilet two to three times after use.
5. Avoid close contact with other—6 feet distance.
6. Avoid contact with infants, children, and pregnant people.
7. Do not share a bed.
8. Avoid public areas.
9. Do not share utensils and/or prepare foods for others.

Thyroid Scan

Description

1. Rapid imaging of thyroid tissue, particularly suspicious nodules, as contrast imaging agent is rapidly taken up by functioning tissue.
2. Useful to diagnose thyroid carcinoma.
3. Contrast media is usually administered via IV line.
   a. Technetium (^{99m}Tc) pertechnetate or ^{123}I is used for best images.
4. Images can be obtained from gamma counter within 20 to 60 minutes.

Nursing and Patient Care Considerations

1. May interfere with serum radioimmunoassay tests; contact laboratory to determine when blood test can be done.
2. Benign adenomas may be visualized as "hot" nodules, indicating increased uptake of iodine, or as "cold" nodules, indicating decreased uptake.
3. Malignant nodules usually take the form of "cold" nodules.
4. No specific measures need to be taken after the test.

GENERAL PROCEDURES AND TREATMENT MODALITIES

See Standards of Care Guidelines 20-1, pages 687 to 688.

STANDARDS OF CARE GUIDELINES 20-1

Endocrine Disorders

When caring for a patient with an endocrine disorder, remember that important metabolic functions may be disrupted, such as fluid and electrolyte balance, glucose and protein metabolism, energy production, calcium ionization, blood pressure (BP) control, thermoregulation, cardiac contractility, intestinal peristalsis, and ability of the body to react to stress.

- Monitor closely for electrolyte imbalance—sodium, potassium, chloride, bicarbonate—by checking laboratory test results, changes in the electrocardiogram (ECG) pattern, and signs of particular excess or deficit (see Chapter 21, page 734).
- Check fingerstick or serum glucose periodically for patients on corticosteroids or for patients with adrenal disease; watch for signs of hyperglycemia (polydipsia, polyphagia, polyuria, blurred vision) or hypoglycemia (nervousness, tremor, difficulty concentrating, lethargy).
- Monitor for hypocalcemia after thyroidectomy, parathyroidectomy, or with hypoparathyroidism by checking serum calcium and phosphorus levels; watch for muscular twitching, anxiety, apprehension, spasms, and tetany. Check Chvostek sign and Trousseau sign.
- Monitor vital signs for heart rate, BP, and presence of arrhythmias.
- Monitor temperature and respiratory rate changes in thyroid and adrenal disease.
- Monitor intake and output, weight changes, and edema.
- Maintain a calm, quiet environment, and provide meticulous care to prevent infection or dehydration in patients with adrenal hypofunction or patients on corticosteroid replacement.

- After surgery, check for bleeding, signs of infection, changes in vital signs. Monitor respiratory status carefully after thyroidectomy.
- Report worsening condition or development of suspicious signs and symptoms promptly to prevent serious complications, such as myxedema coma, thyroid storm, hypocalcemic tetany, and adrenal crisis.
- Provide support, and explain care slowly and repeatedly because patient may have mental slowness, confusion, or lethargy because of their condition. Ask patient to restate important information to verify understanding.

This information should serve as a general guideline only. Each patient situation presents a unique set of clinical factors and requires nursing judgment to guide care, which may include additional or alternative measures and approaches.

Steroid Therapy

Steroid therapy is a treatment used in some endocrine disorders and in various other conditions. Steroids are hormones that affect metabolism and many body processes.

Classification of Steroids

(By major metabolic effects on the body.)

Mineralocorticoids

1. Concerned with sodium and water retention and potassium excretion.
2. Example—aldosterone and 11-desoxycorticosterone.

Glucocorticoids (Corticosteroids, Steroids)

1. Concerned with metabolic effects, including carbohydrate metabolism.
2. Example—cortisol.

Sex Hormones

1. Important when secreted in large amounts or when the growth of hormone-sensitive cancers is stimulated.
2. Examples:
   a. Androgens—testosterone.
   b. Estrogens—estradiol.
   c. Progestins—progesterone.

Effects of Glucocorticoids

1. Antagonize action of insulin; promote gluconeogenesis, which provides glucose.
2. Increase breakdown of protein (inhibit protein synthesis).
3. Increase breakdown of fatty acids.
4. Suppress inflammation, inhibit scar formation, block allergic responses.
5. Decrease number of circulating eosinophils and leukocytes; decrease size of lymphatic tissue.
6. Exert a permissive action (allow the full effects) on catecholamines.
7. Exert a permissive action on functioning of central nervous system (CNS).
8. Inhibit release of adrenocorticotropin.
9. In summary, glucocorticoids are necessary to resist noxious stimuli and environmental change.

Uses of Steroids

1. Physiologically—to correct deficiencies or malfunction of a particular endocrine organ or system (e.g., Addison disease).
2. Diagnostically—to determine proper functioning of the endocrine system.
3. Pharmacologically—to treat the following:
   a. Asthma and obstructive lung disease, moderate to severe cases of COVID-19.
   b. Acute rheumatic fever.
   c. Blood conditions, such as idiopathic thrombocytopenic purpura, leukemia, hemolytic anemia.
   d. Allergic conditions—allergic rhinitis, anaphylaxis (after epinephrine).
   e. Dermatologic problems—drug rashes, contact dermatitis, atopic dermatitis.
   f. Ocular diseases—conjunctivitis, uveitis.
   g. Connective tissue disorders—systemic lupus erythematosus, rheumatoid arthritis.
   h. Gastrointestinal (GI) problems—ulcerative colitis.
   i. Organ transplant recipients—as an immunosuppressive agent.
   j. Neurologic conditions—cerebral edema, multiple sclerosis.

Preparing the Patient to Receive Steroid Therapy

1. Determine contraindications/precautions for such therapy.
   a. Peptic ulcer.
   b. Diabetes mellitus.
   c. Viral infections.
2. Administer a tuberculin test, if indicated, before therapy because steroids may suppress response to the test.
3. Assess the patient's own level of steroid secretion, if possible.
4. Explain the nature of the therapy, what is required of the patient, how long therapy will last, adverse effects to watch for, and answer any questions.

Choice of Steroid and Method of Administration

1. May be given by various methods—orally, parenterally, sublingually, rectally, by inhalation, or by direct application to skin or mucous membrane.
2. Combinations of steroids with other drugs should be avoided.
3. To help avoid steroid adverse effects, alternate-day therapy may be used; dose is taken in the morning.
4. May be given in initial high doses, then reduced; if the patient has been taking steroids for several weeks, doses must be tapered gradually to prevent addisonian crisis.

Nursing Interventions

Preventing Infection

1. Steroids may affect the circulating blood, resulting in decreased eosinophils and lymphocytes, increased red cells, and increased incidence of thrombophlebitis and infection.
2. Encourage the patient to avoid crowds and the possibility of exposure to infection.
3. Encourage exercise to prevent venous stasis.
4. Be aware that signs of infection/inflammation may be masked—fever, redness, swelling.
5. Practice and encourage good handwashing technique and asepsis.

Preventing Nutritional and Metabolism Complications

1. Determine whether the patient needs assistance in dietary control. Steroids may cause weight gain and an increase in appetite.
2. Encourage a high-protein diet. Because steroids affect protein metabolism, there may be negative nitrogen balance.
3. Encourage the patient to take steroids with milk or with food. Because steroids increase secretion of gastric acid and have an inhibiting effect on secretion of mucus in the stomach, they may cause peptic ulcer.
4. Be on guard for early evidence of gastric hemorrhage, such as melena, blood in vomitus.
5. Check fasting blood glucose levels.
   a. Steroids precipitate gluconeogenesis and insulin antagonism, which results in hyperglycemia, glucosuria, decreased carbohydrate tolerance.
   b. Temporary insulin injections may be necessary.

Observing for Bone Complications

1. Be on the alert for the possibility of pathologic fractures. Stress safety measures to prevent injury.
   a. Steroids affect the musculoskeletal system, causing potassium depletion and muscular weakness.
   b. Steroids cause increased output of calcium and phosphorus, which may lead to osteoporosis.
2. Administer a diet high in calcium and protein.
3. Recommend activities of daily living (ADLs) and weight-bearing program; recommend normal range of motion and safe repositioning for those who are bedridden.
4. Obtain baseline dual energy X-ray absorptiometry (DXA) scan, if on long-term steroid use.

Avoiding Electrolyte Disturbance

1. Restrict sodium intake and increase potassium intake.
   a. Mineralocorticoids differ from other steroids, resulting in sodium retention and potassium depletion; edema, weight gain.
   b. Lemon juice is high in potassium and low in sodium.
   c. Avoid saline as a diluent in preparing injectable medications.
2. Check blood pressure (BP) frequently, and weigh the patient daily.
3. Observe for edema.

Monitoring Behavioral Reactions

1. Watch for convulsive seizures (especially in children). Steroids may alter behavior patterns, increase excitability, and may affect the CNS.
2. Avoid overstimulating situations.
3. Recognize and report any mood that deviates from the usual behavior patterns.
4. Report unusual behavior, haunting dreams, withdrawal, or suicidal tendencies.

Preventing Stress Reactions

1. Recommend that the patient carry an identification card that indicates steroid therapy and name of health care provider.
2. Be aware that steroids affect the hypothalamic–pituitary–adrenal system, which affects the patient's ability to respond to stress.
3. Advise the patient to avoid extremes of temperature, infections, and upsetting situations.

Preventing Injury and Promoting Healing

1. Instruct the patient to avoid injury; stress safety precautions. Because steroids interfere with fibroblasts and granulation tissue, altered response to injury results in impaired growth and delayed healing.
2. Observe daily the healing process of wounds, particularly surgical wounds, to recognize the potential for wound dehiscence.

Patient Education and Health Maintenance

1. Teach patient that steroids are valuable and useful medications, but that if taken for longer than 2 weeks, they may produce certain adverse effects.
   a. Acceptable adverse effects may include weight gain (because of increased appetite and water retention), acne, headaches, fatigue, and increased urinary frequency.
   b. Unacceptable adverse effects that are to be reported to the health care provider include dizziness when rising from chair or bed (orthostatic hypotension indicative of adrenal insufficiency), nausea, vomiting, thirst, abdominal pain, or pain of any type.
   c. Additional reportable adverse effects include convulsive seizures, feelings of depression or nervousness, or development of an infection.
2. Advise patient that a fall or an automobile accident may precipitate adrenal failure. This requires an immediate injection of hydrocortisone phosphate.
3. Tell patients on long-term therapy that they should wear a MedicAlert bracelet and carry a kit with hydrocortisone, as prescribed.
4. Instruct patient to inform any provider, dentist, or nurse about steroid therapy.
5. Tell patient that regular follow-up visits to health care provider are required.

Care of the Patient Undergoing Fine Needle Aspiration Biopsy

EVIDENCE BASE Turkkan, E., & Uzum, Y. (2023). Evaluation of thyroid nodules in patients with fine-needle aspiration biopsy. *Cureus, 15*(9), e44569. https://doi.org/10.7759/cureus.44569

Fine needle aspiration (FNA) biopsy is a procedure by which tissue from within a thyroid nodule is removed to detect malignancy. This procedure can easily be performed on an outpatient basis and requires no special patient preparation. Complications are uncommon but may include hematoma, tracheal perforation, and infection.

Preparation and Procedure

1. No special patient preparation activities are necessary for this procedure.
2. The procedure is explained to patient, and consent is obtained.
3. Patient is positioned comfortably on an examination table in the supine position with the neck fully exposed.
4. A rolled towel or sheet is placed beneath the patient's shoulder to hyperextend the neck, allowing ease of access to the biopsy site.
5. The biopsy site area is cleaned with alcohol and/or an antibacterial cleaning agent.
6. One percent lidocaine may be injected intracutaneously for local anesthetic to promote patient comfort.
7. A 25-G needle is inserted into the thyroid nodule and manipulated by the provider until a small amount of bloody material is seen on the hub of the needle.

8. The needle is removed and attached to a syringe. The contents of the needle are expressed onto a clean glass slide. A second slide is placed on top of the first slide and then pulled apart quickly to create a thin smear.
9. The slides are placed in a fixative and transported to a cytologist for interpretation.

Postprocedure Management

1. The biopsy site may be dressed with an adhesive bandage or other small dressing.
2. Follow-up visit for patient should be arranged to discuss results.

Nursing Considerations

1. Prevent infection by making sure that biopsy area is prepped appropriately before procedure.
2. Employ comfort measures during procedure, as necessary.
3. Assure patient that most thyroid nodules are determined to be benign and that most thyroid malignancies have a high cure rate.
4. Advise patient that some soreness at the biopsy site should be expected for a brief time.
5. Make sure that patient follows up for results and definitive treatment.

Care of the Patient Undergoing Thyroidectomy

Thyroidectomy involves the partial or complete removal of the thyroid gland to treat thyroid tumors, recurrent thyroid cysts, hyperthyroidism, or hyperparathyroidism.

Types of Procedures

1. Thyroidectomy can be total (removal of the entire thyroid gland); subtotal (95% of gland removed)—to prevent damage to the parathyroid glands; and partial (one lobe or isthmus removed)—to treat nodular disease.
2. The parathyroid glands are usually spared to prevent hypocalcemia.
3. Indications for thyroidectomy include Graves disease refractory to ^{131}I therapy, large goiters, adenoma (thyroid cancer), recurrent thyroid cysts, and some nodules.

Preoperative Management

1. The patient must be euthyroid at time of surgery, so thioamides are administered to control hyperthyroidism.
2. Iodide is given to increase firmness of the thyroid gland and to reduce its vascularity and blood loss.
3. An attempt is made to counteract the effects of hypermetabolism by maintaining a restful and therapeutic environment and by providing a nutritious diet.
4. The patient is prepared for surgery physically and emotionally in the following ways:
   a. Make a special effort to ensure that patient has a good night's rest preceding surgery.
   b. Explain to patient that speaking is to be minimized immediately postoperatively and that oxygen may be administered to facilitate breathing.
   c. Explain that postoperatively, fluids may be given via intravenous (IV) line to maintain fluid, electrolyte, and nutritional needs; IV glucose may also be given in the hours before the administration of anesthetic agents.

Postoperative Management

1. The patient is monitored for bleeding and respiratory distress that indicates laryngeal edema, secondary to swelling in the area of surgery.
2. Signs of hypocalcemia are watched for—irritability, twitching, spasms of the hands and feet.
   a. Calcium levels are monitored. If in 48 hours level falls below 7 mg/100 mL (3 mEq), IV calcium (gluconate, lactate) replacement is given.
   b. IV calcium is used cautiously in patients who have renal disease or who are taking digoxin.
3. Thyroid function is monitored after surgery.
4. Throat pain that extends to the upper back and shoulders can be treated with analgesics.

Complications

1. Hemorrhage, edema of the glottis, damage to laryngeal nerve, tracheal rupture.
2. Hypothyroidism following subtotal thyroidectomy occurs in 5% of patients in first postoperative year; increases at rate of 2% to 3% per year.
3. Hypoparathyroidism occurs in about 4% of patients and is usually mild and transient; requires calcium supplements via IV administration and orally when more severe.

Nursing Interventions

Observing for Hemorrhage and Airway Edema

1. Administer humidified oxygen, as prescribed, to reduce irritation of airway and to prevent edema.
2. Move patient carefully; provide adequate support to the head so that no tension is placed on the sutures.
3. Place patient in semi-Fowler position, with the head elevated and supported by pillows; avoid flexion of the neck.
4. Monitor vital signs frequently, watching for tachycardia and hypotension, which indicates hemorrhage (most likely between 12 and 24 hours postoperatively).
5. Observe for bleeding at sides and back of the neck, and anteriorly, when patient is in dorsal position.
6. Watch for repeated clearing of the throat or for complaint of smothering or difficulty swallowing, which may be early signs of hemorrhage.
7. Watch for irregular breathing, swelling of the neck, and choking—other signs pointing to the possibility of hemorrhage and tracheal compression.
8. Reinforce dressing, if indicated.
9. Be alert for voice changes, which may indicate damage to laryngeal nerve.
10. Keep a tracheostomy set in patient's room for 48 hours for emergency use.
11. Medicate for pain as needed.

Preventing Tetany

1. Watch for the development of tetany caused by removal or disturbance of parathyroid glands through a progression of signs:
   a. Tingling of toes and fingers and around the mouth; apprehension.
   b. Positive Chvostek sign—spasm of facial muscles caused by tapping on the cheek over the facial nerve; causes a twitch of the lip or side of the face (see Figure 20-1A, page 691).
   c. Positive Trousseau sign—carpopedal spasm induced by occluding circulation in the arm or lower leg with a BP cuff

(20 mm Hg above systolic pressure); within 3 minutes, flexion of the hands at the wrists and of the fingers at the metacarpophalangeal joints and extension of the fingers at the phalangeal joints or the feet are dorsiflexed at the ankles and the toes plantar flexed (see Figure 20-1B).

2. Be prepared to treat hypocalcemic tetany.
   a. Position patient for optimal ventilation; remove pillow to prevent head from bending forward and compressing trachea.
   b. Keep side rails padded and elevated, and position the patient to prevent injury if a seizure occurs; do not use restraints because they only aggravate the patient and may result in muscle strain or fractures.
   c. Have equipment available to treat respiratory difficulties that includes airway suction equipment, tracheostomy, and cardiac arrest equipment.
3. Administer IV calcium, as directed.

Patient Education and Health Maintenance

1. Teach patient about complications to look for if discharge occurs within a day or two of surgery.
2. Advise patient to rest at home and to prevent any strain on suture line, as directed by surgeon.
3. Advise nutritious diet; report difficulty swallowing.
4. Patient may be advised not to drive for up to 7 days.
5. Encourage follow-up for monitoring and thyroid hormone replacement after surgery.

Evaluation: Expected Outcomes

- No signs of hemorrhage or edema.
- No signs of hypocalcemia.

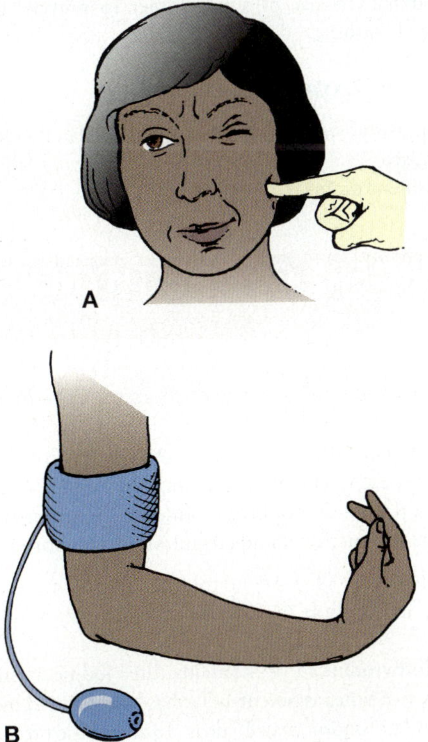

Figure 20-1. **(A)** Chvostek sign. **(B)** Trousseau sign.

Care of the Patient Undergoing Adrenalectomy

Adrenalectomy may be unilateral or bilateral to treat adrenal tumors, Cushing syndrome, or hyperaldosteronism. It is accomplished by an open or minimally invasive procedure—transabdominally, retroperitoneally, or transthoracically. Careful manipulation of the gland is necessary—if surgery is indicated for pheochromocytoma—to prevent excessive release of epinephrine causing hypertensive crisis.

Preoperative Management

1. BP and fluid volume are optimized.
2. Surgical and nursing care is explained to patient. Patient is shown where adrenal glands lie on the top of the kidneys and where incision may be on the abdomen or loin area.
3. BP will be checked frequently before and after surgery, and glucocorticoids will be given to cover period of stress (surgery) because at least one adrenal gland will be removed.
4. The patient will be given prophylactic antibiotics, venous thromboembolism (VTE) prophylaxis, and an antiemetic preoperatively or intraoperatively.
5. Patient is prepared as for major abdominal surgery (see page 512).

Complications

Hemorrhage, adrenal crisis.

Postoperative Management

1. Usual postoperative care for abdominal surgery includes frequent check of vital signs; assessment for hemorrhage; turning, coughing, and deep breathing; early ambulation; slow progression of diet when bowel sounds return; and control of pain with scheduled opioid administration or patient-controlled analgesia (see page 62).
2. IV hydrocortisone is given, as directed, to prevent adrenal crisis.
3. Nonstressful environment is maintained, rest is promoted, and meticulous care is given to protect patient from infection and from other complications that could cause adrenal crisis.
4. Serum sodium, potassium, and glucose are monitored for abnormality.
   a. Sodium and potassium may normalize, or potassium may become elevated (because of transient adrenal insufficiency after surgery).
   b. Electrolyte imbalances may persist for 4 to 18 months after surgery.
   c. Hypertension may persist for 3 to 6 months after surgery.
5. Hydrocortisone treatment causes glucose to rise and worsens control in patients with diabetes; may require additional treatment.

Nursing Interventions

Ensuring Healing

1. Assess dressing for leakage initially, and after it has been changed, assess wound for signs of infection.
2. Perform dressing changes, wound care, and teach family how to do wound care at home.

Providing Patient Education

1. Teach patient with bilateral adrenalectomy that glucocorticoid and mineralocorticoid replacement is necessary for rest of life.

2. Administer additional doses intramuscularly (IM) in times of stress.
3. Administer oral glucocorticoids after unilateral adrenalectomy, and teach patient that this treatment will be needed for 6 months to 2 years after surgery until remaining adrenal gland can compensate.
4. Encourage wearing or carrying a medical alert tag containing this information at all times so that proper treatment can be instituted if patient becomes unconscious.
5. Encourage follow-up to monitor for signs of adrenal insufficiency.

Care of the Patient Undergoing Transsphenoidal Hypophysectomy

Procedure

1. Transsphenoidal approach to pituitary removal is carried out through the nasal cavity, sphenoid sinus, and into the sella turcica (see Figure 20-2).
2. Advantages over intracranial approach to hypophysectomy include:
   a. No need to shave the head.
   b. No visible scar.
   c. Low blood loss, less need for transfusions.
   d. Lower infection rate.
   e. Well tolerated by frail and older patients.
   f. Good visualization of tumor field.
3. Disadvantages include:
   a. Restricted field of surgery.
   b. Potential cerebrospinal fluid (CSF) leak.

Preoperative Management

1. Sinus infection is assessed and treated, if necessary.
2. Hydrocortisone may be given preoperatively because the source of adrenocorticotropic hormone (ACTH) is being removed.
3. The patient is prepared physically and emotionally for surgery.
   a. Deep-breathing exercises.
   b. Avoid coughing and sneezing postoperatively to prevent CSF leak.

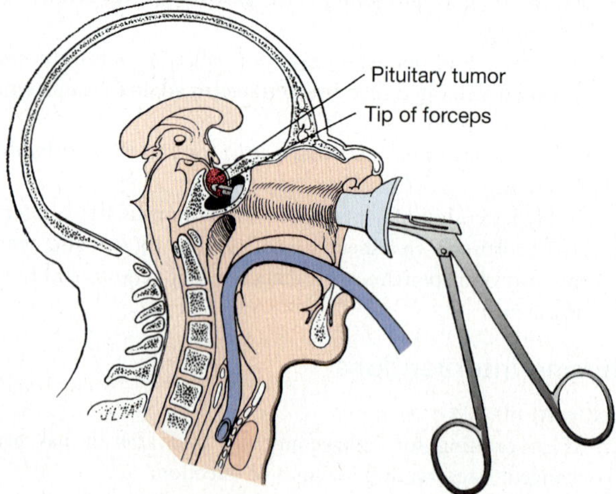

Figure 20-2. Transsphenoidal approach to the pituitary. A special nasal speculum is used to view the sinus cavity. After the dura is opened, the tumor is removed using microcurettes or other specially designed instruments.

Complications

1. CSF leak, sinusitis, meningitis.
2. Transient diabetes insipidus (DI).
3. Syndrome of inappropriate antidiuretic hormone (SIADH).

Postoperative Management

1. Vital signs, visual acuity, and neurologic status are monitored.
2. Urine output and specific gravity and serum electrolytes and osmolality are monitored for development of DI or SIADH.
3. Drainage from nose is monitored for signs of infection or CSF leak (clear fluid).

Nursing Interventions

Protecting Against Complications

1. Patients are generally monitored in the intensive care unit during the immediate postoperative period.
2. Monitor vital signs, visual acuity, and neurologic status frequently for signs of increasing intracranial pressure (see page 336).
3. Monitor fluid intake and output, and report any increase in output and decrease in specific gravity, which may indicate DI.
4. Report persistent clear fluid from nose and increasing headache; could signal CSF leak.
5. Teach patient signs of complications and to report them immediately and to follow up as scheduled.
6. Assess level of pain, and administer analgesic or supervise patient-controlled analgesia.

Preventing Infection

1. Observe for signs of infection. Check incision within inner aspect of upper lip for drainage or bleeding.
2. Note frequency of nasal dressing changes and character of drainage. Prepare patient for packing removal one to several days postoperatively.
3. Encourage the use of a humidifier to prevent drying from mouth breathing.

Evaluation: Expected Outcomes

- Vital signs stable, urine specific gravity 1.010, no clear drainage from nose.
- No purulent drainage noted.

DISORDERS OF THE THYROID GLAND

See additional online content: Nursing Care Plan 20-1

The thyroid gland affects the basal metabolic rate of all tissues, including the speed of chemical reactions, the volume of oxygen consumed, and the amount of heat produced. The stimulating effect is through the production and distribution of two hormones:

1. Levothyroxine (T_4)—contains four iodine atoms; maintains body's metabolism in a steady state; T_4 serves as a precursor of T_3.
2. Triiodothyronine (T_3)—contains three iodine atoms; approximately five times as potent as T_4; has a more rapid metabolic action and utilization than T_4 does. T_3 affects the protein synthesis and substrate by modifying gene transcription in most tissue.

3. Most conversion of T_4 to T_3 occurs at the cellular level in the periphery. Some T_3 is produced in the thyroid gland.

Hypothyroidism

Hypothyroidism is a condition that arises from a deficiency in endogenous production of thyroid hormone in the bloodstream.

Pathophysiology and Etiology

1. Primary hypothyroidism is the most common form of this condition and is generally caused by:
   a. Autoimmune disease—chronic lymphocytic thyroiditis (also known as Hashimoto thyroiditis).
   b. Postpartum thyroiditis.
   c. Use of radioactive iodine.
   d. Destruction, suppression, or removal of all or some of the thyroid tissue by thyroidectomy.
   e. Dietary iodide deficiency.
   f. Subacute granulomatous thyroiditis.
   g. Drug-induced iatrogenic hypothyroidism.
   h. Genetic causes.
2. Secondary hypothyroidism is caused when damage occurs to the hypothalamic–pituitary axis (i.e., tumor, necrosis, head trauma, certain drugs, brain/pituitary irradiation).
3. Inadequate secretion of thyroid hormone leads to a general slowing of all physical and mental processes.
4. General depression of most cellular enzyme systems and oxidative processes occurs.
5. The metabolic activity of all cells of the body decreases, reducing oxygen consumption, decreasing oxidation of nutrients for energy, and producing less body heat.
6. The signs and symptoms of the disorder range from vague, nonspecific complaints that make diagnosis difficult to severe symptoms that may be life threatening if unrecognized and untreated.

Clinical Manifestations

1. Fatigue and lethargy, decreased energy, exhaustion.
2. Weight gain—despite possible decreased appetite.
3. Complaints of cold hands and feet, cold intolerant.
4. Increased blood pressure (BP), decreased pulse.
5. Reduced attention span; impaired short-term memory.
6. Constipation; decreased peristalsis.
7. Generalized appearance of "doughy" thick, puffy skin; subcutaneous swelling in the hands, feet, and eyelids.
8. Thinning hair; loss of the lateral one third of the eyebrow.
9. Dry skin.
10. Enlarged tongue.
11. Depression, other psychological problems.
12. Menorrhagia or amenorrhea; may have difficulty conceiving or may experience spontaneous abortion; decreased libido, erectile dysfunction.
13. Neurologic signs include polyneuropathy, cerebellar ataxia, muscle aches or weakness, clumsiness, prolonged deep tendon reflexes (especially ankle jerk).
14. Hyperlipoproteinemia and hypercholesterolemia.
15. Enlarged heart on chest x-ray.
16. Increased susceptibility to all hypnotic and sedative drugs and anesthetic agents.
17. Syndrome of subclinical hypothyroidism: state in which the patient is asymptomatic and the free T_4 level is within the normal range; however, the thyroid-stimulating hormone (TSH) level is elevated, suggesting impending thyroid gland failure. Therefore, many clinicians may elect to treat this condition as if the patient were symptomatic.

Diagnostic Evaluation

1. Low T_3 and T_4 levels.
2. Elevated TSH levels in primary hypothyroidism.
3. Elevation of serum cholesterol.
4. Electrocardiogram (ECG)—sinus bradycardia, low voltage of QRS complexes, and flat or inverted T waves.
5. Elevation of thyroid peroxidase (TPO) and antithyroglobulin antibodies.

Management

Approach

1. Depends on severity of symptoms; may necessitate replacement therapy in mild cases or lifesaving support and treatment in severe hypothyroidism and myxedema coma.
2. As thyroid hormone levels gradually return to normal, the patient is monitored closely to prevent complications resulting from sudden increases in metabolic rate and oxygen requirements.

Restoration of Normal Metabolic State (Euthyroid)

1. Thyroid hormone: T_4, levothyroxine; T_3, liothyronine; T_3 and T_4 mixed. T_4 replacement therapy is typically the treatment of choice.
   a. In myxedema coma, a loading dose of levothyroxine is administered parenterally (until consciousness is restored) to restore T_4 level. Use of T_3 is controversial, may increase adverse cardiac events.
   b. Later, patient is continued on oral thyroid hormone therapy.
   c. With rapid administration of thyroid hormone, plasma T_4 levels may initiate adrenal insufficiency; hence, steroid therapy may be started.
   d. Mild symptoms in alert patient or asymptomatic cases (with abnormal laboratory results only) require only initiation of low-dose thyroid hormone given orally.
2. Monitoring to anticipate treatment effects.
   a. Diuresis, decreased puffiness.
   b. Improved reflexes and muscle tone.
   c. Accelerated pulse rate.
   d. A slightly higher level of total serum T_4.
   e. All signs of hypothyroidism should disappear in 3 to 12 weeks.
   f. Decreasing TSH level.
   g. Patients on T_4 can have an increase of dose every 4 to 6 weeks until TSH is therapeutic.

POPULATION AWARENESS When starting thyroid hormone replacement, care must be taken with older patients and with those who have coronary ischemia disease, because of increased oxygen demands of the heart. It is preferable to start with much lower doses 25% to 50% lower than needed.

Complications

1. Myxedema coma—hypotension, unresponsiveness, bradycardia, hypoventilation, hyponatremia, (possibly) convulsions, hypothermia, cerebral hypoxia.
2. High mortality in myxedema coma.

Nursing Assessment

1. Obtain history of symptoms, medication program, and past history of thyroid disease, surgery, or treatment.
2. Perform multisystem assessment, including cardiac, respiratory, neurologic, and gastrointestinal (GI) systems.

Nursing Interventions

Increasing Cardiac Output

1. Monitor vital signs frequently to detect changes in cardiovascular status and ability to respond to stress.
2. Monitor ECG tracings to detect arrhythmias and deterioration of cardiovascular status.
3. Prevent chilling to avoid increasing metabolic rate, which, in turn, places strain on the heart. Provide bed socks, bed jacket, warm environment.
4. Avoid rapid rewarming techniques (warmed intravenous [IV] fluids, hypothermia blanket) because the resulting increased oxygen requirements and peripheral vasodilation may worsen cardiac failure.
5. Administer fluids cautiously, even though hyponatremia is present.
6. Administer all prescribed drugs with caution before and after thyroid replacement begins.
   a. Monitor the effects of sedatives, opioids, and anesthetics closely because patient is more sensitive to these agents.
   b. After thyroid replacement is initiated, the thyroid hormones may increase the effects of digoxin (monitor pulse) and anticoagulants (watch for signs of bleeding).
7. Report occurrence of angina and be alert for signs and symptoms of myocardial infarction and cardiac failure.
8. Monitor arterial blood gas levels to assess cardiopulmonary function.

Promoting Normal Bowel Movements

1. Encourage too fluid intake of at least 64 ounces daily, unless contraindicated.
2. Recommend high-fiber food intake, including fresh or frozen fruit and vegetables lightly cooked, whole grains, and beans.
3. Advise patient to increase activity as tolerated and paying attention to the body's natural urge to evacuate the bowel.

Increasing Exercise Tolerance

1. Provide for uninterrupted rest periods between activities to assist with reconditioning.
2. Encourage exercise and walking goals based on patient's age and previous physical conditioning, in consultation with a physical therapist if required.
3. Recommend gradually increasing exercise and activity but stop if short of breath, chest pain, dizziness, or weakness. Report these symptoms if they do not resolve quickly with rest.

Patient Education and Health Maintenance

Instruct the patient about the following:

1. The need to receive lifelong thyroid hormone replacement therapy.
2. How and when to take medications.
3. Signs and symptoms of insufficient and excessive medication; reinforce teaching by providing written instructions.
4. The necessity of having blood evaluations periodically to determine thyroid levels.
5. Energy conservation techniques and the need to increase activity gradually.
6. Fluid intake and use of fiber to prevent constipation.
7. Control of dietary intake to limit calories and reduce weight.
8. Assist patient in identifying sources of information (see Box 20-1) and support available in the community such as local Office on Aging.

Evaluation: Expected Outcomes

- BP and pulse rate stable.
- Soft bowel movement without straining daily.
- Walking 15 minutes three times a day.

Hyperthyroidism

EVIDENCE BASE Ross, D. S., Burch, H. B., Cooper, D. S., Greenlee, M. C., Laurberg, P., Maia, A. L., Rivkees, S. A., Samuels, M., Sosa, J. A., Stan, M. N., & Walter, M. A. (2016). American Thyroid Association guidelines for diagnosis and management of hyperthyroidism and other causes of thyrotoxicosis. *Thyroid, 26*(10), 1343–1421. https://doi.org/10.1089/thy.2016.0229

Hyperthyroidism, a hypermetabolic condition, is characterized by excessive amounts of thyroid hormone in the bloodstream.

Pathophysiology and Etiology

1. More common in females than in males.
2. Graves disease (most prevalent)—diffuse hyperfunction of the thyroid gland with autoimmune etiology and associated with ophthalmopathy.
   a. Thyroid-stimulating immunoglobulin (TSI), an immunoglobulin found in the blood of patients with Graves disease, is capable of reacting with the receptor for TSH on the thyroid plasma membrane and of stimulating thyroid hormone production and secretion.
   b. Most common in younger females; may subside spontaneously.
3. Toxic nodular goiter (single or multiple)—more common preexisting goiter.
4. Toxic adenoma—present in 3% to 5% of thyrotoxicosis cases.
5. Hyperthyroidism is characterized by hypertrophy and hyperplasia of the thyroid gland, which is accompanied by increased vascularity and blood flow and enlargement of the gland.
6. Most of the clinical manifestations result from increased metabolic rate, excessive heat production, increased neuromuscular and cardiovascular activity, and hyperactivity of the sympathetic nervous system.
7. Hyperthyroidism ranges from a mild increase in metabolic rate to the severe hyperactivity known as thyrotoxicosis, thyroid storm, or thyroid crisis.
8. Hyperthyroidism can also be the result of ingestion of excessive amounts of thyroid hormone medication (factitious hyperthyroidism).

Clinical Manifestations

1. Nervousness, emotional lability, irritability, apprehension.
2. Difficulty sitting quietly; anxiety, hyperactivity.
3. Rapid pulse at rest and on exertion (ranges between 90 and 160); palpitations.
4. Heat intolerance; profuse perspiration; flushed skin (e.g., hands may be warm, soft, moist).

5. Fine tremor of hands; change in bowel habits—constipation or diarrhea.
6. Increased appetite and progressive weight loss; frequent stools.
7. Muscle fatigability and weakness; amenorrhea.
8. Atrial fibrillation possible (cardiac decompensation common in older patients).
9. Exophthalmos, periorbital edema, chemosis, diplopia, proptosis suggestive of Graves disease.
10. Thyroid gland may be palpable, and a bruit may be auscultated over gland.
11. Course may be mild, characterized by remissions and exacerbations.
12. May progress to emaciation, extreme nervousness, delirium, disorientation, thyroid storm or crisis, and death.
13. Thyroid storm or crisis, an extreme form of hyperthyroidism, is characterized by hyperpyrexia, diarrhea, dehydration, tachycardia, arrhythmias, extreme irritation, delirium, coma, shock, and death if not adequately treated.
14. Thyroid storm may be precipitated by stress (surgery, infection) or inadequate preparation for surgery in a patient with known hyperthyroidism.

Diagnostic Evaluation

1. Elevated T_3 and T_4.
2. Elevated serum T_3 resin uptake and free thyroid index.
3. Low TSH levels.
4. Presence of TSI antibodies (if Graves disease is the cause).
5. ^{131}I uptake scan may be elevated or below normal depending on the underlying cause of the hyperthyroidism.

Management

Approach to Management

1. Treatment depends on causes, age of patient, severity of disease, and complications.
2. Remission of hyperthyroidism (Graves disease) occurs spontaneously within 1 to 2 years; however, relapse can be expected in half the patients. Antithyroid drugs, radiation, or surgery may be used for treatment.
3. Nodular toxic goiter—surgery or use of radioiodine is preferred.
4. Thyroid carcinoma—surgery or radiation is used.
5. Goal of therapy is to bring the metabolic rate to normal as soon as possible and to maintain it at this level.

Pharmacotherapy

1. Drugs that inhibit hormone formation:
   a. Thioamides—propylthiouracil (PTU) and methimazole.
   b. Act by depressing the synthesis of thyroid hormone by inhibiting thyroid peroxidase.
   c. Propylthiouracil given in divided daily doses; methimazole may be given in a single daily dose.
   d. Duration of treatment is determined by clinical criteria.
      i. Thyroid gland becomes smaller.
      ii. Treatment continued until patient becomes clinically euthyroid; this varies from 3 months to 2 years; if euthyroidism cannot be maintained without therapy, then radiation or surgery is recommended.
      iii. Therapy is withdrawn gradually to prevent exacerbation.
2. Drugs to control peripheral manifestations of hyperthyroidism:
   a. Propranolol, a beta-adrenergic blocking agent.
      i. Inhibits peripheral conversion of T_4 to T_3.
      ii. Abolishes tachycardia, tremor, excess sweating, nervousness.
      iii. Controls hyperthyroid symptoms until antithyroid drugs or radioiodine can take effect.
   b. Glucocorticoids—decrease the peripheral conversion of T_4 to T_3, a more potent thyroid hormone.

Radioactive Iodine

1. Action—limits secretion of thyroid hormone by destroying thyroid tissue.
2. Dosage is calculated to help prevent hypothyroidism.
3. Chief advantage over thioamides is that a lasting remission can be achieved.
4. Chief disadvantage is that permanent hypothyroidism can be produced.

Surgery

1. Used for those with large goiters or for those for whom the use of radioiodine or thioamides is contraindicated.
2. Subtotal thyroidectomy involves removal of most of the thyroid gland (see page 690).

DRUG ALERT Observe the patient for evidence of iodine toxicity: swelling of buccal mucosa, excessive salivation, coryza, skin eruptions. If these occur, iodides are discontinued.

Emergency Management of Thyroid Storm

1. Inhibition of new hormone synthesis with thioamides (PTU and methimazole).
2. Inhibition of thyroid hormone release using a solution of potassium iodine.
3. Inhibition of peripheral effects of thyroid hormones with propranolol, corticosteroids, and PTU.
4. Treatment aimed at systemic effects of thyroid hormones and prevention of decompensation.
   a. Hyperthermia—cooling blanket, acetaminophen.
   b. Dehydration—administration of IV fluids and electrolytes.
5. Treatment of precipitating event.

Complications

1. Thioamide toxicity—agranulocytosis may occur suddenly.
2. Hypothyroidism if overtreated with antithyroid medication or if radiation treatment is used.
3. Radiation thyroiditis (a transient exacerbation of hyperthyroidism) may occur as a result of leakage of thyroid hormone into the circulation from damaged follicles.
4. Infiltrative ophthalmopathy.
   a. Occurs in 50% of patients with Graves disease.
   b. Features include exophthalmos, weakness of extraocular muscles, lid edema, lid lag.

Nursing Assessment

1. Obtain history of symptoms, family history of thyroid disease, medications, any recent physical stress, particularly infection.
2. Perform multisystem assessment that includes cardiac, respiratory, neurologic, and GI systems.
3. Closely monitor patient's temperature for thyroid storm.

Nursing Interventions

Providing Adequate Nutrition

1. Determine patient's food and fluid preferences.
2. Provide high-calorie foods and fluids consistent with the patient's requirements.
3. Provide a quiet, calm environment at meals.
4. Restrict stimulants (tea, coffee, alcohol); explain rationale of requirements and restrictions to patient.
5. Encourage and permit patient to eat alone if embarrassed or if otherwise disturbed by voracious appetite.
6. Monitor IV infusion when prescribed to maintain fluid and electrolyte balance.
7. Monitor fluid and nutritional status by weighing patient daily and by keeping accurate intake and output records.
8. Monitor vital signs to detect changes in fluid volume status.
9. Assess skin turgor, mucous membranes, and neck veins for signs of increased or decreased fluid volume.

Maintaining Skin Integrity

1. Assess skin frequently to detect diaphoresis.
2. Bathe frequently with cool water; change linens when damp.
3. Avoid soap to prevent drying, and apply lubricant skin lotions to pressure points.
4. Protect and relieve pressure from bony prominences while immobilized or while hypothermia blanket is used.

Promoting Normal Thought Processes

1. Explain procedures to patient in an unhurried, calm manner.
2. Limit visitors; avoid stimulating conversations or television programs.
3. Reduce stressors in the environment; reduce noise and lights.
4. Promote sleep and relaxation through use of prescribed medications, massage, and relaxation exercises.
5. Minimize disruption of patient's sleep or rest by clustering nursing activities.
6. Use safety measures to reduce risk of trauma or falls (padded side rails, bed in low position).

Relieving Anxiety

1. Encourage patient to verbalize concerns and fears about illness and treatment.
2. Support patient who is undergoing various diagnostic tests.
   a. Explain the purpose and requirements of each prescribed test.
   b. Explain results of tests if unclear to the patient or if questions arise.
3. Clear up misconceptions about treatment options.

Patient Education and Health Maintenance

1. Instruct patient as follows:
   a. When to take medications.
   b. Signs and symptoms of insufficient and excessive medication.
   c. Necessity of having blood evaluations periodically to determine thyroid levels.
   d. Signs of agranulocytosis (fever, sore throat, upper respiratory infection) or rash, fever, urticaria, or enlarged salivary glands caused by thioamide toxicity.
   e. Signs and symptoms of thyroid storm (i.e., tachycardia, hyperpyrexia, extreme irritation) and predisposing factors to thyroid storm (i.e., infection, surgery, stress, abrupt withdrawal of antithyroid medications and adrenergic blockers).
2. Reinforce teaching by providing written instructions as well.
3. Assist patient in identifying sources of information and support available in the community (see Box 20-1, page 700).

Evaluation: Expected Outcomes

- Food and fluid intake adequate, gaining weight.
- Skin cool, dry, and intact.
- Maintains concentration, follows conversation, and responds appropriately.
- Verbalizes concerns and questions about illness, treatment, and surgery.

Subacute Thyroiditis

Subacute thyroiditis is a self-limiting, painful inflammation of the thyroid gland, usually associated with viral infections.

Pathophysiology and Etiology

1. Affects younger females predominantly.
2. Previous viral infection (2 to 6 weeks earlier) is considered a factor in genetically susceptible individuals. Severe acute respiratory syndrome, often related to COVID-19, may be an additional risk factor.
3. Acute inflammation results in sudden release of preformed T_3 and T_4, commonly causing symptoms of hyperthyroidism initially.
4. A clinical variant of this disorder, "silent thyroiditis," has been described as similar to subacute thyroiditis; however, the symptoms may be milder, and the thyroid gland is not painful.
5. Subacute thyroiditis has been associated with onset within 6 months of the postpartum period.

Clinical Manifestations

1. Pain, swelling, thyroid tenderness last several weeks or months and then disappear.
2. Sore throat.
3. Pain referred to the ear, making swallowing difficult and uncomfortable.
4. Fever, malaise, chills, fatigue, anorexia, and/or myalgia.
5. May develop clinical manifestations of hyperthyroidism (irritability, nervousness, insomnia, and weight loss) or hypothyroidism, depending on the point of time in the natural course of the disease when patient presents.

Diagnostic Evaluation

1. TSH level is low.
2. ^{131}I uptake is low.
3. Serum T_3 and T_4 levels are elevated.
4. Erythrocyte sedimentation rate is increased, usually greater than 50 m/h.
5. C-reactive protein may also be elevated.
6. Ultrasound.

Management

1. Analgesics and mild sedatives.
2. The patient may be placed on beta-adrenergic blockers to reduce the symptoms of thyrotoxicosis.

3. Steroids may be administered for inflammation, pain, fever, and malaise.
4. Aspirin or nonsteroidal anti-inflammatory drugs may be used in mild cases to treat the symptoms of inflammation.

DRUG ALERT Aspirin should be avoided if the patient exhibits signs of hyperthyroidism because it displaces thyroid hormone from its binding site and may increase the amount of free circulating hormone, resulting in exacerbation of the symptoms of hyperthyroidism.

Complications

In about 10% of patients, permanent hypothyroidism occurs, and long-term T_4 therapy is needed.

Nursing Assessment

1. Assess for signs and symptoms of hyperthyroidism (see page 694).
2. Assess for level of discomfort.
3. Evaluate patient's coping skills regarding pain.

Nursing Interventions

Reducing Pain

1. Administer or teach self-administration of pain relief medication, as prescribed.
2. Provide a restful environment, and explain all tests and procedures to patient/family.
3. Assess for degree of pain relief.
4. Notify health care provider if pain relief medications are inadequate for acceptable pain control.

Patient Education and Health Maintenance

1. Explain all medications patient is to continue at home.
2. Reassure patient that subacute thyroiditis usually resolves spontaneously during weeks to months.
3. Teach patient signs and symptoms of hypothyroidism (i.e., fatigue and lethargy, weight gain, cold intolerance) that may be experienced. These should be reported as inflammation of the gland subsides.
4. Assist patient in identifying sources of information and support available in the community (see Box 20-1, page 700).

Evaluation: Expected Outcomes

- Verbalizes acceptable pain relief.

Hashimoto Thyroiditis (Lymphocytic Thyroiditis)

Hashimoto thyroiditis is a chronic progressive autoimmune disease of the thyroid gland caused by infiltration of lymphocytes; it results in progressive destruction of the parenchyma and hypothyroidism if untreated.

Pathophysiology and Etiology

1. Cause is unknown; believed to be an autoimmune disease related to genetic susceptibility, environmental triggers, epigenetic effects, and perhaps related to Graves disease.
2. Ninety-five percent of cases occur in women in their 40s or 50s. Incidence increases with age and is more prevalent in White individuals.
3. Possibly the most common cause of adult hypothyroidism.
4. Appears to be increasing in incidence.

Clinical Manifestations

1. Marked by a slowly developing, firm enlargement of the thyroid gland.
2. Usually, no gross nodules.
3. Local symptoms such as dysphonia, dyspnea, and dysphagia due to compression of anatomic structures of the neck.
4. Basal metabolic rate is usually low.
5. Periods of hyperthyroidism caused by large amounts of T_3 and T_4 being released into bloodstream.

Diagnostic Evaluation

1. T_3 and T_4 may be normal but usually become subnormal as the disease progresses.
2. TSH level is usually elevated.
3. Antithyroglobulin antibodies and antimicrosomal antibodies are virtually always present.
4. Normal or high concentration of thyroglobulin-binding protein.

Management

1. Thyroid medications to maintain a normal level of circulating thyroid hormone; this is done to suppress production of TSH, to prevent enlargement of the thyroid, and to maintain a euthyroid state.
2. Vitamin D supplementation.
3. Surgical resection of goiter if tracheal compression, cough, or hoarseness occurs.
4. Careful follow-up to detect and treat hypothyroidism.

Complications

1. Progressive hypothyroidism.
2. Without treatment, Hashimoto thyroiditis may progress from goiter and hypothyroidism to myxedema.

Nursing Assessment

1. Assess for signs and symptoms of hyperthyroidism and hypothyroidism.
2. Assess size of the thyroid gland and symptoms of compression—neck tightness, cough, hoarseness.

Nursing Interventions

Reducing Anxiety

1. Explain physiology of the disorder and the reason for enlarging gland. Show anatomic pictures of the thyroid gland, if possible.
2. Administer or teach self-administration of thyroid hormone to suppress stimulation on gland and possibly reduce size.
3. Reassure regarding slow progression of gland enlargement (during months) and the option of surgical resection, if necessary.
4. Suggest wearing loose-necked clothing, avoiding jewelry or scarves around the neck, and avoiding excessive neck flexion or hyperextension, which may aggravate feeling of compression.

Patient Education and Health Maintenance

1. Teach signs of tracheal compression that should be reported to health care provider as soon as possible—difficulty breathing, cough, hoarseness.

2. Explain outcome of hypothyroidism and necessity of taking thyroid hormones every day for life.
3. Explain the need for regular medical follow-up visits to monitor thyroid hormone and TSH levels.
4. Assist patient in identifying sources of information and support available in the community (see Box 20-1, page 700).

POPULATION AWARENESS Careful and regular follow-up of older patients with Hashimoto thyroiditis is especially important because the progression to hypothyroidism is usually subtle in older people and is unlikely to be recognized promptly.

Evaluation: Expected Outcomes

- Verbalizes reduced anxiety, appears more relaxed, sleeps better.

Cancer of the Thyroid

Cancer of the thyroid is a malignant neoplasm of the gland.

Pathophysiology and Etiology

1. Incidence in women is three times higher than in males. Usually diagnosed at 30 to 50 years of age but also increasing with females ages 15 to 19 years of age.
2. Exposure to radiation increases risk of thyroid carcinoma significantly. Exposure to Agent Orange also has been associated with higher risk.
3. Papillary and well-differentiated adenocarcinoma (most common, approximately 80%).
   a. Growth is slow, and spread is confined to lymph nodes that surround thyroid area.
   b. Cure rate is excellent after removal of involved areas.
4. Follicular (rapidly growing, widely metastasizing type, approximately 10%).
   a. Occurs predominantly in middle-aged and older persons.
   b. Brief encouraging response may occur with irradiation.
   c. Progression of disease is rapid; high mortality.
5. Parafollicular–medullary thyroid carcinoma.
   a. Rare, inheritable type of thyroid malignancy, which can be detected early by a radioimmunoassay for calcitonin.
6. Undifferentiated anaplastic carcinoma (approximately less than 3%).
   a. The most aggressive and lethal solid tumor found in humans.
   b. Least common of all thyroid cancers.
   c. Usually fatal within months of diagnosis.

Clinical Manifestations

1. On palpation of the thyroid, there may be a firm, irregular, fixed, painless mass or nodule.
2. The occurrence of signs and symptoms of hyperthyroidism is rare.

Diagnostic Evaluation

1. A thyroid uptake and scintigraphy using ^{99m}Tc will detect a "cold" nodule, indicating a nonfunctional thyroid area.
2. Ultrasound-guided fine needle aspiration (FNA) biopsy for diagnostics.
3. Surgical exploration.

Management

1. Surgical removal is extensive, as required.
   a. Postoperative radiation therapy is commonly done to reduce chances of recurrence.
   b. Radioactive iodine (RAI) therapy is administered after total thyroidectomy.
   c. Follow-up includes periodic ^{131}I uptake scan to detect evidence of recurrence along with following other laboratory tests.
2. Thyroid replacement.
   a. Thyroid hormone is administered to suppress secretion of TSH.
   b. Such treatment is continued indefinitely and requires annual checkups.
3. For unresectable cancer, patient is referred for treatment with ^{131}I, chemotherapy, or radiation therapy.

Complications

1. Untreated thyroid carcinoma can be fatal.
2. Removal of the thyroid can disrupt the parathyroid function; calcium levels need to be monitored.

Nursing Assessment

1. Explore risk factors such as exposure to radiation and family history.
2. Explore patient's feelings and concerns regarding the diagnosis, treatment, and prognosis.

Nursing Interventions

Also see "Care of the Patient Undergoing Thyroidectomy," section page 690.

Allaying Anxiety

1. Provide all explanations in a simple, concise manner, and repeat important information, as necessary, because anxiety may interfere with patient's processing of information.
2. Stress the positive aspects of treatment and high cure rate, as outlined by health care provider.
3. Encourage support by significant other, clergy, social worker, nursing staff, as available.

Patient Education and Health Maintenance

1. Instruct the patient on thyroid hormone replacement and follow-up blood tests.
2. Stress the need for periodic evaluation for recurrence of malignancy.
3. Supply additional information or suggest community resources dealing with cancer prevention and treatment.
4. Assist patient in identifying sources of information and support available in the community (see Box 20-1, page 700).

Evaluation: Expected Outcomes

- Discusses concerns with family, hospital, clergy.

DISORDERS OF THE PARATHYROID GLANDS

The *parathyroid glands* are small, pea-size glands embedded in the posterior section of the thyroid gland. Functions include the production, storage, and release of Parathyroid hormone (PTH) in response to the serum level of ionized calcium. PTH increases serum calcium by decreasing elimination of calcium ions in the urine by the kidney, increasing absorption of calcium ions from the gut, and increasing bone contribution of calcium ions to the plasma.

Hyperparathyroidism

Hyperparathyroidism is hypersecretion of PTH.

Pathophysiology and Etiology

1. Disorder is most common among post-menopausal females older than age 50.
2. Primary hyperparathyroidism.
   a. Single parathyroid adenoma is the most common cause (approximately 85% of cases).
   b. Parathyroid hyperplasia accounts for approximately 14% of cases.
   c. Parathyroid carcinoma accounts for less than 1% of cases.
   d. May present asymptomatic but can affect central nervous, cardiac, renal, and gastrointestinal (GI) systems.
3. Secondary hyperparathyroidism.
   a. Primarily the result of chronic kidney disease and renal failure.
4. Excess secretion of PTH results in increased serum calcium levels (see Figure 20-3).

Clinical Manifestations

1. May be asymptomatic with incidental elevated calcium and PTH.
2. Decalcification of bones.
   a. Skeletal pain, backache, pain on weight bearing, pathologic fractures, deformities, formation of bony cysts.
   b. Formation of bone tumors—overgrowth of osteoclasts.
   c. Formation of calcium-containing renal calculi.
3. Depression of neuromuscular function.
   a. The patient may trip, drop objects, show general fatigue, lose memory for recent events, experience emotional instability, have changes in level of consciousness, with stupor and coma.
   b. Cardiac arrhythmias, hypertension, cardiac standstill, palpations, bradycardia, changes in PR and QT intervals on electrocardiogram (ECG), fatigue, irritability.
4. Development of kidney stones.
5. Other signs and symptoms.
   a. Anorexia, nausea, constipation, polydipsia, polyuria, depression, acute pancreatitis, and proximal myopathy weakness.

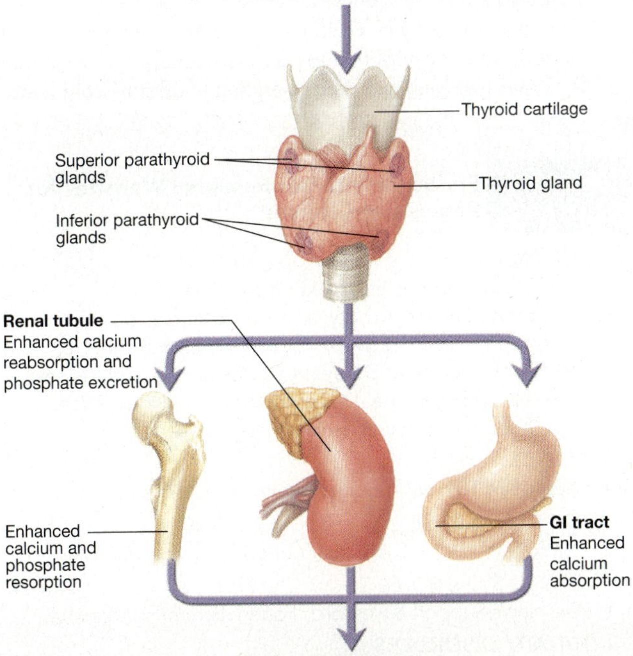

Figure 20-3. Pathogenesis of hyperparathyroidism. GI, gastrointestinal; PTH, parathyroid hormone. (Reprinted with permission from Stewart, J. G. [2017]. *Anatomical chart company atlas of pathophysiology* [4th ed.]. Lippincott Williams & Wilkins.)

Diagnostic Evaluation

1. Persistently elevated serum calcium (11 mg/100 mL); test is performed on at least two occasions to determine consistency of results and albumin level also obtained. If change in serum albumin or pH, ionized calcium is more accurate.
2. Exclusion of other causes of hypercalcemia—malignancy (usually bone or breast), vitamin D excess, multiple myeloma, sarcoidosis, milk-alkali syndrome, such drugs as thiazides, Cushing disease, hyperthyroidism.
3. PTH increased and alkaline phosphatase increased; phosphorus decreased.
4. Twenty-four–hour urine collection to evaluate kidney function.
5. Skeletal changes are revealed by x-ray or dual-energy x-ray absorptiometry (DEXA) test.
6. Cine computed tomography (CT) will disclose parathyroid tumors more readily than x-ray.
7. Sestamibi scan is used to evaluate location of the tumor prior to surgery.

Management

Treatment of Hypercalcemia

1. Hydration with intravenous (IV) saline, loop diuretics such as furosemide and ethacrynic acid—to increase urinary excretion of calcium in patients not in renal failure.
2. Oral phosphate may be used as an antihypercalcemic agent.
3. In patients developing osteoporosis, pamidronate, calcitonin, or etidronate disodium are effective in treating hypercalcemia by inhibiting bone resorption.
4. Dietary calcium is restricted, and all drugs that might cause hypercalcemia (thiazides, lithium, vitamin A&D, canagliflozin, hormone therapy, antacids) may be discontinued.
5. Dialysis may be necessary in patients with resistant hypercalcemia or those with renal failure.
6. Digoxin is reduced because the patient with hypercalcemia is more sensitive to toxic effects of this drug.
7. Monitoring of daily serum calcium, blood urea nitrogen (BUN), potassium, and magnesium levels.
8. Removal of underlying cause.
9. Calcimimetics are a new class of medications that can decrease PTH secretion.

Treatment of Primary Hyperparathyroidism

Surgery for removal of abnormal parathyroid tissue.

Complications

1. Formation of renal calculi, calcification of kidney parenchyma, renal shutdown.
2. Ulceration of upper GI tract, leading to hemorrhage and perforation.
3. Demineralization of bones, cysts, and fibrosis of marrow leads to fractures, especially of vertebral bodies and ribs.
4. Hypoparathyroidism after surgery.

Nursing Assessment

1. Obtain review of systems and perform multisystem examination to detect signs and symptoms of hyperparathyroidism.
2. Closely monitor patient's input and output and serum electrolytes, especially calcium level.
3. Monitor ECG to detect changes secondary to hypercalcemia. (During moderate elevations of serum calcium, QT interval is shortened; with extreme hypercalcemia, widening of the T wave is seen.)

Nursing Interventions

Achieving Fluid and Electrolyte Balance

1. Monitor fluid intake and output.
2. Provide adequate hydration—administer water, glucose, and electrolytes orally or via IV line, as prescribed.
3. Prevent or promptly treat dehydration by reporting vomiting or other sources of fluid loss.
4. Help patient understand why and how to avoid dietary sources of calcium—dairy products, broccoli, calcium-containing antacids.

Promoting Urinary Elimination

1. Strain all urine to observe for calculi.
2. Increase fluid intake to 3,000 mL/day to maintain hydration and prevent precipitation of calcium and formation of calculi.
3. Instruct patient about dietary recommendations for restriction of calcium.
4. Observe for signs of urinary tract infection (UTI), hematuria, and renal colic.
5. Assess renal function through serum creatinine and BUN levels.

Increasing Physical Mobility

1. Assist patient in hygiene and activities if bone pain is severe or if patient experiences musculoskeletal weakness.
2. Protect patient from falls or injury.
3. Turn patient cautiously and handle extremities gently to avoid fractures.
4. Administer analgesia, as prescribed.
5. Assess level of pain and patient's response to analgesia.
6. Encourage patient to participate in mild exercise gradually as symptoms subside.
7. Instruct and demonstrate correct body mechanics to reduce strain, backache, and injury.

Relieving Anxiety

1. Encourage patient to verbalize fears and feelings about upcoming surgery.
2. Explain tests and procedures to patient.
3. Reassure patient about skeletal recovery.
   a. Bone pain diminishes fairly quickly.
   b. Fractures are treated by orthopedic procedures.
4. Prepare patient for surgery as for thyroidectomy (see page 690).

Patient Education and Health Maintenance

1. Instruct patient about calcium-reducing medications.
   a. Calcitonin is given subcutaneously—teach proper technique.
   b. Etidronate disodium—calcium-rich foods should be avoided within 2 hours of dose; therapeutic response may take 1 to 3 months.
   c. Pamidronate—monitor hypercalcemia-related parameters when treatment begins. Adequate intake of calcium and vitamin D is necessary to prevent hypocalcemia. Bisphosphonates should be used with caution in patients with active upper GI problems.
2. Teach signs and symptoms of tetany that patient may experience postoperatively and should report to health care provider (numbness and tingling in extremities or around mouth).
3. Assist patient in identifying sources of information and support available in the community (see Box 20-1, page 700).

Evaluation: Expected Outcomes

- Output equals intake, normal skin turgor, moist mucous membranes.
- No signs and symptoms of renal calculi or UTI; serum creatinine and BUN levels normal.
- Reports less bone and joint pain; uses correct body mechanics, avoid immobilization.
- Verbalizes concerns and fears about surgery; appears less anxious.

Hypoparathyroidism

Hypoparathyroidism is a rare endocrine disorder that results from a deficiency of PTH and is characterized by hypocalcemia and neuromuscular hyperexcitability.

Pathophysiology and Etiology

1. The most common cause is accidental removal or destruction of parathyroid tissue or its blood supply during thyroidectomy or radical neck dissection for malignancy.
2. Decrease in gland function (idiopathic hypoparathyroidism); may be autoimmune or familial in origin.
3. Malignancy or metastasis from a cancer to the parathyroid glands.
4. Genetic causes include DiGeorge Syndrome, autoimmune polyendocrine syndrome type I, autosomal dominant hypocalcemia.
5. Resistance to PTH action.
6. With inadequate PTH secretion, there is decreased resorption of calcium from the renal tubules, decreased absorption of calcium in the GI tract, and decreased resorption of calcium from bone.

Box 20-1 Endocrine Internet Resource Websites for Patients and Nurses

GENERAL
- The Endocrine Society: *www.endocrine.org*
- Endocrine Nurses Society: *www.endo-nurses.org*
- Hormone Health Network: *https://www.hormone.org/*
- National Institute of Diabetes and Digestive and Kidney Diseases—Endocrine Diseases: *https://www.niddk.nih.gov/health-information/endocrine-diseases*

THYROID
- American Thyroid Association: *www.thyroid.org*

ADDISON DISEASE
- National Adrenal Diseases Foundation: *www.nadf.us*

CUSHING SYNDROME
- Cushing's Support & Research Foundation: *https://csrf.net/*

PITUITARY DISORDERS
- Pituitary Network Association: *https://pituitary.org/* Pituitary Foundation: *https://www.pituitary.org.uk/*

7. Blood calcium falls to a low level, causing symptoms of muscular hyperirritability, uncontrolled spasms, and hypocalcemic tetany.
8. In response to decreased serum calcium levels and lack of PTH, the serum phosphate level rises, and phosphate excretion by the kidneys decreases.

Clinical Manifestations

1. Neuromuscular irritability: laryngeal spasm, bronchospasm, muscle cramps, paresthesias, seizures.
2. Tetany—general muscular hypertonia; attempts at voluntary movement result in tremors and spasmodic or uncoordinated movements; fingers assume classic tetanic position; Chvostek and Trousseau signs (see page 690).
3. Neurologic signs and symptoms such as extrapyramidal signs, personality disturbances, irritability, parkinsonism, dystonic spasms.
4. Mental status changes: confusion, psychosis, fatigue, anxiety, poor memory.
5. Ectodermal changes: dry skin, brittle nails, coarse hair, atopic eczema, psoriasis.
6. Cardiac changes: ECG with prolonged QT interval, congestive heart failure, cardiomyopathy.
7. Renal dysfunction: kidney stones, chronic kidney disease.
8. Ophthalmologic changes: subcapsular cataracts, papilledema.

Diagnostic Evaluation

1. Decrease in serum calcium level to a low level (7.5 mg/100 mL or less).
2. Phosphorus level in blood is elevated.
3. May have concurrent hypomagnesemia and/or vitamin D deficiency.
4. Pseudohypocalcemia—total serum calcium level is low, but serum ionized calcium is normal. This is due to calcium binding to protein.
5. PTH levels are low in most cases; may be normal or elevated in pseudohypoparathyroidism.
6. In chronic hypoparathyroidism, bone density may be increased as seen on radiography.
7. Genetic studies may be indicated in those patients who did not have neck surgery, are younger, and have other endocrine abnormalities.

Management

IV Calcium Administration

1. A syringe and an ampule of a calcium solution (calcium chloride, calcium gluceptate, calcium gluconate) are to be kept at the bedside at all times.
2. Most rapidly effective calcium solution is ionized calcium chloride (10%).
3. For rapid use to relieve severe tetany, infusion carried out every 10 minutes.
   a. All IV calcium preparations are administered slowly. It is highly irritating, stings, and causes thrombosis; patient experiences unpleasant burning flush of skin and tongue.
   b. Typical doses are as follows:
      i. Calcium chloride—500 mg to 1 g (5 to 10 mL) as indicated by serum calcium; administer at rate of less than 1 mL/min of 10% solution.
      ii. Calcium gluconate—500 mg to 2 g (10 to 20 mL) at a rate of less than 0.5 mL/min of a 10% solution.
      iii. Calcium gluceptate—1 to 2 g (5 to 10 mL) at a rate of less than 1 mL/min.
4. A slow drip of IV saline containing calcium gluconate is given until control of tetany is ensured; then, IM or oral administration of calcium is prescribed.
5. Later, vitamin D is added to calcium intake—increases absorption of calcium and also induces a high level of calcium in the bloodstream. Thiazide diuretics may also be added because of their calcium-retaining effect on the kidney; doses of calcium and vitamin D may be lowered.
6. Administration of IV calcium seems to cause rapid relief of anxiety.

DRUG ALERT Too rapid calcium administration may cause cardiac arrest.

Other Measures

1. Treat renal calculi.
2. Monitor patient for hypercalciuria.
3. Monitor blood calcium level periodically; variations in vitamin D may affect calcium levels.

Complications

1. Acute complications related to hypocalcemia include seizures, tetany, and mental disorders, all of which can be reversed with calcium therapy.
2. If onset of hypocalcemia is acute, the major concerns are laryngeal spasm, acute airway obstruction, and cardiovascular failure.
3. Long-term complications include subcapsular cataracts, calcification of the basal ganglia, and papilledema (caused by precipitation of calcium out of serum and deposition in tissue); shortening of the fingers and toes; and bowing of the long bones (caused by inadequate PTH and additional genetic abnormalities). Of these complications, only papilledema is reversible.

Nursing Assessment

1. Perform multisystem assessment, focusing on neuromuscular system.
2. Closely monitor patient's input and output and serum electrolytes, especially calcium level.
3. Assess anxiety.

Nursing Interventions

Maintaining Normal Serum Calcium Levels

1. Assess neuromuscular status frequently in patients with hypoparathyroidism and in those at risk for hypocalcemia (patients in the immediate postoperative period after thyroidectomy, parathyroidectomy, radical neck dissection).
2. Check for Trousseau and Chvostek signs, and notify health care provider if test results are positive.
3. Assess respiratory status frequently in acute hypocalcemia and postoperatively.
4. Monitor serum calcium and phosphorus levels.
5. Promote high-calcium diet, if prescribed—dairy products; green, leafy vegetables.
6. Instruct the patient about signs and symptoms of hypo—and hypercalcemia that should be reported.

7. Use caution in administering other drugs to the patient with hypocalcemia.
   a. The patient who is hypocalcemic is sensitive to digoxin; as hypocalcemia is reversed, the patient may rapidly develop digoxin toxicity.
   b. Cimetidine interferes with normal parathyroid function, especially with renal failure, which increases the risk of hypocalcemia.

Patient Education and Health Maintenance

1. Explain to patient and family the function of PTH and the roles of vitamin D and calcium in maintaining good health.
2. Discuss the importance of each medication prescribed for the control of hypocalcemia, including vitamin D, calcium, and thiazide diuretic.
   a. Take medications, as prescribed.
   b. Do not substitute with over-the-counter preparations without the advice and supervision of the health care provider.
3. Provide patient with a written list about hypercalcemia and hypocalcemia, and advise the patient to contact the health care provider immediately should signs of either condition develop.
4. Advise patient to wear a medical alert tag.
5. Explain the need for periodic medical follow-up for life.

Evaluation: Expected Outcome

- Verbalizes understanding of diet and medications; calcium level within normal limits.

DISORDERS OF THE ADRENAL GLANDS

The *adrenal medulla,* or inner portion of the gland, is not necessary to maintain life but enables a person to cope with stress. It secretes two hormones:

- *Epinephrine* (adrenalin) acts on alpha and beta receptors to increase contractility and excitability of heart muscle, leading to increased cardiac output; facilitates blood flow to muscles, brain, and viscera; enhances blood sugar by stimulating conversion of glycogen to glucose in the liver; and inhibits smooth muscle contraction.
- *Norepinephrine* (noradrenaline) acts primarily on alpha receptors to increase peripheral vascular resistance, leading to increases in diastolic and systolic blood pressure (BP).
  - The adrenal cortex, or outer portion of the gland, is essential to life. It secretes adrenocortical hormones—synthesized from cholesterol.
- *Glucocorticoids* (cortisone and hydrocortisone) enhance protein catabolism and inhibit protein synthesis; antagonize action of insulin and increase blood sugar; increase synthesis of glucose by the liver; influence defense mechanism of the body and its reaction to stress; and influence emotional reaction.
- *Mineralocorticoids* (aldosterone and desoxycorticosterone) regulate reabsorption of sodium; regulate excretion of potassium by renal tubules.
- *Adrenosterones* (adrenal androgens) exert minimal effect on sex characteristics and function.

Primary Aldosteronism

Primary aldosteronism refers to excessive secretion of aldosterone by the adrenal cortex.

Pathophysiology and Etiology

1. Excessive secretion of aldosterone results in the conservation of sodium and excretion of potassium, primarily, not only in the renal tubules but also in the sweat glands, salivary glands, and gastrointestinal (GI) tract.
2. Caused primarily by a cortical adenoma, bilateral adrenal hyperplasia, or genetic–familial primary aldosteronism.
3. Secondary aldosteronism occurs in conjunction with heart failure, renal dysfunction, or cirrhosis of the liver.
4. Females constitute 70% of patients with aldosterone-secreting adenomas, and the incidence of primary aldosteronism is four times higher among African Americans than among the general population.

Clinical Manifestations

1. Hypertension (5% to 15% of cases of hypertension are a result of primary aldosteronism, which can usually be treated successfully by surgical removal of the adenoma).
2. A profound decline in blood levels of potassium (hypokalemia) and hydrogen ions (alkalosis) results in muscle weakness and inability of kidneys to acidify or concentrate urine, leading to excess volume of urine (polyuria).
3. A decline in hydrogen ions (alkalosis) results in tetany, paresthesia.
4. An elevation in blood sodium (hypernatremia) results in excessive thirst (polydipsia) and arterial hypertension.

Diagnostic Evaluation

1. Suspected in all patients who are hypertensive with spontaneous hypokalemia; also if hypokalemia develops concurrently with start of diuretics and remains after diuretics are discontinued.
2. The screening test of choice is the aldosterone/renin ratio, which is suggestive of primary aldosteronism if the ratio is greater than 20:1.
3. Serum potassium and estimated glomerular filtration rate (eGFR) are important baseline tests.
4. Salt loading may be used as a confirmatory test—ingestion of at least 200 mEq/day (approximately 12 g salt) for 4 days does not influence the serum potassium level without aldosteronism but will cause a decrease in serum potassium to less than 3.5 mEq/L in a patient with aldosteronism.
5. Computed tomography (CT) scanning to determine and localize cortical adenoma.

Management

1. Laparoscopic adrenalectomy if the tumor is localized to one side—unilateral adrenalectomy.
2. If the cause is bilateral adrenal hyperplasia—spironolactone is used to treat both hypertension and potassium-depleted stages; therapy is needed 4 to 6 weeks before the full effect on BP is seen.
   a. Adverse effects include reduced testosterone in males (decreased libido, impotence, gynecomastia) and GI discomfort.
   b. Amiloride may be used instead in sexually active males or in cases of GI intolerance.
   c. Sodium restriction is necessary—no saline infusions, low-sodium diet.
   d. Potassium supplementation is usually necessary, based on severity of deficit.

3. Addition of antihypertensive agent—thiazide diuretic such as triamterene.
4. Management of underlying causes of secondary aldosteronism.

Complications

Long-term effects of untreated hypertension—stroke, renal failure, heart failure.

Nursing Assessment

1. Obtain history of symptoms, such as muscle weakness, paresthesia, thirst, and polyuria.
2. Perform multisystem physical examination.
3. Evaluate BP.

Nursing Interventions

Also see "Care of the Patient Undergoing Adrenalectomy," section page 691.

Maintaining Normal Fluid and Sodium Balance

1. Monitor fluid intake and output, daily weight, electrocardiogram (ECG) changes for hypokalemia.
2. Teach low-sodium diet, administration of potassium supplements, as ordered; evaluate serum sodium and potassium results.
3. Monitor BP; administer or teach self-administration of antihypertensives, as ordered.
4. Assess for dependent edema; encourage activity, frequent repositioning, and elevation of feet periodically.

Patient Education and Health Maintenance

1. Instruct patient about the nature of illness, the necessary treatment, and the need for continued medical care after discharge.
2. Instruct patient on the importance of following prescribed medical treatments.
   a. For medical management, patient must remain on spironolactone for life.
   b. Patient should report significant adverse effects that interfere with sexual performance and quality of life.
   c. Glucocorticoid administration may be temporary after subtotal or unilateral adrenalectomy, chronic for bilateral adrenalectomy; dose may need to be increased during times of illness or stress.
3. Teach patient and family members how to take BP readings, if indicated.

Evaluation: Expected Outcomes

- Intake equals urine output, daily weight stable.

Cushing Syndrome

Cushing syndrome is a condition in which the plasma cortisol levels are elevated, causing signs and symptoms of hypercortisolism.

Pathophysiology and Etiology

1. Is more common in females than in males.
2. The normal feedback mechanisms that control adrenocortical function are ineffective, resulting in secretion of adrenal cortical hormones despite adequate amounts of these hormones in the circulation.
3. The manifestations of Cushing syndrome are the result of excess hormones (glucocorticoids).
4. Excess of one hormone or all the hormones can occur; the predominant hormone secreted in excess (usually, glucocorticoids) determines the predominant symptoms.
5. Pituitary Cushing syndrome (Cushing disease)—hyperplasia of both adrenal glands caused by overstimulation of the adrenal cortex by adrenocorticotropic hormone (ACTH), usually from a pituitary adenoma or hyperplasia.
   a. Most common cause of Cushing syndrome.
   b. Affects mostly females between ages 20 and 40.
6. Adrenal Cushing syndrome.
   a. Associated with tumors of the adrenal cortex—adenoma or carcinoma.
7. Ectopic—results from autonomous ACTH secretion by extrapituitary neoplasms (such as lung).
8. Iatrogenic Cushing syndrome caused by exogenous glucocorticoid administration.

Clinical Manifestations

Manifestations Caused by Excess Glucocorticoids

1. Weight gain or obesity (see Figure 20-4).
2. Heavy trunk; thin extremities.
3. "Buffalo hump" (fat pad) in neck and supraclavicular area.

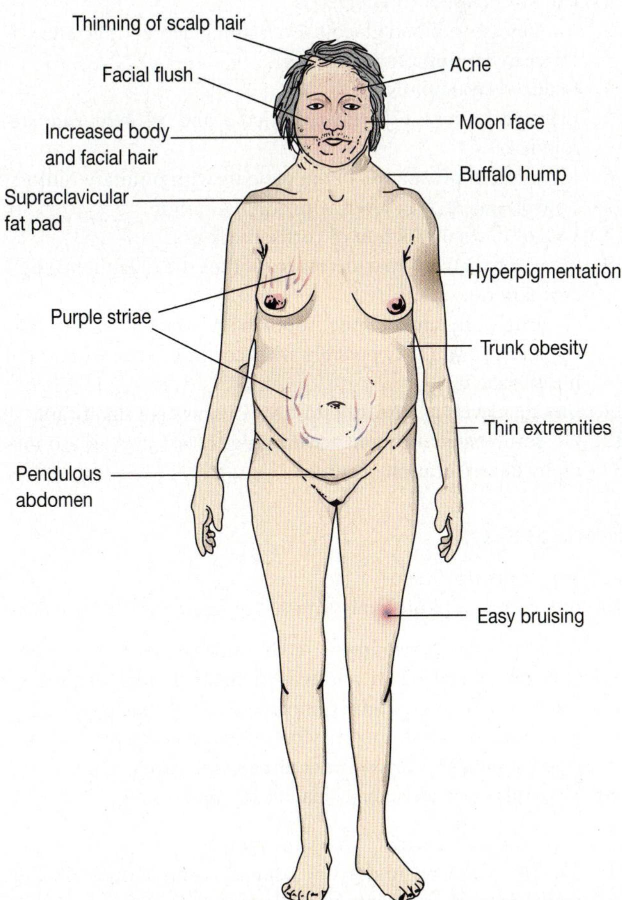

Figure 20-4. Clinical manifestations of Cushing syndrome. (Reprinted with permission from Smeltzer, S., & Bare, B. [2000]. *Brunner and Suddarth's textbook of medical–surgical nursing* [9th ed.]. Lippincott Williams & Wilkins.)

4. Rounded face (moon face); plethoric, oily.
5. Fragile and thin skin, striae and ecchymosis, acne.
6. Muscles wasted because of excessive catabolism.
7. Osteoporosis—characteristic kyphosis, backache.
8. Mental disturbances—mood changes, psychosis.
9. Increased susceptibility to infections.

Manifestations Caused by Excess Mineralocorticoids

1. Hypertension.
2. Hypernatremia, hypokalemia.
3. Weight gain.
4. Expanded blood volume.
5. Edema.

Manifestations Caused by Excess Androgens

1. Females experience virilism (masculinization).
   a. Hirsutism—excessive growth of hair on the face and midline of the trunk.
   b. Breasts—atrophy.
   c. Clitoris—enlargement.
   d. Voice—masculine.
   e. Loss of libido.
2. If exposed in utero—possible hermaphrodite.
3. Males—loss of libido.

Diagnostic Evaluation

1. Excessive plasma cortisol levels.
2. An increase in blood glucose levels and glucose intolerance.
3. Decreased serum potassium level.
4. Reduced eosinophils.
5. Elevated urinary 17-hydroxycorticoid and 17-ketogenic steroid levels.
6. Elevation of plasma ACTH in patients with pituitary tumors.
7. Low plasma ACTH levels with adrenal tumor.
8. Loss of diurnal variation of cortisol secretion.
9. X-rays of the skull may detect erosion of the sella turcica by a pituitary tumor.
10. Overnight dexamethasone suppression test (DST) or 48-hour low-dose DST, possibly with cortisol urinary excretion measurement.
11. Elevated levels of cortisol measured in saliva are significant.
12. CT scan, magnetic resonance imaging (MRI), and ultrasonography detect location of tumor.

Management

Surgery and Radiation

Tumor (adrenal or pituitary) is removed or treated with irradiation.

1. An important development in the management of pituitary Cushing syndrome in adults is transsphenoidal adenomectomy or hypophysectomy (pituitary removal) (see page 692).
2. Transfrontal craniotomy may be necessary when pituitary tumor has enlarged beyond sella turcica (see page 692).
3. Hyperplasia of adrenals—bilateral adrenalectomy.

Replacement Therapy Postoperatively

1. Patients who have undergone adrenalectomy require lifelong replacement therapy with the following:
   a. A glucocorticoid—cortisone.
   b. A mineralocorticoid—fludrocortisone.
2. After pituitary irradiation or hypophysectomy, patient may require adrenal replacement, plus thyroid, posterior pituitary, and gonadal replacement therapy.
3. After transsphenoidal adenomectomy, patient requires hydrocortisone replacement therapy for periods of 12 to 18 months and additional hormones if excessive loss of pituitary function has occurred.
4. Protein anabolic steroids may be given to facilitate protein replacement; potassium replacement is usually required.

Medical Treatment

1. If patients cannot undergo surgery, cortisol synthesis–inhibiting medications may be used.
   a. Mitotane, an agent toxic to the adrenal cortex (dichlorodiphenyltrichloroethane derivative)—known as medical adrenalectomy. Nausea, vomiting, diarrhea, somnolence, and depression may occur with use of this drug.
   b. Metyrapone to control steroid hypersecretion in patients who do not respond to mitotane therapy.
   c. Aminoglutethimide blocks cholesterol conversion to pregnenolone, effectively blocking cortisol production. Adverse effects include GI disturbances, somnolence, and skin rashes.

Complications

Possibility of recurrence in patients with adrenal carcinoma.

Nursing Assessment

1. Observe patient for signs and symptoms of Cushing disease.
2. Perform multisystem physical examination.
3. Monitor intake and output, daily weights, and serum electrolytes.

Nursing Interventions

Maintaining Skin Integrity

1. Assess skin frequently to detect reddened areas, breakdown or tearing of skin, excoriation, infection, or edema.
2. Handle skin and extremities gently to prevent trauma; protect from falls by use of side rails.
3. Avoid use of adhesive tape to reduce risk of trauma to skin on its removal.
4. Encourage patient to turn in bed frequently or to ambulate to reduce pressure on bony prominences and areas of edema.
5. Use meticulous skin care to reduce injury and breakdown.
6. Provide foods low in sodium to minimize edema formation.
7. Assess intake and output and daily weight to evaluate fluid retention.

Encouraging Active Participation in Self-Care

1. Assist patient with ambulation and hygiene when weak and fatigued.
2. Assist patient in planning schedule to permit exercise and rest.
3. Encourage patient to rest when fatigued.
4. Encourage gradual resumption of activities as patient gains strength.
5. Identify for patient the signs and symptoms indicating excessive exertion.
6. Instruct patient in correct body mechanics to avoid pain or injury during activities.
7. Use assistive devices during ambulation to prevent falls and fractures.
8. Encourage foods high in potassium (bananas, orange juice, tomatoes), and administer potassium supplement, as prescribed, to counteract weakness related to hypokalemia.

Strengthening Body Image

1. Encourage patient to verbalize concerns about illness, changes in appearance, and altered role functions.
2. Identify situations that are disturbing to patient, and explore with patient ways to avoid or modify those situations.
3. Be alert for evidence of depression; in some instances, this has progressed to suicide; alert health care provider of mood changes, sleep disturbance, change in activity level, change in appetite, or loss of interest in visitors or other experiences.
4. Refer for counseling, if indicated.
5. Explain to patient who has benign adenoma or hyperplasia that, with proper treatment, evidence of masculinization can be reversed.

Reducing Anxiety

1. Answer questions about surgery and encourage thorough discussion with health care provider if patient is not well informed.
2. Describe nursing care to expect in postoperative period.
3. Prepare the patient for abdominal surgery (see page 512) or hypophysectomy (see page 709) as indicated.

Providing Postoperative Care

1. Provide routine postoperative care for patient with abdominal surgery (see page 512) or hypophysectomy (see page 709).
2. Monitor closely for infection because glucocorticoid administration interferes with immune function; maintain sterile technique, clean environment, and good handwashing.
3. Monitor thyroid function tests and provide hormone replacement therapy (HRT), as ordered, after hypophysectomy.
4. Monitor fluid intake and output and urine specific gravity to detect diabetes insipidus (DI) caused by antidiuretic hormone (ADH) deficiency after hypophysectomy.

Patient Education and Health Maintenance

1. Instruct patient on lifetime HRT and the need to follow up at regular intervals to determine if dosage is appropriate or to detect adverse effects.
2. Instruct patient in proper skin care and in the prompt reporting of trauma or infection for medical treatment.
3. Teach patient to monitor urine or blood glucose or to report for blood glucose tests, as directed, to detect hyperglycemia.
4. Help patient prevent hyperglycemia and obesity by teaching about a low-calorie, low-concentrated carbohydrate, and low-fat diet and to increase activity, as tolerated.
5. Encourage diet high in calcium (dairy products, broccoli) and weight-bearing activity to prevent osteoporosis caused by glucocorticoid replacement.
6. Assist patient in identifying sources of information and support available in the community (see Box 20-1, page 700).

Evaluation: Expected Outcomes

- Skin intact without evidence of breakdown, excoriation, infection, or trauma.
- Participates safely in activities of daily living (ADLs).
- Verbalizes concerns about appearance, interacts well with visitors.
- Verbalizes understanding of surgery.
- Vital signs stable, pain controlled, no signs of infection.

Adrenocortical Insufficiency

Adrenocortical insufficiency occurs with inadequate secretion of the hormones of the adrenal cortex, primarily, the glucocorticoids and mineralocorticoids.

Pathophysiology and Etiology

1. Acquired primary adrenocortical insufficiency (Addison disease)—destruction and subsequent hypofunction of the adrenal cortex, usually caused by autoimmune process. Addison disease is a rare but potentially life-threatening endocrine disorder.
2. Secondary adrenocortical insufficiency—ACTH deficiency from pituitary disease or suppression of hypothalamic–pituitary axis by corticosteroid treatment for nonendocrine disorders causes atrophy of the adrenal cortex.
3. Inadequate aldosterone produces disturbances of sodium, potassium, and water metabolism.
4. Cortisol deficiency produces abnormal fat, protein, and carbohydrate metabolism; no cortisol during a period of stress can precipitate addisonian crisis, an exaggerated state of adrenal cortical insufficiency, and can lead to death.

Clinical Manifestations

1. Clinical manifestations may be insidious and gradual; thus, diagnosis is often delayed until the patient presents in an acute crisis.
2. Hyponatremia, hyperkalemia, and in some cases, anemia.
3. Water loss, dehydration, and hypovolemia.
4. Muscular weakness, fatigue, weight loss.
5. GI problems—anorexia, nausea, vomiting, diarrhea, constipation, abdominal pain.
6. Hypotension, hypoglycemia, low basal metabolic rate, increased insulin sensitivity.
7. Mental changes—depression, irritability, anxiety, apprehension caused by hypoglycemia and hypovolemia.
8. Normal responses to stress lacking.
9. Hyperpigmentation.

Diagnostic Evaluation

1. Blood chemistry—decreased glucose and sodium; increased potassium, calcium, and blood urea nitrogen (BUN) levels.
2. Increased lymphocytes on complete blood count.
3. Low fasting plasma cortisol levels; low aldosterone levels.
4. Twenty-four–hour urine studies—decreased 17-ketosteroid, 17-hydroxycorticoid, and 17-ketogenic steroid levels.
5. ACTH stimulation test—no rise or minimal rise in plasma cortisol and urinary 17-ketosteroid levels.
6. Increased plasma renin activity.
7. In suspected adrenal hemorrhages, an abdominal scan may provide useful information.

Management

1. Restoration of normal fluid and electrolyte balance: high-sodium, low-potassium diet and fluids.
2. Treatment of glucocorticoid deficiency with such agents as hydrocortisone or prednisone. Patients with chronic obstructive pulmonary disease and heart failure may require preparations with low mineralocorticoid activity, such as methylprednisolone, to prevent fluid retention.
3. Mineralocorticoid deficiency is treated with fludrocortisone.
4. Cardiovascular support, if indicated.
5. Immediate treatment if addisonian (adrenal) crisis or circulatory collapse is imminent:
   a. Intravenous (IV) sodium chloride solution to replace sodium ions.
   b. Hydrocortisone.
   c. Injection of circulatory stimulants, such as atropine sulfate, calcium chloride, epinephrine.

6. Diagnosis and treatment of underlying cause of adrenocortical insufficiency or addisonian crisis (e.g., antibiotic therapy to treat infection if this is a factor in crisis).
7. Overtreatment may be manifested by hypertension, edema from sodium and water retention, and weakness caused by potassium loss.

Complications

1. Adrenal crisis—hypotension, nausea, vomiting, weakness, lethargy, fever, confusion, acute abdomen, and possibly coma.
2. May be precipitated by physiologic stress, such as surgery, infection, trauma, dehydration.

Nursing Assessment

1. Obtain recent or past history of corticosteroid therapy, including length of treatment, dosage, and adherence.
2. Review history for sources of stress, such as surgical procedures, infection, or development of other illness.

Perform thorough physical examination for manifestations of adrenocortical insufficiency or contributing factors.

Nursing Interventions

Achieving Normal Fluid and Electrolyte Balance

1. Assess fluid intake and output and serial daily weights.
2. Monitor vital signs frequently; a drop in BP may suggest an impending crisis.
3. Monitor results of serum sodium and potassium.
4. Assess skin turgor and mucous membranes for dehydration.
5. Encourage diet high in sodium and fluid content; administer or teach self-administration of potassium supplements, if prescribed.
6. Administer or teach self-administration of prescribed glucocorticoids and mineralocorticoids; document response.
7. Administer IV infusions of sodium, water, and glucose, as indicated.

Protecting Well-Being

1. Minimize stressful situations.
2. Protect patient from infection.
   a. Control patient's contacts so that infectious organisms are not transmitted.
   b. Protect patient from drafts, dampness, exposure to cold.
   c. Prevent overexertion.
   d. Use meticulous handwashing and sterile techniques.
3. Assess comfort and emotional status of patient.
   a. Control the temperature of the room to avoid sharp deviations in patient's temperature.
   b. Maintain a quiet, peaceful environment; avoid loud talking and noisy radios.
4. Observe and report early signs of addisonian crisis (sudden drop in BP, nausea and vomiting, fever).

Increasing Activity Tolerance

1. Assist the patient with ADLs.
2. Provide for periods of rest and activity to avoid overexertion.
3. Provide for high-calorie, high-protein diet.

Patient Education and Health Maintenance

1. Instruct patient about the necessity for long-term therapy for adrenocortical insufficiency and medical follow-up visits.
   a. Inform patient that therapy must be continued throughout their life.
   b. Emphasize the importance of taking more hormones when under stress.
   c. Suggest that patient carry an identification card that indicates the type of medication being taken and health care provider's telephone number.
2. Educate patient about manifestations of excessive use of medications and reportable symptoms.
3. Identify actions to take to avoid factors that may precipitate addisonian crisis (infection, extremes of temperature, trauma).
4. Assist patient in identifying sources of information and support available in the community (see Box 20-1, page 700).

Evaluation: Expected Outcomes

- Normal skin turgor, moist mucous membranes, stable vital signs.
- No signs of infection or stress.
- Completes daily activities with minimal assistance.

Pheochromocytoma

Pheochromocytoma is a rare catecholamine-secreting neoplasm associated with hyperfunction of the adrenal medulla. It may appear wherever chromaffin cells are located; however, most are found in the adrenal medulla.

Pathophysiology and Etiology

1. Pheochromocytoma can occur at any age but is most common between the ages of 30 and 60; it is uncommon in people older than age 65.
2. Males and females are affected equally.
3. Most pheochromocytoma tumors are benign; 10% are malignant with metastasis into bone, liver, and lymph nodes.
4. Thirty-five percent of extra-adrenal pheochromocytomas are malignant.
5. Tumors located in the adrenal medulla produce both increased epinephrine and norepinephrine; those located outside the adrenal gland tend to produce epinephrine only.
6. May occur as component of multiple endocrine neoplasia IIA, an autosomal dominant syndrome characterized by pheochromocytoma, thyroid cancer, and hyperparathyroidism.

Clinical Manifestations

1. Variation in signs and symptoms depends on the predominance of norepinephrine or epinephrine secretion and on whether secretion is continuous or intermittent.
2. Excess secretion of norepinephrine and epinephrine produces hypertension, hypermetabolism, and hyperglycemia.
3. Hypertension may be paroxysmal (intermittent) or persistent (chronic).
   a. Chronic form mimics essential hypertension; however, antihypertensives are not effective.
   b. Headaches and vision disturbances are common.
4. The hypermetabolic and hyperglycemic effects produce excessive perspiration, tremor, pallor or face flushing, nervousness, elevated blood glucose levels, polyuria, nausea, vomiting, diarrhea, abdominal pain, and paresthesia.
5. Emotional changes, including psychotic behavior, may occur.
6. Symptoms may be triggered by allergic reactions, physical exertion, or emotional upset or may occur without identifiable stimulus.

Diagnostic Evaluation

1. Plasma fractionated or 24-hour urine metanephrine (metabolites of epinephrine and norepinephrine) are elevated.

2. Epinephrine and norepinephrine in urine and blood are elevated while patient is symptomatic.
3. CT scan and MRI of the adrenal glands or of the entire abdomen are done to identify tumor.
4. Nuclear medicine functional imaging.

Management

Medical Control of BP and Preparation for Surgery

1. Alpha-adrenergic blocking agents, such as phentolamine or phenoxybenzamine, inhibit the effects of catecholamines on BP.
   a. Effective control of BP and blood volume may take 1 or 2 weeks.
   b. Surgery is delayed until BP is controlled and blood volume has been expanded.
2. Catecholamine synthesis inhibitors, such as metyrosine, may be used preoperatively or for long-term management of inoperable tumors.
   a. Adverse effects include sedation and crystalluria.

Surgery

Unilateral or bilateral adrenalectomy or other tumor removal.

Complications

Metastasis of tumor.

Nursing Assessment

1. Obtain history of signs and symptoms patient has been experiencing.
2. Assess for predisposing factors that may be triggering signs and symptoms (i.e., physical exertion, emotional upset, allergies).
3. Perform thorough physical examination to determine effects of hypertension.

Nursing Interventions

Reducing Anxiety

1. Remain with patient during acute episodes of hypertension.
2. Ensure bed rest and elevate the head of bed 45 degrees during severe hypertension.
3. Carry out tasks and procedures in calm, unhurried manner when with patient.
4. Instruct patient about use of relaxation exercises.
5. Reduce environmental stressors by providing calm, quiet environment. Restrict visitors.
6. Eliminate stimulants (coffee, tea, cola) from the diet.
7. Reduce events that precipitate episodes of severe hypertension—palpation of the tumor, physical exertion, emotional upset.
8. Administer sedatives, as prescribed, to promote relaxation and rest.
9. Monitor for orthostatic hypotension after administration of phentolamine.
10. Encourage oral fluids and maintain IV infusion preoperatively to ensure adequate volume expansion going into surgery.

Maintaining Tissue Perfusion Postoperatively

1. Monitor vital signs, ECG, arterial BP, neurologic status, and urine output closely postoperatively.
2. Assess for and report complications of hypertension, hypotension, and hyperglycemia.
3. Maintain adequate hydration with IV infusion to prevent hypotension. (Because reduction of catecholamines immediately postoperatively causes vasodilation and enlargement of vascular space, hypotension may occur.)
4. Monitor intake and output and laboratory results for BUN, creatinine, and glucose levels.

Patient Education and Health Maintenance

1. Instruct patient how and when to take medications. Warn patients taking metyrosine of sedation and need to avoid taking other central nervous system (CNS) depressants and participating in activities that require alertness; need to increase fluid intake to at least 2,000 mL/day to prevent renal calculi.
2. Inform patient regarding the need for continued follow-up for:
   a. Recurrence of pheochromocytoma.
   b. Assessment of any residual renal or cardiovascular injury related to preoperative hypertension.
   c. Documentation that catecholamine levels are normal 1 to 3 months postoperatively (by 24-hour urine test).
3. Help patient identify sources of information and support available in the community (see Box 20-1, page 700).

Evaluation: Expected Outcomes

- Reports less anxiety during hypertensive episodes.
- BP stable, adequate urine output.

DISORDERS OF THE PITUITARY GLAND

The pituitary gland (hypophysis) exerts prime control over the body's hormonal functions. It is located in the sella turcica at the base of the brain. Its function is regulated by the hypothalamus. The pituitary consists of two parts that are structurally and functionally separate: the anterior pituitary and the posterior pituitary. Hypothalamic control of the anterior pituitary is mediated by releasing factors secreted by the hypothalamus; the posterior pituitary is regulated through direct neural stimulation. See Table 20-2 for hormones of the pituitary gland.

Diabetes Insipidus

Diabetes insipidus (DI) is a rare disorder of water metabolism caused by deficiency of antidiuretic hormone (ADH), also called vasopressin, secreted by the posterior pituitary (central DI) or by inability of the kidneys to respond to ADH (nephrogenic DI). Prevalence is 1 in 25,000 individuals and affects males and females equally at any age.

Table 20-2 Hormones of the Pituitary Gland

HORMONE	TARGET TISSUE
Anterior Pituitary	
Growth hormone	Multiple sites
Thyroid-stimulating hormone	Thyroid gland
Adrenocorticotropic hormone	Adrenal glands
Prolactin	Breasts
Luteinizing hormone	Ovaries, testes
Follicle-stimulating hormone	Ovaries, testes
Melanocyte-stimulating hormone	Melanocytes (skin)
Posterior Pituitary	
Oxytocin	Uterus, breasts
Antidiuretic hormone	Kidneys

Pathophysiology and Etiology

1. Primary: idiopathic.
2. Secondary: head trauma, neurosurgery, tumors (intracranial or metastatic), vascular disease (aneurysms, infarct), infection (meningitis, encephalitis).
3. Nephrogenic DI: long-standing renal disease, hypokalemia, some medications.
4. Deficiency of ADH results in decreased renal water reabsorption; it may be partial or complete (see Figure 20-5).
5. DI may be transient or permanent.

Clinical Manifestations

1. Marked polyuria—daily output of greater than 3 L for adults, 2 L of dilute urine for children; corresponding to a urine osmolality of less than 250 mOsm/kg.
2. Polydipsia (intense thirst)—drinks 4 to 40 L of fluid daily; has craving for cold water.

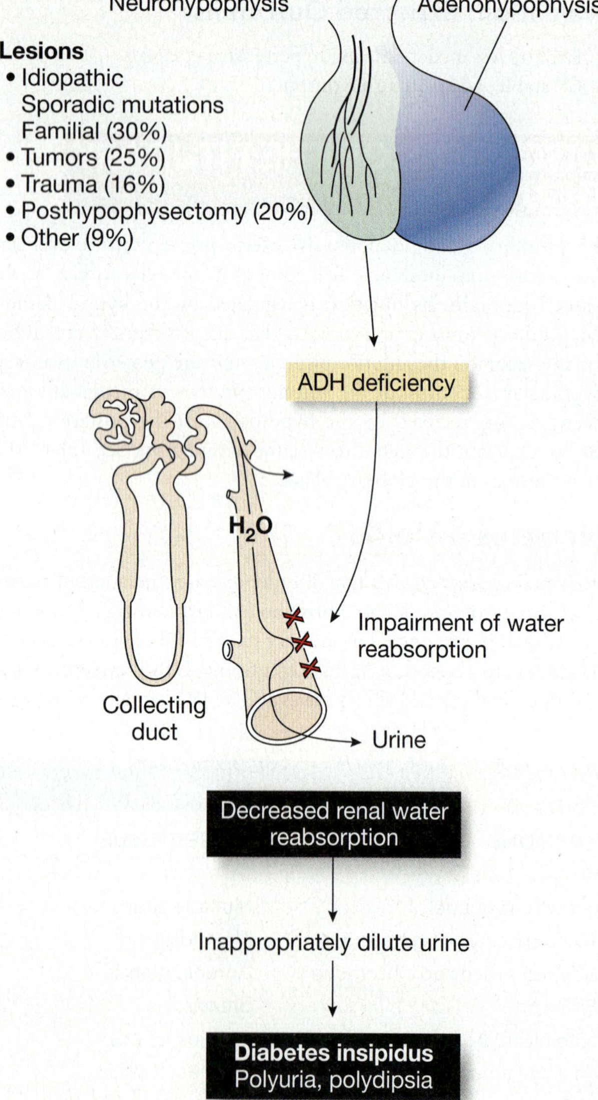

Figure 20-5. The mechanisms of diabetes insipidus. ADH, antidiuretic hormone. (Reprinted with permission from Strayer, D. S., Saffitz, J. E., & Rubin, E. [2022]. *Rubin's pathology: Mechanisms of human disease* [8th ed., Fig. 27-12]. Lippincott Williams & Wilkins.)

3. High serum osmolality (above 295 mOsm) and high serum sodium level (greater than 142 mEq/L).

Diagnostic Evaluation

1. Serum osmolality—high; urine osmolality—low.
2. Water deprivation test determines central and nephrogenic DI.
3. Measurements of serum and urine ADH—decreased to absent.
4. Pituitary magnetic resonance imaging (MRI).

Management

1. Administration of ADH or its derivative.
   a. DDAVP—vasopressin derivative administered intravenously, into the nose through a soft, flexible nasal tube, by nasal spray, or orally in tablet form. Potency varies by form of preparation (e.g., intravenous [IV] form almost 10 times more potent than nasal spray).
      i. Duration of action 8 to 12 hours.
      ii. For patients who have some residual hypothalamic ADH (determined by low levels of circulating ADH).
      iii. Dosage may be reduced in older adults and in individuals with renal impairment.
   b. Chlorpropamide—potentiates action of vasopressin on renal concentrating mechanism.
   c. Tricyclic antidepressants and selective serotonin reuptake inhibitor antidepressants may potentiate the action of DDAVP.
   d. Carbamazepine—potentiates action of endogenous vasopressin (rarely used).
2. For patients with nephrogenic DI—chlorpropamide or thiazide diuretics may be of value. Reversible by discontinuing causative medication if cause is drug related.

Complications

1. If untreated, may result in death.
2. Overtreatment of DDAVP may cause hyponatremia and water intoxication.

POPULATION AWARENESS Older patients are more sensitive to the effects of DDAVP, so make sure that overdosage does not occur, and watch for early signs of hyponatremia and water intoxication—drowsiness, confusion, headache, anuria, weight gain—to prevent seizures, coma, and death.

Nursing Assessment

1. Obtain complete health history to determine possible cause of DI.
2. Assess hydration status.

Nursing Interventions

Maintaining Adequate Fluid Volume

1. Measure fluid intake and output accurately.
2. Obtain daily weights.
3. Monitor hemodynamic status, as indicated, via frequent blood pressure (BP), heart rate, central venous pressure, and other measurements.
4. Provide patient with ample water to drink, and administer IV fluids as indicated.
5. Monitor results of serum and urine osmolality and serum sodium tests.
6. Administer or teach self-administration of medication, as prescribed, and document patient response.

Patient Education and Health Maintenance

1. Inform patient that metabolic status must be monitored on a long-term basis because the severity of DI changes from time to time.
2. Advise patient to avoid limiting fluids to decrease urine output; thirst is a protective function.
3. Advise patient to wear a medical alert tag stating that the wearer has DI.
4. Teach patient to be alert for signs of dehydration—decreased weight, decreased urine output, increased thirst, dry skin and mucous membranes; and overhydration—increased weight and edema; report these to the health care provider.
5. Tell patient to consider eliminating coffee and tea from diet—may have an exaggerated diuretic effect.
6. Give written instruction on vasopressin administration. Have patient demonstrate intranasal and injection technique.

Evaluation: Expected Outcomes

- Fluid intake equals output, weight stable.

Pituitary Tumors

Pituitary tumors represent various cell types. Symptoms reflect tumor effects on target tissues or on local structures surrounding the pituitary gland.

Pathophysiology and Etiology

1. Multiple oncogene abnormalities are thought to be involved with pituitary tumorigenesis.
2. Typically, pituitary tumors are characterized by size and by what hormones, if any, are secreted.
   a. Size.
      i. Microadenoma—less than 10 mm wide.
      ii. Macroadenoma—greater than 10 mm wide.
   b. Functional status.
      i. Hormone secreting—exaggerated hormone activity; may secrete multiple hormones.
      ii. Nonsecreting—usually diminished hormone activity.
3. Malignancy in pituitary tumors is rare.

Clinical Manifestations

1. Mass effects—effects of tumor on surrounding structures.
   a. Nonspecific headache.
   b. Impairment of cranial nerves II, III, IV, and VI on testing because of bilateral hemianopsia, which results from pressure on the optic chiasm.
   c. Vision disturbances, such as visual field defects and diplopia.
2. Endocrine effects—effects of hormone imbalances caused by tumor (see Table 20-3).

Diagnostic Evaluation

1. MRI of the brain and sellar region; computed tomography (CT) can also be done but is inferior.
2. Serum hormone levels to identify suspected abnormalities based on clinical evaluation.
3. Provocative testing to detect hormone secretion abnormalities of the pituitary, such as glucose tolerance test and dexamethasone suppression test (DST).

Management

Hypophysectomy

1. Surgical removal of the pituitary; considered first line of treatment for pituitary adenomas.
2. Transsphenoidal hypophysectomy—direct approach through the sinus and nasal cavity to sella turcica (see page 692).
3. Frontal craniotomy—uncommon approach except where tumor occupies broad area (see page 704).

Other Methods of Pituitary Ablation

1. Cryogenic destruction or stereotaxic radiofrequency coagulation (may be used in conjunction with surgery or drug therapy).
2. Radiation therapy.
3. Drug therapy.
   a. Bromocriptine for prolactinomas and, in some instances, growth hormone (GH)-secreting tumors is given daily.
   b. Cabergoline, a dopamine agonist, is administered twice per week for the treatment of acromegaly.
   c. Somatostatin analogues (octreotide, lanreotide) used in the treatment of acromegaly.
   d. GH antagonist (pegvisomant) used in the treatment of acromegaly.
   e. hormone replacement therapy (HRT) for hypopituitarism.

Complications

1. Hypothyroidism and adrenocortical insufficiency after ablation, requiring hormone replacement.
2. Menstruation ceases and infertility occurs almost always after total or nearly total ablation.
3. Transient or permanent DI after surgery.
4. Without treatment—death or severe disability caused by stroke, blindness, or imbalances of ACTH, thyroid-stimulating hormone (TSH), or ADH.

Nursing Assessment

1. Obtain history of signs and symptoms.
2. Perform thorough neurologic examination and general physical examination to identify signs of hormone deficiency or excess.
3. Assess patient's understanding of the management plan, coping with the diagnosis, and support from others.

Table 20-3 Clinical Manifestations Associated with Hormone Effects of Pituitary Tumors

HORMONE	HYPERPITUITARISM (INCREASED SECRETION)	HYPOPITUITARISM (DIMINISHED SECRETION)
Growth hormone	• Gigantism (child) • Acromegaly (adult)	• Shortness of stature (child) • Silent (adult)
Prolactin	• Infertility and galactorrhea (female)	• Postpartum lactation failure
Adrenocorticotropic hormone	• Cushing disease	• Adrenocortical insufficiency
Thyroid-stimulating hormone	• Hyperthyroidism	• Hypothyroidism
Luteinizing hormone and follicle-stimulating hormone	• Gonadal dysfunction	• Hypogonadism

Nursing Interventions

Also see "Care of the Patient Undergoing Transsphenoidal Hypophysectomy," section page 692.

Reducing Anxiety

1. Provide emotional support through the diagnostic process, and answer questions about treatment options.
2. Prepare patient for surgery or other treatment by describing nursing care thoroughly.
3. Stress likelihood of positive outcome with ablation therapy.

Promoting Management of the Therapeutic Regimen

1. Teach patient the nature of hormonal deficiencies after treatment and the purpose of replacement therapy.
2. Instruct patient about the early signs and symptoms of cortisol or thyroid hormone deficiency or excess and the need to report them.
3. Describe and demonstrate the correct method of administering prescribed medications.
4. Encourage patient in assuming active role in self-care through information seeking and problem solving.

Patient Education and Health Maintenance

1. Advise patient on temporary limitations in activities.
2. Teach patient the need for frequent initial follow-up visits and lifelong medical management when on hormonal therapy.
3. If applicable, advise patient on the need for postsurgery radiation therapy and periodic follow-up MRI and visual field testing.
4. Teach patient to notify health care provider if signs of thyroid or cortisol imbalance become evident.
5. Advise patient to wear medical alert tag.
6. Help patient identify sources of information and support available in the community (see Box 20-1, page 700).

Evaluation: Expected Outcomes

- States rationale for treatment, asks appropriate questions.
- Demonstrates correct medication administration.

SELECTED READINGS

Bergmann, M. L., & Schmedes, A. (2020). Highly sensitive LC-MS/MS analysis of catecholamines in plasma. *Clinical Biochemistry, 82*, 51–57. https://doi.org/10.1016/j.clinbiochem.2020.03.006

Bilezikian, J. P. (2020). Hypoparathyroidism. *The Journal of Clinical Endocrinology and Metabolism, 105*(6), 1722–1736. https://doi.org/10.1210/clinem/dgaa113

Choy, K. W., Fuller, P. J., Russell, G., Li, Q., Leenaerts, M., & Yang, J. (2022). Primary aldosteronism. *BMJ (Clinical Research Ed.), 377*, e065250. https://doi.org/10.1136/bmj-2021-065250

Christ-Crain, M., Winzeler, B., & Refardt, J. (2021). Diagnosis and management of diabetes insipidus for the internist: An update. *Journal of Internal Medicine, 290*(1), 73–87. https://doi.org/10.1111/joim.13261

Durante, C., Hegedüs, L., Czarniecka, A., Paschke, R., Russ, G., Schmitt, F., Soares, P., Solymosi, T., & Papini, E. (2023). 2023 European Thyroid Association clinical practice guidelines for thyroid nodule management. *European Thyroid Journal, 12*(5), e230067. https://doi.org/10.1530/ETJ-23-0067

El-Asmar, N., Rajpal, A., & Arafah, B. M. (2021). Primary hyperaldosteronism: Approach to diagnosis and management. *The Medical Clinics of North America, 105*(6), 1065–1080. https://doi.org/10.1016/j.mcna.2021.06.007

Farrugia, F. A., & Charalampopoulos, A. (2019). Pheochromocytoma. *Endocrine Regulations, 53*(3), 191–212. https://doi.org/10.2478/enr-2019-0020

Fleseriu, M., Auchus, R., Bancos, I., Ben-Shlomo, A., Bertherat, J., Biermasz, N. R., Boguszewski, C. L., Bronstein, M. D., Buchfelder, M., Carmichael, J. D., Casanueva, F. F., Castinetti, F., Chanson, P., Findling, J., Gadelha, M., Geer, E. B., Giustina, A., Grossman, A., Gurnell, M., … Biller, B. M. K. (2021). Consensus on diagnosis and management of Cushing's disease: A guideline update. *The Lancet. Diabetes & Endocrinology, 9*(12), 847–875. https://doi.org/10.1016/S2213-8587(21)00235-7

Haugen, B. R., Alexander, E. K., Bible, K. C., Doherty, G. M., Mandel, S. J., Nikiforov, Y. E., Pacini, F., Randolph, G. W., Sawka, A. M., Schlumberger, M., Schuff, K. G., Sherman, S. I., Sosa, J. A., Steward, D. L., Tuttle, R. M., & Wartofsky, L. (2016). 2015 American Thyroid Association management guidelines for adult patients with thyroid nodules and differentiated thyroid cancer: The American Thyroid Association guidelines task force on thyroid nodules and differentiated thyroid cancer. *Thyroid, 26*(1), 1–133. https://doi.org/10.1089/thy.2015.0020

Iqbal, A., & Rehman, A. (2022). Thyroid uptake and scan. In *StatPearls*. StatPearls Publishing.

Jain, A., Baracco, R., & Kapur, G. (2020). Pheochromocytoma and paraganglioma-an update on diagnosis, evaluation, and management. *Pediatric Nephrology (Berlin, Germany), 35*(4), 581–594. https://doi.org/10.1007/s00467-018-4181-2

Khan, A. A., Bilezikian, J. P., Brandi, M. L., Clarke, B. L., Gittoes, N. J., Pasieka, J. L., Rejnmark, L., Shoback, D. M., Potts, J. T., Guyatt, G. H., & Mannstadt, M. (2022). Evaluation and management of hypoparathyroidism summary statement and guidelines from the Second International Workshop. *Journal of Bone and Mineral Research, 37*(12), 2568–2585. https://doi.org/10.1002/jbmr.4691

Kim, M., & Kim, B. H. (2021). Current guidelines for management of medullary thyroid carcinoma. *Endocrinology and Metabolism (Seoul, Korea), 36*(3), 514–524. https://doi.org/10.3803/EnM.2021.1082

Munir, S., Quintanilla Rodriguez, B. S., Waseem, M., & Haddad, L. M. (2023). Addison disease (nursing). In *StatPearls*. StatPearls Publishing.

Nwariaku, F. (2022) Adrenalectomy techniques. *UpToDate*. Retrieved June 1, 2023, from https://www.uptodate.com/contents/adrenalectomy-techniques

Parasher, A. (2021). COVID-19: Current understanding of its pathophysiology, clinical presentation and treatment. *Postgraduate Medical Journal, 97*(1147), 312–320. https://doi.org/10.1136/postgradmedj-2020-138577

Priya, G., Kalra, S., Dasgupta, A., & Grewal, E. (2021). Diabetes insipidus: A pragmatic approach to management. *Cureus, 13*(1), e12498. https://doi.org/10.7759/cureus.12498

Ralli, M., Angeletti, D., Fiore, M., D'Aguanno, V., Lambiase, A., Artico, M., de Vincentiis, M., & Greco, A. (2020). Hashimoto's thyroiditis: An update on pathogenic mechanisms, diagnostic protocols, therapeutic strategies, and potential malignant transformation. *Autoimmunity Reviews, 19*(10), 102649. https://doi.org/10.1016/j.autrev.2020.102649

Stasiak, M., & Lewiński, A. (2021). New aspects in the pathogenesis and management of subacute thyroiditis. *Reviews in Endocrine & Metabolic Disorders, 22*(4), 1027–1039. https://doi.org/10.1007/s11154-021-09648-y

Thyroidectomy. (2021). *AORN Journal, 113*(3), P12–P14. https://doi.org/10.1002/aorn.12055

Tritos, N. A., & Biller, B. M. K. (2021). Current concepts of the diagnosis of adult growth hormone deficiency. *Reviews in Endocrine & Metabolic Disorders, 22*(1), 109–116. https://doi.org/10.1007/s11154-020-09594-1

Tsiomidou, S., Pamporaki, C., Geroula, A., Van Baal, L., Weber, F., Dralle, H., Schmid, K. W., Führer, D., & Unger, N. (2022). Clonidine suppression test for a reliable diagnosis of pheochromocytoma: When to use. *Clinical Endocrinology, 97*(5), 541–550. https://doi.org/10.1111/cen.14724

Wells, S. A., Asa, S. L., Dralle, H., Elisei, R., Evans, D. B., Gagel, R. F., Lee, N., Machens, A., Moley, J. F., Pacini, F., Raue, F., Frank-Raue, K., Robinson, B., Rosenthal, M. S., Santoro, M., Schlumberger, M., Shah, M., Waguespack, S. G., & American Thyroid Association Guidelines Task Force on Medullary Thyroid Carcinoma. (2015). Revised American Thyroid Association guidelines for the management of medullary thyroid carcinoma. *Thyroid, 25*(6), 567–610. https://doi.org/10.1089/thy.2014.0335

Wilson, S. A., Stem, L. A., & Bruehlman, R. D. (2021). Hypothyroidism: Diagnosis and treatment. *American Family Physician, 103*(10), 605–613. https://pubmed.ncbi.nlm.nih.gov/33983002/

Zhu, C. Y., Sturgeon, C., & Yeh, M. W. (2020). Diagnosis and management of primary hyperparathyroidism. *The Journal of the American Medical Association, 323*(12), 1186–1187. https://doi.org/10.1001/jama.2020.0538

Zubair, A., & Das, J. M. (2022). Transsphenoidal hypophysectomy. In *StatPearls*. StatPearls Publishing.

21 Diabetes Mellitus and Related Disorders*

OVERVIEW AND ASSESSMENT

EVIDENCE BASE Parker, E. D., Lin, J., Mahoney, T., Ume, N., Yang, G., Gabbay, R. A., ElSayed, N. A., & Bannuru, R. R. (2024). Economic costs of diabetes in the U.S. in 2022. *Diabetes Care*, *47*(1), 26–43. https://doi.org/10.2337/dci23-0085

Centers for Disease Control and Prevention. (2023, November 29). *National diabetes statistics report: Estimates of diabetes and its burden in the United States*. https://www.cdc.gov/diabetes/data/statistics-report/

Akinbami, L. J., Chen, T. C., Davy, O., Ogden, C. L., Fink, S., Clark, J., Riddles, M. K., & Mohadjer, L. K. (2022). National Health and Nutrition Examination Survey, 2017–March 2020 prepandemic file: Sample design, estimation, and analytic guidelines. *Vital and Health Statistics. Series. 1. Programs and Collection Procedures*, (190), 1–36. PMID: 35593699.

According to the Centers for Disease Control and Prevention, approximately 38.4 million Americans have diabetes mellitus (DM), affecting 11.6% of the U.S. population. Almost 23% of adults with DM are undiagnosed. Unfortunately, if current trends continue and in the absence of major lifestyle changes, the number of Americans diagnosed with DM will continue to rise.

It is thought that the factors contributing to the explosion of diabetes are an aging population, increased prevalence of type 2 DM in youth, growing numbers of ethnic minorities, and the increasing trend of obesity. According to National Health and Nutrition Examination Survey data, approximately 41.9% of adults aged 20 years and up, and 19.7% of children and adolescents, are obese.

In addition, the cost of caring for people with diabetes is staggering. In 2022, the total estimated cost of diagnosed diabetes in the United States was $412.9 billion, with $306.6 billion of that spent on direct medical care. Those with diabetes spend 2.6 times the health care costs of those without diabetes.

DM is the leading cause of blindness, kidney failure, and lower limb amputations. People with diabetes are two to four times more likely to be diagnosed with heart disease, three times more likely to have dental disease, and twice as more likely to suffer from depression.

This is a very serious disease with even more serious consequences. All nurses must stay current on the latest care recommendations. Screening for this disease is essential because early treatment leads to a reduction of morbidity and mortality.

Insulin Secretion and Function

1. Insulin is a hormone secreted by the beta cells of the islet of Langerhans in the pancreas.
2. Small amounts of insulin are released into the bloodstream in response to changes in blood glucose levels throughout the day (basal secretion).
3. Increased secretion or a bolus of insulin, released during meals, helps maintain euglycemia.
4. Through an internal feedback mechanism that involves the pancreas and the liver, circulating blood glucose levels are maintained at a normal range of 60 to 100 mg/dL.
5. Insulin is essential for the utilization of glucose for cellular metabolism as well as for the proper metabolism of protein and fat.
   a. Carbohydrate metabolism—insulin affects the conversion of glucose into glycogen for storage in the liver and skeletal muscles and allows for the immediate release and utilization of glucose by the cells.
   b. Protein metabolism—amino acid conversion occurs in the presence of insulin to replace muscle tissue or to provide needed glucose (gluconeogenesis).
   c. Fat metabolism—storage of fat in adipose tissue and conversion of fatty acids from excess glucose occurs only in the presence of insulin.

*Please note that the term "male" in this chapter refers to a person assigned male at birth, and the term "female" in this chapter refers to a person assigned female at birth.

6. Glucose can be used in the endothelial and nerve cells without the aid of insulin.
7. Without insulin, plasma glucose concentration rises and glycosuria results.
   a. Absolute deficits in insulin result from decreased production of endogenous insulin by the beta cell of the pancreas.
   b. Relative deficits in insulin are caused by inadequate utilization of insulin by the cell.

Classification of Diabetes

EVIDENCE BASE Blonde, L., Umpierrez, G. E., Reddy, S. S., McGill, J. B., Berga, S. L., Bush, M., Chandrasekaran, S., DeFronzo, R. A., Einhorn, D., Galindo, R. J., Gardner, T. W., Garg, R., Garvey, W. T., Hirsch, I. B., Hurley, D. L., Izuora, K., Kosiborod, M., Olson, D., Patel, S. B., ... Weber, S. L. (2022). American Association of Clinical Endocrinology Clinical Practice Guideline: Developing a diabetes mellitus comprehensive care plan—2022 update. *Endocrine Practice, 28*(10), 923–1049. https://doi.org/10.1016/j.eprac.2022.08.002

American Diabetes Association Professional Practice Committee. (2024). 2. Diagnosis and classification of diabetes: *Standards of care in diabetes—2024. Diabetes Care, 47* (Suppl. 1), S20–S42. https://doi.org/10.2337/dc24-S002

Type 1 Diabetes Mellitus

Type 1 DM, formerly known as insulin-dependent DM or juvenile DM.

1. Little or no endogenous insulin, requiring injections of insulin to control diabetes, prevent ketoacidosis, and sustain life.
2. Only 5% to 10% of all people with diabetes have type 1 DM.
3. Etiology is not well understood: includes autoimmune, viral, and certain histocompatibility antigens as well as genetic components.
4. Clinical manifestation is abrupt with classic symptoms of polydipsia, polyphagia, polyuria, and weight loss.
5. Most commonly seen in patients under age 35 but can be seen in older adults.

Type 2 Diabetes Mellitus

Type 2 DM, formerly known as non–insulin-dependent DM or adult-onset DM.

1. Caused by a combination of insulin resistance and relative insulin deficiency—some individuals have predominantly insulin resistance, whereas others have predominantly deficient insulin secretion, with little insulin resistance.
2. Approximately 90% to 95% of people with diabetes have type 2 DM.
3. Etiology: strong hereditary component, commonly associated with obesity.
4. Usual presentation is slow and typically insidious with symptoms of fatigue, weight loss, poor wound healing, and recurrent infection.
5. Found primarily in adults over age 30; however, it can be found in younger adults and adolescents who are overweight.
6. People with this type of diabetes may be treated with insulin but are still referred to as having type 2 DM.

Gestational Diabetes Mellitus

Gestational diabetes mellitus (GDM) is defined as diabetes diagnosed in the second or third trimester of pregnancy that is not clearly either type 1 or type 2.

1. Affects approximately 8.3% of pregnancies.
2. Patients with GDM have a 20% chance of developing type 2 DM diabetes in the next 10 years and a 60% chance within their lifetime. They should be screened for diabetes 6 to 12 weeks postpartum and continue to have lifelong screening every 1 to 3 years.
3. GDM is associated with significant risk of maternal and fetal complications.
4. Because of the worldwide increases of both obesity and diabetes rates, both the American Association of Clinical Endocrinologists (AACE)/American College of Endocrinology (ACE) and the American Diabetes Association (ADA) recommend that all pregnant patients with risk factors for type 2 DM be screened for the presence of type 2 DM at the initial prenatal visit using the standard diagnostic criteria. Patients who screen positive in the first trimester should be classified as having preexisting pregestational diabetes, not GDM.
5. Pregnant patients who screen negative for type 2 DM in the first trimester should then be screened for GDM at 24 to 28 weeks of gestation. The AACE/ACE recommends using an oral glucose tolerance test (OGTT) with a one-step strategy (see page 713); the American College of Obstetricians and Gynecologists (ACOG) supports using the OGTT with a two-step strategy and following the diagnostic criteria established by either Carpenter and Coustan or the National Diabetes Data Group. The ADA states that either screening method is appropriate.

Diabetes Because of Other Causes

1. Genetic defects of insulin secretion and/or insulin action.
2. Pancreatic diseases (such as cystic fibrosis, pancreatitis, and pheochromocytoma).
3. Drug induced (such as corticosteroids, medications used to treat human immunodeficiency virus [HIV]/acquired immunodeficiency syndrome [AIDS], or those used after organ transplant).

Prediabetes

1. *Prediabetes* is an abnormality in glucose values intermediate between normal and overt diabetes.
2. Associated with obesity, dyslipidemia, and hypertension; prediabetes is a potent risk factor for developing type 2 DM and cardiovascular disease.
3. Every effort should be made to assist the patient with aggressive lifestyle modifications (diet, exercise, and weight loss) to prevent the progression from prediabetes to overt type 2 DM.
4. There are two forms of prediabetes, based on when glucose is elevated. Patients who simultaneously have both forms of prediabetes have a very high risk of developing type 2 DM.
   a. Impaired fasting glucose (IFG)—defined as having fasting blood glucose levels of 100 to 125 mg/dL.
   b. Impaired glucose tolerance (IGT)—defined as blood glucose measurement of 140 to 199 mg/dL using a 2-hour 75-g OGTT.

Laboratory Tests

This section includes the laboratory tests used to diagnose and monitor short- and long-term glucose control as well as the recommended glucose treatment goals for different population groups. See Box 21-1 for information on screening criteria for type 2 DM in nonpregnant adults.

Blood Glucose

Description

1. Fasting blood sugar (FBS), drawn after at least an 8-hour fast, to evaluate circulating amounts of glucose.
2. Postprandial test, drawn usually 2 hours after a well-balanced meal, to evaluate glucose metabolism.
3. Random glucose, drawn at any time, without regard to the time of last caloric intake.

Nursing and Patient Care Considerations

1. For fasting glucose, make sure that patient has maintained 8-hour fast overnight; sips of water are allowed.
2. Advise patient to refrain from smoking before the glucose sampling because this affects the test results.
3. For postprandial glucose, advise patient that no additional food or caloric beverages should be consumed during the 2-hour interval.
4. For random blood glucose, note the time and content of the last meal.

Blood Glucose Values: Diagnostic Criteria and Treatment Goals

1. Diagnostic blood glucose values for DM of all ages (ADA, AACE/ACE, and International Society for Pediatric and Adolescent Diabetes [ISPAD]):
   a. Fasting blood glucose ≥126 mg/dL, confirmed with a repeat test on another day.
   b. Random blood sugar (regardless of time of last caloric intake) ≥200 mg/dL *and* presence of classic symptoms of diabetes (polyuria, polydipsia, polyphagia, and weight loss). This test, when patients present symptomatic as described earlier, does not need to be repeated nor does the diagnosis need to be confirmed with another test.
   c. Fasting blood glucose result of 100 to 125 mg/dL is IFG, which is diagnostic for prediabetes and demands close follow-up and repeat monitoring at least every 3 years.
2. Blood glucose treatment goals for many nonpregnant adults with DM:
   a. Premeal: 80 to 130 mg/dL (ADA) or less than 110 mg/dL (AACE/ACE).
   b. 1 to 2 hours postmeal: less than 180 mg/dL (ADA) or less than 140 mg/dL (AACE/ACE).
3. Blood glucose treatment goals for pregnant patients with gestational diabetes (ADA and AACE/ACE):
   a. Premeal: ≤95 mg/dL.
   b. 1 hour postmeal: ≤140 mg/dL.
   c. 2 hours postmeal: ≤120 mg/dL.
4. Blood glucose treatment goals for pregnant patients with preexisting diabetes:
   a. Premeal, bedtime: 60 to 95 mg/dL (AACE/ACE) or 70 to 95 mg/dL (ADA).
   b. 1 hour postmeal: 100 to 140 mg/dL (AACE/ACE) or 110 to 140 mg/dL (ADA).
   c. 2 hours postmeal: 100 to 120 mg/dL (AACE/ACE/ADA).
5. Blood glucose treatment goals for older adults (ADA):
   a. Healthy, few complications: 80 to 130 mg/dL fasting; 80 to 180 mg/dL bedtime.
   b. Complex with multiple coexisting chronic conditions: 90 to 150 mg/dL fasting; 100 to 180 mg/dL bedtime.
   c. Very complex/frail: 100 to 180 mg/dL fasting; 110 to 200 mg/dL bedtime.
6. Blood glucose treatment goals for hospitalized patients (critically and noncritically ill).
   a. 140 to 180 mg/dL (ADA and AACE/ACE).

BOX 21-1 Risk Factors and Screening for Type 2 Diabetes

Screening should begin at age 35 and should occur at least every 3 yr for adults with normal glucose levels.

Earlier screening should be considered for those with one or more of the following risk factors:

- Family history of diabetes (first-degree relative).
- Sedentary lifestyle/habitual inactivity.
- Ethnicity (i.e., Black, Hispanic American, Native American, Alaskan American, and Pacific Islander) with body mass index (BMI) ≥25, and BMI ≥23 if the patient is Asian American.
- Previous diagnosis of prediabetes (impaired fasting glucose (IFG) or impaired glucose tolerance (IGT) or A1C ≥5.7%)
- History of gestational diabetes mellitus (GDM)
- Blood pressure ≥130/80 mm Hg or on therapy for hypertension.
- High-density lipoprotein (HDL) cholesterol less than 35 mg/dL and/or triglyceride level greater than 250 mg/dL.
- History of insulin resistance (i.e., polycystic ovary disease, acanthosis nigricans, severe obesity).
- History of cardiovascular disease.

CLINICAL JUDGMENT Capillary blood glucose values obtained by fingerstick samples tend to be higher than values in venous samples. Diagnostic tests are always to be conducted in a laboratory using venous samples.

Oral Glucose Tolerance Test

Description

The OGTT evaluates insulin response to glucose loading. FBS is obtained before the ingestion of a glucose load, and blood samples are drawn at timed intervals.

Nursing and Patient Care Considerations

1. Advise patient that for accuracy in results, certain instructions must be followed:
   a. Usual diet and exercise pattern must be followed for 3 days before OGTT.
   b. During OGTT, patient must refrain from smoking and remain seated.
   c. Hormonal contraceptives, salicylates, diuretics, phenytoin, and nicotinic acid can impair results and may be withheld before testing based on the advice of the health care provider.

Diagnostic Criteria Using the 75-g 2-Hour Oral Glucose Tolerance Test (Nonpregnant Adults)

1. ADA and AACE/ACE diagnostic OGTT values when screening for DM in children, adolescents, and nonpregnant adults:
   a. 200 mg/dL or higher at the 2-hour interval.
   b. 140 to 199 mg/dL at the 2-hour interval is prediabetes (IGT) and demands close follow-up and repeat monitoring at least every 3 years.
2. Standard 2-h OGTT: 1.75 g/kg (75 g maximum) oral glucose administration remains the gold standard test for disease staging in type 1 DM (according to ISPAD).
3. See Box 21-2, page 714, for diagnostic criteria using OGTT for gestational diabetes.

Glycated Hemoglobin (Glycohemoglobin, HbA1C, A1C)

Description

Measures glycemic control over a 60- to 120-day period by measuring the irreversible reaction of glucose to hemoglobin through freely permeable erythrocytes during their 120-day life cycle. Currently used to screen for diabetes as well as to monitor control.

Nursing and Patient Care Considerations

1. No prior preparation, such as fasting or withholding insulin/medications, is necessary.
2. Test results can be affected by red blood cell disorders (e.g., thalassemia, sickle cell anemia), room temperature, ionic charges, and ambient blood glucose values.
3. Many methods exist for performing the test, making it necessary to consult the laboratory for normal values.
4. Should be performed at least twice yearly in patients whose diabetes is stable and well controlled. Quarterly (every 3 months) testing is recommended for patients who have had treatment changes/adjustments or whose diabetes is not well controlled.

Diagnostic Criteria and Treatment Goals for A1C Values

1. ADA and AACE/ACE diagnostic A1C values when screening for DM in children, adolescents, and nonpregnant adults.
   a. 6.5% or higher (diagnosis should be confirmed with repeat A1C or a fasting glucose or OGTT).
   b. 5.7% to 6.4% (ADA and AACE/ACE) is considered prediabetes and demands close follow-up and repeat monitoring at least every 3 years.
2. ADA asserts that in general, the A1C goal for nonpregnant adults with diabetes is less than 7%, but that this must be individualized based on life expectancy, duration of diabetes, history of hypoglycemia, presence of microvascular complications, and presence of cardiovascular disease.
3. The ADA and AACE/ACE treatment A1C goal of pregnant patients with preexisting type 1 or type 2 diabetes is less than 6% (if without excessive hypoglycemia).
4. Pregnant patients at high risk should be screened earlier. Abnormal fasting glucose of 110 to 125 mg/dL or A1C of 5.9% to 6.4% should undergo further diagnosis and treatment to advert maternal and neonatal complications.
5. Because GDM is diagnosed late in pregnancy, the A1C is not a reliable marker of control (3-month average), and the fructosamine assay (2- to 3-week average) may be more meaningful.

EVIDENCE BASE Skyler, J. S., Bergenstal, R., Bonow, R. O., Buse, J., Deedwania, P., Gale, E. A., Howard, B. V., Kirkman, M. S., Kosiborod, M., Reaven, P., Sherwin, R. S., American Diabetes Association, American College of Cardiology Foundation, & American Heart Association. (2009). Intensive glycemic control and the prevention of cardiovascular events: Implications of the ACCORD, ADVANCE, and VA diabetes trials: A position statement of the American Diabetes Association and a scientific statement of the American College of Cardiology Foundation and the American Heart Association. *Diabetes Care*, *32*(1), 187–192. https://doi.org/10.2337/dc08-9026

BOX 21-2 Screening and Diagnostic Parameters for Gestational Diabetes

ONE-STEP STRATEGY

WHEN: 24–28 wk of gestation.

HOW: 75-g 2-h oral glucose tolerance test (OGTT) performed in the morning following 8-h fast the night before.

WHAT is diagnostic for gestational diabetes mellitus (GDM) (with any ONE of the following results):

Fasting glucose: ≥92 mg/dL.
1-h interval: ≥180 mg/dL.
2-h interval: ≥153 mg/dL.

TWO-STEP STRATEGY

WHEN: 24–28 wk of gestation.

HOW:

Step 1: nonfasting, 50-g glucose load test; PROCEED to step 2 if 1-h result: ≥130 mg/dL, ≥135 mg/dL, ***or*** ≥140 mg/dL (determined by the provider and patient risk factors).

Step 2: 100-g 3-h OGTT performed in the morning following an 8-h fast the night before.

WHAT is diagnostic for GDM (**two positive results; choose one set of criteria to follow**):

GLUCOSE VALUE	CARPENTER/COUSTAN (MG/DL)	NATIONAL DIABETES DATA GROUP (MG/DL)
Fasting	≥95	≥105
1-h interval	≥180	≥190
2-h interval	≥155	≥165
3-h interval	≥140	≥145

Fructosamine Assay

Description

Glycated protein with a much shorter half-life than glycated hemoglobin, reflecting control over a shorter period, approximately 14 to 21 days. May be advantageous in patients with hemoglobin variants that interfere with the accuracy of glycated hemoglobin tests.

Nursing and Patient Care Considerations

1. Note if patient has hypoalbuminemia or elevated globulins because test may not be reliable.
2. Should not be used as a diagnostic test for DM.
3. No special preparation or fasting is necessary.

C-Peptide Assay (Connecting Peptide Assay)

Description

Cleaved from the proinsulin molecule during its conversion to insulin, C-peptide acts as a marker for endogenous insulin production.

Nursing and Patient Care Considerations

1. Test can be performed after an overnight fast or after stimulation with Sustacal, intravenous (IV) glucose, or 1 mg of glucagon subcutaneous (SQ).
2. Absence of C-peptide indicates no beta-cell function, reflecting possible type 1 DM or insulinopenia in type 2 DM.

Autoantibody Testing

Description

Islet cell autoantibodies cause destruction to the pancreatic beta cells and are strongly associated with the development of type 1 DM. The appearance of autoantibodies to one or several of the autoantigens—GAD65, tyrosine phosphates (IA-2, IA-2β), ZnT8, or insulin—signals an autoimmune pathogenesis of beta-cell destruction. The positivity of any of these autoantibodies in the presence of hyperglycemia is used to confirm the diagnosis of type 1 DM. Because type 1 DM affects such a small number of the population, screening is only recommended for first-degree family members of people diagnosed with type 1 DM. Generalized screening would be costly and, therefore, is not recommended.

Nursing and Patient Care Considerations

1. No special preparation or fasting is necessary.
2. Screen patients with type 1 DM for other autoimmune disorders, such as hypothyroidism and celiac disease.

GENERAL PROCEDURES AND TREATMENT MODALITIES

See additional online content: Procedure Guidelines 21-1 and 21-2.

EVIDENCE BASE American Diabetes Association. (2022). Standards of medical care in diabetes—2023. *Diabetes Care*, 46 (Suppl. 1). https://diabetesjournals.org/care/issue/47/Supplement_1

Glucose Monitoring

EVIDENCE BASE Bailey, T. S., Grunberger, G., Bode, B. W., Handelsman, Y., Hirsch, I. B., Jovanovič, L., Roberts, V. L., Rodbard, D., Tamborlane, W. V., Walsh, J., American Association of Clinical Endocrinologists, & American College of Endocrinology. (2016). American Association of Clinical Endocrinologists and American College of Endocrinology 2016 outpatient glucose monitoring consensus statement. *Endocrine Practice*, *22*(2), 231–261. https://doi.org/10.4158/EP151124.CS

Accurate determination of capillary blood glucose assists patients in the control and daily management of diabetes mellitus (DM). Blood glucose monitoring helps evaluate the effectiveness of medication, reflects glucose excursion after meals, assesses glucose response to exercise regimen, and assists in the evaluation of episodes of hypoglycemia and hyperglycemia to determine appropriate treatment.

Intermittent Glucose Monitoring

1. Procedure varies by the equipment chosen; follow manufacturer's instructions. Ensure that the appropriate glucose strips are used for the glucose meter used.
2. The most appropriate schedule for glucose monitoring is determined by the patient and health care provider.
   a. Medication regimens and meal timing are considered to set the most effective monitoring schedule.
   b. Scheduling of glucose tests should reflect cost-effectiveness for the patient. Medicare and most insurance will approve coverage for more strips if medically necessary.
   c. Glucose monitoring is intensified during times of stress or illness or when changes in therapy are prescribed.
3. Patients with type 2 DM who are not being treated with insulin or other medications that increase the risk of hypoglycemia (i.e., sulfonylureas) should be testing blood glucose using a structured format where information obtained is used to guide treatment. Make sure that patient brings glucose meter and/or log to follow up appointments.
4. Patients with type 1 DM as well as those with type 2 DM who are using a multiple-dose insulin regimen should test blood sugar at least three times a day. Those times should include before/after meals, at bedtime, and, occasionally, at 2:00 to 3:00 a.m.
5. Caution patient about using alternate site testing if there are complaints of painful fingers, and for individuals such as musicians, who use their fingertips for occupational activities. Testing in sites such as the forearm, palm, thigh, and calf have not proved as accurate as fingertip testing in most studies.
   a. If alternate site is used, the area should be rubbed until it is warm before testing.
   b. Do not use an alternate site when:
      i. Glucose levels are rapidly changing (postprandial, hypoglycemia, reaction to exercise/activity).
      ii. Accuracy is critical (hypoglycemia is suspected, before exercise, or before driving).
   c. Check with the glucometer manufacturer to see if it is approved for alternate site testing.

Continuous Glucose Monitoring

1. Continuous glucose monitoring (CGM) is a supplemental tool that has become more readily available to monitor glucose frequently or continuously to make lifestyle modifications. It is especially useful for patients with type 1 DM and type 2 DM who are experiencing frequent hypoglycemia episodes, severe hypoglycemia, and/or hypoglycemia unawareness. CGM used during pregnancy can improve maternal and neonatal outcomes, therefore outweighing the cost of use. CGM measures glucose in the interstitial fluid, rather than capillary blood. Ongoing advances in technology have rendered these readings highly reliable and correlate closely with plasma glucose.
2. CGM systems consist of a sensor inserted into the skin and attached to a transmitter, which remains adherent to the skin for up to 14 days until the sensor needs to be changed. A reader is used to obtain glucose values, or the information can be transmitted to a smartphone.
3. CGM may be integrated with automated insulin delivery (AID) systems. CGM-automated algorithm can adjust insulin delivery and assist with diabetes self-care decision-making. As this technology continues to advance in accuracy, less input will be required by the user.
4. CGM also detects changes in glucose patterns and will alert the user of potentially dangerous rises and falls. This enables the user to be proactive and avert harmful events. All professionals should be aware that certain medications (e.g., high dose of

Table 21-1 Standardized Continuous Glucose Monitoring (CGM) Metrics Over 14 Days

AMBULATORY GLUCOSE PROFILE	GLUCOSE IN MG/DL	PREGNANT PATIENTS	PERCENTAGE OF READINGS
Time in range (TIR)	70–180	63–140	>70
Time in range (TAR): Adults	>180	>140	<25—Level 1 hyperglycemia
TAR: Children	>250	NA	<5—Level 2 hyperglycemia
Time below range (TBR): Adults	<70	<63	<4—Level 1 hypoglycemia
TBR: Children	<54	<54	<1—Level 1 hypoglycemia

vitamin C, acetaminophen, hydroxyurea, mannitol, and tetracycline) may interfere with accuracy of glucose readings.

5. Professional CGM systems available for experienced health care professionals to use as a diagnostic tool, and personal CGM systems are available to patients as either stand-alone devices or in an integrated insulin pump/CGM system.
   a. Real-time CGM does not require scanning but is most beneficial when used daily, while intermittently scanned CGM requires the user to scan at least every 8 hours to prevent gaps in readings.
   b. Readings are evaluated for time in range to guide management decisions. See Table 21-1 for optimal metrics.

Insulin Therapy

EVIDENCE BASE Garber, A. J., Abrahamson, M. J., Barzilay, J. I., Blonde, L., Bloomgarden, Z. T., Bush, M. A., Dagogo-Jack, S., DeFronzo, R. A., Einhorn, D., Fonseca, V. A., Garber, J. R., Garvey, W. T., Grunberger, G., Handelsman, Y., Hirsch, I. B., Jellinger, P. S., McGill, J. B., Mechanick, J. I., Rosenblit, P. D., & Umpierrez, G. E. (2018). Consensus statement by the American Association of Clinical Endocrinologists and American College of Endocrinology on the comprehensive type 2 diabetes management algorithm—2018 executive summary. *Endocrine Practice*, *24*(1), 91–120. https://doi.org/10.4158/CS-2017-0153

Insulin therapy involves the subcutaneous (SQ) injection of rapid-, short-, intermediate-, or long-acting insulin at various times to achieve the desired effect (see Table 21-2). Short-acting regular human insulin as well as some of the rapid-acting analogs can also be administered intravenously. There are many types of insulin currently available in the United States, including the newer biosimilar insulins, and more are being added. Biosimilar insulins are not generic insulins, meaning exact replicas, but they work with the same effect when administered. They are available in different concentrations (U-100, U-200, U-300, U-500) and premixed combinations. Most of the available insulin products are human insulin manufactured synthetically (analogs). Beef and pork insulins are no longer available in the United States.

POPULATION AWARENESS The following insulin types can be used during pregnancy: Human Regular (U-100 and U-500), aspart, lispro (U-100 and U-200), Human NPH. The long-acting insulins detemir and glargine have not been tested extensively in pregnancy but have been found to be safe when used in pregnant patients with already existing type 1 DM or type 2 DM. All others have not been studied in humans or have insufficient data and, therefore, may pose possible risk to the fetus and should not be used during pregnancy if other alternatives are available.

Self-injection of Insulin

1. Teaching of self-injection of insulin should begin as soon as the need for insulin has been established.
2. Teach the patient and another family member or significant other.
3. Use written and verbal instructions and demonstration techniques.
4. Teach injection first because this is the patient's primary concern; then, teach loading the syringe.
5. Almost all insulin preparations are available in prefilled pen devices. These are much easier and safer for the patients to learn and use. It is recommended that pen devices be used whenever possible. These are imperative for patients with dexterity or vision limitation.

Community and Home Care Considerations

1. Reusing insulin syringes is not recommended. However, some patients find the cost of supplies to be a major financial burden. Assist the patient in deciding whether to reuse insulin syringes at home. The patient will need to understand that the newer, finer needles may become dull or bent after one or two injections, causing tearing of tissue, which can lead to lipodystrophy.
   a. Needles should not be reused if painful injection or irritated site results.
   b. Needle should be recapped by patient and stored in a clean place if it is going to be reused.
2. Assist the patient in obtaining the appropriate syringe size and needle length for injections.
   a. Determine whether there are visual or dexterity issues that make a syringe with gradations farther apart more desirable.
   b. There is no medical reason to use needles greater than 8 mm in length, even in patients who are obese. Needle lengths of 4, 5, and 6 mm are reliable to deliver medication into the SQ space. To prevent inadvertent intramuscular injection in patients who are thin, the needle can be inserted at a 45-degree angle (rather than at a 90-degree angle) and/or the skin should be folded prior to needle insertion.
   c. There are now insulin syringes available specifically for the use of u-500 regular insulin that are to be prescribed and dispensed with each vial of u-500 regular insulin. u-500 insulin is also now available in prefilled pen devices. Both the new u-500–specific syringes and the prefilled pens make the administration of this insulin much safer.

CLINICAL JUDGMENT Using a u-100 syringe or tuberculin syringe to dose u-500 regular insulin is not safe and is not recommended.

3. Advise the patient that it is not necessary to use alcohol to wipe off the top of the vial or to prepare the skin before injection.

Table 21-2 Pharmacokinetics of Common Insulin Products

TYPE	ONSET	PEAK	DURATION	ROUTE
Rapid-Acting Analogs				
Insulin aspart (Fiasp)	<5 min	<1 h	<3 h	SQ, IV
Insulin aspart (Novolog)	<15 min	1–2 h	3–4 h	SQ, pump, IV
Insulin glulisine (Apidra)	<15 min	1–2 h	3–4 h	SQ, pump, IV
Insulin lispro (Humalog)	<15 min	1–2 h	3–4 h	SQ, pump
Insulin lispro aabc (Lyumjev) U-100 and U-200	<15 min	1 h	2–4 h	SQ (pump, IV u-100 only)
Afrezza human insulin	<15–30 min	53 min	2 h	Inhaled
Short-Acting Human Insulin				
Humulin R	0.5–1 h	2–4 h	5–7 h	SQ, IV
Novolin R	0.5–1 h	2–4 h	5–7 h	SQ, IV
Intermediate-Acting Basal				
Insulin isophane susp.; NPH*	2–4 h	4–10 h	10–16 h	SQ
Humulin N	2–4 h	4–10 h	10–16 h	SQ
Novolin N				
Long-Acting Basal Analogs				
Insulin detemir (Levemir)**	3–4 h	None	6–24 h	SQ
Insulin glargine (Lantus)	3–4 h	None	<24 h	SQ
Ultra–Long-Acting Basal Analogs				
Insulin glargine u-300 (Toujeo)	6 h	None	>24 h	SQ
Insulin degludec u-100 and u-200 (Tresiba)	30–90 min	None	>40 h	SQ
Premixed Insulin				
Analog Preparations				
Novolog Mix 70/30 (aspart)	<15 min	2–4 h	24 h	SQ
Humalog Mix 75/25 (lispro)	<15 min	0.5–1.5 h	24 h	SQ
Humalog Mix 50/50 (lispro)	<15 min	1 h	16 h	SQ
Ryzodeg 70/30 (degludec + aspart)	<15 min	72 min	>24 h	SQ
NPH and Regular Suspensions				
Humulin 70/30	30 min	2–12 h	24 h	SQ
Novolin 70/30	30 min	2–12 h	24 h	SQ
Biosimilar insulin				
Insulin lispro (Admelog)	<15 min	1 h	2–4 h	SQ, pump, IV
Insulin glargine (Basaglar)	3–4 h	None	12–24 h	SQ
Insulin glargine yfgn (Semglee)	1.5–2 h	None	24 h	SQ
Insulin glargine (Rezvoglar)	1.5–2 h	None	24 h	SQ

IV, intravenous; SQ, subcutaneous.
*Insulin isophane suspension is also known as NPH insulin, which stands for neutral protamine Hagedorn.
**To be discontinued in the US by the Manufacturers.

It has not proved to result in lower rate of infection and adds cost and time to the procedure. The patient should maintain good hygiene (handwashing using soap and water).

4. Instruct the patient to store insulin currently in use in a clean, secure place away from direct sunlight and heat. In-use insulin does not require refrigeration. Check manufacturer's recommendations for when to discard insulin vials and pens; recommendations may vary from 10 to 56 days after initial use. All unopened vials/pens must be stored in the refrigerator until initial use.
5. Check manufacturer's recommendations before teaching the patient how to mix insulin; for example, the patient should know that insulin glargine and insulin detemir must never be mixed with any other insulin. Other manufacturers' websites containing recommendations are Aventis (www.aventis.com), Eli Lilly (www.lilly.com), and Novo Nordisk (www.novonordisk.com).
6. Avoid prefilling syringes if possible because manufacturers have no data on the stability of insulin stored in syringes for long periods. If prefilling is the only option, store in refrigerator or suggest an insulin pen injection device.
7. Help the patient develop a plan for the disposal of needles. There are no federal regulations for discarding needles used at home; however, needles and lancets can pose a risk for injury. The rules and regulations regarding sharps disposal are different in towns and counties around the country, so advise the patient to check with local sanitation or health departments.
   a. Sharps can be placed in a hard plastic or metal container with a tightly secured lid after use (i.e., empty plastic laundry detergent container).
   b. More information on disposal can be obtained by contacting the Coalition for Safe Community Needle Disposal (800-643-1643 or www.safeneedledisposal.org).

Insulin Regimens

See Figure 21-1.

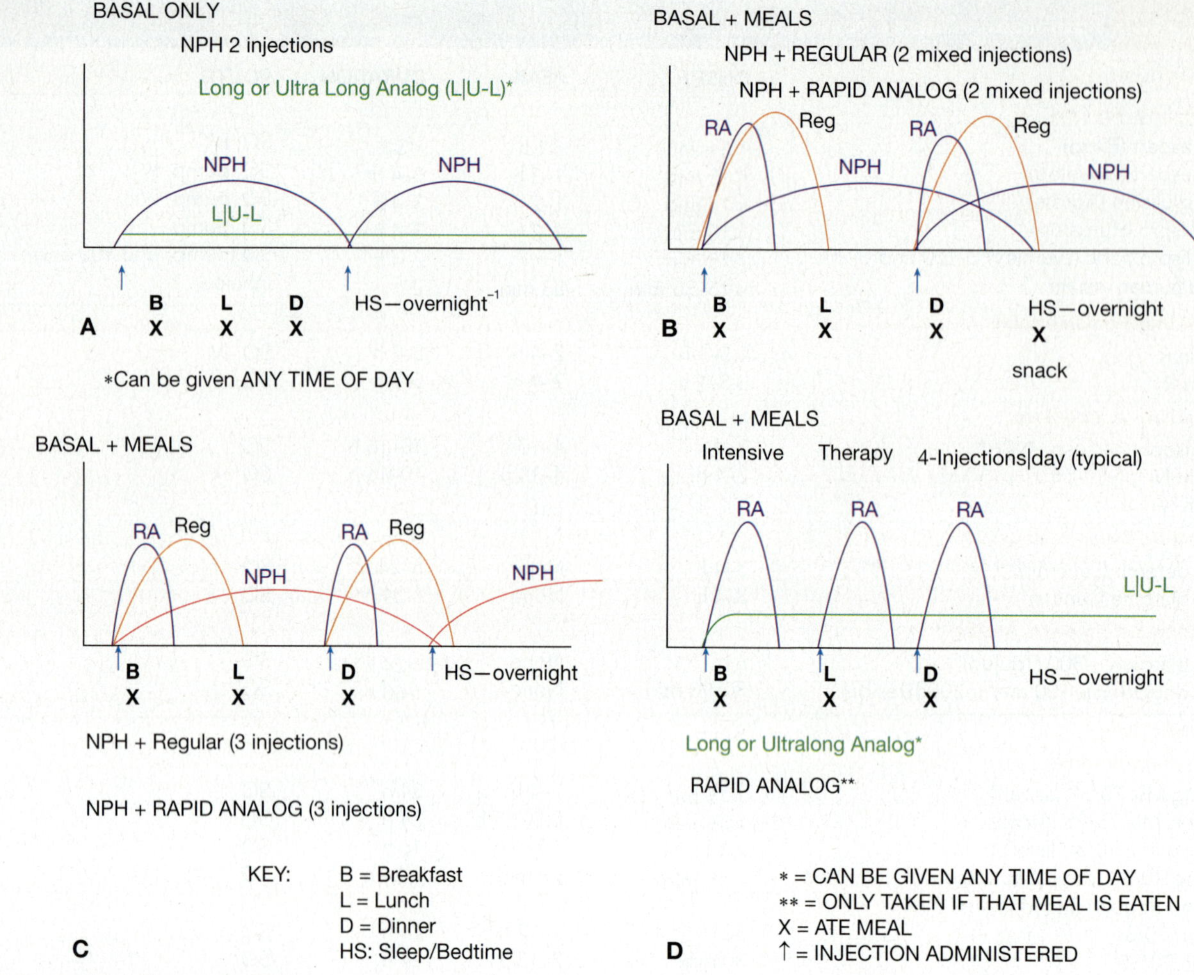

Figure 21-1. **(A–D)** Insulin regimens.

Basal Insulin Only (Figure 21-1A)

1. Either NPH or long-acting analogs may be used as monotherapy only in type 2 DM as a supplement for better glucose control when patients are still capable of producing some exogenous insulin. Patients with type 1 DM will always require mealtime coverage in addition to basal insulin.
2. NPH is not as desirable as a basal insulin because of the availability of the newer analog basal insulins that are more reliable, longer acting, and associated with less hypoglycemia. However, NPH is available without a prescription and may also be the most affordable option for some patients.
3. Basal insulin is traditionally administered at bedtime to assist with controlling early-morning hyperglycemia. Patients may take NPH in addition to a mealtime insulin before dinner and can be mixed in the same syringe. If NPH is taken before dinner, a snack before bed is usually necessary to prevent nocturnal hypoglycemia because of the onset of the peaking action several hours later. Bedtime dosing of NPH typically eliminates the need for a bedtime snack and will better address dawn phenomenon (elevated glucose values upon awakening the following morning).
4. When used as basal insulin, NPH is typically administered twice daily—in the morning to address afternoon hyperglycemia and again at bedtime to provide overnight coverage. Typically, 2/3 to 3/4 of the daily dosage is given before breakfast, and 1/3 to 1/4 is given at bedtime.
5. The longer acting insulin analogs typically allow for once-daily dosing and can be administered at various times of the day, and eating snacks between meals to prevent hypoglycemia is usually not required.

Basal Plus Prandial Insulin (Figure 21-1B, 2 Mixed Injections/Day)

1. Short-acting regular insulin or rapid-acting lispro, glulisine, or aspart insulin is added to NPH to promote postprandial glucose control.
2. Short- or rapid-acting insulin added to morning NPH controls glucose elevations after breakfast.
3. Increased blood glucose levels after supper can be controlled by the addition of short- or rapid-acting insulin before supper.
4. NPH and regular, lispro, glulisine, or aspart insulin given before breakfast and before supper is termed a "split-mix" regimen, providing 24-hour insulin coverage. However, there is an increased risk of nocturnal hypoglycemia (2:00 to 3:00 a.m.) when NPH is given before supper. Therefore, an alternative is to administer the prandial insulin alone before the evening meal and the NPH at bedtime (see Figure 21-1C).

Intensive Insulin Therapy (Figure 21-1D)

1. Designed to mimic the body's normal insulin responses to glucose.

2. Characterized by at least one basal injection daily with additional mealtime injections for every meal and snack consumed. Typically consists of four to five injections of insulin daily.
3. Long-acting (glargine insulin) or ultra–long-acting (glargine u-300 or degludec insulin) analog is used for basal insulin control. These are often administered once daily at bedtime; however, any time of the day (but must be consistently the same time) can be used for the once-daily administration, and this allows for greater patient adherence.
4. Regular insulin acts as a premeal bolus given 30 minutes before each meal. However, analog rapid-acting insulin (lispro, glulisine, or aspart) is now often preferred to regular insulin. The rapid-acting insulin is taken within 1 to 15 minutes before eating. As with NPH, regular human insulin is available without a prescription and is often a more affordable choice for some patients.
5. A 24-hour insulin coverage designed in this way can be flexible to accommodate mealtimes and physical activity.

Sliding Scale Versus Algorithm Therapy

1. Sliding scale therapy uses short- or rapid-acting insulin to retrospectively correct hyperglycemia. Sliding scale dosing is not recommended because it fails to prevent and adequately address hyperglycemia and places patients at significant risk for hypoglycemia hours later.
2. Algorithm therapy prospectively determines short- or rapid-acting insulin dosages, considering meal content, premeal blood glucose level, and physical activity.
3. Individualization of insulin dosages is the most important aspect of sliding scale and algorithm therapy.
   a. The patient is encouraged to test blood glucoses to analyze insulin dose response.
   b. A pattern of increased blood glucose associated with certain foods (e.g., pasta, pizza) can help determine the appropriate regimen of insulin dosage.
   c. Physical activity, which enhances insulin activity and decreases serum glucose, may indicate the need to reduce the dosage of premeal insulin.

Continuous Subcutaneous Insulin Infusion (Insulin Pump Therapy)

Pump therapy is more commonly considered for the treatment of type 1 DM, but it is becoming more common in the treatment of type 2 DM when multiple daily injections/intensive insulin management is required.

1. Continuous subcutaneous insulin infusion (CSII) or insulin pump therapy provides continuous infusion of regular, lispro, glulisine, or aspart insulin via SQ catheter.
2. There are several different pumps available. The type of insulin pump used by the patient is determined by the patient with the guidance of an expert clinician.
3. The catheter should be replaced every 72 hours or sooner if the site becomes painful or inflamed.
   a. Usually, the insulin pump is removed for bathing, and the tubing and catheter can be changed at that time. Other pumps are waterproof and do not need to be disconnected with bathing, showering, or even swimming.
   b. A tube-free pump is available. The patient wears a "pod" filled with enough insulin to last 2 to 3 days. The pod is discarded, and a new pod placed every 2 to 3 days. The delivery of insulin is remotely controlled via a handheld device.
4. Intensive insulin management by pump therapy requires patient motivation to overcome possible disadvantages.
   a. Blood glucose monitoring must be done at least four to six times per day. Most insulin pumps are now available as integrated systems, which utilize CGM (see "Glucose Monitoring" section).
   b. Frequent contact with health care team is necessary to adjust insulin dosage.
   c. Must understand carbohydrate counting and careful consideration of diet and activity when insulin boluses are given through the pump.
   d. Increased cost of insulin pump and infusion set compared to usual syringe method.
   e. Heightened risk of hypoglycemia with tighter glucose control.
   f. Danger of hyperglycemia exists should insulin catheter become kinked or dislodged, and patient then fails to receive appropriate insulin dosage.
   g. Although newer pumps are smaller and more discreet, there is increased awareness of diabetes by others due to visibility of the external device.
5. Advantages of CSII in improving blood glucose control:
   a. Insulin pump can deliver basal insulin at individualized programmed rates throughout a 24-hour period.
   b. Bolus injections of short-acting insulin given 30 minutes before eating or rapid-acting insulin no more than 15 minutes before a meal allow for flexibility in meal content and timing.
   c. Correction supplements of short- or rapid-acting insulin are easily given to rapidly correct elevated glucose levels.

Combination Noninsulin Agents and Insulin Therapy

1. Except for using pramlintide in addition to insulin, all other combinations of insulin with noninsulin agents are only Food and Drug Administration (FDA) approved to be used for patients with type 2 DM.
2. Always refer to the full prescribing information for each noninsulin agent to determine whether and how they are FDA approved for use with insulin therapy.
3. Because of the increased risk for hypoglycemia, concomitant use of insulin and sulfonylureas is not recommended.

DIABETES MELLITUS AND RELATED DISORDERS

See additional online content: Procedure Guidelines 21-3.

Diabetes Mellitus

Diabetes mellitus (DM) is a metabolic disorder characterized by hyperglycemia and results from defective insulin production, secretion, or utilization. Type 1 DM in children is covered in Chapter 50.

Pathophysiology and Etiology

1. There is an absolute or relative lack of insulin produced by beta cells, resulting in hyperglycemia.
2. Defects at the cell level, impaired secretory response of insulin to rises in glucose, and increased nocturnal hepatic glucose production (gluconeogenesis) are seen in type 2 DM.

3. Etiology of type 1 DM is not well understood; viral, autoimmune, and environmental theories are under review.
4. Etiology of type 2 DM involves heredity, genetics, and obesity.
5. Risk factors for type 2 DM in adults and children include family history and ethnicity and a variety of other factors (see page 735).

Clinical Manifestations

1. Onset is usually abrupt with type 1 DM and insidious with type 2 DM.
2. Classic symptoms of hyperglycemia include polyuria, polydipsia, polyphagia, weight loss, fatigue, and blurred vision.
3. Chronic hyperglycemia often presents as disorders of altered tissue response, evidenced by poor wound healing and recurrent infections of the skin and genitourinary (GU) tract.

Diagnostic Evaluation

See page 734.

Management

EVIDENCE BASE Garber, A. J., Abrahamson, M. J., Barzilay, J. I., Blonde, L., Bloomgarden, Z. T., Bush, M. A., Dagogo-Jack, S., DeFronzo, R. A., Einhorn, D., Fonseca, V. A., Garber, J. R., Garvey, W. T., Grunberger, G., Handelsman, Y., Hirsch, I. B., Jellinger, P. S., McGill, J. B., Mechanick, J. I., Rosenblit, P. D., & Umpierrez, G. E. (2018). Consensus statement by the American Association of Clinical Endocrinologists and American College of Endocrinology on the comprehensive type 2 diabetes management algorithm—2018 executive summary. *Endocrine Practice*, *24*(1), 91–120. https://doi.org/10.4158/CS-2017-0153

A multidisciplinary approach, which combines diet, exercise, behavioral/psychosocial therapy, and pharmacologic agents, is required to optimally manage glucose control and the comorbid conditions of hypertension, dyslipidemia, and obesity.

Diet

1. The goal of meal planning is to meet nutritional requirements essential for healthy growth/development, achieve/maintain healthy weight, and control blood glucose and lipid levels (see Table 21-3).
2. Weight reduction is a primary treatment for prediabetes and type 2 DM. A target of greater than 5% weight loss is desired.
3. Medical nutrition therapy should be conducted by a registered dietitian, preferably one who is also a certified diabetes care and education specialist (CDCES).

Exercise

Regularly scheduled, moderate exercise of at least 150 minutes a week, including 30 to 60 minutes at least every other day, promotes

Table 21-3 Meal Planning Guidelines

PRINCIPLE	ACTION
Each meal should consist of a balance of carbohydrates, proteins, and fats.	• Carbohydrates should be varied to include fruits, starches, and vegetables. • Protein selections that are lean will help reduce fat and cholesterol intake. • Fats should be used sparingly with <10% of total calories derived from saturated fats. High in calories, fats contribute to weight gain in type 2 diabetes mellitus.
Consistency in timing of meals and amounts of food eaten on a day-to-day basis help regulate blood glucose levels.	• Avoid skipping or delaying meals. • Measure portion sizes using a scale or measuring cups. • Know the equivalent amounts of commonly used foods within a food group (e.g., 1 slice of bread = ½ cup cooked pasta).
Increase the intake of soluble and insoluble fiber.	• Substitute foods high in fiber for processed foods when possible (e.g., whole-grain bread in place of white bread). • Eat fresh fruits and vegetables in place of juices.
Avoid salt whenever possible.	• Do not season foods with salt or salt-containing spices. • Limit use of foods with "hidden" sodium content (e.g., crackers, pickled foods, cheese, processed meats). • Use salt-containing condiments sparingly (ketchup, soy sauce, gravies, bouillon).
Prepare foods to retain vitamins and minerals and reduce fats.	• Do not fry foods. • Bake, broil, or boil foods and discard fat. • Eat raw fruits and vegetables or steam vegetables to retain fiber. • Avoid adding calories with butter or cream sauces, fatback, and bacon. • Trim all visible fat from meat; skim off fat from stews or other prepared dishes.
Distribute snacks in the meal plan depending on insulin/medication regimens, physical activity, and lifestyle.	• Smaller, more frequent meals may enhance glucose control in type 2 diabetes mellitus. • Unplanned activity may call for an additional snack to avoid hypoglycemia.
Use alcohol only in moderation.	• Always consume alcohol with food to avoid hypoglycemia. • Do not omit food from meal plan in exchange for alcohol. • Limit intake to 1–2 drinks/wk (4 oz. dry wine, 12 oz. beer, or 1.5 oz. distilled liquor = 1 alcohol serving).
Use alternative nonnutritive, noncaloric sweeteners in moderation.	• Limit "diet" soda intake to 2 L/d. • Avoid frequent use of foods and beverages with concentrated sucrose.

the utilization of carbohydrates, assists with weight control, enhances the action of insulin, and improves cardiovascular fitness. The patient should be instructed as follows:

1. Check blood glucose level before starting, during, and after exercise.
2. Avoid vigorous exercise if blood glucose is greater than 270 mg/dL; moderate exercise is acceptable if feeling well.
3. Eat 15 g of carbohydrate before exercising if blood glucose is less than 100 mg/dL.

Psychosocial Care

1. Psychosocial care should be an integrated component of comprehensive diabetes management for all patients with diabetes.
2. Assess for symptoms of diabetes distress, depression, anxiety, disordered eating, and cognitive capacity.
3. Assess for life circumstances that impact patient ability to perform self-care management. Include input from family members/caregivers.
4. Promptly refer to behavioral health specialist when problems are identified.

EVIDENCE BASE Young-Hyman, D., de Groot, M., Hill-Briggs, F., Gonzalez, J. S., Hood, K., & Peyrot, M. (2016). Psychosocial care for people with diabetes: A position statement of the American Diabetes Association. *Diabetes Care*, *39*(12), 2126–2140. https://doi.org/10.2337/dc16-2053

Medication

Both the American Diabetes Association (ADA) and American Association of Clinical Endocrinologists (AACE)/American College of Endocrinology (ACE) treatment algorithms place emphasis on individualizing pharmacologic treatment based on effectiveness, risk of hypoglycemia, risk of weight gain, cost, and patient preferences. Lifestyle management (diet and exercise) will always remain the cornerstone of management even when medications are required. Insulin is always an appropriate therapy for glucose management and should be discussed with the patient early in the disease process to alleviate fears and other stigma associated with its use.

Only insulin and amylin analogs are approved for use in patients with type 1 DM.

1. Oral and injectable antidiabetic agents for patients with type 2 DM who do not achieve glucose control with diet and exercise only (see Table 21-4, pages 722 to 723).
2. Insulin therapy is essential for patients with type 1 DM who require replacement (see pages 716 to 719). Insulin therapy may also be used for type 2 DM when glucose management is unresponsive to diet, exercise, and noninsulin therapy as well as when beta-cell failure progresses or they are unable to tolerate/safely use other diabetes medications.

DRUG ALERT Hypoglycemia may result from insulin therapy as well as rebound hyperglycemia (Somogyi effect). Insulin therapy commonly results in increased appetite and weight gain.

3. Sulfonylurea compounds promote the increased secretion of insulin by the pancreas and partially normalize both receptor and postreceptor defects.
   a. Many drug interactions exist, so patient should alert all health care providers of use.
   b. Potential adverse reactions include hypoglycemia, photosensitivity, gastrointestinal (GI) upset, allergic reaction, reaction to alcohol, cholestatic jaundice, and blood dyscrasias.
4. Metformin, a biguanide compound, appears to diminish insulin resistance. It decreases hepatic glucose production and intestinal reabsorption of glucose and increases insulin reception and glucose transport in cells.
   a. Many drug interactions exist, so patient should alert all health care providers of its use.
   b. Metformin must be used cautiously in renal insufficiency, conditions that may cause dehydration, and hepatic impairment.
   c. Potential adverse reactions include GI disturbances, metallic taste, and lactic acidosis (rare). Riomet is the only formulation available as an oral solution.

DRUG ALERT Lactic acidosis is a rare complication of metformin that prompts caution when dehydration, vomiting, diarrhea, fasting states, hemodynamic instability, heavy alcohol use, and use of iodinated contrast media occur.

5. Alpha glucosidase inhibitors (AGIs) (acarbose and miglitol) delay the digestion and absorption of complex carbohydrates (including sucrose or table sugar) into simple sugars, such as glucose and fructose, thereby lowering postprandial and fasting glucose levels.
   a. Contraindicated in inflammatory bowel disease and other conditions of the intestinal tract. They are used cautiously in renal insufficiency and with several other drugs.
   b. Flatulence, abdominal pain, and diarrhea are common.
   c. If these medications are taken in conjunction with insulin secretagogues (i.e., sulfonylureas) and hypoglycemia occurs, patient must use a monosaccharide (glucose tablets) or milk to treat hypoglycemia because sucrose will not be broken down to an absorbable sugar. Juice will not be effective.
6. Thiazolidinedione (TZD) derivatives (rosiglitazone and pioglitazone) primarily decrease resistance to insulin in skeletal muscle and adipose tissue without increasing insulin secretion. Secondarily, they reduce hepatic glucose production.
   a. They should be used cautiously in liver disease and heart failure. Liver function tests should be monitored periodically.
   b. Ovulation may occur in anovulatory premenopausal patients.
   c. Adverse reactions include edema, weight gain, anemia, elevation in serum transaminases, and increased incidence of bone fracture.
   d. Pioglitazone is associated with increased risk of bladder cancer; therefore, it should not be used in patients with a history of bladder cancer.
   e. TZDs themselves do not cause hypoglycemia; however, when administered with insulin or oral medications that increase the secretion of insulin, the risk for hypoglycemia is increased. Be aware that insulin requirements will reduce with TZD therapy, so glucose monitoring and insulin adjustments should be done regularly.

DRUG ALERT Both pioglitazone and rosiglitazone can cause or worsen heart failure and are contraindicated for use in patients with New York Heart Association class III or class IV heart failure (see page 272).

Table 21-4 Antidiabetic Medications (Noninsulin)

AGENT	ROUTE AND DOSE
Insulin-Secreting Agents	
Second-Generation Sulfonylureas	
• Glyburide	1.25–20 mg PO in single or divided doses with meals
• Glyburide, micronized	0.75–12 mg PO in single or divided dose
• Glipizide	2.5–40 mg PO in single or divided doses with meals
• Glipizide, long-acting	2.5–20 mg PO in single dose, usually before breakfast
• Glimepiride	1–8 mg PO in single dose with first main meal
Meglitinide Analog	
Repaglinide	0.5–16 mg PO in two to four divided doses, 1–30 min before meals Do not take if meal is skipped.
Amino Acid Derivative	
Nateglinide	120–360 mg PO in three divided doses, 1–30 min before meals Do not take if meal is skipped.
Insulin-Sensitizing Agents	
Biguanides	
• Metformin	500–2,550 mg PO in two to three divided doses
• Metformin, long-acting	500–2,000 mg PO in single or two divided doses
Thiazolidinediones	
• Pioglitazone	15–45 mg PO once daily
• Rosiglitazone	4–8 mg PO in single or two divided doses
Glucose Absorption–Delaying Agents	
α Glucosidase Inhibitors	
• Acarbose	50–300 mg PO in three divided doses before meals
• Miglitol	50–300 mg PO in three divided doses before meals
Incretin Agents	
DPP-4 Inhibitors	
• Sitagliptin	25–100 mg PO once daily
• Linagliptin	5 mg PO once daily
• Saxagliptin	2.5–5 mg PO once daily
• Alogliptin	6.25–25 mg PO once daily
GLP-1 and GLP-1 Receptor Agonists	
• Exenatide	5–10 μg subcutaneously twice daily 1–60 min before meals
• Liraglutide	1.2–1.8 mg subcutaneously once daily
• Lixisenatide	10–20 μg subcutaneously once daily
• Exenatide, extended release	2 mg subcutaneously every 7 d
• Albiglutide	20–50 mg subcutaneously every 7 d
• Dulaglutide	0.75–1.5 mg subcutaneously every 7 d
• Semaglutide	0.5–1 mg subcutaneously every 7 d
• Tirzepatide	2.5–15 mg subcutaneously weekly
• Oral Semaglutide (Rybelsus)	3 mg starter dose, increase to 7 mg after 30 d, daily on empty stomach; may increase to 14 mg if needed
Glucose-Excreting Agents	
SGLT2 Inhibitors	
• Canagliflozin	100–300 mg PO once daily
• Empagliflozin	10–25 mg PO once daily
• Dapagliflozin	5–10 mg PO once daily
• Ertugliflozin	5–15 mg PO once daily
• Bexagliflozin	20 mg PO once in morning
Amylin Analog	
Pramlintide	Type 1: 15–60 μg subcutaneously with each main meal Type 2: 60–120 μg subcutaneously with each main meal
Other Agents	
Bile Acid Sequestrant	
Colesevelam	625 mg tablets: 3 tabs PO twice daily or 6 tabs PO once daily

Table 21-4 Antidiabetic Medications (Noninsulin) (*continued*)

AGENT
Combination Agents With Brand Names
• Actoplus Met, Actoplus Met XR (pioglitazone + metformin) • Amaryl M (glimepiride + metformin) • Avandamet (rosiglitazone + metformin) • Avandaryl (rosiglitazone + glimepiride) • Duetact (pioglitazone + glimepiride) • Glucovance (glyburide + metformin) • Glyxambi (linagliptin + empagliflozin) • Invokamet, Invokamet XR (canagliflozin + metformin) • Janumet, Janumet XR (sitagliptin + metformin) • Jentadueto (linagliptin + metformin) • Kazano (alogliptin + metformin) • Kombiglyze XR (saxagliptin + metformin) • Metaglip (glipizide + metformin) • Oseni (alogliptin + pioglitazone) • PrandiMet (repaglinide + metformin) • Qtern (dapagliflozin + saxagliptin) • Soliqua 100/33 (lixisenatide + insulin glargine) • Steglatro (ertugliflozin + metformin) • Steglujan (ertugliflozin + sitagliptin) • Synjardy (empagliflozin + metformin) • Xigduo, Xigduo XR (dapagliflozin + metformin) • Xultophy 100/3.6 (liraglutide + insulin degludec)

DM, diabetes mellitus; DPP-4, dipeptidyl peptidase 4; GLP-1 RA, glucagon-like peptide-1 receptor agonist; PO, by mouth; XR, extended release.

7. Meglitinide analogs (repaglinide) and amino acid derivatives (nateglinide) stimulate pancreatic release of insulin in response to a meal. They have a more rapid onset and shorter duration than sulfonylureas.
   a. Should not be taken when a meal is skipped or missed.
   b. Should be used cautiously in patients with renal and hepatic dysfunction and may cause hypoglycemia.
8. Dipeptidyl peptidase 4 inhibitors (DPP-4i) (sitagliptin, linagliptin, saxagliptin, alogliptin) inhibit the breakdown of glucagon-like peptide-1 (GLP-1). GLP-1 stimulates insulin release from the pancreas and decreases glucagon secretion, which inhibits glycogenolysis and gluconeogenesis. These agents are most effective at controlling postprandial blood glucose and, when used either alone or in combination with metformin or TZD, do not cause hypoglycemia.
   a. Dose is based on renal function.
   b. Generally, well tolerated and weight neutral. Adverse reactions include upper respiratory infections, nasopharyngitis, and headaches.
   c. Can be combined with all other diabetes medication, except for those in the GLP-1 RA (receptor agonist) class.

DRUG ALERT Patients with a history of pancreatitis should not be prescribed either DPP4-i or GLP-1 RA.

9. Sodium glucose cotransporter 2 inhibitors (SGLT2i) (canagliflozin, empagliflozin, dapagliflozin, ertugliflozin) block glucose absorption in the proximal renal tubule by inhibiting SGLT2 receptors. Glucose is excreted in the urine, which leads to modest weight loss and some improvement in systolic blood pressure (BP).
   a. Dose is based on renal function.
   b. These have been known to cause ketoacidosis in the absence of significant glucose elevations (euglycemic diabetic ketoacidosis [DKA]), especially in patients who are ill, suffer trauma, require surgery, or have type 1 DM. These should be stopped and resumed only when patient is stable. Patients should be advised to stop these medications and seek medical assistance immediately if they experience any symptoms consistent with DKA (nausea/vomiting, abdominal pain).
   c. Adverse reactions include urinary tract infections and mycotic infection of the genital tract.
   d. Hold SGLT2 before surgery a minimum of 24 hours (AACE), or at least 3 days according to the U.S. Food and Drug Administration (FDA). The patient must be monitored for acid–base and ketones pre/postoperatively until resuming eating normally.
10. Bile acid sequestrant (colesevelam) is traditionally a cholesterol-lowering agent that is also indicated for the treatment of type 2 DM. The exact mechanism of action is unclear but may have effect on sensitizing the liver to insulin, reducing hepatic glucose production. May also work by reducing intestinal absorption of glucose.
    a. Side effects include nausea, bloating, and constipation.
    b. Causes triglyceride levels to rise and, therefore, should not be used in patients with baseline elevation of triglyceride levels.
11. GLP-1 receptor agonists (GLP-1 RAs) work to lower blood glucose by enhancing first-phase insulin secretion by the pancreas, slowing gastric emptying, suppressing glucagon secretion, and reducing appetite, which can facilitate weight loss.
    a. The long-acting GLP-1 RAs are all injected once weekly. These tend to be better tolerated than the agents requiring more frequent administration.
    b. These are used as add-on therapy to all other diabetes medications (except DPP-4); all but long-acting exenatide are approved for use with insulin.
    c. GLP-1 RAs are not to be used as a substitute for insulin.
    d. GLP-1 RA and insulin (lixisenatide plus insulin glargine; liraglutide plus insulin degludec) are available as daily fixed ratio for combination therapies with long-acting insulin.
    e. Most common adverse effects are nausea and vomiting. Other adverse reactions include GI upset, headache, and pancreatitis.
    f. They have also been associated with medullary thyroid and pancreatic cancer in rats, but not in humans during trials.

DRUG ALERT The class GLP-1 RA has a boxed warning from the FDA that they should not be used if the patient has a personal or familial history of medullary thyroid cancer or multiple endocrine neoplasia syndrome (MENS) type 2a or 2b. They also should not be used in patients with severe GI disorders, such as gastroparesis, and used cautiously when renal impairment is present. Refer to full prescribing information available with each product.

12. Amylin analog (pramlintide). Amylin is co-secreted by the B cells of the pancreas to assist with postprandial glucose control. Its actions are like GLP-1 incretin mimetics (reduced gastric emptying, suppression of glucagon, increased satiety, and weight loss). It is indicated for patients with either type 1 or type 2 diabetes who require a mealtime insulin bolus.
    a. It is not a substitute for insulin but must be administered immediately prior to meals that must consist of at least 250 kcal or at least 30 g of carbohydrates.
    b. If used with insulin, mealtime dose of insulin must be reduced by 50%. Pramlintide cannot be mixed with insulin and must be injected at least 1 in (2.5 cm) away from insulin injection site. It is available in a disposable pen device.
    c. It is contraindicated in patients with confirmed gastroparesis and should be used with caution in patients who require the use of drugs to stimulate gastric motility.
    d. The most common adverse effects are GI related (nausea/vomiting).

DRUG ALERT Pramlintide may cause severe insulin-induced hypoglycemia and is contraindicated in patients with hypoglycemia unawareness.

General Health

In addition to the glycemic and A1C goals discussed previously, prevention and management guidelines have been established for BP, lipid values, and kidney function to prevent complications. Patients with diabetes are at a much higher risk for cardiovascular disease than the general population; therefore, cardiovascular risk factors must be monitored and aggressively treated. Several authoritative groups recommend the following goals of treatment for nonpregnant adults, adolescents, and children with DM.

EVIDENCE BASE Garber, A. J., Abrahamson, M. J., Barzilay, J. I., Blonde, L., Bloomgarden, Z. T., Bush, M. A., Dagogo-Jack, S., DeFronzo, R. A., Einhorn, D., Fonseca, V. A., Garber, J. R., Garvey, W. T., Grunberger, G., Handelsman, Y., Hirsch, I. B., Jellinger, P. S., McGill, J. B., Mechanick, J. I., Rosenblit, P. D., & Umpierrez, G. E. (2018). Consensus statement by the American Association of Clinical Endocrinologists and American College of Endocrinology on the comprehensive type 2 diabetes management algorithm—2018 executive summary. *Endocrine Practice, 24*(1), 91–120. https://doi.org/10.4158/CS-2017-0153

ElSayed, N. A., Aleppo, G., Aroda, V. R., Bannuru, R. R., Brown, F. M., Bruemmer, D., Collins, B. S., Das, S. R., Hilliard, M. E., Isaacs, D., Johnson, E. L., Kahan, S., Khunti, K., Kosiborod, M., Leon, J., Lyons, S. K., Perry, M. L., Prahalad, P., Pratley, R. E., ... on behalf of the American Diabetes Association. (2023). 10. Cardiovascular disease and risk management: *Standards of care in diabetes—2023. Diabetes Care,* 46(Suppl 1), S158–S190. https://doi.org/10.2337/dc23-S010

Adults:

1. BP <140/90 mm Hg (all ages) (ADA); ≤130/80 mm Hg (AACE/ACE); pregnant patients: 140/90 mm Hg is threshold to initiate or titrate therapy with goal of 110 to 135/85 mm Hg.
    a. BP should be measured at every visit; high BP is diagnosed when BP is above referenced threshold measured on ≥2 BP measurements obtained on two and more occasions.
    b. BP goal should be individualized with understanding of risk for cardiovascular complications and potential adverse effect of the medication.
2. Lipid control (all ages).
    a. Low-density lipoprotein (LDL) less than 100 mg/dL.
    b. High-density lipoprotein (HDL) greater than 40 mg/dL (males); greater than 50 mg/dL (females).
    c. Triglycerides less than 150 mg/dL.
    d. Diabetes is considered an independent risk factor for cardiovascular disease; therefore, according to the American College of Cardiology/American Heart Association (ACA/AHA) guidelines, all patients with diabetes between the ages of 45 and 75 years should be prescribed a moderate-intensity statin (without regard to the above-mentioned parameters). More aggressive treatment is recommended if additional cardiovascular risk factors are present. Use careful consideration of benefit/risk ratio when prescribing statin therapy in adults younger than 40 and older than 75 years of age.
    e. Statins are contraindicated during pregnancy; use with extreme caution in all patients of childbearing age.
3. Urinary albumin-to-creatinine ratio (spot urine) less than 30 mg/g creatinine (monitor at least annually).
4. Aspirin (75 to 162 mg/day) for most males and females ≥50 years with at least one additional major cardiovascular risk factor.

Children and adolescents (also see Chapter 46):

1. BP below the 90th percentile for sex assigned at birth, age, and height. If ≥13 years <120/80 mm Hg.
2. Lipid control:
    a. LDL less than 100 mg/dL.
    b. Statin may be required if LDL greater than 160 despite lifestyle modifications.

Complications

Acute

1. Hypoglycemia (blood glucose ≤70 mg/dL) occurs because of an imbalance in food, activity, and insulin/oral antidiabetic agent. Blood glucose less than 54 mg/dL is considered serious, clinically important hypoglycemia.
2. DKA occurs primarily in type 1 diabetes during times of severe insulin deficiency or illness, producing severe hyperglycemia, ketonuria, dehydration, and acidosis (see page 732).
3. Hyperosmolar hyperglycemic state (HHS) primarily affects patients with type 2 diabetes, causing severe dehydration, hyperglycemia, hyperosmolarity, and stupor (see page 734).

Chronic

See Table 21-5.

1. In type 1 diabetes, chronic complications usually appear about 5 years after the initial diagnosis.

Table 21-5 Chronic Complications of Diabetes Mellitus

CONDITION	ASSESSMENT	INTERVENTION	PREVENTION/TEACHING
Macrovascular Complications			
Cerebrovascular Disease			
• *Incidence*: Two to four times more likely in diabetes. • Hypertension, increased lipids, smoking, uncontrolled blood glucose, increase risk of stroke and transient ischemic attack	• Increased BP. • Change in mental status • Hemiparesis. • Aphasia. • Clinical presentation mimics that of a patient who is not diabetic.	• Check blood glucose level to differentiate signs and symptoms of stroke versus hypoglycemia. Monitor for bleeding if aspirin or other antiplatelet/anticoagulant medication is used.	• Maintain target goals of blood glucose, avoiding severe hypoglycemia and hyperglycemia, which predispose the patient to stroke. In hypoglycemia, increased levels of adrenalin and catecholamines can produce cardiac arrhythmias. • Hyperglycemia can lead to dehydration, which affects platelet aggregation.
Coronary Artery Disease			
• *Incidence*: Increased vessel disease with more vessels affected in diabetes. Higher incidence of "silent" myocardial infarctions (MIs). • Hyperglycemia contributes to atherosclerosis and vessel deterioration.	• Severe CAD is commonly asymptomatic, seen only in ECG changes. ECG changes may indicate silent MI. • Symptoms can also present as pain in the jaw, neck, or epigastric area.	• Usual medical treatment for angina prevails—sublingual nitroglycerin, oral nitrates. β-Adrenergic blockers and calcium channel blockers can also be used.	• Emphasis must be placed on reducing cardiac risk factors (e.g., cigarette smoking, hypertension, hyperlipidemia). Avoid wide fluctuations in blood glucose. Patients with autonomic neuropathy, which can cause orthostatic hypotension, should be carefully monitored when cardiac drug therapies are introduced. β-Adrenergic blockers can blunt or eliminate the clinical signs and symptoms of hypoglycemia.
Peripheral Vascular Disease			
• *Incidence*: 60% of non-traumatic amputations are related to diabetes. • Intermittent claudication, absent pedal pulses, and ischemic gangrene are increased in diabetes.	• Physical examination of the lower extremities may reveal changes in skin integrity associated with diminished circulation. • Decreased lower leg hair, absent or decreased anterior tibial or dorsal pedis pulses, poor capillary refill of toenails may occur. The extremity may appear pale/cool. Further examination for neurologic changes is indicated.	• Any lesion, decrease in peripheral pulses, or change in skin color, temperature, or sensation should be evaluated within 24–48 h. To ensure proper healing and prevent infection, treatment should begin as soon as possible and be carefully monitored. Mild antiseptics/antibiotic preparations are used to avoid further damage to the surrounding skin. Avoid the use of surgical tape to skin. Rest affected leg to promote circulation and wound healing.	• Foot care guidelines and smoking cessation must be stressed. Safe exercise guidelines and weight reduction, as appropriate, will further reduce risk of foot injury.
Microvascular Complications			
Retinopathy			
• *Incidence*: Type 1—Will develop after 3–5 yr of diagnosis and by 15–20 yr of diabetes duration almost all patients will have some	• Usually asymptomatic in the early stages. Symptoms occurring with acute visual problems—"floaters," flashing lights, blurred vision— may	• Laser therapy (photocoagulation) can be helpful in macular edema (focal laser) and proliferative retinopathy (panretinal laser). Reduction	• Stress importance of annual eye examination with an ophthalmologist (preferably retina specialist). Optimal glucose control can prevent

(continued)

Table 21-5 Chronic Complications of Diabetes Mellitus (*continued*)

CONDITION	ASSESSMENT	INTERVENTION	PREVENTION/TEACHING
degree of retinopathy. Type 2—~7% present with retinopathy at diagnosis, which increases to 50%–80% after 20 yr. DM is the leading cause of preventable blindness in the United States. • Appearance of hard exudates, blot hemorrhages, and microaneurysms on the retina in background retinopathy. Progresses to neovascularization in proliferative diabetic retinopathy.	indicate hemorrhage or retinal detachment. Funduscopic examination should be done by an ophthalmologist for full retinal visualization. • Type 1 DM initial evaluation should occur after 5 yr. • Type 2 DM initial evaluation at time of diagnosis. • GDM initial evaluation at conception or during first trimester.	of active neovascularization by laser therapy reduces the risk of vitreous hemorrhage. Vitrectomy may be needed to treat retinal detachment or remove vitreous hemorrhage. • During the acute phase, before laser therapy, patients must avoid activities that increase the chances of vitreous hemorrhage (e.g., weight lifting, high-impact aerobics).	or slow the progression of retinopathy. Maintaining normal BP also reduces the risk of retinopathy.
Nephropathy			
• *Incidence*: Up to 50% of people with diabetes will have renal impairment after 15-yr duration of diabetes. • The incidence is higher in Native American people, Hispanic people, and Black people. DM is the leading cause of kidney failure in the United States. • Thickening of the glomerular basement membrane, mesangial expansion, and renal vessel sclerosis are caused by diabetes. • Subsequently, diffuse and nodular intercapillary glomerulosclerosis diminishes renal function.	• Evidence of decreased glomerular filtration rate. • Microalbuminuria is the first clinical sign of renal disease. • Elevation in blood urea nitrogen and creatinine levels indicates advanced renal disease. • Gross proteinuria is a further indication of renal deterioration.	• Hypertension control, blood glucose control, and reduction of protein and sodium are essential. Angiotensin-converting enzyme inhibitors are the drugs of choice to control BP. Calcium channel blockers may also be used. In end-stage renal disease, dialysis or transplantation may be necessary.	• Frequent hypertension screening, noting any deviation from patient's normal reading. Early initiation of BP control to prevent kidney damage. Excellent glucose control with insulin/oral agent adjustment to compensate for reduced kidney function, which predisposes the patient to hypoglycemia. Avoidance of nephrotoxic drugs, dyes, or renal procedures that may cause infection. Immediate treatment for any urinary tract infections.
Peripheral Neuropathy			
• In general, neuropathy affects 60%–70% of persons with diabetes, with nearly 50% asymptomatic. • It can affect almost every organ system with varying specific symptoms. • Distal symmetrical polyneuropathy involving the lower extremities is most commonly seen. • In conjunction with peripheral vascular disease, neuropathy to the feet increases susceptibility to trauma and infection. The more severe forms of peripheral neuropathy are a major contributing cause of lower extremity amputations. • Three clinical syndromes of distal symmetrical polyneuropathy are seen: acute painful, small fiber, and large fiber neuropathy.	• Decreased light touch, vibratory, temperature sensation. Loss of foot proprioception, followed by ataxia, gait disturbances. • Diminished ankle jerk response. • Formation of "hammertoes," Charcot joint disease, which predispose patient to new pressure point areas. • Hypersensitivity or other dysesthetic symptoms are experienced, followed by hypnoanesthesia or anesthesia, which is not reversible.	• All foot wounds or injuries are immediately evaluated. Culture and sensitivity tests ordered for any drainage present. Affected foot is elevated—avoid weight bearing. Wet-to-dry dressings applied as ordered. Avoid use of caustic chemicals, dressing tapes. • Use of systemic antibiotics, as needed. • Medication for painful neuropathy may include use of the tricyclic antidepressant drugs (amitriptyline), a serotonin and epinephrine reuptake inhibitor (duloxetine), or topical application of capsaicin ointment.	• In general, blood glucose control is recommended, avoiding wide fluctuations. In patients who are poorly controlled, care must be taken to correct glucoses slowly to avoid increasing symptoms of neuropathy. • Foot care guidelines. • Smoking cessation. • Frequent evaluation by podiatrist for modified footwear (e.g., orthotics, extra-depth shoes). • Safe exercise guidelines. • Weight reduction, as necessary.

Table 21-5 Chronic Complications of Diabetes Mellitus (*continued*)

CONDITION	ASSESSMENT	INTERVENTION	PREVENTION/TEACHING
Autonomic Neuropathy			
Cardiac Autonomic Neuropathy			
• Affects 30% of patients with type 1 DM after 20 yr and 60% of patients with type 2 DM after 15 yr. • Asymptomatic in early stages. Loss of heart rate variability detected on ECG. • Late stages: resting tachycardia, orthostatic hypotension, exercise intolerance. • Greater than threefold mortality; 38% "silent" MI	• Patients may report episodes of syncope, weakness, or visual impairment, particularly with positional changes. Evaluate BP and pulse in lying and standing position at each visit. BP changes that indicate neuropathic involvement: fall in systolic pressure of >30 mm Hg or fall in diastolic pressure of >10 mm Hg with change from lying to standing position.	• Improvement in blood glucose control to prevent fluid loss from glycosuria. Moderate amounts of sodium may be used in the diet to encourage fluid retention during hot weather or strenuous exercise. Mechanical devices such as support stockings (full hose to waist) may decrease venous pooling. Drugs to enhance volume expansion may be used (e.g., fludrocortisone).	• Encourage increased fluid intake to maintain hydration. • Caution should be used in changing position from lying to standing. Sitting on side of bed with feet dangling is recommended until BP stabilizes. • Avoid standing in one position, which may increase venous pooling. • Observe exercise programs.
Gastroparesis			
• *Incidence*: Occurs in 50% of people with long-standing diabetes. • *Characteristics*: Delayed gastric emptying, prolonged pylorospasms, and loss of the powerful contractions of the distal stomach to grind and mix foods.	• Typical symptoms may include nausea/vomiting, early satiety, abdominal bloating, epigastric pain, change in appetite. Wide fluctuations in blood glucoses and postmeal hypoglycemia caused by poor glucose absorption. Visualization of the gut by upper GI barium series may show retained food after an 8- to 12-h fast.	• Excellent glucose control to avoid hyperglycemia, which interferes with gut contractility. • Avoidance of severe postmeal hypoglycemia by small, frequent meals, low fat, and low fiber. This diet is also helpful in bloating/early satiety. Medication to improve gut motility is metoclopramide.	• Maintenance of excellent glucose control. Regular exercise improves/maintains GI motility. Avoid use of laxatives. Small, frequent meals may help.
Diarrhea			
• *Incidence*: ~20% of patients with diabetes. • *Characteristics*: Frequent, watery movements. • Mild steatorrhea. • Can be intermittent, persistent, or alternate with constipation.	• Diarrhea occurs without warning, frequently at night or after meals. Fecal incontinence may be caused by loss of internal sphincter control and anorectal sensation. Other causes, such as celiac sprue, pancreatic insufficiency, and lactose intolerance, must be investigated. Bacterial overgrowth in the bowel is also suspected.	• Dietary changes may include increased fiber, elimination of milk products. Sphincter-strengthening exercises may help. Medications: For diarrhea, hydrophilic fiber supplement, cholestyramine, or synthetic opiates are used. • Tetracycline and ampicillin are used for bacterial overgrowth.	• Routine bowel elimination habits. • Maintenance of adequate hydration. • Excellent blood glucose control reduces dehydration. • Inclusion of dietary fiber in the daily diet. • Daily exercise program that includes walking or swimming has been effective in encouraging bowel regularity.
Sexual Dysfunction			
• Affects 35%–75% males and 46% females with diabetes. • Sexual dysfunction in all patients can involve changes in libido, ability to achieve orgasm, and sexual satisfaction.	• *Males*: History of poor erectile function despite stimulation. Absence of early-morning erection in response to increased hormonal levels. • *Females*: May experience decreased vaginal lubrication and dyspareunia. • Screening for use of ethanol or other medications associated with impotence (e.g., antidepressants, antihypertensives).	• *Males*: Referral to urologist for full examination is indicated. Treatment options may include injection of alprostadil (a prostaglandin), inflatable penile prosthesis, or oral medications. • *Females*: Increase lubrication with use of water-based lubricant or estrogen creams, which may also help thicken the vaginal mucosa, affecting dyspareunia.	• Reduce consumption of alcohol, which may hasten or contribute to neuropathy. • Maintain target ranges of blood glucose control to reduce likelihood of vaginal infections. • Discuss alternative ways of maintaining intimacy.
Bladder Dysfunction			
• *Incidence:* Affects 37%–50% of people with diabetes, F > M.	• Overflow incontinence is common problem for females. Inquire about use	• Credé maneuver every 4 h. • Bethanechol (10–30 mg three times daily).	• Avoid caloric beverages, which lead to significant hyperglycemia and glucosuria.

(*continued*)

Table 21-5 Chronic Complications of Diabetes Mellitus (*continued*)

CONDITION	ASSESSMENT	INTERVENTION	PREVENTION/TEACHING
• Inability to sense a full bladder, incomplete void/overflow incontinence. Increased frequency of UTI and pyelonephritis leading to or exacerbating renal failure.	of pads in undergarments, which may be clue. • Distended bladder. • Burning/pain with voiding; straining to empty bladder. Nocturia.	• Doxazosin. • Intermittent self-catheterization.	• Avoid caffeine and other bladder irritants (nicotine). • Establish a scheduled routine for attempting to empty bladder to avoid overflow incontinence
Hypoglycemia Unawareness			
• *Incidence*: Severe hypoglycemia occurs most frequently in patients with type 1 DM (30%–40% annual prevalence); however, it will also occur in patients with type 2 DM who are treated with insulin, sulfonylureas, and/or glinides. • Occurs in ~17% of patients with type 1 diabetes and at a rate of two to three times more frequently than those with type 2 DM. • Condition in which the usual warning signs of hypoglycemia are no longer experienced. The symptoms may be different (and therefore not recognized), less pronounced, or even absent. • Can eventually lead to hypoglycemia-associated autonomic failure, which includes both hypoglycemia unawareness and defective glucose counterregulatory hormones. • *Causes*: Long-standing diabetes, reduced glucagon excretion, frequent low blood sugars, alcohol consumption within the previous 12 h, previous low blood sugar within the last 24–48 h, certain medications (i.e., β-adrenergic blockers). • Females more susceptible because of reduced counterregulatory response and reduced symptoms. • More likely to occur in patients with other types of autonomic neuropathy.	• Patients may exhibit irrational thought; unprovoked anger or irritability; insisting that they "feel fine" in the midst of very unusual behavior; inappropriate laughing/silliness/giddiness/crying. • Syncope or Grand mal seizures can occur if hypoglycemia is not recognized and treated.	• Can be reversed by avoiding frequent low blood sugars. Raising target blood sugar (i.e., 140 mg/dL) by easing up on aggressive/intensive insulin treatment for a few weeks will allow the counterregulatory hormone response to return to normal. • Injected glucagon is the best treatment when the patient resists treatment, becomes unconscious, or has seizures because of hypoglycemia.	• Increase frequency of blood glucose monitoring and stay alert to physical warning signs for 48 h following low blood sugar. Keeping a glucose log, or using a continuous glucose monitor (CGM) will help patients predict when lows are more likely to occur. An occasional 2:00 a.m. blood glucose test can help with identifying unrecognized nocturnal hypoglycemia. • Carry glucose tablets/gel at all times to quickly and appropriately raise blood sugar levels. • All patients using intensive insulin management should have glucagon emergency kits and their family members must know how and when to administer. • Patients will need to closely match insulin doses to diet and exercise. They may need to reduce their insulin doses during and for several hours following increased physical activity. • Avoid alcohol or limit to no more than one to two drinks per day, and never drink on an empty stomach. • Patients should wear a medical alert device at all times to facilitate appropriate treatment by emergency personnel.

BP, blood pressure; F, female; CAD, coronary artery disease; ECG, electrocardiography; GI, gastrointestinal; GDM, gestational diabetes mellitus; M, male.

2. The prevalence of microvascular complications (retinopathy, nephropathy, and neuropathy) is higher in type 1 diabetes.
3. Because of its insidious onset, chronic complications can appear at any point in type 2 diabetes. Approximately 50% will have at least one complication at the time of diagnosis.
4. Macrovascular complications (i.e., cardiovascular disease)—occurring in type 1 and type 2 diabetes—are the leading cause of morbidity and mortality among persons with diabetes.

Nursing Assessment

1. Obtain a history of current problems, family history, and general health history.
   a. Has the patient experienced polyuria, polydipsia, polyphagia, and any other symptoms?
   b. Number of years since initial diagnosis of diabetes.
   c. Family members diagnosed with diabetes, their subsequent treatment, and complications.
2. Perform a review of systems and physical examination to assess for signs and symptoms of diabetes, general health of patient, and presence of complications.
   a. General: recent weight loss or gain, increased fatigue, tiredness, anxiety.
   b. Skin: skin lesions, infections, dehydration, evidence of poor wound healing.
   c. Eyes: changes in vision—floaters, halos, blurred vision, dry or burning eyes, cataracts, glaucoma.
   d. Mouth: gingivitis, periodontal disease.
   e. Cardiovascular: orthostatic hypotension, cold extremities, weak pedal pulses, leg claudication.
   f. GI: diarrhea, constipation, early satiety, bloating, increased flatulence, hunger, or thirst.
   g. GU: increased urination, nocturia, impotence, vaginal discharge.
   h. Neurologic: numbness and tingling of the extremities, decreased pain and temperature perception, changes in gait and balance.

Nursing Interventions

See Standards of Care Guidelines 21-1.

STANDARDS OF CARE GUIDELINES 21-1
Caring for Patients With Diabetes Mellitus

When caring for patients with diabetes mellitus:

- Assess level of knowledge of disease and ability to care for self.
- Assess adherence to diet therapy, monitoring procedures, medication treatment, and exercise regimen.
- Assess resources/support system available to patient; involve behavioral health, social work services, and case management as needed.
- Assess for signs of hyperglycemia: polyuria, polydipsia, polyphagia, weight loss, fatigue, blurred vision.
- Assess for signs of hypoglycemia: sweating, tremor, nervousness, tachycardia, lightheadedness, confusion.
- Perform thorough skin and extremity assessment for peripheral neuropathy or peripheral vascular disease and any injury to the feet or lower extremities.
- Assess for trends in blood glucose and other laboratory results.
- Reinforce appropriate insulin dosage is given at the right time and in relation to meals and exercise.
- Assess adequate knowledge of diet, exercise, and medication treatment and cognitive skills to safely adhere to prescribed regimen.
- Immediately report to health care provider any signs of skin or soft tissue infection (redness, swelling, warmth, tenderness, drainage).
- Get help immediately for signs of hypoglycemia that do not respond to usual glucose replacement.
- Get help immediately for patient presenting with signs of either ketoacidosis (nausea and vomiting, Kussmaul respirations, fruity breath odor, hypotension, and altered level of consciousness) or hyperosmolar hyperglycemic nonketotic syndrome (nausea and vomiting, hypothermia, muscle weakness, seizures, stupor, coma).

This information should serve as a general guideline only. Each patient situation presents a unique set of clinical factors and requires nursing judgment to guide care, which may include additional or alternative measures and approaches.

Improving Nutrition

1. Assess current timing and content of meals.
2. Advise patient on the importance of an individualized meal plan in meeting weight loss goals. Reducing intake of carbohydrates may benefit some patients; however, fad diets or diet plans that stress one food group and eliminate another are generally not recommended.
3. Discuss the goals of dietary therapy for the patient. Setting a goal of greater than 5% weight loss over several months is usually achievable and effective in reducing blood sugar and other metabolic parameters.
4. Assist patient to identify problems that may have an impact on dietary adherence and possible solutions to these problems. Emphasize that lifestyle changes should be maintainable for life.
5. Explain the importance of exercise in maintaining/reducing body weight.
   a. Caloric expenditure for energy in exercise.
   b. Carryover of enhanced metabolic rate and efficient food utilization.
6. Assist patient to establish goals for weekly weight loss and incentives to assist in achieving them.
7. Strategize with patient to address the potential difficulties and problem-solving for social situations that may not be conducive to personal goals.

Teaching About Insulin

1. Assist patient to reduce fear of injection by encouraging verbalization of fears regarding insulin injection, conveying a sense of empathy, and identifying supportive coping techniques.
2. Demonstrate and explain thoroughly the procedure for insulin self-injection.
3. Help patient to master technique by taking a step-by-step approach.
   a. Allow patient time to handle insulin and syringe/pen to become familiar with the equipment.
   b. Teach self-injection first to alleviate fear of pain from injection.
   c. Instruct patient in filling syringe when they express confidence in self-injection procedure.

4. Review dosage and time of injections in relation to meals, activity, and bedtime based on patient's individualized insulin regimen.

POPULATION AWARENESS Assess older adults for sensory deficits (e.g., impaired vision, hearing, fine touch), motor challenges (e.g., tremors), and arthritic changes that may have an impact on learning and the ability to self-administer insulin. Explore use of an insulin pen, enhanced lighting, magnifying devices, and video communication with someone to assist with proper daily dosing.

DRUG ALERT For mixed insulin, such as NPH combinations, the pen must be inverted 10 times to ensure mixing before setting the dose.

Preventing Injury Secondary to Hypoglycemia

1. Closely monitor blood glucose levels to detect hypoglycemia (blood glucose ≤70 mg/dL).
2. Instruct patient on the importance of accuracy in insulin preparation, administration, and meal timing to avoid hypoglycemia.
3. Assess patient for signs and symptoms of hypoglycemia.
   a. Adrenergic (early symptoms)—sweating, tremor, pallor, tachycardia, palpitations, nervousness from the release of adrenalin when blood glucose falls rapidly.
   b. Neurologic (later symptoms)—lightheadedness, headache, confusion, irritability, slurred speech, lack of coordination, staggering gait from depression of central nervous system as glucose level progressively falls.
4. Treat hypoglycemia promptly using the 15-g/15-minute rule according to the ADA with 15-g of rapidly absorbed carbohydrates.
   a. One-half cup (4 oz.) juice, one cup skim milk, four glucose tablets, one tablespoon of sugar/honey, or five to six pieces of hard candy may be taken orally.
   b. Wait 15 minutes.
   c. Repeat blood glucose; if less than 70 mg/dL, repeat the treatment.
   d. If greater than 70 mg/dL and more than 3 hours since last dose of rapid-acting insulin, no further treatment required.
   e. If greater than 70 mg/dL but less than 3 hours since last dose of rapid-acting insulin, follow with a snack that contains a carbohydrate and protein source.
   f. If using a "split-mix" or REG/NPH insulins and more than 30 minutes before next planned meal/snack, have meal/snack now.
   g. Glucagon 1 mg (SQ or intramuscular [IM]) is given if severe hypoglycemia (<50 mg/dL) occurs and the patient cannot safely ingest a carbohydrate source. Family member or staff must administer injection. It is also available as a nasal spray.
   h. Intravenous (IV) bolus of 50 mL of 50% dextrose solution can be given if the patient fails to respond to glucagon within 15 minutes.
5. Encourage patient to always carry a carbohydrate source for the treatment of hypoglycemia.
6. Assess patient for cognitive or physical impairments that may interfere with ability to accurately administer insulin.
7. Between-meal snacks as well as extra food taken before exercise should be encouraged to prevent hypoglycemia.
8. Encourage patients to wear an identification bracelet or card that may assist in prompt treatment in a hypoglycemic emergency.
   a. Obtain a commercially available medical alert device.
   b. Identification card may be requested from the ADA (www.diabetes.org).
9. If hypoglycemia occurs frequently, discuss with health care provider. Dose adjustments of insulin and/or oral medications may be necessary.
10. Address safety issues if patient has a hypoglycemic event while driving, operating machinery, or during exertional activity. Cognitive recovery takes 45 to 75 minutes following blood glucose levels of less than 50 mg/dL.

DRUG ALERT Patients taking an AGI must use a monosaccharide (glucose tablets) to treat hypoglycemia because sucrose will not be broken down to an absorbable sugar.

Improving Activity Tolerance

1. Advise patient to assess blood glucose level before and after strenuous exercise.
2. Instruct patient to plan exercises on a regular basis each day.
3. Encourage patient to eat a carbohydrate snack before exercising to avoid hypoglycemia.
4. Advise patient that prolonged strenuous exercise may require increased food at bedtime to avoid nocturnal hypoglycemia.
5. Instruct patient to avoid exercise whenever blood glucose levels exceed 250 mg/day and urine ketones are present. Patient should contact health care provider if levels remain elevated.
6. Counsel patient to inject insulin into the abdominal site on days when arms or legs are exercised.

Providing Information About Noninsulin Agents

1. Identify barriers to learning, such as visual or hearing impairments, low literacy, and distractive environment.
2. Encourage active participation of the patient and family in the educational process.
3. Teach the action, use, and adverse effects of noninsulin agents (see pages 721-723).
4. Identify financial barriers to accessing medications and follow-up care. Offer resources such as Partnership for Prescription Assistance (www.helpingpatients.org).

Maintaining Skin Integrity

1. Assess feet and legs for skin temperature, sensation, soft tissue injuries, corns, calluses, dryness, hammertoe or bunion deformation, hair distribution, pulses, deep tendon reflexes.
   a. Use a monofilament to test sensation of the feet and detect early signs of peripheral neuropathy (see Figure 21-2).
   b. Test vibratory sense over interphalangeal joints of the feet using a low-frequency (128 Hz) tuning fork. Vibratory sense is typically lost before tactile sensation. The test is considered abnormal if the vibratory sensation is felt for less than 10 seconds.
2. Protect skin from dryness and breakdown.
   a. Use heel protectors, special mattresses, and foot cradles for patients on bed rest.
   b. Avoid applying drying agents to skin (e.g., alcohol).
   c. Apply skin moisturizers (preferably creams) to maintain suppleness and prevent cracking and fissures.
3. Instruct patient in foot care.

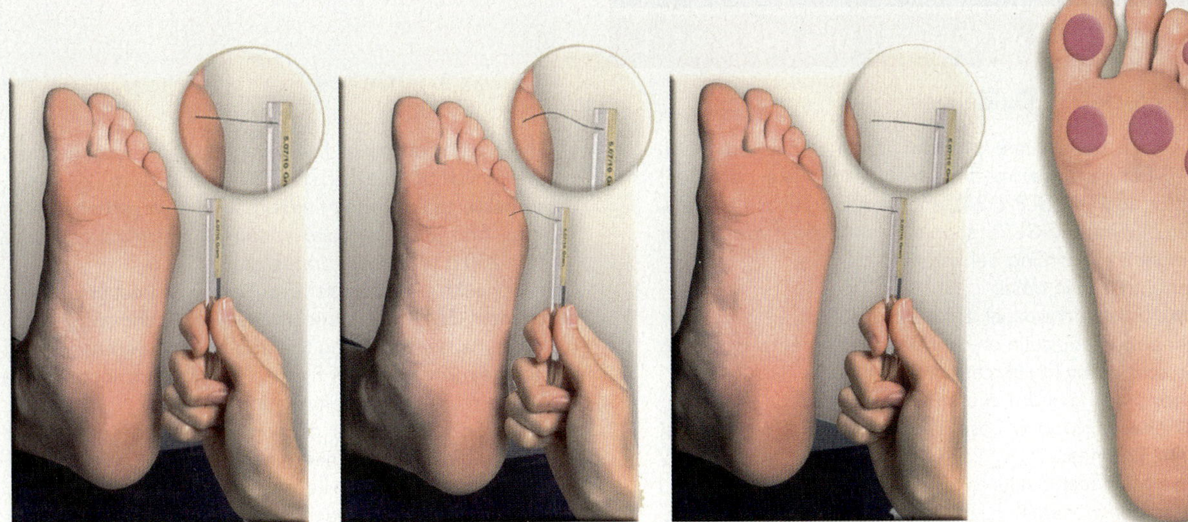

Figure 21-2. The Semmes-Weinstein 5.07 (10-g) monofilament test. (Reprinted with permission from Cameron, B. L. [2002]. Making diabetes management routine. *American Journal of Nursing, 102*[2], 26–33. https://doi.org/10.1097/00000446-200202000-00017)

4. Advise the patient who smokes to stop smoking, or reduce, if possible, to reduce vasoconstriction and enhance peripheral blood flow. Help patient to establish behavior modification techniques and encourage consideration of a smoking cessation program.

Focusing on Transitional Care

1. Begin discharge planning upon admission and update the plan as the patient's needs change or are more clearly understood, with the goal of reducing risk of readmission. People with diabetes are involved in almost 22% of all inpatient hospitalizations, and 13% will have diabetes as the primary reason for admission. Unfortunately, the 30-day readmission rates can be as high as 21% for patients with DM. The risk increases based on comorbidities, if admitted via emergency department, low socioeconomic status, and/or lack of health insurance.

CLINICAL JUDGMENT A1C levels should be obtained on all patients known to have diabetes—even if diabetes was not the primary reason for hospitalization. Be aware that patients with an A1C greater than 9% upon admission are very high risk for poor outcomes and readmission.

2. Ensure patients are being discharged with all medications with correct dose and adequate supplies.
   a. Insulin pens must have pen needles ordered, and if drawing insulin, syringes also need to be ordered.
   b. Make certain that the patient has a functioning glucose meter, test strips, and lancets and is comfortable with the testing procedure. If needed, ensure that order for supplies has been placed with pharmacy or diabetic supply company.
   c. Assess patient understanding of all medications prescribed, including timing with meals or bedtime.
   d. Ensure that patient can afford the out-of-pocket cost of all medications. Implement a social work referral if needed.
   e. Ensure that all chronic medications were not inadvertently stopped; all changes in medications must be made very clear to patient to prevent medication errors.
3. Ensure a 7-day follow-up appointment with the patient's primary care, or specialist provider is scheduled prior to discharge and that the patient has a secured means of transportation.
4. Provide patient with written discharge summary and instructions with symptoms to report and phone number to call.
   a. Teach patient to notify their provider any time their blood sugar is consistently higher than goal (and especially if associated with fever, nausea, vomiting, or diarrhea and positive for urine ketones).
   b. Notify health care provider if two or more occasions of low blood sugar (<70 mg/dL) occur.
5. Notify case manager or a transitional care team nurse to provide postdischarge follow-up phone calls to continue patient education started in the hospital and ensure the patient has resources for self-care at home.
6. Ensure that home health care is ordered for skilled nursing management and education and social work services if needed.

Patient Education and Health Maintenance

Ongoing education should be provided to include advanced skills and rationales for treatment, prevention, and management of complications.

1. Instruct the patient about the signs/symptoms of hypoglycemia and the importance of checking glucose level when symptoms occur or hypoglycemia is suspected. Ensure the patient has a handy source of glucose (15 g carbohydrate) to use if glucose is <70 mg/dL.
2. As long as the home is clean and the patient uses reasonable hygiene, procedures for glucose self-monitoring and insulin injection do not need to be sterile. No alcohol preparation of the skin or insulin vial is needed.
3. Advise the patient that while it is strongly discouraged, insulin syringes may be reused, so long as the needle is clean and no pain or signs of skin irritation develop due to dulling or damaged needle.
4. Review sick-day guidelines for insulin and medication dosage with the patient (see Patient Education Guidelines 21-1).

PATIENT EDUCATION GUIDELINES 21-1

Diabetes Sick-Day Guidelines

- Check with health care provider about noninsulin medication. For instance, metformin, glucagon-like peptide-1 receptor agonist (GLP-1 RA), and sodium glucose cotransporter 2 inhibitor (SGLT2i) should be withheld if vomiting or in danger of becoming dehydrated.
- Never omit insulin dose.
  - Take at least the usual dosage of insulin.
  - Keep regular insulin on hand for supplemental doses, as prescribed by health care provider.
- Monitor blood glucose and urine ketones every 2–4 h.
  - Whenever blood glucose is greater than 240 mg/dL, test urine ketones.
  - Record all test results to report to health care provider if condition worsens.
- Drink plenty of fluids.
  - Six to eight ounce of fluid every hour is recommended; every third hour, the fluid should include sodium (i.e., broth).
  - If unable to eat, drink fluids that contain carbohydrates (e.g., fruit juices, regular soda); patient must consume 150–200 g of carbohydrates/day.
- Contact health care provider or report to nearest emergency department (ED) if illness becomes severe or unmanageable.
  - Fever, nausea, vomiting (greater than one episode), and diarrhea (greater than five episodes or for longer than 6 h) increase risk of dehydration.
  - Signs and symptoms of skin, respiratory, urinary, or other infection—may need immediate attention.
  - Large amount of urine ketones or other signs and symptoms of diabetic ketoacidosis: call health care provider immediately.

5. Review skin care and foot care and encourage regular ophthalmology evaluations.
6. Advise patient to bring the following to follow-up medical appointments: all medications for reconciliation, glucose log for review, and glucometer so that it can be periodically calibrated and checked for correlation with clinic monitor or laboratory glucose result.
7. Ensure that patient understands the importance of periodic laboratory monitoring.
   a. Glycated hemoglobin (Hgb A1C) is followed every 3 to 6 months.
   b. Renal function tests (serum creatinine and estimated glomerular filtration rate) and urine for microalbuminuria or microalbumin/creatinine ratio are monitored at least yearly.
   c. Fasting lipid panel is done at least annually.
8. For additional information and support, refer to organization websites, such as the ADA (*www.diabetes.org*) or Academy of Nutrition and Dietetics (*www.eatright.org*).

Evaluation: Expected Outcomes

- Maintains goal weight.
- Demonstrates correct technique for self-injection of insulin and/or noninsulin agents.
- Signs and symptoms of hypoglycemia identified and treated appropriately.
- Verbalizes understanding of importance of daily exercises.
- Verbalizes appropriate use and action of insulin and noninsulin agents.
- No evidence of skin breakdown and able to verbalize appropriate foot care.
- Verbalizes understanding of discharge instructions and has prescription for medications and supplies as well as follow-up appointment with their provider before leaving hospital.

Diabetic Ketoacidosis

EVIDENCE BASE Eledrisi, M. S., & Elzouki, A. N. (2020). Management of diabetic ketoacidosis in adults: A narrative review. *Saudi Journal of Medicine & Medical Sciences, 8*(3), 165–173. https://doi.org/10.4103/sjmms.sjmms_478_19

Gosmanov, A. R., Gosmanova, E. O., & Kitabchi, A. E. (2021). Hyperglycemic crises: Diabetic ketoacidosis and hyperglycemic hyperosmolar state. In K. R. Feingold, B. Anawalt, M. R. Blackman, et al. (Eds.), *Endotext*. Nih.gov; MDText.com, Inc. https://www.ncbi.nlm.nih.gov/books/NBK279052

DKA is an acute complication of DM that often occurs in people with type 1 diabetes; however, people of African American/Black ancestry, Afro-Caribbean Black ancestry, or Hispanic ancestry with type 2 diabetes also experience DKA. DKA is a result of a lack of circulatory insulin in the body. It is characterized by hyperglycemia, ketonuria, acidosis, dehydration, and insulinopenia. Underlying infection is the most common cause of this acute complication. DKA is the most common cause of death in children and adolescents with type 1 diabetes.

Pathophysiology and Etiology

1. Insulin deficiency prevents glucose from being used for energy, forcing the body to metabolize fat for fuel.
2. Free fatty acids, released from the metabolism of fat, are converted to ketone bodies in the liver.
3. Ketone bodies are organic acids that cause metabolic acidosis.
4. Increase in the secretion of glucagon, catecholamines, growth hormone, and cortisol, in response to the hyperglycemia caused by insulin deficiency, accelerates the development of DKA.
5. Osmotic diuresis caused by hyperglycemia creates a shift in electrolytes, with losses in potassium, sodium, phosphate, and water.
6. Caused by inadequate amounts of endogenous or exogenous insulin.
   a. Commonly occurs due to failure to increase the dose of insulin during periods of stress (e.g., infection, surgery, pregnancy).
   b. May occur in those with undiagnosed or untreated OM.

Clinical Manifestations

Early

1. Polydipsia, polyuria.
2. Fatigue, malaise, drowsiness.
3. Anorexia, nausea, vomiting.
4. Abdominal pain, muscle cramps.

Later

1. Kussmaul respirations (deep respirations).
2. Fruity, sweet breath.
3. Hypotension, weak pulse.
4. Stupor and coma.

Diagnostic Evaluation

1. Serum glucose level is elevated over 250 mg/dL.
2. Serum and urine ketone bodies are present.
3. Serum bicarbonate and pH are decreased because of metabolic acidosis, and partial pressure of carbon dioxide is decreased as a respiratory compensation mechanism.
4. Serum sodium and potassium levels may be low, normal, or high because of fluid shifts and dehydration, despite total body depletion.
5. Blood urea nitrogen (BUN), creatinine, hemoglobin, and hematocrit are elevated because of dehydration.
6. Urine glucose is present in high concentration and specific gravity is increased, reflecting osmotic diuresis and dehydration.

CLINICAL JUDGMENT Severity of DKA is not determined by serum glucose levels; the degree of acidosis determines the severity of DKA.

Management

1. IV fluids to replace losses from osmotic diuresis, vomiting.
2. IV insulin drip to increase glucose utilization and decrease lipolysis. Only use insulin preparations approved for IV administration. Should not be started until serum potassium is greater than 3.3 mEq/L.
3. Electrolyte repletion—sodium chloride and phosphate as required and potassium chloride and bicarbonate based on laboratory results.

Complications

1. Premature discontinuation of IV insulin or the failure to initiate SQ insulin injections prior to discontinuing IV insulin will result in rebound of DKA.
2. Too-rapid infusion of IV fluids in cases of severe dehydration can cause cerebral edema and death.

Nursing Assessment

1. Assess skin for dehydration—poor turgor, flushing, dry mucous membranes.
2. Observe for cardiac changes reflecting dehydration, metabolic acidosis, and electrolyte imbalance—hypotension; tachycardia; weak pulse; electrocardiographic changes, including elevated P wave, flattened T wave, or inverted, prolonged QT interval.
3. Assess respiratory status—Kussmaul respirations, acetone breath characteristic of metabolic acidosis.
4. Perform GI assessment—nausea, vomiting, extreme thirst, abdominal bloating and cramping, diarrhea.
5. Determine GU symptoms—nocturia, polyuria.
6. Observe for neurologic signs—crying, restlessness, twitching, tremors, drowsiness, lethargy, headache, decreased reflexes.
7. Interview family or significant other regarding precipitating events to episode of DKA.
   a. Patient self-care management before hospitalization.
   b. Unusual events that may have precipitated episode (e.g., chest pain, trauma, illness).

Nursing Interventions

Restoring Fluid and Electrolyte Balance

1. Assess BP and heart rate frequently, depending on patient's condition; assess skin turgor and temperature.
2. Monitor intake and output every hour.
3. Replace fluids, as ordered, through peripheral IV line.
4. Monitor urine specific gravity to assess fluid changes.
5. Monitor blood glucose frequently.
6. Assess for symptoms of hypokalemia—fatigue, anorexia, nausea, vomiting, muscle weakness, decreased bowel sounds, paresthesia, arrhythmias, flat T waves, ST-segment depression.
7. Administer replacement electrolytes and insulin, as ordered. Flush the entire IV infusion set with solution containing insulin and discard the first 50 mL because plastic bags and tubing may absorb some insulin and the initial solution may contain decreased concentration of insulin.
8. Monitor serum glucose, bicarbonate, and pH levels periodically.
9. Provide reassurance about improvement of condition and that correction of fluid imbalance will help reduce discomfort.

CLINICAL JUDGMENT Electrolyte levels may not reflect the total body deficit of potassium (primarily) and sodium (to a lesser extent) because of compartment shifts and fluid volume loss. Replacement is necessary despite normal to high values.

DRUG ALERT Premature interruption of IV insulin administration may result in reaccumulation of ketone bodies and worsening acidosis. Glucose will normalize before acidosis resolves, so IV insulin is continued until bicarbonate levels normalize, SQ insulin takes effect, and the patient tolerates oral caloric intake.

Preventing Further Episodes of Diabetic Ketoacidosis

1. Review with patients precipitating events and causes of DKA.
2. Assist patient in identifying warning signs and symptoms of DKA.
3. Instruct patient on sick-day guidelines (see page 732).

Patient Education and Health Maintenance

1. Make sure that patient and caregivers can demonstrate administration of the correct dose of insulin using proper technique, blood glucose monitoring, and urine ketone testing.
2. Make sure that patient and caregivers know whom to notify in the event of hyperglycemia, stressful situation, underlying infection, or symptoms of DKA.

Evaluation: Expected Outcomes

- BP and heart rate stable; glucose and bicarbonate levels improving.
- Verbalizes sick-day guidelines correctly.

Hyperosmolar Hyperglycemic State

EVIDENCE BASE Gosmanov, A. R., Gosmanova, E. O., & Kitabchi, A. E. (2021). Hyperglycemic crises: Diabetic ketoacidosis and hyperglycemic hyperosmolar state. In K. R. Feingold, B. Anawalt, M. R. Blackman, et al. (Eds.), *Endotext*. Nih.gov; MDText.com, Inc. https://www.ncbi.nlm.nih.gov/books/NBK279052

HHS is an acute complication of DM (particularly type 2 diabetes) characterized by hyperglycemia, dehydration, and hyperosmolarity, with little or no ketosis. Underlying infection is the most common cause of this acute complication.

Pathophysiology and Etiology

1. Prolonged hyperglycemia with glucosuria produces osmotic diuresis.
2. Loss of water, sodium, and potassium results in severe dehydration, causing hypovolemia and hemoconcentration.
3. Hyperosmolarity is a result of excessive blood sugar and increasing sodium concentration in dehydration.
4. Insulin continues to be produced at a level that prevents ketosis.
5. Increased blood viscosity decreases blood flow to the organs, creating tissue hypoxia.
6. Intracellular fluid and electrolyte shifts produce neurologic signs and symptoms.
7. Caused by inadequate amounts of endogenous/exogenous insulin to control hyperglycemia.
   a. Precipitating event may occur, such as cardiac failure, burn, or chronic illness that increases need for insulin.
   b. Use of therapeutic agents that increase blood glucose levels (e.g., glucocorticoids, immunosuppressive agents).
   c. Use of therapeutic procedures that cause stress or increase blood glucose levels (e.g., hyperosmolar hyperalimentation, peritoneal dialysis).

Clinical Manifestations

Early

1. Polyuria, dehydration.
2. Fatigue, malaise.
3. Nausea, vomiting.

Later

1. Hypothermia.
2. Muscle weakness.
3. Seizures, stupor, coma.

Diagnostic Evaluation

1. Serum glucose and osmolality are greatly elevated, with glucose values usually greater than 600 mg/dL.
2. Serum and urine ketone bodies are minimal to absent.
3. Serum sodium and potassium levels may be elevated, depending on degree of dehydration, despite total body losses.
4. BUN and creatinine may be elevated because of dehydration.
5. Urine specific gravity is elevated because of dehydration.

Management

1. Correct fluid and electrolyte imbalances with IV fluids.
2. Provide insulin via IV drip to lower plasma glucose.
3. Evaluate complications, such as stupor, seizures, or shock, and treat appropriately.
4. Identify and treat underlying illnesses or events that precipitated HHS.

Complications

1. Too rapid infusion of IV fluids can cause cerebral edema and death.
2. HHS is a medical emergency that, if not treated properly, can cause death (10% to 50% mortality).
3. Patients who become comatose will need nasogastric (NG) tubes to prevent aspiration.

Nursing Assessment

1. Assess level of consciousness (LOC).
2. Assess for dehydration—poor turgor, flushing, dry mucous membranes.
3. Assess cardiovascular status for shock—rapid, thready pulse, cool extremities, hypotension, electrocardiogram changes.
4. Interview family or significant other regarding precipitating events to episode of HHS.
   a. Evaluate patient's self-care regimen before hospitalization.
   b. Determine events, signs of infection, treatments, or drugs that may have caused the event.

Nursing Interventions

Restoring Fluid Balance

1. Assess patient for increasing signs and symptoms of dehydration, hyperglycemia, or electrolyte imbalance.
2. Institute fluid replacement therapy, as ordered (usually normal or half-strength saline initially), maintaining patent IV line.
3. Assess patient for signs and symptoms of fluid overload and cerebral edema as IV therapy progresses.
4. Administer regular insulin IV, as ordered, and add dextrose to IV infusion as blood glucose falls below 300 mg/dL, to prevent hypoglycemia.
5. Monitor hydration status by monitoring hourly intake and output and urine specific gravity.

Preventing Aspiration

1. Assess patient's LOC and ability to handle oral secretions.
   a. Cough and gag reflex.
   b. Ability to swallow.
2. Properly position patient to reduce possibility of aspiration.
   a. Elevate head of bed unless contraindicated.
   b. If nausea is present, use side-lying position.
3. Suction as frequently as needed to maintain patent airway.
4. Withhold oral intake until patient is no longer in danger of aspiration.
5. Insert NG tube as indicated for gastric decompression.
6. Monitor respiratory rate and breath sounds for signs of aspiration pneumonia.
7. Provide mouth care to maintain adequate mucosal hydration.

Patient Education and Health Maintenance

1. Advise patient and family that it may take 3 to 5 days for symptoms to resolve.
2. Instruct patient and family on signs and symptoms of hyperglycemia and use of sick-day guidelines (see page 732).
3. Explain possible causes of HHS.
4. Review changes in medication, activity, meal plan, or glucose monitoring for home care. It may not be necessary to continue insulin therapy following HHS; many patients can be treated with diet and oral agents.

Evaluation: Expected Outcomes

- BP stable, dehydration resolved.
- No evidence of aspiration.

Metabolic Syndrome

Metabolic syndrome (also known as *syndrome X, insulin resistance syndrome*, and *dysmetabolic syndrome*) is a term that has been used to characterize a constellation of related risk factors that increase the risk of developing several significant health problems to include type 2 DM and cardiovascular disease. There has been much discussion and debate in the literature as to whether metabolic syndrome is an actual diagnosis and, if so, which diagnostic criteria should be included when screening. To improve consistency, a "harmonized definition" was set forth in 2009 by the International Diabetes Federation Task Force on Epidemiology and Prevention; National Heart, Lung, and Blood Institute; AHA; World Heart Federation; International Atherosclerosis Society; and International Association for the Study of Obesity.

Three of the following five criteria must be met:

- Increased waist circumference (population- and country-specific criteria) (in the United States, greater than 35 in for females and greater than 40 in for males).
- Hypertriglyceridemia: ≥150 mg/dL.*
- Low HDL cholesterol: less than 40 mg/dL in males and less than 50 mg/dL in females.*
- Elevated BP: systolic BP ≥130 mm Hg or diastolic BP ≥85 mm Hg.*
- Elevated fasting glucose: ≥100 mg/dL.*

EVIDENCE BASE Fahed, G., Aoun, L., Bou Zerdan, M., Allam, S., Bou Zerdan, M., Bouferraa, Y., & Assi, H. I. (2021). Metabolic syndrome: Updates on pathophysiology and management in 2021. *International Journal of Molecular Sciences, 23*(2), 786. https://doi.org/10.3390/ijms23020786

Pathophysiology and Etiology

1. The central feature of this metabolic disorder is the diminished responsiveness of peripheral tissues to circulating insulin (insulin resistance).
2. The typical physiologic response of the body to this condition is the increased production and secretion of insulin, leading to a state of compensatory hyperinsulinemia to maintain glucose homeostasis.
3. Although this response is beneficial from the standpoint of glucose metabolism, it is now understood that the state of hyperinsulinemia necessary to prevent glucose intolerance gives rise to other abnormalities that have significant health consequences.
4. In addition to increased risk of type 2 diabetes associated with insulin resistance, hyperinsulinemia has also been associated with the development of hypertension, dyslipidemia, atherosclerotic cardiovascular disease, cerebrovascular disease, polycystic ovarian syndrome (PCOS), metabolic dysfunction-associated steatotic liver disease (MASLD), and obstructive sleep apnea (OSA).
5. Because these clinical features are associated with insulin resistance, the term "syndrome" has been applied to signify that these conditions are linked to a common problem.
6. Although the pathogenesis of insulin resistance is not fully understood, genetic factors, lifestyle (diet, physical activity), and obesity play an important role in the development and natural course of this condition.

Risk Factors

1. Prediabetes, cardiovascular disease, PCOS, hypertension, hyperlipidemia, or acanthosis nigricans (appearance of dark, velvety patches of skin on back of neck or other skin folds).
2. History of glucose intolerance or gestational diabetes.
3. Family history of type 2 diabetes, cardiovascular disease, or hypertension.
4. Sedentary lifestyle.
5. Obesity.

Management

1. Treatment of metabolic syndrome involves measures that are directed at treating any diagnosed disease resulting from insulin resistance (diabetes, hypertension, dyslipidemia) as well as the underlying insulin resistance. This is accomplished by interventions that improve insulin sensitivity.
2. Nonpharmacologic interventions effective in reducing insulin resistance include lifestyle changes that can have a direct impact on insulin sensitivity and include regular physical activity and nutritional management designed to reduce body weight. Smoking cessation and reduced alcohol intake are also important lifestyle changes.
3. Natural approaches to reducing weight and promoting gut health help to treat metabolic syndrome. The Mediterranean diet is well documented to include foods that lower the risk of cardiovascular disease. Nutraceuticals such as turmeric, garlic, ginger, neem, and bergamot orange act as anti-inflammatories and increase glucose tolerance. Butyrate or high fiber and probiotics for improving gut health have all been reported to help manage metabolic syndrome.
4. No pharmacologic agents have been FDA approved for use in the treatment of metabolic syndrome or prediabetes. However, metformin is being used, especially if the risk for developing type 2 DM is very high. Other agents currently available with known insulin-sensitizing effects (i.e., TZD compounds) have shown effectiveness in treating individuals with PCOS and prediabetes. The potential role of these agents in the management of metabolic syndrome is under investigation.
5. Antiobesity medications are available to treat patients struggling with obesity (body mass index [BMI] greater than 30 kg/m^2). Surgical interventions (i.e., bariatric surgery) are recommended for patients with morbid obesity (BMI greater than 40 kg/m^2 or greater than 35 kg/m^2 with comorbid conditions).

*Or taking medications to address.

Nursing and Patient Care Considerations

1. The primary nursing role is education about the condition, risks if left untreated, importance of monitoring, and therapeutic lifestyle changes.
2. The patient should be encouraged to monitor BP and weigh; and to follow up for routine evaluation of cholesterol profile, glucose, HgbA1C, and other laboratory tests.
3. Resources to assist the patient with weight loss, increased physical activity, smoking cessation, and diet change can be found through the National Library of Medicine, https://medlineplus.gov/metabolicsyndrome.html

SELECTED READINGS

ACCORD (The Action to Control Cardiovascular Risk in Diabetes) Study Group. (2008). Effects of intensive glucose lowering in type 2 diabetes. *New England Journal of Medicine, 358*(24), 2545–2559. https://doi.org/10.1056/nejmoa0802743

ADVANCE (Action in Diabetes and Vascular Disease: Preterax and Diamicron Modified Release Controlled Evaluation) Collaborative Group. (2008). Intensive blood glucose control and vascular outcomes in patients with type 2 diabetes. *New England Journal of Medicine, 358*(24), 2560–2572. https://doi.org/10.1056/nejmoa0802987

American Diabetes Association. (2018). Economic costs of diabetes in the U.S. in 2017. *Diabetes Care, 41*(5), 917–928. https://doi.org/10.2337/dci18-0007

Bailey, T. S., Grunberger, G., Bode, B. W., Handelsman, Y., Hirsch, I. B., Jovanovič, L., Roberts, V. L., Rodbard, D., Tamborlane, W. V., & Walsh, J. (2016). American Association of Clinical Endocrinologists and American College of Endocrinology 2016 Outpatient Glucose Monitoring Consensus Statement. *Endocrine Practice, 22*(2), 231–261. https://doi.org/10.4158/ep151124.cs

Blonde, L., Umpierrez, G. E., Reddy, S. S., McGill, J. B., Berga, S. L., Bush, M., Chandrasekaran, S., DeFronzo, R. A., Einhorn, D., Galindo, R. J., Gardner, T. W., Garg, R., Garvey, W. T., Hirsch, I. B., Hurley, D. L., Izuora, K., Kosiborod, M., Olson, D., Patel, S. B., & Pop-Busui, R. (2022). American Association of Clinical Endocrinology Clinical Practice Guideline: Developing a diabetes mellitus comprehensive care plan—2022 update. *Endocrine Practice, 28*(10). https://doi.org/10.1016/j.eprac.2022.08.002

Centers for Disease Control and Prevention. (2022, July 19). *Diabetes Report Card 2021.* US Department of Health and Human Services. https://archive.cdc.gov/#/details?url=https://www.cdc.gov/diabetes/library/reports/reportcard.html

Centers for Disease Control and Prevention. (2023, January 5). *Obesity and overweight.* CDC/National Center for Health Statistics. https://www.cdc.gov/nchs/fastats/obesity-overweight.htm

Centers for Disease Control and Prevention. (2024, April 15). *Health and Economic Benefits of Diabetes Interventions.* https://www.cdc.gov/nccdphp/priorities/diabetes-interventions.html?CDC_AAref_Val=https://www.cdc.gov/chronicdisease/programs-impact/pop/diabetes.htm

Centers for Disease Control and Prevention. (2024a, January 8). *National Diabetes Statistics Report.* CDC Diabetes. https://www.cdc.gov/diabetes/php/data-research/?CDC_AAref_Val=https://www.cdc.gov/diabetes/data/statistics-report/index.html

Centers for Disease Control and Prevention. (2024b, April 15). *Your Feet and Diabetes.* CDC Diabetes. https://www.cdc.gov/diabetes/diabetes-complications/diabetes-and-your-feet.html?CDC_AAref_Val=https://www.cdc.gov/diabetes/library/features/healthy-feet.html

de Bock, M., Codner, E., Craig, M. E., Huynh, T., Maahs, D. M., Mahmud, F. H., Marcovecchio, L., & DiMeglio, L. A. (2022). ISPAD Clinical Practice Consensus Guidelines 2022: Glycemic targets and glucose monitoring for children, adolescents, and young people with diabetes. *Pediatric Diabetes, 23*(8), 1270–1276. https://doi.org/10.1111/pedi.13455

de Boer, I. H., Bangalore, S., Benetos, A., Davis, A. M., Michos, E. D., Muntner, P., Rossing, P., Zoungas, S., & Bakris, G. (2017). Diabetes and hypertension: A position statement by the American Diabetes Association. *Diabetes Care, 40*(9), 1273–1284. https://doi.org/10.2337/dci17-0026

Duque, A., Mediano, M. F. F., De Lorenzo, A., & Rodrigues, L. F., Jr. (2021). Cardiovascular autonomic neuropathy in diabetes: Pathophysiology, clinical assessment and implications. *World Journal of Diabetes, 12*(6), 855–867. https://doi.org/10.4239/wjd.v12.i6.855

Durnwald, C. (2022, March 18). *UpToDate.* www.uptodate.com; Wolters Kluwer. https://www.uptodate.com/contents/gestational-diabetes-mellitus-glucose-management-and-maternal-prognosis

Eledrisi, M. S., & Elzouki, A.-N. (2020). Management of diabetic ketoacidosis in adults: A narrative review. *Saudi Journal of Medicine & Medical Sciences, 8*(3), 165–173. https://doi.org/10.4103/sjmms.sjmms_478_19

ElSayed, N. A., Aleppo, G., Bannuru, R. R., Beverly, E. A., Bruemmer, D., Collins, B., Darville, A., Ekhlaspour, L., Hassanein, M., Hilliard, M. E., Johnson, E. L., Khunti, K., Lingvay, I., Matfin, G., McCoy, R. G., Perry, M. L., Pilla, S. J., Polsky, S., Prahalad, P., & Pratley, R. E. (2023). 5. Facilitating positive health behaviors and well-being to improve health outcomes: *Standards of Care in Diabetes—2024. Diabetes Care, 47*(Supplement_1), S77–S110. https://doi.org/10.2337/dc24-s005

ElSayed, N. A., Aleppo, G., Bannuru, R. R., Bruemmer, D., Collins, B., Das, S. R., Ekhlaspour, L., Hilliard, M. E., Johnson, E. L., Khunti, K., Kosiborod, M., Lingvay, I., Matfin, G., McCoy, R. G., Perry, M. L., Pilla, S. J., Polsky, S., Prahalad, P., Pratley, R. E., & Segal, A. R. (2023). 10. Cardiovascular disease and risk management: *Standards of Care in Diabetes—2024. Diabetes Care, 47*(Supplement_1), S179–S218. https://doi.org/10.2337/dc24-s010

ElSayed, N. A., Aleppo, G., Bannuru, R. R., Bruemmer, D., Collins, B., Ekhlaspour, L., Gaglia, J. L., Hilliard, M. E., Johnson, E. L., Khunti, K., Lingvay, I., Matfin, G., McCoy, R. G., Perry, M. L., Pilla, S. J., Polsky, S., Prahalad, P., Pratley, R. E., Segal, A. R., & Seley, J. J. (2023a). 2. Diagnosis and classification of diabetes: *Standards of Care in Diabetes—2024. Diabetes Care, 47*(Supplement_1), S20–S42. https://doi.org/10.2337/dc24-s002

ElSayed, N. A., Aleppo, G., Bannuru, R. R., Bruemmer, D., Collins, B., Ekhlaspour, L., Gaglia, J. L., Hilliard, M. E., Johnson, E. L., Khunti, K., Lingvay, I., Matfin, G., McCoy, R. G., Perry, M. L., Pilla, S. J., Polsky, S., Prahalad, P., Pratley, R. E., Segal, A. R., & Seley, J. J. (2023b). 3. Prevention or delay of diabetes and associated comorbidities: *Standards of Care in Diabetes—2024. Diabetes Care, 47*(Supplement_1), S43–S51. https://doi.org/10.2337/dc24-s003

ElSayed, N. A., Aleppo, G., Bannuru, R. R., Bruemmer, D., Collins, B., Ekhlaspour, L., Gaglia, J. L., Hilliard, M. E., Johnson, E. L., Khunti, K., Lingvay, I., Matfin, G., McCoy, R. G., Perry, M. L., Pilla, S. J., Polsky, S., Prahalad, P., Pratley, R. E., Segal, A. R., & Seley, J. J. (2023c). 9. Pharmacologic approaches to glycemic treatment: *Standards of Care in Diabetes—2024. Diabetes Care, 47*(Supplement_1), S158–S178. https://doi.org/10.2337/dc24-s009

ElSayed, N. A., Aleppo, G., Bannuru, R. R., Bruemmer, D., Collins, B., Ekhlaspour, L., Galindo, R. J., Hilliard, M. E., Johnson, E. L., Khunti, K., Lingvay, I., Matfin, G., McCoy, R. G., Perry, M. L., Pilla, S. J., Polsky, S., Prahalad, P., Pratley, R. E., Segal, A. R., & Seley, J. J. (2023). 16. Diabetes care in the hospital: *Standards of Care in Diabetes—2024. Diabetes Care, 47*(Supplement_1), S295–S306. https://doi.org/10.2337/dc24-s016

ElSayed, N. A., Aleppo, G., Bannuru, R. R., Bruemmer, D., Collins, B., Ekhlaspour, L., Gibbons, C. H., Giurini, J. M., Hilliard, M. E., Johnson, E. L., Khunti, K., Lingvay, I., Matfin, G., McCoy, R. G., Perry, M. L., Pilla, S. J., Polsky, S., Prahalad, P., Pratley, R. E., & Segal, A. R. (2023). 12. Retinopathy, neuropathy, and foot care: *Standards of Care in Diabetes—2024. Diabetes Care, 47*(Supplement_1), S231–S243. https://doi.org/10.2337/dc24-s012

ElSayed, N. A., Aleppo, G., Bannuru, R. R., Bruemmer, D., Collins, B., Ekhlaspour, L., Hilliard, M. E., Johnson, E. L., Khunti, K., Lingvay, I., Matfin, G., McCoy, R. G., Perry, M. L., Pilla, S. J., Polsky, S., Prahalad, P., Pratley, R. E., Segal, A. R., Seley, J. J., & Selvin, E. (2023). 6. Glycemic goals and hypoglycemia: *Standards of Care in Diabetes—2024. Diabetes Care, 47*(Supplement_1), S111–S125. https://doi.org/10.2337/dc24-s006

ElSayed, N. A., Aleppo, G., Bannuru, R. R., Bruemmer, D., Collins, B., Ekhlaspour, L., Hilliard, M. E., Johnson, E. L., Khunti, K., Lingvay, I., Matfin, G., McCoy, R. G., Perry, M. L., Pilla, S. J., Polsky, S., Prahalad, P., Pratley, R. E., Segal, A. R., Seley, J. J., & Stanton, R. C. (2023a). 1. Improving care and promoting health in populations: *Standards of Care in Diabetes—2024. Diabetes Care, 47*(Supplement_1), S11–S19. https://doi.org/10.2337/dc24-s001

ElSayed, N. A., Aleppo, G., Bannuru, R. R., Bruemmer, D., Collins, B., Ekhlaspour, L., Hilliard, M. E., Johnson, E. L., Khunti, K., Lingvay, I., Matfin, G., McCoy, R. G., Perry, M. L., Pilla, S. J., Polsky, S., Prahalad, P., Pratley, R. E., Segal, A. R., Seley, J. J., & Stanton, R. C. (2023b). 7. Diabetes technology: *Standards of Care in Diabetes—2024. Diabetes Care, 47*(Supplement_1), S126–S144. https://doi.org/10.2337/dc24-s007

ElSayed, N. A., Aleppo, G., Bannuru, R. R., Bruemmer, D., Collins, B., Ekhlaspour, L., Hilliard, M. E., Johnson, E. L., Khunti, K., Lingvay, I., Matfin, G., McCoy, R. G., Perry, M. L., Pilla, S. J., Polsky, S., Prahalad, P., Pratley, R. E., Segal, A. R., Seley, J. J., & Stanton, R. C. (2023c). 11. Chronic kidney disease and risk management: *Standards of Care in Diabetes—2024. Diabetes Care, 47*(Supplement_1), S219–S230. https://doi.org/10.2337/dc24-s011

ElSayed, N. A., Aleppo, G., Bannuru, R. R., Bruemmer, D., Collins, B., Ekhlaspour, L., Hilliard, M. E., Johnson, E. L., Khunti, K., Lingvay, I., Matfin, G., McCoy, R. G., Perry, M. L., Pilla, S. J., Polsky, S., Prahalad, P., Pratley, R. E., Segal, A. R.,

Seley, J. J., & Stanton, R. C. (2023d). 13. Older adults: *Standards of Care in Diabetes—2024. Diabetes Care, 47*(Supplement_1), S244–S257. https://doi.org/10.2337/dc24-s013

ElSayed, N. A., Aleppo, G., Bannuru, R. R., Bruemmer, D., Collins, B., Ekhlaspour, L., Hilliard, M. E., Johnson, E. L., Khunti, K., Lingvay, I., Matfin, G., McCoy, R. G., Perry, M. L., Pilla, S. J., Polsky, S., Prahalad, P., Pratley, R. E., Segal, A. R., Seley, J. J., & Stanton, R. C. (2023e). 14. Children and adolescents: *Standards of Care in Diabetes—2024. Diabetes Care, 47*(Supplement_1), S258–S281. https://doi.org/10.2337/dc24-s014

ElSayed, N. A., Aleppo, G., Bannuru, R. R., Bruemmer, D., Collins, B., Ekhlaspour, L., Hilliard, M. E., Johnson, E. L., Khunti, K., Lingvay, I., Matfin, G., McCoy, R. G., Perry, M. L., Pilla, S. J., Polsky, S., Prahalad, P., Pratley, R. E., Segal, A. R., Seley, J. J., & Stanton, R. C. (2023f). 15. Management of diabetes in pregnancy: *Standards of Care in Diabetes—2024. Diabetes Care, 47*(Supplement_1), S282–S294. https://doi.org/10.2337/dc24-s015

Fahed, G., Aoun, L., Bou Zerdan, M., Allam, S., Bou Zerdan, M., Bouferraa, Y., & Assi, H. I. (2022). Metabolic syndrome: Updates on pathophysiology and management in 2021. *International Journal of Molecular Sciences, 23*(2), 786. https://doi.org/10.3390/ijms23020786

Flaxel, C. J., Adelman, R. A., Bailey, S. T., Fawzi, A., Lim, J. I., Vemulakonda, G. A., & Ying, G. (2020). Diabetic Retinopathy Preferred Practice Pattern®. *Ophthalmology, 127*(1), P66–P145. https://doi.org/10.1016/j.ophtha.2019.09.025

Garber, A. J., Handelsman, Y., Grunberger, G., Einhorn, D., Abrahamson, M. J., Barzilay, J. I., Blonde, L., Bush, M. A., DeFronzo, R. A., Garber, J. R., Garvey, W. T., Hirsch, I. B., Jellinger, P. S., McGill, J. B., Mechanick, J. I., Perreault, L., Rosenblit, P. D., Samson, S., & Umpierrez, G. E. (2020). Consensus statement by The American Association of Clinical Endocrinologists and American College of Endocrinology on The Comprehensive Type 2 Diabetes Management Algorithm—2020 Executive Summary. *Endocrine Practice, 26*(1), 107–139. https://doi.org/10.4158/cs-2019-0472

Goldberg, R. B., Stone, N. J., & Grundy, S. M. (2020). The 2018 AHA/ACC/AACVPR/AAPA/ABC/ACPM/ADA/AGS/APhA/ASPC/NLA/PCNA Guidelines on the Management of Blood Cholesterol in Diabetes. *Diabetes Care, 43*(8), 1673–1678. https://doi.org/10.2337/dci19-0036

Gosmanov, A. R., Gosmanova, E. O., & Kitabchi, A. E. (2021). *Hyperglycemic crises: Diabetic ketoacidosis (DKA), and hyperglycemic hyperosmolar state (HHS)*. Nih.gov; MDText.com, Inc. https://www.ncbi.nlm.nih.gov/books/NBK279052/

Hinkle, J. (2021). *Brunner & Suddarth's Textbook of Medical-Surgical Nursing* (15th ed.). Lippincott Williams & Wilkins.

Kapoor, D., & Lad, V. (2021). Perioperative implication of sodium-glucose cotransporter-2 inhibitor in a patient following major surgery. *Indian Journal of Critical Care Medicine, 25*(8), 958–959. https://doi.org/10.5005/jp-journals-10071-23929

Khzouz, A., Rickson, M., Sieradzan, R., & Goldman, J. (2021). Injection force variability: An overlooked aspect of proper insulin injection technique. *ADCES in Practice, 9*(2), 42–47. https://doi.org/10.1177/2633559x20972353

Kuźnik, E., Dudkowiak, R., Adamiec, R., & Poniewierka, E. (2020). Diabetic autonomic neuropathy of the gastrointestinal tract. *Gastroenterology Review, 15*(2), 89–93. https://doi.org/10.5114/pg.2020.95554

Lipska, K. (2023, January 20). *UpToDate*. https://www.uptodate.com/contents/exercise-and-medical-care-for-people-with-type-2-diabetes-beyond-the-basics

Mangione, C. M., Barry, M. J., Nicholson, W. K., Cabana, M., Chelmow, D., Coker, T. R., Davidson, K. W., Davis, E. M., Donahue, K. E., Jaén, C. R., Kubik, M., Li, L., Ogedegbe, G., Pbert, L., Ruiz, J. M., Stevermer, J., Tseng, C.-W., & Wong, J. B. (2022). Screening for prediabetes and type 2 diabetes in children and adolescents. *JAMA, 328*(10), 963. https://doi.org/10.1001/jama.2022.14543

Maryland State School Health Services Guideline Management of Diabetes in Schools. (2020). *Management of diabetes in schools*. https://health.maryland.gov/pophealth/Documents/School%20Health%20-%20Guidelines/Management-of-Diabetes-in-Schools-Guideline-Revised-September-2020.pdf

Mayo Clinic. (2022, July 22). *Autonomic neuropathy—Symptoms and causes*. Mayo Clinic Diseases and Conditions. https://www.mayoclinic.org/diseases-conditions/autonomic-neuropathy/symptoms-causes/syc-20369829

Nachawi, N., Rao, P. P., & Makin, V. (2022). The role of GLP-1 receptor agonists in managing type 2 diabetes. *Cleveland Clinic Journal of Medicine, 89*(8), 457–464. https://doi.org/10.3949/ccjm.89a.21110

Office of Disease Prevention and Health Promotion. (2020). *Healthy People 2030*. Health.gov. https://health.gov/healthypeople

Rowley, W. R., Bezold, C., Arikan, Y., Byrne, E., & Krohe, S. (2017). Diabetes 2030: Insights from yesterday, today, and future trends. *Population Health Management, 20*(1), 6–12. https://doi.org/10.1089/pop.2015.0181

Selby, N. M., & Taal, M. W. (2020). An updated overview of diabetic nephropathy: Diagnosis, prognosis, treatment goals and latest guidelines. *Diabetes, Obesity and Metabolism, 22*(S1), 3–15. https://doi.org/10.1111/dom.14007

Sesti, G., Incalzi, R. A., Bonora, E., Consoli, A., Giaccari, A., Maggi, S., Paolisso, G., Purrello, F., Vendemiale, G., & Ferrara, N. (2018). Management of diabetes in older adults. *Nutrition, Metabolism and Cardiovascular Diseases, 28*(3), 206–218. https://doi.org/10.1016/j.numecd.2017.11.007

Sharifi, Y., Ebrahimpur, M., & Tamehrizadeh, S. S. (2022). Hypoglycemic unawareness: Challenges, triggers, and recommendations in patients with hypoglycemic unawareness: A case report. *Journal of Medical Case Reports, 16*(1). https://doi.org/10.1186/s13256-022-03498-1

Shukla, U. V., & Tripathy, K. (2022). *Diabetic Retinopathy*. PubMed; StatPearls Publishing. https://www.ncbi.nlm.nih.gov/books/NBK560805/#:~:text=Ninety-three%20million%20people%20are%20globally%20affected%20by%20diabetic

Sudo, S. Z., Montagnoli, T. L., Rocha, B. de S., Santos, A. D., de Sá, M. P. L., & Zapata-Sudo, G. (2022). Diabetes-induced cardiac autonomic neuropathy: Impact on heart function and prognosis. *Biomedicines, 10*(12), 3258. https://doi.org/10.3390/biomedicines10123258

Todd, B. (2021). The USPSTF recommends earlier screening for prediabetes and type 2 diabetes. *AJN, American Journal of Nursing, 121*(12), 60–60. https://doi.org/10.1097/01.naj.0000803220.83780.07

Valier, M., Elam-Evans, L., Mu, Y., Santibanez, T., Yankey, D., Zhou, T., Pingali, C., & Singleton, J. (2023). *Morbidity and mortality weekly report racial and ethnic differences in COVID-19 vaccination coverage among children and adolescents aged 5–17 years and parental intent to*. https://www.cdc.gov/mmwr/volumes/72/wr/pdfs/mm7201-H.pdf

Wallace, A. S., Wang, D., Shin, J.-I., & Selvin, E. (2020). Screening and diagnosis of prediabetes and diabetes in US children and adolescents. *Pediatrics, 146*(3). https://doi.org/10.1542/peds.2020-0265

Yehl, K. (2018). Back to basics: A recap of the AADE practice paper, teaching injection technique to people with diabetes. *AADE in Practice, 6*(5), 40–42. https://doi.org/10.1177/2325160318789163

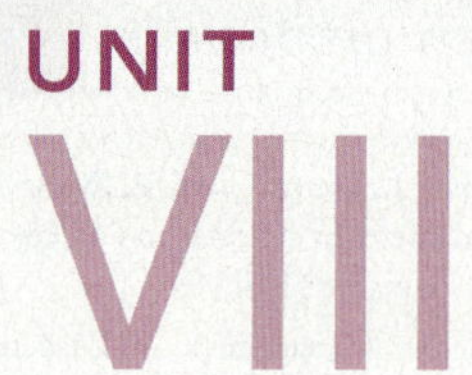

HEMATOLOGIC HEALTH

22 Hematologic Disorders*

OVERVIEW AND ASSESSMENT

See additional online content: Procedure Guidelines 22-1

Blood, the body fluid circulating through the heart, arteries, capillaries, and veins, consists of plasma and cellular components. The average male adult has about 5.5 L of blood and the average female 4.5 L. Plasma, the fluid portion, accounts for 55% of the blood volume and is composed of 92% water, 7% protein, and 1% inorganic salts; nonprotein organic substances such as urea; dissolved gases; hormones; and enzymes. Plasma proteins include albumin, fibrinogen, and globulins. Cellular components include erythrocytes (red blood cells [RBCs]), leukocytes and lymphocytes (white blood cells [WBCs]), and platelets. These cells are derived from pluripotent stem cells in the bone marrow, a process known as *hematopoiesis* (see Figure 22-1). Under normal conditions, only mature cells are found in circulating blood. The cellular components of blood account for 45% of the blood volume.

Characteristics of Cellular Components

Blood has multiple functions that are carried out by plasma or the cellular components (see Table 22-1, page 739).

Erythrocytes (Red Blood Cells)

1. Enucleated, biconcave disc.
2. Approximately 5 million erythrocytes per cubic millimeter of blood.
3. Cell contents consist primarily of hemoglobin, essential for oxygen transport. Whole blood contains 14 to 15 g of hemoglobin per 100 mL of blood.
4. Circulate about 115 to 130 days before elimination by reticuloendothelial system, primarily in the spleen and liver.

Leukocytes (White Blood Cells)

See Table 22-2, page 739.

1. Approximately 5,000 to 10,000 leukocytes (WBCs) per cubic millimeter of blood.
2. Classified as granulocytes or mononuclear leukocytes.
   a. Granulocytes account for about 70% of all WBCs; have abundant granules in cytoplasm; include neutrophils, basophils, and eosinophils.
   b. Mononuclear leukocytes have single-lobed nucleus and granule-free cytoplasm; include monocytes and lymphocytes.

* Please note that the term “male” in this chapter refers to a person assigned male at birth, and the term “female” in this chapter refers to a person assigned female at birth.

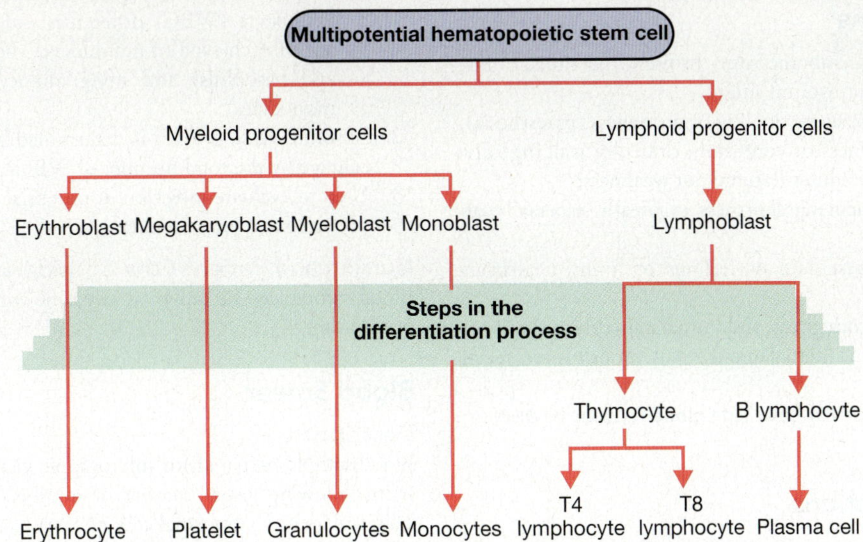

Figure 22-1. Steps in differentiation of blood cells.

Platelets (Thrombocytes)

1. Approximately 150,000 to 450,000 platelets per cubic millimeter of blood.
2. Small particles without nuclei arise as a result of budding from giant cells (megakaryocytes) in bone marrow.
3. Primary function is to control bleeding through hemostasis.

Table 22-1 Functions of Blood

FUNCTION	METHOD INVOLVED	CELLS AND SUBSTANCES
Oxygen and carbon dioxide transport	Binding to hemoglobin; dissolved in plasma	• Erythrocyte • Hemoglobin • Plasma
Nutrient and metabolite transport	Bound to plasma proteins; dissolved in plasma	• Plasma proteins • Plasma
Hormone transport	In plasma	• Plasma
Transport of waste products to kidneys and liver	In plasma	• Plasma
Transport of cells and substances involved in immune reactions	In plasma to site of infection or foreign body	• Granulocytes • Monocytes • Lymphocytes • Immunoglobulins • Other substances
Clotting at breaks in blood vessels	Hemostasis	• Platelets • Clotting factors
Maintenance of fluid balance	Blood volume regulation	• Water • Electrolytes
Body temperature regulation	Peripheral vasoconstriction or dilation	—
Maintenance of acid–base balance	Acid–base regulation	• Electrolytes

Subjective and Objective Data

The patient who presents with a hematologic disorder may have a disruption of the hematologic, immune, or coagulation system, producing a diverse array of symptoms and physical examination findings. Patients commonly present with vague complaints of fatigue, frequent infections, swollen lymph nodes, and abnormal bleeding and/or clotting tendencies. Characterize these complaints and obtain a review of systems, concentrating on the neurologic, respiratory, cardiovascular, gastrointestinal (GI), genitourinary (GU), and integumentary systems to look for more clues of hematologic dysfunction. Perform a systematic physical examination, paying careful attention to the cardiovascular, respiratory, and integumentary systems.

Table 22-2 Characteristics of White Blood Cells

CELL	MAJOR FUNCTION	CHARACTERISTICS OF WHITE BLOOD CELLS
Neutrophil	Ingest and destroy microorganisms (phagocytosis)	Small cell, multilobed nucleus, most plentiful leukocyte
Eosinophil	Host resistance to helminthic infections; also allergic response	Bilobed nucleus; red-staining granules
Basophil	Allergic response	Bilobed nucleus; granules containing heparin and histamine
Monocyte	Phagocytosis	Large cell, kidney-shaped nucleus
B lymphocyte	Produce antibodies (immunoglobulins); humoral immunity	Small, agranular
T lymphocyte	Regulation of immune response; cellular immunity	Small, agranular; include cytotoxic, helper (T4), and suppressor (T8) T cells; identified by surface markers

Review of Systems

1. Skin and mucous membranes: Any bruises, infections, drainage, or bleeding from wound sites?
2. Neurologic: Any dizziness, tingling or numbness (paresthesia), headache, forgetfulness or confusion, difficulty walking (disturbance in gait), tiredness (fatigue), or weakness?
3. Respiratory: Experiencing shortness of breath, especially on exertion?
4. Cardiovascular: Chest pain or feelings of funny heartbeats (palpitations)?
5. GI: Any bleeding from gums, abdominal pain, black stools, or blood-streaked vomit (hematemesis)? Any mouth sores, rectal pain, or diarrhea?
6. GU: Excessive menstrual flow? Any blood in urine or discomfort on urination?

Key History Questions

1. What are your present medications? Do you take over-the-counter (OTC) medications, vitamins, herbals, or nutritional supplements? What else have you taken in the past several months?
2. What medical problems have you had in the past? Any surgeries? Ask specifically about partial or total gastrectomy, splenic injury or splenectomy, tendency to bleed (e.g., with dental procedures), infectious diseases, human immunodeficiency virus (HIV) infection, and cancer.
3. What is your occupation? Ask about exposure to substances such as benzene, pesticides, and ionizing radiation.
4. Do you have a family history of hematologic or malignant disorder?
5. Determine the social history and lifestyle. Do you use illicit drugs or alcohol? What is your pattern of sexual activity?

Key Examination Findings

1. Dyspnea; shiny smooth tongue; ataxia; and pallor of conjunctivae, nail beds, lips, and oral mucosa—suggest anemia.
2. Decreased blood pressure (BP), tachycardia, and, possibly, altered level of consciousness (LOC)—suggest anemia or altered blood clotting.
3. Hematuria, tarry stools, petechiae, and bleeding sites—suggest altered clotting.
4. Fever; tachycardia; abnormal breath sounds; delirium; oral lesions; and erythema, swelling, tenderness, and drainage of the skin—suggest infection.

Laboratory Studies

Laboratory studies routinely done for patients with hematologic disorders include complete blood count (CBC) with differential, blood smear, and iron profile.

Complete Blood Count

Description

1. Generally includes absolute numbers or percentages of erythrocytes, leukocytes, platelets, hemoglobin, and hematocrit in blood sample.
   a. Erythrocyte (RBC) indices—provides information on the size, hemoglobin concentration, and hemoglobin weight of an average RBC; aids in diagnosis and classification of anemias.
   b. Leukocyte (WBC) differential—determines the percentage of each type of granulocyte (neutrophils, eosinophils, and basophils) and nongranulocytes (lymphocytes and monocytes).
2. Absolute value of each is determined by multiplying the percentage by the total number of WBCs.
3. Used to evaluate infection or potential for infection and identify various types of leukemia.

Nursing and Patient Care Considerations

Blood sample can be drawn at any time without fasting or patient preparation.

Blood Smear

Description

Blood sample prepared for microscopic viewing using appropriate stains, allowing visual analysis of numbers and characteristics of cells; can identify abnormal cells of certain anemias, leukemias, and other disorders that affect the bloodstream.

Nursing and Patient Care Considerations

Can be done from blood sample drawn for CBC; no additional sample or patient preparation is necessary.

Iron Profile

Description

Test completed on blood sample that generally includes levels of serum ferritin, iron, total iron-binding capacity, folate, and vitamin B_{12}; used to determine the type and severity of anemia.

Nursing and Patient Care Considerations

Recent administration of chloramphenicol, hormonal contraceptives, iron supplements, and corticotropin may affect results of serum iron and iron-binding capacity. No patient preparation needed.

Other Diagnostic Procedures

Bone Marrow Aspiration and Biopsy

Description

1. Aspiration and biopsy of bone marrow from the iliac crest or (rarely) sternum to obtain specimen for microscopic evaluation. Special needles are inserted into the bone to collect the specimens directly from the bone marrow.
2. Purposes include diagnosis of hematologic disorders; monitoring course of illness and response to treatment; diagnosis of other disorders, such as primary and metastatic tumors, infectious diseases, and certain granulomas; and isolation of bacteria and other pathogens by culture.

Nursing and Patient Care Considerations

1. Give medication for pain and anxiety before or after the procedure, as ordered. A bone marrow aspiration with biopsy is more painful and may require the use of mild-to-moderate sedation with appropriate monitoring.
2. Watch for bleeding and hematoma formation after procedure.

Lymph Node Biopsy

Description

1. Surgical excision or needle aspiration usually of a superficial lymph node in the cervical, supraclavicular, axillary, or inguinal region.

2. Performed to determine the cause of lymph node enlargement, to distinguish between benign and malignant lymph node tumors, and to stage metastatic carcinoma.

Nursing and Patient Care Considerations

1. Local anesthetic is usually given.
2. Specimen is placed in normal saline or 10% formaldehyde solution for transportation to the laboratory for cytologic and histologic evaluation.

GENERAL PROCEDURES AND TREATMENT MODALITIES

See additional online content: Procedure Guidelines 22-2

Splenectomy

The *spleen* is a fist-size organ located in the upper left quadrant of the abdomen. It includes a central "white pulp" where storage and proliferation of some lymphocytes and other leukocytes occurs, and a peripheral "red pulp" involved initially in fetal erythropoiesis and later in erythrocyte destruction and the conversion of hemoglobin to bilirubin. It may be surgically removed because of trauma or to treat certain hemolytic or malignant disorders with accompanying splenomegaly. A laparoscopic technique, usually with a lateral approach, is preferred to remove a normal to slightly enlarged spleen in benign conditions, such as idiopathic thrombocytopenic purpura, hemolytic anemia, or sickle cell disease. Compared with open surgery, laparoscopic splenectomies have a shortened hospital stay, decreased postoperative pain, and decreased risk of wound complications, such as adhesions and infections.

Preoperative Management

1. For general aspects of preoperative nursing management, see Chapter 3.
2. Stabilization of preexisting condition:
   a. For trauma: volume replacement with intravenous (IV) fluids, evacuation of stomach contents via nasogastric tube to prevent aspiration, urinary catheterization to monitor urine output, assessment for pneumothorax or hemothorax, and possible chest tube placement.
   b. For hemolytic or malignant disorders with accompanying thrombocytopenia: coagulation studies, administration of coagulation factors (e.g., vitamin K, fresh frozen plasma, cryoprecipitate), and platelet and red cell transfusions.
3. Preoperative pulmonary evaluation and teaching.
4. For patients undergoing elective splenectomy, vaccination against pneumococcus, *Haemophilus influenzae* type b, and meningococcus are given at least 2 weeks before surgery.

Postoperative Management

1. For general aspects of postoperative nursing management, see Chapter 3.
2. Prevention of respiratory complications: hypoventilation and limited diaphragmatic movement, atelectasis of left lower lobe, pneumonia, and left pleural effusion.
3. Monitoring for hemorrhage.
4. Pharmacologic deep vein thrombosis (DVT) prophylaxis, begun in the operating room or if the patient is at increased bleeding risk, as soon as bleeding risk subsides.
5. Administration of opioids for pain and observance for adverse effects.
6. Monitoring for fever.
   a. Postsplenectomy fever—mild, transient fever is expected.
   b. Persistent fever may indicate subphrenic abscess or hematoma.
7. Monitoring daily platelet count: Thrombocytosis (elevation of platelet count) may appear a few days after splenectomy and may persist during the first 2 weeks.

Potential Complications

1. Pancreatitis and fistula formation: Tail of pancreas is anatomically close to splenic hilum.
2. Hemorrhage.
3. Atelectasis and pneumonia.
4. Overwhelming postsplenectomy infection (OPSI)—increased risk of developing a life-threatening bacterial infection with encapsulated organisms, such as *Streptococcus pneumoniae, Neisseria meningitidis*, or *H. influenzae* type b. The incidence of OPSI is 0.23% to 0.42% per year with a lifetime risk of 5%. An OPSI is a medical emergency and requires immediate IV antibiotics in an intensive care setting. IV immunoglobulins are also used.

CLINICAL JUDGMENT The risk of OPSI is highest soon after splenectomy and in patients whose splenectomy occurred during childhood or for a malignant disease. Early symptoms include fever and malaise; the infection may progress within hours to sepsis and death, with mortality as high as 50% to 70%. Patient education before and after splenectomy is imperative. The nurse should include the risks of OPSI; recognition of early symptoms and prompt medical attention; the use of medical alert identification; immunization against *S. pneumoniae, H. influenzae* type b, and *N. meningitidis*; and, in some cases, prophylactic and standby antibiotics.

Nursing Interventions

Maintaining Effective Breathing

1. Assess breath sounds and report absent, diminished, or adventitious sounds.
2. Assist with aggressive chest physiotherapy and incentive spirometry.
3. Encourage early and progressive mobilization.

Monitoring for Hemorrhage

1. Monitor vital signs frequently and as condition warrants.
2. Measure abdominal girth and report abdominal distention.
3. Assess for pain and report increasing pain.
4. Prepare the patient for surgical reexploration if bleeding is suspected.

Avoiding Thromboembolic Complications

1. Monitor platelet count daily; report abnormal result promptly.
2. Administer DVT prophylaxis, as ordered.
3. Assess for possible thromboembolism.
   a. Assess skin color, temperature, tenderness, and swelling.
   b. Advise the patient to report chest pain, shortness of breath, pain, or weakness.
4. Report signs of thromboembolism immediately.

Preventing Infection

1. Assess vital signs for fever and tachycardia, and surgical incision daily or if increased pain, fever, or foul smell.

2. Maintain meticulous handwashing and change dressings using sterile technique.
3. Teach the patient to report signs of infection (fever, malaise) immediately.
4. Educate the patient and family regarding OPSI, including plan for postsplenectomy immunizations, recognition of symptoms, and the use of prophylactic and standby antibiotics.

Relieving Pain

1. Administer pain medications or teach self-administration, as prescribed and as necessary, to maintain level of comfort.
2. Warn the patient of adverse effects, such as nausea and drowsiness; watch for hypotension and decreased respirations.
3. Teach the use of nonpharmacologic methods, such as music, relaxation breathing, progressive muscle relaxation, distraction, and imagery to help manage pain.
4. Document dosage of medications and response to medication.
5. Make sure the patient has analgesics for use postdischarge.

Patient Education and Health Maintenance

1. Teach care of incision.
2. Encourage to gradually increase activity according to guidelines given by the surgeon.
3. Advise proper rest, nutrition, and stress avoidance while recovering from surgery.
4. Encourage follow-up as directed by the surgeon and primary care provider to maintain immunizations.
5. Encourage the patient to seek prompt medical attention for any infections and to contact health care provider immediately for high fever.

Evaluation: Expected Outcomes

- Respirations unlabored, breath sounds clear.
- Vital signs stable, abdominal girth unchanged.
- No warmth, redness, swelling, or tenderness of extremity.
- Afebrile, no purulent drainage from incision.
- Verbalizes decreased pain.

ANEMIAS

Anemia is the lack of sufficient circulating hemoglobin to deliver oxygen to tissues. Anemia has multiple causes and is commonly associated with other diseases and disorders (e.g., renal disease, cancer, Crohn disease, alcohol use disorder). Anemia may be caused by inadequate production of red blood cells (RBCs), abnormal hemolysis and sequestration of RBCs, or blood loss. Iron-deficiency anemia, pernicious anemia, folic acid deficiency anemia, and aplastic anemia are the anemias most commonly seen in adults. Hereditary hemolytic disorders include spherocytosis, hemoglobinopathies (e.g., sickle cell), and enzymatic deficiencies, such as glucose 6-phosphate dehydrogenase (G6PD). Treatments for anemia include nutritional counseling, supplements, RBC transfusions, and, for some patients, administration of exogenous erythropoietin (epoetin alfa or darbepoetin alfa), a growth factor stimulating production and maturation of erythrocytes. Erythropoietin is used to stimulate RBC production in anemias associated with chronic renal failure, chemotherapy treatment, and human immunodeficiency virus (HIV).

DRUG ALERT Erythropoietin-stimulating agents, such as epoetin alfa and darbepoetin alfa, have been associated with increased risk of death and serious cardiovascular events. Use the lowest possible dose and monitor for potential problems such as hypertension—particularly in patients with chronic kidney disease—and deep venous thrombosis.

Iron-Deficiency Anemia (Microcytic, Hypochromic)

Iron-deficiency anemia is a condition in which the total body iron content is decreased below a normal level, affecting hemoglobin synthesis. RBCs appear pale and are small.

EVIDENCE BASE Shikha, B., & Shalini, A. (2022). Prevalence and approaches to manage iron deficiency anemia (IDA). *Critical Reviews in Food Science and Nutrition, 62*(32), 8815–8828. https://doi.org/10.1080/10408398.2021.1935442

Pathophysiology and Etiology

1. The most common cause is chronic blood loss (gastrointestinal [GI] bleeding including occult colorectal cancers, excessive menstrual bleeding, and hookworm infestation), but anemia may also be caused by insufficient intake of iron (weight loss, inadequate diet), iron malabsorption (end-stage renal disease, small bowel disease, gastroenterostomy), or increased requirements (pregnancy, periods of rapid growth).
2. Decreased hemoglobin may result in insufficient oxygen delivery to body tissues.
3. The incidence of iron-deficiency anemia, the most common type of anemia worldwide, varies widely by age, sex assigned at birth, and ethnicity. In the United States, it is more than twice as common in females as compared to males and often affects lower income populations. It is a major health problem in developing countries.
4. Symptoms generally develop when hemoglobin has fallen to less than 11 g/100 mL.

Clinical Manifestations

1. Headache, dizziness, fatigue, and tinnitus.
2. Palpitations, dyspnea on exertion, and pallor of skin and mucous membranes.
3. In developing world: smooth, sore tongue; cheilosis (lesions at corners of mouth), koilonychia (spoon-shaped fingernails), and pica (craving to eat unusual substances).

Diagnostic Evaluation

1. Complete blood count (CBC) and iron profile—decreased hemoglobin, hematocrit, serum iron, and ferritin; elevated red cell distribution width and normal or elevated total iron-binding capacity (transferrin).
2. Determination of source of chronic blood loss may include sigmoidoscopy, colonoscopy, upper and lower GI studies, and stools and urine for occult blood examination.

Management

1. Diagnosis and correction of chronic blood loss.
2. Oral or parenteral iron therapy.

a. Oral ferrous sulfate preferred and least expensive; treatment continues until hemoglobin level is normalized and iron stores replaced (up to 6 months).
b. Parenteral therapy may be used when the patient cannot tolerate or is nonadherent with oral therapy. There are a variety of iron infusions, such as sodium ferric gluconate, iron sucrose, and iron dextran.

Complications

1. Severe compromise of the oxygen-carrying capacity of the blood may predispose to ischemic organ damage, such as myocardial infarction or stroke.
2. Anaphylaxis to parenteral iron therapy, especially with iron dextran.

Nursing Assessment

1. Obtain a history of symptoms, dietary intake, past history of anemia, and possible sources of blood loss.
2. Examine for tachycardia, pallor, dyspnea, and signs of GI or other bleeding.

Nursing Interventions

Promoting Iron Intake

1. Assess diet for inclusion of foods rich in iron and any barriers to intake, such as dental problems, dysphagia, and religious or personal preferences.
2. Educate patient about the importance of iron in the diet, help develop a nutritional plan, and arrange nutritionist referral, as appropriate.
3. Administer iron infusion or teach self-administration of oral iron replacement, as ordered. Monitor CBC and iron studies, as ordered.

DRUG ALERT Anaphylactic reactions may occur after parenteral iron administration. Monitor the patient closely for hypotension, angioedema, and stridor after injection. Do not administer iron infusions in conjunction with oral iron.

Increasing Activity Tolerance

1. Assess level of fatigue and normal sleep pattern; determine activities that cause fatigue.
2. Assist in developing a schedule of activity, rest periods, and sleep.
3. Encourage conditioning exercises to increase strength and endurance.

Maximizing Tissue Perfusion

1. Assess the patient for palpitations, chest pain, dizziness, and shortness of breath; minimize activities that cause these symptoms.
2. Elevate head of bed and provide supplemental oxygen, as ordered.
3. Monitor vital signs and fluid balance.

Patient Education and Health Maintenance

1. Educate the patient on proper nutrition and good sources of iron: Select a well-balanced diet that includes animal proteins, iron-fortified cereals and bread, beans, dried fruits, legumes, and tofu (see Table 22-3). The daily requirement of iron for adult females ages 19 to 50 years is 18 mg, for males 8 mg; however, more is needed to build iron stores in those who have been anemic and for those who are at risk for anemia.
2. Teach the patient about iron supplementation.
   a. Take iron on empty stomach, with full glass of water or fruit juice.
   b. Liquid forms may stain teeth; mix well with water or fruit juice and use a straw.
   c. Anticipate some epigastric discomfort, change in color of stools to green or black, and, in some cases, nausea, constipation, or diarrhea. Prevent and treat constipation with increased fiber, fluids, and exercise. Report GI intolerance to health care provider.
   d. Keep iron medications away from children as overdose may be fatal.
3. Encourage follow-up laboratory studies and visits to health care provider.

Table 22-3 Dietary Sources of Iron

FOOD	SERVING SIZE	MG PER SERVING
Cereal (fortified)	1 oz	1.8–21
Chicken liver	3.5 oz	12.8
Oatmeal (fortified)	1 cup	10
Soybeans	1 cup	8.8
Beef liver	3 oz	7.5
Lentils	1 cup	6.6
Beans (kidney, lima, navy, pinto)	1 cup	3.6–5.2
Oysters	6 pieces	4.5
Pumpkin seeds, roasted	1 oz	4.2
Beef (various cuts)	3–3.5 oz	2–3.9
Molasses	1 tbsp	3.5
Tofu	1/2 cup	3.4
Spinach, cooked	1/2 cup	3.2
Clams	3/4 cup	3.0
Sardines	3 oz	2.5
Turkey	3.5 oz	1.6–2.3
Macaroni (enriched, cooked)	1 cup	1.9
Bread (enriched)	2 slices	1.8
Rice (cooked)	1 cup	1.8
Apricots (dried)	10 pieces	1.7
Raisins	1/2 cup	1.5
Prune juice	1/2 cup	1.5
Pork	3–3.5 oz	1.2–1.5
Peas	1/2 cup	1.3
Chicken	3–3.5 oz	1.1–1.3

Evaluation: Expected Outcomes

- Incorporates several foods high in iron into diet; takes prescribed iron supplementation, as ordered.
- Tolerates increased activity; obtains sufficient rest.
- Vital signs stable without complaints of chest pain, palpitations, or shortness of breath.

Megaloblastic Anemia: Pernicious (Macrocytic, Normochromic)

A *megaloblast* is a large, nucleated erythrocyte with delayed and abnormal nuclear maturation. *Pernicious anemia* is a type of megaloblastic anemia associated with vitamin B_{12} deficiency.

Pathophysiology and Etiology

1. Vitamin B_{12} is necessary for normal DNA synthesis in maturing RBCs.
2. Pernicious anemia demonstrates familial incidence related to autoimmune gastric mucosal atrophy.
3. Normal gastric mucosa secretes a substance called *intrinsic factor*, necessary for absorption of vitamin B_{12} in the ileum. If a defect exists in the gastric mucosa, or after gastrectomy or small bowel disease, intrinsic factor may not be secreted and orally ingested B_{12} may not be absorbed.
4. Some drugs interfere with B_{12} absorption, notably ascorbic acid, cholestyramine, colchicine, neomycin, cimetidine, metformin, and hormonal contraceptives.
5. Lower serum vitamin B_{12} concentrations are associated with aging, but the evidence linking subnormal vitamin B_{12} to anemia in older people remains limited and inconclusive.
6. Inadequate dietary intake of vitamin B_{12} can also lead to deficiency; this is sometimes seen in those who adhere to vegetarian or vegan diets.

Clinical Manifestations

1. Of anemia—pallor, fatigue, dyspnea on exertion, and palpitations. May lead to angina pectoris and heart failure in older adults or those predisposed to heart disease.
2. Of underlying GI dysfunction—sore mouth, glossitis, anorexia, nausea, vomiting, loss of weight, indigestion, epigastric discomfort, recurring diarrhea, or constipation.
3. Of neuropathy (occurs in high percentage of untreated patients)—paresthesia that involves hands and feet, gait disturbance, bladder and bowel dysfunction, and psychiatric symptoms caused by cerebral dysfunction.

Diagnostic Evaluation

1. CBC and blood smear—decreased hemoglobin and hematocrit; marked variation in size and shape of RBCs with a variable number of unusually large cells.
2. Folic acid (normal) and B_{12} levels (decreased).
3. Gastric analysis—volume and acidity of gastric juice diminished.
4. Schilling test for absorption of vitamin B_{12} uses small amount of radioactive B_{12} orally and 24-hour urine collection to measure uptake—decreased.

Management

Parenteral replacement with hydroxocobalamin or cyanocobalamin (B_{12}) is necessary by intramuscular (IM) injection from health care provider, generally every month.

Complications

Neurologic: Paresthesia, gait disturbances, bowel and bladder dysfunction, and cerebral dysfunction may be persistent.

Nursing Assessment

1. Assess for pallor, tachycardia, dyspnea on exertion, and exercise intolerance to determine the patient's response to anemia.
2. Assess for paresthesia, gait disturbances, changes in bladder or bowel function, and altered thought processes indicating neurologic involvement.
3. Obtain a history of gastric surgery or GI disease.
4. Review nutrition and diet history.

Nursing Interventions

Improving Thought Processes

1. Administer parenteral vitamin B_{12}, as prescribed.
2. Provide the patient with quiet, supportive environment; reorient to time, place, and person, if needed; give instructions and information in short, simple sentences and reinforce frequently.

Minimizing the Effects of Paresthesia

1. Assess the extent and severity of paresthesia, imbalance, or other sensory alterations.
2. Refer the patient for physical therapy and occupational therapy, as appropriate.
3. Provide safe, uncluttered environment; make sure personal belongings are within reach; provide assistance with activities, as needed.

Patient Education and Health Maintenance

1. Advise the patient that monthly vitamin B_{12} administration should be continued for life.
2. Instruct the patient to see health care provider approximately every 6 months for hematologic studies, stool examination for occult blood, gastric cytology and thyroid function studies; patients with pernicious anemia have higher incidence of gastric cancer and thyroid dysfunction.

Evaluation: Expected Outcomes

- Oriented, cooperative, and follows instructions.
- Carries out activities without injury.

Megaloblastic Anemia: Folic Acid Deficiency

Chronic *megaloblastic anemia* is caused by folic acid (folate) deficiency.

Pathophysiology and Etiology

1. Dietary deficiency, malnutrition, marginal diets, excessive cooking of foods; commonly associated with alcohol use disorder.
2. Impaired absorption in jejunum (e.g., with small bowel disease).
3. Increased requirements (e.g., with chronic hemolytic anemia, exfoliative dermatitis, pregnancy).
4. Impaired utilization from folic acid antagonists (methotrexate) and other drugs (phenytoin, broad-spectrum antibiotics, sulfamethoxazole, alcohol, hormonal contraceptives).

Clinical Manifestations

1. Of anemia: fatigue, weakness, pallor, dizziness, headache, tachycardia.
2. Of folic acid deficiency: sore tongue, cracked lips.

Diagnostic Evaluation

1. Vitamin B_{12} and folic acid level—folic acid will be decreased.
2. CBC will show decreased RBC, hemoglobin, and hematocrit with increased mean corpuscular volume and mean corpuscular hemoglobin concentration.

Management

Oral folic acid (folate) replacement on daily basis.

Complications

Folic acid deficiency has been implicated in the etiology of congenitally acquired neural tube defects.

Nursing Assessment

1. Obtain nutritional history.
2. Monitor level of dyspnea, tachycardia, and development of chest pain or shortness of breath for worsening of condition.

Nursing Interventions

Improving Folic Acid Intake

1. Assess diet for inclusion of foods rich in folic acid: beef liver, peanut butter, red beans, oatmeal, broccoli, and asparagus.
2. Arrange nutritionist referral, as appropriate.
3. Administer or teach self-administration of folic acid (folate) supplement.
4. Assist patient with alcohol use disorder to obtain counseling and additional medical care, as needed. Provide information about support groups.

Patient Education and Health Maintenance

1. Teach the patient to select balanced diet that includes green vegetables (asparagus, broccoli, spinach), yeast, liver and other organ meats, and some fresh fruits; avoid overcooking vegetables.
2. Encourage the patient to follow up periodically to monitor CBC.
3. Encourage pregnant patient to maintain prenatal care and to take folic acid supplement.

Evaluation: Expected Outcomes

- Eats nutritious, folate-rich diet; takes folic acid supplements, as prescribed.

Aplastic Anemia

Aplastic anemia is a rare disorder characterized by bone marrow hypoplasia or aplasia, resulting in pancytopenia (insufficient numbers of RBCs, white blood cells [WBCs], and platelets).

Pathophysiology and Etiology

Destruction of hematopoietic stem cells is thought to be through an immune-mediated mechanism.

1. Most often (70% to 80% of patients) characterized as idiopathic because no cause is found.
2. May be caused by exposure to chemical toxins (e.g., benzene); ionizing radiation; viral infections, particularly hepatitis; certain drugs (e.g., chloramphenicol).
3. May be congenital (e.g., Fanconi anemia, Diamond-Blackfan anemia, and Shwachman-Diamond syndrome).
4. Clinical course is variable and dependent on the degree of bone marrow failure; severe aplastic anemia is almost always fatal if untreated.

Clinical Manifestations

1. From anemia: pallor, weakness, fatigue, exertional dyspnea, palpitations.
2. From infections associated with neutropenia: fever, headache, and malaise; adventitious breath sounds; abdominal pain, diarrhea; erythema, pain, exudate at wounds, or sites of invasive procedures.
3. From thrombocytopenia: bleeding from gums, nose, GI or genitourinary (GU) tracts; purpura, petechiae, ecchymoses.

Diagnostic Evaluation

1. CBC and peripheral blood smear show decreased RBC, WBC, and platelets (pancytopenia).
2. Bone marrow aspiration and biopsy: Bone marrow is hypocellular or empty with greatly reduced or absent hematopoiesis.

Management

1. Removal of causative agent or toxin.
2. Allogeneic bone marrow transplantation (BMT)—treatment of choice for patients with severe aplastic anemia (see page 769). This treatment option provides long-term survival for 75% to 90% of patients, depending on the age of the patient, history of prior blood transfusions, and source of marrow.
3. Immunosuppressive treatment with cyclosporine and antithymocyte globulin or cyclophosphamide. This treatment option provides long-term survival for 60% to 70% of patients.
4. Androgens (oxymetholone or testosterone enanthate) may stimulate bone marrow regeneration; significant toxicity encountered. They may be used when other treatments have failed.
5. Supportive treatment includes platelet and RBC transfusions, antibiotics, and antifungals. Blood components should be irradiated for patients eligible for BMT, and this approach is also recommended for patients receiving immunosuppressive therapy.

Complications

1. Untreated severe aplastic anemia is almost always fatal, generally because of overwhelming infection. Even with treatment, morbidity and mortality caused by infections and bleeding are high.
2. Late complications, even after successful treatment, include clonal hematologic diseases such as paroxysmal nocturnal hemoglobinuria, myelodysplasia, and acute myelogenous leukemia (AML).

Nursing Assessment

1. Obtain a thorough history that includes medications, past medical history, occupation, and hobbies.
2. Monitor for signs of bleeding and infection.

Nursing Interventions

Minimizing Risk of Infection

1. Care for patient in protective environment while hospitalized (e.g., private room with strict handwashing and avoidance of any contaminants).
2. Encourage good personal hygiene, including daily shower or bath with mild soap, mouth care, and perirectal care after using the toilet.
3. Monitor vital signs, including temperature, frequently; notify health care provider of oral temperature of 101°F (38.3°C) or higher.
4. Minimize invasive procedures or possible trauma to skin or mucous membranes.
5. Obtain cultures of suspected infected sites or body fluids.

Minimizing Risk of Bleeding

1. Use only soft toothbrush or toothette for mouth care and electric razor for shaving; keep nails short by filing.
2. Avoid IM injections and other invasive procedures.
3. Prevent constipation with stool softeners, as prescribed.
4. Restrict activity based on platelet count and active bleeding.
5. Monitor pad count for menstruating patient; avoid the use of vaginal tampons.
6. Control bleeding by applying pressure to site, using ice packs and prescribed topical hemostatic agents.
7. Administer blood product replacement, as ordered; monitor for allergic reaction, anaphylaxis, and volume overload.

Patient Education and Health Maintenance

1. Teach the patient how to minimize the risk of infection.
   a. Wash hands after contact with possible source of infection.
   b. Immediately clean any abrasion or wound of mucous membranes or skin.
   c. Monitor temperature and report fever or other sign of infection immediately.
   d. Avoid crowds and people with illnesses.
   e. Avoid raw or undercooked foods.
   f. Use condoms and other safe sex practices.
2. Teach the patient how to minimize the risk of bleeding.
   a. Avoid falls or other injury.
   b. Use electric razor rather than plain razor.
   c. Use nail clippers or file rather than scissors.
   d. Avoid blowing nose.
   e. Use soft toothbrush or toothette for mouth care.
   f. Use water-soluble lubricants, as needed, during sexual activity.
3. Advise the patient to avoid exposure to potential bone marrow toxins: solvents, sprays, paints, and pesticides.
4. Teach the patient to take only prescribed medications; avoid aspirin and nonsteroidal anti-inflammatory drugs (NSAIDs), which may interfere with platelet function. As some vitamins and herbs may also affect platelet function, instruct the patient to check with health care provider before using any supplements.
5. Resources for the patient and family include the Aplastic Anemia & MDS International Foundation (www.aamds.org).

Evaluation: Expected Outcomes

- Remains afebrile with no signs or symptoms of infection.
- Episodes of bleeding rapidly controlled.

MYELOPROLIFERATIVE DISORDERS

See additional online content: Patient Education Guidelines 22-1 and 22-2 and Nursing Care Plan 22-1

Myeloproliferative disorders are disorders of the bone marrow that result from abnormal proliferation of cells from the myeloid line of the hematopoietic system. They include polycythemia vera, acute lymphocytic and acute myelogenous leukemia (AML), and chronic myelogenous leukemia (CML).

Polycythemia Vera

Polycythemia vera is a chronic myeloproliferative disorder that involves all bone marrow elements, resulting in an increase in red blood cell (RBC) mass and hemoglobin.

EVIDENCE BASE Duek, A., Berla, M., & Ellis, M. H. (2022). Recent advances in the treatment of polycythemia vera. *Leukemia & Lymphoma*, *63*(8), 1801–1809. https://doi.org/10.1080/10428194.2022.2057491

Pathophysiology and Etiology

1. Hyperplasia of all bone marrow elements results in the following:
   a. Overproduction of all three blood cell lines, most prominently RBCs.
   b. Increased red cell mass.
   c. Increased blood volume and viscosity.
   d. Decreased marrow iron reserve.
   e. Splenomegaly.
2. Increased mass of blood cells increases viscosity and leads to engorgement of blood vessels and possible thrombosis.
3. Underlying cause is unknown.
4. Usually occurs in middle and later years.

Clinical Manifestations

Result from increased blood volume and viscosity.

1. Reddish purple skin and mucosa, pruritus (especially after bathing).
2. Splenomegaly, hepatomegaly.
3. Epigastric discomfort, abdominal discomfort.
4. Painful fingers and toes from arterial and venous insufficiency, paresthesia.
5. Headache, fullness in head, dizziness, visual abnormalities, altered mental status from disturbed cerebral circulation.
6. Weakness, fatigue, night sweats, bleeding tendency.
7. Hyperuricemia from increased formation and destruction of erythrocytes and leukocytes and increased metabolism of nucleic acids.
8. Itching related to histamine release from basophils.

Diagnostic Evaluation

1. Complete blood count (CBC)—elevated RBC and hemoglobin and hematocrit (greater than 60%); elevated platelets.
2. Bone marrow aspirate and biopsy—hyperplasia.
3. Elevated uric acid.

Management

1. Of hyperviscosity: phlebotomy (withdrawal of blood) at intervals determined by CBC results to reduce RBC mass; generally, 250 to 500 mL removed at a time to maintain hematocrit less than 45%. The British Committee for Standards in Hematology recommendations also include aspirin at 75 mg/day unless contraindicated.
2. Of marrow hyperplasia: chronic myelosuppressive therapy, generally using hydroxycarbamide (formerly known as *hydroxyurea*) or intravenous (IV) radioactive phosphorus; biologic response modifier (i.e., alpha-interferon). Aggressive chemotherapy is not recommended because of increased risk of secondary leukemia.
3. Of hyperuricemia: allopurinol.
4. Of pruritus: antihistamines (diphenhydramine, hydroxyzine, cimetidine or cyproheptadine), low-dose aspirin, certain antidepressants (doxepin, paroxetine), phototherapy, cholestyramine, alpha-interferon.

Complications

1. Thromboembolic events caused by hyperviscosity, including deep vein thrombophlebitis, myocardial and cerebral infarction, transient ischemic attacks, pulmonary embolism, retinal vein thrombosis, and thrombotic occlusion of the splenic, hepatic, portal, and mesenteric veins.
2. Spontaneous hemorrhage caused by venous and capillary distention and abnormal platelet function.
3. Gout caused by hyperuricemia.
4. Heart failure caused by increased blood volume and hypertension.
5. Myelofibrosis or acute myeloid leukemia may be terminal complications.

Nursing Assessment

1. Obtain a history of symptoms, including changes in skin, epigastric discomfort, bleeding tendencies, circulatory problems, or painful, swollen joints.
2. Monitor for signs of bleeding or thromboembolism.
3. Monitor for hypertension and signs and symptoms of heart failure, including shortness of breath, distended neck veins.

Nursing Interventions

Preventing Thromboembolic Complications

1. Encourage or assist with ambulation. Employ thromboembolism precautions during periods of immobility.
2. Assess for early signs of thromboembolic complications—swelling of limb, increased warmth, pain, shortness of breath, and chest pain. Report immediately.
3. Monitor CBC and assist with phlebotomy, as ordered.

Patient Education and Health Maintenance

1. Educate the patient about the risk of thrombosis; encourage the patient to maintain normal activity patterns and avoid long periods of bed rest.
2. Advise the patient to avoid taking hot showers or baths because rapid skin cooling worsens pruritus; use skin emollients; take antihistamines, as prescribed; may find starch baths helpful.
3. Instruct the patient to take only prescribed medications.
4. Encourage the patient to report at prescribed intervals for follow-up blood (hematocrit) studies and phlebotomies.
5. Instruct the patient in technique of subcutaneous injection for alpha-interferon.

Evaluation: Expected Outcomes

- Hematocrit less than 45%; no signs or symptoms of thromboembolism, heart failure, or bleeding.

Acute Lymphocytic and Acute Myelogenous Leukemia

Leukemias are malignant disorders of the blood and bone marrow characterized by a loss of regulation of cell division that results in an accumulation of dysfunctional, immature cells. They are classified as acute or chronic based on the development rate of symptoms and further classified by the predominant cell type. Acute leukemias affect immature cells and are characterized by rapid progression of symptoms. When lymphocytes (B or T cell) are the predominant malignant cell, the disorder is *acute lymphocytic leukemia* (ALL); when monocytes or granulocytes are predominant, it is *acute myelogenous leukemia* (AML).

Pathophysiology and Etiology

1. The development of leukemia has been associated with the following:
   a. Exposure to ionizing radiation.
   b. Exposure to certain chemicals and toxins (e.g., benzene, alkylating agents).
   c. Human T-cell leukemia—lymphoma virus (HTLV-1 and HTLV-2) in certain areas of the world, including the Caribbean and southern Japan.
   d. Familial susceptibility.
   e. Genetic disorders (e.g., Down syndrome, Fanconi anemia).
   f. Childhood leukemia is often not associated with a specific cause.
2. Approximately one half of new leukemias are acute. Approximately 85% of acute leukemias in adults are AML. ALL is most common in children, with peak incidence between ages 2 and 9 years.
3. Childhood ALL is usually cured with chemotherapy alone (greater than 75%), whereas only 30% to 40% of adults with ALL are cured.
4. AML is a disease of older people, with a median age at diagnosis of 67. However, it does also occur in children, though much less common than ALL. Even in the younger adults (patients who are younger than age 60), AML is difficult to treat, with a median survival of 5 to 6 months, despite intensive therapy.

Clinical Manifestations

1. Common symptoms include pallor, fatigue, weakness, fever, weight loss, abnormal bleeding and bruising, lymphadenopathy (in ALL), and recurrent infections.
2. Other presenting symptoms may include bone and joint pain, headache, splenomegaly, hepatomegaly, and neurologic dysfunction.

Diagnostic Evaluation

1. CBC and blood smear—peripheral white blood cell (WBC) count varies widely from 1,000 to 100,000/mm^3 and may

include significant numbers of abnormal immature (blast) cells; anemia may be profound; platelet count may be abnormal, and coagulopathies may exist.
2. Bone marrow aspiration and biopsy—cells also studied for chromosomal abnormalities (cytogenetics) and immunologic markers to classify the type of leukemia further.
3. Lumbar puncture and examination of cerebrospinal fluid for leukemic cells (especially in ALL).

Management

1. The National Comprehensive Cancer Network (NCCN; www.nccn.org) guidelines provide recommendations for workup, management, and supportive care of patients with various subtypes of AML. Evidence-based treatment guidelines for management of ALL are published by the National Cancer Institute (www.cancer.gov/cancertopics/pdq/treatment/adultALL/HealthProfessional).
2. Management of AML and ALL is designed to eradicate leukemic cells and allow restoration of normal hematopoiesis.
   a. High-dose chemotherapy given as an induction course to obtain remission (disappearance of abnormal cells in bone marrow and blood) and then in cycles as consolidation or maintenance therapy to prevent recurrence of disease (see Table 22-4).
   b. Leukapheresis (or exchange transfusion in infants) may be used when abnormally high numbers of white cells are present to reduce the risk of leukostasis and tumor burden before chemotherapy.
   c. Radiation, particularly of central nervous system (CNS) in ALL.
   d. Targeted therapies are being developed to stop cancer cell growth by targeting specific genes or proteins; may be used in conjunction with other chemotherapy.
   e. Autologous or allogeneic bone marrow or stem cell transplantation.

Complications

1. Leukostasis: In setting of high numbers (greater than 50,000/mm^3) of circulating leukemic cells (blasts), blood vessel walls are infiltrated and weakened, with high risk of rupture and bleeding, including intracranial hemorrhage.
2. Disseminated intravascular coagulation (DIC).
3. Tumor lysis syndrome: Rapid destruction of large numbers of malignant cells leads to alterations in electrolytes (hyperuricemia, hyperkalemia, hyperphosphatemia, and hypocalcemia), renal failure, and other complications.
4. Infection (sepsis), bleeding, organ damage.

DRUG ALERT Allopurinol and rasburicase are commonly used as part of a regimen to prevent tumor lysis syndrome. In rare cases, they may cause severe, even lethal, skin reactions (toxic epidermolysis syndrome). Allopurinol should be discontinued for any patient who develops a new skin rash.

Table 22-4 Common Chemotherapeutic Drugs Used in Acute Leukemias

DRUG	MAJOR ADVERSE EFFECTS	CLASSIFICATION	PRIMARY USE
All-*trans*-retinoic acid	Dry skin and mucous membranes, headaches, eyesight changes, bone pain, flulike symptoms, bone marrow suppression, and retinoic acid syndrome (includes weight gain, peripheral edema, dyspnea, and fever)	Retinoid	Therapy for AML subtype M3 (APL)
Cyclophosphamide	Bone marrow suppression, alopecia, nausea and vomiting, diarrhea, hemorrhagic cystitis, and cardiomyopathy	Alkylating agent	Induction and consolidation therapy for ALL
Cytarabine	Bone marrow suppression, nausea and vomiting, pulmonary toxicity, mucositis, lethargy, cerebellar toxicity, dermatitis, and keratoconjunctivitis	Antimetabolite	Induction and consolidation therapy for AML
Daunorubicin	Bone marrow suppression, nausea and vomiting, alopecia, cardiotoxicity, and vesicant	Antibiotic	Induction and consolidation therapy for AML
Doxorubicin	Leukopenia, nausea and vomiting, alopecia, cardiotoxicity, photosensitivity, and vesicant	Antibiotic	Induction and consolidation therapy for AML
Imatinib mesylate	Edema, nausea and vomiting, musculoskeletal pain, and rash	Tyrosine kinase inhibitor	Induction and consolidation therapy for Philadelphia chromosome–positive adult ALL
L-Asparaginase	Liver dysfunction, nausea and vomiting, hypersensitivity reaction, depression, and lethargy	Miscellaneous: enzyme	Induction therapy for ALL
6-Mercaptopurine	Mild bone marrow suppression, GI disturbances, and hepatotoxicity	Antimetabolite	Maintenance therapy for ALL
Methotrexate	Bone marrow suppression, stomatitis, nausea, diarrhea, hepatotoxicity, and neurotoxicity with intrathecal doses	Antimetabolite	Intrathecal central nervous system treatment and prophylaxis for ALL; maintenance therapy for ALL
Prednisone	Appetite stimulation, mood alteration, Cushing syndrome, hypertension, diabetes, and peptic ulcer	Corticosteroid	Induction therapy for ALL
Vincristine	Neurotoxicity, alopecia, and vesicant	Plant alkaloid	Induction therapy for ALL

ALL, acute lymphocytic leukemia; AML, acute myelogenous leukemia; APL, acute promyelocytic leukemia; GI, gastrointestinal.

Nursing Assessment

1. Take nursing history, focusing on weight loss, fever, frequency of infections, progressively increasing fatigability, shortness of breath, palpitations, and visual changes (retinal bleeding).
2. Ask about difficulty in swallowing, coughing, and rectal pain.
3. Examine the patient for enlarged lymph nodes, hepatosplenomegaly, evidence of bleeding, abnormal breath sounds, and skin lesions.
4. Look for evidence of infection: mouth, tongue, and throat for reddened areas or white patches. Examine skin for breakdown, which is a potential source of infection.

Nursing Interventions

Preventing Infection

1. Especially monitor for pneumonia, pharyngitis, esophagitis, perianal cellulitis, urinary tract infection, and cellulitis, which are common in leukemia and which carry significant morbidity and mortality.
2. Monitor for fever, flushed appearance, chills, and tachycardia; appearance of white patches in mouth; redness, swelling, heat, or pain of eyes, ears, throat, skin, joints, abdomen, and rectal and perineal areas; cough, changes in sputum; skin rash.
3. Check results of granulocyte counts. Concentrations less than 500/mm^3 put the patient at serious risk for infection. Administer granulocyte- and erythropoiesis-stimulating agents, as ordered (e.g., epoetin alfa or darbepoetin alfa).
4. Avoid invasive procedures and trauma to skin or mucous membrane to prevent entry of microorganisms.
5. Use the following rectal precautions to prevent infection:
   a. Avoid diarrhea and constipation, which can irritate the rectal mucosa.
   b. Avoid the use of rectal thermometers.
   c. Keep the perianal area clean.
6. Care for the patient in private room with strict handwashing practice. Patients with prolonged neutropenia may benefit from high-efficiency particulate air filtration.
7. Encourage and assist the patient with personal hygiene, bathing, and oral care.
8. Obtain cultures and administer antimicrobials promptly, as directed. Prophylactic antimicrobials, antifungals, and antivirals serve to protect the patient from life-threatening infections.

Preventing and Managing Bleeding

1. Watch for signs of minor bleeding, such as petechiae, ecchymosis, conjunctival hemorrhage, epistaxis, bleeding gums, bleeding at puncture sites, vaginal spotting, and heavy menses.
2. Be alert for signs of serious bleeding, such as headache with change in responsiveness, blurred vision, hemoptysis, hematemesis, melena, hypotension, tachycardia, and dizziness.
3. Monitor urine, stools, and emesis for gross and occult blood.
4. Monitor platelet counts daily.
5. Administer blood components, as directed.
6. Keep the patient on bed rest during bleeding episodes.

Patient Education and Health Maintenance

1. Teach infection precautions (see page 746).
2. Teach signs and symptoms of infection and advise whom to notify.
3. Encourage adequate nutrition to prevent emaciation from chemotherapy.
4. Teach avoidance of constipation with increased fluid and fiber and good perianal care.
5. Teach bleeding precautions (see page 746).
6. Encourage regular dental visits to detect and treat dental infections and disease.
7. Provide the patient and family with information about resources in the community, see Box 22-1.

BOX 22-1 Resources for Patients With Hematologic Malignancies

AMERICAN CANCER SOCIETY
250 Williams Street NW
Atlanta, GA 30303
(404) 320-3333 or (800) 227-2345
www.cancer.org
Patient education materials, the *Can Surmount* and *I Can Cope* educational and support programs, and durable medical equipment loans.

CORPORATE ANGEL NETWORK, INC
Westchester County Airport, 1 Loop Road
White Plains, NY 10604
(914) 328-1313 or (866) 328-1313
www.corpangelnetwork.org
Use of corporate aircraft to provide free travel to patients with cancer going to checkups, treatments, or consultations.

LEUKEMIA AND LYMPHOMA SOCIETY
1311 Mamaroneck Avenue
Suite 310
White Plains, NY 10605
(914) 949-5213 or (800) 955-4572
http://www.lls.org
Patient education materials, support groups, financial assistance (patient aid) program for patients with leukemia, Hodgkin and non-Hodgkin lymphoma, and multiple myeloma.

NATIONAL COALITION FOR CANCER SURVIVORSHIP
1010 Wayne Ave., Suite 707
Silver Spring, MD 20910
(301) 650-9127
www.canceradvocacy.org
Network related to survivorship issues, sponsors National Cancer Survivors' Day, publishes Cancer Survivors Almanac of Resources.

NATIONAL MARROW DONOR PROGRAM
3001 Broadway Street NE, Suite 100
Minneapolis, MN 55413
(800) 507-5427
www.bethematch.org
Information for patients and volunteer donors regarding unrelated bone marrow transplant.

NATIONAL CANCER INSTITUTE
National Institutes of Health
Bethesda, MD 20892
(800) 4-CANCER
www.cancer.gov
National telephone hotline for information, patient education materials, and research reports.

BLOOD & MARROW TRANSPLANT INFORMATION NETWORK
2900 Skokie Valley Road, Suite B
Highland Park, IL 60035
(888) 597-7674
www.bmtinfonet.org
Resources, support, and educational materials for patients and families.

Evaluation: Expected Outcomes

- Afebrile, without signs of infection.
- No signs of bleeding.

Chronic Myelogenous Leukemia

CML (i.e., involving more mature cells than acute leukemia) is characterized by proliferation of myeloid cell lines, including granulocytes, monocytes, platelets, and, occasionally, RBCs.

Pathophysiology and Etiology

1. Specific etiology unknown, associated with exposure to ionizing radiation and family history of leukemia. Results from malignant transformation of pluripotent hematopoietic stem cell.
2. First cancer associated with chromosomal abnormality (the Philadelphia [Ph] chromosome), present in more than 90% of patients.
3. Accounts for 25% of adult leukemias and less than 5% of childhood leukemias. Generally presents between ages 25 and 60 years, with peak incidence in the mid-40s.
4. May progress to an accelerated phase or blast crisis, resembling an acute leukemia.

Clinical Manifestations

1. Insidious onset; may be discovered during routine physical examination.
2. About 70% of patients have symptoms at diagnosis, such as fatigue, pallor, activity intolerance, fever, weight loss, night sweats, and abdominal fullness (splenomegaly).

Diagnostic Evaluation

1. CBC and blood smear: Large numbers of granulocytes (usually more than 100,000/mm^3), platelets may be decreased.
2. Bone marrow aspiration and biopsy: hypercellular, usually demonstrates Ph^1 chromosome.

Management

Treatment guidelines for the management of CML are provided by NCCN (www.nccn.org).

EVIDENCE BASE Lipton, J. H., Brümmendorf, T. H., Gambacorti-Passerini, C., Garcia-Gutiérrez, V., Deininger, M. W., & Cortes, J. E. (2022). Long-term safety review of tyrosine kinase inhibitors in chronic myeloid leukemia—What to look for when treatment-free remission is not an option. *Blood Reviews, 56*, 100968. https://doi.org/10.1016/j.blre.2022.100968

Chronic Phase

1. Tyrosine kinase inhibitors are oral agents used as primary treatment for most patients with CML. They include imatinib mesylate, dasatinib, and nilotinib.
   a. These agents work by inhibiting proliferation of abnormal cells and inducing cell death (apoptosis) in abnormal cells.
   b. Adverse effects vary based on the agent used but include edema, diarrhea, headache, muscle cramps, muscle and bone pain, rash, and, rarely, hepatotoxicity, pleural or pericardial effusion, and myelosuppression.
2. For patients who do not respond to tyrosine kinase inhibitors, allogeneic (related or unrelated) bone marrow transplantation (BMT) may be an option.

Accelerated Phase or Blast Crisis

1. High-dose tyrosine kinase inhibitors or chemotherapy (ALL or AML regimens) may be used to attempt to regain chronic phase.
2. Supportive care and palliative care may be appropriate because this phase is usually terminal.

Complications

1. Leukostasis.
2. Infection, bleeding, and organ damage.
3. If untreated, CML is a terminal disease with unpredictable survival, on average 3 years.

Nursing Assessment

1. Obtain health history, focusing on fatigue, weight loss, night sweats, and activity intolerance.
2. Assess for signs of bleeding and infection.
3. Evaluate for splenomegaly and hepatomegaly.
4. Assess for weight gain and edema in patients taking tyrosine kinase inhibitors.

Nursing Interventions

Also see nursing interventions for acute leukemia, page 747.

Managing Fears

1. Encourage appropriate verbalization of feelings and concerns.
2. Provide comprehensive patient teaching about disease, using methods and content appropriate to the patient's needs.
3. Assist the patient in identifying resources and support (e.g., family and friends, spiritual support, community or national organizations, support groups).
4. Facilitate the use of effective coping mechanisms.

Patient Education and Health Maintenance

1. Teach the patient to take medications, as prescribed, and monitor for adverse effects.
2. Teach the patient method of subcutaneous injection for self-administration of alpha-interferon and teach strategies for managing adverse effects, such as fatigue and fever.
3. To avoid delay in evaluation and treatment, provide patient and family with appropriate education before and after discharge regarding the importance of reporting early signs of infection, such as fever, nausea and vomiting, and increasing pain.
4. Provide the patient and family with information about resources in the community (see Box 22-1).

Evaluation: Expected Outcomes

- Demonstrates effective coping skills.

LYMPHOPROLIFERATIVE DISORDERS

Lymphoproliferative disorders result from proliferation of cells from the lymphoid line of the hematopoietic system. They include chronic lymphocytic leukemia, Hodgkin lymphoma, non-Hodgkin lymphoma, and multiple myeloma.

Chronic Lymphocytic Leukemia

Chronic lymphocytic leukemia (CLL) (i.e., involving more mature cells than acute leukemia) is characterized by proliferation of morphologically normal but functionally inert B lymphocytes. In CLL, the abnormal lymphocytes are found in the bone marrow and blood, whereas in *small lymphocytic lymphoma* (SLL), the same abnormal lymphocytes are found predominantly in lymph nodes. The differential diagnosis includes *hairy cell leukemia* and *Waldenström macroglobulinemia*.

Pathophysiology and Etiology

1. Specific etiology unknown. Tends to cluster in families, much more common in Western hemisphere. Male hormones may play role.
2. Most common adult leukemia in the United States and Europe. Disease of later years (90% over age 50); 1.5 times more common in males than in females.
3. Lymphocytes are immunoincompetent and respond poorly to antigenic stimulation.
4. In late stages, organ damage may occur from direct lymphocytic infiltration of tissue.
5. Variable course: may be indolent for years, with gradual transformation to more malignant or aggressive disease with 1- to 2-year course.

Clinical Manifestations

1. Insidious onset; may be discovered during routine physical examination.
2. Early symptoms may include painless lymph node swelling, commonly in cervical area, history of frequent skin or respiratory infections, mild splenomegaly and hepatomegaly, and fatigue.
3. Symptoms of more advanced disease include fever, night sweats, weight loss, pallor, activity intolerance, easy bruising, skin lesions, bone tenderness, and abdominal discomfort.

Diagnostic Evaluation

1. Complete blood count (CBC) and blood smear: large numbers of lymphocytes (10,000 to 150,000/mm^3); may also be anemia, thrombocytopenia, and hypogammaglobulinemia.
2. Bone marrow aspirate and biopsy: lymphocytic infiltration of bone marrow.
3. Lymph node biopsy to detect spread.

Management

Symptom Control and Treatments

1. Patient with newly diagnosed and indolent CLL is generally observed and followed closely until symptoms develop. Treatment is individualized; the National Comprehensive Cancer Network (NCCN) guidelines suggest clinical trial or various chemotherapy and monoclonal antibody combinations (www.nccn.org).
2. Lymphocyte proliferation can be suppressed with chlorambucil, cyclophosphamide, and prednisone.
3. The purine analog fludarabine has significant activity in CLL either alone or in combination with rituximab and/or cyclophosphamide.
4. Monoclonal antibodies, such as alemtuzumab and rituximab, may be used.
5. Hairy cell leukemia, a distinctive type of B-cell leukemia with hairlike projections of cytoplasm from lymphocytes, may be successfully treated with cladribine, pentostatin, or alpha-interferon.
6. Splenic irradiation or splenectomy for painful splenomegaly or platelet sequestration, hemolytic anemia.
7. Irradiation of painful enlarged lymph nodes.
8. Allogeneic bone marrow transplant is also used to treat CLL.

Supportive Care

1. Transfusion therapy to replace platelets and red blood cells (RBCs).
2. Antibiotics, antivirals, and antifungals, as needed, to control infections.
3. Intravenous (IV) immunoglobulins or gamma globulin to treat hypogammaglobulinemia.

Complications

1. Thrombophlebitis from venous or lymphatic obstruction caused by enlarged lymph nodes.
2. Infection, bleeding.
3. Median survival depends on the severity of disease; varies from 2 to 7 years.

Nursing Assessment

1. Obtain health history, focusing on history of infections, fatigue, bruising and bleeding, and swollen lymph nodes.
2. Assess for signs of anemia, bleeding, or infection.
3. Evaluate for splenomegaly, hepatomegaly, and lymphadenopathy.

Nursing Interventions

Reducing Pain

1. Assess the patient frequently for pain and administer or teach the patient to administer analgesics on regular schedule, as prescribed; monitor for adverse effects.
2. Teach the patient the use of nonpharmacologic methods, such as music, relaxation breathing, progressive muscle relaxation, distraction, and imagery to help manage pain.

Improving Activity Tolerance

1. Encourage frequent rest periods alternating with ambulation and light activity, as tolerated.
2. Assist the patient with hygiene and physical care, as necessary.
3. Encourage balanced diet or nutritional supplements, as tolerated.
4. Teach the patient to use energy conservation techniques while performing activities of daily living, such as sitting while bathing, minimizing trips up and down stairs, using shoulder bag or push cart to carry articles.

Patient Education and Health Maintenance

1. Teach the patient to minimize the risk of infection (see page 746).
2. Teach the patient use of medications, as ordered, and possible adverse effects and their management; also teach the patient to avoid aspirin and nonsteroidal anti-inflammatory drugs (NSAIDs), which may interfere with platelet function.
3. Provide the patient and family with information about resources in the community (see page 749).

Evaluation: Expected Outcomes

- States pain relief.
- Performs activities without complaints of fatigue.

Hodgkin Lymphoma

Lymphomas are malignant disorders of the reticuloendothelial system that result in an accumulation of dysfunctional, immature lymphoid-derived cells. They are classified according to the predominant cell type and by the degree of malignant cell maturity (e.g., well differentiated, poorly differentiated, or undifferentiated). Hodgkin lymphoma originates in the lymphoid system and involves predominantly lymph nodes. It accounts for about 12% of all lymphomas.

Pathophysiology and Etiology

1. Etiology is unknown.
2. Characterized by appearance of "Reed–Sternberg" multinucleated giant cell in tumor.
3. Generally spreads via lymphatic channels, involving lymph nodes, spleen, and, ultimately, extralymphatic sites. May also spread via bloodstream to sites such as gastrointestinal (GI) tract, bone marrow, skin, upper air passages, and other organs.
4. Incidence demonstrates two peaks, between ages 20 and 30 and after age 55. Risk is increased in males, for patients with human immunodeficiency virus (HIV), in individuals with previous Epstein-Barr viral infection, and in individuals with first-degree relative with Hodgkin lymphoma.

Clinical Manifestations

1. Common symptoms include painless enlargement of lymph nodes (generally unilateral cervical or supraclavicular), splenomegaly, fever, chills, night sweats, weight loss, and pruritus.
2. Various symptoms may occur with pulmonary involvement, superior vena cava obstruction, and hepatic or bone involvement.

Diagnostic Evaluation

Tests are used to determine the extent of disease involvement before treatment and followed at regular intervals to assess response to treatment.

1. CBC—determines abnormal cells.
2. Lymph node biopsy—determines the type of lymphoma.
3. Bilateral bone marrow aspirate and biopsy—determine whether bone marrow is involved.
4. Radiographic tests (e.g., x-rays, positron emission tomography [PET] scan, computed tomography [CT] scan, magnetic resonance imaging [MRI])—detect deep nodal involvement.
5. Gallium-67 scan—detects areas of active disease and may be used to determine aggressiveness of disease.
6. Liver function tests—determine hepatic involvement; liver biopsy may be indicated if results abnormal.
7. Lymphangiogram—detects size and location of deep nodes involved, including abdominal nodes, which may not be readily seen via CT scan.
8. Surgical staging (laparotomy with splenectomy, liver biopsy, and multiple lymph node biopsies)—in selected patients.

Management

Choice of treatment depends on the extent of disease, histopathologic findings, and prognostic indicators. Hodgkin lymphoma is more readily cured than other lymphomas, with a 5-year survival rate of about 89%. The NCCN guidelines for Hodgkin lymphoma (www.nccn.org) provide recommendations for diagnosis and treatment with chemotherapy, chemotherapy and radiation, and/or hematopoietic stem cell transplant for select patients. Hodgkin lymphoma arising in the presence of HIV requires specialized treatment.

1. Radiation therapy.
   a. Treatment of choice for localized disease.
   b. Areas of body where lymph node chains are located can generally tolerate high radiation doses.
   c. Vital organs are protected with lead shielding during radiation treatments.
2. Chemotherapy.
   a. Initial treatment commonly consists of chemotherapy regimens involving a combination of drugs, including doxorubicin, bleomycin, vinblastine, dacarbazine, nitrogen mustard, vincristine, procarbazine, and prednisone.
   b. Three or four drugs may be given in intermittent or cyclical courses with periods off treatment to allow recovery from toxicities.
3. Immunotherapy.
   a. Immunotherapy medications are specifically designed to help the immune system recognize and destroy the cancer cells.
   b. Medications utilized for Hodgkin lymphoma include monoclonal antibodies and immune checkpoint inhibitors.
4. Autologous or allogeneic bone marrow or stem cell transplantation.

Complications

1. Adverse effects of radiation or chemotherapy (see page 83).
2. Dependent on the location and extent of malignancy but may include splenomegaly, hepatomegaly, thromboembolic complications, and spinal cord compression.

Nursing Assessment

1. Obtain health history, focusing on fatigue, fever, chills, night sweats, and swollen lymph nodes.
2. Evaluate splenomegaly, hepatomegaly, and lymphadenopathy.

Nursing Interventions

Maintaining Tissue Integrity

1. Avoid rubbing, powders, deodorants, lotions, or ointments (unless prescribed) or application of heat and cold to treated area.
2. Encourage the patient to keep the treated area clean and dry, bathing area gently with tepid water and mild soap.
3. Encourage wearing loose-fitting clothes.
4. Advise the patient to protect skin from exposure to sun, chlorine, and temperature extremes.

Preserving Oral and Gastrointestinal Tract Mucous Membranes

1. Encourage frequent small meals, using bland and soft diet at mild temperatures.
2. Teach the patient to avoid irritants, such as alcohol, tobacco, spices, and extreme food temperatures.
3. Administer or teach self-administration of pain medication or antiemetic before eating or drinking, if needed.
4. Encourage mouth care at least twice per day and after meals using gentle flossing, soft toothbrush or toothette, and mild mouth rinse.

5. Assess for ulcers, plaques, or discharge that may be indicative of superimposed infection.
6. For diarrhea, switch to low-residue diet and administer antidiarrheals, as ordered.

Patient Education and Health Maintenance

1. Teach the patient about the risk of infection (see page 746).
2. Teach the patient how to take medications, as ordered, and instruct about possible adverse effects and management.
3. Explain to the patient that radiation therapy may cause sterility; males should be given opportunity for sperm banking before treatment; females may develop ovarian failure and require hormone replacement therapy.
4. Reassure the patient that fatigue will decrease after treatment is completed; encourage frequent naps and rest periods.
5. Provide the patient and family with information about resources in the community (see page 749).

Evaluation: Expected Outcomes

- Skin intact without erythema or swelling.
- Oral mucosa intact, patient eating.

Non-Hodgkin Lymphomas

Non-Hodgkin lymphomas are a group of malignancies of lymphoid tissue arising from T or B lymphocytes or their precursors; it includes both indolent and aggressive forms. In the United States, B-cell lymphomas represent about 80% of all cases. Types of non-Hodgkin lymphomas include CLL or SLL (see page 750), follicular lymphoma, diffuse large B-cell lymphoma, and primary cutaneous B-cell lymphoma.

Pathophysiology and Etiology

1. Association with defective or altered immune system; higher incidence in patients receiving immunosuppression for organ transplant, in HIV-positive people, and in people with some viruses (e.g., HTLV-1 and Epstein-Barr). Other risk factors include family history, male sex assigned at birth, White ethnicity, autoimmune diseases such as rheumatoid arthritis, history of *Helicobacter* gastritis (for gastric B-cell lymphoma), history of Hodgkin lymphoma, history of radiation therapy, diet high in meats and fat, and exposure to certain pesticides.
2. Arise from malignant transformation of lymphocyte at some stage during development; level of differentiation and type of lymphocyte influence course of illness and prognosis.
3. Incidence rises steadily from age 40.

Clinical Manifestations

1. Common symptoms include painless enlargement of lymph nodes (generally unilateral), fever, chills, night sweats, weight loss, unexplained pain in chest, abdomen, or bones. Unlike Hodgkin lymphoma, is more likely to be advanced disease at presentation.
2. Various symptoms may occur with pulmonary involvement, superior vena cava obstruction, and hepatic or bone involvement.

Diagnostic Evaluation

1. Incisional or excisional lymph node biopsy to detect type.
2. CBC, bone marrow aspirate, and biopsy to detect bone marrow involvement.
3. CT scan of the chest, abdomen, and pelvis with oral and intravenous (IV) contrast or PET with CT scan to detect deep nodal involvement.
4. Liver function tests, liver scan to detect liver involvement. Hepatitis B testing is recommended because of risk of reactivation.
5. Lumbar puncture to detect CNS involvement (for some lymphoma types).
6. Surgical staging (laparotomy with splenectomy, liver biopsy, multiple lymph node biopsies).

Management

EVIDENCE BASE Sawalha, Y., & Maddocks, K. J. (2022). Novel treatments in B cell non-Hodgkin's lymphoma. *BMJ, 377*, e063439. https://doi.org/10.1136/bmj-2020-063439

1. The NCCN guidelines for non-Hodgkin lymphomas (www.nccn.org) describe a variety of regimens, using radiation therapy, chemotherapy, monoclonal antibodies, radioimmune therapy, and hematopoietic stem cell transplant. Precise diagnosis and staging is needed to ensure appropriate treatment.
2. Radiation therapy is generally palliative, not curative.
3. Chemotherapy: various regimens available, including medications such as cyclophosphamide, doxorubicin, vincristine, prednisone, and bleomycin.
4. Immunotherapy.
   a. Immunotherapy medications are specifically designed to help an individual's immune system recognize and destroy the cancer cells.
   b. Non-Hodgkin lymphoma treatment often includes monoclonal antibodies, specifically those that target CD19 and CD20, CD52, CD30, and CD79b.
   c. Immune checkpoint inhibitors, immunomodulating drugs, and chimeric antigen receptor (CAR) T-cell therapy are used in treatment as well, depending on the specific case.
5. Autologous or allogeneic bone marrow or stem cell transplantation.

Complications

1. Of radiation therapy and chemotherapy (see page 748).
2. Of disease: depends on the location and extent of malignancy but may include splenomegaly, hepatomegaly, thromboembolic complications, and spinal cord compression.

Nursing Assessment

1. Obtain health history, focusing on fatigue, fever, chills, night sweats, swollen lymph nodes, and history of illness or therapy causing immunosuppression.
2. Evaluate splenomegaly, hepatomegaly, and lymphadenopathy.

Nursing Interventions

Minimizing Risk of Infection

1. Care for patient in protected environment with strict handwashing observed.
2. Avoid invasive procedures, such as urinary catheterization, if possible.
3. Assess temperature and vital signs, breath sounds, level of consciousness (LOC), and skin and mucous membranes frequently for signs of infection.

4. Notify the health care provider of fever greater than 101°F (38.3°C) or change in condition.
5. Obtain cultures of suspected infected sites or body fluids.

Patient Education and Health Maintenance

1. Teach the patient infection precautions (see page 749).
2. Encourage frequent follow-up visits for monitoring of CBC and condition.
3. Provide the patient and family with information about resources in the community (see page 749).

Evaluation: Expected Outcomes

- Remains afebrile with no signs or symptoms of infection.

Multiple Myeloma

Multiple myeloma is a malignant disorder of plasma cells, accounting for approximately 13% of all hematologic malignancies.

Pathophysiology and Etiology

1. Etiology unknown; genetic and environmental factors, such as chronic exposure to low levels of ionizing radiation and agricultural exposures to herbicides, may play a part.
2. Characterized by proliferation of neoplastic plasma cells derived from one B lymphocyte (clone) and producing a homogeneous immunoglobulin (M protein or Bence Jones protein) without any apparent antigenic stimulation.
3. Plasma cells produce osteoclast-activating factor, leading to extensive bone loss, severe pain, and pathologic fractures.
4. Abnormal immunoglobulin affects renal function, platelet function, resistance to infection, and may cause hyperviscosity of blood.
5. Generally affects older people (median age at diagnosis is 68) and is twice as common among African American individuals as among White individuals.

Clinical Manifestations

1. Constant, usually severe bone pain caused by bone lesions and pathologic fractures; sites commonly affected include thoracic and lumbar vertebrae, ribs, skull, pelvis, and proximal long bones.
2. Fatigue and weakness related to anemia caused by crowding of marrow by plasma cells.
3. Proteinuria and renal insufficiency.
4. Electrolyte disturbances, including hypercalcemia (bone destruction) and hyperuricemia (cell death, renal insufficiency).

Diagnostic Evaluation

1. Bone marrow aspiration and biopsy—demonstrate increased number and abnormal form of plasma cells.
2. CBC and blood smear—changes reflect anemia.
3. Urine and serum analysis for the presence and quantity of abnormal immunoglobulin.
4. Skeletal x-rays—osteolytic bone lesions.

Management

1. Patients with "smoldering" multiple myeloma do not require treatment.
2. The NCCN guidelines for symptomatic multiple myeloma (www.nccn.org) and other clinical guidelines often recommend starting with triplet therapy, which includes:
   a. Immunomodulator or chemotherapy agent, or sometimes both.
   b. A targeted therapy agent that is designed to attack a specific feature of the cancer cell, such as a proteasome inhibitor, monoclonal antibody, or CAR T cell.
   c. A corticosteroid, such as dexamethasone.
3. Autologous bone marrow or peripheral blood stem cell transplant in selected cases (usually younger than age 65 with no renal failure, few bone lesions, and good organ function).
4. Supportive care options:
   a. Plasmapheresis to treat hyperviscosity or bleeding.
   b. Radiation therapy for bone lesions.
   c. Bisphosphonates (e.g., pamidronate), potent inhibitors of bone resorption, to treat hypercalcemia and alleviate bone pain.
   d. Allopurinol and fluids to treat hyperuricemia.
   e. Hemodialysis to manage renal failure.
   f. Surgical stabilization and fixation of fractures.

DRUG ALERT Pamidronate and other bisphosphonates may cause transient temperature elevations, hypophosphatemia, hypomagnesemia, hypocalcemia, and local reactions at the site of IV administration, such as thrombophlebitis, pain, and erythema. Bisphosphonates are administered as IV infusions, generally during 4 or more hours; rapid IV administration may cause renal failure. Long-term bisphosphonate use has been associated with jaw osteonecrosis—patients should be monitored closely and advised to maintain good oral health and avoid invasive dental procedures.

Complications

1. Pathologic fractures, spinal cord compression.
2. Recurrent infections, particularly bacterial.
3. Electrolyte abnormalities (hypercalcemia, hypophosphatemia).
4. Renal failure, pyelonephritis.
5. Bleeding.
6. Thromboembolic complications caused by hyperviscosity.
7. Patients with multiple myeloma treated by chemotherapy have a median survival of 2 to 3 years; the impact of newer treatment options on survival is still unknown.

Nursing Assessment

1. Obtain health history, focusing on pain, fatigue.
2. Evaluate for evidence of bone deformities and bone tenderness or pain.
3. Assess the patient's support system and personal coping skills.

Nursing Interventions

Controlling Pain

1. Assess for the presence, location, intensity, and characteristics of pain.
2. Administer pharmacologic agents, as ordered, to control pain. Use adequate doses of regularly scheduled, around-the-clock analgesics.
3. Teach the use of nonpharmacologic methods, such as music, relaxation breathing, progressive muscle relaxation, distraction, and imagery, to help manage pain.
4. Assess effectiveness of analgesics and adjust dosage or drug used, as necessary, to control pain.

Promoting Mobility

1. Encourage the patient to wear a back brace for lumbar lesion.
2. Recommend physical and occupational therapy consultation.
3. Discourage bed rest to prevent hypercalcemia but ensure safety of environment to prevent fractures.
4. Assist the patient with measures to prevent injury and decrease the risk of fractures. Advise avoidance of lifting and straining; use walker and other assistive devices, as appropriate.

Relieving Fear

1. Develop trusting, supportive relationship with the patient and their significant others.
2. Encourage the patient to discuss medical condition and prognosis with the health care provider when the patient is ready.
3. Assure the patient that you are available for support, to provide comfort measures and to answer questions.
4. Encourage the use of the patient's own support network, religious and community services, and national agencies.

Monitoring for Complications

1. Report sudden, severe pain, especially of the back, which could indicate pathologic fracture.
2. Provide assistance, safety precautions, and supervision to prevent injury.
3. Assess patient's home situation and availability of equipment to support reduced mobility and risk of fracture. Encourage the removal of throw rugs and clutter that might lead to falls.
4. Watch for nausea, drowsiness, confusion, polyuria, which could indicate hypercalcemia caused by bony destruction or immobilization. Monitor serum calcium levels.
5. Check results of blood urea nitrogen (BUN) and creatinine and urine protein tests to detect renal insufficiency, caused by nephrotoxicity of abnormal proteins in multiple myeloma.
6. Increase fluid intake, monitor intake and output, and weigh the patient daily.

Patient Education and Health Maintenance

1. Teach the patient about the risk of infection caused by impaired antibody production and chemotherapy (see page 85).
2. Teach the patient to take medications, as prescribed, and monitor for possible adverse effects; avoid aspirin and NSAIDs unless prescribed by health care provider because these drugs may interfere with platelet function.
3. Teach the patient to minimize the risk of fractures. Use proper body mechanics and assistive devices, as appropriate; avoid bed rest, remain ambulatory.
4. Advise the patient to report new onset of pain, new location, or sudden increase in pain intensity immediately. Report new onset or worsening of neurologic symptoms (e.g., changes in sensation) immediately.
5. Encourage the patient to maintain high fluid intake (2 to 3 L/day) to avoid dehydration and prevent renal insufficiency; also not to fast before diagnostic tests.
6. Provide the patient and family with information about resources in the community (see page 749).

Evaluation: Expected Outcomes

- States decreased pain.
- Ambulates without injury.
- Asks questions about disease; contacts support group.
- No development of complications.

BLEEDING DISORDERS

Bleeding disorders may be congenital or acquired and may be caused by dysfunction in any phase of hemostasis (clot formation and dissolution). Bleeding disorders seen in adults include thrombocytopenia, idiopathic thrombocytopenic purpura (ITP), disseminated intravascular coagulation (DIC), and von Willebrand disease.

Thrombocytopenia

Thrombocytopenia is characterized by a decreased platelet count (less than 150,000/mm^3), the most common cause of bleeding disorders.

Pathophysiology and Etiology

Classification by Etiology

1. Decreased platelet production—infiltrative diseases of bone marrow, leukemia, aplastic anemia, myelofibrosis, myelosuppressive therapy, and radiation therapy; may include inherited disorders, such as Fanconi anemia and Wiskott-Aldrich syndrome.
2. Increased platelet destruction—infection (e.g., human immunodeficiency virus [HIV] or hepatitis C), drug induced (e.g., heparin or quinidine), ITP, and DIC.
3. Abnormal distribution or sequestration in spleen.
4. Dilutional thrombocytopenia—after hemorrhage, red blood cell (RBC) transfusions.

Clinical Manifestations

1. Usually asymptomatic.
2. When platelet count drops below 20,000/mm^3:
   a. Petechiae occur spontaneously.
   b. Ecchymoses occur at sites of minor trauma (venipuncture, pressure).
   c. Bleeding may occur from mucosal surfaces, nose, gastrointestinal (GI) and genitourinary (GU) tracts, respiratory system, and within the central nervous system (CNS).
   d. Menorrhagia is common.
3. Excessive bleeding may occur after procedures (dental extractions, minor surgery, biopsies).
4. Thrombotic complications (arterial and venous) and areas of skin necrosis are associated with heparin-*induced thrombocytopenia.*

Diagnostic Evaluation

1. Complete blood count (CBC) with platelet count—decreased hemoglobin, hematocrit, platelets.
2. Bleeding time, prothrombin time (PT), partial thromboplastin time (PTT)—prolonged.
3. Platelet aggregation test for heparin-dependent platelet antibodies—positive.

Management

1. Treat underlying cause.
2. Platelet transfusions.
3. Steroids or intravenous (IV) immunoglobulins may be helpful in selected patients.
4. Heparin-induced thrombocytopenia: Discontinue heparin, use alternate anticoagulant therapy because of high risk of venous

and arterial thromboses in these patients (direct thrombin inhibitors, such as lepirudin or argatroban hirudin), and avoid platelet transfusions. Although incidence varies dependent upon patient population and heparin preparation, any exposure to heparin can precipitate this serious autoimmune syndrome.

Complications

Severe blood loss or bleeding into vital organs may be life-threatening.

Nursing Assessment

1. Obtain health history, focusing on prior illnesses and episodes of bleeding, past surgical experiences, exposure to toxins or ionizing radiation, and family history of bleeding.
2. Obtain list of current and recent medications (including over-the-counter [OTC] preparations, herbal and dietary supplements).
3. Perform complete physical examination for signs of bleeding.

Nursing Interventions

Minimizing Bleeding

1. Institute bleeding precautions.
   a. Avoid the use of plain razor, hard toothbrush or floss, intramuscular (IM) injections, tourniquets, rectal procedures, and suppositories.
   b. Administer stool softeners, as necessary, to prevent constipation.
   c. Restrict activity and exercise when platelet count is less than 20,000/mm^3 or when active bleeding occurs.
2. Monitor pad count and amount of saturation during menses; administer or teach self-administration of hormones to suppress menstruation, as prescribed.
3. Administer blood products, as ordered. Monitor for signs and symptoms of allergic reactions, anaphylaxis, and volume overload.
4. Evaluate urine, stools, and emesis for gross and occult blood.

Patient Education and Health Maintenance

1. Teach the patient bleeding precautions (see page 746).
2. Demonstrate the use of direct, steady pressure at bleeding site if bleeding develops.
3. Encourage routine follow-up for platelet counts.

Evaluation: Expected Outcomes

- Episodes of bleeding rapidly controlled; platelet count maintained at goal (usually 20,000/mm^3).

Idiopathic Thrombocytopenic Purpura

ITP is an acute or chronic bleeding disorder that results from immune destruction of platelets by antiplatelet antibodies.

Pathophysiology and Etiology

1. Proteins on the platelet cell membrane stimulate production of autoantibodies that bind to circulating platelets, leading to destruction of platelets in spleen and liver.
2. Acute disorder more common in childhood, typically following viral illness; has good prognosis, with 80% to 90% recovering uneventfully within 6 months.
3. Chronic disorder (more than 6-month course) most common between ages 20 and 50 years, three times more common in females, may last for years or even indefinitely. May be associated with pregnancy or with development of systemic lupus erythematosus, thyroid disease, and infections (e.g., *Helicobacter pylori*, cytomegalovirus, varicella zoster, hepatitis C, and HIV) or malignancy (e.g., chronic lymphocytic leukemia [CLL]).

Clinical Manifestations

1. Mild disease (platelet counts 30,000 to 100,000/mm^3): may have no signs and symptoms.
2. Moderate-to-severe disease (platelet counts less than 30,000/mm^3): often symptomatic, including bruising, petechiae, bleeding from nares and gums, and menorrhagia.

Diagnostic Evaluation

1. CBC demonstrates platelet count less than 100,000/mm^3; may also be lymphocytosis and eosinophilia.
2. Testing for hepatitis C, HIV, *H. pylori*, and Epstein–Barr virus, which have been found to be associated with ITP.
3. Bone marrow aspirate (not necessary for most patients with typical features of ITP) shows increased numbers of young megakaryocytes, sometimes increased numbers of eosinophils.
4. Assay for platelet autoantibodies sometimes helpful.
5. Bleeding times are typically normal.

Management

1. Supportive care: judicious use of platelet transfusions, control of bleeding.
2. High-dose corticosteroids, IV immunoglobulins, and parenteral anti-D (for Rhesus-positive patients with spleens). Thrombopoietin receptor agonists may be used to treat patients at risk for bleeding with chronic or relapsed ITP.
3. Splenectomy (see page 741) removes potential site for sequestration and destruction of platelets and is used to treat chronic refractory ITP in adults.

Complications

Severe blood loss or bleeding into vital organs may be life-threatening.

Nursing Assessment

1. Obtain a history of bleeding episodes, including bruising and petechiae, bleeding of gums, and heavy menses.
2. Perform physical examination for signs of bleeding.

Nursing Interventions

Minimizing Bleeding

1. Institute bleeding precautions.
2. Monitor pad count and amount of saturation during menses; administer or teach self-administration of hormones to suppress menstruation, as prescribed.
3. Administer blood products, as ordered. Monitor for signs and symptoms of allergic reactions, anaphylaxis, and volume overload.
4. Evaluate all urine and stools for gross and occult blood.

Patient Education and Health Maintenance

1. Teach the patient bleeding precautions (see page 746).
2. Demonstrate the use of direct, steady pressure at bleeding site if bleeding does develop.
3. Encourage routine follow-up for platelet counts.

Evaluation: Expected Outcomes

- Episodes of bleeding rapidly controlled.

Disseminated Intravascular Coagulation

DIC is an acquired thrombotic and hemorrhagic syndrome characterized by abnormal activation of the clotting cascade and accelerated fibrinolysis. This results in widespread clotting in small vessels with consumption of clotting factors and platelets so that bleeding and thrombosis occur simultaneously.

Pathophysiology and Etiology

1. A syndrome arising secondary to an underlying disorder or event.
   a. Overwhelming infections, particularly bacterial sepsis.
   b. Obstetric complications: abruptio placentae, eclampsia, amniotic fluid embolism, retention of dead fetus.
   c. Massive tissue injury: burns, trauma, fractures, major surgery, fat embolism, organ destruction (e.g., severe pancreatitis, hepatic failure).
   d. Malignancy: particularly lung, colon, stomach, and pancreas.
   e. Vascular and circulatory collapse, shock.
   f. Severe toxic or immunologic reactions: hemolytic transfusion reaction, snake bites, recreational drugs.

Clinical Manifestations

1. Signs of abnormal clotting:
   a. Coolness and mottling of extremities.
   b. Acrocyanosis (cold, mottled extremities with clear demarcation from normal tissue).
   c. Dyspnea, adventitious breath sounds.
   d. Altered mental status.
   e. Acute renal failure.
   f. Pain (e.g., related to bowel infarction).
2. Signs of abnormal bleeding:
   a. Oozing, bleeding from sites of procedures, IV catheter insertion sites, suture lines, mucous membranes, and orifices.
   b. Internal bleeding leading to changes in vital organ function, altered vital signs.

Diagnostic Evaluation

1. Platelet count—diminished.
2. PT, PTT, and thrombin time—prolonged.
3. Fibrinogen—decreased level.
4. Fibrin split (degradation) products—increased level.
5. D-Dimer fibrin degradation product—increased level.
6. Antithrombin III—decreased level.
7. Protein C—decreased level.

Management

1. Treat underlying disorder.
2. Replacement therapy for serious hemorrhagic manifestations:
   a. Fresh frozen plasma replaces clotting factors.
   b. Platelet transfusions.
   c. Cryoprecipitate replaces clotting factors and fibrinogen.
3. Supportive measures including fluid replacement, oxygenation, maintenance of blood pressure (BP), and renal perfusion.
4. Heparin or other anticoagulant therapy (controversial) inhibits clotting component of DIC.

Complications

1. Thromboembolic: pulmonary embolism; cerebral, myocardial, splenic, or bowel infarction; acute renal failure; tissue necrosis or gangrene.
2. Hemorrhagic: Cerebral hemorrhage is the most common cause of death in DIC.

Nursing Assessment

1. Be aware that seriously ill patients are at risk; monitor condition closely.
2. Assess for signs of bleeding and thrombosis, including chest pain, shortness of breath, hematuria, abdominal pain, headache, and numbness and coolness of an extremity.

Nursing Interventions

Minimizing Bleeding

1. Institute bleeding precautions.
2. Monitor pad count and amount of saturation during menses; administer or teach self-administration of hormones to suppress menstruation, as prescribed.
3. Administer blood products, as ordered. Monitor for signs and symptoms of allergic reactions, anaphylaxis, and volume overload.
4. Avoid dislodging clots. Apply pressure to sites of bleeding for at least 20 minutes, use topical hemostatic agents. Use tape cautiously.
5. Maintain bed rest during bleeding episode.
6. If internal bleeding is suspected, assess bowel sounds and abdominal girth.
7. Evaluate fluid status and bleeding by frequent measurement of vital signs, central venous pressure, intake, and output.

Promoting Tissue Perfusion

1. Keep the patient warm.
2. Avoid vasoconstrictive agents (systemic or topical).
3. Change the patient's position frequently and perform range of motion exercises.
4. Monitor electrocardiogram and laboratory tests for dysfunction of vital organs caused by ischemia—arrhythmias, abnormal arterial blood gas levels, and increased BUN and creatinine levels.
5. Monitor for signs of vascular occlusion and report immediately.
   a. Brain—decreased level of consciousness (LOC), sensory and motor deficits, seizures, and coma.
   b. Eyes—visual deficits.
   c. Bone—bone pain.
   d. Pulmonary vasculature—chest pain, shortness of breath, tachycardia.
   e. Extremities—cold, mottling, numbness.
   f. Coronary arteries—chest pain, arrhythmias.
   g. Bowel—pain, tenderness, decreased bowel sounds.

Patient Education and Health Maintenance

Explain the syndrome and its management to the patient and family members as part of reassurance and support during this critical illness.

Evaluation: Expected Outcomes

- Episodes of bleeding rapidly controlled.
- Alert, vital signs stable, urine output adequate, and no complaints of chest pain or shortness of breath.

von Willebrand Disease

von Willebrand disease is an inherited (autosomal dominant) or acquired bleeding disorder characterized by decreased level of von Willebrand factor and prolonged bleeding time.

Pathophysiology and Etiology

1. von Willebrand factor synthesized in vascular endothelium, megakaryocytes, and platelets; enhances platelet adhesion as first step in clot formation, also acts as carrier of factor VIII in blood.
2. von Willebrand is the most common inherited bleeding disorder, with estimated incidence of 1% of population in United States; includes multiple subtypes with varying severity; affects all genders.
3. Acquired form is rare, generally appears late in life, typically in association with lymphoma, leukemia, multiple myeloma, or autoimmune disorder.

Clinical Manifestations

1. Mucosal and cutaneous bleeding (e.g., bruising, gingival bleeding, epistaxis, menorrhagia).
2. Prolonged bleeding from cuts or after dental and surgical procedures.

Diagnostic Evaluation

1. Bleeding time—prolonged.
2. Ristocetin cofactor—abnormal.
3. von Willebrand factor—decreased.
4. von Willebrand factor multimers—demonstrate defective von Willebrand factor in some types.
5. Factor VIII—generally decreased.

Management

1. Replacement of von Willebrand factor and factor VIII using clotting factor concentrates.
2. Antifibrinolytic medications (aminocaproic acid, tranexamic acid) to stabilize clot formation before dental procedures and before minor surgery.
3. Desmopressin acetate, a synthetic analog of vasopressin, may be used to manage mild-to-moderate bleeding.
4. Estrogen and progesterone stimulate production of von Willebrand factor and factor VIII and may be particularly helpful in control of menorrhagia.

Complications

Severe blood loss or bleeding into vital organs may be life-threatening.

Nursing Assessment

1. Obtain a history of bleeding episodes, such as menstrual flow. Ask quantitative questions (e.g., how many nosebleeds do you have each year?) as the patient may not realize their experience is abnormal.
2. Perform physical examination for signs of bleeding.

Nursing Interventions

Minimizing Bleeding

1. Institute bleeding precautions:
   a. Avoid the use of plain razor, hard toothbrush, or floss.
   b. Avoid IM injections, tourniquets, rectal procedures, or suppositories.
   c. Administer stool softeners, as necessary, to prevent constipation.
   d. Restrict activity and exercise when platelet count less than 20,000/mm^3 or when active bleeding occurs.
2. Monitor pad count and amount of saturation during menses; administer or teach self-administration of hormones to suppress menstruation, as prescribed.
3. Administer blood products, as ordered. Monitor for signs and symptoms of allergic reactions, anaphylaxis, and volume overload.
4. Use topical hemostatic agents, such as absorbable gelatin, oxidized cellulose, topical adrenaline, or phenylephrine, if pressure and use of ice do not stop bleeding.

Patient Education and Health Maintenance

1. Teach the patient bleeding precautions (see page 746).
2. Demonstrate the use of direct, steady pressure at bleeding site if bleeding develops.

Evaluation: Expected Outcomes

- Episodes of bleeding rapidly controlled.

SELECTED READINGS

Alzanad, F., Feyaza, M., & Chapanduka, Z. C. (2022). A study of patient-reported pain during bone marrow aspiration and biopsy using local anesthesia alone compared with local anesthesia with intravenous midazolam coadministration at a tertiary academic hospital in South Africa. *Health Science Reports, 5*(6), e902. https://doi.org/10.1002/hsr2.902

Bradbury, J., & Bell, J. (2024). The TTP specialist nurse: An advocate for patients and professionals. *British Journal of Nursing, 33*(6), 284–290. https://doi.org/10.12968/bjon.2024.33.6.284

Bussel, J. B., & Garcia, C. A. (2022). Diagnosis of immune thrombocytopenia, including secondary forms, and selection of second-line treatment. *Haematologica, 107*(9), 2018–2036. https://doi.org/10.3324/haematol.2021.279513

Camejo, L., Nandeesha, N., Phan, K., Chharath, K., Tran, T., Ciesla, D. J., & Velanovich, V. (2022). Infectious outcomes after splenectomy for trauma, splenectomy for disease and splenectomy with distal pancreatectomy. *Langenbeck's Archives of Surgery, 407*(4), 1685–1691. https://doi.org/10.1007/s00423-022-02446-3

Giudice, V., & Selleri, C. (2022). Aplastic anemia: Pathophysiology. *Seminars in Hematology, 59*(1), 13–20. https://doi.org/10.1053/j.seminhematol.2021.12.002

Jolles, S., Giralt, S., Kerre, T., Lazarus, H. M., Mustafa, S. S., Ria, R., & Vinh, D. C. (2023). Agents contributing to secondary immunodeficiency development in patients with multiple myeloma, chronic lymphocytic leukemia and non-Hodgkin lymphoma: A systematic literature review. *Frontiers in Oncology, 13*, 1098326. https://doi.org/10.3389/fonc.2023.1098326

Kalot, M. A., Husainat, N., Alayli, A. E., Abughanimeh, O., Diab, O., Tayiem, S., Madoukh, B., Dimassi, A. B., Qureini, A., Ameer, B., Eikenboom, J., Giraud, N., McLintock, C., McRae, S., Montgomery, R. R., O'Donnell, J. S., Scappe, N., Sidonio, R. F., Brignardello-Petersen, R., … Mustafa, R. A. (2022). von

Willebrand factor levels in the diagnosis of von Willebrand disease: A systematic review and meta-analysis. *Blood Advances, 6*(1), 62–71. https://doi.org/10.1182/bloodadvances.2021005430

Luo, X., Zhang, Y., & Chen, Q. (2022). Nursing care plan and management of patients with acute leukemia. *Alternative Therapies in Health & Medicine, 28*(1), 80–85. http://alternative-therapies.com/oa/6996.html

Majeed, H. (2022, September 14). Adverse effects of radiation therapy. In *StatPearls* [Internet]. StatPearls Publishing. https://www.ncbi.nlm.nih.gov/books/NBK563259/

Ogbue, O. D., Bahaj, W., Kewan, T., Ahmed, R., Dima, D., Willimas, N., ... & Maciejewski, J. P. (2024). Splenectomy outcomes in immune cytopenias: Treatment outcomes and determinants of response. *Journal of Internal Medicine, 295*(2), 229–241. https://doi.org/10.1111/joim.13742

Pedersen, M., Engedal, M. S., Tolver, A., Larsen, M. T., Kornblit, B. T., Lomborg, K., & Jarden, M. (2024). Effect of non-pharmacological interventions on symptoms and quality of life in patients with hematological malignancies–a systematic review. *Critical Reviews in Oncology/Hematology,* 104327. https://doi.org/10.1016/j.critrevonc.2024.104327

Popescu, N. I., Lupu, C., & Lupu, F. (2022). Disseminated intravascular coagulation and its immune mechanisms. *Blood, 139*(13), 1973–1986. https://doi.org/10.1182/blood.2020007208

Pourhassan, H., Kareem, W., Agrawal, V., & Aldoss, I. (2024). Important considerations in the intensive care management of acute leukemias. *Journal of Intensive Care Medicine, 39*(4), 291–305. https://doi.org/10.1177/08850666231193955

Rodríguez, M. F. (2022). Diagnosing rare bleeding disorders. *Blood Coagulation & Fibrinolysis, 33*(Suppl 1), S15–S16. https://doi.org/10.1097/mbc.0000000000001092

Rogez, J., Urbanski, G., Vinatier, E., Lavigne, C., Emmanuel, L., Dupin, I., ... & Lacombe, V. (2024). Iron deficiency in pernicious anemia: Specific features of iron deficient patients and preliminary data on response to iron supplementation. *Clinical Nutrition.* https://doi.org/10.7759/cureus.57901

Sarbaz, M., Monazah, F. M., Eslami, S., Kimiafar, K., & Baigi, S. F. M. (2022). Effect of mobile health interventions for side effects management in patients undergoing chemotherapy: A systematic review. *Health Policy and Technology, 11*(4), 100680. https://doi.org/10.1016/j.hlpt.2022.100680

Senapati, J., Jabbour, E., Kantarjian, H., & Short, N. J. (2022). Pathogenesis and management of accelerated and blast phases of chronic myeloid leukemia. *Leukemia, 37*(1), 5–17. https://doi.org/10.1038/s41375-022-01736-5

Shi, Y., Cheng, C., Huang, Y., Xu, Y., Xu, D., Shen, H., Ye, X., Jin, J., Tong, H., Yu, Y., Tang, X., Li, A., Cui, D., & Xie, W. (2022). Global disease burden and trends of leukemia attributable to occupational risk from 1990 to 2019: An observational trend study. *Frontiers in Public Health, 10.* https://doi.org/10.3389/fpubh.2022.1015861

Shi, X., Zhuo, H., Du, Y., Nyhan, K., Ioannidis, J. P. A., & Wallach, J. D. (2022). Environmental risk factors for non-Hodgkin's lymphoma: Umbrella review and comparison of meta-analyses of summary and individual participant data. *BMJ Medicine, 1*(1), e000184. https://doi.org/10.1136/bmjmed-2022-000184

Silver, R., & Abu-Zeinah, G. (2023). Polycythemia vera: Aspects of its current diagnosis and initial treatment. *Expert Review of Hematology, 16*(4), 253–266. https://doi.org/10.1080/17474086.2023.2198698

Sindone, A., Doehner, W., Manito, N., McDonagh, T., Cohen-Solal, A., Damy, T., Núñez, J., Pfister, O., Van Der Meer, P., & Comín-Colet, J. (2022). Practical guidance for diagnosing and treating iron deficiency in patients with heart failure: Why, who and how? *Journal of Clinical Medicine, 11*(11), 2976. https://doi.org/10.3390/jcm11112976

Singh, D., Vaccarella, S., Gini, A., De Paula Silva, N., Steliarova-Foucher, E., & Bray, F. (2022). Global patterns of Hodgkin lymphoma incidence and mortality in 2020 and a prediction of the future burden in 2040. *International Journal of Cancer, 150*(12), 1941–1947. https://doi.org/10.1002/ijc.33948

Skolmowska, D., Głąbska, D., Kołota, A., & Guzek, D. (2022). Effectiveness of dietary interventions to treat iron-deficiency anemia in women: A systematic review of randomized controlled trials. *Nutrients, 14*(13), 2724. https://doi.org/10.3390/nu14132724

Slater, S. J., Lukies, M., Kavnoudias, H., Zia, A., Lee, R. S., Bosco, J. J., Joseph, T., & Clements, W. (2021). Immune function and the role of vaccination after splenic artery embolization for blunt splenic injury. *Injury—International Journal of the Care of the Injured, 53*(1), 112–115. https://doi.org/10.1016/j.injury.2021.09.020

Stemler, J., De Jonge, N. A., Skoetz, N., Sinkó, J., Brüggemann, R. J. M., Busca, A., Ben-Ami, R., Ráčil, Z., Piechotta, V., Lewis, R. E., & Cornely, O. A. (2022). Antifungal prophylaxis in adult patients with acute myeloid leukaemia treated with novel targeted therapies: A systematic review and expert consensus recommendation from the European Hematology Association. *The Lancet Haematology, 9*(5), e361–e373. https://doi.org/10.1016/s2352-3026(22)00073-4

Wacka, E., Nicikowski, J., Jarmuzek, P., & Zembron-Lacny, A. (2024). Anemia and its connections to inflammation in older adults: A review. *Journal of Clinical Medicine, 13*(7), 2049. https://doi.org/10.3390/jcm13072049

23

Transfusion Therapy and Blood and Marrow Stem Cell Transplantation

TRANSFUSION THERAPY

See additional online content: Procedure Guidelines 23-1

Principles of Transfusion Therapy

Because of the potentially life-threatening consequences of blood type ABO incompatibility and disease transmission through blood products, transfusion therapy is limited to occasions when it is absolutely necessary, and stringent screening techniques are required before transfusion begins. Alternatives to transfusion therapy should also be considered, as appropriate, such as erythropoietin-stimulating agents, iron supplementation, blood loss prevention during surgery, and volume replacement with other solutions. Blood product procurement, storage, preparation, and testing are regulated by the Food and Drug Administration (FDA), the American Association of Blood Banks, and The Joint Commission.

Blood Compatibility

Antigens

1. The surface membrane of the red blood cell (RBC) is characterized by glycoproteins known as antigens.
2. More than 700 different antigens have been identified on the RBC membrane.
3. There are fewer than a dozen clinically significant antigens, and of these, only two antigenic systems (ABO and Rh) require routine prospective matching before the transfusion.
4. The ABO blood group system is clinically the most significant because A and B antigens elicit the strongest immune response.
5. The presence or absence of A and B antigens on the RBC membrane determines the person's ABO group (see Table 23-1). The ability to make A or B antigens is inherited.
6. Antibody formation without specific exposure to the antigen is unique to the ABO system. Antibody directed against the missing antigens is produced in neonates by 3 months of age.

Antibodies

1. Antibodies (or immunoglobulins) are proteins produced by B lymphocytes; they consist of two light and two heavy chains that form a Y shape.
2. Antibodies generally have a high degree of specificity and interact only with the antigen that stimulated their production.
3. The five classes of immunoglobulins are determined by differences in their heavy chains: immunoglobulins (Ig) G, IgA, IgM, IgD, and IgE.
4. The interaction of antibodies and antigens triggers the humoral immune response.
5. Antibodies against the A and B antigens are large IgM molecules. When they interact with and coat the A and B antigens on the RBC surface, the antibody/RBC complexes clump together (agglutinate).
6. Antibody/RBC complexes also activate the complement cascade, resulting in the release of numerous active substances and RBC lysis. The large antibody/RBC complexes also become trapped in capillaries, where they may cause thrombotic complications to vital organs, and in the reticuloendothelial system, where they are removed from circulation by the spleen.
7. The extent of the humoral response elicited by anti-A and anti-B interaction with A and B antigens depends on the quantity of antibody and antigen.

Other RBC Antigens

1. Non-ABO RBC antigen–antibody reactions usually do not produce powerful immediate hemolytic reactions, but several have clinical significance.
2. After A and B, D is the most immunogenic antigen. It is part of the rhesus system, which includes C, D, and E antigens.

Table 23-1 Blood Group Antigens and Antibodies of ABO System

BLOOD GROUP	ANTIGEN ON RBC	ANTIBODY IN PLASMA	APPROXIMATE FREQUENCY OF OCCURRENCE IN THE POPULATION (%)
A	A	Anti-B	45
B	B	Anti-A	8
AB	A and B	None	3
O	None	Anti-A and anti-B	44

a. D (Rh)-negative people do not develop anti-D without specific exposure, but have a high incidence of antibody development (alloimmunization) after exposure to D.
b. Two common methods of sensitization to these RBC antigens are by transfusion or fetomaternal hemorrhage during pregnancy and delivery.
c. Anti-D can complicate future transfusions and pregnancies. For the D (Rh)-negative person, exposure to D should be avoided by the use of Rh-negative blood products. In the case of Rh-negative biologic mother and Rh-positive fetus, Rh immunoglobulin (RhoGAM) is used as prophylaxis for exposure to D, preventing anti-D formation.
d. Exposure to RBC antigens from other antigenic systems (such as Lewis, Kidd, or Duffy) may also cause alloimmunization, which becomes clinically significant in people who receive multiple blood products for extended periods of time.

Blood Transfusion Options

Autologous Transfusion

1. Before elective procedures, the patient may donate blood to be set aside for later transfusion. Patients may donate up to 3 days prior to surgery, provided hemoglobin is greater than 11 g/dL.
2. Autologous RBCs can also be salvaged during some surgical procedures or after trauma-induced hemorrhage by use of automated cell-saver devices or by manual suction equipment.
3. Autologous blood products must be clearly labeled and identified.
4. Autologous transfusion eliminates the risks of alloimmunization, immune-mediated transfusion reactions, and transmission of disease, making it the safest transfusion choice.
5. Patients who do not meet standard criteria for blood donation may still be eligible for autologous blood donation before elective surgery.

Homologous Transfusion

1. With this most common option, volunteer donor blood products are assigned to patients randomly.
2. Before donation, volunteer donors receive information about the process, potential adverse effects, tests that will be performed on donated blood, postdonation instructions, and education regarding the risk of human immunodeficiency virus (HIV) infection and signs and symptoms.
3. Donors are screened against eligibility criteria designed to protect donor and recipient (see Table 23-2).

Table 23-2 General Blood Donor Eligibility Criteria

Age	≥17 yr *or* 16 yr with guardian consent if state law allows.
Weight	Minimum 110 lb (49.9 kg) (additional rules apply for donors ≤18 yr).
Vital signs	Afebrile, normotensive, pulse 50–100, blood pressure <180/100 mm Hg.
Hemoglobin	≥12.5 g/dL.
History	Travel, exposures, and past illnesses or events may defer or disallow blood donation. *Examples*: travel to malarial areas, living in areas exposed to bovine spongiform encephalopathy, blood transfusion or tattoo within 12 mo, recent surgery or pregnancy, corneal transplant, history of hepatitis or unexplained jaundice, history of blood cancer or recent cancer, history of behaviors at high risk for human immunodeficiency virus.
Immunizations	Recent attenuated and live vaccines generally result in deferral.
Illnesses	A variety of current illnesses may defer or disallow blood donation. *Examples*: clotting disorders, sickle cell disease, systemic lupus erythematosus, multiple sclerosis, Lyme disease, tuberculosis, chronic fatigue syndrome.
Medications	Blood thinners, such as heparin and warfarin, disallow donation. Some other medications may result in deferral.

EVIDENCE BASE American Red Cross. (2023). *Whole blood donation: Eligibility requirements.* https://www.redcrossblood.org/donate-blood/how-to-donate/types-of-blood-donations/whole-blood-donation.html

Directed Transfusion

1. In directed transfusion, blood products are donated by a person for transfusion to a specified recipient with a compatible blood type.
2. This option may be used in certain circumstances (e.g., a biologic parent who provides sole transfusion support for a child), but in general, no evidence exists that directed donation reduces transfusion risks.

Blood Product Screening

Serologic Testing

1. Routine laboratory testing is performed to assess the compatibility of a particular blood product with the recipient before release of the blood product from the blood bank (see Table 23-3).
   a. ABO group and Rh type: determines the presence of A, B, and D antigens on the surface of the patient's RBCs.
   b. Direct Coombs test: determines the antibody attached to the patient's RBCs.
   c. Crossmatch (compatibility test): detects agglutination of donor RBCs caused by antibodies in the patient's serum.
   d. Indirect Coombs test: identifies lower molecular weight antibodies (IgG) directed against blood group antigens.

Table 23-3 ABO and Rh Compatibility Chart

This chart identifies ABO and Rh compatibility when transfusing whole blood, red blood cells, and plasma. Components suspended in plasma, such as platelets and cryoprecipitate, usually follow plasma compatibility rules if the total volume exceeds 120 mL for an adult patient.

WHOLE BLOOD

	Donor					
Recipient	**A**	**B**	**O**	**AB**	**Rh positive**	**Rh negative**
A	✓					
B		✓				
O			✓			
AB				✓		
Rh positive					✓	✓
Rh negative						✓

RED BLOOD CELLS

	Donor					
Recipient	**A**	**B**	**O**	**AB**	**Rh positive**	**Rh negative**
A	✓		✓			
B		✓	✓			
O			✓	✓		
AB	✓	✓	✓			
Rh positive					✓	✓
Rh negative						✓

PLASMA

	Donor					
Recipient	**A**	**B**	**O**	**AB**	**Rh positive**	**Rh negative**
A	✓			✓		
B		✓		✓		
O	✓	✓	✓	✓		
AB				✓		
Rh positive					✓	✓
Rh negative					✓	✓

Screening for Infectious Diseases

1. Routine laboratory testing is performed to identify antigens or antibodies in donor blood that may indicate prior exposure to specific blood-borne diseases.
2. Such testing supplements other principles of donation designed to decrease the risk of disease transmission via blood products, including the use of volunteer donors, the exclusion of high-risk populations, and the screening of donors via health and social history.
3. Through the use of donor screening and blood testing, the risk of infections transmitted with donated blood is less than 1% and continues to decline.
4. Specific conditions screened for include:
   a. Hepatitis: Per FDA recommendations, each unit of blood is tested for the presence of hepatitis B core antibody, surface antigen, and more recently hepatitis B viral DNA through nucleic acid testing (NAT). Hepatitis C antibody and viral DNA tests (NAT) are also completed.
   b. HIV-1 and HIV-2: tests for prior exposure to the virus.
      i. All blood products in the United States have been screened since the test first became available in 1985. Current tests include testing for antibodies with enzyme-linked immunosorbent assay or enzyme immunoassay or antigen with the P24 test. NAT is becoming more widely used and provides a mechanism to look for the presence of HIV-1 and HIV-2 before antibody formation.
      ii. Because antibody to the virus is not produced until at least 6 weeks after exposure, diligent donor screening and exclusion of high-risk groups remains an important part of preventing transmission of HIV via blood products.
      iii. A low risk of HIV transmission (estimated to be 1/1,467,000) remains.
   c. Cytomegalovirus (CMV): tests for the antibody against CMV.
      i. Approximately 50% to 75% of blood donors have been exposed to CMV, and 10% to 20% carry CMV in their white blood cells (WBCs).
      ii. Patients with impaired immune function (e.g., bone marrow and organ transplant recipients, premature babies) are at risk for CMV infection from transfused blood. It is recommended that these patients receive CMV-seronegative blood or leukoreduced products.
   d. Syphilis: tests for the presence of antibody against the spirochete.
   e. Bacteria: contamination of blood products with bacteria may occur during and after collection of blood. This risk is managed by adherence to sterile technique during phlebotomy and blood-processing procedures, correct storage techniques, visual inspection of blood products, and limitations on shelf life.
   f. Other infections that may be transmitted via blood transfusions include West Nile virus, human T-cell lymphoma virus (HTLV) 1 and 2, human herpesvirus 8 (implicated as the causative agent of Kaposi sarcoma), malaria, babesiosis, Chagas disease, and *Yersinia*. Variant Creutzfeldt–Jakob disease has also been transmitted via blood transfusions, which has led to restrictions on donation by individuals who have lived in areas with bovine spongiform encephalopathy or "mad cow" disease.

Administration of Whole Blood and Blood Components

Whole blood and blood components are administered to increase the amount of oxygen being delivered to the tissues and organs, to prevent or stop bleeding because of platelet defects or because of deficiencies or coagulation abnormalities, and to combat infection caused by decreased or defective WBCs or antibodies. See Standards of Care Guidelines 23-1, page 4.

General Considerations

1. A unit of whole blood is usually separated into its various components shortly after collection.
2. The use of blood components conserves the limited supply of blood, provides optimal therapeutic benefit, and reduces the risk of circulatory overload. Less than 3% of the blood collected nationwide is transfused as whole blood.

STANDARDS OF CARE GUIDELINES 23-1

Blood Transfusion

When administering whole blood or blood components, ensure the following:

- Follow up on results of complete blood count (CBC) and report to health care provider so appropriate blood product can be ordered based on patient's condition.
- Verify informed consent.
- Contact the blood bank with health care provider's order and ensure timely delivery of blood product.
- Establish a patent intravenous (IV) line with compatible IV fluid.
- Use appropriate administration setup, filter, warmer, etc.
- Obtain baseline vital signs.
- Ensure proper blood product is given to the right patient by verifying at least two identifiers (e.g., full name and date of birth) with patient, blood product, and original order.
- Transfuse at a prescribed rate during the prescribed time, as tolerated by patient.
- Observe for acute reactions—allergic, febrile, septic, hemolytic, air embolism, and circulatory overload—by assessing vital signs, breath sounds, edema, flushing, urticaria, vomiting, headache, and back pain.
- Stop transfusion and notify patient's health care provider or available house officer if signs of reaction or other abnormalities occur.
- Be aware of delayed reactions and educate the patient on risk and what to look for: hemolytic, iron overload, graft-versus-host disease, hepatitis, and other infectious diseases.

This information should serve as a general guideline only. Each patient situation presents a unique set of clinical factors and requires nursing judgment to guide care, which may include additional or alternative measures and approaches.

3. Because of the risks, blood components should be administered only with informed consent, meticulous identification procedures, careful protocol, and close monitoring.
4. Crystalloid solutions other than 0.9% saline and all medications are *incompatible* with blood products. Because they may cause agglutination or hemolysis, they are not to be used during transfusions.

CLINICAL JUDGMENT Observe the patient closely and check vital signs at least hourly until 1 hour after transfusion. Observe for fever, chills, flushing, urticaria, difficulty breathing, anxiety, and change in vital signs. Stop transfusion and report signs of adverse effect to health care provider immediately if acute reaction is suspected.

Whole Blood

Description

1. Consists of RBCs, plasma, plasma proteins, and approximately 60-mL anticoagulant/preservative solution in a total volume of approximately 500 mL.
2. Indications include acute, massive blood loss of greater than 1,000 mL, requiring the oxygen-carrying properties of RBCs and the volume expansion provided by plasma. In general, even acute loss of as much as one third of a patient's total blood volume (1,000 to 1,200 mL) can be safely and rapidly replaced with crystalline or colloidal solutions.

Nursing and Patient Care Considerations

1. For rapid infusions of large volumes of whole blood, additional steps may be taken to deliver the product rapidly and safely.
   a. A small-pore (20 to 40 mm) filter may be used to remove microaggregates (platelets, WBCs) that have been identified in the lungs of patients who are massively transfused.
   b. An approved blood warmer may be indicated to prevent hypothermia and cardiac arrhythmias associated with the rapid infusion of refrigerated solutions.
   c. Electromechanical infusion devices to deliver blood at high flow rates can hemolyze RBCs and should be used with caution.
2. Observe closely for the most common acute complication associated with whole blood transfusion—circulatory overload (rise in venous pressure, distended neck veins, dyspnea, cough, crackles at the bases of lungs).

Packed RBCs

Description

1. Consist primarily of RBCs, a small amount of plasma, and approximately 100-mL anticoagulant/preservative solution in a total volume of approximately 250 to 300 mL/unit.
2. Packed RBCs may be contaminated with WBCs that may increase the risk of minor transfusion reactions and alloimmunization. For patients who receive multiple blood products during a specific period (e.g., patients with leukemia or aplastic anemia), packed RBCs may be further manipulated to remove WBCs (leukoreduced) by washing or freezing the product in the blood bank or by the use of small-pore (20 to 40 mm) leukoreduction filters during administration.
3. Indications include restoration or maintenance of adequate organ oxygenation with minimal expansion of blood volume.
4. Dosage: average adult dose administered is two units; pediatric doses are generally calculated as 5 to 15 mL/kg.

Nursing and Patient Care Considerations

1. Infuse at the prescribed rate. Generally, a unit can be given to an adult in 90 to 120 minutes. Pediatric patients are usually transfused at a rate of 2 to 5 mL/kg/h.
2. To reduce the risk of bacterial contamination and sepsis, RBCs must be transfused within 4 hours of leaving the blood bank.
3. Observe closely (particularly during the first 15 to 30 minutes) for the most common acute complications associated with packed RBCs, allergic and febrile transfusion reactions. Signs and symptoms of the more serious, but rare, hemolytic transfusion reactions are usually manifested during infusion of the first 50 mL.

Platelet Concentrates

Description

1. Consist of platelets suspended in plasma. Products vary according to the number of units (each unit is a minimum of 5.5×10^{10} platelets) and the volume of plasma (50 to 400 mL).

2. Platelets may be obtained by centrifuging multiple units of whole blood and expressing off the platelet-rich plasma (multiple-donor platelets) or from a single volunteer platelet donor using automated cell separation techniques (apheresis). The use of single-donor products decreases the number of donor exposures, thus decreasing the risk of alloimmunization and transfusion-transmitted disease.
3. Patients may become alloimmunized to human leukocyte antigens (HLAs) through exposure to multiple platelet products. When this occurs, apheresis products from HLA-matched platelet donors may be necessary. However, HLA-matched transfusions are commonly difficult to obtain because of the vast number of possible HLA combinations among the human population.
4. Indications include prevention or resolution of hemorrhage in patients with thrombocytopenia or platelet dysfunction.
5. Platelet transfusions are generally contraindicated in heparin-induced thrombocytopenia, where they may precipitate arterial thrombosis, and in immune (idiopathic) thrombocytopenia, where they may worsen this autoimmune destruction of platelets.
6. Dosage: average dose is generally 1 unit of platelets for each 10 kg of body weight; however, patients who are actively bleeding or undergoing surgical procedures may require more.

Nursing and Patient Care Considerations

1. Infuse at the rate prescribed. Generally, the infusion can be completed within 20 to 60 minutes, depending on the total volume.
2. Observe closely for the most common acute complications associated with platelet transfusions, allergic and febrile transfusion reactions.
3. Platelets are stored at 68°F to 75°F (20°C to 24°C), a warmer environment than other blood products and more conducive to bacterial growth. This increases the risk of bacterial contamination of a platelet product, which occurs in 4 to 10 per 10,000 units, limiting their shelf life.

Plasma (Fresh or Fresh Frozen)

Description

1. Consists of water (91%), plasma proteins including essential clotting factors (7%), and carbohydrates (2%). Each unit is the volume removed from a unit of whole blood (200 to 250 mL).
2. May be stored in a liquid state or frozen within 6 hours of collection.
3. Indications include treatment of blood loss or blood-clotting disorders related to liver disease and failure, disseminated intravascular coagulation (DIC), overanticoagulation with warfarin, all congenital or acquired clotting factor deficiencies, and dilutional coagulopathy resulting from massive blood replacement. Storage in liquid state results in the loss of labile clotting factors V and VIII, so that only plasma that has been fresh frozen can be used to treat factor V and VIII deficiencies.
4. Dosage: depends on the clinical situation and assessment of prothrombin time, partial thromboplastin time, or specific factor assays.

Nursing and Patient Care Considerations

1. Infuse at the rate prescribed. Generally, the infusion can be completed within 15 to 30 minutes, depending on the total volume.
2. Observe closely for the most common acute complication associated with plasma infusion, volume overload.

Cryoprecipitate

Description

1. Consists of certain clotting factors suspended in 10 to 20 mL plasma. Each unit contains approximately 80 to 120 units of factor VIII (antihemophilic and von Willebrand factors), 250 mg fibrinogen, and 20% to 30% of the factor XIII present in a unit of whole blood.
2. Indications include correction of deficiencies of factor VIII (i.e., hemophilia A and von Willebrand disease), factor XIII, and fibrinogen (i.e., DIC).
3. Dosage: adult dosage is generally 10 units, which may be repeated every 8 to 12 hours until the deficiency is corrected or until hemostasis is achieved.

Nursing and Patient Care Considerations

Infuse at the rate prescribed. Generally, the infusion can be completed within 3 to 15 minutes.

Fractionated Plasma Products

Description

1. Various highly concentrated plasma protein products are commercially prepared by pooling thousands of single plasma units and by extracting the desired protein. Most techniques involve heat or chemical treatments, which eliminate the risk of transmitting blood-borne viruses, such as hepatitis B and HIV.
2. Colloid solutions provide volume expansion in situations where crystalloid solutions are not adequate, such as therapeutic plasma exchange, shock, and massive hemorrhage. They may also be used in the treatment of acute liver failure, burns, and hemolytic disease of the neonate.
    a. Albumin is available as a 5% solution, which is oncotically equivalent to plasma, and as a concentrated 25% solution.
    b. Plasma protein fraction (PPF) is available as a 5% solution. Rapid infusion of PPF has been associated with hypotension.
    c. Albumin and PPF are pasteurized and carry no risk of viral disease. They do not contain preservatives and should be used immediately after opening.
3. Immune serum globulins (ISGs) are concentrated aqueous solutions of gamma globulin that contain high titers of antibody.
    a. Must be administered by deep intramuscular (IM) injection.
    b. Nonspecific ISG is prepared from random donor plasma and is used to increase gamma globulin levels and to enhance the general immune response in mild inherited or acquired immune disorders such as hypogammaglobulinemia.
    c. Specific ISG is prepared from donors who have high antibody titers to known antigens and is used to treat specific disorders or conditions. Hepatitis B immunoglobulin, varicella-zoster immunoglobulin, and Rh immunoglobulin are examples of specific ISGs.
    d. ISGs carry no risk of hepatitis B, HIV, or other blood-borne infections.
    e. Problems associated with use include pain at the injection site, limitations on volume administered, loss of IgG into extravascular tissue, or by degradation at the injection site.
4. Intravenous immunoglobulins (IVIGs) are aqueous solutions of immunoglobulins at a higher concentration and are given in larger volumes than ISGs.

a. Like ISGs, they may be nonspecific or specific.
b. Indications include chronic replacement therapy in patients with congenital or acquired immunodeficiency syndromes, acute autoimmune disorders such as immune (idiopathic) thrombocytopenia, and the treatment of chronic lymphocytic leukemia. Also, there are numerous investigational uses, such as Guillain–Barré syndrome, myasthenia gravis, rheumatoid arthritis, multiple sclerosis, lupus, and viral infections such as CMV, adenovirus, and influenza. IVIGs may also be used to treat platelet alloimmunization.
c. IVIGs do not appear to transmit HIV, but have been reported to transmit hepatitis C.
d. Administration of IVIG should be closely monitored because of the possibility of anaphylactic reactions. Dosage and rate of infusion depend on the manufacturer's formulation.

5. Factor VIII concentrate is a lyophilized concentrate used to treat moderate to severe hemophilia A and severe von Willebrand disease.
6. Factor IX concentrate is a lyophilized concentrate used to treat factor IX deficiency (Christmas disease).

Nursing and Patient Care Considerations

1. These products are often distributed by a pharmacy rather than by a blood bank.
2. Check order and product insert to ensure proper dosage and administration route.

Granulocyte Concentrates

Description

1. Consist of a minimum of 1×10^{10} granulocytes, variable amounts of lymphocytes (usually less than 10% of the total number of WBCs), 6 to 10 units of platelets, 30 to 50 mL RBCs, and 200 to 400 mL plasma.
2. Obtained via apheresis, generally of multiple donors.
3. Indications include treatment of life-threatening bacterial or fungal infection unresponsive to other therapy in a patient with severe neutropenia.
4. Dosage: generally 1 unit daily for approximately 5 to 10 days, discontinuing if no therapeutic response.

Nursing and Patient Care Considerations

1. Product must be ABO compatible and, if possible, Rh compatible because of the high erythrocyte content. Granulocytes are irradiated prior to transfusion to prevent the risk of graft-versus-host disease (GVHD).
2. Transfuse granulocytes as soon as they are available. WBCs have a short survival time, and therapeutic benefit is directly related to dose and viability.
3. Premedicate per order to prevent adverse effects, generally with antihistamine and acetaminophen. A corticosteroid may also be required.
4. Begin the transfusion slowly and increase to the rate prescribed and as tolerated. The recommended length of infusion is 1 to 2 hours.
5. Observe the patient closely throughout the transfusion for signs and symptoms of febrile, allergic, and anaphylactic reactions, which may be severe. Have emergency medications and equipment readily available.
6. Agitate the bag approximately every 15 minutes to prevent granulocytes from clumping at the bottom of the bag.
7. Do not administer amphotericin products immediately before or after granulocyte transfusion because pulmonary insufficiency has been reported with concurrent administration of amphotericin and granulocytes. Many institutions recommend a 4-hour gap to avoid this risk.

Modified Blood Products

Purpose

1. To reduce the risk of specific transfusion-related complications, blood products may receive further processing or treatment.
   a. Leukocytes are removed from blood products through filtration, washing, and freezing to reduce the risk of febrile, nonhemolytic transfusion reactions and alloimmunization to HLA.
   b. Function and proliferation of donor lymphocytes are inhibited by irradiation, to decrease the risk of posttransfusion GVHD in patients who are immunocompromised, including those with oncologic conditions, those who have undergone lung or heart transplant, and pediatric patients under age 6.

Methods

1. Filtration.
   a. Standard filters (170 μm) effectively remove gross fibrin clots.
   b. Microaggregate filters (approximately 40 μm) remove microscopic aggregates of fibrin, platelets, and leukocytes that accumulate in RBC products during storage. Their use is recommended during rapid, massive transfusion of whole blood or packed RBCs to prevent pulmonary complications. They reduce the risk of CMV transmission and may also decrease the incidence of febrile transfusion reactions by removing many of the leukocytes present.
   c. Special leukocyte-depletion filters have been developed for use with platelet products that remove 80% to 95% of leukocytes and that retain 80% of the platelets. These filters also reduce the risk of CMV transmission.
   d. A product may be filtered before release from the blood bank, but more commonly is released with the appropriate filter that must be attached to the standard infusion set at the bedside per manufacturer's or blood bank's instructions.
2. Washing.
   a. Washing RBCs or platelets with a normal saline solution removes 80% to 95% of the WBCs and virtually all of the plasma to reduce the incidence of febrile, nonhemolytic transfusion reactions.
   b. Washing requires an additional hour of processing time, and the shelf life of the product is reduced to 24 hours after this additional manipulation.
3. Freezing.
   a. RBCs can be frozen within 7 days of blood collection and then remain viable for 7 to 10 years.
   b. Removal of the hypertonic freezing preservative (glycerol) before transfusion eliminates all of the plasma and 99% of WBCs.
   c. Thawing and deglycerolization of RBCs require an additional 90 minutes of preparation time and reduce shelf life to 24 hours after this additional manipulation.
   d. Freezing is also an effective method of storing rare blood types and autologous RBCs.

4. Irradiation.
   a. Exposure of blood products to a measured amount of gamma irradiation inhibits lymphocyte function and proliferation without damaging RBCs, platelets, or granulocytes. This eliminates the ability of transfused lymphocytes to engraft in the immunocompromised transfusion recipient and the accompanying risk of posttransfusion GVHD.
   b. Patients at risk for posttransfusion GVHD include those who are bone marrow and peripheral stem cell transplant recipients, those who have undergone lung or heart transplant, premature neonates, and patients with congenital immunodeficiency disorders, Hodgkin and non-Hodgkin lymphomas, and HIV.

Transfusion Reactions

Every transfusion of blood components can result in an adverse effect. Reactions can be placed into two general categories: acute and delayed.

Acute Reactions

1. Acute reactions may occur during the infusion or within minutes to hours after the blood product has been infused.
2. Acute reactions include allergic, febrile, septic, and hemolytic reactions; air embolism; and circulatory overload. Patients who also receive multiple blood products within a short time frame may also be at risk for hyperkalemia, hypocalcemia, and hypothermia.
3. Because reactions may exhibit similar clinical manifestations, every symptom should be considered potentially serious and the transfusion should be discontinued until the cause is determined.
4. When a reaction is suspected, the health care provider should be notified immediately, and blood bags with tubing from all products recently transfused should be returned to the blood bank for evaluation.
5. The following samples should also be obtained if an acute reaction is suspected.
   a. A clotted blood specimen to examine serum for hemoglobin and confirm the RBC group and type.
   b. An anticoagulated blood sample for a direct Coombs test to determine the presence of antibody on the RBCs.
   c. The first-voided urine specimen to test for hemoglobinuria (this does not need to be a clean-catch specimen).
6. Precautions must be taken to avoid the hemolysis of RBCs during venipuncture and sample collection because this could lead to invalid test results. Whenever possible, blood samples should be drawn from a fresh venipuncture and not from existing needles or catheters.
7. If the only symptoms are those resulting from a mild allergic reaction (e.g., urticaria), extensive evaluation may not be necessary. In the event of a severe reaction (e.g., hypotension, tachypnea), more tests may be required to determine the cause of the reaction.
8. Causes, clinical manifestations, management, and prevention of acute reactions are summarized in Table 23-4.

Delayed Reactions

1. Delayed reactions occur days to years after the transfusion.
2. Delayed reactions include delayed hemolytic reactions, iron overload (hemosiderosis), GVHD, and infectious diseases (e.g., hepatitis B, hepatitis C, CMV, Epstein–Barr virus, malaria, HIV, HTLV).
3. Symptoms of a delayed reaction can vary from mild to severe. Diagnosis may be complicated by the long incubation period between transfusion and reaction and the complexity of diagnostic tests.
4. It is important to educate patients about the potential for a delayed blood transfusion reaction at the time of discharge, including signs and symptoms to be on the lookout for and the importance of notifying their health care provider.
5. Causes, clinical manifestations, management, and prevention of delayed reactions are summarized in Table 23-5, pages 9 and 10.

Table 23-4 Acute Reactions to Blood Transfusion

ACUTE REACTION	CAUSE	CLINICAL MANIFESTATIONS	MANAGEMENT	PREVENTION
Allergic	Sensitivity to plasma protein or donor antibody, which reacts with recipient antigen	• Flushing • Itching, rash • Urticaria, hives • Asthmatic wheezing • Laryngeal edema • Anaphylaxis	• Stop transfusion immediately. Keep the vein open (KVO) with normal saline. Notify health care provider and blood bank. • Give antihistamine, as directed (diphenhydramine). • Observe for anaphylaxis—prepare epinephrine if respiratory distress is severe. • If hives are the only clinical manifestation, the transfusion can sometimes continue at a slower rate. • Send blood samples and blood bags to the blood bank. Collect urine specimens for testing.	• Before transfusion, ask patient about past reactions. If patient has history of anaphylaxis, alert health care provider, have emergency drugs available, and remain at bedside for the first 30 min.

Table 23-4 Acute Reactions to Blood Transfusion (*continued*)

ACUTE REACTION	CAUSE	CLINICAL MANIFESTATIONS	MANAGEMENT	PREVENTION
Febrile, nonhemolytic	Hypersensitivity to donor white blood cells, platelets, or plasma proteins	• Sudden chills and fever • Headache • Flushing • Anxiety	• Stop transfusion immediately and KVO with normal saline. Notify health care provider and blood bank. • Send blood samples and blood bags to the blood bank. Collect urine specimens for testing. • Check temperature 30 min after chill and as indicated thereafter. • Give antipyretics, as prescribed—treat symptomatically.	• Give antipyretic (acetaminophen or aspirin) before transfusion as directed. • Leukocyte-poor blood products may be recommended for future transfusions.
Septic reactions	Transfusion of blood or components contaminated with bacteria	• Rapid onset of chills • High fever • Vomiting, diarrhea • Marked hypotension	• Stop transfusion immediately and KVO with normal saline. Notify health care provider and blood bank. • Obtain cultures of patient's blood and return blood bags with administration set to the blood bank for culture. • Treat septicemia, as directed—antibiotics, intravenous (IV) fluids, vasopressors, and steroids.	• Do not permit blood to stand at room temperature longer than necessary. Warm temperatures promote bacterial growth. • Inspect blood for gas bubbles, clotting, or abnormal color before transfusion. • Complete infusions within 4 h. Change administration set after 4 h of use.
Circulatory overload	Fluid administered at a rate or volume greater than the circulatory system can accommodate. Increased blood in pulmonary vessels and decreased lung compliance	• Rise in venous pressure • Distended neck veins • Dyspnea • Cough • Crackles at the base of the lungs	• Stop transfusion and KVO with normal saline. Notify health care provider. • Place patient upright with feet in dependent position. • Administer prescribed diuretics, oxygen, morphine, and aminophylline.	• Concentrated blood products should be given whenever positive. • Transfuse at a rate within the circulatory reserve of the patient. • Monitor central venous pressure of patient with heart disease.
Hemolytic reaction	Infusion of incompatible blood products: • Antibodies in recipient's plasma attach to transfused red blood cells (RBCs), hemolyzing the cells either in circulation or in the reticuloendothelial system • Antibodies in donor plasma attach to recipient RBCs, causing hemolysis (may result from infusion of incompatible plasma—less severe than incompatible RBCs)	• Chills; fever • Lower back pain • Feeling of head fullness; flushing • Oppressive feeling • Tachycardia, tachypnea • Hypotension, vascular collapse • Hemoglobinuria, hemoglobinemia • Bleeding • Acute renal failure	• Stop transfusion immediately—KVO with 0.9% saline. • Notify health care provider and blood bank. • Treat shock, if present. • Draw testing samples; collect urine specimen. • Maintain blood pressure with IV colloid solutions. Give diuretics, as prescribed, to maintain urine flow, glomerular filtration, and renal blood flow. • Insert indwelling catheter to monitor hourly urine output. Patient may require dialysis if renal failure occurs.	• Meticulously verify patient identification—from sample collection to product infusion. • Begin infusion slowly and observe closely for 30 min—consequences are in proportion to the amount of incompatible blood transfused.

Table 23-5 Delayed Reactions to Transfusion Therapy

DELAYED REACTION	CAUSE	CLINICAL MANIFESTATIONS	MANAGEMENT	PREVENTION
Delayed hemolytic reaction	The destruction of transfused red blood cells by antibody not detectable during crossmatch, but formed rapidly after transfusion. Rapid production may occur because of antigen exposure during previous transfusions or pregnancy.	• Fever • Mild jaundice • Decreased hematocrit	• Generally, no acute treatment is required, but hemolysis may be severe enough to cause shock and renal failure. If this occurs, manage as outlined under acute hemolytic reactions.	• The crossmatch blood sample should be drawn within 3 d of blood transfusion. Antibody formation may occur within 90 d of transfusion or pregnancy.
Iron overload (hemosiderosis)	Deposition of iron in the heart, endocrine organs, liver, spleen, skin, and other major organs as a result of multiple, long-term transfusions (aplastic anemia, thalassemia).	• Diabetes • Decreased thyroid function • Arrhythmias • Heart failure and other symptoms related to major organ failure	• Treat symptomatically. • Deferoxamine, which chelates and removes accumulated iron through the kidneys; administered via IV line, IM, or SubQ.	—
Graft-versus-host disease	Engraftment of lymphocytes in the bone marrow of patients who are immunosuppressed, setting up an immune response of the graft against the host.	• Erythematous skin rash • Liver function test abnormalities • Profuse, watery diarrhea • Pruritus • Bone pain	• Immunosuppression with corticosteroids, cyclosporine A. • Symptomatic management of pruritus, pain. • Fluid and electrolyte replacement for diarrhea.	• Transfuse with irradiated blood products.
Hepatitis B	Hepatitis B virus transmitted from blood donor to recipient via infected blood products.	• Elevated liver enzymes (ALT/AST) • Anorexia, malaise • Nausea and vomiting • Fever • Dark urine • Jaundice	• Usually resolves spontaneously within 4–6 wk. Can result in permanent liver damage. Treat symptomatically.	• Screen blood donors, temporarily rejecting those who may have had contact with the virus. Those with a history of hepatitis after age 11 are permanently deferred; pretest all blood products (EIA).
Hepatitis C	Hepatitis C virus transmitted from blood donor to recipient via infected blood products.	• Similar to similar to hepatitis B, but symptoms are usually less severe. Chronic liver disease and cirrhosis may develop	• Symptoms usually mild. Interferon and ribavirin may be used to treat chronic liver disease.	• Pretest all blood donors (ALT, anti-HBc antibody, anti-hepatitis C antibody).
Epstein–Barr virus, cytomegalovirus, malaria	Transmitted through infected blood products.	• Fever • Fatigue • Hepatomegaly • Splenomegaly	• Rest and supportive management.	• Question prospective blood donors regarding colds, flu, and foreign travel.
Acquired immunodeficiency syndrome (AIDS)	Human immunodeficiency virus (HIV) transmitted from blood donor to recipient via infected blood products.	• Night sweats • Unexplained weight loss • Lymphadenopathy • Pneumocystis pneumonia • Kaposi sarcoma • Diarrhea	• Combination antiretroviral therapy.	• Test each donor for HIV antibody. • Reject prospective high-risk donors who have ever had AIDS or tested positive for HIV and those whose sexual contact or needle use increases HIV risk (see https://www.redcrossblood.org/faq.html#eligibility for complete eligibility criteria).

Table 23-5 Delayed Reactions to Transfusion Therapy (*continued*)

DELAYED REACTION	CAUSE	CLINICAL MANIFESTATIONS	MANAGEMENT	PREVENTION
Human T-lymphotropic virus type 1 (HTLV-1)-associated myelopathy and tropical spastic paraparesis (HAM/TSP) Adult T-cell leukemia	HTLV-1 transmitted from blood donor to recipient via blood products.	• Signs of neuromuscular disease • Signs of T-cell leukemia	• HTLV-1-infected individuals have a low risk of developing disease (3%–5%). Incubation period 10–20 yr. • Should disease occur, treat symptomatically.	• Screen all prospective blood donors for anti-HTLV-1 antibody.
Syphilis	Spirochetemia caused by *Treponema pallidum*. Incubation 4–18 wk.	• Presence of chancre • Regional lymphadenopathy • Generalized rash	• Penicillin therapy.	• Test blood before transfusion (rapid plasma reagin). Organism will not remain viable in blood stored 24–48 h at 39.2°F (4°C).

AST, aspartate aminotransferase; ALT, alanine aminotransferase; EIA, enzyme immunoassay; IV, intravenous; IM, intramuscularly; SubQ, subcutaneous.

BLOOD AND MARROW STEM CELL TRANSPLANTATION

Blood and marrow stem cell transplantation is a potentially lifesaving treatment with application in many malignant and nonmalignant disorders. Decades of research have advanced this technology from an experimental treatment of last resort to the preferred method of intervention for selected diseases. Although the basic procedures are now well established, this field continues to grow rapidly through ongoing research in areas such as nonmyeloablative ("mini") allogeneic transplants, the application of biologic response modifiers to modulate the immune response, and the use of donor lymphocyte infusions to prevent or treat posttransplant relapse.

Principles of Blood and Marrow Stem Cell Transplantation

Types of Stem Cell Transplant

The type of transplant selected is contingent on a variety of factors, such as the underlying disorder, the availability of a histocompatible (human leukocyte antigen [HLA]-matched) donor, and the clinical condition of the patient. Stem cells may come from the patient (autologous), an identical twin (syngeneic), or another donor (allogeneic). Stem cells are found in bone marrow, in peripheral blood (especially if the donor is treated to increase the numbers of circulating stem cells), and in umbilical cord blood.

Autologous Bone Marrow Transplantation

1. Bone marrow is removed from the patient during an operative harvesting procedure, frozen, and reinfused after the patient has undergone high-dose chemotherapy and possibly radiotherapy.
2. Advantages: readily available and usually lower morbidity and mortality than allogeneic bone marrow transplantation (BMT).
3. Disadvantages: operative procedure; marrow must be disease free; need to aspirate sufficient quantity of cellular marrow; in most cases has a higher rate of relapse than allogeneic BMT.

Syngeneic BMT

1. Bone marrow is removed from an identical twin during an operative harvesting procedure and infused into the recipient, who has undergone high-dose chemotherapy and possibly radiotherapy.
2. Advantages: recipient's marrow does not need to be harvestable (as in hypocellular or tumor-contaminated bone marrow), generally lower morbidity and mortality than allogeneic BMT.
3. Disadvantages: higher disease relapse rate than in allogeneic BMT.

Allogeneic BMT

1. Bone marrow is removed from a donor who is most commonly a sibling or other close relative (related) but may be a volunteer donor (unrelated).
   a. Identical or mismatched HLA phenotypes may be used, though identical phenotypes are often preferred. HLA mismatches require additional immunosuppression and graft-versus-host disease (GVHD) prophylaxis and can be associated with higher morbidity and mortality.
   b. Bone marrow is removed from the donor during an operative harvesting procedure and infused into the recipient, who has undergone high-dose chemotherapy and possibly radiotherapy.
   c. Allogeneic bone marrow may be treated in various ways before infusion, including removing red blood cells (RBCs) if ABO incompatible and removing T lymphocytes to reduce the risk of GVHD.
2. Advantages: recipient's marrow does not need to be harvestable (as in hypocellular or tumor-contaminated bone marrow) and lowest rate of relapse.
3. Disadvantages: risk for GVHD and generally higher morbidity and mortality than other types of BMT. Unrelated and HLA-mismatched transplants have a higher risk of GVHD and infectious complications and some risk of graft rejection or failure.

Autologous, Syngeneic, or Allogeneic Peripheral Blood Stem Cell Transplantation

1. Although hematopoietic stem cells are primarily found in the bone marrow, they can also be found in the peripheral circulation in smaller numbers.
2. Peripheral blood stem cells are collected using one or more apheresis procedures after the patient or donor has been treated to increase the number of circulating stem cells. This is done by methods such as timed administration of chemotherapy (patient only) and stem cell growth factors. After the collection, the cells are frozen and stored for reinfusion into the patient after high-dose chemotherapy and possibly radiotherapy.
3. Advantages: patient's marrow does not need to be harvestable (as in hypocellular or tumor-contaminated bone marrow); there is no operative risk to the patient or donor.
4. Disadvantages: for allogeneic donors, the long-term risks of boosting healthy bone marrow production with growth factors, and in some cases chemotherapy, are not yet known. Research has shown that allogeneic peripheral blood stem cell transplant may be associated with a higher incidence of chronic GVHD than allogeneic bone marrow transplant.

Umbilical Cord Blood Stem Cell Transplantation

1. Umbilical cord blood is rich in stem cells and may be stored at birth for later autologous use, related allogeneic use, or unrelated allogeneic use. Cord blood transplantation requires less stringent HLA matching because mismatched cord blood stem cells are less likely to cause GVHD than mature stem cells from other sources.
2. Advantages: may provide lifesaving allogeneic stem cells from new sibling to older child at no risk to the donor. Cord blood banks provide options for unrelated donor transplantation when there is an urgent need.
3. Disadvantages: may have a higher risk of graft failure than other types of transplants; the number of stem cells may be insufficient for older patients.

Nonmyeloablative or "Mini" Transplants

1. Conventional conditioning for blood and marrow stem cell transplants requires high doses of chemotherapy and radiotherapy (myeloablative) to destroy existing bone marrow cells. This results in significant morbidity and mortality, particularly in certain patient populations (e.g., older patients, those with poor organ function).
2. Research has demonstrated that under certain conditions, individuals can exist with bone marrow stem cells from two sources (self and allogeneic donor), a state known as *mixed chimerism*. These changes in the immune system appear to enhance the antitumor immune response, creating a desired graft-versus-tumor effect.
3. The goals of nonmyeloablative conditioning regimens are to prevent graft rejection and promote mixed chimerism. The nonmyeloablative preparative regimen uses combinations of agents such as cyclophosphamide, fludarabine, antithymocyte globulin, and low-dose total body irradiation. Alemtuzumab is often considered as well. After the completion of the reduced-intensity regimen, the allogeneic bone marrow or peripheral blood stem cells are then infused.
4. Donor lymphocytes may also be given at specific intervals following transplant to enhance the immune antitumor effect further.
5. Advantages: patients otherwise ineligible for allogeneic transplant because of age, comorbid conditions, or organ function are more likely to tolerate the less-toxic preparative regimen. Patients do not usually experience significant neutropenia, thrombocytopenia, anemia, and other complications that typically accompany myeloablative therapy. Patients generally have shorter episodes of neutropenia and a reduced need for RBC and platelet transfusions, allowing an opportunity for outpatient transplants to be performed.
6. Disadvantages: Increased risk of graft failure.

The HLA System and Transplantation

1. The HLA system is part of the major histocompatibility complex.
2. The immune-mediated recognition of the differences in each individual's HLA system is the first step in the rejection of a transplanted organ or graft or in GVHD.
3. The HLAs are complex proteins expressed on the surface of all nucleated cells (A, B, C antigens—class I) or cells of the immune system (D antigens—class II).
   a. More than 300 different antigens have been identified.
   b. Antigens are classified according to their location on chromosome 6, which encodes them.
   c. A person's genetically inherited mixture of antigens expressed on cell surfaces is their individual phenotype or tissue type.
4. Determination of an individual's HLA type is completed by complex DNA phenotyping or gene sequencing.
   a. The gold standard for HLA typing in BMT is to complete the above testing at high resolution (allelic level), identifying both the class I (A, B, C) and class II (D) groups.
   b. A phenotypically identical donor is considered to be one who matches at all 10 antigens at their associated allelic level—A, B, C, DR, and DQ.
5. Siblings have a 1-in-4 chance of having identical sets of HLAs. With a decreasing national birthrate, however, only 35% of people in the United States can anticipate having an HLA-identical sibling.
6. Because of the complexity of the HLA system, unrelated people have less than a 1-in-5,000 chance of being HLA identical.
7. The National Bone Marrow Donor Program (BeTheMatch Registry), established in 1987, maintains a computerized list of potential HLA-matched peripheral blood stem cell and bone marrow donors, providing assistance to patients who seek an unrelated donor. Information on becoming a volunteer bone marrow donor or on initiating a computerized search for a donor can be obtained by calling the National Marrow Donor Program (1-800-627-7692 or www.bethematch.org), for additional resources for patients undergoing blood and marrow stem cell transplantation.

Indications

1. If an HLA-matched related donor is available, allogeneic bone marrow or stem cell transplantation is generally considered the treatment of choice in certain disorders, including:
   a. Severe aplastic anemia.
   b. Inherited immunodeficiency disorders, such as severe combined immunodeficiency disease and Wiskott–Aldrich syndrome.
   c. Allogeneic bone marrow and peripheral blood stem cell transplantation has also been used with varying success in the treatment of other genetic disorders (e.g., thalassemia, sickle cell disease).
2. Allogeneic, syngeneic, and autologous bone marrow and peripheral blood stem cell transplantation is also widely applied in the treatment of malignancies, where success rates depend

BOX 23-1 Indications for Blood and Marrow Stem Cell Transplantation

ALLOGENEIC

Nonmalignant

- Aplastic anemia.
- Myelofibrosis.
- Wiskott–Aldrich syndrome.
- Thalassemia.
- Severe combined immunodeficiency diseases.
- Mucopolysaccharidoses.
- Sickle cell disease.

Malignant

- Acute myeloid leukemia.
- Acute lymphocytic leukemia.
- Hodgkin lymphoma.
- Non-Hodgkin lymphoma.
- Myelofibrosis.
- Multiple myeloma.
- Selected solid tumors.

AUTOLOGOUS

- Hodgkin lymphoma.
- Non-Hodgkin lymphoma.
- Multiple myeloma.
- Selected solid tumors.

largely on factors such as the age of the patient, disease status at the time of transplant, the extent of prior treatment, and existing comorbidities.

3. Autologous peripheral blood stem cell transplantation is used in the treatment of certain lymphomas, multiple myeloma, and solid tumors such as Ewing sarcoma and neuroblastoma. Allogeneic bone marrow and peripheral blood stem cell transplantation is generally used in the treatment of leukemias as well as certain lymphomas.
4. Diseases and disorders treated with this technology are summarized in Box 23-1.

Harvesting of Bone Marrow and Peripheral Blood Stem Cells

Evaluation of Recipient

1. Eligibility criteria include age (generally younger than age 65 for allogeneic myeloablative transplants and autologous and syngeneic transplants and younger than age 75 for allogeneic nonmyeloablative transplants) and availability of suitable donor and stem cell source.
2. Before undergoing transplantation, an extensive workup is completed to ensure that the patient's disease is treatable with the selected type of transplant and that the patient has no limitations that will increase the risk of mortality.
3. Specific criteria may vary among transplant centers and treatment protocols, but generally include:
   a. Disease-specific evaluation of severity and extent of current disease manifestations.
   b. Adequate cardiac function: generally left ventricular ejection fraction greater than 45%.
   c. Adequate pulmonary function: generally, forced expiratory capacity and forced vital capacity greater than 50%.
   d. Adequate renal function: generally, creatinine less than 2 mg/dL.
   e. Adequate hepatic function: generally, bilirubin less than 2 mg/dL.
   f. No active infections (including human immunodeficiency virus [HIV]).
   g. No coexisting severe or uncontrolled medical conditions.

Evaluation of Blood and Marrow Donors

1. Because bone marrow donation for allogeneic or syngeneic BMT is an elective procedure with no benefit to the donor, great care is taken to ensure that the potential donor is fit for surgery and understands the potential risks. Autologous bone marrow donors must generally meet the same criteria. Evaluation includes:
   a. Thorough medical history and physical examination.
   b. Chest x-ray.
   c. Electrocardiogram.
   d. Laboratory evaluation (complete blood count [CBC]; chemistry profile; testing for cytomegalovirus [CMV], hepatitis B and C, HIV, human T-cell lymphoma virus [HTLV], and syphilis; ABO and Rh determination; coagulation studies).
2. Informed consent including potential donor complications must be obtained.
3. Relatively common complications include:
   a. Bruising.
   b. Pain at aspiration sites.
   c. Mild bleeding.
4. Rare complications include:
   a. Adverse effects of anesthesia (general, spinal, or epidural).
   b. Infection of aspiration sites.
   c. Persistent pain.
   d. Transient neuropathies.
5. Because of the significant loss of blood volume and RBCs during the harvest procedure, donors are advised to give one or two units of autologous blood 1 to 3 weeks before surgery, which may be reinfused during marrow collection, if needed.
6. Evaluation of donors for peripheral blood stem cell transplantation is similar, but less stringent as there is generally no anesthesia required. The apheresis procedure is similar to donating platelets.

Stem Cell Collection Procedure

Bone Marrow Harvest (Autologous, Syngeneic, or Allogeneic)

1. Performed under epidural, spinal, or general anesthesia under sterile conditions in the operating room.
2. An aspiration needle is used to puncture the skin and puncture the iliac crest multiple times without exiting the skin, removing marrow in 2- to 5-mL aliquots (samples).
3. Marrow is drawn up into heparinized syringes and filtered to remove fibrin clots and other debris.
4. Marrow may be infused immediately, treated and infused, or frozen in a preservative solution containing dimethyl sulfoxide (DMSO) until needed.
5. Bone marrow donation is a relatively safe operative procedure with few serious complications.

Postharvest Care of the Bone Marrow Donor

1. Procedure is generally done as same-day care, with discharge after recovery from anesthesia.
2. Observe for potential complications (bleeding, hypotension caused by fluid loss).
3. Instruct patient to resume normal activities gradually during the week after donation.

4. Instruct patient to keep aspiration sites clean and dry and observe for signs of infection (redness, swelling, warmth or discharge at sites, fever, malaise).
5. Provide adequate analgesia and instruct the patient about pain management.
6. Ensure that the donor has a follow-up appointment and understands signs and symptoms that may require medical attention, such as fever, numbness and tingling, or severe pain not responsive to analgesics.

Harvesting of Peripheral Blood Stem Cells

1. Involves donor preparation by "priming" hematopoietic system with timed chemotherapy (autologous stem cell collection only) and sequential growth factor administration to increase the number of circulating stem cells.
2. A large-bore central catheter suitable for apheresis procedures is inserted.
3. One to 10 apheresis procedures may be needed to collect sufficient numbers of suitable cells.
4. Cells are frozen in a preservative solution that contains DMSO until needed.
5. Acute complications of apheresis include citrate toxicity, which may be managed by increasing dietary calcium intake 2 to 3 days before the procedure and by using calcium-based antacids during the procedure. Blood calcium levels are carefully monitored throughout the procedure and intravenous (IV) calcium is given, as needed.

Preparation and Performance of the Transplant

Preparation of Recipient

1. A long-term central catheter is inserted for multiple IV treatments, including blood products, total parenteral nutrition, and blood drawing.
2. High-dose chemotherapy or radiotherapy is administered to:
   a. Destroy residual tumor cells.
   b. Suppress immune response against new stem cells.
   c. Create space within the recipient's marrow for the new stem cells.
3. Symptoms immediately associated with high-dose chemotherapy or radiotherapy regimens used in blood and marrow stem cell transplantation may include:
   a. Severe nausea and vomiting (with most regimens).
   b. Cardiomyopathy and hemorrhagic cystitis (with cyclophosphamide).
   c. Seizures (with busulfan).
   d. Fever, generalized erythema, and parotitis (with total body irradiation).

Infusion of Bone Marrow or Peripheral Blood Stem Cells

Nursing considerations are based on the potential adverse effects of the various types of infusions (see Table 23-6).

CLINICAL JUDGMENT Unlike all other blood products administered to transplant recipients, stem cells should never be irradiated. In addition, infusion pumps and filters should be avoided because they may remove or damage stem cells.

Posttransplant Care

General Considerations

1. Significant complications that require specialized medical and nursing care may occur during the first few weeks and months after blood and marrow stem cell transplantation.
   a. Risk is highest in mismatched unrelated allogeneic BMT.
   b. Followed by matched unrelated and mismatched related allogeneic BMT.

Table 23-6 Infusion Guidelines for Bone Marrow or Peripheral Blood Stem Cells

TYPE OF STEM CELLS	PROCESSING PRIOR TO INFUSION	VOLUME	POTENTIAL ADVERSE EFFECTS	NURSING CONSIDERATIONS
ABO-compatible untreated allogeneic bone marrow	Filtered to remove large particles	500–2,000 mL	Volume overload, allergic reactions, pulmonary compromise (fat emboli, cell aggregates)	Emergency medications available, close monitoring
ABO-incompatible bone marrow	Removal of red blood cells and plasma	200–600 mL	Allergic reactions, intravascular hemolysis (rare)	Prehydrate to ensure adequate renal perfusion and alkaline urine, emergency medications available, close monitoring
Autologous bone marrow	Filtered and frozen with DMSO as preservative, thawed in warm water bath immediately prior to infusion	100–500 mL	Related to DMSO: histamine release reaction (flushing, chest tightness, abdominal cramping, nausea), cardiac arrhythmias, anaphylaxis	Emergency medications available, close monitoring, cardiac monitoring recommended
Peripheral blood stem cells	Frozen with DMSO as preservative, thawed in warm water bath immediately prior to infusion	100–1,000 mL	Related to DMSO: histamine release reaction (flushing, chest tightness, abdominal cramping, nausea), cardiac arrhythmias, anaphylaxis	Administer as tolerated (may be high volume and DMSO content), premedicate with antihistamine and antiemetic, emergency medications available, close monitoring, cardiac monitoring recommended

DMSO, dimethyl sulfoxide.

c. Followed by matched related allogeneic BMT.
d. Followed by syngeneic BMT.
e. Followed by autologous BMT.
f. Followed by autologous peripheral blood stem cell transplantation (lowest risk).

2. Nursing care is aimed at early identification and treatment of problems and includes:
   a. Comprehensive physical and psychosocial assessment.
   b. Immediate notification of health care provider of any abnormal assessment parameters found.
   c. Early recognition and intervention for life-threatening complications, such as sepsis, respiratory failure, gastrointestinal (GI) bleeding, renal and hepatic failure, and veno-occlusive disease (VOD) of the liver.
   d. Prevention of infection.
   e. Prevention of bleeding.
   f. Expert symptom management of problems that may occur after blood and marrow stem cell transplantation, such as nausea, vomiting, diarrhea, pain, fatigue, anxiety, and delirium.

Hematopoietic Complications

1. Patients who have had blood and marrow stem cell transplant, particularly allogeneic recipients, are at risk for life-threatening bacterial, viral, and fungal infections because of their profound neutropenia and prolonged immunosuppression.
   a. Transplant recipients are usually cared for in a protective environment, most commonly single high-efficiency particulate air (HEPA)-filtered rooms.
   b. In an ambulatory or home setting, the patient and family must pay strict attention to methods of preventing infection, including wearing high-filtration masks, handwashing, safe food handling, and avoidance of crowded areas and exposure to illnesses.
   c. Blood and marrow stem cell recipients are at high risk for nosocomial bloodstream infections related to long-term central venous catheters, neutropenia, and immunosuppression. Strict adherence to an evidence-based procedure for insertion and management of central venous catheters is essential in this population.
   d. Colony-stimulating factors such as granulocyte colony-stimulating factor (GCSF) and granulocyte-macrophage colony-stimulating factor (GM-CSF) have been shown to reduce the duration of neutropenia, though the optimal timing for administration has not been determined.
   e. Additional preventive interventions vary widely and include elaborate disinfection procedures, modified or sterile diets, prophylactic antibiotics, antivirals, antifungals, and surveillance cultures.
2. The megakaryocyte is generally the last cell produced by new stem cells, and platelet counts may take months to return to normal.
   a. Patients who have had blood and marrow stem cell transplant require frequent assessment for signs and symptoms of overt or covert bleeding, protection from injury, and support with platelet products.
3. Anemia is a common complication caused by loss of RBCs through aging, destruction, bleeding, and routine phlebotomy. Patients who have undergone blood and marrow stem cell transplant require frequent RBC transfusions. Erythropoietin alfa and darbepoetin alfa may also be used to stimulate RBC production. Delayed erythropoiesis and immune hemolytic anemia are complications of ABO-incompatible allogeneic stem cell transplants.

GI Complications

1. Mucositis may develop because of high-dose chemotherapy and radiation therapy that destroy rapidly dividing cells, including cells lining the mouth, esophagus, and GI tract. Management includes meticulous oral hygiene, local and systemic analgesia, and antimicrobial therapy.
2. Nausea and vomiting may arise from multiple causes, including high-dose chemotherapy, infection, GI bleeding, acute GVHD, and medications. Management includes pharmacologic and nonpharmacologic interventions, adequate replacement of fluids and electrolytes, and support of nutritional requirements.
3. Diarrhea may have multiple causes, including high-dose chemotherapy, infection, GI bleeding, GVHD, and medications. Management includes cautious use of antidiarrheals, adequate replacement of fluids and electrolytes, support of nutritional requirements, and protection of perirectal skin from excoriation.

Renal and Genitourinary Complications

1. Renal failure may arise from multiple factors, including drug toxicity, infection, and ischemia. Management includes maintenance of fluid and electrolyte balance, monitoring of drug levels, and hemodialysis or continuous venovenous hemodialysis.
2. Hemorrhagic cystitis may occur as a result of high-dose cyclophosphamide or with certain viral infections, such as adenovirus and BK Polyomavirus (BKV, named for the first patient). Management includes hydration, blood product support, continuous bladder irrigation, and rare invasive procedures, such as instillation of alum or formalin, or surgery.

Hepatic Complications

Sinusoidal occlusive syndrome (SOS), a type of veno-occlusive disease (VOD) of the liver from high-dose chemotherapy and radiation therapy; incidence is approximately 30%.

1. Signs and symptoms include hepatomegaly (generally painful), hyperbilirubinemia, and weight gain.
2. May progress to hepatic encephalopathy, coagulopathies, coma, and death in up to 50% of patients with VOD.
3. Management is generally aimed at preventing further damage and at treating symptoms. The antithrombotic and thrombolytic agent defibrotide may be administered for severe VOD; however, the risk of bleeding is high with the administration of this agent; other agents being studied include heparin, recombinant tissue plasminogen activator, and ursodeoxycholic acid.

Pulmonary Complications

1. Life-threatening pulmonary infections in stem cell recipients include bacterial pneumonias, fungal infections including aspergillosis, viral infections such as CMV (especially in allogenic recipients), COVID-19, respiratory syncytial virus, parainfluenza, and, less commonly, *Pneumocystis carinii* pneumonia (PCP), Legionnaires' disease, toxoplasmosis, and tuberculosis.
   a. Preventive measures include hand hygiene, encouragement of exercise, deep breathing, and coughing; routine CMV polymerase chain reaction monitoring if recipient or donor is CMV immunoglobulin G (IgG) positive at the time of transplant; administration of CMV-screened and/or leukoreduced blood products, high-dose acyclovir or ganciclovir, and intravenous immunoglobulins (IVIGs) for allogeneic BMT patients at high risk for CMV; and prophylactic co-trimoxazole for patients at risk for PCP.

b. Staff, patient, and family education regarding risk factors and transmission of these infectious agents may help prevent primary and nosocomial infections.
c. Supportive care if symptomatic includes pulmonary hygiene, oxygen therapy, and mechanical ventilation.

2. Noninfectious pulmonary disease includes idiopathic pneumonitis, diffuse alveolar hemorrhage, pulmonary fibrosis, and bronchiolitis obliterans.

Graft-Versus-Host Disease

1. Acute GVHD occurs in 40% to 60% of allogeneic recipients even with HLA matching, generally within the first 3 months after transplant as a manifestation of the immune system's response to activated donor T lymphocytes against the recipient's cells and organs.
   a. Primarily affects the skin, liver, and GI tract; may also affect conjunctivae and lungs.
   b. Severity ranges from mild and self-limited erythematous rash to widespread blistering of the skin, profuse watery diarrhea, and liver failure.
   c. Prophylaxis generally includes immunosuppression with such medications as cyclosporine, tacrolimus, and methotrexate; may also include T-cell depletion of bone marrow.
   d. Recently, research has demonstrated that administration of high-dose cyclophosphamide a few days after the stem cell transplant decreases the rate of acute GVHD.
   e. Treatment generally includes increased doses of routine immunosuppressive drugs and additional drugs, such as corticosteroids, antithymocyte globulin, and monoclonal antibodies.
2. Chronic GVHD occurs in approximately 20% of long-term survivors; usually appears within first year after allogeneic blood and marrow stem cell transplant.
   a. It has many similarities to autoimmune disorders such as scleroderma.
   b. It affects the skin, mouth, salivary glands, eyes, musculoskeletal system, liver, esophagus, GI tract, and vagina.
   c. Treatment generally consists of corticosteroids and other immunosuppressive drugs, such as mycophenolate and thalidomide.
   d. Immune system is frequently suppressed beyond the effects of medications; patient is at risk for infections, particularly from encapsulated bacteria, and should receive prophylaxis with suitable antibiotics such as penicillin.

Long-Term Sequelae and Survivorship Issues

1. Long-term, disease-free survival varies from 5% to 20% for patients with resistant, aggressive leukemias or lymphomas to 75% to 80% for aplastic anemia.
2. Long-term complications of blood and marrow stem cell transplantation include:
   a. Relapse of the original disease.
   b. Secondary malignancy, including skin, oral mucosa, brain, thyroid, bone, and acute leukemia.
   c. Sterility.
   d. Endocrine dysfunction, including reduced levels of human growth hormone, estrogens, and testosterone.
   e. Cataracts (risk increased with radiation therapy, corticosteroids).
   f. Chronic GVHD (allogeneic).
   g. Aseptic necrosis and osteoporosis (risk increased with corticosteroids).
   h. Encephalopathy (risk increased with cranial irradiation and intrathecal chemotherapy).
3. Survivorship issues after this intensive and potentially life-threatening treatment include:
   a. Feelings of isolation, guilt, and loss.
   b. Altered family dynamics.
   c. Delayed puberty, decreased libido, early menopause, and other physical problems that have an impact on sexuality and relationships.
   d. Readjustment to school or work setting.
   e. Financial burden of blood and marrow stem cell transplantation.
   f. Chronic health problems and fatigue.
   g. There may be insurance coverage issues due to preexisting condition.
4. Despite the complex issues blood and marrow stem cell transplant survivors face, several quality-of-life studies have demonstrated that the majority rate their quality of life highly and would choose to undergo transplant again.

SELECTED READINGS

Ackfeld, T., Schmutz, T., Guechi, Y., & Le Terrier, C. (2022). Blood transfusion reactions—A comprehensive review of the literature including a Swiss perspective. *Journal of Clinical Medicine, 11*(10), 2859. https://doi.org/10.3390/jcm11102859

Baumrin, E., Loren, A. W., Falk, S. J., Mays, J. W., & Cowen, E. W. (2024). Chronic graft-versus-host disease. Part I: Epidemiology, pathogenesis, and clinical manifestations. *Journal of the American Academy of Dermatology, 90*(1), 1-16. https://doi.org/10.1016/j.jaad.2022.12.024.

Botteri, M., Celi, S., Perone, G., Prati, E., Bera, P., Villa, G., Mare, C., Sechi, G. M., Zoli, A., & Fagoni, N. (2021). Effectiveness of massive transfusion protocol activation in pre-hospital setting for major trauma. *Injury—International Journal of the Care of the Injured, 53*(5), 1581–1586. https://doi.org/10.1016/j.injury.2021.12.047

Corte, J. R., Candal-Pedreira, C., Ruano-Ravina, A., Pérez-Ríos, M., Rivero-De-Aguilar, A., García, M. M., Porto, L., & Varela-Lema, L. (2022). Home-based blood transfusion therapy: A systematic review. *British Journal of Haematology, 199*(4), 496–506. https://doi.org/10.1111/bjh.18344

Dezan, M. G. F., Cavalcante, L. N., Silva, H. R. C., de Moura Almeida, A., dos Santos de Assis, L. H., de Freitas, T. T.,de Araújo, M. A. S., Cotrim, H. P., & Lyra, A. C. (2024). Hepatobiliary disease after bone marrow transplant: A cross-sectional study of 377 patients. *Alimentary Pharmacology & Therapeutics, 59*(1), 71-79. https://doi.org/10.1111/apt.17756.

DeZern, A. E., Eapen, M., Wu, J., Talano, J., Solh, M., Saldaña, B. J. D., Karanes, C., Horwitz, M. E., Mallhi, K. K., Arai, S., Farhadfar, N., Hexner, E. O., Westervelt, P., Antin, J. H., Deeg, H. J., Leifer, E. S., Brodsky, R. A., Logan, B. R., Horowitz, M. M., … Pulsipher, M. A. (2022). Haploidentical bone marrow transplantation in patients with relapsed or refractory severe aplastic anaemia in the USA (BMT CTN 1502): A multicentre, single-arm, phase 2 trial. *The Lancet Haematology, 9*(9), e660–e669. https://doi.org/10.1016/s2352-3026(22)00206-x

Duarte, L. R. F., Pinho, V., Rezende, B. M., & Teixeira, M. M. (2022). Resolution of inflammation in acute graft-versus-host-disease: Advances and perspectives. *Biomolecules, 12*(1), 75. https://doi.org/10.3390/biom12010075

Farhadfar, N., Kim, Y. S., Bo-Subait, S., Logan, B. R., Stefanski, H. E., Hsu, J. W., Panch, S. R., Confer, D. L., Liu, H. D., Badawy, S. M., Beitinjaneh, A., Diaz, M. A., Hildebrandt, G. C., Kelkar, A. H., Lazarus, H. M., Murthy, H. S., Preussler, J. M., Schears, R. M., Sharma, A., … Switzer, G. E. (2022). The impact of pre-apheresis health related quality of life on peripheral blood progenitor cell yield and donor's health and outcome: Secondary analysis of patient-reported outcome data from the RDSafe and BMT CTN 0201 clinical trials. *Biology of Blood and Marrow Transplantation, 28*(9), 603.e1–603.e7. https://doi.org/10.1016/j.jtct.2022.05.042

Fuchs, E. J., McCurdy, S. R., Solomon, S. D., Wang, T., Herr, M. M., Modi, D., Grunwald, M. R., Nishihori, T., Kuxhausen, M., Fingerson, S., McKallor, C., Bashey, A., Kasamon, Y. L., Bolon, Y., Saad, A., McGuirk, J. P., Paczesny, S., Gadalla, S. M., Marsh, S. G., … Petersdorf, E. W. (2022). HLA informs risk predictions after haploidentical stem cell transplantation with posttransplantation cyclophosphamide. *Blood, 139*(10), 1452–1468. https://doi.org/10.1182/blood.2021013443

Herasevich, S., Schulte, P. J., Hogan, W. J., Alkhateeb, H., Zhang, Z., White, B. A., Khera, N., Roy, V., Gajic, O., & Yadav, H. (2024). Lung injury prediction model in bone marrow transplantation: A multicenter cohort study. *American Journal of Respiratory and Critical Care Medicine, 209*(5), 543-552. https://doi.org/10.1164/rccm.202308-1524OC

Iqbal, K., Iqbal, A., Rathore, S. S., Ahmed, J., Ali, S. A., Farid, E., Hasanain, M., Azeem, Q., Qadar, L. T., Memon, F. R., & Azim, D. (2022). Risk factors for blood transfusion in cesarean section: A systematic review and meta-analysis. *Transfusion Clinique et Biologique, 29*(1), 3–10. https://doi.org/10.1016/j.tracli.2021.09.010

Ito, S., Pandya, A., Hauser, R. G., Krishnamurti, L., Stites, E., Tormey, C., Krumholz, H. M., Hendrickson, J. E., & Goshua, G. (2024). Decreasing alloimmunization-specific mortality in sickle cell disease in the United States: Cost-effectiveness of a shared transfusion resource. *American Journal of Hematology*. https://doi.org/10.1002/ajh.27211

Jacobs, J. M., & Booth, G. S. (2022). Blood shortages and changes to massive transfusion protocols: Survey of hospital practices during the COVID-19 pandemic. *Transfusion and Apheresis Science, 61*(1), 103297. https://doi.org/10.1016/j.transci.2021.103297

Kato, I., Sakaguchi, H., Kato, S., Sato, M., Noguchi, M., Yoshida, N., Koh, K., Koike, T., Yanagimachi, M., Kato, K., Takahashi, Y., Fujita, N., Sato, A., Hashii, Y., Tabuchi, K., Atsuta, Y., Morishima, S., & Kanda, J. (2022). Impact of human leukocyte antigen mismatch on outcomes after unrelated bone marrow transplantation in paediatric patients: A retrospective analysis by the JSTCT HLA working group. *British Journal of Haematology, 199*(3), 392–400. https://doi.org/10.1111/bjh.18425

Malagola, M., Radici, V., Farina, M., Pellizzeri, S., Spoldi, F., Morello, E., Polverelli, N., Buttini, E. A., Bernardi, S., Re, F., Leoni, A., Signorini, L., Caruso, A., & Russo, D. (2024). CMV prophylaxis with letermovir significantly improves graft and relapse free survival following allogeneic stem cell transplantation. *Bone Marrow Transplantation, 59*(1), 138-140. https://doi.org/10.1038/s41409-023-02124-y

Mangada, K. L., Moffet, J., Nishitani, M., Albuquerque, S., & Duncan, C. N. (2022). Interprofessional team-based care of the hematopoietic cell transplantation patient with hepatic veno-occlusive disease/sinusoidal obstruction syndrome. *Journal of Pediatric Hematology Oncology, 45*(1), 12–17. https://doi.org/10.1097/mph.0000000000002594

Mitrus, I., Wilkiewicz, M., Fidyk, W., Ciomber, A., Smagur, A., Glowala-Kosinska, M., Chwieduk, A., Borzdzilowska, P., Sobczyk-Kruszelnicka, M., Mendrek, W., Najda, J., Czerw, T., & Giebel, S. (2022). The impact of blood donation on bone marrow harvest efficiency. *Bone Marrow Transplantation, 57*(3), 507–509. https://doi.org/10.1038/s41409-022-01573-1

Myers, D. J., & Collins, R. A. (2022). *Blood donation*. In *StatPearls* [Internet]. StatPearls Publishing.

Parida, L., Jahan, A., & Singh, S. (2024). Quality Control in Blood Transfusion Services. In *Clinical Laboratory Management* (pp. 161-167). Cham: Springer Nature Switzerland.

Stramer, S. L., Lanteri, M. C., Brodsky, J. P., Foster, G. D., Krysztof, D. E., Groves, J. A., Townsend, R. L., Notari, E. P., Bakkour, S., Stone, M., Simmons, G., Spencer, B. R., Tonnetti, L., & Busch, M. P. (2022). Mitigating the risk of transfusion-transmitted infections with vector-borne agents solely by means of pathogen reduction. *Transfusion, 62*(7), 1388–1398. https://doi.org/10.1111/trf.16950

Suddock, J. T., & Crookston, K. P. (2022). *Transfusion reactions*. In *StatPearls* [Internet]. StatPearls Publishing.

Sun, Z., Yao, B., Xie, H., & Su, X. (2022). Clinical progress and preclinical insights into umbilical cord blood transplantation improvement. *Stem Cells Translational Medicine, 11*(9), 912–926. https://doi.org/10.1093/stcltm/szac056

Wang, Y., Rao, Q., & Li, X. (2022). Adverse transfusion reactions and what we can do. *Expert Review of Hematology, 15*(8), 711–726. https://doi.org/10.1080/17474086.2022.2112564

Wolf, J., Lee, J., Pearce, R., Wilson, M., Snowden, J. A., & Orchard, K. (2022). The impact of COVID-19 on related-donor allogeneic stem cell harvest processes: A British Society of Blood and Marrow Transplantation and Cellular Therapy survey. *British Journal of Haematology, 198*(4), e51–e53. https://doi.org/10.1111/bjh.18299

Wongsa, C., Ghiyassi, N., Cornelius, M., Villamin, C., Tomczak, N., & Bates, T. (2022). A quality approach to reducing the occurrence of occluded leukocyte reduction filters during platelet transfusion. *Journal of Nursing Care Quality, 37*(1), 42–46. https://doi.org/10.1097/ncq.0000000000000573

UNIT

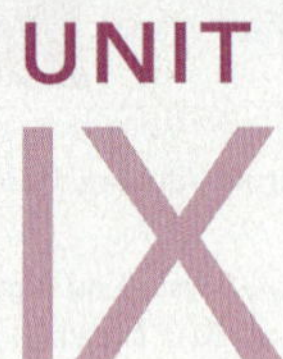

IMMUNOLOGIC HEALTH

24 Asthma and Allergy

OVERVIEW AND ASSESSMENT

See additional online content: Procedure Guidelines 24-1 to 24-2.

The Allergic Reaction

An allergic reaction results from antigen (Ag)–antibody (Ab) reaction on sensitized mast cells or basophils, causing the release of chemical mediators. The reaction may be characterized by inflammation, increased secretions, and bronchoconstriction.

Definitions

1. Ag—a protein that is found on the surface of a pathogen and stimulates an immune reaction, causing the production of antibodies.
2. Ab—immunoglobulin (Ig) (protein) secreted by B cells as a defense mechanism against foreign material, such as Ag.
3. Atopy—ability to produce IgE antibodies to common allergens. The genetic tendency to develop classic allergic disease or hypersensitivity reaction.
4. Immunity:
   a. Humoral—process by which B lymphocytes produce and secrete, circulating antibodies to act against Ags.
   b. Cell mediated—part of the immune system composed of T lymphocytes responsible for Ag-specific cell-mediated immunity (CMI) by activating cytotoxic T cells that identify infectious pathogens, such as virus, bacteria, fungi, and protozoan cells. Cell-mediated response also fights cancers.
5. Mast cell—type of white blood cell (WBC) tissue cell similar to peripheral blood basophil, which contains granules with chemical mediators. Known for its role in allergic and anaphylactic reactions.
6. Basophil—leukocyte with large granules that contain the vasodilator histamine and the anticoagulant heparin.
7. Histamine is a known mediator of allergic reactions, autoimmune conditions, and it also plays a role in gastric acid secretion and hematopoiesis.
8. Hypersensitivity—reaction to an Ag after reexposure; there are four types.
   a. Type I (immediate, IgE)—allergic reactions, such as atopy, anaphylaxis, asthma.
   b. Type IV (delayed, T cells mediated)—occurs 48 to 72 hours after exposure, as in contact dermatitis, tuberculin reaction, and transplant rejection (also considered allergic reaction).
   c. Type 2 (IgM, IgG Ab dependent)—autoimmune hemolytic anemia.
   d. Type 3 (IgG, IgM Ab dependent)—immune complex disease, such as rheumatoid arthritis.

Immunoglobulins

Antibodies that are formed by lymphocytes and plasma cells in response to an immunogenic stimulus comprise a group of serum proteins called *immunoglobulins.*

1. The abbreviation for immunoglobulin is Ig.
2. Antibodies combine with Ags in lock-and-key style.
3. There are five major classes of Igs.
   a. IgM—produced by B cells; constitutes 10% of Ig pool; found mostly in intravascular fluid and primarily engaged in initial defense; levels elevated with recent infection or exposure to Ag.
   b. IgG—major Ig that accounts for 70% to 75% of secondary immune responses and combats tissue infection.

c. IgA—15% to 20% of Igs; predominantly found in seromucous secretions (such as saliva, tears, sweat, and secretions from the gastrointestinal [GI] tract, genitourinary tract, prostate, and respiratory epithelium). It provides a primary defense mechanism.
d. IgD—less than 1% of Ig pool; found on circulating B lymphocytes, and signals B cells to become activated.
e. IgE—only a trace found in serum; attaches to surface membrane of basophils and mast cells; responsible for immediate types of allergic reactions (type 1 hypersensitivity).

Immunologic Reactions

Immediate Hypersensitivity (Type I)

1. Characterized by:
   a. IgE-mediated allergic reaction Mast cells and/or basophils (see Figure 24-1).
   b. Occurs immediately after contact with the Ag (early phase).
   c. Causes release and neo-synthesis of preformed chemical mediators.
   d. Late phase occurs 4 to 8 hours after allergen exposure and is caused by cytokines.
   e. Can occur secondary to medications.
2. Examples—anaphylaxis, allergic rhinitis, urticaria.

Products of Immediate Hypersensitivity (Chemical Mediators)

1. Histamine—bioactive amine stored in granules of mast cells and basophils.
2. Leukotrienes—newly synthesized potent bronchoconstrictors; cause increased venous permeability.
3. Prostaglandins—potent vasodilators and potent bronchoconstrictors.
4. Platelet-activating factor—has many properties; causes the aggregation of platelets.
5. Cytokines—control and regulate Ig functions (e.g., interleukins, tumor necrosis factor, and granulocyte monocyte colony-stimulating factor).
6. Proteases—enzymes, such as tryptase and chymase; increase vascular permeability.
7. Eosinophil chemotactic factor of anaphylaxis—causes an influx of eosinophils into the area of allergic inflammation (fevers, stomatitis, sepsis).
8. Examples—drug-induced hemolytic anemia, drug-induced thrombocytopenia, drug-induced neutropenia.

Effects of Chemical Mediators and Their Manifestations

1. Generalized vasodilation (histamine, nitric oxide, prostaglandin), hypotension, flushing.
2. Increased permeability (histamine, bradykinin, leukotrienes, among others).
   a. Capillaries of the skin—edema.
   b. Mucous membranes—edema.
3. Smooth muscle contraction.
   a. Bronchioles—bronchospasm.
   b. Intestines—abdominal cramps, diarrhea.
4. Increased secretions.
   a. Nasal mucous glands—rhinorrhea.
   b. Bronchioles—increased mucus in airways.
   c. GI—increased gastric secretions.
   d. Lacrimal—tearing.
   e. Salivary—salivation.
5. Pruritus (itching).
   a. Skin.
   b. Mucous membrane.

Delayed Hypersensitivity (Type IV)

1. Characterized by a cell-mediated reaction between Ags and Ag-responsive T lymphocytes (IgG, IgM).
2. Maximal intensity occurs between 24 and 48 hours.
3. Usually consists of erythema and induration.

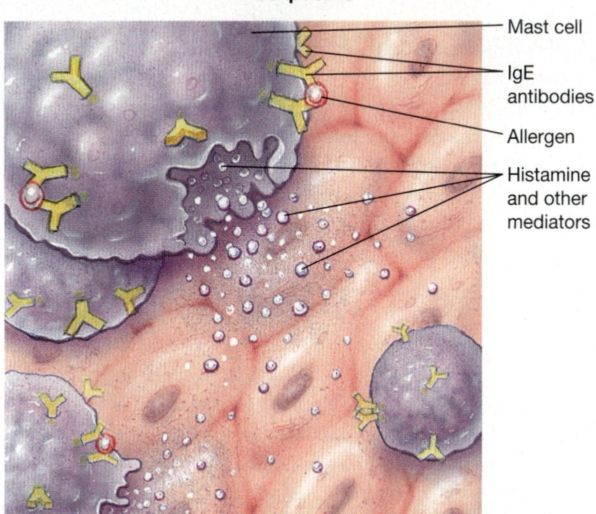

Figure 24-1. Type I immediate hypersensitivity. During the initial exposure, T cells recognize foreign allergens and release chemicals to instruct B cells to produce immunoglobulin (Ig) E. These antibodies attach themselves to mast cells. Upon reexposure, the allergen comes in contact with the IgE antibodies attached to mast cells, causing degranulation and release of chemical mediators. (Reprinted with permission from Stewart, J. G. [2017]. *Anatomical chart company atlas of pathophysiology* [4th ed.]. Lippincott Williams & Wilkins.)

4. Examples—tuberculin skin test, contact dermatitis such as poison ivy, Hashimoto thyroiditis, Stevens-Johnson syndrome.

Allergy Assessment

Subjective and Objective Data

1. Evaluate for symptoms related to hay fever, asthma, skin reactions, insect allergy, and food allergy.
2. Determine exacerbating factors such as contact with pets, outdoor exposure, seasonal allergies, contact with mold, exposure to dust.
3. Obtain complete medical history for past illnesses, medication allergies, family history, medications that have been tried, exercise, smoking, and work environment.
4. Perform physical examination based on patient presentation and specific allergy conditions, usually skin, head, chest, eye, ear, nose, and throat examination.

Skin Testing

The purpose of skin testing is to identify Ags responsible for immediate hypersensitivity. The types of skin tests used in clinical allergy are epicutaneous (prick, puncture, or scratch) and intradermal methods. The skin test remains unequaled as a sensitive, specific, and effective test for the diagnosis of allergies.

Epicutaneous (Prick) Method—Remains the First-Line Approach in Most Instances

1. Advantages:
   a. Efficient—results within 15 minutes.
   b. Little discomfort to the patient/relatively safe.
   c. Only rare instances of anaphylaxis because of minimal systemic absorption.
2. Disadvantages:
   a. Old or thick, leathery skin decreases reactivity.
   b. Lack of standardization and quantification.
   c. Drops have a tendency to run together, which would affect the accuracy of the test.

Intradermal Method

1. Advantages:
   a. Useful to confirm equivocal epicutaneous results with some Ags.
   b. Moderate sensitivity and reproducibility.
2. Disadvantages:
   a. Less specific than prick testing/subjective interpretation.
   b. Increased possibility for anaphylactic reactions.
   c. Requires more time and a higher level of technical expertise and interpretation to perform.
   d. Increased discomfort to the patient/variation in wheal size and erythema.

In Vitro Testing

Description

1. In vitro—using blood samples—tests for IgE antibodies to specific allergens. Instead of looking for a reaction in vivo (with the patient's body—as in skin testing), in vitro testing measures the IgE response to specific Ags added to blood samples.
2. Advantages over skin testing include the following:
   a. Can be done without special knowledge of skin testing or availability of allergen extract.
   b. Patient does not need to stop antihistamine before testing.
   c. Can be done even with severe eczema or other skin-related diseases.
   d. There is no risk of systemic anaphylactic reaction.
3. An immunofluorescent process is preferred for specific IgE testing because of the high degree of sensitivity and specificity.
4. Some laboratories may offer a radioallergosorbent test (RAST); measures the allergen-specific IgE antibodies in serum samples after panel of allergens has been added to samples.

Nursing and Patient Care Considerations

1. Tell the patient that it is allergy testing without the risk of causing a severe allergic reaction.
2. Obtain adequate venous blood for each allergen panel to be tested.
3. A positive result depends on the standards for that particular laboratory. The test does not indicate clinical significance of symptoms and must be interpreted with the patient's history.
4. Arrange for a follow-up visit for the patient with the health care provider to discuss test results.

GENERAL PROCEDURES AND TREATMENT MODALITIES

See additional online content: Procedure Guidelines 24-3.

Immunotherapy

Immunotherapy is the modulation of the immune system to develop tolerance to a known allergen that causes immunoglobulin E (IgE), type I (immediate) hypersensitivity. Given in appropriate doses, it can significantly decrease patient symptoms in most patients. It is indicated for significant symptoms of allergic rhinitis, allergic conjunctivitis, allergic asthma, and stinging insect allergy that cannot be controlled by avoidance of the allergen. Subcutaneous immunotherapy is recommended as an adjunct to standard pharmacotherapy in individuals who have demonstrated allergic sensitization and evidence of worsening asthma symptoms after they have been exposed to the offending antigen(s). Adherence and a considerable time commitment are essential for successful therapy.

Features of Immunotherapy

1. Specific allergens are identified by skin or blood testing.
2. Subcutaneous injections remain the gold standard; however, new approaches are being developed, which include sublingual immunotherapy and intralymphatic immunotherapy.
3. Serial injections are begun that contain extracts from identified allergens (allergy vaccine).
4. Initially, a small amount of dilute allergy vaccine is given, usually at weekly intervals.
5. Amount and concentration are slowly increased to maximum tolerable dose.
6. The maintenance dose is injected every 2 to 4 weeks for a period of several years to achieve maximal benefit.
7. Several allergens are now standardized (dust mite, cat, grass and ragweed pollens, Hymenoptera venoms [yellow jacket, yellow and white-faced hornet, honey bee, wasp]).

Precautions and Considerations

1. Anaphylaxis rarely occurs after injection, but risk remains.
   a. Usually given in health care facility with epinephrine, trained personnel, and emergency equipment available. See Standards of Care Guidelines 24-1, page 779.

STANDARDS OF CARE GUIDELINES 24-1

Immunotherapy

To perform immunotherapy or allergy testing, have epinephrine 1:1,000 available with a 1-mL syringe and a 1-in (2.5 cm) needle.

- Make sure that the patient remains under observation for at least 30 minutes after injection and assess for local reaction and respiratory distress before the patient leaves.
- If a significant reaction occurred after the last injection or if the patient is late for their dosage, follow written protocol for those cases or call the patient's health care provider for instructions.
- Be prepared to inject 0.3 to 0.5 mL (or 0.01 mL/kg for children less than 30 kg) of epinephrine intramuscular (IM) as directed by health care provider present or facility protocol if signs of anaphylaxis develop. Call for immediate help and transfer to an acute care facility.

This information should serve as a general guideline only. Each patient situation presents a unique set of clinical factors and requires nursing judgment to guide care, which may include additional or alternative measures and approaches.

   b. Patient should remain in office for 30 minutes after injection, after which the risk of anaphylaxis is greatly reduced.
   c. If large, local reaction (erythema, induration) occurs after an injection, the next dose should not be increased without checking with prescribing health care provider because a systemic reaction may occur.
2. If several weeks are missed, dosage may need to be decreased to prevent a reaction.
3. Medication, such as antihistamines and decongestants, should be continued until significant symptom relief occurs (may take 12 to 24 months).
4. Immunotherapy should not be administered to those with severe asthma. In addition, immunotherapy should not be initiated, increased, or given as maintenance while any individual has active asthma symptoms.
5. Environmental controls should be maintained to enhance the effectiveness of therapy.

CLINICAL JUDGMENT With immunotherapy (allergy shots), the risk of systemic reaction is always present, occurring in 0.02% of injections. Skin testing can also result in systemic reactions. Have epinephrine 1:1,000 available during these procedures (with syringe and tourniquet) and have the patient remain in office or clinic for at least 30 minutes after administration.

ALLERGIC DISORDERS

Anaphylaxis

Anaphylaxis is an immediate, life-threatening systemic reaction that can occur on exposure to a particular allergen. It can occur within an hour or longer. It is a result of a type I hypersensitivity reaction in which chemical mediators released from mast cells and basophils affect many types of tissue and organ systems. It can be an immunoglobulin E (IgE)-mediated allergen such as immunotherapy or a non–IgE-mediated allergen as in contrast media.

EVIDENCE BASE Curry, S. (2021). Managing anaphylaxis in adults. *British Journal of Nursing (Mark Allen Publishing)*, *30*(19), 1118–1122. https://doi.org/10.12968/bjon.2021.30.19.1118

Pathophysiology and Etiology

1. May be caused by:
   a. Immunotherapy.
   b. Stinging insects such as honeybee, Australian native ants, wasps.
   c. Skin testing.
   d. Medications, most commonly antibiotics, nonsteroidal anti-inflammatory drugs (NSAIDs), and chemotherapeutic agents.
   e. Contrast media infusion.
   f. Foods such as peanuts, tree nuts, seeds, cow's milk, seafood, dairy products, eggs.
   g. Exercise and exposure to cold.
   h. Latex.
   i. Idiopathic.
2. Mast cell activation causes the release of chemical mediators (histamine, leukotrienes, tumor necrosis factor, cytokines), which results in massive vasodilation, increased capillary permeability, smooth muscle contraction, and increased mucosal secretions, which results in bronchoconstriction and decreased peristalsis.

Clinical Manifestations

1. Respiratory—laryngeal edema, bronchospasm, hoarse voice cough, wheezing, stridor dyspnea, hypoxia, respiratory arrest.
2. Cardiovascular—hypotension, tachycardia (as a compensatory response to the hypotension), palpitations, syncope, bradycardia with cardiovascular collapse can occur before cutaneous changes occur.
3. Cutaneous—urticaria (hives), angioedema of deeper tissues: eyelids, lips, tongue, throat, pruritus, patchy erythema (flushing), generalized rash.
4. Gastrointestinal (GI)—nausea, vomiting, diarrhea, abdominal pain, bloating.

DRUG ALERT Before administering any drug, ask if the patient has ever had a reaction to it. Do not rely on the medical record alone.

Management

Prompt identification of signs and symptoms and immediate intervention are essential; a reaction that occurs quickly tends to be more severe.

Immediate Treatment

www.aaaai.org/conditions-and-treatments/allergies/anaphylaxis

1. Place the patient supine and check vital signs.
2. Immediately administer epinephrine 1:1,000—adolescents and adults, 0.3 to 0.5 mL; children, 0.01 mL/kg via intramuscular (IM) route into vastus lateralis muscle. This may be repeated after 5 minutes if no change in condition—causes vasoconstriction, decreases capillary permeability, relaxes airway smooth muscle, and inhibits mast cell mediator release. 1:1,000 intravenous (IV) epinephrine used only in an acute care setting.
3. Monitor vital signs continuously.
4. Administer high-flow oxygen, if needed.

5. A tourniquet is applied above the site of antigen injection (allergy injection, insect sting, etc.) or skin test site to slow the absorption of antigen into the system.

Subsequent Adjunct Treatment

1. An adequate airway is established, and bronchodilator (albuterol or salbutamol) is administered by nebulization (using face mask or handheld mouthpiece), as needed.
2. Hypotension and shock are treated with IV fluids (normal saline) and vasopressors.
3. Additional bronchodilators are given to relax bronchial smooth muscle.
4. Histamine-1 (H_1) antihistamines, such as diphenhydramine, and, possibly, H_2 antihistamines, such as ranitidine, are given to block the effects of histamine by relieving itching and urticaria.
5. Corticosteroids such as methylprednisolone are given to decrease vascular permeability and diminish the migration of inflammatory cells; may be helpful in preventing late-phase responses.

Complications

1. Cardiovascular collapse.
2. Respiratory failure.

Nursing Assessment

1. Promptly assess airway, breathing, and circulation (ABC) with severe presentation and intervene with cardiopulmonary resuscitation, as appropriate.
2. When ABCs are stable, assess vital signs, degree of respiratory distress, and angioedema.
3. Obtain a history of the onset of symptoms and exposure to allergen.

Nursing Interventions

Restoring Effective Breathing

1. Establish and maintain an adequate airway.
   a. If epinephrine has not stabilized bronchospasm, assist with endotracheal intubation, emergency tracheostomy, or cricothyroidotomy, as indicated.
   b. Continually monitor respiratory rate, depth, and breath sounds for decreased work of breathing and effective ventilation.
2. Administer nebulized albuterol or other bronchodilators, as ordered. Monitor heart rate (increased with bronchodilators).
3. Provide high-flow oxygen, as ordered.
4. Administer IV corticosteroids, as ordered.

Increasing Cardiac Output

1. Monitor blood pressure (BP) by continuous automatic cuff, if available.
2. Administer rapid infusion of IV fluids to fill vasodilated circulatory system and raise BP.
3. Monitor central venous pressure (CVP) to ensure adequate fluid volume and to prevent fluid overload.
4. Insert indwelling catheter and monitor urine output hourly to ensure kidney perfusion.
5. Initiate and titrate vasopressor, as ordered, based on BP response.

Reducing Anxiety

1. Provide care in a prompt, calm, and confident manner.
2. Remain responsive to the patient, who may remain alert but not completely coherent because of hypotension, hypoxemia, and effects of medication.
3. Keep family or significant others informed of patient's condition and the treatment being given.
4. When the patient is stable and alert, give a simple, honest explanation of anaphylaxis and the treatment that was given.

Community and Home Care Considerations

1. Make sure that the patient who has experienced anaphylaxis or severe local reactions obtains a prescription for self-injectable epinephrine to have available at all times.
2. Even if treatment is given successfully at home, encourage the patient to follow up with the health care provider immediately.
3. Make sure that the patient with a history of anaphylaxis has access to emergency medical system and does not spend time alone if the risk of reaction is present.

Patient Education and Health Maintenance

1. Teach the patient at risk for anaphylaxis about the potential seriousness of these reactions, avoiding allergens, and identifying early signs and symptoms of anaphylaxis.
2. Instruct the patient and family members on the injection technique upon exposure to known antigen or at the first signs of a systemic reaction.
   a. Provide the patient with information on epinephrine, including dose, drug action, possible adverse effects, and the importance of prompt administration at the first sign of a systemic reaction.
   b. Encourage the patient to check expiration date regularly and obtain replacement of outdated epinephrine.
   c. Ensure day care providers, coworkers, and school personnel are aware of the patient's potential for anaphylaxis and have access to and are able to administer epinephrine.
3. People allergic to venom stings should avoid wearing brightly colored or black clothes, perfumes, and hair spray. Shoes should be worn at all times.
4. For exercise-induced anaphylaxis, the patient should exercise in moderation, preferably with another person, and in a controlled setting, where assistance is readily available.
5. Instruct the patient to wear a medical alert tag at all times.
6. For potential drug allergies, teach the patient to:
   a. Read labels and be familiar with the generic name of the drug thought to cause a reaction.
   b. Discard all unused drugs. Make sure any drug kept in the medicine cabinet is clearly labeled.
   c. Become familiar with drugs that may cross-react with a drug to which the patient is allergic.
   d. Always know the name of every drug taken.
   e. Clear all herbals and nutraceuticals with health care provider.
7. Advise the patient with a known sensitivity to a food product to be extremely careful about everything they eat—allergen compounds may be hidden in a preparation (such as caseinate, lactalbumin).
8. Advise that if food is associated with exercise-induced anaphylaxis, wait at least 2 hours after eating to exercise.

Evaluation: Expected Outcomes

- Respirations unlabored with clear lung fields, minimal wheezing.
- BP and CVP within normal range; urine output adequate.
- Responsive and cooperative.

Allergic Rhinitis

Allergic rhinitis is an inflammation of the nasal mucosa caused by an allergen that affects 10% to 20% of the population and up to 40% of children.

Pathophysiology and Etiology

1. Type I hypersensitivity causes local vasodilation and increased capillary permeability.
2. Caused by airborne allergens.
3. IgE-mediated inflammatory process is now believed to be the same disease process for asthma and allergic rhinitis. IgE antibodies bind to IgE receptors on mast cells in respiratory mucosa. When the patient is exposed to the same allergen, then mast cells activate chemical mediators, resulting in allergic rhinitis.
4. Allergic rhinitis was formerly classified as seasonal or perennial; current classifications are intermittent or persistent.
   a. Intermittent—symptoms present less than 4 days per week and less than 4 weeks per year.
   b. Persistent—symptoms present more than 4 days per week and more than 4 weeks per year.
5. Severity is classified as mild (no interference with daily activities or troublesome symptoms) or moderate-severe (presence of at least one: impaired sleep, daily activity, work, or school; troublesome symptoms).

Clinical Manifestations

1. Nasal—mucous membrane congestion, edema, itching, rhinorrhea with clear secretions, paroxysmal sneezing, nasal obstruction, or nasal drip.
2. Eyes—edema, itching, burning, tearing, redness, dark circles under eyes (allergic shiners).
3. Ears—itching, fullness.
4. Other—postnasal drainage, palatal itching, throat itching, nonproductive cough.

Diagnostic Evaluation

1. Skin testing—confirms a hypersensitivity to certain allergens. Quick and cost-effective.
2. Nasal smear—increased number of eosinophils suggests allergic disease.
3. ImmunoCAP or other in vitro IgE-specific antigen testing—positive test result for offending allergens.
4. Rhinoscopy—allows better visualization of the nasopharynx; helps rule out physical obstruction (septal deviation, nasal polyps).
5. Evaluation for asthma.

Management

Avoidance

1. Patient should minimize contact with offending allergens, regardless of other treatment.
2. Patient may be instructed to reduce dust mite exposure by encasing bed pillows and mattress in allergen-proof covering; however, studies have not shown that this alone improves symptoms. Use of allergen-proof bedding should be carried out in conjunction with broad environmental controls (see Patient Education Guidelines 24-1).

Medications: Antihistamines

H_1 antihistamines—block the effects of histamine on smooth muscle and blood vessels by blocking histamine receptor sites, thereby preventing the symptoms of allergic rhinitis.

1. Loratadine, fexofenadine, and cetirizine are long-acting antihistamines sold over the counter (OTC) and are considered nonsedating (cetirizine is considered less sedating).
2. Long-acting, nonsedating antihistamines available by prescription include desloratadine and levocetirizine.
3. Topical antihistamine nasal spray available by prescription (azelastine or olopatadine).
4. Older, sedating antihistamines (diphenhydramine, chlorpheniramine) are inexpensive, available OTC, short acting, and effective if tolerated by the patient. Older antihistamines are sedating. They also have an anticholinergic effect—inhibit mucous secretions, act as drying agents.

Medications: Controllers

1. Intranasal corticosteroids: beclomethasone, flunisolide, budesonide, mometasone.
   a. Reduce inflammation of nasal mucosa.
   b. Prevent mediator release.

PATIENT EDUCATION GUIDELINES 24-1

Environmental Control for Allergic Rhinitis

The following environmental modifications may help reduce symptoms of allergic rhinitis (hay fever):

- Encase pillows and mattress in allergen-proof covers.
- Wash all bed linens (mattress pad, sheets, blanket, comforter, and bedspread) in hot water weekly.
- Keep clothing in a closet with door shut or in dresser drawers that are kept closed.
- Use easily cleaned shades, blinds, and curtains.
- Avoid stuffed animals and other items that collect dust.
- Vacuum and damp dust weekly; wear a mask while doing it.
- If you have severe symptoms of dust allergy, leave the house during cleaning. Allergic reaction is possible for about 30 minutes after vacuuming because dust mite feces and other allergens become airborne. Fine-filtering face masks may provide some protection.
- Eliminate upholstered furniture, carpets, and draperies.
- Use air conditioning and keep windows closed during high pollen and mold seasons to reduce antigen load indoors.
- Change furnace and air conditioner filters frequently.
- Using a high-efficiency air filtering system may help.
- Avoid smoking and smoke-filled areas.
- Avoid rapid changes in temperature.
- If you are allergic to animal dander, you should not have household pets. If pets are present in your household, keep them out of the bedroom and run a high-efficiency particulate air filter (place on table).
- Avoid mold growth by dehumidification (less than 45% ambient humidity) and use of a fungicide in bathrooms, damp basements, food storage areas, and garbage containers.
- Avoid outdoor activities when pollen or other pollutants are in the air.

c. Can be used safely every day.
d. May be given systemically for a short course during a disabling attack.

2. Mast cell stabilizers—such as intranasal cromolyn sodium or ophthalmic cromolyn and lodoxamide hinder the release of chemical mediators. These medications are used before and during allergen season.
3. Leukotriene receptor antagonists, including montelukast and zafirlukast, are systemic agents used for asthma; montelukast also has an indication in allergic rhinitis and reduces the inflammation, edema, and mucous secretion of allergic rhinitis.

Medications: Symptom Relief

1. Oral corticosteroids may be given systematically for a short course during a disabling attack.
2. Decongestants—shrink nasal mucous membrane by vasoconstriction; oral and topical, many available OTC and in combination with antihistamines, pain relievers, and anticholinergics.
3. Topical eye preparations—sold OTC and by prescription; reduce inflammation and relieve itching and burning.

Immunotherapy

1. Regimen consists of administering subcutaneous injections of increasing amounts of an allergen to which the patient is sensitive to decrease sensitivity and reduce the severity of symptoms (see page 778).
2. Immunotherapy produces the following immunologic changes:
   a. Production of IgG-blocking antibody that combines with antigen before it reacts with IgE antibodies.
   b. Decreases IgE antibodies against specific antigens.
   c. Modulation from T helper (Th) 2 to Th1 T lymphocytes (Th2 associated with allergy).
3. Possible adverse effects of immunotherapy.
   a. Systemic reactions—anaphylaxis is rare but potentially fatal.
   b. Local reactions—consist of erythema and induration at the site of injection.

CLINICAL JUDGMENT Immunotherapy should be administered with caution to patients taking beta-adrenergic blockers and should not be given to patients whose asthma is not controlled.

Complications

1. Allergic asthma.
2. Chronic otitis media, hearing loss.
3. Chronic nasal obstruction, nasal polyps, sinusitis.
4. Orthodontic malocclusion in children.

Nursing Assessment

1. Obtain a history of severity and seasonality of symptoms.
2. Inspect for characteristic tearing, conjunctival erythema, pale nasal mucous membranes with clear discharge, allergic shiners, and mouth breathing.
3. Auscultate lungs for wheezing or prolonged expiration characteristic of asthma.

Nursing Interventions

Facilitating Normal Breathing Pattern

1. Reassure the patient that suffocation will not occur because of nasal obstruction; mouth breathing will occur.
2. Use intranasal saline to soothe irritated mucous membranes and increase oral fluid intake to prevent drying of mucous membranes and increased insensible loss through mouth breathing.
3. Administer and teach self-administration of antihistamines, decongestants, intranasal corticosteroids and antihistamine, and other medications, as directed.
   a. Instruct the patients on the proper use of nasal sprays—clear mucus from nose first, exhale, flex neck to point nose downward, direct spray away from the nasal septum (toward the eye), activate the spray, and gently sniff while releasing medication. Report any nasal irritation or nose bleeds to provider.
   b. Warn the patient to avoid driving or other situations that require alertness if sedating antihistamines, such as diphenhydramine or chlorpheniramine, are being used.
   c. Do not use OTC nasal decongestants for more than 4 to 5 days because their effect is short term and a rebound effect, which causes nasal mucosal edema, commonly occurs.

DRUG ALERT Long-term use of nasal corticosteroids may cause nasal septum rupture. Teach the patients to direct spray or aerosol away from septum.

Patient Education and Health Maintenance

1. Provide information on purpose, administration method, time frame of expected results, and possible risks involved (local reactions, anaphylaxis) with immunotherapy.
2. Inform the patient that close observation for 30 minutes is essential after each injection.
3. Alert the patient to the possibility of a delayed reaction during immunotherapy that should be reported to the nurse or health care provider.
4. Teach lifestyle and environmental changes to reduce exposure to allergens.
5. For additional information and support, refer to the American Academy of Allergy, Asthma, and Immunology (www.aaaai.org), American College of Allergy, Asthma & Immunology (www.acaai.org), and National Institute of Allergy and Infectious Diseases Office of Communications (www.niaid.nih.gov).

Evaluation: Expected Outcomes

Decreased nasal congestion, no mouth breathing, and no complaints of dry mouth.

Urticaria and Angioedema

Urticaria, or hives, may affect 25% of the population at any given time. Lesion is intensely pruritic erythematous. *Angioedema* is a similar lesion but involves deep dermis and subcutaneous tissues. Urticaria and angioedema can occur either individually or in combination.

Pathophysiology and Etiology

1. Acute urticaria:
   a. Hives that last less than 6 weeks.
   b. A detectable cause is often determined.
2. Chronic urticaria:
   a. Hives that last 6 weeks or longer.
   b. Up to 50% of cases may be autoimmune chronic urticaria with autoantibodies against high-affinity IgE receptor or IgE.
   c. At least 50% are idiopathic.

3. Cause may be undetermined or may include:
   a. Ingested substances—food, food additives, latex, drugs (such as penicillins, cephalosporins, vaccinations).
   b. Infections—viral, bacterial, parasitic.
   c. Physical factors—heat, sunlight, cold, pressure, vibration.
   d. Emotional stress.
   e. Insect stings (bees, wasps, hornets, fire ants).

Clinical Manifestations

1. Raised, red, edematous wheals.
2. Intense pruritus.
3. May affect any body region.
4. Diffuse swelling with angioedema, especially of the lips, eyelids, cheeks, hands, and feet.
5. Symptoms may develop within seconds or over 1 to 2 hours and may last up to 24 to 36 hours.

Diagnostic Evaluation

1. Laboratory—serum tryptase is elevated in the acute phase, complement study results can be abnormal, total serum IgE elevated.
2. Challenge testing to determine physical cause.
   a. Dermographism (most common).
   b. Exercise challenge.
   c. Ice cube challenge.
   d. Heat challenge.
   e. Pressure challenge.

Management

Acute Urticaria

1. Identification and elimination of causative factors.
2. Medications.
   a. H_1 antihistamines, such as diphenhydramine and cetirizine.
   b. Corticosteroids—limited to severe cases; unresponsive to antihistamines.
   c. Epinephrine 1:1,000 (0.3 to 0.5 mL IM) for severe angioedema or urticaria.

Chronic Urticaria

1. Avoid causative factors.
2. Documentation of symptoms by patient to help identify triggers.
3. Medications.
   a. H_1 antihistamines.
   b. H_2 antihistamines, such as ranitidine, may be of some value.
   c. Tricyclic antidepressants, such as doxepin, given for antihistaminic effect.
   d. Topical agents to relieve itching (moisturizer or oatmeal baths).
4. Severe, unremitting urticarial treatment may include low-dose cyclosporine, tacrolimus, or omalizumab therapy.

Complications

1. Neurovascular impairment because of swelling.
2. Rarely, edema of the larynx or bronchi.

Nursing Assessment

1. Assess for time frame during which lesions appear and disappear.
2. Assess for triggering factors.
3. Assess for family history of angioedema; may indicate hereditary angioedema rather than allergic reaction.

Nursing Interventions

Relieving Pruritus

1. Administer or teach self-administration of antihistamines, corticosteroids, and additional medications, as prescribed.
2. Encourage the proper use of topical and OTC agents, as directed.
3. Advise the patient to avoid exposure to heat, exercise, sunburn, and alcohol and to promptly control fever and anxiety—factors that may aggravate reactions caused by vasodilation.
4. Warn the patient to avoid identified triggers.
5. Teach relaxation techniques and methods of distraction to enhance coping.
6. Assess the effectiveness of therapy.

Patient Education and Health Maintenance

1. Warn the patient to monitor for symptoms of laryngeal edema and to seek medical intervention immediately if respiratory distress occurs.
2. Instruct the patients with laryngeal edema how to self-administer epinephrine.

Evaluation: Expected Outcomes

- Reports relief of pruritus with antihistamines and distraction methods.

Food Allergies

Food allergies result when the body's immune system overreacts to certain, otherwise harmless, substances. Food allergies occur in 8% of children and in 2% of adults, although the perceived prevalence is much higher because other existing adverse food reactions cause similar symptoms. Symptoms may range from mild to severe, and in some cases, they may cause anaphylaxis.

Pathophysiology and Etiology

1. Food hypersensitivity—a true food allergy is an IgE-mediated response to a food allergen (protein).
2. Food intolerance—an abnormal physical response to a food or additive; may be immunologic, but not IgE mediated.
   a. Toxicity (poisoning)—caused by toxins contained in foods, microorganisms, or parasites.
   b. Metabolic—lactose intolerance.
   c. Pharmacologic (chemical)—such as caffeine.
   d. Idiosyncratic—etiology unknown.
3. Common food allergens include cow's milk, eggs, crustacean shellfish, fish, peanuts, tree nuts, soybean, and wheat.

Clinical Manifestations

1. Respiratory—rhinoconjunctivitis, sneezing, laryngeal edema, wheezing.
2. Cutaneous—urticaria, angioedema, atopic dermatitis.
3. Gastroenteritis—lip swelling, palatal itching, nausea, abdominal cramping, diarrhea, vomiting.
4. Neurologic—migraine headache in some patients.

Diagnostic Evaluation

1. Skin testing.
   a. Limited to those foods suspected of provoking symptoms based on history.

b. Only epicutaneous testing is recommended.
c. Intradermal testing has not been demonstrated to have a high degree of clinical correlation.
2. ImmunoCAP, radioallergosorbent test (RAST), or other IgE-specific antigen in vitro testing—positive result.
3. Oral challenge—the suspected food is given to the patient to identify the allergen by reproducing the symptoms caused by the initial reaction.
a. Open—may be used if the suspected food skin test result is negative; suspected food is openly administered, and the patient is monitored for a reaction.
b. Single blind—suspected food is disguised in capsules, liquids, or other foods and administered to the patient in increasing doses at intervals determined by history and may be interspersed with placebo. Some bias exists, however.
c. Double blind, placebo controlled—the "gold standard" and most definitive technique to confirm or refute food allergy. The suspected food is administered in capsules or via some other vehicle that masks its identity; it is interspersed with placebo so neither the health care provider nor the patient knows whether the suspected food or placebo is being ingested.
4. Elimination diet.
a. To determine whether the patient's symptoms will stop when certain foods are avoided.
b. Restrict one or two foods at a time if certain foods are suspected.
c. If no particular food is suspected, a highly restricted diet for 14 days is preferable.
d. May result in nutritional deficiencies if multiple foods are withheld.

Management

1. Avoidance of specific foods is the only way of effectively preventing food allergy reactions.
2. Medications:
a. Antihistamines—may modify IgE-mediated symptoms but will not eliminate them.
b. Corticosteroids—only used in the treatment of food allergy if associated with eosinophilic gastroenteritis or gastroenteropathy.
c. Epinephrine—if history of anaphylaxis, the patient should carry subcutaneous self-injection at all times.
3. Oral desensitization may be considered under careful observation.

Complications

Anaphylaxis.

Nursing Assessment

1. Assist with assessment for offending foods; encourage the patient to keep a food and symptom diary.
2. Auscultate lungs and document any wheezing.
3. Assess adherence with prescribed diet and relief of symptoms.

Nursing Interventions

Promoting Adequate Nutrition

1. Consult with dietitian to ensure a balanced diet that excludes identified allergens and incorporates the patient's food preferences.
2. Administer dietary supplements, as needed.
3. Discuss alternative food preparation techniques and methods of substitution (such as using extra baking powder in place of eggs).
4. Administer and teach self-administration of medications, if necessary, to reduce abdominal cramping and diarrhea, which may deter food intake.
5. Monitor weight.

Patient Education and Health Maintenance

1. Instruct the patient with a history of anaphylactic reaction about self-injection technique for the administration of epinephrine.
2. Caution highly allergic patient about restaurant food; when eating out, avoid buffets and the patient should request ingredient information; brochures listing ingredients of various dishes are now available in many restaurants, including fast-food establishments.
3. Explain hidden sources of foods to decrease the risk of unexpected exposure to an offending allergen. Some foods may contain allergens not as primary ingredients but as fillers or additives. Likewise, a food that has been prepared or stored in the same container or cooled on the same surface as an allergen-containing food may become contaminated with a sufficient quantity of the allergen to cause a reaction. Encourage label reading.
4. Advise the patient that most young children and about one third of older children and adults lose their food sensitivity after several years of avoidance. Adherence with elimination of these foods from the diet is the key. Sensitivity to shellfish and nuts is rarely lost, however.
5. Provide resource for patient to obtain more information: The Food Allergy & Anaphylaxis Network (www.foodallergy.org).

Evaluation: Expected Outcomes

Decreased frequency and severity of food allergy reactions by log; verbalizes acceptance of diet; weight stable.

Latex Sensitivity

Latex sensitivity is becoming a major health concern for health care workers, patients, and others at risk by occupation. Allergic reaction may be immediate or delayed. Latex is present in approximately 40,000 medical and other products, including household products and toys. The prevalence of latex sensitivity is estimated to be 1% in the general population, 25% in nurses, and is higher among children with spina bifida and other congenital anomalies, such as esophageal atresia, neurologic diseases, and cerebral palsy.

Pathophysiology and Etiology

1. Natural rubber latex, manufactured from the sap of rubber trees, is highly irritating and allergenic in some people.
2. Increased use of latex, in the form of sterile and unsterile gloves, has made latex sensitivity a problem for many health care workers since the inception of Universal Precautions (now called *standard precautions*) in the 1980s.
3. Three types of reactions to latex may occur:
a. Irritant dermatitis—not an allergic reaction.
b. Type IV (cell mediated, delayed) hypersensitivity—a localized contact allergic reaction.

   c. Type I (IgE mediated, immediate)—a systemic allergic reaction.
4. No predictable pattern exists for the progression of reactions; anaphylaxis may occur at any time. More severe reaction occurs with latex contact with mucous membrane than with intact skin.
5. Those at risk include children with spina bifida, health care workers, people with atopic allergies, people with a history of multiple surgeries, and workers in factories that produce latex products.

Clinical Manifestations

1. Irritant dermatitis—may be caused by powder or chemical residue on gloves; erythema and pruritus localized to area of contact; occurs immediately.
2. Type IV (delayed) hypersensitivity—contact allergic reaction; erythema, pruritus, urticaria; possible flushing, localized edema, rhinitis, coughing, and conjunctivitis. Symptoms occur 1 to 48 hours after contact with product.
3. Type I (immediate) hypersensitivity—urticaria, angioedema, conjunctivitis, dyspnea, pharyngeal edema, arrhythmias, and anaphylaxis. Symptoms are immediate and may be moderate to life-threatening in intensity.
4. Latex-fruit syndrome—40% of patients with latex allergy are also known to have a cross-reactivity with food allergens (banana, avocado, chestnut, and kiwifruit).

Diagnostic Evaluation

1. History of symptoms gives presumptive diagnosis, but confirmation is difficult because standardized tests are not yet widely available. History should include the presence or absence of other allergies or prior medical procedures involving latex products.
2. A crude skin prick test uses a fragment of latex glove soaked in saline for 15 minutes as the solution. This is not standardized, but a positive test result is considered proof of latex sensitivity.
3. A challenge test can be done by having the patient wear a latex glove or fingertip of a glove for 15 minutes; look for a reaction. Latex-free gloves can be used as a control. Severe reactions may occur with this test.
4. Standardized skin testing will become more available pending Food and Drug Administration (FDA) approval of standardized latex solution, but the threat of anaphylaxis will still exist.
5. RAST or other IgE in vitro blood testing is safe but expensive and is limited due to both false-positive and false-negative results. Serologic tests have a sensitivity of 70% to 80%.

Management

1. Avoidance is the key. See Box 24-1 for safety and prevention techniques in the health care workplace.
2. For irritant reactions, changing brands of gloves or changing to a powder-free glove may be sufficient.
3. Decreasing length of exposure time or wearing cotton liners in gloves may help, but may not solve the problem.
4. Use of latex-free gloves and products is usually necessary. Although more hospitals and medical offices are making latex-free products available, a job change may be necessary for some people.
5. A latex-free environment is necessary for treatment.
6. Topical corticosteroid creams may be used for local reactions.

BOX 24-1 Latex Safety for Patients and Health Care Workers

- Use latex-free gloves of synthetic rubber, vinyl, nitrile, neoprene, or other material.
- Be aware that removing latex gloves with power may cause latex particles to become aerosolized for up to 5 hours and be carried to other areas on clothing and equipment.
- Do not enter operating room with latex gloves or without having scrubbed after removing latex gloves in another area and remove possibly latex-laden clothing.
- Schedule patients who are latex-sensitive early in the day or as the first surgical case.
- Post signs indicating Latex Allergy or Latex Alert.
- Encourage latex-sensitive individuals to wear identification bracelets.
- Evaluate all equipment for latex prior to use.
- A latex-free cart should accompany a patient who is latex-sensitive throughout the facility.
- Each facility should form a latex allergy task force with representatives from all departments.

7. Oral antihistamines may be used for mild-to-moderate reactions.
8. Epinephrine, oral or parenteral corticosteroids, and IM antihistamines are given for severe reactions.
9. IV fluids, oxygen, and intubation may be needed for cardiovascular and pulmonary support with severe reactions.

Complications

Unpredictable anaphylaxis and death.

Nursing Assessment

1. Assess the patient for a history of risk factors and pattern of suspected reactions.
2. Assess skin for erythema, swelling, vesicles, and other lesions.
3. Assess mucous membranes for conjunctivitis, rhinitis, and other lesions.
4. For suspected systemic reactions, assess vital signs for hypotension, tachycardia, arrhythmia, and respiratory distress.
5. Assess respiratory status for stridor caused by laryngeal edema and breath sounds for wheezing.
6. Assess for signs of internal edema with systemic reaction, such as nausea, vomiting, and diarrhea.

Nursing Interventions and Patient Education

Increasing Knowledge About Latex Avoidance

1. Educate patients about the widespread use of latex; latex-free alternatives are usually available (see Table 24-1).
2. Ensure that patients with a history of type I reaction have self-injectable epinephrine and antihistamines on hand at all times to use at first sign of a reaction.
3. Encourage patients who have had immediate hypersensitivity reactions to wear a medical alert tag.
4. Encourage patients to notify all their health care providers, labs, and clinics before they make a visit, to facilitate the use of latex-free products. These patients should be given the first appointment of the day, and all supplies that contain latex should be removed from the room or covered with a cotton

Table 24-1 Sources of Latex in Health Care Facilities and at Home

HEALTH CARE FACILITY	HOME AND COMMUNITY
Syringes	Mattresses and foam in furniture
Medication vial stoppers	Undergarments and clothing
Intravenous catheters, tubing	Bathmats and rugs
Stopcocks	Pacifiers and diapers
Tourniquet	Toys such as balls and dolls
Tape, dressings, drains	Pet toys
Elastic wraps	Bicycle helmets
Waterproof pads	Cosmetics
Blood pressure cuff	Food storage bags
Stethoscope	Drain stoppers
Reflex hammer	Spatulas
Electrocardiograph electrodes	Earphones
Oximetry sensor	Garden hose
Manual resuscitation bag	Rubber handled tools
Oxygen cannula, mask, tubing	Weather stripping
Airways, endotracheal tube	Plants—rubber, poinsettia, ficus
Urinary catheters	Scratch-off tickets and advertisements
Suction catheters	Raincoats and waterproof boots
Casting materials	Glue, envelopes, stamps

cloth. Only latex-free products should be used, and staff members should be careful to avoid wearing or removing latex gloves in the hall while the patient is in the office.

5. Support the patient who has had a severe reaction in the workplace. Remind the patient that the Americans with Disabilities Act guarantees workers reasonable modifications to the workplace to accommodate a disability. However, the area of latex sensitivity as a disability is controversial.
6. For further information, contact the American Latex Allergy Association (www.latexallergyresources.org) and the National Institute for Occupational Safety and Health (www.cdc.gov/NIOSH/homepage.html).

Evaluation: Expected Outcomes

- Verbalizes signs of reaction and appropriate treatment.

Bronchial Asthma

EVIDENCE BASE Expert Panel Working Group of the National Heart, Lung, and Blood Institute (NHLBI) administered and coordinated National Asthma Education and Prevention Program Coordinating Committee (NAEPPCC), Cloutier, M. M., Baptist, A. P., Blake, K. V., Brooks, E. G., Bryant-Stephens, T., DiMango, E., Dixon, A. E., Elward, K. S., Hartert, T., Krishnan, J. A., Lemanske, R. F., Jr., Ouellette, D. R., Pace, W. D., Schatz, M., Skolnik, N. S., Stout, J. W., Teach, S. J., Umscheid, C. A., & Walsh, C. G. (2020). 2020 focused updates to the asthma management guidelines: A report from the National Asthma Education and Prevention Program Coordinating Committee Expert Panel Working Group. *The Journal of Allergy and Clinical Immunology, 146*(6), 1217–1270. https://doi.org/10.1016/j.jaci.2020.10.003

Mauer, Y., & Taliercio, R. M. (2020). Managing adult asthma: The 2019 GINA guidelines. *Cleveland Clinic Journal of Medicine, 87*(9), 569–575. https://doi.org/10.3949/ccjm.87a.19136

Asthma is a chronic inflammatory disease of the airways, characterized by airflow obstruction, which is at least partially reversible; bronchial hyperreactivity; and mucus production. The course of asthma is highly variable. In 2020, focused updates to the asthma management guidelines: A report from the National Asthma Education and Prevention Program Coordinating Committee Expert Panel Working Group and in 2019 the Global Initiative for Asthma guidelines were updated. These updates are evidence based and continue to recommend treatment that is stepwise and based on severity. These updates address six priority areas, including fractional exhaled nitric oxide testing, indoor allergen mitigation, intermittent inhaled corticosteroids (ICSs), long-acting muscarinic antagonists, immunotherapy in the treatment of allergic asthma, and bronchial thermoplasty. Although severity is best established prior to the use of asthma medications, it may be determined based on the medications necessary to gain control and directs initial therapy.

Asthma therapy is characterized by periodic follow-up visits and continual reassessment. One such factor that is always assessed includes control, which can be measured at home by the patient and family and evaluated and discussed at subsequent visits. The level of control guides adjustment of medications. Nurses can use control assessment to identify patients and families who need more asthma education to gain better control of asthma. In addition, before the escalation of treatment, clinicians should assess whether the patient is consistently and correctly utilizing the prescribed medication regimen and have reduced modifiable triggers. Barriers such as lack of access and financial ability should also be determined prior to escalation of therapy.

Pharmacotherapy for asthma is now based on three age groups: ages 0 to 4 years, ages 5 to 11 (see Chapter 44), and ages 12 and older. It is composed of multiple steps and has expanded to include more medications for asthma, ICSs are now recommended for all patients with asthma taken daily or as needed.

Pathophysiology and Etiology

The basic defect appears to be an abnormality in the host, which intermittently leads to an increased constriction of smooth muscle, hypersecretion of mucus in the bronchial tree, and mucosal edema.

Neuromechanisms (Autonomic Nervous System)

1. Stimulation of the vagus nerve (which is responsible for bronchomotor tone) by viral respiratory infections, air pollutants, and other stimuli causes bronchoconstriction, increased secretion of mucus, and dilation of the pulmonary vessels.
2. Beta-adrenergic receptor cells that line the airways are also responsible for bronchomotor tone. Abnormal functioning of these cells predisposes patients to bronchoconstriction.

Antigen–Antibody Reaction

1. Susceptible individuals form abnormally large amounts of IgE when exposed to certain allergens. Most children and more than half of adults with asthma are sensitized to at least one common inhaled allergen.

2. Antigen-specific IgE fixes itself to the mast cells of the bronchial mucosa.
3. When the person is exposed to certain allergens, the resulting antigen combines with the cell-bound IgE molecules, causing the mast cell and basophil to degranulate and release chemical mediators.
4. These chemical mediators act on bronchial smooth muscle to cause bronchoconstriction, on dilated epithelium to reduce mucociliary clearance, on bronchial glands to cause mucus secretion, on blood vessels to cause vasodilation and increased permeability, and on leukocytes to cause cellular infiltration and inflammation.
5. Late-phase reactions (these occur 4 to 8 hours after the initial response) include the influx of eosinophils, neutrophils, lymphocytes, and monocytes.

Bronchial Inflammation

1. Occurs in both the immediate- and late-phase reactions caused by antigen–antibody response.
2. Factors other than allergens (such as noxious environmental stimuli) cause bronchial inflammation and hyperreactivity by mast cell activation.

Classification

Extrinsic Asthma

1. Hypersensitivity reaction to inhalant allergens (dust mites, animal allergens, cockroaches, pollen, and mold are the major ones).
2. Mediated by IgE.

Intrinsic Asthma

1. No inciting allergen.
2. Infection, typically viral.
3. Environmental stimuli (such as air pollution).

Mixed Asthma

Immediate type I reactivity appears to be combined with intrinsic factors.

Aspirin-Induced Asthma

1. Induced by ingestion of aspirin and related compounds.
2. "Samter Triad" has been described as a combination of aspirin-induced asthma, nasal polyps, and sinusitis.

Exercise-Induced Bronchoconstriction

Symptoms vary from slight chest tightness and cough to severe wheezing and cough and shortness of breath that usually occurs after 5 to 20 minutes of sustained exercise.

Occupational Asthma

Caused by inhalation of industrial fumes, dust, allergens, and gases.

Classification by Severity

1. Asthma severity for purposes of treatment is classified as intermittent, mild persistent, moderate persistent, and severe persistent based on the level of impairment and risk for exacerbation.
2. Level of impairment parameters include degree of symptoms, nighttime awakenings, need to use short-acting beta$_2$-agonist for symptom control, interference with normal activity, and lung function by spirometry.
3. Risk level is based on the number of exacerbations that required oral corticosteroids within the past year and how severe they were.

See details of classifying asthma severity at https://www.nhlbi.nih.gov/files/docs/guidelines/asthma_qrg.pdf

Clinical Manifestations

1. Episodes of coughing.
2. Wheezing.
3. Dyspnea.
4. Feeling of chest tightness.

CLINICAL JUDGMENT Lack of wheezing on auscultation when the patient reports severe shortness of breath may indicate that airflow may be so restricted that wheezing ceases.

Diagnostic Evaluation

1. Pulmonary function testing (spirometry)—more than 12% increase over baseline in forced expiratory volume in first second of exhalation (FEV_1) following inhalation of bronchodilator. Peak flow more than 20% variability between a.m. and p.m. measurements.
2. Bronchial challenge with airborne agent resulting in airway hyperreactivity; a positive challenge is determined by a decrease in FEV_1 from baseline.
   a. Methacholine bronchial challenge (nebulized)—20% decrease in FEV_1.
   b. Mannitol (dry powder inhalation)—15% decrease in FEV_1.
3. Skin testing to identify causative allergens.
4. Fractional exhaled nitric oxide testing—nitric oxide is measured in exhaled breath and can serve as a measure of the level of airway inflammation. In individuals with asthma, fractional exhaled nitric oxide testing may be indicative of the type of asthma present. The following is a statement from the 2020 updates to asthma guidelines regarding this mode of testing: "In individuals ages 5 years and older for whom the diagnosis of asthma is uncertain using history, clinical findings, clinical course, and spirometry, including bronchodilator responsiveness testing, or in whom spirometry cannot be performed, the Expert Panel conditionally recommends the addition of FeNO measurement as an adjunct to the evaluation process."
5. Chest x-ray to exclude other lung diseases in new-onset asthma in adult.

Management

The goal is to allow the person with asthma to live a normal life. The treatment plan should be as simple as possible and individualized to the patient's lifestyle. See Figure 24-2 for stepwise therapy for those aged 12 years and older; see pages 788 and 789, for stepwise therapy for children younger than age 12. See Table 24-2, pages 789 and 790, and Table 24-3, page 790, for medication information. For additional information on treatment and specific dosages, see https://www.nhlbi.nih.gov/files/docs/guidelines/asthma_qrg.pdf

Long-Term Controllers

1. ICSs, such as beclomethasone, budesonide, ciclesonide, flunisolide, fluticasone, mometasone.
2. Long-acting inhaled beta-agonists (LABAs) include salmeterol, formoterol. *Note:* Arformoterol is a LABA that is indicated for long-term control of chronic obstructive pulmonary disease, not asthma.
3. Combination inhalers, such as fluticasone and salmeterol, budesonide and formoterol, mometasone and formoterol.

	Intermittent Asthma	Management of Persistent Asthma in Individuals Aged 12+ Years				
Treatment	**STEP 1**	**STEP 2**	**STEP 3**	**STEP 4**	**STEP 5**	**STEP 6**■
Preferred	PRN SABA	Daily low-dose ICS and PRN SABA or PRN concomitant ICS and SABA▲	Daily and PRN combination low-dose ICS-formoterol▲	Daily and PRN combination medium-dose ICS-formoterol▲	Daily medium-high dose ICS-LABA + LAMA and PRN SABA▲	Daily high-dose ICS-LABA + oral systemic corticosteroids + PRN SABA
Alternative		Daily LTRA* and PRN SABA or Cromolyn,* or Nedocromil,* or Zileuton,* or Theophylline,* and PRN SABA	Daily medium-dose ICS and PRN SABA or Daily low-dose ICS-LABA, or daily low-dose ICS + LAMA,▲ or daily low-dose ICS + LTRA,* and PRN SABA or Daily low-dose ICS + Theophylline* or Zileuton,* and PRN SABA	Daily medium-dose ICS-LABA or daily medium-dose ICS + LAMA, and PRN SABA▲ or Daily medium-dose ICS + LTRA,* or daily medium-dose ICS + Theophylline,* or daily medium-dose ICS + Zileuton,* and PRN SABA	Daily medium-high dose ICS-LABA or daily high-dose ICS + LTRA,* and PRN SABA	
		Steps 2–4: Conditionally recommend the use of subcutaneous immunotherapy as an adjunct treatment to standard pharmacotherapy in individuals ≥ 5 years of age whose asthma is controlled at the initiation, buildup, and maintenance phases of immunotherapy ▲			Consider adding asthma biologics (e.g., anti-IgE, anti-IL5, anti-IL5R, anti-IL4/IL13)**	

Assess Control

- First check adherence, inhaler technique, environmental factors,▲ and comorbid conditions.
- **Step up** if needed; reassess in 2–6 weeks.
- **Step down** if possible (if asthma is well controlled for at least 3 consecutive months).

Consult with asthma specialist if Step 4 or higher is required. Consider consultation at Step 3.

Control assessment is a key element of asthma care. This involves both impairment and risk. Use of objective measures, self-reported control, and health care utilization are complementary and should be employed on an ongoing basis, depending on the individual's clinical situation.

Abbreviations: ICS, inhaled corticosteroid; IgE, immunoglobulin E; IL4, interleukin-4; LABA, long-acting beta2-agonist; LAMA, long-acting muscarinic antagonist; LTRA, leukotriene receptor antagonist; PRN, as needed; SABA, inhaled short-acting beta2-agonist.

Figure 24-2. Stepwise approach for managing asthma in youths aged 12 years or older and adults. (Reprinted from Expert Panel Working Group of the National Heart, Lung, and Blood Institute [NHLBI] administered and coordinated National Asthma Education and Prevention Program Coordinating Committee [NAEPPCC], Cloutier, M. M., Baptist, A. P., Blake, K. V., Brooks, E. G., Bryant-Stephens, T., DiMango, E., Dixon, A. E., Elward, K. S., Hartert, T., Krishnan, J. A., Lemanske, R. F., Jr., Ouellette, D. R., Pace, W. D., Schatz, M., Skolnik, N. S., Stout, J. W., Teach, S. J., Umscheid, C. A., & Walsh, C. G. [2020]. 2020 focused updates to the asthma management guidelines: A report from the National Asthma Education and Prevention Program Coordinating Committee Expert Panel Working Group. *The Journal of Allergy and Clinical Immunology, 146*[6], 1217–1270. https://doi.org/10.1016/j.jaci.2020.10.003)

4. Leukotriene modifiers, such as montelukast; limited availability for use in the United States and may have an increased risk of adverse consequences or required testing that makes their use less desirable. Boxed warning issued in 2020 for montelukast by the FDA.
5. Long-acting oral beta-agonists, such as albuterol extended-release tablets.
6. Oral corticosteroids (maintenance dose).
7. Long-acting muscarinic antagonist (LAMA), namely, tiotropium, as an adjunct therapy.
8. An IgE blocker (omalizumab) can be added to standard maintenance therapy to reduce exacerbations in moderate-to-severe allergic asthma.
   a. It is given by subcutaneous injection every 2 to 4 weeks.
   b. The most common adverse reactions are injection site reactions and viral infection.
9. The most convenient and inexpensive method of aerosol delivery to patients is the metered-dose inhaler (MDI) or dry powder inhaler; however, nebulization offers alternative delivery for those with unreliable inhaler technique.

Table 24-2 Long-Term Control Medications

DRUG/INDICATION	MECHANISM	POTENTIAL ADVERSE EFFECTS
Inhaled Corticosteroids		
Beclomethasone, budesonide, flunisolide, ciclesonide, fluticasone, mometasone *Indications:* In individuals aged 12 yr and older with mild persistent asthma, conditional recommendation of a daily low-dose ICS and an as-needed SABA for quick relief therapy or as-needed ICS and SABA used concurrently. In individuals aged 12 yr and older (already taking low- or medium-dose ICS) with moderate-to-severe persistent asthma, conditional recommendation ICS-formoterol in a single inhaler as daily controller and reliever therapy.	*Anti-inflammatory:* Block late reaction to allergen and reduce airway hyperresponsiveness; inhibit cytokine production, adhesion protein activation, and inflammatory cell migration and activation. Reverse β_2-receptor downregulation. Inhibit microvascular leakage.	Cough, dysphonia, oral candidiasis. In high doses, systemic effects may occur (adrenal suppression, osteoporosis, skin thinning, easy bruising), although studies are not conclusive, and clinical significance has not been established. In low to medium doses, suppression of growth velocity has been observed in children, but this effect may be transient, and the clinical significance has not been established. Individuals taking ICS-salmeterol as maintenance therapy should not take ICS-formoterol as reliever therapy.
Systemic Corticosteroids		
Methylprednisolone, prednisolone, prednisone *Indications:* Short-term burst therapy to gain control of inadequately controlled asthma; long-term prevention of symptoms in severe persistent asthma.	*Anti-inflammatory:* Block late reaction to allergen and reduce airway hyperresponsiveness; inhibit cytokine production, adhesion protein activation, and inflammatory cell migration and activation. Reverse β_2-receptor downregulation. Inhibit microvascular leakage.	Short-term use: Reversible abnormalities in glucose metabolism, increased appetite, fluid retention, weight gain, mood alteration, hypertension, peptic ulcer, and, rarely, aseptic necrosis. Long-term use: Adrenal axis suppression, growth suppression, dermal thinning, hypertension, diabetes, Cushing syndrome, cataracts, muscle weakness, and, rarely, impaired immune function. Consideration should be given to coexisting conditions that could be worsened by systemic corticosteroids, such as herpes virus infections, varicella, tuberculosis, hypertension, peptic ulcer, diabetes mellitus, osteoporosis, and *Strongyloides*.
Mast Cell Stabilizers		
Immunotherapy		
Omalizumab *Indications:* Conditional recommendation as an adjunct treatment to standard pharmacotherapy in individuals ≥ 5 yr of age whose is asthma is controlled at the initiation, buildup, and maintenance phases of immunotherapy.	Binds to circulating IgE, preventing it from binding to high-affinity receptors on basophils and mast cells. Decreases mast cell mediator release from allergen exposure and the number of high-affinity receptors in basophils and submucosal cells.	Pain and bruising at injection sites have been reported in 45% of patients. Anaphylaxis has been reported in 0.2% of treated patients. Malignant neoplasms have been reported in 0.5% of patients compared to 0.2% of patients receiving placebo; however, relationship to drug is unlikely.
Leukotriene Modifiers		
zafirlukast *Indications:* Long-term control and prevention of symptoms in mild persistent asthma; may be used in combination with ICS in moderate persistent asthma. zafirlukast, > age 7.	*Leukotriene receptor antagonist* (zafirlukast): Selective competitive inhibitors of CysLT1 receptor.	With zafirlukast, cases of reversible hepatitis and, rarely, irreversible hepatic failure resulting in liver transplantation and death.
Long-Acting β_2-Agonists		
Formoterol, salmeterol, oral sustained-release albuterol *Indications:* Long-term prevention of symptoms, added to ICS; prevention of exercise-induced bronchospasm. *Note:* Not to be used to treat acute exacerbations; only used in combination with ICA.	*Bronchodilation:* Smooth muscle relaxation following adenylate cyclase activation and increase in cyclic AMP, producing functional antagonism of bronchoconstriction. Compared to SABA, salmeterol (but not formoterol) has slower onset of action (15–30 min). Both salmeterol and formoterol have longer duration (>12 h) compared to SABA.	Tachycardia, skeletal muscle tremor, hypokalemia, prolongation of QTc interval in overdose. A diminished bronchoprotective effect may occur within 1 wk of chronic therapy (clinical significance has not been established). Potential risk of severe, life-threatening, or fatal exacerbation.

(*continued*)

Table 24-2 Long-Term Control Medications (*continued*)

DRUG/INDICATION	MECHANISM	POTENTIAL ADVERSE EFFECTS
Long-Acting Muscarinic Antagonists (Tiotropium Bromide) *Indications:* • In individuals with uncontrolled, persistent asthma, age 12 yr and older there is a conditional recommendation against adding LAMA to ICS compared to combining a LABA to ICS therapy. • In individuals aged 12 yr and older with uncontrolled persistent asthma where a LABA is not used there is a conditional recommendation to add LAMA to ICS controller therapy when compared to continuing the same dose of ICS alone. • In individuals aged 12 yr and older with uncontrolled persistent asthma, there is a conditional recommendation to add a LAMA to the ICS-LABA regimen as compared to continuing with the same dose of ICS-LABA.	Tiotropium acts on M3 muscarinic receptors located in the airways to produce smooth muscle relaxation and bronchodilation. Tiotropium is an antagonist of muscarinic receptors M1 to M5. Inhibition of the M3 receptor in lung smooth muscle leads to relaxation of smooth muscle and results in bronchodilation.	Immediate hypersensitivity, paradoxical bronchospasm, worsening of narrow angle glaucoma, worsening of urinary retention and renal impairment.

AMP, adenosine monophosphate; ICS, inhaled corticosteroid; IgE, immunoglobulin E; LABA, long-acting β-agonist; LAMA, long-acting muscarinic antagonist; SABA, short-acting β-agonist.

Modified from National Heart, Lung, and Blood Institute, National Asthma Education and Prevention Program. (2020). 2020 focused updates to the asthma management guidelines: A report from the National Asthma Education and Prevention Program Coordinating Committee Expert Panel Working Group. www.nhlbi.nih.gov/asthmaguidelines

Table 24-3 Quick-Relief Medications

DRUG/INDICATION	MECHANISM	POTENTIAL ADVERSE EFFECTS
Short-Acting β_2-Agonists		
Albuterol, levalbuterol, pirbuterol *Indications:* Relief of acute symptoms; preventive treatment for exercise-induced bronchospasm prior to exercise.	*Bronchodilation:* Bind to the β_2-adrenergic receptor, producing smooth muscle relaxation following adenylate cyclase activation and increase in cyclic AMP, producing functional antagonism of bronchoconstriction.	Tachycardia, skeletal muscle tremor, hypokalemia, increased lactic acid, headache, hyperglycemia. Inhaled route, in general, causes few systemic adverse effects. Patients with preexisting cardiovascular disease, especially older adults, may have adverse cardiovascular reactions with inhaled therapy.
Anticholinergic		
Ipratropium *Indications:* Acute bronchospasm; reverses only cholinergically mediated bronchospasm; does not modify reaction to antigen; does not block exercise-induced bronchospasm. Multiple doses of ipratropium in the emergency department provide additive effects to SABA. May be an alternative for patients who do not tolerate SABA Treatment of choice for bronchospasm because of β-blocker medication.	*Bronchodilation:* Competitive inhibition of muscarinic cholinergic receptors Reduces intrinsic vagal tone of the airways. May block reflex bronchoconstriction secondary to irritants or to reflux esophagitis. May decrease mucous gland secretion.	Drying of mouth and respiratory secretions, increased wheezing in some individuals, blurred vision if sprayed in eyes. If used in the emergency department, produces less cardiac stimulation than SABAs.

Table 24-3 Quick-Relief Medications (*continued*)

DRUG/INDICATION	MECHANISM	POTENTIAL ADVERSE EFFECTS
Systemic Corticosteroids		
Methylprednisolone, prednisolone, prednisone *Indications:* For moderate or severe exacerbations to prevent progression of exacerbation, reverse inflammation, speed recovery, and reduce rate of relapse.	*Anti-inflammatory:* Block late reaction to allergen and reduce airway hyperresponsiveness; inhibit cytokine production, adhesion protein activation, and inflammatory cell migration and activation. Reverse β_2-receptor downregulation. Inhibit microvascular leakage.	Short-term use: Reversible abnormalities in glucose metabolism, increased appetite, fluid retention, weight gain, facial flushing, mood alteration, hypertension, peptic ulcer, and, rarely, aseptic necrosis. Consideration should be given to coexisting conditions that could be worsened by systemic corticosteroids, such as herpes virus infections, varicella, tuberculosis, hypertension, peptic ulcer, diabetes mellitus, osteoporosis, and *Strongyloides*.

AMP, adenosine monophosphate; SABA, short-acting β-agonist.

DRUG ALERT Nonselective beta-adrenergic blockers, such as propranolol, have the potential to cause bronchoconstriction and should not be given to patients with asthma. Cardiac selective beta-blockers can be used, such as carvedilol.

Quick-Relief Medications

1. Short-acting bronchodilators by inhalation.
   a. Short-acting beta-agonists (SABAs), such as albuterol, pirbuterol, and levalbuterol.
   b. Anticholinergic agent, such as ipratropium bromide.
2. Systemic corticosteroids (short course)—prednisone, prednisolone, and methylprednisolone.

DRUG ALERT Patients should be encouraged to use SABAs appropriately when needed and not to wait for severe symptoms.

Other Measures

1. Environmental control (see page 781).
2. Immunotherapy (see page 778).
3. Avoidance of foods that contain tartrazine (yellow dye number 5) in patients who are aspirin-sensitive.
4. Regular aerobic exercise should be encouraged.
5. Use of an inhaled beta-adrenergic agonist taken 5 to 10 minutes before exercise will decrease exercise-induced bronchoconstriction.
6. Antibiotics are prescribed only during acute exacerbations if signs and symptoms of bacterial infection are present.
7. Alternative and complementary therapies that include acupuncture, herbal preparations, yoga, and chiropractic treatment have been suggested for acute and chronic asthma control; however, none is a substitute for usual medical treatment. In fact, glucosamine and chondroitin have been suspected of causing asthma exacerbation in some patients.

Nursing Assessment

1. Review patient's record: ask about coughing, dyspnea, chest tightness, wheezing, exertional changes, nighttime awakenings with asthma, use of SABA, and recent unscheduled, or emergency department (ED) visits. Use an assessment tool such as the Asthma Control Test, Asthma Control Questionnaire, and Asthma Therapy Assessment Questionnaire. These tools quantify symptoms, quick-relief medication usage, effect of asthma on quality of life, and patient/family perception of control. They can be found at https://www.nhlbi.nih.gov/files/docs/guidelines/asthma_qrg.pdf
2. Observe the patient and assess the rate, depth, and character of respirations, especially on expiration; observe for hyperinflation. Assess peak flow.
3. Auscultate the chest for breath sounds or wheezing.
4. Assess for triggers of asthma that include the following:
   a. Allergens.
   b. Respiratory infections.
   c. Inhalation of irritating substances (dust, fumes, and gases).
   d. Environmental factors (weather, air pollution, and humidity).
   e. Exercise, particularly in cold weather.
   f. Aspirin and its derivatives.
   g. Sulfite-containing agents used as food preservatives.
   h. Emotional factors (stress).
   i. Tobacco smoke.
5. After acute episode subsides, attempt to determine the patient's degree of adherence with medications and management regimen.
6. Observe and correct inhalation technique and discuss care of inhaler (e.g., cleaning, priming).

Nursing Interventions

Attaining Relief of Dyspneic Breathing

1. Monitor vital signs, skin color, retraction, oxygen saturation, and degree of restlessness, which may indicate hypoxia.
2. Provide medication and oxygen therapy, as prescribed.
3. Monitor airway functioning through peak flow meter or spirometry (FEV_1, FEV_1/FVC [forced vital capacity]) to assess the effectiveness of treatment.
4. Encourage intake of fluids to liquefy secretions.
5. Instruct the patient on positioning to facilitate breathing—sitting upright (leaning forward on a table).
6. Encourage the patient to use adaptive breathing techniques (e.g., pursed-lip breathing) to decrease the work of breathing.

Relieving Anxiety

1. Explain rationale for interventions to gain the patient's cooperation. Provide care in prompt, confident manner.

2. Help the patient clarify sources of anxiety; suggest measures to reduce anxiety and to control breathing.
3. Encourage active participation and support efforts to adhere to the management plan.

Preventing Adverse Effects of Drugs

1. Teach the patient to rinse mouth and spit out after using ICS to prevent the growth of fungi and be alert for sore throat or mouth caused by oropharyngeal candidiasis.
2. Suggest a spacer if the patient is prone to candidiasis and ensure proper dosing and inhalation technique. Blood glucose testing may also be indicated to rule out hyperglycemia.
3. Monitor liver function enzymes, as directed, for patients taking zileuton and zafirlukast, and advise the patient to report signs of liver dysfunction: abdominal pain, nausea, itching, and jaundice.
4. Make sure the patient is aware that LABAs are not used for acute symptoms or as anti-inflammatory therapy or monotherapy for asthma. Duration of protection against exercised-induced bronchospasm may decrease with regular use.
5. Warn patients that regular use (greater than 2 days/week) of SABA for symptom control (not prevention of exercise-induced bronchospasm), increasing use, or lack of expected effect indicates inadequate asthma control. For patients frequently using SABA, anti-inflammatory medication should be initiated or intensified.

Community and Home Care Considerations

1. Initiate peak flow monitoring, if indicated. This may be done twice daily by the patient with persistent asthma. Provide written and verbal instruction and have the patient demonstrate the procedure.
2. The patient can buy a peak flow meter from a pharmacy or from a medical supply company.
3. Once optimal asthma control is obtained, daily peak flow measurements in the early morning and early afternoon should be used during a 2- to 3-week period to determine the patient's personal best. The personal best peak flow measurement will be used to monitor control and to guide self-therapy in an individualized action plan.
4. Teach the patient how to obtain peak flow measurement.
   a. Place the indicator at the base of the numbered scale.
   b. Stand (preferably) or sit upright.
   c. Take a deep breath.
   d. Place the meter in mouth and close lips around mouthpiece, with tongue under the mouthpiece.
   e. Blow out as hard and as fast as possible. Coughing or spitting will result in a falsely elevated level.
   f. Note the measurement that the indicator is pointing to on the number scale.
   g. Repeat previous steps twice more and record the highest number.
5. Provide written and verbal instruction on an action plan for self-management of asthma exacerbation as outlined by the health care provider. National Asthma Education and Prevention Program Guidelines suggest the following:
   a. For symptomatic worsening of asthma or asymptomatic decrease in peak flow measurement, use initial inhalation of a short-acting beta-adrenergic agonist by MDI, two to four puffs for up to three treatments at 20-minute intervals, or a single nebulization treatment.
   b. After initial treatment, recheck peak flow; if it is more than 80% of personal best and no wheezing or shortness of breath, continue beta-adrenergic agonist every 3 to 4 hours for 24 to 48 hours. The patient should contact the health care provider for further instructions.
   c. If peak flow is 40% to 80% of personal best, or if the patient has persistent wheezing and shortness of breath, an oral corticosteroid should be initiated and beta-adrenergic agonist should be continued. The patient should contact the health care provider the same day for further instructions.
   d. If peak flow is less than 40% of personal best or if the patient has significant wheezing and shortness of breath, an oral corticosteroid should be started, beta-adrenergic agonist should be repeated immediately, and the patient should proceed to the ED.

Patient Education and Health Maintenance

1. Provide information on the nature of asthma and methods of treatment.
2. Provide information regarding medications, including the difference between long-term controllers and quick-relief medications and the proper use of inhalers and spacer devices; stress avoiding overuse of inhalers and nebulizers. Ensure that the patient understands that long-acting bronchodilating inhalers, such as salmeterol, are not effective for asthma exacerbations.
3. Demonstrate the use of MDIs (see Patient Education Guidelines 24-2) and nebulization equipment.
   a. Inhalers vary widely with hydrofluoroalkane (HFA) propellant and breath-actuated devices currently on the market; familiarize yourself with the manufacturer's instructions to help the patient.
   b. Teach patients how to clean inhalers according to manufacturer's instructions.
   c. Advise patients to count number of inhalations if the inhaler does not have an automatic counter.
4. Help the patient to identify what triggers asthma, warning signs of an impending attack, and strategies for preventing and treating an attack.
5. Teach adaptive breathing techniques and breathing exercises, such as pursed-lip breathing.
6. Discuss environmental control/indoor allergen mitigation.
   a. Avoid people with respiratory infections. Get an annual flu shot.
   b. Avoid substances and situations known to precipitate bronchospasm, such as allergens, irritants, strong odors, gases, fumes, pet dander, and smoke.
   c. Wear a mask if cold weather precipitates bronchospasm.
   d. Stay inside when air pollution is high.
   e. Also see Patient Education Guidelines 24-1, page 781.
7. Promote optimal health practices, including nutrition, rest, and exercise.
   a. Encourage regular exercise to improve cardiorespiratory and musculoskeletal conditioning.
   b. Drink liberal amounts of fluids to keep secretions thin.
   c. Try to avoid upsetting situations.
   d. Use relaxation techniques, biofeedback management.
   e. Use community resources for smoking cessation classes, stress management, exercises for relaxation, asthma support groups.
8. Make sure that the patient knows with whom to follow up and the frequency of follow-up. Discuss with the patient how to overcome any barriers to follow up, such as transportation, limited office or clinic hours, childcare, and work requirements.

PATIENT EDUCATION GUIDELINES 24-2

How to Use an Inhaler and Spacer

Using An Inhaler

1. Make sure that the medication canister is attached to the plastic inhaler and shake well or, if using a dry powder inhaler (DPI) system, load the medication according to the manufacturer's instructions.
2. If recommended, attach a spacer to your metered-dose inhaler (MDI) (see "Using a Spacer").
3. If using the closed-mouth method (recommended for DPI and HFA systems):
   a. Exhale fully and place the mouthpiece of the inhaler in your mouth and close lips tightly around it.
   b. While starting to inhale, use your index finger to press down firmly on the top of the canister.
   c. Continue to inhale for 3 to 5 seconds to obtain a full breath, then hold your breath for 5 to 10 seconds.
   d. Remove the inhaler from your mouth before you exhale and breathe normally.
4. If more than one inhalation of a beta$_2$-agonist is prescribed, wait 30 seconds before taking another inhalation, then repeat steps 1 to 5.
5. Replace the mouthpiece cap after each use.
6. Clean the inhaler according to the manufacturer's instructions.
7. Discard the canister after you have used the labeled number of inhalations. You should not use it beyond this indicated number because the correct dose amount can no longer be guaranteed.
8. For DPIs, use a forceful, rapid inhalation with closed-mouth technique. See the instructions provided by the manufacturer of the device you use.

Using a Spacer

Unless you use your inhaler correctly, much of the medicine can end up on your tongue, on the back of your throat, or in the air. If you experience this problem, your health care provider may recommend using a spacer. Also called a *valved holding chamber*, a spacer is a device that attaches to an MDI. It holds the medicine in its chamber long enough for you to inhale it in one or two slow, deep breaths, thereby enabling you to get your full dose of medicine. It also prevents you from coughing and may prevent a yeast infection in your mouth if you use a steroid inhaler. Several types of spacers are available; these devices may be purchased through your pharmacist.

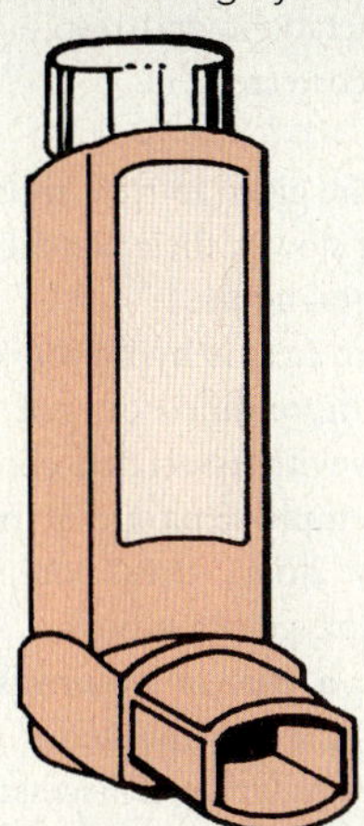

1. Attach the inhaler to the spacer or holding chamber as shown in the product instructions.
2. Shake well.
3. Press the canister on the inhaler, which will put one puff of medicine into the holding chamber.
4. Place the mouthpiece of the spacer into your mouth and inhale slowly.
5. Hold your breath a few seconds, then exhale.

EVIDENCE BASE Center for Disease Control and Prevention. (2018). *Know how to use your asthma inhaler* [multimedia]. https://www.cdc.gov/asthma/inhaler_video/default.htm

9. For additional information and support, refer to the American Academy of Allergy, Asthma and Immunology (www.aaaai.org).

DRUG ALERT Never submerge an inhalation canister in water to determine whether any medication remains. Moisture in the tip will ruin the canister.

Evaluation: Expected Outcomes

- Symptoms (wheezing, coughing, dyspnea, chest tightness) reduced; peak flow improved.
- Verbalizes relief of anxiety.
- No adverse reactions to drug therapy reported.

Status Asthmaticus

Status asthmaticus is a severe form of asthma in which the airway obstruction is unresponsive to usual drug therapy. Up to 20% of patients presenting with an asthma exacerbation require admission to the intensive care unit.

Contributing Factors

1. Infection.
2. Inhalation of air pollutants and allergens to which sensitized.
3. Nonadherence in taking medications, including overuse of bronchodilators.
4. Ingestion of aspirin or related drugs in patient who is aspirin-sensitive.
5. Aspiration of gastric acid.

Clinical Manifestations

1. Tachypnea, labored respirations, with increased effort on exhalation.
2. Suprasternal retractions, use of accessory muscles of respiration.
3. Diminished breath sounds, decreased ability to speak in phrases or sentences.
4. Anxiety, irritability, fatigue, headache, impaired mental functioning.
5. Muscle twitching, somnolence, diaphoresis—from continued carbon dioxide retention.

6. Tachycardia, elevated BP.
7. Heart failure and death from suffocation.

Management and Nursing Interventions

1. Monitor respiratory rate and oxygen saturation continuously; frequently monitor arterial blood gas levels, BP, electrocardiogram.
2. Administer repeated aerosol treatments with $beta_2$-agonist bronchodilators, such as albuterol or levalbuterol; add anticholinergic ipratropium, as prescribed—administer with caution until the metabolic and respiratory acidosis and hypoxemia have been corrected.
3. Monitor IV therapy.
   a. Corticosteroids are given to treat inflammation of airways; because these act slowly, their beneficial effects may not be apparent for several hours.
   b. Fluids are given to treat dehydration and loosen secretions.
4. Provide continuous humidified oxygen via nasal cannula, as prescribed. (Patients with associated chronic obstructive pulmonary disease or emphysema are at risk for depressed hypoxemic ventilatory drive, thus compounding respiratory insufficiency, so use oxygen cautiously.)
5. Prior to intubation, a trial of noninvasive positive pressure ventilation (NIPPV) may be initiated.
6. Initiate mechanical ventilation, if necessary.
7. Assist with mobilization of obstructing bronchial mucus.
   a. Perform chest physiotherapy (chest wall percussion and vibration).
   b. Administer expectorant and mucolytic drugs, as prescribed.
   c. Remove secretions by suctioning or prepare for bronchoscopy, if needed.
8. Provide adequate hydration.
9. Obtain portable chest x-ray and administer antibiotic, as prescribed, to treat any underlying respiratory infection.
10. Alleviate the patient's anxiety and fear by acting calmly and by reassuring the patient during an attack. Stay with the patient until the attack subsides.

CLINICAL JUDGMENT In status asthmaticus, the return to normal or increasing partial pressure of carbon dioxide does not necessarily mean that the patient with asthma is improving—it may indicate a fatigue state that develops just before the patient slips into respiratory failure.

SELECTED READINGS

Ansotegui, I. J., Melioli, G., Canonica, G. W., Caraballo, L., Villa, E., Ebisawa, M., Passalacqua, G., Savi, E., Ebo, D., Gómez, R. M., Luengo Sánchez, O., Oppenheimer, J. J., Jensen-Jarolim, E., Fischer, D. A., Haahtela, T., Antila, M., Bousquet, J. J., Cardona, V., Chiang, W. C., … Zuberbier, T. (2020). IgE allergy diagnostics and other relevant tests in allergy, a World Allergy Organization position paper. *The World Allergy Organization Journal, 13*(2), 100080. https://doi.org/10.1016/j.waojou.2019.100080

Baker, J. A., & Houin, P. R. (2023). Comparison of national and global asthma management guiding documents. *Respiratory Care, 68*(1), 114–128. https://doi.org/10.4187/respcare.10254

Bousquet, J., Humbert, M., Gibson, P. G., Kostikas, K., Jaumont, X., Pfister, P., & Nissen, F. (2021). Real-world effectiveness of omalizumab in severe allergic asthma: A meta-analysis of observational studies. *The Journal of Allergy and Clinical Immunology: In Practice, 9*(7), 2702–2714. https://doi.org/10.1016/j.jaip.2021.01.011

Czech, E. J., Overholser, A., & Schultz, P. (2023). Allergic rhinitis. *Primary Care, 50*(2), 159–178. https://doi.org/10.1016/j.pop.2023.01.003

Dhaliwal, A., & Bajaj, T. (2022). Zafirlukast. In *StatPearls*. StatPearls Publishing.

Dispenza, M. C. (2019). Classification of hypersensitivity reactions. *Allergy and Asthma Proceedings, 40*(6), 470–473. https://doi.org/10.2500/aap.2019.40.4274

Durham, S. R., & Shamji, M. H. (2023). Allergen immunotherapy: Past, present and future. *Nature Reviews. Immunology, 23*(5), 317–328. https://doi.org/10.1038/s41577-022-00786-1

Godwin, H. T., Fix, M. L., Baker, O., Madsen, T., Walls, R. M., & Brown, C. A., 3rd. (2020). Emergency department airway management for status asthmaticus with respiratory failure. *Respiratory Care, 65*(12), 1904–1907. https://doi.org/10.4187/respcare.07723

Hopkinson, K. (2019). The role of patient-reported outcomes in the management of chronic spontaneous urticaria. *British Journal of Nursing (Mark Allen Publishing), 28*(3), 144–150. https://doi.org/10.12968/bjon.2019.28.3.144

Muiser, S., Gosens, R., van den Berge, M., & Kerstjens, H. A. M. (2022). Understanding the role of long-acting muscarinic antagonists in asthma treatment. *Annals of Allergy, Asthma & Immunology: Official Publication of the American College of Allergy, Asthma, & Immunology, 128*(4), 352–360. https://doi.org/10.1016/j.anai.2021.12.020

Parisi, C. A. S., Kelly, K. J., Ansotegui, I. J., Gonzalez-Díaz, S. N., Bilò, M. B., Cardona, V., Park, H. S., Braschi, M. C., Macias-Weinmann, A., Piga, M. A., Acuña-Ortega, N., Sánchez-Borges, M., & Yañez, A. (2021). Update on latex allergy: New insights into an old problem. *The World Allergy Organization Journal, 14*(8), 100569. https://doi.org/10.1016/j.waojou.2021.100569

Patel, R. H., & Mohiuddin, S. S. (2023). Biochemistry, histamine. In *StatPearls*. StatPearls Publishing.

Seth, D., Poowutikul, P., Pansare, M., & Kamat, D. (2020). Food allergy: A review. *Pediatric Annals, 49*(1), e50–e58. https://doi.org/10.3928/19382359-20191206-01

25 HIV Infection and AIDS*

OVERVIEW

Human immunodeficiency virus (HIV) is an RNA retroviral infection that is transmitted from person to person most often through sexual and blood-to-blood contact. HIV interferes with the immune system's ability to coordinate an effective response against infection. Over time, eroded immune function without treatment leads to the stage of disease called *acquired immune deficiency syndrome* (AIDS), which is marked by vulnerability to opportunistic infections. Without antiretroviral therapy (ART), HIV infection is almost universally fatal.

Since the immune deficiency syndrome associated with HIV was first described in 1981, great strides have been made in care and treatment of people living with HIV (PLWH). Potent ART regimens have been simplified into fixed-dose combination tablets with once-daily dosing and long-acting injectable formulations; furthermore, the cost of medication has decreased globally, clearing the way for more widespread access to treatment. There is international will to test and treat more people and prevent new infection among those who are at risk for acquiring HIV, and life expectancy on ART has increased significantly across all income settings of the world. People who take ART and achieve an undetectable level of HIV RNA in plasma testing (viral suppression) are not able to transmit HIV to others. Perinatal transmission of HIV in the United States occurs rarely. Globally, the Joint United Nations Programme on HIV/AIDS (UNAIDS) has rolled out a fast-track strategy to end AIDS by 2030. This framework sets ambitious 95-95-95 goals: 95% of people with HIV will be diagnosed, 95% of them will be on ART, and 95% will be virally suppressed by 2030. Synergy among public and private partner organizations is expanding treatment capacity, expertise, and programmatic infrastructure. There is still no effective vaccine against HIV; however, research programs are investigating several cure strategies.

HIV treatment extends life, reduces morbidity, and prevents new infections. Nevertheless, HIV has claimed more than 40 million lives since the beginning of the epidemic, and approximately 38 million people were living with HIV in 2021 globally. As of 2022, the Centers for Disease Control and Prevention (CDC) estimated that about 1.2 million people were living with HIV in the United States, with 87% knowing their HIV status in 2019. The Patient Protection and Affordable Care Act (ACA) enacted in 2010 has extended opportunities to millions who had been uninsured or underinsured in the United States. In 2019, 66% of PLWH in the United States had received care, and 57% were virally suppressed (see Figure 25-1). The National HIV/AIDS Strategy solidifies political will and sets ambitious societal goals to end the HIV epidemic in the United States by 2030. There is work to do. Nurses are present at each point in the HIV care continuum: preventing new infections, testing, treating, and retaining patients in care. Nursing's role is essential toward achieving these domestic and international goals.

EVIDENCE BASE Centers for Disease Control and Prevention. HIV and AIDS data through December 2019 provided for the Ryan White HIV/AIDS Program, for fiscal year 2021. *HIV Surveillance Supplemental Report*, *27*(1). Published January 2022. Accessed April 11, 2023. http://www.cdc.gov/hiv/library/reports/hivsurveillance.html

UNAIDS. (2021). *Global AIDS strategy 2021–2026—End inequalities*. End AIDS. https://www.unaids.org/en/resources/documents/2021/2021-2026-global-AIDS-strategy

World Health Organization. (2022). *WHO HIV fact sheet*. WHO. https://www.who.int/news-room/fact-sheets/detail/hiv-aids

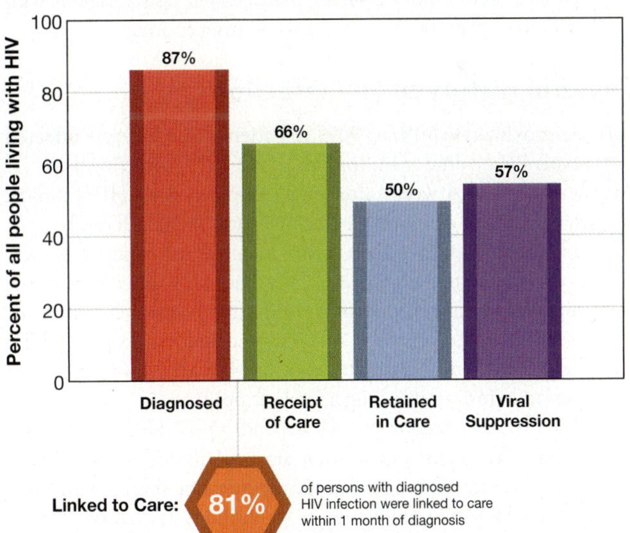

Figure 25-1. Prevalence-based HIV Care Continuum United States and 6 Dependent Areas, 2019. HIV, human immunodeficiency virus. Reprinted from *What is the HIV care continuum?* (2022). https://www.hiv.gov/federal-response/policies-issues/hiv-aids-care-continuum/

*Please note that the term "male" in this chapter refers to a person assigned male at birth, and the term "female" in this chapter refers to a person assigned female at birth.

Transmission and Natural History

Epidemiology and Pathophysiology

1. Today, most new HIV infections are found among men who have sex with men (MSM) (71% of new infections in 2020). Among MSM, adults of underrepresented ethnic groups and adolescent/young adult Black and Hispanic males aged 13 to 34 are disproportionately affected. Heterosexual transmission accounted for 22% of new HIV infections in 2020. The trend in new infections from injection drug use has declined to approximately 7%. Geographical distribution of new infections is uneven across the United States. Between 2015 and 2019, the South represented the highest burden of incident infections (12.4), the Northeast (7.6), the West (8.0), and the Midwest (6.0) per 100,000 people. Ensuring the availability of comprehensive HIV prevention and treatment programs across all regions will be important to preventing new infections and finding and treating people who are living with HIV.
2. HIV enters the body through condomless sexual contact or blood-to-blood transmission from contact with a person with HIV who is not virally suppressed.
3. The virus binds to $CD4^+$ T helper immune cells and gains entry, where HIV uses the T helper cell as a factory to reproduce. Replicating HIV within the host cell ruptures the cell membrane and destroys the T cell, which releases new HIV virions into the plasma that bind to and disable other $CD4^+$ cells at an exponential rate.
4. Antiretroviral (ARV) drugs interfere with viral binding or entry into $CD4^+$ T cells and replication at specific points in the viral life cycle.
5. HIV infection can be viewed as a chronic condition among PLWH who strictly adhere to ART and care. Even though pill burden is low and treatment has few side effects, it is still lifelong therapy. Some patients have difficulty managing highly structured medication and appointment regimens and need encouragement or special interventions to support their treatment plan. Nursing expertise and multidisciplinary management assists patients with tailoring a plan for successful and enduring treatment.

Natural History of HIV Infection

1. Approximately 50% to 90% of patients who become infected experience some symptom of acute HIV seroconversion at around 2 to 4 weeks after being infected with HIV. Typical symptoms of acute HIV seroconversion include fever, lymphadenopathy, sore throat, rash, myalgia/arthralgia, diarrhea, weight loss, and headache. Many new HIV infections evade diagnosis because symptoms overlap with other common illnesses. Seroconversion is marked by a sudden decrease in T4 helper cells and a sharp increase in HIV viral load for a brief period before establishing a viral set point.
2. The time to detection of HIV depends upon the diagnostic test being used. Fourth-generation antigen/antibody combination HIV-1/2 immunoassays detect early infection, because the assay detects HIV p24 antigen prior to antibody formation. If positive, a confirmatory antigen/antibody combination HIV-1/2 immunoassay is performed. If a patient is suspected of being in the window period between the time of exposure and the time when infection can be detected by antibody/antigen testing, then a nucleic acid test (NAT) may be drawn to detect the presence of HIV RNA from approximately 10 days after infection.
3. The CDC provides a case definition for staging HIV infection and defining progression to AIDS (see Table 25-1). A typical $CD4^+$ count is approximately 1,500/mm^3. HIV replication destroys $CD4^+$ T cells, causing the number of CD4 cells to diminish over time.
4. Waning immunity in people who have untreated or undertreated infection or who are on a failing ARV regimen leads to frequent infections, severe opportunistic infections, and malignancies (see Figure 25-2).

Table 25-1 Revised Surveillance Case Definition for HIV Infection Stages in the United States, 2014

	STAGE 1	STAGE 2	STAGE 3
Age <1 yr	≥1,500 μL ≥34% $CD4^+$	750–1,499 μL 26%–33% $CD4^+$	<750 μL <26% $CD4^+$
Age 1–5 yr	≥1,000 μL ≥30% $CD4^+$	500–999 μL 22%–29% $CD4^+$	200–499 μL 14%–25% $CD4^+$
Age 6 yr to adult	≥500 μL ≥26% $CD4^+$	200–499 μL 14%–25% $CD4^+$	<200 μL <14% $CD4^+$

HIV, human immunodeficiency virus
Stages 1 and 2 indicate HIV infection; stage 3 indicates AIDS diagnosis.
Source: Centers for Disease Control and Prevention. (2014). Revised surveillance case definition for HIV infection—United States, 2014. www.cdc.gov/mmwr/preview/mmwrhtml/rr6303a1.htm?s_cid=rr6303a1_e

CLINICAL JUDGMENT The period around acute HIV seroconversion is a time when the patient is highly infectious to others. Elevated HIV viral load is linked to a higher rate of transmission. Counsel patients to use effective measures to prevent transmission through sexual contact and/or needle sharing. Encourage and refer newly diagnosed people into care and treatment. Ask patients to talk with their partner(s) about preexposure prophylaxis (PrEP) or refer them to a PrEP center for advice.

Diagnostic Evaluation

EVIDENCE BASE Sax, P. E. (2022). Acute and early HIV infection: Clinical manifestations and diagnosis. *UpToDate.* Retrieved April 11, 2023, from https://www.uptodate.com/contents/acute-and-early-hiv-infection-clinical-manifestations-and-diagnosis

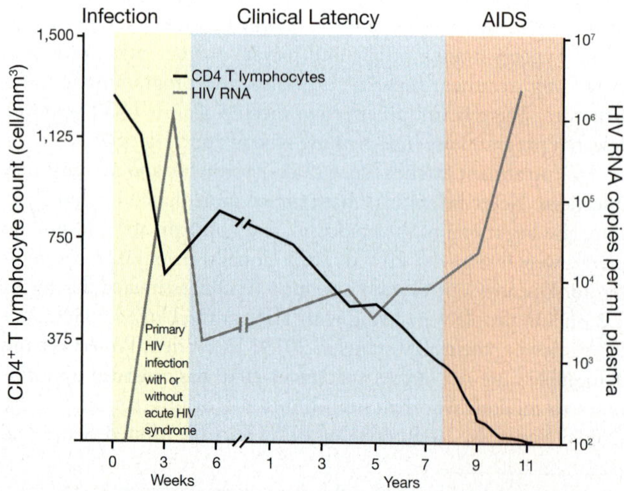

Figure 25-2. Natural history of untreated HIV infection. AIDS, acquired immune deficiency syndrome; HIV, human immunodeficiency virus.

Broholm, C., Yingling, C., & Vail, R. (2022). Preventing HIV with pre-exposure prophylaxis: Current and emerging modalities. *The Journal for Nurse Practitioners, 18*, 62–66.

HIV Testing

Description

1. HIV-1/2 combination antigen/antibody immunoassay.
   a. Third-generation tests detect HIV immunoglobulin M (IgM) and IgG antibody within approximately 20 to 30 days from infection.
   b. Fourth-generation tests detect HIV IgM and IgG antibody and p24 antigen within approximately 15 to 20 days from infection.
2. NAT.
   a. NAT confirms the presence of HIV genetic material (RNA).
   b. HIV RNA can be detected at about 10 days from infection.
   c. A NAT test can be used as a confirmatory test after antibody/antigen testing.
3. Western blot is a confirmatory test that detects HIV IgM and IgG antibody within approximately 45 to 60 days from exposure. Indeterminate results may occur prior to this interval.
4. Quantitative HIV RNA viral load assays detect an HIV RNA level in plasma.
   a. Assays that are sensitive to more than 20 copies/mL can measure viral load within 10 to 15 days of infection.
   b. Ultrasensitive assays that can detect to more than 5 copies/mL may be used while on treatment or in the research setting.
5. The CDC recommends opt-out HIV testing for people aged 13 to 64 years, informing them that screening is routine and affirming that they may decline. Written consent and pretest and post-test counseling are no longer recommended, but consult state law to ensure adherence to local testing requirements.

Other Laboratory Tests

1. Lymphocyte panel may show decreased $CD4^+$ count or $CD4^+$ percentage. In early infection, in long-term nonprogressors, elite controllers, and PLWH who are on ART, $CD4^+$ count may be nearly normal.
2. A complete blood count (CBC) may show anemia, leukopenia, and/or thrombocytopenia.
3. HIV viral load testing measures the level of HIV RNA that is present in plasma. Resistance testing determines whether a patient is infected with or has acquired drug-resistant virus. Genotypic resistance assays amplify HIV virus to reveal mutations in the viral genotype that block or impair the efficacy of specific ARV medications.
4. An undetectable HIV viral load result does not indicate that the patient is cured of HIV. Latent reservoirs exist in lymphoid tissue and resting memory $CD4^+$ T cells indefinitely. These reservoirs are not reached by ARV agents. Therefore, counsel patients that they must still maintain strict adherence to ART.

MANAGEMENT

Pharmacologic Treatment

EVIDENCE BASE Panel on Antiretroviral Guidelines for Adults and Adolescents. (2023). *Guidelines for the use of antiretroviral agents in adults and adolescents with HIV*. Department of Health and Human Services. Accessed April 7, 2023. https://clinicalinfo.hiv.gov/en/guidelines/adult-and-adolescent-arv

Treatment Overview

1. Antiretroviral therapy (ART) serves a four-part purpose: (1) to decrease human immunodeficiency virus (HIV) viral burden and increase immune function, (2) to reduce morbidity and mortality, (3) to increase quality of life and life expectancy, and (4) to prevent HIV transmission. Successful treatment requires strict adherence to medication.
   a. Test-and-treat efforts promote ART initiation very soon after diagnosis to curb the inflammatory effects of ongoing viral replication, reduce morbidity, and prevent transmission to others. Before initiating ART, patients should be assessed for readiness to start; however, some trepidation is expected and is not a complete barrier to initiating treatment.
   b. Test-and-prevent efforts provide a snapshot of a person's HIV status so they have an opportunity to make choices that protect partners if positive, or to remain uninfected if negative.
2. Universal treatment is recommended for all patients who are HIV positive, regardless of CD4 count. If the CD4 count falls below 200 cells/mm^3, some opportunistic infections can be prevented by taking additional prophylactic medication (see Table 25-2).

Table 25-2 Opportunistic Infections (OIs) and Drug Therapies

NAME OF OI	CLINICAL SYMPTOMS	DIAGNOSTIC TESTS	TREATMENT
Pneumocystis jirovecii pneumonia (PCP)	• Low-grade fever • Shortness of breath • Cough: dry or scant white sputum production	• Chest x-ray • Induced sputum specimen • Bronchoscopy • Microscopy • PCR	• Co-trimoxazole (± steroids) • Clindamycin with primaquine ± steroids • Atovaquone
Oral *Candida* and *Candida* esophagitis	• White coating in mouth • White coating down throat • Sensation of food getting caught in throat while swallowing	• Gross observation • Microscopy for hyphae • Endoscopy	• Nystatin • Clotrimazole • Itraconazole • Fluconazole • Liposomal amphotericin B

(continued)

Table 25-2 Opportunistic Infections (OIs) and Drug Therapies (*continued*)

NAME OF OI	CLINICAL SYMPTOMS	DIAGNOSTIC TESTS	TREATMENT
Mycobacterium avium complex (MAC)	• Fever • Weakness • Weight loss • Diarrhea • Bone marrow suppression	• Blood culture for acid-fast bacilli (AFB) • Bone marrow biopsy	• Rifabutin • Ethambutol • Azithromycin • Clarithromycin
Kaposi sarcoma	• Pink, purple, or brown spots or nodules • ± Pain, edema of affected area	• Gross observation • Biopsy	• ART (improved immune function) • Chemotherapy
Toxoplasmosis	• Fever • Headache • Change in mental status • Confusion • Lethargy • Psychosis	• CT • MRI • Serum *Toxoplasma* IgG antibodies	• Pyrimethamine • Sulfadiazine • Folinic acid
Tuberculosis	• Fever • Cough: none, dry or scant frothy white or pink sputum, hemoptysis • Shortness of breath • Weight loss • Lymphadenopathy	• Chest x-ray • Sputum for smear, microscopy, Gene Xpert, and culture • Positive purified protein derivative (PPD) (≥5 mm induration) • Interferon-gamma release assays (IGRAs) • Note that PPD and IGRAs detect evidence of past exposure and are not conclusive for TB disease)	• Rifampin • Isoniazid • Pyrazinamide • Ethambutol • Pyridoxine
Cryptosporidium	• Severe watery diarrhea • Severe abdominal cramping	• Stool microscopy for *Cryptosporidium*	• ART (improved immune function) • Nitazoxanide + aggressive ART
Cryptococcal meningitis	• Headache • Confusion, memory loss • Nausea • Seizures • Change in mental status • Fever • Photophobia	• Serum and CSF cryptococcal antigen • CSF fungal culture	• Liposomal amphotericin B • Flucytosine • Fluconazole
Cytomegalovirus (CMV)	• Visual changes; floaters, flashes or blind spots, and blindness • Difficulty swallowing • Nausea, vomiting • Abdominal cramping • Altered mental status • Adrenal insufficiency	• Ophthalmologic examination • Blood, urine, tissue culture for CMV • PCR • Immunohistochemistry • Histopathology (visualization of characteristic owl's eyes inclusion bodies)	• Valganciclovir • Ganciclovir • Foscarnet • Cidofovir • Intraocular ganciclovir-release device
Herpes simplex virus 1 and 2	• Blisters or ulcerations: mouth, lips, genitalia, perianal area • Ocular changes • Change in mental status, neurologic findings	• PCR • Viral culture • Clinical observation	• Acyclovir • Famciclovir • Valacyclovir
Herpes zoster	• Painful vesicular rash on one or more dermatome(s)	• PCR • Viral culture • Clinical observation	• Famciclovir • Valacyclovir • Acyclovir
Mpox	• Painful or nonpainful firm, circumscribed lesions of the skin, oral mucosa, genital, urethral, perianal, rectal, periorbital areas • Change in mental status, neurologic findings	• PCR • Viral culture	• Tecovirimat • Brincidofovir • Cidofovir, • Trifluridine (ocular dz) • VIGIV

ART, antiretroviral therapy; CSF, cerebrospinal fluid; CT, computed tomography; IgG, immunoglobulin G; IV, intravenous; MRI, magnetic resonance imaging; PCR, polymerase chain reaction; TB, tuberculosis; VIGIV, vaccinia immune globulin intravenous.

a. Patients with a CD4 count less than 200 cells/mm^3 are prescribed prophylaxis against *Pneumocystis jirovecii* pneumonia (PCP).
b. Patients who have a CD4 count less than 100 cells/mm^3 and are *Toxoplasma gondii* serum IgG$^+$ are prescribed prophylaxis against toxoplasmosis.
c. Patients who have a CD4 count less than 50 cells/mm^3 are prescribed prophylaxis against *Mycobacterium avium* complex (MAC), after an initial culture for *M. avium intracellulare* (MAI) is negative.

3. Many patients who are living with HIV are coinfected with hepatitis C virus (HCV), which is curable with 8 to 12 weeks of direct-acting antiviral treatment. Consult the HCV HIV-specific treatment guidelines before initiating HCV therapy.

Initiating ART in Patients Who Are Treatment-Naïve

1. Universal treatment is recommended for all people living with HIV (PLWH), regardless of CD4 count. ART medications belong to drug classifications that interfere with HIV replication at different points in the viral life cycle. To simplify medication taking and reduce pill burden, there is a growing arsenal of multiclass combination formulations and long-acting injectable products.
2. The standard of care for ART is to use drugs from at least two different drug classifications.
3. ART is dynamic, and clinical practice guidelines are updated frequently. Guidelines should be consulted before starting or switching an ART regimen. Expert consultation and multidisciplinary care may be required for patients who are heavily treatment experienced or who have other viral coinfections, complex comorbidities, or social and mental health needs.
4. Classes of antiretroviral (ARV) drugs:
   a. Nucleoside/nucleotide reverse transcriptase inhibitors (NRTIs).
   b. Nonnucleoside reverse transcriptase inhibitors (NNRTIs).
   c. Protease inhibitors (PIs).
   d. Entry/fusion inhibitor.
   e. Entry inhibitor/CCR5 antagonist.
   f. Integrase strand transfer inhibitor (INSTI).
   g. CD4 T-cell postattachment inhibitors.
   h. gp120 attachment inhibitor.
   i. HIV capsid inhibitor.
   j. Multiclass combination products.

Adverse Effects of ARV Medications

EVIDENCE BASE Panel on Antiretroviral Guidelines for Adults and Adolescents. (2023). *Guidelines for the use of antiretroviral agents in adults and adolescents with HIV.* Department of Health and Human Services. Accessed April 7, 2023. https://clinicalinfo.hiv.gov/en/guidelines/adult-and-adolescent-arv

1. Contemporary medications have simplified medication dosing and reduced side effects significantly.
2. Bone density reduction is associated with tenofovir disoproxil fumarate (TDF). Effect can be reduced by switching to the newer formulation tenofovir alafenamide (TAF).
3. Cardiac disease and/or cardiac effects are associated with NRTIs, some NNRTIs, and PIs.
4. Diabetes mellitus and insulin resistance are associated with NRTIs and some PIs.
5. Dyslipidemia is associated with NRTIs, NNRTIs, PIs, and INSTI.
6. Gastrointestinal (GI) effects such as nausea, vomiting, and diarrhea are associated with NRTIs and some PI-containing regimens.
7. Hepatotoxicity can occur with most NRTIs, some NNRTIs, and all PIs. Check hepatitis B status before discontinuing the NRTIs TAF, TDF, lamivudine, or emtricitabine, as discontinuation can cause severe hepatitis B virus (HBV) flares. The PI combination TPV/r is contraindicated in patients with hepatic disease that is characterized as Child-Pugh B or C.
8. Hypersensitivity reaction (HSR) is associated with the NRTI abacavir (ABC), the NNRTI nevirapine (NVP), and the INSTI raltegravir (RAL) and can present with any combination of the following symptoms: fever, rash, malaise, nausea, headache, myalgia, chills, diarrhea, vomiting, abdominal pain, dyspnea, fatigue, blisters, oral lesions, facial swelling, eosinophilia, granulocytopenia, arthralgia, lymphadenopathy, and respiratory symptoms.
9. Lactic acidosis/steatohepatitis occur with some NRTI medications; present with nausea, vomiting, fatigue, and abdominal pain. May progress rapidly to a life-threatening condition.
10. Myopathy and elevated creatinine phosphokinase (CPK) are associated with the NRTI Zidovudine (ZDV) and the INSTI RAL.
11. Central nervous system (CNS) and psychiatric effects are associated with the NRTI d4T, the NNRTI efavirenz (EFV), and all INSTI.
12. Rash is associated with nearly all ARVs.
13. Renal effects such as elevated serum creatinine and kidney stones are associated with the NRTI TDF (elevated creatinine) and some PIs (elevated creatinine and stone/crystal formation).
14. Stevens-Johnson syndrome and toxic epidermal necrosis have been reported among NRTIs, NNRTIs, PIs, and INSTI.
15. Treatment fatigue is an emotional reaction to the need for lifelong treatment, a medication's dosing structure, and adverse effects. Treatment fatigue may be managed effectively by switching to a simplified regimen, if possible, and by offering supportive care. Drug "holidays" are not recommended, since HIV reactivation occurs almost immediately.
16. Weight gain is associated with INSTI.
17. If a patient decides to stop taking ART, then all ARV medications should be stopped at the same time. Taking only some of the ARVs creates resistance to HIV, which could lead to the loss of effective treatment options for this patient in the future. Resistance can develop within a few days to a few weeks of inadequate dosing. Special rules exist for stopping a regimen that contains drugs with a different half-life. Consult with guidelines or seek expert care before a planned treatment interruption or discontinuation, and counsel patients to contact their provider for advice before stopping a regimen on their own.

Health Maintenance

EVIDENCE BASE Panel on Guidelines for the Prevention and Treatment of Opportunistic Infections in Adults and Adolescents with HIV. (2023). *Guidelines for the prevention and treatment of opportunistic infections in adults and adolescents with HIV.* National Institutes of Health, Centers for Disease Control and Prevention, HIV Medicine Association, and Infectious Diseases Society of America. Accessed April 7, 2023. https://clinicalinfo.hiv.gov/en/guidelines/adult-and-adolescent-opportunistic-infection

Patient Education and Health Maintenance

1. Emphasize the importance of ART to improve health, to promote longevity, and to prevent transmission to others.
2. Encourage patient to disclose HIV status to sex partner(s) and/or needle-sharing partner(s).
3. Discuss the risk of acquiring and/or transmitting sexually transmitted infections (STIs) and assist patient in developing a prevention strategy.
4. Discuss advances in hepatitis C treatment that can cure HCV in 8 to 12 weeks.
5. Discuss family planning with all patients, if relevant. Consult drug–drug interaction platforms about specific ART regimens and hormonal contraceptives. Encourage routine health maintenance such as dental care, immunizations, eye examinations, annual cervical Pap smear for females and anal Pap smear for men who have sex with men (MSM), lipid screening, glucose and A1C monitoring, and routine screening for older adult patients.
6. Teach patient to recognize and report a new symptom or complaint.
7. Discuss smoking cessation, alcohol intake, and substance use. Refer to treatment as needed.
8. Ask patient if they use complementary or alternative therapies, such as vitamins, herbs, or teas. Check drug interaction platforms for interactions between ART and specific supplements and herbals.
9. Refer patient to resources such as:
   a. Patient-oriented site with many resources including a list of hotlines for people at risk for acquiring HIV and PLWH, *www.thebody.com.*
   b. Consumer-oriented magazine, which is available at *www.poz.com.*
   c. *100 Question and Answers about HIV and AIDS*, by Joel Gallant, Fourth Edition (2017) (paperback available online and at bookstores). Excellent resource for patients in easy-to-understand language.
   d. Questions and Answers about HIV/AIDS, by the Centers for Disease Control and Prevention, https://www.cdc.gov/hiv/basics/whatishiv.html.
   e. Information about clinical trials that are open to enrollment at ClinicalTrials.gov, *https://clinicaltrials.gov/*
   f. Preexposure prophylaxis. www.cdc.gov/hiv/risk/prep/index.html.
   g. American Liver Foundation. https://liverfoundation.org/

DRUG ALERT Hormonal contraceptives have drug–drug interactions and interact with many ATR regimens. Encourage patient to discuss contraceptive choices with their provider.

DRUG ALERT PI levels are affected by St. John wort and grapefruit. Teach patient to use over-the-counter supplements with caution, disclose usage to their provider, and avoid grapefruit products.

Preventing Opportunistic Infections

1. PCP prophylaxis is started when the $CD4^+$ count is $\leq 200/mm^3$. The most effective medication is trimethoprim/sulfamethoxazole (TMP/SMZ); others are dapsone, atovaquone, and aerosolized pentamidine. To reduce pill burden and prevent unnecessary antibiotic exposure, primary PCP prophylaxis should be discontinued when the CD4 count has increased to ≥ 200 cells/mm^3 for greater than 3 months.
2. Toxoplasmosis prophylaxis is appropriate in patients who are *Toxoplasma* immunoglobulin G (IgG) ab^+ when the $CD4^+$ count is $\leq 100/mm^3$. TMP/SMZ is the preferred agent. Benefit will be conferred when the patient already receives TMP/SMZ PCP prophylaxis using TMP/SMZ. Alternative drug combinations are available for patients who cannot tolerate sulfa drugs, and these combinations are also effective prophylaxis against PCP.
3. MAC prophylaxis is started when the $CD4^+$ count is $\leq 50/mm^3$ and blood cultures for *M. avium* are negative; medications include azithromycin or clarithromycin. Alternative therapy is available for patients who cannot tolerate a macrolide antibiotic.
4. Cytomegalovirus (CMV) end-organ prophylaxis, including for CMV retinitis, is not recommended, owing to high cost and toxicity. Current guidelines recommend immune reconstitution through ART and clinician monitoring for symptoms of disseminated disease as the means for preventing CMV disease.

Immunizations

1. Pneumococcal pneumonia—all patients should receive the most recently recommended pneumococcal vaccine(s).
2. Influenza—all patients should receive the inactivated flu vaccine each fall.
3. Tetanus booster—all patients should receive routine booster every 10 years or, in the case of a wound, after 5 years.
4. Hepatitis A—recommended if at risk and baseline total antibody test is negative.
   a. Risk factors include being a male who has sex with males, being a person who injects drugs, traveling to endemic areas, and being a person with hemophilia.
   b. People who are coinfected with viral hepatitis or who have chronic liver disease should be vaccinated to prevent morbidity and mortality associated with acute hepatitis A infection.
5. Hepatitis B—recommended if baseline antibody test is negative.
6. Human papillomavirus (HPV)—HPV vaccine is recommended up to age 26 in PLWH.
7. Meningococcal—recommended if a risk exists (college freshman living in dormitory, military recruits, asplenia, complement component deficiency, travel to or residence in area with outbreaks, occupational exposure).
8. Measles, mumps, rubella (MMR)—recommended for all patients who are nonimmune with CD4 $\geq 200/mm^3$ (live virus is contraindicated in patients with CD4 $\leq 200/mm^3$).
9. COVID-19 virus—COVID-19 vaccine (all CD4 count) plus booster, especially in people with CD4 $< 200/mm^3$.
10. Mpox—modified vaccinia Ankara as preexposure prophylaxis in high-risk PLWH or as postexposure prophylaxis.

Nursing Management of HIV Infection and AIDS

See Standards of Care Guidelines 25-1.

Nursing Assessment

1. Obtain history of date of HIV diagnosis, $CD4^+$ count at the time of diagnosis, risk factors for infection, constitutional signs and symptoms, recent infections, positive test result for HIV, most recent $CD4^+$ count, and HIV RNA viral load.

STANDARDS OF CARE GUIDELINES 29-1

HIV/AIDS

When caring for patients with HIV infection,

- Practice standard precautions.
- Protect confidentiality.
- Educate the patient about methods that prevent HIV transmission to others.
- Perform a psychosocial assessment and identify mental health needs.
- Develop adherence strategies for patients taking antiretroviral therapy.
- Provide education and interventions for HIV symptom management.
- Assist with tobacco, alcohol, and substance use cessation.

2. Review patient's present complaints, if any.
3. Assess patient's knowledge about HIV/AIDS, including causes, signs and symptoms, modes of transmission, methods for preventing transmission to others, disease progression, and importance of $CD4^+$ count and HIV RNA viral load monitoring.
4. Assess the patient's adherence to medications by reviewing all prescribed drugs, dosing, and frequency. Ask the patient how many times over the last day or week they missed a dose. Encourage honest reporting by acknowledging that missed doses occur.
5. Evaluate nutritional and general health status by assessing weight, body mass index (BMI), anemia, lipid profile, fasting glucose, hemoglobin A1C, and other pertinent labs and anthropometric measures.
6. Assess respiratory rate and depth and auscultate lungs for breath sounds; assess skin color and temperature, palpate lymph nodes, and ask about fever and night sweats.
7. Inspect mouth for hygiene, lesions, and dentition.
8. Examine skin for temperature, condition, and presence of rash, lesions, and other changes.
9. Ask about bowel movement patterns, changes in habits, constipation, abdominal cramping, number and volume of stools, and presence of perianal pain and ulceration.
10. Assess patient's orientation to person, place, time, and situation. Note patient's affect. Ask about any problem with memory and concentration, headaches, seizures, visual changes.
11. Find out as much as possible about patient's lifestyle (assessing for ongoing risk behavior), experience and skills, hobbies, and social support system.

Clinical Manifestations of HIV/AIDS With Advancing Infection

1. Pulmonary manifestations.
   a. Persistent or acute cough, with or without sputum production, shortness of breath, chest pain, fever, hemoptysis.
   b. Possible causes: PCP, bacterial pneumonia (community-acquired pneumonia), *Mycobacterium* tuberculosis, disseminated MAC, *Aspergillus*, *Pseudomonas*, CMV, *Histoplasma*, Kaposi sarcoma, lung cancer, lymphoma, *Cryptococcus*, *Legionella*, or other pathogens and malignancies.
2. GI manifestations.
   a. Diarrhea, weight loss, anorexia, abdominal cramping, feeling of fullness, rectal urgency (tenesmus).
   b. Possible causes: enteric pathogens or malignancies including *Salmonella*, *Shigella*, *Campylobacter*, *Entamoeba histolytica*, *Clostridium difficile*, CMV, MAC, herpes simplex, *Strongyloides*, *Giardia*, *Cryptosporidium*, *Isospora belli*, *Chlamydia*, lymphoma, Kaposi sarcoma, and others.
   c. Difficulty swallowing or substernal pain upon swallowing (feeling of food being stuck), usually caused by *Candida* esophagitis. Also, consider an esophageal ulcer caused by herpes simplex, CMV, or aphthous stomatitis, malignancy, or Mpox.
3. Oral manifestations.
   a. Appearance of oral lesions, white plaques on oral mucosa, particularly in the posterior pharynx, and angular cheilitis from *Candida albicans* of mouth.
   b. Vesicles with ulceration from herpes simplex virus.
   c. White, thickened lesions on lateral margins of tongue from oral hairy leukoplakia.
   d. Oral warts because of HPV.
   e. Periodontitis progressing to gingival necrosis.
   f. Painful, solitary lesions with raised margins may be aphthous ulcers of unclear etiology.
   g. Appearance of flat or nodular purple lesions on the hard or soft palate, buccal mucosa, posterior pharynx from Kaposi sarcoma.
   h. Rubbery, well-circumscribed lesions with or without umbilication may indicate Mpox.
4. CNS manifestations.
   a. Cognitive, motor, and behavioral symptoms may be caused by HIV encephalopathy, acquired immune deficiency syndrome (AIDS) dementia, acute infection, toxicity from alcohol or drugs, adverse reaction to medication, psychiatric condition, and other infectious and malignant causes.
   b. Acute symptoms of infection with fever, malaise, headache, and/or mental status change, seizure, hemiparesis, abnormal gait or speech may be caused by toxoplasmosis, cryptococcal meningitis, herpes virus infections, CMV encephalitis, progressive multifocal leukoencephalopathy, CNS lymphoma, neurosyphilis, or other pathogens and malignancies.
   c. May also have sensory symptoms that present as numbness, tingling, and neuropathic pain of the feet or hands.
5. Ocular manifestations.
   a. Experiencing floaters in the visual field, flashes of light, or sudden loss of a visual field in people who have less than 100 CD4/mm^3, which may be caused by CMV retinitis, a sight-threatening infection that requires urgent evaluation by an ophthalmologist.
   b. Blurry vision, dry eyes, double vision, or swelling of the eyelid or conjunctiva, which may be caused by bacterial or viral conjunctival infection, adverse reaction to medication, syphilis, Kaposi sarcoma, or other pathogens and malignancies.
6. Malignancies.
   a. Kaposi sarcoma.
   b. Non-Hodgkin lymphoma and other lymphomas.
   c. Cervical cancer.
   d. Liver cancer.
   e. Lung cancer.
   f. Anal cancer.
7. Skin manifestations.
   a. Pruritic rash with raised, erythematous papules, located on surfaces that contain hair follicles known as HIV folliculitis. Check for eosinophilia.

b. Abscess caused by methicillin-sensitive and methicillin-resistant *Staphylococcus aureus* infections, *Streptococcus*, or other common skin pathogens.
c. Pruritic nodular rash located on any skin surface, known as prurigo nodularis.
d. Purple, flat, or nodular lesions located on any skin surface including soles of feet, palms of hands, oral mucosa including hard palate might be Kaposi sarcoma and should be biopsied.

Nursing Interventions

Managing ART

1. Assess patient's adherence to medications and clinical appointments; work together to problem-solve a plan to improve adherence.
2. Provide education about prescribed medications before ART is started and periodically thereafter; provide educational materials that the patient can take home.
3. Develop a medication schedule for the patient that incorporates their usual day-to-day activities; place pills in a medication box per the dosing schedule, identify medication reminder tools and apps.
4. Encourage the involvement of a household member or friend during patient education and home medication administration. Continue to monitor for medication adherence after patient has achieved an undetectable viral load.
5. Routinely ask about adverse effects. Encourage patient to report new or ongoing symptoms and teach management of common or expected symptoms.
6. Encourage patient to keep their insurance and prescription drug coverage active and up to date, to prevent lapses in refills and periods without insurance.

DRUG ALERT At every visit, emphasize the importance of medication adherence to achieve viral suppression and prevent resistance. Anticipate and problem-solve barriers to adherence. Develop strategies that anticipate going off course, such as how to manage late or missed doses, change in daily routine, vacation, spending the night away from home, and other life events.

Promoting Dignity and Reducing Fear

1. Maintain a nonjudgmental and positive approach.
2. Anticipate that the patient may pass through a series of stages: initial crisis, transitional stage, acceptance state, and, possibly, preparation for death if treatment options have been exhausted.
3. Allow patient to use some degree of denial as a protective mechanism, which gives some control over when and how the patient will confront the diagnosis and their prognosis.
   a. Expect some displaced anger; avoid being personally affronted by patient's anger.
   b. Allow patient to acknowledge the reality of the situation without giving false assurance.
4. Acknowledge that symptoms of anxiety and depression are common initially but generally improve with time and support. Refer patient to counseling or mental health care, if needed.
5. Anticipate that patients who have a substance use disorder may experience feelings of alienation and isolation. Refer for counseling and treatment.
6. Provide careful discussion and clarification of treatment options.
7. Help patient set realistic goals and expectations.
8. Involve social work expertise for available insurance related, prescription drug and other social resources, and community-based case management.
9. Help patient identify and strengthen personal resources, such as coping skills, relaxation techniques, support network, and self-care.
10. Encourage patient to join an in-person or virtual support community.
11. Observe for mental health changes and intervene or refer to care as needed.
12. Discuss creating advance directives and legal guardianship for minor children as part of routine care for all patients who are engaged in health care. The population of PLWH is aging, with approximately 70% projected to be over age 50 by 2030.
13. Consider the needs of an aging population regarding comorbidities, polypharmacy, health maintenance, socialization, adaptive equipment, and home safety. Consider consultation with a geriatrician.
14. Never assume a patient's family or friends know the patient's HIV status. Always ask the patient who knows of their status. Encourage the patient to share their diagnosis to decrease isolation. Offer to be with the patient when the diagnosis is shared with family or friend(s). Role-playing before disclosing status may be helpful.

Preventing Infection

1. Assess for overt and subtle signs of infection at every visit.
2. Follow standard precautions with all patients.
3. Discuss food safety regarding handling, preparation, and storage.
4. Promote skin care to prevent breaks in the skin.
5. Teach wound care and management; monitor wound for signs of worsening or infection, if applicable.
6. Discuss harm reduction and STI prevention, if relevant.
7. Teach patient to take all antibiotics as directed.
8. Use aseptic techniques when performing invasive procedures.
9. Recommend that someone else clean a cat litter box or bird cage. If no one else is available, then use rubber gloves, wear a mask, change clothes, and wash hands afterward.
10. Ensure that the patient is up to date with immunizations.

Improving Nutritional Status

1. Monitor nutritional status by weighing patient, calculating BMI, and reviewing dietary choices.
2. Consult with a dietitian to develop strategies that optimize nutritional status.
3. Review ART dosing in relation to meal times to optimize ART absorption if the regimen is affected by food. For a patient with oral or esophageal pain:
   a. Administer prescribed antifungal and/or antiviral therapy.
   b. Avoid highly seasoned or acidic foods.
   c. Offer fluids and pureed or soft foods to minimize chewing and ease swallowing and recommend liquid nutritional supplements.
4. Discourage alcohol use because it can impair judgment, affect medication adherence, promote infection, and accelerate liver damage in patients with chronic hepatitis.
5. Refer patient to a community meal delivery program.

Relieving Oral Discomfort

1. Ask about tooth pain, sore throat, dysphagia, and heartburn.
2. Examine mouth and pharynx for oral *Candida* or lesions and teach patient to do the same.
3. Administer antifungal treatment, oral analgesics, and antibacterial oral rinses as indicated.

4. Refer to dental care in the community for routine care, poor dentition, and/or gum disease.

Minimizing the Effects of Diarrhea

1. Diarrhea is common and can have many causes.
2. Review medication list for causative agents.
3. Send new diarrheal stool for ova and parasite studies, polymerase chain reaction (PCR), or culture.
4. Teach patient to monitor stools and report frequency, consistency, and presence of blood.
5. Monitor intake and output; assess skin and mucous membranes for poor turgor and dryness or irritation.
6. Monitor electrolytes. Administer fluids and electrolyte replacement therapy as prescribed.
7. Follow contact precautions and practice strict handwashing.
8. Plan skin care regimen that includes bathing and drying by blotting. Apply ointment or skin barrier cream to the area.
9. Advise patient to eliminate caffeine, alcohol, dairy products, high-fat foods, and acidic juices.
10. Drink liquids at room temperature.
11. Advise patient to avoid foods that increase motility and distention, such as gas-forming fruits and vegetables or dairy.

Managing Altered Mental Status

1. HIV has an affinity for the brain; in patients with advanced HIV infection, the brain is a target organ for opportunistic infections.
2. Take measures to keep the patient safe. Refer outpatients with altered mental status to an acute care appointment or to the emergency department.
3. In inpatients, promote patient safety: bed alarm on, call signal available, assistive devices within reach. Anticipate a plan for toileting. Make frequent checks.
4. Assess for depressive, suicidal, or homicidal ideations or gestures.
5. Provide routine assessment of mental status; monitor for changes in behavior, memory, concentration ability, and motor dysfunction.
6. Check labs and other diagnostic evaluations for abnormalities and examine medication side-effect profiles for possible cause.
7. Maintain a low stimulus environment such as dim lighting and low noise; promote sleep/wake cycle, quiet activities, light socialization, light exercise, and listening to quiet music.
8. Reorient patient frequently: use calendar, clock, family and friends' pictures, lists, white board.
9. Provide reassurance.
10. Anticipate need for advance directives, a health care agent or guardianship, powers of attorney for health care and financial matters, and managing the process of informed consent if patient becomes incapacitated.

Reducing Fever

1. Assess for chills, fever, tachycardia, and tachypnea.
2. Aggressively treat the underlying cause.
3. Encourage increased fluid intake to replace insensible water losses.
4. Administer or teach patient to administer antipyretics as prescribed.

Improving Breathing Pattern

1. Provide supplemental oxygen as ordered. Monitor for increased oxygen demand.
2. Position patient to optimize effective breathing, elevate head of bed, support head and neck to maintain patent airway.
3. To reduce effort, offer soft foods, small portions, bite-size pieces, and nutritional supplements.
4. Monitor for change in respiratory status.
5. Administer or teach patient to take cough medication.
6. Encourage smoking cessation and supplement with nicotine patch to prevent withdrawal during acute phase.
7. Answer questions and provide support if patient has made decision for or against resuscitation and mechanical ventilation.

Community and Home Care Considerations for the Patient With End-Stage AIDS

1. Assist patient, family, or significant other to locate care and support services in the community.
2. If patient is homebound, contact an agency that offers help specifically for PLWH and provides home visits for services such as light housekeeping or food delivery.
3. Assess the home for safety and needs; provide durable medical equipment that can enhance safety and comfort, and optimize function.

Evaluation: Expected Outcomes

- Takes prescribed ART that maintains an undetectable viral load.
- Prevents opportunistic infections.
- Practices safe sex and other harm reduction measures that prevent HIV transmission.
- Eats balanced meals.
- Engages in health maintenance and self-care.
- Participates in activities of daily living.
- Anticipates a full lifespan.

SELECTED READINGS

Archin, N., Bar, K. J., Burdo, T., Caskey, M., Chahroudi, A., Farzan, M., Ho, Y. C., Jones, R. B., Kearney, M., Kuritzkes, D., Margolis, D., Martinez-Picado, J., Okoye, A., Salgado, M., & Stevenson, M. (2023). Highlights from the tenth international workshop on HIV persistence during therapy, December 13–16, 2022, Miami, Florida-USA. *Journal of Virus Eradication, 9*(1), 100315. https://doi.org/10.1016/j.jve.2023.100315

Beichler, H., Grabovac, I., & Dorner, T. E. (2023). Integrated care as a model for interprofessional disease management and the benefits for people living with HIV/AIDS. *International Journal of Environmental Research and Public Health, 20*(4), 3374. https://doi.org/10.3390/ijerph20043374

Centers for Disease Control and Prevention. (2014). *Revised surveillance case definition for HIV infection—United States, 2014.* www.cdc.gov/mmwr/preview/mmwrhtml/rr6303a1.htm?s_cid=rr6303a1_e

Hibberd, P. L., & Garland, J. M. (2022). *Immunizations in persons with HIV. UpToDate.* Retrieved April 14, 2023, from https://www.uptodate.com/contents/immunizations-in-persons-with-hiv

New York State Department of Health AIDS Institute. Clinical Guidelines Program. *PrEP to prevent HIV and promote sexual health.* Accessed April 7, 2023. https://www.hivguidelines.org/prep-for-prevention/

Rao, A. K., Schrodt, C. A., Minhaj, F. S., Waltenburg, M. A., Cash-Goldwasser, S., Yu, Y., Petersen, B. W., Hutson, C., & Damon, I. K. (2023). Interim clinical treatment considerations for severe manifestations of Mpox—United States, February 2023. *Morbidity and Mortality Weekly Report (MMWR), 72*, 232–243. http://dx.doi.org/10.15585/mmwr.mm7209a4

Sax, P. (2024). *100 questions and answers about HIV and AIDS* (6th ed.). Jones & Bartlett.

Schmidt, H. A., Schaefer, R., Nguyen, V. T. T., Radebe, M., Sued, O., Rodolph, M., Ford, N., & Baggaley, R. (2022). Scaling up access to HIV pre-exposure prophylaxis (PrEP): Should nurses do the job? *Lancet HIV, 9*(5), e363–e366. http://doi.org/10.1016/S2352-3018(22)00006-6

Siegler, E. L., Moxley, J. H., & Glesby, M. J. (2021). Aging-related concerns of people living with HIV referred for geriatric consultation. *HIV AIDS (Auckl), 13*, 467–474. http://doi.org/10.2147/HIV.S306532

Wolfe, C. (2019). *Immune reconstitution inflammatory syndrome. UpToDate.* Retrieved April 11, 2023, from https://www.uptodate.com/contents/immune-reconstitution-inflammatory-syndrome?search=immune%20reconstitution%20inflammatory%20syndrome&source=search_result&selectedTitle=1~150&usage_type=default&display_rank=1

Wells, J., Flowers, L., Mehta, C. C., Chandler, R., Knott, R., Holstad, M. M., & Bruner, D. W. (2022). Follow-up to high-resolution anoscopy after abnormal anal cytology in people living with HIV. *AIDS Patient Care and STDs, 36*, 263–271. http://doi.org/10.1089/apc.2022.0057

26 Connective Tissue Disorders*

OVERVIEW AND ASSESSMENT

Connective tissue is a fibrous tissue that supports and connects internal organs, forms bones and the walls of blood vessels, attaches muscles and bones to bones (tendons and ligaments), and replaces tissue following injury (scar tissue). The long fibers of connective tissue contain a protein called *collagen*.

Connective tissue disorders affect the integrity of the musculoskeletal system and may also affect blood vessels, the skin, and a variety of organs. Many connective tissue disorders are rheumatic in nature, meaning that they are characterized by inflammation and pain of the joints, muscles, and fibrous tissue. They may also be autoimmune in nature, meaning that they result from a dysfunctional immune system that misinterprets body cells as a threat, resulting in the attack on body tissues. Many of these conditions are chronic and progressive and may lead to disability; however, they can often be controlled with medication.

Musculoskeletal and Related Assessment

Assessment for connective tissue disorders must be comprehensive and include all body systems. Clues to connective tissue disorders are often found in the skin, eyes, lungs, and gastrointestinal and neurologic systems. Functional assessment is also important; developing a standardized approach to measuring disease activity as well as patient-reported outcomes is a priority of the leading international rheumatic research consortiums and patient care groups, such as the American College of Rheumatology (ACR), the European Alliance of Associations for Rheumatology (EULAR), and the International Consortium of Health Outcome Measurement (ICHOM). Many questionnaires and assessments are available, including the Patient-Reported Outcomes Measurement Information System (PROMIS) program, a free program developed by the National Institutes of Health (available at https://www.healthmeasures.net), the Health Assessment Questionnaire, the RAPID3 (which measures disease activity by asking patients to rate their ability to participate in daily activities, pain on a 0 to 10 scale, and overall health on a 0 to 10 scale), and others.

Subjective Data

Obtain a history of presenting symptoms, including duration and intensity, course of the illness, and impact of symptoms on the patient's life.

1. Musculoskeletal pain—characteristics.
   a. Joint pain.
   b. Joint swelling.
   c. Morning stiffness.
   d. Enthesitis—area of inflammation at the site of attachment of tendon or ligament to bone.
   e. Dactylitis—inflammation of finger or toe, known as "sausage digit."
2. Constitutional symptoms.
   a. Fever.
   b. Weight loss and anorexia.
   c. Fatigue.
3. Involvement of other body symptoms.
   a. Skin—rashes, sun sensitivity, color changes in fingers or toes.
   b. Ocular—dry or red/painful eyes; light sensitivity.
   c. Pulmonary—chronic shortness of breath or cough.
   d. Neurologic—numbness or tingling in fingers or toes, foot drop.
   e. Mucous membranes—dry mouth, oral/nasal or vaginal ulcers.
   f. Gastrointestinal (GI)—chronic diarrhea or history of bloody stool.
   g. Vascular—history of blood clots or miscarriages.

*Please note that the term "male" in this chapter refers to a person assigned male at birth, and the term "female" in this chapter refers to a person assigned female at birth.

4. Depression or psychosis.
5. Self-care activities and functional ability.
6. Social activities and roles.
7. Family history of rheumatic or autoimmune disorders.

Objective Data

1. Musculoskeletal examination:
   a. Pain on palpation or range of motion (ROM).
   b. Joint swelling, warmth, or erythema.
   c. Joint motion restriction.
   d. Pain, swelling, or warmth of soft tissues surrounding joints.
   e. Deformities.
2. Skin:
   a. Skin rash or other abnormalities such as thickening.
   b. Alopecia.
   c. Nail changes such as pitting or lifting.
3. Oral mucosa:
   a. Ulcerations.
   b. Dryness.
4. Ocular:
   a. Conjunctival inflammation.
   b. Dryness.
5. Pulmonary:
   a. Adventitious sounds.
   b. Friction rub.
6. Neurologic:
   a. Foot drop.
   b. Muscle weakness.
   c. Neurologic deficits.

Laboratory Studies

Antinuclear Antibody

Antinuclear antibodies (ANAs) are antibodies directed against certain proteins found in the cell nucleus. A positive ANA can be found in several rheumatic diseases, nonrheumatic diseases, and certain infections. ANA is highly sensitive for detecting systemic lupus erythematosus (SLE) but is nonspecific (high false-positive rate).

Nursing and Patient Care Considerations

1. Be alert for drugs that may cause false-positive results.
2. Results will be reported in a staining pattern (speckled, homogeneous, peripheral, nucleolar) if positive, which correlates to various types of connective tissue disorders and various subsets of SLE (see Table 26-1).
3. Titer will also be reported with positive ANA (when measured by immunofluorescence) but does not reflect disease activity or prognosis. An isolated ANA of <1:160 without supporting clinical findings is not considered diagnostic or clinically relevant.

Anti–Double-Stranded DNA

Anti–double-stranded DNA (anti-dsDNA) is a highly specific marker for diagnosing SLE. This antibody is also useful for monitoring disease progression because anti-dsDNA levels fluctuate with disease activity.

Nursing and Patient Care Considerations

1. High anti-dsDNA levels are associated with the development of lupus nephritis.
2. Other connective tissue disorders (besides SLE) can occasionally result in a positive dsDNA.
3. There is no special preparation for this blood test.

Table 26-1 ANA Staining Patterns and Connective Tissue Disorders

ANA PATTERN	CONNECTIVE TISSUE DISORDER
Peripheral (rim, ring, membranous)	Active SLE, usually with renal disease
Homogenous (diffuse)	SLE, RA
Speckled	SLE, RA, scleroderma, Sjögren syndrome, mixed connective tissue disorder
Nucleolar	Scleroderma

ANA, antinuclear antibody; RA, rheumatoid arthritis; SLE, systemic lupus erythematosus.

Rheumatoid Factor

Rheumatoid factor (RF) is a test for macroglobulin found in the blood of patients with rheumatoid arthritis (RA) and other disorders. RF is a single antibody directed against immunoglobulin G.

Nursing and Patient Care Considerations

1. RF is 60% to 80% sensitive in adult patients with RA. The specificity is 70% to 85%.
2. May also be positive in patients with SLE, Sjögren syndrome, Hashimoto thyroiditis, and multiple sclerosis. May be false positive with endocarditis, tuberculosis, syphilis, sarcoidosis, cancer, hepatitis C, patients with skin or renal allographs, and in some liver, lung, or kidney diseases.
3. Negative RF does not exclude the diagnosis of RA.
4. Certain disease manifestations, such as severe joint involvement and extra-articular manifestations, may be more frequent in those with high-titer RF.

Anticyclic-Citrullinated Peptide

Anticyclic-citrullinated peptide (anti-CCP) is a marker that helps diagnose RA. These autoantibodies are produced as a response to citrullination of amino acids that occurs during periods of inflammation in patients with RA.

Nursing and Patient Care Considerations

1. Anti-CCP is about as sensitive, but more specific (90%), than the RF test. Found in approximately 75% of patients with RA.
2. It may be valuable in cases of early arthritis when symptoms are mild and nonspecific, and aggressive treatment is being contemplated. Anti-CCP antibody is used with the RF as the gold standard in making the diagnosis of RA.
3. No specific preparation is needed for this blood test.

Complement

- *Complement* is a complex cascade system that activates proteins as part of the body's defense against infection.
- Specific components include CH50 (total complement), C3, and C4; measurement helps determine immune complex formation or agammaglobulinemia.
- Complement levels are decreased in certain autoimmune diseases, particularly SLE, because of complement consumption and because of activation of proteolytic enzymes and tissue damage.

Nursing and Patient Care Considerations

1. C3 and C4 are often monitored to evaluate disease activity in SLE.

Table 26-2 Synovial Fluid Analysis

	NORMAL COLOR	WHITE BLOOD CELL COUNT	VISCOSITY	CRYSTALS
Normal	Clear, yellow	200/µm³	Normal	None
Osteoarthritis	Clear, slightly turbid	200–600/µm³	Low	None
Gout	Turbid	2,000–75,000/µm³	Low	Monosodium urate
Inflammatory arthritis (Rheumatoid arthritis, systemic lupus erythematosus, Sjögren syndrome, psoriatic)	Turbid, yellow	2,000–75,000/µm³	Low	None
Septic arthritis	Pus, very turbid	Generally 80,000/µm³	Low	None

2. Obtain venous blood sample and refrigerate; send to laboratory promptly because complement deteriorates at room temperature.
3. Serial measurements may be helpful in monitoring the activity of some rheumatic diseases; decreased levels indicate increased disease activity.

C-Reactive Protein

C-reactive protein (CRP) is produced by the liver and is a nonspecific marker for infection and inflammation.

Nursing and Patient Care Considerations

1. CRP reacts quicker to inflammatory changes than erythrocyte sedimentation rate (ESR); it rises within a few hours of an infection or inflammatory condition and then decreases quickly when inflammation resolves.
2. CRP can be used to differentiate inflammatory from noninflammatory conditions and to monitor the effectiveness of treatment.
3. Normal CRP is usually below 10 mg/L; a level over 100 mg/L usually indicates infection or inflammation; however, some inflammatory conditions can raise CRP by 1000-fold.

Erythrocyte Sedimentation Rate

ESR determines the rate at which red blood cells (RBCs) fall out of unclotted blood in 1 hour. The test is based on the premise that inflammatory and other disease processes create changes in blood proteins, thus causing aggregation of RBCs that makes them heavier. Most beneficial in monitoring inflammatory disease activity.

Nursing and Patient Care Considerations

1. ESR is sometimes, but not always, elevated in rheumatic illnesses.
2. The test is sensitive for inflammatory conditions, but not specific to connective tissue disorders.
   a. Result may be elevated by obesity, pregnancy, menstruation, medications (such as heparin and oral contraceptives), infection, malignancy, anemia, and advanced age.
   b. Result may be reduced by elevated blood levels of glucose, albumin, and phospholipids, or drugs, such as corticosteroids or high-dose aspirin.

Other Tests

Synovial Fluid Analysis

1. A sample of synovial (joint) fluid is analyzed for several components.
   a. Color.
   b. Clarity/turbidity.
   c. Viscosity.
   d. White blood cell (WBC) count with differential.
   e. Crystals and their identification.
2. Arthrocentesis, a sterile procedure, requires antiseptic cleaning agent, local anesthetic, a 20-G needle (an 18-G needle if infected fluid is suspected), and a 10- to 20-mL syringe.

Nursing and Patient Care Considerations

1. Patients are generally apprehensive about having a needle inserted into a joint. They require reassurance and explanation of the importance of information derived from test results.
2. Assist the health care provider with the test by collecting supplies, maintaining a sterile field, sending joint fluid samples for testing, and monitoring for bleeding following the procedure.
3. Results help to differentiate infection, inflammation, and crystal deposition in a painful joint (see Table 26-2).

GENERAL PROCEDURES AND TREATMENT MODALITIES

Pharmacologic Agents

EVIDENCE BASE American College of Rheumatology. (2021). *2021 American College of Rheumatology guideline for the treatment of rheumatoid arthritis.* Author. https://www.rheumatology.org/Practice-Quality/Clinical-Support/Clinical-Practice-Guidelines/Rheumatoid-Arthritis

Fraenkel, L., Bathon, J. M., England, B. R., St Clair, E. W., Arayssi, T., Carandang, K., Deane, K. D., Genovese, M., Huston, K. K., Kerr, G., Kremer, J., Nakamura, M. C., Russell, L. A., Singh, J. A., Smith, B. J., Sparks, J. A., Venkatachalam, S., Weinblatt, M. E., Al-Gibbawi, M., Baker, J. F., Barbour, K. E., Barton, J. L., Cappelli, L., Chamseddine, F., George, M., Johnson, S. R., Kahale, L., Karam, B. S., Khamis, A. M., Navarro-Millán, I., Mirza, R., Schwab, P., Singh, N., Turgunbaev, M., Turner, A. S., Yaacoub, S., & Akl, E. A. (2021). American College of Rheumatology guideline for the treatment of rheumatoid arthritis. *Arthritis Care Res (Hoboken)*, 73(7), 924-939. https://doi.org/10.1002/acr.24596

Connective tissue disorders may be treated with various drugs to relieve pain and to halt or minimize the disease process. Types of agents include nonsteroidal anti-inflammatory drugs (NSAIDs), corticosteroids, and disease-modifying antirheumatic drugs (DMARDs). Drug therapy is typically long term and requires frequent evaluation for adverse effects (see Table 26-3). Patient education information about pharmacologic agents used to treat various disorders can be obtained from the National Institute of Arthritis and Musculoskeletal and Skin Disease (www.niams.nih.gov) or from the American College of Rheumatology (ACR; www.rheumatology.org).

Table 26-3 Drug Therapy for Rheumatic Diseases

DRUG	ACTION	ADVERSE EFFECTS (REPORTED IN >10% PER PRODUCT LABELING UNLESS OTHERWISE NOTED)
Anti-inflammatory agents		
• Salsalate • Trisalicylate		
Salicylates		
• Aspirin (may be buffered or enteric coated)	• Anti-inflammatory, antipyretic, and analgesic effects	• Tinnitus, gastric intolerance or GI bleeding, and purpuric tendencies.
Nonsteroidal anti-inflammatory drugs (NSAIDs)		
• Ibuprofen • Fenoprofen • Naproxen • Tolmetin • Sulindac • Meclofenamate • Ketoprofen • Diclofenac • Nabumetone • Ketorolac • Oxaprozin • Flurbiprofen • Diflunisal • Piroxicam • Etodolac • Indomethacin • Meloxicam	• Anti-inflammatory and analgesic effects • Mechanism of action may be related to inhibition of prostaglandin synthesis (prostaglandins have a role in inflammatory process, pain, and fever). • Nonsteroidal anti-inflammatory agents for adjunctive treatment of rheumatoid arthritis • Sometimes remarkably effective in the control of articular symptoms	• GI irritation: nausea, vomiting, epigastric distress, precipitation and reactivation of peptic ulcer, hepatitis • Hematologic: bone marrow depression, anemia, leukopenia, thrombocytopenia purpura • Decrease in renal function can precipitate renal failure. • Central nervous system: headache, dizziness, drowsiness, aseptic meningitis • Cardiovascular: edema, dyspnea palpitations • Boxed warnings for cardiovascular thrombotic events and serious GI adverse events.
Selective COX-2 inhibitor		
• Celecoxib	• Selective prostaglandin inhibition so that the inflammatory process is reduced without reducing protective prostaglandin effects on gastric mucosa	• Same adverse effects as other NSAIDs • Boxed warnings for cardiovascular thrombotic events and serious GI adverse events.
Disease-modifying anti-rheumatic drugs (DMARDs)		
Antimalarial agents		
• Hydroxychloroquine sulfate • Chloroquine phosphate	• Remission-induction agents for inflammatory arthritis usually in combination with other DMARDs • Used frequently for lupus	• Retinopathy (4%, dose dependent)
Sulfonamides		
• Sulfasalazine	• Salicylate, sulfonamide	• Rash, GI upset, headache
Biologic DMARDs		
• Etanercept • Adalimumab • Golimumab • Certolizumab pegol • Infliximab	• Tumor necrosis factor blocker • SC: etanercept, adalimumab, certolizumab, golimumab • IV: infliximab, golimumab	• Infection, hypersensitivity reactions, diarrhea, rash, +ANA. Other serious adverse effects: demyelinating disorders, activation of latent TB infection, reactivation of hepatitis B, lupus-like syndrome, TNF-induced psoriasis • Use caution in patients with CHF. • Do not use etanercept in patients with previously diagnosed inflammatory eye disease. • Boxed warnings: serious infection, malignancy
• Abatacept	• Selective T-cell costimulation modulator; available as IV or SC	• Nausea, infection, headach
• Tocilizumab • Sarilumab	• Interleukin-6 receptor blocker available as IV (tocilizumab) or SC (tocilizumab, sarilumab)	• Infection, increased cholesterol, constipation, elevated ALT/AST, neutropenia/thrombocytopenia • Use caution in patients with demyelinating disorders, hepatic impairment, history of diverticulitis. • Boxed warning for infections
• Anakinra	• Interleukin-1 receptor agonist (SC)	• Infection, injection site reactions, headache, arthralgia

(continued)

Table 26-3 Drug Therapy for Rheumatic Diseases (*continued*)

DRUG	ACTION	ADVERSE EFFECTS (REPORTED IN >10% PER PRODUCT LABELING UNLESS OTHERWISE NOTED)
• Rituximab	• Selective B-cell–depleting agent (IV)	• Infection, flushing, hypertension, peripheral edema, night sweats, hypogammaglobulinemia, cytopenias, chills, fatigue, headache, insomnia, nausea, cough, muscle spasm • Boxed warnings for infusion-related reactions, mucocutaneous reactions, hepatitis B reactivation, and progressive multifocal leukoencephalopathy
• Secukinumab • Ixekizumab	• Interleukin 17A inhibitors available as SC (ixekizumab and secukinumab) or IV (secukinumab)	• Infection, reactivation of tuberculosis, hypersensitivity reactions, neutropenia • May cause inflammatory bowel disease • Avoid in patients with known inflammatory bowel disease.
• Belimumab	• B-lymphocyte stimulator (BLyS-specific) inhibitor (IV or SC)	• Diarrhea, nausea, infection, hypersensitivity reactions, psychiatric disturbance • Assess patients for depression prior to and during therapy.
• Anifrolumab	• Type 1 interferon receptor antagonist	• Adverse effects are infection and increased risk of herpes zoster
• Ustekinumab	• Interleukin-12/23 inhibitor (SC)	• Infection, hypersensitivity reactions, reactivation of tuberculosis
Small molecules		
• Baricitinib	• JAK1/JAK2 inhibitor (PO)	• Infection • Use caution in patients at risk for GI perforation. • Boxed warning for major adverse cardiovascular events; use caution in patients who smoke, patients with a history of MI/CVA, and/or patients with other risk factors for cardiovascular events. • Boxed warning for thrombus; use caution in patients with cardiovascular risk factors or at risk for clots. • Boxed warning for malignancies
• Tofacitinib	• JAK1/JAK3 inhibitor (PO)	• Infection, hyperlipidemia, hypersensitivity reactions • Use caution in patients with a history or at risk for ILD, patients with hepatic and/or renal impairment. • Boxed warning for major adverse cardiovascular events; use caution in patients who smoke, patients with a history of MI/CVA, and/or patients with other risk factors for cardiovascular events. • Boxed warning for thrombus; use caution in patients with cardiovascular risk factors or at risk for clots • Boxed warning for malignancies
• Upadacitinib	• JAK1 inhibitor PO)	• Infection, acne, hypersensitivity reactions, hyperlipidemia, cytopenias • Use caution in patients at risk for GI perforation. • Boxed warning for major adverse cardiovascular events; use caution in patients who smoke, patients with a history of MI/CVA, and/or patients with other risk factors for cardiovascular events. • Boxed warning for thrombus; use caution in patients with cardiovascular risk factors or at risk for clots • Boxed warning for malignancies
Traditional DMARDs		
• Methotrexate	• Immunosuppressant—antimetabolite	• Diarrhea, nausea, mucocutaneous ulcers, increased AST/ALT, dizziness, fatigue, headache, cough, infection • Pregnancy precautions • Alcohol screening/counselling required prior to and periodically throughout use
• Azathioprine	• Immunosuppressant—antiproliferative agent	• Nausea, vomiting, leukopenia, infection, hepatotoxicity, pancreatitis • Use with caution in patients with renal or hepatic impairment. • Boxed warning for malignancies

Table 26-3 Drug Therapy for Rheumatic Diseases (*continued*)

DRUG	ACTION	ADVERSE EFFECTS (REPORTED IN >10% PER PRODUCT LABELING UNLESS OTHERWISE NOTED)
• Cyclophosphamide	• Immunosuppressant—alkylating agent	• Bone marrow suppression, cardiotoxicity, hemorrhagic cystitis, hepatotoxicity, pulmonary toxicity, secondary primary malignancy
• Cyclosporine	• Immunosuppressant—calcineurin inhibitor	• Edema, skin rash, increased nitrogen, increased triglycerides, abdominal pain, diarrhea, dyspepsia, nausea, headache, pain, parasthesia, muscle cramps, tremor, flu-like symptoms, genital tract disease, hepatotoxicity, hyperkalemia • Boxed warnings: should only be prescribed by experienced health care providers; increased susceptibility to infection and neoplasm; erratic bioavailability; increased risk of skin malignancies; hypertension and nephrotoxicities
• Leflunomide	• Immunosuppressant—pyrimidine synthesis inhibitor	• Alopecia, skin rash, diarrhea, nausea, headache, hypertension, infection • Use with caution in patients with renal impairment. • Boxed warnings: embryo-fetal toxicity, hepatotoxicity
• Mycophenolate mofetil	• Immunosuppressant—antiproliferative agent	• Infections, nausea, abdominal pain, headaches, dizziness, insomnia, tremors, rash • Use with caution in patients with renal impairment. • Boxed warnings: should only be prescribed by experienced health care providers; serious infections; malignancies; embryo-fetal toxicity
Corticosteroids • Prednisone • Prednisolone • Triamcinolone • Betamethasone • Hydrocortisone • Dexamethasone • Methylprednisolone	• Alter immune response by binding to intracellular corticosteroid receptors • Potent anti-inflammatory action • Ideally used for short-term management.	• Osteoporosis, fractures, avascular necrosis • Gastric ulcers, infection susceptibility • Hirsutism, acne, moon facies, abnormal fat deposition, edema, emotional disorders, menstrual disorders • Hyperglycemia, hypokalemia • Hypertension, cataracts

ALT, alanine aminotransferase; ANA, antinuclear antibody; AST, aspartate aminotransferase; CHF, congestive heart failure; COPD, chronic obstructive pulmonary disease; CVA, cerebrovascular accident; GI, gastrointestinal; ILD, interstitial lung disease; IV, intravenous; JAK, Janus kinase; MI, myocardial infarction; PO, by mouth; SC, subcutaneous; TB, tuberculosis; TNF, tumor necrosis factor.

Physical and Occupational Therapy

Physical and occupational therapy provides a multimodal program to help reduce pain and to improve joint function. Many other measures can be taught to patients for home practice. Components of the program may include:

- Joint conservation.
- Energy conservation.
- Splinting (in rare instances).
- Range of motion (ROM) exercises.
- Application of heat and cold.
- Endurance or aerobic conditioning.
- Modification of home and work environment.

Joint Conservation

Teach or reinforce the following practices:

1. Perform activities using good body mechanics.
2. Avoid overuse of joints. Pace task and include rest in long or repetitive activities.
3. Use large joints to perform activities—spread the load over as many joints as possible.
4. Perform activities in smooth movements to avoid trauma induced by abrupt movements.

Energy Conservation

Teach or reinforce the following practices:

1. Organize materials, utensils, and tools.
2. Perform lengthy activities in a seated position.
3. Work at an even pace—avoid rushing.
4. Delegate work to others when possible.

Splinting

1. May be used for wrists and hands.
2. Ensure proper application.
3. Periodically inspect for skin irritation, neurovascular compromise, or improper fit.
4. Usually worn during an acute stage of inflammation to protect the joint.

Exercise

Instruct and reinforce correct method of exercise:

1. Avoid exercising inflamed joints—putting these joints through ROM exercises one to two times per day when inflamed is sufficient.
2. Perform exercises daily, as prescribed.

3. Aerobic conditioning exercises may be indicated when disease activity permits.
4. Walking, biking, swimming, and water walking for 30 minutes, three times per week. Regular exercise three times per week for at least 20 minutes for 6 months has been shown to reduce fatigue and disability in patients with RA compared to those who did not exercise.

Other Measures

1. Reinforce correct use and application of heat and cold.
2. Obtain and teach correct use of assistive devices.
3. Reinforce use of behavior modification and relaxation techniques as adjuncts to therapy.
4. Suggest discussion with health care provider about complementary and alternative therapies. A wide variety of herbal and nutraceutical products have been used and studied, but data remain inconclusive about efficacy (see Table 26-4).
   a. Many herbal and supplemental products are marketed for pain, inflammation, and repair of cartilage; however, scientific evidence for clear-cut treatment benefit is lacking.
   b. Reflexology, tai chi, qi gong, yoga, and acupressure or acupuncture have benefited some patients with arthritis and connective tissue disorders. Assist the patient in finding certified providers in these disciplines, if desired.
   c. Use of magnets to relieve pain has not shown effectiveness in numerous studies since the concept was introduced.
   d. For more information, refer patients to the National Center for Complementary and Integrative Health at https://nccih.nih.gov.
5. Advise patient to modify home and work environments as needed, to install safety devices, and to maintain a safe environment.
6. Advise patient to seek counseling regarding sexuality if joint pain and inflammation are barriers to performance.
7. Reinforce the chronic waxing-and-waning nature of the illness to lessen susceptibility to quackery.

EVIDENCE BASE National Center for Complementary and Alternative Medicine. (2019). *Rheumatoid arthritis: In depth.* Author. https://www.nccih.nih.gov/health/rheumatoid-arthritis-in-depth

DISORDERS

Rheumatoid Arthritis

Rheumatoid arthritis (RA) is a chronic inflammatory disease that affects joints and other organ systems. RA affects 0.5% to 1% of the population worldwide. Diagnostic criteria include synovitis in any joint where no alternative diagnosis can explain the synovitis and a score of 6/10 in four domains: number and site of involved joints, serologic abnormality, elevated acute-phase response (markers of inflammation), and symptom duration. Joint erosions as seen on imaging confirm diagnosis, regardless of score.

EVIDENCE BASE Fraenkel, L., Bathon, J. M., England, B. R., St Clair, E. W., Arayssi, T., Carandang, K., Deane, K. D., Genovese, M., Huston, K. K., Kerr, G., Kremer, J., Nakamura, M. C., Russell, L. A., Singh, J. A., Smith, B. J., Sparks, J. A., Venkatachalam, S., Weinblatt, M. E., Al-Gibbawi, M., ... Akl, E. A. (2021). 2021 American College of Rheumatology guideline for the treatment of rheumatoid arthritis. *Arthritis & Rheumatology, 73*(7), 1108–1123. https://doi.org/10.1002/art.41752

Table 26-4 Complementary and Alternative Drug Therapy for Rheumatic Diseases

DRUG	EFFECT	COMMENTS
Fish oil (omega-3 fatty acid)	May reduce tenderness and stiffness; may reduce the need for NSAIDs	May interact with blood thinners, antihypertensives. Avoid high-dose fish liver oil, which may cause vitamins A and D toxicity.
Gamma-linoleic acid (GLA) (omega-6 fatty acid, evening primrose oil, borage, black currant)	Converted into substances that reduce inflammation to relieve joint pain, stiffness, tenderness, and possibly NSAID use	Appears to be safe but some borage oil preparations contain hepatotoxic chemicals. More research on dose and duration is needed.
Thunder god vine (*Tripterygium wilfordii*)	May fight inflammation and suppress the immune system; may relieve rheumatoid arthritis symptoms.	May cause serious side effects—diarrhea, stomach upset, hair loss, headache, skin rash, menstrual changes, male infertility; long-term use may reduce bone mineral density.
Green tea	Substances might be useful in rheumatoid arthritis, lupus.	High doses have been linked to hepatic dysfunction.
Turmeric (curcumin)	Small studies completed in lupus nephritis.	Generally safe, no adverse effects; however, may cause stomach ulcers in high doses with prolonged use
Cayenne pepper (capsicum)	Thought to deplete substance P, reducing pain transmission	Takes several days to obtain pain relief; do not use with heat application.
	Applied topically to the skin over joints in concentrations of 0.025%-0.25%	

GLA, gamma-linoleic acid; NSAID, nonsteroidal anti-inflammatory drug.

Pathophysiology and Etiology

1. Immunologic processes result in inflammation of synovium, producing antigens and inflammatory by-products that lead to destruction of articular cartilage and bone, synovitis, and production of a granular tissue called *pannus* (see Figure 26-1).
2. Granulation tissue forms adhesions that lead to decreased joint mobility.
3. Similar adhesions can occur in supporting structures, such as ligaments and tendons, and cause contractures and ruptures that further affect joint structure and mobility.
4. The etiology is unknown but is probably a combined effect of environmental, epidemiologic, infectious, and genetic factors. Smoking is known to worsen the symptoms of RA.
5. Females are affected more frequently than males.
6. Differential diagnosis includes reactive arthritis, psoriatic arthritis, and other inflammatory arthritides.

Clinical Manifestations

1. Arthritis—synovitis in any joint (see Figure 26-2, page 811).
2. Skin manifestations.
   a. Rheumatoid nodules—elbows, fingers, and feet.
   b. Vasculitic changes—brown, splinter-like lesions in fingers or nail folds.
3. Cardiac manifestations.
   a. Acute pericarditis.
   b. Conduction defects.
   c. Valvular insufficiency.
   d. Coronary arteritis.
   e. Cardiac tamponade—rare.
   f. Myocardial infarction and sudden death—rare.
4. Pulmonary manifestations.
   a. Bronchiectasis.
   b. Pleural effusion and pleurisy.
   c. Interstitial lung disease—most commonly usual interstitial pneumonia (UIP) or nonspecific interstitial pneumonia (NSIP).
   d. Laryngeal obstruction caused by involvement of the cricoarytenoid joint—rare.
   e. Pulmonary nodules.
5. Neurologic manifestations.
   a. Mononeuritis multiplex—wrist drop and foot drop.
   b. Carpal tunnel syndrome.
   c. Compression of spinal nerve roots (cervical spine only).
   d. Distal sensory neuropathy.

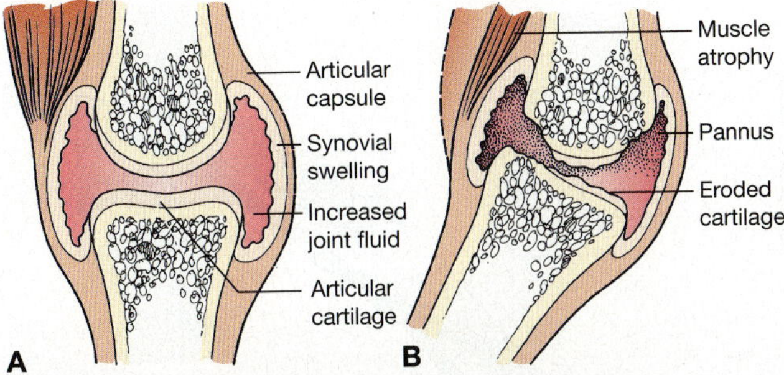

Figure 26-1. Pathophysiology of rheumatoid arthritis. **(A)** Joint structure with synovial swelling and fluid accumulation in the joint. **(B)** Pannus, eroded articular cartilage with joint space narrowing, muscle atrophy, and ankylosis.

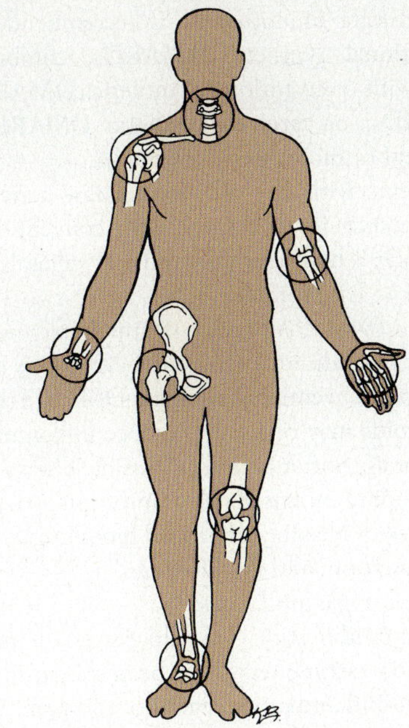

Figure 26-2. Rheumatoid arthritis characteristically involves the joints of the hands, wrist, feet, ankles, knees, and elbows; the glenohumeral and acromioclavicular joints; and the hips. The articulations of the cervical spine are also affected.

6. Other manifestations.
   a. Felty's Syndrome.
   b. Fatigue.
   c. Weight loss.
   d. Episcleritis.

Diagnostic Evaluation

1. Complete blood count (CBC)—normochromic, normocytic anemia of chronic disease; may also have iron deficiency anemia (hypochromic, microcytic); platelets may be elevated with inflammation.
2. Rheumatoid factor (RF)—positive in up to 60% to 80% of patients with RA; cyclic citrullinated peptide (CCP) antibody is more specific for RA than RF testing.
3. Erythrocyte sedimentation rate (ESR) and C-reactive protein (CRP)—may be elevated due to active inflammation.
4. Synovial fluid analysis may be done in acute swollen large joint—see page 806.
5. X-rays—erosive disease may occur in up to 65% of patients. Typically, changes develop within 2 years of symptom onset.
   a. Hands/wrists—marginal erosions of the proximal interphalangeal (PIP), metacarpophalangeal, and carpal joints; generalized osteopenia.
   b. Cervical spine—erosions that produce atlantoaxial subluxation (generally after many years).
6. Magnetic resonance imaging (MRI)—detects spinal cord compression that results from C1 to C2 subluxation and compression of surrounding vascular structures. Also detects erosions earlier than x-ray.
7. Ultrasound—detects synovitis and erosion (very user dependent).

Management

1. Disease-modifying antirheumatic drugs (DMARDs) to reduce disease activity; the goal of treatment is low disease activity or remission to prevent joint damage and disability.

a. Methotrexate monotherapy is recommended over other conventional synthetic DMARDs, combination treatment with conventional synthetic DMARDs, biologic DMARDs, or targeted synthetic DMARDs for initial treatment of moderate-to-severe RA.
b. In patients with RA with low disease activity, the order of preference for treatment with conventional synthetic DMARDs is hydroxychloroquine > sulfasalazine > methotrexate > leflunomide.
c. In patients who do not reach treatment targets, addition of a biologic or traditional synthetic DMARD is recommended over triple conventional synthetic DMARD therapy.

2. Corticosteroids may be used to reduce inflammation. Generally used for as short a period as possible due to multiple side effects, including increased risk of infection, loss of bone mass, increased risk of bleeding, increased blood sugar, higher risk of cataracts, agitation, and mood swings.
3. Nonpharmacologic modalities:
   a. Behavior modification—to reduce stress on inflamed joints.
   b. Relaxation techniques—have been shown to decrease levels of pro-inflammatory cytokines and pain.
4. Surgery:
   a. Synovectomy.
   b. Arthrodesis—joint fusion.
   c. Total joint replacement.

DRUG ALERT The American College of Rheumatology (ACR) publishes management guidelines regarding DMARDs and vaccinations (available at https://www.rheumatology.org/Practice-Quality/Clinical-Support/Clinical-Practice-Guidelines/Vaccinations). Reference these guidelines prior to recommending or giving any vaccines to patients on anti-rheumatic medications.

Complications

1. Loss of joint function because of bony adhesions, erosions, and damage of supporting structures.
2. Interstitial lung disease—affects 10% to 50% of those with RA.
3. Anemia of chronic disease—more common in active disease.
4. Myocardial infarction—RA is an independent risk factor for coronary artery disease.
5. Heart failure—the risk for heart failure in patients with RA is approximately twice that of the general population.

Nursing Assessment

1. Perform joint examination, if indicated, noting which joints affected; range of motion (ROM) of each joint; presence of heat, redness, synovial swelling; and possible joint effusion.
2. Note presence of deformities (see Figure 26-3):
   a. Swan neck—PIP joints hyperextend.
   b. Boutonniere—PIP joints flex.
   c. Ulnar deviation—fingers point toward the ulna.
3. Assess pain using a pain measurement scale such as the visual analog scale (10-cm straight line scored 0 to 100; patient makes a mark indicating intensity of pain).
4. Assess functional status using the ACR revised criteria for classification for global functional status.
   a. Class I—completely able to perform usual activities of daily living (ADLs).
   b. Class II—able to perform usual self-care and vocational activities, but limited in avocational activities.
   c. Class III—able to perform usual self-care activities, but limited in vocational and avocational activities.
   d. Class IV—limited ability to perform usual self-care, vocational, and avocational activities.
5. Assess for adherence to treatment plan, any complementary methods used, and any adverse reactions to medications.

Nursing Interventions

Controlling Pain

1. Apply local heat or cold to affected joints for 15 to 20 minutes, three to four times per day. Avoid temperatures likely to cause skin or tissue damage by checking temperature of warm soaks; always cover cold packs with a towel.
2. Administer or teach self-administration of pharmacologic agents.
   a. Advise patient when to expect pain relief, based on mechanism of action of the drug.
3. Encourage the use of adjunctive pain control measures.
   a. Progressive muscle relaxation.
   b. Biofeedback.
   c. Meditation.
   d. Acupuncture or similar therapies.

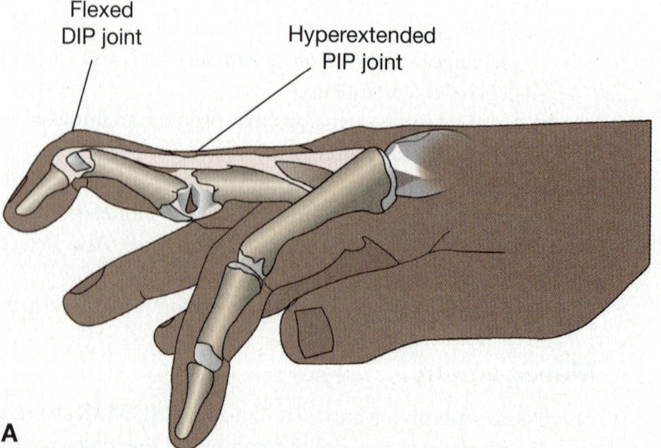

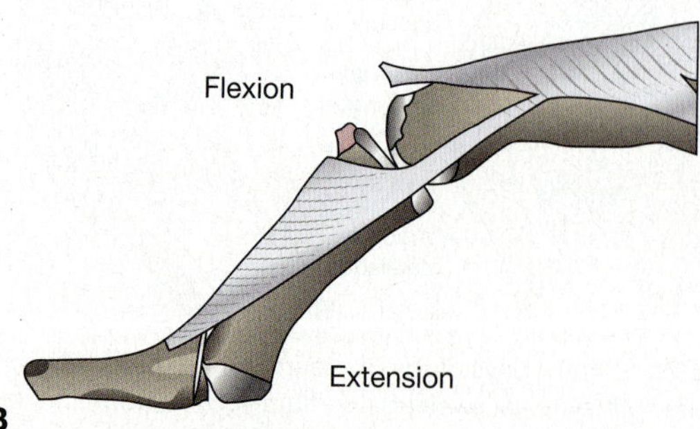

Figure 26-3. Swan neck (A) and boutonniere (B) deformities. DIP, distal interphalangeal; PIP, proximal interphalangeal.

4. Note frequency, location, and degree of pain. Tracking and trending "flares" of disease important in setting plan of care and change in medication regimen.

Optimizing Mobility

1. Encourage warm bath or shower in the morning to decrease morning stiffness.
2. Encourage measures to protect affected joints.
   a. Perform gentle ROM exercises.
   b. Use splints, if necessary.
   c. Assist with ADLs, if necessary.
3. Encourage exercise consistent with the degree of disease activity.
4. Refer to physical therapy and occupational therapy.

Preventing Infection and Adverse Reactions to Drug Therapy

1. Review drug information before administration to ensure that baseline blood work, such as CBC and liver function tests, has been done; there are no drug interactions; and you understand reconstitution and administration information.
2. Ensure that a tuberculin test has been done prior to starting biologics. If positive, treatment for latent tuberculosis (TB) and biologic may be started simultaneously.
   a. In immunocompromised individuals, including those with autoimmune diseases, greater than 5-mm reaction to tuberculin skin test is considered positive.
   b. Interferon-gamma release assays for tuberculosis screening are preferred method of detecting mycobacterial exposure.
3. Know that almost all DMARDs, including conventional synthetic DMARDs such as methotrexate, should be held for 4 weeks following administration of live vaccines. Therefore, no DMARDs should be initiated within 4 weeks of any live vaccine administration. The exceptions are hydroxychloroquine and sulfasalazine.
4. Ensure that the patient has no active or untreated infections. Be aware that latent viral infections, such as hepatitis B, can become reactivated in the presence of certain immunosuppressant medications.
5. Administer or teach patient to administer medication subcutaneously by rotating sites of the abdomen, thigh, and upper arm, as directed.
   a. All biologics, which are approved for home subcutaneous injection, are available in prefilled syringe or pen form.
   b. Methotrexate is available as a prefilled pen as well as in a liquid form that the patient must draw up at home; ensure that the patient/caregiver receives instruction on proper preparation and injection techniques.
   c. Give intravenous (IV) drugs (abatacept, rituximab, infliximab, golimumab, and tocilizumab) by recommended time as identified in the prescribing information, monitoring for side effects as per infusion protocol.

CLINICAL JUDGMENT Teach patients taking biologics the early signs and symptoms of infection and the appropriate action to take (call provider or proceed to emergency department) to reduce the risk of overwhelming infection and hospital admission. Also, teach patients that biologics are generally held when an antibiotic is prescribed.

Promoting Self-Care

1. Provide privacy and an environment conducive to performance of daily activities.
2. Schedule adequate rest periods during flare.
3. Discuss importance of promoting the patient's self-care at an appropriate level with patient and family.
4. Help patient attain appropriate assistive devices, such as raised toilet seats, special eating utensils, and zipper pulls. Contact occupational therapist, social worker, or Arthritis Foundation for information.

Strengthening Coping Skills

1. Be aware of potential job, childcare, home maintenance, and social and family functioning problems that may result from RA.
2. Encourage patient to verbalize problems and feelings.
3. Assist with problem-solving approach to explore options and to gain control of problem areas, such as cost of drugs and medical care and limited resources at home.
   a. Patient assistance programs are available for drug therapy through the manufacturer or Partnership for Prescription Assistance (www.pparx.org). There are also several foundations that may be able to assist with copays and other costs.
   b. Obtain order for home care nursing or physical or occupational therapy for treatment and monitoring, as needed.
   c. Consult social worker, the Arthritis Foundation, or other community resources for additional services, as needed.
4. Reinforce effective coping mechanisms.
5. Refer for therapy to mental health counselor, as needed.

Patient Education and Health Maintenance

1. Instruct patient and family on the nature of disease.
   a. Chronic nature of RA with characteristic exacerbations and remissions with time.
   b. Disease can have systemic effects that result in constitutional symptoms and involvement of other organ systems.
   c. Severity of RA is variable, but with proper treatment, most patients are *not* confined to bed or wheelchair.
   d. RA has no cure; avoid advertised "miracle cures."
2. Educate patient about pharmacologic agents.
   a. Medication must be taken consistently to achieve maximum benefit.
   b. Most medications used in the treatment of RA require periodic laboratory testing, such as CBC and liver functions, to monitor for potential adverse effects.
   c. Advise patient of possible adverse effects of medications and need to report adverse effects to health care provider, including fever, chills, lethargy, rash, difficulty breathing, swelling, worsening of arthritis, and severe diarrhea.
   d. Advise patients to discuss the use of any complementary or alternative therapies with their health care provider.
   e. Reinforce to patient the need for lifelong treatment.
3. During periods of remission, encourage patient to exercise regularly, choosing an activity that is inexpensive, convenient, enjoyable, and not dependent on the weather. Suggest dancing, mall walking, use of stationary bicycle in the home, or contacting the local YMCA about special programs for arthritis.
4. For additional information and support, refer to the Arthritis Foundation (www.arthritis.org) or the ACR (www.rheumatology.org).

Evaluation: Expected Outcomes

- Reports reduction in pain and fatigue.
- Protects joints from overuse.

- No signs of infection and no adverse reactions to drug therapy.
- Maintains independent toiletry, bathing, and feeding.
- Verbalizes concerns about cleaning and cooking; meets with occupational therapist.

Systemic Lupus Erythematosus

Systemic lupus erythematosus (SLE) is a chronic, multisystem autoimmune disease. Discoid lupus is a form of cutaneous lupus. Discoid lupus is a separate entity, which, in 95% of cases, is limited to skin involvement only.

Classification criteria for SLE include an antinuclear antibody (ANA) of at least 1:80 as well as at least one clinical criterion and a score of at least 10 of the additive criterion of the 2019 European Alliance of Associations for Rheumatology (EULAR)/ACR Classification Criteria for SLE.

EVIDENCE BASE Aringer, M., Costenbader, K., Daikh, D., Brinks, R., Mosca, M., Ramsey-Goldman, R., Smolen, J. S., Wofsy, D., Boumpas, D. T., Kamen, D. L., Jayne, D., Cervera, R., Costedoat-Chalumeau, N., Diamond, B., Gladman, D. D., Hahn, B., Hiepe, F., Jacobsen, S., Khanna, D., ... Johnson, S. R. (2019). 2019 European League Against Rheumatism/American College of Rheumatology classification criteria for systemic lupus erythematosus. *Arthritis & Rheumatology, 71*(9), 1400–1412. https://doi.org/10.1002/art.40930

Pathophysiology and Etiology

1. Primarily a disease of immune dysregulation.
2. Both B cells and T cells are inappropriately and persistently activated.
3. Regulatory immune cells ("off-switches") are also dysfunctional, which results in an inability to slow or to halt the production of inappropriate autoantibodies.
4. Autoantibodies may combine with other elements of the immune system to activate immune complexes. These immune complexes and other immune system constituents combine to form complement, which is deposited in organs, causing inflammation and tissue necrosis.
5. In adults, the female-to-male ratio ranges from 7:1 to 15:1.

Clinical Manifestations

1. Skin:
   a. Butterfly-shaped rash of the malar region of the face, characterized by erythema and edema.
   b. Discoid lesions affect only the head in 80% of cases and present as indurated plaques with a scale. They may evolve into disfiguring scars.
   c. Subacute cutaneous lupus lesions present as erythematous, scaly plaques or papules on the neck, arms, and upper trunk.
2. Arthritis:
   a. Generally bilateral and symmetric, involving the hands, wrists, and other joints.
   b. Can resemble RA and may be mistaken for it, especially early in the course of the disease.
   c. Unlike RA, the arthritis is primarily migratory and nonerosive; may (very rarely) be erosive.
   d. Tendon involvement is common and may lead to deformities or tendon rupture.
3. Cardiac:
   a. Pericarditis (with or without effusion) can affect up to 25% of patients with SLE.
   b. Myocarditis.
   c. Endocarditis.
   d. Coronary artery disease.
4. Pulmonary:
   a. Pleuritis (with or without effusion).
   b. Interstitial lung disease
   c. Lupus pneumonitis.
   d. Alveolar hemorrhage.
   e. Pulmonary hypertension.
   f. Shrinking lung.
5. Gastrointestinal (GI):
   a. Oral ulcers.
   b. Hepatitis.
   c. Pancreatitis.
   d. Spontaneous bacterial peritonitis.
   e. Bowel infarction.
6. Renal: occurs in 50% of patients, with as many as 15% of patients developing renal failure. Renal thrombosis is rare. Lupus nephritis is more common.
   a. Mesangial nephritis—mild form, can be reversible, best prognosis.
   b. Focal segmental glomerulonephritis—active necrotic or sclerosing lesions.
   c. Proliferative—may be focal or diffuse; diffuse carries good prognosis.
   d. Membranous nephritis—may persist for years without serious renal function decline; may present as nephrotic syndrome.
   e. Sclerosing nephritis—increase in the amount of matrix material in the glomeruli.
7. Central nervous system:
   a. Neuropsychiatric disorders—depression and psychosis.
   b. Transient ischemic attacks and stroke.
   c. Seizures.
   d. Migraine headache.
   e. Myelopathy.
   f. Guillain-Barré syndrome.
   g. Chorea and other movement disorders.
   h. Poor concentration and "lupus fog."
8. Hematologic:
   a. Hemolytic anemia.
   b. Leukopenia.
   c. Thrombocytopenia.
9. Vascular:
   a. Hypertension.
   b. Raynaud phenomenon.
10. Constitutional:
    a. Fever.
    b. Weight loss.
    c. Fatigue.

Diagnostic Evaluation

1. CBC—leukopenia, anemia (may be hemolytic), and thrombocytopenia.
2. ANA—positive in more than 98% of patients with SLE; predominant pattern is homogeneous.
3. Anti–double-stranded DNA (anti-dsDNA)—97% specific for lupus.
4. Autoantibodies specific for SLE, including Smith, anti-Sjögren syndrome–related antigen A (SSA), and anti-Sjögren syndrome–related antigen B (SSB), and anti-ribosomal P.
5. ESR—generally elevated.
6. Complement levels—generally decreased when disease is active.

7. Urinalysis—hematuria, proteinuria, and active sediment (RBC casts).
8. A 24-hour urine for protein and creatinine clearance.
9. X-ray of hands and wrists—nondestructive arthritis.
10. Computed tomography (CT) or MRI may be clinically indicated.
    a. Brain—to define any neurologic manifestations.
    b. Abdomen/chest—to evaluate abdominal pain and/or for interstitial lung disease.
    c. Cerebral arteriogram—to look for evidence of cerebral vasculitis.
    d. Magnetic resonance angiography—to confirm thrombotic lesions.

Management

EVIDENCE BASE Fanouriakis, A., Tziolos, N., Bertsias, G., & Boumpas, G. T. (2021). Update on the diagnosis and management of systemic lupus erythematosus. *Annals of the Rheumatic Diseases, 80*(1), 14–25. https://doi.org/10.1136/annrheumdis-2020-218272

Pharmacologic

1. Antimalarials to decrease disease activity.
2. Corticosteroids to reduce inflammatory process.
3. Immunosuppressives to suppress immune process and to act as steroid-sparing agents.
   a. Azathioprine, mycophenolate, and/or cyclophosphamide.
   b. Belimumab is a monoclonal antibody that neutralizes the B-cell survival factor and B-lymphocyte stimulator (BLyS). Belimumab is available in SC or IV delivery systems.
   c. Anifrolumab is a monoclonal antibody that blocks the activity of type I interferons by blocking their receptor. It is available as an IV medication only.
4. Antihypertensives and diuretics to treat hypertension and fluid overload, if present due to renal disease.
5. Calcium channel blockers, angiotensin receptor blockers, or sildenafil for Raynaud phenomenon.

Nonpharmacologic

1. Avoid direct exposure to sunlight to reduce the chance of disease flare.
2. Behavior modification to prevent exacerbations and to reduce symptoms.
3. Joint protection and energy conservation.

Other Management

1. Close follow-up for evaluation of cardiac, neurologic, renal, and other body systems.
2. Referral to specialists for systemic manifestations.

Complications

1. Renal failure.
2. Permanent neurologic impairment.
3. Infection.
4. Death caused by disease process.

Nursing Assessment

1. Obtain clinical history, review systems, and perform physical examination for characteristic findings.
2. Assess for signs and symptoms of infection and other adverse effects to medications.
3. Assist with monitoring of urinary and renal status.
   a. Monitor intake and output and urine specific gravity.
   b. Check laboratory test results of serum blood urea nitrogen and creatinine, and urine protein and microalbumin levels.
4. Assess patient's and family's ability to cope with the impact of prolonged disease.

Nursing Interventions

Reducing Pain

1. Administer and teach self-administration of medications.
2. Suggest the use of hot or cold applications, relaxation techniques, and exercise to enhance pain relief.
3. Monitor for adverse reactions to corticosteroids (see page 809).

Increasing Control Over Disease Process

1. Instruct the patient to avoid factors that may exacerbate disease.
   a. Avoid exposure to sunlight and ultraviolet light.
      i. Use sunscreen with sun protection factor of 30 or greater. Avoid prolonged sun exposure.
      ii. Wear protective, lightweight clothing with long sleeves and wide-brimmed hats.
      iii. Avoid the use of tanning beds.
   b. Avoid exposure to any skin irritants.
   c. Discuss any new medications (prescription or over-the-counter [OTC]), vitamins, or supplements with a health care provider before starting.
2. Reinforce the importance of adhering to all prescribed therapies.
3. Encourage good nutrition (Mediterranean diet has been researched and shown to be effective), sleep habits, exercise, rest, and relaxation to improve general health and to help prevent infection.
4. Encourage expression of feelings, counseling, or referrals to social work and occupational therapy, as needed.

EVIDENCE BASE England, B. R., Smith, B. J., Baker, N. A., Barton, J. L., Oatis, C. A., Guyatt, G., Anandarajah, A., Carandang, K., Chan, K. K., Constien, D., Davidson, E., Dodge, C. V., Bemis-Dougherty, A., Everett, S., Fisher, N., Fraenkel, L., Goodman, S. M., Lewis, J., Menzies, V., Moreland, L. W., Navarro-Millan, I., Patterson, S., Phillips, L., Shah, N., Singh, N., White, D., AlHeresh, R., Barbour, K. E., Bye, T., Guglielmo, D., Haberman, R., Johnson, T., Kleiner, A., Lane, C. Y., Li, L. C., Master, H., Pinto, D., Poole, J. L., Steinbarger, K., Sztubinski, D., Thoma, L., Tsaltskan, V., Turgunbaev, M., Wells, C., Turner, A. S., & Treadwell, J. R. (2023). 2022 American College of Rheumatology Guideline for exercise, rehabilitation, diet, and additional integrative interventions for rheumatoid arthritis. *Arthritis Care & Research*, 75, 1603-1615. https://doi.org/10.1002/acr.25117

Maintaining Skin and Mucous Membrane Integrity

1. Apply topical corticosteroids to skin lesions, as ordered.
2. Suggest alternative hairstyles, scarves, and wigs to cover significant areas of alopecia.
3. Encourage good oral hygiene and inspect mouth for oral ulcers.
   a. Avoid hot or spicy foods that may irritate oral ulcers.
   b. Apply topical agents or analgesics to reduce pain and to promote eating.

Reducing Fatigue

1. Advise the patient that fatigue level will fluctuate with disease activity.

2. Encourage the patient to modify schedule to include several rest periods during the day; pace activity and exercise according to body's tolerance; use energy conservation techniques in daily activities.
3. Teach relaxation techniques, such as deep breathing, progressive muscle relaxation, and imagery, to reduce emotional stress that causes fatigue.

Patient Education and Health Maintenance

1. Stress that close follow-up is essential, even in times of remission, to detect early progression of organ involvement and to alter drug therapy.
2. Advise on the use of special cosmetics to cover skin lesions.
3. Advise about reproduction.
   a. Avoid pregnancy during the time of severe disease activity. Should have stable disease for 1 year before planning pregnancy.
   b. Patients of childbearing age should understand implications of treatment medications on fertility and pregnancy. Hydroxychloroquine may be used because it is proven safe during pregnancy.

DRUG ALERT Immunomodulators such as leflunomide, methotrexate, mycophenolate, and cyclophosphamide may have teratogenic effects; use of some drugs for treatment of SLE, such as cyclophosphamide, can result in sterility.

4. Stress that any complementary or alternative therapies should be discussed with the health care provider.
5. For additional information and support, refer to agencies such as the Lupus Foundation (www.lupus.org) or the American Occupational Therapy Association (www.aota.org).

Evaluation: Expected Outcomes

- Reports pain reduction.
- Verbalizes appropriate use of medications, avoidance of sun and chemicals, and need for nutrition and sleep to minimize disease process.
- Reports oral ulcers healing without interference with appetite.
- Reports resting as needed, with adequate energy to carry out activities.

Systemic Sclerosis

Systemic sclerosis (SSc) is a generalized disorder of connective tissue, characterized by hardening and thickening of the skin (scleroderma), blood vessels, synovium, skeletal muscles, and internal organs. Fibrotic, degenerative, and inflammatory changes result in changes in joints and several organ systems. Classification criteria published by ACR and EULAR include eight major criteria and nine subitems.

EVIDENCE BASE van den Hoogen, F., Khanna, D., Fransen, J., Johnson, S. R., Baron, M., Tyndall, A., Matucci-Cerinic, M., Naden, R. P., Medsger, T. A., Jr., Carreira, P. E., Riemekasten, G., Clements, P. J., Denton, C. P., Distler, O., Allanore, Y., Furst, D. E., Gabrielli, A., Mayes, M. D., van Laar, J. M., ... Pope, J. E. (2013). 2013 Classification criteria for systemic sclerosis: An American College of Rheumatology/European League Against Rheumatism collaborative initiative. *Annals of the Rheumatic Diseases, 72*(11), 1747–1755. https://doi.org/10.1136/annrheumdis-2013-204424

Pathophysiology and Etiology

1. The changes seen in the skin and internal organs in SSc are most likely caused by the overproduction of collagen by fibroblasts.
2. The etiology of SSc is unknown.
3. SSc affects three to eight times as many females as males.
4. Major subtypes include:
   a. Diffuse cutaneous SSc—rapidly progressive, generalized skin thickening of the proximal and distal extremities and trunk and tendency toward early internal organ involvement (lung fibrosis, renal crisis, cardiac involvement).
   b. Limited cutaneous SSc, also known as CREST syndrome—skin thickening is limited to the distal extremities and face (CREST stands for calcinosis; Raynaud's phenomenon; esophageal dysfunction; sclerodactyly; and telangiectasia).
   c. SSc *sine* scleroderma—clinical features of SSc and positive autoantibodies, but no skin involvement.
   d. Overlap with other rheumatic diseases (RA, polymyositis, Sjögren syndrome).

Clinical Manifestations

Skin

1. Bilateral symmetric swelling of the hands and, sometimes, the feet.
2. After the edematous phase, the skin becomes hard and thick.
3. Digits, dorsum of the hand, neck, face, and trunk are involved.
4. Normal landmarks in the skin are absent—no skin folds.
5. Increased or decreased skin pigmentation (salt-and-pepper skin).
6. Skin changes may regress after several years.
7. Telangiectasia—on/under the tongue, face, fingers, and lips.
8. Areas of calcinosis—late in the course of disease.
9. Raynaud phenomenon.
10. Decreased oral aperture.

Gastrointestinal

1. Esophageal dysmotility—resulting in reflux and dysphagia.
2. Distal esophageal dilation and esophagitis.
3. Barrett metaplasia—may predispose to adenocarcinoma of the esophagus.
4. Duodenal atrophy dilation—may cause postprandial abdominal pain, malabsorption, diarrhea, and abdominal distention.
5. Colonic hypomotility—results in constipation.

Musculoskeletal

1. Joint pain—large and small joints affected.
2. Carpal tunnel syndrome.
3. Flexion contractures.
4. Inflammatory muscle atrophy.

Cardiac

1. Left ventricular dysfunction.
2. Myocardial involvement—heart failure and atrial and ventricular arrhythmias.
3. Right ventricular involvement—secondary to pulmonary disease.

Pulmonary

1. Interstitial fibrosis.
2. Restrictive lung disease.
3. Pulmonary hypertension.

Renal

Scleroderma renal crisis—rapid malignant hypertension with encephalopathy.

Diagnostic Evaluation

1. CBC and ESR—generally normal.
2. RF—positive in approximately 30% of patients.
3. ANA—generally positive with speckled or nucleolar patterns.
   a. Antitopoisomerase I antibody (Scl-70)—generally associated with diffuse cutaneous disease and severe interstitial lung disease.
   b. Anticentromere antibody—usually associated with limited cutaneous disease.
   c. Anti-RNA polymerase III antibody—typically associated with aggressive diffuse cutaneous SSc as well as the risk for scleroderma renal crisis.
4. Pulmonary function test—decreased diffusion capacity and vital capacity; high-resolution computed tomography (CT) of the chest to evaluate for pulmonary fibrosis.
5. Echocardiogram to evaluate for pulmonary hypertension.
6. Endoscopy, barium swallow, and/or esophageal manometry testing should be guided by patient symptoms.

Management

Pharmacologic

1. Immunosuppressives (methotrexate, mycophenolate) are recommended for patients with progressive skin involvement but no visceral involvement. Cyclophosphamide may be used for refractory disease.
2. Calcium channel blockers, PDE5 inhibitors, or angiotensin II receptor blockers are used to treat Raynaud phenomenon.
3. Nonsteroidal anti-inflammatory drugs (NSAIDs) and/or other analgesics for arthralgias, polyarthritis, and painful calcinosis—renal function must be carefully monitored.
4. Proton pump inhibitors for reflux.
5. Antibiotics for malabsorption because of bacterial overgrowth or secondarily infected skin ulcerations.
6. Antihypertensive agents.
7. For pulmonary involvement, bronchodilators and three classes of medications, which all promote pulmonary vasodilation: PDE5 inhibitors, endothelin receptor antagonists, and prostacyclin pathway agonists.

Nonpharmacologic

1. Skin lubricants and care for ulcerations to promote healing.
2. Lifestyle modification for control of Raynaud phenomenon:
   a. Increased environmental temperature.
   b. Appropriate dress, which keeps the core as well as extremities warm.
   c. Avoidance of handling cold and frozen items without gloves.
   d. Avoidance of wind and exposure to cold weather.
   e. Use of hand and foot warmers.
   f. Smoking cessation.
3. Raynaud attack can possibly be aborted by placing the hand or foot in tepid water.
4. Biofeedback to abort or prevent Raynaud attack.
5. Dietary modifications for GI involvement:
   a. Avoidance of caffeinated beverages.
   b. Eating smaller meals.
   c. Remaining upright after meals for at least 45 to 60 minutes.
   d. Avoidance of alcohol.
   e. Elevating the head of the bed.

Complications

1. Skin ulcers.
2. Malabsorption.
3. Esophageal adenocarcinoma.
4. Pulmonary hypertension.
5. Renal failure.
6. Heart failure.
7. Death caused by disease process.

Nursing Assessment

1. Focus physical assessment on:
   a. Skin ulcers, thickening, subcutaneous (SC) deposits, and secondary infection.
   b. Joint examination—flexion contractures.
   c. Pulmonary examination—for shortness of breath and wheezing.
   d. Blood pressure and renal status.
2. Determine nutritional intake.
3. Assess mood, support system, and coping ability.

Nursing Interventions

Maintaining Tissue Perfusion

1. Teach the patient to identify Raynaud phenomenon.
   a. Characteristic color change of the fingers—white, blue, and red.
   b. Coldness, pallor, numbness, and pain.
2. Teach the patient to reduce factors associated with precipitation or exacerbation of Raynaud phenomenon.
   a. Dress warmly—cover head and extremities; keep trunk warm.
   b. Discontinue tobacco usage.
   c. Avoid prolonged exposure to cold.
      i. Weather.
      ii. Artificially controlled environments (e.g., air conditioning).
      iii. Limit contact with cold food items, such as frozen foods and ice cube trays—use gloves or tongs.
3. Protect ulcerated digits and report signs of infection.
4. Avoid vasoconstricting agents such as decongestants.

Preserving Skin Integrity

1. Use moisturizers on the skin daily.
2. Advise the patient to avoid the use of drying soaps and detergents.
3. Use protective padding (e.g., elbow pads) to protect the skin from friction or trauma.
4. Inspect the skin daily for cracking, ulceration, and signs of infection.
5. Soak ulcerations, apply topical antibiotic, and use occlusive dressings, as directed.

Achieving Optimal Nutritional Status

1. Make sure the patient is in proper position for meals to avoid aspiration (i.e., in chair if possible).
2. Provide smaller, more frequent feedings of a well-balanced diet.

3. Encourage the patient to remain upright after meals for 45 to 60 minutes and raise the head of the bed during sleep to avoid reflux.
4. Administer or teach self-administration of medications to prevent nausea and reflux, as ordered.
5. Encourage good oral hygiene and frequent dental visits.
6. Advise the use of lubricating agents, if necessary, to treat dry mouth and to teach stretching exercises of the mouth to maintain aperture.
7. Weigh weekly and ask the patient to keep food diary.

Strengthening Body Image

1. Encourage the patient to take an active role in treatment plan to feel in control of body changes.
2. Explain that changes may be gradual and slow; although not noticeable, internal organ involvement is even more important than external changes.
3. Suggest continuance of activities that the patient enjoys and foster strong support network.
4. Refer for counseling, as needed.

Patient Education and Health Maintenance

1. Explain diagnostic tests and their purpose in detecting GI, pulmonary, or renal involvement.
2. Teach about drug treatment and adverse effects.
3. Encourage regular follow-up visits and prompt attention to worsening symptoms.
4. Refer to agencies such as the National Scleroderma Foundation (*www.scleroderma.org*).

Evaluation: Expected Outcomes

- Relates factors that precipitate Raynaud phenomenon.
- Reports no skin cracking or ulceration.
- Reports no weight loss.
- Reports participating in community activities and groups.

Gout

Gout is a disorder of purine metabolism, characterized by elevated uric acid levels and deposition of uric acid (also known as urate), usually in the form of crystals, in joints and other tissues. More common in males but may affect postmenopausal females, especially those taking diuretics.

Pathophysiology and Etiology

Gout results from an overabundant accumulation and subsequent deposition of monosodium urate crystals in joints and other connective tissue. This can occur in one of two ways.

Overproduction of Uric Acid (10% of Cases)

1. Inherited enzyme defects.
2. Certain conditions:
   a. Myeloproliferative disorders.
   b. Lymphoproliferative disorders.
   c. Cancer chemotherapy.
   d. Hemolytic anemias.
   e. Psoriasis.

Underexcretion of Uric Acid (90% of Cases)

1. Renal disease.
2. Endocrine disorders.
3. Medications and chemicals:
   a. Diuretics.
   b. Ethanol (alcohol).
   c. Low-dose aspirin.
   d. Cyclosporine, tacrolimus.

Clinical Manifestations

Acute Gouty Arthritis

1. Generally affects one joint—in 50% of cases will be the first metatarsophalangeal joint (called podagra); see Figure 26-4.
2. Other joints can be affected, such as the ankle, tarsals, and knee; upper extremities are less commonly involved.
3. Pain, warmth, erythema, and swelling of tissue surrounding the affected joint.
4. Onset of symptoms is sudden; intensity is severe.
5. Duration of symptoms is self-limiting; lasts approximately 3 to 10 days without treatment.

Intercritical Gout

1. The intercritical stage is the time between acute flares.
2. The patient is still hyperuricemic but asymptomatic.
3. Intercritical stages become shorter in duration as the disease progresses.

Chronic Tophaceous Gout

1. Occurs if acute gout is inadequately treated or if it goes untreated.
2. Characterized by development of tophi or deposits of uric acid in and around joints, cartilage, and soft tissues.
3. Arthritis is more prolonged in nature with discrete attacks less common.
4. Arthritis can produce bone erosions and subsequent bony deformities.

Diagnostic Evaluation

1. Synovial fluid analysis.
   a. Identification of monosodium urate crystals under polarized microscopy.
   b. Synovial white blood cell (WBC) count can range from 2,000 to 100,000/mm^3.
   c. Culture of synovial fluid to rule out infection.
2. A 24-hour urine for uric acid to determine overproduction of uric acid versus underexcretion.
3. ESR—elevated.
4. X-rays of affected joints may show changes consistent with the diagnosis of gout.

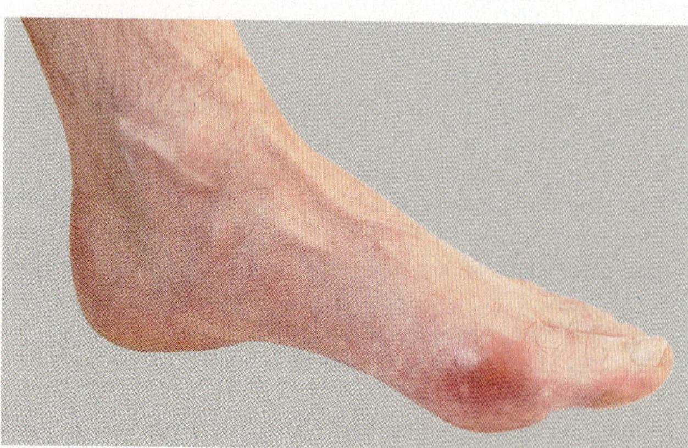

Figure 26-4. Inflammation of the first metatarsal due to acute gout. (Shutterstock/ValDan22)

5. Dual-energy CT scans produce a 3-D image of the affected body part allowing visualization and quantification of monosodium urate crystal deposits.
6. The 2015 ACR/EULAR classification criteria for gout are 92% sensitive and 89% specific and include methods for classifying patients when synovial fluid analysis and/or imaging are not available.

EVIDENCE BASE FitzGerald, J. D., Dalbeth, N., Mikuls, T., Brignardello-Petersen, R., Guyatt, G., Abeles, A. M., Gelber, A. C., Harrold, L. R., Khanna, D., King, C., Levy, G., Libbey, C., Mount, D., Pillinger, M. H., Rosenthal, A., Singh, J. A., Sims, J. E., Smith, B. J., Wenger, N. S., Bae, S. S., Danve, A., Khanna, P. P., Kim, S. C., Lenert, A., Poon, S., Qasim, A., Sehra, S. T., Sharma, T. S. K., Toprover, M., Turgunbaev, M., Zeng, L., Zhang, M. A., Turner, A. S., Neogi, T. (2020). American College of Rheumatology Guideline for the Management of Gout. *Arthritis Care Res* (Hoboken). 72(6), 744-760. https://doi.org/10.1002/acr.24180

Management

Acute Management

1. NSAIDs for acute attacks to relieve pain and swelling; considered first-line therapy.
2. Colchicine for acute treatment and prevention of attacks; considered second-line therapy.
   a. May be given orally at the onset of an attack, taken two to three times a day as tolerated on day 1 of attack only (may cause nausea, cramping, diarrhea).
   b. Taken once to twice a day on continuous basis to prevent attack, usually while transitioning to urate-lowering medications. May be used every other day for patients with chronic kidney disease.
3. Corticosteroids.
   a. Intra-articular if attack confined to one or two joints.
   b. Oral—in short-tapering course if other treatments are contraindicated or if attack involves many joints.
4. Increase fluids (orally because usually treated as outpatient) and rest joint for 48 hours.

Chronic Management

1. Antihyperuricemic agents reduce uric acid. They are taken to prevent progressive articular damage in chronic symptomatic gout, tophaceous gout, and in certain patients with asymptomatic hyperuricemia.
   a. Allopurinol—a xanthine oxidase inhibitor, interferes with conversion of hypoxanthine and xanthine to uric acid. May also be given to prevent renal calculi and kidney disease.
   b. Febuxostat—a selective xanthine oxidase inhibitor, lowers uric acid.
   c. Probenecid—a uricosuric drug. Interferes with tubular reabsorption of uric acid. Should be avoided in patients with a history of kidney stones.
   d. Pegloticase is a pegylated uric acid–specific enzyme indicated for the treatment of chronic gout in adult patients refractory to conventional therapy. Should be coadministered with methotrexate/folic acid, mycophenolate, azathioprine, or leflunomide to prevent infusion reactions.
2. Adverse reactions for these drugs include headache, anorexia, nausea and vomiting, allergic reaction, hemolytic anemia and other blood dyscrasias, and worsening of gout.
3. Rapid increase or decrease in uric acid may precipitate a gout flare, so oral medication is usually started at a low dose and titrated up.
4. Uric acid levels and renal function are monitored during chronic therapy. A small percentage of patients develop elevated liver functions with urate-lowering treatment.

DRUG ALERT Exfoliative dermatitis (sometimes fatal) and liver and biliary dysfunction may occur with use of allopurinol and febuxostat.

Lifestyle Modification

1. Avoidance of obesity and fluctuations in weight.
2. Avoidance of alcohol—can precipitate gout attacks through overproduction and decreased excretion of urate.
3. Low-purine diet leads to only a minor decrease in serum uric acid levels.
4. Moderate coffee consumption has been linked to decreased uric acid levels.

Complications

1. Uric acid renal calculus.
2. Urate nephropathy.
3. Erosive, deforming arthritis/contractures.

Nursing Assessment

1. Obtain a history for factors predisposing to gout, such as malignancy, alcohol use disorder, and renal insufficiency.
2. Perform physical examination.
   a. Inspect the involved joint for pain, swelling, redness, warmth, and effusion.
   b. Observe for tophi, which can occur anywhere but most commonly are found over the pinna of the ear, olecranon bursa, Achilles tendon, and fingertips.
3. Assess pain and pain relief pattern if attack is acute.

Nursing Interventions

Relieving Pain

1. Administer and teach self-administration of pain-relieving medications, as prescribed.
2. Encourage adequate fluid intake to assist with excretion of uric acid and to decrease the likelihood of stone formation.
3. Instruct the patient to take prescribed medications consistently because interruptions in therapy can precipitate acute attacks.
4. Encourage the patient to follow up as directed, usually in 48 hours and then 4 to 8 weeks after acute attack to evaluate for chronic therapy.

Facilitating Activity

1. Elevate and protect the affected joint during acute attack.
2. Assist with ADLs.
3. Encourage exercise and maintenance of routine activity in chronic gout, except during acute attacks.
4. Protect draining tophi by covering and applying antibiotic ointment, as needed.

Patient Education and Health Maintenance

1. Instruct the patient and family about the nature of disease.
   a. Generally, acute attacks are followed by periods of premission.
   b. Once need for chronic treatment has been determined, it will generally be lifelong.
2. Encourage avoidance of alcohol.

3. Avoid rapid weight loss by fasting or crash diets because rapid weight loss results in the production of chemicals that compete with uric acid for excretion from the body, resulting in increased uric acid levels.
4. Advise prompt treatment of acute attack to reduce joint damage associated with repeated attacks.
5. Instruct about signs and symptoms of allopurinol hypersensitivity syndrome and need to report promptly.
6. Advise patients to avoid foods containing purines (i.e., sardines, anchovies, shellfish, organ meats) and, in general, to consume meat, seafood, and high-calorie food in moderation.

Evaluation: Expected Outcomes

- Reports relief from pain.
- Performs ADLs with minimal assistance.

Sjögren Syndrome

Sjögren syndrome is a chronic inflammatory autoimmune process that primarily affects the lacrimal and salivary glands. The disease can be primary or secondary. Secondary Sjögren syndrome is seen most commonly in RA and SLE but can also be seen with other rheumatic diseases. Diagnosis is based on a combination of objective evidence of dry eye or salivary hypofunction along with evidence of an underlying autoimmunity. Diagnosis of primary Sjögren syndrome (not associated with another rheumatic disease) requires a score of at least 4 on the ACR/EULAR classification criteria for primary Sjögren syndrome.

EVIDENCE BASE Shiboski, C. H., Shiboski, S. C., Seror, R., Criswell, L. A., Labetoulle, M., Lietman, T. M., Rasmussen, A., Scofield, H., Vitali, C., Bowman, S. J., Mariette, X., & International Sjögren's Syndrome Criteria Working Group. (2016). 2016 American College of Rheumatology/European League Against Rheumatism classification criteria for primary Sjögren's syndrome: A consensus and data-driven methodology involving three international patient cohorts. *Arthritis & Rheumatology, 69*(1), 35–45. https://doi.org/10.1002/art.39859

Pathophysiology and Etiology

1. The etiology of Sjögren syndrome is unknown but is thought to include several factors: genetic predisposition, immunologic, and environmental.
2. It is thought that antibodies directed at exocrine glands are produced, leading to disturbed function of the involved tissue.
3. Lymphocytes are found infiltrating the affected tissues.
4. Sjögren syndrome occurs most commonly in middle-aged females.

Clinical Manifestations

1. Ocular—xerophthalmia (dry eyes) because of decreased tear formation that leads to keratoconjunctivitis and photophobia, greater than 3 months.
2. Oral—xerostomia (dry mouth) caused by diminished production of saliva, mucosal ulcers, and stomatitis, greater than 3 months. Need for fluids to swallow food.
3. Recurrent or persistent salivary gland enlargement—unilateral or bilateral.
4. Dryness of the skin, vagina, and other tissues may also occur.
5. Extraglandular features include rash, dysphagia, Raynaud phenomenon, arthralgias/arthritis, and myalgias.
6. Less commonly, major organ dysfunction, such as interstitial pneumonitis, glomerulonephritis, vasculitis, thyroid disease, and central and peripheral neuropathy may occur.

Diagnostic Evaluation

1. Schirmer test—filter paper is placed onto the lower conjunctival sac of one eye for 5 minutes to absorb moisture. Gradings on the paper strip indicate if moisture content reaches normal tear production level.
2. Ocular staining—fluorescein dye is inserted into the eye, and a blue light is used to scan the cornea for damage, which may be caused by decreased tear production and used for Sjögren disease classification.
3. CBC—leukopenia and anemia are associated with disease activity.
4. ESR—often elevated.
5. RF—positive in approximately half of patients with primary Sjögren and over 90% of patients with secondary Sjögren.
6. ANA—typically positive.
7. Antibodies to SSA/SSB—detects antibodies to specific nuclear proteins.
   a. SSA (Ro antibody)—positive in approximately 50% of patients with Sjögren syndrome.
   b. SSB (La antibody)—positive in approximately 50% of patients with Sjögren syndrome.
8. Salivary scintigraphy—salivary gland function is measured by determining excretion of radioisotope dye.
9. Salivary gland biopsy—to determine lymphocytic infiltration of tissue and confirm diagnosis; usually done on one of the minor salivary glands in the lower lip.

Management

EVIDENCE BASE Ramos-Casals, M., Brito-Zerón, P., Bombardieri, S., Bootsma, H., De Vita, S., Dörner, T., Fisher, B. A., Gottenberg, J. E., Hernandez-Molina, G., Kocher, A., Kostov, B., Kruize, A. A., Mandl, T., Ng, W. F., Retamozo, S., Seror, R., Shoenfeld, Y., Sisó-Almirall, A., Tzioufas, A. G., ... EULAR-Sjögren Syndrome Task Force Group. (2020). EULAR recommendations for the management of Sjögren's syndrome with topical and systemic therapies. *Annals of the Rheumatic Diseases, 79*, 3–18. https://doi.org/10.1136/annrheumdis-2019-216114

Systemic Drugs

1. Systemic therapy is usually not needed for dry mouth alone; however, pilocarpine and cevimeline are oral medications that act as secretagogues to increase saliva and are taken tid to four times a day.
2. Treatment of extraglandular symptoms (arthritis, rashes, renal involvement, etc.) typically mimics treatment for SLE or RA.

Topical Agents

1. Artificial tears—available OTC; preservative free preferred.
2. Topical cyclosporine, topical steroids, and punctal plugs may be used in patients with moderate-to-severe dry eyes.
3. OTC treatments for dry mouth, including specialized mouthwashes and lozenges. Avoid anything containing sugar.
4. Artificial saliva.

Complications

1. Ocular complications, such as corneal ulceration, corneal opacification, vascularization of the cornea, infection, glaucoma, and cataract formation.
2. Dental caries and tooth loss.
3. Lymphoma, interstitial lung disease, pericarditis, autoimmune hepatitis, primary biliary cholangitis, interstitial nephritis, renal tubular dysfunction, glomerular disease.

Nursing Assessment

1. Obtain a history of signs and symptoms, emphasizing dryness, and how this may be affecting function and quality of life.
2. Perform complete physical examination, focusing on the oral cavity, eyes, skin, lungs, GI, and neurologic systems.
3. Assess nutritional status because decreased saliva may make eating difficult.

Nursing Interventions

Maintaining Mucous Membranes

1. Inspect oral mucosa for oral *Candida*, ulcers, saliva pools, and dental hygiene.
2. Instruct and assist patient in proper oral hygiene.
   a. At least twice daily brushing.
   b. Frequent rinsing with antiseptic mouthwash.
3. Encourage frequent intake of noncaffeinated, nonsugared liquids. Keep pitcher filled with cool water.
4. Promptly report any ulcers or signs of infections.

Protecting Skin Integrity

1. Instruct and assist the patient with daily inspection of the skin for areas of trauma or for potential breakdown.
2. Apply lubricants to the skin daily.
3. Avoid shearing forces and encourage or perform frequent position changes.

Promoting Adequate Nutritional Intake

1. Increase liquid intake with meals.
2. Assist and instruct the patient to avoid choosing spicy or dry foods from menu choices.
3. Suggest small, more frequent meals.
4. Weigh weekly and review diet history for deficiency in basic nutrients.
5. Suggest nutritional supplement beverage as indicated.

Promoting Comfort and Optimal Sexual Functioning

1. Encourage the patient to discuss sexual difficulty and explain its relation to disease process.
2. Advise on proper use of water-soluble vaginal lubrication.
3. Suggest alternative positioning and practices to prevent discomfort.
4. Teach the patient to report symptoms of vaginitis—discharge, irritation, and itching—because infection may result from altered mucosal barrier.

Patient Education and Health Maintenance

1. Advise patient of commercially available artificial saliva preparations, artificial tears, moisturizing nasal sprays, and artificial vaginal moisturizers.
2. Encourage frequent dental visits. Dental cavities and tooth loss are more frequent in Sjögren syndrome.
3. Advise patient to check with health care provider before using any medications because many, such as diuretics, tricyclic antidepressants, and antihistamines, have the adverse effect of dry eyes and mouth.
4. Advise patient to wear protective eyewear while outdoors.
5. Encourage support through Sjögren's Foundation (www.sjogrens.org) or the American College of Rheumatology (www.rheumatology.org).

Evaluation: Expected Outcomes

- Demonstrates proper oral hygiene.
- Reports skin without cracking, scaling, or other lesions.
- Maintains weight.
- Reports vaginal comfort and satisfying sexual activity.

Seronegative Spondyloarthropathies

Seronegative spondyloarthropathies (SpA) are inflammatory conditions with negative RF or other autoantibodies but may be associated with the HLA-B27 gene, which is present in about 7% of the population, but in about 90% of those diagnosed with ankylosing spondylitis (AS) (the most common SpA). Genetic influence (HLA-B27 and other genes) along with environmental exposure to microorganisms and microtrauma triggers inflammation at enthesis (point of bone insertion of tendons and ligaments), which leads to changes in the bone and pathologic new bone formation. SpA include the following:

- AS—characterized by lower back stiffness (sacroiliac involvement), uveitis, cardiac, and decreased chest expansion. Untreated AS may result in fusion of affected joints.
- Reactive arthritis (previously known as Reiter syndrome)—follows an infection and is characterized by the triad of urethritis, arthritis, and conjunctivitis.
- Inflammatory bowel disease (IBD)-associated arthritis—overlap of Crohn disease or ulcerative colitis and axial or peripheral arthritis of the large and small joints, with synovitis.
- Psoriatic arthritis (PsA)—characterized by arthritis with synovitis, enthesitis, and (usually, but not always) the skin lesions of psoriasis.

Clinical Manifestations

1. Inflammatory back or peripheral joint pain.
   a. Axial SpA typically presents with chronic low back pain for more than 3 months.
   b. Peripheral SpA presents with acute onset, asymmetric joint pain (often knee or ankle), enthesitis, and/or dactylitis.
2. Morning stiffness lasting more than an hour, improving with activity, worsening with rest and inactivity.
3. Nonmusculoskeletal features, such as ocular inflammation, preceding GI or genitourinary infection, psoriasis, and signs of IBD.
4. Family history of SpA or other autoimmune disorders.

Diagnosis/Treatment

1. X-rays of the spine and sacroiliac joints—may show structural changes late in disease process.
2. Serologic testing for HLA-B27 typing.
3. Blood testing for inflammatory markers such as ESR and CRP.
4. MRI may be considered to detect earlier signs of inflammation in affected areas.
5. Primary treatment is NSAIDs at maximal dose, except for IBD-associated arthritis or if contraindicated due to other conditions.

6. Certain TNF inhibitors, interleukin-17 and interleukin-12/23 inhibitors, and JAK inhibitors are approved for the treatment of IBD-associated arthritis, or the next step if NSAIDs are ineffective, intolerable, or contraindicated.
7. Certain TNF inhibitors, interleukin-17 and interleukin-12/23 inhibitors, and JAK inhibitors are approved for the treatment of AS and nonradiographic axial spondyloarthritis (nr-axSpA).
8. Certain TNF inhibitors, interleukin-17 and interleukin-12/23 inhibitors, JAK inhibitors, and a T-cell costimulation modulator are approved for the treatment of PsA.
9. Nonbiologic DMARDs such as methotrexate, leflunomide, and sulfasalazine may be effective for peripheral arthritis in some disorders.
10. Corticosteroids are usually ineffective, except in cases of IBD-associated arthritis and severe uveitis.

Nursing and Patient Care Considerations

1. Ensure that complete review of systems and physical examination is done to evaluate extra-articular manifestations.
2. Evaluate the functional impact of SpA on each patient. Utilize physical and occupational therapists to improve comfort and function.
3. Monitor for renal and GI adverse effects of NSAIDs.
4. Be aware that biologics and JAK inhibitors are contraindicated in cases of active infection (including untreated latent tuberculosis). Caution is advised in patients with advanced heart failure, a family history of multiple sclerosis, or a personal history of cancer. In addition, JAK inhibitors are used cautiously with anyone who currently smokes or has a history of myocardial infarction, stroke, or deep vein thrombosis.

Polymyalgia Rheumatica

Polymyalgia rheumatica (PMR) is an inflammatory disease that causes profound stiffness in the shoulders and hips. It is found in people aged 50 years and above and more commonly in females and in White individuals. Cause is unknown but is related to immune-mediated inflammation. It may be triggered by environmental factors, such as viral infections and immunizations. There is an association with a type of vasculitis called giant cell arteritis (GCA).

Clinical Manifestations

1. Myalgia of proximal muscles of upper and lower extremities, usually involving shoulders and hips. Neck also may be involved. Onset is often acute and unilateral, but progressing to bilateral muscle groups and lasting >1 month.
2. Accompanying profound stiffness, lasting 1 hour or more each morning.
3. Strength is preserved; however, pain and stiffness make movement difficult.
4. Joint swelling or limb edema may occur.
5. Systemic symptoms include fever, malaise, weight loss, fatigue, depression.

Diagnosis/Treatment

1. Despite the symptoms, no evidence of inflammation is found on muscle imaging, electrophysiologic testing, or biopsy. Rather, MRI may reveal periarticular inflammation and bursitis.
2. Blood testing may include general markers of inflammation and specific markers of rheumatic and muscle disease.
   a. ESR >40 mm/s, elevated CRP.
   b. RF, ANA, creatine kinase are negative.
3. PMR is considered self-limiting; however, treatment is aimed at controlling pain and stiffness and resolving systemic symptoms.
   a. Oral corticosteroids, usually starting at 15 mg daily and slowly tapering, are effective in quickly resolving symptoms and reducing inflammatory markers, but do not prevent the possible complication of vasculitis.
   b. Biologic therapy with interleukin-6 inhibitors is approved for patients in whom prolonged steroid use is not a viable option or who are not able to taper off steroids after 12 to 18 months of treatment.

Nursing and Patient Care Considerations

1. Encourage ROM and exercise to prevent muscle atrophy and falls due to pain and stiffness.
2. Administer or teach self-administration of pain medications such as NSAIDs if the patient is unable to take corticosteroids, due to diabetes or other conditions.
3. Monitor for elevated glucose associated with corticosteroids, and encourage routine follow-up for checkups and blood work during the long course of treatment (usually 1-2 years) to induce remission (see page 806).
4. Recommend supplemental calcium and vitamin D intake as well as weight-bearing exercise to prevent corticosteroid-induced osteoporosis, and encourage bone mineral density screening. Treatment with a bisphosphonate is often offered while the patient is taking corticosteroids, especially if other risk factors for osteoporosis (e.g., family history, other high-risk medication use) are present.

Giant Cell Arteritis

GCA, also known as temporal arteritis, is a systemic inflammatory vasculitis. It often affects the small- to medium-sized temporal, vertebral, ophthalmic, posterior ciliary, and occipital arteries; the larger aorta, carotid, subclavian, and iliac arteries may also be affected. Cause is unknown but inflammation occurs in the intima, media, and adventitia of the artery wall, along with infiltration of lymphocytes, macrophages, and multinucleated giant cells, possibly resulting in distal ischemia. GCA rarely occurs in people younger than 50 years, is more common in females, and smoking increases risk sixfold.

Clinical Manifestations

1. Constitutional symptoms may present first: malaise, fever, night sweats, anorexia, fatigue.
2. Headache (localized to temporal or occipital area), jaw claudication (pain on chewing or prolonged speaking), visual disturbance, neck pain, and scalp tenderness with involvement of temporal (most commonly involved) and other arteries of the head.
3. Visual disturbances occur in 50% of patients and may be transient and intermittent, such as blurred or double vision; some may experience a sudden visual field deficit, which progresses to complete vision loss over several days.
4. Manifestations of other arteries involved include limb claudication, transient ischemic attacks (TIAs), stroke, aortic rupture, or myocardial infarction.

CLINICAL JUDGMENT Be alert for reports of sudden vision loss or change along with symptoms of headache, tenderness of temples, and jaw pain. Prompt referral to rheumatologist, ophthalmologist, or the emergency department is essential to prevent permanent vision loss.

Diagnosis/Treatment

1. ESR >50 mm/h and elevated CRP.
2. CBC may show mild normocytic anemia and mildly elevated platelet count.
3. Temporal artery biopsy is important to confirm diagnosis in order to commit to a long course of therapy. Color duplex ultrasound is a promising alternative.
4. High-dose corticosteroid therapy (oral or IV) is the universally accepted treatment and should be started immediately upon development of visual symptoms to prevent permanent blindness. Do NOT wait for biopsy or lab results to initiate treatment.
   a. Treatment is tapered very slowly to prevent relapse. ACR/EULAR guidelines recommend trying to taper over 1 year.
   b. Low-dose aspirin is added for patients with large vessel involvement.
   c. Proton pump inhibitors are indicated to prevent GI bleeding.
5. For patients who cannot tolerate high doses of corticosteroids for long periods, methotrexate or tocilizumab may be utilized as steroid-sparing agents.

Nursing and Patient Care Considerations

1. Perform thorough vascular examination including blood pressure in both arms, auscultation of arteries for bruits, and inspection for localized signs of ischemia.
2. Educate patients about the potential adverse effects of high-dose corticosteroids, including hyperglycemia, hypertension, fluid retention, osteoporosis, compression fracture, and mood changes. Encourage close follow-up and monitoring (see page 809).
3. Encourage healthy diet with limited sodium, sugar, and calories; increase physical activity.
4. Advise the patient to report visual disturbance immediately.

Sarcoidosis

Sarcoidosis is a chronic, granulomatous multisystem disorder that most notably affects the lungs and lymph nodes but can mimic rheumatic disease by causing fever, arthritis, uveitis, myositis, and skin lesions. Sarcoidosis also has similarities to tuberculosis, with a possible association with *Mycobacterium* causing granulomas. Cause is unknown but is thought to be a combination of environmental factors, genetic predisposition, and dysregulated immune system (exaggerated T helper 1 immune response).

Clinical Manifestations

1. Sarcoidosis can present in many ways, from asymptomatic to acute presentation with erythema nodosum (painful nodules on anterior legs), bilateral hilar lymphadenopathy, and polyarthritis (known as Lofgren syndrome). See Figure 26-5.
2. General and vague symptoms of fever, fatigue, weight loss, arthralgias, and lymphadenopathy may occur in addition to organ-specific involvement.

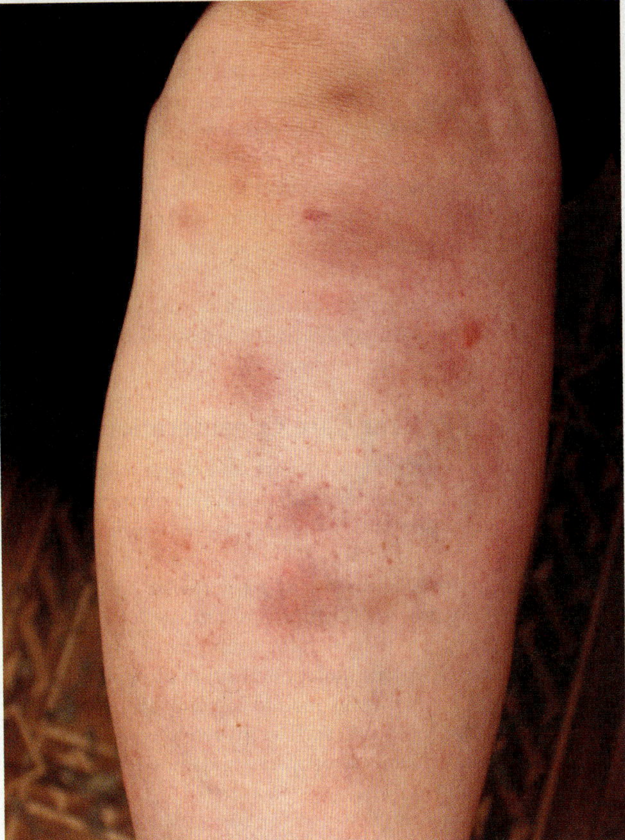

Figure 26-5. Erythema nodosum presenting on lower legs of a patient with sarcoidosis. (Shutterstock/Dermatology11)

3. Chronic sarcoidosis usually consists of chronic lung involvement (mediastinal and hilar lymphadenopathy and pulmonary infiltrates) with possible symptoms of dry cough, wheezing, dyspnea, and chest tightness.
4. Sarcoid-specific skin involvement may present with SC nodules, papules, and plaques, which may be violaceous, pigmented, erythematous, or skin colored. Alopecia and nail changes also may occur.
5. Ocular sarcoidosis presents as various forms of uveitis and can lead to blindness due to adhesions and scarring.
6. Renal, cardiac, neurologic, and other system involvement may also occur.

Diagnosis/Treatment

1. There are several serum markers for sarcoidosis, including angiotensin-converting enzyme (ACE), which have low sensitivity and specificity for sarcoidosis, so may not be helpful in diagnosis. Serum and urine calcium levels, creatinine, and alkaline phosphatase may be elevated with other organ involvement.
2. Diagnosis relies on a combination of biopsy of lesion (external lesions such as skin, eye, peripheral lymph node preferred to surgical biopsy of internal lesions) showing histopathology of noncaseating granuloma, conforming clinical presentation (including chest x-ray showing bilateral hilar lymphadenopathy), and exclusion of other disease-causing granulomatous disease.
3. Spontaneous regression often occurs, so treatment is only necessary when symptoms are severe and disabling,

granulomatous inflammation is progressive, and end-organ failure is impending.
4. Corticosteroids may be used when pulmonary involvement is active and severe, with progressively decreasing lung function, starting with 20 to 40 mg daily and slowly tapering to 5 or 10 mg daily over 1 year; however, relapse may occur. DMARD therapy such as methotrexate, azathioprine, or mycophenolate may be added as corticosteroid-sparing agents.
5. Extrapulmonary disease may be treated with topical or ocular corticosteroids.
6. Immunosuppressants may be needed in some cases. Certain TNF inhibitors have been used for sarcoid arthropathy that does not respond to conventional DMARDs.

Nursing and Patient Care Considerations

1. Assist with assessment of diverse and vague clinical manifestations since diagnosis is often elusive; probe history for general symptoms such as fever, fatigue, weight loss, and arthralgias.
2. Reassure the patient that many cases resolve spontaneously and long-term progressive arthritis is rare.
3. Caution the patient to be alert for symptoms of eye inflammation and to seek ophthalmology evaluation promptly.
4. Educate the patient about monitoring and control of corticosteroid adverse effects, such as hyperglycemia, hypertension, fluid retention, osteoporosis, and mood changes (see page 809).

Other Rheumatic Diseases

Polymyositis (dermatomyositis if rash is present)—an inflammatory disease of striated muscles that most commonly affects the proximal limb girdle, neck, pharynx, proximal third of the esophagus, and, occasionally, the heart. Corticosteroids, DMARDs, immune globulin infusions, and some biologics are used for treatment (most off-label).

Calcium pyrophosphate dihydrate crystal deposition disease, also known as pseudogout—results in crystal deposition in the joint cartilage and menisci, bursae, and periarticular tissue and can present similarly to gout. Treatment is similar to gout and consists of colchicine and NSAIDs (see page 819).

SELECTED READINGS

American College of Rheumatology. (2023). *2022 American College of Rheumatology (ACR) guideline for exercise, rehabilitation, diet, and additional integrative interventions for rheumatoid arthritis: Guideline summary*. Author. https://www.rheumatology.org/Portals/0/Files/Integrative-RA-Treatment-Guideline-Summary.pdf

American Nurses Association and Rheumatology Nurses Society. (2019). *Rheumatology nursing: Scope and standards of practice* (Vol. 2). Author.

Bass, A. R., Chakravarty, E., Akl, E. A., Bingham, C. O., Calabrese, L., Cappelli, L. C., Johnson, S. R., Imundo, L. F., Winthrop, K. L., Arasaratnam, R. J., Baden, L. R., Berard, R., Bridges, S. L., Jr., Cheah, J. T. L., Curtis, J. R., Ferguson, P. J., Hakkarinen, I., Onel, K. B., Schultz, G., … Reston, J. (2023). 2022 American College of Rheumatology guideline for vaccinations in patients with rheumatic and musculoskeletal diseases. *Arthritis Care & Research (Hoboken)*, *75*(3), 449–464. https://doi.org/10.1002/acr.25045

Cena, H., & Calder, P. C. (2020). Defining a healthy diet: Evidence for the role of contemporary dietary patterns in health and disease. *Nutrients*, *12*(2), 334. https://doi.org/10.3390/nu12020334

England, B. R., Tiong, B. K., Bergman, M. J., Curtis, J. R., Kazi, S., Mikuls, T. R., O'Dell, J. R., Ranganath, V. K., Limanni, A., Suter, L. G., & Michaud, K. (2019). 2019 Update of the American College of Rheumatology recommended rheumatoid arthritis disease activity measures. *Arthritis Care & Research (Hoboken)*, *71*(12), 1540–1555. https://doi.org/10.1002/acr.24042

Geenen, R., Overman, C. L., Christensen, R., Åsenlöf, P., Capela, S., Huisinga, K. L., Husebø, M. E. P., Köke, A. J. A., Paskins, Z., Pitsillidou, I. A., Savel, C., Austin, J., Hassett, A. L., Severijns, G., Stoffer-Marx, M., Vlaeyen, J. W. S., Fernández-de-Las-Peñas, C., Ryan, S. J., & Bergman, S. (2018). EULAR recommendations for the health professional's approach to pain management in inflammatory arthritis and osteoarthritis. *Annals of the Rheumatic Diseases*, *77*(6), 797–807. https://doi.org/10.1136/annrheumdis-2017-212662

Nowell, W. B., Gavigan, K., Kannowski, C. L., Cai, Z., Hunter, T., Venkatachalam, S., Birt, J., Workman, J., & Curtis, J. R. (2021). Which patient-reported outcomes do rheumatology patients find important to track digitally? A real-world longitudinal study in ArthritisPower. *Arthritis Research & Therapy*, *23*(1), 53. https://doi.org/10.1186/s13075-021-02430-0

Pope, J. E., Denton, C. P., Johnson, S. R., Fernandez-Codina, A., Hudson, M., & Nevskaya, T. (2023). State-of-the-art evidence in the treatment of systemic sclerosis. *Nature Reviews Rheumatology*, *19*(4), 212–226. https://doi.org/10.1038/s41584-023-00909-5. Epub 2023 Feb 27. PMID: 36849541; PMCID: PMC9970138.

Raleigh, M. F., Stoddard, J., & Darrow, H. J. (2002). Polymyalgia rheumatica and giant cell arteritis: Rapid evidence review. *American Family Physician*. *106*(4), 420–426. PMID: 36260899.

Robinson, P. C. (2018). Gout—An update of aetiology, genetics, co-morbidities and management. *Maturitas*, *118*, 67–73. https://doi.org/10.1016/j.maturitas.2018.10.012

Sammaritano, L. R., Bermas, B. L., Chakravarty, E. E., Chambers, C., Clowse, M. E. B., Lockshin, M. D., Marder, W., Guyatt, G., Branch, D. W., Buyon, J., Christopher-Stine, L., Crow-Hercher, R., Cush, J., Druzin, M., Kavanaugh, A., Laskin, C. A., Plante, L., Salmon, J., Simard, J., Somers, E. C., Steen, V., Tedeschi, S. K., Vinet, E., White, C. W., Yazdany, J., Barbhaiya, M., Bettendorf, B., Eudy, A., Jayatilleke, A., Shah, A. A., Sullivan, N., Tarter, L. L., Birru Talabi, M., Turgunbaev, M., Turner, A., D'Anci, K. E. (2020). American College of Rheumatology Guideline for the Management of Reproductive Health in Rheumatic and Musculoskeletal Diseases. *Arthritis Rheumatology*, *72*(4), 529–556. https://doi.org/10.1002/art.41191. Epub 2020 Feb 23. PMID: 32090480.

Sen, R., Goyal, A., & Hurley, J. A. (n.d.). Seronegative spondyloarthropathy. In *StatPearls* [Internet]. StatPearls Publishing. Updated July 17, 2023. https://www.ncbi.nlm.nih.gov/books/NBK459356/

Sreeja, C., Priyadarshini, A., Premika, & Nachiammai, N. (2022). Sarcoidosis—A review article. *Journal of Oral & Maxillofacial Pathology*, *26*(2), 242–253. https://doi.org/10.4103/jomfp.jomfp_373_21

Tripolino, C., Ciaffi, J., Ruscitti, P., Giacomelli, R., Meliconi, R., & Ursini, F. (2021). Hyperuricemia in psoriatic arthritis: Epidemiology, pathophysiology, and clinical implications. *Frontiers in Medicine (Lausanne)*, *8*, 737573. https://doi.org/10.3389/fmed.2021.737573

Udompanich, S., Chanprapaph, K., & Suchonwanit, P. (2018). Hair and scalp changes in cutaneous and systemic lupus erythematosus. *American Journal of Clinical Dermatology*, *19*(5), 679–694. https://doi.org/10.1007/s40257-018-0363-8

Vij, R., & Strek, M. E. (2013). Diagnosis and treatment of connective tissue disease-associated interstitial lung disease. *Chest*, *143*(3), 814–824. https://doi.org/10.1378/chest.12-0741

Wang, C. R., & Tsai, H. W. (2023). Seronegative spondyloarthropathy-associated inflammatory bowel disease. *World Journal of Gastroenterology*, *29*(3), 450–468. https://doi.org/10.3748/wjg.v29.i3.450

Whiting, P. F. (2010). Systematic review: Accuracy of anti–citrullinated peptide antibodies for diagnosing rheumatoid arthritis. *Annals of Internal Medicine*, *152*(7), 456. https://doi.org/10.7326/0003-4819-152-7-201004060-00010

Yu Erin, & Chang Jessica R. (2022). Giant cell arteritis: Updates and controversies. *Frontiers in Ophthalmology*. https://doi.org/10.3389/fopht.2022.848861

27
Infectious Diseases

OVERVIEW OF INFECTIOUS DISEASES

Infectious diseases have a significant impact on human health. Lower respiratory and diarrheal infectious diseases alone are two of the top 10 leading causes of death globally. Unlike other diseases, infectious diseases are transmissible from the host to others and may spread rapidly. An infection results when a microbe invades a host organism, using its resources to live and replicate. The associated disease, however, occurs when there is a change or impairment of normal tissue function because of the infection.

The Infectious Disease Process

The chain of infection includes six components that must be in succession for any infectious disease to evolve. If one link is eliminated from the chain, then transmission of the pathogen will not occur. Infection prevention strategies are based on breaking the chain of infection. The six components of the chain of infection include the infectious agent, reservoir, portal of exit from reservoir, mode of transmission, portal of entry into host, and susceptible host (Figure 27-1).

Pathogenic Microorganism

Must be able to enter the body and invade or colonize host tissue by attaching to specific host cells, then cause damage to those cells by the production of toxins or destructive enzymes. The pathogen may enter the body through a body orifice or broken skin.

Types

The types of infectious agents are bacteria (including *Mycobacteria*), viruses, fungi, parasites (including protozoa and helminths), and prions. (For more information, see the "Types of Infectious Diseases" section.)

Characteristics

1. Pathogenicity—ability to produce disease.
2. Virulence—disease severity.
3. Infectious dose—number of organisms needed to initiate infection.
4. Toxigenicity—capacity to produce injurious substances that damage the host.
5. Adaptability—ability to adjust to changing conditions, that is, resistance to antimicrobial agents (see Table 27-1).

Reservoir

The environment in which a pathogenic microorganism lives and survives naturally can be human, animal and insects, or environmental, including soil, water, medical equipment, or fomite. Examples of each type include:

1. Human—*Mycobacterium* tuberculosis in human lungs.
2. Animal—Zika virus via *Aedes aegypti* and/or *Aedes albopictus* mosquitoes.
3. Environmental—Legionnaires disease (*Legionella pneumophila*) through water.
4. Fomite (object or material that may harbor infectious agents)—methicillin (oxacillin)-resistant *Staphylococcus aureus* (MRSA) bacteria on a bedside table.

Portal of Exit From Reservoir

The portal of exit are routes in which infectious agents leave their reservoir and include:

1. Droplets or aerosolization from the respiratory tract.
2. Vomitus and feces.
3. Body fluids (except for sweat).

Mode of Transmission

How the pathogenic microorganism is spread to a host by an infectious source.

1. Horizontal transmission is the spread of a pathogen from one individual to another individual.
2. Vertical transmission is infection spreading from birthing parent to offspring via transplacental transmission, contact through the birth canal, or through breastfeeding or close contact after birth.

There are two main types of transmission: direct and indirect.

Direct Transmission

1. Direct contact—by touching the reservoir (e.g., touching a wound infection with MRSA) or sexual contact (e.g., human papillomavirus).
2. Droplet transmission.
   a. Droplets of large particles more than 5 μm in size usually from respiratory secretions.
   b. Transmitted through coughing, sneezing, or talking to an infected person (e.g., human metapneumovirus spread through coughing).

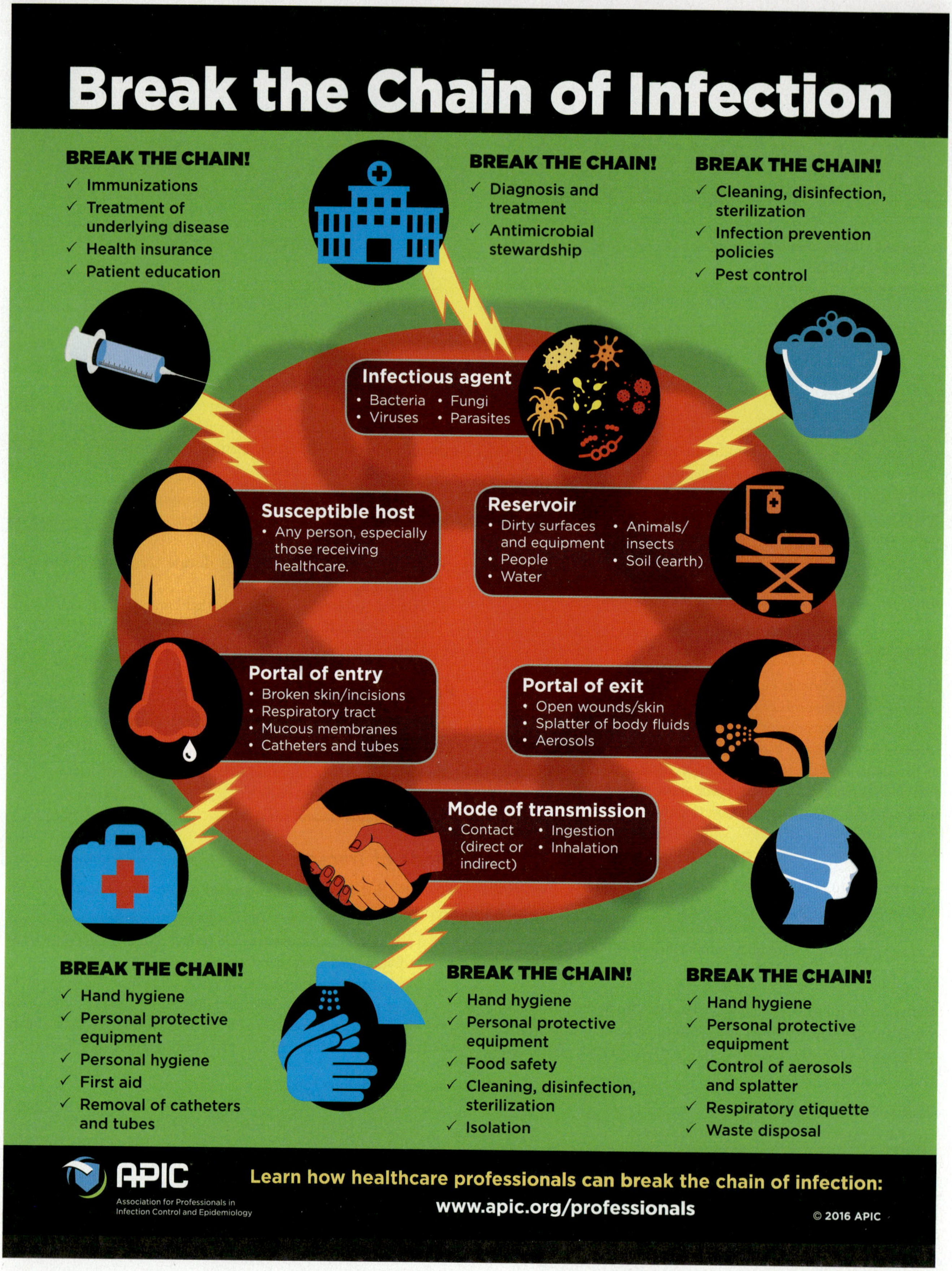

Break the Chain of Infection
BREAK THE CHAIN!
✓ Immunizations
✓ Treatment of underlying disease
✓ Health insurance
✓ Patient education
BREAK THE CHAIN!
✓ Diagnosis and treatment
✓ Antimicrobial stewardship
BREAK THE CHAIN!
✓ Cleaning, disinfection, sterilization
✓ Infection prevention policies
✓ Pest control
Infectious agent
• Bacteria • Fungi
• Viruses • Parasites
Susceptible host
• Any person, especially those receiving healthcare.
Reservoir
• Dirty surfaces and equipment
• People
• Water
• Animals/ insects
• Soil (earth)
Portal of entry
• Broken skin/incisions
• Respiratory tract
• Mucous membranes
• Catheters and tubes
Portal of exit
• Open wounds/skin
• Splatter of body fluids
• Aerosols
Mode of transmission
• Contact (direct or indirect)
• Ingestion
• Inhalation
BREAK THE CHAIN!
✓ Hand hygiene
✓ Personal protective equipment
✓ Personal hygiene
✓ First aid
✓ Removal of catheters and tubes
BREAK THE CHAIN!
✓ Hand hygiene
✓ Personal protective equipment
✓ Food safety
✓ Cleaning, disinfection, sterilization
✓ Isolation
BREAK THE CHAIN!
✓ Hand hygiene
✓ Personal protective equipment
✓ Control of aerosols and splatter
✓ Respiratory etiquette
✓ Waste disposal
APIC
Association for Professionals in Infection Control and Epidemiology
Learn how healthcare professionals can break the chain of infection:
www.apic.org/professionals
© 2016 APIC

Figure 27-1. Chain of infection. (Reprinted from Association for Professionals in Infection Control and Epidemiology. [2016]. *Break the chain of infection: Infection prevention and you.* https://infectionpreventionandyou.org/protect-your-patients/break-the-chain-of-infection/)

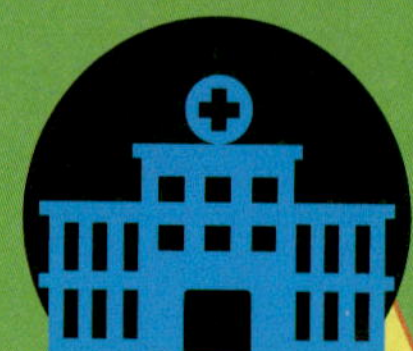

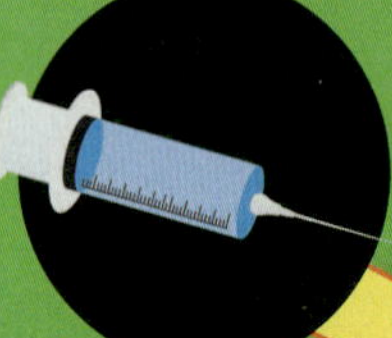

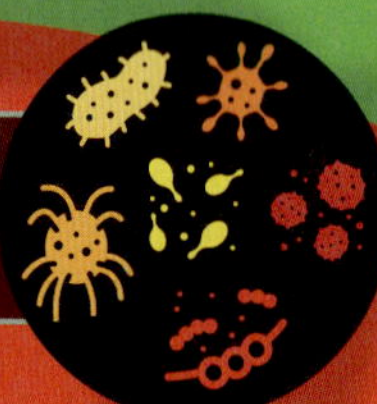

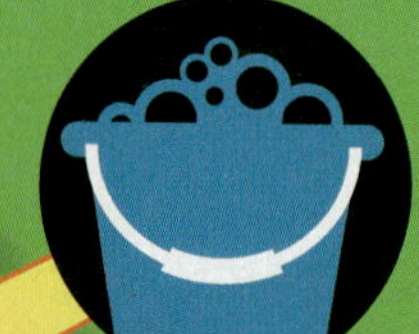

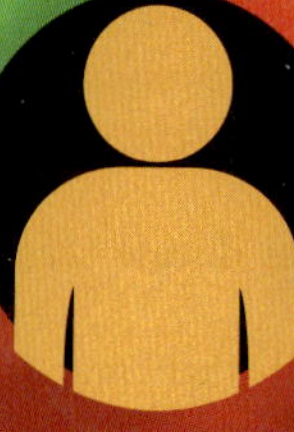

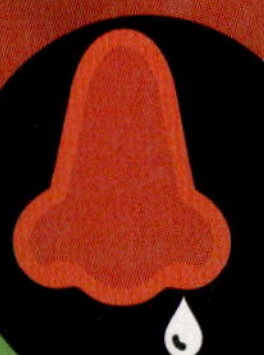

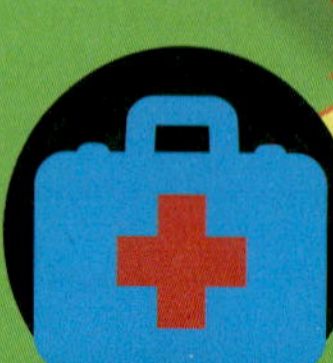

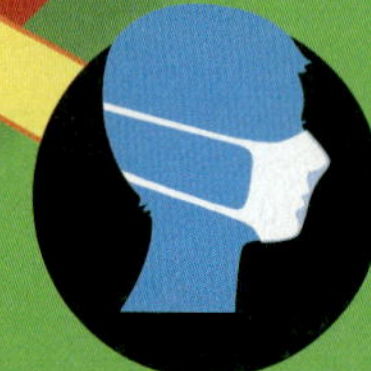

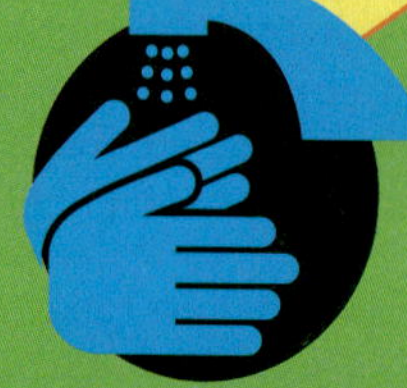

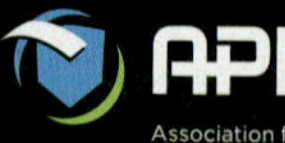

Table 27-1 Antimicrobial-Resistant Organisms

ORGANISM	OVERVIEW AND TRANSMISSION	PREVENTION (ALL)
MRSA	Found in various body sites but especially in nares and on skin. Can produce toxins and invade body tissues. Transmitted via direct and indirect contact. Drug of choice: vancomycin.	• Hand hygiene with soap or alcohol-based hand sanitizer. • Use of gloves and gowns for patient contact. • Isolate patient in private room or cohort patients with the same organisms on contact isolation. • Use disposable equipment or disinfect reusable items after removal from room. • Utilize a system for prompt identification and isolation of patients upon readmission and for discharge planning. • Health care worker, patient, and family education.
VRE	Found in GI tract and female[a] GU tract. Not highly pathogenic but can cause serious illness in immunocompromised persons. If infection occurs, treatment options are limited. Transmitted via direct and indirect contact.	
VISA/VRSA	Transmitted via direct and indirect contact. Must be reported to the CDC and the local health department. Strictly follow contact precautions and dedicate staff for one-to-one care. Treatment options are limited.	
Multidrug-resistant gram-negative rods such as *Escherichia coli*, *Klebsiella pneumoniae*, *Acinetobacter* species, and *Pseudomonas aeruginosa*	Found in various body sites, especially sputum. Spread via direct and indirect contact.	
Emerging MDROs • ESBLs producers • CRE • New Delhi metallo-beta lactamase	Produced by some gram-negative bacteria, making them resistant to multiple antibiotics. Spread via direct and indirect contact. Limited treatment options because of resistance. There is a worldwide concern for growing pan-resistance creating "superbugs."	

CDC, Centers for Disease Control and Prevention; CRE, carbapenem-resistant Enterobacteriaceae; ESBL, extended-spectrum metallo-beta-lactamase; GI, gastrointestinal; GU, genitourinary; MRSA, methicillin-resistant Staphylococcus aureus; MDROs, multidrug-resistant organisms; VISA, vancomycin-intermediate Staphylococcus aureus; VRSA, vancomycin-resistant Staphylococcus aureus; VRE, vancomycin-resistant enterococci.

[a]"Female" refers to a person assigned female at birth.

c. Transmitted through aerosolizing procedures (e.g., sprays of infectious agents during a nebulization treatment or a sputum induction).

3. Airborne transmission.
   a. Droplet nuclei—less than 5 μm that remain suspended in air (e.g., tuberculosis and varicella [primary chickenpox]).
   b. Dust particles in the air containing the infectious agent (e.g., *Aspergillus fungi* through dust).

Indirect Transmission

Touching a fomite that has had direct contact with the reservoir (e.g., touching a tissue of a child with Influenza virus or touching a bedside table contaminated with *Clostridium difficile*).

1. Common vehicle route (through contaminated items).
   a. Food (e.g., Salmonella and Campylobacter).
   b. Water (e.g., *Vibrio cholerae* and *Legionella* species).
   c. Medications (e.g., blood-borne pathogens including hepatitis B virus [HBV], hepatitis C virus [HCV], and human immunodeficiency virus [HIV] from contaminated multidose vials).
2. Vector-borne transmission.
   a. A living creature acts as an intermediary acquiring a pathogen from one living host and transmits the disease agent to another living organism, often an arthropod (fly, mosquito, tick).
   b. Can be mechanical or biological vectors. Mechanical transmission occurs when the vector transports the pathogen on its feet or body surfaces to the host. Biological transmission occurs when the vector takes the pathogen into its body where it develops, produces copies, and then is put in the host by bite or sting, such as the plague transmitted by infected fleas from rats to humans.

Portal of Entry

Defined as how an infectious agent enters a new host. Entry sites include:

1. Respiratory tract.
2. Gastrointestinal/genitourinary.
3. Mucous membranes.
4. Nonintact skin.
5. Blood.

Susceptible Host

Host susceptibility is determined by a complex interrelationship between host and an infectious agent, by factors that influence infection or disease, such as:

1. Pathogenicity—the ability to produce disease in a host. The organism invades a host, enters tissue, colonizes then spreads from host to host while not necessarily causing death to the host.
2. Virulence—the wide range of damage that can occur to the host because of the toxic capabilities of the pathogen. Given that the host–pathogen relationship is fluid, the outcome can be dictated by:
   a. Number of pathogens to which the host is exposed; route and duration of exposure.
   b. Invasiveness of the pathogen and its ability to produce toxins.
   c. Ability to bypass or overcome host defense mechanisms (immunologic response).
3. Host factors—susceptibility of the new host to infection including age, nutritional status, immune status (e.g., vaccination), genetic constitution, and general physical, mental, and emotional health and nutritional status of host.

Types of Infectious Diseases

Infectious diseases are categorized by the type of infectious agent and include bacterial, viral, fungal, parasitic, and prions. Although some microorganisms, called pathogens, can cause infections, the vast majority do not cause disease. Humans are colonized with trillions of microbes. These microbes function as communities in different body sites and are referred to as the microbiome. Microbiomes, along with age, comorbidities, and other factors, significantly impact individual immune systems and susceptibility to infectious disease.

Bacterial

Bacteria are single-cell organisms and differ from eukaryotic cells (as in humans) in that they have a single-circular chromosome (nucleoid) instead of a membrane-bound nucleus. They are often categorized as gram positive or gram negative because of how their cell wall structures appear using the Gram stain. Gram-positive organisms, such as *S. aureus*, contain a thick peptidoglycan layer and will stain purple. Gram-negative organisms, such as *Escherichia coli*, have a thin, inner peptidoglycan layer and outer layer containing proteins, phospholipids, and lipopolysaccharide (LPS) and will stain pink. Some organisms, such as *Bacillus* and *Clostridium*, are defined as gram variable and may appear both pink and purple. Acid-fast bacteria such as *Nocardia* and *Mycobacteria* do not stain well with the traditional Gram stain.

Bacterial pathogens can cause infection in virtually all body sites and are the most common cause of health care–associated infections (HAIs). They can be transmitted by contact (*S. aureus*), droplet (whooping cough [*Bordetella pertussis*]), bacterial meningitis (*Neisseria meningitidis*), airborne (tuberculosis), vectors (ticks: Lyme disease, fleas: Bubonic plague), and/or vehicular (the transmission of pathogens through vehicles such as water, food, and air)/fomites (food: *Salmonella*, fomite: *C. difficile*).

Viral

Viruses are much smaller than bacteria, and unlike bacteria, they require a living cell host to replicate. All viruses contain a genetic component of either RNA or DNA viral genome and a protein coat called a capsid; some also have an envelope of phospholipids. They are classified based on the presence of RNA or DNA and the presence or absence of an envelope. Nonenveloped viruses are more challenging to eliminate from surfaces/equipment.

Like bacterial pathogens, viruses can cause infection in virtually all body sites. They can be transmitted via the fecal-to-oral route (hepatitis A virus [HAV]), blood-borne (HBV, HCV, HIV), droplet (influenza, respiratory syncytial virus [RSV]), airborne (varicella zoster virus [VZV]), vectors (mosquitos: yellow fever, dengue, Zika virus), and vehicular/fomites. Fomites are nonliving entities that participate in the spread of disease, including objects contaminated with a pathogen. Vehicles are also nonliving entities that contribute to the spread of disease, including resources such as air, water, and food.

Fungal

Fungi are eukaryotes and much larger than bacteria. They are divided into yeasts and mold based upon their physical appearance. Yeasts, such as *Candida* spp., are single celled and form smooth colonies on culture plates. Molds, such as *Penicillium* spp., have long-branching filaments of cells called hyphae, which form a mycelium that is visible to the naked eye.

Very few fungi can cause infection in a healthy host, and the vast majority are opportunistic in immunocompromised hosts or after antibiotic exposure. These opportunists are primarily spread by the environment and can cause invasive, systemic infections.

Parasitic (Including Protozoa and Helminths)

Parasites are found in multiple morphologies: single-cell protozoans (*Giardia* and malaria-causing *Plasmodium*), worm-like helminths (tapeworms, hookworms), and arthropods (scabies and lice). Although parasites are not commonly transmitted in the health care setting, parasitic infections impact millions of people each year, particularly in developing countries.

Prions

Transmissible spongiform encephalopathies (TSEs) are rare and a family of progressive neurodegenerative disorders that affect both animals and humans. The causative agent is called a "prion." This pathogen is not well understood but thought to be transmissible and induce abnormal folding of normal proteins called prion proteins, found mostly in the brain. This group of diseases has long incubation periods, associated with neuronal loss and a failure to induce inflammatory response. Once the symptoms begin, it progresses rapidly and is always fatal. Prion diseases in humans include—Creutzfeldt–Jakob disease (CJD), variant Creutzfeldt–Jakob disease (vCJD), Gerstmann–Sträussler–Scheinker syndrome, fatal familial insomnia, and Kuru. Transmission has been reported in 250 cases worldwide and linked to human growth hormone, dura mater and corneal grafts, or neurosurgical equipment. Special considerations are taken with treatments, procedures, or surgeries involving contact with high infectivity tissues (brain, spinal cord, and eyes) of patients thought to have TSEs. The Centers for Disease Control and Prevention (CDC) and World Health Organization (WHO) have developed infection control guidelines for individuals caring for patients with CJD. For more information, see www.cdc.gov/prions/index.html.

Common Infectious Disorders by Body System

Table 27-2 outlines common infectious disease agents by body system. Infectious disorders are covered throughout the book in a variety of body system chapters. Be aware that new data on infectious diseases are emerging daily. For the latest information on infectious diseases including incubation periods, route of transmission, and prevention/treatment, contact your local public health department or the CDC at www.cdc.gov.

INFECTIOUS DISEASE IDENTIFICATION

Collection of Specimens

EVIDENCE BASE Leber, A. L., & Burnham, C.A. (2023). *Clinical microbiology procedures handbook* (5th ed.). American Society for Microbiology Press.

Proper collection and transport of laboratory specimens is important to maximize the outcome of tests for the diagnosis of infectious diseases. A variety of laboratory tests can be performed to make a presumptive or definitive diagnosis so that therapy can begin.

Principles

1. Review local laboratory guidelines for the specimen collection recommendations for each test. These guidelines should be

Table 27-2 Common Infectious Disease Agents by Body System

BODY SYSTEM	INFECTION EXAMPLES	CLINICAL MANIFESTATIONS	BACTERIAL PATHOGENS	VIRAL PATHOGENS	FUNGAL/PARASITIC/ PRION PATHOGENS	NURSING IMPLICATIONS
CNS	Infections include meningitis, encephalitis, brain abscess, and osteomyelitis. Typically occur via spread of infections in distant locations or directly connected to the CNS.	Patients with meningitis often present with neck stiffness, headache, and fever. Other CNS infection symptoms may be nonspecific, including fever and changes in behavior and mental status.	Meningitis: *Neisseria meningitidis, Streptococcus pneumoniae*, group B *Streptococcus* in neonates, *Haemophilus influenzae, Listeria monocytogenes, Escherichia coli*, brain abscess (often polymicrobial): *Streptococcus* species, *Staphylococcus* species	Meningitis: enteroviruses, HSV, CMV Encephalitis: HSV, VZV, arboviruses in Summer months (West Nile virus, Eastern equine encephalitis virus, St. Louis encephalitis virus)	Less common and usually occurs in patients who are immunocompromised, including HIV and transplant populations Fungal meningitis: *Cryptococcus neoformans, Coccidioides immitis, Histoplasma capsulatum* Fungal brain abscess: *Aspergillus* and *Nocardia* in patients who have received transplants Parasitic: toxoplasmosis prions	• Patients with symptoms should wear a surgical mask to prevent transmission. • Implement droplet precautions for all suspected, probable, or confirmed cases of bacterial meningitis until further identification or at least 24 h of effective antibiotic therapy. • For patients with suspected/confirmed prion disease, dedicate surgical instruments for high-risk tissues or follow evidence-based processes to decontaminate. • Stay up to date and encourage patients at high risk to stay up to date on recommended vaccines.
Upper respiratory system	Self-limiting infections involving the upper airway (sinuses/nose, pharynx, larynx) with no signs of pneumonia	Patients often present with congestion, runny nose, sore throat, and/or fever.	Strep throat (strep group A, *Streptococcus pyogenes*)	Very common cause and may include a variety of viruses, such as rhinovirus, adenovirus, coronavirus, enterovirus, parainfluenza virus	Less common	• Patients with symptoms should wear a surgical mask to prevent transmission. • Stay up to date on recommended vaccines. • Implement droplet precautions for all suspected and confirmed cases. • Practice excellent hand hygiene and disinfection of shared equipment. • Educate patients and families on prevention techniques, including vaccination, hand hygiene, and respiratory etiquette.
Lower respiratory system	Infections include bronchitis, bronchiolitis, and pneumonia.	Symptoms may include fever, cough, wheezing, and/or shortness of breath.	Pneumonia, common: *S. pneumoniae, H. influenzae, S. aureus* Atypical causes: *Mycobacteria* (tuberculosis and nontuberculosis, NTM), *Mycoplasma pneumoniae, Legionella* (associated with contaminated water), leptospirosis, *Chlamydia pneumoniae, Chlamydia psittaci*	Bronchitis: most caused by influenza and rhinovirus Bronchiolitis: RSV in infants/children Pneumonia: influenza, coronavirus, adenovirus, RSV	Less common, may often be associated with immunosuppression Fungal: *H. capsulatum, C. immitis, Aspergillus* spp. Parasitic: *Schistosoma, Ascaris lumbricoides*, hookworm	• Patients with symptoms should wear a surgical mask to prevent transmission. • Stay up to date on recommended vaccines. • Implement droplet precautions for all suspected and confirmed cases. • Practice excellent hand hygiene and disinfection of shared equipment. • Educate patients and families on prevention techniques, including vaccination, hand hygiene, and respiratory etiquette.

(continued)

Table 27-2 Common Infectious Disease Agents by Body System (*continued*)

BODY SYSTEM	INFECTION EXAMPLES	CLINICAL MANIFESTATIONS	BACTERIAL PATHOGENS	VIRAL PATHOGENS	FUNGAL/PARASITIC/ PRION PATHOGENS	NURSING IMPLICATIONS
GI system	Infections may occur in the upper or lower GI tract, including the esophagus, stomach, small bowel, and colon.	Symptoms may include nausea, vomiting, diarrhea, fever, abdominal pain, and/or abdominal cramping.	Foodborne: *Salmonella* species, *Shigella* species, STEC, *Campylobacter* species, *Bacillus cereus*, *Listeria*, *Yersinia* Antibiotic associated: *Clostridioides difficile*	Rotavirus, *Norovirus*, hepatitis A	Parasitic: *Giardia lamblia*, *Cryptosporidium*, *Ascaris* Fungal: yeast overgrowth	• Implement contact precautions for all patients requiring diapers or with fecal incontinence. • Follow health care facility diagnostic stewardship protocols when testing for GI pathogens, including *C. difficile*. • Practice excellent hand hygiene and disinfection of shared equipment. • For *C. difficile* and *Norovirus*, soap and water are recommended instead of alcohol-based hand sanitizer. • Educate patients and families on prevention techniques, including food and water safety (especially with travel), vaccination for hepatitis A, and hand hygiene.
Urinary tract	Infections may involve the bladder and kidneys.	Symptoms range from asymptomatic to fever, costovertebral pain, urinary urgency, urinary frequency, and/or dysuria.	Gram-negative bacteria: *E. coli*, *Klebsiella pneumoniae*, *Proteus* Gram-positive bacteria: *Enterococcus*, *Staphylococcus saprophyticus*	Uncommon cause of UTIs may occur in patients who are immunocompromised.	Uncommon cause of UTIs, *Candida* infection may occur in patients who are immunocompromised.	• Follow standard precautions and health care facility diagnostic stewardship protocols. • To prevent catheter-associated UTIs, avoid the use of invasive catheters (consider alternatives first) and remove invasive catheters as soon as clinically feasible.
Skin	Infections can range from minor cellulitis, rashes, and abscesses to severe necrotizing fasciitis.		*S. aureus*, *S. pyogenes* (strep group A, flesh-eating bacteria), Polymicrobial	VZV, measles, rubella, HSV	Fungal: *Tinea corporis* (ringworm), yeast Parasitic: lice, scabies, hookworm (from larvae migration), *Borrelia burgdorferi* (Lyme disease rash)	• Follow standard precautions and contact precautions for draining wounds/abscesses, which cannot be contained. • Rashes should be evaluated. Implement appropriate transmission-based precautions as indicated (i.e., airborne for measles). • Monitor response to prescribed therapy. • Practice meticulous hand hygiene. • Consider testing for coinfections if testing for tickborne illness and rash.
Sexually transmitted	May be transmitted through vaginal, oral, or anal sexual contact	Symptoms vary and infections are often undetected as many people may have no symptoms.	Gonorrhea (*Neisseria gonorrhoeae*), chlamydia (*Chlamydia trachomatis*), syphilis (*Treponema pallidum*)	HSV, HPV, blood-borne pathogens: HBV, HCV, HIV	Parasitic: *Trichomonas vaginalis*, pubic lice	• Follow standard precautions and sharps safety practices to prevent exposure to blood-borne pathogens. • Complete the HBV vaccine series. • Educate patients on safe sexual practices and encourage HBV vaccination. • Monitor for skin lesions.

CMV, cytomegalovirus; CNS, central nervous system; GI, gastrointestinal; HBV, hepatitis B virus; HCV, hepatitis C virus; HIV, human immunodeficiency virus; HPV, human papilloma virus; HSV, herpes simplex virus; NTM, nontuberculous Mycobacteria; RSV, respiratory syncytial virus; STEC, Shiga toxin-producing Escherichia coli; UTI, urinary tract infection; VZV, varicella zoster virus.

From World Health Organization. (2021). Key facts and figures. https://www.who.int/campaigns/world-hand-hygiene-day/2021/key-facts-and-figures; World Health Organization. (2020, December 9). The top 10 causes of death. https://www.who.int/news-room/fact-sheets/detail/the-top-10-causes-of-death

readily available and include information on the appropriate specimen containers, sample size, and transport requirements (temperature, time, etc.).
2. It is imperative that specimens be collected and handled carefully by following standard precautions (see Standards of Care Guidelines 27-1).
3. Specimen collection should occur before the initiation of antibiotic therapy whenever possible.
4. To prevent contamination, specimens should be collected using aseptic technique.
5. Obtain an adequate amount of the specimen necessary for all tests.
6. Label the container properly according to local laboratory protocol with at least two patient identifiers (e.g., patient's name, date of birth, medical record number) and include on a requisition the source of the specimen, date and time collected, test to be performed, and any special instructions.
7. Seal specimen containers tightly and place them in a biohazard bag to transport the specimen to the laboratory as soon as possible according to laboratory guidelines.
8. Be familiar with hospital policy recommending the transport of specified pathogens by staff personnel to the laboratory instead of via a pneumatic tube system.

STANDARDS OF CARE GUIDELINES 27-1

Universal Precautions (Referenced OSHA 1910.1030)

These infection control precautions, mandated by the Occupational Safety and Health Administration (OSHA), recommend that all blood and certain body fluids are treated as potentially infectious for human immunodeficiency virus (HIV), hepatitis B virus (HBV), hepatitis C virus (HCV), and other blood-borne pathogens:

- Employers are required to provide appropriate personal protective equipment (PPE) and other engineering/work practice controls to eliminate or minimize employee exposure to blood-borne pathogens as mandated in OSHA regulation 1910.
- Gloves are to be worn when there is anticipation of contact with blood, other potentially infectious materials, mucous membranes, and nonintact skin.
- Gowns, aprons, or other protective body clothing are to be worn when contamination of clothing with blood or other potentially infectious materials is anticipated.
- Masks in combination with protective eyewear are to be worn when performing procedures likely to generate sprays or splashes of blood or other potentially infectious materials into the eyes, nose, or mouth.
- Hands and other skin surfaces are to be washed immediately if contaminated with blood or other potentially infectious materials.
- Utilize safety devices for needles and other sharps and do not manipulate by hand (e.g., recapping, purposely bending or breaking, or removing from syringes).
- Needles and other sharps are to be placed in puncture-resistant containers for disposal.
- All specimens and items with blood or other potentially infectious materials are to be transported in containers that prevent leakage.
- Blood and body fluid spills are to be cleaned up promptly with an appropriate germicide, such as a bleach solution or phenolic.

Types of Specimen Collection

Blood Culture

1. Normally a sterile body fluid.
2. Specimens obtained by peripheral venipuncture are preferred to sampling from vascular catheters because of contamination of the catheter. Culturing hardware to determine a central line infection is not recommended in the literature.
3. Aseptic technique is essential to avoid contaminating the specimen with organisms colonizing the skin or the collector's hands.
4. Cleanse the venipuncture site with 70% alcohol followed by chlorhexidine gluconate and allow the alcohol to fully dry before inoculating with blood.
5. The diaphragm tops of the culture bottles are not sterile and must be cleaned with alcohol before injection of blood.

Urine Culture

1. Normally a sterile body fluid.
2. A clean-catch, midstream urine collection provides the best method for obtaining a specimen to detect a urinary tract infection.
3. Patients who are catheterized should have the specimen withdrawn using a sterile syringe from the catheter sampling port.
4. Urine specimens must be transported to the laboratory promptly. If sent in a sterile container, the urine must be cultured within 30 minutes if transported at room temperature or should be refrigerated and cultured within 24 hours. Note: It is preferred to collect a urine specimen in a container containing a preservative to prevent overgrowth and preserve the specimen in the event of delays in transport.
5. Other types of urine specimens may be collected, such as a straight in-and-out catheter specimen or suprapubic bladder drainage.

Stool Testing

1. Obtained to detect organisms in patients with gastroenteritis or colitis (e.g., *Salmonella* species, *Shigella* species). Note: Many laboratories have adopted molecular syndromic panel test for detection of bacterial, viral, and parasitic pathogens.
2. Patient should defecate into a sterilized container or bedpan. Stool specimens should not contain urine or water from the toilet bowl. Send specimens in Carey–Blair medium for bacterial stool detection and specialized transport for parasitology testing (e.g., Total Fix).
3. Stool specimens can also be obtained directly from the rectum using an approved swab. Check with the local laboratory to determine which swabs are acceptable.

Sputum Culture

1. Specimen needs to be from the lower respiratory tract, not oropharyngeal secretions. The laboratory will perform a Gram stain on all sputum specimens to determine whether they are representative of pulmonary secretions and appropriately collected. A specimen containing a majority of cells from squamous epithelium may be rejected.
2. The most common method of collection is expectoration from a cooperative patient with a productive cough. Early morning is the optimal time to collect sputum specimens.
3. A sputum specimen can be collected in a sputum trap from patients who have artificial airways and require suctioning.
4. If a patient cannot produce sputum, sputum induction using an aerosol nebulizer may assist with loosening thickened secretions.
5. Bronchoscopy may be required to obtain sputum if induction fails.

Wound Culture

1. Specimens are usually cultured for aerobic and anaerobic organisms.
2. Specimens may be collected by multiple techniques, depending on the depth of the wound, including tissue samples, needle aspiration, and swabbing the surface.
3. Surface cultures are often heavily contaminated and are not representative of deeper infections.
4. To collect a wound culture using a sterile swab, cleanse the surface with 70% alcohol and collect as much exudate as possible from the advancing margin of the lesion. Avoid swabbing surrounding skin.
5. Place the swab immediately in the appropriate transport culture tube and send it to the laboratory.
6. Label with the specific anatomic site.

Throat Culture/Molecular Testing

1. Use a tongue depressor to hold the tongue down.
2. Carefully yet firmly rub swab over areas of exudate or over the tonsils and posterior pharynx, avoiding the cheeks, teeth, and gums.
3. Insert the swab into the packet and follow directions for handling the transport medium.

Laboratory Tests

Microbiologic Evaluation

Microscopy

1. Microscopic examination distinguishes tissue cells from microorganisms.
2. Various stains are used to highlight the structural characteristics of microorganisms (e.g., Gram stain to identify groups of bacteria, acid-fast stains to isolate *Mycobacteria*).
3. Classification is conducted according to physical appearance such as shape, size, or tendency to form chains or clusters and stain reactions such as gram positive versus gram negative.
4. Results of microscopy are usually available within minutes, which permits early initiation of treatment based on a presumptive diagnosis.

Culture

1. Culture was the gold standard for positive identification of many microorganisms, although technological advances have transitioned to molecular and other innovative testing for several microbes.
2. Different culture media are used for suspected pathogens and can be selective (allow growth of only certain microorganisms) and/or differential (distinguish between different bacteria based on different characteristics).
   a. A liquid medium is used for blood specimens because lower numbers of microorganisms are detectable.
   b. A solid medium is used to isolate mixtures of organisms and grow pure cultures of each type of organism found.
3. Recovery of pathogens from culture varies depending on the microorganism type, test selected, and stage of illness.
   a. Most common pathogens, such as staphylococci, streptococci, and enterococci, are often identifiable to genus and species within a few hours.
   b. Fungal organisms may take 10 to 14 days to grow in culture medium.
   c. *Mycobacteria* may take up to 6 weeks to grow in culture medium.

Matrix-Assisted Laser Desorption Ionization-Time of Flight Mass Spectrometry

1. Bacterial or fungal isolates to be identified are inoculated to a target, and a matrix is applied. The target is placed into the mass spectrometry (MS) instrument.
2. Biomolecules absorb energy from a short laser pulse to become ionized, which are then accelerated in an electrical field and collide with a detector. They are then separated based upon their mass-to-charge ratio and lead to molecular detections into mass spectrum.
3. Based upon databases of mass spectrum profiles, identifies a microorganism, including bacteria, *Mycobacteria*, and fungus, to the genus and species level within minutes versus several hours to days with traditional cultures.

Antibiotic Susceptibility Testing

1. Used to determine whether a panel of antimicrobial agents will inhibit organism growth at achievable serum concentrations. Two methods are routinely used in clinical laboratories:
   a. Broth microdilution—determines the minimum inhibitory concentration (MIC), which is the lowest concentration of an antimicrobial drug that will inhibit organism growth and is measured by turbidity in a broth microdilution panel. The first well to demonstrate inhibited growth represents the MIC.
   b. Disk diffusion—a standard inoculum of a specific organism to be tested is applied to a Mueller Hinton agar plate. Disks containing standardized concentrations of antimicrobial agents are then applied to the plate. After overnight incubation, the zone of inhibition of growth is measured and, using Clinical Laboratory Standards Institute (CLSI) documents, is interpreted as resistant (R), susceptible (S), or intermediate (I).

Molecular Testing

1. There are several technologies to detect specific genetic portions of pathogenic organisms or to identify the specific host's response to the presence of the pathogen. Examples include DNA probe testing and polymerase chain reaction (PCR).
2. These tests may be more sensitive for lower amounts of organism and often yield a more rapid result than culture.
3. Some tests, including multiplex PCRs, detect the presence of multiple organisms at once such as respiratory viruses or gastrointestinal infectious agents.

White Blood Cell Count

1. An increase in white blood cell (WBC) count or "leukocytosis" may indicate infection, inflammatory response, tissue necrosis, or bone marrow failure.
2. The total number of circulating leukocytes and the differential (given as a percent of the total WBC count) may change during a bacterial or viral infection.
3. During an acute bacterial infection, the WBC count often increases (greater than 11,000/mm^3), accompanied by increased neutrophils and increased bands (immature neutrophils) in the differential. The shift (to the left) in differential reflects phagocytic activity.

Immunologic Tests

1. Pathogens that are antigenic stimulate antibodies that can be detected in the serum of patients.
2. Detection of antibodies is not necessarily diagnostic of current infection.

3. Antigen–antibody reactions must be evaluated over a period of time.
4. Immunoglobulin M (IgM) antibody production peaks during active infection and decreases during convalescence.
5. IgG antibodies peak during convalescence and persist.
6. A fourfold rise in antibody titer between the acute and convalescence samples indicates recent infection.

PREVENTION AND TREATMENT

Immunity and Immunization

The human body is equipped with defense mechanisms to protect against disease. These include anatomic barriers, such as the skin, and physiologic barriers, such as enzymes in saliva. The normal flora of microorganisms on and in the body also helps to prevent the invasion of pathogens. If these nonspecific defense mechanisms fail, the body's specific immune response usually provides protection. Specific immunity to a particular organism implies that an individual has either generated the appropriate antibody in their own body or received ready-made antibodies from another source. Immunity may be *natural* or *acquired* or *passive* or *active*.

Natural active immunity occurs when antibodies are acquired following an infection. Antibodies are also acquired through *natural passive immunity*, such as from birthing parent to fetus through the placenta or to infant via breast milk.

Passive artificial immunity is achieved through administration of immune globulin or antitoxin. *Active artificial immunity* occurs when antibodies are produced in response to a vaccine or toxoid.

There has been debate over the possibility of a link between childhood vaccines and subsequent development of autism. Public fear and refusal to obtain childhood vaccines for preventable diseases has shown an increase of these diseases in the community. There have been multiple studies in the scientific community to refute these fears (see www.cdc.gov/vaccinesafety/concerns/autism.html).

Vaccines are the best protection against infections that may cause serious complications and possible poor outcomes in children and adults. The Advisory Committee on Immunization Practices (ACIP) posts the most updated recommendations for vaccine schedules for those aged birth to 6 years, those aged 7 to 18 years, those aged 19 years or above, pregnant patients, and other groups. The ACIP group members consist of 15 medical and public health experts who are selected by the Secretary of the U.S. Department of Health and Human Services (DHHS) following a rigorous review of their qualifications and accomplishments to the field. The ACIP meets three times a year and collaborates with 30 highly regarded professional organizations, such as the American Academy of Pediatrics (AAP) and the American Academy of Family Physicians (AAFP) to produce a harmonized annual vaccination schedule. https://www.cdc.gov/vaccines/schedules/index.html

For age-specified vaccine recommendations, see: www.cdc.gov/vaccines/parents/downloads/parent-ver-sch-0-6yrs.pdf

www.cdc.gov/vaccines/schedules/easy-to-read/adolescent-easy-read.html

www.cdc.gov/vaccines/adults/rec-vac/index.html

Infection Prevention in Health Care

Health care–associated infections (HAIs) occur when a patient comes to a health care facility and acquires a new infection during their care or shortly after leaving the facility. Approximately 1 in 31 hospital patients and 1 in 43 nursing home residents has an HAI. During 2021, overall HAIs increased compared to 2019, due to COVID-19–related hospitalizations, resulting in extended length of stay, more comorbidities, and patients with higher acuity levels. Through engagement by local, state, and federal public health agencies in conjunction with hospitals and other health care facilities, these infections are preventable using evidence-based prevention initiatives.

Infection prevention efforts include surveillance and reporting, monitoring transmission of multidrug-resistant organisms (MDROs), hospital-wide hand hygiene adherence, antimicrobial stewardship, and cleaning and disinfection. In addition, occupational health measures include vaccine adherence, staff education, and performance improvement initiatives to reduce HAIs. Infection prevention strategies are aimed at breaking the chain of infection.

HAI Surveillance

1. The four most common HAIs for which hospitals perform surveillance are as follows:
   a. Surgical site infection (SSI).
   b. Central line–associated bloodstream infection (CLABSI).
   c. Ventilator-associated events (VAE).
   d. Catheter-associated urinary tract infection (CAUTI).
2. HAI rates are used as indicators of quality and patient safety in health care facilities.
3. Hospitals are reporting infection rates to the National Health Safety Network (NHSN), part of the Centers for Disease Control and Prevention (CDC), and the data are being published and made available to the public via state/local health department websites and the Centers for Medicare & Medicaid Services' (CMS) hospital site.
4. Each year, the bottom quartile of performers in hospital quality metrics including HAI rates receive a penalty of reduced CMS reimbursement of expenses.

Fundamentals of Standard Precautions

Standard precautions are to be utilized for the care of all patients in any setting, every time. They apply to (1) blood; (2) all body fluids, secretions, and excretions, regardless of whether they contain visible blood; (3) nonintact skin; and (4) mucous membranes. If there is a chance of coming into contact with a potentially infectious material, a barrier is recommended to be placed between the patient and the care provider. The barrier may be a gown, glove, mask, or goggles, depending on the reason and area of contact.

Hand Hygiene

1. Hand hygiene is the single most recommended measure to reduce the risks of transmitting microorganisms. Proper hand hygiene prevents half of preventable HAIs, including to care team members.
2. Hand hygiene should be performed between patient contacts; after contact with blood, body fluids, secretions, excretions, and contaminated equipment or articles; before donning and after removing gloves is vital for infection control. It may be necessary to clean hands between tasks on the same patient to prevent cross-contamination of different body sites.
3. To perform hand hygiene, clean hands with soap and water, applying friction for 20 seconds upon all surfaces of the hands, or applying alcohol-based waterless hand sanitizer covering all surfaces of both hands until completely dry.

4. Waterless hand cleaners are recommended unless there is visible soil on the hands, before eating, after using the restroom, and when there is significant buildup of waterless hand cleaners.
5. If caring for a patient with a spore-producing pathogen such as *Clostridioides difficile*–associated disease (CDAD), then use hand hygiene with soap and water applying friction for 20 seconds, as the spores this organism forms are resistant to alcohol hand gel.
6. Similarly, for other pathogens known or suspected to be resistant to alcohol waterless hand gels—such as *Norovirus*—hand hygiene with soap and water while applying friction for 20 seconds.

Respiratory Hygiene/Cough Etiquette

1. When coughing or sneezing, cover the mouth and nose with a tissue or the fabric of your sleeve.
2. Use the nearest waste receptacle to dispose of the tissue after use.
3. Perform hand hygiene immediately.
4. Apply a mask when coughing or sneezing to contain secretions.
5. Sit at least 6 feet from others.

Transmission-Based Precautions

In addition to standard precautions, the CDC recommends instituting transmission-based precautions when there is a suspicion for, or a laboratory-confirmed case involving, an epidemiologically significant pathogen. There are three types of transmission-based precautions recommended by the CDC: contact, droplet, and airborne. Each type of isolation takes into account the pathogen and its mode of transmission. They are also to be utilized in combination when necessary (i.e., contact and airborne precautions for varicella zoster virus). Always refer to each health care facility's infection prevention policies, as hospitals may be more restrictive than the CDC recommendations influenced by endemic or newly emerging pathogens in that region. Care should be taken when donning and doffing personal protective equipment (PPE) to avoid contamination (see Figure 27-2).

CLINICAL JUDGMENT Standard precautions are recommended for the care of each patient, in all circumstances, even if the patient is already in another type of isolation. When possible, dedicate the use of noncritical patient care equipment to a single patient. Thoroughly clean and disinfect reusable equipment before use on another patient.

Contact Precautions

1. Used for patients known or suspected to be infected or colonized with epidemiologically significant microorganisms, which can be transmitted by direct contact with the patient or indirect contact with environmental surfaces (fomites) or patient care items in the patient's environment.
2. Examples of microorganisms requiring contact precautions:
   a. Methicillin (oxacillin)-resistant *Staphylococcus aureus* (MRSA).
   b. Vancomycin-resistant *Enterococcus*.
   c. Carbapenem-resistant Enterobacteriaceae (CRE).
   d. *C. difficile* (CDIFF).
3. Place the patient in a private room or in a room with a patient who has the same microorganism (cohorting).
4. Wear PPE when entering a room marked as contact isolation, including gloves and a gown (see Box 27-1). Many hospitals encourage visitors to follow the same precautions.
5. All equipment, including intravenous poles, handles on carts, and other devices, should be cleaned, disinfected, and identified as clean prior to transport in halls, elevators, or before provided to a new patient—doing so protects the environment, staff, visitors, and patients from contamination with potentially infectious germs.

Droplet Precautions

1. Designed for care of patients known or suspected to be infected with microorganisms transmitted by large particle droplets generated by the patient when coughing, sneezing, talking, or during the performance of certain procedures, such as sputum induction or nebulization.
2. These large particle droplets fall out of the air 3 to 6 feet from the patient's mouth, so use of surgical mask, eye protection, gown, and gloves is mandatory.
3. Examples of illnesses requiring droplet precautions: *Neisseria meningitidis*, pneumonic plague, scarlet fever, pertussis, adenoviruses, parainfluenza viruses, influenza, respiratory syncytial virus, human metapneumovirus, rhinovirus, mumps, parvovirus B12, rubella.
4. Place the patient in a private room.
   a. When a private room is not available, place patients with the same microorganism together (cohorting).
   b. If neither of these is possible, maintain spatial separation of at least 6 feet between the patient who is infected and other patients and visitors.
5. Special air handling and ventilation are not necessary, and the door may remain open.
6. PPE includes surgical masks; gowns and gloves may also be required based on the disease, refer to the disease-specific hospital policy.
   a. Wear a mask when working within the patient's room/care environment.
   b. To protect the mucous membranes of the eyes, nose, and mouth, masks and goggles or face shields are worn by health care workers during patient care to protect against splashes or sprays of blood, body fluids, or secretions.
7. Limit transport of the patient from the room for essential purposes only. If transport is necessary, minimize dispersal of droplets by masking the patient immediately prior to and during transport. For additional measures, see the later discussion.

Airborne Precautions

1. Designed to reduce the risk of airborne transmission of infectious agents through dissemination of small droplet nuclei less than 5 μm in size, which remain suspended in the air for long periods of time.
2. Certain procedures, including, but not limited to, intubation, extubation, and bronchoscopy, generate aerosols and are referred to as aerosol-generating procedures. This is due to air currents moving across liquid particles. These aerosols can be small in size and can increase the risk of pathogen transmission.
3. Microorganisms can be dispersed widely by air currents and may become inhaled by or deposited on a susceptible host within the same room or over a longer distance from the source patient. Therefore, special air handling, filtration, and ventilation are required.
4. Examples of illnesses requiring airborne precautions: COVID-19, measles, varicella (including disseminated zoster), and tuberculosis.
5. PPE—respirators are required (N95 respirator, a high-efficiency particulate air [HEPA] filter respirator, or a powered air-purifying respirator [PAPR]); gowns and gloves may also be required based on the disease, refer to the disease-specific hospital policy.

SEQUENCE FOR PUTTING ON PERSONAL PROTECTIVE EQUIPMENT (PPE)

The type of PPE used will vary based on the level of precautions required, such as standard and contact, droplet or airborne infection isolation precautions. The procedure for putting on and removing PPE should be tailored to the specific type of PPE.

1. GOWN

- Fully cover torso from neck to knees, arms to end of wrists, and wrap around the back
- Fasten in back of neck and waist

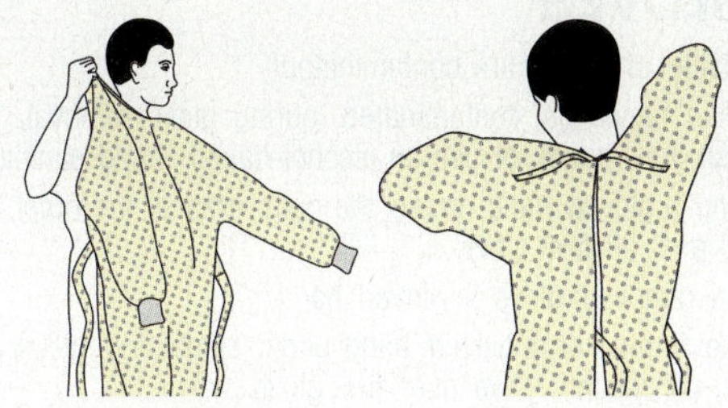

2. MASK OR RESPIRATOR

- Secure ties or elastic bands at middle of head and neck
- Fit flexible band to nose bridge
- Fit snug to face and below chin
- Fit-check respirator

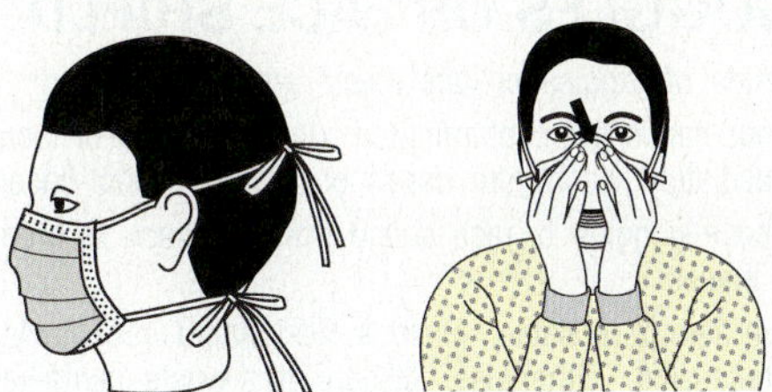

3. GOGGLES OR FACE SHIELD

- Place over face and eyes and adjust to fit

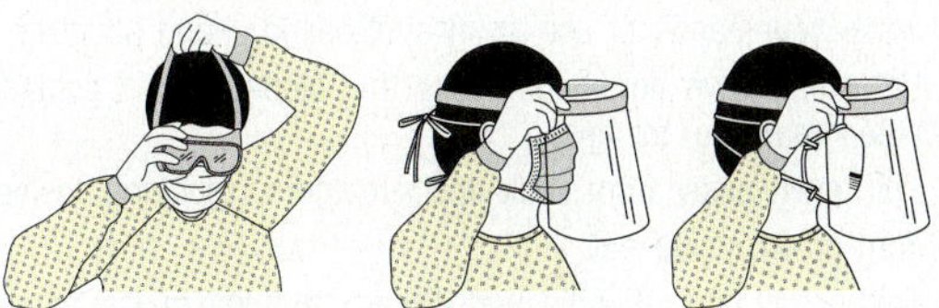

4. GLOVES

- Extend to cover wrist of isolation gown

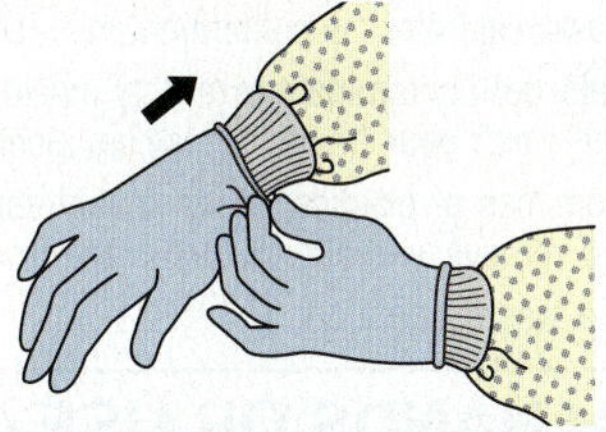

USE SAFE WORK PRACTICES TO PROTECT YOURSELF AND LIMIT THE SPREAD OF CONTAMINATION

- Keep hands away from face
- Limit surfaces touched
- Change gloves when torn or heavily contaminated
- Perform hand hygiene

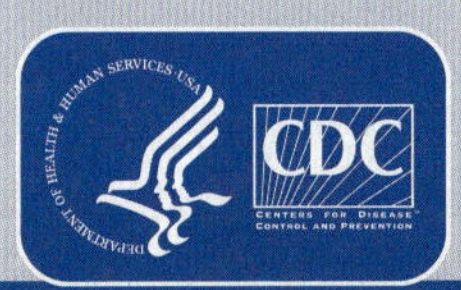

Figure 27-2. The Centers for Disease Control and Prevention guide to donning and doffing PPE. (Reprinted from Centers for Disease Control and Prevention. Sequence for putting on personal protective equipment (PPE). https://www.cdc.gov/hai/pdfs/ppe/ppe-sequence.pdf)

HOW TO SAFELY REMOVE PERSONAL PROTECTIVE EQUIPMENT (PPE) EXAMPLE 1

There are a variety of ways to safely remove PPE without contaminating your clothing, skin, or mucous membranes with potentially infectious materials. Here is one example. **Remove all PPE before exiting the patient room** except a respirator, if worn. Remove the respirator **after** leaving the patient room and closing the door. Remove PPE in the following sequence:

1. GLOVES

- Outside of gloves are contaminated!
- If your hands get contaminated during glove removal, immediately wash your hands or use an alcohol-based hand sanitizer
- Using a gloved hand, grasp the palm area of the other gloved hand and peel off first glove
- Hold removed glove in gloved hand
- Slide fingers of ungloved hand under remaining glove at wrist and peel off second glove over first glove
- Discard gloves in a waste container

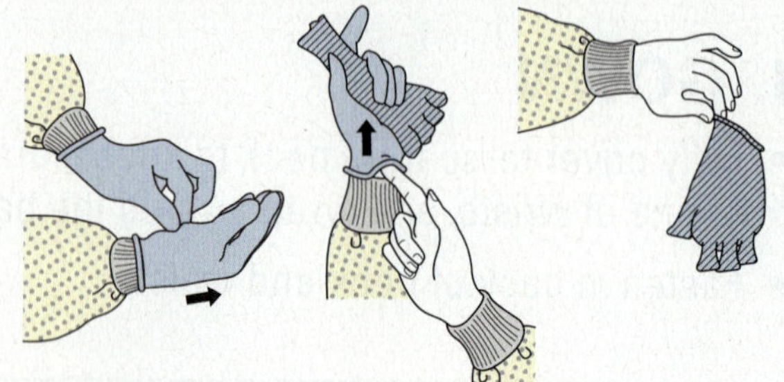

2. GOGGLES OR FACE SHIELD

- Outside of goggles or face shield are contaminated!
- If your hands get contaminated during goggle or face shield removal, immediately wash your hands or use an alcohol-based hand sanitizer
- Remove goggles or face shield from the back by lifting head band or ear pieces
- If the item is reusable, place in designated receptacle for reprocessing. Otherwise, discard in a waste container

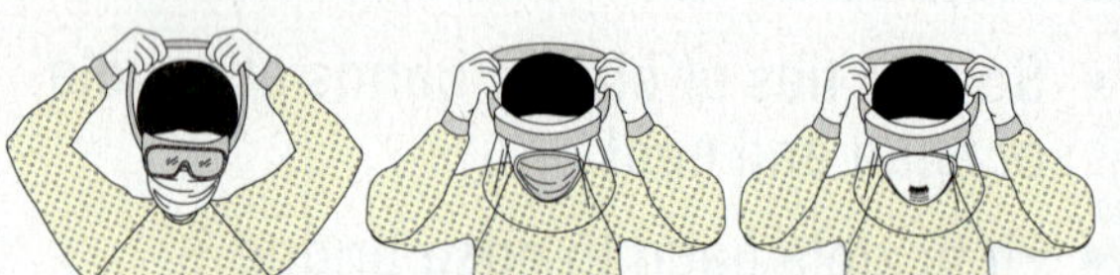

3. GOWN

- Gown front and sleeves are contaminated!
- If your hands get contaminated during gown removal, immediately wash your hands or use an alcohol-based hand sanitizer
- Unfasten gown ties, taking care that sleeves don't contact your body when reaching for ties
- Pull gown away from neck and shoulders, touching inside of gown only
- Turn gown inside out
- Fold or roll into a bundle and discard in a waste container

4. MASK OR RESPIRATOR

- Front of mask/respirator is contaminated — DO NOT TOUCH!
- If your hands get contaminated during mask/respirator removal, immediately wash your hands or use an alcohol-based hand sanitizer
- Grasp bottom ties or elastics of the mask/respirator, then the ones at the top, and remove without touching the front
- Discard in a waste container

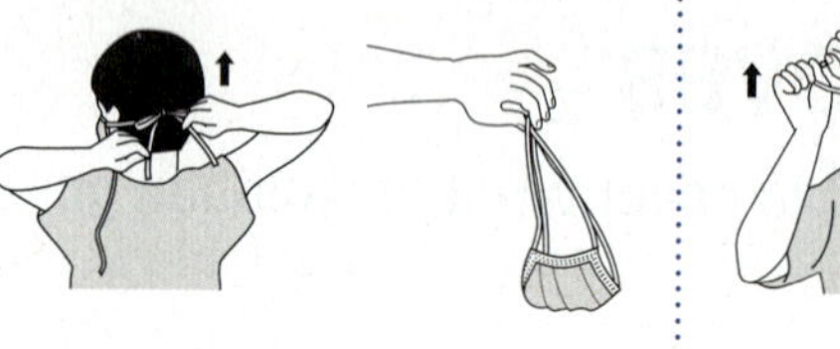

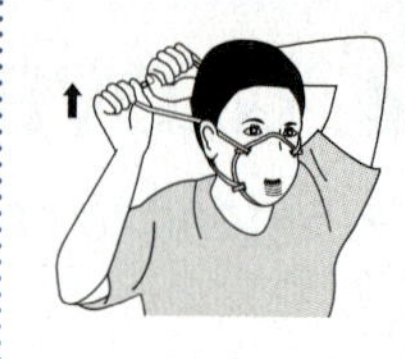

5. WASH HANDS OR USE AN ALCOHOL-BASED HAND SANITIZER IMMEDIATELY AFTER REMOVING ALL PPE

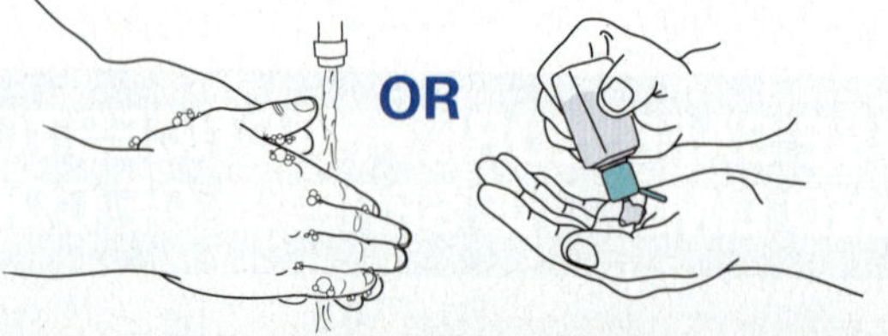

PERFORM HAND HYGIENE BETWEEN STEPS IF HANDS BECOME CONTAMINATED AND IMMEDIATELY AFTER REMOVING ALL PPE

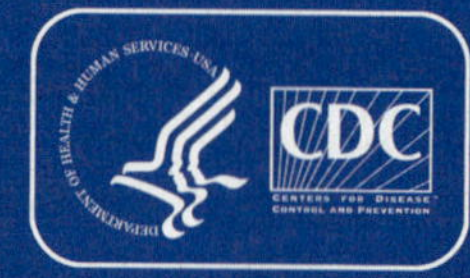

Figure 27-2. *(continued)*

HOW TO SAFELY REMOVE PERSONAL PROTECTIVE EQUIPMENT (PPE) EXAMPLE 2

Here is another way to safely remove PPE without contaminating your clothing, skin, or mucous membranes with potentially infectious materials. **Remove all PPE before exiting the patient room** except a respirator, if worn. Remove the respirator **after** leaving the patient room and closing the door. Remove PPE in the following sequence:

1. GOWN AND GLOVES

- Gown front and sleeves and the outside of gloves are contaminated!
- If your hands get contaminated during gown or glove removal, immediately wash your hands or use an alcohol-based hand sanitizer
- Grasp the gown in the front and pull away from your body so that the ties break, touching outside of gown only with gloved hands
- While removing the gown, fold or roll the gown inside-out into a bundle
- As you are removing the gown, peel off your gloves at the same time, only touching the inside of the gloves and gown with your bare hands. Place the gown and gloves into a waste container

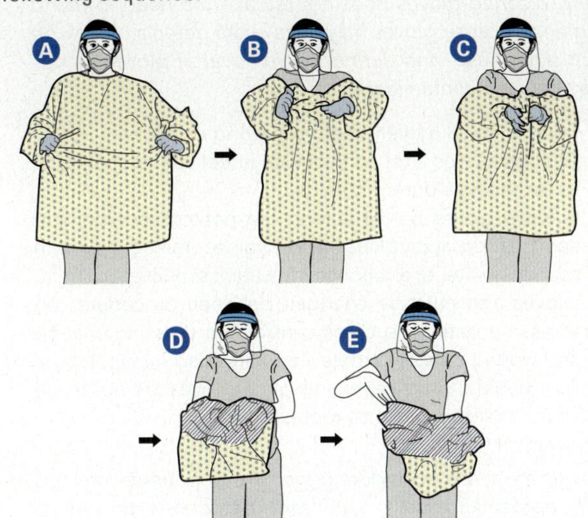

2. GOGGLES OR FACE SHIELD

- Outside of goggles or face shield are contaminated!
- If your hands get contaminated during goggle or face shield removal, immediately wash your hands or use an alcohol-based hand sanitizer
- Remove goggles or face shield from the back by lifting head band and without touching the front of the goggles or face shield
- If the item is reusable, place in designated receptacle for reprocessing. Otherwise, discard in a waste container

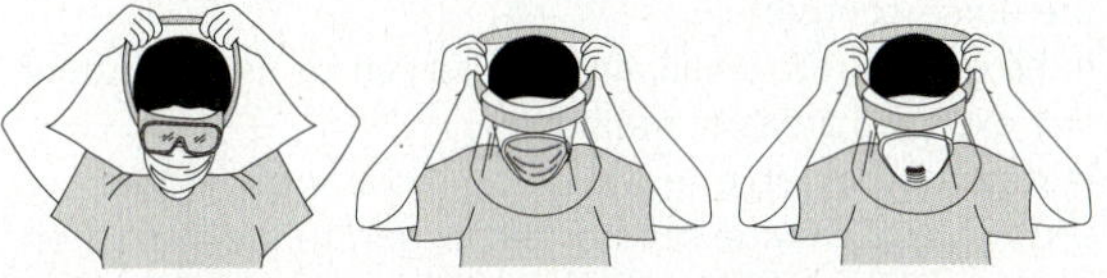

3. MASK OR RESPIRATOR

- Front of mask/respirator is contaminated— DO NOT TOUCH!
- If your hands get contaminated during mask/respirator removal, immediately wash your hands or use an alcohol-based hand sanitizer
- Grasp bottom ties or elastics of the mask/respirator, then the ones at the top, and remove without touching the front
- Discard in a waste container

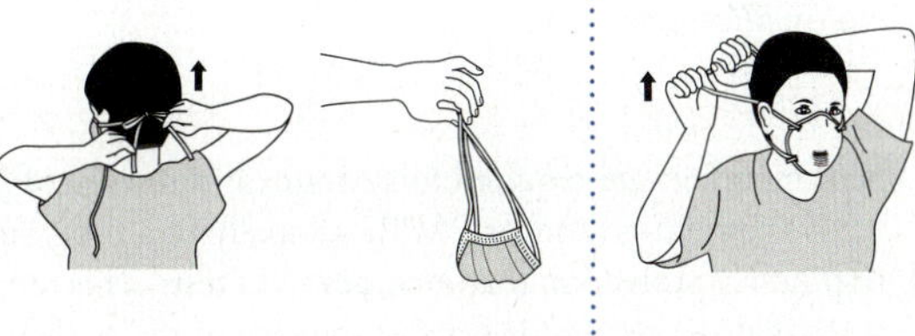

4. WASH HANDS OR USE AN ALCOHOL-BASED HAND SANITIZER IMMEDIATELY AFTER REMOVING ALL PPE

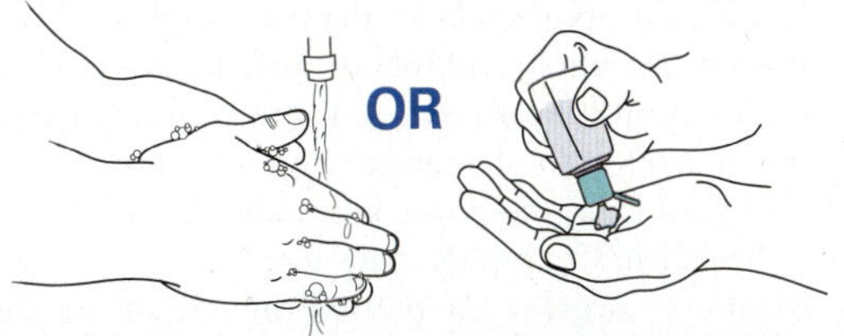

PERFORM HAND HYGIENE BETWEEN STEPS IF HANDS BECOME CONTAMINATED AND IMMEDIATELY AFTER REMOVING ALL PPE

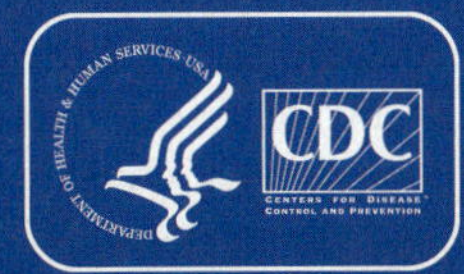

Figure 27-2. *(continued)*

BOX 27-1 Personal Protective Equipment

GLOVES

Gloves are worn to provide a protective barrier and prevent gross contamination of the hands of health care workers; if used properly, they reduce the transmission of microorganisms and help prevent cross-contamination within a patient. Wearing gloves does not replace the need for hand hygiene because gloves may have small defects or may be torn during use, and during the removal of gloves, hands may become contaminated.

- Perform hand hygiene before putting on gloves.
- Change gloves after contact with infective material, such as feces and wound drainage.
- Remove gloves before leaving the patient's environment and perform appropriate hand hygiene immediately with soap and water or alcohol-based waterless antiseptic agent.
- Gloves also must be changed between procedures on the same patient, such as central line dressing change and wound care or catheter drainage bag manipulation.
- As a general practice, examination gloves are not to be worn outside a patient's room.

GOWNS

Gowns are to be worn during the care of patients infected with epidemiologically significant pathogens to reduce contamination of the health care worker's clothing. Contaminated clothing can transmit pathogens to patients.

- The gown must be tied at the neck and sides, covering the nurse completely.
- If the gown is too small, two gowns can be used to cover any exposed areas of the nurse.
- Water-impermeable gowns, leg coverings, boots, or shoe covers provide greater protection to the skin when large splashes of blood or body fluid are possible such as in the operating room (OR).
- Gowns must be removed and discarded prior to leaving the patient's environment, and appropriate hand hygiene must be performed.

   a. Staff members are required to be trained in the use of protective respirators and/or PAPRs annually in a program of respiratory protection that includes a "fit test." This test ensures that the respirator seals to the face of the staff member, teaches the staff member how to use the respirator, and optimizes the protection for the staff member.
   b. Persons immune to rubeola or varicella need not wear a mask but must wear gown and gloves when having exposure to lesions, to prevent carrying contaminants to a patient outside the room who is nonimmune.
6. Place the patient in a private room that has:
   a. Monitored negative air pressure in relation to the surrounding areas.
   b. Preferably 12 air changes per hour.
   c. Appropriate discharge of air outdoors or monitored high-efficiency filtration of room air before recirculation.
   d. Door that is closed at all times with the patient in the room.
7. Limit the transport of the patient from the room to essential purposes only. If transport is necessary, minimize patient dispersal of droplet nuclei by placing a surgical or procedural mask on the patient. For additional measures, see further discussion.

Other Considerations

Limiting the Movement of Patients

1. Limiting the movement of patients with epidemiologically significant microorganisms reduces transmission. Every effort should be made to limit the movement of patients on airborne precautions.
2. When transport is necessary for a patient on contact, droplet, or airborne precautions:
   a. Patient should be in a clean hospital gown with clean linens.
   b. Appropriate barriers (such as masks and impervious dressings) are to be worn by the patient.
   c. Personnel in the area to which the patient is taken need notification with time to collect PPE, prepare a room that will meet specifications for the identified isolation, and communicate with cleaning staff and ensure the patient will not sit in a waiting area with other patients, visitors, and staff.
   d. Unless transporting staff are giving care during the transport, there is no need to wear PPE. If the patient may require care in the hallway, consider having two transporters: one to remain without PPE to open doors, touch elevator buttons, and push the patient, whereas the other person with PPE will only touch the patient.
3. When appropriate, patients are taught how they can assist in preventing transmission.

Attention to Equipment, Linens, and Supplies

1. Medical equipment should be cleaned in between each patient according to the equipment manufacturer's instructions for use (IFUs) according to the Spaulding classification of medical equipment.
   a. Noncritical equipment are devices, such as a stethoscope and blood pressure cuff, used on intact skin. Routine cleaning and low- to intermediate-level disinfection are required.
   b. Semicritical equipment are devices, such as a vaginal speculum or fiberoptic endoscope, used on mucous membranes or nonintact skin. High-level disinfection (HLD) at minimum is required; however, given the complicated steps and cross-contamination challenges with HLD processes, the latest recommendations from the American Association for the Advancement of Medical Instrumentation (AAMI) are to sterilize whenever feasible.
   c. Critical equipment are devices used in sterile body sites, such as the vascular system, and include surgical instrumentation, catheters, and implants. Sterilization of these devices is required.
2. Soiled linen should be handled, transported, and laundered in a manner that avoids transfer of microorganisms to patients, personnel, and environments in accordance with best practice guidelines. With some organisms, such as smallpox or anthrax, care must be taken to not expel the air from plastic linen bags outside airborne patient rooms.
3. There is currently no evidence indicating a need for special precautions for dishes, glasses, cups, or eating utensils because the combination of hot water and detergents used in hospital dishwashers is sufficient for decontamination for most infectious diseases. However, appropriate hand hygiene is required when removing food trays from some isolated rooms.
4. Patient care equipment that is soiled with blood, body fluids, secretions, and excretions must be handled in a manner that

prevents skin and mucous membrane exposures, contamination of clothing, and transfer of microorganisms to other patients and environments.

a. There must be a procedural mechanism in place labeling or otherwise identifying used equipment as not to be used on another patient.
b. Clean and dirty equipment should be stored in separate physical locations.
c. Reusable equipment must be transported in a manner to prevent contamination of the staff, the environment, and visitors until it reaches the area where it will be cleaned, disinfected, and reprocessed appropriately before use for another patient.
d. Single-use items must be discarded properly.

5. Care must be taken to prevent injuries from needles, scalpels, and other sharp objects. Used needles must never be recapped using both hands, removed from syringes, bent, broken, or otherwise manipulated. Used needles and sharps must have the engineered sharps injury protection activated and be disposed of immediately into an Occupational Safety and Health Administration (OSHA) approved puncture-resistant container. These containers should be mounted per the OSHA guidelines and be located as close as is practical to the area of use.
6. Protective mouthpieces, resuscitation bags, or other ventilation devices are used instead of mouth-to-mouth resuscitation methods.

Infection Prevention Bundles

In addition to standard and isolation precautions, hand hygiene, and appropriate equipment/supply handling, there are inclusive, grouped steps called bundles, which are evidence-based practices shown to prevent specific HAIs when all steps are followed. Bundled practices exist for the prevention of CLABSI, CAUTI, CDAD, and VAE. Bundles prevent infection through aseptic/sterile technique at the time of device insertion as well as properly maintaining devices. An essential component is daily review of necessity for indwelling devices and prompt early removal of devices to avoid infection.

Patient Education on Infection Prevention

Education on basic infection prevention practices should be provided for all patients who will be discharged either with devices and caring for them while at home or with antimicrobial-resistant organisms. For example, for central lines, the patient should be taught to wash hands before and after touching the lines; when and how to change dressings; how to shower or bathe with the dressing (depending on the type of supplies used); ongoing monitoring for early signs and symptoms of infection; and to communicate to the health care provider immediately. Proper care of devices and infection prevention practices in the home setting will reduce the risk for the spread of antimicrobial-resistant organisms, infections and other complications, and potential readmission to the hospital.

Treatment

Treatment of infectious diseases varies based upon the pathogen and host factors. Some infectious diseases, such as the common cold and other upper respiratory illnesses, are self-limiting, and treatment beyond supportive therapy may not be indicated. However, for certain infectious diseases and in certain hosts, antimicrobials—including antibiotics, antivirals, antifungals, and antiparasitics—may be indicated. Antimicrobial agents (see Box 27-2) are only effective against the microbial pathogens as indicated by the type of agent; for example, antibiotics are only effective against bacteria, and antivirals are only effective against viruses. When an antimicrobial is prescribed, it should be appropriate for the suspected or confirmed pathogen, susceptibility pattern, and properly dosed. Broad-spectrum antibiotics may be initially appropriate; however, it is best to narrow the antibiotic treatment once the organism and susceptibility patterns become available to avoid overuse of these antibiotics and ensure effective treatment. Antibiograms are a helpful tool to utilize when prescribing as these give an idea of the antimicrobial susceptibility patterns by organisms within a health care or local setting.

BOX 27-2 Antimicrobial Resistance and Antimicrobial Stewardship

Antimicrobial resistance (AMR) occurs when microorganisms (such as bacteria, fungi, viruses, and parasites) evolve or mutate after exposure to antimicrobial drugs (such as antibiotics, antifungals, antivirals, antimalarials, and anthelmintics). Resistance occurs naturally over time; however, it has accelerated due to overuse and misuse of antibiotics. Types of misuse include prescribing antibiotics for viruses such as the common cold or influenza or giving them to animals such as fish or livestock as growth promoters. AMR is found in human and animal populations and in the environment; thus, resistant bacteria are found in rivers, streams, soil, and wildlife.

AMR is an increasing global concern and has been recognized as a major public health threat by the Centers for Disease Control and Prevention (CDC), with 2.8 million antibiotic-resistant infections and >35,000 deaths occurring annually in the United States. In health care, the most urgent threats in the United States are carbapenem-resistant *Acinetobacter, Candida auris, Clostridioides difficile*, carbapenem-resistant Enterobacteriaceae, and drug-resistant *Neisseria gonorrhoeae*.

Antimicrobial stewardship in institutions is the coordinated effort by infectious disease and pharmacy leaders to educate providers, develop treatment strategies, and enact treatment standards to drive the appropriate use of antibiotics based on the established evidence. To slow antibiotic resistance, hospitals were mandated by The Joint Commission (2017) to have an Antibiotic Stewardship Program to target pharmacists and prescribers to reduce unnecessary or incorrect antibiotic use to ultimately help prevent bacterial resistance. Literature supports that nurses, as part of the interdisciplinary team, may be best poised as gatekeepers to positively influence best practices at the bedside; thus, influencing positive outcomes. Nurses can impact AMR by questioning the need for urine cultures, ensuring proper specimen collection technique, questioning daily the need for catheters or other access devices, monitoring daily for discontinuation of antibiotic use as recommended by pharmacy, and advocating for progressing the patient from intravenous to oral antibiotics as soon as tolerated by the patient. Change is best realized with a multidisciplinary team approach using a framework including nurses who are trusted members of the care team.

EVIDENCE BASE American Nurses Association & Centers for Disease Control and Prevention. (2017). *White Paper: Redefining the antibiotic stewardship team: Recommendations from the American Nurses Association/Centers for Disease Control and Prevention workgroup on the role of registered nurses in hospital antibiotic stewardship practices.* American Nurses Association. www.cdc.gov/antibiotic-use/healthcare/pdfs/ana-cdc-whitepaper.pdf

SELECTED READINGS

Association for Professionals in Infection Control and Epidemiology. (2016). *Break the chain of infection: Infection prevention and you.* Retrieved December 4, 2023, from https://infectionpreventionandyou.org/protect-your-patients/break-the-chain-of-infection/

Agency for Healthcare Research and Quality. (2023, March). *AHRQ's Healthcare-Associated Infections Program.* Retrieved March 2023, from http://www.ahrq.gov/professionals/quality-patient-safety/hais/index.html

Baker, S., Shiner, D., Stupak, J., Cohen, V., & Stoner, A. (2022). Reduction of catheter-associated urinary tract infections: A multidisciplinary approach to driving change. *Critical Care Nursing Quarterly, 45*(4), 290–299. https://doi.org/10.1097/CNQ.0000000000000429

Blot, S., Ruppé, E., Harbarth, S., Asehnoune, K., Poulakou, G., Luyt, C. E., Rello, J., Klompas, M., Depuydt, P., Eckmann, C., Martin-Loeches, I., Povoa, P., Bouadma, L., Timsit, J. F., & Zahar, J. R. (2022). Healthcare-associated infections in adult intensive care unit patients: Changes in epidemiology, diagnosis, prevention and contributions of new technologies. *Intensive & Critical Care Nursing, 70,* 103227. https://doi.org/10.1016/j.iccn.2022.103227

Bono, M. J., Leslie, S. W., & Reygaert, W. C. (2022). Urinary tract infection. In *StatPearls* [Internet]. StatPearls Publishing.

Centers for Disease Control and Prevention. (n.d.-a). *2023 recommended immunizations for children from birth through 6 years old.* www.cdc.gov/vaccines/parents/downloads/parent-ver-sch-0-6yrs.pdf

Centers for Disease Control and Prevention. (n.d.-b). *Autism and vaccines.* www.cdc.gov/vaccinesafety/concerns/autism.html

Centers for Disease Control and Prevention. (n.d.-c). *Immunization schedules: Recommended vaccinations for children 7 to 18 years old, parent-friendly version.* www.cdc.gov/vaccines/schedules/easy-to-read/adolescent-easyread.html

Centers for Disease Control and Prevention. (n.d.-d). *Recommended vaccinations for infants and children, parent-friendly version.* Retrieved February 10, 2023, from www.cdc.gov/vaccines/schedules/easy-to-read/child-easyread.html

Centers for Disease Control and Prevention. (n.d.-e). *Show me the science—How to wash your hands.* www.cdc.gov/handwashing/show-me-the-science-handwashing.html

Centers for Disease Control and Prevention. (n.d.-f). https://www.cdc.gov/infectioncontrol/basics/transmission-based-precautions.html

Centers for Disease Control and Prevention. (n.d.-g). *The Advisory Committee on Immunization Practices (ACIP) and the childhood immunization schedule.* www.cdc.gov/vaccines/hcp/conversations/acip-recommendations.html

Centers for Disease Control and Prevention. (n.d.-h). *Vaccine information for adults: What vaccines are recommended for you.* www.cdc.gov/vaccines/adults/rec-vac/index.html

Centers for Disease Control and Prevention. (2019, November 4). *Healthcare facilities: Information about CRE.* Retrieved February 16, 2024, from https://www.cdc.gov/hai/organisms/cre/cre-facilities.html

Centers for Disease Control and Prevention. (2020, January 30). *Hand hygiene in health-care settings.* Retrieved February 16, 2024, from https://www.cdc.gov/handhygiene/providers/guideline.html

Centers for Disease Control and Prevention (2021). *Healthcare-associated infections (HAIs)—Current progress report.* www.cdc.gov/hai/data/portal/progress-report.html

Centers for Disease Control and Prevention. (2021, July 15). *Bacterial meningitis.* Retrieved April 15, 2023, from https://www.cdc.gov/meningitis/bacterial.html

Centers for Disease Control and Prevention. (2021, November 17). *Prion diseases.* Retrieved February 16, 2024 from https://www.cdc.gov/prions/

Centers for Disease Control and Prevention. (2022). *COVID-19: U.S. impact on antimicrobial resistance, special report 2022.* U.S. Department of Health and Human Services. https://www.cdc.gov/drugresistance/covid19.html

Centers for Disease Control and Prevention. (2023, June 16). *Types of fungal diseases.* Retrieved February 16, 2024, from https://www.cdc.gov/fungal/diseases/index.html

Centers for Disease Control and Prevention. (2023, November 15). *Healthcare associated infections: Data portal.* Retrieved February 16, 2024, from https://www.cdc.gov/hai/data/portal/index.html

Centers for Disease Control and Prevention. (2023, November 16). *Adult immunization schedule by age: Recommendations for ages 19 years or older, United States, 2024.* Retrieved February 16, 2024, from https://www.cdc.gov/vaccines/schedules/hcp/imz/adult.html

Clinical and Laboratory Standards Institute. *Principles and procedures for blood cultures* (2nd ed.). CLSI guideline M47. Clinical and Laboratory Standards Institute; 2022.

Cookson, W., Moffatt, M., Rapeport, G., & Quint, J. (2022). A pandemic lesson for global lung diseases: Exacerbations are preventable. *American Journal of Respiratory and Critical Care Medicine, 205*(11), 1271–1280. https://doi.org/10.1164/rccm.202110-2389CI

Cummings, R. D., Hokke, C. H., & Haslam, S. M. (2022). Parasitic infections. In A. Varki, R. D. Cummings, J. D. Esko, P. Stanley, G. W. Hart, M. Aebi, D. Mohnen, T. Kinoshita, N. H. Packer, J. H. Prestegard, R. L. Schnaar, & P. H. Seeberger (Eds.), *Essentials of glycobiology* [Internet] (4th ed.). Cold Spring Harbor Laboratory Press. https://www.ncbi.nlm.nih.gov/books/NBK579956/

Garcia, M. R., Leslie, S. W., & Wray, A. A. (2022). Sexually transmitted infections. In *StatPearls* [Internet]. StatPearls Publishing.

Johnson, S., Lavergne, V., Skinner, A. M., Gonzales-Luna, A. J., Garey, K. W., Kelly, C. P., & Wilcox, M. H. (2021). Clinical practice guideline by the Infectious Diseases Society of America (IDSA) and Society for Healthcare Epidemiology of America (SHEA): 2021 Focused update guidelines on management of Clostridioides difficile infection in adults. *Clinical Infectious Diseases, 73*(5), e1029–e1044. https://doi.org/10.1093/cid/ciab549

Klompas, M., Baker, M., & Rhee, C. (2021). What Is an aerosol-generating procedure? *JAMA Surgery, 156*(2), 113–114. https://doi.org/10.1001/jamasurg.2020.6643

Li, S., Nguyen, I. P., & Urbanczyk, K. (2020). Common infectious diseases of the central nervous system-clinical features and imaging characteristics. *Quantitative Imaging in Medicine and Surgery, 10*(12), 2227–2259. https://doi.org/10.21037/qims-20-886

Manning, M. L., Pogorzelska-Maziarz, M., Hou, C., Nikunj, V., Kraemer, M., Carter, E., & Monsees, E. (2021). *A novel framework to guide antibiotic stewardship nursing practice.* College of Nursing Faculty Papers & Presentations. Paper 112. Retrieved April 15, 2023, from https://jdc.jefferson.edu/cgi/viewcontent.cgi?article=1112&context=nursfp

Martin-Loeches, I., Blake, A., & Collins, D. (2021). Severe infections in neurocritical care. *Current Opinion in Critical Care, 27*(2), 131–138. https://doi.org/10.1097/MCC.0000000000000796

McAteer, J., Lee, J. H., Cosgrove, S. E., Dzintars, K., Fiawoo, S., Heil, E. L., Kendall, R. E., Louie, T., Malani, A. N., Nori, P., Percival, K. M., & Tamma, P. D. (2023). Defining the optimal duration of therapy for hospitalized patients with complicated urinary tract infections and associated bacteremia. *Clinical Infectious Diseases, 76*(9), 1604–1612. https://doi.org/10.1093/cid/ciad009

Murthy, N., Wodi, A. P., Bernstein, H., & Ault, K. A. (2022). Recommended adult immunization schedule, United States, 2022. *Annals of Internal Medicine, 175*(3). www.acpjournals.org/doi/10.7326/M22-0036

Paxton, L. (2022). *Up close: Joint Commission requirements for antimicrobial stewardship programs.* Rpharmy—Safety first blog. Published June 2, 2022, from www.rpharmy.com/blog/antimicrobial_stewardship

Samuel, L. P., Glen, T. H., Kraft, C. S., & Pritt, B. S. (2021). The need for dedicated microbiology leadership in the clinical microbiology laboratory. *Journal of Clinical Microbiology, 59,* e0154919. https://doi.org/10.1128/JCM.01549-19

Thomas, M., & Bomar, P. A. (2023, January). Upper respiratory tract infection. In *StatPearls* [Internet]. StatPearls Publishing. Updated June 27, 2022. https://www.ncbi.nlm.nih.gov/books/NBK532961/

van Huizen, P., Kuhn, L., Russo, P. L., & Connell, C. J. (2021). The nurses' role in antimicrobial stewardship: A scoping review. *International Journal of Nursing Studies, 113,* 103772. https://doi.org/10.1016/j.ijnurstu.2020.103772

Walter, C., Soni, T., Gavin, M. A., Kubes, J., & Paciullo, K. (2022). An interprofessional approach to reducing hospital-onset Clostridioides difficile infections. *American Journal of Infection Control, 50*(12), 1346–1351. https://doi.org/10.1016/j.ajic.2022.02.017

World Health Organization. (2020, December 9). *The top 10 causes of death.* https://www.who.int/news-room/fact-sheets/detail/the-top-10-causes-of-death

World Health Organization. (2021). *Key facts and figures.* https://www.who.int/campaigns/world-hand-hygiene-day/2021/key-facts-and-figures

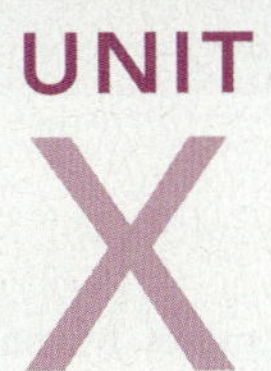

UNIT X

MUSCULOSKELETAL HEALTH

28 Musculoskeletal Disorders*

OVERVIEW AND ASSESSMENT

Subjective Data

Much can be learned about musculoskeletal disorders from subjective data. History of injury, description of symptoms, and associated personal health and family history can give clues to the underlying problem and appropriate care for that problem.

Common Manifestations of Musculoskeletal Problems

Pain

1. Where is the pain located?
   a. Joints, as in osteoarthritis (OA).
   b. Muscles or soft tissue, as in contusions, sprains, or strains.
   c. Bone, as in fractures or tumors.
2. Is it sharp, as in a fracture or sprain, or dull, as in a bone tumor?
3. Does the pain radiate?
   a. To buttocks or legs, as in lower back pain.
   b. To thigh or knee, as in hip fracture, or arm, as in shoulder injury.
4. What makes the pain increase? What makes it better?
5. When was the onset of pain?

Limited Range of Motion

1. Is stiffness present? How long does it last?
   a. Present in the morning for less than 30 minutes or after sitting for long period when due to OA.
   b. May persist and is associated with acute pain when due to spasm of lower back strain.
2. Is swelling present and limiting mobility?
   a. May be due to fracture.
   b. May be soft tissue injury, such as sprain, strain, or contusion.
3. How does limited mobility affect activities of daily living (ADLs)?

Associated Symptoms

1. Any sensory or motor deficits, such as numbness, paresthesias, or weakness, indicating neurovascular compromise?
2. Any weight loss, fever, or malaise, as in bone tumors?
3. Any bony nodules or deformity, as in rheumatoid arthritis (RA)?

History

Mechanism of Injury

1. How did the injury occur? Essential for all trauma, including fractures, contusions, sprains, and strains, to help identify the extent of injury.
2. What was the progression of symptoms?

*Please note that the term "male" in this chapter refers to a person assigned male at birth, and the term "female" in this chapter refers to a person assigned female at birth.

3. If not an acute injury, was there any repetitive movement or strain that may have contributed to problem, as in tendinitis?

Medical History

1. What medications are you taking (include name, dosage schedule, and last time taken—include prescription medications, vitamins, over-the-counter [OTC] medications, and dietary supplements)?
2. Any history of corticosteroid use that predisposes to osteoporosis?
3. Is the patient postmenopausal? On estrogen replacement? If estrogen deficient, may predispose to osteoporosis.
4. Any history of prostate, breast, or lung cancer, which may metastasize to the bone?
5. What are other conditions that may affect immobility imposed by casting, traction, or surgery?
6. Any chronic illnesses such as diabetes that may affect healing?

Social History

1. What are the patient's occupation and specific job activities, which may contribute to lower back strain or OA?
2. Does the patient exercise? What type of exercise is performed, how frequently, and what is the duration of exercise? When was the last time this was performed?
3. What activities or sports does the patient participate in, such as running or tennis, which may cause repetitive injury?
4. Are there risk factors for osteoporosis, such as smoking, inactivity, low calcium intake, or lack of exposure to the sun?
5. Is there a family history of osteoporosis or arthritis?
6. What cultural issues/religious beliefs contribute to this history?
7. Does the patient drink alcohol? If yes, what is the daily alcohol consumption?

Objective Data

Data on current condition and functional abilities are secured through inspection, palpation, and measurement. Always compare with contralateral side (one side of the body to the other).

Musculoskeletal System

Skeletal Component

1. Note deviation from normal structure—bony deformities, length discrepancies, alignment, symmetry, or amputations.
2. Identify abnormal motion and crepitus (grating sensation), as found with fractures.

Joint Component

1. Identify swelling that may be due to inflammation or effusion.
2. Note deformity associated with contractures or dislocations.
3. Evaluate stability, which may be altered.
4. Estimate active and passive range of motion (ROM).

Muscle Component

1. Inspect for size and contour of muscles.
2. Assess coordination of movement.
3. Palpate for muscle tone.
4. Estimate strength through resistance testing using scaled criteria (i.e., 0 = no palpable contraction; 5 = normal ROM against gravity with full resistance).
5. Measure girth to note increases due to swelling or bleeding into muscle or decreases due to atrophy (difference of more than 1 cm is significant).
6. Identify abnormal clonus (rhythmic contraction and relaxation) or fasciculation (contraction of isolated muscle fibers).

Additional Assessment

Neurovascular Component

1. Assess circulatory status of involved extremities by noting skin color and temperature, peripheral pulses, capillary refill response, pain, and edema.
2. Assess neurologic status of involved extremities by the patient's ability to move distal muscles and description of sensation (e.g., paresthesia).
3. Test reflexes of extremities.
4. Compare all to uninjured/unaffected extremity.

Skin Component

1. Inspect traumatic injuries (e.g., cuts, bruises).
2. Assess chronic conditions (e.g., dermatitis, stasis ulcers, scars overlying joints).
3. Note hair distribution and nail condition.
4. Inspect for Heberden or Bouchard nodes.
5. Assess for warmth or coolness of skin.

CLINICAL JUDGMENT The subjective and objective data will help to differentiate acute from chronic processes. Signs and symptoms of infection, neurovascular compromise, and fracture require immediate diagnostic testing.

Radiologic and Imaging Studies

Many radiologic and imaging studies are helpful in evaluating musculoskeletal problems to rule out fracture or skeletal changes and to differentiate soft tissue injury.

DRUG ALERT Many radiologic studies include injection or oral contrast. Check the patient's allergies and make sure a recent creatinine level has been obtained. To prevent contrast-induced nephropathy, make sure that elevated creatinine or reduced estimated glomerular filtration (eGFR) is reported to the radiology department. Ensure that nephrotoxic drugs and metformin are held according to facility protocol (usually if eGFR is less than 30 mL/min, for 24 hours before the procedure and for 48 hours following). The patient should be well hydrated before and after the procedure.

X-rays

1. Of bone—to determine bone density, texture, integrity, erosion, changes in bone relationships.
2. Of cortex—to detect any widening, narrowing, irregularity.
3. Of medullary cavity—to detect any alteration in density.
4. Of involved joint—to show fluid, irregularity, spur formation, narrowing, changes in joint contour.
5. Tomogram—special x-ray technique for detailed view of special plane of bone.

Nursing and Patient Care Considerations

1. Tell the patient that proper positioning is important to obtain a good x-ray, so cooperation is essential.
2. Advise the patient to remove all jewelry, clothing with zippers or snaps, change from pockets, or other items that may interfere with x-ray.
3. Medicate the patient for pain prior to x-ray, as needed.

Bone Scan

A *bone scan* consists of parenteral injection of bone-seeking radiopharmaceutical (such as gallium); concentration of isotope uptake revealed in primary skeletal disease (osteosarcoma), metastatic bone disease, inflammatory skeletal disease (osteomyelitis); fracture.

Nursing and Patient Care Considerations

1. There is usually no special preparation prior to the scan.
2. Injectable radionuclide is given several hours before the scan.
3. Reassure the patient that the procedure will not cause pain and that the scan will take 1 to 2 hours.
4. Analgesics or sedatives may be ordered for patients for whom lying immobile for any length of time is difficult.
5. Breastfeeding should be discontinued for at least 4 weeks after test to prevent radionuclide exposure to infant.
6. Inform the patient that the exposure to radioactive substances is small (dose of radiation is less than a chest x-ray) and that substances are excreted quickly by the body.

Bone Densitometry

Bone densitometry is a noninvasive study that yields an actual measurement of bone density and is diagnostic for osteoporosis (see page 117). It is most often performed on the lower spine and hips; however, simple portable screening tests that analyze the wrist or heel are also available.

Nursing and Patient Care Considerations

1. Calcium supplements should be avoided 24 hours prior to exam.
2. Dual-energy x-ray absorptiometry (DXA) scan should be avoided for 10 to 14 days if the patient recently had a barium examination or has been injected with a contrast material for a computed tomography (CT) scan or radioisotope scan.
3. Have the patient remove clothing and all jewelry or other metal objects.
4. Advise the patient to lie still with hips flexed for 10 to 30 minutes; during test; technician will remain in the room.
5. Reassure the patient that radiation exposure is minimal.

Magnetic Resonance Imaging

Magnetic resonance imaging (MRI) uses magnetic fields to demonstrate differences in hydrogen density of various tissues. Demonstrates tumors and soft tissue (muscle, ligament, tendon) abnormalities. Although it is costlier than CT scans, the cost is typically validated through the diagnostic accuracy. MRI not only clearly defines internal organs but is also able to detect nerve damage and changes, such as edema or bruises, of bone. Bone bruises (osseous contusions) with traumatic injuries have some predictive value for future development of posttraumatic arthritis.

Nursing and Patient Care Considerations

1. Prepare the patient for the need to lie still for about 1 hour; repetitive clanging noise of machine will be heard; patients may feel closed in.
2. Practice relaxation techniques, such as relaxation breathing and imagery, ahead of time.
3. Some patients may need sedation; patients who are claustrophobic may be unable to undergo procedure or may need open MRI.
4. May be contraindicated for patients with some types of metal implants and devices. Notify the technologist or radiologist of any surgical implants, medical devices, or hardware for evaluation prior to MRI.
   a. In general, metal objects used in orthopedic surgery pose no risk during MRI. However, a recently placed artificial joint may require the use of another imaging procedure. If there is any question of their presence, an x-ray may be taken to detect the presence of and identify any metal objects.
   b. Patients who might have metal objects in certain parts of their bodies may also require an x-ray prior to an MRI. Notify the technologist or radiologist of any shrapnel, bullets, or other pieces of metal that may be present because of accidents.
   c. Dyes used in tattoos may contain iron and could heat up during MRI, but this is rarely a problem.
   d. Tooth fillings and braces are usually not affected by the magnetic field, but they may distort images of the facial area or brain, so the radiologist should be aware of them.
   e. Parental caregivers who accompany children into the scanning room also need to remove metal objects and notify the technologist of any medical or electronic devices they may have.

CLINICAL JUDGMENT In most cases, an MRI exam is safe for patients with metal implants, except for a few types. People with the following implants cannot be scanned and should not enter the MRI scanning area unless cleared by a radiologist:

- Internal (implanted) defibrillator or pacemaker
- Cochlear (ear) implant
- Some types of clips used on brain aneurysms
- Some types of metal coils placed within blood vessels

Other Tests

1. CT scan—narrow beam of x-ray that scans the area in successive layers to evaluate disease, bone structure, joint abnormalities, and trauma (fractures).
2. Arthrogram—injection of radiopaque substance or air into joint cavity to outline soft tissue structures (e.g., meniscus) and contour of joint.
3. Myelogram—injection of contrast medium into subarachnoid space at lumbar spine to determine level of disk herniation or site of tumor.
4. Discogram—injection of small amount of contrast medium into lumbar disk abnormalities.
5. Arthrocentesis—insertion of needle into joint and aspiration of synovial fluid for purposes of examination or injection of therapeutic medications.
6. Arthroscopy—endoscopic procedure that allows direct visualization of joint structures (synovium, articular surfaces, menisci, ligaments) through a small needle incision. May be combined with arthrography.
7. Nerve studies—to differentiate nerve root compression, muscle disease (e.g., dystrophy, myositis), peripheral neuropathies, central nervous system—anterior horn cell neuropathies, neuromuscular junction problems.
   a. Electromyography (EMG)—measures electrical potential generated by the muscle during relaxation and contraction.
   b. Nerve conduction velocities—measure the rate of potential generation along specific nerves (speed of impulse conduction).

GENERAL PROCEDURES AND TREATMENT MODALITIES

See additional online content: Procedure Guidelines 28-1 to 28-3

Crutch Walking

Crutches are artificial supports that assist patients who need aid in walking because of disease, injury, or a birth defect.

Preparation for Crutch Walking

The goals are to develop power in the shoulder girdle and upper extremities that bear the patient's weight in crutch walking and strengthen and condition the patient.

Strengthening the Muscles Needed for Ambulation

Instruct the patient as follows:

1. For quadriceps setting:
   a. Contract the quadriceps muscle while attempting to push the popliteal area against the mattress and raise the heel.
   b. Maintain the muscle contraction for a count of 5.
   c. Relax for the count of 5.
   d. Repeat this exercise 10 to 15 times hourly.
2. For gluteal setting:
   a. Contract or pinch the buttocks together for a count of 5.
   b. Relax for the count of 5.
   c. Repeat 10 to 15 times hourly.

Strengthening the Muscles of the Upper Extremities and Shoulder Girdle

Instruct the patient as follows:

1. Flex and extend arms slowly while holding traction weights; gradually increase poundage of weight and number of repetitions to increase strength and endurance.
2. Do push-ups while lying in a prone position.
3. Squeeze rubber ball—increases grasping strength.
4. Raise the head and shoulders from the bed; stretch the hands forward as far as possible.
5. Sit up on bed or chair.
   a. Raise the body from the chair by pushing hands against chair seat (or mattress).
   b. Raise the body out of the seat. Hold. Relax.

Measuring for Crutches

1. When the patient is lying down (an approximate measurement):
   a. Measure from the anterior fold of the axilla to the sole. Then add 2 in (5 cm).
   b. Alternatively, subtract 16 in (40 cm) from the patient's height.
2. When the patient is standing erect:
   a. Stand the patient against the wall with feet slightly apart and away from the wall.
   b. The crutches should be fitted with large rubber suction tips.
   c. The elbow is flexed 30 degrees with the hand resting on the grip.
   d. There should be a two-finger-width insertion between the axillary fold and the underarm piece grip. A foam rubber pad on the underarm piece will relieve pressure on the upper arm and thoracic cage.
   e. The tip of the crutch is placed 6 to 8 in (15 to 20 cm) lateral to the forefoot.

Teaching the Crutch Stance

1. Have the patient wear well-fitting shoes with firm soles.
2. Before using the crutches, have the patient stand by a chair on the unaffected leg to achieve balance.
3. Position the patient against a wall with head in a neutral position.

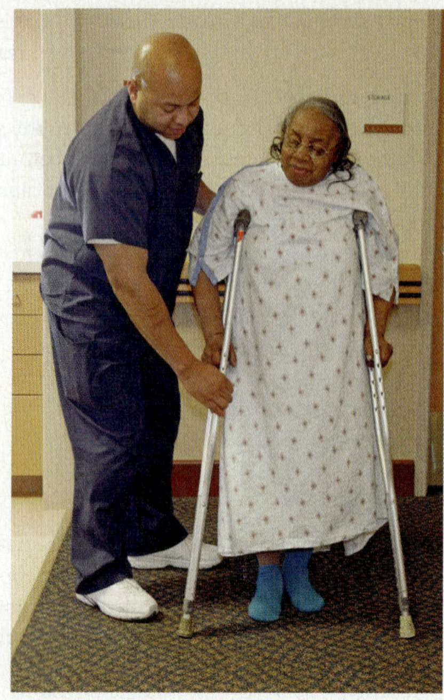

Figure 28-1. For a person walking with crutches, the tripod stance, with crutches out to the sides and in front of the toes, increases stability. (Reprinted with permission from Hinkle, J. L., Cheever, K. H., & Overbaugh, K. [2022]. *Brunner and Suddarth's textbook of medical-surgical nursing* [15th ed., Fig. 2-4]. Wolters Kluwer.)

4. Tripod position—basic crutch stance for balance and support.
   a. Crutches rest approximately 8 to 10 in (20 to 25 cm) in front of and to the side of the patient's toes (see Figure 28-1).
   b. A taller patient requires a wider base, whereas a shorter patient needs a narrower base.
5. Teach the patient to support weight on hands; weight borne on the axillae can damage the brachial plexus nerves and produce "crutch paralysis."

Teaching the Crutch Gait

1. Crutch walking requires balance, coordination, and a high expenditure of energy; these can be acquired with diligent and regular practice.
2. Practice balancing with crutches while leaning against the wall.
3. Practice shifting body weight in different positions while standing with crutches.
4. The selection of the crutch gait depends on the type and severity of the disability, weight-bearing status, and the patient's physical condition, arm and trunk strength, and body balance.
5. Teach the patient at least two gaits—a faster gait to be used for swiftness and a slower one to be used in crowded places.
6. Instruct the patient to change from one gait to another—relieves fatigue because a different combination of muscles is used.

Crutch Gaits

See Figure 28-2 and Patient Education Guidelines 28-1.

Four-Point Gait (Four-Point Alternate Crutch Gait)

1. Four-point gait is a slow but stable gait; the patient's weight is constantly being shifted.

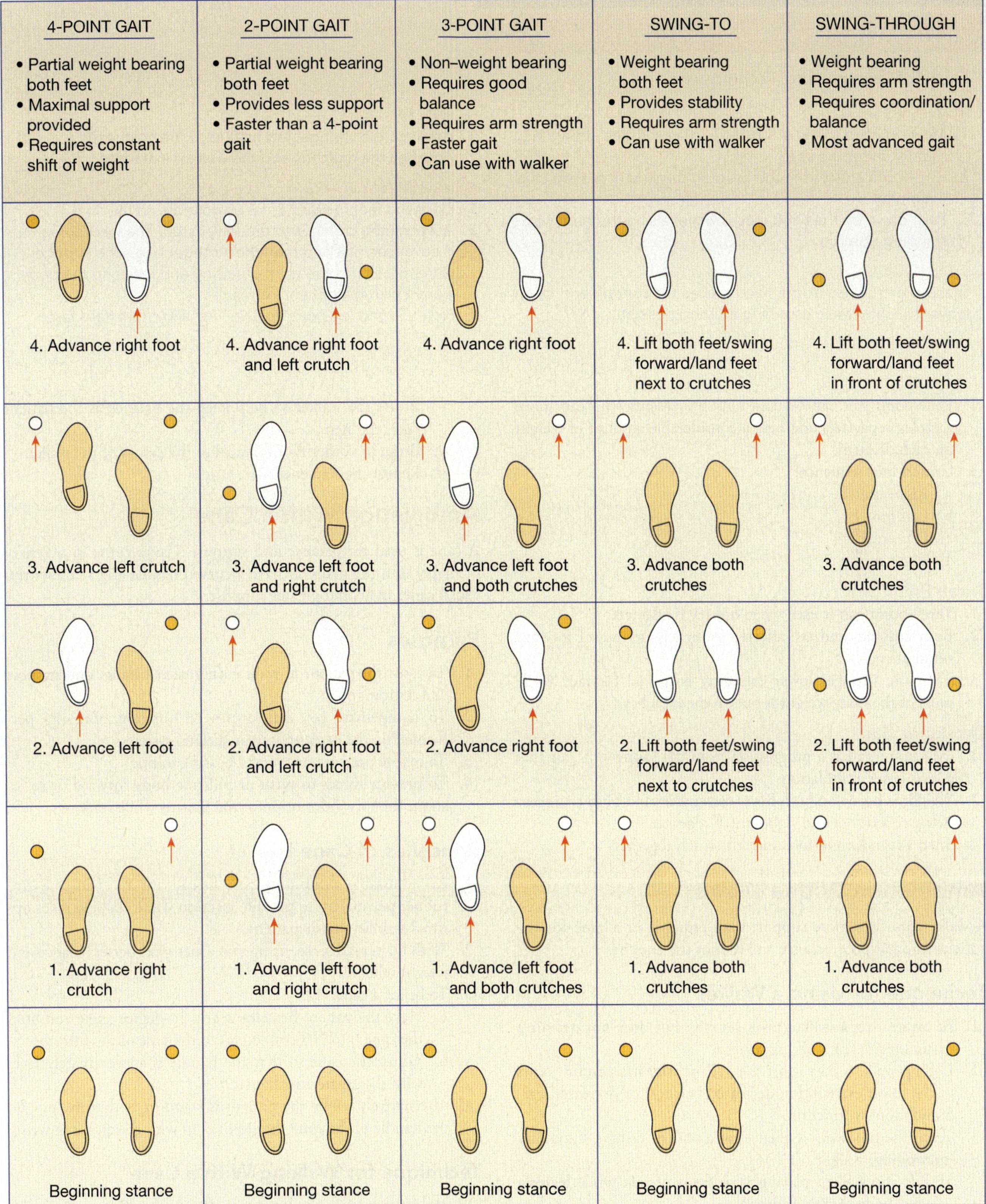

Figure 28-2. Crutch gaits. Shaded areas are weight bearing. Arrow indicates advance of foot or crutch. (Read chart from bottom, starting with beginning stance.) (Reprinted with permission from Hinkle, J. L., Cheever, K. H., & Overbaugh, K. [2022]. *Brunner and Suddarth's textbook of medical-surgical nursing* [15th ed., image in Chart 2-5]. Wolters Kluwer.)

PATIENT EDUCATION GUIDELINES 28-1

Crutch-Maneuvering Techniques

STANDING UP

1. Move forward to the edge of the chair with the strong leg slightly under the seat.
2. Place both crutches in the hand on the side of the affected extremity.
3. Push down on the hand pieces while raising the body to a standing position.

SITTING IN A CHAIR

Grasp the crutches at the hand pieces for control, and bend forward slightly while assuming a sitting position.

GOING UPSTAIRS

1. Advance the stronger leg first up to the next step.
2. Advance the crutches and the weaker extremity.

GOING DOWNSTAIRS

1. Place the feet forward as far as possible on the step.
2. Advance the crutches to the lower step. The weaker leg is advanced first and then the stronger one—the stronger extremity shares the work of raising and lowering the body weight with the patient's arms.

Note: Strong leg goes upstairs first and downstairs last.

2. Four-point gait can be used only by patients who can move each leg separately and bear a considerable amount of weight on each of them.
3. Crutch-foot sequence:
   a. Right crutch.
   b. Left foot.
   c. Left crutch.
   d. Right foot.

Three-Point Gait

1. Three-point gait is used when one leg is affected.
2. Both crutches and the affected lower leg are moved forward simultaneously.
3. Then the stronger lower extremity is moved forward while most of the body weight is put on the crutches.

Two-Point Gait

1. Two-point gait is a progression from the four-point gait that allows faster ambulation.
2. Weight is borne on both lower extremities and both crutches.
3. Advance left foot and right crutch together.
4. Then advance right foot and left crutch together.

Ambulation With a Walker

A walker provides more support than crutches or a cane for the patient who has poor balance and cannot use crutches.

Technique for Using a Walker

1. Be aware that a walker gives stability but does not permit a natural reciprocal walking pattern.
2. Rolling walkers may assist the patient who has painful joints in the lower extremities, decreased balance, or decreased cardiopulmonary function.
3. Teach the following sequence for a patient using a stationary (nonrolling) walker:
   a. Lift the walker, placing it in front of you while leaning your body slightly forward.
   b. Take a step or two into the walker.
   c. Lift the walker and place it in front of you again.
4. Teach the following sequence for a patient using a rolling walker:
   a. Roll the walker and move it forward about 12 in.
   b. If the patient has an injured leg, a new joint, or a weaker side, step forward with that foot first. Instruct the patient to use the walker to help keep the balance as the patient takes the step.
   c. Bring the other foot forward to the center of the walker.
   d. Repeat the sequence.

Ambulation With a Cane

A cane is used for balance and support. Canes come in a variety of shapes, but the majority have a curved handle and a rubber tip. Quad canes may offer greater support.

Purposes

1. To assist the patient to walk with greater balance and support and less fatigue.
2. To compensate for deficiencies of function normally performed by the neuromuscular skeletal system.
3. To relieve pressure on weight-bearing joints.
4. To provide forces to push or pull the body forward or to restrain the forward motion of the patient while walking.

Principles of Cane Use

1. An adjustable aluminum cane fitted with a 1.5-in (3.8-cm) rubber suction tip to provide traction while walking gives optimal stability to the patient.
2. With bilateral disease, using two canes gives better balance and weight relief.
3. To fit for a cane:
   a. Have the patient flex elbow at a 30-degree angle and hold the cane 6 in (15 cm) lateral to the base of the fifth toe.
   b. Adjust the cane so that the handle is approximately level with the greater trochanter.
4. Alternatively, while the patient is standing with arms at side, the handle of the cane should line up with the crease in wrist.

Technique for Walking With a Cane

1. Hold the cane in the hand opposite to the affected extremity (i.e., the cane should be used on the good side)—allows partial weight-bearing relief because the cane is in contact with the floor at the same time as the affected extremity.
2. Advance the cane at the same time that the affected leg is moved forward.
3. Keep the cane fairly close to the body to prevent leaning.

4. If the patient cannot use the cane in the opposite hand, the cane may be carried on the same side and advanced when the affected leg is advanced.
5. To go up and down stairs:
   a. Step up on the unaffected extremity.
   b. Then place the cane and affected extremity on the step.
   c. Reverse this procedure for the descending steps.
   d. The strong leg goes up first and comes down last.
6. When using a quad cane, ensure that all four tips are touching the ground.

Casts

A *cast* is an immobilizing device made up of layers of plaster or fiberglass (water-activated polyurethane resin) bandages molded to the body part that it encases.

Purposes

1. To immobilize and hold bone fragments in reduction.
2. To apply uniform compression of soft tissues.
3. To permit early mobilization.
4. To correct and prevent deformities.
5. To support and stabilize weak joints.

Types of Casts

1. Short arm cast—extends from below the elbow to the proximal palmar crease.
2. Gauntlet cast—extends from below the elbow to the proximal palmar crease, including the thumb (thumb spica).
3. Long arm cast—extends from upper level of axillary fold to proximal palmar crease; elbow usually immobilized at right angle.
4. Short leg cast—extends from below knee to base of toes.
5. Long leg cast—extends from upper thigh to the base of toes; foot is at right angle in a neutral position.
6. Body cast—encircles the trunk stabilizing the spine.
7. Spica cast—incorporates the trunk and extremity.
   a. Shoulder spica cast—a body jacket that encloses trunk, shoulder, and elbow.
   b. Hip spica cast—encloses trunk and a lower extremity.
      i. Single hip spica—extends from nipple line to include pelvis and extends to include pelvis and one thigh.
      ii. Double hip spica—extends from nipple line or upper abdomen to include pelvis and extends to include both thighs and lower legs.
      iii. One-and-a-half hip spica—extends from upper abdomen, includes one entire leg and extends to the knee of the other.
8. Cast brace—external support about a fracture that is constructed with hinges to permit early motion of joints, early mobilization, and independence.
   a. Cast bracing is based on the concept that some weight bearing is physiologic and will promote the formation of bone and contain fluid within a tight compartment that compresses soft tissues, providing a distribution of forces across the fracture site.
   b. Cast brace is applied after initial edema and pain have subsided and there is evidence of fracture stability.
9. Cylinder cast—can be used for upper or lower extremity. Used for fracture or dislocation of knee (lower extremity) or elbow dislocation (upper extremity).

Complications Associated With Casts

1. Pressure of cast on neurovascular and bony structures causes necrosis, pressure injuries, and nerve palsies.
2. Compartment syndrome is a condition resulting from increased progressive pressure within a confined space, thus compromising the circulation and the function of tissues within that space. This is a medical emergency and can be limb threatening. A tight cast, trauma, fracture, prolonged compression of an extremity, bleeding, and edema put patients at risk for compartment syndrome.
3. Immobility and confinement in a cast, particularly a body cast, can result in multisystem problems.
   a. Nausea, vomiting, and abdominal distention associated with cast syndrome (superior mesenteric artery syndrome, resulting in diminished blood flow to the bowel), adynamic ileus, and possible intestinal obstruction.
   b. Acute anxiety reaction symptoms (i.e., behavioral changes and autonomic responses—increased respiratory and heart rate, elevated blood pressure [BP], diaphoresis) associated with confinement in a space.
   c. Thrombophlebitis and possible pulmonary emboli associated with immobility and ineffective circulation (e.g., venous stasis).
   d. Respiratory atelectasis and pneumonia associated with ineffective respiratory effort.
   e. Urinary tract infection—renal and bladder calculi associated with urinary stasis, low fluid intake, and calcium excretion associated with immobility.
   f. Anorexia and constipation associated with decreased activity.
   g. Psychological reaction (e.g., depression) associated with immobility, dependence, and loss of control.

Nursing Assessment

1. Assess neurovascular status of the extremity with a cast for signs of compromise.
   a. Pain (pain out of proportion to injury is an indication of compartment syndrome).
   b. Swelling.
   c. Discoloration—pale or blue.
   d. Cool skin distal to injury.
   e. Tingling or numbness (paresthesia).
   f. Pain on passive extension (muscle stretch).
   g. Slow capillary refill; diminished or absent pulse.
   h. Paralysis.
2. Assess skin integrity of casted extremity. Be alert for the following:
   a. Severe initial pain over bony prominences; this is a warning symptom of an impending pressure injury. Pain increases when ulceration occurs.
   b. Odor.
   c. Drainage on the cast.
3. Carefully assess for positioning and potential pressure sites of the casted extremity (see Figure 28-3).
   a. Lower extremity—heel, malleoli, dorsum of foot, head of fibula, anterior surface of patella.
   b. Upper extremity—medial epicondyle of humerus, ulnar styloid.
   c. Plaster jackets or body spica casts—sacrum, anterior and superior iliac spines, vertebral borders of scapulae.

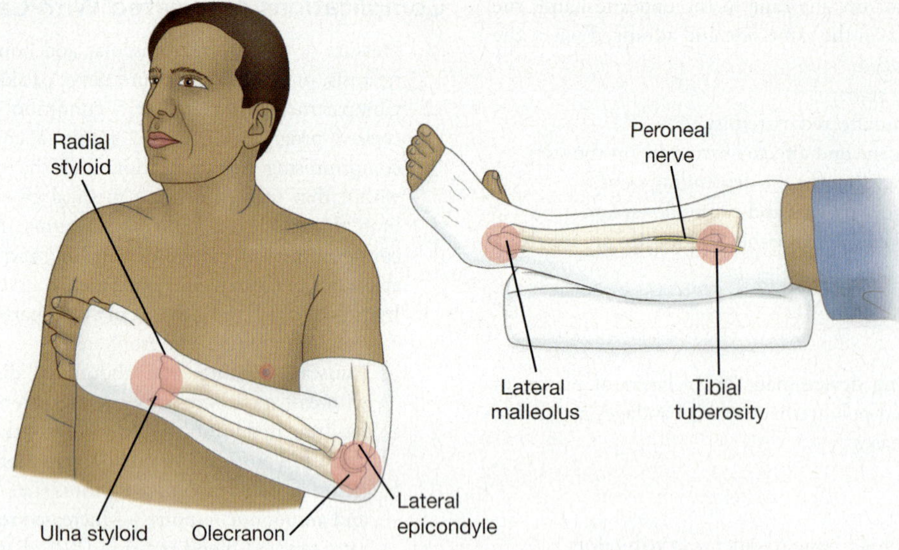

Figure 28-3. Pressure areas in common types of casts. Left, long arm cast. Right, long leg cast. (Reprinted with permission from Hinkle, J. L., Cheever, K. H., & Overbaugh, K. [2022]. *Brunner and Suddarth's textbook of medical-surgical nursing* [15th ed., Fig. 37-8]. Wolters Kluwer.)

4. Assess cardiovascular, respiratory, and gastrointestinal (GI) systems for possible complications of immobility.
5. Assess psychological reaction to illness, cast, and immobility.

CLINICAL JUDGMENT Signs and symptoms of compartment syndrome include pain, paresthesia, pallor, pulselessness, poikilothermia, and paralysis. Pain is the first sign and is usually described as deep, constant, poorly localized, and out of proportion to the injury. The pain is not relieved by analgesia and worsens with stretching of the muscle group. The other signs occur late in the course of compartment syndrome. Unrelenting pain and other signs of compartment syndrome should be reported immediately. The cast may have to be split and removed.

Nursing Interventions

Maintaining Adequate Tissue Perfusion

1. Elevate the extremity on a cloth-covered pillow above the level of the heart. Keep the heel off the mattress.
2. Avoid resting the cast on hard surfaces or sharp edges that can cause denting or flattening of the cast and consequent pressure sores.
3. Handle moist cast with palms of hands.
4. Turn the patient every 2 hours while cast dries, and feel cast for abnormal warm areas when dry.
5. Instruct the patient not to place objects into the cast. Advise the patient of alternative methods of managing itching such as blowing cool air under the cast.
6. Assess neurovascular status hourly during the first 24 hours and then less frequently as condition warrants and swelling resolves.
7. If symptoms of neurovascular compromise occur:
   a. Notify the health care provider immediately.
   b. Bivalve the cast—split cast on each side over its full length into two halves.
   c. Cut the underlying padding—blood-soaked padding may shrink and cause constriction of circulation.
   d. Spread cast sufficiently to relieve constriction.
8. If symptoms of pressure area occur, cast may be "windowed" (hole cut in it) so the skin at the pain point can be examined and treated. The window must be replaced so the tissue does not swell and cause additional pressure problems at window edge.

Minimizing the Effects of Immobility

1. Encourage the patient to move about as normally as possible.
2. Encourage adherence with prescribed exercises to avoid muscle atrophy and loss of strength.
   a. Active range of motion (ROM) for every joint that is not immobilized at regular and frequent intervals.
   b. Isometric exercises for the muscles of the casted extremity. Instruct the patient to alternately contract and relax muscles without moving affected part.
3. Reposition and turn the patient frequently.
4. Avoid pressure behind knees, which reduces venous return and predisposes to thromboembolism.
5. Use antiembolism stockings and sequential compression devices (SCDs), on unaffected limb, as indicated.
6. Administer prophylactic anticoagulants, as prescribed.
7. Encourage deep-breathing exercises and coughing at regular intervals to prevent atelectasis and pneumonia.
8. Encourage the patient to drink liberal quantities of fluid to avoid urinary infection and calculi secondary to immobility.
9. Facilitate patient participation in care planning and activities. Encourage verbalization of feelings and concerns regarding restriction of activities.
10. Provide and encourage diversional activities.
11. Pay special attention to positioning and turning for patients in spica or body cast (see Box 28-1).

CLINICAL JUDGMENT People at high risk for pulmonary emboli include older adults and persons with previous thromboembolism, obesity, heart failure, or multiple trauma. These patients require prophylaxis against thromboembolism.

BOX 28-1 Specific Care for the Patient in Spica or Body Cast

Positioning

1. Place a bed board under the mattress for uniform support of the body.
2. Support the curves of the cast with cloth-covered flexible pillows—prevents cracking and flat spots while cast is drying.
   a. Place three pillows crosswise on bed for body cast.
   b. Place one pillow crosswise at the waist and two pillows lengthwise for affected leg for spica cast. If both legs are involved, use two additional pillows.
3. Encourage the patient to maintain physiologic position by the following:
   a. Using the overhead trapeze.
   b. Placing good foot flat on bed and pushing down while lifting self up on the trapeze.
   c. Avoiding twisting motions.
   d. Avoiding positions that produce pressure on groin, back, chest, and abdomen.

Turning

1. Move the patient to the side of the bed using a steady, even pulling motion.
2. Place pillows along the other side of the bed—one for the chest and two (lengthwise) for the legs.
3. Instruct the patient to place the arms at the side or above the head.
4. Turn the patient as a unit. Avoid twisting the patient in the cast.
5. Turn the patient toward the leg not encased in plaster or toward the unoperated side if both legs are in plaster.
   a. One nurse stands at other side of bed to receive the patient's shoulders.
   b. Second nurse supports leg in plaster, while the third nurse supports the patient's back as they are turned.
   c. Turn the patient in body cast to a prone position twice daily—provides postural drainage of bronchial tree; relieves pressure on back.
6. Keep the cast level by elevating the lumbar sacral area with a small pillow when the head of the bed is elevated.

CLINICAL JUDGMENT Do not grasp crossbar of spica cast to move the patient. The purpose of the bar is to maintain the integrity of the cast.

Other Care

1. Protect cast from soiling.
   a. Cover perineum with a towel. Tuck 4-in (10-cm) strips of thin polyethylene sheeting under perineal area of cast, and tape to cast exterior. Replace when soiling occurs.
   b. Clean outside of soiled cast with a mild powdered cleanser and a *slightly* dampened or dry, clean cloth and pat dry completely, only when necessary.
2. Roll the patient onto fracture bedpan; use small pillow in lumbosacral area for support.
3. Inspect skin for signs of irritation around cast edge, under cast using a flashlight for illumination.
4. Reach up under the cast and massage accessible skin.
5. Protect the toes from the pressure of the bedding.

Preventing Gastrointestinal Impairment

1. Encourage balanced nutritional intake.
   a. Assess the patient's food preferences. Serve small meals.
   b. Provide natural bowel stimulants (e.g., fiber) and good fluid intake.
   c. Monitor bowel movements, bowel sounds, and use a bowel program, if necessary.
2. Observe for symptoms of cast syndrome—nausea, vomiting, abdominal distention, abdominal pain, and decreased bowel sounds.
3. If symptoms of cast syndrome develop, report immediately to the health care provider.
   a. Place the patient in a prone position, if tolerated, to relieve pressure symptoms.
   b. Use nasogastric suction as prescribed.
   c. Maintain electrolyte balance by intravenous (IV) replacement of fluids, as prescribed.
   d. Prepare the patient for removal of the cast or surgical relief of duodenal obstruction, if necessary.

CLINICAL JUDGMENT Cast syndrome (superior mesenteric artery syndrome) is a rare sequela of body cast application, yet it is a potentially fatal complication. It is important to teach patients about this syndrome because this can develop as late as several weeks after cast application.

Patient Education and Health Maintenance

Neurovascular Status

1. Instruct the patient to check neurovascular status and to control swelling.
   a. Watch for signs and symptoms of circulatory disturbance, including blueness or paleness of fingernails or toenails accompanied by pain and tightness, numbness, cold or tingling sensation.
   b. Elevate the affected extremity and wiggle fingers or toes.
   c. Apply ice bags, as prescribed (one third to one half full), to each side of the cast, making sure they do not make indentations in plaster.
   d. Call the health care provider promptly if excessive swelling, paresthesia, persistent pain, pain on passive stretch, or paralysis occurs.
2. Instruct the patient to alternate ambulation with periods of elevation to the cast when seated. Encourage the patient to lie down several times daily with cast elevated.

Skin Irritation

Advise the patient to prevent skin irritation at the cast edge by padding the edges of the cast with moleskin or "petaling" cast edges with strips of tape.

Exercise

1. Instruct the patient to actively exercise every joint that is not immobilized and to perform isometric exercises (contract muscles without moving joint) of those immobilized to maintain muscle strength and to prevent atrophy.
2. Tell the patient to perform hourly when awake:
   a. Leg cast—push down on the popliteal space, hold it, relax, repeat. Move toes back and forth; bend toes down and then pull them back.
   b. Arm cast—make a fist, hold it, relax, repeat. Move shoulders.
3. Encourage ambulation with weight-bearing restrictions.

Cast Care

1. Advise to avoid getting cast wet, especially padding under cast—causes skin breakdown as plaster cast becomes soft.
2. Warn against covering a leg cast with plastic or rubber boots because this causes condensation and wetting of the cast.
3. Instruct to avoid weight bearing or stress on plaster cast for 24 hours.
4. Instruct to report to the health care provider if the cast cracks or breaks; instruct the patient not to try to fix it.
5. Teach how to clean the cast:
   a. Remove surface soil with slightly damp cloth.
   b. Rub soiled areas with mild powder cleanser and slightly dampened cloth, and then pat dry completely.
   c. Wipe off residual moisture.

Teaching Safety Measures

To prevent falls, avoid walking on wet floors or sidewalks. To prevent pressure and injury to the skin, do not place objects inside the cast.

After Cast Removal

1. Instruct to clean skin with mild soap and water, blot dry, and apply emollient lotion to dry skin.
2. Warn against scratching the skin.
3. Advise to continue prescribed exercises. Gradually resume activities and elevate extremity to control swelling.

Evaluation: Expected Outcomes

- No pain, discoloration, or sensory or motor impairment of affected extremity; warm, with good capillary refill.
- Ambulates with assistance; performing active ROM and isometric exercises every 1 to 2 hours.
- No signs of cast syndrome.

Traction

Traction is the force applied in a specific direction. To apply the force needed to overcome the natural force or pull of muscle groups, a system of ropes, pulleys, and weights is used.

Purposes of Traction

1. To reduce and immobilize fracture.
2. To regain normal length and alignment of an injured extremity.
3. To lessen or eliminate muscle spasm.
4. To prevent deformity.
5. To give the patient freedom for "in-bed" activities.
6. To reduce pain.

Types of Traction

Running Traction

1. A form of traction in which the pull is exerted in one plane.
2. May use either skin or skeletal traction.
3. Buck extension traction (see Figure 28-4) is an example of running skin traction.

Balanced Suspension Traction

1. Uses additional weights to counterbalance the traction force and float the extremity in the traction apparatus.
2. The line of pull on the extremity remains fairly constant despite changes in the patient's position.

Application of Traction

Traction may be applied to the skin or to the skeletal system.

Skin Traction

1. Accomplished by applying a light force that pulls on tape, sponge rubber, or special device (boot, cervical halter, pelvic belt) that is in contact with the skin.
2. The pulling force is transmitted to the musculoskeletal structures.
3. Skin traction is used as a temporary measure in adults to control muscle spasm and pain.
4. It is used before surgery in the treatment of hip fracture (Buck extension) and femoral shaft fractures (Russell traction).
5. It may be used definitively to treat fractures in children.

Skeletal Traction

See Figure 28-5.

1. Traction applied by the orthopedic surgeon under aseptic conditions using wires, pins, or tongs placed through bones and provides a strong, steady, continuous pull.
2. Skeletal traction is used most frequently in treating fractures of the femur, humerus (supracondylar fractures), tibia, and cervical spine.

Complications

1. Infection of pin tracts in skeletal traction.
2. Skin breakdown and dermatitis under skin traction.
3. Neurovascular compromise resulting in increased pain, muscle spasms, numbness, tingling, and loss of sensation.

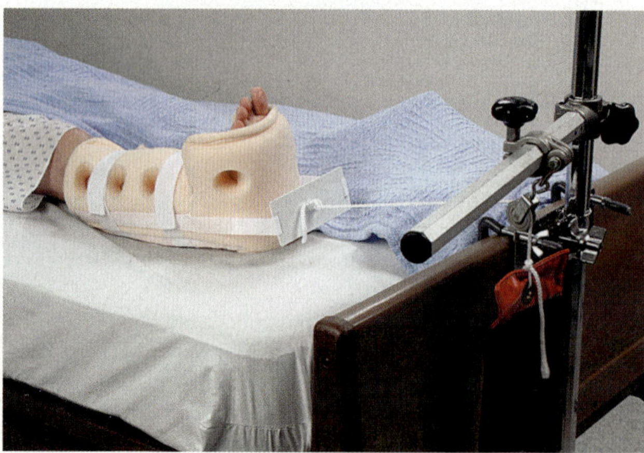

Figure 28-4. Buck extension traction. Lower extremity in unilateral Buck extension traction is aligned in a foam boot and traction applied by the free-hanging weight. The Heelift Traction Boot is shown here. (Photo courtesy of DM Systems, Inc.)

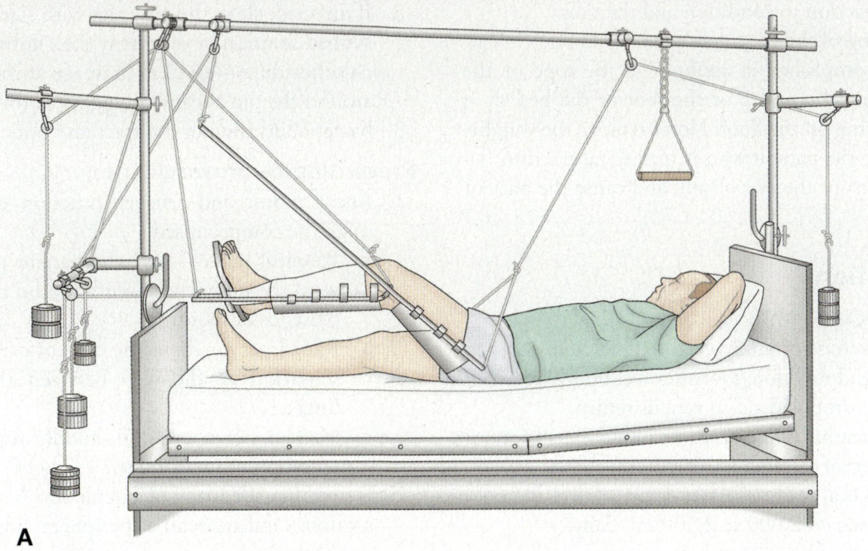

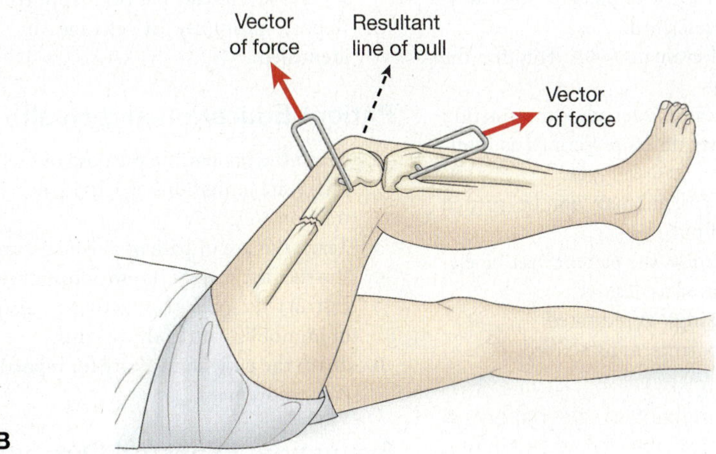

Figure 28-5. **(A)** Balanced suspension skeletal traction with Thomas leg splint. The patient can move vertically as long as the resultant line of pull is maintained. Note the use of overhead trapeze. **(B)** Traction may be applied in different directions to achieve the desired therapeutic line of pull. Adjustments in applied forces may be prescribed over the course of treatment. (Reprinted with permission from Hinkle, J. L., Cheever, K. H., & Overbaugh, K. (2022). *Brunner and Suddarth's textbook of medical-surgical nursing* [15th ed., Figs. 37-12, 37-10]. Wolters Kluwer.)

4. Inadequate fracture alignment resulting in posttreatment arthritis.
5. Complications of immobility include the following:
   a. Stasis pneumonia.
   b. Thrombophlebitis.
   c. Pressure ulcers.
   d. Urinary infection and calculi.
   e. Constipation.

Nursing Assessment

1. Assess for pain, deformity, swelling, motor and sensory function, and circulatory status of the affected extremity.
2. Assess skin condition of the affected extremity, under skin traction and around skeletal traction, as well as over bony prominences throughout the body.
3. Assess for alignment of the affected body part.
4. Assess for signs and symptoms of complications.
5. Assess traction equipment for safety and effectiveness.
   a. The patient is placed on a firm mattress.
   b. The ropes and the pulleys should be in alignment.
   c. The pull should be in line with the long axis of the bone.
   d. Any factor that might reduce the pull or alter its direction must be eliminated.
      i. Weights should hang freely.
      ii. Ropes should be unobstructed and not in contact with the bed or equipment.
      iii. The patient's bed should have an overhead trapeze set up to assist the patient to pull self up in bed at frequent intervals.
   e. The amount of weight applied in skin traction must not exceed the tolerance of the skin. The condition of the skin must be inspected frequently.
   f. Cover exposed sharp ends of skeletal pins with cork or other pin covering to protect the patient and caregivers from injury.

6. Assess emotional reaction to condition and traction.
7. Assess understanding of the treatment plan.
8. Traction is *not* accomplished if the knot in the rope or the footplate is touching the pulley or the foot of the bed or if the weights are resting on the floor. Never remove the weights when repositioning the patient who is in skeletal traction because this will interrupt the line of pull and cause the patient considerable pain.

Nursing Interventions

Minimizing the Effects of Immobility

1. Encourage active exercise of uninvolved muscles and joints to maintain strength and function. Dorsiflex feet hourly to avoid development of footdrop and aid in venous return.
2. Encourage deep breathing hourly to facilitate expansion of lungs and movement of respiratory secretions.
3. Auscultate lung fields at least twice per day.
4. Encourage fluid intake of 2,000 to 2,500 mL daily.
5. Provide balanced high-fiber diet rich in protein; avoid excessive calcium intake.
6. Establish bowel routine through the use of diet and stool softeners, laxatives, and enemas, as prescribed.
7. Prevent pressure on the calf and evaluate twice daily for the development of thrombophlebitis.
8. Check traction apparatus at repeated intervals—the traction must be continuous to be effective, unless prescribed as intermittent, as with pelvic traction.
   a. With running *traction*, the patient may not be turned without disrupting the line of pull.
   b. With *balanced* suspension *traction*, the patient may be elevated, turned slightly, and moved as desired.
9. Use SCDs and compression stockings, as indicated.
10. Administer prophylactic anticoagulants, as prescribed.

CLINICAL JUDGMENT Every complaint of the patient in traction should be investigated immediately to prevent injury.

Maintaining Skin Integrity

1. Examine bony prominences frequently for evidence of pressure or friction irritation.
2. Observe for skin irritation around the traction bandage.
3. Observe for pressure at traction–skin contact points.
4. Report complaint of burning sensation under traction.
5. Relieve pressure without disrupting traction effectiveness.
   a. Make sure that linens and clothing are wrinkle free.
   b. Use lambs' wool pads, heel and elbow protectors, and special mattresses, as needed.
6. Special care must be given to the back every 2 hours because the patient maintains a supine position.
   a. Have the patient use trapeze to pull self up and relieve back pressure.
   b. Provide backrubs.

Avoiding Infection at Pin Site

1. Monitor vital signs for fever or tachycardia.
2. Watch for signs of infection, especially around the pin tract.
   a. The pin should be immobile in the bone, and the skin surrounding the wound should be dry. Small amount of serous oozing from pin site may occur.
   b. If infection is suspected, percuss gently over the tibia; this may elicit pain if infection is developing.
   c. Assess for other signs of infection: heat, redness, fever.
3. If directed, clean the pin tract with sterile applicators and prescribed solution or ointment (i.e., normal saline, sterile water, chlorhexidine)—to clear drainage at the entrance of tract and around the pin because plugging at this site can predispose to bacterial invasion of the tract and bone.

Preventing Neurovascular Injury

1. Assess motor and sensory function of specific nerves that might be compromised.
   a. Peroneal nerve—have the patient point the great toe toward the nose; check sensation on the dorsum of the foot; presence of footdrop.
   b. Radial nerve—have the patient extend the thumb; check sensation in the web between the thumb and index finger.
   c. Median nerve—thumb–middle finger apposition; check sensation of index finger.
2. Determine adequacy of circulation (e.g., color, temperature, motion, capillary refill of peripheral fingers or toes).
   a. With Buck traction, inspect the foot for circulatory difficulties within a few minutes and then periodically after the elastic bandage has been applied.
3. Report promptly if change in neurovascular status is identified.

Patient Education and Health Maintenance

1. Teach the patient the purpose of traction therapy.
2. Delineate limitations of activity necessary to maintain effective traction.
3. Teach the use of patient aids (e.g., trapeze).
4. Instruct the patient not to adjust or modify traction apparatus.
5. Instruct the patient in activities designed to minimize effects of immobility on body systems.
6. Teach the patient necessity for reporting changes in sensations, pain, movement.

Evaluation: Expected Outcomes

- Exercises as instructed; deep breaths hourly; fluid intake 2,000 to 2,500 mL/24 hours.
- No signs of skin breakdown under traction bandage or over bony prominences.
- No drainage, redness, or odor at pin site.
- No motor or sensory impairment; good capillary refill, color, and warmth of extremity.

External Fixation

External fixation is a technique of fracture immobilization in which a series of transfixing pins is inserted through bone and attached to a rigid external metal frame (see Figure 28-6). The method is used mainly in the management of open fractures with severe soft tissue damage.

Advantages

1. Permits rigid support of severely comminuted open fractures, infected nonunions, and infected unstable joints.
2. Facilitates wound care (frequent debridements, irrigations, dressing changes) and soft tissue reconstruction (delayed wound closure, muscle flaps, skin grafts).
3. Allows early function of muscles and joints.
4. Allows early patient comfort.

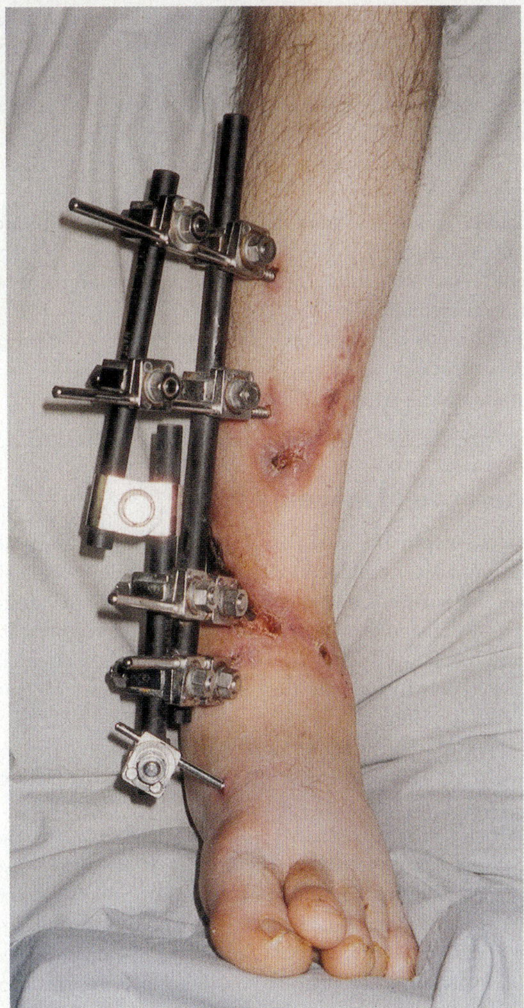

Figure 28-6. External fixation device. Pins are inserted into bone. The fracture is reduced and aligned and then stabilized by attaching the pins to a rigid portable frame. The device facilitates treatment of soft tissue damaged in complex fractures. (Reprinted with permission from Hinkle, J. L., Cheever, K. H., & Overbaugh, K. [2022]. *Brunner and Suddarth's textbook of medical-surgical nursing* [15th ed., Fig. 37-9]. Wolters Kluwer.)

Circular Fixators

Purpose

May be used for limb lengthening, correction of angulation and rotation defects, and in treatment of nonunion.

Components

1. This fixator apparatus consists of through-the-bone tension wires placed above and below the treatment site.
2. The wires are attached to fixator rings surrounding the limb.
3. The rings are connected to one another by telescoping rods.

Management

1. Adjustments are made daily at about 1 mm/day, stimulating callus and bone formation.
2. Patient adherence is essential.
3. Weight bearing is encouraged.
4. When the desired length or correction is achieved, the fixator is left in place without further adjustment until bone healing occurs.

Application of External Fixator

1. Under general anesthesia, the skin is cleaned, and transfixing pins are inserted into the bone through small incisions above and below the fracture.
2. After reduction of the fracture, the appliance is stabilized by adjusting and tightening the bars connecting the sets of pins.
3. The sharp pinheads are covered with plastic, cork, or rubber covers to protect the other extremity and caregivers.

Nursing Assessment

1. Determine the patient's understanding of procedure and fixation device.
2. Evaluate neurovascular status of involved body part.
3. Inspect each pin site for redness, drainage, tenderness, pain, and loosening of the pin.
4. Inspect open wounds for healing, infection, or devitalized tissue.
5. Assess functioning of other body systems affected by injury or immobilization.

Nursing Interventions

Relieving Anxiety

1. If possible, before placement of the device, reassure the patient that, although the fixator appears clumsy and cumbersome, it should not hurt once it is in place.
2. Emphasize the positive aspects of this device in treating complex musculoskeletal problems.
3. Encourage the patient to verbalize reaction to the device.
4. Inform the patient that greater mobility can be achieved with an external fixation device, thereby minimizing the development of other system problems.
5. Involve the patient in care and in the management of external fixator.

Maintaining Intact Neurovascular Status

1. Assess neurovascular status frequently—every 15 minutes to 1 hour while swelling is significant and later, every 2 to 8 hours.
2. Establish baseline of functioning for comparative monitoring. Complex musculoskeletal injuries frequently result in disruption of soft tissue functioning.
3. Elevate extremity to reduce swelling.
4. Report any abnormal findings or change in neurovascular status.

Preventing Infection

1. Provide site and fixator care.
   a. Clean pin sites and remove crusts with sterile cotton applicator, using solution as prescribed, or established standard of care.
      i. Crusts formed by serous drainage can prevent fluid from draining and can cause infection.
      ii. A small amount of serous drainage from the pin sites is normal.
   b. Note and report inflammation, swelling, tenderness, and purulent drainage at pin site.
   c. Note skin tension at pin site—tension can cause discomfort.
   d. Report loosened pins.
   e. Clean fixator with clean cloth and water, as needed.
2. Provide wound care.
   a. The open wounds at the fracture site are usually treated by daily dressing changes.
   b. Use sterile technique.
   c. Note wound appearance. Monitor healing. Report signs of infection.
3. Monitor for local and systemic indicators of infection.

Encouraging Mobility

1. Encourage the patient to participate in care activities.
2. Assure the patient that pain associated with injury will diminish as tissue reactions to injury and manipulation resolve and healing progresses.
3. Inform the patient that the external fixator maintains the fracture in a stable position and that the extremity can be moved. Adjustment of the fixator is done by the health care provider. (The patient is taught how to adjust the circular fixator.)
4. To move the extremity, do not grasp the frame; rather, support the entire extremity, and assist the patient to move. Reassure the patient that the fixator can withstand normal movement.
5. Teach quadriceps exercises and ROM exercises for joints; usually started on first postoperative day.
6. Teach crutch walking when soft tissue swelling has diminished; encourage weight bearing, as prescribed.

Patient Education and Health Maintenance

1. Instruct the patient to inspect around each pin site daily for signs of infection and loosening of pins. Watch for pain, soft tissue swelling, and drainage.
2. Teach the patient how to clean around each pin daily, using aseptic technique. Do not touch the wound with hands.
3. Advise the patient to clean the fixator regularly—to keep it free of dust and contamination.
4. Warn against tampering with clamps or nuts—can alter compression and misalign fracture.
5. Review weight bearing and other restrictions associated with injury and treatment regimen.
6. Encourage the patient to follow rehabilitation regimen.

Evaluation: Expected Outcomes

- Verbalizes understanding of and comfort with fixator device.
- Swelling relieved; neurovascular status intact.
- No drainage or signs of infection at pin sites; pin tracts remain intact; no loosening of pins.
- Ambulating with ambulatory device, as directed.

Orthopedic Surgery

EVIDENCE BASE National Association for Orthopaedic Nursing. (2017). *Orthopaedic surgery manual* (3rd ed.). Author.

Arkin, L. C., Lyons, M. T., McNaughton, M. A., & Quinlan-Colwell, A. (2022). Position Statement: Acute perioperative pain management among patients undergoing orthopedic surgery by the American Society for Pain Management Nursing and The National Association of Orthopaedic Nurses. *Pain Management Nursing: Official Journal of the American Society of Pain Management Nurses, 23*(3), 251–253. https://doi.org/10.1016/j.pmn.2022.01.006

Types of Surgery

1. Open reduction—reduction and alignment of the fracture through surgical incision.
2. Closed reduction—manipulation of bone fragments or joint dislocation without surgical incision.
3. Internal fixation—stabilization of the reduced fracture with the use of metal screw, plates, nails, or pins.
4. Bone graft—placement of autologous or homologous bone tissue to replace, promote healing of, or stabilize diseased bone.
5. Arthroplasty—repair of a joint through realignment or reconstruction; may be done through arthroscope (arthroscopy) or open joint repair.
6. Joint replacement—type of arthroplasty that involves replacement of joint surfaces with metal or plastic materials.
7. Total joint replacement—replacement of both articular surfaces within a joint.
8. Meniscectomy—excision of damaged meniscus (fibrocartilage) of the knee.
9. Tendon transfer—movement of tendon insertion point to improve function.
10. Fasciotomy—cutting muscle fascia to relieve constriction or contracture.
11. Amputation—removal of a body part.

Note: Joint replacement and amputation will be covered separately.

Preoperative Management

1. Hydration, protein, and caloric intake are assessed. The goal is to maximize healing and reduce risk of complications by providing IV fluids, vitamins, and nutritional supplements, as indicated.
2. Prescription and over-the-counter (OTC) medications, as well as dietary supplements are reviewed, and the patient is instructed on which medications should be held prior to surgery and for how long.
   a. Aspirin, anti-inflammatories, anticoagulants, and antiplatelet agents that may affect clotting may be held for up to a week prior to surgery.
   b. If the patient has had previous corticosteroid therapy, it could contribute to current orthopedic condition (aseptic necrosis of the femoral head, osteoporosis) as well as affect the patient's response to anesthesia and the stress of surgery. History of corticosteroid therapy must be documented.
   c. Metformin is usually held for 48 hours prior to surgery to prevent lactic acidosis due to fasting, a rare complication.
   d. Antidepressants, particularly monoamine oxidase inhibitors, and herbals should be explored for interaction with anesthetics.
3. Signs of infection (respiratory, dental, skin, urinary), which could contribute to development of osteomyelitis after surgery, are ruled out.
4. Coughing and deep breathing, frequent vital sign and wound checks, repositioning are described to prepare the patient.
5. Prepare the patient for voiding in bedpan or urinal in recumbent position before surgery, if indicated. This helps reduce the need for postoperative catheterization.
6. The patient is acquainted with traction apparatus and the need for splint or cast, as indicated by type of surgery.
7. Type and cross-match is ordered if there is a potential need for the patient to receive blood products. Autologous blood donation may be done several weeks before surgery.
8. Discharge planning is begun prior to surgery with plan for rehabilitation options postoperatively.

POPULATION AWARENESS Many older patients are at risk for poor healing due to poor nutritional status. Suggest obtaining albumin, prealbumin, and transferrin evaluation and nutrition consult in advance of surgery.

Postoperative Management

1. Neurovascular status is monitored, and swelling caused by edema and bleeding into tissues (causing a hematoma) should be assessed and controlled.

2. The affected area is immobilized and activity limited to protect the operative site and stabilize musculoskeletal structures.
3. Hemorrhage is watched for to prevent hypovolemic shock, which may result from significant blood loss.
4. Complications of immobility are prevented through aggressive and vigilant postoperative care. Deconditioning is limited through isometric and isotonic exercises.

Complications

1. Compartment syndrome.
2. Blood loss, shock, anemia.
3. Atelectasis and pneumonia.
4. Osteomyelitis, wound infections.
5. Venous thromboembolic events.
6. Fat embolus.

Nursing Interventions

Monitoring for Shock and Hemorrhage

1. Evaluate BP and pulse rates frequently—rising pulse rate, widening pulse pressure, or slowly falling BP indicate persistent bleeding or development of a state of shock.
2. Monitor for hemorrhage—orthopedic wounds tend to ooze more than do other surgical wounds.
   a. Measure suction drainage, if used.
   b. Anticipate up to 500 mL of drainage in the first 24 hours, decreasing to less than 30 mL/8 hours within 48 hours, depending on surgical procedure.
   c. Report increased wound drainage or steady increase in pain of the operative area.
3. Administer IV fluids and blood products, as ordered.

Promoting Effective Breathing Pattern

1. Give respiratory depressant drugs cautiously. Monitor respiration depth and rate frequently. Opioid analgesic effects may be cumulative.
2. Change position every 2 hours—mobilizes secretions and helps prevent bronchial obstruction.
3. Encourage the use of incentive spirometer and coughing and deep-breathing exercises every 2 hours.
4. Auscultate the lungs for atelectasis and retention of secretions.

Monitoring Peripheral Neurovascular Status

1. Monitor circulation distal to the part where cast, bandage, or splint has been applied.
2. Prevent constriction leading to interference with blood or nerve supply.
3. Elevate affected extremity and apply covered ice packs, as directed, to reduce swelling and bleeding into tissues.
4. Observe toes and fingers for healthy color and good capillary refill.
5. Check pulses of affected extremity; compare with unaffected extremity.
6. Note skin temperature and sensation.
7. Document observations.

CLINICAL JUDGMENT If neurovascular problems are identified, loosen cast or dressing at once, and notify surgeon.

Relieving Pain

1. Institute comfort measures, as prescribed, as well as nursing measures, as indicated: backrubs; soft light; soft, tranquil music.
2. Be aware that muscle spasms may contribute to discomfort.
3. Use patient-controlled analgesia according to standards of care.
4. Facilitate progression from IV medications to by mouth when tolerated.
5. Prevent constipation due to opioids by obtaining order for bowel regimen and instituting diet regimen.

Preventing Infection

1. Monitor vital signs for fever, tachycardia, or increased respiratory rate, which may indicate infection.
2. Examine incision for redness, increased temperature, swelling, and induration. Document findings.
3. Note and document character of drainage.
4. Evaluate complaints of recurrent or increasing discomfort.
5. Administer antibiotic therapy, as prescribed.
6. Maintain aseptic technique for dressing changes and wound care.

Minimizing the Effects of Immobility

1. Encourage the patient to exercise by self with a planned program of exercise as soon as possible after surgery.
2. Have the patient exercise the unaffected extremity (unless instructed by physical therapist to exercise affected extremity as well): flex knee, extend the knee with hip still flexed, and then lower the extremity to the bed. Passive motion devices may be used to maintain ROM.
3. Encourage the patient to move fingers and toes hourly.
4. Advise the patient to move joints that are not fixed by traction or appliance through their ROM as fully as possible.
5. Suggest muscle-setting exercises (quadriceps setting) if active motion is contraindicated.
6. Apply antiembolism stockings, foot pumps, or SCDs as prescribed by the surgeon.
7. Give prophylactic anticoagulants as directed (e.g., heparin, warfarin, aspirin, a low molecular weight heparin).
8. Encourage early resumption of activity.

Providing Adequate Nutrition

1. Provide a balanced diet, and increase fluids and fiber to promote healing and reduce incidence of constipation associated with immobility.
2. Encourage a high-iron diet, and administer blood products and iron supplements to counteract significant blood loss, as directed.
3. Monitor hemoglobin and hematocrit levels. Report below-normal results to the health care provider.
4. Watch for signs and symptoms of anemia, especially after fracture of long bones:
   a. Fatigue.
   b. Shortness of breath.
   c. Pallor.
   d. Tachycardia.
5. Maintain good fluid intake and urinary output to prevent infection and calculi. Watch for urinary retention—especially in older men with some degree of prostatism who may have difficulty voiding.

Patient Education and Health Maintenance

1. Teach the patient activities that will minimize the development of complications (e.g., turning, ankle pumps, antiembolism stockings, SCDs, coughing, and deep breathing, early mobilization as able).
2. Instruct the patient in dietary considerations to facilitate healing and minimize development of constipation and renal calculi.
3. Inform the patient of techniques that facilitate moving while minimizing associated discomforts (e.g., supporting injured area and practicing smooth, gentle position changes).

4. Encourage long-term follow-up and physical therapy (PT) exercises, as prescribed, to regain maximum functional potential.
5. When working with patients with musculoskeletal disorders, the main focus is the return of function to one's previous physical condition. Upon discharge from the hospital, equipment will be necessary for assistance at home, as well as the help of a caregiver to provide support and safety. Help prepare the patient and caregiver by teaching safe body mechanics and use of mobility aids. Facilitate referrals for durable medical equipment, home health nursing and therapy services, and ongoing caregiver education and support through community resources to help prevent complications and reduce the risk of readmission.

Evaluation: Expected Outcomes

- BP stable; drainage from wound less than 30 mL.
- Respirations, deep; performing effective deep breathing and coughing every 2 hours.
- Extremity beyond operative site neurovascularly intact.
- Verbalizes decreased pain.
- Afebrile; incision without drainage.
- Ambulating as directed.
- Eats a balanced diet high in iron; hemoglobin within normal range.

Arthroplasty and Total Joint Replacement

Arthroplasty is reconstructive surgery to restore joint motion and function and to relieve pain. It generally involves replacement of bony joint structure by a prosthesis. *Total joint arthroplasty* is the replacement of both articular surfaces with metal or plastic components. The most common types of joint replacement (see Figure 28-7) include the following:

Total hip arthroplasty—replacement of a severely damaged hip with an artificial joint. A large number of implants are available, often with a metal femoral component topped by a spherical ball fitted into a plastic acetabular socket. Surgical approach is anterior (muscle sparing) or posterior (involves cutting and reattachment of muscles and longer healing time).

Total knee arthroplasty—implant procedure in which tibial, femoral, and patellar joint surfaces are replaced because of destroyed knee joint.

Total shoulder arthroplasty—replacement of the humeral head and the glenoid surface with prostheses.

Clinical Indications

1. For patients with unremitting pain and irreversibly damaged joints:
   a. Primary osteoarthritis (OA).
   b. Rheumatoid arthritis (RA).
2. Selected fractures (e.g., femoral neck fracture).
3. Failure of previous reconstructive surgery (osteotomy, cup arthroplasty, femoral neck fracture complications—nonunion, avascular necrosis).
4. Congenital hip disease.
5. Pathologic fractures from metastatic cancer.
6. Joint instability.

Considerations

1. The prostheses are of various designs and may be fixed to the remaining bone by cement, press fit, or bone ingrowth.

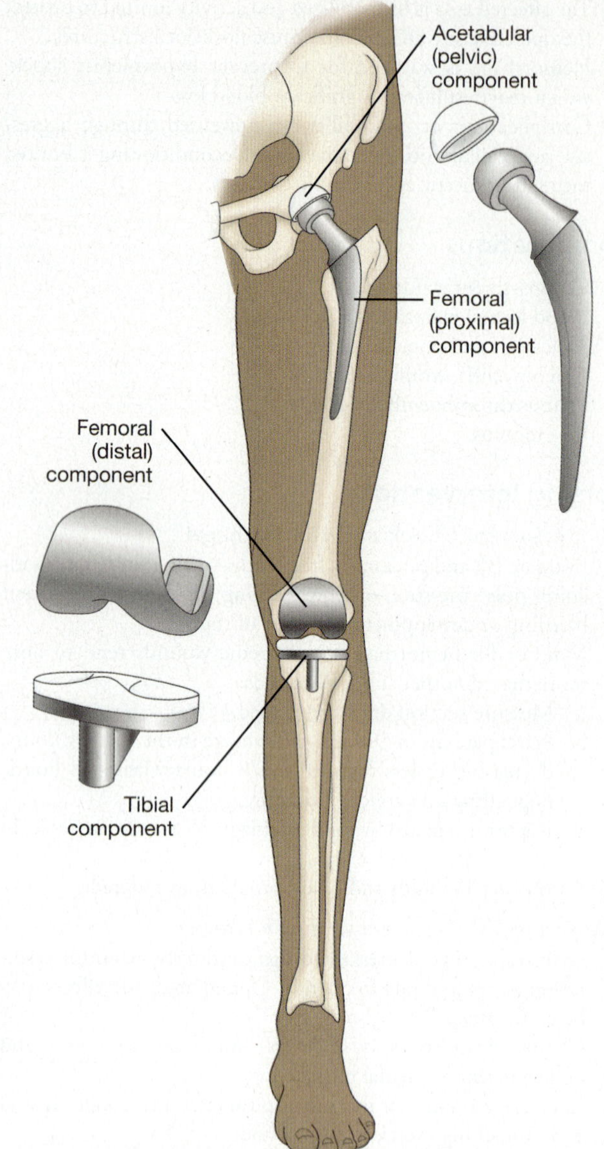

Figure 28-7. Examples of hip and knee replacement. (Reprinted with permission from Hinkle, J. L., Cheever, K. H., & Overbaugh, K. [2022]. *Brunner and Suddarth's textbook of medical-surgical nursing* [15th ed., Fig. 36-9]. Wolters Kluwer.)

2. Selection of the prosthesis and fixation technique depends on the patient's bone structure, joint stability, and other individual characteristics, including age, weight, and activity level.
3. Arthroplasty is an exacting and meticulous procedure. To reduce the risk of an infected prosthesis, special precautions are carried out in the operating room (impermeable operating room attire, clean air system) to reduce particulate matter and bacterial count of the air.

Preoperative Management

1. Infections (urinary, dental, skin, respiratory) are ruled out or treated because they are potential foci of infection for seeding prosthesis infection.
2. Preoperative patient teaching is provided.
   a. Postoperative regimen (e.g., extended exercise program) that will be carried out after surgery is explained; atrophied muscles must be reeducated and strengthened.

   b. Isometric exercises (muscle setting) of quadriceps and gluteal muscles are taught.
   c. Bed-to-wheelchair transfer without going beyond the hip flexion limits (usually 60 to 90 degrees) is taught.
   d. Non–weight- and partial weight–bearing walking with ambulatory aid (walker, crutches) is taught to facilitate postoperative ambulation.
   e. Abduction splint, knee immobilizer, or continuous passive motion is demonstrated if equipment will be used postoperatively.
3. Antiembolism stockings are applied to minimize development of thrombophlebitis.
4. Skin preparation includes antimicrobial solution to reduce skin microorganisms, a potential source of infection.
5. Antibiotics are administered timely, as prescribed, to ensure therapeutic blood level during and immediately after surgery. Antimicrobials are usually given immediately preoperatively, intraoperatively, and postoperatively to reduce incidence of infection.
6. Cardiovascular, respiratory, renal, and hepatic function are assessed, and measures are taken to maximize general health condition.
7. Discharge planning is begun, including rehabilitation options postoperatively.

Postoperative Management

Use of Appropriate Positioning

To prevent dislocation of prosthesis and facilitate healing, numerous modifications are required in positioning these patients postoperatively.

1. After hip arthroplasty (posterior approach):
   a. The patient is usually positioned supine in bed.
   b. The affected extremity is held in slight abduction by either an abduction splint or pillow or Buck extension traction to prevent dislocation of the prosthesis.
   c. Two nurses turn the patient on the unoperated side while supporting the operated hip securely in an abducted position; the entire length of leg is supported by pillows.
      i. Use pillows to keep the leg abducted; place pillow at back for comfort.
      ii. If the bed is equipped, use overhead trapeze to assist with position changes.
   d. The bed is usually not elevated more than 45 to 60 degrees; placing the patient in an upright sitting position puts a strain on the hip joint and may cause dislocation.
   e. A fracture bedpan is used. Instruct the patient to flex the unoperated hip and knee and pull up on the trapeze to lift buttocks onto pan. Instruct the patient *not* to bear down on the operated hip in flexion when getting off the pan.
2. Following anterior hip arthroplasty, the patient can flex the hip and bear weight often within hours. Restrictive positioning is not necessary to prevent dislocation.
3. After knee arthroplasty:
   a. The knee may be immobilized in extension with a firm compression dressing and an adjustable soft extension splint or long-leg plaster cast.
   b. Leg is elevated to control swelling being mindful to ensure that there is nothing causing the knee to remain bent if it is not in an immobilizer.
   c. Alternatively, continuous passive motion may be started to facilitate joint healing and restoration of joint ROM.

CLINICAL JUDGMENT The patient must not adduct the hip or flex it beyond recommended degree, as indicated by the surgeon, as this may lead to subluxation or dislocation of the hip. Signs of joint dislocation include shortened extremity, increasing discomfort, inability to move joints.

Deterring Complications

1. Aggressive care and frequent assessment can reduce the complication rate.
2. Prevent thromboembolism by continuous use of elastic hose and SCD while the patient is in bed. Discontinue SCD when the patient is ambulatory.
3. C-reactive protein and erythrocyte sedimentation rate (ESR) can be used to quantify the risk of periprosthetic joint infection. High serum levels indicate a high risk of infection and require further diagnostic testing or biopsy.

Promoting Early Ambulation

1. Ambulation may begin on the day of surgery or the first postoperative day.
2. Transfers to the chair or ambulation with aids, such as walkers, are encouraged as tolerated and based on the patient's condition and type of prosthesis.
3. Caution is taken in moving the patient to upright position, and the patient is monitored for orthostatic hypotension.

Nursing Interventions

Also see page 854.

Promoting Mobility

After posterior hip arthroplasty:

1. Use an abduction splint or pillows while assisting the patient out of bed.
   a. Keep the hip at maximum extension.
   b. Instruct the patient to pivot on unoperated extremity.
   c. Assess the patient for orthostatic hypotension.
2. When ready to ambulate, teach the patient to advance the walker, and then advance the operated extremity to the walker, permitting weight bearing, as prescribed.
3. With increased stability, assist the patient to use crutches or cane, as prescribed.
4. Encourage practice of PT exercises to strengthen muscles and prevent contractures.
5. Encourage bed mobility by providing an overhead frame/trapeze.

After knee arthroplasty:

1. Assist the patient with transfer out of bed into wheelchair with extension splint in place, if applicable.
2. Encourage weight bearing, as directed by the surgeon.
3. Apply continuous passive motion equipment or carry out passive ROM exercises, as prescribed.

Community and Home Care Considerations

1. Encourage the patient to continue to wear compression stockings after discharge until full activities are resumed.
2. Ensure that the patient avoids excessive hip adduction, flexion, and rotation for 6 weeks after hip arthroplasty (posterior hip precautions).
   a. Avoid sitting in a low chair or toilet seat to avoid flexing the hip more than 90 degrees.
   b. Keep the knees apart; do not cross the legs.

   c. Limit sitting to 30 minutes at a time—to minimize hip flexion and the risk of prosthetic dislocation and to prevent hip stiffness and flexion contracture.
   d. Avoid internal rotation of the hip.
   e. Follow weight-bearing restrictions from the surgeon.
3. Encourage quadriceps setting and ROM exercises, as directed.
   a. Have a daily program of stretching, exercise, and rest throughout lifetime.
   b. Do not participate in any activity placing undue or sudden stress on joint (jogging, jumping, lifting heavy loads, gaining weight, excessive bending and twisting).
   c. Use a cane when taking fairly long walks.
4. Suggest self-help and energy-saving devices.
   a. Handrails by toilet.
   b. Raised toilet seat if there is some residual hip flexion problem.
   c. Bar-type stool for kitchen work.
   d. Occupational therapy (OT) devices for dressing, reaching.
   e. Adequate home lighting to prevent falls.
   f. Removal of scatter rugs.
5. Advise the patient to sleep with two pillows between legs to prevent turning over in sleep. The patient should get out of bed with nonoperative leg.
6. Tell the patient to lie prone when able twice daily for 30 minutes to promote full extension of hip.
7. Monitor for late complications—deep infection, increased pain, or decreased function associated with loosening of prosthetic components, implant wear, dislocation, fracture of components, avascular necrosis or dead bone caused by loss of blood supply; heterotrophic ossification (formation of bone in periprosthetic space).
8. Assess home for safety to prevent falls—long phone cords, scatter rugs, pets that run underfoot, slippery floors.

Patient Education and Health Maintenance

1. Teach the patient use of supportive equipment, such as walkers and raised toilet seat, as prescribed.
2. Advise the patient to notify all health care providers about prosthetic joint because prophylactic antibiotic (to prevent implant infection) will be needed prior to other surgical procedures or any procedure known to cause bacteremia (tooth extraction, manipulation of genitourinary tract). Patients with inflammatory arthropathies, immunosuppressive therapies, and immunocompromising conditions are especially at risk.

EVIDENCE BASE American Association of Orthopaedic Surgeons and American Dental Association. (2012). *Prevention of orthopaedic implant infection in patients undergoing dental procedures: Evidence-based guideline and evidence report.* Author.

Coll, P. P., Lindsay, A., Meng, J., Gopalakrishna, A., Raghavendra, S., Bysani, P., & O'Brien, D. (2020). The prevention of infections in older adults: Oral health. *Journal of the American Geriatrics Society*, *68*(2), 411–416. https://doi.org/10.1111/jgs.16154

3. Avoid MRI studies because of implanted metal component.
4. Advise the patient that metal component in hip or knee may set off metal detectors (airports, some buildings). The patient should carry a medical identification card.
5. New hip or knee is designed for low-impact exercise, such as walking, golf, dancing. High-impact exercises, such as jogging, may cause the prosthesis to loosen.

Evaluation: Expected Outcomes

- Maintains proper positioning without evidence of complications.

Amputation

Amputation is the total or partial surgical removal of digits, foot, lower leg, or forearm. Amputation is considered a surgical reconstructive procedure.

Indications

1. Inadequate tissue perfusion caused by peripheral vascular diseases.
2. Severe trauma.
3. Malignant tumor.
4. Congenital deformity.
5. Osteomyelitis/infection.

Types of Amputation

Open (Guillotine)

1. Used with infection and for patients who are poor surgical risks.
2. Wound heals by granulation over time or secondary closure 1 week later.

Closed (Myoplastic or Flap)

1. Residual limb is covered by a flap of skin.
2. Flap of skin is sutured posteriorly.
3. Most common technique used for vascular disease.

Surgical Considerations

1. The surgeon considers possible limb-salvage techniques.
   a. Revascularization (research is focusing on angiogenesis and stem cell therapy).
   b. Hyperbaric oxygenation.
   c. Tumor resection with bone grafting.
2. Determines level for amputation based on level of maximal viable tissue for wound healing.
3. Develops a functional, nontender, pressure-tolerant residual limb.

Types of Dressings

Soft Dressing

1. Secured with elastic bandage.
2. Permits wound inspection.
3. Used with patients who should avoid early weight bearing (e.g., those with peripheral vascular disease).

Closed, Rigid Plaster Dressing

1. Applied immediately after surgery (i.e., immediate postoperative prosthesis).
2. Controls edema.
3. Supports circulation, promoting healing.
4. Minimizes pain on movement.
5. Shapes residual limb.
6. Permits attachment of prosthetic extension (pylon) and early ambulation.

Preoperative Management

1. Hemodynamic evaluation is performed through testing, such as angiography, arterial blood flow, and xenon 133 scan, to determine optimal amputation level.

2. Culture and sensitivity tests of draining wounds are done to assist in control of infection preoperatively.
3. Evaluation of contralateral extremity is performed to determine functional potential postoperatively.
4. Evaluation of cardiovascular, respiratory, renal, and other body systems is necessary to determine preoperative condition of the patient and reduce the risks of surgery by optimizing function.
5. Nutritional status is evaluated and optimized with adequate protein to enhance wound healing.
6. Exercises are taught to strengthen muscles for the use of ambulatory aids (lower-limb amputee).
   a. Flex and extend arms while holding traction weights.
   b. Do push-ups from a prone position, if feasible.
   c. Do sit-ups from a seated position, if feasible.
7. Use of ambulatory aids taught to maintain mobility, prepare for postoperative status, and instill confidence in ability.
8. Phantom sensation is explained—the patient will continue to "feel" the amputated body part for some time.
9. Emotional support is given.
   a. Support concept of amputation as a surgical reconstructive procedure.
   b. Explore the patient's perception of procedure and effect on lifestyle.
   c. Avoid unrealistic and misleading reassurance—management of prosthesis can be slow and painful.

POPULATION AWARENESS Amputation of the lower extremity can be a life-threatening procedure, especially in patients over age 60 with peripheral vascular disease. Significant morbidity accompanies above-knee amputations because of associated poor health and disease as well as the complications of sepsis and malnutrition and the physiologic insult of amputation.

Postoperative Management

1. The extremity should be in full extension and may be elevated, if possible. An extension splint/immobilizer may be indicated.
2. Complications are monitored—hemorrhage, infection, unrelieved phantom pain, nonhealing wound.
3. Rehabilitation is initiated through PT and prosthetic fitting, if indicated.
4. Optimal treatment is provided for diabetes mellitus, heart disease, infection, stroke, chronic obstructive pulmonary disease, peripheral vascular disease, and age-related deterioration, which are factors limiting rehabilitation.
5. If wound breakdown, infection, or delay in healing of residual limb occurs, therapy is provided to prevent delay in rehabilitation.
6. Acceptance of body image change is promoted.

Nursing Interventions

CLINICAL JUDGMENT Prevention of complications associated with a major operation and facilitation of early rehabilitation are essential to prevent prolonged disability. Frequent monitoring of the patient's physiologic responses to anesthesia, surgery, and immobility is required.

Monitoring Fluid Balance

1. Monitor the patient for systemic symptoms of excessive blood loss—hypotension, widening pulse pressure, tachycardia, diaphoresis, decreased level of consciousness.
2. Watch for excessive wound drainage.
   a. Keep tourniquet (in view) attached to end of bed to apply to residual limb (stump) if excessive bleeding occurs.
   b. Reinforce dressing, as required, using aseptic technique.
   c. Measure suction drainage.
   d. Maintain accurate record of bloody drainage on dressing and in drainage system.
3. Monitor intake and output for fluid balance.

Maintaining Adequate Tissue Perfusion

1. Control edema.
   a. Elevate residual limb to promote venous return.
   b. Use air splint, if prescribed.
2. Maintain pressure dressing.
   a. Reapply, if necessary, using sterile dressing secured with elastic bandage.
   b. Notify the surgeon if rigid cast dressing comes off.

Supporting Effective Coping

1. Accept patient responses to the loss of body part (i.e., depression, withdrawal, denial, frustration).
2. Encourage expression of fears and concerns.
3. Recognize that modification of body image takes time.
4. Encourage participation in rehabilitation planning and self-care.
5. Assist the patient to adapt to changes in self-care activities.
   a. Upper-extremity amputation—encourage independence in one-handed self-care activities using one-handed aids (e.g., one-handed knife), as needed.
   b. Lower-extremity amputation—encourage mobility using transfer assistance and ambulatory aids, as needed.

Controlling Pain

1. Surgical pain.
   a. Assess the patient's pain experience.
   b. Administer prescribed medications, as needed, to control postoperative pain.
   c. Use nonpharmaceutical pain-management techniques, such as progressive muscle relaxation and imagery.
   d. Recognize that increasing discomfort may indicate presence of hematoma, infection, or necrosis.
2. Phantom sensations (pain).
   a. Anticipate complaint of pain and sensation located in the missing limb ("phantom pain").
   b. The use of adjunctive pain medications may be prescribed, such as gabapentin.
   c. Use physical modalities (e.g., wrapping, temperature changes) and transcutaneous electrical nerve stimulation (TENS), if prescribed, in relieving discomfort.
   d. Encourage patient activity to decrease awareness of phantom limb pain.
   e. Reassure the patient that phantom limb pain will diminish over time.
   f. Patients may benefit from cognitive behavioral therapy to assist in pain management. Virtual reality–based interventions may also be effective.

Promoting Physical Activity

1. Encourage frequent repositioning in bed.
2. Teach the patient to avoid long periods in one position.
   a. Avoids dependent edema.
   b. Avoids flexion deformity.
   c. Avoids skin pressure areas.

3. Prevent deformities.
   a. Lower-extremity amputations—hip flexion contracture (avoid placing residual limb on pillow; encourage prone position twice per day) and abduction deformity (use trochanter roll; avoid pillow between legs).
   b. Upper-extremity amputations—postural abnormalities (encourage good posture).
4. Encourage active ROM and muscle-strengthening exercises when prescribed to
   a. Minimize muscle atrophy.
   b. Increase muscle strength.
   c. Prepare residual limb for prosthesis.
5. Promote reestablishment of balance (amputation alters distribution of body weight).
   a. Transfer to chair within 48 hours after surgery.
   b. Instruct and guard lower-limb amputee during balance exercises (i.e., arise from chair; stand on toes holding on to chair; bend knee holding on to chair; balance on one leg without support; hop on one foot while holding on to chair).
6. Supervise ambulation, use of wheelchair, and self-care activities.

Patient Education and Health Maintenance

1. Teach the patient and family how to wrap residual limb with elastic bandage to control edema and to form a firm conical shape for prosthesis fitting (see Figures 28-8 and 28-9).
   a. Wrapping generally begins 1 to 3 days after surgery or after hard plaster dressing is removed.
   b. Use diagonal figure-of-8 bandaging technique.
   c. Wrap distal to proximal to maintain pressure gradient and to control edema.
   d. Begin wrapping with minimal tension, and increase as wound heals and sutures are removed.
   e. Flatten skin at ends of incision to ensure conical stump shape.
   f. Rewrap residual limb a couple of times per day and as necessary to achieve a smooth, graded tension dressing.
   g. Rewrap if the patient complains of more pain—dressing is probably too tight.

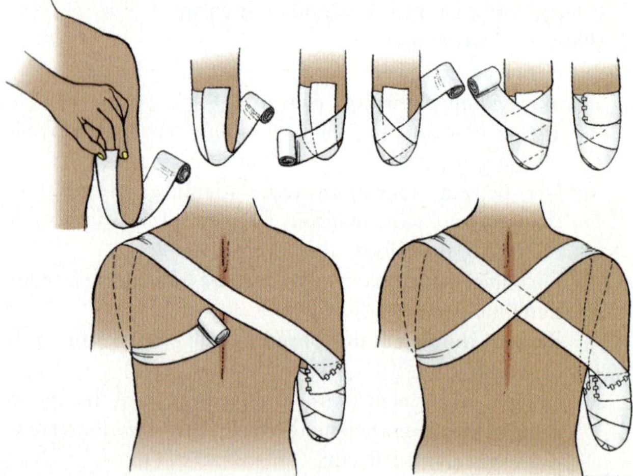

Figure 28-8. Wrapping above-elbow residual limb. Elastic bandaging reduces edema and shapes the residual limb for the prosthesis. Bandage may need to be secured by wrapping across back and shoulders. (Adapted with permission from Smeltzer, S., & Bare, B. [2000]. *Brunner and Suddarth's textbook of medical-surgical nursing* [9th ed.]. Lippincott Williams & Wilkins.)

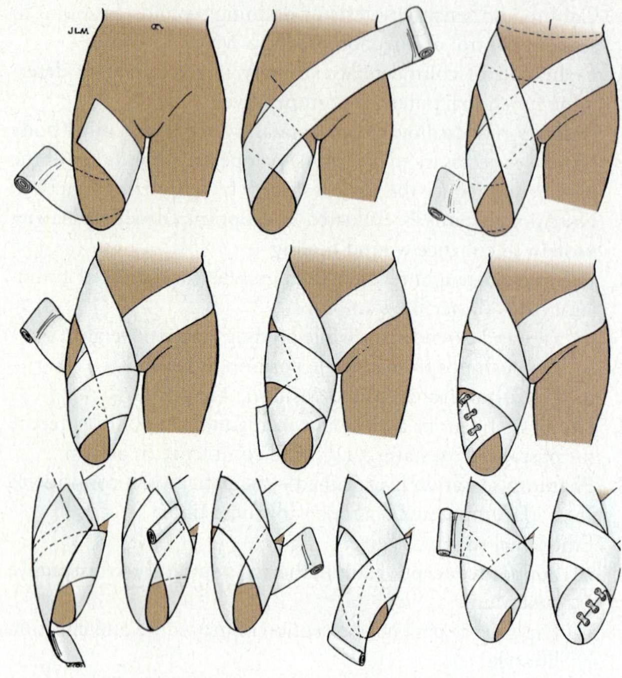

Figure 28-9. Wrapping above-knee residual limb. Elastic bandaging reduces edema and shapes the residual limb in a firm conical form for the prosthesis. (Adapted with permission Smeltzer, S., & Bare, B. [2000]. *Brunner and Suddarth's textbook of medical-surgical nursing* [9th ed.]. Lippincott Williams & Wilkins.)

   h. Keep residual limb wrapped at all times except when bathing (when the patient is cleared for bathing by provider).
2. Teach the patient residual limb conditioning.
   a. Push the residual limb against a soft pillow.
   b. Gradually push residual limb against harder surfaces.
   c. Massage healed residual limb to soften scar, decrease tenderness, and improve vascularity.
3. Fitting of prosthesis.
   a. Note residual limb contour.
   b. Assess for residual limb contraction.
   c. When maximum shrinkage occurs, the prosthetist measures and fits the prosthesis.
   d. Adjustments are made by the prosthetist to minimize skin problems.
4. Continuing care of residual limb and prosthesis.
   a. Instruct the patient to wash and dry the limb thoroughly at least twice per day, removing all soap residue, to prevent skin irritation and infection.
   b. Avoid soaking residual limb because it results in edema.
   c. Inspect residual limb and skin under prosthesis harness daily for pressure, irritation, and actual skin breakdown.
   d. Wear residual limb sock or cotton underwear—to absorb perspiration and to avoid direct contact between the prosthetic socket or harness and skin.
   e. Avoid wrinkles in residual limb sock—potential pressure areas.
   f. Wipe the socket of the prosthesis with a damp cloth when the prosthesis is removed for the evening.
   g. Have the prosthesis checked periodically.
5. Teach the patient to protect the remaining extremity from injury and to secure prompt treatment of problems.

Evaluation: Expected Outcomes

- Vital signs stable; dressing reinforced once in 4 hours.
- Pressure dressing intact; stump elevated without edema.
- Participates in care plan; expresses concerns about independence.
- Verbalizes relief of incisional pain; dull phantom sensation tolerable.
- Performs ROM actively; transfers to wheelchair with assistance; participates in PT and OT activities.

MUSCULOSKELETAL TRAUMA

See Standards of Care Guidelines 28-1.

Contusions, Strains, and Sprains

A *contusion* is an injury to the soft tissue produced by a blunt force (blow, kick, or fall). A *strain* is a microscopic tearing of the muscle caused by excessive force, stretching, or overuse. A *sprain* is an injury to ligamentous structures surrounding a joint; it is usually caused by overstretching, sudden twisting, or hyperextension of the joint, resulting in a decrease in joint stability.

Clinical Manifestations

Contusion

1. Hemorrhage into injured part (ecchymosis)—from rupture of small blood vessels; also associated with fractures.
2. Pain, swelling, and ecchymosis.
3. Hyperkalemia may be present with extensive contusions, resulting in destruction of body tissue and loss of blood.

Strain

1. Hemorrhage into the muscle.
2. Swelling.
3. Tenderness.
4. Pain with isometric contraction.
5. May be associated spasm.

Sprain

1. Rapid swelling—due to extravasation of blood within tissues.
2. Pain on passive movement of joint.
3. Increasing pain during first few hours due to continued swelling.

Management

1. X-ray may be done to rule out fracture.
2. Immobilize in splint, elastic wrap, or compression dressing to support painful structures and control swelling.
3. Apply ice while swelling is present.
4. Analgesics usually include nonsteroidal anti-inflammatory drugs (NSAIDs).
5. Severe sprains may require surgical repair or cast immobilization.
6. The acronym PRICE-M is often used to guide treatment at home for minor injuries: Protection—of the affected part from injury; Rest—to promote healing; Ice—to control swelling (do not use heat until acute swelling is relieved); Compression—with an elastic wrap or splint to control swelling and prevent stiffness, can be removed at night; Elevation—above the level of the heart to reduce swelling; Medication—analgesic and anti-inflammatories, often over the counter.

Nursing Interventions and Patient Education

1. Elevate the affected part to reduce swelling. Maintain splint or immobilization, as prescribed.
2. Apply cold compresses for the first several days (15 to 20 minutes at a time every few hours)—to produce vasoconstriction, decrease edema, and reduce discomfort (do not apply ice directly to skin). Ice may be needed for up to a week to control acute swelling.
3. Assess neurovascular status of contused extremity every 1 to 4 hours as the patient's condition indicates.
4. Instruct the patient on the use of pain medication, as prescribed.
5. Ensure the correct use of crutches or other mobility aid with or without weight bearing, as prescribed.
6. Educate on the need to rest injured part for about a month to allow for healing.
7. Teach the patient to resume activities gradually.
8. Teach the patient to avoid excessive exercise of injured part.
9. Teach the patient to avoid reinjury by "warming up" before exercise and stretching tendons and muscles before and after exercise.
10. Complementary methods, such as acupuncture, biofeedback, and imagery, may contribute to healing by reducing anxiety and pain.

Tendinitis

Tendinitis is an inflammation of a tendon caused by a lack of sufficient lubrication of the tendon sheath. May be caused by acute stress on tendon structure or by chronic overuse.

STANDARDS OF CARE GUIDELINES 28-1

Caring for a Patient With Musculoskeletal Trauma, Surgery, Casting, or Immobilization

When caring for a patient with musculoskeletal trauma, surgery, casting, or immobilization, provide the following care, as indicated:

- Check neurovascular status of involved extremities.
- Palpate for intact and equal pulses bilaterally.
- Palpate for proper warmth of the skin.
- Check for brisk capillary refill.
- Test sensation to light touch and pain.
- Observe for unusual or increased swelling.
- Ensure that the patient can move affected parts.
- Ensure proper positioning for comfort and alignment.
- Determine pressure points and take precautions to prevent pressure injuries.
- Medicate to control pain, particularly before movement, procedures, and PT.
- Provide diversional activities and emotional support during long immobilizations.
- Always document assessments and interventions meticulously, realizing that the patient may be involved in workers' compensation claim or litigation due to accident and that records will be essential to the patient's future well-being.

This information should serve as a general guideline only. Each patient situation presents a unique set of clinical factors and requires nursing judgment to guide care, which may include additional or alternative measures and approaches.

Clinical Manifestations

1. Onset of pain may occur immediately after activity or may be delayed up to a day later. Range of motion (ROM) and resistance testing is painful.
2. Mild swelling occurs, and the tendon sheath is tender to the touch.
3. Sudden onset of sharp pain in extremity and hearing or feeling a "snap" are associated with tendon rupture, as in Achilles tendinitis due to running injuries or stop–start activities such as basketball. Also occurs in gastrocnemius and biceps.

Management

1. X-rays are not usually diagnostic.
2. Thompson test helps with diagnosis of Achilles rupture. The patient kneels on a chair or lies prone. Examiner squeezes the calf of the affected leg. Normal response: foot flexes, denoting intact tendon. If the foot does not move, tendon is assumed to be ruptured.
3. Initial treatment includes protection, rest, ice, compression, elevation (PRICE).
4. Splinting or casting for up to 6 weeks in functional position is usually necessary.
5. Surgical intervention may be necessary if rupture is complete.
6. Physical therapy (PT) to regain strength and function.
7. Corticosteroid injection.
8. NSAIDs for pain and inflammation.

Nursing Interventions and Patient Education

1. Ensure understanding of the need for proper immobilization for full time period even though fracture is not present.
2. Encourage the use of warm compresses after 24 hours to relieve pain and inflammation.
3. Advise the patient not to return to full activity until strength is equal to that of unaffected extremity.
4. Teach proper warm-up before exercise and sports activities (stretching of all major tendons).

Bursitis

Bursitis is a painful inflammation of the bursae, fluid-filled sacs lined with synovium similar to the lining of the joint spaces. Bursae reduce friction between tendons and bones or tendons and ligaments. They are found over joints with bony prominences, such as the trochanter, patella, and olecranon. Friction between skin and musculoskeletal tissues may result in bursitis.

Clinical Manifestations

1. Pain around a joint—commonly the knee, elbow, shoulder, and hip.
2. Varying degrees of redness, warmth, and swelling may be visible.
3. There is point tenderness and limited ROM on examination.

Management and Nursing Interventions

1. Rest and immobilization of affected joint.
2. Ice for the first 48 hours; moist heat every 4 hours thereafter.
3. Nonopioid analgesics such as NSAIDs.
4. ROM exercises.
5. Corticosteroid injection into the area.
6. Surgery indicated when calcified deposits or adhesions have diminished function.

Plantar Fasciitis

Plantar fasciitis is inflammation of the fascia that runs along the bottom of the foot from heel to toes. As the fascia is stretched, microscopic tears develop at the point where fascia attaches to the calcaneus.

Clinical Manifestations

1. Pain along the sole of the foot, usually unilateral but may be bilateral.
2. Worse upon arising, long period of standing, and walking.
3. Tenderness of heel area.

Management and Nursing Interventions

1. Rest—decrease walking, running, exercise, standing.
2. NSAIDs for pain and inflammation.
3. Good supportive footwear.
4. Orthotic devices may be beneficial.
   a. Heel cup to cushion the heel (OTC).
   b. Arch support orthotics for pes planus (flat foot).
   c. Cushioning of arches for pes cavus (high arch).
5. Stretching exercises several times per day.
6. Massage of the bottom of the foot.
7. Steroid injection into the painful area.
8. Low-intensity extracorporeal shock wave therapy, also known as orthotripsy, may be tried when conservative management has failed.
   a. Using a handheld device, shock waves are focused directly at the painful area, causing microtraumas to the tissue causing the plantar fasciitis.
   b. An inflammatory response occurs, causing increased blood supply to the painful area, as well as breaking down injured tissue and calcifications, allowing a natural healing process.
   c. One or more 15-minute treatments take place in the office setting without anesthesia or any special preparation.
9. Surgery for the release of fascia as last resort.

Traumatic Joint Dislocation

Dislocation of a joint occurs when the surfaces of the bones forming the joint are no longer in anatomic contact. This is a medical emergency because of associated disruption of surrounding blood and nerve supplies. Shoulder, fingers, and elbow are the most commonly dislocated joints. Mechanism of injury can be anterior, posterior (most common), lateral, or medial force.

Clinical Manifestations

1. Pain.
2. Deformity.
3. Change in the length of the extremity.
4. Loss of normal movement.
5. X-ray confirmation of dislocation without associated fracture.

Management

1. Immobilize the part while the patient is transported to emergency department, x-ray department, or clinical unit.
2. Secure reduction of dislocation (bring displaced parts into normal position) as soon as possible to prevent circulatory or nerve impairments; usually performed under anesthesia.
3. Stabilize reduction until joint structures are healed to prevent permanently unstable joint or aseptic necrosis of bone.

Nursing Interventions and Patient Education

1. Assess neurovascular status of extremity before and after reduction of dislocation.
2. Administer or teach self-administration of pain medications such as NSAIDs.
3. Ensure proper use of immobilization device after reduction.
4. Review instructions for activity restrictions and need for PT and follow-up.

Knee Injuries

The knee ligaments provide stability to the knee joint. These ligaments promote rotational stability (*anterior cruciate ligament [ACL]* and *posterior cruciate ligament*) and prevent varus and valgus instability (*medial and lateral collateral ligaments*). Pieces of cartilage that stabilize the knee internally are known as the medial and lateral menisci. *ACL injuries* and *medial meniscus tears* are common because of sports injuries.

Clinical Manifestations

1. Severe stresses are applied to the knee during many sports activities (e.g., soccer, skiing, running).
2. Injury to knee structures occurs during rapid position changes involving flexing and twisting of the joint.
3. Torn cartilage (meniscus) causes pain, tenderness, joint effusion, clicking sensations, and decreased ROM.
4. Knee ligaments may be torn, resulting in pain on ambulation, swelling, and joint instability. The patellar tendon may rupture.

Management

1. Special assessment techniques are done to detect ACL injury (see Table 28-1).
2. Magnetic resonance imaging (MRI) shows injury to soft tissue involved.
3. Some injuries may be immobilized (splint, brace, or cast) and treated with PT.
4. ACL reconstruction frequently indicated.
   a. Arthroscopic surgery preferred; synthetic ligaments selected where ligaments failed. Graft rejection is a complication.
   b. Postoperative continuous passive motion used.
   c. Postoperative ACL rehabilitation program includes progressive ROM, bracing (not done with synthetic ligaments).
   d. Long-term bracing during sports controversial.
5. Meniscal injury—damaged cartilage removed.
   a. Arthroscopic or open meniscectomy.
   b. Rehabilitation includes progressive ROM and quadriceps strengthening.

Nursing Interventions and Patient Education

1. After arthroscopic surgery, ensure proper use of crutches, as indicated, and encourage pain control through medications, as prescribed, and RICE.
2. For open joint surgery, see care of the patient undergoing orthopedic surgery, page 854.
3. Teach the patient strengthening exercises for affected extremity.
4. Teach the patient to prevent fatigue through rest periods, conservation of energy.
5. Advise on prevention of injuries using proper equipment and footwear for sports.

Fractures

A *fracture* is a break in the continuity of bone. A fracture occurs when the stress placed on a bone is greater than the bone can absorb. Muscles, blood vessels, nerves, tendons, joints, and other organs may be injured when fracture occurs.

Types of Fractures

1. Complete—involves the entire cross section of the bone, usually displaced (abnormal position).
2. Incomplete—involves a portion of the cross section of the bone or may be longitudinal.
3. Closed (simple)—skin not broken.
4. Open (compound)—skin broken, leading directly to fracture.
   a. Grade I—minimal soft tissue injury.
   b. Grade II—laceration greater than 1 cm without extensive soft tissue flaps.
   c. Grade III—extensive soft tissue injury, including skin, muscle, neurovascular structure, with crushing.
5. Pathologic—through an area of diseased bone (osteoporosis, bone cyst, bone tumor, bony metastasis).

Patterns of Fracture

See Figure 28-10.

1. Greenstick—one side of the bone is broken, and the other side is bent.
2. Transverse—straight across the bone.
3. Oblique—at an angle across the bone.
4. Spiral—twists around the shaft of the bone.

Table 28-1 Assessment Techniques for Anterior Cruciate Ligament Injury

TEST	DESCRIPTION	POSITIVE FINDING
Anterior drawer test	Place the patient supine with knee in 90 degrees of flexion with foot flat on table. Proximal tibia is pulled forward by examiner using two hands.	Tibia subluxes (dislocates) forward on femur.
Lachman test	Place the patient supine with knee in 15–20 degrees of flexion. Examiner grasps distal femur with one hand and the proximal tibia with the other hand and applies forward pressure.	Tibia subluxes forward on femur.
Pivot shift test (evaluates anterolateral rotational stability)	Place the patient supine with knee slightly flexed. The examiner grasps the patient's ankle with one hand and places the palm of the other hand over the lateral aspect of the knee distal to the joint. Lower leg is extended and internally rotated, applying a valgus (lateral) stress to knee.	Tibia subluxes and reduces itself ("pivots and shifts").

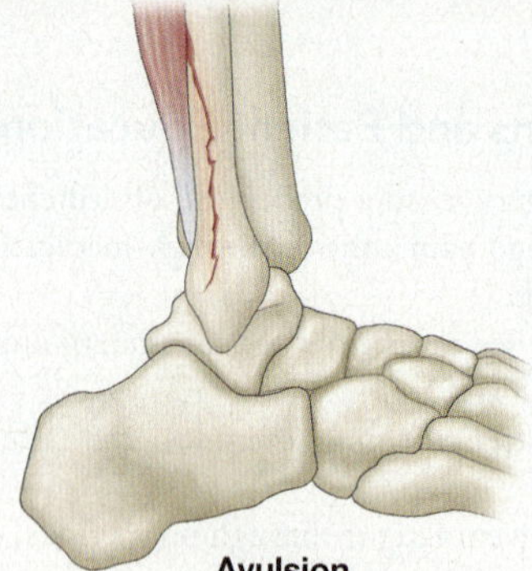

Avulsion
A fracture in which a fragment of bone has been pulled away by a tendon and its attachment

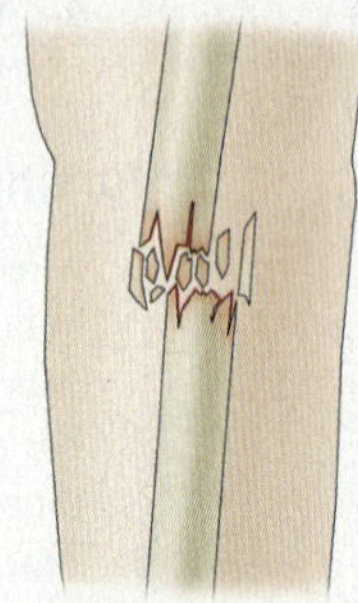

Comminuted
A fracture in which bone has splintered into several fragments

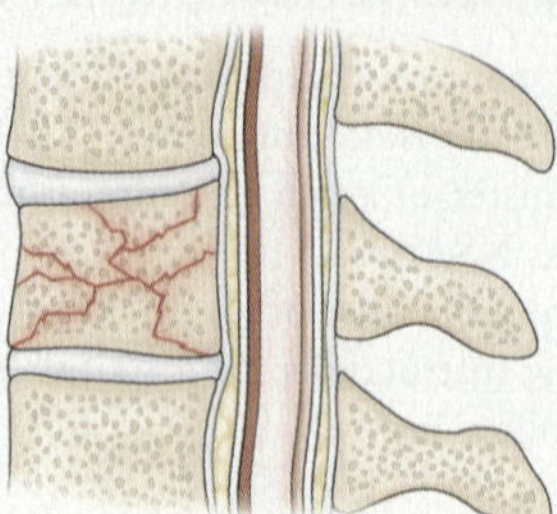

Compression
A fracture in which bone has been compressed (seen in vertebral fractures)

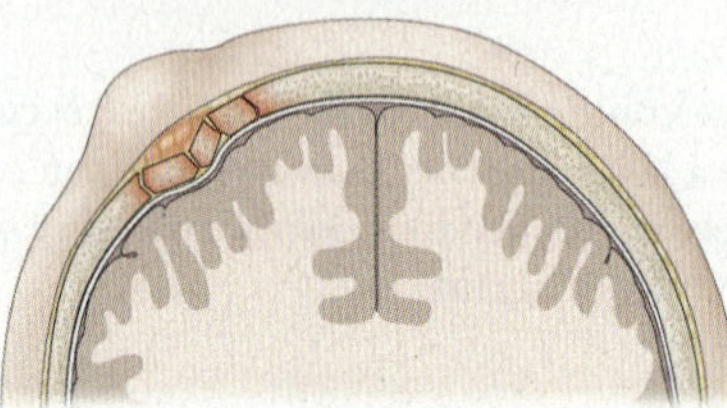

Depressed
A fracture in which fragments are driven inward (seen frequently in fractures of skull and facial bones)

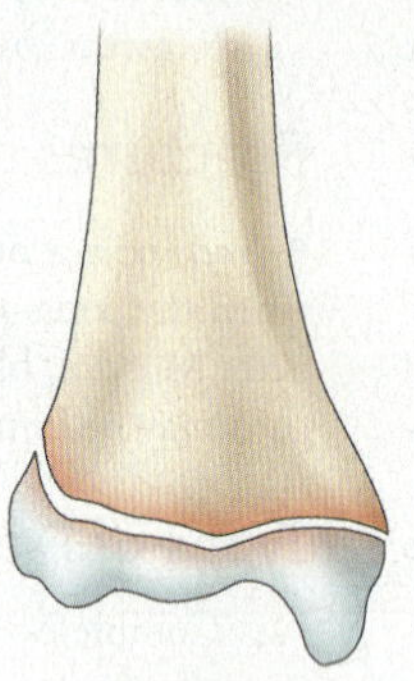

Epiphyseal
A fracture through the epiphysis

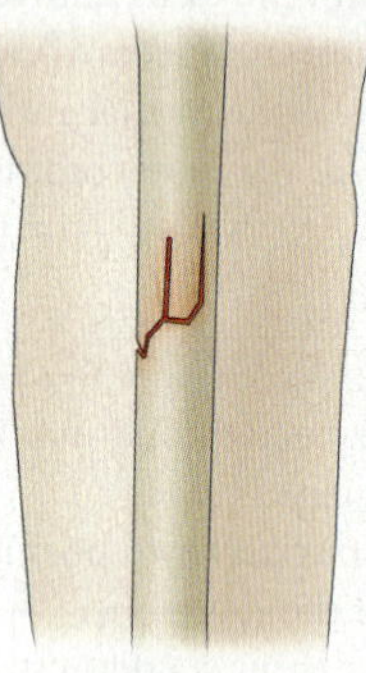

Greenstick
A fracture in which one side of a bone is broken and the other side is bent

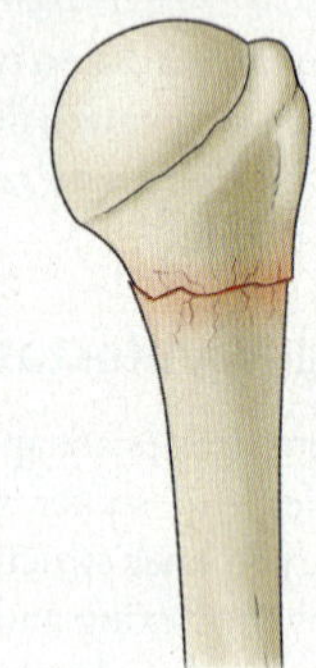

Impacted
A fracture in which a bone fragment is driven into another bone fragment

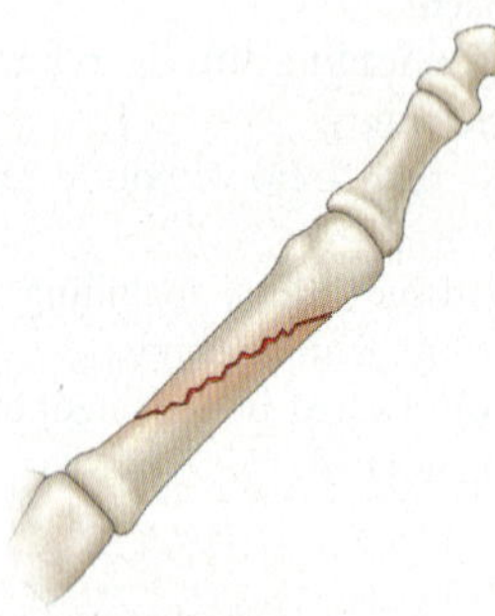

Oblique
A fracture occurring at an angle across the bone (less stable than a transverse fracture)

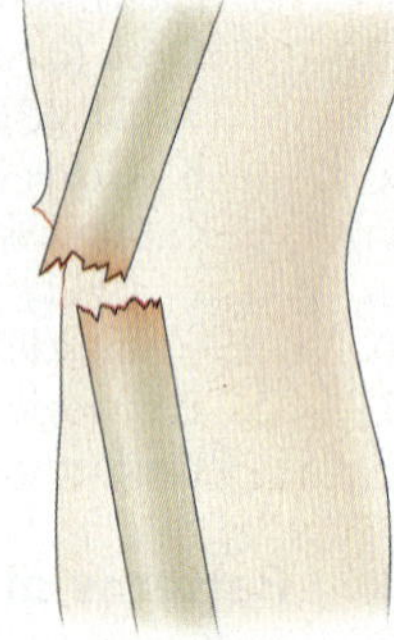

Open
A fracture in which damage also involves the skin or mucous membranes, also called a compound fracture

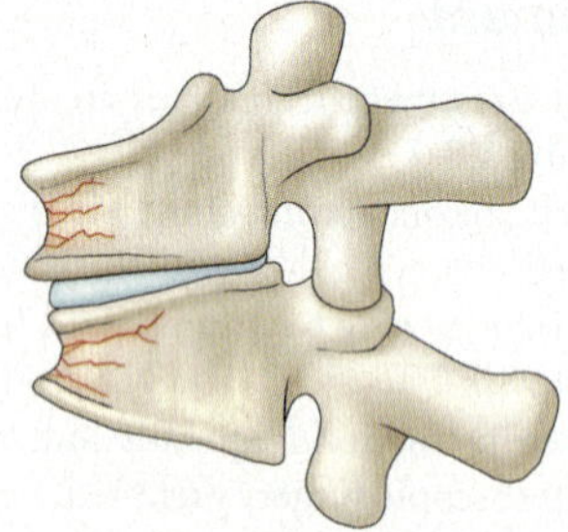

Pathologic
A fracture that occurs through an area of diseased bone (e.g., osteoporosis, bone cyst, Paget disease, bony metastasis, tumor); can occur without trauma or fall

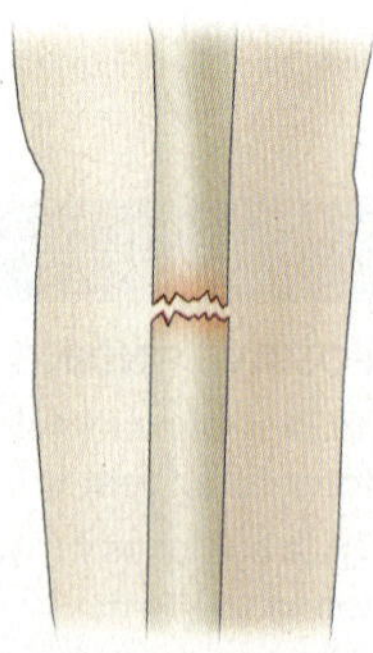

Simple
A fracture that remains contained, with no disruption of the skin integrity

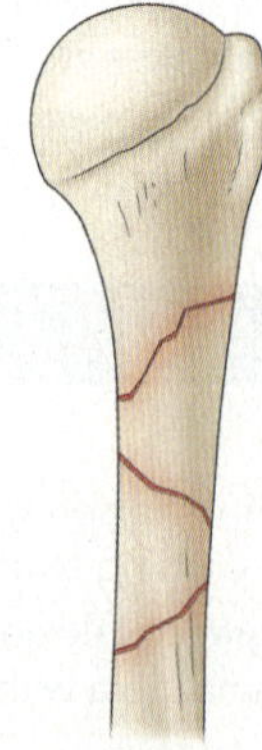

Spiral
A fracture that twists around the shaft of the bone

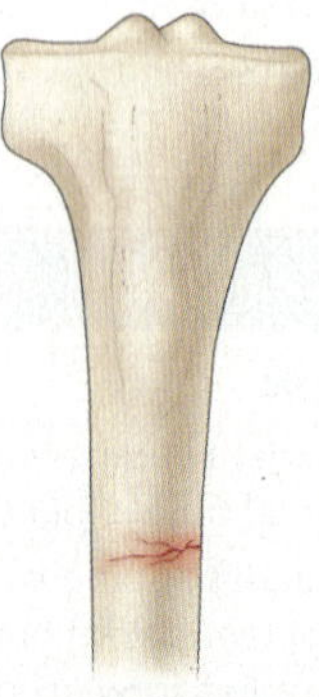

Stress
A fracture that results from repeated loading of bone and muscle

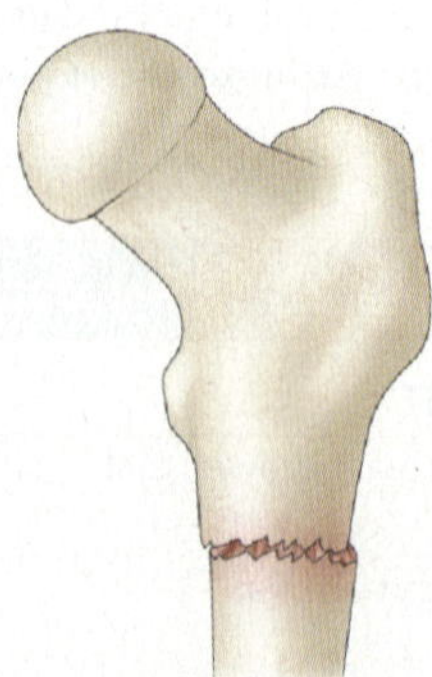

Transverse
A fracture that is straight across the bone shaft

Figure 28-10. Specific types of fractures. (Reprinted with permission from Hinkle, J. L., Cheever, K. H., & Overbaugh, K. (2022). *Brunner and Suddarth's textbook of medical-surgical nursing* [15th ed., Fig. 37-2]. Wolters Kluwer.)

5. Comminuted—bone splintered into more than three fragments.
6. Depressed—fragments are driven inward (seen in fractures of the skull and facial bones).
7. Compression—bone collapses in on itself (seen in vertebral fractures).
8. Avulsion—fragment of bone pulled off by ligament or tendon attachment.
9. Impacted—fragment of bone wedged into other bone fragment.
10. Fracture dislocation—fracture complicated by the bone being out of the joint.
11. Other—described according to anatomic location: epiphyseal (end of large bones containing growth plate), supracondylar (above the articular prominence of a bone), midshaft, intra-articular.

POPULATION AWARENESS Osteoporosis is a major risk for fractures, particularly hip and vertebral compression fractures.

Clinical Manifestations

Physical Findings

1. Pain at the site of injury.
2. Swelling.
3. Tenderness.
4. False motion and crepitus (grating sensation).
5. Deformity.
6. Loss of function.
7. Ecchymosis.
8. Paresthesia.

Altered Neurovascular Status

1. Injured muscle, blood vessels, nerves.
2. Compression of structures, resulting in ischemia.
3. Findings:
   a. Progressive uncontrollable pain.
   b. Pain on passive movement.
   c. Altered sensations (paresthesia).
   d. Loss of active motion.
   e. Diminished capillary refill response, diminished distal pulse.
   f. Pallor.

Shock

1. Bone is very vascular.
2. Overt hemorrhage through open wound.
3. Covert hemorrhage into soft tissues (especially with femoral fracture) or body cavity, as with pelvic fracture.
4. May be fatal if not detected.

Diagnostic Evaluation

1. X-ray and other imaging studies to determine integrity of bone.
2. Blood studies (complete blood count [CBC], electrolytes) with blood loss and extensive muscle damage—may show decreased hemoglobin level and hematocrit.
3. Arthroscopy to detect joint involvement.
4. Angiography if associated with blood vessel injury.
5. Nerve conduction and electromyogram studies to detect nerve injury.

Management

For emergency management, see page 935.

Principles of Management

1. Factors influencing choice of management include the following:
   a. Type, location, and severity of fracture.
   b. Soft tissue damage.
   c. Age and health status of the patient, including type and extent of other injuries.
2. Goals include the following:
   a. To regain and maintain correct position and alignment.
   b. To regain the function of the involved part.
   c. To return the patient to usual activities in the shortest time and at the least expense.
3. The management process is a three-step process:
   a. Reduction—setting the bone; refers to restoration of the fracture fragments into anatomic position and alignment.
   b. Immobilization—maintains reduction until bone healing occurs (see Figures 28-11 and 28-12).
   c. Rehabilitation—regaining normal function of the affected part.

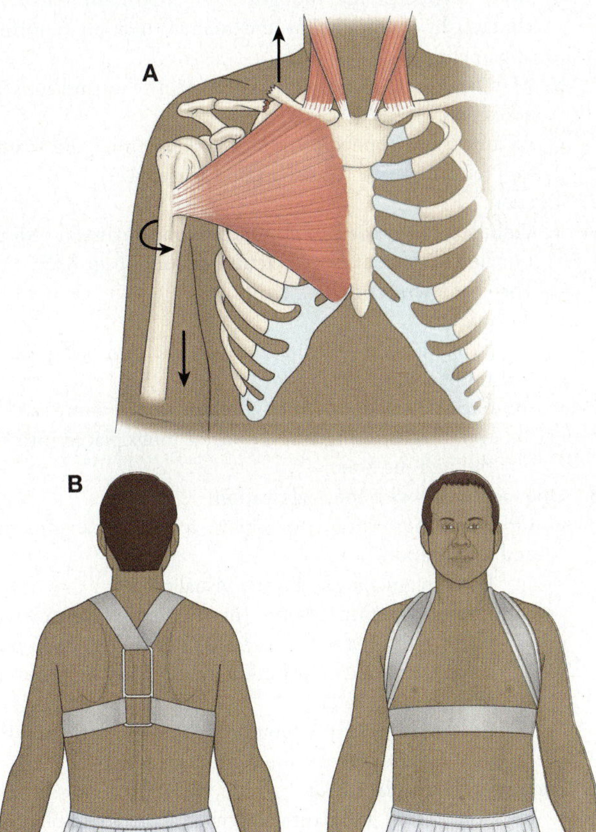

Figure 28-11. Fracture of the clavicle. **(A)** Anteroposterior view shows typical displacement in midclavicular fracture. **(B)** Immobilization is accomplished with a clavicular strap. (Adapted with permission from Hinkle, J. L., Cheever, K. H., & Overbaugh, K. [2022]. *Brunner and Suddarth's textbook of medical-surgical nursing* [15th ed., Fig. 37-13]. Wolters Kluwer.)

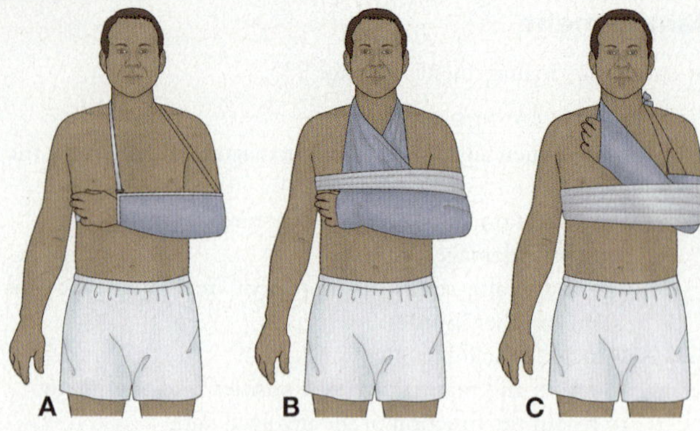

Figure 28-12. Immobilizers for proximal humeral fractures. **(A)** Commercial sling with immobilizing strap permits easy removal for hygiene and is comfortable on the neck. **(B)** Conventional sling and swathe. **(C)** Stockinette Velpeau and swathe are used when there is an unstable surgical neck component. This position relaxes the pectoralis major. (Adapted with permission from Hinkle, J. L., Cheever, K. H., & Overbaugh, K. [2022]. *Brunner and Suddarth's textbook of medical-surgical nursing* [15th ed., Fig. 37-15]. Wolters Kluwer.)

Approaches to Management

Vary by specific site of fracture (see Table 28-2, pages 867-869).

1. Closed reduction.
   a. Bony fragments are brought into apposition (ends in contact) by manipulation and manual traction restoring alignment.
   b. May be done under anesthesia for pain relief and muscle relaxation.
   c. Cast or splint applied to immobilize extremity and maintain reduction (see "Casts" section, page 847).
2. Traction.
   a. Pulling force applied to accomplish and maintain reduction and alignment (see "Traction" section, page 850).
   b. Used for fractures of long bones.
   c. Techniques.
      i. Skin traction—force applied to the skin using foam rubber, tape.
      ii. Skeletal traction—force applied to the bony skeleton directly, using wires, pins, or tongs placed into or through the bone.
3. Open reduction with internal fixation.
   a. Operative intervention to achieve reduction, alignment, and stabilization.
      i. Bone fragments are directly visualized.
      ii. Internal fixation devices (metal pins, wires, screws, plates, nails, rods) used to hold bone fragments in position until solid bone healing occurs (may be removed when bone is healed).
      iii. After closure of the wound, splints or casts may be used for additional stabilization and support.
4. Endoprosthetic replacement.
   a. Replacement of a fracture fragment with an implanted metal device.
   b. Used when fracture disrupts nutrition of the bone or treatment of choice is bony replacement.
5. External fixation device.
   a. Stabilization of complex and open fracture with the use of a metal frame and pin system.
   b. Permits active treatment of injured soft tissue.
      i. Wound may be left open (delayed primary wound closure).
      ii. Repair of damage to blood vessels, soft tissue, muscles, nerves, and tendons, as indicated.
      iii. Reconstructive surgery may be necessary (see "External Fixation" section, page 852).

Complications

Complications Associated With Immobility

1. Muscle atrophy, loss of muscle strength, and endurance.
2. Loss of ROM due to joint contracture.
3. Pressure sores at bony prominences from immobilizing device pressing on skin.
4. Diminished respiratory, cardiovascular, gastrointestinal (GI) function, resulting in possible pooling of respiratory secretions, orthostatic hypotension, ileus, anorexia, and constipation.
5. Psychosocial compromise, resulting in feelings of isolation and depression.

Other Acute Complications

1. Venous stasis and thromboembolism—particularly with fractures of the hip and lower extremities.
2. Neurovascular compromise.
3. Infection, especially with open fractures.
4. Shock due to significant hemorrhage related to trauma or as a postoperative complication.
5. Pulmonary emboli.

Fat Emboli Syndrome

1. Associated with embolization of marrow or tissue fat or platelets and free fatty acids to the pulmonary capillaries, producing rapid onset of symptoms.
2. Clinical manifestations.
   a. Respiratory distress—tachypnea, hypoxemia, crackles, wheezes, acute pulmonary edema, interstitial pneumonitis.
   b. Mental disturbances—irritability, restlessness, confusion, disorientation, stupor, coma due to systemic embolization, and severe hypoxia.
   c. Fever.
   d. Petechiae in buccal membranes, hard palate, conjunctival sacs, chest, anterior axillary folds, due to occlusion of capillaries.

CLINICAL JUDGMENT Restlessness, confusion, irritability, and disorientation may be the first signs of fat embolism syndrome. Confirm hypoxia with arterial blood gas (ABG) analysis. Young adults (age 20 to 30) and older adults (age 60 to 70) with multiple fractures or fractures of long bones or pelvis are particularly susceptible to development of fat emboli.

Bone Union Problems

1. Delayed union (takes longer to heal than average for type of fracture).
2. Nonunion (fractured bone fails to unite).
3. Malunion (union occurs but is faulty—misaligned).

Nursing Assessment

1. Ask the patient how the fracture occurred—mechanism of injury important in determining possible associated injuries.
2. Ask the patient to describe location, character, and intensity of pain to help determine possible source of discomfort.

Table 28-2 Fractures of Specific Sites

SITE AND MECHANISM	MANAGEMENT	NURSING CONSIDERATIONS
Clavicle		
Fall on shoulder	• Closed reduction and immobilization with clavicular strap (see Figure 28-11) figure-of-8 bandage or sling. • ORIF for marked displacement, severely comminuted fracture, and extensive soft tissue injury.	• Pad the axilla to prevent nerve damage from pressure of immobilizer. • Assess neurovascular status of arm. • Teach exercises of elbow, wrist, and fingers. • Teach shoulder exercises through full ROM, as prescribed.
Proximal Humerus		
Fall on outstretched arm; osteoporosis is predisposing factor	• Many remain in alignment and are supported by a sling and swathe or Velpeau bandage for comfort (see Figure 28-12). • If displaced, treated with reduction under x-ray control, open reduction, or replacement of humeral head with prosthesis.	• Place a soft pad under the axilla to prevent skin maceration. • Encourage shoulder ROM exercises after specified period of immobilization to prevent frozen shoulder. • Instruct the patient to lean forward and allow affected arm to abduct and rotate.
Shaft of Humerus		
Direct fall, blow to arm, or auto injury; damage to radial nerve may occur	• Immobilize with sling and swathe, splint, or hanging cast. • A hanging cast is applied for its weight to correct displaced fractures with shortening of the humeral shaft. • ORIF for associated vascular injury or pathologic fracture, followed by support in sling.	• Hanging cast must remain unsupported to maintain traction. • Teach the patient to avoid supporting elbow in lap or arm on pillow. • The patient should sleep in upright position to maintain 24-h traction. • Encourage exercise of fingers immediately after application of cast. • Teach pendulum exercises of arm, as prescribed, to prevent frozen shoulder.
Elbow and Forearm		
Fall on elbow, outstretched hand, or direct blow (sideswipe injury)	• Treatment depends on specific characteristics of fracture—ORIF, arthroplasty, external fixation, casting. • Closed drainage system may be used to decrease hematoma formation and swelling.	• Assess neurovascular status of forearm and hand. • If radial pulse weakens or disappears, report immediately to prevent irreversible ischemia. • Elevate arm to control edema. • Encourage finger and shoulder exercises.
Wrist		
Colles fracture is common (0.5–1 in [1.2–2.5 cm] above the wrist with dorsal displacement of lower fragment); caused by fall on outstretched palm; commonly associated with osteoporosis	• Closed reduction with splint or cast support. • Percutaneous pins and external fixator or plaster cast.	• Elevate arm above level of heart for 48 h after reduction to promote venous and lymphatic return and reduce swelling. • Watch for swelling of fingers and check for constricting bandages or cast. • Teach finger exercises to reduce swelling and stiffness. • Hold the hand above the level of the heart. • Move fingers from full extension to flexion. • Hold and release. • Repeat at least 10 times every half hour when awake for as long as swelling occurs. • Encourage daily-prescribed exercises to restore full extension and supination.
Hand		
Caused by numerous injuries	• Splinting for undisplaced fractures of fingers. • Debridement, irrigation, and Kirchner wire fixation for open fractures. • Reconstructive surgery may be necessary for complex injuries.	• Provide aggressive care and encouragement with rehabilitation plan to regain maximal function of hand.

(continued)

Table 28-2 Fractures of Specific Sites (*continued*)

SITE AND MECHANISM	MANAGEMENT	NURSING CONSIDERATIONS
Hip (Proximal Femur)		
Occur frequently in older adults, females with osteoporosis, and with fall types: • Intracapsular—femoral neck within joint capsule • Extracapsular—femoral neck between greater and lesser trochanter (intertrochanteric) or of femoral shaft • Subtrochanteric—of femur just below level of lesser trochanter	• Hip fracture identified by shortening and external rotation of affected leg; pain in hip or knee; inability to move leg. • Immobilization with Buck extension traction until surgery. • Surgery as soon as medically stable; choice depends on location, character, and patient factors. • Internal fixation with nail, nail–plate combination, multiple pins, screw, or sliding nails. • Femoral prosthetic replacement. • Total hip arthroplasty.	• Provide constant monitoring and nursing care to reduce the risk of complications, such as pneumonia, thrombophlebitis, fat emboli, dislocation of prosthesis, infection, and pressure injuries. • Administer aspirin, warfarin, subcutaneous heparin, or low molecular weight heparin, as ordered. • Use sequential compression devices, as ordered. • Provide meticulous skin care to prevent breakdown. • Use trapeze for the patient to assist with position changes. • Use a special bed or mattress, as indicated. • Inspect heels daily and use heel protection measures. • Prevent UTI by increasing fluids, limiting use of indwelling catheter, and encouraging frequent voiding. • Keep affected leg in abduction and neutral rotation. • Teach quadriceps setting exercise to prevent muscle atrophy of affected leg.
Femoral Shaft		
	• Closed reduction and stabilization with skeletal traction—Thomas leg splint with Pearson attachment; followed by use of orthosis (cast brace) to allow weight bearing. • Open reduction with hardware or with bone grafting may be necessary. • External fixator may be used.	• Marked concealed blood loss may occur; watch for signs of shock initially and anemia later. • Examine skin under the ring of the Thomas splint for signs of pressure.
Knee		
Direct blow to knee area; involve distal shaft of femur (supracondylar), articular surfaces, or patella	• Closed reduction and immobilization through casting, traction, braces, splints. • ORIF. • Goal is to preserve knee mobility.	• Elevate extremity by raising foot gatch of bed. • Evaluate for effusion—report and loosen pressure dressing if pain is severe; prepare for joint aspiration. • Teach quadriceps setting exercises and limited weight bearing, as prescribed.
Tibia and Fibula/Ankle		
Distal tibia or fibula, malleoli, or talus fractures generally result from forceful twisting of ankle and commonly associated with ligament disruption; also, high incidence of open fractures of tibial shaft because tibia lies superficially beneath the skin	• Closed reduction and toe-to-groin cast for closed fractures, later replaced by short leg cast or orthosis. • ORIF may be necessary for some closed fractures. • External fixator for open fracture.	• Elevate lower leg to control edema. • Avoid dependent position of extremity for prolonged periods. • Prepare the patient for long immobilization period, as union is slow (12–16 wk, longer for open and comminuted fractures). • Prepare the patient for stiff ankle joint following immobilization.
Foot		
Metatarsal fracture due to crush injuries of the foot	• Immobilization with cast, splint, or strapping.	• Encourage partial weight bearing, as allowed. • Elevate the foot to control edema.
Thoracic and Lumbar Spine		
Trauma from falls, contact sports, or auto accidents, or excessive loading may cause fracture of vertebral body,	• Suspected with pain that is worsened by movement and coughing and radiates to extremities, abdomen, or intercostal muscles and presence of sensory and motor deficits.	• Use log roll technique to change positions. • Monitor bowel and bladder dysfunction, as paralytic ileus and bladder distention may occur with nerve root injury.

Table 28-2 Fractures of Specific Sites *(continued)*

SITE AND MECHANISM	MANAGEMENT	NURSING CONSIDERATIONS
lamina, spinous and transverse processes; usually stable compression fractures	• Bed rest on firm mattress and pain relief followed by progressive ambulation and back strengthening to treat stable fractures; takes about 6 wk to heal. • ORIF with Harrington rod, body cast, or laminectomy with spinal fusion may be necessary for unstable or displaced fractures.	• Assist the patient to ambulate when pain subsides, no neurologic deficit exists, and x-rays reveal no displacement. • Teach proper body mechanics and back preservation techniques. • Encourage weight reduction. • Teach the patient with osteoporosis the importance of safety measures to avoid falls.
Pelvis		
Sacrum, ilium, pubic, ischium, and coccyx fractures may occur from auto accidents, crush injuries, and falls; most are stable fractures that do not involve the pelvic ring and have minimal displacement	• Emergency management to treat multiple trauma, shock from intraperitoneal hemorrhage, and injury to internal organs is necessary (see pages 936 to 940). • Bed rest for several days followed by progressive weight bearing for stable fracture. • Prolonged bed rest, external fixation, ORIF, skeletal traction, and pelvic sling are options for unstable fracture.	• Monitor and support vital functions, as indicated. • Observe urine output for blood indicating genitourinary injury. • Do not attempt to insert urethral catheter until patency of urethra is known; incidence of urethral injury in males is high with anterior fractures. • Assist the patient being treated in pelvic sling. • Fold sling back over buttocks to enable the patient to use bedpan. • Reach under the sling to give skin care; line the sling with sheepskin. • Loosen sling only as directed.

ORIF, open reduction with internal function; ROM, range of motion; UTI, urinary tract infection.

3. Ask the patient to describe sensations in injured extremity to aid in evaluation of neurovascular status.
4. Observe the patient's ability to change position to assess functional mobility.
5. Note the patient's emotional status and behavior—indicators of ability to cope with stress of injury.
6. Assess the patient's support system; identify current and potential sources of support, assistance, and caregiving.
7. Review findings on past and present health status to aid in formulating care plan.
8. Conduct physical examination.
   a. Examine skin for lacerations, abrasions, ecchymosis, edema, and temperature.
   b. Auscultate lungs to establish baseline assessment of respiratory function.
   c. Assess pulses and BP; assess peripheral tissue perfusion, especially in injured extremity, to establish circulatory status baseline.
   d. Determine neurologic status (sensations and movement) of extremity distal to injury.
   e. Note length, alignment, and immobilization of injured extremity.
   f. Evaluate behavior and cognitive functioning of the patient to determine ability to participate in care planning and patient education activities.

CLINICAL JUDGMENT Change in behavior or cerebral functioning may be an early indicator of cerebral anoxia from shock or pulmonary or fat emboli.

POPULATION AWARENESS Assessment of the patient's health and functional abilities before a fracture along with available support systems facilitates development of realistic rehabilitation and discharge goals.

Nursing Interventions

Evaluating for Hemorrhage and Shock

1. Monitor vital signs as frequently as clinical condition indicates, observing for hypotension, elevated pulse, widening pulse pressure, cold clammy skin, restlessness, pallor.
2. Watch for evidence of hemorrhage on dressings or in drainage containers.
3. Review laboratory data; report abnormal values.
4. Administer prescribed fluids/blood to maintain circulating volume.
5. Monitor intake and output. Goal is to maintain at least 30 mL/h and establish individual's normal voiding pattern.

CLINICAL JUDGMENT Patients with hip and long bone fractures are at high risk for hemorrhage. Frequent checks for hemodynamics, neurovascular status, and drainage should be performed, particularly in patients with other comorbidities who may not tolerate changes in hematocrit and hemoglobin levels.

Monitoring for Impaired Gas Exchange

1. Evaluate changes in mental status and restlessness that may indicate hypoxia.

2. Review diagnostic evaluation data—especially ABG values and chest x-ray.
3. Position to enhance respiratory effort. Report any sudden or progressive changes in respiratory status.
4. Encourage coughing and deep breathing to promote lung expansion and diminish pooling of pulmonary secretions.
5. Monitor pulse oximetry; administer oxygen, as prescribed.
6. Maintain cervical spine precautions if spinal injury is suspected.

Preventing Neurovascular Compromise

1. Monitor neurovascular status for compression of nerve, diminished circulation, development of compartment syndrome.
   a. Pain—progressive, localized, deep throbbing, persistent, unrelieved by immobilization and medications.
   b. Pain on passive stretch.
   c. Weakness progressing to paralysis.
   d. Altered sensation, hypoesthesia, paresthesia.
   e. Poor capillary refill (greater than 3 seconds).
   f. Skin color—pale, cyanotic.
   g. Elevated compartment pressure—palpable tightness of muscle compartment, elevated measured tissue pressure.
   h. Pulselessness—a late sign.
2. Reduce swelling.
   a. Elevate injured extremity (unless compartment syndrome is suspected—may contribute to vascular compromise).
   b. Apply cold to injury, if prescribed.
3. Relieve pressure caused by immobilizing device, as prescribed (such as bivalving cast, rewrapping elastic bandage, or splinting device).
4. Relieve pressure on skin to prevent development of pressure injury.
   a. Frequent repositioning.
   b. Skin care—do not massage bony prominences.
   c. Special mattresses.

CLINICAL JUDGMENT Monitoring the neurovascular integrity of the injured extremity is essential. Development of compartment syndrome (increased tissue pressure causing hypoxemia) leads to permanent loss of function in 6 to 8 hours. This situation must be identified and managed promptly.

Preventing Development of Thromboembolism

1. Encourage active and passive ankle exercises.
2. Use elastic stockings, foot pumps, or sequential compression devices (SCDs), as prescribed.
3. Elevate legs to prevent stasis, avoiding pressure on blood vessels.
4. Encourage mobility; change position frequently; encourage ambulation.
5. Administer anticoagulants, as prescribed.
6. Monitor for development of thrombophlebitis.
   a. Note complaint of pain and tenderness in calf.
   b. Report calf pain.
   c. Report increased size and temperature of calf.
   d. Homans sign has not been proved to be an effective screen for deep vein thrombosis (DVT); therefore, it is no longer an acceptable measure for assessing DVT.

POPULATION AWARENESS Older adults with fractures, trauma, immobility, obesity, or history of thrombophlebitis are at high risk for developing thromboembolism.

Relieving Pain

1. Perform a comprehensive pain assessment.
   a. Have the patient describe the pain, location, characteristics (dull, sharp, continuous, throbbing, bony, radiating, aching).
   b. Ask the patient what causes the pain, makes the pain worse, relieves the pain. Evaluate the patient for proper body alignment, pressure from equipment (casts, traction, splints, appliances).
2. Initiate activities to prevent or modify pain.
   a. Assist the patient with pain-reduction techniques—cutaneous stimulation, distraction, guided imagery, transcutaneous electrical nerve stimulation (TENS), biofeedback.
   b. Immobilize injured part.
   c. Position the patient in correct alignment.
   d. Support splinted fracture above and below fracture when repositioning or moving the patient.
   e. Reposition the patient with slow and steady motion; use additional personnel, as needed.
   f. Elevate painful extremity to diminish venous congestion.
   g. Apply heat or cold modalities, as prescribed. Heat versus cold is controversial. One randomly controlled trial found significantly less edema with cold packs versus heat 3 to 5 days post injury.
   h. Modify environment to facilitate rest and relaxation.
3. Administer prescribed medications, as indicated. Encourage the use of less potent drugs as severity of discomfort decreases.
4. Establish a supportive relationship to assist the patient to deal with discomfort.
5. Encourage the patient to become an active participant in rehabilitative plans.

DRUG ALERT Meperidine may cause toxicity as it breaks down into the metabolite normeperidine, which has a 15- to 20-hour half-life, especially in patients with impaired renal function or older patients.

Monitoring for Development of Infection

1. Clean, debride, and irrigate open fracture wound, as prescribed, as soon as possible to minimize risk of infection.
   a. All open fractures are contaminated.
   b. Begin prescribed antibiotic therapy promptly after wound culture obtained.
2. Use sterile technique during dressing changes to minimize infection of wound, soft tissues, and bone.
3. Evaluate the patient for elevation of temperature every 4 hours as indicated by facility or provider order.
4. Note and report elevated white blood cell (WBC) counts.
5. Report areas of inflammation and swelling around incision or open wound.
6. Report purulent odiferous drainage.
7. Obtain specimens for culture and sensitivity to determine causative organism.

Promoting Adequate Hygiene

1. Encourage participation in care.
2. Arrange the patient area and personal items for patient convenience and to promote independence.
3. Modify activities to facilitate maximum independence within prescribed limits.
4. Allow time for the patient to accomplish the task.
5. Teach safe use of mobility and necessary aids.

6. Assist with activities of daily living (ADLs), as needed.
7. Teach family how to assist the patient while promoting independence in self-care.

Promoting Physical Mobility

1. Perform active and passive exercises to all nonimmobilized joints.
2. Encourage patient participation in frequent position changes, maintaining support to fracture during position changes.
3. Minimize prolonged periods of physical inactivity, encouraging ambulation when prescribed.
4. Administer prescribed analgesics judiciously to decrease pain associated with movement.

Preventing Disuse Syndrome

1. Teach and encourage isometric exercises to diminish muscle atrophy.
2. Encourage the use of immobilized extremity within prescribed limits.

Minimizing the Psychological Effects of Trauma

1. Monitor the patient for symptoms of posttraumatic stress disorder.
   a. Memory of event; anger, helplessness, vulnerability, mood swings, depression, cognitive impairment, sleep disturbance, increased dependency, and social withdrawal.
2. Assist the patient to move through phases of posttraumatic stress (outcry, denial, intrusiveness, working through, completion).
3. Establish trusting therapeutic relationship with the patient.
4. Encourage the patient to express thoughts and feelings about traumatic event.
5. Encourage the patient to participate in decision making to reestablish control and overcome feelings of helplessness.
6. Teach relaxation techniques to decrease anxiety.
7. Encourage development of adaptive responses and participation in support groups.
8. Refer the patient to psychiatric liaison nurse or refer for psychotherapy, as needed.

Community and Home Care Considerations

1. Assist the patient to actively exercise joints above and below the immobilized fracture at frequent intervals.
   a. Isometric exercises of muscles covered by cast—start exercise as soon as possible after cast application.
   b. Increase isometric exercises as fracture stabilizes.
2. After removal of immobilizing device (e.g., cast, splint), have the patient start isotonic exercises and continue with isometric exercises.
3. Assess the home for any fall hazards when the patient ambulates.
4. Obtain PT/occupational therapy (OT) consultation for assistance with ADLs, transferring technique, gait strengthening, and conditioning after lengthy immobilization, as needed.
5. Assess orthostatic BP when the patient begins to ambulate to prevent falls.

Patient Education and Health Maintenance

1. Explain the basis for fracture treatment and need for patient participation in therapeutic regimen.
2. Promote adjustment of usual lifestyle and responsibilities to accommodate limitations imposed by fracture.
3. Instruct the patient on exercises to strengthen upper-extremity muscles if crutch walking is planned.
4. Instruct the patient in methods of safe ambulation—walker, crutches, cane.
5. Emphasize instructions concerning amount of weight bearing that will be permitted on fractured extremity.
6. Discuss prevention of recurrent fractures—safety considerations, avoidance of fatigue, proper footwear.
7. Encourage follow-up medical supervision to monitor for union problems.
8. Teach symptoms needing attention, such as numbness, decreased function, increased pain, elevated temperature.
9. Encourage adequate balanced diet to promote bone and soft tissue healing.

Evaluation: Expected Outcomes

- Vital signs within normal parameters; urine output at least 30 mL/h.
- Respirations unlabored; alert and oriented.
- No signs of neurovascular compromise (i.e., circulation, motor, sensory intact).
- No calf pain reported.
- Reports decreased pain with elevation, ice, and analgesic.
- Afebrile; no wound drainage.
- Performing hygiene and dressing practices with minimal assistance.
- Performing active ROM correctly.
- Using affected extremity for light activity, as allowed.
- Denies acute symptoms of stress; reports working through feelings about trauma.

OTHER MUSCULOSKELETAL DISORDERS

Lower Back Pain

EVIDENCE BASE Qaseem, A., Wilt, T. J., McLean, R. M., & Forciea, M. A.; for the Clinical Guidelines Committee of the American College of Physicians. (2017). Noninvasive treatments for acute, subacute, and chronic low back pain: A clinical practice guideline from the American College of Physicians. *Annals of Internal Medicine*, *166*(7), 514–530. https://doi.org/10.7326/M16-2367

Longtin, C., Décary, S., Cook, C. E., & Tousignant-Laflamme, Y. (2021). What does it take to facilitate the integration of clinical practice guidelines for the management of low back pain into practice? Part 1: A synthesis of recommendation. *Pain Practice: The Official Journal of World Institute of Pain*, *21*(8), 943–954. https://doi.org/10.1111/papr.13033

Lower back pain is characterized by an uncomfortable or acute pain in the lumbosacral area associated with severe spasm of the paraspinal muscles, usually with pain radiating to the lower extremities.

Pathophysiology and Etiology

Acute low back pain lasts up to 4 weeks, subacute low back pain lasts 4 to 12 weeks, and chronic low back pain lasts longer than 12 weeks. There are multiple causes:

1. Mechanical (joint, muscular, or ligamentous sprain).
2. Degenerative disk disease; acute herniation of disks.
3. Lack of physical activity and exercise; weakness of musculature of back.
4. Arthritic conditions.
5. Diseases of bone (osteoporosis, vertebral fracture, Paget disease, metastatic carcinoma).
6. Congenital disorders.
7. Systemic diseases.
8. Infections of disk spaces or vertebrae.
9. Spinal cord tumors.
10. Referred pain from other areas.

Clinical Manifestations

1. Pain localized or radiating to buttocks or to one or both legs.
2. Paresthesias, numbness, and weakness of lower extremities.
3. Spasm in acute phase.
4. Bowel or bladder dysfunction in cauda equina syndrome.

Diagnostic Evaluation

1. X-rays of lumbar spine are usually negative.
2. Computed tomography (CT) of spine—to detect arthritic changes, degenerative disk disease, tumor, and other abnormalities.
3. Myelography—to confirm and localize disk herniation.
4. MRI—to detect pathology, disk herniation, soft tissue injury, stenosis, nerve impingement.
5. EMG of lower extremities—to detect nerve changes related to back pathology.
6. Diskogram—to evaluate herniated disk.

Management

For management of herniated disk, see page 407. For management of spinal cord tumors, see page 396. Guidelines call for conservative, nonpharmacologic management as first-line treatment. Most people with acute and subacute low back pain improve over time.

1. Avoid activities that may strain the back until healed, but bed rest is to be avoided as well because it may significantly decrease the rate of recovery, increase pain and disability, and lengthen time spent absent from work.
2. Exercise, physical therapy (PT), and tai chi may be helpful for chronic pain.
3. Heat or ice is used to relax muscle spasm and relieve discomfort. Follow heat with massage.
4. Medications.
   a. Oral analgesic and anti-inflammatory agent—usually a nonsteroidal anti-inflammatory drugs (NSAID) is first-line agent, unless contraindicated because of history or high risk of gastrointestinal (GI) bleeding, renal insufficiency, or allergy. If there is a high risk of GI bleeding, COX-2 inhibitors may be used unless the patient has a sulfa or aspirin allergy or is in the third trimester of pregnancy.
   b. Painful trigger points may be injected with hydrocortisone/xylocaine for pain relief.
   c. Opioids may be sedating.
   d. Muscle relaxant to relieve spasm and tense muscles. Muscle relaxants may be sedating.
   e. Adjunct medications to reduce chronic neuropathic pain include duloxetine.
5. Lumbosacral support may be used—provides abdominal compression and decreases load on lumbar intervertebral disks.
6. Acupuncture is helpful for acute and chronic pain; transcutaneous electrical nerve stimulation (TENS) may be helpful in relieving chronic pain.
7. Behavioral intervention, such as mindfulness-based stress reduction techniques, is helpful for chronic pain.
   a. Psychotropic medication may be used for treatment of depression and anxiety, which potentiate pain.
   b. Focus on getting back to functional state after long disability.

CLINICAL JUDGMENT Risk factors of chronic low back pain include high severity of pain, depression, lack of positive coping skills, beliefs that the patient cannot control their pain, and high rate of missing work because of low back pain. Cognitive behavioral strategies can be used to help the patient with pain management and strengthen positive coping skills. Screening tools are available to help identify risk factors and guide treatment decisions.

Complications

1. Spinal instability, infection, sensory and motor deficits.
2. Chronic pain.
3. Malingering and other psychosocial reactions.

Nursing Assessment

1. Obtain history to determine when, where, and how the pain occurs; aggravating or relieving factors; relationship of pain to specific activities; presence of numbness or paresthesia.
2. Perform physical examination of neurologic system—spots localized weakness of extremities and reflex and sensory loss.
3. Perform musculoskeletal examination for changes in strength, tone, and range of motion (ROM).
4. If condition is chronic, assess coping ability of the patient and family or significant others.
5. Assess effect of illness on daily living—work, school.

Nursing Interventions

Relieving Pain

1. Advise the patient to stay active and avoid bed rest, in most cases.
2. Keep pillow between flexed knees while in side-lying position—minimizes strain on back muscles.
3. Apply heat or ice, as prescribed.
4. Administer or teach self-administration of pain medications and muscle relaxants, as prescribed.
   a. Give NSAIDs with meals to prevent GI upset and bleeding.
   b. Muscle relaxants and opioids may cause drowsiness.

Coping With Chronic Pain

1. Administer adjunct pain medications, as directed. Explain that medications may not completely relieve pain but will reduce level of discomfort so that the patient can increase daily activities. Encourage adherence to therapy.
2. Teach relaxation techniques such as progressive muscle relaxation and imagery.
3. Encourage balanced diet, exercise program, and avoidance of smoking.
4. Suggest consultation with physical/occupational therapist, psychologist, or pain management clinician, as needed.

Promoting Mobility

1. Encourage ROM of all uninvolved muscle groups.
2. Suggest gradual increase in activities and alternating activities with rest in semi-Fowler position.
3. Avoid prolonged periods of sitting, standing, or lying down.

4. Encourage the patient to discuss problems that may be contributing to backache.
5. Encourage the patient to do prescribed back exercises. Exercise keeps postural muscles strong, helps recondition the back and abdominal musculature, and serves as an outlet for emotional tension.

Patient Education and Health Maintenance

Instruct the patient to avoid recurrences as follows:

1. Standing, sitting, lying, and lifting properly are necessary for a healthy back.
2. Alternate periods of activity with periods of rest.
   a. Avoid prolonged sitting (intradiskal pressure in lumbar spine is higher during sitting), standing, and driving.
   b. Change positions and rest at frequent intervals.
   c. Avoid assuming tense, cramped positions.
   d. Sit in a straight-back chair with the knees slightly higher than the hips. Use a footstool, if necessary.
   e. Flatten the hollow of the back by sitting with the buttocks "tucked under." Pelvic tilt (small of back is pressed against a flat surface) decreases lordosis.
   f. Avoid knee and hip extension. When driving a car, have the seat pushed forward as necessary for comfort. Place a cushion in the small of the back for support.
3. When standing for any length of time, rest one foot on a small stool or platform to relieve lumbar lordosis.
4. Avoid fatigue that contributes to spasm of back muscles.
5. Use good body mechanics when lifting or moving about.
6. Daily exercise is important in the prevention of back problems (see Patient Education Guidelines 28-2).
   a. Do prescribed back exercises twice daily—strengthens back, leg, and abdominal muscles.
   b. Walking outdoors (progressively increasing distance and pace) is recommended.
   c. Reduce weight, if necessary—decreases strain on back muscles.

PATIENT EDUCATION GUIDELINES 28-2

Taking Care of Your Lower Back

Almost everyone has lower back pain at some time. Chronic pain will develop in some, and a few will become disabled because of it. Risk factors for chronic lower back pain include being overweight, being deconditioned (out of shape), having poor posture, and having poor abdominal muscle tone. You can relieve pain and avoid disability by adhering to the following instructions.

DO BACK EXERCISES EVERY DAY

- Lie on your back on the floor or a firm mattress. Bend one knee and bring that leg up toward your chest. Hold it against your chest a few seconds. Then repeat with the other leg. Alternate legs several times.
- Lie on your back with your knees bent and feet flat on the floor. Tighten your abdomen and buttocks, and push your lower back to the floor. Hold for a few seconds, and then relax. Repeat several times.
- Lie on your back with knees bent and feet flat on the floor. Do a partial sit-up by crossing your arms on your chest or behind your head and lifting your shoulders off the floor 6 to 12 in (15 to 30.5 cm). Repeat several times.

BE CAREFUL HOW YOU LIFT

- Move your body close to an object before picking it up.
- Bend at the knees, not the back, to pick up an object that is low.
- Hold the object close to your abdomen and chest.
- Bend at the knees again to put down an object.
- Avoid reaching, twisting, or turning your back as you lift or carry an object.

PROTECT YOUR BACK WHILE SITTING AND STANDING

- Avoid sitting in soft, cushioned chairs too long.
- If you sit for long periods at work, make sure your knees are level with your hips. Use a step stool, if necessary.
- If you stand for long periods, try to put one foot up on a stool and then the other. Walk around and change position periodically.
- Adjust your car seat so there is a bend in your knees. Do not stretch.
- Put a firm pillow behind your lower back if it does not feel supported while you are sitting.

STAY ACTIVE AND IN GOOD HEALTH

- Take a walk every day wearing comfortable, low-heeled shoes.
- Eat a balanced, low-fat diet with plenty of fruits and vegetables to avoid constipation.
- Get plenty of sleep on a firm mattress.
- See your health care provider promptly for worsening pain or new injury.

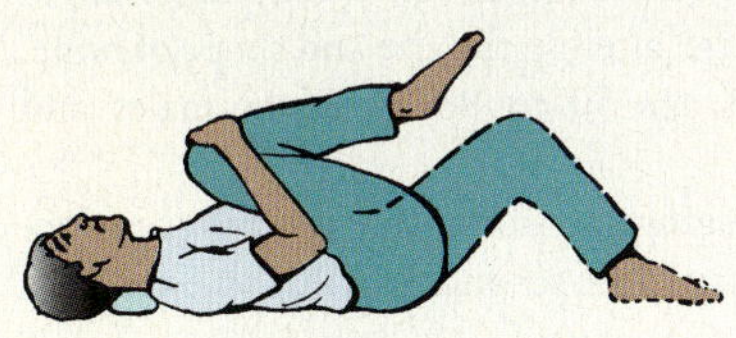

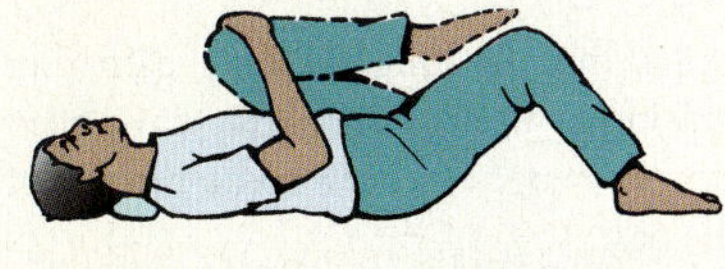

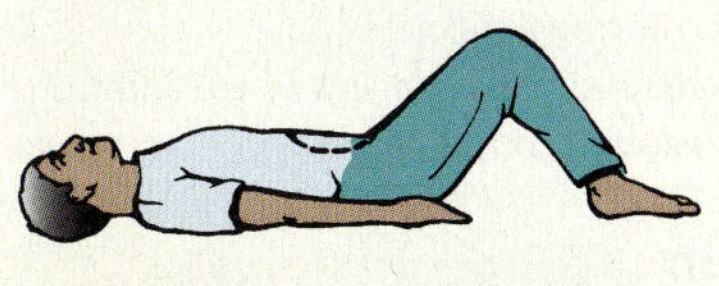

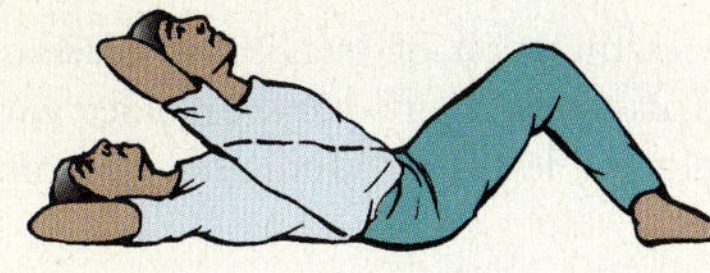

Back exercises to strengthen abdominal and postural muscles, to stretch contracted back muscles, and to maintain flexibility.

Evaluation: Expected Outcomes

- Verbalizes relief of pain with rest and medication.
- Able to participate in activities of daily living (ADLs) with sedation or pain greater than 3/10.
- Performs back exercises correctly.

Osteoarthritis

EVIDENCE BASE Brophy, R. H., & Fillingham, Y. A. (2022). AAOS clinical practice guideline summary: Management of osteoarthritis of the knee (nonarthroplasty), third edition. *The Journal of the American Academy of Orthopaedic Surgeons, 30*(9), e721–e729. https://doi.org/10.5435/JAAOS-D-21-01233

Gibbs, A. J., Gray, B., Wallis, J. A., Taylor, N. F., Kemp, J. L., Hunter, D. J., & Barton, C. J. (2023). Recommendations for the management of hip and knee osteoarthritis: A systematic review of clinical practice guidelines. *Osteoarthritis and Cartilage, 31*(10), 1280–1292. https://doi.org/10.1016/j.joca.2023.05.015

Rees H. W. (2020). Management of osteoarthritis of the hip. *The Journal of the American Academy of Orthopaedic Surgeons, 28*(7), e288–e291. https://doi.org/10.5435/JAAOS-D-19-00416

Osteoarthritis (OA), or degenerative joint disease, is a chronic, noninflammatory, slowly progressing disorder that causes deterioration of articular cartilage. It affects weight-bearing joints (hips and knees) as well as joints of the distal interphalangeal and proximal interphalangeal joints of the fingers.

Pathophysiology and Etiology

1. Changes in articular cartilage occur first; later, secondary soft tissue changes may occur.
2. Progressive wear and tear on cartilage leads to thinning of joint surface and ulceration into bone.
3. Leads to inflammation of the joint and increased blood flow and hypertrophy of subchondral bone.
4. New cartilage and bone formation at joint margins result in osteophytosis (bone spurs), altering the size and shape of bone.
5. Generally affects adults age 50 to 90; equal in males and females.
6. Cause is unknown, but aging and obesity are contributing factors. Previous trauma may cause secondary OA.

Clinical Manifestations

1. Pain in one or more joints, may be long-standing pain that increases with weight bearing or use of joint; may have been a gradual, insidious onset, or may have been some history of trauma to the joint in the past.
2. Less than 30 minutes of morning stiffness.
3. Bony deformity (osteophyte) or enlargement of the joint.
4. Possible crepitation, effusion.

Diagnostic Evaluation

1. No specific laboratory examination or imaging is necessary to make the diagnosis if person is 45 years or older with activity-related joint pain and less than 30 minutes of morning stiffness.
2. X-rays of affected joints show joint space narrowing, osteophytes, and sclerosis.
3. Radionuclide imaging (bone scan) shows increased uptake in affected bones.
4. Analysis of synovial fluid differentiates OA from rheumatoid arthritis (RA).

Management

Conservative Management

1. Exercise for muscle strengthening and general fitness, including low-impact aerobic self-management programs; may involve PT and occupational therapy (OT) to maintain function while preserving the joints. Manipulation and stretching may be added with hip arthritis.
2. Weight loss if patient is overweight or has obesity to reduce stress on joints.
3. Pain management using nonopioid analgesics, particularly NSAIDs, which have proven more effective in many studies than acetaminophen, but side effects must be considered; tramadol may need to be added, and opioids should be avoided unless benefits outweigh risks.
4. Hyaluronate and hylan G-F 20, agents known as viscosupplements, have been approved by the Food and Drug Administration. These drugs are administered over time through intra-articular injections into the knee. However, current guidelines no longer recommend their use because of lack of sufficient improvement for a majority of patients.
5. TENS as adjunct to pain management.
6. Proper nutrition, sleep, and stress reduction to improve well-being.
7. Over-the-counter (OTC) supplements glucosamine and chondroitin sulfate are commonly used but have not proven to be more effective than placebo.

CLINICAL JUDGMENT The patient's body mass index can be used to determine the need for weight loss, a major factor in preventing chronic pain due to OA. Long-term management with a primary care provider or weight-loss specialist may assist the patient in successful weight reduction.

Surgical Intervention

Surgical intervention is considered when the pain becomes intolerable to the patient and mobility is severely compromised. Options include osteotomy, debridement, joint fusion, arthroscopy, and arthroplasty.

Complications

1. Limited mobility.
2. Neurologic deficits associated with spinal involvement.

Nursing Assessment

1. Obtain history of pain and its characteristics, including specific joints involved.
2. Evaluate ROM and strength.
3. Assess effect on ADLs and emotional status.

Nursing Interventions

Relieving Pain

1. Advise the patient to take prescribed NSAIDs or OTC analgesics as directed to relieve inflammation and pain. If tramadol

or opioids are prescribed, ensure that the patient is taking them as directed.

2. Provide rest for involved joints—excessive use aggravates the symptoms and accelerates degeneration.
   a. Use splints, braces, cervical collars, traction, and lumbosacral corsets, as ordered by health care provider.
   b. Have prescribed rest periods in recumbent position.
3. Advise the patient to avoid activities that precipitate pain.
4. Apply heat, as prescribed—relieves muscle spasm and stiffness; avoid prolonged application of heat—may cause increased swelling and flare symptoms.
5. Teach correct posture and body mechanics—postural alterations lead to chronic muscle tension and pain.
6. Advise sleeping with a rolled terry cloth towel under the neck—for relief of cervical OA.
7. Provide crutches, braces, walker, or cane when indicated—to reduce weight-bearing stress on hips and knees. Teach proper use of assistive devices, see page 844.
8. Advise wearing corrective shoes and metatarsal supports for foot disorders—also helps in the treatment of arthritis of the knee.
9. Encourage weight loss to decrease stress on weight-bearing joints.
10. Support the patient undergoing orthopedic surgery for unremitting pain and disabling arthritis of joints (see page 854).

POPULATION AWARENESS Older patients are at greater risk for GI bleeding and renal failure associated with NSAID use. Encourage administration with meals and monitor stool for occult blood. Celecoxib and meloxicam are associated with less risk of GI bleeding but may cause an increased risk of cardiovascular embolic events and deleterious effects on the kidneys.

Increasing Physical Mobility

1. Encourage activity as much as possible without causing pain.
2. Teach ROM exercises to maintain joint mobility and muscle tone for joint support, to prevent capsular and tendon tightening, and to prevent deformities. Avoid flexion and adduction deformities.
3. Teach isometric exercises and graded exercises to improve muscle strength around the involved joint.
4. Advise putting joints through ROM after periods of inactivity (e.g., automobile ride).

Promoting Self-Care

1. Suggest performing important activities in morning, after stiffness has been abated and before fatigue and pain become a problem.
2. Advise on modifications, such as wearing looser clothing without buttons, placing bench in tub or shower for bathing, sitting at table or counter in kitchen to prepare meals.
3. Help with obtaining assistive devices, such as padded handles for utensils and grooming aids, to promote independence.
4. Refer to OT for additional assistance.

Patient Education and Health Maintenance

1. Suggest swimming or water aerobics (offered by the YMCA) as a form of nonstressful exercise to preserve mobility.
2. Encourage adequate diet and sleep to enhance general health.
3. Advise the patient to discuss the use of complementary therapies, such as glucosamine and chondroitin sulfate, with health care provider.
4. For additional information and support, refer to the Arthritis Foundation (www.arthritis.org).

Evaluation: Expected Outcomes

- Reports reduction in pain while ambulatory.
- Performs ROM exercises.
- Dresses, bathes self, and grooms with assistive devices.

Neoplasms of the Musculoskeletal System

Musculoskeletal neoplasms include primary *sarcomas, metastatic bone disease*, and benign tumors (*osteoma, chondroma, osteoclastoma*) of the bone. More than 60% of bone neoplasms are metastatic from other sites of cancer.

Pathophysiology and Etiology

Benign Bone Tumors

Osteoid osteoma, chondroma, and osteoclastoma (benign giant cell tumor) are examples of benign bone tumors. Malignant transformation occurs with some.

Malignant Bone Tumors

1. Chondrosarcoma and osteosarcoma are examples of primary malignant bone tumors.
   a. Tumors develop in areas of rapid growth.
   b. Risk factors include Paget disease, previous radiation therapy to the bone, and other bone diseases.
   c. Hematogenous spread to the lung occurs.
2. Multiple myeloma is a malignant neoplasm arising from the bone marrow.

Metastatic Bone Tumors

1. Metastatic bone tumors are most frequently associated with cancers of the breast, prostate, and lung (primary malignancy site).
2. Bone metastasis most frequently occurs in the vertebrae and results in pathologic fracture.

Clinical Manifestations

1. Pain in the involved bone—from effects of tumor (destruction, erosion, and expansion of tumor).
   a. Generally mild to constant pain, which may be worse at night or with activity.
   b. Pain will be acute with fracture.
   c. Neurologic symptoms may present with nerve root compression.
2. Swelling and limitation of motion and joint effusion.
3. Physical findings.
   a. Palpable, tender, fixed bony mass.
   b. Increase in skin temperature over mass.
   c. Superficial veins dilated and prominent.

Diagnostic Evaluation

1. X-ray will usually reveal bone tumor; may show increased or decreased bone density. Tomograms may be helpful for some benign osseous lesions.
2. CT and MRI demonstrate soft tissue involvement and location of tumors.

3. Bone scan—helpful in detecting initial extent of malignancy, planning therapy, defining level of amputation, and following course of radiation or chemotherapy.
4. Ultrasound may help with identification of the lesion.
5. Serum alkaline phosphatase—usually increased.
6. Bence Jones protein in urine with multiple myeloma.
7. Biopsy of bone—to confirm suspected diagnosis.
8. Chest x-ray and lung scan—to determine if metastasis is present.
9. Arteriography—to assess soft tissue involvement.

Management

A multidisciplinary approach in a cancer center is usually preferred. The basic objective is to halt the progression of the tumor by destroying or removing the lesion. Treatment depends on the type of tumor. Combinations of chemotherapy, surgery, and radiation may be indicated as most appropriate for specific type of tumor.

Surgery

1. Tumor curettage or resection with bone grafting may be used.
2. Limb-salvaging procedures involve resection of affected bone and surrounding normal muscle tissue and reconstruction using metallic prostheses or allografts for bone or joint replacement and skin grafting, as needed.
3. Amputation is necessary in some cases.

Chemotherapy

May be used as preoperative, adjunctive, and palliative treatment.

1. Chemotherapy may be administered before (to shrink the tumor) and after (to destroy metastasis) surgery.
2. Chemotherapy used in combination to achieve a greater patient response at a lower toxicity rate and to minimize potential problems of drug resistance and may be given in varying courses separated by rest periods.

Radiotherapy

1. Tumor irradiation may be used.
2. Prophylactic lung irradiation may be performed—to suppress metastasis.

Other Therapies

1. Immunotherapy—interferon.
2. Hormone therapy may be used with metastatic tumors of the breast and prostate.
3. If pathologic fracture occurs, the fracture is managed with open reduction and internal fixation or other fracture treatment method.

Complications

1. Lack of tumor control and metastases.
2. Pathologic fracture.
3. Hypercalcemia from bone destruction.

Nursing Assessment

1. Obtain history of progression of disease; presence of pain, fever, weight loss, malaise.
2. Examine for painless mass.
3. Review records for evidence of pathologic fracture.
4. Assess knowledge of cancer, experiences with family or others, and present coping.

Nursing Interventions

See also "Orthopedic Surgery" section, page 854, and "Amputation" section, page 858.

Relieving Pain

1. Use multiple approaches to reduce discomfort (see page 1505).
2. Administer pain medications 30 minutes before ambulation or other uncomfortable movement.
3. Support painful extremities on pillows.

Preventing Pathologic Fractures

1. Assist the patient in movement with gentleness and patience.
2. Avoid jarring the patient or bed.
3. Support joints when repositioning the patient.
4. Guard the patient to avoid falls.
5. Create a hazard-free environment.
6. Provide patient education on safety.

Strengthening Coping Ability

1. Create a supportive environment.
2. Use psychological support services, as needed.
3. Answer questions and clear up misconceptions about treatment options.

Patient Education and Health Maintenance

1. Teach about particular treatment selected. See page 77 for information on chemotherapy and page 122 for radiation therapy information.
2. Encourage appropriate follow-up and diagnostic testing for recurrence.
3. Refer for additional information and support to the American Cancer Society *(www.cancer.org)*.

Evaluation: Expected Outcomes

- Reports decreased pain with ambulation.
- No signs or symptoms of fractures.
- Verbalizes understanding of treatment options and strength to make decisions.

Osteomyelitis

Osteomyelitis is a severe pyogenic infection of the bone and surrounding tissues, which requires immediate treatment.

Pathophysiology and Etiology

1. Generally, bacteria gain entry to the bone via three routes:
   a. Bloodstream (hematogenous spread).
   b. Adjacent soft tissue infection (contiguous focus).
   c. Direct introduction of microorganisms into the bone.
2. Bacteria lodge and multiply in bone.
3. Pressure increases as pus collects in confined rigid bone, contributing to ischemia and vascular occlusion and leading to bone necrosis.
4. *Staphylococcus aureus* is the most common infecting microorganism, although others are prevalent: *Escherichia coli*, *Pseudomonas*, *Klebsiella*, *Salmonella*, and *Proteus*.

Clinical Manifestations

1. Infection of long bones with acute pain and signs of sepsis.
2. Localized pain and drainage.
3. Symptoms vary in adults and children according to the site of involvement.

Diagnostic Evaluation

1. Acute osteomyelitis diagnosis made on initial clinical signs (history, physical examination, complete blood count [CBC], erythrocyte sedimentation rate [ESR]).

2. Aerobic and anaerobic cultures of bone and deep tissue to identify the organism. Wound cultures are not reliable.
3. ESR elevated, white blood cell (WBC) and hemoglobin decreased.
4. Radiographic evidence of osteomyelitis lags behind symptoms by up to 14 days.
5. Radionuclide bone scans used to diagnose early acute osteomyelitis.
6. MRI used increasingly—distinguishes between soft tissue and bone marrow. Bone marrow edema is the earliest feature of acute osteomyelitis seen on MRI and can be detected as early as 1 to 2 days after the onset of infection.

Management

1. Acute: full recovery possible with minimal loss of function.
2. Chronic: develops with inadequate or ineffective course of antibiotics or delayed treatment.

Surgical Intervention

1. Needle aspiration or needle biopsy done initially.
2. Surgical intervention may be needed to obtain culture and sensitivity of specimen.
3. Surgical decompression considered when the patient does not improve after 36 to 48 hours of antimicrobial therapy.
4. Debridement may be done or antibiotic-impregnated beads used in wound (removed after 2 to 4 weeks and replaced with bone graft).
5. Hyperbaric oxygen therapy may be used as an adjunctive therapy.

Pharmacologic Intervention

1. Employ quickly after presentation of symptoms to avoid chronicity.
2. Parenteral antimicrobial therapy based on blood/wound cultures.
3. Medications depend on organism but include the following:
   a. Penicillins (penicillin G, penicillin V).
   b. Semisynthetic penicillins (nafcillin, oxacillin, methicillin).
   c. Extended-spectrum penicillins (ampicillin, carbenicillin, amoxicillin).
   d. Beta-lactam agents (imipenem).
   e. Tetracyclines.
   f. Cephalosporins.
   g. Aminoglycosides.
4. Requires 6 to 8 weeks of intravenous (IV) antibiotic therapy, requiring a peripherally inserted central catheter line or other long-term access device and coordination of home care services.

Complications

1. Nonhealing wound.
2. Sepsis.
3. Immobility.
4. Amputation.

Nursing Assessment

1. Obtain detailed history of injury.
2. Assess pain and functional deficits.
3. Be aware that systemic symptoms are acute in children but of varied intensity in adults.
4. Perform general systemic assessment because adults with long bone involvement generally have more systemic septic symptoms.

Nursing Interventions

Relieving Pain

1. Administer opioids for acute pain, nonopioids for chronic pain.
2. Administer medications around the clock versus as necessary to establish a consistent blood level.
3. Report any increase in pain that may indicate worsening infection.

Increasing Knowledge

1. Describe the infectious process and rationale for prolonged treatment with osteomyelitis.
2. Explain IV antibiotic therapy, potential adverse effects, and reactions.
3. Explain strict adherence to infection control practices (sterile technique, handwashing, selection of roommate) to prevent spread of infection in some cases.
4. Initiate home care nursing and infusion service referrals before discharge.

Promoting Rest Without Complications

1. Support the affected extremity (splint, traction) to minimize pain.
2. If the patient is on bed rest, prevent hazards of immobility (passive ROM, position changes, coughing, and deep breathing).
3. Encourage distraction activities.

Patient Education and Health Maintenance

1. Advise the patient to adhere to infection control principles—proper handwashing, disposal of wound drainage, dressings to prevent reinfection or transmission of infection at home.
2. Stress adherence to medication regimen, which may be prolonged, with frequent follow-up visits.
3. Teach care of indwelling device for medication delivery.
4. Educate the patient on signs and symptoms of infection to monitor for and when to notify provider.

Evaluation: Expected Outcomes

- Pain managed with nonopioid analgesics.
- Infectious process minimized.
- Functional status of affected joint intact.

Paget Disease (Osteitis Deformans)

Paget disease of the bone is a skeletal disorder resulting from excessive osteoclastic activity, affecting the long bones, pelvis, lumbar vertebrae, and the skull predominantly.

Pathophysiology and Etiology

1. The cause of this disease is unknown, although there is evidence of familial tendency (25% to 40% have at least one affected relative).
2. More common in males than in females.
3. Rare before age 40 and increases as age does—12% after age 80.
4. May be caused by infection from blood-borne viruses. After acute viremia, osteoclasts become chronically infected, stimulating osteoclastic proliferation. See Figure 28-13.

Clinical Manifestations

1. Generally asymptomatic.
2. Most common symptoms are pain and predisposition to fracture.

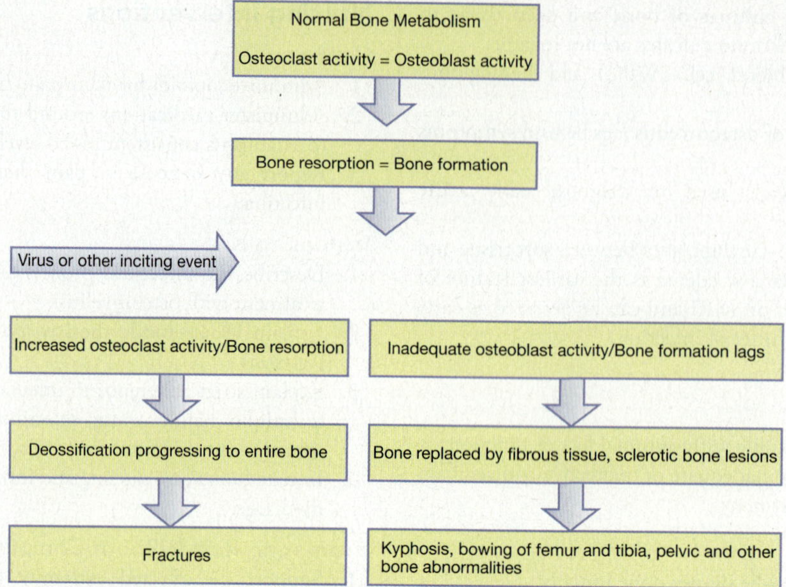

Figure 28-13. Pathophysiology of Paget disease.

3. Pagetic lesions can lead to OA, joint destruction, spinal deformity.
4. Decrease in hearing, tinnitus, and vertigo as a result of skull abnormality.
5. Waddling gait due to abnormality of pelvis.
6. Radiculopathy and nerve palsies due to effects from the vertebral column.
7. Rarely, heart failure and other cardiovascular effects from increased blood supply over abnormal bone.
8. Malignant bone tumors occur in 5% to 10%.

Diagnostic Evaluation

1. Elevated serum alkaline phosphatase and urine hydroxyproline.
2. Serum calcium, phosphorus, and albumin levels usually normal.
3. Generally confirmed with radiologic examinations showing characteristic abnormalities.
4. Bone scans can evaluate rapid bone turnover.
5. Bone biopsy to differentiate from osteomyelitis or bone tumor.

Management

1. No treatment for asymptomatic Paget.
2. Pain management—NSAIDs, aspirin.
3. Medications—calcitonin is the main medication used to suppress bone turnover, reduce pain, and prevent progression.
4. Other medications used to block bone resorption—the bisphosphonates etidronate disodium, alendronate, pamidronate, risedronate; an antineoplastic agent, plicamycin.
5. Tibial osteotomy done to realign knees and relieve pain.

Nursing Assessment

1. Assess pain and functional ability.
2. Observe for bowing (legs) or complaint that hats feel tight.
3. Assess for cardiovascular complications.
4. Assess for auditory symptoms—tinnitus, vertigo, and hearing loss.

Nursing Interventions

Reducing Pain

1. Administer and teach self-administration of analgesics.
2. Avoid sedation due to opioids, which may increase risk of falls.

Preventing Injury

1. Establish exercise protocols through a PT consult to maintain physical abilities and prevent falls.
2. Teach safe transferring, and make sure that the patient can alert nurses if they need help.
3. Assist the patient with activities, as necessary.
4. Provide function and mobility aids such as heel lifts, walking aids, as needed, through an OT consult.

Patient Education and Health Maintenance

1. Teach safety measures in the home—removal of loose rugs and obstacles to prevent falls, good lighting.
2. Provide education about the disease process and medication treatment.
3. Make sure that the patient knows how to use mobility aids.
4. Initiate home care referral, as indicated.
5. Advise the patient that laboratory testing to monitor serum calcium, phosphorous, vitamin D, and kidney function may be ordered.
6. Encourage follow-up for periodic hearing tests and blood work.

Evaluation: Expected Outcomes

- The patient reports reduced pain scale score
- No falls

Hallux Valgus

Also called *bunion, hallux valgus* is a deformity of the foot involving the first metatarsal and great toe. Occurs in females more frequently than in males, and incidence increases with age; may have a genetic predisposition. Commonly occurs with other deformities of the feet, such as hammertoe, mallet toe, and claw toe.

Clinical Manifestations

1. Pain.
2. Possible callus of skin overlying bunion and accompanying toe deformities.
3. Diminished ROM.
4. Generally associated with tight footwear.

Management and Nursing Interventions

Conservative Management

1. Wearing footwear made of soft material with a wider toe box, rounded rather than pointed, and with low heel.
2. Special orthoses can be ordered.
3. Steroid injections to relieve pain.

Surgical Management

Surgical alignment of the great toe by osteotomy of metatarsal or proximal phalanx of the great toe or fusion of the metatarsal–metatarsophalangeal joint.

Postoperative Care

1. Elevation of the foot to reduce pain.
2. Initial non–weight-bearing activity, with very gradual progress in activity.
3. Crutch walking initially, followed by wooden shoe immobilizer for several weeks.
4. NSAIDs and opioid analgesics for pain.
5. Bandages changed by the surgeon initially.

SELECTED READINGS

Alnawafleh, K. A., Abozead, S. E., Khalil, S. S., Elkhalik, E. F.A., Taha, S. H., Alabdallah, E., & Mohammad, W. T. (2023). The Autar deep venous thrombosis risk assessment among orthopedic surgeries' patients. *Journal of Pharmaceutical Negative Results, 14*(2), 55–66. https://doi.org/10.47750/pnr.2023.14.02.008

American Academy of Orthopaedic Surgeons. (2017). *Management of osteoarthritis of the hip evidence-based clinical practice guideline.* Author.

American Academy of Orthopaedic Surgeons. (2021). *Management of hip fractures in older adults: Evidence-based clinical practice guideline.* Author. https://www.aaos.org/globalassets/quality-and-practice-resources/hip-fractures-in-the-elderly/hipfxcpg.pdf

American Academy of Orthopaedic Surgeons. (2022). *Management of anterior cruciate ligament injuries: Evidence-based clinical practice guideline.* Author. https://www.aaos.org/globalassets/quality-and-practice-resources/anterior-cruciate-ligament-injuries/aclcpg.pdf

Anheyer, D., Heidmarie, H., Romy, L., Gustay, D., & Cramer, H. (2022). Yoga for treating low back pain: A systematic review and meta-analysis. *Pain, 162(4)*, e504–e517. https://doi.org/10.1097/*j.pain*.0000000000002416

Fontani, V., Rinaldi, A., Castagna, A., & Rinaldi, S. (2022). Calcific tendinitis of the shoulder: A neuro-psychomotor behavioral diagnostic and therapeutic approach with radioelectric asymmetric conveyer neurobiological stimulation treatments. *Cureus, 14*(7), e26770. https://doi.org/10.7759/cureus.26770

Fullen, B., Morlion, B., Linton, S. J., Roomes, D., van Griensven, J., Abraham, L., Beck, C., Wilhelm, S., Constantinescu, C., & Perrot, S. (2022). Management of chronic low back pain and the impact on patients' personal and professional lives: Results from an international patient survey. *Pain Practice, 22*(4), 463–477. https://doi.org/10.1111/papr.13103

Guo, J., Zhao, X., & Xu, C. (2022). Effects of a continuous nursing care model on elderly patients with total hip arthroplasty: A randomized controlled trial. *Aging Clinical and Experimental Research, 34*(7), 1603–1611. https://doi.org/10.1007/s40520-021-01965-1

Gwynne-Jones, D., Martin, G., & Crane, C. (2017). Enhanced recovery after surgery for hip and knee replacements. *Orthopaedic Nursing, 36*(3), 203–210. https://doi.org/10.1097/NOR.0000000000000351

Morrison, C., Brown, B., Lin, D. Y., Jaarsma, R., & Kroon, H. (2021). Analgesia and anesthesia using the pericapsular nerve group block in hip surgery and hip fracture: A scoping review. *Regional Anesthesia & Pain Medicine, 46*(2), 169–175. https://doi.org/10.1136/rapm-2020-101826

National Association of Orthopaedic Nurses. (2013). *Acute pain management algorithms for the adult orthopaedic patient.* Author.

National Association of Orthopaedic Nurses. (2013). *Clinical practice guideline for surgical site infection prevention.* Author.

National Association of Orthopaedic Nurses. (2015). *Clinical practice guideline for thromboembolic disease prevention.* Author.

National Association of Orthopaedic Nurses. (2016). *Safe patient handling and mobility algorithms for the adult orthopaedic patient.* Author.

National Association of Orthopaedic Nurses. (2018). *An introduction to orthopaedic nursing* (5th ed.). Author.

National Institute for Health and Clinical Excellence. (2020). *Osteoarthritis: Care and management.* Author.

Powell-Cope, G., Thomason, S., Bulat, T., Pippins, K. M., & Young, H. M. (2018). Preventing falls and fall-related injuries at home. *American Journal of Nursing, 118*(1), 58–61. https://doi.org/10.1097/01.NAJ.0000529720.67793.60

Prah, A., Richards, E., Griggs, R., & Simpson, V. (2017). Enhancing osteoporosis efforts through lifestyle modifications and goal-setting techniques. *Journal for Nurse Practitioners, 13*(8), 552–561. https://doi.org/10.1016/j.nurpra.2017.07.015

Slaughter, A., Reynolds, K. A., Jambhekar, K., David, R. M., Hasan, S. A., & Pandey, T. (2014). Clinical orthopedic examination findings in the lower extremity: Correlation with imaging studies and diagnostic efficacy. *RadioGraphics, 34*(2), e41–e55. https://doi.org/10.1148/rg.342125066

Walter, N., Rupp, M., Olesen, U. K., & Alt, V. (2022). Which pin site dressing is the most optimal? A systematic review on current evidence. *Journal of Limb Lengthening & Reconstruction, 8*(Suppl. 1), S36–S43. https://doi.org/10.4103/jllr.jllr_29_21

Zhang, W., Huang, X., & Huang, T. (2023). Individualized management of quality of care in orthopedic nurses based on sensitive indicators. *Computational and Mathematical Methods in Medicine.* https://doi.org/10.1155/2023/1950220

UNIT

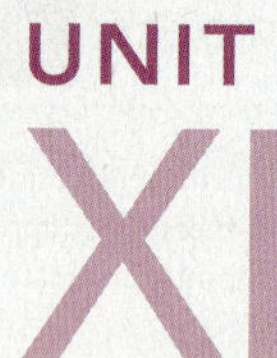

INTEGUMENTARY HEALTH

29 Dermatologic Disorders*

OVERVIEW AND ASSESSMENT

Description of Skin Lesions

The description of dermatologic conditions always includes the morphology of the lesions that appear on the skin (i.e., their size, shape, color, pattern, and distribution; see Figure 29-1).

Primary Lesions

1. Macule—flat, circumscribed discoloration of the skin; may have any size or shape.
2. Papule—solid, elevated lesion less than 1 cm wide.
3. Nodule—raised, solid lesion larger than 1 cm wide.
4. Vesicle—circumscribed elevated lesion less than 0.5 cm, containing fluid.
5. Bulla—a vesicle or blister larger than 0.5 cm wide.
6. Pustule—circumscribed raised lesion that contains pus; may form as a result of purulent changes in a vesicle.
7. Wheal—elevation of the skin that lasts less than 24 hours, caused by edema of the dermis; may be surrounded by erythema or blanching.
8. Plaque—solid, elevated lesion on the skin or mucous membrane, larger than 1 cm in diameter; psoriasis is commonly manifested as plaques on the skin; leukoplakia is an example of plaques on mucous membranes.
9. Cyst—soft or firm mass in the skin, filled with semisolid or with liquid material contained in a sac.

Secondary Lesions

Secondary lesions involve changes that take place in primary lesions that modify them.

1. Scale—heaped-up, horny layer of dead epidermis; may develop as a result of inflammatory changes.
2. Crust—covering formed by the drying of serum, blood, or pus on the skin (scab).
3. Excoriation—linear scratch marks or traumatized areas of the skin.
4. Fissure—linear cracks in the skin, usually from marked drying and long-standing inflammation.
5. Ulcer—lesion formed by local destruction of the epidermis and part or all of the underlying dermis.
6. Lichenification—thickening of the skin accompanied by accentuation of skin markings.
7. Scar/keloid—abnormal new formation of connective tissue that replaces the loss of substance in the dermis as a result of injury or disease. A keloid is a hypertrophic scar that is larger than the original lesion or injury.
8. Atrophy—diminution in size or in loss of skin cells that causes thinning of the skin.

Other Lesions

1. Petechiae—circumscribed deposits of blood or blood pigment 1 to 2 mm wide.
2. Purpura—circumscribed deposits of blood or blood pigment greater than 0.5 cm wide.

*Please note that the term "male" in this chapter refers to a person assigned male at birth, and the term "female" in this chapter refers to a person assigned female at birth.

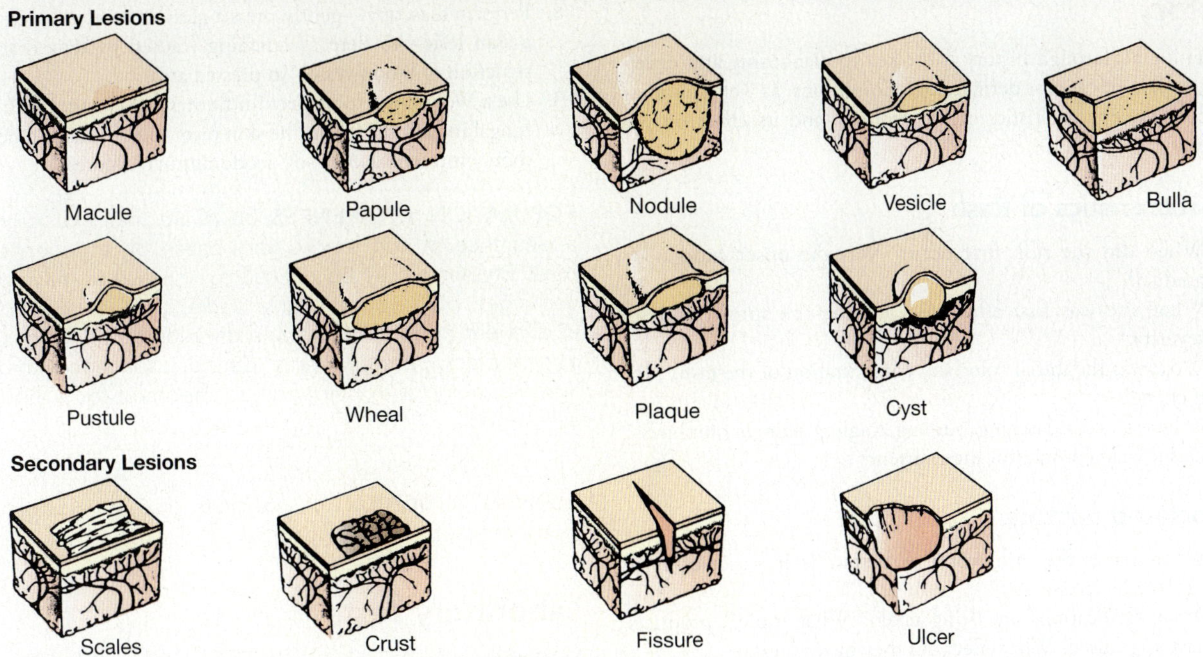

Figure 29-1. Types of skin lesions. (Reprinted with permission from Smeltzer, S., & Bare, B. [2000]. *Brunner and Suddarth's textbook of medical-surgical nursing* [9th ed.]. Lippincott Williams & Wilkins.)

3. Comedones—hair follicle obstructed by a sebum and keratin plug; blackheads and whiteheads.
4. Telangiectasia—small, irregular blood vessels visible in the epidermis.
5. Burrow—linear, irregular, elevated tunnel produced by parasites in the skin.

Shape and Configuration

After the type of lesion is identified, the shape, configuration or arrangement (in relation to each other), and pattern of distribution are noted (see Figure 29-2). The following are descriptions commonly used:

1. Annular—ring shaped.
2. Circinate—circular.
3. Confluent—lesions run together or join.
4. Discoid—disk shaped.
5. Discrete—lesions remain separate.
6. Generalized—widespread eruption.
7. Grouped—clustering of lesions.
8. Guttate—droplike.
9. Herpetiform—grouped vesicles.
10. Iris—ring or a series of concentric circles (bull's eye).
11. Linear—in lines.
12. Nummular—coin-shaped.
13. Polymorphous—occurring in several or many forms.
14. Reticulated—lacelike network.
15. Serpiginous—snakelike or creeping eruption.
16. Telangiectatic—a tiny red, purple, or dark thread or line.
17. Zosteriform or dermatomal—bandlike distribution, limited to one or more dermatomes of the skin.

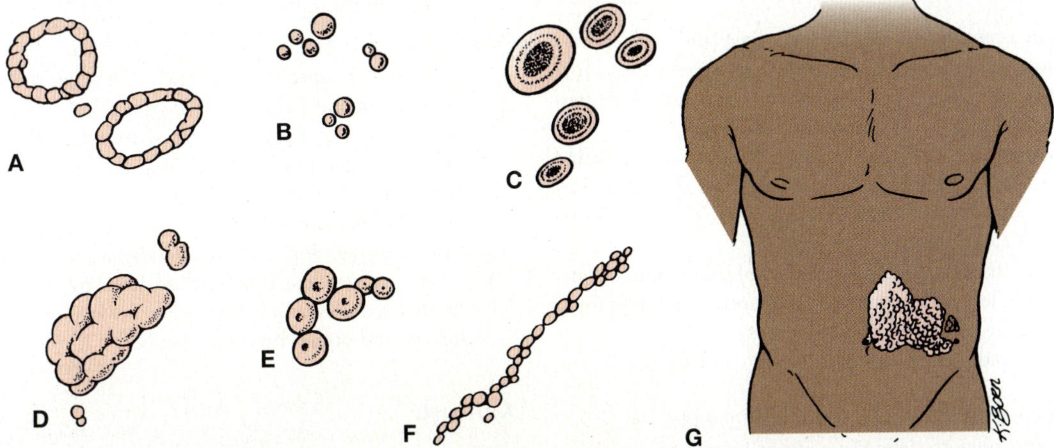

Figure 29-2. Shape and arrangement of skin lesions: **(A)** annular, **(B)** grouped, **(C)** iris, **(D)** confluent, **(E)** herpetiform, **(F)** linear, and **(G)** zosteriform or dermatomal.

History

Obtaining a thorough history is the key to diagnosing and developing a plan of care for dermatologic conditions, as well as understanding the characteristics of the problem and its effect on the patient.

Characteristics of Rash

1. When did the rash first occur? Was the onset sudden or gradual?
2. What site was first affected? Describe the spread and its severity.
3. What was the initial color and configuration of the rash? Has it changed?
4. Is there associated itching, burning, tingling, pain, or numbness?
5. Has it been constant or intermittent?

Associated Factors

1. What makes the rash worse or better? Is it seasonal? Is it affected by stress?
2. What medications are being taken? What topical products have been used? What effect did they have?
3. What skin products are used? What chemicals have come into contact with the skin: such as laundry detergent, cleaning products, insecticides, or nickel?
4. Has there been pet contact?
5. What is the patient's occupation? Any hobbies, such as gardening or hiking, that may have contributed? Are latex gloves worn routinely? Is frequent handwashing required?
6. What is the sexual history and chance of sexually transmitted disease exposure (if relevant)?
7. Any international travel?

Medical History

1. Is there a history of hay fever, asthma, hives, eczema, or allergies?
2. Has the patient had this particular rash or other skin disorders in the past?
3. What is the family history of skin disorders?
4. Are there any long-standing medical problems? Immunosuppressive therapy?

Physical Examination

1. Focus your examination on the skin, hair, and nails. Many dermatologic conditions involve other body systems (e.g., hair loss may be associated with thyroid disease or anemia); perform a general physical examination as necessary.
2. Ask the patient to show you the area of concern and examine the skin surface under good lighting. Patients should be undressed, in a gown, and the skin of the total body should be examined, not just the area affected.
3. Note the distribution and configuration of skin lesions. Compare right and left sides of the body and areas distal, proximal, adjacent and distant to the affected area(s).
4. Inspect the color, shape, border, texture, and surface of the lesions.
5. Palpate the lesions for texture, warmth, and tenderness.
6. Use a metric ruler to determine size of lesions to serve as a baseline for comparison with subsequent measurements.
7. Examine the scalp, nails, lymph nodes, and oral mucosa.
8. Perform diascopy—gently press a glass slide or clear ruler over a skin lesion to detect blanching (caused by temporary obstruction of blood vessels to pressed area).
9. Use a Wood light to inspect for fluorescent changes with some fungal infections. Clean the skin prior to examination because some ointments, soaps, or deodorant may fluoresce.

POPULATION AWARENESS Be aware that the color and appearance of skin lesions vary based on a patient's skin tone. Erythema may be difficult to visualize or may appear very light, black, purple, or a darker than usual skin tone in different people. Brown and discolored skin lesions may appear black, purple, or gray. Careful inspection with direct lighting, along with palpation, is important for a thorough assessment.

CLINICAL JUDGMENT If infectious disease is suspected, follow precautions as indicated.

Laboratory Tests

Some dermatologic conditions can be evaluated by laboratory tests such as microscopy and culture.

Microscopy

Description

1. Sample taken by scraping, swabbing, or aspirating a lesion is transferred to a glass slide for microscopic examination or staining.
   a. Direct visualization of scrapings mixed with mineral oil to detect scabies, mites, or lice nits that cling to the hair.
   b. A Tzanck smear is obtained from vesicular fluid or a moist ulcer and stained to detect characteristics of herpes simplex virus, herpes zoster, and varicella; however, this is not as reliable as other tests due to its low sensitivity for detecting the virus.
   c. Potassium hydroxide may be added to skin scrapings on a glass slide and heated to dissolve skin cells to detect hyphae and spores in fungal infections.
   d. Gram stain may be performed by the laboratory or dermatopathologist to tentatively identify bacteria or fungi in certain skin infections.

Nursing and Patient Care Considerations

1. To obtain the specimen for microscopy, use the side of a glass slide or a scalpel held at a 45-degree angle to gently scrape the active border of a dry lesion or of an inflamed area; only mild discomfort and pinpoint bleeding should occur.
2. For moist or semimoist ulcerations or crusted lesions, roll normal saline–soaked cotton or Dacron-tipped swab over the lesion; for weeping lesions, use a dry swab.
3. For intact vesicles, aspirate fluid from the edge with a 25-G sterile needle; if vesicle is partially broken, gently unroof with forceps and obtain fluid on a swab.

Culture

Description

1. Drainage from lesions may be cultured on specific media to detect causative organism and sensitivity to antimicrobial

therapy; also, portions of the skin, hair, and nails may be submitted for fungal culture.
2. Usually takes 24 to 48 hours for results; fungal cultures may take 4 to 5 weeks.

Nursing and Patient Care Considerations

1. Obtain specimen with cotton- or Dacron-tipped swab and send to laboratory in bacterial culture container clearly labeled, with the patient's name, the date, and the site where the specimen was obtained, or in a viral culture container also clearly labeled. Refrigerate viral culture if laboratory pickup is delayed.
2. To obtain specimen for fungal culture, scrape or clip the affected skin, hair, or nails; then, place into a dry, sterile container for transport or onto a dermatophyte test medium.

Other Tests

Patch Testing

Description

1. *Patch testing* is an office procedure done to determine if patients are sensitive to contact materials.
2. Materials are applied in patches to the skin and checked for reaction 48 hours after application and possibly again in 1 week.
3. Erythema, itching, swelling, papules, and vesicles indicate an allergic contact dermatitis rather than an irritant contact dermatitis or no reaction.

Nursing and Patient Care Considerations

1. Confirm that patient has been off oral corticosteroids and antihistamines at the time of the test; topical corticosteroids should be discontinued 1 to 2 weeks before testing to prevent a weak reaction or false-negative results. Make sure the patient has followed the health care provider's instructions.
2. When patient returns in 48 hours for the first reading, mark the outline of the patch strip on the patient's back; then, remove the strip. A skin marker or an ultraviolet skin pen marker may be used.
3. Wait 30 minutes; then, do the first reading. Document based on the outcome as follows or take a picture for the patient's record:
   a. 1+ Weak reaction. Nonvesicular, but with erythema, induration, and possible papules.
   b. 2+ Strong reaction. Edematous and vesicular, with erythema, edema, papules, and vesicles.
   c. 3+ Extreme reaction. Spreading, bullous, ulcerative irritant reaction (IR).
   d. Negative reaction.

GENERAL PROCEDURES AND TREATMENT MODALITIES

Baths and Wet Dressings

A therapeutic bath is used to apply medication to the entire skin surface and is useful in treating widespread eruptions and general pruritus. Baths soothe, soften, and reduce inflammation and relieve itching and dryness. Wet dressings and soaks are damp compresses that contain water, normal saline solution, aluminum acetate (Burow) solution, or magnesium sulfate solution. They may be sterile or clean, or warm or cool, depending on the skin condition and the area to which they are applied.

Therapeutic Baths

Indications

1. Vesicular disorders, eczema, atopic dermatitis.
2. Acute inflammatory conditions.
3. Erosions and exudative, crusted surfaces.

Nursing and Patient Care Considerations

1. Prepare the bath or teach patient to prepare a lukewarm bath at 90°F to 100°F (32.2°C to 37.8°C); with the tub half-full, add the prescribed quantity of medication and mix thoroughly to prevent sensitivity reaction. Add oatmeal products or oils to emulsifying baths.
   a. Bleach baths may be used for acute and chronic atopic dermatitis.
   b. Add ½ cup of bleach to full tub or ¼ cup to half tub of warm water and soak limbs and torso for 5 to 10 minutes (do not submerge head).
2. Do not rub the skin. Soaking for at least 5 to 10 minutes will promote removal of loosened scales.
3. Keep the room and water at comfortable temperature and humidity level.
4. Tell patient to use a bath mat inside the tub and to use a rug outside the tub when bathing at home because medication may make the tub and other wet surfaces slippery.
5. Blot skin dry with a towel and apply emollient or topical medication to moist skin within 3 minutes. While the skin is wet, apply prescribed steroid to inflamed areas, followed by emollient.

Open Wet Dressings

Indications

1. Bacterial infections that require drainage.
2. Inflammatory and pruritic conditions.
3. Oozing and crusting conditions.

Nursing and Patient Care Considerations

1. Apply dressing to affected area or teach patient to apply. Moisten to the point of slight dripping; remoisten as necessary.
2. Use warm tap water if warming is desired.
3. Application may be from 5 to 15 minutes, three to four times per day, unless otherwise indicated.
4. Keep patient warm and do not treat more than one-third of the body at a time because open wet dressings can cause chilling and hypothermia.
5. Teach patients to prevent burns by measuring the temperature of solution with a bath thermometer or by testing tap water on the wrist before applying compress. Advise them not to use microwave ovens to warm dressings because uneven heating and overheating can occur.

Other Dressings

Occlusive Dressing

An *occlusive dressing* is formed by an airtight plastic or vinyl film applied over medicated areas of the skin (usually with corticosteroids) to enhance absorption of medication and to promote moisture retention.

Indications

Skin conditions with thick scaling, such as psoriasis, eczema, and lichen simplex chronicus.

Nursing and Patient Care Considerations

1. Wash area and pat dry.
2. Apply medication while the skin is still moist.
3. Cover with plastic wrap, vinyl gloves, or plastic bag.
4. Seal with paper tape at edges or cover with other self-adhesive dressings to hold in place.
5. Do not apply to ulcerated or abraded skin; removal is recommended within 12 to 24 hours. High-potency steroids are for short-term use only.

DRUG ALERT Excessive use of occlusive dressings that contain corticosteroids may cause skin atrophy, striae, telangiectasia, folliculitis, nonhealing ulceration, erythema, and systemic absorption of corticosteroids.

Nonocclusive Dressings

Other dressing materials may be used as dry dressings to protect the skin, keep affected areas clean, absorb drainage, cover medication, or hold occlusive dressings in place.

Nursing and Patient Care Considerations

1. Apply dry gauze dressing using clean technique (unless sterile technique is indicated by open wounds).
2. Wrap extremities with elastic or cotton-rolled bandages or apply tape. Avoid constricting circulation.
3. Alternative dressing materials can be used for home care, such as disposable or white cotton gloves for the hands, cotton socks for the feet, sheets or towels for large areas, disposable diapers or towels folded in diaper fashion for the groin, washcloths for the axilla, cotton T-shirt or cotton pajamas for the trunk, turban or plastic shower cap for the scalp, or mask made from gauze for the face, with holes cut for the eyes, mouth, and nose.

Skin Biopsy

Removal of a piece of the skin by shave, punch, or excision technique to detect malignancy or other characteristics of skin disorders.

Types of Biopsy

1. Shave biopsy—scalpel used to remove raised lesions, leaving lower layers of the dermis intact.
2. Punch biopsy—special instrument used to remove round core of lesion, containing all layers of the skin. Biopsy site is usually closed with sutures.
3. Excisional biopsy—scalpel and scissors used to remove the entire lesion, usually with prescribed margins; suturing required.

Nursing and Patient Care Considerations

1. Position patient comfortably with the site exposed; explain that a local anesthetic will be given.
2. Check if patient has any known allergies to local anesthetics.
3. Ask patient what current medication they are taking. Aspirin, some herbal supplements, or anticoagulants may cause increased postoperative bleeding.
4. Explain the procedure.
5. Obtain written consent.
6. After the biopsy, apply hemostatic agent and pressure to the site to stop bleeding, along with an appropriate dressing. Pressure dressing may be required for larger wounds or wounds that are bleeding.
7. Place the biopsy specimen in a clearly labeled container containing 10% formaldehyde. Transport the container to the dermatopathology laboratory for hematoxylin and eosin staining. It is essential that skin biopsies are sent to a specialized dermatopathology laboratory for examination by a dermatopathologist. This ensures the best analysis and provides the most complete information on the histology of the skin disease or lesion.

Patient Education

1. Keep the bandage on the surgery site for 24 to 48 hours. During this time, ensure the site remains clean and dry.
2. After this period, remove the bandage and perform the following steps daily:
   a. Wash the incision with soap and water.
   b. Dry the incision well.
   c. Apply petroleum- or mineral oil–based ointment, such as Vaseline or Aquaphor, one to four times per day to keep the incision moist at all times.
3. After a few days, the dressing is no longer needed, but continue applying ointment one to four times per day to keep the site moist and help reduce scarring.
4. Do not apply makeup directly to the stitches.
5. Repeat wound care for 2 or 3 days after stitches have been removed, unless otherwise instructed.
6. Use caution when shaving around stitches on the face.

DRUG ALERT Many patients are allergic to neomycin, which is a component of Neosporin and triple antibiotic ointment. Petrolatum- or mineral oil–based ointments pose less risk of allergic dermatitis.

Wound Coverage: Grafts and Flaps

Wound coverage, using grafts and flaps, is a type of reconstructive (plastic) surgery performed to improve the skin's appearance and function. These are sometimes used following Mohs micrographic surgery to remove skin cancers, especially on the face, head, and neck.

Skin Graft

1. A section of skin tissue is separated from its blood supply and transferred as free tissue to a distant (recipient) site; it must obtain nourishment from capillaries at the recipient site.
2. In dermatology, skin grafting is used to repair defects that result from excision of skin tumors and to cover areas of denuded skin.
3. Definitions.
   a. Autografts—grafts done with tissue transplanted from the patient's own skin.
   b. Allografts—involve the transplant of tissue from one individual of the same species; these grafts are also called allogenic or homografts.
   c. Xenograft or heterograft—involves the transfer of tissue from another species.
4. Classification by thickness.
   a. Split thickness (thin, intermediate, or thick)—graft that is cut at varying thicknesses and is used to cover large wounds because its total potential donor area is virtually unlimited.

b. Full thickness—graft consists of epidermis and all of the dermis without the underlying fat; used to cover wounds that are too large to close primarily. They are used frequently to cover facial defects because they provide a better contour match and less postoperative contracture.

Skin Flaps

1. A flap is a segment of tissue that has been left attached at one end (called a base or pedicle); the other end has been moved to a recipient area. It is dependent for its survival on functioning arterial and venous blood supplies and on lymphatic drainage in its pedicle or base.
   a. Free-flap or free-tissue transfer—one that is completely severed from the body and is transferred to another site; receives early vascular supply from microvascular anastomosis with vessels at recipient site.
2. Flaps may consist of the skin, mucosa, muscle, adipose tissue, and omentum.
3. Used for wound coverage and to provide bulk, especially when bone, tendon, blood vessels, or nerve tissue are exposed.
4. Flaps offer the best aesthetic solution because a flap retains the color, texture, and thickness match of the donor area.
5. Flaps are classified according to the method of movement, composition, location, or function.

Procedure for Skin Grafts

1. Split-thickness skin graft is obtained by razor blade, skin-grafting knife, or electric or air-powered dermatome or drum dermatome. Most commonly obtained from the inner aspect of the upper arm or outer thigh.
2. A full-thickness skin graft is primarily excised, defatted, and tailored to fit accurately over the defect area.
3. Skin is taken from the donor or host site and applied to the wound or defect site, called the recipient site or graft bed.
4. A bolster (pressure) dressing is applied to the graft to enhance the survival of the skin graft by providing stable approximation of the graft to the recipient bed.
5. The bolster dressing is left in place for 1 week. The process of revascularization and reattachment of the skin graft to the recipient bed is referred to as a take.
6. The donor site is maintained clean and dry.
   a. If Scarlet Red (a single-layer dressing impregnated with epithelial growth promoter) is used on the donor site for split-thickness grafts, it is left in place for 2 to 3 weeks to allow the wound to heal.
   b. Occlusive dressings, such as Omniderm or Allevyn, may also be used to decrease pain, alleviate frequent wound care, and speed healing.
   c. Daily wound care and dressing change with an antimicrobial ointment and nonstick dressing may also be used.

Preoperative Management and Nursing Care

1. Aspirin and nonsteroidal anti-inflammatory drugs (NSAIDs) and vitamin E are discontinued 14 days before the procedure. Coumadin should be held for several days before the procedure, and prothrombin time and international normalized ratio should be measured before the procedure, as ordered. Herbal supplements, such as ginkgo, ginseng, green tea, and vitamin E, can inhibit coagulation.
2. Efforts should be made to enhance wound healing several months to several weeks before the procedure, such as smoking cessation, alcohol avoidance, and proper nutrition.
3. Medical history and examination should include evaluation for latex sensitivity, cardiovascular problems requiring antibiotic prophylaxis for endocarditis, bleeding problems, and high blood pressure (BP).
4. The procedure is usually done under local anesthetic, so no meals are withheld.
5. The operative site should be free from makeup.
6. The patient should have someone available to drive them home after surgery, unless otherwise notified.

Postoperative Management and Nursing Care

Educate the patient with a skin graft on the following care:

1. Initial pressure dressing will be left in place for 24 to 48 hours.
2. If wound begins to ooze, apply firm pressure for 10 to 15 minutes (without peeking). If bleeding persists, contact surgeon.
3. Do not take aspirin or aspirin-containing medication for pain. May take one to two acetaminophen tablets every 4 to 6 hours, as needed.
4. Most skin grafts are held in place by a bolster dressing (cotton ball or foam). Do not remove the bolster dressing during the next week.
5. May clean site and apply ointment to the surrounding area of the bolster dressing.
6. Do not get the bolster dressing wet.
7. When the bolster dressing is removed, may shower, but *do not* let the water hit the graft directly.
8. Keep the graft edges moist with ointment.
9. Protect the graft from the sun. The sun will cause pigmentation changes in the graft. A sunscreen may be used in 2 to 3 weeks.
10. Skin grafts to the lower leg must be kept elevated because the new capillary connections are fragile and excess venous pressure may cause rupture. Keep leg elevated as much as possible during the next week.
11. Inspect the dressing daily. Report unusual drainage or signs of an inflammatory reaction.
12. After 2 to 3 weeks, any water-based moisturizer may be applied to the skin donor site for split-thickness skin grafts.
13. Expect some loss of sensation in the grafted area for a time.
14. Avoid strenuous exercise (jogging, lifting heavy objects). Anything that causes face flushing will raise BP, cause bleeding, and impair healing.

Aesthetic Procedures

Aesthetic procedures (cosmetic surgery) consist of reconstructive (plastic) surgery or the use of injected substances, which may be performed to reconstruct or to alter congenital or acquired defects or to restore or improve the body's appearance. Noninvasive procedures alter the skin surface through the use of light sources or chemical applications.

Types of Procedures

Rhytidectomy

1. Done through various techniques and incisions to alleviate skin folds and wrinkles to improve the appearance of the aging face (face-lift).

2. The correction can last as long as 10 years, but results vary with each individual. The skin relaxes with time and the muscles may also relax, but seldom does the face revert to its preoperative condition.
3. Surgical procedures include:
   a. Operative—standard incisions that are either temporal (hidden in hairline) or submental.
   b. Laser—several laser modalities are now used in facial plastic surgery, including radiofrequency tissue tightening, which causes collagen shrinkage and reduction of deep wrinkles and lines.

Blepharoplasty

1. Removes loose skin, muscle, and excess fat from upper or lower eyelids. It will not remove lines at the lateral corners of the eyes ("crow's feet").
2. The procedure is generally done by either scalpel under local or general anesthetic or by carbon dioxide laser.

Dermabrasion, Chemical Peel, Laser Resurfacing, and Fillers

1. Patients with weathered skin, fine wrinkles (especially at the corners of the eyes and along the vermilion border), or acne pitting and scarring may benefit from these procedures.
2. The use of laser technology allows for a more predictable result and eliminates the porcelain appearance resulting from such chemicals as trichloroacetic acid. There is less risk of hypopigmentation than with dermabrasion.
3. Chemical peels using tretinoin cream and alpha hydroxy acids result in the destruction of portions of the epidermis and dermis, with subsequent regeneration of new tissues.
4. New nonablative laser resurfacing is used for fine wrinkles, smoker lines, sun-damaged skin, and shallow acne scarring with minimal downtime.
5. Contraindications of laser resurfacing include:
   a. History of isotretinoin therapy 6 to 12 months prior to treatment.
   b. Status of postradiation or scleroderma.
   c. History of herpes simplex—requires perioperative treatment.
6. Hyperpigmentation can occur in persons with dark skin.
7. Purified botulinum toxin and fillers (collagen, hyaluronic acid, autologous fat) are used to correct deep wrinkles and facial hollows. Results may last 3 to 12 months.

Liposuction

1. Also called body contouring, liposuction reduces localized deposits of fat not amenable to weight loss with a cannula aided by suction or fitted to a syringe.
2. May be done on the face, neck, breasts, abdomen, flanks, hips, buttocks, and extremities.

Preoperative Management and Nursing Care

1. Local or general anesthetic will be administered. For local anesthetic, patient may eat and drink before surgery. For general anesthetic:
   a. Preoperative assessment may be necessary, depending on health status and patient's age.
   b. No eating or drinking for several hours before surgery.
   c. Patient should have escort and must be reminded not to drive home alone after surgery.
2. Review patient's allergies and medication before surgery.
3. Instruct patient to cleanse the skin with antiseptic agent the night before surgery, if prescribed.
4. Make sure patient thoroughly understands the procedure and has discussed the risks and benefits with the health care provider before surgery.
5. Make sure a consent form is signed before any procedure.
6. Make sure aspirin, warfarin, and NSAIDs have been discontinued for 2 weeks before surgery, unless otherwise indicated. Herbal supplements, such as ginkgo, ginseng, green tea, and vitamin E, can inhibit coagulation.
7. If applicable, instruct the patient to stop smoking for the 2 weeks leading up to rhytidectomy and to continue cessation for 2 weeks postprocedure and permanently, if possible.
8. Be aware of signs of topical lidocaine toxicity (if used)—drowsiness, tingling of lips, and metallic taste—which may lead to seizures.

Postoperative Management and Nursing Care

Rhytidectomy

1. Mild exercise can be resumed in 3 days postoperatively.
2. No strenuous exercise (that will increase the BP) for 1 month.
3. Dressings are usually removed on the first postoperative day. Elastic facial support garment is recommended for 1 to 3 weeks.
4. Eyelid sutures are removed in 3 to 5 days; facial sutures in 7 days.
5. Showering and gentle hair washing may begin on day 2 or 3.
6. The patient is to apply ointment (petroleum or a similar ointment) to all suture lines.
7. Stress to the patient not to remove crusts by "picking" at them along suture lines or scarring may result.
8. Elevate the head at night for 2 weeks after the procedure. Avoid bending and lifting, which may increase edema and provoke bleeding.
9. Expect the face or affected part to be swollen, bruised, and numb for several days to weeks.
10. Be aware that complications include bleeding and hematoma, sloughing of the skin, and possible facial nerve damage. Notify surgeon if the areas become increasingly red or swollen or if they become more tender or painful.

Blepharoplasty

1. Apply iced gauze compresses to eyes for 10 minutes four to six times per day to reduce edema after surgery.
2. Head of bed should be elevated to reduce internal pressure that might cause bleeding.
3. Avoid strenuous exercise for 1 week.
4. Bruising and swelling generally resolve in 2 weeks.
5. Watch for such complications as eyelid hematomas, ocular mobility dysfunction, and postsurgical ectropion (eversion of the edge of the eyelid).

Dermabrasion and Chemical Peel

1. Instruct patients to not pick at crusts because new epithelium will be injured; soak face several times per day and apply emollient, as directed. Crusts form in 2 to 3 days and start to separate by 7 to 10 weeks. Total separation can take up to 3 weeks.
2. Keep treated areas clean and moist.
3. Avoid sun on treated areas. Apply sunscreen with a minimum sun protection factor (SPF) of 30 when outdoors.
4. Manage bruising and swelling from injectables with ice packs.

Laser Resurfacing

1. Dressings, such as hydrogel dressings (see page 117), may be applied to the affected areas immediately and left in place for 24 to 48 hours.
2. Alternately, the open technique involves using petroleum gel and daily face washes with tepid water.

Liposuction

1. After liposuction, increased fluids are required.
2. Aspirin and NSAIDs should be avoided for at least 1 week to prevent bleeding.
3. Wear compression garment, as instructed.
4. Notify the surgeon if increased swelling develops; could indicate development of a seroma.
5. Expect blood-tinged fluids from cannula injection sites for 2 to 3 days.
6. Keep sutured areas moist with ointment, as instructed.
7. Avoid jarring exercise.
8. Complications include development of seromas, lumpiness in treated areas, excessive bruising.

CLINICAL JUDGMENT Advise all postoperative patients to notify health care provider if sudden pain, swelling, or bruising develops; these suggest hematoma or abscess. Do not take aspirin for postoperative discomfort; follow surgeon's orders.

DERMATOLOGIC DISORDERS

Dermatitis

Dermatitis and eczema are broad terms encompassing conditions that cause skin inflammation. The National Eczema Association characterizes seven different types: atopic, contact, dyshidrotic, neurodermatitis, nummular, seborrheic, and stasis. Complications and nursing implications for dermatitis-related disorders in general are presented here. The specific etiology, clinical manifestations, and management of each type are presented in Table 29-1. Diagnosis is generally based on history and clinical assessment, although skin biopsy may be undertaken to confirm diagnosis. Several sets of clinical diagnostic criteria have been set forth; the common criteria among them include pruritus, eczematous changes, xerosis, and personal or family history of atopy.

EVIDENCE BASE Reynolds, M., Gorelick, J., & Bruno, M. (2020). Atopic dermatitis: A review of current diagnostic criteria and a proposed update to management. *Journal of Drugs in Dermatology, 19*(3), https://doi.org/10.36849/JDD.2020.4737

Complications

- Increased risk of secondary infection by bacteria (namely *Staphylococcus aureus*), viruses (such as molluscum contagiosum, papillomaviruses/warts, and herpes simplex), and fungus (tinea and *Candida* species)
- Disturbance in sleep, focus at work/school, and quality of life
- Depression
- Adverse effects from topical corticosteroids and other topical medications (skin atrophy, folliculitis, acne, local reactions)
- Adverse reactions from injectable biologic medications (injection site reactions and pain, conjunctivitis) or immunosuppressant medications (increased risk of infection and malignancy)
- Occupational impact when patient is unable to participate in activities due to unavoidable contact with triggers (high-risk jobs include cleaning, health care, food preparation, hairdressing)

Nursing Assessment

1. Conduct a comprehensive history of the rash focusing on location, onset, duration, previous episodes, and morphology; medications and treatments that were tried and their effects; associated and additional symptoms the patient is experiencing; and known and potential triggers.
2. Ask about the patient's and family's comfort, sleep, mood, stress, and emotional well-being.
3. A thorough history of occupational, recreational, and home exposures should be documented to identify all potential triggers and exposures; be sure to ask about cleansing agents, cosmetics, self-care products, diet, physical activity, hobbies, and medications, including all prescription, over-the-counter, homeopathic, and herbal and dietary supplements.
4. Review the patient's personal and family medical history.
5. Examine the patient for any associated symptoms such as fever, fatigue, scratching, and related atopic symptoms (wheezing, cough, congestion, mouth breathing).
6. Perform a physical examination of the entire skin surface, noting appearance and distribution of lesions, any nonintact areas, drainage, and temperature throughout; and palpate for lymphadenopathy.

Nursing Interventions

Maintaining Skin Integrity

1. Improve skin integrity by preventing and reducing inflammation and dry skin. Administer medications and treatments as ordered.
2. Apply unscented skin emollients several times daily, especially after washing.
3. Apply clean, damp, lukewarm compresses using a soft lightweight cloth to acutely inflamed skin for 20 minutes.
4. After the compress, apply topical corticosteroid (the least potent that provides adequate control) followed by emollient to further reduce inflammation.
5. Use mild, gentle, hydrating cleansers; avoid bathing with hot water; and lubricate skin with unscented emollients within 3 minutes of bathing (when skin is still slightly moist). Creams and ointments are better at preventing evaporation of water from skin and thus are more effective than lotions. Topical medications should be applied under emollients.
6. Use dye-free, fragrance-free detergent and avoid use of fabric softeners, dryer sheets, and fragrances (including those in soaps, lotions, cosmetics, and other self-care products).
7. Maintain a clean, warm, smoke-free environment with 40% humidity. Encourage patient to wear gloves when handling chemicals, cleaning, and doing dishes. Discourage scratching, and implement anti-scratching interventions.

Improving Comfort

1. Administer antipruritic medications and treatments as ordered by the health care provider, monitor for improvement in itching and development of any side effects, and provide medication teaching as needed. Side effects may include drowsiness from oral medications and application site stinging from topical medications.

Table 29-1 Types of Dermatitis

ETIOLOGY	CLINICAL MANIFESTATIONS	MANAGEMENT

Atopic Dermatitis
• Most common
• Involves underlying immunologic, genetic, and environmental factors
• A genetic deficiency of filaggrin (an important skin protein) lends to inherent skin barrier dysfunction
• Exaggerated inflammatory responses due to an overactive immune system
• Triggered by common environmental exposures
	• Intense itching (hallmark)
	• Characterized as acute (marked erythema, vesicles, bullae, weeping crusting), subacute (varying degrees of erythematous, scaly plaques with indistinct borders), and chronic (lichenification, scaling and postinflammatory pigment changes)
	• Involves face (usually spares nose) and upper body, extremities, and flexural surfaces (including eyelids)
	• Most cases appear before 5 yr old but increasingly being recognized in adult populations
		• Medications
		  • Topical corticosteroids
		  • Topical calcineurin inhibitors, tacrolimus, and pimecrolimus
		  • Topical PDE4 inhibitor, crisaborole
		  • Injectable monoclonal antibodies, dupilumab, and tralokinumab
		  • Oral Janus-associated kinases, abrocitinib, and upadacitinib
		  • Older oral, less-targeted immunosuppressants (azathioprine, cyclosporine, methotrexate, mycophenolate mofetil, tacrolimus)
		• Phototherapy
		• Prevent dry skin
		  • Use gentle, nonsoap cleansers
		  • Liberal use of bland emollients, especially after bathing/washing
		  • Open wet dressings
		• Avoid triggers
		  • Stress
		  • Bathing in hot water
		  • Irritants (e.g., fragrances and dyes in soap, detergent, lotion, fabric softener)
		  • Sweating
		  • Environmental allergens
		• Control pruritus

Contact Dermatitis
• Caused by a triggering agent coming into contact with skin
• *Irritant* contact dermatitis (ICD) due to direct toxic effect without induction of a T-cell response
• *Allergic* contact dermatitis (ACD) related to a delayed type IV hypersensitivity reaction (immune-mediated)
	• Acute
	• Erythema, vesicles, bullae, oozing, crusting; may have a sharp geometric border corresponding to the area of contact exposure
	• Subacute
	• Scaly plaques, round erosions, crusts
	• Chronic
	  • Scaling, cracks, lichenification
	• Hands are the most common location for ICD (hand dermatitis)
	• Fingertips can have fissures and desquamation
		• Avoidance of contact with offending agent
		  • For nickel allergy, iron-on patches or clear nail polish can be used to coat belt buckles or metal tabs on clothes
		• Patch testing
		• Access databases that provide lists of safe products free of identified offending agents such as the American Contact Dermatitis Society's Contact Allergen Management Program (contactderm.com) and SkinSAFE (allergyfreeskin.com)
		• Medications
		  • Topical and oral steroids
		  • Antihistamines may be used for treatment of itch
		  • Phototherapy for refractory cases

Dyshidrotic Dermatitis (also known as pompholyx) • Recurrent vesicular eruption on hands and sometimes feet • Specific etiology unknown; can be associated with other types of dermatitis	• Extremely pruritic, small, tense, clear fluid-filled deep-seated vesicles on medial and lateral aspects of the digits (often referred to as "tapioca pudding" appearance) • May involve nail changes (pitting, transverse ridges, thickening) in long-standing disease	• May be triggered by dermatophyte and bacterial infections, hyperhidrosis, hot weather, high dietary intake of nickel or cobalt, emotional stress • Limit handwashing and moisturize hands after washing to decrease frequency of flares • Similar to atopic dermatitis (see earlier)
Neurodermatitis • Repeated scratching, picking, or rubbing of an itchy area of skin in the absence of underlying pathology • Etiology largely unknown, although often starts during times of stress • May be associated with underlying psychiatric disease (obsessive-compulsive disorder, depression, anxiety, and substance use disorder; methamphetamines/crystal meth and pruritus-inducing drugs such as heroin)	• Shallow, linear, round, angulated or otherwise geometric erosions with overlying crusting and surrounding erythema or violaceous hue • Typically distributed on easily accessible and exposed body sites • No lesions at the midline upper back because it is out of reach	• Ensure short clipping of fingernails • Refer to mental health professional • Maintain nonjudgmental and nonconfrontational attitude toward patient • Occlusion of eroded lesions will show gradual healing because of being protected from scratching • No FDA-approved pharmacologic treatment specifically for this condition but SSRIs might help • Cognitive-behavioral interventions

Table 29-1 Types of Dermatitis *(continued)*

ETIOLOGY	CLINICAL MANIFESTATIONS	MANAGEMENT
Nummular Dermatitis • Etiology unknown • May be a form of atopic dermatitis	• Scaly, erythematous coin-shaped plaques often involving dorsal surfaces symmetrically distributed on trunk and extremities • Variable pruritus • Most common in men • Peak incidence 50–65 yr old and 15–25 yr old	• Similar to atopic dermatitis

Seborrheic Dermatitis
Abnormal immune response to Pityrosporum (Malassezia) yeast, which is a common skin commensal, in sebum-rich body
	• Erythematous plaques with loose greasy scale
	• Often involving the scalp, eyebrows, glabella, nasolabial folds, beard area, and ears; but may affect other areas (scale usually not apparent in intertriginous areas)
	• Chronic waxing and waning nature
		• Medications
		  • Topical imidazole treatments (e.g., ketoconazole creams)
		  • High-potency topical corticosteroids (not for use on face or intertriginous areas) such as clobetasol solution, shampoo, foam, gel or lotion
		  • Low potency topical corticosteroids such as desonide or hydrocortisone 2.5% sparingly to facial and intertriginous areas for limited time as needed for acute inflammation
		  • Topical calcineurin inhibitors in place of topical steroids, e.g., pimecrolimus
		  • Zinc pyrithione
		• Rotate medicated shampoos
		  • Salicylic acid shampoos
		  • Tar shampoos (e.g., coal tar or pine tar)
		  • Ketoconazole shampoo
		  • Selenium sulfide shampoo
		  • Pyrithione zinc shampoo
		Oil-based treatments to scalp at bedtime to loosen thick scales

Stasis Dermatitis Due to underlying venous insufficiency causing swelling and pressure on the skin	• Erythematous scaly papules and plaques with erosion and crusting involving the ankle and distal lower leg • Most prevalent in older individuals	• Topical antipruritic medications and emollients • Compression stockings • Referral to vascular specialist for treatment of underlying vascular insufficiency

FDA, U. S. Food and Drug Administration; SSRI, selective serotonin reuptake inhibitor

2. Dress in soft, lightweight cotton clothing and avoid wool and other occlusive synthetic fabrics.
3. Address stressful circumstances as much as possible and assess and meet psychosocial needs.
4. Explain the itch-scratch cycle, and explore possible approaches such as mindfulness, distraction, and breathing techniques that might help the patient decrease the urge to scratch.
5. Prevent secondary infections by maintaining intact skin and addressing scratching per interventions described earlier. Check for lymphadenopathy and signs of viral, bacterial, or fungal infection (discharge, oozing, crusts, increased redness, fever), and report any positive findings.

CLINICAL JUDGMENT Be alert for continued or worsening itching despite interventions. The itch-scratch cycle occurs when itching leads to scratching, which leads to inflammation and worsening itch and then more scratching; and the cycle continues and usually amplifies as time goes on, unless the cycle is broken.

Patient Education and Health Maintenance

1. Explain the itch-scratch cycle and the importance of maintaining healthy skin barrier and not scratching.
2. Provide medication teaching for all topical and systemic medications.
   a. Explain what each topical medication is for and where, when, and how to apply it.
   b. Warn about the side effects of overusing topical steroid medications.
   c. Provide injection training as necessary.
3. Help patient to identify and avoid triggers, such as hot water exposure, harsh soaps, and environmental temperature changes.
4. Teach the importance of moisturizing frequently, especially after bathing; avoiding hot water, harsh soaps and detergents, fragrances, chemicals and fabric softeners; and dressing in soft, lightweight cotton clothing.
5. Instruct patient to avoid exposure to temperature extremes, smoking, and high-humidity environments.

6. Discuss stress-alleviation techniques.
7. Educate about the signs and symptoms of infection.
8. For more information, refer to the National Eczema Association, nationaleczema.org.

Evaluation: Expected Outcomes

- Skin intact with minimal erythema and lichenification and no signs of infection.
- Patient verbalizes less itching, and less scratching is observed.

Cellulitis

Cellulitis is a diffuse inflammation of the deep dermal and subcutaneous tissue that results from an infectious process.

Pathophysiology and Etiology

1. Caused by infection with group A beta-hemolytic streptococci, *S. aureus*, *Haemophilus influenzae*, or other organisms.
2. Usually results from break in the skin that may be as simple as athlete's foot.
3. Infection can spread rapidly through lymphatic system.

CLINICAL JUDGMENT Methicillin-resistant *S. aureus* (MRSA) is a significant problem outside of the hospital as well as within. It is resistant to previously effective antistaphylococcal antibiotics and may be fatal. Be alert for worsening condition despite standard treatment.

Clinical Manifestations

1. Tender, warm, erythematous, and swollen area that is not well demarcated relative to erysipelas (which is bright red and has sharp well-demarcated borders and is sometimes confused with cellulitis).
2. Tender, warm, erythematous streak that extends proximally from the area, indicating lymph vessel involvement.
3. Possible fluctuant abscesses or purulent drainage.
4. Possible fever, chills, headache, malaise.

Diagnostic Evaluation

1. Gram stain and culture of drainage.
2. Blood cultures.

Management

1. Oral antibiotics (penicillinase-resistant penicillins, cephalosporins, quinolones, or sulfa-based) may be adequate to treat small, localized areas of cellulitis of legs or the trunk.
2. Parenteral antibiotics may be needed for cellulitis of the hands, face, or lymphatic or widespread involvement.
3. Surgical drainage and debridement for suppurative areas recommended for MRSA infections.

Complications

1. Tissue necrosis.
2. Septicemia.

Nursing Assessment

1. Obtain history of trauma to the skin, needlestick, insect bite, or wound.
2. Observe for expanding borders and lymphatic streaking; palpate for fluctuance of abscess formation.
3. Watch for signs of antibiotic sensitivity—shortness of breath, urticaria, angioedema, maculopapular rash, or severe skin reaction, such as erythema multiforme or toxic epidermal necrolysis.
4. Assess for patient and caregiver ability to provide care at home, keep affected area clean, and adhere to medication prescribed.

Nursing Interventions

Protecting Skin Integrity

1. Administer or teach patient to administer antibiotics, as prescribed; teach dosage schedule and adverse effects. Assess ability to swallow pills. Recommend crushing or taking with food to avoid stomach irritation, if applicable.
2. Maintain intravenous (IV) infusion or venous access to administer IV antibiotics, if indicated.
3. Elevate affected extremity to promote drainage from area and reduce swelling.
4. Prepare patient for surgical drainage and debridement, if necessary.

Relieving Pain

1. Encourage comfortable position and immobilization of affected area.
2. Administer or teach patient to administer analgesics, as prescribed; monitor for adverse effects.
3. Use bed cradle to relieve pressure from bed covers.

CLINICAL JUDGMENT Inform the health care provider immediately if pain is out of proportion to injury or if progressive skin changes occur. The patient should be assessed for necrotizing fasciitis.

Patient Education and Health Maintenance

1. Make sure that patient understands dosage schedule of antibiotics and the importance of adhering to therapy to prevent complications.
2. Advise patient to notify health care provider immediately if condition worsens; hospitalization may be necessary.
3. Outpatient-treated cellulitis should be observed within 24 to 48 hours of starting antibiotics to determine efficacy.
4. Teach patient with impaired circulation or impaired sensation how to perform proper skin care and how to inspect skin for trauma.

Evaluation: Expected Outcomes

- Skin is normal color and temperature, nontender, nonswollen, and intact.
- Actively moves extremity; verbalizes no pain.

Necrotizing Fasciitis

Necrotizing fasciitis is a type of necrotizing infection of the soft tissue that spreads quickly along fascia. It rapidly progresses toward death if not treated quickly.

Pathophysiology and Etiology

1. Usually caused by group A *Streptococcus*, known as flesh-eating bacteria, but may also be a clostridia or polymicrobial infection. It is emerging as a complication of MRSA infection.
2. May result postoperatively or from local injury with superficial or deep infection.

3. More common in patients with diabetes, those that misuse drugs, and other immunocompromised populations.
4. Spreads along fascia, causing extensive necrosis of the skin and subcutaneous tissue.

Clinical Manifestations

1. Increasing pain or pain out of proportion to local infection or injury; increasing redness, edema, and warmth.
2. Fever, rapid pulse.
3. Tissue appears darkened under the skin.
4. Possible bullae or petechiae or appears hemorrhagic.
5. May be foul odor and drainage (delayed).

Diagnostic Evaluation

1. Surgical excision and debridement are diagnostic to determine extent as well as therapeutic.
2. Gram stain and culture from deep tissue to determine exact etiology.
3. Blood cultures to rule out septicemia.

Management

1. Immediate hospitalization with intensive care support.
2. Prompt and repeated surgical debridement.
3. IV antibiotic regimen using multiple agents, including clindamycin, penicillin G, erythromycin, ceftriaxone, and others.

Complications

1. Muscle gangrene—requires amputation.
2. Loss of tissue and function.
3. Death.

Nursing Assessment

1. After trauma, surgery, or with cellulitis, frequently assess for increasing pain, fever, and changes in skin appearance, which may indicate necrotizing fasciitis.
2. Be aware of underlying conditions that may cause immunocompromise, such as diabetes, alcohol use disorder, malnutrition, IV drug use, cancer and cancer treatment, and HIV/AIDS, which increases the risk and worsens the course of necrotizing fasciitis.
3. Monitor vital signs frequently for any change (rise or fall in blood pressure [BP], temperature, pulse, and respirations) that may indicate worsening condition.
4. Monitor wound dressings after debridement for amount, color, and odor of drainage. Wounds will usually be left open to heal by secondary intention.

Nursing Interventions

Normalizing Body Temperature

1. Administer antipyretics, as directed.
2. Encourage oral fluids and administer IV fluids, as directed.
3. Monitor intake and output to ensure adequate hydration because of fluid loss through fever and insensible loss.
4. Provide cool compresses, sponge baths, and clothing and linen changes as comfort measures.

Relieving Pain

1. Administer analgesics, as directed and based on pain assessment; however, be alert for sedation that may mask signs of worsening condition.
2. Assist patient to position of comfort that will not place pressure on affected area.
3. Administer analgesic 30 to 60 minutes before wound care and dressing changes.

Patient Education and Health Maintenance

1. Make sure that patient can complete wound care at home and will follow-up as directed.
2. Make home care nursing referral, as necessary.
3. Teach patient signs of infection and to notify health care provider immediately if experiencing increasing pain, fever, redness, swelling, warmth, or increased and odorous drainage.
4. Advise patient to eat a balanced diet rich in protein, vitamin C, iron, and zinc for wound healing.

Evaluation: Expected Outcomes

- Core temperature 97.6°F to 98.8°F (36.4°C to 37.1°C).
- Patient turning in bed, verbalizing minimal pain.

Toxic Epidermal Necrolysis

Toxic epidermal necrolysis is a severe, potentially fatal skin disease associated with erythema, blistering, and epidermal sloughing. A less severe form is known as *Stevens-Johnson syndrome*.

Pathophysiology and Etiology

1. Exact mechanism is unknown, but can be induced by various drugs, including sulfonamides, anticonvulsants, nonsteroidal anti-inflammatory drugs (NSAIDs), and allopurinol.
2. Resembles second-degree burns, with sloughing of the skin at epidermal or dermal junction.
3. Mortality ranges from 3.2% to 90%, based on an illness severity score with factors such as age, presence of malignancy, heart rate, and percentage of epidermal detachment.

Clinical Manifestations

1. Malaise, fatigue, vomiting, cough, fever, and diarrhea may be prodromal symptoms.
2. Sudden onset of urticaria and large dark red areas; within 5 to 8 days, large, flaccid bullae appear.
3. Within hours, coma may develop.
4. Bullae become confluent and slough in large sheets, leaving moist, erythematous surface.
5. Positive Nikolsky sign (desquamation of the skin on light pressure).
6. Erosions of mucosal sites, including lips, oral pharynx, or urinary tract.

Diagnostic Evaluation

1. Skin biopsy to determine level of separation.
2. Possible cultures of blood and body fluids to differentiate infection.

Management

1. Treatment in intensive care unit or regional burn center because toxic epidermal necrolysis has similar pathophysiologic characteristics to those of extensive burns (see page 912).
2. Treatment of affected skin.
   a. Wounds are cleaned in operating room under anesthesia; loose skin and blisters are removed, and necrotic areas are debrided to prevent infection.

   b. Temporary biologic dressings (porcine cutaneous xenografts, amnion, collagen-based skin substitute, or plastic semipermeable dressings) applied to prevent secondary skin infection while awaiting reepithelialization.
3. All nonessential drugs are stopped immediately.
4. Fluid replacement therapy, as necessary, and possible enteral nutrition if oral involvement.
5. Topical antimicrobial dressings to enhance reepithelialization.
6. Ophthalmologic examination and removal of corneal adhesions, as necessary.
7. Use of systemic corticosteroids is not recommended and use of human IV immunoglobulin is controversial.

Complications

1. Sepsis.
2. Pneumonia.
3. Blindness.

Nursing Assessment

1. Obtain medication and immunization history.
2. Monitor vital signs and level of consciousness closely because the condition is rapidly progressive.
3. Monitor fluid and nutritional status through daily weight, vital signs, and laboratory test results (electrolytes, especially glucose, bicarbonate, blood urea nitrogen, creatinine, albumin, and total protein).

Nursing Interventions

Restoring Skin Integrity

1. Place patient on warmed air-fluidized bed to distribute weight with minimal shearing forces.
2. Use extreme care in handling patient because the skin is very fragile; obtain assistance to move patient.
3. Gently apply warm, wet compresses of prescribed antiseptic solution to reduce bacterial population of wound surface.
4. Inspect xenograft several times daily for dislodgment or purulence; these will require new xenograft.
5. Watch for new areas of toxic epidermal necrolysis; note and record progression of skin slough and chart progress.
6. Patient should be in private room on reverse isolation to prevent infection.
7. Provide nutritional supplements through enteral feeding to ensure healing.

Maintaining Fluid Balance

1. Monitor vital signs for falling BP or for rising pulse that indicates hypovolemia; use an indwelling arterial catheter to provide continuous measurement while avoiding cuff pressure on the skin.
2. Measure hourly urine output.
3. Weigh patient daily.
4. Give IV fluids, as prescribed.
5. Assess bowel sounds and give oral or enteral fluids, as tolerated.

Reducing Pain

1. If patient cannot verbalize, watch for facial expressions, for guarding, or for increased pulse and respirations to indicate pain.
2. Administer analgesics, as prescribed and as required, possibly around the clock; monitor for adverse effects and document effectiveness.
3. Provide distraction through music or other measures to promote relaxation.
4. Provide emotional support and encouragement. Emotional/psychological support to patient and family is crucial.

Protecting Mucous Membranes

1. Use meticulous oral hygiene.
   a. Inspect oral cavity daily; note any changes.
   b. Rinse mouth with normal saline, diluted hydrogen peroxide, or other solution to remove debris and to cleanse ulcerations.
   c. Apply petroleum jelly or other lubricant/protectant to cracked, swollen lips.
2. Assess urethral, vaginal, and anal regions for ulcerations or bleeding.
3. Inspect eyes and remove crusts from eyelid margins using damp compresses or normal saline-soaked swabs; apply eyedrops as prescribed.

Patient Education and Health Maintenance

1. Encourage follow-up appointments with plastic surgeon and other health care providers as indicated.
2. Encourage adherence to physical therapy, as indicated, to restore function.
3. Advise patient to use sunscreen of at least sun protection factor (SPF) 30, avoid direct sunlight during the healing phase, and continue to use sunscreen.
4. Advise patient to avoid suspected medication in the future.

Evaluation: Expected Outcomes

- New epithelium noted without scarring.
- Output equals input; weight and vital signs remain stable.
- Patient verbalizes reduced pain.
- Oral mucosa intact.

Herpes Zoster

Herpes zoster (varicella–zoster, shingles) is an inflammatory condition in which reactivation of the chickenpox virus produces a vesicular eruption along the distribution of the nerves from one or more dorsal root ganglia (dermatome). The prevalence increases with age. The Centers for Disease Control and Prevention (CDC) recommends two doses of recombinant zoster vaccine (RZV, Shingrix) to prevent shingles and related complications in adults 50 years and older. Shingrix is also recommended for adults 19 years and older who have weakened immune systems because of disease or therapy.

EVIDENCE BASE Centers for Disease Control and Prevention. (2022). *Shingles (herpes zoster).* https://www.cdc.gov/shingles/index.html

Pathophysiology and Etiology

1. Caused by a varicella–zoster virus, which is a member of a group of deoxyribonucleic acid viruses.
2. Virus is identical to the causative agent of varicella (chickenpox). After the primary infection, the varicella–zoster virus may persist in a dormant state in the dorsal nerve root ganglia. The virus may emerge from this site in later years, either spontaneously or in association with immunosuppression, to cause herpes zoster.

Clinical Manifestations

1. Eruption may be accompanied or preceded by fever, malaise, headache, and pain; pain may be burning, lancinating, stabbing, or aching.
2. Inflammation is usually unilateral, involving the cranial, cervical, thoracic, lumbar, or sacral dermatome in a bandlike configuration.
3. Vesicles appear in 3 to 4 days.
   a. Characteristic patches of grouped vesicles appear on erythematous, edematous skin.
   b. Early vesicles contain serum; they later rupture and form crusts; scarring usually does not occur unless the vesicles are deep and they involve the dermis.
   c. If ophthalmic branch of the facial nerve is involved, patient may have a painful eye. (This can be a medical emergency.) Vesicles on the tip of the nose suggest eye involvement.
   d. In healthy host, lesions resolve in 2 to 3 weeks.
4. A susceptible person can acquire chickenpox if there is contact with the infective vesicular fluid of a zoster patient. A person with a history of chickenpox or who has received the immunization is immune and thus is not at risk from infection after exposure to zoster patients.

CLINICAL JUDGMENT Be aware that varicella–zoster virus may be a life-threatening condition to the patient who is immunosuppressed, who is receiving cytotoxic chemotherapy, or who is a bone marrow transplant recipient.

Diagnostic Evaluation

1. Usually diagnosed by clinical presentation.
2. Culture of varicella–zoster virus from lesions or detection by fluorescent antibody techniques, including viral detection that uses monoclonal antibodies or by electron microscopy, to confirm diagnosis.

Management

1. Antiviral drugs such as acyclovir, famciclovir, and valacyclovir interfere with viral replication; may be used in all cases, but especially for treatment of immunosuppressed or debilitated patients. Must be started within 72 hours of onset. If started early (within 48 to 72 hours of onset), may decrease risk of postherpetic neuralgia.
2. Corticosteroids early in illness (controversial)—given for severe herpes zoster if symptomatic measures fail; given for anti-inflammatory effect and for relief of pain.
3. Pain management—aspirin, acetaminophen, NSAIDs, opioids—useful during the acute stage, but not generally effective for postherpetic neuralgia.
4. Postherpetic neuralgia may be treated with anticonvulsant agents, such as gabapentin or pregabalin, and 5% lidocaine patch.

Complications

1. Approximately 20% of patients will experience chronic pain syndrome (postherpetic neuralgia), characterized by constant aching and burning pain or by intermittent lancinating pain or hyperesthesia of affected skin after it has healed.
2. Ophthalmic complications with involvement of ophthalmic branch of trigeminal nerve with keratitis, uveitis, corneal ulceration, and possibly blindness.
3. Facial and auditory nerve involvement, resulting in hearing deficits, vertigo, and facial weakness (Ramsay Hunt syndrome).
4. Visceral dissemination—pneumonitis, esophagitis, enterocolitis, myocarditis, and pancreatitis.

Nursing Interventions

Controlling Pain

1. Assess patient's level of discomfort and medicate, as prescribed; monitor for adverse effects of pain medications.
2. Teach patient to apply wet dressings, such as aluminum acetate (Burow) solution, for soothing effect.
3. Encourage distraction techniques such as music therapy.
4. Teach relaxation techniques, such as deep breathing, progressive muscle relaxation, and imagery, to help control pain.

Improving Skin Integrity

1. Apply wet dressings to cool and dry inflamed areas by means of evaporation.
2. Administer antiviral medication in dosage prescribed (usually high dose); warn the patient of adverse effects such as headache, dizziness, nausea, abdominal pain, change in bowel movements, and change in mood or alertness.

Patient Education and Health Maintenance

1. Teach patient to use proper handwashing technique to avoid spreading herpes zoster virus.
2. Advise patient not to open the blisters to avoid secondary infection and scarring.
3. Advise all persons age 50 and older to talk to health care provider about receiving the herpes zoster vaccine.

POPULATION AWARENESS In older patients, the pain of herpes zoster may be more pronounced and incapacitating, and prolonged if postherpetic neuralgia results. Dysesthesia and skin hypersensitivity are distressing. A caregiver may be required to assist with usual activities of daily living such as dressings and preparing meals.

Evaluation: Expected Outcomes

- Verbalizes decreased pain.
- Reepithelialization of the skin without scarring.

Pemphigus

Pemphigus is a serious autoimmune disease of the skin and of the mucous membranes, characterized by the appearance of flaccid blisters (bullae and vesicles) of various sizes on apparently normal skin and mucous membranes (mouth, esophagus, conjunctiva, or vagina) (see Figure 29-3). Familial benign chronic pemphigus (Hailey-Hailey disease) is a familial type of pemphigus that appears in adults, particularly affecting the axillae and groin.

Pathophysiology and Etiology

1. The exact cause is unknown.
2. Certain drugs, other autoimmune diseases, and genetics may play a role in its development.
3. Many variants of pemphigus exist.

Clinical Manifestations

1. Initial lesions may appear in the oral cavity; flaccid blisters (bullae) may arise on normal or erythematous skin.

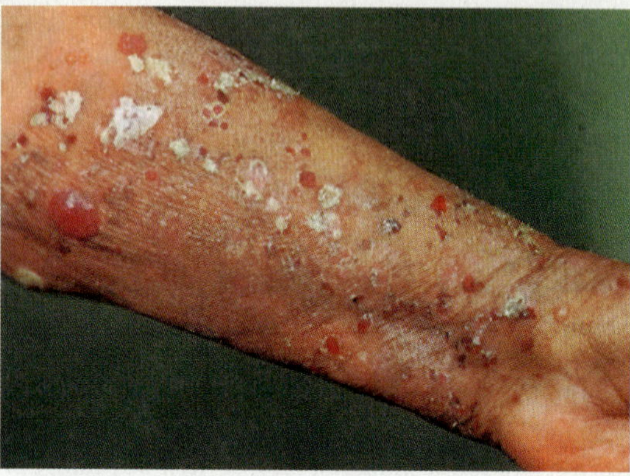

Figure 29-3. Pemphigus vulgaris blisters on the forearm. (Reprinted with permission from Hall, J. C., & Hall, B. J. [2017]. *Sauer's manual of skin diseases* [11th ed., Fig. 46-9B]. Wolters Kluwer.)

a. The bullae enlarge and rupture, forming painful, raw, and denuded areas that eventually become crusted. These areas can become secondarily infected.
b. The eroded skin heals slowly; eventually, widespread areas of the body may become involved.
c. In the mouth, the blisters are usually multiple, of varying size and irregular shape, painful, and persistent. Oral lesions may appear initially, with lesions of the mucous membranes of the pharynx and esophagus; the conjunctivae, larynx, urethra, cervix, and rectum may become affected as well.

2. An offensive odor may emanate from the bullae because of infection.
3. Positive Nikolsky sign—separation of the epidermis when minimal pressure is applied to the skin; downward pressure on a bulla will cause it to expand laterally.

Diagnostic Evaluation

1. Skin biopsies of blisters and surrounding skin—demonstrate acantholysis (separation of epidermal cells from each other).
2. Immunofluorescence of skin cells shows antibodies that bind to the epidermis in a lacy pattern network (pemphigus antibodies).

Management

1. Corticosteroids in large doses to control the disease and keep skin free from blisters.
2. Immunosuppressive agents, such as cyclophosphamide and azathioprine, are used alone or in combination with steroids, for immunosuppressive and steroid-sparing effect.
3. Plasmapheresis—reinfusion of specially treated plasma cells; temporarily decreases serum level of antibodies.
4. Treatment of denuded skin.

Complications

1. Infections (skin, pneumonia, septicemia).
2. Adverse effects from acute and chronic corticosteroids: gastrointestinal (GI) bleeding, secondary infection, psychosis, hyperglycemia, and others (see page 688).

Nursing Assessment

1. Assess for odor or drainage from lesions, which may indicate infection.
2. Assess for fever and signs of systemic infection.
3. Assess for adverse effects of corticosteroids, such as abdominal pain, white patches in the mouth that indicate *Candida* infection, and emotional changes.

Nursing Interventions

Restoring Oral Mucous Membrane Integrity

1. Inspect oral cavity daily; note and report any changes—oral lesions heal slowly.
2. Provide gentle oral care to keep oral mucosa clean and allow regeneration of epithelium.
3. Give topical oral therapy, as directed.
4. Teach patient to apply petrolatum to lips frequently.
5. Use cool mist therapy to humidify environmental air.

Restoring Skin Integrity

1. Keep skin clean and eliminate debris and dead skin—the bullae will clear if epithelium at the base is clean and not infected.
2. Obtain swab of bullous fluid for cultures—most common organism is *S. aureus*.
3. Administer cool, wet dressings or baths or teach patient to administer to soothe and cleanse the skin. Large areas of blistering have a characteristic odor that is lessened when secondary infection is under control.
4. The nursing management of patients with blistering or with bullous skin conditions is similar to that of the patient with a burn (see page 918).

Restoring Fluid Balance

1. Evaluate for fluid and electrolyte imbalance—extensive denudation of the skin leads to fluid and electrolyte imbalance.
   a. Monitor serum albumin and protein levels.
   b. Monitor vital signs for hypotension or tachycardia.
   c. Weigh patient daily.
   d. Monitor intake and output.
2. Administer IV normal saline solutions, as directed.
3. Encourage the patient to maintain hydration; suggest cool, nonirritating fluids.
   a. Suggest soft, high-protein, high-calorie diet or liquid supplements that will not be irritating to oral mucosa but will replace lost protein.

Promoting Positive Body Image

1. Develop a trusting relationship with the patient.
2. Educate patient and family about the disease and its treatment; this reduces uncertainty and clears up misconceptions.
3. Encourage expression of anxieties, embarrassment, and discouragement.
4. Encourage patient to maintain social contacts and activities among support network.

Patient Education and Health Maintenance

Instruct the patient as follows:

1. The disease may be characterized by relapses that require continuing therapy to maintain control.
2. Long-term administration of immunosuppressive drugs is associated with numerous adverse effects and risks—hyperglycemia, osteoporosis, psychosis, adrenal suppression, and increased risk of cancer. Report for health care follow-up visits regularly.
3. Monitor the skin and mouth for recurrence of pemphigus activity.
4. For additional information, refer to the International Pemphigus and Pemphigoid Foundation (pemphigus.org)

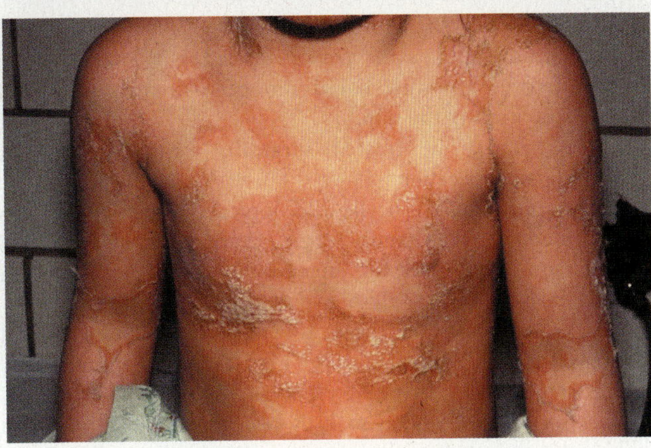

Figure 29-4. The lesions of psoriasis appear as red, raised patches of the skin covered with silvery scales that in time coalesce, forming irregularly shaped patches.

Evaluation: Expected Outcomes

- Oral mucous membranes pink with healing lesions and no signs of infection.
- Skin with intact bullae, healing lesions, and no signs of infection.
- Vital signs stable; urine output adequate.
- Patient expresses concerns and plans activities.

EVIDENCE BASE D'Amiano, N., Lai, J., & Cohen, B. (2023). Pemphigus: Updated review and emerging therapies. *Dermatology Times, 44*(2). https://www.dermatologytimes.com/view/pemphigus-updated-review-and-emerging-therapies

Psoriasis

Psoriasis (see Figure 29-4) is a chronic T-cell–mediated inflammatory disorder causing secondary epidermal turnover, which occurs at a rate six to nine times faster than normal.

Pathophysiology and Etiology

1. Affects 2% to 3% of people.
2. Classified as mild if less than 2% of body surface area affected; moderate, if 2% to 10% affected; and severe, if more than 10%.
3. Types of psoriasis include:
   a. Plaque—most common type (about 80% of cases); occurs on the knees, elbows, scalp, and other areas.
   b. Guttate—droplike pattern occurs on the trunk, arms, or legs; often starts in childhood or young adulthood; comes on suddenly, often triggered by streptococcal infection.
   c. Inverse—affects flexural areas, such as the axilla and groin.
   d. Erythrodermic—scalded appearance that affects most of the body; can lead to protein and fluid loss.
   e. Pustular—primarily seen in adults; exacerbated by the sun; blisters contain purulent material on palms and soles or on widespread area.
   f. Psoriatic arthritis—joint involvement, pain, and other abnormalities accompany skin involvement.
4. Formerly considered idiopathic, now thought to be genetically linked and immune system modulated.
   a. May be caused by some antigenic stimuli that activate cytokines and T cells, thus causing an extreme dermal response.
   b. Genes are being identified that may predispose a person to developing psoriasis.
5. Condition tends to last a person's life span, with flares and remissions. May be exacerbated by infection (particularly beta-hemolytic streptococcal infection), stress, injury, hormonal changes, and drugs, such as lithium, beta-adrenergic blockers, angiotensin-converting enzyme inhibitors, antimalarial drugs, and indomethacin.
6. Recent research may indicate that the inflammatory nature of disease may be associated with increased coronary artery calcification. Appropriate medical follow-up should be recommended.

Clinical Manifestations

1. Characteristic rash.
   a. Plaque type—erythematous plaques with silvery scales, symmetric involvement, may be pruritic and painful; often appears at areas of epidermal injury (Koebner reaction).
   b. Guttate—small, red individual spots, not as thick as plaque psoriasis.
   c. Inverse—bright, red patches that are smooth and shiny, involving skin folds.
   d. Pustular—white blisters and noninfectious pus surrounded by red skin.
   e. Erythrodermic—redness of most of the body, shedding of the skin, severe itching, and signs of systemic illness.
2. Characteristic pitting of nails in 50% of patients.
3. Arthritis in approximately 30% of patients; most frequently occurs between age 30 and 50.

Management

1. Diagnosed by clinical features; rarely, a biopsy may be needed.
2. Coal tar and anthralin preparations inhibit excessive skin turnover.
   a. Applied topically, with no systemic adverse effects.
   b. Application may be messy, odorous, and may stain clothing.
3. Topical corticosteroids are the mainstay topical treatment. Adverse effects may include striae, thinning of the skin, adrenal suppression (rare). Tachyphylaxis may result if used for extended periods.
4. Topical calcipotriene, a vitamin D derivative, used for mild to moderate psoriasis, generally produces no adverse effects.
5. Another topical preparation is tazarotene, a receptor-selective retinoid, which is potentially teratogenic (pregnancy category X).
6. Phototherapy—20 to 30 short treatments. Narrowband ultraviolet B (UVB) light is safer than ultraviolet A (UVA), which carries the risk of sunburn and skin cancer.
   a. Photochemotherapy—ingestion of an oral photosensitizer (psoralen) followed by exposure to UVA light therapy (PUVA).
   b. Cataracts, nausea, and malaise are possible adverse effects of systemic PUVA.
7. Oral methotrexate, the retinoid acitretin, and cyclosporine were the common medications used in the past, but their use is limited by adverse effects.
   a. Hepatotoxicity may occur with methotrexate.
   b. Hypertension and renal failure may occur with cyclosporine.
   c. Acitretin is a potent teratogen and should not be used if any risk of pregnancy up to 3 years posttreatment in females of childbearing age.

8. Biologic agents such as etanercept, infliximab, ustekinumab, certolizumab, adalimumab, ixekizumab, risankizumab, guselkumab, secukinumab are U.S. Food and Drug Administration (FDA)-approved for moderate to severe psoriasis and psoriatic arthritis. They are administered by injection or infusion.
9. Oral medications that are FDA-approved to treat psoriasis are apremilast, which is a systemic phosphodiesterase-4 (PDE4) inhibitor and deucravacitinib, which is tyrosine kinase 2 (TYK2) inhibitor.

EVIDENCE BASE Van Voorhees, A., Feldman, S., Lebwohl, M., Orbai, A., & Ritchlin, C. (2022). *The psoriasis and psoriatic arthritis pocket guide*. National Psoriasis Foundation. psoriasis.org

Nursing Interventions and Patient Education

1. Assist patient, as needed, with daily tub bath to soften scales and plaques.
2. Apply topical preparations after bath and gentle debridement of scale removal.
3. Warn patient that coal tar and anthralin preparations may stain clothing; let it dry before dressing.
4. Advise patient to wear goggles for phototherapy to prevent cataracts and to follow-up with periodic eye examinations.
5. Encourage patient to follow-up closely with primary care provider or with dermatologist and to report for blood work to check renal function and liver function tests as indicated.
6. Reinforce to females of childbearing age that retinoids and methotrexate are teratogenic; must be using birth control.
7. Encourage patients to try to identify triggers that may cause flare-ups and to practice avoidance techniques, such as relaxation therapy, to avoid stress.
8. Teach patients to avoid direct sun exposure by wearing protective clothing and sunscreen, especially on the day of phototherapy.
9. Advise patients to use good lubricants to prevent drying and cracking of the skin, which can lead to hyperkeratinization.
10. Encourage verbalization of frustration of condition, treatment, and impact on social network. For more information, refer to the National Psoriasis Foundation (psoriasis.org).

American Academy of Dermatology Psoriasis Resource Center (aad.org/public/diseases/psoriasis)

Benign Tumors

Benign tumors are common skin growths. Most do not require any treatment but are important to recognize to differentiate from malignant lesions.

Characteristics and Management

Seborrheic Keratoses

1. Lesions are benign and wartlike of varying size and color, ranging from light tan to black that may appear to be stuck on; they are the most common skin tumors in middle-aged and older people.
2. Treatment is usually unnecessary, but lesions can be removed by liquid nitrogen cryotherapy or curettage.

Verrucae (Warts)

1. Common, benign skin tumors caused by human papillomavirus.
2. Often disappear spontaneously without scarring and may not need treatment.
3. Many topical treatment options are available for office and self-treatment, but some may cause scarring.
   a. Cryotherapy with liquid nitrogen—destroys wart and spares rest of the skin.
   b. Area may be treated surgically with curettage or electrodesiccation.
   c. Application of salicylic acid, topical fluorouracil, imiquimod, topical vitamin A acid, cantharidin, or other irritants may be helpful, especially for flat warts, except on the face.
   d. Occlusion with duct tape is controversial. Modest clinical effectiveness has been shown in studies, but not statistically significant.
   e. Apple cider vinegar soak. Apply petroleum ointment on the surrounding skin to protect it. Apply small piece of cotton soaked in vinegar and tape it to the wart overnight and repeat until the wart is gone.
   f. Suggestive therapy (placebo) is not effective for adults but often works with children through age 10.

Hemangiomas

1. Hemangiomas are benign tumors of the capillaries, which present shortly after birth.
2. They grow rapidly for 6 to 18 months, followed by stabilization and subsequent regression. Most hemangiomas resolve by age 9.
3. Surgery is reserved for complicated hemangiomas that may be obstructing the airway.
4. Hemangiomas blocking the visual axis or compressing against the eye are treated with high doses of corticosteroids or interferon.
5. For hemangiomas that do not threaten vision or life, no intervention is preferred.
6. Lasers can be used for ulcerated hemangiomas.
7. For more information, patients can be referred to The Vascular Birthmarks Foundation (birthmark.org).

Pigmented Nevi (Moles)

1. Common skin tumors of various sizes and shapes, ranging from yellowish to brown to black; may be flat, macular lesions, elevated papules, or nodules that occasionally contain hair.
2. Most pigmented nevi are harmless; however, in rare cases, malignant changes supervene and a melanoma develops at the site of the nevus.
3. Nevi at sites subject to repeated irritation from clothing or jewelry can be removed for comfort.
4. Nevi that show change in size, shape, or color become symptomatic (itch or bleed) or develop notched borders that should be removed to determine if malignant changes have occurred. This is especially true for nevi with irregular borders or variations of red, blue, and blue-black.
5. Use "ABCDE" to recall criteria for evaluation of nevi: A = asymmetry, B = border (irregular), C = color (lack of uniform), D = diameter (greater than 6 mm), and E = evolving or changing.

Keloids

1. Benign overgrowths of connective tissue expanding beyond the site of scar or trauma in predisposed individuals.
2. More prevalent among dark-skinned individuals.
3. Usually asymptomatic—may cause disfigurement and cosmetic concern.
4. Management—intralesional corticosteroid therapy, surgical removal, radiation, or silicone gel sheeting.

Premalignant Lesions: Actinic (Solar) Keratoses

1. Premalignant skin lesions appearing as rough, scaly patches with underlying erythema, which develop as a consequence of prolonged exposure to ultraviolet rays.
2. Develop in areas of the body that experience prolonged sun exposure such as the scalp, face, dorsal hands, and arms; may gradually transform into squamous cell carcinoma (SCC).
3. Many topical treatments are available, including the antineoplastic fluorouracil, the immune response modifier imiquimod, liquid nitrogen cryosurgery, and curettage.
4. Photodynamic therapy with application of aminolevulinic acid and exposure to blue light that destroys abnormal cells.

Skin Cancer

Skin cancer is the most common malignancy, accounting for about half of all cancers. Nonmelanoma skin cancers are categorized as basal cell carcinoma (BCC) (80%) or SCC (20%). BCCs are more easily curable because of early diagnosis and slow progression. These cancers are locally invasive and tend not to metastasize. SCCs have an increased potential for metastasis. Conversely, malignant melanomas are least common and have a higher risk of metastasis.

EVIDENCE BASE Machin, C. (2022). Skin cancer: Getting back to basics. *Practice Nursing, 33*(9). https://www.practicenursing.com/content/clinical/skin-cancer-getting-back-to-basics/

Pathophysiology and Etiology

1. Most BCCs and SCCs are located on sun-exposed areas and are directly related to ultraviolet radiation. Sun damage is cumulative.
2. Risk factors for skin cancer include:
   a. Fair complexion, blue eyes, and blond or red hair; Fitzpatrick skin—type I or II (see page 898).
   b. Working outdoors.
   c. Older people with sun-damaged skin.
   d. History of radiation treatment of skin conditions.
   e. Exposure to certain chemical agents (arsenicals, nitrates, tar and pitch, oils, and paraffins).
   f. Burn scars, damaged skin in areas of chronic osteomyelitis, fistulae openings.
   g. Long-term immunosuppressive therapy, including organ transplants.
   h. Genetic susceptibility.
   i. Multiple dysplastic nevi—moles that are larger, irregular, more numerous, or variable colors—or family history of dysplastic nevi.
   j. Congenital nevi that are large (more than 20 cm in size).
   k. Presence of human papillomavirus.
3. Types of skin cancer:
   a. BCC—arises from basal layers of the epidermis or hair follicle; most common type but rarely metastasizes; can be locally invasive.
   b. SCC—arises from the epidermis; metastasis occurs more commonly than with BCC.
   c. Malignant melanoma—a malignancy of melanocytes; can metastasize.

CLINICAL JUDGMENT Although only 3% of skin cancers are melanoma, this form of skin cancer causes the majority of skin cancer deaths. Melanoma incidence is increasing at about 3% per year, so remain vigilant when assessing skin of any patient.

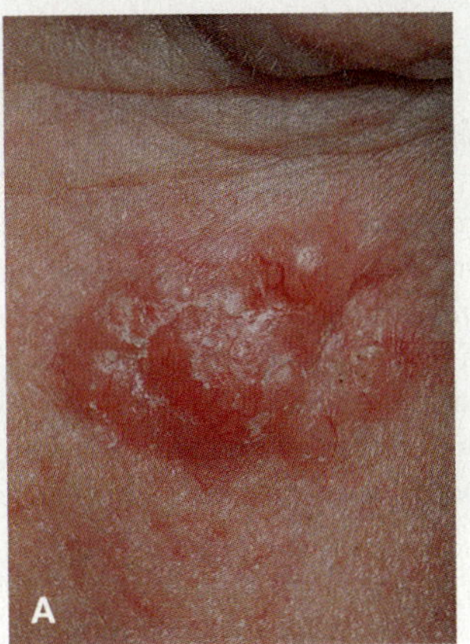

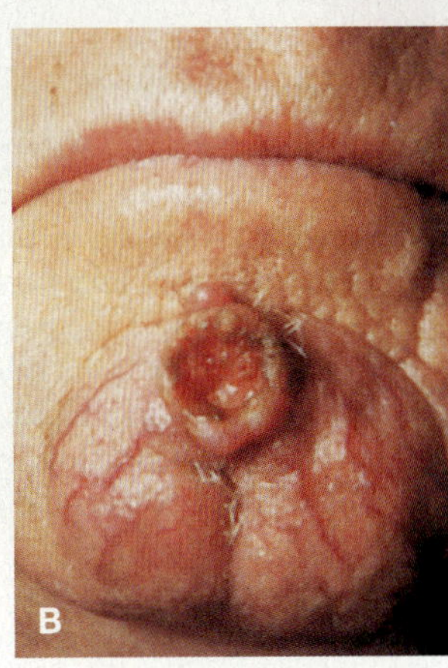

Figure 29-5. **(A)** Basal cell carcinoma and **(B)** squamous cell carcinoma. (Reprinted with permission from Smeltzer, S., & Bare, B. [2000]. *Brunner and Suddarth's textbook of medical-surgical nursing* [9th ed.]. Lippincott Williams & Wilkins.)

Clinical Manifestations

Basal Cell Carcinoma

1. Lesions typically begin as small nodules with a rolled, pearly, translucent border with telangiectasia, crusting, and occasionally ulceration (see Figure 29-5A).
2. Appear most frequently on sun-exposed skin, frequently on the face between the hairline and upper lip or back.
3. If neglected, may cause local destruction, hemorrhage, and infection of adjacent tissues, producing severe functional and cosmetic disabilities.

Squamous Cell Carcinoma

1. Appears as reddish, rough, thickened, scaly lesion with bleeding and soreness—may be asymptomatic; border may be wider, more indurated, and more inflammatory than BCC (see Figure 29-5B).
2. May be preceded by leukoplakia (premalignant lesion of mucous membrane) of the mouth or tongue, actinic keratoses, and scarred or ulcerated lesions.
3. Seen most commonly on the lower lip, rims of ears, head, neck, and backs of the hands.

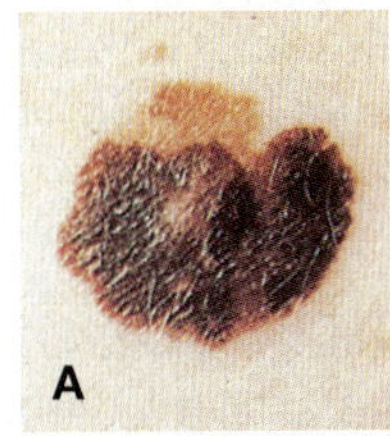

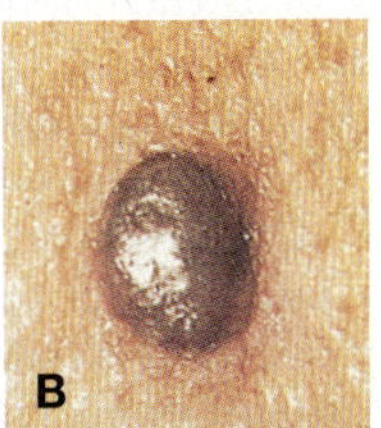

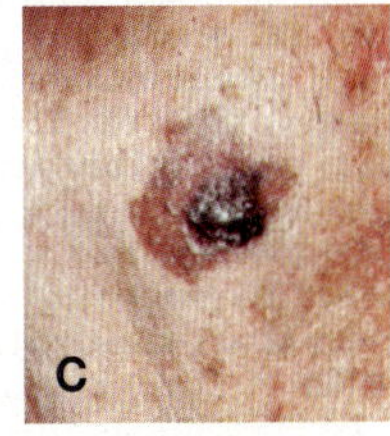

Figure 29-6. **(A)** Superficial spreading melanoma; note irregular border. **(B)** Nodular melanoma. **(C)** Lentigo maligna melanoma; note irregular pigment pattern. (A, B: Reprinted with permission from Hinkle, J. L., Cheever, K. H., & Overbaugh, K. [2022]. *Brunner & Suddarth's textbook of medical-surgical nursing* [15th ed., Fig. 56-9.]. Wolters Kluwer; C: Reprinted with permission from Hall, J. C., & Hall, B. J. [2017]. *Sauer's manual of skin diseases* [11th ed.]. Lippincott Williams & Wilkins.)

Malignant Melanoma

See Figure 29-6.

1. Melanoma in situ; earliest phase, difficult to recognize because clinical changes are minimal.
2. Superficial spreading melanoma (most common).
   a. Circular, with irregular outer portions; the margins may be flat or elevated and palpable.
   b. Has combination of colors—hues of tan, brown, and black mixed with gray, bluish black, or white.
   c. May be dull pink-rose color in a small area within the lesion.
   d. Occurs anywhere on the body; usually affects middle-aged people.
3. Nodular melanoma.
   a. Spherical blueberry-like nodule with relatively smooth surface and uniform blue-black, blue-gray, or reddish-blue color.
   b. May be polypoidal and elevated, with smooth surface of rose-gray or black color.
   c. Occurs commonly on the torso and extremities.
   d. Invades directly into the subjacent dermis (vertical growth) and hence has a poorer prognosis.
4. Lentigo malignant melanoma.
   a. First appears as tan, flat macule—malignant degeneration is manifested by changes in color, size, and topography.
   b. Evolves slowly; occurs on sun-exposed skin surfaces of people in their 40s or 50s.
5. Acrolentiginous melanoma (uncommon).
   a. Irregular pigmented macules, which develop nodules; may become invasive early.
   b. Occurs on palms, soles, nail beds, and rarely on mucous membranes.
   c. Most common type of melanoma in Black people and Asian people.

Diagnostic Evaluation

Excisional biopsy (for histopathologic diagnosis) and microstaging determination of thickness and level of invasion; helps determine treatment and prognosis. Shave biopsy is usually performed for suspected BCC or SCC lesions.

Management

BCC and SCC

Method of treatment depends on tumor location, cell type (location and depth), history of previous treatment, whether it is invasive, or if metastasis has occurred.

1. Curettage followed by electrodesiccation—usually done on small tumors of basal or squamous cell type (less than 1 to 2 cm).
2. Surgical excision by Mohs surgery for larger lesions or for those in areas more likely to recur or located in cosmetically sensitive areas (around the nose, eyes, ears, lips); may be followed by simple closure, flap, or graft.
   a. Microscopically controlled excision, with immediate examination of frozen or chemically fixed sections for evidence of cancer cells.
   b. Layers are removed until a reasonable cancer-free margin is achieved.
3. Radiation therapy—should be reserved for older adults, may be used for extensive malignancies where goal is palliation or when other medical conditions contraindicate other forms of therapy.
4. Other therapeutic regimens—topical fluorouracil, the immune response modifier imiquimod, photodynamic therapy.

Malignant Melanoma

1. Complete excision of lesion. If depth is between 1 and 4 mm or there is ulceration present, sentinel lymph node biopsy may be done at the time of reexcision. Margins of 1 to 2 cm are required on reexcision. Close subsequent follow-up is necessary.
2. Systemic chemotherapy—generally used for recurrence of metastasis or palliation; may be combined with autologous bone marrow transplantation or several agents used in combination.
3. Early detection has a 5-year survival rate approaching 95% for thin (less than 1 mm) lesions in primary melanoma. The 10-year survival rate for lesions of 1.01 to 2 mm in thickness is 89% but drops off to 32% for lesions at greater than 4 mm.

Complications

1. BCC arising around the eyes, nasolabial folds, ear canal, or posterior sulcus may invade deeply and cause extensive destruction into muscle, bone, and dura mater. Hemorrhage may result from eroded vessels.
2. SCC may metastasize in 3% to 4% of cases.
3. If left untreated, melanoma will metastasize over months to years.

Nursing Assessment

1. Have a high index of suspicion for people at risk. Fitzpatrick skin type can be used to assess risk for sun damage to the skin.
   a. Type I: very white skin, always burns.
   b. Type II: white, burns easily, tans with difficulty.
   c. Type III: white to olive, tans after initial burn.
   d. Type IV: light brown, tans easily.
   e. Type V: brown, tans easily.
   f. Type VI: black, does not burn.
2. Ask about sunbathing habits and sunburn history. Question patient about pruritus, tenderness, pain, or bleeding, which are not features of a benign nevus (mole).
3. Ask about changes in preexisting moles or about development of a newly pigmented lesion.
4. Use a magnifying lens or dermatoscope in a brightly lit room to look for variegated color and irregular border and surface in the nevus. Use side lighting to assess subtle elevation.
5. Examine entire skin surface, including the scalp, genital area, gluteal folds, and soles of feet.
6. Examine diameter of mole; melanomas are usually larger than 6 mm; look for lesions situated near the mole.

CLINICAL JUDGMENT Any skin lesion that changes in size or color, bleeds, ulcerates, or becomes infected may be skin cancer. Advise the patient to be evaluated by a dermatologist.

Nursing Interventions

Increasing Knowledge and Awareness

1. Encourage follow-up skin examinations and instruct the patient to examine the skin monthly as follows:
   a. Use a full-length mirror and a small hand mirror to aid in examination.
   b. Learn where moles and birthmarks are located.
   c. Inspect all moles and other pigmented lesions; report any change in color, size, elevation, thickness, or development of itching or bleeding.

2. Teach the patient to use a sunscreen with at least SPF 30 routinely and to avoid becoming sunburned. Reapply sunscreen at least every 2 hours.
   a. Sunlight permanently damages DNA in the skin, and the cumulative effects of the sun may result in skin cancers.
   b. Avoid tanning, especially if the skin burns easily, never tans, or tans poorly.
   c. Avoid unnecessary exposure to the sun, especially during times when ultraviolet radiation is most intense (10:00 a.m. to 3:00 p.m.).
   d. Wear protective clothing (long sleeves, broad-brimmed hat, high collar, long pants). However, clothing does not provide complete protection of UVA rays.
   e. Do not use sunlamps for indoor tanning; avoid commercial tanning salons. Indoor tanning beds are not safe. All sources of ultraviolet light have been determined to be carcinogenic by the World Health Organization.

Reducing Anxiety

1. Provide dressing changes and wound care while teaching patient to take control, as directed, after surgical intervention.
2. Administer chemotherapy with attention to possible adverse effects, as directed.
3. Allow patient to express feelings about the seriousness of diagnosis.
4. Answer questions, clarify information, and correct misconceptions.
5. Emphasize use of positive coping skills and support system.

Patient Education and Health Maintenance

1. Encourage lifelong clinical skin examinations at least annually and self-skin checks monthly.
2. Encourage all individuals to have moles removed that are accessible to repeated friction and irritation, congenital, or suspicious in any way.
3. Teach all individuals the importance of sun protection measures; teach proper use of sunscreen:
   a. Sun protective clothing.
   b. Sunscreens should be used throughout the life span, starting at age 6 months, with UVA and ultraviolet B (UBV) protection, and a minimum SPF of 30.
   c. Sunscreens should be applied before going outdoors to all areas that may be exposed, preferably before dressing. They should be applied liberally to achieve the stated SPF.
   d. Newly developed sunscreens are more resistant to removal by water, clothing, sweating; however, periodic reapplication is necessary when spending prolonged periods outdoors, especially when swimming.
   e. Protect lips with a lip balm that contains a sunscreen with the highest SPF.
4. For more information, refer to any of the following organization:
   The Skin Cancer Foundation (skincancer.org)
   Melanoma Research Foundation (melanoma.org)
   American Cancer Society (cancer.org)
   Melanoma Research Alliance (curemelanoma.org)
   The American Melanoma Foundation (melanomafoundation.org)
   Melanoma Focus (melanomafocus.org)

Evaluation: Expected Outcomes

- Uses sunscreen with an SPF of 30 or greater on a daily basis and reapplies frequently, wears protective clothing, and performs monthly skin examinations.
- Verbalizes decreased anxiety.

Other Dermatologic Disorders

See Table 29-2.

Table 29-2 Other Dermatologic Disorders

NAME AND DESCRIPTION	CLINICAL MANIFESTATIONS	MANAGEMENT	NURSING CONSIDERATIONS
Bacterial Infections			
Folliculitis			
Inflammation of the hair follicle.	• Single or multiple papules or pustules. • Commonly seen from shaving in areas such as the chin or legs.	• Twice daily cleansing with moisturizing soap and/or benzoyl peroxide. • Topical antibiotic treatment, as prescribed by health care provider. • Systemic antibiotics for recurrent or recalcitrant cases.	• Suggest warm compresses to relieve inflammation and promote drainage.
Furunculosis			
Perifollicular abscess (boil) caused by *Staphylococcus aureus*; carbuncles are two or more confluent furuncles.	• Tender, circumscribed, erythematous area whose center may become fluctuant and suppurate. • Commonly occur on the back of the neck, axillae, or buttocks. • Common organism is methicillin-resistant *Staphylococcal aureus* (MRSA).	• Warm compresses to reduce inflammation and promote drainage. • When area becomes fluctuant, incision and drainage can be performed, followed by packing. • Furuncles of the ear canal, nares, upper lip, and nose may require systemic antibiotic treatment because these areas drain directly into cranial venous sinuses.	• Suggest warm compresses. • Warn patient not to squeeze or incise the lesion. • Suggest mild analgesics, if needed. • If severe or recurrent, look for underlying immunosuppression by disorders, such as diabetes, AIDS, alcohol use disorder, or malnutrition.

(continued)

Table 29-2 Other Dermatologic Disorders (*continued*)

NAME AND DESCRIPTION	CLINICAL MANIFESTATIONS	MANAGEMENT	NURSING CONSIDERATIONS
Paronychia			
Inflammation of skin folds surrounding the fingernail; may be bacterial or fungal or both.	• Tender, purulent, erythematous swelling of nail border. • Chronic and recurrent paronychia causes horizontal ridges at the base of the nail.	• Incision and drainage for acutely inflamed paronychia. • Fungicidal or bactericidal ointment for chronic paronychia. • Systemic antibiotic treatment usually is not necessary. • Prevention of trauma and maceration.	• Encourage soaking in warm water for 10–15 min three to four times per day while acutely inflamed to relieve pain and promote drainage. • Identify persons with work-related chronic paronychia (such as bartenders, dishwashers, and housekeepers) and recommend use of rubber gloves over thin cotton gloves when working around moisture.
Erysipelas			
Streptococcal infection involving the superficial dermal lymphatics of the head or extremities, may be *S. aureus* of the face.	• Prodromal—malaise, fever, chills, headache, vomiting, and joint pain. • Local—redness, warmth, swelling, and characteristic raised indurated border. • Leukocytosis. • Advancing edge of the patch with extension. • May vesiculate.	• Oral, IM, or IV antibiotics, usually penicillinase-resistant penicillin derivatives; cephalosporin or macrolide antibiotic may be used.	• Ice or cold compresses may be soothing. • Prompt treatment required in patient with diabetes to prevent extensive spread and necrotizing fasciitis.
Intertrigo			
Superficial inflammation and secondary infection where two skin surfaces are in apposition; may be bacterial or fungal or both.	• Erythematous and macerated rash under breasts, in abdominal skin fold, or in the groin. • Rash may exhibit erosions, fissures, and drainage. • Burning and itching.	• Topical antibacterial and antifungal agents, as prescribed by health care provider.	• Teach patient to prevent skin maceration by separating opposing skin surfaces with gauze or cotton material. • Skin surfaces should be dried thoroughly after bathing with a hair dryer on low setting. • Absorbent powder can be applied lightly to the area after drying as long as no redness or irritation is present. • Loose, air-permeable clothing should be worn.
Mycotic (Fungal) Infections			
Tinea Pedis			
Tinea Pedis—ringworm of the foot Tinea corporis—ringworm of the body Tinea cruris—ringworm of the groin Tinea capitis—ringworm of the scalp	• Caused by the dermatophytes *Trichophyton*, *Epidermophyton*, or *Microsporum*. • Erythematous, inflamed, and vesicular lesions of feet. • Scaling erythematous patches of the body or head with central clearing. • Dull red or brownish rash of upper inner thighs and groin with scaling borders. • Itching and irritation.	• Examination of rash under Wood light differentiates erythrasma, which will fluoresce; most tinea patches will not. • Skin scraping from leading edge shows characteristic spores and hyphae with KOH preparation under microscope. • Treat with topical antifungals or systemic antifungals for severe cases. • Reduction of moisture in the groin, between toes.	• Advise washing one to two times per day with water and mild soap and then applying talcum powder or cornstarch to well-dried area. • Use hair dryer set on low temperature to dry tender areas. • Encourage wearing cotton socks and underwear and light, air-permeable clothing to promote evaporation. • Warn about contamination from feet to the groin or other areas of the body by hands or clothing. • In tinea pedis, encourage use of open shoes or canvas sneakers and avoidance of tight shoes or plastic or rubber-soled shoes or boots. • Wash contaminated clothing in hot water.

Table 29-2 Other Dermatologic Disorders (*continued*)

NAME AND DESCRIPTION	CLINICAL MANIFESTATIONS	MANAGEMENT	NURSING CONSIDERATIONS
DRUG ALERT Oral antifungal agents are associated with significant drug interactions with such agents as warfarin, simvastatin, lovastatin, triazolam, ritonavir, efavirenz, digoxin, cyclosporine, phenytoin, cimetidine, and rifampin. Baseline and periodic liver function test monitoring is recommended. More frequent monitoring of INR or blood levels may be required.			
Tinea Versicolor			
Superficial fungal infection by *Malassezia furfur*	• Patchy macular or mildly scaly rash of the upper trunk and upper arms; yellowish or brownish in light-skinned people, hypopigmented in those with dark skin. • Mild itching and scaling.	• On Wood light examination, may fluoresce and will show hypopigmented patches. • Microscopic examination with KOH preparation of skin scraping shows characteristic "spaghetti and meatball" appearance of hyphae and spores. • Treat with selenium sulfide shampoo (leave on for 40 min before showering) daily for 1 wk. • Topical or systemic antifungal treatment may be used as prescribed by health care provider.	• Common in high-temperature, high-humidity environments. • Advise patient that discoloration may persist after fungus has been eradicated; lost pigmentation will resolve with sun exposure. • Tell patient that recurrence is common after 2–12 wk if prophylactic treatment is not given periodically.
Onychomycosis (Tinea Unguium)			
Fungal infection of the nail	• Discoloration (white, yellow, or darkened) of the nail. • Nail becomes brittle, cracked, irregular, and loosened. • May be some inflammation and pain.	• Identification of offending fungus by microscopic examination of shavings with KOH or by culture. • Treatment with appropriate systemic antifungal for prolonged period—usually at least 6 wk for fingernails and at least 12 wk for toenails. • Surgical removal of the nail may be necessary.	• Encourage patient to adhere to lengthy treatment, as fungal infections of the nail are difficult to treat. • Examine patient for other areas of tinea infection (feet, groin), encourage treatment, and teach patient that infection may be spread from fingernails by scratching. • After nail removal, advise patient to keep hand or foot elevated for several hours and change dressing daily by applying gauze and antibiotic ointment or other prescribed medication until nail bed is free of exudate or blood.
Parasitic and Other Infestations			
Pediculosis			

Pediculosis capitis—head lice
Pediculosis corporis—body lice
Pediculosis pubis—crab louse infestation of the genital region
DRUG ALERT Caution patients who are pregnant and who have pediculosis capitis not to use antiparasitic preparations.
	• Itching is primary complaint.
	• Lice and nits may be seen in seams of clothing (body lice) or clinging to hairs (pubic lice).
	• Skin excoriation in affected area.
	• Erythematous macules or wheals may appear at puncture sites.
	• Gray-blue macules may appear on the trunk or inner thighs with pediculosis pubis.
		• Treatment for pediculosis corporis involves washing with soap and water and washing all infested clothing and linens with hot water. Alternatively, clothes may be dry-cleaned or ironed, paying close attention to the seams.
		• Pediculosis capitis and pubis are treated with a topical antiparasitic preparation, such as lindane or permethrin.
		• Manual removal of nits (eggs) may be performed; retreatment with topical antiparasitic in 3–7 d is recommended.
			• Advise patient that pediculosis pubis is considered a sexually transmitted disease; partners must be examined and treated.
			• Teach patient the proper use of medication:
			  • Apply lotion or cream after bathing to affected hairy and adjacent areas; wash off after 8–12 h.
			  • Alternatively, apply shampoo to affected hairy areas and lather for 4–5 min, rinse, and let hair dry.
			  • Use fine-tooth comb to remove nits.

(*continued*)

Table 29-2 Other Dermatologic Disorders (*continued*)

NAME AND DESCRIPTION	CLINICAL MANIFESTATIONS	MANAGEMENT	NURSING CONSIDERATIONS
		• Petroleum may be applied to eyelashes and then lice and nits removed with swab or tweezers, or pilocarpine drops can be used to paralyze the lice. • Items that cannot be washed or dry-cleaned can be stored for 30 d without use.	• Urge patient to wash all clothing, towels, linens, combs, and hair items by soaking in hot water for 10 min. • Advise patient not to use antiparasitic preparations more frequently than recommended.
Scabies			

Superficial infestation by itch mite; transmitted by close personal contact
POPULATION AWARENESS Infestation with scabies may be a problem in nursing homes, particularly among debilitated patients who require extensive hands-on care.
	• Itching, more intense at night.
	• Small erythematous papules and short, wavy burrows are seen on skin surface.
	• Frequently seen between fingers or in groin area.
	• Spares head and scalp except in children under age 1.
	• Atypical scabies may be found in immunocompromised people and may be resistant to standard treatment.
		• Parasite identified by microscopic examination of skin scraping.
		• Treated with antiparasitic, such as permethrin or crotamiton, and oral treatment with ivermectin 0.2 mg/kg × 1 dose, if indicated.
		• Machine wash and dry clothing and linens on hot cycle.
		• Topical or systemic steroids may be needed to treat symptoms of allergic reaction to mites.
			• Teach proper use of medication:
			  • Apply thin layer from the neck downward, with particular attention to hands, feet, and intertriginous areas; every inch of the skin must be treated because mites are migratory. Apply to dry skin. (Wet skin allows more penetration and the possibility of toxicity.)
			  • Leave medication on for 8–12 h—but no longer, as doing so will irritate the skin. Wash thoroughly.
			• Advise patient to avoid close contact for 24 h after treatment to prevent transmission.
			• Encourage treatment of sexual and close contacts simultaneously.
			• Tell patient that itching may persist for days to weeks following treatment because of an allergic reaction to mites; retreatment is not necessary.

Bedbugs			
Small, nocturnal, blood-sucking insects requiring weekly meals to advance in their life cycle; however can survive up to a year without a meal. Bedbugs hide during the day in seams, crevices, and cracks in mattresses, box springs, walls, and floors.	• Pruritic papules often assume a linear configuration of three to four lesions ("breakfast, lunch, and dinner"). • Found on exposed areas. • Affected individuals often awake in the early morning because of pruritus as this is the time bedbugs are most active. • May be variance in reaction to bedbugs in household members (not all individuals react to bedbug bites to the same degree).	• Bedbug bite lesions will resolve on their own in 1–2 wk. • Treatment aimed at controlling symptoms: oral antihistamines and topical corticosteroids per health care provider.	• Advise close examination of mattress seams for brown spots (excrement of bedbugs), especially when traveling and staying in hotels (to prevent transporting of bedbugs home on luggage) • Advise professional extermination to eradicate infestation • Explain to patient that scratching will make itching worse and may lead to secondary skin infection such as impetigo • Reassure patient that bedbugs do not carry disease and are not associated with uncleanliness.

Table 29-2 Other Dermatologic Disorders (*continued*)

NAME AND DESCRIPTION	CLINICAL MANIFESTATIONS	MANAGEMENT	NURSING CONSIDERATIONS
Viral Infections			
Herpes Simplex Acute vesicular eruption caused by herpes simplex virus type 1 or 2	• Prodromal pain, burning, or tingling, possible fever and malaise. • Tiny vesicles appear on erythematous, swollen base; they rupture, forming painful ulcers and crusting; healing occurs but outbreaks are recurrent. • Can occur anywhere, especially near mucocutaneous junctions. • Viral shedding may occur between symptomatic periods, leading to transmission of the infection.	• Tzanck smear from scraping of ulcer or fluid from vesicle shows characteristic giant cells with intranuclear inclusions but is only 65% sensitive and does not identify type; diagnosed by fluorescent antibody detection or viral culture. • Antiviral treatment with acyclovir, famciclovir, or valacyclovir for acute infection or continuous suppressive therapy to prevent or lessen recurrence. • Analgesics may be needed for widespread and genital eruptions.	• Teach patient that herpes simplex can be transmitted by close and sexual contact; good personal and hand hygiene is required for facial cases; sexual abstinence or condom use is required for genital cases. • Recurrence may be brought on by fever, illness, emotional stress, menses, pregnancy, sunlight, and other factors. • Advise patients with active herpes simplex infection to avoid contact with immunosuppressed individuals, such as those with diabetes, HIV disease, cancer (including those undergoing cancer treatment), alcohol use disorder, and malnutrition, because herpes simplex infection can be severe in these individuals. • Tell patients that lesions usually resolve in 1–2 wk without scarring.
Other Conditions			
Exfoliative Dermatitis Chronic extensive scaling and inflammation of the skin; may be idiopathic or related to preexisting skin conditions, drug reactions, or underlying malignancy	• Starts as patchy erythema, with possible fever, chills, and malaise. • Rapid spread until whole integument is involved. • Skin color changes to scarlet, desquamates, and may ooze serous fluid. • Pruritus, hair loss, and secondary infection.	• Discontinuation of offending drug or treatment of underlying condition. • Systemic corticosteroids should control most cases. • Supportive treatment—bed rest, warm environment, and fluid and electrolyte replacement. • Soothing baths and topical emollients for symptomatic relief • Possible use of immunosuppressants—azathioprine, methotrexate, and cyclophosphamide.	• Monitor fluid balance and electrolyte values. • Watch for signs of secondary infection and report; antimicrobial therapy may be necessary. • Watch for signs of heart failure caused by chronically increased cutaneous blood flow. • Teach patient how to relieve itching with oatmeal baths and emollient creams. • Tell patient to avoid environments with temperature fluctuations to avoid chilling. • Advise patient to avoid all irritants.
Alopecia Hair loss, may be idiopathic (alopecia areata), male-pattern, physiologic, or because of hair pulling (trichotillomania); also because of scarring from other skin or systemic disorders	• Patterned, patchy, or diffuse hair loss. • Inflammation and scarring with some types. • Physiologic alopecia may be associated with hormonal changes, such as childbirth, nutritional factors, or toxin exposure.	• Treatment of underlying causes. • Minoxidil may cause fine hair regrowth in male-pattern baldness and alopecia areata. Finasteride, an oral agent, can be used by only males, with good results. • Other methods of hair replacement—surgical grafting of hair follicles, hair weaving, or hairpieces.	• Explain that alopecia areata and physiologic hair loss are usually temporary and self-limiting. • Encourage patient to change hairstyle or wear hairpieces or turbans, if preferred, until hair grows back after childbirth or temporary condition. • Counsel patient using minoxidil on the slow, limited effects of this treatment, and stress that effects reverse when treatment is stopped.

(*continued*)

Table 29-2 Other Dermatologic Disorders (*continued*)

NAME AND DESCRIPTION	CLINICAL MANIFESTATIONS	MANAGEMENT	NURSING CONSIDERATIONS
Hidradenitis Suppurativa			
Chronic follicular plugging and secondary infection of the apocrine glands of the groin and axilla	• Development of tender red nodules that enlarge, rupture, and suppurate. • Sinus tracts develop with recurrent lesions, leading to continuous inflammation and drainage.	• Initially, prolonged (2 mo or more) administration of an antibiotic, such as tetracycline, clindamycin, or erythromycin, as well as systemic or intralesional corticosteroids; however, progression of the condition is likely. • Surgical treatment necessary when chronic suppuration and fistulas develop. • Incision and drainage or laser stripping. • Cauterization of sinus tracts. • Exteriorization with curettage and electrodesiccation. • Excision with possible skin grafting. • Isotretinoin, antiandrogens, and intralesional or systematic steroid therapy may relieve exacerbations.	• Advise patient to use moisturizing soap and keep axilla and groin dry to reduce bacterial colonization of the skin. • Teach patient the signs of bacterial infection—purulent drainage, odor, pain—that call for notification of health care provider and treatment with antibiotics. • Encourage use of warm compresses to relieve inflammation. • Obesity and cigarette smoking contribute to the disease. Encourage weight loss and smoking cessation, if applicable.
Bullous Pemphigoid			
Chronic bullous disease of autoimmune etiology; occurs in older adults	• Tense vesicles and bullae arise on normal or erythematous skin, rupture, and heal without scarring. • Occurs on flexor aspects of the body, axilla, inguinal areas, abdomen, and, occasionally, on mucous membranes.	• Systemic corticosteroid treatment in widespread involvement. Topical corticosteroids if limited lesions. Immunosuppressant for resistant cases. • Condition may remit within 2–4 yr even without treatment.	• Keep skin clean and dry to reduce chances of secondary infection. • If patient is immobilized, encourage positioning to prevent undue pressure on lesions to avoid risk of premature rupture and secondary infection. • Make sure to differentiate from early pressure injury development and treat pressure injuries appropriately. • Advise patient that lesions usually heal without scarring.
Acne Vulgaris			
Obstruction and inflammation of sebaceous glands and follicles	• Closed comedones (whiteheads). • Open comedones (blackheads). • Papules, pustules, nodules, cysts, or abscesses may develop. • Primary sites are the face, chest, upper back, and shoulders.	• Topical benzoyl peroxide—antibacterial and comedolytic. • Topical retinoic acid, a comedolytic, or adapalene, a more potent synthetic retinoid. • Topical antibiotics—suppress growth of *Propionibacterium acnes* and decrease comedones, papules, and pustules without systemic adverse effects. • Azelaic acid, a topical agent with multiple antiacne effects. • Systemic antibiotics—long-term, low-dose therapy for more inflammatory and extensive cases.	• Advise patient to wash face gently with mild soap and water one to two times per day. • Teach proper application of topical preparation—use sparingly and decrease frequency if irritation and redness develop. • Inform patient about adverse effects of systemic antibiotics. • Ensure that females of childbearing potential are using contraceptives and that a negative pregnancy test has been obtained before starting isotretinoin therapy. Such patients must be on two forms of birth control. All patients must be enrolled in the iPLEDGE system.

Table 29-2 Other Dermatologic Disorders (*continued*)

NAME AND DESCRIPTION	CLINICAL MANIFESTATIONS	MANAGEMENT	NURSING CONSIDERATIONS
		• Retinoid therapy—inhibits sebum production and secretion; for severe, disfiguring cystic acne. • Estrogen therapy—antiandrogenic effect decreases sebum production in females taking oral contraceptives. Spironolactone may be added, if needed, to increase antiandrogenic effect. • Intralesional steroid injection—for inflamed lesions. • Dermabrasion—surgical planning or chemical peels to smooth surface configuration of old scars. Should not be done within 6–12 mo of Accutane use.	• Encourage follow-up and monitoring of laboratory tests during treatment with isotretinoin for elevated liver enzymes, cholesterol, and triglycerides and for decreased HDL. • Advise patient taking isotretinoin to notify health care provider of persistent headache—could signal pseudotumor cerebri. • Tell patient that initiation of therapy may worsen symptoms for several weeks, but to continue treatment. • Advise patient not to squeeze pimples and avoid friction around the face. • Suggest use of water-based and hypoallergenic cosmetics. • Encourage stress management, balanced diet, and avoidance of foods believed to aggravate acne.
Rosacea Erythematous, pustular eruption of the malar cheeks, forehead, nose or around the eyes; most common in adults ages 40–60; unknown cause; may affect the eyes in 20% to 50% of cases	• Diffuse redness, papules, and pustules develop over malar cheeks, forehead, nose, or around the eyes. • Later, dilated blood vessels and flushing are seen. • Rhinophyma (hypertrophic, bulbous nose) may develop. More common in males; rare in females.	• Topical metronidazole gel applied bid. • Oral doxycycline. • Treatment necessary for 4–6 wk and repeated if recurrence. May need long-term suppression with oral antibiotics. • Avoid exercise, stress, hot beverages, and spicy foods.	• Teach patient to avoid flushing by reducing stress, replacing strenuous exercise with low-intensity workouts, staying cool, and avoiding the sun. • Suggest contacting the National Rosacea Society (www.rosacea.org).

AIDS, acquired immunodeficiency syndrome; HDL, high-density lipoprotein; HIV, human immunodeficiency virus; IM, intramuscular; INR, international normalized ratio; IV, intravenous; KOH, potassium hydroxide.

SELECTED READINGS

Aktas, E., Esin, M. H., & Monsen, K. A. (2022). Describing occupational health nursing interventions and outcomes in hair stylist apprentices with hand eczema using the Omaha System as a framework. *Journal of the Dermatology Nurses' Association, 14*(2), 67–75. https://doi.org/10.1097/JDN.0000000000000670

American Academy of Dermatology Association. (2023). *Skin cancer resource center.* https://www.aad.org/public/diseases/skin-cancer

Brown, B., & Hood Watson, K. (2023). Cellulitis. In: *StatPearls*. StatPearls Publishing. https://www.ncbi.nlm.nih.gov/books/NBK549770/

Caro, J. (2022). Alopecia areata exploring the literature. *Journal of the Dermatology Nurses' Association, 14*(5), 214–219. https://doi.org/10.1097/JDN.0000000000000703

Davis, K. (2020). Skin cancer: Back to basics: Basal cell carcinoma. *Journal of the Dermatology Nurses' Association, 12*(2), 78–84. https://doi.org/10.1097/JDN.0000000000000523

Gomez, J., & Admani, S. (2023). Nevus simplex: A review. *Journal of the Dermatology Nurses' Association, 15*(2), 84–85. https://doi.org/10.1097/JDN.0000000000000730

Huang, W., & Ahn, C. (2020). *Clinical manual of dermatology*. Springer. https://doi.org/10.1007/978-3-030-23940-4

Ingold, C. J., & Khan, M. A. B. (2023). Pemphigus vulgaris. In *StatPearls*. StatPearls Publishing. https://www.ncbi.nlm.nih.gov/books/NBK560860/

Jarell, A. (2023). Seborrheic keratosis: The most common reason patients see me. *The Dermatologist, 31*(2), 26–27. https://www.hmpgloballearningnetwork.com/site/thederm/dermatopathologist/seborrheic-keratosis-most-common-reason-patients-see-me

Kohn, M. (2023). *Herpes simplex virus (HSV) in emergency medicine workup*. Medscape. https://emedicine.medscape.com/article/783113-workup

Labib, A., & Milroy, C. (2023). Toxic epidermal necrolysis. In *StatPearls*. StatPearls Publishing. https://www.ncbi.nlm.nih.gov/books/NBK574530/

Litchman, G., Nair, P., Atwater, A., & Bhutta, B. (2023). Contact dermatitis. In *StatPearls*. StatPearls Publishing. https://www.ncbi.nlm.nih.gov/books/NBK459230/

Mastacouris, N., & Mafee, M. (2021). Mohs micrographic surgery: A guide for dermatology nurses. *Journal of the Dermatology Nurses' Association, 13*(4), 201–213. https://doi.org/10.1097/JDN.0000000000000624

National Center for Emerging and Zoonotic Infectious Diseases, Division of Healthcare Quality Promotion. (2020, May). *Skin infections*. Centers for Disease Control and Prevention. https://www.cdc.gov/antibiotic-use/skin-infections.html

Onoday, H. (2021). Skin cancer: Back to basics squamous cell carcinoma. *Journal of the Dermatology Nurses' Association, 13*(1), 28–34. https://doi.org/10.1097/JDN.0000000000000596

Panikkath, D. R., & Sandhu, V. K. (2022). Cutaneous manifestations of systemic lupus erythematosus. *Journal of the Dermatology Nurses' Association, 14*(4), 163–169. https://doi.org/10.1097/JDN.0000000000000692

Rager, T., & Lake, E. (2022). Mycosis fungoides in skin of color. *Journal of Derrmatology Nurses' Association, 14*(6), 261–264. https://doi.org/10.1097/JDN.0000000000000708

Robinson, C. A., Love, L. W., & Farci, F. (2022). Nummular dermatitis. In *StatPearls*. StatPearls Publishing. https://www.ncbi.nlm.nih.gov/books/NBK565878/

Rustad, A., Nickles, M., & Lio, P. (2021). Atopic dermatitis and *Staphylococcus aureus*: A complex relationship with therapeutic implications. *Journal of the Dermatology Nurses' Association, 13*(3), 162–167. https://doi.org/10.1097/JDN.0000000000000619

Simmons, J. (2022). Wound healing and assessment. *Journal of the Dermatology Nurses' Association, 14*(5), 197–202. https://doi.org/10.1097/JDN.0000000000000704

So, J. Y., & Admani, S. (2023). Halo nevi in the pediatric population. *Journal of the Dermatology Nurses' Association, 15*(1), 41–45. https://doi.org/10.1097/JDN.0000000000000719

Stiegler, J., & Brickley, S. (2021). Vitiligo: A comprehensive review. *Journal of the Dermatology Nurses' Association, 13*(1), 18–27. https://doi.org/10.1097/JDN.0000000000000589

Wallace, H. A., & Perera, T. B. (2023). Necrotizing fasciitis. In *StatPearls*. StatPearls Publishing. https://www.ncbi.nlm.nih.gov/books/NBK430756/

Wiley, K. (2021). *Nursing considerations for melanoma survivorship care.* Oncology Nursing Society Voice. https://voice.ons.org/news-and-views/nursing-considerations-for-melanoma-survivorship-care

Zahirsha, Z., & Lake, E. (2020). A ringed enigma: The clinical spectrum of granuloma annulare. *Journal of the Dermatology Nurses' Association, 12*(2), 70–72. https://doi.org/10.1097/JDN.0000000000000525

30 Burns

OVERVIEW AND ASSESSMENT

Burns are a form of traumatic injury caused by thermal, electrical, chemical, or radioactive agents.

Inhalation injury and associated pulmonary complications are a significant factor in mortality and morbidity from burn injury.

Etiology and Pathophysiology

EVIDENCE BASE American Burn Association (2024). *Burn Incidence Fact Sheet.* https://ameriburn.org/resources/burn-incidence-fact-sheet.

American Burn Association (2023). *Annual Burn Injury Summary Report. Analysis of Inpatient Care at Burn Centers 2018-2022.* https://ameriburn.org/quality-care/burn-care-quality-platform-bcqp-registry/bcqp-bisr/

Incidence

1. In the United States, an estimated 398,000 patients seek medical treatment for burn injuries in emergency departments each year, with about 29,000 requiring hospitalization. Approximately 80% of those patients are admitted to burn centers.
2. With an estimated 3,800 fire-related deaths per year, one civilian fire death occurs approximately every 2 hours and 17 minutes. More than 79% of these deaths are from residential fires, with the remaining from motor vehicle fires.
3. The majority of burn-related hospitalizations (52%) are for minor injuries. The mortality rate for patients hospitalized with minor burns is under 1%; for deep burns requiring surgical treatment 2.6%; and for deep burns requiring both surgical intervention and prolonged mechanical ventilation 4.4%. There is nearly a 25% mortality rate for patients who have burn injuries and an inhalation injury. The overall national mortality rate for patients with burns is 3.3%.
4. Flame injury (40%) is the leading cause of burn injuries. Other etiologies include scald (32%), contact with a hot object (43%), electrical injuries (3%), and chemical injuries (9%). Fifty-eight percent of all burns in children are scalds.

Burn Injury

1. A burn injury usually results from energy transfer from a heat source to the body. The type of burn injury may be flame/flash, contact, scald (water, grease), chemical, electrical, inhalation, or any thermal source. Many factors alter the response of body tissues to these sources of heat.
   a. Local tissue conductivity—bone is most resistant to the heat source accumulation. Lesser resistance is seen in nerves, blood vessels, and muscle tissue.
   b. Adequacy of peripheral circulation.
   c. Skin thickness, insulating material of clothing, or dampness of the skin.
2. Physiologic reaction to a burn is dependent on burn size and depth. Smaller burns produce a local response of pain, erythema, and edema at the site of injury. Severe burns, generally described as 20% TBSA or more, may produce a systemic response with widespread hemodynamic and cardiovascular changes.
3. Systemic response to burn injury is a unique combination of distributive and hypovolemic shock. The release of mediators such as tumor necrosis factor-alpha produce a profound effect on the circulatory system. In burns greater than 20% TBSA, there is an intravascular depletion, low pulmonary artery occlusion pressures, elevated systemic vascular resistance, and depressed cardiac output.
   a. Systemic microcirculation loses its vessel wall integrity, and proteins are lost into the interstitium.
   b. Protein loss causes intravascular colloid osmotic pressure to drop and allows fluid to leak from the vessels.
   c. There is an increase of fluid leaking into the interstitium, caused by decreased interstitial pressure and increased capillary permeability to protein.
   d. Over 24 hours, there is a loss of intravascular fluids, electrolytes, and proteins into the interstitium.
   e. The resultant changes are reflected in massive edema formation, loss of circulating plasma volume, hemoconcentration, decreased urine output, and depressed cardiac function.
4. Burns may be superficial thickness (first degree), partial thickness (second degree), or full thickness (third degree) (see Figure 30-1).
   a. Superficial thickness burns are commonly termed first-degree burns. Only the epidermis is involved, remaining intact with no blistering. Local erythema and

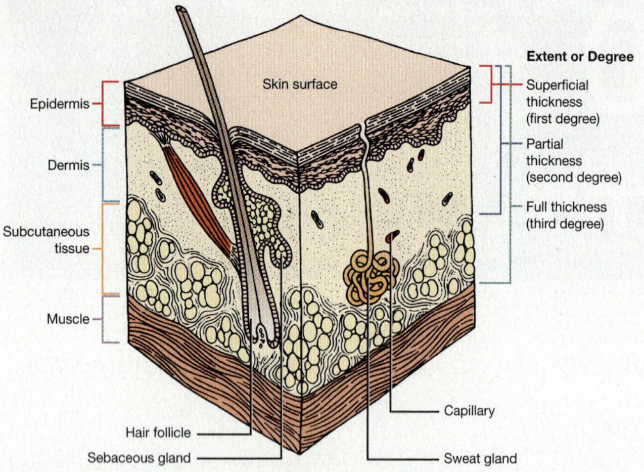

Figure 30-1. Cross-section of the skin depicting blood supply, depth of burn, and relative thickness of skin grafts.

blanching occur similar to a sunburn. Superficial burns are not included in TBSA calculations. Epidermis only injuries usually heal within 5-7 days.

b. Partial-thickness burn injuries, commonly known as second-degree burns, involve the epidermis and upper portions of the dermis. Sweat glands, hair follicles, and nerves remain intact. The wound is moist and very painful. Partial-thickness injuries can be categorized as superficial or deep, depending on how far into the dermis the damage extends. In superficial partial-thickness burns, some of the dermal appendages remain, from which the wound can spontaneously reepithelialize and heal on its own. A deep partial-thickness burn injury can convert to a full-thickness burn injury if patient is underresuscitated or develops an infection. Healing time is 5 to 35 days.

c. Full-thickness injuries, or third-degree or fourth-degree burns, involve all layers of the skin, and sometimes, underlying tissues are destroyed. The burn wound is dry, white, brown, or leathery in appearance. Fourth-degree burns penetrate into or below the subdermal fat and may involve fascia, muscle, or bone. Grafting is usually required to close the wound because dermal appendages are destroyed.

5. Burn depth is directly related to the temperature of the burning agent and the duration of contact with body tissue.
   a. Below 112°F (44.4°C), no local damage occurs unless exposure is for a protracted period.
   b. At 120°F (48.9°C), it takes 5 minutes' exposure to create a full-thickness burn.
   c. At 125°F (51.7°C), the time requirement is 2 minutes, and at 140°F (60°C), only 6 seconds is required.
   d. At 159°F (70.6°C), it takes 1 second to create a full-thickness burn in a healthy adult—less time or temperature in children or older adults.
6. Cellular damage also correlates with duration of exposure to the heat source.
   a. At the core of the burn is the area that was exposed the longest (zone of coagulation). This zone is characterized by coagulation necrosis of cells.
   b. Surrounding the zone of coagulation is the zone of stasis. This area includes injured cells with decreased perfusion.
   c. The zone of hyperemia is an erythematous area surrounding the zone of stasis. This area is likely to recover over approximately 7 to 10 days.
   d. The zones appear in a bull's eye pattern (see Figure 30-2). Underresuscitation or vasoconstriction can lead to further perfusion deficits in the zone of stasis and extend necrosis, causing burn wound conversion and worsening of burn depth.

Inhalation Injury

EVIDENCE BASE Herndon, D. N. (2018). *Total burn care* (5th ed.). Elsevier.

1. Inhalation injury is broadly defined as damage to the airway and pulmonary tissue by heat or chemical irritants. Patients with larger flame burns, and those who were trapped in a burning, enclosed space, are at the highest risk for inhalation injury. Inhalation injuries, combined with extensive cutaneous injury, greatly increase the risk of mortality.
2. Most inhalation injuries that result in death are a result of hypoxia and inhalation of the toxic by-products of combustion.
3. A patient's smoke exposure will contain a variety of poisonous gases, such as cyanide, aldehydes, benzenes, and hydrogen chloride, as a result of the synthetic and natural materials burned near them.
4. Breathing toxic smoke creates a lower airway injury characterized by bronchial casts and constriction, increased pulmonary capillary permeability, and the leakage of protein-filled fluid into the alveolar space.
5. Impaired gas exchange from inhalation injury can be considered a type of acute lung injury (ALI) and may progress to acute respiratory distress syndrome (ARDS).
6. Carbon monoxide toxicity is a complication of inhalation injury and exposure to smoke. Carbon monoxide is a colorless, odorless, tasteless, nonirritating gas produced from incomplete combustion of carbon-containing materials.

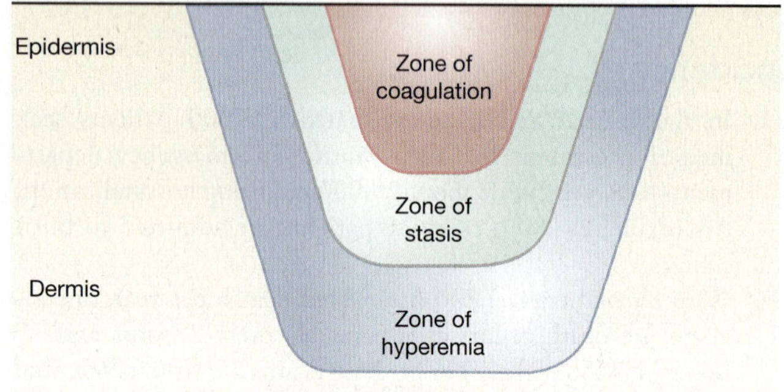

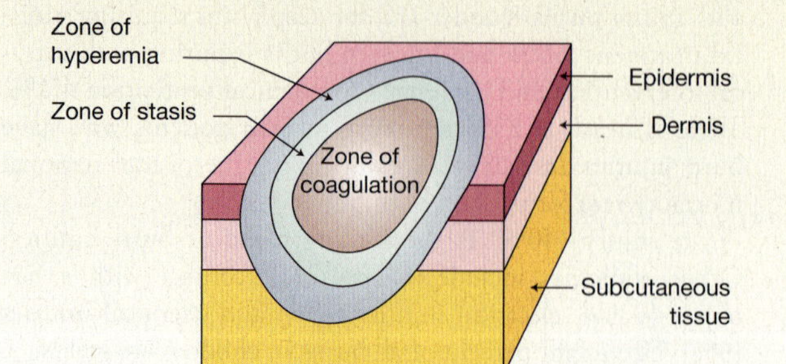

Figure 30-2. **(A)** Cross-section. **(B)** Surface view and depth.

7. Carbon monoxide's affinity for hemoglobin is 200 times greater than oxygen's affinity for hemoglobin.
8. Toxicity depends on concentration of carbon monoxide in inspired air and the length of time of exposure.
9. Although oxygen content of the blood is diminished, the amount of dissolved oxygen in the plasma (PaO_2) is unaffected by carbon monoxide poisoning; therefore, the arterial blood gas (ABG) will appear normal.
10. Pulse oximetry only detects saturated hemoglobin and does not measure carbon monoxide; therefore, the pulse oximetry will appear normal.
11. A serum carboxyhemoglobin level must be measured in any patient with possible exposure to carbon monoxide in a fire.
    a. A carboxyhemoglobin level of less than 10% is not a cause for alarm. Normal carboxyhemoglobin in patients who do not smoke is less than 5%, and patients who smoke can have carboxyhemoglobin levels as high as 10%.
    b. From 10% to 20%, severe headache, flushing, and dilation of skin vessels occur.
    c. Levels of 30% to 50% can produce disorientation, nausea, irritability, dizziness, vomiting, prostration, tachypnea, and tachycardia.
    d. Levels above 50% result in coma, seizures, convulsions, and Cheyne-Stokes respirations, and death is possible.

Systemic Changes in Major Burns

EVIDENCE BASE Cartotto, R., Burmeister, D. M., & Kubasiak, J. C. (2022). Burn shock and resuscitation: Review and state of the science. *Journal of Burn Care & Research, 43*(3), 567-585. https://doi.org/10.1093/jbcr/irac025

CLINICAL JUDGMENT Smaller burn injuries (TBSA less than 20%) are typically characterized by a local response of pain, erythema, and edema at the site of injury. Major burns involving more than 20% TBSA are at risk for exhibiting systemic cardiovascular and hemodynamic changes resulting in burn shock. Act quickly to assess and monitor these patients.

Fluid Shifts

1. The water vapor barrier for the body is the outermost layer of the epidermis. When it is rendered nonfunctioning, severe systemic reactions from fluid losses can occur.
2. Fluid volume deficit is directly proportional to the extent and depth of burn injury.
3. Capillary permeability increases, permitting fluid and protein to move from vascular to interstitial spaces (edema results) for the first 24 to 36 hours, peaking at 12 hours postburn. Protein-rich fluid is lost in blebs of the burned tissues as well as by weeping of second-degree wounds and surface of full-thickness wounds. With reduced vascular volume, the patient will go into shock if untreated.
4. Capillary permeability starts to change in about 48 hours, but protein lost in interstitial spaces may remain there for 5 days to 2 weeks before returning to the vascular system.
    a. When fluid mobilizes (moves from interstitial spaces back to vascular compartment), patients with good cardiac and renal function will diurese.
    b. Patients with impaired cardiac or renal function are in danger of fluid overload and pulmonary edema at this time.
5. Red blood cell (RBC) mass is also diminished because of thrombosis, sludging, and RBC death from thermal injury; as fluid escapes from capillary walls, however, blood concentrates and the hematocrit rises, causing sluggish flow (see Figure 30-3).
6. Capillary stasis may cause ischemia and even necrosis.
7. The body attempts to compensate for losses of plasma volume.
    a. Constriction of vessels.
    b. Withdrawal of fluid from undamaged extracellular space.
    c. Patient thirst.
8. Electrolyte imbalance may also occur.
    a. Hyponatremia usually occurs during the 3rd to 10th day because of fluid shift.
    b. The burn injury also causes hyperkalemia initially because of cell destruction, followed by hypokalemia as fluid shifts occur if potassium is not replaced.

Hemodynamic Changes

1. The initial systemic inflammatory response results in decreased intravascular volume, capillary leak, and edema formation.
2. Compensatory mechanisms, such as an increase in circulating catecholamines, increases heart rate and systemic vascular resistance.
3. Prolonged compensatory responses, increased myocardial oxygen demands, and fluid loss lead to reduced cardiac function that can increase morbidity and mortality.
4. All of these factors result in inadequate tissue perfusion, which may, in turn, cause metabolic acidosis, renal failure, and irreversible burn shock.

Metabolic Demands

1. The initial metabolic response is thought to be activated by proinflammatory cytokines. The release of catecholamines, cortisol, glucagon, renin–angiotensin, antidiuretic hormone, and aldosterone is also increased. The major fuel source is stored glycogen. Major hypermetabolism and catabolism occur immediately postburn. The degree of the response is directly proportionate to the size of the burn injury.

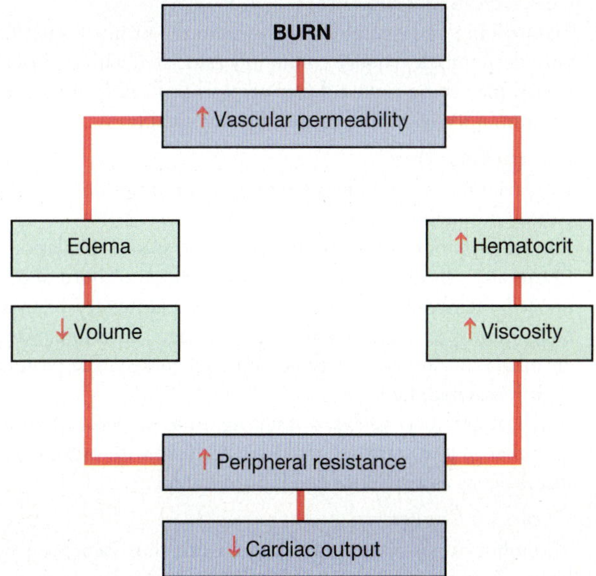

Figure 30-3. Hemodynamic changes in burn injury.

2. Tachycardia, ranging from 100 to 120 beats/min, is common and results from persistent elevation of catecholamine levels.
3. Hyperthermia (usually seen during the first week) is common and is dependent on depth of burn and percentage of TBSA involved.
4. Total body glucose stores are limited and stored liver and muscle glycogen is exhausted within the first few days postburn, hepatic glucose synthesis (gluconeogenesis) increases, and patients with glucose intolerance (patients with obesity and older adults) usually develop hyperglycemia.
5. Increased catabolism leads to increased urea production, especially in nutritionally depleted patients.
6. Body levels of protein begin to decrease as high levels of cortisol and inflammatory cytokines continue to circulate. Skeletal and visceral proteins are mobilized to meet increased nutritional demands. This can lead to muscular weakness, decreased wound healing, and further weakening of the immune system.
7. With adequate fluid resuscitations, the patient's weight will increase during the first few days. Fluid mobilization will result in weight loss, as will the catabolic response. Nutritional support in the form of enteral or total parenteral nutrition (TPN) may be necessary. Weight loss from fluid mobilization usually starts within 3 to 4 days postresuscitation.
8. Despite all nutritional support, it is almost impossible to counteract a negative nitrogen balance; the sooner a burn wound is closed, the more rapidly a positive nitrogen balance is reached.
9. The resting metabolic expenditure increases linearly with the amount of TBSA.
10. The adult patient with burn injury may require 3,000 to 5,000 calories or more per day.
    a. A burn of less than 10% usually requires minimal supplementation.
    b. A high-protein, high-calorie diet is necessary for a 10% to 20% burn.
    c. For burns 20% and greater, beginning enteral nutrition within 24 hours of the injury is recommended.

Renal Needs

1. Glomerular filtration may be decreased in extensive injury.
2. Without resuscitation or with delay, decreased renal blood flow may lead to high output or oliguric renal failure and decreased creatinine clearance.
3. Hemoglobin and myoglobin, present in the urine of patients with deep muscle damage commonly associated with electrical injury, may cause acute tubular necrosis and call for a greater amount of initial fluid therapy and osmotic diuresis.

Pulmonary Changes

1. Hyperventilation and increased oxygen consumption are associated with major burns.
2. The majority of deaths from fire are due to smoke inhalation.
3. Overzealous fluid resuscitation and the effects of burn shock on cell membrane potential may cause pulmonary edema, contributing to decreased alveolar exchange. Therefore, with an inhalation injury, it may be necessary to keep the patient slightly less hydrated.
4. Initial respiratory alkalosis resulting from hyperventilation may change to respiratory acidosis associated with pulmonary insufficiency as a result of major burn trauma.

Hematologic Changes

1. Thrombocytopenia, abnormal platelet function, depressed fibrinogen levels, inhibition of fibrinolysis, and a deficit in several plasma clotting factors occur postburn.
2. Anemia results from the direct effect of destruction of RBCs because of burn injury, reduced life span of surviving RBCs, and blood loss during diagnostic and therapeutic procedures.

Immunologic Activity

1. The loss of the skin barrier and presence of eschar favor bacterial growth.
2. Polymorphonuclear chemotactic activity is suppressed, which results in decreased oxygen consumption and impaired bactericidal activity.
3. Abnormal inflammatory response after burn injury causes a decreased delivery of antibiotics, white blood cells, and oxygen to the injured area.
4. Hypoxia, acidosis, and thrombosis of vessels in the wound area impair host resistance to pathogenic bacteria.
5. Sera IgA, IgM, and IgG are depressed, reflecting depressed B-cell function.
6. Depressed cellular immunity is reflected by lymphocytopenia, delayed skin sensitivity, decreased allograft rejection potential, depletion of thymus-dependent lymphoid tissue, and increased susceptibility to fungi, viruses, and gram-negative organisms.
7. Burn wound sepsis.
    a. After colonization of the burn wound surface by bacteria, subeschar and intrafollicular colonization develops. Intraeschar and subeschar colonization may progress to invasion of subadjacent, nonburned, previously viable tissue.
    b. A bacterial count of 10^5 per gram of tissue, as determined by burn wound biopsy (quantitative culture), indicates burn wound sepsis. Usually, only a swab culture is done of the wound surface, however.
    c. The wound is fully colonized in 3 to 5 days.
8. Seeding of bacteria from the wound may give rise to systemic septicemia.

Gastrointestinal System Impact

1. As a result of sympathetic nervous system response to trauma, peristalsis decreases and gastric distention, nausea, vomiting, and paralytic ileus may occur.
2. Ischemia of the gastric mucosa and other etiologic factors put the patient with burn injury at risk for duodenal and gastric ulcers. Curling ulcers are gastric ulcers associated with severe burn injuries and well-known for causing life-threatening bleeding. The incidence of Curling ulcers has decreased due to the early enteral feeding and gastrointestinal (GI) ulcer prophylaxis now routinely given to patients with severe burns.

Immediate Assessment

Immediate assessment of the burned patient is imperative, particularly to determine burn size and depth, as fluid resuscitation is a hallmark for initial management of severe burns. As with all trauma patients, it is important to start with both the primary and secondary trauma surveys. Avoid becoming distracted by the visual appearance of the burn injury. Instead, consider the mechanism of injury and assess for any concomitant traumatic injuries.

Severity of Burns

Severity of burns is determined by:

1. Depth: first, second (partial-thickness), and third degree (full-thickness). Patients with deeper burns may experience a

greater systemic response. Full-thickness injuries require surgical excision and grafting.
2. Extent: percentage of TBSA. The higher the TBSA, the higher the risk of a systemic response and burn shock.
3. Age: mortality rate increases with age.
4. Area of the body burned: face, hand, feet, perineum, and circumferential burns require special care.
5. Medical history and concomitant injuries and illness. Preexisting conditions such as diabetes, renal failure, and congestive heart failure can complicate the management of even a small burn injury.
6. Inhalation injury.

Assessment for Inhalation Injury

1. If patient was burned in an enclosed space, there should be a high index of suspicion that smoke inhalation has occurred.
2. Evaluate all patients in closed-space fires for symptoms of carbon monoxide poisoning—headache, visual changes, confusion, irritability, decreased judgment, nausea, ataxia, and collapse (see Table 30-1).
3. Observe for upper body burn erythema or blistering of lips, buccal mucosa, or pharynx; singed nasal hair; soot in the oropharynx; and dark gray or black sputum (see Figure 30-4).
4. Listen for hoarseness and crackles. Increasing hoarseness, stridor, and drooling are indicators of increasing need for intubation.
5. Obtain ABGs and carboxyhemoglobin levels.
6. Direct visualization of the vocal cords may be necessary. Further visualization may be accomplished through bronchoscopy, if needed.
7. A chest x-ray should be obtained as a baseline.

Extent of Body Surface Area Burned

1. Anatomic location: burns affecting hands, feet, face, and perineum require specialized care. Circumferential burns also require special attention, and may require escharotomy.

TABLE 30-1 Signs and Symptoms of Toxicity From Carbon Monoxide

CO BLOOD LEVEL	MANIFESTATIONS
0%–10%	• None. • Patients who smoke may have 10% carbon monoxide level or greater.
10%–20%	• Headache, vision disturbance, angina in patients with cardiovascular disease, and slowed mental function.
20%–40%	• Tight feeling in the head, rapid fatigue from muscular effort, decreased muscular coordination, confusion, irritability, ataxia, nausea, vomiting, increased pulse rate, decreased blood pressure, and dysrhythmias.
40%–60%	• Pulmonary and cardiac dysfunction, collapse, coma, and convulsions.
>60%	• Commonly fatal.

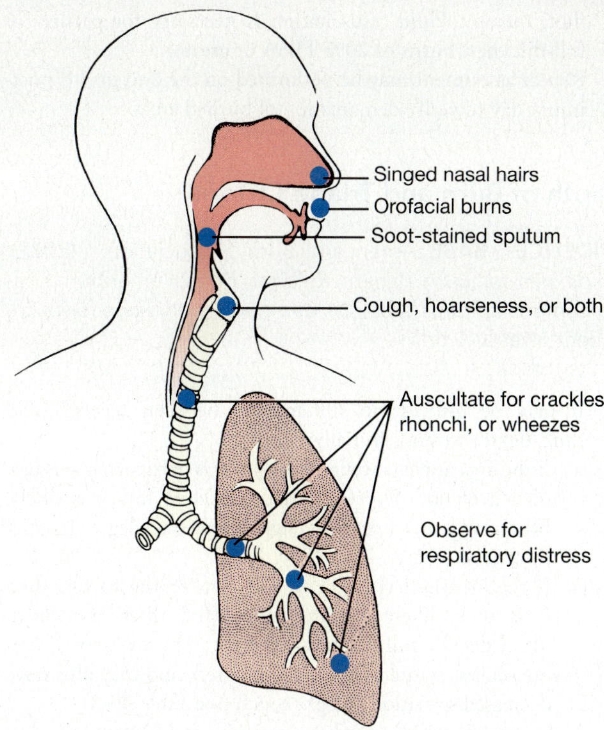

Figure 30-4. Respiratory system signs of inhalation injury.

2. Determination is based on body location and assessments tools, such as the rule of nines (see Figure 30-5), Lund and Browder chart (most accurate; see page 1429), and the rule of palm (approximately 1% of the patient's TBSA). Calculation of the percentage of TBSA burned serves as a guide for

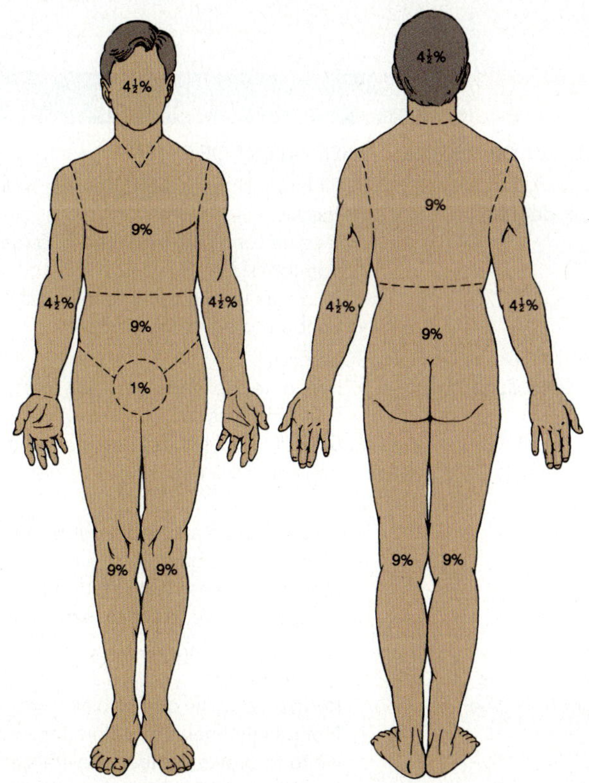

Figure 30-5. Rule of nines for calculating total burn surface area (TBSA).

fluid therapy. Fluid resuscitation is necessary for partial- or full-thickness burns of 20% TBSA or greater.

3. Repeat assessment may be performed on the 2nd or 3rd post-injury day to verify demarcation of burned areas.

Depth of Burn and Triage Criteria

EVIDENCE BASE American Burn Association. (2022). *Guidelines for Burn Patient Referral*. https://ameriburn.org/wp-content/uploads/2024/04/one-page-guidelines-for-burn-patient-referral-1.pdf

1. It may be difficult to differentiate between second- and third-degree wounds initially.
   a. If the area appears wet and pink and is particularly sensate, then a second-degree (partial thickness) injury is likely. Blistering is another classic sign of a second-degree (partial thickness) injury.
   b. If the area is dry, leathery, and firm to the touch, then it is most likely a third-degree (full thickness) burn. Third-degree (full thickness) burns can be a variety of colors such as white, mottled, or charred, and may also have decreased sensation to light touch (see Table 30-2).
2. Melanocytes, which produce melanin and determine skin tone, are found in the epidermal layer. Differences in healthy versus burned skin may be difficult to determine in patients with darker skin tones.
   a. Inflammatory hyperpigmentation may appear rather than erythema.
   b. Patient assessment should be conducted with ambient or natural lighting, and a comparison of the injured and noninjured skin must be made to decipher differences.
   c. Careful assessment and reassessment are necessary to ensure accurate determination of burn depth and TBSA.
3. Reassess daily for the first few days because a partial-thickness burn can convert or progress to a full-thickness burn injury.
4. Patients with partial-thickness burns greater than 10% TBSA, full-thickness burns greater than 5% TBSA, chemical burns, electrical burns, burns of certain areas of the body, and any airway or inhalation injury should be transferred to a regional burn center (see Box 30-1).
5. Telemedicine consultation with the burn center is also recommended in many cases.

BOX 30-1 Burn Center Referral Criteria

- Partial-thickness burns of greater than 10% total body surface area (TBSA).
- Involvement of the face, hands, feet, and genitalia.
- Third-degree burns.
- Electrical burns.
- Chemical burns.
- Inhalation injury.
- Preexisting medical conditions that could complicate management.
- Concomitant trauma where burn injury poses greatest risk.
- Children with burns where facilities lack qualified staff and equipment.
- Patients who require special social, emotional, or rehabilitative intervention.

TABLE 30-2 Assessment of Burn Injury

EXTENT OR DEGREE	ASSESSMENT OF EXTENT	REPARATIVE PROCESS
Superficial Thickness (first degree)	• Pink to red tone; slight edema, which subsides quickly. • Deeper tone may be found in patients with darker skin tones. • Pain may last up to 48 h; relieved by cooling. • Sunburn is a typical example.	• In about 5 d, epidermis peels and heals spontaneously. • Itching and erythema persist for about 1 wk. • No scarring. • If burn does not become infected, heals spontaneously within 5-14 d.
Partial Thickness (second degree)	Superficial: • Pink or red; blisters (vesicles) form; weeping, edematous, and elastic. • Superficial layers of the skin are destroyed; wound is moist and painful.	• Heals in 2–3 wk. • Little to no scarring.
	Deep dermal: • Mottled white and red; edematous reddened areas blanch on pressure. • May be yellowish but soft and elastic—may or may not be sensitive to touch; sensitive to cold air.	• Takes several weeks to heal. • Scarring may occur.
Full Thickness (third degree or fourth degree)	• Destruction of epithelial cells—epidermis and dermis destroyed. • Reddened areas do not blanch with pressure. • Not painful; inelastic; coloration varies from waxy white to brown; leathery devitalized tissue is called eschar. • Destruction of epithelium, fat, muscles, and bone.	• Eschar must be removed. Granulation tissue forms to nearest epithelium from wound margins or support graft. • For areas larger than 1¼–2 in (3–5 cm), grafting is required. • Expect scarring and loss of skin function. • Area requires debridement, formation of granulation tissue, and grafting.

MANAGEMENT

Management of the acute burn injury includes hemodynamic stabilization, metabolic support, wound debridement, use of topical antimicrobial therapy, biologic dressings, and wound closure. Prevention and treatment of complications, including infection and pulmonary damage, and rehabilitation considerations, including physical and occupational therapy and psychiatric and nutritional support, are of major importance.

Hemodynamic Stabilization

Intravenous Fluid Therapy

EVIDENCE BASE American Burn Association. (2018). *Advanced burn life support course. Provider manual 2018 update.* https://ameriburn.org/wp-content/uploads/2019/08/2018-abls-providermanual.pdf

1. The goal of fluid resuscitation is to maintain tissue perfusion and organ function. Careful and continuous fluid management is critical to minimize complications associated with overresuscitation and underresuscitation.
   a. Overzealous fluid resuscitation has been associated with acute coronary syndrome, compartment syndrome of the extremities and abdomen, acute respiratory distress syndrome (ARDS), airway obstruction, and pulmonary edema.
   b. Underresuscitation may lead to inadequate organ and cellular perfusion, stress ulcer development, acute tubular necrosis, and conversion of deep partial-thickness burns to full-thickness burns.
2. The American Burn Association recommends fluid resuscitation for partial-thickness and full-thickness burns exceeding 20% total body surface area (TBSA).
   a. Immediate intravenous (IV) fluid resuscitation is indicated for patients with electrical injury, older patients, or those with cardiac or pulmonary disease.
   b. These patients require meticulous monitoring and may require a modification of fluid requirements.
3. Two large-bore peripheral IV catheters are established for fluid resuscitation and pain management, preferably through nonburned skin. If unable to obtain peripheral IV access, intraosseous or central line catheters may be used.
4. Generally, a crystalloid (lactated Ringer) solution is used for fluid resuscitation. One of several formulas may be used to determine the amount of fluid to be given in the first 48 hours.
   a. Any formula that is used is only a guide and a starting point. Some patients will require more or less fluid depending on their response.
   b. The consensus formula is most commonly used.
   c. Several regional burn centers have developed protocols for fluid resuscitation and a number of computer-driven algorithms have been developed, using technology to more precisely guide fluid management.
5. Traditionally, fluid resuscitation is guided by the consensus formula.
   a. First 24 hours: 2 to 4 mL of lactated Ringer × weight in kg × % TBSA.
   b. One-half amount of fluid is given in the first 8 hours, calculated from the time of injury. If the starting of fluids is delayed, then the same amount of fluid is given over the remaining time. Remember to deduct any fluids given in the prehospital setting.
   c. The remaining half of the fluid is given over the next 16 hours.
   d. Example:
      Patient's weight: 70 kg; % TBSA: 80%.
      4 mL × 70 kg × 80% TBSA = 22,400 mL of lactated Ringer.
      First 8 hours: 11,200 mL or 1,400 mL/h.
      Second 16 hours: 11,200 mL or 700 mL/h.
6. The American Burn Association now recommends specific resuscitation formulas based on burn mechanism and patient age/weight.
   a. Flame/scald injury
      - Adults/children ≥14: 2 mL/kg/TBSA.
      - Children ≤14: 3 mL/kg/TBSA.
      - Infants and young children (≤30 kg): 3 mL/kg/TBSA plus dextrose 5% in lactated Ringer (D5LR) at maintenance rate.
   b. Electrical injury (all ages)
      - 4 mL/kg/TBSA plus D5LR at maintenance rate for infants and young children (≤30 kg).
7. Adjustment to fluid rates should be made based on patient response (i.e., urine output and physiologic response).

Wound Care

Diligent wound care is essential to getting the burn wound healed as soon as possible. Treatment of the partial-thickness burn wounds includes daily or twice-daily wound cleansing with gentle debridement or hydrotherapy (tubbing/showering) and dressing changes. Treatment of deep partial-thickness and full-thickness burns requires early surgical excision of eschar, skin grafting, and postoperative wound care.

Cleansing and Debridement

1. Burn wounds must be cleansed initially and usually daily with a mild antibacterial cleansing agent and saline solution or water.
   a. May be done in the hydrotherapy tub, in the bathtub or shower, or at the bedside.
   b. See "Hydrotherapy Process," later.
2. Nonviable tissue (eschar) may be removed through natural, enzymatic, mechanical, and/or surgical debridement.
3. Burn eschar will begin to separate from the underlying viable tissue by a natural process of bacterial growth, which causes a lysis of protein at the viable–nonviable tissue interface.
4. Loose eschar, dried blood, and exudate can be debrided at the time of wound cleansing.

Hydrotherapy Principles

1. Hydrotherapy is bathing of the patient with burn injury in a tub of water or with a water shower to facilitate cleansing and debridement of the burned area. Even ventilator-dependent patients can be safely bathed when a shower table is used.
2. Advantages
   a. Topical medications, adherent dressings, and eschar are more easily removed.
   b. Provides an opportunity for the patient to practice range-of-motion (ROM) exercises.
   c. Total assessment of the burn area is facilitated; total body cleansing can be achieved.
3. Disadvantages
   a. Loss of body heat; loss of sodium.
   b. Uncomfortable and, at times, painful for the patient.

c. Maintenance of IV lines and ventilator care may be difficult during bathing and showering.

CLINICAL JUDGMENT Adequately premedicating the patient with an opioid and anxiolytic, as prescribed, allows the patient to participate in and tolerate the bathing and dressing change process.

Hydrotherapy Process

1. Describe the procedure to the patient who is experiencing hydrotherapy for the first time.
2. Select the time for future hydrotherapy sessions in collaboration with the patient; administer a pain control medication, as prescribed, before the treatment so that maximum benefit is realized. The use of nonpharmacologic nursing interventions can also reduce the pain experience.
3. If the patient has an indwelling catheter, drain and plug it or maintain a closed system to avoid contamination.
4. Sterile technique is adhered to as closely as possible in preparing the patient for hydrotherapy, during hydrotherapy, and in redressing the patient's wounds after therapy.
5. During hydrotherapy, after cleansing of the wounds, debride wound, shave adjacent areas at health care provider's direction, shampoo hair, and gently wash unburned skin.
6. Limit hydrotherapy to as brief a time as possible to decrease the loss of body temperature and subsequent chilling.
7. Never leave the patient unattended in the tub.
8. Respect the patient's feelings and expressions of stress, pain, cold, and fatigue.
9. After treatment, the patient may be weighed before being carefully dressed and returned to the unit/room.
10. Document significant data, including status of the wound.

Topical Antimicrobials

1. Topical medications are used to cover burn areas and to reduce the number of organisms. See Table 30-3. Identifying the most

TABLE 30-3 Topical Antimicrobial Agents for Burns

TOPICAL AGENT	DESCRIPTION AND INDICATIONS	DISADVANTAGES	NURSING CONSIDERATIONS
Silver Sulfadiazine 1%			
	• White, crystalline, highly insoluble compound in an opaque, odorless, water-miscible cream. • Exerts antimicrobial effect against gram-negative and gram-positive bacteria and yeasts at level of cell membrane and cell wall. • Systemic absorption is rare. • Most widely used agent and least common incidence of adverse effects.	• May cause transient leukopenia that disappears after 2–3 d of treatment. • May increase possibility of kernicterus; should not be used in pregnant patients in the last trimester, premature neonates, or infants younger than age 2 mo. • Impairment of hepatic and renal function that results in decreased excretion of drug constituents may preclude therapeutic benefits of continued silver sulfadiazine administration. • Exposure to sunlight produces gray discoloration. • Crystalluria and methemoglobinemia are rare toxic effects. • Protracted use may be associated with emergence of sulfadiazine resistance.	• Use with open treatment or with light or occlusive dressings. • Apply with sterile gloved hand directly to the wound or to gauze dressing 1/16 in (0.2 cm) thick, once or twice per day after a thorough wound cleansing. • Silver sulfadiazine will be discontinued if white blood cell (WBC) count is <1,500 in an adult or <2,000 in a child; WBC count usually returns to normal in 2–4 d, after which application may be resumed.
Mafenide Acetate			
About 10% cream or 5% solution	• Usually supplied in water-miscible, hydroscopic cream base. • Active against gram-positive and gram-negative organisms and some anaerobes. • Not significantly bound by protein and wound exudate. • Good penetrating power and useful for control of established invasive burn wound infection.	• Painful during and for a short period following application. • A potent carbonic anhydrase inhibitor resulting in metabolic acidosis, therefore not used if total body surface area is >20%. • Brisk alkaline diuresis and inappropriate polyuria may result when used on patients with a large burn surface area. • Compensatory hyperventilation and pulmonary failure may ensue if mafenide is not discontinued. • Hemolytic anemia is a rare complication.	• Cream is applied without dressing, if possible and must be reapplied every 12 h to maintain therapeutic effectiveness. • Therapeutic solution concentration is maintained with bulky wet dressings; rewet every 2–4 h. • Application is associated with significant pain. • Hypersensitivity evidenced by maculopapular rash; it is treated with antihistamines or by discontinuing use. • Requires careful monitoring of pulmonary status and acid–base and fluid balance.

TABLE 30-3 Topical Antimicrobial Agents for Burns (*continued*)

TOPICAL AGENT	DESCRIPTION AND INDICATIONS	DISADVANTAGES	NURSING CONSIDERATIONS
Silver Nitrate (0.5% solution)	• Clear solution with low toxicity and significant antimicrobial effect against common burn wound pathogens. • Active against gram-positive and gram-negative organisms, and yeasts. • Absorption is minimal because of the insolubility of its chloride and other salts. • Nonallergenic and not usually painful on application.	• Can cause electrolyte abnormalities by depleting serum sodium, chloride, potassium, and magnesium. • Methemoglobinemia is a rare complication. • Stains everything (including skin) brown or black. • Does not penetrate deeply into eschar.	• Monitor electrolyte balance carefully; supplementation with sodium and potassium salts is routinely needed for patients with extensive burns. • Use bulky dressings; rewet every 2–4 h to maintain therapeutic concentration. • Maintain patient warmth and minimize transcutaneous evaporative water loss with dry top layer, such as stockinette or bath blanket.
Mupirocin 2% Ointment	Active against gram-positive and methicillin-resistant *Staphylococcus aureus* (MRSA).	• Allergy is a major contraindication. • Prolonged use may result in superinfection.	• May be ordered based on culture or prophylactically. • Apply two to three times daily.
Silver Impregnated Dressings	• Silver impregnated on a neutral backing.	• Cannot be moistened until time of application. • Moisten with sterile water only; saline deactivates the silver. • Need to keep moist with sterile water every 8 h.	• Dressing change required only every 4–7 d, reducing pain. • Can be used on an outpatient basis. • Benefit over silver sulfadiazine related to decreased wound pain.
Bacitracin, Polymyxin B, and Neomycin	• Bacitracin ointment (petroleum based) helps maintain moist environment; is active against gram-positive organisms; no action against gram-negative organisms or yeast. • Polymyxin B ointment is active against gram-negative organism; limited action against gram-positive. • Neomycin ointment is active against gram-negative and gram-positive organisms. • Combination topical agents (e.g., Polysporin [Bacitracin/Polymyxin B], Neosporin [Bacitracin/Polymyxin B/Neomycin]) overcome limited spectrum of microbial coverage of single-drug ointments.	• Primary use in superficial burns. • May lead to fungal superinfection with prolonged use. • Polymyxin B may lead to systemic absorption with large total body surface area (TBSA) burns. • Neomycin: resistance is more common. Local skin irritation is more common. When used with a large TBSA burn nephrotoxicity and ototoxicity is more common.	• All agents: • Discontinue use after wound healing. • Clean affected area before use and apply small amounts. • May be left open to air or be covered with a dressing.

effective topical antimicrobial and dressing medium is an essential aspect in promoting wound closure.

2. Factors such as location of burn, burn depth, ease of application and removal, pain, frequency of dressing changes, and cost need to be considered.
3. Topical antimicrobials are applied directly to the burn area as ointments, creams, or solutions, or they may be incorporated in single-layer dressings that do not stick to the wound but permit drainage.
4. Dressings may take the form of commercial multilayered pads, standard 4 × 4-gauze pads, or several layers of stretch bandage (Kerlix type).
5. If gauze or pads are used, they may be held in place by stretch gauze or net tube dressings.

6. When wet dressings are used, that is, after a surgical procedure, then the same dressings are maintained. They are remoistened every 4 to 6 hours, as ordered. Heat loss may be prevented by limiting evaporative loss with a dry blanket and by warming the bed and room. When wet dressings are used, 20-ply gauze will help retain solution at the proper concentration if rewet every 4 hours. A dry top layer of stockinette or a cotton bath blanket prevents evaporative heat loss.
7. Desired characteristics in a topical antimicrobial:
   a. Demonstrates action against a broad spectrum of bacteria.
   b. Has the ability to diffuse through the wound and penetrate the eschar.
   c. Nontoxic and noninjurious to body tissue.
   d. Is inexpensive, is pleasant to use, is odorless or has pleasant odor; will not stain the skin or clothing.
   e. Will not cause resistant strains of pathogenic organisms to develop.
8. Generally, all of the previously applied topical cream should be removed and the wound gently cleansed before applying new cream with each dressing change. Extremity dressings should be wrapped distally to proximally, taking care to avoid circulatory compromise when edema occurs or dressing is too tight.
9. Some silver-based dressings can be left in place on second-degree (partial thickness) wounds or donor sites for several days. Most require an outer wrap to secure the dressing in place and this can be changed as needed.
10. Identifying the best evidence on dressings for superficial and partial-thickness burn injuries has produced limited results. There is a need for more well-developed, high-quality studies evaluating the multitude of dressing options for burn care and wounds in general.

EVIDENCE BASE Sangha, M. S., Deroide, F., & Meys, R. (2024). Wound healing, scarring and management. *Clinical and Experimental Dermatology, 49*(4), 325-335. https://doi.org/10.1093/ced/llad410

Surgical Management

Early excision and skin grafting are the goal to early wound closure for deep partial-thickness and full-thickness burn injuries. For types of burn wound coverings, see Table 30-4, page 916.

TABLE 30-4 Burn Wound Coverings

COVERING AND DESCRIPTION	INDICATIONS	SOURCE OR FORM	NURSING CONSIDERATIONS
Allograft/Homograft			
• Human cadaver skin, about 0.015 in thick. • Preferred biologic dressing.	• Debridement and coverage option. • To protect granulation tissue after escharotomy. • To cover excised wound immediately. • To serve as test graft before autograft.	Fresh, cryopreserved homografts available from tissue banks throughout the United States.	• Length of time dressing is left in place varies greatly. • Observe for exudate; also, watch for local and systemic signs of infection and rejection.
Xenograft Heterograft			
• Pigskin similar to human skin, harvested after slaughter, then cryopreserved, or lyophilized for long-term storage.	• Same as for homograft. • To cover meshed autografts. • To protect exposed tendons. • To cover partial-thickness burns that are eschar-free and clean or only slightly contaminated.	Available in fresh, frozen, or lyophilized form, in rolls or sheets; also available meshed and impregnated with silver sulfadiazine.	• Change every 2–5 d; wound may be dressed or left open. • Observe for signs of infection.
Biobrane			
• Nylon fabric bonded to silicon rubber membrane, containing collagenous porcine peptides. • Elastic and durable; adheres to wound surface until removed or sloughed by spontaneous re-epithelialization.	• To cover donor graft sites. • To protect clean, superficial, partial-thickness burns and excised wounds awaiting autografts. • To cover meshed autografts.	Individually packaged sterile sheets of various sizes; also in glove-shaped form for hand burns.	Useful for wounds awaiting autograft because it can be left in place 3–14 d and is permeable to antimicrobials, which can be applied over it.
DuoDERM			
• Hydroactive dressing that interacts with moisture on the skin, creating bond that makes it adhere. • Interacts with wound exudate to produce soft, moist gel, facilitating removal.	• To cover small partial-thickness burns. • To prevent bacterial contamination.	Individual, peelable, "blister" packages containing sheets of various sizes (from 3 × 3 in to 8 × 12 in).	• Use size that allows dressing to extend beyond wound onto healthy skin. • Be careful to distinguish pus from liquefied material that normally remains in the wound. • Used until it falls off, usually 7–10 d.

TABLE 30-4 Burn Wound Coverings *(continued)*

COVERING AND DESCRIPTION	INDICATIONS	SOURCE OR FORM	NURSING CONSIDERATIONS
Integra Artificial Skin			
• Permanent bilayer membrane composed of a dermal portion consisting of a porous lattice of fibers of cross-linked bovine collagen and glycosaminoglycan composite and an epidermal layer of synthetic polysiloxane polymer.	• To create a template for dermal regeneration by formation of a "neodermis." Provides an immediate post-excisional physiologic wound closure. Allows use of a thinner autograft.	Sterile individual sheets.	• Dermal regeneration layer is very soft and fragile. No hydrotherapy immersion should occur while the silicone layer is still in place. • Change outer dressing every 4–5 d. • Removal of the silicon layer is usually done in 14–21 d.
Silver Releasing Dressings (Acticoat, Aquacel AG)			
• Nanocrystalline dressings when moistened produce a sustained release of silver ions. • Hydrocolloid dressings have silver bound to the dressing and gradually release silver with the absorption of fluid. • Activated charcoal dressings absorb bacteria into the dressing to be destroyed by silver. • Some silver foam dressings are available.	• Provide wound coverage or a temporary layer of protection with antimicrobial protection. • Benefit over silver sulfadiazine related to decreased wound pain.	• Sterile individual sheets or rolls.	• Follow manufacturer's guidelines for application, care, and removal as directed by a provider.

General Considerations

1. Early surgical intervention reduces the potential for wound infection and potentially reduces the length of stay.
2. Operative excision is very stressful metabolically and incurs significant blood loss; therefore, more conservative measures may be indicated for some patients.
3. With tangential excision, a special blade is used to remove thin layers of damaged skin until live tissue is evidenced by capillary bleeding. It is commonly used with deep partial-thickness burns and full-thickness burns and followed with immediate coverage with a biosynthetic or biologic dressing or an autograft.
4. With fascial (primary) excision, the skin, lymphatics, and subcutaneous tissue are removed down to fascia, with either immediate autografting or temporary coverage with biologic or biosynthetic dressings. This is repeated until all deep burn areas are removed.

Biologic Dressings

1. Biologic dressings are used to temporarily cover large surfaces of the body. Usually, they are split-thickness grafts harvested either from human cadavers or from other mammalian donors such as pigs.
   a. An allograft is a graft of the skin taken from a person other than the patient with burn injury and applied to a burn wound (most common type of biologic dressing). A cadaver is the most common source. Other sources may be live donors having a panniculectomy or other surgery.
   b. A xenograft or heterograft is a segment of the skin taken from an animal such as a pig.
2. Allograft can provide temporary wound closure for large surface area burns when there is not enough healthy skin available for autografting. They typically adhere for 2 to 3 weeks before sloughing off.
   a. Skin color is unimportant because it is only a temporary graft.
   b. Donor should be an adult, free from infection. All donated skin must be tested and free from contagious diseases before it can be used for donation.

Purpose and Benefits

1. Decreases heat, fluid, and protein losses.
2. Reduces bacterial proliferation.
3. Closes wound temporarily; enhances production and protection of granulation tissue.
4. Protects exposed neurovascular and muscle tissue as well as tendons.
5. Reduces pain and facilitates patient comfort.
6. Acts as a test graft to determine when granulating wounds will accept autograft successfully.
7. Provides an effective donor site dressing.

Clinical Procedures

1. Devitalized tissue is first removed surgically or enzymatically.
2. Allograft is applied directly (shiny side down) to the denuded area. Before applying, it may be dipped in saline solution. It may be trimmed to fit the wound.
3. Grafts are usually secured with adhesive strips or with staples or sutures. The graft is covered with wet nonadherent gauze (antibiotic solution or saline) and covered with stretch gauze; this is again wet down with the appropriate solution.
4. The wound remains unchanged initially for 3 to 5 days, during which time it is wet down every 4 to 6 hours. Sheet grafts do not require the wet-down procedure.
5. After the initial takedown (typically known as the first postoperative dressing removal), dressings are changed daily.

6. If allograft or xenograft is used, the wound bed may be prepared for permanent autografting.

Biosynthetic Dressings

1. Temporary biosynthetic dressings help prevent bacterial contamination.
2. Used when permanent autograft is unavailable or unnecessary (as when partial-thickness wounds will heal spontaneously over time).
3. Biobrane (Woodruff Laboratories) consists of a custom-knit nylon fabric mechanically bonded to an ultrathin silicone rubber membrane, to which collagenous peptides of porcine skin are covalently bonded.
   a. Has a longer shelf life and lower cost than biologic dressings such as pigskin.
   b. Is widely used for coverage of shallow wounds awaiting epithelialization, excised wounds awaiting autografts, widely meshed autografts until closure of interstices, and donor sites awaiting healing.

Artificial Dermis

1. Method being studied in selected burn centers to improve survival of patients with massive burns and little donor skin available.
2. Composed of a porous collagen–chondroitin 6-sulfate fibrillar mat covered with a thin Silastic sheet.
3. Used with an epidermal graft to provide a permanent cover that is at least as satisfactory as other available grafting techniques.
4. Used with donor sites that are thinner and that heal faster; seems to result in less hypertrophic scarring than the usual grafting methods.

Wound Closure

1. Skin grafting is usually required or preferred with full-thickness burns or in deep partial-thickness wounds or in areas of function.
2. After gradual eschar removal and development of a base of granulating tissue or in the presence of viable tissue after excision, grafts of the patient's own skin (autografts) are applied.
3. Sheet grafts or meshed grafts, providing wider expansion from donor sites, may be used.
4. Blood flow is established by the 3rd or 4th day, and postgrafting, vascular continuity, and wound closure have been established by the 7th to 10th day.
5. Definitive wound closure in patients with extensive full-thickness injuries may require multiple operations over many weeks or even months. To hasten healing, cultured epithelial autografts (cultured skin) may be used for patients with large burns and little available donor skin.
6. Many partial-thickness burn wounds will heal spontaneously within a few weeks, provided they are protected from infection.
7. The donor site requires meticulous care and may be covered with a synthetic dressing, silver sheeting, or an antimicrobial cream such as silver sulfadiazine 1%, among other dressings.

Other Interventions

Pain Management

1. Pain relief should be considered in the primary assessment of all initial burn injuries. A burn injury is one of the most feared painful injuries; all burn injuries are painful.
2. Initial pain medications should be given via the IV route. Pain medication that is given intramuscularly may not be metabolized properly through burned tissue. Acceptable IV pain medications are morphine, hydromorphone, and fentanyl.
3. Careful administration of opioids for pediatrics, older adults, and patients with higher pain tolerances to avoid respiratory suppression or overdose.

Nutrition Support

1. Initially, institute nothing-by-mouth (NPO) status until bowel sounds return (1 to 2 days). However, isotonic enteral tube feedings are typically started within 24 hours to help maintain a functioning gastrointestinal (GI) tract. Small amounts of erythromycin may be used to encourage GI motility.
2. Reduce metabolic stress by allaying pain, fear, and anxiety and maintaining a warm environment.
3. Nutritional management must be aggressive to combat acute nutritional deficiency and weight loss; a positive nitrogen balance should be the goal throughout postburn care.
4. When bowel sounds return, administer oral fluids and advance diet, as tolerated.
5. Offer more solid food after 2 to 3 days postburn as tolerance to food improves.
   a. Build up daily caloric intake to match daily caloric expenditure.
   b. Provide 3-g protein/kg body weight: 20% of needed calories in the form of fats; remainder in carbohydrates.
6. Oral anabolic steroids have shown good results in helping to maintain lean muscle mass.
7. When caloric requirements cannot be met by enteral feedings, it may be necessary to initiate total parenteral nutrition (TPN) (amino acids, carbohydrates, and fat emulsions).
8. Provide potassium and vitamin and mineral supplements (zinc, iron, and vitamin C).

Prevention and Treatment of Complications

Primary causes of morbidity and mortality in patients with burn injuries are those related to infection and pulmonary problems.

1. Topical antibacterial agents help to slow the proliferation of pathogenic organisms until wound closure occurs spontaneously or through surgical intervention.
2. Broad-spectrum antibiotics may be necessary to treat systemic gram-positive and gram-negative infections and sometimes fungal infection.
3. Critical diagnostic parameters include observing for signs of burn wound sepsis, obtaining quantitative and qualitative wound biopsy, assessing for signs of systemic septicemia, and taking blood for cultures.
4. Meticulous pulmonary care is essential because pneumonia is common.
5. Severe inhalation injury, including ARDS, can contribute significantly to mortality, even though the burn wound size may be small.

Nursing Management of the Patient With Burn Injury

Nursing Assessment

1. Obtain a thorough history, including:
   a. Causative agent: hot water, chemical, gasoline, flame, tar, radiation PUVA (Psoralen plus ultraviolet A) light, and so on.

b. Duration of exposure.
c. Circumstances of injury, including whether in closed or open space, accidental or intentional, or self-inflicted.
d. Initial treatment, including first aid, prefacility emergency care (including fluids, intubation), or care rendered in another facility (emergency department, etc.).
e. Patient's age and preexisting medical problems, for example, heart disease, human immunodeficiency virus, substance use disorder, diabetes, chronic obstructive pulmonary disease (COPD), or hepatitis.
f. Current medications: include both prescription and over the counter.
g. Concomitant injuries (e.g., from fall, explosions, assaults).
h. Evidence of inhalation injury.
i. Medication and food allergies and tetanus immunization status.
j. Height and weight.

2. Perform ongoing assessment of hemodynamic and respiratory status, condition of wounds, and signs of infection.
3. Perform pain assessment using simple pain scale and observing for signs of pain.

Nursing Interventions

EVIDENCE BASE Carey, M. G., Valcin, E. K., Lent, D., & White, M. (2021). Nursing care for the initial resuscitation of burn patients. *Critical Care Clinics of North America, 33*, 275–285. https://doi.org/10.1016/j.cnc.2021.05.004

Achieving Adequate Oxygenation and Respiratory Function

1. Provide humidified 100% oxygen until carbon monoxide level is known. (*Caution:* Adjust oxygen flow rate for patient with COPD, as prescribed.) If the patient is stable, try to get the initial arterial blood gas (ABG) on room air.
2. Assess for signs of hypoxemia (anxiousness, tachypnea, tachycardia) and differentiate this from pain.
3. Suspect respiratory injury if burn occurred in an enclosed space.
4. Observe for and report erythema or blistering of the buccal mucosa; singed nasal hairs; burns of lips, face, or neck; and increasing hoarseness.
5. Monitor respiratory rate, depth, rhythm, and cough.
6. Auscultate chest and note breath sounds.
7. Note character and amount of respiratory secretions; report carbonaceous sputum.
8. Observe for signs of inadequate ventilation and begin serial monitoring of ABG levels and oxygen saturation.
9. Keep intubation equipment nearby and be alert for signs of airway obstruction.
10. Provide mechanical ventilation, continuous positive airway pressure, or positive end-expiratory pressure, if requested.
11. In mild inhalation injury:
    a. Provide humidification of inspired air.
    b. Encourage coughing and deep breathing.
    c. Promote clearance of secretions through chest physical therapy (see page 154) or intrapulmonary percussive ventilation.
12. In moderate to severe inhalation injury:
    a. Initiate more frequent bronchial suctioning.
    b. Closely monitor vital signs, urine output, and ABG levels.
    c. Administer bronchodilator treatments, as ordered.
    d. It may be necessary to have patient intubated and placed on mechanical ventilation.
13. Document all observations and particularly note trends in vital sign changes.

CLINICAL JUDGMENT Be prepared to assist with early intubation if inhalation injury is suspected, as progressive airway edema is expected in the first 24 hours of inhalation injury.

Maintaining Adequate Tidal Volume and Unrestricted Chest Movement

1. Observe rate and quality of breathing; report if progressively more rapid and shallow.
2. Assess tidal volume; report decreasing volume to health care provider.
3. Encourage deep breathing and incentive spirometry (may use sigh control on ventilator, as needed).
4. Place patient in semi-Fowler position to permit maximal chest excursions if there are no contraindications, such as hypotension or trauma.
5. Make sure that chest dressings are not constricting.
6. Prepare the patient for chest escharotomy and assist, as indicated.
7. Document all observations and particularly note trends in vital sign changes.

Supporting Cardiac Output

1. Position the patient to increase venous return.
2. Administer fluids, as prescribed.
3. Monitor vital signs, including apical pulse and respirations, and urine output at least hourly.
4. Monitor invasive hemodynamic parameters (central venous pressure, pulmonary artery pressures, and cardiac output) as requested.
5. Monitor sensorium.
6. Document all observations and particularly note trends in vital sign changes.

Promoting Peripheral Circulation

1. Remove all jewelry and clothing.
2. Elevate extremities.
3. Monitor peripheral pulses hourly; use Doppler, as necessary.
4. Prepare the patient for extremity escharotomy if circulation is impaired.
5. Avoid tight, constrictive dressings.

Facilitating Fluid Balance

1. Titrate fluid intake, as tolerated and per order/protocol. The initial resuscitation formula is only a base.
2. Maintain accurate intake and output records.
3. Weigh the patient daily with dressings removed.
4. Monitor results of serum potassium and other electrolytes.
5. Be alert to signs of fluid overload and heart failure, especially during initial fluid resuscitation and immediately afterward, when fluid mobilization is occurring.

POPULATION AWARENESS Older patients and those with impaired renal function, cardiovascular disease, and pulmonary disease are more likely to develop fluid overload. Proceed with caution.

Protecting and Reestablishing Skin Integrity

1. Cleanse wounds and change dressings one to two times per day. Use an antimicrobial solution or mild soap and water. Dry gently. This may be done in the hydrotherapy tank, bathtub, shower, or at the bedside.
2. Debridement may be performed at this time. Monitor patient tolerance and limit as appropriate. Additional analgesia may be necessary.
3. Apply topical bacteriostatic agents, as directed. Cream or ointment is applied 1/8 in (3 mm) thick.
4. Dress wounds, as appropriate, using conventional burn pads, gauze rolls, or any combination. Dressings may be held in place with gauze rolls or netting.
5. For grafted areas, use extreme caution in removing dressings; observe for and report serous or sanguineous blebs or purulent drainage. Redress grafted areas according to facility protocol/per provider order.
6. Observe all wounds daily and document wound status on the patient's record. Report any odor, drainage, bleeding, or signs of infection or cellulitis.
7. Promote healing of donor sites by:
   a. Preventing contamination of donor sites that are clean wounds.
   b. Opening to air for drying postoperatively if gauze or impregnated gauze dressing is used.
   c. Following health care provider's or manufacturer's instructions for care of sites dressed with synthetic materials.
   d. Allowing dressing to peel off spontaneously.
   e. Cleansing healing donor site with mild soap and water when dressings are removed; lubricating site twice daily and as needed.

Preventing Urinary Infection

1. Follow institutional protocols to avoid catheter-associated urinary tract infection.
   a. Maintain closed urinary drainage system and ensure patency. Use a catheter impregnated with an antimicrobial agent whenever possible.
   b. Empty drainage bag per facility protocol.
   c. Provider catheter care per facility protocol.
2. Frequently observe color, clarity, and amount of urine.
3. Encourage removal of catheter and use of urinal, bed pan, or commode as soon as frequent urine output determinations are not required.

Promoting Stable Body Temperature

1. Be efficient in care; do not expose wounds unnecessarily.
2. Maintain warm ambient temperatures.
3. Use radiant warmers, warming blankets, or adjustment of the room temperature to keep the patient warm.
4. Provide a dry top layer for wet dressings to reduce evaporative heat loss.
5. Warm wound cleansing and dressing solutions to body temperature.
6. Use blankets in transporting patient to other areas of the hospital.
7. Obtain urine, sputum, and blood cultures for temperatures above 102°F (38.9°C) rectal or core temperature or if chills are present.
8. Administer antipyretics, as prescribed.

Avoiding Wound and Systemic Infection

1. Wash hands with antibacterial cleansing agent before and after all patient contact.
2. Use barrier garments—isolation gown or plastic apron—for all care requiring contact with the patient or the patient's bed.
3. Cover hair and wear mask when wounds are exposed or when performing a sterile procedure.
4. Use sterile examination gloves for all dressing changes and all care involving patient contact.
5. Maintain proper concentration of topical antibacterial agents used in wound care.
6. Be alert for reservoirs of infection and sources of cross-contamination in equipment and assignment of personnel. Use single use and dedicated patient equipment when able.
7. Check history of tetanus immunization and provide passive or active tetanus prophylaxis as prescribed.
8. Change IV tubing and central line catheters according to the recommendations of the Centers for Disease Control and Prevention.
9. Administer antibiotics, as prescribed, and be alert for toxic effects and incompatibilities.
10. Assess wounds daily for local signs of infection—swelling and erythema around wound edges, purulent drainage, discoloration, and loss of grafts.
11. Be alert for early signs of septicemia, including changes in mentation, tachypnea, and decreased peristalsis, as well as later signs, such as increased pulse, decreased blood pressure (BP), increased or decreased urine output, facial flushing, increased or decreased temperatures, increasing hyperglycemia, and malaise. Report to health care provider promptly.
12. Promote optimal personal hygiene for the patient, including daily cleansing of unburned areas, meticulous care of teeth and mouth, shampooing of hair every other day, shaving of hair in or near burned areas, and meticulous care of IV and urinary catheter sites.
13. Inspect the skin carefully for signs of pressure injury and skin breakdown.
14. Observe for and report signs of thrombophlebitis or catheter-induced infections.
15. Prevent atelectasis and pneumonia through chest physical therapy, postural drainage, meticulous pulmonary technique, and, if indicated, tracheostomy care.

Promoting Mobility and Ability to Perform Activities of Daily Living (ADLs)

1. Ensure consultation with physical and occupational therapists.
2. Encourage the patient to be as active as possible and to perform active ROM exercises throughout the day.
3. Maintain splints in proper position as prescribed by occupational therapist; remove splints on regular schedule, and observe for signs of skin irritation before reapplying.
4. Position the patient to decrease edema and avoid flexion of burned joints.
5. Coordinate pain management and other care to allow optimal effort during periods of physical exercise.
6. Initiate passive and active ROM and breathing exercises during early postburn period.
7. Plan for a conditioning regimen that gradually increases energy expenditure and tolerance for activity with therapists.
8. Act as advocate for the patient's need for rest by coordinating the patient's therapeutic and social activities and prioritizing interventions and visits.
9. Help the patient achieve adequate relaxation and sleep through medication and nonpharmacologic methods.

Ensuring Adequate Nutrition

1. Weigh the patient daily with dressings removed.
2. Obtain consultation from dietitian for calculation of nutritional needs based on age, weight, height, and burn size.
3. Administer vitamins and mineral supplements, as prescribed. Deficiencies in zinc, copper, and selenium can occur after a burn.
4. Minimize metabolic stress by allaying fears, pain, and anxiety and by maintaining a warm environmental temperature.
5. Generally, for burns less than 10% TBSA, a well-balanced diet with emphasis on protein intake is necessary. For 10% to 20% TBSA, a high-protein, high-calorie diet is ordered. For 20% TBSA and greater, early enteral nutrition is believed to decrease the metabolic response and improve outcomes. When the patient is ready for oral fluids, observe tolerance and advance the diet, as tolerated.
6. Provide enteral tube feeding, as prescribed.
7. Administer IV hyperalimentation and fat emulsions prescribed with usual nursing precautions.
8. Keep record of caloric intake.
9. Encourage the patient to feed self.
10. Supplement meals with between-meal high-protein, high-calorie snacks, such as milkshakes or foods brought from home according to patient's preference.

Preventing Paralytic Ileus and Stress Ulcer

1. Keep on NPO status until bowel sounds resume.
2. Assess bowel sounds every 2 to 4 hours while acutely ill. (Decreased peristalsis may be an early sign of septicemia.)
3. Recent practice now encourages beginning tube feeds within 24 hours of the initial injury to help preserve the function of the gut and prevent paralytic ileus or stress ulcer.
4. Administer stress ulcer prophylaxis with a proton pump inhibitor or histamine-2 blocker, as prescribed.
5. Assess for abdominal distention, tube placement, and residual aspirate while administering enteral tube feeding.
6. Provide oral care every 2 hours while intubated.

EVIDENCE BASE Anne-Françoise, R., Olivier, P., & Heyland, D. K. (2023). Nutrition after severe burn injury. *Current Opinion in Clinical Nutrition and Metabolic Care, 26*(2), 99-104. https://doi.org/10.1097/MCO.0000000000000904

Reducing Pain

1. Assess for pain hourly and as needed; do not wait for complaints of pain to intervene. Common opioids used include morphine, fentanyl, hydromorphone, and propofol administered via IV line or by patient-controlled analgesia. Oral agents such as oxycodone, hydrocodone, and long-acting continuous-release agents are appropriate once the patient is tolerating PO food and fluids.
2. Determine previous experience with pain, the patient's response, and coping mechanisms.
3. Offer analgesics before wound care or before particularly painful treatments. Analgesia given orally should be administered 30 to 45 minutes before the procedure. Ketamine IV is now more commonly used than before. It is also becoming more popular to use conscious sedation for dressing changes (requirement for specialized training or anesthesiologist in attendance is dependent on state board of nursing regulations and facility policies).
4. Change the patient's position when possible, supporting extremities with pillows.
5. Teach relaxation techniques, such as imagery, breathing exercises, and progressive muscle relaxation, to help the patient cope with pain.
6. Allow the patient to make choices regarding care whenever possible, thus allowing some measure of input and control in care.
7. Greater emphasis is now focusing on pain management both from an inpatient and an outpatient perspective. Midrange analgesics are often used rather than just morphine. Pain and sedation guidelines should be followed for patients who are ventilated. It is not always possible to make a conscious patient completely pain-free, but increased comfort is the goal.

Enhancing Coping

1. Assess the patient's coping mechanisms from past history and current behavior.
2. Provide opportunities for the patient to express thoughts, feelings, fears, and anxieties regarding injury.
3. Explore with the patient alternative mechanisms for coping with the burn injury and its consequences.
4. Assure the patient of the normality of responses and the effect that time and healing will likely have on current concerns.
5. Interpret patient behavior to concerned family members and significant others.
6. Respect current coping mechanisms and discourage them only when an appropriate alternative can be provided.
7. Support family and friends' communications and visits if this is noted to help the patient.
8. Assess need for mental health consultation.
9. Offer antianxiety medications, as prescribed.

Preserving Positive Body Image

1. Gather data on the patient's preburn self-image and lifestyle.
2. When ready, encourage the patient to express concerns regarding changes in self-image or lifestyle that may result from burn injury.
3. Be honest, but positive, in responding to the patient and family.
4. Positively reinforce appropriate, effective coping mechanisms.
5. Arrange for the patient to see face (if burned) with appropriate supportive personnel before being placed/transferred to a room with access to a mirror.
6. Arrange for the patient to talk with other patients who have had a similar injury and are progressing satisfactorily.
7. Encourage participation in a burn survivor's group such as the Phoenix Society or other local support group.
8. Use and emphasize the concept of being a burn survivor. Survivors continue onward. Avoid the use of the term "burn victim" because it enhances the sick role.
9. Refer to psychological services, as needed. Consider other areas of the patient's traumatic experience that may require intervention as well.

Promoting Sleep

1. Assess patient's pain level at hour of sleep and administer pain medications, as needed.
2. Ensure comfort with room temperature and splints.
3. Administer sleep medications, as prescribed.
4. Schedule dressing changes accordingly to accommodate patient's sleep–wake cycle.
5. Establish a calming pre-sleep routine and ensure low lighting and sound throughout the night to maintain sleep hygiene.

Ensuring Safe Home Care

1. Demonstrate and explain wound care procedures to be continued after discharge:
   a. Wash hands.
   b. Clean small open wounds with mild soap in tub or shower.
   c. Rinse well with tap water.
   d. Pat dry with clean towel.
   e. Apply prescribed topical agent and dressing.
2. Assess for and teach patient to observe for local signs of wound infection:
   a. Increased erythema of unburned skin around burn area.
   b. Increased or purulent drainage.
   c. Increased pain and foul odor in burn area.
   d. Elevated body temperature.
3. Coordinate physical therapy consultation and encourage patient to develop a schedule to incorporate exercise regimen, as prescribed by physical therapist.
   a. Suggest scheduling exercises immediately after wound cleansing and application of topical agent because the skin may be more pliable and less sensitive to stretching then.
4. Instruct the patient in use and care of splints and pressure garments.
   a. Cleanse with mild soap and rinse well daily.
   b. Keep away from heat; dry garment by laying it flat on towels.
   c. Wear pressure garment, as prescribed. This is usually 23 out of 24 hours/day. The garment is usually worn for 1 to 1½ years.
   d. Small open wounds should be covered with a light dressing under splints or pressure garments.
   e. Observe for signs of skin breakdown. Reassure the patient that small blister formation is normal and generally lessens after the first year.
   f. Wear/bring splints and pressure garments to follow-up visits to be checked for proper fit.

CLINICAL JUDGMENT Ensure the patient or family member is able to demonstrate how they will perform a dressing change from start to finish prior to going home. Confidence with wound care upon discharge may decrease the risk of the patient returning with an infection because of fear of changing the dressings on their own. Provide reteaching using additional education tools and home health resources as needed.

Patient Education and Health Maintenance

Health education is closely related to rehabilitation as the patient with burn injury prepares to return to a productive place in society. Functional and cosmetic reconstruction is accomplished, and the patient attempts to integrate a new self-concept into social realities. Broadly viewed, health education focuses on biologic, psychological, and social parameters.

1. Assist the patient in transition from dependence on the health team to independence by assisting the patient to communicate needs and functional abilities to others.
2. Guide the patient in thinking positively about self. Promote ability to redirect others' attention from the scarred body to the self within.
3. Instruct the patient in measures to lubricate and enhance comfort of healing skin:
   a. After cleaning, use moisturizers such as cocoa butter or other nonperfumed hand lotion at least twice per day or more frequently, as needed.
   b. Wear clean white underwear and clothing free from irritating dyes until wounds are well healed.
   c. Take antipruritics, as prescribed.
   d. Stay in a cool environment if itching occurs.
   e. Protect the skin from further trauma; use a sunscreen with a sun protection factor of 24 or higher.
   f. Discuss summer precautions, which should include a hat with a full, wide brim if there were facial or neck burns. Also, limit exposure to sun because the affected areas will sunburn more easily and tan more deeply.
   g. Advise the patient that if wearing a pressure vest with or without sleeves, or tights, the Occupational Safety and Health Administration standards for work in a hot environment should be used. The patient should also be aware of the need for oral fluid replacement.
4. Review with the patient and family common emotional responses during convalescence (depression, withdrawal, grieving, dreaming, anxiety, guilt, excessive sensitivity, emotional lability, insomnia, and fear of future), and discuss usual temporary nature of these as well as effective coping mechanisms.
   a. There may be some psychological sequelae that will require long-term intervention, such as image adjustment disorders or posttraumatic stress issues. If not already in place, psychological referral is appropriate as an outpatient.
   b. Make sure that the patient has a phone number or referral to the counselor to make follow-up appointments, if desired.
5. Make sure that information has been given about follow-up evaluations and home health care services, as needed, in the interim.
6. Offer to connect the patient with a peer support program for burn survivors if available.
7. For additional information and support, contact agencies such as the American Burn Association (www.ameriburn.org) or the Phoenix Society for Burn Survivors (www.phoenix-society.org). The Phoenix Society is a national foundation with local chapters and whose primary function is support of other burn survivors. It has a toll-free number that burn survivors may use: (800) 888-BURN (2876).

Evaluation: Expected Outcomes

- Carboxyhemoglobin level below 10%, ABG levels within normal limits, and respiratory rate 12 to 28 breaths/min.
- Tidal volume within normal limits.
- Pulse 110 to 120 mm Hg or below and BP stable.
- Peripheral pulses strong.
- Weight stable, no edema, and lungs clear.
- Wounds clean and granulating.
- Catheter patent, urine clear, and quantity sufficient.
- Temperature normal to low-grade fever; no chills.
- No signs of infection.
- Normal ROM achieved and performing ADLs independently.
- Less than 5% weight loss from baseline.
- No gastric distention, and both gastric aspirate and stool Hemoccult tests are negative.
- Reports minimal pain after analgesic administration.
- Uses appropriate coping mechanisms.
- Verbalizes fears and concerns after viewing self in mirror.
- Sleeping 2- to 4-hour intervals; falls back to sleep easily.
- Demonstrates appropriate dressing change.

SELECTED READINGS

Abazari, M., Ghaffari, A., Rashidzadeh, H., Badeleh, S. M., & Maleki, Y. (2022). A systematic review on classification, identification, and healing process of burn wound healing. *International Journal of Lower Extremity Wounds, 21*(1), 18–30. https://doi.org/10.1177/1534734620924857

American Burn Association (2023). *Advanced Burn Life Support Course Manual. 2023 Update*. www.ameriburn.org

American Burn Association (2023). *Annual Burn Injury Summary Report. Analysis of Inpatient Care at Burn Centers 2018-2022.* https://ameriburn.org/quality-care/burn-care-quality-platform-bcqp-registry/bcqp-bisr/

Bettencourt, A. P., Romanowski, K. S., Joe, V., Jeng, J., Carter, J. E., Cartotto, R., Craig, C. K., Rabia, R., Vercruysse, G. A., Hickerson, W. L., Liu, Y., Ryan, C. M., & Shulz, J. (2020). Updating the burn center referral criteria: Results from the 2018 eDelphi Consensus Study. *Journal of Burn Care & Resuscitation, 41*(5), 1052–1062. https://doi.org/10.1093/jbcr/iraa038

Grieve, B., Shapiro, G. D., Wibbenmeyer, L., Acton, A., Lee, A., Marino, M., Jette, A., Schneider, J. C., Kazis, L. E., Ryan, C. M., & LIBRE Advisory Board. (2020). Long-term social reintegration outcomes for burn survivors with and without peer support attendance: A Life Impact Burn Recovery Evaluation (LIBRE) Study. *Archives of Physical Medicine and Rehabilitation, 101*(1S), S92–S98. https://doi.org/10.1016/j.apmr.2017.10.007

Herndon, D., Zhang, F., & Lineaweaver, W. (2022). Metabolic responses to severe burn injury. *Annals of Plastic Surgery, 88*(Suppl. 2), S128–S131. https://doi.org/10.1097/SAP.0000000000003142

Jeschke, M. G., van Baar, M. E., Choudhry, M. A., Chung, K. K., Gibran, N. S., & Logsetty, S. (2020). Burn injury. *Nature Reviews Disease Primers, 6*, 11. https://doi.org/10.1038/s41572-020-0145-5

Lanham, J. S., Nelson, N. K., Hendren, B., & Jordan, T. S. (2020). Outpatient burn care: Prevention and treatment. *American Family Physician, 101*(8), 463-470. https://www.aafp.org/pubs/afp/issues/2020/0415/p463.html#treatment

Masch, J. L., Bhutiani, N., & Bozeman, M. C. (2019). Feeding during resuscitation after burn injury. *Nutrition in Clinical Practice, 34*(5), 666–671. https://doi.org/10.1002/ncp.10400

Pusey-Reid, E., Quinn, L., Samost, M. E., & Reidy, P. A. (2023). Skin assessment in patients with dark skin tone. *American Journal of Nursing, 123*(3), 36–43. https://doi.org/10.1097/01.NAJ.0000921800.61980.7e

Rivas, E., Foster, J., Crandall, C. G., Finnerty, C. C., & Suman-Vejas, O. E. (2023). Key exercise concepts in the rehabilitation from severe burns. *Physical Medicine and Rehabilitation Clinics of North America, 34*(4), 811–824. https://doi.org/10.1016/j.pmr.2023.05.003

Tapking, C., Popp, D., Herndon, D. N., Branski, L. K., Hundeshagen, G., Armenta, A. M., Busch, M., Most, P., & Kinsky, M. P. (2020). Cardiac dysfunction in severely burned patients: Current understanding of etiology, pathophysiology, and treatment. *Shock, 53*(6), 699–678. https://doi.org/10.1097/SHK.0000000000001465

Tejiram, S., Tranchina, S. P., Travis, T. E., & Shupp, J. W. (2023). The first 24 hours: Burn shock resuscitation and early complications. *Surgical Clinics of North America, 103*, 403–413. https://doi.org/10.1016/j.suc.2023.02.002

Weller, C. D., Team, V., & Sussman, G. (2020). First-line interactive wound dressing update: A comprehensive review of the evidence. *Frontiers in Pharmacology, 11*, 55. https://doi.org/10.3389/fphar.2020.00155

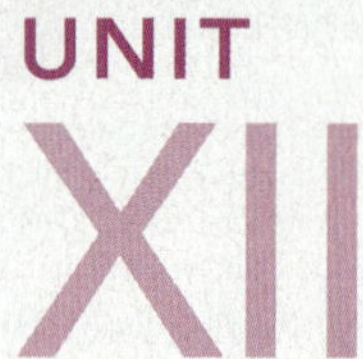

UNIT XII EMERGENCY NURSING

31 Emergent Conditions*

OVERVIEW AND ASSESSMENT

Emergency medicine is the care, diagnosis, and treatment of unforeseen illness or injury. It is provided to patients with conditions ranging from minor to serious or life-threatening. The philosophy of emergency care includes the concept that an emergency is whatever the patient or family considers it to be. Emergency nursing is a dynamic and evolving practice that deals with patients who are unstable, undiagnosed, and usually presenting unexpectedly. See Standards of Care Guidelines 31-1 (see page 925).

Emergency Assessment

When a patient presents with an emergency, it is essential that a systematic approach is used to ensure all factors are identified. The primary and secondary surveys provide the emergency nurse with a methodical approach to help identify and prioritize patient needs.

Primary Survey

The initial, rapid ABCD (**a**irway, **b**reathing, **c**irculation, and neurologic **d**isability) assessment of the patient is meant to identify life-threatening problems. If conditions are identified that present an immediate threat to life, the health care provider or team must stop and take corrective action prior to moving on to the next steps.

ABCD–AVPU

1. **A**—Airway: Does the patient have an open airway? Is the patient able to speak, swallow, or cry? Check for airway obstructions such as loose teeth, foreign objects, bleeding, vomitus, or other secretions. Immediately treat anything that compromises the airway. Never do a blind finger sweep of an airway.
2. **B**—Breathing: Is the patient breathing adequately? Assess for equal rise and fall of the chest (check for bilateral breath sounds), respiratory rate and pattern, skin color, use of accessory muscles, adventitious breath sounds, integrity of the chest wall, and position of the trachea. All patients with major trauma require supplemental oxygen via a nonrebreather mask at 12 to 15 L/min. Dress any penetrating chest injuries with occlusive dressings.
3. **C**—Circulation: Is circulation adequate? Can you palpate central and peripheral pulses? What is the quality of the pulses (strong, weak, slow, rapid)? Is the skin warm and dry? Is the

*Please note that the term "male" in this chapter refers to a person assigned male at birth, and the term "female" in this chapter refers to a person assigned female at birth.

STANDARDS OF CARE GUIDELINES 31-1

Emergency Assessment and Intervention

When a patient presents with a potentially life-threatening condition, proceed swiftly with the following:

- Call for help.
- Ensure the area is safe for you to enter, with no live electric current, hazardous materials, dangerous persons, or other threats.
- Remove the patient from potential source of danger, such as live electric current, water, or fire. If hazardous materials are present, consult protocols from the Occupational Safety and Health Association (OSHA) for decontamination procedures.
- Determine whether patient is conscious.
- Assess for adequate airway, breathing, and circulation in systematic manner. If any of these are absent, or inadequate, begin basic life support.
- Assess pupillary reaction and level of responsiveness to voice or touch, as indicated.
- If the patient is unconscious or has sustained a significant head injury, assume there is a spinal cord injury and maintain C-spine stabilization.
- Remove clothing to assess for wounds and skin lesions as indicated. Control any hemorrhage, as needed.
- When help arrives, assist with further assessment and transport, as needed.

This information should serve as a general guideline only. Each patient situation presents a unique set of clinical factors and requires nursing judgment to guide care, which may include additional or alternative measures and approaches.

skin color normal? What is the capillary refill? Obtain a blood pressure (BP; in both arms if chest trauma or dissecting aortic aneurysm is suspected). Is there any major bleeding?

4. **D**—Disability: Assess level of consciousness (LOC) and pupils (a more thorough neurologic survey will be completed in the secondary survey). Assess LOC using the AVPU scale:
   a. **A**—Is the patient alert? Are they looking at you and responding?
   b. **V**—Does the patient respond to voice? Do they open their eyes or respond when you call them?
   c. **P**—Does the patient respond to painful stimulus? Do they respond to sternal rub or nail bed pressure?
   d. **U**—The patient is unresponsive even to painful stimulus.

Secondary Assessment

The secondary assessment is a brief, but thorough, systematic assessment designed to identify all injuries. The steps include *expose/environmental* control, *full* set of vital signs, *five* interventions, *facilitate* family presence, and *give* comfort measures. If your emergency department (ED) has enough staff, these interventions may be assigned to multiple staff members and performed simultaneously.

1. Expose/environmental control: It is necessary to remove all of the patient's clothing to identify all injuries. You must then prevent heat loss by using warm blankets, overhead warmers, and warmed intravenous (IV) fluids unless induced hypothermia is indicated. If your facility has a dedicated trauma or resuscitation room, keep the ambient temperature elevated to prevent heat loss.
2. Full set of vital signs:
   a. Obtain a full set of vital signs including BP, heart rate, respiratory rate, temperature, and oxygen saturation.
   b. As stated previously, obtain BP in both arms if chest trauma or dissecting aortic aneurysm is suspected.
   c. Institute continuous cardiac monitoring.
   d. Assess Glasgow Coma Scale (GCS) (see page 334) and pain scores.
3. Five potential interventions:
   a. Vascular access with two large-bore IV catheters, if possible.
   b. Pulse oximetry to measure the oxygen saturation; consider capnography to measure end-tidal carbon dioxide ($EtCO_2$), noninvasive ultrasonic cardiac output monitor, and 12-lead electrocardiogram (ECG).
   c. Indwelling urinary catheter (do not insert if blood is noted at the meatus, if there is blood in the scrotum, or if a pelvic fracture is suspected).
   d. Gastric tube (if there is evidence of facial fractures, insert the tube orally rather than nasally).
   e. Laboratory studies may include type and cross-matching, complete blood count (CBC), coagulation panel, urine drug screen, blood alcohol, electrolytes, prothrombin time and partial thromboplastin time, arterial blood gas (ABG), venous blood gases (VBG), lactate, lipase, amylase, and pregnancy test, if applicable.
4. Facilitate family presence: Family presence is important during unexpected, potentially life-threatening events. They often have information that is critical in formulating the correct treatment plan. It is important to assess and respect the family's needs and wishes. Resuscitation rooms are often loud and appear chaotic. Assigning a staff member to any family wishing to be present can do much to alleviate their anxiety and assure them that everything is being done to help their loved one. If a family member does not wish to be present, providing them with a quiet area to wait and assigning a staff member as a contact person or liaison can be helpful.
5. Give comfort measures including pain management and verbal reassurance: Do not forget to give comfort measures to the family as well as the patient during the resuscitation process.

History

1. Obtain prehospital information from emergency personnel, patient, family, or bystanders using the mnemonic MIVT.

   M—Mechanism of injury: It is helpful to understand the mechanism of injury to anticipate probable injuries. It is particularly helpful in motor vehicle accidents to know such information as speed of vehicle prior to impact (high vs. low vs. stopped), external and internal damage to the vehicle (or at least if the vehicle was drivable after the accident), if the patient was ejected, if they were wearing a seat belt, if airbags were deployed, if the patient was ambulatory at the scene, and the period of time elapsed before the patient received medical attention.

   I—Injuries sustained or suspected: Ask prehospital personnel to list any injuries that they have identified. Most prehospital providers will have completed a rapid trauma survey, including looking for DCAP/BTLS (deformities, contusions, abrasions, punctures/burns, tenderness, lacerations, and swelling).

V—Vital signs: What were the prehospital vital signs?
T—Treatment: What treatment did the patient receive before arriving at the hospital and what was the patient's response to those interventions?

2. If the patient is conscious, it is essential to ask what happened. How did the accident occur? Why did it happen? A fall, for example, may not be a simple fall—perhaps, the patient blacked out and then fell. If the patient is conscious and time permits, explore the chief complaint through the OPQRST mnemonic.
   O—Onset: When did they first notice symptoms? Was today the first time? Has it been ongoing? Is it getting progressively worse?
   P—Provokes, Palliates, and Precipitates: What makes the symptoms better or worse?
   Q—Quality: How would they describe the discomfort? Burning, stabbing, throbbing, aching, and like an electric shock are all commonly used to describe the quality of pain.
   R—Region and Radiates: Can the patient point to their pain with one finger? Does it radiate (move) or shoot anywhere?
   S—Severity and Associated Symptoms: How do they rate their symptom? Is it accompanied by anything else such as numbness, tingling, or nausea?
   T—Timing: Have the symptoms been constant or do they come and go? How often?
3. Obtain past medical history from the patient or a family member or friend; it may be helpful to utilize the mnemonic SAMPLE to assist in organizing history information:
   S—Signs and symptoms, including chief complaint and OPQRST.
   A—Allergies to foods and medications.
   M—Medications, including herbal supplements and over-the-counter (OTC) medications.
   P—Past medical and surgical history.
   L—Last oral intake.
   E—Events leading up to the incident.
4. History of alcohol or substance use disorder.
5. To obtain a good descriptive history, use open-ended questioning.

Head-to-Toe Assessment

The head-to-toe assessment begins with assessment of the patient's general appearance, including body position guarding, or any posturing. Work from the head down, systematically assessing one body area at a time.

1. Head and face.
   a. Inspect for any lacerations, abrasions, contusions, avulsions, puncture wounds, impaled objects, ecchymosis, or edema. Ecchymosis around the eyes is known as raccoon eyes and can signify a basilar skull fracture. Hair can obscure injuries, so take time to do a thorough inspection. Scalp lacerations also tend to bleed profusely, further obstructing the area during quick inspections.
   b. Gently palpate for crepitus, crackling, or bony deformities.
   c. Inspect ears and nares for any bleeding or drainage; if present, check for halo sign (occurs when blood mixes with cerebral spinal fluid; result is a dark spot in center [blood] with a lighter colored ring ["halo"] around it). Check for ecchymosis in skin overlying the mastoid process, known as Battle sign that can signify a basilar skull fracture.
2. Neck (ensure proper C-spine stabilization is maintained).
   a. Inspect for any punctures, lacerations, contusions, swelling, tracheal deviation, jugular venous distention (JVD), or subcutaneous emphysema.
   b. Check for stomas or medical alert devices.
   c. Gently palpate for midline cervical tenderness.
3. Chest.
   a. Inspect for breathing effectiveness, paradoxical (uneven) chest wall movement, and disruptions in chest wall integrity (lacerations, punctures, subcutaneous emphysema).
   b. Auscultate for bilateral breath sounds and adventitious breath sounds.
   c. Auscultate for muffled heart tones.
   d. Gently palpate for bony crepitus or deformities.
4. Abdomen/flanks.
   a. Inspect for lacerations, abrasions, contusions, avulsions, puncture wounds, impaled objects, ecchymosis, edema, scars, eviscerations, or distention.
   b. Auscultate for the presence of bowel sounds.
   c. Gently palpate for rigidity, guarding, masses, or areas of tenderness.
5. Pelvis/perineum.
   a. Inspect for lacerations, abrasions, contusions, avulsions, puncture wounds, impaled objects, ecchymosis, edema, or scars. Look for blood at the urinary meatus and vagina in females. Look for priapism in males (which could indicate spinal cord injury).
   b. Gently palpate for pelvic instability or tenderness (do not rock the pelvis).
6. Neurologic/spinal (maintaining proper stabilization).
   a. Reassess mental status.
   b. Gently palpate for midline bony spinal tenderness.
   c. Check for paresthesias and determine sensory level.
   d. Check motor function and sphincter tone.
7. Extremities.
   a. Inspect skin color and temperature. Look for signs of injury and bleeding. Does the patient have movement in all four extremities? Touch the patient on a distal extremity and ask them to identify the part you are touching.
   b. Gently palpate peripheral pulses, any bony crepitus, or areas of tenderness.
   c. Check capillary refill.
   d. Gently palpate extremities for compartment firmness or signs of compartment syndrome.
8. Pregnancy presents a unique set of challenges. While performing assessments and interventions, a towel or roll should be placed under the right side of the backboard, tipping the patient slightly to the left and preventing fetal compression of the inferior vena cava and decreased blood return to the heart.

CLINICAL JUDGMENT Any penetrating chest wound has the potential to rapidly cause a life-threatening tension pneumothorax and must be treated immediately.

Focused Assessment

Any injuries that were identified during the primary and secondary surveys require a detailed assessment, which will typically include a team approach and radiographic studies.

Emergency Triage

Triage is a French verb meaning "to sort." Emergency triage is a subspecialty of emergency nursing, which requires specific, comprehensive educational preparation. The goal of an efficient triage system is to rapidly connect a patient with the proper level of care and the correct resources in the shortest amount of time.

Upon entering an ED, patients are greeted by a triage nurse, who will perform a rapid assessment, to include a general impression, chief complaint, immediate or potential life threats, and pertinent history, and then make a decision about the patient's acuity and the resources needed. These decisions can often be difficult if the patient is nonverbal, developmentally delayed, cognitively impaired, has an altered mental status, is intoxicated, or is otherwise impaired. Thus, the primary role of the triage nurse is to make acuity and disposition decisions and set priorities while maintaining awareness for potentially violent or communicable disease situations. Secondary triage decisions involve the initiation of triage-extended protocols and practices, such as the ordering of standardized laboratories or radiology studies. With the waiting times in EDs because of overcrowding becoming an increasing problem, the accuracy of the triage nurse in assigning acuity level is of critical importance. With extended wait times, triage is an ongoing process, with the triage nurse frequently reevaluating those who are waiting for changes in condition and updating their status, as needed.

Priorities of Care and Triage Categories

Standardized five-level triage systems, such as the Australasian Triage Scale, the Canadian Triage and Acuity Scale, and the Emergency Severity Index, have been developed and proven through research to possess utility, validity, reliability, and safety. All three systems utilize similar time frames and are evidence based (the Manchester Triage System is a consensus-based algorithm approach, which utilizes longer time frames).

Triage Level 1: Immediately Life-Threatening or Resuscitation

1. Conditions requiring immediate clinician assessment. Any delay in treatment is potentially life-threatening or limb-threatening. These are the patients who are in active danger of dying if there is no immediate intervention.
2. Conditions include (but are not limited to):
   a. Airway or severe respiratory compromise.
   b. Cardiac arrest.
   c. Severe shock.
   d. Symptomatic cervical spine injury.
   e. Multisystem trauma.
   f. Altered LOC (GCS less than 10).
   g. Eclampsia.
   h. Acute mental status changes or unresponsiveness.

Triage Level 2: Imminently Life-Threatening or Emergent

1. These are conditions that are not immediately dangerous but have the potential to deteriorate rapidly if not treated.
2. Conditions include (but are not limited to):
   a. Head injuries.
   b. Trauma.
   c. Conscious overdose.
   d. Severe allergic reaction without airway compromise.
   e. Chemical exposure to the eyes.
   f. Chest pain without hemodynamic instability.
   g. Back pain with sensory or motor deficits.
   h. Gastrointestinal (GI) bleed with unstable vital signs.
   i. Stroke with deficit.
   j. Severe asthma without airway compromise.
   k. Abdominal pain in patients older than age 50.
   l. Vomiting and diarrhea with dehydration.
   m. Fever in infants younger than age 3 months.
   n. Acute psychotic episode.
   o. Severe headache.
   p. Pain greater than 7 on a scale of 1 to 10.
   q. Sexual assault.
   r. Neonates age 7 days or younger.

Triage Level 3: Potentially Life-Threatening/Time Critical or Urgent

1. These are conditions requiring urgent care-level activities with stable vital signs but have the potential to deteriorate and utilize multiple resources.
2. Conditions include (but are not limited to):
   a. Alert head injury with vomiting.
   b. Mild to moderate asthma.
   c. Moderate trauma.
   d. Abuse or neglect.
   e. GI bleed with stable vital signs.
   f. History of seizure and alert on arrival.

Triage Level 4: Potentially Life-Serious/Situational Urgency or Semi-urgent

1. These are stable conditions that use few resources.
2. Conditions include (but are not limited to):
   a. Alert head injury without vomiting.
   b. Minor trauma.
   c. Vomiting and diarrhea in patient older than age 2 without evidence of dehydration.
   d. Earache.
   e. Minor allergic reaction.
   f. Corneal foreign body.
   g. Chronic back pain.

Triage Level 5: Less/Nonurgent

1. These are stable conditions that utilize little to no resources.
2. Conditions include (but are not limited to):
   a. Minor trauma such as minor cuts, abrasions, bruises, and so on.
   b. Minor symptoms such as rhinorrhea, sneezing, conjunctivitis, and so on.

CLINICAL JUDGMENT When working with pediatric patients in a triage setting, it is important to remember that they can deteriorate rapidly. Pediatric patients should be triaged by those experienced in identifying the subtle clues that often precede this rapid deterioration.

Psychological Considerations

Serious illness or trauma is an insult to physiologic and psychological homeostasis; it requires both physiologic and psychological healing. Both patients and families experience high levels of anxiety when being treated in the ED. It is important for the emergency nurse to recognize, understand, and alleviate these anxieties whenever possible.

Approach to the Patient

1. Understand and accept the basic anxieties of the patient who is acutely ill or traumatized. Be aware of the patient's fear of death, disablement, and isolation.
   a. Personalize the situation as much as possible. Speak, react, and respond in a warm manner; give reassurance. Look directly at the patient when speaking or listening to them.

b. Give explanations on a level that the patient can understand. An informed patient can cope with psychological/physiologic stress in a more positive manner.
c. Accept the rights of the patient and family to have and display their own feelings.
d. Maintain a calm and reassuring manner—help the patient or family who are emotionally distressed to mobilize their psychological resources.
e. Include the patient's family or significant others if the patient wishes.
f. Encourage the patient or family to reach out to their support system. Often friends, other family members, or clergy can be of great comfort.

2. Understand and support the patient's feelings concerning loss of control (emotional, physical, and intellectual). Whenever possible, give the patient options and choices. This can help alleviate some of their feelings of helplessness.
3. Speak to the patient who is unconscious. Touch, call by name, and explain every procedure that is done. Avoid making negative comments about the patient's condition.
   a. Orient the patient to person, time, and place as soon as they are conscious; reinforce by repeating this information.
   b. Bring the patient back to reality in a calm and reassuring way.
   c. Encourage the family, when possible, to touch the patient and aid in orienting the patient to reality.
4. Be prepared to handle all aspects of acute illness and trauma; know what to expect and what to do. When in doubt, stop, take a deep breath, and refocus. This will help alleviate the nurse's anxiety and increase the patient's confidence.

Approach to the Family

1. Inform the family where the patient is and give as much information as possible about the treatment they are receiving.
2. Allow a family member to be present during the resuscitation. Assign a staff person to the family member to explain procedures and offer comfort.
3. Recognize the anxiety of the family and allow them to talk about their feelings. Acknowledge expressions of remorse, anger, guilt, and criticism.
4. Allow the family to relive the events, actions, and feelings preceding admission to the ED.
5. Deal with reality as gently and quickly as possible; avoid encouraging and supporting denial.
6. Assist the family to cope with sudden and unexpected death. Some helpful measures include the following:
   a. Take the family to a private place.
   b. Talk to the entire family together so they can mourn together.
   c. Assure the family that everything possible was done; inform them of the treatment rendered.
   d. Avoid using euphemisms such as "passed on."
   e. Allow family to talk about the deceased—permits ventilation of feelings of loss. Encourage family to talk about events preceding admission to the ED.
   f. Encourage family to support each other and to express emotions freely—grief, loss, anger, helplessness, tears, and disbelief.
   g. Avoid volunteering unnecessary information (e.g., patient was drinking).
   h. Ensure diversity, equity, and inclusion. Be certain that nursing care and practice provide for all persons in a nonjudgmental manner. Be cognizant of cultural and religious beliefs and needs.
   i. Encourage family members to view the body if they wish—doing so helps to integrate the loss (cover mutilated areas, if necessary).
      i. Prepare the family for visual images and explain any legal requirements.
      ii. Accompany the family to see the body.
      iii. Show acceptance of the body by touching to give the family permission to touch and talk to the body.
      iv. Spend a few minutes with the family, listening to them.
      v. Allow the family some private time with the body, if appropriate (no forensic issues).
7. Encourage the ED staff to discuss among themselves their reactions to the event, sharing intense feelings for review and for group support. Organize a formal debriefing session for staff if warranted by the circumstances of the event.

Pain Management

Pain is an unpleasant sensory and emotional experience associated with actual or potential tissue damage and is also associated with significant morbidity. Pain inhibits immune function and has detrimental effects on cardiovascular, respiratory, GI, and other body systems. Over 60% of patients report pain upon arrival at the ED, making pain the most common patient complaint. It is imperative to adequately assess, monitor, and relieve pain (to the extent that is possible) in the ED. Despite this, significant evidence–practice gaps continue to be identified with underestimation and undertreatment of pain, as well as gaps in pain documentation, despite available clinical practice guidelines. In general, adult patients aged 65 and older and pediatric patients tend to have their pain underestimated and undertreated more frequently than adults under age 65 do. Pain may be somatic or visceral, acute or chronic, or centrally or peripherally generated. Pain relief is moral, humane, and physiologically and psychologically imperative. Pain assessment includes whatever the patient states their pain level is, along with objective assessments made by the nurse.

Primary Assessment

1. ABCD.
2. Evaluate pain using the OPQRST mnemonic.
3. Assess pain score using a pain rating tool, such as the numeric rating scale, PAINAD scale (pain assessment in advanced dementia scale), CPOT scale (critical care pain observation tool), visual analogue scale, Wong–Baker FACES pain scale (see page 1146), FLACC (faces, legs, activity, cry, and consolability) behavioral scale, verbal rating scale, or Abbey pain scale.

Primary Interventions

1. Pain is whatever the patient states it is. Never doubt that a patient has pain based on how they look.
2. Establish a supportive relationship with the patient.
3. Respect the patient's response to pain and its management.
4. Educate the patient regarding methods of pain relief, preventive measures, and expectations.
5. Establish a baseline pain level, as well as a pain level the patient would consider tolerable.
6. Administer pharmaceutical and nonpharmaceutical pain control.
7. Monitor the patient's response to and effectiveness of treatment.

8. If initial interventions do not bring pain down to the tolerable level, explore other options.
9. Always reassure your patient and let them know you take their pain seriously.

CARDIOPULMONARY RESUSCITATION AND AIRWAY MANAGEMENT

See additional online content: Procedure Guidelines 31-1 to 31-4

EVIDENCE BASE American Heart Association. (2020). American Heart Association 2020 guidelines for CRP and ECC. *Circulation, 142*(16, Suppl. 2). https://cpr.heart.org/en/resuscitation-science/cpr-and-ecc-guidelines

Mathiesen, C., McPherson, D., Ordway, C., & Smith, M. (2015). Caring for patients treated with therapeutic hypothermia. *Critical Care Nurse, 35*(5), e1–e12. https://doi.org/10.4037/ccn2015168

Cardiopulmonary Resuscitation

Cardiopulmonary resuscitation (CPR) is a technique of basic life support for the purpose of oxygenating the brain and heart until appropriate, definitive medical treatment can restore normal heart and ventilatory action. Management of foreign-body airway obstruction or cricothyroidotomy may be necessary to open the airway while CPR is performed.

Over the years, many changes have been made to the CPR guidelines. The emphasis is now on performing good, high-quality chest compressions, with minimum interruptions, in an effort to not only preserve life but prevent anoxic brain injuries as well. The traditional "look–listen and feel" for breathing has been eliminated, as well as the A–B–C order for assessing the patient who is unresponsive. For the lay public, the focus has changed to a compressions-only resuscitation model, with no interruptions to deliver breaths. For the professional provider, airway, breathing, and circulation are still important parts of the resuscitation effort; however, A–B–C has become C–A–B, or circulation, airway, and then breathing. All efforts begin with good, high-quality chest compressions.

Indications

1. Cardiac arrest.
   a. Ventricular fibrillation.
   b. Ventricular tachycardia.
   c. Asystole.
   d. Pulseless electrical activity.
2. Respiratory arrest.
   a. Drowning.
   b. Stroke.
   c. Foreign-body airway obstruction.
   d. Smoke inhalation.
   e. Drug overdose.
   f. Electrocution/injury by lightning.
   g. Suffocation.
   h. Accident/injury.
   i. Coma.
   j. Epiglottitis.

Assessment

1. Loss of consciousness.
2. Absence of palpable carotid or femoral pulse; pulselessness in large arteries.
3. Absence of breath sounds or air movement through the nose or mouth.

Interventions

1. Kneel as close to the side of the patient's chest as possible, placing the heel of one hand on the lower half of the sternum, taking care to avoid the xiphoid process. Fingers may be interlaced or extended, but care must be taken to keep them off the chest.
2. Keep your arms straight and your elbows locked. Ensure your shoulders are directly over your hands, and quickly and forcefully depress the patient's sternum straight down to a depth of at least 2 in.
3. Deliver 30 compressions at a rate of at least 100 compressions a minute. Always allow for complete chest recoil after each compression without taking your hands off of the chest between compressions.
4. Taking no more than 10 seconds, open the airway and deliver 2 breaths.
5. Continue resuscitation at a rate of 30:2 with one or two rescuers.
6. Utilize the automatic external defibrillator according to audio instructions (see page 219).

Complications

1. Postresuscitation distress syndrome (secondary derangements in multiple organs).
2. Neurologic impairment and brain damage.
3. The patient who has been resuscitated is at risk for another episode of cardiac arrest.

Induced Hypothermia Postcardiac Arrest

In adults with persistent coma (postcardiac arrest), initiating induced hypothermia to a temperature of 89°F to 93°F (32°C to 34°C) for 12 to 24 hours results in neuroprotection, improving neurologic function, and decreasing mortality. It is also associated with beneficial hemodynamic, renal, and acid–base effects. Hypothermia should be initiated within 6 hours of collapse.

Indications

1. Persistent coma in the adult patient following cardiac arrest and return of spontaneous circulation (ROSC).
2. Traumatically induced cerebral anoxia with or without cardiac arrest.
3. Time frame from cardiac arrest to ROSC is less than 60 minutes.
4. Systolic blood pressure (SBP) greater than 90 mm Hg with a mean arterial pressure (MAP) greater than 60 mm Hg, with or without pressors.

CLINICAL JUDGMENT The patient who responds to verbal stimuli after cardiac arrest should not be treated with induced hypothermia.

Assessment

1. Institute continuous cardiac monitoring. Monitor for bradycardia caused by cooling or other dysrhythmias.
2. Institute continuous temperature monitoring, preferably core temperature.
3. Frequently monitor blood pressure (BP) to avoid hypotension, particularly during rewarming.
4. Monitor complete blood count (CBC) for signs of infection, because temperature will not be an accurate sign. Monitor electrolyte panel for hypokalemia caused by hypothermia. Arterial blood gas (ABG) levels should be analyzed at patient's actual body temperature.
5. Assess the skin every 2 hours for pressure and cold injury.
6. Monitor pupils every hour and consider continuous electroencephalogram (EEG) monitoring.

Interventions

1. Apply cold packs to the groin, axillae, sides of the chest, and neck, or apply cooling device according to manufacturer's instructions. There are a number of commercially available cooling devices, including cooling blankets, cooling gel pads applied to the skin, and centrally inserted heat exchange catheters.
2. Instill 30 mL/kg of refrigerated lactated Ringer's solution over 30 minutes through a femoral line (if patient is not in acute pulmonary edema).
3. Remove cold packs once temperature is less than 91°F (33°C). Target temperature is 91.4°F (32°C).
4. Replace cold packs and consider further ice-cold lactated Ringer's solution if temperature remains above 92.3°F (33.5°C).
5. Use nondepolarizing neuromuscular blockade to prevent shivering. Provide sedation according to standard intensive care unit (ICU) protocol.
6. Maintain patient at target temperature for a period of 12 to 24 hours once temperature is reached.
7. After the targeted time has elapsed, allow passive rewarming slowly over 8 to 12 hours.

Complications

1. Shivering—patient will require sedation and neuromuscular blockade to relieve shivering, which will interfere with hypothermia.
2. Seizures—continuous neuromuscular blockade may mask postcardiac arrest seizure activity.
3. Ileus because of slowing of metabolic processes.
4. Hypotension because of vasodilation.

Foreign-Body Airway Obstruction

Foreign-body obstruction of the airway may be either partial or complete. Abdominal thrusts (the Heimlich maneuver) are recommended for relieving foreign-body airway obstruction in the conscious adult. Back blows and chest thrusts are used in the conscious infant or toddler.

Assessment

1. Weak, ineffective cough.
2. High-pitched noises on inspiration.
3. Respiratory distress.
4. Inability to speak or breathe.
5. Cyanosis.
6. Hands at the throat (universal choking sign).

Interventions

1. If the patient is conscious, stand behind the patient; wrap your arms around patient's waist, and proceed as follows:
   a. Make a fist with one hand, placing the thumb side of the fist against the patient's abdomen in the midline, slightly above the navel and well below the xiphoid process. Grasp the fist with your other hand.
   b. Press your fist into the patient's abdomen with a quick upward thrust. Each new thrust should be a separate and distinct maneuver.
   c. Continue until the obstruction is cleared, help arrives, or the patient becomes unresponsive.
   d. Should the patient become unresponsive, immediately begin CPR, checking the airway after each set of compressions and prior to attempting ventilations.
2. If the patient is pregnant or has obesity, do not do abdominal compressions. Follow these steps:
   a. Stand behind the patient with your arms under the axillae to encircle the chest.
   b. Place the thumb side of your fist on the middle of the patient's sternum, taking care to avoid the xiphoid process and rib cage margins.
   c. Grasp your fist with your other hand and perform backward thrusts until the foreign body is expelled. If the patient becomes unconscious, stop and begin CPR.

Cricothyroidotomy

Cricothyroidotomy is the puncture or incision of the cricothyroid membrane to establish an emergency airway in certain emergency situations when placement of an endotracheal tube or laryngeal mask airway is not possible or is contraindicated and when adequate oxygenation cannot be maintained utilizing a bag-valve-mask device with 100% oxygen.

Indications

1. Compromised airway and inability to intubate or perform tracheostomy:
   a. Complete foreign-body airway obstruction.
   b. Trauma to the head and neck.
2. Allergic reaction causing laryngeal edema.

Contraindications

1. Laryngeal fracture.
2. Tracheal rupture.
3. Tracheal transection with distal tracheal retraction into the mediastinum.

Interventions

Assist the physician or emergency health care provider as follows:

1. Preoxygenate the patient, if possible.
2. Extend the patient's neck. Place a towel roll beneath the shoulders.
3. Attach a 10-mL syringe containing 5 mL of saline to the insertion catheter.
4. Identify the prominent thyroid cartilage (Adam apple), and allow your finger to descend in the midline to the depression

between the lower border of the thyroid cartilage and the upper border of the cricoid cartilage.
5. Scrub insertion site and maintain sterility throughout procedure.
6. Provide skin tension and hold the trachea in place with the nondominant hand, using the index finger to palpate the cricothyroid membrane.
7. Place the catheter at the inferior margin of the cricothyroid membrane, in the midline of the neck, and direct it caudally at a 30- to 45-degree angle.
8. While maintaining negative pressure on the syringe, advance the catheter through the skin and tissue until air bubbles are seen in the syringe.
9. Thread the catheter off of the needle until the hub rests on the skin surface and withdraw the needle.
10. Listen for air passing back and forth through the needle synchronously with the patient's respirations.
11. Secure the needle with adhesive tape or sutures.
12. Ventilate with a bag-valve-mask device, allowing for prolonged exhalation time.

Complications

1. Bleeding.
2. Aspiration.
3. Subcutaneous emphysema.

INJURIES TO THE HEAD, SPINE, AND FACE

Head Injuries

Head injuries can include fractures to the skull and face, direct injuries to the brain (as from a bullet), and indirect injuries to the brain (such as a concussion, contusion, or intracranial hemorrhage). Head injuries commonly occur from motor vehicle accidents, assaults, or falls.

Concussion: a mild diffuse axonal injury resulting in a transient disturbance of neurologic function that may or may not include a loss of consciousness.

Contusion: a focal injury resulting in bruising of the brain tissue. Actual small amounts of bleeding into the brain tissue associated with edema formation and possible tissue necrosis and infarction.

Intracranial hemorrhage: significant bleeding into a space or a potential space between the skull and the brain. This is a serious complication of a head injury with a high mortality because of rising intracranial pressure (ICP) and the potential for brain herniation. Intracranial hemorrhages can be classified as *epidural hematomas*, *subdural hematomas*, or *subarachnoid hemorrhages*, depending on the site of bleeding.

CLINICAL JUDGMENT Always assume a cervical spine fracture for any patient with a significant head injury until proven otherwise.

Primary Assessment

1. Airway: assess for vomitus, bleeding, and foreign objects. Ensure cervical spine immobilization.
2. Breathing: assess for abnormally slow or shallow respirations. An elevated carbon dioxide partial pressure can worsen cerebral edema.
3. Circulation: assess pulse and bleeding.
4. Disability: assess the patient's neurologic status.

Primary Interventions

1. To protect the cervical spine, open the airway using the jaw-thrust technique without head tilt. Oral suction equipment (to handle heavy vomitus) should be at hand. Avoid stimulating the gag reflex as this can cause increases in ICP.
2. Administer high-flow oxygen, preferably with a nonrebreather face mask.
3. Assist inadequate respirations with a bag-valve-mask, as necessary. Prophylactic hyperventilation is contraindicated.
4. Control bleeding—do not apply pressure to the injury site. Apply a bulky, loose dressing.
5. Initiate two intravenous (IV) lines. The administration of fluid and rate of flow should be determined by the patient's hemodynamic status.

Subsequent Assessment

1. History.
   a. Mechanism of injury.
   b. Presence and duration of loss of consciousness.
   c. Amnesia of the event.
   d. Position found.
2. Level of consciousness (LOC).
   a. Change in mental status is a very reliable indicator of a change in the patient's condition.
   b. Glasgow Coma Scale (GCS) (see page 334).
3. Vital signs.
   a. Hypertension and bradycardia are late signs of increasing ICP.
   b. Patients with a head injury may have associated cardiac dysrhythmias, noted by an irregular or rapid pulse.
   c. Changing patterns of respiration or apnea may indicate a head injury.
   d. Elevated temperature—high temperatures may be associated with head injury.
4. Unequal or unresponsive pupils.
5. Confusion or personality changes.
6. Impaired vision.
7. One or both eyes appear sunken.
8. Seizure activity.
9. Periauricular ecchymosis—"Battle sign," ecchymosis on the mastoid process and or "Raccoon eyes," periorbital ecchymosis (indicate a possible basal skull fracture).
10. Rhinorrhea or otorrhea (indicative of leakage of cerebrospinal fluid [CSF]).

CLINICAL JUDGMENT If basilar skull fracture or severe midface fractures are suspected, a nasogastric (NG) tube is contraindicated. An orogastric (OG) tube may be considered for insertion.

General Interventions

1. Keep the neck in a neutral position with the cervical spine immobilized.
2. Establish an IV line of normal saline or lactated Ringer's solution—fluid volume should be based on the patient's hemodynamic status.

3. Be prepared to manage seizures—if seizures occur, they should be controlled immediately.
4. Maintain normothermia.
5. Pharmacologic interventions may include:
   a. Anticonvulsants—to control seizures.
   b. Mannitol or hypertonic saline—to reduce cerebral edema and decrease ICP.
   c. Antibiotics.
   d. Antipyretics to control hyperthermia.

Cervical Spine Injuries

Injuries to the cervical spine are serious because the crushing, stretching, and rotational shear forces exerted on the cord at the time of trauma can produce severe neurologic deficits. Edema and cord swelling contribute further to the loss of spinal cord function.

Any person with a head, neck, or back injury or fractures to the upper leg bones or to the pelvis should be suspected of having a potential spinal cord injury until proven otherwise.

Primary Assessment

1. Provide immediate immobilization of the spine and maintain immobilization throughout assessment.
2. Airway—determine patency.
3. Breathing.
   a. Intercostal paralysis with diaphragmatic breathing indicates cervical spinal cord injury.
   b. In conscious patient, observe for increased respiratory rate and difficulty in speaking because of shortness of breath.
4. Circulation—heart rate, BP, presence and quality of pulses, and capillary refill.
5. Disability—assess neurologic status.

Primary Interventions

1. Immobilize the cervical spine.
2. Open the airway using the jaw-thrust technique without head tilt.
3. If the patient needs to be intubated, consider nasal intubation.
4. If respirations are shallow, assist with a bag-valve-mask.
5. Administer high-flow oxygen to minimize potential hypoxic spinal cord damage.

Subsequent Assessment

1. Assess the position of the patient when found; this may indicate the type of injury incurred.
2. Hypotension and bradycardia accompanied by warm, dry skin—suggests spinal shock.
3. Neck and back pain/extremity pain or burning sensation to the skin.
4. History of unconsciousness.
5. Total sensory loss and motor paralysis below level of injury.
6. Loss of bowel and bladder control; usually urinary retention and bladder distention.
7. Loss of sweating and vasomotor tone below level of cord lesion.
8. Priapism—persistent erection of the penis.
9. Hypothermia—because of the inability to constrict peripheral blood vessels and conserve body heat.
10. Loss of rectal tone.

General Interventions

CLINICAL JUDGMENT A spinal cord injury can be made worse during the acute phase of injury, resulting in permanent neurologic damage. Proper positioning and movement of the patient is an immediate priority.

1. Ensure adequacy of airway, breathing, and circulation. Frequently monitor vital signs.
2. Insert an NG/OG tube.
3. Keep the patient normothermic.
4. Initiate IV access.
5. Insert an indwelling urinary catheter to avoid bladder distention.
6. Continue with repeated neurologic examinations to determine if there is deterioration of the spinal cord injury.
7. Be prepared to manage seizures if head injury is also suspected.
8. Pharmacologic interventions: possible steroids or antiepileptics.

CLINICAL JUDGMENT Patients with spinal cord injuries can experience autonomic dysreflexia, an exaggerated sympathetic response to noxious stimuli. It has the potential to be life-threatening if signs are not immediately recognized and treated, along with the removal of the offending stimuli. Signs are vasospasm, hypertension, skin pallor, bradycardia, flushed skin, profuse sweating above level of injury, headache, and anxious/restless feeling. Common offending stimuli are a full bladder or rectum, and pain receptor stimulation.

Maxillofacial Trauma

Injuries to the head frequently result in facial lacerations and fractures of the facial bones (i.e., nasal fractures, orbital fractures, maxillary fractures, and mandibular fractures).

Primary Assessment

1. Maintain immobilization of the spine while performing assessment.
2. Airway—obstruction can occur due to tongue swelling, bleeding, or broken or missing teeth.
3. Breathing—have suction ready to prevent aspiration of blood or broken teeth.
4. Circulation—control bleeding; monitor vital signs for signs of instability.
5. Disability—neuro assessment.

Primary Interventions

1. Establish and maintain an airway. Apply high-flow oxygen and assist with intubation. Oral and nasopharyngeal airways should be used with caution. Do not use a nasopharyngeal airway if there is evidence of nasal fractures or CSF leakage from the nose.
2. Control bleeding—do not apply pressure to the injury site. Apply a bulky, loose dressing.

Subsequent Assessment

1. Examine the mouth for broken or missing teeth.
2. Assess for a potential eye injury, vision loss, double vision, or pain in the eye.

3. Examine the eye for disconjugate gaze—uncoordinated eye movements.
4. Paralysis of the upward gaze is indicative of an inferior orbit fracture (known as a blow-out fracture).
5. Crepitus or a crackling feeling on palpation around the nose usually indicates a nasal fracture.
6. Malocclusion of the teeth is indicative of a maxilla or mandible fracture.
7. A palpable flattening of the cheek and a loss of sensation below the orbit may indicate a zygoma (cheek bone) fracture.
8. Spasms of the jaw (trismus) and mobility of the jaw indicate a maxilla fracture.
9. Rhinorrhea or otorrhea (may be indicative of leakage of CSF).

General Interventions

1. Gently apply cold pack to areas of swelling or ecchymosis. This may reduce further swelling and pain. However, if you suspect an injury to the eye itself, do not apply the cold pack.
2. If other injuries permit, elevate the head of the bed.
3. Possible pharmacologic interventions:
   a. Pain management.
   b. Sedation.
4. With the potential for a CSF leak, the patient should be instructed not to blow the nose because of the potential for transmitting infection to the brain or eyes.

INJURIES TO SOFT TISSUE, BONES, AND JOINTS

Soft Tissue Injuries

Soft tissue injuries involve the skin and underlying subcutaneous tissue and muscles. They can be classified as closed or open injuries. A *closed wound* is an injury to the soft tissue but without an associated break in the skin. Closed wounds include:

1. Contusion—bleeding beneath the skin into the subcutaneous tissue. Discoloration, swelling, and pain may be present.
2. Hematoma—well-defined pocket of blood and fluid beneath the skin resulting from a disruption of the deeper veins and arteries. Hematomas present as an appreciable soft mass on palpation.

An *open wound* is an injury to soft tissue with an associated break in the skin. Generally, they are more serious than closed injuries because of the potential for blood loss and infection. Open wounds include:

1. Abrasion—superficial loss of the skin resulting from rubbing or scraping the skin over a rough or uneven surface.
2. Laceration—a tear or cut in the skin. They can be a partial- or full-thickness cut, incisional or jagged.
3. Puncture—occurs when the skin is penetrated by a pointed object. Can be penetrating (entrance wound only) or perforating (entrance and exit wound). Generally, puncture wounds do not cause serious external bleeding, but there may be significant internal bleeding and damage to vital organs, as well as significant risk of infection.
4. Avulsion—involves a tearing off or loss of a full-thickness flap of the skin.
5. Amputation—traumatic cutting or tearing off of an appendage (e.g., finger, toe, arm, or leg).
6. Burn—tissue injury that results from thermal, chemical, electrical, or radiation energy.

Primary Assessment

1. Always ensure the adequacy of airway, breathing, and circulation.
2. If the bleeding from the injury has been significant, be aware of the clinical signs and symptoms of shock.
   a. Restlessness, confusion, and anxiety.
   b. Skin pale, mottled, cold, and diaphoretic.
   c. Tachycardia (rapid pulse).
   d. Tachypnea (rapid, shallow breathing).
   e. Hypotension (falling blood pressure [BP] is a late sign of shock).
3. Assess for arterial or venous bleeding. Arterial bleeding is bright red and usually spurts from the wound. Venous bleeding is darker red and will flow steadily from a wound.

Primary Interventions

The primary goal and nursing intervention are to control severe bleeding.

CLINICAL JUDGMENT Wounds that result in severe arterial bleeding should be considered life-threatening, and treatment is second only to cardiopulmonary resuscitation (CPR).

Direct Pressure

1. Most external bleeding can be controlled with firm direct pressure.
2. Cover the injury with sterile dressings.
3. While maintaining pressure, assess for distal pulses.
4. Pressure should be maintained until the bleeding stops, a pressure dressing is applied, or definitive treatment is undertaken.
5. If the dressing becomes saturated, reinforce the dressing; do not remove the dressing.
6. After bleeding has stopped, apply a pressure dressing.
   a. A pressure bandage is made by securing several gauze pads over the injury with a rolled gauze bandage.
   b. A pressure dressing allows the nurse freedom to continue assessing the patient or attend to other injuries.
   c. After applying a pressure dressing, always ensure that the patient has a pulse distal to the dressing. If no pulse is present, the dressing may be too tight.

Elevation

1. Elevating the injured area while applying direct pressure helps to control bleeding. This measure uses gravity to slow the blood flow.
2. If possible, the injured area should be elevated above the level of the heart.
3. Do not raise a limb if a fracture is suspected or if elevation causes the patient pain or discomfort.

Pressure Points

1. Pressure points are used when direct pressure and elevation alone cannot control bleeding or when direct pressure cannot be applied to a bleeding site because of a protruding bone or an embedded object.
2. Pressure points are located between the site of injury and the heart, where a main artery passes over a bone or underlying muscle mass (see Figure 31-1).

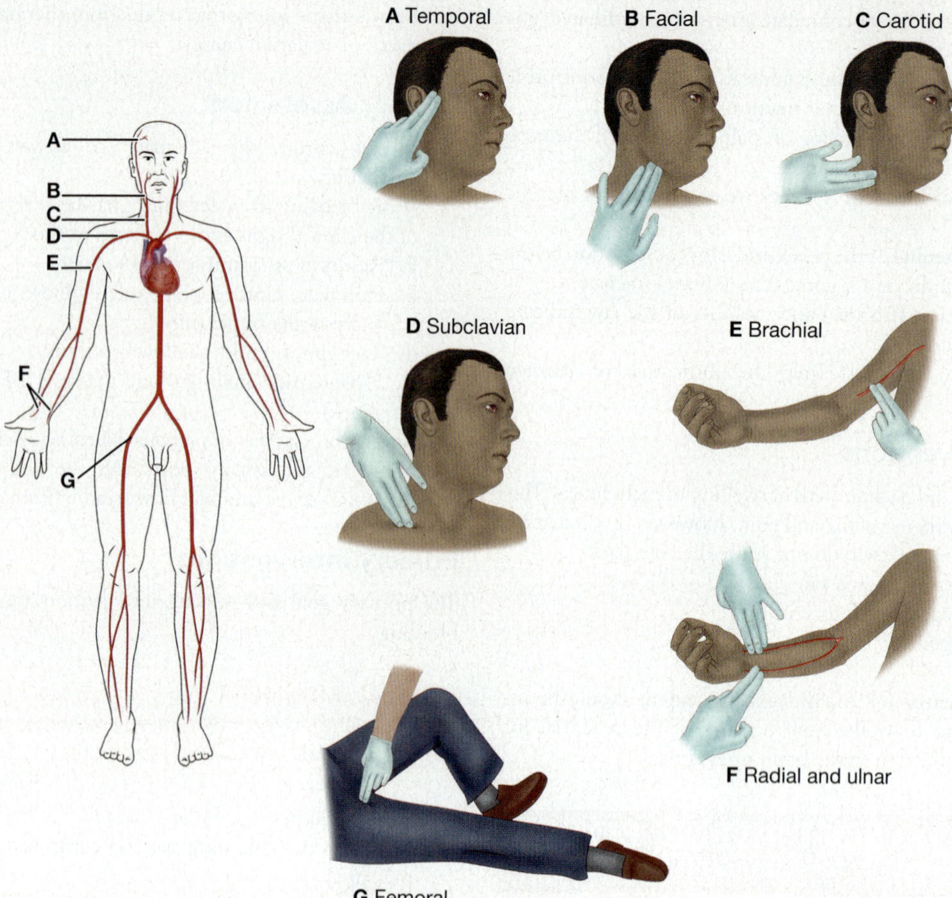

Figure 31-1. (A–G) Pressure points for control of hemorrhage. (Adapted with permission from Hinkle, J. L., Cheever, K. H., & Overbaugh, K. [2022]. *Brunner and Suddarth's textbook of medical–surgical nursing* [15th ed., Fig. 67-3]. Wolters Kluwer.)

3. Locate the pressure point and apply firm, steady pressure with the heel of the hand.
4. If heavy bleeding is still not controlled, the patient may risk exsanguination, in which case a tourniquet should be used or a vascular clamp can be applied to the artery.

Subsequent Assessment

1. Expose the wound by cutting away clothing if necessary. Secure any impaled objects in place.
2. Assess for the presence of concomitant injuries. The obvious wound is not necessarily the most life-threatening.
3. Assess vascular status distal to the injury and compare it to the uninjured extremity.
   a. Color of the injured extremity—pallor suggests poor arterial perfusion and cyanosis suggests venous congestion.
   b. Test capillary refill time by depressing the nail bed until it blanches and seeing how long until the nail bed returns to pink. A capillary refill time greater than 2 seconds (assuming ambient temperature) suggests decreased capillary perfusion.
   c. Test pulses distal to the injury—generally, they should be full and strong.
4. Perform a neurologic assessment of the injured extremity to determine peripheral nerve insult, possibly caused by direct injury, compression, or edema.
   a. Sensory function—while the patient's eyes are closed, lightly touch the area distal to the injury and ask them to identify the area being touched. Have them discriminate between sharp and dull touch.
   b. Motor function—have patient move extremity distal to the injury.
5. Determine tetanus immunization status.
6. History of the injury, including when and how the wound occurred. Any wound on the body that is more than 18 hours old and any facial wounds older than 24 hours are considered at high risk for infection, and primary closure by suturing may not be an option.
7. Allergies to local anesthesia, epinephrine, and antibiotics.

General Interventions

Wound Preparation

1. Shaving of body hair is not recommended.
2. Irrigate gently and copiously with isotonic sterile saline solution to remove dirt and debris. All wounds must be thoroughly explored for retained foreign objects before closure. If the wound is grossly contaminated, it may need to be cleansed with a surgical scrub sponge and then irrigated. If the patient is in pain, anesthetize the wound prior to cleansing and irrigating.
3. Topical anesthetic may be applied to the wound (prior to infiltration with local anesthetic) intradermally through the wound margins or by regional nerve block.

4. Devitalized tissue and foreign matter are removed—devitalized tissue inhibits wound healing and increases the chance of bacterial infection.

Wound Closure

1. Closure by primary intent.
   a. Wound is repaired without delay after the injury; yields the fastest healing.
   b. Primary closure may be with sutures, wound closure strips, staples, or tissue adhesives. Location and size of the wound are key factors in determining closure material used.
2. Closure by secondary intent.
   a. Wound is allowed to granulate on its own without surgical closure.
   b. Wound is cleaned and covered with a sterile dressing.
3. Closure by secondary intent with delayed closure.
   a. Wound is cleaned and dressed.
   b. Patient returns in 3 to 4 days for definitive closure.

Wound Dressing

1. Dressing should be applied in three layers.
   a. The first layer is the contact layer. This should consist of a nonabsorbent hydrophilic dressing that will allow exudate to pass through to the second layer without wetting the contact layer. An examples of a contact layer dressing is petroleum.
   b. The second layer is the absorbent layer and is usually constructed of surgical dressing pads or 4 × 4-gauze dressings.
   c. The third layer is the outer wrap that holds the dressing in place. The outer wrap may consist of rolled gauze and tape.
2. There are many different proprietary dressings available for application.

Pharmacologic Interventions

1. Give antimicrobial treatment, as directed, depending on how the injury occurred, age of wound, presence of soil, and infection potential.
2. Give tetanus prophylaxis, as indicated, based on patient's immunization status, and wound.
3. Rabies prophylaxis, as indicated. For more information on four-dose postexposure rabies prophylaxis, go to www.cdc.gov/vaccines/hcp/acip-recs/vacc-specific/rabies.html

Patient Education

1. Inform the patient that pain should subside over the course of the next 24 to 48 hours.
2. Explain that acetaminophen, ibuprofen, or prescribed analgesic is to be taken for the first 24 hours after a simple laceration.
3. Recommend that the wound be monitored for signs of infection: fever/chills, persistent or worsening pain, purulent discharge, foul odor, erythema and warmth surrounding the wound, red streaking from the extremity, increase in swelling. If any of these signs occur, patient should contact a health care provider.

Injuries to Bones and Joints

Injuries to bones and joints are common. *Fractures* may be caused by direct trauma (e.g., projectiles, crush injuries) or by indirect trauma (i.e., bones being pulled apart or rotational forces). In addition, bones may fracture due to pathologic reasons. A pathologic fracture occurs due to weakness in the bone secondary to a disease process such as metastatic cancer. For the classification of fractures, see page 1412.

Other injuries include:

1. Dislocation—complete displacement or separation of a bone from its normal place of articulation. It may be associated with tearing of the ligaments. The shoulder, elbow, fingers, hips, and ankles are the joints most frequently affected.
2. Subluxation—partial disruption of the articulating surfaces.
3. Sprains—injuries in which ligaments are partially torn or stretched. These injuries are usually caused by twisting a joint beyond its normal range of motion. The severity can range from mild to severe. The more seriously injured ligaments may resemble a fracture.
4. Strains—stretching or tearing of muscle and tendon fibers, usually caused by overexertion or overextension.

Primary Assessment

1. Always ensure the adequacy of the airway, breathing, and circulation before initiating treatment.
2. Occult blood loss into a closed space from the fracture may be significant enough to produce hypovolemic shock (more common with pelvic and femur fractures). Estimated blood loss in adults from closed fractures in liters:
   a. Tibia—1.5 L.
   b. Femur—2 L.
   c. Pelvis—6 L.
   d. Humerus—2 L.
3. A fractured cervical spine, pelvic fracture, or fractured femur may cause life-threatening injuries. Posterior dislocations of the hip are life-threatening and limb-threatening emergencies because of the potential for blood loss and disruption in blood supply to the head of the femur. Unless this dislocation is promptly reduced, the patient may develop avascular necrosis of the femoral head and subsequently may require a hip replacement.

Primary Interventions

1. Support airway, breathing, and circulation, if compromised.
2. Initiate intravenous (IV) line and treat for shock, if evident.
3. Assess circulation distal to the site of injury (skin color and temperature, pulses). Loss of distal pulses requires immediate intervention.
4. Protect injured part from movement or further trauma by splinting.
5. Understand that pain management is essential.

Subsequent Assessment

1. Seek information on the mechanism of injury.
   a. How did the injury occur and when did the injury occur?
   b. In what position was the limb after the injury?
   c. If the mechanism of injury was a fall, how many feet did the person fall, and what type of surface did they land on?
   d. If the mechanism was a motor vehicle accident, where was the patient? What was the direction and amount of force? Were the airbags in the vehicle deployed? Certain musculoskeletal injuries commonly occur together.
2. Assess for the presence of concomitant injuries.
   a. A fractured calcaneus as the result of a fall from a great height may also include a compression fracture of the spine.

b. A person with a fractured patella from a motor vehicle accident may also have a fractured or dislocated femur.
c. A fractured pelvis may occur with lumbosacral spine fractures and bladder injuries.
3. Perform a neurovascular assessment to include the area above and below the injury.
a. Assess for ischemia to the extremity.
b. Pallor suggests poor arterial perfusion, whereas cyanosis suggests venous congestion.
i. A capillary refill time greater than 2 seconds suggests decreased arterial capillary perfusion.
c. Assess neurologic supply of the injured extremity to determine peripheral nerve insult. Damage to a peripheral nerve can be the result of a direct injury, compression, stretching, or edema.
i. Test sensory function—with the patient's eyes closed, lightly touch the area distal to the injury. Ask the patient to identify the area being touched.
ii. Test motor function—have patient move extremity distal to the injury.
iii. Numbness or paralysis indicates pressure on the nerves and may require immediate medical intervention.
4. Examine the bones and joints adjacent to the injury. If there was enough force to produce one injury, there may be other injuries.
5. Signs and symptoms of fractures:
a. Pain and tenderness over the fracture site, called "point tenderness."
b. A grating or crepitus over the fracture site.
c. Swelling because of internal bleeding and edema.
d. Deformity, unnatural position, or movement where there is no joint.
e. Loss of use or guarding.
f. Discoloration because of bleeding into the surrounding tissue.
g. Shortening of an extremity or rotation of the extremity.
6. Signs and symptoms of dislocations:
a. Loss of joint motion—the joint may appear "frozen."
b. Obvious deformity—lump, ridge, or excavation.
c. Pain.
7. Signs and symptoms of sprains:
a. Pain in the joint area.
b. Swelling.
c. Limited use or movement.
d. Ecchymosis.
8. Signs and symptoms of strains:
a. Pain located in a muscle or its tendon, not a bone or a joint.
b. Swelling is usually minimal.
9. Closely monitor vital signs.

General Interventions

Interventions for the Patient Who Are Severely Injured

1. Ensure the adequacy of the airway, breathing, and circulation. Closely monitor vital signs.
2. Initiate two IV lines and start volume replacement with lactated Ringer's solution or normal saline.
3. Immobilize the injury—this will prevent further damage and will help to relieve the pain.
4. Prepare the patient for the possibility of needing to go to the operating room (OR)—keep the patient nothing by mouth (NPO).
5. Antibiotics may be started if warranted.

Other Interventions

1. Elevate to prevent or limit swelling.
2. Apply cold packs; cold packs should not be placed directly on the skin.
3. Open fractures: If bone is protruding, do not attempt to tuck the ends of the bone under the skin. Cover with a sterile dressing moistened with normal saline.
4. Splint the extremity in as good alignment as possible until definitive care is complete. Immobilize the joint above and below the fracture.
5. Handle the injured part gently and as little as possible.
6. Pain management may include cold packs, simple or opioid analgesics, nonsteroidal anti-inflammatory drugs, or regional nerve blocks.
7. High-flow oxygen should be administered to patients with pelvic or femoral fractures, compartment syndrome, or signs of shock.

Assess for Compartment Syndrome

1. Increased pressure within an extremity resulting from bleeding and swelling into a closed space, causing pressure on vital structures.
2. The six Ps (signs and symptoms) of compartment syndrome are:
a. Pain—development of a different type of pain, the return of pain after treatment/splinting had caused pain relief, or pain out of proportion to the severity of the injury.
b. Pallor—deterioration in skin color and an increase in the capillary refill time.
c. Pulselessness.
d. Paresthesias.
e. Paralysis—late sign.
f. Puffiness—late sign.
3. Patients with long bone or pelvic fractures are at risk for developing fat emboli and should be monitored closely.

CLINICAL JUDGMENT Compartment syndrome is a limb-threatening event; therefore, if suspected, do not elevate limb above the level of the heart. This may decrease perfusion to the compromised extremity. Emergent fasciotomy is often required.

SHOCK AND INTERNAL INJURIES

Shock

Shock is the common denominator in a wide variety of disease processes that present as an immediate threat to life. Simply defined, *shock* is inadequate tissue perfusion with oxygen and metabolic substrates. This inadequate tissue perfusion is the result of failure of one or more of the following: (1) the heart–pump failure, (2) blood volume, (3) arterial resistance vessels, and (4) the capacity of the venous beds. Any condition that significantly affects any of the aforementioned may precipitate a shock state. Shock can be classified as compensated (hemodynamically stable) or uncompensated (hemodynamically unstable).

Types of shock are as follows:

1. Hypovolemic shock—occurs when a significant amount of fluid is lost from the intravascular space. May result from hemorrhage, burns, gastrointestinal (GI) losses, or fluid shifts.

2. Cardiogenic shock—occurs when the heart fails as a pump. Primary causes of this failure are myocardial infarction (MI), serious cardiac dysrhythmias, and myocardial depression from diseases such as myocarditis, endocarditis, and pericarditis. Secondary causes include mechanical restriction of cardiac function or venous obstruction, as occurs with cardiac tamponade, vena cava obstruction, or tension pneumothorax.
3. Distributive—occurs as a result of a loss of vascular tone. It may be anaphylactic, septic, neurogenic, or due to acute adrenal insufficiency. Septic shock may occur with or without an infection. Sepsis is characterized by a systemic inflammatory response in the presence of suspected or confirmed infection. Systemic inflammatory response syndrome (SIRS) is the body's systemic clinical response to an insult with an acute inflammatory reaction. See Table 31-1, for defining characteristics of SIRS and sepsis.
4. Obstructive—caused by a physical obstruction in blood flow into and out of the heart. It can be divided into two main categories: mechanical and pulmonary vascular. Mechanical causes may include tension pneumothorax, pericarditis, superior vena cava syndrome, and pericardial tamponade. Pulmonary vascular causes include severe pulmonary hypertension and pulmonary embolism.

Primary Assessment and Interventions

1. Rapid recognition and prompt intervention are essential to increase the chance of survival because a downward spiral of physiologic responses culminating in multiorgan dysfunction syndrome and eventual death will occur if shock is not treated.
2. The initial priorities in the assessment are the same for all types of shock.
   a. Is the airway open?
   b. Is the patient breathing?
   c. Is there a circulation problem?
3. Initiate immediate interventions, as indicated.
   a. Resuscitate as necessary. Fluid replacement with isotonic fluids and eventually blood products is essential.
   b. Administer oxygen.
   c. Start cardiac monitoring.
   d. Control hemorrhage or other fluid loss, if present.
4. Pain management is essential.

Subsequent Assessment

1. Assess level of consciousness (LOC)—important indicator of shock because it reflects cerebral perfusion. Changes may include:
   a. Confusion.
   b. Irritability.
   c. Anxiety.
   d. Agitation.
   e. Inability to concentrate.
2. Watch for increasing lethargy progressing to obtundation and coma, indicating progression of shock.
3. Monitor arterial blood pressure (BP).
   a. If the patient can compensate for the shock state, the BP may initially rise approximately 20%. A significant decrease in BP may not occur until late in the shock state.
   b. Narrowing pulse pressure—early in shock, the diastolic pressure may rise due to an initial vasoconstriction produced by release of catecholamines from the sympathetic nervous system.
   c. Fall in the systolic pressure—there is no absolute value in BP that indicates a shock state. It is the deviation from normal that is important. However, it is generally accepted that a systolic pressure below 80 mm Hg or a mean arterial pressure below 60 mm Hg is indicative of shock.
4. Assess pulse quality and rate change.
   a. The rate is usually increased.
   b. Weak, thready pulse because of decreased cardiac output and increased peripheral vascular resistance.
5. Assess urine output.
   a. A decrease in renal blood flow or pressure will result in decreased urine output.
   b. Ideally in an adult, the urine output should be 0.5 mL/kg/h.

Table 31-1 Defining Characteristics of Sepsis

SEPTIC CONDITION	CHARACTERISTICS
SIRS, two or more of:	Temperature >100.4°F (38°C) or <96.8°F (36°C) HR >90 bpm RR >20 breaths/min or $PaCO_2$ <32 mm Hg WBC >12,000/µL or <4,000/µL
Sepsis	The presence of an infection with two or more SIRS criteria
Severe sepsis—organ dysfunction or tissue hypoperfusion	Hypotension—systolic BP <100 mm Hg, MAP <65 mm Hg, or a reduction of >40 mm Hg from usual reading Serum lactate >4 mmol/L Altered mental state Hyperglycemia in the absence of diabetes Hypoxemia, oxygen saturation <93% Urine output <0.5 mL/kg/h and/or an elevated urea or creatinine Coagulopathy, INR >1.5
Septic shock—multiple organ failure	Refractory hypotension and lactate that does not improve with adequate fluid resuscitation (40 mL/kg)

BP, blood pressure; bpm, beats per minute; HR, heart rate; INR, international normalized ratio; MAP, mean arterial pressure; $PaCO_2$, partial pressure of carbon dioxide; RR, respiratory rate; SIRS, systemic inflammatory response syndrome; WBC, white blood cell.

6. Assess capillary perfusion.
    a. Pale, ashen, mottled, cold, and diaphoretic skin indicates potent vasoconstriction.
    b. Capillary refill greater than 2 seconds indicates vasoconstriction.
7. Also assess for:
    a. Subjective feeling of impending doom.
    b. Metabolic acidosis secondary to anaerobic metabolism within the cells.
    c. Excessive thirst.
8. Rapid identification and treatment of SIRS or sepsis are essential in the treatment of septic shock. Although a source of infection may not be identified, signs include fever, tachypnea, tachycardia, and leukocytosis.

General Interventions

1. Administer 100% O_2 by nonrebreather face mask to maintain the partial pressure of arterial oxygen at 90% to 100%.
2. Assist with intubation if the patient is unable to maintain airway.
3. Fluid resuscitation.
    a. Two large-bore intravenous (IV) lines should be established.
    b. Administer IV fluids—lactated Ringer's or normal saline. Rate of infusion depends on severity of blood loss and clinical evidence of hypovolemia.
    c. Packed red blood cells or whole blood are infused when there is hypovolemic shock secondary to blood loss and when shock is refractory to isotonic fluid boluses.
    d. Additional platelets and coagulation factors are given when large amounts of blood are needed because replacement blood is deficient in clotting factors.
    e. Warm the blood and fluids using a commercial fluid warmer—massive fluid replacement has a cooling effect that can cause cardiac dysrhythmias, paradoxical hypotension, decreased oxyhemoglobin dissociation, or cardiac arrest.
4. Insert an indwelling urinary catheter.
    a. Record urine output minimally every hour until patient is hemodynamically stable.
    b. Urinary volume reveals adequacy of kidney and visceral perfusion.
5. Maintain patient in supine position with the legs slightly elevated. (This position is contraindicated in patients with head injuries.)
6. Electrocardiogram (ECG) monitoring—dysrhythmias may contribute to shock.
7. Maintain ongoing nursing surveillance of total patient—LOC, BP, heart rate, respiratory rate, temperature, color, central venous pressure (CVP), arterial blood gas (ABG) levels, urine output, ECG, hematocrit, hemoglobin, coagulation profiles, and electrolytes—to assess patient response to treatment.
8. Immobilize fractures to minimize blood loss.
9. Maintain normothermia.
    a. Overwarming produces vasodilatation, which counteracts the body's compensatory mechanism of vasoconstriction and also increases fluid loss through perspiration.
    b. A patient who is in septic shock should be kept cool because high fever will increase the cellular metabolic effects of shock.
10. Provide pharmacologic interventions:
    a. Vasopressors may be indicated, but they should not be used in place of volume replacement except as dictated by cardiogenic or neurogenic shock states.
    b. Antibiotics—broad spectrum for septic shock.
11. Be aware that Trendelenburg position is no longer recommended because of the potential for respiratory compromise caused by pressure from abdominal organs.

Abdominal Injuries

Abdominal injuries account for a large percentage of trauma-related injuries and deaths. The visceral organs contained within the abdomen can be classified as either hollow or solid. Damage to a hollow organ can result in acute peritonitis, leading to shock within a few hours, and damage to a solid organ can result in lethal hemorrhage. Abdominal injuries may be classified as either penetrating or blunt. Examples of penetrating abdominal injury are gunshot wounds or stab wounds. The mechanism that caused the penetrating abdominal trauma may cross the diaphragm and enter the chest. The opposite can also occur. Common causes of blunt abdominal injury are motor vehicle accidents and falls. Trauma to the abdomen is commonly associated with extra-abdominal injuries (i.e., chest, head, and extremity injuries) and severe concomitant trauma to multiple intraperitoneal organs. Blunt abdominal injury is often associated with delayed complications, especially if there is injury to the liver, spleen, or blood vessels, which can lead to substantial blood loss into the peritoneal cavity.

Primary Assessment and Interventions

1. Assess airway, breathing, and circulation.
2. Initiate resuscitation, as indicated.
3. Control bleeding and be prepared to treat shock.
4. If there is an impaled object in the abdomen, do not remove it. Stabilize the object in place with bulky dressings along the sides of the object.

Subsequent Assessment

1. Obtain a history of the mechanism of the injury, type of weapon, and estimated amount of blood loss.
    a. If the patient was stabbed, what were they stabbed with? If a knife, what kind and how long was the blade?
    b. Was the person who stabbed the patient a male or a female?
        i. Males usually hold a knife underhand and stab/thrust upward.
        ii. Females usually will stab/thrust downward with an overhand motion.
    c. If the patient sustained a gunshot wound, attempt to ascertain the type of gun and range at which shot.
    d. Time of injury/onset of symptoms.
    e. Passenger location (driver frequently sustains spleen/liver rupture). Were seat belts worn? Did the airbag deploy? Were there any other injured parties or fatalities involved in the same accident?
2. Inspect the abdomen for obvious signs of injury (penetrating injury, bruising, seat belt marks).
3. Evaluate for signs and symptoms of hemorrhage—usually accompanies abdominal injury, especially if the liver and spleen have been traumatized.
4. Note tenderness, rebound tenderness, guarding, rigidity, and spasm.
    a. Firmly press, with the whole hand, the area of maximal tenderness (let the patient point to the area).
    b. Remove the fingers quickly to check for rebound tenderness; pain at suspected point indicates peritoneal irritation.

5. Ask about referred pain, such as Kehr sign—pain radiating to the left shoulder may be a sign of blood beneath the left diaphragm and can signify a splenic laceration or rupture; pain in the right shoulder can result from laceration of the liver. The patient must be lying flat for this type of shoulder pain to occur.
6. Look for increasing abdominal distention. Measure abdominal girth at the umbilical level early in your assessment—this serves as a baseline from which changes can be determined. Making a mark where you measured can also assist in ensuring that the same place is measured each time.
7. Auscultate—a silent abdomen accompanies peritoneal irritation or ileus. The presence of bowel sounds *in the chest* indicates a ruptured diaphragm. Bruits over the aorta or other large arteries may indicate disrupted arterial blood flow.
8. Percuss—tympani over solid organs (liver, spleen) indicates the presence of free air; dullness over regions normally containing gas may indicate the presence of blood or other fluids.
9. Look for chest injuries, which frequently accompany intra-abdominal injuries.
10. Cullen sign, a slight bluish discoloration around the navel, indicates blood in the abdominal wall. Grey Turner sign, or flank ecchymosis, is indicative of renal injuries or retroperitoneal bleeding.
11. Pain is a poor indicator of the extent of an abdominal injury. Rebound tenderness and board-like rigidity are indicative of a significant intra-abdominal injury.
12. A rectal examination and examination of the perineum should be done on all patients. The presence of blood may be indicative of trauma.
13. Continuously assess vital signs, urine output, CVP readings, hematocrit values, and neurologic status. Tachypnea, tachycardia, and hypotension may be clues to intra-abdominal bleeding.

General Interventions

1. Assess adequacy of airway, breathing, and circulation. Reassess frequently.
2. Goals are to control bleeding, maintain blood volume, and prevent infection.
3. Keep the patient quiet and on the stretcher because movement may fragment or dislodge a clot in a large vessel and produce massive hemorrhage.
4. Cut the clothing away from the wound. Do not cut through bullet holes or stab marks. These will be needed by law enforcement authorities as forensic evidence.
5. Count the number of wounds.
6. Look for entrance and exit wounds.
7. If the patient is comatose, immobilize the cervical spine until after cervical films are taken and cleared.
8. Apply compression to external bleeding.
9. Insert two large-bore IV lines and infuse fluid as dictated by the patient's hemodynamic status.
10. Be prepared to insert a nasogastric (NG) tube to decompress the abdomen. This will serve to empty the stomach, relieve gastric distention, and facilitate abdominal assessment. In addition, if blood is found, it may indicate stomach injury or esophageal injury.
11. Cover protruding abdominal viscera; do not attempt to replace the protruding organs into the abdomen. Use sterile saline dressings to protect viscera from drying.
12. Cover open wounds with dry dressings.
13. Withhold oral fluids to prevent increased peristalsis and vomiting.
14. Insert an indwelling urethral catheter to ascertain the presence of hematuria and to monitor urine output. If a fracture of the pelvis is suspected, a catheter should not be placed until the integrity of the urethra is ensured.
15. Pharmacologic interventions.
    a. Analgesics.
    b. Tetanus prophylaxis.
    c. Broad-spectrum antibiotics because bacterial contamination is a frequent complication (depending on history and nature of wound).
16. Prepare for focused ultrasound when there is uncertainty about intraperitoneal bleeding. Focused assessment with sonography in trauma (FAST) is a standard for rapid bedside assessment using ultrasound performed by providers to identify free fluid in the abdomen, pericardium, or peritoneum.
17. Prepare for surgery if the patient shows evidence of unexplained shock, unstable vital signs, peritoneal irritation, bowel protrusion or evisceration, significant penetrating injury, significant GI bleeding, or peritoneal air.
18. Prepare the patient for diagnostic procedures.
    a. Catheterization and urinalysis—as a guide to possible urinary tract injury and to monitor urine output.
    b. Type and crossmatch and serial hemoglobin and hematocrit levels—their trend reflects presence or absence of bleeding.
    c. Complete blood count (CBC)—white blood cell count is generally elevated with trauma.
    d. Serum amylase elevation usually indicates pancreatic injury or perforations of the GI tract.
    e. Computed tomography (CT) scans permit detailed evaluation of abdominal and retroperitoneal injuries.
    f. Abdominal and chest x-rays may reveal free air beneath the diaphragm, indicating a ruptured hollow viscus.

Multiple Injuries

The patient with multiple injuries requires rapid and definitive assessment and interventions during the first hour after trauma to increase the chance of survival; this first hour has been called the "golden hour." During this time, multiple assessments and interventions are performed simultaneously by the health care team.

Primary Assessment and Interventions

Airway

1. Assume a cervical spine injury and open the airway using the jaw-thrust technique without head tilt.
2. Apply suction to clear the trachea and bronchial tree. Remove debris from the mouth (i.e., broken teeth, mucus).
3. Insert an oropharyngeal airway—to prevent occlusion by the tongue. Oropharyngeal airways are used only in patients who are unconscious to prevent stimulation of the gag reflex.
4. Prepare for endotracheal intubation if adequate airway cannot be maintained.
5. If upper airway trauma or edema exists, a cricothyroidotomy may be indicated.

Breathing

1. Note the character and symmetry of chest wall motion and pattern of breathing. Assess for open wounds, deformity, and flail segments.

2. Auscultate the lungs and assess for tracheal deviation. If a tension pneumothorax is present, the trachea will shift away from the injury. Tracheal deviation is a late sign.
3. Ask the patient who is conscious if they are experiencing difficulty breathing or chest pain while breathing.
4. Administer oxygen by 100% nonrebreather mask or, if ventilation is inadequate, assist the patient's ventilations by bag-valve-mask.
5. Suspect serious intrathoracic injuries if respiratory distress continues after adequate airway has been established.
6. Assess the overall effectiveness of ventilations.

Circulation

1. Assess cardiac function and treat cardiac arrest (hypoxia, metabolic acidosis, and chest trauma may precipitate cardiac arrest).
2. If pulseless (cardiac arrest), begin chest compressions (cardiopulmonary resuscitation [CPR]).
3. Control hemorrhage.
   a. Apply direct pressure over bleeding points, if able.
   b. Expect significant blood loss in patients with fractures to the shaft of the femur, multiple fractures, or pelvic trauma.
   c. Use tourniquet(s) for massive arterial bleeding from extremities that cannot be halted with pressure.
   d. Prepare for immediate surgical intervention if patient is bleeding internally.
4. Palpate the carotid pulse and note its rate and quality. Palpate both central and peripheral pulses and compare their quality. Patients will lose their peripheral pulses before losing their central pulse. In addition, assess the femoral and radial pulses to determine an approximate systolic pressure.
   a. If the carotid pulse is present, the systolic pressure is at least 60 mm Hg.
   b. If the femoral pulse is present, the systolic pressure is at least 70 mm Hg.
   c. If the radial pulse is present, the systolic pressure is at least 80 mm Hg.
5. Prevent and treat hypovolemic shock.
   a. Insert two large-bore IV lines.
   b. If indicated, place a central venous catheter to monitor the patient's response to fluid infusion—to prevent fluid overload and as a route for fluid infusion.
   c. Fluid resuscitation—lactated Ringer's solution or normal saline is given for volume replacement until blood is available.
   d. Administer warmed blood—massive transfusions of unwarmed blood have a cooling effect that can cause cardiac irritability and arrest.
6. Note presence or absence of pulses in fractured extremities.

Neurologic

1. Assess level of responsiveness, pupil size and reactivity, strength, and reflexes.
2. Determine a Glasgow Coma Score as a baseline (see page 334).
3. If signs of increased intracranial pressure (ICP) exist, ICP monitoring may be instituted.
4. Agitation or other mental status changes are often the first sign of impending problems.

Subsequent Assessment and Interventions

1. The goals are rapid determination of the extent of the injuries and treatment prioritization.
2. Monitor ECG—to detect life-threatening dysrhythmias.
3. Insert indwelling urethral catheter and monitor urine output to aid in diagnosis of shock as well as monitor effectiveness of therapy. If unable to insert catheter, do not force—the patient may have a ruptured urethra.
4. Perform an ongoing clinical evaluation to observe for improvement or deterioration, such as changes in vital signs, improvement in level of responsiveness, skin warmth, and speed of capillary filling.
5. Prepare for immediate surgical intervention if the patient does not respond to fluids or blood. Inability to restore BP and circulatory volume in the patient usually indicates major internal bleeding.
6. Splint extremity fractures; this will prevent further trauma to soft tissues and blood vessels and to relieve pain.
7. Examine the patient for abdominal pain, rigidity, tenderness, rebound tenderness, diminished bowel sounds, hypotension, and shock.
8. Prepare for FAST examination or CT scan to assess for intraperitoneal bleeding.
9. Draw blood for laboratory studies (type and cross-matching, hemoglobin, hematocrit, baseline CBC, electrolytes, blood urea nitrogen [BUN], glucose, coagulation studies).
10. Insert an NG tube to prevent vomiting and aspiration.
11. Prepare for laparotomy if the patient shows continuing signs of hemorrhage and deterioration.
12. Continue to monitor urine output every 30 minutes—reflects cardiac output and state of perfusion of vital organs; assess for hematuria and oliguria.
13. Evaluate the patient for other injuries and institute appropriate treatment, including tetanus immunization.
14. Perform a more thorough physical examination after resuscitation and management of the aforementioned priorities.

ENVIRONMENTAL EMERGENCIES

Heat Exhaustion

Heat exhaustion is the inadequacy or the collapse of peripheral circulation because of volume and electrolyte depletion. Heat exhaustion is one condition in the spectrum of heat-related illnesses, including heat rash, heat edema, heat cramps, and heat syncope. Untreated heat exhaustion may progress to heatstroke.

Primary Assessment and Interventions

1. Expect the patient to be alert without significant cardiorespiratory or neurologic compromise.
2. If vital functions are significantly impaired, suspect secondary condition, such as myocardial infarction (MI) or stroke.

Subsequent Assessment

1. Ask patient about headache, fatigue, dizziness, muscle cramping, and nausea.
2. Inspect the skin—usually pale, ashen, and moist.
3. The temperature may be normal, slightly elevated, or as high as 104°F (40°C).
4. Measure vital signs for hypotension, orthostatic changes, tachycardia, and tachypnea.
5. The patient will be awake but may give a history of syncope or confusion.

6. Laboratory analysis will show hemoconcentration and hyponatremia (if sodium depletion is the primary problem) or hypernatremia (if water depletion is the primary problem).
7. The electrocardiogram (ECG) may show dysrhythmias without evidence of infarction.

General Interventions

1. Move the patient to a cool environment and remove all clothing.
2. Position the patient supine with feet slightly elevated.
3. If the patient complains of nausea or vomiting, do not give fluids by mouth.
4. Start an intravenous (IV) line with normal saline until electrolyte results are confirmed.
5. Monitor the patient for changes in the cardiac rhythm and vital signs. Vital signs should be taken at least every 15 minutes until the patient is stable.
6. Provide fans and cool sponge baths as cooling methods.
7. Provide patient education.
   a. Advise the patient to avoid immediate re-exposure to high temperatures; the patient may remain hypersensitive to high temperatures for a considerable length of time.
   b. Emphasize the importance of maintaining an adequate fluid intake, wearing loose clothing, and reducing activity in hot weather.
   c. Athletes should monitor fluid losses, replace fluids, and use a gradual approach to physical conditioning, allowing sufficient time for acclimatization.
8. Identify those at increased risk for heat exhaustion and heatstroke so preventive measures can be taken. Risk factors include underlying conditions such as cardiovascular disease, alcohol misuse, malnutrition, diabetes, skin diseases, as well as major burn scarring. Other risk factors include very young or very old age, and the use of drugs such as anticholinergics, phenothiazines, diuretics, antihistamines, antidepressants, and beta-adrenergic blockers. Also behaviors such as working outdoors, wearing inappropriate clothing, inadequate fluid intake, and living in poor environmental conditions can increase the risk.

Heatstroke

Heatstroke is a medical emergency that can result in significant morbidity and mortality. It is defined as the combination of hyperpyrexia greater than 104°F (40°C) and neurologic symptoms. Heatstroke is caused by a shutdown or failure of the heat-regulating mechanisms of the body. It can be classified as exertional or nonexertional.

Primary Assessment and Interventions

1. Assess airway, breathing, and circulation.
2. Level of consciousness (LOC) may be altered.
3. Expect to intervene immediately if cardiovascular collapse occurs.

Subsequent Assessment

1. Obtain a history from accompanying person about environmental conditions, activity, underlying health, and medications that may have contributed to heatstroke.
2. Perform a neurologic assessment.
   a. Initially, the patient may exhibit abnormal behavior or irritability. This may progress to confusion, combativeness, deliriousness, and coma.
   b. Other central nervous system (CNS) disturbances include tremors, seizures, fixed and dilated pupils, and decerebrate or decorticate posturing.
3. Assess vital signs.
   a. Temperature greater than 104°F (40°C).
   b. Hypotension.
   c. Rapid pulse; may be bounding or weak.
   d. Tachypnea.
4. The skin may appear flushed and hot; in early heatstroke, the skin may be moist, but, as the heatstroke progresses, the skin will become dry as the body loses its ability to sweat.
5. Arterial blood gas (ABG) values show metabolic acidosis.

General Interventions

1. Protect the airway in patients with deteriorating mental status or absent gag reflex.
2. Provide cooling measures. When the diagnosis of heatstroke is made or suspected, it is imperative to reduce the patient's temperature.
   a. Reduce the core (internal) temperature to 102°F (38.9°C) as rapidly as possible.
   b. Evaporative cooling is the most efficient. Spray tepid water on the skin while electric fans are used to blow continuously over the patient to augment heat dissipation.
   c. Apply cold packs to the neck, groin, axillae, and scalp (areas of maximal heat transfer).
   d. Soak sheets/towels in ice water and place on patient, using fans to accelerate evaporation/cooling rate.
   e. Immersion in cold or ice water is contraindicated.
   f. If the temperature fails to decrease, initiate core cooling: iced saline gastric lavage, cool fluid peritoneal dialysis, cool fluid bladder irrigation, or cool fluid chest irrigation.
   g. Cooling blankets may be used after the temperature is stabilized.
   h. Discontinue active cooling when the temperature reaches 102°F (38.9°C). In most cases, this will reduce the chance of overcooling because the body temperature will continue to fall after cessation of cooling.
3. Oxygenate the patient to supply tissue needs that are exaggerated by the hypermetabolic condition: 100% nonrebreather mask or intubate the patient, if necessary, to support a failing cardiorespiratory system.
4. Monitor condition.
   a. Monitor and record the core temperature continually during cooling process to avoid hypothermia; also, hyperthermia may recur spontaneously within 3 to 4 hours.
   b. Monitor the vital signs continuously. Assess rhythm with continuous cardiac monitoring.
   c. Perform frequent (every 30 minutes) neurologic assessments.
   d. Monitor laboratory values for signs of coagulopathy and liver or renal damage.
5. Replace fluids.
   a. Start IV infusion using normal saline solution to replace fluid losses, maintain adequate circulation, and facilitate cooling.
   b. If possible, a central line should be established with monitoring of central venous pressure (CVP).
   c. Fluid replacement is based on the patient's response and laboratory results.
6. Other potential measures:
   a. Dialysis for renal failure.
   b. Diuretics, such as mannitol, to promote diuresis.

c. Anticonvulsant agents to control seizures.
d. Potassium for hypokalemia and sodium bicarbonate to correct metabolic acidosis, depending on laboratory results.
e. Antipyretics are not useful in treating heatstroke. They may contribute to the complications of coagulopathy and hepatic damage.
f. Intense shivering may be controlled by diazepam. Shivering will generate heat and increase the metabolic rate.
g. Patients with depleted clotting factors may be treated with platelets or fresh frozen plasma.
7. Monitor urine output, likely with an indwelling catheter—acute tubular necrosis is a complication of heatstroke.
8. Perform continuous ECG monitoring and frequent cardiovascular assessments for possible ischemia, infarction, and dysrhythmias.
9. Perform serial laboratory testing (coagulation studies, electrolytes, glucose, and serum enzymes).
10. The patient should be admitted to an intensive care unit (ICU); complications can occur, including heart failure, cardiovascular collapse, hepatic failure, renal failure, disseminated intravascular coagulation, and rhabdomyolysis.
11. Monitor the patient for the development of seizures and provide for a safe environment in case of seizures.

POPULATION AWARENESS Proceed cautiously with patients aged 65 and older. Vigorous fluid replacement in older adults or those with underlying cardiovascular disease may cause pulmonary edema.

Frostbite

Frostbite is trauma because of exposure to very low temperatures that cause freezing of tissue fluids in the cell and intracellular spaces, resulting in vascular damage. The areas of the body most likely to develop frostbite include the ear lobes, cheeks, nose, fingers, and toes. Frostbite can be classified into three categories: frostnip (initial response to cold, reversible), superficial frostbite, and deep frostbite.

Primary Assessment and Interventions

1. Assess airway, breathing, and circulation.
2. Deficits may indicate coexisting hypothermia or underlying condition.
3. Protect frostbitten tissue while performing other interventions.

Subsequent Assessment

Frostnip

1. History of gradual onset.
2. The skin appears pale.
3. Complaints of numbness or tingling.

Superficial Frostbite

1. Damage is limited to the skin and subcutaneous tissue.
2. The skin will appear white and waxy.
3. On palpation, the skin will feel stiff, but the underlying tissue will be pliable and soft and have its normal "bounce."
4. Sensation is absent.

Deep Frostbite

1. The skin will appear white, yellow–white, or mottled blue–white.
2. On palpation, the surface will feel frozen, and the underlying tissue will feel frozen and hard.
3. The affected part is completely insensitive to touch.

General Interventions

1. Frostnip may be treated by placing a warm hand over the chilled area.
2. Leave the frostbitten area alone until definitive rewarming is undertaken. Pad the extremity to prevent damage from trauma.
3. Handle the part gently to avoid further mechanical injury.
4. Remove all constricting clothing that can impair circulation, including watchbands and rings.
5. Rewarming: when definitive rewarming of a frostbitten extremity has started, it must not be stopped. Refreezing of a partially thawed extremity may increase tissue damage and loss.
6. Rewarming:
   a. Rewarm the extremity by controlled and rapid rewarming. Rewarm in a tepid water bath (temperature between 98.6°F to 104°F or 37°C to 40°C) where the part can be fully immersed without touching the side or bottom. If clothing, socks, or gloves are frozen to the extremity, they should be left on and removed after rewarming.
   b. More warm water may be added to the container by removing some cooled water and adding warm water.
   c. Slow rewarming is less effective and may increase tissue damage.
   d. Dry heat is not recommended for rewarming.
   e. The rewarming procedure may take 20 to 30 minutes.
   f. Rewarming is considered complete when the area feels warm to the touch and appears pink or flushed. Changes in black and brown skin may be difficult to assess.
   g. Do not rub or massage a frostbitten extremity. The ice crystals in the tissue will lacerate delicate tissue.
7. Pharmacologic interventions:
   a. Opioids or nonsteroidals for pain control.
   b. Antibiotics if there is an open wound.
   c. Tetanus prophylaxis.

Post-Rewarming Care

1. Protect the thawed part from infection. Large blisters may develop in 1 hour to a few days after rewarming; these blisters should not be broken. If necessary, fluid may be aspirated from the blister with a sterile needle.
2. Place sterile gauze or cotton between affected fingers/toes to absorb moisture.
3. Use sterile technique during dressing changes.
4. Elevate the part to help control swelling. Make sure dressings are applied loosely.
5. Use a foot cradle to prevent contact with bedding if the feet are involved—to prevent further tissue injury.
6. Perform a physical assessment to look for concomitant injury (soft tissue injury, dehydration, alcohol coma, fat embolism because of fracture, immobility).
7. Restore electrolyte balance; dehydration and hypovolemia are common in frostbite patients.
8. Whirlpool bath for the affected extremity—to aid circulation, debride dead tissue, and help prevent infection.
9. Potential escharotomy (incision through the eschar)—to prevent further tissue damage, allow for normal circulation, and permit joint motion.

10. Potential fasciotomy (incision in fascia to release pressure on the muscles, nerves, blood vessels)—to treat compartment syndrome.
11. Encourage hourly active motion of the affected digits to promote maximum restoration of function and to prevent contractures.
12. Advise patient not to use tobacco because of the vasoconstrictive effects of nicotine, which further reduce the already deficient blood supply to injured tissues.
13. Perform serial laboratory testing (urinalysis, electrolytes, and serum enzymes) to monitor for the complications of rhabdomyolysis and subsequent renal failure.

Hypothermia

Hypothermia is a condition in which the core (internal) temperature of the body is less than 95°F (35°C) as a result of exposure to cold or a loss of thermoregulation. In response to a decreased core temperature, the body will attempt to produce or conserve more heat by (1) shivering, which produces heat through muscular activity; (2) peripheral vasoconstriction, to decrease heat loss; and (3) raising the basal metabolic rate. Hypothermia may be classified as mild, moderate, or severe.

POPULATION AWARENESS Older patients are at greater risk for hypothermia because of altered compensatory mechanisms.

Primary Assessment and Interventions

1. Assess airway and breathing.
   a. Spontaneous respirations may be extremely slow and imperceptible.
   b. Assist breathing and oxygenation with supplemental oxygen at 100% or a bag-valve-mask device.
   c. If intubation is necessary, extreme caution should be used because ventricular fibrillation may be precipitated.
2. Assess circulation.
   a. If the body temperature falls below 86°F (30°C), the heart sounds may not be audible even if the heart is still beating. Tissues conduct sound poorly at low temperatures.
   b. Blood pressure (BP) readings may be extremely difficult to hear because cold tissue conducts sound waves poorly.
   c. Pupil reflexes may be blocked by a decrease in cerebral blood flow, so the pupils may appear fixed and dilated.
   d. A patient with severe hypothermia may present like a patient in cardiac arrest with fixed dilated pupils, no pulse or perfusing rhythm, and no BP. If there is any doubt about whether a pulse is present, begin cardiopulmonary resuscitation (CPR).

Subsequent Assessment

1. Progressive deterioration is marked by apathy, poor judgment, ataxia, dysarthria, drowsiness, and, eventually, coma.
2. Speech is slow and may be slurred.
3. Shivering may be suppressed below a temperature of 90°F (32.2°C).
4. Cardiac dysrhythmias—cold disrupts the conduction system of the heart, and a variety of dysrhythmias may be seen. A hypothermic heart is extremely susceptible to conduction delays. Ventricular fibrillation may occur if the temperature falls below 81°F (25°C). Patients with core temperatures below 86°F (30°C) do not respond to drugs or defibrillation.
5. The heartbeat and the BP may become so weak that peripheral pulsations become undetectable. Always check for a central pulse.
6. Urine output may increase in response to peripheral vasoconstriction—cold diuresis.
7. Initial tachypnea is usually followed by slow and shallow respirations, possibly two or three per minute in severe hypothermia.

General Interventions

The goal is to rewarm patients without precipitating cardiac dysrhythmias. Extreme caution should be exercised in moving or transporting patients with hypothermia because of the increased risk of cardiac dysrhythmias.

Supportive Measures

1. Handle the patient carefully and gently—to avoid triggering arrhythmias.
2. Continuously monitor core temperatures with a low-reading rectal thermometer.
3. Continuously monitor ECG and central pulses. Loss of a central pulse indicates a nonperfusing rhythm and the need for immediate CPR and advanced cardiac life support (ACLS) interventions.
4. Monitor the patient's condition through vital signs, CVP, urine output, ABG values, and blood chemistry determinations.
5. Maintain an arterial line for recording BP and to facilitate blood sampling—this allows rapid detection of acid–base disturbances and assessment of adequacy of ventilation and oxygenation.
6. Start IV therapy with warmed normal saline. Lactated Ringer's solution is not recommended because the cold liver may not be able to metabolize the lactate.

Rewarming Techniques

The type of rewarming depends on the degree of hypothermia. Rewarming should be continued until the core temperature reaches 93.2°F (34°C). Death in hypothermia is defined as the failure to revive after rewarming.

1. Passive external rewarming (mild hypothermia).
   a. Remove all the wet or cold clothing and replace with warm clothing.
   b. Provide insulation by wrapping the patient in several warmed blankets.
   c. Provide warmed fluids to drink.
   d. Disadvantage: slow process.
2. Active external rewarming (moderate to severe hypothermia or hemodynamic instability).
   a. Provide external heat for the patient—external warming devices, warmed blankets, or warm hot water bottles placed in the armpits, neck, or groin. (Do not apply hot water bottles directly to the skin.)
   b. Warm water immersion.
   c. Disadvantages:
      i. Causes peripheral vasodilation, returning cool blood to the core, causing an initial lowering of the core temperature.
      ii. Induces acidosis because of the "washing out" of lactic acid from the peripheral tissues.
      iii. Leads to an increase in metabolic demands before the heart is warmed to meet these needs.

iv. A combination of active external rewarming and active core rewarming can be used to minimize rewarming shock.

3. Active core rewarming (severe hypothermia less than 82.4°F [less than 28°C]).
   a. Inhalation of warmed, humidified oxygen by mask or ventilator.
   b. Warmed IV fluids.
   c. Peritoneal dialysis with warmed standard dialysis solution.
   d. Mediastinal irrigation through open thoracotomy has been used successfully but carries serious complications.
   e. Cardiopulmonary bypass.
   f. Disadvantage: invasiveness of the procedures.

TOXICOLOGIC EMERGENCIES

Toxicology is the study of the harmful effect of various substances on the body. Toxins are substances that are harmful to the body, no matter how much or in what manner they enter the body. Drugs become toxic when taken in excessive quantities or manners that are not therapeutic. Alcohol is considered a drug. The treatment goals of toxicologic emergencies are threefold: first, to provide support; second, to prevent or minimize absorption; and third, to administer an antidote.

Ingested Poisons

Ingested poisons can produce immediate or delayed effects. Immediate injury is caused when the poison is caustic to the body tissues (i.e., a strong acid or a strong alkali). Other ingested poisons must be absorbed into the bloodstream before they become harmful. Ingested poisoning may be accidental or intentional.

Primary Assessment and Interventions

1. Maintain an open airway—some ingested substances may cause soft tissue swelling of the airway.
2. Attain control of the airway, ventilation, and oxygenation; in the absence of cerebral or renal damage, the patient's prognosis depends largely on successful management and support of vital functions.

Subsequent Assessment

1. Identify the poison.
   a. Try to determine the product taken: where, when, why, how much, who witnessed the event, and the time since ingestion. Histories obtained from the patient are often inaccurate and should be confirmed if possible.
   b. Always contact the local poison control center for assistance in identifying the toxin if unknown, treatment recommendations, and antidote information. In the United States, local poison control centers can all be reached by calling (800) 222-1222.
2. Continue the focused assessment, observing any significant deviations from normal. Different poisons will affect the body in different ways.
3. Obtain blood and urine tests for toxicology screening. Gastric contents may also be sent for toxicology screening in serious ingestions.
4. Monitor neurologic status, including mentation; monitor the course of vital signs and neurologic status over time.
5. Monitor for fluid and electrolyte imbalance.

General Interventions

Supportive Care

1. Assess and protect the patient's airway, as needed.
2. Administer oxygen and assist ventilations, as needed.
3. Monitor and treat shock.
4. Insert two large-bore intravenous (IV) lines.
5. Give supportive care to maintain vital organ systems.
6. Insert an indwelling urinary catheter to monitor renal function.
7. Support the patient having seizures; many poisons excite the central nervous system (CNS) or the patient may convulse from oxygen deprivation.
8. Monitor and treat for complications: hypotension, coma, cardiac dysrhythmias, and seizures.
9. Psychiatric evaluations should be done after the patient is stabilized.

Minimizing Absorption

1. The primary method for preventing or minimizing absorption is to administer activated charcoal. Newer super activated charcoals can reduce absorption of a toxic substance by as much as 50%. Administering activated charcoal alone is recommended. Insertion of a large-bore orogastric tube and gastric lavage are no longer recommended. The routine use of a cathartic in combination with activated charcoal is also no longer recommended.
   a. Administration of premixed oral-activated charcoal adsorbs the poison on the surface of its particles and allows it to pass with the stool. Multiple doses may be administered.
   b. A routine nasogastric (NG) tube may be inserted to facilitate emptying of stomach contents (without lavage) within 30 minutes of ingestion or to instill charcoal if the patient is unable to drink the mixture.
   c. Contact your local poison control center for recommendations on giving charcoal. Do not give charcoal if the patient may not be able to maintain airway unless you have an artificial airway established.
2. Gastric lavage is contraindicated due to poor outcomes and complications.
3. Procedures to enhance the removal of the ingested substance if the patient is deteriorating.
   a. Forced diuresis with urine pH alteration—to enhance renal clearance.
   b. Hemoperfusion (process of passing blood through an extracorporeal circuit and a cartridge containing an adsorbent, such as charcoal, after which the detoxified blood is returned to patient).
   c. Hemodialysis—used in selected patients to purify blood and accelerate the elimination of circulating toxins.
   d. Repeated doses of charcoal—for binding nonabsorbed drugs/toxins.
4. Do not induce emesis after ingestion of caustic substances (hydrocarbons, iodides, silver nitrates, strychnine, or petroleum distillates), or in a patient having seizures or in a pregnant patient.

Providing an Antidote

1. An antidote is a chemical or physiologic antagonist that neutralizes the poison.
2. Administer the specific antidote as early as possible to reverse or diminish effects of the toxin.
3. Repeated antidote doses may be necessary.
4. Follow the recommendations of your poison control center.

Carbon Monoxide Poisoning

Carbon monoxide poisoning is an example of an inhaled poison and results from the inhalation of the byproducts of incomplete hydrocarbon combustion. It may occur as an industrial or household accident or as an attempted suicide. Carbon monoxide exerts its toxic effect by binding to circulating hemoglobin, reducing the oxygen-carrying capacity of the blood. The affinity between carbon monoxide and hemoglobin is 200 to 250 times more than that between oxygen and hemoglobin. (Carbon monoxide combines with hemoglobin to form carboxyhemoglobin.) As a result, tissue anoxia occurs.

Primary Assessment

1. Assess airway and breathing. Assist with ventilations, as needed.
   a. Respiratory depression may be present.
   b. If carbon monoxide poisoning is due to smoke inhalation, stridor (indicative of laryngeal edema because of thermal injury) may be present. Check for soot on the back of the hard palate or pharynx if smoke inhalation is suspected.

Primary Interventions

1. Provide 100% oxygen via non-rebreather mask that fits snugly to the patient's face. (The elimination half-life of carboxyhemoglobin in serum for a person breathing room air is 5 hours and 20 minutes. If the patient breathes 100% oxygen, the half-life is reduced to 80 minutes; 100% oxygen in a hyperbaric chamber will reduce the half-life to 23 minutes [treatment of choice].)
2. Intubate, if necessary, to protect the airway.

Subsequent Assessment

1. A thorough history is important: determine the type and length of exposure as well as the possibility of other fumes being inhaled. An underlying anemia, cardiac disease, or pulmonary disease may place a person at higher risk.
2. Determine the level of consciousness (LOC)—the patient may appear intoxicated from cerebral hypoxia; confusion may rapidly progress to coma.
3. Assess complaints of headache, muscular weakness, palpitation, and dizziness.
4. Inspect the skin: it may appear pink, cherry red, or cyanotic and pale—skin color is not a reliable sign.
5. Monitor vital signs: increased respiratory and pulse rates are generally present. Be alert for altered breathing patterns and respiratory failure.
6. Listen for rales or wheezes in the lungs (with smoke inhalation, indicating acute respiratory distress syndrome).
7. Obtain arterial or venous blood samples for carboxyhemoglobin levels.
   a. Normal levels for a patient who does not smoke are less than 3%. For a patient who smokes one to two packs per day, 4% to 5%, and for those who smoke two or more packs per day, 8% to 10%.
   b. Toxic concentrations are considered to be greater than 20%.

General Interventions

1. History of exposure to carbon monoxide justifies immediate treatment.
2. The goals are to reverse cerebral and myocardial hypoxia and to hasten carbon monoxide elimination.
3. Give 100% oxygen at atmospheric or hyperbaric pressures to reverse hypoxia and accelerate the elimination of carbon monoxide. Patients should receive hyperbaric oxygen if available, especially for CNS or cardiovascular system dysfunction.
4. Use continuous electrocardiogram (ECG) monitoring, treat dysrhythmias, and correct acid–base and electrolyte abnormalities.
5. Observe the patient constantly—psychoses, spastic paralysis, vision disturbances, and deterioration of personality may persist after resuscitation and could be symptoms of permanent CNS damage.

Insect Stings

Insect stings or bites are injected poisons that can produce either local or systemic reactions. Local reactions are characterized by pain, erythema, and edema at the site of injury. Systemic reactions usually begin within minutes and can produce mild to severe and life-threatening reactions.

Primary Assessment and Interventions

1. Assess airway, breathing, and circulation.
2. Anaphylactic reactions may result in unconsciousness, laryngeal edema, and cardiovascular collapse.
3. Epinephrine is the drug of choice—the dosage and route depend on the severity of the reaction.
4. Administer a bronchodilator to help relieve the bronchospasm.
5. Initiate an IV line with an isotonic IV solution.
6. Prepare for cardiopulmonary resuscitation (CPR).

Subsequent Assessment

1. Obtain history of insect sting, previous exposure, and allergies.
2. Inspect the skin for local reaction—erythema, edema, and pain at site of injury—as well as generalized pruritus, urticaria, and angioedema.
3. Continue to monitor blood pressure (BP) and respiratory status for dyspnea, wheezing, and stridor.

General Interventions

1. Apply ice packs to affected area to relieve pain.
2. Elevate extremity if there is a large edematous local reaction.
3. Administer oral antihistamine.
4. Clean the wound thoroughly with soap and water or an antiseptic solution.
5. Administer tetanus prophylaxis if not up to date.
6. Provide patient education.
   a. If an epinephrine auto-injector is prescribed, the patient should always have it with them and be instructed on its use.
   b. Wear a medical alert device indicating hypersensitivity.
   c. Instructions when sting occurs:
      i. Take epinephrine immediately if stung.
      ii. Remove the stinger with one quick scrape of a fingernail.
      iii. Do not squeeze the venom sac because this may cause additional venom to be injected.
      iv. Report to the nearest health care facility for observation.

d. Avoid exposure.
   i. Avoid locales with stinging insects (camp and picnic sites).
   ii. Stay away from insect-feeding areas—flower beds, ripe fruit orchards, garbage, and fields of clover.
   iii. Avoid going barefoot outdoors—yellow jackets may nest on the ground.
   iv. Avoid perfumes, scented soaps, and bright colors, which attract bees.
   v. Keep car windows closed.
   vi. Spray garbage cans with rapid-acting insecticide and keep areas meticulously clean.

Snakebites

The majority of snakes in the United States are not poisonous. Some poisonous varieties include pit vipers (rattlesnakes and copperheads) and coral snakes. Bites from these snakes may result in envenomation, an injected poisoning. Other parts of the world have many snakes capable of delivering lethal bites. Snakebites can cause neurotoxic muscle paralysis, coagulopathy, and hemolysis. Therefore, knowledge of snakes indigenous to your area is important for swift and appropriate treatment.

Primary Assessment and Interventions

1. Assess airway, breathing, and circulation.
2. Severe envenomation may lead to neurotoxicity with respiratory paralysis, shock, coma, and death.
3. Be prepared to resuscitate and provide advanced life support.

Subsequent Assessment

1. Get a description of the snake, the time of the snakebite, and the location of the bite. Bites to the head and trunk may progress more rapidly and be more severe.
   a. Pit vipers have triangular heads, vertical pupils, indentations between the eyes and nostrils, and long fangs.
   b. Coral snakes are small and brightly colored, with short fangs and teeth behind them, and a series of bands of yellow, red, yellow, and black (in that order).
   c. Venom detection kits are available in some areas of the world, such as Australia, where venomous snakes are not uncommon. Specific antivenom may be available.
2. Assess for local reactions—burning, pain, swelling, and numbness at the site. Local reactions to coral snakebites may be delayed by several hours and may be very mild.
3. A few hours after the bite, hemorrhagic blisters may occur at the site, and the entire extremity may become edematous.
4. Watch for signs of systemic reactions, including nausea, sweating, weakness, light-headedness, initial euphoria followed by drowsiness, difficulty in swallowing, paralysis of various muscle groups, signs of shock, seizures, and coma.
5. Monitor vital signs closely because tachycardia or bradycardia may develop.

CLINICAL JUDGMENT Patients will, on occasion, bring the snake that bit them into the emergency department (ED) for identification. Even if dead, a snake can reflexively bite for several hours. Caution should be used to avoid becoming a second patient.

General Interventions

1. Keep the patient calm and at rest in a recumbent position with the affected extremity immobilized. Remove jewelry or other constricting items, as the area may become edematous.
2. Administer oxygen.
3. Start an IV line with normal saline or lactated Ringer's solution.
4. Administer antivenin and be alert to allergic reactions.
5. Administer vasopressors for the treatment of shock.
6. Monitor for bleeding and administer blood products for coagulopathies.

Drug Intoxication

Substance misuse includes the use of specific substances that are intended to alter mood or behavior.

Drug misuse is the use of drugs for purposes other than legitimate medical reasons. There is a growing tendency among patients with substance use disorder to take a variety of drugs simultaneously (polypharmacy misuse), including alcohol, sedatives, hypnotics, and marijuana, which may have addictive effects. The clinical manifestations may vary with the drug used (see Table 31-2), but the underlying principles of management are essentially the same.

Overdose refers to the toxic effects that occur when a drug is taken in a larger-than-normal dose.

Primary Assessment and Interventions

1. Assess airway, breathing, and circulation.
2. Attain control of the airway, ventilation, and oxygenation.
3. Intubate and provide assisted ventilation in patients with severe respiratory depression or in patients lacking gag or cough reflexes. If possible, intubation should be held off until a trial dose of naloxone is given.
4. Begin CPR in the absence of pulse.

Subsequent Assessment

1. Do a thorough physical examination to rule out insulin shock, meningitis, head injury, stroke, or trauma.
2. If the patient is unconscious, consider all possible causes of loss of consciousness.
3. Monitor LOC continuously.
4. Monitor vital signs frequently—some drugs will cause depressed vital signs; others will elevate the vital signs.
5. Monitor the pupils: extreme miosis (pinpoint pupils) may indicate opioid overdose.
6. Look for needle marks and external evidence of trauma.
7. Perform a rapid neurologic survey: level of responsiveness, pupil size and reactivity, reflexes, and focal neurologic findings; these can all give clues for identifying the drug taken.
8. Keep in mind that many patients with substance use disorder take multiple drugs simultaneously.
9. Practice the use of standard precautions—there is an increased incidence of human immunodeficiency virus (HIV), tuberculosis, and infectious hepatitis among patients with substance use disorder.
10. Examine the patient's breath for characteristic odor of alcohol or acetone.
11. Obtain a history of drug experiences (from the person accompanying the patient or from the patient, if possible).

Table 31-2 Specific Drug Overdose Presentations and Interventions

TYPE OF DRUG	PRESENTATION	INTERVENTIONS
CNS Stimulants • Amphetamines • Designer drugs (MDMA, ecstasy, ice, Eve, bath salts) • Cocaine (can be smoked in free-base or crack form, snorted, or injected)	Palpitations, feeling of impending doom, tachycardia, hypertension, dysrhythmia, myocardial ischemia or infarction, euphoria, agitation, combativeness, confusion, hallucinations, paranoia, aggressive or violent behavior, suicide attempts, hyperpyrexia, and seizures. When the drug wears off, depression, exhaustion, irritability, and sleeplessness.	• Secure airway, breathing, and circulation. • Monitor ECG and provide oxygen for ischemia. • Sedate, as necessary. • Administer antiarrhythmics for ventricular dysrhythmia. • Administer diazepam for seizures. • Closely monitor hemodynamic status and provide IV fluids, as indicated.
Hallucinogens • Lysergic acid diethylamide (LSD) • Phencyclidine HCl (PCP) • Mescaline • Psilocybin mushrooms • Jimson weed seeds • Salvia	Marked anxiety bordering on panic, confusion, incoherence, hyperactivity, hallucinations, hazardous behavior, convulsions, coma, circulatory collapse, and death. Flashbacks may occur months to years after initial drug use.	• Reduce sensory stimuli, encourage patient to keep eyes open, and stay with patient. • Monitor for hypertensive crisis and evidence of trauma. • Sedate if hyperactivity cannot be controlled and place patient in a protected environment.
Opioids • Heroin (may be cut with other ingredients in 20:1–200:1 ratios) • Morphine and its derivatives • Codeine and its derivatives • Fentanyl	Pinpoint pupils, cold and clammy skin, cyanosis, coma, hypoxia and respiratory failure leading to death.	• Administer naloxone 0.4–2 mg via IV line or by endotracheal tube (effective in 1–2 min). • Maintain an open airway but defer intubation until naloxone is given, if possible. • Monitor for reappearance of symptoms and re-administer naloxone. • Protect the patient from harm (may be combative on awakening).
Sedatives • Barbiturates, such as amobarbital and secobarbital • Benzodiazepines, such as diazepam and flurazepam • Other sedative/hypnotics, such as chloral hydrate and glutethimide	Incoordination, ataxia, impaired thinking and speech, lethargy to coma, early miosis; later, fixed and dilated pupils, hypoventilation, hypotension, hypothermia, and decreased reflexes.	• Administer flumazenil to reverse or diminish effects of benzodiazepines. • Administer activated charcoal. • Protect the airway. • For hypotension, infuse with lactated Ringer's solution and give vasopressors.
Alcohol Intoxication generally occurs with blood levels >100 mg/dL. Levels more than 400 mg/dL are due to rapid consumption of alcohol and represent a medical emergency.	Slurred speech, incoordination, ataxia, belligerent behavior progressing to stupor and coma, odor of alcohol on breath and clothing, and respiratory depression.	• Protect the airway. • Closely monitor for CNS and respiratory depression. • Draw blood for ethanol concentration, electrolytes, glucose, and drug screen, using nonalcohol skin cleanser. • Assess for head injury and other trauma, as well as organic disease. • Administer IV fluids, magnesium sulfate (to reduce risk of seizures), thiamine (to prevent Wernicke–Korsakoff syndrome), and glucose (to treat hypoglycemia).

CNS, central nervous system; ECG, electrocardiogram; IV, intravenous; MDMA, methylenedioxymethamphetamine.

General Interventions

1. Goals:
   a. Support the respiratory and cardiovascular functions.
   b. Give definitive treatment for drug overdose, such as naloxone.
   c. Prevent further absorption, enhance drug elimination, and reduce its toxicity.
2. Measure arterial blood gas (ABG) values for hypoxia because of hypoventilation or for acid–base derangements.
3. Continuously monitor ECG.

4. Draw blood samples and test for glucose, electrolytes, blood urea nitrogen (BUN), creatinine, and appropriate toxicology screen.
5. Initiate IV fluids.
6. Administer oxygen.
7. Pharmacologic interventions:
   a. Give specific drug antagonist if drug is known.
   b. Naloxone for CNS depression because of opioids.
   c. Dextrose 50% IV to rule out hypoglycemic coma.
8. If the drug was taken by mouth, the primary method for preventing or minimizing absorption is to administer activated charcoal. Multiple doses may be administered. A routine NG tube may be inserted to facilitate emptying of stomach contents (without lavage) within 30 minutes of ingestion, or charcoal may be instilled if the patient is unable to drink.
9. In patients who are unconscious or semiconscious and who lack or may lack gag or cough reflexes, use an NG tube only after intubation with a cuffed endotracheal tube to prevent aspiration of charcoal stomach contents.
10. Take rectal temperature—extremes of thermoregulation (hyperthermia/hypothermia) must be recognized and treated.
11. Treat seizures with diazepam.
12. Assist with hemodialysis/peritoneal dialysis for potentially lethal poisoning.
13. Obtain urine sample for a toxicology screen—drugs or their metabolites are excreted in the urine.
14. Do not leave the patient alone; there is a potential for the patient to harm themselves or ED staff.
15. Anticipate complications—sudden death from cerebral hypoxia, dysrhythmias, seizures, respiratory arrest, and myocardial infarction (MI).
16. Always suspect mixtures of medications and alcohol.

DRUG ALERT Antidotes generally have a shorter half-life than the drugs they are used to treat. Repeated dosing is often necessary.

CLINICAL JUDGMENT Many drugs will not or cannot be detected in a standard toxicology screen. A negative drug screen does not mean an overdose is not the cause of the emergency.

Alcohol Withdrawal Delirium

Alcohol withdrawal delirium (*delirium tremens* or *alcoholic hallucinosis*) is an acute toxic state that follows a prolonged bout of steady drinking or sudden withdrawal from prolonged intake of alcohol. It may be precipitated by acute injury or infection. Symptoms can begin as early as 4 hours after a reduction of alcohol intake and usually peak at 24 to 48 hours, but may last up to 2 weeks. Alcohol withdrawal delirium is a serious complication of inadequate withdrawal management and is life-threatening.

Primary Assessment and Interventions

1. Patient may present alert, unless experiencing a seizure.
2. Ensure adequacy of airway, breathing, and circulation.

Subsequent Assessment

1. Assess for major symptoms—may occur independently or in combination.
   a. Nausea.
   b. Tremors.
   c. Paroxysmal sweating.
   d. Anxiety.
   e. Agitation.
   f. Headache.
   g. Mental status.
   h. Hallucinations (may be tactile, visual, or auditory).
2. Utilizing a standard Clinical Institute Withdrawal Assessment for Alcohol scale may assist in identifying those at risk for withdrawal problems and guide treatment. See Box 31-1.
   a. Each category is given a score and the total is added. The cumulative score provides a basis for treatment. Generally, a score of 8 to 10 or higher is the threshold for treatment to alleviate symptoms and prevent seizures.
   b. Reassess frequently during the first 48 hours, and discontinue treatment and assessments when three subsequent determinations fall below the threshold.
3. Obtain drinking history, including the severity of past withdrawal episodes and any recent drug intake. Be aware that individuals may underestimate their drinking habits.
4. Perform a thorough examination for signs of autonomic hyperreactivity—tachycardia, diaphoresis, elevated temperature, and dilated but reactive pupils—as well as any coexisting illnesses or injuries (head injury, pneumonia, metabolic disturbances).
5. Observe behavior for talkativeness, restlessness, agitation, or preoccupation.

General Interventions

1. Protect the patient from injury. Not all patients hallucinate; however, if they do, the hallucinations may be visual, tactile, or auditory and are frequently frightening. Seizures may also occur.
2. Using a nonalcoholic skin preparation, draw blood for measurement of ethanol concentration, toxicology screen for illicit drugs, and other tests, as directed.
3. Pharmacologic interventions:
   a. Diazepam or chlordiazepoxide for sedation. Sedate the patient with sufficient dosage of medication to induce adequate relaxation, reduce agitation, prevent exhaustion, and promote sleep without compromising the airway.
   b. Diazepam, lorazepam, or phenytoin for seizure control.
4. Monitor vital signs every 30 minutes.
5. Maintain close observation.
6. Maintain electrolyte balance and hydration through oral or IV route—fluid losses may be extreme because of profuse perspiration, vomiting, and agitation.
7. Assess the respiratory, hepatic, and cardiovascular status of the patient—pneumonia, liver disease, and cardiac failure are potential complications.
8. Observe for hypoglycemia and treat appropriately. Hypoglycemia may accompany alcoholic withdrawal because alcohol depletes liver glycogen stores and impairs gluconeogenesis; many patients also suffer from malnutrition. Thiamine, or vitamin B_1, is commonly administered because chronic alcohol consumption reduces the availability of this essential nutrient to the cells of the brain.

BOX 31-1 Clinical Institute of Withdrawal From Alcohol Scale Revised (CIWA-Ar)

NAUSEA AND VOMITING

Ask: "Do you feel sick to your stomach? Have you vomited?"

0 = No nausea, no vomiting
1 = Mild nausea with no retching or vomiting
4 = Intermittent nausea with dry heaves
7 = Constant nausea, frequent dry heaves, and/or vomiting

TREMOR

Arms extended and fingers spread apart.

0 = No tremor
1 = Not visible, but can be felt fingertip to fingertip
4 = Moderate with patients arm extended
7 = Severe, even with arms not extended

SWEATING

0 = No sweat visible
1 = Barely perceptible sweating, palms moist
4 = Beads of sweat obvious on the forehead
7 = Drenching sweat over the face and chest

ANXIETY

Ask, "Do you feel nervous?"

0 = No anxiety, at ease
1 = Mildly anxious
4 = Moderately anxious or guarded, so anxiety is inferred
7 = Equivalent to acute panic states, as seen in severe delirium or acute schizophrenic reaction

AGITATION

0 = Normal activity
1 = Somewhat more than normal activity (may move legs up and down, shift position occasionally)
4 = Moderately fidgety and restless, shifting position frequently
7 = Paces back and forth or constantly thrashes about

TACTILE DISTURBANCES

Ask, "Have you any itching, pins-and-needles sensation, burning or numbness, or do you feel bugs crawling on or under your skin?"

0 = None
1 = Very mild
2 = Mild
3 = Moderate
4 = Moderately severe hallucinations
5 = Severe hallucinations
6 = Extremely severe hallucinations
7 = Continuous hallucinations

AUDITORY DISTURBANCES

Ask, "Are you more aware of the sounds around you? Are they harsh? Do they frighten you? Are you hearing anything disturbing? Are you hearing things you know are not there?"

0 = Not present hallucinations
1 = Very mild
2 = Mild
3 = Moderate
4 = Moderately severe
5 = Severe hallucinations
6 = Extremely severe hallucinations
7 = Continuous hallucinations

VISUAL DISTURBANCES

Ask, "Does the light appear to be too bright? Is its color different? Does it hurt your eyes? Are you seeing anything disturbing to you? Are you seeing things you know are not there?"

0 = Not present
1 = Very mild
2 = Mild
3 = Moderate
4 = Moderately severe
5 = Severe hallucinations
6 = Extremely severe hallucinations
7 = Continuous hallucinations

HEADACHE, FULLNESS IN HEAD

Ask, "Does your head feel different? Does it feel like there is a band around your head?" Do not rate dizziness or light-headedness. Otherwise, rate severity.

0 = Not present
1 = Very mild
2 = Mild
3 = Moderate
4 = Moderately severe
5 = Severe
6 = Very severe
7 = Extremely severe

ORIENTATION AND CLOUDING OF SENSORIUM

Ask, "What day is this? Where are you? Who am I?"

0 = Oriented and can do serial additions
1 = Cannot do serial additions or is uncertain about date
2 = Disoriented for date by no more than 2 calendar days
3 = Disoriented for date by more than 2 calendar days
4 = Disoriented for place and/or person

Assessment is made in each category and cumulative score is used to determine treatment (institutional protocols vary).

The CIWA-Ar is not copyrighted and may be reproduced freely. This assessment for monitoring withdrawal symptoms requires approximately 5 minutes to administer. The maximum score is 67 (see instrument). Patients scoring less than 10 do not usually need additional medication for withdrawal. Reprinted from Sullivan, J. T., Sykora, K., Schneiderman, J., Naranjo, C. A., & Sellers, E. M. (1989). Assessment of alcohol withdrawal: The revised Clinical Institute Withdrawal Assessment for Alcohol scale (CIWA-Ar). British Journal of Addiction, 84(11), 1373–1357. https://doi.org/10.1111/j.1360-0443.1989.tb00737.x

BEHAVIORAL EMERGENCIES

A *behavioral emergency* is an urgent, serious disturbance of behavior, affect, or thought that makes the patient unable to cope with their life situation and interpersonal relationships. A patient presenting with a psychiatric emergency may exhibit overactivity or violence, depression, or suicidal tendencies.

Patients Who Are Violent

Violent and aggressive behavior is usually episodic and is a means of expressing feelings of anger, fear, or hopelessness about a situation.

Assessment

1. Assess for overactivity, aggression, or anger out of proportion to the circumstances.
2. Determine risk factors for violence, including:
   a. Intoxicated with drugs/alcohol.
   b. Going through drug or alcohol withdrawal.
   c. Acute paranoid schizophrenic states, acute organic brain syndrome, acute psychosis, paranoia, or borderline personality.
3. Obtain psychiatric assessment.

General Interventions

1. The goals are to bring violence under control and protect both the patient and staff from harm.
2. Establish control.
   a. Keep room door open, and be in clear view of the staff. Always leave a clear exit pathway. Never allow the patient to be between you and safety.
   b. Help the patient bring violence under control.
      i. Give patient space; do not make sudden moves.
      ii. Avoid touching patients who are agitated or standing close.
      iii. Ask if the patient has a weapon; request that it be placed in a neutral area.
      iv. If the patient will not surrender their weapon, leave the room and allow security personnel/police to handle the situation.
   c. Try not to leave the patient alone unless your safety is in jeopardy; this may be interpreted as rejection, or the patient may attempt self-harm.
   d. Adopt a calm nonconfrontational approach and remain in control of the situation. External calm and structure may help the patient gain control.
   e. Offer the patient choices and options about treatments or the timing of events whenever possible.
3. Provide emotional support.
   a. Talk and listen to the patient.
   b. Crisis intervention is best done with an attitude of interest in the patient's well-being and with an attempt to "tune in" to the patient while remaining firm.
   c. Acknowledge the patient's state of agitation (e.g., "I want to work with you to relieve your distress").
   d. Give the patient the opportunity to ventilate anger verbally; avoid challenging the delusional state.
   e. Try to hear what the patient is saying.
   f. Convey the expectation of appropriate behavior and make the patient aware that help is available for them to gain control.
   g. Administer prescribed medications to reduce anxiety and hyperactivity if verbal management techniques fail to attenuate the patient's tension.
4. Secure assistance.
   a. Allow security personnel/police to intervene if patient does not become calm.
   b. Use of a dedicated safe room is encouraged. The room should be free of cords, cables, or any object capable of being used as a weapon and easily seen by staff. Shatterproof windows and/or cameras are encouraged. Use restraints only when absolutely necessary and per the facility's policy.
   c. Have a specific plan and enough well-trained personnel available when applying restraints; if patient is intoxicated, restrain them in a left lateral position and monitor closely for aspiration.
   d. Talk reassuringly while applying restraints; use empathic and supportive verbal interactions.
   e. Monitor patient continuously after restraints are applied; check circulation of restrained extremities.

Depression

Depression may present as the primary condition at the health care facility or may be masked by the presentation of anxiety and somatic complaints.

Assessment

1. Observe for sadness, apathy, feelings of worthlessness, self-blame, suicidal thoughts, desire to escape, worsening of mood in the morning, anorexia, weight loss, sleeplessness, lessening interest in sex, reduction of activity, or ceaseless activity.
2. The person who is agitated or depressed may exhibit motor restlessness and severe anxiety.

General Interventions

1. Listen to the patient in a calm, unhurried manner.
2. The patient will benefit from ventilation of feelings.
3. Give the patient an opportunity to talk about problems.
4. Anticipate that the patient may be suicidal.
5. Attempt to find out if the patient has thought about or attempted suicide and the lethality of the suicide plan.
   a. "Have you ever thought about taking your own life?" "Do you have a plan?"
   b. The patient is generally relieved because of the opportunity to discuss feelings.
6. Find out if there is an illness, perceived or real.
7. Assess whether there has been sudden worsening of depression.
8. Notify relatives about a patient who is seriously depressed. Do not leave the patient alone because suicide is usually an act committed in solitude.
9. Give antidepressant and antianxiety agents, as prescribed.
10. Point out to the patient that depression is treatable.
11. Be aware of crisis and supportive services in the community: telephone counseling and referral, suicide prevention centers, group therapy, marital and family counseling, drug/alcohol counseling, adolescent counseling, or befriending programs.
12. Refer for psychiatric consultation or to psychiatric unit.

Suicide Ideation

According to the Centers for Disease Control and Prevention (CDC), suicide is the 11th leading cause of death in the United

States and the third most common cause of death in adolescents aged 15 to 19 years.

Assessment

1. Assess for risk factors:
   a. Associated psychiatric illness (affective disorders and substance use disorders in adults; conduct disorders and depression in young people).
   b. Personality traits, such as aggression, impulsivity, depression, hopelessness, borderline personality disorder, or antisocial personality.
   c. Persons who have experienced early loss, decreased social support, chronic illness, or recent divorce.
   d. Genetic and familial factors: family history of suicide, certain psychiatric disorders or alcoholism, alcohol and substance misuse.
2. Determine whether patient has communicated suicidal intent, such as preoccupation with death or talking about someone else's suicide.
3. Determine whether patient has ever attempted suicide—the risk is much greater in these people.
4. Determine whether there is a specific plan for suicide and a means to carry out the plan.

General Interventions

1. Treat the consequences of the suicide attempt, if one has been made.
2. After the patient has been stabilized, or if there was no active attempt made, use crisis intervention (a form of brief psychotherapy) to determine suicide potential, discover areas of depression and conflict, find out about the patient's support system, and determine whether hospitalization, psychiatric referral, and so forth are warranted.
3. Prevent further self-injury—a patient who has made a suicide gesture may do so again.
4. Arrange follow-up care, or admit to hospital or psychiatric unit, depending on assessment of suicide potential.

SEXUAL ASSAULT

Rape

Rape is defined as any form of penetration of another person without their consent. This definition includes both males and females, as well as the use of objects, not just body parts. Lack of consent is the key. *Lack of consent* can imply either force or the incapacity or inability to consent. Children, individuals with intellectual disabilities, and persons who are intoxicated or drugged are all considered incapable of consenting to sexual acts. While management of the sexual assault is important, immediate physical health should be ensured first. A complete primary and focused assessment should take place, being alert for signs of internal hemorrhage, shock, or respiratory distress. If the patient has suffered trauma in the form of physical assault (e.g., choking, or head or abdominal trauma), the trauma should be managed in the order of established priorities.

Assessment

Initiating a Supportive Relationship

1. The manner in which the patient is received and treated in the emergency department (ED) is important for their future psychological well-being. Many areas have sexual assault nurse examiners. These nurses have specialized education and clinical experience to prepare them for forensic examinations of sexual assault patients. Some areas of the country have a designated center for the treatment of sexual assault patients. If this is true in your area, the patient should have any life-threatening injuries stabilized in the ED and then be transferred to the dedicated facility for examination.
   a. Call a rape crisis intervention counselor (if available), who will meet the patient/family in the ED.
   b. Do not leave patient alone. Accept the emotional reactions of the patient (hysteria, stoicism, overwhelmed feeling, etc.).
2. Emotional trauma may be present for weeks, months, or years. Patients may experience complex posttraumatic stress disorder or rape trauma syndrome. Patients may go through phases of psychological reactions:
   a. Acute phase (disorganization)—shock, disbelief, fear, anxiety, guilt, humiliation, and suppression of feelings—may be for a few days to several weeks.
   b. Outward adjustment phase—patient resumes what appears to be a normal life but internally faces continued turmoil, manifested as fear, flashbacks, sleep disturbances, hyper alertness, and psychosomatic reactions.
   c. Resolution phase—the rape is no longer the central focus of the patient's life and they are able to move on from the incident.

Interviewing the Patient

1. Consent should be obtained for the examination, the collecting of cultures/evidence, and for release of information to law enforcement agencies.
2. Record history of event in the patient's own words.
3. Ask if the patient has bathed, douched, gargled or brushed teeth, changed clothes, or urinated or defecated since attack and record their response—may alter interpretation of subsequent findings.
4. Record time of admission, time of examination, date and time of sexual assault, and the general appearance of the patient.
   a. Document any evidence of trauma—discoloration, bruises, lacerations, secretions, and torn and bloody clothing.
   b. Record emotional state.

Interventions

Preparing for Physical Examination

1. Most EDs have commercially prepared rape evidence collection kits as well as written protocols for the treatment of injuries, legal documentation, prevention of sexually transmitted infection (STI), human immunodeficiency virus (HIV) testing and postexposure prophylaxis, and pregnancy prevention. Remember that the evidence collection kit is meant to preserve forensic evidence.
2. Assist the patient to undress over a sheet/large piece of paper to obtain debris.
3. Place each item of clothing in a separate paper bag (plastic bags promote moisture retention which can destroy DNA evidence).
4. Label bags appropriately; give to appropriate law enforcement authority.
5. Advise the patient of the nature and necessity of each procedure; give the rationale for each question asked.

Physical Examination

1. Examine the patient (from head to toe) for injuries, especially to the head, neck, breasts, thighs, back, and buttocks.
2. Assess for external evidence of trauma (bruises, contusions, lacerations, stab wounds).
3. Assess for dried semen stains (appearing as crusted, flaking areas) on the patient's body.
4. Inspect fingers for broken nails and tissue and foreign materials under nails. Obtain scrapings or clippings of fingernails.
   a. Conduct an oral examination looking for any contusions and petechiae, and obtain swabs for DNA testing.
5. Document evidence of trauma with body diagrams and photographs if available.

Pelvic and Rectal Examinations

1. Examine the perineum and thighs with an ultraviolet light (Wood lamp) if available. Areas that are found to fluoresce may indicate semen stains. Urine and other stains may also fluoresce.
2. Note color and consistency of any discharge present.
3. Examine external vaginal area and rectum for any bleeding, contusion, ecchymosis, erythema, lacerations, scars, or any other injuries or abnormalities.
4. Use water-moistened vaginal speculum for examination; do not use lubricant (contains chemicals that may interfere with later forensic testing of specimens and acid phosphatase determinations).

Obtaining Laboratory Specimens

1. Obtain separate swabs from the oral, labial, vaginal, and anal areas.
2. Obtain swabs of body orifices for gonorrhea and chlamydia testing, or send a urine sample to test for gonorrhea, chlamydia, and trichomonas if the facility has that testing capability.
3. Comb and trim areas of pubic hair suspected of containing semen; obtain several pubic hairs with follicles; place in separate containers and identify these as patient's pubic hairs.
4. Obtain blood sample for syphilis and hepatitis B and C, and offer the patient HIV testing.
5. Collect foreign material or debris (leaves, grass, dirt, loose hair, string) and place in appropriate container.
6. Conduct a pregnancy test on all females of child-bearing capability.
7. Label all specimens with name of patient, date, time of collection, body area from which specimen was obtained, and names of personnel collecting specimens to preserve chain of evidence; give to designated person (e.g., crime laboratory), and document who you gave the collected evidence to in the medical record.
8. Photographs, if taken, should be preserved according to facility policy.

Other Interventions

1. Treat physical trauma as with any patient.
2. Offer the patient treatment for STIs, pregnancy prevention, and HIV postexposure prophylaxis. Centers for Disease Control and Prevention (CDC) recommendations for prophylactic treatment following a sexual assault are:
   Ceftriaxone 500 mg intramuscular (IM) in a single dose.
   plus
   Metronidazole 500 mg orally twice a day for 7 days.
   plus
   Doxycycline 100 mg orally twice a day for 7 days.
3. Protect patient against pregnancy.
   a. It is important to determine whether pregnancy existed before the attack.
   b. Negative pregnancy test should be obtained before administering postcoital therapy.
   c. Hormonal treatment to prevent pregnancy—morning-after pill, as indicated, with patient's consent.
4. Provide the patient with cleansing facilities, including a cleansing douche, shower, and mouthwash after forensic examination is completed.

Providing for Follow-Up Services

1. Ensure the patient has follow-up for results of her STI cultures, HIV test, and any other laboratory testing that was done.
2. Ensure the patient has follow-up with counseling services. This is imperative to prevent long-term psychological effects of the assault. Families of the patient may need counseling services as well. Stress to the patient the importance of post-assault counseling to return to her previous level of functioning.
3. Provide support to the patient in their decision to involve law enforcement.
4. Ensure a safety plan for the patient prior to discharge. The patient should be accompanied by a family member or friend when leaving the health care facility.

BIOLOGIC WEAPONS AND PREPAREDNESS

Following the September 11, 2001, terrorist attacks on the United States, bioterrorism has become a real possibility. As frontline responders, emergency nurses must be aware of possible acts of bioterrorism and be familiar with their facilities' policies regarding such emergencies.

Biologic Agents

Terrorism may consist of the intentional release of a chemical, biologic, radiologic, nuclear, or explosive device intended to cause widespread illness or death. Explosive devices tend to announce themselves rather quickly and definitively. Bioterrorism, however, can have a slow, insidious onset, leaving the population with little idea they have been the patient of an attack. The emergency nurse should be on the alert for possible signs of terrorism:

1. Large numbers of people with similar disease.
2. Cases of unexplained illness or death.
3. More severe illness than would normally be expected for a specific pathogen.
4. An illness that is resistant to usual treatment.
5. Unusual routes of exposure for a specific pathogen.
6. Disease that is unusual for an area.
7. A single case of unusual disease (smallpox, hemorrhagic fever).
8. Disease unusual for an age group.

For specific agents of bioterrorism, such as smallpox, anthrax, plague, and botulism, see Table 31-3.

For additional information regarding bioterrorism, please visit the following website:

- Centers for Disease Control and Prevention, Emergency Preparedness and Response: https://emergency.cdc.gov/bioterrorism/prep.asp

Table 31-3 Potential Biologic Weapons

AGENT AND METHOD OF TRANSMISSION	CLINICAL MANIFESTATIONS	MANAGEMENT
Smallpox		
Transmitted by inhalation or direct contact with the variola virus; has a 2-wk incubation period.	High fever, fatigue, muscle aches, and rash that progresses to blisters after 3 d. The rash first develops on the face and around the wrists and then spreads to the trunk. Smallpox lesions progress at the same rate, unlike lesions of chickenpox, which may be seen in various stages of progression.	The patient should be isolated (preferably at home) until all of the scabs have fallen off. Management includes IV hydration. Health care providers should use masks, gowns, and gloves when caring for these patients and should receive smallpox vaccination within 2–3 d of exposure. Persons who have had contact with the patient should be isolated for 17 d.
Anthrax		
Transmitted through consumption of contaminated animal products, ingestion of raw meat, or inhalation of airborne spores of *Bacillus anthracis*, a gram-positive, spore-forming bacterium. The incubation period is 1–6 d.	Fever, fatigue, cough, chest discomfort, widened mediastinum on chest x-ray, and respiratory distress.	Ensure that standard precautions are observed and that all surfaces are disinfected. Persons who have had contact with the patient should be started on the vaccine schedule and treated with ciprofloxacin or doxycycline.
Pneumonic Plague		
Transmitted by inhalation of *Yersinia pestis*. The incubation period is 2–6 d.	Fever, headache, weakness, and upper respiratory symptoms often including hemoptysis.	Treatment must begin within 24 h and should include gentamicin or streptomycin drug. Isolate the patient for 48 h after antibiotics are started. Postexposure prophylaxis consists of tetracycline or doxycycline for 7 d.
Botulism		
Transmitted primarily by ingestion of food contaminated with a preformed toxin produced by *Clostridium botulinum*. An inhalation form has been developed specifically as a biologic agent.	Blurred or double vision, slurred speech, nausea, vomiting, diarrhea, and descending muscle weakness.	An antitoxin is effective if used early in the disease. Standard precautions are satisfactory; botulism is not contagious.
Viral Hemorrhagic Fevers (Lassa, Ebola, and Marburg Viruses, and Machupo Virus)		
Caused by viruses that are members of the Filoviridae and Arenaviridae families. Bats and rodents are typical reservoirs. Direct contact through bodily fluids. May be a potential biologic weapon through aerosolization.	Characterized by abrupt onset of fevers, myalgias, headache, abdominal pain, nausea, vomiting and diarrhea. Symptoms may progress to hepatic and renal failure, multisystem organ failure, and shock.	Patients should be isolated and supportive measures should be implemented. Monoclonal antibodies are currently under investigation for treatment.
Tularemia		
A zoonotic disease caused by the bacterium *Francisella tularensis*. Domestic rabbits serve as the primary source of human infection through direct contact. Aerosolized dispersal could lead to a severe form of pneumonia.	Sudden fever, chills, headache, diarrhea, muscle aches, joint pain, dry cough, progressive weakness. Severe cases may lead to pneumonia and respiratory failure.	Treated by selected antibiotics. Isolation is not generally required due to the lack of person-to-person transmission.

SELECTED READINGS

American Heart Association. (2020). *Advanced cardiovascular life support provider manual 2020*. Author.

Claus, B. (2022). Alcohol withdrawal syndrome: Early screening equals early intervention. *MEDSURG Nursing, 31*(6), 361–366. https://web-p-ebscohost-com.ezproxy.niagara.edu/ehost/pdfviewer/pdfviewer?vid=1&sid=c09362f6-19d0-4f19-87b5-ec420f545641%40redis

Colls Garrido, C., Riquelme Gallego, B., Sánchez Garcia, J. C., Cortés Martin, J., Montiel Troya, M., & Rodríguez Blanque, R. (2021). The effect of therapeutic hypothermia after cardiac arrest on the neurological outcome and survival—A systematic review of RCTs published between 2016 and 2020. *International Journal of Environmental Research and Public Health, 18*(22), 11817. https://doi.org/10.3390/ijerph182211817

Couper, K., Hassan, A., Ohri, V., Patterson, E., Tang, H., Bingham, R., Olasveengen, T., & Perkins, G. (2020). Removal of foreign body airway obstruction: A systematic review of interventions. *Resuscitation, 156*, 174–181. https://doi.org/10.1016/j.resuscitation.2020.09.007

Dankiewicz, J., Cronberg, T., Lilja, G., Jakobsen, J. C., Belohlavek, J., Callaway, C., Cariou, A., Eastwood, G., Erlinge, D., Jovdenes, J., Joannidis, M., Kirkegaard, H., Kuiper, M., Levin, H., Morgan, M., Nichol, A., Oddo, P., Pelosi, P., Rylander, C., … Nielsen, N. (2019). Targeted hypothermia versus targeted normothermia after out-of-hospital cardiac arrest (TTM2): A randomized clinical trial—Rationale and design. *American Heart Journal, 217*, 23–31. https://doi.org/10.1016/j.ahj.2019.06.012

Dankiewicz, J., Cronberg, T., Liljia, G., Jakobsen, J., Levin, H., Ullen, S., Rylander, C., Wide, M., Oddo, M., Cariou, A., Belohlavek, J., Hovdenes, J., Saxena, M., Kirkegaard, H., Young, P. J., Pelosi, P., Storm, C., Taccone, F., Joannidis, M., … Nielsen, N. (2021). Hypothermia versus normothermia after out-of-hospital cardiac arrest. *The New England Journal of Medicine, 383*(24), 2283–2294. https://doi.org/10.1056/NEJMoa2100591

Day, E., & Daly, C. (2022). Clinical management of the alcohol withdrawal syndrome. *Addiction, 117*, 804–813. https://doi.org/10.1111/add.15647

Donaldson, A. E. (2020). New Zealand emergency nurses knowledge about forensic science and its application to practice. *International Emergency Nursing, 53*, 100854. https://doi.org/10.1016/j.ienj.2020.100854

Emergency Nurses Association. (2017). *Emergency nursing core curriculum* (7th ed.). W.B. Saunders.

Emergency Nurses Association. (2023). *Trauma nursing core course* (9th ed.). Author.

Farrokh, S., Roles, C., Owusu, K., Nelson, S., & Cook, A. (2021). Alcohol withdrawal syndrome in neurocritical care unit: Assessment and treatment challenges. *Neurocritical Care, 34*, 593–607. https://doi.org/10.1007/s12028-020-01061-8

Gaieski, D., & Mikkelsen, M. (2023). *Definition, classification, etiology, and pathophysiology of shock in adults. UpToDate.* Retrieved June 25, 2023, from https://www.uptodate.com/contents/definition-classification-etiology-and-pathophysiology-of-shock-in-adults

Guidelines 2020/CPR and ECC. (2020). *Channing Bete Company, South Deerfield, MA.* https://cpr.heart.org/en/resuscitation-science/cpr-and-ecc-guidelines

Holstege, C. P., & King, J. D. (2022). Toxicologic emergencies. *Emergency Medicine Clinics of North America, 40*(2), 193–442. https://www.google.com/books/edition/Toxicology_Emergencies_An_Issue_of_Emerg/QEVtEAAAQBAJ?hl=en&gbpv=1&dq=https://doi.org/10.1016/j.emc+.2022.03.002&pg=PR13&printsec=frontcover

Moore, W. R., Vermuelen, A., Taylor, R., Kihara, D., & Wahome, E. (2019). Improving 3-hour sepsis bundled care outcomes: Implementation of a nurse-driven sepsis protocol in the emergency department. *Journal of Emergency Nursing, 45*(6), 690–698. https://doi.org/10.1016/j.jen.2019.05.005

Pribék, I. K., Kovács, I., Kádár, B. K., Kovács, C. S., Richman, M. J., Janka, Z., Andó, B., & Lázár, B. (2021). Evaluation of the course and treatment of alcohol withdrawal syndrome with the clinical institute withdrawal assessment for alcohol—Revised: A systematic review-based meta-analysis. *Drug and Alcohol Dependence, 220*, 108536. https://doi.org/10.1016/j.drugalcdep.2021.108536

Proffitt, R. D., & Hooper, G. (2020). Evaluation of the (qSOFA) tool in the emergency department setting: Nurse perception and the impact on patient care. *Advanced Emergency Nursing Journal, 42*(1), 54–62. https://doi.org/10.1097/TME.0000000000000281

Rahman, N. I. A., Chan, C. M., Zakaria, M. I., & Jaafar, M. J. (2019). Knowledge and attitude towards identification of systemic inflammatory response syndrome (SIRS) and sepsis among emergency personnel in tertiary teaching hospital. *Australasian Emergency Care, 22*(1), 13–21. https://doi.org/10.1016/j.auec.2018.11.002

Rajan, J. J., & Rodzevik, T. (2021). Sepsis awareness to enhance early identification of sepsis in emergency departments. *Journal of Continuing Education in Nursing, 52*(1), 39–42. https://doi.org/10.3928/00220124-20201215-10

Rathjen, N. A., & Shahbodaghi, S. D. (2021). Bioterrorism. *American Family Physician, 104*(4), 376–385. aafp.org/pubs/afp/issues/2021/1000/p376.pdf

Sandean, D. (2020). Management of acute spinal cord injury: A summary of the evidence pertaining to the acute management, operative and non-operative management. *World Journal of Orthopedics, 11*(12), 573–583. https://doi.org/10.5312/wjo.v11.i12.573

Simpson, H., Tomlinson, J., Wass, J., Dean, J., & Arlt, W. (2020). Guidance for the prevention and emergency management of adult patients with adrenal insufficiency. *Clinical Medicine, 20*(4), 371–378. https://doi.org/10.7861/clinmed.2019-0324

Tiglao, S. M., Meisenheimer, E. S., & Oh, R. C. (2021). Alcohol withdrawal syndrome: Outpatient management. *American Family Physician, 104*(2), 253–262. https://www.aafp.org/pubs/afp/issues/2021/0900/p253.html

Tiwari, A. K., Jamshed, N., Sahu, A. K., Kumar, A., Aggarwal, P., Bhoi, S., Mathew, R., & Ekka, M. (2023). Performance of qSOFA score as a screening tool for sepsis in the emergency department. *Journal of Emergencies, Trauma, and Shock, 16*(1), 3–7. https://doi.org/10.4103/jets.jets_99_22

Uffen, J. W., Oosterheert, J. J., Schweitzer, V. A., Thursky, K., Kaasjager, H. A. H., & Ekkelenkamp, M. B. (2021). Interventions for rapid recognition and treatment of sepsis in the emergency department: A narrative review. *Clinical Microbiology and Infection, 27*(2), 192–203. https://doi.org/10.1016/j.cmi.2020.02.022

Walter, K. (2023). Fentanyl overdose. *JAMA, 329*(2), 184. https://doi.org/10.1001/jama.2022.22462

Wolf, C., Curry, A., Nacht, J., & Simpson, S. A. (2020). Management of alcohol withdrawal in the emergency department: current perspectives. *Open Access Emergency Medicine, 12*, 53–65. https://doi.org/10.2147/OAEM.S235288

Yost, J. S., Loveless, J. P., Shahane, A. A., & Clayton, A. H. (2022). An innovative model of behavior management to address behavioral emergencies in the acute medical inpatient setting: Pilot data. *Journal of Clinical Psychology in Medical Settings, 29*(1), 54–61. https://doi.org/10.1007/s10880-021-09775-3

Part Two

Maternity and Neonatal Nursing

32 Maternal and Fetal Health*

INTRODUCTION TO MATERNITY NURSING

According to the World Health Organization (WHO), social determinants of health (SDOH)—where people are born, grow, live, work, and age—will impact health outcomes. The WHO also notes that SDOH directly impacts maternal–fetal outcomes. This presents evolving challenges for nurses and for the achievement of optimal birth outcomes. In addition to SDOH, pregnancies complicated by preexisting health conditions such as obesity, diabetes, hypertension, extremes of age, lifestyle factors (e.g., substance use disorders), as well as late or no prenatal care increase the risks associated with pregnancy and childbirth. Today's childbearing families are more diverse with unique social and cultural structures that impact reproduction and parenting. Furthermore, advances in assisted reproductive technologies (ARTs) have afforded opportunities for pregnancy once thought impossible; however, these pregnancies may experience additional inherent risks that also impact maternal–fetal outcomes.

Childbirth occurs in traditional hospital settings, birthing centers, or in the home with providers that include physicians, certified registered nurse midwives, and/or community midwives. Birth-related choices commonly include various birthing positions and analgesic methods; alternative pain-relief strategies, such as hydrotherapy; and the decision to allow children and others to be present during labor and delivery. Regionalization of obstetric services has provided childbearing families with access to technological advances and skilled personnel capable of managing pregnancy or neonatal complications. The combination of advancing technology, pregnancy risk factors, and the current economic climate for health care challenges the nurse to be proficient in areas of neonatal resuscitation, fetal monitoring, maternal and neonatal assessment, and interprofessional communication.

EVIDENCE BASE American College of Obstetricians and Gynecologists. (2018, reaffirmed 2021). Importance of social determinants of health and cultural awareness in the delivery of reproductive health care (Committee Opinion, no. 729). *Obstetrics & Gynecology*, *131*(1), e43–e48. https://www.acog.org/clinical/clinical-guidance/committee-opinion/articles/2018/01/importance-of-social-determinants-of-health-and-cultural-awareness-in-the-delivery-of-reproductive-health-care

Association of Women's Health, Obstetric and Neonatal Nurses. (2022). Respectful maternity care framework and evidence-based clinical practice guideline. *Nursing for Women's Health*, *26*(2), S1–S52. https:/doi.org/10.1016/j.nwh.2022.01.001

Terminology Used in Maternity Nursing

1. Gestation—pregnancy or maternal condition of having a developing fetus in the body.
2. Embryo—human conceptus up to the 10th week of gestation (eighth week postconception).
3. Fetus—human conceptus from 10th week of gestation (eighth week postconception) until delivery.
4. Periviability—alternately termed the *limit of viability*; is considered the stage of fetal maturity needed for extrauterine survival between 20 0/7 and 25 6/7 weeks of gestation.

EVIDENCE BASE American College of Obstetricians and Gynecologists and Society for Fetal Medicine. (2017, reaffirmed 2021). Periviable birth: Obstetric care consensus (Number 6). *Obstetrics & Gynecology*, *130*(4), e187–e199. https://www.acog.org/clinical/clinical-guidance/obstetric-care-consensus/articles/2017/10/periviable-birth

5. Gravida (G)—a person who is or has been pregnant, regardless of pregnancy outcome.
6. Nulligravida—a person who is not now and never has been pregnant.
7. Primigravida—a person pregnant for the first time.
8. Multigravida—a person who has been pregnant more than once.
9. Para (P)—refers to past pregnancies that have reached viability.
10. Nullipara—a person who has never completed a pregnancy to the period of viability. The person may or may not have experienced an abortion.
11. Primipara—a person who has completed one pregnancy to the period of viability, regardless of the number of infants delivered and the number of infant being live-born or stillborn.

*Please note that the term "male" in this chapter refers to a person assigned male at birth, and the term "female" in this chapter refers to a person assigned female at birth.

12. Multipara—a person who has completed two or more pregnancies to the stage of viability.
13. Living children—refers to the number of children delivered who are living.

A person who is pregnant for the first time is a primigravida and is described as gravida 1, para 0 (G1P0). A person who delivered one fetus carried to the period of viability and who is pregnant again is described as gravida 2, para 1. A person with two pregnancies ending in abortions (spontaneous and/or elective) and no viable children is gravida 2, para 0.

Obstetric History

TPAL

In some obstetric services, a person's obstetric history is summarized by a series of four numbers, such as 5-0-2-5. These numbers correspond with the abbreviation TPAL.

1. **T**—represents full-term deliveries, 37 completed weeks or more.
2. **P**—represents preterm deliveries, 20 to less than 37 completed weeks.
3. **A**—represents abortions, elective or spontaneous loss (miscarriage) of a pregnancy before the period of viability.
4. **L**—represents the number of children living. If a child has died, further explanation is needed for clarification.
5. For example, if an obstetric history is summarized as G7, P5-0-2-5, a person has been pregnant seven times, had five term deliveries, zero preterm deliveries, two abortions (spontaneous and/or elective), and five living children.

GTPALM

In some institutions, obstetric history can also be summarized as GTPALM, especially when multiple gestations or births are involved.

1. **G**—represents gravida.
2. **T**—represents full-term deliveries, 37 completed weeks or more.
3. **P**—represents preterm deliveries, 20 to less than 37 completed weeks.
4. **A**—represents abortions, elective or spontaneous loss of a pregnancy before the period of viability.
5. **L**—represents the number of children living. If a child has died, further explanation is needed for clarification.
6. **M**—represents the number of multiple gestations and births (not the number of neonates delivered).

For example, if an obstetric history is summarized as G5, P5-0-0-6-1, a person has been pregnant five times, had five term deliveries, zero preterm deliveries, zero abortions, six living children, and one multiple gestation/birth.

THE PATIENT WHO IS PREGNANT

EVIDENCE BASE Blackburn, S. T. (2021). Physiologic changes of pregnancy. In K. R. Simpson, P. A. Creehan, N. O'Brien-Abel, C. K. Roth, & A. J. Rohan (Eds.), *Perinatal nursing* (5th ed., pp. 48–65). Wolters Kluwer.

Bodnar, L. M., & Himes, K. P. (2023). Maternal nutrition. In C. J. Lockwood, J. A. Copel, L. Dugoff, J. Louis, T. R. Morre, R. M. Silver, & R. Resnick (Eds.), *Creasy & Resnick's maternal–fetal medicine: Principles and practice* (9th ed., pp. 143–149). Elsevier.

Records, K., & Clark, A. (2024). Physiology of pregnancy. In B. Baker & J. Janke (Eds.), *Core curriculum for maternal-newborn nursing* (6th ed., pp. 98–116). Elsevier.

Manifestations of Pregnancy

Pregnancy may be determined by the cessation of menses, enlargement of the uterus, ultrasound, and/or a positive human chorionic gonadotropin (hCG) test. Manifestations of pregnancy are classified into three groups: presumptive, probable, and positive.

Presumptive Signs and Symptoms

Presumptive physical signs and symptoms suggest pregnancy, but they do not prove pregnancy.

1. Abrupt cessation of menses—pregnancy is suspected if more than 10 days have elapsed since the time of the expected onset in a healthy person who previously had predictable menstrual periods.
2. Breast changes:
   a. Breasts enlarge and become tender. Veins in breasts become increasingly visible.
   b. Nipples become larger and more pigmented. Nipple tingling may also be present.
   c. Colostrum—a thin, milky fluid—may be expressed in the second half of pregnancy.
   d. Montgomery glands—small elevations on the areolae—may appear.
3. Skin pigmentation changes:
   a. Chloasma or melasma gravidarum (the mask of pregnancy)—brownish pigmentation appearing on the face in a butterfly pattern in 50% to 70% of patients that is progressive throughout the pregnancy; usually symmetric and distributed on the forehead, cheeks, and nose; more common in those with dark hair and brown eyes.
   b. Linea nigra—dark vertical line on the abdomen between the sternum and the symphysis pubis.
   c. Striae gravidarum (stretch marks)—reddish or purplish linear markings sometimes appearing on the breasts, abdomen, and buttocks, because of the stretching, rupture, and atrophy of the deep connective tissue of the skin.
4. Nausea (morning sickness)—with or without vomiting occurs mainly in the morning but may occur at any time of the day, lasting a few hours. Begins between 2 and 6 weeks after conception and usually disappears spontaneously near the end of the first trimester (12 weeks).
5. Urinary frequency:
   a. Caused by the pressure of the expanding uterus on the bladder.
   b. Decreases when the uterus rises out of the pelvis (around 12 weeks).
   c. Reappears when the fetal head engages in the pelvis at the end of pregnancy.
6. Constipation—because of the decreased absorption of fluid by the gut.
7. Fatigue—characteristic of early pregnancy in response to increased hormonal levels.

Probable Signs and Symptoms

Objective findings detected by 12 to 16 weeks of gestation.

1. Enlargement of the abdomen—at about 12 weeks of gestation, the uterus can be felt through the abdominal wall, just above the symphysis pubis.
2. Uterine changes:
   a. Uterus enlarges, elongates, and decreases in thickness as pregnancy progresses. The uterus changes from a pear shape to a globe shape.
   b. Hegar sign—lower uterine segment softens 6 to 8 weeks after the onset of the last menstrual period (LMP).
3. Cervical changes:
   a. Chadwick sign—bluish or purplish discoloration of the cervix and vaginal wall.
   b. Goodell sign—softening of the cervix; may occur as early as 4 weeks.
   c. With inflammation and carcinoma during pregnancy, the cervix may remain firm.
4. Braxton-Hicks contractions—intermittent contractions of the uterus generally painless, palpable contractions occurring at irregular intervals, more frequently felt after 28 weeks. They usually disappear with walking or exercise.
5. Ballottement—sinking and rebounding of the fetus in its surrounding amniotic fluid in response to a sudden tap on the uterus (occurs near mid-pregnancy).
6. Leukorrhea—increase in vaginal discharge.
7. Quickening—the sensations of fetal movement in the abdomen occurring between the 16th and 20th week after the onset of the last menses.
8. Positive hCG—laboratory (urine or serum) test for pregnancy.

Positive Signs and Symptoms

Diagnostic of Pregnancy

1. Fetal heart tones (FHTs)—usually heard between the 16th and 20th week of gestation with a fetoscope or the 10th and 12th week of gestation with a Doppler stethoscope.
2. Fetal movements felt by the examiner (after about 20 weeks of gestation).
3. Outlining of the fetal body through the maternal abdomen in the second half of pregnancy with Leopold maneuvers.
4. Sonographic evidence (after 4 weeks of gestation) using vaginal ultrasound. Fetal cardiac motion can be detected by 6 weeks of gestation.

Maternal Physiology During Pregnancy

Duration of Pregnancy

1. Averages 280 days or 40 weeks (10 lunar months, 9 calendar months) from the first day of the last normal menses.
2. Duration may also be divided into three equal parts, or trimesters, of slightly more than 13 weeks or 3 calendar months each.
3. Estimated date of confinement (EDC), more commonly referred to as *estimated date of delivery* (EDD), is calculated by adding 7 days to the date of the first day of the last menses and counting back 3 months (Nägele rule). In addition, most antenatal clinics have obstetric wheels where the outer wheel has markings for the calendar and an inner, sliding wheel with weeks and days of gestation. These wheels facilitate the estimation of gestational age (GA) and the calculation of the EDD. The accuracy of these wheels may vary.
   a. For example, if the LMP began on September 10, 2024, the EDC would be June 17, 2025. The calculation would start with September 10, 2024, plus 7 days (September 17, 2025), minus 3 months (June 17, 2025). If the date of the LMP begins after March 31, an additional year must be added to give a correct EDD.
   b. Another method of calculating the EDD is the McDonald rule—the fundal height measurement corresponds to the week of gestation, plus 2 to 4 weeks, after 24 weeks of gestation.
   c. The most accurate assessment of the EDD uses ultrasound technology, preferably in the first trimester. GA in the first trimester is usually calculated from the fetal crown–rump length (CRL). This is the longest demonstrable length of the embryo or fetus, excluding the limbs and the yolk sac. The correlation between CRL and GA is excellent until about 12 weeks of gestation, and the estimate has a 95% confidence interval of plus or minus 6 days.

Reproductive Tract Changes

Uterus

1. Enlargement during pregnancy involves stretching and marked hypertrophy of existing muscle cells secondary to increased estrogen and progesterone levels. Enlargement and thickening of the uterine wall are most marked in the fundus.
2. An increase in fibrous tissue and elastic tissue occurs, and the size and number of blood vessels and lymphatics increase.
3. By the end of the third month (12 weeks), the uterus is too large to be contained within the pelvic cavity and can now be palpated above the pubis.
4. As the uterus rises out of the pelvis, it rotates a bit to the right because of the presence of the rectosigmoid colon on the left side of the pelvis.
5. By 20 weeks of gestation, the fundus has reached the level of the umbilicus.
6. By 36 weeks, the fundus has reached the xiphoid process.
7. By the end of the fifth month, the myometrium hypertrophy ends and the walls of the uterus become thinner, allowing palpation of the fetus.
8. During the last 3 weeks of pregnancy, the uterus descends slightly because of fetal descent into the pelvis.
9. Changes in contractility occur from the first trimester, with irregular painless contractions beginning later in the second trimester.
10. There is a progressive increase in uteroplacental blood flow during pregnancy.

Cervix

1. Pronounced softening and cyanosis because of increased vascularity, edema, hypertrophy, and hyperplasia of the cervical glands.
2. Endocervical glands secrete thick mucus that forms a cervical plug and obstructs the cervical canal. This plug prevents bacteria and other substances from entering and ascending into the uterus.
3. Erosions of the cervix that are common during pregnancy represent an extension of proliferating endocervical glands and columnar endocervical epithelium.
4. Evidence of Chadwick sign, the bluish, purplish coloring of the cervix, is due to the increased vascularity and hyperemia caused by increased estrogen levels.

Ovaries

1. Ovulation ceases during pregnancy, and maturation of new follicles is suspended.
2. The corpus luteum functions during early pregnancy (first 10 to 12 weeks), producing progesterone. However, small levels of estrogen and relaxin are also produced by the corpus luteum.
3. After 8 weeks of gestation, the corpus luteum remains the source for the hormone relaxin. Relaxin is not required for a successful pregnancy outcome and normal delivery.

Vagina and Outlet

1. Increased vascularity, hyperemia, and softening of connective tissue occur in skin and muscles of the perineum and vulva.
2. Vaginal walls prepare for labor as mucosa increases in thickness, connective tissue loosens, and small muscle cells cause hypertrophy. Secretions are thick, white, and acidic in nature and play a major role in the prevention of infections.
3. Vaginal secretions increase; pH is 3.5 to 6—because of increased production of lactic acid from glycogen in the vaginal epithelium by *Lactobacillus acidophilus*. (Acid pH probably aids in keeping vagina relatively free of pathogenic bacteria.)
4. Hypertrophy of the structures and fat deposits causes the labia majora to close and cover the vaginal introitus (vaginal opening).

Abdominal Changes

1. Striae gravidarum (stretch marks) may develop on the skin of the abdomen, breast, and thighs (become glistening silvery lines after pregnancy).
2. Linea nigra may form characterized by a line of dark pigment extending from the umbilicus down the midline to the symphysis. Commonly seen in the first pregnancy, the linea nigra occurs at the height of the uterus. During subsequent pregnancies, the entire line may be present early in gestation.
3. Diastasis recti may occur as muscles (rectus) separate. If severe, a part of the anterior uterine wall may be covered by only a layer of skin, fascia, and peritoneum.

Breast Changes

1. Tenderness and tingling occur in the early weeks of pregnancy.
2. Increase in size by the second month because of the hypertrophy of mammary alveoli. Veins become more prominent, and striae may develop as the breasts enlarge.
3. Nipples become larger, more deeply pigmented, and more erectile early in pregnancy.
4. Colostrum, a yellow secretion rich in antibodies, may be expressed by the second trimester.
5. Areolae become broader and more deeply pigmented. The depth of pigmentation varies with the patient's pigmentation.
6. Glands of Montgomery are hypertrophic sebaceous glands scattered through the areola surrounding the nipple.
7. Lactation is suppressed in pregnancy because progesterone inhibits prolactin production.

Metabolic Changes

Numerous and concentrated changes occur in response to a rapidly growing fetus and placenta.

Weight Gain Average

Twenty-five to 35 lb (11.5 to 16 kg) (see Table 32-1).

Table 32-1 Components of Weight Gain

AREA	KG	POUND
Fetus	3.2–3.4	7–7.5
Placenta	0.5–0.7	1–1.5
Amniotic fluid	0.9	2
Uterus	1.1	2.5
Breast tissue	0.7–1.4	1.5–3
Blood volume	1.6–2.3	3.5–5
Maternal stores	1.8–4.3	4–9.5

Water Metabolism

1. Total body water increases to 6 to 8 L during the pregnancy because of hormonal influence with approximately 4 to 6 L of fluid moving to the extracellular fluid (ECF) resulting in an increase in blood volume.
2. Many people experience a normal accumulation of fluid in their legs and ankles at the end of the day during pregnancy. This is most common in the third trimester and is referred to as *physiologic edema*.
3. Additional sodium is required during pregnancy to meet the need for increased intravascular and ECF volumes and to maintain a normal isotonic state. The limitation of sodium is discouraged in pregnancy because it can result in decreased kidney function, resulting in decreased urine output and a potential adverse outcome.
4. Sodium excretion is similar to the nonpregnant state.
5. Sodium retention is usually directly proportional to the amount of water accumulated during the pregnancy. However, pregnancy lends itself toward sodium depletion, making sodium regulation more difficult.

Protein Metabolism

1. The fetus, uterus, and maternal blood are rich in protein rather than in fat or carbohydrates.
2. At term, the fetus and placenta contain approximately 500 g of protein or approximately half of the total protein increase in pregnancy.
3. Approximately 500 g more of protein is added to the uterus, breasts, and maternal blood in the form of hemoglobin and plasma proteins.

Carbohydrate Metabolism

1. Carbohydrate metabolism during pregnancy is controlled by glucose levels in the plasma and the metabolism of glucose in the cells.
2. The liver controls the plasma glucose level. Not only does it store glucose as glycogen, but also it converts it into glucose when blood glucose levels are low.
3. Early in pregnancy, the effects of estrogen and progesterone can induce a state of hyperinsulinemia. As pregnancy advances, there is increased tissue resistance partnered with increased hyperinsulinemia.
4. Approximately 2% to 3% of patients will develop gestational diabetes mellitus during pregnancy, regardless of if they have a history of carbohydrate intolerance.
5. Those with preexisting diabetes mellitus (type 1 or 2) may experience a worsening of the disease attributed to hormonal changes occurring with pregnancy.

6. During pregnancy, there is a "sparing" of glucose used by maternal tissues and shunting of glucose to the placenta for use by the fetus.
7. Human placental lactogen (hPL) promoting lipolysis increases plasma-free fatty acids, thereby providing alternative maternal fuel sources.
8. Estrogen, progesterone, hPL, and cortisol oppose the action of insulin during pregnancy and promote maternal lipolysis as well.

Fat Metabolism

1. Lipid metabolism during pregnancy causes an accumulation of fat stores, mostly cholesterol, phospholipids, and triglycerides.
2. This accumulation of fat stores has no negligible effect on the fetus.
3. Fat storage occurs before the 30th week of gestation. After 30 weeks of gestation, fat mobilization occurs correlating with increased utilization of glucose and amino acids by the fetus.

Nutrient Requirements

Caloric Requirements

1. Additional calories are usually not required during the first trimester because of the limited metabolic demands.
2. During the second trimester, maternal calorie intake should increase by 340 calories per day; and in the third trimester, caloric intake should increase by 452 calories daily. However, because of varying individual needs, the exact caloric requirements need to be established on an individual basis.
3. Caloric expenditure varies throughout pregnancy. There is a slight increase in early pregnancy and a sharp increase near the end of the first trimester, continuing throughout pregnancy.

Protein Requirements

1. Protein is required for adequate amino acids to accommodate the normal development of the fetus, blood volume expansion, and growth of maternal breast and uterine tissue. During pregnancy, 60 to 80 g of protein should be consumed daily.
2. The ratio of low-density proteins to high-density proteins is increased during pregnancy.

Carbohydrate and Fat Requirements

1. As in the nonpregnant person, carbohydrates should supply 55% to 60% of calories in the diet and should be in the form of complex carbohydrates, such as whole-grain cereal products, starchy vegetables, and legumes.
2. Fat intake should not exceed 30% of the diet. Saturated fats should not exceed 10% of the total calories.

Iron Requirements

1. Total circulating red blood cells (RBCs) increase about 20% to 30% (250 to 450 mL) during pregnancy; therefore, iron requirements are increased to 500 mg of iron needed: 270 mg by fetus; 90 mg by the placenta. This equates to 0.8 g/day in early pregnancy and 7.5 mg/day by term. This usually exceeds dietary intake.
2. Supplemental iron is valuable and necessary during pregnancy and for several weeks after pregnancy or lactation.
3. During the last half of pregnancy, iron is transferred to the fetus and stored in the fetal liver. This store lasts 3 to 6 months.

Other Nutritional Requirements

1. If folic acid intake has not already been increased in preparation for conception, a pregnant person should increase folic acid intake from 400 to 800 μg/day.
2. Vitamin D deficiency is the most common nutritional deficit globally. In addition, vitamin D deficiency has been associated with increased rates of preeclampsia and cesarean births; therefore, pregnant persons should take 400 IU (10 μg) daily. Many manufactured prenatal vitamins increase vitamin D levels.

POPULATION AWARENESS Because of the increasing rates of obesity, diabetes, and hypertension in younger people of reproductive age, it is essential for nurses to focus on maternal and fetal well-being to include nutritional education and appropriate weight gain during pregnancy. The promotion of healthy behaviors may decrease the risk for hospitalization and improve maternal and fetal outcomes.

Cardiovascular System Changes

Heart

1. The diaphragm progressively elevates during pregnancy, causing displacement of the heart to the left and upward with the apex moved laterally.
2. Heart sounds are exaggerated, splitting of the first heart sound with a loud, easily heard third sound.
3. Heart murmurs—systolic murmurs are common and usually disappear after delivery.

Blood Volume Changes

1. Cardiac output increases by 30% to 50% (1,450 to 1,750 mL), beginning as early as 6 weeks and peaking by 28 to 34 weeks of gestation, causing slight hypertrophy of the heart and increased cardiac output. Multiple gestation may cause even higher cardiac outputs, especially after 20 weeks of gestation.
2. Cardiac output peaks in the second trimester and plateaus until term, reaching a volume of 6 to 7 L/min by term.
3. Position greatly influences cardiac output, especially in the third trimester.
   a. In the supine position, the large uterus compresses the venous return from the lower half of the body to the heart. This may cause arterial hypotension, referred to as *supine hypotensive syndrome*.
   b. Turning from supine to lateral position (either left or right side) increases cardiac output by 25% to 30%, with an increase in uterine and renal blood flow.
4. Femoral venous pressure increases due to the slowing of blood flow from the lower extremities as a result of pressure of the enlarged uterus on pelvic veins and inferior vena cava.
5. Increased cutaneous blood flow dissipates excess heat caused by increased metabolism of pregnancy.
6. Plasma volume increases 40% to 60% (1,200 to 1,600 mL) by term, resulting in hemodilution, more commonly referred to as *physiologic anemia of pregnancy* or *physiologic dilutional anemia*. This "anemic" state is not a true pathologic state and decreases the risk of thrombosis. It is due to the rapid increase in plasma volume and the later increase in RBC volume.

Blood Pressure Changes

1. Blood pressure (BP)—during the first half of pregnancy, there is a slight (5 to 10 mm Hg) decrease in systolic BP (SBP) and diastolic BP (DBP), with the lowest point occurring in the second trimester. By the third trimester, the BP gradually returns to prepregnancy levels.
2. Maternal position influences BP: The highest reading is obtained in the sitting position, the lowest reading is obtained in the left lateral position, and an intermediate reading is

obtained in the supine position. Sitting or standing positions show minimal change in SBP readings; however, they can decrease the DBP by about 10 to 15 mm Hg.

3. Maternal BP will also rise with uterine contractions and returns to the baseline level after the uterine contraction is over.
4. Hypertensive disease affects up to 22% of pregnancies and is associated with maternal and fetal death. According to the National Institutes of Health, those with hypertension in pregnancy should be referred to as having hypertensive disorders of pregnancy. In addition, the term "gestational hypertension" replaces the term "pregnancy-induced hypertension" to describe cases in which elevated BP without proteinuria occurs in a person beyond 20 weeks of gestation who previously had a normal BP. Essentially, gestational hypertension is an elevated BP past 20 weeks of gestation without proteinuria. See page 1041.

Hematologic Changes

1. Total volume of circulating RBCs increases 17% to 33%; hemoglobin concentration at term averages 12 to 16 g/dL; hematocrit concentration at term averages 37% to 47%.
2. Average leukocyte (white blood cell [WBC]) count in the third trimester is 5 to 12,000/mm^3. WBC count can be elevated as high as 30,000 or more during labor—cause unknown; probably represents the reappearance in the circulation of leukocytes previously shunted from active circulation.
3. Pregnancy is a hypercoagulable state because of the increased levels of essential coagulation factors, including factor I (fibrinogen) by 50%, factor V (proaccelerin or labile factor), factor VII (proconvertin or serum prothrombin conversion accelerator), factor VIII (antihemophilic factor or antihemophilic globulin), factor IX (plasma thromboplastin component or Christmas factor), factor X (Stuart or Prower factor), factor XII (Hageman or glass or contact factor), and von Willebrand factor (vWF antigen). Factor II (prothrombin) increases slightly, whereas factors XI (plasma thromboplastin antecedent) and XIII (fibrin-stabilizing factor) decrease during pregnancy.
4. There is no significant change in the number, appearance, or function of platelets. Average platelet count is 150,000 to 400,000/mm^3.
5. Pregnancy increases the risk for venous thrombosis.

Respiratory Tract Changes

1. Nasal stuffiness and epistaxis (nosebleeds) are also common during pregnancy, secondary to vascular congestion caused by the increased estrogen levels.
2. Approximately 60% to 70% of patients experience shortness of breath during pregnancy.
3. Diaphragm is elevated (about 4 cm) during pregnancy—chiefly by the enlarging uterus that decreases the length of the lungs. Breathing is more diaphragmatic rather than costal.
4. Thoracic cage expands its anteroposterior diameter (by 2 cm). The increased pressure from the uterus also widens the substernal angle by about 50%, causing slight flaring of the ribs—result of increased mobility of rib attachments.
5. Oxygen consumption increases by 15% to 20% and as much as 300% in labor. This increase leads to increased maternal alveolar and arterial oxygen partial pressure levels.
6. Hyperventilation—an increase in respiratory rate, tidal volume (amount of air inspired and expired with normal breath) increases by 30% to 40%, and minute ventilation (amount of air inspired in 1 minute) increases by 40%.
7. Total lung volume (amount of air in lungs at maximum inspiration) decreases by about 5%. Residual volume (amount of air in lungs after maximum expiration), respiratory reserve volume (maximum amount of air expired during rest), and functional residual capacity (amount of air remaining in lungs at rest and allowing for gas exchange) drop by about 18% to 20%.
8. Increased total volume lowers partial pressure of arterial carbon dioxide ($PaCO_2$), causing mild respiratory alkalosis that is compensated for by lowering of the bicarbonate concentration.
9. Partial pressure of arterial oxygen (PaO_2) elevates to 106 to 108 mm Hg in the first trimester and 101 to 104 mm Hg at term. $PaCO_2$ is decreased to 27 to 32 mm Hg. Bicarbonate decreases to 18 to 21 mEq/L. Normal pH during pregnancy is 7.40 to 7.45. These changes allow for removal of fetal carbon dioxide via passive diffusion in the placenta.

Renal System Changes

1. Ureters dilate and elongate during pregnancy because of mechanical pressure and perhaps because of the effects of progesterone. When the uterus rises out of the uterine cavity, it rests on the ureters, compressing them at the pelvic brim. Dilation is greater on the right side—the left side is cushioned by the sigmoid colon.
2. Renal plasma flow (RPF) increases by 60% to 80% by the end of the first trimester because of the increases in blood volume and cardiac output as well as a decrease in systemic vascular resistance due to the effects of progesterone. RPF increases early in pregnancy and decreases to nonpregnant levels in the third trimester. These changes may be due to hPL.
3. Glomerular filtration rate (GFR) increases 40% to 50% by the second trimester and persists almost to term. Glucosuria may be a result of an increase in GFR without an increase in tubular resorptive capacity for filtered glucose.
4. Protein excretion is also increased to a rate not always handled by the kidneys' tubular resorptive capability. Therefore, protein can spill into the urine. However, protein in the urine should not be considered an abnormal finding until 24-hour urine values exceed 300 mg/dL.
5. Toward the end of pregnancy, pressure of the presenting part impedes drainage of blood and lymph from the bladder base, typically leaving the area edematous, easily traumatized, and more susceptible to infection.
6. Because of the increased RPF and GFR, the amount of glucose the kidneys filter increases 10- to 100-fold. The kidneys cannot always keep up with this increase; therefore, whatever glucose that is not filtered is lost in the urine, contributing to glycosuria.

Gastrointestinal Tract Changes

1. Gums may become hyperemic and soft; bleeding easily.
2. *Epulis of pregnancy*—a localized vascular swelling of the gums may appear.
3. Stomach and intestines are displaced upward and laterally by the enlarging uterus. Heartburn (pyrosis) is commonly caused by reflux of acid secretions in the lower esophagus.
4. Peptic ulcer formation or exacerbation is uncommon during pregnancy because of decreased hydrochloric acid (caused by increased estrogen levels).
5. Tone and motility of gastrointestinal (GI) tract decrease, leading to prolonged gastric emptying because of the large amount

of progesterone produced by the placenta. Decreased motility, mechanical obstruction by the fetus, and decreased water absorption from the colon lead to constipation.
6. Hemorrhoids are common because of elevated pressure in veins below the level of the large uterus and constipation.
7. Distention and hypotonia of the gallbladder are common, causing stasis of bile. In addition, there is a decrease in emptying time and the thickening of bile, resulting in hypercholesterolemia and gallstone formation.
8. Liver function tests are altered with pregnancy: bilirubin, aspartate aminotransferase, and alanine aminotransferase values are unchanged; prothrombin time may show a slight increase or be unchanged. Liver size and morphology are unchanged.
9. The appendix is pushed superiorly.

Endocrine Changes

1. Anterior pituitary gland enlarges in both weight (30% increase) and volume (twofold increase). Its shape also changes from convex to dome shaped; posterior pituitary gland remains unchanged.
2. Thyroid is moderately enlarged because of hyperplasia of glandular tissue and increased vascularity.
   a. Basal metabolic rate increases progressively during normal pregnancy (as much as 25%) because of metabolic activity of fetus.
   b. Level of protein-bound iodine and thyroxine rises sharply and is maintained until after delivery because of increased circulatory estrogen and hCG.
   c. Hyperthyroidism during pregnancy is rare. Although the levels of thyroxine (T_4) and triiodothyronine (T_3) are elevated by as much as 40% to 100% by term, this is a result of estrogen, hCG, and increased urinary iodide secretion, resulting in "euthyroid hyperthyroxinemia."
3. Parathyroid gland size is known to increase, but there is a decrease in the parathyroid hormone (PTH) during pregnancy. This decrease is balanced by the increased production of PTH by the fetus and placenta.
4. Adrenal secretions considerably increased—amount of aldosterone increases as early as the 15th week to accommodate for the increased sodium excretion.
5. Pancreas—because of the fetal glucose needs for fetal growth, there are alterations in maternal insulin production and usage.
   a. Estrogen, progesterone, cortisol, and hPL decrease the maternal utilization of glucose.
   b. Cortisol also increases maternal insulin production.
   c. Insulinase, an enzyme produced by the placenta, deactivates maternal insulin.
   d. These changes cause an increased demand for insulin, triggering the islets of Langerhans to increase production of insulin.

Integumentary Changes

1. Pigment changes occur because of melanocyte-stimulating hormone as a result of increased estrogen and progesterone and is elevated from the second month of pregnancy until term.
2. Striae gravidarum appear in later months of pregnancy as reddish, slightly depressed streaks in the skin of the abdomen and occasionally over the breasts and thighs and occur in as much as 50% of all patients who are pregnant.
3. Linea nigra—a brownish black line of pigment is usually formed in the midline of the abdominal skin.
4. Chloasma or melasma (mask of pregnancy)—brownish patches of pigment may form on the face. Chloasma usually disappears after pregnancy but can reappear with excessive exposure to the sun or with oral contraceptive treatment.
5. Angiomas (vascular spider nevus)—minute red elevations commonly on the skin of the face, neck, upper chest, legs, and arms may develop.
6. Palmar erythema—reddening of the palms may also occur.
7. Increased warmth to the skin and variation in hair and nail growth occur.

Musculoskeletal Changes

1. The increasing mobility of sacroiliac, sacrococcygeal, and pelvic joints during pregnancy is a result of hormonal changes, specifically the hormone relaxin.
2. The center of gravity shifts secondary to increased weight gain, fluid retention, lordosis, and mobile ligaments. This mobility and the change in the center of gravity contribute to alteration of maternal posture and to back pain.
3. Late in pregnancy, aching, numbness, and weakness in the upper extremities may occur because of lordosis and paresthesia, which ultimately produces traction on the ulnar and median nerves.
4. Separation of the rectus muscles because of the pressure of the growing uterus creates what is called a *diastasis recti*. If this is severe, a portion of the anterior uterine wall is covered by only a layer of skin, fascia, and peritoneum.

Neurologic Changes

1. Usually no system changes.
2. Mild frontal headaches are common in the first and second trimesters and are usually related to tension or hormonal changes.
3. Dizziness is common and related to vasomotor instability, postural hypotension, or hypoglycemia following long periods of standing or sitting.
4. Tingling sensations in the hands are common and are due to excessive hyperventilation, which decreases maternal $PaCO_2$ levels.

Hormonal Changes

Steroid Hormones

1. Estrogen:
   a. Secreted by the ovaries in early pregnancy, with over half of the estrogen secreted by the placenta by 7 weeks of gestation.
   b. The three classic estrogens during pregnancy are estrone, estradiol, and estriol. More than 90% of the estrogen secreted during pregnancy is estriol.
   c. Estrogens also ensure uterine growth and development, maintenance of uterine elasticity and contractility, maintenance of breast growth and its ductal structures, and enlargement of the external genitalia.
2. Progesterone:
   a. Is initially secreted by the corpus luteum and later by the placenta playing a critical role in the maintenance of the pregnancy by suppressing the maternal immunologic response to the fetus and the rejection of the trophoblasts.
   b. Progesterone helps maintain the endometrium, inhibits uterine contractility, helps in the development of breast lobules for lactation, stimulates the maternal respiratory center, and relaxes smooth muscle.

Placental Protein Hormones

1. hCG:
   a. Secreted by the syncytiotrophoblasts and stimulates the production by the corpus luteum of progesterone and estrogen until the fully developed placenta takes over.
   b. In multiple gestations, hCG can be twice as high as in a single pregnancy.
   c. hCG levels peak around 10 weeks of gestation (50,000 to 100,000 mIU/mL), then decrease to 10,000 to 20,000 mIU/mL by 20 weeks of gestation.
2. Human chorionic somatomammotropin (hCS) also called *human placental lactogen* (hPL) is produced by the syncytiotrophoblasts of the placenta; detected in maternal serum as early as 6 weeks of gestation.
   a. Serum hCS levels rise concomitantly with placental growth.
   b. hCS is an antagonist of insulin. It increases the amount of free fatty acids available to the fetus for metabolic needs and decreases the maternal metabolism of glucose, allowing for protein synthesis. This action allows the fetus to have the needed nutrients despite variation in the timing of maternal nutrient intake.

Other Hormones

1. Prostaglandins:
   a. Exact function is still unknown but is essential for the cardiovascular adaptation to pregnancy, cervical ripening, and initiation of labor.
   b. Affect smooth muscle contractility, with increased levels leading to vasodilation.
2. Relaxin:
   a. Secreted primarily by the corpus luteum and be secreted in small amounts by the decidua and the placenta.
   b. Inhibits uterine activity and decreases the strength of uterine contractions and cervical ripening.
3. Prolactin:
   a. Released from the anterior pituitary gland and responsible for sustaining milk protein, casein, fatty acids, lactose, and the volume of milk secretion during lactation.

Structure of the Pelvis

Bones of the Pelvis

The pelvis is composed of four bones:

1. Two innominate bones (hip bones) form the sides and front.
2. Sacrum and coccyx form the back.
3. Pelvic bones are held together by fibrocartilage of the symphysis pubis and several ligaments.

Divisions of the Pelvis

1. False pelvis—lies above an imaginary line called the *linea terminalis* or *pelvic brim* (see Figure 32-1). Function of the false pelvis is to support the enlarged uterus.
2. True pelvis lies below the pelvic brim or linea terminalis; it is the bony canal through which the fetus must pass. It is divided into three planes: the inlet, the midpelvis, and the outlet.
   a. Inlet:
      i. Upper boundary of the true pelvis—bound by the upper margin of symphysis pubis in the front, linea terminalis on the sides, and sacral promontory (first sacral vertebra) in the back.
      ii. Largest diameter of inlet is transverse (see Figure 32-2).
      iii. Smallest diameter of inlet is anteroposterior.
      iv. Anteroposterior diameter is the most important diameter of inlet: measured clinically by diagonal conjugate—distance from the lower margin of symphysis to the sacral promontory (usually 5½ in [14 cm]) (see Figure 32-3).
      v. Obstetric (true) conjugate—distance between inner surface of symphysis and sacral promontory measured by subtracting ½ to ¾ in (1.5 to 2 cm) (thickness of symphysis) from the diagonal conjugate. Adequate diameter is usually 4½ in (11.5 cm). This is the shortest anteroposterior diameter through which the fetus must pass.
   b. Midpelvis:
      i. Bounded by inlet above and outlet below—true bony cavity. Midpelvis contains the narrowest portion of the pelvis.
      ii. Diameters cannot be measured clinically.
      iii. Clinical evaluation of adequacy is made by noting the ischial spines. Prominent spines that protrude into the cavity indicate a contracted midpelvic space. The interspinous diameter is 4 in (10 cm).
   c. Outlet:
      i. Lowest boundary of the true pelvis.
      ii. Bounded by the lower margin of symphysis in the front, ischial tuberosities on the sides, and tip of sacrum posteriorly.
      iii. Most important diameter clinically is the distance between the tuberosities (greater than 4 in).

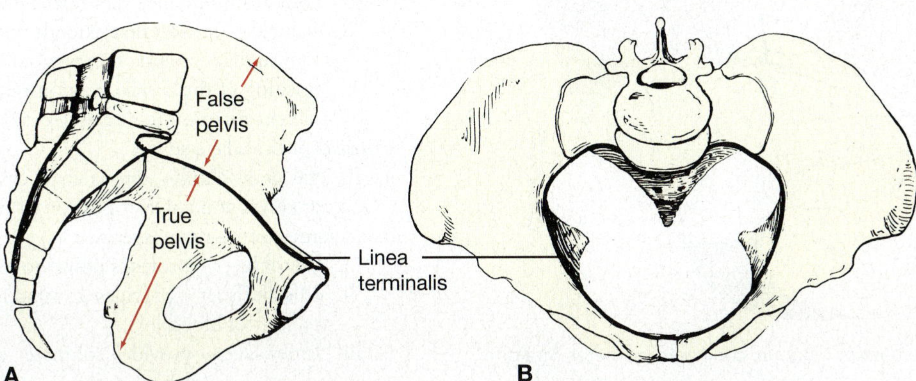

Figure 32-1. **(A)** Side view of the true and false pelvis. **(B)** Front view showing linea terminalis (pelvic brim).

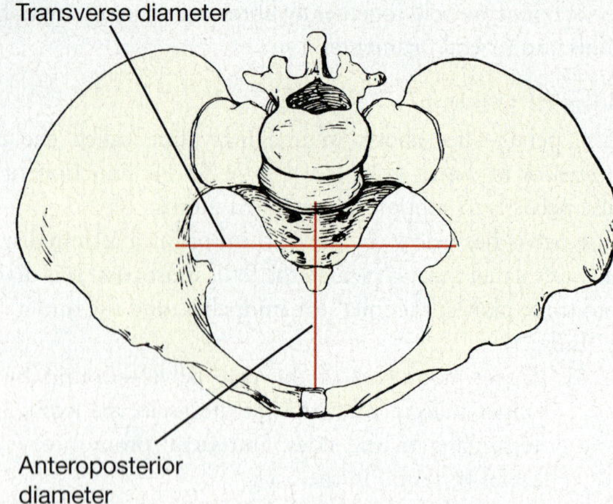

Figure 32-2. Inlet of usual female pelvis showing transverse and anteroposterior diameters.

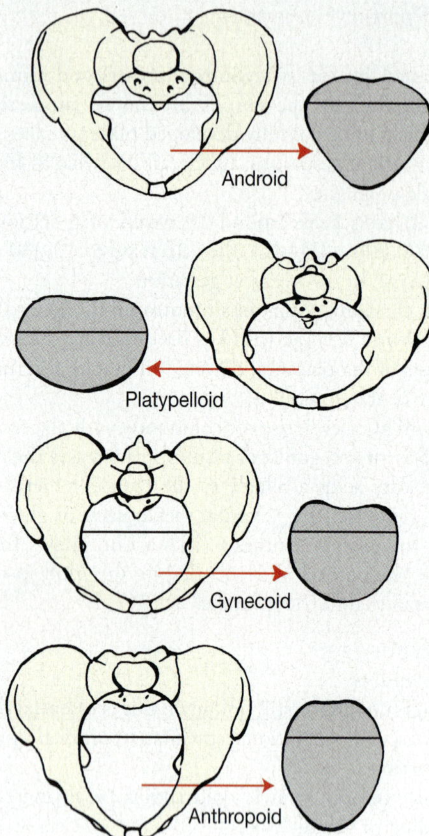

Figure 32-4. Four types of female pelvises. *Android*—male-type pelvis. *Platypelloid*—broad pelvis with shortened anteroposterior diameter and flattened, oval, transverse shape. *Gynecoid*—usual female pelvis in which inlet is round instead of oval. *Anthropoid*—pelvis in which anteroposterior diameter is equal to or greater than the transverse diameter.

Shapes of the Pelvis

There are four main types of pelvic shapes (see Figure 32-4).

1. Gynecoid (usual female pelvis, about 50%); optimal diameters in all three planes for fetal descent.
2. Android (usual male pelvis, about 20%); posterior segments are decreased in all three planes; deep transverse arrest of descent and failure of rotation of the fetus are common.
3. Anthropoid (long anteroposterior diameter, about 25%); may allow for easy delivery of an occiput-posterior presentation of the fetus.
4. Platypelloid (flat pelvis with wide transverse diameter, about 5%); arrest of fetal descent at the pelvic inlet with poor labor progress is common.

Structure of the Uterus

1. Located behind the symphysis pubis between the bladder and the rectum, increasing in size after childbirth.

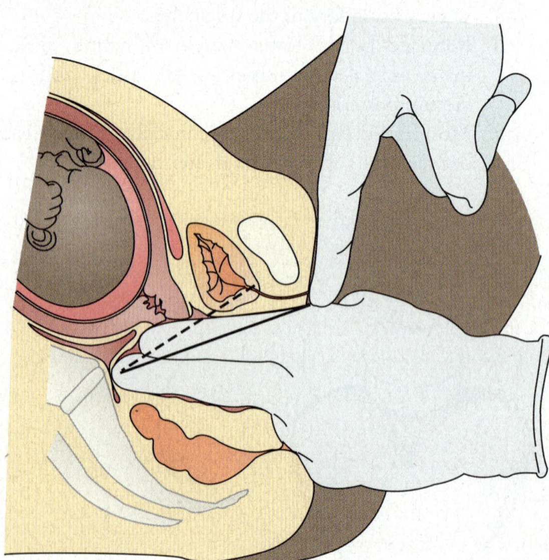

Figure 32-3. Measurement of diagonal conjugate diameter. Straight line shows diagonal conjugate; dotted line shows true conjugate.

2. Consists of four parts:
   a. Fundus—upper rounded segment that extends above the insertion of the fallopian tubes; fetal growth is measured by fundal height in centimeters correlating with weeks of gestation.
   b. Body (corpus)—main portion between cervix and fundus.
   c. Isthmus (neck)—lower uterine segment.
   d. Cervix—divided into two sections:
      i. Supravaginal—portion that extends inside the uterus; contains internal os that opens into the uterine cavity.
      ii. Vaginal—portion that extends outside the uterus into the vagina; contains the external os that is the visible opening of the cervix; portion that is felt during vaginal examination in assessing cervical dilation.
3. Consists of three layers:
   a. Parietal peritoneum—serous coat; covers most of uterus, except cervix and anterior portion of body.
   b. Myometrium—three layers:
      i. Outer layer—provides power to expel the fetus.
      ii. Middle layer—provides contractions after childbirth to control blood loss.
      iii. Inner layer—provides sphincter action to help keep cervix closed during pregnancy.

c. Endometrium—highly vascular mucous membrane; responds to hormonal stimulation with hypertrophy and secretion; sloughs if pregnancy does not occur.

Prenatal Assessment

EVIDENCE BASE Lyndon, A., & Wisner, K. (2021). *Fetal heart monitoring: Principles and practices* (6th ed.). Association of Women's Health, Obstetric, Neonatal Nurses.

Health History

Age

The reproductive life cycle extends for many years, with extremes defined as younger than 19 years and older than 35 years. These extremes carry an increased risk of prematurity, congenital anomalies, as well as other risks of pregnancy.

1. Pregnant adolescents have an increased incidence of anemia, gestational hypertension, preterm labor (PTL), small-for-gestational age (SGA) infants, intrauterine growth–restricted infants, cephalopelvic disproportion, and dystocia.
2. Advanced maternal age (AMA) results in an increased incidence of hypertension with pregnancies complicated by underlying medical problems such as diabetes, multiple gestation, and infants with genetic abnormalities.

Family History

Includes maternal and paternal history for conditions such as congenital disorders, hereditary diseases, multiple pregnancies, diabetes, heart disease, hypertension, intellectual disability, renal disease, and any recent global travel destinations.

Maternal Medical History

1. Childhood diseases and immunization records especially rubella, measles, and chickenpox.
2. Major illnesses, surgery (especially of the reproductive tract, spinal surgery, or appendectomy, which may have resulted in adhesions), blood transfusions.
3. Existing medical conditions, such as epilepsy, cardiac disease, endocrine disorders (e.g., diabetes, thyroid disease), asthma, and hypertension.
4. Drug, food, and environmental allergies.
5. Urinary tract infections (UTIs) and sexually transmitted infections (STIs).
6. Menstrual history (onset of menarche, length, amount, regularity, and dysmenorrhea). Also, assess for bleeding between menses.
7. Gynecologic history (reproductive history, contraceptive use, and sexual history).
8. Use of medications (prescription, herbal, and over the counter [OTC]), recreational drugs, alcohol, nicotine, tobacco, and caffeine.
9. History of tuberculosis, hepatitis, group B beta-hemolytic *Streptococcus* (GBS), or human immunodeficiency virus (HIV).

Maternal Nutritional History

1. Adherence to special dietary practices (religious, social, or cultural preferences).
2. History of eating disorders (obesity, bulimia, anorexia nervosa), gastric bypass, absorption problems (e.g., phenylketonuria [PKU] and celiac disease), and food allergies.
3. Eating patterns (times and frequency of eating daily), number of servings of food from the five food groups, calories, protein, vitamins, and minerals consumed daily.
4. Additional factors to be considered include where the food was eaten, the quantity of food eaten, how food was prepared (i.e., fried, baked), and which foods are limited and why.
5. The U.S. Department of Agriculture provides an online interactive diet program, Daily Food Plan for Moms, specifically tailored to people who are pregnant or breastfeeding. This program gives a personalized plan for nutrition for pregnancy, including multiples and lactation. See https://www.myplate.gov/life-stages/pregnancy-and-breastfeeding
6. Weight gain of less than 10 pounds (4.5 kg) or loss of more than 5 pounds (2.3 kg).

EVIDENCE BASE United States Department of Agriculture and United States Department of Health and Human Services. (2020). *Dietary guidelines for Americans 2020–2025* (9th ed.). Author. https://www.dietaryguidelines.gov

Past Obstetric History

1. Infertility issues, dates of previous pregnancies and deliveries, infant weights, length of labors, types of deliveries, anesthesia use, multiple births, abortions, stillbirths, and maternal, fetal, and neonatal complications. Include a history of infertility to include treatments, medications, and conceived or lost pregnancies.
2. Last delivery less than 1 year before present conception.
3. Patient's perception of past pregnancy, labor, and delivery experience for self and effect on family.

Current Obstetric Experience

1. Gravidity, parity.
2. Date of last menses.
3. Estimated date of birth—EDC/EDD.
4. Signs and symptoms of pregnancy—amenorrhea, breast changes, nausea and vomiting, fetal movement, fatigue, urinary frequency, and skin pigment changes.
5. Expectations for present pregnancy, labor, and delivery.
6. Expectations for health care providers and perception of relationship with nurse.
7. Rest and sleep patterns—length, quality, and regularity of rest and sleep.
8. Activity and employment—exercise patterns, type and hours of employment, exposure to hazardous material (occupational hazards), and plans for continued employment.
9. Sexual activity and contraceptive practices.
10. Inadequate prenatal care, intrauterine growth problems, Rh sensitization, or PTL.

Psychosocial History

1. Psychiatric and mental status history: history of mood or anxiety disorders; mental illness; medications or treatments for psychiatric or mental problems. Past history of depression, with or without an association with pregnancy.
2. Self-concept or self-esteem issues.
3. Current social support systems available.
4. Screening for intimate partner violence.
5. Current use of local community, regional or federal support services (i.e., CareNet; Women, Infants, and Children [WIC; https://www.fns.usda.gov/wic]; Moms on Medicaid [MOMS]).

6. Stressors: personal, financial, and occupational stressors that may affect the pregnancy, including current coping strategies.
7. Emotional changes and adjustment to pregnancy.
8. Utilize an evidence-based screening tool to identify factors impacting physical and mental health that could interfere with the continuity of prenatal care. Any negative responses require further investigation and intervention. The National Institute for Health and Care Excellence recommends a mental health assessment within 2 weeks and treatment within 6 weeks of risk identification.

EVIDENCE BASE Beck, C. T. (2021). Perinatal mood and anxiety disorders: Research and implications for nursing care. *Journal of Obstetric, Gynecologic & Neonatal Nursing, 50*(4), e1–e46. https://doi.org/10.1016/j.jogn.2021.02.007

Howard, L. M., & Khalifeh, H. (2020). Perinatal mental health: A review of progress and challenges. *World Psychiatry, 19*(3), 313–327. https://doi.org/10.1002/wps.20769

Román-Gálvez, R. M., Martín-Peláez, S., Martínez-Galiano, J. M., Khan, K. S., & Bueno-Cavanillas, A. (2021). Prevalence of intimate partner violence in pregnancy: An umbrella review. *International Journal of Environmental Research and Public Health, 18*(2), 707. https://doi.org/10.3390/ijerph18020707

Laboratory Data

Urinalysis

1. Urine is tested for glucose, ketones, and protein. Urine is usually collected by a clean-catch, midstream technique.
2. Glucose (glucosuria) may be present in small amounts because the GFR is increased without the same increase in kidney tubular reabsorption. Glucosuria should be investigated to rule out diabetes.
3. Protein in the urine that exceeds 300 mg/dL/24-hour urine collection should be reported because it may be a sign of preeclampsia, renal problems, or UTI.
4. Ketones in the urine should be reported because ketonuria may be a sign of excessive weight loss, dehydration, or electrolyte imbalance. Ketonuria is commonly secondary to nausea and vomiting of pregnancy.
5. If the urine is cloudy and bacteria or leukocytes are present (more than four leukocytes per high-power field), a urine culture is performed.
6. The presence of bilirubin is indicative of liver or gallbladder disease or the breakdown of RBCs.
7. The presence of blood in the urine (hematuria) is suggestive of UTI, kidney disease, or vaginal contamination.

Complete Blood Count

1. Determination of hematocrit and hemoglobin levels and description of the morphology of the RBCs are done to find evidence of anemias, such as sickle cell or thalassemia.
2. Hemoglobin levels average 12 to 16 g/dL.

Blood Type and Screening

1. Blood type, Rh factor, and antibody screen—if the patient who is pregnant is found to be Rh negative or to have a positive antibody screen, the partner is screened and a maternal antibody titer is drawn, as indicated.
   a. Coombs test—retested at 28 weeks in the Rh-negative patient who is pregnant for detection of antibodies.
   b. Rh_0 (D) immune globulin (RhoGAM) given at 28 weeks, as indicated. Also administered following chorionic villus sampling (CVS), percutaneous umbilical sampling, amniocentesis, trauma, or placental separation (abruptio placentae or placenta previa).
   c. Administered within 72 hours following birth to maternal patient who is Rho (D) or Du^-, without antibodies and the newborn is Rh positive blood type
2. Glucose testing—if average risk, diabetic screening is conducted at 24 to 28 weeks using a 1-hour 50-g glucose load test. According to the American Diabetes Association, average risk includes age 25 or above, obesity at any age, family history of diabetes mellitus in a first-degree relative, previous delivery resulting in an infant with macrosomia, member of an ethnic group with a high prevalence of diabetes (Hispanic, Black, Pacific Islander, Native American, Asian American), history of abnormal glucose tolerance, and history of poor obstetric outcome.
3. Maternal serum alpha-fetoprotein (MS-AFP)—may be done at 15 to 18 weeks primarily to screen for neural tube defects. High maternal levels may indicate an open neural tube defect in the fetus; low levels have been associated with Down syndrome. It is important to stress to the patient that the MS-AFP is only a screening tool and that further testing is needed for a definitive diagnosis.
4. Non-Invasive Prenatal Screening (NIPS)—a cell-free DNA blood test can be obtained at any time during gestation after 9 to 10 weeks. NIPS is recommended over traditional screening methods for all patients who are pregnant with singleton and twin gestations for fetal trisomies 21, 18, and 13. In addition, NIPS is recommended to screen for fetal sex chromosome aneuploidy.

EVIDENCE BASE Dungan, J. S., Klugman, S., Darilek, S., Malinowski, J., Akkari, Y., Monaghan, K. G., Erwin, A., & Best R. G. (2023). Noninvasive prenatal screening (NIPS) for fetal chromosome abnormalities in a general-risk population: An evidence-based clinical guideline of the American College of Medical Genetics and Genomics (ACMG). *Genetics in Medicine, 25*(2), 1–12. https://doi.org/10.1016/j.gim.2022.11.004

Infection

1. Rapid plasma reagin (RPR), Venereal Disease Research Laboratory (VDRL), or fluorescent treponemal antibody absorption test for syphilis is done on the initial visit; repeat testing at 32 weeks, as indicated.
2. Gonorrhea—cervical cultures are usually done at the initial visit and when symptoms are present.
3. HSV—all visible lesions are cultured, and the cervix is cultured weekly, beginning 4 to 8 weeks before delivery.
4. Chlamydia—done at the initial visit and when symptoms are present.
5. Rubella titer—immunity is 10 IU/mL or greater.
6. Hepatitis B surface antigen.
7. HIV—screening is recommended in all pregnancies.

Other Tests

1. Toxoplasmosis—done as indicated for those at risk.
2. Tuberculin skin tests—done as indicated for symptoms, contact, or high risk.
3. Papanicolaou (Pap) smear—done unless recent results are available.
4. Sickle cell screen—done to detect the presence of sickle hemoglobin in those at risk.

5. Group B beta *Streptococcus* (rectovaginal swab)—done to detect carriers or active GBS.
6. Drug screen—done to decrease possible neonatal abstinence syndrome.

Physical Assessment

General Examination

1. Voiding before the examination will enhance comfort and facilitate palpation of the uterus and pelvic organs during the vaginal examination.
2. Evaluation of weight and BP.
3. Examination of the eyes, ears, and nose—nasal congestion during pregnancy may occur as a result of peripheral vasodilation.
4. Examination of the mouth, teeth, throat, and thyroid—the gums may be hyperemic and softened because of increased progesterone.
5. Inspection of breasts and nipples—the breasts may be enlarged and tender; nipple and areolar pigment may be darkened.
6. Auscultation of the heart.
7. Auscultation and percussion of the lungs.

Abdominal Examination

1. Examination for scars or striations, diastasis recti (separation of the rectus muscle), or umbilical hernia.
2. Palpation of the abdomen for fundal height (palpable after 13 weeks of pregnancy); measurement recorded and used as a guideline for subsequent calculations.
3. Palpation of the abdomen for fetal outline and position (Leopold maneuvers)—third trimester.
4. Check for FHTs—FHTs are audible with a Doppler after 10 to 12 weeks and at 18 to 20 weeks with a fetoscope.
5. Record fetal position, presentation, and FHTs.

Pelvic Examination

1. The patient is placed in the lithotomy position.
2. Inspection of external genitalia.
3. Vaginal examination—done to rule out abnormalities of the birth canal and to obtain cytologic smear (Pap and, if indicated, smears for gonorrhea, vaginal trichomoniasis, candidiasis, herpes, group B beta *Streptococcus*, and chlamydia) (see Figure 32-5).
4. Examination of the cervix for position, size, mobility, and consistency. Cervix is softened and bluish (increased vascularity) during pregnancy.
5. Identification of the ovaries (size, shape, and position).
6. Rectovaginal exploration to identify hemorrhoids, fissures, herniation, or masses.
7. Evaluation of pelvic inlet—anteroposterior diameter by measuring the diagonal conjugate (see Figure 32-3, page 964).

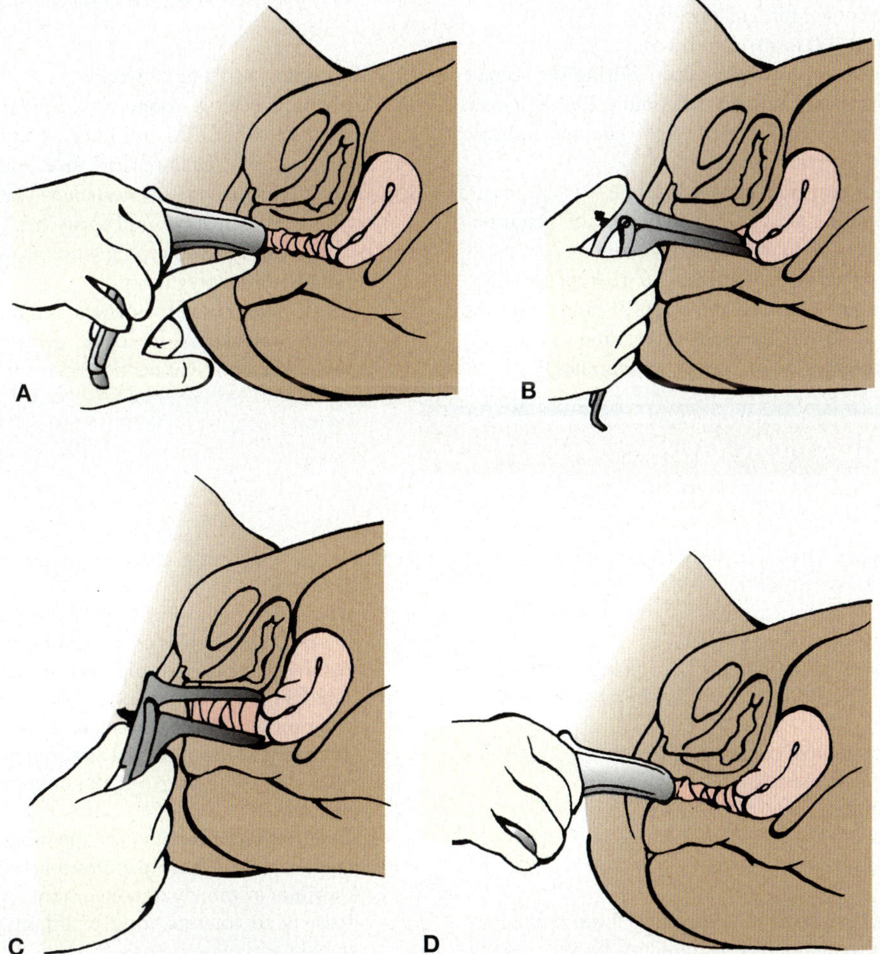

Figure 32-5. Vaginal speculum examination. **(A)** Blades held obliquely on entering the introitus. **(B)** Blades rotated to horizontal position and pushed toward the cervix. **(C)** Blades separated to encircle the cervix. **(D)** Blades removed with gentle pulling.

8. Evaluation of midpelvis—prominence of the ischial spines.
9. Evaluation of pelvic outlet—distance between ischial tuberosities and mobility of coccyx.

Subsequent Prenatal Assessments

1. Uterine growth and estimated fetal growth (see Figure 32-6).
   a. Fundus at symphysis pubis indicates 12 weeks of gestation.
   b. Fundus at umbilicus indicates 20 weeks of gestation.
   c. Fundal height corresponds to GA between 22 and 34 weeks.
   d. Fundus at the lower border of rib cage indicates 36 weeks of gestation.
   e. Uterus becomes globular and drop indicates 40 weeks of gestation.
2. A greater fundal height suggests:
   a. Multiple pregnancy.
   b. Miscalculated due date.
   c. Hydramnios (excessive amniotic fluid).
   d. Gestational trophoblastic disease (degeneration of villi into grapelike clusters; fetus does not usually develop).
   e. Uterine fibroids.
3. A lesser fundal height suggests:
   a. Intrauterine fetal growth restriction.
   b. Error in estimating gestation.
   c. Fetal or amniotic fluid abnormalities.
   d. Intrauterine fetal death.
   e. SGA.
4. FHTs—palpate abdomen for fetal position.
   a. Normal—110 to 160 beats/min (bpm).
5. Weight—major increase in weight occurs during the second half of pregnancy; usually between 0.5 pound (0.2 kg)/week and 1 pound (0.5 kg)/week. Greater weight gain may indicate fluid retention and hypertensive disorder.
6. BP—should remain near prepregnant baseline.
7. Complete blood count at 28 and 32 weeks of gestation; VDRL—rechecked at 36 to 40 weeks of gestation.
8. Antibody serology screen if Rh negative at 36 weeks of gestation.
9. Culture smears for gonorrhea, chlamydia, GBS, and herpes, as indicated; usually at 36 and 40 weeks of gestation.
10. Urinalysis—for protein, glucose, blood, and nitrates.

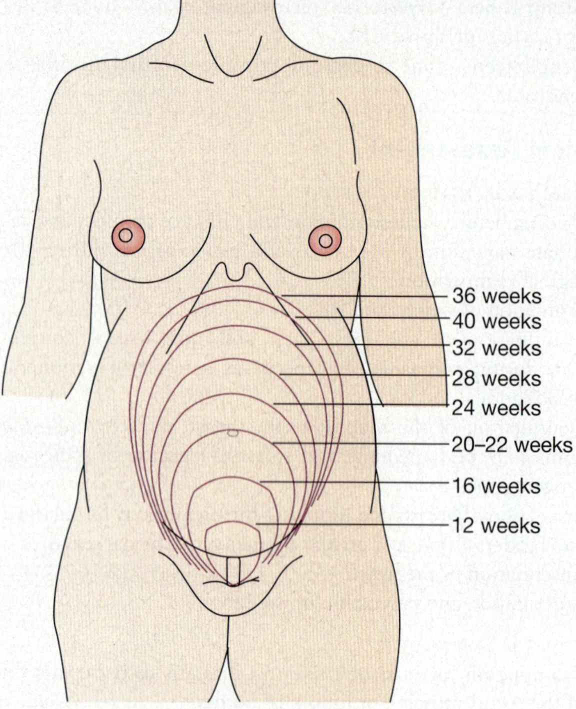

Figure 32-6. Height of fundus. (LifeART image copyright [c] 2024. Lippincott Williams & Wilkins. All rights reserved.)

11. AFP—done at 15 to 20 weeks.
12. Diabetic screening—done, as indicated, at 24 to 28 weeks.
13. Administer RhoGAM, as indicated, at 28 weeks.
14. Edema—check the lower legs, face, and hands.
15. Evaluate discomforts of pregnancy—fatigue, heartburn, hemorrhoids, constipation, and backache.
16. Evaluate eating and sleeping patterns, general adjustment and coping with the pregnancy.
17. Evaluate concerns of the patient and family.
18. Evaluate preparation for labor, delivery, and caregiving. See Patient Education Guidelines 32-1.

PATIENT EDUCATION GUIDELINES 32-1

Prenatal Care

- It is important to keep scheduled prenatal care appointments:
  - Weeks 1 to 28: Every month.
  - Weeks 28 to 36: Every 2 weeks.
  - Weeks 36 to delivery: Every week.
- Expect the following discomforts of pregnancy, and speak with your nurse or health care provider about strategies for relief:
  - Back pain, leg cramps, breast tenderness.
  - Morning sickness, heartburn.
  - Frequent urination.
  - Constipation.
  - Swelling of legs, varicose veins.
  - Fatigue.
- Follow a healthy, balanced diet equal to three meals per day and take prenatal vitamins as directed by your health care provider.
- Get regular exercise and use proper body mechanics to avoid injury.
- Be aware of danger symptoms of pregnancy; these must be reported to your health care provider promptly:
  - Vision disturbances—blurring, spots, or double vision.
  - Vaginal bleeding, new or old blood.
  - Edema of the face, fingers, and sacrum.
  - Headaches—frequent, severe, or continuous.
  - Fluid discharge from vagina; unusual or severe abdominal pain.
  - Chills, fever, or burning on urination.
  - Epigastric pain (severe stomachache).
  - Muscular irritability or convulsions.
  - Inability to tolerate food or liquids, leading to severe nausea and hyperemesis.

Nursing Management

Nursing Interventions and Patient Education

Minimizing Pain

1. Teach patient to use good body mechanics—wear comfortable, low-heeled shoes with good arch support; try the use of a maternity girdle.
2. Instruct patient on the technique for pelvic-rocking exercises.
3. Encourage patient to take rest periods with legs elevated.
4. Inform patient that adequate calcium intake may decrease leg cramps.
5. Instruct patient to dorsiflex the foot while applying pressure to the knee to straighten the leg for immediate relief of leg cramps.
6. Instruct patient to wear a fitted, supportive bra.
7. Instruct patient to wash breasts and nipples with water only.
8. Instruct patient to apply vitamin E or lanolin cream to the breast and nipple area. Lanolin is contraindicated for those with allergies to lamb's wool.

Minimizing Morning Sickness and Heartburn and Maintaining Adequate Nutrition

1. Encourage patient to eat a few bites of a soda cracker or dry toast before getting out of bed in the morning.
2. Instruct patient to rise from bed slowly.
3. Encourage patient to eat low-fat protein foods and dry carbohydrates, such as toast and crackers.
4. Encourage patient to eat small, frequent meals to equal three regular meals, if necessary, to maintain nutrition.
5. Advise patient to eat slowly.
6. Teach patient the importance of good nutrition for self and fetus. Review the basic food groups with appropriate daily servings for essential vitamins and nutrients.
   a. Seven servings of protein-rich foods, including one serving of a vegetable protein.
   b. Three servings of dairy products or other calcium-rich foods.
   c. Seven servings of grain products.
   d. Two or more servings of vitamin C–rich vegetable or fruit.
   e. Three servings of other fruits and vegetables.
   f. Three servings of unsaturated fats.
   g. Two or more servings of other fruits and vegetables.
7. Encourage patient to drink soups and liquids between meals to avoid stomach distention and dehydration.
8. Instruct patient in the use of antacids; caution against the use of sodium bicarbonate because it results in the absorption of excess sodium and fluid retention.
9. Instruct patient to avoid brushing teeth soon after eating.
10. Instruct patient to avoid foods or cooking odors that may trigger nausea.
11. Recommended dietary reference intakes for pregnancy can be obtained from https://www.nal.usda.gov/human-nutrition-and-food-safety/dri-calculator. If vegetarian, assess food intake.
    a. Two broad groups of vegetarians:
       i. Traditional—cultural or religious affiliation prescribes their diet.
       ii. New—adopted vegetarian dietary patterns as a personal or philosophical choice.
    b. Subgroups exist within these two groups:
       i. Vegan—eat foods from a plant origin; eat no animal foods or anything derived from an animal (i.e., eggs, milk, cream, etc.).
       ii. Lacto—eat milk/dairy products, but eat no meat, poultry, fish, seafood, or eggs.
       iii. Lacto-ovo—eat milk/dairy products and eggs, but eat no meat, poultry, fish, or seafood.
       iv. Pesce—eat foods from a plant origin and fish or cheese, but no meat, poultry, or eggs.
    c. Partial vegetarians may exclude a specific type of animal food, usually meat, but may consume fish and poultry.
    d. Recommend iron and folic acid supplements.
12. Inform patient that average weight gain in pregnancy is 25 to 35 pounds (11 to 16 kg). About 2 to 5 pounds (0.9 to 2.3 kg) are gained in the first trimester and about 1 pound (0.5 kg) per week for the remainder of the gestation.
    a. Average weight gain if patient has obesity is 15 pounds (6.8 kg).
    b. Adolescent weight gain should be about 5 pounds (2.3 kg) more than for adult if within 2 years of starting menses.
    c. Multiple pregnancies should gain between 35 and 45 pounds (16 and 20 kg).
    d. Average weight gain if underweight is 28 to 40 pounds (13 to 18 kg).
    e. Assess for any cultural or religious times of fasting (e.g., Lent or Ramadan).
13. Advise patient to limit the use of caffeine.
14. Inform patient that alcohol should be eliminated during pregnancy because no safe level of intake has been established.
15. Inform patient that smoking should be eliminated or severely reduced during pregnancy related to the increased risk of spontaneous abortion, fetal death, low birth weight, and neonatal death.
16. Inform patient that ingesting any drug during pregnancy may affect fetal growth and should be discussed with health care provider.
17. Social support is available from the WIC Special Supplemental Feeding Program, breastfeeding groups (La Leche League https://www.llli.org/), and other support groups.

Minimizing Urinary Frequency and Promoting Elimination

1. Instruct patient to limit fluid intake in the evening and to void before going to bed.
2. Encourage patient to void after meals, with the urge to void, and after sexual intercourse.
3. Encourage patient to wear loose-fitting cotton underwear.
4. Cranberry or blueberry juice may be recommended to help prevent UTIs.
5. Caffeine should be avoided.

Avoiding Constipation

1. Instruct patient to increase fluid intake to at least eight glasses of water per day. One to 2 quarts of fluid per day is desirable.
2. Encourage daily intake of foods high in fiber.
3. Encourage patient to establish regular patterns of elimination.
4. Encourage daily exercise, such as walking.
5. Inform patient that OTC laxatives should be avoided. Providers may recommend stool softeners or bulk-forming agents as indicated.

Maintaining Tissue Integrity

1. Encourage frequent rest periods with legs elevated.
2. Teach the patient how to don support stockings and wear loose-fitting clothing for leg varicosities.

3. Instruct patient to avoid constipation, apply cold compresses, take sitz baths, and use topical anesthetics, such as Tucks, for the relief of anal varicosities (hemorrhoids).

Reducing Anxiety and Fear and Promoting Preparation for Labor, Delivery, and Postpartum Considerations

Those who attended childbirth preparation have reported increased satisfaction with their birth experience. Additional benefits to childbirth preparation include improved breastfeeding rates and decreased use of pharmacologic pain management. The nurse should facilitate education related to the following:

1. Current knowledge, perceptions, cultural values, and expectations of the labor and delivery process and caregiving.
2. Availability of childbirth preparation classes that include infant care, breastfeeding, and caregiving and encourage attendance.
3. Availability of sibling and grandparent preparation, as indicated.
4. A tour of the birth facility.
5. Common procedures that may be performed during labor and birth.
6. Creating a personalized birth plan to include coping and relaxation techniques and pain management options both nonpharmacologic and pharmacologic, for labor and birth.
7. General guidelines for coming to the birth facility.
8. Preparations for the infant, such as a sleeping space, clothing, feeding, changing, and bathing equipment.

Enhancing Role Changes

1. Encourage discussion of feelings and concerns regarding new parental roles.
2. Provide emotional support to the patient and partner regarding the altered family roles.
3. Discuss physiologic causes for changes in sexual relationships, such as fatigue, loss of interest, and discomfort from advancing pregnancy. Some patients experience heightened sexual activity during the second trimester.
4. Teach the patient that there are no contraindications to intercourse or masturbation or orgasm, provided the membranes are intact, there is no vaginal bleeding, and there are no current problems or history of premature labor.
5. Teach the patient and partner that maternal superior or side-lying positions are usually more comfortable in the latter half of pregnancy.

Minimizing Fatigue

1. Teach the patient reasons for fatigue and encourage the scheduling of adequate rest.
   a. Fatigue in the first trimester is due to increased progesterone and its effects on the sleep center.
   b. Fatigue in the third trimester is due mainly to carrying the increased weight of the pregnancy.
   c. About 8 hours of rest are recommended with frequent 15- to 30-minute rest periods to avoid overfatigue.
   d. Whenever possible, the patient should work while sitting with legs elevated.
   e. The patient should avoid standing for prolonged periods, especially during the third trimester.
   f. To promote placental perfusion, the patient should not lie flat on the back—left lateral position provides the best placental perfusion; however, either side is acceptable. In the third trimester of pregnancy, sleeping with a small pillow under the abdomen may enhance comfort.
2. Help the patient plan for adequate exercise (if not contraindicated).
   a. Exercise during pregnancy should be in keeping with prepregnancy exercise patterns and type.
   b. Activities or sports that have a risk of bodily harm (skiing, snowmobiling, ice skating, inline skating, horseback riding) should be avoided.
   c. During pregnancy, endurance during exercise may be decreased.
   d. Exercise classes during pregnancy that concentrate on toning and stretching have resulted in enhanced physical condition, increased self-esteem, and greater social support as a result of being in the exercise group.
   e. Contraindications to aerobic exercise during pregnancy include hemodynamically significant heart disease, restrictive lung disease, incompetent cervix, cerclage, multiple gestations at risk for PTL, persistent second- or third-trimester bleeding, placenta previa after 26 weeks of gestation, ruptured membranes, PTL in current pregnancy, and preeclampsia.

CLINICAL JUDGMENT Exercise in pregnancy benefits both the patient and the fetus by enhancing overall health and fitness by promoting adequate weight gain, strengthened muscle tone, and reduced blood sugar. Outcomes demonstrate a decrease in operative delivery, gestational diabetes, and hypertension. Encourage regular exercise for all who are able. Identify those activities that may increase the risk of injury and those patients with pregnancy complications in whom exercise may be contraindicated.

EVIDENCE BASE American College of Obstetricians and Gynecologists. (2020). Physical activity and exercise during pregnancy and the postpartum period: Committee Opinion, Number 804. *Obstetrics and Gynecology*, *135*(4), e178–e188. https://doi.org/10.1097/AOG.0000000000003772

Alternative Therapies

General Measures

1. Be aware that alternative therapies range from nutrition and lifestyle changes to mind and body programs.
   a. Physical activities—maintaining an active lifestyle and healthy diet. Some use macrobiotic diets and isometric exercise.
   b. Attitudinal activities—maintaining a positive attitude and self-image; have fun and laugh.
   c. Relational activities—maintaining social relationships—friends, pets, and family.
   d. Spiritual activities—having faith, hope, prayer, and music and meditating as an active part of daily life.
   e. Self-caring activities—taking care of self, balancing life, personal integrity, knowing and trusting self, and own time management.
   f. Help-seeking activities—seeking assistance in health care ranging from prescribed treatments to biomedicine (self-healing touch). Help-seeking activities include ethnomedicine (Chinese herbal medicine and acupuncture), structure/energy therapies (therapeutic touch and osteopathy), pharmacologic/biologic treatments (antioxidants), biofeedback, guided imagery, music therapy, meditation, and prayer.
2. Encourage patient to discuss options with health care provider, and consult a credentialed naturopath, acupuncturist, or another complementary practitioner.

Alternative Therapies Specific to the Prenatal Period

1. Advise the patient to discuss the use of herbs with the obstetric provider before use, become familiar with manufacturers, and ask questions. Although herbs are natural, they can be harmful if misused. Herbs should be used with the same respect as medications.
2. Advise the patient to become aware that herbs come in different forms—capsules, tablets, extracts, tinctures, powders, dried and prepared as teas or juices, in combinations, and as external preparations. It is important to understand the dosage of a particular product based on form.
3. Become familiar with herbal therapies that are Food and Drug Administration approved, which include:
   a. Aloe, cascara (sacred bark, bitter bark), psyllium (plantago seed), and senna, which are used as a laxative.
   b. Capsicum or cayenne pepper (chili pepper, red pepper) as a topical analgesic; marketed as a cream and used topically.
   c. Slippery elm (red elm) as an oral demulcent; marketed as throat lozenges.
4. Be aware of other herbal preparations and their uses.
   a. Catnip, fennel, lobelia, papaya, spearmint, and wild yams decrease colic, stomach cramps, gas, and heartburn. They also improve appetite.
   b. Cranberry or blueberry juices are used for UTI prevention.
   c. Nausea is sometimes attributed to vitamin B deficiencies but does not always improve with simple vitamin supplements. Red raspberry, peppermint, spearmint, or chamomile tea and ginger root or ginger ale may be used to alleviate nausea. To increase the effectiveness of red raspberry tea, alfalfa may be added to the tea.
5. Refer for acupressure or acupuncture, which may assist with the relief of nausea.
6. Refer for other therapies to increase well-being, including therapeutic touch and yoga.

EVIDENCE BASE National Center for Complementary and Integrative Health. (2020). *Be an informed consumer.* https://www.nccih.nih.gov/health/be-an-informed-consumer

Evaluation: Expected Outcomes

- Verbalizes understanding of proper body mechanics and wears low-heeled shoes.
- Identifies the basic food groups and describes meals to include needed servings for pregnancy.
- Reports limited fluid intake in the evening.
- Describes foods high in fiber.
- Wears support stockings and loose-fitting clothing.
- Discusses expectations for attending educational classes, labor, delivery, postpartum period, and newborn care.
- Verbalizes an understanding of the physiologic causes that may change the sexual relationship.
- Reports engaging in regular exercise.

Psychosocial Adaptation of Pregnancy

EVIDENCE BASE Ruyak, S. L. (2024). Psychology of pregnancy. In B. Baker & J. Janke (Eds.), *Core curriculum for maternal-newborn nursing* (6th ed., pp. 117–126). Elsevier.

Rubin's Framework for Maternal Role Attainment

1. Attainment of the maternal role occurs with each pregnancy.
2. Involves a series of cognitive operations:
   a. Mimicry—observing and modeling behavior of others who are pregnant.
   b. Role-play—acting out behaviors of the maternal role (e.g., rocking a baby to sleep).
   c. Searching for a role "fit"—perceptions of how the maternal role will be; observes others' behaviors to determine how well they fit with expectations of the maternal role.
   d. Grief work—experiences a sense of loss of "old" self as preparing to begin new maternal role.
3. Maternal tasks—commonly divided by trimesters.
   a. First trimester:
      i. Acceptance of pregnancy—moves from a state of conflict and ambivalence to one of acceptance of the pregnancy, the child, and the maternal role.
      ii. Realignment of roles—begins to realign their roles and responsibilities as they relate to the child.
      iii. Safe passage—although they seek to ensure a safe passage for their fetus and self throughout pregnancy, the main focus during this trimester is on self-safety.
   b. Second trimester:
      i. Safe passage—in this trimester, the main focus is on appropriate nutrition and exercise.
      ii. Acceptance by others—acceptance of the child by each family member.
      iii. Binding-in to the child—maternal perception of the child as a real person.
   c. Third trimester:
      i. Safe passage—during this trimester, the main focus is on the safety of the fetus and is inseparable from self-safety.
      ii. Giving of oneself—the most complex task; they learn to place the fetus's needs in relation to their own needs.
      iii. Critical to this trimester is the preparation of the nursery because it solidifies the acceptance of the unborn child.

Rubin's Framework for Paternal Role Attainment

1. The paternal role can also be attained with the pregnancy.
2. Paternal tasks can also be divided by trimesters.
   a. First trimester:
      i. Announcement and realization of the pregnancy—exhibits excitement over the announcement of the pregnancy and is more interested in maternal changes. Usually, insists on accompanying the patient to each prenatal appointment.
      ii. May begin to experience the same signs and symptoms of pregnancy experienced in the maternal role. This is commonly referred to as *couvade syndrome.*
   b. Second trimester:
      i. Anticipation—anticipates and adapts to the paternal role.
      ii. Fantasy and exploration—along with partner, begins to imagine what the child will look like and may also begin to think about the child's future talents and attributes.
      iii. Adjustment of sexual expression to accommodate the pregnancy.

c. Third trimester:
   i. Preparation—now, serious preparation for the forthcoming child includes preparation of the nursery and childbirth education courses to prepare for labor and delivery.
   ii. Reassurance—provided to ease their anxious partner's fears regarding labor and delivery.

THE FETUS

EVIDENCE BASE Founds, S. A., & Baker, B. (2024). Fetal and placental development and functioning. In B. Baker & J. Janke (Eds.), *Core curriculum for maternal-newborn nursing* (6th ed., pp. 27–44). Elsevier.

Fetal Growth and Development

Advances in knowledge and technology have provided newer methods for assessing fetal well-being and maturity. Improved methods for assessment and diagnosis enable early intervention for improved outcomes. See Figure 32-7 for critical periods of fetal growth.

Stages of Growth and Development

The growth and development of the fetus is typically divided into three stages.

Preembryonic Stage: Fertilization to 2 to 3 Weeks

1. Rapid cell division and differentiation.
2. Develop embryonic membranes and germ layers.

Embryonic Stage: 4 to 8 Weeks of Gestation

1. Most critical stage of physical development.
2. Organogenesis.

Fetal Stage: 9 Weeks to Birth

1. Every organ system and external structure present.
2. Refinement of fetus and organ function occurs.

Development by Month

First Lunar Month

1. Fertilization to 2 weeks of embryonic growth.
2. Implantation is complete.
3. Primary chorionic villi forming.
4. Embryo develops into two cell layers (trophoblast and blastocyst).
5. Amniotic cavity appears.

Second Lunar Month

1. Three to 6 weeks of embryonic growth.
2. At the end of 6 weeks of growth, the embryo is approximately ½ in (1.3 cm) long.
3. Arm and leg buds are visible; arm buds are more developed, with finger ridges beginning to appear.
4. Rudiments of the eyes, ears, and nose appear.
5. Lung buds are developing.
6. Primitive intestinal tract is developing.
7. Primitive cardiovascular system is functioning.
8. Neural tube, which forms the brain and spinal cord, closes by the fourth week.

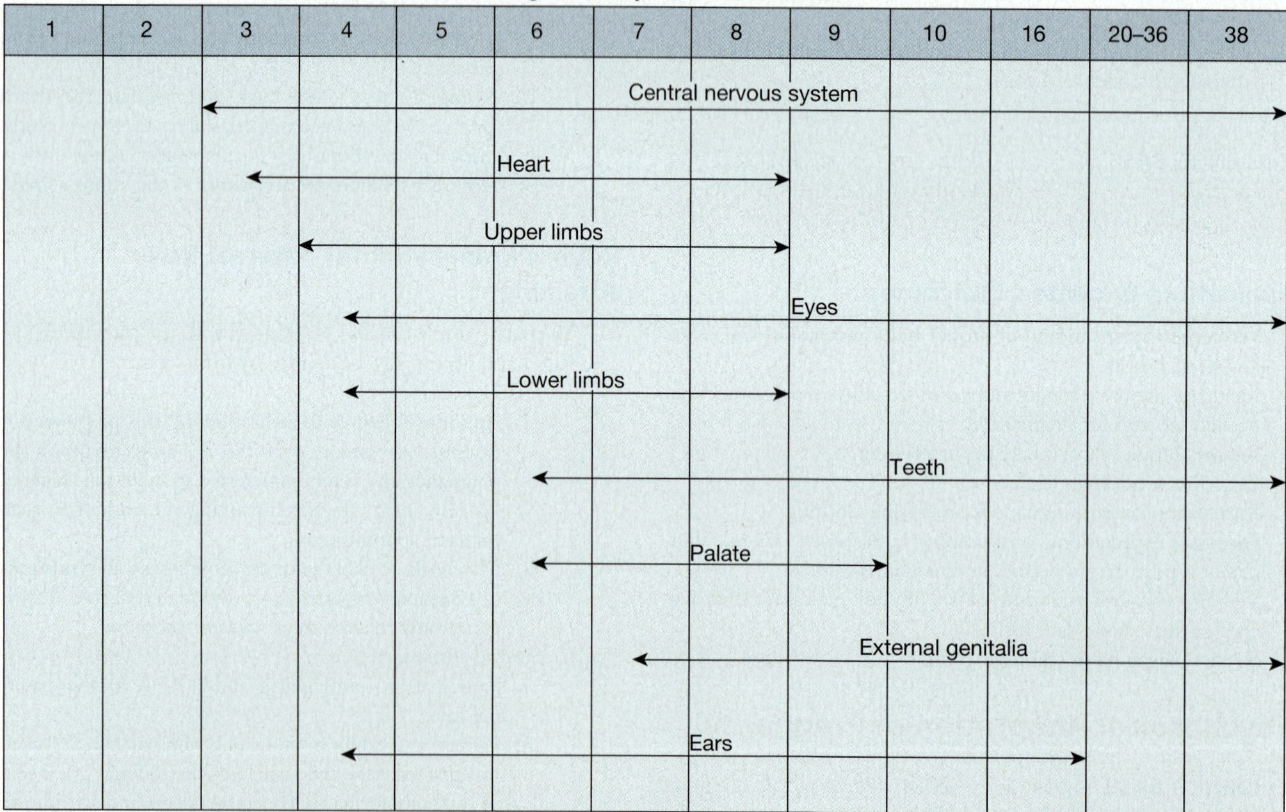

Figure 32-7. Critical periods of fetal growth. (Reprinted with permission from Silbert-Flagg, J. (2023). *Maternal and child health nursing* (9th ed., Fig. 9-4). Lippincott Williams & Wilkins.)

Third Lunar Month

1. Seven to 10 weeks of growth.
2. The middle of this period (9 weeks) marks the end of the embryonic period and the beginning of the fetal period.
3. At the end of 10 weeks of growth, the fetus is approximately 2½ in (6.3 cm) from crown to rump and weighs ½ oz (14 g).
4. Appearance of external genitalia.
5. By the middle of this month, all major organ systems have formed.
6. The membrane over the anus has broken down.
7. The heart has formed four chambers (by the seventh week).
8. The fetus assumes a human appearance.
9. Bone ossification begins.
10. Rudimentary kidney begins to secrete urine.

Fourth Lunar Month

1. Eleven- to 14-week-old fetus.
2. At the end of 14 weeks of growth, the fetus is approximately 4¾ in (12 cm) crown–rump length and 3¾ oz (110 g).
3. Head erect; lower extremities well developed.
4. Hard palate and nasal septum have fused.
5. External genitalia of male and female can now be differentiated.
6. Eyelids are sealed.

Fifth Lunar Month

1. Fifteen- to 18-week-old fetus.
2. At the end of 18 weeks of growth, the fetus is approximately 6¼ in (16 cm) crown–rump length and 11¼ oz (320 g).
3. Ossification of fetal skeleton can be seen on x-ray.
4. Ears stand out from head.
5. Meconium is present in the intestinal tract.
6. Fetus makes sucking motions and swallows amniotic fluid.
7. Fetal movements may be felt by the patient (end of month).

Sixth Lunar Month

1. Nineteen- to 22-week-old fetus.
2. At the end of 22 weeks of growth, the fetus is approximately 8¼ in (21 cm) crown–rump length and 1 pound, 6¼ oz (630 g).
3. Vernix caseosa covers the skin.
4. Head and body (lanugo) hair visible.
5. Skin is wrinkled and red.
6. Brown fat, an important site of heat production, is present in the neck and sternal area.
7. Nipples are apparent on the breasts.

Seventh Lunar Month

1. Twenty-three- to 26-week-old fetus.
2. At the end of 26 weeks of growth, the fetus is approximately 10 in (25 cm) crown–rump length and 2 pounds, 3¼ oz (1,000 g).
3. Fingernails present.
4. Lean body.
5. Eyes partially open; eyelashes present.
6. Bronchioles are present; primitive alveoli are forming.
7. Skin begins to thicken on hands and feet.
8. Startle reflex present; grasp reflex is strong.

Eighth Lunar Month

1. Twenty seven- to 30-week-old fetus.
2. At the end of 30 weeks of growth, the fetus is approximately 11 in (28 cm) crown–rump length and 3 pounds, 12 oz (1,700 g).
3. Eyes open.
4. Ample hair on head; lanugo begins to fade.
5. Skin slightly wrinkled.
6. Toenails present.
7. Testes in inguinal canal begin descent to scrotal sac.
8. Surfactant coats much of the alveolar epithelium.

Ninth Lunar Month

1. Thirty one- to 34-week-old fetus.
2. At the end of 34 weeks of growth, the fetus is approximately 12½ in (32 cm) crown–rump length and 5 pounds (2,267 g), 8 oz (2,500 g).
3. Fingernails reach fingertips.
4. Skin appears smooth rather than wrinkled.
5. Testes in scrotal sac.

Tenth Lunar Month

1. Thirty five- to 38-week-old fetus; end of this month is also 40 weeks from onset of last menses.
2. At the end of 38 weeks of growth, fetus is approximately 14½ in (37 cm) crown–rump length and 6.6 pounds (2,900 g), 8 oz (3,400 g).
3. Ample subcutaneous fat.
4. Lanugo almost absent.
5. Toenails reach toe tips.
6. Testes in scrotum.
7. Vernix caseosa mainly on the back.
8. Breasts are firm.

Fetal Circulation

See Figure 32-8.

Assessment of Fetal Maturity and Well-Being

EVIDENCE BASE American College of Obstetricians and Gynecologists. (2021). Antepartum fetal surveillance (Practice Bulletin, no. 229). *Obstetrics and Gynecology, 137*(6), e116–e127. https://doi.org/10.1097/AOG.0000000000004410

American College of Obstetricians and Gynecologists. (2020). Screening for fetal chromosomal abnormalities (Practice Bulletin, no. 226). *Obstetrics and Gynecology, 136*(4), e48–e69. https://doi.org/10.1097/AOG.0000000000004084

Maternal History and Examination

1. Comprehensive family medical history, personal medical history, and reproductive health history, including previous pregnancy experience/outcomes and sexually transmitted infections (STIs).
2. Comprehensive physical examination, history of current pregnancy, and identified risk factors.
3. Routine prenatal labs.
4. Fetal assessment after the first trimester and individualized fetal surveillance, as indicated.

Fetal Heart Tones

Description

Fetal heart tones (FHTs) represent the fetal heart rate (FHR) and are an indicator of oxygen perfusion to the fetal brain, heart, and adrenals. The evaluation of FHTs is indicated in routine assessment of fetal well-being, in determining gestational age, and in cases of threatened abortion or other abnormalities. FHTs can be heard using techniques that amplify sound.

1. Doppler at approximately 10 to 12 weeks of fetal gestation.
2. Fetoscope (fetal stethoscope) at approximately 18 to 20 weeks of fetal gestation.

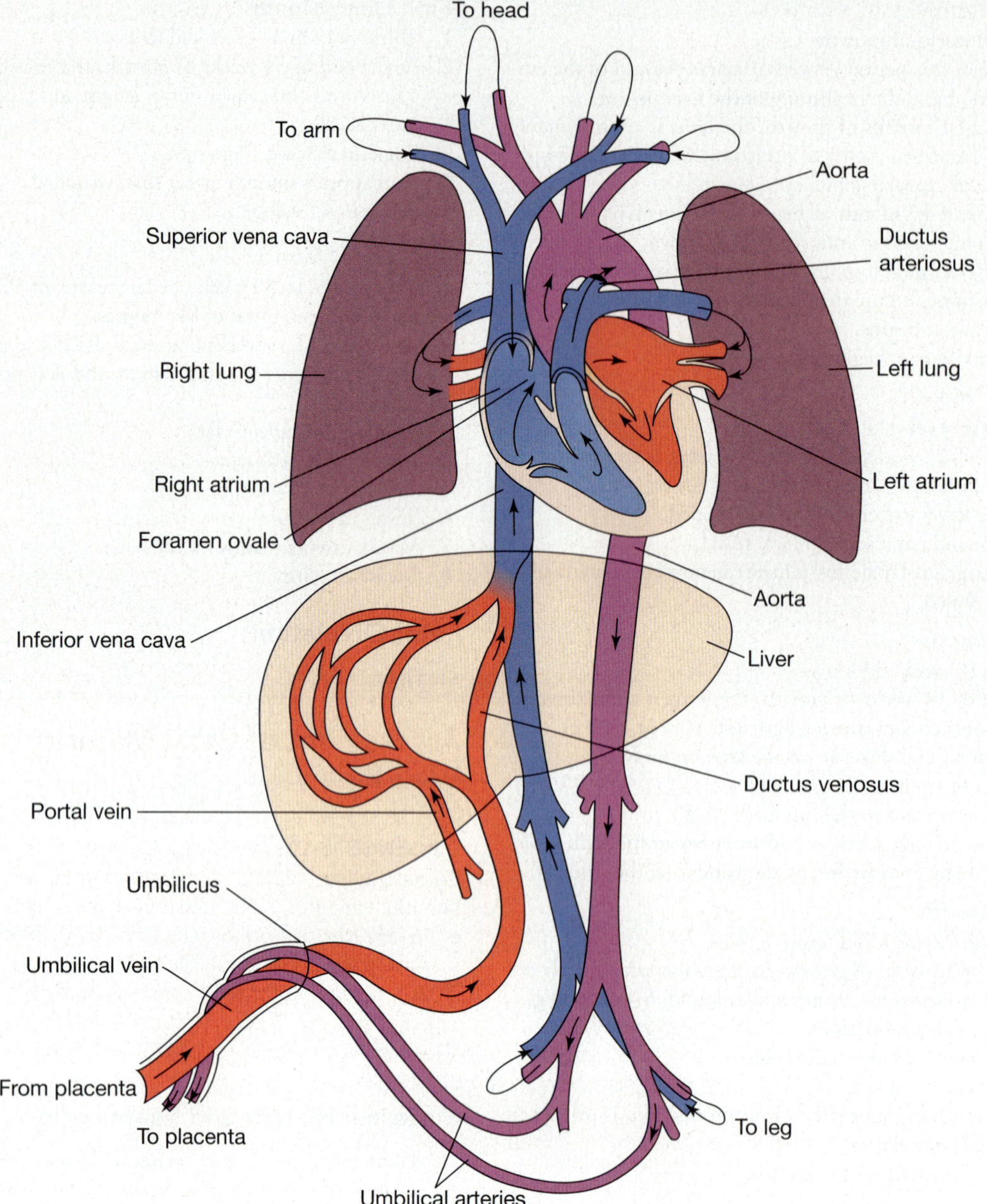

Figure 32-8. Diagram of the fetal circulation shortly before birth. Arrows indicate course of blood. (Reprinted with permission from Silbert-Flagg, J. (2023). *Maternal and child health nursing* (9th ed., Fig. 9-5). Lippincott Williams & Wilkins.)

3. Electronic fetal monitoring testing is usually done when the fetus is considered viable, around 24 weeks of gestation.
4. Rate—between 110 and 160 beats/min (bpm).
5. In the later months of pregnancy, fetal heart sounds found:
   a. Near the pregnant patient's midline in fetal occipit-anterior (OA) positions.
   b. Lateral to midline in fetal occipit-transverse (OT) positions.
   c. In the patient's flank in fetal occipit-posterior (OP) positions.
   d. Below the patient's umbilicus in cephalic presentations.
   e. At or above the patient's umbilicus in breech presentations.
   f. Position may affect the ability to clearly hear the heart tones.
6. Failure to hear FHTs at the expected time may be due to maternal obesity, polyhydramnios, error in date calculation, or fetal death.

Nursing and Patient Care Considerations

1. Explain the equipment, purpose, and procedure to the patient.
2. Assist patient to a side-lying or semi-Fowler position. Perform Leopold maneuvers.
3. Document findings in the patient's chart with date, time, activity level, medications, and other information per facility's guidelines.
4. Discontinue electronic fetal monitoring, as indicated, according to facility guidelines.
5. Document and communicate appropriate information in the patient record to the patient and provider.
6. Ensure that fetal tracings remain part of the records of the neonate and of the patient who is pregnant. They are legal documents that may be used in litigation. When electronic documentation is unavailable for archiving the patient record, paper record must be saved.

Assessment of Fetal Movement

Description

Fetal movement or "kick counts" may be evaluated daily by the patient who is pregnant to provide reassurance of fetal well-being. Several methods are used in practice, but study comparisons do not provide sufficient evidence to influence practice related to the ideal number of kicks or the ideal interval for movement counting. Methods are facility specific, and policy should be standardized for consistency. Testing can be as short as 5 minutes or as long as 2 hours.

Nursing and Patient Care Considerations

1. Instruct patient to lie on the side in a quiet place with no distractions. Have the patient place hands on the largest part of the abdomen and concentrate on fetal movement.
2. Instruct patient to use a clock and record the movements felt. Once the 10th movement is felt, the testing is stopped. If fewer than 10 movements are felt in 2 hours or if the time it takes to get the 10 movements takes longer to achieve than earlier testing, the patient should contact obstetric provider.
3. Instruct patient that fetal movements are best assessed after meals, after or with light abdominal massage, or after short walks; advise the patient to avoid smoking for the last 2 hours prior to assessment.
4. Instruct patient that the fetus can sleep for up to 40 minutes.
5. Request patient to explain the procedure so understanding is ensured.

Alpha-Fetoprotein

Description

Alpha-fetoprotein (AFP) is produced by the fetus' liver and present in amniotic fluid. Small amounts cross the placenta into the maternal circulation.

1. Maternal serum alpha-fetoprotein (MS-AFP) levels are analyzed at 15 to 20 weeks of gestation to primarily identify neural tube defects of anencephaly and open spinal defects and may be tested either alone or with a triple or quad screening. This testing is not diagnostic, and further diagnostic testing may be indicated.
   a. Elevated MS-AFP levels may be associated with congenital anomalies and chromosomal abnormalities, such as open neural tube defects, open abdominal defects, and congenital nephrosis. Also associated with Rh isoimmunization, multiple gestation, maternal diabetes mellitus, and fetoplacental dysfunction.
   b. Decreased levels have been associated with Down syndrome and other chromosomal anomalies (e.g., gestational trophoblastic disease) but are not diagnostic.
   c. Follow-up for abnormal high or low levels includes ultrasound examination and amniocentesis.
2. Triple marker screening (TMS) can also be used for the evaluation of trisomies 18 and 21 and neural tube defects. This test is costly when compared to MS-AFP; thus, it is limited in its use. The TMS evaluates unconjugated estriol and human chorionic gonadotropin (hCG): Down syndrome shows increased hCG and decreased estriol levels; trisomy 18 shows decreased hCG and decreased estriol levels.
3. The quadruple screen, which includes a measurement of the substance dimeric inhibin A, provides a more sensitive and accurate detection of trisomy 21.

Nursing and Patient Care Considerations

1. Obtain health and pregnancy history, including the date of patient's last menses and risk factors. Accurate dating of the pregnancy is crucial to interpret the results of the serum levels.
2. Explain the purpose and procedure for the test.
3. Explain that the testing is for screening purposes only and not diagnostic. If an abnormal result is detected, further testing may be recommended.
4. Discuss patient's concerns.

Ultrasound and Doppler Studies

Description

Ultrasonography is a noninvasive, safe technique that uses reflected sound waves as they travel in tissue to produce a picture. In the abdominal approach, a clear gel is applied to the patient's abdomen or to the transducer, and the transducer is moved along the abdomen by the examiner. Images are produced on a screen. During the early weeks of gestation, when the uterus remains a pelvic organ, a full bladder may be necessary to facilitate visualization. In the transvaginal approach, a lubricated transducer probe is inserted (either by the patient or by the examiner) into the vagina. No full bladder is necessary, and this technique is especially useful during the early weeks of pregnancy or when cervical evaluation is important (i.e., for assessment of preterm labor [PTL]). Three-dimensional (3D) ultrasonography is a newer technology that is believed to offer improved assessment of fetal growth and weight parameters.

1. Indications for a first trimester (prior to 13 6/7 weeks of gestation) ultrasonography:
   a. Early confirmation of intrauterine pregnancy.
   b. To confirm cardiac activity.
   c. Estimated date of confinement.
   d. Estimate gestational age.
   e. To evaluate for an ectopic pregnancy or gestational trophoblastic disease.
   f. Detection of an intrauterine device.
   g. Evaluation of placental location.
   h. Diagnosis of multiple gestation.
   i. Guidance for chorionic villous sampling (CVS) between 10 and 13 weeks requiring a small sample of placental tissue for prenatal diagnosis of certain chromosomal abnormalities when early diagnosis is preferred.
   j. Nuchal translucency at 11 to 14 weeks to screen for fetal aneuploidy.
2. Indications for second- and third-trimester ultrasonography that may be standard, limited, or specialized as necessary:
   a. Fetal survey for anatomy, growth, weight, gestational age, and anomalies.
   b. Evaluation of the placenta position and attachment.
   c. Evaluation of fetal presentation and position.
   d. Evaluation of fetal viability and cardiac activity.
   e. Biophysical profile (BPP).
   f. Evaluation of amniotic fluid volume.
   g. Guidance for amniocentesis or fetal blood sampling.
3. Doppler flow study, also known as *Doppler velocimetry*, is a noninvasive way to analyze uteroplacental blood flow within the umbilical, uterine, and cerebral arteries. The use of this technology primarily focuses on placental analysis to identify patients at risk for increased perinatal mortality. Systolic and diastolic ratios are measured within the arteries. If the ratios

rise above normal, it means that blood flow to the placenta is decreased.

4. 3D and 4D ultrasonography evaluates major and superficial vessels of the placenta, including the cord, fetal physiologic development, and fetal behavior. There are a number of advantages to 3D and 4D ultrasonography over Doppler velocimetry, such as decreased time of fetal exposure to ultrasound beam (2 to 5 minutes for 3D vs. 15 to 30 minutes for velocimetry), off-line image processing, and identification of placental anastomoses, to mention a few.

Nursing and Patient Care Considerations

1. Explain the purpose and procedure to patient, emphasizing the need to remain still.
2. Inform patient of the need for a full bladder, if indicated, before the procedure.
3. When indicated, instruct patient to drink three to four glasses of water if the bladder is not full.
4. Instruct patient not to void until the procedure is over.
5. Remove the lubricant from patient's abdomen after the procedure or provide perineal cleaning products, as needed.

Note: Nurse can perform ultrasound if credentialed in limited ultrasound.

Amniocentesis

Description

Amniocentesis is a diagnostic procedure requiring informed consent, in which amniotic fluid is removed from the uterine cavity by insertion of a needle through the abdominal and uterine walls and into the amniotic sac. When performed before 20 weeks of gestation, the procedure is used for genetic evaluation. In later pregnancy, amniocentesis is performed for the assessment of fetal lung maturity and to treat hydramnios (also called *polyhydramnios*). Risks are associated with the procedure such as miscarriage (1:300 to 500 procedures), chorioamnionitis, and preterm premature rupture of membranes. In determination of genetic or metabolic diseases, the procedure is performed between 16 and 18 weeks of gestation. It is useful at age 35 years or above; for those with a family history of metabolic disease, a previous child with a chromosomal abnormality, or a family history of chromosomal abnormality; a patient or partner with a chromosomal abnormality; or a possible female carrier of an X-linked disease.

1. In determination of lung maturity, the lecithin/sphingomyelin (L/S) ratio of the amniotic fluid is analyzed.
   a. When the L/S ratio is 2:1 or greater, the fetal lung is considered mature and the incidence of respiratory distress syndrome in the neonate is low.
   b. Results may be less reliable with maternal diabetes or if the fluid is contaminated with blood or meconium.
2. The presence of phosphatidylglycerol (PG), one of the last lung surfactants to develop, is the most reliable indicator of fetal lung maturity. PG is not present until 36 weeks of gestation and is measured as being present or absent. Unlike the L/S ratio, PG is not affected by hypoglycemia, hypoxia, or hypothermia.
3. In the treatment of hydramnios (2,000 mL amniotic fluid or greater than 25 cm amniotic fluid index [AFI]), amniocentesis may be performed to drain excess fluid and relieve pressure. Hydramnios can be associated with specific fetal abnormalities, such as trisomy 18, anencephaly, spina bifida, and esophageal atresia or tracheoesophageal fistula.

Nursing and Patient Care Considerations

1. Reduce anxiety related to the procedure.
   a. Reduce the patient's and partner's anxiety by determining their understanding of the procedure and the meaning it holds for them.
   b. Reexplain the procedure before it begins and answer any questions they have. Ensure informed consent is signed.
   c. Provide explanations during the procedure, correct misinformation they may have, and make sure they know when the results will be available and how they may obtain the results as soon as possible.
2. Reduce pain and discomfort related to the procedure.
   a. Reduce discomfort by having patient lie supine with hands tucked under pillow at the head. Relaxation and controlled breathing may help.
   b. Ensure adequate time between infiltration of local anesthetic and introduction of needle into the amniotic sac.
3. Provide for intravenous (IV) access in accordance with facility policy. Tocolytics such as terbutaline may be administered per facility policy.
4. Reduce potential for traumatic injury to fetus, placenta, or maternal structures.
   a. Have patient empty bladder if the fetus is more than 20 weeks of gestation to avoid injury to the patient's bladder. If the fetus is less than 20 weeks of gestation, the patient's full bladder will hold the uterus steady and out of the pelvis. The placenta is localized with the use of ultrasound.
   b. Obtain maternal vital signs and a 20-minute FHR tracing to serve as a baseline to evaluate possible complications.
   c. Monitor patient during and after the procedure for signs of premature labor or bleeding.
   d. Tell patient to report signs of bleeding, unusual fetal activity or abdominal pain, cramping, or fever while at home after the procedure.
   e. If patient in Rh negative, may need to administer Rh_o (D) immune globulin (RhoGAM).

Chorionic Villus Sampling

Description

CVS involves obtaining samples of chorionic villus (placental tissue [fetal origin]) to test for chromosomal (via DNA) and enzymatic disorders of the fetus. CVS is ideally performed between 10 and 14 weeks of gestation.

1. Using ultrasound, a catheter is passed vaginally into the uterus, where a specimen of chorionic villus tissue is removed.
2. Complications include rupture of membranes, intrauterine infection, spontaneous abortion, hematoma, fetal trauma, or maternal tissue contamination.
3. Incidence of fetal loss is about 2% to 5%.

Nursing and Patient Care Considerations

1. Obtain maternal vital signs.
2. Instruct patient to void.
3. Offer reassurance and compassionate presence during the procedure.
4. If patient is Rh negative, may need to administer RhoGAM.
5. Inform patient that a small amount of spotting is normal, but heavy bleeding or passing clots or tissue should be reported to provider immediately. Also report fluid leaking from the vagina.
6. Instruct patient to rest at home for a few hours after the procedure.

Percutaneous Umbilical Blood Sampling

Description

Percutaneous umbilical blood sampling (PUBS), or *cordocentesis*, involves a puncture of the umbilical cord (vein) for aspiration of fetal blood under ultrasound guidance.

1. It is used in the diagnosis of fetal blood disorders, infections, Rh isoimmunization, metabolic disorders, and karyotyping.
2. Transfusion to the fetus may be conducted with this procedure.
3. Using ultrasound picture, the provider inserts a needle (guided by ultrasound) into one of the umbilical vessels. A small amount of blood is withdrawn.
4. Can also be used for fetal therapies, such as red blood cell (RBC) and platelet transfusion.

Nursing and Patient Care Considerations

1. Explain the procedure to patient.
2. Provide support to patient during the procedure.
3. Monitor patient after the procedure for uterine contractions and the FHR for distress.
4. If patient is Rh negative, may need to administer RhoGAM.

Fetal Fibronectin

Description

1. *Fetal fibronectin* (fFN) is a protein that is secreted by the trophoblast of the implanted egg. The exact function is unknown; however, this protein is thought to play a key role in placental–uterine attachment. It is used to help predict risk for PTL. It is considered a better biomarker for those who will *not* go into PTL, rather than those who *will* go into PTL.
2. Normally present in cervical or vaginal fluid before 20 weeks of gestation.
3. After 20 weeks of gestation, the presence of fFN can indicate a detachment of the fetal membranes and should be evaluated as an early marker for preterm birth.
4. Specimen is collected no earlier than 24 weeks and no later than 34 weeks and 6 days.
5. A positive finding for fFN alone is not predictive of PTL.

Nursing and Patient Care Considerations

1. Explain the procedure to patient.
2. Collect specimen with a Dacron swab placed in the posterior fornix of the vagina and rotated for 10 seconds. Sexual activity within 24 hours of sample collection, recent cervical examination, and vaginal bleeding may result in a false-positive test.
3. Provide support to patient during the procedure.

EVIDENCE BASE American College of Obstetricians and Gynecologists. (2021). Prediction and prevention of spontaneous preterm birth (Practice Bulletin, no. 234). *Obstetrics and Gynecology, 138*(2), e65–e90. https://doi.org/10.1097/AOG.0000000000004479

Nonstress Test

Description

The *nonstress test* (NST) is used to evaluate fetal well-being by assessing FHR accelerations that normally occur in response to fetal activity as a measure of uteroplacental function. Accelerations are indicative of an intact central and autonomic nervous system and are a sign of fetal well-being. Absence of FHR accelerations in response to fetal movements may be associated with hypoxia, acidosis, drugs (analgesics, barbiturates), fetal sleep pattern, and some fetal anomalies.

1. Maternal indications include postdates, Rh sensitization, maternal age 35 or above, chronic renal disease, hypertension, collagen disease, sickle cell disease, diabetes, premature rupture of membranes, history of stillbirth, trauma, and vaginal bleeding in the second and third trimesters.
2. There are no contraindications or known adverse effects associated with the NST.
3. Fetal indications include decreased fetal movement, intrauterine growth restriction, fetal evaluation after an amniocentesis, external cephalic version, oligohydramnios, or hydramnios.
   a. Criteria for a reactive NST for a fetus greater than 32 weeks of gestation include two accelerations within 20 minutes, each lasting at least 15 seconds with an FHR increased by 15 bpm above baseline in response to fetal activity. The quality of the tracing is an important factor in the test interpretation.
   b. Criteria for a reactive NST in a preterm fetus (less than 32 completed weeks of gestation) include two accelerations within 20 minutes, each lasting at least 10 seconds with an FHR increased by 10 bpm above baseline in response to fetal activity.
   c. In a nonreactive NST, the abovementioned criteria are not met. Further testing with a BPP may be warranted.
4. Significance/management.
   a. Reactive NST—is reassuring and suggests a less than 1% chance of fetal death within 1 week of the NST. However, nonpreventable fetal death for abruptio placentae, sepsis, and cord accidents are excluded.
   b. Nonreactive NST—suggests a fetus that may be compromised, and there needs to be further follow-up with a BPP, modified BPP, contraction stress test (CST), or oxytocin challenge test (OCT).

Nursing and Patient Care Considerations

1. Explain the procedure and equipment to the patient. Make sure the patient has had adequate nutrition and fluid intake and, if the patient smokes, has not been smoking within the past 2 hours.
2. Instruct the patient to void prior to NST for comfort.
3. Assist patient to a semi-Fowler position in bed. Perform Leopold maneuvers, and apply the external fetal and uterine monitors.
4. Event markers do not need to be used unless the fetal movement is not observed on the fetal monitor. If fetal movement not observed, instruct patient to make a mark on the monitor strip each time fetal movement is felt. The nurse will do this if the patient cannot.
5. Evaluate the response of the FHR immediately after fetal activity.
6. Monitor patient's blood pressure (BP) and uterine activity during the procedure.

Fetal Acoustic Stimulation Test and Vibroacoustic Stimulation Test

Description

Acoustic (sound) and vibroacoustic stimulation (VAS) are sound plus vibration involving the use of handheld battery-operated devices (usually a laryngeal stimulator) placed over the patient's abdomen near the fetal head. This technique produces a low-frequency vibration and a buzzing tone intended to induce fetal movement along with associated FHR accelerations. The sound stimulus should last for up to 3 seconds. The *fetal acoustic stimulation test* (FAST) and *vibroacoustic stimulation test* (VST) are used as an adjunct following a nonreactive NST; these tests may also be used with fetuses that exhibit a nonreassuring FHR cardiotocographic (CTG) tracing during labor. If no FHR accelerations occur in response to the stimulus, it is repeated at 1-minute intervals up to three times (total of 6 seconds). If the FHR tracing remains nonreactive, further evaluation with BPP or CST is indicated. In the light of advanced ultrasound technology, this test is being used less frequently. However, there are still facilities that do not have the ultrasound capabilities; therefore, this testing is appropriate.

1. It is not known whether the fetus responds more to the sound or to the vibration.
2. Both methods of testing are noninvasive, easy to perform, and yield rapid results.
3. No adverse neurologic or auditory effects noted in the fetus after testing.

Nursing and Patient Care Considerations

1. Explain procedure, equipment, and purpose to patient.
2. Instruct the patient to void prior to NST for comfort.
3. Assist patient to a semi-Fowler position in bed.
4. Apply external fetal monitors to patient.
5. Demonstrate how the stimulus may feel on patient's forearm or leg.
6. Observe for reactivity.

Contraction Stress Test (Oxytocin Challenge Test)

Description

CST or OCT is used to evaluate the ability of the fetus to withstand the stress of uterine contractions as would occur during labor.

1. The test is generally used when a patient has a nonreactive NST or FAST/VST, although in many areas, the CST has been replaced by the BPP.
2. The test is contraindicated with third-trimester bleeding, multiple gestation, incompetent cervix, placenta previa, previous classic uterine incision, hydramnios, history of PTL, or premature rupture of membranes.
3. Contractions may occur spontaneously (unusual), or they may be induced endogenously, producing oxytocin with nipple or breast stimulation.
4. The OCT utilizes exogenous oxytocin, which is administered by titrated IV infusion with continuous fetal monitoring.

Nursing and Patient Care Considerations

1. Obtain maternal vital signs, especially BP.
2. Instruct patient to void for comfort.
3. Assist patient to a semi-Fowler or side-lying position in bed.
4. Obtain a 20-minute strip of the FHR and uterine activity for baseline data.
5. For CST:
   a. Apply warm packs to the breasts for 10 minutes before the CST.
   b. Instruct patient on nipple stimulation. Instruct the patient to brush or roll the nipple, using the palmar surface of the index finger and thumb. The patient can do this through clothes or skin to skin. If using skin to skin, provide the patient with some lubricant to use on fingers to ease stimulation. Stimulation occurs in four cycles of 2 minutes *on* and 2 to 5 minutes off (*for ease of memory: 1 cycle = 2 minutes on and 2 minutes off*). The nipple is stimulated until contractions begin *or* 2 minutes have passed.
   c. If contractions occur during stimulation, instruct the patient to stop the stimulation; the patient can begin the stimulation again when the contraction is over. If no contractions after four cycles, two different methods can be used:
      i. Let the patient rest for 5 to 10 minutes, then begin bilateral continuous stimulation for 5 to 10 minutes, stopping when contractions begin (have the patient resume stimulation when contraction ends).
      ii. Let the patient rest for 5 to 10 minutes, then begin stimulation again, alternating nipples, stopping when contractions begin (have the patient resume stimulation when contraction ends).
   d. Stop the stimulation if:
      i. Three or more contractions occur within 10 minutes that last more than or equal to 40 seconds.
      ii. Hyperstimulation or tachysystole occurs.
      iii. Unsuccessful nipple stimulation (two rounds of four cycles without contractions). Notify health care provider and prepare for OCT, BPP, or modified BPP.
6. For OCT: Follow steps 1 through 4. In addition:
   a. Administer low-dose oxytocin infusion using a pump, as indicated, until three contractions occur within 10 minutes and last ≥40 seconds. Maintain mainline IV fluids in accordance with facility policy.
   b. Discontinue the infusion when:
      i. Criteria are met.
      ii. Maximum dose of 16 milliunits per minute has been achieved.
      iii. Hyperstimulation or tachysystole occurs. Prolonged deceleration, bradycardia, or late decelerations are observed.

Interpretation of Contraction Stress Test/Oxytocin Challenge Test

1. Negative (normal/reassuring)—absence of late or variable decelerations.
2. Positive (abnormal/nonreassuring)—late decelerations with more than 50% of uterine contractions even if frequency is less than three contractions in 10 minutes; usually associated with absent or minimal variability.
3. Equivocal—intermittent late decelerations (less than 50% of uterine contractions) or significant variables.
4. Unsatisfactory—quality of tracing inadequate to assess or less than three contractions in 10 minutes or contractions less than 40 seconds in duration.
5. Equivocal and unsatisfactory results can be repeated in 24 hours or sooner unless indication for delivery is present.
6. Regardless of the result, if variable decelerations are present, a BPP may be needed to assess AFI.

Biophysical Profile

Description

The *BPP* uses ultrasonography and NST to assess five biophysical variables in determining fetal well-being. A BPP is performed during a 30-minute time frame by someone credentialed in ultrasonography.

1. For each variable, if the criteria are met, a score of 2 is given. For an abnormal observation, a score of 0 is given.

2. A score of 8 to 10 is reassuring, 6 is equivocal and requires further evaluation, and 4 or less is nonreassuring and requires further evaluation and delivery may be considered.
   a. NST—assessing for FHR acceleration (fetal reactivity) in relation to fetal movements.
   b. AFI—assessing for one or more pockets of amniotic fluid measuring at least (2 cm) or more in two perpendicular planes.
   c. Fetal breathing movements—one or more episodes lasting at least 30 seconds within 30 minutes.
   d. Gross fetal body movements—three or more body or limb movements, in 30 minutes.
   e. Fetal muscle tone—one or more episodes of active extension with return to flexion of spine, hand, or limbs within 30 minutes.

Nursing and Patient Care Considerations

1. Explain the purpose and procedure to the patient; provide emotional support.
2. Instruct patient to empty bladder for comfort.
3. Assist patient onto the examination table and assume a position of comfort.
4. Remove the lubricant from patient's abdomen after the procedure.
5. Assist patient in rising from the examination table.

Modified Biophysical Profile

Description

The modified BPP is used more commonly today than the BPP. It consists of an NST and an assessment of AFI. The modified BPP performed twice per week provides the same predictive results as the weekly CST.

1. Normal interpretation is a reactive NST with an AFI greater than 5 cm. A normal AFI is 9 to 25 cm, with a borderline "normal" being 5 to 8 cm.
2. An abnormal AFI of less than 5 cm of amniotic fluid (oligohydramnios) requires a full ultrasound evaluation, and the fetus is evaluated for functioning renal tissue.

Nursing and Patient Care Considerations

1. Explain NST and AFI check in accordance with previously stated guidelines, as noted earlier.
2. Document findings in patient's prenatal record.

SELECTED READINGS

Adams, E. D. (2021). Antenatal care. In K. R. Simpson, P. A. Creehan, N. O'Brien-Abel, C. K. Roth, & A. J. Rohan (Eds.), *Perinatal nursing* (5th ed., pp. 66–97). Wolters Kluwer.

American College of Obstetricians and Gynecologists, Committee on Obstetric Practice. (2013, reaffirmed 2020). Weight gain during pregnancy: Committee Opinion, Number 548. *Obstetrics and Gynecology, 121*(1), 210–212. https://www.acog.org/clinical/clinical-guidance/committee-opinion/articles/2013/01/weight-gain-during-pregnancy

American College of Obstetricians and Gynecologists, Committee on Obstetric Practice. (2021). Indications for outpatient antenatal fetal surveillance: ACOG Committee Opinion, Number 828. *Obstetrics and Gynecology, 137*(6), e177–e197. https://doi.org/10.1097/AOG.0000000000004407

Auerbach, M. (2021). *Anemia in pregnancy. UpToDate.* https://www.uptodate.com/contents/anemia-in-pregnancy

Baker, B., & Janke, J. (2024). *Core curriculum for maternal-newborn nursing* (6th ed.). Elsevier.

Bellussi, F., Po', G., Livi, A., Saccone, G., De Vivo, V., Oliver, E. A., & Berghella, V. (2020). Fetal movement counting and perinatal mortality: A systematic review and meta-analysis. *Obstetrics and Gynecology, 135*(2), 453–462. https://doi.org/10.1097/AOG.0000000000003645

Coppola, J. S. (2024). Reproductive anatomy, physiology, and the menstrual cycle. In B. Baker & J. Janke (Eds.), *Core curriculum for maternal-newborn nursing* (6th ed., pp. 1–14). Elsevier.

Cypher, R. L. (2024). Prenatal testing and antepartum fetal surveillance. In B. Baker & J. Janke (Eds.), *Core curriculum for maternal-newborn nursing* (6th ed., pp. 53–70). Elsevier.

Goldberg, A. E., & Allen, K. R. (2022). "I'm not just the nonbiological parent": Encountering, strategizing, and resisting asymmetry and invalidation in genetic/gestational parent status among LGBTQ parents. *Journal of Family Nursing, 28*(4), 381–395. https://doi.org/10.1177/10748407221123062

Hoyert, D. L. (2021). *Maternal mortality rates in the United States, 2019.* https://www.cdc.gov/nchs/data/hestat/maternal-mortality-2021/E-Stat-Maternal-Mortality-Rates-H.pdf

Kaimal, A. J. (2023). Assessment of fetal health. In M. F. Greene, R. K. Creasy, J. D. Resnick, J. D. Iams, C. J. Lockwood, & T. Moore (Eds.), *Maternal–fetal medicine: Principles and practice* (9th ed., pp. 560–573). Elsevier.

Kyozuka, H., Murata, T., Sato, T., Suzuki, S., Yamaguchi, A., & Fujimori, K. (2019). Utility of cervical length and quantitative fetal fibronectin for predicting spontaneous preterm delivery among symptomatic nulliparous women. *International Journal of Gynecology and Obstetrics, 145*(3), 331–336. https://doi.org/10.1002/ijgo.12821

Luxion, K. (2020). LGBTQ reproduction and parenting. In N. A. Naples *(Ed.), Companion to sexuality studies* (pp. 179–203). Wiley Online Library. https://doi.org/10.1002/9781119315049.ch10

Mastrobattista, J. M., & Monga, M. (2023). Maternal cardiovascular, respiratory, and renal adaptation to pregnancy. In C. J. Lockwood, J. A. Copel, L. Dugoff, J. Louis, T. R. Morre, R. M. Silver, & R. Resnick (Eds.), *Creasy & Resnick's maternal–fetal medicine: Principles and practice* (9th ed., pp. 143–149). Elsevier.

Perry, S. E., Lowdermilk, D. L., Cashion, K., Alden, K. R., Olshansky, E., & Hockenberry, M. J. (2020). The family, culture, and home care. In *Maternity & women's health care* (12th ed., pp. 14–30). Elsevier.

Ricci, S. S. (2021). *Essentials of maternity, newborn, and women's health nursing* (5th ed.). Wolters Kluwer.

Rubin, R. (1984). *Maternal identity and the maternal experience.* Springer.

Saarikko, J., Niela-Vilén, H., Rahmani, A. M., & Axelin, A. (2021). Identifying target behaviors for weight management interventions for women who are overweight during pregnancy and the postpartum period: A qualitative study informed by the Behaviour Change Wheel. *BMC Pregnancy and Childbirth, 21*(200), 1–12. https://doi.org/10.1186/s12884-021-03689-6

Sagi-Dain, L. (2021). Obesity in pregnancy: ACOG Practice Bulletin, Number 230. *Obstetrics and Gynecology, 138*(3), 489. https://doi.org/10.1097/AOG.0000000000004527

Sarecka-Hujar, B., & Szulc-Musioł, B. (2022). Herbal medicines—Are they effective and safe during pregnancy? *Pharmaceutics, 14*(1), 171. https://doi.org/10.3390/pharmaceutics14010171

Simpson, K. R., Creehan, P. A., O'Brien-Abel, N., Roth, C. K., & Rohan, A. J. (2021). *Perinatal nursing* (5th ed.). Wolters Kluwer.

Wang, E., Glazer, K. B., Howell, E. A., & Janevic, T. M. (2020). Social determinants of pregnancy-related mortality and morbidity in the United States: A systematic review. *Obstetrics and Gynecology, 135*(4), 896–915. https://doi.org/10.1097/AOG.0000000000003762

33 Nursing Management During Labor and Delivery

THE LABOR PROCESS

The phases of pregnancy, labor, and birth are normal physiologic processes. The patient who is pregnant typically approaches the birth process with concerns of personal well-being, the well-being of the fetus, and fear of labor pain. Addressing these concerns, minimizing discomfort, optimizing patient safety, and respecting sociocultural factors should be paramount to all participants involved in the care of the patient and fetus during the intrapartum period.

General Considerations

EVIDENCE BASE Baker, B., & Janke, J. (2024). *Core curriculum for maternal-newborn nursing* (6th ed.). Elsevier.

Murray, S., McKinney, E., Holub, K. S., Jones, R., & Scheffer, K. L. (2023). *Foundations of maternal-newborn and women's health nursing* (8th ed.). Elsevier.

Prepared Childbirth

Historically, the term *natural childbirth* has evolved to mean (1) delivery outside in nature, (2) home birth, (3) nonhospital birth (birthing center), (4) facility birth—no medical intervention (e.g., no intravenous [IV] medications)—and, most recently, (5) facility birth without analgesia or anesthesia. Preparation through education and training prior to labor gives the patient who is pregnant a method of coping with the discomforts of labor and delivery. This method is known as *prepared childbirth* and incorporates analgesia and anesthesia into the process. Variances in prepared childbirth are outlined.

Psychoprophylactic or Lamaze Method

1. Psychoprophylactic childbirth has a rationale based on Pavlov's concept of pain perception and his theory of conditioned reflexes (the substitution of favorable conditioned reflexes for unfavorable ones). The Lamaze method is an example of this technique.
2. The patient learns to replace responses of restlessness, fear, and loss of control with more controlled measures, which can excite the cerebral cortex efficiently to inhibit other stimuli such as pain in labor.
3. The patient learns exercises that strengthen the abdominal muscles and relax the perineum.
4. The patient/partner/support person learns various breathing techniques to help maintain focus and a sense of control during the labor process.
5. The patient learns to respond with respiratory measures and dissociation or relaxation of the uninvolved muscles while controlling the patient's perception of the stimuli associated with labor.

The Bradley Method of Delivery

1. Commonly referred to as "partner-coached childbirth." A coach may be *any* significant other designated by the patient.
2. Involves the concepts of leading, guiding, supporting, caring, and fostering specific skills and confidence.
3. Coaches attend classes and learn to help the patient prior to labor.
4. The coach serves as a conditioned stimulus using the sound of their voice, use of particular words, and repetition of practice.
5. Relaxation is the core component, and medications are not encouraged for pain relief. Increased tolerance to pain is accomplished by decreased mental anxiety and fear, which ultimately decreases the awareness of the pain stimulus. This occurs through cognitive and physical rehearsal.

Planned Home Birth

EVIDENCE BASE American College of Obstetricians and Gynecologists. (2017). Committee Opinion No. 697: Planned home birth. *Obstetrics & Gynecology, 129*(4), e117–e122. https://doi.org/10.1097/AOG.0000000000002024

Association of Women's Health, Obstetric and Neonatal Nurses. (2022). Respectful maternity care framework and evidence-based clinical practice guideline. *Nursing for Women's Health, 26*(2), S1–S52. https://doi.org/10.1016/j.nwh.2022.01.001

1. Motivations for home delivery:
   a. Increases patient choices and flexibility during the birth process while decreasing patient separation and fear of medical intervention.
   b. Desire to avoid medical intervention, such as anesthesia and operative procedures.
2. Contraindications:
   a. High-risk pregnancies, such as placental abnormalities, multiple gestation, preeclampsia, and gestational diabetes.
   b. History of premature or postdate delivery in previous or current pregnancy or previous cesarean delivery.
   c. Known fetal abnormalities.
3. Alternatives to home delivery:
   a. Family-centered hospital setting.
   b. Birthing centers with adequate facilities for emergency care for low-risk patients.

POPULATION AWARENESS Giving birth is an intimately unique experience. How the patient chooses to incorporate the myriad of options for the birth experience should be through informed and respectful decision-making. For example, patients with low obstetrical risk could plan a home birth that includes consideration for maternal and neonatal outcomes. Accounting for cultural preferences and offering childbirth education provide all patients with the resources that foster informed decision-making.

Initiation of Labor

EVIDENCE BASE Cunningham, F. G., Leveno, K. J., Bloom, S. J., Dashe, J. S., Hoffman, B. L., Casey, B. M., & Spong, C. Y. (2022). *Williams obstetrics* (26th ed.). McGraw Hill.

Minehart, R. D., & Minnich, M. E. (2020). Childbirth preparation and nonpharmacologic analgesia. In D. Chestnut, C. Wong, L. Tsen, D. Warwick, Y. Beilin, J. Mhyre, & B. Bateman (Eds.), *Chestnut's obstetric anesthesia: Principles and practice* (6th ed.). Elsevier.

Parturition is a multifactorial physiologic process, and the exact mechanism initiating labor is unknown. The inhibition of labor during pregnancy is maintained by a constant release of progesterone and other uterotonic inhibitors (e.g., prostaglandin I_2 [PGI_2], relaxin, nitric oxide, and parathyroid hormone). Progesterone is the primary hormone of pregnancy, which prevents uterine contractility during pregnancy. As the pregnancy approaches term, progesterone levels begin to decrease and estrogen levels increase, reciprocally stimulating uterine contractility. Labor onset involves both maternal and fetal influences as outlined:

1. Maternal factors:
   a. Prostaglandin (PG) is released as the uterus stretches to accommodate the fetus.
   b. The posterior pituitary releases oxytocin because of pressure on the cervix.
   c. Oxytocin and PG jointly aid in the inhibition of calcium binding in muscle cells, thus increasing the calcium levels intracellularly causing uterine contractions.
2. Placental and fetal factors:
   a. Placental maturation triggers the onset of contractions.
   b. The concentration of fetal cortisol increases in response to the increase in maternal oxytocin.

Factors Affecting Labor Process

The five Ps: The success of labor and delivery depends on five factors: *passageway (birth canal)*, *passenger (fetus)*, *powers (contractions)*, *position (maternal)*, and *psychological response*.

EVIDENCE BASE Ricci, S. S. (2021). *Essentials of maternity, newborn, and women's health nursing* (5th ed.). Wolters Kluwer.

Passageway: Pelvic Dimensions

1. Pelvic inlet (anteroposterior diameter): The obstetric conjugate anteroposterior measurement is typically more than 10 cm. A gynecoid-shaped pelvis accommodates proper descent (see page 964).
2. Mid-pelvis (ischial spines): Interspinous diameter is typically more than 10 cm; protrusion of the spines into the birthing canal may complicate descent.
3. Pelvic outlet (intertuberous diameter plus suprapubic arch): Dimensions are estimated as the anteroposterior diameter from the coccyx to the symphysis pubis. This is typically 13 cm in length, but one must subtract 1.5 to 2 cm from the calculation because of the thickness of the symphysis. A prominent coccyx may impede descent.

Passenger: Fetal Dimensions

1. Size—assessed via palpation using Leopold maneuvers or ultrasound. Excessive size may lead to inadequate or asynclitic (asymmetrical position of the head) descent, labor dystocia, shoulder dystocia, or postpartum hemorrhage (PPH).
2. Attitude—typically, the fetal head and extremities are flexed while the back is rounded. Flexion of the head allows for the smallest diameter (occiput) to present and pass through the birth canal with ease (see Figure 33-1). Nonflexed presentations may increase the risk of asynclitic conditions.
3. Lie—constitutes the comparison of the fetal long axis to the maternal long axis. Variances include transverse, longitudinal, or oblique; 99% of fetuses present as a longitudinal lie parallel to the birthing parent's spine. This improves ease of access into the birth canal.
4. Presentation—the fetal body part presenting into the birth canal first and is felt on vaginal examination (see Figure 33-2).
   a. Cephalic (head)—occiput, sinciput, brow, face, or chin (mentum).
   b. Breech (feet)—frank, complete, or footling (single or double).
   c. Shoulder (transverse).
   d. Compound—two or more parts presenting at the same time.
5. Position—specific landmark of fetal presenting part (occiput, mentum, sacrum, scapula) in comparison to the anterior, posterior, or transverse portion of the patient's pelvis and the maternal left or right side; designated by a three-letter abbreviation.
   a. The first letter L or R represents the side (right or left) in the maternal pelvis the presenting part is facing.

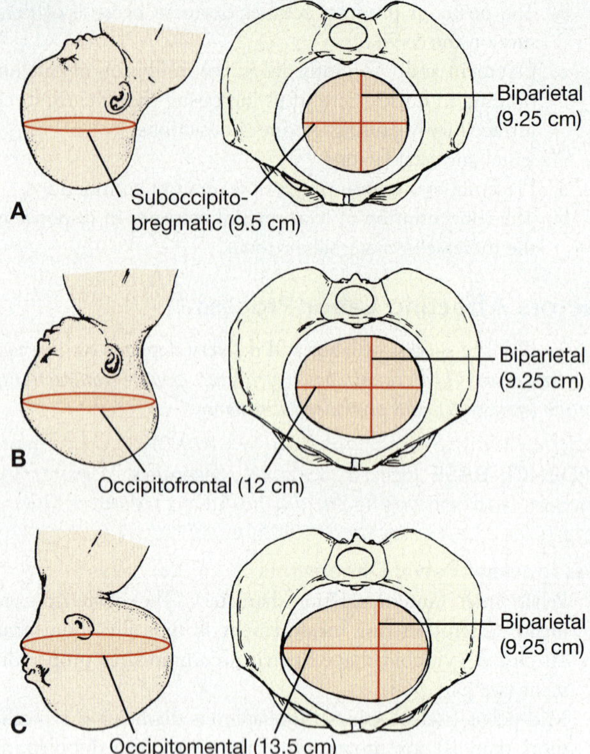

Figure 33-1. **(A)** Complete flexion allows smallest diameter of the head to enter the pelvis. **(B)** Moderate extension causes larger diameter to enter the pelvis. **(C)** Marked extension forces largest diameter against pelvic brim, but the head is too large to enter the pelvis.

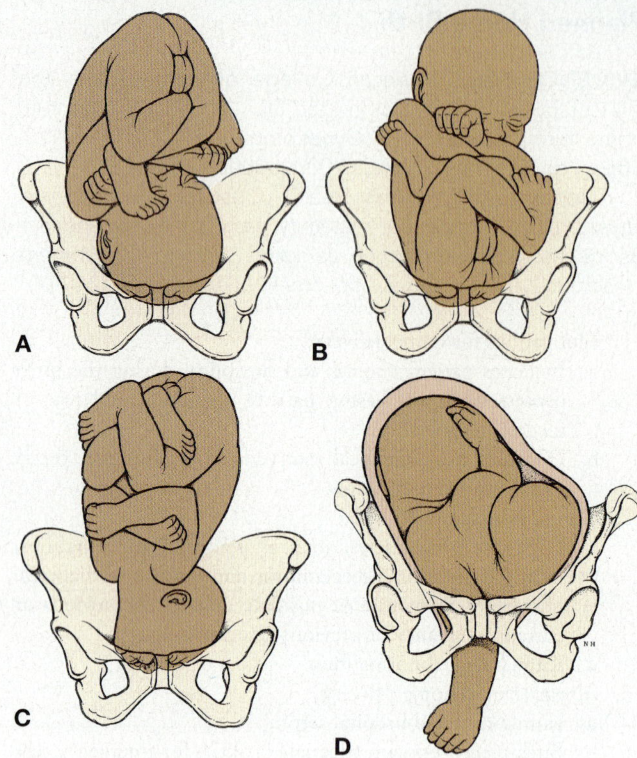

Figure 33-2. Fetal presentations. **(A)** Cephalic; **(B)** breech; **(C)** face; **(D)** transverse.

   b. The second letter represents the landmark that is presenting: O for occiput, M for mentum (chin), S for sacrum, and Sc for scapula or shoulder.
   c. The third letter represents the direction (anterior [A], posterior [P], or transverse [T]) the presenting part is facing in the pelvis.
   d. For example, the fetus with the head presenting and facing toward the maternal right anterior pelvis is right occiput anterior (ROA).

EVIDENCE BASE Hurst, H. M., & Baker, B. (2024). Essential forces and factors in labor. In B. Baker & J. Janke (Eds.), *Core curriculum for maternal-newborn nursing* (6th ed., pp. 127–141). Elsevier.

Passenger: Fetal Head (Vertex)

In approximately 95% of all births, the fetal head (vertex) presents first. Sutures and fontanelles provide important landmarks for determining fetal position during a vaginal examination (see Figure 33-3).

1. Bones of the fetal skull:
   a. One occipital bone posteriorly.
   b. Two parietal bones bilaterally.
   c. Two temporal bones bilaterally (not palpable during a vaginal examination).
   d. Two frontal bones anteriorly.
2. Sutures of the fetal skull—membranous spaces between the bones of the fetal skull:
   a. Frontal—between the two frontal bones.
   b. Sagittal—between the two parietal bones.
   c. Coronal—between the frontal and parietal bones.
   d. Lambdoidal—between the back of the parietal bones and the margin of the occipital bone.
3. Fontanelles of the fetal skull—irregular spaces formed where two or more sutures meet. Sutures and fontanelles allow fetal skull bones to overlap to pass through the maternal pelvis.
   a. Anterior—largest fontanelle; junction of the sagittal, frontal, and coronal sutures; closes by age 18 to 24 months; "diamond" shaped.
   b. Posterior—located where the sagittal suture meets the lambdoidal suture (smaller than anterior); closes by 1 year; "triangle" shaped.

Powers: Uterine Contractions

Successful labor depends on regular uterine contractions of adequate intensity that lead to cervical advancement and

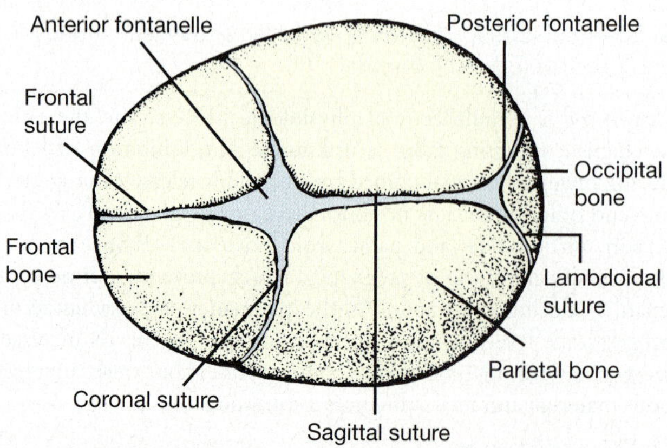

Figure 33-3. Fetal head.

facilitate fetal descent. The following are characteristics of labor contractions:

a. Uterine contractions typically increase in intensity, frequency, and duration as labor progresses.
b. Uterine contractions may cause vasoconstriction of the umbilical cord, leading to potential alterations in the fetal heart rate (i.e., variable decelerations).
c. The active upper portion of the uterus (fundus) stimulates activation of contractions during labor (referred to as *fundal dominance*).
d. At the completion of a contraction, the upper uterine segment retains its shortened, thickened cell size, and, with each succeeding contraction, becomes thicker and shorter. As a result, the upper uterine segment never totally relaxes during labor. Cells of the lower uterine segment become thinner and longer with each contraction. This mechanism is greatly responsible for the progress of the fetus through the birth canal.
e. The differentiation point between the upper and lower uterine segment is known as the "physiologic retraction ring."
f. Intra-abdominal pressure increases with voluntary maternal pushing efforts during the second stage of labor.

Position (Maternal)

1. The maternal position may influence pelvic size and contour and fetal position and assist fetal rotation.
2. The upright position may facilitate a shortened first and second stage.
3. Allows for the use of gravity for fetal decent.

Psychological Responses

1. A patient's psyche is essential to the labor process in the following ways:
   a. To maintain a sense of well-being and control.
   b. Assists the patient in facing the challenge of labor and sense of accomplishment.

Events Leading to Labor

1. Lightening is the settling of the fetus in the lower uterine segment occurring 2 to 3 weeks before term in the primigravida and typically during labor in the multigravida.
   a. Breathing becomes easier as the fetus falls away from the diaphragm.
   b. Lordosis of the spine is increased as the fetus enters the pelvis and moves more anteriorly. Walking may become more difficult as leg cramping may increase.
   c. Urinary frequency occurs due to pressure on the adjacent bladder.
2. Vaginal secretions may increase due to hormonal changes.
3. Mucus plug may be discharged from the cervix along with a small amount of blood from surrounding capillaries—referred to as "bloody show."
4. The cervix softens and effaces (shortens and thins) and gradually moves from a posterior to an anterior position.
5. Membranes may rupture spontaneously.
6. False labor contractions (Braxton-Hicks) may occur (see Table 33-1) in preparation for true labor.
7. Backaches may occur due to fetal size and lightening.
8. Gastrointestinal alterations (e.g., diarrhea) and weight loss of 1 to 3 pounds (0.5 to 1.5 kg) may occur with advanced pregnancy.
9. Energy may increase (referred to as "nesting") or decrease in the last few weeks.

Table 33-1 True and False Labor Contractions

TRUE LABOR CONTRACTIONS	FALSE LABOR CONTRACTIONS
Result in progressive cervical dilation and effacement	Do not result in progressive cervical dilation and effacement
Occur at regular intervals	Occur at irregular intervals
Interval between contractions decreases	Interval between contractions remains the same or increases.
Frequency, duration, and intensity increase	Intensity decreases or remains the same.
Located mainly in the back and abdomen	Located mainly in the lower abdomen and groin
Generally intensified by walking	Generally unaffected by walking
Not easily disrupted by medications	Generally relieved by mild sedation

Stages of Labor

First Stage of Labor (Labor Onset to Full Cervical Dilation and Effacement)

1. Begins with regular and rhythmic true labor contractions and ends with complete effacement (100%) and dilation of the cervix (10 cm).
2. The length of the first stage varies and is almost double in a primiparous patient; this stage of labor consists of two phases:
   a. Latent phase (early):
      i. Effacement is the shortening and thinning of the cervix that occurs at the end of pregnancy.
      ii. Dilation from 0 to 5 cm; contractions are typically mild by palpation and occur every 5 minutes at the beginning of the latent phase.
      iii. Dilation and contractions gradually increase and at the end of the latent phase; contractions typically occur regularly every 2 to 5 minutes and are moderate to strong by palpation.
   b. Active phase:
      i. Effacement evolves over this period to 100%.
      ii. Dilation from 6 to 10 cm; dilation averages 1.2 cm/h in the nullipara and 1.5 cm/h in the multipara.
      iii. Contractions increase in frequency to every 2 to 5 minutes, lasting 40 to 60 seconds. Intensity may be moderate to strong by palpation or 60 to 80 mm Hg when an internal uterine pressure catheter (IUPC) is in use.
      iv. Contractions continue to increase in intensity and duration at the end of the active phase, occurring every 2 to 3 minutes, lasting 60 to 90 seconds with strong intensity by palpation or 70 to 90 mm Hg with an IUPC.

Second Stage of Labor (Fetal Expulsion)

1. Begins with complete effacement and dilation ending with delivery of the fetus.
2. The second stage may last from 1 to 4 hours in the nullipara and typically less than 1 hour in the multipara. Variance in time depends on maternal pushing efforts, contraction pattern, anesthesia, and fetal descent and position.

Third Stage of Labor (Placental Expulsion)

1. Begins with delivery of the fetus and ends with delivery of the placenta.
2. The third stage may last from a few minutes to 30 minutes typically. Prolonged periods may be attributable to abnormal placentation (i.e., placenta accreta) and may require further evaluation and intervention related to the increased risk of hemorrhage.

Fourth Stage (Immediate Postpartum)

This period lasts from delivery of the placenta until the patient's postpartum condition has become stabilized. With the increase for improved outcomes related to hemorrhage, the fourth stage of labor lasts at least the first 2 hours and may require further assessment and evaluation based on maternal status.

Seven Cardinal Fetal Movements of Labor

Once the fetus enters the pelvis, seven "cardinal movements" occur to facilitate passage through the maternal pelvis during labor and birth (see Figure 33-4).

Engagement

Engagement begins when the biparietal diameter (BPD) of the fetal head, which is the largest transverse diameter, descends into the pelvic inlet, and 0 station.

Descent

1. The downward movement of the fetus through the birth canal is accomplished by the force of uterine contractions and pressure of the amniotic fluid; during the second stage of labor, "maternal bearing-down" efforts increase intra-abdominal pressure, thus augmenting effects of uterine contractions.
2. *Station* refers to the relationship of the presenting part to the ischial spines. Subsequently, station has a direct correlation to the degree of descent, as described later (see Figure 33-5):
   a. Floating—fetal presenting part is not engaged in pelvic inlet; may be ballotable via cervical examination.
   b. Engagement—fetal presenting part enters the pelvis as the BPD passes through the inlet.
   c. The pelvis is divided into sections measured in centimeters; a 5-cm scale is used (see Figure 33-6).

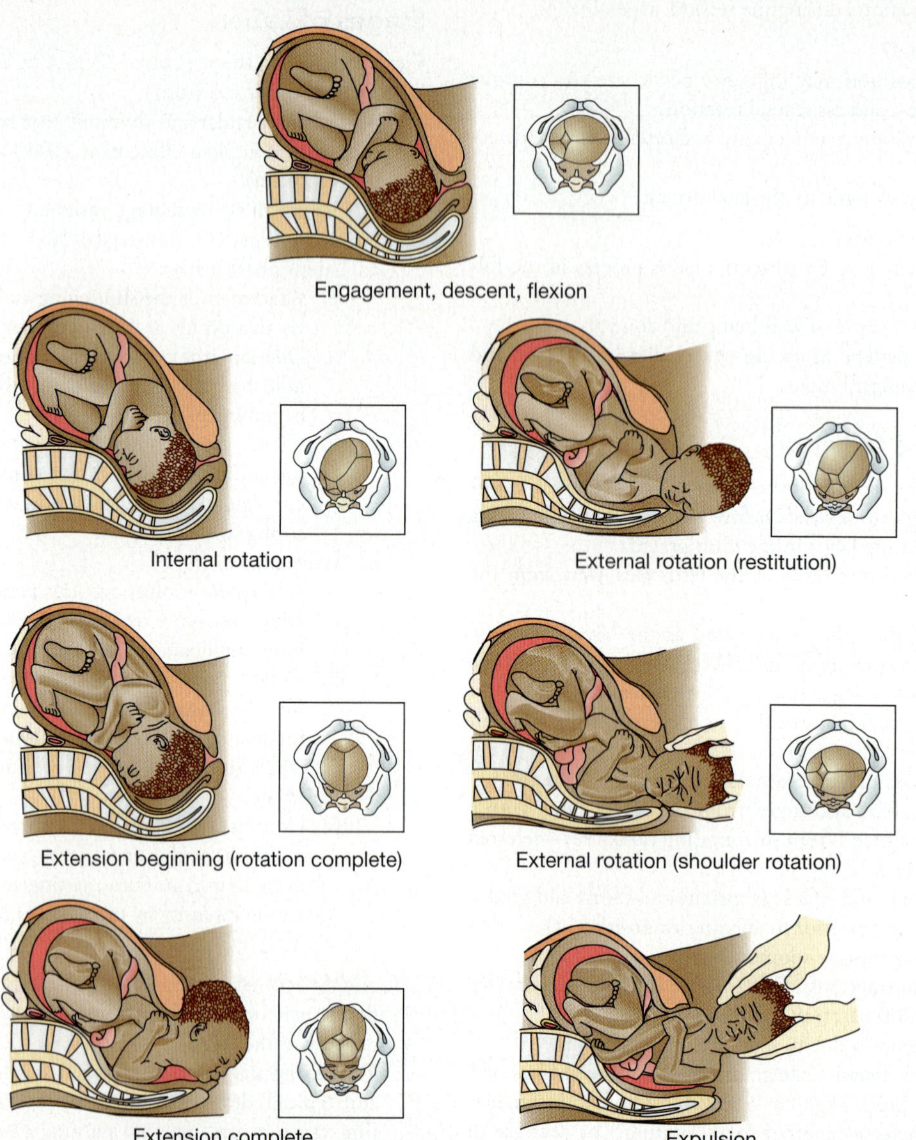

Figure 33-4. Seven fetal cardinal movements of labor (vertex presentation). (Reprinted with permission from Silbert-Flagg, J. (2023). *Maternal and child health nursing* (9th ed., Fig. 15-8). Lippincott Williams & Wilkins.)

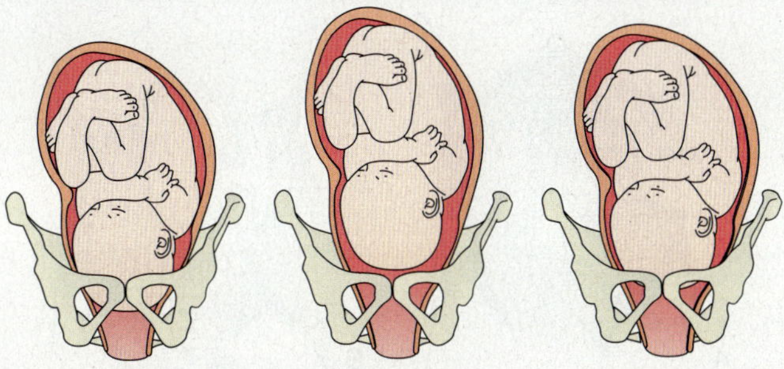

Figure 33-5. Engagement, floating, and dipping.

Flexion

Resistance to descent causes the fetal head to flex down, leading to convergence onto the chest.

1. Flexion results in the smallest head diameter, the suboccipitobregmatic, to present through the canal.
2. This position relocates the posterior fontanelle to the center of the cervix, easily palpable on vaginal examination.
3. Flexion begins at the pelvic inlet and continues until the fetal head (or presenting part) reaches the pelvic floor.

Internal Rotation

To accommodate the birth canal, the fetal occiput rotates 45 or 90 degrees from its original position toward the symphysis.

1. The rotation is usually anteriorly; however, if the pelvis cannot accommodate the occiput anteriorly because of a narrow forepelvis, it will rotate posteriorly, resulting in an occipitoposterior (OP) position of the fetus.
2. This movement results from the shape of the fetal head and maternal pelvis, as well as the contour of the perineal muscles.
3. The ischial spines project into the mid-pelvis, causing the fetal head to rotate anteriorly to accommodate the available space.

Extension

1. As the fetal head meets the pelvic floor, it meets resistance from the perineal muscles and is forced to extend up and outward.

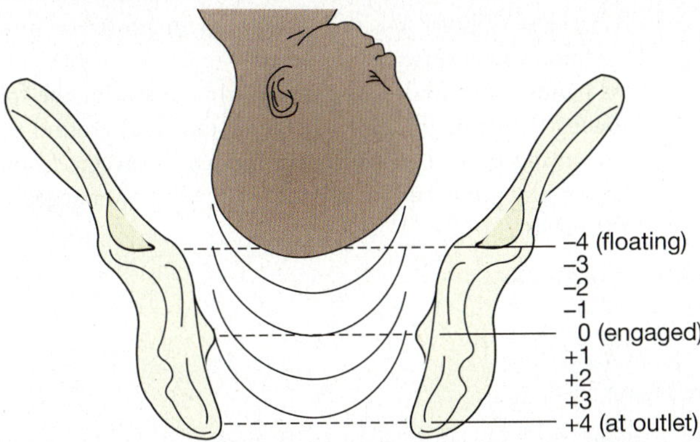

Figure 33-6. Stations of presenting part. The location of the presenting part in relation to the level of the ischial spines is designated station and indicates the degree of advancement of the presenting part through the pelvis. Stations are expressed in centimeters above (minus) or below (plus) the level of the ischial spines (zero). (Reprinted with permission from Silbert-Flagg, J. (2023). *Maternal and child health nursing* (9th ed., Fig. 15.7). Lippincott Williams & Wilkins.)

2. The fetal head becomes visible at the vulvovaginal ring; its largest diameter is encircled (crowning) and later emerges from the vagina.

External Rotation

1. Initial phase is called *restitution*. Once the fetal head realigns with the shoulders, restitution is complete.
2. The second phase of external rotation occurs as the body rotates so that the shoulders are in the anteroposterior diameter of the pelvis.

Expulsion

1. After delivery of the fetal head and internal rotation of the shoulders, the anterior shoulder resets beneath the symphysis pubis.
2. The posterior shoulder is expelled, followed by the anterior shoulder, leading to total body expulsion.

NURSING ASSESSMENT AND INTERVENTIONS

Initiation of Labor

Nursing responsibilities begin with an initial assessment once a patient presents in labor.

Collection of History and Baseline Data

EVIDENCE BASE Baker, B., & Janke, J. (2024). *Core curriculum for maternal-newborn nursing* (6th ed.). Elsevier.

Simpson, K. R., & O'Brien-Abel, N. (2021). Labor and birth. In K. R. Simpson, P. A. Creehan, N. O'Brien-Abel, C. K. Roth, & A. J. Rohan (Eds.), *AWHONN's perinatal nursing* (5th ed., pp. 326–412). Wolters Kluwer.

1. Introduce yourself; maintain eye contact as culturally appropriate; ask for name of patient's health care provider; inquire if the provider has been notified about the patient coming to the facility or birth center; ask about presenting complaints/concerns; orient the patient and partner to surroundings and explain the plan of care.
   a. Establish baseline obstetric, medical, and surgical information. Inquire and validate patient information with the prenatal care record, if available. Complete a brief review of past medical (including allergies), surgical, and obstetric history.
   b. Obtain a history of the current pregnancy: gravidity, parity, expected date of delivery or confinement, complications, fetal growth, antepartum testing results, sexually transmitted infections, recent travel abroad, and group beta *Streptococcus* status if tested.
   c. Inquire about current labor status and validate uterine contraction data with palpation: when did contractions begin, frequency, intensity, and duration; fetal movement; bloody show; have the membranes ruptured, time of rupture, color, consistency, amount of fluid, and any odor?
   d. Assess patient's comfort level.
   e. Inquire about a birth plan, participation in childbirth preparation classes, and pain management plans.
   f. Last oral intake of solids and liquids.
   g. Medications taken—prescription, over the counter (OTC), illicit drugs, herbals, or supplements?
   h. Inquire about the patient's support system.

2. Obtain baseline maternal and fetal vital signs.
   a. Temperature—elevation more than 100.0°F (37.8°C) suggests a possible infection or dehydration.
   b. Pulse—elevated over the resting rate during contractions; may be elevated between contractions because of medications, bleeding, or drug use; goal: 60 to 100 bpm.
   c. Respirations—increase as labor progresses; goal: 12 to 24 breaths/min.
   d. Blood pressure (BP)—slight elevation over baseline may be attributed to anxiety and pain.
      i. BP more than 140 systolic or 90 diastolic (mm Hg) may be suggestive of hypertensive disorder of pregnancy and requires further evaluation and notification to the provider.
      ii. BP of more than 160/110 requires immediate attention and notification of the provider because of the potential for stroke or seizure (see page 1040).
      iii. Goal: systolic more than 90 and less than 140 mm Hg; diastolic more than 60 and less than 90 mm Hg; mean arterial pressure (MAP) less than 100.
   e. Complete fetal heart rate (FHR) assessment; if a fetal monitor is to be used, run a 20- to 30-minute strip for baseline data and assessment of fetal well-being.
   f. Physical assessment—may include heart and lung sounds and deep tendon reflexes as indicated based on history.
3. Obtain a urine specimen—if indicated for symptoms of urinary tract infection or in cases of hypertension to check protein.

Methods for Determining Fetal Presentation

Leopold Maneuvers

The manual manipulation of the maternal abdomen to determine fetal placement in relation to maternal structures (see Figure 33-7).

1. First maneuver (fundal grip) (see Figure 33-7A)—determines fetal parts (fetal head or breech) located in the uterine fundus.
   a. While facing the patient, place both hands laterally on each side of the fundus and palpate; note the size, shape, and consistency.
   b. A head feels smooth, hard/firm, and round, mobile, and ballotable (movable on palpation); breech position feels irregular, rounded, soft, and not independently mobile.
2. Second maneuver (lateral grip) (see Figure 33-7B)—identifies the relationship of the fetal back and the small parts to the front, back, or sides of the maternal abdomen (fetal lie).
   a. In the same position, lower hands bilaterally along the lateral borders of the maternal abdomen.
   b. Select one hand to stabilize one side of the uterus while the opposite hand palpates downward over the opposite side. Repeat on the opposing side.
   c. Determine fetal anatomy by palpated contents: firm, smooth, and a hard continuous structure = fetal back; if small, knobby, irregular, protruding, and moving = fetal extremities.
3. Third maneuver (first pelvic grip) (see Figure 33-7C)—determines the portion of the fetus that is presenting into the pelvic inlet (fetal presentation). This maneuver is also known as *Pallach's maneuver or grip.*
   a. Grasp the part of the fetal presenting part situated in the lower uterine segment between the thumb and the middle finger of one hand.
   b. Assess contents as described in the first maneuver; findings should be opposite of information found in the fundus.

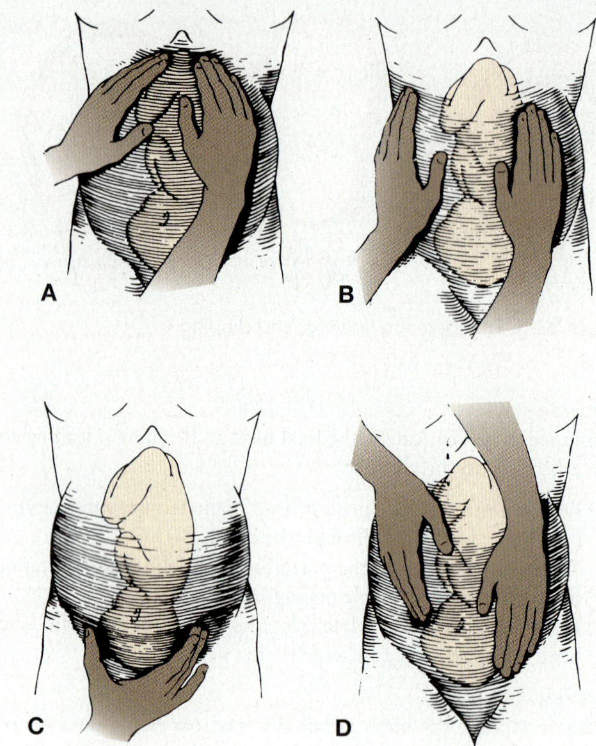

Figure 33-7. Leopold maneuvers (description below).

4. Fourth maneuver (second pelvic grip) (see Figure 33-7D)—determines flexion or attitude of the fetal vertex or the greatest prominence of the fetal head over the pelvic brim.
   a. Face patient's feet and place hands on each side of the uterus, below the umbilicus and pointing toward the symphysis pubis.
   b. Press deeply with the fingertips toward the symphysis pubis, locating the cephalic prominence.
      i. If the cephalic prominence is felt on the same side as the small parts, sinciput, fetal vertex is flexed.
      ii. If the cephalic prominence is felt on the same side as the back, occiput, fetal vertex is flexed.
      iii. If the cephalic prominence is felt equally on both sides, military position (common in posterior position), fetal vertex is nonflexed.
   c. As hands move toward the pelvic brim, assess for the following: If the hands converge (come together) around the presenting part, it is floating; if the hands diverge (move apart), the presenting part is either dipping or engaged in the pelvis.

Ultrasonography

See page 975.

Vaginal Examination

See Figure 33-8.

1. Explain the procedure and assist patient to a lithotomy position.
2. Keep the patient covered as much as possible to maintain privacy.
3. Conduct an examination gently using a sterile glove.
4. Perineum—visually assess the perineum for lesions, ulcerations, bruising, discharge, odor, rupture of membranes (ROMs), or bleeding. If an infection is suspected (i.e., syphilis

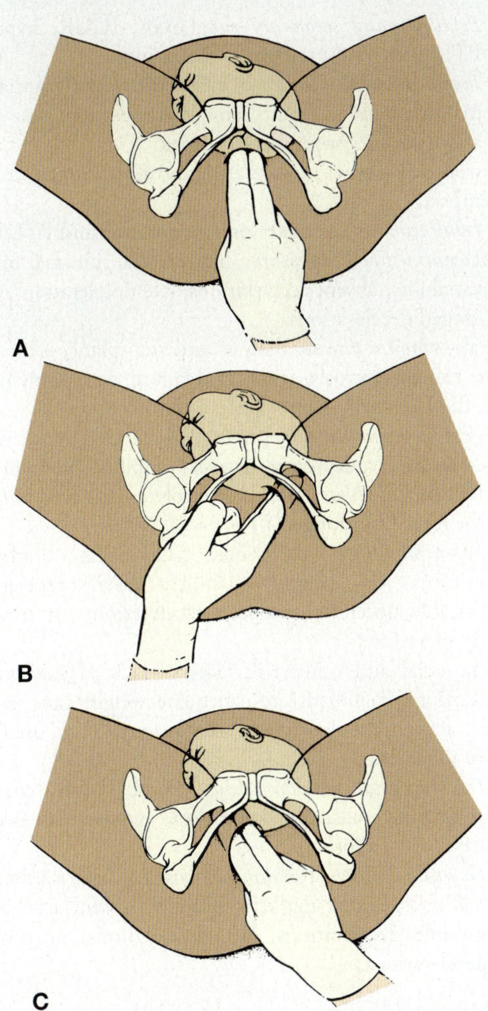

Figure 33-8. Vaginal examination. **(A)** Determining the station and palpating the sagittal suture. **(B)** Identifying the posterior fontanelle. **(C)** Identifying the anterior fontanelle.

or genital herpes) or active bleeding exists, stop the examination and notify the health care provider for further evaluation.

5. Perform manual examination with the dominant hand (may use the nondominant hand over fundus to stabilize fetal presenting part against the cervix):
   a. Cervical assessment.
      i. Location: posterior, mid, or anterior (facing the introitus and aligned parallel to the vagina).
      ii. Hard or soft: The cervix softens during latent phase of labor.
      iii. Long or short? As effacement occurs, the cervix shortens and thins. Measured in percentages from 0% to 100%.
      iv. Open or closed: measure degree of dilation in centimeters from 1 to 10 cm (complete).
   b. Presentation.
      i. Breech, cephalic/vertex face, shoulder, transverse, or compound.
      ii. Caput succedaneum (edema occurring in and under fetal scalp) present (mild, moderate, severe) or absent.
      iii. Station identified: signifies descent in relation to maternal pelvis (−5 to +5).
   c. Position.
      i. Cephalic presentation (in relation to maternal pelvis anterior, posterior, transverse).
      ii. Location of fontanelles.
   d. Membranes—intact or ruptured.
      i. Amount, color, and any odor of fluid.
      ii. Passage of meconium and consistency.

Sterile Speculum Examination

In some situations (e.g., premature ROMs, or positive group beta *Streptococcus*), a vaginal examination may be deferred, and a sterile speculum examination may be required or preferred.

1. Explain the procedure, ask patient to empty the bladder and remove all clothing from the waist down, and provide a sheet as cover.
2. Assist the patient into a lithotomy position (place hip roll under one hip to displace the uterus).
3. Drape legs and abdomen and adjust lighting at the perineum.
4. After selecting a sterile speculum, utilizing sterile technique, open the package.
5. Put on sterile gloves using proper technique.
6. Ask patient to relax the legs for proper visualization.
7. Explain each step of the procedure to decrease anticipatory anxiety of the patient.
8. With the nondominant hand separating the labia, place two fingers just inside the introitus, and gently press down on the base of the vagina. Next, insert the closed speculum past the fingers at a 45-degree downward angle such that the handle is perpendicular to the introitus.
9. Once the speculum enters the vagina, remove your fingers and turn the blades of the speculum into a horizontal position with the handle now parallel to the introitus; maintain a moderate and constant downward pressure (alleviates pain to the urethra).
10. As the speculum enters the posterior fornix, gently open the blades to visualize the cervix. If you still cannot visualize, close the blades, withdraw the speculum slightly, and move the blades toward the back of the vagina and try again. Once the cervix is in view, tighten the thumbscrew to maintain the blades in an open position. Complete a visual cervical assessment and obtain any samples necessary.
11. When the examination is complete, release the thumbscrew and withdraw in reverse order of placement.
12. Wipe any moisture or discharge from the perineal area and tell the patient the procedure is over; assist to a comfortable position.

Fetal Heart Assessment

EVIDENCE BASE Lyndon, A., & Wisner, K. (2021). *Fetal heart monitoring: Principles and practices* (6th ed.). Association of Women's Health, Obstetric, Neonatal Nurses.

Association of Women's Health, Obstetric and Neonatal Nurses. (2022). Standards for professional registered nurse staffing for perinatal units. *Journal of Obstetric, Gynecologic, & Neonatal Nursing, 51*(4), e5–e98. https://doi.org/10.1016/j.jogn.2022.02.003

Providers caring for patients during labor and delivery must be skilled in utilizing correct instrumentation for the current clinical scenario, interpreting FHR characteristics and patterns, applying appropriate interventions, and communicating both routine and critical data to the perinatal team as the conditions of the patient and fetus warrant. The Eunice Kennedy Shriver National Institute of Child Health and Human Development (NICHD) standardized the nomenclature of FHR to the use of categories of FHR interpretation to enhance interpretation, understanding, and communication among providers. Categories are as follows:

Category I tracings are *normal*

- Strongly predictive of normal acid–base status at the time of observation.
- Can be followed in a routine manner.
- No specific action required.

Category II tracings are *indeterminate*

- Not predictive of abnormal fetal acid–base status.
- Require evaluation and continued surveillance and reevaluation.
- Need to consider entire associated clinical circumstances.

Category III tracings are *abnormal*

- Predictive of abnormal fetal acid–base status at the time of observation.
- Depending on the clinical situation, efforts to expeditiously resolve the abnormal FHR pattern may include, but are not limited to:
  - Provision of oxygen.
  - Change in maternal position.
  - Discontinuation of labor stimulation.
  - Treatment of maternal hypotension.
- Intrauterine resuscitation may be necessary.

Maternal Risk Factors, Fetal/Neonatal Risks, and Fetal Heart Rate Implications

One cannot sufficiently interpret FHR variances without considering the impact of maternal physiology and pathophysiology during gestation. The large majority of maternal and fetal dyads tolerate physiologic challenges of pregnancy, labor, and birth without consequence. Conditions that may negatively impact maternal oxygenation and perfusion may lead to oxygen deprivation and hypoxemia in the fetus. Under extreme conditions (i.e., asthma attack, seizure, hemorrhage), the maternal blood flow and oxygen shunt to maternal vital organs (heart, brain, kidneys), which then negatively impacts nonvital uteroplacental blood flow to the fetus. Several maternal conditions outlined later explain risk factors to the fetus and subsequent FHR changes possibly witnessed during the intrapartum period.

1. Cardiovascular—acquired or congenital cardiac disease, anemias (sickle cell), or hypertensive disorders (most common).
   a. *Fetal/neonatal secondary risks*: small for gestational age (SGA), intrauterine growth restriction (IUGR), hydrops fetalis, hypoxemia, decreased amniotic fluid volume (AFV), preterm labor (PTL)/birth, and placental abruption.
   b. *Potential FHR alterations*: tachycardia, bradycardia, minimal or absent variability, absent accelerations, late decelerations, variable decelerations, prolonged decelerations, or sinusoidal patterns.
2. Respiratory—*chronic disease*: asthma and smoking; *acute disease*: status asthmaticus, acute respiratory distress syndrome, pulmonary embolus, sickle cell crisis, amniotic fluid embolus, or infections.
   a. *Fetal/neonatal secondary risks*: SGA, IUGR, hypoxemia, PTL/birth, and presence of meconium.
   b. *Potential FHR alterations*: tachycardia, bradycardia, minimal or absent variability, absent accelerations, late decelerations, or prolonged decelerations.
3. Neurologic—*chronic disease*: epilepsy; *acute disease*: stroke and eclampsia.
   a. *Fetal/neonatal secondary risks*: hypoxemia and PTL/birth.
   b. *Potential FHR alterations*: bradycardia, minimal or absent variability, absent accelerations, late decelerations, or prolonged decelerations.
4. Renal—*chronic disease*: dialysis and transplant; *acute disease*: acute tubular necrosis, acute renal failure, development of calculi, fluid/electrolyte imbalance, and infection.
   a. *Fetal/neonatal secondary risks*: SGA, IUGR, hypoxemia, decreased AFV, decreased/reversed umbilical blood flow, and PTL/birth. (*Note*: Altered electrolytes may adversely affect the fetus if prolonged.)
   b. *Potential FHR alterations*: tachycardia, bradycardia, minimal or absent variability, absent accelerations, variable decelerations, late decelerations, or prolonged decelerations.
5. Psychosocial and other risk factors—lack of prenatal care, medications, malnutrition/inadequate weight gain, excessive stress, domestic violence, and substance use (e.g., use of alcohol or illicit drugs).
   a. *Fetal/neonatal secondary risks*: SGA, IUGR, congenital anomalies, placental anomalies, hypoxemia, decreased AFV, or PTL/birth.
   b. *Potential FHR alterations*: tachycardia, bradycardia, minimal or absent or marked variability, absent accelerations, variable decelerations, late decelerations, or prolonged decelerations.

Fetal Heart Monitoring: External and Internal Options

Fetal Heart Rate Assessment by Auscultation

1. *Auscultation* is the use of a fetoscope or Doppler to count the FHR over a specified time frame (see Table 33-2).
2. Interpretation of data includes FHR baseline (FHRB) rate, rhythm, and accelerations and decelerations in the FHR.
3. Benefits:
   a. Neonatal outcomes comparable to the use of an electronic fetal monitor (EFM), in low-risk populations and with 1:1 nurse–patient ratio.
   b. Noninvasive, easy to use, and most methods require no electricity.
   c. Patient has increased freedom of movement and ambulation.
4. Limitations:
   a. Subjective data collection; variances between practitioners may exist.
   b. Conditions may limit the practitioner's ability to assess the FHR (obesity, increased fetal movement, or hydramnios).
   c. Cannot assess FHR variability (FHRV) or periodic/episodic decelerations or accelerations.
   d. Lack of continuous recording from monitor for visual comparative analysis.
   e. Requires a 1:1 nurse–patient ratio during intrapartum; therefore, may create the need to increase or realign labor and delivery staff.

Table 33-2 Frequency of Auscultation: Recommended Assessment and Documentation

ORGANIZATION	FIRST STAGE, LATENT PHASE	FIRST STAGE, ACTIVE PHASE	SECOND STAGE
ACOG			
Low risk	—	q30min	q15min
High risk	—	q15min	q5min
AWHONN			
Low risk	—	q30min	q15min
High risk	—	q15min	q5min
SOGC	Regularly after rupture of membranes or clinically significant change	q15min	q5min when pushing is initiated

Assess fetal heart rate (FHR) before initiation of labor-enhancing procedures, ambulation, administration of medications, administration or initiation of analgesia or anesthesia, and transfer or discharge of patient.
Assess FHR after admission of patient, artificial or spontaneous rupture of membranes, ambulation, recognition of abnormal uterine activity patterns, and administration of medications.
ACOG, American College of Obstetricians and Gynecologists; AWHONN, Association of Women's Health, Obstetric and Neonatal Nurses; SOGC, Society of Obstetrics and Gynecology of Canada; q, every.

5. Procedure:
   a. Position the patient in a semi-Fowler or lateral position; place hip roll on one side to displace the uterus; explain the procedure to the patient and support persons.
   b. Palpate the maternal abdomen to locate the fetal back by using Leopold maneuvers (see page 986). Figure 33-9 outlines FHR locations and corresponding fetal positions.
   c. When using Doppler device, apply conduction gel to the underside of device.
   d. Position the bell of the fetoscope or Doppler on the area of the abdomen where maximum fetal heart sounds can be heard, usually over the back or chest of fetus. If using a fetoscope, use firm pressure. If using Doppler device, avoid friction noises caused by fingers on the abdominal surface area.
   e. Assess and compare maternal heart rate (radial pulse/pulse oximeter) against the FHR; confirm differentiation.
   f. Palpate uterine contractions simultaneously and compare with FHR data.

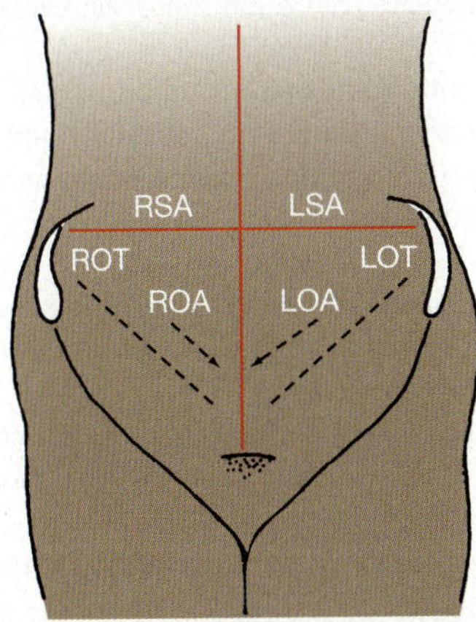

Figure 33-9. Fetal heart tone locations on the abdominal wall indicating possible corresponding fetal positions and the effects of the internal rotation of the fetus. LOA, left occiput anterior; LOT, left occiput transverse LSA, left sacrum anterior; ROA, right occiput anterior; ROT, right occiput transverse; RSA, right sacrum anterior.

   g. Differentiate between FHR/tone and other abdominal sounds.
      i. FHR—a rapid crisp ticking or galloping sound.
      ii. Uterine bruit—a soft murmur, caused by the passage of blood through dilated uterine vessels; synchronous with maternal pulse.
      iii. Funic souffle (uterine souffle)—a hissing sound produced by passage of blood through the umbilical arteries; synchronous with the FHR.
   h. Count the FHR between contractions for at least 30 to 60 seconds.
      Interpret findings to include FHRB rate, rhythm, and increases or decreases in FHR. Further evaluation via EFM is indicated if FHRB less than 110 or more than 160, irregular rhythm, and abrupt or gradual decreases in FHR during, immediately after, or 30 seconds after a contraction.
   i. Document and communicate findings with the patient and support person.
   j. Communicate abnormal findings to the provider immediately.
6. Troubleshooting interventions:
   a. Verify placement; utilize Leopold maneuvers to verify fetal position.
   b. Assess all four quadrants of the maternal abdomen slowly; fetal malpresentation or demise may exist.
   c. Reposition the patient to try to reposition the fetus.
   d. Reaffirm and compare data to the maternal pulse.
   e. Use alternative equipment options (i.e., EFM) if unable to assess.
   f. Consult with other members of the perinatal team (patient care team) and notify the provider as warranted.
7. Multiple fetuses require a keen sense of auscultation; each FHR should be documented by location. For example, baby A/#1 = left lower quadrant, 150 beats/min (bpm); baby B/#2 = right upper quadrant, 120 bpm. Ultrasound may be warranted to discern two separate FHRs.

Fetal Heart Rate Assessment by Ultrasound Transducer

1. Monitoring the FHR via ultrasound transducer allows detection of the FHR baseline rate, variability, accelerations, and decelerations.

2. Benefits:
   a. Noninvasive.
   b. ROMs not required.
   c. Provides permanent record for review and collaboration.
3. Limitations:
   a. Signal transmission may be influenced by maternal obesity, polyhydramnios, or anterior placental placement providing a weak, absent, or false signal.
   b. Restricts maternal mobility.
   c. Episodic maternal and fetal movement may interfere with continuous recording.
   d. Half or double counting of FHR may occur, especially with fetal tachycardia or bradycardia.
   e. May document maternal pulse with undiagnosed intrauterine fetal demise; always validate and compare data to maternal pulse.
4. Procedure:
   a. Perform Leopold maneuvers to locate the fetal back or chest (point of maximum intensity [PMI]).
   b. Lubricate the face of the transducer with a thin layer of ultrasonic gel to aid in the transmission of sounds. Place the transducer over the PMI.
   c. Readjust the device periodically to maximize signal quality. Maintain a constant strip of FHR data as diligently as possible during the course of labor.

Fetal Heart Assessment by Fetal Spiral Electrode

1. The use of the *fetal spiral electrode* (FSE) to monitor the FHR allows for detection of FHR baseline rate, variability, accelerations, decelerations, and FHR dysrhythmias. Indications for use during labor include FHR not detected or abnormal findings via an external device.
2. Contraindications:
   a. Face, shoulder, compound, or footling breech presentations.
   b. Unable to identify the presenting part.
   c. Presence of placenta previa; active vaginal or cervical herpes; active hepatitis, or human immunodeficiency virus (HIV) infection; active vaginal bleeding; or category III FHR pattern.
3. Benefits:
   a. Ability to detect FHR characteristics to include dysrhythmias and direct FHRV.
   b. Maternal position change does not alter the quality of tracing.
   c. Continuous detection of FHR; permanent recording in health record.
   d. Enhanced maternal comfort with removal of abdominal belt from external device.
4. Limitations:
   a. Invasive procedure; requires ruptured membranes, cervical dilation, and accessible/appropriate fetal presenting part.
   b. Potentially small risk of fetal hemorrhage, injury, or infection.
   c. May record maternal heart rate in the presence of fetal demise.
   d. Electronic interference and artifact may occur (i.e., may become twisted in fetal hair).
5. Procedure:
   a. Perform EFM test if turning on EFM for the first time.
   b. Open FSE package utilizing sterile technique and place sterile glove on dominant hand.
   c. Following completion of a cervical examination, secure hand inside the cervix with the second and third fingers pressed against the presenting part, avoiding the face, genitalia, and fontanelles.
   d. Press catheter against the presenting part and turn clockwise one full turn, pinch locking device at the end, remove introducer, and attach to the EFM while securing to the maternal abdomen or inner thigh.
   e. Interpret and document data.

Uterine Contraction Monitoring External and Internal Options

Uterine Contraction Assessment by Palpation

1. Uterine palpation is performed periodically throughout labor to validate labor adequacy and progression; if applicable, palpation is also utilized to validate information received from internal equipment (e.g., intrauterine pressure catheter [IUPC]).
2. Intensity may be described as follows (this may be taught to patient and labor coach):
   a. Able to easily indent the uterus: feels like the tip of the nose (mild intensity).
   b. Able to slightly indent the uterus: feels like the chin (moderate intensity).
   c. Unable to indent the uterus: feels like the forehead (strong intensity).
3. Uterine contraction data include:
   a. Frequency: beginning of one contraction to the beginning of the next.
   b. Duration: beginning of one contraction to the end of the same contraction.
   c. Intensity: peak pressure of a contraction.
   d. Resting tone: pressure of the uterus at rest or between contractions.
4. Benefits:
   a. Noninvasive; increases provider–patient interaction; direct assessment; easy to use/teach.
   b. Provides information regarding relative frequency, duration, strength, and resting tone.
   c. Allows freedom of movement and ambulation.
5. Limitations:
   a. Subjective information that leads to potential practitioner variance.
   b. No permanent record for visual comparison analysis or collaboration.
   c. Clinical conditions that may limit or alter data collection: overextended uterus (e.g., multiple gestation), polyhydramnios (hydramnios), macrosomia, uterine fibroids, or maternal obesity.
6. Procedure:
   a. Position patient in semi-Fowler or lateral position; place hip roll on one side to displace the uterus; explain the procedure to the patient.
   b. Place the pads of your fingers on the patient's abdomen in the area of the fundus and at the PMI (this is not always midline).
   c. Assess uterine contraction frequency, duration, intensity, and resting tone.
      i. Normal findings/intrapartum active phase: frequency, less than or equal to five contractions in 10 minutes, averaged over a 30-minute period; duration, less than 90 to 120 seconds.
      ii. Abnormal findings—tachysystole, more than five contractions in 10 minutes; hypertonus, intensity. When

compared with IUPC intensity (see page 1052), greater than 80 mm Hg; resting tone greater than 20 to 25 mm Hg or Montevideo units (MVUs) greater than 400.

Uterine Contraction Assessment by Tocodynamometer

1. A *tocodynamometer* (TOCO, tocotransducer) detects changes in tension or muscular tone over the fundus on the outside layer of the maternal abdomen. The electronic data are then converted into a number and printed on the lower half of the EFM paper. However, proper placement is key for accuracy:
   a. If patient is at term—place over the PMI in the fundal region of the maternal abdomen.
   b. If patient is preterm—place over the lower uterine segment below the umbilicus, typically beside the ultrasound device if the fetus is vertex.
2. Benefits:
   a. Noninvasive and easy to use.
   b. Detects relative uterine resting tone, frequency, intensity, and duration of uterine contraction.
   c. Does not require ruptured amniotic membranes.
   d. Generates a tracing for future assessment and permanent record keeping.
3. Limitations:
   a. Nonspecific data are gathered, particularly intensity and resting tone. External uterine monitoring identifies contraction frequency and duration. Contraction intensity is subjectively identified by patient and manual palpation.
   b. Difficult to obtain data in patients with the following conditions: obesity, polyhydramnios, macrosomia, PTL, maternal vomiting, and maternal bearing-down efforts/pushing during the second stage or during procedures.
   c. Location sensitive; placement may result in false or inadequate information.
   d. Sensitive to maternal and fetal movement—may be superimposed on contraction waveform.
   e. May limit maternal movement and ambulation during labor.
4. Procedure:
   a. Position patient in a semi-Fowler or lateral position; place hip roll on one side to displace the uterus; explain the procedure to the patient and support persons.
   b. Palpate the PMI over the fundus and secure belt.
   c. Press the uterine activity (UA) reference button on the EFM between contractions to set the resting tone between 5 and 15 mm Hg.
   d. Palpate the fundus and compare printed data.
   e. Reposition the device periodically, as needed, for patient comfort and during labor as the fetus descends.
   f. Interpret data and document and communicate findings.

Uterine Contraction Assessment by Intrauterine Pressure Catheter

An IUPC is the most objective technique to evaluate all uterine contraction characteristics and patterns. The device may be utilized for amniotic fluid testing and to perform an intrapartum amnioinfusion. IUPCs are either fluid-filled or solid-tipped catheters. Currently, there is no absolute indication for the use of the IUPC in labor. Although not required, many practitioners utilize this device during labor of a patient with a previous uterine scar (e.g., vaginal birth after cesarean).

1. IUPCs are typically placed by the health care provider.
   a. Two types: transducer and sensor-tipped catheters.
   b. UA (frequency, duration, intensity, and resting tone) can be calculated using MVUs. MVUs are calculated by subtracting the resting tone of the uterus (20 mm Hg) from the peak pressure of each contraction (in mm Hg) occurring in a 10-minute period. These resultant numbers are then added together for the total number of MVUs during that 10-minute period. Two hundred MVUs is considered adequate labor and uterine function.

CLINICAL JUDGMENT IUPC data should also be periodically checked against manual palpation until delivery.

2. Benefits:
   a. Assists in the interpretation of the FHR (i.e., comparison of a variable vs late deceleration).
   b. Tracing generated as a permanent part of the medical record.
   c. Allows for amniotic fluid collection and amnioinfusion.
3. Limitations:
   a. ROMs and adequate cervical dilation are required for insertion.
   b. Invasive procedure.
   c. Increased risk of uterine infection.
   d. Improper insertion can lead to maternal or fetal trauma (i.e., uterine perforation, uterine cord prolapse).
   e. Limits maternal ambulation during labor.
   f. May be contraindicated in the presence of vaginal bleeding.
   g. Differences may occur in readings between transducer and sensor-tipped catheters.
4. Contraindications: placenta previa, active vaginal bleeding.

Interpretation of Fetal Heart Rate

EVIDENCE BASE Lyndon, A., & O'Brien-Abel. (2021). Fetal heart rate interpretation. In A. Lyndon & K. Wisner (Eds.), *Fetal heart rate monitoring: Principles and practices* (6th ed.). Kendall-Hunt.

American College of Obstetricians and Gynecologists. (2019). Practice Bulletin No. 116: Management of intrapartum fetal heart rate tracings. *Obstetrics & Gynecology, 116*(5), 1232–1240. https://doi.org/10.1097/AOG.0b013e3182004fa9

Obstetric health care providers utilize the standardized NICHD terminology for enhanced understanding, collaboration, and teamwork to optimize patient safety.

Fetal Heart Rate

FHRB is the approximate mean FHR rounded to increments of 5 bpm during a 10-minute segment and excluding periodic/episodic changes, periods of marked FHRV, and segments of the baseline that differ by more than 25 bpm; interpretation between contractions is recommended, but not required.

1. Documented as a single number.
2. Normal FHRB, 110 to 160 bpm; tachycardia, more than 160 bpm for 10 minutes or greater; bradycardia, less than 110 bpm for 10 minutes or greater.
3. In any 10-minute window, the minimum baseline duration must be at least 2 minutes, or the baseline for that period is indeterminate. In this case, one may need to refer to the previous

10-minute segment for determination of the baseline. Two consecutive minutes are recommended, but not required.
4. FHRB is calculated by determining the range of FHRV first and then calculating the mean in increments of 5 (if FHRV equals 10 [i.e., 140 to 150], mean FHRB = 145; if FHRV equals 15 [i.e., 120 to 135], mean = 7.5, round up to FHRB of 130).
5. Variations from the normal baseline rate are tachycardia, bradycardia, and sinusoidal patterns.

Tachycardia

1. Etiology—maternal causes:
   a. Maternal fever.
   b. Maternal infection.
   c. Dehydration.
   d. Hyperthyroidism.
   e. Endogenous adrenaline or anxiety.
   f. Medications.
      i. Sympathomimetics (e.g., terbutaline, albuterol, epinephrine, ephedrine).
      ii. Parasympathomimetics (i.e., atropine, hydralazine, phenothiazines, hydroxyzine).
      iii. Selected positive inotropic agents (dobutamine and positive chronotropic drugs).
      iv. OTC medications (decongestants, appetite suppressants, and caffeine).
      v. Illicit drugs (cocaine, methamphetamines, and heroin).
      vi. Nicotine (if inhaled, nicotine may increase FHR; if absorbed through a nicotine patch, it may decrease FHR).
      vii. Labor enhancement agents (i.e., oxytocin, misoprostol), leading to persistent abnormal uterine contraction patterns.
2. Etiology—fetal causes:
   a. Infection.
   b. Fetal activity or stimulation.
   c. Compensatory response to early/acute hypoxemia.
   d. Fetal hyperthyroidism.
   e. Fetal tachyarrhythmias (supraventricular tachycardia).
   f. Prematurity.
   g. Congenital anomalies—cardiac abnormalities or heart failure.
   h. Anemia.
3. Interventions:
   a. Monitor vital signs: maternal temperature and pulse; compare to FHR data.
   b. Assess maternal hydration (initiate or increase intravenous [IV] fluids, as needed).
   c. Decrease maternal temperature, if elevated, via an antipyretic, as ordered.
   d. Decrease maternal anxiety, give explanations for treatment measures, provide comfort measures, and assist with breathing/relaxation techniques.
   e. Assess additional FHR characteristics: If decelerations exist, consider the need to:
      i. Change patient to a lateral position.
      ii. Administer oxygen via face mask (8 to 10 L/min); prolonged use discouraged.
      iii. Assess medication history and use.
      iv. Assess for tachydysrhythmia.
      v. If auscultating, apply EFM, as needed.
      vi. Notify the primary health care provider and perinatal team.

Bradycardia

Bradycardia in the fetus may result from maternal or fetal conditions and defined as less than 110 bpm for 10 minutes or greater. *Severe bradycardia* is defined as FHR less than 60 bpm. Sudden and sustained bradycardia accompanied by absent FHRV has the highest risk of fetal and neonatal morbidity or mortality.

1. Etiology—maternal causes:
   a. Beta-blocking agents (propranolol).
   b. Connective tissue disease (systemic lupus erythema).
   c. Prolonged maternal hypoglycemia.
   d. Maternal hypotension (r/t supine positioning, hypovolemia).
   e. Hypothermia.
   f. Anesthetics (epidural, spinal, pudendal, or paracervical).
   g. Conditions that may cause acute maternal cardiopulmonary compromise (amniotic fluid embolus, pulmonary embolus, cerebral vascular ischemia, hemorrhage, uterine rupture, trauma).
2. Etiology—fetal causes:
   a. Congenital heart block.
   b. Mature parasympathetic nervous system (postgestation).
   c. Acute hypoxemia.
   d. Cardiac structural defects.
   e. Impaired fetal oxygenation (e.g., umbilical cord occlusion, cord prolapse, uterine rupture, abruptio placentae).
   f. Maternal or fetal sentinel event precipitating hypoxia.
3. Hypoxic causes: umbilical cord prolapse or compression, uterine rupture, maternal hemorrhage, prolonged maternal hypoglycemia, placental abruption, maternal trauma, and persistent abnormal uterine contraction patterns (i.e., tachysystole). An FHR category III pattern of lengthy and severe bradycardia accompanied by absent FHRV may lead to permanent central nervous system (CNS) injury or death in the fetus or neonate.
4. Interventions:
   a. If using intermittent auscultation, change to continuous fetal monitoring.
   b. Confirm the FHR versus maternal heart rate with pulse oximetry.
   c. Perform vaginal examination to assess for umbilical cord prolapse.
   d. Perform frequent assessment of maternal vital signs to rule out maternal-fetal perfusion etiologies. Increase IV fluids as indicated.
   e. Assess FHRV and other FHR characteristics—consider:
      i. Maternal lateral position change.
      ii. Discontinue oxytocin administration or augmentation agents.
      iii. Modify maternal pushing techniques or stop pushing during the second stage of labor until FHR resolves.
   f. Administer oxygen via face mask (8 to 10 L/min) as necessary.
   g. Notify the health care provider and perinatal team.

Sinusoidal

1. This pattern differs from variability in that it has a smooth, sine wavelike pattern (equal deflections above and below the FHRB) of regular frequency and amplitude and is excluded in the definition of variability; described as *sinusoidal* or *pseudosinusoidal (medication induced)*.
2. Etiology:
   a. Severe fetal anemia: Rh isoimmunization.
   b. Fetal–maternal hemorrhage.

c. Severe fetal hypoxia or asphyxia.
d. Maternal opioid administration; may lead to pseudosinusoidal pattern.

3. Interventions:
   a. Lateral positioning.
   b. Administer IV infusion (IVF) of lactated Ringer's or normal saline.
   c. Administer oxygen via face mask (8 to 10 L/min).
   d. Assess patient for hemorrhage and treat accordingly.
   e. Notify the health care provider and perinatal team.
   f. If etiology necessitates, consider:
      i. Kleihauer–Betke test to assess for fetal red cell detection in maternal blood for identification of transplacental hemorrhage, to determine fetal versus maternal bleeding origin, and to allow patients who are Rh negative to receive Rhogam for the prevention of isoimmunization.
      ii. Expeditious delivery.

Fetal Heart Rate Variability

See Figure 33-10.

1. FHRV is the result of electrical impulses received by the cardiac muscle from the brainstem's medulla oblongata. The medulla oblongata receives information from both the parasympathetic (slow) and sympathetic (fast) nervous systems; the combined effect leads to a cyclic push and pull of the heart rate over time (heart rates are never static unless permanent CNS damage has occurred). Oxygenation must remain constant for communication to occur between the CNS and the cardiac muscle.
2. At the time of observation, variability indicates adequate oxygenation of the fetal CNS.
3. *Fetal heart rate variability* is defined as fluctuations in the FHRB. These fluctuations are irregular in amplitude and frequency and are visually quantified as the *amplitude of the peak-to-trough range* in beats per minute as follows:
   a. Absent FHRV—undetectable.
   b. Minimal FHRV—more than undetectable but less than or equal to 5 bpm.
   c. Moderate FHRV—6 to 25 bpm.
   d. Marked FHRV—more than 25 bpm.
4. Calculation of FHRV range is determined by the mean peak-to-trough range rounded to increments of 5 bpm (i.e., 120 to 135, 115 to 130, 150 to 155); the mean is reported as the FHRB.
5. Absent or minimal variability may be due to preterm gestation (less than 28 to 32 weeks), alteration in nervous system function, medications, abnormal uterine contraction patterns, or inadequate oxygenation.
6. Normal sleep and wake states, medications, alcohol, and illicit drugs that cause fetal neurologic damage; morphine; methadone; anomalies; and previous insults that have damaged the fetal brain can affect the baseline variability.
7. Moderate FHRV, even in the presence of decelerations, is strongly associated (98%) with an umbilical pH of more than 7.2 (nonacidemic) or newborn vigor (Apgar score ≥7 at 5 minutes).
8. Abnormal findings: prolonged periods of absent, minimal, or marked FHRV; if absent FHRV is accompanied by recurrent decelerations (late, variable, or prolonged), fetal or neonatal morbidity or mortality may result.
9. Interventions for category III pattern: recurrent late, variable, or prolonged decelerations accompanied by absent FHRV (caused by CNS dysfunction, hypoxia, asphyxia):
   a. Notification to provider and perinatal team for expeditious delivery.

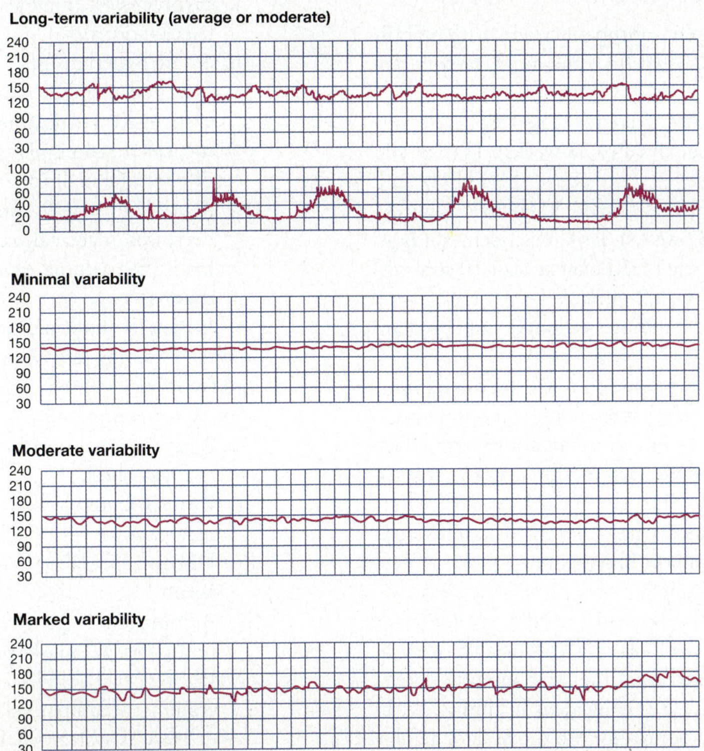

Figure 33-10. Fetal heart rate variability. (Reprinted with permission from Ricci, S. [2021]. *Essentials of maternity, newborn, and women's health nursing* [5th ed., Fig. 14-7]. Wolters Kluwer.)

   b. Prepare for expeditious and immediate delivery; route dependent on clinical conditions.
   c. Discontinue oxytocin administration, if applicable.
   d. Assess maternal vital signs (initiate/increase IVF, as needed).
   e. Administer oxygen via face mask (8 to 10 L/min).
   f. Change maternal lateral position.
10. Interventions for minimal FHRV (caused by sleep state, medications, hypoxia, CNS dysfunction, dysrhythmias):
   a. Rule out nonhypoxic causes: sleep state and medications.
   b. If minimal FHRV is accompanied by recurrent late, variable, or prolonged decelerations, extended time to complete all interventions outlined in 9a to f (previous paragraph) is afforded.
   c. If pattern does not resolve within 60 to 90 minutes, delivery via the most expeditious route is recommended.
11. Interventions for marked FHRV (possibly caused by cord entanglement, excessive release of fetal catecholamines, asphyxia): same as for minimal FHRV.

Periodic/Episodic Fetal Heart Rate Patterns

Periodic or episodic changes are visually apparent increases or decreases in the FHRB in the form of an acceleration or deceleration. Their duration is greater than 15 seconds and less than 2 minutes. After 2 minutes, they are considered prolonged. If duration exceeds 10 minutes, a baseline rate change has occurred. *Periodic* patterns occur simultaneously with contractions, and *episodic* patterns occur in the absence of contractions. Periodic and episodic patterns are distinguished on the basis of waveforms, currently accepted as "abrupt" (onset to peak or nadir [lowest point] is less than 30 seconds) or "gradual" (onset to nadir is greater than or equal to 30 seconds). *Decelerations* are defined as recurrent if they appear with 50% or greater of uterine contractions in any 20-minute period, or intermittent, if they occur with less than 50% of uterine contractions, in any 20-minute period.

1. Acceleration: visually apparent, abrupt increase in the FHR above the baseline rate; calculated from the most recently determined FHRB.
   a. The following criteria reflect gestational age implications:
      i. Term (greater than or equal to 32 weeks): Peak of acceleration is 15 bpm or more above the FHRB and 15 seconds or more in duration but less than 2 minutes.
      ii. Preterm (less than 32 weeks): Peak of acceleration is at least 10 bpm above the FHRB and at least 10 seconds in duration but less than 2 minutes.
      iii. Prolonged: duration 2 minutes or longer but less than 10 minutes.
   b. Etiology: fetal movement, uterine contraction, partial umbilical cord occlusion, breech presentation, occiput posterior in vertex position, vaginal examination, fetal scalp stimulation, following application of vibroacoustic stimulator, and application of FSE.
   c. Accelerations are associated with a nonhypoxic fetus and normal fetal pH at the time of observation.
   d. Interventions—none required.
2. Early deceleration—visually apparent, usually symmetrical gradual decrease and return of the FHR associated with a uterine contraction; calculated from the most recently determined portion of the FHRB. It is coincident in timing, with the nadir of the deceleration occurring with the peak of a contraction. In most cases, the onset, nadir, and recovery of the deceleration occur with the beginning, peak, and end of the contraction, respectively.
   a. Physiology—head compression causing increased intracranial pressure (ICP) that leads to a vagal response. This is a benign, nonhypoxic occurrence.
   b. Interventions—none required.
3. Late decelerations—visually apparent, usually symmetrical gradual decrease and return of the FHR associated with a uterine contraction. The decrease in FHR is calculated from the onset to the nadir of the deceleration. The deceleration is delayed in timing, with the nadir of the deceleration occurring after the peak of the contraction. In most cases, the onset, nadir, and recovery of the deceleration occur after the beginning, peak, and ending of the contraction, respectively.
   a. Physiology.
      i. Reflex—chemoreceptor stimulation leading to the transient decrease in FHR accompanied by normal FHRB and moderate variability. Prolonged supine positioning may precipitate reflex late decelerations; repositioning patient laterally often resolves pattern.
      ii. Myocardial depression—decreased oxygen transfer at the placental interface may lead to uteroplacental insufficiency (UPI). Prolonged periods of UPI may lead to progressive fetal hypoxia and metabolic acidosis. Metabolic acidosis can directly influence the electrical conduction and performance of the fetal heart, causing direct myocardial depression. These late decelerations are "myocardial mediated" and may be accompanied by a change in the fetal heart baseline (tachycardia or bradycardia), absent or minimal variability, and the absence of accelerations, usually indicative of a fetus in metabolic acidemia. A category III FHR pattern of recurrent late decelerations accompanied by absent FHRV requires immediate delivery via the most expeditious route.
   b. Maternal factors that may promote UPI:
      i. Hypotension (may also be associated with reflex late decelerations).
      ii. Severe hypertension.
      iii. Placental changes that may affect uteroplacental gas exchange (i.e., postmaturity, premature placental aging, calcification, placental abruption, placenta previa, or placental malformations).
      iv. Physiologic conditions that may be associated with decreased maternal oxygen saturation or hemoglobin levels (i.e., asthma attack, cardiopulmonary disease, or trauma).
      v. Persistent abnormal uterine contraction patterns (i.e., tachysystole, tetany, or hypertonus).
   c. Interventions—aimed at increasing uteroplacental perfusion by correcting cause.
      i. Alter maternal position: lateral position (right or left) or knee–chest.
      ii. Correct maternal hypotension with hydration and/or medication.
      iii. Discontinue labor stimulation or cervical ripening agents.
      iv. Administer oxygen by face mask at 10 L/min via a nonrebreather mask; prolonged use discouraged.
      v. If category III FHR pattern of recurrent late decelerations accompanied by absent FHRV, immediate delivery is warranted by the most expeditious route. Notification of the primary health care provider and perinatal team is indicated. Preparations for emergent delivery are warranted.

4. Variable deceleration—visually apparent abrupt decrease in FHR from the onset of the deceleration to the beginning of the FHR nadir is less than 30 seconds. When variable decelerations are associated with uterine contractions, their onset, depth, and duration commonly vary with successive uterine contractions. It is important to note that variable decelerations vary in shape, timing, and return to baseline. Severe variable decelerations last more than 60 seconds yet less than 2 minutes and fall more than 70 beats below the FHRB. Therefore, deceleration depth correlates with the degree of acidemia.
   a. Physiology—decreased umbilical cord perfusion, resulting from compression or stretch. Compression may result from maternal positioning, prolapsed cord, cord entanglement, second-stage labor, short cord, and a true knot in the cord.
   b. Interventions.
      i. Change maternal position, which may dislodge an occluded cord.
      ii. Perform a vaginal examination to assess for cord prolapse or imminent delivery.
      iii. If prolapse, elevate the presenting part of the cord while palpating for an umbilical pulse and FHR.
      iv. Amnioinfusion, if appropriate.
      v. Decrease or discontinue oxytocin, if appropriate.
      vi. Provide oxygen by face mask at 8 to 10 L/min; prolonged use discouraged.
      vii. Discontinue or alter second-stage pushing technique if repetitive, severe variables occur in the second stage.
      viii. If category III FHR pattern of recurrent variable decelerations accompanied by absent FHRV, immediate delivery is warranted by the most expeditious route. Notification of the primary practitioner and perinatal team is indicated. Preparations for emergent delivery are warranted.
5. Prolonged deceleration—visually apparent decrease in FHR of at least 15 bpm or more below the baseline and lasting more than 2 minutes but less than 10.
   a. Physiology—causes may reflect similar pathophysiology of late or variable deceleration.
   b. Interventions—if more than 4 to 5 minutes and causes unknown or unresolved, perinatal team should prepare for an emergent delivery.
6. Document all findings and classify patterns as normal (category I FHR), indeterminate (category II FHR), or abnormal (category III FHR) per NICHD guidelines (see Table 33-3).

Table 33-3 Three-Tier Fetal Heart Rate Interpretation System

CATEGORY	FHR PATTERNS
Category I: normal patterns	Baseline rate: 110–160 beats/min Baseline FHR variability: moderate Late or variable decelerations: absent Early decelerations: present or absent Accelerations: present or absent
Category II: indeterminate patterns (includes all tracings not categorized in category I or III)	Bradycardia not accompanied by absent baseline variability Tachycardia Minimal variability Absent variability not accompanied by recurrent decelerations Marked variability Absence of induced accelerations after fetal stimulation Recurrent variable decelerations accompanied by minimal or moderate variability Prolonged decelerations Recurrent late decelerations with moderate variability Variable decelerations with other characteristics, such as slow return to baseline, overshoots, or "shoulders"
Category III: abnormal patterns	Absent variability plus any of the following: Recurrent late or variable decelerations Bradycardia Sinusoidal pattern

EVIDENCE BASE American College of Obstetricians and Gynecologists. (2019). ACOG Committee Opinion No. 766: Approaches to limit intervention during labor and birth. *Obstetrics and Gynecology, 133*(2), e164–e173. https://doi.org/10.1097/AOG.0000000000003074

Lothian, J. (2024). Normal childbirth. In B. Baker & J. Janke (Eds.), *Core curriculum for maternal-newborn nursing* (6th ed., pp. 142–157). Elsevier.

First Stage of Labor: Latent Phase (0 to 5 cm)

Obstetric units should have comprehensive policies and procedures in place detailing evidence-based labor and delivery supportive practices based on the Association of Women's Health, Obstetric and Neonatal Nurses (AWHONN) and American College of Obstetricians and Gynecologists (ACOG) guidelines. Research supports that maternal–fetal outcomes, hospital readmission rates, and patient satisfaction with the birth experience are improved with continuous nursing support.

Nursing Interventions

Maintaining Nutrition and Hydration

1. Provide clear liquids and ice chips, as allowed.
2. Initiate IV access and infuse fluids, if ordered.
3. Assess intake and output, and evaluate urine for ketones and glucose, per facility policy.

Relieving Anxiety

1. Establish a relationship with the patient and support persons.
2. Inform the patient/partner/support persons of maternal status, fetal status, and labor progress periodically during the labor process. Ensure appropriate permission for information sharing.
3. Explain all procedures and equipment used during labor; answer questions and offer support.
4. Review birth plan and explain rationales for necessary revisions, if applicable.
5. Promote partner/support persons' participation in the labor experience.
6. Monitor maternal vital signs as the patient's condition warrants.
   a. Temperature every 2 to 4 hours, unless elevated or membranes ruptured, and then every 1 to 2 hours per facility policy.
   b. Pulse and respirations, as indicated by facility policy, medical condition, or medication administration (e.g., oxytocin or magnesium sulfate infusions).

c. BP is obtained typically every hour unless hypertension or hypotension exists or patient has received pain medication or anesthesia; then, evaluate more frequently based on findings or as indicated.

7. Monitor FHR periodically per facility policy (refer to Table 33-2, page 989).

Promoting Comfort

1. Encourage ambulation and frequent repositioning, as tolerated.
2. Encourage diversional activities, such as reading, talking, watching TV, playing cards, and listening to music.
3. Review, evaluate, and teach proper breathing techniques:
   a. Slow chest breathing (slow paced)—relax, take one deep cleansing breath, and exhale slowly and completely. Breathe deeply, slowly, rhythmically throughout the contraction. Average 10 to 12 breaths/min. Breathe slowly and deeply in through the nose and out through the nose or slightly pursed lips.
   b. Modified-paced breathing—used when slow chest breathing no longer effective, typically as labor progresses. Take one deep breath and exhale slowly and completely. As contractions intensify, breathe with more frequent shallow breaths during a contraction. At conclusion of contraction, take a deep breath and exhale slowly. Maintain a pace not to exceed twice the patient's average respiratory rate or less than 24 breaths/min. Encourage HOOT–HOUT breathing with emphasis on a "crisp T" for exhalation.
   c. Patterned-paced breathing (pant–blow breathing)—utilized in later stages of labor as contractions intensify and deep long breaths are not obtainable. Concentrate on breathing in a controlled manner. Take a deep breath and exhale slowly and completely. Then, take four shallow breaths through the mouth, making a "hee" or "heh" sound; maintain steady rhythm. Finish with a deep cleansing breath at the end of contraction. This breathing pattern is most commonly used during transition prior to active pushing.
4. Teach effleurage—light touch and massage over maternal skin, typically the abdomen, with fingertips; can be used with slow chest and modified-paced breathing. Start at the pubic bone and move hands slowly up to the sides of the abdomen in wide circular sweep; during exhalation, move fingertips down the center of the abdomen. Usually performed by laboring birthing parent, but can be done with one hand if side lying or coach assisted (see Figure 33-11).
5. Encourage a warm shower or whirlpool, if approved by primary practitioner.
6. Provide comfort measures.
   a. Give back or foot rubs.
   b. Assist patient with position changes. Walking, rocking chairs, squatting, hands-and-knees position, kneeling, standing, side lying, or sitting on the toilet assist fetal descent and alleviate pain. Side-lying position or hands-and-knees position will assist to rotate a persistent OP position to an anterior position.

Educate for Safe and Effective Use of Alternative Therapies

1. Provide information and clear up misconceptions about alternative therapies if patient is interested, on topics such as the following:
   a. Birthing balls—sturdy inflatable vinyl balls approximately 2½ feet (0.8 m) in diameter. The laboring patient can sit on the ball and sway from side to side, or may kneel and lean forward resting on the birthing ball to assist in fetal descent.
   b. Acupressure, massage—may be helpful for some, as it assists in decreasing pain sensation and promotes the release of endorphins.
2. Educate about herbal therapies—although many of the herbs used are not approved by the Food and Drug Administration, they have been researched and found to be effective during labor and are documented in medical and nursing references.
   a. Evening primrose oil—rubbed on the abdomen in prelabor to stimulate UA.
   b. Corn silk—stimulates sluggish labor.
   c. Nutmeg—enhances uterine contractions; if added, cayenne and bayberry help to reduce bleeding after delivery.
   d. Nutmeg with yarrow, mistletoe, and corn silk—utilized as a treatment for PPH.

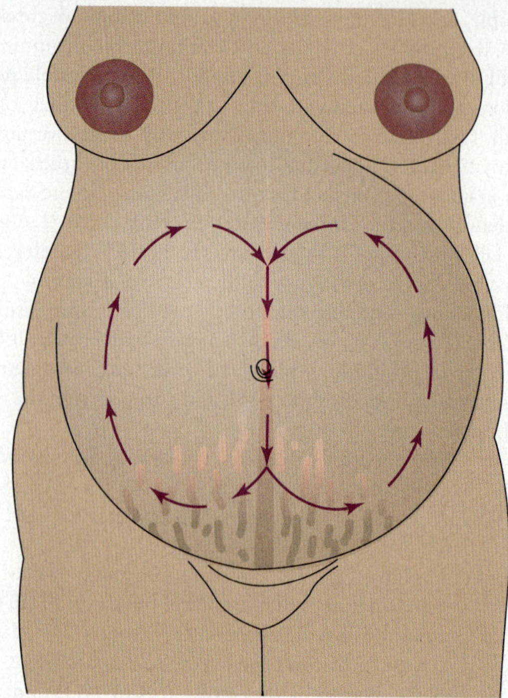

Figure 33-11. Effleurage patterns. During uterine contractions, a patient traces a pattern on the bare abdomen with the fingers. (Adapted with permission from Silbert-Flagg, J., & Pillitteri, A. [2018]. *Maternal and child health nursing: Care of the childbearing and childrearing family* [8th ed., Fig. 14-7]. Lippincott Williams & Wilkins.)

EVIDENCE BASE Abdurahman, A., Alchalidi, A., Lina, L., Nora, N., & Mutia, C. (2022). Analysis of the use of herbal therapy to reduce labor pain. *Macedonian Journal of Medical Sciences, 10*(F), 556–562. https://doi.org/10.3889/oamjms.2022.9651

Evaluation: Expected Outcomes

- Tolerates fluids well and urine negative for ketones and glucose.
- Verbalizes positive statements about self and fetus.
- Reports pain decreased from comfort strategies.
- Use of birthing ball and evening primrose oil with provider consent and partner assistance.

First Stage of Labor: Active Phase (6 to 10 cm)

EVIDENCE BASE Davidson, M. W., London, M. L., & Ladeweig, P. W. (2020). *Old's maternal–newborn nursing and women's health across the lifespan* (11th ed.). Pearson.

Shokry, S., Shabana, K., Farouk, O., & Mohamed, R. (2022). Effect of supportive measures guidelines on nurses' practices during labor. *Open Journal of Obstetrics and Gynecology, 12*, 482–497. https://doi.org/10.4236/ojog.2022.125042

Nursing Interventions

Relieving Anxiety

1. Monitor maternal vital signs every hour if low-risk pregnancy or every 30 minutes if high-risk pregnancy; assess FHR as outlined in Table 33-2, page 989. Reassure birthing parent of progress and of the fetus's well-being.
2. Provide encouragement and continuous labor support, and involve the patient/partner/support persons in the maternal–fetal plan of care.

Minimizing Pain

1. Encourage frequent position changes for comfort.
2. Assist the patient with breathing and relaxation techniques, as needed.
3. Provide back, leg, and shoulder massage, as needed.
4. Evaluate cervical status as needed to monitor progression. Cervical checks should be kept to a minimum with ROM and positive beta *Streptococcus* status.
5. Assist with preparation for analgesia and anesthesia following patient request (see Table 33-4).
6. Intervene for analgesia as follows:
   a. Confirm known allergies.
   b. Assess and document baseline temperature, BP, pulse, and respiratory rate.
   c. Monitor FHR before and after intramuscular (IM) or IV administration of analgesic medication.
   d. Assess efficacy of analgesics.
   e. Monitor FHR, continuous or intermittent, per facility policy and patient status.
7. Intervene for regional anesthesia as follows:
   a. Communicate maternal health information, laboratory results, labor status, and current obstetric complications with members of the health care team.

Table 33-4 Obstetric Analgesia and Anesthesia

DRUG	COMMENTS
Analgesics/Parenteral Opioids	
Butorphanol Nalbuphine Fentanyl Morphine sulfate	Decreases fear and anxiety, promotes physical relaxation and rest between contractions; may cause nausea and vomiting; respiratory depression is the main adverse effect and is seen primarily in the neonate. Most commonly given via IV line or IM every 3–4 h. Nalbuphine and butorphanol have opioid agonist and antagonist effect; avoid use if history of opioid dependency and may lead to a rapid withdrawal response.
Antiemetics/Antihistamines	
Promethazine Hydroxyzine	May be used in combination with opioids; potentiates opioids; may be used as an antiemetic. Used in latent and active first stage of labor to relieve anxiety, increase sedation and rest, and decrease nausea and vomiting.
Sedatives	
Sodium pentobarbital Sodium secobarbital Zolpidem tartrate	Produces sedation and hypnosis. Used for latent stage of labor to decrease anxiety, inhibit uterine contractions, and allow for rest. Does not relieve pain. Given orally or IM. Secobarbital has long half-life, up to 40 h after administration.
Regional Anesthesia/Analgesia	
Epidural opioids	Used with a local anesthetic to provide pain relief with a decreased motor block in labor. Used postoperatively to promote long-acting analgesia.
Epidural block	Used for labor to provide a sensory block up to the T10–T12 level. Medication is given through the epidural catheter. Used for cesarean delivery and postpartum tubal ligation by increasing the level of anesthesia up to T4–T6.
Subarachnoid block (spinal/intrathecal)	Used for surgical procedures such as a cesarean delivery and postpartum tubal ligation. The procedure is quicker and easier to perform. There is no catheter left in place for the procedure. Medication lasts for a finite period.
Local anesthesia	Used for pain control of the perineal area for an episiotomy or repair during a vaginal delivery.
Pudendal block	Used during the second stage of labor just before delivery to numb the lower vaginal canal, vulva, and the perineum for delivery. May also be used to provide pain relief for a forceps delivery if the patient does not have an epidural and for perineal repair.
General anesthesia	Used for emergency delivery involving cesarean delivery; if the patient refuses regional anesthesia; if regional anesthesia cannot be performed.

IM, intramuscular; IV, intravenous.

b. Administer IV fluid bolus of lactated Ringer's solution (500 to 1,000 mL) as directed, if not contraindicated (i.e., severe preeclampsia, pulmonary edema).
c. Assist anesthesia care provider by helping to position and hold patient for catheter insertion (lateral decubitus or sitting with feet supported, head flexed forward, elbows resting on knees with feet supported on a stool).
d. Monitor maternal BP, pulse, and respiratory rate after initiation or rebolus of regional anesthesia per facility protocol; typically every 5 minutes for the first 15 minutes.

8. Support patient to comfortable position as labor progresses—lateral or semi-Fowler position, side of bed with legs dangling, or Taylor sitting position with uterine displacement.
9. Intervene for maternal hypotension by assisting to lateral positioning; infusing additional IV fluids, as directed; and administering ephedrine per facility protocol.
10. Monitor for adverse reactions from IV injection of local anesthetic: maternal tachycardia or bradycardia, hypertension, dizziness, tinnitus, metallic taste in the mouth, loss of consciousness, or cardiopulmonary collapse.
11. Monitor for adverse effects of opioids or anesthetics:
    a. Pruritus (itching on the chest, face, and arms), especially during the first hour after medication administration (usually begins within 30 to 60 minutes and decreases during the next hour).
    b. Nausea/emesis—can occur in up to 50% of patients who are pregnant; administer medications to help with nausea/emesis, as directed by provider.
    c. Headache (pain in the frontal/occipital regions or radiating to the neck, stiff neck); increases in upright position and may decrease in horizontal position; relieved by abdominal compression; and may be accompanied by nausea/vomiting, ocular symptoms (photophobia, diplopia, difficulty in accommodation), and auditory symptoms (hearing loss, hyperacusis, tinnitus).
    d. Urine retention—observe for bladder distention; may utilize straight or indwelling catheter to empty the bladder if patient loses the ability to sense fullness.
12. Assess dermatomes following procedure and periodically as indicated.
13. Periodically evaluate and document maternal pain level on a continuum using pain assessment tools in accordance with facility policy.
14. Evaluate labor progress; anesthetics may slow labor progression; realize that augmentation agents may be necessary.
15. Following delivery, assess neonate for effects of analgesia or anesthesia (neurobehavioral change, such as decreased motor tone and decreased respiratory rate). Initiate neonatal resuscitation, as indicated.

Encouraging Bladder Emptying

1. Encourage the patient to void every 2 hours at least 100 mL, if possible.
2. Palpate the lower abdomen; evaluate for a distended bladder periodically throughout labor.
3. Provide privacy to the patient to complete task. Running water or providing a perineal bottle of warm water to squirt against perineum may assist success.
4. Catheterize patient if unable to void voluntarily.
5. Monitor intake and output per facility policy, particularly for certain medical conditions or following medication administration of IV oxytocin or magnesium sulfate.

Strengthening Coping With Active Labor and Transition

1. Assist the patient with breathing and relaxation techniques.
2. Encourage partner/support persons to assist with coping strategies.
3. Provide comfort measures, which may include:
    a. Effleurage, back rubs, and leg stroking.
    b. Cool cloth to the face, neck, abdomen, or back.
    c. Ice chips to moisten the mouth.
    d. Peri care and change pads and linens, as needed.
    e. Quiet, calm environment.
    f. Repositioning frequently for comfort with pillow and blanket.
4. Assist patient to pace self and to deal with one contraction at a time.
5. Provide information on the contraction's ascent, peak, and descent; encourage resting between contractions. Anticipatory guidance helps to assist with the patient's ability to tolerate labor.
6. Encourage the patient not to push with feelings of rectal pressure until complete cervical dilation has occurred. Short panting breaths may assist to divert bearing-down sensation.

Preventing Intrauterine Infection

1. Assess temperature every 2 hours if membranes are not ruptured. If ruptured, assess temperature every hour.
2. Periodically change pads and linens when wet or soiled.
3. Provide perineal care after voiding and as needed.
4. Discourage the use of perineal pads or folded towels against the perineum because they create a warm, moist environment for bacteria.
5. Minimize vaginal examinations.
6. Observe for fetal tachycardia and warmth of maternal skin as signs of infection.
7. Assess complete blood count, as indicated and available.

Maintaining Mobility

1. Provide information regarding limitations and opportunities for movement with EFM.
2. Encourage ambulation or sitting in a chair while being monitored, if appropriate.
3. Encourage frequent upright or lateral position changes.

Encouraging Effective Breathing Techniques

1. Assist the patient to alter breathing and utilize relaxation techniques, as needed, to maintain pain control.
2. Inform the patient that the urge to push is common during transition and occurs as the fetal presenting part meets the perineal floor muscles. Pushing with feelings of rectal pressure before complete cervical dilation should be avoided due to the risks of increasing cervical edema and lacerations.
3. Assist the patient to avoid pushing prematurely by:
    a. Maintaining close eye contact during breathing and keeping patient focused.
    b. Breathing with the patient and encouraging strong, short breaths while blowing out (pant–blow).

Evaluation: Expected Outcomes

- Verbalizes positive statements about self and fetus.
- Reports pain decreased from comfort strategies and medical interventions.
- The bladder remains nondistended.

- Directs strategies for decreasing discomfort.
- Absence of fever and signs of infection.
- Changes position during labor.
- Utilizes patterned breathing techniques during contractions.

Second Stage of Labor

The second stage of labor is typically the most maternal and fetal challenging stage. As contractions become more frequent and increase in intensity, perineal pressure is heightened as the fetus completes the last few cardinal movements through the birth canal. Breathing techniques and positioning may either help or hinder descent and oxygenation. It is important for the nurse to assist the maternal–fetal couplet with strategies to optimize oxygenation, encouragement, descent, and patient safety.

Positioning

1. It is most beneficial to encourage the patient to utilize upright positions to facilitate fetal descent.
2. Research supports that the most successful position is the squat; additional options exist (i.e., standing, upright kneeling, leaning against a wall).
   a. Advanced imaging techniques have verified an increase in the pelvic outlet during squat positioning of approximately 1 to 2 cm.
   b. Subsequent findings also conclude that a squat position is accompanied by a shorter second stage, higher Apgar scores, reduced pain, decreased perineal trauma, and decreased need for neonatal resuscitation intervention.
   c. With advancements in anesthesia preparations and dosing, patients have increased mobility during anesthetic infusions. Therefore, encouraging and assisting the epidural-induced patient into a squat position is achievable.
3. Additional positions are available to encourage fetal rotation and descent: side lying, knee–chest, hands-and-knees, and forward lean accompanied by a pelvic tilt or pelvic rocking.
4. Supine positioning is inappropriate during labor—at all stages—as it promotes maternal aortocaval compression syndrome with subsequent maternal and fetal deoxygenation and reduced perfusion.

Pushing Techniques

For optimum success, pushing techniques should be initiated once the cervix is fully dilated, fetal presenting part is on the pelvic floor (+1, +2, or greater than station), and the patient has a sense to push/bear down (Ferguson reflex). Because of the expanded use and effects of anesthetics during labor and birth, some patients lose sensitivity to perineal pressure, requiring guidance and instruction with pushing efforts. Two methods of pushing exist: passive pushing or laboring down, and active pushing.

1. Passive pushing ("laboring down"/"rest and descend")—this technique offers no active participation by the patient or practitioner to facilitate descent; strength of second-stage labor contractions moves the fetus down the birth canal. Reasons that may necessitate the need for this method include the following:
   a. Because of epidural anesthesia/analgesia, the patient does not feel the urge to push.
   b. Maternal clinical conditions such as cardiac disease, respiratory distress, or trauma.
   c. Fetal clinical conditions such as category III FHR or persistent abnormal UA data.
   d. Maternal exhaustion; need for periods of rest during prolonged second stage.
   e. Lack of nursing personnel to provide 1:1 support.
   f. Absence or unavailability of primary provider to assist with delivery.
2. Active pushing—this technique involves active participation (breathing techniques and positioning) by the patient and practitioner to assist in fetal descent. It is essential to facilitate pushing efforts through spontaneous pushing and supporting the patient's preferred pushing choice. Closed-glottis pushing (i.e., breath holding) is no longer recommended during the second stage as it limits oxygenation and encourages CO_2 retention. If prolonged, this technique may negatively impact the fetus and potentially lead to abnormal FHR patterns. Strategies that promote oxygen exchange in the birthing parent include:
   a. Open-glottis pushing—this technique allows the patient to maintain a patent airway for gas exchange while enhancing bearing-down efforts with several short, quick breaths over the duration of a contraction (60 to 90 seconds). The method includes several short, quick breaths of 4 to 6 seconds accompanied by bearing-down efforts that utilize muscles in the upper abdomen; improves maternal–fetal oxygenation.
   b. Tug of war—utilization of a gown or short sheet tied in a knot at both ends. Feeling the urge to push, the patient grabs one end of the gown or short sheet and pulls while the coach or nurse provides resistance by holding the other end (alternative way is to tie knot in one end and tie the other end to squat bar of labor bed); relaxes the perineum and has been found to decrease the second stage of labor by as much as 20 minutes.
3. Birthing aids—birthing balls, squat bars, birthing stools, and cushions may also be utilized to support the patient and fetus at this time.

Nursing Interventions

Minimizing Fear and Anxiety

1. Monitor maternal vital signs per facility policy.
2. Assess FHR and contraction every 5 to 15 minutes per facility policy and patient status.
3. Explain procedures, breathing technique, and equipment during the delivery process.
4. Keep the patient informed of progress and alterations in care plan.
5. Provide frequent, positive encouragement and utilize a mirror to assist the patient to see progress.
6. Assist with positioning and pushing, as outlined earlier.

Promoting Comfort

1. Change positions frequently to increase comfort and promote fetal descent.
2. Evaluate bladder fullness and encourage voiding or catheterizing, as needed.
3. Evaluate the effectiveness of analgesia or anesthesia, as indicated; notify if alterations in dosing are needed to facilitate progression while maintaining pain control.

Facilitating an Uncomplicated Delivery Process

1. Explain delivery process and equipment to patient/partner/support persons.

2. Prepare the delivery equipment maintaining sterile technique, and prepare the delivery area to maximize work area and accessibility of equipment.
3. Prepare the infant resuscitation equipment and preheat radiant warmer; notify pediatric personnel, per facility policy as appropriate; if category III pattern, have two practitioners available to administer neonatal resuscitation, as indicated.
4. Notify necessary obstetric personnel and primary practitioner to prepare for delivery.
5. If delivery room is to be used, safely transfer the patient to the delivery bed before the birth is imminent.
6. If delivering in a birthing room, prepare labor bed for delivery.
7. Position the patient for vaginal birth in a semi-Fowler position (C-position) supported by pillows for head, back, and shoulders. Positioning may vary by patient preference, practitioner, and facility.
   a. If used, gently place legs in padded stirrups or footrests symmetrically to avoid ligament strain, backache, or injury.
   b. Under-buttock drapes are recommended to evaluate blood loss during birth process. Accurate blood loss should be assessed and documented at every birth.
   c. Follow facility protocol or provider preference for cleansing the perineal area.
8. Support and guide the patient step by step during the delivery process. When the birth is imminent, encourage the patient to breath and maintain focus. Controlled pushing may decrease the risk of lacerations, tears, and episiotomy. Evidence-based criteria do not support routine use of episiotomy to facilitate the second stage of labor; however, clinical judgment is the best guide based on individualized patient and fetal status.
   a. An episiotomy may be performed when the fetal head is encircled by the vulvovaginal ring.
   b. Once the head is delivered, the patient is instructed to stop pushing. Mucus is wiped from the infant's face and then mouth and nose. A bulb syringe may be used. Neonatal resuscitation guidelines no longer recommend suctioning of any kind on the perineum for the presence of meconium.
   c. Nuchal cord intervention—loops of umbilical cord found around the neonate's neck are loosened and slipped over the head, whenever possible. If the cord cannot be slipped over the head, it is clamped with two clamps and cut between the two clamps.
   d. Next, the patient is instructed to give a gentle push to assist with delivery of the neonate's body and placed skin to skin on the maternal abdomen as the neonatal condition allows.
   e. Cord clamping—depending on the newborn's condition, some providers may delay clamping until the umbilical cord stops pulsating. This is done primarily to increase neonatal weight and hemoglobin and iron stores. The cord is clamped with two cord clamps and cut between the two clamps. It is common for the patient's partner or support person to cut the cord with assistance from the provider.
   f. If color and tone are adequate and accompanied by a vigorous cry, basic neonatal care can be delayed to support skin-to-skin contact and family bonding. If additional resuscitative support is indicated, the baby is passed to the neonatal team for immediate care.
9. Practice standard precautions during labor and delivery.

CLINICAL JUDGMENT Evidence clearly supports the routine implementation of uninterrupted skin-to-skin contact during the "Golden Hour" for physiologic stabilization between the patient and a healthy newborn. Studies demonstrate improved neonatal outcomes with respect to cardiorespiratory status, thermoregulation, and blood glucose stabilization. Maternal benefits include improved breastfeeding, pain management, and reduced anxiety. Nurses should make this a routine process after delivery as the neonate's condition allows and perform all initial assessments without interrupting contact. Discharge instruction should include continued skin-to-skin contact.

Evaluation: Expected Outcomes

- Verbalizes positive statements about delivery outcome.
- Reports decreased pain from proper positioning.
- Infant is delivered without complications.

Third Stage of Labor: Delivery of the Placenta

Nursing Interventions

Promoting Tissue Integrity

1. Observe for signs of placental separation (see Figure 33-12):
   a. The uterus becomes globular in shape and rises upward in the abdomen.
   b. Umbilical cord lengthens.
   c. Small amount (gush) of blood appears.
2. Once signs of placental separation are observed, instruct the patient to assist delivery of the placenta with gentle bearing-down efforts. Be aware that delivery of the placenta typically occurs within the first 5 to 10 minutes, but may persist past 30 minutes, particularly in preterm gestations.
3. Administer and titrate oxytocin as directed to maintain uterine tone. Once the neonate has been delivered, oxytocin 10 units IM or 10 to 40 units IV per 1,000 mL is often utilized as the first line of treatment to prevent obstetric hemorrhage because of uterine atony.

CLINICAL JUDGMENT PPH is a leading cause of maternal mortality and morbidity. Nurses should anticipate the risk of PPH during the intrapartum period and be prepared to quickly intervene. Induction and/or augmentation with oxytocics has been identified as a potential risk for PPH. PPH protocols are recommended in obstetrical units for immediate intervention to improve maternal outcomes.

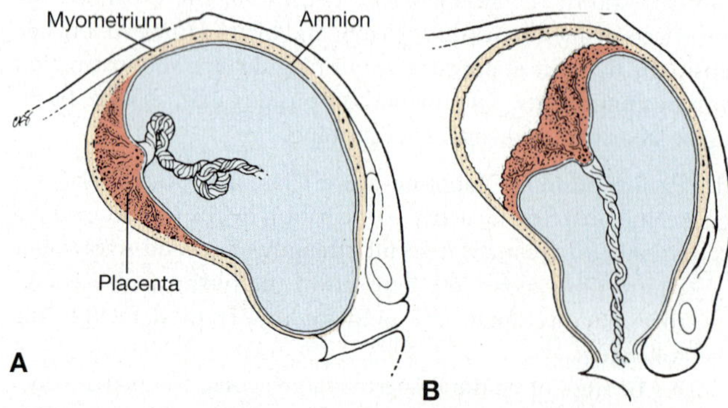

Figure 33-12. Placental separation. **(A)** Placenta attached to uterine wall. **(B)** Placenta separated from uterine wall. (LifeART image copyright (c) 2024. Lippincott Williams & Wilkins. All rights reserved.)

DRUG ALERT Oxytocin should never be administered IV push as it can cause cardiac dysrhythmias and death.

4. Inspect the placenta for size, shape, insertion site of cord, and intact cotyledons. The presence of even one cotyledon remaining intact within the uterus may lead to a PPH. Umbilical cord should be inspected for true/false knots, clots, length, and a three-vessel cord. Abnormalities in the placenta, cord, or foul odor should be documented in the labor record and may necessitate the provider to request the placenta be sent for pathology.

Fourth Stage of Labor: Immediate Postpartum

EVIDENCE BASE Association of Women's Health, Obstetric and Neonatal Nurses. (2021). Quantification of blood loss: AWHONN Practice Brief Number 13. *Nursing for Women's Health, 25*(4), e5–e7. https://doi.org/10.1016/j.nwh.2021.04.005

Promoting Normal Involution and Controlled Bleeding

Also, see postpartum hemorrhage, page 1065.

1. Monitor BP, pulse, respirations, and oxygen saturation every 15 minutes for the first 2 hours after delivery with a temperature every 1 hour. Depending on the patient's condition, fundal and lochia checks and vital signs may be assessed more frequently as needed. Ongoing assessment in postpartum patients should follow facility policy.

CLINICAL JUDGMENT Nurses must be aware that maternal tachycardia is an early indicator of PPH and should always be evaluated. Hypotension is a late sign of hypovolemia and requires immediate evaluation and intervention.

2. Immediately after delivery of the placenta, assess uterine fundal tone, height, and position every 15 minutes for 2 hours. Place a hand over the lower uterine segment above the symphysis pubis to inhibit uterine inversion and gently massage the fundus with the other hand. Visual inspection of the perineum should occur simultaneously to assess lochia.
3. Note that the uterus is firm at or around the level of the umbilicus and midline. If deviated to the side (usually the right side), it is indicative of a full bladder. Assist the patient to void spontaneously or utilize a straight catheter to empty bladder if anesthesia effects remain.
4. Gently massage uterine fundus at least every 15 minutes for 2 hours to promote firmness and expression of clots to decrease the risk of hemorrhage. Also, teach the patient self-massage of the uterus. Uterine massage may be performed with a bimanual technique, when indicated, by a provider.
5. Utilize an under-buttock drape after the placenta is delivered to improve accuracy of blood loss calculation and identify obstetrical hemorrhage. Quantitative blood loss (QBL) versus estimated blood loss (EBL) is facility dependent.
6. Assess and document vaginal bleeding (lochia):
   a. Scant—blood only on tissue when wiped or less than 1-in (2.5-cm) stain on perineal pad.
   b. Small/light—less than 4-in (10.2-cm) stain on perineal pad.
   c. Moderate—less than 6-in (15.2-cm) stain on perineal pad.
   d. Heavy—saturated perineal pad.
   e. Clots—note size and frequency; weigh for blood loss.
7. Assess the perineum for pain, edema, discoloration, bleeding, odor, or hematoma formation, if excessive perineal pain.
8. Assess episiotomy/lacerations for approximation, drainage, bleeding, or infection.
9. Report and document all assessments.
   a. The patient is stable if the fundus remains firm or firms quickly with massage and there is small to moderate amount of lochia. If the patient continues to saturate perineal pads or pass large clots, massage fundus, quantify blood loss, and notify the provider.
   b. The patient is unstable if MAP is less than 60, has a systolic BP less than 90, or a 15% drop from normal baseline BP (clinical indicators of obstetrical hemorrhage).
   c. Severe tachycardia (≥120) and severe tachypnea (greater than 30/min) are signs of impending compromise and require immediate evaluation and intervention by a provider.

Maintaining Fluid Volume

1. Maintain IV fluids as clinical condition warrants. Administer oxytocin as earlier if not given in the third stage.
2. Maintain accurate measurement of intake and output during the immediate postpartum.
3. Provide oral fluids and a snack or meal, as tolerated, if vital signs are stable and bleeding is controlled.

Relieving Discomfort and Fatigue

1. Apply a covered ice pack to the perineum immediately after delivery and periodically during the first 24 hours for an episiotomy, perineal laceration, or edema.
2. Administer analgesics, as indicated. Excessive perineal pain unrelieved by medications suggests hematoma formation and mandates careful examination of the vulva, vagina, and rectum.
3. Ensure that epidural catheter has been removed by anesthesia provider, if appropriate.
4. Assist the patient in finding comfortable positions.
5. Assist the patient with a partial bath and perineal care. Periodically change linens and pads, as necessary.
6. Allow for privacy and promote rest periods between postpartum checks.
7. Provide warm blankets and reassure the patient that tremors are common during this period because of intravascular fluid shifts.

Encouraging Bladder Emptying

1. Evaluate the bladder for distention.
2. Encourage the patient to void periodically.
   a. Provide adequate time and privacy.
   b. The sound of running water may stimulate voiding.
   c. Gently squirting tepid water on the perineum may facilitate voiding.
3. Catheterize the patient if the bladder is full and unable to void.
   a. Birth trauma, anesthesia, and pain from lacerations and episiotomy may reduce or alter the voiding reflex.
   b. Bladder distention may displace the uterus upward and to the right side, impairing tone.

Preventing Injury Pending Return of Sensation

1. Evaluate mobility and sensation of the lower extremities.
2. Evaluate vital signs.

3. Remain with the patient and assist out of bed for the first time. Evaluate the patient's ability to support weight and ambulate safely.

Promoting Caregiving

1. Once stable, bring the neonate to the patient and partner immediately after birth.
2. Encourage them to hold the infant as soon as possible.
3. Assist and teach them to hold the neonate close to their faces, about 8 to 12 in (20.5 to 30.5 cm) to engage the neonate.
4. Assist them to inspect the infant's body to familiarize themselves with their child.
5. Assist with breastfeeding as soon as possible once maternal and newborn stability is established. This is typically a period of quiet alert time for the neonate often optimizing successful breastfeeding.
6. Document appropriate and inappropriate bonding; notify primary provider and social services if suspect lack of or inappropriate response in patient, partner, or any other potential caregiver.

Evaluation: Expected Outcomes

- Vital signs remain stable, vaginal bleeding remains light to moderate, and the uterus remains firm at the midline below the umbilicus.
- Tolerates fluids and food well after delivery.
- Verbalizes decreased perineal pain and feels rested.
- Voids within 2 hours of delivery.
- Ambulates without assistance.
- Appropriate parental interaction with the neonate.

Immediate Care of the Neonate

EVIDENCE BASE Ricci, S. S. (2021). *Essentials of maternity, newborn, and women's health nursing* (5th ed.). Wolters Kluwer.

American Academy of Pediatrics & American Heart Association. (2021). *Textbook of neonatal resuscitation* (7th ed.). American Academy of Pediatrics.

Nursing Interventions

Promoting Airway Clearance and Transitioning of the Neonate

1. Closely observe all neonates for a minimum of 4 to 6 hours after birth. Over 90% of newborns complete intrauterine to extrauterine transition without compromise or assistance.
2. Clean mucus from the face, mouth, and nose. Aspirate with a bulb syringe, as necessary.
   a. Neonatal resuscitation protocols no longer require suctioning on the perineum if meconium is present in the amniotic fluid.
   b. A vigorous newborn demonstrating strong respiratory effort, good muscle tone and a heart rate greater than 100 may only require bulb suctioning of the mouth and nose if needed.
   c. In the presence of meconium-stained amniotic fluid and a nonvigorous infant, deep suctioning of the mouth and trachea may be necessary to prevent aspiration.
3. Assess neonate's transition using the Apgar scoring system (see Table 33-5) at 1 and 5 minutes after birth. When the 5-minute score is less than 7, scoring continues every 5 minutes up to 20 minutes after delivery. An Apgar score of 0 to 3 at 20 minutes is associated with increased neonatal morbidity. Wear gloves at all times when handling an unbathed newborn and maintain standard precautions.

Promoting Thermoregulation

1. Dry the neonate immediately after delivery, remove wet towels, and place skin to skin on the maternal abdomen, if the neonate is vigorous, and cover with a blanket and hat to prevent heat loss.

CLINICAL JUDGMENT If a newborn is nonvigorous, place under a prewarmed radiant warmer for further evaluation. A neonate can lose up to 200 cal/kg/min through evaporation, convection, conduction, and radiation. Double wrap the neonate in warm blankets, with hat, and return to patient after stabilization.

2. Provide a warm, draft-free environment for the neonate.
3. Assess neonate's axillary temperature—a normal temperature is between 97.7°F and 99.3°F (36.5°C and 37.4°C, respectively).

Preventing Infection and Other Complications

1. Provide phylactic eye care: Administer a 1-cm ribbon of erythromycin 0.5% or tetracycline 1% ophthalmic ointment to the lower conjunctival sac to prevent ophthalmia neonatorum (gonorrheal or chlamydial). This can be delayed up to 1 hour after birth to facilitate breastfeeding and parental bonding. Ointment may be gently wiped away after 1 minute with a sterile cotton ball.
   a. If maternal gonococcal or chlamydial culture is positive, the neonate will require further treatment.
   b. Prophylaxis is mandatory in all states.
2. Administer vitamin K: Administer a single prophylactic dose of vitamin K_1 (phytonadione) 0.5 to 1 mg IM to the vastus lateralis and document site.
   a. Given to prevent a vitamin K–dependent hemorrhagic disease of the newborn.
   b. If the caregivers decline vitamin K administration, inform the caregivers that if they desire a circumcision, it may not be performed related to the increased risk of bleeding.
   c. Inform caregivers that vitamin K levels will reach their peak (without neonatal injection) at 8 days after birth.
3. Ensure security and identification: Place identical maternal and neonatal identification bracelets per facility policy. An additional electronic security device may also be secured at this time to prevent infant abduction.
   a. Information on bands may include maternal name, hospital/admission number, neonate's sex assigned at birth, primary health care provider, and date and time of birth and other information specified in the facility's policy.
   b. An additional identification bracelet with the same information may also be worn by the patient's partner or a designated person, according to facility policy.
   c. Footprinting and fingerprinting of the neonate are not adequate methods of patient identification and may or may not be performed based on facility policy.
   d. Complete all identification procedures before the infant leaves the delivery room.
4. Perform measurements: Weigh and measure the infant shortly after birth.
   a. Average neonate weight is 5 to 8 pounds (2,500 to 4,000 g).
   b. Average neonate length is 18 to 22 in (46 to 56 cm).
   c. Head, chest, and abdominal circumferences are also measured (facility dependent).

Table 33-5 Apgar Scoring Chart

SIGN	SCORING 0	1	2	INTERPRETATION
Activity (muscle tone)	Floppy	Flexed arms and legs	Active	0–3: severely depressed 4–6: moderately depressed 7–10: reassuring
Pulse	Absent	<100	>100	
Grimace (reflex irritability)	No response	Minimal response to stimuli	Prompt response to stimuli	
Appearance (skin color[a])	Blue, pale	Pink body, blue extremities	Pink	
Respirations	Absent	Slow and irregular	Vigorous cry	

[a]*May not be applicable for all ethnicities; palms, soles, and nailbeds more reliable.*

5. After birth, evaluate the neonate's status and assess risks of birth trauma or injury.
6. Administer hepatitis B virus (HBV) vaccine according to your facility's policy.
   a. Vaccination of all infants born in the United States is recommended, regardless of maternal hepatitis status. If maternal hepatitis B surface antigen (HBsAg) status is negative, the vaccine is given within 12 hours of birth to age 2 months and then again at 1 to 2 months after the initial dose, with the final vaccine (#3) given at 6 to 18 months. The vaccine is given for the prevention of acute and chronic hepatitis B infection.
   b. If maternal HBsAg positive, the infant will receive hepatitis B immunoglobulin (HBIG) and the HBV vaccine at birth to within 12 hours. In addition, these infants will receive HBV vaccine at ages 1 to 2 months and age 6 months.
   c. If maternal hepatitis screening is not done, the neonate will receive the HBV vaccine within 12 hours of birth. If later, maternal hepatitis B testing is positive, the neonate will also receive HBIG (0.5 mL) IM as soon as possible, but no later than 1 week after birth. The infant will also receive HBV vaccine at 1 to 2 months and another injection at 6 to 18 months.

Home Birth Considerations

1. Issues regarding promoting airway clearance, transitioning, and thermoregulation promotion are essentially unchanged for home births; Apgar scores are not always given at home deliveries.
2. Eye prophylaxis is required using an antimicrobial ointment (i.e., erythromycin) to prevent ophthalmia neonatorum.
3. Vitamin K administration is not a requirement for home deliveries. Vitamin K levels naturally increase at 8 days of life. If caregivers desire circumcision (removal of foreskin from the penis), the procedure is withheld until after day 8.
4. Make sure attendants are familiar with neonatal resuscitation and that emergency numbers and procedures are readily available.
5. Identification procedures are not required for home births, although required state paperwork must be completed by the health care provider.

Evaluation: Expected Outcomes

- Neonate transitions appropriately, as evidenced by Apgar score between 7 and 10.
- Temperature remains between 97.5°F and 99°F (36.4°C and 37.2°C).
- Eye prophylaxis and other procedures completed following delivery.

SPECIAL CONSIDERATIONS

Precipitous Delivery or Delivery in the Absence of Health Care Provider (Nurse Assisted)

A precipitous delivery is an emergent event. Coordination to prevent maternal and fetal infection, injury, and hemorrhage is key.

Interventions

1. Provide reassurance and instruct the patient in a calm, controlled manner. Sustain eye contact and assist the patient to utilize pant–blow breathing until told to push.
2. Position patient for comfort and enhance visualization of the perineum.
3. Wash hands, put on gloves, and clean the perineum as time permits.
4. Exert gentle pressure against the head of the fetus, using pads of the thumb, index finger, and middle fingers or cupped palm of the hand, to control progress and prevent precipitous delivery; this prevents undue stretching of the perineum and sudden expulsion through the vulva with subsequent infant and maternal complications.
5. Encourage the patient to pant–blow at this time to prevent bearing down.
6. If membranes are intact at the time of delivery, rupture can be achieved by applying pressure to the membranes.
7. Wipe the infant's face and mouth with a clean towel. Suction the mouth and nose with a bulb syringe, if available.
8. Check for nuchal cord and reduce, if possible. If the cord is too tight to permit slipping over the infant's head, it must be clamped in two places and cut between the clamps before the rest of the body is delivered.
9. Allow head to restitute (return to normal alignment). Place one hand over each ear bilaterally to support the infant's head; gently exert downward pressure toward the floor, thus slipping the anterior shoulder under the symphysis pubis.
10. As soon as the anterior shoulder is delivered, provide upward, outward traction to the head to deliver the posterior shoulder.
11. Support the infant's body and head in the lower hand. As the body is delivered, place skin to skin on maternal abdomen.
12. Gently rub the infant's back, if needed, to stimulate breathing.
13. Cover the maternal-neonate dyad with warm blankets.
14. Watch for signs of placental separation (gush of dark blood from introitus, lengthening of umbilical cord, change in uterine contour). Avoid pulling on the cord, which might break and cause hemorrhage.

15. Clamp and cut the cord after pulsation ceases.
16. Assess fundal tone and massage the uterus.
17. Put the newborn to breast to promote oxytocin release.
18. Place identification bands on both.
19. Encourage maternal hydration.
20. Teach self-fundal massage.
21. Record the time and date of birth, as well as:
    a. Notifications and preparations for the birth.
    b. Fetal presentation and position.
    c. Presence of nuchal or body cord.
    d. ROMs: character, color, odor, and amount of amniotic fluid.
    e. Time of placental expulsion.
    f. Placental appearance.
    g. Maternal condition.
    h. Unusual occurrences during birth (i.e., shoulder dystocia).
22. Assist and transport as necessary.

Neonatal Resuscitation

EVIDENCE BASE American Academy of Pediatrics & American Heart Association. (2021). *Textbook of neonatal resuscitation* (8th ed.). American Academy of Pediatrics.

Neonatal resuscitation is most effective with an organized and efficient team. At every delivery, there should be at least one person whose primary responsibility is the neonate and who is capable of initiating neonatal resuscitation. Any high-risk delivery (requiring more advanced neonatal resuscitation) requires at least two people to be present to manage the resuscitation—one with complete resuscitation skills (intubation and umbilical catheter placement) and one to assist.

Causes

Perinatal asphyxia is the main cause for neonatal resuscitation. When the infant is deprived of oxygen, an initial period of rapid respirations occurs, followed by apnea, decreased heart rate, and decreased neuromuscular tone.

Primary Apnea

1. Intrauterine asphyxia may result in passage of meconium, fetal tachycardia, absent variability, recurrent late or variable decelerations, or prolonged bradycardia.
2. Infants born with primary apnea will need sensory stimuli (tactile or positive-pressure ventilation [PPV]) to initiate respirations.
3. May occur in utero or after birth.

Secondary Apnea

1. Secondary apnea occurs when primary apnea is unresolved. The heart rate continues to drop lower (begins to drop about the same time the infant enters into primary apnea), the blood pressure (BP) drops, the infant becomes flaccid, and spontaneous gasps occur.
2. May occur in utero or after birth.
3. At birth, these infants are pale, flaccid, and bradycardia.

CLINICAL JUDGMENT Anticipation and preparation of neonatal resuscitation should occur at every birth. When the infant is apneic at birth, it is difficult to distinguish between primary and secondary apnea; therefore, one must assume secondary apnea, and resuscitation must begin immediately.

Initial Steps

Remember A: Airway, B: Breathing, and C: Circulation. Performing the initial steps should take no more than 30 seconds.

1. Call for assistance, if needed.
2. Place the infant on a warm, dry radiant warmer.
3. Dry the infant thoroughly with warmed towels, dispose of wet towels, and stimulate the infant by rubbing back or slapping the soles of feet, if necessary.
4. Assess respirations (rise and fall of the chest, air moving in the lungs) and pulse (heart rate more than 100 bpm).
5. If apnea or the heart rate is less than 100 bpm, begin PPV (bag and mask ventilation) and SpO_2 monitoring. Breaths are administered at a rate of 40 to 60 per minute. Resuscitation starts with room air (21%) and increases are made to the concentration of oxygen based upon the neonate's oxygen saturation.
    a. Observe chest movement and auscultate for air movement in all lung fields.
    b. To prevent air filling in the stomach during PPV, an orogastric tube can be inserted orally.
6. If the heart rate is less than 60 bpm, even with 30 seconds of positive ventilation, start chest compressions. Current recommendations are to ensure adequate ventilation is established prior to beginning chest compressions to improve circulation of oxygenated blood; endotracheal intubation may be necessary. One cycle of events consists of three compressions plus one ventilation, resulting in 120 "events" per 60 seconds or 90 compressions plus 30 breaths.
    a. If the heart rate increases to above 60 bpm, cease chest compressions and maintain ventilation at a rate of 40 to 60 breaths/min.
    b. Once the heart rate exceeds 100 and spontaneous breathing resumes, gradually decrease the rate of PPV.
7. Assist with endotracheal intubation, if needed.
8. Assist with insertion of an umbilical catheter for administration of medications and fluids, if needed. If the heart rate remains below 60 bpm for over 60 seconds of PPV and chest compressions, medications (e.g., epinephrine) should be considered and administered intravenously (IV) via an umbilical catheter or endotracheally.
9. Continue to assess the neonate periodically once stabilization is reestablished and transport accordingly.

SELECTED READINGS

Alliance for Innovation on Maternal Health. (2023). *Patient safety bundles.* https://saferbirth.org

American College of Obstetricians and Gynecologists. (2018). ACOG Practice Bulletin No. 198: Prevention and management of obstetric lacerations at vaginal delivery. *Obstetrics and Gynecology, 132*(3), e87–e102. https://doi.org/10.1097/AOG.0000000000002841

American College of Obstetricians and Gynecologists. (2019). ACOG Practice Bulletin No. 106: Intrapartum fetal heart rate monitoring: Nomenclature, interpretation, and general management principles. *Obstetrics & Gynecology, 114*(1), 192–202. https://doi.org/10.1097/AOG.0b013e3181aef106

American College of Obstetricians and Gynecologists. (2019). ACOG Practice Bulletin No. 209: Obstetric analgesia and anesthesia. *Obstetrics and Gynecology, 133*(3), e208–e225. https://doi.org/10.1097/AOG.0000000000003132

American College of Obstetricians and Gynecologists. (2020). Delayed umbilical cord clamping after birth (ACOG Committee Opinion, Number 814). *Obstetrics & Gynecology, 136*(6), e100–e106. https://doi.org/10.1097/aog.0000000000004167

Association of Women's Health, Obstetric and Neonatal Nurses. (2019). *Evidence-based clinical practice guideline: Nursing care and management of the second stage of labor* (3rd ed.). Author.

Association of Women's Health, Obstetric and Neonatal Nurses. (2019). Fetal heart monitoring (AWHONN Position Statement). *Journal of Obstetric, Gynecologic, & Neonatal Nursing, 47*(6), 874–877. https://doi.org/10.1016/j.jogn.2018.09.007

Association of Women's Health, Obstetric and Neonatal Nurses. (2020). Role of the registered nurse in the care of the pregnant woman receiving analgesia and anesthesia by catheter techniques: AWHONN position statement. *Journal of Obstetric, Gynecologic, and Neonatal Nurses, 49*(3), 327–329. https://doi.org/10.1016/j.jogn.2020.02.002

Blosser, C., Smith, A., & Poole, A. T. (2021). Quantification of blood loss improves detection of postpartum hemorrhage and accuracy of postpartum hemorrhage rates: A retrospective cohort study. *Cureus, 13*(2), e13591. https://doi.org/10.7759/cureus.13591

Burke, C. (2021). Pain in labor: Nonpharmacologic and pharmacologic management. In K. Simpson, P. Creehan, N. O'Brien-Abel, C. Roth, & A. Rohan (Eds.), *AWHONN's perinatal nursing* (5th ed., pp. 466–508). Wolters Kluwer.

Cypher, R. (2019). Shared decision-making: A model for effective communication and patient satisfaction. *The Journal of Perinatal & Neonatal Nursing, 33*(4), 285–287. https://doi.org/10.1097/JPN.0000000000000441

Dore, S., & Ehman, W. (2020). No. 396—Fetal health surveillance: Intrapartum consensus guideline. *Journal of Obstetrics and Gynaecology Canada, 42*(3), 316–348. https://doi.org/10.1016/j/jogc.2019.05.007

Fraser, D. (2021). Newborn adaptations to extrauterine life. In K. R. Simpson, P. A. Creehan, N. O'Brien-Abel, C. K. Roth, & A. J. Rohan (Eds.), *AWHONN's perinatal nursing* (5th ed., pp. 564–578). Wolters Kluwer.

Gee, S. E., Maayeh, M., Ward, C., Buhimschi, C., Klebanoff, M., & Rood, K. (2020). Intrauterine pressure catheter use is associated with an increased risk of postcesarean surgical site infections. *American Journal of Perinatology, 37*(6), 557–561. https://doi.org/10.1055/s-0039-1700861

Grünebaum, A., Bornstein, E., Dudenhausen, J. W., Lenchner, E., De Four Jones, M., Varrey, A., Lewis, D., & Chervenak, F. A. (2023). Hidden in plain sight in the delivery room—The Apgar score is biased. *Journal of Perinatal Medicine, 51*(5), 628–633. https://doi.org/10.1515/jpm-2022-0550

Heuser, C. C. (2020). Physiology of fetal heart rate monitoring. *Clinical Obstetrics and Gynecology, 63*(3), 607–615. https://doi.org/10.1097/GRF.0000000000000553

Kibuka, M., Price, A., Onakpoya, I., Tierney, S., & Clarke, M. (2021). Evaluating the effects of maternal positions in childbirth: An overview of Cochrane Systematic Reviews. *European Journal of Midwifery, 5*, 1–14. https://doi.org/10.18332/ejm/142781

Lamaze International. (2021). *Lamaze healthy birth practices*. https://www.lamaze.org/childbirth-practices

Liyanage, S. K., Nina, K., & McDonald, S. D. (2020). Guidelines on deferred cord clamping and cord milking: A systematic review. *Pediatrics, 146*(5), e20201429. https://doi.org/10.1542/peds.2020-1429

Macones, G. A., Hankins, G. D., Spong, C. Y., Hauth, J., & Moore, T. (2008). The 2008 National Institute of Child Health and Human Development workshop report on electronic fetal monitoring: Update on definitions, interpretation, and research guidelines. *Obstetrics and Gynecology, 112*(3), 661–666. https://doi.org/10.1097/AOG.0b013e3181841395

Miller, L. A., Miller, D. A., & Cypher, R. L. (2021). *Mosby's pocket guide to fetal monitoring: A multidisciplinary approach* (9th ed.). Elsevier.

Mohamed, F. Z., & Aboelmagd, A. N. (2020). Effect of early skin to skin contact between mother and her neonate on initiation of breastfeeding and neonate physiological parameters. *International Journal of Research in Paediatric Nursing, 2*(1), 55–62. https://www.researchgate.net/publication/343510745_Effect_of_early_skin_to_skin_contact_between_mother_and_her_neonate_on_initiation_of_breast_feeding_and_neonate_physiological_parameters

Mueller, C. G., Webb, P. J., & Morgan, S. (2020). The effects of childbirth education on maternity outcomes and maternal satisfaction. *The Journal of Perinatal Education, 29*(1), 16–22. https://doi.org/10.1891/1058-1243.29.1.16

O'Brien-Abel, N. (2020). Clinical implications of fetal heart rate interpretation based on underlying physiology. *MCN: The American Journal of Maternal/Child Nursing, 45*(2), 82–91. https://doi.org/10.1097/NMC.0000000000000596

Pusey-Reid, E., Quinn, L., Samost, M. E., & Reidy, P. A. (2023). Skin assessment in patients with dark skin tone. *American Journal of Nursing, 123*(3), 36–43. https://doi.org/10.1097/01.NAJ.0000921800.61980.7e

Raghurman, N., Temming, L. A., Doering, M. M., Stoll, C. R., Palanisamy, A., Stout, M. J., & Tuuli, M. G. (2021). Maternal oxygen supplementation compared with room air for intrauterine resuscitation: A systematic review and meta-analysis. *JAMA Pediatrics, 175*(4), 368–376. https://doi.org/10.1001/jamapediatrics.2020.5351

Simpson, K. R., Creehan, P. A., O'Brien-Abel, N., Roth, C. K., & Rohan, A. J. (2021). *AWHONN's perinatal nursing* (5th ed.). Wolters Kluwer.

Suplee, P. D., & Janke, J. (2020). *AWHONN compendium of postpartum care* (3rd ed.). Association of Women's Health, Obstetric and Neonatal Nurses.

True, B. A., & Sleutel, M. R. (2020). On analgesia and anesthesia in the intrapartum period: Evidence-based clinical practice guideline. *Journal of Obstetric, Gynecologic & Neonatal Nursing, 49*(3), 227–229. https://doi.org/10.1016/j.jogn.2020.03.003

Wong, C. A. (2020). Epidural and spinal analgesia/anesthesia for labor and delivery. In D. Chestnut, C. Wong, L. Tsen, D. Warwick, Y. Beilin, J. Mhyre, & B. Bateman (Eds.), *Chestnut's obstetric anesthesia: Principles and practice* (6th ed.). Elsevier.

34

Maternal and Neonatal Care During the Postpartum Period*

MATERNAL CARE

The Puerperium

The *puerperium* begins after the expulsion of the placenta and lasts approximately 6 weeks as the body returns to the nonpregnant state. During this time, there are physiologic and psychological transitions as outlined further on (see Standards of Care Guidelines 34-1, page 1007).

Physiologic Changes of the Puerperium

EVIDENCE BASE Baker, B., & Janke, J. (2024). *Core curriculum for maternal-newborn nursing* (6th ed.). Elsevier.

Cunningham, F. G., Leveno, K. J., Bloom, S. J., Dashe, J. S., Hoffman, B. L., Casey, B. M., & Spong, C. Y. (2022). *Williams's obstetrics* (26th ed.). McGraw-Hill.

1. Uterine changes.
   a. Uterine involution begins immediately after delivery where the fundus is palpable two fingerbreadths below the umbilicus (U-2) at the midline.
   b. At 1 hour postpartum, the fundus is usually level with or slightly below the level of the umbilicus.
   c. At 12 hours postpartum, the fundus may be ½ inch (1.3 cm) above the umbilicus.
   d. After 12 hours, the level of the fundus descends approximately 1 fingerbreadth (or ½ inch) each day; by the 10th to 14th day, it has descended into the pelvic cavity and can no longer be palpated (see Figure 34-1).
   e. Uterine involution is complete at approximately 6 weeks postpartum.
2. Lochia—vaginal discharge which is described by color and quantity. Lochial flow can be scant (less than 2.5 cm stain [1 inch]/h), light (less than 10 cm stain [4 inches]/h), moderate (less than 15.2 cm stain [6 inches]/h), or heavy (one pad saturated within 1 hour). See Figure 34-2.
   a. Lochia consists of fatty epithelial cells, shreds of membrane, decidua, and blood—it is described as lochia rubra (red), lasting approximately 2 to 3 days. Lochial flow is considered excessive if the perineal pad becomes saturated in less than 15 minutes.
   b. Lochia then progresses to lochia serosa, which is pale pink or brown-tinged in color and of serosanguineous consistency; it lasts 4 to 10 days.
   c. Lochia alba, which is a whitish or yellowish color, follows in the 10th to 14th day. Lochia usually ceases by 2 to 4 weeks, and the placental site is completely healed by the sixth week.

CLINICAL JUDGMENT Immediate assessment for possible postpartum hemorrhage (PPH) is needed if bright red vaginal bleeding returns after lochia rubra has subsided. PPH is a leading cause of maternal morbidity and mortality. Blood loss from vaginal birth averages 200 to 500 mL and 600 to 1,000 mL from Cesarean birth. The American College of Obstetrics and Gynecology (ACOG) defines PPH as greater than 1,000 mL blood loss regardless of mode of delivery.

*Please note that the term "male" in this chapter refers to a person assigned male at birth, and the term "female" in this chapter refers to a person assigned female at birth.

STANDARDS OF CARE GUIDELINES 34-1

Postpartum Care

- Perform focused assessment regularly using the BUBBLE-HE acronym—breasts, uterus (size and consistency), bladder (distention), bowel elimination, lochia, episiotomy (lacerations), Homans sign, and emotional status/bonding.
- Notify health care provider immediately if abnormalities are present:
  - Tachycardia, tachypnea, hypotension, and orthostatic changes may indicate hemorrhage.
  - Elevated blood pressure (BP), visual changes, headache, and brisk reflexes may indicate preeclampsia.
  - Heavy vaginal bleeding (saturation of peripad within 1 hour for 2 or more hours) or excessive bleeding (saturating a peripad in 15 minutes), expulsion of large clots, or steady increase in vaginal bleeding is abnormal and indicates hemorrhage.
  - Boggy uterine fundus that does not become firm and remain firm with massage, indicating atony.
  - Inability to void and bladder distention, which may displace uterus, leading to uterine atony.
  - Decreased urine output, which may indicate hemorrhage.
  - Elevated temperature, increased pain, swelling, and redness from incisions, indicating infection.
  - Calf tenderness, swelling, redness, or warmth, which may indicate a blood clot.
  - Excessive irritability, crying, moodiness, withdrawal, insomnia, and loss of interest in activities, which may indicate postpartum depression (PPD).
- Encourage rest, nutrition, and bonding with the infant.
- Provide education on feeding, bathing, changing, safety measures, signs of illness, and when to call infant's pediatric care provider with questions.

This information should serve as a general guideline only. Each patient situation and facility policy presents a unique set of clinical factors and requires nursing judgment to guide care, which may include additional or alternative measures and approaches.

3. Cervical and vaginal changes.
   a. Immediately after delivery of the placenta, the cervix has little tone.
   b. After approximately 2 to 3 days, the cervix appears more like the prepregnant state and is dilated to 2 to 3 cm.
   c. By the end of the first postpartum week, it is approximately 1 cm in diameter.
   d. The cervical opening will remain more slit-like than the prepregnant dimple, unless the cervix was never dilated during the birth process.
   e. Immediately after delivery, the vaginal walls are smooth and swollen because the vaginal rugae are absent. Rugae reappear approximately 3 weeks postpartum.
   f. The vaginal walls, uterine ligaments, and muscles of the pelvic floor and abdominal wall regain most of their tone during the puerperium.
4. Breasts—after delivery of the placenta, circulating levels of estrogen and progesterone decrease, and levels of prolactin increase, initiating lactogenesis.
   a. *Colostrum*—a thick, yellowish fluid that contains more minerals and protein but less sugar and fat than mature breast milk and that has a laxative effect on the infant—is secreted for the first 2 days postpartum.
   b. Breast engorgement is the result of milk production and venous and lymphatic stasis occurring 3 to 5 days postpartum. Breasts will be swollen, tense, and tender.
   c. Milk secretion usually presents by the third to fifth day postpartum. Galactopoiesis (maintenance of lactation) is established, and mature breast milk is present by the 2nd week postpartum.
5. Endocrine/metabolic function.
   a. Human chorionic gonadotropin (HCG) declines rapidly and is nonexistent by the end of the first postpartum week.
   b. Thyroid hormone levels are normal by 4 to 6 weeks postpartum.
   c. Glucose levels are low secondary to the decrease in human placental lactogen (HpL), cortisol, estrogen, and growth hormone.
   d. Blood glucose levels for patients with gestational diabetes mellitus (GDM) may return to normal limits shortly after birth. However, ACOG and the Centers for Disease Control and Prevention (CDC) recommend that all patients

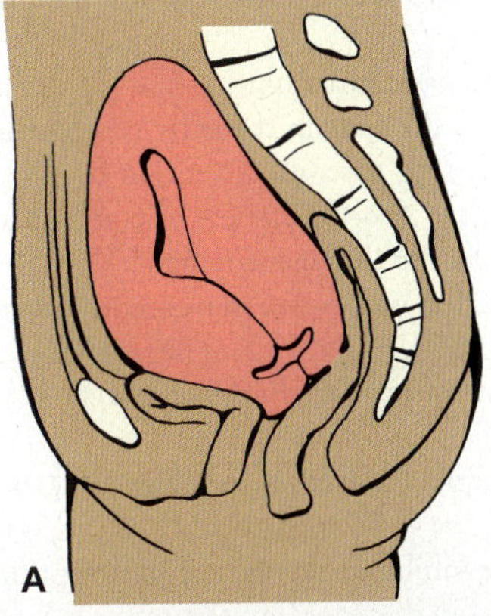

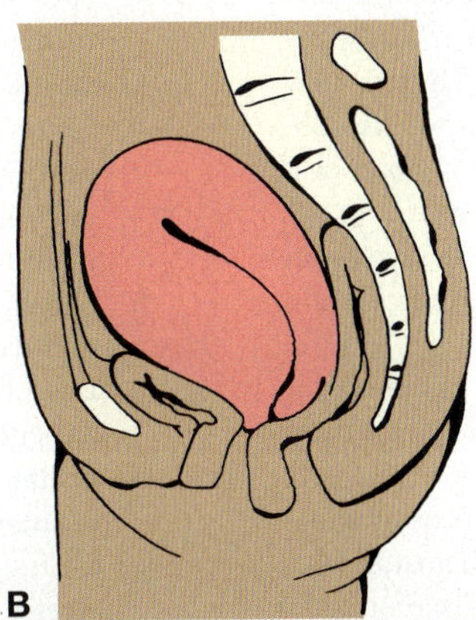

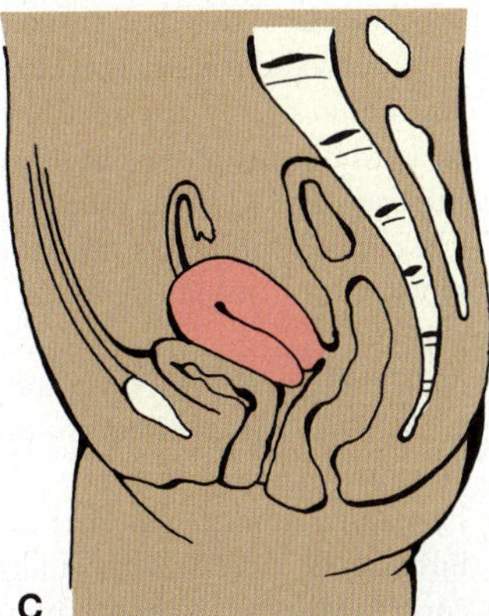

Figure 34-1. Changes in uterine size and shape following delivery. (**A**) Uterus after delivery. (**B**) Uterus at sixth day. (**C**) Nongravid uterus. (Adapted with permission from Reeder, S., Martin, L., & Koniak-Griffin, D. [1997]. *Maternity nursing: Family newborn, and women's health care* [18th ed.]. Lippincott-Raven Publishers.)

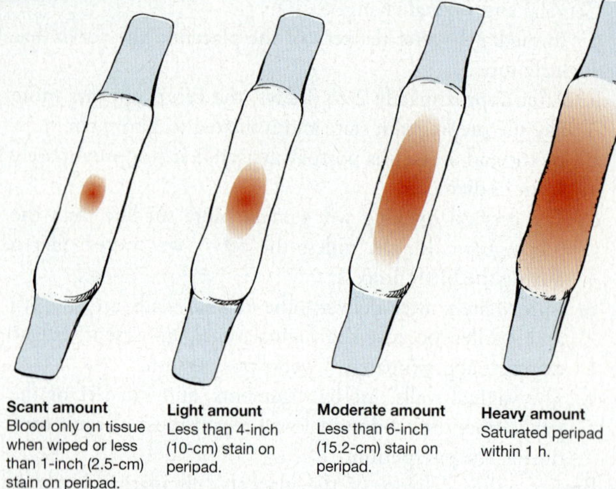

Figure 34-2. Assessing the volume of lochia by peripad saturation.

with GDM should have glucose tested 6 to 12 weeks postpartum and screened for diabetes every 1 to 3 years for early identification of type 2 diabetes mellitus.

6. Ovarian function.
   a. Estrogen and progesterone levels decrease rapidly after delivery of the placenta and are usually their lowest by the seventh postpartum day.
   b. Estrogen reaches the follicular phase by 3 weeks after birth in patients who are nonlactating.
   c. Ovulation may occur as early as 27 days after delivery. However, in patients who are exclusively breastfeeding, ovulation may be delayed 70 to 190 days. Patients should be counseled that ovulation can still occur without accompanying menses.
   d. The start of menses after delivery is individualized. Usually, the first menses occurs approximately 7 to 9 weeks after delivery in patients who are nonlactating, although patients who are breastfeeding may not start menses up to 18 months after delivery.
7. Urinary function.
   a. Spontaneous voiding should return by 6 to 8 hours postpartum. Bladder tone returns between 5 and 7 days postpartum.
   b. Postpartum diuresis begins within 12 hours after birth and continues for 2 to 5 days postpartum, as extracellular water accumulated during pregnancy is excreted. (Diuresis may also occur shortly after delivery if urine output was obstructed because of the pressure of the presenting part or if intravenous (IV) fluids were given during labor.)
   c. The catabolic process of involution can cause an increase in blood urea nitrogen (BUN) levels during the postpartum period.
   d. Mild proteinuria (+1 on urine dipstick) is common for 1 to 2 days after delivery in 40% to 50% of postpartum patients.
   e. Hematuria immediately after normal spontaneous vaginal birth can be indicative of bladder trauma. If hematuria occurs after the first 24 hours, it may be indicative of urinary tract infection (UTI).
   f. Stress incontinence is common during the first 6 weeks postpartum, and Kegel exercises should be encouraged.
8. Neurologic function
   a. Discomfort and fatigue are common. Discomfort (also called "afterpains") is due to the involution process, delivery, lacerations, episiotomy, and muscle aches that are common for the first 2 to 3 days postpartum.
   b. Frontal and temporal headaches are common and generally caused by fluid shifts in the first week postpartum. Further assessment and evaluation is indicated in a patient complaining of headache unrelieved by analgesia to rule out preeclampsia and a spinal headache (if regional anesthesia was used).
   c. An eclamptic seizure can occur during the intrapartum period and within 48 hours after delivery. However, seizures can occur as late as 4 weeks postpartum. Seizures are commonly preceded by severe headache and/or visual disturbances. Discharge teaching should include signs and symptoms of preeclampsia and seizures, especially in patients with prenatal diagnosis of preeclampsia or hypertension.
   d. Carpal tunnel syndrome, if present during pregnancy, is usually relieved by postpartum diuresis.
9. Cardiovascular function.
   a. Most dramatic changes occur between 6 and 12 weeks to return to the prepregnant state.
   b. Cardiac output generally decreases to prelabor parameters within 1 hour postpartum and may be dependent on multiple factors, including use of anesthesia and method of delivery. However, it can remain elevated for as much as 48 hours postpartum. Cardiac output returns to prepregnant parameters by 6 to 12 weeks postpartum.
   c. Hematocrit increases, increasing the risk of clotting, and the increased red blood cell (RBC) production of pregnancy stops.
   d. Leukocytosis (increased white blood cells [WBCs]) is common during the first postpartum week.

CLINICAL JUDGMENT A positive Homans sign or an increase in calf size may indicate thrombophlebitis and should be reported to the health care provider. Avoid any massage of the legs.

10. Respiratory function.
    a. Patients should not experience tachypnea, shortness of breath, or adventitious lung sounds.
    b. Any acute change is considered abnormal and requires immediate intervention.
11. Gastrointestinal (GI)/hepatic function.
    a. GI tone and motility decrease in the early postpartum period, commonly causing gaseous distention of the abdomen and constipation. Stool softeners, dietary fiber, and increased fluid intake should be encouraged.
    b. Normal bowel function and bowel movements return in 2 to 3 days postpartum.
    c. Liver function returns to normal approximately 10 to 14 days postpartum.
    d. Gallbladder contractility increases to allow for expulsion of small gallstones.
    e. GI function can be inhibited by surgical intervention, analgesia, anesthesia, and decreased muscle tone.
12. Musculoskeletal function.
    a. Generalized fatigue and weakness are common.
    b. Decreased abdominal tone is common.

c. Diastasis recti may resolve spontaneously by 8 weeks postpartum. Starting any exercise regimen should be discussed with the health care provider.
d. Joint instability returns to normal between 6 and 8 weeks postpartum.

13. Integumentary function.
    a. Striae gravidarum fade and melasma usually resolve by 6 weeks postpartum.
    b. Hair loss can increase for the first 4 to 20 weeks postpartum. With hair regrowth, hair may not be as thick as it was before pregnancy.
14. The acronym **BUBBLE-HE** is commonly used to assess postpartum changes:
    a. **B**—Breast
    b. **U**—Uterus
    c. **B**—Bladder
    d. **B**—Bowels
    e. **L**—Lochia
    f. **E**—Episiotomy/lacerations/perineum
    g. **H**—Homans sign/extremities
    h. **E**—Emotional status/bonding

Emotional and Behavioral (Psychosocial) Status

EVIDENCE BASE Beck, C. T. (2021). Perinatal mood and anxiety disorders: Research and implications for nursing care. *Nursing for Womens Health*, *25*(4), e8-e53. htptps://doi.org/10.1016/j.nwh.2021.02.003

American College of Obstetricians and Gynecologists. (2018). Optimizing postpartum care (Committee Opinion #736). *Obstetrics and Gynecology*, *131*(5), e140–e150. https://doi.org/10.1097/AOG.0000000000002633

1. Reva Rubin, the noted nursing theorist, developed the developmental tasks of pregnancy documenting maternal changes and role attainment. After delivery, the patient may progress through Rubin's stages of taking in, taking hold, and letting go.
    a. Taking in (extends over first 24 hours postpartum):
        i. May begin with a refreshing sleep after delivery. Restorative sleep should occur within first 24 hours postdelivery.
        ii. Patient exhibits passive, dependent behavior.
        iii. Patient is concerned with sleep and the intake of food, mainly for self.
    b. Taking hold (if not in the first 24 hours postpartum, then between days 2 and 4 postpartum):
        i. Patient begins to initiate action and to function more independently. The first sign is alert interest in the infant.
        ii. Patient may require more explanation and reassurance that they are functioning well, especially in caring for the infant.
        iii. Openness to teaching on care of self and neonate.
        iv. With the current trend toward early discharge, attainment may be impacted.
    c. Letting go:
        i. May begin near the end of the first week; no specific end time noted.
        ii. Is influenced by cultural beliefs.
        iii. Reestablishment of couple relationship.
        iv. As maternal adjustment to the new role progresses, concerns extend to other family members and activities.
2. Some patients may experience euphoria in the first few days after delivery and set unrealistic goals for activities after discharge.
3. Many patients may experience temporary mood swings during this period because of the discomfort, fatigue, and exhaustion following labor and delivery and because of hormonal changes after delivery. Nursing research findings indicate that postpartum patients commonly identify postpartum needs such as coping with:
    a. The physical changes and discomforts of the puerperium, including a need to regain their prepregnancy figure.
    b. Changing family relationships and meeting the needs of family members, including the infant.
    c. Fatigue, emotional stress, feelings of isolation, and being tied down.
    d. A lack of time for personal needs and interests
    e. Up to 60% to 80% of postpartum patients may experience a transient period of depression termed postpartum blues. The blues can last for 10 to 14 days and may include symptoms such as irritability, poor appetite, insomnia, tearfulness, or crying. This is a normal, transient reaction to the physiologic and psychological shifts that occur postdelivery.
    f. Postpartum depression (PPD) affects as many as 20% of postpartum patients (see page 1069).
        i. A prenatal diagnosis of depression is considered a significant risk factor for PPD.
        ii. A postpartum patient may experience an increase in the manifestations listed previously as well as inability to adequately care for themselves and the baby.
        iii. Astute assessment and cultural awareness is imperative when working with the postpartum population as cultural and ethnic influences may have an impact.

Nursing Assessment

EVIDENCE BASE Olshansky, E. F. (2023). The family, culture, and home care. In S. E. Perry, K. Cashion, K. R. Alden, E. F. Olshansky, D. L. Lowdermilk, & M. Hockenberry (Eds.), *Maternity & women's health care* (7th ed., pp. 14–30). Elsevier.

Immediate Postpartum Assessment

The first 2 hours after the delivery of the placenta (fourth stage of labor) is a critical period, and postpartum hemorrhage is most likely to occur during this period (see page 1065).

Subsequent Postpartum Assessment

1. Assess the fundus at regular intervals for tone and location. Perform fundal massage if the uterus is boggy (not firm) (see Figure 34-3).
2. Teach patient self-fundal massage and warning signs to report, such as gushing of vaginal bleeding and vertigo.
    a. Inspect the perineum regularly for bleeding. Note color, amount, clots, and odor of the lochia as well as swelling and ecchymosis.
3. Weigh perineal pads as necessary. Assess patient's ability to perform self-care. Provide support and education as needed.
4. Assess vital signs at least twice daily and more frequently, if indicated.
5. Assess bowel and bladder elimination.

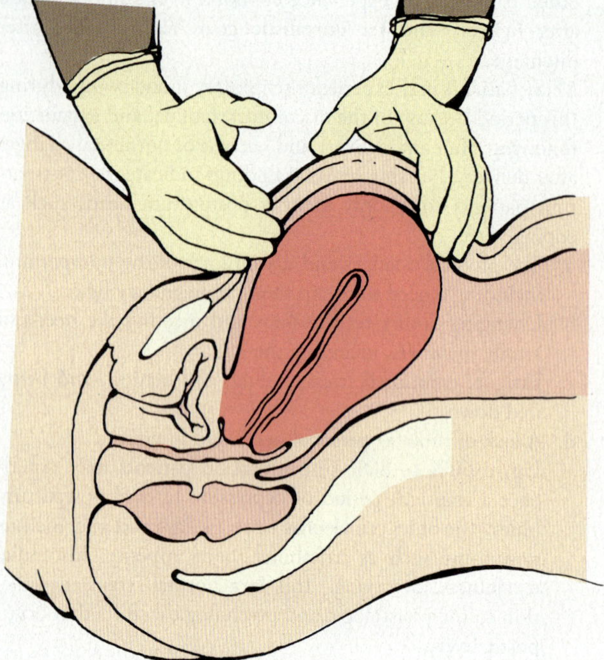

Figure 34-3. Fundal massage. With hands correctly positioned, gentle fundal massage stimulates the uterine muscles to contract, helping to restore normal tone and control bleeding. (Adapted with permission from Reeder, S., Martin, L., & Koniak-Griffin, D. [1997]. *Maternity nursing: Family newborn, and women's health care* [18th ed.]. Lippincott-Raven Publishers.)

6. Evaluate interaction and the new family's ability to provide care to the newborn. Provide support and education as needed.
7. Assess breasts for colostrum, milk production, engorgement, and condition of the nipples if breastfeeding.
8. Assess Homans sign and calf swelling for possible thrombophlebitis.
9. Assess any incision for signs of infection and healing. If perineal sutures are used, they will usually dissolve in 2 to 6 weeks.
10. Assess the perineum using the REEDA acronym. REEDA is based on a 3-point scale. A score of 3 indicates an assessment of very poor wound healing. On the first postpartum day, the REEDA score may range from 0 to 3; by the second postpartum week, the score should be 0 to 1.
    a. **R**—Redness
    b. **E**—Edema
    c. **E**—Ecchymosis (purplish patch of blood flow)
    d. **D**—Discharge
    e. **A**—Approximation or the closeness of the skin edges
11. If the patient is Rh negative, evaluate the need for Rho(D) immune globulin (RhoGAM) based on the neonate's Rh status. If the newborn is Rh positive, administer the RhoGAM within 72 hours of delivery.
12. If the patient is rubella and/or varicella nonimmune, these vaccinations may be administered at discharge. Note: If the rubella vaccine is administered at discharge, educate the patient to avoid pregnancy for 1 month to minimize fetal risks of congenital anomalies.
13. During the flu season, the influenza vaccine should also be offered if the patient has not been previously immunized during the pregnancy.
14. A tetanus toxoid, reduced diphtheria toxoid, and acellular pertussis (Tdap) vaccine should be administered if needed.
15. Depending on the facility, a COVID-19 vaccine may be offered.

Nursing Management

EVIDENCE BASE American College of Obstetricians and Gynecologists. (2018). Optimizing postpartum care (Committee Opinion #736). *Obstetrics and Gynecology, 131*(5), e140–e150. https://doi.org/10.1097/AOG.0000000000002633

Association of Women's Health, Obstetric, and Neonatal Nurses. (2017). *Post birth warning signs.* https://www.awhonn.org/education/hospital-products/post-birth-warning-signs-education-program/

Baker, B., & Janke, J. (2024). *Core curriculum for maternal-newborn nursing* (6th ed.). Elsevier.

Nursing Interventions

Monitoring for Complications Through Postpartum Assessment

1. Monitor vital signs every 4 hours during the first 24 hours and then every 8 to 12 hours or per facility policy.
    a. Assess lung function. Increased respiratory rate greater than 24 breaths/min may be caused by increased blood loss, pulmonary edema, or a pulmonary embolus.
    b. Assess perfusion. Increased pulse rate greater than 100 beats/min (bpm) may occur in response to increased blood loss, fever, pain, or infection.
    c. Assess blood pressure. Decrease in blood pressure (BP) 15 to 20 mm Hg below baseline pressures may indicate decreased fluid volume, increasing blood loss, or additional complications. Capillary refill should be less than 3 seconds.
    d. Assess for light-headedness and dizziness when sitting upright or before ambulating the patient.
    e. Evaluate orthostatic BP if symptoms persist, and maintain bedrest if indicated.
2. Assist out of bed until stable, and emphasize the need to call for assistance.
3. Evaluate lower extremity sensory function and motor function before ambulation if regional anesthesia was used.
    a. Assess epidural/spinal site if applicable.
    b. Before ambulation, assess lower extremity strength by plantar dorsiflexion.
4. Assess lochia for amount and presence of clots.
5. Maintain IV access and infusion, as ordered, and if Rhogam is indicated.
6. Monitor postpartum complete blood count (CBC) and chemistries as ordered.
7. Encourage oral fluids.

Promoting Urinary Elimination

1. Assess for voiding within 6 to 8 hours after delivery.
2. Palpate the abdomen for bladder distention if unable to void or with complaints of bladder fullness. Uterine displacement from the midline suggests bladder distention.
    a. Frequent voiding of small amounts of urine suggests urine retention.
    b. Bladder distention may lead to uterine atony.
3. Utilize a bladder scanner if available to assess retained urine volume.

4. Perform urinary catheterization if indicated.
5. Encourage the patient to void every 4 hours to keep the bladder empty.

Promoting Bowel Function

1. Explain that bowel activity is sluggish because of decreased abdominal muscle tone, anesthetic effects, effects of progesterone, decreased solid food intake during labor, and opioid use.
2. Explain that pain from hemorrhoids, lacerations, and episiotomies may cause patient to delay first bowel movement.
3. Encourage adequate intake of fiber through fresh fruit, vegetables, and at least eight glasses of water daily.
4. Encourage frequent ambulation.
5. Administer stool softeners, hydrocortisone, and/or witch hazel pads, as indicated.

Preventing Infection

1. Educate the patient about the care of the perineum, including the need to change peripads frequently and use cleansing peri bottle with warm water. Ice packs may help to reduce swelling and enhance comfort.
2. Observe for elevated temperature above 100.4°F (38°C).
3. Evaluate episiotomy/perineum using the REEDA scale.
4. Assess for pain, burning, and frequency with urination.
5. Assess epidural/spinal site.

Reducing Fatigue

1. Provide a quiet environment and minimize disruptions by clustering care of the couplet (maternal–neonatal dyad).
2. Encourage the patient to sleep while the baby is sleeping.

Adequate Pain Management

1. Instruct patient how to apply ice packs to perineal area for the first 24 hours for perineal trauma or edema and then to apply heat to the area. Commercial or handmade packs may be used.
2. Initiate the use of warm water sitz baths for 15 to 20 minutes for perineal discomfort after the first 24 hours as needed.
3. Assist with positioning for comfort.
4. Encourage frequent perineal cleansing.
5. Provide witch hazel pads, or topical creams and/or ointments for hemorrhoids, as indicated.
6. Administer analgesics such as acetaminophen and ibuprofen as indicated. If opioids are used, assess for decreased respiratory rate below 12 breaths/min.
7. Assess breasts for signs of engorgement (swollen, tender, tense, shiny breast tissue).
   a. If breastfeeding, educate on the following:
      i. Nurse the infant on both breasts to ensure adequate emptying of breasts.
      ii. If desired, apply cold packs to breasts after feeding.
      iii. Encourage a warm-to-hot shower water to flow over the breasts to improve comfort; alternatively, warm compresses on the breasts may improve comfort while feeding.
      iv. Express some milk manually or by breast pump to improve comfort and to make the nipple more available for infant feeding.
      v. Be aware that over-the-counter (OTC) analgesics may be used to enhance comfort.
   b. If engorgement occurs in patients who are nonbreastfeeding, instruct on the following:
      i. Wear a snug and supportive bra at all times.
      ii. Avoid any stimulation to breasts, including warm water falling on breasts during showers, because the heat stimulates milk production.
      iii. Apply ice or cold cabbage leaves to the breasts to provide comfort.
      iv. Take OTC analgesics as needed

Promoting Postpartum Health Maintenance

1. Teach perineal care or sitz baths using warm water over the perineum after each voiding and/or bowel movement (aiming water front to back) to promote comfort, cleanliness, and healing. Peripads should be changed after any elimination to avoid infection.
2. Provide good breast care.
   a. Assess the condition of the breasts and nipples for intactness, reddening, ecchymosis, fissures, and pain.
   b. Encourage and demonstrate proper latching technique and the use of different breastfeeding positions to reduce nipple soreness.
   c. Advise the expression of colostrum and air-drying nipples after feeding.
   d. Advise that commercially prepared lanolin-based creams and ointments may also enhance comfort. It is important to read the label in the event that the cream/ointment needs to be removed prior to feeding.
   e. Teach the patient to avoid the use of soaps on the breast and nipples to maintain the protective skin oils and avoid dryness and cracking.
   f. Encourage wearing a support bra without underwires for comfort.
3. Encourage good nutrition.
   a. Encourage foods from all food groups with three to four servings of protein; four to six servings of dairy; and four servings each of fruits, grains, and vegetables.
   b. Advise that occasional use of caffeine is acceptable.
   c. Advise taking prenatal vitamins until the 6-week follow-up appointment. The World Health Organization (WHO) recommends that patients who are lactating continue taking a prenatal/postnatal vitamin while breastfeeding; consult with provider.
   d. Increase fluid intake to maintain straw-colored urine.
   e. Instruct patients who are lactating to add 300 to 500 additional calories daily for milk production.
4. Encourage activity, but realize that anatomic and physiologic changes during pregnancy must be considered before beginning an exercise program.
   a. Note that with uncomplicated pregnancies, activity may be resumed as tolerated to maintain a healthy lifestyle.
   b. Advise patients with medical and surgical complications to consult with their providers before beginning any exercise program.
   c. Teach patients that common exercises for all postpartum patients may include Kegel exercises, short walks that gradually increase in duration, stationary cycling, low-impact aerobics, and modified yoga.

Promoting Breastfeeding

1. Assist the patient and infant with the breastfeeding process.
   a. Encourage hand hygiene prior to breastfeeding.
   b. Encourage comfortable positioning such as sitting upright in the bed or in a chair or side-lying and to hold the baby close to prevent back, shoulder, and arm strain.
   c. Instruct the patient to place the infant in the "tummy-to-tummy" position, where the infant's nose touches the breast. Common positions include cradle hold, with the baby's head and body supported against the

patient's arm, with buttocks resting in the hand; the football hold, in which the baby's body and legs are supported under the patient's arm and the head is at the breast, resting in the patient's hand; and side-lying facing each other.

d. Cup the breast in the hand in a C-position, with the bottom of the breast in the palm of the hand and the thumb on top, or the U position, with the fingers and the thumb to the sides of the breast and the breast resting in the palm of the hand.
e. Place the nipple against the side of the baby's mouth, and when the mouth opens, guide the nipple and the areola into the mouth. The baby should latch on to as much of the areola as possible for an adequate deep latch. If the baby has latched on to the nipple only or a shallow latch causing pain, break the latch by putting the tip of the patient's finger in the corner of the baby's mouth to break the suction, and then reposition on the breast to prevent nipple pain and trauma.
f. Encourage alternating breasts when beginning a feeding to ensure stimulation and emptying of both breasts for maintaining milk supply.
g. Advise the patient to use each breast at each feeding. Begin with at least 10 minutes at each breast, and then increase the duration as necessary to ensure an adequate feeding. Although there is no time limit on each breastfeeding session, it is recommended to last at least 10 to 15 minutes on each breast.
h. Breastfeed infants every 2 to 3 hours and on demand (8 to 12 times/24 hours) to maintain the milk supply.
i. Following the feeding, advise expressing colostrum/milk and applying to nipples; then, air-dry for approximately 15 to 20 minutes after feeding to help prevent nipple trauma.

2. Encourage burping between feeding on each breast and at the end of the feeding. Changing the infant's diaper will assist in waking the baby to feed on the other breast.
3. Alert the patient that uterine cramping (afterpains) may occur, because of the release of oxytocin needed for milk ejection during feeding. Multiparous patients may experience increased discomfort related to decreased uterine tone.
4. Encourage adequate rest periods and nutrition as well as avoiding stress, which can inhibit the let-down reflex and make breast milk less available at feeding.
5. Instruct the patient to consult the provider prior to taking any OTC and prescription medications for their effect on milk production or the infant.
6. Provide resources to obtain a breast pump and referrals to community agencies for lactation and women, infant and children (WIC) as needed.

Evaluation: Expected Outcomes

- Vital signs within normal limits; decreasing color and amount of lochia.
- Voids freely and without discomfort.
- Lack of constipation; eats high-fiber foods and uses stool softeners.
- Afebrile, no abnormal redness of the perineum, no purulent discharge or foul-smelling lochia.
- Verbalizes feeling rested.
- Verbalizes decreased pain.
- Incorporates postpartum care into activities of daily living.
- Demonstrates successful breastfeeding; breasts and nipples intact and without redness or cracks.

Postpartum Discharge Teaching

1. **Provider Follow-up:** Stress the importance of provider follow-up within 2 to 4 weeks to evaluate physical and psychological transition in the postpartum period. Some patients may require an earlier appointment.
2. **Involution:** Educate the patient on the normal involution process and change in lochial flow that occurs over a 6-week period.
3. **Menses:** Advise that menses may return within 4 to 8 weeks if bottle-feeding; if breastfeeding, menses is delayed and may return between 2 and 18 months postpartum. Additionally, ovulation may occur without menses; thus, some form of contraception should be utilized if pregnancy is to be avoided.
4. **Nutrition:** Encourage a well-balanced diet from all food groups, especially protein and iron-rich foods and increased fluid intake.
5. **Activity:** May resume physical activity as tolerated and instructed by provider. Pelvic floor muscle exercises are encouraged. Abdominal muscle exercises should be postponed for 4 weeks with operative delivery. To minimize fatigue, rest when the baby sleeps.
6. **Sexuality**
   a. Encourage the couple to provide times to reestablish their own relationship and to renew their social interests and relationships apart from the infant.
   b. Inform that intercourse may be resumed when perineal/abdominal areas have healed and when vaginal bleeding has stopped.
   c. Advise that normal vaginal secretions may not occur for up to 6 months and use of vaginal lubricants may be helpful.
   d. Advise that sexual arousal and desire may be diminished due to infant needs and fatigue for the first 3 months after delivery.
   e. Encourage breastfeeding the infant prior to sexual activity as arousal may cause milk ejection.
   f. Review contraception and family planning options, and stress that breastfeeding is not a reliable method of contraception.
7. **Postbirth Warnings:**
   Report to the provider any of the following:
   - Excessive bleeding, soaking a peripad every hour, passing clots larger than a golf ball, or foul odor.
   - Shortness of breath, chest pain, pain or swelling in the calf.
   - Signs and symptoms of infection: poor wound healing, temperature ≥100.4°F, purulent drainage, pain.
   - Headache that does not resolve with analgesia, visual disturbances, seizures.
   - Thoughts of harming yourself or others.

NEONATAL CARE

EVIDENCE BASE Perry, S. E., Lowdermilk, D. L., Cashion, K., Alden, K. R., Olshansky, E. F., & Hockenberry, M. J. (2023). *Maternity & women's health care* (7th ed.). Elsevier.

Verklan, M. T., Walden, M., & Forest, S. (2020). *Core curriculum for neonatal intensive care nursing* (6th ed.). Elsevier.

Physiology of the Neonate

The first 24 hours of life is a highly vulnerable time, when the infant makes major physiologic adjustments to extrauterine life. Most neonates transition without difficulty within the first 6 to 10 hours of life.

Transitional Stages

During the period of postnatal transition, six overlapping stages have been identified:

- Stage 1. Receives stimulation (during labor) from the pressure of the uterine contractions and from changes in pressure when the membranes rupture.
- Stage 2. Encounters various foreign stimuli—light, cold, gravity, and sound.
- Stage 3. Initiates breathing.
- Stage 4. Changes from fetal circulation to neonatal circulation.
- Stage 5. Undergoes alteration in metabolic processes, with activation of the liver and gastrointestinal (GI) tract for passage of meconium.
- Stage 6. Achieves a steady level of equilibrium in metabolic processes (production of enzymes, increased blood oxygen saturation, decrease in acidosis associated with birth, and recovery of the neurologic system from the trauma of labor and delivery).

Respiratory Changes

Factors Initiating Respiration

1. Mechanical—pressure changes (e.g., compression of the fetal chest with delivery) from intrauterine life to extrauterine life produce stimulation to initiate respirations.
2. Chemical—changes in the blood related to transitory asphyxia include:
   a. Cessation of placental blood flow.
   b. Lowered oxygen level.
   c. Increased carbon dioxide level.
   d. Lowered pH—if asphyxia is prolonged, depression of the respiratory center (rather than stimulation) occurs, and resuscitation is necessary.
3. Sensory—light (visual), sound (auditory), olfactory, and tactile stimulation, beginning in utero with uterine contraction and when the infant is touched and dried, contribute to the initiation of respiration by stimulating the neonate's respiratory center in the brain.
4. Thermal—a drop in environmental temperature produced by sudden chilling of the moist infant stimulates the respiratory center in the brain.
5. First breath—maximum effort is required to expand the lungs and to fill the collapsed alveoli.
   a. Surface tension in the respiratory tract and resistance in lung tissue, thorax, diaphragm, and respiratory muscles must be overcome.
   b. First active inspiration comes from a strong contraction of the diaphragm, which creates a high negative intrathoracic pressure, causing a marked retraction of the ribs and distention of the alveolar space. Any remaining fetal fluid is reabsorbed rapidly if the pulmonary capillary blood flow is adequate because the fluid is hypotonic and passes easily into the capillaries.
6. Contributing factors, such as pulmonary blood flow, surfactant production, and respiratory musculature, also increase the respiratory effort of the neonate.

Character of Normal Respirations

1. First period of reactivity occurs immediately after birth. Vigorous, diffuse, purposeless movements alternate with periods of relative immobility/inactivity.
2. Respirations are rapid, as frequent as 80 breaths/min, accompanied by tachycardia, 160 to 180 breaths/min. Respirations will then reduce to 30 to 60 breaths/min and become quiet and shallow; respiration is carried out by the diaphragm and abdominal muscles.
3. Period of dyspnea and cyanosis may occur suddenly in an infant who is breathing normally; this may indicate an anomaly or a pathologic condition.
4. Pauses in respirations of less than 20 seconds are normal in the neonatal period.
5. Relaxation occurs and the infant usually sleeps; the infant then awakes to a second period of activity. Oral mucus may be a major problem during this period.

Circulatory Changes

1. Cord clamping causes increased systemic vascular resistance (SVR), an increase in blood pressure (BP), and increased pressures in the left side of the heart.
2. Functional closure of the ductus venosus shunt and anatomic closure the first week of life (see page 1202).
3. With the neonate's first breath, the foramen ovale shunt functionally closes. Permanent closure occurs by 3 months of age.
4. Increased SVR, falling pulmonary vascular resistance (PVR), and increased sensitivity to rising arterial oxygen concentrations in the blood = closure of ductus arteriosus shunt. The shunt is completely closed in all infants by 96 hours of age, with permanent closure within 3 weeks to 3 months of age.
5. Blood volume can be as high as 300 mL/kg immediately after birth and then decrease to 80 to 85 mL/kg shortly after birth. Factors that influence blood volume:
   a. Maternal blood volume (affected by maternal diseases and iron intake).
   b. Placental function.
   c. Uterine contractions during labor.
   d. Amount of blood loss associated with delivery.
   e. Placental transfusion at birth with delayed cord clamping—increase in blood volume of 60% if cord is clamped and cut after pulsation ceases.
6. Acrocyanosis (cyanosis in hands and feet) is a normal finding related to sluggish peripheral circulation in the first 24 hours after birth.
7. Normal apical pulse rate 110 to 160 bpm; may rise to 180 bpm when the infant is crying or drop to 80 to 110 bpm during deep sleep.
8. BP in the full-term newborn ranges from 60 to 80 mm Hg systolic and 30 to 60 mm Hg diastolic at birth and varies with gestational age, weight, activity, and appropriate cuff size (slightly higher in legs).
   a. A systolic BP in the upper extremities that is 20 mm Hg greater than in the lower extremities strongly suggests coarctation of the aorta.
   b. BP measurement is best accomplished with an automated noninvasive blood pressure (NIBP) device while the infant is at rest.
9. Coagulation is temporarily diminished due to immature liver function and a vitamin K deficiency related to a sterile GI tract. Vitamin K synthesis begins after 5 hours of bacterial colonization in the intestinal tract.
10. Values for blood components in the neonate:
    a. Hemoglobin, 14.5 to 22 g/dL.
    b. Hematocrit, 14% to 72%.
    c. Reticulocytes, 4% to 6%.
    d. Leukocytes, 9,000 to 34,000/mm^3.

Temperature Regulation

1. Temperature instability in the full-term newborn can be the result of anatomic and physiologic factors such as a thin subcutaneous adipose tissue, blood vessels closer to the skin, and larger body surface to body weight ratio.
2. Heat loss in full-term newborns may occur at birth by radiation, convection, evaporation, and conduction.
   a. Radiation—transfer of heat from neonate to cooler object not in direct contact with the infant.
   b. Convection—transfer of heat when flow of cool air passes over infant's skin.
   c. Evaporation—loss of heat when water on infant's skin is converted to vapor.
   d. Conduction—transfer of heat when neonate comes into direct contact with cooler surface/object.
3. Infants respond readily to environmental heat and cold stimuli and develop mechanisms to counterbalance heat loss.
   a. Vasoconstriction—blood directed away from skin surfaces.
   b. Insulation—from subcutaneous adipose tissue.
   c. Heat production—by nonshivering thermogenesis (brown fat metabolism) elicited by the sympathetic nervous system's response to decreased temperatures; activated by adrenaline.
   d. Fetal position—by assuming a flexed position.

Basal Metabolism

1. Surface area of infant, especially the head, is large in comparison to weight.
2. Basal metabolism per kilogram of body weight is higher than that of an adult.
3. Calorie requirements are high—110 to 130 calories/kg of body weight per day.

Renal Function

Neonatal kidneys have functional deficiency in concentrating urine and coping with fluid and electrolyte fluctuations. Low arterial BP and increased renal vascular resistance lead to the following effects:

1. Decreased ability to concentrate urine because of low tubular resorption rate and low levels of antidiuretic hormone.
2. Limited ability to maintain water balance by excretion of excess water or retention of needed water.
3. Decreased ability to maintain acid–base mechanism; slower excretion of electrolytes, especially sodium and hydrogen ions, results in accumulation of these substances, which predisposes the infant to dehydration, acidosis, and hyperkalemia.
4. Excretion of large amount of uric acid during neonatal period—appears as brick dust stain on diaper.

Hepatic Function

Function limited because of lack of GI tract activity, deficiency in forming plasma proteins, and limited blood supply; consequences include the following:

1. Decreased ability to conjugate bilirubin (rationale for physiologic jaundice).
2. Decreased ability to regulate blood glucose concentration (less glycogen stores) (rationale for neonatal hypoglycemia).
3. Deficient production of prothrombin and other coagulation factors that depend on vitamin K for synthesis (rationale for neonate's predisposition to hemorrhage).

Endocrine Function

Endocrine glands are better organized than other systems: disturbances are most commonly related to maternally provided hormones. This can cause the following:

1. Vaginal discharge or bleeding (pseudomenstruation) in female infants.
2. Enlargement of mammary glands (breast engorgement) in all infants—related to increased estrogen, luteal, and prolactin activity. Milky secretions may occur.
3. Disturbances related to postpartum patient endocrine pathology (e.g., patient with diabetes or with inadequate iodine intake).

GI Changes

The neonate's intestinal tract is proportionately longer than the adult's; however, elastic tissue and musculature are not fully developed, and neurologic control is variable and inadequate.

1. Most digestive enzymes are present, with the exception of pancreatic amylase and lipase. Protein and carbohydrates are easily absorbed, but fat absorption is poor.
2. Limitations relate primarily to anatomic structures and neutrality of the gastric contents.
3. Limited production of pancreatic amylase leads to inadequate utilization of complex carbohydrates.
4. Immaturity of the cardiac and pharyngoesophageal sphincters and neurologic control causes mild regurgitation or slight vomiting.
5. Irregularities in peristaltic motility slow stomach emptying.
6. Peristalsis increases in the lower ileum, resulting in stool frequency—one to six stools per day. Absence of stools within 48 hours after birth may be indicative of intestinal obstruction such as imperforate anus.

Neurologic Changes

Neurologic mechanisms are immature; they are not fully developed anatomically or physiologically. As a result, uncoordinated movements, labile temperature regulation, and poor control over musculature are characteristic of the infant. Reflexes are important indicators of infant neural development (see page 1018).

Nursing Assessment and Management

In caring for the neonate, the nurse establishes an ongoing care plan for the infant and the family until discharge. The nurse's assessment of the neonate includes observing and recording vital signs, daily weight gain or loss, bowel and bladder function, activity and sleep patterns, and thermoregulation. Observation for potential problems in the neonate, ensuring safety, and the prevention of infection are the main goals of nursing care. Delivery of effective neonatal care is enhanced by effective communication of information about the maternal-infant dyad with the interprofessional team.

Another main component of care is to assist with establishing a healthy family unit and promoting health maintenance. This can be accomplished by teaching feeding methods and demonstrating infant care techniques, such as diapering, bathing, and circumcision care. The nurse provides health counseling and education and responds to questions to enable the caregivers to gain confidence, control, and satisfaction in caring for their infant at home. Referrals to community agencies are also important for families to know where they can access assistance outside the hospital setting.

Pertinent Maternal History

1. Social determinants of health, including age, socioeconomic status, ethnic or cultural group, educational level, marital status, social and community context, food security, and health care access.
2. Family medical history.
3. Past obstetric history.
4. Prenatal history with current pregnancy includes review of preexisting medical conditions, rubella status, hepatitis B testing, mental health history (depression and anxiety), drug screening (prescribed and/or recreational), domestic violence, or history of previous child abuse or neglect and also includes other maternal testing relevant to neonatal care (i.e., human immunodeficiency virus [HIV] test results and colonization with group B hemolytic streptococci, sexually transmitted infections [STIs]).
5. Labor and delivery history.

Physical Assessment Findings and Physiologic Functioning

Posture

1. Full-term neonate assumes symmetric posture; face turns to side with full mobility; flexed extremities; hands tightly fisted with thumb covered by fingers.
2. Asymmetric movement may be caused by fractures of the clavicle and humerus or nerve injuries (commonly of the brachial plexus).
3. Infants born in the breech position may keep knees and legs straightened or in frog position, depending on the type of breech presentation.

Length

Newborn (full-term) length ranges from 18 to 22 inches (46 to 56 cm) with an average of 20 inches (51 cm).

Weight

Full-term infant weight ranges from 2,500 to 4,000 g (5 pounds 8 ounces to 8 pounds 13 ounces).

Skin

Infants should be examined under natural light and observed for the following:

1. Hair distribution—full-term infant will have some lanugo over back; most of the lanugo will have disappeared on extremities and other areas of the body.
2. Turgor—full-term infant should have good skin turgor (i.e., after gently pinching small portion of the skin and releasing it, the skin should return to its original position).
3. Color.
   a. Acrocyanosis is bluish discoloration of the hands and feet related to vasoconstriction and sluggish peripheral circulation. It is a normal, transient finding and may be exacerbated by cold temperatures.
   b. Central cyanosis is an indication of reduced arterial oxygen saturation. Persistent central cyanosis requires immediate intervention.
   c. Pallor—may indicate cold, stress, anemia, or cardiac failure.
   d. Plethora—reddish (ruddy) coloration may be caused by a high level of red blood cells (RBCs) to total blood volume from intrauterine intravascular transfusion (twins), cardiac disease, or maternal diabetes.
   e. Jaundice—physiologic jaundice caused by immaturity of the liver is common beginning on day 2, peaking at 1 week, and disappearing by the 2nd week. It first appears in the skin over the face or upper body and then progresses over a larger area; it can also be seen in conjunctivae of the eyes.
   f. Meconium staining of the skin, fingernails, and umbilical cord indicates passage of meconium in utero (possibly caused by fetal hypoxia in utero).
4. Dryness/peeling—marked scaling and desquamation are signs of postmaturity.
5. Vernix—in full-term infants may be found in skin folds under the arms and in the groin under the scrotum (in males) and in the labia (in females). Increased amounts of vernix may indicate prematurity.
6. Nails—reach end of fingertips and be well developed in the full-term infant. There should be no evidence of pits, ridges, aplasia, or hypertrophy.
7. Edema—some edema may occur over buttocks, back, and occiput if the infant has been supine; pitting edema may be caused by erythroblastosis, heart failure, and electrolyte imbalance.
8. Ecchymosis—may appear over the presenting part in a precipitous or prolonged delivery; may also indicate infection or a bleeding problem.
9. Petechiae—pinpoint hemorrhages on the skin caused by increased intravascular pressure, infection, or thrombocytopenia; usually resolves within 48 hours.
10. Erythema toxicum (newborn rash)—small white, yellow, or pink to red papular rash that appears on the trunk, face, and extremities.
11. Hemangiomas—vascular lesions present at birth; some may fade, but others may be permanent.
    a. Strawberry (nevus vasculosus)—bright red, raised, lobulated tumor that occurs on the head, neck, trunk, or extremities; soft, palpable, with sharp demarcated margins; increases in size for approximately 6 months and then regresses after several years.
    b. Cavernous—larger, more mature vascular elements; involves dermis and subcutaneous tissues; soft, palpable, with poorly defined margins; increases in size the first 6 to 12 months and then involutes spontaneously.
12. Telangiectatic nevi (stork bites)—flat red or purple lesions most commonly found on the back of the neck, lower occiput, upper eyelid, and bridge of the nose; regress by age 2, although the ones on the neck may persist through adulthood.
13. Milia—enlarged sebaceous glands found on the nose, chin, cheeks, brow, and forehead; regress in several days to a few weeks. They appear as multiple yellow or pearly white papules, approximately 1 mm in diameter. When found in the mouth, they are referred to as Epstein pearls.
14. Congenital dermal melanocytosis (CDM)—blue-green or gray pigmentation on the lower back, sacrum, and buttocks (also known as Mongolian spots); common in Black, Asian, and Hispanic populations. May be mistaken for signs of child abuse.
15. Café au lait spots—tan or light brown macules or patches. When less than 1¼ inches (3 cm) in length and less than 6 in number, there is no pathologic significance; if greater than 1¼ inches or more than 6 in number, it may indicate cutaneous neurofibromatosis.
16. Harlequin color change—when on side, dependent half turns red and upper half pale; caused by gravity and vasomotor instability.

17. Abrasions or lacerations can result from internal monitoring and instruments used at birth.
18. Cutis marmorata—bluish mottling or marbling of the skin in response to chilling, stress, or overstimulation.
19. Port-wine nevus (nevus flammeus)—flat pink or reddish-purple lesion consisting of dilated, congested capillaries directly beneath the epidermis; does not blanch.

Head

1. Examine the head and face for symmetry, paralysis, shape, swelling, movement.
   a. Caput succedaneum—swelling of soft tissues of the scalp because of pressure; swelling crosses suture lines. May be associated with vacuum-assisted birth or prolonged second stage of labor (pushing).
   b. Cephalohematoma—subperiosteal hemorrhage with collection of blood between the periosteum and bone; swelling does not cross suture lines. May result from vacuum-assisted birth or prolonged second stage of labor.
   c. Molding—overlapping of skull bones, caused by compression during labor and delivery (disappears in a few days).
   d. Examine symmetry of facial movements.
   e. Forceps marks—U-shaped bruising usually on the cheeks following forceps delivery.
2. Measure head circumference—13 to 14 inches (33 to 35.5 cm), approximately ¾ inch (2 cm) larger than the chest. Measure just above the eyebrows and over the occiput.
3. Fontanelles—area where more than two skull bones meet; covered with strong band of connective tissue; also called the soft spot.
   a. Enlarged or bulging—may indicate increased intracranial pressure (ICP).
   b. Sunken—commonly indicates dehydration.
   c. Size—posterior may be obliterated because of molding; closes in 2 to 3 months. Anterior is palpable; closes in 12 to 18 months.
4. Sutures—junctions of adjoining skull bones.
   a. Overriding—caused by molding during labor and delivery.
   b. Separation—extensive separation may be found in malnourished infants and with increased ICP.

Face

1. Eyes
   a. Color—the sclera in most full-term infants is white; subconjunctival hemorrhages are common from the birth process; blue sclera is indicative of osteogenesis imperfecta. Eye color is usually slate gray, brown, or dark blue; final eye color is evident by 6 to 12 months.
   b. Hemorrhagic areas—subconjunctival hemorrhages may appear as a red band from pressure during delivery; regress within 2 weeks.
   c. Edema—edema of the eyelids may be caused by pressure on the head and face during labor and delivery.
   d. Conjunctivitis or discharge—may be caused by eye prophylaxis or infections from organisms, such as staphylococcus, chlamydia trachomatis, or gonococcus. Tear formation does not usually begin until age 2 to 3 months.
   e. Jaundice—may be seen in the sclera because of physiologic or pathologic jaundice.
   f. Pupils—equal in size and should constrict equally in bright light.
   g. Infant can see and discriminate patterns; limited by imperfect oculomotor coordination and inability to accommodate for varying distances.
   h. Red reflex—red-orange color seen when light from an ophthalmoscope is reflected from the retina. No red reflex indicates cataracts.
   i. Brushfield spots—white or yellow pinpoint areas on the iris that may indicate trisomy 21 or even a normal variant.
   j. Abnormal placement of eyes or small eye openings can signify a syndrome or chromosomal anomaly.
   k. Strabismus—cross-eyed appearance that is common; nystagmus (constant, rapid, involuntary movement of the eye) is also common and disappears by age 4 months.
2. Nose
   a. Patency—necessary because infants are obligate nose breathers.
   b. Nasal flaring—abnormal and may indicate respiratory distress. Check for appropriate size and shape of the nose; should be placed vertically midline in the face.
   c. Discharge—stuffiness is normal unless chronic nasal discharge is present; may be caused by possible infection.
   d. Sense of smell—infants will turn toward familiar odors and away from noxious odors.
   e. Septum should be midline; low nasal bridge with broad base may be associated with Down syndrome.
   f. Periodic sneezing is common to clear nasal passages. Excessive sneezing may be an indication of neonatal abstinence syndrome (NAS).
3. Ears—Formation: large, flabby ears that slant forward may indicate abnormalities of the kidney or other parts of the urinary tract.
   a. Position in relation to the eye—helix (top of the ear) on the same plane as the eye; low-set ears may indicate chromosomal or renal abnormalities.
   b. Cartilage—full-term infant has sufficient cartilage to make the ear feel firm.
   c. Hearing—auditory canals may be congested for a day or 2 after birth; the infant should hear well in a few days. Hearing screening may be performed prior to discharge.
   d. Observe for skin tags; preauricular sinus located in front of the ear may be normal or may be associated with genetic disorders.
4. Mouth
   a. Size—small mouth found in trisomy 18 and 21; corners of the mouth turn down (fish mouth) in fetal alcohol syndrome. Mucous membranes should be pink.
   b. Palate—examine hard and soft palate for closure.
   c. Size of the tongue in relation to the mouth—normally does not extend much past the margin of gums. Excessively large tongue seen in congenital anomalies, such as cretinism and trisomy 21.
   d. Teeth—predeciduous teeth are found on rare occasions; if they interfere with feeding or pose an aspiration risk, they may be removed.
   e. Epstein pearls—small white nodules found on sides of hard palate (commonly mistaken for teeth); regress in a few weeks.
   f. Ankyloglossia—thin or thick ridge of tissue running from base of the tongue along undersurface to the tip of the tongue. Most require no intervention, but, depending on the extent of ankyloglossia, breastfeeding and speech may be impacted and require further evaluation.
   g. Sucking blisters (labial tuberales)—thickened areas on midline of the upper lip that may be filled with fluid or callous; no treatment necessary.

h. Infections—thrush, caused by *Candida albicans*, may appear as white patches on the tongue and/or insides of cheeks that do not wash away with fluids; treated with nystatin suspension.

Neck

1. Mobility—can the infant move the head from side to side; palpate for lymph nodes; palpate the clavicle for fractures, especially after a difficult delivery.
2. Torticollis—observe for spasmodic, one-sided contraction of neck muscles; generally from a shortened sternocleidomastoid muscle; physical therapy may be indicated.
3. Excessive skin folds may be associated with congenital abnormalities such as trisomy 21.
4. Stiffness and hyperextension may be caused by trauma or infection.
5. Clavicle—assess for intactness, fractures, and masses such as cystic hygroma, soft and usually seen laterally or over the clavicle.

Chest

1. Circumference and symmetry—average circumference is 12 to 13 inches (30.5 to 33 cm), approximately ¾ inch (2 cm) smaller than head circumference.
2. Breast.
   a. Engorgement—may occur at day 3 because of maternal hormones, especially estrogen; no treatment required. Regresses in 2 weeks.
   b. Nipples and areolae—less formed and pronounced in preterm infants.

Respiratory System

1. Rate—normally between 30 and 60 breaths/min; influenced by sleep–wake status, hunger, medication, and temperature.
2. Rhythm—respirations may be shallow with irregular rhythm.
   a. Respiratory movements are symmetric and mainly diaphragmatic because of weak thoracic muscles. For example, the lower thorax pulls in, and the abdomen bulges with each respiration.
   b. Periodic breathing—resumption of respiration after a 5- to 15-second period without respiration; decreases with time; more common in preterm infants. Substernal retractions, if accompanied by gasps or stridor, are indicative of upper airway obstruction.
   c. Observe for abnormal respiratory signs.
3. Breath sounds
   a. Bronchial sounds are heard over most of the chest with auscultation.
   b. Crackles may be heard immediately after birth.
   c. Expiratory grunting may be indicative of respiratory distress.

Cardiovascular System

1. Rate—normal between 110 and 160 bpm (80 to 110 normal with deep sleep); influenced by behavioral state, environmental temperature, and medication; take apical count for 1 minute.
2. Rhythm—common to find periods of deceleration followed by periods of acceleration.
3. Heart sounds—second sound higher in pitch and sharper than first; third and fourth sounds rarely heard; murmurs common; majority are transitory and benign.
4. Pulses—examine bilateral quality and strength of brachial, radial, pedal, and femoral pulses; lack of femoral pulses indicative of inadequate aortic blood flow (coarctation).
5. Cyanosis—examine for central cyanosis. Record location of any cyanosis and color changes with time and when crying.
6. Blood pressure—BP in the full-term newborn ranges from 60 to 80 mm Hg systolic and 30 to 60 mm Hg diastolic at birth and varies with gestational age, weight, activity, and appropriate cuff size. BP is usually higher in the lower extremities than in the upper extremities. BP assessment may not be conducted routinely on healthy neonates. Measurement of BP and mean arterial blood pressure (>40 mm Hg) is essential for infants who show signs of distress, are premature, or are suspected of having a cardiac anomaly.

Abdomen

1. Shape—cylindrical, protrudes slightly, moves synchronously with chest in respiration. Diastasis recti is a common occurrence in the newborn and characterized by a separation of the right and left sides of the rectus abdominis muscle.
2. Distention may be caused by bowel obstruction, organ enlargement, or infection.
3. Palpate the abdomen for masses; palpate the liver and spleen.
   a. The liver has decreased ability to conjugate bilirubin (rationale for physiologic jaundice).
   b. The liver has decreased production of prothrombin and factors that depend on vitamin K for synthesis, resulting in the neonate's predisposition to hemorrhage.
4. Auscultate abdomen in all four quadrants for bowel sounds; usually bowel sounds occur 1 hour after delivery.
5. Kidneys—palpate kidneys for size and shape.
   a. Infant has decreased ability of the kidney to concentrate urine, excrete a solute load, and maintain water and electrolyte balance.
   b. Urine may contain uric acid crystals, which appear on diaper as reddish stains. Uric acid crystals may yield false-positive result when the infant's urine is tested for protein.
6. Umbilical cord.
   a. Consists of two arteries, one vein; a single umbilical artery is associated with renal and other congenital abnormalities.
   b. Signs of infection (omphalitis) around insertion into abdominal wall—redness, discharge.
   c. Meconium staining—associated with intrauterine compromise or postmaturity.
   d. Cord will dry over 24 hours and fall off in approximately 10 to 14 days.
   e. Umbilical hernia—defect in abdominal wall.
7. Genitalia.
   a. Female:
      i. Labia majora cover labia minora and clitoris in full-term female infants.
      ii. Hymenal tag (tissue) may protrude from the vagina—regresses within several weeks.
      iii. Vaginal discharge—white mucus discharge common; pink-tinged or bloody mucus discharge (pseudomenstruation) may be present because of the drop in maternal hormones; no treatment necessary.
   b. Male:
      i. Full-term—testes in scrotal sac; scrotal sac appears markedly wrinkled because of rugae.
      ii. Edema may be present in scrotal sac if the infant was born in breech presentation; a collection of fluid in the scrotal sac is a hydrocele—regresses in approximately a month.

iii. Examine glans penis for urethral opening—normally central; opening ventral (hypospadias); opening dorsally (epispadias); abnormally adherent foreskin (phimosis).

c. Check for patent anus—infant should stool within 24 hours after delivery.

Back

1. Examine spinal column for normal curvature, closure, and pilonidal dimple or sinus; also for fluid-filled sac, exposed nerves, or other skin abnormality seen with spinal bifida.
2. Examine anal area for position, anal opening, response of anal sphincter (anal wink reflex), and fissures.

Musculoskeletal System

1. Examine extremities for fractures, paralysis, range of motion, and irregular position.
2. Examine fingers and toes for number and separation: extra digits (polydactyly) and fused digits (syndactyly).
3. Examine hips for dislocation—with the infant in supine position, flex knees and abduct hips to side and down to table surface; clicking sound (Ortolani sign) and clunking sound (Barlow sign) indicate dislocation or subluxation. Asymmetric gluteal folds may also indicate congenital hip dislocation.
4. Examine feet for structural and positional deformities, that is, club foot (talipes equinovarus) or metatarsus adductus (inward turning of the foot).

Neurologic System

1. Neurologic mechanisms are immature anatomically and physiologically; as a result, uncoordinated movements, temperature instability, and lack of control over musculature are characteristic of the infant.
2. Examine muscle tone, head control, and reflexes.
3. Two types of reflexes are present in the neonate:
   a. Protective in nature (blink, cough, sneeze, gag)—remain throughout life.
   b. Primitive in nature (rooting/sucking, Moro, startle, tonic neck, stepping, and palmar/plantar grasp)—either disappear within months or become highly developed and voluntary (sucking and grasping) (see Figure 34-4, page 1019).

Behavioral Assessment

Response to Stimulation

1. Neonates exhibit predictable, directed responses in social interactions with nurturing adults or in response to attractive auditory or visual stimuli.
2. Neonate responses are influenced by states of consciousness, such as:
   a. Quiet, deep sleep (sleep state)—no spontaneous activity, eyes closed, and respirations regular, with delayed response to external stimuli.
   b. Light, active sleep (sleep state)—random startles, eyes closed, rapid eye movements (REMs), and frequent change of state with response to stimulation.
   c. Drowsy awake (transitional state)—eyes open or closed, appearing dull and heavy lidded, eyelids flutter, variable activity level, mild startles periodically, and delayed response to stimulation.
   d. Quiet alert (awake state)—eyes open, little motor activity, focuses on source of stimulation. Interacts most with environment; respirations regular.
   e. Alert active (awake state)—eyes open, less bright and attentive, much motor activity, and increase in startles in response to stimulation.
   f. Crying (awake state)—intense crying that is difficult to interrupt with stimulation; increased motor activity and color changes.

Sleeping Pattern

1. Length of sleep cycles (REM, active and quiet sleep) changes with maturation of the central nervous system (CNS).
2. Quiet sleep should increase with time in relation to REM sleep.
3. Neonates usually sleep 20 hours/day.
4. Safe sleep positions should be discussed with families.
5. Prone positioning has been shown to increase the risk of sudden infant death syndrome. The American Academy of Pediatrics (AAP) recommends that all healthy infants be positioned supine for sleep.

Feeding Pattern

1. Most breastfed neonates feed every 2 to 3 hours (10 to 12 times per day) and on demand; a regular feeding pattern is generally established in approximately 2 weeks. Formula-fed babies eat every 3 to 4 hours.
2. Caloric requirements are high—110 to 130 calories/kg of body weight daily.
3. Most digestive enzymes are present at birth.
4. Immaturity of the cardiac and pharyngoesophageal sphincters and neurologic control causes mild regurgitation or slight vomiting.

Pattern of Elimination

1. Stools.
   a. Meconium is usually passed in 24 to 48 hours.
   b. Passage of meconium (tarry green-black stools) continues for about 72 hours, followed by transitional stools (greenish brown to yellowish brown; thin; may contain milk curds). Milk stools (for breastfed, yellow to golden; pasty; odor like sour milk; for formula-fed, pale yellow to light brown; firmer; more offensive odor) are passed by day 4 to 5.
   c. Neonate has up to six stools per day in the first few weeks after birth.
2. Voiding.
   a. Neonate voids within first 24 hours.
   b. After first few days, infant voids from at least six to eight times per day.

Temperature Regulation

1. Infant's body responds readily to changes in environmental temperature.
2. Heat loss at birth may occur through evaporation, convection, conduction, and radiation.
3. Physiologic mechanisms to avoid heat loss include:
   a. Vasoconstriction.
   b. Nonshivering thermogenesis elicited by sympathetic nervous system in response to decreased temperature.
   c. Adipose tissue contains many small blood vessels, fat vacuoles, and mitochondria and is a site of heat production. Brown fat is found between scapulae, around the neck and thorax, behind the sternum, and around kidneys and adrenals.
   d. Flexed position of full-term neonate.

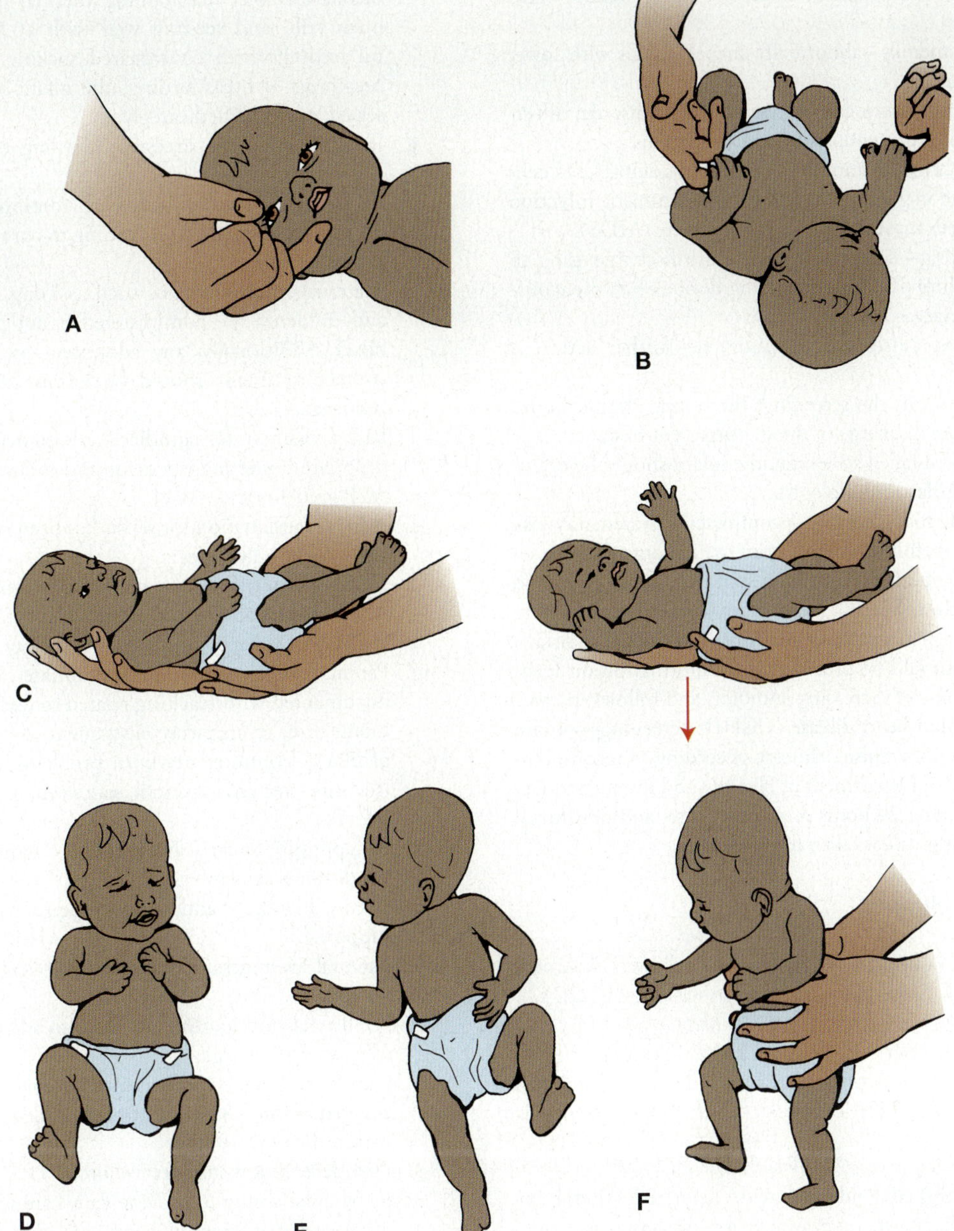

Figure 34-4. Newborn reflexes. (A) Rooting. (B) Grasp. (C) Moro. (D) Startle. (E) Tonic neck. (F) Stepping. (Reprinted with permission from Reeder, S., Martin, L., & Koniak-Griffin, D. [1997]. *Maternity nursing: Family newborn, and women's health care* [18th ed.]. Lippincott-Raven Publishers.)

Universal Newborn Screening

EVIDENCE BASE Lin, H. J., & Vera, M. (2021). Newborn screening. In C. Berkowitz (Ed.), *Berkowitz's pediatrics: A primary care approach* (6th ed., pp. 161–166). American Academy of Pediatrics. https://doi.org/10.1542/9781610023733-25

Public health law requires newborn screening for disorders caused by inborn errors of metabolism, hemoglobinopathies, infectious diseases, and specific genetic and endocrine disorders. In addition, infants are screened for hearing loss, hyperbilirubinemia, and cardiac defects.

1. Blood spot testing—obtain blood by heel stick for the following conditions.
   a. Phenylketonuria—inability of the infant to metabolize phenylalanine; scheduled after 24 hours of protein feedings.
   b. Galactosemia—inborn error of carbohydrate metabolism, in which galactose and lactose cannot be converted to glucose.
   c. Hypothyroidism—thyroid hormone deficiency.
   d. Maple syrup urine disease—inability to metabolize leucine, isoleucine, and valine.

e. Homocystinuria—inborn error of sulfur amino acid metabolism.
f. Sickle cell anemia—abnormally shaped RBCs with lower oxygen solubility.
g. Cystic fibrosis—autosomal recessive genetic disorder affecting the respiratory, endocrine, and GI systems.
h. HIV—weakens the immune system by reducing CD4 cells (T cells) and increasing the risk for opportunistic infection and acquired immunodeficiency syndrome (AIDS).

2. Hearing screening—screen newborn before discharge using an automated auditory brainstem hearing device or an otoacoustic emission device.
   a. If the infant passes the screening, no further action is needed.
   b. If the infant fails the screening, the testing should be repeated before discharge or on an outpatient basis.
   c. With repeated failed screening, the infant should be evaluated by a pediatric audiologist.
3. Hyperbilirubinemia screening—complete a systematic risk screening for hyperbilirubinemia prior to discharge. Use the serum bilirubin result from the blood spot metabolic screen and plot it on the Hour-Specific Nomogram (*https://bilitool.org*).
   a. A treatment plan should be identified for infants at risk.
   b. Caregivers should be provided with information on feeding, symptoms of increasing jaundice, and follow-up care.
4. Critical congenital heart disease (CCHD) screening—obtain oxygen saturation by pulse oximetry, according to recommendation by the U.S. Department of Health and Human Services (HHS). Screen after 24 hours of age using pre- and postductal oxygen saturation values taken for 60 seconds.

Discharge Readiness

EVIDENCE BASE American Academy of Pediatrics & American College of Obstetricians and Gynecologists. (2017). *Guidelines for perinatal care* (8th ed.). Author.

Stewart, D. L., & Barfield, W. D. (2019). Updates on an at-risk population: Late-preterm and early-term infants. *Pediatrics, 144*(5), e20192760. https://doi.org/10.1542/peds.2019-2760

1. The AAP established guidelines with suggested criteria for newborn discharge where readiness for discharge is determined in consultation with the maternal and newborn providers and the postpartum patient. The following criteria apply to the full-term newborn (37 0/7 to 41 6/7 weeks' gestation):
   a. Family, environmental, and social risk factors have been assessed for safety.
   b. Physical assessment and clinical course were unremarkable for abnormalities.
   c. The newborn is stable with documented vital signs within normal ranges for 12 hours prior to discharge; temperature 36.5°C to 37.4°C (97.7°F to 99.3°F); respirations below 60 bpm; no signs of respiratory distress; heart rate 100 to 190 while awake.
   d. Pertinent laboratory data have been reviewed and within normal limits for postpartum patient and neonate. Cord or infant blood type and direct Coombs results (if required) have been reviewed.
   e. Neonate has passed at least one stool spontaneously and urinated.
   f. Neonate stable, maintaining thermal homeostasis in an open crib, and feeding well with at least two successful feedings with coordinated sucking, swallowing, and breathing. If breastfeeding, the infant latch has been assessed by a qualified caregiver.
   g. If circumcised, no excessive bleeding from circumcision site for 2 hours post procedure.
   h. All necessary vaccines have been administered to the newborn (e.g., hepatitis B) according to current AAP immunization schedules.
   i. Maternal immunizations such as Tdap, varicella, rubella, and influenza are administered if not previously immunized. Additionally, any adolescent or adults with close contact to infant should be immunized for Tdap and influenza.
   j. Risk assessment for jaundice has been determined with appropriate home management and follow-up according to AAP guidelines.
   k. Adequate evaluation for sepsis has been completed according to AAP guidelines.
   l. Hearing screening, congenital hip dysplasia screening, newborn metabolic screening, and pulse oximetry for CCHD have been completed per facility protocol.
   m. Parental ability to provide appropriate care to newborn is documented with teaching related to feeding, elimination, infant care, temperature assessment, signs and symptoms of illness, common newborn problems, and infant safety (nicotine-free environment, safe sleep, car seat, and sibling safety).
   n. An appropriate car seat for infant's maturity and medical condition is available at discharge.
   o. Family members and support persons are available for support.
   p. Parental awareness of possible complications for self and neonate.
   q. Facility has mechanisms in place to address patient questions after discharge.
   r. Plan for follow-up medical care is in place. For infants discharged before 48 hours of birth, follow-up should occur within the next 48 hours.
   s. Provide lactation support resources.
2. Assess parental ability to provide daily care of the infant.
   a. Advise participation in baby care classes offered during their stay at the birth facility.
   b. Assess ability to bathe and diaper the infant, perform circumcision care, and initiate either breast- or bottle-feeding.
   c. Assess bonding and encourage skin-to-skin contact, infant eye contact, and talking to and touching the infant.
3. Assess caregivers' knowledge of signs of illness and when to notify health care provider.
   a. Fever above 100.4°F (37.8°C).
   b. Loss of appetite for two consecutive feedings.
   c. Inability to awaken the baby to usual activity state.
   d. Vomiting all or part of two feedings.
   e. Diarrhea—three watery stools.
   f. Extreme irritability or inconsolable crying.
4. Assess parental ability to properly place infant in car seat.
5. Provide positive reinforcement and reassurance.
6. Further assess any knowledge gaps, and provide written instructions and educational material on discharge.

CLINICAL JUDGMENT Be aware that newborn readmission to the hospital increases with primiparity, maternal morbidity, prematurity, operative vaginal delivery, and small for gestational age infants. Recent changes in gestational age terminology such as early term (prior to 37 0/7 weeks' gestation) and late preterm (38 6/7 weeks' gestation) infants have also impacted morbidity in these at-risk groups. Discharge readiness should be assessed by the interprofessional team. Discharge instructions should include a thorough discussion of the infant's sleeping, feeding, metabolic processes, activity, and response patterns for the first month of life. Ensure that caregivers have the ability to remain alert for signs and symptoms of illness, including when to call the provider.

PROBLEMS OF THE NEWBORN

See additional online content: Procedure Guidelines 34-1.

Premature Infant

EVIDENCE BASE American College of Obstetricians and Gynecologists' Committee on Obstetric Practice, Society for Maternal-Fetal Medicine. (2021). Medically indicated late-preterm and early-term deliveries (Committee Opinion #831). *Obstetrics and Gynecology, 138*(1), e35–e39. https://doi.org/10.1097/AOG.0000000000004447

Verklan, M. T., Walden, M., & Forest, S. (2020). *Core curriculum for neonatal intensive care nursing* (6th ed.). Elsevier.

The *premature neonate* is a neonate born before the completion of 37 weeks' gestation. Other classifications include moderately preterm (32 to 36 weeks), late preterm (34 0/7 to 36 6/7 weeks), early term (37 0/7 to 38 6/7 weeks), and very preterm birth (less than 32 weeks). The greatest threat to the preterm neonate is decreased production of surfactant related to the gestational age.

Birth weight is a factor in assessing the premature neonate. Low birth weight is defined as less than 2,500 g (5 pounds, 8 ounces) regardless of gestational age. A very-low-birth-weight neonate is one whose birth weight is below 1,500 (3 pounds, 5 ounces), regardless of gestational age. An extremely-low-birth-weight neonate is one whose birth weight is below 1,000 g (2 pounds, 2 ounces), regardless of gestational age.

Pathophysiology and Etiology

1. A wide range of maternal factors is associated with prematurity.
2. Maternal risk factors associated with prematurity include, but are not limited to:
   a. Chronic health problems, such as hypertension, obesity, or diabetes.
   b. Behavioral and environmental risks, such as late or no prenatal care, smoking, substance misuse, domestic violence, stress, or lack of social support.
   c. Demographic risks, such as being non-Hispanic Black, younger than age 17, older than age 35, or low socioeconomic status.
   d. Genetic endowment.
   e. Assisted reproductive technologies (ARTs).
   f. Current pregnancy risk factors, such as preeclampsia or gestational hypertension, bleeding, placenta previa or abruptio placentae, uterine or cervical anomalies (incompetent cervix), premature rupture of membranes, preterm premature rupture of membranes, polyhydramnios or oligohydramnios, infection, or periodontal disease.
   g. Changes in delivery practices, concern about postmaturity complications, or risk of stillbirth (late preterm).
3. Fetal factors associated with prematurity include:
   a. Chromosomal abnormalities.
   b. Anatomic abnormalities, such as tracheoesophageal atresia or fistula and intestinal obstruction.
   c. Fetoplacental unit dysfunction.
4. The premature infant has altered physiology because of immature and typically poorly developed systems. The severity of any problem that occurs depends on the gestational age of the infant. Systems and situations that are most likely to cause problems in the premature infant include:
   a. Respiratory system
   b. Digestive system
   c. Thermoregulation
   d. Immune system
   e. Neurologic system

Nursing Assessment

1. Notice physical characteristics of the premature neonate:
   a. Hair—lanugo, fluffy.
   b. Poor ear cartilage.
   c. Skin—thin; capillaries are visible (may be red and wrinkled).
   d. Lack of subcutaneous fat.
   e. Sole of the foot is smooth.
      i. 36 weeks' gestation—anterior one third of the foot is creased.
      ii. 38 weeks' gestation—two thirds of the foot is creased.
   f. Breast buds.
      i. 36 weeks' gestation—none.
      ii. 38 weeks' gestation—1¼ inches (3 cm).
   g. Testes—undescended.
   h. Labia majora—undeveloped.
   i. Rugae of scrotum—fine.
   j. Fingernails—soft.
   k. Abdomen—relatively large.
   l. Thorax—relatively small.
   m. Head—appears disproportionately large.
   n. Muscle tone poor and possibly weak reflexes.
2. Obtain accurate body measurements.
   a. Head circumference—frontal–occipital circumference one finger above eyebrows, using parallel lines of tape around the head.
   b. Abdominal girth—one finger above umbilicus, mark location.
   c. Heel to crown.
   d. Shoulder to umbilicus—used to calculate proper length of catheter for umbilical catheter placement.
   e. Weight in grams.
3. Assess gestational age (see Figure 34-5) using a tool such as the New Ballard scoring system (recommended by the Committee of Fetus and Newborn of American Academy of Pediatrics [AAP]):
   a. Observation of physical and neurologic characteristics that change predictably with growth and maturation. Ideally done in the first 12 to 24 hours of life.

	0	1	2	3	4	5
SKIN	gelatinous red, trans-parent	smooth pink, visible veins	superficial peeling and/or rash, few veins	cracking pale area, rare veins	parchment, deep cracking, no vessels	leathery, cracked, wrinkled
LANUGO	none	abundant	thinning	bald areas	mostly bald	
PLANTAR CREASES	no crease	faint red marks	anterior transverse crease only	creases ant. 2/3	creases cover entire sole	
BREAST	barely percept.	flat areola, no bud	stippled areola, 1–2 mm bud	raised areola, 3–4 mm bud	full areola, 5–10 mm bud	
EAR	pinna flat, stays folded	sl. curved pinna, soft with slow recoil	well-curv. pinna, soft but ready recoil	formed and firm with instant recoil	thick cartilage, ear stiff	
GENITALS Male	scrotum empty, no rugae		testes descend-ing, few rugae	testes down, good rugae	testes pendulous, deep rugae	
GENITALS Female	prominent clitoris and labia minora		majora and minora equally prominent	majora large, minora small	clitoris and minora completely covered	

	0	1	2	3	4	5
Posture						
Square Window (Wrist)	90°	60°	45°	30°	0°	
Arm Recoil	180°		100°-180°	90°-100°	<90°	
Popliteal Angle	180°	160°	130°	110°	90°	<90°
Scarf Sign						
Heel to Ear						

Score	Wks
5	26
10	28
15	30
20	32
25	34
30	36
35	38
40	40
45	42
50	44

Figure 34-5. Ballard assessment of gestational age criteria. (Reprinted from Ballard, J. L., Khoury, J. C., Wedig, K., Eilers-Walsman, L., & Lipp, R. [1991]. New Ballard score, expanded to include extremely premature infants. *Journal of Pediatrics, 119*[3], 417–423. https://doi.org/10.1016/s0022-3476(05)82056-6. Copyright 1991, with permission from Elsevier.)

b. Later, adjusted, or corrected age will be determined once the neonate reaches term (40 weeks after conception). Chronologic age is adjusted for prematurity by taking gestational age − 40 + chronologic age = developmental or corrected age. This is the age the neonate would have been if they had been born at 40 weeks' gestation.

Nursing Interventions

Initial Nursing Care

1. Assist with laboratory testing, as indicated, for blood gases, blood glucose, complete blood count (CBC) or hemoglobin and hematocrit, electrolytes, calcium, and bilirubin.
2. Monitor closely for respiratory or cardiac complications.
   a. Respirations above 60 per minute and an oxygen saturation below 92% may indicate respiratory difficulty.
   b. Assess for cyanosis (other than acrocyanosis) and other signs of respiratory distress.
   c. Increased (greater than 180 bpm) or irregular heart rate may indicate cardiac or circulatory difficulties.
   d. Muscle tone and activity should be evaluated.
   e. Hypotension may be caused by hypovolemia.
   f. Hypoglycemia may result from inadequate glycogen stores, respiratory distress, and cold stress.

CLINICAL JUDGMENT In addition to tachypnea and reduced oxygen saturation, be alert for subtle signs of respiratory compromise, such as expiratory grunting, retractions, chest lag, or nasal flaring. These should be reported immediately. Respiratory distress syndrome (RDS) is a common complication of prematurity where the etiologic cause is the decreased level of surfactant production.

3. Institute cardiac monitoring and care for infant in an isolette or radiant heater. Defer bathing until infant's temperature has stabilized. Temperature instability is a risk factor for hypoglycemia and sepsis.
4. Observe for early signs of jaundice and check maternal history for any blood incompatibilities. Also, be aware of maternal factors that can lead to additional complications, such as drug use, diabetes, and infection.
5. Once the infant is admitted to the nursery, be aware that the first 24 to 48 hours after birth is a critical time, requiring constant observation and intensive care management. Assess for the following:
   a. Carefully monitor cardiopulmonary status, increased work of breathing, oxygen saturation, and report vital signs to the interprofessional team as necessary.
   b. Color—cyanosis, jaundice, rashes, paleness, and ruddiness.
   c. Umbilicus—if umbilical lines are in use, observe for bleeding—apply pressure and notify provider.
   d. Urinary output—first void within 24 hours and monitor every 2 to 4 hours. Stools—abdominal distention and lack of stools may indicate intestinal obstruction or other intestinal tract anomalies. Measure abdominal girth at regular intervals.
   e. Activity and behavior—look for sucking movement and hand-to-mouth maneuver, which can help to determine oral feeding initiation depending on gestational age.
   f. Observe for a tense and bulging fontanelle; palpate suture lines, noting separation—may indicate intracranial hemorrhage. Be alert to twitching and seizures.
6. Have resuscitative equipment, oxygen, and suction available.
   a. A bulb syringe is used for clearing the mouth and nose.
   b. Frequent suctioning of the pharynx may not be necessary and should be used judiciously.
   c. May need to assist with intubation for administration of exogenous surfactant depending on the infant's gestational age and clinical presentation.
7. Position to optimize ventilation, with careful attention to maintaining body alignment nesting extremities with blankets.
   a. Elevate head and trunk to decrease pressure on the diaphragm from abdominal organs.
   b. Change position from side to side.
   c. Prone positioning offers some advantage for oxygenation in preterm neonate with respiratory compromise. During the initial phase of illness, these infants are cared for with

cardiorespiratory monitoring and may be placed prone according to the facility's policy.

8. Provide humidified oxygen therapy in percentages necessary to maintain appropriate oxygen saturation and/or blood gas values.
   a. Continuous oxygen saturation monitoring is recommended when oxygen is in use and until infant is stable.
   b. Continuous cardiac monitoring is recommended to assess for apnea and bradycardia episodes.
9. Monitor for apnea (pauses more than 20 seconds) versus periodic breathing (regular repetition of breathing pauses of less than 15 seconds, alternating with breaths of regularly increasing then decreasing amplitude for 10 to 15 seconds). Medications (i.e., theophylline and caffeine) may be given to reduce apneic episodes.

Ongoing Nursing Care

1. Protect the infant from infection by maintaining standard and aseptic practices at all times. Follow facility policies related to visitation by family members.
2. Provide meticulous skin care avoiding adhesives and providing adequate hydration.
3. Avoid deformational plagiocephaly (misshapen head) by frequent repositioning and facility-approved devices such as the "cranial cup" or gel pads.
4. Protect the neonate's eyes from bright lights.
5. Continue to provide intravenous (IV) and oral feedings according to neonate's needs. Assist with maternal breast pumping, and encourage holding and feeding of infant based on infant status.
6. Continue to monitor for complications, such as hypo/hyperglycemia, RDS (see page 1183), apnea, pneumothorax, infection, hypocalcemia, cardiac abnormalities, necrotizing enterocolitis (NEC), intracranial hemorrhage, and hyperbilirubinemia.
7. Make every effort to include biological parents and designated caregivers in their infant's care, and update them frequently on the infant's condition.
8. Prior to discharge, start to transition the neonate to a supine position for sleep with alternating head position in adherence with safe sleep recommendations. Safe sleep positioning should be reinforced. Prone and side-lying positions should be used when the infant is awake and supervised.
9. Work with the health care team to formulate a discharge plan that includes long-term follow-up and support. Provide help for coping with possible long-term complications, including retinopathy of prematurity, chronic lung disease, hearing loss, and learning disabilities.

The Postterm Infant

The postterm newborn infant is one whose gestation is 42 weeks or longer and who may show signs of weight loss with placental insufficiency.

EVIDENCE BASE American Academy of Pediatrics, & American Heart Association. (2021). *Textbook of neonatal resuscitation* (7th ed.). American Academy of Pediatrics.

Pathophysiology and Etiology

1. Cause is not known in many cases. Maternal factors associated with postmaturity include nulliparity, a prior postterm pregnancy, carrying a male fetus, and maternal obesity.
2. Anencephaly and placental sulfatase deficiency are disorders associated with postterm delivery.
3. Maternal risks include:
   a. Trauma to the perineum related to possible fetal macrosomia.
   b. Increased risk of infection, hemorrhage, operative vaginal delivery (forceps, vacuum), and cesarean delivery.
   c. Psychological stress and anxiety.
4. Fetal risks include:
   a. Increased risk of mortality and morbidity.
   b. Increased risk of hypoxia related to an aging placenta and decreased amount of amniotic fluid.
   c. Increased risk of meconium aspiration syndrome (MAS).
   d. Increased risk of trauma related to macrosomia and shoulder dystocia.
   e. Increased risk of seizures.
   f. Increased risk of an Apgar score of less than 4 at 5 minutes of life.

Nursing Assessment

1. Be alert for the physical appearance of a postterm neonate. The following characteristics are most commonly seen in a postterm neonate:
   a. Reduced subcutaneous tissue—loose skin, especially of buttocks and thighs.
   b. Long, curved fingernails and toenails.
   c. Minimal amount of vernix caseosa.
   d. Abundant scalp hair.
   e. Wrinkled, macerated skin; possibly pale, peeling skin.
   f. Having the alert appearance of a 2- to 3-week-old neonate after delivery.
   g. Greenish-yellow staining of the skin, fingernails, or cord may indicate fetal stress in utero.
2. Determine gestational age by physical examination and New Ballard Scale (see page 1022). Measure weight, length, and head circumference.
3. Monitor blood glucose per facility policy; below 40 mg/100 mL indicates hypoglycemia.
4. Assess for asphyxia neonatorum by Apgar score and blood gas analysis.
5. Assess for meconium aspiration; signs include:
   a. Thick meconium in amniotic fluid at delivery.
   b. Tachypnea, increasing signs of cyanosis; difficulty breathing, with need for ventilation.
   c. Tachycardia.
   d. Inspiratory nasal flaring and retraction of the chest.
   e. Expiratory grunting.
   f. Increased anteroposterior diameter of the chest.
   g. Crackles and rhonchi on chest auscultation.
   h. Concomitant cerebral irritation—jitteriness, hypotonia, and seizures.
   i. X-ray changes—classic coarse, patchy, streaky areas with irregular pulmonary infiltrates ranging in severity.
   j. Additional signs: metabolic acidosis, hypotension, hypoglycemia, and hypocalcemia.

Nursing Interventions

1. Provide supportive care for the prevention of MAS. The consistency of the meconium in the amniotic fluid (thin vs thick) is no longer used to determine the need for tracheal suctioning.
   a. The indication for *selective* intubation and tracheal suctioning for infants exposed to meconium-stained amniotic fluid is a nonvigorous infant.

b. The neonatal resuscitation program (NRP) defines nonvigorous as an infant with one or more of the following conditions: depressed respirations, depressed muscle tone, or heart rate below 100 beats/min.
c. Selective intubation and tracheal suctioning is contraindicated in a vigorous infant with strong respiratory effort, good muscle tone, or heart rate above 100 beats/min.

2. Provide supportive care measures, including the following:
   a. Warmth—maintain a thermoregulated environment to reduce oxygen and calorie consumption and preserve glycogen stores.
   b. Adequate humidified oxygenation to maintain oxygen saturation ≥94%.
   c. Respiratory support with a ventilator may be necessary.
   d. Adequate administration of calories and fluid.
   e. Accurate monitoring of vital signs and intake and output—to assess possible alteration in kidney function caused by hypoxia.
   f. Administration of antibiotics prophylactically.
3. Provide oral feeding of glucose or IV dextrose soon after birth to treat or prevent hypoglycemia. If oral feedings are not contraindicated, they can begin 1 to 2 hours after birth. Monitor blood sugar until condition stabilizes per facility policy.
4. Be alert for persistent pulmonary hypertension of the newborn (PPHN)—physiologic disorder characterized by severe, labile cyanosis arising from persistent or return to suprasystemic pulmonary vascular resistance (PVR) and pressure normally found in the fetus.
   a. Cyanosis, pronounced respiratory distress, murmur, and heart failure.
   b. Treatment is aggressive respiratory support in a tertiary care nursery.
5. Provide psychological support to the family and encourage participation in infant's care.

Infant of a Diabetic Mother

This condition occurs due to diagnosis of diabetes prior to pregnancy, unrecognized preexisting diabetes, or gestational diabetes mellitus (GDM). The neonate is commonly termed infant of a diabetic mother (IDM). The severity of neonatal problems will depend on maternal control of blood glucose prenatally and perinatally.

Pathophysiology and Etiology

Poor maternal glycemic control will impact the fetus throughout the pregnancy and will depend on the trimester affected.

1. There is an increased incidence of congenital anomalies, which may be caused by:
   a. Genetic anomaly.
   b. High glucose concentrations in first trimester pregnancy.
   c. Episodes of ketoacidosis in first trimester pregnancy.
2. Common anomalies are renal and central nervous system (CNS) anomalies, caudal regression syndrome, small colon syndrome, cleft lip/palate, and cardiac defects such as patent ductus arteriosus, transposition of the great vessels, and ventricular septal defect.
3. Lung maturity
   a. Fetal hyperinsulinemia can occur with poorly controlled maternal glucose levels and result in decreased surfactant production necessary for lung maturation.
   b. Insufficient surfactant levels and delayed fetal lung maturity may predispose preterm and full-term neonates to RDS.
   c. Prematurity and/or small for gestational age may be associated with placental insufficiency.
4. Infection can lead to:
   a. Prematurity and decreased passive immunity.
   b. Maternal urinary tract infection (UTI) and chorioamnionitis risks are increased.
5. Macrosomia/large for gestational age (LGA):
   a. Fetal hyperinsulinemia acts as a growth hormone that results in increased fetal size.
   b. Large trunk and chest increase risk of shoulder dystocia and birth trauma such as clavicle fracture and cephalohematoma.
   c. Increased amount of body fat and total body water is reduced at birth.
   d. High urine output during the first 2 days of life, likely from diuresis of intracellular water.
6. Hypoglycemia
   a. Hypoglycemia is defined as a serum glucose less than 40 mg/dL.
   b. In utero, fetal glucose levels are 70% to 80% of maternal glucose levels.
   c. In utero, the fetus produces insulin to metabolize glucose independently of maternal endocrine function.
   d. With the cessation of maternal glucose transfer at birth, fetal hyperinsulinemia may result in hypoglycemia. Occurs within first 12 hours of life; may occur within minutes after birth.
   e. The neonate's response to glucose may be labile (i.e., insulin blood level has a slight elevation, will drop, and then peak within 1 hour).
   f. Neonate may be asymptomatic; therefore, careful assessment for hypoglycemia is essential to improve outcomes.
   g. When hypoglycemia is present, symptoms may include: lethargy, jitteriness, poor feeding, temperature instability, vomiting, pallor, apnea, irregular respirations, hypotonia, tremors, seizure activity, and high-pitched cry.
7. Hypocalcemia (less than 7 mg/dL).
   a. Associated with prematurity, difficult labor and delivery, asphyxia at birth, and decreased functioning of parathyroid glands.
   b. Generally occurs during the first 24 to 72 hours of life.
   c. Tremors are characteristic and may be secondary to prematurity or stress during pregnancy, labor, and birth.
   d. The infant may also have hypomagnesemia (less than 1.4 mg/dL) resulting from functional hypoparathyroidism because of maternal magnesium loss.
8. Polycythemia and hyperbilirubinemia—hyperinsulinemia results in polycythemia without concurrent organ system maturation.
   a. Polycythemia increases the risks of occurrence of jaundice, renal vein thrombosis, respiratory distress, hypoglycemia, and hypocalcemia.
   b. Serum hematocrit levels greater than 65% or hemoglobin 22 g/dL.
   c. Hematocrit is higher and extracellular volume is decreased.
   d. Immature liver results in inability to conjugate bilirubin (byproduct of hemoglobin breakdown) and increases the risk of hyperbilirubinemia.

Nursing Assessment

1. Assess for characteristics of IDM—macrosomia, large chest and shoulders, cardiomegaly, hepatomegaly, large umbilical cord and placenta, plethora, full-face, LGA (some may be normal weight or small for gestational age), abundant fat,

abundant hair, liberally coated with vernix caseosa, and hypertrichosis pinnae (excessive hair growth on the external ear).
2. Obtain maternal history of diabetes.
3. Perform assessment for determination of gestational age.
4. Assist with obtaining laboratory tests—serum glucose, calcium, phosphorus, magnesium, electrolytes, bilirubin, arterial blood gas analysis, blood hemoglobin, and hematocrit as ordered.
5. Monitor for hypoglycemia.
    a. Monitor serum glucose levels every 30 to 60 minutes beginning immediately after birth and then every 4 to 8 hours once stabilized. Continue monitoring blood glucose (BGs) for 24 to 48 hours per facility policy.
    b. May be asymptomatic or may exhibit jitteriness, tremors, convulsions, sweating, cyanosis, weak or high-pitched cry, uncoordinated and/or diminished suck/swallow reflex, hypotonia, apnea, and temperature instability.

Nursing Interventions

1. Treatment will depend on neonatal symptomatology. Administer glucose gel and encourage early feeding (breast and/or formula) as ordered.
2. If persistent hypoglycemia, administer IV infusion of 10% dextrose to maintain serum glucose concentrations above 40 mg/dL according to facility protocol.
3. Monitor neonate closely for changes in acid–base status, respiratory distress, temperature instability, hypocalcemia, and sepsis.
4. Observe for herperbilirubinemia due to greater risk of related to depleted glycogen stores and energy production. Bilirubin levels may rise within 24 to 72 hours after birth.
5. Observe for possible cardiac anomalies and secondary heart failure.
6. Observe for other complications, including RDS, renal vein thrombosis, infection, hypermagnesemia or hypomagnesemia, birth injuries (cephalohematomas, facial nerve paralysis, fractured clavicles, brachial nerve plexus injuries), prematurity, asphyxia neonatorum, and organomegaly.
7. Provide supportive care to the family, and encourage full participation in care.

Jaundice in the Newborn (Hyperbilirubinemia)

EVIDENCE BASE American Academy of Pediatrics. (2022). Clinical practice guideline revision: Management of hyperbilirubinemia in the newborn infant 35 or more weeks of gestation. *Pediatrics, 150*(3), e2022058859. https://doi.org/10.1542/peds.2022-058859

Hyperbilirubinemia (jaundice) in the neonate is an accumulation of serum bilirubin above normal levels. It can be characterized as physiologic or pathologic.

Physiologic jaundice occurs after 24 hours postdelivery as excess hemoglobin breaks down. Once the neonate is born and pulmonary function is established, excess fetal hemoglobin is no longer necessary for oxygenation. The breakdown of fetal hemoglobin results in the by-product bilirubin. Bilirubin must be conjugated by the liver, which does not have the full maturity to manage the influx of bilirubin. Approximately 60% of full-term newborns will experience some degree of physiologic jaundice.

Pathologic jaundice occurs before 24 hours postdelivery due to additional pathologic causes. Total serum bilirubin (TSB) usually increases greater than 5 mg/dL/day; TSB greater than 12.9 mg/dL in full-term infant or 15 mg/dL in preterm infant. Direct serum bilirubin usually exceeds 1 to 2 mg/dL.

Onset of clinical jaundice (yellowish discoloration evident on physical exam) is seen when TSB levels are 5 to 7 mg/dL. A transcutaneous bilirubin (TcB) tool can be used as a noninvasive measurement of hyperbilirubinemia. A TSB should be drawn for confirmation if TcB levels are significantly elevated. Jaundice appears first on the face and progresses to the lower body as serum bilirubin levels increase. Bilirubin levels above 20 mg/dL cross the blood–brain barrier.

Kernicterus is the yellow discoloration of specific areas of brain tissue by unconjugated bilirubin and can be confirmed only after death by autopsy. Bilirubin encephalopathy best describes the occurrence of the syndrome and the accompanying neurologic sequela in neonates.

Pathophysiology and Etiology

Causes

1. Increased bilirubin load, due to the following:
    a. Hemolytic disease—Rh and ABO incompatibility.
    b. Morphologic abnormalities of red blood cells (RBCs).
    c. RBC enzyme defects.
    d. Polycythemia.
    e. Sepsis.
    f. Hypoglycemia.
    g. Poor feeding.
2. Extravascular blood collections.
    a. Cephalohematoma.
    b. Pulmonary or cerebral hemorrhage.
    c. Any enclosed occult blood.
3. Decrease or inhibition of bilirubin conjugation.
    a. Immature liver to conjugate bilirubin
    b. Inherited bilirubin conjugation defect: Crigler–Najjar syndrome (deficiency of glucuronyl transferase needed to conjugate bilirubin).
    c. Acquired bilirubin conjugation defect: breast milk jaundice, Lucey–Driscoll syndrome, IDM, asphyxiated infant with respiratory distress.
4. Increased extrahepatic circulation.
    a. Intestinal obstruction.
    b. Ileus.
5. Polycythemia.
    a. Twin–twin transfusion.
    b. Maternal–fetal transfusion.
    c. IDM.
    d. Infant small for gestational age.
6. Hypothyroidism.
7. Familial or genetic history of inherited RBC disorders such as glucose-6-phosphate dehydrogenase (G6PD) deficiency
8. Down syndrome.
9. Obstructive disorders (i.e., biliary atresia).
10. Intrauterine infection.
11. Postterm infants.
12. Breast milk jaundice syndrome.

Physiologic Jaundice

1. Related to increased bilirubin load for conjugation on immature liver cells related to in utero shunting through the ductus venosus.

a. Increased bilirubin production related to rapid hemolysis because of higher level of circulating RBCs per kg of body weight and a shorter RBC life span.
b. Enterohepatic circulation—reabsorption of unconjugated bilirubin.

2. Decreased clearance of bilirubin from plasma.
   a. Predominant bilirubin-binding protein in liver cells may be deficient in the first few days of life.
   b. Glucuronyl transferase enzyme activity may be decreased, resulting in impaired conjugation of bilirubin.
   c. Decreased ability of the liver to excrete large amounts of conjugated bilirubin.
3. Physiologic jaundice occurs 2 to 5 days after birth.
   a. Increase in unconjugated bilirubin levels; levels should not exceed 5 mg/dL/day with physiologic jaundice.
   b. Full-term infant peak levels are reached 48 to 72 hours after birth; clinical jaundice generally declines in 1 week.
   c. Premature infant peak levels are reached by 5 to 6 days of age; clinical jaundice declines in 2 weeks.
   d. Jaundice progresses in head-to-toe fashion. A yellow hue can be seen on the face and on the abdomen with levels of 10 to 15 mg/dL and on the soles of the feet with levels of 20 mg/dL or more.
   e. Risk of developing significant hyperbilirubinemia is dependent on the rapid rate of rise (ROR) in the TSB or TcB. The American Academy of Pediatrics provides an online tool for recommended treatment guidelines (https://bilitool.org).

Erythrocyte Destruction

1. Erythroblastosis fetalis (isoimmunization caused by Rh factor or ABO incompatibility).
   a. Immune hemolysis or Rh/ABO blood group incompatibility; the biological mother's and fetus's blood are different. Rh factor; different ABO blood groups (see Coombs test, page 761).
   b. Fetal cells frequently cross the placenta and may cause the biological mother to produce antibodies against the antigen of the fetus's blood.
   c. Antibodies of the biological mother's blood are in the infant's blood at birth, causing hemolysis of the neonate's RBCs, leading to a rising level of indirect bilirubin.
2. Glucose-6-phosphate dehydrogenase deficiency—nonimmune hemolytic disease (erythrocyte biochemical factor).
   a. Deficiency results in reduced stability to oxidative destruction from substances that act as oxidizing agents (i.e., vitamin K, naphthalene, salicylates).
   b. X-linked recessive disease that affects primarily Black and Mediterranean Asian groups.
   c. Screen maternal blood for carrier state, and screen neonatal blood in high-risk groups.
3. Other conditions associated with increased erythrocyte destruction:
   a. Infection—bacterial, viral, or protozoan.
   b. Structural abnormal erythrocyte.
   c. Sequestered blood (i.e., cephalohematoma, ecchymoses).

Nursing Assessment

1. Assess for risk factors that may increase risk of hyperbilirubinemia as well as signs and symptoms of jaundice:
   a. Sclerae appear yellow before the skin appears yellow.
   b. The skin appears light to bright yellow or orange.
   c. Lethargy.
   d. Dark amber, concentrated urine.
   e. Poor feeding.
   f. Meconium stools.
2. Ensure that observations are made in adequate lighting.
   a. Press the skin areas during the observation to clear away capillary coloration: forehead, cheeks, and clavicle sites allow for clear view.
   b. Be alert to the neonate's age in connection with the appearance of jaundice.
   c. With dark-skinned neonates, observing the color of the sclera, buccal mucosa, palms, and soles of feet is useful.
   d. If available, utilize the TcB monitor to trend bilirubin levels.
3. Monitor serum bilirubin levels as ordered.
   a. Utilize the Hour-specific Nomogram for Risk Stratification on the BiliTool website (*https://bilitool.org*) to evaluate treatment needs.

Nursing Interventions

1. Assist with the following treatment:
   a. Fluids—ensure adequate hydration and increase elimination. Encourage frequent feeding to facilitate excretion of bilirubin.
      i. Breastfeeding every 2 to 3 hours; may require supplementation with formula.
      ii. Avoid the use of water or oral dextrose water.
   b. Phototherapy—uses blue light to convert bilirubin molecules into water-soluble isomers for excretion. Therapy will depend on infant's age in hours, serum bilirubin level, and risk zones identified by neurotoxicity risks (see *www.bilitool.org*).
   c. Exchange transfusion—mechanically removes bilirubin.
2. Provide nursing care related to phototherapy.
   a. Photoisomerization of tissue bilirubin occurs when the neonate is exposed to blue light-emitting diodes. The number of lights used will depend on the clinical presentation of the infant.
   b. Check light intensity for therapeutic range daily with a phototherapy radiometer to ensure adequate light intensity.
   c. Undress infant to expose maximum skin surface to light. A small diaper may be used to cover genitalia.
   d. Keep the neonate's eyes covered with a size-appropriate mask, to protect from constant exposure to high-intensity light, which may cause retinal injury.
   e. Develop a systematic schedule of turning neonate so all body surfaces are exposed (i.e., every 2 hours).
   f. Maintain thermoregulation of infant to prevent cold stress—lights may affect the ambient temperature.
   g. Obtain bilirubin levels, as ordered. Lights should be turned off when blood is being collected to eliminate false-low bilirubin levels. The diminishing icterus (i.e., the diminishing yellowness of the skin) does not reflect the serum bilirubin concentration.
   h. During feedings, remove the neonate from under the lights, remove eye covers, and encourage caregiver participation.
   i. Note that a fiberoptic blanket (biliblanket) delivers continuous phototherapy by wrapping light around the neonate's torso. This method allows the neonate to remain in the birthing parent's room in an open crib. Encourage the patient to remove the infant from the biliblanket and hold for feedings. An eye mask is not required when using the biliblanket.

Septicemia Neonatorum

Septicemia neonatorum (sepsis of the neonate) is a generalized infection that is characterized by the proliferation of bacteria in the bloodstream and commonly involves the meninges (as distinguished from simple bacteremia, congenital infection, septicemia after major diseases or surgery, or major congenital anomalies). Mortality is high.

Pathophysiology and Etiology

1. The distribution of etiologic agents varies from year to year and from facility to facility.
   a. Gram-negative organisms include *Escherichia coli*, *Klebsiella* (Enterobacteriaceae), *Pseudomonas*, *Proteus*, *Salmonella*, and *Haemophilus influenzae*.
   b. Gram-positive organisms include group B beta-hemolytic *Streptococcus*, *Listeria monocytogenes*, *Staphylococcus aureus* (coagulase-negative and coagulase-positive), *Staphylococcus epidermidis*, *Streptococcus pneumoniae*, and *Streptococcus faecalis*.
2. Preterm infants are at increased risk for fungal infections from the organism *Candida albicans* because of immature immune system and diminished integumentary integrity.
3. Predisposing factors include a wide range of maternal perinatal complications such as chorioamnionitis; iatrogenic factors, such as use of catheters, oxygen, and resuscitative equipment; and infant complications, such as prematurity, congenital anomalies, RDS, skin infections, and asphyxia.
4. Infection occurs because of a temporary breakdown or depression of the neonate's defense mechanism for an unknown reason.
5. Risk factors for bacterial infection: prematurity, prolonged rupture of membranes ($\geq$18 hours), foul-smelling amniotic fluid, maternal temperature, urinary tract infection with group B *Streptococci*, chorioamnionitis, low socioeconomic status, no or limited prenatal care, or antenatal or intrapartum asphyxia.

Nursing Assessment

1. Assess for early signs of sepsis, which are vague and subtle.
   a. Poor feeding; gastric retention; weak sucking.
   b. Lethargy, limpness; weak crying, irritability.
   c. Temperature instability—generally hypothermia, but infant may have hyperthermia.
   d. Hypoglycemia or hyperglycemia.
   e. Tachycardia (because of inability to change contractility of the heart).
   f. Decreased perfusion and pulses.
2. Assist with diagnostic testing.
   a. Cultures from the blood, urine, cerebral spinal fluid (CSF), skin lesions, nose, throat, rectum, and gastric fluid may be obtained.
   b. CBC, including white blood cell (WBC) and differential. Be alert for neutrophils less than 5,000 cells/mm^3 or greater than 25,000 cells/mm^3; absolute neutrophil count less than 1,800 cells mm^3; immature/total neutrophils greater than 0.2; platelets less than 150,000.
   c. Blood chemistries—glucose, calcium, pH, electrolytes, acid–base studies, bilirubin.
   d. C-reactive protein (CRP) and erythrocyte sedimentation rate (ESR).
   e. Lactate—elevated.
   f. TORCH (toxoplasmosis–rubella–cytomegalic inclusion virus–herpes–other) detects antibodies against common intrauterine-infective agents.
   g. Arterial blood gases.
   h. Chest x-ray—may demonstrate pulmonary infection.
   i. Urinalysis.
   j. CSF: look for protein 150 to 200 mg/L in full-term neonates and 300 mg/L in preterm neonates; glucose, 50% to 60% or more of blood glucose level.

Nursing Interventions

1. Assist with treatment.
   a. Administer IV antibiotics as directed. Before the specific organism is identified and after cultures have been obtained, the use of broad-spectrum antibiotic therapy is based on common causative agents.
   b. Supportive therapy includes observation, standard precautions, hydration, nutrition, oxygenation, and thermoregulation.
2. Maintain constant surveillance and observe for complications, such as septic shock, adrenal hemorrhage, disseminated intravascular coagulation (DIC), PPHN, seizures, pneumonia, UTI, and heart failure.

Neonatal Abstinence Syndrome

Maternal misuse of such substances as drugs, alcohol, and tobacco may have an impact on the growth, development, and well-being of the fetus and neonate. Drugs and alcohol cross the placental barrier to enter the fetal circulation. The substance supply to the neonate is abruptly terminated at delivery, which may lead to withdrawal symptoms.

Substance use in females of reproductive age has significantly increased over the last three decades, impacting maternal and neonatal outcomes.

Pathophysiology and Etiology

Mechanisms include direct toxic effects on fetal circulation and CNS (heroin/cocaine/fentanyl), indirect toxic and vasoconstrictive effects impacting maternal and placental perfusion (tobacco/alcohol/marijuana/cocaine), and both direct and indirect toxic effects (polysubstance use).

1. Alcohol is a CNS depressant, and fetal alcohol spectrum disorders (FASD) are caused by direct ethanol toxicity to the developing fetus. Additional effects on the fetus come from maternal malnutrition, maternal hypoglycemia, smoking, and alcohol-induced illness. Infants and children with FASD may develop intellectual impairment, poor fine motor control, difficulty feeding, hyperactivity, delay of gross motor skills, and brain dysfunction. FASD symptoms may include:
   a. Difficulty establishing respirations.
   b. Metabolic problems.
   c. Irritability.
   d. Increased muscle tone, tremulousness.
   e. Lethargy.
   f. Opisthotonos.
   g. Poor sucking reflex.
   h. Abdominal distention.
   i. Seizure activity.
   j. Facial abnormalities.
2. Cocaine is a CNS stimulant that produces increased norepinephrine levels resulting in vasoconstriction, tachycardia, hypertension, and uterine contractions, which may lead to cerebral hemorrhage and placental abruption. This can result in complications such as decreased uterine blood flow, intrauterine growth restriction, increased fetal mean arterial pressure, increased fetal heart rate, decreased fetal oxygen, and damage to fetal brain transmitters. Complications of cocaine use include spontaneous abortion, premature labor, abruptio placentae, uterine rupture, meconium staining, congenital

anomalies, and neonatal death. Symptoms may not occur for several days, and the infant may exhibit:
   a. Mild tremulousness.
   b. Increased irritability and startle response.
   c. Muscular rigidity.
   d. Difficulty in being consoled.
   e. Pronounced state of lability.
   f. Tachycardia and tachypnea.
   g. Poor tolerance for oral feedings, diarrhea.
   h. Disturbed sleep pattern.

CLINICAL JUDGMENT Be alert for cocaine withdrawal symptoms several days after birth—the neonate does not appear to experience classic neonatal abstinence syndrome (NAS), because cocaine metabolites are stored in the fetal liver compartment.

3. Opioids are morphine derivatives with three sources of dependence: pain management (misuse of prescribed opioids), an untreated opioid use disorder (heroin dependency), and pharmacologically supported dependence with methadone, buprenorphine, and naloxone. The long-term biologic effects on the neonate of maternal drug-dependency are not fully known. These children are at risk for:
   a. Abnormal psychomotor development associated with intrauterine growth restriction.
   b. Behavioral disturbances, such as hyperactivity, brief attention spans, temper tantrums, and seizures.
   c. Fetal anoxia and meconium aspiration, prematurity, and a wide variety of complications, including, but not limited to, limb reduction defects, uterine tract anomalies such as urethral obstruction malformation, prune belly syndrome, or hydronephrosis.
   d. Neurodevelopmental abnormalities because of damage to the fetal brain neurotransmitters, which may be permanent.

Nursing Assessment

Treatment of a newborn with NAS requires a multidisciplinary approach to care and will depend on the infant's gestational age, clinical presentation, length of exposure, and type of drug misused. Hallmark signs of neonatal withdrawal include excessive high-pitched cry, reduced quality and length of sleep following a feeding, hypertonia, hyperthermia, tremors, and convulsions. Autonomic dysregulation may be present with sweating, frequent yawning and sneezing, and increased respirations. Gastrointestinal manifestations with excessive sucking, poor feeding, regurgitation, or vomiting, and loose or watery stools may also be present.

1. Obtain maternal history of drug, dosage, time of last dose, and length of use.
2. Monitor laboratory testing for drug screen confirmation, as necessary. Collect urine and/or meconium for toxicology screen within 24 hours after birth.
3. Be alert and assess for onset of withdrawal symptoms that vary by drug of choice. Educate caregivers about the possible delayed onset of withdrawal symptoms.
   a. Heroin—several hours after birth to 3 to 4 days of life.
   b. Methadone—7 to 10 days after birth to several weeks of life.
   c. Alcohol—3 to 12 hours after birth.
   d. Barbiturates—1 to 14 days after birth with a mean of 4 to 7 days.
   e. Sedative hypnotics—withdrawal can begin as late as 12 days (diazepam) to 21 days (chlordiazepoxide).
   f. Tobacco—1 to 7 days after birth.
4. Assess infant for NAS using the Neonatal Abstinence Scoring System (NASS) (see Figure 34-6).
   a. Assessment and scoring of the neonate, utilizing the NASS tool, should be every 2 hours for the first 2 days following birth and then decreased to every 8 hours as long as withdrawal symptoms continue.
   b. Scoring is based on observations of the neonates' psychomotor behavior. The use of a scoring tool provides a more objective approach when determining a plan of care.
   c. When a neonate receives a score greater than 8 on three consecutive screenings and nursing interventions implemented have not assisted in decreasing the neonates' withdrawal behaviors, initiation of medications should be considered.
5. Monitor vital signs, oxygen saturation, blood glucose as indicated.
6. Weigh the newborn daily.

Nursing Interventions

1. Provide nursing care to support infants and families to relieve withdrawal symptoms. The "Eat, Sleep, Console" (ESC) model of care for NAS has proven an effective, nonpharmacologic, family-centered approach that decreases medication use, length of hospitalization, and cost. This method encourages feeding the newborn on demand, promptly consoling the infant when irritable, and encouraging sleep (at least 1 hour) between feedings. Additional interventions are as follows:
   a. Safety—keep bulb syringe in crib for use with airway obstruction. Avoid overuse.
   b. Avoid overstimulation by clustering care and decreasing environmental stimuli (light, noise) during care and feedings.
   c. Swaddle newborn with arms and legs flexed toward the body to mimic snug in utero environment.
   d. Encourage skin-to-skin contact using a snug blanket or maternal clothing.
   e. Encourage gentle rocking and using shushing sounds to console infant.
   f. Feed (breast or formula) on demand to maintain adequate fluid and caloric intake.
   g. Burp frequently.
   h. Monitor intake and output.
   i. Positioning—Reposition frequently. Upright position after feeding may help to minimize regurgitation. Supervise prone and side-lying positions while infant is awake.
   j. Provide a pacifier between feedings for sucking.
   k. Skin care—Maintain clean, dry skin, and protect from chin excoriation, abrasions, and irritation by keeping blankets snug and away from the face.
2. Administer medications with feedings, as directed.
   a. Opioid antagonist such as naloxone for opioid-induced respiratory depression at birth.
   b. Drug therapy for alleviation of signs of withdrawal. Duration of therapy using decreasing dosages will depend on clinical presentation.
      i. Morphine.
      ii. Tincture of opium.
      iii. Phenobarbital.
      iv. Chlorpromazine.
      v. Diazepam.
      vi. Methadone.
      vii. Lorazepam.
3. Provide supportive care to caregivers to promote bonding; nonjudgmental, therapeutic communication is essential. Teaching should include infant care, bathing, and feeding. Referral for maternal substance use is essential.

NEONATAL ABSTINENCE SCORING SYSTEM															
SYSTEM	SIGNS AND SYMPTOMS	SCORE		A^M						P^M					COMMENTS
CENTRAL NERVOUS SYSTEM DISTURBANCES	Excessive High Pitched (Or other) Cry	2													Daily Weight
	Continuous High Pitched (Or other) Cry	3													
	Sleeps <1 h. After Feeding	3													
	Sleeps <2 h. After Feeding	2													
	Sleeps <3 h. After Feeding	1													
	Hyperactive Moro Reflex	2													
	Markedly Hyperactive Moro Reflex	3													
	Mild Tremors Disturbed	1													
	Moderate-Severe Tremors Disturbed	2													
	Mild Tremors Undisturbed	3													
	Moderate-Severe Tremors Undisturbed	4													
	Increased Muscle Tone	2													
	Excoriation (Specific Area)	1													
	Myoclonic Jerks	3													
	Generalized Convulsions	5													
METABOLIC/VASOMOTOR/RESPIRATORY DISTURBANCES	Seating	1													
	Fever <101 (99–100.8°F/37.2–38.2°C)	1													
	Fever >101 (38.4°C and Higher)	2													
	Frequent Yawning (>3–4 Times/ Interval)	1													
	Mottling	1													
	Nasal Stuffiness	1													
	Sneezing (>3–4 Times/Interval)	1													
	Nasal Flaring	2													
	Respiratory Rate >60/min	1													
	Respiratory Rate >60/min with Retractions	2													
GASTROINTESTIONAL DISTURBANCES	Excessive Sucking	1													
	Poor Feeding	2													
	Regurgitation	2													
	Projectile Vomiting	3													
	Loose Stools	2													
	Watery Stools	3													
TOTAL SCORE															
INITIALS OF SCORES															

Figure 34-6. Neonatal abstinence scoring system. (Reprinted with permission from Finnegan, L. P. [1986]. Neonatal abstinence syndrome: Assessment and pharmacotherapy. In F. F. Rubaltelli & B. Granati [Eds.], *Neonatal therapy: An update* [pp. 122–146]. Excerpta Medica.)

SELECTED READINGS

Abramowski, A., Ward, R., & Handman, A. H. (2020). Neonatal hypoglycemia. In *StatPearls*. StatPearls Publishing. https://www.ncbi.nlm.nih.gov/books/NBK537105/

American Academy of Pediatrics. (2023). *Neonatal care: A compendium of AAP practice guidelines and policies* (2nd ed.). Author. https://doi.org/10.1542/9781610024167

American Academy of Pediatrics, Committee on Infectious Diseases, & Committee on Fetus and Newborn. (2017). Elimination of perinatal hepatitis B: Providing the first vaccine dose within 24 hours of birth. *Pediatrics, 140*(3), e20171870. https://doi.org/10.1542/peds.2017-1870.

American College of Obstetricians and Gynecologists. (2018). Gestational diabetes mellitus (#190). *Obstetrics and Gynecology, 131*(2), e49–e64. https://doi.org/10.1097/AOG.0000000000002501

American College of Obstetricians and Gynecologists. (2018). *Quantitative blood loss in obstetrical hemorrhage (Committee Opinion #794)*. Author.

American College of Obstetricians and Gynecologists. (2018). *Screening for perinatal depression (ACOG Committee Opinion #757)*. Author.

American College of Obstetricians and Gynecologists. (2020). *Management of late-term and postterm pregnancies (Practice Bulletin #146)*. Author.

American College of Obstetricians and Gynecologists. (2020). *Prevention of group B streptococcal early-onset disease in newborns (Committee Opinion #797)*. Author.

American College of Obstetricians and Gynecologists. (2021). Fetal growth restriction (Practice Bulletin #227). *Obstetrics and Gynecology, 137*(2), e16–e28. https://doi.org/10.1097/AOG.0000000000004251

American College of Obstetricians and Gynecologists. (2021). *Medically indicated late-preterm and early-term deliveries (Committee Opinion #831)*. Author.

American College of Obstetricians and Gynecologists. (2022). *Use of psychiatric medications during pregnancy and lactation (Practice Bulletin #92)*. Author.

American College of Obstetricians and Gynecologists. (2023). *Tobacco and nicotine cessation during pregnancy (Committee Opinion # 807)*. Author.

Amin, A., Frazie, M., Thompson, S. & Patel, A. (2023). Assessing the Eat, Sleep, Console model for neonatal abstinence syndrome management at a regional referral center. *Journal of Perinatology, 43*, 916–922. https://doi.org/10.1038/s41372-023-01666-9

Anbalagan, S., & Mendez, M. D. (2023). Neonatal abstinence syndrome. In *StatPearls*. StatPearls Publishing. https://www.ncbi.nlm.nih.gov/books/NBK551498/

Association of Women's Health, Obstetric and Neonatal Nurses. (2021). Quantification of blood loss: AWHONN practice brief number 13. *Nursing for Women's Health Journal, 25*(4), e5–e7. https://doi.org/10.1016/j.nwh.2021.04.005.

Association of Women's Health, Obstetric, and Neonatal Nurses. (2022). Newborn screening: Position statement. *Journal of Obstetric, Gynecologic, and Neonatal Nursing, 51*(5), e3–e5. https://doi.org/10.1016/j.jogn.2022.07.004

Balaram, K., & Marwaha, R. (2021). Postpartum blues. In *StatPearls*. StatPearls Publishing. https://www.ncbi.nlm.nih.gov/books/NBK554546/

Ballard, J. L., Khoury, J. C., Wedig, K., Eilers-Walsman, L., & Lipp, R. (1991). New Ballard score, expanded to include extremely premature infants. *Journal of Pediatrics, 119*(3), 417–423. https://doi.org/10.1016/s0022-3476(05)82056-6

Berkowitz, C. (2021). *Berkowitz's pediatrics: A primary care approach* (6th ed). American Academy of Pediatrics. https://doi.org/10.1542/9781610023733-25

Callister, L. C. (2021). Integrating cultural beliefs and practices when caring for childbearing women and families. In K. Simpson & P. Creehan (Eds.), *AWHONN's perinatal nursing* (5th ed.). Elsevier.

Centers for Disease Control and Prevention. (2021). *Guidelines for vaccinating pregnant women*. https://www.cdc.gov/vaccines/pregnancy/index.html

Centers for Disease Control and Prevention. (2022). *Gestational diabetes and pregnancy*. https://www.cdc.gov/pregnancy/diabetes-gestational.html

Davidson, M. W., London, M. L., & Ladeweig, P. W. (2020). *Old's maternal–newborn nursing and women's health across the lifespan* (11th ed.). Pearson.

DiCioccio, H. C., Ady, C., Bena, J. F., & Albert, N. M. (2019). Initiative to improve breastfeeding by delaying the newborn bath. *Journal of Obstetric, Gynecologic & & Neonatal Nursing, 48*, 189–196. https://doi.org/10.1016/j.jogn.2018.12.008

DiTomasso, D., & Cloud, M. (2019). A systematic review of expected weight changes in full term breastfed newborns after birth. *Journal of Obstetric, Gynecologic, and Neonatal Nursing, 48*, 593–603. https://doi.org/10.1016/j.jogn.2019.09.004.

Egge, J. A, Anderson, R. H., & Schimelpfenig, M. D. (2022). Care of the well newborn. *Pediatrics in Review, 43*(12), 676–690. https://doi.org/10.1542/pir.2022-005511

Ende, H. B., Lozada, M. J., Chestnut, D. H., Osmundson, S. S., Walden, R. L., Shotwell, M. S., & Bauchat, J. R. (2021). Risk factors for atonic postpartum hemorrhage: A systematic review and meta-analysis. *Obstetrics and Gynecology, 137*(2), 305–323. https://doi.org/10.1097/AOG.0000000000004228

Finnegan, L. P. (1990). Neonatal abstinence syndrome: Assessment and pharmacotherapy. In N. Nelson (Ed.), *Current therapy in neonatal–perinatal medicine* (2nd ed.). Mosby.

Hein, S., Clouser, B., Tamim, M., Lockett, D., Brauer, K., & Cooper, L. (2021). Eat, sleep, console and adjunctive buprenorphine improved outcomes in neonatal opioid withdrawal syndrome. *Advances in Neonatal Care, 21*(1), 4–48. https://doi.org/10.1097/ANC.0000000000000824

Jilani, S. M., Jordan, C. J., Jansson, L. M., & Davis, J. M. (2021). Definitions of neonatal abstinence syndrome in clinical studies of mothers and infants: An expert literature review. *Journal of Perinatology, 41*(6), 1364–1371. https://doi.org/10.1038/s41372-020-00893-8

Kaiser Permanente Research. (2019). *Neonatal sepsis risk calculator*. Author. https://neonatalsepsiscalculator.kaiserpermanente.org/

Kenner, C., Altimier, L. B., & Boykova, M. V. (2020). *Comprehensive neonatal nursing care* (6th ed.). Springer.

Lockwood, C. J., Copel, J. A., Dugoff, L., Louis, J., Moore, T. R., Silver, R. M., & Resnik, R. (2023). *Creasy and Resnick's maternal-fetal medicine: Principles and practice* (9th ed.). Elsevier.

Moon, R. Y., Carlin, R. F., & Hand, I. (2022). Sleep related infant deaths: Updated 2022 recommendations for reducing infant deaths in the sleep environment. *Pediatrics, 150*(1), e2022057990. https://doi.org/10.1542/peds.2022-057990

Murray, S., McKinney, E., Holub, K. S., Jones, R., & Scheffer, K. L. (2023). *Foundations of maternal-newborn and women's health nursing* (8th ed.). Elsevier.

National Center for Chronic Disease Prevention and Health Promotion. (2022). *Urgent Maternal Warning Signs*. https://www.cdc.gov/hearher/maternal-warning-signs/index.html

Ozkaya, M. & Korukcu, O. (2023). Effect of cold cabbage leaf application on breast engorgement and pain in the postpartum period: A systematic review and meta-analysis, *Health Care for Women International*, (3), 328–334. https://doi.org/10.1080/07399332.2022.2090567

Patrick, S. W., Barfield, W. D., Poindexter, B. B., Committee on Fetus and Newborn, & Committee on Substance Use and Prevention. (2020). Neonatal opioid withdrawal syndrome. *Pediatrics, 145*(5), e2020029074. https://doi.org/10.1542/peds.2020-029074

Ricci, S. S. (2021). *Essentials of maternity, newborn, and women's health nursing* (5th ed.). Wolters Kluwer.

Rogers, T. P., Fathi, O., & Sánchez, P. J. (2023). Neonatologists and vitamin K hesitancy. *Journal of Perinatology, 43*, 1067–1071. https://doi.org/10.1038/s41372-023-01611-w

Rubin, R. (1975). Maternal tasks in pregnancy. *Maternal-Child Nursing Journal, 4*(3), 143–153.

Rubin, R. (1984). *Maternal identity and the maternal experience*. Springer.

Simpson, K. R, Creehan, P. A., O'Brien-Abel, N., Roth, C. K., & Rohan, A. J. (2021). *AWHONN's perinatal nursing* (5th ed.). Wolters Kluwer.

Taylor, K., & Maguire, D. (2020). A review of feeding practices in infants with neonatal opioid withdrawal. *Advances in Neonatal Care, 20*(6), 430–439. https://doi.org/10.1097/ANC.0000000000000780

Theoharakis, M., Feldman, E. & Friedman, S. (2022). Circumcision. *Pediatrics in Review, 44*(2), 728–730. https://doi.org/10.1542/pir.2022-005536

Wambach, K., & Spencer, B. (2021). *Breastfeeding and human lactation* (6th ed.). Jones and Bartlett.

Widstrom, A., Brimdyr, K., Svensson, K., Cadwell, K., & Nissen, E. (2019). Skin-to skin contact for the first hour after birth, underlying implications and clinical practice. *Acta Pediatrics, 108*(7), 1192–1204. https://doi.org/10.1111/apa.14754.

35 Complications of the Childbearing Experience

ANTEPARTUM/OBSTETRIC COMPLICATIONS

POPULATION AWARENESS Maternal mortality rates have been rising in the United States for a variety of reasons including cardiovascular conditions leading to hypertension, hemorrhage, rising obesity rates, trauma, and lack of access to quality care. Moreover, the Black maternal population has seen a significant rise in maternal death during pregnancy and in the year following childbirth. Maternal morbidity and mortality is a complex issue, and nurses need to be acutely aware of the subtle physiologic changes that occur with pregnancy and childbirth. Astute nursing assessment and early intervention can improve outcomes for the maternal population.

EVIDENCE BASE Simpson, K. R., Creehan, P. A., O'Brien-Abel, N., Roth, C. K., & Rohan, A. J. (2021). *AWHONN's perinatal nursing* (5th ed.). Wolters Kluwer.

Petersen, E. E., Davis, N. L., Goodman, D., Cox, S., Syverson, C., Seed, K., Shapiro-Mendoza, C., Callaghan, W. M., & Barfield, W. (2019). Racial/ethnic disparities in pregnancy-related deaths—United States, 2007–2016. *MMWR: Morbidity and Mortality Weekly Report, 68*(35), 762–765. https://doi.org/10.15585/mmwr.mm6835a3

Ectopic Pregnancy

Ectopic pregnancy occurs when a fertilized ovum implants outside the uterine cavity. Locations include the fallopian tube (97%), ovary, cervix, or abdominal cavity (Figure 35-1). Most ectopic pregnancies occur in the distal (ampullary) two thirds of the fallopian tube while some are located in the proximal portion of the extrauterine part of the tube (isthmic).

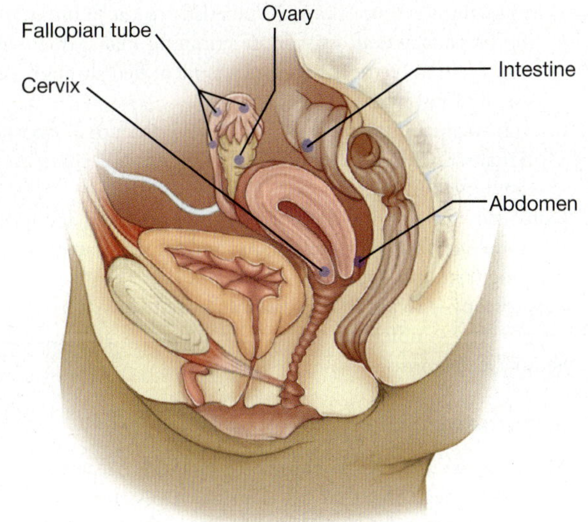

Figure 35-1. Possible sites for implantation with an ectopic pregnancy. (Adapted with permission from Ricci, S. S. [2021]. *Essentials of maternity, newborn, and women's health nursing* [5th ed., Fig. 19.1]. Wolters Kluwer.)

Pathophysiology and Etiology

1. Clinical risk or structural factors that prevent or delay the passage of the fertilized ovum:
   a. Pelvic inflammatory disease.
   b. History of previous ectopic pregnancy, tubal surgery, and/or ligation.
   c. Multiple induced abortions.
   d. Endometriosis.
   e. Sexually transmitted infections (chlamydia and gonorrhea).

2. Assisted reproduction technologies (ART), particularly with multiple embryo transfer, may also lead to ectopic pregnancy.
3. Consequences of a growing ectopic pregnancy may lead to inflammation, rupture, hemorrhage, peritonitis, or death.

Clinical Manifestations

1. Abdominal or pelvic pain (typically unilateral). Pain may become severe if the fallopian tube ruptures, and the clinical presentation will evolve into shock.
2. Irregular vaginal bleeding—usually scanty and dark (most common).
3. Amenorrhea.
4. Abdominal tenderness on palpation.
5. Radiating shoulder pain is the result of bleeding that irritates nerves in the peritoneal cavity.
6. Increased pulse and anxiety.
7. Nausea, vomiting, faintness, vertigo, or syncope.
8. Pelvic examination may reveal a pelvic mass, posterior or lateral to the uterus, adnexal tenderness, and cervical pain with movement of the cervix.

Diagnostic Evaluation

1. Serial quantitative levels of the beta subunit of human chorionic gonadotropin (beta-hCG) can be used in combination with ultrasound in most instances to confirm diagnosis.
   a. Serum beta-hCG (produced by trophoblastic cells)—serial evaluations will not show characteristic rise as in intrauterine pregnancy and assist in determining management of care when an ectopic pregnancy is identified through the use of ultrasound.
   b. Transvaginal ultrasound—identifies the absence of a gestational sac within the uterus and is the most accurate and rapid method of diagnosis.
2. Culdocentesis—bloody aspirate from the pouch of Douglas, the posterior fornix of the vagina, indicates intraperitoneal bleeding from tubal rupture.
3. Laparoscopy—abdominal visualization of tubal.
4. Laparotomy—indication for surgery if there is any question about the diagnosis.

Management

1. Methotrexate (MTX) is considered first-line treatment for an ectopic pregnancy that will depend on gestational age, an intact fallopian tube, no active bleeding, and hemodynamic stability. MTX, a chemotherapeutic agent, interferes with the processing of folic acid and inhibits rapid cell division. The treatment goal is to resolve the ectopic pregnancy while preserving tubal patency and reproductive function.
   a. Contraindications to MTX include breastfeeding, immunodeficiency, alcohol use disorder, liver disease, pulmonary disease, peptic ulcer disease, renal dysfunction, or blood dyscrasias.
   b. MTX is administered intramuscularly (IM), and dosage is weight based (50 mg/m^2). The volume of the dose may need to be divided into two syringes for safe administration.
   c. Additional doses of MTX may be necessary if hCG levels remain elevated.
   d. Absorption of the pregnancy will take approximately 4 to 6 weeks after successful treatment.
2. When MTX is not an option, surgical intervention is recommended and will depend on the extent of tubal involvement and if rupture has occurred.
   a. Salpingostomy (opening of the fallopian tube) to remove the fertilized ovum is the preferred choice to preserve future fertility.
   b. If the fallopian tube is not salvageable, a salpingectomy (removal of the fallopian tube) is performed.
   c. Additional surgical options range from removal of ectopic pregnancy with tubal resection, salpingostomy, and possibly salpingo-oophorectomy (removal of tube and ovary on the affected side) depending on the extent of involvement.
3. Treat shock and hemorrhage accordingly, as clinical condition warrants.
4. Administer Rho(D) immune globulin (RhIG) if the patient is Rh-negative.

Complications

1. Infertility.
2. Hemorrhage and death.

Nursing Assessment

1. Obtain history for the following:
   a. Date of last menses.
   b. Presence of positive pregnancy test.
   c. Rh type.
2. Monitor and trend the following:
   a. Maternal vital signs.
   b. Presence and amount of vaginal bleeding.
   c. Amount, type, and evolving intensity of pain.
   d. Presence of abdominal tenderness on palpation accompanied by radiating shoulder pain.

Nursing Interventions

Maintaining Fluid Volume

1. Establish an intravenous (IV) line with a large-bore catheter (16G to 18G) for IV fluids and blood components as the clinical condition warrants.
2. Obtain complete blood count (CBC) and type and screen, as directed.
3. Monitor intake and output.

Promoting Comfort

1. Administer analgesics, as needed.
2. Encourage rest and relaxation techniques.

Providing Support Through the Grieving Process

1. Provide emotional support to patient and family.
2. Offer compassionate presence and empathy, which are essential.
3. Offer bereavement resources.

Patient Education and Health Maintenance

1. Teach signs and symptoms of ectopic pregnancy to patients at risk: increased vaginal bleeding, moderate to severe abdominal pain (typically unilateral and low), shoulder pain, nausea, and vomiting.
2. Instruct patient to report signs and symptoms to the provider or emergency department immediately.
3. Encourage grief counseling and supportive care at home.

4. If MTX was administered, be aware that the recommendation is to avoid pregnancy for 3 months due to the potential for teratogenic effects. Instruct the patient about the need for reliable birth control.

Evaluation: Expected Outcomes

- Vital signs stable.
- Verbalizes pain relief.
- Patient and support person express appropriate response.

Gestational Trophoblastic Disease

EVIDENCE BASE Soper, J. T. (2021). Gestational trophoblastic disease: Current evaluation and management. *Obstetrics and Gynecology, 137*(2), 355–370. https://doi.org/10.1097/AOG.0000000000004240

Gestational trophoblastic disease (GTD) ("molar pregnancy") comprises a myriad of interrelated conditions, originating from anomalous development of the placenta that can be uterine or extrauterine (rare). It is characterized by the conversion of the chorionic villi into a mass of clear vesicles (moles). GTD is observed in one in every 1,000 to 1,200 pregnancies. Molar pregnancies are usually diagnosed during the first trimester of pregnancy and classified as incomplete (partial) or complete. In a complete GTD pregnancy, the fetus, placenta, and amniotic membranes or fluid are absent. Incomplete molar pregnancies may contain embryonic or fetal parts and an amniotic sac. The majority of patients experiencing a molar pregnancy will not have invasive malignant moles; however, 20% will develop a malignancy. The use of chemotherapy will be dependent on presentation and pathology.

Pathophysiology and Etiology

1. GTD occurs due to an excess of paternal chromosomes.
   a. Complete homozygous moles are generally the result of abnormal fertilization of an ovum devoid of genetic material (empty egg without DNA) with a single sperm containing a haploid set (single set of unpaired chromosomes) of 23X chromosomes (80%) that duplicates to 46XX.
   b. A heterozygous mole (20% of complete moles) occurs when two sperm fertilize an empty egg (46XX/46XY).
   c. Partial moles are triploid and occur due to two paternal sperm cells fertilizing the ovum. The mole has a karyotype of 69XXX, 69XXY, or 69XYY.
2. Malignancy results from one of the following: invasive hydatidiform mole (most common), choriocarcinoma, placental trophoblastic tumor, or an epithelioid trophoblastic tumor.
3. Complete moles account for approximately 50% of all choriocarcinomas, with the heterozygous mole presenting the greater risk of developing a malignancy.

Clinical Manifestations

1. First-trimester vaginal bleeding.
2. Absence of fetal heart tones and fetal structures.
3. Uterine enlargement greater than dates (size may double if complete mole exists).
4. Beta-hCG titers greater than expected for gestational age.
5. Expulsion of the vesicles.
6. Hyperemesis gravidarum (severe nausea and vomiting).
7. Early onset of preeclampsia before 24 weeks of gestation.

Diagnostic Evaluation

1. Beta-hCG levels—excessive elevations.
2. Ultrasound—a diffuse mixed echogenic pattern replaces the placenta and may be described as villous cavitation—clear "grapelike" structures fill the uterine cavity and a fetus is absent.

Management

1. Chest radiography should be taken prior to evacuation of the molar to detect metastasis.
2. Suction curettage is the method of choice for immediate evacuation of the mole with the possibility of laparotomy; hysterectomy may be an option but is rare.
3. Serial quantitative beta-hCG should be performed to confirm resolution to baseline values (≤5 mIU/mL). Persistent elevations indicate malignant postmolar GTD.
4. Hormonal contraception during beta-hCG monitoring is advised.
5. Chemotherapy for patients with a malignant invasive GTD.
6. Administer RhIG per your facility's policy if patient is Rh-negative.

Complications

1. Significant blood loss.
2. Malignancy (10% to 20%).
3. Infertility.

Nursing Assessment

1. Monitor vital signs; note symptoms of early-onset preeclampsia before 24 weeks of gestation (see page 1041).
2. Assess the amount and type of vaginal bleeding; note the presence of other vaginal discharge.
3. Determine the date of the last menstrual period (LMP) and the date of positive pregnancy test.
4. Measure fundal height (FH) and compare to LMP.
5. Evaluate CBC results and Rh type.

Nursing Interventions

Maintaining Fluid Volume

1. Obtain blood for CBC and type and screen; blood products may be indicated.
2. Establish and maintain peripheral IV access with a large-gauge IV catheter (16G to 18G).
3. Assess maternal vital signs and evaluate bleeding.
4. Monitor laboratory results.
5. Administer blood products as ordered.

Decreasing Anxiety

1. Explain preoperative and postoperative care.
2. Educate patient and family about the acute and chronic aspects of GTD.
3. Allow the family to grieve over the loss of pregnancy and possible infertility.

Patient Education and Health Maintenance

1. Discuss the importance of continuous follow-up care, including serial evaluation of beta-hCG until levels return to normal and remain normal for 3 weeks, then monthly monitoring for 6 months.

2. Provide reinforcement of follow-up, which typically lasts at least a year postdiagnosis.
3. Encourage ongoing discussion of care and fertility options with health care provider.

Evaluation: Expected Outcomes

- Vital signs stable; laboratory work within normal limits.
- Verbalizes understanding of procedures and reduced anxiety.

Spontaneous Abortion

EVIDENCE BASE American College of Obstetricians and Gynecologists' Committee on Practice Bulletins—Gynecology, Society of Family Planning. (2020). Medication abortion up to 70 days of gestation: ACOG Practice Bulletin, Number 225. *Obstetrics and Gynecology, 136*(4), e31–e47. https://doi.org/10.1097/AOG.0000000000004082

Spontaneous abortion occurs as a natural termination of pregnancy prior to 20 weeks. Variations are outlined in Table 35-1. Medical termination of a pregnancy is known as a *therapeutic* (maternal or fetal indications) accomplished through medication administration or surgical intervention.

Pathophysiology and Etiology

1. Natural causes are commonly unknown; however, 50% are due to chromosomal anomalies.
2. Exposure or contact with teratogenic agents.
3. Poor maternal nutritional status.
4. Maternal illness with specific bacterial infections or viruses, such as rubella, cytomegalovirus, varicella, active herpes, and toxoplasmosis.
5. Endocrine imbalance: luteal phase defect, insulin-dependent diabetes mellitus, thyroid disease.
6. Systemic lupus erythematosus and other immunologic factors: antiphospholipid antibodies.
7. Smoking, substance use disorder, and high caffeine intake.
8. Genetic factors.
9. Morbid obesity.
10. Abnormal uterine development or structural defect in the maternal reproductive system (i.e., incompetent cervix, uterine fibroids, bicornuate uterus).
11. Presence of intrauterine device.
12. Environmental factors such as chemicals, radiation, or trauma.
13. Bleeding during the first trimester.

Table 35-1 Types of Spontaneous Abortions

CLASSIFICATION	CLINICAL MANIFESTATIONS	MANAGEMENT
Threatened	• Vaginal bleeding or spotting. • Mild cramps. • Tenderness over uterus, simulates mild labor or persistent lower backache with feeling of pelvic pressure. • Cervix closed or slightly dilated. • Symptoms subside or develop into inevitable abortion.	• Vaginal examination. • Bed rest (some clinicians do not believe that bedrest will make a difference in the outcome). • Pad count.
Inevitable	• Bleeding more profuse. • Cervix dilated. • Membranes rupture. • Painful uterine contractions.	• Embryo delivered, followed by dilatation and evacuation (D & E).
Habitual	• Spontaneous abortion occurs in successive pregnancies (three or more).	• D & E. • Treatment of possible causes: hormonal imbalance, tumors, thyroid dysfunction, abnormal uterus, incompetent cervix; with treatment, 70%–80% carry a pregnancy successfully. • Hysterogram to rule out uterine abnormalities, infections. • Surgical suturing of the cervix if incompetent cervix is a causative factor.
Incomplete	• Fetus usually expelled. • Placenta and membranes retained.	• D & E.
Missed	• Fetus dies in utero and is retained. • Maceration of fetus. • No symptoms of abortion, but symptoms of pregnancy regress (uterine size, breast changes).	• Real-time ultrasound, and if second trimester, fetal monitoring to determine if fetus has died. • D & E if early pregnancy. • If fetus is not passed after diagnosis, oxytocin induction may be used; retained dead fetus may lead to development of disseminated intravascular coagulation (DIC) or infection. • Fibrinogen concentrations should be measured weekly.

Clinical Manifestations

1. Uterine cramping and lower back pain.
2. Vaginal bleeding may begin with dark spotting and progress to frank bleeding.
3. hCG levels may be elevated for as long as 2 weeks after the loss of embryo.

Diagnostic Evaluation

1. Ultrasound (external/transvaginal) evaluation of the uterus for a gestational sac or embryo.
2. Visualization of the cervix for dilation or tissue expulsion.

Complications

1. Hemorrhage.
2. Uterine infection.
3. Septicemia may occur due to missed/undiagnosed abortion.
4. Disseminated intravascular coagulation (DIC) is rare but may occur with a missed abortion.

Nursing Assessment

1. Determine the date of LMP and the date of positive pregnancy test.
2. Monitor maternal vital signs.
3. Assess for hemorrhage and/or infection.
4. Evaluate blood loss: initiation, duration, estimated total amount, and precipitating factors.
5. Evaluate any blood clot or tissue for the presence of amniotic membranes, placenta, or fetus.

Nursing Interventions

Maintaining Fluid Volume

1. Obtain CBC and type and screen.
2. Assess and report signs of hemorrhage: tachycardia, hypotension, hyperventilation, altered level of consciousness (LOC), diaphoresis, or pallor.
3. Establish and maintain an IV access with a large-gauge catheter (16G to 18G) for fluid replacement and possible blood products; two IV lines may be warranted.
4. Inspect all expelled tissue and assess for completeness; retained products of conception may lead to further bleeding and possibly hemorrhage if not completely expelled.
5. Administer RhIG as indicated for a patient who is Rh-negative.

Providing Support Through the Grieving Process

1. Evaluate the need for grief counseling; offer emotional support to patient and family.
2. Acknowledge the loss and allow grieving. Every pregnancy, irrespective of gestational age, deserves recognition, respect, and acknowledgment. Treat the fetus reverently and call by name if one was chosen.
3. Provide time alone for the couple/family to discuss their feelings and to grieve.
4. Allow the patient and family to discuss the possibility of future pregnancy if desired.
5. Provide an opportunity for viewing the fetus if desired.
6. Screen for signs and symptoms of depression.
7. Inquire about faith-based practices and offer spiritual support; provide referral for social worker and community resources.

Preventing Infection and Hemorrhage

1. Monitor vital signs including temperature.
2. Assess vaginal bleeding for increased amount and odor; may indicate infection.
3. Educate and encourage perineal care after each urination and defecation to prevent infection.
4. Educate the patient on the signs of infection (fever, pelvic pain, change in character, and amount of vaginal discharge) and advise to report to the provider immediately.

Promoting Comfort

1. Instruct and encourage the use of relaxation techniques.
2. Administer pain medications, as needed and prescribed.

Patient Education and Health Maintenance

1. For patients experiencing possible spontaneous abortion at home who are seeking telephone advice, educate them to seek medical treatment if hemorrhage occurs, and to collect any expelled products of conception and bring them to facility for evaluation.
2. Provide the names of local bereavement support groups; Resolve Through Sharing (https://www.resolvethroughsharing.org/) groups may be available.
3. Discuss the desired method of contraception to be used.
4. Inform the patient to discuss the timing of the next pregnancy with the provider, if desired. A 2- to 4-month interval may be advised.
5. Provide information regarding genetic testing of the products of conception, if indicated; send the specimen according to facility policy.

Evaluation: Expected Outcomes

- Normal vital signs; minimal blood loss.
- Expresses feelings regarding the loss of the pregnancy by demonstrating appropriate coping.
- No signs of infection, temperature normal, performs perineal care.
- Verbalizes relief of pain and discomfort.

Nausea and Vomiting of Pregnancy (Hyperemesis Gravidarum)

EVIDENCE BASE American College of Obstetricians and Gynecologists. (2021). Nausea and vomiting of pregnancy (Practice Bulletin #189). *Obstetrics and Gynecology, 131*(1), e15–e30. https://doi.org/10.1097/AOG.0000000000002456

Nausea and vomiting are commonly associated with pregnancy in the first trimester. *Hyperemesis gravidarum* is the excessive and persistent nausea and vomiting that occurs during pregnancy and is the most common indication for hospitalization during the antepartum period. The clinical diagnosis of exclusion is based on the presentation in the absence of any other disease processes, such as gastrointestinal (GI) conditions, metabolic disease, neurologic disorders, drug use, or acute fatty liver or preeclampsia during pregnancy. Early identification and treatment at the onset of nausea and vomiting may decrease the incidence of developing hyperemesis gravidarum.

Pathophysiology and Etiology

1. Typically occurs during the first 16 weeks' gestation but may last into the third trimester in severe cases.

2. Etiology is unknown; however, hormonal stimulus (high levels of beta-hCG or estrogen), evolutionary adaptation, and a psychological predisposition are possible hypotheses.
3. Risk factors: large placental mass (GTD), multiple gestation, history of hyperemesis in previous pregnancies, motion sickness, migraine headaches, genetic predisposition, and carrying a female fetus.
4. Persistent vomiting may result in fluid and electrolyte imbalances, dehydration, jaundice, and elevation of serum transaminase.

Clinical Manifestations

1. Persistent vomiting; inability to tolerate anything by mouth.
2. Dehydration—fever, dry skin, decreased urine output, ketonuria.
3. Weight loss (up to 5% to 10% of body weight).
4. Severity of symptoms commonly increases as the condition progresses.

Diagnostic Evaluation

1. Testing to rule out other conditions causing vomiting (cholecystitis, appendicitis, pancreatitis, thyroid disease, or hepatitis).
2. Elevated liver enzymes: lactate dehydrogenase (LDH), aspartate transaminase (AST), and alanine transaminase (ALT).
3. Elevated serum bilirubin.
4. CBC may indicate anemia.
5. Blood urea nitrogen (BUN) and creatinine—may be slightly elevated.
6. Serum electrolytes—may result in hypokalemia, hyponatremia, or hypernatremia; loss of hydrogen and chloride.
7. Urine is positive for ketones and elevated specific gravity.
8. Ultrasound may be considered to identify multiple gestation or GTD pregnancy.

Management

1. Maintain nothing by mouth (NPO) status for 24 to 48 hours or until vomiting stops. Advance diet as tolerated, encouraging small, frequent meals.
2. Nonpharmacologic therapies:
   a. Aromatherapy, acupressure, and acupuncture have been used.
   b. Mindfulness-based cognitive therapy and hypnosis have been proven effective options for some patients.
3. Pharmacologic therapies:
   a. Pyridoxine (vitamin B_6) with or without doxylamine—first line of treatment for nausea and vomiting of pregnancy.
   b. Ginger capsules, 250 mg four times daily, have been shown to be more effective than placebo and cause fewer side effects than other medications.
   c. With persistent symptoms, antiemetics such as dimenhydrinate, diphenhydramine, prochlorperazine, or promethazine may be added to the treatment regimen.
   d. If no dehydration is present, metoclopramide, ondansetron, promethazine, or trimethobenzamide are additional options.
4. If dehydration occurs, treatment with IV fluids—typically 1 to 3 L of dextrose solution with electrolytes and vitamins, as needed. Most patients respond quickly to initially restricting oral intake followed by IV fluid and electrolyte replacement and the pharmacologic therapies outlined above. However, in rare incidences, an enteral feeding tube or total parenteral nutrition (TPN) may be necessary.

Complications

1. Hypovolemia and renal insufficiency.
2. Electrolyte imbalance.
3. Malnutrition.
4. In rare instances, esophageal rupture, pneumothorax, acute tubular necrosis, liver failure, Wernicke encephalopathy, and splenic avulsion have occurred.
5. Small for gestational age (SGA) or low-birth-weight (LBW) neonate.

Nursing Assessment

1. Monitor dietary intake.
2. Assess for dehydration—concentrated urine, dry mucous membranes.
3. Evaluate environmental factors that may affect appetite.
4. Assess for pica (ingestion of nonfood substances such as starch, clay, or toothpaste).
5. Monitor vital signs for tachycardia, hypotension, and fever.

Nursing Interventions

Maintaining Fluid Volume

1. Establish an IV access and administer IV fluids, as prescribed.
2. Monitor and trend weight loss.
3. Monitor serum electrolytes and report abnormalities.
4. Administer medications as prescribed. Maintain NPO status for 24 to 48 hours or until vomiting stops.
5. Monitor intake and output, urine-specific gravity and ketones, vital signs, skin turgor.
6. Maintain fetal surveillance as indicated by gestational age.

Encouraging Adequate Nutrition

1. Advance diet as tolerated, encouraging small, frequent meals.
2. Avoid greasy, gas-producing, and spicy foods.
3. Encourage an environment conducive to eating.
4. Administer medications as prescribed.
5. Seek dietary consult, as indicated.

Strengthening Coping Mechanisms

1. Therapeutic communication and compassionate presence allow patients to verbalize feelings regarding this pregnancy and associated stressors.
2. Refer the patient to social service and counseling services, as needed.

Patient Education and Health Maintenance

1. Educate the patient regarding diet, nutrition, and healthy weight gain.
2. Educate the patient on the proper use of prescribed medications.

Evaluation: Expected Outcomes

- Demonstrates adequate hydration.
- Tolerates oral intake without vomiting.
- Verbalizes concerns and stresses related to pregnancy.

Placenta Previa

Placenta previa is the abnormal implantation of the placenta in the lower uterine segment that may partially or completely cover the internal cervical os (Figure 35-2). The classification of a previa may change over the course of the pregnancy as the lower

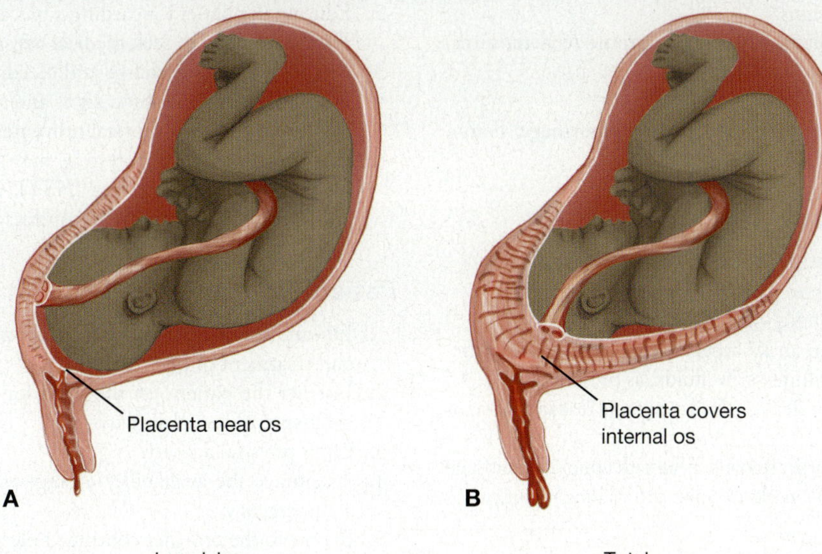

Figure 35-2. Classification of placenta previa. **(A)** Low-lying. **(B)** Total. (Adapted with permission from Ricci, S. S. [2021]. *Essentials of maternity, newborn, and women's health nursing* [5th ed., Fig. 19-4]. Wolters Kluwer.)

uterine segment stretches and thins. Placenta previa is associated with intrauterine growth restriction (IUGR) and increased risk for hemorrhage. The improvement in ultrasound technology has increased the accuracy of assessing the placental location and cervical os.

EVIDENCE BASE American College of Obstetricians and Gynecologists & Society for Maternal-Fetal Medicine. (2018). Obstetric Care Consensus No. 7: Placenta accreta spectrum. *Obstetrics and Gynecology*, *132*(6), e259–e275. https://doi.org/10.1097/AOG.0000000000002983

Pathophysiology and Etiology

1. *Classifications* of placenta previa:
   a. Total: placenta covers the entire cervical os.
   b. Low-lying: placental implantation in the lower uterine segment next to the cervical os; the placenta may migrate upward and away from the os as the uterus stretches and grows during the course of the pregnancy.
2. *Causation* is unknown, but risk factors include:
   a. Previous myomectomy.
   b. Endometritis.
   c. Scarred uterus to include vaginal birth after cesarean delivery (VBAC).
   d. Induced or spontaneous abortions involving suction curettage.
   e. Advanced maternal age, multiparity, cigarette smoking.
   f. Previous placenta previa.

Clinical Manifestations

1. Cardinal sign of placenta previa is the sudden onset of painless bright red vaginal bleeding during the second or third trimester; some patients may not exhibit bleeding until labor starts.
2. Initial episode of bleeding is rarely life-threatening and usually stops spontaneously. Bleeding can be intermittent or continuous.
3. With a complete placenta previa, bleeding typically occurs earlier in the pregnancy.

Diagnostic Evaluation

1. Ultrasound (transabdominal or transvaginal) is the method of choice to identify the location of placental implantation.

Management

1. Conservative management is usually possible with immature fetus and maternal stability.
2. Avoid vaginal examinations in patients with active vaginal bleeding as this may aggravate the condition.
3. Once viable and fetal lung maturity is established, delivery may be attempted based on maternal–fetal status. Continuous maternal and fetal monitoring may be necessary.
4. If repeated episodes or heavy bleeding, IV access should be established immediately, along with CBC, blood type, screen, and cross-match, as indicated.
5. Cesarean delivery is usually indicated if maternal–fetal status is unstable or complete previa.
6. Vaginal delivery may be attempted in a marginal or low-lying placenta without active bleeding. Operating room and neonatal teams should be available.

Complications

1. Placenta accreta (placenta abnormally adherent to uterine wall, difficult to expel); increased incidence if placenta previa exists with maternal history of uterine surgery.
2. Placenta increta (placenta attaches very deeply into the muscle layer of uterus) and placenta percreta (placenta grows through the uterus possibly to surrounding organs).
3. Immediate hemorrhage, possible shock, and maternal death.
4. Postpartum hemorrhage.
5. Uterine rupture.
6. Fetal malpresentation.
7. Prematurity.

Nursing Assessment

1. Assess blood loss.
2. Assess for pain in association with the bleeding.

3. Assess maternal vital signs.
4. Maintain fetal surveillance through electronic fetal monitoring (EFM).
5. Assess for symptoms of labor.
6. Review laboratory data to assess signs of hemorrhage: hemoglobin and hematocrit.

Nursing Interventions

Promoting Tissue Perfusion

1. Monitor vital signs as the patient's condition warrants.
2. Maintain EFM if the fetus viable.
3. Establish and maintain an IV access with a large-gauge catheter (16G to 18G). Administer IV fluids, as prescribed.
4. Prepare for emergency delivery and neonatal resuscitation, as needed.
5. Administer antenatal corticosteroids (betamethasone) if gestational age is between 24 and 34 weeks to enhance fetal lung maturity.

Maintaining Fluid Volume

1. Establish and maintain IV access as indicated.
2. Obtain CBC, type and screen/cross for blood replacement, platelets, prothrombin time (PT)/partial thromboplastin time (PTT), and fibrinogen. Repeat periodically as the patient's condition warrants.
3. Assess bleeding frequently to note changes in frequency and volume.
4. Note that activity may be restricted while hospitalized based on patient and fetal condition.
5. Administer blood products as prescribed.

Decreasing Anxiety

1. Explain all treatments and procedures; answer related questions to patient satisfaction.
2. Offer compassionate presence and emotional support.

Maintaining Care at Home

1. Home care for patients with placenta previa and other antenatal bleeding disorders can occur if the following criteria are met:
    a. No active bleeding.
    b. No signs and symptoms of preterm labor (PTL).
    c. Follow-up plan with health care team in place.
    d. Emergency support readily available.
2. Educate the patient regarding signs and symptoms of hemorrhage and when to seek medical assistance.
3. Monitor vaginal discharge and bleeding.
4. Educate the patient about signs and symptoms of labor.
5. Educate the patient on fetal movement counts (kick counts).
6. Additional antepartum testing may include biophysical profile (BPP), nonstress testing (NST), and amniotic fluid index (AFI); may be ordered to be conducted weekly.

Patient Education and Health Maintenance

1. Educate the patient and family about the diagnosis, etiology, and treatment of placenta previa.
2. Instruct the patient on the need for pelvic rest, stressing the avoidance of sexual activity.
3. Limit physical activity.
4. Encourage the availability of support people in the event of an emergency.
5. Report to the provider continued bleeding, more than six uterine contractions per hour, and/or decreased fetal movement.

Evaluation: Expected Outcomes

- Fetal condition stable.
- Absence of shock, stable vital signs, absence of bleeding.
- Verbalizes concerns and understanding of procedures and treatments.
- Maintains rest at home.

Abruptio Placentae

Abruptio placentae results from the premature separation of a normally implanted placenta before the birth of the fetus; typically occurs after 20 weeks of gestation. Classifications include partial abruption with concealed hemorrhage, partial abruption with apparent hemorrhage, and complete abruption with concealed hemorrhage (Figure 35-3). Hemorrhage may be obvious or concealed (occult/hidden behind the placenta) and is accompanied by constant cramping or general abdominal pain. Prompt intervention is essential as placental abruption can be life-threatening to the patient and fetus.

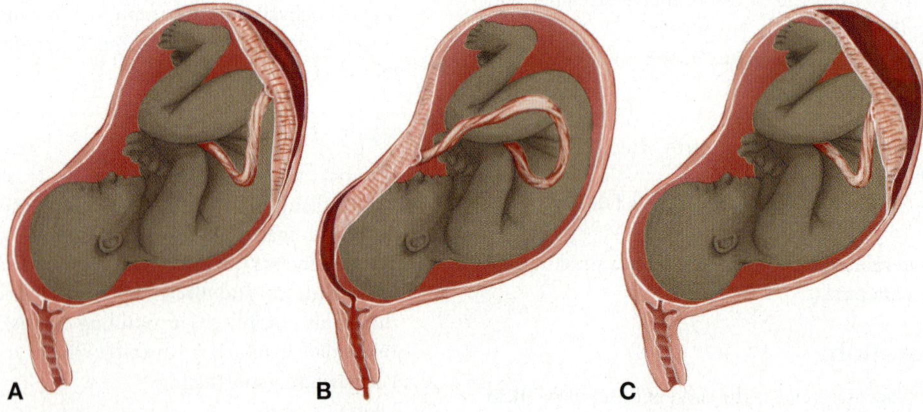

Figure 35-3. Classifications of placental abruption. **(A)** Partial abruption with concealed hemorrhage. **(B)** Partial abruption with apparent hemorrhage. **(C)** Complete abruption with concealed hemorrhage. (Adapted with permission from Ricci, S. S. [2021]. *Essentials of maternity, newborn, and women's health nursing* [5th ed., Fig. 19-5]. Wolters Kluwer.)

Pathophysiology and Etiology

1. The etiology is unknown, but risks include:
   a. History of abdominal trauma, prior cesarean birth, uterine anomalies (fibroids, septum).
   b. Maternal hypertension: 50% of placental abruptions are associated with some form of hypertension.
   c. Cigarette smoking; cocaine or amphetamine use.
   d. Thrombophilias, such as Factor V Leiden or antiphospholipid antibody.
   e. Previous history of abruptio placentae or partial abruption in current pregnancy.
   f. Rapid decompression of the uterus (reduction of fluid with polyhydramnios).
   g. Preterm prelabor rupture of membranes (PPROM): less than 34 weeks.
   h. Maternal autoimmune disease.
2. Hemorrhage occurs into the decidua basalis behind the placenta and forms a hematoma. This hematoma will expand as bleeding increases; enlargement further detaches the placenta from the uterine wall.

Clinical Manifestations

1. Sudden-onset, intense, constant, generalized abdominal pain/tenderness with obvious or occult vaginal bleeding. The abdomen is firm and boardlike.
2. Signs and symptoms of shock.
3. Uterine contractions are typically low amplitude and high frequency. Uterine baseline resting tone may be elevated over course of evolving abruption.
4. Patient may exhibit signs and symptoms of rapid labor progress and delivery.
5. Changes in the fetal heart rate (FHR) may commonly be the first sign of maternal hemodynamic instability. Category II or III FHR tracings may present with tachycardia or bradycardia, and recurrent late decelerations with minimal or absent variability.
   a. Fetal response depends on the amount of blood loss and extent of uteroplacental insufficiency present.
   b. Without prompt intervention, increased maternal and fetal morbidity and mortality may occur.

Diagnostic Evaluation

1. Clinical diagnosis is based on maternal history, physical examination, laboratory studies, EFM data, and signs and symptoms to include vaginal bleeding, abdominal pain, uterine contractions, uterine tenderness, and/or maternal–fetal distress. Presentations vary per patient.
2. Ultrasound is performed to exclude placenta previa but may not be sensitive enough to diagnose or rule out abruptio placentae; EFM is frequently more accurate.
3. A serum Kleihauer–Betke may be ordered to detect fetal cells in the maternal circulation.

Management

1. Management depends on the maternal and fetal status and degree of abruption. Teamwork and effective communication are essential for optimal maternal and fetal outcomes.
2. IV fluids to maintain hemodynamic stability.
3. Active transfusion protocol may be activated.
4. Continuous EFM is indicated until delivery.
5. In the event of fetal compromise, severe hemorrhage, coagulopathy, or increasing uterine activity dysfunction, emergent cesarean delivery is highly recommended.
6. Team members should be assembled to manage the neonate at delivery.

Complications

1. Postpartum hemorrhage.
2. Maternal shock.
3. Coagulopathy—DIC.
4. Hysterectomy.
5. Sheehan syndrome (postpartum pituitary necrosis).
6. Acute renal tubular necrosis.
7. Acute kidney injury.
8. Precipitous labor and delivery.
9. Anaphylactoid syndrome of pregnancy (formerly amniotic fluid embolism).
10. Maternal death.
11. Fetal prematurity, acute respiratory distress syndrome, IUGR, exsanguination, and/or demise.

Nursing Assessment

See Table 35-2.

1. Assess qualitative blood loss (QBL).
2. Assess for pain with the type of bleeding.
3. Monitor maternal vital signs.

Table 35-2 Characteristics of Abruptio Placentae and Placenta Previa

CHARACTERISTIC	ABRUPTIO PLACENTAE	PLACENTA PREVIA
Onset	Third trimester	Third trimester (commonly at 32–36 wk)
Bleeding	May be concealed, external dark hemorrhage, or bloody amniotic fluid	Mostly external, small to profuse in amount, bright red
Pain and uterine tenderness	Usually present; irritable uterus, progresses to boardlike consistency	Usually absent; uterus soft
Fetal heart tone	May be irregular or absent	Usually normal
Presenting part	May be engaged	Usually not engaged
Shock	Moderate to severe depending on extent of concealed and external hemorrhage	Usually not present unless bleeding is excessive
Delivery	Immediate delivery, usually cesarean delivery	Delivery may be delayed, depending on size of fetus and amount of bleeding

4. Maintain fetal surveillance with continuous EFM.
5. Palpate the abdomen for firmness and uterine relaxation.
6. Measure and record FH periodically to evaluate accumulation of concealed bleeding.

Nursing Interventions

Maintaining Fluid Volume and Tissue Perfusion

1. Monitor CBC results for drop in hemoglobin and hematocrit, and coagulation studies as directed.
2. Position the patient in a lateral position.
3. Administer oxygen via facemask at 8 to 10 L/min. Maintain oxygen saturation level above 90% to 95%.
4. Evaluate fetal status with continuous external fetal monitoring.
5. Establish IV access and administer rapid infusion of parenteral crystalloids (lactated Ringer's [LR] and/or normal saline [NS]) or colloids (Plasmanate).
6. Monitor vaginal bleeding and evaluate FH to detect an increase in bleeding.
7. Prepare for possible cesarean delivery if maternal or fetal compromise is evident.

Reducing Anxiety and Fear

1. Inform the patient and family about maternal–fetal status frequently.
2. Explain all procedures in advance when possible or as they are performed.
3. Answer questions in a calm manner, using simple terms.
4. Encourage the presence of a support person.
5. Encourage relaxation techniques.

Patient Education and Health Maintenance

1. Provide information regarding etiology and treatment for abruptio placentae.
2. Encourage involvement from the neonatal team regarding education related to fetal/neonatal outcome.
3. Instruct patient to report to labor and delivery immediately should excessive bleeding or constant pain occur at home.
4. Instruct patient to have emergency plan in place for transport to medical facility.

Evaluation: Expected Outcomes

- FHR remains as category I or II with minimal fetal deterioration noted.
- Absence of shock, demonstrated by stable maternal vital signs after initiation of treatment.
- Verbalizes concerns; asks questions.

Hypertensive Disorders of Pregnancy

EVIDENCE BASE American College of Obstetricians and Gynecologists. (2020). Gestational hypertension and preeclampsia (Practice Bulletin #222). *Obstetrics and Gynecology, 135*(6), e237–e260. https://doi.org/10.1097/AOG.0000000000003891

Hypertensive disorders of pregnancy (HDP) are a leading cause of maternal and fetal morbidity and mortality in the United States, complicating approximately 8% to 10% of pregnancies according to the American College of Obstetricians and Gynecologists (ACOG). Hypertensive disorders are categorized as chronic hypertension, gestational hypertension, or preeclampsia (superimposed, with or without severe features, and eclampsia). Any HDP can negatively impact maternal and fetal outcomes due to the increased risk of maternal stroke, impaired uteroplacental perfusion, placental abruption, and postpartum hemorrhage. It is essential that nurses have the knowledge and expertise to recognize changes that may suggest disease progression to mitigate injury.

Classification

Table 35-3 outlines the classification of HDP.

Chronic Hypertension

1. *Hypertension* is defined as mild, systolic blood pressure (BP) greater than or equal to 140 mm Hg *or* diastolic BP greater than or equal to 90 mm Hg, or severe, systolic BP greater than or equal to 160 mm Hg *or* diastolic BP greater than or equal to 110 mm Hg. The condition may be observable before pregnancy, diagnosed before the 20th week of gestation, or persisting beyond 12 weeks postpartum.
2. Patients with chronic hypertension may develop superimposed preeclampsia based on the presence of one or more of the following before 20 weeks' gestation:
   a. New onset of proteinuria.
   b. Sudden increase in proteinuria.
   c. Sudden increase in hypertension.
   d. Development of HELLP (Hemolysis, Elevated Liver enzymes, Low Platelets) syndrome (Box 35-1).

Table 35-3 Hypertensive Disorders of Pregnancy

CATEGORY	CHRONIC HYPERTENSION	GESTATIONAL HYPERTENSION	PREECLAMPSIA Without severe features	PREECLAMPSIA With severe features
Clinical parameters	Prepregnancy or before 20 weeks' gestation • Mild: BP ≥140/90 • Severe: BP ≥160/110	Hypertension after 20 weeks' gestation • BP ≥140/90	Hypertension after 20 weeks' gestation • BP ≥140/90 with proteinuria: ≥300 mg in 24-h urine; protein/creatinine ratio ≥0.3 g; urine dipstick >1+ protein	Hypertension after 20 weeks' gestation • BP ≥160/110, worsening cerebral irritability, proteinuria ≥5 g, oliguria, pulmonary edema, and/or HELLP syndrome
Preeclampsia/ eclampsia	**Superimposed preeclampsia** With or without severe features can occur with an increase in BP, proteinuria, and/or HELLP syndrome		**Eclampsia** Seizures with preeclampsia related to cerebral irritation/ edema/vasospasm	

BP, blood pressure; HELLP, Hemolysis, Elevated Liver enzymes, Low Platelets.

BOX 35-1 HELLP Syndrome

HELLP syndrome—consisting of Hemolysis of red blood cells (RBCs), Elevated Liver enzymes, and Low Platelets (<100,000 mm^3)—is a severe complication with or without preeclampsia.

- These findings are commonly associated with disseminated intravascular coagulation (DIC) and, in fact, may be diagnosed as DIC.
- The hemolysis of erythrocytes is seen in the abnormal morphology of the cells.
- The elevated liver enzyme measurement is associated with decreased blood flow to the liver as a result of fibrin thrombi.
- The low platelet count is related to vasospasm and platelet adhesions.
- Treatment is similar to treatment for preeclampsia with close monitoring of liver function and bleeding.
- These patients are at increased risk for postpartum hemorrhage.
- Complaints range from malaise, epigastric pain, and nausea and vomiting to nonspecific viral syndromelike symptoms.

Gestational Hypertension

1. New onset of hypertension (systolic BP ≥140 mm Hg *or* diastolic BP ≥90 mm Hg), generally after 20 weeks' gestation in the absence of gestational proteinuria.
2. BP typically normalizes to prepregnancy values by 12 weeks postpartum; if it remains elevated past 12 weeks, then a diagnosis of chronic hypertension is confirmed.

Preeclampsia and Eclampsia

1. Preeclampsia without severe features is defined as hypertension after 20 weeks' gestation accompanied by proteinuria.
   a. Gestational proteinuria >300 mg on a random specimen or greater than 1+ on a dipstick.
   b. Urinary excretion greater than or equal to 0.3 g protein in a 24-hour specimen (24-hour specimens are recommended for diagnosis).
2. Preeclampsia with severe features is diagnosed in patients with preeclampsia with the presence of any of the following conditions:
   a. Systolic BP greater than or equal to 160 mm Hg; diastolic BP greater than or equal to 110 mm Hg.
   b. Proteinuria 5 g or greater in a 24-hour specimen or 3+ on two or more random urine specimens.
   c. Renal dysfunction—oliguria of less than 500 mL/24 h; elevated creatinine, uric acid.
   d. Cerebral or visual disturbances.
   e. Epigastric or right upper quadrant pain.
   f. Hepatic dysfunction—HELLP Syndrome—***H****emolysis* (anemia), ***E****levated* ***L****iver enzymes* (AST/serum glutamic-oxaloacetic transaminase [SGOT], ALT/serum glutamic pyruvic transaminase [SGPT], or LDH), ***L****ow* ***P****latelets* (thrombocytopenia—≤150,000/mm^3); elevated indirect bilirubin (refer to Box 35-1).
   g. Pulmonary edema.
   h. IUGR.
3. Eclampsia is a complication of preeclampsia and a medical emergency. Eclampsia is characterized by the new onset of generalized tonic–clonic seizure activity or coma without any other underlying pathology. The etiologic cause of the seizures is cerebral edema, vasospasm, and/or stroke.

Pathophysiology and Etiology

1. Etiology is unknown though many theories include immunologic, genetic, and endocrine factors. A common characteristic of preeclampsia is impaired placentation related to inadequate trophoblastic invasion of uterine spiral arteries. Microangiopathy causing endothelial dysfunction, systemic inflammatory response, vasoconstriction, vascular occlusion and leakage, and subsequent increased capillary permeability resulting in hypertension, proteinuria, and edema. Clinical manifestations include:
   a. Headache—related to vasoconstriction, cerebral edema.
   b. Visual disturbances—related to retinal artery spasm, cerebral edema.
   c. Epigastric pain—right-sided pain related to liver involvement.
2. Risk factors:
   a. Nulliparity.
   b. First pregnancy with a new partner.
   c. History of preeclampsia.
   d. Black ethnicity.
   e. Chronic hypertension.
   f. GTD.
   g. Multifetal gestation.
   h. Polyhydramnios.
   i. Preexisting cardiovascular disease.
   j. Pregestational obesity (body mass index [BMI] 30 or greater).
   k. Diabetes mellitus, including pregestational and gestational diabetes.
   l. Social determinants of health.
   m. Periodontal disease.
   n. Maternal age younger than age 19 and older than age 40 are at higher risk.
   o. Preexisting collagen/vascular disease—lupus.
   p. Antiphospholipid antibody syndrome.
   q. Renal disease.
   r. Obstructive sleep apnea.
   s. Thrombophilia.
   t. ART.

Diagnostic Evaluation

1. Evaluate BP with the patient in a comfortable sitting position with legs uncrossed and feet flat on the floor after 10 minutes of rest. An appropriately sized cuff should be placed at the level of the heart and directly on the skin for accuracy.
2. Laboratory workup to include:
   a. CBC and platelets.
   b. Serum BUN, creatinine, uric acid, and glomerular filtration rate evaluate renal function and disease progression.
   c. A 24-hour urine for protein–creatinine ratio is recommended to confirm diagnosis of preeclampsia.
3. Serum liver function testing (AST, ALT, LDH, bilirubin) to assess for organ dysfunction and disease progression.
4. Surveillance for fetal well-being with BPP, ultrasound and NST to assess fetal growth, amniotic fluid volume, and placental implantation and function.
5. Deep tendon reflexes (DTRs) and clonus evaluation to assess for hyperreflexia and evolving disease symptomatology that may impact treatment protocol.

Management

Management of HDP is individualized and determined by maternal/fetal status and gestational age. The focus of treatment (expectant management) is to maintain optimal maternal health, an intrauterine environment for adequate fetal well-being, and pregnancy prolongation as the maternal/fetal status allows. Delivery is recommended by 37 0/7 weeks; however, earlier delivery may be indicated for maternal/fetal indications. Note: ACOG recommends treating patients who are hypertensive without proteinuria but who have severe BP range with the same management as a patient diagnosed with severe preeclampsia.

Expectant Management

Expectant management is considered for the following:

1. Maternal factors:
   a. Controlled hypertension.
   b. Urinary protein less than 0.3 g/L.
   c. Adequate renal and liver function.
2. Fetal factors:
   a. BPP greater than 6.
   b. AFI greater than 2 cm.
   c. Ultrasound fetal weight greater than 5th percentile.

Delivery

Delivery may be considered if any of the following occur:

1. Maternal factors:
   a. Uncontrolled hypertension: persistently greater than or equal to 160/100 mm Hg.
   b. Eclampsia.
   c. Thrombocytopenia: platelets less than 100,000/mm^3.
   d. Compromised renal and/or liver function.
   e. Pulmonary edema.
   f. Abruptio placentae.
   g. Persistent and unresolved severe headache or visual changes.
2. Fetal factors:
   a. Evolving category II patterns or category III FHR patterns (see page 995).
   b. BPP less than 4 on two occasions, 4 hours apart.
   c. AFI less than 2 cm.
   d. Ultrasound fetal weight less than 5th percentile.
   e. Reverse umbilical artery diastolic flow.
   f. Evidence of acute placental abruption.

Antihypertensive Drug Therapy

Acute and persistent (>15 minutes) onset of preeclampsia with severe features, systolic greater than 160 or diastolic greater than 110, is considered a hypertensive emergency warranting prompt medical management. A clinical relationship between severe systolic hypertension and risk of hemorrhagic stroke has been observed in pregnant and nonpregnant adults. Therefore, a systolic BP of 160 mm Hg or greater is widely adopted as the definition of severe hypertension in pregnant or postpartum people. The goal of antihypertensive therapy is not to achieve normotension but to reduce risk of stroke and coma.

1. Hydralazine—relaxes vascular arterioles and stimulates cardiac output via direct peripheral vasodilation.
   a. Dosage: 5 to 10 mg IV push over 2 minutes every 15 to 20 minutes to a maximum dose of 20 mg; dose cautiously and avoid hypotension. Monitor BP and heart rate; cardiac monitoring is not required. Oral dosing will depend on clinical presentation.
   b. Onset of action can occur in 10 to 20 minutes, with peak action in 20 minutes; duration of the drug can last 3 to 8 hours.
   c. Monitor BP and pulse closely. If desired response is not achieved within a 20-minute time frame after the administration, consider changing therapeutic agents or hemodynamic monitoring.
   d. Adverse effects: flushing, headache, tachycardia, palpitations, postural hypotension, uteroplacental insufficiency with subsequent fetal tachycardia, late decelerations, and worsening hypertension (if due to elevated cardiac output). Rebound hypotension is possible if hydralazine is given too rapidly.
2. Labetalol—alpha/beta-adrenergic blocker that decreases systemic vascular resistance without reflex tachycardia and slows the maternal heart rate.
   a. Contraindicated in patients with asthma, heart failure, and/or heart block and bradycardia.
   b. Initial dosing is 10 to 20 mg IV bolus over at least 2 minutes with cardiac monitoring. If no effect, follow with 40mg; if no effect in 10 minutes, then give 80mg every 10 minutes. If ineffective, consider alternative treatment. Monitor BP and heart rate; cardiac monitoring is not required. Oral dosing will depend on clinical presentation. Hold labetalol if maternal pulse is less than 60 beats/min.
   c. Onset of action is 1 to 2 minutes, with peak of action at 5 minutes; duration of drug effect lasts 2 to 6 hours after IV administration.
   d. Adverse effects: Maternal bradycardia, hypotension, and hypoglycemia, transient fetal and neonatal hypotension, bradycardia, and hypoglycemia.
3. Nifedipine—a calcium channel blocker that inhibits calcium reuptake and smooth-muscle cell contractility.
   a. Administer 10 to 20 mg orally.
   b. Onset of action is 20 minutes, may repeat ×1 if necessary.
   c. Sublingual route is contraindicated due to risk of excessive hypotension and acute myocardial ischemia and death. Monitor BP and heart rate; cardiac monitoring is not required.
   d. Adverse effects: maternal hypotension, flushing, reflex tachycardia, and headache.

Anticonvulsant Therapy

1. Magnesium sulfate is the primary therapy for the prophylactic treatment of seizure activity. It may be administered IV or IM; however, the IV route is preferred. IM administration is reserved for patients with eclampsia without IV access. Contraindications: myasthenia gravis and renal disease.
   a. A 4- to 6-g loading dose of magnesium sulfate is administered IV over 15 to 20 minutes followed by a maintenance dose (secondary infusion) of 1 to 2 g/h. Magnesium sulfate should have its own separate IV bag and primary IV tubing that is piggybacked into the maintenance IV fluids at the lowest port on an IV infusion pump.
   b. Therapeutic level for serum magnesium sulfate is 4 to 7 mEq/dL. Periodic laboratory analysis of serum levels is required.
   c. Actions: decreases neuromuscular irritability and blocks release of acetylcholine at the neuromuscular junction; depresses vasomotor center; depresses central nervous system (CNS) irritability.
   d. Signs of magnesium sulfate toxicity include serum magnesium sulfate level greater than 8 mEq/dL, loss of DTRs, including patellar reflex, respiratory depression, oliguria, respiratory arrest, and cardiac arrest.
   e. Calcium gluconate should be immediately available in a secured area as an antidote for magnesium toxicity; administer 1 g (10 mL of 10% solution) by slow IV push.

f. Potential maternal adverse effects: flushing, lethargy, headache, muscle weakness, diminished DTR, diplopia, dry mouth, pulmonary edema, and cardiac arrest.
g. Potential fetal adverse effects: lethargy, hypotonia, respiratory depression, and demineralization with prolonged use.

2. Phenytoin, although proposed for eclampsia prophylaxis, is considered second-line therapy in the United States; preferred for patients with kidney dysfunction.

Complications

Complications of preeclampsia affect many organ systems, including cardiovascular, renal, hematologic, neurologic, hepatic, and uteroplacental.

1. Abruptio placentae.
2. DIC.
3. HELLP syndrome.
4. Maternal or fetal death.
5. Hypertensive crisis, hemorrhagic stroke, or coma.
6. Pulmonary edema; cerebral edema.
7. Oliguria; acute renal dysfunction or failure.
8. Thrombocytopenia; acute liver dysfunction or failure.
9. Postpartum hemorrhage.
10. Blindness; retinal detachment.
11. Fetal intolerance of labor; evolving category II or category III patterns.
12. Hypoglycemia.
13. Hepatocellular dysfunction; hepatic rupture.
14. Prematurity.
15. Growth restriction and placental dysfunction.

DRUG ALERT Magnesium sulfate administration requires specific education, training, and resources to respond to potential adverse events of treatment. The Agency for Healthcare Research and Quality (AHRQ) Safety Program for Perinatal Care developed a tool for the safe administration of magnesium sulfate. The tool includes an outline of key elements of therapy, staff responsibilities, standard dosing parameters, packaging and infusion criteria as well as hospital policy recommendations for all practitioners (providers, nurses, pharmacists, laboratory personnel) involved in its administration. For enhanced safety, nurses should use a two-person verification system when magnesium sulfate administration is initiated or whenever there is a need for a rate adjustment.

Source: Agency for Healthcare Research and Quality. (2018). *Safe medication administration: Magnesium sulfate.* https:// www.ahrq.gov/patient-safety/settings/labor-delivery/perinatal-care/modules/strategies/medication/safe-medication-slides.html

Nursing Assessment

1. Assess vital signs and evaluate BP with appropriate cuff size and placement.
2. Assess urine output and proteinuria.
3. Auscultate lung sounds.
4. Assess DTRs and clonus.
5. Assess LOC and neurologic status.
6. Maintain fetal surveillance with EFM (continuous/intermittent) per facility policy.
7. Evaluate uterine activity assessing for complications such as PTL or placental abruption.
8. Monitor laboratory data including a CBC with platelets, chemistry, coagulation profile, liver enzymes, urine protein/creatinine, and serum magnesium levels as ordered.
9. Assist with additional diagnostic testing such as NST, fetal movement (kick) counts, BPP, contraction stress test (CST), and serial ultrasound with or without Doppler flow velocimetry for fetal tolerance.

CLINICAL JUDGMENT Vigilant nursing assessment of maternal/fetal changes are critical to prevent seizures but also to identify subtle changes in status, which may be related to magnesium toxicity, including absent patellar reflex, respiratory depression, somnolence, and pulmonary edema. Progressing disease may involve deteriorating laboratory data and continued signs and symptoms of preeclampsia such as worsening headache, clonus, and hyperreflexia. Remain alert and report subtle changes promptly.

Nursing Interventions

Maintaining Fluid Balance

1. Monitor vital signs per facility protocol and as the patient's condition warrants.
2. Auscultate lung sounds at regular intervals; report signs of pulmonary edema (i.e., wheezing, crackles, shortness of breath, tachycardia, increased respiratory rate, or reduced SpO_2 saturation).
3. Maintain strict intake and output—control IV fluid intake using an infusion pump. Foley catheter with urometer for strict assessment of output may be ordered. Notify provider if urine output is less than 30 mL/h or less than 500 mL in 24 hours.

Promoting Adequate Tissue Perfusion

1. Limit activity with possible bed rest. Position laterally to optimize maternal and placental perfusion.
2. Evaluate continuous EFM to determine fetal status.

Preventing Injury

1. Instruct patient on importance of reporting signs of advancing disease: headaches, visual changes, dizziness, respiratory distress, and/or epigastric pain.
2. Keep the environment quiet and calm as possible, minimizing visitors.
3. Implement seizure precautions with padded side rails and maintain safe environment.
4. Closely monitor all ordered diagnostic testing.
5. Ensure that hospitalized patients have oxygen, suction, and emergency medications immediately available for seizure management.
6. Communicate the plan of care and patient status with the interprofessional team to optimize management of care to include the neonate.

Decreasing Anxiety and Increasing Knowledge

1. Explain disease process and plan of care including treatment, expectations, and signs and symptoms of evolving disease.
2. Encourage patient and family to ask questions and express feelings regarding the diagnosis and treatment plan.

Maintaining Cardiac Output

1. Monitor maternal vital signs and pulse oximetry. Report abnormalities to provider.
2. Maintain strict intake and output.
3. Ensure cautious use of parenteral therapy with magnesium sulfate infusion.

4. Assess for edema: peripheral and pulmonary. Report pitting edema of +2 or less or evidence of pulmonary edema to primary care provider immediately.
5. Monitor EFM for moderate variability and accelerations.

Patient Education and Health Maintenance

1. Instruct the patient regarding prescribed medications with potential side effects and the importance of following the provider's activity and positioning recommendations.
2. Instruct the patient to call the provider if experiencing any change in health status.
3. Preeclampsia without severe features may be considered for home care based on maternal/fetal status and provider discretion. Periodic home visits by nurses may be warranted.
   a. Educate the patient and family regarding the signs and symptoms of evolving disease.
   b. Note that monitoring of home BP, weight, and urine output is recommended.
   c. Instruct the patient on how to perform a daily fetal movement (kick) counts; arrange for weekly NST, if indicated.

Evaluation: Expected Outcomes

- BP and other vital parameters stable.
- Absence of evolving category II or category III FHR patterns.
- No seizure activity.
- Expresses concern for self and fetus.
- No evidence of pulmonary edema; urine output adequate.

Hydramnios

Hydramnios (or poly*hydramnios*) is excess amniotic fluid and occurs in 1% to 5% of pregnancies; volume typically exceeds 2 L between 32 and 36 weeks' gestation. Although about 50% of cases result in normal outcomes, hydramnios often leads to preterm delivery, fetal malpresentation, and umbilical cord prolapse.

Pathophysiology and Etiology

1. Amniotic fluid is 98% to 99% water, with the remainder consisting of proteins, carbohydrates, fats, electrolytes, enzymes, hormones, urinary by-products, fetal cells, lanugo, and vernix.
   a. Amniotic fluid volume is influenced by fetal urination and fetal lung liquid production.
   b. Volume facilitates normal lung and neuromuscular maturity.
   c. A fetus near term will produce 500 to 1,200 mL of urine and swallow 210 to 760 mL of amniotic fluid daily.
   d. At 36 weeks' gestation, approximately 1 L of fluid is present with subsequent decreases over the duration of gestation.
2. Hydramnios is idiopathic in 60% of patients but may be associated with multiple gestation, immune and nonimmune hydrops fetalis, chromosomal anomalies such as Down syndrome, and fetal GI–cardiac–neural tube abnormalities.

Clinical Manifestations

1. Excessive weight gain, dyspnea.
2. Abdomen may be tense and shiny.
3. Edema of the vulva, legs, and lower extremities may be evident.
4. Increased uterine size for gestational age; usually accompanied by difficulty in palpating fetal parts or auscultation of the FHR.
5. Possible evolving category II or category III FHR patterns.

Diagnostic Evaluation

1. Ultrasound evaluation: AFI greater than 20 cm or single deepest pocket depth greater than 8 cm or total volume greater than 2 L.
2. Difficult to palpate fetus or auscultate FHR.
3. FH greater than age of gestation.

Management

1. Treatment is based on severity and underlying conditions; may include direct fetal therapy, such as amnioreduction or administration of prostaglandin inhibitors such as indomethacin.
2. Indomethacin decreases fetal urine output through the constriction of the renal arteries. Used cautiously after 30 weeks' gestation to prevent premature closure of the patent ductus arteriosus.
3. Amnioreduction:
   a. Accomplished with amniocentesis where fluid is slowly removed under ultrasound-guided needle aspiration; rapid removal can result in a premature separation of the placenta.
   b. Usually 500 to 1,000 mL of fluid is removed during one procedure. Fluid should be removed slowly, no faster than 1,000 mL over 20 minutes.

Complications

1. Potential for dysfunctional labor with increased risk for cesarean delivery.
2. Postpartum hemorrhage because of uterine atony from prolonged gross distention of the uterus.
3. Acute fetal hypoxia secondary to prolapsed cord or trauma.
4. Potential for preterm delivery.

Nursing Assessment

1. Evaluate maternal respiratory status; dyspnea may be present as hydramnios increases.
2. Evaluate EFM to assess fetal status.
3. Inspect abdomen and evaluate fundal height and compare with previous findings.
4. Evaluate for abdominal pain, edema, varicosities of lower extremities, and vulva.

Nursing Interventions

Promoting Effective Maternal Oxygenation and Mobility

1. Assist with positioning to alleviate dyspnea.
2. Limit exertional activities but encourage short walks and frequent position changes, alternating with frequent rest periods.
3. Encourage the patient to wear comfortable clothing, shoes with support, and abdominal support binder if necessary.

Decreasing Anxiety

1. Explain probable causes of hydramnios, if known, and all procedures and treatments, focusing on positive outcomes.
2. Encourage the patient and family to ask questions and express feelings regarding any treatment or procedure.
3. Prepare patient for mode of delivery that is anticipated and for the expected findings at the time of delivery.
4. Encourage presence and participation of support person in plan of care.

Preventing Hemorrhage During Labor and Postpartum

1. Notify provider of inadequate or abnormal labor curve.
2. Maintain IV access and administer parenteral fluids as ordered (LR).

3. Administer uterotonic medications as prescribed to decrease postpartum bleeding, as necessary (see Postpartum Hemorrhage section, page 1065).
4. Observe for alterations in vital signs indicating excessive blood loss.

Patient Education and Health Maintenance

1. Instruct the patient to notify provider if experiencing respiratory distress, contractions, or bleeding.
2. Teach the patient to seek care immediately if spontaneous rupture of membranes occurs due to risk of umbilical cord prolapse.

Evaluation: Expected Outcomes

- Unlabored breathing; verbalizes improved comfort with light activity.
- Discusses pregnancy outcome realistically; asks questions regarding treatment for self and fetus.
- Normal labor progression and involution occurs without hemorrhage.

Oligohydramnios

Oligohydramnios is the marked decrease of amniotic fluid of less than 500 mL in the amniotic sac; it is less common than hydramnios.

Pathophysiology and Etiology

1. Commonly related to amnion abnormalities, placental insufficiency, severe preeclampsia, prelabor rupture of membranes (PROM), and any condition that prevents the formation of urine or the entry of urine into the amniotic sac. Fetal urine problems include obstruction in the urinary tract, renal agenesis, pulmonary hypoplasia (Potter syndrome), and IUGR.
2. Commonly seen in postdate pregnancies.

Clinical Manifestations

1. Prominent fetal parts on palpation of the abdomen.
2. Small-for-date uterine size.
3. FHR variable decelerations (sporadic or repetitive) may present on EFM tracing due to cord compression. FHR may exhibit late decelerations if cord compression is not alleviated.

Diagnostic Evaluation

1. Ultrasound evaluation of the AFI—decrease of amniotic fluid in all four vertical plane quadrants of the uterus of less than 500 mL, single deep pocket depth less than 2 cm, or AFI less than 5 cm at term.

Management

1. Frequent evaluation of fetal status through NST, AFI, BPP, CST, as indicated.
2. Periodic ultrasound evaluations performed to evaluate fetal renal dysfunction and abnormal fetal growth.
3. During labor, an amnioinfusion may be used to alleviate fetal cord compression or particulate meconium. An amnioinfusion is the installation of IV fluid (LR or NS) into the uterus through an internal uterine pressure catheter (IUPC).
4. Delivery may be indicated for such conditions as IUGR or fetal compromise.

Complications

1. Preterm delivery.
2. Umbilical cord compression.
3. Passage of meconium possibly leading to meconium aspiration syndrome (MAS).
4. Fetal/neonatal death.
5. Neonatal respiratory distress because of pulmonary hypoplasia related to fetal compression and growth restriction.

Nursing Interventions and Patient Education

1. Evaluate maternal vital signs per facility protocol; note signs of infection, especially if oligohydramnios is secondary to PROM.
2. Evaluate fetal status with EFM. Changing maternal position to left lateral may assist in improving FHR pattern.
3. Monitor amnioinfusion, as indicated.
4. Evaluate neonate after birth for signs of respiratory complications and congenital anomalies.
5. Maintain communication with the interprofessional team to optimize management of care to optimize maternal/fetal outcomes.
6. Keep patient and family informed of any interventions and include them in plan of care.

Multiple Gestation

Multiple gestation or *multifetal pregnancy* results when two or more fetuses are present in the uterus at the same time. According to the National Vital Statistics System, there was a dramatic increase in the twin birth rate from 1980 to 2009 and an even greater increase in triplet and high-order multiple gestation rate in the 1980s and 1990s because of advanced maternal age and ART. Rates have been declining slightly since then, with 32.6 twins per 1,000 live births and 93.0 triplet and higher order multiples per 1,000 live births in 2018. Multiple gestation is not a complication of pregnancy; rather, it is a condition that presents an increased risk of morbidity and mortality for pregnant patient and neonates.

EVIDENCE BASE American College of Obstetricians and Gynecologists. (2021). *Multifetal gestations: Twin, triplet, and higher-order multifetal pregnancies* (Practice Bulletin #231). *Obstetrics and Gynecology, 137*(6), e145–e162. https://doi.org/10.1097/AOG.0000000000004397

Pathophysiology and Etiology

1. Types of twinning (Figure 35-4): The degree to which structures are shared (amnion, chorion, placenta) is related to the time of zygotic division after conception (within 72 hours).
   a. Monozygotic (identical)—one ovum fertilizes with one sperm, later dividing early in gestation resulting in two embryos. Each embryo has identical genetic makeup and sex but may vary in size because of unequal splitting of the cytoplasm; etiology unclear; rarest type of twinning with increased risk of twin-to-twin transfusion syndrome.
   b. Dizygotic, trizygotic (fraternal, nonidentical)—two or more ova are fertilized by two or more separate sperm. The twins do not always share same genetic makeup or sex.
2. Artificially induced ovulation, as well as in vitro fertilization with multiple embryos transferred into the uterus, increases risk of multiple gestation.

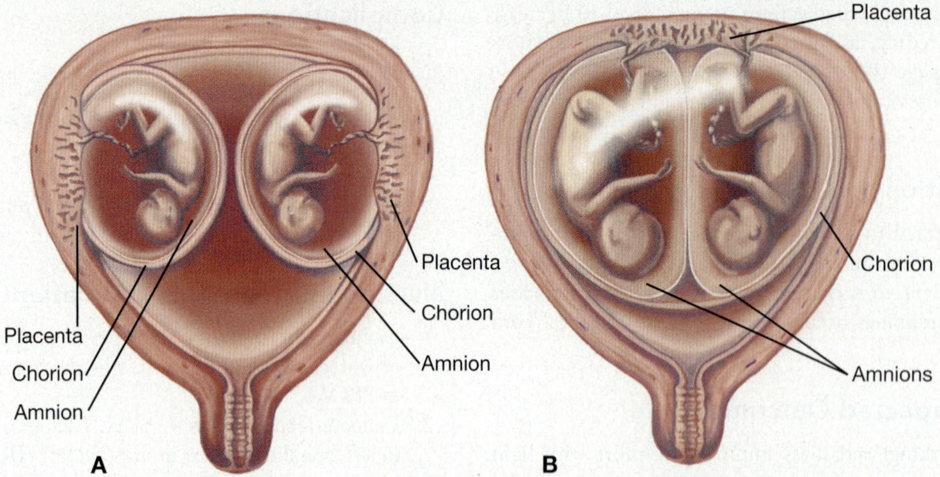

Figure 35-4. Multiple gestation with twins. **(A)** Dizygotic twins: each fetus has its own placenta, chorion, and amnion. **(B)** Monozygotic twins: the fetuses share one placenta, two amnions, and one chorion. (Reprinted with permission from Ricci, S. S. [2021]. *Essentials of maternity, newborn, and women's health nursing* [5th ed., Fig. 19.6.]. Wolters Kluwer.)

3. Increasing maternal age and parity increase odds of twinning.
4. Other terminology:
   a. Monochorionic—one chorionic membrane.
   b. Monoamniotic—one amniotic sac.
   c. Dichorionic—two chorionic membranes.
   d. Diamniotic—two amniotic sacs.

Clinical Manifestations

1. Uterine size is large for gestational age. FH is typically 2 cm larger than normal.
2. Auscultation of two or more distinct and separate fetal hearts may occur with a Doppler late in the first trimester or with a fetoscope after 20 weeks' gestation.
3. Ultrasound is the primary diagnostic tool. Gestational sacs can be identified as early as 6 to 8 weeks.
4. High initial quantitative beta-hCG is an early indictor; however, ultrasound should be used to confirm the diagnosis due to the potential for a false positive result.

Complications

1. Maternal cardiopulmonary compromise.
   a. Pulmonary edema.
   b. Complications from tocolytic drugs to inhibit labor, such as hypotension and tachycardia.
   c. Hypertension or preeclampsia.
   d. Aortocaval compression syndrome.
   e. Peripartum and postpartum cardiomyopathy.
2. Maternal liver disease.
   a. Acute fatty liver of pregnancy.
   b. Cholestasis of pregnancy.
3. Maternal anemia.
4. Obstetric complications.
   a. PTL or preterm birth.
   b. Incompetent cervix.
   c. Increased incidence of cesarean delivery.
   d. Increased use of tocolysis.
   e. Antepartum and postpartum hemorrhage.
   f. Abruptio placentae.
   g. Uterine rupture.
   h. Gestational diabetes.
   i. Hydramnios or oligohydramnios common with twins.
   j. Spontaneous abortion.
   k. IUGR.
   l. Umbilical cord problems, such as entanglement, cord prolapse, or vasa previa.
5. Fetal risks—structural abnormalities, such as congenital heart defects, intestinal tract anomalies, neural tube defects, hydrocephaly, craniofacial defects, skeletal defects, anencephaly, and encephalocele.
6. Conjoined twins.
7. Twin-to-twin transfusion syndrome leads to anastomoses of placental vessels; increased risk with one placenta. Disparate fetal growth between the fetuses may result.

Management and Nursing Interventions

1. Nutritional counseling—increased caloric and protein intake as well as vitamin supplements are needed to meet demands of multiple fetuses.
2. Fetal evaluation:
   a. NSTs, BPPs, and serial ultrasounds to evaluate growth and development.
   b. Amniocentesis for fetal lung maturity.
   c. Percutaneous umbilical cord sampling may be used to establish fetal well-being if twin-to-twin transfusion is suspected.
3. PTL prevention:
   a. Encourage modified activity and hydration.
   b. Tocolytic therapy, when indicated.
   c. Hospitalization for fetal surveillance may be required.
4. Mode of delivery—dependent on the presentation of the twins, maternal and fetal status, and gestational age. Cesarean delivery is commonly used for multiples other than twins.
5. Intrapartum management—vaginal delivery of multiples is recommended to occur in the operation room in the event an emergency operative birth is indicated.
   a. Establish IV access.
   b. Provide for EFM for each fetus; may need ultrasound availability during delivery.
   c. Separate equipment setups to provide for care and possible resuscitation of neonates.

   d. Guidelines for vaginal birth of twins—surgical suite immediately available and adequate staffing of the healthcare team to meet the needs of the patient and neonates.
   e. Pitocin induction/augmentation may be required secondary to labor dystocia.
   f. An increased risk of postpartum hemorrhage exists; postpartum hemorrhage kit needs to be readily available.
6. Emotional support—encourage family to discuss feelings about multiple births and plan of care.

Patient Education and Health Maintenance

1. Discuss the warning signs of PTL and when to call the provider.
2. Explain that home care may include nursing visits and fetal assessments.
3. Ensure provider contact information is available.

INTRAPARTUM COMPLICATIONS OF LABOR

Preterm Labor

Preterm labor (PTL) is defined as regular contractions associated with cervical change between 20 0/7 and 36 6/7 weeks of gestation. Uterine irritability without cervical change is not PTL.

Preterm birth (PTB) is the delivery of a neonate between 20 0/7 and 36 6/7 weeks of gestation. The PTB rate in the United States was 10.5% in 2021 and is a leading cause of infant morbidity and mortality; however, advances in technologies and improvements in neonatal care have dramatically impacted outcomes for the preterm population.

Low birth weight (LBW) is not synonymous with PTB and refers to birth weight alone regardless of gestational age.

Pathophysiology and Etiology

1. The exact etiology for PTL remains unknown, but may include:
   a. Placental abruption.
   b. Mechanical factors such as uterine overdistention (hydramnios, multiple gestation) or cervical incompetence.
   c. Hormonal dysfunction.
   d. Anatomic and structural abnormalities.
   e. Infectious etiology (e.g., bacterial vaginosis, group B streptococci [GBS]).
   f. Chronic stress.
2. Physiologic alterations occur with onset of spontaneous labor.
   a. Cervical changes occur: softening, shortening, and location.
   b. Oxytocin receptors present in the myometrium respond to circulating levels.
   c. Prostaglandin levels in the amniotic fluid rise.

Risk Factors for PTL

1. Medical/obstetric complications (predating the current pregnancy):
   a. Prior PTB triples risk in a current pregnancy.
   b. Habitual abortions.
   c. Uterine/cervical abnormalities.
   d. Parity (0 or >4).
   e. Hypertension.
   f. Diabetes.
   g. Obesity or low prepregnancy weight.
2. Current pregnancy complications:
   a. Anemia.
   b. Multiple gestation.
   c. Placenta previa.
   d. Abruptio placentae.
   e. Fetal anomaly.
   f. Hydramnios.
   g. Abdominal surgery.
   h. Infection.
   i. Bleeding in first trimester.
   j. Short interpregnancy interval.
   k. Prelabor rupture of membranes (PROM).
   l. Cervical incompetence.
   m. UTIs/pyelonephritis.
   n. Periodontal disease.
3. Demographic data:
   a. Maternal age younger than 17 or older than 35.
   b. Non-Hispanic Black ethnicity (doubles the risk).
   c. Social determinants of health (e.g., low socioeconomic status).
4. Behavioral and environmental:
   a. Smoking (especially if more than 11 cigarettes/day).
   b. Poor nutrition or excessive stress.
   c. Substance use disorder.
   d. Late or no prenatal care.
   e. Intimate partner violence.

Clinical Manifestations

1. Uterine cramping (menstrual-like, intermittent, or constant).
2. Uterine contractions occurring at intervals of 10 minutes or less.
3. Low abdominal pain or pressure (pelvic pressure).
4. Dull low backache (intermittent or constant).
5. Increase or change in vaginal discharge.
6. Feeling that baby is "pushing down" or that "something" is in the vagina.

Diagnostic Evaluation

1. Transvaginal cervical ultrasound can estimate cervical length and direct internal changes.
2. Fetal fibronectin (fFN) is a protein produced by fetal membranes and functions as an adhesive to hold membranes against the uterine myometrium. It is normally absent in cervical secretions after 16 to 20 weeks and reappears after 34 weeks. Therefore, a mid-trimester assay with positive fFN is an indicator of risk for PTL/PTB and possible infection (see Chapter 32).
3. Screening for infection.

Management

Management of PTL is focused on early education, prevention, and limiting neonatal morbidity.

Preconception Care

1. Baseline assessment of health and risks; advise patient to decrease risks attributable to PTL/PTB.
2. Pregnancy planning and identification of barriers to care.
3. Periodontal care.
4. Adjustment of prescribed and over-the-counter medications that may pose a threat to the developing fetus.
5. Nutritional counseling, as needed.

Antepartum Treatment

1. Educate patient regarding signs/symptoms of PTL.
2. Instruct patient and provide resources for lifestyle modifications:
   a. If applicable, encourage smoking cessation classes.
   b. Discuss aspects of a healthy diet and adequate maternal weight gain during pregnancy.
3. Early therapy options may include limiting activity which may include bed rest, hydration, and abstention from intercourse and orgasm; effectiveness of each method is uncertain.

Tocolytics and Pharmacologic Therapies

If conservative management is unsuccessful, pharmacologic therapies may be implemented, with no one medication recognized as primary to stop PTL. Pharmacologic treatment will be individualized and based on maternal condition, potential drug side effects, and gestational age where the potential benefit to the fetus outweighs the potential risk. Pharmacologic intervention is not a long-term option; however, it is advantageous to allow time to administer corticosteroids to enhance fetal lung development and patient transfer to a higher level of care.

1. Terbutaline: is a betamimetic that acts on $beta_2$ receptor cells located in smooth muscle, inhibiting uterine contractions. Administered subcutaneously and should not be used for prolonged treatment (beyond 48 to 72 hours) of PTL in either the hospital or outpatient setting because of the potential for serious maternal heart problems and death. In addition, oral terbutaline should not be used because it has not been shown to be effective and has similar safety concerns.
   a. Withhold medication for a maternal pulse greater than 120 bpm or fetal heart rate (FHR) greater than 180 bpm.
   b. Contraindications: cardiac dysrhythmias and preeclampsia with severe features.
   c. Potential maternal adverse effects: tachycardia, cardiac dysrhythmias, pulmonary edema, myocardial ischemia, hypotension, and death.
   d. Potential fetal adverse effects: tachycardia, hyperinsulinemia, hyperglycemia, myocardial or septal hypertrophy, myocardial ischemia.
2. Magnesium sulfate: interferes with smooth-muscle contractility and blocks neuromuscular transmission by decreasing acetylcholine release. Contraindications: myasthenia gravis and renal disease.
   a. A 4- to 6-g loading dose of magnesium sulfate is administered intravenous (IV) over 15 to 20 minutes followed by a maintenance dose (secondary infusion) of 1 to 2 g/h.
   b. Magnesium sulfate should have its own separate IV bag and primary IV tubing that is piggybacked into the maintenance IV fluids at the lowest port on an IV infusion pump.
   c. Therapeutic level for serum magnesium sulfate is 4 to 7 mEq/dL. Periodic laboratory analysis of serum levels is required.
   d. Signs of magnesium sulfate toxicity include serum magnesium sulfate level greater than 8 mEq/dL; loss of deep tendon reflexes (DTRs), including patellar reflex; respiratory depression; oliguria; respiratory arrest; and cardiac arrest.

DRUG ALERT Calcium gluconate should be immediately available in a secured area as an antidote for magnesium toxicity. Administer 1 g (10 mL of 10% solution) by slow IV push if signs of toxicity develop.

   e. Potential maternal adverse effects: flushing, lethargy, headache, muscle weakness, diminished DTR, diplopia, dry mouth, pulmonary edema, and cardiac arrest.
   f. Potential fetal adverse effects: lethargy, hypotonia, respiratory depression, and demineralization with prolonged use.
3. Indomethacin: inhibits prostaglandin stimulation of contractions. Use should be limited to less than 32 weeks' gestation; may cause premature closure of the fetal ductus arteriosus.
   a. Dosage: 50 to 100 mg loading dose orally and then 25 mg orally every 6 hours for 48 hours maximum.
   b. Contraindications: poorly controlled hypertension.
   c. Potential maternal adverse effects: nausea, heartburn, postpartum hemorrhage.
   d. Potential fetal adverse effects: constriction of the ductus arteriosus, pulmonary hypertension, reversible decreased renal function with oligohydramnios, intraventricular hemorrhage (IVH), hyperbilirubinemia, necrotizing enterocolitis (NEC).
4. Nifedipine: a calcium channel blocker that relaxes smooth muscle by inhibiting the transport of calcium mitigating contraction formation.
   a. Recommended dosage: 30 mg loading dose orally followed by 10 to 20 mg every 4 to 6 hours. Dose should not exceed 180 mg/day.
   b. Contraindications: cardiac disease; use caution with renal disease, maternal hypotension (≤90/50 mm Hg); avoid concomitant use with magnesium sulfate.
   c. Potential maternal adverse effects: flushing, dizziness, headache, nausea, transient hypotension.
   d. Potential fetal adverse effects: none currently known.
5. Antibiotic therapy: several regimens exist for intrapartum antimicrobial prophylaxis for perinatal GBS disease prevention. Treatment should be started as presumptive positive for GBS. Screening and treatment for bacterial vaginosis should also be considered.

General Contraindications to Tocolytic and Pharmacologic Therapies

1. Category III FHR patterns.
2. Intra-amniotic infection.
3. Preeclampsia with severe features and eclampsia.
4. Fetal demise.
5. Fetal maturity.
6. Maternal hemodynamic instability.
7. Severe bleeding of any cause.
8. Fetal anomaly incompatible with life.
9. Severe intrauterine growth restriction (IUGR).
10. Cervical dilation greater than 5 cm.

Acceleration of Fetal Lung Maturity

1. Corticosteroid administration—betamethasone or dexamethasone.
   a. Given to potential PTL patients between 24 and 34 weeks' gestation.
   b. Betamethasone is given intramuscularly (IM) in two doses of 12 mg each, 24 hours apart.
   c. Dexamethasone is given IM in four doses of 6 mg each, every 12 hours.
      i. Decreases complications and mortality that may be a result of prematurity.
   d. Timely administration is essential; given before delivery to patient when postponing delivery for administration is an option.

Complications

1. Prematurity and associated neonatal complications include:
   a. Intraventricular hemorrhage.
   b. Respiratory distress syndrome (RDS) because of lung immaturity related to lack of surfactant production.
   c. Patent ductus arteriosus (PDA).
   d. Necrotizing enterocolitis.

Nursing Assessment

During tocolytic therapy, assess the following:

1. Maternal vital signs.
2. Fetal and maternal surveillance for FHR and uterine activity.
3. Respiratory status (pulmonary edema is an adverse effect).
4. Tremors.
5. DTRs.
6. Palpitations.
7. Dizziness/lightheadedness.
8. Urine output.
9. Patient understanding of signs and symptoms of PTL.
10. Patient understanding of signs and symptoms of infection.

Nursing Interventions

Decreasing Anxiety

1. Explain the purpose and common adverse effects of tocolytic therapy.
2. Provide accurate information on the status of the fetus and progressive labor.
3. Allow the patient and support person to verbalize feelings.

Minimizing Injury to Fetus

1. Encourage use of lateral positions to enhance placental perfusion.
2. Monitor fetal status and labor progress.
3. Notify the interprofessional team of progressing labor.
4. Assist with delivery of infant, as needed.

Minimizing Risk of Drug-Related Complications

1. Maintain accurate intake and output.
2. Assess maternal vital signs. Notify the provider if maternal pulse greater than 120 bpm or FHR greater than 180 bpm.
3. Assess for signs and symptoms of pulmonary edema.
4. Assess DTRs noting hyporeflexia.
5. Discontinue infusion if adverse effects occur; notify provider.
6. Make sure calcium gluconate is readily available when magnesium sulfate is in use.

Promoting Maternal–Family Coping

1. Provide support and encourage private time for patient and support person.
2. Encourage asking questions and verbalization of feelings.
3. Facilitate social work/care management referral as needed. Ensure communication and information sharing with home health staff if home care is ordered.

Patient Education and Health Maintenance

1. Educate the patient and family about PTL/PTB and the plan of care.
2. Encourage adherence to treatment regimen, nutrition, and hydration.
3. Teach the patient signs and symptoms of infection and PTL and when to notify provider.

Evaluation: Expected Outcomes

- Patient verbalized understanding of the plan of care.
- PTL ceases.
- Maternal vital signs stable.
- Reassuring fetal surveillance.

Prelabor Rupture of Membranes

PROM is defined as rupture of the amniotic membranes before the onset of labor. PROM is independent of gestational age and is also described as premature rupture of membranes. When PROM occurs prior to 37 0/7 weeks, it is referred to as preterm prelabor rupture of membranes (PPROM) and is associated with one of the most common occurrences for PTBs. PROM increases the risk of variable decelerations in the FHR tracing related to decreased amniotic fluid volume. Pregnancies with PROM are at increased risk for fetal perinatal morbidity and mortality.

EVIDENCE BASE American College of Obstetricians and Gynecologists. (2020). *Prelabor rupture of membranes* (Practice Bulletin #217). *Obstetrics and Gynecology, 135*(3), e80–e102. https://doi.org/10.1097/AOG.0000000000003700

Pathophysiology and Etiology

1. Rupture of membranes normally occurs during the course of labor. The exact etiology of PROM is not clearly understood, although nonpathologic causes, such as the combination of stretching of the membranes and biochemical changes, are suspected to contribute; infection has commonly been found to be a primary cause.
2. PROM is manifested by a gush of amniotic fluid or leaking of fluid through the vagina, which usually persists; flow may decrease in the sitting or supine position.

Diagnostic Evaluation

1. Patient history and physical exam.
2. Sterile speculum examination for identification of "pooling" of fluid in the vagina, cervicitis, umbilical or fetal prolapse, and cervical advancement. Collect cultures as appropriate.
3. Vaginal fluid assessment—vaginal fluid sample is tested with nitrazine paper to assess pH; will turn blue for pH greater than 6.0 to 6.5, indicating amniotic fluid. False-positives may result when blood, semen, alkaline antiseptics, and bacterial vaginosis are present.
4. Fern test—swab of the posterior vaginal fornix is taken to obtain amniotic fluid. Positive test will reveal arborization or "ferning" (visually appears as a fern leaf) on a slide viewed under a microscope.
5. Ultrasound to assess amniotic fluid volume and oliguria.

Management (>34 Weeks)

1. When PROM is confirmed, the gestational age, fetal presentation, and well-being will determine if hospitalization is warranted.
2. At any gestational age, a patient with evident intrauterine infection, placental abruption, or evidence of category III FHR pattern is best cared for by expeditious delivery.
3. If immediate delivery is not indicated, cultures of the cervix should be obtained to identify best antibiotic management (to treat chlamydia, gonorrhea, and GBS, if appropriate).
4. If plan of care is conservative management based on increased risk for neonatal mortality and morbidity, care should be provided in

a facility that has resources for emergent delivery such as placenta abruptio, prolapsed umbilical cord, or fetal stress.

5. Expectant management: offer adequate time for the latent phase of labor to progress (may be as long as hours to days or at the discretion of the primary practitioner) and electronic fetal monitoring (EFM).
   a. Vaginal examinations are kept to a minimum to prevent infection.
   b. Once the decision to deliver is made, GBS prophylaxis should be initiated based on prior culture results or risk factors.
6. Active management: oxytocin induction/augmentation may be initiated at the time of presentation to reduce the risk for perinatal morbidity and mortality.
   a. GBS screening and prophylaxis if indicated.
   b. Administer corticosteroids if indicated.
   c. Antibiotic regimen if indicated.

Complications

1. Maternal infection—chorioamnionitis (intrapartum) and endometritis (postpartum).
2. Potential increased rates of cesarean delivery.
3. Fetal/neonatal infection or compromise.

Nursing Assessment

1. Note the time of PROM, odor, and color.
2. Evaluate maternal blood pressure (BP), respirations, pulse, and temperature per facility policy. Temperatures should be done every 2 hours. If temperature or pulse is elevated, continue monitoring more frequently.
3. Monitor the amount and type of leaking amniotic fluid. Observe for purulent, foul-smelling discharge and report immediately.
4. Assess for diffuse abdominal pain or pain on palpation, signs of infection.
5. Evaluate complete blood count (CBC) with differential results as ordered; any shift to the left (i.e., increase of immature forms of neutrophils/white blood cells [WBCs]) signals infection.
6. Communicate signs of infection to the provider.
7. Fetal surveillance with EFM per facility policy; recognize maternal infection is the primary cause of fetal tachycardia.

Nursing Interventions

Preventing Infection

1. Ensure that vaginal exams with sterile gloves are kept to a minimum.
2. Educate on the need for good hand hygiene particularly after urination and defecation.
3. Administer GBS prophylaxis and other antibiotics, as indicated.

Evaluation: Expected Outcomes

- No signs of infection.

Induction and Augmentation of Labor

EVIDENCE BASE American College of Obstetricians and Gynecologists. (2019). Induction of labor (Practice Bulletin #107). *Obstetrics and Gynecology, 114*(2 Pt 1), 386–397. https://doi.org/10.1097/AOG.0b013e3181b48ef5

Simpson, K. R. (2020). AWHONN Practice Monograph: Cervical ripening and labor induction and augmentation, 5th edition. *Nursing for Women's Health, 24*(4), S1–S41. https://doi.org/10.1016/j.nwh.2020.04.005

Induction of labor (IOL) refers to utilization of exogenous labor enhancement agents or procedures, resulting in rhythmic contractions and spontaneous onset of labor. Cervical ripening utilizes pharmacologic and/or mechanical methods to affect the physical properties (softening and dilation) of the cervix in preparation for labor and delivery. Benefits of induction must outweigh the risks to the maternal–fetal unit. Inductions may be medically indicated or elective. Elective inductions prior to 39 completed weeks of gestation are contraindicated.

Augmentation refers to the administration of uterine stimulants once labor dystocia (dysfunction) ensues. Dysfunctional labor may result for several reasons (outlined in the next section) and remains the number one cause for primary cesarean deliveries. Similar medications are utilized for induction, augmentation, and sometimes cervical ripening.

Indications for Induction

Medically Indicated

1. Abruptio placentae.
2. Chorioamnionitis (intra-amniotic infection).
3. Fetal demise.
4. Hypertensive disorders of pregnancy: chronic, gestational, preeclampsia with severe features, or eclampsia.
5. PROM.
6. Postterm pregnancy.
7. Maternal medical conditions: diabetes mellitus, renal disease, chronic pulmonary disease, or underlying cardiac disease.
8. Fetal conditions: IUGR, anomalies, isoimmunization, oligohydramnios.

Considerations for Elective Induction

1. Recommended gestational age for IOL is 39 weeks.
2. Patient or provider preference.
3. Logistic reasons: risk of rapid labor, distance from hospital.
4. Psychosocial indications.
5. Evaluation of fetal lung maturity should be established prior to the induction.
6. Risks associated with elective IOL should be discussed with the patient and family. Some facilities may obtain informed consent.

Contraindications for Induction

1. Vaginal bleeding, known placenta previa or vasa previa.
2. Abnormal presentation: transverse or funic (cord).
3. Previous transfundal ("classic") uterine incision or extensive myomectomy.
4. Acute fetal distress.
5. Active genital herpes infection.
6. Umbilical cord prolapse.
7. Fetal presenting part above pelvic inlet.
8. Category III FHR pattern.

Indications for Augmentation

1. Uterine hypocontractility.
2. Labor dystocia (slow, abnormal progression of labor).
3. Augmentation should be considered in the absence of cervical change if the frequency of contractions is less than 3 over 10 minutes or the intensity of contractions is less than 25 mm Hg above baseline with intrauterine pressure catheter (IUPC) or both.

Contraindications for Augmentation

1. Same as induction.

Cervical Ripening

Cervical ripening is performed if induction is indicated and the cervix is unfavorable.

Bishop score refers to a scoring system that documents cervical favorability, giving a score of 0 to 3 for each of five parameters: dilation, position of cervix, effacement, station, and cervical consistency. With a Bishop score of 8 or greater, the likelihood of a vaginal delivery is similar to spontaneous labor. A Bishop score should be documented along with fetal presentation prior to IOL.

Cervical Ripening Management

1. Mechanical methods:
   a. Hygroscopic/osmotic dilators—a seaweed preparation that is inserted directly into and dilates the cervix by absorption of vaginal/cervical fluids. An increased risk of intrapartum infection has been associated.
   b. Transcervical balloon catheter is inserted through the cervix, balloon is inflated (30 to 80 mL NS), with gentle traction and secured to the patient's leg to dilate the cervix. Once the balloon spontaneously releases, the cervix is 2 to 3 cm dilated.
   c. Membrane stripping—during a cervical exam, membranes are separated digitally from the lower uterine segment, without rupturing the membranes, to stimulate labor. Complications include maternal–fetal infection, PPROM, umbilical cord prolapse, precipitous labor and birth, and maternal discomfort.
   d. Amniotomy—mechanical method of induction through artificial rupture of membranes (AROM) using an amnihook.
      i. Data show when amniotomy is used alone, the results are unpredictable, often with long intervals before the onset of labor and increased risk of infection.
      ii. Utilized with oxytocin at onset, induction to delivery is shorter than with amniotomy alone.
      iii. Monitor with EFM per facility policy. An FHR should be documented after AROM as well as a description of the amniotic fluid (color and amount).
      iv. Complications include umbilical cord prolapse or compression and possible maternal and/or fetal infection, evolving Category II or III FHR tracing.

Pharmacologic Methods of Induction

1. Dinoprostone (Prostaglandin E_2 [PGE_2])—time-released 10 mg insert placed into the vagina and can be removed for excessively frequent uterine contractions (tachysystole) or fetal intolerance (evolving FHR category II or category III pattern).
   a. Requires continuous fetal monitoring with EFM.
   b. Keep frozen until immediately prior to use; unstable at room temperature; stable up to 3 years when frozen.
   c. Patient is to remain supine for 2 hours after insertion; may ambulate after 2 hours when continuous EFM by telemetry is available.
   d. Removal after 12 hours or at onset of labor; oxytocin should be delayed at least 30 to 60 minutes after removal.
2. Misoprostol (Prostaglandin E_1) is an off-label use for cervical ripening or labor induction.
   a. Dosing of 25 to 50 mcg administered orally or intravaginally—every 4 hours is commonly prescribed. Lower doses are associated with less uterine tachysystole.
   b. Adverse effects include shivering, backache, vomiting, diarrhea, shortness of breath, uterine hypertonus, or uterine rupture.
   c. Misoprostol will be discontinued with tachysystole, adequate cervical ripening (cervix 80% effaced and 3 cm dilated), active labor, or FHR category II or III pattern.
   d. Patient should be observed for up to 2 hours after spontaneous rupture of membranes. If the cervix remains unfavorable, the uterine activity is minimal, there is absence of category II/III FHR pattern, and the last dose was given at least 3 hours, redosing is acceptable.
   e. Oxytocin can be initiated 4 hours after the last dose.

DRUG ALERT Misoprostol is contraindicated in patients with a previous history of cesarean birth or uterine surgery through myometrium related to the increased risk of uterine rupture.

CLINICAL JUDGMENT The administration of pharmacologic agents for cervical ripening, induction, and/or augmentation of labor requires requisite competency, training, and staffing resources to respond to potential adverse events. The Association of Women's Health, Obstetric and Neonatal Nurses (AWHONN) has published safe staffing recommendations for perinatal units as a framework to provide safe, quality nursing care to patients and babies for improved outcomes.

Source: Association of Women's Health, Obstetric and Neonatal Nurses. (2022). Standards for professional registered nurse staffing for perinatal units. *Journal of Obstetric, Gynecologic & Neonatal Nursing, 51*(4), e5–e98. https://doi.org/10.1016/j.jogn.2022.02.003

3. Oxytocin is a naturally produced peptide hormone by the hypothalamus and released by the posterior pituitary. Synthetic oxytocin stimulates a uterine response within 3 to 5 minutes of infusion and reaches a steady state in 40 minutes; however, patient sensitivity varies. Cervical dilation, parity, and gestational age impact the dosing response of oxytocin.
   a. Oxytocin infusion is administered through a separate IV bag and primary IV tubing that is piggybacked into the maintenance IV fluids at the lowest port on an IV infusion pump.
   b. Solution concentrations vary and may be mixed by pharmacy or on labor and delivery by a staff registered nurse per facility policy.
   c. Typical dosing starts at 1 to 2 milliunits/min (mU) increasing 1 to 2 mU/min every 30 to 60 minutes until an adequate contraction pattern is achieved with the goal of establishing regular uterine contractions leading to cervical change and fetal descent.
      i. Cervical dilation of 0.5 to 1 cm/h in the active phase of labor.
      ii. Contractions occurring every 2 to 3 minutes lasting 60 to 90 seconds and an intensity of 50 to 70 mm Hg (moderate) or greater than 180 Montevideo units but less than 400. (Montevideo units are measured using an IUPC.)
   d. Assessment including maternal vital signs, lung sounds, FHR, and uterine activity must be documented prior to oxytocin administration and any titration. Continuous monitoring of maternal and fetal status with EFM is required during ongoing administration.

e. Due to the antidiuretic property of oxytocin, water intoxication may occur, which can lead to heart failure. Symptoms include headache, nausea and vomiting, mental confusion, decreased urine output, hypotension, tachycardia, and cardiac dysrhythmia.
f. If oxytocin is discontinued for less than 20 to 30 minutes, once reassuring uterine activity and FHR data are established, oxytocin may be restarted at half the prior rate of infusion; the rate of administration may be slowly increased based on fetal/maternal status facility/provider protocols. However, if the oxytocin has been discontinued for over 30 to 40 minutes, it must be restarted at the initial dose.
g. Complications of oxytocin include:
   i. Uterine tachysystole (more than 5 contractions in 10 minutes). Uterine tachysystole accompanied by fetal bradycardia may be treated with tocolytics such as terbutaline 0.25 mg subcutaneous to assist in resolving uterine tachysystole if indicated.
   ii. Uterine hypertonus (resting tone greater than 20 to 25 mm Hg, depending on the type of IUPC; intensity >80 mm Hg).
   iii. Contractions longer than 2 minutes in duration.
   iv. Increased incidence of cesarean delivery.
   v. Hypotension with rapid infusion.
   vi. Fetal intolerance.

Nursing Assessment

CLINICAL JUDGMENT IOL requires nurses to perform continuous, skilled assessment before, during, and after the labor process. Nurses must demonstrate competency in EFM assessment. The risk of injury and adverse events such as uterine rupture, placenta abruptio, and postpartum hemorrhage can greatly impact maternal/fetal outcomes. Astute recognition of symptoms and prompt intervention are essential to optimize outcomes.

Prior to Induction of Labor

1. Obtain a nonstress testing (NST) to assess fetal well-being.
2. Evaluate maternal vital signs, especially BP.
3. Place an IV and evaluate patency prior to initiation.
4. Document fetal presentation, Bishop score, and fetal assessment according to facility policy.
5. Note time of any cervical ripening agents that have been administered and follow appropriate protocols as required prior to beginning oxytocin administration.

CLINICAL JUDGMENT Assess maternal lung sounds prior to the administration of oxytocin as a baseline and then throughout the infusion. Although acute pulmonary edema during pregnancy and postpartum is a rare event, most cases are attributable to tocolytic therapy, cardiac disease, preeclampsia, or iatrogenic volume overload. Cardiomyopathy can occur during or after delivery, and subtle symptoms such as fatigue and shortness of breath may not be recognized because they are seen as common in the last trimester or early postpartum period.

During Administration of Oxytocin

1. Assess and document FHR and uterine activity every 30 minutes and as indicated per facility policy.
2. Assess maternal vital signs per facility policy; BP and pulse should be assessed at each dose titration.
3. Monitor intake and output.

Nursing Interventions

Decreasing Anxiety

1. Review hospital protocols for IOL and plan of care with patient and family.
2. Ask for feedback related to birth plan and cultural preferences.
3. Teach or review the use of relaxation and distraction techniques.
4. Answer questions and offer emotional support.

Enhancing Uteroplacental Oxygenation

1. Assess fetal status and uterine contractions per facility policy. Assess for tachysystole and signs of uteroplacental insufficiency: minimal-absent variability, abnormal baseline FHR, recurrent or repetitive late or variable decelerations.
2. With persistent hyperstimulation and/or nonreassuring FHR characteristics (evolving category II or category III FHR pattern), implement the following:
   a. Discontinue the oxytocin infusion immediately.
   b. Place patient in lateral position and assess vital signs; increase IV fluids if hypotension occurs.
   c. Administer oxygen (8 to 10 L/min by nonrebreather facemask).
   d. Notify provider and communicate the plan of care and patient status with the interprofessional team to optimize management of care to include the neonate.
3. Administer tocolytics, as ordered, and prepare for possible emergent cesarean delivery.

Controlling Pain

1. Encourage use of breathing/relaxation techniques, distraction, positioning, and nonpharmacologic comfort measures.
2. Encourage active partner participation.
3. Administer analgesia/anesthesia as requested and prescribed.
4. Support patient and partner through the process with presence and empathy.

Evaluation: Expected Outcomes

- Verbalizes understanding of the induction process and shows effective coping through labor.
- No evidence of uterine hyperstimulation or category III FHR pattern.
- Verbalizes adequate pain control.

Dystocia

Dystocia is characterized by slow, abnormal labor progression typically resulting from abnormal uterine activity patterns or maternal expulsive forces. Dystocia is the leading indication for augmentation and primary cesarean delivery. Causes of labor dystocia include problems with the ***power*** (contractions), ***passageway*** (pelvis), and/or or ***passenger*** (fetus) (refer to Chapter 33).

Pathophysiology and Etiology

Power Abnormalities

1. Inadequate contractions impair labor progression and slow fetal descent. Common causes include increased uterine tone, abnormal contraction pressure, hypotonic labor (prolonged latent phase, protracted or arrested active phase, or prolonged second stage of labor), and abnormal contraction pressure.
2. Problems with the force of labor result in ineffective contractions or bearing-down efforts (pushing) during the second stage of labor.

3. Etiology of abnormalities in the force of labor includes:
   a. Early or excessive use of analgesia.
   b. Overdistention of the uterus (hydramnios, macrosomia, multiple gestation).
   c. Grand multiparity (>6).

Passageway Abnormalities

1. Abnormalities in the passageway may be the result of pelvic or soft tissue anomalies.
2. Pelvic abnormalities that interfere with the engagement, descent, and expulsion of the fetus include:
   a. Size and shape of the pelvis.
   b. Obstruction from soft tissue problems, such as a uterine or ovarian fibromyoma, and obesity.
   c. Cervical abnormalities.
3. Contracted pelvic inlet (of genetic origin or as a result of rickets) may prevent descent if the interaxial dimension is less than 10 cm or the greatest transverse diameter is less than 12 cm.
4. Cephalopelvic disproportion (CPD) is the disparity between the size of the maternal pelvis and fetal head that prevents fetal descent and subsequent vaginal birth; cesarean birth is indicated if unresolved.

Passenger Abnormalities

1. Breech presentations occur in approximately 3% of all deliveries.
   a. More common in multiple gestations, increased parity, hydramnios, congenital dislocated hip, placenta previa, and preterm neonates.
   b. Generally, cesarean delivery is the method of choice for delivery.
2. A transverse lie (shoulder) presentation occurs when the infant lies perpendicular to the maternal spine and cervical os.
3. A large fetus increases the risk of trauma, both maternal and fetal; CPD may result.
4. External cephalic version (ECV) may be attempted after careful review of maternal and fetal status and likelihood of success. If a version is unsuccessful or not an option, a cesarean delivery is warranted.

Diagnostic Evaluation

1. Labor progress is assessed by vaginal examination to determine cervical effacement, dilation, or descent of the presenting part.
2. Comparison of serial evaluations of labor progress using Friedman curve criteria, if available.
   a. A prolonged latent phase in the primigravida is greater than 20 hours and greater than 14 hours in the multigravida.
   b. During the active phase, the cervix of a primigravida will normally dilate at a rate of 1.2 cm/h and a multigravida 1.5 cm/h. In addition, the fetus generally descends at a rate of 1 cm/h in a primigravida and 2 cm/h for a multigravida.

Management

1. Labor dystocia will be managed with augmentation of contractions with mechanical and/or pharmacologic methods depending on the stage of labor and maternal/fetal status (see IOL, page 1053).
2. An IUPC may be inserted into the uterus through the vagina for accurate assessment of uterine contraction strength.
   a. An IUPC can be implemented for uterine assessment and/or amnioinfusion in the case of recurrent variable decelerations, oligohydramnios, or meconium-stained fluid.
   b. Use should be limited due to the increased risk of maternal fever and infection.

Complications

1. Infection.
2. Postpartum hemorrhage.
3. Fetal intolerance: evolving category II or category III FHR patterns.
4. Fetal or maternal trauma from operative vaginal delivery.

Nursing Assessment

1. Perform Leopold maneuvers and evaluate fetal presentation, position, and size.
2. Using Friedman labor curve, periodically evaluate progress of labor.
3. Monitor FHR and contraction status per facility policy.

Nursing Interventions

Promoting Comfort

1. Demonstrate and encourage controlled breathing and relaxation techniques.
2. Encourage frequent change of position (lateral, hands and knees, throne).
3. Encourage voiding at regular intervals to decompress the bladder.
4. Demonstrate or provide comfort measures such as massage, sacral pressure, effleurage. Encourage participation from labor support person.
5. Offer ice chips and clear fluids as permitted.
6. Provide frequent encouragement to the patient and support person.
7. Administer analgesia and/or assist with the administration of regional analgesia as indicated.

Decreasing Anxiety

1. Provide anticipatory guidance regarding labor process and progress, medication use for pain relief and/or augmentation, equipment, procedures, and potential for cesarean delivery.
2. Elicit feedback from patient and support person about their questions, concerns, and anxieties.

Evaluation: Expected Outcomes

- Verbalizes increased comfort.
- Verbalizes understanding and coping through labor progression.

Shoulder Dystocia

Shoulder dystocia is the dysfunctional descent and expulsion of the fetal shoulders, resulting in impaction of the anterior shoulder behind the maternal pubis symphysis or posterior shoulder on the sacral promontory during the second stage (pushing) of labor. This condition is often relieved with gentle manipulation but may rapidly progress to an obstetric emergency. Attributable risk factors include maternal diabetes, obesity, fetal macrosomia, and IOL; however, approximately 50% of all shoulder dystocias occur without identifiable risk factors.

Pathophysiology and Etiology

1. Antepartum risk factors:
   a. Fetal macrosomia more than 4,500 g.
   b. Maternal diabetes (type 1, 2, or gestational).
   c. Postterm gestation.
   d. Previous history of shoulder dystocia, macrosomia, or postterm pregnancy.

2. Intrapartum factors:
   a. Labor induction.
   b. Regional anesthesia.
   c. Dystocia or arrest of labor.
   d. Prolonged second stage.
   e. Operative vaginal delivery.
3. None of the risk factors noted earlier individually or collectively can predict shoulder dystocia. Facilities should develop interprofessional protocols to effectively manage and anticipate shoulder dystocia at every delivery. Simulation exercises are recommended to enhance team communication and function during this emergency.

Management

1. Compare labor progression to Friedman labor curve.
2. Communicate labor progression concerns to the provider.

CLINICAL JUDGMENT Communicate the plan of care and patient status with the interprofessional team to optimize management of care to include the neonate if risks are identified.

3. Keep in mind that prevention is the key because shoulder dystocia is difficult to predict.
   a. Early identification and treatment of gestational diabetes mellitus.
   b. Antepartum glucose control of insulin-dependent diabetes mellitus.
   c. Periodic estimated fetal weight measurements; third-trimester ultrasound measurements are significantly inaccurate.
   d. Avoid postterm deliveries.
   e. Manage labor dystocia in a timely manner.
   f. Promote adequate maternal weight gain.
4. Once shoulder dystocia is identified, the following interventions may be indicated, based on individual clinical conditions and facility protocols:
   a. Call for assistance to support delivery and postpartum management.
   b. Document the delivery of the fetal head.
   c. Document the time shoulder dystocia is called.
5. Perform appropriate nursing maneuvers. Fundal pressure is contraindicated as it may further impact the shoulder.
   a. McRoberts maneuver—exaggerated flexion of the pregnant patient's legs, simulating a supine squat position, which can flatten the sacrum and aid the delivery of fetal shoulder altering the correlation of the maternal spine and pelvis.
   b. Suprapubic pressure—place the heel or palm of one hand over the suprapubic area and press firmly down and to the left or right, as directed by the primary practitioner, to assist in dislodging the anterior shoulder under the maternal pubic bone. Have a step stool available to assist position of staff.
   c. Gaskin maneuver—hands-and-knees position; assist the patient onto hands and knees in an "all-fours" position; it is suspected the anterior shoulder drops posteriorly in this position, releasing the dystocia and resulting in delivery. This may be difficult but obtainable in the patient with epidural anesthesia.
6. Assist with medical maneuvers, if applicable. Although episiotomies are not routinely performed, an episiotomy may be advantageous to assist the provider in performing necessary maneuvers for delivery.
   a. Rotation of the anterior shoulder to oblique position.
   b. Barnum maneuver—delivery of posterior arm across fetal chest.
   c. Rubin technique—displacement of the posterior shoulder anteriorly, with respect to fetus.
   d. Wood screw maneuver—rotation of the shoulders to an oblique position.
   e. Zavanelli maneuver—replacement of the head by reverse cardinal movements into the vagina and delivery by cesarean.
7. Notify staff and provider so they will be available to manage the neonate at delivery.
8. Document throughout the process.
   a. Document time from the delivery of the fetal head to delivery of the body to determine length of shoulder dystocia.
   b. Document all maneuvers performed, time of application, and person(s) performing the intervention(s).
   c. Document postpartum complications and management.
   d. Document newborn initial transition, response, and resuscitation interventions if applicable.
9. Assess newborn carefully, particularly the clavicles, movement of upper extremities, and bruising.

Complications

Fetal

1. Fetal hypoxia and asphyxia.
2. Neonatal hypoxia.
3. Brachial plexus injury.
4. Fractured clavicle or humerus.
5. Facial nerve paralysis.
6. Cognitive deficits.
7. Neonatal death.

Maternal

1. Postpartum hemorrhage.
2. Vaginal lacerations.
3. Cervical lacerations.

Nursing Assessment

1. Continuously evaluate labor curve for signs of dystocia.
2. Maintain EFM until delivery is successful.

Nursing Interventions

Reducing Fear and Anxiety

1. Coach patient on pushing efforts and positioning.
2. Maintain communication, provide support, and answer any questions for patient and family after delivery in a calm and controlled manner.
3. Educate the patient about increased risk for shoulder dystocia in future deliveries.

Decreasing Pain

1. Maintain appropriate anesthesia/analgesia for pain relief during maneuvers.
2. Offer additional anesthesia/analgesia after delivery, as needed or indicated.

Reducing Risk of Injury

1. Provide nursing interventions, assist with medical maneuvers, maintain team communication, and document as outlined previously.

Evaluation: Expected Outcomes

- Verbalizes understanding of the situation; is focused on pushing.
- Pain is controlled
- Absence of maternal or neonatal injury.

Uterine Rupture

EVIDENCE BASE American College of Obstetricians and Gynecologists. (2019). Vaginal birth after cesarean (Clinical Management Guidelines #205). *Obstetrics and Gynecology, 133*(2), e110–e127. https://doi.org/10.1097/AOG.0000000000003078

Uterine rupture is a spontaneous or traumatic tear in the uterus exposing the internal uterine compartment to the peritoneal cavity; extrusion of the umbilical cord, fetus, or fetal parts may occur. *Uterine dehiscence* occurs due to partial separation of an old scar prior to full rupture. Uterine rupture is a rare, catastrophic event with significant risk of maternal, fetal, and neonatal morbidity and mortality.

Pathophysiology and Etiology

Risk factors include:

1. Number of prior cesarean births and scar type (vertical uterine incision).
2. Hydramnios, multifetal gestation, or fetal malpresentation, which cause the uterus to become overdistended.
3. Trial of labor after cesarean (TOLAC). Misoprostol is contraindicated for labor induction/augmentation if patient had a previous cesarean birth.
4. History of uterine rupture.
5. Abdominal trauma.
6. Obstetric maneuvers.

Clinical Manifestations

Clinical manifestations depend on location, size, and duration of rupture. Clinical conditions may evolve rapidly during the intrapartum period requiring immediate interventions. Signs and symptoms may be absent or present individually or collectively as listed below:

1. Constant abdominal pain and tenderness (may be dulled by anesthesia or analgesia).
2. Uterine hypertonus and/or tachysystole.
3. Vaginal or abdominal bleeding into the peritoneal cavity.
4. Nausea/vomiting.
5. Syncope.
6. Hemodynamic instability: early (tachycardia, tachypnea, hypertension); late (signs of shock: rapid, weak pulse); hypotension; cold, clammy skin; pale color.
7. Uteroplacental insufficiency as evidenced by evolving category II or category III FHR patterns.
8. Clinical signs of placental abruption or cord prolapse (sudden onset of FHR variable decelerations).

Management

1. Immediate stabilization of maternal hemodynamics with IV access and fluid replacement.
2. Emergent cesarean delivery. If the uterus cannot be repaired, a hysterectomy may be performed.
3. Manage newborn as condition warrants.
4. Anticipatory preparation should include the risk of significant blood loss and the potential of a massive transfusion protocol (MTP) administration.

Complications

Maternal:

1. Urologic injury.
2. Hysterectomy.
3. Concurrent complete or partial abruptio placentae.
4. Hemorrhage.
5. Hypovolemic shock.
6. Bowel laceration, with possibility of peritonitis.
7. Infection.
8. Death.

Fetal:

1. Hypoxia leading to fetal acidosis and perinatal asphyxia.
2. Hypoxic–ischemic encephalopathy; neonatal brain injury.
3. Death.

Nursing Assessment

1. Continuously evaluate maternal vital signs for clinical triggers of decompensation.
2. Observe for signs and symptoms of impending rupture periodically during labor progression, particularly during vaginal birth after cesarean (VBAC) delivery or a history of uterine surgery (see Box 35-2).
3. Assess fetal status by continuous EFM.

Nursing Interventions

Maintaining Fluid Volume

1. Maintain primary IV line and start a secondary line, as indicated, with lactated Ringer's or normal saline via rapid infusion.
2. Monitor vital signs frequently to observe for maternal decompensation.
3. Monitor central venous access lines, if used, to monitor hemodynamics.
4. Place indwelling urinary catheter and monitor urine output hourly or as indicated.

BOX 35-2 Vaginal Birth After Cesarean

- Selection criteria to identify patients eligible for vaginal birth after cesarean (VBAC):
  - One or two low-transverse cesarean births.
  - Clinically adequate pelvis.
  - No other uterine scars or previous rupture.
  - Primary provider (capable of monitoring labor and performing an emergent cesarean delivery) is immediately available throughout active labor.
  - Anesthesia and surgical team available for emergent cesarean delivery.
- Contraindications for VBAC (because of high risk of uterine rupture):
  - Prior classic or T-shaped incision or other transfundal uterine surgery.
  - Contracted pelvis.
  - Medical or obstetric complication that prevents/precludes vaginal delivery.
  - Inability to perform emergency cesarean delivery because of unavailability of surgeon, anesthesia provider, sufficient personnel, primary provider capable of performing cesarean delivery, or sufficient facility.

5. Administer blood component therapy as prescribed.
6. Monitor for signs of disseminated intravascular coagulation (DIC)—spontaneous bleeding from IV sites, oral mucous membranes, and vagina; bruising.

Maintaining Maternal Vital Organ and Fetal Tissue Perfusion

1. Continually monitor maternal vital signs with oximetry.
2. Maintain continuous EFM to assess fetal status.
3. Administer oxygen via facemask at 8 to 10 L/min, as needed.
4. Monitor arterial blood gas levels, hemoglobin and hematocrit, and serum electrolyte levels, as indicated.
5. Monitor quantitative blood loss (QBL).

Reducing Fear

1. Provide explanation and answer questions of events and procedures to patient and support person.
2. Maintain a quiet and calm atmosphere to enhance relaxation.
3. Communicate with family and debrief them on events, following stabilization of patient and newborn, as Health Insurance Portability and Accountability Act (HIPAA) allows.
4. Provide support if patient and/or fetus do not survive.

Patient Education and Health Maintenance

1. Provide information and support regarding the possibility for future pregnancies.
2. Encourage iron-rich foods and increased protein intake. Iron supplementation should be taken with vitamin C for optimal absorption.
3. Inform patient of the postoperative risk reduction for thrombophlebitis, pneumonia, and infection.
4. Advise on prescribed pain management.
5. Encourage the support of family and provide referral for grief counseling, if needed.

Evaluation: Expected Outcomes

- Vital signs stable; no evidence of shock.
- Hemoglobin and hematocrit stable.
- Verbalizes concerns about self and fetus.

Anaphylactoid Syndrome of Pregnancy

Anaphylactoid syndrome of pregnancy (ASP), also called *amniotic fluid embolism,* is an unpredictable and unpreventable catastrophic event characterized by sudden cardiovascular collapse during the intrapartum or postpartum period. The incidence is estimated as 2 to 8 per 100,000 deliveries with a mortality rate of 8% to 10%. However, those who survive are often left with mild to severe physical and cognitive deficits. If the ASP occurs prior to delivery, outcomes are poor.

Pathophysiology and Etiology

1. The etiology of ASP is unknown. Amniotic fluid and fetal debris (meconium, hair, skin cells) enter the maternal circulation due to a disruption of the placenta–amniotic interface (uterine incision, site of placental attachment, cervical vessels).
2. Once the fluid and debris enter the maternal vasculature, the maternal system may stimulate an immunologic (allergic) response to the foreign substance similar to rejection of a transplanted organ or infusion of the wrong blood type.
3. It is postulated that this immunologic response triggers coagulopathy resulting in DIC (see Figure 35-5).
4. Debris may be large enough to block perfusion through the pulmonary artery, leading to pulmonary hypertension and right-sided heart failure; subsequent left-sided heart failure may ensue, accompanied by hypoxia and acidosis.

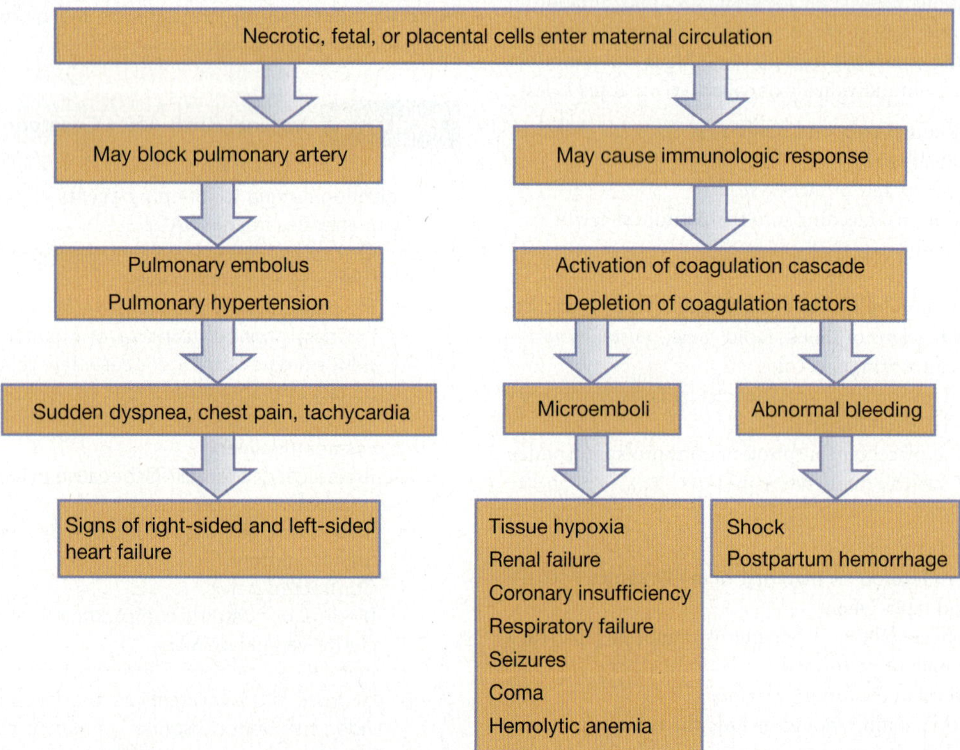

Figure 35-5. Pathogenesis of disseminated intravascular coagulation from amniotic fluid embolism.

5. Although ASP is unpredictable, the following conditions have a higher association to ASP.
   a. Placenta previa.
   b. IOL.
   c. Cesarean delivery.
   d. Preeclampsia/eclampsia.
   e. Multiparity.
   f. Advanced maternal age.
   g. Male fetus.
   h. Trauma.
   i. Abruptio placentae.
   j. Cardiovascular and cerebrovascular disease comorbidities.
   k. Multiple gestations.
   l. Renal disease.
   m. Chorioamnionitis.
   n. Hydramnios.

Clinical Manifestations

1. Sudden dyspnea and chest pain.
2. Cyanosis, tachycardia.
3. Pulmonary edema.
4. Seizures.
5. Increasing restlessness and anxiety.
6. Feeling of impending doom.
7. DIC.
8. Cardiac dysrhythmias.
9. Cardiopulmonary collapse.

Diagnostic Evaluation

1. Clinical picture of sudden onset of respiratory collapse, shock, and cardiopulmonary arrest.
2. DIC confirmed by coagulation studies: prolonged prothrombin time (PT), and partial thromboplastin time (PPT); decreased factors V, VIII, and X; decreased platelets; increased fibrin split products.
3. Pulmonary aspirate evaluation for fetal cells.
4. Autopsy evaluation to confirm fetal cells and debris in maternal pulmonary artery blood.

Management

Also see Disseminated Intravascular Coagulation, page 757.

1. Respiratory support with oxygen therapy and intubation, as necessary.
2. Administration of IV crystalloid fluids in the treatment of shock.
3. Administration of blood component therapy for hemorrhage, shock, and DIC.
4. Central line insertion, if appropriate.
5. Cardiopulmonary resuscitation (CPR) may be necessary; place patient in a wedge position or displace abdomen if undelivered. If the patient requires ongoing CPR, a bedside cesarean delivery may be necessary to enhance maternal vital organ perfusion.
6. A perimortem cesarean delivery should be initiated immediately in the event of maternal cardiopulmonary collapse to maximize maternal and fetal outcomes.

Nursing Assessment and Interventions

See page 758 for additional nursing care.

1. Assess for signs and symptoms of ASP identify patients at risk (see above risk factors).
2. Assess maternal vital signs for signs of shock.
3. Monitor EFM per facility policy if undelivered. Administer oxygen to assist respiratory status.
4. Alert the interprofessional team immediately and assist with emergency procedures, such as delivery and CPR, as needed.
5. Provide information and comfort to the family or support people as the situation allows.

Umbilical Cord Prolapse

Umbilical cord prolapse occurs when the umbilical cord precedes the presenting part of the fetus or lies adjacent to the primary presenting part. Types of cord prolapse include:

Complete—the cord completely and significantly precedes the primary fetal presenting part; may be in the vagina or visible outside the introitus.

Occult—the cord is beside or just in front of the presenting part of the fetus (hidden).

Funic—the cord can be felt on vaginal examination through intact membranes preceding the fetal presenting part.

Pathophysiology and Etiology

Predisposing factors include:

1. Rupture of membranes before the presenting part is engaged in the pelvis.
2. More common in abnormal fetal positions, such as shoulder and foot presentations.
3. Prematurity.
4. Hydramnios.
5. Multifetal gestation.
6. CPD.
7. Abnormally long umbilical cord.
8. Result of interventions or maneuvers (i.e., ECV or amniotomy).
9. Low-lying placenta.

Clinical Manifestations

1. Cord may be seen protruding from vagina or palpated in the vagina or through the cervix.
2. Compression of the cord may cause variable decelerations; prolonged decelerations or bradycardia may develop over time.

CLINICAL JUDGMENT A prolapsed cord should be suspected when an FHR tracing shows prolonged deceleration or bradycardia immediately after spontaneous or AROM. When a prolapsed umbilical cord is identified or suspected, the priority is to reduce pressure on the cord from the fetal presenting part to increased uteroplacental perfusion. Rapid intervention can be facilitated by positioning the patient in the knee–chest or Trendelenburg position or by inserting a gloved hand into the vagina to elevate the presenting fetal part off the cord.

Management

1. Deliver fetus as soon as possible via the most expeditious route.
2. When prolapsed cord is identified, relieve pressure off the umbilical cord by positioning the cord between your two examination fingers and elevating the fetal presenting part up and off the cord.
3. Change maternal positions to potentially alleviate compression (typically knee–chest position or side-lying is adequate).
4. Prepare for emergent delivery.

Complications

Maternal:

1. Infection.
2. Risk of increased perineal trauma from emergency operative delivery.

Fetal:

1. Prematurity.
2. Hypoxia and perinatal asphyxia.
3. Meconium aspiration.
4. Fetal death.

Nursing Assessment and Interventions

1. Observe for variable or prolonged FHR deceleration following spontaneous or AROM.
2. Perform vaginal exam with sterile gloves; if cord is palpated, call for assistance and prepare for emergent delivery. Keep pressure off the cord as described earlier. Do not remove hand from vagina (see Figure 35-6).
3. If lack of additional staff to assist, remove hand and place patient in a Trendelenburg position with buttocks elevated, or turn the patient on all four extremities for a knee–chest position. These positions will help to alleviate pressure on the cord from the fetal head while preparing for emergent delivery.
4. An umbilical cord exposed to room air may exhibit a reflexive constriction of the umbilical blood vessels, further restricting oxygen and blood flow to the fetus. Do not pinch or squeeze the umbilical cord as spasm may occur, decreasing oxygen transport to the fetus.
5. Explain the situation and procedures as much as possible to the patient and support person during this emergent situation.
6. Administer oxygen at 8 to 10 L/min via nonrebreather mask.

Uterine Inversion

Uterine inversion is an unpredictable obstetric complication characterized by collapse of the fundus into the uterine cavity during the third stage of labor (delivery of placenta) that may occur before, during, or after placental detachment. Uterine inversion is a rare occurrence with a greater risk of maternal morbidity and mortality due to hemorrhage and shock. It is important to note that the incidence of uterine inversion has decreased with active management of the third stage of labor with uterotonics (oxytocin).

Uterine inversions may be classified as:

Incomplete—the fundus of uterus inverts but not beyond the cervical os.

Complete—internal lining of the fundus inverts and passes through the cervical os. There is no palpable fundus in the abdomen.

Prolapse—the entire uterus inverts through the cervical os and through the introitus.

Pathophysiology and Etiology

1. The two most common causes are excessive traction (pulling) on the umbilical cord with fundal attachment of the placenta and fundal pressure in the presence of a relaxed uterus. However, most instances of uterine inversion are unpredictable with no identifiable risk factors or cause.
2. Uterine inversion may also be associated with:
   a. Precipitous labor and delivery.
   b. Adherent placenta (accrete or increta).
   c. Placenta previa.
   d. Fundal placentation.
   e. Manual removal of placenta.
   f. Short umbilical cord.
   g. Prolonged labor.
   h. Hydramnios.
   i. Nulliparity.
   j. Fetal macrosomia.
   k. Use of uterine relaxants.
   l. Connective tissue disorders (Marfan syndrome and Ehlers-Danlos syndrome).

Clinical Manifestations

1. Sudden onset of maternal hemorrhage, shock, and hemodynamic instability that may be disproportionate to the amount of blood loss.
2. Severe pelvic pain (regional anesthesia may be necessary to dull pain sensation).

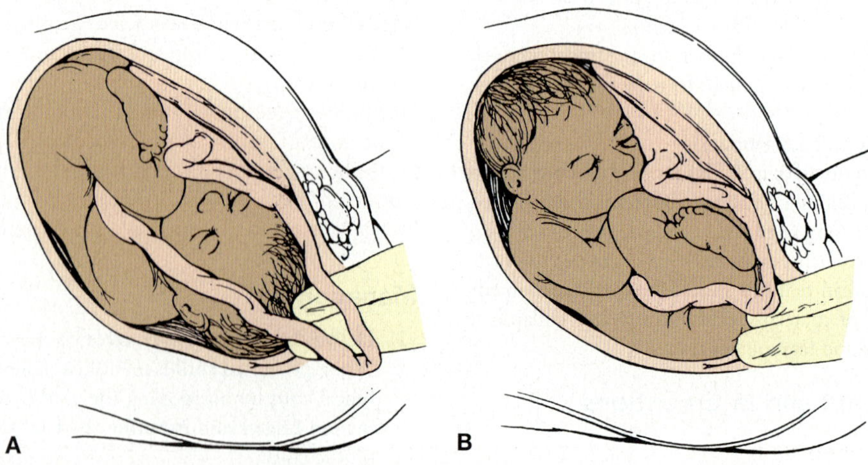

Figure 35-6. Prolapsed cord. Reduction of cord compression using gloved examiner's hand in vagina to elevate presenting part. **(A)** Vertex. **(B)** Breech. (Adapted with permission from Reeder, S., Martin, L., & Koniak-Griffin, D. [1997]. *Maternity nursing: Family newborn, and women's health care* [18th ed.]. Lippincott-Raven Publishers.)

3. Inability to palpate fundus in the abdomen in association with other clinical manifestations.
4. Confirmed with bimanual examination and/or ultrasound.

Management

1. Prevention is the most effective therapy, through active management of the third stage of labor.
2. Immediate identification and interventions are essential, with the goal of manually restoring the uterus to its normal position.
3. The interprofessional team should be assembled immediately for timely intervention.
4. Anesthesia will be needed to complete manual manipulation and to alleviate associated pain.
5. If manipulation is difficult or lengthy, the administration of tocolytics such as terbutaline or magnesium sulfate may be needed.
6. After the uterus has been restored, uterotonic agents (oxytocin, methylergonovine, misoprostol) are administered to maintain uterine contractility.
7. If manual replacement is unsuccessful, surgical intervention may be necessary.

Complications

1. Anemia.
2. Infection.
3. Hemorrhagic shock.
4. DIC.
5. Hysterectomy—loss of fertility.
6. Death.

Nursing Assessment and Interventions

Also see page 937 for additional nursing care.

Before Correction of the Inversion

1. Continuous monitoring for hemodynamic stability of vital signs with pulse oximetry and evaluation of blood loss.
2. Assist health care provider, as needed, for manual replacement.
3. Administer oxygen, as needed.
4. Maintain primary IV line and establish a second line with a 16G or 18G catheter for administration of fluids, blood products, and/or medications. Administer crystalloid solutions (lactated Ringer's and normal saline) to maintain BP.
5. Administer a broad-spectrum antibiotic, as ordered, to prevent infection.
6. If replacement of the uterus is unsuccessful, prepare the patient and support people for surgery.

After Correction of the Inversion

1. Continuously monitor vital signs, and remain alert for signs of hemorrhage and infection.
2. Monitor CBC for anemia related to blood loss as well as coagulation studies for possible DIC.
3. Maintain IV fluid administration as ordered.
4. Administer oxytocin and any additional uterotonic agents as ordered. Note: methylergonovine is contraindicated with hypertensive disorders.
5. Measure accurate QBL by weighing pads.
6. Monitor intake and output.
7. Evaluate fundus carefully for position and tone, avoiding vigorous massage.
8. Maintain indwelling catheter for bladder decompression if ordered.
9. If blood products are administered, evaluate for transfusion reactions (i.e., itching, wheezing, anaphylaxis).
10. Administer antibiotics, as ordered, to minimize risk of infection.
11. Provide support to the patient and encourage expression of feelings.
12. Instruct patient that if future fertility is desired, a cesarean delivery may be necessary because of the potential for recurrence and/or uterine rupture if surgical intervention was required to restore the uterus.

OPERATIVE OBSTETRICS

See additional online content: Procedure Guidelines 35-1

Episiotomy

EVIDENCE BASE American College of Obstetricians and Gynecologists. (2018). *Prevention and management of obstetric lacerations at vaginal delivery* (Practice Bulletin #198). *Obstetrics and Gynecology, 132*(3), e87–e97. https://doi.org/10.1097/AOG.0000000000002841

An *episiotomy* is a surgical incision of the perineum implemented to increase the vaginal opening for delivery of the fetus during the second stage of labor. In the United States, episiotomies occur at a rate of 12% of vaginal births. They are no longer the routine recommendation in current practice. Median or mediolateral episiotomies are generally recommended for such maternal or fetal indications as avoiding severe maternal lacerations and/or expediting the delivery of the fetus under urgent circumstances.

Types of Episiotomies

See Figure 35-7.

Median (Midline)

1. Incision is made midline downward on the perineum toward the anus.
2. This method heals with few complications, is more comfortable for the patient during healing, is easy to repair, and is associated with minimal blood loss and decreased postpartum dyspareunia.
3. Increases the risk of third- and fourth-degree lacerations.

Mediolateral

1. Incision is made at a 45- to 60-degree angle laterally to avoid the anal sphincter musculature.
2. Patients report more discomfort, and healing occurs over a longer time frame.
3. More challenging to repair and associated with increased blood loss.

Management

1. Some research suggests that the application of warm compresses to the perineum and perineal massage during the second stage of labor has demonstrated a reduction in third- and fourth-degree lacerations.

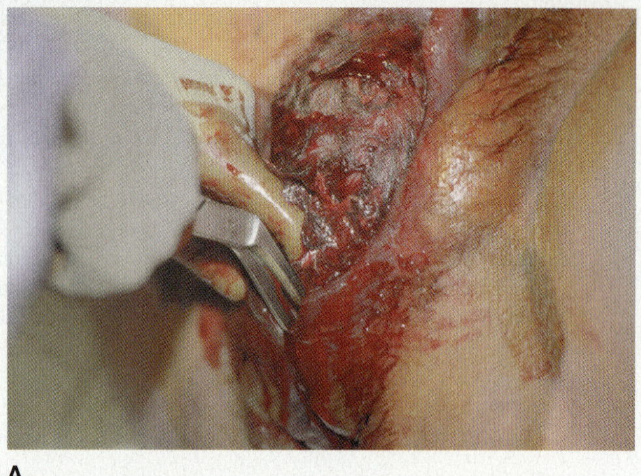

A

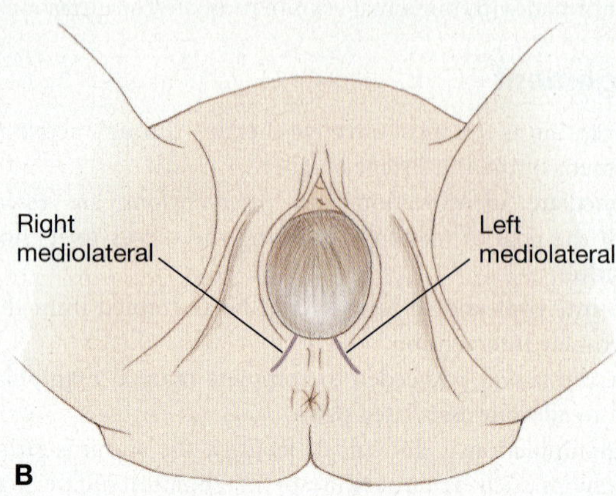

B

Figure 35-7. Location of an episiotomy. **(A)** Midline episiotomy. **(B)** Right and left mediolateral episiotomies. (Reprinted with permission from Ricci, S. S. [2021]. *Essentials of maternity, newborn, and women's health nursing* [5th ed., Fig. 14-14]. Wolters Kluwer.)

2. Pain relief.
   a. The stretching of the perineum and pressure from the fetal head during the second stage of labor may provide a natural numbing effect.
   b. Local perineal infiltration with lidocaine provides anesthesia for performing and repairing the episiotomy.
   c. A pudendal block provides anesthesia to the lower two thirds of the perineum and vagina using lidocaine injection into the vaginal walls.
   d. Epidural anesthesia provides anesthesia from the level of the umbilicus to the midthigh area.
3. An episiotomy is performed when the fetal head is 3 to 4 cm visible with a contraction.

Complications

1. Infection.
2. Bleeding.
3. Third- and fourth-degree lacerations.
4. Pain.
5. Hematoma.
6. Dyspareunia (painful intercourse).

Nursing Assessment

1. During the recovery period, inspect and assess the episiotomy periodically.
2. Describe and document the degree of healing.
3. Assess for signs of infection: edema, redness, purulent drainage at the site, and/or increased temperature.
4. Monitor for hematoma formation.

Nursing Interventions

Preventing Infection

1. Explain the importance of proper handwashing before and after perineal care.
2. Provide instructions on perineal care.
   a. Provide a peri bottle; teach patient to squirt warm water gently on the perineum after voiding or defecating.
   b. Direction of flow of water should be from front to back.
   c. Gently blot dry from front to back.
3. Instruct patient to change the perineal pad after any urination and defecation; dispose of in proper biohazard receptacle.
4. Notify health care provider of signs of infection or excessive bleeding at site.
5. Encourage a diet that is high in fiber, protein, and vitamin C and encourage hydration.

Promoting Comfort

1. Apply covered ice packs to the perineal area for the first 24 hours after delivery. The ice packs should not remain in place longer than 20 minutes at a time to get the maximum benefit from the treatment.
2. Encourage sitz baths with either warm or cool water.
3. Administer or teach self-administration of pain medication and topical anesthetics, as ordered.
4. Remind patient to sit on one buttock and roll gently to a full sitting position to avoid discomfort from the ice pack.
5. Encourage isometric exercises (Kegel) as tolerated to strengthen perineal floor.
6. Instruct patient to abstain from sexual intercourse until healing is complete, typically 4 to 6 weeks. Encourage the use of lubricants as needed.

Evaluation: Expected Outcomes

- No evidence of infection.
- Verbalizes increase in comfort.

Operative Vaginal Delivery: Forceps

Obstetric forceps (see Table 35-4) are used to facilitate delivery of the fetal head during the second stage and expedite a safe vaginal delivery when indicated for maternal and fetal health. Most forceps are placed on each side of the fetal vertex and others are utilized for special considerations (pipers: vaginal breech birth). Forceps consist of two pieces: a right blade, which is slipped into the right side of the patient's pelvis, and a left blade, which is slipped into the left side. Forceps increase the diameter of the presenting part and may hinder delivery. Special training and skill are required.

Table 35-4 Representative Types of Forceps

MAJOR CLASSIFICATIONS	USE
Simpson—separated shanks	
(e.g., DeLee forceps)	Extract fetus with elongated, molded head; commonly used with nulliparas who have long labors
Elliot—overlapping shanks	
(e.g., Tucker-McLean)	Extract fetus with unmolded, rounder heads; commonly used with multiparas who have briefer labors
Specialized types	
Piper	Deliver aftercoming head in a breech presentation
Kielland	Rotate head from transverse or posterior position to an anterior position; used with patients with anthropoid pelvises
Barton	Rotate head from transverse to an anterior position; designed for use in patients with flat pelvises

There are more than 600 types of forceps.

Types of Forceps Deliveries

American College of Obstetricians and Gynecologists (ACOG) definitions for obstetric forceps:

Outlet Forceps

1. Scalp is visible at the introitus without separating labia.
2. Fetal skull has reached pelvic floor.
3. Sagittal suture in anteroposterior diameter or right or left occiput anterior or posterior position.
4. Fetal head is at or on perineum.
5. Rotation does not exceed 45 degrees.

Low Forceps

1. Leading point of fetal skull is at station +2 cm or above and not on the pelvic floor.
   a. Rotation is less than 45 degrees (left or right occiput anterior to occiput anterior or left or right occiput posterior to occiput posterior).
   b. Rotation is greater than 45 degrees.

Indications for Forceps Delivery

1. The fetal head must be engaged and the cervix fully dilated.
2. Suspicion of immediate or potential fetal compromise.
3. Shortening of the second stage of labor for maternal or fetal benefit.
4. Prolonged second-stage labor.
   a. Nulliparous patient: lack of progress for 3 hours with regional anesthesia or 2 hours without regional anesthesia.
   b. Multiparous patient: lack of progress for 2 hours with regional anesthesia or 1 hour without regional anesthesia.
5. Category II or III fetal heart rate (FHR) pattern and clinical judgment of provider.
6. Maternal cardiac or neurologic disease.

Contraindications

1. Malpresentations: face or brow presentation.
2. Incomplete dilation of the cervix.
3. Unengaged fetal head.
4. Gestational age less than 34 weeks.
5. Live fetus with bone demineralization.
6. Fetal coagulopathies.
7. Inexperience of practitioner or unavailable operative personnel.

Management

1. Lithotomy position is achieved and the bladder must be emptied (urinary catheter is generally used).
2. Local or regional anesthesia may be used.
3. Neonatal staff in attendance at delivery.
4. An episiotomy should not be routinely performed for an operative delivery.
5. Each blade is placed bilaterally over the fetal ear, avoiding the face.
6. Gentle traction is administered in a downward motion with maternal expulsion efforts during contractions.

Complications

Maternal

1. Perineal trauma: lacerations of the vulva, cervix, vagina, and rectum; coccyx fracture.
2. Extensions of an episiotomy into the rectum: fourth-degree laceration.
3. Bladder trauma, uterine rupture.
4. Postpartum infection, postpartum hemorrhage secondary to uterine atony.
5. Anemia secondary to uterine atony/hemorrhage.
6. Urinary or fecal incontinence; fistula formation.

Fetal

1. Bruising.
2. Cephalohematoma.
3. Nerve injuries.
4. Facial lacerations and facial nerve palsy.
5. Skull fracture.
6. Ocular trauma.
7. Intracranial hemorrhage.

Nursing Assessment

1. After application of forceps, the FHR should be evaluated frequently per facility policy until delivery.

Nursing Interventions

Decreasing Anxiety

1. Provide education and support for the patient and support person when use of a vaginal assisted birth is expected.
2. Explain that a sensation of pressure will be felt.
3. Stay with the patient and provide guidance during the delivery process.
4. Prepare for delivery and possible neonatal resuscitation.
5. Assemble additional team members for immediate assistance for patient and infant.
6. Document placement, time, and number of pulls required to deliver the fetal head.
7. Keep the delivery provider apprised of FHR status through the delivery process.

Promoting Comfort

1. Encourage use of breathing and relaxation techniques.
2. Make sure indwelling catheter is draining and that bladder is completely empty.
3. Encourage relaxation between contractions and use of abdominal muscles and pushing with the contractions.
4. Use blankets and pillows for support when positioning the patient for delivery.

Evaluation: Expected Outcomes

- Verbalizes concerns regarding forceps; responds to instructions.
- Demonstrates increased level of comfort.

Vacuum Extraction

Vacuum extraction applies suction to the fetal vertex, which is slowly increased to assist in delivery. Advantages include ease of application with a decrease in intensity to the fetal vertex. It is also associated with less maternal trauma, decreased injuries to fetus, and less need for general or regional anesthesia.

Indications

1. Same as forceps.

Contraindications

1. Same as forceps.

Management

1. Fetus is in vertex presentation.
2. Fetus should not be below 34 weeks' gestation.
3. The patient is in the lithotomy position.
4. The bladder is emptied by catheterization.
5. Pressure is applied during contractions and released between contractions. Fetal descent should occur with maternal expulsion efforts during uterine contraction.
6. Anesthesia may be indicated.
7. Unsuccessful extraction is followed by a cesarean delivery.
8. Neonatal staff is in attendance at delivery.

Complications

Complications are usually less frequent and less severe with vacuum extraction than with forceps.

Maternal

1. Lacerations of the cervix or vagina.
2. Pain.
3. Infection.
4. Bladder trauma.
5. Hemorrhage.

Fetal

1. Cephalohematoma.
2. Caput succedaneum (swelling of the scalp) from the vacuum.
3. Intracranial hemorrhage.
4. Retinal hemorrhage.
5. Abrasions and lacerations to scalp.
6. Subgaleal (scalp) hemorrhage with hematoma formation.

Nursing Assessment

1. After application of the vacuum extractor, the FHR should be assessed frequently per facility policy until delivery.
2. Evaluate maternal sensation.
3. Monitor the vacuum pressure of the equipment according to your facility's protocol and document maternal–fetal response during procedure.
4. Monitor "pop-offs" (vacuum extractor cup pops off the fetal head) and vacuum applications; if three pop-offs have occurred or greater than 20 minutes have passed, other options should be considered.

Nursing Interventions

Same as for forceps delivery, pages 1060–1062.

Cesarean Delivery

Cesarean delivery is the surgical removal of the fetus from the uterus through an abdominal and uterine incision. The overall cesarean birth rate in the United States is comprised of both primary and repeat cesarean deliveries and was 32.1% in 2021. Recent trends demonstrate an increase in the primary cesarean rate and a decline in repeat cesarean deliveries. The decision to perform a cesarean section is determined to optimize maternal and neonatal outcomes. ACOG recommends the fetal gestational age of 39 weeks be confirmed prior to an elective cesarean delivery.

Types of Cesarean Delivery

Uterine Incisions

Incision choice is based on the clinical scenario and future fertility.

1. Low transverse—transverse incision made across the lower uterine segment.
   a. First-line choice of incision in most clinical scenarios.
   b. Incision is made across the thickest section and away from uterine activity (fundus); minimizes blood loss and improves the integrity of the scar, decreasing risk of future dehiscence or rupture.
   c. Incidence of postoperative adhesions and danger of intestinal obstruction are reduced.
2. Classic or vertical incision from the fundus down the body of the uterus to the lower uterine segment; may be utilized for emergent or preterm deliveries.
   a. Useful when bladder and lower segment are involved in extensive adhesions.
   b. Surgery of choice with a diagnosed anterior placenta previa, which inhibits the use of the low-transverse incision.
   c. Increased blood loss versus low transverse.
   d. Increased risk of uterine rupture in subsequent deliveries.

Indications for Cesarean Delivery

1. Maternal medical complications, such as asthma, chronic hypertension, diabetes, cardiac disease, and active herpes infection.
2. Labor complications: dystocia, malpresentation, cephalopelvic disproportion (CPD), category II or III FHR pattern, prolonged or arrest of first or second stage of labor, early labor induction prior to cervical ripening.
3. Obstetric complications: placenta previa, breech, elective induction of nulliparous (50% higher risk than spontaneous labor).
4. Possible indications for cesarean hysterectomy:
   a. Ruptured uterus.
   b. Intrauterine infection.
   c. Postpartum hemorrhage: unresponsive to conservative management options.

d. Laceration of major uterine vessel.
e. Severe dysplasia or carcinoma in situ of the cervix.
f. Placenta accreta.
g. Gross multiple fibromyomas.
h. Uterine inversion unresponsive to manual replacement.

Management

Preoperative

1. Surgery should be delayed for 8 hours following last meal unless emergent.
2. Complete blood count (CBC), blood type and screen, and additional laboratory work based on the patient's clinical presentation should be obtained.
3. Anesthesia, regional or general, depends on indication for surgery.
4. Informed consents signed and witnessed.
5. A large-gauge intravenous (IV) is established with lactated Ringer's (LR). Bolus (1,000 mL) is administered prior to regional anesthesia.
6. Indwelling urinary catheter is placed, often after anesthesia to minimize discomfort.
7. Antacid is given orally to reduce gastric acidity, limiting complications should aspiration occur.
8. Pubic hair may be clipped downward toward the mons pubis prior to the incision per provider and facility guidelines.
9. Antimicrobial wash (usually chlorhexidine) is used per facility protocol to cleanse the incision area.
10. Vaginal preparation with antiseptic solution has been shown to reduce endometritis, especially if membranes are ruptured.

EVIDENCE BASE Haas, D. M., Morgan, S., Contreras, K., & Kimball, S. (2020). Vaginal preparation with antiseptic solution before cesarean section for preventing postoperative infections. *Cochrane Database of Systematic Reviews*, (4), Article CD007892. https://doi.org/10.1002/14651858.CD007892.pub7

11. Prophylactic antibiotic therapy to decrease surgical site infection (SSI) per facility guidelines.

Intraoperative

1. Patient is moved to the operating room and time documented.
2. Application of pneumatic compression devices is recommended.
3. Grounding pad applied per manufacturer's instructions.
4. Application of monitors (cardiorespiratory).
5. Facility verification process is completed prior to beginning of procedure, including "Time Out" per facility policy.
6. Lower abdominal cleansing with the United States Food and Drug Administration (FDA)–approved antiseptic agent, such as isopropyl alcohol, based on provider preference and facility policy. May be done by provider or designated personnel.
7. Instrument, needle/knife, and lap pad counts should be performed periodically: before, during, and after surgery.
8. Neonatal resuscitation equipment should be readily accessible and radiant warmers preheated.
9. Receive newborn and perform neonatal assessment; maintain asepsis.
10. Encourage skin-to-skin contact with the patient, which is recommended once the neonate is stable.
11. Provide hand-off communication per facility policy.

Postoperative

In addition to routine postoperative recovery room care (see page 59), fundal checks must be performed as with the fourth stage of labor (page 984).

Complications

1. Hemorrhage.
2. Endometritis.
3. Paralytic ileus (intestinal obstruction).
4. Pulmonary embolism.
5. Thrombophlebitis.
6. Anesthesia complications.
7. Bowel or bladder injury.
8. Incisional hernia.
9. Wound dehiscence.
10. Potential for placenta previa or uterine rupture with future pregnancy.
11. Respiratory depression of the infant from anesthetic drugs.
12. Possible delay in caregiver–infant bonding.

Nursing Assessment

Before Delivery

1. Assess patient's knowledge of procedure; assess feelings and clear up misconceptions.
2. Perform admission assessment.
3. Obtain 20- to 30-minute fetal tracing strip to assess fetal and uterine status.
4. Obtain maternal vital signs.
5. Identify drug allergies; identify other allergies (e.g., latex, iodine, tape).

After Delivery (also see Chapter 33)

1. Assess maternal vital signs every 15 minutes the first 2 hours or more frequently as the patient's condition warrants.
   a. Respiratory status: airway patency, oxygen needs, rate/quality/depth of respirations, auscultation of breath sounds, oxygen saturation readings.
   b. Circulation: blood pressure (BP), pulse, electrocardiogram monitoring for assessing dysrhythmias, color; assess dressing for drainage.
   c. Level of consciousness (LOC): orientation and response to verbal/tactile/painful stimulation.
2. Assess mobility and sensation of extremities if regional anesthesia is used.
3. Assess postpartum status (same intervals for assessment): fundal position and contractions, condition of incision and abdominal dressing, maternal–neonatal attachment, lochia (color, amount), neonate condition (if applicable), feeding preferences.
4. Assess hourly intake and output and reestablishment of bowel sounds.
5. Perform pain assessment: evaluate the level of anesthesia, medications given (amount/time/results).
6. Assess knowledge and performance of breastfeeding.

Nursing Interventions

Relieving Anxiety

1. Explain the purpose of all interventions and answer questions.
2. Allow the support person to attend the birth, if appropriate.

Promoting Comfort

1. Encourage use of relaxation techniques after medication has been given for pain.

2. Monitor for respiratory depression up to 24 hours after epidural opioid administration.
3. Monitor and instruct patient on the use of a patient-controlled anesthesia pump, as applicable.
4. Use a backrub and a quiet environment to promote the effectiveness of the medication.
5. Support and splint the abdominal incision when moving or coughing and deep breathing.
6. Encourage frequent rest periods.
7. To reduce pain caused by gas, encourage ambulation or use of a rocking chair.
8. Administer pain medications (opioids, nonsteroidal anti-inflammatory drugs [NSAIDs], acetaminophen) as ordered. Research demonstrates a decrease in opioid use when nonopioid analgesics such as NSAIDs and acetaminophen are scheduled at regular intervals around the clock.

DRUG ALERT Do not administer parenteral opioids if patient is receiving epidural opioids unless ordered by the anesthesia provider.

Preventing Infection and Other Complications

1. Adhere to appropriate hand hygiene.
2. Establish protocol to decrease surgical site infection per national guidelines.
3. Maintain sterile technique during surgery and use sterile technique when changing dressings postoperatively.
4. Monitor vital signs and report tachycardia and hyperthermia, which may indicate infection.
5. Provide perineal care every 4 hours or as needed.
6. Remove urinary catheter per provider or facility protocol as soon as possible. Provide catheter care per facility protocol.
7. Utilize incentive spirometer for deep breathing and coughing every hour while awake.
8. Implement pneumatic compression devices and anticoagulation therapy per provider order.
9. Encourage early ambulation.

Promoting Effective Family Unit

1. Encourage neonate bonding and skin-to-skin contact as soon as possible.
2. Emphasize the positive outcomes of the operative delivery—safe delivery to avoid maternal/fetal complications.
3. Provide patient education and family time as tolerated by the postpartum patient.
4. Emphasize to patient that adjustments under any circumstances are necessary and normal.
5. Encourage partner participation until patient can assist in newborn care.

Patient Education and Health Maintenance

1. Teach and assist the patient with breastfeeding positioning; "football hold" alleviates pressure on the abdominal incision.
2. Teach incisional care per facility policy and instruct to observe for signs of infection (foul-smelling lochia, elevated temperature, increased pain, redness, and edema at the incision site) and to report them immediately through 12 weeks' postpartum.
3. Assist the patient in managing expectations and encourage openness to assistance from friends and family during the immediate postpartum period.
4. Encourage a diet of iron-rich foods, fiber, protein, and fluids. The patient should continue taking prenatal vitamins. Iron supplementation may be necessary. Increase calories by 300 to 500 calories if breastfeeding.
5. Encourage rest periods.

Evaluation: Expected Outcomes

- Verbalizes an understanding of the cesarean delivery procedure and postdelivery care.
- Vital signs normal, no signs of infection.
- Reports ability to care for self and neonate.

POSTPARTUM COMPLICATIONS

Postpartum Infection

Postpartum (puerperal) infection should be suspected if the patient's temperature exceeds 100°F (37.8°C) on two occasions at least 6 hours apart during the first 10 days postpartum. This fever is exclusive of the first 24 hours postpartum. The infection may be localized or extend to various parts of the body such as connective tissue by lymphatic dissemination (parametritis). The broad ligament is the main pathway for systemic infection.

Pathophysiology and Etiology

The most common cause of puerperal infection is ascending bacteria to the uterus from the lower genital tract.

1. Types of infection include:
   a. Endometritis: inflammation of the endometrium.
   b. Endomyometritis: inflammation of the endometrium and myometrium.
   c. Parametritis: inflammation of the endometrium and parametrial tissue.
2. Other infections include:
   a. Wound.
   b. Cystitis, urinary tract.
   c. Pneumonia.
   d. Mastitis.
   e. Pelvic thrombophlebitis.
   f. Necrotizing fasciitis.
3. Risk factors:
   a. Operative birth.
   b. Prolonged labor or rupture of membranes.
   c. Use of invasive procedures (i.e., internal monitoring, amnioinfusion).
   d. Multiple pelvic examinations.
   e. Excessive blood loss.
   f. Pyelonephritis or diabetes.
   g. Socioeconomic and nutritional factors compromising host defense mechanisms.
   h. Anemia and systemic illness.
   i. Smoking.
   j. Mastitis-specific risk factors: infrequent breastfeeding, incomplete breast emptying, plugged milk duct, cracked or bleeding nipples (may be secondary to improper latch-on and removal).

Clinical Manifestations

Endometritis Postpartum

1. Fever occurring around third day postpartum is the most important finding.
2. Uterus usually larger than expected for postdelivery day and tender.

3. Lochia may be profuse, bloody, and foul-smelling.
4. Chills, malaise, and fever occur if lochial discharge is obstructed by clots.
5. White blood cells (WBCs) greater than 20,000/mm^3 with increased neutrophils.
6. Infection may spread to myometrium (endomyometritis), parametrium, fallopian tubes, peritoneum, and blood.

Parametritis (Pelvic Cellulitis)

1. Chills, fever (38.9°C to 40°C [102°F to 104°F]), tachycardia.
2. Severe unilateral or bilateral pain in lower abdomen.
3. Enlarged, tender uterus.
4. Uterine position may become fixed as it is displaced by the exudate along the broad ligament.

Diagnostic Evaluation and Management

1. Obtain urinalysis and urine culture to rule out urinary tract infection (UTI).
2. Obtain blood sample for complete blood count (CBC) with differential and report results; assess for leukocytosis more than 20,000/mm^3.
3. Antibiotic therapy: obtain cultures to identify causative agent prior to administration of broad-spectrum antibiotics including penicillins, cephalosporins (cefoxitin, cefazolin), clindamycin, and aminoglycosides (gentamicin, tobramycin). Antibiotics are given until the patient is afebrile for 48 hours (maternal response usually occurs within 48 to 72 hours) and may include home therapy. Stress the importance of completing the full course of antibiotics.
4. Increase daily fluid intake.
5. Encourage increased intake of 300 to 500 calories if lactating; diet should include a variety of foods, usually high in protein, iron, and vitamin C to promote wound healing.
6. Encourage hydration and ensure adequate urine output (30 mL/h).

Complications

1. Thrombophlebitis may result from a venous postpartum infection or immobility.
   a. Femoral thrombophlebitis—appears 10 to 20 days after delivery as pain in calf, fever, edema; affected leg circumference is 2 cm greater than unaffected leg.
   b. Pelvic thrombophlebitis—infection of the veins of uterine wall and broad ligament usually caused by anaerobic streptococci; presents 14 days after delivery with severe chills and wide range of temperature changes.
   c. Treatment may include bed rest, compression stockings anticoagulants, and antibiotics.
2. Pulmonary embolus may occur—respiratory distress and chest pain.
3. Peritonitis—spread of infection through lymphatic channels.

Nursing Assessment

1. Perform postpartum assessment: note uterine tenderness on palpation and the color, amount, and odor of lochia; assess for proper breastfeeding techniques.
2. Monitor vital signs for signs of infection.
3. Monitor ordered laboratory work and report abnormalities to provider.

Nursing Interventions

Restoring Normothermia

1. Stress importance of adequate hand hygiene.
2. Provide for adequate rest periods.
3. Increase fluid intake to make up for insensible loss.
4. Position in high-Fowler position to promote drainage.
5. Administer or teach self-administration of antibiotics and analgesics, as ordered.
6. Explain importance of pericare; proper cleaning (front to back) after voiding or defecation, and changing peripads after every occurrence.
7. Observe for signs of septic shock: severe tachycardia, hypotension, tachypnea, changes in level of consciousness (LOC), and decreased urine output. Report to interprofessional team.

Promoting Infant Attachment

1. Encourage minimal separation from the neonate and continuation of breastfeeding, as able.
2. Promote hand hygiene for the patient before contact with the neonate.
3. Encourage partner and family participation in care of patient/baby unit.

Evaluation

- Afebrile, tolerating antibiotics well, using good hand hygiene.
- Bonding time uninterrupted.

Postpartum Hemorrhage

Postpartum hemorrhage (PPH), also known as *obstetric hemorrhage (OH),* reflects a blood loss of greater than 1,000 mL regardless of method of delivery and is the primary cause of maternal morbidity and mortality worldwide. Blood loss of greater than 500 mL with vaginal delivery should be considered abnormal and warrants further evaluation. Primary PPH occurs in the first 24 hours; secondary occurs after 24 hours up until 12 weeks after birth. The greatest risk is during the first hour following delivery. Hemorrhage may also be defined as a decrease in hematocrit of at least 10%, but determinations of hemoglobin and hematocrit concentrations may not reflect current hematologic status.

EVIDENCE BASE American College of Obstetricians and Gynecologists. (2022). Quantitative blood loss in obstetric hemorrhage (Committee Opinion #794). *Obstetrics and Gynecology, 134*(6), e151–e156. https://doi.org/10.1097/AOG.0000000000003564

Association of Women's Health, Obstetric and Neonatal Nurses. (2021). Quantification of blood loss: AWHONN Practice Brief Number 13. *Nursing for Women's Health, 25*(4), e5–e7. https://doi.org/10.1016/j.nwh.2021.04.005

Pathophysiology and Etiology

Excessive bleeding from a point between the uterus and perineum (see Table 35-5).

Primary PPH

1. Uterine atony (80% of cases) is the main cause of PPH and is defined as the relaxation of the uterus secondary to:
   a. Overdistention of uterus secondary to multiple pregnancy, hydramnios, and/or macrosomia.
   b. High parity (greater than six pregnancies).
   c. Prolonged labor.
   d. Medications—oxytocin, magnesium sulfate, tocolytics, anesthetics.
   e. Fibroids—space occupying preventing the uterus from contracting.

Table 35-5 Factors Placing a Patient at Risk for Postpartum Hemorrhage

CLINICAL RISK FACTORS	ASSOCIATED CLINICAL CONDITIONS
Tone (abnormalities of uterine contractions)	
Overdistention of uterus	Polyhydramnios Multifetal gestation Macrosomia
Uterine muscle exhaustion	Rapid labor Prolonged labor Oxytocin use
Uterine infection	Maternal fever Prolonged rupture of membranes
Tissue (retained in uterus)	
Products of conception	Incomplete placenta at birth
Retained blood clots	Atonic uterus
Trauma (of the genital tract)	
Lacerations anywhere	Precipitate birth or operative birth
Laceration extensions	Malposition of fetus Previous uterine surgery
Uterine inversion	Forceful pulling when placenta isn't separated yet; traction on the cord when uterus isn't contracted
Thrombin (coagulation abnormalities)	
Preexisting conditions	Hereditary inheritance Hemophilia von Willebrand disease History of previous PPH Acquired in pregnancy Idiopathic thrombocytopenia purpura Bruising, elevated blood pressure Disseminated intravascular coagulation
Traction on umbilical cord	Strong traction placed on umbilical cord prior to its separation from the uterine wall may lead to hemorrhage

PPH, postpartum hemorrhage.
Source: Ricci, S. (2021). Essentials of maternity, newborn, and women's health nursing (5th ed., Table 22.2). Wolters Kluwer; Centers for Disease Control and Prevention. (2019). What is von Willebrand disease? Retrieved June 16, 2020, from https://www.cdc.gov/ncbddd/vwd/facts.html; Kadir, R. A., James, P. D., & Lee, C. A. (2019). Inherited bleeding disorders in women (2nd ed.). John Wiley & Sons; and Smith, J. R. (2019). Postpartum hemorrhage treatment and management. eMedicine. Retrieved June 27, 2018, from https://emedicine.medscape.com/article/275038-treatment#d10

f. Retained placental fragments—result from manual removal of placenta, succenturiate (additional) lobe, abnormally adherent placenta (placenta accreta), or spontaneous Duncan placenta delivery (periphery detaches first instead of central detachment).

2. Uterine inversion.
3. Coagulopathies (e.g., disseminated intravascular coagulation [DIC]).
4. Trauma, laceration, or hematomas of the vagina, cervix, or perineum secondary to:
   a. Forceps delivery, especially rotation forceps.
   b. Macrosomia.
   c. Multiple gestation.
5. Prolonged third stage of labor; aggressive fundal manipulation or cord traction.
6. Chorioamnionitis; sepsis.
7. Uterine rupture.
8. Uterine inversion.
9. Other risk factors include augmented or induced labor, rapid labor, history of PPH, preeclampsia, or Asian or Hispanic ethnicity.

Secondary PPH

1. Retained placental fragments is the main cause of secondary PPH.
2. Infection.
3. Subinvolution (delayed healing) of placental site.

Clinical Manifestations

Primary PPH

1. Uterine atony—uterus is soft or boggy, usually difficult to palpate, and will not remain contracted leading to excessive vaginal bleeding.
2. Lacerations of the vagina, cervix, or perineum cause bright red, continuous bleeding even when the fundus is firm.
3. Tachycardia, hypotension, dizziness, pallor, and decreased urine output occur after loss of 10% total blood volume.

Secondary PPH

1. Uterus is soft or boggy.
2. Slow, oozing, or heavy rubra bleeding (first 6 weeks postdelivery).
3. Low persistent backache.
4. Abdominal pain or tenderness.
5. Fatigue.
6. Loss of appetite.

CLINICAL JUDGMENT It is estimated that approximately 50% of deaths from a PPH were preventable and the result of ineffective medical management. Early assessment, identification, and intervention in the event of a PPH is essential to improving obstetric outcomes.

Management

The goals of treatment are to stop hemorrhage by alleviating the cause, correct hypovolemia, and return maternal hemostasis. These goals are accomplished through identification of risk factors with early identification and treatment of the underlying cause of PPH. Visual estimates of blood loss are frequently imprecise and inaccurate, delaying diagnosis and treatment.

1. Prompt notification and communication to the interprofessional team, including anesthesia provider, primary care provider, nursing and operating room personnel, as indicated by the patient's condition.
2. Continue fundal massage and bimanual massage if indicated.
3. Maintain IV access with lactated Ringer's infusion and add a secondary line with 16G to 18G catheter for severe loss.
4. Obtain ordered laboratory work (CBC, type and screen, cross-match). For each 450 to 500 mL of blood loss, there will be a decrease in the hematocrit of 2% to 4% and a decrease in the hemoglobin of 1 to 1.5 g/dL.
5. Notify blood bank, as indicated; order 4 to 6 units, as needed.

POPULATION AWARENESS When anticipating administration of blood products or transfusions, it is important to recognize that some patients may decline them based on religious beliefs. It is important to identify the patient's cultural and religious practices upon admission and communicate to the interprofessional team.

6. Administer medications, as ordered.
   a. Administration of oxytocin, IV or intramuscularly (IM), is first-line therapy for uterine atony; however, if ineffective to control bleeding, anticipate the need for additional medications to treat PPH:
   b. Methylergonovine 0.2 mg IM every 2 to 4 hours for sustained uterine contraction (contraindicated in patients with hypertension, Raynaud syndrome, scleroderma).
   c. Misoprostol 800 to 1,000 mcg per rectum (single dose); may cause fever, tachycardia, and rigors.
   d. Carboprost tromethamine 0.25 mg IM every 15 to 90 minutes (8 dose maximum)—contraindicated in patients with asthma, active cardiac, hepatic, or renal disease; may cause fever, chills, nausea, vomiting, diarrhea.
   e. Tranexamic acid (TXA) (antifibrinolytic agent) 1 g (100 mg/mL) IV at 1 mL/min. If bleeding continues after 30 min or medication is stopped and restarted within 24 h of the first dose, a second dose of 1 g can be given.
      i. Adverse effects include seizures, headaches, backache, abdominal pain, nausea, vomiting, diarrhea, fatigue, pulmonary embolism, deep vein thrombosis, anaphylaxis, impaired color vision, and other visual disturbances.
      ii. Contraindications: intracranial bleeding, known defective color vision, history of venous or arterial thromboembolism, or active thromboembolic disease.
7. In the presence of continuous bleeding and a firm uterus, notify the provider for evaluation and possible intervention.
   a. Repair of lacerations, transfusion of blood products, dilation and curettage, B-lynch suture, uterine tamponade, and selective arterial embolization.
   b. Intrauterine balloon tamponade using, for example, the Bakri SOS (surgical obstetric silicone) to control bleeding (see Figure 35-8).

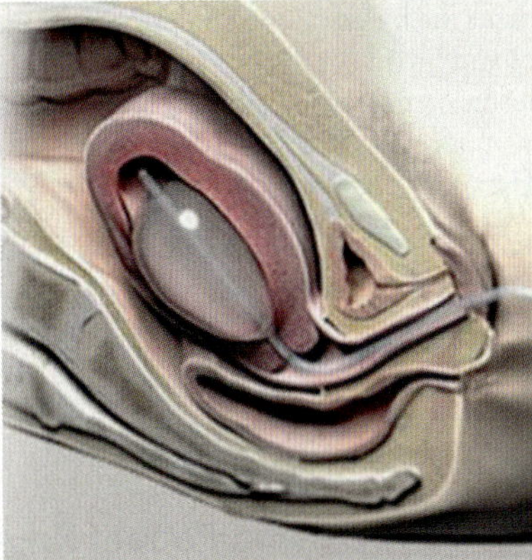

Figure 35-8. The Bakri SOS provides balloon tamponade to stop postpartum hemorrhage. SOS, surgical obstetric silicone.

      i. About 250 to 500 mL of saline is introduced into the balloon to maintain pressure against the uterine walls. Pooled blood above the balloon is removed through the drainage port of the catheter.
      ii. Vaginal packing is also placed to increase the tamponade effect on the lower uterine segment, and a urinary catheter is placed for bladder drainage.
8. Opioid analgesics may be needed for pain control.
9. Emergency hysterectomy may be necessary.

Complications

1. Hypovolemic shock.
2. Hysterectomy.
3. Death.

Nursing Assessment

1. Assess patient for known PPH risk factors, plan accordingly, and communicate to the perinatal team.
2. Document quantitative blood loss (QBL) during the postpartum period. See Box 35-3 for blood loss estimates.
3. Evaluate for presence of clots expelled or passed during voiding; note number of pads saturated in 1 hour or shorter time frame, if applicable. Weigh pads, as necessary, to determine loss.
4. Assess vital signs, pulse pressure, and oxygen saturation per facility policy and increase assessments if the patient shows signs of instability—tachycardia, hypotension, pallor, diaphoresis, altered LOC, tachypnea, nausea and vomiting, feelings of impending doom; all may indicate hypovolemic shock.
   a. Normal vital signs are not an indication that the patient is *not* in shock. Traditional signs of hypovolemic shock are not evident until approximately 15% to 20% of total maternal blood volume is lost.
   b. Continuous blood pressure (BP) monitor readings may falsely lower diastolic and raise systolic readings. Assessments more frequent than 2 minutes apart may not allow for reperfusion of the vessels within the extremity.

BOX 35-3 Estimation of Blood Loss

Accurate evaluation of blood loss is critical to maternal outcomes. Studies validate the inaccuracy of blood loss estimation with visual inspection. The use of under buttock drapes to collect blood loss during delivery has been valuable in improving the ability to measure blood loss during childbirth. Estimation by weight using a scale is desirable. Follow these steps:

- Obtain the dry weight (in grams) of commonly used items such as disposable underpad, perineal pad, 4 × 4).
- Weigh the saturated items and subtract the dry weight of the items to determine blood loss.
- 1-g weight = 1 mL of blood. In the absence of a scale, the following estimations may be utilized:
  - Saturated 12-ply surgical sponge (4 × 4 in) = 5 mL.
  - Standard perineal pad 50% saturated = 25 mL.
  - Saturated 18 × 18 inch surgical laparotomy pad = 100 mL.
  - Clot the size of a golf ball = 50 mL.
  - Clot the size of a tennis ball = 140 mL.

5. Assess intake and output (maintain >25 mL/h), including a cumulative total of all labor and delivery infusions as well as any fluids administered during surgery, such as with cesarean delivery.
6. Assess location and firmness of uterine fundus.
7. Percuss and palpate for bladder distention, which may interfere with contracting of the uterus. Foley catheter may be used for bladder decompression.
8. Inspect the perineum for swelling, ecchymosis, intactness, and approximation.
9. Assess lung sounds for signs of pulmonary edema.

Nursing Interventions

Decreasing Anxiety

1. Maintain a quiet and calm atmosphere; provide emotional support.
2. Provide information about the current clinical situation; answer questions.
3. Encourage the presence of a support person.
4. Explain changes to care plan.

Maintaining Fluid Volume

1. Maintain primary IV access and place a second large-gauge 16G to 18G catheter for infusing crystalloids and blood products, as indicated.
2. Monitor CBC and additional ordered laboratory work.
3. Administer uterotonic agents and pain relief medications, as ordered.
4. Monitor and maintain accurate intake and output.
5. Ensure cross-matched blood is available; administer per facility protocol when necessary.
6. Provide supplemental oxygen by facemask; monitor oxygen saturation with pulse oximetry.
7. Change patient positions to facilitate perfusion to vital organs: elevate legs 20 to 30 degrees.

Preventing Infection

1. Maintain standard precautions, asepsis, and hand hygiene.
2. Evaluate for symptoms of infection: chills, elevated temperature, increased WBCs, uterine tenderness, and odor of lochia.
3. Administer antibiotics, as prescribed.
4. Maintain adequate rest and proper nutrition.

Patient Education and Health Maintenance

1. Educate the patient about the cause of hemorrhage.
2. Teach the patient the importance of eating a balanced diet high in iron-rich food options and taking vitamin supplements. Iron supplements should be taken with vitamin C for optimal absorption.
3. Advise the patient that it is not unusual to feel tired and fatigued and to schedule daily rest periods.
4. Teach patient and family signs and symptoms of hemorrhage for home care.
5. Advise the patient to notify the provider of increased bleeding or other changes in status.

Evaluation: Expected Outcomes

- Verbalizes concerns about well-being and understanding of treatment plan.
- Vital signs stable, urine output adequate, stable hematocrit.
- Remains afebrile, WBC count within normal limits.

Postpartum Hematomas

Postpartum hematomas are localized collections of blood in loose connective tissue beneath the skin of external genitalia and in the potential space that exists adjacent to the vaginal wall mucosa. Hematomas generally occur without laceration of the overlying tissue.

Pathophysiology and Etiology

1. Bleeding occurs in the subcutaneous tissue of external genitalia or walls of vaginal mucosa and can expand to the vulva and extraperitoneal space that is bound by the bladder, rectum, uterus, and broad ligament.
2. Caused by trauma during spontaneous labor or operative (forceps) vaginal delivery.
3. Risk factors include the following:
   a. Hypertensive disorders of pregnancy.
   b. Preexisting coagulopathy.
   c. Macrosomia.
   d. Precipitous delivery.
   e. Nulliparity.
   f. Vulvar varicosities.
   g. Inadequate suturing of an episiotomy or laceration.
   h. Prolonged second stage of labor

Clinical Manifestations

1. Complaints of pressure and pain; pain may be verbalized as excruciating.
2. Discolored skin that is tight, full feeling, and painful to the touch.
3. Possible decrease in BP, tachycardia.
4. Decrease or absence of lochia flow if the vaginal opening is impeded.
5. Inability to spontaneously void or defecate.

CLINICAL JUDGMENT Excessive perineal pain unrelieved by analgesics suggests hematoma formation and mandates careful examination of the vulva, vagina, perineum, and rectum. Due to the concealed nature of a hematoma, blood loss can be substantial. Early recognition and intervention is needed to optimize maternal outcomes.

Management

1. Small, nonexpanding hematomas (≤3 cm) are left to resolve on their own—ice packs, warm sitz baths, and analgesics may also increase comfort.
2. Large, expanding hematomas (>3 cm) may require surgical evacuation of the blood and ligation of blood vessels.
3. Analgesics and broad-spectrum antibiotics may be ordered.
4. Blood transfusion may be indicated for hemodynamic instability.

Complications

1. Hypovolemia and shock from extreme blood loss.
2. Anemia, infection.
3. Increased length of postpartum recovery period.
4. Sepsis.
5. Calcification and scar tissue.
6. Dyspareunia (painful intercourse).

Nursing Interventions and Patient Education

1. Inspect perineal and vulvar area for signs of a hematoma routinely during the postpartum period.

2. Inspect vaginal area for signs of a hematoma if patient is unable to void.
3. Monitor vital signs and evaluate for signs of shock.
4. Relieve pain of a hematoma by applying an ice pack intermittently to perineal area, medicating with mild analgesics, and positioning for comfort to decrease pressure on the affected area.
5. Help relieve voiding problems by assisting to bathroom if able to ambulate. If patient is unable to ambulate, then assist patient on to a bedpan with legs over side of bed. Provide privacy and run water while the patient is attempting to void.
6. Catheterize patient if prolonged inability to void.
7. Teach the patient the importance of eating a balanced diet and to include food high in iron.
8. Encourage the patient to take vitamin supplements and to take all medications, as ordered.
9. Instruct the patient on the use of a sitz bath to provide perineal comfort after the first 24 hours and at home.
10. Encourage stool softeners at home if needed to prevent or relieve constipation.

Postpartum Depression

EVIDENCE BASE Beck, C. T. (2021). Perinatal mood and anxiety disorders: Research and implications for nursing care. *Journal of Obstetric, Gynecologic & Neonatal Nursing, 50*(4), e1–e46. https://doi.org/10.1016/j.jogn.2021.02.007

There is no consensus regarding the classification of postpartum depression. It is estimated to complicate 13% to 19% of pregnancies. The severity and presenting symptoms vary from patient to patient.

Pathophysiology and Etiology

Social, cultural, physiologic, and psychological factors may contribute to postpartum depression. Predisposing factors include:

1. Stressful life events during pregnancy or the postpartum period.
   a. Loss of loved one (fetus, neonate, partner, or other child).
   b. Illness of loved one.
   c. Financial difficulties.
   d. Loss of job.
   e. Move to new area, home, or job.
   f. Previous mental health history.
2. Poor interpersonal relationships.
3. Inadequate support.
4. History of sexual abuse or domestic violence.
5. High levels of anxiety, neurotic behavior, and depression or emotional distress.
6. Personal or family history of psychopathology, especially depression.

Common Presentations

1. Maternity blues; postpartum blues; baby blues; or 3rd-, 4th-, or 10th-day blues.
2. Postpartum or postnatal depression.
3. Postpartum or puerperal psychosis.
4. Postpartum panic disorder.
5. Postpartum obsessive–compulsive disorder.

Clinical Manifestations

1. Confusion.
2. Exaggerated and prolonged periods of irritability, moodiness, hostility, and fatigue.
3. Ineffective coping.
4. Withdrawal and inappropriate response to the infant or family.
5. Loss of interest in activities.
6. Insomnia or sleep disturbances.
7. Headache.
8. Constipation or other gastrointestinal symptoms.
9. Hair loss.
10. Dysmenorrhea.
11. Difficulties with lactation.
12. Decreased sexual responsiveness.

Diagnostic Evaluation and Management

1. Signs and symptoms may be overlooked, making the diagnosis of depression difficult. Several assessment tools, designed to screen for patients who may need further evaluation for postpartum depression, are available. The psychosocial screening tool recommended by the American College of Obstetricians and Gynecologists (ACOG) can be used by the nurse or health care provider as a means of communication. Questions should be worded empathically and nonjudgmentally to stimulate an honest response from the postpartum patient.
2. Counseling with a mental health professional, medication, and continuous support from family and friends may be helpful in managing the patient with postpartum depression. If untreated, the patient may possibly harm the neonate, self, or others.
3. The use of psychotropic medications during breastfeeding remains a controversial issue. All of the major classes of psychotropic drugs are expressed in breast milk. Use will depend on the risk versus benefits of treatment. Consultation with the interprofessional team including lactation consultant is recommended.
4. Any indication of suicide or harm to neonate requires immediate intervention to relieve the danger and referral to mental health professional.

Nursing Interventions and Patient Education

1. Actively listen to the patient regarding adjustment to role of caregiver and observe for any clinical manifestations suggesting depression.
2. Teaching related to signs and symptoms should include the patient and partner.
3. Provide multimedia resources if available.
4. Ask the patient about the neonate's behavior. Negative statements about the neonate may suggest that the patient is having difficulty coping. Notify the patient's obstetric or primary care provider.
5. Consult or refer patient to health care provider and other resources skilled in postpartum depression, as indicated. Refer patients to Postpartum Support International (https://www.postpartum.net).
6. Provide support and encourage family and friends to support and assist with the neonate and patient. Physical support as well as emotional support may be indicated.
7. Educate the patient that treatment may help alleviate symptoms and allow for better self-care and care of neonate.
8. Encourage the patient to engage in activities that enhance attachment: rooming-in, breastfeeding, and becoming involved in the medical examination of the neonate.
9. Realize that effective attachment behaviors differ from culture to culture and do not necessarily indicate maladaptive caregiving behaviors.

SELECTED READINGS

American College of Obstetricians and Gynecologists. (2020a). Antenatal corticosteroid therapy for fetal maturation (Committee Opinion # 713). *Obstetrics and Gynecology, 130*(2), e102–e109. https://doi.org/10.1097/AOG.0000000000002237

American College of Obstetricians and Gynecologists. (2020b). External cephalic version (Practice Bulletin #221). *Obstetrics and Gynecology, 135*(5), e203–e212. https://doi.org/10.1097/AOG.0000000000003837

American College of Obstetricians and Gynecologists. (2020c). Macrosomia (Practice Bulletin #216). *Obstetrics and Gynecology, 135*(1), e18–e35. https://doi.org/10.1097/AOG.0000000000003606

American College of Obstetricians and Gynecologists. (2020d). Management of late-term and postterm pregnancies (Practice Bulletin #146). *Obstetrics and Gynecology, 124*(2), 390–396. https://doi.org/10.1097/01.AOG.0000452744.06088.48

American College of Obstetricians and Gynecologists. (2020e). *Management of preterm labor* (Practice Bulletin #171). *Obstetrics and Gynecology, 128*(4), e155–e164. https://doi.org/10.1097/AOG.0000000000001711

American College of Obstetricians and Gynecologists. (2020f). Prevention of group B streptococcal early-onset disease in newborns (Committee Opinion #797). *Obstetrics and Gynecology, 135*(2), e51–e72. https://doi.org/10.1097/AOG.0000000000003668

American College of Obstetricians and Gynecologists. (2020g). Shoulder dystocia (Practice Bulletin #178). *Obstetrics and Gynecology, 129*(5), e123–e133. https://doi.org/10.1097/AOG.0000000000002043

American College of Obstetricians and Gynecologists. (2021). Antepartum fetal surveillance (Practice Bulletin #229). *Obstetrics and Gynecology, 137*(6), e116–e127. https://doi.org/10.1097/AOG.0000000000004410

American College of Obstetricians and Gynecologists. (2022). *Use of psychiatric medications during pregnancy and lactation* (Practice Bulletin #92). Author.

Anca, R., Schumacher, A., Tomassetti, J., Jean, M., Penna, S., & Iannacone, J. (2021). A nurse-driven initiative to educate an interprofessional team about postpartum hemorrhage emergency responses. *Journal of Obstetric, Gynecologic & Neonatal Nursing, 50*(5), s5–s6. https://doi.org/10.1016/j.jogn.2021.08.022

Baker, B., & Janke, J. (2024). *Core curriculum for maternal-newborn nursing* (6th ed.). Elsevier.

Baradaran, K. (2021). Risk of uterine rupture with vaginal birth after cesarean in twin gestations. *Obstetrics and Gynecology International, 2021*, 6693142. https://doi.org/10.1155/2021/6693142

Bixel, K., Ramaswamy, B., Christian, B., & Cohen, D. E. (2023). Malignancy and pregnancy. In C. J. Lockwood, J. A. Copel, L. L. Dugoff, J. Louis, T. R. Moore, R. M. Silver, & R. Resnik (Eds.), *Creasy and Resnick's maternal-fetal medicine: Principles and practice* (9th ed., pp. 1070–1087). Elsevier.

Blosser, C., Smith, A., & Poole, A. T. (2021). Quantification of blood loss improves detection of postpartum hemorrhage and accuracy of postpartum hemorrhage rates: A retrospective cohort study. *Cureus, 13*(2), e13591. https://doi.org/10.7759/cureus.13591

Cai, J., Ribkoff, J., Olson, S., Raghunathan, V., Al-Samkari, H., DeLoughery, T. G., & Shatzel, J. J. (2020). The many roles of tranexamic acid: An overview of the clinical indications for TXA in medical and surgical patients. *European Journal of Haematology, 104*(2), 79–87. https://doi.org/10.1111/ejh.13348

Chaemsaithong, P., Sahota, D. S., & Poon, L. C. (2022). First trimester preeclampsia screening and prediction. *American Journal of Obstetrics and Gynecology, 226*(2S), S1071–S1097.e2. https://doi.org/10.1016/j.ajog.2020.07.020

Cunningham, F. G., Leveno, K. J., Bloom, S. J., Dashe, J. S., Hoffman, B. L., Casey, B. M., & Spong, C. Y. (2022). *Williams's obstetrics* (26th ed.). McGraw-Hill.

Deckers, G. W. F., Broeren, M. A. C., Truijens, S. E. M., Kop, W. J., & Pop, V. J. M. (2020). Hormonal and psychological factors in nausea and vomiting during pregnancy. *Psychological Medicine, 50*(2), 229–236. https://doi.org/10.1017/S0033291718004105

Griggs, K. M., Hrelic, D. A., Williams, N., McEwen-Campbell, M., & Cypher, R. (2020). Preterm labor and birth: A clinical review. *MCN: The American Journal of Maternal/Child Nursing, 45*(6), 328–337. https://doi.org/10.1097/NMC.0000000000000656

Harden, R., Dawkins, D., Stallings-Saints, K., Hampton, M. D., & DeLilly, C. (2023). A multimodal protocol to limit opioid exposure and effectively manage postoperative cesarean birth pain. *MCN: The American Journal of Maternal/Child Nursing, 48*(2), 69–75. https://doi.org/10.1097/NMC.0000000000000899

Hauspurg, A., & Jeyabalan, A. (2022). Postpartum preeclampsia or eclampsia: Defining its place and management among the hypertensive disorders of pregnancy. *American Journal of Obstetrics and Gynecology, 226*(2), S1211–S1221. https://doi.org/10.1016/j.ajog.2020.10.027

Hoffman, E., Wilburn-Wren, K., Dillon, S. J., Barahona, A., McIntire, D. D., & Nelson, D. B. (2022). Impact of implementation of the maternal-fetal triage index on patients presenting with severe hypertension. *American Journal of Obstetrics and Gynecology, 227*(3), 521.e1–528.e8. https://doi.org/10.1016/j.ajog.2022.06.006

Horowitz, N. S., Eskander, R. N., Adelman, M. R., &, Burke, W. (2021). Epidemiology, diagnosis, and treatment of gestational trophoblastic disease: A Society of Gynecologic Oncology evidenced-based review and recommendation. *Gynecologic Oncology, 163*(3), 605–613. https://doi.org/10.1016/j.ygyno.2021.10.003

Joseph, N. T., Worell, N. H., Collins, J., Schmidt, M., Sobers, G., Hutchins, K., Chahine, E. B., Faya, C., Lewis, L., Green, V. L., Castellano, P. Z., & Lindsay, M. K. (2020). Implementation of a postpartum hemorrhage safety bundle at an urban safety-net hospital. *American Journal of Perinatology Reports, 10*(03), e255–e261. https://doi.org/10.1055/s-0040-1714713

Karadağ, C., & Çalışkan, E. (2020). Ectopic pregnancy risk with assisted reproductive technology. *Current Obstetrics and Gynecology Report, 9*, 153–157. https://doi.org/10.1007/s13669-020-00292-y

Khorasani, F., Hossein, A., Sobhi, A., Aryan, R., Abavi-Sani, A., Ghazanfarpour, M., Saidi, M., & Dizavandi, F. R. (2020). A systematic review of the efficacy of alternative medicine in the treatment of nausea and vomiting of pregnancy. *Journal of Obstetrics and Gynecology, 40*(1), 10–19. https://doi.org/10.1080/01443615.2019.1587392

Kinney, M. T., Quinney, S. K., Trussell, H. K., Silva, L. L., Ibrahim, S. A., & Haas, D. M. (2021). Do maternal demographics and prenatal history impact the efficacy of betamethasone therapy for threatened preterm labor? *BMC Pregnancy and Childbirth, 21*, 1–7. https://doi.org/10.1186/s12884-021-03949-5

Krywko, D. M., Sheraton, M., & Presley, B. (n.d.). Perimortem cesarean. In *StatPearls* [Internet]. StatPearls Publishing. Updated April 10, 2023. https://www.ncbi.nlm.nih.gov/books/NBK459265/

Landon, M. B., Galan, H. L., Jauniaux, R. M., Driscoll, D. A., Berghella, V., Grobman, W. A., Kilpatrick, S., & Cahill, A. (Eds.). (2021). *Gabbe's obstetrics: Normal and problem pregnancies* (8th ed.). Elsevier.

Murray, S., McKinney, E., Holub, K. S., Jones, R., & Scheffer, K. L. (2023). *Foundations of maternal-newborn and women's health nursing* (8th ed.). Elsevier.

Osterman, M. J. (2022). *Changes in primary and repeat cesarean delivery: United States, 2016–2021.* National Center for Health Statistics Report 21. https://www.cdc.gov/nchs/data/vsrr/vsrr021.pdf

Padda, J., Khalid, K., Colaco, L. B., Padda, S., Boddeti, N. L., Khan, A. S., Cooper, A. C., & Jean-Charles, G. (2021). Efficacy of magnesium sulfate on maternal mortality in eclampsia. *Cureus, 13*(8), e17322. https://doi.org/10.7759/cureus.17322

Sinha, S., Agarwal, M., & Singh, S. (2023). Large vaginal hematoma in a puerperium patient: Treating a delayed diagnosis & management caused by an incomplete clinical examination. *Cureus, 15*(1), e33386. https://doi.org/10.7759/cureus.33386

Thakur, M., & Thakur, A. (n.d.). Uterine inversion. In *StatPearls* [Internet]. StatPearls Publishing. Updated November 28, 2022. https://www.ncbi.nlm.nih.gov/books/NBK525971/

Vikhareva, O., Nedopekina, E., Kristensen, K., Dahlbäck, C., Pihlsgård, M., Skott Rickle, G., & Herbst, A. (2022). Strategies to increase the rate of vaginal deliveries after cesarean without negative impact on outcomes. *Midwifery, 106*, 103247. https://doi.org/10.1016/j.midw.2021.103247

Part Three

Pediatric Nursing

UNIT

XIII GENERAL PRACTICE CONSIDERATIONS

36 Pediatric Growth and Development*

GROWTH AND DEVELOPMENT

Infant to Adolescent Growth and Development

Growth and development begin with birth. As infants and children grow and mature, they pass through predictable stages of development. Knowledge and assessment of growth and development help the nurse provide screening for physical and emotional problems, offer anticipatory guidance to parental caregivers, develop a rapport with the child to enhance the provision of health care, and provide education to the family to build a healthy lifestyle for the future. For assessment of the neonate, see Chapter 34, pages 1012–1021. This chapter covers the beginning of infancy (age 1 month) to adolescence (ages 12 to 14). See Table 36-1, for further details.

Developmental Screening

Assessment tools have been created to determine the overall developmental age of a child or to detect specific areas of development that may be lacking. The most widely used developmental screening tool is the Denver II Developmental Screening Test (Denver II). This tool provides for a quick overview of development in children from birth to age 6 years and identifies areas of strength and weakness relative to age norms. Denver II test forms and an instruction manual can be accessed from www.denverii.com. This test has been criticized for a lack of sensitivity in detecting children with more subtle developmental delays. The American Academy of Pediatrics recommends that developmental surveillance be conducted at all well-child examinations and screening tests administered at the 9-, 18-, and 30-month visits. However, they do not recommend a specific test.

Another method for developmental screening involves interviewing the parental caregivers about the attainment of developmental milestones. Persistent deficits or deficits in multiple areas indicate a more serious problem than deficits in a single area (Table 36-2, pages 1083 and 1084).

*Please note that the term "male" in this chapter refers to a person assigned male at birth, and the term "female" in this chapter refers to a person assigned female at birth.

Table 36-1 Infant to Adolescent Growth and Development

AGE AND PHYSICAL CHARACTERISTICS	BEHAVIOR PATTERNS	NURSING CONSIDERATIONS
Birth to 4 wk (1 mo) • Significant neurologic disorganization. • Strong Moro reflex. • Sleep cycle disorganized. • GI system too immature for solid foods.	***Motor development*** • Momentary visual fixation on objects and human face. • Eyes follow bright moving objects. • Lies awake on back. • Immediately drops objects placed in hands. • Responds to sounds of a bell and other similar noises. • Keeps hands fisted. ***Socialization and vocalization*** • Mews and makes throaty noises. • Shows interest in human face. ***Cognitive and emotional development*** • Reflexive. • External stimuli are meaningless. • Responses are generally limited to tension states or discomfort. • Gains satisfaction from feeding and being held, rocked, fondled, and cuddled. • Has an intense need for sucking pleasure. • Quiets when picked up.	***Play stimulation*** • Use human face—smile and talk. • Dangle bright moving object (e.g., mobile) in field of vision. • Hold, touch, caress, fondle, and kiss. • Rock, pat, and change position. • Play soft music or have infant listen to ticking clock or sing. • Talk to infant; call by name. ***Parental caregiver guidance*** • Begin to expose infant to different household sounds. • Change crib location in the room. • Use brightly colored clothing and linens. • For safety, put infant to sleep on back at all times until old enough to roll. • Keep infant nearby. • Play with infant when awake. • Hold during feeding.
4–8 wk (2 mo) • Crossed extensor reflex disappears. • Tonic neck reflex begins to fade.	***Motor development*** • Reflexive behavior is slowly being replaced by voluntary movements. • Turns from side to back. • Begins to lift head momentarily from prone position. • Shows improved eye coordination. • If a bell is sounded nearby, infant will stop activity and listen. • Eyes more accurately follow vertical and horizontal alignment. Focuses well. ***Socialization and vocalization*** • Begins vocalization—coos, especially to a voice. • Crying becomes differentiated. • Visually looks for sounds. • May squeal with delight when stimulated by touching, talking, or singing. • Begins to smile socially. • Eyes follow person or object more intently. ***Cognitive and emotional development*** • Recognizes familiar face. • Becomes more aware and interested in environment. • Anticipates being fed when in feeding position. • Enjoys sucking—puts hand in the mouth.	***Play stimulation*** • Securely arrange mobile over crib. • Hang wind chimes near infant. • Hang brightly colored pictures on the wall. • Use cradle gym and infant seat. • Use rattles. • Hold infant and walk around the room. • Allow freedom of kicking with clothes off. ***Parental caregiver guidance*** • Talk to infant and smile; get excited when infant coos. • Place infant seat on a secure surface (e.g., floor, center of a table—never near the edge of the table) near parental caregiver's activities. • Put infant in prone position in bed or on floor for supervised periods. • Expose infant to different textures. • Exercise infant's arms and legs. • Sing to infant. • Provide tactile experience during bathing, diapering, and feeding.
8–12 wk (2–3 mo) • Landau reflex appears at 3–4 mo. • Positive support reflex disappears. • Posterior fontanelle closes. • Increase in body fluids—real tears appear, drooling and GI juices increase.	***Motor development*** • When prone, will rest on forearms and keeps head in midline—makes crawling movements with legs, arches back, and holds head high; may get chest off the surface. • Indicates preference for prone or supine. • Discovers hands—bats objects with hands. • Holds objects in the hands and brings to the mouth. • Has fairly good head control. ***Socialization and vocalization*** • Smiles more readily, babbles, and coos. • Stops crying when parental caregiver enters the room or when caressed.	***Play stimulation*** • Encourage socialization, smiling, and laughing. • Place on mat on the floor. • Continue to introduce new sounds. ***Parental caregiver guidance*** • Take outdoors with proper clothing (similar warmth as that of adults), a hat, and PABA-free sunscreen of at least SPF 15, reapplied every 30 min of sun exposure. • Bounce on bed.

(continued)

Table 36-1 Infant to Adolescent Growth and Development (*continued*)

	• Enjoys playing during feeding. • Stays awake longer without crying. • Turns head to follow familiar person. ***Cognitive and emotional development*** • Shows active interest in environment. • Recognizes familiar faces and objects. • Focuses and follows objects. • Shows repetitiveness in play activity. • Is aware of strange situations. • Derives pleasure from sucking—purposefully gets hand to the mouth. • Begins to establish routine preceding sleep.	• Play with infant during feeding. • Rattles can be used effectively for visual following and for handplay. • Encourage older siblings to "make faces," sing, and talk to infant.
12–16 wk (3–4 mo) • Moro reflex fades. • Stepping reflex disappears. • Rooting reflex disappears. • By 4–5 mo, infant's weight approximately doubles birth weight. • Average weekly weight gain, 4–7 ounces (113.5–198.5 g). • Average monthly height gain, 1 in (2.5 cm). • Pulse rate slows to 100–140 beats/min. • Respirations, 20–40 breaths/min. • Grasp becomes voluntary. • Sucking becomes voluntary.	***Motor development*** • Eyes focus on small objects; may pick a dangling ring. • Holds head up (when being pulled to sitting position). • Becomes more interested in environment. • Hand comes to meet rattle. • Listens—turns head to familiar sound. • Sits with minimal support. • Intentional rolling over, back to side. • Reaches for offered objects. • Grasps objects with both hands and everything goes into the mouth. ***Socialization and vocalization*** • Laughs and chuckles socially. • Demands social attention by fussing. • Recognizes parental caregiver. • Begins to respond to "No, no." • Enjoys being propped in sitting position. ***Cognitive and emotional development*** • Actively interested in environment. • Enjoys attention; becomes bored when alone for long periods. • Recognizes bottle. • More interested in parental caregiver. • Indicates increasing trust and security. • Sleeps through the night; has defined nap time.	***Play stimulation*** • Encourage mirror play. • Provide soft squeeze toys in vivid colors of varying textures. • Allow infant to splash in bath. • Infant still enjoys holding and playing with rattles. • Enjoys old-fashioned clothespins and playing pat-a-cake and peekaboo. ***Parental caregiver guidance*** • Be certain button eyes on toys and other small objects cannot be pulled off. • Hold rattle and let infant reach and grasp it. • Secure infant in high chair or infant seat. • Move mobile out of reach—infant may grab it and cause injury. • Repeat child's sounds. • Talk in varying degrees of loudness. • Begin looking at and naming pictures in book. • Begin physically active play by all adult caregivers. • Give space in playpen or on sheet on the floor to practice rolling over. • Place on the abdomen for part of playtime.
16–26 wk (4–7 mo) • By 5–6 mo, tonic neck reflex disappears. • By 6–7 mo, palmar grasp disappears. • Two central lower incisors erupt. • Spine "C-shaped"—lacks lordotic and lumbar curves. • Eustachian tube short and horizontal, which may be a factor in ear infections. • GI system mature enough for solid foods.	***Motor development*** • Shows momentary sitting with hand support. • Bounces and bears some weight when held in standing position. • Transfers and mouths objects in one hand. • Discovers feet. • Bangs objects together. • Rolls over well. • May begin some form of mobility. ***Socialization and vocalization*** • Discriminates between strangers and familiar people. • Crows and squeals. • Starts to say "Ma," and "Da." • Play is self-contained. • Laughs out loud. • Makes "talking" sounds in response to others' talking. ***Cognitive and emotional development*** • Secures objects by pulling on string. • Searches for lost objects that are out of sight.	***Play stimulation*** • Enjoys social games, hide-and-seek with adult, toys, and large blocks. • Likes to bang objects. • Plays in bounce chair and walker. • Enjoys large nesting toys (round rather than square). • Likes to drop and retrieve things. • Likes metal cups, wooden spoons, and things to bang with. • Loves crumpled paper. • Enjoys squeeze toys in bath. • Likes peekaboo, bye-bye, and pat-a-cake. ***Parental caregiver guidance*** • Will play as long as you can. • Let play with extra spoon at feeding. • Give soft finger foods in small amounts.

Table 36-1 Infant to Adolescent Growth and Development (*continued*)

	• Inspects objects; localizes sounds. • Likes to sit in high chair. • Drops and picks up objects. • Displays exploratory behavior with food. • Exhibits beginning fear of strangers. • Becomes fretful when parental caregiver leaves. • Shows much mouthing and biting.	• Because infant puts everything in the mouth, use safety precautions. • Keep small items away from infant, which could choke on them. • Show excitement at achievements. • Supply safe kitchen items for toys.
26–40 wk (7–10 mo) • By 7–9 mo, develops eye-to-eye contact while talking; engages in social games. • Four upper incisors erupt around 7–9 mo. • By 9–12 mo, plantar reflex disappears. • By 9–12 mo, neck righting reflex disappears. **6–12 mo** • Average weekly weight gain, 3–5 ounces (85–141.7 g). • Average monthly height gain, ½ in (1.25 cm).	***Motor development*** • Sits without support. • Recovers balance. • Manipulates objects with hands. • Unwraps objects. • Creeps. • Pulls self upright at crib rails. • Uses index finger and thumb to hold objects. • Rings a bell. • Can feed self a cracker and can hold a bottle. Chewing reflex develops. • Can control lips around cup. • Does not like supine position. • Can hold index finger and thumb in opposition. ***Socialization and vocalization*** • Claps hands on request. • Responds to own name. • Is very aware of social environment. • Imitates gestures, facial expressions, and sounds. • Smiles at image in the mirror. • Offers toy to adult, but does not release it. • Begins to test parental caregiver reaction during feeding and at bedtime. • Will entertain self for long periods. • Begins fear of strangers, 8½–10 mo. ***Cognitive and emotional development*** • Begins to imitate. • Shows more interest in picture books. • Enjoys achievements. • Has strong urge toward independence—locomotion, feeding, and dressing.	***Play stimulation*** • Encourage use of motion toys—rocking horse and stroller. • Supervised water play. • Imitate animal sounds. • Allow exploration outdoors. • Provide for learning by imitation. • Offer new objects (blocks). • Child likes freedom of creeping and walking, but closeness of family is important. • Good toys: plastic milk carton; beanbag for tossing; fabric books; things to move around, fill up, and empty out; pileup and knockdown toys. ***Parental caregiver guidance*** • Protect from dangerous objects—cover electrical outlets, block stairs, and remove breakable objects from tables. • Have child with family at mealtime. • Offer cup. • Talk and sing to infant.

10–12 mo (1 yr)
• Develops lordotic and lumbar curves to make walking possible.
• Weight should approximately triple birth weight.
• Two lower lateral incisors appear.
• Four first molars appear by 14 mo.
Child development theories
• Freud: behavior.
  • Birth to 1 yr—oral stage.
• Erikson: emotion/personality.
  • Birth to 1 yr—sense of trust vs. mistrust.
	Motor development
	• Cruises around furniture.
	• Beginning to stand alone and toddle.
	• Turns pages in book.
	• Tries tossing object.
	• Shows hand dominance.
	• Navigates stairs; climbs on chairs.
	• Builds a tower of two blocks.
	• Puts balls in the box.
	• May use spoon.
	• Can release objects at will.
	• Has regular bowel movements.
	Socialization and vocalization
	• Uses jargon.
	• Points to indicate wants.
	• Loves give-and-take game.
	• Responds to music.
	• Enjoys being center of attention and will repeat laughed-at activities.
		Play stimulation
		• Ball play.
		• Cloth doll.
		• Motion objects and toys.
		• Transporting objects.
		• Name and points to body parts.
		• "Put-in" and "take-out" toys.
		• Sandbox with spoons and other simple objects.
		• Blocks.
		• Music.
		Parental caregiver guidance
		• Allow self-directed play rather than adult-directed play.
		• Continue to expose to foods of different texture, taste, smell, and substance.
		• Offer cup.
		• Show affection and encourage child to return affection.

(*continued*)

Table 36-1 Infant to Adolescent Growth and Development (*continued*)

• Piaget: intellectual activity (thought process) • Birth to 2 yr—sensorimotor period.	***Cognitive and emotional development*** • Shows fear, anger, affection, jealousy, anxiety, and sympathy. • Experiments to reach new goals. • Displays intense determination to remove barriers to action. • Begins to develop concepts of space, time, and causality. • Has increased attention span.	• Safety teaching: child gets into everything within reach. Place medications in safe, locked place. Create a safe environment for child. Use stair guards, faucet protectors, and drawer locks. Have poison control center phone number readily available.
12–18 mo • *Note:* Between ages 1 and 3 yr, the child is called a "toddler." • By 12–24 mo, Landau reflex disappears. • Anterior fontanelle closes. • The abdomen protrudes; arms and legs lengthen. • Large muscles become well developed. • Four cuspids appear by 18 mo. • Fine muscle coordination begins to develop. • Average yearly weight gain, 4½–6½ pounds (2–3 kg). • Average height gain during second year, 4¾ in (12 cm).	***Motor development*** • Walks up stairs with help and creeps downstairs. • Walks without support and with balance. • Falls less frequently. • Throws ball. • Stoops to pick up toys and looks at bug. • Turns pages of book. • Holds and lifts cup. • Builds three-block tower. • Picks up and places small beads in a container. • Begins to use spoon. ***Cognitive and emotional development*** • Has vocabulary of 10 words that have meanings. • Uses phrases and imitates words. • Points to objects named by adult. • Follows directions and requests. • Imitates adult behavior. • Retrieves toy from several hiding places. ***Psychosocial development*** • Develops new awareness of strangers. • Wants to explore everything in reach. • Plays alone, but near others. • Is dependent on parental caregivers, but begins to reach out for autonomy. • Finds security in a blanket, toy, or thumb-sucking.	***Play stimulation*** • Allow unrestricted motor activity (within safety limits). • Offer push–pull toys. • Child selects favorite toy. • Child likes blocks, pyramid toys, teddy bears, dolls, pots and pans, cloth picture books with large colorful pictures, telephone, musical top, and nested blocks. ***Parental caregiver guidance*** • Begin to teach toothbrushing to establish good dental habits; however, continue to brush child's teeth with specially formulated pediatric toothpaste. • Establish limits to give toddler sense of security, but encourage exploration. • Reinforce safety teaching.
1½–2 yr • Protruding abdomen less noticeable. • During first 2 yr, 14 in (35 cm) is added to height. • Slight bowing of legs with a wide-based walk. • Hand preference may become apparent.	***Motor development*** • Walks up and down the stairs. • Opens doors; turns knobs. • Has steady gait. • Holds drinking cup well with one hand. • Uses spoon without spilling food (may prefer fingers). • Kicks a ball in front of them without support. • Builds a tower of four to six blocks. • Scribbles. • Rides tricycle or kiddie car (without pedals). ***Cognitive development*** • Has 200–300 words in vocabulary. • Begins to use short sentences. • Refers to self by pronoun. • Obeys simple commands. • Does not know right from wrong. • Begins to learn about time sequences. ***Psychosocial development*** • Uses word "mine" constantly. • Is possessive with toys. • Displays negativism—uses "no" as assertion of self. • Routine and rituals are important. • May begin cooperation in toilet training. • Resists restrictions on freedom. • Has fear of parental caregivers leaving.	***Play stimulation*** • Shows parallel play, although enjoys having other children around. • Has very short attention span. • Enjoys same toys as child of 18 mo. • Likes doll play and balls. • Imitates parental caregivers in domestic activities. • Likes swing, hammering, paper, and large crayons. ***Parental caregiver guidance*** • Has need for peer companionship (parallel play) although displays immaturity by inability to share and take turns. • A decrease in appetite normally occurs at this stage. • Toilet training readiness should be assessed and started if appropriate (each child follows own pattern). • Begin to have child eat meals with family if not already doing so. • Begin to read to child; child likes storybooks with large pictures.

Table 36-1 Infant to Adolescent Growth and Development (*continued*)

	• Shows parallel play. • Dawdles. • Resists bedtime—uses transitional objects (blanket, toy). • Vacillates between dependence and independence.	

2–3 yr
• Height approximates one-half adult height.
• Legs are about 34% of body length.
• Begins 5 pounds (2.3 kg) or more weight gain per year until age 5 yr.
• At 2½ yr, has full set (20) of baby teeth.
• Four second molars appear by 2½ yr.
• Height gain, 2⅜–3¼ in (6–8 cm).
• Lordosis and protuberant abdomen of toddler disappear.
 	
Child development theories
• Freud:
  • 1–3 yr—anal stage.
• Erikson:
  • 1–3 yr—sense of autonomy vs. shame and doubt.
• Piaget:
  • 2–7 yr—preoperational period; shows egocentrism and centering.
	Motor development
	• Throws objects overhead.
	• Pedals tricycle.
	• Walks backward.
	• Washes and dries hands.
	• Begins to use scissors.
	• Can string large beads.
	• Can undress on their own.
	• Feeds themselves well.
	• Tries to dance.
	• Jumps in place.
	• Builds tower of eight blocks.
	• Balances on one foot.
	• Swings and climbs.
	• Can eat an ice cream cone.
	• Drinks from a straw.
	• Chews gum without swallowing it.
	
	Cognitive development
	• Shows increased attention span.
	• Gives first and last name.
	• Begins to ask "why."
	• Is egocentric in thought and behavior.
	• Beginning ability to reflect on own behavior.
	• Talks in short sentences.
	• Uses plurals.
	• May attempt to sing simple songs.
	• Has vocabulary of 900 words.
	• Begins fantasy.
	• Begins to understand what it means to take turns.
	• Can repeat three numbers.
	• Shows interest in colors.
	
	Psychosocial development
	• Negativism grows out of child's sense of developing independence—says "no" to every command.
	• Ritualism is important to toddler for security (follows certain pattern, especially at bedtime).
	• Temper tantrums may result from toddler's frustration in wanting to do everything for self.
	• Shows parallel play as well as beginning interaction with others.
	• Engages in associative play.
	• Fears become pronounced.
	• Continues to react to separation from parental caregivers but shows increasing ability to handle short periods of separation.
	• Has daytime bladder control and is beginning to develop nighttime bladder control.
	• Becomes more independent.
	• Begins to identify gender roles.
	• Explores environment outside the home.
	• Can create different ways of getting desired outcome.
		Play stimulation
		• Plays simple games with other children.
		• Enjoys storytelling and dress-up play.
		• Plays "house."
		• Uses colors.
		• Uses scissors and paper.
		• Rides tricycle.
		• Reads simple books to child.
		• Will assist in developing memory skills, visual discrimination skills, and language.
		
		Parental caregiver guidance
		• From 2–3 yr, the child develops a seeming maturity; do not expect more than child is able to do.
		• Arrange first visit to the dentist to have teeth checked if not done prior.
		• Be aware that negativistic and ritualistic behavior is normal.
		• Be consistent in discipline.
		• Control temper tantrums.
		• Begin to teach stranger, animal, and traffic safety.
		• Supervise outdoor play.

(*continued*)

Table 36-1 Infant to Adolescent Growth and Development (*continued*)

3–4 yr *Note:* Between ages 3 and 5 yr, the child is called a "preschooler." May appear "knock-kneed."	***Motor development*** • Drawings have form and meaning, not detail. • Copies a circle and a cross. • Buttons front and side of clothes. • Laces shoes. • Bathes self, but needs direction. • Brushes teeth. • Shows continuous movement going up and down the stairs. • Climbs and jumps well. • Attempts to print letters. ***Cognitive development*** • Awareness of body is more stable; child becomes more aware of own vulnerability. • Is less negativistic. • Learns some number concepts. • Begins naming colors. • Can identify longer of two lines. • Has vocabulary of 1,500 words. • Uses mild profanities and name-calling. • Uses language aggressively. • Asks many questions. • May not be abstract enough to understand body parts that cannot be seen or felt. • Can be given simple explanation as to cause and effect. • Thinks very concretely; demonstrates irreversibility of thought. • Immature concept of death—believes it is reversible. • Has beginning understanding of past and future. • Is egocentric in thought.	***Play stimulation*** • Plays and interacts with other children. • Shows creativity. • Likes ring-around-the-rosy. • "Helps" adults. • Likes costumes and enjoys dramatic play. • Toys and games: record player, nursery rhymes, housekeeping toys, transportation toys (tricycle, trucks, cars, wagon), blocks, hammer and peg bench, floor trains, blackboard and chalk, easel and brushes, clay, crayon and finger paints, outside toys (sandbox, swing, small slide), books (short stories, action stories), drum, and scrapbook. ***Parental caregiver guidance*** • Base your expectations within child's limitations. • Provide limited frustrations from environment to assist in coping. • Give small tasks to do around the house (putting silverware on table, drying an unbreakable dish). • Expand child's world with trips to the zoo, to the supermarket, to restaurant, etc. • Prevent accidents. ***Psychosocial development*** • Is more active with peers and engages in cooperative play. • Performs simple tasks. • Frequently has imaginary companion. • Dramatizes experiences. • Is proud of accomplishments. • Exaggerates, boasts, and tattles on others. • Can tolerate separation from parental caregiver longer without feeling anxiety. • Is keen observer. • Has good sense of "mine" and "yours." • Behavior still frequently ritualistic. • Becomes curious about life and sex. Often masturbates. • Provide for brief nonthreatening separation from parental caregivers and home. • Reinforce correct use of language. • Use opportunities for simple sexual education as child's needs arise. • Accept masturbation as a normal phenomenon to be discouraged in public. • Provide consistent discipline, motivated by love rather than anger. • Consider nursery school/preschool opportunities.

Table 36-1 Infant to Adolescent Growth and Development (*continued*)

4–5 yr
• By 2–5 yr, adds 9½ in (25 cm) to height.
• At age 4, legs comprise about 44% of body length.
 	
Child development theories
• Freud:
  • 3–6 yr—phallic stage.
• Erikson:
  • 3–6 yr—sense of initiative vs. guilt.
• Piaget:
  • 2–7 yr—preoperational period; shows egocentrism and centering.
	Motor development
	• Hops two or more times.
	• Dresses without supervision.
	• Has good motor control—climbs and jumps well.
	• Walks up stairs without grasping handrail.
	• Walks backward.
	• Washes self without wetting clothes.
	• Prints first name and other words.
	• Adds three or more details in drawings.
	• Draws a square.
	
	Cognitive development
	• Has 2,100-word vocabulary.
	• Talks constantly.
	• Uses adult speech forms.
	• Participates in conversations.
	• Asks for definitions.
	• Knows age and residence.
	• Identifies heavier of two objects.
	• Knows weeks as time units.
	• Names days of the week.
	• Begins to understand kinship.
	• Knows primary colors.
	• Can count to 10.
	• Can copy a triangle.
	• Has a high degree of imagination.
	• Questioning is at a peak.
	• Begins to develop power of reasoning.
	
	Psychosocial development
	• May have an imaginary companion.
	• Has a sense of order (likes to finish what was started).
	• Is obedient and reliable.
	• Is protective toward younger children.
	• Begins to develop an elementary conscience with some influence in governing behavior.
	• Has increased self-confidence.
	• Accepts responsibility for acts.
	• Is less rebellious.
	• Has dreams and nightmares.
	• Is cooperative and sympathetic.
	• Shows generosity with toys.
	• Begins to question parental caregivers' thinking.
	• Identifies strongly with parent caregiver(s) of same gender.
		Play stimulation
		• Demonstrates gross motor activity—likes to jump rope, skip, climb on jungle gym, etc.
		• Prefers group play and cooperates in projects.
		• Plays simple letter, number, form, and picture games.
		• Plays with cars and trucks.
		• Still likes being read to.
		• Continues to enjoy fantasy play.
		
		Parental caregiver guidance
		• Child may no longer require an afternoon nap.
		• Prepare child for kindergarten.
		• Tell them stories.
		• Provide opportunities and reassurance for group play; have their friends visit for lunch and an afternoon of playing.
		• Prevent accidents.
		• Encourage child's participation in household activities.

Middle Childhood (5–9 yr) • Growth rate is slow and steady. • Gains an average of 7 pounds (3.2 kg) per year. Height increases approximately 2½ in (6.3 cm) per year. • Among children, there is considerable variation in height and weight. • Appears taller and slimmer. • Early lordosis disappears. • Begins to lose baby teeth; permanent teeth appear at a rate of about four teeth per year from 7–14 yr.	***Motor development*** *6 yr* • Is active and impulsive. • Balance improves. • Uses hands as manipulative tools in cutting, pasting, and hammering. • Can draw large letters or figures. *7 yr* • Has lower activity level. • Capable of fine hand movements; can print sentences. • Nervous habits, such as nail biting, are common. • Muscular skills, such as ball throwing, have improved. *8 yr* • Moves with less restlessness. • Has developed grace and balance, even in active sports. • Has developed coordination of fine muscles, allowing child to write in script.	***Parental caregiver guidance*** • Family atmosphere continues to have an impact on the child's emotional development and future response within the family. • The child needs ongoing guidance in an open, inviting atmosphere. Limits should be set with conviction. Deal with only one incident at a time. When punishment is necessary, the child should not be humiliated. Child should know that it was the act that the adult found undesirable, not the child.

(*continued*)

Table 36-1 Infant to Adolescent Growth and Development (*continued*)

Neuromuscular and skeletal development allows improved coordination.

- Eyes become fully developed; vision approaches 20/20.
- Handedness should be well developed.

Child development theories

- Freud:
  - 5–9 yr—beginning of latency period.
- Erikson:
  - 5–9 yr—industry vs. inferiority.
- Piaget:
  - 5–9 yr—enters stage of concrete operations.

9 yr

- Uses both hands independently.
- Has become skillful in manual activities because of improved eye–hand coordination.

Cognitive development

6 yr

- Begins to learn to read. Defines objects in terms of use. Time sense is as much in past as present.
- Is interested in relationship between home and neighborhood; knows some streets.
- Uses sentences well; uses language to share others' experiences; may swear or use slang.
- Distinguishes morning from afternoon.

7 yr

- More reflective and has deeper understanding of meanings.
- Interested in conclusions and logical endings. Begins to have scientific interests in cause and effect.
- More responsible in relation to time, more punctual. Sense of space is more realistic; child wants some space of own.
- Knows value of coins.
- Concept of death maturing—includes idea of irreversibility.

8 yr

- Thinking is less animistic. Is aware of impersonal forces of nature. Begins to understand logical reasoning, conclusions, and implications.
- Less self-centered in thinking. Personal space is expanding; goes places on own. Aware of time; plans events of the day. Understands right from left.

9 yr

- Intellectually energetic and curious. Realistic; reasonable in thinking. Able to plan in advance. Breaks complex activities into steps.
- Focuses on detail.
- Sense of space includes the entire earth.
- Participates in family discussions.
- Likes to have secrets.

Psychosocial development

5–9 yr

- Still requires parental caregiver support, but pulls away from overt signs of affection.
- Peer groups provide companionship in widening circle of persons outside the home. Child learns more about self as they learn about others.
- "Chum" stage occurs at about age 9 or 10. Child chooses a special friend of same gender and age in whom to confide. This is usually child's first love relationship outside of home, when someone becomes as important to them as themselves.
- Play teaches the child new ideas and independence. Child progressively uses tools of competition, compromise, cooperation, and beginning collaboration.
- Body image and self-concept are fluid because of rapid physical, emotional, and social changes.
- Latency-stage sexual drive is controlled and repressed. Emphasis is on the development of skills and talent.

Patterns of play

6–7 yr

- Child acts out ideas of family and occupational groups with which they have contact.

- Needs assistance in adjusting to new experiences and demands of school. Should be able to share experiences with family. Parental caregivers need to have communication with the teacher to work together for the health of the child.
- Convey love and caring in communication. The child understands language directed at feelings better than at intellect. Get down to eye level with the child.
- Focus attention on child's abilities and accomplishments rather than shortcomings and limitations.
- The child is sex-conscious and should be able to discuss questions at home rather than with friends. Requires simple, honest answers to questions.
- Common problems include teasing, quarreling, nail biting, enuresis, whining, poor manners, swearing, lying, cheating, and stealing. These are usually fleeting phases and should not be handled negatively. The causes for such behavior should be investigated and dealt with constructively.
- The child needs order and consistency to help in coping with doubts, fears, unacceptable impulses, and unfamiliar experiences.
- Encourage peer activities as well as home responsibilities and give recognition to child's accomplishments and unique talents.
- Television may stimulate learning in several spheres, but should be monitored.
- Accidents are a major cause of disability and death. Safety practices should be continued. (Refer to "Safety" section, page 1123.)
- Exercise is essential to promote motor and psychosocial development. The child should have a safe place to play and simple pieces of equipment.
- A school health program should be available and concerned with the child's physical, emotional, mental, and social health. This should be augmented by information and example at home.
- Medical supervision should continue with yearly examination to detect developmental delay and disease. Appropriate immunizations should be administered.
- The child frequently has "quiet days"—periods of shyness, which should be tolerated as part of growing up and deciding who they are.

Table 36-1 Infant to Adolescent Growth and Development (*continued*)

	• Painting, pasting, reading, simple games, watching television, digging, running games, skating, riding bicycle, and swimming are all enjoyed activities. *8 yr* • Child enjoys collections; loosely formed, short-lived clubs, table games, card games, books, television, and music.	• The child may be subject to nightmares, a situation that requires reassurance and understanding. • Parental caregivers, teachers, and health professionals should be available and able to provide information and answer questions about the physical changes that occur.

Late Childhood (9–12 yr)
• Vital signs approach adult values.
• Loses childish appearance of face and takes on features that will characterize individual as an adult.
• Growth spurt occurs, and some secondary sex characteristics appear: in females between ages 10 and 12 yr and in males between ages 12 and 14 yr.
Physical changes of puberty
• Increased height and weight, increased perspiration and activity of sebaceous glands; vasomotor instability; increased fat deposition.
• **Females:** the pelvis increases in transverse diameter; hips broaden; tenderness in developing breast tissue; enlargement of areola diameter; appearance of pubic hair.
• **Males:** size of testes increases; scrotum color changes; breasts enlarge, temporarily; height and shoulder breadth increase.
• Appearance of lightly pigmented hair at the base of the penis.
• Increase in length and width of the penis.
Child development theories
• Freud:
  • 9–12 yr—latency period continues.
• Erikson:
  • 9–12 yr—industry vs. inferiority continues.
• Piaget:
  • 9–12 yr—stage of concrete operations continues.
	Motor development
	• Energetic, restless, active movements such as finger drumming or foot tapping appear.
	• Has skillful manipulative movements nearly equal to those of adults.
	• Works hard to perfect physical skills.
	Cognitive development
	10 yr
	• Likes to reason and enjoys learning.
	• Thinking is concrete and matter of fact.
	• Wants to measure up to challenge.
	• Likes to memorize and identify facts.
	• Attention span may be short. Space is rather specific (i.e., where things are).
	• Can write for relatively long time with speed.
	• Likes action in learning.
	• Concentrates well when working competitively.
	• Can understand relational terms, such as weight and size.
	• Perceives space as nothingness that goes on forever.
	• Can discuss problems.
	• Can conceptualize symbolically enough to understand body parts.
	• Can describe some abstract terms.
	12 yr
	• Enjoys learning.
	• Considers all aspects of a situation.
	• Motivated more by inner drive than by competition.
	• Able to classify, arrange, and generalize.
	• Likes to discuss and debate.
	• Begins conceptual thinking.
	• Verbal, formal reasoning now possible.
	• Can recognize moral of a story.
	• Defines time as duration; likes to plan ahead.
	• Understands that space is abstract.
	• Can be critical of own work.
	Psychosocial development
	• Gang becomes important and gang code takes precedence over nearly everything. Gang codes are typically characterized by collective action against the mores of the adult world. Here, children begin to work out their own social patterns without adult interference. Early gangs may include people of more than one gender; later gangs are separated by gender.
	• May strive for unreasonable independence from adult control.
	• Usually interested in religion and morality.
	• Has increased interest in sexuality.
	• May reach puberty; resurgence of sexual drives causes recapitulation of Oedipal struggle.
	Patterns of play
	• Continues to enjoy reading, TV, and table games.
	• More interested in active sports as a means to improve skills.
		Parental caregiver guidance
		• Continue appropriate interventions related to early childhood.
		• Continue sex education and preparation for adolescent body changes.
		• Understanding is important.
		• Encourage participation in organized clubs and youth groups.
		• Democratic guidance is essential as child works through a conflict between dependence (on parental caregivers) and independence. The child needs realistic limits set.
		• Needs help channeling energy in proper direction—work and sports.
		• Requires adequate explanation of body changes prior to changes appearing. Special understanding is required for the child who lags in physical development compared to peers or to those who develop significantly earlier than peers.
		• Continue consistent disciplinary style.

(*continued*)

Table 36-1 Infant to Adolescent Growth and Development (*continued*)

	• Creative talents may appear; may enjoy drawing and modeling clay. By age 10, gender differences in preferred play activities may be more pronounced. • Occasional privacy is important. • Begins to have vocational aspirations, may be seemingly unrealistic and frequently changing.	

Early Adolescence (12–14 yr)
• Phase of development begins when reproductive organs become functionally operative; the phase ends when physical growth is completed.
• Skeletal system grows faster than supporting muscles.
• Hands and feet grow proportionately faster than the rest of the body.
• Large muscles develop more quickly than small muscles.
• **Females:** physical changes include beginning of menarche, growth of axillary and perineal hair, deepened voice, ovulation, and further development of breasts.
• Nutritional need for iron and calcium increases dramatically.
• **Males:** physical changes include growth of axillary, perineal, facial, chest hair, deepening of voice, production of spermatozoa, and nocturnal emissions.
Child development theories
• Freud:
  • 12–14 yr—begins stage of sexuality.
• Erikson:
  • 12–14 yr—identity vs. role diffusion.
• Piaget:
  • 12–14 yr—begins stage of formal operations.
	Motor development
	• Usually uncoordinated; has poor posture.
	• Tires easily.
	Cognitive development
	• Mind has great ability to acquire and use knowledge.
	• Abstract thinking is sufficient to learn multivariable ideas such as the influence of hormones on emotions.
	• Categorizes thoughts into usable forms.
	• May project thinking into the future.
	• Is capable of highly imaginative thinking.
	Psychosocial development
	• Interest in people of other genders increases.
	• Often revolts from adult authority to conform to peer–group standards.
	• Continues to rework feelings for all caregivers and to unravel the ambivalence toward parental caregiver of same gender.
	• Affection may turn temporarily to an adult outside of the family (e.g., crush on family friend, neighbor, or teacher).
	• Uses peer–group dialect—highly informal language or specially coined terminology.
	• Peer groups are especially important and help adolescent to define own identity, to adapt to changing body image, to establish more mature relationships with others, and to deal with heightened sexual feelings. Cliques may develop.
	• Dating generally progresses from groups of couples to double dates and finally single couples.
	• Teenage "hangouts" become important centers of activity.
	• Begins questioning existing moral values
		Parental caregiver guidance
		• Stresses frequently result from conflicting value systems between generations. The parental caregivers may need help to see that the adolescent is a product of the times and that actions reflect what is happening around the adolescent.
		• The parental caregivers' limits and rules should be realistic and consistent. They should convey the parental caregiver's love and concern and should be a source of comfort and reassurance, protecting the child from activities for which they are not ready.
		• The home should be an accepting, emotionally stable environment.
		• Continue sex education, including discussion of ovulation, fertilization, menstruation, pregnancy, contraception, masturbation, nocturnal emissions, and hygiene.
		• Adolescents have an increased need for rest and sleep because they are expending large amounts of energy and are functioning with an inadequate oxygen supply.
		• Recreational interests should be fostered. Favorite activities include sports, dating, dancing, reading, hobbies, and social media. Socializing via telephone or computer and listening to music are favorite pastimes.
		• Adolescent health problems that require preventive education are accidents, obesity, acne, pregnancy, sexually transmitted disease, and drug use.
		• Allow the adolescent to handle their own affairs as much as possible, but be aware of physical and psychosocial problems that may require help. Encourage independence but allow child to seek support and guidance from parental caregivers or trusted adults when frightened or unable to attain goals.
		• Adolescents with special problems should have access to specialists, such as adolescent clinics and psychologists.
		• Requires reassurance and help in accepting a changing body image. Parental caregivers should make the most of the child's positive qualities.

Table 36-1 Infant to Adolescent Growth and Development (*continued*)

		• Give gentle encouragement and guidance regarding dating. Avoid strong pressures in either direction. • Understand conflicts as the child attempts to deal with social, moral, and intellectual issues.

GI, gastrointestinal; PABA, para-aminobenzoic acid; SPF, sun protection factor.

Table 36-2 Developmental Milestones

AGE	GROSS MOTOR	VISUAL–MOTOR/ PROBLEM-SOLVING	LANGUAGE	SOCIAL/ADAPTIVE
1 mo	Raises head slightly from prone, makes crawling movements	*Birth:* visually fixes *1 mo:* has tight grasp, follows to midline	Alerts to sound	Regards face
2 mo	Holds head in midline, lifts chest off table	No longer clenches fist tightly, follows object past midline	Smiles socially (after being stroked or talked to)	Recognizes parental caregiver
3 mo	Supports on forearms in prone, holds head up steadily	Holds hands open at rest, follows in circular fashion, responds to visual threat	Coos (produces long vowel sounds in musical fashion)	Reaches for familiar people or objects, anticipates feeding
4 mo	Rolls front to back, supports on wrists, and shifts weight	Reaches with arms in unison, brings hands to midline	Laughs, orients to voice	Enjoys looking around environment
5 mo	Rolls back to front, sits supported	Transfers objects	Says "ah-goo," blows raspberries, orients to bell (localizes laterally)	—
6 mo	Sits unsupported, puts feet in the mouth in supine position	Unilateral reach, uses raking grasp	Babbles	Recognizes strangers
7 mo	Creeps	—	Orients to bell (localized indirectly)	—
8 mo	Comes to sit, crawls	Inspects objects	"Dada" indiscriminately	Finger-feeds
9 mo	Pivots when sitting, pulls to stand, cruises	Uses pincer grasp, probes with forefinger, holds bottle, throws objects	"Mama" indiscriminately, gestures, waves bye-bye, inhibits to "no"	Starts to explore environment; plays gesture games (e.g., pat-a-cake)
10 mo	Walks when led with both hands held	—	"Dada/mama" discriminately; orients to bell (directly)	—
11 mo	Walks when led with one hand held	—	One word other than "dada/mama," follows one-step command with gesture	—
12 mo	Walks alone	Uses mature pincer grasp, releases voluntarily, marks paper with pencil	Uses two words other than "dada/mama," immature jargoning (runs several unintelligible syllables together)	Imitates actions, comes when called, cooperates with dressing
13 mo	—	—	Uses three words	—
14 mo	—	—	Follows one-step command without gesture	—
15 mo	Creeps up stairs, walks backward	Scribbles in imitation, builds tower of two blocks in imitation	Uses four to six words	*15–18 mo:* uses spoon, uses cup independently
17 mo	—	—	Uses 7–20 words, points to five body parts, uses mature jargoning (includes intelligible words in jargoning)	—

(*continued*)

Table 36-2 Developmental Milestones (*continued*)

AGE	GROSS MOTOR	VISUAL–MOTOR/ PROBLEM-SOLVING	LANGUAGE	SOCIAL/ADAPTIVE
18 mo	Runs, throws objects from standing without falling	Scribbles spontaneously, builds tower of three blocks, turns two to three pages at a time	Uses two-word combinations	Copies parental caregiver in tasks (sweeping, dusting), plays in company of other children
19 mo	—	—	Knows eight body parts	—
21 mo	Squats in play, goes up steps	Builds tower of five blocks	Uses 50 words, two-word sentences	Asks to have food and to go to toilet
24 mo	Walks up and down steps without help	Imitates stroke with pencil, builds tower of seven blocks, turns pages one at a time, removes shoes, pants, etc.	Uses pronouns (*I*, *you*, *me*) inappropriately, follows two-step commands	Parallel play
30 mo	Jumps with both feet off the floor, throws ball overhand	Holds pencil in adult fashion, performs horizontal and vertical strokes, unbuttons	Uses pronouns appropriately, understands concept of "1," repeats two digits forward	Tells first and last names when asked; gets self drink without help
3 yr	Can alternate feet when going up steps, pedals tricycle	Copies a circle, undresses completely, dresses partially, dries hands if reminded	Uses minimum 250 words, three-word sentences; uses plurals, past tense; knows all pronouns; understands concept of "2"	Group play, shares toys, takes turns, plays well with others, knows full name, age, gender
4 yr	Hops, skips, alternates feet going down steps	Copies a square, buttons clothing, dresses self completely, catches ball	Knows colors, says song or poem from memory, asks questions	Tells "tall tales," plays cooperatively with a group of children
5 yr	Skips alternating feet, jumps over low obstacles	Copies triangle, ties shoes, spreads with knife	Prints first name, asks what a word means	Plays competitive games, abides by rules, likes to help in household tasks

SELECTED READINGS

Albert, P., Romski, M. A., Rose, A., & Morris, R. (2021). Patterns of cognition, communication, and adaptive behavior in children with developmental disabilities. *American Journal on Intellectual & Developmental Disabilities, 126*(4), 324–340. https://doi.org/10.1352/1944-7558-126.4.324

Augustyn, M., & Zuckerman, B. (2018). *The Zuckerman Parker handbook of developmental and behavioral pediatrics: A handbook for primary care* (4th ed.). Lippincott Williams & Wilkins.

Azzano, A., Ward, R., Vause, T., & Feldman, M. (2022). Parent-mediated targeted intervention for young children at risk for autism spectrum disorder. *Infants & Young Children: An Interdisciplinary Journal of Early Childhood Intervention, 35*(4), 320–338. https://doi.org/10.1097/IYC.0000000000000226

Coffield, C., Harris, J., Janvier, Y., Lopez, M., Gonzalez, N., & Jimenez, M. (2020). Parental concerns of underserved young children at risk for autism. *Journal of Health Care for the Poor & Underserved, 31*(2), 742–755. https://doi.org/10.1353/hpu.2020.0058

DeCandia, C., Volk, K., Unick, G., & Donegan, L. (2020). Developing a screening tool for young children using an ecological framework. *Infants & Young Children: An Interdisciplinary Journal of Early Childhood Intervention, 33*(4), 237–258. https://doi.org/10.1097/iyc.0000000000000173

Garzon, D., Starr, N., Brady, M., Gaylord, N., Driessnack, M., & Duderstadt, K. (2021). *Burns' pediatric primary care* (7th ed.). Elsevier.

Hine, J., Allin, J., Allman, A., Black, M., Browning, B., Ramsey, B., Sawnson, A., Warren, Z., Zawoyski, A., & Allen, W. (2020). Increasing access to autism spectrum disorder diagnostic consultation in rural and underserved communities: Streamlined evaluation within primary care. *Journal of Developmental and Behavioral Pediatrics, 41*(1), 16–22. https://doi.org/10.1097/DBP.0000000000000727

Johns Hopkins Hospital; Kleinman, K., McDaniel, L., & Molloy, M. (Eds.). (2021). *The Harriet Lane handbook* (22nd ed.). Elsevier.

Kim, S. (2022). Worldwide national intervention of developmental screening programs in infant and early childhood. *Clinical and Experimental Pediatrics, 65*(1), 10–20. https://doi.org/10.3345/cep.2021.00248

Kyle, T. (Ed.). (2020). *Essentials of pediatric nursing* (4th ed.). Wolters Kluwer Health.

Landi, I., Giannotti, M., Venuti, P., & Simona, F. (2020). Maternal and family predictors of infant psychological development in at-risk families: A multilevel longitudinal study. *Research in Nursing & Allied Health, 43*(1), 17–27. https://doi.org/10.1002/nur.21989

Lane, A. (2020). Practitioner Review: Effective management of functional difficulties associated with sensory symptoms in children and adolescents. *Journal of Child Psychology & Psychiatry, 61*(9), 943–958. https://doi.org/10.1111/jcpp.13230

Lipkin, P., & Macias, M. (2020). Promoting optimal development: Identifying infants and young children with developmental disorders through developmental surveillance and screening. *Pediatrics, 145*(1), e20193449. https://doi.org/10.1542/peds.2019-3449

Martin-Herz, S., Buyesse, C., DeBattista, A., & Feldman, H. (2020). Colocated developmental-behavioral pediatrics in primary care: Improved outcome across settings. *Journal of Developmental & Behavioral Pediatrics, 41*(5), 340–348. https://doi.org/10.1097/DBP.0000000000000789

McNeilly, L. (2022). Speech, language, and feeding of children birth to 5 years old and the use of developmental milestone checklists. *Zero to Three, 43*(1), 66–69. https://eric.ed.gov/?id=EJ1352443

Minde, M., Remmerswaal, M., Raat, H., Steegers, E., & Kroon, M. (2020). Innovative postnatal risk assessment in preventive child health care: A study protocol. *Journal of Advanced Nursing, 76*(12), 3654–3661. https://doi.org/10.1111/jan.14547

Moser, M., Mullner, C., Ferro, P., Albermann, K., Jenni, O., & von Rhin, M. (2023). The role of well-child visits in detecting developmental delay in preschool children. *BMC Pediatrics, 23*, 180. https://doi.org/10.1186/s12887-023-04005-1

Murray, C., Hastings, R., & Totsika, V. (2021). Clinical utility of the parent-reported Strengths and Difficulties Questionnaire as a screen for emotional and behavioral difficulties in children and adolescents with intellectual disability. *British Journal of Psychiatry, 218* (6), 323–325. https://doi.org/10.1192/bjp.2020.224

Obusanya, B., Storbeck, C., Cheung, V., & Hadders-Lagra, M. (2023). Disabilities in early childhood: A global health perspective. *Children, 10*(1), 155. https://doi.org/10.3390/children10010155

Rooner, T., Stern, Y., Hampton, L., Grauzer, J., Hobson, A., Levin, A., Jones, M., Kaat, A., & Roberts, M. (2022). Screening for autism in 2-year-old children: The application of the systematic observation of red flags to the screening tool for autism in toddlers and young children. *American Journal of Speech-Language Pathology, 31*(6), 2759–2769. https://doi.org/10.1044/2022_AJSLP-22-00132

Sullivan, M., Lynch, E., & Msall, M. (2020). Late adolescent & young adult functioning and participation outcomes after prematurity. *Seminars in Fetal & Neonatal Medicine, 25*(3), 101118. https://doi.org/10.1016/j.siny.2020.101118

Vermij, B., Wiefferink, C., Scholte, R., & Knoors, H. (2021). Language development and behaviour problems in toddlers indicated to have a developmental language disorder. *International Journal of Language & Communication Disorders, 56*(6), 1249–1262. https://doi.org/10.1111/1460-6984.12665

Whitmore Schanzembach, D., & Thorn, B. (2020). Supporting development through child nutrition. *Future of Children, 30*(2), 115–141. https://eric.ed.gov/?id=EJ1293600

37 Pediatric Physical Assessment*

HISTORY

Obtaining a History

A history of the child is obtained to establish a relationship with the child and family, to assess family understanding about the child's health, to formulate an individual care plan, and to correct misinformation the family may have.

Focus on specific topics in the history, depending on the child's age, including:

- Infant—prenatal and postnatal history, nutrition, development.
- Toddler—home environment, safety issues, development, caregiver's response to child's interactions.
- School age—school, friends, reaction to previous hospitalizations.
- Adolescent—alcohol, drugs, friends, sexual history, relationships with caregivers, identity.

Identifying Information

Type of Information Needed

1. Date and time.
2. Health care provider's name and telephone number, if known.
3. Insurance data.
4. Patient's name, address, telephone number, birth date.
5. Referring health care source (e.g., school, other health care provider, clinic).

Note: Permission from the legal guardian must be obtained to treat a child unless it is an emergency.

Method of Collecting Data

1. Identify the caregiver in charge of the patient by name and relationship to the patient; obtain a relative's or alternate caregiver's address and home, cell, and work telephone numbers, if different from those of the primary caregiver.
2. To make the caregiver feel more at ease, the questions should begin in a friendly, nonthreatening manner. Questions addressed to the caregiver should be phrased appropriately.
3. Casual, friendly responses or remarks on the part of the interviewer may also help break the ice, such as:
   a. "Whoever takes care of this baby certainly does a good job."
   b. "That is a lovely outfit the baby is wearing." (Remember that families will usually put good clothes on a child for a visit to a health care agency.)
4. Sometimes, repeat the information to verify data. This will give you a better judgment of the caregiver's cooperation and reliability.
5. If age appropriate, get some data directly from the child.

Chief Complaint

Method of Recording

1. Record who arrived with the child and write an exact description of the complaint.
2. Use quotation marks to clearly indicate that the informant's words are being used. It is helpful to explain to the caregiver that this is what you're recording and why:
   a. "I will write it down so there will be no mistake."
   b. "Let me read this back to you to make sure it is correct."
3. Quotation of the caregiver's exact words may give an indication of how they feel about the symptoms; it may reflect fear, guilt, or defensiveness.

Method of Collecting Information

1. Begin with a helpful, open-ended question:
   a. "How have things been going?"
   b. "Please tell me the reason for your coming here today."
   c. "Do you have any particular worries or concerns about the baby?"
2. Then, proceed to more specific questions.

Duration of Complaint

1. The information obtained may indicate the natural history of the disease, if one is present, and its gradual evolution. Pursue the information with a series of probing questions.
   a. "How long has the baby (child) had this problem?"
   b. If the informant cannot remember, try another route: "When did the child last act well? Before summer vacation? Last Christmas? Did the baby have the trouble then?"
2. Write down the responses; try to assess, as more questions are asked, how accurate the informant's answers may be.

*Please note that the term "male" in this chapter refers to a person assigned male at birth, and the term "female" in this chapter refers to a person assigned female at birth.

Remember, a child who is a reliable historian may be the most accurate source of information regarding their health history, treatments, and other health needs.

History of Present Illness

Type of Information Needed

For an infant, a preverbal, or a nonverbal child, information will consist mainly of what the informant has been able to observe. Having established what the chief complaint is, identify further problems, if any. Obtain the following information for each problem:

1. Body location—of pain, itching, weakness.
2. Quality and quantity of complaint—both type (a burning pain) and severity (knifelike, comes and goes).
3. Degree of symptom—for example, pain, how severe; cough, day and night; eye drainage, amount.
4. Chronology—indicate time sequence and whether the problem is episodic (lasts for a while and then clears up completely).
5. Environment or setting—where and when the symptoms occur.
6. Aggravating and alleviating factors—what makes the pain worse or better.
7. Associated manifestations or symptoms—accompanied by vomiting, blurred vision.

Importance of Detail

1. Typically, a carefully written description of a symptom will be the source of a future diagnosis and will serve all who are involved in helping the patient.
2. Do not worry that you are taking too many notes.
3. You will be able to recheck this information when you do the review of systems.

Family History

1. Family members—caregivers' age and state of health, siblings ("who is at home with you?")
2. Family health history:
   a. Eyes, ears, nose, throat—nosebleeds, sinus problems, glaucoma, cataracts, myopia, strabismus, other problems of eyes, ears, nose, throat.
   b. Cardiorespiratory—tuberculosis, asthma, hay fever, hypertension, heart murmurs, heart attacks, strokes, rheumatic fever, pneumonia, emphysema, other problems.
   c. Gastrointestinal—ulcers, colitis, vomiting, diarrhea, other problems.
   d. Genitourinary—kidney infections, bladder problems, congenital abnormalities.
   e. Musculoskeletal—congenital hip or foot problems, muscular dystrophy, arthritis, other problems.
   f. Neurologic—seizures, epilepsy, nervous disorder, intellectual disability, emotional problems, comas, headaches, others.
   g. Chronic disease—diabetes, liver disease, cancer, tumors, anemia, thyroid problems, congenital disorder.
   h. Sensory deficits—anyone deaf or blind or with significant deficits in visual or auditory perception.
   i. Miscellaneous—other medical problems not mentioned.
3. Family social history:
   a. Residence—apartment or house and size. Yard, stairs, proximity to transportation, shopping, playground, school, safe neighborhood? City or well water?
   b. Financial situation—who works, where employed, occupation, public assistance programs.
   c. Other primary caregiver—babysitters, day care center.
   d. Family interrelationships—happy, cooperative, antagonistic, chaotic, multiproblem, violent.

Past History

Prenatal

1. Pregnancy—planned or not; source of care; approximate date of seeking care; birth order of this pregnancy, including miscarriages. This area of the history may be one of great sensitivity. Try to make the questions gentle and supportive:
   a. "Did you plan a baby around this time?"
   b. "When was your first checkup for the pregnancy?"
   c. "Were there any unusual problems related to your pregnancy or delivery?"
2. Maternal health—includes illnesses and dates, abnormal symptoms (e.g., fever, rash, vaginal bleeding, edema, hypertension, urine abnormalities, sexually transmitted disease). Avoid technical words, if possible.
   a. "Were the doctors or nurses worried about your health?"
   b. "Were your rings or shoes tight?"
   c. "Do you know if your blood pressure went up?"
   d. "Did you have trouble with your urine?"
3. Weight gain—validate by trying to get a figure for nonpregnant weight and weight at delivery.
4. Medications taken—for example, vitamins, iron, calcium, aspirin, cold preparations, tranquilizers (which patients might refer to as "nerve medicine"), antibiotics; use of ointments, hormones, injections during pregnancy; special or unusual diet; radiation exposure; sonography; and amniocentesis.
5. Quality of the fetal movements—when felt?
6. Use of alcohol, tobacco, or drugs during pregnancy.

Natal

1. Expected date of delivery and approximate duration of pregnancy.
2. Place of delivery and name of the person who conducted the delivery.
3. Labor—spontaneous or induced, duration, and intensity.
4. Analgesia or anesthesia.
5. Type of delivery—vaginal (breech or vertex presentation); cesarean delivery; forceps delivery.
6. Complications (e.g., need for blood transfusion or delay in delivery).

Neonatal

1. Condition of infant.
2. Color (if seen) at delivery.
3. Activity of infant.
4. Type of crying heard.
5. Breathing abnormality.
6. Birth weight and length.
7. Problems that occurred immediately at birth.

Postnatal

1. Duration of hospitalization of the birthing parent and infant.
2. Problems with baby's breathing or feeding.
3. Need for supportive care (e.g., oxygen, incubator, special care nursery, isolation, medications).
4. Weight changes, weight at discharge, if known.
5. Color—cyanosis or jaundice.
6. Bowel movements—when.
7. Problems—seizures, deformities identified, consultation required.

8. Hearing—was a hearing screen conducted in the nursery? The U.S. Preventative Services Task Force recommends universal screening for all newborns using otoacoustic emissions and/or auditory brain stem response testing. The guideline is available online at www.guideline.gov/summaries/summary/47317/preventive-services-for-children-and-adolescents?q=newborns+otoacoustic.
9. Birthing parent's contact with the baby and their first impression:
   a. "What was it like when you first saw your baby?"
   b. "What did the baby do when you were first together?"

Nutrition

1. Breast- or bottle fed? What formula? How prepared?
2. Amounts offered and consumed.
3. Frequency of feeding—weight gain.
4. Addition of juice or solid foods.
5. Food preferences or allergies.
6. Feeding problems—variations in appetite.
7. Age of weaning.
8. Vitamins—type, amount, regularity.
9. Pattern of weight gain.
10. Current diet—frequency and content of meals.

Growth and Development

1. Past weights and lengths, if available.
2. Milestones—sat alone unsupported; walked alone; used words, then sentences.
3. Teeth—eruption, difficulty, cavities, brushing, flossing.
4. Toilet training.
5. Current motor, social, and language skills.
6. Sexual development.
   a. Infant—swollen breast tissue, vaginal discharge, hypertrophy of the labia.
   b. Toddler or school-age child—early development of breasts or pubic hair.
   c. Prepubertal or pubertal child—in females, time of development of breasts and pubic hair and onset of menstruation. In males, time of enlargement of testes and penis, development of pubic and facial hair, and voice changes.

Health Maintenance

1. Immunizations—rubella, rubeola, mumps, polio, diphtheria, pertussis, tetanus toxoid, varicella, pneumococcal, Bacillus Calmette–Guérin, influenza, *Haemophilus influenzae* type b, hepatitis A and B, meningococcal conjugate, human papillomavirus, and rotavirus. Indicate the number and dates. Recommended immunization schedules are available online at https://www.cdc.gov/vaccines/schedules/hcp/imz/child-adolescent.html.
2. Screening procedures—hematocrit or hemoglobin level, urinalysis, tuberculin testing, visual and auditory acuity, color vision, lead testing, cholesterol screening, syphilis testing, human immunodeficiency virus (HIV) testing, gonorrhea, and Chlamydia screening.
3. Dental care—source and frequency of care, dental hygienist visits, fillings, extractions, last checkup.

Acute Infectious Diseases

Rubella, rubeola, mumps, chickenpox, group A beta-hemolytic pharyngitis, parvovirus B19 (fifth disease), hepatitis, infectious mononucleosis, sexually transmitted disease, tuberculosis, influenza. Recent exposure to a communicable disease.

Hospitalizations and Surgeries

1. Dates, hospital, health care provider.
2. Indications, diagnosis, procedures.
3. Complications.
4. Reactions to previous hospitalizations.

Injuries

1. Emergency department or urgent care visits—frequency and diagnosis.
2. Fractures, injuries, burns—location and treatment.
3. Ingestions.
4. Ask the caregivers about provision of a safe environment; for example, cleaning supplies out of reach, electrical outlets with appropriate covers, guns in the house unloaded and kept in a locked room or cabinet, and water safety education (bathtub and pools). Ask about use of safety equipment, such as seat belts, bike helmets, childproof safety caps on medications, smoke and carbon monoxide detectors in the home.

Medications

1. For general use, such as vitamins, antihistamines, laxatives.
2. Special or fad diets.
3. Recent antibiotics.
4. Herbal or complementary remedies.
5. Routine use of aspirin.
6. Hormonal contraceptives—types, dose, duration.
7. Drugs, opioids, marijuana, hallucinogens, mood elevators, tranquilizers, alcohol.
8. Determine when the last dose of medication was taken; is the medication with the patient? How does the child take the medication?
9. Allergy or adverse reaction to medication?

School History

Type of Information Needed

1. Present and past schooling, attendance, grade, and performance.
2. Favored and least-favored subjects.
3. School-related behavior—anxious to go, anxious to stay home.
4. General attitude toward school and career plans.
5. General attitude toward peer groups, attempt to avoid or be included.

Method of Collecting Data

1. Straightforward questions to a child (e.g., "What grade are you in?" "Who are your friends?").
2. Questions about wishes asked to the child:
   a. "If your birthday were here, what would you ask for?"
   b. "If you could be anyone, who would it be?"
   c. "What would be the best thing that could happen to you?"
3. Questions about friends:
   a. To child:
      i. "Do you have friends?"
      ii. "Who is your best friend?"
   b. To parental caregivers:
      i. "Do you know the friends your child identified?"
4. Adolescents—interviews with older children and teens may start with the caregivers present, but the child should also be provided with some private time with the nurse, away from the caregivers, to discuss concerns. The caregivers should also be allowed a brief time with the nurse, away from their child, to voice any concerns.
5. Emphasize the positive (e.g., "What is your best subject?").

Social History

Type of Information Needed

1. Environment—rural, urban.
2. Housing—type, location, heating, sewage, water supply, family pets, other animal exposure.
3. Primary adult caregivers' occupations (employment) and marital status.
4. Number of individuals living in home and sleeping arrangements.
5. Religious affiliations, if any.
6. Previous utilization of social agencies.
7. Health insurance and usual source of care.
8. After assuring older children of the confidentiality of their answers, inquire about risk-taking behaviors, such as cigarette smoking, vaping, alcohol and drug use (including cannabis), drinking and driving, and sexual history.

Method of Collecting Data

Caregivers are proud, so use tact and diplomacy when asking some questions. Ask permission.

1. "Can you tell me a little bit about your home?"
2. "To help you with your child's problem, I need to know more about how you live."

Personal History

Type of Information Needed

1. Hygiene.
2. Exercise.
3. Sleep habits.
4. Elimination habits.
5. Activities, hobbies, special talents.
6. Relationships with friends and teacher.
7. Relationships with siblings (if any) and caregivers.
8. Expression of emotions.
   a. Loses temper easily.
   b. Quiet.
9. Idiosyncratic behavior and habits (e.g., thumb-sucking, nail-biting, temper tantrums, head banging, pica, breath-holding, rituals, tics).
10. Emotional issues, such as school avoidance, somatic complaints.

Review of Systems

Type of Information Needed

1. General—activity, appetite, affect, sleep patterns, weight changes, edema, fever, behavior.
2. Allergy—eczema, hay fever, asthma, hives, food or drug allergy, sinus disorders.
3. Skin—rash or eruption, nodules, pigmentation or texture change, sweating or dryness, infection, hair growth, itching.
4. Head—headache, head trauma, dizziness.
5. Eyes—visual acuity, corrective lenses, strabismus, lacrimation, discharge, itching, redness, photophobia.
6. Ears—auditory acuity, earaches (frequency, ages, response to specific medications), infection, drainage.
7. Nose—colds and runny nose (frequency), infection, drainage.
8. Teeth—hygiene practices, frequency of brushing, general condition, cavities, malocclusions.
9. Throat—sore throat, tonsillitis, difficulty swallowing.
10. Speech—peculiarity of or change in voice, hoarseness, clarity, enunciation, stuttering, development of articulation, vocabulary, use of sentences.
11. Respiratory—difficulty breathing, shortness of breath, chest pain, cough, wheezing, croup, pneumonia, tuberculosis or exposure.
12. Cardiovascular—cyanosis, fainting, exercise intolerance, palpitations, murmurs.
13. Hematologic—pallor, anemia, tendency to bruise or bleed.
14. Gastrointestinal—appetite (amount, frequency, cravings), nausea, vomiting, abdominal pain, abnormal size, bowel habits and nature of stools, parasites, encopresis (incontinence of feces), colic.
15. Genitourinary—age of toilet training, frequency of urination, straining, dysuria, hematuria (or unusual color or odor of infant's soiled diaper), previous urinary tract infection, enuresis (age of onset; day or nighttime), urethral or vaginal discharge. Prepubertal and young females: age at menarche, last menses, cramps, changes in interval and duration.
16. Musculoskeletal—deformities, fractures, sprains, joint pains or swelling, limited motion, abnormality of nails.
17. Neurologic—weakness or clumsiness, coordination, balance, gait, dominance, fatigability, tone, tremor, seizures or paroxysmal behavior, personality changes.

PHYSICAL EXAMINATION

General Principles

1. Establish the order of all data collection according to the needs of the patient. For example:
   a. An exhausted caregiver with a screaming baby will not give a careful, comprehensive history.
   b. Alternative care may not be available for preschoolers when the neonate comes in for their first checkup.
2. If the caregiver has come in with more than one child, try to organize some supervision of the other children so that you can have a little time alone with the caregiver.
3. Remember that the safest place for a young child is on the caregiver's lap. Privacy may not be possible when other children are present.
4. Attempt to develop rapport with the young patient from the moment you first see or meet them.
5. Explain to the school-age child or teenager what you are looking for as you proceed with the examination, and provide feedback.

APPROACH TO THE PATIENT

1. Offer the young child a choice of being examined on the caregiver's lap or on your "special table."
2. Start with examination of the lungs and heart. You will need to listen for at least 15 seconds. Consider the use of a pacifier for a crying infant.
3. The part to be examined should be completely exposed, but if an apprehensive child objects to having clothes removed, slip your stethoscope under the shirt.
4. After listening to the heart, begin with parts of the body that are already exposed.
5. Start with either the head or the toes and work thoroughly and systematically toward the other end.

6. Gradually remove the child's clothes (may best be done by the usual caregiver); look for asymmetry very carefully in the bodies of all children.
7. Develop a pattern appropriate to the patient's age.
   a. With infants, it may be wise to leave the diaper area until last.
   b. Adolescents and school-age children are usually embarrassed at the genital examination—you may want to leave this until last, covering areas already examined.
8. Using a cold stethoscope may result in a frightened, crying child, so clean and warm the stethoscope before bringing it into contact with the child.
9. Some children are less frightened if allowed to hold the examination equipment first.
10. Show the child the procedure by demonstrating it on the caregiver first.
11. Many young children enjoy listening to their own hearts.
12. Toddlers and preschoolers enjoy blowing the otoscope light out.

PEDIATRIC PHYSICAL ASSESSMENT

VITAL SIGNS

Technique

1. Obtain temperature, pulse rate, respiratory rate, and blood pressure as often as necessary, based on the child's condition.
2. Measure core temperature, whenever possible, via rectal or ear route. An electronic thermometer will alert the user when the temperature is accurately registered. Avoid taking temperature via oral route following fluid or food intake.
3. Obtain apical pulse rate on an infant or small child; radial, temporal, or carotid pulse may be measured on an older child. Pulse may be counted for 30 sec and multiplied by 2.
4. Count respirations on an infant for 1 full minute; observe the chest as well as the abdomen. Respirations may be counted for 30 sec and multiplied by 2 in an older child.
5. Obtain blood pressure by auscultatory method, rather than palpation method, whenever possible. Make sure the cuff covers no less than ½ and no more than ⅔ the length of the upper arm or leg.

Findings

Temperature

Oral	*Rectal*	*Axillary*
97.6°F–99.3°F (36.4°C–37.4°C)	97°F–100°F (36.1°C–37.8°C)	96.6°F–98°F (35.9°C–36.7°C)

Pulse and respiratory rates

Age	Pulse	Respirations
Neonate	70–170	30–50
11 mo	80–160	26–40
2 yr	80–130	20–30
4 yr	80–120	20–30
6 yr	75–115	20–26
8 yr	70–110	18–24
10 yr	70–110	18–24
Adolescent	60–110	12–20

Blood pressure

Varies with age, height, and weight of child

STANDING HEIGHT, HEAD CIRCUMFERENCE, AND CHEST CIRCUMFERENCE

Technique

1. Use a tape measure to obtain accurate head circumference (see Figure 37-1). Measure the widest part of the head.

Findings

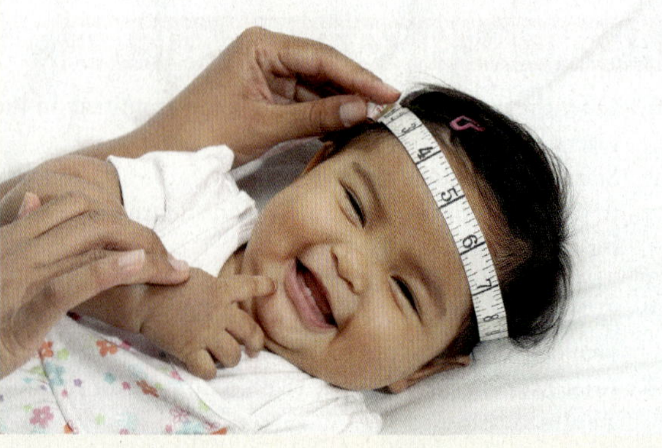

Figure 37-1. Measuring head circumference. (Shutterstock/Marlon Lopez MMG1 Design)

PEDIATRIC PHYSICAL ASSESSMENT *(continued)*

2. Measure the chest at the level of the nipples.

3. Record height and weight at each visit. Plot on the growth chart.

3. A variety of clinical growth charts on which to record length, head, circumference, BMI, and weight can be downloaded from https://www.cdc.gov/growthcharts/index.htm. Trends in growth are as important as the basic measurements.

4. Calculate body mass index (BMI) and plot it on the appropriate chart.

4. BMI is calculated by following the formula on page 548, or for online pediatric BMI calculator, https://www.cdc.gov/healthyweight/bmi/calculator.html.

GENERAL APPEARANCE

Technique	Findings
1. Begin your observations with the first contact with the patient, remembering to also observe the caregiver's interaction with the child.	1. If the child is easily distracted or sleepy, it may be nap time.
2. The patient's interaction with the caregiver, whether it be the mother, father, a babysitter, an older sibling, a friend of the family, or someone else, is vital in the assessment of the child. As you observe for sex assigned at birth, general physical development, nutritional state, mental alertness, evidence of pain, restlessness, body position, clothes, apparent age, hygiene, and grooming, remember that many of these things are a measure of the caregiver's caretaking.	2. Careful observation of the general state of the child will provide many clues about the child's relationship with the family and its response to the child.

SKIN AND LYMPHATICS

Technique	Findings
Examine as you move through each body region (include hair and skin).	
Inspection	
Inspection of the skin is the same as for the adult.	
1. Observe for skin color, pigmentation, lesions, jaundice, cyanosis, scars, superficial vascularity, moisture, edema, color of mucous membranes, hair distribution.	1. In young infants, the skin is soft, smooth, and velvety in texture.
2. Describe any variation in color, particularly in children with increased pigmentation. For children with a dark skin tone, not if no pigment, or vitiligo, is found.	2. Pigmentations vary in children and will change as the child gets older.
3. Birthmarks of any type are recorded. (May change as the child grows older.)	3. A suntan, freckles, and small, light-brown patches or *café-au-lait* spots may occur.
4. Bruises or unusual marks, wounds or insect bites, scratch marks, or scars may have particular significance.	4. Bruises are particularly important because of the possibility of reoccurring injury and/or child abuse.
5. Draw a picture of anything unusual such as a scar and measure the dimensions of the lesion when recording the findings.	5. If you have difficulty describing something, use ordinary words rather than inaccurate technical terms.
6. To ascertain suspected jaundice, take the child to the window, if possible, to get a true picture of the color of the skin. (A room with yellow walls and artificial lighting may create a wrong impression when jaundice is suspected.)	6. Carotenemia, which causes the nose and palms to have a yellowish tinge, may lead the caregivers to suspect jaundice; however, carotenemia is caused by eating a large amount of yellow vegetables (sweet potatoes, squash, carrots). In carotenemia, the sclerae are clear; this is not the case in jaundice.
7. The skin of neonates will still be covered with vernix caseosa, the oily material that covers the fetus's body while in utero.	7. Swollen sebaceous glands over the nose and chin are commonly seen immediately after birth and are called *milia*.
8. Postmature infants may have scaliness or peeling that persists for several weeks after birth, particularly around the feet. The color of the skin may change as the child gets a little older.	8. The blotchy, pink patches over the eyelid, bridge of the nose, and the back of the neck may persist until the child is almost 2 yr of age.

(continued)

PEDIATRIC PHYSICAL ASSESSMENT *(continued)*

9. Note striae.

   9. May indicate rapid weight gain or loss.

10. Dark-skinned children may have congenital dermal melanocytosis (formerly called Mongolian spots) at the base of the spine or elsewhere.

    10. Important to distinguish from child abuse.

Palpation

1. Use the tips of your fingers to palpate—fingertips are more sensitive.
2. Check the tension of the skin by pinching up a fold of skin (see Figure 37-2)—normal skin quickly falls back, but dehydrated skin remains in a pinched position.

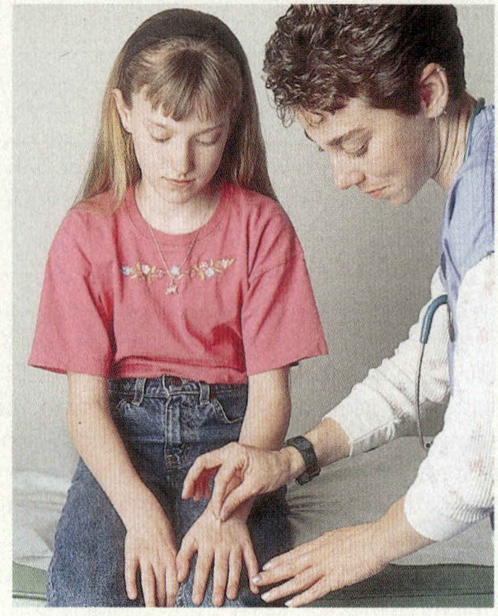

Figure 37-2. Checking skin tension.

3. Feel the skin for texture, moisture, temperature, turgor, elasticity, masses, tenderness.

   3. Skin that is rough and dry in texture may actually have a discrete rash that can be felt but not seen.

Lymph

1. Observe and palpate for lymph node enlargement in lymph chain areas.
   a. Neck.
   b. Axilla.
   c. Inguinal.
   d. Epitrochlear.

   1. May be large or readily palpable, but should be nontender, mobile, and slightly spongy.

2. Note tenderness, size, and consistency.

Nails

1. Observe for color, shape, irregularities in surface, and general nail care; cleanliness, evidence of biting.

   1. Nail beds should be pink, nails convex.

2. Palpate the skin around the fingernails for firmness. Palpate any part that appears inflamed.

   2. General care of the child is frequently reflected in good care of nails.

Hair

1. Observe for color and distribution.
   a. Note according to the age of the child and race.
   b. Be aware that tufts of hair over the spine or sacral area may mark an underlying abnormality.

   1. *Neonate*: Normally varies from no hair to a thick bush. Infant: lanugo, a soft, downy covering commonly seen over the shoulders, back, arms, face, and sacral area, especially in dark-skinned children; lanugo is present for the first 1–2 mo, after which it disappears.

2. Note changes in pigmentation.

   2. Remember, children may experiment with hair dye or rinse.

3. Palpate the hair for texture and thickness.

   3. Texture may be thick or thin, coarse or fine, straight or curly.

4. Examine to see if there are patches on the head where hair is missing.

   4. May denote underlying skin infection; however, some children pull their hair out; sometimes, the hair is braided so tightly that it falls out. Infants who sleep consistently on their backs may have thinning or absent hair in the occiput.

5. Separate thick hair on the head to get a good view of the scalp. Check for dandruff or scaliness in older children.

   5. Look carefully for broken hairs, for scaliness on the scalp, or cradle cap in infants.

PEDIATRIC PHYSICAL ASSESSMENT *(continued)*

Technique	Findings
6. Check scalp for signs of lice infestation.	6. Nits (louse eggs) appear on the hair as little white dots. Lice may be seen on the scalp; they move quickly and may jump.
7. Inspect the axillae and over the pubis and the extremities for hair and its quantity, to gauge the development and level of puberty.	7. The child does not need to be totally undressed at one time; a prepubertal child will usually be embarrassed if all clothes are removed.

HEAD AND NECK

Technique	Findings
1. Unless specifically requested, examine the eyes and ears last, especially in the younger child.	
2. Also, examine the throat toward the end of the examination, unless the child exhibits concern about the "throat stick." It is then best to examine the throat right away to "get it over with." If a child cries or can open their mouth widely with encouragement, you may be able to avoid using a tongue depressor.	
3. To avoid frightening the child when palpating the head, make a game out of it—ask, "Where is your nose?" "Where are your eyes?"	
Inspection	
1. Observe the face and skull for asymmetry, deformity, and abnormal or limited movements.	1. An infant's head may be asymmetrical because of pressure during pregnancy and delivery. The rounded head of an infant born by breech delivery contrasts with the long, pointed head of an infant who is a firstborn and whose head was molded during a prolonged labor.
2. Closely observe facial expressions and blinking if the child is not crying. This may be one of your few moments to see the child when they are not crying. If you are examining a crying infant, watch particularly for asymmetry of the face.	2. In an infant born by forceps delivery, there may be signs of weakness of the facial nerve caused by pressure of the forceps over the front of the ear where the facial nerve emerges. When the infant cries, the involved side will show weakness and down turning of the mouth.
3. Observe the movement of the head on the neck as the infant looks around. When turning an infant over, observe the head for control, position, and movement.	3. There should be very little head lag after age 3 months.
4. Because an infant's neck is typically short and there are usually several folds of skin under the chin, it is necessary to lift the chin a little to observe the skin completely—to see that it is clear and free from perspiration rash or irritation.	4. In the back, the neck should be free of webbing or extra folds of skin extending from just beneath the ear toward the shoulder.
Palpation	
1. Palpate the skull for the suture lines. Feel the face for masses, noting size, consistency, surface, temperature, and tenderness (see Figure 37-3).	1. The suture lines of the skull may be felt to override as a result of the pressure applied when contractions occurred during labor. This is usually most marked between the frontal and the parietal bones, where the coronal suture is located (see Figure 37-4).

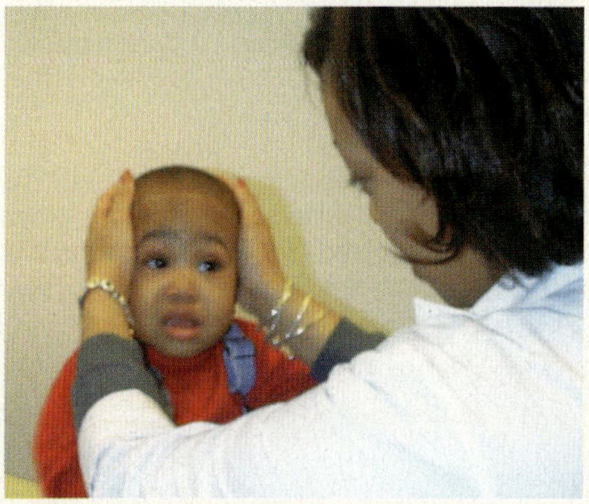

Figure 37-3. Palpation of the head.

(continued)

PEDIATRIC PHYSICAL ASSESSMENT (continued)

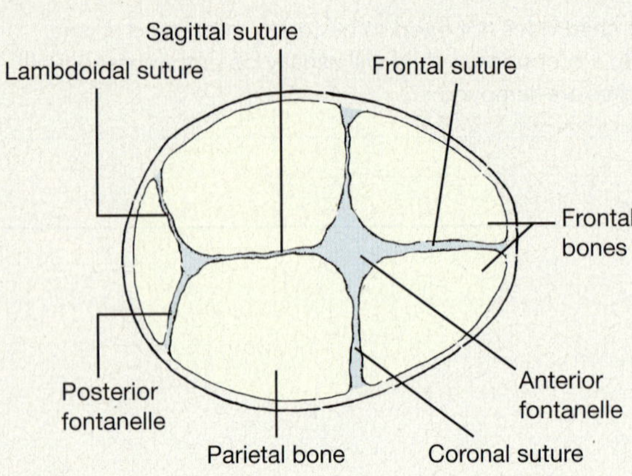

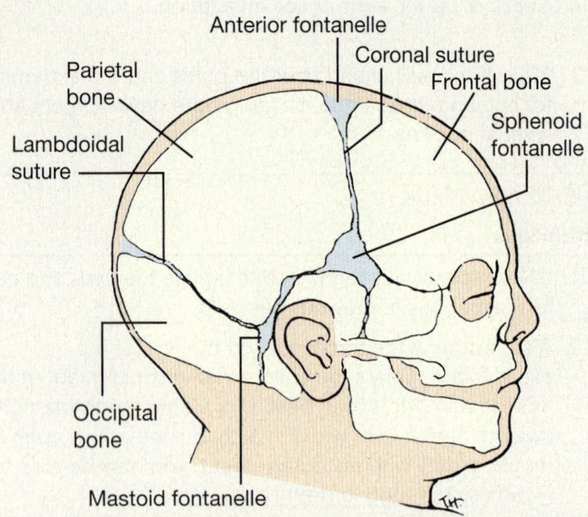

Figure 37-4. The bones and suture lines of the skull.

2. Palpate the anterior and posterior fontanelles.

2. The fontanelles are soft and flat when the child is quiet. Tense or bulging fontanelles may indicate hydrocephalus. Depressed fontanelles are often a sign of dehydration. The posterior fontanelle usually closes by 1–2 months; anterior fontanelle by 18 months.

3. Palpate along the lambdoidal suture at the back of the head between the parietal bones and the occipital bone.

4. Palpate the neck for swollen lymph nodes, noting tenderness, mobility, location, and consistency (see Figures 37-5 and 37-6).

4. Palpation of the lymph nodes may reveal slightly enlarged nodes in the anterior cervical chain secondary to sore throat.

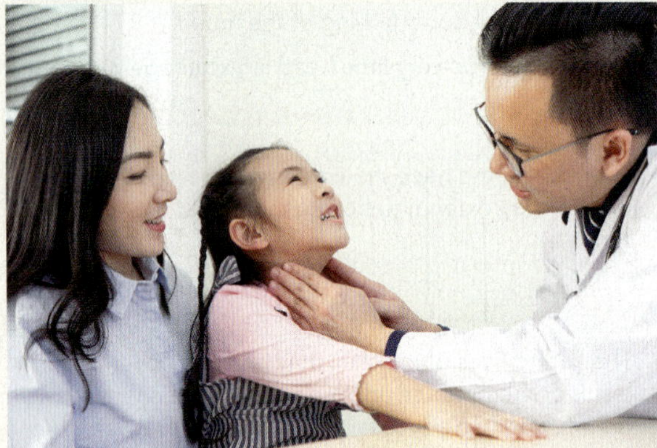

Figure 37-5. Palpation of the neck. (Shutterstock/plo)

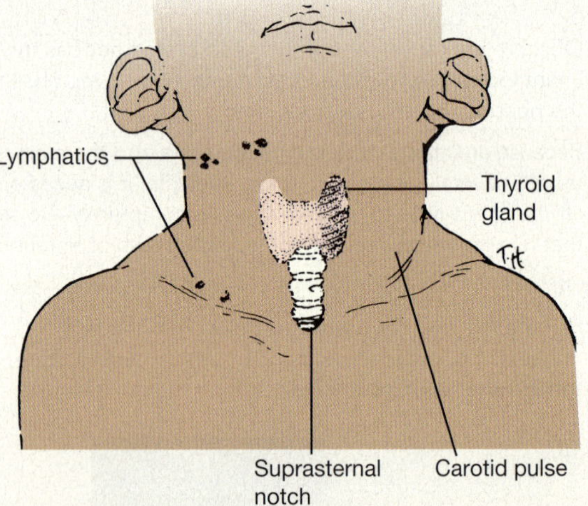

Figure 37-6. Internal structures of the neck.

5. Note that there are other nodes, which are normally not palpable.

5. These include the preauricular and postauricular, the posterior cervical (behind the sternomastoid), the submental and submandibular (under the jaw), the supraclavicular, and the occipital nodes (along the prominence of the occiput).

6. Feel the pulses in the neck for location, strength, and equality.

7. Check the thyroid for enlargement, position, texture, and tenderness.

PEDIATRIC PHYSICAL ASSESSMENT *(continued)*

Technique	Findings
8. Locate the trachea in the suprasternal notch for position in the center of the neck.	
9. Palpate the sternocleidomastoids, making sure they are equal in size.	
Percussion	
1. Percussion of the face may elicit tenderness over the sinuses.	1. Tenderness may be caused by a tooth cavity or by a sinus infection.
2. Percuss over the head and neck directly with the fingertips, usually the middle finger of the right hand.	2. Gentle tapping over the skull elicits a typical sound when the sutures are open and elicits a different sound when the sutures are closed.
3. Percuss over the forehead for tenderness in the sinuses and across the zygoma or cheek bone.	3. Determines underlying tenderness in the frontal or maxillary sinus.
Auscultation	
Auscultate the skull and carotid arteries in the neck.	To determine bruits.

EYES AND VISION

Technique	Findings
Inspection	
Similar to adult examination; see pages 4 to 32.	
1. Pay particular attention to the lacrimal duct and excessive tearing.	1. Discharge from the eyes along the lower lid or from the lacrimal duct can occur as a result of infection or reaction to silver nitrate administered to the neonate.
2. Note the distance between the eyes and the distribution of the eyebrows.	2. Hypertelorism denotes a wider than normal area between the eyes. Excessively long and full eyebrows that meet in the midline and extra-long eyelashes may signify a developmental abnormality from a genetic disorder.
3. Test the eyes for light perception.	3. It is difficult to prevent children from blinking their eyes or closing them when testing light response.
4. Do cover–uncover test.	4. To discover strabismus.
5. Beginning at about age 3 yr, a visual acuity screen using an age-appropriate chart should be attempted at every well-child checkup.	5. Ensure that the child is able to identify and communicate their answers to the evaluator.
Palpation	
If the child is old enough, have them squeeze the eyes tightly (not possible in younger children) while you try to open them.	Weakness of the muscles around the eyes is difficult to demonstrate in the young child. Muscle strength or weakness can be evaluated when the child cries.
Funduscopic examination (see Figure 37-7)	

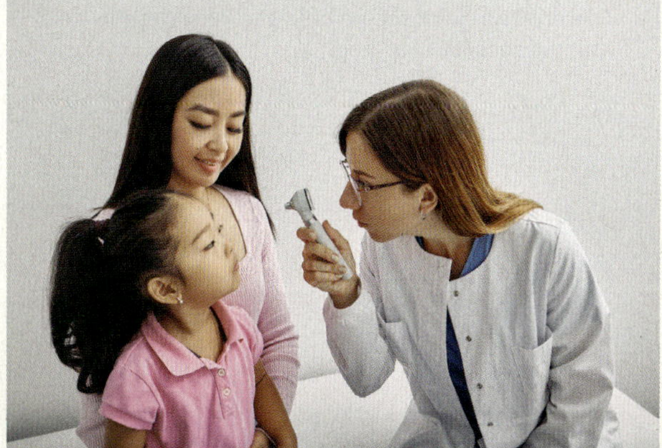

Figure 37-7. Funduscopic examination. (Shutterstock/Peakstock)

(continued)

PEDIATRIC PHYSICAL ASSESSMENT (continued)

Technique	Findings
1. Check to see that the child's eyes move in a conjugate fashion. Ask the caregiver if they have noticed signs of squinting, especially when the child is tired.	1. Loss of vision can occur if the eyes are not working together properly. Squinting can indicate vision problems.
2. This is a difficult examination to conduct because children tend to watch the light and stare directly at you, which constricts their pupils. If the child cannot follow your instructions, it may be necessary to dilate the pupil to see the fundus. (This is only infrequently necessary and will likely require referral to a specialist.)	2. A picture can be pinned to the wall opposite the child, who is then instructed to look at the picture during the examination. If the child is examined while lying down, a picture can be placed on the ceiling.
3. Start your examination at about 1 foot (0.3 m) from the patient. Look for the red reflex, which should be readily observable.	3. The corneal light reflex and red reflex should be symmetrical.
4. Look for opacities and then slowly approach the patient, turning the ophthalmoscope dial to the smaller plus (+) numbers. Start originally at +8 to +10.	4. The red reflex is diminished if there is something obstructing your view. A cataract or opacity in the retina can cause this, as would a tumor filling the posterior chamber. If there is any paleness in the red reflex or difficulty in identifying it, a consultation should be sought immediately. The red reflex may also be absent, and the abnormality is obvious in photographs of patients with ocular tumors or congenital cataracts.
5. To help guide your gaze, put your hand on top of the child's head or at the side, with your thumb at the corner of the eye at the outer edge. If you lose the fundus, you can return to your thumb and get your bearings by directing your gaze medial to the tip of your thumbnail.	

EARS AND HEARING

Technique	Findings
Equipment	
• Otoscope with insufflator (pneumatic bulb and tubing). • Varying sizes of ear speculum. • Fresh batteries to ensure a bright light.	
Inspection	
1. When examining the external ear, the auricle, or the pinna, be sure to note the position of the ear.	1. The top of the ear should cross an imaginary line drawn between the edge of the eye and the back of the occiput. If the ear is positioned more obliquely or is low set, some underlying abnormality, particularly of the genitourinary system, may be present.
2. If you cannot get the child to cooperate by offering an explanation or by playing a game, the child will need to be restrained. Many children will enjoy watching the light on their legs or seeing the red glow of their fingers with the light shining through or blowing the light out. If restraint is needed: a. The child can be seated on the caregiver's knee, facing them, with arms and legs wrapped around the them. The caregiver can then use one hand to hold the child's head firmly against the caregiver's chest and the other hand to hold the child's back. b. An older child may be held in a supine position, with the caregiver controlling the head by holding the child's arms above their head.	2. If the child is in a supine position, be sure to remove the child's shoes because some children will kick when frightened. a. This allows a good secure hold and provides the child with the security of a "hug."
Inspection with otoscope	
1. Attach the insufflator, a small bulb and tube device, to the otoscope. Hold the otoscope gently with the handle between the thumb and forefinger. This will enable you to control the head of the otoscope while keeping your hand steady on the child's head.	1. Small children move abruptly, so be careful not to push the speculum into the eardrum. The insufflator allows assessment of mobility of the tympanic membrane.

PEDIATRIC PHYSICAL ASSESSMENT *(continued)*

Technique	Findings
2. With your free hand, pull the pinna back and slightly upward to straighten the canal. Examine the canal.	2. Cerumen or wax may interfere with your view of the eardrum. You may need to remove the wax with an ear curette or warm water instillation.
3. Use the insufflator to inspect the eardrum and test for mobility. Do not use an insufflator if there is any suspicion of a perforated eardrum.	3. The normal eardrum moves slightly when air is introduced into the ear canal.
Palpation	
Palpate behind the ear over the mastoid process.	Tenderness behind the ear may denote infection. Sometimes, a lymph node can be felt in this area.
Special testing	
1. Most children will be able to respond to a test of gross hearing.	1. A small bell, or a cell phone application of a similar sound, can be used to determine hearing ability by noting if the child stops moving when the bell is rung and turns their head toward the sound.
2. More specific tests using an electrical screening device are used before school age.	

NOSE AND SINUSES

Technique	Findings
Equipment	
• Nasoscope • Small speculum	
Inspection	
1. Observe for general deformity.	
2. With a nasoscope, examine the nasal septum, mucous membranes, and turbinates and observe for discharge and nasal obstruction (see "Adult Physical Examination," pages 4–32).	2. Dry mucous membranes may bleed and cause clots of blood to form in the nares. Scratches may also occur if the child picks at their nose or scratches when itching occurs.
3. Check for the presence of a foreign body. Always remember that a foul odor may indicate a foreign body in the nose, ear, or any other body orifice including the anus or the vagina.	3. A foreign body in the nose will cause a foul odor, purulent discharge, and possibly cause bleeding.
4. Observe for nasal flaring.	4. Indicates respiratory distress.
Palpation	
Palpate the sinuses, remembering the order of development.	Sinuses develop in a set order; the ethmoid and maxillary sinuses are present at birth. The frontal sinuses begin to develop at about 7 yr and are fully formed by adolescence. The sphenoid sinuses develop after puberty.

MOUTH AND THROAT

Technique	Findings
Equipment	
• Penlight • Tongue blade	
Inspection	
Note: The child may gag when the tongue blade is placed on the tongue. The use of the tongue blade may be avoided by encouraging the child to open widely, or perform oral inspection if a young child is crying during ear exam (lying in supine position on exam table).	

(continued)

PEDIATRIC PHYSICAL ASSESSMENT (continued)

1. Observe the lips, noting the color. (Remember that cyanosis is difficult to detect in a Black child.)

1. *Infants*: There may be a protuberance on the upper lip, the so-called sucking blister.
Children: May have dry lips and redness around the lips caused by allergy.

2. Count the teeth (see Figure 37-8) and note any extra or missing teeth and any evidence of caries, staining, tartar, and malocclusion.

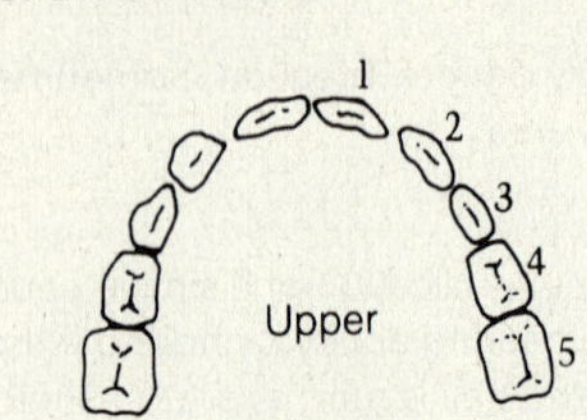

PRIMARY

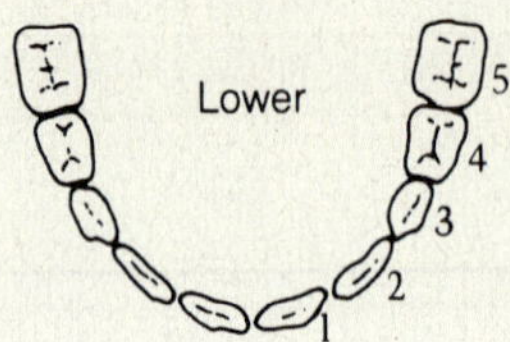

	(Upper)	(Lower)
1 Central incisor	8 to 12 months	5 to 9 months
2 Lateral incisor	8 to 12 months	12 to 18 months
3 Cuspid	18 to 24 months	18 to 24 months
4 First molar	12 to 18 months	12 to 18 months
5 Second molar	24 to 30 months	24 to 30 months

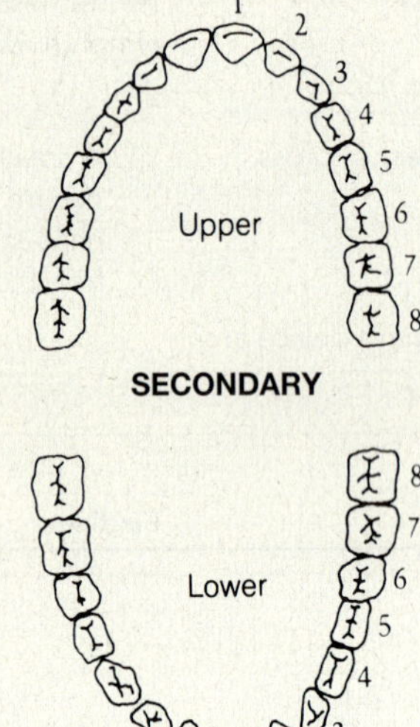

	(Upper)	(Lower)
1 Central incisor	6 to 7 years	7 to 8 years
2 Lateral incisor	7 to 8 years	8 to 9 years
3 Cuspid	9 to 10 years	11 to 12 years
4 First bicuspid	10 to 11 years	10 to 11 years
5 Second bicuspid	11 to 12 years	10 to 12 years
6 First molar	6 to 7 years	6 to 7 years
7 Second molar	11 to 13 years	12 to 13 years
8 Third molar	17 years	17 to 18 years

Figure 37-8. Diagram of the usual progression of eruption for teeth in children.

3. Check the gums for swelling and signs of easy bleeding. Also note mouth odor.

4. Check the tongue for movement, color, and taste buds on the surface. Check to see that the frenulum under the tongue is the proper length.

4. If the frenulum is too short, the child may be tongue-tied (meaning that they cannot advance the tip of the tongue beyond the lips), which may interfere with sucking or speech.

5. As the gag reflex is elicited, note how the palate moves upward and the uvula springs into view.

5. It should be midline and single, although occasionally, it will be divided or bifurcated.

6. Examine the roof of the mouth.

6. Whitish lesions, called Epstein pearls, may be noted on the roof of the mouth at the junction of the hard and soft palate and persist through infancy.

7. Inspect the height of the arch of the palate.

7. With experience, an unusually high arch is easily recognizable.

8. Note the tonsils on each side of the uvula and immediately posterior to it for position, surface, size, equality, and color.

8. Any coating with pus or ulcers or a pocket or cryptic appearance should be recorded.

9. As the child cries, note the odor of the breath and any hoarseness of the voice; note difficulty on inspiration, as in croup, or wheezing on expiration.

9. These signs may indicate throat and chest disturbances.

Palpation

1. Palpate the lips and cheeks manually using a finger cot or glove.

1. By comparing one side with the other, differences caused by abnormality can be detected.

2. Note evidence of swelling.

3. Palpate for submucous cleft.

3. Submucous cleft may indicate a genetic disposition toward cleft palate.

PEDIATRIC PHYSICAL ASSESSMENT *(continued)*

BREAST

Technique	Findings
1. Realize that a child may be resistant to examination because of not wanting to remove clothes.	1. Resistance may be due to modesty or fear of being exposed.
2. The following approaches may help overcome this problem: a. Distract the child by having them listen to a few heartbeats. b. Have the caregiver (while the child is sitting on their knee) remove the child's underclothing while you stand by. c. For an older child entering puberty, provide an examination sheet or gown.	
Inspection	
1. Check to see if there are any small extra nipples present.	1. These would appear along a line extending from the anterior axillary line through the normal nipple down toward the symphysis pubis.
2. In the neonate, the nipples appear a little darker than normal, and breast tissue underneath may form a small knot with occasional leakage of fluid.	2. This leakage is a secondary effect of the hormone level in the birthing parent; instruct them not to try to express the fluid because of the danger of infection.
3. In the child, a lump may be found under or near one or both nipples in either males or females, causing caregivers to worry about cancer.	3. Such lumps are almost always secondary to hormone stimulation and occur toward puberty or during the neonatal period.
4. Occasionally, the breasts begin to develop earlier than normal, at about age 5 or 6 yr.	4. This may indicate the need for referral to an endocrinologist.

THORAX

Technique	Findings
Inspection	
1. Observe the entire thorax as the child breathes; note symmetry and equal expansion of both sides as the lungs inflate.	1. Diaphragm excursion is more marked than intercostal expansion in infants (especially an infant lying on the caregiver's knee) and young children. Thus, the abdomen goes up and down more than the chest expands.
2. Confirm the respiratory rate as you observe the child with shirt off.	
3. Observe for substernal, suprasternal, and intercostal retractions.	3. Indicates respiratory distress.
Percussion	
Percussion of the child's chest is difficult. Because the underlying structures are crowded, little information is gathered. The heart edge is difficult to outline.	Light percussion is necessary; a hyperresonant note may be elicited over air, particularly of a stomach bubble that projects up into the left side of the chest.
Palpation	
1. Use warmed hands as you palpate the shape and angle of the sternum. Note if there is depression of the sternum.	1. The shape of the sternum may vary, although a large depression of the sternum (funnel sternum) may cause subsequent trouble because of pressure on underlying structures.
2. Palpate the costochondral junctions for tenderness and enlargement.	2. May suggest an underlying inflammatory response.
3. As you palpate, vibration may be felt through your hands as the child cries.	3. Normal inspiration and expiration do not give a sensation under the fingers, except for the expansion of the chest.
4. Vocal fremitus is difficult to elicit in the smaller child since it is difficult to have them make repetitive sounds on command.	4. In the older child, it is worth trying to obtain transmission of sound through the lung tissue (see page 17).

(continued)

PEDIATRIC PHYSICAL ASSESSMENT (continued)

Auscultation

1. Try to examine the child before crying begins.
   - Note, however, that crying increases lung expansion.
2. Warm the stethoscope before using by rubbing it between your hands.
   - A cold stethoscope will startle the child.
3. Be aware that breathing is louder in younger children with slightly increased length of inspiration, almost to the point of bronchovesicular breathing in the adult.
   - Bronchial breathing with equal inspiration and expiration is very loud and easy to hear in children with respiratory tract infections.
4. Crackles (discontinuous; interrupted, explosive sounds) may be heard more easily in children.
   - Added coarse-quality sounds in the chest are commonly associated with mucus in the trachea or in the back of the nose and usually clear with cough.
5. Wheezes.
   - Recurrent wheeze is an important finding in children.

HEART

Technique / **Findings**

Inspection

In thin children, the apical beat or the point of maximal impulse can easily be seen, particularly if you look obliquely across the chest wall.

Findings: Measurement and documentation of the distance from the midline and the exact rib space are worth noting.

Palpation

The apical beat may be felt in the sixth intercostal space about 2 inches (5 cm) from the midline in the school-age child. It is more difficult to feel in the infant, particularly a plump child, and would not be so far out toward the anterior axillary line.

Findings: The apical beat will be deviated to the left with cardiac enlargement or a collapsed lung on that side. The apical pulse could be pushed toward the right by a tumor or a collapsed lung on the right. Pneumothorax under tension will push the heart away from the side of the increased pressure.

Auscultation (see Figure 37-9)

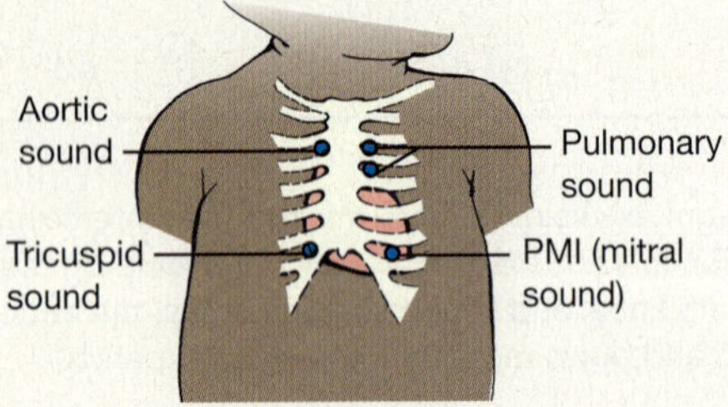

Figure 37-9. Positions of heart sound auscultation. PMI, point of maximal impulse.

1. Identify the first heart sound (S_1) (occurs during systole).
   a. Locate the apical beat (closing of the mitral valve) by placing the stethoscope over the maximum impulse area, concentrating on the first heart sound. (As the ventricle on the left contracts, pushing the blood up into the aorta, the sound of the mitral valve closing is heard.)
   b. That sound can be identified by placing the thumb on the carotid pulse of the neck, which will coincide very closely with the heart sounds.

   Findings: 1. Consists of the "lub" portion of the "lub–dub" heart sound.

2. Identify the second heart sound (S_2).
   a. Move the stethoscope up toward the sternum and to the left.
   b. At the base of the heart, both over the aortic and pulmonic areas, S_2 is louder than S_1.

   Findings: 2. Represents the "dub" portion of the "lub–dub" heart sound.
   a. In a child, S_2 can be heard as two heart sounds because the two valves in the aorta and pulmonary vessels do not close at the same time. This split will increase with inspiration and decrease with expiration.

3. Move the stethoscope in small jumps from the apical area medially toward the sternum. Go up to the left side of the sternum, listening at each interspace next to the sternum.

   Findings: 3. Represents the area of maximum intensity of sound of the pulmonary vessels.

PEDIATRIC PHYSICAL ASSESSMENT (*continued*)

4. Move next to the child's right second intercostal space—again next to the sternum.	4. It is at this area that you will hear the aortic sound best.
5. Listen to only one sound; concentrate on that to the exclusion of all others. Can you identify this sound? Is it clear? Compare it with your own heart sound or that of the caregiver.	5. The child will enjoy this comparison if allowed to listen.
6. If there is question of a heart murmur or added sounds, refer to the health care provider.	
7. As you listen to the heart sounds, you are also listening to the rhythm to confirm your findings on pulse. a. If the child breathes in and out deeply, a sinus arrhythmia may be detected. b. If the child holds their breath, the sinus arrhythmia will disappear.	7. The typical rhythm of a child is called *sinus arrhythmia*. As the heart speeds up, the child is breathing in; the heart slows down on expiration.
8. Be sure to note a rapid heart rate that is present even when the child is at rest and quiet.	8. This may be indicative of a tachycardia that requires further investigation.
9. In the infant, heart sounds are just a series of taps; they occur so fast that it may be very difficult to determine which sound is S_1.	9. In the infant, the S_1 and S_2 are equal in intensity.

ABDOMEN

Technique	Findings
1. For examination of the abdomen, the child should be lying down, relaxed, and not crying. Placing a small child, particularly those between ages 1 and 3 years, on a high table on cold paper can be frightening; as a result, the abdomen will not be relaxed.	1. The abdomen needs to be relaxed to palpate abnormal masses or enlarged liver or spleen as well as to auscultate for abnormal sounds.
2. Infants up to age 1 years do not seem to be bothered and will usually lie down and cooperate as long as they can see the caregiver, who should be stationed at the head of the child while you examine the abdomen.	
3. Having the child lie across the caregiver's knees with the legs dangling on one side and the head cradled in their arms will enable you to feel the abdomen quite well. a. You may find that with the infant's head in the caregiver's left arm, you can use your left hand to examine the infant's abdomen on the right, feeling up under the right costal margin and into the right hypochondrium. b. You may need to turn the infant around and use your right hand to examine the left side of the infant's abdomen.	
Inspection	
1. Observe the abdomen for contour and any markings while the child is standing and when lying down. As you inspect, you may see some abdominal movement with respiration. (Remember that the diaphragm, as it goes up and down, will move the contents of the abdomen.)	1. Sometimes superficial veins are seen on the abdomen, particularly in a very blond infant. Striae are commonly noticed on the flank following rapid loss or gain of weight.
2. Check for early signs of puberty as evidenced by pubic hair over the symphysis pubis.	2. Early pubic hair in younger children (ages 8–10 yr) may appear long, light, and silky. This will ultimately become curly and darker toward the onset of puberty.
3. Carefully inspect the umbilicus for cleanliness and the presence of scar tissue.	3. A deep umbilicus may be difficult to keep clean. Immediately after the cord has dropped off, a granuloma may occur.

(*continued*)

PEDIATRIC PHYSICAL ASSESSMENT (*continued*)

Auscultation

1. Because percussion and palpation may stimulate the small bowel and increase bowel sounds, auscultation should precede these two techniques.
2. To obtain the child's cooperation, you can conduct a running commentary as you listen, saying such things as, "I can hear the Cheerios in there."

1. Bowel sounds are heard as tinkling, irregular sounds that indicate that fluid is moving from one section of the bowel to the next.
2. In a quiet infant who has just eaten, not many bowel sounds will be heard. In a hungry child, noisy bowel sounds can be heard, even without a stethoscope.

Percussion

1. On the right side, percuss for the liver. Confirm on palpation.
2. Percuss over the left upper quadrant (LUQ).
3. Percuss the lower abdomen, particularly above the symphysis pubis.

1. Liver dullness can frequently be outlined to determine size of the liver.
2. Percussion over a gas-filled bowel or stomach results in a high-pitched, hollow sound.
3. Above the symphysis pubis, a filled bladder can produce a duller sound, as does a pregnant uterus. (A mass in the abdomen of a female older than age 10 yr may be related to pregnancy.)
   a. The liver is frequently felt about ¾ inch (1 cm) below the right costal margin and in some instances as low as ¾ inch (2 cm). This is a common finding in the neonate and through the early school-age years.

Palpation

1. Divide the abdomen into imaginary quadrants, palpating each with the fingertips.
2. In the right upper quadrant, palpate for the liver edge.
   a. Although the liver is easily palpable in many children, you may have to press quite firmly.
3. In the LUQ, palpate for the spleen. Less resistance is encountered as you feel up under the left costal margin.
4. In the upper quadrants, also try to palpate for the kidneys. Deep palpation for both kidneys should routinely be a part of the examination to make sure there is no enlargement of the kidney. Normally, the kidney is not palpable.
5. In the iliac fossa or the left lower quadrant (LLQ) (see Figure 37-10B), palpate for the descending bowel.
6. Palpate on the right lower quadrant (RLQ) (see Figure 37-10A), where the appendix is located.

3. Typically, only the tip of the spleen can be felt in the outer LUQ in the early months of life and in very thin children of preschool age.
4. Kidney palpation is difficult, but during the neonatal period, the lower pole of the right kidney may be felt and sometimes the left as well. (This applies to the period immediately after delivery, when the neonate's abdomen is relaxed and the bowel is not distended.)
5. The descending colon can be felt, particularly if it's filled with firm stool and the child is quiet. It may be slightly tender, but it should not cause severe pain on gentle palpation.
6. In the RLQ, usually, the only sensation is that of gas-filled bowel. Tenderness in this area could be related to an inflamed appendix.

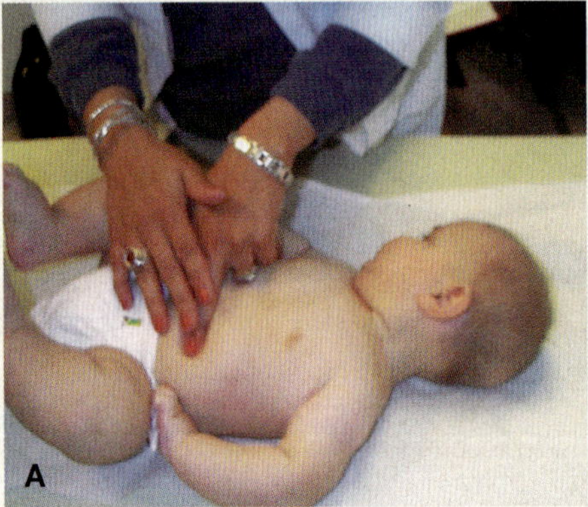

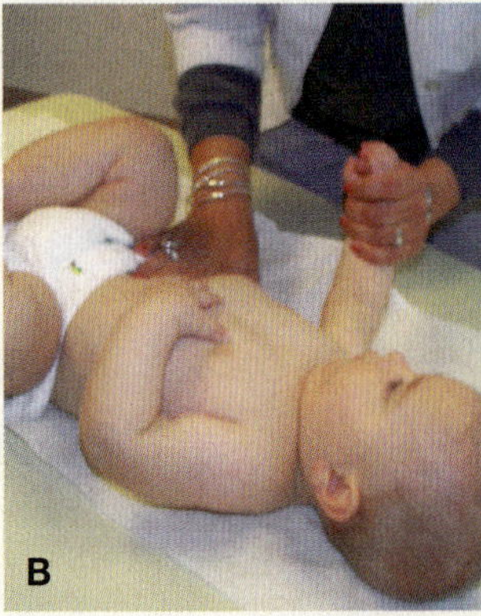

Figure 37-10. Palpation of the right lower quadrant (**A**) and the left lower quadrant (**B**) of the abdomen.

PEDIATRIC PHYSICAL ASSESSMENT *(continued)*

7. If the child has pain in any area or has pointed to the umbilicus when asked to show where the pain is, avoid the area demonstrated and leave it until last. Note whether the pain is with pressure or rebound.

7. If the painful area is palpated first, the child may tense up when the other areas of the abdomen are examined.

8. Palpate around the umbilicus for any masses that may indicate a hernia, especially in preterm and Black children. As you press over the protruding hernia, you can feel the sensation of gurgling under your fingers as the bowel returns to the abdomen.

8. Most of these hernias heal naturally by age 6 years. A hernia above the umbilicus can be revealed by asking the child to lift their head from the table. (Widening of the muscles above the umbilicus is called *diastasis recti*.)

RECTUM AND ANUS

1. Rectal examinations are rarely necessary in infants and young children.
2. If the child will be examined by another health care provider, it is not necessary to duplicate this part of the examination.
3. Rectal examinations are embarrassing and uncomfortable for most children. Explain the procedure before performing the examination.
4. Positioning for a rectal examination:
   a. Infants can be placed on their abdomens, sides, or backs with their legs raised to their chests.
   b. Young children and teenagers can be positioned on their sides.

Inspection

1. When examining an infant or toddler, place the child on a flat surface so that the weight is evenly distributed on the front of the pelvis. As the infant moves about on the abdomen, observe the entire back, the lower back, the upper thigh, and the tightening of the buttocks.

1. If one buttock is larger than the other, you will see that side projected above the other. Weakness of one side will be obvious as the infant moves around, although a child in the early stages of crawling will tend to use one knee as a predominant leader, dragging the other.

2. Check particularly the lower part of the back for hairiness or a mass.

2. This may indicate an underlying abnormality of the vertebrae in spina bifida.

3. As the child moves away, part the buttocks and look at the cleft between them.

3. A pilonidal dimple or sinus may be seen over the lower back. This is a common finding, but caregivers should be told about it for cleaning purposes. Make sure there is no drainage.

4. Pay careful attention to the outer appearance of the anus and the perineum, the underside of the scrotum in the male, and the labia majora in the female.

4. The anus is inspected for blood, fissures, or splitting in the external tissue, redness, swelling, or pads of extra flesh. On occasion, small white pinworms may be seen adhering to the anal skin. This requires further evaluation and treatment.

Palpation

1. Consider the child's age and feelings; ask the caregiver to assist, if necessary. This part of the examination is not always needed.

2. Start by parting the buttocks with the left hand and introducing a well-lubricated finger (with finger cot) into the anus.

2. When an infant is being examined, the small finger should be used.

3. Gently apply pressure on the anal sphincter to allow the muscles to relax and the fingertip to slide into the rectum.

3. Apply pressure with pulp of the finger rather than jab at the anus with the fingertip.

4. Gently palpate the inner ring, feeling for areas of thickening and tenderness and simultaneously judging the sphincter tone.

4. As the perianal area is pressed on from the inside, tenderness will be elicited if a deep fissure exists or if an infection has occurred around a fissure.

5. If the rectum is full of stool, it will be impossible to feel any other mass.

5. In a young child, particularly an infant, dilation provided by the finger may result in a bowel movement. In an older child, a suppository or even an enema may be required.

6. Palpate the walls of the rectum.

6. The mucosal walls should be smooth, and deep palpation should elicit mild tenderness and no acute pain.

(continued)

PEDIATRIC PHYSICAL ASSESSMENT (*continued*)

7. In the adolescent male, gently turn your finger through 180 degrees and feel the posterior surface of the prostate. Note size, consistency, tenderness, and contour.

   Findings: 7. This exam should be performed only if indicated. It is unusual in a pediatric patient.

8. In the female, perform a bimanual examination and palpate the cervix.

   Findings: 8. This exam should be performed only if indicated. It is unusual in a pediatric patient. It may be necessary for providers to perform this exam under sedation or general anesthesia in the operating room.

EXAMINING MALE GENITALIA

Technique / **Findings**

1. This part of the examination requires a direct, matter-of-fact approach. Acknowledge that it is normal to feel embarrassed during an examination of the genitals. Explain what you are looking for as you proceed through the examination with a teenager.
2. Reassure the child after the examination that the genitals are normal. This decreases anxiety.
3. When examining the testes in a prepubertal male, you may need to block the canals to prevent them from retracting into the abdomen.

Scrotum and Testes

Inspection

1. Before touching the child, determine by observation of the testes whether they are in the scrotum.

   Findings: 1. Retraction of the testes into the abdomen occurs frequently in young children; the development of the scrotum depends on the presence of the testes.

2. Observe the skin over the scrotum for color and surface appearance, noting the presence of wrinkles or rugae.

   Findings: 2. The skin over the scrotum varies in color, being a darker brown to black in children with darker skin tones and reddish in children with lighter complexions. The wrinkles, or rugae, are more developed as the child grows older.

Palpation

1. Check the scrotum wall for swelling or sensitivity. Gently feel the testes, palpating across the upper pole and feeling for the epididymis. (Remember the scrotum is extremely sensitive to pressure.)

   Findings: 1. The epididymis is a ridge of soft, bumpy tissue extending from the superior pole and running down and behind the testis.

2. Estimate the size of the testes and identify the spermatic cord, tracing it from the testis up toward the groin.

   Findings: 2. The spermatic cord, with the vas deferens, feels firm and is accompanied by softer nerves, arteries, veins, and a few muscle fibers.

3. Make a special effort to locate the testis in a young child whose testes may be retracted into the abdomen via a hyperactive cremasteric reflex. You may need to have the child in a sitting or standing position. Occasionally, you may need to ask a caregiver to check at home with the child sitting in a warm bathtub.
   a. If the testes cannot be felt in the scrotum, gently run the skin of the upper scrotum between your fingers, moving superiorly and approaching the external inguinal ring.
   b. Try to milk the testis down toward the scrotum from above with your hand.
   c. If this fails, have the child sit cross-legged to abolish the reflex of the cremaster muscle.

   Findings: 3. Ascertaining the presence of the testes in the scrotum is vital in older infant or toddler. Failure of the testes to descend requires further evaluation.
   a. During this period, the testis is about ½–¾ inch (1.5–2 cm) in length. In the quiescent period before puberty, the male genitalia remain fairly infantile.

4. When examining a male in the early stages of puberty, it is important to note the size of the testis as well as the greater number of rugae on the scrotum and the appearance of pubic hair around the penis. If appropriate, discuss importance of self-testicular exam.

   Findings: 4. In early puberty, the testes start to grow. Onset of puberty varies, occurring between the ages of 10 and 14 years. In most teenagers, the findings are similar to those in adults.

PEDIATRIC PHYSICAL ASSESSMENT (continued)

Penis

1. Evaluate the penis on all sides by lifting up the shaft.

1. The shaft of the penis contains the urethra on the under, or ventral, surface and is easily palpable.

2. If the child is not circumcised, partially retract the foreskin to observe the glans and meatus.

2. The foreskin may adhere to the glans for the first few years of life. It is not necessary for the caregiver to "stretch" the foreskin by retraction.

3. Observe the position of the meatus and evert the lips of the meatus to reveal an adequate orifice.

3. The meatus may be positioned off center. If the meatus is located on the dorsal or ventral surface of the shaft, the child should be evaluated by a pediatric urologist.

Whitish discharge around the glans under the foreskin is normal and not a sign of infection. The foreskin should completely encircle the glans.

4. In the older child, inspect the penis for ulcers, sores, or discharge from the meatus.

4. Consider sexually transmitted infections in children of all ages; the possibility of sexual abuse must be considered.

Inguinal Area

Palpation

1. Palpate for a hernia over the external inguinal ring (see Figure 37-11). Have the child cough to enhance your observation.

1. Having the child stand with the caregiver either holding them or placing them against the caregiver's knee will help you in locating a hernia in the inguinal area.

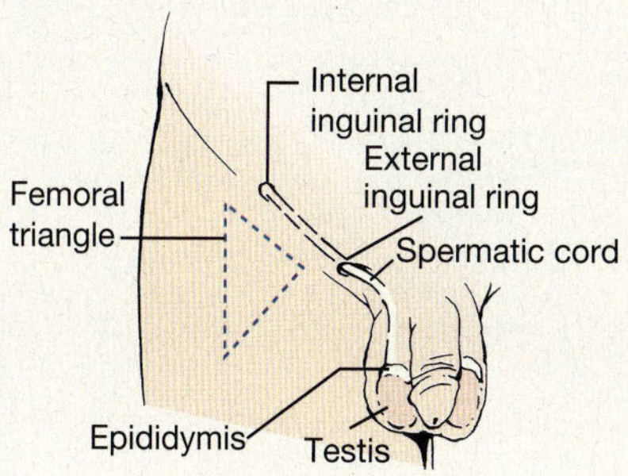

Figure 37-11. External and internal structures of the male genitalia.

2. An increased cough reflex or swelling in the area should be checked by carefully placing a finger on the scrotal skin and invaginating the skin over your fingers toward the external ring. You are trying to follow the course of a hernia that would descend into the scrotum while you feel the external ring from below. A hernia in the inguinal region presents as a bulge that can be either seen or felt from below by placing the finger in the scrotum pointing up toward the external inguinal ring.

3. Also palpate for the inguinal lymph nodes.

3. The inguinal lymph nodes in an infant are palpable as small and "shotty." Anything more than this should alert you to possible infection because the perianal area drains into the superficial inguinal lymph nodes. For example, diaper rash may explain enlargement of the lymph nodes, which should be noted and reported.

(continued)

PEDIATRIC PHYSICAL ASSESSMENT (*continued*)

Femoral Area

Palpation

Palpate the femoral triangle carefully for a hernia and for lymph nodes.

In the femoral area, a swelling that can be reduced with a gurgling sound is an unusual finding.

Auscultation

If you are trying to reduce a mass, listen over the scrotum to determine if there is a gurgling sound.

This will locate the bowel and confirm a hernia.

Transillumination

1. To locate the testis, darken the room and shine a bright light from behind the scrotum. In a normal child, the testis will stand out as a darker area.
2. Transilluminate any suspicious mass to help locate a hernia.

Findings:

1. A scrotal sac that is swollen by fluid (hydrocele) will transilluminate. Fluid around the testes or cord must be differentiated from a hernia.
2. Any mass in this area must be reported to a health care provider immediately.

EXAMINING FEMALE GENITALIA

Technique

1. If the child will be examined by a health care provider, it is not necessary to duplicate this part of the examination.
2. Place the infant or toddler on the table or on the caregiver's knee while the caregiver holds the child's knees in an abducted and flexed position.
3. A preschool child can be allowed to lean over the caregiver's knee. However, remember that the structures are being visualized upside down.
4. The older child or teenager should be draped as an adult would and should be placed in a lithotomy position with the aid of stirrups.

Equipment

- Disposable gloves
- Speculum
- Light source

1. Carefully inspect the perineal area for cleanliness, inflammation, and abnormality (see Figure 37-12).

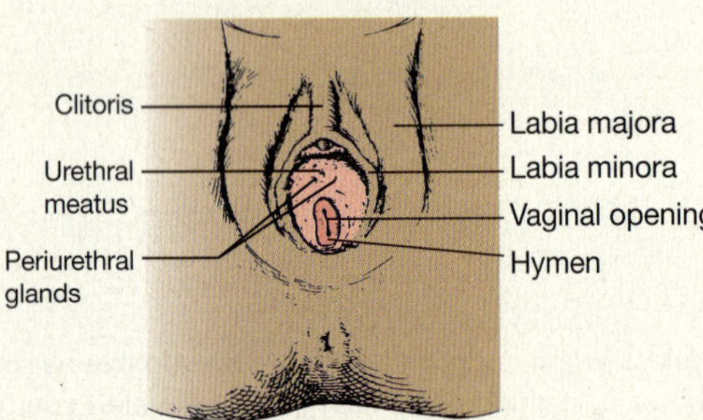

Figure 37-12. External structures of the female genitalia.

Findings

1. This includes the mons pubis, clitoris, labia, urethra, and perineum. The labia minora are seen as two slender folds of tissue inside the labia majora. In some instances, adhesions of the labia minora occur because of the lack of natural hormones.

PEDIATRIC PHYSICAL ASSESSMENT (*continued*)

2. If the caregiver of a neonate has noted a bloody discharge from the infant's vagina during the first few days of life, reassure them that this is sometimes noted and is benign and self-limiting; the discharge will disappear, as will swelling of the labia majora and clitoris and enlargement of the infant's breasts.

2. Hormone stimulation from the birthing parent's body accounts for this occurrence. The discharge usually stops after the hormones are excreted. The bloody appearance on the diaper may be confused with the presence of urates, which are also orange-red and appear normally in urine.

3. Note the vaginal opening, which may vary in size because of the presence of a thin membrane, the hymen. The hymen varies in appearance according to the child's age.

3. The lack of an opening into the vagina may result in the retention of menstrual fluid when the child reaches puberty. In the sexually active adolescent, vestigial remains on the hymen may appear as small particles (caruncles) at the fringe of the vagina.
   The possibility of sexual abuse should always be considered and, if necessary, the child referred to a specialist in sexual abuse.

4. In the young child, it is usually unnecessary to examine inside the vagina. If a young child requires an extensive vaginal exam, it is frequently done under sedation.

4. A foreign body or sexually transmitted infection may be suspected if there is a vaginal discharge, bleeding, or odor.

MUSCULOSKELETAL SYSTEM

Technique	Findings

1. Evaluation of the musculoskeletal system can be done both in an informal manner, while watching the child at rest and at play, and in a formal manner as specific findings are methodically checked.
2. In the neonate, observe the position of the extremities during sleep and the quality of movement when the child is awake.
3. Various aspects of size, shape, and movement are evaluated as the child is observed pushing up on their arms and turning their head toward the caregiver.
4. A child in the early stages of walking offers many opportunities for evaluation of muscle strength and movement.
5. At the same time, rapport with the caregiver can be reinforced by your admiring the child's ability and by inquiring if they are concerned about the way the child is walking.
6. A more mobile child can be evaluated as you watch them play and explore the room.
7. Having the older child reach for crayons, run after a ball, or walk around the room enables you to evaluate the musculoskeletal system and the child's sense of balance.

Upper Extremities

1. In the infant, evaluate the status of the clavicles when examining the skull and neck.

1. During a difficult delivery, the clavicle that has been exposed to traction may snap. A lump can be felt on the bone at about age 3 weeks.

2. Carefully examine the hands to note the shape of the hand, shape and length of the fingers, changes in the nails, and creases on the palms.

2. Variation in the hands or unusual length of the fingers should be noted. An incurved little finger or low-set thumb with the single palmar crease may reflect Down syndrome.

Lower Extremities

1. Examine the appearance of the infant's foot, noting arch formation.

1. The foot of an infant is usually flat and appears broad because the arch on the inside of the foot is covered by a fat pad. Caregivers may need reassurance about this.

(*continued*)

PEDIATRIC PHYSICAL ASSESSMENT (*continued*)

2. Inspect the angle of the foot and lower leg and then manipulate the ankle to evaluate the range of motion.

2. Full flexibility of the foot (plantar flexion) rules out underlying abnormality. The foot should return to the neutral position after manipulation. Typically, the foot will turn in or adduct. Such a finding should be recorded.

3. Place the legs together and see how far the ankles and knees are separated.

3. Toddlers typically have external hip rotation and internal knee rotation, which results in a "bowed" appearance. The preschooler has a normally knock-kneed walk, but with knees touching, ankles should be no more than two fingerbreadths apart.

4. Evaluate the child's ability to walk, noting the appearance of their legs and foot placement. Remember to look at the child's shoes and see which area of the sole is worn down.

4. Infants commonly appear to be bowlegged when they first start to walk because the feet are kept wide apart and turn slightly in. The ankles appear curved when viewed from behind.

Hip

When examining children younger than age 1 year, check for signs of hip dislocation. See pages 1417 and 1418.

Spine

1. Check the spine for signs of abnormal curvature (scoliosis; see Figure 37-13B).

1. The normal young child has a curve inward at the lumbar region (lordosis), but this should not be exaggerated. It is normally more exaggerated in Black children.

2. Observe the child from the side and back in the standing position to see forward curving of the shoulders (kyphosis; see Figure 37-13A).

2. These appear most commonly during school-age years and adolescence.

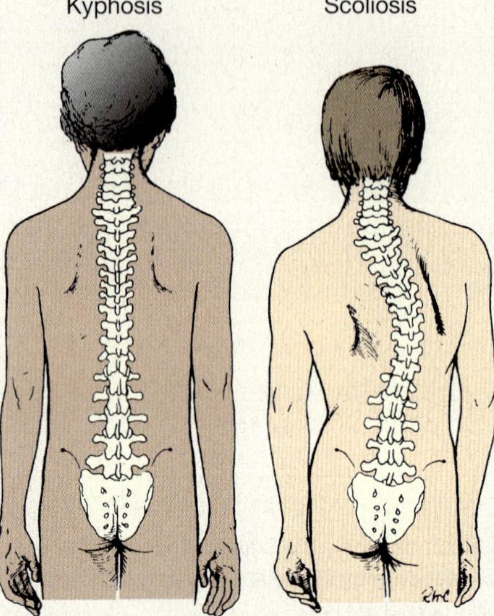

Figure 37-13. (**A**) Kyphosis: forward curvature of the shoulders. (**B**) Scoliosis: side-to-side curvature of the spine.

PEDIATRIC PHYSICAL ASSESSMENT *(continued)*

3. Have the child bend forward with the arms hanging down. A unilateral rib prominence is seen in children with scoliosis (see Figure 37-14).

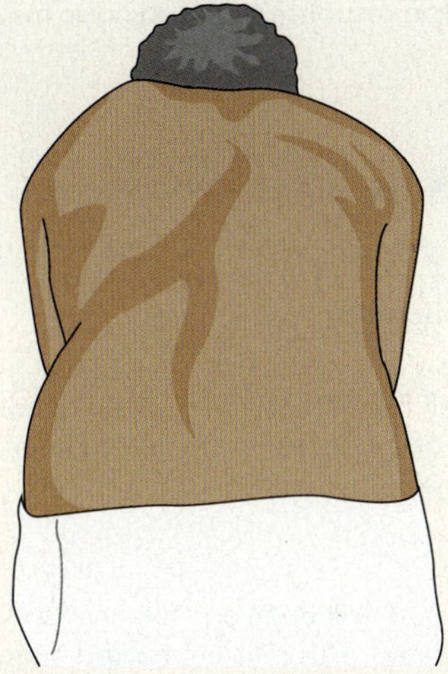

Figure 37-14. A unilateral rib prominence is seen in children with scoliosis.

NEUROLOGIC EXAMINATION

Technique	Findings
1. The neurologic system at birth is different from that in an infant age 3 months. There is an even greater contrast between the infant and children and adults.	
2. The central nervous system at birth is underdeveloped, and the functions tested are below the level of the cortex.	

Equipment

- Flashlight
- Noisemaker
- Ophthalmoscope
- Tongue depressor
- Tuning fork

Procedure for the Neonate and Young Infant

Technique	Findings
1. Observe the neonate for general appearance, positioning, activity, crying, and alertness. Take note of the posture—including head, neck, and extremities.	1. Stiffness of the neck or marked extension of the head will cause a position of opisthotonos and necessitates referral.
2. Note the pitch, volume, and character of their cry.	2. The high-pitched cry of the infant who has intracranial irritation is distinctive.
3. Observe the infant's facial expression and facial symmetry when crying or sucking.	3. Poor sucking, with dribbling, is abnormal. Transient weakness of the mouth caused by cranial nerve VII paralysis is commonly seen as a result of a forceps delivery in which the forceps is pressed on the facial nerve where it emerges from the ear.
4. Most of the cranial nerves are difficult to check at this early age.	

(continued)

PEDIATRIC PHYSICAL ASSESSMENT (continued)

Automatic Reflexes

Technique	Findings
1. *Blinking reflex because of loud noise* Clap your hands or produce a loud clicking noise. Be careful not to clap near the infant to prevent a wave of air from causing a blinking of the eyes.	1. Lack of a blink in response to a loud noise may indicate deafness.
2. *Blinking reflex because of bright light* Shine a bright light into the infant's eyes to elicit the blinking reflex.	2. Failure to blink may indicate blindness.
3. *Cranial nerve X* can be checked by using a tongue blade to gag the infant.	3. Palate moves upward.
4. *Palmar grasp reflex* Place your fingers across the infant's palm from the ulnar side. The infant needs to be in a relaxed position with head in a central position. Reinforcement may be offered by having the infant suck on a bottle at the same time.	4. Both hands will flex and can be compared for strength. Weakness on one side may be indicated by a failure to grasp when the palm is stimulated.
5. *Rooting reflex* Touch the edge of the infant's mouth.	5. The infant's mouth will open and the head will turn toward the side stimulated. This reflex is marked during the early weeks of life.
6. *Incurving of the trunk (Galant reflex)* Hold the infant horizontally and prone in one arm while using the other hand to stimulate one side of the infant's back from the shoulders to the buttocks (see Figure 37-15). The trunk curves toward the stimulated side as the shoulders and pelvis move toward the stroking hand (persists until the infant is about age 2 mo).	

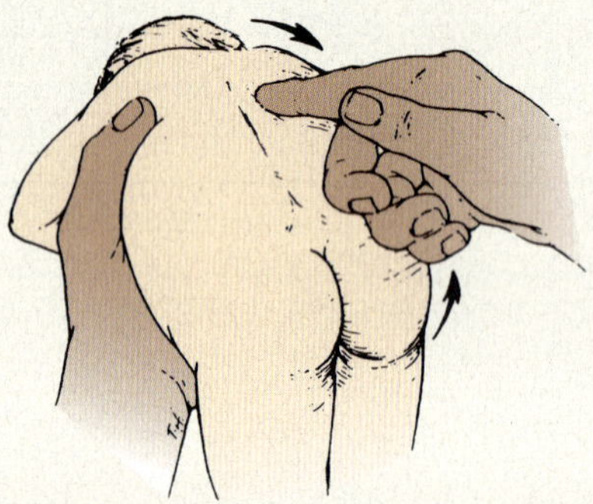

Figure 37-15. Galant reflex.

Technique	Findings
7. *Vertical suspension position* Place your hands under the infant's axillae with thumbs supporting the back of the head and hold the infant upright.	7. The legs flex at the hips and knees (persists for about 4 mo).
8. *Stepping response* Hold the infant under its axillae with thumbs supporting the back of the head. Allow the infant's foot to touch a firm surface.	8. Normally, the infant responds by lifting one knee and hip into a flexed position and moving the opposite leg forward—making a series of stepping movements (see Figure 37-16A). a. Difficulty with the stepping reflex and stiffness or spasticity connected with crossing of the feet and scissoring (see Figure 37-16B) is indicative of spastic paraplegia or diplegia.

PEDIATRIC PHYSICAL ASSESSMENT (continued)

b. It should be noted that the stepping response may be affected by breech delivery. (It may also be affected by weakness.)

c. The stepping response is evident toward the end of the first week after birth and persists for a variable time.

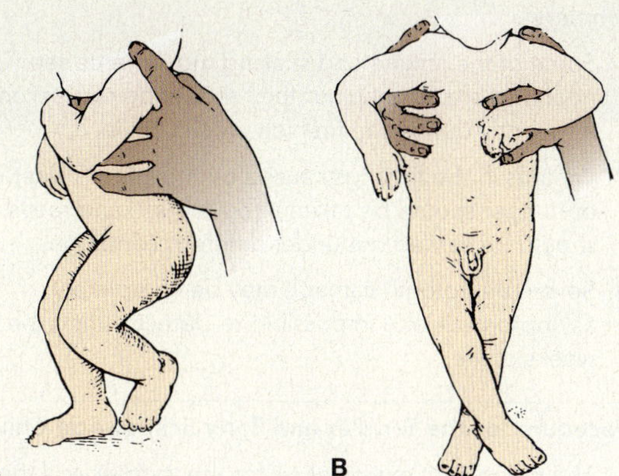

Figure 37-16. Stepping response (**A**) typical and (**B**) spastic paraplegia or diplegia.

9. *Tonic neck reflex*
   Hold the infant in a supine position with the head turned to one side and the jaw held in place over the shoulder (see Figure 37-17).

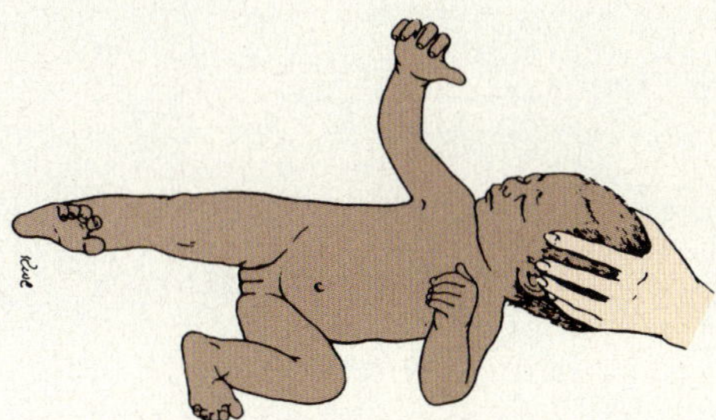

Figure 37-17. Tonic neck reflex.

9.
   a. The arm and leg on the side to which the head is turned will extend, whereas those on the other side will flex (the so-called fencing reflex).
   b. This reflex persists for about 5–6 months; it may be present at birth or delayed until the infant is age 6 or 8 weeks.
   c. Persistence beyond 6 mo suggests major cerebral damage.

10. *Mass reflexes (Moro or startle reflex)*
    Hold the infant along your arm with the other hand below the lower legs. Lower the feet and body in a sudden motion (see Figure 37-18).

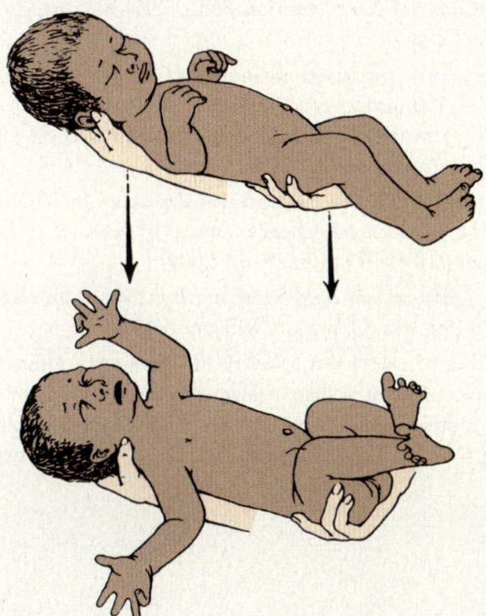

Figure 37-18. Moro reflex.

10. The arms will spring up and out, abducting and extending; the fingers are also extended. The arms then return forward over the body with a clasping motion. At the same time, the legs flex slightly and the hips abduct.
    a. The Moro reflex is present at birth and disappears at approximately the end of the third month. Persistence beyond 6 mo is significant.
    b. Asymmetrical response may be caused by paralysis of the arm after difficult delivery, tension and injury to the brachial plexus, or a fracture of the clavicle or humerus. A dislocated hip would produce an asymmetrical response in the lower extremities.

(continued)

PEDIATRIC PHYSICAL ASSESSMENT (*continued*)

11. *Perez reflex*
    Hold the infant in a prone position along your arm; place the thumb of the other hand on the sacrum and move it firmly toward the head, along the entire length of the spine.

11. The head and spine will extend and the knees will flex upward.

Summary

1. Some of the jerking and shaking movements seen in neonates are normal, but they should be rechecked frequently during the first few weeks of life.
2. Variants in the findings caused by the infant's sleepiness or hunger should be taken into account, and reevaluations should be carried out under different conditions.
3. Severe neurologic damage may be completely asymptomatic and impossible to detect during the first few weeks of life.

Procedure for the Toddler and Early School-Age Child

1. The neurologic examination for the toddler and the early school-age child is similar to that for the adult (see pages 29–32).
2. The Draw-A-Person Test and the Denver Developmental Assessment are both well-accepted methods for testing areas in the development of the child.

2. See www.denverii.com https://www.ccmedical.org/forms/1428352937_171971.pdf for instructions and findings of the Denver Development Assessment. Refer to Chapter 36 for additional information on developmental assessment.

3. Beyond the neonatal period, specific gross and fine motor coordination testing, accompanied by appropriate evaluation of the Denver test, will assist in assessing the child's level of development.
4. These tests also assess social and language development and are important screening devices.
5. Interview techniques can also be useful in assessing development in the preschool child.

SELECTED READINGS

American Academy of Pediatrics. (2011). *Bright futures: Nutrition* (3rd ed.). American Academy of Pediatrics.

American Academy of Pediatrics. (2017). *Bright futures: Guidelines for health supervision of infants, children, and adolescents* (4th ed.). American Academy of Pediatrics.

Bickley, L. (2020). *Bates' guide to physical examination and history taking* (13th ed.). Lippincott Williams & Wilkins.

Centers for Disease Control and Prevention. (2010). *Growth charts.* Centers for Disease Control and Prevention. www.cdc.gov/growthcharts/

Duderstadt, K. G. (2019). *Pediatric physical examination: An illustrated handbook* (3rd ed.). Mosby Elsevier.

Garzon, D., Starr, N., Brady, M., Gaylord, N., Driessnack, M., & Duderstadt, K. (2021). *Burns' pediatric primary care* (7th ed.). Elsevier.

Guerrerp, N., Small, A., Schwei, R., & Jacobs, E. (2018). Informing physician strategies to overcome language barriers in encounters with pediatric patients. *Patient Education & Counseling, 101*(4), 653–658. https://doi.org/10.1016/j.pec.2017.10.018

Johns Hopkins Hospital; Kleinman, K., McDaniel, L., & Molloy, M. (Eds.). (2021). *The Harriet Lane handbook* (22nd ed.). Elsevier.

Lobelo, F., Muth, N., Hanson, S., & Nemeth, B. (2020). Physical activity assessment and counseling in pediatric clinical settings. *Pediatrics, 145*(3), 1–21. https://doi.org/10.1542/peds.2019-3992

Martinez, L., & Constantinides, S. (2021). Sleep assessment for sleep problems in children. *Nursing Clinics of North America, 56*(2), 299–309. https://doi.org/10.1016/j.cnur.2021.02.008

Matek, K. (2021). The pre-participation examination in a COVID-19 world. *Pediatric Nursing, 47*(6), 299–300. https://ezproxy.niagara.edu/login?url=https://www.proquest.com/scholarly-journals/pre-participation-examination-covid-19-world/docview/2615893181/se-2?accountid=28213

McDonald, K., & Eckhardt, A. (2017). Evidence-based practice in action: Ensuring quality of pediatric assessment frequency. *Journal of Pediatric Nursing, 35*, 134–138. https://doi.org/10.1016/j.pedn.2016.12.009

Silbert-Flagg, J. (2022). *Maternal and child health nursing: Care of the childbearing and childrearing family* (9th ed.). Lippincott Williams & Wilkins.

Wagner, R., Lima, T., Silva, M., Rabha, A., Ricieri, M., Fachi, M., Alfonso, R., & Motta, F. (2023). Assessment of pediatric telemedicine using remote physical examinations with a mobile medical device: A nonrandomized controlled trial. *JAMA Open Network, 6*(1), e2252570. https://doi.org/10.1001/jamanetworkopen.2022.52570

38 Pediatric Primary Care*

HEALTH MAINTENANCE

See additional online content: Patient Education Guidelines 38-1 and Procedure Guidelines 38-1

Pediatric primary care includes health promotion and disease prevention interventions that will positively affect the well-being of children and their families. The goal of pediatric primary care is to achieve physical, emotional, and developmental health for all children. Primary prevention—through immunizations, proper nutrition, and safety counseling—is an essential component of pediatric health care.

Immunizations

Disease prevention through immunizations has significantly reduced childhood morbidity and mortality from infectious diseases. However, despite effective immunization availability, vaccine-preventable diseases are still present in the United States and continue to pose significant public health problems. The rate of immunization in the United States exceeds 85% for children aged 19 to 35 months for poliovirus vaccine; measles, mumps, rubella (MMR); hepatitis B vaccine (HBV); and varicella vaccine. However, rates vary by state and decrease after this age. In 2022, 89.9% of adolescents aged 13 to 17 years have received at least one tetanus toxoid, diphtheria, and acellular pertussis (Tdap) dose, 88.6% have received at least one for meningococcal protection, and 76% have received at least one dose for human papillomavirus (HPV) protection (CDC, 2023).

Nurses are in a vital position to promote child health by assessing, recommending, and administering immunizations. In addition, nurses are frequently asked to provide documentation (to parental caregivers) of the immunizations that have been administered to facilitate children's enrollment in day care, school programs, and summer camp participation. A review of immunizations and administration of needed vaccines should be done at every health care visit.

EVIDENCE BASE Lewandowska, A., Lewandowski, T., Rudzki, G., Rudzki, S., & Laskowska, B. (2020). Opinions and knowledge of parents regarding preventive vaccinations of children and causes of reluctance toward preventive vaccinations. *International Journal of Environmental Research and Public Health*, *17*(10), 3694. https://doi.org/10.3390/ijerph17103694

Hill, H. A., Chen, M., Elam-Evans, L. D., Yankey, D., & Singleton, J. A. (2023). Vaccination coverage by age 24 months among children born during 2018–2019—National Immunization Survey-Child, United States, 2019–2021. *Morbidity and Mortality Weekly Report*, *72*(2), 33–38. https://doi.org/10.15585/mmwr.mm7202a3

Barriers to Vaccination

EVIDENCE BASE Daley, M. F., Reifler, L. M., Shoup, J. A., Narwaney, K. J., Kharbanda, E. O., Groom, H. C., Jackson, M. L., Jacobsen, S. J., McLean, H. Q., Klein, N. P., Williams, J. T. B., Weintraub, E. S., McNeil, M. M., & Glanz, J. M. (2021). Temporal trends in undervaccination: A population-based cohort study. *American Journal of Preventive Medicine*, *61*(1), 64–72. https://doi.org/10.1016/j.amepre.2021.01.037

Chellapandian, P., Myneni, S., Ravikumar, D., Padmanaban, P., James, K. M., Kunasekaran, V. M., Manickaraj, R. G. J., Puthota Arokiasamy, C., Sivagananam, P., Balu, P., Meesala Chelladurai, U., Veeraraghavan, V. P., Baluswamy, G., Nalinakumari Sreekandan, R., Kamaraj, D., Deiva Suga, S. S., Kullappan, M., Mallavarapu Ambrose, J., Kamineni, S. R. T., & Surapaneni, K. M. (2021). Knowledge on cervical cancer and perceived barriers to the uptake of HPV vaccination among health professionals. *BMC Women's Health*, *321*(1), 65. https://doi.org/10.1186/s12905-021-01205-8

*Please note that the term "male" in this chapter refers to a person assigned male at birth, and the term "female" in this chapter refers to a person assigned female at birth.

There are many reasons that parental caregivers may give to refuse vaccinations for their children.

1. Safety concerns, such as concerns that the child may develop learning disabilities. Information about vaccine safety can be obtained from the Centers for Disease Control and Prevention (CDC) at https://www.cdc.gov/vaccinesafety/concerns/index.html
2. Concern for the pain inflicted on the child.
3. Because of the success of vaccine programs for many years, many parental caregivers have no memory or knowledge of the serious vaccine-preventable illnesses that have been nearly eradicated.
4. Unfortunately, many parental caregivers may be influenced by high-impact negative media information regarding vaccinations despite the fact that most is not supported by evidence.

CLINICAL JUDGMENT Nurses can be instrumental in assisting parental caregivers in discerning factual information from myths and erroneous information that may be presented in the media.

General Considerations

Requirements of National Childhood Vaccine Injury Act (Effective 1988)

1. This act mandated providers to notify all patients and parental caregivers about the risks and benefits associated with vaccines.
2. The patient, parental caregiver, or legal guardian should be informed about the benefits and risks of immunizations. Before administration of the vaccine, they must be provided with the current Vaccine Information Statement (VIS), developed by the CDC. Health care providers must record the name of the VIS publication (e.g., polio), the date of VIS publication, and the date the VIS was given to the patient or their family on the child's medical record.
3. Federal law mandates that all health care providers must record the following information in the patient's permanent medical record: month, day, and year of administration; vaccine or other biologic administered; manufacturer, lot number, and expiration date; and name, address, and title of the health care provider administering the vaccine.
4. In addition, the site and route of administration should be documented in the patient's record.
5. Health care providers are required to report selected events occurring after vaccination to the Vaccine Adverse Events Reporting System, part of the CDC Immunization Safety Office, which monitors and investigates possible vaccine adverse effects.

Routine Vaccinations for Children in the United States

The Advisory Committee on Immunization Practices (ACIP) annually develops written recommendations for the CDC regarding the routine administration of vaccines, along with schedules detailing the appropriate timing, dosage, and contraindications for children and adults in the civilian population in the United States. The most recent recommendations are reviewed, but complete immunization schedules can be found at www.cdc.gov/vaccines.

Childhood-recommended vaccines (ages 0 to 6 years) include diphtheria, tetanus toxoid, and acellular pertussis (DTaP); inactivated poliovirus vaccine (IPV); MMR; *Haemophilus influenzae* type b (Hib) vaccine; HBV; *Varicella*; pneumococcal conjugate vaccine (PCV7 and PCV13); rotavirus (Rota); hepatitis A (HepA); and meningococcal vaccine (MCV4). Influenza and coronavirus disease 2019 (COVID-19) vaccines are recommended to be given annually to healthy people aged 6 months to 19 years. In many areas of the United States, influenza vaccine is a requirement for day care attendance.

The recommended immunization schedule for persons aged 7 to 18 years includes Tdap; HPV vaccine; MCV4; pneumococcal polysaccharide vaccine (PPV)—to certain groups at high risk; annual influenza vaccine (trivalent inactivated influenza vaccine [TIV]); HepA—for certain groups of children; HBV; MMR; *Varicella*; and IPV, if necessary, to equal a total of four doses. COVID-19 immunizations are also recommended for children greater than 6 months of age. While not required by schools, the HPV vaccine is recommended to start by age 9 years but can be given until age 26 years. If the child receives the vaccine before age 14 years, they need only a two-dose vaccine series; after age 14 years, three doses of the vaccine are required.

Immunization Schedules

1. Routine immunizations are started in infancy. However, if a child is not immunized in infancy, immunizations may be started at any age, and a slightly different schedule may be followed, depending on the child's age and the prevalence of specific diseases at that time.
2. Usually, an interrupted primary series of immunizations does not need to be restarted; rather, the original series should be resumed, regardless of the length of time that has elapsed.
3. In special circumstances involving some cancer treatments and severe immunologic disorders, immunization schedules will require adjustment.
4. The immune response is limited in a significant proportion of infants, and the recommended booster doses are designed to ensure and maintain immunity.
5. When using a combination vaccine, if there is a contraindication to any of the components, do not vaccinate.

Contraindications and Precautions

It is important to read the manufacturer's insert for each vaccine before administration.

1. Contraindications to all vaccines:
   a. Anaphylactic reaction to a vaccine or a vaccine constituent.
   b. Moderate or severe illnesses with or without a fever. Children with moderate or severe illnesses, with or without fever, can be vaccinated as soon as they are recovering and no longer acutely ill.
2. All live virus vaccines (live oral poliovirus vaccine [OPV], MMR, *Varicella*) are contraindicated in pregnancy, immunosuppression or immunodeficiency, and household or close contact with those who are immunosuppressed or immunodeficient.
   a. MMR vaccine should be considered for all symptomatic human immunodeficiency virus (HIV)-infected persons who do not have evidence of severe immunosuppression or evidence of measles immunity.
   b. *Varicella* vaccine should be considered for asymptomatic or mildly symptomatic HIV-infected children.
3. Diphtheria, tetanus, and pertussis (DTP)/DTaP—encephalopathy within 7 days of administration of the previous dose of DTP/DTaP.
   a. Infants and children with stable neurologic conditions, including well-controlled seizures, may be vaccinated; however, such vaccination should be decided on an individual basis.

4. IPV—anaphylactic reaction to neomycin, streptomycin, or polymyxin B.
5. MMR and *Varicella*—anaphylactic reactions to neomycin or gelatin.
6. Influenza—anaphylactic reaction to eggs or egg protein. Persons with asthma, reactive airway disease, or other chronic pulmonary or cardiovascular disorders should not receive live attenuated influenza vaccine (LAIV).
7. HBV—anaphylactic reaction to baker's yeast.
8. MCVs—can be given to pregnant people; should not be administered with other vaccines for children with sickle cell disease or those without a functioning spleen.

Misconceptions Concerning Vaccine Contraindications

1. Some health care providers and parental caregivers inappropriately consider certain conditions or circumstances to be contraindications to vaccination. Conditions most commonly regarded as such include the following:
   a. Mild acute illness with a low-grade fever or mild diarrheal illness in an otherwise well child.
   b. Current antimicrobial therapy or the convalescent phase of illness.
   c. Reaction to a previous DTaP dose that involved only mild pain, redness, swelling in the immediate vicinity of the vaccination site, or temperature of less than 105°F (40.5°C).
   d. Prematurity.
   e. Person using aerosolized steroids, short course of oral steroids (less than 14 days), or topical steroids.
   f. Pregnancy of patient or other household contact.
   g. Recent exposure to an infectious disease.
   h. Breastfeeding.
   i. History of nonspecific allergies or relatives with allergies.
   j. Allergies to penicillin or other antibiotic, except anaphylactic reactions to neomycin or streptomycin.
   k. Allergies to duck meat or duck feathers.
   l. Family history of seizures in people considered for pertussis or measles vaccination.
   m. Family history of sudden infant death syndrome in children considered for DTaP vaccination.
   n. Family history of an adverse event, unrelated to immunosuppression, after vaccination.
   o. Malnutrition.
2. In most cases, children with the abovementioned conditions can still be immunized.

Vaccine Administration Considerations

1. Strict adherence to the manufacturer's storage and handling recommendation is vital. Failure to observe these precautions and recommendations may reduce the potency and effectiveness of vaccines.
2. Health care personnel administering vaccines should be immunized against MMR, hepatitis B, influenza, tetanus, pertussis, and diphtheria. *Varicella* vaccine is recommended for health care providers with no serologic proof of immunity, prior vaccination, or previous disease. Gloves should be worn when administering vaccines. Good handwashing technique is mandatory before and after vaccine administration.
3. Sterile, disposable needles and syringes should be discarded promptly in appropriate biohazard containers. Do not recap needles.
4. Parenteral vaccines should be administered in the anterolateral aspect of the upper thigh in infants and in the deltoid area of the upper arm in older children and adolescents. Recommended routes of administration are included in the package inserts of vaccines.
5. Before administering a subsequent dose of any vaccine, question patients and parental caregivers about adverse effects and possible reactions from previous doses.
6. Routine vaccines can be safely and effectively administered simultaneously in most healthy children.

Specific Immunizations

COVID-19 Vaccine

1. With the COVID-19 pandemic and persistent infections, COVID-19 vaccine is approved and recommended for children aged 6 months and above.
2. The vaccine helps prevent children from getting COVID-19. Although children often get less sick than adults, many children have been hospitalized from COVID-19 or have long-term effects from "long COVID." Vaccination helps prevent more serious infections.
3. The 2023-2024 formulation for all COVID-19 vaccines licensed or authorized in the United States (Moderna, Novavax, and Pfizer-BioNTech) has been updated to a monovalent vaccine based on the Omicron XBB.1.5 sublineage of a severe acute respiratory syndrome coronavirus 2 (SARS-CoV-2). The original monovalent and bivalent formulations should no longer be used. There are different formulations in the Moderna and Pfizer-BioNTech COVID-19 vaccine preparations for children aged 6 months to 11 years and those aged 12 years and above. Novavax COVID-19 vaccine adjuvant is approved for those aged 12 years and above.
4. Children aged 11 years and below will receive a child's dose, and those aged 12 years and above will receive the full adult dose.
5. The COVID-19 vaccines are administered intramuscularly (IM). The vaccine is a series, with the second being administered at least 3 weeks after the initial dose for children aged 6 months to 4 years. Children aged 5 years and above can receive one dose of the updated vaccine.
6. Side effects from the vaccines vary from child to child; they tend to be mild and temporary. They are more common after the second dose and can include pain or swelling at the injection site, fatigue, headache, muscle or joint pain, chills, and swollen lymph nodes.
7. The CDC recommends one bivalent booster dose in children aged 6 months or above if they have completed the primary vaccine series and if it has been at least **2 months** since their last dose.

Diphtheria, Tetanus Toxoid, and Acellular Pertussis

1. Administered IM.
2. A time lapse of 8 weeks is recommended between the first three DTaP injections for desirable maximum effects.
3. Administration of acetaminophen at the time of immunization and 4 and 8 hours after immunization decreases the incidence of febrile and local reactions.
4. Tdap is recommended for children over age 7 years. As of 2006, vaccination guidelines recommend that Tdap be routinely used in adolescents aged 11 to 18 years and single doses for adults aged 19 to 64 years in attempts to control recent pertussis outbreaks.
5. For contaminated wounds, a booster dose of tetanus should be given if more than 5 years have elapsed since the last dose.

6. For infant pertussis protection, the ACIP has recommended that Tdap be given during each pregnancy between 27 and 36 weeks of gestation to maximize the maternal antibody response and passive antibody transfer to the infant.

Tuberculin Skin Test

1. It is recommended that, if indicated, the tuberculin test be given before or at the time of the MMR vaccine. The measles vaccine may temporarily suppress tuberculin reactivity for 4 to 6 weeks, so the results may not be accurate during that time frame.
2. The frequency of repeated tuberculin testing depends on the following:
   a. Risk of tuberculosis (TB) exposure to the child.
   b. Prevalence of TB in the population group.
   c. Presence of underlying host factors in the child (immunosuppressive conditions or HIV infection).
3. Children who have immigrated or been adopted from another country may have received an immunization for TB (Bacillus Calmette–Guérin [BCG] vaccine). It is not recommended in the United States because of low effectiveness.
   a. BCG may cause a false-positive TB skin test; however, screening for TB should still occur.
   b. Interferon-gamma release assays (IGRAs) are the preferred method of TB testing in those immunized with BCG. An IGRA measures how strongly a person's immune system reacts to TB bacteria by testing the person's blood in a laboratory. This testing method is not influenced by BCG administration.
   c. Chest x-ray confirms pulmonary disease.

EVIDENCE BASE Cameron, L., & Cruz, A. (2022). Childhood tuberculosis. *Current Opinion in Infectious Diseases, 35* (5), 477–483. https://doi.org/10.1097/QCO.0000000000000866

Measles Vaccine

1. Usually given between ages 12 and 15 months, but should be given at 12 months in high-risk areas. Second dose is recommended between ages 4 and 6 years.
2. Administered subcutaneously.
3. During an outbreak, infants as young as age 6 months can be immunized. A second dose should be given between ages 12 and 15 months and again at school entry.
4. Mild postimmunization symptoms include transient skin rashes and fever up to 2 weeks after vaccination.
5. Immunoglobulin preparations will interfere with the serologic response to measles vaccine; therefore, wait the specified time after administration for vaccination.

Meningococcal Vaccine

1. Usually given between the ages of 11 and 12 years, with a booster dose at age 16 years for healthy children. Is administered earlier (minimum age of 9 months) for some children with underlying conditions or children who are resident or travel to countries with epidemic disease.
2. Administer the MPSV4 vaccine subcutaneously into the fatty tissue of the arm. The MCV4 vaccines are given IM.
3. Mild postimmunization symptoms such as local discomfort may occur. A small percentage of those who receive the vaccine may develop a fever. Severe reactions (such as an allergic reaction) are very rare.

Meningococcal B Vaccine

1. Adolescents and young adults (age 16 through 23 years) may receive serogroup B meningococcal (MenB) vaccine.
2. The CDC recommends that individuals who are at high risk of contracting meningococcal B be vaccinated.
   a. These groups include individuals with certain medical conditions, those with functional anatomic asplenia (including sickle cell disease), those taking complement inhibitors, individuals working in professional settings where they are exposed, and individuals who are part of a community at risk for outbreaks, such as college campuses.
3. There are two MenB vaccines available. Once starting vaccination, individuals should receive the same vaccine for the entire series.
4. The MenB vaccines require multiple doses.
   a. Bexsero: two doses at least 1 month apart.
   b. Trumenba: two to three doses, with the first two doses 1 month apart and the third dose at least 6 months later.
5. Individuals with the medical conditions listed earlier should receive the initial series of vaccines and then a booster 1 year after the initial series and then every 2 to 3 years.
6. Common side effects can include pain at the injection site, fever, and headache. These side effects usually resolve on their own within 3 to 5 days after vaccination.

Mumps Vaccine

1. Usually administered in combination with measles and rubella vaccine between ages 12 and 15 months.
2. Second dose administered as MMR is important because a substantial number of cases have occurred in people with previous immunizations.
3. Important to immunize susceptible children approaching puberty, adolescents, and adults.

Rubella Vaccine

1. Two doses of rubella vaccine are recommended to avoid consequences such as congenital rubella syndrome; usually administered in combination with mumps and measles.
2. Important to immunize postpubertal individuals, especially college students and military recruits.
3. Females should avoid pregnancy within 3 months of vaccine because of the theoretical risk to the fetus.

Polio Vaccine

1. Two types of trivalent vaccines have been developed—OPV and IPV (given IM or subcutaneously). Both are effective in preventing poliomyelitis; however, as of 2000, both the ACIP and CDC recommend exclusive use of IPV for infants and children in the United States, to reduce the risk of vaccine-induced polio from OPV.
2. Because live OPV is excreted in the stool for up to 1 month after vaccination, vaccine-induced polio is a risk to both the nonimmune child and any immunosuppressed contact.

Haemophilus influenzae Type B Vaccine

1. Incidence of invasive disease caused by Hib has declined dramatically since the introduction of the conjugate vaccine.
2. Several different types of Hib vaccines are available. Different vaccines have different schedules.
3. Minimal adverse reactions (pain, redness, or swelling at the immunization site for less than 24 hours).

Hepatitis B Vaccine

1. There are two schedules for this vaccine. Infants born to hepatitis B surface antigen (HBsAg)-negative birthing parents should receive the routine schedule. Infants born to HBsAg-positive birthing parents should be on an accelerated vaccination schedule.
2. Recommended for all infants born to HBsAg-negative birthing parents. Three-dose schedule is initiated in neonatal period or by age 2 months; the second dose is given 1 to 2 months later; the third dose given 6 to 18 months later.
3. All infants born to HBsAg-positive birthing parents, including premature neonates, should receive hepatitis B immunoglobulin and HBV within 12 hours after birth. The second dose is given between ages 1 and 2 months; the third dose is given at age 6 months.
4. Preterm neonates weighing less than 2,000 g may have lower seroconversion rates. Initiation of HBV should be delayed until just before hospital discharge if the infant weighs 2,000 g or more or until about age 2 months when other routine immunizations are given.
5. All children and adolescents who have not had HBV should be immunized.
6. Administered IM.

Pneumococcal Vaccines

1. There are two types of pneumococcal vaccines:
   a. PCV7/Prevnar (must be administered IM).
   b. 23-Valent PPV/Pneumovax (may be given IM or subcutaneously).
2. The pneumococcal is included in the recommended childhood vaccines for all children aged 2 to 23 months and for certain children aged 2 to 5 years.
3. Efficacy for the vaccine is 97%, and the adverse effects are mild (fever and localized tenderness and redness at the injection site).
4. PPV is recommended for children aged 2 to 5 years in certain high-risk groups (sickle cell disease, functional or anatomic asplenia, nephrotic syndrome, chronic renal failure, immunosuppressive disorders, HIV infection, and cerebrospinal fluid leak).

Influenza Vaccine

1. The influenza vaccine known as TIV or LAIV contains three virus strains and is changed yearly, based on predictions of predominate strains expected to circulate in the upcoming influenza season. LAIV is approved for use in those aged 2 through 49 years in the United States and is administered intranasally. TIV is available in both pediatric and adult formulations and is administered IM.
2. The influenza vaccine should be given annually to children aged 6 months through 18 years. The "Recommended Immunization Schedule" provides more specifics.
3. This vaccine is given annually, before influenza season, usually in October, November, or December.
4. In children aged 8 years and below, the first time influenza vaccine is administered, two doses should be given 1 month apart. In subsequent years, only one dose is needed.
5. TIV should be used for children with asthma, children aged 2 to 4 years who had wheezing in the past 12 months, or children who have any other underlying medical contraindications to the LAIV.
6. When available, LAIV is recommended for children aged 2 to 8 years.

Rotavirus Vaccine

1. A live, oral vaccine—RotaTeq—is licensed. In the United States, routine vaccination of infants—with three doses of rotavirus vaccine administered at 2, 4, and 6 months—is recommended.

Varicella Virus Vaccine

1. *Varicella* virus vaccine contains live attenuated virus; approved for children aged 12 months and above and for adults.
2. Administered subcutaneously at 12 to 15 months old; second dose at 4 to 6 years (or at least 3 months after the first dose).
3. May be given to older children and adults who do not have immunity. In those older than age 13, the second dose may be delayed only 4 weeks following the first dose.

CLINICAL JUDGMENT Millions of children travel overseas every year, risking exposure to infectious diseases not covered by routine immunizations. Refer families to their local public health department or retail travel clinic for special immunizations and malaria prophylaxis.

Nutrition in Children

The nutritional status of the child is an important aspect of health maintenance. A balanced diet influences child growth and psychosocial development. Feeding provides emotional and psychological benefits in addition to nutritional needs. In the United States, obesity in childhood has become a major problem, and in developing countries, undernutrition—due to scarcity of nutrient-rich foods—leads to malnutrition and illness. In addition, anorexia, bulimia, and other purposeful or unintentional dietary restrictions may place children and adolescents at risk for serious health consequences. Good eating habits, nutrient-rich foods, and physical activity introduced early in life can help foster good nutrition practices into adulthood. Nurses can be instrumental in providing factual information to both parental caregivers and children on typical nutritional needs and those required for specific sport participation. Table 38-1 presents nutritional guidelines based on age and developmental maturation.

EVIDENCE BASE Hossain, Z., Qasem, W. A., Friel, J. K., & Omri, A. (2021). Effects of total enteral nutrition on early growth immunity and neuronal development of preterm infants. *Nutrients*, *13*(8), 2755. https://doi.org/10.3390/nu13082755

Breastfeeding

Breastfeeding is the natural and ideal nourishment that will supply an infant with adequate nutrition as well as immunologic and anti-infection properties. With breast milk being at the proper temperature, it may prevent other gastrointestinal (GI) disturbances as well. The development of allergies is reduced in breastfed babies.

1. Breastfeeding is recommended solely for infants up to 6 months of age. As the infant grows and develops, the breast milk properties change with respect to the amounts of fat, carbohydrates, and protein as well as physical properties such as pH needed for the respective age of the infant.
2. Breastfeeding provides psychological and emotional satisfaction for the infant and breastfeeding parent and can promote

Table 38-1 Nutrition in Children

AGE AND DEVELOPMENTAL INFLUENCE ON NUTRITIONAL REQUIREMENTS AND FEEDING PATTERNS	FEEDING PATTERN AND DIET	NURSING CONSIDERATIONS AND PARENTAL GUIDANCE
Neonate		

Birth–4 wk
• Neonate's rapid growth makes infant especially vulnerable to dietary inadequacies, dehydration, and iron deficiency anemia.
• Feeding process is the basis for infant's first human relationship, formation of trust.
• Neonates require more fluid relative to their size than do adults.
• Sucking ability is influenced by individual neuromuscular maturity.
Infant
1–3 mo
• Infants consume more formula or breast milk with each feeding and sleep for longer periods.
• Infants have increased interaction during feeding because of cooing and development of a social milestone.
• Bowel movements become less frequent. Breastfed infants may not have a bowel movement after each feeding.
	• Breast milk or formula is generally given in six to eight feedings per day, spaced 2–4 h apart.
	• Feeding schedules should be individualized according to infant's needs.
	• Breastfed infants should receive 400 IU of supplemental vitamin D daily, beginning in the first few days of life. Supplementation should continue until baby is weaned to at least 1 qt (1 L) of whole milk per day. Whole milk should not be used until after 12 mo of age.
	• Human milk contains little iron, so infants who are exclusively breastfed are at increased risk of iron deficiency after 4 mo of age. It is recommended that infants be given 1 mg/kg/day of a liquid iron supplement until iron-containing solid foods are introduced at about 6 mo of age.
	• Infant formula should be iron fortified to prevent anemia.
	• All formulas sold in the United States have at least 400 IU/L of vitamin D; if baby is drinking at least 32 oz of formula, vitamin D supplementation is not needed.
		• Provide information to help parental caregivers make decision concerning breastfeeding or bottle-feeding.
		• Support parental caregivers in their decision.
		Breastfed infant:
		• Help breastfeeding parent assume comfortable and satisfying position for self and baby.
		• Help breastfeeding parent to determine schedule, timing, and when infant is satisfied.
		• Provide specific information about:
		  • Feeding technique: position, "bubbling/burping"
		  • Care of breasts
		  • Manual expression of milk from breast
		• Maternal diet
		Bottle-fed infant:
		• Provide specific information about:
		  • Type of formula
		  • Preparation of formula: measuring and sterilization
		  • Equipment—types of bottles and nipples
		  • Sterilization of equipment
		  • Technique of feeding: position, "bubbling/burping"
		• Help breastfeeding parent to determine when infant is satisfied; develop schedule for feeding.
		• Provide information about normal characteristics of stools, signs of dehydration, constipation, colic, milk allergy.
		• Discuss need for prescribed supplements and how to administer (by dropper).
		• Discuss need for additional fluids during periods of hot weather and with fever, diarrhea, and vomiting.
		• Observe for evidence of common problems and intervene accordingly:
		  • Overfeeding
		  • Underfeeding
		  • Difficulty digesting formula because of its composition
		  • Improper feeding technique; holes in nipples too large or too small; formula too hot or too cold; uncomfortable feeding position; failure to "bubble/burp"; improper sterilization; bottle propping
		  • Bottles should never be given to infants to take to bed.

3 mo–1 yr overview • Increased neuromuscular development allows infant to make transition from a totally liquid diet to a diet of milk and solid foods as well as to more active participation in the feeding process. **3–6 mo** • Sucking reflex becomes voluntary and chewing action begins; infant can approximate lips to rim and cup and may begin drinking from cup at 6 mo.	• Number of feedings per day decreases through the first year. • By ages 4–6 mo, generally ready to begin strained foods. The usual sequence of foods is cereal followed by vegetables and fruits. Meats may be started between 8 and 9 mo. Sequence may vary according to preferences of the family and health care provider.	• The person feeding should be calm, gentle, relaxed, and patient in approach. • When first offered puréed foods with a spoon, the child expects and wants to suck. The protrusion of the tongue, which is needed in sucking, makes it appear as if the child is pushing the food out of the mouth. This response should not be interpreted as dislike for the food; it is a result of immature muscle coordination and surprise at the taste and feel of the new food. • The baby foods selected should be high in nutrients without providing excessive calories. Personal and cultural preferences should be considered. Iron-fortified formulas and cereals are needed to prevent physiologic anemia. • New foods should be offered one at a time and early in the feeding while the infant is still hungry. Allow 3–5 d between new foods to assess for any allergic reaction.

6–12 mo
• Loses maternal iron stores at 6 mo; first tooth erupts between ages 6 and 9 mo; eyes and hands can work together; infant can sit without support and has developed grasp; can feed self a biscuit; bangs objects on table; able to hold own bottle between ages 9 and 12 mo; can "pincer" grasp food; able to be weaned from bottle as child becomes developmentally able to take sufficient fluids from the cup.
• Food provides the infant with a variety of learning experiences; motor control and coordination in self-feeding; recognition of shape, texture, and color; stimulation of speech movement through use of mouth muscles.
• Mealtime allows the infant to continue development of trust in a consistent, loving atmosphere. The infant is forming lifetime eating habits; it is, therefore, important to make mealtime a positive experience.
	• Mashed table foods or junior foods are generally started between ages 6 and 8 mo, when infant begins chewing action.
	• Infant begins to enjoy finger foods between ages 10 and 12 mo.
	• The transition from iron-fortified formula or breast milk to cow's milk is usually advised at about age 12 mo.
	• By age 1 yr, most infants are satisfied with three meals and additional fluids throughout the day.
		• Infants should be observed for allergic reactions when new foods are added. Common allergies are to citrus juices, egg whites, and cow's milk. These foods should be avoided until age 12 mo. Research has shown early introduction of peanuts into the diet of pregnant person and infants at high risk of peanut allergy can play a role in the prevention of peanut allergies. Health care providers may recommend introducing peanut-containing products into the diets of infants between ages 4 and 11 mo.
		• Honey should be avoided until age 12 mo because of the risk of infantile botulism.
		• Finger foods should be selected for their nutritional value. Good choices include teething biscuits, cooked vegetables, bananas, cheese sticks, and enriched cereals. Avoid nuts, raisins, and raw vegetables, which can cause choking.
		• Parental caregivers can be taught to prepare their own strained or junior foods using a commercial baby food grinder or blender.
		• Weaning is a gradual process.
		  • Assist parental caregivers to recognize indications of readiness.
		  • Do not expect the infant to completely drop old pattern of behavior while learning a new one; allow overlap of old and new techniques.

(*continued*)

Table 38-1 Nutrition in Children (*continued*)

AGE AND DEVELOPMENTAL INFLUENCE ON NUTRITIONAL REQUIREMENTS AND FEEDING PATTERNS	FEEDING PATTERN AND DIET	NURSING CONSIDERATIONS AND PARENTAL GUIDANCE
		• Evening feedings are usually the most difficult to eliminate because the infant is tired and in need of sucking comfort. • During illness or household disorganization, the infant may regress and return to sucking to relieve their discomfort and frustration. **CLINICAL JUDGMENT** Obtain a thorough nursing history for the hospitalized infant that includes feeding pattern and schedule; types of foods that have been introduced; likes and dislikes; breastfed or bottle-fed, type of bottle; and temperature at which infant prefers foods and fluids.

Toddler
1–3 yr
• Growth slows at the end of the first year. The slower growth rate is reflected in a decreased appetite.
• The toddler has a total of 14–16 teeth, making them more able to chew foods.
• Increased self-awareness causes the toddler to want to do more for self. Refusal of food and refusal of assistance in feedings are common ways in which the toddler asserts self.
• Because body tissues, especially muscles, continue to grow quite rapidly, protein needs are high.
	• Transition from a bottle to a cup before, or at the age of 1 is recommended to prevent tooth decay.
	• Appetite is sporadic; specific foods may be favored exclusively or refused from time to time.
	• Child may be ritualistic concerning food preferences, schedule, and manner of eating.
	• Diet should include a full range of foods: milk, meat, fruits, vegetables, breads, and cereals. Iron-fortified dry cereals (rice, barley) are an excellent source of iron during the second year of life.
	• Older toddler can be expected to consume about one half the amount of food than an adult consumes.
	• Whole milk is recommended up to age 2 yr.
		• Provide foods with a variety of colors, textures, and flavors. Toddlers need to experience the feel of foods.
		• Offer small portions. It is fun for the child to ask for more. It is more effective to give small helpings than to insist that they eat a specific amount.
		• Maintain a regular mealtime schedule.
		• Provide appropriate mealtime equipment:
		  • Silverware scaled to size
		  • Dishes—colorful, unbreakable; shallow, round bowls are preferable to flat plates.
		  • Plastic bibs, placemats, and floor coverings permit a relaxed attitude toward child's self-feeding attempts.
		  • Comfortable seating at good height and distance from table
		• Adults who help toddlers at mealtime should be calm and relaxed. Avoid bribes or force-feeding because this reinforces negative behavior and may lead to a dislike for mealtime. Encourage independence, but provide assistance when necessary. Do not be concerned about table manners.
		• Avoid the use of soda or "sweets" as rewards or between-meal snacks. Instead, substitute fruit or cereal.
		• Toddlers who show little interest in eggs, meat, or vegetables should not be permitted to appease their appetite with carbohydrates or milk because this may lead to iron deficiency anemia. Milk should be limited to 24 oz a day and should be offered after solid foods.
		
		CLINICAL JUDGMENT Nursing history for the hospitalized toddler should include feeding pattern and schedule; food likes and dislikes; food allergies; special eating equipment and utensils; whether child is weaned; and what child is fed when ill.

<table>
<tr>
<td>Preschooler
3–5 yr
• Increased manual dexterity enables child to have complete independence at mealtime.
• Psychosocially, this is a period of increased imitation. The preschooler identifies with parental caregivers at the table and will enjoy what parental caregivers enjoy.
• Additional nutritional habits are developed that become part of the child's lifetime practices.
• Slower growth rate and increased interest in exploring their environment may decrease the preschooler's interest in eating.
• Eating assumes increasing social significance. Mealtime promotes socialization and provides the preschooler with opportunities to learn appropriate mealtime behavior, language skills, and understanding of family rituals.

CLINICAL JUDGMENT Consider cultural differences. Allow parental caregivers to bring in favorite foods or eating utensils from home for the hospitalized preschooler. Encourage family members to be present at mealtime.</td>
<td>• Appetite tends to be sporadic.
• Child requires the same basic four food groups as the adult, but in smaller quantities.
• Generally likes to eat one food from plate at a time
• Likes vegetables that are crisp, raw, and cut into finger-sized pieces. Often dislikes strong-tasting foods</td>
<td>• Emphasis should be placed on the quality rather than the amount of food ingested.
• Foods should be attractively served, mildly flavored, plain, as well as separated and distinctly identifiable in flavor and appearance.
• Nutritional foods (e.g., crackers and cheese, yogurt, fruit) should be offered as snacks.
• Desserts should be nutritious and a natural part of the meal, not used as a reward for finishing the meal or omitted as punishment.
• Unless they persist, periods of overeating or not wanting to eat certain foods should not cause concern. The overall eating pattern from month to month is more pertinent to assess.
• Frequent causes of insufficient eating:
  • Unhappy atmosphere at mealtime
  • Overeating between meals
  • Parental example
  • Attention seeking
  • Excessive parental expectations
  • Inadequate variety or quantity of foods
  • Tooth decay
  • Physical illness
  • Fatigue
  • Emotional disturbance
• Measures to increase food intake:
  • Allow child to help with preparations, planning menu, setting table, and other simple chores.
  • Maintain calm environment with no distractions.
  • Avoid between-meal snacks.
  • Provide rest period before meal.
  • Avoid coaxing, bribing, threatening.
• Place children in small groups, preferably at tables during mealtime. Use nursing history to determine likes and provide simple foods in small portions. Peanut butter and jelly sandwiches are often favorites. Allow and encourage children to feed themselves. Do not punish children who refuse to eat. Offer alternative foods.</td>
</tr>
<tr>
<td>School-Aged Child
• Slowed growth rate during middle childhood results in gradual decline in food requirements per unit of body weight.
• The preadolescent growth spurt occurs about age 10 in females and about age 12 in males. At this time, energy needs increase and approach those of the adult. Intake is particularly important because reserves are laid down for the demands of adolescence.</td>
<td>• By this time, food practices are generally well established, a product of the eating experiences of the toddler and preschool period.
• Many children are too busy with other affairs to take time out to eat. Play readily takes priority unless a firm understanding is reached and mealtime is relaxed and enjoyable.</td>
<td>• Nutrition education should help the child to select foods wisely and to begin to plan and prepare meals.
• Parental attitudes continue to be important as the child copies parental behavior (e.g., skipping breakfast, not eating certain foods, consuming fast foods frequently).</td>
</tr>
</table>

(continued)

Table 38-1 Nutrition in Children (*continued*)

AGE AND DEVELOPMENTAL INFLUENCE ON NUTRITIONAL REQUIREMENTS AND FEEDING PATTERNS	FEEDING PATTERN AND DIET	NURSING CONSIDERATIONS AND PARENTAL GUIDANCE
• The child becomes dependent on peers for approval and makes food choices accordingly. • The child experiences increased socialization and independence through opportunities to eat away from home (e.g., at school and homes of peers).		• Most children require a nutritious breakfast to avoid lassitude in late morning. • Mealtime should continue to be relaxed and enjoyable. Diversions, such as television, should be avoided. • Calcium and vitamin D intake warrant special consideration. They must be adequate to support the rapid enlargement of bones. • Parental caregivers and health care professionals should be alert to signs of developing obesity. Intake should be altered accordingly. • Table manners should not be overemphasized. The young child typically stuffs mouth, spills food, and chatters incessantly while eating. Time and experience will improve habits. • Provide some companionship and conversation at the child's level during meals. Peers should be invited occasionally for meals. **CLINICAL JUDGMENT** Nursing history of the hospitalized child should include food preferences; mealtime patterns and snacks; food allergies; and food preferences when ill. Provide opportunities for children to eat in small groups at tables. Consider cultural differences. Allow parental caregivers to bring in favorite foods from home. Allow child to order their own meal.

Adolescent
11–17 yr
• Dietary requirements vary according to stage of sexual maturation, rate of physical growth, and extent of athletic and social activity.
• When rapid growth of puberty appears, there is a corresponding increase in energy requirements and appetite.
• Menstruating teen is particularly susceptible to iron deficiency anemia.
	• Previously learned dietary patterns are difficult to change.
	• Food choices and eating habits may be quite unusual and are related to the adolescent's psychological and social milieu.
	• Generally, a significant percentage of the daily caloric intake of the adolescent comes from snacking.
		• Continue nutrition education, with emphasis on:
		  • Selecting nutritious foods high in iron
		  • Nutritional needs related to growth
		  • Preparing favorite "adolescent foods"
		  • Foods and physical fitness
		• Informal sessions are generally more effective than lectures on nutrition.
		• Special problems requiring intervention:
		  • Obesity
		  • Excessive dieting
		  • Extreme fads—eccentric and grossly restricted diets
		  • Anorexia nervosa and bulimia
		  • Adolescent pregnancy
		  • Iron deficiency anemia
		• Provide nutritious foods relevant to the adolescent's lifestyle.
		• Discourage cigarette smoking, which may contribute to poor nutritional status by decreasing appetite and increasing the body's metabolic rate.
		
		CLINICAL JUDGMENT Allow hospitalized adolescent to choose own foods, especially if on a special diet. Provide a refrigerator in the recreation room for snacks or utilize a snack cart. Serve foods that appeal to adolescents. Use a nursing history similar to that for the school-aged child.

bonding. The physical closeness may also provide comfort after a frightening or painful procedure.
3. Breastfeeding can be continued through most illnesses and hospitalizations of the infant. In times of stress, the infant may cope with breastfeeding better than bottle-feeding. Because breast milk is more easily and quickly digested, shorter periods without food preoperatively and postoperatively may be necessary. Attempts should be made to maintain the breastfeeding bond and routines of the child and breastfeeding parent.
   a. Supplemental artificial formula can be given to the infant if the breastfeeding parent is not available.
   b. The breastfeeding parent can pump the breasts so that milk can be given to the infant by way of bottle when that parental caregiver is not available.
   c. Breast milk can be frozen for up to 6 months (check the facility's specific policy).
   d. Thaw frozen breast milk for use in tepid water. Do not use a microwave, which may destroy vitamins and nutritional properties as well as result in extreme overheating of portions of the breast milk.
4. Stress of new parenthood or illness in the infant or breastfeeding parent may decrease the milk supply and inhibit the "let-down" reflex, as well as increase or decrease the infant's desire to suckle. Pumping may be initiated to help stimulate the milk supply. An electronic pump may be necessary if prolonged pumping is expected or if manual pumping is not successful.
5. Education and encouragement should be offered to all new breastfeeding parents and those having difficulty or concerns about breastfeeding.

Bottle-Feeding

1. Bottle-feeding is a method of supplying nutrition to the infant by oral feedings, using a bottle and nipple setup.
2. Bottle-feeding can supplement breastfeeding with formula or water or can be the sole means of nutritional intake for the infant.
3. Bottle-feeding can also provide intermittent feedings of expressed breast milk when the breastfeeding parent cannot be present at the time of the feeding.
4. Bottle-feeding can be a time of bonding between the breastfeeding parent and the infant. The nonbreastfeeding parent or other capable members of the family should be taught bottle-feeding techniques as well.
5. Some birthing parents may have chosen bottle-feeding for a variety of reasons, ranging from poor milk production, discomfort (psychological or physical) with breastfeeding, or drug treatment not compatible with breastfeeding. It is important that health care providers offer information on all methods of feeding, but not be judgmental when the birthing parent chooses one method over another.

Safety

Safety is an important aspect of child's health and well-being. Injuries are the leading cause of death for children in the United States. In addition, injury is a significant cause of childhood morbidity. Although childhood deaths from other causes have decreased, deaths from injuries remain constant.

Role of the Nurse

1. Identify environmental hazards and act to reduce or eliminate them.
2. Identify behavioral characteristics of individual children that may be related to accidental liability and caution parental caregivers accordingly. Pay particular attention to children who show the following:
   a. Characteristics that increase exposure to hazards, such as excessive curiosity, inability to delay gratification, hyperactivity, and daringness.
   b. Characteristics that reduce the child's ability to cope with hazards, such as aggressiveness, stubbornness, poor concentration, low frustration threshold, poor impulse control, and lack of self-control.
3. Provide anticipatory guidance about child development as it relates to accidents. Direct preventive teaching toward the intended audience, be it individuals or groups, children, or adults.
4. Participate in policy setting for accident prevention, with great emphasis on effective public health measures.

Principles of Safety

1. The type of accident likely to occur is influenced by the child's age and developmental level. Parental caregivers who have knowledge of their own child's typical behavior patterns may foresee potential accident situations. This information should be relayed to individuals who provide frequent supervision to the child (day care, etc.) to ensure their safety when the parental caregivers are not present.
2. Children are naturally curious, impulsive, and impatient. The young child needs to touch, feel, and investigate. Consistent adult supervision will enable children to learn in a safe environment.
3. Children copy the behavior of their parental caregivers and absorb their attitudes. Parental caregivers and other adults should be a role model for using proper and safe methods.
4. Children become less careful and less willing to listen to warnings and to observe routine safety precautions when they are tired or hungry.
5. An estimated 90% of all accidents are preventable.

General Areas of Adult Responsibility for Child Safety

Motor Vehicle

EVIDENCE BASE American Academy of Pediatrics. (2023). *Car seats: Information for families.* https://healthychildren.org/English/safety-prevention/on-the-go/Pages/Car-Safety-Seats-Information-for-Families.aspx

1. Automobiles should be in good mechanical condition.
2. Use properly fitted and installed car seats and seat belts. Be aware of the guidelines for restraints based on the child's age, weight, and height.
   a. Rear-facing car seat until age 2 years, or if the child has outgrown the manufacturer's recommendation for maximum height and weight.
   b. Front-facing car seat from age 2 years until the child has outgrown the manufacturer's recommendation for maximum height and weight.
   c. Belt-positioning booster seat until the vehicle seat belt fits properly, typically when the child has reached 4 feet, 9 in in height, between 8 and 12 years of age.
3. All children younger than 13 years should be restrained in the rear seats of vehicles (when the vehicle has a rear seat with lap

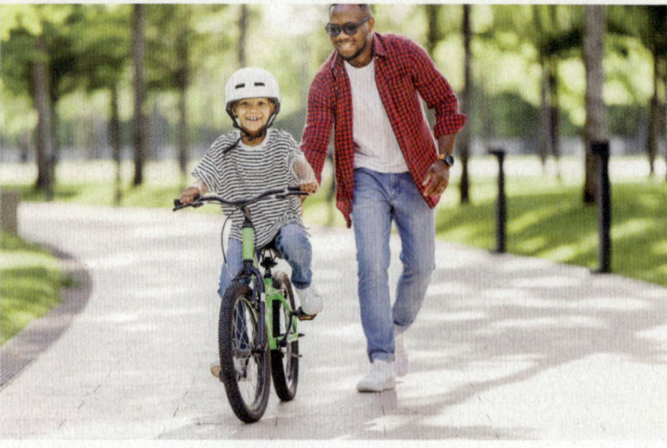

Figure 38-1. Use of bike helmets by all children for safety. (Shutterstock/Evgeny Atamanenko.)

and shoulder belts) for optimal protection. The center rear seat is the safest seat for a child.

4. The driver should look carefully in front and back of the car before getting into the car.
5. Lock all car doors.
6. Never leave young children in a car alone.
7. Do not place heavy or sharp objects on the same seat with a child.

Sports and Recreation

1. Keep equipment in good condition and proper working order.
2. Ensure that children are aware of the correct use of sports equipment.
3. Encourage the routine use of bike helmets (see Figure 38-1).
4. Wear appropriate clothing and safety equipment for the activity (see Figure 38-2).
5. Do not attempt activities beyond one's physical endurance.
6. Keep firearms and ammunition locked in different locations.

Electrical and Mechanical Equipment

1. Only underwriter-approved devices should be installed; they should be inspected periodically.
2. Dry hands before touching appliances. Keep radios, transportable heaters, and hair dryers out of the bathroom.
3. Disconnect appliances after each use and before attempting minor repairs.

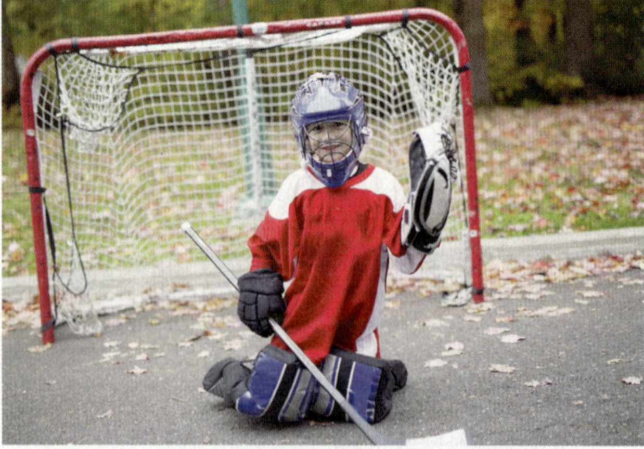

Figure 38-2. Use of appropriate pads and helmets for safety. (Shutterstock/Lopolo.)

4. Keep garden equipment and machinery in a restricted area. Teach proper use of the equipment as soon as the child is old enough.
5. Avoid overloading electrical circuits.
6. Discourage children from playing with or being in an area where appliances or power tools (e.g., washing machine, clothes dryer, saw, lawn mower) are in operation.

Prevention of Falls

1. Keep stairs well lit and free from clutter.
2. Use gates at tops and bottoms of stairways where toddlers have access.
3. Provide sturdy railings.
4. Anchor small rugs securely.
5. Use rubber mats in the bathtub and shower.
6. Use only sturdy ladders for climbing.
7. The American Academy of Pediatrics and the National Association of Children's Hospitals and Related Institutions have recommended that baby walkers be banned as most injuries using these walkers will occur even when adults are present (rolling down stairs, burns, drowning, reaching unsafe objects because of greater stability provided by walkers).

Poisonings and Ingestions

1. Do not mix bleaches with ammonia, vinegar, and other household cleaners.
2. See section on ingested poisons and pediatric poisoning (see page 944).
3. Label poisonous household materials, and keep them out of child's reach.
4. Become familiar with the telephone number for poison control centers where available. Post the local poison control phone number in an easily accessible location (e.g., refrigerator door).

Fire

1. Maintain an adequate fire escape plan and routinely conduct home fire drills. Teach children to escape routes as soon as they are old enough. Identify a safe place (e.g., neighbor's yard) where the family should all meet if they become separated in a fire.
2. Keep a pressure-type, handheld fire extinguisher on each floor. Regularly check expiration or necessary inspection dates. Consider additional units in areas where there are higher risks of fires (kitchen, laundry room, garage). Instruct all family members who are old enough in its use.
3. Fit fireplaces with snug fireplace screens.
4. Store gasoline and other flammable fluids in tightly covered containers that are clearly labeled, away from heat and sparks, and out of reach.
5. Dispose of paint and oil-soaked cloths promptly.
6. Use flame-retardant sleepwear.
7. Mark children's rooms so they are obvious to firefighters.
8. Teach children about the danger of smoke inhalation.
9. Teach children to stop, drop, and roll if their clothing catches fire.
10. Maintain smoke and carbon monoxide detectors in working order.
11. Keep lighters and matches out of the reach of children.
12. Keep children away from heated oven, stovetop, and outdoor grill.

Swimming Pools

1. Completely enclose the pool with a fence that complies with local regulations. The gate should be self-closing and have a lock.

2. Indicate water depth with numbers on the edge of the pool. Place a safety float line where the bottom of the slope begins to deepen.
3. Install at least one ladder at each end of the pool. Ladders should have handrails on both sides, and the diameter of the rails should be small enough for a child to grasp.
4. Use nonslip materials on ladders, deck, and diving boards.
5. If the pool is used at night, install underwater lighting as well as outdoor lights.
6. Install a ground fault circuit interrupter on the pool circuit to cut off electrical power and thus prevent electrocutions should electrical fault occur.
7. Instruct children about safety rules, such as not swimming alone, need for adult supervision, not running around the pool, and not pushing others. Avoid using radios or other electrical appliances around the pool.
8. Warn children not to attempt to walk on any remaining pool water after the season—frozen water or pool-covering equipment.
9. Keep essential rescue devices and first-aid equipment close to the pool and within easy reach.

Emergency Precautions

1. Record emergency telephone numbers in an obvious and easily accessible place.
2. Keep a well-stocked first-aid kit immediately available for emergencies. It is helpful to also carry a small first-aid kit in family vehicles.
3. Give instruction in principles of first aid to all family members who are old enough.
   a. Responsible adults should enroll in first-aid courses offered by the American Red Cross and adult education programs.
   b. Be aware of first-aid procedures for the following conditions: burns, electric shock, poisoning, bites and stings, wounds, near drowning, fractures, cardiopulmonary arrest.
   c. Teach children safety precautions concerning bicycles, answering the telephone or door, strangers outside the home, and street safety.
4. Know the location of gas, water, and electrical switches and how to turn them off in an emergency.
5. Teach children their addresses and telephone numbers and how to dial 911 in case of emergency.

Miscellaneous

1. Take advantage of preventive health care.
   a. Obtain recommended immunizations.
   b. Have regular physical and dental examinations.
2. Seek immediate treatment of all diseases and health problems.
3. Balance periods of work, rest, and exercise in daily living.

PEDIATRIC CARE TECHNIQUES

Nursing Management of the Child With Fever

EVIDENCE BASE Alsofyani, B. A., & Hassanien, N. S. (2022). Factors affecting parental caregiver practice regarding the management of children's fever. *Cureus*, *14*(6), e25658. https://doi.org/10.7759/cureus.25658

Fever is an abnormal elevation of body temperature. Prolonged elevation of temperature above 104°F (40°C) may produce dehydration and harmful effects on the central nervous system (CNS).

General Considerations

1. Consider basic principles related to temperature regulation in pediatric patients.
   a. Usually, an infant's temperature does not stabilize before age 1 week. A neonate's temperature varies with the temperature of the environment.
   b. The degree of fever does not always reflect the severity of the disease. A child may have a serious illness with a normal or subnormal temperature.
   c. Febrile seizures may occur in some children when the temperature rises rapidly.
   d. The range for normal temperature varies widely in children. A common explanation for "fever" is misinterpretation of a normal temperature reading.
   e. A child's temperature is influenced by activity and by the time of day; temperatures are highest in the late afternoon.
2. Temperature interpretation depends on accurate temperature measurement in a child. The mode should be appropriate for the child's age and condition, and the thermometer should be left in place for the required time period. Parental caregivers should be taught the appropriate assessment of temperature as the child grows.

Causes of Fever in Children

1. Infection.
2. Inflammatory disease.
3. Dehydration.
4. Tumors.
5. Disturbance of temperature-regulating center.
6. Extravasation of blood into the tissues.
7. Drugs or toxins.

Nursing Assessment

1. Assess the history of the present illness for the source of fever.
   a. Age of the child.
   b. Pattern of the fever.
   c. Length of the illness.
   d. Change in normal patterns of eating, elimination, and recreation.
   e. Other symptoms—poor feeding, cough, earache, diarrhea, vomiting, and rash.
   f. Exposure to any illness.
   g. Recent immunizations or drugs.
   h. Treatment of fever and effectiveness of treatment, including appropriate dosing of antipyretic medications.
   i. Previous experiences with fever and its control.
2. Assess the general appearance of the child.
3. Perform a systematic physical assessment.
   a. Inspection of the skin for rashes, sores, or flushed appearance.
   b. Inspection of eyes, ears, nose, and throat for redness and drainage.
   c. Auscultation of the lungs for abnormal sounds.
   d. Neurologic observation for changes in state of consciousness, pupillary reaction, strength of grip, abnormal muscle movement, or lack of movement.
   e. Inspection of external genitals for redness and drainage.
   f. Presence of abdominal or flank tenderness.
4. Assist with laboratory tests, as indicated. Initial tests typically include complete blood count; urinalysis; cultures of the

throat, nasopharynx, urine, blood, and spinal fluid; and chest x-ray.

5. Attempt to identify the pattern of the fever. Take the child's temperature by the same method every hour until stable, then every 2 hours until normal, then every 4 hours for 24 hours.

Nursing Measures to Reduce Fever

Fever does not necessarily require treatment. The presence of fever should not be obscured by the indiscriminate use of antipyretic measures. However, if the child is uncomfortable or appears toxic because of fever, an attempt should be made to reduce it by any of the following nursing measures or by a combination of these measures:

1. Increase the child's fluid intake to prevent dehydration.
2. Expose the skin to the air by leaving the child lightly dressed in absorbent material. Avoid warm, binding clothing, and blankets.
3. Administer antipyretic drugs, as prescribed. Avoid aspirin/acetylsalicylic acid as its use is known to result in Reye syndrome (encephalopathy, fatty degeneration of the liver with associated hypoglycemia) in some children. Children aged 4 to 12 years with a viral illness are at greatest risk for Reye syndrome.
4. Use a tepid tub or sponge bath or a hypothermia blanket. Do not allow the child to shiver, as that may increase the body temperature.

Administering Medications to Children

Administration of medication can be traumatic for children. The proper approach to administration can facilitate the process and enhance the child's understanding of the importance of taking medications.

Important Considerations

1. The manner of approach should indicate that the nurse firmly expects the child to take the medication. This manner usually convinces the child of the necessity of the procedure.
2. Establishing a positive relationship with the child will allow expression of feelings, concerns, and misconceptions regarding medications.
3. Explanation about medication should be directed to the child's level of understanding (i.e., through play or comparison to something familiar).
4. The nurse must mask their own feelings regarding the medication.
5. Always be truthful when the child asks, "Does it taste bad?" or "Will it hurt?" Respond by saying, "The medication does not taste good, but I will give you some juice as soon as you swallow it," or "It will hurt for just a minute."
6. It is typically necessary to mix distasteful medications or crushed pills with a small amount of carbonated drink, cherry syrup, ice cream, or applesauce. After mixing, monitor to ensure that the child finishes the preparation.
7. Never threaten a child with an injection when refusing oral medication.
8. Do not mix medications with large quantities of food or with any food that is taken regularly (e.g., milk).
9. Avoid giving medications to a child at mealtime unless specifically prescribed.
10. For each medication administered, the nurse should know the common use, safe dosage based on the child's weight, contraindications, adverse effects, and toxic effects.
11. The child must be accurately identified before medication is given.
12. When preparing intramuscular (IM) injections, draw 0.2 mL of air into the syringe, in addition to the correct amount of medication. This clears the medication from the needle on injection and prevents backflow and the depositing of medication in subcutaneous (SC) fat when the needle is withdrawn.
13. Physical intervention (through swaddling, side or stomach position, shushing, swinging, sucking) and oral sucrose administration have been shown through research to reduce pain reactions in infants aged 2 and 4 months during vaccine injections.

Calculating the Pediatric Dosage

General Principles

1. The nurse is responsible for knowing the safe dosage range for the medication the nurse administers.
2. Factors determining the amount of drug prescribed include the following:
   a. Action, absorption, detoxification, and excretion of the drug are related to the maturity and metabolic rate of the child.
   b. Neonates and premature neonates require a reduced dosage because of:
      i. Deficient or absent detoxifying enzymes.
      ii. Decreased effective renal function.
      iii. Altered blood–brain barrier and protein-binding capacity.
   c. Dosage recommendations based on age groups are not satisfactory because a child may be much smaller or larger than the average child in the age group.
   d. Dosages based on child's weight are more accurate; however, these calculations have limitations.
3. Consult drug references for recommended dosage and other information, and be alert for prescription that would be inappropriate for a child.
4. Advise parental caregivers not to save unused medications that are unneeded or outdated, and do not give one child's prescription to another child.

Calculating by Body Surface Area

The following formulas are used to estimate the pediatric dosage based on the child's body surface area (BSA). BSA calculations are generally preferred because many physiologic processes in the child (e.g., blood volume, glomerular filtration) are related to BSA.

1. Surface area in square meters × dose per square meter = approximate child dose.
2. Surface area of child/surface area of adult × dose of adult = approximate child dose.
3. Surface area of child in square meters/1.75 × adult dose = child dose.

Calculating by Clark Rule

Clark rule may be used as an estimate of the pediatric dosage based on the child's weight with respect to the adult dose of the drug:

Child's weight in pounds/150 × adult dose = approximate dose for child.

CLINICAL JUDGMENT Ensure proper identification of all patients via the identification bracelet before administration of medication.

Oral Medications

Infants

1. Draw up medication in a plastic dropper or disposable syringe.
2. Elevate the infant's head and shoulders; depress the chin with a thumb to open the mouth.
3. Place a dropper or syringe on the middle of the tongue and slowly drop the medication on the tongue.
4. Release the thumb and allow the child to swallow.
5. When the correct amount of medication has been measured, it can be placed in a nipple and the infant can suck the medication through the nipple.
6. If the nurse feels comfortable managing the infant in their lap, it is acceptable to hold the infant for medication administration.

Toddlers

1. Draw up liquid medications in a syringe or measure into a medicine cup. Medications may be placed in a medicine cup or spoon after being measured accurately in a syringe.
2. Elevate the child's head and shoulders.
3. Squeeze the cup and put it to the child's lips or place the syringe (without needle) in the child's mouth, positioning the syringe tip in the space between the cheek mucosa and gum, and slowly expel the medicine. The child may prefer using a familiar teaspoon.
4. Allow the child time to swallow.
5. Allow the child to hold the medicine cup if able and to drink it at their own pace. (This may be a more agreeable method.) Offer a favorite drink as a "chaser," if not contraindicated.
6. The small, safe medicine cups can be given to the child for play.

School-Aged Children

1. When a child is old enough to take medicine in pill or capsule form, teach the child to place the pill near the back of the tongue and immediately swallow fluid, such as water or fruit juice. If swallowing of the fluid is emphasized, the child will no longer think about the pill.
2. Always give praise after a child takes medication.
3. If the child finds it particularly difficult to take oral medications, express understanding and offer help.

Subcutaneous and Intramuscular Medications

For sites and techniques for IM injections, see Figures 38-3 and 38-4.

General Considerations

1. After the medication to be given IM is drawn from the vial, draw up an additional 0.2 to 0.3 mL of air into the syringe, thus clearing the needle of medication and preventing medication seepage from the injection site.
2. When injecting less than 1 mL of medication, use a tuberculin syringe for accuracy.
3. Clean site thoroughly, using friction with an antiseptic solution; let the site dry.
4. Establish anatomic landmarks and prepare to position the needle at a 45-degree angle for SC injection and a 90-degree angle for IM injection (see Figure 38-3). Alternate injection sites and keep record at bedside or on medication card.
5. With IM injections, after penetrating site, aspirate to check for blood vessel puncture. If this occurs, withdraw the needle, discard the medicine, and start again.
6. After injection, massage site (unless contraindicated). When multiple injections are being administered, complications such as fibrosis and contracture of the muscle can be diminished by massage, warm soaks, and range of motion exercises to disrupt and stretch immature scar tissue.

Infants

1. Acceptable sites for IM injections include the rectus femoris (anterior thigh, middle third), vastus lateralis (lateral thigh, middle third), or ventrogluteal, as these sites are relatively free from major nerves and blood vessels. The gluteus maximus

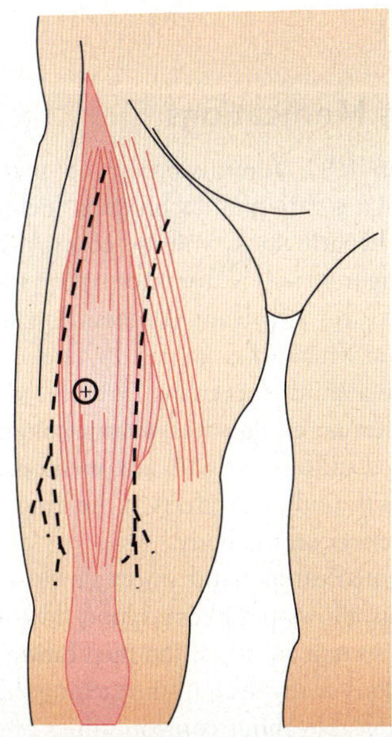

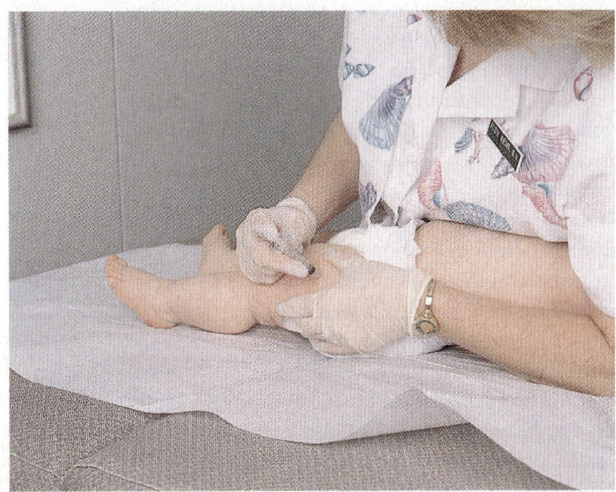

Figure 38-3. (A) For infants under walking age, use the vastus lateralis muscle for intramuscular injections. (B) The technique for administering an intramuscular injection to an infant. Note the way the nurse uses their body to restrain and stabilize the infant. (Reprinted with permission from Silbert-Flagg, J. [2023]. *Maternal and child health nursing: Care of the childbearing and childrearing family* [9th ed., Fig. 38-5]. Wolters Kluwer.)

and deltoid muscles are underdeveloped in the infant, and the use of these sites can result in nerve damage.

2. Rectus femoris injection.
   a. Place the child in a secure position to prevent movement of the extremity.
   b. Do not use a needle longer than 1 in.
   c. Bunch the muscle between your thumb and forefinger.
   d. Insert needle at a 90-degree angle or slightly toward the knee.
3. Vastus lateralis injection.
   a. Place the child in a prone or supine position.
   b. Area is a narrow strip of muscle extending along a line from the greater trochanter to lateral femoral condyle below.
   c. Insert needle at a 90-degree angle, ¾ to 1½ in (2 to 4 cm) deep.
4. Ventrogluteal injection.
   a. This site provides a dense muscle mass that is relatively free from the danger of injuring the nervous and vascular systems.
   b. The disadvantage is that the injection site is visible to the child.
   c. Administration.
      i. Position the child supine.
      ii. Place the index finger on the anterosuperior spine.
      iii. With the middle finger moving dorsally, locate the iliac crest; drop finger below the crest. The triangle formed by the iliac crest, index finger, and middle finger is the injection site.
      iv. Inject needle perpendicular to the surface on which the child is lying.
5. After administration of medication, hold and cuddle the infant.
6. Administer SC injection in the fatty tissue over the anterolateral thigh.

Toddlers and School-Aged Children

1. Posterogluteal injection—upper outer quadrant for IM injection.
   a. Gluteal muscles do not develop until a child begins to walk; they should be used only when the child has been walking for 1 year or more. Complications include sciatic nerve injury or SC injury (because of medication being injected) and poor absorption.
   b. Upper outer quadrant of the young child's buttock is smaller in diameter than that of an adult; thus, accuracy in determining the area constituting the upper outer quadrant is essential.
   c. Administration.
      i. Do not use a needle longer than 1 in.
      ii. Position the child in a prone position.
      iii. Place thumb on the trochanter.
      iv. Place middle finger on the iliac crest.
      v. Let index finger drop at a point midway between the thumb and the middle finger to the upper outer quadrant of the buttock. This is the injection site.
      vi. Insert needle perpendicular to the surface on which the child is lying, not to the skin.
2. Ventrogluteal injection for IM injection.
   a. May be used for the older child who is difficult to restrain.
   b. See description given earlier.
3. Deltoid injection for IM injection.
   a. May be used for older, larger children.
   b. Inaccurate site injection can result in damage to the radial nerve or brachial artery.
   c. Determine injection site by palpating the acromion process of the shoulder and placing two fingers down from the acromion process.
   d. Inject needle at a 90-degree angle or slightly toward the shoulder.
4. Lateral and anterior aspects of the thigh for IM injection.
   a. Do not use a needle longer than 1 in.
   b. Use the upper outer quadrant of the thigh.
   c. Insert needle at a 45-degree angle in a downward direction, toward the knee.
5. Administer SC injection in the fatty tissue over the anterolateral thigh or outer aspect of the upper arm.
6. Nursing support of toddlers and older children.
   a. Prepare all equipment before approaching the child.
   b. Explain to the child where you are going to give the injection (site) and why you are giving it.
   c. Allow the child to express fears.
   d. Carry out the procedure quickly and gently. Have needle and syringe completely prepared and ready before contact with the child.
   e. Numb the site of injection by rubbing the skin firmly with cleaning swab or with ice (older children may assist with this). Minimize pain of an IM injection by injecting the needle into the muscle with a quick, darting motion.
   f. Always secure the assistance of a second nurse or a family member to help immobilize the child and divert their attention as well as to offer support and comfort.
   g. Praise the child for behavior after the injection. Allowing the child to assist with applying an elastic bandage will give some feeling of comfort.
   h. Also encourage activity that will use the muscle site of the injection, this promotes dispersal of medication and decreases soreness. This can also be done by firmly massaging the muscle after injection, unless contraindicated.
   i. Accurately record the injection site to ensure proper site rotation.

Intravenous Medications

1. Intravenous (IV) administration of medications may be done through a variety of techniques, including piggyback or through a heparin lock, volume control set, or implantable port. See pages 36 and 37 for information on these techniques.
2. Prepare mixtures aseptically (laminar flow hood) and use sterile technique when accessing the IV line. (Sepsis is a constant threat when a child is receiving IV medications.)
3. Be aware that an exaggerated pharmacologic effect may exist with IV medications. As with any medication, know the use, adverse effects, and toxic effects of the drug as well as the pharmacologic effect on the body.
4. Dilute IV medications and inject slowly—never less than 1 minute (this allows peripheral blood flow through the entire circulating system to dilute the medication and prevent high concentrations of the drug from reaching the brain and heart).
5. Be knowledgeable about compatibilities of drugs, electrolytes in IV solutions, and the fluid itself.
6. Observe the IV site frequently. Restrain the child, as needed, to prevent infiltration. Infiltration of fluids containing medications can cause rapid and severe tissue necrosis.

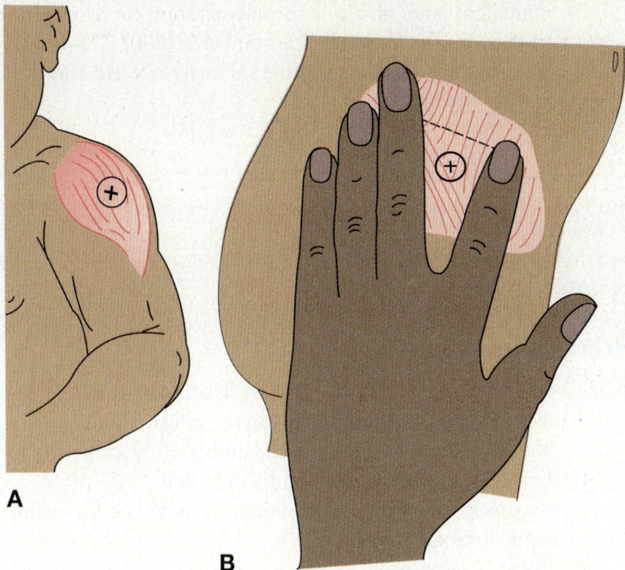

Figure 38-4. Sites for intramuscular injection. (**A**) In older children, the deltoid muscle is an acceptable site. (**B**) A ventrogluteal site may also be used in older children. Place the heel of the hand on the greater trochanter with the index finger angled toward the child's anterosuperior iliac crest, spreading the middle finger along the crest posteriorly. The triangle formed by the space between the index and the middle fingers is the correct site. (Adapted with permission from Silbert-Flagg, J. [2023]. *Maternal and child health nursing: Care of the childbearing and childrearing family* [9th ed., Fig. 38-6]. Wolters Kluwer.)

SPECIAL CONSIDERATIONS IN PEDIATRIC PRIMARY CARE

Acute Poisoning

Exposure to poisons can occur by ingestion, inhalation, or skin or mucous membrane contact. This section focuses on the most common poisoning, toxic ingestions. Poisoning by ingestion refers to the oral intake of a harmful substance that, even in a small amount, can damage tissues, disturb body functions, and, possibly, cause death. The substances may include medications such as acetaminophen and iron, household products, and plants.

Children are at risk for acute poisoning. According to the Centers for Disease Control and Prevention (CDC), every day more than 300 children aged 0 to 19 years are treated in an emergency department in the United States, and two children will die daily as a result of being poisoned. The most common agents ingested by children younger than age 6 include cosmetics and personal care products; cleaning products, analgesics, plants, pesticides, vitamins, and cough and cold medications also pose a risk.

Pathophysiology and Etiology

1. Improper or dangerous storage of potentially toxic substances.
2. Poor lighting—causes errors in reading.
3. Human factors:
   a. Failure to read the label properly.
   b. Failure to return poisons to their proper place.
   c. Failure to recognize the material as poisonous.
   d. Lack of supervision of the child.
   e. Purposeful use of poison.
4. Toxin is ingested and may have limited local effects or continue to a stage of absorption and interference with metabolic processes and organ function.
5. Typically occurs in children younger than age 6 years, with a peak incidence between 12 and 24 months.
6. Acute poisoning may result in arrhythmias or permanent multiorgan damage due to initial loss of airway, breathing, and circulation (ABCs) and specific organ toxicity.

Poisoning With Acetaminophen

Acetaminophen is a common drug poisoning agent in children because of its replacement of salicylates and the pleasant taste of the preparations developed to facilitate administration. Ingestion by adolescents is frequently intentional. Acetaminophen is toxic to the liver, resulting in cell necrosis and, possibly, cell death.

Clinical Manifestations

Phase I (first 24 hours after ingestion):

1. May be asymptomatic.
2. Anorexia.
3. Nausea and vomiting.
4. Diaphoresis.
5. Malaise.
6. Pallor.

Phase II (24 to 48 hours after ingestion):

1. Symptoms of phase I diminish or disappear.
2. Right upper quadrant pain due to liver damage.
3. Liver enlargement with elevated bilirubin and hepatic enzymes and prolonged prothrombin time.
4. Oliguria.

Phase III (days 3 to 5 after ingestion):

1. Signs of hepatic failure, such as jaundice, hypoglycemia, coagulopathy, and encephalopathy.
2. Peak liver function abnormalities.
3. Anorexia, nausea, vomiting, and malaise may reappear.
4. Renal failure and cardiomyopathy may occur.

Phase IV:

1. Associated with recovery or progression to complete liver failure and death.

Diagnostic Evaluation

1. Serum acetaminophen level 4 hours after ingestion.
2. Serial liver function tests.
3. Urine and serum chemistry studies for renal function.

Management

1. Activated charcoal should be given if treatment is instituted within 6 to 8 hours after ingestion; if treatment is begun after this time frame, activated charcoal is not used unless another toxic substance was ingested.
2. *N*-Acetylcysteine as an antidote given orally or via intravenous (IV) line. This is the most extensively studied regimen for acetaminophen overdose.
3. As with all poisons, ABCs and treatment of shock are always the priority in management.

Iron Poisoning

Iron poisoning occurs frequently in childhood because of the prevalence of iron-containing preparations. The severity of iron poisoning is related to the amount of elemental iron absorbed. The range of potential toxicity is between 50 and 60 mg/kg.

Clinical Manifestations

1. 30 minutes to 2 hours after ingestion:
   a. Local necrosis and hemorrhage of gastrointestinal (GI) tract.
   b. Nausea and vomiting, including hematemesis.
   c. Abdominal pain.
   d. Diarrhea, usually bloody.
   e. Severe hypotension.
   f. Symptoms subside after 6 to 12 hours.
2. 6 to 24 hours—period of apparent recovery.
3. 24 to 40 hours:
   a. Systemic toxicity with cardiovascular collapse, shock, hepatic and renal failure, seizures, coma, and, possibly, death.
   b. Metabolic acidosis.
4. 2 to 4 weeks after ingestion:
   a. Pyloric and duodenal stenosis.
   b. Hepatic cirrhosis.

Diagnostic Evaluation

1. Measurement of serum-free iron.
   a. Total serum iron.
   b. Total serum iron-binding capacity.
2. Abdominal x-ray to visualize iron tablets; limited use for visualizing liquid toxins.

Management

1. Gastric lavage may be of some benefit because iron is not absorbed by activated charcoal; however, a wide lumen must be used, which may not be possible in small children.
2. Whole-bowel irrigation reduces the absorption of iron and sustained-release drugs.
3. Administration of deferoxamine for severe cases—iron-chelating agent that binds with iron and is excreted in urine (urine will be bright red).

Primary Assessment in Acute Poisoning

1. Initial assessment should include evaluation of ABCs, level of consciousness, vital signs, and neurologic assessment.
2. Assess for symptomatic effects of poisoning by systems.
   a. GI—common in metallic acid, alkali, and bacterial poisoning. These may include nausea and vomiting, diarrhea, abdominal pain or cramping, and anorexia.
   b. Central nervous system (CNS)—may include seizures (especially with CNS depressants, such as alcohol, chloral hydrate, barbiturates) and behavioral changes. Dilated or pinpoint pupils may be noted.
   c. Skin—rashes; burns to the mouth, esophagus, and stomach; eye inflammation; skin irritations; stains around the mouth; lesions of the mucous membranes. Cyanosis may be visible, especially with cyanide and strychnine.
   d. Cardiopulmonary—dyspnea (especially with aspiration of hydrocarbons) and cardiopulmonary depression or arrest.
   e. Other—odor around the mouth.
3. Identify the poison when possible.
   a. Determine the nature of the ingested substance from the child's history or by reading the label on the container. Nursing intervention may need to be implemented immediately after this assessment.
   b. Call the nearest poison control center or toxicology section of the medical examiner's office to identify the toxic ingredient and obtain recommendations for emergency treatment. The U.S. toll-free number is (800) 222-1222.
   c. Save vomitus, stool, and urine for analysis when the child reaches the hospital.

CLINICAL JUDGMENT It may be necessary to initiate emergency respiratory and circulatory support at this time. If needed, obtain venous access, maintain safety during seizure activity, and treat shock. Otherwise, continue with assessment.

Primary Interventions

Assisting the Family by Telephone Management

1. Calmly obtain and record the following information:
   a. Name, address, and telephone number of the caller.
   b. Evaluation of the severity of the ingestion.
   c. Age, weight, and signs and symptoms of the child, including neurologic status.
   d. Route of exposure.
   e. Name of the ingested product, approximate amount ingested, and time of ingestion.
   f. Brief past medical history.
   g. Caller's relationship to patient.
2. Instruct the caller about appropriate emergency actions or refer to (800) 222-1222.
3. Direct the patient to the nearest emergency department. Dispatch an ambulance, if necessary.
4. Instruct the caller to clear the child's mouth of any unswallowed poison.
5. Identify what treatments have already been initiated.
6. Instruct the parental caregivers to save vomitus, unswallowed liquid or pills, and the container and to bring them to the hospital as aids in identifying the poison.
7. Identify whether other children were involved in the poisoning to initiate treatment for them also.

DRUG ALERT Do not administer household neutralizing foods or products (unless recommended by poison control specialist) because the heat generated by the chemical reaction could result in a burn (or exacerbation of an existing burn).

Intervention Related to the Patient's Condition

Support ABCs, as needed.

Removing the Poison From the Body

1. If the poison is nonpharmaceutical, have the child drink 100 to 200 mL of water if told to do so by poison control. If a medication was ingested, do not dilute with water, as this may speed absorption.
2. For skin or eye contact, remove contaminated clothing and flush with water for 15 to 20 minutes.
3. For inhalation of poisons, remove from the exposed site.
4. Administer gastric lavage if the toxin is not bound by charcoal (most effective within 50 minutes after ingestion).
5. Follow lavage with a cathartic and activated charcoal to hasten removal of the poison from the GI tract. Use cautiously with young children.
6. Be aware of the dangers associated with lavage.
   a. Esophageal perforation—may occur in corrosive poisoning.
   b. Gastric hemorrhage.

c. Impaired pulmonary function resulting from aspiration.
d. Cardiac arrest.
e. Seizures—may result from stimulation in strychnine ingestion.

7. Follow lavage (if performed) with activated charcoal (preferably within 1 hour after ingestion) to hasten removal of the poison from the GI tract.
   a. Charcoal poorly absorbs most electrolytes, iron, lithium, mineral acids and bases, alcohols, cyanide, most solvents, and hydrocarbons.
   b. Administer 30 to 50 g for an adolescent, in 6 to 8 ounces (180 to 240 mL) of water with sweetener.
   c. It is sometimes easier to administer in an opaque beverage container as some children are hesitant to drink the charcoal because of its unusual dark color.

EVIDENCE BASE Gummin, D. D., Mowry, J. B., Beuhler, M. C., Spyker, D. A., Bronstein, A. C., Rivers, L. J., Pham, N. P. T., & Weber, J. (2021). 2020 Annual report of the American Association of Poison Control Centers' National Poison Data System (NPDS): 38th annual report. *Clinical Toxicology, 59*(12), 1282–1501. https://doi.org/10.1080/15563650.2021.1989785

Reducing the Effect of the Poison by Administering an Antidote

1. An antidote may either react with the poison to prevent its absorption or counteract the effects of the poison after its absorption.
2. Not all poisons have specific antidotes.
3. Information about appropriate antidotes for specific poisons is available through all poison control centers. Antidotes for the most common poisons should be listed in the emergency department of the hospital.
4. Effectiveness of the antidote usually depends on the amount of time that elapses between ingestion of the poison and administration of the antidote.

Eliminating the Absorbed Poison

1. Force dieresis.
   a. Administer large quantities of fluid either orally or via IV line.
   b. Carefully monitor intake and output.
2. Assist with kidney dialysis, which may be necessary if the child's kidneys are not functioning effectively.
3. Assist with exchange transfusion if this method is indicated for removing the poison.

Providing Emotional Support

1. Remain calm and efficient while working rapidly.
2. Reassure the child and their family that therapeutic measures are being taken immediately.
3. Discourage anxious parental caregivers from holding, caressing, and overstimulating the child.

Subsequent Nursing Assessment and Interventions

Observing the Child for Progression of Symptoms

1. CNS involvement.
   a. Observe for restlessness, confusion, delirium, seizures, lethargy, stupor, or coma.
   b. Administer sedation with caution—to avoid CNS depression and masking of symptoms.
   c. Avoid excessive manipulation of the child.
   d. See nursing care of the child with seizures, page 1134.
   e. See nursing care of the patient who is unconscious, Chapter 11.
2. Respiratory involvement.
   a. Observe for respiratory depression, obstruction, pulmonary edema, pneumonia, or tachypnea.
   b. Have artificial airway and tracheostomy set available.
   c. Be prepared to administer oxygen and provide artificial respiration.
   d. Other nursing concerns:
      i. Nursing care for mechanical ventilation, see page 1163.
      ii. Procedures for administration of oxygen, see page 146.
      iii. Procedure for cardiopulmonary resuscitation, see page 929.
3. Cardiovascular involvement.
   a. Observe for peripheral circulatory collapse, disturbances of heart rate and rhythm, or heart failure.
   b. Maintain IV therapy, as directed, to prevent shock. Assess for complications of overhydration.
   c. Be prepared for cardiac arrest.
4. GI involvement.
   a. Observe for nausea, pain, abdominal distention, and difficulty swallowing.
   b. Maintain IV therapy to replace water and electrolyte losses.
   c. Offer a diet that is easily swallowed and digested.
      i. Begin with clear liquids.
      ii. Progress to full liquids, soft foods, and then a regular diet as the child's condition improves.
5. Kidney involvement.
   a. Observe the child for decreased urine output. Record oral and IV intake and urine output exactly.
   b. Observe for hypertension.
   c. Insert indwelling catheter, if necessary, for urinary retention.
   d. Administer appropriate amounts of fluids and electrolytes.
   e. See nursing care of child with renal failure, page 1321.
   f. Correct and monitor acid–base balance.

Providing Supportive Care

1. Maintain adequate caloric, fluid, and vitamin intake. Oral fluids are preferable if they can be retained.
2. Avoid hypothermia or hyperthermia. (Control of body temperature is impaired in many types of poisoning.) Monitor the child's temperature frequently.
3. Observe closely for inflammation and tissue irritation.
   a. This is especially important in ingestion of kerosene or other hydrocarbons, which cause chemical pneumonitis.
   b. Isolate the patient from other children, especially those with respiratory infections.
   c. Administer antibiotics, as prescribed by the health care provider.
4. Counsel parental caregivers who typically feel guilty about the accident.
   a. Encourage parental caregivers to talk about the poisoning.
   b. Emphasize how their quick action in getting treatment for the child has helped.
   c. Discuss ways that they can be supportive to their child during the hospitalization.
   d. Do not allow prolonged periods of self-incrimination to continue. Refer parental caregivers to a psychologist for assistance in resolving these feelings, if necessary.

5. Involve the young child in therapeutic play to determine how they view the situation.
   a. The child commonly sees nursing measures as punishments for misdeeds involving the poisoning.
   b. Explain treatment and correct misinterpretations in a manner appropriate for child's age.
6. Initiate a community health nursing referral for any childhood poisoning incident. A home assessment should be made to identify any potential or actual problems and provide proper poisoning prevention interventions and education.

Family Education and Health Maintenance

Stressing Prevention

1. Information concerning poison prevention should be available in every hospital pediatric unit and during every child health care visit.
   a. Many free booklets and home safety checklists are available from sources such as insurance companies and drug companies.
   b. Teaching may be done with any parental caregivers, regardless of the reason for the child's hospitalization or office visit.
2. Teach the following precautions:
   a. Keep medicines and poisons out of the reach of children.
   b. Provide locked storage for highly toxic substances; select a cabinet that is higher than the child can reach or climb.
   c. Do not store poisons in the same areas as foods.
   d. Make sure all containers are properly marked and labeled. Keep medicines, drugs, and household chemicals in their original containers.
   e. Do not discard poisonous substances in receptacles where children can reach them; however, do discard used containers of poisonous substances.
   f. Teach children not to taste or eat unfamiliar substances.
   g. Clean out medicine cabinets periodically.
   h. Keep medications in childproof containers that are securely closed.
   i. Read all labels carefully before each use.
   j. Do not give medicines prescribed for one child to another.
   k. Never refer to drugs as candy or bribe children with such inducements.
   l. Never give or take medications in the dark.
   m. Encourage parental caregivers not to take medication in front of young children because children role-play adult behavior.
   n. Suggest that parental caregivers avoid keeping medications in their purses or on the kitchen table.
   o. Keep baby creams and ointments away from young children.
   p. Never puncture or heat aerosol containers.
   q. Store lawn and garden pesticides in a separate place under lock and key outside the house; do not store large quantities of cleaning products or pesticides.
3. Advise parental caregivers to dispose of syrup of ipecac if they keep it in the household. According to the American Academy of Pediatrics, there is no evidence supporting improved outcomes of poisonings with the use of ipecac. In addition, there is potential for misuse of ipecac with bulimic or anorexic teenagers; therefore, the recommendation for keeping ipecac on hand to induce vomiting has been rescinded.
4. Tell family to keep a list of emergency telephone numbers, including the poison control center, health care provider's number, nearest hospital, and ambulance service.
5. Reinforce the need for vigilance and consistent supervision of infants and young children because of their increased mobility, increased curiosity, and increased dexterity.

Teaching Emergency Actions

1. Suspect poisoning with the occurrence of sudden, bizarre symptoms or peculiar behavior in toddlers and preschoolers.
2. Read label on the ingested product or call the health care provider, hospital, or poison control center for instructions about treatment for the poisoning. Give all relevant information about the child, condition, and substance ingested.
3. Maintain an adequate airway in a child who is convulsing or who is not fully conscious.
4. Dilute the poison with 100 to 200 mL of water, if advised by poison control or other medical providers.
5. Transport the child promptly to the nearest medical facility.
   a. Wrap the child in a blanket to prevent chilling.
   b. Bring the container and any vomitus or urine to the hospital with the child.
6. Avoid excessive manipulation of the child.
7. Act promptly but calmly.
8. Do not assume the child is safe simply because the emesis shows no trace of the poison or because the child appears well. The poison may have produced a delayed reaction or may have reached the small intestine where it is still being absorbed.

Lead Poisoning

There are approximately half a million children with elevated blood lead levels (greater than 5 µg/dL) in the United States. Lead poisoning, referred to as *plumbism*, results from some form of lead consumption. Blood lead levels even lower than the prior accepted level of 10 µg/dL can affect intellectual functioning in children. This has resulted in the acceptable lead level being lowered to 5 from 10 µg/dL as of 2017.

Millions of children live in housing built before 1950, which contains the highest surface soil level and internal household dust contaminated with lead. Normal hand-to-mouth activities of children may introduce leaded household dust, soil, and nonfood items into their GI tract. Pica (eating nonfood substances, particularly leaded paint chips) is generally associated with more severe degrees of lead poisoning.

Pathophysiology and Etiology

Etiologic Factors

1. Multiple episodes of chewing on, sucking, or ingestion of nonfood substances.
   a. Toys, furniture, windowsills, household fixtures, and plaster painted with lead-containing paint.
   b. Cigarette butts and ashes.
   c. Acidic juices or foods served in lead-based earthenware pottery made with lead glazes.
   d. Colored paints used in newspapers, magazines, children's books, matches, playing cards, and food wrappers.
   e. Water from lead pipes.
   f. Fruit treated with insecticides.
   g. Dirt containing lead fallout from automobile exhaust.
   h. Antique pewter, especially when used to serve acidic juices or foods.
   i. Lead weights (curtain weights, fishing sinkers).
   j. Continuous proximity to lead-processing center.
   k. Occupations or hobbies that use lead.

l. Imported folk remedies, cosmetics, food, or cookware that contains lead.
2. Inhalation of fumes containing lead (less common cause in children).
   a. Leaded gasoline.
   b. Burning storage batteries.
   c. Dust containing lead salts.
   d. Dust in the air at shooting galleries and in enclosed firing ranges with poor ventilation.
   e. Cigarette smoke.
3. Highest incidence in children between ages 1 and 6 years, especially those between ages 1 and 3 years.
   a. High incidence in individuals living in old homes or deteriorated housing conditions.
   b. No significant difference in incidence by sex assigned at birth.
   c. High incidence among siblings.
4. Symptomatic lead poisoning occurs most frequently in summer months.

CLINICAL JUDGMENT Legislation stipulates that toys, children's furniture, and the interior of homes be painted with lead-free paint; however, the problem arises when deeper layers of paint and plaster on older products are contaminated with lead. One paint chip contains much more lead than is considered safe.

Systemic Effects

1. Lead absorption from GI tract is affected by age, diet, and nutritional deficiency. Young children absorb 40% to 50% and retain 20% to 25% of dietary lead.
2. It takes the body twice as long to excrete lead as it does to absorb lead.
3. Lead is stored in two places in the body:
   a. Bone.
   b. Soft tissue.
4. Principal toxic effects occur in the nervous system, bone marrow, and kidneys.
5. Nervous system.
   a. Brain—increased capillary permeability results in edema, increased intracranial pressure (ICP), and vascular damage; destruction of brain cells causes seizures, intellectual disability, paralysis, blindness, and learning disabilities.
   b. Neurologic damage cannot be reversed.
   c. CNS of young children and fetuses is most sensitive to lead.
6. Bone marrow.
   a. Lead attaches to red blood cells (RBCs).
   b. Inhibition of a number of steps in the biosynthesis of heme, thus reducing the number of RBCs, increasing fragility, and reducing half-life.
   c. The decreased production of hemoglobin results in anemia and respiratory distress.
7. Kidneys—injury to the cells of the proximal tubules, causing increased excretion of amino acids, protein, glucose, and phosphate.
8. Recurrence rate is high, especially if the lead is not removed from the home environment.

Clinical Manifestations

Symptoms in young children may develop insidiously and may abate spontaneously.

1. GI—anorexia, sporadic vomiting, intermittent abdominal pain (colic), constipation.
2. CNS—hyperirritability; decreased activity; personality changes; loss of recently acquired developmental skills; falling, clumsiness, loss of coordination (ataxia); local paralysis; peripheral nerve palsies.
3. Hematologic—anemia, pallor.
4. Cardiovascular—hypertension, bradycardia.

Diagnostic Evaluation

1. Detailed history with emphasis on the presence or absence of clinical symptoms; evidence of pica; family history of lead poisoning; possible source of exposure to lead; recent change in behavior, developmental delay, or behavior problems; recent change of address; or recent renovations in the home.
2. Assess serum lead level and repeat confirmatory, preferably by way of venipuncture. Recent changes in screening recommendations have been made to include targeted screening of all Medicaid-enrolled and Medicaid-eligible children. In addition, all children born outside the United States should be screened.
   a. For levels greater than 5 μg/dL, a more extensive environmental history should be reviewed.
   b. For levels between 10 and 14 μg/dL, the level should be confirmed and repeated in 3 months. Education on decreasing exposure and limiting absorption of lead should be done on all levels greater than 10 μg/dL.
   c. Levels between 15 and 19 μg/dL should be repeated within 2 months, while an environmental history additionally is reviewed.
   d. Levels between 20 and 44 μg/dL should be repeated within 2 days and referred to the local health department plus a thorough medical history and physical examination added to education as noted earlier.
   e. Levels between 45 and 69 μg/dL should be confirmed immediately, referred to the local health department, and should be considered for chelation therapy in consultation with an expert.
   f. Immediate hospitalization is required for levels greater than 70 μg/dL.
3. Hematologic evaluation for iron deficiency anemia.
4. Flat plate of abdomen—may reveal radiopaque material if lead has been ingested during the preceding 24 to 36 hours.
5. Erythrocyte protoporphyrin level—not sensitive enough for identifying lead levels below 25 mg/dL. Can be used to follow levels after medical and environmental interventions for poisoned children have occurred. A progressive decline in erythrocyte protoporphyrin levels indicates that management is successful.
6. 24-hour urine—more accurate than a single-voided specimen in determining elevated urinary components that correspond with elevated blood lead levels.
7. Radiologic examination of long bones—unreliable for diagnosis of acute lead poisoning; may provide some indication of past lead poisoning or length of time poisoning has occurred.
8. Edetate calcium disodium provocation chelation test—used only in selected medical centers treating large numbers of lead-poisoned children; demonstrates increased lead levels in urine over an 8-hour period after injection of edetate disodium.

CLINICAL JUDGMENT Venous sampling is the best method for assessing the level of lead in the blood as it limits cutaneous contamination. If a fingerstick sample is being used, careful collection should include a free-flowing specimen.

EVIDENCE BASE American Academy of Pediatrics. (2020). Prevention of childhood lead toxicity. *Pediatrics, 145*(6), e20201014. https://doi.org/10.1542/peds.2020-1014

Management

Removal of Lead From the Environment

1. Remove leaded paint and paint chips or objects containing lead from the child's environment.
2. Remove child from environment during lead abatement process.

Nutritional Considerations

1. Consume adequate amounts of iron. Iron supplementation may be indicated to correct anemia.
2. Reduced-fat diet and small, frequent meals will reduce the GI absorption of lead.
3. Encourage foods high in vitamin C (such as fruits and juices) and calcium (such as milk, yogurt, and ice cream).

Chelation Therapy

According to the CDC, although chelation therapy is considered a mainstay in the medical management of children with blood lead levels greater than 45 mg/dL, it should be used with caution. An expert in the management of lead chemotherapy should be consulted prior to using chelation agents. State lead poisoning programs, local poison control centers, or the Lead Poisoning Prevention Branch at the CDC can be used as resources to identify accessible experts.

EVIDENCE BASE Lead Hazard Control and Healthy Homes. (2022). *Federal Grants & Contracts, 46*(15), 6–7. https://doi.org/10.1002/fgc.32470

Complications

1. Severe and usually permanent mental, emotional, and physical impairment.
2. Neurologic deficits.
   a. Learning disabilities.
   b. Intellectual disability.
   c. Seizures.
   d. Encephalopathy.

Nursing Assessment

1. Partake in primary prevention through screening for lead poisoning—should target high-risk groups. This includes children:
   a. Who live in homes built before 1950.
   b. With iron deficiency anemia.
   c. Who are exposed to contaminated dust or soil.
   d. Who have developmental delays.
   e. Who are sufferers of abuse or neglect.
   f. Whose parental caregivers are exposed to lead through occupational hazards or hobbies.
   g. Who live in low-income families.
2. Screening should also be targeted at children who live in communities with more than 27% of houses built before 1950 or in populations where 12% or more of the children have elevated lead levels.
3. Assess all children for signs of lead toxicity, including hyperactivity, developmental delay, constipation, anorexia, colicky abdominal pain, clumsiness, and pallor.
4. Inquire about the presence of pica behavior in children younger than age 6 years.
5. Assess the child's level of development. The Denver Developmental Screening Test II or other standardized developmental assessment tools may be useful for this purpose and will help detect delays possibly caused by lead poisoning.

Nursing Interventions

Protecting the Child With Seizures and Encephalopathy

1. Maintain seizure precautions.
   a. Crib or bed rails elevated and padded.
   b. Tongue blade (if indicated per institutional guidelines) and suction equipment at bedside.
2. Be aware that encephalopathy may occur 4 to 6 weeks after the first symptoms:
   a. Sudden onset of persistent vomiting.
   b. Severe ataxia.
   c. Altered state of consciousness.
   d. Coma.
   e. Seizures.
   f. Massive cerebral edema in younger children.
3. Observe for signs of increased ICP in the child with encephalopathy:
   a. Rising blood pressure.
   b. Papilledema.
   c. Slow pulse.
   d. Seizures.
   e. Unconsciousness.
4. Provide supportive care to maintain vital functions.

Reducing Pain Associated With Chelation Therapy

1. Plan appropriate play activities to prepare the child for the injections and as an outlet for the pain and anger the child feels.
2. Implement measures to decrease pain at the injection site.
   a. Rotate injection sites.
   b. Apply warm packs to the site to decrease pain.
   c. Move painful areas slowly.
3. Provide diversion activities, fluids, and meals between injections.
4. Monitor intake and output and blood studies, such as electrolytes and liver and renal function tests, as directed.

Promoting Growth and Development

1. Provide and encourage activities that will help the child to learn and progress from their present developmental state to meet the next appropriate milestone.
2. Initiate appropriate referrals in cases of obvious developmental delays or learning difficulties. The referrals may be to professionals such as psychologists, psychiatrists, and specialists in early child education.
3. Share the results of developmental testing with the parental caregivers and discuss ways to provide stimulation for the child at home.

Strengthening Family Coping

1. Use sensitivity in interviewing and teaching to avoid causing or increasing guilt feelings about the poisoning and to establish a positive, trusting relationship between the family and the health care facility.
2. Explain the treatment and its purpose because parental caregivers are commonly faced with putting an asymptomatic child through painful treatments.
3. Encourage frequent visits by parental caregivers and siblings and facilitate family involvement.

Community and Home Care Considerations

1. Carry out lead screening in the community. It is recommended that all high-risk children be screened for high lead levels between ages 9 and 12 months and, if feasible, again at 24 months. Screening policies, universal or targeted, are determined by local departments of health, based on the prevalence of risk factors in the community.
2. Coordinate community care efforts to return the child to a safe home. Communicate with community outreach workers so that environmental case management is conducted. Lead abatement must be conducted by experts, not untrained parental caregivers, property owners, or contractors.
3. Suggest periodic, focused household cleaning to remove the lead dust; use a wet mop.
4. Encourage handwashing before meals and at bedtime to eliminate lead consumption from normal hand-to-mouth activity.
5. Observe the child and other children in the home for pica.
   a. Observe and record the child's eating habits and food preferences.
   b. Report any attempted eating of nonfood substances.
   c. Encourage parental caregivers to provide regular meals and make mealtime a pleasurable time for the child.
   d. Teach parental caregivers to discourage oral activity and to substitute activity that contributes to play, social skills, and ego development.
   e. Refer the family for additional social or psychiatric casework, if indicated, to reduce economic and other factors that result in pica in the child.
6. Screen siblings and playmates of known cases immediately.
7. Make sure that the family is able to provide close supervision of the child or assist them to make arrangements to ensure that the child is adequately supervised at home.

Family Education and Health Maintenance

Ensuring Long-Term Follow-Up

1. Teach the parental caregivers why long-term follow-up is important. Tell them that residual lead is liberated gradually after treatment and:
   a. May result in the renewal of symptoms.
   b. May increase serum lead to a dangerous level.
   c. May cause additional damage to the CNS, which may not become apparent for several months.
2. Stress that acute infections must be recognized and treated promptly because these may reactivate the disease.
3. Teach that iron supplementation may be continued to treat anemia. Advise the parental caregivers about medication administration and adverse effects and periodic complete blood count monitoring.

Preventing Reexposure of the Child to Lead

1. Advise the parental caregivers that the single most important factor in managing childhood lead poisoning is reducing the child's reexposure to lead.
2. Instruct the parental caregivers about the seriousness of repeated lead exposure.
3. Initiate referrals to home health nursing and community agencies, as indicated.

CLINICAL JUDGMENT Children should not return home until their home environment is lead free.

Providing Community Education

1. Initiate and support educational campaigns through schools, day care centers, and news media to alert parental caregivers and children to hazards and symptoms of lead poisoning.
2. Provide literature in clinics, waiting rooms, and other appropriate settings that stress the hazards of lead, sources of lead, and signs of lead intoxication.
3. Support legislation to study the nature and extent of the lead poisoning problem and to eliminate the causes of lead poisoning.
4. Include the topic of pica and lead poisoning in nutritional teaching.
5. For additional information, contact the state or local health department or CDC (www.cdc.gov).

Evaluation: Expected Outcomes

- Seizure precautions maintained; no signs of increased ICP.
- Tolerates chelation therapy injections; expresses anger through doll play.
- Parental caregivers provide appropriate play and stimulation for development.
- Family involved in care; provides support to the child.

Communicable Diseases

With the dramatic success of immunizations, many childhood diseases have decreased in frequency. However, a number of communicable diseases still cause significant morbidity in children (see Table 38-2). Many other infections that occur in childhood are covered elsewhere in the book, such as Chapter 27, Infectious Diseases, or the chapters of each body system.

Child Abuse and Neglect

EVIDENCE BASE Tiyyagura, G., Asnes, A. G., & Leventhal, J. M. (2023). Improving child abuse recognition and management: Moving forward with clinical decision support. *The Journal of Pediatrics, 252*, 11–13. https://doi.org/10.1016/j.jpeds.2022.08.020

Child abuse is any type of maltreatment of children or adolescents by their parental caregivers or guardians. It is considered a major problem worldwide, with most countries tracking the problem and allocating some resources toward services to prevent and treat child abuse. Child abuse includes physical or emotional abuse, injury, trauma, neglect, or sexual abuse of a child that is intentional and nonaccidental. Abuse includes the following:

- Battering—physical injury.
- Substance use—intentional administration of harmful drugs, especially during pregnancy.
- Sexual abuse.
- Sexual assault or molestation (non–family member).
- Incest (family offender).
- Emotional abuse—scapegoating, belittling, humiliating, lack of caregiving.

Neglect is the omission of certain appropriate behaviors, with such omission having detrimental physical or psychological effects on development. Neglect includes:

- Child abandonment.
- Lack of provision of the basic needs of survival, including shelter, clothing, stimulation, medical care, food, love, supervision, education, attention, emotional nurturing, and safety.

Table 38-2 Communicable Diseases

DISEASE, AGENT, MODE OF TRANSMISSION, AGE WHEN MOST COMMON	INCUBATION AND COMMUNICABILITY PERIODS	SYMPTOMS	TREATMENT	COMPLICATIONS	NURSING CONSIDERATIONS
Chickenpox					
Varicella-zoster virus • Highly communicable; acquired in direct contact, droplet spread, and airborne transmission • 2–9 yr; January to May *Diagnostic tests:* Tzanck smear shows multinucleated giant cells; a culture may be done for confirmation.	*Incubation (I):* 11–21 d after exposure. *Communicability (C):* onset of fever (1–2 d before the first lesion) until the last vesicle is dried (5–7 d)	• General malaise, low-grade fever, and anorexia for 24 h • Rash—macules to papules and vesicles to crusts within several hours • Pruritus of lesions may be severe and scratching may cause scarring. • *Rash characteristics:* rash appears first on the head and mucous membranes and then becomes concentrated on body and sparse on extremities, papulovesicular eruption.	• Symptomatic: shorten fingernails to prevent scratching • Daily antiseptic baths • Oral antihistamines to decrease pruritus • Treatment of itching: baking soda (sodium bicarbonate) or oatmeal baths, calamine lotion to lesions • Isolation until all lesions have crusted • Acyclovir by mouth (PO) within first 24 h • Avoid salicylates.	• Complications are rare in otherwise healthy children. • Secondary bacterial infection of lesions • Hemorrhagic varicella, pneumonia, encephalitis, and thrombocytopenia are not common, but they can occur. • Reye syndrome	• Severe in neonate and pregnant people • Varicella-zoster immune globulin is available for high-risk susceptible children who have been exposed to varicella zoster. • Prevention through immunization is the best practice.
Rubella (German 3-D Measles)					
Rubella virus; RNA toga virus • Oral droplet or transplacentally • School aged, young adults; spring, winter *Diagnostic tests:* tissue culture of throat, blood, or urine; latex agglutination, enzyme immunoassay, passive hemagglutination, fluorescent immunoassay tests *Passive immunity:* birth to age 6 mo from maternal antibodies	*I:* 14–21 d after exposure. *C:* virus can be passed from 7 d before to 5 d after rash appears.	• Enlarged lymph nodes in postauricular, auricular, suboccipital, and cervical areas 24 h before rash develops • Enanthem: discrete rose spots on soft palate • Exanthem: variable; begins on face, spreads quickly over entire body; usually maculopapular; clears by the third day	• Symptomatic—isolation	• In adolescent females: arthritis; arthralgias • Encephalitis • Thrombocytopenia	• Exposure of nonimmune pregnant people in the first trimester results in a high percentage of affected fetuses and infants born with various birth defects: cataracts, deafness, growth retardation, congenital heart disease, intellectual disability. • Prevention is the best practice.

Roseola Infantum (Exanthem Subitum)					
Human herpesvirus 6 • Direct contact or droplet • 6–24 mo; late fall to early spring	*I:* 5–15 d. *C:* not known—believed not to be highly contagious	• Fever of 103°F–106°F (39.4°C–41.1°C), either intermittent or sustained 3–4 d with no clinical findings • Fever suddenly drops and macular or maculopapular rash develops on trunk, spreading to arms and neck; mild involvement of face and legs; rash fades quickly.	• Symptomatic—antipyretic	• Seizures due to high fever • Encephalitis (rare)	• Reassure family that this is a self-limiting illness.
Rubeola (Hard, Red, 7-D Measles)					
Measles virus, RNA-containing paramyxovirus • Direct contact with droplets from infected persons, respiratory route • *Diagnostic tests:* serologic procedures not routinely done • *Passive immunity:* birth to between ages 4 and 6 mo if birthing parent is immune before pregnancy • 5–10 yr, adolescents; spring	*I:* 10–12 d. *C:* fifth day of incubation to fourth day of rash	• Fever, lethargy, cough, coryza, and conjunctivitis • 2–3 d later; Koplik spots on buccal pharyngeal mucosa (grayish white spots with reddish areolae), which disappear within 12–18 h • 2 d later: maculopapular rash appears at hairline and spreads to feet in 1 d; rash begins to clear after 3–4 d.	• Symptomatic: • Sedatives • Antipyretic • Bed rest in humid, comfortably warm room • Dark room for photophobia • Adequate fluids	• Otitis media • Pneumonia, laryngitis • Mastoiditis, encephalitis • Appendicitis	• Provide symptomatic care and respiratory isolation. • Prevention through immunization is the best practice.
Mumps					
Mumps virus, paramyxovirus • Direct contact, through families, airborne droplets, saliva, and possibly urine • School aged; all seasons but slightly more frequent in late winter and early spring *Diagnostic tests:* serologic testing and viral culture from throat swab *Passive immunity:* birth to age 6 mo if birthing parent is immune before pregnancy	*I:* 16–18 d. *C:* 3 d before to 9 d after swelling appears; virus in saliva greatest just before and after parotitis onset	• Headache, anorexia, generalized malaise; fever 1 d before glandular swelling; fever lasts 1–6 d • Glandular swelling usually of parotid—one side or bilaterally • Enlargement and reddening of Wharton duct and Stensen duct • Subclinical infection may occur.	• Isolation until swelling has subsided • Symptomatic: • Analgesics • Hydration • Alimentation • Antipyretics • Rest	• Meningoencephalitis • Orchitis, epididymitis • Auditory nerve involvement, resulting in unilateral deafness	• Provide symptomatic care. • Prevention through immunization is the best practice.

(continued)

Table 38-2 Communicable Diseases (*continued*)

DISEASE, AGENT, MODE OF TRANSMISSION, AGE WHEN MOST COMMON	INCUBATION AND COMMUNICABILITY PERIODS	SYMPTOMS	TREATMENT	COMPLICATIONS	NURSING CONSIDERATIONS
Diphtheria					

Corynebacterium diphtheriae
• Acquired through secretions of carrier or infected individual by direct contact with contaminated articles and environment
• Unimmunized children under 15 yr old; incidence increased in autumn and winter
Diagnostic tests: cultures of nose and throat
	I: 2–4 d. *C:* 2–4 wk untreated; 1–2 d with antibiotic treatment	**Nasal diphtheria**
		• Coryza with increasing viscosity, possibly epistaxis, low-grade fever
		• Whitish gray membrane may appear over nasal septum.
		Pharyngeal and tonsillar diphtheria
		• General malaise, low-grade fever, anorexia
		• 1–2 d later, whitish gray membranous patch on tonsils, soft palate, and uvula
		• Lymph node swelling, fever, rapid pulse, "bull's neck"
		Laryngeal diphtheria
		• Usually spread from pharynx to larynx
		• Fever, harsh voice, stridor, barking cough; respiratory difficulty with inspiratory retraction
		Nonrespiratory diphtheria
		• Affects eye, ear, genitals, or, rarely, skin
			• Diphtheria antitoxin via IV line or IM
			• Antibiotic therapy (penicillin, erythromycin)
			• Supportive treatment:
			  • Respiratory support and cardiac monitoring
			  • Isolation until three cultures are negative after antibiotic therapy is completed
			  • Bed rest for 2–3 wk
			  • Hydration
			  • Immunization with diphtheria toxoid after recovery
				• Myocarditis
				• Neuritis
				• Paralysis
				• Toxic neurosis and hyaline degeneration of heart, liver, adrenal glands, and kidneys
				• Gastritis, hepatitis
				• Nephritis
					• Identify close contacts and monitor for illness; culture nose, throat, and cutaneous lesions and administer prophylactic antimicrobial therapy.
					• Prevention through immunization is the best practice.

Pertussis (Whooping Cough)					

Bordetella pertussis
• Direct contact or respiratory droplet spread
• Infants and young children; females more than males
Diagnostic tests: culture of nasopharyngeal mucus
	I: 3–12 d; mean of 7 d. *C:* 7 d after exposure (greatest just before catarrhal stage) to 3 wk after onset of paroxysms or until cough has ceased	**Stage I (catarrhal stage)**
		• Lasts 1–2 wk
		• Rhinorrhea, conjunctival injection, lacrimation, mild cough, and low-grade fever
		Stage II (paroxysmal stage)
		• Lasts 2–4 wk or longer
		• Frequent severe, violent coughing attacks occurring in clusters, leading to vomiting, cyanosis, and exhaustion
		Stage III (convalescent stage)
		• Lasts 2 wk to several months
		• Coughing attacks decrease, but may return with each respiratory infection.
		• Duration: 9 mo to 2 yr
			• Specific:
			  • Erythromycin estolate
			  • Azithromycin
			  • Clarithromycin
			• Supportive:
			  • Antipyretics
			  • Bed rest
			  • Quiet environment to reduce coughing
			  • Gentle suctioning
			  • Increase fluid intake
			  • Oxygen
				• Respiratory: pneumonia, atelectasis, emphysema, aspiration pneumonia, pneumothorax
				• CNS: convulsions, encephalopathy, coma
				• Death may occur among the unvaccinated.
					• Erythromycin should be given to all close and household contacts for 14 d.
					• Neither immunization nor natural disease confers complete or lifelong immunity.

Staphylococcal Scalded Skin Syndrome (Ritter Disease)					

Group II phage-type *Staphylococcus aureus*
• Disseminated from a primary infection site (usually nose or around eyes)
• Infants and children under 10 yr old
Diagnostic tests: cultures of skin, conjunctiva, nasopharynx, stools, and blood. Biopsy of exfoliated epidermis
	I: few days. *C:* onset of rash until after antibiotics initiated	• Malaise, fever, irritability, or asymptomatic
		• Rash develops in three phases:
		  • Erythematous—macular involving face, neck, axilla, and groin
		  • Exfoliative—upper layer of epidermis becomes wrinkled and can be removed by light stroking (Nikolsky sign); crusting around eyes, mouth, and nose produces characteristic "sunburst," radial pattern; irritable because of extreme tenderness of skin.
		  • Desquamative—epidermis peels away, leaving moist areas that dry quickly and heal in 10–14 d.
			• Specific:
			  • Therapy with penicillinase-resistant penicillin PO, IM, or via IV line
			• Symptomatic:
			  • Gentle cleaning of skin with compresses
				• Excessive fluid loss, electrolyte imbalance, pneumonia, septicemia, cellulitis	• Provide symptomatic care.

(continued)

Table 38-2 Communicable Diseases (*continued*)

DISEASE, AGENT, MODE OF TRANSMISSION, AGE WHEN MOST COMMON	INCUBATION AND COMMUNICABILITY PERIODS	SYMPTOMS	TREATMENT	COMPLICATIONS	NURSING CONSIDERATIONS
Erythema Infectiosum (Fifth Disease or Slapped Cheek)					

Parvovirus B19
• Respiratory route
• School-age children
Diagnostic tests: not widely available; IgM antibody test, polymerase chain reaction detection test
	I: 6–14 d. *C:* until rash develops	• Mild fever, chills, fatigue, or nonpruritic rash develops in three stages:
		  • Sudden appearance of bright erythema on cheeks
		  • Erythematous, maculopapular rash on trunk and extremities
		  • Rash on body fades with central clearing, giving a lacy or reticulated appearance.
		• Rash lasts 2–39 d; frequently pruritic without desquamation.
		• Occasional joint arthropathy
			• Symptomatic treatment
			• Immunoglobulin for patients who are immunocompromised
				• Complications are rare among otherwise healthy children.
				• Children with abnormal RBCs (sickle cell disease, hereditary spherocytosis, and thalassemia) can develop transient aplastic anemia and may require multiple transfusions.
				• Patients who are immunocompromised may develop severe, chronic anemia.
					• Avoid contact of child with pregnant person (<5% of exposed fetuses will have severe anemia; rare chance of miscarriage).

Rotavirus					
Reoviridae group A • Most common agent responsible for infantile diarrhea • Fecal–oral route • Ages 6 mo to 2 yr; most common in winter in temperate climates *Diagnostic tests:* enzyme-linked immunosorbent assay	*I:* 1–3 d. *C:* until 2–5 d after diarrhea	• Fever • Vomiting • Profuse, watery, non-foul-smelling diarrhea	• Oral fluid and electrohydrate solution	• Isotonic dehydration with acidosis • Malnourished infants may develop malabsorption dehydration and die.	• Excellent hygiene (handwashing) is necessary to avoid spreading disease. • Current vaccine will prevent 74% of all cases and 98% of severe cases.
Hand, Foot, Mouth Disease					
Coxsackie virus A16 or other enteroviruses • Moderately contagious by direct contact with nose and throat secretions, fluid from blisters, and stool • Most common in children under age 10 during summer and fall *Diagnostic tests:* throat swab or stool culture for virus; rarely indicated	*I:* 3–7 d. *C:* first week of illness	• Mild fever, poor appetite, malaise, and sore throat • Painful sores develop in the mouth 1–2 d after fever begins (usually on the tongue, gums, and buccal mucosa). A nonpruritic rash follows on the palms and soles, occasionally on the buttocks.	• Symptomatic for fever, aches, and mouth lesions	• Rare, asymptomatic meningitis	• Provide pain relief and monitor fluid intake to prevent dehydration from not eating.

CNS, central nervous system; IgM, immunoglobulin M; IM, intramuscular; IV, intravenous.

Etiology and Incidence

EVIDENCE BASE Palusci, V. J., Schnitzer, P. G., & Collier, A. (2023). Social and demographic characteristics of child maltreatment fatalities among children 5–17 years. *Child Abuse & Neglect, 136*, 106002. https://doi.org/10.1016/j.chiabu.2022.106002

The cause of child abuse and maltreatment is multidimensional. The abuse may be related to the combined presence of three factors: special kind of child, special kind of parental caregiver, and special circumstances of crisis. Abuse occurs in all ethnic, geographic, religious, educational, occupational, and socioeconomic groups.

1. In 2021, more than 3 million children in the United States were followed by child welfare agencies; most were reported sufferers of child abuse and neglect. There were 1820 reported deaths of children from abuse and neglect in 2021.
2. In 2021, 1770 children in the United States died due to maltreatment (HHS, 2023).

Contributing Factors

1. Incidents of child abuse may develop as a result of disciplinary action taken by the person who abuses their child who responds in uncontrolled anger to real or perceived misconduct of the child. The parental caregivers may confuse punishment with discipline. "Good caregiving" may be equated with physical contact to eradicate child behavior. The person who abuses their child may be a stern, authoritarian disciplinarian.
2. Incidents of child abuse may develop out of a disagreement between parental caregivers. The child may come to the aid of one parental caregiver and may be entered into the midst of the quarrel; discord between the parental caregivers is common.
3. The person who abuses their child may be under a great deal of stress because of life circumstances (debt, poverty, illness) and may thus resort to child abuse. Crisis and stress may be ongoing. They may have a low frustration tolerance level and may not have a well-developed means of coping with stress in general.
4. The person who abuses their child may be intoxicated with alcohol or drugs at the time of the abuse; only 10% of people who abuse their children have a history of mental illness.
5. Child abuse may occur by a surrogate caregiver, such as a babysitter or boyfriend.
6. Lack of effective caregiving, inappropriate parental caregiver–child bonding, and punitive treatment of a child may contribute to the parental caregiver becoming a person who abuses their child.
7. Specific characteristics evident in many parental caregivers who abuse their child include:
   a. Low self-esteem—a sense of incompetence in role, unworthiness, unimportance, or having difficulty controlling aggressive impulses; commonly living in social isolation.
   b. Unrealistic attitudes and expectations of the child, little regard for the child's own needs and age-appropriate abilities, lack of knowledge related to caregiving skills.
   c. Fear of rejection—a deep need to feel wanted and loved, but a feeling of rejection when love is not obvious; a crying infant may elicit a feeling of rejection.
   d. Inability to accept help—isolation from the community, loneliness.
   e. Unhappiness due to unsatisfactory relationships; may look to child for satisfaction of own emotional needs.
   f. People who abuse their children are commonly the children of abuse or sufferers of spousal abuse.
8. Incidents of child abuse may develop from a general attitude or resentment or rejection on the part of the person who abuses toward the child.
9. Atypical child behavior (e.g., hyperactivity or a technology-dependent child who needs additional care) may unintentionally provoke the person who abuses their child.
10. The degree of the family crisis is not usually in proportion to the degree of abuse.

Clinical Manifestations

Characteristics of the Child That Should Raise Suspicion

1. The child is usually younger than age 3 years. School-aged children and adolescents are also subject to abuse. The average age of a sexually abused child is 9 years.
2. General health of the child indicates neglect (diaper rash, poor hygiene, malnutrition, unattended physical problem).
3. Characteristic distribution of fractures (scattered over many parts of body).
4. Disproportionate amount of soft tissue injury.
5. Evidence that injuries occurred at different times (healed and new fractures, resolving and fresh bruises).
6. Cause of recent trauma in question.
7. History of similar episodes in the past.
8. No new lesions during the child's stay in the hospital.
9. May show a wide range of reactions—may be either very withdrawn or overactive. The child may be anxious, tense, or nervous or show regressive behavior.
10. The child may show unusual affection for strangers or may be overly fearful of adults and avoid any physical contact with them.
11. For sexual abuse: The child may fear no one will believe them; may experience self-blame; most know the person who is abusing them.
12. Children may not "tell" about abuse from parental caregivers, fearing a loss of security; "a bad parental caregiver is better than none at all."
13. Behavior problems, depression, acting-out behaviors, and aggression toward younger children may result.
14. For abuse that occurs in school or day care, the child may exhibit fear of the teacher, have nightmares, decrease school attendance, or develop psychosomatic illnesses.

Injuries or Types of Abuse That May Occur

1. Bruises, welts (linear or loop-like).
2. Abrasions, contusions, lacerations (most common).
3. Wounds, cuts, punctures.
4. Burns (cigarette, radiator), scalding—stocking or glove distribution.
5. Bone fractures.
6. Sprains, dislocations.
7. Subdural hemorrhage or hematoma; "shaken baby syndrome."
8. Brain damage.
9. Internal injuries.
10. Drug intoxication.
11. Malnutrition (deliberately inflicted).
12. Freezing, exposure.
13. Whiplash-type injury.
14. Eye injuries, periorbital injuries, ear bruises.
15. Dirty, infected wounds or rashes.

16. Unexplained coma in infant.
17. Failure to thrive—developmental delay, malnutrition with decreased muscle mass, decreased interaction with environment and with others, dental caries, listlessness, behavior problems.
18. Sexually transmitted infections—genital trauma, recurrent urinary tract infection, pregnancy.

CLINICAL JUDGMENT Factitious disorder imposed on another (previously called *Munchausen syndrome by proxy*) is a condition in which symptoms are induced in a child by the actions of a parental caregiver. A wide range of methods have been noted as the basis for the fabricated illness, with most falling into one of four general categories: poisoning, bleeding, infections, and injuries. Many of the conditions cannot be observed by a health care provider nor can diagnosis be confirmed by further evaluation. Factitious disorder imposed on another is a serious form of child abuse and is associated with a high rate of morbidity and mortality. It is important for nurses to obtain thorough histories of any illness or injury and be extremely observant in unusual cases.

Management

1. The goal of treatment is to ensure the physical and emotional safety of the child. Therefore, treatment is inclusive of other family members and caregivers and is often focused on the parental caregivers. A team approach is employed to determine the most effective use of community resources to protect the child and help the parental caregivers.
2. It is estimated that 80% to 90% of parental caregivers who abuse their children can be rehabilitated. The ideal approach is to return the child to the parental caregivers after treatment concludes.
3. Counseling is offered to help parental caregivers do the following:
   a. Understand and redirect their anger.
   b. Develop an adequate parental caregiver–child relationship.
   c. See their child as an individual with their own needs and differences.
   d. Understand child development and normal behaviors of developing children.
   e. Learn about effective discipline techniques.
   f. Enjoy the child.
   g. Develop realistic expectations of their child.
   h. Decrease their use of criticism.
   i. Increase parental caregivers' self-esteem and confidence.
   j. Establish supportive relationships with others.
   k. Improve their economic situation (if appropriate).
   l. Show progress toward the physical, emotional, and intellectual development of their child.

Nursing Assessment

1. Identify family or child at risk.
   a. Person who misuses alcohol or drugs.
   b. Adolescent parental caregiver.
   c. Low-income, single-parental caregiver family.
   d. Multiple births.
   e. Unwanted child.
   f. Sickly and more demanding child.
   g. Premature child with long separation from birthing parent at birth.
2. Inspect for evidence of possible abuse.
   a. Describe completely on the medical record all bruises, lacerations, and similar lesions as to location and state of healing. Look carefully at areas generally covered with clothing (i.e., buttocks, underarms, behind knees, bottom of feet).
   b. Ask how injuries occurred and record descriptions of the injury, including the date, time, and place of the event.
3. Collect necessary specimens for identification of organisms, sperm, or semen.
4. Take color photographs, as indicated.
5. Assess developmental level of the child.
6. Observe for behaviors common in abusing or neglecting parental caregivers. Be aware that not all abusing parental caregivers exhibit these behaviors but be alert for the parental caregiver who:
   a. Anxiously volunteers information or withholds information related to an injury.
   b. Gives explanation of the injury that does not fit the condition or gets story confused concerning the injury.
   c. Shows inappropriate reaction or concern to the severity of injury.
   d. Becomes irritable about questions being asked.
   e. Seldom touches or speaks to the child; does not respond to child. May be critical or indicate unreal expectations of child (or may be over solicitous to the child).
   f. Delays seeking medical help; refuses to sign permit for diagnostic studies; frequently changes hospitals or health care providers.
   g. Shows no involvement in the care of the hospitalized child; does not inquire about the child.
   h. Obtains little or no prenatal care and shows inappropriate response to the neonate; acts disinterested or unhappy with the child.
7. Assess the parental caregiver–child relationship in the areas of appropriate involvement in care, show of affection, reaction to arrival and leaving, expectations, role portrayal.
8. Assess for signs of sexual abuse. Sexual abuse should be suspected when the young, prepubertal child presents with:
   a. Genital trauma not readily explained.
   b. Gonorrhea, syphilis, or other sexually transmitted infections.
   c. Blood in urine or stool.
   d. Painful urination or defecation.
   e. Penile or vaginal infection or itch.
   f. Penile or vaginal discharge.
   g. Report of increased, excessive masturbation.
   h. Report of increased, unusual fears.
   i. Trauma to genitalia, inner thigh, breast.
9. Establish a relationship with the child based on mutual respect, empathy, and sensitivity to facilitate further investigation.
   a. Consideration of the child's emotions in conjunction with a good relationship may encourage the child to express feelings either verbally or through drawings or play.
   b. Prepare the child physically and psychologically for the necessary physical and pelvic examination.
   c. Talk with the child without the presence of the parental caregivers, especially when incest is possible.
10. Report suspicion of child abuse based on your assessment. All states (as well as the District of Columbia) have mandatory reporting laws. All states provide statutory immunity for those who report real or suspected child abuse. There is no immunity from civil or criminal liability for failure to report such. Notify the appropriate officials.

CLINICAL JUDGMENT If the alleged sexual abuse occurred within 72 hours of the health care visit, or if trauma or bleeding is present, an immediate physical examination should be done. Assessment and evidence collection are very important, and every attempt should be made to enlist the assistance of a health care provider experienced in this task. Many emergency departments have SANE-Ps (Sexual Abuse Nurse Examiners–Pediatric) who have had extensive training in the acute management of sexual abuse and also in managing the long-term needs of the abused child. If more than 72 hours have passed since the alleged sexual abuse, the physical examination might be delayed. After child abuse has been reported, additional children in the family may be examined as well.

CLINICAL JUDGMENT Every nurse is morally and legally responsible to report and provide protective services for the abused child. Become familiar with laws, procedures, and protective services in your community and state.

Nursing Interventions

Relieving Fear and Fostering Trust

1. Be aware that some of these children have never learned how to trust an adult; they are fearful of giving affection for fear of rejection.
2. Assign one nurse to care for the child over a period of time so that a therapeutic relationship can be established.
3. Make no threatening moves toward the child. The child will indicate readiness and awareness of the environment by verbal or facial expressions.
4. Touch the child gently.
5. Provide nonthreatening physical contact (hold and frequently cuddle the child). Pick up and carry child around; encourage any exploration of your face and hair.
6. Provide appropriate opportunities for play.
7. Set limits for the child.
8. Provide therapeutic play to allow the child to express fears and anger in a nonverbal manner; be nonjudgmental and supportive with expression of feelings; correct misconceptions.
9. Provide additional help in these areas:
   a. Having ambivalent feelings toward the parental caregivers or any adult caretaker.
   b. Overcoming low self-image and the fear that something is wrong with them.
   c. Fearing future abuse upon their return home or for misbehavior in the hospital.

Providing Support in Parenting

1. Assume an attitude that is neither punitive nor threatening. Convey a desire to help the parental caregivers through the healing process.
2. Refrain from questioning them about the incident of abuse. The health care provider, social worker, and investigative authority will interview the person suspected of abusing their child.
3. Include the parental caregivers in the hospital experience (i.e., orient them to the unit and to any procedure to be done to the child). Serve as a role model in the management of the child's behavior as well as their own. Try to give the parental caregivers as much information as possible about the care of their child. Listen to what they are saying.
4. Refrain from challenging all the information they may give.
5. Express appropriate concern and kindness. Remain objective, yet empathic. This will help foster the parental caregivers' self-respect and improve their self-image and dignity.
6. Discuss the reporting to the authorities with them because of the widespread nature of the problem and the need for education and assistance.
7. Support the parental caregivers who may have feelings of guilt, anger, and helplessness. Explain to them the extent of trauma and educate them. Allow them to express their feelings. Support their parental role in handling the child (e.g., allow the child to talk about or play out the incident, but do not force it).
8. Build a relationship by working with the parental caregivers' strengths rather than their weaknesses. Use compliments as positive reinforcement.
9. Assist the parental caregivers to learn safe and appropriate parenting skills.
   a. Remember that many of these parental caregivers were abused as children and have no role models or personal experience with nurturing behaviors.
   b. Foster attachment between child and parental caregivers, not between child and nurse, when the parental caregivers are present; the latter would increase their feelings of incompetence in the parenting role.
   c. Correct erroneous expectations as to what is appropriate behavior for a particular age group.
   d. Encourage the parental caregivers to take time out from caring for their children to meet their own needs; assist them in identifying safe and appropriate resources for their child's care.
10. Provide the parental caregivers with psychological support and reinforcement for appropriate parenting behaviors.
11. Work with the parental caregivers in planning for the child's future care.
12. Determine the areas in which the parental caregivers need help. Does the infant cry often? How does this make the parental caregivers feel? How do the parental caregivers comfort the child? Is there someone the parental caregivers can call for help?

CLINICAL JUDGMENT A critical part of working in this area is learning to recognize, examine, and work with your own feelings of anger, disgust, and contempt toward the parental caregivers. It may help to do the following:

1. Realize that most abusive parental caregivers do love their children and want the best for them despite their ambivalent feelings toward their children.
2. Understand the dynamics of child abuse and neglect. This crisis is due to stress, with which the parental caregivers are unable to cope, and to deprivations they have themselves suffered in the past.

Community and Home Care Considerations

Nurses typically provide home care visits as part of a multidisciplinary team engaging in extensive community follow-up. Education and continued assessment are the focus.

1. Teach the parental caregivers about normal growth and development (see Chapter 36).
   a. Give specific information about and examples of the types of behavior to expect at the various stages of development. Point out in a nonthreatening way the normal behavior exhibited by their child.

   b. Provide specific strategies for dealing with whatever behavior the child exhibits.
   c. Serve as a role model and teacher; minimize intensity when the parental caregivers become threatened.
2. Teach the parental caregivers how to use discipline without resorting to physical force.
   a. Discipline must be consistent. Offer suggestions for alternative ways of handling undesirable behavior (e.g., time-out).
   b. Suggest using a reward system for acceptable behavior (e.g., a trip to the zoo, staying up later than usual for a special television show, a special treat).
   c. Instruct the parental caregivers to withhold rewards for unacceptable behavior.
3. Teach children how to avoid being the sufferers of abuse.
   a. Teach them about "good touch" and "bad touch."
   b. Emphasize that they can say no to anyone who wants to touch their body.
   c. Provide names or places where they can go if they feel they are being abused.
   d. Assist them in dealing with their fears that their parental caregivers will be sent to jail or that they will be removed from the home.
4. Be alert for signs of abuse in the school. If a teacher is suspected of child abuse, the child may:
   a. Display increased fear of the teacher.
   b. Decrease school attendance.
   c. Develop psychosomatic symptoms during school days.
   d. Develop nightmares.
   e. Worry excessively over school performance.

Bullying

Bullying is a form of abuse, frequently initiated among children. It is defined by the CDC as unwanted aggressive behaviors against a youth, initiated by another youth or groups of youths. Bullying can take many forms and can include physical, verbal, or social aggression. These behaviors can be direct with actual violence with verbal and/or physical results or indirect involving social media (spreading rumors). Bullying can cause physical and/or psychological symptoms in the sufferers of this abuse. Nurses should be aware of the possibility of bullying and refer to a primary health care provider, mental health counselor, or social worker for further care.

Family Education and Health Maintenance

1. Teach the parental caregivers and child (if age is appropriate) any specific instructions relative to injury and follow-up care.
2. Ensure that the family knows where and when to follow up.
3. Review schedule for well-child visits and immunizations so the family can keep up with routine care.
4. Make known to the parental caregivers your continued concern and your availability as a source of help. Help them to use resources in the community, including the home health nurse, social worker, and therapists.
5. Refer those interested in learning more about abuse to the following agencies: Prevent Child Abuse America (www.preventchildabuse.org, 1-800-CHILDREN) and Child Welfare Information Gateway (www.childwelfare.gov).

Evaluation: Expected Outcomes

- Exhibits appropriate developmental behavior.
- Both parental caregivers participate in feeding and playing with child.

TELEMEDICINE IN PEDIATRIC PRIMARY CARE

Historically, pediatric primary care practices have felt that the best approach to care required seeing the child and family face to face for in-office visits. Prior to the coronavirus disease 2019 (COVID-19) pandemic, telemedicine visits in pediatrics were largely utilized by subspecialty clinics to increase access to quality care. With the onset of the COVID-19 pandemic, many families were reluctant to bring children into office settings for fear of exposure. As practices have attempted to keep offices virus free, telehealth has become a means by which children with fever, cough, or known COVID-19 exposure could be evaluated. Similarly, video visits have also been used to assess injury before sending a family to an emergency department or other facility for care. Pediatric primary care practices are also now using telehealth to provide follow-up visits for treatments for attention deficit disorder, reproductive health, asthma, and other conditions.

The utilization of virtual visits has decreased the need for patients and families to go elsewhere, such as nonpractice-based telehealth services, urgent care facilities, and emergency departments, thereby promoting continuity of care and ease of follow-up treatment, as needed. Many have accepted in-practice telemedicine visits because it has enabled the child to see known providers who readily have access to the child's medical records.

SELECTED READINGS

American Academy of Pediatrics. (2023). *COVID-19 vaccine for children.* https://www.aap.org/en/pages/2019-novel-coronavirus-covid-19-infections/covid-19-vaccine-for-children/

Bono, S. A., Siau, C. S., Chen, W. S., Low, W. Y., Faria de Moura Villela, E., Pengpid, S., Hasan, M. T., Sessou, P., Ditekemena, J. D., Amodan, B. O., Hosseinipour, M. C., Dolo, H., Siewe Fodjo, J. N., & Colebunders, R. (2021). Adults' acceptance of COVID-19 vaccine for children in selected lower- and middle-income countries. *Vaccines, 10*(1), 11. https://doi.org/10.3390/vaccines10010011

Centers for Disease Control and Prevention. (2021a). *Injuries Among Children and Teens.* https://www.cdc.gov/injury/features/child-injury/index.html

Centers for Disease Control and Prevention. (2021b). *Meningococcal vaccine recommendations.* https://www.cdc.gov/vaccines/vpd/mening/hcp/recommendations.html

Centers for Disease Control and Prevention. (2022a). *Child and adolescent immunization schedule by age.* https://www.cdc.gov/vaccines/schedules/hcp/imz/child-adolescent.html

Centers for Disease Control and Prevention. (2022b). *TB Testing & diagnosis.* www.cdc.gov/tb/topic/testing/default.htm#bcg

Centers for Disease Control and Prevention. (2024). *Interim clinical considerations for use of COVID-19 vaccines in the United States.* https://www.cdc.gov/vaccines/covid-19/clinical-considerations/interim-considerations-us.html

Chaney, S. C., Mechael, P., Thu, N. M., Diallo, M. S., & Gachen, C. (2021). Every child on the map: A theory of change framework for improving childhood immunization coverage and equity using geospatial data and technologies. *Journal of Medical Internet Research, 23*(8), e29759. https://doi.org/10.2196/29759

Chesnel, M. J., Healy, M., & McNeill, J. (2022). Experiences that influence how trained providers support women with breastfeeding: A systematic review of qualitative evidence. *PLoS One, 17*(10), e0275608. https://doi.org/10.1371/journal.pone.0275608

Cosenza, G., & Sanna, L. (2021). The origins of the alleged correlation between vaccines and autism. A semiotic approach. *Social Epistemology, 37*(2), 150–163. https://doi.org/10.1080/02691728.2021.1954716

Elam-Evans, L. D., Yankey, D., Singleton, J. A., Sterrett, N., Markowitz, L. E., Williams, C. L., Fredua, B., McNamara, L., & Stokley, S. (2020). National, regional, state, and selected local area vaccination coverage among adolescents aged 13–17 years—United States, 2019. *Morbidity and Mortality Weekly Report, 69*(33), 1109–1116. https://doi.org/10.15585/mmwr.mm6933a1

Fisher, W. A., Gilca, V., Murti, M., Orth, A., Garfield, H., Roumeliotis, P., Rampakakis, E., Brown, V., Yaremko, J., Van Buynder, P., Boikos, C., & Mansi, J. A. (2022). Clinicians are not able to infer parental intentions to vaccinate infants with a seasonal influenza vaccine, and perhaps they should not try: Findings from the Pediatric Influenza Vaccination Optimization Trial (PIVOT)-IV. *Vaccines, 10*(11), 1955. https://doi.org/10.3390/vaccines10111955

Fitzgerald, M., Bhatt, A., Thompson, L. A., Schwartz, A., Thomas, A. O., Schinasi, D. A., Otero, J., Carpenter, P., Thomas, J. S., & Black, N. P. (2021). Telemedicine in pediatric training: A national needs assessment of the current state of telemedicine education in pediatric training. *Academic Pediatrics, 22*(5), 713–717. https://doi.org/10.1016/j.acap.2021.10.009

Fraguas, D., Díaz-Caneja, C. M., Ayora, M., Durán-Cutilla, M., Abregú-Crespo, R., Ezquiaga-Bravo, I., Martín-Babarro, J., & Arango, C. (2021). Assessment of school anti-bullying interventions: A meta-analysis of randomized clinical trials. *JAMA Pediatrics, 175*(1), 44–55. https://doi.org/10.1001/jamapediatrics.2020.3541

Gabrielli, S., Rizzi, S., Carbone, S., & Piras, E. M. (2021). School interventions for bullying-cyberbullying prevention in adolescents: Insights from the UPRIGHT and CREEP projects. *International Journal of Environmental Research and Public Health, 18*(21), 11697. https://doi.org/10.3390/ijerph182111697

Gaffney, G. R., Bereznicki, L. R., & Bereznicki, B. J. (2021). Knowledge, beliefs and management of childhood fever among nurses and other health professionals: A cross-sectional survey. *Nurse Education Today, 97*, 104731. https://doi.org/10.1016/j.nedt.2020.104731

Gallo, M., Eleftheriou, G., Giampreti, A., Contessa, M. G., Faraoni, L., Sangiovanni, A., Negri, G., Butera, R., & Bacis, G. (2020). Drugs of abuse in breastfeeding: the old and new psychoactive substances. *Reproductive Toxicology, 97*, 3. https://doi.org/10.1016/j.reprotox.2020.04.066

Goin-Kochel, R., Fombonne, E., Mire, S. S., Minard, C. G., Sahni, L. C., Cunningham, R. M., & Boom, J. A. (2020). Beliefs about causes of autism and vaccine hesitancy among parents of children with autism spectrum disorder. *Vaccine, 38*(40), 6327–6333. https://doi.org/10.1016/j.vaccine.2020.07.034

Grigoryan, Z., McPherson, R., Harutyunyan, T., Truzyan, N., & Sahakyan, S. (2022). Factors influencing treatment adherence among drug-sensitive tuberculosis (DS-TB) patients in Armenia: A qualitative study. *Patient Preference and Adherence, 16*, 2399–2408. https://doi.org/10.2147/PPA.S370520

He, K., Mack, W. J., Neely, M., Lewis, L., & Anand, V. (2022). Parental perspectives on immunizations: Impact of the COVID-19 pandemic on childhood vaccine hesitancy. *Journal of Community Health, 47*, 39–52. https://doi.org/10.1007/s10900-021-01017-9

Kleinman, K., McDaniel, L., & Molloy, M. (Eds.). (2020). *The Harriet Lane handbook* (22nd ed.). Elsevier.

Leeb, R. T., Danielson, M. L., Bitsko, R. H., Cree, R. A., Godfred-Cato, S., Hughes, M. M., Powell, P., Firchow, B., Hart, L. C., & Lebrun-Harris, L. A. (2020). Support for transition from adolescent to adult health care among adolescents with and without mental, behavioral, and developmental disorders—United States, 2016–2017. *Morbidity and Mortality Weekly Report, 69*(34), 1156–1160. https://doi.org/10.15585/mmwr.mm6934a2

Lin, C., Mullen, J., Smith, D., Kotarba, M., Kaplan, S. J., & Tu, P. (2021). Healthcare providers' vaccine perceptions, hesitancy, and recommendation to patients: A systematic review. *Vaccines, 9*(7), 713. https://doi.org/10.3390/vaccines9070713

Malek, L., Duffy, G., Fowler, H., & Katzer, L. (2020). Use and understanding of labelling information when preparing infant formula: Evidence from interviews and eye tracking. *Food Policy, 93*, 101892. https://doi.org/10.1016/j.foodpol.2020.101892

Meek, J. Y., & Noble, L. (2022). Policy statement: Breastfeeding and the use of human milk. *Pediatrics, 150*(1), e2022057988. https://doi.org/10.1542/peds.2022-057988

Myers, H. A., Batten, S., & Brewer, T. L. (2021). Breastfeeding: An evidence-based intervention for neonatal abstinence syndrome. *Worldviews on Evidence-Based Nursing, 18*(6), 350–351. https://doi.org/10.1111/wvn.12520

Newman, N. C., Knapke, J. M., Kniiyalocts, R., Belt, J., & Haynes, E. (2023). Evaluation of academic detailing to educated clinicians regarding childhood lead poisoning prevention: A pilot study. *Journal of Osteopathic Medicine, 123*(3), 159–165. https://doi.org/10.1515/jom-2022-0125

Parks, E. P., Shaikhkhalil, A., Sainath, N. N., Mitchell, J. A., Brownell, J. N., & Stallings, V. A. (2020). Feeding healthy infants, children, and adolescents. In R. Kliegman, B. Stanton, J. St Geme III, & N. Schor (Eds.), *Nelson's textbook of pediatrics* (21st ed., pp. 321–331). Elsevier.

Pingali, C., Yankey, D., Elam-Evans, L., Markowitz, L., Valier, M., Fredua, B., Crowe, S., DeSisto, C., Stokley, S., & Singleton, J. (2023). Vaccination coverage among adolescents aged 13-17 years-National Immunization Survey-Teen, United States, 2022. *MMWR, 72*(34). https://cdc.gov/mmwr/volumes/72/wr/pdfs/mm7234a3-H.pdf.

Pop, C. F., Coblisan, P., Capalna, L., Panța, P. C., Buzoianu, A. D., & Bocsan, I. C. (2023). Safety of vaccination within first year of life-the experience of one general medicine center. *Children (Basel, Switzerland), 10*(1), 104. https://doi.org/10.3390/children10010104

ProQuest. (2022, April 26). *Delivery of a preparation containing diphtheria toxoid, acellular pertussis vaccine and tetanus toxoid for children* (MENA report). https://www.proquest.com/wire-feeds/delivery-preparation-containing-diphtheria-toxoid/docview/2655316420/se-2

Sharley, V. (2020). Identifying and responding to child neglect within schools: Differing perspectives and the implications for inter-agency practice. *Child Indicators Research, 13*(2), 551–571. https://doi.org/10.1007/s12187-019-09681-z

U.S. Department of Health and Human Services, Administration for Children and Families, Children's Bureau. (2022). *Child maltreatment 2020.* Author. https://www.acf.hhs.gov/cb/report/child-maltreatment-2020

U.S. Department of Health & Human Services, Administration for Children and Families, Administration on Children, Youth and Families, Children's Bureau. (2023). *Child Maltreatment 2021.* https://www.acf.hhs.gov/cb/data-research/child-maltreatment.

39 Care of the Sick or Hospitalized Child

GENERAL PRINCIPLES

Hospitalization of a child brings about a range of emotions in the child and their family. To care for the hospitalized child, one must take into consideration the child's development and family coping skills. Being hospitalized versus receiving care at home affects the child's response to their illness. In addition, family presence is often an integral part of pediatric patient care. Facilitating family-centered care allows the family to fully support the child during their hospitalization. Knowledge of these aspects will assist the registered nurse in providing appropriate pediatric patient care.

Pain Management

EVIDENCE BASE Gai, N., Naser, B., Hanley, J., Peliowski, A., Hayes, J., & Aoyama, K. (2020). A practical guide to acute pain management in children. *Journal of Anesthesia*, *34*(3), 421–433. https://doi.org/10.1007/s00540-020-02767-x

Accurate assessment and timely management of pain in children is an important and challenging nursing responsibility because infants and young children cannot express their pain, as adults can.

General Considerations

1. Pain experienced by infants and children often is not effectively identified or managed by health care providers.
2. There are still misunderstandings about the ways pain is experienced and expressed by infants and children. Studies have shown that long-term effects can occur from inadequately treated pain.
3. Behavioral and physiologic cues are used to assess pain in infants. Special rating tools are available to involve children in assessing the intensity of their pain, including the pain experience inventory, CRIES neonatal postoperative pain measurement scale, Oucher pain rating scale, numerical or visual analog scale, Face, Legs, Activity, Cry, and Consolability Scale (FLACC) behavioral pain assessment scale, and the Wong-Baker FACES Pain Rating Scale.
4. Pain caused by a condition is not always proportional to the seriousness of the illness or injury. For example, a relatively minor illness, such as an earache, is a very painful experience, whereas an enlarging tumor may not cause pain in early stages.
5. It is important to consider pain when a child is noncommunicative, has decreased consciousness, is intubated, or whose chosen language is not understood by the health caregivers. Changes in vital signs (such as heart rate, respiratory rate, and blood pressure) may indicate pain.
6. It is equally important to consider pain when a child requires an injection, blood test, or noninvasive or invasive diagnostic test.
7. Consider parental caregivers when assessing and managing the pain of their child. Parental caregivers are important influences on their children.
   a. Consider the way in which the parental caregivers view the situation experienced by the child and work with them to intervene effectively.
   b. Presence of the parental caregivers during a procedure can be very positive, especially when the family has been prepared.
   c. At other times, it is recommended that the parental caregivers mutually agree to wait in a nearby area.
   d. Arbitrary rules against parental caregiver presence are often designed to meet the needs of staff, not the needs of the child and their parental caregivers.

Nursing Interventions

1. Anticipate pain and intervene early.
2. Use a rating scale that the child can understand and use it consistently with that child for initial pain assessment and to determine the effectiveness of interventions. Attempt to introduce the pain rating scale to the child prior to the surgery or procedure.
3. Use self as therapeutic presence to help ease pain.
4. Teach self-regulation and self-control techniques.
5. Utilize distraction by sounds, music, audio images, and movies.
6. Allow self-soothing maneuvers (thumb-sucking, clinging to blanket, rocking).
7. Reposition patient, as needed.

8. Decrease environmental light and noise when possible.
9. Consider referral for self-hypnosis and conscious relaxation techniques.
10. Utilize medication delivered by way of noninvasive routes where possible.
11. Administer premedication—anesthetizing, antianxiety, and antiemetic medications. Utilize a multimodal approach whenever possible.
12. Assist with conscious sedation when indicated, following standards of practice related to assessment, staffing, care, and documentation.
13. Reassess the patient's response to the intervention and document appropriately. This is important to evaluate effectiveness and identify possible new pain issues.

The Child Undergoing Surgery

EVIDENCE BASE Mansson, M., Forsner, M., & Heden, L. (2023). Children need to know: A follow-up study two decades later on informing and preparing children for clinical examinations and procedures. *Pediatric Nursing, 49*(1), 1–10https://www.proquest.com/openview/5165e7d96cf5935239d13aef28106d73/1?pq-origsite=gscholar&cbl=47659.

Romito, B., Jewell, J., & Jackson, M. (2021). Child life services. *Pediatrics, 147*(1). e2020040261. https://doi.org/10.1542/peds.2020-040261

Physical and emotional preparation for surgery will minimize stress and help the child and family cope effectively with surgery. Also, see Chapter 3.

Psychological Preparation and Support

1. Potential threats for the hospitalized child anticipating surgery are as follows:
   a. Physical harm—bodily injury, pain, mutilation, death.
   b. Separation from parental caregivers; peers for the older child or adolescent.
   c. The strange and unknown—possibility of surprise.
   d. Confusion and uncertainty about limits and expected behavior.
   e. Relative loss of control of their world, loss of autonomy.
   f. Fear of anesthesia.
   g. Fear of the surgical procedure itself.
   h. Misinterpretation of medical jargon (e.g., *dye/die*).
2. The attitudes of the parental caregivers toward hospitalization and surgery largely determine the attitudes of their child.
   a. The experience may be emotionally distressing.
   b. Parental caregivers may have feelings of fear or guilt.
   c. The preparation and support should be integrated for parental caregiver, child, and family unit.
   d. Give individual attention to parental caregivers; explore and clarify their feelings and thoughts; provide accurate information and appropriate reassurance.
   e. Stress parental caregivers' importance to the child. Help parental caregivers understand how they can care for their child.

Preoperative Teaching

1. All preparation and support must be based on the child's age, developmental stage, personality, past history and experience with health professionals and hospitals, and background including religion, socioeconomic circumstances, culture, and family attitudes and dynamics. Anxiety level and coping skills should be taken into consideration.
2. Inquire as to what information the child has already received.
3. Determine what the child knows or expects; identify family myths and possible misunderstandings.
4. Additional guidelines in preparation include the following:
   a. Use illustration or model of a child's body, concrete examples, and simple terms (not medical jargon).
   b. Identify changes that may occur as a result of the procedure, in both body and daily routine.
   c. Give explanations slowly and clearly, saving anxiety-producing aspects until the end. Repeat as needed.
   d. Make use of the child's creative ability and logical thinking powers to aid in preparation for procedures.
   e. Involve parental caregivers, as indicated, depending on the situation.
   f. Allow and encourage the child to participate as able.
   g. Suggest ways for the child to cope—crying is okay.
   h. Offer constant reassurance; speak in a calm manner.
   i. Evaluate the child's understanding of your teaching. Repeat and correct information, as necessary.
5. Orient the patient and family to the unit, room, location of playroom, operating room, and recovery room (if applicable) and introduce them to appropriate personnel. Make arrangements for the child to meet the anesthesiologist as well as the operating room nurse and recovery room nurse.
6. Allow and encourage questions. Give honest answers.
   a. Such questions will give the nurse a better understanding of the child's fears and perceptions of what is happening.
   b. Infants and young children need to form a trusting relationship with those who care for them.
   c. The older the child, the more reassuring information can be.
7. Provide opportunity for the child and parental caregivers to work out concerns and feelings (play, talk). Such supportive care should result in less upset behavior and more cooperation.
8. Prepare the child for what to expect postoperatively (i.e., equipment to be used or attached to child, where the child will wake up, how the child will feel, what the child will be expected to do, diet, any physical restrictions). Be honest about what pain they may experience.
9. Educate parental caregivers regarding the option to be with their child, if available at the facility, during induction of anesthesia to reduce separation anxiety and fear.

Physical Preparation

1. Assist with necessary laboratory studies. Explain to the child what is going to happen before the procedure and how they may respond. Give continual support during the procedure.
2. See that the patient has nothing by mouth (NPO). Explain to the child and their parental caregivers what NPO means and the importance of it. Place signs on the patient's hospital door indicating the NPO status to ensure that nonfamily members and nonstaff members do not give the patient food.
3. Assist with fever reduction.
   a. Fever can result from some surgical problems (e.g., intestinal obstruction).
   b. Fever increases the risk of anesthesia and the need for fluids and calories.
4. Administer appropriate medications, as prescribed. Sedatives and drugs to dry the secretions are often given on the unit preoperatively.

5. Establish good hydration. Parenteral therapy may be necessary to hydrate the child, especially if the child is NPO, vomiting, or febrile.
6. With the parental caregivers in attendance, assist the surgeon with marking the patient's intended surgical site, as recommended by The Joint Commission as part of the National Safety Goals.
7. Allow the child to carry a toy or other comfort item to the preoperative area.

Immediate Postoperative Care

1. Maintain a patent airway and prevent aspiration.
   a. Position the child as ordered depending on their surgical procedure; position as needed to allow secretions to drain and to prevent the tongue from obstructing the pharynx.
   b. Suction any secretions present. Avoid causing a gag reflex or spasm during suctioning.
2. Make frequent observations of general condition and vital signs. Postoperative protocols may vary per procedure and facility.
   a. Take vital signs every 15 minutes until the child is awake and their condition is stable.
   b. Note temperature, respiratory rate and quality, pulse rate and quality, blood pressure, and skin color.
   c. Watch for signs of shock.
      i. Children in shock may have signs of pallor, coldness, increased pulse, and irregular respiration.
      ii. Older children have decreased blood pressure and respiration.
   d. Change in vital signs may indicate airway obstruction or compromise, hemorrhage, atelectasis, and altered hemodynamics.
   e. Restlessness may indicate pain or hypoxia. Medication for pain is not usually given until anesthesia has worn off. Give analgesics and sedatives per the pain management team orders.
   f. Check dressings for drainage, constriction, and pressure. Perform dressing changes per protocol.
3. See that all drainage tubes are connected and functioning properly. Gastric decompression relieves abdominal distention and decreases the possibility of respiratory compromise. Chest tubes evacuate pleural air and fluid. Ensure all tubes are secure to prevent accidental removal.
4. Monitor parenteral fluids, as prescribed.
5. Be physically near as the child awakens to offer soothing words and a gentle touch. Reunite the parental caregivers and child as soon as possible after the child recovers from anesthesia. If a language barrier exists, the parental caregivers should be with the child during recovery from anesthesia and an interpreter should be present when medical explanations are being given to the parental caregivers or child.

After Recovery From Anesthesia

After undergoing simple surgery and receiving a small amount of anesthesia, the child may be ready to play and eat in a few hours. More complicated and extensive surgery debilitates the child for a longer period of time.

1. Continue to make frequent and astute observations in regard to behavior, comfort level and pain control, vital signs, dressings or operative site, and special apparatus (intravenous [IV] lines, chest tubes, oxygen, nasogastric tubes).
   a. Note signs of dehydration—dry skin and membranes, sunken eyes, poor skin turgor, sunken fontanelle in an infant, poor urine output.
   b. Record any passage of flatus or stool and bowel sounds. Observe for intestinal ileus. Gastric distention may be caused by swallowed air in the crying child.
   c. Record vomiting including time, amount, and characteristics.
2. Assess behavior for signs of pain and medicate appropriately.
3. Record intake and output accurately.
   a. Parenteral fluids and oral intake.
   b. Drainage from gastric tubes or chest tubes, colostomy, wound, and urinary output.
   c. Parenteral fluid is evaluated and prescribed by considering output and intake. It is usually maintained until the child is taking adequate oral fluids.
4. Advance diet as tolerated, according to the child's age and the health care provider's directions.
   a. First feedings are usually clear fluids; if tolerated, advance slowly to full diet for age. Note any vomiting or abdominal distention.
   b. Because anorexia may occur, offer what the child likes in small amounts and in an attractive manner.
5. Prevent infection.
   a. Keep the child away from other children or personnel with respiratory or other infections.
   b. Change the child's position every 2 to 4 hours; support infant with a blanket roll.
   c. Encourage the child to cough and breathe deeply; let the infant cry for short periods of time, unless contraindicated. Offer older children incentive spirometry every hour while awake.
   d. Keep operative site clean—change dressing, as ordered; in infant, keep the diaper away from the wound.
   e. Enforce diligent handwashing by family members and staff before any contact with the patient.
   f. Do not cohort surgical patients with patients with a proven or presumptive infection.
   g. Administer prophylactic antibiotics, as ordered.
6. Provide good general hygiene and opportunities for exercise and diversional activity; encourage sleep and rest.
7. Provide emotional support and psychological security. Reassure the child that things are going well; if there are complications, offer honest information based on the patient's health and developmental stage and the parental caregivers' willingness to share this information with their child. Talk about going home, if appropriate.
8. Hospitalization can be anxiety provoking for both the child and parental caregivers. Identify parental caregivers early, and try to coordinate nursing care and education with their visits. This includes teaching special procedures, providing written instructions, and arranging for home nursing and/or supplies.
9. Ensure that parental caregivers have access to and adequate time to secure necessary medical supplies and medications to provide adequate care. If this cannot be ensured, supplies may have to be dispensed through the hospital for discharge.

The Child Who Is Dying

The nursing role is to assist the child and family to cope with the experience in such a way that it will promote growth rather than destroy family integrity and emotional well-being.

Table 39-1 Stages of Dying as Identified by Dr. Elisabeth Kübler-Ross

STAGE	NURSING CONSIDERATIONS
i. Denial, shock, disbelief	• Accept denial, but function within a reality sphere. Do not tear down the child's (or family's) defenses. • Be aware that denial usually breaks down in the early morning when it may be dark and lonely. • Be certain that it is the child or family who is using denial, not the staff.
ii. Anger, rage, hostility	• Accept anger and help the child express it through positive channels. • Be aware that anger may be expressed toward other family members, health care providers, and other persons involved. • Help families recognize that it is normal for children to express anger for what they are losing.
iii. Bargaining (from "No, not me," to "Yes, me, but …")	• Recognize this period as a time for the child and family to regain strength. • Encourage the family to finish any unfinished business with the child. This is the time to do things such as take a promised trip or buy a promised toy.
iv. Depression (the child and/or family experiences silent grief and mourns past and future losses)	• Recognize this as a normal reaction and expression of strength. • Help families to accept the child who does not want to talk and excludes help. This is the usual pattern of behavior. • Reassure the child that you can understand their feelings.
v. Acceptance	• Assist families to provide significant loving human contact with their child and one another.

EVIDENCE BASE Kübler-Ross, E. (1997). *On death and dying*. Scribner.

Linebarger, J. S., Johnson, V., & Boss, R. D. (2022). Guidance for pediatric end-of-life care. *Pediatrics, 149*(5), e2022057011. https://doi.org/10.1542/peds.2022-057011

Recognize the Stages of Dying

See Table 39-1.

1. Be aware that the patient, their family, and the health care providers all progress through these stages, not necessarily at the same time.
2. Children experience the stages with much variation. They tend to pass more quickly through the stages and may merge some of these stages.
3. The nursing goal is to accept the child and their family at whatever stage they are experiencing, not to push them through the stages.
4. Understand the meaning of illness and death at various stages of growth and development (see Table 39-2).
5. Be aware of other factors that influence a child's personal concept of death. Of particular importance are the following:
   a. The amount and type of direct exposure a child has had to death.
   b. Cultural values, beliefs, and patterns of bereavement.
   c. Religious beliefs about death and an afterlife.
6. Meet with the parental caregivers separately from the child and discuss their wishes regarding dissemination of information to their child.

Communicate With the Child About Death

Research indicates that children generally can cope with more than adults will allow and that children appreciate the opportunity to know and understand what is happening to them. It is important that the child's questions be answered simply but truthfully. The answers should be based on the child's particular level of understanding. The following responses have been suggested by Easson in *The Dying Child: The Management of the Child or Adolescent Who Is Dying* and may be useful as a guide:

Preschool-Age Child

1. When the child at this age is comfortable enough to ask questions about illness, questions should be answered. When death is anticipated at some future time and the child asks, "Am I going to die?," a response might be, "We will all die someday, but you are not going to die today or tomorrow."
2. When death is imminent and the child asks, "Am I going to die?," the response might be, "Yes, you are going to die, but we will take care of you and stay with you."

Table 39-2 Stages in the Development of a Child's Concept of Death

AGE OF CHILD	STAGE OF DEVELOPMENT
Child up to age 3	• At this stage, the child cannot comprehend the relationship of life to death because the child has not developed the concept of infinite time. • The child fears separation from protecting and comforting adults. • The child perceives death as a reversible act.
Preschool child	• At this age, the child has no real understanding of the meaning of death; the child feels safe and secure with parental caregivers. • The child may view death as something that happens to others. • The child may interpret the separation that occurs with hospitalization as punishment; the painful tests and procedures that the child is subjected to support this idea. • The child may become depressed because of not being able to correct these wrongdoings and regain the grace of adults. • The concept may be connected with magical thoughts of mystery.

(continued)

Table 39-2 Stages in the Development of a Child's Concept of Death *(continued)*

AGE OF CHILD	STAGE OF DEVELOPMENT
School-age child	• The child at this age sees death as the cessation of life; child understands that they are alive and can become "not alive"; child fears dying. • The child differentiates death from sleep. Unlike sleep, the horror of death is in pain, progressive mutilation, and mystery. • The child is vulnerable to guilt feelings related to death because of difficulty in differentiating death wishes and the actual event. • The child believes death may be caused by angry feelings or bad thoughts. • The child learns the meaning of death from own personal experiences, such as the death of pets, family members, and public figures. • Television and movies have contributed to the concept of death and understanding of the meaning of illness. There may be more knowledge in the meaning of the diagnosis and an awareness that death may occur violently.
Adolescent	• The adolescent comprehends the permanence of death as the adult does, although the adolescent may not comprehend death as an event occurring to persons close to self. • The adolescent wants to live—sees death as thwarting pursuit of goals: independence, success, achievement, physical improvement, and self-image. • The adolescent fears death before fulfillment. • The adolescent may become depressed and resentful because of bodily changes that may occur, dependency, and the loss of social environment. • The adolescent may feel isolated and rejected because adolescent friends may withdraw when faced with impending death of a friend. • The adolescent may express rage, bitterness, and resentment; especially resents the fact that fate is to die.

3. When the child asks, "Will it hurt?," the response should be truthful and factual.
4. Death should never be described as a form of sleep. Some children may fear sleep as the result of this type of explanation. Anesthesia is sometimes called a "special sleep" so it is not currently recommended to refer to death as "sleep."
5. Parental caregivers can express to the child the fact that they do not want the child to go and that they will miss the child very much; they feel sad, too, that they are going to be separated.

School-Age Child

1. Responses to the school-age child's questions about death should be answered truthfully. The child looks for support from those they trust.
2. The school-age child should be given a simple explanation of their diagnosis and its meaning; the child should also receive an explanation of all treatments and procedures.
3. The child should be given no specific time in terms of days or months because each individual and each illness is different.
4. When the school-age child asks, "Am I going to die?" and death is inevitable, the child should be told the truth. The school-age child has the emotional ability to look to parental caregivers and those they trust for comfort and support.
5. The school-age child believes in their parental caregivers. The child should be allowed to die in the comfort and security of their family.
6. The school-age child knows death means final separation and what will be missed. The child must be allowed to mourn this loss. The child who is dying may be sad and bitter and demonstrate aggressive behavior. The child must be allowed the opportunity to verbalize this if able to do so.

Adolescent

1. The adolescent should be given an explanation of their illness and all necessary treatments and procedures.
2. The adolescent feels deprived and reasonably resentful regarding their illness because they want to live and reach fulfillment.
3. As death approaches, the adolescent becomes emotionally closer to the family.
4. The adolescent should be allowed to maintain emotional defenses—including absolute denial. The adolescent will indicate by questions what types of answers are desired.
5. An adolescent who states, "I am not going to die" is pleading for support. Be truthful and state, "No, you are not going to die right now."
6. The adolescent may ask, "How long do I have to live?" Adolescents are able to face reality more directly and can tolerate more direct answers. No absolute time should be given because that blocks all hope. If an adolescent has what is felt to be a prognosis of approximately 3 months, the response might be, "People with an illness like yours may die in 3 to 6 months, but some may live much longer."

Support Parental Caregivers' Adaptation to Child's Death

1. Develop a care plan that includes this approach:
   a. The primary responsibility for communicating with the parental caregivers should be designated to one nurse.
   b. Information regarding the parental caregivers' concerns should be communicated to all staff members and should be included in the patient's care plan.
2. Accept parental caregivers' feelings about the child's anticipated death and help them deal with these feelings.
   a. It is not unusual for parental caregivers to reach the point of wishing the child dead and to experience guilt and self-blame because of this thought.
   b. The parental caregivers may withdraw emotional attachments to the child if the process of dying is lengthy. This

occurs because the parental caregivers complete most of the mourning process before the child reaches biologic death. They may relate to the child as if they were already dead.

3. Provide anticipatory guidance regarding the child's actual death and immediate decisions and responsibilities afterward.
   a. Describe what the death will probably be like and how to know when it is imminent. This is necessary to dispel the horrifying fantasies that many parental caregivers have. Reassure the parental caregivers that all measures will be taken to keep the child comfortable at the time of death. (*Note:* Certain diseases, despite appropriate medical interventions, may cause an uncomfortable or painful death. Parental caregivers should be promised complete comfort for their child only if this expectation is realistic.)
   b. Clarify the parental caregivers' wishes about being present at the child's death and respect their desires. See if they want to hold the child—before, during, or after the death.
   c. If appropriate, allow the parental caregivers to discuss their feelings about issues such as autopsy and organ donation in order that they may make appropriate decisions. Do not make them feel guilty if they do not consent.
   d. If necessary, assist the parental caregivers to think about funeral arrangements.
4. Be aware of factors that affect the family's capacity to cope with fatal illness, especially social and cultural features of the family system, previous experiences with death, present stage of family development, and resources available to them.
5. Contact the appropriate clergy if the family desires. Contact other extended family members for support if they wish.
6. During final hours, do not leave the family alone, unless they request it.
7. Encourage parental caregivers and siblings to share their thoughts with the child who is dying.
8. Provide information on bereavement support groups, usually available through hospital or church.

PEDIATRIC PROCEDURES

See additional online content: Procedure Guidelines 39-1 to 39-7

Restraints

EVIDENCE BASE Dalton, E., & Doupnik, S. (2024). Envisioning zero: A path to eliminating restraint use in children's hospitals. *Pediatrics, 153*(1), e2023064054. https://doi.org/10.1542/peds.2023-064054

Dalton, E., Herndon, A., Cundiff, A., Fuchs, D. C., & Hart, S. (2021). Decreasing the use of restraints on children admitted for behavioral health conditions. *Pediatrics, 148*(1), e2020003939. https://doi.org/10.1542/peds.2020-003939

Protective measures to limit movement may be necessary for restraining children in the health care setting (see Figure 39-1). They can be a short-term restraint to facilitate examination and minimize the child's discomfort during special tests, procedures, and specimen collections. Restraints can also be used for a longer period of time to maintain the child's safety, protect them from injury, and/or to protect medically necessary devices.

General Considerations

1. Protective devices should be used only when necessary and after all other considerations are exhausted, never as a substitute for careful observation of the child.
2. Protective devices cannot be used on a continuous basis without an order. Continuous use requires justification and full documentation of the type of restraint used, reason for use, and the effectiveness of the restraint used. Ongoing monitoring, documentation, and renewal of the order, with the length of time the restraint will be in place, are required.
3. The reason for using the protective device should be explained to the child and parental caregivers to prevent misinterpretation and to ensure their cooperation with the procedure. Children often interpret restraints as punishment.
4. Teach the child and family about specific devices they may be using in the hospital (i.e., side rails) and after discharge (i.e., mitts, elbow restraints).
5. Any protective device should be checked frequently to make sure it is effective and is not causing any ill side effects. It should be removed periodically to prevent skin irritation or circulation impairment. Provide range of motion and skin care routinely.
6. Do not cover an intravenous (IV) site with a restraint when possible. If it is necessary to use a restraint that covers an IV site, it must be accessible for frequent assessment.
7. Protective devices should always be applied in a manner that maintains proper body alignment and ensures the child's comfort.
8. Any protective device that requires attachment to the child's bed should be secured to the bed springs or frame, never the mattress or side rails. This allows the side rails to be adjusted without removing the restraint or injuring the child's extremity.
9. Any required knots should be tied in a manner that permits their quick release. This is a safety precaution.
10. When a child must be immobilized, an attempt should be made to replace the lost activity with another form of motion. For example, although restrained, a child can be moved in a stroller, in a wheelchair, or in bed. When arms are restrained, the child may be allowed to play kicking games. Water play, mirrors, body games, and blowing bubbles are helpful replacements.
11. Restraints should be removed as soon as the child is no longer considered a danger to self or others or when medical devices are no longer in place.

CLINICAL JUDGMENT An order from a health care provider is needed to initiate continuous restraints. Proper documentation is required when restraints are in use. Do not secure restraints to bed rails or mattresses. Hourly assessment of the restrained extremity is needed to ensure there has been no impairment of circulation and constriction or respiratory compromise with chest restraints. Ensure that facility policies for restraint use are followed and documented.

Mummy Device

The *mummy device* involves securing a sheet or blanket around the child's body in such a way that the arms are held to the sides and leg movements are restricted (see Figure 39-1A). This short-term type of restraint is used on infants and small children during treatments and examinations involving the head and neck.

Equipment

Small sheet or blanket.

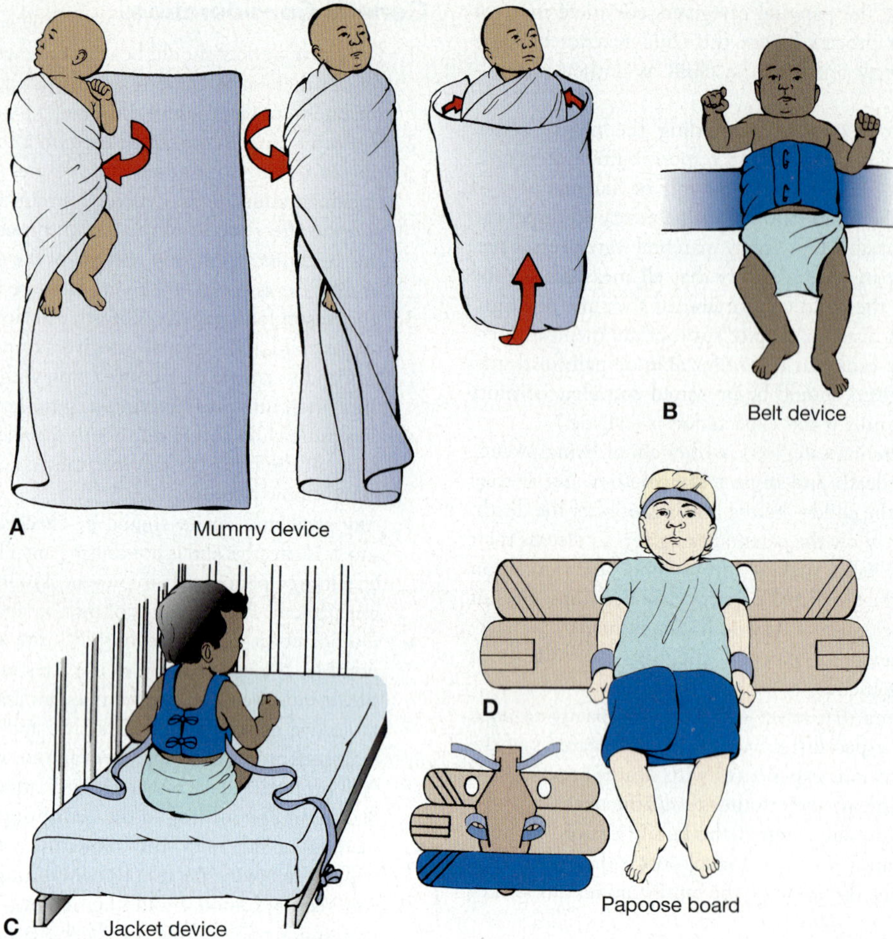

Figure 39-1. Types of restraints.

Nursing Action

1. Place the blanket or sheet flat on the bed.
2. Fold over one corner of the blanket.
3. Place the child on the blanket with shoulder at the edge of the fold.
4. Pull the right side of the blanket firmly over the child's right shoulder.
5. Tuck the remainder of the right side of the blanket under the left side of the child's body.
6. Repeat the procedure with the left side of the blanket.
7. Separate the corners of the bottom portion of the sheet and fold it up toward the child's neck.
8. Tuck both sides of the sheet under the child's body.
9. Secure by crossing one side over the other in the back and tucking in the excess or by pinning or taping the blanket in place.

Special Precautions

Make certain the child's extremities are in a comfortable position during this procedure. Make sure that the restraint is not obstructing the child's airway.

Jacket Device

The *jacket device* is a piece of material that fits the child like a jacket or halter. Long tapes are attached to the sides of the jacket (see Figure 39-1C). Jacket device restraints are used to keep the child in a wheelchair, high chair, or crib.

Nursing Action

1. Put the jacket on the child so the opening is in the back.
2. Tie the strings securely with a knot that can be easily released, if necessary.
3. Position the child in a wheelchair, high chair, or crib.
4. Secure the long tapes appropriately:
   a. Under the arm supports of a chair.
   b. Around the back of the wheelchair or high chair.
   c. To the springs or frame of a crib.

Special Precautions

Children in cribs must be observed frequently to make certain they do not become entangled in the long tapes of the jacket device. Release, reposition, and perform range-of-motion exercises as per hospital policy.

Belt Device

The *belt device* is exactly like the jacket method of restraining, except that the material fits the child like a wide belt with buckles in the front (see Figure 39-1B).

Elbow Device

The *elbow device* is a plastic device that fits around the arm at the elbow bend and is secured with a Velcro strap. This type of restraint prevents flexion of the elbow. It is especially useful for pediatric patients receiving IV therapy, those with eczema or other skin rashes, and those following a cleft lip repair, eye surgery, or any other type of procedure or surgery in which touching the upper extremities, head, or neck should be prevented.

Equipment

1. Elbow device.
2. Skin protective material for under the device (long-sleeved shirt or gauze).

Nursing Action

1. Cover the elbow with a long-sleeved shirt or gauze if irritation or sweating is expected.
2. Place the child's arm in the center of the appropriately sized elbow restraint.
3. Wrap the restraint around the child's arm.
4. Secure with Velcro.

Special Precautions

1. The child's fingers should be observed frequently for coldness or discoloration and the skin under the device should be checked for signs of irritation.
2. The device should be removed periodically according to facility policy or standards of care to provide skin care and range of motion.

Devices to Limit Movement of the Extremities

Many different kinds of devices are available to limit motion of one or more extremities. One commercial variety consists of a piece of material with tapes on both ends to be secured to the frame of the bed. The material also has two small flaps sewn to it for securing the child's ankles or wrists. Similar devices are available that use sheepskin flaps. These should be used when the device will be necessary over a prolonged period or for children with sensitive skin. This restraining device may be used to restrain infants and young children for procedures, such as IV therapies and urine collection.

Equipment

1. Extremity restraint of appropriate size for the child (small, medium, or large).

Nursing Action

1. Secure the device to the crib or bed frame.
2. Velcro the small flaps securely around the child's ankles or wrists.

Special Precautions

1. The child's fingers or toes should be observed frequently for coldness or discoloration and the skin under the device should be checked for signs of irritation.
2. The device should be removed periodically according to policy or standards of care to provide skin care and range-of-motion exercises and documentation should be completed.

Abdominal Device

The *abdominal device* is used for restraining a small child in a crib. It operates exactly like the method described for limiting the movements of extremities. However, the strip of material is wider and has only one wide flap sewn in the center for fastening around the child's abdomen.

Mitts

Mitts are used to prevent a child from injuring self with their hands and from removing tubes or IV lines. They are especially useful for children with dermatologic conditions such as eczema or burns and for those with nasogastric or nasojejunal (NJ) feeding tubes. Mitts can be purchased commercially or made by wrapping the child's hands in Kling gauze or by covering the child's hands with a pair of clean socks and securing them to the wrist with tape.

CLINICAL JUDGMENT Mitts should be removed at least every 4 hours to permit skin care and to allow the child to exercise fingers.

Crib Top Device

A *crib top device* is used to prevent an infant or small child from climbing over the crib sides. Several types of commercial devices are available, including nets, plastic tops, and domes. A crib top device should be applied to the crib of a child capable of climbing over the crib sides (usually between 1 and 4 years of age).

CLINICAL JUDGMENT In all instances, it is essential to be certain that the crib sides are kept all of the way up and latched securely.

Papoose Board

A papoose board is a restraint device to be used for procedures of the head, chest, and abdomen. Straps restrain the child or infant at the forehead, lower arms, and thighs (see Figure 39-1D, page 1152).

Specimen Collection

Evaluation of specimens such as blood, urine, and stool is important in determining the status of the child. The nurse should be adept in the techniques for obtaining specimens, as well as meticulous in labeling and recording them.

KEY DECISION POINT Anticipate bleeding if venipuncture was difficult. Hold pressure over the area until oozing has stopped (longer if the child is being treated with aspirin or an anticoagulant). Assess frequently and reapply pressure, if needed; report continued oozing or hematoma formation.

EVIDENCE BASE Bowden, V. R., & Greenberg, C. S. (2016). *Pediatric nursing procedures* (4th ed.). Lippincott Williams & Wilkins.

For catheterization of the urinary bladder, refer to Chapter 17. For infants and children, the catheter size is 6 to 10 Fr, depending on the size of the child.

EVIDENCE BASE Fleet, S., & Duggan, C. (2022). Overview of enteral nutrition in infants and children. *UpToDate*. Retrieved May 21, 2022, from www.uptodate.com/contents/overview-of-enteral-nutrition-in-infants-and-children

Malekiantaghi, A., AsnaAshari, K., Shabani-Mirzaee, H., Vigeh, M., Sadatinezhad, M., & Eftekhari, K. (2022). Evaluation of the risk of malnutrition in hospitalized children by PYMS, STAMP, and STRONGkids tools and comparison with their anthropometric indices: A cross-sectional study. *BMC Nutrition, 8*, 1–7. https://doi.org/10.1186/s40795-022-00525-8

Feeding and Nutrition

Nutritional requirements may increase while the infant or child is ill, but the ability to feed naturally may be impaired by illness or the child's response to illness. If existing feeding patterns cannot be maintained, alternate methods may be necessary. The ability to feed enterally is preferred over parenteral nutrition because of decreased risk of complications as well as improved physiologic response.

Gavage Feeding

KEY DECISION POINT If improper placement occurs and the catheter enters the trachea, the patient may cough, struggle, and become cyanotic. Remove the catheter immediately and allow the patient to rest before attempting to insert the tube again.

KEY DECISION POINT If bradycardia occurs, remove tube and allow the patient to relax. If the child appears to be in distress, follow basic life support protocols and contact the health care provider. When the patient's vital signs normalize, reattempt tube replacement.

EVIDENCE BASE Northington, L., Kemper, C., Rempel, G., Lyman, B., Pauley, R., Visscher, D., Moore, C., & Guenter, P. (2022). Evaluation of methods used to verify nasogastric feeding tube placement in hospitalized infants and children—A follow-up study. *Journal of Pediatric Nursing, 63*, 72–77. https://doi.org/10.1016/j.pedn.2021.10.018

1. *Gavage feeding* is a means of providing food by way of a catheter passed through the nares or mouth, past the pharynx, down the esophagus, and into the stomach, slightly beyond the cardiac sphincter. Feedings may be continuous or intermittent.
2. Gavage feedings can provide a method of feeding or administering medications that require minimal patient effort when the child is unable to suck or swallow adequately.
3. Gavage feedings can be used to administer supplemental calories to a patient who is unable to meet their caloric needs by mouth. They also can be used to provide full calories to those unable to tolerate oral intake.
4. Gavage feedings can prevent fatigue or cyanosis that can occur from bottle-feeding in susceptible infants. They can provide supplements for an infant who is a poor bottle-feeder.
5. Gavage feedings can provide a safe method of feeding patients with hypotonia, patients experiencing respiratory distress, patients with uncoordinated suck and swallow, patients that are intubated, patients with a debilitation, and patients with anomalies of the digestive tract.

Gastrostomy Feeding

KEY DECISION POINT If the gastrostomy tube becomes dislodged and if it is newly placed (less than 6 weeks), replace tube (if allowed in scope of practice) with gastrostomy tube or Foley catheter and secure tube. Frequently, a smaller size must be used if the stoma is closing. Notify health care provider before using the tube, as oftentimes imaging will be needed to confirm correct tube placement, and accurately record events.

If gastrostomy tube is established (more than 6 weeks) and dislodged, replace with a Foley catheter or comparable-sized gastrostomy tube and aspirate the tube for gastric contents. If gastric contents are obtained, feeds may be resumed. If there is difficulty verifying placement, notify the health care provider.

1. Gastrostomy feeding is a means of providing nourishment and fluids by way of a tube that is surgically inserted through an incision made through the abdominal wall into the stomach. A gastrostomy tube may also be placed surgically or by endoscopy using interventional radiology. Gastrostomy placement is the method of choice for those requiring tube feedings for an extended period of time (usually longer than 4 to 6 months).
2. Gastrostomy feedings provide a safe method of feeding a hypotonic or debilitated patient or one who cannot tolerate alternative methods. Prolonged feeding problems occur frequently in those with physical disabilities, prematurity, and chronic disease. Gastrostomy feedings may provide a route that allows adequate calorie or fluid intake in a child with chronic lung disease or in one who does not have continuity of the gastrointestinal (GI) tract, such as in esophageal atresia, chronic reflux, or aspiration processes.
3. Gastrostomy tubes can also allow better decompression of the stomach because of larger tube size.

Community and Home Care Considerations

1. If gastrostomy feedings are likely to be ordered upon discharge, involve parental caregivers in early education. Ensure that home health team is ready to support patient and family immediately upon discharge.
2. Teach the child (if age appropriate) and parental caregivers about the gastrostomy tube and feeding regimen.
   a. Anatomy of tube placement.
   b. Type of gastrostomy tube (button or tube).
   c. Amount and timing of feedings.
   d. Signs and symptoms of problems—tube obstruction or displacement, distended stomach, infection.
   e. Appropriate actions to be taken if problems occur—call home care nurse or health care provider.
3. Teach use of equipment: syringes, feeding bag, feeding tubing.
4. Teach the use of feeding pump (for continuous feedings or slow boluses).
5. Teach care of the gastrostomy tube—how to clamp, observe for leakage, determine amount of water in the balloon, and change a gastrostomy tube at home, if the site is mature and family is willing to learn.
6. Teach stoma care—clean area with soap and water, observe for breakdown, and apply skin barrier cream or powder, as appropriate.
7. Instruct about formula—proper mixing if not reconstituted; need to refrigerate if opened; discard any unused and nonrefrigerated formula after 4 hours.
8. Teach measures to take in an emergency.
   a. Procedure to follow if the tube falls out—replace tube (gastrostomy or Foley catheter), secure and cover site with gauze dressing, and call health care provider or proceed to emergency room if the tube has been in place less than 6 weeks. If tube has been in place for longer than 6 weeks, the tube may be replaced by the family or home care nurse.

b. Troubleshooting for nonfunctioning equipment—ensure that the pump is plugged in and turned on; tubing is unclamped, not kinked; and abdomen is not distended.
c. Proper phone numbers available to have as a resource or to obtain assistance.

9. Perform regular home visits as prescribed to assess nutritional and hydration status of the child, check tube placement and stoma site, and modify the care plan, as needed.

Nasojejunal and Nasoduodenal Feedings

KEY DECISION POINT If abdominal pain, distention, diarrhea, or vomiting occurs, stop feeds and check emesis and stools for gross blood and report to health care provider immediately—this may be a sign of necrotizing enterocolitis.

1. NJ or nasoduodenal (ND) feedings are means of providing full enteral feedings by way of a catheter passed through the nares, past the pharynx, down the esophagus, through the stomach, through the pylorus into the duodenum or jejunum.
2. Duodenal or jejunal feedings may decrease the risk of aspiration and can minimize regurgitation and gastric distention because the feeding bypasses the stomach and pylorus.
3. ND and NJ feedings provide a route that allows for adequate calorie or fluid intake (a full enteral feeding) by way of continuous drip.
4. ND or NJ feedings may also provide a route for administration of enteral medications.
5. ND or NJ feedings can provide a method of feeding that requires minimal patient effort when the child or infant is unable to tolerate alternative feeding methods (low birth weight, increased respiratory effort, and intubated patient).
6. ND or NJ feeding tubes may be placed under fluoroscopy, endoscopically, or at the bedside.

Fluid and Electrolyte Balance

EVIDENCE BASE Zieg, J., Narla, D., Gonsorcikova, L., & Raina, R. (2024). Fluid management in children with volume depletion. *Pediatric Nephrology, 39*(2), 423–434. https://doi.org/10.1007/s00467-023-06080-z

Rooholamini, S., Jennings, B., Zhou, C., Kaiser, S., & Garber, M. (2022). Effect of a quality improvement bundle to standardize the use of intravenous fluids for hospitalized pediatric patients: A stepped-wedge, cluster randomized clinical trial. *JAMA Pediatrics, 176* (1), 26–33. https://doi.org/10.1001/jamapediatrics.2021.4267

Basic Principles

1. Infants and small children have different proportions of body water (see Table 39-3) and body fat than adults.
   a. The body water of a neonate is approximately 75% of body weight compared with that of an average adult person assigned male at birth, which is approximately 60%.
   b. The typical neonate demonstrates a rapid physiologic decline in the ratio of body weight to body water during the immediate postpartum period.
   c. Proportion of body water declines more slowly throughout infancy and reaches the characteristic value for adults by about age 2 years.

Table 39-3 Body Fluids Expressed as Percentage of Body Weight

	ADULT		INFANT
FLUID	MALE[a] (%)	FEMALE[a] (%)	MALE OR FEMALE[a] (%)
Total body fluids	60	54	75
Intracellular	40	36	35
Extracellular	20	18	40

[a]*Please note that the term "male" in this table refers to a person assigned male at birth, and the term "female" in this table refers to a person assigned female at birth.*

2. Compared with adults, a greater percentage of the body water of infants and small children is contained in the extracellular compartment.
   a. Infants—approximately one half of the body water is extracellular.
   b. Adults—approximately one third of the body water is extracellular.
3. Compared with adults, the water turnover rate per unit of body weight is three or more times greater in infants and small children.
   a. The child has more body surface in relation to weight.
   b. The immaturity of kidney function in infants may impair their ability to conserve water.
4. Electrolyte balance depends on fluid balance and cardiovascular, renal, adrenal, pituitary, parathyroid, and pulmonary regulatory mechanisms (see Table 39-4).
5. Infants and children are more vulnerable to dehydration than adults.
   a. The basic principles relating to fluid balance in children make the magnitude of fluid losses considerably greater in children than in adults.
   b. Children are prone to severe disturbances of the GI tract that result in diarrhea and vomiting.
   c. Young children cannot independently respond to increased losses by increased intake. They depend on others to provide them with adequate fluid.

Common Fluid and Electrolyte Therapy

1. Repair of preexisting deficits that may occur with prolonged or severe diarrhea or vomiting.
   a. Deficits are estimated and corrected as soon and as safely as possible.
   b. Initial therapy is aimed at restoring intravascular and intracellular fluid volume to relieve or prevent shock and restore renal function.
   c. Intracellular deficits are replaced slowly over an 8- to 12-hour period after the circulatory status is improved.
2. Provision of maintenance requirements.
   a. Maintenance requirements occur as a result of normal expenditures of water and electrolytes because of metabolism.
   b. Maintenance requirements bear a close relationship to metabolic rate and are ideally formulated in terms of caloric expenditure.

Table 39-4 Common Anomalies of Fluid and Electrolyte Metabolism

SUBSTANCE AND MAJOR FUNCTION	ANOMALY	CAUSE	CLINICAL MANIFESTATION	LABORATORY DATA
Water				
Medium of body fluids, chemical changes, body temperature, lubricant	Volume deficit	• Primary—inadequate water intake • Secondary—loss following vomiting, diarrhea, and GI obstruction	Oliguria, weight loss, signs of dehydration including dry skin and mucous membranes, lassitude, sunken fontanelles, lack of tear formation, increased pulse rate, decreased blood pressure	Concentrated urine; azotemia; elevated hematocrit, hemoglobin level, erythrocyte count, and sodium level
	Volume excess	• Failure to excrete water in the presence of normal intake, such as in cardiac disease or failure or renal disease • Water intake in excess of output	Weight gain, peripheral edema, signs of pulmonary congestion	Variable urine volume, low specific gravity of urine, decreased hematocrit
Potassium				
Intracellular fluid balance, regular heart rhythm, muscle and nerve irritability	Potassium deficit	• Excessive loss of potassium because of vomiting, diarrhea, prolonged cortisone, corticotropin or diuretic therapy, diabetic acidosis • Shift of potassium into the cells, such as occurs with the healing phase of burns, recovery from diabetic acidosis	Signs and symptoms variable, including weakness, lethargy, irritability, abdominal distention, and, eventually, cardiac arrhythmias	Low plasma potassium level (<3.5 mEq/L) may be normal in some situations; hypochloremic alkalosis; ECG changes
	Potassium excess	• Excessive administration of potassium-containing solutions, excessive release of potassium because of burns, severe kidney disease, adrenal insufficiency • β-blocker therapy	Variable, including listlessness, confusion, heaviness of the legs, nausea, diarrhea, abdominal cramping, ECG changes, and, ultimately, paralysis and cardiac arrest	Elevated potassium plasma level; decreased arterial pH; ECG anomalies
Sodium				
Osmotic pressure, muscle and nerve irritability	Sodium deficit	• Water intake in excess of excretory capacity, replacement of fluid loss without sufficient sodium; excessive sodium losses	Headache, nausea, abdominal cramps, confusion alternating with stupor, diarrhea, lacrimation, salivation, later hypotension; early polyuria, later oliguria	Sodium plasma level may be normal or low (<135 mEq/L).
	Sodium excess	• Inadequate water intake especially in the presence of fever or sweating; increased intake without increased output; decreased output	Thirst, oliguria, weakness, muscular pain, excitement, dry mucous membranes, hypotension, tachycardia, fever, agitation	Elevated sodium plasma level (>148 mEq/L), high plasma volume
Bicarbonate				
Acid–base balance	Primary bicarbonate deficit	• Diarrhea (especially in infants), diabetes mellitus, starvation, infectious disease, shock or cardiac failure producing tissue anoxia and renal failure	Progressively increasing rate and depth of respiration—ultimately becoming Kussmaul respiration; flushed, warm skin; weakness; disorientation progressive to coma	• Urine pH usually <6.0 • Plasma bicarbonate <20 mEq/L • Plasma pH <7.35
	Primary bicarbonate excess	• Loss of chloride through vomiting, gastric suction, or the use of excessive diuretics; excessive ingestion of alkali	Depressed respiration, muscle hypertonicity, hyperactive reflexes, tingling of fingers and toes, tetany, and, sometimes, convulsions	Urine pH usually >7, plasma bicarbonate >26 mEq/L (30 mEq/L in adults), plasma pH >7.45

ECG, electrocardiographic; GI, gastrointestinal.

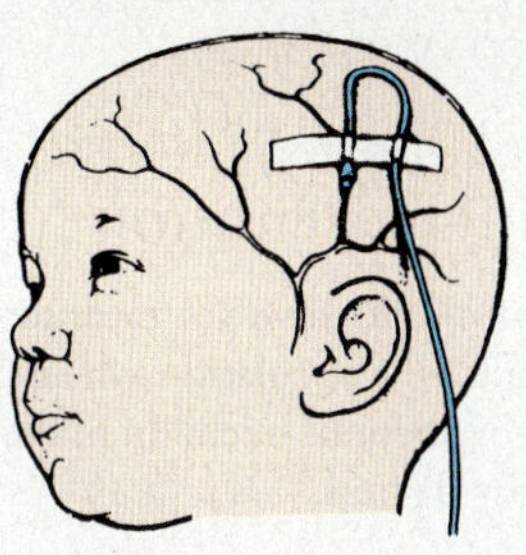
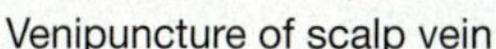

Venipuncture of scalp vein

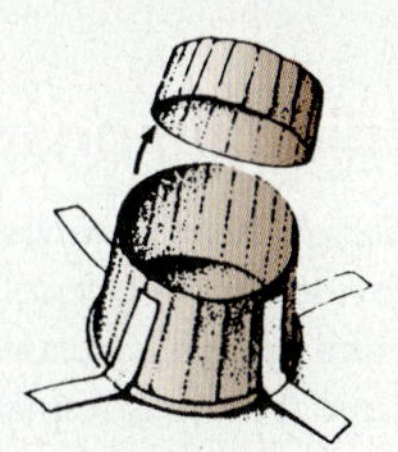

Paper cup taped over venipuncture site for protection. A clear plastic cup may also be used.

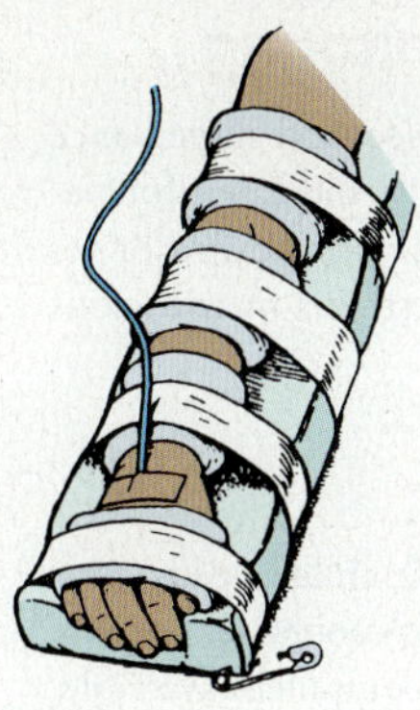

Restraint of arm when hand is site of infusion

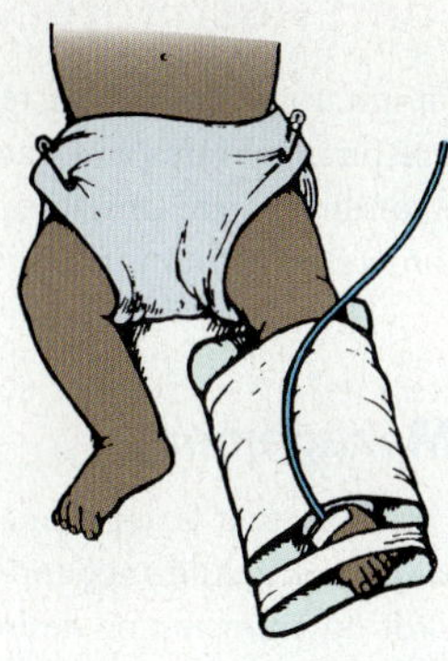

Infant's leg taped to sandbag for immobilization (IV site should be visible)

Figure 39-2. Intravenous (IV) fluid therapy.

3. Correction of concurrent losses that may occur by way of the GI tract as a result of vomiting, diarrhea, or drainage of secretions.
4. Replacement should be similar in type and amount to the fluid being lost.
5. Replacement is usually formulated as milliliters of fluid and milliequivalents of electrolytes lost.

Intravenous Fluid Therapy

IV therapy refers to the infusion of fluids directly into the venous system. This may be accomplished through the use of a needle or by venous cut down and insertion of a small catheter directly into the vein (see Figure 39-2). IV therapy is used to restore and maintain the child's fluid and electrolyte balance and body homeostasis when oral intake is inadequate to serve this purpose.

1. Infusion pumps are often used in pediatrics to provide a controlled, constant rate of infusion.
2. Because infants and children are vulnerable to fluid shifts, the rates need to be monitored carefully.
3. During an IV infusion, every hour, check the following:
   a. Rate of infusion.
   b. Volume delivered.
   c. IV site for infiltration, because many pumps will continue to infuse solution even if infiltration has occurred.

See Standards of Care Guidelines 39-1.

STANDARDS OF CARE GUIDELINES 39-1

Pediatric IV Therapy

When caring for a child undergoing IV therapy:

- Check IV site hourly, noting skin color and evidence of swelling. Compare to the opposite extremity or look for asymmetry. Feel area for sponginess. Observe for leakage.
- Check the IV tubing and equipment hourly. Stop the infusion if any cracks are noted in the tubing or there is discoloration of the IV fluid.
- Record the reading on the container or reservoir, amount of fluid absorbed in the hour, flow rate.
- Check for blood return in the tube by stopping IV fluid flow. It may be normal not to see blood return due to small catheter size.
- Check function of pump rate set versus amount infused.
- Maintain accurate intake and output record and 24-hour totals.
- Describe consistency and approximate volume of all stools and vomitus.
- Weigh child at regular intervals, using the same scale each time. An increase or decrease of 5% body weight in a relatively brief time period is usually significant.
- Monitor electrolytes (see Table 39-4, page 1156).
- Report evidence of electrolyte imbalances: decreased skin turgor, marked increase or decrease in urination, fever, sunken or bulging fontanelles, sudden change in vital signs, diarrhea, weakness, lethargy, apathy, pyrogenic reactions, and arrhythmias.
- If the child is experiencing severe reactions, the IV should be discontinued and the solution saved for possible analysis.
- Change the IV container and tubing every 24 hours or as per facility policy.
- If infiltration occurs, remove the IV, raise the affected extremity, apply heat to the site, and restart the IV at an alternative site. Notify the health care provider if irritation develops or toxic medication has infiltrated.

This information should serve as a general guideline only. Each patient situation presents a unique set of clinical factors and requires nursing judgment to guide care, which may include additional or alternative measures and approaches.

IV, intravenous.

Cardiac and Respiratory Monitoring

Cardiac and respiratory monitoring refers to electrical surveillance of heart and respiratory rates and patterns. It is indicated for patients whose conditions are unstable, patients with cardiac or respiratory disorders, and patients receiving anesthesia or conscious sedation.

Nursing Management

1. Select a monitor that is appropriate for the child's needs. This will depend on the child's age and ability to cooperate, purpose for monitoring, information desired, and equipment available.
2. Stabilize the device to reduce the amount of mechanical noise and for safety considerations. Ensure the equipment is functioning well and there are no frayed cords. Plug into an emergency power outlet.
3. Reduce the child's anxiety:
   a. Provide age-appropriate explanations of the equipment.
   b. When possible, involve the child in care, including change of electrodes.
4. Select lead placement sites according to equipment specifications:
   a. Cardiac monitors frequently use three leads located at:
      i. Right upper chest wall below the clavicle.
      ii. Left lower chest wall in the anterior axillary line.
      iii. Left upper chest wall below the clavicle.
   b. Respiratory monitors frequently use three electrodes located:
      i. On either side of the chest (anterior axillary line in fourth or fifth intercostal space).
      ii. A reference electrode placed on the manubrium or other suitable distal point.
5. Apply electrodes by:
   a. Cleaning the appropriate areas on the chest with soap and water.
   b. Placing pre-gelled, disposable electrodes to dry skin.
6. Plug the leads into the lead cable at appropriate insertion points.
7. Make sure that the monitor alarms are in the "on" position. High- and low-alarm limits should be set according to the child's age and condition so that apnea, tachypnea, bradycardia, and tachycardia can be readily detected.
8. Avoid skin breakdown by changing lead placement sites, as needed. Clean and dry old sites and expose them to air.
9. Check integrity of the entire system at least once per shift.
   a. Carefully inspect lead wires and cable for breaks and proper attachment.
   b. If malfunction is suspected, change equipment and notify the engineering department or manufacturer immediately.
10. Continue to count respiratory and apical rates at least once per shift.
   a. Compare with monitor rates to verify accuracy of equipment.
   b. It must be remembered that monitors cannot substitute for close observation and nursing assessments of the child.

EVIDENCE BASE Topjian, A., Raymond, T., Atkins, D., Chan, M., Duff, J., Joyner, B., Lasa, J., Lavonas, E., Levy, A., Mahgoub, M., Meckler, G., Roberts, K., Sutton, R., & Schexnayder, S. (2020). Part 4: Pediatric basic and advanced life support: 2020 American Heart Association Guidelines for cardiopulmonary resuscitation and emergency cardiovascular care. *Circulation, 142*(16_Suppl_2), S469–S523. https://doi.org/10.1161/CIR.0000000000000901.

Cardiopulmonary Resuscitation

Cardiopulmonary resuscitation (CPR) involves measures instituted to provide effective ventilation and circulation when the patient's heart and lungs have ceased to function. In children, the most common initial cause is respiratory distress.

Underlying Considerations

Cardiac Arrest

1. Signs—absence of heartbeat and absence of carotid and femoral pulses.
2. Causes—asystole, ventricular fibrillation, cardiovascular collapse, shock, or progression of respiratory failure.

Respiratory Arrest

1. Signs—apnea and cyanosis.
2. Causes—obstructed airway, depression of the central nervous system, neuromuscular paralysis.

Emergency Preparation

1. Every hospital should have a well-defined and organized plan to be carried out in the event of cardiac or respiratory arrest.
2. Emergency carts should be placed in strategic locations in the hospital and checked daily to ensure that all equipment is available.
3. Personnel should be trained in up-to-date CPR maneuvers and be certified in basic life support at least every 2 years.

Equipment

1. Emergency cart—assembled and ready for use.
2. Positive pressure breathing bag with nonrebreathing valve and universal 15-mm adapter.
3. Mask (premature neonate, child, adult sizes).
4. Oropharyngeal airway tubes, sizes 0 to 4.
5. Laryngoscope with blades of various sizes.
6. Extra batteries and light bulbs for laryngoscope.
7. Endotracheal tubes with connectors (complete sterile set, 2.5- to 8-mm inner diameter).
8. Portable suction equipment and sterile catheters of various sizes.
9. Bulb syringe, DeLee trap.
10. Oxygen source—portable supply, gauge, and tubing.
11. Cardiac board (30 × 50 cm).
12. Emergency drugs:
   a. Sodium bicarbonate.
   b. Epinephrine.
   c. Isoproterenol.
   d. Normal saline solution (for dilution).
   e. Diphenhydramine.
   f. Diazepam.
   g. Hydrocortisone sodium succinate.
   h. Digoxin.
   i. Naloxone.
   j. Calcium gluconate.
   k. Calcium chloride 10%.
   l. Dextrose 50%.
   m. Lidocaine.
   n. Atropine.

o. Phenytoin.
p. Insulin.
q. Procainamide.
r. Propranolol.
s. Dopamine.
t. Bretylium tosylate.
u. Volume expanders (lactated Ringer's solution, normal saline solution).
v. Vasopressin.
w. Amiodarone.
x. Magnesium sulfate.
y. Vecuronium.

13. Intracardiac needles, 20G and 22G, 2 to 3 in long.
14. IV equipment, including infusion set, IV fluids.
15. Tourniquet, arm boards, and tape.
16. Scalp vein needles of various sizes.
17. Gloves, mask, gown, other protective barriers.
18. Nasogastric tubes of various sizes.
19. Syringes and syringe needles of various sizes.
20. Intraosseous needles.
21. Long dwell catheters of various sizes.
22. Three-way stopcock.
23. Cutdown set.
24. Alcohol wipes.
25. Tongue blades.
26. Sterile 4" × 4" gauze pads.
27. Sterile hemostat.
28. Sterile scissors.
29. Blood specimen tubes.
30. Electrocardiograph (ECG) monitor, lead wires.
31. Defibrillator and paddles (pediatric and adult), lubricating jelly.
32. Arrest documentation record and patient-specific labels.

Artificial Ventilation

Mouth-to-Mouth Technique

1. Infants:
   a. Slightly extend neck by gently pulling chin up and forward and the head back by pressing forehead into a neutral position (known as head tilt–chin lift; use jaw thrust if cervical trauma is suspected). Place a rolled towel or diaper under the infant's shoulder or use one hand to support the neck in an extended position. Do not hyperextend the neck because this narrows the airway.
   b. Check the mouth and throat, and clear mucus or vomitus with finger or suction, if visible.
   c. Take a breath.
   d. Make a tight seal with your mouth over the infant's mouth and nose.
   e. Gently blow air from the cheeks and observe for chest rise. Give a total of two slow breaths.
   f. Remove your mouth from infant's mouth and nose and allow the infant to exhale.
   g. If spontaneous respiration does not return, continue breathing at a rate and volume appropriate for the size of the infant (usually 12 to 20 times/min or 1 breath every 3 to 5 seconds).
2. Children older than 1 year:
   a. Clear mouth of mucus or vomitus with fingers or suction.
   b. Extend neck with one hand or a rolled towel (head tilt, chin lift, or jaw thrust, if cervical trauma is suspected).
   c. Clamp the nostrils with the fingers of one hand, which also continues to exert pressure on the forehead to maintain the neck extension.
   d. Take a deep breath.
   e. Make a tight seal with your mouth over the child's mouth.
   f. Force air into the lungs until chest expansion is observed.
   g. Release your mouth from the child's mouth and release nostrils to allow the child to exhale passively. Give a total of two slow breaths.
   h. Repeat approximately 10 to 12 times/min or 1 breath every 5 to 6 seconds if spontaneous breathing does not occur.

Hand-Operated Ventilation Devices

1. Remove secretions from mouth and throat and move chin forward.
2. Appropriately extend the neck with one hand or place a diaper roll behind the neck.
3. Select an appropriate-sized mask to obtain an adequate seal and connect mask to bag.
4. Hold the mask snugly over the mouth and nose, holding the chin forward and the neck in extension.
5. Squeeze the bag, noting inflation of the lungs by chest expansion. If there is no chest expansion, realign the patient's head and adjust the mask; retry.
6. Release the bag, which will expand spontaneously. The child will exhale and the chest will fall.
7. Repeat 12 to 20 times/min (depending on the size of the child).
8. Because this technique is commonly difficult to master, it should be practiced in advance, under supervision.

Indications of Effective Technique

1. Patient's chest rises and falls.
2. Rescuer can feel in their own airway the resistance and compliance of the patient's lungs as they expand.
3. Rescuer can hear and feel the air escape during exhalation.
4. Patient's color improves.

Management of Complications

1. Gastric distention (occurs frequently if excessive pressure is used for inflation).
   a. Turn patient's head and shoulders to one side.
   b. Exert moderate pressure over the epigastrium between the umbilicus and the rib cage.
   c. A nasogastric tube may be used to decompress the stomach.
2. Vomiting.
   a. Turn patient on side for drainage.
   b. Clear the airway with finger or suction.
   c. Resume ventilations after the airway is clear and patent.

Artificial Circulation

General Principles Related to Artificial Circulation

See Table 39-5, page 1160. See also Figure 39-3, page 1161.

1. A backward tilt of the head lifts the back in infants and small children. A firm support beneath the back is therefore essential if external cardiac compression is to be effective.
2. A supine position on a firm surface is mandatory. Only in this position can chest compression squeeze the heart against the immobile spine enough to force blood into the systemic circulation.
3. Because most infant/child cardiac arrests are the result of respiratory failure or shock, there is a decrease in the oxygen levels in the blood prior to the arrest. Thus, chest compressions alone

Table 39-5 Technique of Artificial Circulation

SIZE OF CHILD	PREPARATORY PHASE	ACTION PHASE	COMPRESSION	RATE
Neonate, premature, or otherwise small infant	1. Place in supine position. 2. Encircle the chest with the hands, with thumbs over the midsternum. *or* Use method for a larger infant.	Compress midsternum with both thumbs, gently but firmly.	1/3 the depth of the chest (~1½ in)	At least 100/min
Larger infant	1. Place on a firm, flat surface. 2. Support the back with one hand or use a small blanket under the shoulders. 3. Place the tips of the index and middle fingers of one hand over the midsternum, just below the nipple line.	1. Compress the midsternum with the tips of the index and middle fingers.	1/3 the depth of the chest (~1½–2 in)	At least 100/min
Small child	1. Place on a firm, flat surface. 2. Support the back by slipping one hand beneath it, or use a small blanket. 3. Place the heel of one hand over the midsternum, parallel with the long axis of the body (at the nipple line).	1. Apply a rapid downward thrust to the midsternum, keeping the elbow straight. 2. Instantly and completely release the pressure so the chest wall can recoil. 3. Do not remove the heel of the hand from the chest.	1/3 the depth of the chest (~2 in)	At least 100/min
Larger child, adolescent	1. Place on a flat, firm surface, or place a board under the thorax. 2. Place the heel of one hand on the lower half of the sternum, about 1–1½ in (2.5–3.8 cm) from the tip of the xiphoid process and parallel with the long axis of the body. 3. Place the other hand on top of the first one (may interlock fingers). 4. Place shoulders directly over child's sternum, to use own weight in application of pressure.	1. Exert pressure vertically downward to depress lower sternum, keeping elbows straight. 2. Instantly and completely release the pressure so the chest wall can recoil. 3. Do not remove the hands from the chest.	2 in (5 cm)	At least 100/min

are not an effective method for delivering oxygen to the heart and brain.

4. This is different from cardiac arrest in an adult, in which the blood usually has a high level of oxygen and compressions alone are an effective way to deliver oxygen to the heart and brain.
5. Compressions must be regular, smooth, and uninterrupted. Avoid sudden or jerking movements. Push hard and push fast. Compressions should be done at a rate of at least 100 compressions/min.
6. The chest must recoil (return to normal position) fully after each compression.
7. Between compressions, the fingers or heel of the hand must completely release their pressure but should remain in constant contact with the chest. This allows for complete recoil of the chest while minimizing interruptions to the compressions.
8. Fingers should not rest on the patient's ribs during compression. Pressure with fingers on the ribs or lateral pressure increases the possibility of fractured ribs and costochondral separation.
9. Never compress the xiphoid process at the tip of the sternum. Pressure on it may cause laceration of the liver.
10. Indications of effective technique include the following:
    a. A palpable femoral or carotid pulse.
    b. Decrease in size of pupils.
    c. Improvement in the patient's color.

Nursing Management

1. Recognize cardiac and respiratory arrest.
2. Send for assistance and note time.
3. Initiate CPR:
    a. Check for responsiveness and breathing; if the patient is unresponsive and not breathing, palpate a pulse. Checking for a pulse should not take more than 10 seconds.
    b. If no pulse is felt, institute artificial circulation using appropriate technique.
    c. For an infant or child, each cycle contains a ratio of 30 compressions to two breaths, starting with compressions.
    d. Continue repeating this cycle until help arrives.
    e. If alone, perform CPR as previously described for five cycles or 2 minutes of CPR, then call for help. After call, resume CPR until help arrives.
4. When help arrives:
    a. One rescuer performs mouth-to-mouth resuscitation or institutes bag breathing.

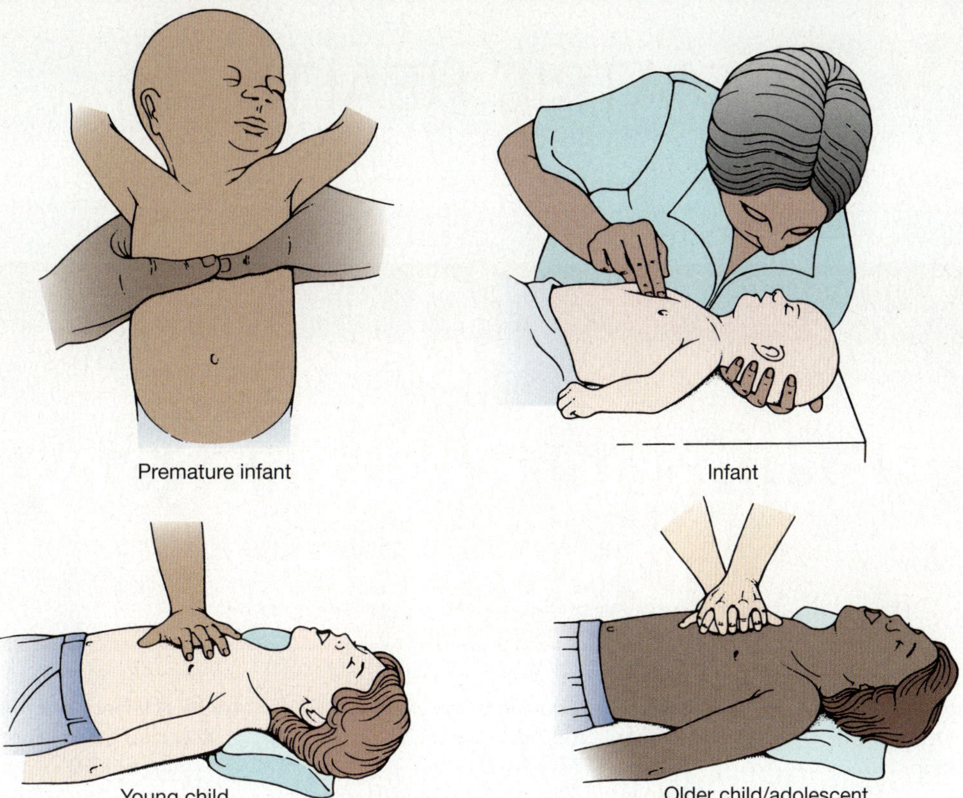

Figure 39-3. Cardiopulmonary resuscitation in children. In the premature infant, encircle the chest with the hands, with thumbs over the midsternum. In the infant, place the tips of the index and middle fingers of one hand over the midsternum, just below the nipple line. In the young child, the heel of the hand is placed over the lower sternum at the nipple line. In older children and adolescents, both hands are used.

   b. Another rescuer performs cardiac compressions.
   c. A ratio of 15 compressions to two breaths is maintained for both infants and children.
   d. Cardiac compression should not be stopped for respiration. Breaths should be interposed on the upstroke of each fifth cardiac compression.
5. Anticipate and assist with emergency procedures.
   a. Assist with intubation, monitoring, placement of intravascular access, administration of IV fluids, defibrillation, and other definitive measures.
   b. Prepare and administer emergency medications, as prescribed. Record dose and time.
   c. Notify family of current management and CPR.
6. After resuscitation:
   a. Care for the child, as required.
   b. Determine if family members have been notified and are being cared for.
   c. Record all events.
   d. Restock emergency cart.

SELECTED READINGS

Anderson, C., Shikofski, N., Kapoor, S., Lee, C., Mark, T., & The Johns Hopkins Hospital. (2023). *The Harriet Lane handbook* (23rd ed.). Elsevier.

Easson, W. (1981). *The dying child: The management of the child or adolescent who is dying* (2nd ed.). Charles C. Thomas Publishing.

Edwards, F. (2020). National children's hospitals bereavement network standards for supporting families following the death of a child. *Nursing Children and Young People, 32*(6), 14–18. https://doi.org/10.7748/ncyp.2020.e1336

Ernst, K. (2020). Resources recommended for the care of pediatric patients in hospitals. *Pediatrics, 145*(4), e20200204. https://doi.org/10.1542/peds.2020-0204

Feld, L., Neuspiel. D., Foster, B., Leu, M., Garber,M., Austin, K., Basu, R., Conway, E., Fehr, J., Hawkins, C., Kaplan, R., Rowe, E., Waseem, M., & Moritz, M. (2018). Clinical practice guideline: Maintenance intravenous fluids in children. *Pediatrics, 142*(6), e20183083. https://doi.org/10.1542/peds.2018-3083.

Friedrichsdorf, S. J., & Goubert, L. (2020). Pediatric pain treatment and prevention for hospitalized children. *PAIN Reports, 5*(1), e804. https://doi.org/10.1097/pr9.0000000000000804

Halpern, L. (2021). New guidelines for prescribing opioids to children and teens after surgery. *American Journal of Nursing, 121*(3), 18–19. https://doi.org/10.1097/01.NAJ.0000737268.29194.7d

Kennedy, M., & Howlin, F. (2022). Preparation of children for elective surgery and hospitalisation: A parental perspective. *Journal of Child Health Care, 26*(4), 568–580. https://doi.org/10.1177/13674935211032804

Larson, S. (2022). Vascular access in children: Background, indications, options for vascular access. *EMedicine*. https://emedicine.medscape.com/article/1018395-overview#a3

Lombart, B., De Stefano, C., Dupont, D., Nadji, L., & Galinski, M. (2020). Caregivers blinded by the care: A qualitative study of physical restraint in pediatric care. *Nursing Ethics, 27*(1), 230–246. https://doi.org/10.1177/0969733019833128

Mitchell, E., Jones, P., & Snelling, P. (2022). Ultrasound for pediatric peripheral intravenous catheter insertion: A systematic review. *Pediatrics, 149*(5), e2021055523. https://doi.org/10.1542/peds.2021-055523

Ring, L., Rana, M., & Deutsch, N. (2023). Implementation of a non-sedated procedural pain management practice guideline order set. *Pediatric Nursing, 49*(1), 12–20. https://www.proquest.com/openview/b5abd4651d823ebd1272a3b0ed6e9f2d/1?pq-origsite=gscholar&cbl=47659

Schondelmeyer, A., Dewan, M., Brady, P., Timmon, K., Cable, R., & Britto, M. (2020). Cardiorespiratory and pulse oximetry in hospitalized children: A Delphi process. *Pediatrics, 146*(2), 1–10. https://doi.org/10.1542/peds.2019-3336

Wathen, B., McNeely, H., Peyton, C., Pan, Z., Thomas, R., Callahan, C., Fidanza, S., Brown, J., & Neu, M. (2021). Comparison of electromagnetic guided imagery to standard confirmatory methods for ascertaining nasogastric tube placement in children. *Journal for Specialists in Pediatric Nursing, 26*(4), 1–9. https://doi.org/10.1111/jspn.12338

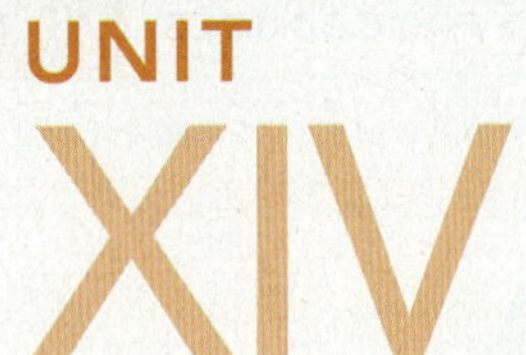

PEDIATRIC HEALTH

40 Pediatric Respiratory Disorders

PEDIATRIC RESPIRATORY PROCEDURES

See additional online content: Procedure Guidelines 40-1

Oxygen Therapy

Children with respiratory problems may receive oxygen therapy via nasal cannula, mask, face tent, high-flow nasal cannula, endotracheal (ET) tube, or tracheostomy device (see pages 146 to 148). An Isolette or oxygen hood may also be used for infants and young children.

Mechanical Ventilation

Infants and children requiring mechanical ventilation need specialized care. These patients are typically treated in facilities that focus on providing a safe environment for technology-dependent children, with care provided by highly skilled nurses, nurse practitioners, respiratory therapists, and pediatricians. Specific nursing procedures and interventions and management of technology-dependent infants and children are beyond the scope of this book. General considerations are as follows.

Maintenance of a Patent Airway

1. Artificial airway options include nasotracheal, orotracheal, and tracheostomy. ET and tracheostomy tubes are available in several sizes, cuffed and uncuffed, for the pediatric population.
   a. Several methods are available to determine the appropriate size, such as ET tube size = age in years + 16 divided by 4 (consult facility policy).
2. The patient should be closely monitored for hypoxia and bradycardia during intubation.
   a. Only experienced and highly trained and skilled practitioners should perform intubation.
   b. Resuscitation and reintubation equipment and access to oxygen and suction equipment must always be readily available.
   c. An appropriately sized self-inflating bag with reservoir for oxygenation and mask should remain with the patient.
3. Action should be taken to prevent dislodgement of the artificial airway (especially during movement of the child) and obstruction of the airway.
   a. Pediatric ET tubes have small diameters and are easily obstructed by thick secretions.
   b. Adequate humidification will loosen secretions, and suctioning will prevent airway obstruction.
   c. Frequent vital signs and respiratory assessments are necessary. Cardiorespiratory monitors, pulse oximeter, end-tidal carbon dioxide, or transcutaneous carbon dioxide monitors are also necessary.
4. Nursing care should address issues of hydration, nutrition, sedation, skin integrity, tissue perfusion, infection control, communication, safety, and parental caregiver support and education.
5. Available ventilators for pediatric use have a wide range of capabilities, versatility, and clinical application. Some are more suitable for use with infants; others with older children.

a. Nurses must be well acquainted with the characteristics of the particular ventilator being used and the meaning of the settings and alarms on each of the various machines.

Nursing Management

See Chapter 6, page 150. In addition, the nurse who is caring for a pediatric patient should remember the following:

Setting Controls

In setting controls, inspiratory flow rate will be less and the respiratory rate greater than in the adult patient. These parameters depend on the patient's size and condition and are determined by the health care provider or respiratory therapist.

Humidification

During ventilation of an infant in an incubator, the amount of ventilator tubing outside the incubator should be kept to a minimum. The warm temperature inside the incubator helps decrease the amount of condensation in the tubing and thus provides higher water content in the inspired gas.

Oxygen Concentration

1. In infants, inspired concentrations of oxygen should always be kept as low as possible (while still providing for physiologic requirements) to prevent the development of retinopathy of prematurity or pulmonary oxygen toxicity.
2. The oxygen concentration should be checked periodically with an analyzer.

Blood Gases

1. Blood gas analysis, via arterial puncture, umbilical or arterial lines, is necessary to monitor oxygenation.
2. The arterialized capillary sample method is inaccurate for infants in respiratory distress because the constricted peripheral circulation may not reflect the arterial blood gases (ABGs) levels accurately.

Sterile Precautions

The neonate has only those antibodies transferred across the placenta from the birthing parent. Therefore, sterile precautions are essential.

1. Ventilator tubing should be changed every 24 hours or per hospital policy.
2. Routine cultures should be taken after intubation; may include frequent Gram staining of secretions.
3. Suctioning requires aseptic technique.

Tubing Support

1. Special frames are available to support ventilator tubing; this helps to prevent accidental decannulation in infants and small children, especially when using uncuffed ET tubes.
2. Infants may require support or padding on either side and at the top of their heads to decrease mobility and fill space between the head and the frame.

Monitoring the Ventilator

1. Pressure gauges should be checked at frequent intervals as this gives an indication of changing compliance or increased airway resistance.
2. Volume measurements are difficult to obtain in infants because most spirometers incorporated into ventilators and meters do not read accurately at low volumes and flows. However, they are helpful with older children.
3. Measure respiratory rates of the machine and the patient at least every hour and record.

DISORDERS

See additional online content: Procedure Guidelines 40-2

Common Pediatric Respiratory Infections

Respiratory tract infection is a frequent cause of acute illness in infants and children. Many pediatric respiratory infections are seasonal. The child's response to the infection will vary based on the age of the child, causative organism, general health of the child, and existence of chronic medical conditions. Information about specific respiratory infections, including bacterial pneumonia, viral pneumonia, *Pneumocystis* pneumonia, *Mycoplasma* pneumonia, bronchiolitis, croup, and epiglottitis, may be found in Figure 40-1 and Table 40-1, pages 1163 to 1173.

Nursing Assessment

Determine the severity of the respiratory distress that the child is experiencing. Make an initial nursing assessment.

1. Observe the respiratory rate and pattern. Count the respirations for 1 full minute, document, and note level of activity, such as awake or asleep. Determine if the rate is appropriate for the child's age (see page 1090).
2. Observe respiratory rhythm and depth. Rhythm is described as regular, irregular, or periodic. Depth is normal, hypopnea or too shallow, and hyperpnea or too deep.
3. Auscultate breath sounds for a full cycle of inspiration and expiration over all lung fields. Note airflow and presence of adventitious sounds such as crackles, wheeze, or stridor.
4. Observe degree of respiratory effort—normal, difficult, or labored. Normal breathing is effortless and easy.
5. Document character of dyspnea or labored breathing; continuous, intermittent, worsening, or sudden onset. Note relation

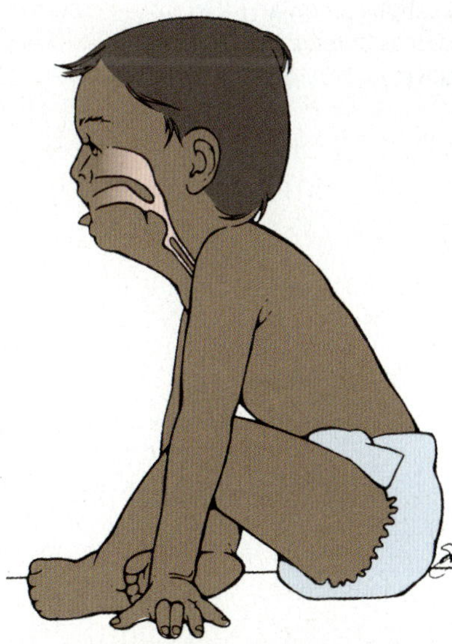

Figure 40-1. Characteristic posture of a child with acute epiglottitis: leaning forward on hands, in the "tripod" position; mouth open, tongue out, head forward, and tilted up in a sniffing position in an effort to relieve the acute airway obstruction secondary to swollen epiglottis.

Table 40-1 Common Pediatric Respiratory Infections

CONDITION AND CAUSATIVE AGENT	AGE AND INCIDENCE	CLINICAL MANIFESTATIONS
Bacterial Pneumonia Bacterial infection of the lung parenchyma General considerations: In the normal child, bacterial pneumonias are not common. A viral respiratory infection commonly occurs before bacterial pneumonia. The initial viral infection alters the lungs' defense mechanisms.		
Pneumococcal pneumonia The most common causative agent is *Streptococcus pneumoniae.*	• Responsible for the majority of bacterial pneumonias in ages 1 mo through 6 yr. However, it is seen in all age groups. • The incidence has declined because of the use of the vaccine. • Most common in winter and spring **CLINICAL JUDGMENT** Pneumococcal polysaccharide vaccine provides protection from 23 types of *S. pneumoniae.* It is recommended for children age 2 yr and older with sickle cell disease, functional or anatomic asplenia, nephrotic syndrome, human immunodeficiency virus (HIV) infection, and Hodgkin disease before beginning cytoreduction therapy.	• *Infants:* Mild URI of several days' duration, poor feeding, decreased appetite • Abrupt onset of fever 102.2°F (39°C) or higher; restlessness, respiratory distress, air hunger, pallor, cyanosis (common), nasal flaring, retractions, grunting, tachypnea, tachycardia, irritability; may see abdominal distention due to swallowed air or ileus. • *Older child:* Mild URI, followed by fever up to 104.9°F (40.5°C), shaking chills, headache, decreased appetite, abdominal pain, vomiting, drowsiness, restlessness, irritability, lethargy, rhonchi, fine crackles, dry hacking cough, increased respirations, anxiety, occasionally circumoral cyanosis, pleuritic pain, diminished breath sounds; may develop a pleural effusion, empyema.
Streptococcal pneumonia • β-hemolytic Streptococcus group A	• Ages 3–5 yr. Uncommon, serious • An endemic influenza predisposes to streptococcal pneumonia and tracheobronchitis.	• Sudden onset, high fever, chills, worsening cough, pleuritic pain, respiratory distress, grunting, retractions, altered mental status, signs of shock, decreased capillary refill, tachycardia • May be insidious, mildly ill, low-grade fever • Severe infections—toxic shock syndrome with erythematous rash, desquamation, hypotension, hepatic dysfunction, renal involvement, vomiting and diarrhea, hematologic abnormalities, acute respiratory distress syndrome
Staphylococcal pneumonia • *Staphylococcus aureus,* gram-positive	• Most common in children ages 6 mo to 1 yr., October–May (rare)	• Predisposing factors: cystic fibrosis, maternal infection, immunodeficiency. • Usually preceded by a viral URI. Changes abruptly to high fever, cough, respiratory distress, tachypnea, grunting, nasal flaring, cyanosis, retractions. • Anxiety, lethargic, occasionally vomiting, diarrhea, anorexia, abdominal distention, toxic appearance.

DIAGNOSTIC EVALUATION	TREATMENT	NURSING CONSIDERATIONS	COMPLICATIONS
• Chest x-ray: Commonly does not correspond to clinical findings. • *Infants:* Patchy, diffuse areas follow a bronchial distribution, many limited areas of consolidation around smaller airways. • *Young and older child:* Lobar or segmental consolidation; pleural fluid may be present. • WBC count elevated, ABG analysis indicates hypoxemia. • *Cultures:* Sputum, nasopharyngeal secretions, pleural fluid, blood	• Oxygen • Penicillin G; penicillin allergy: erythromycin, trimethoprim–sulfamethoxazole, alternately amoxicillin, ampicillin, cefuroxime, cefotaxime, ceftriaxone, clindamycin, chloramphenicol • Because of the increased incidence of penicillinase-resistant pneumococci, all pneumococcal isolates should be tested for resistance. Vancomycin has been recommended for penicillin-resistant strains. • Bronchodilators	• Bed rest; monitor fluids, intake and output. Give oral fluids cautiously to avoid aspiration. Do not give oral fluids to a child in respiratory distress. • Administer oxygen with humidification. Perform frequent, thorough respiratory assessment. • Administer antipyretics as prescribed. • Change position frequently. Isolation procedures, as ordered or per facility policy	• Rare, but include bacteremia, empyema, pleural effusion, otitis media, sinusitis, meningitis, hemolytic uremic syndrome, lung abscess, necrotizing pneumonia
• Initial chest x-ray may be normal or slightly abnormal. Within 24 h, chest x-ray worsens. • Unilateral lobar disease, bilateral diffuse infiltrates with severe disease • Blood cultures, nasopharyngeal secretions cultured, throat swab, culture pleural fluid and lung aspirate • Leukocytosis, sedimentation rate increased, elevated serum ASO titer	• β-lactam antibiotics (amoxicillin, cefuroxime, cefdinir) are preferred for outpatient management. Macrolides antibiotics (azithromycin, clarithromycin) are useful in most school-aged children and adolescents.	• Administer antipyretics. • Provide humidified oxygen, as needed. Rest. Monitor intake and output.	• Empyema, toxic shock syndrome, severe respiratory compromise, pneumatoceles; can be life threatening.
• *Older infant/young child:* Elevated WBC count, especially polymorphonuclear cells • *Young infant:* WBC count may be normal, mild to moderate anemia. • Cultures—pleural fluid, lung aspirate, sputum, gastric aspirate, blood • If pulmonary fluid is purulent and of a large amount, closed chest drainage may be utilized. • Chest x-ray: Patchy infiltrate, may involve entire lobe or hemithorax Right lung involvement common; bilateral involvement is also seen. Pleural effusion, empyema, pyopneumothorax, pneumatoceles, pneumothorax, lung abscesses	• Thoracentesis • Nafcillin, oxacillin, methicillin, cefazolin, clindamycin, vancomycin. MRSA exists, especially in long-term care facilities or in patients with a prolonged hospital stay.	• Isolation per policy, check for MRSA, prevent nosocomial infection. • Rapid treatment is important. Administer antibiotics as soon as possible. Monitor for signs of tension pneumothorax. Monitor fluid status closely. • Strict handwashing • Staphylococcal pneumonia is rare and must be treated aggressively because of rapid onset and deterioration.	• Empyema, tension pneumothorax, abscess, fibrothorax, bronchiectasis, osteomyelitis, staphylococcal pericarditis; consider screening infants for cystic fibrosis and immunodeficiency.

(continued)

Table 40-1 Common Pediatric Respiratory Infections (*continued*)

CONDITION AND CAUSATIVE AGENT	AGE AND INCIDENCE	CLINICAL MANIFESTATIONS
***Haemophilus influenzae*, type B**	• Majority of children younger than age 4 yr • Infants and children who are not immunized • Winter and spring	• Usually preceded by URI Associated with otitis media, epiglottitis, and meningitis; appears toxic • Insidious onset; cough, febrile, tachypneic, nasal flaring, retractions
Viral Pneumonia		
• Respiratory syncytial virus (RSV); parainfluenza virus types 1, 2, 3; adenovirus types 1, 2, 5, 6 and types 3, 7, 11, 21; influenza A and B	• Peak age for bronchiolitis is within the first year of life. Peak age for viral pneumonia is age 2.3 yr. • Typically seen in the winter months	• Usually preceded by URI with symptoms of cough, rhinitis, and mild fever. Progressing to tachypnea, poor feeding in infants and retractions (suprasternal, intercostal, subcostal, and substernal), leading to nasal flaring. Along with use of accessory muscles, wheezing, severe cough, cyanosis, and respiratory fatigue. • Viral pneumonia may present concurrently with bacterial pneumonia. Adenovirus types 3, 7, 11, and 21 may cause severe necrotizing pneumonia in infants.
• RSV subgroup A (more virulent, associated with more severe disease); RSV subgroup B	• In infants, RSV is the most common cause of pneumonia, bronchiolitis, and hospitalizations. • Severity of RSV infection decreases with age and subsequent infections. • Peak age is 2–7 mo, October–April.	• Typically begins with URI, rhinorrhea, fever usually <102°F (38.9°C), otitis media, and conjunctivitis. • Progressing to coughing, wheezing, tachypnea (>70 breaths/min), intercostal and subcostal retractions, poor air exchange, hypoxia, decreased breath sounds, cyanosis, lethargy, listless apneic episodes, and irritability. Infants will present with poor feeding, inability to suck and breathe.

DIAGNOSTIC EVALUATION	TREATMENT	NURSING CONSIDERATIONS	COMPLICATIONS
• Chest x-ray: usually lobar infiltrates; however, segmental, single, or multiple lobe infiltrates are also seen. Pleural effusion, pneumatocele CBC: elevated WBC, lymphopenia • Cultures: blood, pleural fluid, lung aspirates, and nasal secretions; in the absence of a positive culture, a positive urine latex agglutination can confirm diagnosis. • If atelectasis is present, bronchoscopy to rule out foreign body.	• Patients may present receiving antibiotics for otitis media. • Ceftriaxone and other cephalosporins, ampicillin, chloramphenicol, azithromycin	• Administer antibiotics on time. • Ensure adequate hydration. Monitor for signs of upper respiratory impairment, drooling, stridor, and dusky color. • Respiratory isolation until 24 h after appropriate antibiotic therapy is initiated • Rifampin prophylaxis should be considered for close household contacts if there are: • Incomplete or unvaccinated members younger than age 2 yr • Immunocompromised child • Day care setting with two or more cases of invasive disease within 2 mo and incompletely vaccinated children in attendance • Not recommended for pregnant people	• Frequently in young infants, bacteremia, pericarditis, cellulitis, empyema, meningitis, pyarthrosis
• Chest x-ray shows patchy infiltrates, transient lobular infiltration, and hyperinflation • CBC: slightly elevated WBC count • Cultures: blood and nasopharyngeal secretions • Viral antigens for rapid diagnosis	• If bacterial pneumonia is suspected, administer antibiotics. • Supportive measures: IV fluids, antipyretics, humidified oxygen, assisted ventilation • Avoid aspirin because of risk of Reye syndrome. • Oseltamivir or zanamivir for influenza infection	• Monitor closely for signs of respiratory fatigue or distress. • Monitor oxygen saturation levels and response to oxygen therapy if hypoxic. • Close cardiac monitoring may be indicated. • Monitor for adequate hydration and nutritional status. Elevate infants up to an angle of 10–30 degrees to ease breathing. Infants and children who require mechanical ventilation require close supervision and frequent monitoring. Institute contact precautions with strict handwashing. • Prevention: influenza vaccine and RSV vaccine for those that qualify.	• Influenza: severe fulminant pneumonia with hemorrhagic exudate; death may result. Severe disease may be seen in children with cardiopulmonary disease, cystic fibrosis, bronchopulmonary dysplasia, and neurovascular disease. • Type B—myositis.
• Nasopharyngeal secretions for rapid antibody or assay for RSV antigen detection. • Chest x-ray: chest hyperexpanded, air trapping, multiple lobe infiltrates, atelectasis • ABG analysis • Pulse oximetry	• Supportive measures, such as oxygen, respiratory support, hydration • Bronchodilators should not be used routinely. • Racemic epinephrine can be effective in bronchiolitis. • Glucocorticoids and ribavirin are not supported in the literature. • Antibiotics only if a secondary bacterial infection is suspected	• Prevent nosocomial spread. Institute contact isolation. Strict handwashing • Patients who are RSV positive should not be in contact with other patient who are at high risk, such as those with chronic cardiac or respiratory illness or patient who are immunocompromised. • Assess frequently for signs of respiratory failure. • Use noninvasive oxygen monitoring.	• RSV can be fatal, especially in children with chronic cardiac and respiratory diseases, premature infants, and those with underlying neuromuscular or immunologic diseases. • Respiratory failure, intubation, and mechanical ventilation • In older children with asthma, RSV can cause an acute asthmatic episode.

(continued)

Table 40-1 Common Pediatric Respiratory Infections (*continued*)

CONDITION AND CAUSATIVE AGENT	AGE AND INCIDENCE	CLINICAL MANIFESTATIONS
***Pneumocystis carinii* Pneumonia (PCP)**		
• *P. carinii*, also known as *P. jirovecii*, is a fungus with similarities to protozoa. The organism exists in three forms in the tissues: trophozoite, sporozoite, and cyst.	• Most healthy humans are infected before age 4 yr and are asymptomatic. • Life-threatening pneumonia is seen in the immunosuppressed host. PCP in severely immunocompromised children with acquired or congenital immunodeficiency disorders, malignancies, organ transplant recipients, and debilitated, malnourished, and premature infants. In HIV-infected children, it most commonly occurs between ages 3 and 6 mo. PCP can occur during remission or relapse in patients with leukemia or lymphoma.	• Slow onset, tachypnea, retractions, and nasal flaring cyanosis • Sporadic form in patients who are immunocompromised. Signs may vary; onset may be acute or fulminant. • Fever, tachypnea, dyspnea, cough, nasal flaring, cyanosis, subacute, diffuse pneumonitis with dyspnea at rest, tachypnea and decreasing oxygen saturation Extrapulmonary sites rarely occur and usually produce no symptoms.
Mycoplasma Pneumonia		
• *Mycoplasma pneumoniae*, microorganisms with properties between bacteria and viruses	• Fall and winter • Crowded living conditions. Seen frequently in school-age children and adolescents.	• Slow onset; 2- to 3-wk incubation period Coryza, malaise, headache, anorexia, normal temp or low-grade fever, sore throat, muscle pain, vomiting, subacute tracheobronchitis, shortness of breath, dry cough that progresses to mucopurulent cough, mild chest pain, wheezing. May present with maculopapular rash.
Bronchiolitis		
• Inflammation of the bronchioles. Causative agents: RSV, adenovirus, parainfluenza type 1 or 3, influenza virus, and *M. pneumoniae*.	• Winter and spring • Most common in infants younger than 6 months old, may occur up to age 2 yr • Greater incidence in people assigned male at birth • Increased in day care centers	• Gradual onset after exposure to an individual with URI Coryza, tachypnea, respiratory rate >50 bpm, retractions, wheezing, paroxysmal cough, fever, cyanosis, dehydration, poor feeding, vomiting, tachycardia, irritability, dyspnea • Apnea may be first sign in infants with RSV. Decreased breath sounds with prolonged expiratory phase Hypoxemia may persist for 4–6 wk.

DIAGNOSTIC EVALUATION	TREATMENT	NURSING CONSIDERATIONS	COMPLICATIONS
	• Early detection is important in patient who are hospitalized. Institute contact precautions with strict handwashing. RSV immune globulin (RSV-IGIV) and palivizumab may be given to prevent infection in select patient populations. Consult AAP Guidelines for specific information.	• In patients with tachypnea and those in respiratory distress, oral fluids are contraindicated because of risk of aspiration.	
• Chest x-ray: Bilateral, diffuse, alveolar disease with a granular pattern, initially perihilar densities, which progress to peripheral and apical areas • Organism cannot be cultured from routine specimens. • Open lung biopsy is the most reliable method. • Bronchoalveolar lavage is also utilized to obtain samples. Needle aspiration of the lung. IgM-ELISA: elevated. CBC: mild leukocytosis, moderate eosinophilia.	• PCP mortality is 5%–40% in patients who are immunocompromised; if untreated, 100%. • Trimethoprim–sulfamethoxazole; rate of adverse reactions is high in patients who are HIV infected. • Pentamidine, parenterally or aerosolized IV form associated with increased risk of adverse reactions. Aerosolized for children ages 5 and older • Corticosteroids recommended for children older than age 13, may be used in younger children.	• Close monitoring of respiratory status, hydration, and nutrition • Monitor for adverse reactions to therapy: vomiting, nausea, rash. • Respiratory isolation should be instituted for 48 h after initiation of therapy. • PCP prophylaxis (see page 1387).	—
• Chest x-ray: bronchopneumonic, diffuse bilateral infiltrates • Complement fixation test: increased Cold agglutinins: increased Immunofluorescent and enzyme immunoassay tests • Positive sputum culture.	• Erythromycin, azithromycin, clarithromycin, tetracycline, and doxycycline may be used in children ages 8 and older. Rule out pregnancy prior to use.	• Children should be on secretion precautions. • Monitor fever. • Assess need for cough suppressants.	• May be fatal if infection becomes systemic or if the child has a preexisting chronic lung disease, sickle cell anemia, immunodeficiencies, or cardiac disease. Those with Down syndrome can develop severe pneumonia. • Pleural effusions.
• Chest x-ray: patchy or peribronchial infiltrates, hyperinflation of lungs with flattening of diaphragms Some will present with a normal chest x-ray. • Nasopharyngeal viral cultures • Serologic studies for specific organisms ABG analysis for children with respiratory distress	• Humidified oxygen, ventilatory assistance as needed (Note treatment for RSV above regarding bronchodilators, glucocorticoids, antibiotics.) • Antipyretics for fever • Continuous cardiac monitoring for apnea or bradycardia • Pulse oximetry	• Avoid high-density humidity; may cause bronchospasm. • Monitor fluid and electrolyte balance closely. Place infant on apnea monitor. • Keep nasal passages free of secretions; infants are obligate nose breathers. • Position patient upright to facilitate breathing. Monitor closely for signs of impending respiratory failure. • There is a high risk of cross-contamination to noninfected children. Institute contact precautions and respiratory isolation. • Monitor oxygenation levels with noninvasive monitoring.	• Increasing respiratory distress, resulting in the need for mechanical ventilation • Secondary bacterial infection • Pneumothorax and pneumomediastinum Apneic episodes, may be life-threatening in children with chronic respiratory or cardiac disease. • Some infants demonstrate abnormal lung functions months after infection.

(continued)

Table 40-1 Common Pediatric Respiratory Infections (*continued*)

CONDITION AND CAUSATIVE AGENT	AGE AND INCIDENCE	CLINICAL MANIFESTATIONS
Croup Syndromes		
Croup syndromes refer to infections of the supraglottis, glottis, subglottis, and trachea.		
Acute laryngotracheobronchitis (subglottic croup) • Parainfluenza types 1, 2, 3; RSV; influenza A and B; adenovirus; measles **CLINICAL JUDGMENT** If ABG analysis is done, a normal partial pressure of arterial carbon dioxide may not indicate decreased severity. By the time hypercapnia is seen, intubation will be required. Children decompensate very quickly.	• Ages 3 mo to 5 yr. Peak ages 1–2 yr. • Greater incidence in people assigned male at birth. • Late autumn, early winter.	• Usually, a preceding URI is seen. Initially, a mild brassy or barking cough, hoarse, intermittent stridor, progresses to continuous stridor. • Nasal flaring, suprasternal, infrasternal, intercostals, retractions • Breathing labored, prolonged expiratory phase Temperature slightly elevated. • Crying and agitation aggravate signs. • Child prefers to be held upright or sit up in bed. Symptoms are worse at night. • Severe croup: restlessness, air hunger, decreased breath sounds, hypoxemia, hypercapnia, anxiety, cyanosis, tachycardia, and cessation of breathing
Spasmodic croup and acute spasmodic laryngitis • No infectious agents seen. Thought to be related to spasm of laryngeal muscle. • Cause may be viral in a few cases, allergic or psychological.	• Ages 1–6 yr. • Peak incidence 7–36 mo.	• Similar to acute laryngotracheobronchitis. Symptoms are sudden, in the evening. • Afebrile, barking, brassy cough, hoarse, stridor Child may be anxious and frightened. • Breathing is noisy on inspiration, slow, and labored; respiratory distresses • Tachycardia; skin cool, moist; dyspnea is worse with excitement. • Cyanosis is rare; severity decreases over time. Patient appears well in the morning, may cough or sound hoarse. The symptoms may recur for subsequent nights; however, they will be less severe.
Bacterial tracheitis (pseudomembranous croup) • Tracheal inflammation in the subglottic region • *S. aureus, H. influenzae,* streptococci groups A and B, *Escherichia coli, Klebsiella, Moraxella catarrhalis, Pseudomonas, Chlamydia trachomatis,* and *Corynebacterium diphtheriae* should be considered in the patient who is nonvaccinated.	• No season variation • Age is variable, 1 mo to 6 yr; however, most are younger than age 3 yr.	• Usually follows a viral illness. Slow or sudden deterioration, child appears toxic. • High fever, stridor, hoarse, respiratory distress Thick, purulent, copious airway secretions • Mucosal necrosis, brassy or barking cough Epiglottitis may coexist. May cause life-threatening airway obstruction.
Acute epiglottitis • Supraglottitis, inflammation of the epiglottis and edema of the arytenoepiglottic folds • *H. influenzae type B, most common. S. pneumoniae, S. aureus, group A.* β*-hemolytic streptococcus, Streptococcus pyogenes, Moraxella catarrhalis, and Candida albicans* (in the immunocompromised).	• Range ages 2–7 yr; peak ages 3–5 yr • Autumn and winter • Incidence significantly decreased because of the routine use of the *H. influenzae* vaccine.	• Sudden fulminating course, high fever, toxic appearance, sore throat, drooling, dysphagia, aphonia, retractions, air hunger, anxiety, tachycardia, hoarseness, irritability, restlessness, rapid progression to respiratory distress • Sitting forward, neck hyperextended, mouth open, tongue protruding Older child will sit in tripod position. Drooling, agitation, and absence of spontaneous cough are predictive of epiglottitis. • Absence of croupy cough.

DIAGNOSTIC EVALUATION	TREATMENT	NURSING CONSIDERATIONS	COMPLICATIONS
• Diagnosis is made by clinical evaluation and careful history. A croup score may be assigned to grade severity. Lateral neck x-ray: subglottic edema, narrowing with normal supraglottic structures. Anterior/posterior neck film: steeple sign • Lower airway involvement	• Racemic epinephrine nebulized with oxygen. Monitor pulse and cardiac rhythm. • Severe airway edema may require intubation. • Corticosteroid therapy • Antibiotic therapy	• Maintain a calm environment, avoid agitating the child, and disturb as little as possible. Monitor oxygenation with noninvasive pulse oximeter. Monitor respiratory status closely and frequently. Closely observe response to racemic epinephrine. Have intubation equipment at bedside and available during transport. Increasing tachypnea may be first sign of hypoxia. If severe distress does not respond to initial treatment, ABG analysis should be obtained. In a patient who is hypoxic, pale, cyanotic, or obtunded, do not manipulate larynx, and do not examine with a tongue blade; it may lead to sudden cardiopulmonary arrest.	• Dehydration, intubation, airway obstruction, death
• CBC is normal, x-ray: subglottic narrowing. • Endoscopic exam: inflammation of the arytenoids cartilage, epithelium intact, pale mucosa	• Corticosteroid therapy • Racemic epinephrine, nebulized	• Same as for acute laryngotracheobronchitis (above) • Allow the parental caregiver to hold the child, remain in upright position. • Use racemic epinephrine with caution, and provide cardiac monitoring, because of possible tachycardia.	
• Neck x-ray: subglottic narrowing, large epiglottis, thick arytenoepiglottic folds, pseudomembrane in trachea • Tracheal culture Laryngoscopy, CBC, leukocytosis, bandemia	• Humidified oxygen as required, mist, antibiotic therapy, cephalosporin, antipyretics • Admit to the intensive care unit (ICU), intubation, and frequent suctioning • Racemic epinephrine ineffective	• Monitor closely for airway obstruction.	• Airway obstruction, death, tracheostomy, pneumothorax, toxic shock syndrome
• Clinical evaluation and history, determining the onset of symptoms • Monitor oxygen saturation level. • Lateral neck films: while sitting in parental caregiver's lap with portable radiology, swollen epiglottis	• Medical emergency • Establish a stable artificial airway first. Approach child in a calm manner; emotional upset and agitation may result in complete airway obstruction.	• Allow the parental caregivers to remain with and hold the child. Before transport to the operating room, observe closely for signs of airway obstruction. Allow the child to maintain a position of comfort (not supine).	• Airway obstruction, death, tracheostomy, pneumothorax, toxic shock syndrome

CLINICAL JUDGMENT
Do not attempt to visualize the epiglottis with a tongue blade or take a throat culture. May cause laryngospasm and airway obstruction. Have intubation equipment ready.

(continued)

Table 40-1 Common Pediatric Respiratory Infections (*continued*)

CONDITION AND CAUSATIVE AGENT	AGE AND INCIDENCE	CLINICAL MANIFESTATIONS
		• Complete fatal airway obstruction and death may occur within hours if not treated. In group A β-hemolytic streptococcus and *H. influenzae*, patient will present with acute respiratory distress. • Stridor and breath sounds decrease as child begins to tire. • A brief episode of air hunger with restlessness and agitation may rapidly progress into increasing cyanosis, coma, and death.

ABG, arterial blood gas; ASO, antistreptolysin; CBC, complete blood count; HIV, human immunodeficiency virus; MRSA, methicillin-resistant S. aureus; RSV, respiratory syncytial virus; URI, upper respiratory infection.

to activity, such as rest, exertion, crying, feeding, and association with pain, positioning, or orthopnea.

6. Note presence of additional signs of respiratory distress: nasal flaring, grunting, and retractions. Note location of retractions (see Figure 40-2) and character (mild, moderate, or severe).
7. Observe for head bobbing, usually noted in a sleeping or exhausted infant. The infant should be held by the parental caregiver with head supported on the parental caregiver's arm at the suboccipital area. The head bobs forward with each inspiration.
8. Observe the child's color. Note the presence and location of cyanosis—peripheral, perioral, facial, and trunk. Note degree of color changes, duration, and association with activity such as crying, feeding, and sleeping.
9. Observe the presence of cough, noting type and duration, such as dry, barking, paroxysmal, or productive. Note any pattern, such as time of day or night, association with activity, physical exertion, or feeding. Severity of croup may be determined by cough and signs of respiratory effort.
   a. Mild croup—occasional barking cough, no audible stridor at rest and either mild or no suprasternal or intercostal retractions.
   b. Moderate croup—frequent barking cough, easily audible stridor at rest, and suprasternal and sternal retractions at rest, but little or no agitation.
   c. Severe croup—frequent barking cough, prominent inspiratory and occasional expiratory stridor, marked sternal retractions, and agitation and distress.
   d. Impending respiratory failure—barking cough (often not prominent), audible stridor at rest (may be hard to hear), sternal retractions (may be marked), lethargy or decreased level of consciousness, and often dusky appearance in the absence of supplemental oxygen.

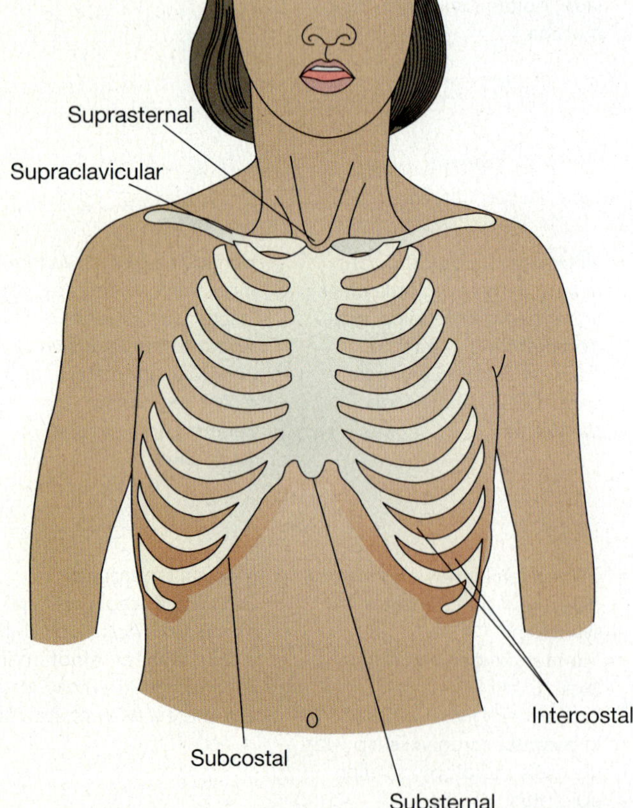

Figure 40-2. Sites of respiratory retractions. (Reprinted with permission from Silbert-Flagg, J. [2023]. *Maternal and child health nursing: Care of the childbearing and childrearing family* [9th ed., Fig. 40-2]. Wolters Kluwer.)

DIAGNOSTIC EVALUATION	TREATMENT	NURSING CONSIDERATIONS	COMPLICATIONS
• Direct exam or laryngoscopy: large, swollen cherry-red epiglottis, edema of arytenoepiglottic folds CBC, cultures, IV catheters must be done after intubation.	• Proceed to the operating room or ICU with personnel skilled and equipped to intubate or perform a percutaneous tracheostomy. • Lateral neck films should be done in the operating room or ICU after airway is established. • Antibiotics: intravenous cefotaxime, ceftriaxone, ampicillin with sulbactam • Supplemental humidified oxygen; mechanical ventilation, if necessary • If epiglottitis is strongly suspected, examination of the throat is contraindicated; because of reflex laryngospasm, acute airway obstruction, aspiration, and cardiopulmonary arrest during or immediately after examination of the pharynx with a tongue blade. Do not attempt throat culture.	• Equipment for intubation and tracheostomy must remain with the patient at all times. A practitioner skilled in intubation and tracheostomy procedures must accompany the child to the operating room or ICU. After intubation, the child should remain in the ICU with frequent assessment of oxygenation levels and need for mechanical ventilation. Prevent self-extubation; use arm boards or restraints to prevent arm movements, extubation, and death. After intubation, administer sedation, as needed. When the decision is made to extubate the child, emergency tracheostomy and intubation equipment must be at bedside.	

10. Note the presence of sputum, including color, amount, consistency, and frequency.
11. Observe the child's fingernails and toenails for cyanosis and the presence and degree of clubbing, which indicate underlying chronic respiratory disease.
12. Evaluate the child's degree of restlessness, apprehension, level of responsiveness, and muscle tone.
13. Note the presence or complaint of chest pain and its location, whether it is local or generalized, dull or sharp, and associated with respiration or grunting.
14. Assess for signs of infection, such as elevated temperature; enlarged cervical lymph glands; purulent discharge from nose or ears; sputum; or inflamed mucous membranes.

EVIDENCE BASE Choi, Y. Y., Kim, Y. S., Lee, S. Y., Sim, J., Choe, Y. J., & Han, M. S. (2022). Croup as a manifestation of SARS-CoV-2 omicron variant infection in young children. *Journal of Korean Medical Science*, *37*(20), e140. https://doi.org/10.3346/jkms.2022.37.e140

Nursing Interventions

Promoting Effective Airway Clearance

1. Provide a humidified environment enriched with oxygen to combat hypoxia and to liquefy secretions.
2. Advise the parental caregivers to use a jet or ultrasonic nebulizer at home if prescribed and to encourage fluids, as tolerated.
3. Keep nasal passages free of secretions. Infants are obligate nose breathers. Use a bulb syringe to clear nares and oropharynx.

Improving Breathing Pattern

1. Place the child in a comfortable position to promote easier ventilation.
   a. Maintain semi-Fowler position—use infant seat or elevate head of bed.
   b. Do not place the infant in prone position. Occasional side or abdominal position will aid drainage of liquefied secretions.
   c. Do not position the child in severe respiratory distress in a supine position. Allow the child to assume a position of comfort, but continue to visualize and monitor airway.
2. Provide measures to improve ventilation of the affected portion of the lung.
   a. Change position frequently.
   b. Provide postural drainage, if prescribed.
   c. Relieve nasal obstruction that contributes to breathing difficulty. Instill normal saline solution or prescribed nose drops, and apply nasal suctioning.
   d. Quiet prolonged crying, which can irritate the airway, by soothing the child; however, crying may be an effective way to inflate the lungs.
   e. Realize that coughing is a normal tracheobronchial cleansing procedure, but temporarily relieve coughing by allowing the child to sip water; use extreme caution to prevent aspiration.
   f. Insert a nasogastric tube, as ordered, to relieve abdominal distention, which can limit diaphragmatic excursion.
3. Ensure that the child's oxygen input is not compromised.
   a. Monitor oxygen saturations, as indicated; pulse oximetry should be performed if hypoxia is suspected.
   b. If compressed air or oxygen is to be administered to a small infant, use a method that is best tolerated, monitoring excess carbon dioxide concentrations and increased respiratory rate.
4. Administer appropriate antibiotic or antiviral therapy.
   a. Observe for drug sensitivity.
   b. Observe the child's response to therapy.

5. Administer specific treatment for respiratory syncytial virus (RSV), if ordered.
   a. There is currently no evidence that supports the use of ribavirin or inhaled corticosteroids in acute bronchiolitis; however, some health care providers do consider these options in the management of RSV, especially in high-risk populations such as children who have undergone a stem cell transplant.
6. The American Academy of Pediatrics no longer routinely recommends ribavirin therapy for RSV, except in specific cases in very high-risk patients. If the decision is made to initiate ribavirin therapy, appropriate precautions should be implemented to protect personnel and parental caregivers.
   a. Information about the potential but unknown risk of exposure to ribavirin.
   b. Pregnant people should not provide direct care to patients who are receiving ribavirin therapy; also, they should not enter the patient's room while ribavirin is being administered.
   c. Methods to reduce environmental exposure to ribavirin should be employed:
      i. Stop aerosol administration before opening hood or tent.
      ii. Use room with adequate ventilation of at least six air exchanges per hour. Place the patient in a negative pressure room if indicated by organizational policy.
      iii. Consider the use of scavenger devices to help decrease the escape of ribavirin into the air.
      iv. Gowns and N95 face masks should be used for the duration of the time the nebulizer is in use.
7. For cases of severe respiratory distress, assist with intubation or tracheostomy and mechanical ventilation.
   a. Tracheostomy and endotracheal (ET) tubes are generally not cuffed for infants and small children because the tube itself is big enough relative to the size of the trachea to act as its own sealer.
   b. Position the infant with a tracheostomy with the neck extended by placing a small roll under the shoulders to prevent occlusion of the tube by the chin. Support their head and neck carefully when moving the infant to prevent dislodgement of the tube.
   c. When feeding, cover the tracheostomy with a moist piece of gauze, or use a bib for older infants or young children.
   d. See pages 1162 and 1163 in this chapter as well as Chapter 10 for care of the patient on mechanical ventilation.

EVIDENCE BASE Zhu, G., Xu, D., Zhang, Y., Wang, T., Zhang, L., Gu, W., & Shen, M. (2021). Epidemiological characteristics of four common respiratory viral infections in children. *Virology Journal*, *18*(1), 10. https://doi.org/10.1186/s12985-020-01475-y

Wollny, K., Pitt, T., Brenner, D., & Metcalfe, A. (2022). Predicting prolonged length of stay in hospitalized children with respiratory syncytial virus. *Pediatric Research*, *92*(6), 1780–1786. https://doi.org/10.1038/s41390-022-02008-9

CLINICAL JUDGMENT Infants with a history of very low birth weight (VLBW) and bronchopulmonary dysplasia (BPD) may have chronic, compensated carbon dioxide retention. Careful attention must be given to oxygen administration to avoid respiratory depression by suppressing their hypoxic drive.

Promoting Adequate Hydration

1. Administer fluids via intravenous (IV) route at the prescribed rate.
2. To prevent aspiration, withhold oral food and fluids if the child is in severe respiratory distress.
3. Offer the child small sips of clear fluid when respiratory status improves.
   a. Note any vomiting or abdominal distention after the oral fluid is given.
   b. As the child begins to take more fluid by mouth, notify the health care provider and modify the IV fluid rate to prevent fluid overload.
   c. Do not force the child to take fluids orally as this may cause increased distress and possibly vomiting. Anorexia will subside as the condition improves.
4. Assist in the control of fever to reduce respiratory rate and fluid loss.
   a. Give antipyretics, as prescribed.
5. Record the child's intake and output, and monitor urine-specific gravity.
6. Provide mouth care or offer mouth rinse if child is able to perform this safely.

Promoting Adequate Rest

1. Disturb the child as little as possible by organizing nursing care, and protect the child from unnecessary interruptions.
2. Be aware of the age and level of development of the child, and be familiar with the level of growth and development as it applies to hospitalization.
3. Encourage the parental caregivers to stay with the child as much as possible to provide comfort and security.
4. Provide opportunities for quiet play as the child's condition improves.

Reducing Anxiety

1. Explain procedures and hospital routine to the child as appropriate for age.
2. Provide a quiet, stress-free environment.
3. Observe the child's response to the oxygen therapy environment such as a mist tent or head box, and provide reassurance.
   a. The child may experience fear of confinement or suffocation.
   b. Vision is distorted through the plastic.
   c. The environment is noisy and damp.
   d. Physical and diversional activities are restricted.
   e. Parental caregiver contact is decreased.
   f. The environment is often uncomfortable.
4. Avoid the use of sedatives and opiates, which may obscure restlessness. Restlessness may be a sign of increasing respiratory distress or obstruction.
5. Allow the child to assume a position of comfort, but continue to monitor the airway and breathing.

Strengthening the Parental Caregivers' Role

1. Help the parental caregivers understand the purpose of the oxygen therapy/humidifier and how to work with it.

2. Discuss their fears and concerns about the child's therapy.
3. Include the parental caregivers in planning for the child's care. Promote their participation in caring for the child.
4. Recognize that the parental caregivers will need rest periods. Encourage them to take breaks and eat on a regular basis.

Family Education and Health Maintenance

1. Teach the importance of good hygiene. Include information on handwashing and appropriate ways to handle respiratory secretions at home.
2. Teach the family when it is appropriate to keep the child home from school or day care (any fever, coughing up secretions, and significant runny nose in toddler or younger child).
3. Teach methods to keep the ill child well hydrated.
   a. Provide small amounts of fluids frequently.
   b. Offer clear liquids and prepared electrolyte preparations.
   c. Offer frozen juice pops.
   d. Avoid juices with a high sugar content.
4. Teach methods to assess the child's hydration status at home.
   a. Decreased number of wet diapers or number of times the child urinates per day.
   b. Decreased activity level.
   c. Dry lips and mucous membranes.
   d. No tears when the child cries.
5. Teach the parental caregivers when to contact their health care provider—signs of respiratory distress, recurrent fever, decreased appetite and activity, and signs of dehydration.
6. Teach about medications and follow-up.
7. If a tracheostomy was required, teach care of the tracheostomy, use of equipment, safety, and referral for home nursing care before discharge.

Evaluation: Expected Outcomes

- Breath sounds clear and equal.
- Easy, regular, unlabored respirations on room air (or back to baseline if the child is on oxygen).
- Mucous membranes moist; urine output adequate.
- Bathing and feeding tolerated well.
- Child calm and interacts appropriately with family and staff.
- Parental caregivers participate in the child's care.

Disorders Requiring Surgery of the Tonsils and Adenoids

EVIDENCE BASE Cui, X., Zhang, J., Gao, Z., Sun, L., & Zhang, F. (2022). A randomized, double-blinded, placebo-controlled, single dose analgesic study of preoperative intravenous ibuprofen for tonsillectomy in children. *Frontiers in Pediatrics, 10*, 956660. https://doi.org/10.3389/fped.2022.956660

Tonsillectomy and *adenoidectomy* are the surgical removal of the adenoidal and tonsillar structures, part of the lymphoid tissue that encircles the pharynx. These are among the most frequently performed surgical procedures in the child. The most common disease processes that require tonsillectomy and adenoidectomy are obstructive sleep apnea; chronic, persistent tonsillitis or adenoiditis; and chronic persistent otitis media.

Pathophysiology and Etiology

Function of Tonsils and Adenoids

1. They are a first line of defense against respiratory infections.
2. Because the growth of the tonsils and adenoids in the first 10 years of life exceeds general somatic growth, these structures are proportionally larger in the child.
3. The natural process of involution of tonsillar and adenoidal lymphoid tissue in the prepubertal years is associated with decreased frequency of throat and ear infections.

Obstructive Sleep Apnea

1. Adenotonsillar hypertrophy causes airway obstruction, leading to persistent hypoventilation during sleep.
2. Peak incidence in children is between ages 3 and 6 years.
3. Incidence is increased in children with Down syndrome.

Tonsillitis and Adenoiditis

1. In tonsillitis and adenoiditis, structures that are already large become inflamed because of an infectious agent and cause airway obstruction, decreased appetite, and pain.
2. Infection may be caused by bacterial or viral organisms, with viral organisms most commonly implicated.
3. Group A *Streptococcus, Mycoplasma pneumoniae,* and *Haemophilus influenzae* type B are common bacterial causes of tonsillitis and adenoiditis. Common viral causes include Epstein–Barr virus and adenovirus.
4. Enlarged adenoids may block nasal passages, resulting in persistent mouth breathing.
5. Chronic adenoiditis without tonsillitis is typically seen in children younger than age 4 years.

Otitis Media

1. Otitis media often develops after a viral respiratory tract infection. Bacterial infection is caused most commonly by *Streptococcus pneumoniae* or *H. influenzae.*
2. Chronic infection may be associated with enlarged adenoids that block drainage from the eustachian tubes.
3. Breastfeeding until 6 months of age can reduce the risk of otitis media.

Clinical Manifestations

Obstructive Sleep Apnea

1. Loud snoring or noisy breathing in sleep.
2. Excessive daytime sleepiness.
3. Mouth breathing.

Chronic Infection of Tonsils and Adenoids

1. Mouth breathing or difficulty breathing.
2. Frequent sore throat.
3. Anorexia, decreased growth velocity.
4. Fever.
5. Obstruction to swallowing or breathing.
6. Nasal, muffled voice.
7. Night cough.
8. Offensive breath.

Chronic Otitis Media

1. Ear pain or general irritability in young children.
2. Alterations in hearing.
3. Fever.
4. Enlarged lymph nodes.
5. Anorexia.

Diagnostic Evaluation

1. Thorough ear, nose, and throat examination and appropriate cultures to determine presence and source of infection.
2. Preoperative blood studies to determine risk of bleeding—clotting time, smear for platelets, prothrombin time, and partial thromboplastin time.

Management

Appropriate antibiotics are given, and the decision is made to perform surgery. Tonsillectomy and adenoidectomy may be performed together or separately. Debate continues over indications for and benefits of surgery.

Indications for Tonsillectomy

1. Conservative.
   a. Recurrent or persistent tonsillitis; the widely accepted criteria for surgery are seven episodes of tonsillitis in the previous 12 months or five episodes in each of the preceding 2 years.
   b. Marked hypertrophy of tonsils, which distorts speech, causes swallowing difficulties, and causes subsequent weight loss.
   c. Tonsillar malignancy.
   d. Diphtheria carrier.
   e. Cor pulmonale due to obstruction.
2. Controversial.
   a. Peritonsillar abscess or retrotonsillar abscess.
   b. Suppurative cervical adenitis with tonsillar focus.
   c. Persistent hyperemia of anterior pillars.
   d. Enlarged cervical lymph nodes.

Indications for Adenoidectomy

1. Conservative.
   a. Adenoid hypertrophy resulting in obstruction of airway, leading to hypoxia, pulmonary hypertension, and cor pulmonale.
   b. Hypertrophy with nasal obstruction accompanied by breathing difficulty and severe speech distortion.
   c. Hypertrophy associated with chronic suppurative or serous otitis media and sensorineural or conductive hearing loss, chronic mastoiditis, or cholesteatoma.
   d. Mouth breathing due to hypertrophied adenoids.
2. Controversial.
   a. Enlarged adenoids.
   b. Chronic otitis media and no evidence of complications.
   c. Child younger than age 4 years, unless life-threatening situation.

Contraindications to Surgery

1. Bleeding or coagulation disorders.
2. Uncontrolled systemic disorders (e.g., diabetes, rheumatic fever, cardiac or renal disease).
3. Presence of upper respiratory infection in the child or immediate family.
4. Specific for adenoidectomy—certain palate abnormalities (i.e., cleft palate or submucous cleft palate).

Complications

1. If untreated, obstructive sleep apnea in the child may result in pulmonary hypertension, cor pulmonale, failure to thrive, respiratory failure, attention-deficit disorders, and cardiac arrhythmias.
2. Untreated chronic tonsillitis may result in failure to thrive, peritonsillar or retropharyngeal abscess, difficulty swallowing, and poor eating.
3. Untreated chronic otitis media may result in hearing loss, scarring of the eardrum (tympanosclerosis), mastoiditis, and meningitis. Hearing loss may result in delayed language development.
4. Complications of surgery include hemorrhage, reactions to anesthesia, otitis media, and bacteremia.

Nursing Assessment

Preoperative Assessment

1. Assess the child's developmental level. Preschool children are especially vulnerable to psychological trauma as a result of surgical procedures or hospitalization.
2. Assess the parental caregivers' and child's understanding of the surgical procedure.
3. Assess psychological preparation of the child for hospitalization and surgery.
   a. Does the child understand what will happen?
   b. Do the parental caregivers know the importance of telling the child the truth, and do they have a good understanding of the procedure?
   c. Does the child have preconceived ideas that may pose a threat?
4. Obtain thorough nursing history from the child and parental caregivers to gather any pertinent information that would impact the child's care.
   a. Has the child had a recent infection? It is desirable for the child to be free of respiratory infection for at least 2 weeks.
   b. Has the child recently been exposed to any communicable diseases?
   c. Does the child have any loose teeth or dental appliances that may pose the threat of aspiration?
   d. Are there any bleeding tendencies in the child or family?
   e. Are there any family members with a history of adverse reactions to anesthesia?
5. Obtain the child's baseline vital signs along with their height and weight.
6. Assess the child's hydration status.

Postoperative Assessment

1. Assess respiratory status and pain often.
2. Assess frequently for signs of postoperative bleeding; monitor vital signs, as warranted.
3. Assess oral intake.
4. Assess for indications of negative psychological sequelae related to the surgery and hospitalization.

Nursing Interventions

Reducing Fear

1. Prepare the child and parental caregivers by encouraging participation in hospital tours and preadmission programs specifically for children.
2. Share information with the child, commensurate with their development stage and cognitive ability, as well as the family.
3. Prepare the child specifically for what to expect postoperatively, using techniques appropriate to the child's developmental level (books, dolls, drawings). Include the following:
   a. Where the child will wake up.

b. Temporary sore throat, emesis of blood, position, and foul taste and smell in mouth.
c. Medications.
d. Fluid regimen and possible IV infusion.
4. Talk to the child about the new things to be seen in the operating room, and clear up any misconceptions. Whenever possible, allow the child to see, touch, and examine equipment, such as thermometers, beds, tubing, and suction equipment.
5. Where available, involve the play specialist in the preparation.

Relieving Parental Caregiver Anxiety

1. Help the parental caregivers prepare the child by talking at first in general terms about surgery and progressing to more specific information.
2. Reassure the parental caregivers that complication rates are low and that recovery is usually swift.
3. Encourage the parental caregivers to stay with the child, and help provide care.

Maintaining Adequate Fluid Volume

1. Assess the child frequently for postoperative bleeding. Check all secretions and emesis for the presence of fresh blood. These are indications of hemorrhage:
   a. Increased pulse.
   b. Frequent swallowing while awake and asleep.
   c. Pallor.
   d. Restlessness.
   e. Clearing of throat and vomiting of blood.
   f. Continuous slight oozing of blood over a number of hours.
   g. Oozing of blood in back of throat.
2. Have suction equipment, oxygen, and packing material readily available in case of emergency.
3. Provide adequate fluid intake.
   a. Give small ice cubes 1 to 2 hours after awakening form anesthesia
   b. When vomiting has ceased, cautiously advance to clear liquids.
   c. Offer cool fruit juices without pulp at first because they are best tolerated; then offer ice pops and cool water for the first 12 to 24 hours. Avoid fluids or medications that are red, purple, or brown fluids.
   d. There is some debate regarding the intake of milk and ice cream the evening of surgery. It can be soothing and can reduce swelling; however, it coats the mouth and throat, causing the child to clear the throat more often, which may initiate bleeding.

CLINICAL JUDGMENT Notify the surgeon immediately if bleeding is suspected.

Promoting Effective Airway Clearance

1. Assist the child in maintaining a patent airway by draining secretions and preventing aspiration of vomitus.
2. Assess the child for signs and symptoms of airway obstruction and respiratory distress (stridor, drooling, restlessness, agitation, tachypnea, and cyanosis), which may result from edema or the accumulation of secretions.
   a. Place the child prone or semiprone with their head turned to a side while still under the effects of anesthesia.
   b. Allow the child to assume a position of comfort when alert. (The parental caregiver may hold the child.)
   c. The child may vomit old blood initially. If suctioning is necessary, avoid trauma to the oropharynx.
   d. Remind the child not to cough, clear throat, or blow nose.

Improving Comfort

1. Give analgesics, as ordered, parenteral or rectally.
2. Rinse the child's mouth with cool water or alkaline solution.
3. Keep the child and environment free from blood-tinged drainage to help decrease anxiety.
4. Encourage the parental caregivers to be with the child when the child awakens.
5. When the parental caregivers must leave, reassure the child that they will return.

Family Education and Health Maintenance

1. Explain and provide written instructions concerning the care of the child at home after discharge.
   a. Diet should still consist of large amounts of fluids and soft, cool, nonirritating foods. (Supply a list of suggestions for the family.)
   b. Eating helps promote healing because it increases the blood supply to the tissues.
   c. Bed rest should be maintained for 1 to 2 days and then daily rest periods for about 1 week. Resume normal eating and activities within 2 weeks after surgery.
   d. Avoid contact with people with infections.
   e. Discourage the child from blowing nose and frequent coughing and clearing of their throat.
   f. Avoid gargling. Mouth odor may be present for a few days after surgery; only mouth rinsing is acceptable.
   g. Discourage use of red dye–enhanced foods or analgesics if possible—can be difficult to differentiate from bleeding.
2. Advise the parental caregivers to call the health care provider if the following occur. (Ensure that the parental caregivers have the phone numbers of the health care provider and hospital emergency department.)
   a. Earache accompanied by fever.
   b. Any bleeding, often indicated only by frequent swallowing; most common between the 5th and 10th postoperative days when membrane sloughs from surgical site.
3. Teach about medications prescribed or suggested for pain relief.
4. Discuss with the parental caregivers what results they can expect from the surgery.
   a. Decreased number of sore throats.
   b. Lessened evidence of obstructive symptoms.
   c. Decreased incidence of cervical lymphadenitis.
   d. Improvement in nutritional status.
   e. No improvement in nasal allergies.
   f. No improvement in secretory otitis media.
5. Guide the parental caregivers in helping the child think of the experience as a positive one after the surgery is over, to make subsequent health care experiences easier.
   a. Talk about what happened and the positive outcomes.
   b. Let the child play out their feelings.

Evaluation: Expected Outcomes

- Acts out surgery with dolls, asks questions.
- Parental caregivers interact with the child and ask appropriate questions.
- Takes fluids well; no signs of bleeding.
- No vomiting; breathing without difficulty.
- Verbalizes reduced pain.

Asthma

Asthma is a chronic, inflammatory disease of the airways, characterized by airflow obstruction, bronchial hyperreactivity, and increased mucus production. The course of asthma is highly variable. Many cells and mediators play a role, including mast cells, eosinophils, neutrophils, and epithelial cells. Classic signs and symptoms include cough, wheezing, shortness of breath/dyspnea, and chest tightness. Children may also report stomach pain when they are experiencing an asthma exacerbation. Provide evidence-based categorization, treatment, and ongoing control information.

Assessment of Asthma Control

1. Although severity is best evaluated prior to the use of asthma medications, it can be established based on the medications necessary to gain control and direct initial therapy.
2. Two domains of asthma control are assessed at each encounter: risk and impairment.
   a. Risk is measured by exacerbations.
   b. Impairment is determined both on initial diagnosis and ongoing assessment.
3. Factors that affect impairment include the following:
   a. Day and nighttime asthma symptoms.
   b. Use of quick-relief medication.
   c. Pulmonary function tests/peak flow measurements if the child is capable.
   d. Limitations of daily activities.
   e. Adverse effects of medications.
   f. Progression of lung disease.
4. Several validated tools are available for patients aged 12 years and older to complete, including the Asthma Control Test, Asthma Control Questionnaire, and Asthma Therapy Assessment Questionnaire.
   a. These tools quantify symptoms, quick-relief medication usage, effect of asthma on quality of life, and patient/family perception of control.
   b. To assist in the diagnosis of asthma, particularly in very small children who cannot perform lung function tests, an asthma predictive index can help identify children likely to have asthma.
5. Level of control guides adjustment of medications, and nurses can use this assessment to identify patients/families who need more asthma education for better control of asthma.

EVIDENCE BASE Avery, C., Perrin, E. M., & Lang, J. E. (2021). Updates to the pediatrics asthma management guidelines. *JAMA Pediatrics*, *175*(9), 966–967. https://doi.org/10.1001/jamapediatrics.2021.1494

Variations of Asthma

Cough Variant Asthma

Cough variant asthma is typically seen in children, where cough (especially at night or during exercise) is the principal symptom. The child may never wheeze. Although the symptoms are chronic and commonly mild in many children, severe exacerbations (attacks) may arise, even resulting in respiratory failure and death.

Exercise-Induced Bronchospasm

Exercise-induced bronchospasm refers to symptoms of cough, shortness of breath, chest pain, tightness, wheezing, and endurance problems during or after vigorous activity. Typically, symptoms begin during exercise and peak 5 to 10 minutes after stopping; they may resolve spontaneously within 20 to 30 minutes. Diagnosis is confirmed by documenting a decrease in peak expiratory flow (PEF) or forced expiratory volume in 1 second (FEV_1), before and after exercise and at 5-minute intervals for 20 to 30 minutes. This condition may occur without chronic asthma and has a different pathophysiology from asthma that is triggered by exercise. The preferred treatment consists of short-acting beta-2 agonists, taken 15 minutes prior to exercise. Ipratropium is an inhaled medication that relaxes the airway that may be effective in some patients.

Factors that Increase Risk of Asthma Death

EVIDENCE BASE Hopp, R. J., Wilson, M. C., & Pasha, M. A. (2022). Small airway disease in pediatric asthma: The who, what, when, where, why, and how to remediate. A review and commentary. *Clinical Reviews in Allergy & Immunology*, *62*(1), 145–159. https://doi.org/10.1007/s12016-020-08818-1

Stern, J., Pier, J., & Litonjua, A. (2020). Asthma epidemiology and risk factors. *Seminars in Immunopathology*, *42*(1), 5–15. https://doi.org/10.1007/s00281-020-00785-1

1. Previous severe exacerbation (intubation or intensive care admission).
2. Hospitalization two or more times within the year, three or more emergency department (ED) visits in the last year.
3. Use of more than two canisters per month of short-acting beta-adrenergic (SABA).
4. Difficulty perceiving airway obstruction or the severity of worsening asthma.
5. Low socioeconomic status or inner-city residence.
6. Illicit drug use.
7. Major psychological problems or psychiatric disease.
8. Comorbidity, such as cardiovascular disease or other chronic lung disease.
9. Other factors, lack of asthma action plan, sensitivity to *Alternaria*.

Management

The Stepwise Approach to Managing Asthma, developed by the National Asthma Education Program, identifies classifications of asthma according to symptoms and suggests pharmacologic options for the control of asthma. Medications may be "stepped up or down" depending on the patient's response to therapy. See Tables 40-2 and 40-3, pages 1179–1181, for the recommended management of asthma for infants and children age 0 to 4 and 5 to 12 years. The management of children greater than 12 years of age will be referenced to the pages in the Adult Respiratory Chapter 7 on asthma management.

Acute Exacerbation

1. Be alert for severe asthma exacerbation. Exacerbations may be associated with viral respiratory infections.
2. In a severe exacerbation, the child is short of breath, may be audibly wheezing with a prolonged expiratory phase, restless, apprehensive, anxious, diaphoretic, and tachycardic; color may be pale or flushed, and lips may be dark red or cyanotic. Cyanosis of the lips and nail beds is an ominous sign.
   a. There are signs of respiratory distress, such as nasal flaring, use of accessory muscles, retractions, one- to two-word dyspnea (speaking in short phrases), tachypnea, hypoxemia, and respiratory alkalosis progressing to respiratory acidosis.
   b. Breath sounds may be decreased, and there may be decreased level of consciousness. Absence of wheezing,

Table 40-2 Stepwise Approach for Managing Asthma in Children 0–4 Years of Age

AGES 0–4 YEARS: STEPWISE APPROACH FOR MANAGEMENT OF ASTHMA

Treatment	Intermittent Asthma	Management of Persistent Asthma in Individuals Ages 0–4 Years				
	STEP 1	STEP 2	STEP 3	STEP 4	STEP 5	STEP 6
Preferred	PRN SABA and At the start of RTI: Add short course daily ICS▲	Daily low-dose ICS and PRN SABA	Daily medium-dose ICS and PRN SABA	Daily medium-dose ICS-LABA and PRN SABA	Daily high-dose ICS-LABA and PRN SABA	Daily high-dose ICS-LABA + oral systemic corticosteroid and PRN SABA
Alternative		Daily montelukast* or Cromolyn,* and PRN SABA		Daily medium-dose ICS + montelukast* and PRN SABA	Daily high-dose ICS + montelukast* and PRN SABA	Daily high-dose ICS + montelukast*+ oral systemic corticosteroid and PRN SABA
			For children age 4 years only, see Step 3 and Step 4 on Management of Persistent Asthma in Individuals Ages 5–11 Years diagram.			

Assess Control

- First check adherence, inhaler technique, environmental factors,▲ and comorbid conditions.
- **Step up** if needed; reassess in 4–6 weeks
- **Step down** if possible (if asthma is well controlled for at least 3 consecutive months)

Consult with asthma specialist if Step 3 or higher is required. Consider consultation at Step 2.

Control assessment is a key element of asthma care. This involves both impairment and risk. Use of objective measures, self-reported control, and health care utilization are complementary and should be employed on an ongoing basis, depending on the individual's clinical situation.

Abbreviations: ICS, inhaled corticosteroid; LABA: long-acting-beta$_2$-agonist; SABA: short-acting-beta$_2$-agonist; RTI, respiratory tract infection; PRN, as needed

▲ Updated based on the 2020 guidelines.

* Cromolyn and montelukast were not considered for this update and/or have limited availability for use in the United States. The FDA issued a Boxed Warning for montelukast in March 2020.

NOTES FOR INDIVIDUALS AGES 0–4 YEARS DIAGRAM

Quick-relief medications	• Use SABA as needed for symptoms. The intensity of treatment depends on severity of symptoms: up to 3 treatments at 20-minute intervals as needed. • **Caution:** Increasing use of SABA or use >2 days a week for symptom relief (not prevention of EIB) generally indicates inadequate control and may require a step up in treatment. • Consider short course of oral systemic corticosteroid if exacerbation is severe or individual has history of previous severe exacerbations.
Each step: Assess environmental factors, provide patient education, and manage comorbidities▲	• In individuals with sensitization (or symptoms) related to exposure to pests‡: conditionally recommend integrated pest management as a single or multicomponent allergen-specific mitigation intervention.▲ • In individuals with sensitization (or symptoms) related to exposure to identified indoor allergens, conditionally recommend a multicomponent allergen-specific mitigation strategy.▲ • In individuals with sensitization (or symptoms) related to exposure to dust mites, conditionally recommend impermeable pillow/mattress covers only as part of a multicomponent allergen-specific mitigation intervention but not as a single-component intervention. ▲
Notes	• If clear benefit is not observed within 4–6 weeks and the medication technique and adherence are satisfactory, the clinician should consider adjusting therapy or alternative diagnoses.
Abbreviations	EIB, exercise-induced bronchoconstriction; SABA, inhaled short-acting beta$_2$-agonist. ▲Updated based on the 2020 guidelines. ‡ Refers to mice and cockroaches, which were specifically examined in the Agency for Healthcare Research and Quality systematic review.

Reprinted from National Heart, Lung and Blood Institute, National Asthma Education and Prevention Program. (2020). 2020 focused updates to the asthma management guidelines: Clinician's guide. https://www.nhlbi.nih.gov/sites/default/files/publications/Asthma%20Clinicians%20Guide%20508_02-03-21.pdf

decreased breaths sounds, and inability to blow a PEF requires immediate intervention. Respiratory failure tends to progress quickly and is difficult to reverse.

c. A young child will assume tripod position; an older child will sit upright with shoulders hunched.

3. Signs of respiratory distress in infants include use of accessory muscles, inspiratory and expiratory wheezing, paradoxical breathing, cyanosis, respiratory rate greater than 60, and oxygen saturation less than 90%. These infants are at greater risk of respiratory failure.
4. The goals of emergency management are to quickly reverse airflow obstruction, to correct hypoxemia, and to reduce the likelihood of recurrence.
5. Assess PEF rate or FEV_1 on arrival; assess degree of respiratory distress or fatigue.
6. Obtain an oxygen saturation level by pulse oximetry.
7. Obtain arterial or capillary blood gas levels in infants with an oxygen saturation of 90% or less and in a child with moderate to severe respiratory distress.
8. Deliver humidified oxygen via nasal cannula, hood, or face mask at lowest level necessary to maintain adequate oxygenation. Obtain a brief history and physical, and focus on prior treatment and possible triggers of the episode, such as respiratory infection or lack of medication.
9. Administer emergency treatment, as indicated.
    a. SABA with ipratropium, either by nebulization or by metered dose inhalers (MDIs) with spacer (with face mask in young child).
    b. Systemic corticosteroids should be administered early in treatment.
    c. Adjunctive treatments include IV leukotriene modifiers, heliox, and magnesium sulfate.

Table 40-3 Stepwise Approach for Managing Asthma in Children 5–11 Years of Age

AGES 5–11 YEARS: STEPWISE APPROACH FOR MANAGEMENT OF ASTHMA

	Intermittent Asthma	Management of Persistent Asthma in Individuals Ages 5-11 Years				
Treatment	**STEP 1**	**STEP 2**	**STEP 3**	**STEP 4**	**STEP 5**	**STEP 6**
Preferred	PRN SABA	Daily low-dose ICS and PRN SABA	Daily and PRN combination low-dose ICS-formoterol▲	Daily and PRN combination medium-dose ICS-formoterol▲	Daily high-dose ICS-LABA and PRN SABA	Daily high-dose ICS-LABA + oral systemic corticosteroid and PRN SABA
Alternative		Daily LTRA,* or Cromolyn,* or Nedocromil,* or Theophylline,* and PRN SABA	Daily medium-dose ICS and PRN SABA or Daily low-dose ICS-LABA, or daily low-dose ICS + LTRA,* or daily low-dose ICS +Theophylline,* and PRN SABA	Daily medium-dose ICS-LABA and PRN SABA or Daily medium-dose ICS + LTRA* or daily medium-dose ICS + Theophylline,* and PRN SABA	Daily high-dose ICS + LTRA* or daily high-dose ICS + Theophylline,* and PRN SABA	Daily high-dose ICS + LTRA* + oral systemic corticosteroid or daily high-dose ICS + Theophylline* + oral systemic corticosteroid, and PRN SABA
		Steps 2–4: Conditionally recommend the use of subcutaneous immunotherapy as an adjunct treatment to standard pharmacotherapy in individuals ≥ 5 years of age whose asthma is controlled at the initiation, buildup, and maintenance phases of immunotherapy ▲			Consider Omalizumab**▲	

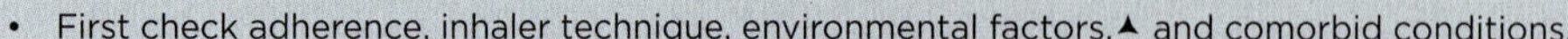

Assess Control

- First check adherence, inhaler technique, environmental factors,▲ and comorbid conditions.
- **Step up** if needed; reassess in 2–6 weeks
- **Step down** if possible (if asthma is well controlled for at least 3 consecutive months)

Consult with asthma specialist if Step 4 or higher is required. Consider consultation at Step 3.

Control assessment is a key element of asthma care. This involves both impairment and risk. Use of objective measures, self-reported control, and health care utilization are complementary and should be employed on an ongoing basis, depending on the individual's clinical situation.

Abbreviations: ICS, inhaled corticosteroid; LABA, long-acting $beta_2$-agonist; LTRA, leukotriene receptor antagonist; SABA, inhaled short-acting $beta_2$-agonist

▲ Updated based on the 2020 guidelines.

* Cromolyn, Nedocromil, LTRAs including montelukast, and Theophylline were not considered in this update and/or have limited availability for use in the United States, and/or have an increased risk of adverse consequences and need for monitoring that make their use less desirable. The FDA issued a Boxed Warning for montelukast in March 2020.

** Omalizumab is the only asthma biologic currently FDA-approved for this age range.

(continued)

Table 40-3 Stepwise Approach for Managing Asthma in Children 5–11 Years of Age *(continued)*

NOTES FOR INDIVIDUALS AGES 5–11 YEARS DIAGRAM

Quick-relief medications	• Use SABA as needed for symptoms. The intensity of treatment depends on severity of symptoms: up to 3 treatments at 20-minute intervals as needed. • In Steps 3 and 4, the preferred option includes the use of ICS-formoterol 1 to 2 puffs as needed up to a maximum total daily maintenance and rescue dose of 8 puffs (36 μg).▲ • **Caution:** Increasing use of SABA or use >2 days a week for symptom relief (not prevention of EIB) generally indicates inadequate control and may require a step-up in treatment.
Each step: Assess environmental factors, provide patient education, and manage comorbidities▲	• In individuals with sensitization (or symptoms) related to exposure to pests‡: conditionally recommend integrated pest management as a single or multicomponent allergen-specific mitigation intervention.▲ • In individuals with sensitization (or symptoms) related to exposure to identified indoor allergens, conditionally recommend a multicomponent allergen-specific mitigation strategy.▲ • In individuals with sensitization (or symptoms) related to exposure to dust mites, conditionally recommend impermeable pillow/mattress covers only as part of a multicomponent allergen-specific mitigation intervention, but not as a single component intervention.▲
Notes	• The terms ICS-LABA and ICS-formoterol indicate combination therapy with both an ICS and a LABA, usually and preferably in a single inhaler. • Where formoterol is specified in the steps, it is because the evidence is based on studies specific to formoterol. • In individuals ages 5–11 years with persistent allergic asthma in which there is uncertainty in choosing, monitoring, or adjusting anti-inflammatory therapies based on history, clinical findings, and spirometry, FeNO measurement is conditionally recommended as part of an ongoing asthma monitoring and management strategy that includes frequent assessment.
Abbreviations	EIB (exercise-induced bronchoconstriction); FeNO (fractional exhaled nitric oxide); ICS (inhaled corticosteroid); LABA (long-acting beta$_2$-agonist); SABA (inhaled short-acting beta$_2$-agonist). ▲Updated based on the 2020 guidelines. ‡ Refers to mice and cockroaches, which were specifically examined in the Agency for Healthcare Research and Quality systematic review.

Reprinted from National Heart, Lung and Blood Institute, National Asthma Education and Prevention Program. (2020). 2020 focused updates to the asthma management guidelines: Clinician's guide. https://www.nhlbi.nih.gov/sites/default/files/publications/Asthma%20Clinicians%20Guide%20508_02-03-21.pdf

d. Antibiotics are generally not used unless there is evidence of bacterial infection.

10. Hospitalized patients will need frequent assessment, repeat or continuous SABA treatments, corticosteroids, and treatment of any comorbid condition, such as sinusitis.
11. Discharge planning for patients with exacerbations should include an action plan for medications, recognition and treatment of acute asthma, and plans for follow-up.
12. Children in severe status asthmaticus unresponsive to the aforementioned therapy may require the following:
    a. Intubation and mechanical ventilation with 100% oxygen for impending or actual respiratory distress, decreased mental alertness, increased fatigue, or partial pressure of arterial carbon dioxide ($PaCO_2$) greater than or equal to 42 mm Hg.
    b. Nebulized beta-2 agonist, hourly or continuously.
    c. Anticholinergic such as ipratropium, although generally limited to the emergency department.
    d. IV corticosteroid therapy.
    e. Admission to intensive care unit (ICU).
    f. Pharmacologic paralysis to ventilate effectively.
    g. Cardiopulmonary monitoring of the child's response to treatment.
    h. Placement of an arterial line for blood monitoring.
    i. Therapies not recommended for treating an exacerbation; subcutaneous beta-2 agonist provides no advantage over inhaled medication.
    j. Theophylline or aminophylline therapy is not recommended in the ED. It does not provide additional benefit to short-acting beta-2 agonists; it may produce adverse effects.
    k. Chest physiotherapy (CPT) and mucolytics.

l. Antibiotics are not recommended for asthma treatment. However, antibiotics may be needed in patients with fever, purulent sputum, and evidence of bacterial pneumonia.
m. Anxiolytic and hypnotic drugs are contraindicated.
n. Aggressive hydration is not recommended in older children. Assess fluid status; make corrections, as needed, for infants and young children to decrease risk of dehydration.

Asthma hospitalization readmissions do occur. To prevent readmission for acute asthma exacerbation in the period from hospitalization to outpatient/community care, strategies prior to discharge should target medication adherence and parental caregiver knowledge of asthma. Care providers and school personnel should be aware of the child's treatment plan if an exacerbation occurs in these environments. Adherence to treatment plan has been cited as the most important factor in preventing readmission.

Long-Term Management

1. As the child becomes stabilized, begin to develop a home and school management plan. Components of the plan should include the following:
   a. The use of quick-relief medications (SABA); expected effect and side effects.
   b. The use of long-term controllers, which include corticosteroids, leukotriene modifiers, mast cell stabilizers, and long-acting beta agonists (LABAs). See pages 789 and 790 for mechanism and adverse reactions. Note: LABA should be prescribed only in the case of poor control with other medications due to increased risk of asthma-related deaths.
   c. Inhalation technique with nebulizer or MDI with spacer (see Figure 40-3).
   d. Peak flow and symptom monitoring.
   e. Use of PEF zone system, if indicated (see further on).
   f. Identification of triggers (e.g., exercise, weather change, infection, allergen exposure [pollen, mold, dust mite, animal dander, cockroach or mouse exposure]).
   g. Environmental control by removal of suspected stimuli.
   h. Hydration, nutrition, rest, and exercise regimens.
   i. Emergency action plans.
2. Plan a team conference involving the child, parental caregivers, school nurse, and teacher, if possible. Ideally, the plan should be clear and easy for the child and family to follow, adapted to their lifestyle, and using the least amount of medications necessary to control and prevent the child's asthma symptoms. A written action plan should be submitted to the school (or day care), including information on medications (possible self-medication by the adolescent), identified triggers, steps in an emergency plan, and emergency contact information. Emergency action plans may need to include multiple family caregivers, residences, or coaches if the child is involved in sports. An example of this form can be found at https://www.nhlbi.nih.gov/resources/asthma-action-plan-2020. Emphasize that, without exception, no smoking should be permitted in the home or car of a child with asthma. Even if the child is out of the home, the residual odor will cause symptoms. Opening windows or using sprays and air cleaners is not an acceptable alternative.
3. Encourage the parental caregivers to pay particular attention to environmental control in the child's bedroom, including elimination of dust, not allowing any pets, and avoidance of any strong smells or sprays. If using wood stoves in the home, find out if there is an alternative source of heat.
4. Obtain more information from the National Asthma Education Program (https://www.nhlbi.nih.gov/science/national-asthma-education-and-prevention-program-naepp) the American Academy of Allergy, Asthma and Immunology (www.aaaai.org), or the American Lung Association (http://lung.org).

Peak Expiratory Flow Monitoring and the Zone System

1. Teach the family and child about PEF monitoring at home as well as other important indicators, as directed (see Figure 40-4).
   a. PEF monitoring is not emphasized as much in current guidelines as in the past.
   b. Other indicators of severity include symptom assessment, need for medication, and measures of control such as the asthma control questionnaire.
2. A PEF meter measures the PEF rate that can be produced during a forced expiration. It measures airflow through the large airways; the result is effort dependent. PEF measurements can be initiated in children as young as age 5 years of age. Given time and practice, consistent readings will be produced. (See page 792 for directions on use of PEF meter.)
3. A table of predicted PEF values should be included in the packaging of the home PEF meter. These values are based on age and height. A few patients may find their readings above or below the published values. Therefore, each child should

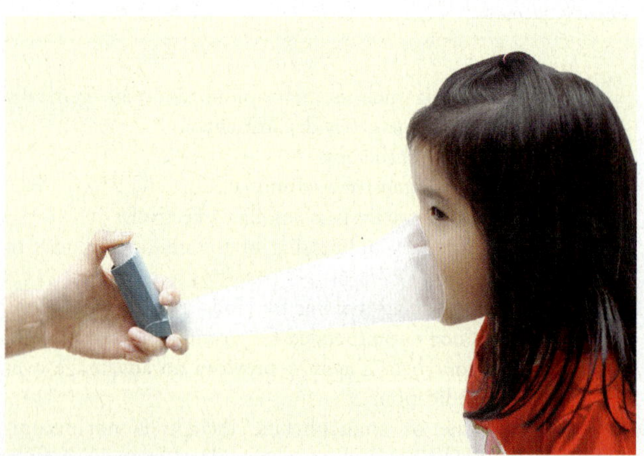

Figure 40-3. Multidose inhaler use with spacers. (Shutterstock/wk1003mike)

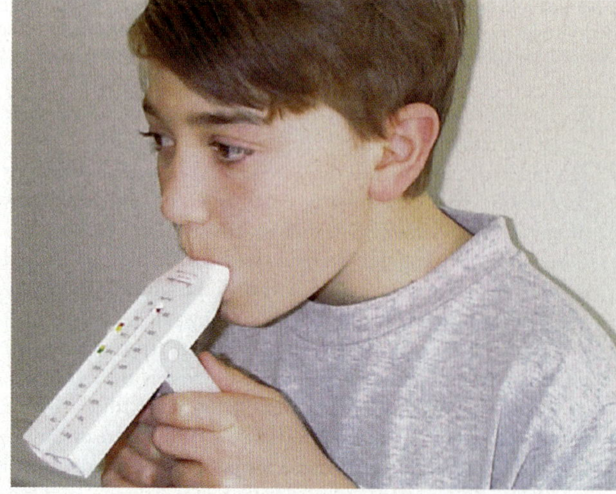

Figure 40-4. Peak flow monitoring.

establish a personal best PEF value. Ideally, this should be implemented during a time when the child is symptom free. If PEF readings are consistently below predicted values, the health care provider should be contacted, and additional medications may be necessary.

4. Use of the PEF zone system along with a home asthma management plan can assist families in the proper use of medications and assists in decision making regarding the degree of airflow obstruction. After the personal best PEF value is identified, teach the patient that subsequent PEF measurements can be classified into three zones that will dictate a home management plan.
   a. Green Zone = 80% to 100% of personal best. No asthma symptoms are present. Continue usual medications.
   b. Yellow Zone = 50% to less than 79% of personal best; signals caution; may be experiencing an asthma episode or day-to-day control is suboptimal; need to use short-acting inhaled beta-2 agonist, follow emergency plan, and contact health care provider for further instructions.
   c. Red Zone = less than 50% of personal best value. This zone signals danger. a short-acting inhaled beta-2 agonist must be taken immediately, and if PEF does not return to yellow or green zone, contact health care provider or proceed to the ED immediately.

Respiratory Distress Syndrome (Hyaline Membrane Disease)

Respiratory distress syndrome (RDS), formerly known as hyaline membrane disease, is a syndrome of premature neonates that is characterized by progressive and usually fatal respiratory failure resulting from atelectasis and immaturity of the lungs. RDS occurs most commonly in premature neonates (primarily weighing between 1,000 and 1,500 g) and between 28 and 37 weeks' gestation. In neonates of 26 to 28 weeks' gestation, the incidence is 50% to 70% and increases with degree of prematurity. RDS can be fatal; those who survive are at risk for chronic respiratory and neurologic complications.

Pathophysiology and Etiology

1. Adequate pulmonary function at birth depends on the following:
   a. An adequate amount of surfactant (a lipoprotein mixture) lining the alveolar cells, which allows for alveolar stability and prevents alveolar collapse at the end of expiration.
   b. An adequate surface area in air spaces to allow for gas exchange (i.e., sufficient pulmonary capillary bed in contact with this alveolar surface area).
2. RDS is ultimately the result of decreased pulmonary surfactant, incomplete structural development of lung, and a highly compliant chest wall.
3. Contributing factors are any factor that decreases surfactant, such as the following:
   a. Prematurity and immature alveolar lining cells.
   b. Acidosis.
   c. Hypothermia.
   d. Hypoxia.
   e. Hypovolemia.
   f. Diabetes.
   g. Elective cesarean delivery.
   h. Fetal or intrapartum stress that compromises blood supply to fetal lungs: vaginal bleeding, maternal hypertension, difficult resuscitation associated with birth asphyxia. (Some situations, such as steroid therapy or a birthing parent dependent on heroin, result in the acceleration of surfactant.)
   i. RDS due to nonpulmonary factors such as cardiac defects, sepsis, airway obstruction, intraventricular hemorrhage, hypoglycemia, and acute blood loss.
4. Surfactant production is deficient by type II alveolar cells. (Although some surfactant may be present at birth, it may not be regenerated at an adequate rate.) Surfactant production may be reduced because of the following:
   a. Extreme immaturity of alveolar lining cells.
   b. Diminished or impaired production rate resulting from fetal or early neonatal stress.
   c. Impairment of release mechanism for phospholipid from type II alveolar cells.
   d. Death of many of these cells responsible for decreased surfactant production.
5. Intra-alveolar surface tension is increased, and alveoli are unstable and collapse at the end of expiration. Functional reserve capacity—the amount of air left in the lungs after expiration—is decreased; thus, the next breath requires almost as much effort as the first breath after birth.
6. More oxygen and energy are required to expand the alveoli with each breath, causing fatigue.
7. The number of alveoli that expand progressively decreases, leading to alveolar instability and atelectasis.
8. Pulmonary vascular resistance increases, causing hypoperfusion of lung.
9. Persistence of fetal circulation right-to-left shunt results, leading to hypoxemia and hypercapnia, which lead to respiratory and metabolic acidosis.
10. Hypoxemia and pulmonary vascular pressure cause ischemia in the alveoli, leading to transudate in the alveoli and formation of a membranous layer (see Figure 40-5).
11. Gas exchange becomes inhibited. Lungs become stiff (decreased compliance), requiring more pressure to expand them.
12. Airway obstruction leads to increased hypoxia and vasoconstriction, and the cycle continues.
13. RDS is usually a self-limiting disease, and symptoms peak in about 3 to 4 days, at which time surfactant synthesis begins to accelerate and pulmonary function and clinical appearance begin to improve.
    a. Moderately ill infants or those who do not require assisted ventilation usually show slow improvement by about 48 hours and rapid recovery over 3 to 4 days, with few complications.
    b. Severely ill and very immature infants who require some ventilatory assistance usually demonstrate rapid deterioration, such as decreased cardiac inflow, decreased arterial pressure, apneic episodes, cyanosis, pallor, and flaccid, unresponsive shocklike state. Ventilatory assistance may be required for several days, and chronic lung disease and other complications are common.

Clinical Manifestations

Symptoms are usually observed soon after birth and may include those listed here and increase in severity over the first 2 days of life.

Primary Signs and Symptoms

1. Expiratory grunting.
2. Sternal, suprasternal, substernal, and intercostal retractions progressing to paradoxical seesaw respirations.

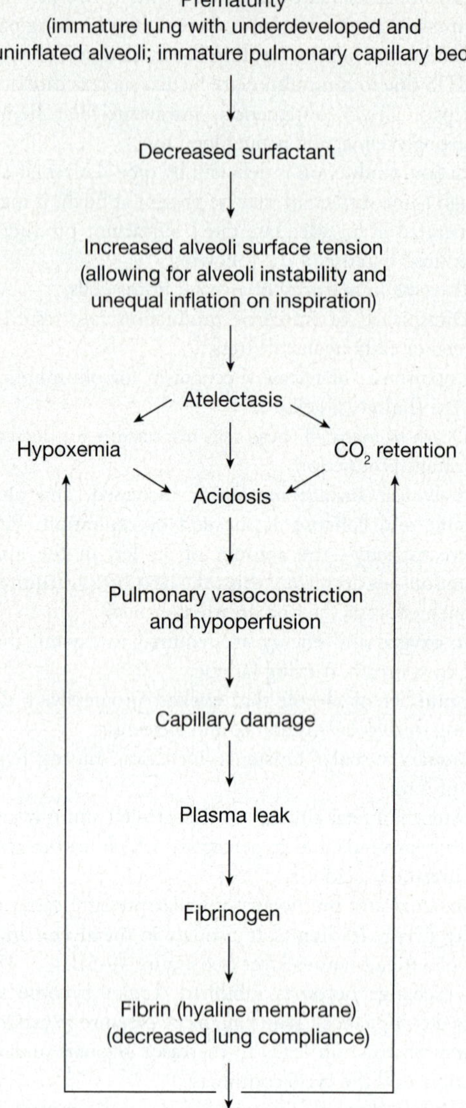

Figure 40-5. Schematic outline of respiratory distress syndrome.

3. Inspiratory nasal flaring.
4. Tachypnea greater than 60 breaths/min.
5. Hypothermia.
6. Cyanosis when child is in room air (infants with severe disease may be cyanotic even when given oxygen), increasing need for oxygen.
7. Decreased breath sounds and dry "sandpaper" breath sounds.
8. Pulmonary edema.
9. As the disease progresses:
   a. Seesaw retractions become pronounced with marked abdominal protrusion on expiration.
   b. Peripheral edema increases.
   c. Muscle tone decreases.
   d. Cyanosis increases.
   e. Body temperature drops.
   f. Short periods of apnea occur.
   g. Bradycardia may occur.
   h. Changes in distribution of blood throughout the body result in pale gray skin color.
   i. Diminished breath sounds.

Secondary Signs and Symptoms

1. Hypotension.
2. Edema of the hands and feet.
3. Absent bowel sounds early in the illness.
4. Decreased urine output.

Diagnostic Evaluation

1. Prenatal diagnosis: evaluation of amniotic fluids to assess fetal lung maturity.
   a. Lecithin/sphingomyelin ratio—tests of surfactant phospholipids in amniotic fluid.
   b. Phosphatidylcholine and phosphatidylglycerol (PG)—phospholipids that stabilize surfactant.
   c. Fetal maturity assay—determines PG levels in amniotic fluid or neonatal tracheal aspirates.
   d. Lamellar bodies test—measures a storage form of surfactant in amniotic fluids.
2. Laboratory tests:
   a. $PaCO_2$—elevated.
   b. Partial pressure of arterial oxygen (PaO_2)—low.
   c. Blood pH—low because of metabolic acidosis.
   d. Calcium—low.
   e. Serum glucose—low.
3. Chest x-ray—diffuse, fine granularity; "whiteout," very heavy, uniform granularity, reflecting fluid-filled alveoli and atelectasis of some alveoli, surrounded by hyperdistended bronchioles; "ground glass" appearance with prominent air bronchogram extending into periphery of lung fields; pulmonary interstitial emphysema is observed in premature neonates with RDS because of overdistention of distal airways.
4. Pulmonary function studies—stiff lung with a reduced effective pulmonary blood flow.

Management

EVIDENCE BASE Cucerea, M., Moscalu, M., Moldovan, E., Santa, R., Gall, Z., Suciu, L. M., & Simon, M. (2023). Early surfactant therapy for respiratory distress syndrome in very preterm infants. *Healthcare (Basel, Switzerland)*, *11*(3), 439. https://doi.org/10.3390/healthcare11030439

Tana, M., Tiron, C., Aurilia, C., Lio, A., Paladini, A., Fattore, S., Esposito, A., De Tomaso, D., & Vento, G. (2023). Respiratory management of the preterm infant: Supporting evidence-based practice at the bedside. *Children (Basel, Switzerland)*, *10*(3), 535. https://doi.org/10.3390/children10030535

Early recognition is imperative so that treatment may be initiated to halt the progression of RDS. In fact, treatment should begin prior to birth if the pregnant person is at risk for delivering the baby preterm. Transportation to a facility providing specialized care is desirable, when possible.

Supportive

1. Maintenance of oxygenation—PaO_2 at 60 to 80 mm Hg to prevent hypoxia; frequent arterial pH and blood gas measurements and use of a pulse oximeter.
2. Maintenance of respiration with ventilatory support, if necessary.
   a. Intermittent mandatory ventilations delivered via ET tube; allows the infant to breathe spontaneously at their own rate

while the ventilator provides a preset cycle of respirations and pressure.
   b. Positive end-expiratory pressure (PEEP) via ET tube. The ventilator is pressure or volume limited; provides increased PEEP during expiration to prevent alveolar collapse; residual airway pressure is maintained.
   c. Continuous positive airway pressure (CPAP) delivered via mask, nasal prongs or RAM cannula; used in spontaneous respiration to improve oxygenation by preventing collapse of the alveoli and increasing diffusion time.
   d. Synchronized intermittent mandatory ventilation allows the infant to breathe spontaneously between mechanical breaths. In assist or control mode, mechanical breaths are delivered at a regular rate if spontaneous breaths are not detected.
3. Maintenance of normal body temperature.
4. Maintenance of fluid, electrolyte, and acid–base balance—metabolic acidosis buffered with sodium bicarbonate.
5. Maintenance of nutrition—IV fluids, as prescribed.
6. Antibiotics, as needed, to treat infection.
7. Constant observation for complications—pneumothorax, disseminated intravascular coagulation (DIC), patent ductus arteriosus (PDA) with heart failure, chronic lung disease.
8. Care appropriate for a small, premature neonate.
9. Prevent hypotension.
10. Maintain a hematocrit of 40% to 45%.

Aggressive (Offered in Tertiary Care Centers)

1. Administration of exogenous surfactant into lungs early in the disease.
   a. Especially beneficial in the VLBW infant.
   b. May be given preventively to VLBW infants at birth.
   c. Available preparations are natural (derived from animal lungs) and synthetic (protein free): bovine and synthetic surfactant.
   d. Administered into the ET tube.
2. Surfactant replacement therapy.
   a. Prophylactic surfactant therapy: infants at increased risk for RDS, infants of less than 27 weeks' gestational age, and infants with a birth weight of less than 1,250 g.
   b. Treatment initiated after infant is stabilized in the delivery room or within 15 minutes of life.
   c. Rescue surfactant therapy: infants with moderate to severe RDS, requiring ventilatory assistance, with an oxygen requirement greater than 40%.
   d. Benefits of surfactant: decreases oxygen requirement and mean airway pressure; decreases pulmonary leaks.
   e. Complications observed in surfactant administration: pulmonary hemorrhage, PDA, mucus plugging.
   f. Nursing assessment with surfactant administration: suctioning delayed for 1 hour or as indicated by protocol. Assist with delivery of surfactant, collection and monitoring of arterial blood gas (ABG) studies, meticulous monitoring of oxygenation status with pulse oximeter or transcutaneous monitor ($TcpCO_2$).
   g. Assess the infant's tolerance of the procedure: increase in respiratory compliance, which will require adjustments of the ventilator.
3. High-frequency ventilation—mechanical ventilation that uses rapid rates (can be greater than 900 breaths/min) and tidal volumes near and, commonly, less than anatomic dead spaces.
   a. Jet ventilator delivers short burst of gases at high flow.
      i. Exhalation is passive.
      ii. Necrotizing tracheitis is a significant complication, along with hypotension and pneumopericardium.
   b. Oscillator ventilator delivers gases by vibrating columns of air.
      i. Exhalation is active.
      ii. The child appears to shake on the bed, which may be frightening for the parental caregivers.
4. Extracorporeal membrane oxygenation (ECMO)—indicated in infants with reversible cardiac or respiratory failure. ECMO is a modified heart–lung bypass machine used to allow gas exchange outside the body.
   a. Blood is removed from the venous system by a catheter placed in the internal jugular vein or right atrium.
   b. Oxygen is added and carbon dioxide is removed with a membrane oxygenator.
   c. Oxygenated blood is returned by way of the right common carotid (in venoarterial ECMO) or the femoral vein (in venovenous ECMO).
   d. The infant must be heparinized for the procedure, increasing the risk of intraventricular hemorrhage. For this reason, VLBW infants or infants of decreased gestational age are usually not candidates for the procedure.
   e. One nurse and one ECMO specialist must be present at the bedside at all times to monitor the patient and equipment. The patient will receive paralytic agents as well as analgesia and sedation; therefore, diligent continuous monitoring is required.
   f. Cannula dislodgement or tubing separation will result in immediate hemorrhage. Tubing and cannula must be secured and visible.
   g. Administration of vasoactive medications may be required to support alteration in cardiac output and blood pressure.
   h. Blood transfusions may be indicated because of blood loss from frequent sampling or anemia of prematurity.
5. Ventilatory support modalities for RDS currently under study: nitric oxide, liquid ventilation (tidal or partial), and perfluorocarbon-assisted gas exchange.

Complications

1. Complications related to respiratory therapy are as follows:
   a. Air leak: pneumothorax, pneumomediastinum, pneumopericardium, and pneumoperitoneum.
   b. Pneumonia, especially gram-negative organisms.
   c. Pulmonary interstitial emphysema.
2. PDA or heart failure.
3. Hypotension.
4. Intraventricular hemorrhage—typically seen in infants weighing less than 1,500 g.
5. DIC.
6. Chronic problems associated with long-term use of oxygen:
   a. BPD—cystic-appearing lungs with hyperinfiltration, obstructive bronchiolitis, dysplastic changes, and pulmonary fibrosis.
   b. Chronic respiratory infections.
7. Necrotizing enterocolitis.
8. Tracheal stenosis.
9. Retinopathy of prematurity (retrolental fibroplasia).
10. Other complications related to prematurity.
11. Renal failure requiring use of dialysis.

Nursing Assessment

1. Review the birth history.
   a. Apgar scores 1 and 5 minutes after birth.
   b. Type of resuscitation required.
   c. Treatments or medications administered.

   d. Medications or anesthesia administered to the pregnant patient during labor.
   e. Estimated gestational age.
   f. Maternal history—contributing factors or complications.
2. Carefully assess the infant's respiratory status to determine the degree of respiratory distress.
   a. Determine the degree and severity of retractions.
   b. Count the respiratory rate for 1 full minute, note level of activity, and determine if they are regular or irregular.
   c. Identify periods of apnea, length, and type of stimulation necessary.
   d. Listen for expiratory grunting or whining sounds from the infant when quiet. This indicates an attempt to maintain PEEP and prevent alveoli from collapse.
   e. Note nasal flaring.
   f. Note cyanosis—location, improvement with oxygen.
   g. Auscultate chest for diminished breath sounds and presence of crackles.
3. Determine the infant's cardiac rate and rhythm.
   a. Count the apical pulse for 1 full minute.
   b. Note irregularities in the rate or bounding pulses.
4. Observe the infant's general activity.
   a. Lethargic or listless.
   b. Active and responds to stimuli.
   c. Infant's cry.
5. Assess the skin for cyanosis, jaundice, mottling, paleness or grayness, and edema.

Nursing Interventions

Promoting Adequate Gas Exchange

1. Have emergency equipment readily available for use in the event of cardiac or respiratory arrest.
2. Institute cardiorespiratory monitoring to continuously monitor heart and respiratory rates.
3. Administer supplemental oxygen.
   a. Incubator with oxygen at prescribed concentration.
   b. Plastic hood with oxygen at prescribed concentration when using radiant warmer.
   c. CPAP, if indicated, using nasal prongs or ET tube.
4. Assist with ET intubation and maintain mechanical ventilation, as indicated.
5. Measure oxygen concentration every hour and record.
6. Monitor ABG levels, as appropriate. Obtain sample of blood through indwelling umbilical line, arterial puncture, or capillary puncture. (Capillary gas analysis for monitoring $PaCO_2$ and pH but not PaO_2.)
7. Institute pulse oximetry, if available, for continuous monitoring of the blood's arterial oxygen saturation (SaO_2).
   a. Avoid using adhesive to secure the sensor when the infant is active. Wrap it snugly enough to reduce sensitivity to movement but not tight enough to constrict blood flow.
   b. If transcutaneous PaO_2 monitor is used, reposition the probe every 3 to 4 hours to avoid burns caused by heating the probe to achieve sufficient arterialization.
8. Observe the infant's response to oxygen.
   a. Observe for improvement in color, respiratory rate and pattern, and nasal flaring.
   b. Note response by improvement in arterial or capillary blood gas levels.
   c. Observe closely for apnea.
9. Stimulate the infant if apnea occurs. If unable to produce spontaneous respiration with stimulation within 15 to 30 seconds, initiate resuscitation.
10. Position the infant to allow for maximal lung expansion.
   a. Prone position provides for a larger lung volume because of the position of the diaphragm, decreases energy expenditure, and increases the time spent in quiet sleep; however, it may be contraindicated because of placement of the umbilical catheter. The risk of sudden infant death syndrome (SIDS) is increased, but the infant is continuously monitored.
   b. Change position frequently.
11. Suction, as needed, because the gag reflex is weak and cough is ineffective.
12. Try to minimize time spent on procedures and interventions, and monitor effects on respiratory status. (Infants undergoing multiple procedures lasting 45 minutes to 1 hour have shown a moderate decrease in PaO_2.)
13. The decision to suction should be based on assessment of the infant, such as auscultation of chest, decrease in oxygenation, excessive moisture in the ET tube, and irritability.
   a. Nasopharyngeal, tracheal, or ET tube suctioning should be done gently, quickly, 5 seconds or less, with intermittent suction applied as the catheter is withdrawn.
   b. To prevent hypoxemia, observe oximeter before, during, and after the procedure.
   c. Suctioning of the ET tube is done to maintain a patent airway. The practice of inducing a catheter into the tube until resistance is met and then withdrawn has been shown to cause trauma to the tracheal wall. Instead, the suction catheter should be premeasured according to the size of the infant's ET tube length and documented. When suctioning, do not insert the catheter beyond this predetermined length. This will prevent damage to the mucosa.
14. Observe for complications of suctioning: bronchospasm, vagal nerve stimulation, bradycardia, hypoxia, increased intracranial pressure, trauma to airway, infection, and pneumothoraces.
15. VLBW and extremely low birth weight neonates cannot tolerate percussion and vibration. Trendelenburg position is contraindicated in premature neonates and may result in increased intracranial pressure.
16. Record all nursing observations.

CLINICAL JUDGMENT Prone position may present several problems: Turning head to side can compromise upper airway and increase airflow resistance; observation of chest is obstructed, making retractions difficult to detect; and abdominal distention is more difficult to recognize.

Promoting Adequate Nutrition and Hydration

1. Administer IV fluids or enteral feeding, as ordered, and observe infusion rate closely to prevent fluid overload.
2. Observe IV sites for infiltration or infection; use meticulous technique to prevent sepsis.
3. If umbilical artery catheter is in place, observe for bleeding.
4. Provide adequate caloric intake (80 to 120 kcal/kg/24 hours) through the following:
   a. Nasojejunal tube (best tolerated by VLBW neonates).
   b. Nasogastric tube.
   c. Parenteral nutrition—$D_{10}W$ or hyperalimentation fluid usually required, especially in the acute phase of illness.

5. Monitor for hypoglycemia, which is especially common during stress. Maintain serum glucose greater than 45 mg/dL.
6. Monitor intake and output closely.
   a. Include amount of blood drawn (small infants can become anemic because of frequent blood sampling).
   b. Apply urine collection bag to obtain sample of urine, and measure specific gravity periodically.
7. Weigh the infant daily and record.

Maintaining Thermoregulation

1. Provide a neutral thermal environment to maintain the infant's abdominal skin temperature between 97°F and 98°F (36.1°C and 36.7°C) to prevent hypothermia, which may result in vasoconstriction and acidosis.
2. Adjust incubator or radiant warmer to obtain desired skin temperature. For the infant weighing less than 1,250 g, the radiant warmer should be used with caution because of increased water loss and potential for hypoglycemia.
3. Prevent frequent opening of incubator.
4. Ensure that oxygen is warmed to a temperature between 87.6°F and 93.2°F (30.9°C and 34°C) with 60% to 80% humidity.

Encouraging Parental Caregiver Attachment

1. Identify factors that may prohibit the parental caregivers' visitation and communication: geographic distance, lack of transportation, care of siblings, employment restrictions, economic issues, lack of telephone in the home, and fear. Refer to social services for assistance and intervention, if required.
2. If the neonate was transported to a tertiary care center immediately after birth, send the birthing parent a photograph of the neonate.
3. Call the parental caregivers daily to update them on the infant's condition until they are able to visit the child. Emphasize positive aspects of the infant's status.
4. Refer to the child by their first name when speaking with the parental caregivers.
5. Prepare the parental caregivers for the neonatal intensive care unit (NICU) environment and how their child will appear before their first visit.
6. Assist the parental caregivers to participate in the child's care, as appropriate.
7. Demonstrate for the parental caregivers how they can touch and speak to the child while the child is in an Isolette/incubator.
8. Allow the parental caregivers to hold the infant as soon as possible.
9. If breastfeeding is planned, assist with expressing the milk, and use the breast milk to feed the infant when enteral feedings are initiated.
10. If the infant has siblings, provide the parental caregivers with information on how to discuss the infant's illness with them.
11. If unit policies allow and the situation is appropriate, encourage sibling visitation with adequate preparation.
12. Provide the parental caregivers with information concerning the disease process, expected outcomes, and usual course of the NICU stay. Encourage the parental caregivers to ask questions and participate in the care plan.
13. Help parental caregivers work through their distress at the birth of a premature child.
14. Assess parental caregivers' support mechanisms (e.g., grandparents, friends).

Family Education and Health Management

1. Prepare the family for long-term follow-up, as appropriate. Infants with BPD may eventually go home on oxygen therapy.
2. Stress the importance of regular health care, periodic eye examinations, and developmental follow-up with the parental caregivers.
3. Ensure that the family receives information on routine well-baby care.
4. Before discharge, parental caregivers should feel comfortable in their abilities to care for the infant. Referrals for home nursing visits should be completed and a provider identified for follow-up care.

Evaluation: Expected Outcomes

- Respiratory rate within normal range for age; pattern regular and unlabored.
- Tolerates enteral feedings well; weight gain noted.
- Maintains temperature within normal limits.
- Parental caregivers interact with infant, participate in care, and ask appropriate questions.

Cystic Fibrosis

EVIDENCE BASE De Boeck, K. (2020). Cystic fibrosis in the year 2020: A disease with a new face. *Acta Paediatrica (Oslo, Norway: 1992), 109*(5), 893–899. https://doi.org/10.1111/apa.15155

Endres, T. M., & Konstan, M. W. (2022). What is cystic fibrosis? *JAMA, 327*(2), 191. https://doi.org/10.1001/jama.2021.23280

Cystic fibrosis (CF) is an autosomal recessive disorder affecting the exocrine glands, causing abnormal viscosity of secretions. It primarily affects the pulmonary and GI systems. Approximately 4% to 5% of White individuals are symptomless carriers of the CF gene. Slightly more people assigned male at birth than people assigned female at birth are affected. Incidence is estimated at approximately 1 in 2,500 to 3,500 live births of White newborns. CF is found in all racial groups. The median survival age is around 47 years, compared with a life expectancy of less than 1 year in the 1950s.

Pathophysiology and Etiology

1. CF is caused by a genetic defect in a single gene located on the long arm of chromosome 7 that encodes the cystic fibrosis transmembrane conductance regulator (CFTR).
2. The variations in the onset of the disease, symptomatology, and clinical presentation within the CF population are attributed to the over 1,000 mutations of the CF gene. CFTR is responsible for the fluid balance across epithelial cells.
3. The malfunction of CFTR results in the following:
   a. Decreased chloride secretion into the airway lumen.
   b. Increased sodium reabsorption, which leads to decreased airway surface liquid volume.
   c. Thickened mucus, impaired mucociliary clearance, chronic infection, plugged bronchi.
   d. Chronic inflammation, airway damage, atelectasis, and hyperinflation of lungs.
   e. Progressive bronchiectasis, irreversible fibrotic changes in lungs.
4. GI and pancreatic involvement includes the following:
   a. Acini and ducts of pancreas become filled with thick mucus and are obstructed.
   b. Trypsin, chymotrypsin, lipase, and amylase do not reach the small intestine.

c. Digestion is impaired. Interruption of the enterohepatic circulation of bile acids probably results in interference with normal pancreatic lipolysis and fat absorption through the intestinal wall.
d. Stools are abnormal and indicate malabsorption syndrome.
e. Meconium ileus often occurs in infants, indicating that bowel is obstructed by thick intestinal secretions.
f. Biliary cirrhosis occurs because the intrahepatic biliary tract is obstructed by thick secretions.
g. In 30% of CF patients, the gallbladder is small, with suboptimal function. Gallstones develop in up to 10% of patients.

5. Sweat gland involvement includes the following:
   a. Secretions contain excessive amount of sodium and chloride, leading to excessive loss, especially with hot weather, fever, or exertion.
   b. Saliva also contains an excess of sodium and chloride.

Clinical Manifestations

Presentation usually occurs younger than age 6 months but may occur at any age. Signs and symptoms and severity of the disease vary and change over time as the disease progresses.

Respiratory Manifestations

1. Recurrent pulmonary infections—*H. influenza, Staphylococcus aureus, Pseudomonas aeruginosa.*
2. Cough, dry to productive. Chronic clearing of throat may indicate increased mucus production.
3. Wheezing, crackles on auscultation are indicative of respiratory exacerbation.
4. Dyspnea.
5. Barrel-shaped chest (increased anteroposterior chest diameter).
6. Cyanosis.
7. Clubbing of fingers and toes.
8. Nasal polyps and pansinusitis.
9. Progressive chronic obstructive pulmonary disease (COPD). A 10% drop in FEV_1 is a sign of an acute exacerbation or worsening lung disease.
   a. Mild form of CF—slightly decreased FEV_1 (70% to 90%).
   b. Moderate CF—FEV_1 of 40% to 69%
   c. Severe forms of CF—life-threatening pulmonary disease with FEV_1 of less than 40%

GI Manifestations

1. Meconium ileus found in neonates.
2. Failure to thrive and failure to gain weight in the presence of a good appetite.
3. Abdominal distention.
4. Vomiting, dehydration, and electrolyte imbalance.
5. Maldigestion, steatorrhea (fatty stools, loss of fat-soluble vitamins).
6. Rectal prolapse.
7. Distal intestinal obstructive syndrome.
8. Biliary cirrhosis, obstructive jaundice.
9. Pancreatitis.

Other Manifestations

1. Thin extremities, sallow skin, wasted buttocks.
2. Hyperglycemia, glucosuria, polyuria, weight loss.
3. Salty taste when parental caregivers kiss skin.
4. Sterility in people assigned male at birth.
5. Hypoproteinemia and anemia.
6. Bleeding diathesis.
7. Hyponatremia and heat prostration.
8. Kyphosis.

Diagnostic Evaluation

1. Quantitative sweat chloride test; pilocarpine iontophoresis, performed at a CF Foundation accredited center by skilled personnel; measures sodium and chloride content in sweat.
   a. Chloride level greater than 60 mEq/L is virtually diagnostic.
   b. Chloride of 40 to 60 mEq/L is borderline and should be repeated, followed by genotype for the most frequent CFTR mutations.
   c. Sodium level greater than 60 mEq/L is diagnostic.
2. Measurement of trypsin concentration in duodenal secretions; absence of normal concentration virtually diagnostic.
3. Analysis of digestive enzymes (trypsin and chymotrypsin) in stool—reduced, used for initial screening for CF.
4. Chest x-ray—may be normal initially; later shows areas of infection, overinflation, bronchial thickening and plugging, atelectasis, fibrosis, and emphysema.
5. Sinus radiograph or computed tomography shows mucus plugging.
6. Analysis of stool for steatorrhea.
7. Meconium strip test for stool includes lactose and protein content and is used for screening.
8. Sputum or throat cultures to rule out infection.
9. Pulmonary function studies (after age 4 years).
   a. Decreased vital capacity and flow rates.
   b. Increased residual volume or increased total lung capacity.
10. Diagnosis made when a positive sweat test is seen in conjunction with one or more of the following:
    a. Positive family history for CF.
    b. Typical COPD.
    c. Documented exocrine pancreatic insufficiency.
    d. Failure to thrive.
    e. History of frequent respiratory infections.
11. Prenatal diagnostic tests—prenatal genetic screening for families affected with CF:
    a. Chorionic villus sampling at approximately 12 weeks' gestation.
    b. Deoxyribonucleic acid (DNA) probes.
    c. Microvillar enzymes.
12. Neonatal screening: immunoreactive trypsinogen; if elevated, DNA assay for single and multiple CFTR mutations.

Management

Goals of treatment are to prevent and minimize pulmonary complications, ensure adequate nutrition for growth, and assist the family and child to adapt to chronic disease.

Pulmonary Interventions

1. Antimicrobial therapy, as indicated, for pulmonary infection.
   a. Oral antibiotics may be given prophylactically or when symptomatic.
   b. IV antibiotics are given when the child fails to respond to oral antibiotics; this may be inpatient or at-home therapy.
   c. Inhaled antibiotics such as tobramycin may be used to prevent infection and colonization of organisms. Recently, some practitioners advocate using nebulized antibiotics earlier in therapy.
   d. Patients with CF metabolize antibiotics rapidly; if drug dosage is higher than normal, monitor for signs of toxicity.
2. Bronchodilators to increase the airway size and assist with mucociliary clearance. Many CF patients also have airway hyperreactivity.
3. Long-term clinical improvement with inhaled bronchodilators has not been well supported in the literature; aerosols, expectorants, and mucolytic agents to decrease viscosity of secretions.

a. Recombinant human DNase administered via nebulizer improves pulmonary function and decreases sputum viscosity and pulmonary exacerbations.
b. Hypertonic saline solution 3% to 7%.
c. Improves airway clearance and lung function, although it is not as effective as recombinant human DNase.
d. Acetylcysteine solution is not recommended because of irritant effect on airways.

4. CPT for bronchial drainage, especially during acute exacerbations.
   a. Postural drainage (see Figure 40-6).
   b. Some patients use a vibrating vest that utilizes a shaking motion rather than manual postural drainage.

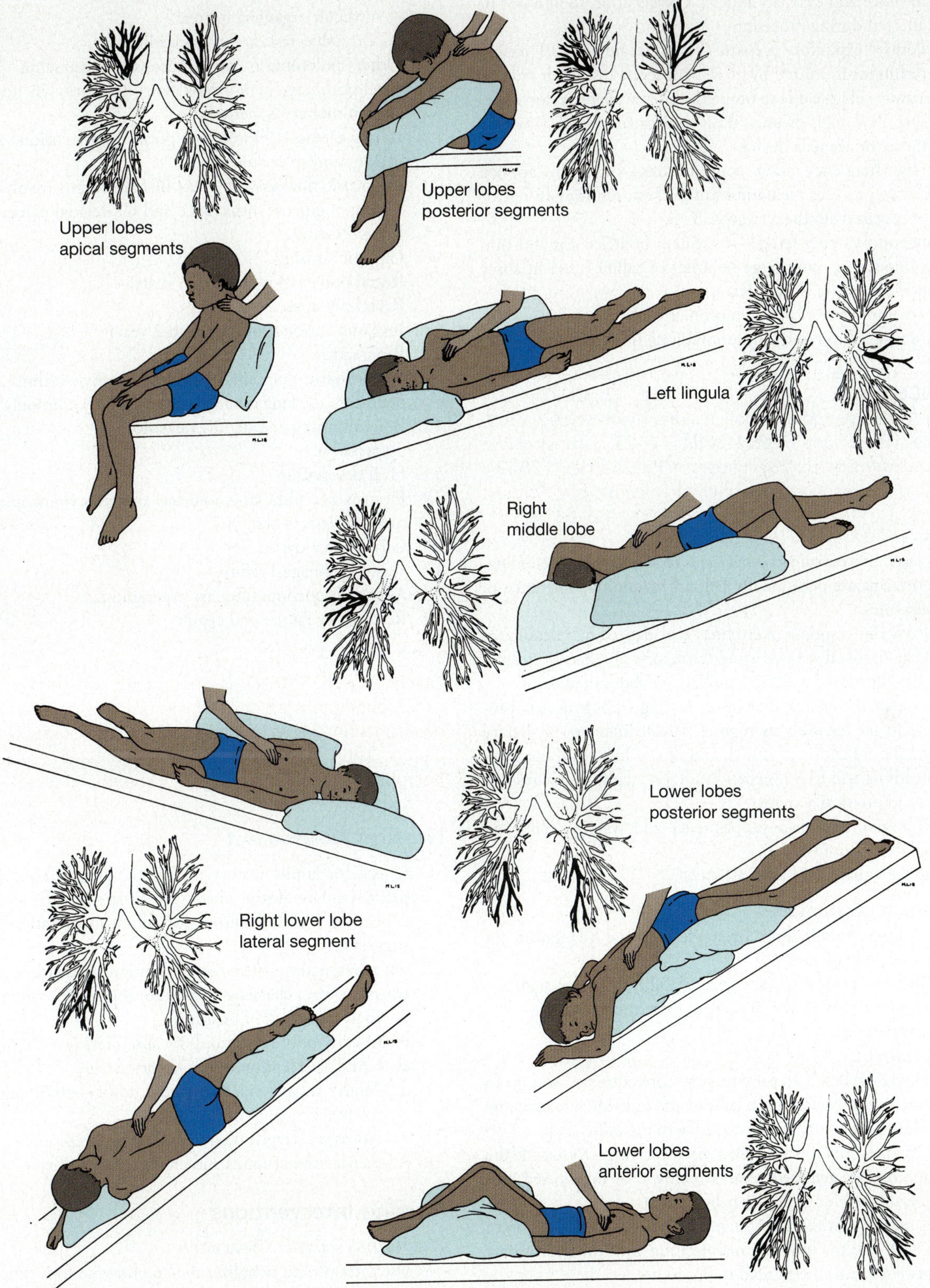

Figure 40-6. Positions for postural drainage.

c. Coughing and deep-breathing exercises; huffing helps move secretions from smaller airways.
d. Increase physical activity—aerobic activity.
e. Active cycle of breathing, a new technique, improves lung function without decreasing oxygenation. Consists of breathing control, thoracic expansion, forced expiratory technique, and huffing. An assistant is not required.
f. Autogenic drainage—breathing at various lung volumes to move and evacuate mucus. Oxygenation should not be affected during procedure.
g. Positive expiratory pressure (PEP) and flutter; PEP airway technique is utilized by those with severe disease. It reduces airway collapse due to bronchiectasis; available as low-pressure PEP, high-pressure PEP, and oscillating PEP with a flutter or acapella device.
h. High-frequency chest compressions—externally applied device provides oscillation to the chest, resulting in release of mucus from the airway wall.

5. Bronchopulmonary lavage—treatment of atelectasis and mucoid impaction using large volumes of saline (used in some institutions in the United States).
6. Lobectomy—resection of symptomatic lobar bronchiectasis to retard progression of lesion to total lung involvement.

EVIDENCE BASE Patel,D., & Gaillard, E. (2022). Optimising the management of children with cystic fibrosis. *The Practitioner, 266*(1855), 17-21. https://www.thepractitioner.co.uk//Symposium/Paediatrics/12843-/Optimising-the-management-of-children-with-cystic-fibrosis

GI Interventions

1. Pancreatic enzyme supplementation is provided with each feeding.
   a. Antacids are occasionally helpful to improve tolerance of enzymes.
   b. Favorable response to enzymes is evidenced by tolerance of fatty foods, decreased stool frequency, absence of steatorrhea, improved appetite, and lack of abdominal pain.
2. Provide a high-energy diet by increasing carbohydrates, protein, and fat (possibly as high as 40%). Increases in dietary intake should consider growth and repair, infection, the work of breathing and energy expenditure for coughing, malabsorption, and physical activity.
3. Provide zinc and iron supplements and water-soluble and fat-soluble vitamins.
4. Ensure adequate fluid and salt intake.

Experimental Treatments

1. Heart–lung, double-lung, or single-lung transplantation for end-stage lung disease.
   a. This treatment is limited by availability of donor organs.
   b. Long-term survival at 5 years is approximately 50%.
2. Liver transplant.
3. Gene therapy.
   a. Therapy is based on somatic gene correction; an attempt to correct the defect in the cells of the individual is made by adding the correct gene sequence to the cells.
   b. One trial method will use a virus carrying DNA with the appropriate gene sequence, which will be introduced into the affected lung cells by nebulization.
   c. A second method being investigated is the introduction of DNA into the lungs by nebulization with the appropriate gene sequence suspended in liposomes.
   d. It is thought that the treatment will need to be repeated at regular intervals.
4. *P. aeruginosa* genome is complete, which should lead to the development of new medications to combat this common lung infection in CF.

Complications

1. Pulmonary infections:
   a. Most frequently caused by *P. aeruginosa, S. aureus, H. influenzae*, and *Burkholderia cepacia. Pseudomonas* is the most difficult organism to treat.
   b. Bronchiectasis and bronchiolitis.
2. Other pulmonary complications—emphysema, atelectasis, pneumothorax, hemoptysis (seen primarily in adolescents), and pulmonary hypertension.
3. Biliary cirrhosis, leading to portal hypertension, esophageal varices, and splenomegaly.
4. Pancreatic fibrosis with islets of Langerhans involvement, resulting in glucose intolerance and CF-related diabetes.
5. Cor pulmonale.
6. Chronic sinusitis.
7. Rectal polyps (3 months to 3 years).
8. Rectal prolapse.
9. Intussusception (younger than 2 years).
10. Pancreatitis.
11. Hypertrophic pulmonary osteoarthropathy—arthritis, clubbing, periostitis; the long tubular bones are most commonly involved.
12. Bone thinning and demineralization.
13. Depression.
14. Heat prostration.
15. Fibrosis of epididymis and vas deferens in people assigned male at birth; aspermia.
16. Growth retardation.
17. Gastroesophageal reflux.
18. Allergic bronchopulmonary aspergillosis.
19. Respiratory failure and death.

CLINICAL JUDGMENT *B. cepacia* affects approximately 5% of CF patients, is associated with a rapid decline in pulmonary function, and is multiple antibiotic resistant. Twenty percent of colonized patients develop fulminant septicemia and necrotizing pneumonia, leading to death.

Nursing Assessment

1. Check for family history of CF, failure to thrive, and unexplained infant death; check the child's history and physical condition. Carefully listen for subtle information that may suggest CF.
2. Assess respiratory status—respiratory rate, presence of tachypnea, wheeze, cough, character of sputum, and oxygen saturation level.
   a. Increased work of breathing.
   b. Quality of breath sounds by auscultation.
   c. Child's perception of respiratory status.
   d. Ability to participate in activities of daily living, exercise tolerance, quality of sleep.
   e. Assess for oxygen desaturation with sleep.
3. Assess nutritional status and characteristics of stool.

Nursing Interventions

Promoting Airway Clearance

1. Use intermittent nebulizer therapy three to four times per day when child is symptomatic.
   a. Use pretreatment postural drainage.

b. Administer bronchodilators and other medications, diluted in normal saline, in aerosol form to penetrate respiratory tract. Proper technique is necessary to deliver the correct dose of medication. If using a face mask, it should fit snugly; movement of the mask by ¾ in (2 cm) could decrease the delivery of medication by 85%.

2. Perform CPT three to four times per day after nebulizer therapy; perform more frequently if infection is present.
   a. Perform prior to meals or 1 hour after eating to prevent vomiting or discomfort.
   b. Place the child in a position that gives the greatest access to the affected lobes of the lung and facilitates gravity drainage of mucus from specific lung areas.
   c. Children with gastroesophageal reflux should not use the head-down position during CPT.
3. Help the child to relax to cough more easily after postural drainage.
4. Suction the infant or young child when necessary if they are unable to cough.
5. Teach child breathing exercises using pursed lips to increase duration of exhalation.
6. Monitor child's oxygen saturation levels during procedures.
7. Maintain cautious oxygen therapy because of chronic carbon dioxide retention.
8. Monitor for signs and symptoms of pneumothorax, such as tachypnea, tachycardia, pallor, dyspnea, and cyanosis.
9. Monitor for hemoptysis, which requires immediate treatment and may be life threatening.
10. Provide treatment of hemoptysis: bed rest, cough suppressants, and antibiotics.
    a. Bronchoscopy is used to locate the site, cauterize, or embolize.
    b. Administer vitamin K, as directed.

CLINICAL JUDGMENT Mist therapy is no longer recommended because water droplets may cause bronchospasm in some patients, and the equipment required to deliver the therapy is frequently contaminated with opportunistic organisms.

Preventing Infection

Adherence to infection control procedures must be enforced to prevent the spread of nosocomial infections.

1. Provide frequent mouth care to reduce the chance of infection because mucus is present.
2. Restrict contact with people with respiratory infections.
3. Administer antibiotics, as prescribed, to treat specific organisms when the child is symptomatic.
4. Follow institutional guidelines on replacing nebulizers for hospitalized CF patients. Evidence varies with recommendations from each use to every 1 to 3 days.
5. Monitor closely for deteriorating respiratory status.
6. Provide good skin care and position changes to prevent skin breakdown of malnourished child.
7. Change diapers promptly to prevent diaper rash and superimposed infection.

CLINICAL JUDGMENT To decrease the risk of transmission of *B. cepacia* within the hospital setting, children who test positive for the pathogen are placed on room isolation.

Promoting Adequate Nutrition

1. Refer to dietitian for dietary assessment.
2. Encourage diet composed of foods high in calories and protein and moderate to high in fat because absorption of food is incomplete. Provide 120% to 150% of recommended dietary allowances because only 80% to 85% of intake is absorbed.
3. Administer fat-soluble vitamins in water-miscible solution in two to three times the normal dose, as prescribed, to counteract malabsorption.
   a. Give vitamins A, D, and E on a daily basis.
   b. Give vitamin K when the child has an infection or is being treated with antibiotics.
4. Administer pancreatic enzymes with each meal and snack. Dose is based on the child's weight, weight gain, growth, food intake, and number and character of bowel movements.
   a. Mix capsule, granules, or powder with small portion of food for infant or small child; do not mix with formula, which may not be finished.
   b. Offer the older child capsules or tablets.
   c. Withhold enzymes, as ordered, if the child is taking only clear liquid diet or enteral feedings.
   d. Beads should not be chewed or crushed.
   e. The CF Foundation discourages the use of generic enzymes.
5. Increase salt intake during hot weather, fever, or excessive exercise to prevent sodium depletion and cardiovascular compromise.
6. To prevent vomiting, allow ample time for feeding, especially if irritable because of not feeling well and coughing.
7. Check weights at least weekly to assess nutritional interventions. Document and plot height and weight every 3 months.
8. Infants who are breastfed will need enzyme supplementation. If supplementation with formula is necessary, choose a high-calorie preparation.
9. Administer supplemental parenteral or enteral feedings, as required.
10. Constipation, due to malabsorption, decreased gastric motility; viscous intestinal secretions may be treated with laxatives, stool softeners, or rectal administration of x-ray contrast material.

Enhancing Self-esteem and Body Image

1. Explain each procedure, medication, and treatment to the child as appropriate for age.
2. Allow the child to show frustrations, fears, and feelings by talking, complaining, or crying.
3. Support and comfort the child by talking to and holding them.
4. Provide diversional activities related to the child's interests, and praise the child for their accomplishments.
5. Encourage the older child to take an active role in their self-management and be involved in the care plan.
6. Help the child to identify strengths and limitations and to feel good about self.
7. Help to redirect feelings of anger, fear, or frustration to increase adherence to CPT.
8. Encourage regular exercise and activity to foster a sense of accomplishment and independence and improve pulmonary function. Consent from health care provider is necessary prior to the initiation of an exercise program. Oxygenation status during exercise should be assessed.

Enhancing Family Processes

1. Provide opportunities for the parental caregivers to learn all aspects of care for the child.
2. Provide education and support during hospitalization to make home care easier.
3. Encourage maintenance of family activities and involvement with other children.
4. Initiate social work referral, as needed.
5. Encourage information sharing about CF with friends, teachers, and relatives. Explain that one of the most important things people can do to help a child with CF is to treat them just as they would any other child.

6. Help family share and interpret feelings about CF and its impact on all of their lives.
7. Encourage families to foster the older child's independence when the time comes.

Family Education and Health Maintenance

1. Teach parental caregivers to have a thorough understanding of the dietary regimen and special need for calories, fat, and vitamins. Consultation with a registered dietitian is recommended.
2. Discuss the child's need for salt replacement and free access to salt as well as the increased need for salt during hot weather or in the presence of fever, vomiting, or diarrhea.
3. Help the parental caregivers to become skilled at CPT and other pulmonary treatments. Demonstrate and explain procedures and evaluate their return demonstration.
4. Help the family to schedule care for the child within the framework of family life.
   a. CPT should be done at least 1 hour after meals.
   b. Nebulizer treatments should be done before CPT.
   c. Mild exercise and activity are beneficial to the child.
   d. Vacations and major family outings can be planned for remission of the child's symptoms.
5. Help the parental caregivers to provide emotional support to their child. The child needs love, understanding, and security, not overprotection.
6. Stress the importance of regular medical care.
   a. Routine immunizations.
   b. Prompt attention to infection.
   c. Continued evaluation and supervision in home management.
   d. Attention to developments through research that may change therapy.
   e. Prevention or early detection of complications.
7. Stress the importance of following up with regular health care provider for routine follow-up according to Cystic Fibrosis Foundation.
   a. Outpatient visits, four per year.
   b. Pulmonary function tests, two or more per year.
   c. Respiratory cultures, at least one per year.
   d. Creatinine level, every year.
   e. Glucose level, every year if older than age 13
   f. Liver enzymes, every year.
8. Discuss with parental caregivers the limitations and expectations for the child.
   a. With proper care, the child will most likely live to adulthood but may be smaller and shorter than peers.
   b. Play and school participation depends on severity of illness.
   c. Involve teachers and school nurses in planning of the child's day.
9. Suggest parental caregivers and child meet other CF families. Investigate location and participation in summer camps for children with CF.
10. Investigate home care options for families, especially respite services for parental caregivers.
11. After the diagnosis is confirmed, refer the parental caregivers to genetic counseling. It is important for the parental caregivers to realize that the affected child inherits the mutated gene from both biological parents. Each pregnancy will result in a 25% chance that the infant will have CF, a 50% chance that it will be a carrier of the CF gene and *not* have CF, and a 25% chance that the infant will neither be a carrier of the CF gene nor have CF.
12. Refer families for additional information and support to agencies such as Cystic Fibrosis Foundation (www.cff.org). Most areas have local chapters of the organization.
13. The pediatric health care team should discuss with the patient and parental caregivers the concept of eventual transitioning of care from a pediatric CF center to an adult CF center as early as possible—an important issue that should not be left until adolescence. Facilitate a planned, efficient, and smooth transition by
    a. Encouraging the child to gradually assume responsibility for health care.
    b. Encouraging the parental caregivers to foster the adolescent's independence.
    c. Providing patient and family time to adjust and educate themselves about the transitioning process.
    d. Identifying and introducing the child and their family to members of the adult care team.
    e. Advocating for the patient in regard to any restrictions superimposed by the patient's health insurance plan.
14. Sadly, at some point, it will become apparent to the health care team that the time has arrived to discuss end-of-life issues. Use a family-centered approach to provide care for the child and family facing a life-threatening illness or death. Discuss hospice care and other available services with the family (see page 93).

EVIDENCE BASE Kapnadak, S. G., Dimango, E., Hadjiliadis, D., Hempstead, S. E., Tallarico, E., Pilewski, J. M., Faro, A., Albright, J., Benden, C., Blair, S., Dellon, E. P., Gochenour, D., Michelson, P., Moshiree, B., Neuringer, I., Riedy, C., Schindler, T., Singer, L. G., Young, D., ... Simon, R. H. (2020). Cystic Fibrosis Foundation consensus guidelines for the care of individuals with advanced cystic fibrosis lung disease. *Journal of Cystic Fibrosis, 19*(3), 344–354. https://doi.org/10.1016/j.jcf.2020.02.015

Bell, J., Alexander, L., Carson, J., Crossan, A., McCaughan, J., Mills, H., O'Neill, D., Moore, J. E., & Millar, B. C. (2020). Nebuliser hygiene in cystic fibrosis: Evidence-based recommendations. *Breath, 16* (2), 190328. https://doi.org/10.1183/20734735.0328-2019

Dongarwar, D., Garcia, B. Y., Miller, K., & Salihu, H. M. (2022). Assessment of hospitalization rates, factors associated with hospitalization and in-patient mortality in pediatric patients with cystic fibrosis. *Journal of the National Medical Association, 113*(6), 683–692. https://doi.org/10.1016/j.jnma.2021.08.038

Kavalieratos, D., Georgiopoulos, A., Dhingra, L., Basile, M., Rabinowitz, E., Hempstead, S. E., Faro, A., & Dellon, E. P. (2021). Models of palliative care delivery for individuals with cystic fibrosis: Cystic Fibrosis Foundation evidence-informed consensus guidelines. *Journal of Palliative Medicine, 24*(1), 18–30. https://doi.org/10.1089/jpm.2020.0311

Evaluation: Expected Outcomes

- Tolerates CPT four times per day for 30 minutes with stable oxygen saturation.
- No signs of respiratory infection.
- Eats well with no vomiting; weight stable.
- Plays, interacts appropriately.
- Parental caregivers ask questions; meet, as necessary, with a social worker; and take part in care of their child.

Apnea of Infancy and Brief Resolved Unexplained Events in Infants

Apnea of infancy (AOI) is defined as an unexplained episode of cessation of breathing for 20 seconds or longer or a shorter respiratory pause associated with bradycardia, cyanosis, pallor, and marked hypotonia in an infant of 37 weeks' gestation or more at the onset of apnea.

Apnea of prematurity (AOP) is defined as sudden cessation of breathing that lasts for 20 seconds and may or may not be accompanied by bradycardia and cyanosis in an infant younger than 37 weeks' gestation.

Brief Resolved Unexplained Event in Infants (BRUE) are defined as an episode that is frightening to the observer and is characterized by some combination of apnea (central or obstructive), color change, cyanosis, pallor or plethora, marked change in muscle tone, extreme limpness, choking, or gagging. This was formerly referred to as ALTE (Apparent Life Threatening Event).

Pathophysiology and Etiology

1. Cause is often unknown—may result from many different pathologic processes; may be idiopathic.
2. Apnea may be related to organic disorders, such as seizure disorders, sepsis, severe infection, hypoglycemia, and impaired regulation of breathing while sleeping or feeding, gastroesophageal reflux, upper airway abnormalities, metabolic disorders, or abuse.
3. Abnormal properties of surfactant have been reported in some children with recurrent BRUE.
4. A diagnosis of AOI is made when no identifiable cause of BRUE is found.
5. AOP is related to immature neurologic and respiratory control mechanisms.

Clinical Manifestations

1. The infant may be found by parental caregivers to be limp, cyanotic, and pale with no respiration. Skin is cool to the touch.
2. Some form of resuscitation may be required.
3. The infant usually exhibits symptoms when asleep, although the syndrome may occur during waking hours.
4. Types of AOP are as follows:
   a. Central or diaphragmatic—chest movement ceases, airflow is absent.
   b. Obstructive—chest and diaphragm move, but there is no air exchange.
   c. Mixed—cessation of airflow and chest movement, followed by respiratory effort without airflow.

Diagnostic Evaluation

Complete history, physical examination, and diagnostic tests are aimed at ruling out other medical problems that could result in respiratory failure as a secondary cause.

1. Complete blood count with differential, serum glucose, electrolytes, calcium, phosphate, magnesium, and ABG levels, as indicated.
2. Chest x-ray.
3. Electrocardiogram.
4. Electroencephalogram (may not be routine) and neurologic examination.
5. Respiratory studies—a 12-to-24-hour pneumogram recording of small changes in electrical resistance with each breath or respiratory pattern; multichannel sleep test with continuous printout, monitoring heart rate, chest impedance, nasal airflow, and oxygen saturation.
6. Continuous cardiac and apnea monitoring for recurrence of event, prolonged apnea, or bradycardia.
7. pH probe test for GERD (gastroesophageal reflux disease).
8. Because of hypoxemia that may have occurred, the child should be assessed for learning difficulties, discrete neurologic impairments, impaired hearing or vision, and personality disorders.
9. Polysomnograph—records brain waves, eye movements, esophageal manometry, and end-tidal carbon dioxide.

Management

1. BRUE may require hospitalization and cardiorespiratory monitoring.
2. Specific treatment of the underlying cause, if identified.
3. Theophylline is no longer recommended for management of AOP. Caffeine (caffeine citrate), which also acts as a central nervous system stimulant for breathing, may be given as a loading dose of 20 mg/kg, followed by a daily maintenance dose of 5 to 10 mg/kg (IV or orally). It is preferred over theophylline due to its longer half-life, wider margin of safety, and lower frequency of adverse effects. Blood level measurements of caffeine levels are no longer routinely recommended.
4. Long-term follow-up for physiologic and neurologic behavioral functions.
5. Prevention of SIDS: the most effective method of prevention is public education to avoid prone sleeping. More education is needed, with an emphasis on poor, underserved areas (see Box 40-1).

CLINICAL JUDGMENT Infants who have experienced apnea may be at risk for recurrent apnea, hypoxia, and sudden death and should be monitored closely. Research has shown that SIDS is more likely in infants sleeping prone. It is now recommended that all infants be put to sleep on their backs.

Nursing Assessment

1. Obtain a nursing history, including the parental caregivers' description of the events that preceded the hospitalization and their understanding of prolonged apnea.
   a. This information may provide clues for factors to observe during hospitalization and provides data for the development of a teaching plan.
   b. It allows for the correction of misinformation and misconceptions.
2. Have the parental caregivers describe sleep patterns, feeding habits, prior health problems, immunizations, and medications; this may provide data regarding possible influencing factors or causes of the condition.
3. Have the parental caregivers describe a typical day in the life of the infant and the family unit. This provides important data on how home monitoring may affect family life and contributes to the effective development of home management and family teaching plans; it also provides a basis for continuity of care for the infant.

Nursing Interventions

Maintaining Breathing Pattern

1. Be prepared for the infant's admission, and have all equipment, including apnea monitor, ready for use. Continuous cardiac monitoring is also recommended.

BOX 40-1 Sudden Infant Death Syndrome

EVIDENCE BASE Stiffler, D., Matemachani, S., & Crane, L. (2020). Considerations in Safe to Sleep® messaging: Learning from African-American mothers. *Journal for Specialists in Pediatric Nursing, 25*(1), e12277. https://doi.org/10.1111/jspn.12277

Sudden infant death syndrome (SIDS) is sudden death of an infant under the age of 1 year, which remains unexplained after a thorough case investigation, including performance of a complete autopsy, examination of the death scene, and review of clinical history.

The peak incidence occurs between 2 and 3 months of age. In addition, it has been found that there is a higher rate of incidence, two to three times the national average, in children who are Black or American Indian or of Alaskan origin. Additional infant risk factors include being a person assigned male at birth, prematurity, preterm birth or low birth weight, low Apgar scores, prone sleeping position, overheating, sleeping on soft surfaces, and twin victim of SIDS. Maternal risk factors include young maternal age, late or no prenatal care, smoking or exposure to smoking during pregnancy, history of sexually transmitted infection or urinary tract infection, anemia, and poverty.

There has generally been a reduction in death rate, with 1.2 deaths per 1,000 live births reported in 1992 and 0.5% deaths per 1,000 live births in 2002. However, since 2001, there has been a slightly higher proportion of deaths occurring in the neonatal period and after 6 months of age, possibly due to classification.

Current theories on the cause of SIDS focus on abnormalities of the brain stem and its network. Recent autopsy results from victims of SIDS have indicated deficits in serotonin receptors in this network, which are responsible for breathing, body temperature, blood pressure, and arousal.

The American Academy of Pediatrics' Task Force on Sudden Infant Death Syndrome introduced a policy statement in July 2022 that put forth a number of recommendations that were developed to reduce the risk of SIDS.

The recommendations are as follows:

- Infants should be placed in the supine position for sleep.
- A firm sleep surface should be used. For example, soft items, such as quilts or pillows, should not be placed under the infant.
- Soft objects and loose bedding should not be part of the infant's sleeping environment.
- Smoking and exposure to passive smoke during pregnancy should be avoided.
- Infants should not share the same bed as adults.
- Overheating should be avoided.
- Using a pacifier, when placing the infant down to sleep, should be considered.
- Home monitors should not be used as a strategy to reduce the risk of SIDS as there is no evidence that proves their effectiveness for this purpose. This is only suggested for infants who have had an apparent life-threatening event.

   a. Select a room that is clearly visible from the nursing station; the room should be quiet to reduce sensory stimulation, which may reduce the likelihood of a recurring episode.
   b. Be aware that the family has just experienced the extreme stress of feeling that their infant has almost died. Reassure them with empathy and efficiency at the time of admission.
2. Continuously monitor respirations. Document apnea along with state of consciousness; sleep state; color; position of infant; muscle tone; respiratory effort before, during, and after event; relationship to activity (e.g., feeding); and intervention necessary (nothing, gentle stimulation, vigorous stimulation, resuscitation).
3. Administer theophylline, if prescribed. Observe for signs of toxicity: apical rate above 200, vomiting, and agitation. Concentration of theophylline for apnea is lower than the concentration for bronchospasm.
4. Continue the infant's normal activities whenever possible (e.g., holding them for feedings, playing with them, disconnecting from monitor for bathing); allow for continuation of usual eating or sleeping patterns. Simulating the home environment as much as possible will encourage deep sleep patterns, which may stimulate apnea and provide valuable diagnostic information.

Minimizing Anxiety

1. Encourage the parental caregivers to continue involvement in infant care during hospitalization.
2. Clarify any misconceptions about apnea and SIDS.
3. Allow ventilation of feelings and concerns.
4. Assess family dynamics for any conflicts or maladapted responses; intervene or refer, as appropriate.
5. Use anticipatory guidance in preparing the parental caregivers for emotional responses to home monitoring.
   a. Increased anxiety or tension.
   b. Constant worry about the alarm even when it does not go off.
   c. Fatigue.
   d. Financial and emotional burdens encountered by the family.
   e. Perceived loss of "normal, healthy child"; parental caregivers may grieve when given the diagnosis.

Increasing Confidence in Home Monitoring

1. Demonstrate operation and maintenance of the monitor. Reinforce teaching by equipment supplier. Provide information on contacting a monitor technician. Teach parental caregivers proper electrode and belt placement and skin care.
   a. Do not adjust monitor to eliminate false alarms.
   b. Maintain an unobstructed view of the monitor. Plug power cord directly into outlet—do not use extension cords. Check battery and charger. Place monitor on firm surface.
   c. Monitored infant should not share their bed.
2. Identify the presence of a telephone in the home, and, if not, devise an alternative plan in the event of an emergency.
3. Describe how to record apnea in relation to activity and position and when to report apnea to health care provider.
4. Teach methods of responding to alarms; what to observe and document in diary (e.g., color, presence or absence of breathing) and how to respond (gentle vs. vigorous stimulation, cardiopulmonary resuscitation [CPR]). Never vigorously shake the child.

5. Discuss the necessary adjustments in daily living and anticipated changes.
   a. Emphasize that responsibility must be shared by family members.
   b. Discuss the possible impact on siblings.
   c. Advise the parental caregivers to eliminate noises that would interfere with their ability to hear the alarm (e.g., showering, vacuuming). Someone must always be available to hear and respond to the alarm. Be aware of electrical interference from appliances or cellular phones and in public places such as airports.
   d. Avoid traveling long distances alone with the infant.
   e. Encourage the parental caregivers to enlist the assistance of a third person who is willing to learn CPR and to help care for the infant and provide the parental caregivers with an opportunity for respite time.
6. Emphasize the healthy aspects of the infant. Encourage the parental caregivers to continue as many usual routines as possible. Provide specific things parental caregivers can do to encourage normal development and a healthy parental caregiver–child relationship.
7. Encourage the parental caregivers to provide total care for their infant 24 hours before discharge so they regain confidence in caring for their child.

Family Education and Health Maintenance

1. Advise the family to keep emergency numbers near the telephone or set on speed dial.
2. Educate about feeding precautions: frequent burping, no bottle in bed, upright position after feeding, positioning the infant on their back instead of their abdomen. Avoid soft, moldable sleeping surfaces and pillows; toys and stuffed animals should be removed from the crib.
3. Have parental caregivers contact local emergency service to inform them about their infant and to be certain that they have infant resuscitation equipment. Arrange for notification of the utility company to plan for the event of a power outage.
4. Instruct the parental caregivers in the administration of any new medications.
5. Teach CPR to all those involved in providing care for the infant (including day care workers and babysitters).
6. Refer the family to a home care agency for home nursing visits, additional teaching, and support.

Evaluation: Expected Outcomes

- Monitoring maintained; respirations regular without apnea.
- Parental caregivers verbalize concern over infant's well-being.
- Parental caregivers demonstrate correct operation of respiratory monitor and response to alarms.

CLINICAL JUDGMENT Respiratory disorders are among the most common conditions in the pediatric population due to their developing airways and their potential for rapid decompensation. Children being discharged with respiratory disorders may require oxygen therapy, suction procedures, and numerous medications delivered via many routes (oral, nebulizer, etc.). Families should have thorough written (and if necessary to assist understanding, pictorial) instructions on signs and symptoms to monitor for worsening of status. Nurses responsible for discharging children should ensure that families understand (and can demonstrate if possible) proper use of necessary treatments.

EVIDENCE BASE Ramgopal, S., Colgan, J., Roland, D., Pitetti, R. D., & Katsogridakis, Y. (2022). Brief resolved unexplained events: A new diagnosis, with implications for evaluation and management. *European Journal of Pediatrics, 181*(2), 463–470. https://doi.org/10.1007/s00431-021-04234-5

SELECTED READINGS

American Academy of Pediatrics. (2021). Pediatric acute care. In R. E. Kleinman (Ed.), *Pediatrics* (6th ed., pp. 26–36). Elsevier.

Friedrichsdorf, S. (2020). Pediatric pain treatment and prevention for hospitalized children. *PAIN Reports, 5*(1), pe804. https://doi.org/10.1097/PR9.000000000000804.

Mamaril, M. E. (2020). Preoperative risk factors associated with PACU pediatric respiratory complications: An integrative review. *Journal of PeriAnesthesia Nursing, 35*(2), 125–134. https://doi.org/10.1016/j.jopan.2019.09.002

McClure, N., Catrambone, C., Carlson, E., & Phillippi, J. (2020). Maximizing the role of the nurse: Strategies to address gaps in asthma care in Schools. *Journal of Pediatric Nursing, 53*, 52-56. https://doi.org/10.1016/j.pedn.2020.05.003

Moscovich, D., Averbuch, D., Kerem, E., Cohen-Cymberknoh, M., Berkun, Y., Brooks, R., Reiff, S., Bar Meir, M., Wolf, D., & Breuer, O. (2023). Pediatric respiratory admissions and related viral infections during the COVID-19 pandemic. *Pediatric Pulmonology, 58*(7), 2076-2084. https://doi.org/10.1002/ppul.26434

Ong, T., & Ramsey, B. (2023). Cystic fibrosis: A review. *JAMA, 329*(21), 1859-1871. https://doi.org/10.1001/jama.2023.8120

Pomiato,E., Perrone, M., Palmieri, R., & Gagliardi,M. (2022). Pediatric myocarditis: What have we learnt so far? *Journal of Cardiovascular Development and Disease, 9*(5), 143. https://doi.org/10.3390/jcdd9050143"10.3390/jcdd9050143

Ramachandran, H. J., Jiang, Y., Shan, C. H., Tam, W. W. S., & Wang, W. (2021). A systematic review and meta-analysis on the effectiveness of swimming on lung function and asthma control in children with asthma. *International Journal of Nursing Studies, 120*, 103953. https://doi.org/10.1016/j.ijnurstu.2021.103953

Rowan, C., Klein, M., Hsing, D., Dahmer, M., Spinella,P., Emeriaud, G., Hassinger, A., Pineres-Olave, B., Flori, H., Haileselassie, B., Lopez-Fernandez, Y., Chima, R., Shein, S., Maddux, A., Lillie, J., Izquierdo, L., Kneyber, M., Smith, L., Khemani, R., & Thomas, N. et al. (2020). Early use of adjunctive therapies for pediatric acute respiratory distress syndrome: A PARDIE study. *American Journal of Respiratory Critical Care Medicine, 201*(11), 1389-1397. https://doi.org/10.1164%2Frccm.201909-1807OC"10.1164/rccm.201909-1807OC

Smith, J. C., & Lofland, G. (2023). Pediatric acute bronchiolitis. In R. M. Kliegman, B. F. Stanton, & N. F. Schor (Eds.), *Nelson textbook of pediatrics* (21st ed., pp. 1471–1476). Elsevier.

Stevens, R., & Kelsall-Knight, L. (2022). Clinical Assessment and Management of Children with Bronchiolitis. *Nursing of Children and Young People, 34*(2), 13-21. https://doi.org/10.7748/ncyp.2022.e1430

Subramonian, A., & Featherstone, R. (2020). *Interventions for the prevention of sudden infant death syndrome and sudden unexplained death in infancy: A review of guidelines.* Canadian Agency for Drugs and Technologies in Health.

41

Pediatric Cardiovascular Disorders*

CARDIAC PROCEDURES

Cardiac Catheterization

Cardiac catheterization is an invasive procedure used to identify cardiac anatomy; measure intracardiac pressures, shunts, and oxygen saturations; and calculate systemic and pulmonary vascular resistance.

Procedure

1. Catheter insertion sites include femoral vein or artery, umbilical vein or artery, brachial vein, or internal jugular vein.
2. Under fluoroscopy, catheters are guided through the heart, collecting pressure measurements and oxygen saturations.
3. Contrast dye is injected through the catheters to visualize blood flow patterns and structural abnormalities.
4. Cardiac catheterization is usually an outpatient procedure for children who undergo an elective procedure. After interventional procedures, some children are observed in the hospital for 12 to 24 hours.

Indications

1. To confirm or establish the diagnosis.
2. To measure cardiac output.
3. To measure pressures and oxygen saturations.
4. To calculate intracardiac shunting and pulmonary and systemic vascular resistance.
5. To visualize coronary arteries.
6. To assess for myocarditis or rejection following heart transplantation.
7. To intervene in congenital heart disease (CHD) (see Box 41-1 for definitions of abbreviations):
   a. Balloon atrial septostomy (Rashkind) for restrictive atrial septum.
   b. Balloon valvuloplasty (aortic stenosis [AS], pulmonary stenosis [PS]) and angioplasty (recurrent coarctation of the aorta [CoA]).
   c. Endomyocardial biopsy.
   d. To occlude vessels (coil embolization) or defects (atrial septal defect [ASD], ventricular septal defect [VSD], or patent ductus arteriosus [PDA] closure devices).
   e. To stent vessels open (branch pulmonary artery [PA] stenosis, recurrent CoA).
   f. To dilate stenotic valves (mitral, pulmonary, tricuspid).
   g. To dilate right ventricular (RV) outflow tracts in native and previously placed conduits in the pulmonary position.

Complications

1. Arrhythmias (usually catheter induced).
2. Infection.
3. Bleeding at catheter insertion site; large hematoma.
4. Allergic reaction to contrast material.
5. Loss of pulse in the extremity used for cannulation.
6. Perforation of heart or vessels.
7. Stroke.
8. Dislodgment of coils, closure devices, or stents.
9. Death.

Nursing Interventions

Reducing Fear in Child and Caregivers

1. Provide specific instructions in a nonthreatening manner:
   a. Day and time of the procedure.
   b. Nothing-by-mouth (NPO) guidelines.
   c. Sedation versus general anesthesia.
   d. Site of the planned arterial and venous puncture.
   e. Routine postprocedure care.

*Please note that the term “male” in this chapter refers to a person assigned male at birth, and the term “female” in this chapter refers to a person assigned female at birth.

BOX 41-1 Abbreviations Used for Congenital Heart Disease

ASD	Atrial septal defect
AV	Atrioventricular
CoA	Coarctation of the aorta
HLHS	Hypoplastic left heart syndrome
IAA	Interrupted aortic arch
IVC	Inferior vena cava
LVOTO	Left ventricular outflow tract obstruction
PA	Pulmonary artery
PAPVR	Partial anomalous pulmonary venous return
PDA	Patent ductus arteriosus
PFO	Patent foramen ovale
PS	Pulmonary stenosis
PVR	Pulmonary vascular resistance
SVC	Superior vena cava
TA	Tricuspid atresia
TAPVR	Total anomalous pulmonary venous return
TGA	Transposition of great arteries
TOF	Tetralogy of Fallot
VSD	Ventricular septal defect

2. Provide appropriate teaching geared toward the child's age and level of cognitive development. Use diagrams and models, as appropriate.
3. Provide caregivers an opportunity, without the child present, to discuss the procedure, risks, benefits, and alternative choices.
4. Give the child an opportunity to express fears and ask questions.
5. Provide tour of the cardiac catheterization laboratory and recovery area, if appropriate.
6. Use of child life specialist, if available, to prepare for procedure and aid in insertion of IV.

Explaining and Providing Nursing Care

1. Obtain baseline set of vital signs: heart rate, blood pressure (BP), respiratory rate, and oxygen saturation.
2. Measure and record the child's height and weight.
3. Note the time of last oral intake: solids and liquids.
4. Identify known allergies.
5. List current medications and note the time last taken.
6. Help the child change into a hospital gown.
7. Start peripheral IV, as needed.
8. Administer sedation, as prescribed.
9. Assess and mark the location of pulses (dorsalis pedis, posterior tibial).

Observe for and Prevent Complications

1. Monitor and record routine vital signs (q 15 min × 4, q 30 min × 2, then q 1 h); extremity temperature, color, and pulse check with vital signs.
2. Notify health care provider for:
   a. Heart rate, respiratory rate, or BP outside normal parameters for age.
   b. Bleeding or increasing hematoma at puncture site.
   c. Change in oxygen saturations.
   d. Fever.
   e. Cool, pulseless extremity.
3. Observe puncture site for redness, pain, swelling, or induration.
4. Maintain the child in a reclining position for 4 to 6 hours after the procedure, with no ambulation.
5. Offer fluids as soon as the child is able to tolerate.

Family Education and Health Maintenance

1. Provide discharge information:
   a. Care of incision or puncture site (keep dry for 48 hours).
   b. Activity restrictions (usually for multiple weeks following placement of closure devices).
   c. Observe for and report late complications: redness, swelling, drainage from puncture site.
   d. Follow-up medical care.
   e. Reinforce infective endocarditis precautions.
2. If cardiac catheterization was a preoperative procedure, use the recovery time to teach the child and family about upcoming hospital stay.

Evaluation: Expected Outcomes

- Child describes the procedure in their own words; caregivers and child discuss the procedure and ask appropriate questions.
- Child cooperative with preoperative nursing care.
- Insertion site intact without drainage, redness, or hematoma.

Cardiac Surgery

The ultimate goal of treatment of cardiovascular disease in children is to restore normal heart structure and function. Most types of CHDs can be palliated or definitively repaired.

Procedures

Closed-Heart Surgery

1. Surgical approach: lateral thoracotomy or mediastinal incision.
2. Indications:
   a. PDA ligation.
   b. PA banding.
   c. CoA repair.
   d. Vascular ring repair.
   e. Blalock–Taussig (BT) shunt placement.
   f. Occasionally, Glenn and Fontan procedures.

Open-Heart Surgery

1. Surgery is done through a mediastinal incision.
2. With the use of cardiopulmonary bypass, the surgeon can stop the heart and operate inside to repair the defects.
3. Deep hypothermia with circulatory arrest, and/or aortic cross-clamping, allows the surgeon to safely stop cardiopulmonary bypass and remove arterial or venous cannulas to better visualize and repair the defects.
4. Indications:
   a. Anomalous coronary arterial anatomy.
   b. ASD, VSD, atrioventricular (AV) canal defect.
   c. Aortic stenosis, PS.
   d. Tetralogy of Fallot (TOF).
   e. Transposition of great arteries (TGA).
   f. Tricuspid atresia.
   g. Total anomalous pulmonary venous return (TAPVR) or partial APVR.

h. Truncus arteriosus.
i. Hypoplastic left heart syndrome (HLHS).
j. Complex single ventricle.

Potential Complications of Specific Surgeries

1. PDA ligation: laryngeal nerve damage, phrenic nerve damage, diaphragm paralysis, thoracic duct injury.
2. CoA: rebound hypertension, mesenteric arteritis (abdominal pain), coarctation restenosis.
3. Aorta-pulmonary shunt (modified BT shunt): shunt occlusion, PA distortion, pulmonary overcirculation.
4. ASD: atrial arrhythmias, sinoatrial node dysfunction.
5. VSD: transient or permanent heart block, residual VSD, ventricular dysfunction.
6. TOF: low cardiac output, residual right ventricular outflow tract obstruction (RVOTO) or VSD, ectopic junctional tachycardia or arrhythmias, thoracic duct injury.
7. D-TGA (dextro-transposition of the great arteries): arterial switch operation—coronary artery injury, ventricular dysfunction, suprapulmonary stenosis.
8. L-TGA (levo-transposition of the great arteries): atrial switch operation—baffle obstruction, RV failure, atrial arrhythmias.
9. Valvotomy (for valve stenosis): valve insufficiency.
10. Bidirectional Glenn shunt: superior vena cava (SVC) syndrome, low cardiac output, hypoxia, pleural effusions.
11. Fontan completion: low cardiac output, pleural effusions, ventricular dysfunction, thrombus formation, arrhythmias, hepatic dysfunction, lymphatic dysfunction.

Cardiac Transplant Surgery

Cardiac transplantation is a treatment option for children with progressive congestive heart failure (CHF) or certain cardiac diseases not amenable to conventional medical–surgical therapy. Children who cannot grow and meet developmental milestones or who have unacceptable quality-of-life issues may benefit from cardiac transplant surgery. However, approximately one in four children dies while waiting for an organ donor. Those children who receive a donor heart can develop significant complications and must take lifelong immunosuppression medications to prevent organ rejection.

Indications for Cardiac Transplantation

1. End-stage cardiomyopathy.
2. Untreatable complex CHD.
3. Malignant arrhythmia.
4. Retransplant for cardiac graft failure.

Immunosuppressive Medications

EVIDENCE BASE Velleca, A., Shullo, M. A., Dhital, K., Azeka, E., Colvin, M., DePasquale, E., Farrero, M., Garcia-Guereta, L., Jamero, G., Khush, K., Lavee, J., Pouch, S., Patel, J., Michaud, C. J., Shullo, M. A., Schubert, S., Angelini, A., Carlos, L., Mirabet, S., ... Reinhardt, Z. (2023). The International Society for Heart and Lung Transplantation (ISHLT) guidelines for the care of heart transplant recipients. *Journal of Heart and Lung Transplantation*. https://doi.org/10.1016/j.healun.2022.09.023

Mechanical Circulatory Support Before and After Transplant

Most pediatric patients undergoing cardiac transplant require preoperative management for end-stage heart failure. Mechanical circulatory support is used to manage these patients while they await transplantation as well as postoperatively to stabilize the patient who is newly transplanted. These devices can include extracorporeal membrane oxygenation (ECMO), ventricular assist devices (VADs), and most recently, the Berlin Heart (Bearl, 2022).

Immunosuppressive therapy is divided into two phases: induction and maintenance. Induction therapies reduce early rejection and may help to reduce the child's overall exposure to corticosteroids. Combination therapy is usually used in the maintenance phase to ensure ongoing protection against rejection.

1. Phase I: induction.
   a. Polyclonal antibodies.
      i. Antibodies harvested from equine (Atgam) or rabbit (thymoglobulin).
      ii. Interleukin-2 receptor antibodies.
         1. Daclizumab.
         2. Basiliximab.
2. Phase II: maintenance therapies.
   a. Calcineurin inhibitors.
      i. Cyclosporine.
      ii. Tacrolimus.
   b. Antiproliferative agent.
      i. Azathioprine.
      ii. Mycophenolate mofetil.
   c. Mammalian target of rapamycin (mTOR) inhibitors.
      i. Sirolimus.
      ii. Everolimus.
      iii. Less nephrotoxic than calcineurin inhibitors.
   d. Corticosteroids.
   e. Oral prednisone and prednisolone most common.
      i. Used in higher doses early posttransplant, gradually tapering over time.
      ii. Short-burst IV doses of methylprednisolone can be used in acute rejection.

Complications

1. Organ rejection: routine surveillance endomyocardial biopsies are performed to assess for rejection.
   a. With mild to moderate rejection, children may initially be without symptoms.
   b. With severe rejection, children are usually symptomatic with hemodynamic instability.
2. Infection.
3. Adverse effects of immunosuppressive agents:
   a. Polyclonal antibodies—fever, chills, urticaria, headaches, severe hypotension, abdominal pain, leukopenia, and thrombocytopenia.
   b. Reactions can be minimized by premedicating with corticosteroids, acetaminophen, diphenhydramine.
   c. Calcineurin inhibitors:
      i. Ciclosporin—nephrotoxicity, hypertension, diabetes mellitus, hirsutism, gingival hyperplasia, tremor.
      ii. Tacrolimus—nephrotoxicity, diabetes mellitus, hypertension, hyperkalemia, hypomagnesemia, tremor.
   d. Antiproliferative agent:
      i. Azathioprine—leukopenia, thrombocytopenia, nausea, hepatic dysfunction, pancreatitis.
      ii. Mycophenolate mofetil—leukopenia, nausea, vomiting, diarrhea, anorexia.
   e. mTOR—hyperlipidemia, thrombocytopenia, anemia, leukopenia, interference with wound healing, oral lesions.
   f. Prednisone—hypertension, Cushing syndrome, growth retardation.

4. Graft dysfunction/failure:
   a. Leading cause of death posttransplant.
   b. The most severe cases become apparent in the immediate postoperative period.
   c. Treat with inotropic drugs, short-term mechanical circulatory support with ECMO or VAD, eventual retransplantation.
5. Cardiac allograft vasculopathy (CAV):
   a. Occurs late after transplant.
   b. Unique and progressive atherosclerosis affecting only transplanted hearts.
   c. Treat with mechanical circulatory support, discontinuation of all immunosuppressive agents.
6. Posttransplant lymphoproliferative disease.

Routine Follow-Up

1. Routine well-child care visits to primary care provider:
   a. Transplant children should not receive any live virus immunizations (oral polio, measles–mumps–rubella, varicella). Monitor for adverse effects of chronic steroids and immunosuppressive medications.
2. Routine cardiology clinic visits:
   a. Laboratory studies: chemistry, hematology, therapeutic drug levels.
   b. Vital signs.
   c. Electrocardiogram (ECG).
   d. Echocardiography.
3. Serial cardiac catheterizations and endomyocardial biopsies.
4. Yearly coronary angiography.

Nursing Assessment

Baseline Assessment on the Day of Surgery

1. Measure and record height and weight.
2. Document vital signs: heart rate, respiratory rate, BP, and oxygen saturation.
3. Assess for preoperative infection: fever, signs of upper respiratory infection (URI) (cough, runny nose, crackles), vomiting, or diarrhea might necessitate delaying surgery.
4. Document the last oral intake.
5. Void on call to the operating room.

Nursing Interventions

Preparing the Child and Family and Reducing Fear

1. Be honest and use nonthreatening language the child can understand.
2. The following are frequently asked questions from caregivers. Address them with the caregivers:
   a. What to tell the child.
   b. When to tell the child.
   c. What to bring to the hospital.
   d. Anticipated hospital course: how long in the operating room; how many days in the intensive care unit (ICU); how many days in the general care unit; visiting policy, rooming-in accommodations.
3. Review preoperative instructions.
   a. NPO guidelines.
   b. Where to report on the day of the surgery.
   c. Time to arrive at the hospital; time of surgery.
   d. Preoperative medications (injection, liquid, inhalation).
   e. What the operating room looks like; what the people wear in the operating room (hats, gowns, and masks).
4. Explain the preoperative period.
   a. Change into a hospital gown.
   b. Caregivers stay with the child.
   c. Transportation to the operating room (walking, wheelchair, or stretcher).
5. Explain the operative period.
   a. Operating room waiting room.
   b. Updates during the surgery will come from the surgical scrub nurses.
   c. Surgeon will meet the family after surgery to review the surgical findings and to describe the operation.
6. Explain the postoperative period. Use models and diagrams.
   a. Pediatric ICU routines and procedures.
   b. Monitoring lines and equipment.
   c. Ventilators, oxygen therapy.
   d. Protective restraints.
7. Offer medical equipment to handle and play with (ECG leads, facemask, BP cuff), age-appropriate books about surgery and hospital stays, and tour of the ICU and surgical area, as available.
8. Prehospital tour of the pediatric ICU and general pediatric care unit.
9. Allow an opportunity for the child and family to ask questions, express their concern, or ask for more detail.

Observing for and Preventing Complications

1. Assess respiratory status and maintain respiratory support.
   a. Maintain ventilatory support, as needed.
   b. Maintain patent airway with routine endotracheal suctioning.
   c. Auscultate breath sounds frequently. Decreased breath sounds may indicate pleural effusions, atelectasis, pneumothorax, or hemothorax.
   d. Report results of routine chest x-ray.
   e. Perform frequent position changes: side-back-side.
   f. Monitor arterial blood gas levels and oxygen saturations.
   g. Assess chest or mediastinal tube drainage; examine characteristics and quantify hourly in the initial postoperative period.
   h. Identify those patients at risk for pulmonary hypertension in the postoperative period.
   i. Treatment includes oxygen, analgesia and sedation, prevention of acidosis, chemical paralysis, and inhaled nitric oxide.
   j. Extubate when hemodynamically stable and when patient meets extubation criteria.
   k. Administer oxygen therapy, as needed, after extubation.
2. Assess cardiac status.
   a. Monitor vital signs and oxygen saturations.
   b. Auscultate heart sounds immediately upon admission, noting the quality and presence of any residual murmurs.
   c. If patient has had a BT shunt placed, frequently assess shunt murmur presence and volume. Sudden or progressive muting of this could indicate shunt occlusion and is an emergency.
   d. Maintain continuous ECG monitoring.
      i. Daily 12-lead ECG to assess rhythm.
      ii. Temporary epicardial pacemaker wires available for atrial and/or ventricular pacing, as needed.
      iii. In the presence of these, keep pacer located at the bedside.
   e. Continuous BP monitoring (arterial line).

f. Monitor intracardiac pressures (central venous pressure [CVP], left atrial [LA], PA).
g. Monitor peripheral perfusion, capillary refill, and toe temperature.
h. Titrate vasopressors (dopamine, dobutamine, epinephrine, milrinone), as prescribed.

3. Assess fluid status.
   a. Record hourly intake (IV fluids, blood products, fluid boluses).
   b. Record hourly output (urine, chest/mediastinal tube drainage, nasogastric drainage).
   c. Concerning if chest/mediastinal tube output exceeds 5 to 10 mL/kg/h.
   d. Take note if chest/mediastinal tube drainage suddenly decreases, concern for obstruction in tube with resultant pericardial or pleural effusion.
   e. Perform daily weights.
   f. Administer diuretics, as prescribed, noting the response.
4. Assess neurologic status.
   a. Monitor level of responsiveness, response to verbal commands, and response to pain.
   b. Check pupil size and reactivity to light.
   c. Document movement of all extremities.
   d. Monitor all invasive lines for air bubbles and potential air embolism.
   e. Observe for signs of neurologic injury related to hypoperfusion or embolism.
5. Monitor for potential specific complications related to particular surgery for CHD.
6. Assess for postoperative pain.
   a. Monitor the level of responsiveness, agitation.
   b. Implement pediatric pain scale rating to assist the child in identifying the severity of pain. Use this choice consistently throughout the hospital stay.
   c. Administer pain and anxiolytic medication, as prescribed: continuous IV infusion and IV boluses, as necessary to control pain and hypertension related to pain and anxiety.
   d. Utilize patient-controlled analgesia continuous pump, as appropriate.
7. Assess serum electrolyte balance. Obtain blood tests and report results. Treat deficits with supplements, paying particular attention to potassium, calcium, and magnesium levels.
8. Assess packed cell volume, platelet count, and coagulation studies.
   a. Low hematocrit (less than 30%): consider directed donor transfusion or blood bank transfusion.
   b. Low platelet count: continue to monitor; if bleeding persists, transfuse platelets.
   c. Prolonged coagulation studies: continue to monitor; if bleeding or oozing persists, give fresh-frozen plasma, protamine.

Enhancing Adjustment Postoperatively

1. Provide continuity of care (primary nursing and consistent medical team).
2. Explain all procedures and routines to the child and caregivers to minimize fear.
3. Explain to the caregivers a child's typical reactions to stressful events.
   a. Regression—temporary loss of developmental milestones.
   b. Fear of any medical personnel (white coat anxiety).
   c. Sibling jealousy that one child is receiving a lot of attention.
   d. Withdrawal—related to stimulation overload and lack of undisturbed sleep.
   e. Nightmares.
   f. Increased dependency; clinging behavior.
4. Suggest caregiver and patient support groups, Child Life Therapy, community resources, and counseling, as needed.

Family Education and Health Maintenance

1. Provide the child and family with oral and written discharge instructions and recommendations.
   a. Medications.
   b. Activity restrictions.
   c. Sternal precautions.
      i. No strenuous activity or contact sports for 6 to 8 weeks after surgery.
      ii. Most children are ready to return to school at least part time about 2 weeks after surgery.
      iii. If child needs prolonged recovery time at home, may need to consider home tutoring.
      iv. No gym class until full recovery.
   d. Care of the incision.
   e. Dietary recommendations.
   f. Bathing or showering guidelines.
2. Provide the child and family with a list of potential signs of complications and instructions to notify the health care provider.
   a. Fever greater than or equal to 101.5°F (38.6°C).
   b. Any redness, swelling, or drainage from chest incision.
   c. Partial opening of the chest incision.
   d. Poor appetite, nausea, vomiting.
   e. Breathing difficulties, shortness of breath.
   f. Lethargy, sustained.
   g. For neonates and infants, increased fussiness or sudden inconsolability, decreased feeding, consistent weight loss.
3. Provide the family with the names and phone numbers of people to call for questions and emergencies.
4. Make follow-up appointments for the child to be seen by their primary care provider 2 to 3 days after discharge from the hospital and 10 to 14 days to be seen by their pediatric cardiologist.
5. Review the American Heart Association's recommendations for infective endocarditis prophylaxis. In children with CHD, prophylaxis is indicated only for patients who:
   a. Have cyanotic heart disease that has not been fully repaired.
   b. Have prosthetic material or device for the first 6 months postoperatively.
   c. Have residual cardiac lesions even after repair, such as abnormal flow or regurgitation at patches or valves.

Community and Home Care Considerations

1. Arrange skilled home nursing visits, as needed, to:
   a. Review medications.
   b. Assess wound healing.
   c. Monitor vital signs and oxygen saturations.
   d. Monitor growth for single ventricle and complex CHD infants postoperatively, during the interstage period (between staged palliative surgeries); optimize nutrition.
   e. Assess oral intake; nutritional status.
   f. Resource for family.
2. Make referral to community agencies, as needed (infant and toddler program).
3. Arrange for home medical equipment (oxygen, feeding pump, and supplies), as needed.

4. Review safety precautions in the home:
   a. Childproof medication bottles.
   b. Poison control phone number for inadvertent medication overdose.
   c. Infant and child cardiopulmonary resuscitation (CPR) techniques.
   d. Bleeding precautions for children on anticoagulation therapy. No aspirin or ibuprofen products. Be sure to read the labels on over-the-counter cold and cough syrups. Avoid activities with a high risk of injury. All head injuries need to be evaluated by a primary provider. Signs of bleeding:
      i. Blood in the urine.
      ii. Black tarry stools.
      iii. Prolonged nosebleeds.
      iv. Bleeding gums.
      v. Bruising for no known trauma.
      vi. Spitting or coughing up blood.
      vii. Any unusual swelling or pain.
   e. Medical alert device or tags.
5. Discuss developmental issues with the family.
   a. A child on diuretics may have difficulty with toilet training.
   b. Disciplining, establishing behavioral expectations, and setting limits in a child with CHD should be similar to those for a child without CHD.
6. Discuss the need for home schooling or tutoring during recovery time. Return to the classroom as soon as the child is ready.
7. Discuss infants with CHD in daycare situations—address each case individually. Daycare programs usually have an increased risk of URIs and other communicable diseases.
8. Encourage routine dental visits to prevent dental caries (dental caries predispose to bacteremia and endocarditis).
9. Encourage heart-healthy eating and exercise routines.
10. Encourage age-appropriate activities. A few children will need exercise restrictions. Children with CHD should be allowed to participate in activities with rest periods, as needed. Children with pacemakers and children on anticoagulation therapy should refrain from contact sports.
11. Maintain a standard childhood immunization schedule. Delay vaccines around the perioperative time until fully recovered from surgery (no immunizations for 6 weeks postoperatively). The COVID-19 vaccine can be safely administered, except in immediate post-op patients and those on certain immune-suppressing drugs.
12. Encourage yearly influenza vaccine for children with unrepaired or complex CHD.
13. Encourage respiratory syncytial virus (RSV) immunization for children younger than age 2 with complex CHD and those at risk of CHF or pulmonary hypertension.

Evaluation: Expected Outcomes

- Child describes procedure without fear; caregivers and child discuss the procedure and ask appropriate questions.
- Vital signs stable, no signs of infection.
- Caregivers offer support to child.

CONGENITAL HEART DISEASE

Overview

EVIDENCE BASE Liu, A., Gerhard-Paul, D., Moons, P., Daniels, C. J., Jenkins, K. J., & Marelli, A. (2023). Changing epidemiology of congenital heart disease: Effect on outcomes and quality of care in adults. *Nature Reviews Cardiology, 20*, 126–137. https://doi.org/10.1038/s41569-022-00749-y

Congenital heart disease (or *defects*) *(CHD)* is one of the most common forms of congenital anomalies. It involves the chambers, valves, and vessels arising from the heart (see Figure 41-1, page 1202). In most cases, the cause of CHD is not known. Some infants and children with CHD may appear perfectly healthy, whereas others may present as critically ill. Most infants and children with CHD can be successfully managed with medications and surgeries.

Etiology and Incidence

1. CHD affects 8 of every 1,000 live births (range from 3 to 10).
2. Exact cause of CHD is unknown in approximately 85% of cases.
3. The heart begins as a single cell and develops into a four-chambered pumping system during the 3rd to 8th weeks of gestation.
4. Associated factors for CHD include:
   a. Fetal or maternal infection during the first trimester (rubella).
   b. Chromosomal abnormalities (trisomy 21, 18, 13).
   c. Maternal insulin-dependent diabetes.
   d. Phenylketonuria.
   e. Systemic lupus erythematosus.
   f. Teratogenic effects of drugs and alcohol.
      i. Lithium—Ebstein anomaly.
      ii. Phenytoin—aortic and pulmonic stenosis.
      iii. Alcohol—atrial septal defect (ASD) and ventricular septal defect (VSD).
5. Syndromes that include CHD:
   a. Marfan syndrome—mitral valve prolapse (MVP), dilated aortic root.
   b. Turner syndrome—aortic valve stenosis (AVS), coarctation of the aorta (CoA).
   c. Noonan syndrome—dysplastic pulmonary valve.
   d. William syndrome—supravalvular pulmonary stenosis (PS).
   e. DiGeorge syndrome—interrupted aortic arch (IAA), truncus arteriosus, transposition of the great arteries (TGA), and Tetralogy of Fallot (TOF).
   f. Down syndrome (trisomy 21)—endocardial cushion can develop abnormally, commonly atrioventricular (AV) canal defect, VSD. About 50% of children with Down syndrome have a CHD.

DRUG ALERT Teratogenic drugs also include amphetamines, estrogen, progesterone, retinoic acid, selective serotonin reuptake inhibitors, trimethadione, and valproic acid.

Common Congenital Heart Malformations

Congenital heart defects can be classified into three categories: obstruction to blood flow, increased pulmonary blood flow (acyanotic lesions), and decreased pulmonary blood flow (cyanotic lesions).

1. Obstructive lesions:
   a. aortic stenosis (AS)—valvular, subvalvular, or supravalvular.
   b. CoA.
   c. PS—valvular, subvalvular, or supravalvular.
   d. IAA.

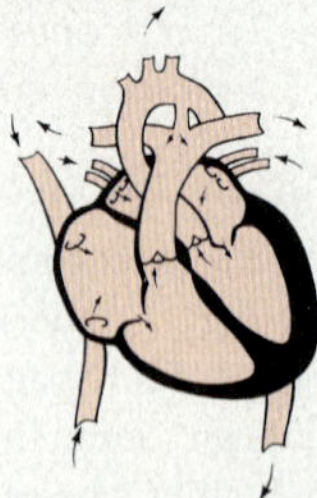

Patent Ductus Arteriosus

Patent ductus arteriosus (PDA) is a vascular connection that, during fetal life, shunts blood from the pulmonary artery to the aorta. Functional closure of the ductus normally occurs soon after birth. If the ductus remains patent after birth, the direction of blood flow in the ductus is reversed from aorta to pulmonary circuit by the higher pressure in the aorta.

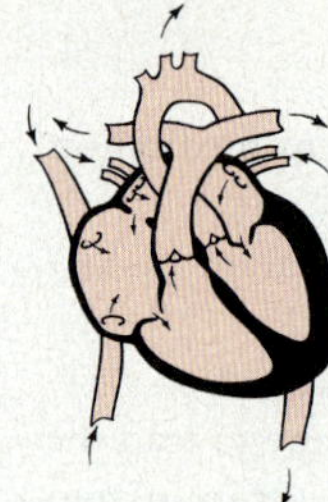

Tetralogy of Fallot

Tetralogy of Fallot (TOF) is characterized by the combination of four defects: (1) pulmonary stenosis, (2) ventricular septal defects, (3) overriding aorta, and (4) hypertrophy of right ventricle. It is the most common defect causing cyanosis in patients surviving past age 2. The severity of symptoms depends on the degree of pulmonary stenosis, the size of the VSD, and the degree to which the aorta overrides the ventricular septal defect.

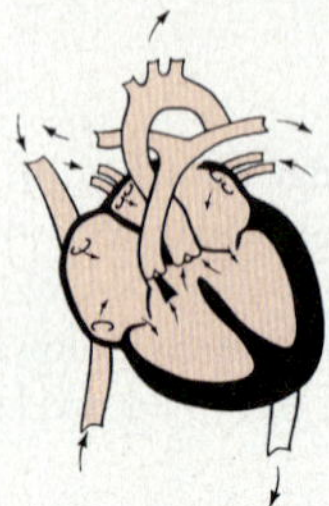

Ventricular Septal Defect

Ventricular septal defect (VSD) is an abnormal opening between the right and left ventricle. VSDs vary in size and may occur in either the membranous or muscular portion of the ventricular septum. Due to the higher pressure in the left ventricle, a shunting of blood from the left to right ventricle occurs during systole. If pulmonary hypertension or obstruction to pulmonary flow exists, the shunt of blood is then reversed from the right to the left ventricle, with cyanosis resulting.

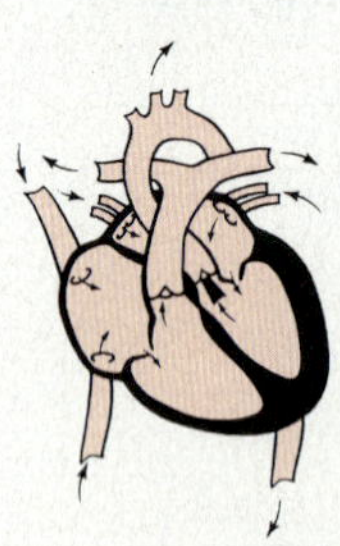

Transposition of the Great Arteries

In *transposition of the great arteries (TGA)*, the aorta originates from the right ventricle and the pulmonary artery from the left ventricle. An abnormal communication between the two circulations (atrial septal defect [ASD] or VSD) must be present to sustain life.

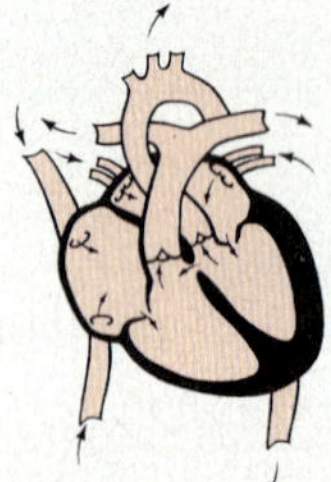

Pulmonary Stenosis

Pulmonary stenosis refers to any lesion that obstructs the blood flow from the right ventricle to the pulmonary artery. This obstruction may cause right ventricular hypertrophy and eventual right-sided heart failure.

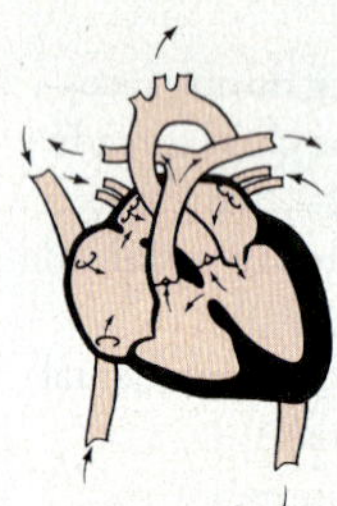

Atrial Septal Defect

An atrial septal defect (ASD) is an abnormal opening between the right and left atria. Basically, three types of abnormalities result from incorrect development of the atrial septum: (1) sinus venosus at the top of the atrial septum, (2) ostium secundum at the middle of the atrial septum, and (3) ostium primum at the bottom of the atrial septum. In general, left-to-right shunting of blood occurs in all ASDs.

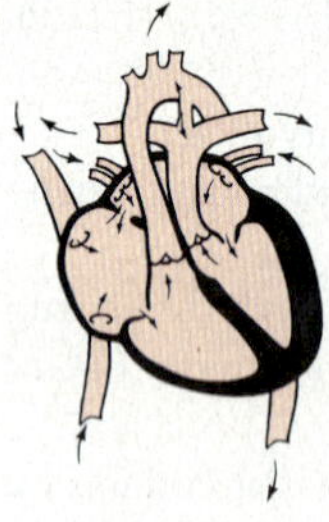

Aortic Stenosis

Aortic stenosis may be at the subvalvular, valvular (with thickening or fusion of the cusps), or supravalvular level. Subaortic stenosis is caused by a fibrous ring below the aortic valve in the outflow tract of the left ventricle. At times, valvular and subaortic stenosis exist in combination. The obstruction presents an increased workload for the normal output of the left ventricular blood and results in left ventricular enlargement.

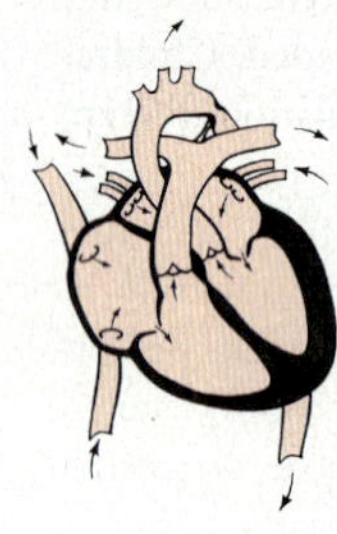

Tricuspid Atresia

Tricuspid atresia (TA) is characterized by absence of the tricuspid valve, a small right ventricle, and usually diminished pulmonary circulation. Cyanosis is present because blood from the right atrium passes through an ASD into the left atrium, mixes with oxygenated blood returning from the lungs, flows into the left ventricle, and is propelled into the systemic circulation. The lungs may receive blood through one of three routes: (1) VSD, (2) PDA, and (3) collateral aortopulmonary vessels.

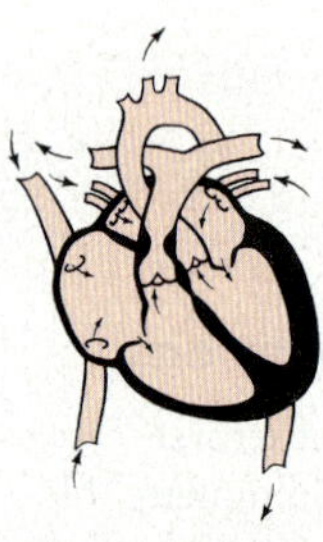

Coarctation of the Aorta

Coarctation of the aorta is characterized by a narrowed aortic lumen. It normally occurs in the juxtaductal position. Coarctations exist with great variation in anatomic features. The lesion produces an obstruction to the flow of blood through the aorta, causing increased left ventricular pressure and workload.

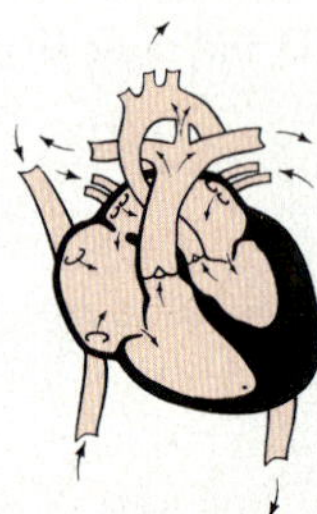

Hypoplastic Left Heart Syndrome

In *hypoplastic left heart syndrome (HLHS)*, a collection of complex congenital heart lesions results in the abnormal development of the left side of the heart. These lesions include: (1) mitral stenosis/atresia, (2) aortic stenosis or atresia, (3) aortic arch hypoplasia, and (4) hypoplastic left ventricle. The right ventricle pumps blood through the pulmonary and systemic circulations. A patent foramen ovale allows a left-to-right shunt and blood is shunted from left atrium back to right atrium. A PDA is often the sole supply of blood to the systemic circulation.

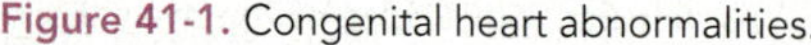

Figure 41-1. Congenital heart abnormalities.

2. Increased pulmonary blood flow (acyanotic):
   a. Patent ductus arteriosus (PDA).
   b. ASD.
   c. VSD.
   d. AV canal (balanced or unbalanced).
   e. Partial anomalous pulmonary venous return (PAPVR).
3. Decreased pulmonary blood flow (cyanotic):
   a. TOF.
   b. Tricuspid atresia (TA).
   c. Total anomalous pulmonary venous return (TAPVR).
   d. TGA.
   e. Truncus arteriosus.
   f. Hypoplastic left heart syndrome (HLHS).
   g. Double outlet right ventricle (DORV).

Aortic Stenosis

EVIDENCE BASE Boe, B. A., & Gajarski, R. J. (2022). Aortic stenosis. In R. E. Shaddy, D. J. Penny, T. F. Feltes, F. Cetta, & S. Mital (Eds.), *Moss and Adams' heart disease in infants, children, and adolescents: Including the fetus and young adult* (10th ed., pp. 1049–1066). Lippincott Williams & Wilkins.

Congenital *aortic stenosis (AS)* is a left ventricular outflow tract obstructive lesion. It may be caused by a bicuspid aortic valve with fused commissures that does not open completely, by a hypoplastic aortic valve annulus, or by stenosis above or below the aortic valve (subvalvular or supravalvular stenosis). The result is turbulent blood flow across the aortic valve and into the ascending aorta. Patients with AS must be evaluated for additional left heart lesions that include CoA, mitral valve stenosis, hypertrophic cardiomyopathy, and hypoplastic left heart. AS is the most common form of left ventricular outflow tract obstruction (LVOTO). It accounts for 3% to 6% of CHDs. AS may present at any age, and it occurs more commonly in males.

Pathophysiology and Etiology

1. Blood flows at an increased velocity across the obstructive valve or stenotic area and into the aorta.
2. During systole, left ventricular pressure rises dramatically to overcome the increased resistance at the aortic valve.
3. Myocardial ischemia may occur because of an imbalance between the increased oxygen requirements related to the hypertrophied left ventricle (LV) and the amount of oxygen that can be supplied.
4. A consistent increased pressure load on the LV causes pathologic ventricular remodeling. Progression to left-sided heart failure and eventual cellular changes are reflected in clinical signs of failure.

Clinical Manifestations

Neonate

Onset of symptoms occurs quickly with critical AS, upon the closure of the ductus arteriosus.

1. Severe congestive heart failure (CHF).
2. Metabolic acidosis.
3. Tachypnea.
4. Faint peripheral pulses, poor perfusion, poor capillary refill, cool skin.
5. Poor feeding and feeding intolerance.

Child and Adolescent

Symptoms may be slower to progress and develop over time.

1. Chest pain on exertion, decreased exercise tolerance.
2. Dyspnea, fatigue, shortness of breath.
3. Syncope, lightheadedness.
4. Palpitations.
5. Sudden death.

Diagnostic Evaluation

1. Auscultation.
   a. Systolic ejection murmur heard best at the right upper sternal border, radiates to neck.
   b. Ejection click. May be absent with severe stenosis.
   c. S_2 splits normally or narrowly.
2. Four-limb blood pressure (BP).
   a. Systolic BP normally 5 to 10 mm higher in lower extremities.
   b. For patients with supravalvar aortic stenosis, right arm may have a 15- to 20-mm Hg increase in systolic pressure as compared to left arm.
3. Palpation.
   a. Thrill may be palpable over suprasternal notch with mild valvar aortic stenosis, right upper sternal border in moderate or worse stenosis.
4. Auscultation.
   a. May hear harsh crescendo–decrescendo systolic ejection murmur at the right upper sternal border for valvar and supravalvar stenosis, at the left mid-sternal border for subvalvar stenosis.
5. Electrocardiogram (ECG): left ventricular hypertrophy (LVH) with a strain pattern may be seen in severe cases.
6. Chest x-ray: increased cardiac silhouette, increased pulmonary vascular markings. A prominent aortic knob may be seen occasionally from poststenotic dilatation with valvular AS.
7. Echocardiogram: two-dimensional echocardiogram with Doppler study and color flow mapping to visualize the anatomy and to estimate the gradient across the valve and through the aorta.

Management

Neonate

1. Stabilize with prostaglandin E_1 (PGE_1) infusion to maintain cardiac output through the PDA.
2. Inotropic support, as needed.
3. Intubation and ventilation, as needed.
4. Cardiac catheterization after initial stabilization: aortic balloon valvuloplasty or aortic balloon angioplasty.
5. Surgical valvotomy, commissurotomy, or myectomy/myotomy.

Child and Adolescent

1. Medical management with close follow-up to monitor increasing gradient across the aortic valve or through the aorta.
2. Continued hypertension can significantly dilate the aortic root over time.
3. Exercise testing to determine the recommended level of activity. Those who have more abnormal results and/or ECG changes should stay away from sports with a high aerobic component.
4. Aortic balloon valvuloplasty or aortic balloon angioplasty.
5. Surgical intervention.
   a. Surgical valvotomy, commissurotomy, or myectomy/myotomy.

b. In neonates with critical aortic stenosis, success of a biventricular repair has to be determined, gauging the strength of the LV and its associated structures. If the damage is too great, then a single ventricle staged repair approach may be used.
c. Aortic valve replacement.
   i. Mechanical prosthesis (St. Jude valve).
   ii. Ross procedure (pulmonary autograft, placement of right ventricle [RV] to pulmonary artery [PA] conduit).

Complications

1. CHF and pulmonary edema.
2. Dizziness, lightheadedness, and syncope.
3. Palpitations, arrhythmias.
4. Infective endocarditis.
5. Sudden death.

Coarctation of the Aorta

EVIDENCE BASE Backer, C. L., Dearani, J. A., & Mavroudis, C. (2023). Coarctation of the aorta. In C. Mavroudis & C. Backer (Eds.), *Pediatric cardiac surgery* (pp. 249–277). https://doi.org/10.1002/9781119282327.ch13

CoA is a discrete narrowing or a long segment hypoplasia of the aortic arch, usually in the juxtaductal position. It accounts for 6% to 8% of CHDs and is two to five times more common in males. Thirty percent of infants with Turner syndrome have CoA. Commonly associated defects include VSD, mitral valve stenosis, and bicuspid aortic valve.

Pathophysiology and Etiology

1. The discrete narrowing or hypoplastic segment of the aorta increases the workload of the LV (increased LV systolic pressure).
2. In a neonate with critical CoA, lower body blood flow occurs through the PDA (right-to-left shunting).
3. In the older child, collateral vessels grow and bypass the coarctation to perfuse the lower body.

Clinical Manifestations

1. The neonate with critical CoA (ductal dependent lesion):
   a. Without symptoms until the PDA begins to close, rapid decompensation at 7 to 10 days of life.
   b. After PDA closure: severe CHF, poor lower body perfusion, tachypnea, acidosis, progressive circulatory shock, absent femoral and pedal pulses.
2. The child or adolescent with CoA:
   a. Usually without symptoms—normal growth and development.
   b. Hypertension in the upper extremities, with absent or weak femoral pulses.
   c. Murmur present.
   d. Nosebleeds, headaches, leg cramps with exercise.

Diagnostic Evaluation

1. Auscultation—varies; nonspecific systolic ejection murmur. Murmur may be heard over the base or posteriorly in the left scapular region. Single S_2 loud S_3 gallop is usually present.
2. Four-limb BP.
   a. Systolic BP elevated in upper extremities, proximal to coarctation, as compared to lower extremities. A significant gradient exists between the two.
3. Chest x-ray—cardiomegaly and pulmonary edema or pulmonary venous congestion.
4. ECG—varies; normal or right ventricular hypertrophy (RVH) in infants and LVH in older children.
5. Two-dimensional echocardiography with Doppler and color flow mapping identifies the area of aortic arch narrowing and potentially associated lesions (bicuspid aortic valve, VSD, PDA), left ventricular size and function.
6. Invasive studies (cardiac catheterization) usually not needed to make the initial diagnosis; may need aortic angiography to identify the presence of collateral vessels before surgery.
7. Cardiac magnetic resonance imaging may be done to noninvasively assess the location and degree of narrowing and identify collateral vessels.

Management

Critical Coarctation in the Neonate

1. Medical management:
   a. Resuscitation and stabilization with PGE_1 infusion: monitor for complications related to PGE_1 therapy (fever, apnea).
   b. Intubation and ventilation, as needed.
   c. Anticongestive therapy (digoxin and Lasix) and inotropic support, as needed.
   d. Assessment of renal, hepatic, and neurologic function.
2. Balloon angioplasty may be indicated for infants who are at high surgical risk.
3. Surgical intervention: usually performed as soon as the diagnosis is made.
   a. Subclavian flap repair (Waldhausen procedure).
   b. End-to-end anastomosis.
   c. Dacron patch repair.
   d. Stent implantation.

Coarctation in the Child or Adolescent

1. Surgical intervention.
   a. End-to-end anastomosis.
   b. Dacron patch.
   c. Stent implantation.
2. Medical management for hypertension (beta-adrenergic blockers).

Recurrent Coarctation in the Child or Adult

More common in the patient who underwent repair in infancy.

1. Balloon angioplasty in the cardiac catheterization laboratory.
2. Redo surgical intervention.

Complications

1. Systemic hypertension.
2. CHF—occurs in 20% to 30% of all infants with CoA by age 3 months.
3. Intracranial hemorrhage.
4. Left ventricular failure.
5. Aortic aneurysm.

Pulmonary Stenosis

EVIDENCE BASE Sekhon, S., Barger, P. M., & Abarbanell, A. M. (2021). Outcomes 60 years after surgical valvotomy for isolated congenital pulmonary valve stenosis. *Journal of Cardiac Surgery, 36*(4), 1531–1533. https://doi.org/10.1111/jocs.15276

The pulmonary valve opens during systole to let blood flow from the RV into the main PA. Obstruction to flow can occur at three levels: subvalvular, valvular, or supravalvular. The most common cause of RV outflow tract obstruction is PS. PS accounts for 8% to 10% of CHDs.

Pathophysiology and Etiology

1. Critical PS in the neonate: blood flows into the right atrium (RA), across a patent foramen ovale (PFO) into the left side of heart; pulmonary blood flow comes from a left-to-right shunt through a PDA.
2. Right ventricular pressure increases to pump blood across the obstructive pulmonary valve.
3. RVH develops in response to the increased pressure gradient across the pulmonary valve.
4. Signs of right-sided heart failure include hepatic congestion, neck vein distention, and elevated central venous pressure (CVP).

Clinical Manifestations

Critical PS in the Neonate

1. Hypoxia.
2. Tachypnea.
3. RV failure.

Mild to Moderate PS in the Child and Adolescent

1. Without symptoms.
2. Decreased exercise tolerance, fatigue, exertional dyspnea.
3. Chest pain.

Diagnostic Evaluation

1. Auscultation: systolic ejection murmur heard best at the left upper sternal border; ejection click.
2. ECG: varies; normal in mild cases and RVH in moderate to severe cases.
3. Chest x-ray: varies; may show right ventricular enlargement; poststenotic dilatation of PA.
4. Two-dimensional echocardiography with Doppler study and color flow mapping to visualize the sites of obstruction, observe the degree of RVH, and estimate the pressure gradient across the valve.
5. Cardiac catheterization is usually not needed for the initial diagnosis.

Management

Neonate With Critical PS

1. Medical management:
   a. Stabilize and improve oxygen saturations with PGE_1 infusion.
   b. Intubation and ventilation, as needed.
   c. Inotropic support, as needed.
2. Balloon pulmonary valvuloplasty.
3. Blalock–Taussig (BT) shunt (Gore-Tex graft between the subclavian artery and the PA to supply pulmonary blood flow), as initial intervention.

Child and Adolescent With PS

1. Medical management:
   a. Close follow-up to monitor and record RV-to-PA gradient and assess RV function.
   b. Restrict strenuous exercise.
   c. Refer for intervention when RV pressure is greater than two thirds of the systemic pressure.
2. Balloon pulmonary valvuloplasty in the cardiac catheterization laboratory.
3. Surgical intervention:
   a. Valvotomy or valvectomy for dysplastic pulmonary valve.
   b. Patch repair of the right ventricular outflow tract.
   c. Placement of an RV-to-PA conduit.

Complications

1. Cyanosis (critical PS in the neonate as a result of suprasystemic pulmonary pressures through anatomic shunt).
2. Arrhythmia; sudden death.
3. Infective endocarditis.
4. Right ventricular failure.

Patent Ductus Arteriosus

EVIDENCE BASE Parkerson, S., Philip, R., Talati, A., & Sathanandam, S. (2021). Management of patent ductus arteriosus in premature infants in 2020. *Frontiers in Pediatrics, 8*, 590578. https://doi.org/10.3389/fped.2020.590578

The *ductus arteriosus* is a normal fetal connection between the left PA and the descending aorta. During fetal life, blood flow is shunted away from the lungs through the ductus arteriosus and directly into the systemic circulation. PDAs occur in up to 60% of premature neonates who weigh less than 1,000 g. In term infants, PDAs account for 5% to 10% of CHDs; the male-to-female ratio is 1:2.

Pathophysiology and Etiology

1. During fetal life, the ductus arteriosus allows blood to bypass the pulmonary circulation (fetus receives oxygen from the placenta) and flow directly into the systemic circulation.
2. After birth, the ductus arteriosus is no longer needed. Functional closure usually occurs within 24 to 72 hours after birth. Anatomic closure is completed by age 2 to 3 weeks.
3. When the ductus arteriosus fails to close, blood from the aorta (high pressure) flows into the low-pressure PA, resulting in pulmonary overcirculation.
4. Increased pulmonary blood flow leads to a volume-loaded LV.

Clinical Presentation

Small- to Moderate-Sized PDA

Usually without symptoms.

Large PDA

1. CHF, tachypnea, frequent respiratory tract infections.
2. Poor weight gain, failure to thrive.
3. Feeding difficulties.
4. Decreased exercise tolerance.
5. Infective endocarditis.

Diagnostic Evaluation

1. Auscultation: continuous murmur heard best at left upper sternal border. Hyperactive precordium with large PDAs.
2. Wide pulse pressure; bounding pulses.
3. Chest x-ray: varies; normal or cardiomegaly with increased pulmonary vascular markings.
4. ECG: varies; normal, LVH, or RVH.
5. Two-dimensional echocardiogram with Doppler study and color flow mapping to visualize the PDA with left-to-right blood flow.

6. Elevated levels of N-terminal pro-B-type natriuretic peptide and cardiac troponin T.
7. Cardiac catheterization is not needed for the initial diagnosis.

Management

1. In the symptomatic premature neonate—nonsteroidal anti-inflammatory drug (NSAIDs) (indomethacin) are given via intravenous (IV) line. These drugs are not effective in term infants.
2. Medical management:
   a. Monitor growth and development.
   b. Reassess for spontaneous PDA closure.
   c. Diuretics (furosemide, chlorothiazide) for pulmonary congestion.
   d. Increase caloric intake as needed to maintain normal weight gain.
   e. Infective endocarditis prophylaxis for 6 months after surgery or coil occlusion.
3. Cardiac catheterization:
   a. For small PDAs, coil occlusion.
   b. For larger PDAs, a closure device may be used.
4. Surgical management through PDA ligation.

Complications

1. CHF, pulmonary edema.
2. Infective endocarditis.
3. Pulmonary hypertension/pulmonary vascular occlusive disease.
4. Recurrent pneumonia.

Atrial Septal Defect

EVIDENCE BASE Parthiban, A., & Sachdeva, R. (2022). Atrial septal defects. In R. E. Shaddy, D. J. Penny, T. F. Feltes, F. Cetta, & S. Mital (Eds.), *Moss and Adams' heart disease in infants, children, and adolescents: Including the fetus and young adult* (10th ed., pp. 703–720). Lippincott Williams & Wilkins.

ASD is an abnormal communication between the left and right atria. ASDs account for 8% to 10% of CHDs. There are four types:

1. Ostium secundum ASD: most common type of ASD (accounts for 50% to 70%); abnormal opening in the middle of the atrial septum.
2. Ostium primum ASD (accounts for 30%): abnormal opening at the bottom of the atrial septum; increased association with cleft mitral valve and AV defects.
3. Sinus venosus ASD (accounts for 10%): abnormal opening at the top of the atrial septum; increased association with PAPVR.
4. Coronary sinus defect (rare): abnormal opening between coronary sinus and left atrium (LA).

Pathophysiology and Etiology

1. Blood flows from the higher pressure LA across the ASD into the lower pressure RA (left-to-right shunt).
2. Increased blood return to the right side of the heart leads to right ventricular volume overload and right ventricular dilation.
3. Increased pulmonary blood flow leads to elevated PA pressures.

Clinical Manifestations

1. Usually without symptoms.
2. Clinical symptoms vary depending on the type of associated defects and degree of shunting:
   a. CHF (usually not until the third or fourth decade of life).
   b. Frequent upper respiratory infections (URIs).
   c. Poor weight gain.
   d. Decreased exercise tolerance.
   e. Dyspnea and fatigue.

Diagnostic Evaluation

1. Auscultation: soft systolic ejection murmur heard best at the left upper sternal border; widely split, fixed second heart sound.
2. Prominent systolic impulse.
3. Chest x-ray: varies; normal to right atrial and ventricular dilation, increased pulmonary markings.
4. ECG: varies; right-axis deviation and mild RVH or right bundle-branch block. Alterations are present only when the shunt is large and the pulmonary resistance to systemic resistance ratio is greater than 1.5:1 (Qp:Qs > 1.5:1).
5. Two-dimensional echocardiogram with Doppler study and color flow mapping to identify the site of the ASD and associated lesions and document left-to-right flow across the atrial septum.
6. Cardiac catheterization is usually not needed for initial diagnosis; performed if the defect can be closed using an atrial occlusion device (device can be used only in ostium secundum defects).

Management

1. Medical management:
   a. Monitor and reassess (spontaneous closure rate is small but may occur up to age 2 years).
   b. Treatment with diuretics may be necessary if signs of CHF are present (usually not until the third to fourth decade of life if ASD unrepaired).
   c. Infective endocarditis prophylaxis for 6 months after surgery or atrial occlusion device is used.
2. Cardiac catheterization for placement of an atrial occlusion device for ostium secundum defects.
3. Surgical intervention:
   a. Primary repair: suture closure of the ASD.
   b. Patch repair of the ASD.

Complications

1. CHF (rare).
2. Infective endocarditis.
3. Embolic stroke.
4. Pulmonary hypertension.
5. Atrial arrhythmias.

Ventricular Septal Defect

EVIDENCE BASE Cohen, M. S., & Lopez, L. (2022). Ventricular septal defects. In R. E. Shaddy, D. J. Penny, T. F. Feltes, F. Cetta, & S. Mital (Eds.), *Moss and Adams' heart disease in infants, children, and adolescents: Including the fetus and young adult* (10th ed., pp. 746–764). Lippincott Williams & Wilkins.

A *VSD* is an abnormal communication between the RV and LV. It is the most common type of CHD, accounting for up to 40% of CHDs. VSD is slightly more common in females and is the most common lesion found in chromosomal syndromes (Trisomy 13, 18, 21). VSDs vary in size (small and restrictive to large and nonrestrictive), number (single vs. multiple), and type (perimembranous or muscular).

Pathophysiology and Etiology

1. Blood flows from the high-pressure LV across the VSD into the low-pressure RV and into the PA, resulting in pulmonary overcirculation. The size of the defect determines the physiologic effect on the infant.
2. A left-to-right shunt because of a VSD results in increased right ventricular pressure and increased PA pressure.
3. The increased pulmonary venous return to the left side of the heart results in left atrial dilation.
4. Long-standing pulmonary overcirculation causes a change in the pulmonary arterial bed, leading to increased pulmonary vascular resistance (PVR). High PVR can reverse the blood flow pattern that leads to a right-to-left shunt across the VSD (Eisenmenger syndrome), resulting in cyanosis. Once this develops, the child is no longer a candidate for surgical repair.

Clinical Manifestations

1. Small VSDs—usually without symptoms; high spontaneous closure rate during the first year of life. Ongoing risk of endocarditis.
2. Moderate VSDs—present with similar symptoms as the larger VSDs, but in milder form that is not quite as pronounced or significant.
3. Large VSDs—typical presentation at 4 to 8 weeks of age.
   a. CHF: tachypnea, tachycardia, excessive sweating associated with feeding, hepatomegaly.
   b. Frequent URIs.
   c. Poor weight gain, failure to thrive presenting at age 2 to 3 months.
   d. Feeding difficulties.
   e. Fatigue.

Diagnostic Evaluation

1. Auscultation: harsh systolic regurgitant murmur heard best at the lower left sternal border (LLSB); systolic thrill felt at LLSB, narrowly split S_2. The murmur may radiate toward the head along the left parasternal border or to the right of the sternum.
2. Chest x-ray: varies; normal or cardiomegaly and increased pulmonary vascular markings. Pulmonary vascular markings are directly proportionate to the amount of left-to-right shunting.
3. ECG: varies; normal to biventricular hypertrophy.
4. Two-dimensional echocardiogram with Doppler study and color flow mapping to identify the size, number, and sites of the defects; estimate PA pressure; and identify associated lesions.
5. Cardiac catheterization usually not needed for initial diagnosis; may be needed to calculate the size of the shunt or to assess PVR. May be performed if the defect can be closed using a ventricular occlusion device (device can be used only in muscular defects).

Management

Small VSD

1. Medical management:
   a. Usually no anticongestive therapy is needed.
   b. Infective endocarditis prophylaxis for 6 months after surgical implantation of a ventricular occlusion device.
2. Cardiac catheterization for placement of a ventricular occlusion device for muscular defects (for Qp:Qs > 1.5:1).
3. Surgical intervention is usually not necessary.

Moderate to Large VSD

1. Medical management:
   a. CHF management: digoxin, angiotensin-converting enzyme (ACE) inhibitors, and diuretics.
   b. Avoid oxygen; oxygen is a potent pulmonary vasodilator and will increase blood flow into the PA.
   c. Maximize nutrition: increase caloric intake by fortifying formula or breast milk to make 24 to 30 cal/ounce; supplemental nasogastric feeds, as needed.
   d. Infective endocarditis prophylaxis for 6 months after surgery/ventricular device occluder.
2. Cardiac catheterization for placement of a ventricular occlusion device for muscular defects (for Qp:Qs > 1.5:1).
3. Refer for surgical intervention.
   a. Usually repaired before age 2.
   b. Patch closure of VSD.

Long-Term Follow-Up

1. Monitor ventricular function.
2. Monitor for subaortic membrane and double-chamber RV.
3. Monitor for the formation of residual VSD following patch closure.

Complications

1. CHF.
2. Frequent URIs.
3. Failure to thrive; poor weight gain.
4. Infective endocarditis.
5. Arrhythmias (right bundle-branch block, transient complete heart block in postop period).
6. Eisenmenger syndrome.
7. Pulmonary hypertension.
8. Aortic insufficiency.

Tetralogy of Fallot

EVIDENCE BASE Wald, R. M., & Redington, A. N. (2022). Tetralogy of Fallot with pulmonary stenosis, pulmonary atresia, and absent pulmonary valve. In R. E. Shaddy, D. J. Penny, T. F. Feltes, F. Cetta, & S. Mital (Eds.), *Moss and Adams' heart disease in infants, children, and adolescents: Including the fetus and young adult* (10th ed., pp. 983–1008). Lippincott Williams & Wilkins.

TOF is the most common complex CHD. The four abnormalities of TOF include:

1. A large, nonrestrictive VSD.
2. Overriding aorta.
3. Pulmonary stenosis (right ventricular outflow tract obstruction [RVOTO]).
4. RVH.

Pathophysiology and Etiology

1. Degree of cyanosis depends on the size of the VSD and the degree of RVOTO.
2. Obstruction of blood flow from the RV to the PA results in deoxygenated blood being shunted across the VSD and into the aorta (right-to-left shunt causes cyanosis).
3. RVOTO can occur at any or all of three levels: PS, infundibular stenosis, or supravalvular stenosis.
4. The RV becomes hypertrophied as a result of the increased gradient across the right ventricular outflow tract (RVOT).
5. Minimal RVOTO results in a pink TOF variant, with the physiology behaving more like a large, nonrestrictive VSD. As PVR decreases, signs/symptoms may become more apparent as a result of increased shunting.

Clinical Manifestations

1. Clinical manifestations are variable and depend on the size of the VSD and the degree of RVOTO.
2. Cyanosis.
   a. Neonate may have normal oxygen saturations; as the infant grows, the RVOTO increases and the oxygen saturation falls.
   b. Neonate with unacceptably low oxygen saturation needs PGE_1 infusion to maintain ductal patency and adequate oxygen saturation (necessary for the TOF with pulmonary atresia).
   c. Cyanosis may initially be observed only with crying and with exertion (increasing PVR and right-to-left shunting).
3. Loud second heart sound with a harsh systolic ejection murmur.
4. Polycythemia.
5. Decreased exercise tolerance.
6. A common clinical manifestation years ago was squatting, a posture characteristically assumed by older children to increase systemic vascular resistance and to encourage increased pulmonary blood flow. Squatting is rarely seen currently, however, because TOF is now surgically repaired during the first year of life.
7. Hypercyanotic spells (formerly known as Tet spells): life-threatening hypoxic event with a dramatic decrease in oxygen saturations; mechanism is usually infundibular spasm, which further obstructs pulmonary blood flow and increases right-to-left flow across the VSD.
   a. Typical hypoxic spells occur in the morning soon after awakening; during or after a crying episode; during or after a feeding; and during painful procedures such as blood draws.
   b. Typical scenario includes tachypnea, irritability, and increasing cyanosis, followed by flaccidity and loss of consciousness.
   c. Home treatment for the caregiver: soothe the infant and place them in a knee–chest position; notify the health care provider immediately.
   d. Hospital treatment includes knee–chest position, sedation (morphine), oxygen, beta-adrenergic blockers (propranolol) to relax the infundibulum, and administration of medications to increase systemic vascular resistance (phenylephrine, norepinephrine).
   e. Intubation and ventilation as needed to reduce work of breathing and oxygen consumption.
   f. Hypercyanotic spells usually prompt the cardiologist to refer for surgical intervention.

Diagnostic Evaluation

1. Auscultation: harsh systolic ejection murmur heard best at the upper left sternal border (RVOT murmur); single loud second heart sound; aortic ejection click. Murmur is caused by pulmonary stenosis—in mild stenosis, the murmur is louder and longer than when stenosis is more severe; during a hypercyanotic spell, the murmur disappears.
2. Palpation: systolic thrill palpable along left lower and left middle sternal border (50% of cases). RV tap at left sternal border.
3. Chest x-ray: varies; normal or decreased pulmonary vascular markings. The heart may appear "boot shaped" because of a concave main PA with an upturned apex resulting from RVH.
4. ECG: varies; normal or RVH.
5. Two-dimensional echocardiogram with Doppler study and color flow mapping to identify the structural abnormalities, estimate the degree of RVOTO, and assess the coronary artery pattern.
6. Cardiac catheterization is usually not needed for the initial diagnosis. May be performed before surgical intervention to identify the location and number of VSDs, the PVR, the degree of RVOTO, and the presence of any coronary abnormalities.

Management

1. Medical management:
   a. Monitor oxygen saturation level.
   b. Monitor growth and development.
   c. Monitor for hypercyanotic spells (many spells go unnoticed by caregivers).
   d. Infective endocarditis prophylaxis (lifelong).
   e. Restrict strenuous activity and participation in competitive sports.
2. Balloon pulmonary angioplasty (rarely).
3. Infants with severe pulmonary stenosis may require PGE_1 to maintain ductal patency.
4. Surgical intervention: palliative versus definitive repair.
   a. Many medical centers prefer definitive, one-stage repair.
   b. Potential obstacles for one-stage repair: abnormal coronary artery distribution (left anterior descending arises from right coronary artery and crosses RVOT); multiple VSDs; hypoplastic branch pulmonary arteries; small infant weighing less than 5.5 pounds (2.5 kg).
   c. Palliative surgery: modified BT shunt-tube Gore-Tex graft between the left subclavian artery and the PA; increased pulmonary blood flow results in higher oxygen saturations.
   d. Reparative surgery: patch closure of VSD, relief of RVOTO; with or without transannular patch across the pulmonary valve.
   e. For patients with pulmonary atresia, an RV-to-PA conduit is placed, bypassing the atretic RVOT. As the patient grows, this conduit will need to be upsized surgically, up to several times throughout childhood, and/or dilated by transcatheter pulmonary valve implantation.
5. Long-Term Follow-Up
   a. Assess RV outflow tract, monitor the degree of pulmonary insufficiency.
   b. Monitor RV function and exercise tolerance.

c. Monitor for arrhythmias.
d. Continue monitoring for incompletely understood sequelae of long-term effects of repaired physiology, extending to adulthood.

Complications

1. Hypoxia.
2. Hypercyanotic spells.
3. Polycythemia.
4. CHF: rare; associated with pink TOF.
5. Right ventricular dysfunction.
6. Ventricular arrhythmias.
7. Infective endocarditis.

Transposition of the Great Arteries

EVIDENCE BASE Qureshi, A. M., Justino, H., & Heinle, J. S. (2022). Transposition of the great arteries. In R. E. Shaddy, D. J. Penny, T. F. Feltes, F. Cetta, & S. Mital (Eds.), *Moss and Adams' heart disease in infants, children, and adolescents: Including the fetus and young adult* (10th ed., pp. 703–720). Lippincott Williams & Wilkins.

TGA occurs when the PA arises off the LV and the aorta arises off the RV. It accounts for 5% of CHDs and is more common in males. The most commonly associated additional lesion is a VSD. Ten percent of infants with TGA also have noncardiac malformations.

Pathophysiology and Etiology

1. This defect results in two parallel circulations:
   a. The RA receives deoxygenated blood from the inferior vena cava (IVC) and superior vena cava (SVC); blood flow continues through the tricuspid valve into the RV and is pumped back to the aorta.
   b. The LA receives richly oxygenated blood from the pulmonary veins; blood flow continues through the mitral valve into the LV and is pumped back into the PA.
2. To sustain life, there must be an accompanying defect that allows mixing of deoxygenated blood and oxygenated blood between the two circuits, such as PDA, ASD, PFO, or VSD.
3. Neonates born with TGA with an intact ventricular system are usually more cyanotic and sicker than neonates born with TGA and a VSD.

Clinical Manifestations

Symptoms evident soon after birth; clinical scenario and varying degrees of clinical manifestations are influenced by the extent of intercirculatory mixing (presence or absence of intact ventricular septum).

1. Cyanosis.
2. Tachypnea.
3. Metabolic acidosis.
4. CHF.
5. Feeding difficulties.

Diagnostic Evaluation

1. Auscultation: varies; no murmur or a murmur related to an associated defect, single loud S_2.
2. Chest x-ray: varies; neonate chest x-ray usually normal; cardiomegaly with a narrow mediastinum (egg-shaped cardiac silhouette) and increased pulmonary markings; or decreased pulmonary markings with pulmonary stenosis.
3. ECG: right atrial enlargement, RVH, or biventricular hypertrophy.
4. Two-dimensional echocardiogram with Doppler study and color flow mapping identifies the structural abnormalities: transposed vessels, coronary artery pattern, and degree of mixing across the atrial septum plus associated lesions.

Management

Medical Management

1. Stabilize with PGE_1 infusion.
2. Correct metabolic acidosis.
3. Supplemental oxygen to decrease PVR.
4. Treat pulmonary overcirculation with digoxin and diuretics, as needed.
5. Intubate and ventilate, as needed.
6. Inotropic support, as needed.

Cardiac Catheterization

1. Balloon atrial septostomy (Rashkind) is indicated for severe hypoxia to create or improve atrial level mixing, for those patients who have an intact ventricular septum.

Surgical Management

1. Arterial switch operation (Jatene)—procedure of choice:
   a. Ideally performed during the first 1 to 2 weeks of life—center-specific timing.
   b. Consideration of level of severity of pulmonary hypertension prior to surgery factors into surgical timing.
   c. The aorta and PA are switched back to their anatomically correct ventricle above the level of the valve.
   d. Coronary arteries are transferred to the new aorta.
   e. Associated lesions are also repaired at this time.
2. Rastelli operation—performed for TGA, VSD, and PS.
   a. Repaired during the first year of life.
   b. VSD patch repaired to include LV to aortic outflow continuity with pulmonary blood flow provided via an RV-to-PA homograft.
3. Atrial switch operation—Mustard or Senning procedure:
   a. Rerouting of atrial blood flow: RA → mitral valve → LV → PA and LA → tricuspid valve → RV → aorta.
   b. Restores oxygenated blood into the systemic system and deoxygenated blood guided to the pulmonary system.
   c. Disadvantages:
      i. RV is left as the systemic ventricle—will develop RV dysfunction.
      ii. Increased incidence of atrial dysrhythmias and baffle obstruction.

Complications

1. Severe hypoxia.
2. Multiorgan ischemia.
3. Arrhythmias.
4. RV dysfunction.
5. Coronary artery obstruction leading to myocardial ischemia or death.
6. Long-term follow-up is necessary for pediatric and adult patients, regardless of surgical repair technique.

Tricuspid Atresia

EVIDENCE BASE Cetta, F., Dearani, J. A., & O'Leary, P. W. (2022). Tricuspid valve disorders: Atresia, dysplasia, and Ebstein anomaly. In R. E. Shaddy, D. J. Penny, T. F. Feltes, F. Cetta, & S. Mital (Eds.), *Moss and Adams' heart disease in infants, children, and adolescents: Including the fetus and young adult* (10th ed., pp. 914–939). Lippincott Williams & Wilkins.

TA involves the absence of the tricuspid valve and hypoplasia of the RV. Such associated defects as ASD, VSD, or PDA are necessary for survival. TA accounts for about 3% of CHDs.

Pathophysiology and Etiology

1. With TA, systemic venous return enters the RA and cannot continue into the RV; blood flows across an atrial septal opening into the LA.
2. Pulmonary blood flow occurs through a PDA or VSD.

Clinical Manifestations

1. Cyanosis.
2. Tachypnea.
3. Feeding difficulties.
4. Additional signs of failure.

Diagnostic Evaluation

1. Auscultation: murmurs vary depending on the associated lesions; single S_2.
2. Palpation: if a restrictive VSD is present, a thrill may be palpated.
3. Chest x-ray: pulmonary vascular markings related to the amount of pulmonary blood flow (usually decreased); normal to slightly increased cardiac silhouette.
4. ECG: superior axis; right and left atrial hypertrophy; LVH. First-degree AV block can be common.
5. Two-dimensional echocardiogram identifies the atretic tricuspid valve and hypoplastic RV; Doppler study and color flow mapping document the right-to-left atrial shunt and the size of the PDA or VSD.
6. Cardiac catheterization may be necessary to delineate anatomy.

Management

Medical Management

1. Stabilize with PGE_1 infusion.
2. Maintain oxygen saturation at greater than 75%.
3. Intubate and ventilate, as needed.
4. Inotropic support, as needed.

Surgical Management

1. First surgery—neonate:
   a. BT/modified BT shunt—indicated if pulmonary blood flow is insufficient.
   b. PA band—indicated if pulmonary blood flow is excessive.
   c. No treatment is required if pulmonary blood flow is balanced.
   d. If the great arteries are transposed, Damus–Kaye–Stansel (DKS) may be performed—placement of a modified BT shunt as well as joining of the aorta and main PA.
2. Second surgery—ages 6 to 9 months:
   a. Bidirectional Glenn shunt: end-to-side anastomosis of the SVC to the right PA.
3. Third surgery—ages approximately 3 to 4 years.
   a. Fontan completion: IVC to PA connection (extracardiac conduit with or without fenestration or intracardiac baffle).

Complications

1. CHF.
2. Persistent pleural effusion (especially after stage II and stage III repairs).
3. Thrombus formation in the systemic venous system.
4. Infective endocarditis.
5. Rarely, heart block.
6. Eventual Fontan circulation can result in lifelong multisystem complications, to varying degrees, in childhood, as well as adulthood.

Hypoplastic Left Heart Syndrome

EVIDENCE BASE Jacobs, J. P. (2022). Hypoplastic left heart syndrome: Definition, morphology, and classification. *World Journal for Pediatric and Congenital Heart Surgery, 13*(5), 559–564. https://doi.org/10.1177/21501351221114770

Tweddell, J. S., Hoffman, G. M., Ghanayem, N. S., Frommel, M. A., Mussatto, K. A., & Berger, S. (2022). Hypoplastic left heart syndrome. In R. E. Shaddy, D. J. Penny, T. F. Feltes, F. Cetta, & S. Mital (Eds.), *Moss and Adams' heart disease in infants, children, and adolescents: Including the fetus and young adult* (10th ed., pp. 1083–1121). Lippincott Williams & Wilkins.

HLHS is a constellation of left-sided heart abnormalities that include:

1. Critical mitral stenosis or atresia.
2. Hypoplastic LV.
3. Critical aortic stenosis or atresia.
4. Hypoplastic ascending aorta with severe CoA.
5. Associated anomalies include CoA (75%), ASD (15%), and VSD (10%).

HLHS accounts for 1.4% to 3.8% of all CHDs. It is the most common cause of death from cardiac defects in the first month of life.

Pathophysiology and Etiology

1. The left side of the heart is underdeveloped and essentially nonfunctional.
2. The RV supports the pulmonary and systemic circulations.
3. An ASD allows blood to flow from the LA into the right heart.
4. Blood flows right to left across the PDA and into the descending aorta to deliver oxygen and nutrients to the body.

Clinical Manifestations

1. Neonate may appear completely well initially but becomes critically ill when the PDA closes.
2. Once the PDA begins to close:
   a. Tachypnea due to CHF.
   b. Decreased urine output.
   c. Poor feeding and feeding intolerance.

d. Lethargic; change in level of alertness.
e. Pallor; gray.
f. Weak peripheral pulses.
g. Cyanosis.
h. Metabolic acidosis.

Diagnostic Evaluation

1. Auscultation: single S_2; usually no heart murmur is present, but occasionally, a soft systolic ejection murmur may be heard. As CHF develops, gallop rhythm may be heard.
2. Chest x-ray: cardiac silhouette varies (normal to increased size); increased pulmonary markings and pulmonary edema.
3. ECG: RV hypertrophy; decreased electrical forces in V_5 and V_6.
4. Two-dimensional echocardiogram with Doppler study and color flow mapping identifies the structural abnormalities and the altered blood flow patterns.
5. A cardiac catheterization is usually not needed for initial diagnosis. It may be performed if a balloon atrial septostomy is needed to improve oxygenation.

Management

Medical Management

1. Resuscitation and stabilization with PGE_1 infusion.
2. Inotropic support, as needed (dopamine, dobutamine).
3. Intubate and ventilate, as needed.
4. Correct metabolic acidosis.
5. Assess hepatic, renal, and neurologic function.
6. Infective endocarditis prophylaxis (lifelong).
7. Refer for surgical intervention.

Cardiac Catheterization

1. May need balloon atrial septostomy to allow unrestrictive LA to RA blood flow.
2. Hybrid approach to first-stage palliation, combining both catheterization and surgery; often consists of stenting the PDA and placement of bilateral PA bands. Institution-specific criteria for high-risk surgical candidates.

Surgical Management

1. Palliative, staged repair:
   a. Stage I Norwood (neonate): reconstruction of the hypoplastic aorta using the PA and an aortic or pulmonary allograft, an atrial septectomy, repair of the coarctation, and placement of a BT shunt or RV-PA conduit (Sano modification).
   b. Postoperatively, desire to have a balanced systemic and pulmonary circulation, maintaining oxygen saturations at approximately 75% to 85%.
   c. Stage II bidirectional Glenn shunt (ages 6 to 9 months): transect the SVC off the RA and directly suture end to side to right PA; ligate BT shunt.
   d. Expect goal oxygen saturations postoperatively to be approximately 75% to 85%.
   e. Stage III Fontan (ages 18 months to 4 years): IVC to PA connection (extracardiac conduit with or without fenestration or intracardiac baffle).
   f. Expect goal oxygen saturations postoperatively to be greater than 85%, increasing to near normal postdischarge.
   g. Fontan circulation is not meant to be a permanent curative procedure, and the child will eventually progress to failure with multiple body system involvement in later childhood, adolescence, and adulthood without further intervention.
2. Cardiac transplantation.

Complications

1. Cyanosis.
2. Metabolic acidosis.
3. Persistent pleural effusion (especially after stage II or III repair).
4. Thrombus formation in the systemic venous system.
5. Infective endocarditis.
6. Cardiovascular collapse, multisystem failure, possible death.
7. Interstage period, between stages I and II of surgical repair, has been identified as a vulnerable period for neonates, the second highest risk for mortality. As a result, most programs have adopted interstage monitoring, consisting of oxygen saturation and weight checks, designed to be completed in the home. This may identify top risk factors that can be recognized early and treated during this time.

Nursing Care of the Child With CHD

EVIDENCE BASE Ding, X., Wen, J., Yue, X., Zhao, Y., Qi, C., Wang, D., & Wei, X. (2022). Effect of comprehensive nursing intervention for congenital heart disease in children: A meta-analysis. *Medicine, 101*(41), e31184. https://doi.org/10.1097/MD.0000000000031184

LaRonde, M. P., Connor, J. A., Cerrato, B., Chiloyan, A., & Lisanti, A. (2022). Individualized family-centered developmental care for infants with congenital heart disease in the intensive care unit. *American Journal of Critical Care, 31*(1), e10–e19. https://doi.org/10.4037/ajcc2022124

Nursing Assessment

1. Obtain a thorough nursing history.
2. Discuss the care plan with the health care team (cardiologist, cardiac surgeon, nursing case manager, social worker, and nutritionist). Discuss the care plan with the patient, primary caregivers, and other caregivers.
3. Measure and record height and weight and plot on a growth chart.
4. Record vital signs and oxygen saturations.
   a. Measure vital signs at a time when the infant/child is quiet.
   b. Choose an appropriate-size BP cuff.
   c. Check four extremity BP × 1.
5. Assess and record:
   a. Skin color: pink, cyanotic, mottled.
   b. Mucous membranes: moist, dry, cyanotic.
   c. Extremities: check peripheral pulses for quality and symmetry; dependent edema; capillary refill; color and temperature.
6. Assess for clubbing (cyanotic heart disease).
7. Assess chest wall for deformities; prominent precordial activity.
8. Assess respiratory pattern.
   a. Before disturbing the child, stand back and count the respiratory rate.
   b. Loosen or remove clothing to directly observe chest movement.
   c. Assess for signs of respiratory distress: increased respiratory rate, grunting, retractions, and nasal flaring.
   d. Auscultate for crackles, wheezing, congestion, and stridor.
9. Assess heart sounds.
   a. Determine rate (bradycardia, tachycardia, or normal for age) and rhythm (regular or irregular).
   b. Identify murmur (type, location, and grade).

10. Assess fluid status.
    a. Daily weights.
    b. Strict intake and output (number of wet diapers; urine output).
11. Assess and record the child's level of activity.
    a. Observe the infant while feeding. Does the infant need frequent breaks or do they fall asleep during feeding? Assess for sweating, color change, or respiratory distress while feeding.
    b. Observe the child at play. Is play interrupted to rest? Ask the caregiver if the child keeps up with peers while at play.
    c. Assess and record findings relevant to the child's developmental level: age-appropriate behavior, cognitive skills, gross and fine motor skills.

Nursing Interventions

Relieving Respiratory Distress

1. Position the child in a reclining, semi-upright position.
2. Suction oral and nasal secretions, as needed.
3. Identify target oxygen saturations and administer oxygen, as prescribed.
4. Administer prescribed medications and document response to medications (improved, no change, or worsening respiratory status).
    a. Diuretics.
    b. Bronchodilators.
5. May need to change oral feedings to nasogastric feedings because of the increased risk of aspiration with respiratory distress.

Improving Cardiac Output

See Table 41-1.

1. Organize nursing care and medication schedule to provide periods of uninterrupted rest.
2. Provide play or educational activities that can be done in bed with minimal exertion.
3. Maintain normothermia.
4. Administer diuretics (furosemide, spironolactone), as prescribed.
    a. Give the medication at the same time each day. For older children, do not give a dose right before bedtime.
    b. Monitor the effectiveness of the dose: measure and record urine output.
    c. Monitor serum electrolytes. May experience hypokalemia and hypocalcemia with diuretic use.
5. Administer digoxin, as prescribed.
    a. Check heart rate for 1 minute. Withhold the dose and notify the physician for bradycardia (heart rate less than 90 beats/minute).
    b. Lead II rhythm strip may be ordered for PR interval monitoring. Prolonged PR interval indicates first-degree heart block (dose of digoxin may be withheld).
    c. Give medication at the same time each day. For infants and children, digoxin is usually divided and given twice per day.
    d. Monitor serum electrolytes. Increased incidence of digoxin toxicity associated with hypokalemia.
6. Administer afterload-reducing medications (captopril, enalapril), as prescribed.
    a. When initiating medication for the first time: check BP immediately before and 1 hour after dose.
    b. Monitor for signs of hypotension: syncope, lightheadedness, and faint pulses.
    c. Withhold medication and notify the physician according to ordered parameters.

Improving Oxygenation and Activity Tolerance

1. Place pulse oximeter probe (continuous monitoring or measure with vital signs) on the finger, earlobe, or toe. Preductal

Table 41-1 Common Cardiac Drugs

DRUG CLASSIFICATION	MECHANISM OF ACTION	EXAMPLES
β-Adrenergic blockers	Antagonize epinephrine receptors resulting in decreased cardiac contractility and decreased heart rate	Propranolol, esmolol, atenolol
Angiotensin-converting enzyme (ACE) inhibitor	Lowers blood pressure by decreasing blood vessel tone (reduces afterload)	Captopril, enalapril
Angiotensin II receptor blockers	Decrease blood pressure by causing dilation of blood vessels	Losartan, valsartan
Calcium channel blockers	Decrease intracellular calcium leading to reduced cardiac and vascular smooth muscle contraction and lower blood pressure	Amlodipine, diltiazem, felodipine, isradipine, intravenous nicardipine, nifedipine, and verapamil
Vasopressors	Increase cardiac contractility and vascular muscle tone resulting in increased blood pressure	Dopamine, dobutamine, milrinone, epinephrine
Diuretics	Reduce blood volume by increasing urinary output Used to treat high blood pressure and congestive heart failure	Furosemide, spironolactone, chlorothiazide, metolazone
Antiarrhythmics	Various classifications used to treat cardiac dysrhythmias	Lidocaine, amiodarone, disopyramide adenosine
Cardiac glycosides	Strengthens cardiac contractility and decreases heart rate Used to treat congestive heart failure	Digoxin
Pulmonary vasodilators	Reduce elevated pressure in pulmonary vasculature, treatment of pulmonary hypertension	Sildenafil, inhaled nitric oxide, bosentan

and postductal saturation monitoring provides the most comprehensive information about oxygenation.
2. Administer oxygen, as needed.
3. Titrate the amount of oxygen to reach target oxygen saturations.
4. Assess response to oxygen therapy: increase in baseline oxygen saturations, improved work of breathing, and change in patient comfort.
5. Explain to the child how oxygen will help. If possible, give the child the choice for facemask oxygen or nasal cannula oxygen.

Providing Adequate Nutrition

1. For the infant:
   a. Small, frequent feedings.
   b. Fortified formula or breast milk (up to 30 cal/ounce).
   c. Limit oral feeding time to 15 to 20 minutes.
   d. Supplement oral feeds with nasogastric feedings, as needed, to provide weight gain (i.e., continuous nasogastric feedings at night with ad-lib by-mouth feeds during the day).
2. For the child:
   a. Small, frequent meals.
   b. High-calorie, nutritional supplements.
   c. Determine child's likes and dislikes and plan meals accordingly.
   d. Allow the caregivers to bring the child's favorite foods to the hospital.
3. Report feeding intolerance: nausea, vomiting, and diarrhea.
4. Document daily weight (same time of day, same scale, same clothing).
5. Record accurate intake and output; assess for fluid retention.
6. Fluid restriction not usually needed for children; manage excess fluid with diuretics.

Preventing Infection

1. Maintain a routine childhood immunization schedule. With the exception of respiratory syncytial virus (RSV) and influenza, immunizations should not be given for 6 weeks after cardiovascular surgery.
2. Administer yearly influenza vaccine.
3. Administer RSV immunization for children younger than age 2 with complex CHD and those at risk for CHF or pulmonary hypertension.
4. Prevent exposure to communicable diseases.
5. Good handwashing.
6. Report fevers.
7. Report signs of URI: runny nose, cough, and increase in nasal secretions.
8. Report signs of gastrointestinal (GI) illness: diarrhea, abdominal pain, and irritability.

Reducing Fear and Anxiety

1. Educate the patient and family.
2. Provide the family with contact phone numbers: how to schedule a follow-up visit; how to reach a cardiologist during the work week, evenings, weekends, and holidays.

Family Education and Health Maintenance

1. Instruct the family on necessary measures to maintain the child's health:
   a. Complete immunization.
   b. Adequate diet and rest.
   c. Prevention and control of infections.
   d. Regular medical and dental checkups. The child should be protected against infective endocarditis when undergoing certain dental procedures.
   e. Regular cardiac follow-up appointments.
2. Teach the family about the defect and its treatment.
   a. Provide patients and families with written and verbal information regarding the CHD. Offer appropriate internet resources for information about CHD and medical and surgical treatment options.
   b. Provide individualized resources for caregivers and patient if applicable. Visual aid of current physiology as well as repair, medication list, and emergency action cards, upon discharge.
   c. Signs and symptoms of CHF (see pages 1213–1215).
   d. Signs of hypercyanotic spells associated with cyanotic defects and need to place child in knee–chest position.
   e. Need to prevent dehydration, which increases the risk of thrombotic complications.
   f. Emergency precautions related to hypercyanotic spells, pulmonary edema, cardiac arrest (if appropriate).
   g. Special home care equipment, monitors, oxygen.
3. Encourage the caregivers and others (teachers, peers) to treat the child in as normal a manner as possible.
   a. Avoid overprotection and overindulgence.
   b. Avoid rejection.
   c. Promote growth and development with modifications. Facilitate performance of the usual developmental tasks within the limits of the child's physiologic state.
   d. Prevent adults from projecting their fears and anxieties onto the child.
   e. Help family deal with anger, guilt, and concerns related to the child who is disabled.
4. Initiate a community health nursing referral, if indicated.
5. Stress the need for follow-up care.
6. Encourage attendance in support groups for patients and families.

Evaluation: Expected Outcomes

- Improved oxygenation evidenced by easy, comfortable respirations.
- Improved cardiac output demonstrated by stable vital signs, adequate peripheral perfusion, and adequate urine output.
- Increased activity level.
- Maximal nutritional status demonstrated by weight gain and increase in growth curve percentile.
- No signs or symptoms of infection.
- Caregivers discuss diagnosis and treatment together and with the child.

Congestive Heart Failure

EVIDENCE BASE Ahmed, H., & VanderPluym, C. (2021). Medical management of pediatric heart failure. *Cardiovascular Diagnosis and Therapy, 11*(1), 323–335. https://doi.org/10.21037/cdt-20-358

O'Connor, M. J., & Kantor, P. F. (2022). Chronic heart failure in children. In R. E. Shaddy, D. J. Penny, T. F. Feltes, F. Cetta, & S. Mital (Eds.), *Moss and Adams' heart disease in infants, children, and adolescents: Including the fetus and young adult* (10th ed., pp. 1652–1673). Lippincott Williams & Wilkins.

CHF occurs when cardiac output cannot meet the metabolic demands of the body.

Pathophysiology and Etiology

1. May result from:
   a. CHDs with a volume or pressure overload (moderate to large left-to-right shunt [PDA, VSD], AV valve insufficiency, or outflow obstruction [HLHS, CoA]).
   b. Acquired heart disease: myocarditis, cardiomyopathy, acute rheumatic fever.
   c. Chronic pulmonary disease: cor pulmonale, bronchopulmonary dysplasia.
   d. Arrhythmias: prolonged supraventricular tachycardia (SVT), complete heart block.
   e. Anemia.
   f. Iatrogenic fluid overload.
2. In an attempt to meet the metabolic needs of the body, the heart rate increases to increase cardiac output.
   a. Cardiac output = heart rate × stroke volume.
   b. Stroke volume is the amount of blood (mL) ejected from the heart with each heartbeat; it depends on preload and vascular resistance.
3. Preload (CVP) increases as the failing heart contracts poorly.
4. With decreased cardiac output, the systemic vascular resistance increases to maintain BP. This increase in afterload limits cardiac output.
5. With decreased blood flow to the kidneys, the glomerular filtration rate decreases as tubular reabsorption increases sodium and water retention, resulting in decreased urine output.
6. In the long term, these compensatory mechanisms are detrimental to the failing myocardium. The chronic increase in preload and afterload contributes to chamber dilation and myocardial hypertrophy, leading to progressive CHF.

Clinical Manifestations

1. Impaired myocardial function.
   a. Tachycardia, S_3 gallop.
   b. Poor peripheral perfusion: weak peripheral pulses, cool extremities, delayed capillary refill.
   c. Pallor.
   d. Exercise or activity intolerance.
2. Pulmonary congestion.
   a. Tachypnea.
   b. Cyanosis.
   c. Retractions, nasal flaring, grunting.
   d. Cough.
3. Systemic venous congestion.
   a. Hepatomegaly.
   b. Peripheral edema: scrotal and orbital.
   c. Water weight gain.
   d. Decreased urine output.

Diagnostic Evaluation

1. Characteristic physical examination findings.
2. Chest x-ray shows cardiomegaly and pulmonary congestion.
3. B-type natriuretic peptide (BNP) as a biomarker for diagnostic, prognostic, and therapeutic monitoring use for pediatric patients with CHD, cardiomyopathy.

Management

1. Diuretics to reduce intravascular volume (furosemide, spironolactone).
2. Digoxin to increase myocardial contractility for symptomatic patients with low ejection fraction. Not necessary for those patients with left ventricular dysfunction without symptoms.
3. Afterload reduction to decrease the workload of the ailing myocardium (ACE inhibitors—captopril, enalapril, lisinopril).
4. Beta-adrenergic blockers to counteract increased sympathetic activity and reduce systemic vascular resistance (metoprolol, carvedilol).
5. Angiotensin II receptor blockers (ARBs) for patients who are intolerant of ACE inhibitors, but who can benefit from renin–angiotensin–aldosterone system (RAAS) blockade.
6. Inotropic support, as needed.
7. Mechanical circulatory support (see above information in the section on cardiac transplantation).

Complications

1. Pulmonary edema.
2. Metabolic acidosis.
3. Failure to thrive.
4. URIs.
5. Arrhythmia.
6. Death.

Nursing Assessment

1. Assess response to medical treatment plan.
2. Document vital signs and oxygen saturations.
3. Observe infant or child during feeding or activity. Assess for diaphoresis, need for frequent rest periods, and inability to keep up with peers.
4. Follow the growth curve.

Nursing Interventions

Improving Myocardial Efficiency

1. Administer digoxin, as prescribed.
   a. Measure heart rate. Hold medication and notify health care provider for heart rate less than 90 beats/min.
   b. Check the most recent potassium level. Hold medication and notify health care provider for potassium less than 3.5 mEq/L.
   c. Run lead II ECG, if ordered, to monitor PR interval. If first-degree AV block occurs, notify the health care provider and hold medication, as directed.
   d. Report signs of possible digoxin toxicity: vomiting, nausea, visual changes, and bradycardia.
   e. Double-check the dose of digoxin with another nurse before administering the dose. Make sure the digoxin order has two signatures.
2. Administer afterload reduction medications, as prescribed.
   a. Measure BP before and after giving the patient the medication. Hold the medication and notify the health care provider for low BP (greater than a 15-mm Hg drop from baseline).
   b. Observe for other signs of hypotension: dizziness, lightheadedness, and syncope.

Maintaining Fluid and Electrolyte Balance

1. Administer diuretics, as prescribed.
   a. Obtain daily weights.
   b. Keep strict intake and output record.
   c. Monitor serum electrolytes. Provide potassium supplements, as needed.

2. Sodium restriction: not usually needed in children; provide dietary assistance, as needed.
3. Fluid restriction: not usually needed in children.

Relieving Respiratory Distress

1. Administer oxygen therapy, as prescribed.
2. Elevate the head of bed; infants may be more comfortable in an upright infant seat.

Promoting Activity Tolerance

1. Organize nursing care to provide periods of uninterrupted sleep/rest.
2. Avoid unnecessary activities.
3. Respond efficiently to a crying infant. Provide comfort and treat the source of distress: wet or dirty diaper, hunger.
4. Provide diversional activities that require limited expenditure of energy.
5. Provide small, frequent feedings.

Decreasing Risk of Infection

1. Ensure good handwashing by everyone.
2. Avoid exposure to ill children or caregivers.
3. Monitor signs of infection: fever, cough, runny nose, diarrhea, and vomiting.

Providing Adequate Nutrition

1. For the older child: provide nutritious foods that the child likes, along with supplemental high-calorie snacks (milkshake, pudding).
2. For the infant:
   a. High-calorie formula (24 to 30 cal/ounce).
   b. Supplement oral intake with nasogastric feedings. Allow ad-lib oral intake through the day with continuous nasogastric feedings at night.

Reducing Anxiety and Fear

1. Communicate the care plan to the child and family.
2. Educate the family about CHF and provide home care nursing referral to reinforce teaching after discharge.
3. Encourage questions; answer questions as able or refer to another member of the health care team.

Family Education and Health Maintenance

1. Teach the signs and symptoms of CHF.
2. Teach medications: brand name and generic name, expected effects, adverse effects, and dose.
3. Demonstrate medication administration.
4. With the family, design a medication administration time schedule.
5. Provide guidelines for when to seek medical help.
6. Teach infant and child cardiopulmonary resuscitation (CPR), as needed.
7. Reinforce dietary guidelines; provide a recipe to the caregiver on how to make high-calorie formula.
8. Reinforce ways to prevent infection.
9. Make sure that follow-up visit with health care providers is scheduled, prior to discharge.
10. Educate the patient and family on infective endocarditis guidelines and provide them with written materials. Standard general prophylaxis for children at risk: amoxicillin 50 mg/kg (maximum dose = 2 g) given orally 1 hour before the procedure.

Evaluation: Expected Outcomes

- Heart rate within normal range for age; adequate urine output.
- No unexpected weight gain.
- Clear lungs; normal respiratory rate and effort.
- Participates in quiet diversional activities.
- No signs or symptoms of infection.
- Adequate intake of small, frequent feedings.
- Caregivers express understanding of disease process and treatment.

ACQUIRED HEART DISEASE

Note: Kawasaki disease is discussed in Chapter 49.

Acute Rheumatic Fever

EVIDENCE BASE de Loizaga, S. R., Arthur, L., Arya, B., Beckman, B., Belay, W., Brokamp, C., Hyun Choi, N., Connolly, S., Dasgupta, S., Dibert, T., Dryer, M. M., Hahn, L. R. G., Greene, E. A., Kernizan, D., Khalid, O., Klein, J., Kobayashi, R., Lahiri, S., Lorenzoni, R. P., … Beaton, A. (2021). Rheumatic heart disease in the United States: Forgotten but not gone: Results of a 10 year multicenter review. *Journal of the American Heart Association, 10*(16), e020992. https://doi.org/10.1161/JAHA.120.020992

Acute rheumatic fever (ARF) is an acute autoimmune disease that occurs as a sequela of group A beta-hemolytic streptococcal infection. In the United States, the incidence is <2 cases per 100,000 in school-age children. Rates are significantly higher in countries stricken by lack of resources and a high rate of poverty. It is characterized by inflammatory lesions of connective tissue and endothelial tissue, primarily affecting the joints and heart.

Pathophysiology and Etiology

1. Most initial attacks of ARF occur 1 to 5 weeks (average 3 weeks) after a streptococcal infection of the throat or of the upper respiratory tract.
2. Peak incidence occurs in children ages 5 to 15 years. Incidence after a mild streptococcal pharyngeal infection is 0.3%; after a severe streptococcal infection, 1% to 3%.
3. Family history of rheumatic fever is usually positive.
4. Streptococcal infection abates with or without treatment; however, autoantibodies attack the myocardium, pericardium, and cardiac valves.
   a. Aschoff bodies (fibrin deposits) develop on the valves, possibly leading to permanent valve dysfunction, especially of the mitral and aortic valves.
   b. Severe myocarditis may cause dilation of the heart and congestive heart failure (CHF).
5. Inflammation of the large joints causes painful arthritis that may last 6 to 8 weeks.
6. Involvement of the nervous system causes chorea (sudden involuntary movements).

Clinical Manifestations

Documented or undocumented group A beta-hemolytic streptococcal infection is usually followed (within several weeks) by fever, malaise, and anorexia. Major symptoms of ARF may appear several weeks to several months after initial infection.

Major Manifestations (Jones Criteria)

1. Carditis—manifested by sinus tachycardia, a soft-blowing pansystolic murmur, prolonged PR and QT intervals on electrocardiogram (ECG), and possibly by signs of CHF (see pages 1213-1215).
2. Polyarthritis—pain and limited movement of two or more joints; joints are swollen, red, warm, and tender.
3. Chorea—purposeless, involuntary, rapid movements commonly associated with muscle weakness, involuntary facial grimaces, speech disturbance, and emotional lability.
4. Erythema marginatum—nonpruritic pink, macular rash mostly of the trunk with pale central areas; migratory.
5. Subcutaneous nodules—firm, painless nodules over the scalp, extensor surface of joints, such as wrists, elbows, knees, and vertebral column.

Minor Manifestations

1. History of previous rheumatic fever or evidence of preexisting rheumatic heart disease.
2. Arthralgia—pain in one or more joints without evidence of inflammation, tenderness, or limited movement.
3. Fever—temperature greater than 100.4°F (38°C).
4. Laboratory abnormalities—elevated erythrocyte sedimentation rate, positive C-reactive protein, elevated white blood cell count.
5. ECG changes—prolonged PR interval.

Diagnostic Evaluation

1. Diagnosed clinically through use of the Jones criteria from the American Heart Association—presence of two major manifestations or one major and two minor manifestations (as listed earlier), with supporting evidence of a recent streptococcal infection.
2. ECG to evaluate PR interval and other changes.
3. Laboratory tests listed previously. In addition, group A streptococcal culture and/or antistreptolysin-O titer to detect streptococcal antibodies from recent infection.
4. Chest x-ray for cardiomegaly, pulmonary congestion, or edema.

Management

1. Course of antibiotic therapy to completely eradicate streptococcal infection (may be given despite previous treatment).
   a. Usually, benzathine penicillin is given intramuscularly (IM) in a single dose or a 10-day course of oral penicillin V.
   b. Oral erythromycin may be used for children who are allergic to penicillin.
2. Nonsteroidal anti-inflammatory drugs (naproxen sodium) usually used to control pain and inflammation of arthritis. Aspirin for acute carditis.
3. Corticosteroids may be used in severe cases to try to control cardiac inflammation; however, there is limited evidence to support their use.
4. Phenobarbital, diazepam, or other neurologic agent to control chorea.
5. Bed rest during the acute phase to rest the heart. Gradual return to activities is recommended once acute symptoms resolve.
6. Mitral valve replacement may be necessary in some cases.
7. Secondary prevention of recurrent ARF:
   a. Risk of recurrence greatest within first 5 years, with multiple episodes of ARF, and with rheumatic heart disease. Prophylactic antibiotic treatment may be lifelong.
   b. For those at low risk for recurrence, antibiotic prophylaxis may be continued for 5 years or longer.
   c. Antibiotic regimens may include:
      i. Benzathine penicillin IM once.
      ii. Penicillin V 250 mg orally twice per day for children less than 27 kg, 500 mg orally twice per day for patients greater than 27 kg.
      iii. Patients with penicillin allergies may be prescribed cephalosporin, clindamycin, azithromycin, or clarithromycin.

Complications

1. CHF.
2. Pericarditis, pericardial effusion.
3. Permanent damage to the aortic or mitral valve, possibly requiring valve replacement.

Nursing Assessment

1. Assess for signs of cardiac involvement by auscultation of the heart for murmur and cardiac monitoring for prolonged PR interval.
2. Monitor pulse for 1 full minute to determine heart rate.
3. Assess temperature for elevation.
4. Observe for involuntary movements: stick out tongue or smile; garbled or hesitant speech when asked to recite numbers or the ABCs; hyperextension of the wrists and fingers when trying to extend arms.
5. Assess child's ability to feed self, dress, and do other activities if chorea or arthritis present.
6. Assess pain level using a scale appropriate for child's age.
7. Assess caregivers' ability to cope with illness and care for child.
8. Assess the need for homeschooling while the patient is on bed rest.

Nursing Interventions

Improving Cardiac Output

1. Explain to the child and family the need for bed rest during the acute phase and as long as CHF is present. In milder cases, light indoor activity is allowed.
2. In severe cases, organize care to minimize exertion and provide uninterrupted rest.
3. Maintain cardiac monitoring, if indicated.
4. Administer course of antibiotics, as directed. Be alert to adverse effects, such as nausea, vomiting, and gastrointestinal (GI) distress.
5. Administer medications for CHF, as directed. Monitor blood pressure (BP), intake and output, and heart rate.

Relieving Pain

1. Administer anti-inflammatory medication, analgesics, and antipyretics, as directed.
   a. Monitor for side effects of corticosteroid use—GI distress, acne, weight gain, and emotional disturbances—or long-term effects, such as rounded face, ulcer formation, and decreased resistance to infection.
   b. Administer all anti-inflammatory medications with food to reduce GI injury.

c. Be aware that anti-inflammatories may not alter the course of myocardial injury.
2. Teach family the importance of maintaining a dosage schedule, continuing medication until all signs and symptoms of the ARF have gone, and tapering the dose, as directed by health care provider.
3. Assist child with positioning for comfort and protecting inflamed joints.
4. Suggest diversional activities that do not require the use of painful joints.

Protecting the Child With Chorea

1. Use padded side rails if chorea is severe.
2. Assist with feeding and other fine motor activities, as needed.
3. Assist with ambulation if weak.
4. Avoid the use of straws and sharp utensils if chorea involves the face.
5. Make sure that the child consumes a nutritious diet with recommended vitamins, protein, and calories.
6. Be patient if speech is affected and offer emotional support.
7. Protect the child from stress.
8. Administer phenobarbital or other medication for chorea, as directed. Observe for drowsiness.

Family Education and Health Maintenance

1. Teach the appropriate administration of all medications, including prophylactic antibiotic.
2. Encourage all family and household members to be screened for streptococcus and receive the appropriate treatment.
3. Instruct on additional prophylaxis for endocarditis with dental procedures and surgery, as indicated.
4. Encourage following activity restrictions, resuming activity gradually, and resting whenever tired.
5. Encourage keeping appointments for follow-up evaluation by cardiologist and other health care providers.
6. Advise the caregivers that child cannot return to school until the health care provider assesses that all disease activity is gone. Caregivers may need to discuss with teachers how the child can catch up with schoolwork.
7. Instruct on follow-up with usual health care provider for immunizations, well-child evaluations, hearing and vision screening, and other health maintenance needs.

Provide general health education about early identification and treatment seeking for any possible streptococcal infection (fever, sore throat). Adherence to 10 to 14 days of antibiotics can greatly reduce the risk of ARF and other poststreptococcal sequelae.

Evaluation: Expected Outcomes

- Heart rate and PR interval within the normal range for age; no signs of CHF.
- Adherent to anti-inflammatory therapy; reports pain as 1 to 2 on a scale of 1 to 10.
- Feeds self, washes face and hands, and ambulates to the bathroom without injury.

Cardiomyopathy

EVIDENCE BASE Rossano, J. W., Kantor, P. F., Shaddy, R. E., Shi, L., Wilkinson, J. D., Jeffries, J. L., Czachor, J. D., Razoky, H., Wirtz, H. S., Depre, C., & Lipshultz, S. E. (2020). Elevated heart rate and survival in children with dilated cardiomyopathy: A multicenter study from the pediatric cardiomyopathy registry. *Journal of the American Heart Association*, 9(15), e015916. https://doi.org/10.1161/JAHA.119.015916

According to the type of myocardial changes, *cardiomyopathy* can be classified into three categories: dilated, hypertrophic, and restrictive. The most common type in children is dilated cardiomyopathy. Hypertrophic cardiomyopathy is a leading cause of death in young athletes.

Pathophysiology and Etiology

1. Familial (family history, genetic predisposition) tendency.
2. Idiopathic in most cases.
3. May be related to:
   a. Nutritional deficiency (carnitine or selenium).
   b. Viral infection (myocarditis), human immunodeficiency virus.
   c. Collagen vascular disease (systemic lupus erythematosus).
   d. Cardiotoxic drugs (doxorubicin).
   e. Cocaine use.
   f. Infants of birthing parents who have diabetes.
   g. Ion channelopathies.
   h. Catecholamine surge; hyperthyroidism.
4. Dilated cardiomyopathy involves dilatation of one or both ventricles associated with normal septal and left ventricle (LV) free wall thickness.
5. Decreased systolic function (contractility) results in CHF.
6. Increasing end-systolic dimension results in atrioventricular (AV) valve insufficiency, further worsening CHF.

Clinical Manifestations

1. Signs of CHF—tachycardia, tachypnea, dyspnea, crackles, hepatosplenomegaly.
2. Decreased exercise tolerance, fatigue, sweating.
3. Poor weight gain, nausea, abdominal tenderness.
4. Ventricular arrhythmia.
5. Chest pain.
6. Syncope.

Diagnostic Evaluation

1. Auscultation: systolic regurgitant murmur (if mitral or tricuspid insufficiency is present), S_2 is normal or narrowly split, prominent S_3 gallop.
2. ECG: tachycardia, abnormal ST segments, arrhythmia, ectopic atrial tachycardia, deep Q waves, left ventricular hypertrophy (LVH).
3. Chest x-ray: cardiomegaly, pulmonary congestion.
4. Two-dimensional echocardiogram: increased wall thickness, poor ventricular systolic function, dilated heart chambers; AV valve insufficiency.
5. Cardiac magnetic resonance imaging (MRI) will provide useful information on cardiac function and may demonstrate ventricular hypertrophy or fibrosis.
6. Cardiac catheterization: not needed for initial diagnosis; endomyocardial biopsy (to rule out myocarditis); assess pulmonary vascular resistance (PVR).

Management

General Measures

1. Identify and treat the underlying cause.
2. Maximize caloric intake: fortify formula; supplemental nasogastric feedings.
3. Supplemental oxygen, as needed.
4. Activity restriction (usually self-imposed by the younger child and infant). Restrict participation in strenuous and competitive sports.

Treatment of Systolic Dysfunction With Dilated Cardiomyopathy

1. Diuretics: furosemide, spironolactone.
2. Inotropes for patients with poor perfusion: milrinone, dopamine, epinephrine.
3. Afterload reduction: captopril, enalapril, lisinopril.
4. Anticoagulation: warfarin, low-molecular-weight heparin (enoxaparin).
5. Antiarrhythmics.
6. Placement of an automatic implantable cardioverter defibrillator.
7. Biventricular pacing.
8. Cardiac transplant.

Treatment of Diastolic Dysfunction With Hypertrophic Cardiomyopathy

1. Beta-adrenergic blockers: propranolol.
2. Calcium channel blockers: verapamil.
3. AV sequential pacing.
4. Myomectomy or myotomy.

Treatment of Diastolic Dysfunction With Restrictive Cardiomyopathy

1. Diuretics.
2. Anticoagulation.
3. Permanent pacemaker for advanced heart block.

Complications

1. Severe CHF.
2. Increased PVR.
3. Intracardiac thrombus.
4. Embolus.
5. Malignant arrhythmias.
6. Sudden death.

Nursing Assessment

Perform a thorough nursing assessment as for congenital heart disease (CHD) (see page 1211).

Nursing Interventions

Maximizing Cardiac Output

1. Monitor vital signs; notify the physician for hypotension, tachycardia, arrhythmia; increasing tachypnea.
2. Administer oxygen therapy, as prescribed.
3. Administer medications, as prescribed.
   a. Maintain bleeding precautions for patients who are anticoagulated.
   b. Document response to diuretics; monitor intake and output.
4. Monitor electrolytes.
5. Restrict the level of activity.

Providing Maximal Nutritional Support

1. Encourage frequent, small meals. Provide foods the child likes.
2. Provide high-calorie supplements (milkshakes, pudding).
3. Administer supplemental tube feedings if nutritional needs are not being met.
4. Administer parenteral hyperalimentation and intralipids, as directed (rarely needed).

Promoting Effective Coping and Control Within the Family

1. Organize a family meeting with various members of the health care team to review the child's medical condition and to explain the treatment plan.
2. Allow the child and family to express their questions, fears, and concerns.
3. Identify support systems and services for the child and family: extended family members, clergy, support groups, community resources.

Family Education and Health Maintenance

1. Health literacy assessment of primary caregivers should be completed before the creation of a teaching plan. Methods of instruction can include written, illustrated visuals, and video recorded instructions on care routine and signs and symptoms to monitor.
2. Teach child and family medication administration: purpose of the drug, drug dosage, drug schedule, and adverse effects.
3. Help family design a realistic medication schedule.
   a. Identify usual wake-up time and bedtime. Schedule medications accordingly.
   b. Do not give a diuretic right before bedtime or nap time.
   c. If possible, avoid having to give medications at school.
4. Teach bleeding precautions if the child is on anticoagulation agents (coumadin).
   a. Monitor prothrombin international normalized ratio regularly.
   b. Observe for signs of bleeding.
   c. Counsel regarding menses and pregnancy.
   d. Instruct on foods and medications that interfere with coumadin.
5. Give guidelines for notifying the physician.
   a. Worsening shortness of breath.
   b. Irregular pulse; palpitations.
   c. Syncope, dizziness, or lightheadedness.
   d. Increasing fatigue, exercise intolerance.
6. Teach infant and child cardiopulmonary resuscitation (CPR) to family members and other caregivers.

Evaluation: Expected Outcomes

- Stable vital signs.
- Maximal nutritional status, as evidenced by weight gain and growth.
- Understanding of treatment plan, prognosis, consistent attendance of follow-up visits.

Pediatric patients with some previous or preexisting cardiovascular conditions may be associated with increased severity of COVID-19 symptoms, especially those younger than 12 years of age with a history of previous cardiac arrest.

Research is ongoing to ascertain which pediatric patients with heart disease (acquired or congenital) are at greatest risk of post-COVID-19 complications (Ehwerhemuepha et al., 2022).

TRANSITIONAL CARE ALERT Many children discharged from the hospital diagnosed with a complex cardiac condition will have extensive discharge needs. Families will need support in the transition to home or another aftercare location. It is crucial that they have complete and understandable care instructions on home care, medications, and follow-up appointments. If arrangements have been made for nursing care in the home, families should be aware of the agency providing services and when they can expect communication regarding care arrangements. Instructions should include a clear understanding of acceptable discharge expectations as many children may be in different phases if a surgical repair is necessary. Caregivers should be aware of when and where they should seek further emergency care if the child's condition deteriorates.

SELECTED READINGS

Baizabal-Carvallo, J., & Cardoso, F. (2020). Chorea in children: Etiology, diagnostic approach and management. *Journal of Neural Transmission, 127*, 1323–1342. https://doi.org/10.1007/s00702-020-02238-3

Bearl, D. (2022). The importance of mechanical circulatory support on pediatric waitlist and post heart transplant survival: A narrative review. *Pediatric Medicine, 5*(25), 1–9. https://doi.org/10.21037/pm-21-10

Boyd, R., McMullen, H., Beqaj, H., & Kalfa, D. (2021). Environmental exposures and congenital heart disease. *Pediatrics, 149*(1), e2021052151. https://doi.org/10.1542/peds.2021-052151

Cox, D., & Tani, L. (2020). Pediatric infective endocarditis: A clinical update. *Pediatric Clinics of North America, 67*(5), 875–888. https://doi.org/10.1016/j.pcl.2020.06.011

Dore-Stites, D., Lopez, M., Magee, J., Bucuvalas, J., Campbell, K., Shieck, V., Well, A., & Fredericks, E. (2020). Health literacy and its association with adherence in pediatric liver transplant recipients and their parents. *Pediatric Transplantation, 24*(5), e13726. https://doi.org/10.1111/petr.13726

Dykes, J., Rosenthal, D., Bernstein, D., McElhinney, D., Chrisant, M., Daly, K., Ameduri, R., Knecht, K., Richmond, M., Lin, K., Urschel, S., Simmonds, J., Simpson, K., Albers, E., Khan, A., Schumacher, K., Almond, C., Chen, S., & Pediatric Heart Transplant Society. (2021). Clinical and hemodynamic characteristics of the pediatric failing Fontan. *The Journal of Heart and Lung Transplantation, 40*(12), 1529–1539. https://doi.org/10.1016/j.healun.2021.07.017

Ehwerhemuepha, L., Roth, B., Patel, A. K., Heutlinger, O., Heffernan, C., Arrieta, A. C., Sanger, T., Cooper, D. M., Shahbaba, B., Chang, A. C., Feaster, W., Taraman, S., Morizono, H., & Marano, R. (2022). Association of congenital and acquired cardiovascular conditions with COVID-19 severity among pediatric patients in the US. *JAMA Network Open, 5*(5), e2211967. https://doi.org/10.1001/jamanetworkopen.2022.11967

Gonzalez, V., Kimbro, R., Cutitta, K., Shabosky, J., Bilal, M., Penny, D., & Lopez, K. (2021). Mental health disorders in children with congenital heart disease. *Pediatrics, 147*(2), e20201693. https://doi.org/10.1542/peds.2020-1693

Gurvitz, M., Lui, G., & Marelli, A. (2020). Adult congenital heart disease: Preparing for the changing work force demand. *Cardiology Clinics, 38*(3), 283–294. https://doi.org/10.1016/j.ccl.2020.04.011

Lawrence, P., Feinberg, I., & Spratling, R. (2021). The relationship of parental health literacy to health outcomes of children with medical complexity. *Journal of Pediatric Nursing, 60*, 65–70. https://doi.org/10.1016/j.pedn.2021.02.014

Levy, E., Dearani, J., Blumenthal, J., Johnson, J., Overman, D., Stephens, E., & Chiotos, K. (2022). COVID-19 FAQs in pediatric cardiac surgery: 2022 perspective and updates. *World Journal for Pediatric and Congenital Heart Surgery, 13*(3), 287–292. https://doi.org/10.1177/21501351221085966

Morton, S. U., Quiat, D., Seidman, J. G., & Seidman, C. E. (2022). Genomic frontiers in congenital heart disease. *Nature Reviews Cardiology, 19*, 26–42. https://doi.org/10.1038/s41569-021-00587-4

Nakagawa, N. (2023). Infective endocarditis in congenital heart disease. *IntechOpen.* https://doi.org/10.5772/intechopen.107877

O'Byrne, M., Huang, J., Asztalos, I., Smith, C., Dori, Y., Gillespie, M., Rome, J., & Glatz, A. (2020). Pediatric congenital cardiac catheterization quality: An analysis of existing metrics. *Journal of American College of Cardiology: Cardiovascular Interventions, 13*(24), 2853–2864. https://doi.org/10.1016/j.jcin.2020.09.002

Ommen, S. R., Mital, S., Burke, M. A., Day, S. M., Deswal, A., Elliott, P., Evanovich, L. L., Hung, J., Joglar, J. A., Kantor, P., Kimmelstiel, C., Kittleson, M., Link, M. S., Maron, M. S., Martinez, M. W., Miyake, C. Y., Schaff, H. V., Semsarian, C., & Sorajja, P. (2020). 2020 AHA/ACC guideline for the diagnosis and treatment of patients with hypertrophic cardiomyopathy: Executive summary: A report of the American College of Cardiology/American Heart Association Joint Committee on clinical practice guidelines. *Journal of the American College of Cardiology, 76*(25), 3022–3055. https://doi.org/10.1016/j.jacc.2020.08.044

Samayoa, J., Boucek, D., McCarthy, E., Riley, M., Ou, Z., Tani, L., Hoskoppal, A., Gray, R., & Martin, M. (2022). Echocardiographic assessment of Melody versus Sapien valves following transcatheter pulmonary valve replacement. *Journal of American College of Cardiology: Cardiovascular Interventions, 15*(2), 176–178. https://doi.org/10.1016/j.jcin.2021.11.002

VandenEynde, J., Pompeu, M., Vervoort, D., Roever, L., Meyns, B., Budts, W., Gewillig, M., Ruhparwar, A., Zhigalov, K., & Weymann, A. (2022). Pulmonary valve replacement in Tetralogy of Fallot: An updated meta-analysis. *The Annals of Thoracic Surgery, 113*(3), 1036–1046. https://doi.org/10.1016/j.athoracsur.2020.11.040

42 Pediatric Neurologic Disorders*

NEUROLOGIC AND NEUROSURGICAL DISORDERS

It is essential to have a strong knowledge of growth and development and to use physical assessment skills while caring for a child with a neurologic or neurosurgical condition. Children are not little adults. They have their own unique physiology, which is important to consider when assessing and understanding the manifestation of neurologic conditions in children. Young children often cannot either speak or express how they feel; therefore, a complete ongoing physical assessment is essential. Caregivers are an invaluable source of information and know their child the best and should always be included in all aspects of care delivery.

Cerebral Palsy

Cerebral palsy (CP) is a nonprogressive disorder of posture, muscle tone, and movement. There are a number of causes, but CP is a result of abnormalities of the developing brain. CP is the most common movement disorder in children, affecting approximately 3 out of every 1,000 children, with a higher prevalence in preterm and low-birthweight infants. Preterm infants account for less than half of all cases of CP.

Pathophysiology and Etiology

1. Prematurity.
2. Perinatal hypoxic–ischemic injury.
3. Congenital abnormalities.
4. Genetic susceptibility.
5. Multiple births.
6. Stroke.
7. Intracranial hemorrhage.
8. Intrauterine postnatal causes.

Classification of Cerebral Palsy

Spastic Subtypes

1. Spastic Diplegia
   a. 13% to 25% of CP cases.
   b. Most commonly associated with periventricular leukomalacia.
   c. Lower limbs more affected than upper limbs.
   d. Presence of flexion, adduction, and internal rotation of the hips with contractures of hip flexors and hamstring muscles.
   e. Variable degrees of flexion at elbows and knees.
   f. Reduced limb length and muscle bulk in lower extremities.
2. Spastic Hemiplegia
   a. 21% to 40%
   b. One side of the body affected.
   c. The arm typically more affected than the leg.
   d. The arm adducted at the shoulder and flexed at the elbow, with forearm pronated with the wrist and fingers flexed with hand closed.
   e. The hip is partially flexed and adducted, the knee and ankle are flexed, and the foot may be in equinovarus or calcaneovalgus position.
   f. Sensory deficits present in most children.
   g. Postural abnormalities more apparent during walking or running in mildly affected children; walking occurs at appropriate developmental stage unless in the presence of intellectual disability.
3. Spastic Quadriplegia
   a. 20% to 43%.
   b. All limbs affected.
   c. Upper limbs may be equally or more involved than lower limbs.
   d. Children often severely affected.
   e. Feeding difficulties, chronic respiratory insufficiency, and seizure disorders are common.

*Please note that the term "male" in this chapter refers to a person assigned male at birth, and the term "female" in this chapter refers to a person assigned female at birth.

Dyskinetic Subtypes

1. 12% to 14%.
2. Involuntary movements.
3. Contractures not common but may evolve later in life.
4. Variable degree of dysarthria and intellectual disability.
5. Choreoathetotic CP
   a. Rapid, irregular, unpredictable contractions of individual muscles or small muscle groups that involve the face, bulbar muscles, proximal extremities, fingers, and toes.
   b. Athetosis—slow, smooth, writhing movements involving the distal muscles.
      i. Movements may be induced or may be heightened by emotions or change in posture.
      ii. Very obvious during reaching.
      iii. Chorea may be aggravated by fever, stress, or excitement.
      iv. Persistent primitive reflexes.
      v. Commonly seen are oropharyngeal difficulties.
6. Dystonic CP
   a. Slow or rapid repetitive, patterned, twisting, and sustained movements of the trunk and limbs.
   b. May have pyramidal signs and anarthria.
   c. Sudden involuntary increase (tension) in tone may affect flexor and extensor muscles during attempted movement or with emotion.
   d. It may be difficult to elicit tendon reflexes or they may be normal.
   e. Absence of clonus and extensor plantar responses.
7. Ataxic CP
   a. 4% to 13%.
   b. Ataxic movements.
   c. Widespread disorder of motor function.
   d. Over time, ataxia will usually improve.
   e. Speech is slow, jerky, and explosive.

Clinical Manifestations

Common associated findings include:

1. Pain (50% to 75%).
2. Intellectual disability (50%).
3. Speech–language disorders (40%).
4. Epilepsy (25% to 40%).
5. Visual impairment (30%).
6. Hip displacement (30%).
7. Behavior disorder (25%).
8. Bladder control problems (30% to 60%).
9. Sleep disorder (20%).
10. Drooling (20%).
11. Hearing impairment (10% to 20%).
12. Gastrostomy tube dependence (7%).

Diagnostic Evaluation

Diagnosis is based on clinical examination and history. Various diagnostic tests also help determine the cause and evaluate for associated problems, such as cognitive impairment, epilepsy, sensory impairment, and behavioral difficulties.

History and Physical Examination

1. Review of prenatal and birth history.
2. Review of newborn screening results.
3. Review of family history
   a. Intellectual disability/developmental disabilities.
   b. Seizures.
   c. CP.
   d. Neuromotor/movement disorders.
   e. Neurobehavioral disorders.
   f. Joint contractures/stiffness.
   g. Thromboses/vascular accidents.
   h. Congenital anomalies.
   i. Infertility.
   j. Recurrent miscarriages/stillborn.
   k. Adult-onset neurodegenerative conditions.

Diagnostic Tests

Although CP is diagnosed based on clinical findings, diagnostic evaluation should be completed to identify underlying causes of CP and to rule out other conditions. According to the American Academy of Pediatrics (2022), early identification and diagnosis of CP is essential to ensure close developmental monitoring and developmental screenings for delays.

1. Magnetic resonance imaging (MRI) of the brain
   a. Should be obtained in all children with CP of undetermined etiology.
   b. MRI is preferred to computed tomography (CT) because its diagnostic yield is higher and it can help determine etiology and timing of insult.
   c. Abnormalities on MRI seen in patients with CP include hypoxic–ischemic lesions (periventricular leukomalacia or PVL), cortical malformations, and lesions in the basal ganglia.
2. Electroencephalography (EEG) should be obtained in children who are suspected of having seizure activity.
   a. 40% of children with CP have seizures.
3. Lumbar puncture (LP) should be obtained in children with drug-resistant seizures or movement disorders such as ataxic–spastic gait or dyskinesias.
   a. Screening is done for pediatric neurotransmitter disorders to evaluate low cerebrospinal fluid (CSF) glucose concentration, which may be caused by glucose transporter deficiency (GLUT1).
4. Metabolic and genetic testing should be done if:
   a. The history reveals features that are atypical for CP but suggestive of a genetic or metabolic etiology (e.g., history of progressive encephalopathy, metabolic decompensation, family history of childhood neurologic disorder associated with CP, and a history of consanguinity).
   b. There is a developmental brain malformation on brain imaging (e.g., lissencephaly, schizencephaly, pachygyria) or frontal/temporal atrophy.
   c. No etiology has been identified on history and physical examination and on neuroimaging.
   d. There are atypical symptoms or a brain malformation on MRI.
5. Thrombophilia screening should be done in children with hemiplegic CP or MRI evidence of a cerebral infarction.
   a. 50% to 60% of patients with hemiplegic CP have at least one prothrombotic coagulation abnormality.
   b. Test for factor V Leiden mutation, prothrombin 202210 mutation, antithrombin deficiency, protein C deficiency, protein S deficiency, hyperhomocysteinemia, antiphospholipid antibodies, and elevated factor VIII.

Management

Management of CP requires a multidisciplinary team that will look at medical, psychological, educational, social, and therapeutic needs. Management of CP includes the following:

Functional Evaluation

1. Important in planning treatment as functional evaluation is based on the limitations of the patient with respect to body structure and function.
2. Treatment is guided by standardized measurement of functional status such as the Gross Motor Function Classification System (GMFCS), Modified Ashworth Scale, Manual Ability Classification System (MACS), and Communication Function Classification System (CFCS), and Pediatric Evaluation of Disability Inventory.

Management of Spasticity

1. Botulinum toxin injections of botulinum type A (BTXA) into affected muscles
   a. Most commonly used in calf muscles in patients with diplegia or hemiplegia.
   b. To maintain efficacy, injections are repeated every 3 to 8 months.
   c. Used to treat children who have increased muscle tone that negatively affects function, which, over time with growth, will likely result in formation of contractures.
2. Antispastic drugs
   a. Although less effective than Botox, oral antispastic drugs such as baclofen, benzodiazepines (e.g., diazepam), and dantrolene are sometimes used to treat spasticity in CP.

Intrathecal Baclofen (Muscle Relaxant)

1. Administered via the intrathecal route via pump to achieve higher CSF drug levels as opposed to oral administration, which results in lower CSF drug levels.
2. Reduces spasticity in severely affected children. Appropriate for children with chronic, severe stiffness or uncontrolled body movements.
3. Medication can be titrated via pump if muscle tone is worse during certain times of the day/night.
4. Has significant complications and is therefore reserved for children with severe spasticity that is unresponsive to other treatment modalities.

Surgical Treatment

1. Selective dorsal rhizotomy (SDR) is the primary surgical intervention used in the treatment of spasticity when more conservative treatments have failed.
2. Deep brain stimulation (DBS) is an emerging therapy that has been used in the treatment of severe primary dystonia in adults who have failed to respond to pharmacotherapy such as Botox; however, further studies are needed to establish efficacy in treating dyskinetic CP.

Orthopedic Interventions

1. Gait analysis is utilized in identifying muscles that may benefit from surgical lengthening and is used postoperatively to evaluate surgical outcomes on function.
   a. Gait analysis is typically used in children aged 6 to 10 years who have a mature gait.
   b. Ankle–foot orthoses are often used to try to stabilize or improve range of motion (ROM) or gait.
2. Casting
   a. Serial casting is often used to stretch and shorten muscles in lower limbs as well as improve ROM.
3. Muscle–Tendon Surgery
   a. To reduce restrictions in joint motion or malalignment, surgical intervention to release or recess limb muscles and tendons is performed when function is affected by fixed contractures.
4. Surgical Treatment of Hip Disorders
   a. Children with spastic CP commonly have hip disorders, including subluxation, dislocation, and dislocation with degeneration and pain.
   b. Soft tissue lengthening is done to correct hip subluxation, whereas reconstructive hip surgery is done in children younger than 4 years who are more severely affected but who have not developed degenerative changes of the femoral head.

Physical Therapy

1. Physical therapy is a vital component of treatment programs for the management of CP and includes establishing methods to promote posture, mobility, and transfer and to allow for effective methods of promoting activities of daily living (ADL).
2. Bimanual training for hemiplegic CP.
   a. The child is trained to use two hands together through repetitive tasks.
   b. Constraint-induced movement therapy (CIMT)—used in children who have hemiplegic CP to promote limb function through the use of intermittent restraint of the unaffected limb during therapeutic tasks and often involves casting of the unaffected limb.
   c. Context-focused therapy—the task or environment is changed to promote successful task performance rather than changing the child's approach.
   d. Goal-directed/functional training—promotes the focus of activities that are based on goals set by the child using a motor learning approach.
3. Occupational therapy for the upper limbs—involves physical therapy approaches and can be done concurrently with botulinum toxin treatment.

Feeding and Nutrition

Children with CP often have oromotor difficulties and feeding problems. Infants should be assessed for their ability to suck and for swallowing difficulties. School-age children should be assessed for their height and weight status, as well as for any difficulty feeding, need for assistance with feeding, duration of feeding time, choking, and/or frequent vomiting and their nutritional status to ensure they receive adequate intake. Gastrostomy feeding should be considered in children with failure to thrive or who have chronic aspiration.

Management of Drooling

1. Children with CP who have oromotor dysfunction often drool. Management of drooling includes medication, behavior therapy, and surgery. Noninvasive methods such as behavior therapy and medications are often tried before surgical intervention.
2. Medications to manage drooling include anticholinergic agents such as benzhexol hydrochloride, scopolamine, or glycopyrrolate.
3. Botox injections into the salivary glands to decrease the flow of saliva are often used.
4. Surgical treatment of drooling targets the reduction of salivary production.
5. Behavior management includes behavior management techniques and biofeedback techniques.

Management of Osteopenia

1. For children with CP who have severe reductions in bone mineral density and/or pathologic extremity fractures or vertebral compression, treatment with bisphosphonates is employed.

Urinary Incontinence

1. Anticholinergic medication is often used to treat urinary incontinence.
2. Children with CP who have a neurogenic bladder are managed with anticholinergic medication, modification of the toileting schedule or environment, and/or intermittent catheterization, which is contingent on features of a neurogenic bladder.

EVIDENCE BASE Evensen, K. A., Ustad, T., Tikanmäki, M., Haaramo, P., & Kajantie, E. (2020). Long-term motor outcomes of very preterm and/or very low birth weight individuals without cerebral palsy: A review of the current evidence. *Seminars in Fetal and Neonatal Medicine*, *25*(3), 101116. https://doi.org/10.1016/j.siny.2020.101116

DRUG ALERT Intrathecal baclofen lowers the seizure threshold. Children may develop severe withdrawal syndrome characterized by fever, hypertension, tachycardia, agitation, and hallucinations, which may occur in situations of pump malfunction, catheter breakage, or improper filling of pump.

EVIDENCE BASE Galindo-Zavala, R., Bou-Torrent, R., Magallares-Lopez, B., Mir-Perello, C., Palmou-Fontana, N., Sevilla-Perez, B., Medrano-San, I., Gonzalez-Fernandez, M., Roman-Pascual, A., Alcaniz-Rodriguez, P., Nieto-Gonzalez, J., Lopez-Corbeto, M., & Grana-Gil, J. (2020). Expert panel consensus recommendations for diagnosis and treatment of secondary osteoporosis in children. *Online Journal of Pediatric Rheumatology*, *18*(1), 20. https://doi.org/10.1186/s12969-020-0411-9

Complications

1. Contractures.
2. Hip subluxation/dislocation.
3. Malnutrition.
4. Scoliosis.
5. Osteopenia/fractures.
6. Gastroesophageal reflux.
7. Constipation.
8. Seizures.
9. Spasticity.
10. Pain.

Nursing Assessment

1. Perform a functional assessment; determine ability to perform ADL.
2. Perform a developmental assessment; use Denver II developmental or other screening tools.
3. Evaluate ability to protect airway—gag reflex and swallowing.
4. Assess nutritional status—growth (height, weight, head circumference, ideal body weight), signs of nutritional deficiency, risk of aspiration, length of time it takes to feed, food diary to determine quantify of food and fluid consumed, and hydration.
5. Assess neuromuscular function and mobility—ROM, spasticity, coordination, and scoliosis.
6. Assess speech, hearing, and vision.
7. Evaluate caregiver–child interaction.
8. Determine caregivers' understanding of and adherence with treatment plan.
9. Assess the skin for pressure injuries, especially in areas of friction (splints).
10. Assess for the presence of pain (chronic or acute because of hip subluxation, dislocation).

Nursing Interventions

Increasing Mobility and Minimizing Deformity

1. Teach the caregivers to carry out appropriate exercises under the direction of the physical therapist and occupational therapist, and encourage them to incorporate this into their child's daily routine. Ensure they understand the rationale/importance of completing the exercises.
2. Use splints and braces to facilitate muscle control and improve body functioning.
   a. Apply, as directed.
   b. Remove for recommended time.
   c. Inspect the underlying skin for redness, irritation, skin breakdown, and signs of improper application or fit of splints or orthoses.
   d. Regularly inspect orthoses for cracks, loose screws, or broken Velcro straps.
   e. Use splint as directed for constraint-induced therapy in children with unilateral CP.
3. Use assistive devices, such as adapted grooming tools, writing implements, and utensils, to enhance independence. Handles for toothbrushes, spoons, and forks can be built up with sponges or specially curved to make holding easier.
4. Encourage self-dressing with easy pull-on pants, large sweatshirts, Velcro closures, and other loose clothing.
5. Use play, such as board games, ball games, pegboards, puzzles, computers, and tablets, to improve coordination.
6. Maintain good body alignment to prevent contractures.
7. Provide adequate rest periods.
   a. Employ good sleep hygiene practices.
   b. Administer or teach caregivers about side effects of medications and how to administer medications safely, as prescribed.

Maximizing Growth and Development

1. Evaluate the child's developmental level, and then assist with age-appropriate tasks.
2. Provide for continuity of care at home, day care, therapy centers, and the hospital.
   a. Obtain a thorough history from the caregivers regarding the child's usual home routines, weaknesses and strengths, and likes and dislikes.
   b. Communicate with representatives from all disciplines involved in the child's care to ensure that the specific needs of the child are identified.
   c. Formulate a consistent care plan that incorporates the goals of all related disciplines and aligns with the goals of the child and family. Include in the care plan guidelines for the following:
      i. Feeding.
      ii. Sleeping.
      iii. Physical therapy/occupational therapy.
      iv. Play.
      v. Other ways to foster growth and development.
      vi. Medications.
      vii. Psychosocial needs.
      viii. Family needs.
      ix. Pain assessment/management.
3. During feeding, maintain a pleasant, distraction-free environment.
   a. Provide a comfortable chair.
   b. Serve the child alone, initially. After the child begins to master the task of eating, encourage the child to eat with other children.
   c. Do not attempt feedings if the child is very fatigued.

d. Find the eating position in which the child can be most self-sufficient.
e. Allow the child to hold the spoon even if self-feeding is minimal.
f. Stand behind and reach over the child's shoulder to guide the spoon from the plate to the child's mouth.
g. Serve foods that stick to the spoon, such as thick applesauce or mashed potatoes.
h. Encourage finger foods that the child can handle to self-feed.
i. Provide appropriate assistive devices for independent feeding, such as a spoon and fork with special handles, plate and glass holders, and a special feeding chair.
j. Disregard "messy" eating; use a large plastic bib, smock, or towel to protect the child's clothes.

4. If the child requires assistance with feeding, do so slowly and carefully. Be aware of difficulty sucking and swallowing caused by poor muscle control. Cut large pieces of food into small pieces, or serve pureed foods.
5. Be alert for associated sensory deficits that delay development and could be corrected.
   a. Hearing, speech, and vision.
   b. Squinting, failure to follow objects, or bringing objects very close to the face.

Strengthening Family Processes

1. Assess caregiver coping and provide anticipatory guidance, emotional support, access to peer support, and contact with social worker, as needed.
2. Help the caregivers to recognize immediate needs, and identify short-term goals that can be integrated into the long-term plan.
3. Assess for caregiver burden because of the numerous challenges of daily care, and link with appropriate resources (e.g., home care, respite, funding) and provide access to social work for assistance in obtaining such support.
4. Provide positive feedback for effective caregiving skills and positive approaches to caring for the child.
5. Assist the caregivers to deal with siblings' responses to the child who is disabled.
   a. Encourage caregivers to find time to spend with each sibling separately.
   b. Encourage family to maintain contact with friends and community and engage in outside activities as much as possible.
   c. Suggest family counseling.
6. Assist caregivers to find local resources to help in the child's care.
   a. Contact hospital social worker or discharge planner for information about local CP organizations, chapters, funding sources, community supports, or charities.
   b. Help to navigate through the national and regional programs that may have local chapters.

Protecting the Child from Injury

1. Evaluate the child's need for specific safety equipment, such as a suction machine, helmet, and walker, and modify the environment as appropriate to ensure the child's safety.
2. Provide for frequent position changes and adequate fit on orthotics, wheelchairs, and walking or standing devices to prevent skin breakdown. Assess skin integrity regularly.

Community and Home Care Considerations

1. Assess the home environment for safety. Stairs should be gated, and paths should be cleared for walking with assistive devices or for adequate passage of wheelchairs, walkers, and so on.
2. Assist caregivers in arranging for equipment that may be required in the home (e.g., wheelchair, pump for intermittent G-tube feedings, walkers, home suction machine).
3. Check all adaptive equipment, braces, and walkers for correct fit. Arrange for replacement, as needed.

Family Education and Health Maintenance

1. Instruct the caregivers in all areas of the child's physical care.
2. Encourage regular medical and dental evaluations.
3. Advise caregivers that the child needs discipline to feel secure.
4. Refer caregivers to such agencies as the United Cerebral Palsy Association of America (www.ucp.org).
5. Connect families with other families who have a child with CP so that they may provide a supportive network.
6. Encourage maintenance of good nutritional status.
7. Help the child engage in regular exercise to maintain health.

Evaluation: Expected Outcomes

- Dresses and feeds self as independently as possible; minimal contractures noted.
- Consistent growth curve maintained; sequential developmental milestones consistent with condition achieved.
- Family participates in usual school and community activities; uses respite care when available.
- Safety equipment used; no injury reported.

Hydrocephalus

Hydrocephalus is characterized by an increased volume of CSF that accumulates in the ventricles and/or subarachnoid spaces and is associated with progressive ventricular dilatation. There are two main categories of hydrocephalus: communicating and noncommunicating. Hydrocephalus occurs with such conditions as tumors, infections, congenital malformations, and hemorrhage. The incidence of hydrocephalus is 0.5 to 4 per 1,000 live births.

Pathophysiology and Etiology

1. Noncommunicating hydrocephalus—obstruction of CSF flow within the ventricular system or blockage of CSF flow from the ventricular system to the subarachnoid space.
   a. May be partial, intermittent, or complete.
   b. More common than communicating type.
   c. Congenital causes.
      i. Aqueductal stenosis.
      ii. Congenital lesions (vein of Galen malformation, congenital tumors).
      iii. Arachnoid cyst.
      iv. Chiari malformations (with or without myelomeningocele).
      v. X-linked hydrocephalus.
      vi. Dandy–Walker malformation.
   d. Acquired causes.
      i. Aqueductal gliosis (posthemorrhagic or postinfectious).
      ii. Space-occupying lesions (tumors or cysts).
      iii. Head injuries.
2. Communicating hydrocephalus—CSF circulates through the ventricular system into the subarachnoid space with no obstruction.
   a. Congenital causes.
      i. Achondroplasia.
      ii. Arachnoid cyst.
      iii. Craniofacial syndromes.

b. Acquired causes.
   i. Posthemorrhagic (intraventricular or subarachnoid).
   ii. Choroid plexus papilloma or choroid plexus carcinoma.
   iii. Venous obstruction (e.g., superior vena cava syndrome).
   iv. Postinfectious.

Clinical Manifestations

May be rapid, slow and steadily advancing, or intermittent. Clinical signs depend on the age of the child, whether the anterior fontanelle has closed, whether the cranial sutures have fused, and the type and duration of hydrocephalus.

Infants

1. Excessive head growth (may be seen up to age 3 years).
2. Delayed closure of the anterior fontanelle.
3. Fontanelle tense and elevated above the surface of the skull.
4. Signs of increased intracranial pressure (ICP) (see Box 42-1).
5. Alteration of muscle tone of the extremities, including clonus or spasticity.
6. Later physical signs:
   a. Forehead becomes prominent ("bossing").
   b. Scalp appears shiny with prominent scalp veins.
   c. Eyebrows and eyelids may be drawn upward, exposing the sclera above the iris.
   d. Infant cannot gaze upward, causing "sunset eyes."
   e. Strabismus, nystagmus, and optic atrophy may occur.
   f. Infant has difficulty holding head up.
   g. Child may experience physical or mental developmental lag.
7. Pseudobulbar palsy (difficulty sucking, feeding, and phonation, which leads to regurgitation, drooling, and aspiration).

CLINICAL JUDGMENT It is important to measure head circumference because the infant's skull is highly elastic and can accommodate an increase in ventricular size. Ventriculomegaly may progress without obvious signs of increased ICP.

BOX 42-1 Signs and Symptoms of Increased Intracranial Pressure in Infants and Children

- Vomiting.
- Restlessness and irritability.
- High-pitched, shrill cry (infants).
- Rapid increase in head circumference (infants).
- Tense, bulging fontanelle (infants).
- Changes in vital signs:
  - Increased systolic blood pressure (BP).
  - Decreased pulse.
  - Decreased and irregular respirations.
  - Increased temperature.
- Pupillary changes.
- Papilledema.
- Possible seizures.
- Lethargy, stupor, and coma.
- Older children may also experience:
  - Headache, especially on awakening.
  - Lethargy, fatigue, and apathy.
  - Personality changes.
  - Separation of cranial sutures (may be seen in children up to age 10).
  - Visual changes such as double vision.

Older Children

Older children have closed sutures and present with signs of increased ICP.

Diagnostic Evaluation

1. Percussion of the infant's skull near the junction of the frontal, temporal, and parietal bones may produce a typical "cracked pot" sound (Macewen sign).
2. Ophthalmoscopy may reveal papilledema.
3. MRI is the diagnostic tool of choice.
4. CT is also used for diagnosis in cases where sedation poses added risk because of need for general anesthetic or in situations in which MRI is not available.
5. Ultrasonography is also used.

Management

Hydrocephalus can be treated through a variety of surgical procedures, including direct operation on the lesion causing the obstruction, such as a tumor; intracranial shunts for selected cases of noncommunicating hydrocephalus to divert fluid from the obstructed segment of the ventricular system to the subarachnoid space; and extracranial shunts (most common) to divert fluid from the ventricular system to an extracranial compartment, frequently the peritoneum or right atrium. CSF production may also be reduced by medication or surgical intervention.

Extracranial Shunt Procedures

1. Ventriculoperitoneal (VP) shunt (see Figure 42-1):
   a. Diverts CSF from a lateral ventricle or the spinal subarachnoid space to the peritoneal cavity.
   b. A tube is passed from the lateral ventricle through an occipital burr hole subcutaneously through the posterior aspect of the neck and paraspinal region to the peritoneal cavity through a small incision in the right lower quadrant.

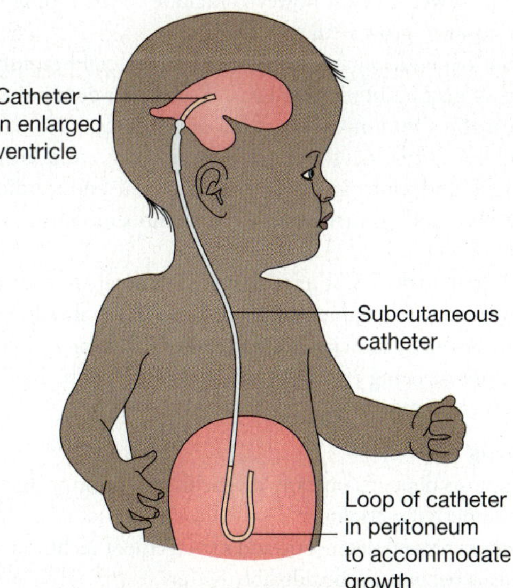

Figure 42-1. A ventriculoperitoneal shunt removes excessive cerebrospinal fluid from the ventricles and shunts it to the peritoneum. A one-way valve is present in the tubing behind the ear. (Adapted with permission from Silbert-Flagg, J. [2023]. *Maternal and child health nursing: Care of the childbearing and childrearing family* [9th ed., Fig. 27-16]. Wolters Kluwer.)

   c. A ventricular access device is an implanted reservoir and catheter used for premature neonates <1,500 g in lieu of a shunt. The catheter drains fluid from the ventricles into the reservoir, which can then be emptied using aseptic technique. When infant weight exceeds 1,500 g, a shunt is usually placed.
2. Ventriculoatrial (VA) shunt:
   a. A tube is passed from the dilated lateral ventricle through a burr hole in the parietal region of the skull.
   b. It is then passed under the skin behind the ear and into a vein down to a point where it discharges into the right atrium or superior vena cava.
   c. A one-way pressure-sensitive valve will close to prevent reflux of blood into the ventricle and open as ventricular pressure rises, allowing fluid to pass from the ventricle into the bloodstream.
3. Ventriculopleural shunt:
   a. Diverts CSF to the pleural cavity.
   b. Indicated when the VP or VA route cannot be used.
4. Ventricle–gall bladder shunt:
   a. Diverts CSF to the common bile duct.
   b. Used when all other routes are unavailable.
5. Most shunts have the following components:
   a. Ventricular tubing.
   b. A one-way or unidirectional pressure-sensitive flow valve.
   c. A pumping chamber.
   d. Distal tubing.
6. Programmable shunts are available. These can be programmed to a certain flow pressure, and pressure settings can be readjusted based on patient response. A magnetic device is used to adjust the pressure setting of the shunt valve. The use of a programmable shunt eliminates the need for multiple surgeries or hospital visits to adjust shunt pressure.

Shunt Complications

1. Need for shunt revision frequently occurs because of occlusion, infection, or malfunction, especially in the first year of life.
2. Shunt revision may be necessary because of growth of the child. Newer models, however, include coiled tubing to allow the shunt to grow with the child.
3. Shunt dependency frequently occurs. The child rapidly manifests symptoms of increased ICP if the shunt does not function optimally. Onset may be sudden or insidious.
4. Children with VA shunts may experience endocardial contusions and clotting, leading to bacterial endocarditis, bacteremia, and ventriculitis or thromboembolism and cor pulmonale.
5. Children with VA shunts require biannual or annual chest x-ray to check length of tubing. Chest x-ray is also done during growth spurts, especially during puberty. When tubing is short or close to being out of the right atrium, shunt replacement needs to be scheduled.

Prognosis

1. Prognosis depends on early diagnosis and prompt therapy and the underlying etiology.
2. With improved diagnostic and management techniques, prognosis is becoming considerably better.
   a. Many children experience normal motor and intellectual development.
   b. The severity of neurologic deficits is directly proportional to the interval between onset of hydrocephalus and the time of diagnosis.
3. If they do not receive surgical treatment, approximately 50% of patients will die before age 3 years, and 80% will die before adulthood.
4. Surgery reduces mortality and decreases morbidity, with a survival rate of >90%.

Complications

1. Seizures and headaches.
2. Herniation of the brain.
3. Spontaneous arrest because of natural compensatory mechanisms, persistent increased ICP, and brain herniation.
4. Developmental delays.
5. Depression in adolescents is common.
6. Shunt malfunctions.

Nursing Assessment

Infants

1. Assess head circumference.
   a. Measure at the occipitofrontal circumference—point of largest measurement.
   b. Measure the head at approximately the same time each day.
   c. Use a centimeter measure for greatest accuracy.
2. Palpate fontanelle for firmness and bulging.
3. Assess pupillary response.
4. Assess level of consciousness (LOC).
5. Evaluate breathing patterns and effectiveness.
6. Assess feeding patterns and patterns of emesis.
7. Assess motor function.
8. Assess developmental milestones.

Older Children

1. Measure vital signs for signs of increased ICP.
2. Assess patterns of headache and emesis.
3. Determine pupillary response.
4. Evaluate LOC using the Glasgow Coma Scale.
5. Assess motor function.
6. Evaluate attainment of milestones and school performance.
7. Assess for behavioral changes.

Nursing Interventions

Maintaining Cerebral Perfusion

1. Observe for evidence of increased ICP and report immediately.
2. Assist with diagnostic procedures to determine cause of hydrocephalus and indication for surgical intervention.
   a. Explain the procedure to the child and caregivers at their levels of comprehension.
   b. Administer prescribed sedatives 30 minutes before the procedure to ensure their effectiveness.
   c. Organize activities so that the child is permitted to rest after administration of the sedative.
   d. Observe closely after ventriculography for the following:
      i. Leaking CSF from the sites of subdural or ventricular taps. These tap holes should be covered with a small piece of gauze or other dressing per institutional policy.
      ii. Reactions to the sedative, especially respiratory depression.
      iii. Changes in vital signs indicative of shock.
      iv. Signs of increased ICP, which may occur if air has been injected into the ventricles.

CLINICAL JUDGMENT Brain stem herniation can occur with increased ICP. The patient should be closely monitored for any signs of increased cranial pressure. Failure to intervene may result in respiratory arrest. Prepare for emergency resuscitation and corrective measures, as directed.

DRUG ALERT Sedatives are contraindicated in many cases because increased ICP predisposes the child to hypoventilation or respiratory arrest. If they are administered, the child should be observed very closely for evidence of respiratory depression.

Providing Adequate Nutrition

1. Be aware that feeding is frequently difficult because the child may be listless, have a diminished appetite, and be prone to vomiting.
2. Complete nursing care and treatments before feeding so that the child will not be disturbed during feeding.
3. Hold the infant in a semireclined position with head well supported during feeding. Allow ample time for burping.
4. Offer small, frequent feedings.
5. Place the child on side with head elevated after feeding to prevent aspiration.

Maintaining Skin Integrity

1. Prevent pressure injuries (pressure injuries of the head are a frequent problem) by placing the child on a sponge rubber or lamb's wool pad or an alternating-pressure or egg crate mattress to keep weight evenly distributed. Be mindful of latex allergies and the type of padding used.
2. Keep the scalp clean and dry.
3. Turn the child's head frequently; change position at least every 2 hours.
   a. When turning the child, rotate head and body together to prevent strain on the neck.
   b. A firm pillow may be placed under the child's head and shoulders for further support when lifting the child.
   c. Keep weight off incision during immediate postoperative period.
4. Provide meticulous skin care to all parts of the body, and observe the skin for signs of breakdown or pressure.
5. Give passive ROM exercises to the extremities, especially the legs.
6. Keep the eyes moistened with artificial tears if the child is unable to close the eyelids normally. This prevents corneal ulcerations and infections.

Reducing Anxiety

1. Prepare the caregivers for their child's surgery by answering questions, describing what nursing care will take place postoperatively, and explaining how the shunt will work.
2. Encourage the caregivers to discuss all the risks and benefits with the surgeon. Help them to understand the prognosis and what to expect of the child's neurologic and cognitive development.
3. Prepare the child for surgery by using dolls or other forms of play to describe what interventions will occur, or solicit the help of a child life specialist to prepare the child for surgery through play.

Improving Cerebral Tissue Perfusion Postoperatively

1. Monitor the child's temperature, pulse, respiration, blood pressure (BP), and pupillary size and reaction every 15 minutes until stable; then, monitor every 1 to 2 hours or as indicated by child's condition and institutional policy.
2. Maintain normothermia.
   a. Provide appropriate blankets or covers, an Isolette or infant warmer, or hypothermia blanket.
   b. Administer a tepid sponge bath or antipyretic medication for temperature elevation.
3. Aspirate mucus from the nose and throat, as necessary, to prevent respiratory difficulty.
4. Turn the child frequently.
5. Promote optimal drainage of CSF through the shunt by positioning the child, as directed.
   a. Gradually elevate the head of child's bed to 30 to 45 degrees, as ordered. Initially, the child will be positioned flat to prevent excessive CSF drainage.
6. Assess for excessive drainage of CSF.
   a. Sunken fontanelle, agitation, and restlessness (infant).
   b. Decreased LOC (older child).
7. Assess closely for increased ICP, indicating shunt malfunction.
   a. Note, especially, change in LOC, change in vital signs (increased systolic BP, decreased pulse rate, decreased or irregular respirations), vomiting, and pupillary changes.
   b. Report these changes immediately to prevent cerebral hypoxia and possible brain herniation.
8. Prevent excessive pressure on the skin overlying shunt by placing cotton behind and over the ears under the head dressing and avoiding positioning the child on the area of the valve or the incision until the wound is healed.

Maintaining Fluid Balance

1. Accurately measure and record total fluid intake and output.
2. Administer intravenous (IV) fluids, as prescribed; carefully monitor infusion rate to prevent fluid overload.
3. Use a nasogastric tube, if necessary, for abdominal distention. This is most frequently used when a VP shunt has been performed.
   a. Measure the drainage and record the amount and color.
   b. Monitor for return of bowel sounds after nasogastric suction has been disconnected for at least 30 minutes.
4. Give frequent mouth care while the child is to have nothing by mouth.
5. Begin oral feedings when the child is fully recovered from the anesthetic and displays interest.
   a. Begin with small amounts of dextrose 5% in water.
   b. Gradually introduce formula.
   c. Introduce solid foods suitable to the child's age and tolerance.
   d. Encourage a high-protein diet.
   e. Observe for and report any decrease in urine output, increased urine specific gravity, diminished skin turgor, dryness of mucous membranes, or lethargy, indicating dehydration.

Preventing Infection

1. Assess for fever (temperature normally fluctuates during the first 24 hours after surgery), purulent drainage from the incision, or swelling, redness, and tenderness along the shunt tract.
2. Administer prescribed prophylactic antibiotics.

CLINICAL JUDGMENT All children who have had surgery require assessments for pain. Although pain management is institution specific, acetaminophen is often the medication of choice. Also, use alternative modes of pain management, such as developmentally appropriate distraction and relaxation techniques, and ensure a quiet environment.

Strengthening Family Coping

1. Begin discharge planning early, including specific techniques for care of the shunt and suggested methods for providing daily care.
   a. Turning, holding, and positioning.
   b. Skin care over the shunt.
   c. Exercises to strengthen muscles—incorporated with play.
   d. Feeding techniques and schedule.
   e. Pumping the shunt.
2. Accompany all instructions with reassurance necessary to prevent the caregivers from becoming anxious or fearful about assuming the care of the child.
3. Offer opportunities for care by caregiver during hospitalization so that caregivers may become familiar and capable of care delivery in the home setting through practice.
4. Help the caregivers to assist siblings to understand hydrocephalus and the child's special needs. Encourage caregivers to spend individual time with siblings. Suggest family counseling and social work support, if needed.
5. Assist caregivers in locating additional resources.
   a. Social worker, discharge planner, or department of social services.
   b. Visiting or home health nurses or aides.
   c. Caregiver groups.
   d. Community agencies.
   e. Special programs at school.

Community and Home Care Considerations

1. Follow the community and home care considerations listed under "Cerebral Palsy" on page 1224. Check shunt functioning regularly, and reinforce caregiver performance of shunt checks and assessment for shunt malfunction and increased ICP.
2. Perform total physical assessment regularly, looking for signs of trauma or skin breakdown.
3. Patient should wear a medical alert bracelet when they start to attend school or day care.
4. Ensure caregivers are certified in cardiopulmonary resuscitation (CPR).

Family Education and Health Maintenance

1. Stress the importance of recognizing symptoms of increased ICP and reporting them immediately.
2. Advise caregivers to report shunt malfunction or infection immediately to prevent increased ICP.
3. Teach caregivers that illnesses that cause vomiting and diarrhea or illnesses that prevent an adequate fluid intake are a great threat to the child who has had a shunt procedure. Advise caregivers to consult with the child's health care provider about immediate treatment of fever, control of vomiting and diarrhea, and replacement of fluids.
4. Tell the caregivers that few restrictions are required for children with shunts and to consult with the health care provider about specific concerns.
5. Alert caregivers that additional information and support are available from the Hydrocephalus Association (www.hydroassoc.org).

Evaluation: Expected Outcomes

- No changes in vital signs, LOC, or head size; no vomiting; pupils equal and responsive.
- Feeds every 4 hours without vomiting; no significant weight loss.
- No erythema, blanching, or skin breakdown; wound healing evident.
- Caregivers have an understanding of operative procedure, risks, and benefits.
- Shunt pumping without resistance; stable LOC and vital signs.
- Urine output equal to intake; skin turgor normal; electrolytes within normal limits.
- Afebrile; no drainage from shunt site.
- Caregivers actively seeking resources.

Spina Bifida

Spina bifida, also called *spinal dysraphia*, is a malformation of the spine in which the posterior portion of the laminae of the vertebrae fails to close. It occurs in approximately 1 per 2,000 live births in the United States and is the most common developmental defect of the central nervous system (CNS). Of all ethnicities, it is most common in Hispanics, with 3.8 per 10,000 children affected. The incidence of spina bifida defects has been declining in the United States and United Kingdom because of antenatal screening and changes in environmental factors such as the consumption of folic acid in early pregnancy.

Several types of spina bifida are recognized, of which the following three are most common (see Figure 42-2).

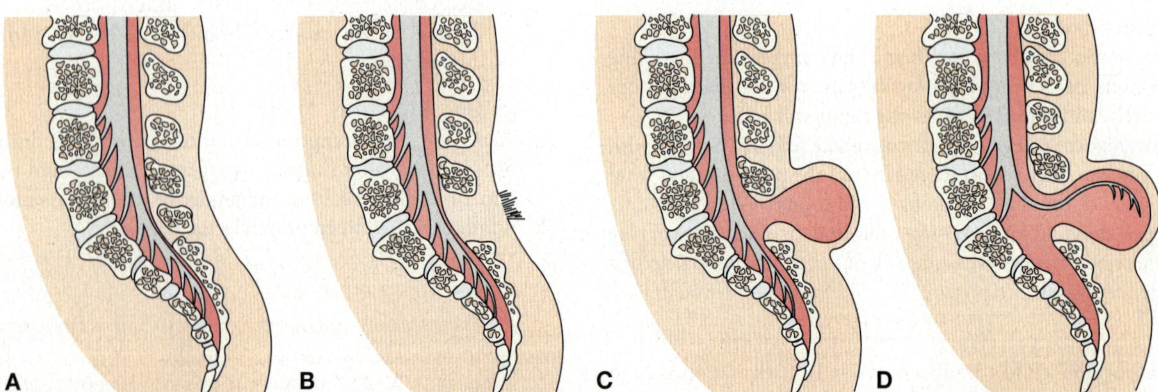

Figure 42-2. Spina bifida. **(A)** Normal spine. **(B)** Spina bifida occulta. **(C)** Spina bifida with meningocele. **(D)** Spina bifida with myelomeningocele. (Reprinted with permission from Silbert-Flagg, J. [2023]. *Maternal and child health nursing: Care of the childbearing and childrearing family* [9th ed., Fig. 27-18]. Wolters Kluwer.)

Spina Bifida Occulta

Spina bifida occulta is seen in 10% to 20% of the US population. It is a result of the posterior vertebral arches failing to fuse. A fat pad, dermal sinus, hairy tuft, or dimple in the lower back/lumbosacral region is often seen.

Meningocele

Meningocele is a herniation of the meninges through the defective posterior arches. The sac does not contain neural elements.

Myelomeningocele (or Meningomyelocele)

The spinal nerve roots and cord membranes protrude through the defect in the laminae of the vertebral column. Myelomeningoceles are covered by a thin membrane.

Pathophysiology and Etiology

1. Unknown etiology, but generally thought to result from genetic predisposition as well as a combination of nutritional and environmental influences.
   a. Certain drugs, including valproic acid, have been known to cause neural tube defects if administered during pregnancy.
   b. Females who have spina bifida and caregivers who have one affected child have an increased risk of producing children with neural tube defects.
2. Involves an arrest in the orderly formation of the vertebral arches and spinal cord that occurs between the 4th and 6th weeks of embryogenesis.
3. Theories of causation include:
   a. Incomplete closure of the neural tube during the 4th week of embryonic life.
   b. The neural tube forms adequately and then ruptures.
4. In spina bifida occulta, the bony defect may range from a very thin slit separating one lamina from the spinous process to a complete absence of the spine and laminae.
   a. A thin, fibrous membrane sometimes covers the defect.
   b. The spinal cord and its meninges may be connected with a fistulous tract extending to and opening onto the surface of the skin.
5. In meningocele, the defect may occur anywhere on the cord. Higher defects (from the thorax and upward) are usually meningoceles.
   a. Surgical correction is necessary to prevent rupture of the sac and subsequent infection.
   b. Prognosis is good with surgical correction.
6. In myelomeningocele (meningomyelocele), the lesion contains both the spinal cord and cord membranes.
   a. A bluish area may be evident on the top because of exposed neural tissue.
   b. The sac may leak in utero or may rupture after birth, allowing free drainage of CSF. This renders the child highly susceptible to meningitis.
   c. Of all defects known as spina bifida cystica, 95% are myelomeningoceles and 5% are meningoceles.

DRUG ALERT Maternal periconceptional use of folic acid supplementation reduces by 50% or more the incidence of neural tube defects in pregnancies at risk. The U.S. Food and Drug Administration (FDA) approved the voluntary addition of folic acid to corn masa flour to assist pregnant Hispanic/Latina people to increase their intake of folic acid. The recommended dose of folic acid is 4 mg/day and can be found in prenatal vitamins.

Clinical Manifestations

Spina Bifida Occulta

1. Most patients have no symptoms.
   a. They may have a dimple in the skin or a growth of hair over the malformed vertebra.
   b. There is no externally visible sac.
2. With growth, the child may develop foot weakness or bowel and bladder sphincter disturbances.
3. This condition is occasionally associated with more significant developmental abnormalities of the spinal cord, including syringomyelia and tethered cord.

Meningocele

1. An external cystic defect can be seen in the spinal cord, usually in the midline.
   a. The sac is composed only of meninges and is filled with CSF.
   b. The cord and nerve roots are usually normal.
2. There is seldom evidence of weakness of the legs or lack of sphincter control.

Myelomeningocele

1. A round, raised, and poorly epithelialized area may be noted at any level of the spinal column. However, the highest incidence of the lesion occurs in the lumbosacral area.
2. Hydrocephalus occurs in approximately 90% of children with myelomeningocele because of associated Arnold–Chiari malformation, which causes a block in the flow of CSF through the ventricles.
3. Loss of motor control and sensation below the level of the lesion can occur. These conditions are highly variable and depend on the size of the lesion and its position on the cord.
   a. A low thoracic lesion may cause total flaccid paralysis below the waist.
   b. A small sacral lesion may cause only patchy spots of decreased sensation in the feet.
4. Contractures may occur in the ankles, knees, or hips. Hips may become dislocated.
   a. Nature and degree of involvement depend on size and location of the lesion.
   b. This occurs because some fibers of innervation get through. One side of a hip, knee, or ankle may be innervated, whereas the opposing side may not be. The unopposed side then becomes pulled out of position.
5. Clubfeet are a common accompanying anomaly; thought to be related to the position of paraplegic feet in the uterus.
6. Bladder dysfunction occurs because of how the sacral nerves that innervate the bladder are affected. The bladder fails to respond to normal messages that it is time to void and simply fills and overflows, causing incontinence and susceptibility to urinary tract infections (UTIs) because of incomplete emptying.
7. Fecal incontinence and constipation are caused by poor innervation of the anal sphincter and bowel musculature.
8. Most children have average intellectual ability despite hydrocephalus. Developmental disabilities include the following:
   a. Gross motor development—children will need assistance in gaining and maintaining mobility.
   b. Most children are able to learn in a "mainstream" school environment, provided they are able to overcome other barriers (architectural and attitudinal).

Diagnostic Evaluation

1. Prenatal detection is done through prenatal ultrasound and fetal MRI. This testing should be offered to all patients at risk

(i.e., those who are affected or who have had other affected children).
2. Maternal serum alpha fetoprotein (MSAFP) screen can be done in the second trimester.
3. Postnatal diagnosis is based primarily on clinical manifestations.
4. CT scan and MRI may be performed to further evaluate the brain and spinal cord.

Management

Surgical Intervention

1. Prenatal surgery to close the defect has demonstrated improved outcomes compared to children who had postnatal surgery. In recent research, results demonstrated that prenatal repair can offer significantly better results than traditional postnatal repair. Babies with spina bifida who received prenatal surgery were better able to walk 2.5 years after surgery than those operated on after birth and had better overall motor function. They were also less likely to need a shunt.
2. Procedure: laminectomy and closure of the open lesion or removal of the sac can usually be done within the first few days after birth.
3. Purpose:
   a. To prevent further deterioration of neural function.
   b. To minimize the danger of rupture and infection, especially meningitis.
   c. To improve cosmetic effect.
   d. To facilitate handling of the infant.

Multidisciplinary Follow-Up for Associated Problems

1. A coordinated team approach will help maximize the physical and intellectual potential of each affected child.
2. The team may include a neurologist, neurosurgeon, orthopedic surgeon, urologist, primary care provider, social worker, physical therapist, occupational therapist, nurse practitioners, and a variety of community-based and hospital staff nurses, and the child and family.
3. Numerous neurosurgical, orthopedic, and urologic procedures may be necessary to help the child achieve maximum function.

Prognosis

1. Influenced by the site of the lesion and the presence and degree of associated hydrocephalus. Generally, the higher the defect, the greater the extent of neurologic deficit and the greater the likelihood of hydrocephalus.
2. In the absence of treatment, most infants with meningomyelocele die early in infancy.
3. Surgical intervention is most effective if it is done early in the neonatal period, preferably within the first few days of life.
4. Even with surgical intervention, infants can be expected to manifest associated neurosurgical, orthopedic, or urologic problems.
5. New techniques of treatment, intensive research, and improved services have increased life expectancy and have greatly enhanced the quality of life for most children who receive treatment.

Complications

1. Hydrocephalus associated with meningocele; may be aggravated by surgical repair.
2. Scoliosis, contractures, and joint dislocation.
3. Skin breakdown in sensory denervated areas and under braces.

Nursing Assessment

1. Assess sensory and motor response of lower extremities.
2. Assess ability to void spontaneously, retention of urine, and symptoms of UTI.
3. Assess usual stooling patterns and need for medications to facilitate elimination.
4. Assess mobility and use of orthoses, casts, and other special equipment.

Nursing Interventions

Protecting Skin Integrity

1. Avoid positioning on the infant's back to prevent pressure on the sac. Check position at least once every hour.
2. Do not place a diaper or other covering directly over the sac.
3. Observe the sac frequently for evidence of irritation or leakage of CSF.
4. Use prone positioning and prevent hip flexion to decrease tension on the sac.
5. Place a foam rubber pad covered with a soft cloth between the infant's legs to maintain the hips in abduction and to prevent or counteract subluxation. A diaper roll or small pillow may be used in place of the foam rubber pad.
6. Allow the infant's feet to hang freely over the pads or mattress edge to prevent aggravation of foot deformities.
7. Provide meticulous skin care to all areas of the body, especially ankles, knees, tip of the nose, cheeks, and chin.
8. Provide passive ROM exercises for muscles and joints that the infant does not use spontaneously. Avoid hip exercises because of common hip dislocation, unless otherwise recommended.
9. Use a foam or fleece pad to reduce pressure of the mattress against the infant's skin.
10. Avoid pressure on the infant's back during feeding by holding the infant with your elbow rotated to avoid touching the sac or feeding while infant is lying on side or prone on your lap. Encourage the caregivers to use these positions to provide infant stimulation and bonding.

Preventing Infection

1. Be aware that infection of the sac is most commonly caused by contamination by urine and feces.
2. Keep the infant's buttocks and genitalia scrupulously clean.
   a. Do not diaper the infant if the defect is in the lower portion of the spine.
   b. Use a small plastic drape taped between the defect and the anus to help prevent contamination.
3. Apply a sterile gauze pad or towel or a sterile, moistened dressing over the sac, as directed.
   a. When the sterile covering is used, it should be changed frequently to keep the area free from exudate and to maintain sterility.
   b. Care must be taken to prevent the covering from adhering to and damaging the sac.
4. Monitor and report immediately any signs of infection.
   a. Oozing of fluid or pus from the sac.
   b. Fever.
   c. Irritability or listlessness.
   d. Seizure.

Promoting Urinary Elimination

1. Ensure fluid intake to dilute the urine.
2. Administer prescribed prophylactic antibiotics.
3. Monitor and report concentrated or foul-smelling urine.

Maintaining Cerebral Tissue Perfusion

1. Monitor for signs of hydrocephalus and report immediately.
   a. Irritability.
   b. Feeding difficulty, vomiting, and decreased appetite.
   c. Temperature fluctuation.
   d. Decreased alertness.
   e. Tense fontanelle.
   f. Increased head circumference.

Reducing Fear

1. Encourage caregivers to express feelings of guilt, fear, lack of control, or helplessness.
2. Provide accurate information about spina bifida and what to expect postoperatively.
3. Include the caregivers in all of infant's care and encourage private bonding time.

Maintaining Thermoregulation and Preventing Complications

1. Frequently monitor temperature, pulse, respirations, color, and level of responsiveness postoperatively, based on the infant's stability.
2. Use an Isolette or infant warmer to prevent temperature fluctuation.
3. Prevent respiratory complications.
   a. Periodically reposition the infant to promote lung expansion.
   b. Watch for abdominal distention, which could interfere with breathing.
   c. Have oxygen available.
4. Maintain hydration and nutritional intake.
   a. Administer IV fluids, as ordered; keep accurate intake and output log.
   b. Administer gavage feedings, as ordered.
   c. Begin bottle-feeding when infant is responsive and tolerating feedings. Give small, frequent feedings slowly so air can be expelled naturally without bubbling.
5. Keep the surgical dressing clean and dry and observe for drainage. Avoid pressure to the area and diapers that cover the incision until healed.
6. Monitor for and teach caregivers to recognize signs of hydrocephalus. Report immediately.
7. Limit or prevent direct contact of the child with products routinely used that contain latex, because of risk of latex allergy and severe reaction. Latex products include BP cuffs, tourniquets, tape, indwelling catheters, gloves, and IV tubing injection ports. Develop protocols specifying modification of care for children at risk for latex allergy.

CLINICAL JUDGMENT Be aware that children with spina bifida have a far greater risk of latex allergy than the general population. It is estimated that up to 50% of spina bifida patients have a latex allergy. Symptoms include hives, itching, wheezing, and anaphylaxis. Incidence increases with time and may be related to repeated exposure to products containing latex.

Achieving Continence

1. Teach caregivers that continence can usually be achieved with clean, intermittent self-catheterization.
   a. Children can generally be taught to catheterize themselves by age 6 or 7.
   b. Caregivers can catheterize younger children.
2. Teach the following procedure:
   a. Gather equipment: catheter, water-soluble lubricant, soap and water, and urine collection container.
   b. Wash hands.
   c. Position patient.
   d. Clean the area around the urethral meatus.
   e. Lubricate the catheter tip.
   f. Insert the catheter until urine starts to flow. Have urine collection container or diaper available.
   g. Remove catheter when urine is drained from the bladder.
   h. Clean any lubricant off the child.
   i. Dispose of urine.
   j. Wash hands.
3. Teach about the action of medications, such as imipramine and ephedrine, if prescribed, which are used to help children retain urine rather than dribbling. When used with self-catheterization, many children can stay dry for 3 to 4 hours at a time.
4. Teach the signs of UTI (concentrated, foul-smelling urine; irritability; pain or burning; and fever) and the proper administration of antibiotics either prophylactically or when prescribed for infection.
5. For children who cannot achieve urinary continence through intermittent catheterization, provide information about options, such as surgically implanted mechanical urinary sphincters and bladder pacemakers, indwelling catheters, external collecting devices, and urinary diversion (may be necessary in some cases).

Achieving Regular Bowel Elimination

1. Assist with bowel training program to compensate for decreased sacral sensation.
   a. Children are placed on a toileting schedule and are taught to push.
   b. Medications, such as stool softeners, suppositories, or enemas, may be used initially to help determine scheduling.
2. To prevent constipation and enhance bowel control, encourage intake of high-fiber, high-fluid diet. Such medications as psyllium may be used to increase bulk or soften stool.

Fostering Positive Body Image

1. Emphasize rehabilitation that makes use of the child's strengths and minimizes disabilities.
2. Continually reassess functional abilities and offer suggestions to increase independence. Periodically consult with physical or occupational therapists to help maximize function.
3. Encourage the use of braces and specialized equipment to enhance ambulation while minimizing the appearance of the equipment. For example, wear pants instead of dresses or shorts to cover leg braces; choose a compact wheelchair that can be decorated or personalized for the child.
4. Encourage participation with peer group and in activities that build on strengths, such as cognitive abilities and interest in music or art.
5. Periodically reassess bowel and bladder programs. The ability to stay dry for reasonable time intervals is one of the greatest factors in enhancing self-esteem and positive body image.

Community and Home Care Considerations

1. Follow the community and home care considerations listed under "Cerebral Palsy" on page 1224.
2. Survey the home environment for latex and substitute products obtained, if possible. Toys and equipment for children,

such as nipples, pacifiers, and elastic on the legs of disposable diapers, also contain latex. Teach the caregivers how to recognize latex allergy and to notify the child's health care provider.
3. Teach the family how to clean and reuse urinary catheters. The catheter should be washed in warm, soapy water and rinsed well in warm water. The catheter should be air-dried and, when completely dried, placed in a clean jar or plastic bag. A catheter should be replaced when it becomes dry, cracked, and stiff or if the child develops a UTI.
4. Instruct the caregivers to notify the health care provider for signs of associated problems, such as hydrocephalus, meningitis, UTI, and latex sensitivity.

CLINICAL JUDGMENT Ensure there is an emergency epinephrine injection available in case of inadvertent latex exposure.

Family Education and Health Maintenance

1. Prepare the caregivers to feed, hold, and stimulate their infant as naturally as possible.
2. Teach the caregivers the special techniques that may be required for holding and positioning, feeding, caring for the incision, emptying the bladder, and exercising muscles.
3. Alert the caregivers to safety needs of the child with decreased sensation, such as protection from prolonged pressure, the risk of burns because of bathwater that is too warm, and avoidance of trauma from contact with sharp objects.
4. Urge continued follow-up and health maintenance, including immunizations and evaluation of growth and development.
5. Advise caregivers that children with paralysis are at risk for becoming overweight because of inactivity, so they should provide a low-fat, balanced diet; control snacking; and encourage as much activity as possible.
6. For additional resources, refer families to agencies such as the Spina Bifida Association of America www.spinabifidaassociation.org.

Evaluation: Expected Outcomes

- No signs of meningeal sac or skin breakdown.
- Afebrile, alert, and active.
- Clear urine without odor; adequate elimination; no infection.
- Fontanelle soft; head circumference stable.
- Caregivers asking questions about surgery, showing affection for infant.
- Vital signs stable; incisional dressing dry and intact.
- Caregivers or child demonstrates proper catheterization technique.
- Passes stool once per day; adequate elimination; no constipation.
- Verbalizes participation in school and other social activities.

Muscular Dystrophy

Muscular dystrophy (MD) refers to a group of genetically determined, progressive, degenerative myopathies affecting a variety of muscle groups—most patients are children. The most common pediatric muscular dystrophies include Duchenne MD (DMD) and Becker MD (BMD). A 2022 US report estimated the prevalence of DMD and BMD at approximately 1 per 1,000. Most with DMD rarely survive beyond ages 20 to 25.

Pathophysiology and Etiology

1. Inherited; may be X-linked, autosomal dominant, or recessive trait affecting males more than females.
2. Genetic coding defect causes abnormal muscle development and function—mutations of the dystrophin gene in DMD and BMD are termed dystrophinopathies.
3. Degeneration and loss of skeletal muscle fibers but no associated structural abnormalities in peripheral nerves or spinal cord.
4. Marked reduction of dystrophin, a protein vital to muscle function. The amount of dystrophin levels varies with the type of MD.

Clinical Manifestations

1. Progressive muscular weakness, calf enlargement (hallmark sign), and leg pain (see Table 42-1).
2. Delayed walking to 18 months, walking on toes, frequent falls.
3. Delayed speech and emotional/behavioral difficulties.
4. Gower sign is a hallmark feature of DMD, characterized by a child's difficulty rising from the floor. The child must take the following steps to assume a standing position:
   a. Roll onto hands and knees.
   b. Bear weight with legs by creating a wide base of support, while using hands on the floor to support some weight.
   c. Use arms to climb up legs.
   d. Push torso to an upright stance with legs remaining wide apart.
5. Heart muscle weakens and tachycardia develops.
6. Respiratory muscles weaken, causing ineffective cough and frequent infections.
7. May have mild cognitive impairment in DMD.

Diagnostic Evaluation

1. Nerve conduction test and electromyography show abnormalities.
2. Serum creatinine kinase—elevated.
3. Deoxyribonucleic acid (DNA) analysis of blood.
4. Muscle biopsy may provide definitive diagnosis.
5. Electrocardiogram and echocardiogram to determine degree of cardiomyopathy.

Management

1. Goals of treatment are directed toward maintaining mobility, quality of life, and prevention of complications.
2. Medications to control symptoms, such as antiarrhythmics and bronchodilators.
3. Promotion of ambulation with appropriate aid after loss of ability to walk.
4. Provision of spinal orthotic supports.
5. Surgical tendon releasing to treat contractures.
6. Physical therapy, such as passive stretching, to preserve function.
7. Vigorous respiratory therapy, such as chest percussion, inspirometry, and assisted cough.
8. Pulmonary function monitoring.
9. Carrier detection and genetic counseling to explain implications of MD to caregivers and detect sibling carriers.
10. Glucocorticoids for patients with DMD 4 years of age and older to delay the progression of muscle weakness.
11. May require early surgical intervention to correct scoliosis.
12. Nutritional management to prevent obesity is necessary as this may affect quality of life, life expectancy, and burden of care.
13. Frequent surveillance of cardiac function.

Table 42-1 Clinical Manifestations of Muscular Dystrophies

TYPE	ONSET	CLINICAL MANIFESTATIONS	OTHER INFORMATION
Duchenne	Age 2–6 yr	Muscle atrophy and weakness over time affecting the pelvis, thighs, upper arms, and eventually, all voluntary muscles; waddling gait, need for wheelchair by age 12; pulmonary and cardiac abnormalities; survival beyond age 20 is rare	Affects only males Most common type of MD in children
Becker	Age 2–16 yr	Similar to Duchenne, but less severe, very mild in some cases; slower progression. Survival into middle age	Affects only males
Limb–girdle	Late teen to adult	Progressive weakness of the pelvic and shoulder girdles and then arms and legs. Walking becomes difficult over a 20-yr period. Survival may be to late adulthood	Affects males and females Most common type overall
Facioscapulohumeral	Teen to early adult	Weakness of fascial muscles, wasting of shoulders and upper arms; slow progression with short periods of rapid deterioration. Causes problems with chewing, swallowing, speaking; characteristic "Popeye" arms and scapular winging. Survival well into adulthood	Affects males and females Severity varies widely
Congenital	At birth	General muscle weakness; possible joint deformities because of contractures; slow progression. Seizures and other brain abnormalities with Fukuyama type. Shortened life span	Affects males and females Several types have been identified
Emery–Dreifuss	Childhood to early teen	Slowly progressive weakness and atrophy of the shoulder, upper arm, and lower leg muscles; joint deformities; possible cardiac problems causing sudden death. Cardiac problems may affect carriers (including females)	Affects males only Rare form

MD, muscular dystrophy.

Complications

1. Infections (pulmonary, urinary, systemic).
2. Cardiac dysrhythmias.
3. Respiratory insufficiency and failure secondary to weakness of the diaphragm and chest muscles.
4. Aspiration pneumonia because of oropharyngeal dysfunction.
5. Depression.
6. Orthopedic deformities—contractures, lordosis, and scoliosis.
7. Learning and behavioral disorders.
8. Malignant hyperthermia—may develop in a few children with mild or nonapparent muscle disease.
9. Osteopenia related to immobility.

Nursing Assessment

1. Assess muscle strength, atrophy, gait, age-related motor development, and progressive loss of function.
2. Evaluate respiratory and cardiac status—breath sounds, heart sounds, pulse rate and rhythm, BP, and peripheral perfusion.
3. Evaluate ADLs.
4. Assess degree of pain.
5. Identify psychosocial issues, such as altered self-concept, decreased socialization, and family discord.

Nursing Interventions

Maintaining Breathing Pattern

1. Encourage upright positioning to provide for maximum chest excursion.
2. Encourage energy conservation techniques and avoidance of exertion.
3. Teach deep breathing exercises to strengthen respiratory muscles.
4. Assess rate, depth, and pattern of respirations; listen to breath sounds; and report any change in condition.
5. Note results of arterial blood gas levels, sputum cultures, and chest x-rays.
6. Encourage coughing and deep breathing or perform chest physiotherapy, as indicated.

Preserving Optimal Motor Function

1. Refer to physical therapy for stretching and strengthening exercises to optimize remaining motor function.
2. Perform ROM exercises to preserve mobility and prevent atrophy.
3. Schedule activity with consideration to energy highs throughout the day.
4. Consult with occupational therapist for assistive devices to maintain independence.
5. Apply braces and splints to prevent contractures.
6. Ensure adequate pain management.

Improving Cardiac Output

1. Monitor vital signs, cardiac rhythm, and signs of heart failure, such as edema, adventitious breath sounds, and weight gain.
2. Monitor intake and output and maintain IV or oral fluid intake, as ordered.

Monitoring Swallowing Function

1. Assess cranial nerve function for swallowing (gag reflex) and chewing.
2. Provide a diet that the patient can handle; a pureed diet may be necessary.
3. Diet should be high protein and controlled calories to provide optimal nutritional value.

4. Encourage eating in upright position without talking, and encourage consumption of smaller, frequent meals.
5. Administer alternative enteral feeding if gag reflex is diminished.

Encouraging Diversional Activities

1. Encourage diversional activities that prevent overexertion and frustration, but discourage long periods of bed rest and inactivity such as TV watching.
2. If upper extremities are mostly affected, suggest walking or riding a stationary bike; if lower extremities are mostly affected, encourage use of a wheelchair to promote mobility and performing simple crafts.
3. Discuss patient's interests and assist with preferred activities.
4. Investigate with the patient various methods of stress management to deal with frustration.
5. Administer analgesics and antidepressants, as ordered, to facilitate participation in activities.

Community and Home Care Considerations

1. Follow the community and home care considerations listed under "Cerebral Palsy" on page 1224.
2. Obtain services and devices that will promote maximal functioning, such as wheelchair ramp, wheelchair van for transportation, and assistive devices.
3. Explore physical and recreational activities with family such as Special Olympics.
4. Assess child's educational progress and ability to attend school versus home schooling.
5. Collaborate with patient and family to establish daily plan of activities that incorporates patient's interests, ability, and need for rest periods.

Family Education and Health Maintenance

1. Offer genetic counseling, if indicated, to determine options of family planning.
2. Instruct the patient and family in ROM exercises, pulmonary care, and methods of transfer and locomotion.
3. Refer to community respite and counseling services.
4. Stress the importance of fluids to decrease risk of urinary/pulmonary infection and minimize constipation.
5. Advise patient or family to report signs of respiratory infection immediately to obtain treatment and prevent heart failure.
6. Refer patient and family to agencies such as the Muscular Dystrophy Association (www.mda.org).

Evaluation: Expected Outcomes

- Deep, unlabored respirations with clear breath sounds.
- Ambulates unassisted; no contractures noted.
- Vital signs stable; no edema.
- Tolerates small pureed feeds without aspiration.
- Out of bed most of day; engages in diversional and social activities.

Bacterial Meningitis

Bacterial meningitis is an inflammation of the meninges that follows the invasion of the spinal fluid by a bacterial agent. Inflammation occurs in the leptomeninges and tissues surrounding the brain and spinal cord. Since the introduction of the *Haemophilus influenzae* type B (1990) and pneumococcal conjugate (2000) vaccines to the pediatric immunization schedule, the incidence of bacterial meningitis has decreased in all age groups except in children under 2 months old. Newborns are at increased risk for bacterial meningitis along with adolescents 16 to 23 years of age. Since the introduction of the meningococcal conjugate vaccine MenACWY in 2005, incidence of bacterial meningitis in this age group has decreased by 90%. In 2015, a vaccine to protect against meningococcal group B (MenB) disease was introduced for adolescents and young adults ages 16 to 23.

Pathophysiology and Etiology

1. The proportion of cases because of a specific organism varies from year to year; there is also considerable geographic difference. The organisms most commonly causing bacterial meningitis in different age groups include:
   a. ≥1 month and <3 months: *Escherichia coli*, *Streptococcus* group B, *Listeria monocytogenes*, *Pseudomonas aeruginosa*, *Staphylococcus* species, *Streptococcus pneumoniae*, *Neisseria meningitidis*, and gram-negative bacilli.
   b. ≥3 months to <3 years: *S. pneumoniae*, *N. meningitidis* (meningococcal meningitis), and group B *Streptococcus*.
   c. ≥3 years to <10 years: *S. pneumoniae and N. meningitidis*.
   d. ≥10 years and <19 years: *N. meningitidis*.
2. Bacterial meningitis is frequently preceded by an upper respiratory infection, which is complicated by bacteremia. Bacteria in the circulating blood then invade the CSF.
   a. Less commonly, bacterial meningitis may occur as an extension of a local bacterial infection, such as otitis media, mastoiditis, or sinusitis.
   b. Bacteria may also gain direct entry through a penetrating wound, spinal tap, surgery, or anatomic abnormality.
3. The infective process results in inflammation, exudation, and varying degrees of tissue damage in the brain.

Clinical Manifestations

1. Signs and symptoms are variable, depending on the patient's age, the etiologic agent, and the duration of the illness when diagnosed. Onset may be insidious or fulminant.
2. Infants younger than age 2 months usually display irritability, lethargy, vomiting, lack of appetite, temperature instability (fever or hypothermia), respiratory distress, poor tone, tremors, seizures, high-pitched cry, and full (possibly bulging) fontanelle.
3. Infants up to age 2 years manifest symptoms similar to those of the young infant and may have a rash, altered sleep patterns, fever, tenseness of the fontanelle, nuchal rigidity, and positive Kernig or Brudzinski signs (see page 360).
4. Children older than age 2 years initially have vomiting, headache, fever, mental confusion, lethargy, irritability, and photophobia. Later symptoms include nuchal rigidity within 12 to 24 hours after onset, positive Kernig or Brudzinski sign, seizures, and progressive decline in responsiveness.
5. Petechiae or purpura may develop.
   a. Characteristic skin lesions are most commonly observed in cases of meningococcal or *Pseudomonas* infection.
   b. Hemorrhagic rashes may occur in any child with overwhelming bacterial sepsis because of disseminated intravascular coagulation (DIC).
6. Septic arthritis suggests either meningococcal or *H. influenzae* infection.

Diagnostic Evaluation

1. Diagnosis is usually established through LP and examination of CSF.
   a. Cloudy or turbid appearance.
   b. Elevated CSF pressure.
   c. High cell count with mostly polymorphonuclear cells.
   d. Low glucose level.
   e. Elevated protein level (also may be normal).
   f. Positive Gram stain and cultures (identifies the causative organism).
2. Additional laboratory studies include:
   a. Complete blood count (CBC)—total white blood cell count usually increased, with a preponderance of young neutrophils in the differential blood count (known as "shift to the left").
   b. Blood, urine, and nasopharyngeal cultures to look for source of infection.
   c. Platelet count, serum electrolytes, glucose, blood urea nitrogen and creatinine, and urinalysis usually done to monitor patient who is critically ill as well as clotting function if petechiae or purpuric lesions are noted.

Management

1. IV administration of the appropriate antimicrobial agents to promote rapid destruction of the bacteria and to suppress the emergence of resistant strains. The first dose of antibiotics should be administered as soon as possible (cultures should be taken before an antibiotic is given).
2. Recognition and treatment of hyponatremia caused by syndrome of inappropriate antidiuretic hormone (SIADH).
3. Supportive management of the comatose child or the child with seizures, including neuroprotective measures.
4. Appropriate prophylactic treatment provided for contacts when indicated.

Complications

1. Acute—seizures, cerebral edema and increased ICP, shock, ischemia, infected subdural effusion, disseminated illness (septic arthritis, pericarditis), and SIADH.
2. Long term—sensorineural hearing loss, hydrocephalus, blindness, learning disabilities, or developmental delays.
3. DIC.

Nursing Assessment

1. Obtain a history from the caregivers about recent upper respiratory or other infection.
2. Assess LOC and neurologic status.
   a. Evaluate for *Kernig sign*—with the child in the supine position and knees flexed, flex the leg at the hip so the thigh is brought to a position perpendicular to the trunk. Attempt to extend the knee. If meningeal irritation is present, this cannot be done, and attempts to extend the knee result in pain.
   b. Evaluate for *Brudzinski sign*—flex the patient's neck. Spontaneous flexion of the lower extremities indicates meningeal irritation.
3. Monitor breathing pattern and circulatory status.

Nursing Interventions

See Standards of Care Guidelines 42-1, page 1235.

STANDARDS OF CARE GUIDELINES 42-1
Caring for a Child With Neurologic Dysfunction

- Monitor vital signs, LOC, pupillary reaction, and behavior, as indicated, and observe for signs of increased ICP; report significant changes immediately.
- Make sure that the patient receives all seizure medications and antibiotics, as directed, and that any deviation from dosage schedule or change in therapeutic serum drug levels is reported immediately.
- Assess for adequate elimination: ability of the child to urinate, or caregiver or child to do catheterization. Report deviation from normal pattern, and take measures to prevent constipation and stool impaction.
- Assess for signs of secondary infection: postoperative incision infection; shunt malfunction and infection; pneumonia; skin breakdown. Report abnormality in timely fashion.
- Monitor for seizures and maintain safety. Document and report all seizures, including type, time of onset, duration, and behavior afterward. Administer medications, as needed, and as directed.
- Make sure that any assistive devices fit adequately to avoid tissue breakdown. Check more frequently if child is restless.
- Observe and assist with ambulation for safety.
- Train all caregivers in standards of home safety, including CPR, seizure control, and accident prevention.
- Make sure that the patient and family are aware of all community resources, including respite and support groups, educational assistance, and social services.
- Teach caregivers to do ROM exercises to prevent contractures. Utilize physical and occupational therapy, as needed.
- Encourage regular health maintenance visits to monitor growth, development, and general health.

This information should serve as a general guideline only. Each patient situation presents a unique set of clinical factors and requires nursing judgment to guide care, which may include additional or alternative measures and approaches.

Maintaining Cerebral Tissue Perfusion

1. Administer antimicrobial agents at specified time intervals to obtain optimal serum levels. Obtain blood studies for peak and trough levels, as ordered.
2. Maintain patent IV line for medication administration; observe for signs of infiltration and phlebitis.
3. Monitor closely for signs of complications affecting cerebral perfusion.
   a. Monitor vital signs, LOC, and neurologic status at frequent intervals.
   b. Monitor intake and output, weight, and head circumference daily to assess for hydrocephalus.
   c. Be especially alert for lethargy or subtle changes in condition, which may indicate cerebral edema.
   d. Accurately chart child's behavior and clinical signs.

Reducing Fever

1. Administer antipyretics, tepid sponge baths, and hypothermia blanket, as ordered, to reduce fever. Fever increases metabolic rate and energy requirements by the brain; this may lead to

hypoxemia and brain damage in the child with cerebral vascular compromise.

2. Monitor for seizures and use seizure precautions in the febrile child.
   a. There is an increased potential for seizures in the febrile child.
   b. Ensure safety by using padded bed or crib rails and having airway and suction equipment on hand.

Relieving Pain and Irritability

1. Reduce the general noise level around the child and prevent sudden loud noises.
2. Organize nursing care to provide for periods of uninterrupted rest.
3. Keep general handling of the child at a minimum. When necessary, approach the child slowly and gently.
4. Maintain subdued lighting as much as possible.
5. Speak in a low, well-modulated tone of voice.
6. Medicate for pain, as ordered, avoiding opioids that cause CNS and respiratory depression.

Preventing Transmission of Infection

Use infection control precautions at all times to prevent transmission of infection. Transmission occurs through droplets from the mouth and nose, requiring droplet and contact precautions.

1. Practice careful handwashing technique.
2. Explain the use of all protective equipment and procedures to child and family to allay anxiety.
3. Make sure that personnel with colds or other infections avoid contact with infants with meningitis and wear a mask when it is necessary to enter the nursery.
4. Teach caregivers and other visitors proper handwashing and gown techniques.
5. Maintain sterile technique for procedures, when indicated.
6. Identify close contacts of the child with meningitis caused by *H. influenzae* or *N. meningitidis* who might benefit from prophylactic treatment.

Avoiding Complications

1. Monitor for and report any of the following:
   a. Decreased respirations, decreased pulse rate, increased systolic BP, pupillary changes, or decreased responsiveness, which may indicate increased ICP.
   b. Decreased urine volume and increased body weight, which may indicate SIADH.
   c. Sudden appearance of a skin rash and bleeding from other sites, which may indicate DIC.
   d. Persistent or recurring fever, bulging fontanelle, signs of increased ICP, focal neurologic signs, seizures, or increased head circumference, which may indicate subdural effusion.
   e. Hearing disturbances and apparent deafness, indicating cranial nerve involvement.
2. Observe for episodes of apnea, and initiate measures to stimulate respiration.
   a. Institute respiratory monitoring.
   b. Stimulate the infant when apnea does occur.
      i. Pinch feet and provide more vigorous stimulation, if necessary.
      ii. When spontaneous respiration does not occur within 15 to 20 seconds, provide bag or mask ventilation.
   c. Report any periods of apnea.
   d. Record length of apneic episode and response to stimulation.

Managing Caregiver Anxiety

1. Encourage the caregivers to engage in quiet activities with their child, such as reading or listening to soft music.
2. Provide the caregivers with an opportunity to express their concerns and answer questions they may have regarding the child's progress and care.
3. Engage the caregivers in the supportive care of the child so they may feel some control over the situation.

Family Education and Health Maintenance

1. Provide caregivers with appropriate information if they and other family members are to receive antibiotic prophylaxis.
2. Discuss symptoms for which the caregivers should watch as signs of possible latent complications, especially hydrocephalus.
3. Give specific instructions about medications to be administered at home.
4. Encourage regular health maintenance visits to chart growth and development, and assess for any delays.
5. Caregivers can obtain more information about meningitis at http://kidshealth.org/en/parents/meningitis.html.
6. Educate caregivers regarding the importance of staying up to date with vaccinations for prevention.

Evaluation: Expected Outcomes

- Alert without signs of increased ICP.
- Fever below 101°F (38.3°C); no subsequent infection.
- Resting comfortably; verbalizing reduced pain.
- Child expresses understanding of infection precautions.
- Vital signs stable; breathing pattern regular without apnea.
- Caregivers participate in child's care and ask questions.

Seizures and Epilepsy

Neonates, infants, and children with epilepsy differ from adults in many ways because of their immature brains: variances are noted in the etiology of seizures, clinical manifestations, responses to antiepileptic medications, and electroencephalogram (EEG) patterns. Although the immature brain is more prone to seizures, as the child grows and develops, some seizures may change and even disappear. In a nationally representative sample of US children, the estimated lifetime prevalence of epilepsy/seizure disorder was 10.2/1,000 (1%), and that of current reported epilepsy/seizure disorder was 6.3/1,000. It is estimated that 1% of US children and teens will have at least one afebrile seizure by age 14 years.

Obtaining a thorough history and physical examination is crucial because the diagnosis of epilepsy is based primarily on clinical features.

The terms seizures and epilepsy are often used interchangeably. A seizure is a physical manifestation of abnormal, excessive, synchronous neuronal discharges generated primarily from the cerebral cortex. The discharges are intermittent in nature and often self-limited and may last for several seconds to minutes.

Epilepsy is diagnosed when any one of the following exists:

- At least two unprovoked (or reflex) seizures that occur more than 24 hours apart.
- One unprovoked (or reflex) seizure with the likelihood of further seizures with a similar recurrence risk after two unprovoked seizures, occurring over the next 10 years (e.g., in cases of remote structural lesions related to CNS infection, stroke, or certain types of traumatic brain injury).

Classification of Epilepsy Syndrome

1. A recent update to the International League Against Epilepsy (ILAE) Classification of the Epilepsies was published in Spring 2022 along with the revised ILAE 2022 Classification of Seizure Types.
2. This new classification of the epilepsies has three levels of diagnosis: seizure type, epilepsy type, and epilepsy syndrome.
3. The ILAE is aware that neonatal seizures may have motor manifestations, and minimal or no behavioral manifestations. A Neonatal Seizure Task Force is currently developing a separate classification of neonatal seizures.

Seizure Type

1. The first step is to rule out another type of paroxysmal event and provide a definitive diagnosis of an epileptic seizure type based on the initial manifestation of the seizure.
2. There are three seizure types:
   a. Focal.
   b. Generalized.
   c. Unknown.

Epilepsy Based on Seizure Type

The second level of diagnosis for patients with epilepsy includes four categories, two are new categories.

a. Focal.
b. Generalized.
c. Combined generalized and focal.
d. Unknown.

Epilepsy Syndromes

1. An epilepsy syndrome refers to a group of findings that occur together and define a clinically recognizable seizure disorder.
2. This cluster of findings includes certain seizure types, imaging, and EEG features along with particular ages of onset, triggers, comorbidities, and prognoses, which may have specific treatment recommendations.
3. A new ILAE educational website EpilepsyDiagnosis.org provides diagnostic guidelines, videos of seizure types, and more relevant information on epilepsy syndromes.
4. Epilepsy syndromes recognized in the neonatal period include:
   a. Benign neonatal seizures.
   b. Benign familial neonatal epilepsy.
   c. Early myoclonic encephalopathy.
   d. Ohtahara syndrome.
5. Epilepsy syndromes of infancy (onset under 2 years) include:
   a. West syndrome.
   b. Dravet syndrome.
   c. Epilepsy of infancy with migrating focal seizures.
   d. Benign infantile epilepsy.
   e. Benign familial infantile epilepsy.
   f. Febrile seizures plus.
6. Epilepsy syndromes of childhood include:
   a. Lennox–Gastaut syndrome.
   b. Landau–Kleffner syndrome.
   c. Epileptic encephalopathy with continuous spike and wave during sleep (CSWS).
   d. Febrile seizures plus (may start in infancy).
   e. Childhood absence epilepsy.
   f. Epilepsy with myoclonic absences.
   g. Late-onset childhood occipital epilepsy (Gastaut type).
   h. Panayiotopoulos syndrome (early childhood onset occipital epilepsy).
   i. Epilepsy with myoclonic atonic (previously astatic) seizures.
   j. Benign epilepsy with centrotemporal spikes.
7. Epilepsy syndromes of adolescence to adulthood include:
   a. Juvenile absence epilepsy (JAE).
   b. Juvenile myoclonic epilepsy (JME).

Infantile Spasms

1. These seizures occur in infants; they are second in incidence only to generalized seizures in this age group.
2. Children with infantile spasms (IS) typically develop epileptic spasms with an associated EEG pattern known as hypsarrhythmia.
3. The triad of spasms, hypsarrhythmia, and developmental regression is known as West syndrome.
4. Peak incidence is in children between ages 3 and 7 months; onset after age 2 years is rare.
5. Clinical signs include the following:
   a. Sudden, forceful, myoclonic contractions involving the musculature of the trunk, neck, and extremities.
      i. Flexor type—infant adducts and flexes the extremities, drops the head, and doubles on themselves.
      ii. Extensor type—infant extends neck, spreads out arms, and bends body backward in a position described as "spread eagle."
      iii. Mixed—combination of the preceding two types, occurring in clusters or volleys of each.
   b. A cry or grunt may accompany severe attacks.
   c. The infant may grimace, laugh, or appear fearful during or after the attack.
6. Duration is momentary (usually <1 minute).
7. Frequency varies from a few attacks per day to hundreds per day.
8. Almost always associated with cerebral abnormalities. Intellectual disability usually accompanies this disorder in 95% of cases.
9. Usually, this type of seizure disappears spontaneously by the time the child reaches age 4 years. Subsequent generalized or other types of seizures usually develop.

CLINICAL JUDGMENT Occurrence of IS is a pediatric emergency. Delay in treatment could lead to permanent cognitive impairment and developmental delay.

Pathophysiology and Etiology

Etiologic Factors

1. *Structural etiology* refers to abnormalities seen on structural neuroimaging where the imaging along with the electroclinical findings indicates the abnormality is the probable cause of the seizures, such as hippocampal sclerosis. Structural abnormalities can be congenital, such as tuberous sclerosis and cortical dysplasia or acquired by hypoxic–ischemic encephalopathy, infection, stroke, trauma, tumors, neurosurgery, and genetic cortical malformations.
2. *Genetic etiology* refers to a pathogenic genetic variant (mutation) of significant effect that causes epilepsy. A large number of epilepsy gene mutations have been identified in both severe and mild epilepsies, many being de novo mutations. Examples of genetic etiologies in children include SCN1A mutations associated with Dravet syndrome and genetic/generalized epilepsy with febrile seizures plus (GEFS+) and mutations in the potassium channel genes KCNQ2 and KCNQ3 (benign familial neonatal epilepsy).

3. *Infectious etiology* refers to epilepsy resulting from a known infection, including tuberculosis, cerebral malaria, HIV, neurocysticercosis, congenital infections (Zika virus, cytomegalovirus), cerebral toxoplasmosis, and subacute sclerosing panencephalitis (SSPE). Epilepsy, which develops after an acute infectious illness, may also fall into this category.
4. *Metabolic etiology* refers to epilepsy, which results directly from a presumed or known metabolic disorder, in which seizures are a main symptom. Often, metabolic disorders and epilepsies will be related to a genetic mutation, but some might be acquired. An example in children is pyridoxine deficiency.
5. *Immune etiology* refers to epilepsy, which results directly from a presumed or known immune disorder, in which seizures are a main symptom and where autoimmune-mediated CNS inflammation is noted. An example of this is anti-NMDA receptor encephalitis.
6. *Unknown etiology* refers to epilepsy in which the cause is not yet determined.

Altered Physiology

1. The basic mechanism for all seizures appears to be prolonged depolarization and other chemical changes, causing neurons to discharge in an uncontrolled manner.
2. This paroxysmal burst of electrical energy spreads to adjacent areas of the brain or may jump to distant areas of the CNS, resulting in a seizure.
3. Some seizures appear to occur under the influence of a triggering factor.
   a. Hormonal factors, such as those related to the menstrual period, menarche, and menopause.
   b. Nonsensory factors, such as hyperthermia; hyperventilation; metabolic disorders such as hypoglycemia, hyponatremia, and hypocalcemia; sleep deprivation; emotional disturbances; and physical stress.
   c. Sensory factors, such as those related to vision, hearing, touch, the startle reaction, and those that are self-induced.

Clinical Manifestation Based on the ILAE 2022 Classification of Seizure Types

Focal Onset Seizures

1. Focal onset seizures originate in networks limited to one hemisphere and include focal aware and focal impaired awareness seizures.
   a. Focal aware seizures were formerly known as simple partial seizures.
      i. No impairment of consciousness; retains awareness of self and environment even if immobile.
      ii. Caused by abnormal activation of a limited number of neurons that allow for localization of the epileptic focus.
   b. Focal impaired awareness seizures
      i. Includes all seizures with impaired consciousness during any portion of the event.
      ii. Formerly known as complex partial seizures.
2. Focal seizures are also subgrouped into those with motor or nonmotor signs and symptoms at the onset and can be further classified by the earliest prominent motor-onset or non–motor-onset characteristic:
   a. Motor Onset seizures
      i. Automatisms—mouth movements (i.e., chewing, lip smacking), hand movements (i.e., picking at clothing, "pill rolling," grasping at objects), rubbing genitalia, eye blinking, head turning, and raising of arms.
      ii. Atonic—loss of tone (degree of awareness usually not specified).
      iii. Clonic—jerking of limbs, often asymmetric and irregular.
      iv. Epileptic spasms—spasms of muscles of the neck, trunk, and extremities (degree of awareness usually not specified).
      v. Hyperkinetic.
      vi. Myoclonic—brief synchronous jerks of one or more muscle groups.
      vii. Tonic—sustained muscle contraction with no clonic phase.
   b. Nonmotor Onset
      i. Autonomic—changes in skin color, BP, heart rate, pupil size, piloerection, drooling, rising epigastric sensation, retching, and vomiting.
      ii. Behavioral arrest.
      iii. Emotional—fear, depression, anger, and irritability.
      iv. Sensory—tingling or numbness, simple visual phenomenon, hallucinations (visual, auditory, gustatory, olfactory), illusions of perception (size [macro- or micropsia], shape, weight, distance, sound), dysphasia, or aphasia.
3. Focal to Bilateral Tonic–Clonic Seizure:
   a. Formerly known as partial-onset seizure with secondary generalization.
   b. A special seizure type, which indicates a propagation pattern of a seizure.

Generalized Onset Seizures

1. Generalized onset seizures are characterized by global synchronized activation of neurons resulting in impaired consciousness, bilateral motor changes, and EEG abnormalities.
   a. Motor
      i. Tonic–clonic—consists of tonic phase (10 to 30 seconds), clonic phase (30 to 60 seconds), and postictal phase (2 to 30 minutes); postictal phase consists of confusion and fatigue.
      ii. Clonic—jerking that is often asymmetric and irregular; occurs more frequently in neonates, infants, and young children.
      iii. Tonic—sustained muscle contractions with no clonic phase, can occur at any age, frequently seen in children with diffuse cerebral damage and Lennox-Gastaut syndrome.
      iv. Myoclonic—brief involuntary muscle contractions of one or several muscle groups; may be triggered by action, noise, percussion, being startled, or photic stimulation; may occur alone or in clusters.
      v. Myoclonic–tonic–clonic—combination of three seizure manifestations.
      vi. Myoclonic–atonic—brief involuntary muscle contractions of one or several muscle groups and then sudden loss of tone.
      vii. Atonic—sudden loss of tone.
      viii. Epileptic spasms—involve spasms of muscles of the neck, trunk, and extremities.
   b. Nonmotor (Absence)
      i. Typical—abrupt onset of activity arrest, brief loss of consciousness, may have eye flickering, lasts 10 seconds,

easily provoked by hyperventilation or photic stimulation, no postictal phase with resumption of normal activity, may occur in clusters.

ii. Atypical—frequently associated with symptomatic epilepsies and mixed seizure disorders, may have aura or automatisms; partial impairment of consciousness, may last several minutes; postictal headache, confusion, and emotional disturbances are common.

iii. Myoclonic—brief involuntary muscle contractions of one or several muscle groups; may be triggered by action, noise, percussion, being startled, or photic stimulation.

iv. Eyelid myoclonia.

Unknown Onset and Unclassified Seizures

1. Unknown onset seizures are those in which there is an absence of knowledge of the seizure's onset, but it can be provisionally classified based on key characteristics.
   a. Motor
      i. Tonic–clonic—consists of tonic phase (10 to 30 seconds), clonic phase (30 to 60 seconds), and postictal phase (2 to 30 minutes); postictal phase consists of confusion and fatigue.
      ii. Epileptic spasms—involve spasms of muscles of the neck, trunk, and extremities.
   b. Nonmotor
      i. Behavioral arrest—abrupt onset of activity arrest.
2. Unclassified—this category is for seizures for which there is a lack of or inadequate information or if the seizure cannot be placed in other categories because of its unusual presentation.

Status Epilepticus

1. A prolonged seizure or repeated seizures lasting longer than 30 minutes with no interictal recovery.
2. Most common pediatric neurologic emergency, possibly resulting in permanent neurologic sequelae.
3. May be overt seizure activity (convulsive) or subclinical (nonconvulsive).
4. Generalized tonic–clonic status epilepticus is life-threatening.
5. Causes include new acute illness, progressive neurologic disease, loss of seizure control in an epileptic, or a febrile seizure in a child who is otherwise in good health.
6. Recurrence occurs more often in children who have other neurologic abnormalities; recurrence is rare in children who experience febrile seizures.
7. Absence and complex partial status epilepticus are often difficult to identify, and children often appear to be in a mildly confused state.

Psychogenic Nonepileptic Seizures

1. Previously known as "hysterical" or "pseudoseizures" and are usually a method of seeking attention and secondary gain.
2. Occur most frequently in adolescents and more often in females than males (3:1). Rates before 12 years of age are equal between females and males.
3. History of sexual abuse is common in females with nonepileptic seizures.
4. May occur in people with true seizures that have come under control.
5. Difficult to distinguish by observation alone.
6. Most episodes of psychogenic nonepileptic seizures (PNES) occur in front of witnesses and tend not to occur during sleep.
7. Forced eye closure suggests PNES, because eyes are usually open during the ictus of an epileptic seizure.
8. Often include three broad patterns:
   a. Unilateral or bilateral motor activity that may include tonic posturing or tremulousness—movements are thrashing or jerking, rather than tonic–clonic, and often different movements occur simultaneously.
   b. Behavioral or emotional changes—distress or discomfort, followed by semipurposeless—but not stereotyped—behaviors and may include walking or fumbling with objects.
   c. Periods of unresponsiveness with precipitation or cessation of the attack occurring after suggestion—no self-harm occurs, with no associated incontinence during these episodes.

Diagnostic Evaluation

Electroencephalogram

1. Used to confirm the clinical diagnosis, classify type of epilepsy, localize the area of epileptic focus, and determine when it is safe to discontinue treatment.
2. A normal EEG does not preclude the diagnosis of epilepsy. Indeed, about 10% to 20% of children who have epilepsy have a normal EEG.

Brain Imaging

1. CT scan and MRI—provide an anatomic picture of the brain; essential in ruling out the presence of a lesion. MRI is the gold standard in evaluation of epilepsy, although CT scan is used when MRI is not available.
2. Single-photon emission CT, positron emission tomography (PET), and functional MRI (fMRI)—brain imaging techniques that measure local vascular or metabolic changes associated with neuronal activity; they can also map cortical function when resective surgery is being planned.
3. Magnetoencephalography (MEG)—noninvasive technology that helps map the sensory and language cortex when resective surgery is being planned.

Neuropsychological Evaluation

1. Used to evaluate the specific learning needs of children with epilepsy because many have learning difficulties.
2. Part of the presurgical workup is to determine cognitive deficits and predict long-term consequences of epilepsy, particularly when surgery is performed in an eloquent area.
3. WADA testing (named after its inventor, Juhn Wada) evaluates hemisphere dominance for language and memory when resective surgery is being planned.
   a. Involves the intracarotid administration of amobarbital to anesthetize each hemisphere of the brain separately.
   b. The patient is then shown objects to name and recall over a short period of time.
   c. Some facilities now use alternative anesthetic agents such as etomidate because amobarbital has not been readily available (i.e., "eSAM"—etomidate speech and memory test).

Laboratory Studies

1. Serum electrolytes, magnesium, calcium, and fasting blood sugar to rule out metabolic causes.
2. Toxicology screen—drug overdoses may cause seizures.
3. Blood cultures—fever and CNS infections may cause seizures.
4. LP may be done if fever is present.
5. Serum levels of seizure medications should follow therapy.
6. Metabolic workup in infants or children with developmental delay.
7. Genetic testing to determine underlying epilepsy syndrome.

Management

Pharmacologic Management

1. Selection of the most effective drug depends on correct identification of the clinical seizure type (see Table 42-2).
2. A desirable drug level is one that will prevent seizures without producing undesirable adverse effects.
3. Dosages are adjusted according to blood level, clinical signs, and the child's weight.
4. Accurate timing is essential to prevent seizures. This is especially true when the child tends to have seizures at a certain time each day.
5. Enteric-coated tablets, which have a delayed effect, should be used for children who are prone to attacks during sleep.
6. Most anticonvulsants are available in liquid form and in capsules or tablets. Some drugs are less well absorbed in liquid form.
7. It may take several months to find the best combination of medications and the best dosages of each to control the child's seizures. Monotherapy is attempted initially. If this is not successful, a second drug may be tried or added on.
8. Symptoms may not be controlled 100% in every patient.
9. Dosage adjustments may be required from time to time because of the child's growth and clinical progress.
10. Blood counts, urinalysis, therapeutic drug levels, and liver function studies are done at regular intervals in children receiving certain anticonvulsants.
11. Medication is commonly not discontinued until 2 to 3 years after the last seizure and if the EEG is normal.
12. Weaning from medication should always be gradual, with stepwise reduction of dosage and withdrawal of one drug at a time.
13. There is some evidence to suggest that long-term use of some antiepileptic agents may cause intellectual impairment in children with epilepsy.
14. Monitor bone health and provide calcium supplementation if calcium intake is inadequate.

Surgical Management

1. If a cerebral lesion, such as a tumor, is found, surgical removal is the treatment of choice.
2. Surgical treatment, such as hemispherectomy, resection of localized seizure focus/epileptogenic zone, or corpus callosotomy, may be performed in children with severe, medically intractable seizure disorders.

Ketogenic Diet Therapy

1. The ketogenic diet is a high-fat, adequate protein, and low-carbohydrate diet that is used for control of seizures refractory to medications. The diet consists of precisely calculated portions of protein, fat, and carbohydrates. The diet causes the child to become ketotic because fats are used for fuel rather than carbohydrates. It has been proposed that ketones may inhibit seizures, although the mechanism of action is not completely understood.
2. There are several ketogenic diet types: classic, medium-chain triglyceride (MCT), modified Atkins, and the low glycemic index diet.
3. Children on this diet should not be given IV fluids with dextrose.
4. All medications should be in sugar-free and carbohydrate-free suspensions, tablets, or capsules.
5. The child will be on strict fluid restriction.
6. This diet must be carefully monitored by a dietitian. Ongoing surveillance monitors the child's growth and nutritional status as well as other parameters, including kidney functions and lipid and micronutrient levels.
7. There is some evidence that this diet may put the child at increased risk for developing kidney stones. The risk may be increased when the child receives concomitant therapy with topiramate. Renal and abdominal ultrasounds are done periodically to monitor for stones.
8. Periodic electrocardiograms are performed to monitor for heart rhythm abnormalities.
9. Another form of the ketogenic diet is the MCT diet. The MCT diet allows for consumption of more carbohydrates than the classic ketogenic diet, reducing the side effects of vomiting and lack of energy.
10. Valproic acid must be weaned off prior to commencing treatment with the MCT ketogenic diet to prevent hepatic toxicity.

EVIDENCE BASE Ko, A., Kwon, H. E., & Kim, H. D. (2022). Updates on the ketogenic diet therapy for pediatric epilepsy. *Biomedical Journal, 45*(1), 19–26. https://doi.org/10.1016/j.bj.2021.11.003

Modified Atkins Diet

1. Less restrictive form of ketogenic diet for seizure control in cases of drug-resistant epilepsy.
2. Carbohydrates are restricted to 10 to 20 g per day, with no restriction of protein, fluid, or calories.
3. Hospital admission is not required to initiate the diet. The diet is often self-administered.

Vagal Nerve Stimulation

The vagal nerve stimulator is a pacemaker-like device that is surgically implanted into the chest and attached to coiled electrodes, which are tunneled to the left cervical vagus nerve. The generator emits a programmed stimulus to stop seizures of long duration (usually 1 minute or longer), and children/families may activate the generator to allow for additional stimulus at times of seizure activity. Vagal nerve stimulation is an adjunctive treatment for intractable epilepsy—although the mechanism of action is unknown, studies have shown that VNS therapy reduces seizure frequency and is well tolerated.

EVIDENCE BASE Hajtovic, S., LoPresti, M. A., Zhang, L., Katlowitz, K. A., Kizek, D. J., & Lam, S. (2022). The role of vagus nerve stimulation in genetic etiologies of drug-resistant epilepsy: A meta-analysis. *Journal of Neurosurgery Pediatrics, 29*(6), 667–680. Retrieved March 15, 2023, from https://thejns.org/pediatrics/view/journals/j-neurosurg-pediatr/29/6/article-p667.xml

Behavioral Management

1. Psychiatric disorders, especially attention deficit hyperactivity disorder, depression, and anxiety, are common in children and adolescents who have epilepsy. They are more prevalent in this population than in children and adolescents in the general population or children who have other chronic conditions. Psychosis occurs infrequently.
2. It is important to monitor children with epilepsy for these disorders to ensure early recognition and treatment to minimize lifelong negative sequelae.
3. Further studies are needed to identify the most effective treatments.

Table 42-2 Drugs Used to Treat Seizures in Children

DRUGS AND DOSAGE	ADVANTAGES	ADVERSE EFFECTS	NURSING CONSIDERATIONS
Phenobarbital			
Maintenance dosage: 3–5 mg/kg given qid or bid *Status epilepticus:* 10–20 mg/kg, may repeat to maximum 40 mg/kg	Relatively safe and inexpensive	Excitement, hyperactivity, rash, GI distress, dizziness, ataxia, worsening of psychomotor seizures, drowsiness; toxicity causing respiratory depression, circulatory collapse, and renal impairment	• Contraindicated in hepatic or renal dysfunction, hypersensitivity • IM or IV loading dose can be given • IV rate should not exceed 1 mg/kg/min
Phenytoin			
Loading dose: 20 mg/kg *Maintenance:* 3–9 mg/kg given qid or bid	Safest drug for psychomotor seizures; does not cause drowsiness	Hypertrophy of gums, hirsutism, rickets, nystagmus, ataxia, rash; may accentuate absence seizures; toxicity may cause blood dyscrasias and liver damage	• May interact with a wide variety of drugs because of extensive protein binding • Daily gum massage may prevent gum disease • Avoid IM administration • If given IV, do not exceed rate of 0.5 mg/kg/min • Dilute with normal saline to prevent formation of precipitant
Ethosuximide			
Maintenance: 20–40 mg/kg given qid by oral route only	Used for absence seizures	Drowsiness, GI distress, lethargy, euphoria; may aggravate generalized seizures; toxicity causes blood dyscrasias and psychiatric symptoms	• This is contraindicated in hepatic or renal disease • Dosage should not be increased more frequently than every 4–7 d
Primidone			
Children younger than age 8 yr: 10–25 mg/kg given tid *Children older than age 8 yr:* 750–1,500 mg tid or qid by oral route only	May control generalized seizures not responsive to treatment by other drugs	Ataxia, vertigo, GI symptoms; megaloblastic anemia is a rare idiosyncratic reaction; drowsiness in breast-fed infants of treated mothers; Stevens-Johnson syndrome, gum hypertrophy, night terrors	• Contraindicated in those hypersensitive to phenobarbital and those with porphyria • Commonly used with other drugs for mixed seizure • Dosage increases are usually done weekly until effect is seen
Diazepam			
IV dosage: 0.04–0.2 mg/kg to maximum of 10 mg if age 5 yr or older; maximum of 5 mg if younger than age 5 yr *Rectal dosage:* 0.5 mg/kg	Given IV, IM, or rectally for status epilepticus or as adjunct therapy	Ataxia, drowsiness, fatigue, venous thrombosis or phlebitis at injection site, confusion, depression, headache; tonic status epilepticus when given IV for absence seizures; toxicity may cause somnolence, confusion, diminished reflexes, hypotension, coma, apnea, cardiac arrest	• If administered IV, give no faster than 1 mg/min. Drug used cautiously in children with limited pulmonary reserve • Monitor respiratory status closely
Carbamazepine			
20–30 mg/kg tid or qid *Maximum dose:* 1,000 mg/d if older than age 12 yr; 100 mg bid if ages 6–12 yr; 20 mg/kg/d if younger than age 6 yr	Especially useful for major motor and psychomotor seizures	Most likely to occur during initiation of therapy: dizziness, drowsiness, nausea, and vomiting; toxicity may cause bone marrow depression (fever, sore throat, oral ulcers, easy bruising)	• Administration with phenytoin reduces half-life of phenytoin; higher dose of phenytoin may be needed • Contraindicated in previous bone marrow depression and is used cautiously in patients with cardiac, hepatic, or renal problems • Erythromycin increases plasma levels • Give with food
Lorazepam			
0.05–0.1 mg/kg q 10–15 min *Maximum dose:* 4 mg	Given IV or rectally for status epilepticus; longer acting; may cause less respiratory depression	Sedation, dizziness, respiratory depression, hypotension, ataxia, weakness	• Use with caution in patients with hepatic or renal dysfunction • Monitor respiratory status closely

(continued)

Table 42-2 Drugs Used to Treat Seizures in Children (*continued*)

DRUGS AND DOSAGE	ADVANTAGES	ADVERSE EFFECTS	NURSING CONSIDERATIONS
Valproic Acid			
Loading dose: 10 mg/kg/d *Maximum dose:* 30–60 mg/kg tid or qid	Adjunct for poor seizure control; some success with behavioral problems	Nausea, vomiting, anorexia, amenorrhea, sedation tremor, weight gain, alopecia, hepatotoxicity	• Use caution with hepatic dysfunction. Increases serum levels of phenytoin, phenobarbital, and primidone
Gabapentin			
Loading dose: 10–15 mg/kg/d in three divided doses *Maximum dose:* 25–40 mg/kg/d in three divided doses	Recommended for add-on therapy in children over age 3 with refractory partial seizures	May interfere with the action of other drugs, including cimetidine; nausea/dizziness	• Must exercise caution in patients with renal impairment
Topiramate			
Loading dose: 25 mg/d at bedtime for the first week *Maximum dose:* 200–400 mg/d in two divided doses	Recommended for patients aged 2–16 with partial-onset seizures and those seizures related to Lennox–Gastaut syndrome	Most commonly associated with fatigue, dizziness, sleepiness	• Must exercise caution in patients with renal impairment • Interacts with other anticonvulsants, altering drug concentrations; may interfere with effectiveness of hormonal contraceptives
Oxcarbazepine			
Loading dose: 8–10 mg/kg/d in two divided doses *Maximum dose:* children 2 to <4 yr—60 mg/kg/d; children 4–16 yr—900 to 1,800 mg/d based on weight	Adjunctive therapy in children aged 4–16 yr for partial seizures	Fatigue, abnormal gait, sedation, difficulty in concentration, and memory impairment	• Need to monitor serum sodium • May interfere with other anticonvulsants by increasing serum concentration; decreases the effectiveness of hormonal contraceptives
Zonisamide			
Loading dose: 2–4 mg/kg/d *Maximum dose:* 12 mg/kg/d in two to three divided doses	Adjunctive therapy in children older than age 16; especially effective in refractive seizures, such as absence, Lennox–Gastaut syndrome, or infantile spasms	Drowsiness, ataxia, loss of appetite, GI upset, and slowing of mental activity, psychiatric symptoms (i.e., depression, psychosis)	• Must exercise caution in patients with renal and/or hepatic impairment, and patients with sensitivity to sulfonamides • Pediatric patients may be at increased risk and may have more severe metabolic acidosis
Lacosamide			
Adolescents ≥17 yr, monotherapy initial dose 100 mg bid, adjunctive therapy initial dose: 50 mg bid; maintenance dose: 200–400 mg/d *Children and adolescents under <17 yr:* 1–2 mg/kg/d divided bid, may titrate to 1 mg/kg/d weekly to effect	Adjunctive therapy in the treatment of partial-onset seizures and severe refractory seizures in children <17 yr	Dizziness, ataxia, light-headedness, excessive drowsiness, headaches, nausea, vomiting, tremors, change in vision or multiorgan sensitivity reactions Report signs of suicide ideation or depression	• Carbamazepine, fosphenytoin, phenobarbital, and phenytoin may decrease lacosamide serum concentration • May prolong PR interval (patients with conduction problems or severe cardiac disease should have ECG tracing prior to/during treatment)

Clobazam			
Lennox–Gastaut (adjunctive), US labeling: *Children ≥2 yr:* refer to adult dosing Epilepsy (monotherapy or adjunctive), oral: *children <2 yr, initial dose*: 0.5–1 mg/kg/d; *Children 2–16 yr, initial dose*: 5 mg/d; *maximum*: 40 mg/d	Adjunctive treatment of seizures associated with Lennox–Gastaut syndrome (FDA-approved in ages ≥ 2 yr and adults); has also been used as monotherapy and adjunctive treatment for other forms of epilepsy	Somnolence, fever, lethargy, upper respiratory tract infection, GI issues, muscle weakness, paradoxical reactions including hyperactive or aggressive behavior, anterograde amnesia, suicidal ideation **US Boxed Warning: Risks from concomitant use of benzodiazepines and opioids**	• May be administered with or without food • Tablets can be crushed and mixed in applesauce • Tolerance and loss of seizure control have been reported with chronic administration • Rebound or withdrawal symptoms may occur following abrupt discontinuation or large decreases in dose • Use caution, adjust dose in patients with hepatic impairment, respiratory disease, and preexisting muscle weakness (Canadian labeling contraindicates use in myasthenia gravis)
Rufinamide, Oral			
Lennox–Gastaut syndrome: *Children ≥4 yr, initial dose*: 10 mg/kg/d in two equally divided doses; *target dose*: 45 mg/kg/d; *maximum dose*: 3,200 mg/d	Adjunctive therapy of seizures associated with Lennox–Gastaut syndrome (FDA-approved in ages ≥4 yr and adults)	Cardiovascular: QT shortening (46%–65%; may be dose-related), headache, somnolence, dizziness, fatigue, aggression, anxiety, ataxia/gait disturbance, vertigo, tremor, attention disturbance, back pain, hyperactivity, seizures, status epilepticus, suicidal thinking, pruritus, rash, frequent urination, anemia, leucopenia; visual, respiratory or GI disturbances	• Contraindicated in patients with familial short QT syndrome • Administer with food • Monitor for signs and symptoms of anxiety, depression, unusual mood or behavior changes, suicide ideation
Vigabatrin			
FDA approved in ages ≥ 10 yr and adults: *Children, oral, initial dose*: 40 mg/kg/d in two divided doses, maintenance dosages based on patient weight Infantile spasms: *FDA approved in children 1 mo to 2 yr, initial dose*: 50 mg/kg/d in two divided doses; *maximum dose*: 150 mg/kg/d	Treatment of infantile spasms; adjunct therapy for refractory complex partial seizures in patients with inadequate response to several alternative treatments and for whom the potential benefits outweigh the potential risk of vision loss	Anemia, somnolence, headache, fatigue, irritability, sedation, nystagmus, tremor, insomnia, GI issues, weight gain, edema, peripheral neuropathy, neurotoxicity, suicidal ideation, vision loss, abnormal MRI changes have been reported in some infants **US Boxed Warning: Permanent Vision Loss** Only available in the United States under the Sabril REMS Program	• May be administered without regard to meals • Assess vision prior to initiating therapy or within 4 wk from start, at least every 3 mo during therapy and at 3–6 mo after therapy has been discontinued • Assess for CNS depression, changes in behavior, and suicidal tendencies
Levetiracetam			
Partial-onset seizures: *Children 1 to <6 mo, initial dose:* 7 mg/kg bid; *maximum dose*: 21 mg/kg bid *Children 6 mo to <4 yr, initial dose*: 10 mg/kg bid; *maximum dose*: 25 mg/kg bid *Children 4 to <16 yr, initial dose*: 10 mg/kg/d bid; *maximum dose*:	Adjunctive therapy in the treatment of partial-onset, myoclonic, and/or primary generalized tonic–clonic seizures	Behavioral/psychiatric symptoms, agitation, amnesia, anxiety, somnolence, fatigue, anorexia and other GI symptoms, ataxia and coordination problems, hypertension	• Be aware of neuropsychiatric adverse events as incidence of behavioral abnormalities and psychiatric symptoms may be increased in children • Use with caution and decrease dose in patients with renal dysfunction • May be administered without regard to meals

(continued)

Table 42-2 Drugs Used to Treat Seizures in Children *(continued)*

DRUGS AND DOSAGE	ADVANTAGES	ADVERSE EFFECTS	NURSING CONSIDERATIONS
30 mg/kg/d bid (*maximum daily dose*: 3,000 mg/d) Tonic–clonic seizures: *Children 6 to <16 yr, initial dose*: 10 mg/kg bid; *recommended dose*: 30 mg/kg twice daily.			
Stiripentol			
Children ≥3 yr and adults, in conjunction with clobazam and valproic acid: increased over 3 d to a final dose of 50 mg/kg/d in 2–3 divided doses with food	Treatment of refractory generalized tonic–clonic seizures in conjunction with clobazam and valproic acid in patients with severe myoclonic epilepsy in infancy (Dravet syndrome) whose seizures are not adequately controlled with clobazam and valproic acid alone	Clobazam concentrations have increased two to threefold when given with stiripentol; a clobazam dosage reduction of 25% per week may be required in the presence of clobazam toxicity (drowsiness, hypotonia, and irritability)	• Product available in various countries; not currently available in the United States • Should be given with food, excluding fruit juice, dairy, or caffeinated or carbonated products
Perampanel			
Children ≥ 12 yr and adolescents—with no enzyme inducing AEDs: initial dose 2 mg HS, increase by 2 mg/wk to recommended dose 8–12 mg; *with enzyme-inducing AEDs*: initial dose 4 mg HS, increase by 2 mg/wk to 8–12 mg HS	Adjunctive therapy in treatment of partial-onset seizures with or without secondarily generalized seizures	Headache, nausea, vomiting, abdominal pain, fatigue, loss of strength and energy, back pain or weight gain, dizziness, passing out, change in balance or abnormal gait **US Boxed Warning: Serious psychiatric and behavioral reactions** such as depression, suicidal ideation, illogical thinking, aggression, anger, hostility, homicidal ideation	• Not recommended (not studied) in cases of severe renal and hepatic impairment; with mild to moderate renal and hepatic impairment, use caution and lower doses with slower titration • To be administered once daily at hour of sleep (HS)
Midazolam			
Infants 1–5 mo: 0.2 mg/kg single dose; *infants ≥ 6 mo, children and adolescents*: 0.2–0.3 mg/kg, maximum single dose 10 mg (intranasal dosing parameters)	For acute treatment of prolonged seizures	Antegrade amnesia, potential respiratory depression, and respiratory arrest if used with other CNS depressants; hypotension, CNS depression, paradoxical reactions such as agitation hyperactive or aggressive behavior **US Boxed Warning: Respiratory depression; IV dosing; neonates (injection); risk from concomitant use with opioids**	• Use a mucosal atomisation device (MAD) nasal drug delivery device to administer intranasal • Maximum 1 mL per nostril (0.5 mL for infants <1 yr old) • Vial can be stored in cool, dry area at room temperature; an open vial can be stored up to 28 d and then must be discarded • Use with caution in children with cardiac, lung, hepatic, or renal impairment

bid, twice a day; CNS, central nervous system; ECG, electrocardiogram; FDA, U.S. Food and Drug Administration; GI, gastrointestinal; IM, intramuscular; IV, intravenous; MRI, magnetic resonance imaging; qid, four times a day; tid, three times a day.

General Prognosis

1. General prognosis depends on type and severity of seizure disorder, coexisting intellectual disability, organic disorders, and the type of medical management.
2. Medically treated seizures—spontaneous cessation of seizures may occur. Drugs may be gradually discontinued when the child has been free from seizures for an extensive period and the EEG pattern has reverted to normal.
3. Untreated epilepsy—seizures tend to become more numerous.

Complications

1. Apnea/hypoventilation.
2. Hypoglycemia in status epilepticus.
3. Injuries sustained during a seizure.
4. Sudden unexpected death in epilepsy (SUDEP).
5. Osteopenia—because of restrictions in physical activity as a result of seizures or other conditions, such as CP, or treatment with antiepileptic medications, such as valproic acid and carbamazepine.

Nursing Assessment

1. During a seizure, assess the following:
   a. Indications of difficulties with airway or breathing.
   b. Significant preseizure events, such as noise, excitement, and lethargy.
   c. Behavior before the seizure, aura.
   d. Types of movements observed.
   e. Time seizure began and ended.
   f. Site where twitching or contraction began.
   g. Areas of the body involved.
   h. Movements of the eyes and changes in pupil size.
   i. Incontinence.
   j. Color change—pallor, cyanosis, and flushing.
   k. Mouth—teeth clenched, abnormal movements, and tongue bitten.
   l. Degree of consciousness during the seizure.
2. After a seizure, assess the following:
   a. Degree of memory for recent events.
   b. Types of speech.
   c. Coordination, paralysis, or weakness.
   d. Length of time the child is postictal.
   e. Pupillary reaction.

CLINICAL JUDGMENT A devastating phenomenon of epilepsy is SUDEP. The American Academy of Neurology and the American Epilepsy Society have created a practice guideline that directs clinicians to incorporate the following in their discussions:

- The incidence in children is 1 in 4,500 annually.
- For those children who have active generalized tonic–clonic seizures, they are strongly encouraged to pursue therapies to manage their epilepsy while incorporating individual treatment preferences in the context of a risk/benefit approach.
- Inform patients and families that freedom from generalized tonic–clonic seizures greatly decreases the risk of SUDEP.

Nursing Interventions

Ensuring Safety during a Seizure

1. Remove hard toys from the bed.
2. Pad the sides of the crib or side rails of the bed.
3. Assess LOC.
4. Make sure the child can be readily observed.
5. During a seizure, monitor vital signs and assess neurologic status frequently.
6. After a seizure, check the child frequently and report the following:
   a. Behavior changes.
   b. Irritability.
   c. Restlessness.
   d. Listlessness.
   e. Neurologic signs.

Preventing Respiratory Arrest and Aspiration

1. During a seizure, take the following emergency actions:
   a. Clear the area around the child.
   b. Do not restrain the child.
   c. Loosen the clothing around the neck.
   d. Turn the child on side so saliva can flow out of the mouth.
   e. Place a small, folded blanket under the head to prevent trauma if the seizure occurs when the child is on the floor.
2. Do not give anything by mouth or attempt to place anything in the mouth.
3. After the seizure, place the child in a side-lying position.

Promoting Socialization

1. Advise the caregivers that the child should be in an environment that is as normal as possible.
2. Encourage regular attendance at school after the school nurse and teachers have been notified and emergency treatment of seizures is understood.
3. Encourage the child to participate in organizations and outside activities with limited restrictions.
   a. Each child must be treated individually; the kind of activity depends on the degree of seizure control.
   b. Generally, children with seizure disorders should not be allowed to climb in high places or to swim alone.
   c. Responsible adults should be made aware of the child's disorder.
   d. Children with seizures should wear a medical alert device at all times.

Strengthening Self-esteem

1. Offer reassurance and praise to the caregivers and child for coping effectively with seizures.
2. Observe caregiver–child interactions for evidence of rejection or overprotection.
   a. Tell the caregivers that the child should not be made to feel that they can never be left alone.
   b. Advise the caregivers that the child needs to be disciplined as any other child and should not gain attention directly or indirectly by having seizures.
3. Help the child gain more control by providing education about seizure disorders.
   a. Include the child in treatment planning.
   b. Allow the opportunity to ask questions and answer them honestly.
   c. Make sure the child is aware of restrictions and can deal with them.

d. Encourage caregivers gradually to give the child responsibility for taking medications.
4. Help the older child or adolescent to achieve independence.
   a. Encourage the caregivers to give the older child the opportunity for privacy to discuss concerns with the provider.
   b. Encourage caregivers to allow the older child to use their own judgment in making decisions.
   c. Help the older child to develop realistic educational and career goals.
5. Help caregivers deal with a nonadherent child. Refusal to take medications requires prompt intervention. Children need to be reassured that they are not abnormal but that they do require medication to control seizures. Children need to be taught that they are normal and can have normal lives. This is most commonly seen during adolescence. Family counseling may be necessary.
6. Teach the caregivers and child seizure safety.

Community and Home Care Considerations

1. Follow community and home care considerations listed under "Cerebral Palsy" on page 1224.
2. Make sure that the home environment is safe, especially where the child sleeps and plays. Remove toys with sharp edges or parts or small pieces the child could choke on if they are put in the mouth, and cover very hard surfaces, such as the floor, against which the child could fall.
3. Reinforce caregivers' knowledge and ability to dispense seizure medications.
4. Help the family acquire a medical alert tag that the child should wear at all times, especially when attending day care or school.
5. Make sure that caregivers know the seizure type, name of all medications, when to call the health care provider, and when to call 911.
   a. The health care provider should be notified of an increased frequency of seizures or new onset of symptoms.
   b. Emergency response should be activated when the child has been seizing for longer than 5 minutes or is unresponsive after a seizure.
6. Make sure that caregivers are trained in CPR and seizure management.

Family Education and Health Maintenance

1. Describe completely any examinations, evaluations, and treatments that the child is receiving.
2. Provide information regarding the disorder itself.
   a. Epilepsy is not contagious, is seldom dangerous, and does not indicate insanity or intellectual disability.
   b. Most children with epilepsy have infrequent seizures and can completely control their convulsions with medications.
   c. The child may have normal intelligence and can live a useful and productive life.
3. Prepare the caregivers for the fact that it may take several months of regulating drug dosages before adequate control is obtained.
4. Encourage caregivers and older children to obtain genetic counseling.
   a. As genetic research progresses, an increasing number of mutations have been found in patients with both sporadic and inherited epilepsy syndromes. There is a genetic predisposition with certain types of seizures, such as absence, febrile, and juvenile myoclonic seizures.
   b. It is impossible to predict accurately the possibility of the seizure disorder appearing in siblings or offspring of the affected child.
5. Teach the caregivers and child factors that may precipitate a seizure.
   a. The child should be kept in optimal physical condition with routine immunizations, medical care, dental care, and eye care and should receive prompt evaluation and treatment of infections.
   b. Excessive fatigue, dehydration, and sleep deprivation should be avoided.
   c. Irregular, fluctuating schedules are detrimental. Advise the caregivers to maintain a daily routine.
   d. Fever or illness of any kind can trigger seizures in children diagnosed with epilepsy even though their seizures may otherwise be under control.
6. For additional resources, refer families to https://www.aboutkidshealth.ca/Article?contentid=2123&language=English&hub=epilepsy.

Evaluation: Expected Outcomes

- Padded bed rails in place.
- Breathing unlabored after seizure, with lungs clear.
- Caregivers and child verbalize understanding of child's ability to participate in activities.
- Child participates in treatment plan and takes medications as ordered without reminders; serum drug levels are therapeutic.

Febrile Seizures

Febrile seizures occur in childhood after 1 month of age and are associated with a febrile illness that is not caused by an infection of the CNS. There is no history of a previous neonatal seizure or a previous unprovoked seizure, and the child does not have an acute symptomatic seizure. Most febrile seizures occur between 6 and 36 months of age, with the peak incidence at 12 to 18 months. In North America, up to 5% of all children will have at least one febrile seizure before age 5 years, and onset after 6 years of age is unusual.

Febrile seizures may be simple or complex:

- Simple febrile seizures—brief, last <10 minutes; tonic–clonic convulsion occurs once in 24 hours; absence of focal features; resolve spontaneously; 70% to 75% of febrile seizures are simple.
- Complex febrile seizures—prolonged, last more than 10 to 15 minutes; focal in nature; may recur within the same febrile illness over 24 hours; approximately 20% of febrile seizures are complex in most series.

Pathophysiology and Etiology

1. Febrile seizures are associated with first- or second-degree relatives with a history of febrile seizure, day care attendance, developmental delay, influenza A viral infection, herpes virus-6 infection, metapneumovirus, and iron-deficiency anemia.
2. Seizures often accompany intercurrent infections, especially viral illness, tonsillitis, pharyngitis, and otitis.
3. They appear to occur in a familial pattern, although the exact pattern of inheritance is not completely understood. Children with a positive family history of febrile seizures have a greater risk of recurrent febrile seizures.

4. Clinical studies have now demonstrated that it is the actual maximum temperature attained, rather than the rate of rise, that is the determinant of risk in febrile seizures. One key variable that alters fever effect is seizure threshold, which is lower in infants.
5. Most febrile seizures consist of generalized tonic–clonic seizures, and the majority occur on the first day of illness (see above). It is believed that fever increases neuronal excitability and lowers the seizure threshold.

Clinical Manifestations

1. Fever is usually more than 101.8°F (38.8°C) rectally, with most occurring with a temperature of 102.2°F (39°C).
2. Seizures usually occur near the onset of fever rather than after prolonged fever.

Diagnostic Evaluation

Measures are directed toward delineating the cause of any seizure as precisely as possible so its implications and prognosis may be discussed with the caregivers. Diagnostic methods may include the following:

1. Careful history taking and physical examination.
2. CSF examination to detect CNS infection—strongly recommended in children experiencing their first febrile seizure, especially in children age <12 months, those who have had a prolonged seizure including febrile status epilepticus, if there are any meningeal signs, if the child is on antibiotics (could mask meningitis signs and symptoms), and for seizures that occur after the second day of febrile illness.
3. CBC and urinalysis to detect signs of infection.
4. Cultures of nasopharynx, blood, or urine, as appropriate, to determine cause of fever.
5. Blood glucose, calcium, and electrolyte levels to detect abnormalities that may cause seizures.
6. EEG (for atypical seizures or for a child at risk for epilepsy).
   a. Demonstrates mild, postictal slowing soon after the attack.
   b. Pattern is generally normal after a few days.

Management

The goals of treatment are to control seizures and decrease temperature.

1. Administration of antipyretics and other cooling measures. Rectal administration of acetaminophen every 6 hours for 24 hours decreases the likelihood of short-term recurrence of seizures.
2. Prevention of febrile seizures with anticonvulsants is not common practice. Prompt control of fevers is the desired course of action.
3. Rectal diazepam gel is the preferred method of acute seizure management for prolonged seizures >5 minutes or for someone who is at risk for status epilepticus. It is used only in extreme cases.
   a. Intermittent therapy with phenobarbital during febrile episodes is apparently of no value because of the length of time required to achieve therapeutic serum levels of the drug.
4. Airway management, as required.
5. Prognosis—likelihood of recurrence is about 40% in those who have had two febrile seizures. The younger the child is at the time of the first seizure, the greater the risk of additional febrile seizures.
6. The risk of development of nonfebrile seizures is relatively low (about 5%). At risk are children who demonstrate the following characteristics:
   a. Prolonged or complex febrile seizures.
   b. Abnormal or suspected abnormal development before the first seizure.
   c. Family history of nonfebrile seizures.
   d. Persistent EEG abnormalities.

Complications

Injury may occur during seizure.

Nursing Assessment and Interventions

Nursing assessment and interventions are the same as for seizure disorders, page 402.

Family Education and Health Maintenance

1. Reinforce realistic, reassuring information, such as the following:
   a. A seizure does not necessarily imply that the underlying disease is serious.
   b. Febrile seizures are relatively common in children.
   c. The prognosis depends on the cause of the seizure.
      i. A single febrile seizure does not indicate later chronic epilepsy.
      ii. Children usually outgrow the tendency to develop febrile seizures by age 4 or 5 years of age.
      iii. Occasional or brief seizures are thought to have no effect on the child's overall development, although this is controversial.
2. Discuss and demonstrate emergency management of seizures.
   a. The child should be positioned on the side, on a flat surface from which they cannot fall.
   b. The surface should be padded, if possible, to prevent injury.
   c. An adult should stay with the child to monitor the airway and breathing until the seizure is complete.
   d. If the child vomits, immediately clear the mouth of all foreign material.
3. Stress that medical evaluation is indicated as soon as the child develops a fever.
   a. Review technique of temperature measurement.
   b. Prompt administration of antipyretic measures is necessary when the child is febrile but may not prevent a febrile seizure.
4. Review administration schedule, adverse reactions, and appropriate follow-up regarding anticonvulsant therapy.
5. Let the family know that when a child is diagnosed with febrile seizures, future events can be adequately managed at home and do not require emergency transport if <5 minutes in duration. However, caregivers should notify pediatrician of febrile illness and seizure occurrence.

Subdural Hematoma

Subdural hematoma refers to an accumulation of fluid, blood, and its degradation products within the potential space between the dura and arachnoid membranes (subdural space). Subdural hematomas are classified as acute or chronic, depending on the time between injury and the onset of symptoms. The incidence of subdural hematoma is approximately 20 to 25 per 100,000, with an estimated 42% to 82% resulting from child abuse. The outcome of pediatric subdural hematoma, with mortality rates ranging from 42% to 90%, is worse than that of epidural hematoma. When subdural hematoma is associated with child abuse, there is a 20% mortality rate and a 50% rate of neurologic morbidity.

Also, see Chapter 11, Neurologic Disorders, for care of patient who is unconscious, ICP monitoring, and other neurologic care.

Pathophysiology and Etiology

Causes

1. Direct or indirect trauma to the head:
   a. Birth trauma.
   b. Accidental causes.
   c. Purposeful violence, as in cases of child abuse.
2. Meningitis.

Classification

1. Acute syndrome—presents as an acute problem, closely related to the time of presumed injury.
2. Chronic:
   a. Signs and symptoms are nonlocalizing and subacute.
   b. This is the most common type of subdural hematoma in children.
   c. It is usually difficult to delineate the exact time and type of injury because the precipitating episode may appear relatively insignificant.

Altered Physiology

1. Trauma to the head causes tearing of the delicate subdural veins, resulting in small hemorrhages into the subdural space. (Bleeding may be of arterial origin in cases of acute subdural hematoma.)
2. As the blood breaks down, there is an increased capillary permeability and effusion of blood cells and protein into the subdural space.
3. The breakdown products of blood stimulate the growth of connective tissue and capillaries largely from the dura.
4. A membrane is formed that usually extends frontally and laterally over the hemispheres, surrounding the clot.
5. Fluid accumulates within the membrane and increases the width of the subdural space.
6. Further hemorrhages occur.
7. The lesion enlarges, compressing the brain and expanding the skull, and, if unrelieved, ultimately causes cerebral atrophy or death from compression and herniation.
8. The lesion may arrest spontaneously at any point.
9. Further bleeding may occur into an already existing sac and may increase symptoms.
10. In long-standing subdural hematoma, the fluid may disappear, leaving a constricting membrane that prevents normal brain growth.

Clinical Manifestations

Acute

1. Typically present with continuous unconsciousness from the time of injury, but child may present with a lucid interval.
2. Ensuing manifestations include deterioration of LOC, progressive hemiplegia, focal seizures, and signs of brain stem involvement and herniation (pupillary enlargement, changes in vital signs, decerebrate posturing, and respiratory failure; see Figure 42-3).

Chronic

This has a slow, gradual onset; symptoms are variable and are related to the age of the child.

1. Infants—early signs:
   a. Anorexia, difficulty feeding, and vomiting.
   b. Irritability.
   c. Low-grade fever.
   d. Retinal hemorrhages.
   e. Failure to gain weight.
2. Infants—later signs:
   a. Enlargement of the head.
   b. Bulging and pulsation of the anterior fontanelle.
   c. Tight, glossy scalp with dilated scalp veins.
   d. Strabismus, pupillary inequality, and ocular palsies (rare).

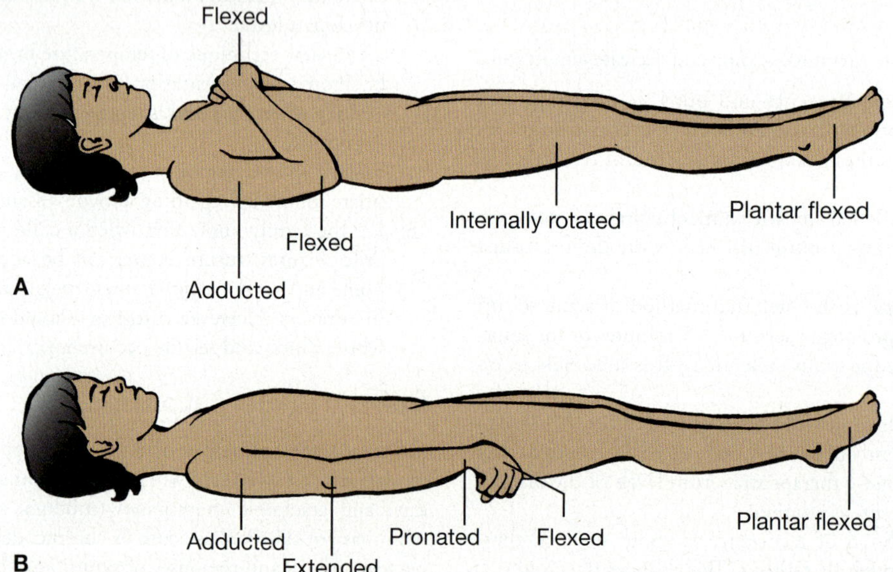

Figure 42-3. Primitive posturing in unconscious states because of loss of motor control. **(A)** Decorticate posturing occurs when cortical loss is present. **(B)** Decerebrate posturing occurs when the midbrain is involved. (Adapted with permission from Silbert-Flagg, J. [2023]. *Maternal and child health nursing: Care of the childbearing and childrearing family* [9th ed., Fig. 49-4]. Wolters Kluwer.)

   e. Hyperactive reflexes.
   f. Seizures.
   g. Delayed motor development.
3. Older children—early signs:
   a. Lethargy and anorexia.
   b. Symptoms of increased ICP (vomiting, irritability, headache).
4. Older children—later signs (may also occur immediately if bleeding takes place rapidly):
   a. Seizures.
   b. Coma.

Diagnostic Evaluation

1. Clinical features.
   a. In infants who are irritable, have failed to gain weight, and have developed an enlarged and tense fontanelle, chronic subdural hematoma should be suspected.
   b. Biparietal bulge of the head.
2. Imaging.
   a. Diagnosis and size of hematoma are confirmed by CT and, if necessary, by MRI.

Management

Acute Subdural Hematoma

This requires evacuation of the clot through a burr hole or craniotomy.

Chronic Subdural Hematoma

1. Repeated subdural taps are done to remove the collecting fluid.
   a. In infants, the needle can be inserted through the fontanelle or suture line.
   b. In older children, burr holes into the skull are necessary before the needle can be inserted.
   c. Subdural taps may be the only treatment required if the fluid disappears entirely and symptoms do not recur.
   d. Concurrently, treatment is instituted to correct anemia, electrolyte imbalance, and malnutrition.
2. Shunting procedure may be indicated if repeated taps fail to significantly reduce the volume or protein content of the subdural collections. Shunting is usually to the peritoneal cavity.

Prognosis

1. Treatment is usually successful when the diagnosis is made before cerebral atrophy and a fixed neurologic deficit have occurred. In such cases, subsequent development is normal.
2. Prognosis depends on the effect of the initial trauma on the brain and the effect of continued fluid collection.
3. Mortality in massive, acute subdural bleeding is very high, even if promptly diagnosed.

Complications

1. Intellectual disability.
2. Ocular abnormalities.
3. Seizures.
4. Spasticity and paralysis.
5. Brain stem herniation and death.
6. Neurologic impairment (cognitive or physical).

Nursing Assessment

Assess the child's neurologic status to evaluate the effectiveness of treatment or to identify disease progress.

1. Observe general behavior, especially irritability, lethargy, and evidence of personality changes. It is important to obtain a thorough history from the caregivers regarding normal behavior and level of functioning so abnormalities can be more easily recognized.
2. Evaluate appetite and feeding difficulties, including vomiting.
3. Assess vital signs for signs of increased ICP—be alert for the following:
   a. Increased systolic BP.
   b. Widened pulse pressure.
   c. Decreased pulse or irregularities.
   d. Changes in respiratory rate or difficulty breathing.
4. Assess LOC; describe response explicitly, including what type of stimulus was required to elicit a response.
5. Assess pupillary and visual changes, especially dilated pupil, double vision, lack of response to light, alterations in visual acuity, and nonsymmetric or abnormal eye movements.
6. Monitor for seizures.
7. Evaluate motor function, including ability to move all extremities. The ability to grasp should be checked and compared bilaterally.
8. Inspect for drainage of CSF from the nose or ears, indicating fractured skull with CSF leak.

Nursing Interventions

Maintaining Cerebral Tissue Perfusion

1. Avoid additional increase in ICP.
   a. Maintain a quiet environment.
   b. Avoid sudden changes in position.
   c. Organize nursing activities to allow for long periods of uninterrupted rest.
   d. Carefully regulate fluid administration to avoid danger of fluid overload.
   e. Measure urine output and record specific gravity.
   f. Administer laxatives or suppositories to prevent straining during a bowel movement.
2. Assist with subdural taps.
   a. Protect and restrain the child, as needed (see page 1151).
   b. Apply a local anesthetic cream as ordered.
   c. Hold the child securely to avoid injury caused by sudden movement.
   d. Apply firm pressure over the puncture site for a few minutes after the tap has been completed to prevent fluid leakage along the needle tract.
   e. Observe the child frequently after the procedure for shock or drainage from the site of the tap.
   f. Note whether there is serous drainage or frank blood.
   g. Reinforce the dressing, as needed, to prevent contamination of the wound.
   h. Monitor temperature frequently and monitor for signs of developing infection.
   i. Report purulent drainage from the site of the subdural tap.
3. Avoid discussing the child's condition near the bed. Even though comatose, the child may be able to hear.
4. Have emergency equipment available for resuscitation.

Preventing Complications of Immobility

1. Change the child's position frequently, and provide meticulous skin care to prevent hypostatic pneumonia and decubitus ulcers.
2. Prevent contractures.
   a. Apply passive ROM exercises to all extremities.

   b. Place pillows appropriately to support the child's body in good alignment.
   c. Use splints designed by physical therapy, as instructed.
3. Suction the child as necessary to remove secretions in the mouth and nasopharynx.
4. Observe for signs of respiratory or urinary infection related to stasis.
5. Keep the child's eyes well lubricated to prevent corneal damage.

Maintaining Nutritional Status

1. Provide nutrition and fluids through nasogastric feedings, as ordered. Observe for gastric distention.
2. Monitor urine output and specific gravity daily.
3. Monitor electrolyte and protein levels on laboratory work.
4. Do not neglect mouth care, even if child is not eating.

Strengthening Family Coping

1. Encourage the caregivers to hold and cuddle their child as much as possible.
2. Encourage the caregivers to bring diversional activities from home.
   a. Infants—mobiles or musical toys.
   b. Older children—quiet games, books, and dolls.
3. Provide emotional support to the caregivers.
   a. Encourage as much caregiver participation in the child's care as possible.
   b. Support caregivers and suggest pastoral counseling, as indicated.
4. Be nonjudgmental in cases caused by intentional or accidental trauma.
5. Make sure that cases of suspected child abuse have been reported to the appropriate agency and that caregivers have been referred for counseling.
6. Encourage visitation by siblings.

Community and Home Care Considerations

1. Follow community and home care considerations listed under "Cerebral Palsy" on page 1224.
2. Perform periodic developmental assessments, and reinforce the need to report any signs of developmental delay to the health care provider.
3. Discuss return-to-activity/play as the child progresses, as directed by the health care provider.

Family Education and Health

1. Reinforce explanations in the following areas:
   a. Condition.
   b. Causes of the child's specific symptoms.
   c. Need and rationale for treatment.
   d. Postoperative and recovery expectations.
2. Encourage caregivers to keep all follow-up appointments for medical evaluation and physical and occupational therapy.
3. Teach caregivers safety measures to prevent injuries in the future.
4. Assist caregivers in seeking additional support and resources through social work department, church groups, community agencies, or private counseling.

Evaluation: Expected Outcomes

- Drowsy but responsive to verbal stimuli; pupils equal and reactive to light; vital signs stable; ventricular tap site without drainage.
- Skin without signs of erythema or breakdown; full ROM of all joints; functional position maintained.
- Tolerates nasogastric feedings without distention; urine output sufficient.
- Caregivers participate in child's care, hold, and read to child; caregivers receive counseling.

SELECTED READINGS

Binder, H., Tiefenboeck, T. M., Majdan, M., Komjati, M., Schuster, R., Hajdu, S., & Leitgeb, J. (2020). Management and outcome of traumatic subdural hematoma in 47 infants and children from a single center. *Wiener Klinische Wochenschrift, 132*(17–18), 499–505. https://doi.org/10.1007/s00508-020-01648-3

Bitton, J. Y., Desnous, B., Sauerwein, H. C., Connolly, M., Weiss, S. K., Donner, E. J., Whiting, S., Mohamed, I. S., Wirrell, E. C., Ronen, G. M., & Lortie, A. (2021). Cognitive outcome in children with infantile spasms using a standardized treatment protocol. A five-year longitudinal study. *Seizure, 89*, 73–80. https://doi.org/10.1016/j.seizure.2021.04.027

Caynes, K., Rose, T., Theodoros, D., Burmester, D., Ware, R., & Johnston, L. (2019). The Functional Communication Classification System: Extended reliability and concurrent validity for children with cerebral palsy aged 5 to 18 years. *Developmental Medicine and Child Neurology, 61*(7), 805–812.

Connors, R., Sackett, V., Machipisa, C., Tan, K., Pharande, P., Zhou, L., & Malhotra, A. (2022). Assessing the utility of neonatal screening assessments in early diagnosis of cerebral palsy in preterm infants. *Brain Sciences, 12*(7), 847. https://doi.org/10.3390/brainsci12070847

Datta, N., & Ghosh, P. S. (2020). Update on muscular dystrophies with focus on novel treatments and biomarkers. *Current Neurology and Neuroscience Reports, 20*(6), 14. https://doi.org/10.1007/s11910-020-01034-6

Desli, E., Spilioti, M., Evangeliou, A., Styllas, F., Magkos, F., & Dalamaga, M. (2022). The efficacy and safety of ketogenic diets in drug-resistant epilepsy in children and adolescents: A systematic review of randomized controlled trials. *Current Nutrition Reports, 11*(2), 102–116. https://doi.org/10.1007/s13668-022-00405-4

Dwyer, E. R., Filion, K. B., MacFarlane, A. J., Platt, R. W., & Mehrabadi, A. (2022). Who should consume high-dose folic acid supplements before and during early pregnancy for the prevention of neural tube defects? *British Medical Journal*, 377, e067728. https://doi.org/10.1136/bmj-2021-067728

Fisher, R. S., Cross, J. H., French, J. A., Higurashi, N., Hirsch, E., Jansen, F. E., Lagae, L., Moshé, S. L., Peltola, J., Perez, E. R., Scheffer, I. E., & Zuberi, S. M. (2017). Operational classification of seizure types by the International League against Epilepsy: Position paper of the ILAE Commission for Classification and Terminology. *Epilepsia, 58*(4), 522–530.

Gonzalez-Viana, E., Sen, A., Bonnon, A., & Cross, J. H. (2022). Epilepsies in children, young people, and adults: Summary of updated nice guidance. *British Medical Journal, 378*, o1446. https://doi.org/10.1136/bmj.o1446

Houtrow, A., MacPherson, C., Jackson-Coty, J., Rivera, M., Flynn, L., Burrows, P., Adzick, N. S., Fletcher, J., Gupta, N., Howell, L., Brock, J., Lee, H., Walker, W., & Thom, E. (2020). Prenatal repair and physical functioning among children with myelomeningocele: A secondary analysis of a randomized clinical trial. *JAMA Pediatrics, 175*(4), e205674. https://doi.org/10.1001/jamapediatrics.2020.5674

Jackman, M., Sakzewski, L., Morgan, C., Boyd, R. N., Brennan, S. E., Langdon, K., Toovey, R. A., Greaves, S., Thorley, M., & Novak, I. (2021). Interventions to improve physical function for children and young people with cerebral palsy: International Clinical Practice Guideline. *Developmental Medicine & Child Neurology, 64*(5), 536–549. https://doi.org/10.1111/dmcn.15055

Jenkins, K. (2023). AAP issues clinical update to cerebral palsy guidelines: Most common neuromotor disorder of childhood. *Pediatric News, 57*(1), 4. https://www.mdedge.com/pediatrics/article/259731/neurology/aap-issues-clinical-update-cerebral-palsy-guidelines

Koleva, M., & De Jesus, O. (2022). Hydrocephalus. [Updated 2022 Jul 25]. In *StatPearls [Internet]*. StatPearls Publishing. https://www.ncbi.nlm.nih.gov/books/NBK560875/

Kourakis, S., Timpani, C. A., Campelj, D. G., Hafner, P., Gueven, N., Fischer, D., & Rybalka, E. (2021). Standard of care versus new-wave corticosteroids in the treatment of Duchenne muscular dystrophy: Can we do better? *Orphanet Journal of Rare Diseases, 16*(1), 117. https://doi.org/10.1186/s13023-021-01758-9

Lim, G. Y., Chen, C. L., & Chan Wei Shih, D. (2021). Utility and safety of perampanel in pediatric FIRES and other drug-resistant epilepsies. *Child Neurology Open, 8*, 2329048X211055335. https://doi.org/10.1177/2329048X211055335

McCartney, E. (2019). The Functional Communication Classification System for children with cerebral palsy: The potential of a new measure. *Developmental Medicine & Child Neurology, 61*(7), 741.

Ng, Y.-T. (2022). Maximizing quality of life in children with epilepsy. *Children, 10*(1), 65. https://doi.org/10.3390/children10010065

Nguyen, K., & Kohli, A. (2022). *Latex allergy*. National Center for Biotechnology Information. Retrieved March 15, 2023, from https://pubmed.ncbi.nlm.nih.gov/31424748/

Ozdemir, N., & Yilmaz, M. (2022). Examination of the relationship between the mental status and social support of parents of children with epilepsy. *Journal of Education and Research in Nursing, 19*(3), 320–327. https://doi.org/10.5152/jern.2022.76743

Patel, D. R., Neelakantan, M., Pandher, K., & Merrick, J. (2020). Cerebral palsy in children: A clinical overview. *Translational Pediatrics, 9*(S1), S125–S135. https://doi.org/10.21037/tp.2020.01.01

Pavone, P., Gulizia, C., Le Pira, A., Greco, F., Parisi, P., Di Cara, G., Falsaperla, R., Lubrano, R., Minardi, C., Spalice, A., & Ruggieri, M. (2020). Cerebral palsy and epilepsy in children: Clinical perspectives on a common comorbidity. *Children (Basel, Switzerland), 8*(1), 16. https://doi.org/10.3390/children8010016

Pellinen, J., Tafuro, E., Baehr, A., Barnard, S., Holmes, M., & French, J. (2020). The impact of clinical seizure characteristics on recognition and treatment of new-onset focal epilepsy in emergency departments. *Academic Emergency Medicine, 28*(4), 412–420. https://doi.org/10.1111/acem.14114

Pickering, C. (2021). Epilepsy: Recognition and management of seizures in children and young people. *British Journal of Child Health, 2*(3), 136–142.

Ricci, G., Bello, L., Torri, F., Schirinzi, E., Pegoraro, E., & Siciliano, G. (2022). Therapeutic opportunities and clinical outcome measures in Duchenne muscular dystrophy. *Neurological Sciences, 43*(S2), 625–633. https://doi.org/10.1007/s10072-022-06085-w

Rivera, S. R., Jhamb, S. K., Abdel-Hamid, H. Z., Acsadi, G., Brandsema, J., Ciafaloni, E., Darras, B. T., Iannaccone, S. T., Konersman, C. G., Kuntz, N. L., McDonald, C. M., Parsons, J. A., Tesi Rocha, C., Zaidman, C. M., Butterfield, R. J., Connolly, A. M., & Mathews, K. D. (2020). Medical management of muscle weakness in Duchenne muscular dystrophy. *PLoS One, 15*(10), e0240687. https://doi.org/10.1371/journal.pone.0240687

Sawires, R., Buttery, J., & Fahey, M. (2022). A review of febrile seizures: Recent advances in understanding of febrile seizure pathophysiology and commonly implicated viral triggers. *Frontiers in Pediatrics, 9*, 801321. https://doi.org/10.3389/fped.2021.801321

Şengül, Y., & Kurudirek, F. (2022). Perceived stigma and self-esteem for children with epilepsy. *Epilepsy Research, 186*, 107017. https://doi.org/10.1016/j.eplepsyres.2022.107017

Sharma, W., & Ramachandrannair, R. (2023). Sudden unexpected death in epilepsy in children. *Developmental Medicine and Child Neurology, 65*(9), 1150–1156.

Stiles-Shields, C., Shirkey, K. C., Winning, A. M., Smith, Z. R., Wartman, E., & Holmbeck, G. N. (2020). Social skills and medical responsibility across development in youth with spina bifida. *Journal of Pediatric Psychology, 46*(3), 341–350. https://doi.org/10.1093/jpepsy/jsaa113

U.S. Department of Health and Human Services. (2023). *Cerebral palsy*. National Institute of Neurological Disorders and Stroke. Retrieved March 15, 2023, from https://www.ninds.nih.gov/health-information/disorders/cerebral-palsy#toc-how-is-cerebral-palsy-diagnosed-and-treated-

U.S. Department of Health and Human Services. (2023). *Spina bifida*. National Institute of Neurological Disorders and Stroke. Retrieved March 15, 2023, from https://www.ninds.nih.gov/health-information/disorders/spina-bifida#:~:text=Diagnosing%20spina%20bifida&text=The%20most%20common%20screening%20methods,also%20perform%20an%20amniocentesis%20test

VanDerhoef, K. F., Bergmann, K., Kaila, R., Shanley, R., & Louie, J. P. (2023). A retrospective report on simple febrile seizure management in a pediatric emergency department. *Clinical Pediatrics*, 99228231188607. Advance Online Publication. https://doi.org/10.1177/00099228231188607

Venugopal, V., & Pavlakis, S. (2022). Duchenne muscular dystrophy. [Updated 2022 Jul 11]. In *StatPearls* [Internet]. StatPearls Publishing. https://www.ncbi.nlm.nih.gov/books/NBK482346/

Wolan-Nieroda, A., Łukasiewicz, A., Leszczak, J., Drużbicki, M., & Guzik, A. (2022). Assessment of functional performance in children with cerebral palsy receiving treatment in a day care facility: An observational study. *Medical Science Monitor, 28*, e936207. https://doi.org/10.12659/MSM.936207

Young, S. M., & Saguil, A. (2022). Bacterial meningitis in children. *American Family Physician, 105*(3), 311–312.

Zainel, A., Mitchell, H., & Sadarangani, M. (2021). Bacterial meningitis in children: Neurological complications, associated risk factors, and prevention. *Microorganisms, 9*(3), 535. https://doi.org/10.3390/microorganisms9030535

Zhang, Y., Mann, J. R,, James, K. A., McDermott, S., Conway, K. M., Paramsothy, P., Smith, T., & Cai, B.; MD STARnet. (2021). Duchenne and Becker muscular dystrophies' prevalence in MD STARnet surveillance sites: An examination of racial and ethnic differences. *Neuroepidemiology, 55*(1), 47–55.

43 Pediatric Eye and Ear Disorders

COMMON EYE PROBLEMS

The eye at birth is not fully developed and has limited function. From birth to 6 months of age is a critical and rapid period of development. The eye continues to develop throughout infancy and childhood and reaches visual maturity at about 10 years of age. There are many common eye problems that are inherited, idiopathic, congenital, or the result of infection or injury. Structure and function of the eye are affected. Many times, eye inflammation can be an indicator of systemic disease. See Chapter 12 for additional information on eye problems.

Infectious Processes

Infectious processes of the eye include conjunctivitis, cellulitis, hordeolum (stye), and chalazion. Signs and symptoms that occur with eye infections are red eye, tearing, discharge, pain and foreign body sensation, photophobia, abnormal red reflex, and visual disturbances.

Pathophysiology and Etiology

1. Microbes are introduced into the eye or surrounding structures including eyelids, eyebrows, and cheeks by direct contact with infected objects. Preseptal cellulitis can occur from a localized injury such as an abrasion or insect bite of the eyelid or may spread from other areas of the eye that are infected, such as hordeolum or dacryocystitis. Respiratory infections and otitis media (OM) can contribute to developing cellulitis.
2. Postseptal cellulitis occurs secondary to paranasal sinus infection, focal eye infection (infected hordeolum, dacryocystitis, dental infection), trauma to orbit such as fracture or penetrating injury, and hematogenous spread from bacteremia.
3. An inflammatory response develops with engorgement and dilation of conjunctival blood vessels with or without discharge and chemosis (edema) of the conjunctiva.
4. Common bacterial agents include *Haemophilus influenzae*, *Streptococcus pneumoniae*, *Staphylococcus aureus*, and *Moraxella catarrhalis*. Pathogens in neonates and adolescents can include *Neisseria gonorrhoeae* and *Chlamydia trachomatis*.
5. Viral infections are common and are usually caused by adenoviruses. Less commonly, coxsackievirus, enterovirus, Zika, and herpesvirus infections may occur.
6. The infecting agents are contagious and easily spread via hand-to-eye contact from infected objects (fomites). Outbreaks in which multiple children in the same family, classroom, or community are infected may occur.
7. Environmental allergens such as pollen are major contributors to conjunctivitis.

Clinical Manifestations

The normal appearance of the bulbar conjunctivae that cover the eyeballs should be clear and transparent, allowing the white sclerae to be seen. The palpebral conjunctivae that line the inner eyelids should be pink and shiny. When there is redness, it can arise from within or outside the globe. Causes range from minor eye dryness to life-threatening systemic illness. It is important to differentiate the causes of red eye because not all red eyes are caused by conjunctivitis (see Table 43-1).

Conjunctivitis

1. Acute onset of inflammation of palpebral and bulbar conjunctival layer leads to dilation of the blood vessels. Appears pink or red on inspection. Usually starts in one eye and may involve the second eye a few days later.
2. Eyelid and conjunctiva edema.
3. Excessive tearing or exudate.
4. Gritty or burning feeling in the eye and itching.
5. Photophobia with fluctuating blurring and cloudy vision.
6. May be accompanied by preauricular lymphadenopathy.

Preseptal Cellulitis

1. Unilateral swelling, redness, warmth, and tenderness of the eyelid and surrounding tissues that does not involve eyeball or internal structures.
2. No significant fever.
3. No pain with or limitation of eye movement.
4. No impaired vision.
5. Age younger than 5 years.

Table 43-1 Common Causes of Eye Redness in Children

CAUSE	ASSOCIATED SYMPTOMS	MANAGEMENT
Conjunctivitis		
Viral	Associated with other symptoms of systemic viral illness, watery discharge, burning, irritation, tearing	Hygiene (see page 1254), rest, cool compresses, artificial tears
Bacterial	Redness, thick purulent discharge, eyelids stick together after sleep, foreign body sensation	Antibiotic eyedrops or ointment, hygiene
Chlamydial	Cough, stringy mucus discharge, history of maternal infection	Systemic antibiotic
Herpetic	Pain, photophobia, vesicular skin lesions on erythematous base	Evaluation by specialist, antiviral agents
Allergic	Itching, bilateral, watery discharge, seasonal onset, other allergic symptoms (rhinorrhea, allergic shiners), cobblestoning of inner eyelids	Topical mast cell stabilizer/antihistamine eyedrops, oral antihistamines, avoidance of allergens, cool compresses several times per day
Chemical	Watery discharge, onset of symptoms when exposed to cigarettes or other irritants	Avoidance of irritating substances
Trauma	Pain, photophobia, increased tear production	May require eye protection, referral to a specialist
Congenital glaucoma	Increased tear production, cloudiness of the cornea	Referral to specialist

Postseptal Cellulitis (Orbital)

1. Red eye. Infection involves eyeball and structures posterior to orbital septum.
2. Pain of the eye area; also sinus, headache, tooth pain.
3. Proptosis (bulging eyeball).
4. Purulent discharge from the eye, nasal congestion
5. Fever.
6. Limited mobility of the eye (reduced visual acuity in advanced cases)
7. Age older than 5 years.

Hordeolum (Stye)

1. Acute inflammation of lubricating glands (glands of Zeis) of eyelids and eyelashes.
2. Begin as diffuse swelling of the area that develops into a nodule of eyelash follicle, accompanied by tenderness.
3. Treat with warm compresses applied four to six times a day. May take weeks to resolve.

Chalazion

1. Deeper, internal inflammation due to obstruction of Meibomian gland opening. Eyelid swelling and erythema.
2. "Lump under the eyelid."
3. Treat with warm compresses applied four to six times a day.

Diagnostic Evaluation

1. Treatment is usually based on clinical signs and symptoms. Laboratory studies and cultures are not routinely obtained.
2. Inspect eye. Screen for visual acuity, assess red reflex, assess eye movement.
3. A dendritic ulcer caused by herpesvirus can be visualized by instilling fluorescein dye and examining the cornea with a cobalt-filtered blue light, looking for the dendrite lesion.
4. Clinical evaluation and computed tomography (CT) scan are the best methods to distinguish preseptal from postseptal cellulitis.
5. In newborns, obtain culture swabs for *N. gonorrheae*, *C. trachomatis* and *herpes simplex virus (HSV)*. Do not delay treatment.

CLINICAL JUDGMENT A child who has a painful red eye should be referred immediately for medical evaluation because this could indicate an infectious process, exposure to a chemical or foreign body, or other traumatic etiology.

Management

1. Allergic conjunctivitis may respond to removal of the underlying allergen and avoidance of eye rubbing. Treatment includes systemic or topical agents such as antihistamines, mast cell stabilizers, and/or corticosteroids.
2. Antibiotic eyedrops or ointment—such as erythromycin, trimethoprim sulfate and polymyxin B, sulfacetamide, ciprofloxacin, tobramycin, azithromycin, or doxycycline—will shorten the course of bacterial conjunctivitis and make the child more comfortable.
3. Hordeolum and chalazion resolve without antibiotic treatment. Warm compresses applied four times daily are recommended. Lid washes of diluted baby shampoo in water aid with drainage. Incision and drainage may be necessary to promote healing of long-standing chalazion.
4. Postseptal (orbital) cellulitis is vision- and life threatening. Admission to the hospital and treatment with systemic antibiotics are recommended for 48 to 72 hours followed by a 1- to 3-week course of oral antibiotics. Treatment of community-acquired methicillin-resistant *S. aureus* (CA-MRSA) must be considered in severe cases of postseptal cellulitis. A multidisciplinary approach—including an ophthalmologist, infectious disease specialist, otorhinolaryngologist, and a neurosurgeon—is indicated.

DRUG ALERT Topical corticosteroids should only be prescribed as needed when a herpetic infection has definitively been ruled out. Topical corticosteroids can aggravate a herpetic infection.

Complications

1. Permanent scarring of the cornea and visual impairment with *HSV, N. gonorrhoeae*, and *C. trachomatis*.
2. Spread of postseptal cellulitis to the central nervous system, with optic nerve damage, vision loss, ptosis, and strabismus.
3. Eyelid deformity.
4. Septicemia.

Nursing Assessment

1. Assess nature and extent of symptoms and their effect on child's activities.
2. Assess visual acuity.
3. Determine resources available to the family for treatment and rehabilitation.

Nursing Interventions

Preventing Spread of Infection

1. Perform or teach proper cleansing of drainage.
   a. Use warm water or saline and a disposable applicator, such as cotton balls or gauze.
   b. Use a separate applicator for each eye.
   c. Wipe from inner to outer canthus to avoid contamination of the other eye.
2. Teach self-care measures to prevent spread to others.
   a. Observe good handwashing practices.
   b. Wipe eyes and nose with tissues and dispose promptly. Do not wipe the nose and then eyes with the same tissue.
   c. Avoid rubbing eyes to prevent spread.
3. Administer and teach proper instillation of eyedrops or ointment (see pages 415 and 417).
4. Administer oral or intravenous (IV) antibiotics, as prescribed.
5. Advise caregivers to only use eyedrops prescribed or recommended by a health care provider and dispose of leftover medication at the end of treatment period.

Minimizing Pain

1. Apply warm compresses to the affected area.
2. Suggest darkened room and sunglasses for patients with photophobia.
3. Administer an analgesic, as prescribed.
4. Administer lubricating eyedrops and ointment, as needed.
5. Minimize environmental stimulation.

Family Education and Health Maintenance

1. Educate to prevent modes of transmission.
   a. Handwashing is the most important factor in infection control.
   b. Do not share washcloths, towels, or handkerchiefs.
   c. Change pillowcases frequently.
   d. Avoid swimming until the infection is resolved.
   e. Return child to school only after having received antibiotic treatment for 24 hours.
   f. Dispose of contaminated items in proper receptacles.
   g. Discontinue use of contact lenses until the infection is cleared.
2. Advise caregivers of indications for reevaluation by health care provider.
   a. Lack of response to antibiotic treatment.
   b. Increased swelling and tenderness; any eye pain.
   c. Worsening of visual acuity.
   d. Identification of dry eye.
   e. Development of additional symptoms such as fever.
3. Encourage routine follow-up visits and vision evaluation.
4. Advise about proper detection and early treatment of sinus, dental, and other infections.
5. Recommend updated immunization, including the *H. influenzae* type B vaccine in children.

Evaluation: Expected Outcomes

- Caregivers perform treatment correctly; hygiene procedures followed.
- Patient verbalizes less pain; tolerates bright light.

Congenital Problems

Congenital problems of the eye include structural defects present at birth or developing soon thereafter. These include cataract, dacryostenosis, glaucoma, ptosis, and strabismus. See Table 43-2 for pathophysiology, clinical manifestations, and management of each.

Nursing Assessment

1. Assess for red light reflex, especially in neonates and infants. Absence or asymmetry of the red light reflex may indicate congenital cataract or an intraocular tumor or other eye disease.
2. Inspect the eyes for redness of the conjunctiva, cloudiness of the cornea, excessive tearing, drooping eyelids that partially occlude the pupil, or obvious misalignment, which provide clues to congenital eye problems.
3. Assess visual acuity routinely in infants and children. Changes in acuity may be the first manifestation of a problem or indication of effectiveness of treatment. Prompt referral to a specialist is necessary.
4. Perform pupillary light reflex test using a penlight or "muscle light" or use a distant light source to help detect strabismus.
   a. Hirschberg test for symmetry of the pupillary light reflexes—normally, the light reflexes are in the same position in each pupil when a light is shone on the bridge of the nose, but asymmetrical reflection will occur with strabismus (positive Hirschberg test).
5. Perform the cover–uncover test to detect latent strabismus caused by weak eye muscles. When the patient is fixated on an object approximately 12 inches (30.5 cm) away, cover one eye. The eye with weak muscles will drift when covered and will snap back when uncovered. An eye with normal muscles will remain straight.

Nursing Interventions

Minimizing Effects of Vision Loss

1. Participate in visual acuity problem identification and encourage prompt treatment to minimize functional impairment. Accurate assessment of (corrected) monocular visual acuity is the single most important element in an examination.
   a. Effective newborn screening in the nursery helps to detect congenital eye problems.
   b. All children should be screened for visual acuity and strabismus. In young children, this is accomplished by physical examination and assessment of developmental milestones (i.e., looks at caregiver's face, smiles responsively, reaches for objects). Instrument-based photoscreening can assess preverbal children. Special assessment tools are available to assess preverbal children. By age 3 to 5 years, most children can cooperate for performance of accurate visual acuity screening tests.

Table 43-2 Congenital Eye Problems

CONDITION AND DESCRIPTION	CLINICAL MANIFESTATIONS	MANAGEMENT
Congenital Cataract		
Opacity of the lens. Possible causes include abnormal embryonic development, intrauterine infection, metabolic disorders, and retinopathy of prematurity. Incidence is 1 in 250 neonates.	• Absence of red reflex. • Visible clouding of lens. • Varying impairment of vision, depending on size, location, and density of the cataract. • May result in amblyopia.	• Surgical removal within first 3 mo to promote visual stimulation. • Postoperative care: sedation for first 24 h to prevent crying, vomiting, and increased IOP; dilating eyedrops; antibiotic and steroid ointments to prevent infection; eye patch and shield for several days. • Aggressive optical therapy and patching of nonoperative eye; monitoring for IOP.
Dacryostenosis		
Relatively common obstruction of the nasolacrimal duct caused by incomplete duct development and persistence of membrane at the lower end of duct. Tears cannot exit via the duct into the nasal cavity and continuously spill over onto the cheek. May be unilateral or bilateral.	• Excessive tearing and spilling onto cheek. • Crusted eyelashes and lids. • Excoriated cheek. • Normal-appearing eye structures and vision. • Possible episodes of secondary conjunctivitis and lacrimal duct infection. • Increased risk of dacryocystitis.	• Resolves spontaneously in 90% of infants in the first year of life. • Gentle massage of lacrimal duct four times daily. • Topical antibiotics for secondary infection. • Surgical probing of duct if persists beyond age 12 mo; more complex surgery if probing unsuccessful.
Glaucoma		
Rare, congenital, or acquired abnormality in which the balance between aqueous fluid production and outflow is disrupted. Increased pressure of fluid in the anterior chamber causes damage to the retina, cornea, and other structures.	• Corneal enlargement. • Haziness of the cornea. • Photophobia and intolerance to ordinary light. • Excessive tearing. • Decreased visual acuity (symptoms present in 35% at birth). • Amblyopia and permanent loss may result without treatment.	• Early diagnosis is essential. • Monitoring of IOP by tonometry and central corneal thickness by pachymetry and fundoscopy. • Medical therapy. • Surgical intervention is first-line treatment. • Postoperatively, a patch and shield may be worn for several days to protect sutures. • Lifetime follow-up.
Ptosis		
Drooping of the upper eyelid caused by weakness of levator palpebrae or, less frequently, Müller muscle. May be congenital or acquired. Affects either the muscle or the nerve that innervates it. Particularly challenging to treat if amblyopia is also present.	• Drooping is visible on inspection. • Vision may be impaired if eyelid covers the pupil. • May be unilateral or bilateral. • If unilateral, amblyopia may result without treatment.	• Surgical correction to raise the eyelid and increase visual field. • Patching not necessary postoperatively. • Nonsurgical modalities, such as the use of "crutch" glasses to support the eyelid.
Strabismus		
Malalignment of the eyes caused by muscle imbalance or by paralysis, which prevents both eyes from focusing correctly on the same image. Affects 2%–5% of the preschool population. Can cause visual and psychological disability.	• Asymmetric pupillary light reflexes. • Asymmetric extraocular movements. • Diplopia, impaired depth. • Tendency to close one eye or tilt head during vision testing. • Amblyopia may result without treatment.	• Early and rigorous amblyopic occlusion therapy (patching of the stronger eye for a prescribed period each day may correct latent strabismus by exercising the muscles of the weaker eye). • Correction of refractive error. • Surgical repositioning of the extraocular muscles for severe or fixed cases. • Postoperatively: antibiotic ointment, no eye patch.

IOP, intraocular pressure.

2. Encourage and assist caregivers in obtaining corrective lenses for the child.
3. Advise and encourage caregivers to adhere to the postoperative treatment plan, such as occlusion therapy following cataract surgery or proper use of eyedrops after glaucoma surgery.
4. Encourage and assist caregivers in providing normal experiences for child to achieve maximum potential:
   a. Assist caregivers in locating and accessing resources, such as financial assistance, special education in Braille, or caregiver support groups.
   b. Remind caregivers of their child's right to an education.

Minimizing Body Image Disturbance

1. Encourage caregivers to focus on normalization rather than on overprotection. Place expectations on the child's abilities rather than disabilities, provide opportunities for interaction with peers, and make the child's life as normal as possible.
2. Encourage acceptance of appearance and emphasize the positive aspects of treatment.

Preventing Injury

1. Encourage the family to be aware of safety in the home, school, and community.
   a. Suggest the use of impact-resistant polycarbonate eyeglasses and devices to keep eyeglasses in place.
   b. Advise the family to maintain a consistent and uncluttered furniture arrangement; notify the child of planned changes.
   c. Instruct child in the use of a cane or other assistive device, if warranted.
   d. Teach traffic safety and personal security measures.
2. Orient visually impaired children to their immediate environment.
   a. Orient child to food placement on meal trays.
   b. Assist child with ambulation, and use side rails on bed or crib to prevent falls.

Promoting Normal Growth and Development

1. Encourage caregivers to provide many sensory opportunities, such as manipulating objects, hearing various sounds, noting the smells in the environment, and tasting an assortment of substances.
2. Allow the child to perform activities of daily living (ADLs) as independently as possible.

Family Education and Health Maintenance

Postoperative Teaching

1. In the interest of hygiene and safety, the patient (if older) and caregiver should be taught correct handwashing techniques before and after instilling eye medication, particularly eyedrops. This must be reinforced before discharge.
2. Teach about instillation of medications and use of eye shield to prevent injury to the operative eye after surgery.
3. Teach about activity restrictions after glaucoma surgery.
   a. Bed rest may be required immediately postoperatively.
   b. Older children should not engage in strenuous activity or contact sports for 2 weeks.
4. Advise that activity is not usually restricted after the repair of ptosis.
5. Following strabismus repair, strenuous activity, contact sports, and swimming are restricted for 2 to 4 weeks.
6. After cataract surgery because of inflammatory reaction, encourage behaviors to reduce the risk of damage to sutures from increased intraocular pressure (IOP):
   a. Prevent vomiting.
   b. Minimize crying.
   c. Encourage intense occlusion therapy and use of optical correction with glasses or contact lenses as advised.
7. Encourage caregivers to remove eye discharge or crusts on lashes regularly by wiping the eyes with warm water. Separate washcloths should be used for each eye and each child. Moistened cotton balls may be used.
8. Advise and encourage about the importance of keeping postoperative follow-up appointments.
9. Advise of indications that would require reevaluation by health care provider:
   a. Worsening of visual acuity.
   b. Evidence of inflammation and infection, such as pain, redness, swelling, drainage, and increased temperature.
10. Refer family to Prevent Blindness America (www.preventblindness.org) for information on eye disease and safety measures. For patients with cataracts or glaucoma, refer to the Pediatric Glaucoma and Cataract Family Association (www.pgcfa.org). Lighthouse International (www.lighthouse.org) aids with rehabilitation of visual impairment.

Evaluation: Expected Outcomes

- Child wears glasses or contact lenses, as prescribed; good visual outcome with adequate optical rehabilitation.
- Caregivers and child report involvement in activities, satisfactory school performance, and positive peer interactions.
- No injuries reported.
- Achieves age-appropriate developmental milestones.

Eye Trauma

EVIDENCE BASE Gervasio, K., & Peck, T. (2022). *The Wills Eye Manual: Office and emergency room diagnosis and treatment of eye disease* (8th ed.). Wolters Kluwer.

Eye trauma causes structural damage to the eye and is produced by mechanical force or contact with a corrosive chemical. Common types of eye trauma are corneal abrasions, blunt trauma, perforating injuries, and chemical injuries. Eye injuries are common among children and are usually related to their involvement in vigorous play activities.

Pathophysiology and Etiology

Corneal Abrasion

1. Injury to corneal epithelium.
2. This may happen when a foreign object becomes lodged in the eye (e.g., dust particle; contact lens rubbing against the eye because of inadequate tear production; injury from a fingernail, tree branch, or other sharp object entering the eye, and scraping the cornea).
3. May occur from the effects of general anesthetic, which cause decreased tear production, decreased eyelid reflexes, decreased perception of pain, and failure of the eye to close properly.
4. May result from corneal exposure with such conditions as ptosis or pressure on the globe, especially in the presence of dry eyes.
5. May result from contact with household or industrial chemicals.

Blunt Trauma

1. Occurs when the eye or surrounding tissues are struck by a blunt object such as a ball, a hockey puck, a bat, a stick, or an air gun. May occur with airbag deployment in a motor vehicle accident.
2. The resulting injury depends on the size, hardness, and velocity of the blunt object and the force imparted. Injury may include tissue swelling and seepage of blood into the surrounding tissues.
3. The bony structures surrounding the eye may be fractured.
4. Subconjunctival hemorrhage, lens dislocation, hyphema (blood in the anterior chamber of the eye), and a retinal detachment may occur.

Perforating Injury

1. When an object penetrates the eyeball, there may be loss of vitreous material and/or damage to the internal structures of the eye—vitreous hemorrhage, choroidal rupture, retinal tears, retinal detachment, and ruptured globe.
2. Bacteria may also be introduced into the interior of the eye causing infection.

Chemical Injury

1. Corrosive chemicals burn the delicate tissues of the cornea and may penetrate into deeper layers of the eye.
2. Healing may occur with scarring.

CLINICAL JUDGMENT A chemical injury is a medical emergency.

Clinical Manifestations

1. Pain or sensation of a foreign body in the affected eye—because of the high concentration of nerve endings in the cornea from the ciliary body.
2. Increased tear production—one of the eye's defenses against injury or irritation.
3. Enlargement of the blood vessels of the cornea—increase of blood flow to the cornea is another protective mechanism; most likely seen with foreign bodies, abrasions, or chemical burns that affect the cornea.
4. Impaired visual acuity caused by:
   a. Swelling of the cornea, reducing its clarity.
   b. Swelling of the soft tissues surrounding the eye, causing the eye to partially or completely close.
   c. Excessive tear production, impairing vision.
   d. Damage to internal structures of the eye, altering or obstructing visual pathways.
5. Visible signs of injury—bruising, swelling, or a foreign object visible in the eye.

CLINICAL JUDGMENT At times, pain may be useful in distinguishing a serious eye problem from a self-limiting condition.

Diagnostic Evaluation

1. Thorough inspection of the eye, including eversion of the upper lid to inspect for a foreign object.
2. A slit-lamp examination to determine the extent of the corneal abrasion.
3. Fundoscopic examination may detect abnormalities, such as a dislodged lens, retinal hemorrhage, retinal detachment, or papilledema with increased IOP.
4. Staining with fluorescein dye reveals lesions of the cornea such as abrasions.
5. Assessment of eye function, including near and far acuity, extraocular movements, and visual field testing.
6. Computed tomography (CT) scan of orbit(s) and brain if concern for fracture or brain hemorrhage.

Management

Early detection and prompt intervention may help reduce the incidence of ocular morbidity.

Corneal Abrasion

1. Removal of the offending foreign body, such as contact lens.
2. Antibiotic drops or ointment for superficial abrasion.
3. For infected or inflamed abrasion, antibiotic eyedrops or ointment to prevent infection and anti-inflammatory drops to decrease inflammation.
4. Follow up for any recurrent symptoms because recurrent corneal erosion can occur months or years following injury because of spontaneous disruption of corneal epithelium that occurs near the site of the corneal abrasion.

CLINICAL JUDGMENT Avoid use of topical anesthetic for pain after the initial examination because this will slow down the healing process. Avoid the use of contact lens until the abrasion has healed. Patching is no longer recommended because it reduces the removal of pathogens by the tear film.

Blunt Trauma

1. The head should be elevated 45 degrees to facilitate settling of hyphema, if present.
2. Hospitalization may be necessary for patients who are nonadherent, patients with blood disorders such as sickle cell trait or disease, or if child abuse is suspected.
3. Surgery may be required because of damage to underlying bones or eye structures.

Perforating Injury

1. Surgery is usually necessary to remove the object and reconstruct damaged tissues.
2. The head should be elevated 30 degrees. Avoid sneezing, nose blowing, and any activity.
3. The child should be kept on nothing-by-mouth status in preparation for surgery. Avoid topical medications. Tetanus toxoid should be given if older than 5 years since the last dose or unknown immunization status.

CLINICAL JUDGMENT Never remove a penetrating object from the eye. It should be stabilized, and the eye should be shielded with a Fox shield, with no pressure applied. In an emergency, use a foam cup with part of the bottom cut off, if necessary, to support the object.

Chemical Injury

1. Continuous, gentle flushing of the affected eye(s) with any available water until able to change to normal saline solution or Ringer lactate solution for at least 30 minutes (see pages 415 and 417) to help remove the offending chemical. Evert the eyelids and flush from the inner aspect of the eye outward to prevent contaminated water from flowing into the other eye. Wash the patient's face and hands.

2. Measure pH every 10 to 15 minutes, should be 6.5 to 7.5
3. Further management depends on the nature and extent of the injury.

CLINICAL JUDGMENT Acid chemicals coagulate the conjunctival protein, leaving the blood vessels undamaged. Alkaline chemicals rapidly permeate the eye's structure, thus causing more damage.

Complications

1. Infection.
2. Bleeding.
3. Refractive problems because of corneal scar, cataract, glaucoma, shrinkage of the affected eye, and inflammation of the unaffected eye may result in vision impairment or loss of vision.
4. Disfigurement may result from severe or extensive tissue damage.

Nursing Assessment

1. Obtain history of injury, including the child's account of how the injury occurred, and a description of symptoms experienced.
2. Inspect for location and extent of swelling and bruising, asymmetry, or abnormality in appearance of any part of the eye.
3. Obtain visual history preinjury. Assess visual acuity. This should include near and far acuity in each eye. If the patient cannot see well enough to read a Snellen chart, assess the ability to count fingers or perceive light. Compare findings with preinjury visual history.

Nursing Interventions

Minimizing Pain

1. Apply cold compresses to the affected area to help reduce swelling and discomfort.
2. Keep the child's room as dark as possible to help reduce pain for patients with photophobia.
3. Administer analgesics, as prescribed.
4. Encourage quiet activities to act as a distraction to pain.

Preventing Injury

1. Enforce safety measures:
   a. Use of bedside rails.
   b. Assistance with ambulation.
   c. Close observation.

Maintaining ADLs

1. Provide assistance with eating, bathing, toileting, and other ADLs, as needed.
2. Teach child location of self-care items and positioning of food on tray to promote independence.
3. Encourage the child to attempt self-care and offer praise even if unsuccessful.

Family Education and Health Maintenance

1. Teach indications for reevaluation by health care provider.
   a. Increase in swelling, tenderness, discoloration, or pain.
   b. Worsening of visual acuity.
   c. Development of additional symptoms, such as fever, alteration in sensorium, or other indications of neurologic injury.
2. Provide safety education to all families to prevent common causes of injury. Encourage families to use protective eyewear when participating in sports or other activities; proper placement of infant car seat, booster seat, and seat belt; proper storage of household chemicals.
3. Provide families with information and support as they cope with having a visually impaired child in the home. The American Council of the Blind has multiple resources for families on its website (https://acb.org).

Evaluation: Expected Outcomes

- Demonstrates decreased pain.
- No injuries reported.
- Dressing and feeding self with minimal assistance.

Functional Problems

Normal visual development requires stimuli from both eyes and the brain's ability to fuse a focused image from each eye into a single image. Any alteration in function between the brain and the eyes during this period of early development may result in a reduction of visual acuity known as amblyopia. Treatment of amblyopia involves identifying and correcting the cause during the early critical period of visual development. There are three subtypes of amblyopia: strabismic, refractive, and deprivation.

Pathophysiology and Etiology

1. Strabismic amblyopia is a condition of eyeball misalignment that results in the inability of both eyes to fixate on the same object, causing two images. The brain suppresses one image to prevent double vision, causing reduced visual acuity in the nonfixating eye.
2. Refractive amblyopia is a result of unequal refractive errors between the two eyes. Each retina is presented with different image clarity. One image is focused and the other is not. Amblyopia may develop in the eye with an unfocused image.
   a. In an elongated or shortened eyeball, the visual image is focused either in front of or behind the retina, resulting in unclear images.
   b. The child with myopia (nearsightedness) can see near objects, such as print in schoolbooks, but cannot focus clearly on far objects, such as words on large classroom viewing devices including chalkboards (with dark backgrounds) and smart board screens.
   c. The child with hyperopia (farsightedness) can see far objects clearly but has difficulty seeing near objects.
   d. May be unilateral or bilateral.
3. Deprivation amblyopia results from deprivation of visual stimuli, disrupting the normal ability to form images at an early age. Cataracts, ptosis, corneal diseases, and vitreous hemorrhage can cause deprivation amblyopia.

Clinical Manifestations

Children usually do not verbalize that they cannot see well but may exhibit other signs of vision problems, including:

1. Poor academic performance or behavioral problems in school.
2. Dislike for reading.
3. Head tilting.
4. Headaches.
5. Squinting.

6. Sitting close to the television or holding reading materials close to the face.
7. Refusal or resistance to covering one eye during vision screening.

Diagnostic Evaluation

1. Standardized vision screening tests using optotype (shapes, symbols) for preschool children such as LEA which uses 4 shapes - apple, house, square, circle. HOTV using the letters H T O V
   a. Tests can be administered to children as young as age 3 years.
   b. Each eye should be tested separately, making sure the nontested eye is occluded.
   c. A two-line difference between eyes requires referral to an ophthalmologist.
2. The Snellen vision acuity test is a letter chart. It is the gold standard for testing visual acuity in children who are able to verbalize and identify the letters of the alphabet.

Management

1. Most visual acuity problems can be treated by the use of corrective lenses or refractive surgery.
2. Amblyopia management focuses on prevention through early identification and treatment of conditions that caused it.
   a. Strabismus is treated by patching the stronger eye to strengthen the weaker eye. Glasses may also be prescribed to improve the vision. In some cases, however, surgery may be required.
   b. Topical miotic drops may be used if the child is not able to tolerate the daily patching required to correct amblyopia.
   c. Surgery may also be required to correct ptosis.
   d. Acuity problems because of refractive error are usually managed with the use of corrective lenses.
3. Optimal outcome is accomplished when treatment is begun early in life, whereas visual pathways are still developing. However, some visual functions may be recovered even if the problem is treated in adolescence or adulthood. Ideally, the problem can be prevented by early identification and treatment of factors that may cause it.

EVIDENCE BASE Sen, S., Singh, P., & Saxena, R. (2022). Management of amblyopia in pediatric patients: Current insights. *Eye, 36*, 44–56.

Complications

Injuries caused by visual impairment.

Nursing Assessment

1. Begin visual acuity screening early, in the preschool years, and whenever a child displays behaviors suggestive of visual acuity problems.
2. Children at risk for vision problems include those with a history of prematurity, family history of congenital eye problems, significant developmental delay, and systemic disease associated with eye problems.
3. Assess Hirschberg test for symmetry of the pupillary light reflexes routinely, beginning at birth.
4. Perform the cover–uncover test as part of routine eye assessment.
5. Assess the effect of the functional deficit on the child's overall function, including academic progress, self-esteem, and safety.

Nursing Interventions

Minimizing Effects of Sensory Deficits

1. Encourage the consistent use of corrective lenses, as prescribed.
2. Teach caregivers ways to help develop the child's skills in interpreting information through the senses of hearing, smell, and touch.
   a. Familiarize the child with common sounds and smells in the environment. Also, orient the child to traffic sounds and sounds associated with danger, such as animals and speeding vehicles, and instruct the child how to respond.
   b. Use voice or touch, rather than facial expressions or gestures, to express emotion.
   c. Speak to the child before touching to reduce startling.
   d. Allow the child to touch and handle unfamiliar objects to learn about them.
   e. Have the child practice such things as retelling stories and giving the home telephone number and address.
   f. Explain unfamiliar sounds and smells to the hospitalized child.

Preventing Injury

1. Recommend the use of shatterproof eyeglasses with flexible frames.
2. Recommend the use of eye protection on a routine basis because eye trauma can occur unexpectedly. This is especially important for children who rely on only one eye.
3. Suggest extra protection, such as shatterproof goggles or shields, when participating in contact or ball sports and activities.
4. Maintain a stable arrangement of furniture in the home, adequate lighting, and an uncluttered environment to minimize falls.
5. Orient hospitalized children to the hospital room and offer assistance when walking.

Promoting a Positive Sense of Self-esteem

1. Provide opportunities for mastery of developmentally appropriate activities such as tablet computer applications.
2. Encourage interactions with sighted children to decrease feelings of isolation. Also, suggest interactions with children with similar alterations in vision.
3. Encourage the child to discuss feelings and strategies for coping with negative peer reactions such as teasing.
4. Encourage independence in self-care activities to promote autonomy, such as dressing, cooking, feeding, and use of bathroom.
5. Assist the patient and family with effective coping mechanisms to promote family stability.

Community and Home Care Considerations

1. Perform a safety inspection of the home environment and make changes as necessary to help prevent falls and other injuries.
2. Assist family with access to financial and social resources, as needed.
3. Make sure that the child is receiving early intervention services and individualized educational resources.

Family Education and Health Maintenance

1. Teach the importance of patching for amblyopia and the wearing of corrective lenses, as prescribed, and their proper care.

2. Refer families of blind children to community resources that can help their child learn special skills, such as reading Braille, using a cane, or developing self-care skills. Information can be obtained from agencies such as the American Foundation for the Blind (www.afb.org).

Evaluation: Expected Outcomes

- Identifies common sounds.
- No injury reported; wears protective eyeglasses.
- Reports good school performance and participation in extracurricular activities; can eat and dress independently.

COMMON EAR PROBLEMS

Also see Chapter 13 for additional information on ear, nose, and throat problems.

Eustachian Tube Dysfunction

The eustachian tube connects the middle ear to the nasopharynx. *Eustachian tube dysfunction (ETD)* is a term describing disorders that arise from the opening and closing of the eustachian tube, which ventilates the middle ear to equalize pressure on both sides of the tympanic membrane. The eustachian tube also protects the middle ear from infection because its ciliated epithelium enables clearance of middle ear secretions and acts as a barrier to the reflux of pathogens from the nasopharynx. ETD is often associated with otitis media with effusion (OME), also known as serous otitis; acute otitis media (AOM) and recurrent otitis media (OM). Approximately 90% of children experience one or more episodes of middle ear effusion by age 2 years.

Pathophysiology and Etiology

1. Inflammation of the eustachian tube lining is caused by an acute upper respiratory infection, an allergic response, trauma, or inflammation of the middle ear mucosa.
   a. Infected secretions may pass through the tube from the nasal area into the middle ear.
   b. When inflammation and swelling cause the eustachian tube to become obstructed, the passage of air into and out of the middle ear is prevented.
   c. The air in the middle ear is absorbed into the middle ear lining, and a vacuum is created.
   d. The vacuum is filled by serous fluid that seeps out of the middle ear lining.
   e. The warm, moist environment of the middle ear and nutrients in the serous fluid are conducive to the growth of viruses or bacteria that may be present in the middle ear cavity.
2. Children are predisposed to the development of AOM because their short, floppy, horizontal eustachian tubes more easily allow the passage of infected nasal secretions into the middle ear cavity. See Box 43-1 for additional risk factors.
3. Viruses account for 15% to 20% of AOM cases. In 30% of AOM cases, there is no identifiable bacterial pathogen. The most common bacterial agents include:
   a. *Streptococcus pneumoniae.*
   b. Nontypeable *Haemophilus influenzae.*
   c. *Moraxella catarrhalis.*
4. Barotrauma, caused by sudden changes in atmospheric pressure (as occur in deep underwater swimming and air travel), may also lead to the closure of the eustachian tube and to the development of serous otitis and hemotympanum. Barotrauma is less likely to involve the introduction of microorganisms through infected nasal secretions; development of AOM is less common.

BOX 43-1 Risk Factors for Eustachian Tube Dysfunction

- Frequent episodes of upper respiratory infections in younger children.
- Nasal allergies.
- Genetic predisposition to floppy eustachian tube.
- Native American or Eskimo heritage.
- Craniofacial abnormalities such as cleft lip and palate and Down syndrome.
- Enlarged adenoids.
- Lower socioeconomic status.
- Exposure to tobacco smoke.
- Bottle-feeding.
- Being a person assigned male at birth.
- Day care attendance with greater than six attendees.
- Caregiver or biologic sibling history of otitis media (OM).
- Immune deficiencies such as cystic fibrosis.

EVIDENCE BASE Maddineni, S., & Ahmad, I. (2022). Updates in eustachian tube dysfunction. *Otolaryngologic Clinics of North America, 55*(6), 1151–1164. https://doi.org/10.1016/j.otc.2022.07.010

Clinical Manifestations

1. OME—decreased hearing, sensation of fullness in the affected ear(s) without pain or fever.
2. AOM—ear pain (otalgia) and signs of infection fever, fussiness, or decreased appetite.
3. ETD—popping sensations in the affected ear(s).

Diagnostic Evaluation

1. Otoscopic examination.
   a. OME—nonpurulent mucoid or serous effusion, prominent bony landmarks, a diffuse light reflex, and decreased mobility of tympanic membrane.
   b. AOM—inflamed tympanic membrane with purulent effusion and decreased or absent mobility; bulging of the tympanic membrane may obscure the bony landmarks and light reflex.
2. Tympanometry—quick and simple way to assess tympanic membrane mobility in children over 7 months of age.
   a. A probe occludes the ear canal while pressure is varied and a test sound is emitted. The test produces a graphic display that shows the mobility of the tympanic membrane at various air pressures. A normal reading has a distinct peak in the middle of the graph.
   b. A flat tympanogram (no peak) indicates a lack of mobility of the tympanic membrane, usually caused by serous otitis or AOM.
   c. A peak to the left of the center indicates negative pressure in the middle ear.

Management

EVIDENCE BASE Otteson, T. (2022). Otitis media and tympanostomy tubes. *Pediatric Clinics of North America, 69*(2), 203–219. https://doi.org/10.1016/j.pcl.2022.01.001

Otitis Media With Effusion

1. Usually resolves spontaneously, but 30% to 40% of patients have repeated episodes, and approximately 25% have persistent effusion after 3 months.
2. OME is the leading cause of hearing loss, so interval visits for reexamination and hearing testing should be done. Hearing levels (HLs) of 40 dB or above require an immediate, complete audiologic evaluation and may indicate pressure equalization tubes (PETs). Persistent effusions of greater than 3 months and any concern for speech and language delay indicate the need for referral to an otolaryngologist.
3. Patients younger than 4 years of age with persistent OME should have PETs placed, and patients 4 years of age and older should have PETs placed with or without adenoidectomy.
4. Hearing evaluation should be obtained if OME persists for 3 months or longer *or* prior to surgery when the child is a candidate for tube placement.
5. Pharmacologic treatment with medications such as antihistamines, decongestants, antimicrobials, and corticosteroids is not indicated.
6. Tonsillectomy is not recommended.

EVIDENCE BASE Spoialâ, E. L., Stanciu, G. D., Bild, V., Ababei, D. C., & Gavrilovici, C. (2021). From evidence to clinical guidelines in antibiotic treatment in acute otitis media in children. *Antibiotics, 10*(1), 52. https://doi.org/10.3390/antibiotics10010052

Hoberman, A., Preciado, D., Paradise, J. L., Chi, D. H., Haralam, M. A., Block, S. L., Kearney, D. H., Bhatnager, S., Muniz Pujalt, G. B., Shope, T. R., Martin, J. M., Felten, D. E., Kurs-Lasky, M. S., Liu, H., Yahner, K., Jeong, J.-H., Cohen, N. L., Czervionke, B., Nagg, J. P., ... Shaikh, N. (2021). Tympanostomy tubes or medical management for recurrent acute otitis media. *The New England Journal of Medicine, 384*(19), 1789–1799. https://doi.org/10.1056/NEJMoa2027278

Acute Otitis Media

1. All infants and children should be assessed for pain and inflammation of the inner ear.
2. All infants younger than age 6 months with presumed or certain AOM should be treated with antibiotics and analgesics.
3. Children ages 6 to 24 months with certain AOM accompanied by acute onset, moderate or severe otalgia, or temperature 39°C (102.2°F) or higher should be treated. Infants with unilateral AOM but no severe symptoms may be observed. Those with bilateral AOM or severe symptoms should receive antibiotic therapy.
4. For children older than age 2 years, observation may be considered for those with certain AOM but who do not have severe illness.
5. If not treating, the clinician should ensure that an adult caregiver is able to observe the child, recognize signs of serious illness, and be able to provide prompt access to medical care if improvement does not occur. If there is a worsening of illness or no improvement in 48 to 72 hours, antibacterial therapy should be considered.
6. First-line treatment includes amoxicillin (80 to 90 mg/kg divided in two divided doses) or, for children allergic to penicillin, cefdinir (14 mg/kg in one or two doses), cefuroxime (30 mg/kg in two divided doses), or cefpodoxime (10 mg/kg in two divided doses) for 10 days.
7. Children who have received amoxicillin in the past 30 days, have concurrent purulent conjunctivitis, or have a history of recurrent AOM unresponsive to amoxicillin should receive high-dose amoxicillin–clavulanate (90 mg/kg/day of amoxicillin with 6.4 mg/kg/day of clavulanate in two divided doses).
8. Alternative antibiotics for treatment failures include ceftriaxone (50 mg/kg/day intramuscular [IM] or intravenous [IV] for 3 days) or clindamycin (30 to 40 mg/kg/day in three divided doses), with or without a second- or third-generation cephalosporin.

Recurrent Otitis Media

1. Placement of ventilating tubes by myringotomy (incision into the tympanic membrane) may be considered for children who experience three or more episodes in 6 months or four or more episodes per year and who have unilateral or bilateral middle ear effusion at the time of assessment for tube placement (see Figure 43-1).

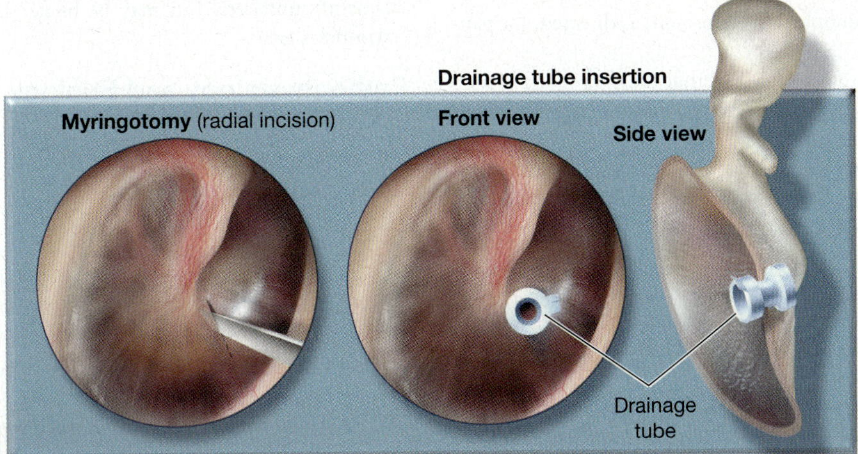

Figure 43-1. Myringotomy with pressure-equalizing tubes. Pressure-equalizing tubes inserted into the myringotomy incision to prevent buildup of fluid in the middle ear. (Asset provided by Anatomical Chart Co.)

Complications

1. Perforations of the tympanic membrane, scarring because of healed perforations, or damage to the ossicles of the middle ear may occur; permanent hearing loss is a rare complication.
2. Delayed speech and language development.
3. Mastoiditis, meningitis, lateral sinus thrombosis, or intracranial abscess; spread of bacterial infection may occur, although all are uncommon.

Nursing Assessment

1. Assess for etiologic factors that contribute to ETD.
2. Assess risk factors for the development of recurrent AOM—age, genetic predisposition, craniofacial abnormalities, daycare attendance, tobacco smoke exposure, and seasonal respiratory infections.
3. Assess for symptoms of serous otitis and AOM to identify and to document the nature and severity of the illness.
4. Assess hearing after the middle ear effusion is resolved. Promptly identify any hearing loss that may have social and educational consequences.
5. Assess speech and language development in children who experience recurrent or prolonged infections to determine deficits.
6. Assess for effects of illness on family, such as sleep deprivation of caregivers caused by staying up with the child at night or decreased attendance at work caused by keeping the child out of school.

CLINICAL JUDGMENT Prompt identification of speech and language delays is important in young children because speech and language development is quite rapid at this time. Young children may demonstrate either rapid regression or failure of progression of speech and language skills.

Nursing Interventions

Minimizing Discomfort

1. Administer and teach caregivers to administer antibiotics. Provide instruction in:
   a. Measurement of correct dosage.
   b. Time of doses.
   c. Importance of administering all doses.
   d. Proper storage and disposal of unused medication.
   e. Adverse effects.
2. Administer acetaminophen or ibuprofen, as directed, for pain or fever.
3. Apply warm compresses to the external ear.
4. Advise elevation of the head to facilitate drainage of fluid from the middle ear into the pharynx.
5. Teach older children to stimulate the opening of their eustachian tubes by yawning or performing Valsalva maneuver.

Facilitating Verbal Communication

1. Assess hearing, speech, and language development regularly.
2. Alert caregivers to report signs of hearing difficulty or delayed speech immediately to ensure early intervention.
3. Refer to a specialist for evaluation and treatment, if necessary.

Family Education and Health Maintenance

1. Teach caregivers that episodes of otitis may be minimized by:
   a. Breast feeding.
   b. Placing older infants who are bottle-fed in a sitting position during feeding.
   c. Identifying and eliminating allergens, such as particular foods, molds, and dust.
   d. Not exposing the child to cigarette smoke.
   e. Immunization with pneumococcal and influenza vaccines.
2. Teach the importance of taking antibiotics at prescribed times for the indicated length of therapy to prevent partial treatment and the development of resistance.
3. Teach all caregivers the difference between viral and bacterial infections, emphasizing that overuse of antibiotics for viral infections contributes to the development of resistant bacteria.
4. If ventilating tubes are placed, instruct caregivers to do the following.
   a. Understand that avoidance of swimming or water sports is unnecessary. Water precautions (preventing water or other fluids from entering the ear canal by use of earplugs) are to be used only when the child has an AOM with ear tube or is prone to AOM with ear tube.
   b. Discourage instillation of eardrops or other medications in the external ear unless they have been prescribed by the health care provider.
   c. Be aware that tubes will fall out of the ear spontaneously, usually in 6 to 12 months.

EVIDENCE BASE Rosenfeld, R. M., Tunkel, D. E., Schwartz, S. R., Anne, S., Bishop, C. E., Chelius, D. C., Hackell, J., Hunter, L. L., Keppel, K. L., Kim, A. H., Kim, T. W., Levine, J. M., Maksimoski, M. T., Moore, D. J., Preciado, D. A., Raol, N. P, Vaughan, W. K., Walker, E. A., & Monjur, T. M. (2022). Clinical practice guideline: Tympanostomy tubes in children (update). *American Academy of Otolaryngology—Head and Neck Surgery Foundation, 166*(1S), S1–S55. https://doi.org/10.1177/01945998211065662

Evaluation: Expected Outcomes

- Demonstrates improved comfort; family states proper treatment regimen.
- Speech and language development appropriate for age; reports regular assessment; receives therapy from specialist, if indicated.

External Otitis

Acute *otitis externa* is inflammation in the external ear canal. It is frequently unilateral but may be bilateral. Commonly known as "swimmer's ear."

Pathophysiology and Etiology

1. Caused by bacteria or fungi. Common pathogens include:
   a. *Pseudomonas aeruginosa.*
   b. *Staphylococcus aureus.*
   c. *Proteus mirabilis.*
   d. *Streptococcus pyogenes.*
   e. Fungi *(Candida, Aspergillus).*
2. Risk factors include:
   a. Frequent swimming.
   b. Insertion of objects, such as cotton swabs, into the ear canals.
   c. AOM with perforation of the tympanic membrane.
   d. Ventilation tubes with drainage.
   e. Poorly fitting earplugs.
3. When water remains in the external ear canal, a warm, moist environment is created.

4. Skin lining the canal is irritated, causing breakdown of its protective barrier.
5. Bacteria or fungi overgrow in a conducive environment and cause symptoms of inflammation and infection in 1 to 2 days.
6. Breakdown of protective barrier and introduction and proliferation of infectious organisms can also occur through trauma to the ear canal, such as cleaning the ear with an inappropriate object or using an improper technique.

Clinical Manifestations

1. Intense ear pain, itching, and white, yellow, or greenish drainage.
2. Inflammation of the external ear canal and structures.
3. Pain when the ear pinna is manipulated.

Diagnostic Evaluation

1. Otoscopic examination may be difficult because of severe pain and swelling; redness, swelling, and drainage in external canal are noted while the tympanic membrane appears normal.
2. Ear pain may be severe.
3. Cellulitis of the surrounding structures can result in displacement of the external ear out and away from the head.
4. Cultures are usually not necessary.

Management

1. Ear pain may be severe, and appropriate analgesia should be provided.
2. Effective topical treatments include diluted acetic acid (vinegar) or boric acid solutions, which dry and modify the pH of the ear canal.
3. Topical antibiotic solution, possibly combined with a steroid to reduce significant discomfort and swelling.
4. Ear canal may be gently cleansed with curette, cotton swab, mild suctioning, or irrigation to remove drainage.
5. An ear wick may be used to aid in medication getting to the lining of the deeper ear canal.
6. Oral antibiotics may be used in addition to topical medications in severe cases or if cellulitis extends beyond the external canal.

Nursing Assessment

1. Assess severity of symptoms and need for pain relief.
2. Assess ear hygiene and the need for earplugs.

Nursing Interventions

Relieving Pain

1. Administer eardrops or teach caregivers administration, as prescribed.
   a. Have the child lie on side with the affected ear upward.
   b. Instill drops, using caution not to contaminate dropper, and press gently on tragus.
   c. Have the child maintain the position for 5 minutes to facilitate penetration of medication into ear canal.
   d. Repeat on the other side, if ordered.
2. Administer analgesics, such as acetaminophen or ibuprofen, as directed.
3. Suggest application of warm or cold compresses to outer ear to relieve discomfort.
4. Frequently clean drainage from the area surrounding the opening of the ear canal to relieve irritation.

Family Education and Health Maintenance

1. Teach proper ear hygiene.
   a. Insert nothing into the ear canal for cleaning or scratching.
   b. Clean the outer area with a washcloth only.
   c. Drain water promptly from the ear by leaning the child over and pulling auricle slightly downward and outward.
2. Instruct in the use of well-fitting earplugs, if necessary.
3. Instruct in the use of routine diluted acetic acid (vinegar) solution instillation after water activity, if prescribed.

Evaluation: Expected Outcomes

- Reports pain relieved; uses compresses and analgesics, if necessary.

Functional Hearing Disorders

Functional hearing disorders arise from problems in the function of the ear. Children with normal hearing can hear tones between 0 and 15 dB (decibels). Categories of hearing impairment include slight, 16 to 25 dB; mild, 26 to 40 dB; moderate, 41 to 55 dB; moderate-severe, 56 to 70 dB; and severe or profound loss, 71 dB or higher. In the United States, moderate to profound bilateral sensorineural hearing loss occurs in 0.5 to 1.0 per 1,000 live births each year. Factors that place an infant at high risk for hearing loss include low birth weight, in utero infections (e.g., cytomegalovirus [CMV], herpes, rubella, syphilis, and toxoplasmosis), developmental delay, craniofacial anomalies, ototoxic medication exposure, family history of hereditary childhood hearing loss, and postnatal infections such as bacterial and viral meningitis.

Pathophysiology and Etiology

1. Hearing loss may be conductive, sensorineural, or mixed.
2. Conductive loss occurs when sound transmission through the outer and/or middle ear is blocked, caused by impaction of cerumen in the external ear canal, fluid in the middle ear cavity, or scarring of the tympanic membrane.
   a. A mechanical obstruction, such as cerumen or a foreign object blocking the external ear canal, may block the passage of sound waves to the tympanic membrane.
   b. With OM or OME, fluid in the middle ear cavity does not transmit sound as well as air.
   c. A scarred or perforated tympanic membrane has lost its normal mobility and does not transmit sound as well as a normal one.
   d. Most cases of conductive hearing loss in children are reversible and produce no permanent effect.
3. Sensorineural hearing loss is related to a defect in the transmission of sound from damage to the cochlear hair cells or auditory nerve. The loss can be congenital (present at birth) or acquired. Both congenital and acquired loss can be hereditary and nonhereditary. Examples include damage caused by ototoxic drugs, damage resulting from prenatal infections, and damage caused by prolonged exposure to loud noise.
   a. Damage to the auditory nerve prevents transmission of sound impulses to the brain for interpretation.
   b. Damage to hair cells of the cochlea may be caused by prolonged exposure to loud noise, resulting in hearing loss, especially pronounced for high-pitched sounds.
   c. Sensorineural problems are usually irreversible.

Clinical Manifestations

1. Infants may be noted to be inconsistent in response to sounds. Response to sound, however, is not sufficiently reliable as a screening method, especially for high-risk infants.
2. Children usually do not verbalize that they cannot hear well. They may exhibit other signs of hearing problems, including:
   a. Poor academic performance or behavior problems in school.
   b. Lack of response to sounds.
   c. Delayed language development.
   d. Listening to the television or radio at a loud volume.
   e. Speaking loudly.

Diagnostic Evaluation

EVIDENCE BASE Raven, S., Mott, N., Ibrahim, N., Cole, C., Munzer, T., Handelsman, J., Vereb, A., Hashikawa, A., & Bohm, L. (2023). Hearing loss in children: Critical medical education delivered as massive open online course. *Perspectives of the ASHA Special Interest Groups, 8*(5), 1003–1010.

Wen, C., Zhao, X., Li, Y., Yu, Y., Cheng, X., Li, X., Deng, K., Yuan, X., & Huang, L. (2022). A systematic review of newborn and childhood hearing screening around the world: Comparison and quality assessment of guidelines. *BMC Pediatrics, 22*, 160. https://doi.org/10.1186/s12887-022-03234-0

1. Universal newborn hearing evaluation requires all newborns to be evaluated for hearing loss prior to discharge. This involves objective methods initially with otoacoustic emission (OAE) testing. If indicated, an automated auditory brain response (ABR) test is used to confirm a positive OAE result.
2. The goal of early hearing and detection and intervention (EHDI) is to identify and confirm hearing loss by 3 months of age and intervention by 6 months of age.
3. Infants who fail their initial evaluation need a follow-up evaluation at 1 month of age. Any infants with a second abnormal result should be evaluated by an audiologist as soon as possible. Infants with high-risk factors require a repeat hearing evaluation at 3 months of age.
4. Infants with documented hearing loss need a referral to specialists (otolaryngology and ophthalmology) by 3 months of age. Referral to other subspecialists (genetics, nephrology, neurology, etc.) may be necessary. The infant should be enrolled in Early Intervention Services (Part C) through the local school system no later than 6 months of age, which will provide physical therapy, occupational therapy, speech therapy, and visual intervention, as indicated.
5. Infants whose initial hearing evaluation is normal should be routinely assessed for their response to sound and achievement of developmental speech language milestones.
6. Routine audiometric screening should be completed as soon as the child can cooperate and follow instructions (between ages 3 and 5 years). It is important that the child be screened and hearing deficits addressed before entry into school.

Management

1. Treatment of the underlying problem, such as impacted cerumen or OM.
2. Hearing aids may be helpful for both conductive and sensorineural hearing loss.
3. Cochlear implants help some children with sensorineural hearing loss.
   a. Consists of an external microphone and speech processor, which sends radio signals to an internal electrode array implanted in the cochlea.
   b. Most effective in the young child who has had shorter hearing deprivation but requires a long period of rehabilitation.
4. If the problem cannot be corrected, the focus of treatment is on the development of adaptive skills through special education, sign language or other communication alternatives, and/or technical devices for the hearing impaired.

Complications

1. Speech and language delays.
2. Inadequate social development.
3. Academic failure.

Nursing Assessment

1. Periodically assess hearing in the child with an identified hearing impairment to follow up promptly on changes in the ability to hear.
2. Assess speech and language development frequently so that children may obtain special assistance, as indicated.
3. Assess social development and academic progress periodically, so that counseling and intervention can be instituted.

Nursing Interventions

Minimizing Effects of Hearing Loss

1. Face the child, use appropriate facial expressions, and make sure the child can see your face clearly when communicating.
2. Approach the child so that you can be seen; touch the deaf child on the shoulder to get attention.
3. Assist the child in utilizing a hearing aid, as prescribed, or assistive technology.

Promoting Effective Communication

1. Determine the usual method of communication: ability to write, using verbal cues, or reading lips. Do not depend on gestures to communicate with a child or with a third party who does not know sign language.
2. Obtain an interpreter, when necessary, for children who communicate using sign language. Adequate communication is especially important when providing health education or when treating children who may have been abused.
3. Help the caregivers of a young child to stimulate and communicate with them using visual language.
   a. Teach them to use gestures, mime, and nonverbal communication.
   b. Teach them to help the infant to develop watching behavior by giving rewards of pleasure and praise.
   c. Teach them to talk to the child while looking directly into their eyes and using appropriate facial expressions.

Preventing Injury

1. Advise caregivers that home safety devices, such as smoke detectors, may require visual or tactile alarms (flashing lights or vibration) rather than auditory alarms.
2. Encourage the use of other senses to compensate for the inability to hear. For example, the child should be especially careful to look in all directions when crossing the street.
3. Do not leave the child alone in an unfamiliar environment without means of communication.

4. Provide close surveillance and frequent visual contact for the hospitalized child.

Increasing Self-esteem

1. Inform families of the child's right to a public education in the least restrictive setting and promote the use of augmented communication devices.
2. Encourage interaction with hearing and nonhearing children to promote integration.
3. Encourage mastery of developmental milestones and skills through self-care activities and play.
4. Help caregivers understand that the child may not be able to express anxiety or frustration and may act out instead.
5. Teach them to be consistent in their use of discipline and to provide alternative ways for the child to gain attention or to relieve stress.
6. Praise the child for accomplishments and attempts at social interaction.

Family Education and Health Maintenance

1. Encourage families to learn sign language and alternative methods of communication with the child.
2. Advise on proper hearing aid cleaning and maintenance.
3. Encourage attention to health maintenance needs, such as immunizations and well-child visits.
4. For additional support and information, refer to groups such as the American Society for Deaf Children (*deafchildren.org*).

Evaluation: Expected Outcomes

- Responds appropriately to environmental stimuli.
- Communicates effectively through sign language, interpreter, and visual cues.
- Reports no injuries.
- Reports adequate progress in school and participation in extracurricular activities.

SELECTED READINGS

Anosike, B. I., Ganapathy, V., & Nakamura, M. M. (2022). Epidemiology and management of orbital cellulitis in children. *Journal of the Pediatric Infectious Diseases Society, 11*(5), 214–220. https://doi.org/10.1093/jpids/piac006

Bajorski, P., Fuji, N., Kaur, R., & Pichichero, M. E. (2023). Window of susceptibility to acute otitis media infection. *Pediatrics, 151*(2), e2022058556.

Chang Pitter, J. Y., Zhong, L., Hamdy, R. F., Preciado, D., Behzadpour, H., & Hamburger, E. K. (2022). Ceftriaxone use for acute otitis media: Associated factors in a large U.S. primary care population. *International Journal of Pediatric Otorhinolaryngology, 160*, 111211. https://doi.org/10.1016/j.ijporl.2022.111211

Cleere, E. F., Crotty, T. J., Lang, J., Young, O., & Keogh, I. J. (2023). Clinical decision making in paediatric otitis media: A pilot quality improvement study. *International Journal of Pediatric Otorhinolaryngology, 164*, 111395. https://doi.org/10.1016/j.ijporl.2022.111395

Dull, K. (2023). *Approach to the pediatric patient with acute vision change. UpToDate.* Retrieved February 8, 2023, from https://www.uptodate.com/contents/approach-to-the-pediatric-patient-with-acute-vision-change

Franz, L., Gallo, C., Marioni, G., de Filippis, C., & Lovato, A. (2021). Idiopathic sudden sensorineural hearing loss in children: A systematic review and meta-analysis. *Otolaryngology-Head and Neck Surgery, 165*(2), 244–254. https://doi.org/10.1177/0194599820976571

Gavrilovici, C., Spoiala, E.-L., Miron, I.-C., Starcea, I. M., Halitchi, C. O. I., Zetu, I. N., Lupu, V. V., & Panzaru, C. (2022). Acute otitis media in children—Challenges of antibiotic resistance in the post-vaccination era. *Microorganisms, 10*(8), 1598. https://doi.org/10.3390/microorganisms10081598

Henriquez-Recine, Noval; S., Zafra, B., De Manuel, S., & Contreras, I. (2020). Ocular emergencies in children: Demographics, origin, symptoms, and most frequent diagnoses. *Journal of Ophthalmology, 2020*, 6820454. https://doi.org/10.1155/2020/6820454

Homoe, P., Heidemann, C. H., Damoiseaux, R. A., Lailach, S., Lieu, J. E. C., Phillips, J. S., & Venekamp, R. P. (2020). Panel 5: Impact of otitis media on quality of life and development. *International Journal of Pediatric Otorhinolaryngology, 130*(Suppl. 1), 109837. https://doi.org/10.1016/j.ijporl.2019.109837

Honkila, M., Koskela, U., Kontiokari, T., Mattila, M. L., Kristo, A., Valtonen, R., Sarlin, S., Paalanne, N., Ikaheimo, I., Pokka, T., Uhari, M., Renko, M., & Tapiainen, T. (2022). Effect of topical antibiotics on duration of acute infective conjunctivitis in children: A randomized clinical trial and a systematic review and meta-analysis. *JAMA Network Open, 5*(10), e2234459. https://doi.org/10.1001/jamanetworkopen.2022.34459

Jacobs, D. S. (2022). *Conjunctivitis. UpToDate.* Retrieved February 8, 2023, from https://www.uptodate.com/contents/conjunctivitis

Nassrallah, F., Whittingham, J., Sun, H., & Fitzpatrick, E. M. (2023). Speech-language outcomes of children with unilateral and mild/moderate hearing loss. *Deafness & Education International, 25*(1), 40–58.

Poe, D., & Corrales, C. E. (2023). *Eustachian tube dysfunction. UpToDate.* Retrieved February 8, 2023, from https://www.uptodate.com/contents/eustachian-tube-dysfunction

Ramsay, C., Murchison, A. P., & Bilyk, J. R. (2021). Pediatric eye emergency department visits: Retrospective review and evaluation. *Journal of Pediatric Ophthalmology & Strabismus, 58*(2), 84–92. https://doi.org/10.3928/01913913-20201118-01

Rosenfeld, R. M., Shin, J. J., Schwartz, S. R., Coggins, R., Gagnon, L. Hackell, J. M., Hoelting, D., Hunter, L. L., Kummer, A. W., Payne, S. C., Poe, D. S., Veling, M., Vila, P. M., Walsh, S. A., & Corrigan, M. D. (2016). Clinical practice guideline: Otitis media with effusion (update). *Otolaryngology-Head and Neck Surgery, 154*(Suppl. 1), S1–S41. https://doi.org/10.1177/0194599815623467

Saniasiaya, J., Kulasegarah, J., & Narayanan, P. (2022). Outcome of eustachian tube balloon dilation in children: A systematic review. *Annals of Otology, Rhinology, & Laryngology, 131*(7), 797–804. https://doi.org/10.117/00034894211041340

Shave, S., Botti, C., & Kwong, K. (2022). Congenital sensorineural hearing loss. *Pediatric Clinics of North America, 69*(2), 221–234. https://doi.org/10.1016/j.pcl.2021.12.006

Smolinski, N. E., Antonelli, P. J., & Winterstein, A. G. (2022). Watchful waiting for acute otitis media. *Pediatrics, 150*(1), e2021055613. https://doi.org/10.1542/peds.2021-055613

Tolhurst-Cleaver, M., Evans, J., Waterfield, T., Adamson, J., Marlow, R., Lyttle, R., & Roland, D. (2022). Periorbital and orbital cellulitis in children: A survey of emergency physicians and analysis of clinical practice guidelines across the PERUKI network. *Emergency Medicine Journal. 39*(10), 766–770

Yeager, L. (2019). The pediatric eye exam. In D. S. Casper, & G. A. Cioffi (Eds.), *The Columbia guide to basic elements of eye care: A manual for healthcare professionals* (531 pp.). Springer.

44

Pediatric Gastrointestinal and Nutritional Disorders*

*Please note that the term "male" in this chapter refers to a person assigned male at birth, and the term "female" in this chapter refers to a person assigned female at birth.

CLEFT LIP AND PALATE

Cleft lip and palate are congenital anomalies, known as *orofacial clefts*, resulting in structural facial malformation. These anomalies are usually present in early fetal development, are one of the most common birth anomalies in the United States, and are associated with any of more than 400 syndromes. The lip, or the lip and palate, fails to close in approximately 1 in every 1,000 neonates. This equals approximately 7,000 infants born each year in the United States. About 1 in every 1,600 babies is born with cleft lip with cleft palate, and about 1 in every 2,800 babies is born with cleft lip without cleft palate (nidcr.nih.gov).

Cleft lip and palate are most prevalent among Native American people. Cleft lip (with or without cleft palate) occurs more frequently in males, and isolated cleft palate is more frequent in females. The chance of having a child with an orofacial cleft increases if one or both biological parents have an anomaly and if there is a sibling born with an anomaly.

EVIDENCE BASE Vyas, T., Gupta, P., Kumar, S., Gupta, R., Gupta, T., & Singh, H. P. (2020). Cleft of lip and palate: A review. *Journal of Family Medicine and Primary Care, 9*(6), 2621–2625. https://doi.org/10.4103/jfmpc.jfmpc_472_20

Pathophysiology and Etiology

EVIDENCE BASE Omori, M. A., Gerber, J. T., Marañón-Vásquez, G. A., Matsumoto, M. A. N., Weiss, S. G., Do Nascimento, M. A., Araújo, M. T. S., Stuani, M. B. S., Nelson-Filho, P., Scariot, R., & Küchler, E. C. (2020). Possible association between craniofacial dimensions and genetic markers in *ESR1* and *ESR2*. *Journal of Orthodontics, 47*(1), 65–71. https://doi.org/10.1177/1465312520901725

1. A failure of fusion of lip/palate tissue between 5 and 7 weeks of gestation, resulting in an anomaly in morphogenesis. It involves patterns of DNA signaling, gene and biochemical organizers, nuclear and cellular differentiation, proliferation, and migration. A major impact is at the level of the neural crest cell.
2. Although the syndrome is not well understood, genetic/hereditary factors may play a role; a fetus with an affected biological parent or biological sibling has a 3% to 5% risk of being affected.
3. In 2004, a gene variant was identified as being a major contributor to orofacial clefts. This gene variant may triple the risk of developing the anomaly in signaling and transcription proteins that are involved in development and differentiation. There is a 50% risk in monozygotic twins.
4. Environmental factors may include the following:
   a. Vitamin B and folic acid deficiency. Some studies have shown that consumption of multivitamins with folic acid prior to conception and during the first trimester may lower the incidence of cleft lip and palate. Current recommendations during pregnancy advise taking a multivitamin containing 400 μg of folic acid. New data suggest a correlation between vitamins A and D and cleft palate phenotypes.
   b. Medications taken during pregnancy, including antiseizure drugs and corticosteroids.
   c. Maternal alcohol and smoking.
   d. Infections.
   e. Diabetes.

EVIDENCE BASE Myhre, A., Råbu, M., & Feragen, K. J. B. (2021). The need to belong: Subjective experiences of living with craniofacial conditions and undergoing appearance-altering surgery. *Body Image, 38*, 334–345. https://doi.org/10.1016/j.bodyim.2021.05.008

Types of Anomalies

1. Cleft lip—prealveolar cleft (see Figure 44-1):
   a. Varies from a notch in the lip to complete separation of the lip into the nose.
   b. May be unilateral or bilateral.
   c. Failure of maxillary process to fuse with nasal elevations on frontal prominence; normally occurs during the fifth and sixth weeks of gestation.
   d. Merging of upper lip at midline complete between the seventh and eighth weeks of gestation.
2. Isolated cleft palate—postalveolar cleft:
   a. Cleft of uvula.
   b. Cleft of soft palate.
   c. Cleft of both soft and hard palates through the roof of mouth.
   d. Unilateral or bilateral.
   e. Failure of mesodermal masses of lateral palatine process to meet and fuse; normally occurs between the seventh and 12th weeks of gestation.
3. Submucous cleft:
   a. Muscles of soft palate not joined.
   b. Not recognized until child talks; cannot be seen at birth.
4. Pierre Robin syndrome—cleft palate, glossoptosis (tongue lays back on pharynx), and micrognathia (underdeveloped mandible):
   a. This causes feeding difficulties, potential airway obstruction by tongue, slow weight gain, and ear infections.
   b. By age 3 to 4 months, the mandible has grown enough to accommodate the tongue, and respiratory difficulty is greatly diminished.

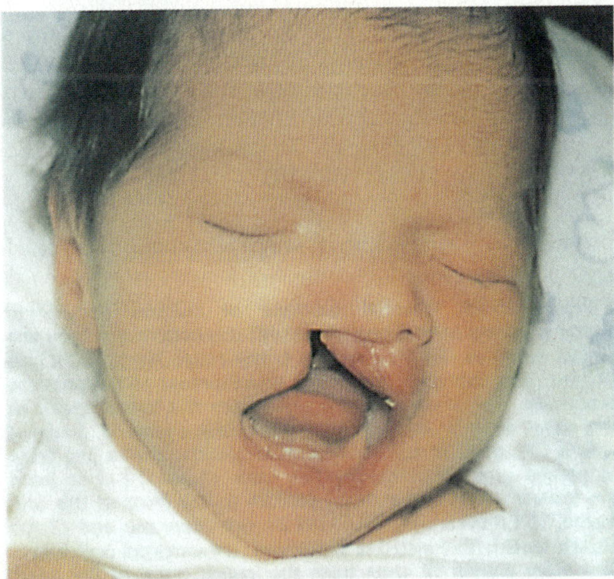

Figure 44-1. Cleft lip. (Reprinted with permission from Nath, J. [2016]. *Stedman's medical terminology* [2nd ed.]. Lippincott Williams & Wilkins.)

Clinical Manifestations

1. Physical appearance of cleft lip or palate:
   a. Incompletely formed lip—varies from slight notch in vermilion to complete separation of lip.
   b. Opening in roof of mouth felt with examiner's finger on palate.
2. Eating difficulty:
   a. Suction cannot be created for effective sucking.
   b. Food returns through the nose.
3. Nasal speech.
4. Increased incidence of otitis media, which may lead to mild-to-moderate hearing loss.
5. Speech delay secondary to lip anomaly as well as related to chronic otitis media.
6. Dental problems.

Diagnostic Evaluation

EVIDENCE BASE Thompson, R. L., Thorson, H. L., Chinnadurai, S., Tibesar, R. J., & Roby, B. B. (2023). Prenatal consultation outcomes for infants with cleft lip with and without cleft palate. *The Cleft Palate-Craniofacial Journal, 60*(9), 1071–1077. https://doi.org/10.1177/10556656221093174

1. Prenatal ultrasonography to detect cleft lips and some cleft palates in utero.
2. Magnetic resonance imaging (MRI) and three-dimensional computed tomography to evaluate the extent of anomaly before treatment.
3. Photography to document the anomaly.
4. Serial x-rays before and after treatment.
5. Dental impressions for expansion prosthesis.
6. Genetic evaluation to determine recurrence risk.

Management

EVIDENCE BASE Padovano, W. M., Snyder-Warwick, A. K., Skolnick, G. B., Pfeifauf, K. D., Menezes, M. D., Grames, L. M., Cheung, S., Kim, A. M., Cradock, M. M., Naidoo, S. D., & Patel, K. B. (2020). Evaluation of multidisciplinary team clinic for patients with isolated cleft lip. *The Cleft Palate-Craniofacial Journal, 57*(7), 900–908. https://doi.org/10.1177/1055665619900625

Interdisciplinary approach begins early and continues into late adolescence. Craniofacial team consists of a plastic surgeon, otolaryngologist, pediatric dentist, prosthodontist, orthodontist, feeding specialist, speech pathologist, audiologist, geneticist, psychologist, and community health nurse. Each team member has a role at some point in the child's care.

1. General management is focused on proper growth and nutrition, closure of the clefts, prevention of complications, oral–motor rehabilitation, and facilitation of normal growth and development of the child.
2. Patients with isolated cleft lips have a greater chance of overcoming feeding difficulties than do those with combined anomalies.
3. The cleft lip is repaired before the palate anomaly, generally around age 3 months.
   a. Techniques performed include the Millard repair, which results in a zigzag scar on the lip, or placement of sutures where the line of the columella would have been.
   b. The surgical goals are adherence and the most cosmetically pleasing and naturally appearing lip.
4. Cleft palate repair may be done any time between ages 6 and 18 months. Surgery and timing are based on the degree of deformity, width of oropharynx, neuromuscular function of palate and pharynx, and surgeon's preference. Some children may require more than one reconstructive surgery.
   a. Palatoplasty is the reconstruction of the palatal musculature.
   b. The surgical goal is adherence, development of normal speech pattern, and safe/appropriate eating skills. In addition, it should decrease the incidence of otitis media.
   c. Surgery may be performed by craniofacial or plastic surgeon in conjunction with other specialists, including oral surgeon and dentist.

Complications

1. Respiratory distress.
2. Infection.
3. Palatal fistulas.
4. Dehydration and electrolyte imbalance.
5. Bleeding.

Nursing Assessment

1. If the newborn has a cleft lip, assess for cleft palate by direct visualization and palpation with finger.
2. Obtain family history of cleft lip or palate.
3. Evaluate feeding abilities.
   a. Effectiveness of suck and swallow.
   b. Amount taken.
   c. Vomiting, regurgitation, or formula coming from nose.
4. Observe for other syndromic features, such as small jaw, abnormal facies, microcephaly/macrocephaly, heart murmur, anal–rectal anomalies.

Nursing Interventions

EVIDENCE BASE Penny, C., McGuire, C., & Bezuhly, M. (2022). A systematic review of feeding interventions for infants with cleft palate. *The Cleft Palate Craniofacial Journal, 59*(12), 1527–1536. https://doi.org/10.1177/10556656211051216

Maintaining Adequate Nutrition

1. Facilitate nutrition and speech therapy for all infants.
2. Encourage the birthing parent to begin feeding the infant as soon as possible to enhance bonding and to strengthen the oral structures needed for mastication and speech production.
3. If sucking is permitted:
   a. Encourage breastfeeding.
   b. Encourage and demonstrate breast pump.
   c. Use a soft nipple with crosscut to facilitate feeding.
4. If sucking is ineffective because of the inability to create a vacuum, try alternate oral feeding methods.
   a. Feeding devices include preemie nipple, crosscut nipple, NUK nipple, Ross Cleft Palate Nurser, Mead Johnson Cleft Palate Nurser, Pidgeon nipple bottle system, Haberman Feeder, or palatal obturator.

b. Avoid enlarging nipple holes because of infant's inability to control flow of milk, which will result in choking. Crosscut nipples allow milk to flow only when infant squeezes the crosscut open.
c. Using a squeezable bottle (e.g., Mead Johnson Cleft Palate Nurser) or plastic liner can be helpful by applying rhythmic pressure along with the infant's normal sucking and swallowing.
d. Rubber-tipped Asepto syringe or dropper; the rubber extension should be long enough to extend back into the mouth to prevent regurgitation through the nose. Direct tip to the side of mouth and feed slowly.

5. Feed infant in an upright, sitting position or the upright side-lying position if airway support is needed. This decreases possibility of fluid being aspirated or returned through the nose or back to the auditory canal.
   a. Feeding is usually easier if the nipple is angled to the side of the mouth away from the cleft so that the infant's tongue can press the nipple against the upper gum or dental arch.
   b. Feed slowly over approximately 18 to 30 minutes. Feedings longer than 45 minutes expend too many calories and tire the infant.
   c. Smaller but more frequent feedings may be necessary if the infant tires or requires extended time to eat.
   d. Burp frequently during feeding to decrease the amount of air swallowed.
   e. If micrognathia exists, the use of the pinky finger under the chin for support aids in improved sucking ability.
   f. Feed the infant before they become too hungry. If the infant is too agitated, feeding becomes a problem.
6. Administer enteral tube feedings if nipple feeding is to be delayed.
7. Advance diet as appropriate for age and needs of infant. Eating usually improves when solids are introduced because they are easier for the infant to manipulate.
8. Assess and calculate adequate nutritional intake.

Preventing Infection

1. Protect the child from infection so that surgery will not be delayed.
   a. Use and teach good handwashing practice.
   b. Avoid patient contact with anyone who has an infection.
   c. Provide frequent assessment for otitis media.
2. Clean the cleft after each feeding with water and a cotton-tipped applicator.
3. Observe for fever, irritability, redness, or drainage around cleft and report promptly.
4. Monitor vital signs; report temperature greater than 101°F (38.3°C).

Promoting Acceptance and Adjustment

1. Show acceptance of the infant; maintain composure and do not show negative emotion when handling the infant. The manner in which the nurse handles the infant can make a lasting impression on the parental caregivers.
2. Support parental caregivers when showing a neonate for the first time. Demonstrate acceptance of the infant's and the parental caregivers' feelings. Parental caregivers may be grieving about the infant's cosmetic imperfections and may harbor ambivalent feelings.
3. Offer information and answer any questions in a simple, matter-of-fact manner. The better informed the family, the easier it will be for them to see the infant as a normal child with a physical difference that will require surgery, dental work, and, possibly, speech therapy.
4. Be aware that the usual sequence of parental caregiver responses may include shock, disbelief, worry, grief, and anger and then proceed to a state of equilibrium and reorganization.
5. Encourage parental caregiver involvement in infant's care: frequent holding, cuddling, and playing.

Preventing Aspiration and Airway Obstruction

1. Prevent respiratory obstruction by the tongue, especially on inspiration and when the infant is quiet.
   a. Positioning: elevated and side lying.
   b. Tilt head back as tolerated by the infant, and elevate upper trunk slightly.
   c. Tongue/lip suture may be placed by otolaryngologist to prevent the tongue from interfering with airway. Assess for slippage, infection, pain, interference with eating.
   d. Suction nasopharynx, as needed.
2. Infants with Pierre Robin syndrome are at greater risk for airway compromise, especially when feeding.
   a. Feeding can be done with a nursing bottle (feeding techniques similar to those used for cleft palate).
   b. Generally use orthopneic position—vertical and slightly forward; this allows the infant to push the jaw forward to suck and allows the feeder a clear view of the infant.
   c. Use gentle finger pressure at mandibular attachment to bring the jaw forward.

Preparing for Home Management

1. Prepare family for home feedings by providing several days to practice feeding and to become familiar with the infant's feeding pattern.
2. Alert the caregiver to difficulties with feeding and how to manage them.
   a. Nasal regurgitation: Feed in more upright position or stop feeding and allow the infant to cough and clear the airway; then continue with smaller feedings.
   b. Respiratory distress: Feed slowly, give smaller feedings. Observe for signs of aspiration, such as coughing, color changes, increased respiration, fever, and/or formula coming from nose.
   c. Prolonged feeding: If oral feedings take longer than 20 to 30 minutes, energy expenditure increases. Smaller, more frequent feedings are indicated, or enteral tube feeding supplements may be warranted.
3. Suggest that about 1 week before scheduled admission for surgery, the birthing parent begin using feeding techniques preferred by multidisciplinary team. Infants who feed well prior to surgery may do better postoperatively than poor feeders.
4. Encourage the parental caregivers to prepare siblings at home for the arrival of the infant. Suggest they show a picture of the new infant.
5. Offer parental caregivers available resources regarding children with cleft lip and palate.
6. Encourage parental caregiver involvement with local self-help groups that provide information and contact with others in the same situation.

7. Initiate referrals, as indicated, for additional support and financial assistance and early intervention programs.
8. Describe and reinforce surgical treatment plans to the parental caregivers to promote communication and hope.
9. Stress adherence with follow-up care with the pediatrician, plastic surgeon, dentist, orthodontist, psychologist, and speech therapist to prevent chronic otitis media, hearing loss, speech impairment, and emotional problems.
10. Initiate a community nurse referral to continue emotional support and teaching progress at home.

Providing Preoperative Care and Allaying Fear in the Child Undergoing Surgery

1. Prepare the infant or toddler for the postoperative experience to decrease fear and increase cooperation.
   a. Practice the feeding measure that will be used postoperatively—cup, side of spoon, or syringe.
   b. Use elbow immobilizers for short periods; allow the child to play with them and the caregiver to use them. Check your facility's policy regarding the use of immobilizers because this is considered a form of restraint but may be deemed medically necessary.
   c. Demonstrate and practice mouth irrigation because it will be done postoperatively for cleft palate repair; allow the child to assist if age appropriate.
2. Prepare the parental caregivers emotionally for the postoperative appearance of the child.
   a. Explain the use of the Logan bow (a curved metal wire that prevents stress on the suture line for cleft lip repair) and restraints.
   b. Encourage a parental caregiver to be with the child, especially when awakening from anesthesia, to offer security and comfort.
3. Address and explain pain management, collaborating with the parental caregivers as to what comforts their child.

Providing Postoperative Care

1. Protect surgical site:
   a. Apply elbow immobilizers to prevent hands from reaching the mouth while still allowing some freedom of movement; follow your institution's policy regarding medical restraints.
      i. Assess the patient's skin and/or intravenous (IV) line every 2 hours or per institutional policy while the immobilizer is in place.
      ii. Remove the immobilizer to exercise the arms.
      iii. Do not allow anything in the child's mouth, such as straw, eating utensils, or fingers.
2. Maintain adherence device: Check that Logan bow or other device is intact and maintaining adherence of lip repair.
   a. Prevent wetting tape or it will loosen.
   b. Observe for and report bleeding or dislodgement of Logan bow.
3. Prevent the child from stressing the suture site—not crying, blowing, sucking, talking, or laughing.
4. Assess and manage pain.
   a. Consult institution's pain management team, if necessary.
   b. Use pain medications appropriate for age, weight, and condition.
   c. Use pain assessment tools appropriate for age.
   d. Recognize signs of pain, such as crying, agitation, poor feeding, increased vital signs.
   e. Discourage pacifiers until cleared by surgeon.
   f. Encourage the birthing parent to hold the infant, swaddle, and use security/comfort items from home.
5. Positioning—elevated head of bed and side lying.
   a. An infant seat may be useful for variation of position, comfort, and entertainment and to prevent interference with suture line.
   b. Provide for appropriate diversional activity, hanging toys, and mobiles.
   c. If only cleft palate was repaired, child may lie on abdomen.
6. Monitor respiratory effort after cleft palate repair.
   a. Be aware that breathing with a closed palate is different from the child's customary way of breathing; the child must also contend with increased mucus production.
   b. Provide humidified air, if needed, to provide moisture to mucous membranes that may become dry from mouth breathing.
7. Prevent infection.
   a. Clean suture line after every feeding.
   b. Gently wipe lip incision with cotton-tipped applicator and solution of choice, such as water, saline, or diluted hydrogen peroxide. Gently pat dry and apply antibiotic ointment or petroleum jelly, if ordered.
   c. Rinse the mouth with water or offer a drink of water after each feeding.
   d. Irrigate the mouth with normal saline solution or water after cleft palate repair. Technique may vary based on the preference of surgeon. You can direct a gentle stream over the suture line using an ear bulb syringe with the child in a sitting position with head forward.
8. Avoid tension on the suture line during feeding for several days after lip repair.
   a. Use dropper or syringe with a rubber tip and insert from the side to avoid suture line or to avoid stimulating sucking.
   b. Use side of spoon. Never put spoon into the mouth.
   c. Perform enteral tube feedings, if prescribed; usually, this is the last treatment of choice.
   d. Advance slowly to nipple feeding, as directed. The infant should be able to suck more efficiently after the lip is repaired.
   e. After palate repair, feed the child in the manner used preoperatively (cup, side of spoon, or rubber-tipped syringe). Never use straw, nipple, or plain syringe.
   f. Consult with speech/occupational therapy if feeding/swallowing continues to be difficult.
9. Facilitate adequate nutrition.
   a. Obtain nutrition consult, if indicated.
   b. Diet progresses from clear liquids to full liquids to soft foods.
   c. Soft foods are usually continued for about 1 month after surgery, at which time a regular diet is started, but excludes hard food.
   d. Ensure that the child is receiving adequate calories.
   e. Weigh daily and plot on growth charts (www.cdc.gov/growthcharts/).
   f. Early feeding intervention relates to appropriate growth.
10. Administer an antibiotic, if prescribed, to prevent infection, as the mouth and skin contain bacteria.

Community and Home Care Considerations

1. As the patient's advocate, alert members of the craniofacial team when a family is overwhelmed by too many appointments and interventions. Act as liaison to case manager, social worker, and home care agency.
2. Continue to assess weight gain, feeding behavior, overall development, parental caregiver–child bonding and interactions.
3. Advise the parental caregivers to discuss the child's problem with teachers and other responsible adults in close contact with the child.
   a. Aesthetic touch-up and bone graft surgery performed later may interfere with schooling.
   b. Speech differences require early identification and intervention.
   c. Monitor for reading and learning problems related to speech and language delays.
   d. Hypernasality may develop at ages 10 to 14 years because of normal shrinkage of adenoid tissue occurring at this time.
4. Assess the child's self-perception and coping skills. Assess the family's support systems and coping mechanisms.
5. Help school-aged children deal with teasing (as a result of being "different" from their peers) by allowing them to express their feelings and guiding their response: ignoring the remark, responding with a joke or good-natured tease, or educating the teaser.
6. The school nurse can also help by performing frequent hearing evaluations, communicating with staff, and educating the school community on the child's condition and individual needs.

EVIDENCE BASE Çınar, S., Ay, A., Boztepe, H., & Gürlen, E. (2021). "Unexpected event": Having an infant with cleft lip and/or palate. *Congenital Anomalies*, *61*(2), 38–45. https://doi.org/10.1111/cga.12398

Family Education and Health Maintenance

1. Instruct on continued protection of the mouth after surgery. Child cannot put anything in mouth, including lollipops.
2. Demonstrate how to rinse mouth after eating.
3. Advise parental caregivers on the introduction of solid foods; semi-upright position or upright position; avoid spicy or acidic foods, which may irritate the oral and nasal cavities; avoid hard, sharp-edged foods, such as raw carrots or potato chips.
4. Advise on increased risk of ear infections and need to seek medical attention for colds, ear pain, fever, or other signs and symptoms. Frequent hearing screens and tympanometry should be done to monitor the effects of middle ear pathology. *Note:* Hearing should be monitored at least every 6 months during the first year of life and then annually to prevent hearing impairment.
5. Encourage modeling "good speech" by providing a stimulating language environment, and encourage spontaneous imitations of sounds at home.
6. Stress the importance of speech therapy and practicing exercises as directed by the speech therapist.
7. Encourage thorough brushing of teeth, regular dental examinations, and fluoride treatment as indicated because of the risk of tooth decay related to defective enamel and abnormally positioned teeth with clefts.
8. Advise the parental caregivers on current therapies available: bone grafting providing permanent teeth support, dental implants to replace missing teeth, and speech prosthesis for incomplete velopharyngeal closure.
9. Help the parental caregivers realize that, although rehabilitation is extensive, their child can live a full life.
10. For additional information and support, refer patients and family to the American Cleft Palate-Craniofacial Association (apacares.org).
11. Refer families to companies that manufacture bottles for cleft palate: Enfamil (Mead Johnson) Cleft Palate Nurser, 1-800-BABY123; Medela Haberman Feeder, 1-800-995-7867; Pigeon Bottle www.pigeon.com

Evaluation: Expected Outcomes

- Infant feeds with appropriate feeding device in small amounts every 2 to 3 hours.
- No signs of infection.
- Parental caregivers involved with care; demonstrate contact with infant as seen by holding and talking to infant.
- Proper positioning maintained, no signs of aspiration.
- Parental caregivers demonstrate proper feeding technique as evidenced by adequate nutrition and weight gain.
- Parental caregivers and child prepared for surgery.
- Parental caregivers express understanding of postoperative home care procedures and identify supportive resources.

ESOPHAGEAL ATRESIA WITH TRACHEOESOPHAGEAL FISTULA

EVIDENCE BASE Krishnan, U., Mousa, H., Dall'Oglio, L., Homaira, N., Rosen, R., Faure, C., & Gottrand, F. (2016). ESPGHAN-NASPGHAN guidelines for the evaluation and treatment of gastrointestinal and nutritional complications in children with esophageal atresia-tracheoesophageal fistula. *Journal of Pediatric Gastroenterology and Nutrition*, *63*(5), 550–570. https://doi.org/10.1097/MPG.0000000000001401

Almog, A., & Zani, A. (2022). Postoperative complications and long-term outcomes of tracheoesophageal fistula repair. *Current Challenges in Thoracic Surgery*, *4*, 1–12. https://doi.org/10.21037/ccts-21-15

O'Donnell, J. E. M., Purcell, M., Mousa, H., Dall'Oglio, L., Rosen, R., Faure, C., Gottrand, F., & Krishnan, U. (2021). Clinician knowledge of societal guidelines on management of gastrointestinal complications in esophageal atresia. *Journal of Pediatric Gastroenterology and Nutrition*, *72*(2), 232–238. https://doi.org/10.1097/MPG.0000000000002945

Esophageal atresia (EA) is failure of the esophagus to form a continuous passage from the pharynx to the stomach during embryonic development. EA can occur with *tracheoesophageal fistula* (TEF), which is an abnormal connection between the trachea and the esophagus. EA/TEF occurs in approximately 1 in 3,500 births.

Clinically, EA/TEF is divided equally into isolated EA and syndromic EA. Additional anomalies vary in severity, with cardiac anomalies as the most common (14.7% to 28%) and life-threatening. Currently, an overall survival of 85% to 90% has been reported from developed countries. In developing countries, however, several factors contribute to higher mortality rates, including prematurity, delay in diagnosis with an increased incidence of aspiration pneumonia, and a shortage of qualified nurses.

Pathophysiology and Etiology

1. Cause is unknown in most cases and likely multifactorial. Possible influences include:
   a. Low evidence for inheritable genetic factor.
   b. 6% to 10% due to chromosomal (structural) abnormalities, including trisomies (12, 18, 21), and partial deletions such as 13q13-qter, 22q11.2.
   c. Teratogenic stimuli, such as the anticancer drug adriamycin and diethylstilbestrol (DES).
2. Failure of proper separation of the embryonic channel into the esophagus and trachea occurring during the fourth and fifth weeks of gestation.
3. EA can be classified as follows (see Figure 44-2):
   a. *Type I* (type A): Proximal and distal segments of esophagus are blind; there is no connection to trachea; accounts for approximately 7% of cases; second most common.
   b. *Type II* (type B): Proximal segment of esophagus opens into trachea by a fistula; distal segment is blind; rare, 0.8% of cases.
   c. *Type III* (type C): Proximal segment of esophagus has blind end; distal segment of esophagus connects into trachea by a fistula; most common, with 86% of cases. (Discussion is limited to this type.)
   d. *Type IV* (type D): EA with fistula between proximal and distal ends of trachea and esophagus (rare, 0.7% of cases).
   e. *Type V* (type E): Proximal and distal segments of esophagus open into trachea by a fistula; no EA but sometimes referred to as an H-type fistula; occurs in 4.2% of cases; not usually diagnosed at birth.
4. Associations:
   a. Down syndrome.
   b. VACTERL (vertebral anomalies, anal atresia, cardiac anomaly, TEF fistula with EA, renal anomalies, and radial limb dysplasia) syndrome.
   c. Feingold syndrome.

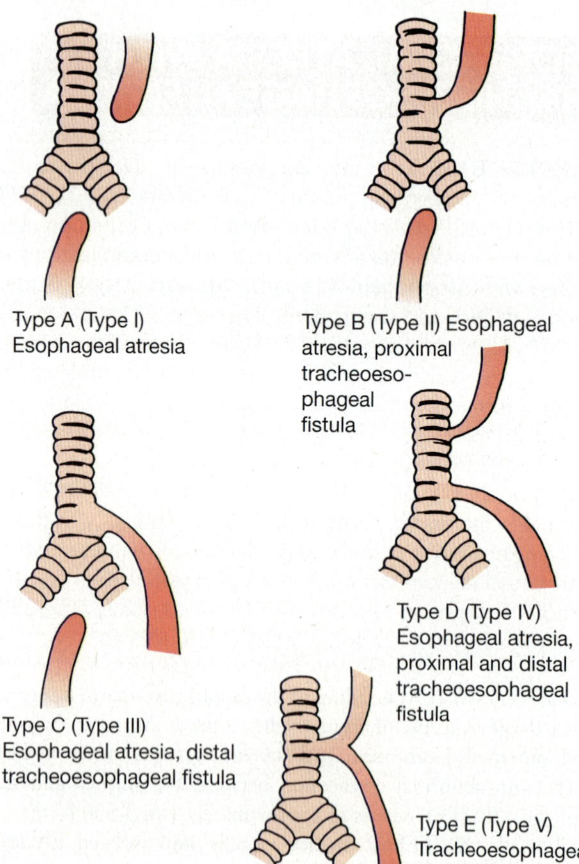

Figure 44-2. Types of esophageal atresia: esophageal atresia and tracheoesophageal fistula.

Clinical Manifestations

These appear soon after birth.

1. Excessive secretions.
   a. Constant drooling.
   b. Large amount of secretions from nose.
   c. Saliva or formula accumulates in upper esophageal pouch and is aspirated into airway.
2. Intermittent, unexplained cyanosis and laryngospasm.
   a. Caused by aspiration of accumulated saliva in blind pouch.
   b. Gastric acid is regurgitated through distal fistula.
3. Abdominal distention.
   a. Occurs as a result of air entering the lower esophagus through the fistula and passing into the stomach, especially when the child is crying.
4. Violent response after the first or second swallow of feeding.
   a. Infant coughs and chokes.
   b. Fluid returns through nose and mouth.
   c. Cyanosis occurs.
   d. Infant struggles.
5. Poor feeding.
6. Inability to pass catheter through nose or mouth into stomach; tip of catheter stops at blind pouch, or atresia. *Note:* Be aware of coiling of catheter; coiling may make catheter appear to be descending into stomach.
7. Infant can be premature, and pregnancy complicated by polyhydramnios. Look for other birth anomalies.

Diagnostic Evaluation

1. Ultrasound scanning techniques enable TEF to be identified in utero for some infants.
2. Failure to pass a 10-F catheter (smaller catheters may coil) into the stomach through nose or mouth. Catheter is left in situ, while an x-ray confirms the diagnosis.
3. pH of tracheal secretions is acidic.
4. Flat plate x-ray of the abdomen and chest may reveal the presence of gas in stomach and catheter coiled in the blind pouch. Barium x-ray may be used in some cases.
5. Electrocardiogram and echocardiogram are performed because there is a high association with cardiac anomalies.

Management

Immediate Treatment

1. Propping infant at 30-degree angle, supine or side lying, to prevent reflux of gastric contents.

2. Nasogastric (NG) tube remains in the esophagus and is aspirated frequently to prevent aspiration until continuous low suction is applied.
3. Pouch is washed out with normal saline to prevent thick mucus from blocking the tube.
4. Gastrostomy to decompress stomach and prevent aspiration; later used for feedings.
5. Nothing by mouth (NPO); intravenous (IV) fluids.
6. Comorbidities, such as pneumonitis and heart failure, are treated.
7. Supportive therapy includes meeting nutritional requirements, IV fluids, antibiotics, respiratory support, and maintaining thermally neutral environment.

Surgery

1. Prompt primary repair: Fistula found by bronchoscopy is divided, followed by esophageal anastomosis of proximal and distal segments if infant weight permits and is without pneumonia.
2. Short-term delay: Subsequent primary repair is used to stabilize infant and prevent deterioration when the patient's condition contraindicates immediate surgery.
3. Staging: Initially, fistula division and gastrostomy are performed with later secondary esophageal anastomosis or colonic transposition performed approximately 1 year later to effect total repair. Approach may be used with a very small, premature infant or a very sick neonate or when severe congenital anomalies exist.
4. Circular esophagomyotomy may be performed on proximal pouch to gain length and allow for primary anastomosis at the initial surgery.
5. Cervical esophagostomy: When the ends of esophagus are too widely separated, esophageal replacement with segment of intestine (colonic transposition) is done at ages 18 to 24 months.
6. Fiberoptic tracheoscopy–assisted repair of TEF can expedite and facilitate surgery on ventilated patients.
7. Staged repair resulted in least amount of gastrointestinal (GI) dysmotility postoperatively.

EVIDENCE BASE Rozensztrauch, A., Śmigiel, R., Bloch, M., & Patkowski, D. (2020). The impact of congenital esophageal atresia on the family functioning. *Journal of Pediatric Nursing, 50*, e85–e90. https://doi.org/10.1016/j.pedn.2019.04.009

Complications

Note: Higher rates of complications occur in patients with cardiac anomalies and low birth weight.

1. Death from asphyxia.
2. Pneumonitis/pneumonia secondary to salivary aspiration and/or gastric acid reflux.
3. Leak at anastomosis site: most common and dangerous complication (15% to 20%).
4. Recurrent fistulas.
5. Esophageal strictures (30% to 40%).
6. Abnormal function of distal esophagus sphincter. (Gastroesophageal reflux [GER] can be found in approximately 50% of these infants.)
7. Esophagitis.
8. Tracheomalacia (10% to 20% of these patients).
9. Gastroesophageal reflux disease (GERD) (40% to 65%).
10. Feeding problems with older children due to esophageal dysmotility (95%).

Nursing Assessment

Assessment begins immediately after birth.

1. Be alert for risk factors of polyhydramnios and prematurity.
2. Suspect in infant with the following:
   a. Excessive amount of mucus.
   b. Difficulty with secretions.
   c. Cyanotic episodes (unexplained).
3. Report suspicion to health care provider immediately.

Nursing Interventions

Preventing Aspiration

1. Position the infant supine with head and chest elevated 20 to 30 degrees to prevent or decrease reflux of gastric juices into the tracheobronchial tree.
   a. This position may also ease respiratory effort by dropping the distended intestines away from the diaphragm.
   b. Side-lying position can be used if the risk of aspiration from being supine is greater than the risk of sudden infant death syndrome (SIDS); supine positioning is preferred to reduce the risk of SIDS.
   c. Turn frequently to prevent atelectasis and pneumonia.
2. Perform intermittent nasopharyngeal suctioning or maintain indwelling Sump tube with constant suction to remove secretions from esophageal blind pouch.
   a. Tip of tube is placed in the blind pouch.
   b. Sump tube allows air to be drawn in through a second lumen and prevents tube obstruction by mucous membrane of pouch.
   c. Maintain indwelling tube patency by irrigating with 1-mL normal saline solution frequently.
3. Place the infant in an isolette or under a radiant warmer with high humidity to aid in liquefying secretions and thick mucus. Maintain the infant's temperature in thermoneutral zone and ensure environmental isolation to prevent infection using isolette.
4. Administer oxygen, as needed.
5. Suction mouth to keep it clear of secretions and prevent aspiration. Provide mouth care.
6. Be alert for indications of respiratory distress.
   a. Retractions.
   b. Circumoral cyanosis.
   c. Restlessness.
   d. Nasal flaring.
   e. Increased respiration and heart rate.
7. Maintain NPO status.
8. Administer antibiotics, as ordered, to prevent or treat associated pneumonitis.
9. Observe infant carefully for any change in condition; report changes immediately.
   a. Check vital signs, color and amount of secretions, abdominal distention, and respiratory distress.
   b. Evaluate for complications that can occur in any neonate or premature infant.
10. Be available and recognize the need for emergency care or resuscitation.
    a. Have resuscitation equipment on hand.
    b. Accompany the infant to other departments and the operating room in isolette with portable oxygen and suction equipment.

11. Monitor for signs or symptoms that may indicate additional congenital anomalies or complications.
12. Gastrostomy tube (GT) may be placed before definitive surgery to aid in gastric decompression, prevention of reflux, or nutrition.

Preventing Dehydration

1. Administer parenteral fluids and electrolytes as prescribed.
2. Monitor vital signs frequently for changes in blood pressure (BP) and pulse, which may indicate dehydration or fluid volume overload.
3. Record intake and output, including gastric drainage (if GT for decompression is present) and weight of diapers.

Reducing Parental Caregiver Anxiety

1. Explain procedures and necessary events to parental caregivers as soon as possible.
2. Orient parental caregivers to the hospital and intensive care nursery environment.
3. Allow family to hold and assist in caring for the infant.
4. Offer reassurance and encouragement to family frequently. Provide for additional support by social worker, clergy, and counselor, as needed.

Maintaining Patent Airway

1. Keep endotracheal (ET) tube patent by frequent lavage and suction. *Note:* Reintubation could damage the anastomosis.
2. Suction frequently; every 5 to 10 minutes may be necessary, but at least every 1 to 2 hours.
3. Observe for signs of obstructed airway. Ventilatory support is continued until clinically stable (usually 24 to 48 hours).
4. Request that the surgeon mark a suction catheter, indicating how far the catheter can be safely inserted without disturbing the anastomosis (usually 2 to 3 cm).
5. Administer chest physiotherapy, as prescribed.
   a. Change the infant's position by turning; stimulate crying to promote full expansion of lungs.
   b. Elevate head and shoulders 20 to 30 degrees.
   c. Use mechanical vibrator 2 to 3 days postoperatively (to minimize trauma to anastomosis), followed by more vigorous physical therapy after the third day.
6. Continue use of isolette or radiant warmer with humidity.
7. Be prepared for an emergency: Have emergency equipment available, including suction machine, catheter, oxygen, laryngoscope, ET tubes in varying sizes.

CLINICAL JUDGMENT Care should be taken not to hyperextend the neck, causing stress to the operative site.

Providing Adequate Nutrition

Feedings may be given NPO, by gastrostomy, or (rarely) by a feeding tube into the esophagus, depending on the type of operation performed and the infant's condition.

1. The gastrostomy is generally attached to gravity drainage postoperatively, then elevated and left open to allow for air to escape and gastric secretions to pass into the duodenum before feedings are begun.
2. Practice patterns differ regarding when to start feedings but generally minimal enteral nutrition is beneficial in promoting gut motility, decreasing bacterial overgrowth, and decreasing the stress on the liver; these "trickle" feedings are given at a rate of 5 to 20 mL/kg/day.
3. Give the infant a pacifier to suck during feedings, unless contraindicated.
4. Use care to prevent air from entering the stomach, thereby causing gastric distention and possible reflux.
5. Continue gastrostomy feedings until the infant can tolerate full feedings orally.

Providing Comfort Measures

1. Position comfortably.
2. Avoid restraints when possible.
3. Administer mouth care frequently.
4. Offer a pacifier frequently.
5. Assess for pain and administer analgesics, as ordered (see page 1146).
6. Caress and speak or sing to the infant frequently. Handling should be kept to a gentle minimum.

Maintaining Chest Drainage

1. Assess the type of chest drainage present (determined by surgical approach). Report saliva or hemorrhage.
   a. Retropleural—small tube in posterior mediastinum; may be left open for drainage.
   b. Transthoracic—chest tube placed in pleural space and connected to suction.
2. Keep tubing patent: free from clots, unkinked, and without tension.
3. If a break occurs in the closed drainage system, immediately clamp tubing close to the infant to prevent pneumothorax.

Observing for Complications

1. Inspect for leak at the anastomosis, causing mediastinitis, pneumothorax, and saliva in chest tube: hypothermia or hyperthermia, severe respiratory distress, cyanosis, restlessness, and weak pulses.
2. Continue to monitor for complications during the recovery process.
   a. Stricture at the anastomosis: difficulty in swallowing, vomiting, or spitting up of ingested fluid; refusing to eat; fever secondary to aspiration and pneumonia.
   b. Recurrent fistula: coughing, choking, and cyanosis associated with feeding; excessive salivation; difficulty in swallowing associated with abnormal distention; repeated episodes of pneumonitis; general poor physical condition (no weight gain).
   c. Atelectasis or pneumonitis: aspiration, respiratory distress.
3. Provide meticulous care for cervical esophagostomy—artificial opening in the neck that allows for drainage of the upper esophagus.
   a. Keep the area clean of saliva.
   b. Wash with clear water.
   c. Place an absorbent pad over the area.
4. As soon as possible, allow the infant to suck a few milliliters of milk at the same time gastrostomy feeding is being done. Advance the infant to solid foods, as appropriate, if esophagostomy is maintained for a few months.
   a. Encourage sucking and swallowing.
   b. Familiarize the infant with food so that when able to eat orally, infant will be used to it.

5. Begin oral feedings 10 to 14 days postoperatively after anastomosis, as directed.
   a. Feed slowly to allow the infant time to swallow.
   b. Use upright sitting position to avoid the risk of regurgitation.
   c. Burp frequently or vent GT.
   d. Do not allow the infant to become overtired at feeding time. Note heart rate.
   e. Try to make each feeding a pleasant experience for the infant. Use a consistent approach and patience. Encourage parental caregiver involvement.

Stimulating Parental Caregiver–Infant Attachment

1. Gently hold and cuddle the infant for feedings and after feedings.
2. Encourage parental caregivers to cuddle and talk to the infant.
3. Provide for visual, auditory, and tactile stimulation, as appropriate, for the infant's physical condition and age.
4. Provide opportunities for the parental caregivers to learn all aspects of care of their infant.
5. Encourage the parental caregivers to talk about their feelings, fears, and concerns.
6. Help to develop a healthy parental caregiver–child relationship through flexible visiting, frequent phone calls, and encouraging physical contact between child and parental caregivers.

Community and Home Care Considerations

EVIDENCE BASE Örnö Ax, S., Dellenmark-Blom, M., Abrahamsson, K., Jonsson, L., & Gatzinsky, V. (2023). The association of feeding difficulties and generic health-related quality of life among children born with esophageal atresia. *Orphanet Journal of Rare Diseases, 18*(1), 237. https://doi.org/10.1186/s13023-023-02836-w

1. Teach carefully and thoroughly all procedures to be done at home. Show the parental caregivers how to do them and then watch return demonstration of the following procedures:
   a. Gastrostomy feedings and care.
   b. Esophagostomy care with feeding technique.
   c. Suctioning.
   d. Identifying signs of respiratory distress.
2. Advise parental caregivers that esophageal motility will be affected for many years, because of the narrowed abnormal esophagus emptying slowly and tension in the stomach from the anastomosis.
3. Reflux may increase after surgery and thus should be maximally treated because of the risk of developing esophageal strictures.
4. Monitor weight gain and developmental progress.
5. Observe the feeding technique of the parental caregiver.
6. Encourage parental caregivers to discuss child's condition with day care workers, teachers, school nurse, or other responsible adults in close contact with the child so that they will be able to recognize possible problems and reinforce good eating habits.
7. To compensate for altered motility, encourage cutting food into small pieces, chewing food well, swallowing food with fluid, and sitting upright while eating.
8. Observe parental caregiver–child interaction to assess for overprotection and appropriate coping skills.

Family Education and Health Maintenance

EVIDENCE BASE Bevilacqua, F., Ragni, B., Conforti, A., Gentile, S., Zaccara, A., Dotta, A., Bagolan, P., & Aite, L. (2020). Fixed the gap, solved the problem? Eating skills in esophageal atresia patients at 3 years. *Diseases of the Esophagus, 33*(1), 1–6. https://doi.org/10.1093/dote/doz102

1. Help the parental caregivers understand the psychological needs of the infant for sucking, warmth, comfort, stimulation, and affection. Suggest that activity be appropriate for age.
2. Encourage the parental caregivers to continue close medical follow-up, and help them learn to recognize possible problems.
   a. Eating problems may occur, especially when solids are introduced.
   b. Repeated respiratory tract infection should be reported.
   c. Occurrence of stricture at the site of anastomosis weeks to months later may be recognized by difficulty in swallowing, spitting of ingested fluid, and fever. Continue all reflux medications until advised otherwise. Medications should be adjusted by weight as infant grows.
   d. Dilatation of esophagus may be necessary to treat stricture at the site of the anastomosis.
   e. Signs of fistula leakage are dusky color or choking with feeding.
3. Help the parental caregivers understand the need for good nutrition and the need to follow the diet regimen suggested by the health care provider.
4. Reassure parental caregivers that an infant's raspy cough is normal and will gradually diminish as the infant's trachea becomes stronger over 6 to 24 months (most infants have some tracheomalacia).
5. Teach parental caregivers to guard against the child swallowing foreign objects.
6. Help and support can be given by introducing the parental caregivers to others in the same situation.
7. For additional information and support, refer parental caregivers to Birth Defect Research for Children (www.birthdefects.org), International Foundation for Functional Gastrointestinal Disorders (www.aboutkidsgi.org), Boston Children's Hospital (www.childrenshospital.org), or the March of Dimes Foundation (www.marchofdimes.org).

Evaluation: Expected Outcomes

- No cyanosis or respiratory distress.
- Hydrated; urine output adequate.
- Parental caregivers hold and talk to the infant; express concerns.
- Postoperatively, tolerates gastrostomy feedings without distention or regurgitation.
- Infant thrives, with adequate weight gain.
- Infant sleeps and rests without irritability or pain.
- Chest tube in place with minimal drainage.
- Feeds without regurgitation 12 days postoperatively.
- Parental caregivers caring for infant postoperatively and assisting with feedings.

GASTROESOPHAGEAL REFLUX AND GASTROESOPHAGEAL REFLUX DISEASE

EVIDENCE BASE Pados, B. F., & Davitt, E. S. (2020). Pathophysiology of gastroesophageal reflux disease in infants and nonpharmacologic strategies for symptom management. *Nursing for Women's Health, 24*(2), 101–114. https://doi.org/10.1016/j.nwh.2020.01.005

Gastroesophageal reflux (GER) is the passage of gastric contents into the esophagus. The barrier between the stomach and the esophagus is controlled primarily by pressure at the lower esophageal sphincter (LES). GER is a normal physiologic process and occurs in all healthy infants and children, usually several times a day, without symptoms or sequelae. Of all infants with GER, 50% will be symptomatic (vomiting or regurgitation) during the first 3 months of life; 67% of infants aged 4 to 9 months will have symptoms; and 5% of infants aged 10 to 12 months will have symptoms. Symptomatic GER often self-resolves by 12 to 14 months of age.

Gastroesophageal reflux disease (GERD) is defined as the symptom complex that results as a complication of GER. GERD is used to describe a condition when this reflux process causes bothersome symptoms and complications, such as significant discomfort and altered feeding and sleeping patterns. Clinical manifestations include vomiting, dysphagia, food refusal, poor weight gain, failure to thrive (FTT), esophagitis, irritability/excessive crying, abdominal pain, substernal pain, respiratory disorders, asthma, and apparent life-threatening events (ALTEs) or apnea.

The North American Society for Pediatric Gastroenterology, Hepatology, and Nutrition has formulated guidelines for the diagnosis and management of GER and GERD in infants and children; however, these guidelines are not intended for the management of neonates less than 72 hours old, premature neonates, or infants/children with neurologic or anatomic abnormalities of the upper gastrointestinal (GI) tract. The American Academy of Pediatrics has also endorsed these guidelines.

Supportive care by nurses and other health care staff regarding feeding techniques and nutrition is often sufficient for patients with GER. GERD may require additional interventions, such as changes to feeding regimen or medication therapy.

Pathophysiology and Etiology

Gastroesophageal Reflux

1. The LES is a physiologic, rather than an anatomic, segment that forms an antireflux barrier.
   a. 2 to 5 cm in length.
   b. Characterized by a pressure greater than that found proximally in the esophagus or distally in the stomach.
   c. Constitutes an effective barrier to protect the esophageal mucosa and airway passages from damage by gastric contents (acid, pepsin, bile salts, food).
   d. Neuromuscular connection is weak in infants, and GER peaks at age 6 months and usually resolves by 12 months.

Gastroesophageal Reflux Disease

1. Episodes of GERD with aspiration of refluxed material are more likely to occur during the nocturnal period—when the esophagus and stomach are leveled and the swallowing response to reflux and airway protection mechanisms are blunted by sleep.
2. Cause is undetermined in most patients; however, possible causes include:
   a. Delayed neuromuscular development.
   b. Cerebral anomalies.
   c. Obstruction at or just below the pylorus (e.g., pyloric stenosis, malrotation).
   d. Physiologic immaturity.
   e. Increased abdominal pressure.
   f. Obesity.
   g. Cystic fibrosis.
   h. Congenital esophageal disease.
3. Associated conditions that contribute to reflux include:
   a. Chronic lung disease—there is a higher incidence of reflux in infants with this condition. It appears to be related to the duration of the episode and how proximal the reflux occurs, possibly contributing to poor clearance.
   b. Trauma/mechanical causes that affect the LES.
      i. Indwelling orogastric/nasogastric (NG) enteric feeding tube.
      ii. Surgery on the esophagus or stomach.
      iii. Mechanical ventilation.
      iv. Extreme changes in position; lying completely flat; seating devices for infants greater than a 30% incline (increases intra-abdominal pressure).
      v. Hiatal hernia.
   c. Studies show a reduced incidence of reflux in the prone position versus the supine position; however, the American Academy of Pediatrics' "Back to Sleep" program discourages prone positioning because of the increased incidence of SIDS.
   d. Protein allergy: increased inflammation in the mucosa of the esophagus and stomach, altering motility.
   e. Medications/drugs that affect LES and increase gastric acidity, such as bronchodilators, antihypertensives, diazepam, meperidine, morphine, prostaglandins, calcium channel blockers, nitrate heart medications, anticholinergics, adrenergic drugs, caffeine, alcohol, and nicotine.
   f. Cystic fibrosis, cardiac disease, and other chronic illnesses.

Clinical Manifestations of Gastroesophageal Reflux Disease

Infants

1. Vomiting or regurgitation of formula or breast milk.
2. Irritability, excessive crying with or without association with vomiting.
3. Sleep disturbances.
4. Arching, stiffening.
5. It is recommended that the infant be referred to a pediatric gastroenterologist if the following manifestations occur:
   a. Refusal to eat.
   b. Weight loss or failure to gain weight.
   c. Dehydration.
   d. Recurrent respiratory symptoms, such as cough, wheezing, stridor, pneumonia, otitis media, bronchitis.
   e. BRUE (brief, resolved, unexplained event): blue spell, decreased responsiveness, limp, apnea, bradycardia. (*Note:* The exact relationship between GER and BRUE is not

clear despite continued investigation. Indeed, both apnea and reflux are common in premature neonates.)

f. Eructation (belching).
g. Sandifer syndrome (rare)—dystonic posturing caused by reflux.
h. Anemia (from chronic esophagitis).
i. Hematemesis (vomitus with blood).
j. Occult blood in stool.
k. Hypoproteinemia: low albumin due to severe inflammation and protein losses in the GI tract; can be seen with or without malnutrition and FTT.

Older Children

1. Intermittent vomiting.
2. Chronic heartburn or regurgitation.
3. Upper abdominal discomfort; pressure or "squeezing" feeling.
4. Chronic respiratory/airway symptoms, such as cough, stridor, otitis media, bronchitis, asthma.
5. Food refusal.
6. Dysphagia: difficulty swallowing.
7. Odynophagia: painful swallowing.
8. Anemia (from chronic esophagitis).
9. Hematemesis.
10. Hypoproteinemia.
11. Occult blood in stool.

Diagnostic Evaluation

1. History and physical examination can diagnose most cases.
2. Multiple intraluminal impedance and esophageal pH monitoring can be performed on all ages; no sedation necessary.
   a. Performed over 24 hours but does not indicate whether aspiration is occurring.
   b. Used as an index of esophageal acid exposure; however, esophageal impedance studies have been found to be more accurate, especially in the neurologically impaired child.
   c. The child must be off acid-suppressing medications for 48 to 72 hours so that acid pH can be detected.
   d. Gastric motility medications may or may not be held depending on the reason for performing the study.
   e. Most centers allow the patient to go home and return 24 hours later. Exceptions include the fragile child, premature infant, infant with active respiratory symptoms, or the child with significant symptoms who requires close observation because reflux may exacerbate while off reflux medications.
   f. Not indicated in the infant/child who is vomiting, unable to tolerate bolus feedings, or acutely ill. Because the probe is inserted in nares, infant/children with oxygen requirements may not tolerate the study.
3. Endoscopy and biopsy allow for visualization of esophageal, gastric, and duodenal mucosa.
   a. Indicated for severe GERD or failure of medical management.
   b. Biopsy can determine cause: allergy (eosinophilic), inflammation, chemical injury, or Barrett esophagus.
   c. Mechanical problems such as strictures, webs, and duplication/cysts will be visualized.
   d. For this procedure, sedation and anesthesia are necessary.
   e. Reflux medications do not have to be discontinued for the study.
   f. Can be done on the child who is not tolerating feedings. However, the severity of illness may prevent the study from being performed because of the risk associated with procedure, such as with anesthesia, infection, bleeding, and cardiac.
4. Technetium scintigraphy (milk/emptying scan) to assess gastric emptying and associated aspiration. This is not a reliable test for determining GERD.
   a. Sedation is not necessary, and the study can be performed on children of all ages.
   b. Involves drinking/eating food with radionuclide, followed by dynamic sequenced imaging.
   c. Not indicated in the infant/child who is vomiting, unable to tolerate bolus feedings, or acutely ill.
   d. Acid suppression medications do not interfere with the study.
5. Modified barium swallow—also called *video fluoroscopy*.
   a. Assesses oral pharyngeal function and potential for aspiration from oral intake using several consistencies of feedings. This is not a reliable test for determining GERD.
   b. Sedation is not necessary for this procedure but does require cooperation with eating.
   c. Should not be performed on the infant/child with acute respiratory symptoms or one identified by speech therapy or occupational therapy as being at risk for aspiration.
   d. Reflux medications do not have to be discontinued for the study.
   e. Speech therapist can be present for the examination to offer detailed assessment of oral–motor skills and swallowing.
6. Esophageal manometry to measure pressure inside the LES.
   a. It is a cooperative, nonsedated procedure and can only be used on an older child.
   b. Reflux medications generally do not have to be discontinued for the study.
7. Intraluminal esophageal impedance to detect the flow of liquids and gas through the esophagus may be used in combination with manometry.
8. Polysomnography may be used for evaluation of infant apnea and sleep apnea.

Complications

Complications result from frequent and sustained reflux of gastric contents into lower esophagus.

1. Recurrent pulmonary disease.
2. Chronic esophagitis.
3. FTT.
4. Anemia.
5. ALTE, although evidence is not strong.
6. Esophageal stricture from scarring.
7. Barrett esophagus: the replacement of distal esophageal mucosa with a potentially malignant metaplastic epithelium caused by chronic exposure to acid.
8. Chronic sinusitis/otitis media.
9. There is an unclear relationship between GERD and dental erosion/caries.

Management

Goal of treatment is to alleviate and relieve symptoms and prevent complications. May be treated medically through careful positioning, feeding techniques, and medication or surgically.

Positioning for Gastroesophageal Reflux

1. Esophageal monitoring has demonstrated that infants have significantly fewer episodes of GER when prone. Several studies support less incidence of reflux episodes in the prone and left-side sleeping position; however, the North American Society for Pediatric Gastroenterology, Hepatology, and Nutrition, along with the American Academy of Pediatrics, endorses the following recommendations:
   a. Place infant with head elevation or left lateral position after feeding when awake, not for sleep.
   b. Handle the infant gently, with minimal movement during and after feeding.

Feeding for Gastroesophageal Reflux

1. Small, frequent feedings followed by upright positioning with infant held over the shoulder.
2. Thickened feedings with dry rice cereal (1 tbsp per ounce of formula) or commercial thickening agent may be used. Thickening does not decrease episodes of reflux but does decrease episodes of vomiting. Commercial formulas thickened with rice starch are now available, but no studies regarding their efficacy have been published. Thickening of breast milk may be necessary in infants with poor weight gain.
3. Continuance of breastfeeding with the birthing parent eliminating milk and soy products is encouraged, as allergen sensitivity can contribute to GER. No studies support the need for dietary restriction in people who breastfeed, but in anecdotal reports, infants appear to improve when dairy products are reduced. A 2- to 4-week trial of partially hydrolyzed formula is useful for refractory symptoms or for those infants/children with signs of allergy, anemia, constipation, occult positive stools, and vomiting. Hypoallergenic (elemental) formula may be used if symptoms persist.
4. Pectin liquid partially decreases GER, as measured by esophageal pH monitoring, and might improve vomiting and respiratory symptoms in children with cerebral palsy.
5. Concentrating formula is a method of increasing calories for the volume-sensitive infant.
6. Avoid constant feeding (grazing), which reduces appetite and, ultimately, caloric intake.
7. Comfort the infant to reduce crying before and after meals, which increases intra-abdominal pressure and swallowing of air, increasing the likelihood of reflux.
8. Use a pacifier for nonnutritive sucking after eating to avoid overeating.

Feeding for Gastroesophageal Reflux Disease

1. Transgastric (transpyloric) enteric feeding tube used for infants when reflux medical management fails and symptoms persist; can reduce the number of reflux episodes, but has not been shown to significantly reduce episodes of apnea.
   a. There are concerns regarding using these feeding tubes in neonates; however, the rate of complications does not appear to be statistically significant in recent reports.
   b. The procedure should be performed by a skilled pediatric radiologist or neonatal intensive care nurse, using a small caliber soft polyurethane nonweighted feeding tube.
   c. Considered a temporary feeding method (to help infant/child gain weight and improve respiratory symptoms) until further options can be explored, such as surgery—Nissen fundoplication or jejunostomy.
   d. To prevent clogging, tubes should be flushed at least four to six times per day and before and after medication administration. If the tube clogs or dislodges, the family must return to a qualified center for reinsertion.
   e. If feeding difficulty persists, consult dietitian and speech and/or occupational therapist.
2. Older child:
   a. Nothing to eat 2 hours before bedtime.
   b. Avoid spicy and acidic foods (onions, citrus products, apple juice, tomatoes), esophageal irritants (chocolate, caffeinated beverages, peppermint, and secondhand smoke), and carbonated beverages.
   c. Chew gum (stimulates parotid secretions, which augment esophageal clearance and provide a buffering effect).

Other Lifestyle Changes for Gastroesophageal Reflux Disease

1. Prevent obesity.
2. Avoid tight or constrictive clothing.
3. Avoid nonsteroidal anti-inflammatory drugs, especially at bedtime.

Drug Therapy for Gastroesophageal Reflux Disease

1. Often used in combination with lifestyle changes. Prescribed for a 4- to 8-week trial and can be tapered and discontinued if symptoms resolve.
2. Antacids—buffer existing acids and also increase serum gastrin levels, leading to an increase in LES pressure (symptomatic relief). Chronic antacid therapy is generally not recommended unless ordered by a gastroenterologist.
3. Histamine-2 (H_2) receptor antagonists—act by reducing hydrochloric acid and pepsinogen secretion by blocking histamine receptors on the parietal cells.
   a. Cimetidine, ranitidine, famotidine, nizatidine.
   b. Oral dosing of three times (tid) versus two times (bid) per day has demonstrated improved duration of acid suppression in one study of infants (44% vs. 90%).
   c. Tolerance to intravenous (IV) dosing within 6 weeks of usage has been observed.
4. Proton-pump inhibitors (PPIs)—block all gastric acid secretion by binding and deactivating the H^+/K^+ ATPase enzyme pumps. To be activated, PPIs require acid in the parietal cell canaliculus; therefore, they are most effective when the parietal cells are stimulated by a meal following a fast.
   a. Omeprazole, lansoprazole, pantoprazole, esomeprazole, rabeprazole.
   b. Generally given 15 to 30 minutes before a meal, once to bid per day.
   c. Generally not recommended in combination with H_2-antagonists because of interference with absorption (H_2 reduces the acid necessary for PPI to work).
   d. Reserved for infants and children resistant to H_2-antagonist therapy. Gastroenterology specialist should be involved. Data on the pharmacology in infants and children are limited.
   e. Dominant regurgitation in neonates and infants responds poorly to PPIs.

5. Prokinetic agents—enhance esophageal peristalsis and accelerate gastric emptying. However, there is insufficient evidence of efficacy in GERD.
   a. Metoclopramide—an antidopaminergic agent whose efficacy is not well observed in clinical trials. Adverse effects include parkinsonian reactions, tardive dyskinesia, irritability, sleeplessness, and lowered seizure threshold.
   b. Erythromycin at low dose: motility receptor agonist. Can be associated with dysrhythmia and increased incidence of hypertrophic pyloric stenosis. Contraindicated in some patients with preexisting cardiac conditions.
6. A surface agent sucralfate may be used—an aluminum complex that acts by adhering to mucosal lesions, reducing symptoms, and promoting healing.
   a. May be used as an adjunct to an H_2-blocker or PPI, and usually for a period of several weeks or less.
   b. If used for esophagitis, should be made into a liquid preparation.
   c. If used for ulcer or gastritis, it is inhibited by H_2 blockers and PPIs because of the need for an acidic environment.

DRUG ALERT All acid-altering medications may affect the efficacy of pH-dependent medications. In addition, PPIs are metabolized to varying degrees by the hepatic cytochrome P450 enzymatic system and may alter drug metabolism by induction or inhibition of the cytochrome P enzymes.

DRUG ALERT The potential adverse effects of aluminum in infants and children should be considered before administering sucralfate; data on its efficacy and safety in children are not fully substantiated.

Surgical Management for Gastroesophageal Reflux Disease

EVIDENCE BASE Tindal, E. W., Willis, M., Recinos Soto, A., Coyle, M. G., Herzlinger, M., Luks, F. I., & Renaud, E. J. (2023). How many tests does it take? Minimizing preoperative testing prior to surgical placement of gastrostomy tubes in children. *Nutrition in Clinical Practice, 38*(2), 434–441. https://doi.org/10.1002/ncp.10949

1. Nissen fundoplication is the most commonly used surgical method to treat moderate-to-severe GERD that is unresponsive to medication therapy. Decisions concerning appropriate long-term feeding access must be individualized.
   a. Involves wrapping of the fundus around the LES (see Figure 44-3).
   b. Overall complication rate ranges from 2.2% to 45%.
   c. Other surgical approaches include ventral (Thal) or dorsal (Toupet) semifundoplication.
   d. In some studies, recurrence of reflux in the child who is neurodisabled is as high as 46%.
   e. Simultaneous gastrostomy is usually performed for feeding purposes or as a temporary measure to decompress the stomach.
   f. The most commonly reported complications of surgery include breakdown of the wrap, small bowel obstruction, gas bloat syndrome, infection, perforation, leaking at the anastomosis site, persistent esophageal stricture, esophageal obstruction, dumping syndrome, incisional hernia, and gastroparesis.
   g. Reoperation rates range from 3% to 18%.
   h. The greater the complexity of the infant or child's health status, the greater the chance of complications.

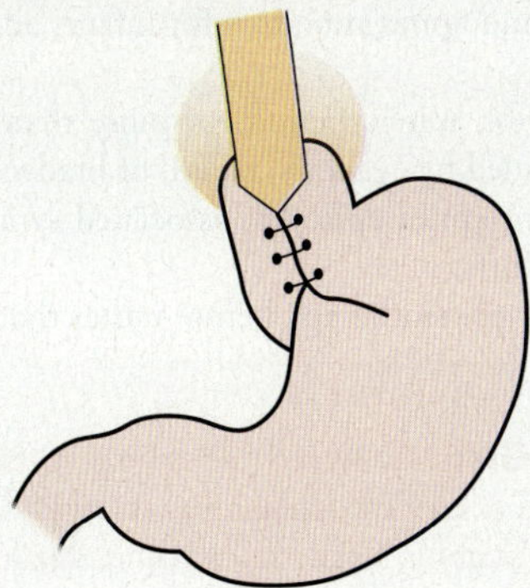

Figure 44-3. Nissan fundoplication for gastroesophageal reflux disease.

2. Jejunostomy feeding tubes can be placed but are usually restricted to severe cases of recurrent GERD and/or failed Nissen procedure.
   a. Most surgeons use either a standard gastrostomy tube (GT) or a low-profile tube (button).
   b. Complications include intestinal obstruction and leaking.

Other Treatments Under Investigation

Investigation is underway to identify pathways and mechanisms that interfere or control the transient relaxation of the LES. Future understanding of this mechanism will aid in the development of lifestyle changes and medical management, which will assist in inhibiting transient relaxations. Reduction of gastric mechanoreceptor signaling to the brain has emerged as one of the likely sites of action for new reflux inhibitor drugs. The most promising among these appear to be the $GABA_B$ receptor agonists and metabotropic glutamate receptor 5 (mGluR5).

Nursing Assessment

1. Obtain a history of infant's or child's eating habits, including formula history, food allergies, volume tolerated at each meal.
2. Obtain a history of complications from GER (i.e., recurrent respiratory infections, asthma, poor weight gain).
3. Observe infant's or child's feeding behaviors. (Does child eat with a bottle, spoon, fingers? Can child feed self?)
4. Assess general appearance, skin integrity, and growth and development.

Nursing Interventions

Preventing Aspiration

1. Administer medications via IV line until tolerating enteral feedings.
   a. Administer prokinetics (motility agents) and acid suppressants 30 minutes before meals when bolus feeding schedule is instituted. Monitor for adverse effects.
   b. Unless abnormal gastric dysmotility prior to surgery, most prokinetics are discontinued after Nissen fundoplication.
2. Maintain positioning, as stated earlier.

3. Use cardiac and apnea monitors for infants and children with severe reflux.
   a. Observe for apneic periods of more than 20 seconds or accompanied by cyanosis, pallor, or bradycardia.
   b. Document apnea episodes, associated symptoms, and recovery efforts.
4. Provide chest physiotherapy before rather than after meals, if ordered.

CLINICAL JUDGMENT Avoid slouching position because this may change angle of esophagus in relation to stomach, increase intra-abdominal pressure, and facilitate reflux of stomach contents.

Maintaining Adequate Nutrition

See also section on feeding, page 1278.

1. Provide concentrated formula if volume cannot be tolerated.
2. Seek nutrition consult if patient continues to have difficulty feeding.
3. Monitor for fatigue during feeding; increased effort to suck requires higher energy expenditures. If noted, referral to occupational/speech therapy and possible modified barium swallow study are advised.
4. Monitor weight on the same scale.
5. Accurately record activity of infant.
   a. Amount of feeding taken; whether retained.
   b. Any change in behavior as a result of feeding technique.
6. Explain to the breastfeeding parent that feeding modifications may need to be made, especially in infants with poor weight gain. Assist them to express milk, quantitate volume, thicken with cereal, and fortify breast milk with formula, as needed.
7. Follow postoperative instructions on initiation of feedings.
8. If the child has a GT:
   a. Usually elevated and vented until return of bowel function.
   b. Monitor drainage, avoid kinking, and follow orders for positioning for straight drainage, elevation, or clamping.

Maintaining Fluid and Electrolyte Balance

1. Monitor vital signs and assess skin turgor for signs of dehydration.
2. Observe and record accurately urine output.
   a. Weigh diapers.
   b. Measure amount, frequency, color, and concentration of voided urine.
   c. Check specific gravity, if possible.
3. Monitor IV therapy, if ordered.
4. Monitor serum electrolytes, magnesium, phosphorus, and calcium. Replace, as ordered. Particular close monitoring is warranted if infant/child has draining gastrostomy.
5. Promote good skin care to prevent lesions of dry and delicate tissues.
   a. Change position frequently.
   b. Change soiled diapers promptly.
   c. Apply lotion and gently massage any reddened areas.

CLINICAL JUDGMENT If patient is malnourished, monitor for refeeding syndrome until laboratory studies are stable. Refeeding syndrome can cause intracellular shifting of electrolytes including calcium, magnesium, and phosphorus, resulting in death. Laboratory studies should be monitored daily or more frequently if abnormal.

Reducing Fear of Eating

1. Provide thickened feedings to increase satisfaction for the infant.
2. Identify and attempt to reduce stress, especially around mealtime.
3. Feed the child in a quiet, calm environment.
4. Children like routines; feed at routine intervals by the person with whom the child is familiar and comfortable.
5. For the older child, encourage participation in family dinnertime so the child observes eating as a pleasurable experience.
6. Advise parental caregivers that clinical specialists in feeding disorders are available.

Community and Home Care Considerations

1. Recognize that home health care referral is appropriate for the following situations:
   a. FTT: medication teaching and monitoring, teaching of formula preparation, positioning, weight.
   b. Respiratory complications/ALTE: medication teaching and monitoring, assessment of respiratory status, teaching of monitor/cardiopulmonary resuscitation (CPR), use of nebulizer.
   c. Nissen fundoplication (with GT): medication teaching and monitoring; wound assessment; monitoring of bloating; dumping syndrome; formula intolerance; GT teaching, including pump teaching, venting, medication administration, tube changing.
2. Recommend careful feeding and behavioral diary to monitor symptoms and improvements.
3. Recognize that school and community activities may affect adherence for older children; work with the family to devise individualized management strategies.
4. Assist parental caregivers to discuss medication and lunchtime behaviors with teacher and school nurse so consistency can be maintained.
5. Assess need for community services, such as respite care, especially for single parental caregiver.

Family Education and Health Maintenance

EVIDENCE BASE Farou, N., Lucas, C., & Olympia, R. (2021). School nurses on the front lines of healthcare: Children with medical devices—A "BOLUS" of information about gastrostomy tube malfunctions and infections. *NASN School Nurse, 36*(3), 144–148. https://doi.org/10.1177/1942602X20940026

1. Plan a program of intensive parental caregiver teaching on how to handle and care for the infant. Explain rationale to parental caregivers. Make sure that they have proper equipment for propping the infant. Help the parental caregivers understand that it is not necessary to keep infant in infant seat or propped up at all times.
   a. Bathe or play with the infant before feeding.
   b. Change position about 1 hour after feeding.
   c. During the night after feeding, the infant can sleep in a semi-reclining (30 degrees) position.
   d. Expect occasional small amounts of vomiting.
2. Offer clear, concise instructions. Focus on fears of the parental caregiver. Discuss techniques to promote development of

infants while facilitating bonding and typical parental caregiver behavior.

3. If infant or child is not demonstrating complication of GER (i.e., GERD), assist parental caregivers in understanding that GER is self-limited; symptoms usually disappear within 12 months.
4. If complications exist (GERD), referral to pediatric gastroenterology and nutrition specialists is recommended.
5. If Nissen fundoplication has been performed:
   a. Teach gastrostomy care, if applicable (see page 1154). Make sure that the parental caregivers know how to use, clear, vent, assess, and replace the tube. Help them to understand the purpose of GT placement (feedings, venting, medications) and the need for surgical or gastroenterology follow-up care.
   b. Explain about potential complications and when to call the health care provider. Such complications include gagging, retching, bloating, abdominal distention, fever, vomiting, diaphoresis, lethargy, diarrhea, and weight loss. Generally, the family should contact the surgeon within the first 6 weeks postoperatively, whereas eventual follow-up is with the gastroenterologist.
   c. It usually takes 12 weeks to heal; if the GT becomes dislodged in this period, the patient should be taken to the emergency department immediately.
   d. Complications of a dislodged GT in the early postoperative period include peritonitis and bacteremia.
6. Help the parental caregivers understand the importance of follow-up for assessment of weight gain and development.
7. Assist with community resource planning (e.g., education, advocacy, and financial assistance). Identify support groups.
8. Instruct parental caregivers in CPR training before discharge of infant, if indicated.
9. Provide written and verbal instructions for medications and adverse effects.
10. Advise parental caregivers on when to call their health care provider in regard to their child's symptoms. Danger signs of dehydration include a decrease in wet diapers, listlessness, lethargy, reduced appetite, sunken fontanelle; those for aspiration include respiratory distress and cyanotic spells, fever.
11. Encourage family to contact their health care provider immediately with treatment concerns or problems.
12. For additional information and support, contact the North American Society of Pediatric Gastroenterology, Hepatology, and Nutrition (www.naspghan.org), the United Ostomy Association (www.ostomy.org), or the Pediatric/Adolescent Gastroesophageal Reflux Association (www.reflux.org).

Evaluation: Expected Outcomes

- Mild regurgitation immediately after feeding; no apnea or cyanosis noted.
- Takes regular feedings without significant symptoms; weight gain noted.
- Urine output adequate.
- Exhibits pleasure in eating.

FAILURE TO THRIVE/ MALNUTRITION

EVIDENCE BASE Reed, M., Mullaney, K., Ruhmann, C., March, P., Conte, V. H., Noyes, L., & Bleazard, M. (2020). Screening Tool for the Assessment of Malnutrition in Pediatrics (STAMP) in the electronic health record: A validation study. *Nutrition in Clinical Practice*, *35*(6), 1087–1093. https://doi.org/10.1002/ncp.10562

Failure to thrive (FTT), or *malnutrition*, is the inadequate physical development of an infant or child manifested as a deceleration in weight gain, a low weight/height ratio, or a low weight/height/head circumference ratio. The exact prevalence is unknown, although research suggests FTT accounts for 3% to 5% of pediatric hospital admissions. Children with FTT are at risk for adverse outcomes, such as short stature, behavior problems, and developmental delay. The Agency for Healthcare Research and Quality has an evidence-based practice program on which clinical guidelines can be developed. The primary causative factors of FTT are insufficient nutrition availability, inadequate absorption and/or utilization of nutrients, and added metabolic requirements.

Previously, practitioners diagnosed FTT when a child's weight for age falls below the fifth percentile of the standard National Center for Health Statistics growth chart or if it crosses two major percentile lines. Recent research has validated using *z* scores, or standard deviations from the mean, of weight for height or body mass index to classify malnutrition:

Mild malnutrition: *z* score −1 to −1.9
Moderate malnutrition: *z* score −2 to −2.9
Severe malnutrition: *z* score −3 or greater

About 25% of normal infants will shift to a lower growth percentile in the first 2 years of life and then follow that percentile; this should not be diagnosed as FTT (see Standards of Care Guidelines 44-1, page 1281).

STANDARDS OF CARE GUIDELINES 44-1

Care of a Child With a Gastrointestinal or Nutritional Disorder

When caring for a child with a GI or nutritional disorder:

- Monitor weight.
- Monitor urinary and bowel elimination.
- Monitor intake and output.
- Assess developmental milestone attainment.
- Provide and teach appropriate feeding products and techniques.
- Use most efficient position for feeding.
- Facilitate a calm, pleasant environment for feeding.
- Avoid foods that may inhibit absorption of nutrients or cause symptoms such as gas.
- Encourage and support parental caregiver involvement in care and feeding of the child.
- Encourage and support normal play and other activities for the child as condition allows.
- Identify and respond to signs and symptoms that may indicate lack of adequate nutrition or sign of complications.

This information should serve as a general guideline only. Each patient situation presents a unique set of clinical factors and requires nursing judgment to guide care, which may include additional or alternative measures and approaches.

Pathophysiology and Etiology

1. FTT is a nutritional disorder having organic and nonorganic components.
   a. Organic FTT implies a major illness or organ system dysfunction as the etiology of the growth failure. It occurs equally in all populations and accounts for approximately 25% of FTT cases.
   b. Nonorganic FTT is the result of multiple psychosocial factors, including disturbances in parental caregiver–child interaction. This type accounts for 50% of cases of FTT and is most common among the psychosocially and economically deprived.
   c. The remaining 25% of cases represent mixed etiology.
2. Organic FTT has a pathophysiologic cause that reduces the availability of nutrients for maintenance and growth and is best divided into three categories:
   a. Insufficient nutrition because of the child's inability to feed properly, which may be a result of severe neurologic dysfunction, gastroesophageal reflux (GER), or cleft palate/lip.
   b. Nutrition is adequate but poorly absorbed and/or utilized (malabsorption syndromes), which may result from chronic ileocecal intussusception, GER, milk protein allergy, malrotation of the colon, hypoplastic stomach, short bowel syndrome (anatomic and functional), pancreatic insufficiency (including cystic fibrosis), pyloric stenosis, inflammatory bowel disease, and acquired immunodeficiency syndrome.
   c. Associated disorders include asthma, cardiac failure, thyroiditis, congenital heart disease, neurologic lesions, hydronephrosis, adrenal hyperplasia, diabetes insipidus, cystic fibrosis, chronic or recurrent urinary tract infection (UTI), hypothyroidism, autoimmune disorders, and immunodeficiency.
3. Nonorganic FTT occurs in the absence of gastrointestinal (GI), endocrine, congenital, or chronic diseases. It is usually associated with psychological deprivation but can also be related to behavioral or economic problems. Multiple features of the parental caregivers, child, and environment interact over time, resulting in parental caregiver–child interaction that ultimately leads to undernutrition and under nurturance of the child.

Clinical Manifestations

Organic Failure to Thrive

1. Retarded growth accompanied by manifestations of the underlying disease.
2. Weight loss in early stages. If poor intake continues, linear growth slows down or ceases. In latent stage, head circumference growth is retarded, indicating compromised brain development.
3. Developmental delays.
4. Infant stress—irritability, fussiness, jitteriness.
5. Feeding disorders—ineffective sucking, difficulty chewing, difficulty swallowing.
6. Clinical symptoms can include vomiting, hypothermia, lethargy, muscle wasting, decreased subcutaneous tissue, hypoalbuminemia, eczema, hair loss, and diarrhea.

Nonorganic Failure to Thrive

1. Retarded growth.
2. Infant stress—irritability, fussiness, jitteriness.
3. Feeding disorders—ineffective sucking, difficulty chewing, difficulty swallowing.
4. Reduced energy level.
5. Difficult temperament.
6. Fitful sleep.
7. Reduced responsiveness and interaction with the environment.
8. Social isolation, lack of vocalization.
9. Spasticity or rigidity when touched.
10. Inability to make eye contact or smile.
11. Refusal to eat; rejection of foods.
12. Spits up, gags, coughs with feeding, rumination.

Parental Caregiver Characteristics

1. Characteristics associated with parental caregivers of children with nonorganic FTT include lack of social and financial support, maladaptive relationships, alcohol or drug use, history of anxiety or depression, lack of caregiving skills, family stress and crisis, absence of a parental caregiver.
2. Postnatal depression corresponds to a higher association of FTT, but on its own, depression does not contribute to a higher incidence of FTT.

Diagnostic Evaluation

Comprehensive Assessment

1. FTT suggested if a child is falling off a previously established growth curve or falls below the fifth percentile. If FTT is of recent onset, weight but not height will fall below accepted standards. Depression of weight and height indicates chronic malnutrition.
2. Technique for evaluating growth—look at growth percentage of the median for that age. Divide the actual value of height or weight by median value for that age. For example, a 12-month-old female weighs 15 pounds (6.8 kg); the median for age is 21 1/2 pounds (9.8 kg). Child is 70% of median for age.
3. Complete health and dietary history—feeding, eating patterns, 3-day calorie count.
4. Physical examination for evidence of organic causes, with particular attention to ears, facial structure, mouth, heart, lungs, abdomen, and neurologic system.
5. Assessment of prenatal, perinatal, and postnatal infections.
6. Developmental assessment.
7. Family assessment—family short stature syndrome, family dynamics.
   a. With the assistance of endocrinologist and dietitian, calculate the midparental height of the biological parents:

{(biological father's height in cm + biological mother's height in cm) + 13 cm} divided by 2

Note: Subtract 13 cm for females and add 13 cm for males. For example, if the biological father is 180 cm and the biological mother is 167 cm, the biological daughter's equation would be $\{(180 + 167) - 13\} \div 2$.

CLINICAL JUDGMENT Children whose weight is less than 60% of the median value for age or less than 70% for height are in acute danger of severe morbidity and malnutrition.

Tests to Rule Out Organic Conditions

1. Complete blood count (CBC) with differential and indices, sedimentation rate to rule out anemia or hematologic or inflammatory cause.
2. Blood cultures if fever present.

3. Urinalysis and urine culture as baseline for bladder and renal function.
4. Thyroid-stimulating hormone and free thyroxine to rule out hypothyroidism.
5. Blood chemistry: provide data on electrolyte balance, renal function, and skeletal disorders.
6. Neonate screening tests, TORCH studies.
7. Stool screening tests to be ordered if diarrhea/abnormal stools are present:
   a. Infection: culture, ova and parasite, *Clostridium difficile*, white blood cell (WBC) count (may have false-negative results if recently on antibiotics).
   b. Protein malabsorption: alpha-one antitrypsin (may have false-negative results if not fed during collection).
   c. Carbohydrate malabsorption: pH, reducing substances (time sensitive, need to be fresh stool; may have false-negative results if not fed during collection).
   d. Fat malabsorption: random qualitative fecal fat (one-time sample); if needed, a 72-hour quantitative fecal fat should be collected. Results are more accurate when sample is collected while patient is receiving adequate nutrition.
   e. Pancreatic sufficiency: stool pancreatic elastase, stool chymotrypsin, and serum trypsin to detect primary or secondary pancreatic insufficiency.
8. Radiologic studies including upper GI series, barium swallow, reflux workup, upper endoscopy, and sweat test.

CLINICAL JUDGMENT One of the best tests to distinguish organic from nonorganic FTT is through observed feedings or enteral tube feedings to assess weight gain and caloric intake.

Management

1. Immediate treatment is directed at reversing malnutrition.
2. All children with FTT need additional calories for catch-up growth (typically 150% of the caloric requirement for their expected, not actual, weight).
3. Nutritional treatment is aimed at providing sufficient calories to support "catch-up" growth to restore deficits in weight and height. Protein and energy requirements for the typical child and the child with FTT are outlined in Table 44-1.
   a. This may require nasogastric (NG) tube feedings for safe refeeding.
   b. If fat malabsorption present, may need formula with high level of medium-chain triglycerides for direct absorption of fat.

Table 44-1 Protein and Energy Requirements

	THE TYPICAL CHILD		THE CHILD WITH FTT	
AGE (YEARS)	PROTEIN (G/KG)	ENERGY (KCAL/KG)	PROTEIN (G/KG)	ENERGY (KCAL/KG)
0–0.5	2.2	0.08	3.2	150–250
0.5–1	1.6	98	3.2	150–250
1–3	1.2	102	2.5	150–250
4–6	1.1	90	2.5	150–250
7–10	1.0	70	2.5	150–250

4. Multivitamin supplementation containing zinc and iron is usually recommended, fat-soluble vitamins (A, D, E, K) if fat malabsorption is present.
5. If cause is organic, the underlying disease entity is treated or managed.
6. In nonorganic FTT, hospitalization is avoided (unless the child is in imminent danger) because it further disrupts the parental caregiver–child relationship. Therefore, frequent home or clinic visits are necessary. Referral to feeding disorder clinic or rehabilitation center may be necessary.
7. Developmental interventions through occupational and physical therapy are instituted, if necessary, to prevent further delay.
8. Support, education, and financial assistance are offered to the family.
9. Nutrition, occupational therapy, and physical therapy consults are indicated.

Complications

Studies are inconsistent regarding the long-term complications of FTT.

1. Anemia, fatigue, hypothermia.
2. Vulnerability to infection.
3. Delayed healing.
4. Behavior problems, poor academic performance.
5. Developmental, speech, and language delays.
6. Perceptual difficulties.

Nursing Assessment

1. Obtain accurate anthropometric measurements.
   a. Weight of children younger than age 3 should be done unclothed in a supine position using a calibrated beam scale. Children older than age 3 should be done standing on a standard scale wearing same clothing each time. Effort should be made to use the same scale each time.
   b. Height should be recumbent up to age 2. All children should be measured without shoes.
   c. Head circumference is measured each visit until age 2 with a nonstretchable tape placed firmly from maximal occipital prominence to just above the eyebrow.
   d. All measurements need to be corrected for prematurity up to the second birthday by subtracting the number of weeks premature from the chronological age.
   e. Measurements should be plotted on growth chart using a straight edge or plot grid. Birth measurements should be obtained and entered for comparison.
2. Obtain nutritional history regarding eating patterns; nutritional beliefs for food allocation; 24-hour recall; who normally feeds the child; the type, amount, and frequency of feedings; the amount of time and effort required for meals; the child's reactions (physiologic and psychological) to feedings; food likes and dislikes; and environmental factors.
3. Observe parental caregiver–child interactions, such as sensitivity to child's needs, eye-to-eye contact, if and how the infant is held, and how the parental caregiver speaks to the child.
4. If possible, observe the parental caregiver feeding the child. Assess child's overall tone, sucking pattern, oral sensitivity (gag reflex), lip and tongue function, and swallowing ability. A videotape of the child eating in the home can be reviewed later to reduce the chance of observer distraction.
5. Assess neurologic and cardiovascular status for alertness, attentiveness, developmental delays, cardiac arrhythmias, or murmurs.

6. Assess skin, hair, and musculoskeletal system.
7. Assess developmental status using a Denver II developmental tool, as indicated.

Nursing Interventions

Promoting Adequate Nutrition

1. Facilitate nutritional consultation.
2. If hospitalized, provide a primary core of staff to feed the child. Ask the parental caregivers to do so when present in a nonthreatening manner.
3. Develop individualized teaching plan to instruct parental caregivers of child's dietary needs. Specify type of diet, essential nutrients, serving sizes, and method of preparation.
4. Provide a quiet, nonstimulating environment for eating.
5. Demonstrate proper feeding techniques including details on how to hold and how long to feed the child.
6. Administer multivitamin supplements, as prescribed.
7. Encourage nutritious, high-calorie, and fortified fluids to increase nutrient density. For infants, use 24 to 30 cal/ounce rather than 20 cal/ounce. For older children, suggest fruit smoothies using whole milk and ice cream.
8. Refeed the malnourished child with caution, monitoring electrolytes, calcium, magnesium, and phosphorus daily or more frequently, if abnormal.
   a. Gradually increase nutrients and use small, frequent feedings with adequate fluids to ensure hydration.
   b. Monitor intake and output.
9. Maintain high-nutrient diet until weight is appropriate for height (usually age 4 to 9 months).
10. Advise family that some nutritional intervention will be continued until appropriate height for age is reached.

CLINICAL JUDGMENT If patient is malnourished, monitor for refeeding syndrome until laboratory studies are stable. Refeeding syndrome can cause intracellular shifting of electrolytes, calcium, magnesium, and phosphorus, resulting in death. Laboratory studies should be monitored daily or more frequently, if abnormal.

CLINICAL JUDGMENT Be alert for signs of dehydration due to sudden change to a high-calorie, high-protein diet. A dramatic increase in protein can increase renal solute load to the point that a child is at risk for dehydration.

Promoting Adequate Growth and Development

1. Obtain accurate weight at every visit or every day, if hospitalized.
2. Assess child's growth by using age- and gender-appropriate growth charts. Extremely low-birth-weight infants born with major anomalies have nearly twice the risk of neurodevelopmental impairment and increased risk of poor growth.
3. Assess child's development by interviewing the parental caregiver or using developmental screening tests, such as the Denver II (Denver Developmental Materials, Inc., http://denverii.com/denverii/).
4. Observe interactions between parental caregivers and child and among family members, including eye contact, communication patterns, and coping ability.
5. Provide the infant with visual and auditory stimulation by exposing to bright colors, shapes, and music. Provide the older child with age-appropriate stimulation, such as books, games, and toys. Place the infant prone, while awake, on the floor to encourage trunk control.
6. Encourage periods of scheduled rest and sleep.

EVIDENCE BASE Atwal, K. (2023). Prevention of malnutrition and faltering growth in children and young people. *Nursing Children and Young People, 35*(2), 34–42. https://doi.org/10.7748/ncyp.2022.e1436

Promoting Effective Caregiving

1. Teach the parental caregiver caregiving skills by demonstrating proper holding, stroking, feeding, and communication using age-appropriate words and gestures.
2. If hospitalized, encourage and facilitate the parental caregivers to spend as much time as possible with the child.
3. Educate the parental caregivers to recognize and respond to the child's distress and hunger calls.
4. Help the parental caregivers to develop organizational skills—write down daily schedule with mealtimes, time for shopping, and so forth.
5. Refer for counseling, if necessary, to help parental caregivers overcome feelings of mistrust or neglect resulting from adverse personal childhood experiences.
6. Refer to social services to help resolve any social and financial difficulties that might interfere with providing a nurturing environment.
7. Monitor parental caregivers' progress and provide positive reinforcement.

Community and Home Care Considerations

Early intervention home visiting has been shown to reduce the long-term complications associated with FTT. This may be due to promotion of maternal sensitivity and helping children build strong work habits that enables them to flourish at school.

1. Make regular home visits to:
   a. Observe for continued parental caregiver–child interaction.
   b. Encourage continued developmentally appropriate play.
   c. Monitor feeding status and assess intake amount.
   d. Determine frequency of voiding and stooling.
   e. Assess child's weight, height, and head circumference.
   f. Monitor vital signs and watch for signs of dehydration.
   g. Auscultate bowel sounds.
   h. Assess muscle tone and vigor of activity.
   i. Assess family dynamics and use of support systems.
2. Inform parental caregivers of community resources, such as Women in Crisis program, food banks, and support groups.
3. Make sure that day care providers can meet child's special needs in terms of diet, feeding, and developmentally appropriate play. Day care may be beneficial in the presence of family dysfunction by providing structure.
4. Make referrals to social work and occupational or physical therapy, as needed.

Family Education and Health Maintenance

1. Reinforce the need for a quiet, nonthreatening, nurturing environment.

2. Encourage the parental caregivers to be consistent with feedings. Although forced feeding is avoided, strict adherence to appropriate feeding is essential for growth.
3. Advise the parental caregivers to introduce new foods slowly and follow the child's rhythm of feeding.
4. Review the importance of providing a routine rest schedule in an environment that is conducive to sleep.
5. Review development, stressing need for visual, auditory, and tactile stimulation and age-appropriate toys for continued development.
6. Reinforce the need for follow-up care, well-child visits, and immunizations.

Evaluation: Expected Outcomes

- Increases weight steadily.
- Attains developmental milestones at appropriate age.
- Parental caregivers participating in child's care, using appropriate feeding technique.

HYPERTROPHIC PYLORIC STENOSIS

EVIDENCE BASE Vinycomb, T. I., Laslett, K., Gwini, S. M., Teague, W., & Nataraja, R. M. (2019). Presentation and outcomes in hypertrophic pyloric stenosis: An 11-year review. *Journal of Paediatrics and Child Health*, *55*(10), 1183–1187. https://doi.org/10.1111/jpc.14372

Hypertrophic pyloric stenosis is an acquired condition in which the circumferential muscle of the pyloric sphincter becomes thickened, causing a high-grade gastric outlet obstruction that results in dilation, hypertrophy, and hyperperistalsis of the stomach. It is the second most common condition (after inguinal hernia) requiring surgery, which rarely occurs before age 2 weeks or later than age 5 months. Incidence is 1 in 250 live births and is predominant in males (5:1) and more common in first-born males. Incidence peaks in spring and fall. It is more likely to affect a full-term infant than a premature infant.

Pathophysiology and Etiology

1. Unknown cause, although new research has identified several genetic markers associated with the condition. Multiple theories of etiology exist, including immature or degenerated pyloric neural elements, variations in infant feeding regimens, excessive production of gastrin (maternal or infant), dyscoordination between gastric peristalsis and pyloric relaxation, deficiency of nitric acid, abnormalities in enteric nervous system, and abnormalities in neurotransmitters.
2. Current studies of combined imaging (pressure recordings, magnetic resonance imaging [MRI], ultrasound, and fluid mechanical analysis) have offered new understanding of the role of the pylorus in gastric emptying and digestion. Other studies have shown that persistent duodenal hyperacidity can lead to increased incidence of pyloric stenosis. This is associated with repeated contractions of the pylorus.
3. The use of erythromycin to treat reflux and gastric dysmotility has led to research regarding the association with pyloric stenosis. The published evidence has concluded that young infants exposed to erythromycin in the first few weeks of life are at greater risk for developing hypertrophic pyloric stenosis. The highest risk seems to be in the first 2 weeks of life in term or near-term infants, with a course of more than 14 days.
4. Increase in size of the circular musculature of the pylorus with thickening (size and shape of an olive). The pylorus muscle becomes elongated and thickened and is enlarged to about twice the usual size. On clinical examination, palpation of an "olive" is diagnostic.
5. Hypertrophy of the pylorus musculature occurs with narrowing of the pyloric lumen.
6. Constriction of the lumen of the pyloric canal (at the distal end of the stomach) causes the stomach to become dilated.
7. Gastric emptying is delayed.

EVIDENCE BASE Obaid, Y. Y., Toubasi, A. A., Albustanji, F. H., & Al-Qawasmeh, A. R. (2023). Perinatal risk factors for infantile hypertrophic pyloric stenosis: A systematic review and meta-analysis. *Journal of Pediatric Surgery*, *58*(3), 458–466. https://doi.org/10.1016/j.jpedsurg.2022.08.016

DRUG ALERT Erythromycin should only be used in young infants (less than 4 weeks) when the therapeutic benefits outweigh the risks and no alternative agent is available.

Clinical Manifestations

Onset usually occurs between ages 3 and 12 weeks.

1. Cardinal sign is projectile, nonbilious vomiting.
   a. Initially, occasional regurgitation (similar to gastroesophageal reflux [GER]) may be present, but eventually vomiting increases in frequency and intensity.
   b. Vomitus contains milk and gastric juices; however, it may be blood streaked or have a "coffee-ground" appearance.
   c. Emesis occurs just after or near the end of a feeding.
2. Constipation or decreased quantity of stools.
3. Loss of weight or failure to gain weight.
4. Epigastric distention.
5. Visible gastric peristaltic waves, left to right, seen just after infant vomits.
6. Excessive hunger—willingness to eat immediately after vomiting.
7. Dehydration—electrolyte disturbance with alkalosis, hypoglycemia, hypochloremia.
8. Decreased urine output.
9. Palpable pyloric mass in upper right quadrant of abdomen, to the right of the umbilicus and best felt during feeding or immediately after vomiting.
10. Jaundice.

Diagnostic Evaluation

1. Palpation of pyloric mass ("olive") in conjunction with persistent, projectile vomiting is pathognomonic.
2. Ultrasound evaluation—broadly used, noninvasive method to evaluate the length and diameter of the pyloric muscle.
   a. Criteria for a positive diagnosis: pyloric muscle thickness (PMT) ≥ 3 mm and pyloric muscle length (PML) ≥ 17 mm.
   b. Sensitivity and specificity of PMT, 91% and 85%, respectively; for PML, 76% and 85%, respectively.
   c. No significant correlation among age, weight, or prematurity and a sonographic diagnosis of infantile hypertrophic pyloric stenosis; therefore, the same ultrasound criteria should apply irrespective of prematurity, age, or weight. Borderline PMT and PML measurements necessitate repeat ultrasound or alternative imaging.

3. Barium upper gastrointestinal (GI) series—indicated if ultrasound is inconclusive.
4. Flat film of abdomen—dilated, air-filled stomach; nondilated pyloric canal.
5. Tests for metabolic alkalosis (seen in less than 10% because of more prompt diagnosis over the past 20 years).
6. Urinalysis—urine alkaline and concentrated.
7. Blood hemoglobin and hematocrit—elevated due to hemoconcentration.

EVIDENCE BASE Piotto, L., & Gent, R. (2023). Ultrasound evaluation of the stomach and pylorus in the neonate and baby. *Sonography, 10*(2), 86–93. https://doi.org/10.1002/sono.12345

Management

EVIDENCE BASE Zaghal, A., El-Majzoub, N., Jaafar, R., Aoun, B., & Jradi, N. (2021). Brief overview and updates on infantile hypertrophic pyloric stenosis: Focus on perioperative management. *Pediatric Annals, 50*(3), e136–e141. https://doi.org/10.3928/19382359-20210215-01

1. Considered a medical emergency because of dehydration and electrolyte imbalance, with initial treatment to rehydrate to correct electrolytes and alkalosis.
2. Surgical treatment is corrective and takes place when electrolytes are stable—Ramstedt pyloromyotomy is procedure of choice, performed through a short transverse incision in the right upper quadrant over the rectus muscle at or above the liver edge. Laparoscopic pyloromyotomy may also be done, but the open procedure continues to be the most performed technique.
   a. Hypertrophy of the pyloric muscle regresses to normal size about 12 weeks postoperatively.
   b. Some postoperative vomiting is expected but should decrease over 48 hours. If persistent vomiting continues, a contrast study should be completed to rule out gastric leak, fluid collection obstructing the gastric outlet, or other causes of obstruction. If these are ruled out, incomplete pyloromyotomy should be considered.
   c. Postoperative complications include duodenal perforation, gastric leak, wound infection, small bowel obstruction, and postoperative vomiting.
3. Good outcomes following surgery appear to be strongly related to the qualifications of the pediatric surgeon, the use of pediatric certified anesthesiologists, qualified pediatric nurses, adequate correction of fluids and electrolytes preoperatively.

Complications

1. Starvation.
2. Dehydration.
3. Severe electrolyte imbalance.
4. Hematemesis.

Nursing Assessment

1. Obtain a thorough history of infant's feeding behaviors and history of vomiting.
2. Assess hydration status and for signs and symptoms of electrolyte imbalance.
3. Assess and chart growth and development parameters.

Nursing Interventions

Maintaining Fluid and Electrolyte Balance

1. Administer intravenous (IV) therapy, as ordered, to treat dehydration, metabolic alkalosis, and electrolyte deficiency.
2. Carefully monitor output, including amount and characteristics of urine (check specific gravity), vomiting, and stools.
3. Accurately measure daily weight as a guide for calculating the need for parenteral fluid.
4. Monitor laboratory data for serum electrolytes.
5. Position infants to prevent interference with fluid therapy.
6. Provide a pacifier for infants who are given by mouth (NPO).
7. Monitor vital signs, as indicated by condition. Watch for tachycardia, hypotension, change in respirations.

CLINICAL JUDGMENT Irregular respiratory rate with apnea may be a sign of severe alkalosis.

Maintaining Nutrition

EVIDENCE BASE Chuang, Y. H., Chao, H. C., Yeh, H. Y., Lai, M. W., & Chen, C. C. (2022). Factors associated with pyloric hypertrophy severity and post-operative feeding and nutritional recovery in infantile hypertrophic pyloric stenosis. *Biomedical Journal, 45*(6), 948–956. https://doi.org/10.1016/j.bj.2021.12.011

1. Emphasize rehydration, electrolyte balance, and replacement of body fat and protein stores. This depends on the severity of depletion and may require total parenteral nutrition for several days or weeks before surgery to reduce surgical risk.
2. Maintain NPO status with indwelling nasogastric (NG) tube (inserted to remove any residual barium and retained formula), as ordered. Ensure placement, position, and patency. Record drainage type, color, and amount.
3. If oral feedings are to be continued, do the following:
   a. Provide small, frequent feedings, given slowly.
   b. Burp frequently before, during, and after feeding.
   c. Allow breastfeeding, as tolerated.
4. Prop the patient in 30-degree upright position (see Figure 44-4).
5. Handle gently and minimally after feeding.

Providing Comfort

1. Provide mouth care and wet lips frequently if NPO.
2. Let the infant suck on a pacifier.
3. Provide for physical contact or nearness without excessive stimulation.
4. Provide for audio and visual stimulation that may be soothing.
5. Do not palpate pyloric "olive" to decrease risk of postoperative wound infection from bruising abdominal wall and excoriating tissue in operative site.
6. Administer analgesics, as ordered.

Alleviating Parental Caregiver Anxiety

1. Assess understanding of diagnosis and care plan.
2. Help minimize guilt feelings by providing adequate, specific information and clarifying any misconceptions.
3. Prepare the parental caregivers for the surgery of their child.
   a. Be honest with them.
   b. Prepare them for the expected postoperative appearance of the infant.

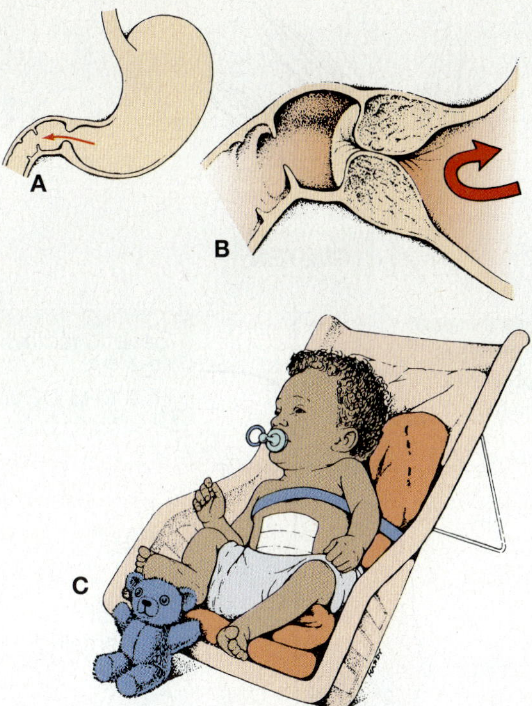

Figure 44-4. Pyloric stenosis. **(A)** Normal passage through pyloric sphincter. **(B)** Stoppage of flow due to stenotic sphincter. **(C)** Postoperative treatment: child propped upright, slightly on right side, aids in gastric emptying.

c. Show them where the operating room and recovery room are located and where to wait during surgery.
4. Allow them to hold the infant to maintain bonding.
5. Encourage them to rest to care better for the infant postoperatively.
6. Accept and explore negative displays of emotion, which may be due to fatigue and frustration because of the extensive care given to the child before hospitalization.
7. Reassure them that surgery is considered curative and normal feeding should resume shortly afterward.

Preventing Complications

1. Assess vital signs to evaluate for fluid and electrolyte imbalances.
2. Assess skin and mucous membranes for hydration status.
3. Weigh daily to assess gain or loss.
4. Elevate head slightly.
5. If placed intraoperatively, maintain patent NG tube to prevent gastric distention. Record losses.
6. Monitor blood glucose levels to prevent hypoglycemia.

Maintaining Hydration

1. Administer IV fluids until adequate intake has been established.
2. Resume oral feeding 2 to 8 hours (standard is 6 hours) after surgery when infant is alert or as ordered.
3. After surgery, infants may progress to ad-lib feedings within 12 to 16 hours, provided they did not have a prolonged preoperative course.
4. Start with small, frequent feedings of glucose water and slowly advance to full-strength (FS) formula and regular diet, as tolerated. An example of a postoperative feeding schedule includes:
   a. NPO for 6 hours.
   b. Sugar water solution orally 30 mL every 2 hours for two feedings.
   c. Then half-strength formula 30 mL every 2 hours for two feedings.
   d. Then FS formula 45 mL every 2 hours for two feedings.
   e. Then FS formula 60 mL every 3 hours for two feedings.
   f. Then formula ad lib every 4 hours.
5. Report any vomiting—amount and characteristics. Feeding schedule may be withheld 2 hours and then reinitiated.
6. Feed slowly and burp frequently.
7. Note how feeding is taken and if it is retained.
8. Increase the amount of feeding as the time interval between feedings is lengthened.
9. Allow breastfeeding to resume, as tolerated, if permitted by the operating surgeon, beginning with limited nursing of 5 to 8 minutes and gradually increase.
10. Continue to elevate the infant's head and shoulders after feeding for 45 to 60 minutes for several feedings after surgery. Place on the right side to aid gastric emptying.
11. Expect that regurgitation may continue for a short period after surgery.

Promoting Healing

1. Provide analgesia and comfort measures, such as a pacifier, rocking, and other soothing stimulation to keep infant quiet and prevent tension on incision.
2. Involve parental caregivers in care of infant postoperatively to prepare them for care of wound after discharge.
3. Observe for drainage or signs of inflammation at incision site and provide care to incision, as ordered.
4. Note that poor nutritional status may delay wound healing.

Community and Home Care Considerations

1. Teach proper care of the operative site.
   a. Check for signs and symptoms of inflammation.
   b. Observe for drainage.
   c. Provide specific care of site, as ordered by provider.
2. Monitor weight and feeding behavior. Encourage close follow-up for growth and development.
3. Observe for signs of delayed gastric emptying or GER.
4. Assess parental caregiver–infant interaction and parental coping.

Family Education and Health Maintenance

1. Teach feeding technique to be continued at home; length of feeding technique varies depending on wound healing, nutritional status, and growth.
2. Provide written and verbal instructions as to infant's care and follow-up schedule.
3. Review with family when medical attention is needed and appropriate resources:
   a. Signs of infection.
   b. Frequent vomiting, vomiting longer than 5 days, or poor feeding with signs of dehydration.
   c. Abdominal distention.

Evaluation: Expected Outcomes

- Vital signs stable; urine output adequate.
- Tolerates 1- to 2-ounce feedings in upright position without vomiting.
- Rests quietly with a pacifier.

- Parental caregivers verbalize understanding of surgery and postoperative care.
- Vital signs stable; blood glucose within normal limits.
- No signs of dehydration.
- Incision healing without signs of infection.

CELIAC DISEASE

EVIDENCE BASE Bingham, S. M., & Bates, M. D. (2020). Pediatric celiac disease: A review for non-gastroenterologists. *Current Problems in Pediatric and Adolescent Health Care, 50*(5), 100786. https://doi.org/10.1016/j.cppeds.2020.100786

Celiac disease (CD), or *gluten-sensitive enteropathy*, is a complex autoimmune genetic disorder with multiple contributing genes. CD affects the small intestine and is characterized by a permanent inability to tolerate dietary gluten; however, it can have systemic manifestations as well. Gluten is a protein found in wheat, rye, and barley (see Figure 44-5). The disease process is reversible with strict adherence to a gluten-free diet.

CD occurs more frequently in White people; however, it is found in all ethnic groups. In the United States and Europe, the prevalence of CD in the pediatric population is between 1 in 300 and 1 in 80, respectively. It is thought to be grossly underdiagnosed.

Pathophysiology and Etiology

1. CD is an immune-mediated disease. The two necessary components of the disease are exposure to gluten and a genetic predisposition resulting in immune activation to gluten. Linkage studies have identified several genomic regions that probably contain CD susceptibility genes.
   a. The genes implicated in CD are HLA-DQ2 and HLA-DQ8. However, these genes can be found in 30% of the normal population as well.
   b. A familial connection is found in 5% to 15% of celiac patients, with an 83% to 86% concordance rate among monozygotic twins.
2. The disease results in inflammation in the mucosa of the small bowel, especially the duodenum and jejunum. This results in damage to the villi, which can be shortened or totally lost.
3. The mucosal damage results in deficiency of enzymes on the mucosal surface, such as disaccharidase and peptidase. This, along with a reduced surface area, leads to malabsorption.
4. The body may be unable to absorb fats, fat-soluble vitamins (A, D, E, and K), minerals, and some protein and carbohydrates.
5. The severity of symptoms depends on the extent of affected intestine. If involvement is focal and limited to the proximal bowel, gastrointestinal (GI) symptoms may be absent.
6. A number of conditions may be associated with CD, including:
   a. Type 1 diabetes mellitus.
   b. Mucocutaneous manifestations, dermatitis herpetiformis.
   c. Cystic fibrosis, seizures, peripheral neuropathy.
   d. Autoimmune thyroiditis, adrenal insufficiency.
   e. Systemic lupus erythematosus, rheumatoid arthritis, and other connective tissue disorders.
   f. Sclerosing cholangitis.
   g. Trisomy 21.
   h. Unexplained folate or iron deficiency, refractory to treatment.
   i. Alopecia areata.
   j. Dental enamel hypoplasia.
   k. Risk of thromboembolism.

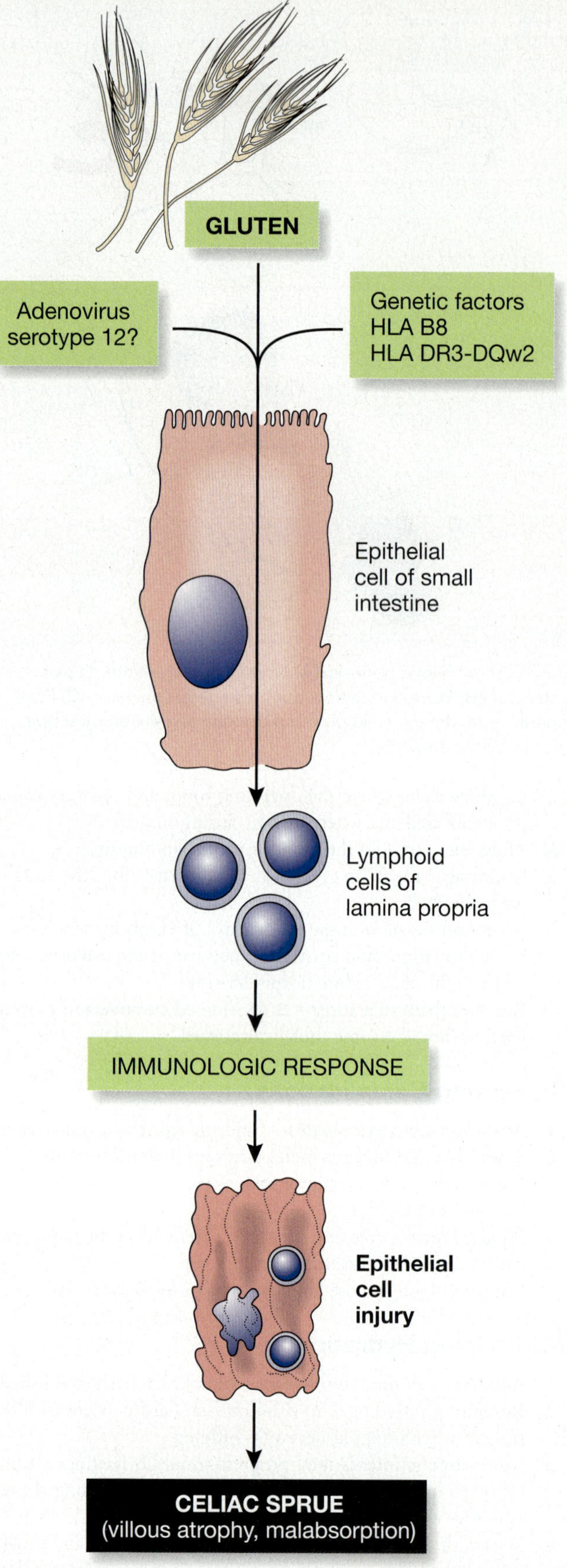

Figure 44-5. Mechanisms in the pathogenesis of celiac disease. (Reprinted with permission from Strayer, D. S., Saffitz, J. E., & Rubin, E. [2020]. *Rubin's pathology: Mechanisms of human disease* [8th ed., Fig. 19-44]. Wolters Kluwer.)

Clinical Manifestations

The age and mode of presenting signs and symptoms are extremely variable. Diagnosis may be made by ages 6 to 24 months when infants are introduced to cereal; however, more subtle GI and extraintestinal symptoms often lead to diagnosis much later in life.

Ages 6 to 18 Months

Presentation may include the following:

1. Impaired growth.
   a. Normal growth during early months of life.
   b. Slackening of weight followed by weight loss.
2. Diarrhea—more frequent, pale, soft, bulky, greasy (steatorrhea) with offensive odor.
3. Recalcitrant constipation (occasionally).
4. Abdominal distention.
5. Anorexia.
6. Muscle wasting—most obvious in buttocks and proximal parts of extremities.
7. Vomiting.
8. Seizures.
9. Loss of tooth enamel.
10. Painful/pruritic skin rash called "dermatitis herpetiformis."

Older Children

1. Complications of malabsorption:
   a. Anemia, vitamin deficiency.
   b. Hypoproteinemia (hypoalbuminemia) with edema.
   c. Hypocalcemia, hypokalemia, hypomagnesemia.
   d. Hypoprothrombinemia resulting from impaired vitamin K absorption.
   e. Disaccharide intolerance—with acid sugar–containing stools (secondary to the altered small bowel mucosa).
   f. Low bone density, osteoporosis secondary to decreased calcium absorption.
2. Diarrhea or constipation.
3. Overweight status.
4. Linear growth delay.
5. Abdominal pain.
6. Fatigue.

EVIDENCE BASE Cyrkot, S., Gidrewicz, D., Anders, S., Marcon, M., Turner, J. M., & Mager, D. R. (2022). Food environment and youth intake may influence uptake of gluten-free food guide recommendations in celiac disease. *Canadian Journal of Dietetic Practice and Research, 83*(4), 186–192. https://doi.org/10.3148/cjdpr-2022-011

Diagnostic Evaluation

EVIDENCE BASE Wessels, M., Dolinsek, J., Castillejo, G., Donat, E., Riznik, P., Roca, M., Valitutti, F., Veenvliet, A., & Mearin, M. L. (2022). Follow-up practices for children and adolescents with celiac disease: results of an international survey. *European Journal of Pediatrics, 181*(3), 1213–1220. https://doi.org/10.1007/s00431-021-04318-2

Ahmadipour, S., Nejad, M. R., Soleimani, S., Mahmoudvand, G., Angari, K., & Rouzbahani, A. K. (2023). Celiac disease screening in the siblings of pediatric patients with a confirmed diagnosis: A cross-sectional study. *Journal of Comprehensive Pediatrics, 14*(1), 1–7. https://doi.org/10.5812/compreped-132834

1. Thorough history, including family history of autoimmune disorders, diabetes, dietary history, growth history, and general status of the child.
2. Serologic testing is done to screen the individual at risk. It has been recommended that all short-stature children be screened irrespective of GI symptoms. Assays detect immunoglobulin (Ig) A antibody to endomysium or tissue transglutaminase. These antibodies have a very high sensitivity and specificity for CD; however, they may be falsely low in a child with IgA deficiency. Therefore, the total IgA level must also be checked. Maintain usual diet during testing.
3. An upper endoscopy is the gold standard test to confirm the diagnosis and must be done in all individuals whose serologic screening is positive. It might show infiltration of the mucosa with lymphocytes and variable degrees of flattened villi.
4. Videocapsule endoscopy shows good sensitivity and excellent specificity for the detection of villous atrophy in patients with suspected CD but is not often practical in the pediatric population; the gold standard of diagnosis remains the small intestinal biopsy.

CLINICAL JUDGMENT Age 3 to 6 months is too early to be able to detect CD with testing because of the length of time of gluten exposure.

Management

EVIDENCE BASE Martín-Masot, R., Jiménez-Muñoz, M., Herrador-López, M., Flor-Alemany, M., Navas-López, V. M., & Nestares, T. (2023). The importance of an early evaluation after establishing a gluten-free diet in children with celiac disease. *Nutrients, 15*(7), 1761–1773. https://doi.org/10.3390/nu15071761

1. Lifelong gluten-free diet.
   a. Avoid all foods containing wheat, rye, and barley and their derivatives because even a small amount, such as a trace contaminant, may cause a pathologic response. Oats are naturally gluten free; however, they are often cross-contaminated during the manufacturing process, so their exclusion may be recommended.
   b. The small intestinal mucosa will always respond abnormally to dietary gluten, although clinical signs may not be immediately evident.
   c. Biopsy and serologic screening revert to normal with appropriate diet.
   d. Clinical signs of improvement are often seen days to weeks after proper diet is initiated but can take up to 1 year in the case of more insidious symptoms, such as delayed linear growth.
2. Adequate caloric and nutrient intake.
3. Supplemental vitamins and minerals may be used when clinically indicated. Folic acid may be used if low level is suspected or detected.
   a. Vitamins A and D.
   b. Iron supplements until anemia resolves.
   c. Vitamin K if evidence of hypoprothrombinemia and bleeding.
   d. Calcium if milk is restricted.

4. Temporary restriction of lactose and sucrose (disaccharidases) from diet for 6 to 8 weeks may be indicated in some cases, if these products are shown to worsen symptoms.
5. Enzyme therapy that protects the mucosal lining from gluten exposure is being investigated in clinical trials.

Complications

1. Nutritional deficiencies (most important short-term risks, which can lead to anemia, osteoporosis, and growth failure).
2. Long-term risks of untreated CD include increased risk of lymphoma and adenocarcinoma of small intestine.
3. Refractory CD.
4. Seizures related to inadequate absorption of folic acid and buildup of calcium deposits on the brain.

Nursing Assessment

1. Obtain family dietary history as it relates to the onset of symptoms.
2. Assess child's nutritional status.
3. Check for signs of infection.
4. Assess growth and developmental parameters.

Nursing Interventions

Provide Adequate Nutrition and Dietary Restrictions

1. Provide gluten-free diet, being careful to avoid accidental exposure via cross-contamination while food is prepared and/or cooked.
2. An initial diet high in protein, relatively low in fat, low in lactose, and free from gluten may be necessary if the newly diagnosed child exhibits severe malabsorption.
   a. Initiate a referral with a dietitian for precise diet recommendations.
   b. Soy milk or Lactaid drops may be indicated if the patient is exhibiting signs of lactose intolerance.
   c. Watch for fat intolerance in infants and young children.
3. Maintain by mouth (NPO) status during the initial treatment of celiac crisis or during diagnostic testing. Take special precautions to ensure proper restriction if the child is ambulatory.
4. Encourage small, frequent, appetizing meals, but do not force eating if the child has anorexia.
5. Note the child's reaction to food. Close observation of the child's responses to food may reveal other intolerances. Note and record:
   a. Foods taken and refused.
   b. Appetite.
   c. Change in behavior after eating.
   d. Characteristics and frequency of stools.
   e. General disposition—behavior improvement commonly seen within 2 to 3 days after diet control is initiated.
6. Be prepared to temporarily eliminate new food introduced if symptoms increase.
7. A gluten-challenged diet is not routinely indicated.
8. Provide the family with assistance to obtain a variety of gluten-free foods. Studies demonstrate that poor availability and expense of gluten-free foods lead to dietary nonadherence.

EVIDENCE BASE Kreutz, J. M., Heynen, L., & Vreugdenhil, A. C. E. (2023). Nutrient deficiencies in children with celiac disease during long term follow-up. *Clinical Nutrition*, *42*(7), 1175–1180. https://doi.org/10.1016/j.clnu.2023.05.003

Promoting Effective Caregiving

1. Teach the parental caregivers to develop an awareness of the child's behavior; recognize changes and care for child accordingly.
2. Explain that diet and eating have a direct effect on behavior and that behavior may indicate how the child is feeling.
3. Help the parental caregivers recognize and understand mood swings, from having temper tantrums to being very timid, nervous, or unstable.
4. Advise the parental caregivers to allow the child to express feelings freely through safe and age-appropriate media.
5. Encourage parental caregivers to define limits of behavior for the child and convey them to all family members.
6. Encourage patience, routines, and consistency.
7. Advise parental caregivers to record changes in behavior, especially in relation to eating and diet, to document effectiveness of therapy.
8. Help the parental caregivers to maintain a balance between the child with CD, the other family members, and additional roles and responsibilities.
9. If the child is withdrawn, advise providing opportunity for play with other children, especially when the child begins to feel better.
10. Explain that the toddler may cling to infantile habits for security. Allow this behavior; it may disappear as physical condition improves.
11. Suggest offering the child other sensory stimulation to compensate for lack of eating pleasure.
12. Help the parental caregivers to understand that, after initial rapid weight gain, further improvement may be slow.
13. Provide emotional support for the child and parental caregivers.
14. Refer for counseling, if indicated.

Family Education and Health Maintenance

1. Teach parental caregivers about CD and how it is controlled by diet. Help them to understand that severe, long-term damage to the intestinal lining has occurred and must be controlled to allow for normal growth and development.
2. Long-term follow-up with a qualified dietitian has been shown to improve adherence based on symptoms and follow-up serologic testing.
3. Provide a specific list of restricted and acceptable foods to get the family started; because there is much variation among brands of packaged foods, it is best for the family to check with the manufacturers.
4. Teach the parental caregivers how to read labels on foods to identify those containing wheat, rye, and barley glutens, thus avoiding them.
   a. Advise that any ingredient of unknown or unspecified grain origin should be assumed to contain gluten, unless the manufacturer confirms that it is gluten free.
   b. Advise that medications should also be checked; filler and excipients, such as alcohol in cough medication, may be wheat based.
   c. Advise parental caregivers that gluten is found in many manufactured products as a filler or thickener, such as gravy powder.
5. Provide information on substitutes for wheat, rye, and barley, such as corn, rice, potato, soybean flour, and gluten-free starch.

6. Help the parental caregivers become comfortable in situation problem solving (e.g., supplying gluten-free cupcakes for birthday party to which child has been invited).
7. Initiate referral to dietitian to ensure that nutrient and energy requirements are being met. There is no standardized vitamin regimen.
8. Discuss the importance of continued adherence to gluten-free diet, even though the child is feeling well, eating well, and has normal stools. Encourage the child to become involved in diet.
9. Adolescent adherence may be variable. Encourage support and understanding.
10. Alteration in diet may have significant cultural, ethnic, and religious implications. Help parental caregivers identify how adjustments can be made.
11. Advise parental caregivers on eating out—check ahead of time with fast-food chains and restaurant chefs or management to determine whether they can ensure gluten-free items. (Be aware that even a gluten-free hamburger cooked on a grill with a breaded chicken breast cannot be considered gluten free.)
    a. Many gluten-free menus at chain restaurants can be found on the internet by searching keyword "gluten free."
    b. Inform friends before visiting and bring gluten-free products, if necessary.
    c. If necessary, consider implementation of formalized plan of necessary dietary restrictions for appropriate accommodations in school settings.
12. Advise parental caregivers to investigate support groups, internet companies, natural food stores, and major food brands that offer information and sell gluten-free products.
13. Tell parental caregivers that common problems with long-term gluten-free diet are constipation due to low dietary fiber intake and weight gain due to now normal absorption; therefore, encourage regular physical activity and avoidance of high-calorie foods.
14. Impress on the parental caregivers the importance of regular medical follow-up.
15. Encourage the parental caregivers to practice good hygiene to prevent infection because the child may be especially prone to infection if malnutrition and/or anemia are present.
16. Advise the family that patients with CD have a predisposition to nonresponse of the hepatitis B vaccine; therefore, titers should be considered.
17. Help the parental caregivers to understand that the emotional climate in the home and around the child is vitally important in maintaining the child's medical and physical stability. Stress the importance of not making the child feel abnormal or a nuisance to the family. Family support is invaluable in facilitating acceptance of the diet.
18. Stress that the disorder is lifelong; however, changes in the mucosal lining of the intestine and the general clinical condition of the child are reversible when dietary gluten is avoided.
19. Advise screening for all first-degree relatives, because of hereditary nature of the disease.
20. For additional information and support, refer to Celiac Sprue Association (www.csaceliacs.org), Canadian Celiac Association (www.celiac.ca), or Celiac Disease Foundation (www.celiac.org).

Evaluation: Expected Outcomes

- Tolerates gluten-free diet well. Poor growth is not the symptom for every child; therefore, gaining weight is not an appropriate expected outcome for each child.
- Parental caregivers setting limits with child and documenting behavior in relation to meals.

DIARRHEA

Diarrhea is the rapid movement of fecal matter through the intestine, resulting in an excessive loss of water and electrolytes and producing more frequent loose, unformed, or watery stools. It is a symptom of many conditions and may be caused by many diseases (see Table 44-2). Commonly, the cause is difficult to determine; occasionally, it is unknown. Worldwide, approximately 1.8 million children die from diarrhea annually. Studies show that approximately 40% of cases of diarrhea have no direct cause, although some viruses have yet to be identified.

Pathophysiology and Etiology

EVIDENCE BASE Levine, A. C., O'Connell, K. J., Schnadower, D., VanBuren, T. J. M., Mahajan, P., Hurley, K. F., Tarr, P., Olsen, C. S., Poonai, N., Schuh, S., Powell, E. C., Farion, K. J., Sapien, R. E., Roskind, C. G., Rogers, A. J., Bhatt, S., Gouin, S., Vance, C., Freedman, S. B., & Pediatric Emergency Research Canada (PERC) the Pediatric Emergency Care Applied Research Network (PECARN) (2022). Derivation of the pediatric acute gastroenteritis risk score to predict moderate-to-severe acute gastroenteritis. *Journal of Pediatric Gastroenterology and Nutrition, 74*(4), 446–453. https://doi.org/10.1097/MPG.0000000000003395

Mechanisms of Diarrhea

1. Secretory—decreased absorption, increased secretion.
2. Osmotic—maldigestion, transport anomalies, ingestion of unabsorbable solute.
3. Intestinal dysmotility—intact absorption with decreased intestinal transit time.
4. Inflammatory—malabsorption; can be caused by infectious or noninfectious agents.

Physiologic Effects of Diarrhea

1. Dehydration (extracellular fluid [ECF] loss).
    a. Large loss of fluid and electrolytes in watery stools.
    b. May be compounded by vomiting, decreased fluid intake, and increased insensible loss due to fever and rapid respirations.
2. Electrolyte imbalance.
    a. Potassium—may be hyperkalemic or hypokalemic.
    b. Sodium and chloride are directly related and may be increased or decreased.
        i. Hypernatremic hyperchloremic (hypertonic) dehydration occurs with acute diarrhea.
        ii. Hyponatremic hypochloremic (hypotonic) hypervolemia occurs with too rapid fluid replacement.
3. Acid–base imbalance—metabolic acidosis.
    a. From large losses of potassium, sodium, and bicarbonate in stools.
    b. From impaired renal function.
4. Monosaccharide intolerance and protein hypersensitivity.

Pathogenic Etiology

1. Bacteria—*Escherichia coli* O157:H7, *Salmonella*, *Shigella*, *Yersinia enterocolitica*, *Campylobacter jejuni*, *Clostridium difficile*, dysentery, cholera.
2. Antibiotic-associated diarrhea, such as *C. difficile* diarrhea, is a leading cause of nosocomial outbreaks.

Table 44-2 Differential Diagnosis of Diarrhea

	INFANT	CHILD	ADOLESCENT
Acute			
Common	• Gastroenteritis • Systemic infection • Antibiotic associated • Overfeeding	• Gastroenteritis • Food poisoning • Systemic infection • Antibiotic associated	• Gastroenteritis • Food poisoning • Antibiotic associated
Rare	• Primary disaccharidase deficiency • Hirschsprung toxic colitis • Adrenogenital syndrome	• Toxic ingestion	• Hyperthyroidism
Chronic			
Common	• Postinfectious secondary lactase deficiency • Cow's milk or soy protein intolerance • Chronic nonspecific diarrhea of infancy • Celiac disease • Cystic fibrosis • AIDS enteropathy	• Postinfectious secondary lactase deficiency • Irritable bowel syndrome • Celiac disease • Lactose intolerance • Giardiasis • Inflammatory bowel disease • AIDS enteropathy	• Irritable bowel syndrome • Inflammatory bowel disease • Lactose intolerance • Giardiasis • Laxative misuse (anorexia nervosa)
Rare	• Primary immune anomalies • Familial villous atrophy • Secretory tumors • Acrodermatitis enteropathica • Lymphangiectasia • Abetalipoproteinemia • Eosinophilic gastroenteritis • Short-bowel syndrome • Intractable diarrhea syndrome • Autoimmune enteropathy	• Acquired immune anomalies • Secretory tumors • Pseudo-obstruction	• Secretory tumor • Primary bowel tumor • Anal intercourse (inflammation confined to the rectum) • Kaposi sarcoma–associated diarrhea

AIDS, acquired immunodeficiency syndrome.

3. Viral—rotavirus (most common; peaks during winter months), enteroviruses (echovirus), adenoviruses, human Reovirus-like agent, Norwalk virus.
4. Fungal—*Candida enteritis.*
5. Parasitic—*Giardia lamblia, Cryptosporidium parvum.*
6. Protozoal.

Noninfectious Etiologic Factors

1. Malabsorption—lactase deficiency, cow's milk protein allergy, food protein-induced enteropathy, celiac disease, cystic fibrosis, microvillus inclusion disease.
2. Inflammatory bowel disease—ulcerative colitis, Crohn disease, rare in infants.
3. Immune deficiency—severe combined immunodeficiency, immunoglobulin A (IgA) deficiency.
4. Infant exposed to overeating.
5. Direct irritation of gastrointestinal (GI) tract by foods, medications, chemicals, radiation.
6. Inappropriate use of laxatives and purgatives.
7. Mechanical disorders—malrotation, incomplete small bowel obstruction, intermittent volvulus.
8. Congenital anomalies (e.g., Hirschsprung disease–related enterocolitis).
9. Drug consumption—increases the risk of colitis, especially in predisposed persons; some agents may just exacerbate underlying colitis.
10. Functional—diagnosis of exclusion, although etiology may be a virus that has not been identified. For example, child exposed to excessive stress, emotional excitement, and fatigue.

Acute Diarrhea

1. Sudden increase in frequency of stools.
2. Usually self-limited but can result in dehydration.

Chronic or Persistent Diarrhea

1. Defined as three loose or liquid bowel movements a day for at least 2 to 4 weeks and a stool weight greater than 200 g/day.
2. Associated with disorders of malabsorption, anatomic anomalies, abnormal bowel motility, hypersensitivity reaction, or a long-term inflammatory response.
3. May be due to behaviors that continue to expose children to pathogens as well as increased resistance of bacteria to commonly used antibacterial agents.

CLINICAL JUDGMENT Infants and young children in day care centers may be at an increased risk for diarrhea due to *Shigella*, *Salmonella*, rotavirus, endopathogenic *E. coli*, and giardiasis. Handwashing is the major preventive measure. These infections are usually reportable to the health department. Bloody diarrhea should be immediately referred for medical evaluation.

Risk Factors for Diarrhea

EVIDENCE BASE Tashiro, S., Mihara, T., Okawa, R., Tanaka, Y., Samura, M., Enoki, Y., Taguchi, K., Matsumoto, K., & Yamagishi, Y. (2023). Optimal therapeutic recommendation for *Clostridioides difficile* infection in pediatric and adolescent populations: a systematic review and meta-analysis. *European Journal of Pediatrics, 182*(6), 2673–2681. https://doi.org/10.1007/s00431-023-04944-y

1. Age—the younger the child, the greater the susceptibility and severity.
   a. ECF volume is proportionately larger in the infant and young child.
   b. Nutritional reserves are relatively smaller in the young child.
2. Impaired health—susceptibility is increased in the malnourished or debilitated child.
3. Climate—susceptibility is increased in warm weather.
4. Environment—frequency is increased where there is overcrowding, poor sanitation, inadequate refrigeration of food, and inadequate health care and education.
5. Virulence of a potential pathogen affects severity.
6. Internationally adopted child.

Clinical Manifestations

Symptoms vary with severity, specific cause, and type of onset (insidious vs. acute).

1. Low-grade fever to 100°F (37.8°C).
2. Anorexia.
3. Vomiting (can precede diarrhea by several days); mild and intermittent to severe.
4. Stools—appearance of diarrhea from a few hours to 3 days.
   a. Loose and fluid consistency.
   b. Greenish or yellow green, although can be any color.
   c. May contain mucus, pus, or blood.
   d. Frequency varies from 3 to 20 per day.
   e. Expelled with force; may be preceded by pain.
5. Behavioral changes.
   a. Irritability and restlessness.
   b. Weakness.
   c. Extreme prostration.
   d. Stupor and convulsions.
   e. Flaccidity.
6. Physical changes.
   a. Little to extreme loss of subcutaneous fat.
   b. Up to 50% total body weight loss.
   c. Poor skin turgor; capillary refill longer than 2 seconds.
   d. Dry mucous membranes and dry, cracked lips.
   e. Pallor.
   f. Sunken fontanelles and eyes.
   g. Petechiae may be seen with bacterial infections.
   h. Excoriated buttocks and perineum.
   i. Urine with blood.
7. Vital sign and urine output changes (signal imminent cardiovascular collapse).
   a. Low blood pressure (BP).
   b. High pulse rate.
   c. Respirations rapid and hyperpneic.
   d. Decreased or absent urine output.

Diagnostic Evaluation

Studies to Evaluate Condition

1. Thorough history and physical examination to determine hydration status.
2. Electrolyte and kidney function tests—serum sodium, chloride, potassium, and blood urea nitrogen variable.
3. Acid–base balance—serum carbon dioxide; arterial pH and carbon dioxide possibly abnormal.
4. Complete blood count (CBC) to determine plasma volume by hematocrit; infection by white blood cell (WBC) count and differential.
5. Sedimentation rate—elevated in infection and inflammation.

CLINICAL JUDGMENT A postural change in heart rate and BP is a useful clue in assessing the fluid state of a toddler (or any child). An increase greater than 20 beats/min when moving from lying to standing is an indicator of hypovolemia. A decrease of at least 20 mm Hg in systolic BP or a decrease of at least 10 mm Hg in diastolic BP when moving from lying to standing is considered orthostatic and likely indicates hypovolemia.

Studies to Determine Cause

1. Thorough history to determine recent contact or exposure, contact with potentially contaminated water (swimming in lakes and ponds, well water), travel to at-risk countries, antibiotic therapy, and possible immunosuppression.
2. Enzyme immunoassay tests such as Rotazyme to test stool for rotavirus.
3. Multiple stool and rectal swab for bacterial cultures, ova and parasites, and *C. difficile*. Some labs require the sample specify for *Giardia* profile, *Cryptosporidium*, and *E. coli* O157:H7 serotyping. If immunosuppressed, add *Microsporidian*, *Cryptosporidium*, and *G. lamblia* antigen 65.
4. Stool for WBC count, calprotectin or lactoferrin, to screen for colitis that may be of a bacterial or inflammatory nature.
5. Stool pH, reducing substances—decreased pH may indicate various noninfectious causes; acid stool containing sugar is characteristic of disaccharide intolerance, anomaly of bile salt reabsorption.
6. Blood cultures can rule out septicemia.
7. Serologic studies can detect viral pathogens.
8. Breath hydrogen test can determine carbohydrate malabsorption and bacterial overgrowth.
9. Urinalysis can exclude urinary tract infection (UTI) as cause of nonspecific diarrhea and screen for blood, which may be part of hemolytic uremic syndrome associated with *E. coli* O157:H7 infection.

Management

EVIDENCE BASE Congdon, M., Schnell, S. A., Londoño Gentile, T., Faerber, J. A., Bonafide, C. P., Blackstone, M. M., & Johnson, T. J. (2021). Impact of patient race/ethnicity on emergency department management of pediatric gastroenteritis in the setting of a clinical pathway. *Academic Emergency Medicine, 28*(9), 1035–1042. https://doi.org/10.1111/acem.14255

Treatment is based on the degree of dehydration; mild (loss of less than 5% of body weight), moderate (5% to 10% loss), and severe (greater than 10% loss) (see Table 44-3).

1. Goal is to prevent spread of disease; communicable disease is suspected until proved otherwise; enteric precautions are followed.
2. Bowel rest may be required based on the degree of diarrhea and vomiting, if blood present, or electrolyte abnormalities.
3. For mild-to-moderate dehydration, oral rehydration solution is given to maintain fluid and electrolyte balance (World Health

Table 44-3 Assessment for Dehydration in Children

CLINICAL SIGNS	DEGREE OF DEHYDRATION		
	MILD	MODERATE	SEVERE
General			
Infant's behavior	Thirsty, alert, restless	Restless or lethargic; irritable to touch	Limp, drowsy; cyanotic extremities
Child's behavior	Thirsty, alert, restless	Thirsty, alert; postural hypotension	Usually conscious; cyanotic extremities
Respirations	Slightly increased	Increased	Deep and rapid
Pulse	Slightly increased	Increased	Rapid
Blood pressure	Normal	Decreased	May be unrecordable
Capillary refill	2 sec	2–3 sec	≥3 sec
Skin turgor	Normal	Slightly reduced	Reduced
Skin color	Pale	Gray	Mottled
Weight loss	Up to 5%	Up to 10%	Up to 15%
Mucous membrane	Tacky	Tacky/dry	Parched
Anterior fontanelle	Flat	Slightly depressed	Sunken
Urine volume	Small	Oliguria	Oliguria/anuria
Specific gravity	1.020	1.030	1.035

Organization [WHO] solution, Pedialyte, Infalyte). BRAT (banana, rice, apple, tea) diet is no longer recommended, as it is nutritionally suboptimal.
   a. For oral rehydration, 100 mL/kg over 4 hours, with additional fluids after each liquid bowel movement.
   b. Candidates for oral rehydration include mild-to-moderate dehydration, older than age 4 months, no persistent vomiting, and probable gastroenteritis.
4. For moderate-to-severe dehydration, intravenous (IV) fluid and electrolyte replacement are given slowly, as ordered (usually 20 mL/kg), usually over 2 days to prevent hypotonic hypervolemia (water intoxication). Administration of larger amounts of IV dextrose is associated with reduced return visits in children with gastroenteritis and dehydration.
5. Supportive care is given: monitoring oral and IV fluid intake, output from all sources, and patient's response to treatment.
6. Specific antimicrobial therapy may be given in some cases, such as immunosuppression, bacteremia, documented *C. difficile*, and traveler's diarrhea.
   a. Metronidazole 30 mg/kg/day in divided doses orally or via IV line may be used to treat *C. difficile* infection, although IV dosing may be less efficacious.
   b. Vancomycin orally (PO) for resistant *C. difficile*. Fidaxomicin PO is another antimicrobial Food and Drug Administration (FDA)-approved treatment for *C. difficile*–associated diarrhea in adults, but its use is not yet approved in children.
   c. Rifampin has been shown to be effective in traveler's diarrhea without associated side effects.
7. Probiotics (*Saccharomyces boulardii*, *Lactobacillus rhamnosus* GG, and probiotic mixtures) significantly reduced the development of antibiotic-associated diarrhea. *S. boulardii* was effective for *C. difficile* infection.
8. The WHO and the American Academy of Pediatrics discourage the use of antidiarrheal agents in children. In children who are younger than age 3 years, malnourished, moderately or severely dehydrated, systemically ill, or who have bloody diarrhea, adverse events outweigh benefits. In children who are older than age 3 years, with no/minimal dehydration, loperamide may be a useful adjunct to oral rehydration and early refeeding.

EVIDENCE BASE Szajewska, H., Guarino, A., Hojsak, I., Indrio, F., Kolacek, S., Orel, R., Salvatore, S., Shamir, R., van Goudoever, J. B., Vandenplas, Y., Weizman, Z., Zalewski, B. M., & Working Group on Probiotics and Prebiotics of the European Society for Paediatric Gastroenterology, Hepatology and Nutrition. (2020). Use of probiotics for the management of acute gastroenteritis in children: An update. *Journal of Pediatric Gastroenterology and Nutrition*, *71*(2), 261–269. https://doi.org/10.1097/MPG.0000000000002751

Complications

1. Severe dehydration and acid–base derangements with acidosis.
2. Shock.

Nursing Assessment

1. Obtain accurate history of signs and symptoms: nature and frequency of stools, type of onset, length of illness, and associated symptoms.
2. Assess degree of dehydration (see Table 44-3).
3. Monitor intake and output including oral and IV fluids, fluid loss from diarrhea, urine output, and vomitus; monitor weight.
4. Note color and consistency of stool and vomitus.
5. Successful rehydration (at 4 hours) is defined as resolution of moderate dehydration, production of urine, weight gain, and the absence of severe emesis (≥5 mL/kg).

CLINICAL JUDGMENT Assess child's behavior to determine comfort level. Crying or legs drawn up to abdomen usually indicates pain.

Nursing Interventions

Restoring Fluid Balance

1. Monitor amount and rate of IV fluid therapy, which have been calculated by the health care provider. Fluid needs are based on fluid deficit, ongoing losses, and body weight.

2. Prevent overload of circulatory system.
   a. Check flow rate and amount absorbed hourly and totally.
   b. Adhere to prescribed volume carefully when oral feedings are given in conjunction with IV fluid.
   c. Never administer IV fluids to pediatric patient without safeguard of a volume-control infusion device or pump.
   d. Observe for signs of fluid overload: edema, increased BP, bounding pulse, labored respirations, and crackles in lung fields.
3. Check IV site for infiltration or improper flow, so site can be changed as necessary.
4. Use appropriate protective devices to prevent the child from injuring involved extremity or causing IV to malfunction.
5. Weigh the patient daily as a guide for fluid needs and patient status.
6. Monitor urine output and keep accurate intake and output record, including vomitus and liquid stools.
7. If NPO, provide frequent mouth care and nonnutritive sucking with a pacifier. Continue to burp infant to expel air swallowed while crying or sucking.
8. If oral rehydration solution is used, reassess hydration status every 2 to 4 hours; once rehydrated, continue for 8 to 12 hours, then resume breastfeeding with increased frequency of feedings or formula at full strength or increased frequency if half strength.

Note: Unless vomiting is severe, do not deprive the patient of nutrition for longer than 1 or 2 days. If adequate nutrition cannot be provided, parenteral nutrition should be instituted.

CLINICAL JUDGMENT Diluted fruit juices and soft drinks are not recommended. High disaccharide content aggravates diarrhea by osmotic effect.

Preventing Spread of Infection

1. Ensure adherence to good handwashing and gown technique protocols for all people having contact with infant or child.
2. Follow your facility's policy on care of diapers.
3. Handle specimens collected using universal precautions and transport to laboratories in appropriate containers per policy. Collect stool sample for culture before instituting antibiotic therapy.
4. Teach good hygiene measures to older children.

Preventing Skin Impairment

1. Protect infant's diaper area from becoming excoriated by making frequent diaper changes.
2. Expose to air and light as much as possible.
3. Avoid commercial baby wipes, which contain alcohol and may sting inflamed or excoriated diaper area. Use mild soap and water, place infant in tub of water or baking soda bath (soothing and neutralizing) for cleaning.
4. Prevent scratching or rubbing of the irritated area. Holding the infant on the parental caregiver's protected lap may provide comfort and stimulation for the parental caregiver and infant.
5. Use protective barrier creams, such as zinc oxide; if excoriated, soak off cream and pat dry—do not rub. Not all cream barrier has to be removed because this can denude skin.
6. Leave diaper area open to air until thoroughly dried.

Resuming Adequate Nutritional Intake

1. After rehydration, advance slowly from clear liquids to half-strength formula, to regular diet.
   a. If chronic diarrhea, bloody diarrhea, or secretory diarrhea, limit milk products containing lactose.
   b. In older infants and children, offer lactose-free, bland, carbohydrate-rich foods shortly after successful rehydration.
2. As diet is advanced, note any vomiting or increase in stools and report it immediately. Oral feedings should not be resumed too early or advanced too rapidly because diarrhea may recur.

Reducing Fear and Anxiety

1. Acknowledge that hospitalization is frightening, especially when it is sudden, as with diarrhea.
2. Many treatments and procedures may be painful. Give reassurance to the child before, during, and after treatment.
   a. Explain treatment in age-appropriate language.
   b. Include family in care and treatments when possible.
3. Explain to family that intermittent abdominal cramps may be painful and provide support.
4. Provide some means of pleasant stimulation, entertainment, or diversion, especially while child remains in bed.
   a. Infant—mobile, musical toy.
   b. Young child—books, tapes.
   c. Older child—television, videos.
5. Provide physical closeness to provide comfort, if child displays interest.
   a. Petting, stroking.
   b. Holding, rocking.

Community and Home Care Considerations

1. Infants and young children in day care centers may be at increased risk for diarrhea due to *Shigella*, *Salmonella*, rotavirus, *E. coli*, *Cryptosporidium*, *Campylobacter*, *C. difficile*, and *Giardia*. Good handwashing is the major preventive measure. This is especially important with rotavirus because it can be excreted for as long as 57 days in some cases.
2. If infectious agent is identified, it should be reported because other children may be at risk.
   a. Encourage parental caregivers to contact the child day care center and report.
   b. A child with diarrhea containing blood or mucus should be excluded from day care and medically evaluated. Exclusion from day care should occur until the diarrhea resolves.
   c. Stool cultures positive for *E. coli* O157:H7 or *Shigella* are reportable to the county health department, and the child should be excluded until the diarrhea resolves and two cultures, from two different stools, are negative for these organisms.
3. Assess sanitation and hygiene practices in the home or day care center for overcrowding, number of working toilets in the home for number of people, availability of working sinks with soap and towels in the bathrooms and their proximity to food preparation areas, disposal of diapers, and handwashing practices of caregivers and children.
4. Because most treatment for diarrhea is done on an outpatient basis, nurses in the community need to be available to answer questions.

Family Education and Health Maintenance

1. After the cause of the diarrhea is determined, it may be necessary to teach proper hygiene, formula or food preparation, handling, and storage.
   a. Use handwashing before bottle and food preparation.
   b. Use disposable bottles or sterilize or use dishwasher for reusable bottles.
   c. Refrigerate reconstituted formula and all other fluids between uses. Milk may become contaminated within 1 hour if left out at room temperature; juice becomes contaminated within several hours.
   d. Discard small amounts of food or fluid from containers already used.
2. Explain the fecal–oral mode of transmission of infectious diarrheal illnesses.
3. Explain the early symptoms of a diarrheal illness and of dehydration, which requires notification of the health care provider.
4. Discourage the use of antiemetics and antidiarrheal medications for infants and children with gastroenteritis; they have little effect on infantile diarrhea, may cause toxicity, and can mask signs and symptoms of more serious illness.
5. Advise parental caregivers when traveling internationally with their children to eat and drink only boiled, bottled, or carbonated water, be aware of drinks with ice cubes, food rinsed with water, and make sure all food is well cooked.
6. Help parental caregivers understand the importance of medical care and general good hygiene.
7. For additional information and support, refer to National Institute of Diabetes and Digestive and Kidney Diseases (www.niddk.nih.gov).

DRUG ALERT Bismuth subsalicylate, an over-the-counter drug that is readily available, has shown only modest beneficial effects in children and may increase the risk of Reye syndrome due to salicylate absorption.

Evaluation: Expected Outcomes

- Vital signs stable; urine output adequate.
- Family, staff members handwashing properly and frequently.
- No redness or excoriation of diaper area.
- Tolerates small feedings of clear liquids without diarrhea or vomiting.
- No signs or symptoms of pain or discomfort.

HIRSCHSPRUNG DISEASE

EVIDENCE BASE Hong, M., Li, X., Li, Y., Zhou, Y., Li, Y., Chi, S., Cao, G., Li, S., & Tang, S. (2022). Hirschsprung's disease: Key microRNAs and target genes. *Pediatric Research*, *92*(3), 737–747. https://doi.org/10.1038/s41390-021-01872-1

Hirschsprung disease (congenital aganglionic megacolon) is a form of chronic intestinal obstruction affecting primarily full-term infants.

It occurs because of the congenital absence of the parasympathetic ganglion nerve cells from within the muscle wall of the intestinal tract, usually at the distal end of the colon. Ganglion cells are located throughout the intestinal tract from the mouth down to the rectum. It occurs in 1 in 5,000 (ranges 1:4,400 to 1:7,000) live births with no racial predilection.

The male:female ratio is reported as 2:1, except in long-segment disease, in which it is closer to 1:1, possibly favoring females. Strong evidence supports a genetic component and the association of other congenital anomalies such as Down syndrome, small/large intestinal atresias, trisomy 18, and other rare disorders.

Pathophysiology and Etiology

1. An arrest in embryologic development affecting the migration of parasympathetic nerve innervation of the intestine.
   a. Normally, the nerve cells migrate to the upper end of the alimentary tract and then proceed in the caudal direction, with migration to the distal colon complete by 12 weeks.
   b. Migration occurs first in the intermuscular layer, called *Auerbach plexus*, and then moves into the submucosal plexus, moving along the gastrointestinal (GI) tract in a descending manner.
2. The process of aganglionosis is almost always continuous within the affected segment, ending in proximal segment with ganglion cells. Intermittent ganglion cells in the colon have been reported, but this is extremely unusual.
   a. Most commonly affected site is the rectosigmoid colon (referred to as *short-segment disease*) (80%).
   b. Long-segment disease extends to the upper descending colon and transverse colon (10%) and occasionally throughout the entire colon, involving the small bowel (5%).
   c. Total angiogliosis of the bowel, involving the entire small and large bowel, is rare.
3. No peristalsis occurs in the affected portion of intestine (i.e., spastic and contracted). This section is usually narrow; therefore, no fecal material passes through it.
4. Proximal to the narrow affected section, the colon is dilated (see Figure 44-6).
   a. Filled with fecal material and gas.
   b. Hypertrophy of muscular coating.
   c. Ulceration of mucosa may be seen in neonate.

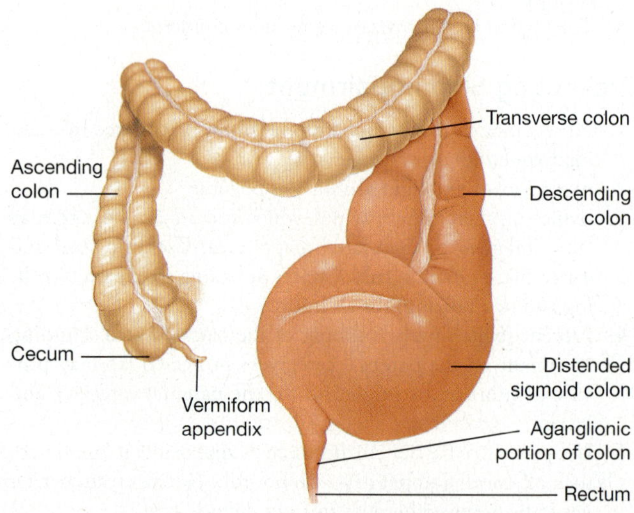

Figure 44-6. Bowel dilation in Hirschsprung disease. (Reprinted with permission from Anatomical Chart Company.)

5. The internal rectal sphincter fails to relax, and evacuation of fecal material and gas is prevented. Abdominal distention and constipation result.

Clinical Manifestations

Clinical manifestations vary depending on the degree of involved bowel.

1. Neonate—symptoms appearing at birth or within the first weeks of life.
   a. No meconium passed in the first 48 hours of life.
   b. Vomiting—bile stained or fecal.
   c. Abdominal distention.
   d. Constipation—occurs in 100% of patients.
   e. Overflow-type diarrhea.
   f. Dehydration; failure to thrive (FTT).
   g. Temporary relief of symptoms with enema.
   h. Bowel perforation—uncommon presentation.
2. Older child—symptoms not prominent at birth. Short-segment disease commonly presents later.
   a. History of obstipation at birth.
   b. Progressive abdominal distention.
   c. Peristaltic activity observable over abdomen.
   d. Absence of retentive posturing (ability to contract the internal and external sphincter to purposefully avoid defecation).
   e. Constipation—unresponsive to conventional remedies.
   f. Presence of encopresis.
   g. Ribbon-like, fluid-like, or pellet stools.
   h. Failure to grow—loss of subcutaneous fat; appears malnourished, stunted growth.
   i. Presentation insidious or catastrophic as with enterocolitis.
3. Enterocolitis—consists of severe toxemia and a proliferation of bacteria in the colonic lumen.
   a. Abdominal distention.
   b. Explosive diarrhea.
   c. Vomiting.
   d. Fever.
   e. Lethargy.
   f. Rectal bleeding.
   g. Shock.

Diagnostic Evaluation

1. Supportive findings on history and physical examination indicate Hirschsprung disease.
2. Digital rectal examination—reveals a tight anal sphincter and a rectum that is narrow and empty of stool (in long-segment disease). In short-segment disease, rectal impaction may be present; removal of finger may be associated with a rush of stool as the obstruction is relieved.
3. Plain films—show severe gaseous distention of the bowel, with absence of air in the rectum.
4. Barium enema—used to demonstrate a transition zone between the proximal dilated, normal innervated colon and the distal, narrow, aganglionic colon.
   a. May be nondiagnostic in young infants who have not had sufficient time to develop a transition zone.
   b. Delayed passage of barium is suggestive but not definitive for Hirschsprung disease.
   c. Must be an unprepped study, as results may be falsely negative if laxatives or rectal stimulation has been used to facilitate defecation.
5. Anorectal manometry—demonstrates failure of the intestinal sphincter to relax in response to transient rectal distention. Requires cooperation of the child.
6. Full-thickness or suction rectal biopsy—absence or reduced number of ganglion nerve cells; definitive diagnosis.
7. Radiopaque markers, ingested, measure intestinal transit time. Use of these markers is not part of the standard diagnostic workup for Hirschsprung disease; however, children with short-segment disease retain the markers in the rectum for long periods.

Management

Definitive treatment is removal of the aganglionic, nonfunctioning, dilated segment of the bowel, followed by anastomosis and improved functioning of internal rectal sphincter.

1. Initially, a colostomy or ileostomy is performed to decompress intestine, divert fecal stream, and rest the normal bowel.
2. Definitive surgery includes the following reconstructive procedures:
   a. Swenson—abdominoperineal pull-through leaving the smallest amount of aganglionic bowel remaining.
   b. Duhamel—retrorectal transanal pull-through creating a neorectum with aganglionic anterior wall and ganglionic posterior wall.
   c. Soave—endorectal pull-through in which the ganglionic segment is pulled through the aganglionic muscular cuff, preserving the internal sphincter; may be done laparoscopically. May be delayed until infant is age 9 to 12 months or until weight reaches 15 to 20 pounds (6.5 to 9 kg).
3. Many surgeons are now performing the endorectal pull-through without colostomy in neonates. This depends on the degree of anomaly, degree of dilatation of the colon, and the clinical status of the infant.
4. In older child whose symptoms are chronic but not severe, treatment may consist of isotonic enemas, stool softeners, and low-residue diet until surgery is performed.
5. Treatment of enterocolitis.
   a. Broad-spectrum intravenous (IV) antibiotics.
   b. Colonic irrigation and decompression with saline solution is initial emergency treatment. Hypertonic phosphate enemas are contraindicated because they may be retained, leading to electrolyte abnormalities.
   c. Surgical decompression colostomy.
   d. At least 1 month after, abdominal perineal pull-through.

CLINICAL JUDGMENT Enterocolitis is a potentially life-threatening event. Notify health care provider immediately if change in abdominal distention occurs in an infant or child with Hirschsprung disease (whether preoperatively or postoperatively), especially if accompanied by fever, diarrhea, vomiting, or lethargy.

Complications

EVIDENCE BASE Berrios, C., Bollinger, J., Yan, J., Biesecker, B., & Chakravarti, A. (2022). Identifying needs, challenges, and benefits among adults and parents of children with Hirschsprung disease. *Journal of Pediatric Gastroenterology and Nutrition*, 74(5), e103–e108. https://doi.org/10.1097/MPG.0000000000003411

1. Preoperative.
   a. Enterocolitis—a major cause of death.
   b. Hydroureter or hydronephrosis.
   c. Water intoxication from tap water enemas.
   d. Bowel perforation.
2. Postoperative.
   a. Enterocolitis: remains the major cause of morbidity and mortality (mortality 6% to 30%).
   b. Diarrhea (69%).
   c. Vomiting (51%).
   d. Fever (34%).
   e. Lethargy (27%).
   f. Leaking of anastomosis and pelvic abscess.
   g. Stenosis, sudden inability to evacuate colon.
   h. Intestinal obstruction from adhesions, volvulus, or intussusception can develop late.
   i. Fecal incontinence is common but can improve with a proper bowel regimen.
   j. Adverse reaction to foods.
   k. Enuresis.

Nursing Assessment

1. Observe neonate for constipation.
2. Obtain parental caregivers' history, especially on infant's bowel and feeding habits.
   a. Onset of constipation.
   b. Character of stools (ribbon like or fluid filled).
   c. Frequency of bowel movements.
   d. Enemas needed.
   e. Suppositories or laxatives needed.
3. Observe for irritability, feeding difficulty, distended abdomen, and signs of malnutrition (pallor, muscle weakness, thin extremities, fatigue).

CLINICAL JUDGMENT Diagnosis of Hirschsprung disease should be suspected in any infant who fails to pass meconium within the first 24 hours and requires repeated rectal stimulation to induce bowel movements.

Nursing Interventions

Improving Breathing Pattern

1. Monitor for respiratory compromise that may result from abdominal distention; watch for rapid, shallow respirations; cyanosis; sternal retractions.
2. Elevate the infant's head and chest by tilting the mattress to facilitate an open airway
3. Administer oxygen, as ordered, to support respiratory status.

Relieving Pain

1. Note the degree of abdominal tenderness.
   a. Infant's legs drawn up.
   b. Chest breathing.
2. Note the color of the abdomen and presence of gastric waves; take sequential measurements of abdominal girth for evidence of changes.
3. Assist in emptying the bowel by giving repeated colonic irrigations.
   a. Procedure for irrigation in an infant is similar to that in an older child, except that less fluid and pressure are used.
   b. Physiologic saline solution (warmed) should be used for irrigations. Tap water may result in large quantities of water being absorbed and in water intoxication.
4. Administer medications (antibiotics), as ordered, to reduce the bacterial flora of the bowel.
5. Note any change in the degree of distention before and after irrigation. Record if the location of distention changes (i.e., upper or lower abdomen).
6. Record all intake and output of irrigant and drainage. Report marked discrepancies in retention or loss of fluid.
7. Insert rectal tube for escape of accumulated fluid and gas, as ordered.
8. If abdominal distention is not relieved by irrigation and decompression and discomfort is significant, insert a nasogastric (NG) tube, as ordered.
   a. Note drainage from NG tube and chart characteristics.
   b. Check for patency; saline irrigations may be requested. Carefully record intake and output.
   c. Perform frequent mouth care.
   d. Alternate nares when changing NG tube, and use minimal amount of tape to prevent skin irritation.
9. Offer a pacifier for nonnutritive sucking if by mouth (NPO), on parenteral fluids.
10. Encourage parental caregivers to hold and rock infant.
11. Maintain position of comfort with head elevated. Offer soothing stimulation (e.g., music, touch, play therapy).

Providing Adequate Nutrition

1. Obtain a dietary history regarding food and eating habits.
   a. Discuss history with dietitian to facilitate potential dietary alterations.
   b. Explain to parental caregivers that eating problems are common with Hirschsprung disease.
2. Monitor IV fluids appropriately; measure all output.
3. Offer small, frequent feedings.
   a. Feed the child slowly.
   b. Provide as comfortable a position as possible for the child during feedings.
4. Inform parental caregivers that anomaly can be corrected, but it may take some time for the child's physical status and feeding habits to improve.
   a. Feeding may cause additional discomfort because of distention and nausea.
   b. Parenteral nutrition may be necessary.

Controlling Constipation in the Older Child

1. Note and record the frequency and characteristics of stools (constipation is likely to occur).
2. Provide demonstration and written and verbal instructions to family for saline enema administration and use of stool softeners.
3. Obtain dietary consultation for teaching of dietary alterations.

Preventing Complications Related to Colostomy

1. Monitor vital signs and respiratory status closely.
2. Monitor for proper functioning of colostomy, if present.
   a. Note drainage from colostomy: characteristics, frequency, fecal material, or liquid drainage.
   b. Record stoma color, size, and return of function.
   c. Note abdominal distention.

   d. Measure fluid loss from colostomy because the amount will affect fluid replacement.
3. Report signs of obstruction from peritonitis, paralytic ileus, handling bowel during surgery, or swelling.
   a. No output from colostomy.
   b. Increased abdominal tenderness.
   c. Irritability.
   d. Vomiting.
   e. Increased temperature.
   f. Firm abdomen.
4. Place the child in a lateral position on a flat or only slightly elevated bed. When the head of the bed is elevated, the residual carbon dioxide in the child's abdominal cavity may cause referred pain in neck and shoulder.
5. Differentiate type and cause of pain to determine appropriate pain management interventions. Proper positioning, patent catheters and tubes, and timely administration of analgesics are key to ensuring patient comfort.
6. "Nothing per rectum" sign should be placed at the head of the bed so that no rectal temperatures, rectal medications, or digital rectal examinations are done.

CLINICAL JUDGMENT Prevent injury to rectal mucosa by taking axillary or external ear temperature.

CLINICAL JUDGMENT Any rectal examination or procedure has the potential to cause serious harm to the patient and surgical site.

Preventing Postoperative Infections

1. Change wound dressing using sterile technique. If done laparoscopically, wound is minimal.
2. Prevent contamination from diaper.
   a. Apply diaper below dressing.
   b. Change diaper frequently.
3. Be aware that 7 to 10 stools per day may be passed postoperatively via ostomy bag. When cleared by surgery, prevent perianal and anal excoriation by thorough cleansing sitz baths and application of zinc oxide paste after soiling.
4. If skin is denuded and moist, apply a skin barrier, and provide specific instruction to the family to prevent further damage to skin with aggressive removal.
5. Use careful handwashing technique.
6. Report wound redness, swelling or drainage, evisceration, or dehiscence immediately.
7. Suction secretions frequently to prevent infection of the tracheobronchial tree and lungs.
8. Encourage frequent coughing and deep breathing to maintain respiratory status.
9. Allow the infant to cry for short periods to prevent atelectasis.
10. Change the infant's position frequently to increase circulation and allow for aeration of all lung areas.

Preventing Abdominal Distention

1. Maintain patency of NG tube immediately postoperatively.
   a. NG suction, as ordered, for 24 to 48 hours or until adequate bowel sounds, gas from rectum or gas from ostomy.
   b. Watch for increasing abdominal distention; measure abdominal girth.
   c. Measure fluid loss because the amount will affect fluid replacement.
2. Maintain NPO status until bowel sounds return, and the bowel is ready for feedings as determined by provider.
3. Administer fluids to maintain hydration and replace lost electrolytes.
4. Maintain Foley catheter for 24 to 48 hours, as ordered.
5. Provide frequent oral hygiene while NPO.
6. Begin oral feedings, as ordered.
   a. Avoid overfeeding.
   b. Burp frequently during feeding.
   c. Turn head to side or elevate after feeding to prevent aspiration.

Supporting the Parental Caregivers

1. Acknowledge that even a temporary colostomy can be a difficult procedure to accept and learn to manage.
   a. Initiate ostomy referral.
   b. Support the parental caregivers when teaching them to care for the colostomy.
   c. Include the parental caregivers in dressing changes and any other appropriate activities soon after surgery.
   d. Assist and encourage the parental caregivers to treat the infant or child as normally as possible.
   e. Reassure parental caregivers that colostomy will not cause delay in the child's normal development.
2. Encourage the parental caregivers to talk about their fears and anxieties. Anticipating future surgery for resection may be confusing and frightening.
3. Initiate community nurse referral to help the parental caregivers care for the child at home away from the comforting situation of the hospital and obtain necessary equipment.
4. Initiate a genetic counseling referral, especially if the parental caregivers plan to have more children.

Ostomy Care in Children

EVIDENCE BASE Uzsen, H., Yaz, S. B., & Gumus, M. (2021). The effect of ostomy on pediatric patient and family in nursing: A systematic review. *Journal of Pediatric Surgical Nursing, 10*(4), 153–158. https://doi.org/10.1097/JPS.0000000000000313

Care of the colostomy and ileostomy in the infant and young child is based on the same principles and is essentially the same as that for an adult (see Chapter 18), with the following exceptions:

1. Colostomy irrigation is not part of management in small children. Irrigation is primarily for the purpose of regulating the colostomy to empty at regular intervals. Because children have bowel movements at more frequent intervals, this type of control is not feasible. Irrigation may be done only in preparation for tests or surgery and occasionally for the treatment of constipation.
2. Dehydration occurs quickly in the infant or small child; therefore, it is particularly important to observe drainage for amount and characteristics. Drainage should be measured to provide an accurate basis for computation of fluid replacement.
3. Prevention and treatment of skin excoriation around the stoma are of primary concern. With the advent of better skin

shields and equipment designed especially for the pediatric patient, keeping an ostomy appliance in place is now less difficult. Through careful application and trying different types of pouches until a proper fit is obtained, most children can be kept clean and dry for at least 24 hours between changes. This is a significant factor in preventing skin breakdown and subsequent infections in the peristomal area. Remember, however, that infant dressings must be checked frequently.
   a. Check ostomy bag for leakage every 2 hours and change bag as soon as leakage is suspected.
   b. Teach the parental caregivers the importance of emptying the bag, when it is one quarter to one-third full.
   c. Skin breakdown is more frequent. Reinforce to parental caregivers to treat breakdown with method and products recommended by ostomy nurse.
   d. Be aware that infant elimination is more frequent than in the older child.
4. For older children with ostomies:
   a. "Potty training" may be achieved for colostomy pouch emptying. This will not be possible for a child with an ileostomy.
   b. Pouching optimizes socialization and developmental activities.
   c. Encourage a matter-of-fact and accepting attitude to help build child's self-confidence.
   d. Encourage the child to participate in ostomy care.
   e. Encourage the child to join age-appropriate ostomy support group.
5. Additional information and support can be obtained from the United Ostomy Associations of America (www.ostomy.org).

Community and Home Care Considerations

1. Begin early teaching about the colostomy (preoperatively, before discharge, and at home), including how it works and how to care for it and the child. Explanations should be thorough and in accordance with family readiness. Encourage care of the ostomy as part of normal activities of daily living.
2. Arrange frequent home visits to carry out a comprehensive teaching plan. Consult with ostomy nurse, as needed, for any skin breakdown or other ostomy problems.
3. Involve the entire family in teaching colostomy care to enhance acceptance of body change of the child. An older child should become totally responsible for their own colostomy care.
4. Assess family's self-care of the ostomy, including procedures such as preparation of skin, application of collecting appliance, care of appliance, and control of odor.
5. Observe for and teach family about signs of stomal complications, including ribbon-like stool, diarrhea, failure of evacuation of stool or flatus, and bleeding.
6. Assess hydration status and teach increased fluid intake because colon absorption is decreased or may be absent if an ileostomy is present.
7. Review gastrostomy tube (GT) feeding techniques, if ordered.
8. Assist family to discuss the child's needs with day care workers, teachers, and school nurse, as applicable. Review care of ostomy with child's care providers.
9. Assist with preoperative preparation for colostomy closure when the time comes.

Family Education and Health Maintenance

1. Instruct the parental caregivers to serve small, frequent meals to the child and be alert for and eliminate foods that cause gas and diarrhea, such as cabbage, spicy foods, beans, Brussels sprouts, fruits, and fruit juices.
2. Advise parental caregivers that colds or viruses may cause loose stools, which increases the risk of dehydration, especially in long-segment disease, so as to increase fluids in these situations.
3. Alert parental caregivers of common postoperative problems, including bacterial overgrowth, colitis or enterocolitis, and lactose intolerance. Advise parental caregivers to contact their health care provider if persistent diarrhea, abdominal distention, abdominal pain, fever, vomiting, or constipation occurs.
4. Encourage parental caregivers to practice all procedures long before the infant is to be discharged.
5. Emphasize the importance of treating the child as normally as possible to prevent behavior problems later.
6. Teach the basics of good nutrition and diet. Involve the dietitian, as necessary.
7. Encourage close medical follow-up and general good health and hygiene.
   a. Safety.
   b. General growth and development.
   c. Immunizations.
8. Advise older children without colostomies that fecal staining may occur, but this will improve with time.

Evaluation: Expected Outcomes

- Respirations unlabored; no cyanosis.
- Abdominal girth decreased; resting comfortably.
- Tolerates 1- to 2-ounce feedings every hour, depending on the age of the child.
- Passes stool at least every 2 days spontaneously or after enema.
- Vital signs within normal limits, afebrile, no abdominal distention.
- Stoma pink without drainage, redness, warmth, and tenderness.
- Bowel sounds present, NG tube discontinued.
- Parental caregivers listen, ask questions about care of child, and demonstrate adequate care/technique for device care/maintenance.

INTUSSUSCEPTION

EVIDENCE BASE Lee, J. Y., Kim, J. H., Choi, S. J., Lee, J. S., & Ryu, J. M. (2020). Point-of-care ultrasound may be useful for detecting pediatric intussusception at an early stage. *BMC Pediatrics*, *20*(1), 155. https://doi.org/10.1186/s12887-020-02060-6

Intussusception is the invagination or telescoping of a portion of the intestine into an adjacent, more distal section of the intestine, which creates a mechanical obstruction. Intussusception is one of the most common causes of intestinal obstruction in infancy. It can occur at any time in life but most commonly occurs in children younger than age 3, with the greatest incidence between ages 5 and 10 months. It is twice as common in male infants as in female infants. Incidence in the United States is 1.5 to 4 cases per 1,000 births. Intussusception should be high on the differential list when a child younger than age 1 presents with sudden onset of abdominal pain.

Pathophysiology and Etiology

1. The cause can fall into one of three categories: idiopathic, lead point, or postoperative.
   a. Idiopathic: This is the most common type, with no identifiable cause. It is not unusual, however, to obtain a history of a recent upper respiratory or gastrointestinal (GI) virus. It is hypothesized that hypertrophy of Peyer patches creates a thickened segment. It is most common in infants.
   b. Lead point: An identifiable change in the intestinal mucosa can be discovered, usually during surgical treatment, and is most common in children aged 2 to 3. Malformations include polyps, cysts, tumors, Meckel diverticulum, and hematomas (seen in Henoch-Schönlein purpura). Children with cystic fibrosis are at risk for lead point intussusception due to mucus and thick stool.
   c. Postoperative: uncommon but can occur after surgery of the abdomen and even the chest. It may be due to interrupted motility from anesthesia or direct handling of the intestine. It can also occur from placing long tubes into the bowel.
2. Invagination results in complete intestinal obstruction.
   a. Mesentery/lymphatics/blood vessels pulled into intestine when invagination occurs.
   b. Intestine becomes curved, sausage like; blood supply is cut off.
   c. Bowel begins to swell; hemorrhage may occur.
   d. Necrosis of involved segment occurs.
   e. If not recognized and treated, bowel death occurs, possibly resulting in significant loss of intestine, shock, and death.
3. Classification of location:
   a. Ileocecal (most common): when ileum and the attached mesentery, lymphatic tissue, and blood vessels invaginate into the cecum (see Figure 44-7).

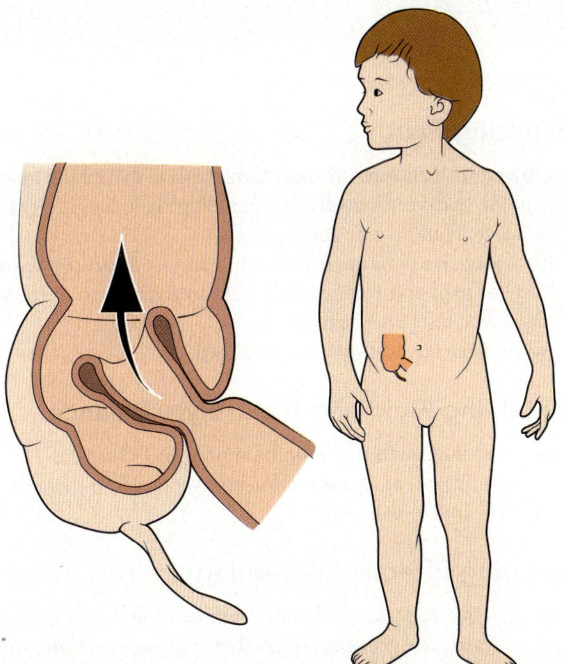

Figure 44-7. Intussusception. A portion of the ileum has been pushed into the lumen of the adjoining cecum. (LifeART image copyright © 2024. Lippincott Williams & Wilkins. All rights reserved.)

   b. Ileocolic: Ileum invaginates into colon.
   c. Colocolic: Colon invaginates into colon.
   d. Ileo–ileo (enteroenteric): Small bowel invaginates into small bowel.
4. An increase in cases of intussusception was noted after the introduction of the first rotavirus vaccine (RotaShield), so this vaccine was taken off the market. The second generation of rotavirus vaccines (RotaTeq and Rotarix) carries a much lower (though not zero) risk of intussusception. It is felt that the small risk is outweighed by the benefit of the vaccine.

EVIDENCE BASE Bergman, H., Henschke, N., Hungerford, D., Pitan, F., Ndwandwe, D., Cunliffe, N., & Soares-Weiser, K. (2021). Vaccines for preventing rotavirus diarrhoea: Vaccines in use. *The Cochrane Database of Systematic Reviews, 11*(11), CD008521. https://doi.org/10.1002/14651858.CD008521.pub6

Clinical Manifestations

1. Classic four signs of intussusception—vomiting, abdominal pain, bloody/red currant jelly–like stool, and abdominal mass—only occur in about 45% of children.
2. Pain is usually paroxysmal.
   a. "Attacks of pain" that awaken child from sleep; inconsolable, drawing up legs, colicky.
   b. Cyclic repetition of symptoms at approximately 5- to 30-minute intervals.
   c. Between episodes, child may act normal.
3. Stool may be like currant jelly—sloughed mucosa of dark red color with a mucoid consistency.
4. Vomiting may begin with decreased appetite and progress to bilious vomiting.
5. Bowel sounds vary:
   a. During a crisis of pain, bowel sounds may be hyperperistaltic rushes (borborygmi).
   b. Ileus/peritonitis: Bowel sounds are diminished or absent.
6. Decreasing frequency of bowel movements.
7. Increasing abdominal distention and tenderness.
8. Sausage-like mass palpable in the abdomen. This is pathognomonic and is known as *Dance sign*—elongated mass in the right upper quadrant of the abdomen with absence of bowel sounds in the right lower quadrant.
9. Unusual-looking anus; may look like rectal prolapse.
10. Dehydration, fever, lethargy; shock-like state with rapid pulse, pallor, marked sweating.
11. Hematochezia (maroon-colored stools)—not always present.
    a. Rectal examination is significant if bloody mucus on examiner's finger.
    b. Occult or gross blood on rectal examination in 60% to 90% of patients.
12. The groin should be inspected for incarcerated hernia or torsion of testicle or ovary as differential diagnosis.

CLINICAL JUDGMENT Currant jelly–like stool indicates damage to the intestine and can be a late sign. *Any* gross blood in the stool should raise suspicion of intussusception, especially when associated with abdominal pain; one should not wait for currant jelly–like stool to report.

Diagnostic Evaluation

EVIDENCE BASE Tonson la Tour, A., Desjardins, M. P., & Gravel, J. (2021). Evaluation of bedside sonography performed by emergency physicians to detect intussusception in children in the emergency department. *Academic Emergency Medicine*, *28*(8), 866–872. https://doi.org/10.1111/acem.14226

1. X-ray examination.
   a. Supine and upright abdomen film. Early course may be normal, but as it progresses, absence of gas in the colon is found. Can also have finding of the right upper quadrant mass and/or the meniscus/crescent sign.
   b. If no intraperitoneal air found on abdominal film, an air or barium enema is attempted.
   c. Commonly, a concave filling anomaly is seen in the transverse colon that can be reduced to the cecum.
2. Ultrasonogram to locate area of telescoped bowel and color Doppler sonography used to determine whether reducible. Absence of blood flow (color) indicates ischemia, and therefore, enema reduction should be avoided. Ultrasound will usually be obtained prior to contrast enema because of the low risk and excellent accuracy.

CLINICAL JUDGMENT Enemas are contraindicated in cases involving clinical findings of peritonitis, shock, or signs of perforation on abdominal x-ray.

Management

EVIDENCE BASE Plut, D., Phillips, G. S., Johnston, P. R., & Lee, E. Y. (2020). Practical imaging strategies for intussusception in children. *American Journal of Roentgenology*, *215*(6), 1449–1463. https://doi.org/10.2214/AJR.19.22445

1. Air or barium enema—both for diagnosis and treatment (hydrostatic reduction) in reducing intussusception.
   a. A surgeon should be present during the barium enema because of risk of perforation.
   b. A noninflatable tube is passed into rectum; contrast enters by gravity under fluoroscopic guidance. If air is used, it is delivered under constant pressure.
   c. As the intussusception is reduced, the contrast or air should reflux freely into the small intestine; this radiographic evidence is needed to confirm a successful reduction.
   d. Success ranges from 70% to 90%. Recurrence is the most common complication, but perforation can also occur.
   e. Nonoperative reduction using air enema or other hydrostatic reduction methods has been the standard treatment in most cases. The success rate can be as high as 84%. However, if nonoperative method is not indicated or fails, open surgery is still necessary.
2. Surgical reduction of intussusception may be necessary when radiologic reduction is unsuccessful, a pathologic lead point or peritonitis is suspected or with multiple recurrences. Factors associated with increased risk of intestinal resection include abdominal distension (32%), bowel obstruction on abdominal x-ray (27%), and hypovolemic shock (40%).
3. Surgery involves a laparotomy—manual milking out of the intussuscepted segment from the distal to proximal end, followed by resection of the nonviable bowel and, commonly, an incidental appendectomy. Up to 86% is successful in reduction.
4. Recurrence is 5% to 7%, regardless of the type of treatment undertaken.

EVIDENCE BASE Lampl, B. S., Glaab, J., Ayyala, R. S., Kanchi, R., & Ruzal-Shapiro, C. B. (2019). Is intussusception a middle-of-the-night emergency? *Pediatric Emergency Care*, *35*(10), 684–686. https://doi.org/10.1097/PEC.0000000000001246

Complications

1. Perforation.
2. Peritonitis.
3. Shock.
4. Loss of bowel resulting in short bowel syndrome.

Nursing Assessment

1. Obtain careful history of infant's or child's physical and behavioral symptoms, including any recent or chronic illness.
2. Perform physical examination, which may reveal a well-developed, well-nourished, afebrile infant with abdominal tenderness and distention.
3. Observe for dehydration; may be mild or severe. Poor capillary refill, decreased mental status, and decreased urine output are reliable indicators of shock in children.

CLINICAL JUDGMENT Report of episodic, severe, colicky abdominal pain combined with vomiting suggests intussusception.

Nursing Interventions

Minimizing Pain

1. Observe behavior as an indicator of pain; the infant may be irritable and very sensitive to handling or lethargic or unresponsive. Handle very gently.
2. Encourage family to participate in comfort measures. Explain cause of pain and reassure parental caregivers as to purpose of diagnostic tests and treatments.
3. Administer medications, as prescribed.

Maintaining Fluid and Electrolyte Balance

1. Monitor fluids and maintain by mouth (NPO) status.
2. Restrain infant, as necessary, for intravenous (IV) therapy.
3. Monitor intake and output.

Promoting Effective Breathing

1. Be alert for respiratory distress because of abdominal distention. Watch for grunting or shallow and rapid respirations if in shock-like state.
2. Insert nasogastric (NG) tube, if ordered, to decompress stomach.
   a. Irrigate, as ordered
   b. Note drainage and return from irrigation.

3. Maintain NPO status, as ordered.
   a. Wet lips and perform mouth care.
   b. Give infant pacifier to suck.
4. Continually reassess condition because disordered breathing or respiratory distress may indicate progression of disease process.

CLINICAL JUDGMENT Passage of one normal brown stool may occur, clearing the colon distal to the intussusception. Passage of more than one normal brown stool may indicate that the intussusception has reduced itself. Report any stools immediately to the provider.

Preparing for Surgery

1. Offer support to the parental caregivers during time of crisis and fear.
2. Offer specific teaching to parental caregivers.
   a. Compare intussusception to a collapsible telescope or antenna or by drawing a picture.
   b. Visual aids, such as a rubber glove with one finger into itself, may be helpful. Reduction can be demonstrated by filling glove with water until the inverted finger resumes its normal position.
3. Children need brief, simple explanations in age-appropriate language.

Preventing Infection and Other Postoperative Complications

1. Monitor vital signs and general condition and notify health care provider of any change or unexpected trend.
2. Assess temperature and administer antipyretics and other cooling measures. Fever may be present from the translocation of bacteria into the bloodstream through the damaged intestinal wall.
3. Assess for abdominal tenderness, bowel sounds, and distention of the abdomen. Maintain NG suction, as ordered.
4. Assess pain and level of consciousness.
5. When able to take fluids, assess tolerance carefully, and advance intake slowly.

Family Education and Health Maintenance

1. Explain that recurrences may occur and usually occur within 24 to 48 hours after reduction. Review signs and symptoms with parental caregivers.
2. Review activity restrictions with parental caregivers (e.g., positioning on back or side, quiet play, and avoidance of water sports until wound heals).
3. Encourage follow-up care.
4. Provide anticipatory guidance for developmental age of the child.
5. Encourage awareness of symptoms that require prompt medical attention among day care centers and other childcare providers (e.g., paroxysmal abdominal pain, blood or mucus in stool).

Evaluation: Expected Outcomes

- Decreased irritability/pain.
- Urine output adequate.
- Respirations unlabored; abdominal distention relieved.
- Parental caregivers verbalize understanding of condition and surgery.
- Postoperative vital signs stable; audible bowel sounds; passes stool postoperatively.

ANORECTAL MALFORMATIONS

The term *anorectal malformation* encompasses multiple congenital anomalies of the rectum, urinary tract, and reproductive system. Incidence is 1 in 2,500 to 1 in 4,000 live births, with a slight male predominance. Complexity varies from isolated imperforate anus to the extremely rare cloacal exstrophy (occurs in males and females 1 in every 250,000 births).

Pathophysiology and Etiology

EVIDENCE BASE Nakamura, H., & Puri, P. (2020). Concurrent Hirschsprung's disease and anorectal malformation: a systematic review. *Pediatric Surgery International*, *36*(1), 21–24. https://doi.org/10.1007/s00383-019-04580-4

1. An arrest in embryologic development of the anus, lower rectum, and urogenital tract at the sixth week of embryonic life; however, cause is unknown.
2. Approximately 40% of infants with anorectal malformations have associated major anomalies, including:
   a. Down syndrome.
   b. VACTERL (vertebral anomalies, anal atresia, cardiac anomaly, tracheoesophageal fistula with esophageal atresia, renal anomalies, and radial limb dysplasia) syndrome.
   c. Congenital heart disease.
   d. Renal abnormalities.
   e. Cryptorchidism.
   f. Esophageal atresia.
   g. Malformation of the spine.
   h. Variant of infantile hemangioma occurring in the extremity.
3. Abnormal development of the terminal hindgut ranges from mild anal stenosis, corrected by simple dilatation, to complex deformities, such as rectal atresia and fistula, with varying degrees of fecal and urinary incontinence.
4. *BMP4* and *Hox* genes may play a role.

Types

See Figure 44-8.

1. Imperforate anal membrane—infant fails to pass meconium; greenish, bulging membrane is seen; bowel and sphincter return to normal after excision.
2. Rectoperineal fistula—rectum opens into the perineum; excellent function.
3. Anal atresia and stenosis—complete obstruction (atresia) or stenosis (decrease in caliber) is present approximately 2 cm above the anal opening.
4. Imperforate anus without fistula (anal agenesis)—rectum is completely blind, ending 2 cm from perineum; intestinal obstruction occurs if no associated fistula.
5. Anorectal malformation with rectourinary fistula in males (present in 80% of males with anorectal malformations).
   a. Rectourethral bulbar fistula.
   b. Rectourethral prostatic fistula.
   c. Rectobladder neck fistula.

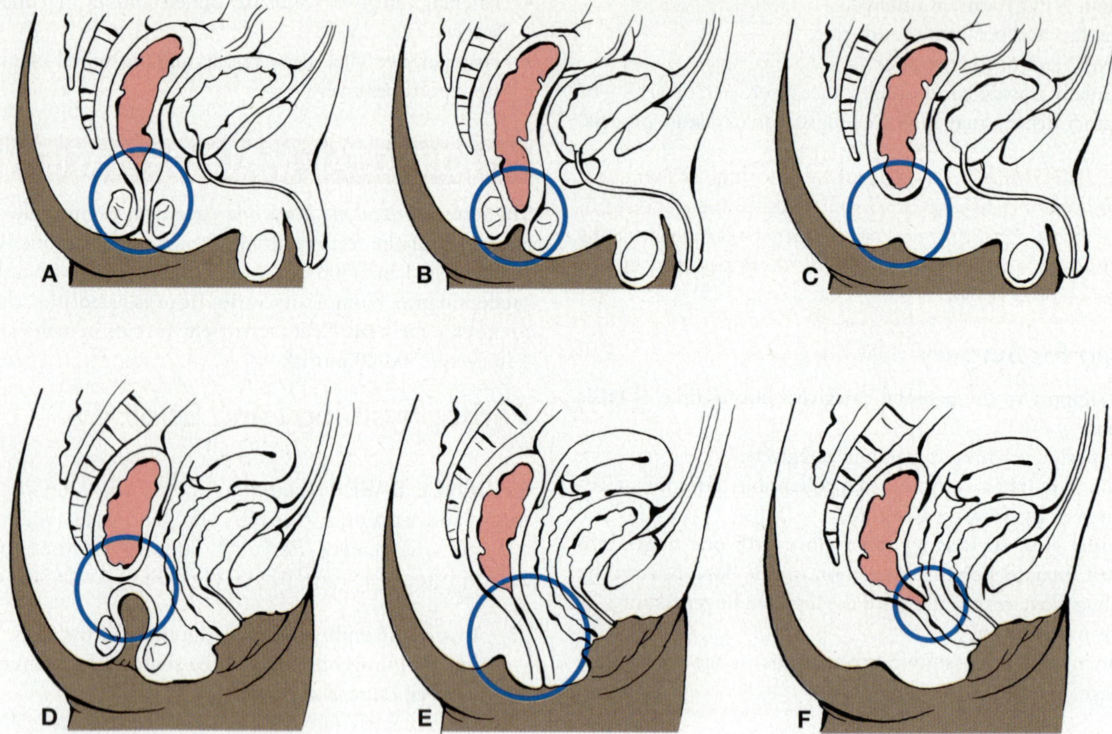

Figure 44-8. Anorectal malformations. **(A)** Anal stenosis. **(B)** Imperforate anal membrane. **(C)** Anal agenesis. **(D)** Rectal agenesis. **(E)** Recto-perineal fistula. **(F)** Small orifice located in the perineum. (Adapted with permission from Wong, D. L. [1995]. *Whaley and Wong's nursing care of infants and children* [5th ed.]. Mosby.)

6. Anorectal malformation with fistula and cloaca in females.
   a. Vestibular fistula—rectum opens through an abnormal narrow orifice located in the vestibule of the genitalia outside the hymen; most common anomalies in females.
   b. Vagina fistula—rectum opens via fistula into vagina; exceptionally rare malformation.
   c. Persistent cloaca—complex anomaly in which the rectum, vagina, and urinary tract are fused together into one common channel ending in a single perineal orifice at the site of the urethra; requires colostomy, urinary diversion, or vaginal diversion.
7. Cloacal exstrophy—complex anorectal anomaly that includes omphalocele, two exstrophied hemibladders with cecum between them, imperforate anus, and abnormalities of sexual structures; rare; occurs in males and females.
8. Ectopic anus—mild displacement of the anus, which causes constipation. It is not a true anorectal malformation but may require dilatations or surgery. The anal position can be measured using the anal position index, which is the ratio of anus–fourchette distance in females and anus–scrotum distance in males to the distance between coccyx and fourchette/scrotum.

Degree of Incontinence

1. It may be difficult to absolutely predict what pediatric patients will obtain bowel and bladder continence for those with congenital gastrointestinal/genitourinary (GI/GU) abnormalities or those who have suffered an injury to the area.
2. Bowel and bladder incontinence can be caused by damage to the nerves that control the sphincter muscles that control the outflow or damage to the muscle wall itself.
3. Complications may also occur from extensive surgical repairs required for surgery of the GI or urologic system.
4. Gender and the type of anomaly will impact the likelihood of continence.
5. Some disorders such as perineal fistula, rectal atresia, and rectal stenosis frequently result in 100% of patients having neither bowel nor bladder control.
6. Disorders such as rectobladder neck fistulas usually cause incontinence of urine but allow for bowel control.

Clinical Manifestations

1. Absence of anal opening; stimulation of perineum leads to puckering.
2. Displaced anal opening.
3. Anal opening near vaginal opening in female.
4. Thermometer, small finger, or rectal tube cannot be inserted into the rectum.
5. Meconium stool is absent or delayed.
6. Stool passed by way of the vagina or urethra may appear as green-tinged urine.
7. Progressive abdominal distention.
8. Fistula is likely to be present.
9. Vomiting if infant is fed.

Diagnostic Evaluation

1. Urine examination for the presence of meconium and epithelial debris indicates the presence of fistula.
2. Cross-table lateral abdominal x-ray—infant in prone position with pelvis elevated.

a. Gas in blind rectum gives a radiolucent image.
b. Measurement from the skin (radiopaque marker) and the blind rectum allow estimate of the height of the anomaly.
3. Abdominal ultrasound to detect urinary obstruction and locate rectal pouch.
4. Voiding cystourethrogram to detect commonly associated urinary tract anomalies such as vesicoureteral reflux.
5. Magnetic resonance imaging (MRI).

Management

EVIDENCE BASE Uzsen, H., Yaz, S. B., & Gumus, M. (2021). The effect of ostomy on pediatric patient and family in nursing: A systematic review. *Journal of Pediatric Surgical Nursing, 10*(4), 153–158. https://doi.org/10.1097/JPS.0000000000000313

Imperforate Anal Membrane

1. Internal and external sphincters are intact, so usually requires only a membrane excision from the anal opening.
2. Repaired at birth; no colostomy required.

Anal Stenosis

1. Internal and external sphincters are intact, so usually treated with anal dilation.
2. Occasionally requires myotomy (cutting of anal muscle).
3. Treated at birth; no colostomy required.

Imperforate Anus (Anal Agenesis)

1. Low lesion.
   a. Can usually be repaired with perineal anoplasty, which creates an anal opening for passage of stool.
   b. Usually accompanied by fistulas that need to be closed at the same time.
   c. Repaired at birth; colostomy usually not needed unless a fistula is present or more time for healing is needed.
2. High lesion.
   a. Requires more extensive surgery because of missing innervation.
   b. Usually requires a two-stage procedure, occasionally three-stage if complex anomaly is present.
   c. First step is a colostomy.
   d. Second step is anal repair, colon/rectum anastomosis, possible colostomy closure.
      i. Posterior sagittal anorectoplasty, also known as the *Pena procedure* (after the surgeon who developed it). The rectum is "pulled down" and sewn into a newly made anal opening in the perineum.
      ii. Most surgeons wait 4 to 6 months to complete it to allow for growth.
   e. Third step is colostomy closure if anomaly is complex and more healing time is needed.

Complex Fistulas and Cloaca

1. Complex rectal, urologic, and vaginal reconstruction are necessary.
2. Urinary diversion is performed in the neonate if a urologic emergency is apparent.

Note: Rectal dilation may be needed for any condition after the final surgery.

Complications

1. Infection.
2. Intestinal obstruction.
3. Loss of bladder or urinary sphincter control.

CLINICAL JUDGMENT Condition is usually discovered immediately after birth or within several hours. A delay in diagnosis is not uncommon and can significantly increase the risk of serious early complications and death.

Nursing Assessment

1. Perform physical assessment of neonate for abnormalities.
   a. Presence of perineal fistula.
   b. Meconium from vagina or presence of meconium-stained urine.
   c. No anal opening or inability to pass thermometer into rectum.
2. Perform thorough examination for other congenital anomalies.
3. Assess parental caregivers' level of understanding of condition and ability to cope with infant's surgery.

CLINICAL JUDGMENT A neonate who does not pass a stool in the first 24 hours after birth requires further assessment.

Nursing Interventions

Maintaining Stability Before Surgery

1. Maintain by mouth (NPO) status. Note any vomiting: color and amount.
2. Minimize energy expenditure due to altered nutritional status.
3. Maintain nasogastric (NG) tube passed to decompress the stomach, as ordered. Measure abdominal girth.
4. Observe the patient carefully for any signs of distress and report. Check vital signs frequently.
5. Use an isolette or radiant warmer to maintain temperature stability.
6. Minimal handling; cluster procedures together to encourage rest and sleep.
7. Keep fistula area clean to prevent urinary tract infection (UTI).
8. Administer good oral care.

Preventing Infection of Suture Line

1. Following anoplasty, do not put anything in the rectum.
   a. Position the infant for easy access to perineum for cleansing and minimal irritation to site (i.e., place the infant on their abdomen, possibly with hips elevated, to prevent pressure on perineal surfaces; turn side to side).
   b. Expose the perineum to air.
   c. Observe incision site for redness, drainage, poor healing.
   d. Apply antibiotic ointment to perineum, as directed.
2. Following colostomy, observe wound and stoma for redness, drainage, poor healing.
3. Administer intravenous (IV) antibiotics, as directed (usually 2 to 3 days).

Preventing Skin Breakdown

See "Ostomy Care in Children," page 1299.

Maintaining Fluid and Electrolyte Balance

1. Monitor for return of peristalsis; NG tube may be discontinued by the health care provider when bowel sounds present.
2. Start oral feedings, as ordered.
   a. Anoplasty: usually within hours.
   b. Colostomy: when bowel sounds present and colostomy has output.
3. Monitor parenteral fluids and discontinue when oral intake is sustained.
4. Report vomiting.
5. Describe stool frequency, consistency, and character. Report blood in stool or lack of stool output.
6. Monitor urine output, particularly important with urethral anomalies (including cloaca).

Strengthening Coping

1. Assure the parental caregivers that colostomy is temporary (unless complex surgery performed).
2. Encourage the parental caregivers to participate in care of the child and to provide emotional security for the child.
3. Provide thorough teaching program for special care needed at home.
   a. Colostomy care.
   b. Anal dilatation to prevent a stricture at site of anastomosis from scar tissue (after instructions by health care provider).
4. Initiate referral to community nurse, especially if the parental caregivers are particularly anxious about caring for the child at home.
5. Encourage the parental caregivers to talk about their concerns.
6. Enlist help of enterostomal nurse specialist before the child leaves the hospital and for continued home care needs.
7. Assist breastfeeding parent to maintain milk supply through frequent pumping.

Maximizing Recovery Following Definitive Pull-Through Surgery

1. Maintain gastrostomy tube (GT) or NG tube decompression until peristalsis returns.
2. If a bladder catheter is used, provide care, as directed, and measure urine output accurately.
3. Observe carefully for abdominal distention, bleeding from perineum, and respiratory compromise. Report immediately.
4. Carry out perineal care.

Family Education and Health Maintenance

1. Review special care and procedures to be continued at home. Involve parental caregivers and other caregivers in teaching. Advise parental caregivers to make day care providers, teachers, and school nurse aware of child's needs.
2. It is important that the family understands the rationale and technique for anal dilation as indicated by the surgeon. Provide written instructions and assess their understanding of the procedure.
3. Help the parental caregivers to understand situations that may be encountered as a result of anorectal malformation repair as the infant gets older.
   a. Fecal impaction due to lack of sensation to defecate.
   b. Future surgery if primary repair was not done or anomaly complicated.
   c. Toilet training—may be delayed, especially after a pull-through procedure.
   d. Inability to control fecal seepage from rectum.
4. Offer practical guidelines to help parental caregivers cope.
   a. Fecal control may not be achieved until age 10; however, about 85% of children achieve normal or socially acceptable continence if anomaly limited to imperforate anus.
   b. If incontinence occurs, anorectal manometric evaluation in postoperative period can give more realistic information about future incontinence.
   c. Encourage bowel habit training or patterning of defecation (e.g., after breakfast).
   d. Promote diet modifications; teach foods that produce laxative effect (plums, prunes, chocolate, nuts, corn) and foods that have binding effect (peanut butter, hot cereal, cheese).
   e. Stool softeners or antidiarrheal medication as ordered by the health care provider.
   f. Rectal inertia may cause fecal impaction in rectosigmoid colon with soiling from fluid overflow. Bisacodyl suppository or cleansing enema provides assistance in management.
5. Antegrade continence enema procedures may allow for continence in children without anal sphincter function.
6. Encourage mutual support from other families who have a child with an anorectal malformation.
7. For additional information and support, refer the parental caregivers to the National Organization for Rare Disorders (www.rarediseases.org) or the United Ostomy Associations of America (www.ostomy.org).

DRUG ALERT Antidiarrheal medications should be used with caution in children.

Evaluation: Expected Outcomes

- Vital signs stable, abdominal girth stable.
- No signs of infection of suture line.
- Skin intact surrounding ostomy.
- Bowel sounds present; oral feeding tolerated without vomiting; NG tube discontinued.
- Family discusses plans for home care with enterostomal therapist.

Children discharged to home with a GI disorder may require a complex level of care by family caregivers. Ensure that the caregivers understand procedures and outcomes for nutritional support. It is crucial that nurses discharging these patients ensure that the families have the financial means and access to secure necessary nutritional requirements as well as the ability to store items (if refrigeration is required). GI disorders frequently cause alteration in means of elimination, or incontinence. Ensure that all necessary equipment is available to maintain optimal hygiene and infection disease containment. This is also crucial for the child (who has successfully toilet trained) to maintain social interactions without embarrassment. If long-term management is expected for nutrition and elimination in the school-aged child, the nurse may be called on to assist in training and education of school personnel to assist in the care.

SELECTED READING

Wilson, K. (2023). Infant feeding issues related to gastrointestinal conditions: Assessment and management. *Primary Health Care, 33,* 35–42. https://doi.org/10.7748/phc.2023.e1781

45 Pediatric Renal and Genitourinary Disorders*

ACUTE DISORDERS

Acute Glomerulonephritis

Postinfectious glomerulonephritis is a broad term used to describe several disease processes that result in glomerular injury. Specifically, in poststreptococcal glomerulonephritis, the glomerular injury is the result of antigen–antibody deposits within the glomeruli. It occurs most frequently in school-aged children, is rare in children younger than age 2 years, and occurs more frequently in males than in females (2:1).

Pathophysiology and Etiology

1. Presumed cause—antigen–antibody reaction secondary to nephritogenic strains of group A beta-hemolytic *Streptococcus*.
2. The initial infection is usually either an upper respiratory infection (URI) or a skin infection.
3. It is speculated that the streptococcal antigen can bind to glomeruli and activate complement via the lectin pathway, thus overactivating the immune system.
4. Antibodies produced to fight the invading organism also react against the glomerular tissue, thus forming immune complexes.
5. The immune complexes become trapped in the glomerular loop and cause an inflammatory reaction in the affected glomeruli.
6. Changes in the glomerular capillaries reduce the amount of the glomerular filtrate, allow passage of blood cells and protein into the filtrate, and reduce the amount of sodium and water that is passed to the tubules for reabsorption.
7. General vascular disturbances, including loss of capillary integrity and spasm of arterioles, are secondary.

Clinical Manifestations

Onset

1. Usually 7 to 15 days after acute pharyngitis. In streptococcal skin infections, the latency period may be as long as 4 to 6 weeks.
2. May be abrupt and severe or mild and detected only by laboratory measures.

Signs and Symptoms

1. Urinary symptoms:
   a. Decreased urine output.
   b. Bloody or brown-colored urine.
2. Edema.
   a. Present in most patients.
   b. Usually mild.
   c. Commonly manifested by periorbital edema in the morning.
   d. May appear only as rapid weight gain.
   e. May be generalized and influenced by posture.
3. Hypertension.
   a. Present in up to 70% of those hospitalized with glomerulonephritis.
   b. Usually mild.
   c. Rise in blood pressure (BP) may be sudden.
   d. Usually appears during the first 4 to 5 days of the illness.
4. Pallor.
5. Malaise, lethargy.
6. Low-grade fever.
7. Mild headache.
8. Gastrointestinal (GI) disturbances, especially anorexia and vomiting.

Diagnostic Evaluation

1. Urinalysis:
   a. Decreased output (oliguria)—may approach anuria.

* Please note that the term "male" in this chapter refers to a person assigned male at birth, and the term "female" in this chapter refers to a person assigned female at birth.

b. Microscopic or gross hematuria (noted in 30% to 70% of all cases).
c. Specific gravity—moderately elevated.
d. Proteinuria may be mild to severe.
e. Microscopic—red blood cells, leukocytes, epithelial cells, and casts.
f. Low urinary sodium may be noted.
2. Blood urea nitrogen (BUN) and creatinine—usually mildly to moderately elevated; however, normal in 50% of cases.
3. Antistreptolysin-O titer—elevated initially.
4. Anti-DNase B titer elevated.
5. Erythrocyte sedimentation rate elevated.
6. Complement C3 and complement C4—depressed.
7. If chest x-ray indicated—may show pulmonary congestion, cardiac enlargement during the edematous phase.

Management

1. Antibiotic therapy may be initiated if there is any concern that streptococci or other organisms are still present.
2. Other management is mostly symptomatic; in most patients, spontaneous recovery is expected. Hospitalization is usually not necessary.
3. Salt and fluid intake should be restricted during the acute phase of the disease.
4. Diuretics should be administered if significant edema or hypertension develops.
5. A renal biopsy may be indicated if the child does not recover from apparent acute poststreptococcal glomerulonephritis.

Complications

The following complications occur infrequently.
1. Circulatory congestion—if severe can lead to pulmonary edema.
2. Hypertensive encephalopathy.
3. Acute renal failure.
4. Anemia.

Nursing Assessment

1. Obtain history regarding recent streptococcal infection.
2. Obtain appropriate cultures and assess for current infection.
3. Measure urine output and degree of hematuria and proteinuria.
4. Weigh the child and document the areas and extent of edema.
5. Obtain baseline BP reading to assess for hypertension.

Nursing Interventions

Promoting Normal Urine Output

1. Monitor daily intake and output.
2. Test and record urine for hematuria and proteinuria, as directed. Note the color of urine.
3. Monitor daily weight.

Reducing Excess Fluid Volume

1. Provide a no-salt-added diet during the acute phase of the illness. Other restrictions may be indicated if renal function is impaired. Protein intake is not usually restricted because of the possible risk of malnutrition.
2. Communicate dietary restrictions in clear and understandable terms per institutional policies so that staff and visitors will be aware of special needs. This may involve placing a sign on the child's bed.
3. Restrict fluids in children with hypertension, edema, heart failure, or renal failure.
4. With fluid restrictions, offer small amounts of fluids spaced at regular intervals throughout the day and evening. Use an appropriate-sized cup for the amount of fluid being offered.
5. Check BP, as ordered or needed, and observe for signs of hypertension (e.g., headache, blurry vision, fussy, fatigue). Administer antihypertensive and diuretic drugs, as ordered by health care provider.

Promoting Diversional Activity

1. Explain fluid restriction at an age-appropriate level and direct the child's focus away from restrictions.
2. Provide the child with diversional activity and play therapy.
3. Encourage activity, as tolerated.

Providing Information

1. Explain all aspects of the diagnostic tests and treatment in terms the family can understand.
2. Explain the purpose of all medications and the restricted diet, including a review of high-sodium foods and liquids to avoid and sample menus.
3. Encourage family participation in the child's care.
4. Help the family plan for adaptation of the child's nursing care to the home environment.
5. Arrange appointments for continued medical supervision and initiate referrals when appropriate.

Family Education and Health Maintenance

1. Reinforce medical explanation of the disease process.
   a. Alert the family to signs and symptoms of disease recurrence.
   b. Be aware that microscopic hematuria may persist for several months.
2. Reinforce activity recommendation; usually not restricted.
3. Advise that tonsillectomy or other oral surgery is not recommended for several months after the acute phase of glomerulonephritis.
   a. If this type of surgery is necessary, penicillin may be recommended before and after the procedure to prevent bacterial infection.
   b. Obtain information regarding drug allergies before administering penicillin.

Evaluation: Expected Outcomes

- Output remains adequate.
- Weight returns to/close to baseline.
- Child does age-appropriate activities, as tolerated, and does not complain of thirst.
- Parental caregivers and the child can state the rationale for treatment.

Nephrotic Syndrome

Nephrotic syndrome is characterized by heavy proteinuria, hypoalbuminemia, hyperlipidemia, and edema. The syndrome can be subdivided into congenital, primary, and secondary types. Primary nephrotic syndrome includes idiopathic, minimal change, and childhood types. Approximately 85% to 95% of primary cases in preadolescents are classified as minimal change nephrotic syndrome (MCNS) and are associated with minimal histologic change in the glomeruli. Nephrotic syndrome afflicts approximately 16 per 100,000 children younger than age 16 in the United States annually; in young children, it is slightly more common in males than in females, but it disappears in teenagers and adults. The most common age for presentation is 2 years, and 70% to 80% of cases occur in children younger than age 6 years.

Pathophysiology and Etiology

1. Underlying defect is thought to be caused by the loss of charge selectivity of the glomerular basement membrane, which permits negatively charged proteins, primarily albumin, to pass easily through the capillary walls into the urine.
2. Excessive urinary loss of protein and catabolization by the kidney of circulating albumin lead to a decrease in serum protein (hypoalbuminemia).
3. The colloidal osmotic pressure that holds water in the vascular compartments is reduced because of the decrease in the amount of serum albumin. This allows fluid to flow from the capillaries into the interstitial spaces, thus producing edema.
4. The shift of fluid from the plasma to the interstitial spaces reduces the vascular fluid volume (hypovolemia), which, in turn, stimulates the renin–angiotensin system and the secretion of antidiuretic hormone and aldosterone.
5. Tubular reabsorption of sodium and water is increased for intravascular volume.
6. The loss of proteins, particularly immunoglobulins, predisposes the child to infection.

Clinical Manifestations

1. Onset is insidious. It is likely to be caused by immune system disturbances because it commonly occurs after a mild URI.
2. Edema is typically the presenting symptom.
   a. Edema may be minimal or massive.
   b. Edema is usually first apparent around the eyes.
   c. Dependent edema occurs in areas of the body, such as the hands, ankles, feet, and genitalia.
   d. Fluid that accumulates in the body spaces may give rise to ascites and pleural effusions.
   e. Striae may appear on the skin from overstretching.
3. Profound weight gain caused by edema; the child may actually double normal weight.
4. Decreased urine output during the edematous phase—urine appears concentrated and frothy.
5. Pallor, irritability, lethargy, and fatigue.
6. GI disturbances, including vomiting, diarrhea, abdominal pain, and anorexia caused by edema of the intestinal mucosa.

Diagnostic Evaluation

1. Urinalysis:
   a. Proteinuria (tests for albumin)—2+ (greater than 1.0 g/L) on urine dipstick; should be sent for urine protein to creatinine ratio (first voided or random spot urine) to confirm. Considered nephrotic range if greater than 200 to 250 mg/mmol.
   b. Blood—gross hematuria is not present, but microscopic hematuria may be found in about 20% of patients.
2. A 24-hour urine collection is the gold standard for quantification of urine protein—nephrotic range greater than 40 mg/m^2/h.
3. Blood tests.
   a. Total protein—reduced.
   b. Albumin—less than 2.5 g/dL.
   c. Complete blood count may show increased hemoglobin, suggesting hemoconcentration.
   d. BUN may be elevated, indicating general renal dysfunction.
   e. Creatinine—usually normal but may be increased if intravascularly depleted.
   f. Electrolytes—may have sodium, potassium, CO_2, and calcium imbalances.
   g. Increased serum cholesterol and triglycerides—due to reactive protein synthesis by the liver in response to hypoproteinemia.
4. Renal biopsy is indicated to look for other causes of renal dysfunction if the patient has persistent proteinuria after 4 to 8 weeks of steroid therapy (median time to remission is 10 days—negative or trace proteinuria for 3 consecutive days). Biopsy also indicated if atypical presentation such as persistent renal failure, age less than 1 year or greater than 10 years, use of nephrotoxic drugs, or persistent hematuria.

Management

Steroid Therapy

1. Corticosteroid therapy—prednisone and prednisolone are drugs of choice because of lower cost and are less likely to induce salt retention and potassium loss. Use intravenous (IV) formulation in hospitalized patients to improve absorption due to intestinal edema. Pediatric patients frequently resist the oral liquid preparations due to taste.
2. No standard program of therapy exists; however, the 2021 Kidney Disease: Improving Global Outcomes guidelines recommend the following:
   a. Corticosteroid therapy be given for at least 12 weeks.
   b. Oral prednisone be administered as a single daily dose starting at 60 mg/m^2/day or 2 mg/kg/day to a maximum of 60 mg/day.
   c. Daily oral prednisone be given for 4 to 6 weeks followed by alternate-day medication as a single daily dose starting at 40 mg/m^2 or 1.5 mg/kg (maximum 40 mg on alternate days) and continued for 2 to 5 months with tapering of the dose.
3. Corticosteroid therapy should be discontinued slowly to avoid complications of steroid withdrawal, particularly benign intracranial hypertension.
4. Children with nephrotic syndrome may respond to steroid therapy in several ways:
   a. Steroid sensitive: achieving remission within 28 days of the start of corticosteroid therapy.
   b. Steroid dependent: relapses on alternate-day dosing or relapses within 14 days of corticosteroid discontinuation.
   c. Steroid resistant: persistent proteinuria after 8 weeks of corticosteroid therapy.
5. Children with steroid-responsive MCNS have a favorable long-term prognosis.

EVIDENCE BASE Kidney Disease: Improving Global Outcomes (KIDGO) Diabetes Work Group. (2022). KDIGO 2022 clinical practice guideline for diabetes management in chronic kidney disease. *Kidney International, 102*(5S), S1–S127. https://doi.org/10.1016/j.kint.2022.06.008. PMID: 36272764.

Intravenous Albumin 25%

1. To shift fluid from interstitial space into the vascular system.
2. Only a temporary treatment to relieve edema but may be used in severe cases of edema that cause respiratory distress or severe discomfort.

3. Diuretic therapy is used in combination with IV albumin to help relieve edema. In cases of hypovolemia, diuretics may not be indicated.

Alternative Drug Therapies

1. Should be considered when children relapse frequently (greater than four relapses in 1 year or two relapses in 6 months), become steroid resistant or steroid dependent, or demonstrate unacceptable adverse effects of steroid therapy (steroid toxicity). The decision to use alternative therapy in conjunction with steroids should be made by an experienced pediatric nephrologist.
2. Immunosuppressants (Figure 45-1).
   a. Cyclophosphamide.
   b. Cyclosporin A.
   c. Tacrolimus.
   d. Mycophenolate mofetil.
   e. Rituximab.

Complications

1. Infections:
   a. Peritonitis, most commonly caused by *Streptococcus pneumoniae* but may also be caused by *Escherichia coli* and *Haemophilus influenzae.*
   b. Gram-negative septicemia.
   c. Staphylococcal cellulitis.
2. Thromboembolic events.
3. Hypertension.
4. Hyperlipidemia.
5. Pulmonary edema.
6. Bone disease secondary to corticosteroid therapy.
7. Acute renal failure.

Nursing Assessment

1. Obtain a history of the onset of illness and symptoms.
   a. Precipitating events.
   b. Recent immunizations.
   c. Recent URIs.
   d. Flulike symptoms.
   e. Time of onset and location of edema.
   f. Urinary pattern changes.
2. Perform physical examination focusing on vital signs; auscultation of breath sounds to determine adventitious sounds; areas and extent of edema, especially periorbital region, extremities, genitalia, abdomen; and peripheral perfusion, including pulses, color, and warmth of extremities.

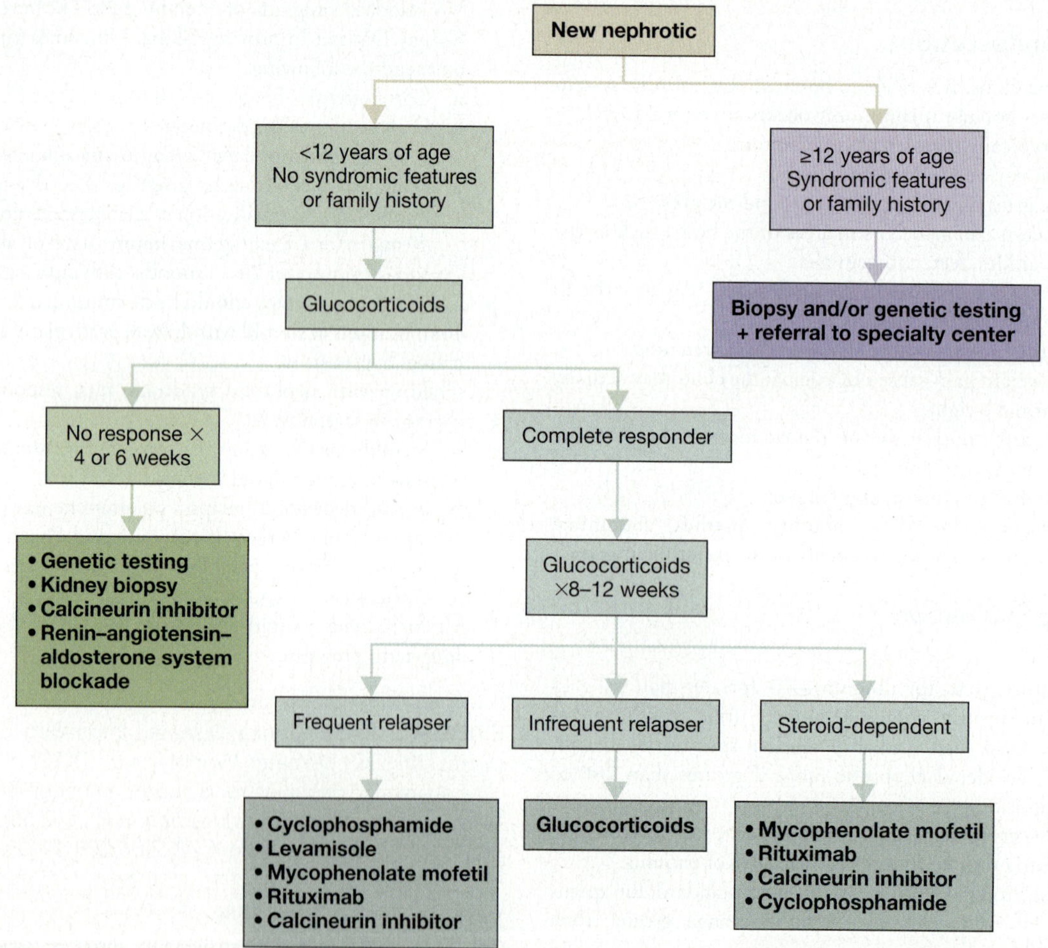

Figure 45-1. Management of glomerular diseases. (Reprinted with permission from Kidney Disease: Improving Global Outcomes [KDIGO] Glomerular Diseases Work Group. [2021]. KDIGO 2021 clinical practice guideline for the management of glomerular diseases. *Kidney International, 100*[4S], S1–S276. https://doi.org/10.1016/j.kint.2021.05.021)

Nursing Interventions

Relieving Excess Fluid

1. Administer corticosteroids, as directed.
   a. Observe for adverse effects and complications of therapy, such as Cushing syndrome—increased body hair (hirsutism), rounding of the face ("moon face"), abdominal distention, striae, increased appetite with weight gain, cataracts, and aggravation of adolescent acne.
   b. Stress that some physical changes are not harmful or permanent and that some will disappear after the steroid treatment is stopped.
   c. Observe for serious adverse effects and uncommon complications of corticosteroids (see pages 688 and 689).
2. Administer immunosuppressive drugs, as prescribed.
   a. Make sure that the patient and parental caregivers understand the desired and adverse effects of therapy.
   b. Observe for complications of therapy, such as decreased white blood cell (WBC) count, increased susceptibility to infection, hair loss or increased hair growth (hirsutism), gingival hyperplasia, and hemorrhagic cystitis.
3. Administer diuretics, as prescribed.
   a. Be aware of those diuretics that may cause potassium depletion.
   b. Offer foods high in potassium, such as orange juice, bananas, and dried fruits (e.g., raisins, apricots).
   c. Administer supplemental potassium chloride, as ordered, and if the urine output is adequate.
4. Encourage activity, as tolerated.
5. Restrict fluids as ordered (usually only during the extreme edematous phases).
   a. Restriction is carefully calculated at frequent intervals, based on the urine output of the previous day plus estimated insensible losses.
   b. Offer small amounts of fluids spaced at regular intervals throughout the day and evening. Use a cup of appropriate size for the amount of fluid being offered.
   c. Measure fluids accurately in graduated containers. Do not estimate fluid intake or output.
   d. Place a sign on the child's bed to make sure that no urine is accidentally discarded and that all intake is recorded.
   e. Determine total intake and output every 8 hours. In children who are not toilet trained, a fairly accurate record of output can be obtained by weighing diapers before and after voiding.
   f. Record other causes of fluid loss, such as the number of stools per day, perspiration.
6. In refractory or extreme cases, assist with abdominal paracentesis; this may be required because of marked ascites. During the procedure, fluid is withdrawn from the peritoneal cavity to relieve pressure symptoms and respiratory distress.
7. Restrict sodium, as ordered (usually done while the child is on corticosteroid therapy). A starting point is 1.5 to 2 g/day.
   a. Use a low-sodium menu when ordering meals from the hospital.
   b. Assist family in making food choices that are low in sodium.
   c. Foods that should be limited include cured, salted, canned, or smoked meats; processed cheese; regular canned or frozen soups and bouillon cubes; and salted crackers and other snack foods.

CLINICAL JUDGMENT No live vaccinations or immunizations should be given during active episodes of nephrosis or while the child receives immunosuppressive therapy.

DRUG ALERT Administer cyclophosphamide in the morning, with large volumes of fluid, to prevent concentration of the drug in the urine and increased susceptibility to cystitis.

Preventing Infection

1. Monitor complete blood count for decreased WBC count and neutropenia.
2. Closely observe the child who takes corticosteroids for signs of infection. Be aware that fever and other symptoms may be masked.
3. Provide meticulous skin care to edematous areas of the body.
   a. Bathe the child frequently and apply appropriate skin preparations to prevent breakdown. Areas of concern are moist parts of the body and edematous male genitalia.
   b. Position the child so that edematous skin surfaces are not in contact. Place a pillow between the child's legs when lying on side.
   c. Elevate the child's head to reduce edema.
4. If possible, avoid invasive procedures, such as femoral venipunctures and intramuscular (IM) injections, to decrease the chance of introducing pathogens. Venipuncture of the lower extremities may also predispose the child to thromboembolism because of hypovolemia, stasis, and increased plasma concentration of clotting factors.
5. Educate the parental caregivers regarding signs and symptoms of possible infections.

Enhancing Nutritional Status

1. Assess nutritional intake, growth, and development as appropriate for age.
2. Provide a diet low in sodium, fat, and sugar. Advise visitors that any additional food or fluids must not be consumed by the child without approval and documentation by nursing personnel.
3. Provide food choices that appeal to the child and that are easy to eat according to the stage of development.
4. Provide nutritional supplements, as needed.

Providing Emotional Support

1. Encourage frequent visits and allow as much parental caregiver participation in the child's care as possible. Hospitalization, if necessary, is usually brief.
2. Allow the child as much activity as tolerated.
   a. Balance periods of rest, recreation, and quiet activities during the convalescent phase.
   b. Allow the child to eat meals with family or other children.
3. Encourage the child and family to verbalize fears, frustrations, and questions.
   a. Be aware that young children frequently fear abandonment by their parental caregivers.
   b. Allow parental caregivers to express frustrations regarding the uncertainties associated with the cause of the disease, the clinical course, and the prognosis.
4. Help the child adjust to changes in body image, such as cushingoid appearance, by explaining changes ahead of time.
5. Discuss the problems of discipline with the parental caregivers. Encourage them to set consistent limits and reasonable expectations of their child's behavior.
6. Suggest parental caregivers get involved with a support group for families of children with chronic illnesses, as needed.

Family Education and Health Maintenance

1. Prepare the family for home management of the child's care plan.
   a. Have the dietitian discuss special diets with the parental caregivers.
   b. Teach the parental caregivers about the child's medication—the desired effects and the potential adverse effects.
   c. Demonstrate urine testing for protein.
   d. Initiate a community health nursing referral, if necessary, for reassessment and reinforcement of teaching.
2. Encourage continued medical follow-up visits.
3. Emphasize the necessity of taking medication according to the prescribed schedule and for an extended time. Discuss complications encountered with steroid therapy.
4. Teach prevention and recognition of signs and symptoms of infection.
5. Advise family on necessary activity restrictions during hospitalization, after discharge, or specific restrictions before or after procedures (e.g., biopsy).
6. Teach signs and symptoms of relapse (proteinuria 3+ on 3 consecutive days on urine dipstick at home, increased edema, and decreased urine output) and whom and when to call with questions.
7. Teach signs and symptoms of fluid imbalances (excess or dehydration).

Evaluation: Expected Outcomes

- Decreased edema and ascites; adequate urine output.
- Exhibits no signs of infection.
- Family verbalizes and follows dietary restrictions as demonstrated by appropriate weight gain/loss.
- Family verbalizes concerns regarding child's illness as demonstrated by open communication with staff and other family members.

Urinary Tract Infection

EVIDENCE BASE Mattoo, T. K., Shaikh, N., & Nelson, C. P. (2021). Contemporary management of urinary tract infection in children. *Pediatrics, 147*(2), e2020012138. https://doi.org/10.1542/peds.2020-012138

Urinary tract infection (UTI) is defined as bacteria that exist anywhere between the renal cortex and the urethral meatus. Because it is usually difficult to determine the exact location of the infection, the term *urinary tract infection* is used to explain microorganisms anywhere within the urinary tract. UTIs are categorized as cystitis or urethritis (located in the bladder or urethra), upper tract (located in the ureters or collecting system), and pyelonephritis (renal parenchyma). The greatest incidence of UTI in males occurs in the first year of life (most common in uncircumcised males), after which it rapidly declines, remaining low through childhood and adolescence. Incidence in females is also highest in the first year of life and steadily declines through adolescence but remains higher than the incidence for males at a rate of 10:1.

Pathophysiology and Etiology

1. Causative organisms—*E. coli* (85% to 90%), *Klebsiella* species, *Proteus* species, *Staphylococcus saprophyticus* (female adolescents and sexually active females), *Enterococcus* species, *Streptococcus* group B (neonates), *Pseudomonas aeruginosa*.
2. Route of entry:
   a. Ascent from the urethra (most common).
   b. Circulating blood (rare).
3. Contributing causes:
   a. Female specific.
      i. Perineal location of urethral orifice and shorter urethra.
      ii. Sexual intercourse (mechanics of vaginal penetration).
      iii. Vaginal voiding—reflux of urine into the vagina while voiding, with subsequent dribbling of urine.
   b. Male specific—foreskin (prepuce can be a reservoir for bacteria).
   c. Abnormal bladder or voiding with or without incontinence.
      i. High pressures in the bladder.
      ii. Incomplete bladder emptying, infrequent voiding.
      iii. Difficulty relaxing pelvic floor.
   d. Constipation and bowel/bladder dysfunction.
   e. Congenital urinary tract anomalies—vesicoureteral reflux (VUR), posterior urethral valves, prune belly syndrome, hydronephrosis, bladder exstrophy.
   f. Neurogenic bladder (spina bifida, spinal injury).
   g. Catheterization, urinary drains/tubes.
   h. Bacterial colonization.
   i. Alteration in periurethral flora by antibiotic therapy.
4. Pathophysiology—colonization of uropathogens in the periurethral area that ascend into the bladder via the urethra, affecting portions of the urinary tract, spreading from the bladder to kidneys through the ureter (pyelonephritis) and, possibly, to the bloodstream (bacteremia).
   a. Clumps of bacteria may be present.
   b. Inflammation results in urine retention and stasis of urine in the bladder.
   c. Backflow of urine into the kidneys may occur through the ureters; this is called *vesicoureteral reflux*.
   d. Inflammatory changes in the renal pelvis, and throughout the kidney, occur when the kidney is involved.
   e. Scarring of the kidney parenchyma occurs in chronic infection and interferes with kidney function, particularly with the ability to concentrate urine.
   f. If pyelonephritis is left untreated, the kidney tissue may be destroyed, and renal function could fail.

Clinical Manifestations

1. Onset may be abrupt or gradual; may be asymptomatic.
2. Failure to thrive in infancy.
3. Young children: may be nonspecific (vomiting, irritability, poor feeding, diarrhea); fever is often the only presenting complaint.
4. Older children and adolescents: urinary frequency, urgency or voiding hesitancy, dysuria, suprapubic tenderness, dribbling, and nocturnal enuresis (more common in lower UTI).
5. Hematuria: often occurs with viral cystitis.
6. Fever.
   a. May be moderate or severe.
   b. May fluctuate rapidly.
   c. May be accompanied by chills or rigors.
7. Anorexia and general malaise.
8. Foul odor or change in the appearance of urine.
9. Abdominal or suprapubic pain (more common in upper tract disease).
10. Tenderness over one or both kidneys.
11. Systemic symptoms: Flank pain, fever, chills, nausea, and vomiting may occur with pyelonephritis.

Diagnostic Evaluation

1. Urinalysis:
   a. Leukocytes, nitrites suggestive, but not indicative.
   b. Casts, especially WBC casts, may be present and are indicative of intrarenal infection.
   c. Hematuria—occurs occasionally.
   d. Decreased specific gravity due to decreased renal concentrating ability.
2. Urine culture:
   a. Urinalysis for proteinuria and bacteriuria should be obtained as part of the general medical evaluation. If the urinalysis indicates an infection, both urine culture and sensitivity are recommended.
   b. Documentation of a single pathogenic organism in the urine is the only means of definitive diagnosis. Multiple organisms found in the culture are suspicious of perineal flora contamination and warrant repeat culture.
   c. A urine culture demonstrating more than 100,000 bacteria per mL indicates significant bacteriuria.
   d. A catheterized urine specimen, with growth greater than 50,000 colonies of bacteria per mL, is considered significant and required in the non–toilet-trained child to prevent contamination from perineal flora.
   e. To avoid contamination, discard the first few milliliters of urine (if quantity is sufficient). A new catheter should be used for each subsequent attempt if unsuccessful.
3. Urologic and radiologic studies to identify anatomic abnormalities or renal changes that stem from recurrent infections—renal bladder ultrasound (ensure the child is well hydrated with distended bladder), voiding cystourethrogram (VCUG).
   f. Dimercaptosuccinic acid (DMSA) scan—evaluates renal function and scarring.

Management

See Table 45-1.

1. Treatment depends on the child's age, severity of infection, and antimicrobial resistance rates in the community.
2. Oral antibiotic therapy for uncomplicated UTI. Usually 7- to 10-day antibiotic therapy for febrile UTIs.
3. IV antibiotics for complicated UTI—infections that do not respond to oral therapy or that develop into pyelonephritis or those that appear septic or dehydrated.
4. Repeat culture following therapy if still symptomatic, has chronic renal disease, or has known colonization of bacteria.

Complications

1. A tendency for recurrent infection exists.
2. Children with obstructive lesions of the urinary tract and those with severe VUR are at highest risk for kidney damage. These patients may need prophylactic oral antibacterial therapy.

Nursing Assessment

1. Obtain history to determine whether UTI is initial or recurrent and to determine whether there may be other disease processes contributing to this infection.
2. Focus assessment on identifying clinical manifestations and determining location of infection, such as presence and appearance of urethral discharge, high-grade fever (more common with upper UTI), or low-grade fever (more common with lower UTI).
3. Determine urinary pattern (i.e., amount and frequency) and associated discomfort.
4. Determine bowel pattern and possibility of constipation.

Nursing Interventions

Promoting Urinary Elimination

1. Obtain a clean urine specimen for urinalysis or culture (see pages 569 and 572).
   a. Obtain freshly voided early morning specimen, if possible (most accurate). This urine is usually acidic and concentrated, which tends to preserve the formed elements.
   b. Provide fluids to help the child void.
   c. Perform catheterization, if necessary, to obtain a sterile specimen; however, this procedure may cause emotional trauma and the accidental introduction of additional bacteria. In females, pulling the labia majora out versus splaying them will help identify the meatus and prevent

Table 45-1 Antimicrobial Agents Commonly Used in the Management of Childhood Urinary Tract Infection

DRUG	ADVERSE EFFECTS	NURSING CONSIDERATIONS
Amoxicillin	• Occasional nausea, vomiting, diarrhea • Hypersensitivity reactions of skin	• Readily absorbed. • May be taken with food.
Ampicillin	• Diarrhea, urticaria • Anaphylactic reaction	• Contraindicated in penicillin-sensitive children. Package insert should be consulted regarding reconstitution, administration, and storage of IM and IV preparation. Absorption of oral preparations may be decreased with food. Dose must be repeated q6h to ensure therapeutic blood level.
Cephalexin	• Diarrhea, nausea, vomiting	• May be taken with food. Dose should be reduced if renal function is impaired.
Gentamicin	• Renal and auditory toxicity; respiratory paralysis	• Toxic effects can be minimized by slow IV infusion (over 1 h).
Nitrofurantoin	• Fever, nausea, vomiting, peripheral neuropathy	• Recommended for prolonged use. Give with food or milk to decrease GI adverse effect May cause urine to be amber or brown in color. Contraindicated in renal failure and in infants younger than 3 mo old.
Co-trimoxazole	• Nausea, vomiting, fever, rash, photosensitivity	• Commonly used if bacterial resistance is anticipated or the child fails to respond to initial therapy.

GI, gastrointestinal; IM, intramuscular; IV, intravenous; q, every.

catheter insertion into the vagina. In the event that there is inadvertent catheterization of the vagina, leaving the catheter in situ and using a new sterile catheter should prevent recatheterization of the vagina. In males, pulling back the foreskin is required to identify the location of the meatal opening.

d. Send urine to the laboratory immediately or refrigerate to avoid a falsely high bacterial count.

2. Administer antibiotics, as ordered by the health care provider (after specimen has been obtained for culture).
   a. Antibiotic therapy is generally determined by the results of the urine cultures and sensitivities and by the child's response to therapy; however, empirical therapy may be started before culture results are back.
   b. Become familiar with the toxic effects of antimicrobial agents and assess the child regularly for any signs and symptoms.

Maintaining Comfort and Providing Symptomatic Relief

1. Administer analgesics and antipyretics, as ordered.
2. Maintain the child on bed rest while febrile.
3. Encourage fluids to reduce the fever and dilute the concentration of the urine. (Water is the best clear fluid.)
4. Administer IV fluids, if necessary.

Promoting Self-esteem

1. Reinforce medical explanations of the disease and its therapy.
2. Explain all diagnostic tests and procedures to the child, allowing time for questions and answers.
3. Encourage verbalizing. Correct any misconceptions and particularly address concerns about the functioning of the urinary tract and sexual function. Reassure the child that they did not cause the problem.
4. Maintain privacy for the child as much as possible.
5. Provide an environment that is as close to normal as possible during hospitalization. Include opportunities for the child to play.
6. Prepare the child and family for discharge and begin discussions of rest, fluids, and medications.

Family Education and Health Maintenance

1. Review long-term antibiotic therapy, if prescribed, to prevent recurrence of UTI. Schedules for prolonged therapy vary from several months to continuous prophylaxis.
2. Encourage scheduled follow-up visits because of the possibility of disease recurrence.
   a. Emphasize that even though this disease may have few symptoms, it can lead to serious, permanent disability.
   b. Advise family that subsequent suspected UTIs should be assessed and followed by health care provider.
3. Teach measures of prevention:
   a. Minimize the spread of bacteria from the anal and vaginal areas to the urethra in female children by cleansing the perianal area from the urethra back toward the anus.
   b. Encourage adequate fluid intake, especially water.
   c. Avoid carbonated and caffeinated beverages because of their irritative effect on bladder mucosa.
   d. Encourage the child to void frequently and to empty the bladder completely with each voiding (double voiding).
   e. Encourage a high-fiber diet to avoid constipation.

Evaluation: Expected Outcomes

- Voids regularly in adequate amounts.
- No complaints of pain during or after voiding; afebrile.
- Shows less anxiety about hospitalization; appears more relaxed about appearance, body image, tests.

ABNORMALITIES OF THE GENITOURINARY TRACT THAT REQUIRE SURGERY

See Figure 45-2 for congenital abnormalities of the urinary tract, exstrophy of the bladder, and hypospadias.

Exstrophy of the Bladder

Bladder exstrophy is an abnormality present at birth in which the bladder and associated structures are improperly formed. Rather

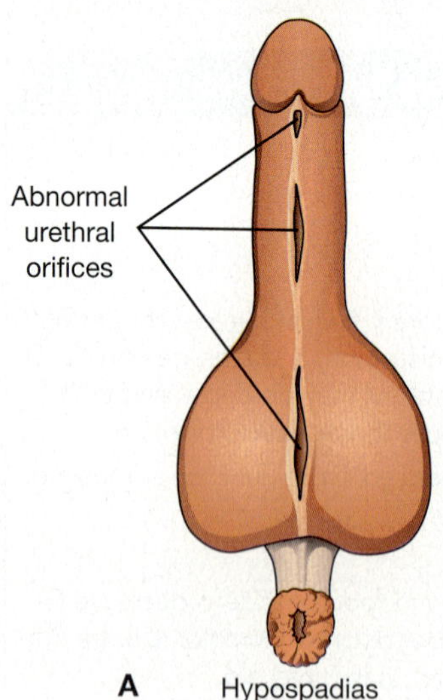

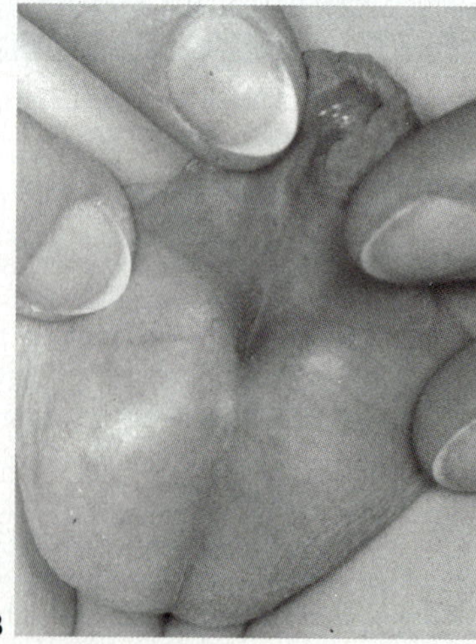

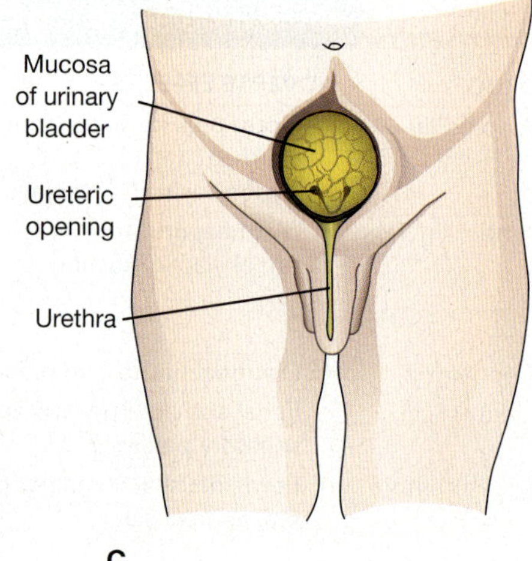

Figure 45-2. **(A)** Hypospadias showing the various locations of abnormal urethral orifices. **(B)** Patient with hypospadias. The urethra is open on the ventral surface of the penis. **(C)** Epispadias combined with exstrophy of the bladder. Bladder mucosa is exposed. (**A** and **C**: Reprinted with permission from Sadler, T. W. [2023]. *Langman's medical embryology* [15th ed., Fig. 16-37A and D]. Wolters Kluwer.)

than being its normal round shape, the bladder is flattened. The skin, muscle, and pelvic bones joining the lower part of the abdomen did not form properly, so the inside of the bladder is exposed outside the abdomen. There are also associated deficiencies of the abdominal muscles and pelvic bones. These occur at a rate of 1:10,000 to 50,000 live births. It is more common in males. Recent published evidence suggests that the risk of bladder exstrophy in children born as a result of assisted fertility techniques is seven times greater than in children conceived naturally without assistance. Evidence exists on genetic predisposition in the likelihood of exstrophy parental caregiver with a 1 in 70 chance of having a child with bladder exstrophy and a reoccurrence probability of 1 in 100.

Pathophysiology and Etiology

1. Results from failure of the abdominal wall and its underlying structures to fuse in utero during the third to fourth weeks of gestation. Presumed cause is persistence of cloacal membrane during fetal development that ruptures to produce exstrophy.
2. In classic exstrophy (about 60% of bladder anomalies), the posterior bladder wall is externalized and lies open on the lower part of the abdomen with an epispadial urethra, allowing constant passage of urine to the outside.
3. Epispadias may occur without exstrophy (about 30% of bladder anomalies); the bladder remains an internal organ, but the urethra is laid open, possibly with a split glans penis and the meatus located proximally.
4. Cloacal anomalies (about 10% of bladder anomalies) involve externalization of the bladder and portions of the gastrointestinal (GI) tract.

Clinical Manifestations

1. Urine dribbles constantly.
2. Infection and ulceration of the bladder mucosa may occur.
3. Genitalia may be ambiguous.
4. Affected children may walk with a waddling or an unsteady gait due to diastasis (separation) of pelvic bones.

Diagnostic Evaluation

1. May be diagnosed prenatally by ultrasound.
2. Newborn inspection is the most important tool in evaluation. The obvious anomaly may involve multiple systems.
3. Diagnostic procedures, such as radiography, ultrasound, magnetic resonance imaging, and urodynamic testing, determine the extent of the anomaly.
4. Spinal ultrasound for infant with sacral dimples to rule out spinal cord tethering.

Management

1. Surgical closure of the bladder within the first 24 to 48 hours of life by means of primary complete bladder closure and epispadias repair. This approach allows for maximal continence postrepair.
2. Urinary diversion should be rare.

Complications

1. Skin excoriation, infection.
2. Trauma to the bladder mucosa.

Nursing Assessment

1. Assess for growth and development milestones during reconstruction.
2. Assess the family for coping ability.

Nursing Interventions

Facilitating Urine Output Preoperatively

1. Protect the bladder area from trauma and infection.
   a. Apply smooth common kitchen plastic wrap.
   b. Warm sterile saline can be squirted over the bladder to keep tissue moist.
   c. Position on back or side.
   d. Ensure umbilical cord is sutured and not clamped.
2. Observe the infant closely for signs of infection.
3. Involve other members of the health care team for parental caregiver support because of the psychosocial implications of a child who has special needs.
4. Assist the parental caregivers in dealing with their emotional reactions regarding the child's defect.
5. Prepare child and parental caregivers for the proposed surgery (see page 1147).
6. While previously repaired at birth, recent trend includes delayed closure to 3 months for better care outcomes including physiologic testosterone surge for penile growth in male patients.

Providing Postoperative Care to Prevent Infection

1. Goal of reconstruction is to preserve renal function, urinary continence and volitional voiding, functional and cosmetically acceptable external genitalia.
2. Provide care for the ureteral and urethral catheters. Observe and record the amount of urinary drainage, catheter positions, and bladder spasms.
3. Care for dressings, castings, stents, and/or skin traction as necessary.
4. Provide care and instruction for an ileal conduit, as necessary (see page 579).
5. Antibiotic prophylaxis and pain control as ordered.
6. Observe for complications.
   a. Urinary or incisional infections.
   b. Fistulae in the suprapubic or penile incisions.
7. Recommend long-term support for children and families to help them deal with concerns about the appearance of genitalia, sexual function, reproduction, and rejection by peers.

Family Education and Health Maintenance

1. Specific teaching and preparation depending on the type of closure (primary or staged). Staged closures will likely require additional surgery at 4 to 5 years of age.
2. Provide community nursing referral, as needed, to support family and make sure that the family understands the importance of follow-up with the various specialists.
3. Act as a liaison, as necessary, to coordinate care.
4. For more information and support, refer families to the following resources:
   a. Association for the Bladder Exstrophy Community (ABC) (www.bladderexstrophy.com).
   b. Book: *A Story about you ... and your special bladder* (male and female versions available). Available directly through ABC.

Evaluation: Expected Outcomes

- No skin breakdown or infection.
- Incision healing well without infection or fistula; eventually, voiding without difficulty.

Vesicoureteral Reflux

EVIDENCE BASE Walker, J., Morin, J., Peard, L., & Saltzman, A. (2021). Vesicoureteral reflux and bladder diverticulum. In P. Godbole, D. T. Wilcox, & M. Koyle (Eds.), *Practical pediatric urology: An evidence based approach* (pp. 263–276). Springer International Publishing.

Vesicoureteral reflux (VUR) is the abnormal retrograde flow of urine from the bladder into the upper urinary tract. In the absence of bacterial infection, VUR is not considered to be critical. In the presence of bacteria, however, VUR is a risk factor for the development of urinary tract infections (UTIs) and pyelonephritis, which can lead to renal damage and scarring. With linear growth, spontaneous resolution of VUR occurs in most children.

Pathophysiology and Etiology

VUR occurs as a result of congenital deficiency in the formation of the ureterovesical junction, resulting in a laterally displaced ureteral orifice. Secondary VUR is acquired as a result of increased bladder pressure.

Clinical Manifestations

1. Febrile UTI—culture confirmed, catheterized specimen for non–toilet-trained child.
2. Unexplained febrile illnesses.
3. Associated urogenital anomalies (bladder exstrophy, posterior urethral valves, neurogenic bladder).
4. Prenatal diagnosis (hydronephrosis detected on prenatal screening ultrasounds).

Diagnostic Evaluation

1. Voiding cystourethrogram (VCUG)—to establish the diagnosis of VUR but should not be performed routinely after the first febrile UTI. It is indicated after ultrasound reveals hydronephrosis, scarring or findings of high-grade VUR or obstructive uropathy, recurrent UTI, or atypical complex clinical circumstances.
2. Renal ultrasound—to assess for renal damage, associated hydronephrosis.
3. Dimercaptosuccinic acid (DMSA)—recommended when renal ultrasound is abnormal w/greater concern for scarring (breakthrough UTI, grade 3 to 4 VUR, elevated creatinine).

Management

1. The goals of medical and/or surgical management are to prevent pyelonephritis, recurrent UTIs, and the formation of renal cortical scarring.
2. Continuous prophylactic antibiotic recommended for some children based on age, history of febrile UTI, and degree of VUR.
3. Surgical intervention is indicated when medical therapy is unsuccessful.
   a. Circumcision offered for infant males with VUR protective for babies before 1 year of age.
   b. Endoscopic polymer injection into the ureter(s)—83% success rate.
   c. Ureter reimplantation—98.1% success rate.
4. Yearly ultrasounds to monitor renal growth and kidney parenchymal scarring.

Complications

1. Recurrent UTI can lead to renal damage and failure.
2. Recurrence of VUR following surgical intervention—postoperative UTI in children close to or toilet-trained age is strongly associated with the incidence of preoperative UTI and the presence of bladder bowel dysfunction (BBD).
3. Postoperative renal obstruction rate of 0.4%.

Family Education and Health Maintenance

1. Association of bowel/bladder dysfunction.
2. General routine evaluation for patients with renal scarring prior to VUR resolution or recurrent UTI after resolution of VUR—blood pressure (BP), height, weight, and urinalysis for protein screening for patients with abnormal ultrasound/DMSA.
3. Communication of long-term concerns of hypertension (especially in pregnancy), renal function loss, recurrent UTI, and familial VUR in siblings and offspring to be discussed when the child is at an appropriate age.
4. Evidence-based study conducted (RIVUR), concluding that prophylaxis reduces the risk of recurrent UTI, but not renal scarring.

For nursing assessment, diagnoses, and interventions, see "Care of the Child Who Undergoes Urologic Surgery" section, page 1319.

Obstructive Lesions of the Lower Urinary Tract

Obstruction of the lower urinary tract may be caused by structural lesions, such as posterior or anterior urethral valves, bladder neck obstruction, meatal stricture, and urolithiasis (stones), or by functional lesions, such as neuromuscular dysfunction. The effect of obstruction on ureteral and renal function depends on the degree and duration of obstruction, the rate of urine formation, and whether infection exists.

Pathophysiology and Etiology

Types of Obstruction

1. Urethral valves—filamentous valves that obstruct urine flow.
2. Congenital narrowing of the urethra.
3. Bladder neck obstruction—most common site of lower urinary tract obstruction.
4. Meatal stricture.
5. Neuromuscular dysfunction.
6. Severe phimosis (rare).
7. Inflammatory processes.
8. Neoplasia.
9. Urolithiasis.
10. Trauma.

Effects of Obstruction

1. Urinary tract becomes distended, proximal to the point of obstruction.
2. The bladder dilates and hypertrophies.

3. Stasis of urine occurs.
4. The ureters become elongated, dilated, and tortuous.
5. Hydronephrosis and destruction of kidney tissue inevitably result if left untreated.

Clinical Manifestations

1. Abnormal urination.
   a. Dysuria, frequency.
   b. Enuresis, dribbling.
   c. Reduced force of urine stream.
   d. Difficulty starting urine stream.
   e. Straining during urination.
   f. Abrupt cessation during urination.
2. Signs of infection—fever, pain, irritability, and, occasionally, hematuria.
3. Lower obstruction: suprapubic pain, prolapse via urethra in females (ureterocele) presenting as bulging vulvar mass in females.

Diagnostic Evaluation

1. Physical examination may reveal abdominal mass.
2. Laboratory findings depend on the degree that renal function is compromised.
3. Renal ultrasound may show hydronephrosis.
4. Radionuclide scanning.
5. Endoscopic examination.
6. Ureteroscopy.
7. Urodynamic examination.

Management

1. Prevention or eradication of infection with antibiotics.
2. Dilation of urethral stenosis or stricture.
3. Urinary diversion may be necessary.
4. Surgical relief of the obstruction.

Complications

1. Urinary stasis and recurrent UTI could lead to renal failure.
2. Severe and recurrent UTI.
3. Recurrence of the obstruction.

For nursing assessment, diagnoses, and interventions, see "Care of the Child Who Undergoes Urologic Surgery" section, page 1319.

Obstructive Lesions of the Upper Urinary Tract

Obstructive lesions of the upper urinary tract include ureteropelvic junction obstruction, ureterovesical junction obstruction, ureteral stricture, congenital absence or duplication of a ureter, and urolithiasis. These obstructive lesions are primarily congenital.

Pathophysiology and Etiology

1. Congenital anomalies develop in the upper urinary tract.
   a. Ureteropelvic junction obstruction.
   b. Ureterovesical junction obstruction.
   c. Stricture of a ureter.
   d. Congenital absence of one ureter.
   e. Duplication of the ureter of one kidney.
2. Urolithiasis (renal calculi) is rare in children but may be associated with metabolic disease, such as cystinosis or oxalosis.

Clinical Manifestations

1. Hydronephrosis may present as an abdominal mass.
2. Commonly asymptomatic (seldom any problem with voiding).
3. Vague signs, such as failure to thrive, may be present.
4. UTIs may be frequent.
5. Hypertension may occur.

Diagnostic Evaluation

1. Laboratory tests to determine renal function.
2. Renal ultrasound, radionuclide imaging, and ureteroscopy to determine the extent of the lesion.

Management

1. Prevention or eradication of infection.
2. Surgical correction of the obstruction.

Complications

Renal failure.

For nursing assessment, diagnoses, and interventions, see "Care of the Child Who Undergoes Urologic Surgery" section, page 1319.

Hypospadias

EVIDENCE BASE Imizcoz, F. L., Velazquez, E. R., & Mushtaq, I. (2021). Hypospadias. In P. Godbole, D. T. Wilcox, & M. Koyle (Eds.), *Practical pediatric urology: An evidence based approach* (pp. 319–332). Springer International Publishing.

Binion, K., Rode, A., Norley, G., Miller, A., Misseri, R., Kaefer, M., Ross, S., Preisser, J., Hu, D., & Chan, K. (2023). A multi-site pilot study of a parent-centered tool to promote shared decision-making in hypospadias care. *Journal of Pediatric Urology, 19*(3), 290.e1–290.e10.

Hypospadias is a congenital defect of the penis, resulting in the incomplete development of the anterior urethra, corpora cavernosa, and prepuce (foreskin). Hypospadias is also associated with penile ventral curvature (chordee), which, depending on the severity of the defect, may result in infertility secondary to difficulty in semen delivery. Hypospadias is a common birth defect, occurring in one out of every 150 to 300 males. The goal of treatment is to achieve cosmetic and functional repair. See Figure 45-2 on page 1314.

Pathophysiology and Etiology

1. In utero, before 1 month, the genitalia looks the same for both female and male fetuses. After about a month, because of the increased exposure to testosterone for male fetuses, the genitalia changes to resemble that of a male and is identifiable as such. By the end of the first trimester, the penile urethra and foreskin are completely formed. Abnormalities in this development, such as subsequent, decreased testosterone production, can lead to hypospadias.
2. Classification is determined by the location of the urethral meatus.
3. The majority of cases have no known etiology but may show genetic inheritability—14% incidence in siblings; 8% incidence in offspring.
4. Undescended testicle, hydrocele, or inguinal hernia may be associated.

Clinical Manifestations

1. Inability to void with penis in normal elevated position.
2. Spraying of urine when voiding.
3. 70% urethral meatus located distal on penile shaft.
4. 30% proximal location and often more complex.
5. In case of concomitant unilateral or bilateral undescended testis, endocrine evaluation advised to exclude disorders of sexual differentiation.

Diagnostic Evaluation

1. Usually not difficult to diagnose because of visual anomaly. Assess glans penis for possible hypospadias before circumcision.
2. Severe cases require genotypic/phenotypic sex determination, chromosomal, and hormonal studies.

Management

Surgical reconstruction between ages 6 and 18 months, if possible (to minimize psychological issues surrounding toileting and genital awareness), and before circumcision because foreskin is essential for most complex repairs. Phalloplasty is also considered a surgical option for removal of dorsal hooded foreskin in mild hypospadias.

Post-op temporary stent in situ for complex hypospadias repair that is typically removed/falls out in 7 to 10 days to allow newly created urethra and opening to heal.

Dressings are typically removed within the first few days at home, and bathing is encouraged to keep incision site clean and prevent bacteria from developing.

Complications

1. Urethrocutaneous fistula.
2. Meatal stenosis.
3. Urethral diverticulum.
4. Residual penile curvature.
5. Wound dehiscence or infection.
6. Urinary tract symptoms.
7. Esthetic result.

Family Education and Health Maintenance

Follow-up postreconstruction is typically few months after reconstruction, 1 year after the repair, after toilet training, and after puberty to ensure satisfaction and understanding of congenital anomaly. Complications are seen as needed.

For nursing assessment, diagnoses, and interventions, see "Care of the Child Who Undergoes Urologic Surgery" section.

Cryptorchidism

EVIDENCE BASE Elamo, H. P, Virtanen, H. E., & Toppari, J. (2022). Genetics of cryptorchidism and testicular regression. *Best Practice and Research Clinical Endocrinology and Metabolism, 36*, 1–12. https://doi.org/10.1016/j.beem.2022.101619

Echeverria Sepúlveda, M. P., Yankovic Barceló, F., & Lopez Egaña, P. J. (2022). The undescended testis in children and adolescents. Part 1: Pathophysiology, classification, and fertility- and cancer-related controversies. *Pediatric Surgery International, 38*(6), 781–787. https://doi.org/10.1007/s00383-022-05110-5

Echeverria Sepúlveda, M. P., Yankovic Barceló, F., & Lopez Egaña, P. J. (2022). The undescended testis in children and adolescents. Part 2: Evaluation and therapeutic approach. *Pediatric Surgery International, 38*(6), 789–799. https://doi.org/10.1007/s00383-022-05111-4

Cryptorchidism refers to the failure of one or both testes to descend through the inguinal canal to the normal position in the scrotum. A testis is considered undescended if, on examination, the testicle is palpable elsewhere and cannot be brought down into the scrotum. It is more common in premature infants and is the most common surgical problem in pediatric urology.

Pathophysiology and Etiology

1. Possibly caused by delayed descent, prevention of descent by mechanical lesion, or endocrine disorder (rare).
2. Testicular and ductal development are abnormal. It is unclear whether this is because of congenital dysplasia or because of underdevelopment.
3. Degeneration of the sperm-forming cells occurs after puberty because of the higher temperatures of the abdomen, compared with normal location in the scrotum.

Clinical Manifestations

Testicle nonpalpable within the scrotum.

Spontaneous descent of the testes may occur in the first corrected 6 months of life.

Diagnostic Evaluation

1. Imaging for cryptorchidism is not recommended prior to referral. Ultrasonography may reveal undescended testicle but is not as reliable as physical examination.
2. Serum testosterone measurements may be decreased.

Management

Complications for cryptorchidism can include testicular malignancy later in life, potential impairment in fertility, testicular torsion, trauma to testicle, and associate hernias.

1. Specialist referral should ensure surgical evaluation by 6 months of age because of low probability of descent and probable damage should the testes remain in a nonscrotal location.
2. Bilateral nonpalpable testicles require immediate urology consultation to evaluate for possible disorder of sex development (DSD).
3. Surgical laparoscopic exploration must be performed after examination under anesthesia confirms that testicles are not palpable on all patients with nonpalpable unilateral and bilateral cryptorchidism. Open approach is used for palpable testicles.
4. Orchiopexy surgery to achieve permanent fixation of the testis in the scrotum. Surgery should be performed between ages 6 and 15 months to prevent damage to the tissues and to lessen emotional concerns related to body image.
5. Surgical placement of testicular prosthesis, if testicle(s) absent.
6. Lack of evidence in long-term success of testicular descent in administration of human chorionic gonadotropin and has noted low response rates.

Family Education and Health

1. Primary care provider should palpate testes with every well-child visit for quality and position.

2. Retractile testes are at increased risk for secondary testicular ascent due to hyperactive cremasteric reflex, short patent processus vaginalis, or entrapping adhesions.
3. Previously cryptorchid males should be assessed with each well-child visit for quality and position postoperatively and eventually taught how to perform monthly testicular self-examination after puberty to facilitate early cancer detection.
4. Former bilateral cryptorchid males have a greatly reduced fertility compared to males with a history of unilateral cryptorchidism and general male population.

For nursing assessment, diagnoses, and interventions, see "Care of the Child Who Undergoes Urologic Surgery" section.

Care of the Child Who Undergoes Urologic Surgery

Also see Chapter 17, pages 577 to 582, for a discussion of kidney surgery and urinary diversion.

Nursing Assessment

1. Obtain history from prenatal and birth record, family, and child.
2. Assess feeding and crying patterns, indicating potential obstruction or abdominal pain.
3. Assess urinary elimination pattern to determine the degree of disorder.
4. Assess for associated congenital defects.
5. Assess for failure to thrive.
6. Determine family's response to body image changes. Expect anxieties regarding sterility and gender identity and perceptions of the child as defective or inadequate.
7. Measure and record vital signs, height, weight, abdominal girth, and compare with previous measurements, if available. Renal insufficiency may alter growth. Fever may be indicative of infection.
8. Visually and manually inspect genitalia and record abnormalities (e.g., if bladder mucosa is visible, describe signs of irritation).
9. Palpate abdomen; note masses.
10. Obtain urine for culture and sensitivity. Note color, amount, odor, and degree of cloudiness.
11. Review results of all laboratory and diagnostic procedures.

Nursing Interventions

Promoting Understanding of Surgical Treatment

1. Determine the child's expectation regarding illness and hospitalization through discussion and play therapy.
2. Explain the anatomy and physiology of the urinary system in terms the child can understand.
   a. Use a body outline appropriate for the age of the child.
   b. Explain how the child differs from the normal. Relate defect to symptoms whenever possible.
3. Explain all diagnostic tests before their occurrence. These may include urinalysis, 24-hour urine collections, intravenous (IV), retrograde pyelography, ultrasound, and/or VCUG. Descriptions should include the following information:
   a. Preparation required—fasting, enemas, catheterization.
   b. Location of the test—operating room, radiology department.
   c. Appearance and attire of personnel.
   d. Positioning.
   e. Anesthesia.
   f. Pain or discomfort.
   g. Expectations after the procedure—diet, rest, urine collections.
4. Determine the child's understanding of the procedure.
   a. Ask simple, direct questions.
   b. Allow the child to perform the procedure on a doll or to demonstrate it on a diagram.
5. Explain the surgical procedure, including the following:
   a. Preparation required—fasting, enemas.
   b. Description of the operating room, including the appearance of the personnel.
   c. Anesthesia.
   d. Postoperative appearance—urinary drainage tubing and collection devices, appearance of urine, sutures, bandages, IV infusion.
6. Reassess the child's understanding of the surgery and reinforce teaching when necessary.
7. Emphasize additional points:
   a. The child is in no way to blame for illness.
   b. No other part of the body will be operated on.

Promoting Normal Urine Output

1. Monitor daily intake and output.
2. Encourage adequate fluids and monitor daily weight.
3. Care for all catheters and urinary tubes according to facility policy. Maintain appropriate position of tubes.
4. Observe and record the amount and appearance of urinary drainage, occurrence of bladder spasms, and symptoms of urinary or incisional infection.

Providing Emotional Support Regarding Body Image

1. Continue reassurance about the appearance of genitalia.
2. Maintain discussions regarding reactions. This may need to be done with patient and family alone as well as the family unit.
3. If additional surgical intervention is required, discuss plans for interim period from initial surgery until secondary or reconstructive procedures can be performed.
4. Initiate independence of care.
5. Focus on activities the child can perform and accomplish.

Preventing Infection

1. Administer antibiotics and IV fluids, as ordered.
2. Maintain patency of catheters. Provide catheter care, as directed.
3. Administer wound care using aseptic technique. Inspect incision for drainage or signs of infection.

Maintaining Fluid Volume

1. Administer fluids, as ordered.
2. Monitor vital signs for hypotension or tachycardia.
3. Assess patient's skin turgor and mucous membranes for signs of dehydration.
4. Measure and record accurate intake and output.

Promoting Comfort

1. Administer analgesics, as ordered and according to the assessment of complaints of pain, restlessness, crying, or withdrawal.
2. Administer antispasmodics, as ordered, for bladder spasm.
3. Provide distraction and comfort measures.

Family Education and Health Maintenance

1. Advise the family about follow-up appointments, additional surgeries, or procedures.
2. Teach care of incision and catheter, signs of infection.

3. Advise on avoidance of straddle toys or positioning for 6 weeks to promote healing.
4. Encourage good nutrition to promote healing and to prevent infection.
5. Provide contact names and phone numbers for families to call to update on status with complications, urgent concerns, and where to go in the case of an emergency.

Evaluation: Expected Outcomes

- Child and family verbalize understanding of surgery.
- Clear urine draining via catheter.
- Incision without drainage or signs of infection.
- Vital signs stable; urine output adequate.
- Decreased crying and increased restful periods and sleep noted.

RENAL FAILURE AND DIALYSIS

Acute Renal Failure

Acute renal failure is a sudden, usually reversible deterioration in normal renal function. This results in fluid and electrolyte imbalance and accumulation of metabolic toxins. Nursing care of children with acute renal failure is generally the same as that of adults (see pages 584 to 587), although there are special considerations for pediatric patients.

Pathophysiology and Etiology

1. Causes are divided into *prerenal* (problem occurs in blood supply to the kidneys), *intrarenal* (problem is within the kidney or kidneys), and *postrenal* (problem occurs in urinary system after the kidneys).
   a. Prerenal causes: Conditions causing hypovolemia (dehydration, shock, trauma, or burns) cause decreased blood flow to the kidneys. The nephrons, however, are structurally and functionally intact.
   b. Intrarenal causes: conditions causing a reduction in glomerular filtration rate (GFR), renal ischemia, and tubular damage. May be due to vascular diseases (hemolytic uremic syndrome, thrombosis), tubular nephropathies (myoglobinuria, hemoglobinuria, toxins), or interstitial nephritis (penicillins, allergies). These are the largest group to require extended medical management.
   c. Postrenal causes: conditions causing obstruction to urine flow. Uncommon, except for obstructive uropathies in the first year of life. Renal function is restored with relief of the obstruction.
2. The exact pathophysiology of acute renal failure is not always known. Three phases of acute renal failure are recognized in children:
   a. Initiating phase: begins when the kidney is injured and lasts from hours to days. Signs and symptoms of renal impairment are present.
   b. Oliguric phase: usually lasts 5 to 15 days but can persist for weeks; shorter in infants and young children (3 to 5 days) and longer in older children and adolescents (10 to 14 days). Not all patients have an oliguric phase.
   c. Diuretic phase: highly variable, from mild and lasting only a few days to profound.
3. Trauma, burns, and nephrotoxic agents may cause acute tubular necrosis and temporary cessation of renal function. Myoglobin (a protein released from muscle when injury occurs) and hemoglobin are released, causing renal toxicity, ischemia, or both.
4. Severe transfusion reactions may result in hemoglobin that filters through the kidney glomeruli. This becomes concentrated in the kidney tubules. Resulting precipitation interferes with the excretion of urine.
5. Nonsteroidal anti-inflammatory drugs (NSAIDs) interfere with prostaglandins that normally protect renal blood flow, decreasing GFR.

DRUG ALERT Nephrotoxic agents include aminoglycosides, penicillins, cephalosporins, sulfonamides, calcineurin inhibitor immunosuppressives, NSAIDs, and certain antineoplastic drugs. Large doses of vitamin A, chemicals that contain arsenic, and mercury are also nephrotoxic.

Clinical Manifestations

1. Nausea and vomiting.
2. Diarrhea.
3. Decreased tissue turgor.
4. Dry mucous membranes.
5. Lethargy.
6. Difficulty in voiding; changes in urine flow; decreased urine output.
7. Steady rise in serum creatinine.
8. Fever.
9. Edema—periorbital, pitting lower leg edema, ascites.
10. Changes in mental status or mood.
11. Headaches and blurry vision due to hypertension.
12. Seizures.

Diagnostic Evaluation

1. Serum creatinine level—the most reliable measure of the GFR, found to be rising.
2. Radionuclide studies—evaluate GFR and renal blood flow and distribution.
3. Urinalysis—reveals proteinuria, hematuria, casts.
4. Ultrasonography—determines anatomic abnormalities.

Management

1. 75% of children with acute renal failure attain complete recovery.
2. Treatment is directed toward the underlying cause.
3. Correction of any reversible cause of acute renal failure (i.e., surgical relief of obstruction).
4. Correction and control of fluid and electrolyte imbalances.
5. Restoration and maintenance of stable vital signs.
6. Maintenance of nutrition with low sodium, low potassium, and low phosphate.
7. Initiation of dialysis (hemodialysis, peritoneal dialysis, or continuous venovenous hemofiltration) for patients with life-threatening complications.

Complications

1. Fluid and electrolyte imbalance, especially hyperkalemia—when GFR is reduced, the patient cannot excrete potassium.
2. Metabolic acidosis, caused by decreased acid excretion and reduced bicarbonate reabsorption (see Box 45-1).
3. Insufficient nutritional intake because of metabolic abnormalities and symptoms, such as nausea and vomiting.

BOX 45-1 Clinical Manifestations of Metabolic Acidosis

GASTROINTESTINAL
- Anorexia.
- Nausea and vomiting.
- Abdominal pain.

NEUROLOGIC
- Lethargy.
- Stupor.
- Coma.

CARDIOVASCULAR
- Decreased heart rate.
- Cardiac dysrhythmias.
- Peripheral vasodilation.

OTHER MANIFESTATIONS
- Warm and flushed skin.
- Weakness and malaise.
- Bone resorption (with chronic acidosis).
- Increased rate and depth of respirations (Kussmaul breathing due to compensation).

LABORATORY FINDINGS
- Decreased pH.
- Decreased HCO_3^- (initially).
- Decreased PCO_2 (compensatory).
- Hyperkalemia.
- Acidic urine (compensatory).

Nursing Assessment

1. Obtain a history of all medications, recent and past illnesses or injuries, allergies, and potential exposure to toxic substances.
2. Measure intake and output. Insert indwelling urinary catheter, as indicated.
3. Monitor vital signs, especially blood pressure (BP). Institute cardiac monitoring, as indicated.
4. Assess for edema and fluid overload (cardiac and respiratory assessment).
5. Monitor urine specific gravity, as directed. Fixed specific gravity of 1.010 indicates the kidneys' inability to concentrate or dilute urine.

Nursing Interventions

Maintaining Fluid Volume

1. Administer intravenous (IV) fluids slowly to prevent heart failure.
2. Maintain fluid restriction, as ordered.
3. Keep strict intake and output records.
4. Weigh child daily.
5. Promptly report signs of heart failure—edema, bounding pulse, third heart sound, shortness of breath, and adventitious breath sounds.

Preventing Severe Electrolyte Disturbance

1. Monitor blood test results (creatinine, blood urea nitrogen [BUN], electrolytes, calcium) and notify health care provider promptly of abnormal levels.
2. Watch for signs of hyperkalemia—weak, irregular pulse, abdominal cramps, and muscle weakness.
3. Do not administer IV fluids with potassium while renal function is impaired.
4. Maintain low-potassium, low-sodium, and high-carbohydrate diet.
5. Administer treatments for hyperkalemia, as ordered, such as IV sodium bicarbonate and IV glucose and insulin (requires careful glucose monitoring), both of which drive potassium into cells and temporarily out of the bloodstream.
6. Administer cation exchange medications to reduce potassium, as ordered.
7. Watch for signs of hypocalcemia—muscle twitching and tetany.

Family Education and Health Maintenance

1. Explain all steps of the diagnostic and treatment process to the family.
2. Teach about dialysis if this becomes necessary.
3. Explain that as kidney function resumes, diuresis may occur to eliminate excess fluid the body was storing.
4. Educate about prompt medical attention for illnesses that may cause dehydration to prevent renal injury in the future.
5. Avoid nephrotoxins, including NSAIDs during recovery period.
6. Set family expectations for long-term follow-up after acute kidney injury.

Evaluation: Expected Outcomes

- No signs of heart failure.
- Potassium remains within normal range; kidney function returns to baseline.

Chronic Renal Failure

Chronic renal failure (CRF) is irreversible destruction of nephrons so that they are no longer capable of maintaining normal fluid and electrolyte balance. *Chronic kidney disease* (CKD) refers to kidney damage with a decreased GFR of less than 60 mL/min/1.73 m^2 for 3 months or greater. Nursing care of children with CRF is similar to that of adults (see pages 587–589). The following considerations are important for pediatric patients.

Pathophysiology and Etiology

1. Congenital renal and urinary tract abnormalities are the most common causes in children younger than age 5 (e.g., polycystic kidney disease, congenital nephrotic syndrome, renal dysplasia).
2. Most common causes in ages 5 to 15 years:
   a. Glomerular disease (e.g., glomerulonephritis).
   b. Urologic abnormalities.
   c. Cystic kidney disease.
3. Similar progression regardless of cause.
   a. Nephron damage that results in hypertrophy and hyperplasia of remaining nephrons.
   b. Overload results in decreased ability for nephrons to excrete effectively.
   c. Results in azotemia and clinical uremia.
   d. Inability of kidney to excrete phosphate causes hypocalcemia, which results in osteodystrophy.
   e. Kidneys cannot synthesize vitamin D, thus impairing calcium absorption. Bones may become so calcium depleted that growth halts and bones become brittle (renal rickets).
   f. Kidneys cannot synthesize erythropoietin, thus resulting in anemia.
   g. Excretion of nitrogenous waste through sweat causes pruritus.
   h. Overload of fluid results in edema and hypertension.
4. Severity of CRF is indicated by GFR. The lower the GFR, the greater the loss of renal function.

Clinical Manifestations

Variable and not chronological.

1. Nausea and vomiting, decreased appetite, and energy level.
2. Initial polyuria caused by kidneys' inability to concentrate urine; later oliguria and anuria.
3. Bone or joint pain.
4. Dryness and itching of skin.
5. Poor growth.
6. Fatigue, lethargy due to anemia.

Diagnostic Evaluation

1. Serum studies:
   a. Anemia and iron studies: decreased hemoglobin, hematocrit, iron levels.
   b. Decreased Na^+, Ca^{++}, and CO_2 (metabolic acidosis); increased K^+ and phosphorus.
   c. As renal function declines, BUN, uric acid, and creatinine values continue to climb.
   d. Elevated parathyroid hormone (PTH).
2. Urine studies:
   a. Specific gravity—increased or decreased.
   b. A 24-hour urine for creatinine clearance is decreased (increased creatinine in urine), thus reflecting decreased GFR.
   c. Changes in total output (may initially be polyuric because of difficulty concentrating urine, then oliguric).
   d. Proteinuria.
3. Many other tests may be ordered to evaluate other systems and extent of disease (e.g., chest x-ray, echocardiogram, bone age).

Management

1. Correction of calcium–phosphorus imbalance. Initiate low-phosphorus diet. Administer activated vitamin D to increase calcium absorption and phosphate binders with meals to bind phosphate in the gastrointestinal (GI) tract.
2. Correction of acidosis with buffers, such as sodium bicarbonate tablets.
3. Correction of hyperkalemia through low-potassium diet or administration of potassium-lowering agents, such as sodium polystyrene.
4. Diets should meet caloric needs of the child and contain adequate protein for development (0.9 to 1.5 g/kg/day).
5. Correction of anemia through the use of oral iron and erythropoietin administered subcutaneously at home.
6. BP should be managed with appropriate antihypertensive medications (angiotensin-converting enzyme inhibitors, angiotensin receptor blockers, calcium channel blockers, or diuretics).
7. Growth retardation should be evaluated for possible use of growth hormone. Consult dietitian to ensure optimal nutrition for use of growth hormone.
8. Renal replacement options for end-stage renal disease include hemodialysis, peritoneal dialysis, transplantation, or no treatment, typically initiated when GFR <15 mL/min/1.73 m^2.
9. Dialysis, while renal transplant workup is in progress.

Complications

1. Growth retardation.
2. Delayed or absent sexual maturation.
3. Severe anemia—kidneys cannot stimulate erythropoietin; uremic toxins deplete erythrocytes; nutritional deficiencies.
4. Hypertension—renal ischemia stimulates renin–angiotensin system.
5. Cardiovascular disease (left ventricular hypertrophy, heart failure, vascular calcification due to hyperphosphatemia).
6. Renal osteodystrophy due to vitamin D deficiency and secondary hyperparathyroidism.
7. Azotemia/uremia—nitrogen waste products accumulate in blood. Toxic levels manifest themselves in many ways, such as headache, GI disturbances, neuromuscular disturbances, and coma.
8. Neurodevelopmental delay due to uremic effects.
9. Metabolic acidosis, which may cause poor growth, confusion, dull headache, and lethargy.
10. Electrolyte imbalance—hypocalcemia, hyperkalemia.

Nursing Assessment

1. Perform a comprehensive, multisystem assessment to help in planning care.
2. Assess nutrition, growth, and developmental status.
3. Assess coping, support systems, and other resources.

Nursing Interventions

Ensuring Safety

1. Protect the child from the effects of decreased level of consciousness and involuntary movements by maintaining crib or bedside rails up and padded, as necessary.
2. Monitor for seizure activity and have airway or tongue blade and suction equipment on hand.
3. Monitor BUN, creatinine, electrolyte, and calcium levels and report abnormalities promptly.

Promoting Fluid Balance

See "Acute Renal Failure" section, pages 1320 and 1321.

Ensuring Adequate Nutrition

1. Ensure adequate protein in diet. Obtain consultation from a registered dietitian.
2. Encourage appropriate fluid intake between meals.
3. Consult with dietitian regarding appropriate milk intake and alternatives because of high phosphate, sodium, and potassium content. Instead, administer feedings high in calories and low in wastes, as directed.

Increasing Activity Tolerance

1. Plan activities when the child is rested.
2. Encourage activity as tolerated.
3. Administer blood transfusions or IV iron therapy, as ordered (if the patient is resistant to erythropoietin therapy and unable to tolerate oral iron supplementation).

Enhancing Coping

Because numerous issues may interfere with the child's psychological and social development and education, help the child and family to cope with:

1. Uncertainty regarding the course of the disease and ultimate prognosis.
2. Abnormal lifestyle necessitated by dialysis (including interference with school).
3. Burden of dialysis and continuous administration of medications.
4. Problems of adjustment related to growth failure.
5. Fear of death, present in most children, adolescents, and family members.

6. Possible kidney transplantation, involving major surgery and prolonged hospitalization, followed by altered body image that is caused by high-dose steroids and potential for rejection, which may threaten survival.

Family Education and Health Maintenance

1. Teach the child to avoid high-sodium foods, such as chips, pretzels, and popcorn; luncheon meats; canned foods; and fast foods, if sodium is restricted.
2. Encourage follow-up as advised by kidney specialist and primary health care provider.
3. Encourage family to keep up with regular dental care, immunizations, and health assessments to help prevent infections, problems with growth, and more severe childhood diseases.
4. Teach about medications and support the child who may be taking multiple medications—calcium, phosphate binder, acid neutralizer, recombinant erythropoietin, antihypertensives, and others.
5. Teach about maintaining good hygiene and peritoneal dialysis catheter care.
6. Advise the family about support services and media resources available—for example, *Children & Teens with Kidney Disease,* by the National Kidney Foundation (www.kidney.org).

Evaluation: Expected Outcomes

- Side rails up with airway and suction at bedside.
- Fluid restriction maintained, weight stable, no signs of heart failure.
- Taking 100% of renal diet.
- Engaging in play without shortness of breath.
- Parental caregivers asking questions and discussing treatment with the child.
- In later school-aged children and adolescents, the child initiates questions regarding diagnosis and care.

The Child Who Undergoes Dialysis

Dialysis is the passage of a solute through a semipermeable membrane. The purpose of dialysis is to preserve life by replacing some of the normal kidney functions. See pages 575 to 577 for a complete description of different types of dialysis.

General Considerations

The following principles should be considered by the nurse who works with pediatric patients:

1. Peritoneal dialysis:
   a. This mode of dialysis continues to be the favored mode in young children.
   b. Because of the child's small size, the volume of dialysate is 1,100 to 1,400 mL/m^2.
   c. The child can be expected to participate at a developmentally appropriate level with their own care.
   d. Peritoneal dialysis is a therapy that continuously removes metabolic wastes and fluid through a catheter placed in the peritoneum and runs over a 7- to 10-hour period, usually overnight.
2. Hemodialysis:
   a. In hemodialysis, metabolic wastes and fluid are removed through an arteriovenous fistula or a centrally placed catheter in an artery in the upper chest. This therapy is performed for 4 hours for three to four treatments a week.

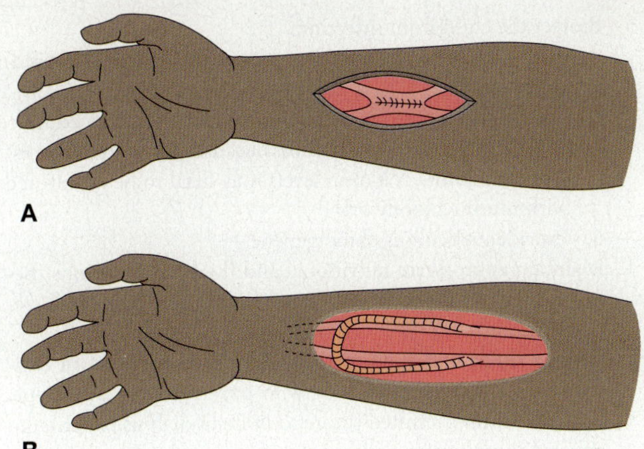

Figure 45-3. (A) An internal arteriovenous fistula. **(B)** An internal arteriovenous graft. (Reprinted with permission from Silbert-Flagg, J. [2023]. *Maternal and child health nursing: Care of the childbearing and childrearing family* [9th ed., Fig. 46-5]. Wolters Kluwer.)

   b. When possible, subcutaneous or intramuscular (IM) injections are avoided because the child is anticoagulated with heparin.
   c. BP cuff and tourniquets should not be applied to a limb with a fistula, and peripheral IVs should not be placed in a limb with a graft or fistula.
3. Specific care for the child during dialysis is generally provided by specially trained personnel in a dialysis unit. However, the following considerations should be noted:
   d. Choice for vascular access depends on patient size and availability of peripheral blood vessels of suitable size (see Figure 45-3). A central venous catheter may also be used.
   b. Extracorporeal blood volume (blood outside the body at any given time) should be as small as possible. It should not exceed 8% to 10% of the child's total blood volume.
   c. Efficiency or adequacy of the dialyzer, relative to the child's weight, should be noted and blood pump speed adjusted accordingly.
   d. External catheter should be secured to make sure catheter is not traumatized.

Nursing Care of the Child Who Undergoes Dialysis

1. Prepare the child for the procedure. Dialysis is threatening to most children and may evoke fears of pain, mutilation, immobilization, helplessness, and dependency. Many children have fears of losing all of their blood during hemodialysis. A child who is well prepared will be less frightened and better able to cooperate during the procedure.
   a. Explain the procedure in terms that the child can understand.
   b. Allow the child to handle equipment similar to that which will be used during dialysis.
   c. Encourage the child to express fears so that misinterpretations can be corrected.
   d. Provide simple pictures and diagrams, if appropriate.
   e. Allow the child to talk with peers who have undergone dialysis.
2. Explain the procedure to family members and answer questions so that they will be in the best position to support the child.

3. Protect the child from infection.
   a. Keep the dressings and area around the catheter (if used) clean and dry.
   b. Use aseptic technique throughout the dialysis procedure.
   c. Provide supplemental vitamins because dialysis removes essential vitamins. Vitamin levels may need to be monitored with routine bloodwork.
   d. Provide meticulous daily hygiene.
4. Maintain appropriate nutritional and fluid modifications. Because anorexia is commonly seen in CRF, provide small frequent meals.
5. Restrict fluids and sodium to prevent fluid overload in children who are hypertensive or who have minimal urine output. Potassium is limited (more so in hemodialysis patients) to prevent complications related to hyperkalemia. The child may see dietary restrictions as a punishment and must be helped to realize the purpose of restrictions.
6. Do not restrict protein, which is vital to allow for normal growth and development.
7. Maintain careful records of intake and output, vital signs, BP, and daily weight. These provide valuable information about the effectiveness of the therapy.
8. Support the child during the dialysis procedure.
   a. Provide symptomatic relief of nausea, vomiting, malaise, muscle cramping, or headache. Notify the health care provider if these symptoms are severe.
   b. Involve the child in diversional activities, such as play therapy, crafts, television, and books.
   c. Encourage the family to bring in articles that will make the child's room appear more homelike (e.g., pictures, posters).
   d. Encourage the child to be as independent as possible in daily care.
9. Help the child to keep up with schoolwork by initiating a referral to a tutor and providing study times.

Community and Home Care Considerations

1. Be aware that although life is preserved, it is by no means normal during the time on dialysis or between dialysis treatments. These measures may increase the child's feeling of self-esteem and diminish regression and social isolation. By serving as role models, health professionals may encourage parental caregivers to recognize and foster the normal, healthy aspects of the child's daily life.
2. Offer appropriate support to the family.
   a. Provide opportunity for family members to discuss their feelings, fears, and frustrations and to ask questions.
   b. Allow family members to become involved in the child's care.
   c. Provide for continuity of personnel.
   d. Initiate appropriate referrals and provide resources. These may include referrals to a social worker, psychiatrist, dietitian, community health agency, or other families who are coping with dialysis.
3. Be aware that families usually need extensive support from many health professionals to cope with the physical, psychological, financial, and logistical aspects of renal failure and dialysis. Attention must be focused on siblings and parental caregivers because sibling relationships are usually strained and difficult.
4. Teach the child and family about all of the important aspects of renal failure and dialysis, including the following:
   a. Protection from infection.
   b. Dietary restrictions and recommendations; ways of incorporating the special diet into the family meal plan.
   c. Dialysis schedule.
   d. Medications.
   e. Emergency procedures.
   f. Reintegration into the community and school.
5. Empower the family to care for the child at home. Learning about the child's care also helps restore some sense of control in a frightening situation.

Renal Transplantation

Renal (kidney) transplantation is the optimal therapeutic modality for end-stage renal disease in the pediatric age group. With successful transplantation, there is a greater likelihood of optimum rehabilitation than with any other form of dialytic therapy. The potential for normal growth and pubertal development is significantly increased after transplantation. However, it should be noted that posttransplant growth is affected by many variables: age of onset of chronic renal disease, caloric intake, corticosteroid dosage, bone age at transplantation, transplant function, and rejection episodes. Requirements of preoperative management and nursing care of children or teens for renal transplantation are similar to that of adults (see pages 577–579). However, they are also more exhaustive because the recipient as well as the parental caregivers must be included. The emotional, psychological, and financial needs of the recipient and the family must be evaluated. An appropriate care plan must then be designed to address identified needs; this care plan must be appropriate for the developmental age of the recipient.

Evaluation of Recipient

The major issues that must be evaluated when considering renal transplantation in children are as follows:

1. Patient age and size.
2. Primary renal disease.
3. Psychological status.
4. Live versus deceased donor allograft.
5. Optimal immunosuppressive regimen.
6. Maximization of growth and pubertal development.

Donor Selection (by Priority)

A tissue-compatible transplantation from a relative is 90% successful.

1. Identical twin sibling.
2. Siblings cannot be used as donors until they are of legal age to give consent for removal of a kidney.
3. Parental caregiver.
4. Other relative.
5. Unrelated live donor, such as a family friend.
6. Deceased donor.

Operative Procedure

A child who weighs more than 22 pounds (10 kg) usually receives the kidney of an adult. In a very small child, the kidney transplant is placed within the abdomen, with vessel anastomosis to the aorta and superior vena cava.

Potential Emotional Concerns of Children With Transplants

1. The concept of a foreign body, especially a cadaver kidney, inside one's own body may be disturbing.

2. Fear that the kidney may wear out sooner if it is from an older person.
3. Altered body image because of growth failure and the effects of steroid therapy.
4. Guilt feelings if a live donor transplant fails, especially that of a family donor.

Nursing Interventions

Also see "After kidney transplantation," pages 578 and 579.

1. Support the child and family through the preoperative phase, including diagnostic testing and blood transfusions.
2. After surgery, maintain strict infection precautions.
3. Administer immunosuppressants and other medications, as directed.
4. Continue support through dialysis, if necessary.
5. Monitor urine output, bloodwork results, and urine specific gravity.
6. Watch for signs of rejection—fever, oliguria, proteinuria, weight gain, hypertension, and tenderness over transplanted kidney. Acute rejection usually occurs in the first 3 months after transplant. Chronic rejection may develop at any time. It occurs slowly over months to years and leads to progressive loss of renal function.
7. Watch for signs of infection: fever, leukopenia, neutropenia.
8. Infection can be bacterial (most common are pneumonia and UTIs) or viral (cytomegalovirus and Epstein–Barr virus are the most common infections).

Community and Home Care Considerations

The practice of discharging patients from an in-hospital setting as quickly as possible is also true for the pediatric transplant recipient. Community and home care nurses must have:

1. The knowledge to care for a child who receives IV and immunosuppressive medications.
2. The ability to access and heparinize central venous lines and peripheral IV catheters.
3. The ability to aid in reinforcing discharge teaching, aid in BP monitoring, and assess medication adherence.

Family Education and Health Maintenance

1. Teach families about the signs of rejection and infection.
2. Encourage close follow-up for proper dosing of immunosuppressants.
3. Education, communication, and employ strategies to promote medication adherence.
4. Advise family that close medical surveillance will always be necessary because the incidence of malignant disease is six times more likely in transplant recipients than in the general population.
5. Teach parental caregivers not to overprotect the child. When the child has healed from surgery, regular activity can be resumed. This includes returning to school; however, the school needs to be aware of the patient's immunosuppressive status.
6. Teach families and patients the importance of good handwashing.
7. Encourage patient to wear a medical alert device or necklace, and inform the community emergency services of transplant status.
8. Advise parental caregivers that no live vaccine should be given to the child who is immunosuppressed.
9. Advise the family about resources available.

SELECTED READINGS

Angeletti, A., Lugani, F., La Porta, E., Verrina, E., Caridi, G., & Ghiggeri, G. M. (2022). Vaccines and nephrotic syndrome: efficacy and safety. *Pediatric Nephrology, 38*, 2915–2928. https://doi.org/10.1007/s00467-022-05835-4

Bévier, A., Novel-Catin, E., Blond, E., Pelletier, S., Parant, F., Koppe, L., & Fouque, D. (2022). Water-soluble vitamins and trace elements losses during on-line hemodiafiltration. *Nutrients, 14*(17), 3454. https://doi.org/10.3390/nu14173454

Jönsson, A., Hellmark, T., & Forsberg, A. (2020). Persons' experiences of suffering from nephrotic syndrome. *Journal of Renal Care, 46*(1), 45–51. https://doi.org/10.1111/jorc.12307

Kallash, M., & Mahan, J. D. (2021). Mechanisms and management of edema in pediatric nephrotic syndrome. *Pediatric Nephrology (Berlin, Germany), 36*(7), 1719–1730. https://doi.org/10.1007/s00467-020-04779-x

Kazi, A. M., & Hashmi, M. F. (2022). Glomerulonephritis. In *StatPearls*. StatPearls Publishing. PMID: 32809479.

Khalighi, M. A., & Chang, A. (2021). Infection-related glomerulonephritis. *Glomerular Disease, 1*(2), 82–91. https://doi.org/10.1159/000515461

Lemoine, C. P., Pozo, M. E., & Superina, R. A. (2022). Overview of pediatric kidney transplantation. *Seminars in Pediatric Surgery, 31*(3), 151194. https://doi.org/10.1016/j.sempedsurg.2022.151194

McAlister, L., Pugh, P., Greenbaum, L., Haffner, D., Rees, L., Anderson, C., Desloovere, A., Nelms, C., Oosterveld, M., Paglialonga, F., Polderman, N., Qizalbash, L., Renken-Terhaerdt, J., Tuokkola, J., Warady, B., Walle, J. V., Shaw, V., & Shroff, R. (2020). The dietary management of calcium and phosphate in children with CKD stages 2–5 and on dialysis-clinical practice recommendation from the pediatric renal nutrition taskforce. *Pediatric Nephrology (Berlin, Germany), 35*(3), 501–518. https://doi.org/10.1007/s00467-019-04370-z

Patino, E., & Akchurin, O. (2022). Erythropoiesis-independent effects of iron in chronic kidney disease. *Pediatric Nephroogy, 37*(4), 777–788. https://doi.org/10.1007/s00467-021-05191-9

Santos, J. D., Rickard, M., & Lorenzo, A. (2021). Office pediatric urology. In P. Godbole, D. T. Wilcox, & M. Koyle (Eds.), *Practical pediatric urology: An evidence based approach* (1st ed., pp. 55–82). Springer International Publishing.

Scialla, J. J., Kendrick, J., Uribarri, J., Kovesdy, C. P., Gutiérrez, O. M., Jimenez, E. Y., & Kramer, H. J. (2021). State-of-the-art management of hyperphosphatemia in patients with CKD: An NKF-KDOQI controversies perspective. *American Journal of Kidney Diseases, 77*(1), 132–141. https://doi.org/10.1053/j.ajkd.2020.05.025

Sethi, S., De Vriese, A. S., & Fervenza, F. C. (2022). Acute glomerulonephritis. *The Lancet (British Edition), 399*(10335), 1646–1663. https://doi.org/10.1016/S0140-6736(22)00461-5

Sohail, M. A., Vachharajani, T. J., & Anvari, E. (2021). Central venous catheters for hemodialysis-the myth and the evidence. *Kidney International Reports, 6*(12), 2958–2968. https://doi.org/10.1016/j.ekir.2021.09.009

Teitelbaum, I. (2021). Peritoneal dialysis. *The New England Journal of Medicine, 385*(19), 1786–1795. https://doi.org/10.1056/NEJMra2100152

Trautmann, A., Boyer, O., Hodson, E., Bagga, A., Gipson, D. S., Samuel, S., Wetzels, J., Alhasan, K., Banerjee, S., Bhimma, R., Bonilla-Felix, M., Cano, F., Christian, M., Hahn, D., Kang, H. G., Nakanishi, K., Safouh, H., Trachtman, H., Xu, H., Cook, W., … International Pediatric Nephrology Association. (2023). IPNA clinical practice recommendations for the diagnosis and management of children with steroid-sensitive nephrotic syndrome. *Pediatric Nephrology, 38*(3), 877–919. https://doi.org/10.1007/s00467-022-05739-3

Warady, B. A., Alexander, S. R., & Schaefer, F. (2021). *Pediatric dialysis*. Springer International Publishing.

46 Pediatric Metabolic and Endocrine Disorders*

OVERVIEW AND ASSESSMENT

Common Nursing Assessment for Growth and Development

Endocrine dysfunction in children frequently leads to altered growth and development. Accurate nursing assessment can help detect variations in growth and developmental patterns, identify factors such as diet and medications that may have an impact on growth and development, and obtain information about adherence to medication regimen and understanding of treatment.

Evaluation of Growth Patterns

1. Perform frequent and accurate measurements of height and weight.
2. Accurately plot measurements on appropriate growth curve for absolute chronologic age.
3. Assess growth pattern for any deviation from the child's percentile or from the parallel of the growth curve for age (includes both an upward and a downward deviation).
4. Calculate growth velocity—take the difference of current height from previous height and divide by the time period. Growth rate for a prepubertal child should be 2 to 3 in (5 to 7 cm) on an annual basis.
5. Report any child whose pattern deviates from the expected pattern for age to health care provider.

General Health History

1. Dietary history—what is the child's meal frequency, volume, and food preferences? Be vigilant while obtaining the history of a child when anorexia may be possible—growth velocity will usually be low, in addition to poor weight gain.
2. History of major illnesses or surgeries that have altered the child's growth and development.
3. Family history—is there a family history of growth or developmental issues? Is there a family history of delayed puberty? Are family members unusually short or tall in stature, or is there obvious dysmorphology?
4. Clothing—outgrowing clothing and shoes?
5. Social history relative to friendships.
6. Academic and school performance—recent changes?
7. Activity—activities the child participates in? Intensity and type of exercise?

Medication History and Adherence

1. Is the child on any steroid medications (such as prednisone) that would suppress growth? Inquire about over-the-counter medications or herbal supplementation.
2. When pubertal signs are present on physical examination, does the child have access to any gonadal steroids, such as birth control pills, or anabolic steroids?
3. Do the child and family understand treatment medication indication and usage instructions?
4. Are the child and family able to take medications as prescribed? Do they know the dose, frequency, and route? Is medication stored properly?
5. If the child is taking oral medication, is it being taken with food, if indicated? If pills are being chewed, are teeth being brushed soon after, which could be rinsing out the medications?
6. If injectable, are injection sites being rotated appropriately? Review technique.

Physical Examination Relative to Development

1. Dental development—eruption of teeth and presence of permanent teeth (see page 1098).
2. Pubertal development—Tanner staging of pubic hair and gonadal development (see Table 46-1).
3. Presence of genetic dysmorphology—such as short-limbed dwarfism and various atypical stigmata.

*Please note that the term "male" in this chapter refers to a person assigned male at birth, and the term "female" in this chapter refers to a person assigned female at birth.

Table 46-1 Tanner Staging of Puberty

MALE[a] GENITAL DEVELOPMENT	FEMALE[a] BREAST DEVELOPMENT	MALE AND FEMALE[a]: PUBIC HAIR
Stage I		
Preadolescent. Testes, scrotum, and penis are of about the same size and proportion as in early childhood. 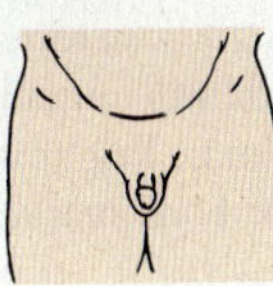	Preadolescent. Elevation of papilla only. 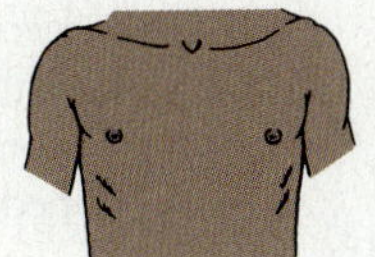 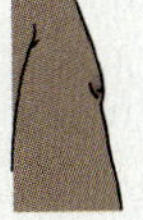	Preadolescent. The vellus over the pubis is not further developed than that over the abdominal wall (i.e., no pubic hair). 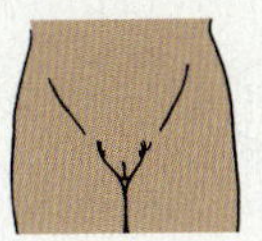 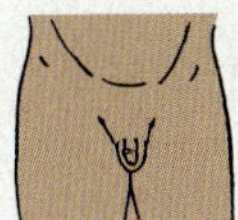
Stage II		
Enlargement of scrotum and testes. Skin of scrotum reddens and changes in texture. Little or no enlargement of penis at this time. 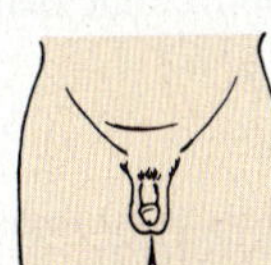	Breast bud stage. Elevation of breast and papilla as small mound. Enlargement of areola diameter. 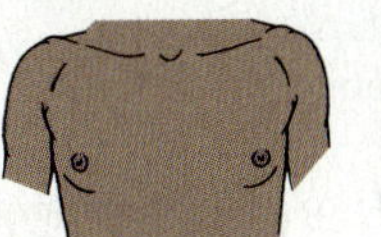 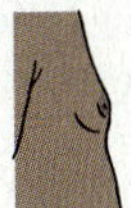	Sparse growth of long, slightly pigmented downy hair. Straight or slightly curled at base of penis or along labia. 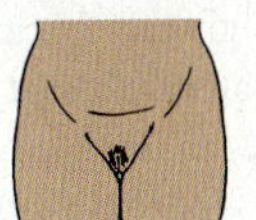 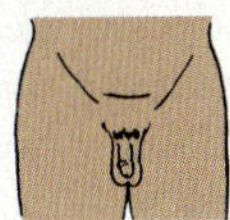
Stage III		
Enlargement of penis that occurs at first mainly in length. Further growth of testes and scrotum. 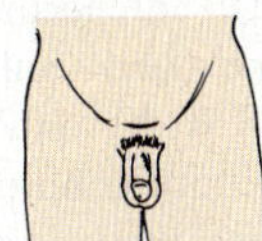	Further enlargement and elevation of breast and areola with no separation of their contours. 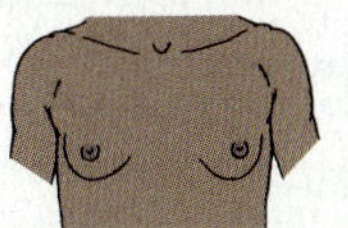 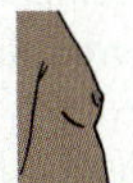	Considerably darker, coarser, and more curled. The hair spreads sparsely over the symphysis pubis. 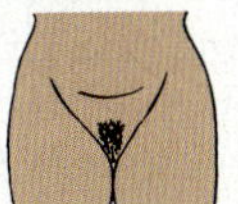 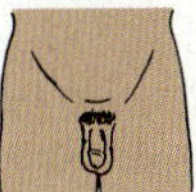
Stage IV		
Increased size of penis with growth in breadth and development of glans. Testes and scrotum larger; scrotal skin darkened. 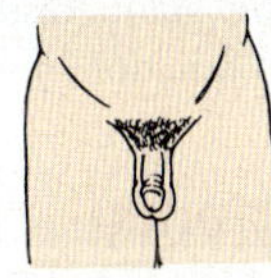	Projection of areola and papilla to form a secondary mound above level of the breast. 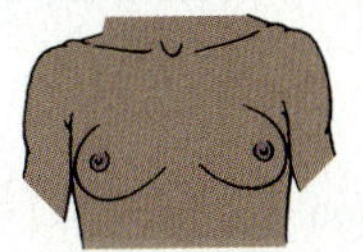 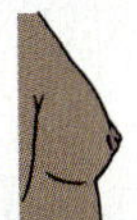	Hair now adult in type, but area covered is still considerably smaller than in adult. No spread to medial surface of thighs. 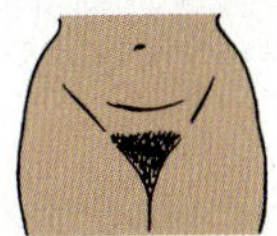 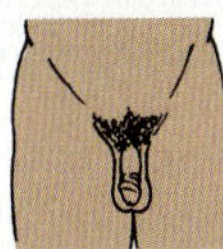
Stage V		
Genitalia adult in size and shape. 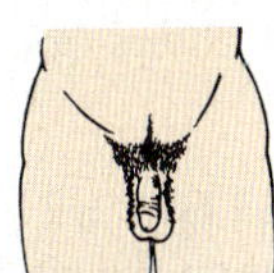	Mature stage: projection of papilla only, due to recession of the areola to the general contour of the breast. 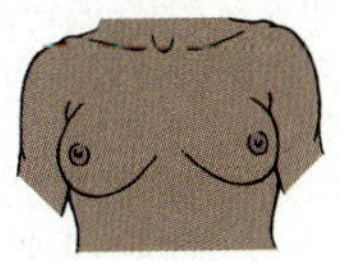 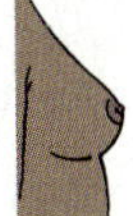	Adult in quantity and type; distribution of the horizontal pattern. Spread to medial surface of thighs or above base of the inverse triangle occurs late (stage VI). 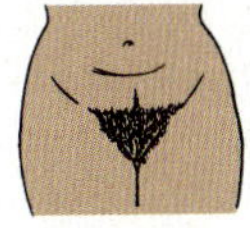 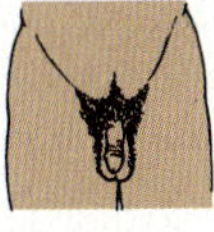

[a]*Note that the term "male" in this table refers to people assigned male at birth and that the term "female" in this chapter refers to people assigned female at birth.*
Adapted from Tanner, J. M. (1975). Growth and endocrinology of the adolescent. In L. Gardner (Ed.), Endocrine and genetic diseases of childhood and adolescence (2nd ed.). W.B. Saunders.

Causes of Disorders of Growth and Stature

It is important to realize that growth and stature problems are caused by a wide variety of factors. Thorough history, physical examination, and diagnostic testing can help reveal the underlying cause. Many of the disorders are associated with other anomalies, such as intellectual disability, cardiac problems, metabolic issues, and secondary sex characteristic abnormalities. The cause may be treatable to resolve the growth problem, may be amenable to growth hormone (GH) supplementation, or may be untreatable because of genetic cause.

Short Stature and Growth Failure

Genetic Causes

1. Familial short stature—short target height relative to U.S. standards; however, growth rate is normal.
2. Constitutional delay—short stature with retarded linear growth beginning in the first 3 years of life followed by short stature relative to peers; however, final height normal upon completion of pubertal development. Puberty is usually delayed.
3. Genetic disorders:
   a. Dwarfism—multiple types and causes relative to chondrodysplasias.
   b. Turner syndrome—occurs in about 1 in 2,500 female births worldwide. Characterized by short stature, ovarian dysgenesis (underdeveloped, degenerate ovaries), and, in some cases, unusual physical appearance (see pages 1454–1456).
   c. Russell–Silver syndrome—occurs in 1 in 15,000 to 100,000 births. Characterized by unilateral poor growth, short stature, characteristic facies, and mental delays. Whenever unilateral change in growth is present, abdominal tumor needs to be ruled out.
   d. Prader–Willi syndrome—occurs in 1 in 10,000 to 30,000 live births and is a rare syndrome characterized by below-normal intelligence, small stature, hypogonadism (see page 558), failure to thrive in infancy followed by obesity and insatiable appetite, binge-type eating behaviors.
   e. Down syndrome—occurs in 1 in 500 live births; characterized by growth retardation and developmental delays (see page 1452).
   f. Cystic fibrosis—occurs in 1 in 2,500 live births. In addition to respiratory and gastrointestinal (GI) symptoms, growth retardation occurs (see page 1187).

Endocrine Disorders

1. Hypothyroidism.
2. GH deficiency.
3. Glucocorticoid excess—Cushing syndrome.

Nonendocrine Disorders

1. Glucocorticoid (prednisone) therapy for asthma, prevention of transplant rejection, adjunct medication in cancer chemotherapy, and severe dermatologic disorders.
2. Nutritional deficiency.
3. Psychosocial issues.
4. Chronic diseases—cardiovascular, renal, hematologic, pulmonary, malabsorptive disorders, and inborn errors of metabolism.
5. Medical interventions—surgical tumor resection and radiation for brain tumors.

Tall Stature and Excessive Growth

Genetic Causes

1. Familial tall stature—tall stature relative to U.S. standards; however, normal for family. Growth rate is usually normal.
2. Genetic disorders:
   a. Marfan syndrome—occurs in 1 in 3,000 to 5,000 births. Characterized by increased height, long extremities, long fingers and toes; cardiac and other anomalies.
   b. Klinefelter syndrome—occurs in 1 in 1 to 2.5 per 1,000 males. Characterized by increased height, slim build, underweight, gynecomastia, small, firm testicles, infertile.

Endocrine Disorders

1. Congenital adrenal hyperplasia.
2. Precocious puberty (see page 1338).
3. Hyperthyroidism (see page 1333).
4. Acromegaly—overproduction of GH usually related to pituitary tumors; very rare in children.

Nonendocrine Disorders

1. Exogenous use of androgens (i.e., testosterone injections):
   a. Although stature and growth will initially be above the normal expected for age, ultimate height will be decreased because of undue advance of bone maturation at growth plate.
   b. The child will ultimately end up shorter than genetically determined.
2. Sotos syndrome (cerebral gigantism)—usually large at birth with rapid growth in the first year of life, intellectual impairment. Hypothesized to be a hypothalamic defect; normal endocrine function.

DISORDERS OF THE ANTERIOR PITUITARY

The anterior pituitary is under the control of the hypothalamus and secretes six specific hormones: growth hormone (GH), thyroid-stimulating hormone (TSH), adrenocorticotropic hormone (ACTH), luteinizing hormone (LH), follicle-stimulating hormone (FSH), and prolactin. GH is the only hormone that does not have a target gland to induce further hormonal secretion. Hypopituitarism is a deficiency of one, some, or all of the hormones secreted by the pituitary gland. With the exception of GH, decreased secretion results in hypofunction of the consequential target gland.

TSH deficiency, ACTH deficiency, and LH/FSH deficiency are discussed under disorders of the thyroid gland, disorders of the adrenal glands, and disorders of gonadal function, respectively.

Growth Hormone Deficiency

EVIDENCE BASE Hage, C., Gan, H.-W., Ibba, A., Patti, G., Dattani, M., Loche, S., Maghnie, M., & Salvatori, R. (2021). Advances in differential diagnosis and management of growth hormone deficiency in children. *Nature Reviews Endocrinology, 17*(10), 608–624. https://doi.org/10.1038/s41574-021-00539-5

Insufficient secretion of GH is caused by a lack of pituitary production or hypothalamic stimulation on the pituitary. Incidence is approximately 1 in 3,800 for classic GH insufficiency and is unknown for varying degrees of insufficiency.

Pathophysiology and Etiology

1. The lack of GH impairs the body's ability to perform the following functions:
   a. Protein metabolism—growth through increased protein synthesis; nitrogen, phosphorus, and potassium storage.
   b. Fat metabolism—increases lipolysis and oxidation of fat.
   c. Carbohydrate metabolism—decreases conversion of glucose to fat in adipose tissue.

2. Organic etiology:
   a. Intracranial cyst.
   b. Central nervous system (CNS) tumor (hypothalamic–pituitary structural lesions).
   c. CNS irradiation.
   d. Exogenous (head trauma from various causes such as birth injury, infection, pituitary infarction, or aneurysm).
   e. Histiocytosis X.
   f. Septo-optic dysplasia (abnormal forebrain development).
3. Idiopathic causes:
   a. Isolated GH deficiency; aplasia.
   b. Traumatic birth or breech delivery.
   c. Genetic (GH gene deletion).
   d. Nutritional deprivation; psychosocial issues.
4. Genetic cause—Turner syndrome:
   a. The pituitary and hypothalamus are not abnormal in Turner syndrome, and GH secretion measurement is usually normal; however, GH is bioinactive because of binding problems.
   b. Hypothyroidism is common with Turner syndrome and Down syndrome.
   c. Growth rate usually declines within the first year of life.
   d. Treatment with GH is a commonly accepted therapy to restore growth.

Clinical Manifestations

1. Hypoglycemia, prolonged jaundice, microphallus (small penis); usually in the neonate.
2. Growth velocity is usually less than the fifth percentile for chronologic age.
3. Delayed skeletal maturation—bone age at least 1 year delayed from chronologic age.
4. "Chubby" when the weight age (50% for weight) exceeds the height age (50% for height).
5. Frequently delayed eruption of primary and secondary teeth (not as severe as in hypothyroidism).
6. Delayed or lack of sexual development.
7. In young adulthood after epiphyseal fusion, the following symptoms may develop, requiring evaluation from an adult endocrinologist:
   a. Altered body composition (increased fat mass, decreased lean body mass).
   b. Reduced aerobic exercise capacity or performance.
   c. Decreased muscle strength.
   d. Abnormal blood lipid (fat and cholesterol) concentrations.
   e. Decreased bone mineral density or content.
   f. Impaired cardiac function.
   g. Impaired health-related quality of life (low energy level, decreased physical mobility, difficulties with concentration and memory, increased emotional lability, irritability, difficulty relating to others, or increased social isolation).

Diagnostic Evaluation

1. In the neonate with hypoglycemia, always draw blood for cortisol and GH *before* initiating corrective action for the hypoglycemia. Early detection and diagnosis will protect the child from future episodes if related to hypopituitarism.
2. Rule out organic, nonendocrine causes of short stature (i.e., chronic illness, nutritional deficiencies, genetic disorders, psychosocial factors).
3. Calculate growth velocity. (Does growth pattern parallel or deviate from the growth curve?)
4. Bone age assessment (usually left wrist and hand), ascertain age of physical development; usually delayed.
5. General physical examination—physical development that of a younger-appearing child, microphallus in the neonate.
6. Chromosome testing of females (rule out Turner syndrome).
7. Thyroid function tests to rule out hypothyroidism.
8. GH secretion laboratory indicators: IGF-1 (insulin-like growth factor 1), IGF-binding protein 3 is decreased. (Malnutrition can cause low IGF-1.)
9. Subnormal secretion of GH in response to two provocative stimuli:
   a. Insulin-induced hypoglycemia.
   b. Abnormal stimulatory response to arginine infusion, L-dopa, clonidine, or glucagon—all of which have specific actions resulting in GH secretion from pituitary. Pharmacologic agent is given, followed by blood sampling for GH response; GH levels less than 10 ng/mL are abnormal.
10. In the neonate with hypoglycemia, GH release is reduced at the time of documented hypoglycemia (concomitant GH level relative to documented hypoglycemia is abnormally low).
11. GH has been associated with reduction in serum levels of free thyroxine (T_4). Patients starting on GH should have their thyroid function monitored in the first 6 months of treatment.
12. Magnetic resonance imaging (MRI) of the head to rule out tumor. (MRI is the gold standard.)

Management

1. Goal of treatment is to restore normal growth and development, as well as to maximize growth potential and prevent hypoglycemia.
2. Replacement of deficiency uses recombinant deoxyribonucleic acid–derived GH given as subcutaneous injection.
3. Typical dose is 0.2 to 0.3 mg/kg per week divided in six or seven doses weekly until final height is achieved. In treatment of Turner syndrome, dose is generally 0.375 mg/kg per week divided in doses as earlier. Note: Administration three times per week is not as effective as six to seven times per week.
4. Therapy is being recommended for adult replacement. Depending on the degree of insufficiency, continued treatment into adulthood may be useful. Dosing recommendations range from less than 0.006 mg/kg/day to as high as 0.0125 mg/kg/day after epiphyseal fusion has occurred.

EVIDENCE BASE Collin, J., Whitehead, A., & Walker, J. (2016). Educating children and families about growth hormone deficiency and its management: Part 1. *Nursing Children & Young People, 28*(1), 32–37. https://doi.org/10.7748/ncyp.28.1.32.s30

Collin, J., Whitehead, A., & Walker, J. (2016). Educating children and families about growth hormone deficiency and its management: Part 2. *Nursing Children and Young People, 28*(2), 30–36. https://doi.org/10.7748/ncyp.28.2.30.s23

Complications

1. Altered carbohydrate, protein, and fat metabolism.
2. Hypoglycemia—seizures/death in neonates.
3. Adverse effects of therapy.
   a. Leukemia.
   b. Recurrence of CNS tumors.
   c. Pseudotumor cerebri.
   d. Slipped capital femoral epiphysis.
   e. Glucose intolerance/diabetes.

Nursing Assessment

1. See "Common nursing assessment for growth and development," page 1326.
2. Obtain family history related to heights and ages of pubertal maturation of biological parents.

Nursing Interventions

Providing Education and Evaluation

1. Teach method of injecting GH through written and verbal instructions. Give demonstration and encourage return demonstration.
2. Encourage rotation of sites in the subcutaneous tissue of the upper arms or thighs to prevent skin irritation and hypertrophy.
3. Document growth every 3 to 6 months while on therapy.
4. If poor growth response, evaluate for appropriate dose, adherence, and injection technique. There may be initial "catch-up" growth that will be exhibited by a growth velocity above normal.
5. Instruct patient and family to report adverse effects: severe headache, hip and knee pain, limp, and increased thirst and urination.

Encouraging Social Interaction

1. Encourage the child to verbalize feelings regarding short stature.
2. Have the child describe what they like about certain people to help the child understand that friendships and social value are based on personality traits rather than absolute height.
3. Suggest involvement in activities that do not use height as an advantage, such as music, art, and gymnastics.
4. Ask the child to identify behaviors that may deter socialization (may or may not be related to short stature) and find ways to change behavior.

Strengthening Self-esteem

1. Help the child and caregivers to identify age-appropriate behaviors and develop a plan for maintaining consistent behaviors in the home and socially.
2. Make sure the caregivers have realistic expectations of the child.
3. Encourage the use of positive feedback rather than punishment.

Community and Home Care Considerations

1. Become familiar with the GH preparation being used and develop a teaching plan for home injection (mixing and injection technique). Provide periodic evaluation and ongoing support.
2. If home injections are difficult relative to family learning or caregiver availability, attempt to include school nurse in administering daily injections.
3. Review storage and stability of GH product relative to manufacturer's specifications for the home, as well as use in travel.

Family Education and Health Maintenance

1. Tell the child and family that short stature is not a "disease."
   a. Growth often catches up with peers usually when peers have stopped growing.
   b. After initial startup of treatment, growth rate should be 4 to 5 in (10 to 12 cm) per year in year 1 and 2¾ to 3½ in (7 to 9 cm) per year over the next 2 years. Growth will slow after that.
   c. Treatment is not to make the child tall; rather, its purpose is to optimize final height potential.
2. Review medication dosage and injection technique periodically.
3. Advise family to think of GH as a replacement that is essential rather than a medication; therefore, it should always be given, regardless of illness or other medication therapies.
4. Encourage regular follow-up for growth evaluation and maintenance of therapy.
5. Discuss potential lifelong therapy, which may be necessary depending on the degree of deficiency. Many patients with hypopituitary condition require lifelong replacement therapy.
6. Recommend counseling about probable infertility for female with Turner syndrome. This should be done with a genetic counselor, if available.

Evaluation: Expected Outcomes

- Growth rate in the initial 2 years of therapy should be two to four times pretreatment growth velocity with a final gain of one to two standard deviations in height.
- The child reports interest in school activities and playing with friends.
- Caregivers report more positive behavior relative to self-esteem.

DISORDERS OF THE POSTERIOR PITUITARY

The posterior pituitary is under the control of the hypothalamus and secretes two hormones, vasopressin (antidiuretic hormone [ADH]) and oxytocin. Abnormality of ADH function is the most common disorder seen in children. The function of ADH is to conserve water at the distal tubules and collecting ducts of the kidney and to act on smooth muscle to increase blood pressure (BP).

Diabetes Insipidus

EVIDENCE BASE Korkmaz, H. A., Kapoor, R. R., Kalitsi, J., Aylwin, S. J., Buchanan, C. R., & Arya, V. B. (2022). Central diabetes insipidus in children and adolescents: Twenty-six year experience from a single centre. *International Journal of Endocrinology, 2022*, 9397130. https://doi.org/10.1155/2022/9397130

Diabetes insipidus (DI) is failure of the body to conserve water due to a deficiency of ADH, decreased renal sensitivity to ADH, or suppression of ADH secondary to excessive ingestion of fluids (primary polydipsia).

Pathophysiology and Etiology

1. The function of water metabolism in the body is to maintain a constant plasma osmolality near the mean level of 287 mOsm/kg.
2. Intake and output of water are governed by the centers in the hypothalamus to control thirst and synthesis of ADH.
3. Thirst ensures adequate intake of water, and ADH prevents water loss through the kidney.
4. Patients with DI are unable to produce appropriate levels or action of ADH, leading to polyuria, increased plasma osmolality, and increased thirst (see Figure 46-1).
5. Classified as central or nephrogenic DI:
   a. Central DI—low levels of ADH; may be congenital or acquired.

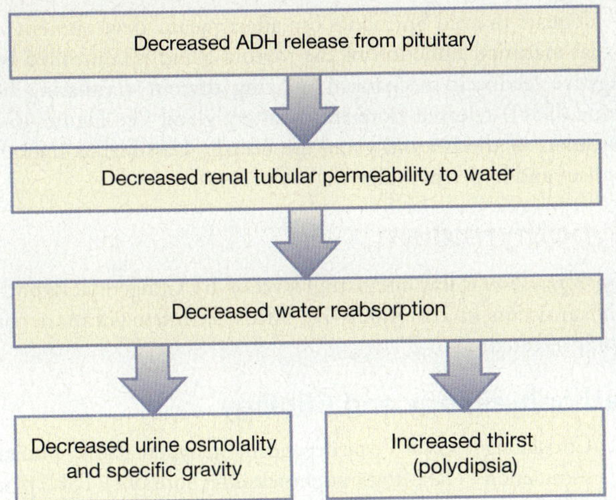

Figure 46-1. Mechanism of antidiuretic hormone (ADH) deficiency in diabetes insipidus.

i. Congenital causes—central nervous system (CNS) defects, hereditary.
ii. Acquired causes—CNS tumors, head trauma (orbital trauma), infections, vascular disorders, idiopathic.

b. Nephrogenic DI—renal unresponsiveness to vasopressin; usually caused by chronic renal disease.
c. Acquired causes—dietary abnormalities such as primary polydipsia, decreased sodium chloride intake, severe protein restriction or depletion, sickle cell disease, drugs (alcohol, lithium, diuretics, medications such as tetracycline).

Clinical Manifestations

1. Sudden onset of excessive thirst and polyuria.
2. In infants:
   a. Excessive crying—quieted with water more than milk feeding.
   b. Rapid weight loss—caloric loss due to water preference over feedings.
   c. Constipation.
   d. Growth failure—weight loss, failure to thrive.
   e. Dehydration—sunken fontanelle, rapid heart rate, headache, fever, low BP.
3. In children:
   a. More abrupt onset, excessive thirst and drinking, preference for ice water.
   b. Polyuria (usually more than 2 L/day) with nocturia and enuresis.
   c. Pale, dry skin with reduced sweating.
   d. Lethargy.

Diagnostic Evaluation

Tests document inability to produce ADH in the face of hyperosmolality of plasma.

1. Urine-specific gravity, sodium, and osmolality are decreased.
2. Serum osmolality and sodium are elevated.
3. Serum measurement of ADH is low in conjunction with high plasma osmolality.
4. Water deprivation test (potentially dangerous):
   a. Fluids are restricted, and the urinary volumes and concentrations are monitored hourly along with the child's weight.
   b. Test is terminated if the child loses more than 3% to 5% of body weight. Serum sodium and osmolality are measured at the completion of test and are high; urine osmolality remains lower.
   c. Test is completed by giving the child a dose of ADH, which should stop the abnormal diuresis. If it does not, the child may have nephrogenic DI.
5. Assess for underlying cause:
   a. Magnetic resonance imaging (MRI) of hypothalamic–pituitary region.
   b. High incidence of associated anterior pituitary disorders.

Management

1. Daily replacement of ADH using desmopressin (DDAVP), a synthetic analog.
2. Available as a metered nasal spray, measured insufflation (nasal) tube, or tablets. In children with cleft lip and palate, sublingual administration has been shown to be effective.
3. Thiazide diuretics in nephrogenic DI.

Complications

1. Dehydration.
2. Hypernatremia.
3. Adverse reactions to DDAVP therapy—hyponatremia and hypertension.

Nursing Assessment

1. Assess children with complaints or behaviors of polyuria and polydipsia for dehydration.
2. Obtain a thorough history of symptoms and behaviors—specific attention to changes in sleep patterns (may be caused by enuresis) and choices of fluids, including sources of water (e.g., does child drink from toilet bowls or dog dishes?).
3. Evaluate height and weight—assess for weight loss related to possible decrease in calories due to excessive drinking, which decreases appetite.
4. For the child on treatment, assess for hydration status. Obtain a history of fluid intake and output from the caregivers to assess appropriate dosage, frequency, and administration of medication.

Nursing Interventions

Regaining Fluid Balance

1. Assess for and teach caregivers assessment of dehydration—dry mucous membranes, weight loss, increased pulse, listlessness or irritability, sunken fontanelle in infants, fever, and poor skin turgor.
2. Administer fluid via intravenous (IV) route, as ordered, if acutely dehydrated.
3. Monitor intake and output and teach caregivers to maintain record of fluid intake and output in child. Reduced output may require restriction of fluids to prevent hyponatremia if overdosage of DDAVP is suspected.
4. Monitor and record daily weights.
5. Family education of DDAVP administration includes nurse demonstration and family administration. Proper management should eliminate symptoms.
6. Teach caregivers to provide free access to fluid (water) sources at all times. However, caution caregivers that the child is unprotected from water excess.
7. Calculate general estimated total daily (24 hours) fluid requirements based on body size to assess fluid replacement

versus excess: 100 mL/kg for first 10 kg of body weight, 50 mL/kg for second 10 kg of body weight, and 20 mL/kg for each additional kilogram.
8. Watch for and report signs of water intoxication due to excess free water and hyponatremia—drowsiness, listlessness, headache, confusion, anuria, and weight gain. Hold DDAVP to prevent seizures, coma, and death.

Maintaining Adequate Nutrition

1. Make sure that adequate formula is ingested between plain water bottles.
2. For older child, provide liquid nutritional supplements.
3. Stress to caregivers the importance of providing nutritional requirements with fluids to ensure meeting caloric demands for growth.
4. Consult with dietitian about need for vitamin or other supplements.
5. Monitor length and weight and developmental milestones at regular intervals.

Normalizing Sleep Pattern

1. Ensure adequate evening administration of DDAVP to prevent nighttime water craving and enuresis.
2. Suggest the use of diapers at night and plastic padding on bed to make controlling bedwetting easier until optimum management of condition is attained.
3. Encourage easy access to fluids and toilet or commode for older child during night.

Family Education and Health Maintenance

1. Teach family insufflation method (for infants and young children):
   a. Correct dose is measured and drawn up into catheter.
   b. Catheter is inserted into patient's nostril.
   c. Caregiver or patient inserts other end of catheter into mouth and gently blows.
   d. Older children may be able to inhale the solution.
2. Advise that nostrils should be as clear as possible before administration of dose.
3. Advise that, if dose is thought to be swallowed, do not readminister because of potential overdosage. Split the dose into both nares if swallowing is occurring.
4. Tell family to store drug away from heat and direct light and moisture (not in bathroom).
5. Advise caregivers that children should wear medical alert device for DI.
6. Tell caregivers that school or daycare personnel should be aware of condition and symptoms needing attention (water intoxication).
7. Advise routine follow-up; treatment may be temporary or lifelong, depending on cause.

Evaluation: Expected Outcomes

- No signs of dehydration; intake equals output.
- No weight loss, growth curve maintained.
- Child sleeping through night.

DISORDERS OF THE THYROID GLAND

Under hypothalamic–pituitary regulation, the thyroid gland secretes thyroxine (T_4) and triiodothyronine (T_3). The action of these hormones promotes cellular growth and differentiation, protein synthesis, and lipid metabolism (cholesterol turnover). Lack of adequate thyroid hormones can affect mental development and sexual maturity. Function of the thyroid gland is controlled by a negative feedback mechanism utilizing thyroid-stimulating hormone (TSH) released from the pituitary gland (see Figure 46-2). Disorders of the thyroid gland are broadly classified as hypothyroidism and hyperthyroidism.

Hypothyroidism

Hypothyroidism is low circulating level of T_4. Congenital hypothyroidism occurs in 1 in 4,000 live births, with females more commonly affected.

Pathophysiology and Etiology

1. Circulating levels of T_4 are dependent on hypothalamic–pituitary stimulation (TRH [thyrotropin-releasing hormone]/TSH) of the thyroid gland.
2. Low levels of T_4 cause an increase in TSH level.
3. Absent or decreased levels of T_4 result in abnormal development of the central nervous system (CNS) of the neonate.
4. In older children, hypothyroidism results in a decrease in metabolism, growth, and physical maturation.
5. Congenital causes:
   a. Thyroid agenesis or dysgenesis.
   b. Hormone synthesis defect.
   c. Maternal thyroid antibodies crossing placenta.
   d. Iodine deficiency.
   e. Drug-induced destruction (thioamides for treatment of hyperthyroidism, iodide excess).
   f. Peripheral T_4 resistance.
6. Acquired (postnatal) causes:
   a. Autoimmune thyroiditis (Hashimoto disease or chronic lymphocytic thyroiditis).

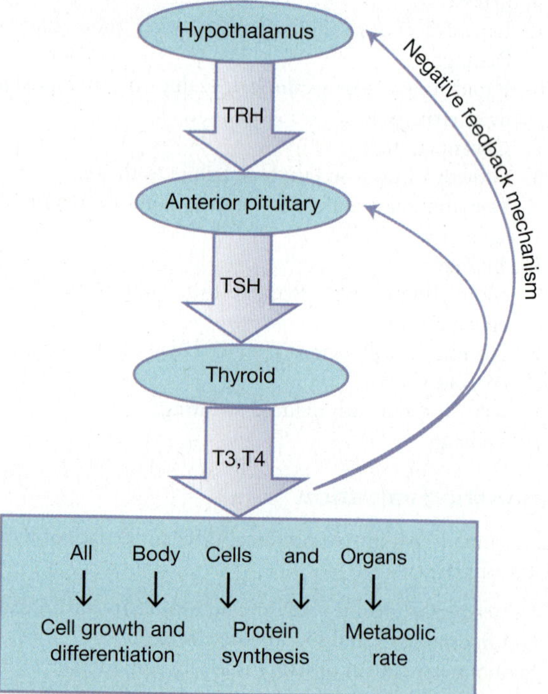

Figure 46-2. Normal thyroid hormone function. TRH, thyrotropin-releasing hormone; TSH, thyroid-stimulating hormone; T_3, triiodothyronine; T_4, thyroxine.

b. Cranial/spinal radiation.
c. Surgical ablation (thyroidectomy).
d. Antithyroid drugs.
e. Iodine deficiency.
f. Central hypothyroidism (TRH/TSH deficiency).

Clinical Manifestations

Neonates

1. Very subtle physical signs, if any.
2. Markedly open posterior fontanelle.
3. Prolonged physiologic jaundice.
4. Feeding difficulties.
5. Skin cool to touch, mottled.
6. Poor muscle tone—hypotonia, umbilical hernia.

After Age 6 Months

1. Growth failure.
2. Large, protruding tongue.
3. Coarse facial features.
4. Poor feeding and constipation.

Acquired Cases

1. Growth retardation—slow growth rate, increased weight gain.
2. Lethargy—obedient, nonaggressive, somnolent.
3. Cold intolerance.
4. Possible poor school performance.
5. Constipation.

Diagnostic Evaluation

1. Neonatal screening of TSH with reflex to T_4; elevation of TSH or a low T_4 may indicate congenital hypothyroidism.
   a. Testing is ideally done at 2 to 4 days of life or immediately before the neonate is discharged from the hospital. TSH levels in the first 24 to 28 hours of life may be falsely elevated.
   b. Abnormal screening test should be confirmed, and treatment begun within 2 weeks after birth.
2. Thyroid nuclear scan—reduced uptake.
3. Abnormal growth rate.
4. Bone age x-ray; delayed.
5. Blood studies:
   a. Free T_4 decreased; TSH elevated.
   b. Thyroid antibodies—elevated in autoimmune thyroiditis.

EVIDENCE BASE Rodriguez, L., Dinauer, C., & Francis, G. (2022). Treatment of hypothyroidism in infants, children and adolescents. *Trends in Endocrinology & Metabolism, 33*(7), 522–532. https://doi.org/10.1016/j.tem.2022.04.007

Management

1. Replacement of thyroid hormone: levothyroxine.
2. Treatment must not be delayed.
3. Therapy goal is to maintain normalcy of thyroid function tests (free T_4, T_4, and T_3 concentrations) in the upper half of normal range.

Complications

1. Developmental delays in neonate who is undiagnosed or untreated.
2. Short stature, growth failure, and delayed physical maturation and development in the older child.

Nursing Assessment

1. Assess the neonate for clinical manifestations listed earlier.
2. Perform behavioral assessment to include sleeping, eating, bowel patterns, level of alertness, and school performance.
3. Assess growth patterns: growth velocity (rate of growth over time), weight gain, and head circumference.

Nursing Interventions

EVIDENCE BASE Rose, S. R., Wassner, A. J., Wintergerst, K. A., Yayah-Jones, N.-H., Hopkin, R. J., Chuang, J., Smith, J. R., Abell, K., & LaFranchi, S. H. (2023). Congenital hypothyroidism: Screening and management. *Pediatrics, 151*(1), e2022060419. https://doi.org/10.1542/peds.2022-060419

Promoting Growth and Development

1. Administer or teach caregivers to administer thyroid hormone replacement daily.
2. Discourage mixing thyroid medication with liquid in bottle that may not be completely finished during a feeding; instead, mix with small amount of fluid and give with dropper or syringe or crush tablet and place in teaspoon of infant food. Do not mix with soy formula.
3. If thyroid pill is being chewed rather than swallowed, have the patient avoid brushing the teeth immediately after to protect against rinsing away dose.
4. Monitor growth and developmental milestones at regular intervals.

Increasing Knowledge

1. Encourage the caregivers to verbalize feelings about the child and the condition.
2. Educate the caregivers as to the importance of the therapy so the child will grow and develop normally.
3. Stress that with replacement therapy, the child can participate in all usual activities.

Family Education and Health Maintenance

1. Encourage follow-up by a primary care provider or pediatric endocrinologist for blood studies to assess and monitor thyroid levels and evaluation of neurologic development to ensure adequate treatment and optimal cognitive development.
2. Make sure the family understands that therapy is usually lifelong. May do a 6-week trial off medication after age 3 years under health care provider's supervision.
3. Support the caregivers and refer child for special testing and therapy if developmental delays are suspected.
4. Teach family the importance of avoiding overdosage of levothyroxine and of being alert for signs of overdosage (weight loss, restlessness, heat intolerance, fatigue, muscle weakness, tachycardia).

Evaluation: Expected Outcomes

- Growth curve and developmental milestones appropriate for age.
- Caregivers verbalize understanding and acceptance of therapy.

Hyperthyroidism

Hyperthyroidism is a disorder of the thyroid gland in which a high circulating level of T_4 results in abnormally increased body metabolism (thyrotoxicosis).

Pathophysiology and Etiology

1. May be caused by autoimmune process—thyrotropin receptor antibodies of a stimulating nature are produced.
   a. Graves disease—most common cause of hyperthyroidism in children, affecting 1% to 2% of school-aged children.
   b. Chronic thyroiditis—Hashimoto disease; usually short-term hyperthyroidism (6 to 18 months duration) before developing hypothyroidism.
2. Autoantibodies stimulate thyroid gland to produce and secrete T_4.
3. Elevated circulating thyroid hormone increases the body's metabolic rate, causing an increase in excitability of the neuromuscular, cardiovascular, and sympathetic nervous systems.
4. May also be caused by ingestion or overdosage of thyroid medication (iatrogenic) or pituitary adenoma (TSH initiated).

Clinical Manifestations

1. Thyromegaly—enlargement of the thyroid, possibly with a bruit.
2. Polyphagia with weight loss.
3. Exophthalmos, proptosis, lid retraction.
4. Hyperactivity—restlessness, nervousness, hand tremors, perspiration, sleeping disturbances, emotional lability; inability to concentrate, decreased school performance.
5. Heat intolerance, excessive diaphoresis.
6. Fatigue (proximal), muscle weakness.
7. Tachycardia, palpitations, wide pulse pressure.
8. Tall stature, underweight for height.

Diagnostic Evaluation

1. Serum thyroid function tests—elevated T_4, T_3 resin uptake with a suppressed TSH.
2. Microsomal antibodies—positive.
3. Thyroid radionuclide scan of goiter—rules out cold nodules that could indicate thyroid carcinoma.

Management

1. Propranolol, a beta-adrenergic blocking agent, for cardiac effects, antipyretics, and anxiolytics.
2. Inorganic iodide preparation, such as propylthiouracil or methimazole, to block the release of thyroid hormone. Adverse effects include headache, nausea, diarrhea, skin rash, itching, liver disease, jaundice, arthralgia, and, rarely, agranulocytosis (severe leukopenia).
3. Radioactive ablation of thyroid gland using radioiodine—preferred to thyroidectomy. This is chosen when medical management is ineffective and results in permanent hypothyroidism that requires treatment.

Complications

1. Development of a goiter (glandular enlargement due to overstimulation).
2. Cardiac problems of tachycardia and hypertension.
3. Exophthalmos—abnormal protrusion of the eyeball.

Nursing Assessment

1. Perform physical assessment to include temperature, heart rate, blood pressure (BP), height, and weight.
2. Obtain history of symptoms specific to onset and subsequent development of symptoms.
3. Elicit history of any changes in behavior, school performance, emotions, or sleep patterns.
4. Assess for presence of goiter—pain with swallowing or talking, palpation of thyroid.

Nursing Interventions

Improving Activity Tolerance

1. Administer and teach caregivers to administer medications and adhere to treatment to gradually lower the metabolic rate and improve activity tolerance.
2. Assess activity tolerance periodically. Determine whether fatigue is present at rest, with activities of daily living, or with exercise. Promote relaxation and rest between activities.
3. Avoid overactivity.

Ensuring Adequate Diet

1. Encourage high-calorie, nutritious diet until thyroid hormone levels are stabilized to try to maintain weight.
2. Advise the caregivers that effective treatment will lower metabolic rate and facilitate appropriate weight gain.
3. Periodically assess growth and development parameters.

Normalizing Sleep Pattern

1. Assess sleep pattern, including naps and sleeping through the night.
2. Adjust schedule to allow maximum amount of rest until sleeping through the night.
3. Allow short naps, as needed.

Reducing Fear

1. Encourage the caregivers and child to verbalize fears related to the thyroid ablation.
2. Teach them about the procedure and clear up misconceptions.
   a. Ablation is accomplished through radioactive destruction of thyroid tissue by administration of a radioactive iodine pill.
   b. The thyroid gland is the only tissue in the body that absorbs iodine; therefore, the radiation only destroys thyroid tissue.
   c. Radiation will be eliminated through the child's urine and feces; precautions for disposal must be followed according to nuclear medicine department policies.
3. Tell them that the resultant effect will most likely be hypothyroidism, which can be managed with lifelong treatment of T_4 replacement.

Family Education and Health Maintenance

1. Review prescribed medications and their functions. Stress the importance of adherence.
2. Advise about periodic blood testing and monitoring for adverse effects of antithyroid medication.
3. Educate family about possibility of oversuppression, from which hypothyroidism could develop.
4. If midday dose of medication is necessary, have family contact school nurse to coordinate dosing.
5. If gland is radioactively ablated, be certain family and other caregivers are appropriately instructed on storage and disposal of human waste after ablative therapy.
6. Encourage follow-up to monitor treatment through blood tests, growth and development evaluation, and size of thyroid gland.

7. Antihyperthyroid medications may cause agranulocytosis (severe leukopenia), thrombocytopenia, and aplastic anemia. Periodic blood testing is necessary to monitor blood counts. Agranulocytosis may present with sore throat and fever. Drug should be discontinued immediately, and health care provider notified.

Evaluation: Expected Outcomes

- The child can play normally without early fatigue.
- No weight loss noted.
- The child displays normal sleep patterns through the night as well as during naps.
- Caregivers and child verbalize understanding of radiation procedure and its rationale.

DISORDERS OF THE ADRENAL GLANDS

The adrenal glands are responsible for the life-sustaining production of mineralocorticoids (aldosterone) for sodium retention, glucocorticoids (cortisol) for blood glucose regulation, and androgens (dehydroepiandrosterone [DHEA], androstenedione) for phallic and secondary sex characteristic development (adrenarche).

Adrenocortical insufficiency is the inability of the adrenal gland to produce aldosterone and cortisol due to adrenal failure or lack of adrenal stimulation. With the exception of congenital adrenal hyperplasia (CAH) (discussed later), pediatric adrenocortical insufficiency is similar in adults (see page 705).

Hyperadrenalism, although rare in children, does occur, causing tissue to be exposed to excessive glucocorticoids (cortisol). This is commonly called *Cushing syndrome.* In addition, hyperfunction of the adrenal medulla, in which epinephrine, norepinephrine, and other catecholamines are secreted, is commonly seen in the disorder of pheochromocytoma. See pages 703 and 706 for a discussion of these conditions.

Congenital Adrenal Hyperplasia

CAH is the most common type of adrenocortical insufficiency in children. Adrenal dysfunction is a result of an enzyme deficiency in the steroid pathway converting cholesterol to cortisol, resulting in overproduction of androgens (sex hormones). The most common form of the condition is life-threatening and requires diagnosis and treatment soon after birth.

Pathophysiology and Etiology

1. Production of adrenal mineralocorticoids and glucocorticoids is blocked by an enzyme deficiency in the steroid pathway. "Blocks" may be severe or partial.
   a. Deficiency of 21-hydroxylase (90% to 95% of CAH cases)—insufficiency in cortisol and usually aldosterone production.
   b. Deficiency of 11-beta-hydroxylase (5% to 8%)—insufficiency of cortisol and aldosterone; however, precursor block to aldosterone is a potent mineralocorticoid.
   c. Deficiency of 3-beta-hydroxysteroid dehydrogenase (5%)—insufficiency in cortisol, aldosterone, and androgen production.
2. Because of lack of feedback suppression, adrenocorticotropic hormone (ACTH) and renin are secreted to stimulate adrenal gland production, causing hyperplasia of the gland.
3. Aldosterone insufficiency results in fluid and electrolyte imbalance.
   a. Loss of sodium at the kidney results in loss of fluid and an increase in serum potassium (cation exchange).
   b. Depletion of extracellular fluid leads to decreased BP.
   c. Low BP stimulates renin in the kidney to activate the adrenal aldosterone pathway.
4. Cortisol insufficiency results in diminished hepatic gluconeogenesis and tissue glucose uptake.
   a. Diminished production/secretion results in low blood sugar levels—more pronounced in times of stress.
   b. Low blood sugar, stress, or low cortisol stimulates feedback to hypothalamic–pituitary axis to release ACTH to stimulate adrenal activity, which also stimulates the release of melanocyte-stimulating hormone (MSH).
   c. Constant ACTH stimulation of gland causes overproduction and "backup" of blocked steroid pathways, resulting in "spillover" production of adrenal androgens.
5. Depending on etiology, overproduction of androgens will virilize female external genitalia or underproduction of androgens will block virilization of male external genitalia.

Clinical Manifestations

1. Ambiguous female genitalia—varying degrees of virilization due to exposure of androgens during development in utero:
   a. Clitoromegaly (may be penile shaped).
   b. Labial fusion (partial or complete).
   c. Rugated labia-appearing scrotal.
   d. Vagina may be incomplete, ending in a blind pouch.
2. Ambiguous male genitalia (3-beta-dehydrogenase)—incomplete virilization development of external genitalia:
   a. Small phallic development.
   b. Incomplete scrotal fusion.
3. Hyperpigmentation (due to MSH secretion).
4. Dehydration.
5. Vomiting/poor feeding.
6. Shock.
7. Latent signs—basal cortisol levels are normal because of compensated chronic ACTH stimulation:
   a. Weakness, fatigue.
   b. Anorexia, nausea, diarrhea.
   c. Weight loss (failure to thrive).
   d. Hyperpigmentation.
   e. Hypotension/postural dizziness.
   f. Rapid growth rate—adrenal androgen effect.
   g. Premature adrenarche—pubic hair, axillary hair, acne, body odor.

Diagnostic Evaluation

Neonates

1. Pelvic ultrasound for identification of uterus, ovaries, or testes to determine sex assigned at birth (internal development of sex-specific organs depends on the presence or absence of Y chromosomal activity; external genital development depends on the presence or absence of androgens).
2. Karyotyping.
3. Serum electrolytes—sodium depletion.
4. Serum glucose levels—hypoglycemia.
5. Serum 17-hydroxyprogesterone (most common precursor to 21-hydroxylase)—elevated.

Latent Diagnosis

1. Rapid growth velocity, premature adrenarche.
2. Advanced bone age x-ray for chronologic age.
3. Elevated serum 17-hydroxyprogesterone.
4. Elevated plasma renin activity—compensated prevention of salt loss.

Management

1. Glucocorticoid replacement—physiologic production of cortisol is 15 to 20 mg/m^2/day. Doses are individually dependent. Replacement is with hydrocortisone twice or three times per day or prednisone once per day when final growth has been achieved.
2. Mineralocorticoid replacement—aldosterone is replaced with fludrocortisone tablets at 0.05 to 0.20 mg daily.
3. Added salt to the diet of neonates if salt loss is severe.
4. Surgical correction of ambiguous genitalia—can require multiple corrections over time.
5. Overdosage of chronic corticosteroid use will result in growth failure. If child fails to grow and exhibits excessive hunger, corticosteroid dosing should be reviewed.

Complications

1. Aldosterone insufficiency:
   a. Hyponatremia, hyperkalemia.
   b. Hypotension.
   c. Shock.
   d. Hypertension in 11-beta-hydroxylase insufficiency in which aldosterone precursor is potent mineralocorticoid.
2. Cortisol insufficiency—hypoglycemia.

Nursing Assessment

Neonates

1. Assess genitalia for ambiguity.
2. In male-appearing genitals, at least one testis must be palpated; if not, assumption must be that child is female with severe virilization. Notify health care provider so diagnostic evaluation can be initiated.
3. Assess for signs of hypoglycemia, hyponatremia, and hyperkalemia (see Box 46-1).
4. Assess feeding pattern of the neonate.
5. Look for hyperpigmentation—may be subjective.

BOX 46-1 Manifestations of Hyponatremia and Hyperkalemia

HYPONATREMIA

- Caused by dilution of sodium (Na^+) when water intake exceeds output. Signs and symptoms occur when Na^+ level falls below 120 mEq/L.
- Gradual fall: anorexia, apathy, mild nausea, and vomiting.
- Rapid fall: headache, mental confusion, muscular irritability, delirium, convulsions

HYPERKALEMIA

- Caused by a shift of potassium out of cells to compensate for decreased Na^+ caused by an oliguric state. Usually asymptomatic, except for electrocardiogram (ECG) changes.
- ECG characteristics: (progressive) shortened QT interval; tall, peaked T waves; ventricular arrhythmias; degeneration of QRS complex; ventricular asystole or fibrillation.

Latent Diagnosis of Child on Treatment

1. Assess growth and development.
2. Monitor vital signs; include sitting and recumbent BP for orthostatic changes.
3. Assess skin for hyperpigmentation.
4. Obtain history to include level of activity/fatigue, dietary history, salt craving, behavior, and school performance.

Nursing Interventions

Minimizing Fatigue

1. Administer glucocorticoids and emphasize adherence to increase energy level.
2. Encourage frequent rest periods and prevent overactivity.
3. Assess activity tolerance to determine adequacy of replacement therapy.
4. Tell the family that the child's activity level as well as growth rate should be normalized on therapy.
   a. If growth rate is too high, review corticosteroid dose and adherence with family.
   b. If growth rate is too low, overdosage of corticosteroid should be suspected.
   c. Review dosing with family.

Maintaining Fluid Balance

1. Assess fluid status and review history of fluid intake and output for appropriate volumes. Assess the hydration status of the child.
2. If the child is vomiting and unable to take oral fluids and mineralocorticoids, administer intravenous (IV) fluids. Start with 5% dextrose in normal saline and monitor serum sodium level.
3. Emphasize adherence with mineralocorticoid replacement.

CLINICAL JUDGMENT No less than 0.5% normal saline should be infused in the child who is aldosterone deficient, because of the inability to retain mineralocorticoid replacement.

Preventing Acute Adrenocortical Insufficiency

1. Identify times of stress, such as acute infections, surgical procedures, or extreme emotional stress, which require increased corticosteroid replacement.
2. Teach the caregivers how to use and give intramuscular (IM) injections of hydrocortisone for stress management, when oral supplementation is not possible because of vomiting.
3. Make sure that the child is evaluated by the primary care provider and treated for the cause of stress.

Reducing Anxiety

1. Encourage the caregivers to verbalize feelings regarding diagnosis, gender decisions or changes, and treatment plans.
2. Explain to the caregivers that the ambiguity is a result of the development process not being completed, rather than being a "mistake."

Family Education and Health Maintenance

1. Stress and reinforce the function of and need for constant replacement of adrenal steroid therapy to maintain normal daily activities.
2. Encourage the caregivers to obtain a medical alert device, which indicates steroid dependency, for the child.

3. Facilitate instructions to the school nurse to notify the caregivers and health care provider of signs of illness and for emergency injection of hydrocortisone should it become necessary.
4. Explain to the caregivers and child why pubic hair may be developing and encourage discussion with teachers and school officials to prevent embarrassment of child in the locker room and other situations.

Evaluation: Expected Outcomes

- Caregivers report the child is more active.
- No signs of dehydration.
- Caregivers verbalize understanding when to call health care provider or when to use emergency hydrocortisone injection; caregivers also demonstrate correct technique for hydrocortisone injection.
- Caregivers verbalize understanding of disorder and need for reconstructive surgery.

DISORDERS OF GONADAL FUNCTION

Proper gonadal function is necessary for developing sexual maturation (puberty). The process involves the hypothalamic release of gonadotropin-releasing hormone (GnRH), which, in turn, stimulates the pituitary to release luteinizing hormone (LH) and follicle-stimulating hormone (FSH). In turn, these stimulate the gonads to produce and release the gonadal steroid testosterone from the testes in males or estrogen from the ovaries in females. The actions of these steroids lead to the development of secondary sexual characteristics and maturation.

Delayed Sexual Development

EVIDENCE BASE Harrington, J., & Palmert, M. R. (2022). An approach to the patient with delayed puberty. *The Journal of Clinical Endocrinology and Metabolism, 107*(6), 1739–1750. https://doi.org/10.1210/clinem/dgac054

Chioma, L., & Cappa, M. (2023). Hypogonadism in male infants and adolescents: New androgen formulations. *Hormone Research in Paediatrics, 96*(6), 581–589. https://doi.org/10.1159/000521455

Delayed sexual development is the lack of pubertal development or progression.

Pathophysiology and Etiology

1. Lack of production or secretion of gonadal steroids from the testes (testosterone) or ovaries (estrogen), due either to the lack of pituitary stimulation (secondary delayed sexual development) or to gonad dysfunction (primary delayed sexual development).
2. Primary delayed sexual development—absence or dysfunction of the gonads.
   a. 45,XO Turner syndrome (chromosomal variants).
   b. Sporadic gonadal dysgenesis.
   c. Bilateral gonadal failure due to radiation, chemotherapy, infection, defect in gonadal steroid synthesis, trauma.
3. Secondary delayed sexual development—lack of hypothalamic–pituitary stimulation to gonads.
   a. Hypothalamic lesions due to infections, trauma, irradiation, or isolated deficiency of GnRH (Kallmann syndrome).
   b. Pituitary lesions due to infection, trauma, or irradiation; also hypopituitarism or isolated LH and FSH deficiencies.
4. Failure of end organs to respond to circulating gonadal steroid—androgen insensitivity.
5. Other causes include chronic illness, anorexia nervosa, and autoimmune atrophy.
6. Resultant effect is failure to achieve sexual maturity.

Clinical Manifestations

1. Females—lack of breast bud development by age 13 years or failure to progress through puberty.
2. Males—lack of testicular enlargement by age 14 years or failure to progress through puberty.
3. Emotional lability.

Diagnostic Evaluation

1. Bone age x-ray to determine physical age—pubertal delay is not consistent with bone age.
2. Laboratory measurement of sex steroids (testosterone and estrogen) and gonadotropins (LH, FSH).
   a. Gonadal failure will show elevated LH and FSH with low estrogen.
   b. No diagnostic test is available to distinguish isolated gonadotropin deficiency (LH or FSH).
3. End-organ insensitivity (lack of gonadal steroid receptor)—sex steroid and gonadotropins will be elevated. Hypothalamic receptors for feedback inhibition are the same as the end-organ receptors; therefore, there is no hypothalamic "shutoff."
4. Abdominal ultrasound to view internal organ structure and development.

Management

1. Replacement of gonadal steroid—should be as close to the physiologic level as possible; however, maximal adult height may be compromised because of potential adverse effect of acceleration of skeletal maturation.
   a. Males—testosterone supplement; 25 to 50 mg by injection every 4 weeks for 6 months, then titrated 50 mg every 6 to 12 months until the dose of 150 to 200 mg every 4 weeks, then decrease interval to every 2 weeks as adult dose.
   b. Females—conjugated estrogen 0.3 to 0.625 mg daily by oral tablet. When appropriate, a progestational agent is added to the therapy for normal periods to occur. An alternative is the use of birth control pills that have the combination of estrogen and progesterone.
2. There is no pituitary or hypothalamic agent for use in secondary gonadal failure.

Complications

1. Sterility.
2. Ambiguity—in androgen insensitivity, male genital development does not respond to circulating level of testosterone from testes; may result in mistaken sex assigned at birth.
3. Potential for dysfunctional dormant gonad to become malignant.

Nursing Assessment

1. Assess growth and development, particularly height.
2. Assess sexual development at regular intervals.

Nursing Interventions

Promoting Sexual Development

1. Administer or teach self-administration of medication, as prescribed.
2. Teach technique for intramuscular (IM) injections of testosterone enanthate. Verify with return demonstration.

3. Stress adherence with prescribed dose and not to exceed recommended dose. Excessive use of testosterone will stunt potential statural growth.

Improving Body Image

1. Discuss strategies for assisting the child to become more comfortable with appearance and ways that may minimize appearance of physical delay in sex characteristics.
2. Stress the importance of the need for slow initiation of therapy to prevent loss of potential height and the fact that this will make sexual development a slow process.

Improving Self-esteem

1. Encourage the child to discuss self-concept; list positive and negative characteristics.
2. Explore ways to strengthen and add to positive characteristics.
3. Encourage participation in age-appropriate activities and social functions.

Family Education and Health Maintenance

1. Teach the patient about adverse effects of testosterone replacement—possible behavioral changes (aggressiveness, moodiness) and an increase in acne.
   a. Suggest over-the-counter acne products or referral to dermatologist if indicated.
   b. Alert the family to report behavioral changes to the health care provider.
2. Teach the patient taking estrogen replacement the importance of daily adherence. Missed doses could result in breakthrough bleeding or spotting due to decreased circulatory estrogen levels. Alert patient to notify health care provider if spotting does occur with estrogen replacement.
3. In both treatments, stress to child and caregivers not to exceed prescribed dose to prevent loss of final adult height.

Evaluation: Expected Outcomes

- At follow-up visit, there is an increase in height and progression of sexual development.
- Child verbalizes improved feelings of body image.
- Child lists more positive concepts of self.

Advanced Sexual Development and Precocious Puberty

Advanced sexual development is secondary sexual development earlier than the normal timing for a child's maturation. There is abnormal early production and secretion of the gonadal steroids or adrenal androgens. Normal pubertal development occurs abnormally early. Skeletal maturation is also advanced under the presence of sex steroids and adrenal androgens.

Pathophysiology and Etiology

Central Precocious Puberty

1. Central precocious puberty (CPP)—early activation of the hypothalamic–pituitary gonadotropin axis.
2. May be idiopathic or caused by:
   a. Tumors of hypothalamus/pituitary.
   b. Cranial irradiation.
   c. Trauma.
   d. Infection—meningitis.
   e. Hydrocephalus.
3. Most common form of precocious puberty.

Peripheral Precocious Puberty

1. Peripheral precocious puberty (PPP)—sex hormone production at the glandular level, independent of central stimulation.
2. Ovarian PPP caused by estrogen-producing tumors or cysts.
3. Testicular PPP caused by androgen- and estrogen-producing tumors or autonomous production of testosterone.
4. Adrenal PPP caused by enzyme defects (congenital adrenal hyperplasia [CAH]) or androgen- and estrogen-producing tumors.

Other Causes

1. Hypothyroidism.
2. Exogenous estrogen or androgen exposure.

Clinical Manifestations

1. Males:
   a. Testicular enlargement (4 mL): younger than age 9½ years.
   b. Tanner stage II pubic hair: younger than age 9 years.
   c. Tanner stage III pubic hair: younger than age 10 years.
2. Females:
   a. Breast bud (stage II): younger than age 8 years.
   b. Tanner stage III pubic hair: younger than age 8½ years.
   c. Menarche: younger than age 9½ years.
3. Both males and females: rapid growth (increased growth velocity) evident.

Diagnostic Evaluation

1. Physical assessment—Tanner staging:
   a. If adrenarche is present without thelarche (breast development) or testicular enlargement, adrenal cause is likely.
   b. In females, if only thelarche is present, ovarian or exogenous estrogen involvement is likely.
   c. If adrenarche and pubarche (gonadal signs) are present, central cause is likely.
2. Skeletal x-ray for bone age—usually advanced. Pubertal stage development is usually commensurate with bone age maturation.
3. Laboratory analysis:
   a. Gonadal steroid levels—may be elevated; however, secretion is diurnal early in development.
   b. Elevated gonadotropins to GnRH stimulation if CPP. Basal levels are frequently unreliable. Lack of elevation of gonadotropins may indicate peripheral source.
   c. Thyroid function to rule out hypothyroidism.
4. Magnetic resonance imaging (MRI) of the head to rule out central etiology.
5. Ultrasound of the abdomen, pelvis, testes for the presence of cysts or tumors.

Management

For CPP, most common form of advanced sexual development in children.

1. Goal is to inhibit puberty to preserve psychosocial well-being and to delay epiphyseal closure to maximize adult height.
2. GnRH agonist—downregulates GnRH receptors of the pituitary against endogenous GnRH.
   a. Nafarelin—intranasal spray, twice daily.
   b. Leuprolide—daily subcutaneous injection.
   c. Depot-leuprolide—monthly IM injection.
   d. Histrelin—subcutaneous daily injection.
3. Progestins.
   a. Medroxyprogesterone injections—biweekly IM injections.
   b. Medroxyprogesterone tablets—oral daily dosing.

DRUG ALERT IM injections of leuprolide have, rarely, been linked to sterile abscesses. The site should not be reused, and the health care provider should be notified immediately if abscess occurs.

Complications

1. Complications of underlying tumor.
2. Behavioral problems.
3. Short stature for final height due to early epiphyseal closure.

Nursing Assessment

1. Assess sexual development using Tanner scale.
2. Obtain history of when signs and symptoms began with specific attention to chronology of events.
3. Perform psychosocial assessment relative to peer relations.
4. While the child is on treatment, perform ongoing assessment of height and sexual characteristics.

Nursing Interventions

Fostering Positive Body Image

1. Encourage the child to verbalize concerns regarding body development changes.
2. Stress to child that the changes are normal events that peers will go through; however, they are occurring early.
3. Teach the child that therapy will halt the process and soon peers will catch up.

Teaching About the Effects of Treatment

1. Assist and encourage caregivers to teach the child about sexual development to reduce fear of the unknown.
2. Encourage proper hygiene practices for body odor, hair growth, and menses.
3. Teach administration techniques for medication treatment, including intranasal, IM, or subcutaneous administration, as indicated.
4. In GnRH-agonist treatment in females, instruct child and caregivers that it takes 10 to 12 days to fully downregulate the pituitary receptors. The suppression results in a fall of estrogen and may cause breakthrough bleeding or even a period to occur. This will happen only once if child remains suppressed on therapy.

Promoting Sense of Identity

1. Encourage the child and caregivers to discuss normal age-related behaviors and identify inappropriate behaviors that are associated with society's expectations of advanced height and development.
2. Encourage the child to wear age-appropriate clothing, participate in age-appropriate activities, and socialize with peers.
3. Suggest counseling, as needed.

Family Education and Health Maintenance

1. Encourage follow-up at regular intervals while on treatment and, if condition is not treated, to monitor progress and address behavioral issues.
2. Discuss with caregivers that child may act out relative to advancing pubertal development. (This may include masturbation.) This behavior needs to be dealt with in an understanding way, not necessarily through punishment.
3. Encourage caregivers to meet with school personnel regarding potential embarrassment in a locker room situation; alternatives to changing clothes in front of peers may be necessary.
4. Prepare family for the start of menstruation if puberty is advanced. The school nurse may need to assist with hygiene during menses. Caregivers may need to meet with the nurse to plan for assistance during school days.
5. Teach family to inspect injection sites and notify health care provider immediately upon noticing a hard, painful, reddened area, which may be a sterile abscess from Lupron injections and require treatment.
6. Teach family to maintain strict adherence to hormonal therapy. Failure to maintain suppression of gonadotropins can result in relative rise in estrogen. Subsequent suppression may cause breakthrough bleeding.

Evaluation: Expected Outcomes

- Child accepts body changes through verbalization at follow-up visits.
- Caregivers or child give adequate return demonstration of IM injection; verbalizes understanding of sexual development.
- Child participates in school activities and socializes with peers of same age.

DISORDERS OF THE PANCREAS

The pancreas manufactures powerful enzymes for digestion as well as the hormones insulin and glucagon. These hormones are manufactured and secreted from cell clusters called the islets of Langerhans. Glucagon and insulin regulate the amount of sugar that is present in the bloodstream. Glucagon is a potent counterregulatory hormone that raises the blood sugar by fostering the release of glucose from stores in the liver. Insulin stimulates glucose uptake by peripheral tissues, inhibits lipolysis, and inhibits hepatic glucose production.

Diabetes Mellitus

EVIDENCE BASE Limbert, C., Tinti, D., Malik, F., Kosteria, I., Messer, L., Jalaludin, M. Y., Benitez-Aguirre, P., Biester, S., Corathers, S., von Sengbusch, S., & Marcovecchio, M. L. (2022). ISPAD Clinical Practice Consensus Guidelines 2022: The delivery of ambulatory diabetes care to children and adolescents with diabetes. *Pediatric Diabetes, 23*(8), 1243–1269. https://doi.org/10.1111/pedi.13417

Lindholm Olinder, A., DeAbreu, M., Greene, S., Haugstvedt, A., Lange, K., Majaliwa, E. S., Pais, V., Pelicand, J., Town, M., & Mahmud, F. H. (2022). ISPAD Clinical Practice Consensus Guidelines 2022: Diabetes education in children and adolescents. *Pediatric Diabetes, 23*(8), 1229–1242. https://doi.org.10.1111/pedi.13418

Diabetes mellitus (DM) is a disorder of glucose intolerance caused by deficiency in insulin production and action, resulting in hyperglycemia and abnormal carbohydrate, protein, and fat metabolism. In younger and school-aged children, most cases are type 1, formerly called juvenile-onset or insulin-dependent DM. Type 2 DM (formerly called adult-onset or noninsulin-dependent DM) traditionally was found in only about 2% of cases of diabetes in children and adolescents. Type 1 DM affects as many as 1 in 400 children. Cases of type 1 and type 2 diabetes are surging among youth in the United States. From 2001 to 2017, the number of people under age 20 living with type 1 diabetes increased by 45%, and the number living with type 2 diabetes grew by 95%. Females and males are equally impacted. The prevalence of type 1 diabetes varies with ethnicity. The incidence is highest in non-Hispanic White children.

Type 2 diabetes now accounts for up to 40% of cases of diabetes diagnosed in adolescents. Etiology suggests morbid obesity, sedentary lifestyle, high caloric intake, and family history of diabetes. There is also an increased risk in Black, Hispanic, and Native American populations. The onset of pubertal development and the insulin resistance that is characteristic of puberty may be a factor in the onset of type 2 diabetes in susceptible adolescents. Type 2 DM is discussed in Chapter 21.

Pathophysiology and Etiology

1. Etiology for type 1 DM suggests genetic and environmental or acquired factors, association with certain human leukocyte antigen types, and abnormal immune responses, including autoimmune reactions.
2. Autoimmune destruction of the islets of Langerhans in the pancreas that secrete insulin, resulting in insulin deficiency.
3. Because insulin facilitates glucose transport into cells, glucose builds up in the bloodstream, causing hyperglycemia.
4. As the kidneys attempt to lower blood glucose levels, glycosuria and polyuria result, with electrolyte excretion.
5. Because the body cells are unable to use glucose for energy, protein and fat are broken down.
6. Fat metabolism results in a buildup of ketones and acidosis.
7. Diabetic ketoacidosis (DKA) occurs in 20% to 40% of patients at the time of diagnosis. Also, DKA at diagnosis is more common in children under 5 years of age and in children who have limited or no access to medical care. It is a potentially fatal condition characterized by hyperglycemia, ketonemia, ketonuria, and metabolic acidosis (pH less than 7.3, bicarbonate less than 15 mEq/L) and caused by insulin deficiency. In children with established Type 1 DM, there is an increased incidence of DKA in those individuals with poor metabolic control, children who omit insulin doses or when caregivers omit doses of their child's insulin, children with psychiatric or eating disorders, peripubertal or adolescent females, and interruption or failure of insulin pump therapy.

Clinical Manifestations

Onset is rapid (usually over a period of a few weeks).

Major Symptoms

1. Increased thirst (polydipsia).
2. Increased urination (polyuria), enuresis, nocturia.
3. Increased food ingestion (polyphagia).
4. Weight loss.
5. Fatigue, lethargy

Minor Symptoms

1. Skin infections.
2. Dry skin, poor wound healing.
3. Monilial vaginitis in adolescent females.

Diabetic Ketoacidosis

1. Hyperglycemia, polyuria, and polydipsia.
2. Dehydration, decreased skin turgor.
3. Nausea, vomiting, generalized malaise, weakness.
4. Kussmaul respirations (rapid, deep, sighing), fruity or acetone breath odor, altered level of consciousness (LOC), confusion.

Diagnostic Evaluation

1. Criteria for diagnosis of type 1 and type 2 DM are the same: fasting blood glucose of more than 126 mg/dL on two occasions (different day); random blood glucose of more than 200 in the presence of symptoms (polydipsia, polyphagia, polyuria); glucose greater than 200 following 2-hour oral glucose tolerance test; random hemoglobin A1C 6.5% or higher (less sensitive and has not been validated in children).
2. Glycosuria or ketonuria on routine examination may arouse suspicion of diabetes.
3. Evaluation for metabolic acidosis with acute presentation (pH less than 7.3 and bicarbonate less than 14 mEq/L).
4. Hemoglobin A1C testing every 3 months to determine long-term plasma glucose control is dependent on age. Children, especially young children, are at high risk for hypoglycemia and are at low risk for complications prior to puberty.
   a. A1C goals must be individualized and reassessed over time. An A1C of less than 7% is appropriate for many children
   b. Less stringent A1C goals (such as less than 7.5%) may be appropriate for patients who cannot articulate symptoms of hypoglycemia; have hypoglycemia unawareness; lack access to analog insulins, advanced insulin delivery technology, and/or continuous glucose monitors; cannot check blood glucose regularly; or have nonglycemic factors that increase A1C.
   c. Even less stringent A1C goals (such as less than 8%) may be appropriate for patients with a history of severe hypoglycemia, limited life expectancy, or extensive comorbid conditions.
   d. Providers may reasonably suggest more stringent A1C goals (such as less than 6.5) for select individual patients if such goals can be achieved without significant hypoglycemia, negative impacts on well-being, or undue burden of care, or in those who have nonglycemic factors that decrease A1C (e.g., lower erythrocyte lifespan). Lower targets may also be appropriate during the honeymoon phase.
5. Screening for celiac disease should be done at the time of diagnosis, and if disease is detected, child should be referred to a pediatric gastroenterologist. A gluten-free diet is the only treatment for children with celiac disease, regardless of symptoms.
6. Thyroid function and screening for autoimmune thyroid disease is also recommended at the time of diagnosis.

EVIDENCE BASE de Bock, M., Codner, E., Craig, M. E., Huynh, T., Maahs, D. M., Mahmud, F. H., Marcovecchio, L., & DiMeglio, L. A. (2022). ISPAD Clinical Practice Consensus Guidelines 2022: Glycemic targets and glucose monitoring for children, adolescents, and young people with diabetes. *Pediatric Diabetes, 23*(8), 1270–1276. https://doi.org/10.1111/pedi.13455

Redondo, M. J., Libman, I., Maahs, D. M., Lyons, S. K., Saraco, M., Reusch, J., Rodriguez, H., & DiMeglio, L. A. (2021). The evolution of hemoglobin A_{1c} targets for youth with type 1 diabetes: Rationale and supporting evidence. *Diabetes Care, 44*(2), 301–312. https://doi.org/10.2337/dc20-1978

Management

1. Insulin therapy (see Table 46-2).
   a. New insulin analogs provide more options for insulin duration and frequency of administration. Longer acting basal insulins, such as U300 glargine and degludec, provide a duration of up to 42 hours without a pronounced peak of action. Rapid-acting insulins (e.g., lispro, glulisine, and aspart), ultrarapid-acting insulins (e.g., insulin lispro-aabc), and faster acting insulin aspart offer rapid onset with shorter duration.
   b. Dosage needs are based on the child's weight, diet, and level of activity. Dosages are adjusted through daily monitoring of blood glucose levels.
   c. Continuous glucose monitors (CGMs) (see Figure 46-3) should be considered in all children and adolescents with type 1 diabetes; the benefits of CGM correlate with adherence to ongoing use of the device.
   d. Insulin pump therapy, consisting of a continuous subcutaneous infusion of insulin that can be programmed to give bolus and basal rates, may be used by some children.
   e. Automated insulin delivery (AID) systems should be offered for diabetes management to youth with type 1 diabetes who are capable of using the device safely (either by themselves or with caregivers). These systems combine CGM with insulin pump and adjust basal insulin based on predicted glucose values.
2. Treatment of DKA (see Box 46-2).
   a. Intravenous (IV) fluid therapy to increase perfusion and glucose uptake in the periphery, which will reduce hyperglycemia; also increases glomerular filtration and reverses acidosis.
   b. Regular IV insulin administration at a rate of 0.1 U/kg/h after initial fluid replacement. Provide IV dextrose solution as plasma glucose decreases, titrate rate of insulin infusion to achieve a rate of glucose decline of 50 to 150 mg/dL/h.
   c. Bicarbonate is not indicated; acidosis will correct with adequate insulin infusion.
   d. Close monitoring of vital signs, electrocardiogram, mental status, and neurologic system.
   e. Replacement of electrolytes—sodium, potassium, ionized calcium.
3. Balanced diet with controlled carbohydrates and adequate protein and fat to meet energy and growth requirements.

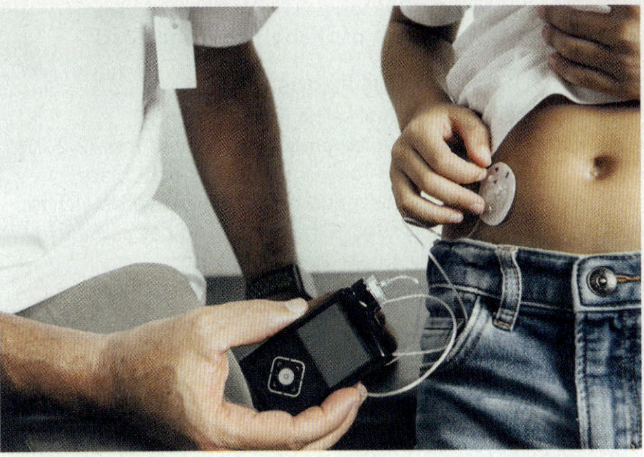

Figure 46-3. | Child with continuous glucose monitor. (Shutterstock/Click and Photo).

EVIDENCE BASE Glaser, N., Fritsch, M., Priyambada, L., Rewers, A., Cherubini, V., Estrada, S., Wolfsdorf, J. I., & Codner, E. (2022). ISPAD clinical practice consensus guidelines 2022: Diabetic ketoacidosis and hyperglycemic hyperosmolar state. *Pediatric Diabetes, 23*(7), 835–856. https://doi.org/10.1111/pedi.13406

Complications

Acute

1. Usually reversible.
2. DKA accounting for 70% of diabetes-related deaths in children younger than age 10 years.
3. Cerebral edema—related to treatment of DKA; thought to be due to a rapid decline in blood glucose, causing a fluid shift in the brain.
4. Hyperglycemia (untreated or undertreated).
5. Hypoglycemia (insulin reaction).

Subacute

Develops over a short period.

1. Lipohypertrophy (localized tissue buildup from giving injections in the same site)—repeated injections in the same area; can cause abnormal absorption.
2. Skeletal and joint abnormalities—limited joint mobility.
3. Growth failure and delayed sexual maturation due to underinsulinization.

Table 46-2 Types of Insulin and Their Effects

TYPE OF INSULIN	ONSET	MAXIMAL ACTIVITY (HOURS)	DURATION (HOURS)
Ultrarapid acting: faster aspart, lispro-aabc	1–15 min	1–2	3–6
Rapid acting: glulisine, aspart, lispro	5–15 min	1–2	4–6
Regular	30–60 min	2–4	6–8
NPH	120 min	4–12	24
Detemir	1–2 h	NA	14–24
Glargine	3–4 h	NA	24
U300 glargine	6 h	NA	30–36
Degludec	1–2 h	NA	>40

NA, not applicable.

BOX 46-2 Treatment of Diabetic Ketoacidosis

INITIATE INTRAVENOUS FLUIDS

- Start with 0.9% normal saline (NS) solution.
- Estimate fluid deficit by amount of weight loss (2.2 lb [1 kg] equals 1 L of fluid). Infuse fluids to replace one half of estimated loss plus maintenance needs (10 to 20 mL/kg) over first 8 to 12 hours; second half plus maintenance needs over next 16 to 36 hours.
- When blood glucose falls below 250 mg/dL, change to 5% glucose in 0.45% NS solution.
- Closely monitor vital signs, electrocardiogram (ECG), and intake and output, and obtain laboratory values, including urine and blood glucose, electrolytes, blood urea nitrogen and creatinine, serum osmolarity, arterial or venous pH, serum and urine ketones, calcium, and phosphorus every 1 to 4 hours as condition warrants.

CLINICAL JUDGMENT Avoid infusion of hypertonic solutions because ketoacidosis is accompanied by a profound free water deficit. Replace fluids slowly to prevent rapid decline in serum osmolarity, which may precipitate cerebral edema.

ADMINISTER INSULIN

- Give IV bolus of 0.1 unit/kg of regular insulin if no intermediate-acting insulin has been given in the past 6 to 8 hours.
- Provide continuous IV drip of regular insulin at rate of 0.1 U/kg/h.
- Continue IV insulin until metabolic acidosis is corrected (pH greater than 7.3 and bicarbonate greater than 13 to 15), bowel sounds have returned, and oral fluids can be taken.
- When meals are tolerated, begin subcutaneous rapid-acting insulin at least 30 minutes before discontinuing IV insulin.
- When stabilized, return to previous insulin regimen or begin therapy using basal-bolus therapy (basal insulin with rapid-acting insulin).

CLINICAL JUDGMENT Flush IV tubing with insulin solution before infusion and change tubing with each bag because insulin will bind to the plastic tubing, changing concentration.

POTASSIUM AND BICARBONATE REPLACEMENT

- Initial serum K levels will be normal or high, even though intracellular levels are low. Serum levels will fall as insulin therapy drives K into the cells.
- Begin replacement of K when urine output and renal function have been established.
- Add KCl 20 to 40 mEq to each liter of fluid.
- Monitor T waves on ECG for peaking (hyperkalemia) or flattening (hypokalemia).
- Bicarbonate administration is controversial in correcting acidosis but may be indicated for respiratory depression, decreased myocardial contractility, or refractory, severe acidosis.

Chronic

Very rarely seen in children, but develops after years to decades with inadequate treatment.

1. Retinopathy/cataracts—may cause blindness.
2. Neuropathy—peripheral and autonomic.
3. Nephropathy—proteinuria/renal failure.
4. Cardiopathy—heart failure.

Nursing Assessment

1. When the child first presents with suspected DM:
   a. Obtain history of onset of signs and symptoms of clinical manifestations.
   b. Assess for levels of dehydration and weight loss with level of appetite.
   c. Check for sores that are slow to heal.
   d. Identify any fruity smell to breath—acetone breath due to ketosis.
   e. Assess abdominal pain—may mimic appendicitis.
2. For child with DKA:
   a. Assess for potential cerebral edema (diminished LOC) on presentation and when fluid replacement is initiated. Fluid replacements precede and are then concurrent with insulin therapy.
   b. Assess cardiac function—tachycardia with dehydration, arrhythmias related to potassium imbalances.
   c. Assess renal function—urine output with intake and output, ketonuria, glycosuria.
   d. Watch for hypoglycemia—overtreatment of insulin; glucose level correction should be slow. IV replacements frequently contain glucose to prevent large osmotic fluid shifts, leading to cerebral edema.
3. During treatment/routine follow-up:
   a. Assess growth parameters—excessive weight gain may indicate overtreatment of insulin (child eats because of constant hunger). Loss or lack of weight gain may indicate underinsulinization (losing calories that are not metabolized).
   b. Review blood glucose diaries and glucose monitor for level of control and need for insulin adjustments. (Check for appropriate adjustments of insulin made by caregivers.) Glucose should be checked before meals (preprandial) and at bedtime. Optimal levels are age related.
   c. Fingerstick capillary glucose (self-monitoring of blood glucose [SMBG]) should be assessed at least six times a day for a person with diabetes taking insulin.
   d. Recommended target glucose values are between 70 and 180 mg/dL, with a narrower fasting target range of 70 to 144 mg/dL.
   e. Where available, CGM should be initiated in all children, adolescents, and young adults with type 1 DM as soon as possible after diagnosis to improve glycemic outcomes.
   f. CGM target time in range:
      i. More than 70%: between 70 and 180 mg/dL.
      ii. Less than 4%: less than 70 mg/dL.
      iii. Less than 1%: less than 54 mg/dL.
      iv. Less than 25%: greater than 180 mg/dL.
      v. Less than 5%: greater than 250 mg/dL.
      vi. Glycemic variability (coefficient of variation, %CV target 36% or less).
   g. Obtain history of any hypoglycemic reactions—be specific to time of day, dietary record, and exercise and activity.
   h. Assess injection sites—look for signs of lipohypertrophy.
   i. Assess for signs of hyperglycemia—polyuria, polydipsia. Does the child need to get up during the night to go to the bathroom?

Nursing Interventions

Restoring Fluid Balance

1. Administer IV fluids, as ordered.
2. Monitor intake and output, blood pressure (BP), serum electrolyte results, and daily weight.
3. Report abnormal sodium and potassium results promptly.
4. Assess for signs of dehydration—dry skin and mucous membranes, constipation.
5. Encourage oral fluids when able.

Meeting Nutritional Requirements

1. Provide an adequate diet for the child and teach the family about the diet.
   a. Dietary recommendations for young people with diabetes are based on population healthy eating recommendations and, therefore, are suitable for the whole family.
   b. The most common meal plan is one based on carbohydrate counting. This type of meal plan offers flexibility and a wide variety of choices. Total carbohydrate requirements will be calculated, then labels can be read and charts consulted to determine grams of carbohydrate per serving of food eaten. Insulin dosage is based on the total amount of carbohydrates eaten; for example, 1 unit of short- or rapid-acting insulin for every 15 g of carbohydrate.
   c. Occasionally, a more rigid, strictly controlled diet is necessary.
      i. The diet should be composed of approximately 55% carbohydrate, 30% fat, and 15% protein. The fat content of the diet should be less than 10% saturated fat and trans fatty acids. Foods with high fiber content should be encouraged.
      ii. All diets must supply sufficient caloric intake for activity and growth, sufficient protein for growth, and the required vitamins and minerals.
   d. Foods are distributed throughout the day to accommodate varying peak action of insulin. Distribution may be adjusted for increased or decreased amounts of exercise.
   e. Determine the child's usual dietary habits so that insulin can be matched with the type of meal and amount of food. Consider family cultural norms when suggesting dietary choices.
   f. Include the child and caregivers in meal planning as soon as possible.
   g. Allow the child normal activity while hospitalized so that the observed result of the dietary control will be valid. Because the child's activity level usually decreases during the hospital stay, the child and family must understand that the insulin and dietary needs will require reassessment on discharge.
   h. Allow the child to eat with other children.
   i. Refer family to a dietitian for additional planning and education.

Increasing Knowledge About Insulin Administration

1. Insulin should be given as directed. Ultrarapid-acting and rapid-acting insulin analogs are absorbed quickly and should be given right before the meal. If taking regular insulin, the child should not eat until 20 to 30 minutes after injection is given.
2. Be aware of the major types of insulin and their effects.
3. Develop a systematic plan for injections that emphasizes rotation of sites (Figure 46-4).
   a. The upper arms, thighs, upper buttocks, or abdomen are all sites for injection in children.
   b. Subsequent injections are given about 1 in (2.5 cm) apart.
   c. Guidelines for site location:
      i. Arms—begin below the deltoid muscle and end one handbreadth above the elbow. Begin at the midline and progress outward laterally, using the external surface only.
      ii. Thighs—begin one handbreadth below the hip and end one handbreadth above the knee. Begin at the midline and progress outward laterally, using only the outer, anterior surface.
      iii. Abdomen—avoid the beltline and 1 in (2.5 cm) around the umbilicus.
      iv. Buttocks—use the upper outer quadrant of the buttocks.
4. Mix insulin solutions, such as NPH (neutral protamine Hagedorn) and 70/30, by slowly rolling the bottle or pen between hands or gently tipping the bottle over a few times. Never shake the bottle vigorously.

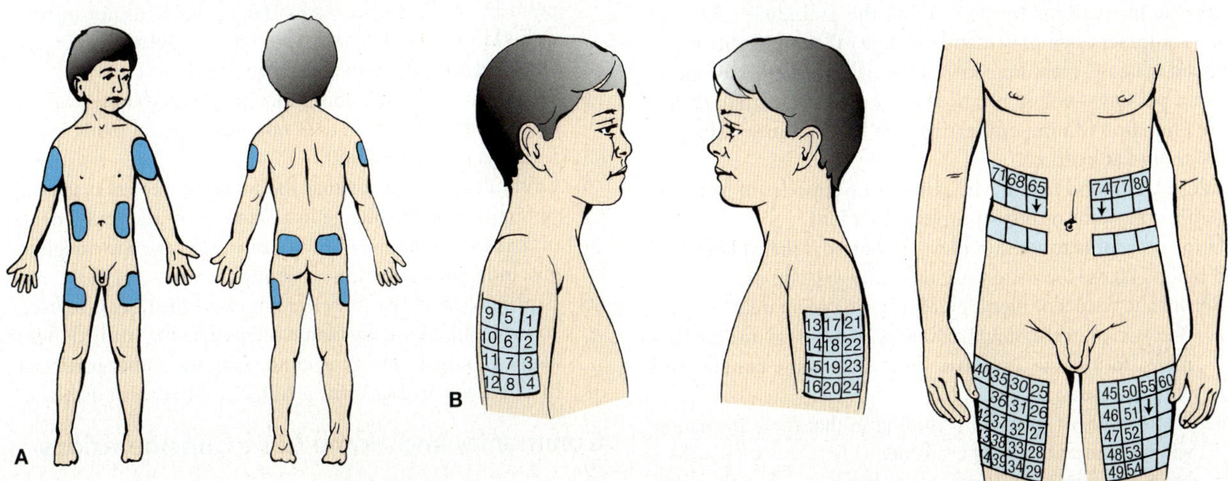

Figure 46-4. **(A)** Insulin injection sites are the upper outer portions of the arms, the buttocks, the thighs, and the abdominal area. **(B)** Injection sites are rotated, with subsequent injections given about 1 in (2.5 cm) apart.

5. All insulin pens require an "air shot" (clearing air from pen) prior to giving *each* dose.
6. Administer insulin subcutaneously. Do not aspirate.
7. Observe the skin closely for signs of irritation. Avoid the injection site for several weeks if signs of local irritation are observed.
8. Observe the skin for a rash indicating an allergic reaction to insulin (rare with newer preparations). Notify the health care provider immediately if there is an allergic reaction.
9. Be aware of factors that vary the need for and utilization of insulin, particularly exercise and infection.
   a. Exercise tends to lower the blood sugar level. Encourage normal activity; insulin and carbohydrates should be regulated to encourage activity.
   b. Infection or illness increases the child's insulin requirement (insulin is still administered during illness). Be alert for signs of infection and dehydration.
10. Observe the following storage requirements:
    a. Opened bottles of insulin may be stored at room temperature or in the refrigerator. Opened insulin pens should not be returned to the refrigerator.
    b. Opened bottles and insulin pens should be discarded based on the type and brand of insulin. Some insulins have a shelf life as long as 8 weeks out of the refrigerator.
    c. Extra bottles and insulin pens should be stored in the refrigerator.
11. Encourage the child to express feelings about the injections. The child may be helped to master fear of injections by gaining control of the situation through play and active participation in the procedure.

DRUG ALERT None of the basal insulins (degludec, detemir, or glargine) have been approved by the Food and Drug Administration for mixing with any other insulin.

Providing Information About Blood Glucose Monitoring

1. Teach family about monitoring options, including SMBG and CGM.
2. Teach child and caregivers the chosen method for blood glucose monitoring. Every child using CGM needs an SMBG monitor as backup.
3. The SMBG procedure requires a drop of blood (obtained by fingerstick), a reagent strip, and a glucometer.
4. Specific instructions for performing the procedure vary with the equipment being used and must be followed explicitly.
5. Blood glucose measurements are usually made six or more times per day—before meals, after meals when carbohydrates are estimated (dining out, eating new foods), during/after exercise, and at bedtime.
6. Additional blood tests are helpful during episodes of hypoglycemic symptoms or other problem situations.
7. Urine tests for ketones should be performed if the child is ill or if blood glucose level is greater than 240 mg/100 dL.
8. Record the results of blood glucose testing accurately.
   a. The use of technology to upload data from the SMBG meter to a cloud improves discussions with families and reduces disease burden.
   b. Use a standard form for recording so that the information will be clear and readily available.
   c. Help the family understand the behaviors that the child can perform at specific age ranges to improve engagement and long-term understanding of the disease.

Identifying and Controlling Hypoglycemia

1. Have glucagon available for injection or nasal administration if a hypoglycemic reaction occurs and the child is unconscious, has a seizure or is unable to swallow liquids safely, or is combative. Administer 0.5 to 1 mg IM or subcutaneously or 1 mg nasally and assess response.
2. Teach family the causes, signs and symptoms, and treatment for hypoglycemia.
   a. Common causes:
      i. Overdose of insulin.
      ii. Reduction in diet or increased exercise without sufficient caloric coverage.
   b. Symptoms:
      i. Trembling, shaking, dizziness.
      ii. Sweating, apprehension.
      iii. Tachycardia.
      iv. Hunger, weakness.
      v. Drowsiness, unusual behavior.
      vi. Mental confusion.
      vii. Seizures, coma.
   c. Be prepared to give glucose tablets, orange juice, sugar cubes, or another food containing readily available simple sugars.
3. Watch for a pattern of activity or time of day that precedes hypoglycemic reactions and work with family to alter insulin, carbohydrates, or behavior to prevent reactions.
4. If prescribed, teach the child and family how to use emergency glucagon.
5. If glucagon is not available and the child is unresponsive, activate the emergency response system (911).

Reducing Fear and Anxiety

1. Explain the need and purpose of every test to child and caregivers. Allow child to vent feelings and cry if fearful. When appropriate, demonstrate procedures on yourself first (e.g., fingersticks for glucose testing, allowing caregiver to give saline injection for practice of insulin injection).
2. Teach family the pathophysiology of diabetes. Understanding the disease process aids in understanding the treatment and signs and symptoms. Assess knowledge level of teaching by having family verbalize knowledge of disease management.
3. Allow caregivers to verbalize feelings related to the expectations of their performance. Stress that the learning is through the actual "hands-on" management. Assist the caregivers in performing the needed tasks (fingersticks, insulin injections) to build their confidence. Give the caregivers clear objectives and directions for home management.
4. Stress that the child's condition is now the family's condition as well. Stress that child does not need "special foods" different from the rest of the family.
5. Caution the caregivers that the focus on the child may cause sibling rivalry. Encourage involvement by all family members in making the home a healthy one and urge the caregivers to give individual attention to siblings as well.
6. Explain to child that they did not cause the disease to occur—young children usually blame themselves for "bad" things that happen to them. Help the child understand that participating in all usual activities is the goal for children with diabetes.

Community and Home Care Considerations

1. Perform home assessment for adequate nutritional resources.
2. Reteach and assess family's adherence to insulin administration and blood glucose monitoring.

3. Reteach and assess family's ability to respond to hypoglycemia.
4. Make sure that school is able to follow-through with management plan for insulin administration, planned exercise and mealtimes, and responding to hypoglycemia.
5. When child is ill, evaluate for dehydration, hyperglycemia, and ketonuria. Teach family how to monitor condition, maintain insulin coverage, and notify the health care provider. (See "Diabetes sick-day guidelines," page 732.)

Family Education and Health Maintenance

Patient or caregiver education is one of the most important aspects in the nursing care of the child with diabetes. Thorough instruction is essential in the following areas:

1. Influence of exercise, emotional stress, and other illnesses on insulin and diet needs.
2. Recognition of the symptoms of insulin shock and diabetic acidosis and knowledge of related emergency management.
3. Discussion of individual goals such as A1C, CGM, SMBG at every visit.
4. Contact with other children/families with type 1 DM for support.
5. Psychosocial screening and referrals to social worker or psychologist as needed.
6. Precautionary measures:
    a. Have the child carry an identifying card that states that they have diabetes and includes name, address, telephone number, and health care provider's name and telephone number.
    b. Suggest a simple, convenient source of glucose that can be carried easily by the child or caregivers to have available for hypoglycemic symptoms. Good examples include glucose tablets, glucose gel, or cake-decorating gel that comes in a tube.
    c. Help the family discuss the child's disease with the school nurse and other responsible adults who are in close contact with the child (e.g., teachers, extracurricular leaders, coaches).
    d. Advise caregivers that vials of insulin and insulin pens should be kept on one's person when traveling because baggage may be subjected to extreme temperatures and pressures incompatible with the stability of insulin.
7. Follow up with the primary care provider or pediatrician for immunizations, all regular health checkups, and growth and development evaluations.
8. For additional information and support, refer to the following agencies:
    a. American Diabetes Association, ATTN: National Call Center, 2451 Crystal Drive, Suite 900 Arlington, VA 22202, 1-800-DIABETES (800-342-2383), www.diabetes.org.
    b. Juvenile Diabetes Research Foundation International, 26 Broadway, 14th floor, New York, NY 10004; 800-JDF-CURE (212-785-9595), *www.jdrf.org.*

Evaluation: Expected Outcomes

- No signs of dehydration.
- Caregivers and child describe consistent meal plan.
- Child and caregivers demonstrate correct insulin administration technique.
- Child and caregivers demonstrate correct glucose monitoring technique.
- Child and caregivers verbalize causes, signs and symptoms, and treatment for hypoglycemia.
- Child and caregivers speak openly about diabetes, ask appropriate questions.

SELECTED READINGS

Ahmed, S. F., Achermann, J., Alderson, J., Crouch, N. S., Elford, S., Hughes, I. A., Krone, N., McGowan, R., Mushtaq, T., O'Toole, S., Perry, L., Rodie, M. E., Skae, M., & Turner, H. E. (2021). Society for Endocrinology UK Guidance on the initial evaluation of a suspected difference or disorder of sex development (Revised 2021*). Clinical Endocrinology, 95*(6), 818–840. https://doi.org/10.1111/cen.14528

Aly, J., & Kruszka, P. (2022). Novel insights in Turner syndrome. *Current Opinion in Pediatrics, 34*(4), 447–460. https://doi.org/10.1097/MOP.0000000000001135

Besser, R. E. J., Bell, K. J., Couper, J. J., Ziegler, A., Wherrett, D. K., Knip, M., Speake, C., Casteels, K., Driscoll, K. A., Jacobsen, L., Craig, M. E., & Haller, M. J. (2022). ISPAD Clinical Practice Consensus Guidelines 2022: Stages of type 1 diabetes in children and adolescents. *Pediatric Diabetes, 23*(8), 1175–1187. https://doi.org/10.1111/pedi.13410

Brady, J., Cannupp, A., Myers, J., & Jnah, A. J. (2021). Congenital hypothyroidism. *Neonatal Network, 40*(6), 377–385. https://doi.org/10.1891/11-T-699

Cengiz, E., Danne, T., Ahmad, T., Ayyavoo, A., Beran, D., Ehtisham, S., Fairchild, J., Jarosz-Chobot, P., Ng, S. M., Paterson, M., & Codner, E. (2022). ISPAD Clinical Practice Consensus Guidelines 2022: Insulin treatment in children and adolescents with diabetes. *Pediatric Diabetes, 23*(8), 1277–1296. https://doi.org/10.1111/pedi.13442

Cerbone, M., Visser, J., Bulwer, C., Ederies, A., Vallabhaneni, K., Ball, S., Kamaly-Asl, I., Grossman, A., Gleeson, H., Korbonits, M., Nanduri, V., Tziaferi, V., Jacques, T., & Spoudeas, H. A. (2021). Management of children and young people with idiopathic pituitary stalk thickening, central diabetes insipidus, or both: A national clinical practice consensus guideline. *The Lancet Child & Adolescent Health, 5*(9), 662–676. https://doi.org/10.1016/S2352-4642(21)00088-2

Chen, Z., Wang, J., Carru, C., Coradduzza, D., & Li, Z. (2023). The prevalence of depression among parents of children/adolescents with type 1 diabetes: A systematic review and meta-analysis. *Frontiers in Endocrinology, 14,* 1095729. https://doi.org/10.3389/fendo.2023.1095729

Cheng, T. S., Ong, K. K., & Biro, F. M. (2022). Trends toward earlier puberty timing in girls and its likely mechanisms. *Journal of Pediatric and Adolescent Gynecology, 35*(5), 527–531. https://doi.org/10.1016/j.jpag.2022.04.009

Chin-Jung, L., Hsiao-Yean, C., Yeu-Hui, C., Kuan-Chia, L., & Hui-Chuan, H. (2021). Effects of mobile health interventions on improving glycemic stability and quality of life in patients with type 1 diabetes: A meta-analysis. *Research in Nursing & Health, 44*(1), 187–200. https://doi.org/10.1002/nur.22094

Collett-Solberg, P. F., Ambler, G., Backeljauw, P. F., Bidlingmaier, M., Biller, B. M. K., Boguszewski, M. C. S., Cheung, P. T., Choong, C. S. Y., Cohen, L. E., Cohen, P., Dauber, A., Deal, C. L., Gong, C., Hasegawa, Y., Hoffman, A. R., Hofman, P. L., Horikawa, R., Jorge, A. A. L., Juul, A., … Woelfle, J. (2019). Diagnosis, genetics, and therapy of short stature in children: A Growth Hormone Research Society International Perspective. *Hormone Research in Paediatrics, 92*(1), 1–14. https://doi.org/10.1159/000502231

Cools, M., Nordenström, A., Robeva, R., Hall, J., Westerveld, P., Flück, C., Köhler, B., Berra, M., Springer, A., Schweizer, K., Pasterski, V., & Cost Action Bm1303 Working Group 1. (2018). Caring for individuals with a difference of sex development (DSD): A Consensus Statement. *Nature Reviews Endocrinology, 14*(7), 415–429. https://doi.org/10.1038/s41574-018-0010-8

Danowitz, M., & Grimberg, A. (2022). Clinical Indications for Growth Hormone Therapy. *Advances in Pediatrics, 69*(1), 203–217. https://doi.org/10.1016/j.yapd.2022.03.005

Duan, R., Qiao, T., Chen, Y., Chen, M., Xue, H., Zhou, X., Yang, M., Liu, Y., Zhao, L., Libuda, L., & Cheng, G. (2021). The overall diet quality in childhood is prospectively associated with the timing of puberty. *European Journal of Nutrition, 60*(5), 2423–2434. https://doi.org/10.1007/s00394-020-02425-8

El-Remessy, A. B. (2022). Diabetic ketoacidosis management: Updates and challenges for specific patient population. *Endocrines, 3*(4), 801–812. https://doi.org/10.3390/endocrines3040066

ElSayed, N. A., Aleppo, G., Aroda, V. R., Bannuru, R. R., Brown, F. M., Bruemmer, D., Collins, B. S., Hilliard, M. E., Isaacs, D., Johnson, E. L., Kahan, S., Khunti, K., Leon, J., Lyons, S. K., Perry, M. L., Prahalad, P., Pratley, R. E., Seley, J. J., Stanton, R. C., … on behalf of the American Diabetees Association. (2023). 14. Children and adolescents: Standards of care in diabetes—2023. *Diabetes Care, 46,* S230–S253. https://doi.org/10.2337/dc23-S014

ElSayed, N. A., Aleppo, G., Aroda, V. R., Bannuru, R. R., Brown, F. M., Bruemmer, D., Collins, B. S., Hilliard, M. E., Isaacs, D., Johnson, E. L., Kahan, S., Khunti, K., Leon, J., Lyons, S. K., Perry, M. L., Prahalad, P., Pratley, R. E., Seley, J. J., Stanton, R. C., & Gabbay, R. A. (2023). 6. Glycemic targets: Standards of care in diabetes—2023. *Diabetes Care, 46*, S97–S110. https://doi.org/10.2337/dc23-S006

Gravholt, C. H., Viuff, M. H., Brun, S., Stochholm, K., & Andersen, N. H. (2019). Turner syndrome: Mechanisms and management. *Nature Reviews Endocrinology, 15*(10), 601–614. https://doi.org/10.1038/s41574-019-0224-4

Gregory, J., Cameron, F. J., Joshi, K., Eiswirth, M., Garrett, C., Garvey, K., Agarwal, S., & Codner, E. (2022). ISPAD Clinical Practice Consensus Guidelines 2022: Diabetes in adolescence. *Pediatric Diabetes, 23*, 857–871. https://doi.org/10.1111/pedi.13408

Gutierrez-Colina, A. M., Corathers, S., Beal, S., Baugh, H., Nause, K., & Kichler, J. C. (2020). Young adults with type 1 diabetes preparing to transition to adult care: Psychosocial functioning and associations with self-management and health outcomes. *Diabetes Spectrum, 33*(3), 255–263. https://doi.org/10.2337/ds19-0050

Hamdan, M. A., Gomez, R., & Chalew, S. A. (2020). Mean blood glucose-independent HbA1c racial disparity and iron status in youth with type 1 DM. *Pediatric Diabetes, 21*(4), 615–620. https://doi.org/10.1111/pedi.13002

He, Q.-X., Zhao, L., Tong, J.-S., Liang, X.-Y., Li, R.-N., Zhang, P., & Liang, X.-H. (2022). The impact of obesity epidemic on type 2 diabetes in children and adolescents: A systematic review and meta-analysis. *Primary Care Diabetes, 16*(6), 736–744. https://doi.org/10.1016/j.pcd.2022.09.006

Hemesath, T. P., de Paula, L. C. P., Carvalho, C. G., Leite, J. C. L., Guaragna-Filho, G., & Costa, E. C. (2019). Controversies on timing of sex assignment and surgery in individuals with disorders of sex development: A perspective. *Frontiers in Pediatrics, 6*, 419. https:doi.org/10.3389/fped.2018.00419

Jordan, T. L., Klabunde, M., Green, T., Hong, D. S., Ross, J. L., Jo, B., & Reiss, A. L. (2023). Longitudinal investigation of cognition, social competence, and anxiety in children and adolescents with Turner syndrome. *Hormones and Behavior, 149*, 105300. https://doi.org/10.1016/j.yhbeh.2022.105300

Karter, A. J., Parker, M. M., Moffet, H., & Gilliam, L. (2023). Racial and ethnic differences in the association between mean glucose and hemoglobin A1c. *Diabetes Technology & Therapeutics, 25*(10), 697–704. https://doi.org/10.1089/dia.2023.0153

Kecskemeti, K. L., & Reis-Dennis, S. (2021). The ethics of elective growth hormone therapy in children with idiopathic short stature. *Journal of Clinical Ethics, 32*(3), 206–214. https://doi.org/10.1086/jce2021323206

Klein, K. O., & Phillips, S. A. (2019). Review of hormone replacement therapy in girls and adolescents with hypogonadism. *Journal of Pediatric and Adolescent Gynecology, 32*(5), 460–468. https://doi.org/10.1016/j.jpag.2019.04.010

Libman, I., Haynes, A., Lyons, S., Pradeep, P., Rwagasor, E., Tung, J. Y.-L., Jefferies, C. A., Oram, R. A., Dabelea, D., & Craig, M. E. (2022). ISPAD Clinical Practice Consensus Guidelines 2022: Definition, epidemiology, and classification of diabetes in children and adolescents. *Pediatric Diabetes, 23*(8), 1160–1174. https://doi.org/10.1111/pedi.13454

Maxwell, A. R., Jones, N.-H. Y., Taylor, S., Corathers, S. D., Rasnick, E., Brokamp, C., Riley, C. L., Parsons, A., Kichler, J. C., & Beck, A. F. (2021). Socioeconomic and racial disparities in diabetic ketoacidosis admissions in youth with type 1 diabetes. *Journal of Hospital Medicine, 16*(9), 517–523. https://doi.org/10.12788/jhm.3664

McDowell, M. E., Litchman, M. L., & Guo, J. (2020). The transition experiences of adolescents with type 1 diabetes from paediatric to adult care providers. *Child: Care, Health & Development, 46*(6), 692–702. https://doi.org/10.1111/cch.12798

Murata, Y., Takita, M., & Kami, M. (2022). Closed-loop control in very young children with type 1 diabetes. *The New England Journal of Medicine, 386*(15), 1482. https://doi.org/10.1056/NEJMc2202163

Nagasaki, K., Minamitani, K., Nakamura, A., Kobayashi, H., Numakura, C., Itoh, M., Mushimoto, Y., Fujikura, K., Fukushi, M., & Tajima, T. (2023). Guidelines for newborn screening of congenital hypothyroidism (2021 revision). *Clinical Pediatric Endocrinology, 32*(1), 26–51. https://doi.org/10.1297/cpe.2022-0063

Ortiz La Banca, R., Pirahanchi, Y., Volkening, L. K., Guo, Z., Cartaya, J., & Laffel, L. M. (2021). Blood glucose monitoring (BGM) still matters for many: Associations of BGM frequency and glycemic control in youth with type 1 diabetes. *Primary Care Diabetes, 15*(5), 832–836. https://doi.org/10.1016/j.pcd.2021.05.006

Shah, A. S., Nadeau, K. J., Dabelea, D., & Redondo, M. J. (2022). Spectrum of phenotypes and causes of type 2 diabetes in children. *Annual Review of Medicine, 73*, 501–515. https://doi.org/10.1146/annurev-med-042120-012033

Shah, A. S., Zeitler, P. S., Wong, J., Pena, A. S., Wicklow, B., Arslanian, S., Chang, N., Fu, J., Dabadghao, P., Pinhas, H. O., Urakami, T., & Craig, M. E. (2022). ISPAD Clinical Practice Consensus Guidelines 2022: Type 2 diabetes in children and adolescents. *Pediatric Diabetes, 23*(7), 872–902. https://doi.org/10.1111/pedi.13409

Sherr, J. L., Schoelwer, M., Dos Santos, T. J., Reddy, L., Biester, T., Galderisi, A., van Dyk, J. C., Hilliard, M. E., Berget, C., & DiMeglio, L. A. (2022). ISPAD Clinical Practice Consensus Guidelines 2022: Diabetes technologies: Insulin delivery. *Pediatric Diabetes, 23*(8), 1406–1431. https://doi.org/10.1111/pedi.13421

Silva, C. T., & Navarro, O. M. (2020). Pearls and pitfalls in pediatric thyroid imaging. *Seminars in Ultrasound, CT, and MR, 41*(5), 421–432. https://doi.org/10.1053/j.sult.2020.05.007

Taraban, L., Wasserman, R., Cao, V. T., Eshtehardi, S. S., Anderson, B. J., Thompson, D., Marrero, D. G., & Hilliard, M. E. (2022). Diabetes-related worries and coping among youth and young adults with type 1 diabetes. *Journal of Pediatric Psychology, 47*(10), 1145–1155. https://doi.org/10.1093/jpepsy/jsac055

Tauschmann, M., Forlenza, G., Hood, K., Cardona-Hernandez, R., Giani, E., Hendrieckx, C., DeSalvo, D. J., Laffel, L. M., Saboo, B., Wheeler, B. J., Latpev, D. N., Yarhere, I., & DiMeglio, L. A. (2022). ISPAD Clinical Practice Consensus Guidelines 2022: Diabetes technologies: Glucose monitoring. *Pediatric Diabetes, 23*(8), 1390–1405. https://doi.org/10.1111/pedi.13451

Zimmerman, J. J., & Rotta, A. T. (2021). *Fuhrman & Zimmerman's pediatric critical care e-book*. Elsevier Health Sciences.

47
Pediatric Oncology*

PEDIATRIC ONCOLOGIC DISORDERS

EVIDENCE BASE American Cancer Society. (2023). *Cancer facts and figures.* https://www.cancer.org/cancer/cancer-in-children/key-statistics.html

Cancer is the leading cause of death from disease in children under the age of 15 years. Cancer incidence in the United States among children aged 1 to 14 years has slightly increased over the past few decades, with an estimated 9,620 new cases predicted in 2024. Cancer deaths have declined over the past few decades; approximately 1,050 children were expected to die from disease in 2022. In the mid-1970s, the 5-year survival rate for pediatric cancer was 58%, but major treatment advances have improved the 5-year overall survival rate to 85%. It is important to note that long-term sequelae from treatment often lead to chronic, lifelong health issues for childhood cancer survivors. In fact, 50% to 75% of pediatric cancer survivors have at least one chronic medical condition or disability that directly resulted from their cancer treatment. There are few known risk factors for childhood cancer; however, the incidence of specific cancers is related to age, gender, ethnic background, and geographical region.

Common types of cancer in children (in order of frequency) include leukemia (the most common types being acute lymphocytic leukemia [ALL] and acute myeloid leukemia [AML]); brain and central nervous system (CNS) cancers are the second most common, followed by lymphoma, neuroblastoma, Wilms tumor, rhabdomyosarcoma (RMS) osteosarcoma, retinoblastoma, and bone cancer. Childhood cancers are treated with surgery, radiation, chemotherapy, blood and marrow transplant, immunotherapy, and gene therapy.

Cancers in adolescents (15 to 19 years) differ somewhat from those in younger children in terms of type and distribution. For example, brain and other nervous system tumors (21%) and lymphoma (20%) are equally common. Leukemia is the third, followed by germ cell and gonadal tumors and thyroid carcinoma.

Acute Lymphocytic Leukemia

EVIDENCE BASE Brown, P., Inaba, H., Annesley, C., Beck, J., Colace, S., Dallas, M., DeSantes, K., Kelly, K., Kitko, C., Lacayo, N., Larrier, N., Maese, L., Mahadeo, K., Nanda, R., Nardi, V., Rodriguez, V., Rossoff, J., Schuettpelz, L., Silverman, L., ... Ogba, N. (2020). Pediatric acute lymphoblastic leukemia, version 2.2020, NCCN clinical practice guidelines in oncology. *Journal of the National Comprehensive Cancer Network, 18*(1), 81–112.

ALL is a primary disorder of the bone marrow in which the normal marrow elements are replaced by immature or undifferentiated blast cells. When the quantity of normal marrow is depleted below the level necessary to maintain peripheral blood elements within normal ranges, anemia, neutropenia, and thrombocytopenia occur. ALL is the most common malignancy in children, representing 75% to 80% of acute leukemias in children. The median age at diagnosis is 15 years. The age-adjusted incidence of ALL (ages 0 to 19 years) within the United States is 3.5 per 100,000 individuals per year; almost 6,000 new cases were estimated in 2023. The use of allogeneic stem cell transplantation, improved understanding of molecular genetics, new targeted and immunotherapy agents (see Table 47-1), as well as risk-adapted therapy are credited with an improved 5-year overall survival rate of 89%. It is more common among White and Hispanic children and is more common in males than in females.

Pathophysiology and Etiology

1. The exact cause of ALL is unknown.
2. Environmental factors, as well as genetic factors and chromosomal anomalies, are suspected in some cases.

TABLE 47-1 Immunotherapeutic Agents Used in Pediatric Cancer

IMMUNOTHERAPEUTIC AGENT	COMMON SIDE EFFECTS
Monoclonal Antibodies	
Blinatumomab Rituximab	Cytokine release syndrome: low blood pressure, capillary leak with pleural or cardiac effusions
Targeted Therapy	
Imatinib Dasatinib	Bone marrow suppression Cardiac dysfunction Fluid retention
CAR T cell (tisagenlecleucel)	Life-threatening cytokine release syndrome

*Please note that the term "male" in this chapter refers to a person assigned male at birth, and the term "female" in this chapter refers to a person assigned female at birth.

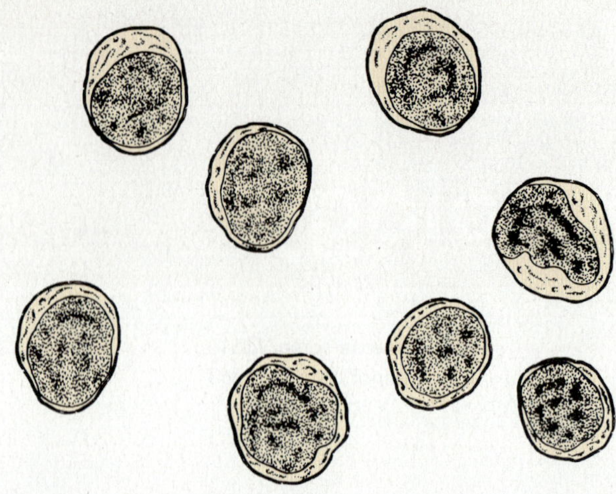

Figure 47-1. Abnormal lymphoblast in acute lymphocytic leukemia.

3. ALL results from the growth of an abnormal type of nongranular, fragile leukocyte in the blood-forming tissues, particularly in the bone marrow, spleen, and lymph nodes.
4. The abnormal lymphoblast has little cytoplasm and a round, homogeneous nucleus (see Figure 47-1).
5. ALL is classified according to the cell type involved: T-lymphoblastic leukemia or B-lymphoblastic leukemia.
6. Normal bone marrow elements may be displaced or replaced in this type of leukemia.
7. The changes in the blood and bone marrow result from the accumulation of leukemic cells and from the deficiency of normal cells.
   a. Red blood cell (RBC) precursors and megakaryocytes from which platelets are formed are decreased, causing anemia, prolonged and unusual bleeding, tendency to bruise easily, and petechiae.
   b. Normal white blood cells (WBCs) are significantly decreased, predisposing the child to infection.
   c. The bone marrow is hyperplastic, with a uniform appearance caused by leukemic cells.
8. Leukemic cells may infiltrate into lymph nodes, spleen, and liver, causing diffuse adenopathy and hepatosplenomegaly.
9. Expansion of marrow or infiltration of leukemic cells into bone causes bone and joint pain.
10. Invasion of the CNS by leukemic cells may cause headache, vomiting, cranial nerve palsies, convulsions, coma, papilledema, and blurred or double vision.
11. Weight loss, muscle wasting, and fatigue may occur when the body cells are deprived of nutrients because of the immense metabolic needs of the proliferating leukemic cells.

Clinical Manifestations

1. Manifestations depend on the degree to which the bone marrow has been compromised and the location and extent of extramedullary infiltration.
2. Presenting symptoms:
   a. Fatigability.
   b. General malaise, listlessness.
   c. Persistent fever of unknown cause.
   d. Recurrent infection.
   e. Petechiae, purpura, and ecchymosis after minor trauma.
   f. Pallor.
   g. Generalized lymphadenopathy.
   h. Abdominal pain caused by organomegaly.
   i. Bone and joint pain.
   j. Headache and vomiting (with CNS involvement).
3. Presenting symptoms may be either isolated or in any combination or sequence.

Diagnostic Evaluation

1. May have altered peripheral blood counts. Blood studies may show the following:
   a. Low hemoglobin level, RBC count, hematocrit, and platelet count.
   b. Decreased, elevated, or normal WBC count.
2. Bone marrow examination and stained peripheral smear examination show large numbers of lymphoblasts and lymphocytes.
3. Lumbar puncture to assess for lymphoblasts in CNS to determine CNS involvement.
4. Renal and liver function studies determine contraindications or precautions for chemotherapy.
5. Chest x-ray determines whether a mediastinal mass or pneumonia is present.
6. Varicella and cytomegalovirus titer determine the risk of infection.
7. The CNS and testes are sites of "sanctuary"; CNS surveillance and treatment are standard, and testes are evaluated with physical examinations.
8. Tumor cytogenetics—a laboratory study of the arrangement of chromosomes that looks for mutations, rearrangements, and missing or broken chromosomes—influences whether biological therapy is indicated.

Management

1. Supportive therapy is indicated to control disease complications, such as hyperuricemia, electrolyte imbalance, infection, anemia, bleeding, pain, nausea/vomiting, and fatigue.
2. Specific therapy is warranted to eradicate malignant cells and to restore normal marrow function.
3. Chemotherapy is used to achieve complete remission, with restoration of normal peripheral blood and physical findings; it is administered through an indwelling central catheter or implantable port (see Table 47-2).
4. Biological (or immunotherapeutic) agents may be used in patients with certain types of cytogenetic anomalies and/or in patients with relapsed disease (see Tables 47-1 and 47-2).
5. Although no universally accepted standard therapy for the treatment of children with ALL exists, most facilities have similar protocols that use a combination of drugs.
6. Components of therapy:
   a. Induction, the initial course of therapy designed to achieve complete remission, usually lasts 4 to 6 weeks. For those who do not achieve complete remission by the end of induction therapy, an allogeneic bone marrow transplant is usually pursued. Induction usually includes a combination of vincristine, L-asparaginase, and corticosteroids. A fourth drug, such as daunorubicin, doxorubicin, or cytosine arabinoside, may be added.
   b. Consolidation treatment, a period of intensified treatment immediately after remission induction, attempts total eradication of residual leukemic cells. Consolidation treatment usually lasts approximately 6 to 9 months but can vary in length based on different protocols. It usually includes

TABLE 47-2 Commonly Used Chemotherapeutic and Biotherapy Agents to Treat Acute Lymphocytic Leukemia

CHEMOTHERAPEUTIC AGENT	COMMON SIDE EFFECTS
Asparaginase	Pain at injection site Allergic reaction Increased plasma ammonia level Clotting factor anomalies Fatigue, weakness Diarrhea
Cytarabine	Nausea, vomiting Fever Headache
Methotrexate	Nausea, vomiting Headache Elevated liver enzymes Mucositis Nephrotoxicity
Vincristine	Hair loss Neuropathy Constipation
Daunorubicin Doxorubicin	Nausea, vomiting Hair loss Red urine Bone marrow suppression Cardiac dysfunction
Cytoxan	Nausea, vomiting Hair loss Loss of appetite Gonadal dysfunction Bone marrow suppression Nephrotoxicity
Mercaptopurine	Bone marrow suppression
Thioguanine	Bone marrow suppression

a combination of methotrexate, 6-mercaptopurine, etoposide, thioguanine, cytosine arabinoside, cyclophosphamide, prednisone, vincristine, L-asparaginase, and doxorubicin or daunorubicin.

c. Maintenance or continuation therapy is the final and often longest stage of treatment in childhood ALL. The goal of maintenance therapy is to lower the risk of relapse once remission has been achieved and typically lasts 2 to 3 years. Males may require longer maintenance therapy to prevent testicular relapse. It usually includes daily oral administration of 6-mercaptopurine and weekly oral administration of methotrexate with intermittent administration of other drugs, such as monthly vincristine, corticosteroids, cyclophosphamide, cytosine arabinoside, or daunorubicin.
d. Reinduction therapy induces remission if relapse occurs and may include new agents along with some of the same initial drugs.
e. If testicular relapse occurs, along with systemic chemotherapy, either radiation therapy to the testicles is administered or orchiectomy is performed.
f. CNS disease prophylaxis generally consists of intrathecal administration of methotrexate, hydrocortisone, and/or cytarabine in combination with systemic therapy that can cross the blood–brain barrier. Craniospinal irradiation may also be used to treat CNS disease.
g. The role of allogeneic hematopoietic stem cell transplant (HSCT) is considered for those patients with a very high risk of relapse and/or treatment failure. Components of this therapy may include total body irradiation (TBI) in combination with chemotherapy and immunotherapy agents followed by stem cell transplant from a matched sibling or alternative donor source. Other donor sources include matched or closely matched unrelated donor and haploidentical (half-matched) familial donor.

7. Current standards of treatment are designed on risk-based criteria; patients with worse prognostic indicators receive more intensive therapy.
8. Blood and marrow transplantation has been used successfully to treat children who fail to respond to conventional treatment.
9. Biological therapy including, but not limited to, blinatumomab, imatinib, and dasatinib are Food and Drug Administration (FDA) approved for the treatment of some types of ALL. Many other biotherapy agents are being tested in clinical trials in pediatrics. (See "Immunotherapy" section in Chapter 4 for further information about types of immunotherapy.) Participation in clinical trials has been instrumental in the improved success of clinical outcomes for pediatric patients with oncologic conditions and will continue to be crucial in consideration for optimal care.

DRUG ALERT Assess the patient and monitor vital signs after administration of asparaginase-type drugs for signs of anaphylaxis. Have emergency drugs and equipment at the bedside (oxygen, epinephrine, antihistamines, and steroids). If administering in the outpatient setting, observe the patients for at least 1 hour.

Prognosis

1. At least 98% of children with ALL are expected to achieve an initial remission if treated in a specialized facility.
2. Overall 5-year survival is 90%.
3. The prognosis becomes poorer with each relapse the child experiences.
4. Relapse is rare after 7 years from diagnosis.
5. Factors associated with prognosis:
   a. Initial WBC count (WBC count greater than 50,000 has worse prognosis).
   b. Age (younger than age 1 year and older than 10 years have a poorer prognosis).
   c. Extramedullary involvement (poorer prognosis).
   d. Leukemia subtype (cytogenetic/genetic and immunophenotypic features).
   f. Response to initial therapy (failed induction confers poorer prognosis).

Complications

1. Infection—most frequently occurs in the blood, lungs, gastrointestinal (GI) tract, or skin. Patients with central lines are at increased risk.
2. Hemorrhage—caused by thrombocytopenia.
3. Hepatic dysfunction, which may be transient or chronic
4. CNS complications, such as stroke, seizure, and neuropathies.
5. Testicular involvement and treatment, which may lead to sub- or absent fertility.

6. Renal dysfunction (rarely seen, except in induction).
7. Acute complications of treatment (e.g., cardiomyopathy).
8. Late effects of treatment (treatment specific). Most frequent long-term complication is neurocognitive dysfunction causing school difficulty.

Nursing Assessment

1. Obtain a history.
   a. When taking the history, focus on symptoms that led to the diagnosis and previous symptoms for the past 2 weeks. For example, inquire about fatigue, headache, nausea, vomiting, pallor, bleeding, pain, or fever.
   b. Ask about past history of varicella zoster infection (chickenpox), which could lead to disseminated infection if acquired during immunosuppression. Also ask about recent exposures, including sibling exposures.
2. Perform a physical examination, including:
   a. Examination of skin for petechiae, purpura, and ecchymosis.
   b. Palpation of lymph nodes for enlargement, tenderness, and mobility.
   c. Palpation of spleen and liver for enlargement.
   d. Inspection of skin for areas of infection, including indwelling catheter sites and perineal area.
   e. Auscultation of lungs for crackles or rhonchi, indicative of pneumonia.
   f. Temperature for fever.
   g. Testicular examination for enlargement, unilateral or bilateral.
3. Assess family coping mechanisms and use of resources, such as support systems.

CLINICAL JUDGMENT Report changes in behavior or personality, persistent nausea, vomiting, headache, lethargy, irritability, dizziness, ataxia, convulsions, or alterations in state of consciousness. These may be signs of CNS disease or relapse. CNS relapse is usually detected during routine lumbar puncture.

Nursing Interventions

Decreasing Parental Caregiver Anxiety

1. Be available to the parental caregivers when they want to discuss their feelings.
2. Offer kindness, concern, consideration, and sincerity toward the child and parental caregivers; be a source of consolation.
3. Contact the family's clergyman or the hospital chaplain.
4. Obtain the services of a social worker, as appropriate, to help the family use appropriate community resources.
5. Provide information about treatment and expected side effects in a realistic yet hopeful manner.
6. Have parental caregivers speak with parental caregivers of a child currently on therapy.
7. Encourage parental caregivers to participate in activities of daily living to help them feel a part of their child's care.
8. Assess family dynamics and coping mechanisms and plan interventions accordingly.
9. Help the parental caregivers to deal with anticipatory grief.
10. Help the parental caregivers to deal with other family members and friends.
11. Encourage the parental caregivers to discuss concerns about limiting their child's activities, protecting the child from infection, disciplining the child, and having anxieties about the illness.
12. Facilitate communication with the clinic nurse or clinical specialist who may interact with the child during the entire course of illness.
13. Provide realistic expectations about continuing established family patterns, including school attendance, social life, and family activities, as medically indicated.

Preventing Infection and Hemorrhage

EVIDENCE BASE Ardura, M., Bibart, M., Mayer, L., Guinipero, T., Stanek, J., Olshefski, R. S., & Auletta, J. J. (2021). Impact of a best practice prevention bundle on Central Line-Associated Bloodstream Infection (CLABSI) rates and outcomes in pediatric hematology, oncology, and hematopoietic cell transplantation patients in inpatient and ambulatory settings. *Journal of Hematology/Oncology, 43*(1), e64–e72.

1. Monitor complete blood count (CBC), and administer blood products as ordered.
2. Provide adequate hydration.
   a. Oral and enteral hydration is preferred.
   b. Maintain parenteral fluids when indicated.
3. Observe renal function carefully.
   a. Measure and record urine output.
   b. Observe the urine for evidence of gross bleeding.
   c. Obtain urinalysis to assess for microscopic hematuria, specific gravity, and pH.
   d. Monitor weight daily for signs of fluid overload.
4. Protect the child from infection sources.
   a. Never use a rectal thermometer, suppositories, or enemas when caring for a patient with neutropenia.
   b. Family, friends, personnel, and other patients who have infections should not visit or care for the child. Discuss care of siblings while the child is on therapy.
   c. Private rooms are preferred, but if it is necessary to share, do not place a child with an infection in the same room with a child with leukemia.
   d. Good handwashing is the most effective way to prevent infection.
   e. Encourage family members and close contacts to receive influenza and coronavirus disease 2019 (COVID-19) vaccinations.
   f. Ensure strict adherence to central line maintenance bundles including recommendations for use of personal protective equipment (PPE), dressing/cap changes, personal hygiene, and environmental measures.
5. Observe the child closely and be alert for signs of impending infection.
   a. Observe broken skin or mucous membrane for signs of infection.
   b. Report fever of more than 100.4°F (38°C).
   c. Assess central line site for redness, drainage, or tenderness.
6. Administer growth factors, such as granulocyte colony–stimulating factor, to stimulate the production of neutrophils and to decrease the incidence of severe infections in the child after high-dose chemotherapy.
7. Administer preemptive and treatment intravenous (IV) antibiotics, antivirals, and antifungals.
8. Administer *Pneumocystis jirovecii* pneumonia (PJP) prophylaxis such as cotrimoxazole, if ordered, twice daily three times per week to prevent infection with *P. jirovecii*. (For patients unable to take cotrimoxazole, dapsone and pentamidine may also be given.)

9. Record vital signs and report changes such as the following, which may indicate infection:
   a. Tachycardia.
   b. Lowered blood pressure (BP).
   c. Pallor.
   d. Diaphoresis.
   e. Increasing anxiety and restlessness.
10. Observe for GI bleeding and test all emesis and stool for blood.
11. Move and turn the child gently because hemarthrosis may occur and may cause pain.
   a. Handle the child in a gentle manner.
   b. Turn the child frequently to prevent pressure injuries.
   c. Place the child in proper body alignment in a comfortable position.
   d. Allow the child to be out of bed in a chair if this position is more comfortable.
   e. Encourage the child to ambulate, when possible.
12. Avoid intramuscular (IM) injections, if possible; if not possible, ensure platelet count has been obtained prior to injection and hold direct pressure to the area for at least 5 minutes.
13. Handle catheters and drainage and suction tubes carefully to prevent mucosal bleeding.
14. Protect the child from injury by monitoring activities and exposure to environmental hazards, such as slippery floors or uneven surfaces.
15. Be aware of emergency procedures for control of bleeding:
   a. Apply local pressure carefully so as not to interfere with clot formation.
   b. Administer leukocyte-poor, irradiated, packed RBCs and platelets, as ordered.
   c. If epistaxis occurs, apply pressure to the bridge of the nose; may require ENT consult to pack the affected nares if bleeding does not cease within 5 minutes.

CLINICAL JUDGMENT Patients with low WBC count may not respond to infection with usual signs and symptoms (i.e., fever and purulent drainage from infected wound). Monitor closely for subtle changes in vital signs that may indicate hemodynamic instability.

Promoting Acceptance of Body Changes

1. Prepare the patient for potential changes in body image (alopecia, weight loss, muscle wasting) and help the child cope with related feelings.
2. Engage child life therapist for medical play and support.
3. Contact the school nurse and teacher to help them prepare for the child's return to school. Discuss the bodily changes that have occurred and that may happen in the future.

Promoting Optimal Nutrition

EVIDENCE BASE 2022. Ringwald-Smith, K., Hill, R., Evanoff, L., Martin, J., & Sacks, N. (2022). When reality and research collide: Guidelines are essential for optimal nutrition care in pediatric oncology. *Journal of Pediatric Hematology/Oncology, 44*(1), e144–e151.

1. Provide a highly nutritious diet as tolerated by the child.
   a. Consult registered dietician to develop and implement nutrition care plans
   b. Determine the child's food likes and dislikes.
   c. Offer frequent, small meals.
   d. Offer high-calorie, high-protein supplemental feedings.
   e. Encourage the parental caregivers to assist at mealtime.
   f. Avoid foods high in salt while the child is taking steroids.
   g. Administer enteral and parenteral feeds, as ordered.
   h. Administer appetite stimulants and oral supplements.
2. Give careful oral hygiene; the gums and mucous membranes of the mouth may bleed easily.
   a. Use a soft toothbrush.
   b. If the child's mouth is bleeding or painful, clean the teeth and mouth with a moistened cotton swab or sponge-tipped swab.
   c. Use a nonirritating rinse for the mouth (no alcohol-containing mouthwash).
   d. Apply nonpetroleum lip balm to dry, cracked lips.
   e. Assess for mucositis and provide pain medication when indicated.
   f. To reduce the incidence of mucositis, implement cryotherapy for chemotherapy infusions, such as melphalan, busulfan, and methotrexate.
3. Be alert for nausea and vomiting; review patients' past experiences.
   a. Administer antiemetic drugs on a round-the-clock, regular schedule (e.g., serotonin antagonist, histamine blockers, dexamethasone).
   b. Become knowledgeable about chemotherapeutic agents and adjust antiemetic therapy for those drugs with delayed nausea and vomiting (cisplatin).
   c. Monitor strict intake and output and obtain daily weight.
   d. Maintain parenteral fluid administration and assess for signs of dehydration or fluid overload.
   e. Administer antiemetic drugs for patients who receive chemotherapy and/or radiation to the chest, abdomen, pelvis, or craniospinal axis.
   d. Suggest relaxation techniques or guided imagery for patients who experience anticipatory nausea and vomiting.

Relieving Pain

EVIDENCE BASE Uhl, K., Burns, M., Hale, A., & Coakley, R. (2020). The critical role of parents in pediatric cancer-related pain management: A review and call to action. *Current Oncology Reports, 22*(4), 37. https://doi.org/10.1007/s11912-020-0899-7

1. Position the child for comfort.
2. Assess the child's pain using a developmentally appropriate pain scale at regular intervals.
3. Administer drugs on a preventive schedule before pain becomes intense. Continuous infusion pumps for opioid administration are commonly used.
4. Prepare the child for treatment and diagnostic procedures.
   a. Use knowledge of growth and development to prepare the child for procedures such as central line insertion, bone marrow aspirations, spinal taps, blood transfusions, and chemotherapy.
   b. Provide a means for talking about the experience. Play, storytelling, or role-playing may be helpful.
   c. Convey to the child that it is acceptable for them to express fear and anger.
   d. Use anesthetic cream at spinal tap, injection, and bone marrow sites to decrease pain.
   e. Administer conscious sedation before procedures and monitor pulse, BP, respirations, and pulse oximetry during and after procedures.

5. Implement complementary and alternative medicine (CAM) interventions for pain control as well as for the management of side effects and anxiety. Include parental caregivers in developing mind–body pain modulation skills to help reduce their own distress as well as that of their child. CAM strategies include the following:
   a. Hypnosis/self-hypnosis.
   b. Imagery.
   c. Distraction/relaxation techniques.
   d. Cognitive-behavioral therapy.
   e. Music therapy.
   f. Massage.

Conserving Energy

1. Assess the child's energy level and space needed for activities accordingly. Allow the child to rest, if necessary.
2. Encourage the child to limit strenuous activity after diagnostic procedures.

Reducing the Child's Anxiety

1. Provide for continuity of care.
2. Encourage family-centered care.
3. Facilitate play activities for the child and use opportunities to communicate through play.
4. Maintain some discipline, placing calm limitations on unacceptable behavior.
5. Provide appropriate diversional activities.
6. Encourage independence and provide opportunities that allow the child to control their environment.
7. Explain the diagnosis and treatment in age-appropriate terms.

Community and Home Care Considerations

EVIDENCE BASE Roug, L., Jarden, M., Wahlberg, A., Hjalgrim, L. L., & Hansson, H. (2023). Ambiguous expectations of parent caregiving for the child and adolescent with cancer at the hospital and at home—An ethnographic study. *Journal of Pediatric Hematology/Oncology*, *40*(2), 100–110.

1. Begin to develop a home care plan before the child leaves the hospital.
2. Communicate with health care provider, hospital nurses, family, and others familiar with the case to gather information about the child's illness, treatment plan, and specific needs in the home.
3. Arrange schedule for blood draws and how results will be managed.
4. Contact the child's school and arrange a meeting with the school nurse, principal, appropriate teachers, and other relevant school personnel to explain child's diagnosis, treatment, and potential time away from school.
5. Discuss with patient the possibility of making a visit to the classroom; explain about cancer and the adverse effects of chemotherapy to facilitate school reentry in a manner that would be understood by classmates.
6. Collaborate with primary care provider regarding immunization schedule and the contraindication for children on immunosuppressive therapy.
7. Make sure that parental caregivers can demonstrate the proper technique for care of venous access, such as dressing changes, flushing, and assessing for infection.
8. Ensure parental caregivers receive education for home medications, including medication schedule, side effects, and indications for scheduled and as-needed (PRN) medications.

Family Education and Health Maintenance

1. Teach parental caregivers about normal CBC values and expected variations caused by therapy.
2. Instruct parental caregivers about leukemia and adverse effects of chemotherapy.
3. Tell parental caregivers to call the health care provider if the child has a fever of more than 100.4°F (38°C), which may indicate overwhelming infection and impending septic shock, bleeding, and signs of infection. Parental caregivers should also immediately report if the child has been exposed to chickenpox. Immunosuppressed children are in danger of developing disseminated varicella and may be treated prophylactically with varicella immune globulin.
4. Teach preventive measures, such as handwashing and isolation from children with communicable diseases, screening of home visitors for viral illness.
5. Reinforce that parental caregivers are *never* to use a rectal thermometer.
6. Provide parental caregivers with a list of support agencies that may be helpful; include both local resources and national organizations.

Evaluation: Expected Outcomes

1. Parental caregivers discuss their feelings about the child's diagnosis and treatment.
2. Remains afebrile, no signs of localized infection or bleeding.
3. Maintains a positive body image.
4. Eats or is provided enough calories to maintain weight.
5. Experiences relief from pain (no crying or expression of pain).
6. Rests at intervals.
7. Acts out feelings in play; participates in age-appropriate activities.

Brain Tumors in Children

EVIDENCE BASE PDQ® Pediatric Treatment Editorial Board. (2022). *PDQ childhood astrocytomas treatment*. National Cancer Institute. Retrieved January 15, 2023, from https://www.cancer.gov/types/brain/hp/child-astrocytoma-treament-pdq

Brain tumors are abnormal and uncontrollable growth of cells in the brain. Approximately 25% of the malignant tumors that occur in children are brain tumors, with an incidence rate according to the National Cancer Institute of 3.2 per 100,000 children aged 0 to 19 years. Tumors occurring in the CNS are the most common cause of death from childhood cancers. Of the children who do survive a brain tumor, approximately 60% will be left with a life-altering disability. Four main types of brain tumors appear in children. Glial cell tumors, including *astrocytoma* and *diffuse pontine glioma*, can grow at any location in the brain and account for approximately 30% to 40% of all pediatric brain tumors. *Medulloblastoma* is a type of embryonal tumor, which is highly malignant and rapidly growing, usually found in the cerebellum. Embryonal tumors are the most common tumors of the CNS in children. *Ependymoma* is a tumor derived from the ependyma or lining of the central canal of the spinal cord and cerebral ventricles. It frequently arises on the floor of the fourth ventricle, causing obstruction of the flow of cerebrospinal fluid (CSF). Ependymomas represent approximately 5% to 10% of all primary childhood CNS tumors. *Germ cell tumors* are midline tumors typically diagnosed in children aged 6 to 14 years with a higher incidence in parts of Asia, specifically Japan.

Pathophysiology and Etiology

1. The etiology of brain tumors is unknown. Triggers that are found to be associated with an increased risk of brain tumors include certain genetic syndromes and environmental factors.
2. Symptoms are associated with the location of the tumor, size of the tumor, rate of growth, and chronological and developmental age of the child.
3. Astrocytoma typically present in the infratentorial region, producing increased intracranial pressure (ICP). It is classified according to its malignancy, from grade I (least malignant) to grade IV (most malignant). More than 80% of astrocytoma located in the cerebellum are low grade I. Surgery and radiation are the primary therapies.
4. Medulloblastoma grows rapidly and produces evidence of increased ICP progressing during several weeks. It is classified as standard risk or high risk depending on tumor histology. Combination therapy of surgery, radiation, and chemotherapy is usually required.
5. Germ cell tumors grow in the midline of the brain and the majority present in the suprasellar or pineal regions. The growth rate varies, but frequently, symptoms precede diagnosis by several months.
6. Ependymomas grow with varying speed. Because of location, tumors can invade the cardiorespiratory center, cerebellum, and spinal cord. They are graded according to the degree of differentiation.

Clinical Manifestations

Glial Cell Tumors

Onset and growth are related to stage of tumor.

1. Evidence of increased ICP—especially ataxia, vomiting, or headache.
2. Cerebellar signs—ataxia, dysmetria (inability to control the range of muscular movement), and nystagmus.
3. Behavioral changes.
4. Seizures.
5. Precocious puberty.
6. Vision and hearing problems.

Medulloblastoma

Fast growing, malignant, and invasive.

1. The child may present with unsteady gait, anorexia, vomiting, and early morning headache.
2. May later develop ataxia, nystagmus, papilledema, drowsiness, increased head circumference, head tilt, and cranial nerve palsies. May develop obstructive hydrocephalus.

Germ Cell Tumor

Signs of midline shifts.

1. Visual disturbances.
2. Personality and sleep pattern alterations.
3. Dramatic weight loss.
4. Hydrocephalus.
5. Endocrinopathies.
6. Seizures.
7. Unusual thirst and frequent urination.

Ependymoma of the Fourth Ventricle

1. Signs of increased ICP.
   a. Nausea or vomiting.
   b. Headache.
2. Unsteady gait or ataxia; dysmetria.
3. Focal motor weakness, vision disturbances, seizures.

Diagnostic Evaluation

Determined by the type of tumor that is suspected; usually includes many or all of the following procedures to localize and determine extent of the tumor:

1. Computed tomography (CT).
2. Magnetic resonance imaging (MRI) with or without fluid-attenuated inversion recovery imaging (FLAIR)
3. Positron emission tomography (PET).
4. Lumbar puncture with CSF cytologic evaluation.
5. Angiography (occasional).

Management

1. Surgery is performed to determine the type of tumor, to assess the extent of invasiveness, and to excise as much of the lesion as possible.
2. When indicated, radiation therapy is initiated as soon as the diagnosis is established and the surgical wound is healed.
3. Chemotherapy is used to treat chemoresponsive tumors and is particularly important in children who are too young to receive radiation therapy.
4. A ventriculoperitoneal shunt is usually necessary for children who develop hydrocephalus.
5. Some immunotherapy has been approved to treat childhood brain tumors; others are being investigated for potential for future treatment.
6. Prognosis is improved in cases that involve early diagnosis and adequate therapy. Five-year survivors are increasing, especially in children with low-grade astrocytomas or ependymomas. However, there are still tumors such as diffuse intrinsic pontine glioma that have no known cure.

Complications

1. Brainstem herniation.
2. Hydrocephalus.
3. Permanent neurologic disabilities.
4. Increased risk for bone fractures.
5. Increased risk of developing other tumors later in life.

Nursing Assessment

Assess the child's neurologic status to help locate the site of the tumor and the extent of involvement as well as to identify signs of disease progression.

1. Obtain a comprehensive nursing history from the child and parental caregivers, particularly data related to normal behavioral patterns and presenting symptoms.
2. Perform portions of the neurologic examination, as appropriate. Assess muscle strength, coordination, gait, posture, and how well the senses and reflexes work.
3. Observe for the appearance or disappearance of the clinical manifestations previously described. Report these to the health care provider and record each of the following in detail:
   a. Headache—onset, beneficial and provoking factors, duration, location, severity, and impact.
   b. Vomiting—onset, amount, presence of blood, color, frequency, and foods eaten in the past 24 hours.
   c. Seizures—activity before seizure, type of seizure, areas of body involved, behavior and level of consciousness (LOC) during and after seizure, duration, changes to skin, heart rate, and respiratory status.

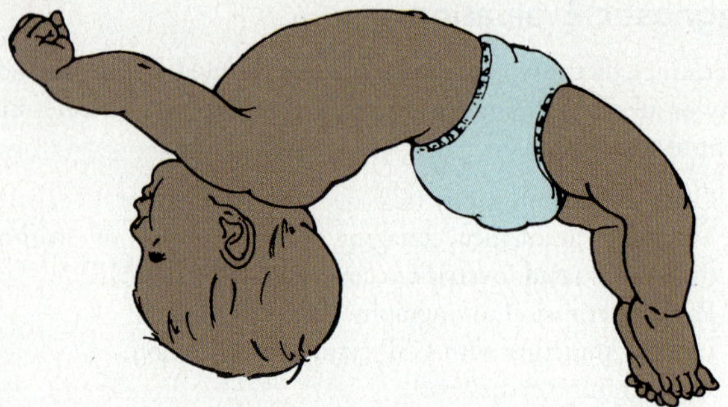

Figure 47-2. Opisthotonos, a sign of brainstem herniation.

4. Monitor vital signs frequently, including BP and pupillary reaction.
5. Monitor ocular signs. Check pupils for size, equality, reaction to light, and accommodation.
6. Observe for signs of brainstem herniation—should be considered a neurosurgical emergency. This complication occurs when brain tissue, CSF, and blood vessels are pressed or shifted from their usual position inside the skull.
   a. Abnormal posturing (opisthotonos) caused by muscle spasms (see Figure 47-2).
   b. Tilting of the head; neck stiffness.
   c. Poorly reactive and dilated pupils.
   d. Increased BP; widened pulse pressure.
   e. Change in respiratory rate and nature of respirations.
   f. Irregular or decreased pulse rate.
   g. Alterations of body temperature.

CLINICAL JUDGMENT Signs of brainstem herniation, especially opisthotonos, are ominous and considered a medical emergency. The health care provider should be called immediately, and the child should be prepared for ventricular tap to relieve pressure. Resuscitation equipment needs to be readily available.

Nursing Interventions

Reducing Parental Caregivers' Anxiety

1. Continue to keep the parental caregivers updated about their child's progress and be honest about differential diagnoses.
2. Encourage the parental caregivers to ask questions and to understand fully the risks and benefits of surgery and other interventions.
3. Prepare the parental caregivers for the postoperative appearance of their child and for the fact that the child might be comatose immediately following surgery.
4. Provide emotional support for the parental caregivers during the postoperative period. They may be frightened, shocked, anxious, and upset by the appearance of their child and by necessary emergency procedures.
5. Facilitate the return of normal parental caregiver–child relationships.
   a. The parental caregivers may be overprotective.
   b. Help the parental caregivers to see the child's increasing capabilities and clinical progression.
   c. Encourage parental caregivers to foster independence with their child.
   d. Help the parental caregiver prepare to adjust to the transition from an inpatient setting to outpatient, follow-up care.
   e. Direct the parental caregiver to services and resources that may support them with the financial costs associated with care and treatment.

EVIDENCE BASE Thornton, C., Semerjian, C., Carey, L., Milla, K., Ruble, K., Pare-Blagoev, J., & Jacobsen, L. (2023). Why psychosocial care matters: Parent preparedness and understanding predict psychosocial function when children return to school after cancer. *Journal of Pediatric Hematology/Oncology Nursing, 40*(4), 226–234.

POPULATION AWARENESS It is important for children with cancer to return to school as soon as they can because it provides them with a clear message that they have a future and the potential for full recovery. Their lives become more normal, and it allows opportunity for social interaction with peers.

Reducing the Child's Fear

1. Prepare the child for surgery in realistic terms, but at the appropriate developmental level. Involve the child life therapist and social worker in the preparation process.
2. Encourage the child to ask questions and express concerns.
3. Determine the plan regarding shaving of the child's head, bandages, and other procedures. Prepare the child accordingly.
4. Prepare the child for postoperative expectations (e.g., may feel sleepy, have a headache, will need to remain flat, and will see IV tubes, drainage tubes, and machines attached to them). Arrange visit to pediatric intensive care unit before surgery to prepare for environment.
5. Bring a comfort item (e.g., special blanket or favorite toy) for the child to have in possession postoperatively.

Reducing Pain Postoperatively

1. Administer opioids, as ordered, in the immediate postoperative period, assessing the child's LOC prior to administration as well as the child's response to opioid administration.
2. Keep the child as comfortable as possible by repositioning.
3. Apply nonpharmacologic techniques for pain management in combination with opioid administration.

Maintaining Nutritional Status

1. Allow the child to participate in the selection of foods.
2. Maintain IV hydration or hyperalimentation and intralipids, if indicated.
3. Encourage the child to eat progressively larger meals as they recover.
4. If the child cannot eat, provide tube feedings. A gastrostomy tube may be inserted.
5. Be aware that children taking steroids to decrease swelling may have increased appetite.
6. Monitor weight and laboratory values daily to ensure the efficacy of nutritional support.

Preventing Infection and Other Complications Postoperatively

1. Position the child according to surgeon's request—usually on unaffected side with head level with body.
   a. Raising the foot of the bed may increase ICP and bleeding.
   b. Post a sign above the bed, noting the exact position of the head.
2. Check the dressing for bleeding and for drainage of CSF.
3. Monitor the child's temperature closely.

a. A significant rise in temperature may be caused by trauma, disturbance of the heat-regulating center, or intracranial edema.
b. If hyperthermia occurs, administer antipyretics and use cooling techniques, as ordered. Temperature should not be reduced too rapidly.

4. Observe the child closely for signs of shock, increased ICP, seizure activity, and alterations in LOC.
5. Assess the child for edema of the head, face, and neck.
6. Carefully regulate fluid administration and BP to prevent increased cerebral edema.
7. Change the child's position frequently and provide meticulous skin care to prevent hypostatic pneumonia and pressure injuries.
   a. Move the child carefully and slowly, being certain to move the head in line with the body.
   b. Support paralyzed or spastic extremities with pillows, rolls, or other devices.
8. Have equipment readily available for cardiopulmonary resuscitation, respiratory assistance, oxygen inhalation, blood transfusion, ventricular tap, and other potential emergency situations.
9. Report fever or signs of infection.
10. If the child is receiving chemotherapy or radiation, assess for fever greater than 100.4°F (38°C) or nausea and vomiting unrelated to chemotherapy.

Promoting Acceptance of Body Changes

1. Encourage the child to express feelings regarding the threat to body image.
2. Reassure the child that a wig or a hat can be worn after recovery. Refer parental caregivers to www.locksoflove.org or www.wigsforkids.org.
3. Reassure the child that hair will grow back after surgery and chemotherapy (hair does not grow back at site of radiation therapy).
4. Prepare the child and family for cushingoid changes (moon face, edema) if long-term steroids are required.

Family Education and Health Maintenance

1. Provide parental caregivers with written information regarding the child's needs—medications, activity, care of the incision, and follow-up appointments.
2. Teach the parental caregivers about radiation and chemotherapy and their adverse effects.
3. If a child has a ventriculoperitoneal shunt, teach parental caregivers to report fever, nausea, vomiting, irritability, or a bulging anterior fontanelle.
4. Initiate a referral to a home health nurse to provide care and teaching at home and to maintain therapeutic support for the family.
5. Encourage parental caregivers to contact the child's teacher and the school nurse before the child returns to school so that they can prepare classmates for child's return and help them to deal with their feelings.
6. Provide the parental caregivers with the phone number of the clinic or nursing unit so that they may call if questions occur after discharge. For additional resources, refer family to agencies such as the American Brain Tumor Association (www.abta.org), Mikey's Way (www.mikeysway.org), Children's Tumor Foundation (www.ctf.org), The Lily Fund (www.thelilyfund.org), or Children's Oncology Group (https://childrensoncologygroup.org/patients-and-families).

Evaluation: Expected Outcomes

- Parental caregivers discuss feelings about the child's diagnosis and surgery.
- Child demonstrates decreased fear and anxiety through verbalization, play, or other age-appropriate activities.
- Child verbalizes relief from pain.
- Child maintains weight through adequate intake.
- Vital signs are stable, afebrile, and lungs are clear.
- Child verbalizes acceptance of physical appearance and desire to visit with friends.

Neuroblastoma

EVIDENCE BASE PDQ® Pediatric Treatment Editorial Board. (2022). *PDQ neuroblastoma treatment.* National Cancer Institute. Retrieved January 15, 2023, from https://www.cancer.gov/types/neuroblastoma/hp/neuroblastoma-treatment-pdq

Irwin, M. S., Naranjo, A., Zhang, F. F., Cohn, S. L., London, W. B., Gastier-Foster, J. M., Ramirez, N. C., Pfau, R., Reshmi, S., Wagner, E., Nuchtern, J., Asgharzadeh, S., Shimada, H., Maris, J. M., Bagatell, R., Park, J. R., & Hogarty, M. D. (2021). Revised neuroblastoma risk classification system: A report from the children's oncology group. *Journal of Clinical Oncology, 39*(29), 3229–3241. https://doi.org/10.1200/JCO.21.00278

Chung, C., Boterberg, T., Lucas, J., Panoff, J., Valteau-Couanet, D., Hero, B., Bagatell, R., & Hill-Kayser, C. E. (2021). Neuroblastoma. *Pediatric Blood & Cancer, 68* (Suppl 2), e28473. https://doi.org/10.1002/pbc.28473

Neuroblastoma refers to a malignant tumor that arises from the sympathetic nervous system. It is the third most common childhood cancer, with a prevalence of 1 in 7,000 children in the United States. It primarily affects infants and young children under the age of 5 years, with the highest rate of diagnosis in the first month of life. Neuroblastoma occurs slightly more frequently in males than in females and is more fatal in Black individuals.

Pathophysiology and Etiology

1. Etiology is unknown; no strong risk factors have been identified.
2. Tumors arise from embryonic neural crest cells anywhere along the craniospinal axis. A type of small, round, blue cell tumor.
3. Histologic picture varies greatly from tumor to tumor and even within the same tumor; racial differences in tumor biology.

TABLE 47-3 INRG Staging System

INRG STAGE	DEFINITION
L1	Localized disease without image-defined risk factors
L2	Localized disease with image-defined risk factors
M	Metastatic disease that does not fall into the MS category (i.e., all older patients with distant metastases)
MS	Age less than 18 mo with metastatic disease limited to liver, bone marrow, or skin

INRG, International Neuroblastoma Risk Group.

4. Tumors are staged primarily by the extent of disease according to the International Neuroblastoma Risk Group (INRG) Staging System (see Table 47-3).
5. Neuroblastoma is one of the few tumors that may demonstrate spontaneous remission.

Clinical Manifestations

1. Symptoms depend on the location of the tumor and the stage of the disease.
2. Most tumors are located within the abdomen and present as firm, nontender, irregular masses that may or may not cross the midline.
3. Other common signs:
   a. Bowel or bladder dysfunction that results from compression by a paraspinal or pelvic tumor.
   b. Neurologic symptoms, such as paralysis and Horner syndrome, because of compression by the tumor on nerve roots or because of tumor extension.
   c. Supraorbital ecchymosis, periorbital edema, and exophthalmos that results from metastases to the skull bones and retrobulbar soft tissue.
   d. Lymphadenopathy, especially in the cervical area.
   e. Bone pain with skeletal involvement.
   f. Swelling of the neck or face, wheezing, dyspnea, and cough with thoracic masses.
   g. Symptoms of bone marrow failure, such as anemia, bleeding, or infection.
   h. General symptoms of pallor, bluish skin discoloration, anorexia, fever, weight loss, and weakness with widespread metastasis.

Diagnostic Evaluation

Workup done to document the extent of the disease throughout the body include:

1. Chest and skeletal x-rays.
2. Bone scan.
3. Bone marrow aspiration and biopsy.
4. CBC, platelet count, ferritin.
5. A 24-hour urine collection—elevated excretion of homovanillic acid (HVA) and vanillylmandelic acid (VMA).
6. Liver and kidney function tests.
7. Histologic confirmation.
8. Additional studies:
   a. CT of primary site and chest.
   b. MRI—areas above diaphragm.
   c. Ultrasound examination.
   d. Liver and spleen scan.
   e. Metaiodobenzylguanidine (MIBG) scan.
9. Genetic indicators of poor prognosis include n-myc oncogene amplification, hyperdiploid karyotype, *ALK* gene alterations, and chromosome deletion.

Management

1. Management of disease varies widely by stage. When complete surgical resection of a low-risk tumor is possible, this may be the only treatment required. In contrast, high-risk disease requires treatment with induction chemotherapy, surgery, high-dose chemotherapy followed by autologous stem cell transplant, radiation, and immunotherapy including monoclonal antibody (dinutuximab) and differentiating agents (isotretinoin). These intensive treatment protocols have dramatically improved overall survival in patients with high-risk neuroblastoma.
2. Drugs of choice include vincristine, topotecan, irinotecan, cyclophosphamide, doxorubicin, cisplatin, carboplatin, ifosfamide, and etoposide (see Table 47-4). Immunotherapy includes dinutuximab and 13-*cis*-retinoic acid.
3. Overall survival rate is 75% to 85% for low-risk disease and less than 50% for high-risk disease.
4. Influencing factors for prognosis:
   a. Stage of disease—the earlier the stage, the better the prognosis.
   b. Age—infants younger than age 1 demonstrate the best survival.

TABLE 47-4 Commonly Used Chemotherapeutic and Immunotherapeutic Agents to Treat Neuroblastoma

AGENT	COMMON SIDE EFFECTS
Chemotherapeutic Agents	
Carboplatin	Nausea, vomiting Bone marrow suppression Electrolyte imbalance
Cyclophosphamide	Nausea, vomiting Hair loss Loss of appetite Gonadal dysfunction Bone marrow suppression Nephrotoxicity
Doxorubicin	Nausea, vomiting Hair loss Red urine Bone marrow suppression Cardiac dysfunction
Etoposide	Nausea, vomiting Hair loss Weakness Bone marrow suppression Nephrotoxicity Hepatotoxicity
Irinotecan	Diarrhea, abdominal cramping, runny nose, tearing, salivation, sweating, photophobia Nausea, vomiting Loss of appetite Bone marrow suppression Fever Weakness Elevated liver enzymes Elevated eosinophils
Temozolomide	Bone marrow suppression Nausea, vomiting Constipation Loss of appetite
Immunotherapeutic Agents	
Monoclonal antibody	
Dinutuximab	Cytokine release syndrome Nerve pain Hypotension
Differentiating agent	
Isotretinoin	Allergic reactions Rash Pain

c. Site of primary tumor—children with tumors above the diaphragm appear to do better than children with abdominal tumors.
d. Pattern of metastasis—children with locoregional disease have superior outcomes compared to those with distant metastasis.
e. Genetic and histologic factors.

Complications

1. Metastasis to the liver, soft tissue, bones, lymph nodes, bone marrow, and skin.
2. Neurologic deficits due to nerve compression.
3. Toxicity associated with intensive treatment, including chemotherapy, radiation, and biotherapy.

Nursing Assessment

1. Obtain a history.
   a. Inquire about when symptoms began. Focus on a decrease in appetite, weakness, pain, abdominal distention, or change in bowel and bladder function.
   b. Symptoms exhibited depend on the location of the primary tumor.
2. Perform a physical examination, including:
   a. Examination of skin for signs of increased bruising or petechiae.
   b. Palpation of liver and spleen for enlargement.
   c. Palpation of abdominal mass or another primary site of tumor.
   d. Auscultation of lungs.
   e. Palpation of lymph nodes.
   f. BP monitoring for detection of hypertension.
   g. Temperature for fever caused by infection or disease.
   h. Assessment of bones and joints for pain or swelling.
   i. Neurologic examination for signs of compression by tumor. Nerves involved depend on the location of tumor.
3. Assess coping mechanisms of family.

Nursing Interventions

Reducing Parental Caregivers' Anxiety

See previous sections, page 1354.

Reducing Child's Anxiety and Fear

See previous section, page 1354.

Increasing Activity Tolerance

See previous section, page 1352.

Regaining Normal Bowel and Bladder Function

1. Assess normal elimination patterns the child had before the illness began.
2. Keep careful intake and output records.
3. Assess for urinary overflow incontinence and loss of bowel function, depending on the child's age.
4. Notify health care provider if these should occur.

Preventing Infection

See previous section, page 1354.

Observe the surgical incision for erythema, drainage, or separation of the incision. Report these changes.

Relieving Pain

See previous section, page 1354.

Monitor for increasing or new location of pain, indicating progression of disease (e.g., fracture due to bone involvement).

Promoting Acceptance of Body Changes

See previous section, page 1355.

Family Education and Health Maintenance

1. Teach parental caregivers about the laboratory tests and imaging studies needed at diagnosis and periodically throughout therapy.
2. Instruct parental caregivers about chemotherapy drugs used and their potential adverse effects.
3. Inform parental caregivers about potential treatment methods, such as radiation therapy and bone marrow transplantation.
4. Advise parental caregivers to use good handwashing technique and to prevent exposure to children with communicable diseases.
5. Refer families to resources such as Children's Oncology Group (https://childrensoncologygroup.org/index.php/patients-and-families).

Evaluation: Expected Outcomes

- Parental caregivers and child discuss their feelings about diagnosis and treatment.
- Participates in play and expresses feelings through play.
- Maintains normal activity level.
- Resumes normal voiding and bowel patterns.
- Remains afebrile, lungs clear, no signs of localized infections.
- Rests without crying or guarding of surgical incision; good pain control according to developmentally appropriate scale.
- Interacts with others, seems comfortable with self.

Rhabdomyosarcoma

EVIDENCE BASE Rogers, T. N., & Dasgupta, R. (2021). Management of rhabdomyosarcoma in pediatric patients. *Surgical Oncology Clinics of North America*, *30*(2), 339–353. https://doi.org/10.1016/j.soc.2020.11.003

PDQ® Pediatric Treatment Editorial Board. (2023). *PDQ childhood rhabdomyosarcoma treatment.* National Cancer Institute. Retrieved January 18, 2023, from https://www.cancer.gov/types/soft-tissue-sarcoma/hp/rhabdomyosarcoma-treatment-pdq

RMS is a highly malignant soft tissue tumor that arises from the immature mesenchymal cells that form striated muscle. The incidence is approximately 4.6 per 1 million children in the United States, and RMS accounts for 2.7% of all malignant disease in children younger than age 14 years and 1.4% of the cases among adolescents and young adults aged 15 to 19 years. Outcomes for localized RMS have improved and reach a survival rate of almost 80%, but metastatic and relapsed disease outcomes have not improved and confer a dismal prognosis (<30% survival). Children aged 1 to 9 years have the best prognosis, whereas those younger and older fare less well. RMS can occur anywhere in the body; the most common sites are the head and neck, genitourinary (GU) tract, and extremities.

Pathophysiology and Etiology

1. Etiology is unknown in most cases.
2. Certain genetic and environmental factors have been associated with its development.
3. The two major subtypes are:
   a. PAX fusion–negative RMS (previously known as *embryonal RMS*), which is most common, occurring in 70%.
   b. PAX fusion–positive RMS (previously called *alveolar RMS*).

PAX fusion–negative disease status is associated with better outcomes than PAX fusion–positive disease.

4. Tumor spreads either by local extension or by metastasis via the venous and lymphatic system.
5. The lung is the most common site of metastasis.
   a. Tumor staging is complex and is based on tumor size, lymph node involvement and presence of metastatic disease, as well as the extent of the initial surgical resection. Tumor biology, tumor site, and patient age also factor into staging of disease and therapy choice.

Clinical Manifestations

1. Commonly presents as an asymptomatic painless lump noted by the patient or parental caregiver.
2. Signs and symptoms are variable and reflect the location of the tumor and metastasis.
   d. Orbit—ptosis, ocular paralysis, exophthalmos, impaired vision.
   e. Nasopharynx—epistaxis, pain, dysphagia, nasal voice, airway obstruction.
   f. Sinuses—swelling, pain, discharge, sinusitis.
   g. Middle ear—pain, chronic otitis, facial nerve palsy.
   h. Neck—hoarseness, dysphagia.
   i. Trunk, extremities, testicular areas—enlarging soft tissue masses.
   j. Prostate, bladder—urinary tract symptoms.
   k. Retroperitoneal tumors—GI and urinary tract obstruction, weakness, paresthesia, pain.
   c. Vaginal—abnormal vaginal bleeding or mass.

Diagnostic Evaluation

To document the extent of the disease and to provide objective criteria for measuring response to therapy:

1. Core needle or incisional biopsy of the primary tumor is preferred diagnostic procedure unless complete excision without loss of function can be ensured.
2. MRI—optimal imaging modality.
3. CT best for assessing bone involvement.
4. Bone marrow aspiration and biopsy.
5. Bone scan or skeletal survey.
6. Ultrasonography.
7. Chest x-ray.
8. PET.
9. CBC, liver and renal function tests, electrolytes, serum calcium and phosphorus, uric acid.
10. Monoclonal antibody assays.
11. Urinalysis.
12. Lumbar puncture—for children with parameningeal lesions.

Management

1. Management of RMS is multimodal and includes chemotherapy, radiation, and surgery. Treatment duration and intensity depend on the risk assignment of the disease.
2. Surgery and biopsy of the lesion—determines the stage of the disease and completely removes or reduces the primary tumor. Chemotherapy and radiation therapy may be used before surgery to avoid the disability associated with radical surgery.
3. Radiation—high-dose radiation to the primary tumor and sites of metastasis is recommended in 85% of patients.
4. Chemotherapy:
   a. Used for all patients, usually in combination with irradiation (see Table 47-5).
5. Commonly used drugs include vincristine, dactinomycin, cyclophosphamide, irinotecan, doxorubicin, and vinorelbine and ifosfamide. Survival rates have improved considerably in recent years in localized disease (to 80% survival), but survival rates in metastatic disease have not dramatically improved in decades (<30% survival).

Complications

1. Direct tumor extension to CNS with cranial nerve palsy, brainstem compromise with bradypnea and bradycardia.
2. Metastasis to the bone, bone marrow, lung.

Nursing Assessment

1. Obtain a history.
   a. Ask about recent illness history and when the child became symptomatic.
   b. Obtain review of systems to help identify the primary tumor and metastasis present.
2. Perform physical examination, including:
   a. Palpation of lymph nodes for enlargement, tenderness, and mobility.
   b. Palpation of the liver and spleen to detect hepatosplenomegaly.
   c. Palpation of primary site of tumor and suspected areas of metastasis.

TABLE 47-5 Commonly Used Chemotherapeutic Agents to Treat Rhabdomyosarcoma

CHEMOTHERAPEUTIC AGENT	COMMON SIDE EFFECTS
Cyclophosphamide	Nausea, vomiting Hair loss Loss of appetite Gonadal dysfunction Bone marrow suppression Nephrotoxicity
Dactinomycin	Nausea, vomiting Bone marrow suppression
Ifosfamide	Nausea, vomiting Hair loss Bone marrow suppression Gonadal dysfunction Renal dysfunction
Irinotecan	Diarrhea, abdominal cramping, runny nose, tearing, salivation, sweating, photophobia Nausea, vomiting Loss of appetite Bone marrow suppression Fever Weakness Elevated liver enzymes Elevated eosinophils
Vincristine	Hair loss Neuropathy Constipation

d. Auscultation of lungs to assess breath sounds or anomaly caused by the spread of the tumor.

3. Assess family coping, resources, and emotional state of the child and parental caregivers.

Nursing Interventions

Reducing Parental Caregivers' Anxiety

See previous section, page 1354.

Reducing the Child's Fear and Anxiety

See previous section, page 1354.

Promoting Optimal Nutrition

See previous section, page 1354.

Relieving Pain

See previous section, page 1354.

Promoting Acceptance of Body Changes

See previous section, page 1355.

Preventing Infection

See previous section, page 1354.

Family Education and Health Maintenance

1. Teach the parental caregivers about laboratory diagnostic tests that will be done periodically to follow the child's condition.
2. Instruct the parental caregivers about treatment methods, including chemotherapy and radiation protocols postoperatively, and their adverse effects.
3. Stress the importance of follow-up care so that recurrence can be detected early and appropriate treatment can be instituted.
4. Refer families to resources such as Children's Oncology Group (https://childrensoncologygroup.org/patients-and-families).
5. Assist patients in coordinating care with an orthopedic surgeon, a medical or pediatric oncologist, a radiation oncologist, a pathologist, and a physiatrist.

Evaluation: Expected Outcomes

- Parental caregivers verbalize understanding of diagnosis.
- Child plays, interacts with others, and asks questions.
- Eats sufficient calories to maintain weight.
- Verbalizes reduced pain.
- Verbalizes acceptance of self; looks in mirror.
- Remains afebrile, no signs of localized infection.

Wilms Tumor

EVIDENCE BASE PDQ® Pediatric Treatment Editorial Board. *PDQ Wilms tumor and other childhood kidney tumors treatment.* National Cancer Institute. Retrieved January 10, 2023, from https://www.cancer.gov/types/kidney/hp/wilms-treatment-pdq

Wilms tumor, also known as *nephroblastoma*, is a malignant renal tumor and is the most common renal neoplasm in children. It constitutes approximately 5% of all childhood tumors. Incidence is approximately eight cases per 100,000 children younger than age 15 years. About 500 to 600 cases are diagnosed each year in the United States; 75% of cases occur before the child is age 5 years. The average age a diagnosis is 3 to 4 years. Most commonly a unilateral disease, but in 5% to 10%, both kidneys are involved. It may appear as swelling in the abdomen below the costal margin. In the United States, girls have a slightly higher risk of Wilms tumor than do males, and the risk is slightly higher in African American children and lowest among Asian American children.

Pathophysiology and Etiology

1. The etiology is not known.
2. Genetic inheritance has been documented in 1% to 2% of cases.
3. Children with Wilms tumor may have associated anomalies.
4. Wilms tumor has a capacity for rapid growth and usually grows to a large size before it is diagnosed.
5. The effect of the tumor on the kidney depends on the site of the tumor.
6. In most cases, the tumor expands the renal parenchyma, and the capsule of the kidney becomes stretched over the surface of the tumor, which is encapsulated at the time of surgery.
7. Wilms tumors present various histologic patterns and are grouped into two general categories: favorable histology and anaplastic histology; those with anaplastic histology tend to be more difficult to treat.
8. The neoplasms metastasize either by direct extension or by way of the bloodstream. They may invade perirenal tissues, lymph nodes, the liver, the diaphragm, abdominal muscles, and the lungs. Invasions of bone and brain are less common.
9. Staging of Wilms tumor is done based on clinical and anatomic findings. It ranges from stage I (tumor is limited to the kidney and is completely excised) to stage IV (metastasis to organs away from the kidney, such as liver, lung, bone, or brain). Stage V includes those cases that include bilateral involvement, either initially or subsequently.

Clinical Manifestations

1. A firm, nontender upper quadrant abdominal mass is usually the presenting sign; it may be on either side. (It is usually first observed by the parental caregivers.)
2. Abdominal pain, which is related to rapid growth of the tumor, may occur. As the tumor enlarges, pressure may cause constipation, vomiting, abdominal distress, anorexia, weight loss, and dyspnea.
3. Less common are hypertension, fever, hematuria, and anemia.
4. Associated anomalies:
   a. Hemihypertrophy.
   b. Aniridia (without the iris of the eyes).
   c. GU tract anomalies.
   d. Overgrowth syndromes (Beckwith-Wiedemann syndrome).
   e. Intellectual disability.

Diagnostic Evaluation

1. Abdominal ultrasound to show the tumor and assess the status of the opposite kidney.
2. Radiography of the chest to identify metastases.
3. CBC and peripheral smear to determine baseline data.
4. Urinalysis to detect for hematuria.
5. Blood chemistries, especially serum electrolytes, uric acid, renal function tests (blood urea nitrogen and creatinine), and liver function tests (bilirubin, alanine aminotransferase, aspartate aminotransferase, lactate dehydrogenase [LD], total protein, albumin, and alkaline phosphatase) may show anomalies.
6. Urinary VMA and HVA to distinguish from neuroblastoma.

7. MRI or CT of the abdomen to evaluate local spread to lymph nodes or adjacent organs.
8. Renal biopsy to confirm diagnosis.
9. Real-time ultrasonography.

Management

1. Accurate staging and assessment of tumor spread is first conducted.
2. The standard treatment for stages I and II tumors is surgery (e.g., partial nephrectomy, simply nephrectomy, or radical nephrectomy), followed by chemotherapy.
3. The standard treatment for stages III and IV is the same as for stages I and II but includes radiation.
4. If both kidneys are removed, which is the treatment for stage V, the patient will require dialysis until a transplant is possible.
5. Radiation or chemotherapy may be administered preoperatively to patients with advanced tumors or risky intravascular extension to reduce tumor burden.
6. Radiation therapy may be given to the tumor bed postoperatively to render nonviable all cells that have escaped locally from the excised tumor. Children who have stage III and IV Wilms tumor, or who have an anaplastic histology, usually receive this treatment.
7. Whole-lung radiation is used to treat stage IV tumors with lung metastasis.
8. Late effects of radiation therapy to the abdomen include scoliosis and underdevelopment of soft tissues and possible organ dysfunction in radiation field.
9. Chemotherapy is initiated postoperatively to achieve complete eradication of tumor cells (see Table 47-6).
10. Overall survival rates for Wilms tumor are among the highest for all childhood cancers—greater than 90% survival at 4 years.
11. Prognosis is based on histologic tumor features (favorable vs. anaplastic histology), stage of disease, and possible chromosomal factors.

Complications

1. Metastasis to the lungs, lymph nodes, liver, bone, and brain.
2. Complications from treatment include heart and lung problems, pregnancy and fertility problems, kidney failure, scoliosis, and dental issues.
3. Cumulative incidence of second malignancy is 1.6% after 15 years, with radiation being the greatest risk factor.

TABLE 47-6 Commonly Used Chemotherapeutic Agents to Treat Wilms Tumor

CHEMOTHERAPEUTIC AGENT	COMMON SIDE EFFECTS
Vincristine	Hair loss Neuropathy Constipation
Dactinomycin	Nausea, vomiting Bone marrow suppression
Doxorubicin	Nausea, vomiting Hair loss Red urine Bone marrow suppression Cardiac dysfunction

Nursing Assessment

1. Obtain a history.
   a. Ask how tumor was first discovered.
   b. Ask whether the child has history of other GU anomalies or whether there is a family history of cancer.
   c. Determine whether the child has had hematuria, dysuria, constipation, abdominal pain, decreased appetite, or fever before hospitalization and ask how these were treated.
2. Perform a physical examination that includes the following:
   a. Assessment for associated anomalies: aniridia, hemihypertrophy of the spine, or cryptorchidism.
   b. Palpation of lymph nodes for enlargement, tenderness, and mobility.
   c. Palpation of the liver and spleen for enlargement.
   d. Palpation of the abdomen to determine the size and location of the tumor.
   e. Auscultation of the lungs to assess breath sounds or anomaly because of spread of tumor.
3. Assess coping, resources, and emotional state of the family.

CLINICAL JUDGMENT Avoid indiscriminate manipulation of the abdomen preoperatively and postoperatively to decrease the danger of metastasis. Because the tumor is soft and highly vascular, seeding may occur with excessive palpation or handling of the child's abdomen.

Nursing Interventions

Reducing Parental Caregivers' Anxiety

See previous section, page 1354.

Reducing the Child's Fear and Anxiety

See previous section, page 1354.

Preventing Fluid Volume Deficit and Other Complications

1. Insert a nasogastric tube, as ordered. Many children require gastric suction postoperatively to prevent distention or vomiting.
2. Monitor gastric output accurately and replace it with the appropriate IV fluids, as ordered.
3. When bowel sounds have returned, begin with small amounts of clear fluids.
4. Keep accurate intake and output record.
5. Monitor vital signs as the child's condition warrants and check the surgical dressing frequently for drainage.

Relieving Pain

See previous section, page 1354.

Promoting Optimal Nutrition

See previous section, page 1354.

Promoting Acceptance of Body Changes

See previous section, page 1355.

Increasing Activity Tolerance

See previous section, page 1352.

Preventing Infection

See previous section, page 1354.

Family Education and Health Maintenance

1. Teach parental caregivers of children with one kidney the signs and symptoms of kidney disease.

2. Advise parental caregivers to call the health care provider if the child has a fever of more than 100.4°F (38°C), bleeding, signs of infections, or has been exposed to chickenpox.
3. Teach measures to prevent infection, such as handwashing and isolation from children with communicable disease.
4. Refer families to resources such as Children's Oncology Group (https://childrensoncologygroup.org/patients-and-families).

Evaluation: Expected Outcomes

- Parental caregivers discuss their feelings about diagnosis and treatment.
- Expresses feelings during play and participates in playroom activities.
- Has no abdominal distention or vomiting, vital signs stable.
- Verbalizes relief from pain.
- Eats adequate calories to maintain weight, nausea relieved by antiemetics.
- Plays with others without notice to alopecia.
- Participates in all normal daily activities without fatigue.
- Remains afebrile, no signs of local infection.

Osteosarcoma

EVIDENCE BASE American Cancer Society. (2020). *Osteosarcoma: Early detection, diagnosis, and staging.* https://www.cancer.org/cancer/osteosarcoma/detection-diagnosis-staging.html

Eaton, B. R., Schwarz, R., Vatner, R., Yeh, B., Claude, L., Indelicato, D. J., & Laack, N. (2021). Osteosarcoma. *Pediatric Blood & Cancer, 68*(Suppl 2), e28352. https://doi.org/10.1002/pbc.28352

Osteosarcoma is a malignant tumor of the bone. It is the most commonly diagnosed primary malignant bone cancer in pediatrics, affecting about 500 children and adolescents in the United States annually. The incidence of osteosarcoma increases with age throughout childhood and adolescents but then decreases. It commonly affects adolescents during the growth spurt when bones and soft tissue are already vulnerable because of the developmental process, with the majority of cases occurring between the ages of 10 and 30 years. The 5-year relative survival rate of osteosarcoma (all stages) is 60%. It is the most common secondary malignancy among retinoblastoma survivors. The incidence of osteosarcoma is slightly higher in males than in females and also higher in African American and Latino children compared with White and Asian/Pacific Islander children. It is somewhat more likely to affect males than females.

Pathophysiology and Etiology

1. Etiology is unknown. Risk factors may include prior radiation treatment for another tumor, taller children, and genetic syndromes.
2. Presumably arises from bone-forming mesenchymal tissue.
3. Produces malignant spindle cell stroma, which gives rise to malignant osteoid tissue.
4. Common sites of occurrence are in the metaphysis of long bones, such as distal femur, proximal tibia, and proximal humerus. Less common sites include the skull, pelvis, phalanges, and jaw.
5. Most commonly metastasizes to lungs and other bones.

Clinical Manifestations

1. Sporadic pain in the affected site, frequently causing limp, stiffness, or limited range of motion.
2. Pain may worsen at night or with activity.
3. A painless swelling or noticeable and palpable, tender, fixed bony mass often in the arm or leg.
4. A broken bone that occurs without injury.
5. Additional symptoms related to the site of metastasis, if present.

Diagnostic Evaluation

1. Radiographic examination of lesion is conducted to visualize the tumor.
2. A biopsy of the lesion is conducted to confirm the diagnosis and to provide histologic data for the selection of a treatment plan.
3. CT and MRI are helpful to assess internal tumor composition and to evaluate local extent of disease prior to surgery.
4. Chest x-ray may be done to detect pulmonary metastases.
5. Bone scan is helpful in detecting the initial extent of malignancy, planning therapy, and evaluating effects of treatment.
6. Renal and liver function tests should be monitored to observe for elevated serum LD.
7. Arteriography may be a possibility if limb salvage procedure is a consideration.

Management

1. Surgery—procedures fall into two categories:
   a. Limb salvage procedure is priority—greater than 80% of tumors can be treated with limb salvage surgery.
   b. Radical amputation of the affected extremity and, commonly, the joint proximal to the involved area. Due to improved chemotherapy treatment regimens and limb salvage procedures, this is less frequently required.
2. The type of surgery performed depends on tumor location, size, extramedullary extent, distant metastasis, age of child, skeletal development, as well as preferences regarding lifestyle and quality of life.
3. Chemotherapy is necessary following surgery because most patients treated with local therapy alone develop distant metastases within several years. Chemotherapy agents, such as methotrexate with leucovorin, cyclophosphamide, cisplatin, doxorubicin, and ifosfamide, are also used preoperatively for patients who undergo resection surgery and for the treatment of metastatic disease (see Table 47-7).
4. Radiation may be used for incomplete resection or unresectable disease, but not as a first-line definitive treatment approach.
5. Survival has greatly improved with the aggressive use of multimodal therapy.
6. With current treatment, the 5-year survival rate for people with localized osteosarcoma is approximately 77% for those who undergo surgery followed by chemotherapy.
7. Important prognostic factors are extent of disease at diagnosis, age, gender, serum D, and amount of tumor necrosis at the time of surgery. Osteosarcomas arising in previously irradiated areas have a worse prognosis.
8. Limb salvage surgery has improved the quality of life for many survivors.
9. Patients with relapse to lung may still be curable with surgical excision.

TABLE 47-7 Commonly Used Chemotherapeutic Agents to Treat Osteosarcoma

CHEMOTHERAPY	COMMON SIDE EFFECTS
Doxorubicin	Nausea, vomiting Hair loss Red urine Bone marrow suppression Cardiac dysfunction
Cisplatin	Nausea, vomiting Bone marrow suppression Hypomagnesemia Loss of appetite Hearing loss Renal dysfunction
Methotrexate	Elevated liver enzymes Mucositis Nephrotoxicity
Etoposide	Nausea, vomiting Hair loss Weakness Bone marrow suppression
Ifosfamide	Nausea, vomiting Hair loss Bone marrow suppression Gonadal dysfunction Renal dysfunction

Complications

1. Metastasis to the lung and bones.
2. Later metastasis to the CNS and lymph nodes.
3. Treatment-induced hearing loss.
4. Physical limitations resulting from surgical resection.

Nursing Assessment

1. Obtain a history.
   a. Inquire about how and when symptoms first presented as well as the duration of symptoms.
   b. Determine whether the child has pain or limitation of motion in the affected area.
2. Perform a physical examination, including:
   a. Palpation of the mass to determine the size and location. (Determine whether the mass is tender or is fixed to the bone.)
   b. Palpation of other bones to check for metastasis.
   c. Auscultation of the lungs to assess breath sounds or other anomalies caused by spread of tumor.
3. Assess family coping, resources such as support systems, and emotional state of the patient and parental caregivers.
4. Assess the degree of mobility, especially for lower extremity tumors.

Nursing Interventions

Reducing Parental Caregivers' Anxiety

1. Involve the parental caregivers in the teaching plan and make sure they know what to expect before going to surgery.
2. Explain to the parental caregiver about the disease process and available treatment options.
3. Provide parental caregivers with strategies related to effective coping with the diagnosis and postoperative care.
4. Provide parental caregivers with positive reinforcement, honesty, and transparency in the care process.
5. Encourage the parental caregiver to participate in the care process to prepare for discharge.

Reducing the Adolescent's Fear and Anxiety

1. Consider the adolescent's developmental level when explaining diagnostic tests and postoperative care.
2. Support and prepare the child for routine surgical care or care of the amputated limb.
3. If an amputation will be done, teach the child about the need for physical therapy for exercises and to learn crutch walking and the need for a prosthesis.
4. If limb salvage surgery will be done, reinforce the importance of physical therapy exercises following surgery to restore as much function as possible to the affected bone and/or joint.
5. Nursing care of the adolescent with osteosarcoma is the same as care of the adult.

Promoting Acceptance of New Self-Image

1. Understand that adolescents need time and support to accept the diagnosis and surgery and to grieve for their lost body part if an amputation is done.
2. Try to introduce the adolescent to another adolescent with the same diagnosis who has undergone similar treatment.
3. Suggest the selection of clothing that will camouflage the prosthesis and be fashionable and appealing.
4. Suggest wigs, scarves, or hats for adolescents who experience hair loss because of chemotherapy.
5. Encourage visits by peers and help the child to deal with questions and reactions from peers.

Relieving Pain

See previous section, page 1354.

Promoting Optimal Nutrition

See previous section, page 1354.

Preventing Infection and Hemorrhage

See previous section, page 1354.

Community and Home Care Considerations

1. Assess the home for accessibility of adolescent who has had an amputation.
2. Educate parental caregivers about changes they may need to make in the home.
3. Encourage the parental caregivers to contact the school system to arrange for a tutor for a student who needs to remain out of school for a lengthy period.
4. Assist the parental caregivers in contacting the school nurse to facilitate reentry into the classroom.
5. Identify any financial concerns that may be associated with care and treatment and refer patients to a social worker or case manager to access community services and resources.

Family Education and Health Maintenance

1. Teach adolescents and parental caregivers about infection control measures, such as good handwashing and preventing exposure to children with communicable diseases, because chemotherapy is usually long term.
2. Parental caregivers and adolescents should be instructed about chemotherapy medications used and their potential adverse effects.

3. Teach parental caregivers and adolescents about the radiation procedure and effects.
4. Advise the adolescent to protect a leg that has received radiation treatment by avoiding excessive pressure on the leg through sports. Consult orthopedic specialist for appropriate activity limitations.
5. Teach parental caregivers measures to ensure safety of patient throughout treatment and convalescence.
6. Refer families to resources such as Children's Oncology Group (https://childrensoncologygroup.org/patients-and-families).

Evaluation: Expected Outcomes

- Parental caregivers and child (if age appropriate) discuss feelings about surgery and chemotherapy treatments.
- Parental caregivers and child (if age appropriate) verbalize feelings about surgery and ask questions.
- Looks in mirror, touches amputation site.
- Parental caregivers and child (if age appropriate) verbalize relief from pain.
- Maintains an adequate eating pattern, nausea relieved by antiemetics.
- Remains afebrile, vital signs stable, no signs of bleeding.
- Maintains skin integrity.

Retinoblastoma

EVIDENCE BASE Ancona-Lezama, D., Dalvin, L. A., & Shields, C. L. (2020). Modern treatment of retinoblastoma: A 2020 review. *Indian Journal of Ophthalmology, 68*(11), 2356–2365. https://doi.org/10.4103/ijo.IJO_721_20

PDQ® Pediatric Treatment Editorial Board. (2022). *PDQ retinoblastoma treatment.* National Cancer Institute. https://www.cancer.gov/types/retinoblastoma/hp/retinoblastoma-treatment-pdq

Retinoblastoma is a malignant, congenital tumor, arising in the retina of one or both eyes. It accounts for about 6% of the cancers occurring in children less than 5 years old, and in the United States, the incidence is 11.8 per million live births. It occurs equally in males and females and is most commonly diagnosed under the age of 4 years. Presentation can be bilateral or unilateral and is categorized based on whether the mutation is germline or somatic.

Pathophysiology and Etiology

1. Most cases appear sporadically, but there is also an inherited form of the disease.
   a. Nonhereditary (somatic) mutations account for approximately 70% of all retinoblastomas; mutations almost always demonstrate unilateral involvement.
   b. Most bilateral cases are heritable (germline mutations).
      i. Mode of inheritance is autosomal dominant.
      ii. Offspring of affected individuals have a 50% chance of inheriting the disease.
2. Can be associated with chromosomal aberrations.
3. Usually arise in multiple foci rather than a single tumor from any of the nucleated retinal layers.
4. Some tumors (endophytic type) arise in the internal nuclear layers of the retina and grow forward into the vitreous cavity.
5. Some tumors (exophytic type) arise in the external nuclear layer and grow into the subretinal space, with detachment of the retina.
6. Most tumors have a combination of endophytic and exophytic growth.
7. Extension of the tumor may occur into the choroid, sclera, and optic nerve.
8. "Trilateral retinoblastoma" is the presence of bilateral retinoblastoma in addition to an intracranial midline neuroblastic tumor.
9. Hematogenous spread of the tumor may occur to the bone marrow, skeleton, lymph nodes, and liver.
10. Most oncologists stage disease using the International Classification for Intraocular Retinoblastoma. Based on the extent of disease and the chances the eye can be saved with current treatment regimens, retinoblastoma is divided into five groups labeled A through E.

Clinical Manifestations

1. Signs and symptoms of an intraocular tumor depend on its size and position.
2. "Cat's-eye reflex"—whitish appearance of the pupil (leukocoria) represents visualization of the tumor through the lens as light falls on the tumor mass—most common sign. Also characterized by the absence of red reflex on photographs.
3. Strabismus—second most common presenting sign.
4. Other occasional presenting signs:
   a. Orbital inflammation, eye pain.
   b. Hyphemia, bulging of the eye.
   c. Fixed pupil.
   d. Heterochromia iridis—different colors of each iris or in the same iris.
5. Vision loss is not a symptom because young children do not complain of unilaterally decreased vision.
6. Symptoms of distant metastasis—anorexia, weight loss, vomiting, headache, bone pain.

Diagnostic Evaluation

1. Bilateral indirect ophthalmoscopy under general anesthesia.
2. Ultrasonography and CT or MRI of head and eyes to visualize tumor.
3. Bone marrow aspiration and lumbar puncture under anesthesia to determine metastasis.

Management

1. Depends on the stage of the disease at the time of diagnosis.
2. Most unilateral tumors are treated with systemic chemotherapy. Newer approaches including intra-arterial chemotherapy (chemotherapy administered into the ophthalmic artery that delivers blood supply to the eye) or intravitreal chemotherapy (chemotherapy injected directly into the vitreous humor of the eye) are showing promise, with fewer side effects than systemic chemotherapy.
   a. Goal of treatment is to eradicate the tumors, prevent systemic metastasis, promote resolution of retinal detachment, preserve useful vision, if possible, and control the malignancy to prevent enucleation or eye removal.
   b. Most common chemotherapies are cisplatin or carboplatin, cyclophosphamide, doxorubicin, and vincristine (see Table 47-8). Melphalan and topotecan are often the agents of choice for intra-arterial or intravitreal chemotherapy for children with advanced disease.
3. Surgery (enucleation) is reserved for eyes with large tumor burden or disease that is not responsive to standard treatment.

TABLE 47-8 Commonly Used Chemotherapeutic Agents to Treat Retinoblastoma

CHEMOTHERAPEUTIC AGENT	COMMON SIDE EFFECTS
Carboplatin	Nausea, vomiting Bone marrow suppression Electrolyte imbalance
Vincristine	Hair loss Neuropathy Constipation

4. Bilateral disease usually requires a combination of chemotherapy followed by focal treatments and sometimes surgery.
   a. Every attempt is made to salvage whatever vision there may be.
   b. Bilateral enucleation may be recommended with extensive bilateral retinoblastoma when no hope of vision exists.
5. Very small tumors can be treated with local therapy. Laser photocoagulation uses laser heat to destroy the blood vessels surrounding the tumor. Transpupillary thermotherapy uses an infrared laser to target and kill the tumor cell directly. Cryotherapy uses a metal probe to freeze the tumor cells but can only be used in tumors toward the front of the eye.
6. External beam radiotherapy can be used to treat eyes unresponsive to other treatments.
7. Gene therapy is a type of therapy that introduces a viral or bacterial gene into tumor cells, thus allowing the conversion of a nontoxic compound into a lethal drug to kill the tumor cells. However, it is unlikely that this type of gene therapy could be used as first-line treatment for retinoblastoma.
8. Many immunotherapy agents are undergoing clinical trials for efficacy in treating retinoblastoma.
9. Overall 5-year survival rate is high (80% to 90%).
10. Heritable retinoblastoma and bilateral retinoblastoma are associated with a high incidence of spontaneous and radiation-related new tumors, particularly sarcomas.

Complications

1. Spread to brain and other eye.
2. Metastasis to bone, bone marrow, liver, and lymph nodes.
3. Risk for secondary tumors, including osteosarcomas, soft tissue sarcomas, and melanomas.

Nursing Assessment

1. Obtain a history.
   a. Ask about a family history that is positive for retinoblastoma or other types of cancer.
   b. Inquire about when symptoms began and strabismus, cat's-eye reflex, orbital inflammation, vomiting, or headache.
2. Perform a physical examination.
   a. Assess pupils for reactivity of light, size, and leukocoria.
   b. Evaluate strabismus when checking muscle balance.
   c. Assess eyes for associated signs, such as erythema, inflammation of the orbit, hyphema, and heterochromia iridis.
3. Assess family's ability to cope, to use support systems, and to communicate feelings.

Nursing Interventions

Decreasing Parental Caregiver Anxiety and Guilt

1. Listen to the parental caregiver feelings of guilt about transmitting the disease to the child or because they did not notice symptoms earlier.
2. Discuss the benefit of consultation about the probability of having another affected child.
   a. Risk ranges from approximately 1% to 10%, depending on family history and whether the affected child had unilateral or bilateral disease.
   b. The reportedly high lifelong cancer burden among patients with retinoblastoma may also be important to parental caregivers in making informed decisions.
   c. Refer for genetic counseling and support parental caregiver decisions regarding future pregnancies.
3. Encourage the parental caregivers to seek genetic counseling for the affected child when they reach puberty.
   a. The risk to offspring is from 1% to 50%, depending on family history and whether disease was unilateral or bilateral.
   b. Among affected offspring, there is a high probability (greater than 50%) of bilateral disease.

Preserving Tissue Integrity

1. Administer sedatives or assist with anesthesia for intraocular chemotherapy, if necessary.
   a. Administer the medication in a timely manner so that sedation is adequate for positioning of the child.
2. Observe for possible adverse effects of chemotherapy and prepare the parental caregivers for their occurrence.
   a. Swelling and edema surrounding the intraocular chemotherapy site.
   b. Nausea and vomiting with systemic chemotherapy.

Reducing the Child's Anxiety and Fear

See also previous sections about reducing child's anxiety and fear.

1. Encourage the parental caregivers to room in and participate in the child's care to minimize separation anxiety.
2. Prepare the child and parental caregivers for all diagnostic procedures.
3. Describe the surgery and anticipated postoperative appearance of the child. Draw pictures or use a doll, if one is available.
   a. A surgically implanted sphere maintains the shape of the eyeball.
   b. The child's face may be edematous and ecchymotic.
4. Offer the family the opportunity to talk with another parental caregiver who has gone through the experience or to see pictures of another child with an artificial eye.
5. See "Nursing management of eye enucleation," page 419.

Promoting Acceptance of Prosthesis

1. Explain to the child the changes related to losing the diseased eye, having a bandaged orbit until it heals after surgery, and receiving a prosthetic eye.
2. Explain that the prosthesis will be made for them and will look like the removed eye.
3. Tell parental caregivers to expect the child to grieve the loss and to help them by talking about it, but to treat the child as the same person.

Minimizing Effects of Vision Loss

1. Maintain a safe, uncluttered environment for the child.
2. Orient the child to the surrounding environment.

3. Hold the child frequently and stand close, within child's field of vision, while speaking or providing care.
4. Encourage the use of touch and other senses for exploring.
5. Set environmental limits so that the child feels safe and can obtain help easily.

Family Education and Health Maintenance

1. Teach care of the orbit.
2. Teach care of the prosthesis—initial instructions are provided by the ocularist and should be reinforced by the nurse.
3. Advise protection of the remaining eye from accidental injury, such as wearing safety glass for sports, not putting sharp objects near eye, treating eye infections promptly.
4. Encourage maintenance of routine checkups for eye and medical care.
5. Stress need to have subsequent children carefully evaluated for retinoblastoma.
   a. An ophthalmologic examination under anesthesia is usually recommended at approximately age 2 months.
   b. The child should receive frequent examinations thereafter until judged safe from developing retinoblastoma, usually approximately age 4 years.
6. Refer families to resources such as Children's Oncology Group.

Evaluation: Expected Outcomes

- Parental caregivers discuss feelings openly, show affection to the child.
- Parental caregivers describe possible adverse effects of radiation and how to care for skin around eyes.
- Demonstrates lessened anxiety by participating in age-appropriate activities.
- Shows acceptance of the prosthesis and not inhibited in behavior.
- Moves about environment with ease.

SELECTED READINGS

Breakey, V., Gupta, A., Johnston, D., Portwine, C., Laverdiere, C., May, S., Dick, B., Hundert, A., Nishat, F., Killackey, T., Nguyen, C., Lalloo, C., & Stinson, J. (2022). A pilot randomized control trial of teens taking charge: A web-based self-management program for adolescents with cancer. *Journal of Pediatric Hematology/Oncology Nursing, 39*(6), 366–378.

Cohen, J., Goddard, E., Brierly, M., Bramley, L., & Beck, E. (2021). Poor diet quality in children with cancer during treatment. *Journal of Pediatric Oncology Nursing, 38*(5), 313–321.

Hockenberry, M., Haugen, M., Slaven, A., Skeens, M., Patton, L., Montgomery, K., Trimble, K., Coyne, K., Hancock, D., Ahmad, A., Daut, E., Glover, L., Brown, L., St. Pierre, S., Shay, A., Maloney, J., Burke, M., Hatch, D., & Arthur, M. (2021). Pediatric education discharge support strategies for newly diagnosed children with cancer. *Cancer Nursing, 44*(6), E520–E530.

Kelly, P. M., & Pottenger, E. (2022). Bone health issues in the pediatric oncology patient. *Seminars in Oncology Nursing, 38*(2), 151275.

Leclerc, R., & Olin, J. (2020). An overview of retinoblastoma and enucleation in pediatric patients. *AORN Journal, 111*(1), 69–79.

Taam, B., & Lim, F. (2023). Best practices in pediatric oncology pain management. *The American Journal of Nursing, 123*(5), 52–58.

48 Pediatric Hematologic Disorders*

PEDIATRIC HEMATOLOGIC DISORDERS

Anemia

EVIDENCE BASE Gallagher, P. G. (2022). Anemia in the pediatric patient. *Blood, 140*(6), 571–593. https://doi.org/10.1182/blood.2020006479

Anemia refers to a lower than normal number of red blood cells (RBCs) or hemoglobin (Hb) in the blood. Hb is a main part of the RBC and binds oxygen. Anemia results in decreased oxygen-carrying capacity of the RBC. It is the most frequent hematologic disorder encountered in children. The World Health Organization (WHO) estimates a quarter of the world's population has anemia, including almost half of preschool children. Anemia is associated with increased morbidity—including neurologic complications, increased risk of low birth weight, infection, and heart failure—as well as increased mortality.

Pathophysiology and Etiology

1. RBCs and Hb are normally formed at the same rate at which they are destroyed. The function of the RBC is to deliver oxygen from the lungs to the tissues and carbon dioxide from the tissues to the lung. This is accomplished by the use of Hb. In anemia, there is a decrease in the number of RBCs transporting oxygen and carbon dioxide.
2. May be caused by blood loss related to:
   a. Trauma and ulceration.
   b. Decreased production of platelets.
   c. Increased destruction of platelets.
   d. Decreased number of clotting factors.
3. May be caused by impairment of RBC production caused by nutritional deficiency. This impairment includes poverty, malnutrition (including strict vegan and vegetarian diets), and certain intestinal/medical conditions.
   a. Iron deficiency—the most common type of anemia in ages 6 months to 3 years.
   b. Folate deficiency—causes formation of large RBCs with abnormal nuclear maturation (megaloblastic anemia).
   c. Vitamin B_{12} deficiency—causes megaloblastic anemia (deficiency in vitamin B_{12}, folate, or both); called *pernicious anemia* because of lack of intrinsic factor for absorption of vitamin B_{12}.
   d. Vitamin B_6 deficiency.
   e. Excessive milk intake.
   f. Certain prescription medications (i.e., antiseizure drugs, antacids).
   g. Lead poisoning—lead absorbed by the bone marrow attaches to newly formed RBCs and inhibits synthesis of heme. This results in a decrease in circulating Hb.
   h. Vitamin C deficiency.
4. May be caused by decreased erythrocyte production. This occurs in the bone marrow and stem cells.
   a. Pure RBC anemia.
   b. Secondary hemolytic anemias associated with chronic infection, renal disease, and drugs. In anemia of chronic infection and inflammation, the lifespan of the RBC is moderately decreased, and the ability of the bone marrow to produce RBCs is significantly decreased.
   c. Bone marrow depression—leukemia, aplastic anemias, and transient erythrocytopenia of childhood.
5. May be caused by increased erythrocyte destruction.
   a. Extrinsic factors:
      i. Drugs and chemicals (i.e., acetaminophen, ibuprofen, antibiotic such as penicillins).
      ii. Infections—transient erythroblastopenia of childhood caused by parvovirus (fifth disease), usually between ages 6 months and 4 years.
      iii. Antibody reactions—passively acquired antibodies against Rh, A, or B isoimmunization (transfusion of ABO-incompatible blood), autoimmune disorders, burns, and poisons (including lead poisoning).
   b. Intrinsic factors:
      i. Abnormalities of the RBC membrane.
      ii. Enzymatic defects—glucose-6-phosphate dehydrogenase deficiency.

*Please note that the term "male" in this chapter refers to a person assigned male at birth, and the term "female" in this chapter refers to a person assigned female at birth.

Table 48-1 Blood Tests in Anemia by Cause

	MCV	MCHC	RETICULOCYTE	FERRITIN	FEP
Iron deficiency	Low	Low	Low	Low	High
Lead poisoning	Low	Low	Low	Normal	High
Beta-thalassemia	Low	Low	Low	Normal	Normal
Folate deficiency	High	Normal	Low	Normal	Normal
B_{12} deficiency	High	Normal	Low	Normal	Normal
Sickle cell disease	Normal	Normal	High	Normal	Normal

FEP, free erythrocyte protoporphyrin; MCHC, mean corpuscular hemoglobin concentration; MCV, mean corpuscular volume.

iii. Abnormal Hb synthesis—sickle cell disease and thalassemia syndromes. These result in defective RBC production.
iv. Malabsorption syndromes such as celiac disease.

c. In hemolytic anemias, the RBCs are destroyed at abnormally high rates, primarily by the spleen. The normal lifespan of an RBC is 120 days. RBCs are sequestered and destroyed in the spleen.
   i. The activity of the bone marrow increases to compensate for the shortened survival time of the RBCs.
   ii. The bone marrow hypertrophies and occupies a larger than normal share of the inner structure of the bones.
   iii. Products of RBC breakdown increase with hemolysis. If chronic, this may lead to increased excretion of bilirubin into the biliary tract, causing gallstones.
   iv. Jaundice results when the conversion of Hb to bilirubin exceeds the liver's capacity.
   v. Iron builds up (hemosiderosis) and may deposit on body tissues.

6. May result from chronic illness such as rheumatoid arthritis, Crohn disease, lupus, and other inflammatory disorders (anemia of chronic disease).
7. May result from gastroesophageal reflux disease secondary to the acidic pH, which can cause erosion.
8. "Physiologic anemia" occurs in term infants at ages 8 to 12 weeks; Hb should be between 9 and 11 g/dL. In mild anemia of prematurity, recovery may occur 3 to 6 months after birth.

Clinical Manifestations

1. Condition may be acute or chronic. The slower the onset of anemia, the less likely the patient will be symptomatic.
2. Early symptoms:
   a. Fatigue and loss of energy.
   b. Dizziness or lightheadedness.
   c. Low appetite.
3. Late symptoms:
   a. Pallor.
   b. Weakness.
   c. Tachycardia.
   d. Palpitations.
   e. Tachypnea and shortness of breath on exertion.
   f. Pica.
   g. Insomnia.
   h. Cold hands and feet.
   i. Leg cramps.
   j. Tingling or numbness in hands and/or feet.
   k. Jaundice (with hemolytic anemias).
   l. Increase in dental caries.
   m. Infection.
   n. Heart failure.
   o. Dysmorphic features.
   p. Increased morbidity.

Diagnostic Evaluation

1. Complete blood count (CBC) with mean corpuscular volume (MCV), mean corpuscular hemoglobin concentration (MCHC), and iron indices—vary with types of anemia (see Table 48-1).
2. Serum iron and total iron-binding capacity (TIBC)—ratio of less than 0.2.
3. Serum ferritin—less than 12 g/dL.
4. Lead—greater than 10 g/dL.
5. Free erythrocyte protoporphyrin—greater than 35 g/dL.
6. B_{12}, B_6, and folate levels—may be decreased.
7. Hb electrophoresis—may show Hb S or other abnormalities.
8. Parvovirus B_{19} titer—may be elevated in transient erythroblastopenia.
9. Coombs test—shows whether your body is making antibodies to destroy RBCs.
10. Haptoglobin, bilirubin, and liver function tests (LFTs).
11. Testing for G6PD deficiency.
12. Hb electrophoresis.
13. Certain novel genetic testing can assist in the diagnosis of certain anemias.

Management

Iron-Deficiency Anemia

1. Oral iron is dosed by age (see Table 48-2). Reticulocyte count should increase in 7 to 10 days; hematocrit (Hct) increases in approximately 4 weeks. Should not be given on an empty stomach; should be given 1 to 2 hours before or after meals; do not give with milk. Vitamin C–containing juice may improve

Table 48-2 Elemental Iron Dosing in Children With Anemia

Age of child	6–23 mo	24–59 mo	5–12 yr	Menstruating, nonpregnant adolescent females
Dose of iron	10–12.5 mg daily	30 mg daily	30–60 mg daily	30–60 mg daily

absorption but is not essential. Avoid medications that reduce gastric acidity.
2. Dietary: decrease milk intake to 16 to 24 ounces per day; include iron-fortified cereals and bread products; increase consumption of red meat; include foods rich in vitamin C; increase green, leafy vegetables.
3. Good sources of iron: red meat, beans, egg yolks, whole grain products, nuts, seafood, spinach, and dark green leafy vegetables.
4. Typically requires a minimum of 3 months of therapy. Treatment on average is 3 to 6 months.
5. Blood transfusion through an intravenous (IV) is not recommended in the setting of chronic anemia other than in patients with hemoglobinopathy (genetic mutation of Hb molecule).
6. Novel pharmacologic agents and advances in gene therapy–based therapeutics trials have the potential to ameliorate anemia-associated disease and provide treatment strategies even in the most difficult and complex cases.

Anemia of Chronic Lead Poisoning

See page 1366.

1. Early detection of high lead levels through patient questionnaires and blood tests. The Centers for Disease Control and Prevention (CDC) defines elevated blood level as 3.5 mg/dL or higher.
2. Maintenance of a well-balanced diet, high in calcium and vitamin D.
3. Administration of chelating agents such as edetate disodium calcium, dimercaprol, or succimer according to recommendations of the CDC. Only used when blood levels are greater than 45 secondary to depletion of essential nutrients, such as calcium, iron, and zinc.
4. Use of lead-free paints and gasoline. (Lead paint was predominantly used in homes built between 1940 and 1959.)
5. Testing of house and soil.
6. Testing of water supply for lead levels.
7. Removal of individuals from unsafe environment.
8. Universal screening of children in vulnerable populations (i.e., children who are Medicaid eligible).

Megaloblastic Anemia

1. Folate deficiency—administration of folic acid orally.
2. B_{12} deficiency—administration of B_{12} (cyanocobalamin) intramuscularly (IM).

Hemoglobinopathies

1. Sickle cell anemia (see page 1370).
2. Thalassemia (see page 1376).

Transient Erythroblastopenia of Childhood

1. Median age of presentation is 18 to 26 months and occurs in children under the age of 4 years.
2. Spontaneous recovery in 4 to 8 weeks.
3. Packed RBC (PRBC) transfusion recommended in patients with severe signs of clinical decompensation including hemodynamic instability, exercise intolerance, or altered mental status.
4. Usually, unless cardiac failure occurs, supportive care, not therapy, is provided.

Anemia From Blood Loss or Bone Marrow Suppression

PRBC transfusions may be necessary (see page 762).

Complications

1. Mental sluggishness, as a result of decreased oxygen and energy for normal neural activity, usually associated with a decreased attention span, decreased intelligence, and lethargy.
2. Decrease in IQ and neurologic development.
3. Long-term behavioral changes.
4. Growth retardation related to anorexia and decreased cellular metabolism.
5. Delayed puberty related to growth retardation.
6. Iron overload.
7. Aplastic crises (in patients with chronic hemolytic anemia).
8. Hypersplenism.
9. Cerebral infarction.
10. Ischemic stroke—most prevalent in children with sickle cell disease.
11. Cardiac enlargement related to muscle hypertrophy because of increased strain on the heart, attempting to compensate for increased oxygen demand by the tissues, and eventually results in heart failure.
12. Studies suggest prolonged lead poisoning can lead to violent and criminal behavior later in life.
13. Death from cardiac failure related to circulatory collapse and shock.

Nursing Assessment

1. Obtain a history of potential causes.
   a. Dietary history: including the amount of milk and meat consumed, including primarily plant-based diets, lack of red meat, animal products, or green leafy vegetables.
   b. Family history for genetic causes, including blood disorders or diseases.
   c. Medication history: Some medications can increase risk of gastrointestinal (GI) blood loss; some can cause vitamin deficiencies.
   d. Past medical history including chronic diseases that can cause anemia.
   e. Persistent infection, fever, or chronic disease.
   f. Symptoms of shortness of breath, palpitations, fatigue, and headache.
   g. Exercise and athletic endeavors/intolerance.
   h. Cold intolerance.
   i. Pica—craving and consuming nonfood items (e.g., paint chips, paper).
   j. Changes in bowel movement habits—constipation, diarrhea, and changes in color and consistency of stool.
   k. Prolonged or heavy menstrual bleeding.
   l. In older children and adolescents—history of alcohol intake.
   m. Socioeconomic status—most common in individuals with low socioeconomic status.
2. Obtain a baseline assessment.
   a. Observe skin and mucous membranes for pallor, dryness, sores, temperature, and jaundice.
   b. Obtain height and weight and plot on growth curve.
   c. Measure vital signs, including blood pressure (BP), heart rate, and respirations.
   d. Assess child's functional level exercise tolerance/intolerance and mental functioning.
   e. Assess attainment of developmental milestones.
   f. Review medication history.
   g. Review history of recent illnesses and surgeries.
3. Observe for fatigue, listlessness, and irritability.
4. Observe for blood loss: bruising, bleeding, hematuria, or hematochezia (blood in stool). Assess for excessive menstrual bleeding in adolescent females.

CLINICAL JUDGMENT Be alert for children at risk for iron-deficiency anemia—children in rapid growth stages (toddlers and adolescents) and pregnant or lactating adolescents. Be mindful of signs and symptoms that caregivers may verbalize that may not necessarily be most prominent in your nursing diagnosis.

Nursing Interventions

Minimizing Fatigue

1. Plan nursing care to allow for lengthy periods when the child is not disturbed by hospital routines, procedures, and treatments; set priorities.
2. Observe for early signs of fatigue, such as irritability, hyperactivity, and listlessness.
3. Establish a balance between activities and rest.
4. Maintain a well-balanced diet.
5. Maintain hydration by drinking water throughout the day and with exercise. Water and sports drinks (during exercise) prevent dehydration, electrolyte loss, and muscle fatigue.
6. Gradually increased endurance and intensity of exercise.
7. Allow for rest and recovery after exercising.
8. Administer oxygen and position upright if dyspnea is present.
9. Transfuse PRBCs, as directed.

CLINICAL JUDGMENT Monitor transfusion for signs and symptoms of transfusion reaction: headache, anxiety, chills, dyspnea, chest pain, hypotension, flank pain, rash, hives, bronchospasm, pruritus, hypertension, and more than 1-degree increase in baseline temperature. If reaction occurs, stop transfusion and initiate facility's emergency protocol for transfusion reaction.

Providing Adequate Nutritional Intake

1. Be aware of the child's food preferences and plan diet accordingly.
2. Provide nutritional guidance as to foods that are rich in iron.
3. Offer small amounts of food at frequent intervals.
4. Reward the child for positive attempts to eat.
5. Allow the child to participate in the selection of foods.
6. Avoid tiring activities and unpleasant procedures at mealtime.
7. Make mealtime as pleasurable as possible.
8. If iron is ordered, give between meals (2 hours before or after meals) and with orange juice (iron is absorbed best in an acidic environment).
9. Limit milk and milk products to 16 to 24 ounces per day. Milk products inhibit the absorption of oral iron.
10. Administer liquid iron with a dropper or straw or dilute with water or fruit juice to prevent staining the teeth.
    a. If administered by dropper, deposit iron in the back of the mouth.
    b. Dental stains can be removed by brushing the teeth with baking soda paste. If the child is resistant, you can put baking soda on a washcloth and rub on the teeth.
11. Be alert for adverse effects of iron supplements—gastric distress, colicky pain, diarrhea, or constipation; may call for decreased dose.
12. Advise the family that the child's stool may turn dark green or black.
13. Stress the importance of continuing iron therapy according to health care provider's directions, even though the child may not appear to be ill.
14. Inform caregivers that iron overdoses can be harmful or fatal.

Preventing Infection

1. Teach and assist with good hygiene practices, such as handwashing and mouth care.
2. Avoid exposure to others with colds and infections.
3. Wash vegetable and fruits well before eating.
4. Cook meat until it is well done.
5. Make sure that staff, family, and visitors always wash hands thoroughly.
6. Keep children away from turtles, snakes, and lizards, which can carry *Salmonella*.
7. Keep immunizations up to date.
8. Report temperature elevation or other signs of infection.

Impaired Gas Exchange

1. Monitor respiratory rate, depth, and effort.
2. Monitor behavior and mental status for restlessness, agitation, or confusion.
3. Monitor oxygen saturation.
4. Position the child with the head of the bed elevated to improve perfusion.
5. Encourage use of oxygen when necessary.

Ineffective Breathing Pattern

1. Assess for signs and symptoms of ineffective breathing pattern, that is, shallow respirations and tachypnea.
2. Provide a calm and restful environment to reduce fear and anxiety.
3. Provide analgesics if the child is in pain.
4. Teach deep breathing techniques through the use of incentive spirometer or bubbles.
5. Increase activity as tolerated.
6. Consult a respiratory therapist if necessary.

Reduce Anxiety

1. Provide a calm and supportive environment.
2. Allow the child to handle equipment used for tests and procedures (tourniquets, syringes).
3. Explain all tests, procedures, and the treatment plan in age-appropriate manner.
4. Encourage verbalization of fear and anxiety.
5. Include caregivers in teaching sessions to encourage their support of the child.

Promoting Normal Growth and Development

1. Make sure that nutrition is adequate for age and activity level.
2. Encourage participation in age-related activities.
3. Encourage bedtime ritual and appropriate hours of sleep.
4. Encourage doing homework and tutored activities.
5. Encourage peer socialization.
6. Promote age-appropriate play and therapeutic play.
7. Provide a support system for child and caregivers.
8. Perform periodic growth chart evaluation and developmental testing.
    a. Share results with caregivers and explain the association between diet/anemia and growth and development.
    b. Notify health care provider and make referrals, as indicated.

Family Education and Health Maintenance

1. Stress to the caregivers the importance of continuing the iron therapy according to the provider's directions, even though the child may not appear ill.
2. Stress the need for regular medical and laboratory follow-up to evaluate disease progression and response to therapy.

3. Initiate and reinforce good dietary habits.
   a. Foods rich in iron include dark green leafy vegetables, fortified cereals, dried fruits, nuts, and red meats.
   b. Limit milk intake to 16 to 24 ounces per day. Promote iron-containing foods.
   c. Provide vitamin supplements, if necessary. Vitamin C appears to enhance the absorption of iron.
   d. Explain the reasons for diet change to caregivers and child in a language they can understand. Visual aids and pictures may be helpful.
   e. Assist the caregivers to select iron-rich foods that are acceptable to the child, within the family's food budget, and culturally acceptable.
   f. Recognize cultural aspects related to food preference and preparation.
4. Initiate a nutritional consultation, as indicated.
5. Discuss with caregivers any of the social, economic, and environmental problems that may contribute to the child's disease.
6. Emphasize to the caregivers the benefits of a referral to a community health nurse if it appears that the family will need support in dealing with the child's chronic disease.
7. Discuss general health measures, including adequate rest, diet, sunshine, and fresh air activity.
8. Encourage regular medical and dental evaluations. Encourage the need for immunizations according to the recommended schedule.
9. Educate regarding infection prevention.
10. Teach the caregivers how to administer medication.
11. Alert the caregivers to signs of disease progression—increased fatigue, pallor, weakness, developmental delays, and poor performance in school and activities.
12. Prepare for possible adverse GI effects, including constipation and change in stool color.

DRUG ALERT Much variation exists in elemental iron content of commercially available liquid preparations that contain iron. For clarity, dosages should be expressed in terms of elemental iron to ensure proper amounts.

Evaluation: Expected Outcomes

- Increasing activity without fatigue noted.
- Nutritional intake will provide a more balanced, iron-containing diet.
- Remains free from infection; normal temperature.
- Maintains growth curve; manages age-appropriate developmental activities.
- Cognitive performance at school and job (for older adolescents) will improve.
- Attendance at school, job (for older adolescents), and other social obligations will improve.
- Maintain adherence with medication regimen and lab monitoring.

Sickle Cell Disease (Sickle Cell Anemia)

EVIDENCE BASE Coco, M., Henderson, W. A., Park, C. L., & Starkweather, A. R. (2023). Growing beyond sickle cell disease: A metasynthesis of children, adolescents, and young adult experiences living with sickle cell disease. *Research in Nursing & Health, 46*(3), 299–312. https://doi.org/10.1002/nur.22310.

Sickle cell disease, a group of inherited RBC disorders, is a severe autosomal recessive genetic defect in Hb. It is a form of anemia in which a mutational form of Hb distorts the RBCs into a crescent shape at low oxygen levels. The crescent-shaped "sickled" cell blocks the flow of cells through the blood vessels and interrupts the delivery of oxygen to the tissues. The most common form of sickle cell disease in North America is homozygous Hb SS disease. In the United States, approximately 100,000 people have sickle cell disease. It occurs in about 16,300 Hispanic American births and in 1 in 365 Black American births. Due to the influx of immigrants, sickle cell disease is seen in a more diverse group of patients. For example, a New York State newborn screening program estimates the incidence of sickle cell disease in the White population at 1 in 40,000. Approximately one in three Black or African Americans has sickle cell trait, accounting for about 3 million people.

Pathophysiology and Etiology

1. Genetically determined and inherited as an autosomal recessive condition (see Figure 48-1).
2. Each person inherits one gene from each biological parent, which governs the synthesis of Hb (see Table 48-3).
3. The sickle cell mutation reflects a single change in the amino acid–building blocks of Hb.
4. Hb is a complex protein molecule made up of four subunits of globin.
5. Hb has two proteins that allow it to carry and release oxygen, alpha-globin, and beta-globin.
6. The alpha-globin is normal in sickle cell disease. The beta-globin has the amino acid valine at position 6 instead of glutamic acid.
7. If only one of the beta genes is the sickled gene and the other is normal, the person is a carrier and has sickle cell trait.
8. If both beta gene codes are sickled, the person has sickle cell disease.
9. Sickle cell Hb aggregates into elongated crystals under conditions of low oxygen concentration, acidosis, and dehydration.
10. This distorts the membrane of the RBC, causing it to assume a crescent or sickle shape. The cells easily become entangled and

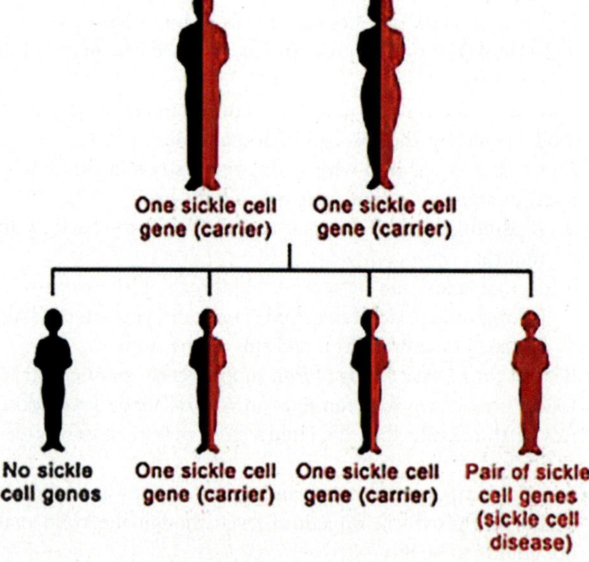

Figure 48-1. Transmission of sickle cell disease.

Table 48-3 Transmission of Sickle Cell Disease

GENOTYPE OF BIOLOGICAL PARENTS	PROBABILITY OF SICKLE CELL DISEASE IN OFFSPRING		
	UNAFFECTED (%)	CARRIER (%)	DISEASE (%)
One biological parent with trait	50	50	0
Both biological parents with trait	25	50	25
One biological parent with trait; one biological parent with disease	0	50	50
Both biological parents with disease	0	0	100

enmeshed, leading to increased blood viscosity, vessel occlusion, and tissue necrosis.

11. Sickled RBCs are fragile and are rapidly destroyed in the circulation; they can live as little as 4 days versus 120 days for normal RBCs.
12. Anemia results when the rate of destruction of RBCs is greater than the rate of production.
13. Increased sequestration of RBCs occurs in the spleen.
14. Surgery.
15. Pregnancy.

Clinical Manifestations

Usually present since the first year of life. Affected infants do not develop symptoms in the first few months of life because the Hb produced by the developing fetus, fetal Hb, protects RBCs from sickling. The fetal Hb is absent in RBCs produced after birth so that by 5 months of age, sickling of RBCs is prominent and symptoms can begin.

Prenatal diagnosis is possible using amniocentesis or chorionic villus sampling. All 50 states, the District of Columbia, and all U.S. territories require every baby be tested for sickle cell anemia on the newborn screening.

Signs of Anemia

Vary from person to person and may change over time.

1. Hb level—6 to 9 g/dL, average of 8 g/dL.
2. Loss of appetite.
3. Pallor.
4. Tiredness.
5. Easily fatigued.
6. Irritability.
7. Shortness of breath.
8. Have a feeling of heart racing.
9. Jaundice; increased hemolysis results in hemosiderosis (increased iron storage in the liver).

Precipitating Factors of Crisis

1. Dehydration.
2. Infection.
3. Stress.
4. Strenuous physical exertion.
5. Extreme fatigue.
6. Cold exposure.
7. Temperature extremes.
8. Humidity.
9. Air quality.
10. Nutritional deficiencies.
11. High altitude.
12. Exposure to low doses of carbon monoxide.
13. Socioeconomic factors.

Sickle Cell (Vaso-occlusive) Crisis

1. Most common form of crisis. Typically lasts 3 to 14 days. Most common sites are the lower back, leg, hip, abdomen, or chest. Usually occurs in one or more locations. Most hospitalizations are seen in children aged 16 to 20 years.
   a. Small blood vessels are occluded by the sickle-shaped cells, causing distal ischemia and infarction. This can cause severe pain and permanent damage to the brain, heart, lungs, kidney, liver, bones, and spleen (see Figure 48-2).
2. Extremities:
   a. Bony destruction—related to erythroid hyperplasia of the marrow, leading to osteoporosis or ischemic necrosis.
   b. Aseptic necrosis—results from poor blood supply to an area of the bone, causing localized bone death.

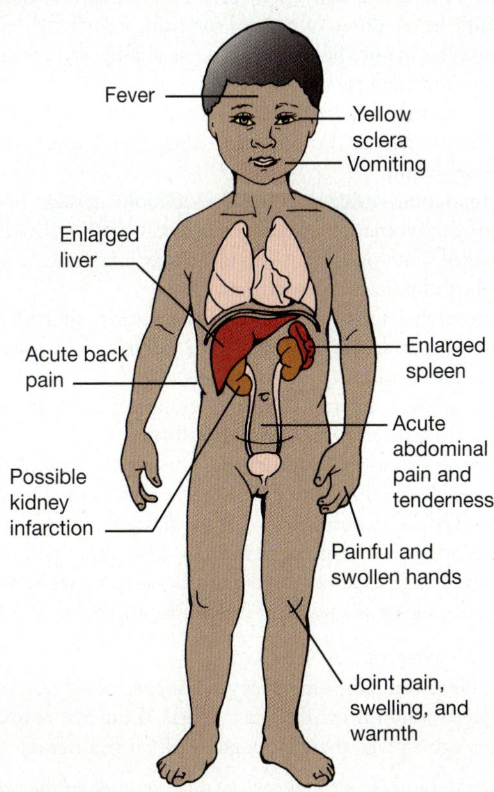

Figure 48-2. Sickle cell crisis signs and symptoms.

c. Bone infarction—bone tissue dies due to lack of sufficient blood supply.
d. Dactylitis ("hand–foot" syndrome)—swelling and inflammation of hands and feet caused by injury to the bones of affected digits by repeated episodes of inadequate blood circulation; commonly first vaso-occlusive event seen in infants and toddlers and children up to age 8 years.
e. Arthritis—can accompany dactylitis—presents with pain, swelling, tenderness, and limited range of motion (ROM).

3. Spleen:
   a. Abdominal pain.
   b. Splenomegaly—initially enlarges because of increased activity at the site of RBC hemolysis; increased size results in discomfort. The spleen usually does not work after 4 to 6 months of age. Enlargement is usually seen up to 5 years of age.
   c. After multiple episodes of splenic vaso-occlusion, the spleen becomes fibrotic and atrophied.
   d. Decreased splenic function increases the risk of infection.
   e. Important for protection against germs; serious, life-threatening infections occur secondary to damage to the spleen.
4. Cerebral occlusion:
   a. Stroke—most common killer of patients over age 3 years; between 8% and 10% of patients have had a stroke, typically at around age 7 years.
   b. Hemiplegia.
   c. Retinal damage, leading to blindness.
   d. Seizures.
   e. Aneurysms—common and often located where they cannot be surgically treated.
5. Pulmonary:
   a. Acute chest syndrome—more likely to occur after infection, sickle cell crisis, general anesthesia, blood clot, and heavy doses of opiates for pain; lowers the levels of oxygen in the blood; and can cause lung damage and be life-threatening.
   b. Pulmonary hypertension—occurs when pressure in the arteries of the lungs increases; seen mostly in adult population.
   c. Infarction—triggered by dehydration; results in cycle of deoxygenation, which exacerbates sickling, leading to small vessel occlusions and ultimately infarction of areas of the pulmonary parenchyma.
6. Altered renal function—enuresis, hematuria, difficulty concentrating urine, protein loss in the urine, and increased risk of kidney disease.
7. Impaired liver function—may develop iron overload secondary to frequent need for blood transfusion.
8. Priapism—abnormal, recurrent, prolonged, painful penile erection; blood flow out of the erect penis is blocked by sickled cells; can lead to permanent damage and impotence.
9. Infections—most common include *Chlamydia pneumoniae*, *Mycoplasma pneumoniae*, and gram-negative bacteria; may develop leg ulcers as a result of infectious process.

Splenic Sequestration Crisis

Can be a life-threatening emergency. Most commonly seen in children between 5 months and 5 years of age. If the first episode occurs under age 2 years, there is a higher risk for recurrence.

1. Large amounts of sickled cells become trapped in the spleen.
2. The spleen becomes massively enlarged.
3. Hb decreases by at least 2 g/dL secondary to sudden, large drop in blood count.
4. Increase in reticulocytes.
5. Signs of circulatory collapse (e.g., shock and hypotension) develop rapidly.
6. Frequent cause of death in infants with sickle cell disease.
7. Restore circulating blood volume; bolus 10 to 20 mL/kg of normal saline while awaiting PRBCs; transfuse 10 mL/kg PRBCs; do not transfuse higher than baseline Hb.
8. Sequestered blood will eventually reenter circulation, increasing the risk for hyperviscosity and strokes.

Aplastic Crisis

1. Increased risk with parvovirus.
2. Bone marrow ceases production of RBCs only.
3. Results in low reticulocyte counts.
4. After a few days, the bone marrow usually recovers on its own.
5. Blood transfusion may be necessary.

Chronic Symptoms

Chronic organ damage results in organ dysfunction.

1. Jaundice.
2. Gallstones.
3. Progressive impairment of kidney function.
4. High risk of infection.
5. Growth retardation of the long bones and spine deformities.
6. Delayed growth and puberty.
7. Cardiac decompensation related to chronic anemia (may develop heart failure).
8. Chronic, painful leg ulcers related to decreased peripheral circulation and unrelated to injury; may take months to heal or may not heal without intense therapy, including blood transfusions and grafting.
9. Deep vein thromboses.
10. Pulmonary emboli.
11. Stroke.
12. Malnutrition.
13. Increased risk of renal medullary carcinoma later in life.
14. Altered bony structures—aseptic necrosis of the bones, especially the femoral and humoral heads.
15. Decreased lifespan.

Diagnostic Evaluation

1. Ante-/perinatal testing via amniocentesis or chorionic villus sampling.
2. Newborn screening—done in all 50 states, the District of Columbia, and all U.S. territories. Normally performed in the hospital prior to discharge. For home births, performed at first pediatric appointment.
3. Those needing further testing:
   a. Immigrants who were not tested in their home country.
   b. Children moving state to state who have not been tested.
   c. Anyone displaying symptoms.
4. HbS solubility test and sodium metabisulfite test.
   a. Done by finger or heel stick.
5. Hemoglobinopathy evaluation.
   a. Hb electrophoresis.
   b. Hb fractionation by high-performance liquid chromatography (HPLC).
   c. Isoelectric focusing—highly sensitive, used at large laboratories

6. DNA analysis—used to investigate alterations and mutations in the genes that produce Hb components.
   a. Requires venipuncture.

Management

Preventing Sickling

1. Promote adequate oxygenation and hemodilution.
   a. Encourage increased intake of fluids—at least eight 8-ounce glasses of water daily.
   b. Avoid high altitudes and other low-oxygen environments.
   c. Exercise regularly but not so much that you become really tired.
   d. Reduce or avoid stress.
   e. Avoid extreme heat or cold. Wear warm clothes in cold weather, stay in air conditioning in hot weather, and do not swim in cold water.
   f. Treat infection as soon as it occurs.
   g. Only travel in commercial pressurized airplanes.
   h. Avoid alcohol, soda, and caffeine because these substances increase the risk of dehydration.
   i. Do not smoke, and avoid passive smoke exposure.
   j. Prophylactic blood transfusions (increase number of normal RBCs) (see page 762). Lowers the Hb S circulating in the blood.

Acute Management

Supportive and symptomatic care depends on the type of crisis.

1. Aplastic episode—supportive care and blood transfusions to maintain adequate Hct until marrow activity is restored.
2. Splenic sequestration—IV fluids and transfusion required to maintain intravascular volume. One or more episodes may require splenectomy, though this is still debated.
3. Hemolytic episode—usually requires only hydration. May occur with splenic sequestration, aplastic, and painful episodes, which are then treated accordingly. Transfusions are required if a significant drop in Hb occurs.
4. Vaso-occlusive or painful episode—must determine whether the painful event is a manifestation of an underlying illness (infection) or of an inflammatory condition. Most commonly caused by increased sickling, resulting from hypoxemia and acidosis. Often requires an inpatient stay.
   a. Hydration—this is accomplished by increased oral and parenteral fluid intake of up to two times (bid) of fluid maintenance needs.
   b. Analgesics—administered on fixed schedule, not to extend beyond the duration of the pharmacologic effect. IV opioids, such as morphine, are preferred for severe pain, either as a continuous infusion or on a patient-controlled analgesia pump to reach desired effects. Other agents, such as nonsteroidal anti-inflammatory drugs (NSAIDs) and acetaminophen, are used for milder pain or to increase the analgesic effects of opioids.
   c. Alternative pain management techniques—behavior modification programs, relaxation therapy, hypnosis, music therapy, and massage.
   d. Those with chronic or severe vaso-occlusive crises may benefit from monthly blood transfusions, which will improve anemia and decrease total amount of sickle Hb; however, iron overload is a possible complication.
   e. Use of hydroxyurea on a daily basis—hydroxyurea increased the amount of fetal Hb in RBCs, allowing the cells to travel more easily through the blood vessels; best used on patients who have had recurrent episodes of pain crises.
   f. If there is a human leukocyte antigen (HLA)-matched sibling without sickle cell disease, an allogeneic transplant is standard of care prior to the presentation of symptoms and disease complications. If there is no HLA-matched sibling, haploidentical transplants from a family member (preferably the child's biological mother) are commonly performed.
   g. Gene therapy options are now in trials, including the use of progenitor cells transduced with a lovo-cel vector. These cells, which are administered via autologous hematopoietic stem transplantation, produce antisickling Hb.
5. Infection—most common cause of morbidity and mortality.
   a. Most serious include *Streptococcus pneumoniae*, *Haemophilus influenzae*, *Salmonella* species, *M. pneumoniae*, *C. pneumoniae*, *Escherichia coli*, and *Klebsiella pneumoniae*.
   b. Infection of any type is more difficult to eradicate in patients with sickle cell and commonly exacerbates crises such as aplastic episodes caused by parvovirus (fifth disease), increases the rate of hemolysis, and precipitates vaso-occlusive episodes.
   c. Prevention is most important—give usual primary immunizations as well as pneumococcal, *Haemophilus* b conjugate, hepatitis, meningococcal, and trivalent influenza vaccines.
   d. Antibiotic prophylaxis—penicillin prophylaxis is recommended in children less than 5 years of age and older children with a previous history of severe pneumococcal infection or have functional/surgical asplenia.
   e. Patients with unexplained fever should be cultured thoroughly. If clinical condition suggests septicemia, broad-spectrum antibiotics should be initiated after complete culturing. Patients with septicemia can expire in only a few hours.
6. Stroke prevention:
   a. Transcranial Doppler (TCD) screening for all children with sickle cell anemia from age 2 to 16 years. TCD should be repeated annually if normal and every 6 months if questionable.
   b. Children with abnormal TCD should be kept on a chronic maintenance transfusion program to keep their Hb S less than 30%.
   c. Stroke risk has decreased from 11% to 1% with use of TCD.

Complications

1. Chronic hemolytic anemia. Characterized by anemia, jaundice, periodic crises, splenomegaly, and gallstones. Symptoms worsen during crises.
2. Main causes of death in children from sickle cell anemia were infection and acute splenic sequestration. Deaths are most common before the age of 2 years.
3. Common causes of death for older individuals with sickle cell anemia are intercurrent infections, acute chest syndrome, pulmonary emboli, infarction of a vital organ, and renal failure.
4. Life expectancy is variable; however, it is improving with new forms of treatment. Survival on average is 42 years for males and 48 years for females.

Nursing Assessment

1. Observe for pallor and jaundice, changes in vital signs (elevated temperature, tachycardia, hypotension, tachypnea), change in mental status, swelling of extremities, ulcers or skin lesions,

or signs of dehydration (decreased elasticity of the skin, dry mucous membranes, decreased urine output, increased urine concentration, and specific gravity).
2. Examine for enlarged liver and spleen and tenderness of hands or feet.
3. Discuss symptoms and duration of pain, dyspnea, fever, pallor, and lethargy.
4. Discuss precipitating factors for crises, that is, fever, travel, and procedures.
5. Discuss the history of chest crises and management.
6. Discuss any comorbidities that may exist, for example, asthma.
7. Discuss usual treatment protocol, including chronic transfusions and use of hydroxyurea.
8. Evaluate growth and development.

CLINICAL JUDGMENT Be aware of your personal biases with regard to pain and pain management. Pain is often misunderstood, dismissed, or overlooked. Nurses need to take the time to listen to their patients' values, cultural traditions, and perception of pain. It is a multifaceted concern for patient and caregiver alike.

EVIDENCE BASE Osunkwo, I., O'Connor, H. F., & Saah, E. (2020). Optimizing the management of chronic pain in sickle cell disease. *Hematology. American Society of Hematology Education Program, 2020*(1), 562–569. https://doi.org/10.1182/hematology.2020000143

Relieving Pain

1. Utilize a multidisciplinary approach, including the hematologist as well as psychosocial and mental health providers; this allows for a holistic, patient-centered approach.
2. Identify and use effective measures to alleviate pain, such as:
   a. Carefully position and support painful areas. Joints and extremities can be extremely painful.
   b. Hold or rock the infant; handle gently.
   c. Provide distractions by singing, reading stories, providing appropriate play activities, or television or videos.
   d. Provide familiar objects.
   e. Bathe the child in warm water, applying local heat or providing massage.
   f. Administer opioid analgesics as ordered. Continuous IV infusion is used for the duration of a painful crisis.
   g. Utilize virtual reality, audiovisual relaxation techniques, and transcutaneous electrical nerve stimulation (TENS), if appropriate.
3. Communicate effective methods of reducing pain with other staff members and family.
4. Patients with chronic pain may not display typical pain behavior; remember, "pain is what the patient says it is."
5. Virtual reality.
6. Audiovisual relaxation.
7. TENS.
8. Assess physical and psychological effectiveness of intervention.
9. Develop an individualized pain management plan for each patient.

Increasing Tissue Perfusion

1. Avoid physical exertion, emotional stress, and low-oxygen environments to reduce the body's need for oxygen.
2. Administer blood transfusions as ordered.
3. Perform caregiving activities in groups to provide for optimum rest.
4. Administer oxygen to increase diffusion of gas across membranes.
5. Educate the family regarding the need for prophylactic transfusions to lower the risk of cardiovascular accident.

Risk of Dehydration

1. Calculate and educate the family with regard to child's daily fluid requirements.
2. Assess mucous membranes for signs of dehydration.
3. Record daily intake and output to ensure adequate fluid intake.

Reducing Infection

1. Ensure adequate nutrition through high-calorie, high-protein diet.
2. Ensure immunizations are up to date.
3. Isolate the child from sources of infection if possible.
4. Administer antibiotics, as prescribed.
5. Provide meticulous care to leg ulcers and other open wounds.
6. Use and demonstrate good handwashing and meticulous technique with all procedures.

Activity Intolerance

1. Assess the child's level of mobility and activity tolerance.
2. Encourage adequate rest periods throughout the day.
3. Prioritize tasks when episodes of activity intolerance occur.
4. Encourage good eating habits, sleep, and relaxation.
5. Encourage verbalization of feelings regarding limitations.

Normalizing Family Processes

1. Encourage caregivers to talk about their child, the illness, and how they feel about it.
2. Expect feelings such as guilt, shock, frustration, depression, and resentment.
3. Accept negative feelings, but try to build on positive coping mechanisms.
4. Provide factual information to the child and caregivers about their concerns.
5. Encourage role-playing and play activities to identify fears.
6. Ensure adolescents that although sexual development is delayed, they will eventually catch up with their peers.
7. Stress the normalcy of the child despite having sickle cell disease.
   a. Sickle cell disease does not affect intelligence; the child should go to school and keep up with classwork while stable.
   b. Between periods of crisis, the child can usually participate in peer group activities, with the exception of some strenuous sports.
   c. The child needs the same discipline as other children in the family.

Knowledge Deficit

1. Review basics of sickle cell disease with family and child.
2. Teach the family about signs and symptoms of crises.
3. Educate the family as to when immediate medical care is essential.
4. Teach the importance of balanced, healthy nutrition, hydration, sleep, and periods of rest.
5. Arrange for genetic counseling and testing for sickle cell trait in family members.

Community and Home Care Considerations

Home care nurses and school nurses can be instrumental in the care of patients with sickle cell anemia by ensuring that their primary health care needs are met. A reliable medical home is essential for patients with sickle cell anemia.

1. The following examinations should be done as indicated:
   a. Regularly scheduled medical checkups: every 2 to 4 months from birth to 24 months, every 3 to 4 months from 2 to 12 years of age, and every 6 months from age 12 and above. Each visit should include height, weight, head circumference (up to age 2), vital signs (including BP), and oxygen saturation level.
   b. CBC—yearly.
   c. Quantitative electrophoresis—at birth, repeat between ages 1 and 2 years.
   d. RBC antigen testing—between ages 1 and 2 years or prior to the first transfusion.
   e. LFTs/bilirubin/renal bloodwork—annually.
   f. Urinalysis—annually in older children and adolescents.
   g. Ophthalmology examinations—annually after age 10.
   h. Hearing tests—only if clinical concern, secondary to prolonged and frequent use of antibiotics.
   i. Pulmonary function tests (PFTs)—oxygen saturation testing at each visit and baseline PFT in adolescence.
   j. A tuberculin skin test every 2 to 3 years (every year in at-risk populations). Any positive findings should be followed up promptly.
   k. All routine childhood immunizations, as well as the hepatitis B series, pneumococcal conjugate vaccine, pneumococcal polysaccharide vaccine, meningococcal, *H. influenzae* type B, COVID-19 vaccine, and yearly trivalent influenza.
   l. Dental checkups and teeth cleaning every 6 months.
2. Educate caregivers, teachers, and daycare providers involved in the care of children with sickle cell disease about their common problems and special needs:
   a. Frequent absences because of pain and illness.
   b. Fatigue and inattention, caused by anemia or ischemia of central nervous system tissue.
   c. Need for adequate hydration throughout the course of the day.
   d. Inability to concentrate urine, requiring frequent restroom breaks.
   e. Permanent learning disabilities or delays, requiring individualized teaching plans.
   f. Need for a controlled environment to prevent sickling, avoiding temperature extremes, dehydration, and excessive stress.
   g. Need for moderate physical exercise, with avoidance of rough contact sports and activities.
   h. Desire to feel "normal" and have opportunities and environmental stimulation similar to other children their age.
3. Assess the child's home environment for protection from infection and injury, adequate nutritional resources, transportation to medical appointments, and emotional support. Initiate social service and other referrals, as needed.
4. Consider/explore possible complementary and alternative therapies.

Family Education and Health Maintenance

1. Discuss the genetic implications of sickle cell disease and offer genetic counseling to the family.
2. Instruct the caregivers in ways that they can help their child to avoid sickling episodes.
   a. Do not allow the child to become chilled or to wear tight clothing that might impede circulation.
   b. Provide adequate fluids and notify health care provider if excessive fluids are lost through vomiting, diarrhea, fever, and excessive sweating.
   c. Limit excessive exercise and offer frequent breaks with activity.
   d. Avoid extreme temperature settings.
3. Instruct caregivers how to recognize signs of dehydration (dry skin and mucous membranes, decreased urine output; irritability or listlessness in the infant).
4. Encourage caregivers to seek prompt treatment of lacerations, wounds, and insect bites and to notify the health care provider if the child is exposed to a communicable disease.
5. Encourage good dental hygiene and twice yearly dental checkups to avoid infections.
6. Instruct on preventive care, including all the recommended childhood immunizations and screening tests.
7. Encourage a calm, emotionally stable environment.
8. Warn against trips to the mountains or against trips in unpressurized airplanes that will decrease oxygen concentration.
9. Provide sexually active adolescents with information on contraception and sexually transmitted diseases.
10. Teach signs of a mild crisis:
    a. Fatigue.
    b. Yellowish color of the skin and whites of eyes.
    c. Decreased appetite.
    d. Irritability.
    e. Low-grade fever.
    f. Painful swelling of hands and/or feet.
    g. Teach caregivers to palpate the spleen.
11. Instruct on home management of mild crisis.
    a. Encourage fluids.
    b. Administer antipyretic medications, as directed by health care provider.
    c. Encourage rest.
    d. Keep the child warm.
    e. Apply warm compresses to the painful area.
    f. Hospitalization may be required for the child if pain becomes severe or if IV hydration is required.
12. Teach the signs of severe crisis and whom to notify:
    a. Pallor.
    b. Lethargy and listlessness.
    c. Severe pain in the abdomen, chest, bones, and/or joints.
    d. Swelling in hands and feet.
    e. Abdominal swelling.
    f. Weakness is the face, arms, or legs.
    g. Trouble walking or talking.
    h. Visual disturbance.
    i. Numbness.
    j. Fever of 102°F (38.9°C)—report immediately.
    k. Decreased appetite and dehydration.
13. Instruct the caregivers to have emergency information available to those involved in the child's care (school nurse, teacher, babysitter, family members).
    a. Name and phone number of health care provider or clinic.
    b. Closest emergency facility and ambulance phone number.
    c. Child's blood type, allergies, medications, and medical records number.
    d. Name of informed neighbor or relative to be notified in an emergency.
14. Stress the benefit of wearing a medical alert device.
15. For additional information and support, refer to Sickle Cell Foundation (*www.scdfc.org*).

Evaluation: Expected Outcomes

- Able to drink enough fluids and eat a well-balanced diet.
- Pain well controlled or absent.
- Less pallor without the need for oxygen.
- Afebrile without signs of infection.
- Respirations within normal limits for age; uses incentive spirometer hourly.
- Ambulates throughout the day for short intervals with minimal or no pain.
- Caregivers verbalize concerns about chronic illness.

Thalassemia Major (Cooley Anemia)

EVIDENCE BASE Liang, H., Pan, L., Xie, Y., Fan, J., Zhai, L., Liang, S., Zhang, Z., & Lai, Y. (2022). Health-related quality of life in pediatric patients with beta thalassemia major after hematopoietic stem cell transplantation. *Bone Marrow Transplantation, 57*(7), 1108–1115. https://doi.org/10.1038/s41409-022-01663-0

Thalassemia major is the most severe of the beta-thalassemia syndromes and represents the homozygous form of the disease. Beta-thalassemia refers to a group of inherited genetic disorders characterized by a reduction or absence of the beta-globulin chain in Hb synthesis. Classification and severity grading are based on spontaneous Hb level and clinical tolerance. Patients with thalassemia major have Hb concentrations between 3 and 7 g/dL and exhibit severe anemia. It was first discovered in the Mediterranean basin and is highly prevalent in countries also affected by malaria. It mainly affects people of Mediterranean, Southern Asia, Southeast Asia, and Middle Eastern origin. In the United States, it affects approximately 1 in 10,000 people.

Pathophysiology and Etiology

1. Genetically determined, inherited autosomal recessive disorder (see Figure 48-3).
2. Defect can be a complete absence of the beta-globin protein or severely reduced synthesis of the beta-globin protein. Severity of the disease is based on the amount of beta-globin production.
3. Determined by reduced production of beta chains and excess accumulation of alpha chains.

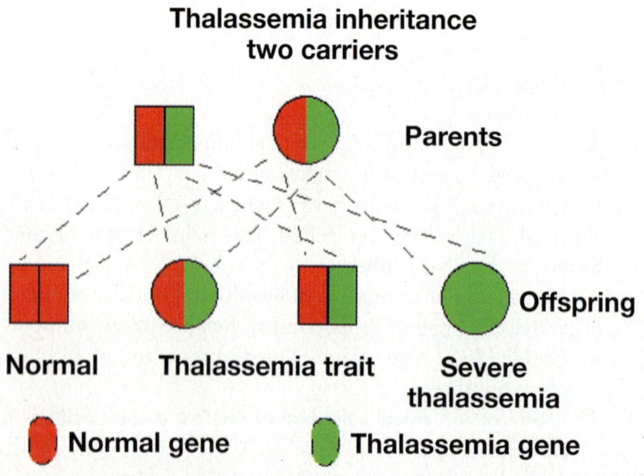

Figure 48-3. Transmission of thalassemia. Note: In this figure, "parents" means biological parents.

4. The resulting RBCs are abnormally small, are not produced in normal amounts, and do not contain enough functional Hb, leading to severe hemolytic anemia and resultant chronic hypoxia.
5. The abnormalities result in quantitative changes in globins as opposed to the qualitative or functional changes seen in hemoglobinopathies.
6. Erythroid activity is significantly increased in an attempt to overcome the increased rate of destruction. This results in:
   a. An enormous expansion of the bone marrow and thinning of the bony cortex.
   b. Skeletal deformities: frontal and maxillary bossing.
   c. Growth retardation.
   d. Deformities of the long bones of the leg.
   e. Massive hepatosplenomegaly.
7. Decreased erythropoietin drive and increased iron load result in higher hepcidin levels. These higher levels moderate dietary absorption and cause macrophages to retain iron. This causes body iron stores to increase because of the inability to excrete the iron and leads to tissue damage.
8. Hb F amounts to less than 1% of Hb by 6 to 12 months of age: In genetic disorders such as thalassemia major, there is a persistent presence of Hb F because of alteration of the beta-globin cluster; Hb F does not hold oxygen well.

Clinical Manifestations

1. Infants exhibit symptoms within the first 2 years of life, often between 3 and 6 months after birth.
2. Symptoms are primarily related to progressive anemia, expansion of the marrow cavities of the bone, hepatosplenomegaly, and extramedullary hematopoiesis in the chest and abdomen.
3. Early symptoms commonly include failure to thrive, feeding difficulties, pallor, diarrhea, irritability or fussiness, dark urine from hemolysis, recurrent fevers, and mild jaundice.
4. Further signs of progressive anemia include headache, bone pain, exercise intolerance, jaundice, and protuberant abdomen caused by hepatosplenomegaly.
5. If untreated, it can cause abnormal expansion of the bone marrow, causing bones to become thinner, wider, and brittle; this can cause frontal bossing, prominent malar eminence, and depressed bridge of the nose and hypertrophy of maxilla; also see increased risk of fracture of the long bones. Furthermore, there is an increased risk of osteopenia and osteoporosis.
6. Growth impairment is evident with delay in adolescent growth spurt.
7. Late symptoms can affect the heart, liver, and endocrine systems.

Diagnostic Evaluation

1. CBC with differential—determines number of RBCs and how much Hb is in them; evaluates red cell indices, including MCV.
2. Peripheral blood smear—looks at a layer of the blood with a microscope and can assess number and type of white blood cells, platelets, and RBCs.
3. Iron studies—iron, ferritin, unsaturated iron-binding capacity (UIBC), TIBC, and percent saturation of transferrin.
4. DNA analysis—confirms mutation in the alpha- and beta-globin–producing gene.
5. Amniocentesis—can be done perinatally if increased risk is a concern.

Management

1. Children with little to no globin chain production have little Hb A and are thus transfusion dependent.
2. Frequent and regular blood transfusions of PRBCs to maintain Hb levels between 9 and 10 g/dL.
   a. All children starting regular transfusions should be vaccinated against hepatitis B as early as possible.
   b. Children on chronic transfusion regimens should have an extended red cell phenotype/genotype prior to or as soon as possible after commencing therapy.
   c. RBC component of transfusions: In children less than 4 months of age, PRBCs should be compatible with maternal and neonatal ABO and D group and clinically significant maternal antibodies; in children over 4 months of age, PRBCs should be compatible with recipients ABO and D group and any red cell alloantibodies.
   d. Washed PRBCs are usually used to minimize the possibility of transfusion reactions. If unavailable, leuko-filtered cells can be substituted.
   e. Goal of transfusion is to shut off erythropoiesis as much as possible; should be given at 3- to 4-week interval.
   f. Target Hb should be between 9 and 10 g/dL; in patients with cardiac insufficiency, higher levels of 10 to 12 g/dL should be maintained.
3. Iron overload is common in conditions that require chronic blood transfusions. Manifestations of this include growth impairment, metabolic and endocrine abnormalities, heart failure and arrhythmias, pulmonary abnormalities, thrombosis, leg ulcers, and certain types of cancer.
4. Iron chelation therapy reduces the toxic adverse effects of excess iron and increases iron excretion through urine and feces. Iron chelation is usually started at 2 to 4 years of age after 20 to 25 units of PRBCs is transfused and a serum ferritin level of greater than 1,000 μg/dL and a liver iron concentration (LIC) of greater than 3 mg/iron/g dry weight measured by liver biopsy or hepatic T2 magnetic resonance imaging (MRI) are achieved.
   a. Deferoxamine: IV, IM, or subcutaneous (SQ) formulation of iron-chelating agent; in IV formulations, it is administered over at least 8 to 12 hours for 5 to 7 days per week—should not exceed 60 mg/kg/day; if given SQ, administered at 30 to 60 mg/kg/day over 8 to 12 hours for 5 to 7 days per week; vitamin C increases the excretion of iron in the presence of deferoxamine—after 1 month of chelation therapy, should take 2 to 4 mg/kg/day of vitamin C soon after infusion is complete.
   b. Deferasirox: oral iron chelation agent; initial dosing at 10 mg/kg/day—can be adjusted up to 40 mg/kg/day; must be mixed in apple juice, orange juice, or water—for dosing less than 1,000 mg, mix in ½ cup fluid, and in dosing greater than 1,000 mg, must be mixed in 1 cup of fluid; no antacids containing aluminum should be given while on deferasirox.
   c. The tablet formulation of deferasirox (Jadenu) has demonstrated improved adherence with therapy.
5. Splenectomy. Optimal clinical management from the time of diagnosis may delay or prevent hypersplenism. Increased efficiency of transfusion therapy may reduce the need for splenectomy. Splenectomy should be considered if:
   a. Annual blood requirement is greater than 1.5 times that of patients who have had a splenectomy.
   b. Increased iron stores despite good chelation therapy.
   c. Splenic enlargement is accompanied by left upper quadrant pain, early satiety, or concern for splenic rupture.
   d. Leucopenia or thrombocytopenia because of hypersplenism causes recurrent bacterial infections or bleeding.
   e. Prior to splenectomy, the child should be immunized against *S. pneumoniae*, *H. influenzae* B, and *Neisseria meningitidis*.
   f. Oral penicillin prophylaxis is necessary (250 mg bid) postsplenectomy.
   g. Family should be educated that urgent medical attention is required for fever greater than 101°F (38.3°C).
   h. Should be avoided under age 5 years secondary to increased risk for fulminant postsplenectomy sepsis.
6. Supportive management of complications.
7. Hematopoietic stem cell transplants are the only known cure. Young patients with few complications are the best candidates. Over the past several years, novel strategies have improved outcomes and decreased transplant related risks such as graft versus host disease.
8. Prognosis is poor; life expectancy is 17 years of age, and most children with thalassemia major die before age 30.

Complications

1. Splenomegaly—usually requires splenectomy; major long-term risk after splenectomy is overwhelming sepsis.
2. Growth retardation in the second decade. Growth is usually normal until 9 to 10 years of age. Multifactorial including hemosiderosis-induced damage of the endocrine glands, chronic anemia, hypoxia, chronic liver disease, vitamin and nutritional deficiencies, use of chelating agents, endocrinopathies, low insulin-like growth factor 1 (IGF-1) levels, and emotional factors.
3. Endocrine abnormalities:
   a. Hypogonadism—most obvious clinical consequence of iron overload.
   b. Delayed puberty.
   c. Hypothyroidism.
   d. Disturbed calcium homeostasis—results in osteopenia and/or osteoporosis.
   e. Hypoparathyroidism.
   f. Growth hormone deficiency.
   g. Diabetes mellitus—presents after the age of 10 years.
   h. Adrenal insufficiency.
4. Skeletal complications—become less common because of early transfusion therapy and maintenance of Hb levels above 10 g/dL:
   a. Frontal and parietal bossing (enlarging).
   b. Maxillary hypertrophy, leading to malocclusion.
   c. Increased risk of osteopenia and osteoporosis.
   d. Pathologic fractures of the long bones and vertebral collapse, especially in the lumbar region.
5. Cardiac complications:
   a. Arrhythmias—electrocardiogram (ECG) changes specifically increased QTc and leftward shift of the T-wave axis.
   b. Cardiomyopathy secondary to cardiac iron overload.
   c. Increase in left ventricular septal and posterior wall thickness.
   d. Premature vascular aging including abnormal vascular stiffening noted as patients live longer.
   e. Heart failure—usual cause of death.

6. Liver disease:
   a. Chronic infection develops in 70% to 80% of patients, leading to chronic liver disease.
   b. Liver fibrosis and cirrhosis.
   c. Hepatocellular carcinoma—develops in 1% to 5% of individuals over the age of 20.
7. Gallbladder disease—gallstones develop secondary to chronic anemia. Up to two thirds of patients with thalassemia major develop gallstones; most patients remain asymptomatic; cholecystectomy is rarely required.
8. Megaloblastic anemia—caused by sporadic folic acid and vitamin B_{12} deficiency from increased use by hyperplastic marrow. Folic acid supplementation is recommended for all patients.
9. Skin—pruritus and xerosis seen frequently and jaundice secondary to iron overload.
10. Leg ulcers.

Nursing Assessment

1. Review family medical history, especially those associated with anemia.
2. Perform whole-body examination to assess for anemia and systemic complications of thalassemia.
3. Observe for signs and symptoms of anemia.
4. Measure growth and development parameters.

Nursing Interventions

Inadequate Tissue Perfusion

1. Blood transfusion:
   a. Mainstay of treatment.
   b. Prevents most of the serious complications associated with thalassemia.
   c. Signs and symptoms indicative of the need for transfusion include increased cardiac effort or tachycardia, sweating, poor appetite, poor growth, and inability to maintain daily activities.
   d. Must rule out infectious/septic etiology.
   e. Observe for signs of transfusion reaction (increased chance caused by frequency):
      i. Fever.
      ii. Chills.
      iii. Hives.
      iv. Edema.
      v. Pain or burning in the abdomen, chest, or back.
      vi. Sense of doom.
      vii. Breathing problems.
      viii. Swelling/bruising at transfusion site.
      ix. Nausea, vomiting, and/or diarrhea.
   f. Reaction may occur within 15 to 20 minutes of start of transfusion, although delayed reactions may occur up to several months later.
2. Monitor cardiovascular status for complications.
   a. Monitor vital signs: apical pulse, BP, and respirations.
   b. Assess for edema.
   c. Auscultate heart sounds for gallop and lungs for rales.
   d. Assess extremities for ulcer formation.
   e. Increased risk of pulmonary hypertension.
   f. Major complication of transfusions is iron overload in the heart. Starting chelation early is essential in preventing life-threatening complications.

Chronic Bone Pain

1. Bone pain is a characteristic feature of thalassemia major.
2. Monitor CBC for Hb values less than 10 g/dL.
3. Use warm packs—can reduce muscle spasms and reduce inflammation.
4. Eat a healthy diet that includes calcium and vitamin D to help keep bones strong.
5. Administer and teach proper administration of NSAIDs, such as ibuprofen or naproxen. Use carefully and monitor liver enzymes in patients with liver complications.

Activity Intolerance

1. Encourage participation in activities that do not require significant strenuous activity. Full participation in some activities, especially with peers, will increase self-esteem. Allow for periods of rest during such activities.
2. Facilitate physical and occupational therapy to develop an acceptable exercise plan.
3. Involve the caregivers and the child's school in developing a plan of gym activities, classes, and rest periods that allow the greatest level of participation and slowly develop endurance.
4. Advise caregivers that during the week of the scheduled transfusion, the fatigue will be greatest, so gym and other exertional activities should be modified.
5. Discourage participation in contact or other sports that increase the child's risk of a fracture (skateboarding, football, soccer).

Infection Risk

1. Maintain and teach good handwashing techniques.
2. Minimize exposure to infectious illnesses.
3. After splenectomy, the child has increased susceptibility to infection and should be maintained on oral penicillin prophylaxis.
4. Vaccinate child against *H. influenzae*, pneumococcal, and meningococcal infections before splenectomy and encourage yearly trivalent influenza vaccination.
5. Encourage prompt medical attention for fever or signs of infection. Fever of 102°F (38.9°C) should be reported immediately, and IV broad-spectrum antibiotics initiated.

Knowledge Deficit

1. Explain the importance of chelating (binding) agents to decrease iron deposits in tissues and to increase iron excretion through urine and feces.
2. Administer IV deferoxamine as prescribed:
   a. Infuse slowly, over 8 to 24 hours, through peripheral line or implanted infusion device or via volumetric pump.
   b. Have emergency resuscitation equipment nearby in case a severe allergic reaction occurs.
3. Review administration of oral deferasirox and encourage adherence to the medication schedule.
4. Ocular and auditory disturbances are seen in long-term use. Periodic visual and audiometric testing is recommended.

CLINICAL JUDGMENT Secondary to the excess iron deposition in children with thalassemia, dietary iron should be decreased as much as possible.

Improving Body Image

1. Explore the child's feelings of being different from other children.
2. Encourage the child to express feelings through the use of play: art and role-playing.

3. Give positive reinforcement regarding appearance.
4. Encourage socialization and peer interaction.
5. Encourage endocrine consultation for delayed growth and puberty.
6. Encourage craniofacial specialist evaluation for bony abnormalities.
7. Suggest support group or individual counseling, as needed.

Improving Family Coping Strategies

1. Alleviate the child's anxieties about illness by providing explanation based on developmental level.
2. Use role-playing and play activities to identify concerns.
3. Assist in strengthening coping mechanisms, such as support network and problem-solving.
4. Help identify resources for financial support, medical supplies, respite care, and so on.
5. Encourage involvement in school and after-school activities.
6. Encourage caregivers to set limits and to provide discipline for the child that is consistent with that for other children in the family.
7. Provide supportive care to the dying child.
8. Encourage bereavement support for caregivers, siblings, and family.

Family Education and Health Maintenance

1. Discuss the genetic implications of thalassemia and refer for genetic counseling.
2. Provide a detailed instruction about:
   a. Prevention and prompt treatment of infections.
   b. Medications.
   c. Home chelation therapy.
   d. Dietary modifications to limit iron intake.
   e. Activity restrictions, including avoidance of activities that increase the risk of fractures.
   f. Signs of complications.
3. Encourage caregivers to provide information about the child's condition to significant adults who are involved with the child (teacher, school nurse, babysitter, scout leader).
4. For additional information and support, refer to Cooley's Anemia Foundation (*www.thalassemia.org*).

Evaluation: Expected Outcomes

- Vital signs stable.
- Skin integrity intact without evident edema.
- No edema evident.
- Rates pain as less than 4 out of 10 on developmentally appropriate scale.
- Attends school on a regular basis.
- Reports increased participation in activity and less fatigue.
- No febrile illnesses reported. Immunizations up to date.
- Caregiver has good understanding of and is proficient in administration of chelation agents.
- Child verbalizes interest in appearance and positive statements about self.
- Family participates in support groups.
- Caregivers discuss illness with child and siblings.

Hemophilia

EVIDENCE BASE Zhao, Y., Weyand, A. C., & Shavit, J. A. (2021). Novel treatments for hemophilia through rebalancing of the coagulation cascade. *Pediatric Blood and Cancer, 68*(5), e28934. https://doi.org/10.1002/pbc.28934

Hemophilia is one of a group of inherited X-linked recessive bleeding disorders that cause abnormal or exaggerated bleeding and poor blood clotting. It is most commonly used to refer to two specific conditions, hemophilia A and hemophilia B. Hemophilia A is caused by a deficiency of clotting factor VIII. Hemophilia B is caused by a deficiency of clotting factor IX. Males are commonly affected, and females are usually carriers of the disease. Hemophilia A occurs in 1 in 15,000 to 1 in 30,000 live male births and is four times as common as hemophilia B. There are an estimated 20,000 individuals in the United States with hemophilia. Worldwide incidence is estimated at more than 400,000.

- 80% to 85% have factor VIII deficiency or hemophilia A (classic hemophilia).
- 15% to 20% have factor IX deficiency or hemophilia B (Christmas disease).

Sites of bleeding differ based on age:

- Infants—often seen in the central nervous system such as cephalohematoma, and sites of medical interventions (i.e., blood draws and circumcision).
- Children—musculoskeletal areas and joints; oral injuries are seen in the toddler age group.
- Adolescents—often seen in the joints, muscles, central nervous system, and oral or GI tract.

EVIDENCE BASE Connell, N. T., James, P. D., Brignardello-Petersen, R., Abdul-Kadir, R., Ameer, B., Arapshian, A., Couper, S., Di Paola, J., Eikenboom, J., Giraud, N., Grow, J. M., Haberichter, S., Jacobs-Pratt, V., Konkle, B. A., Kouides, P., Laffan, M., Lavin, M., Leebeek, F. W. G., McLintock, C., ... Flood, V. H. (2021). Von Willebrand disease: Proposing definitions for future research. *Blood Advances, 5*(2)565–569. https://doi.org/10.1182/bloodadvances.2020003620

von Willebrand disease (pseudohemophilia) is the most common inherited bleeding disorder (in the hemophilia category) caused by deficiency or abnormality in von Willebrand factor (VWF), a key protein that helps clotting. von Willebrand disease shows no geographical or ethnic predilection. Males and females inherit the genetic mutation with equal frequency, although females outnumber males (2:1). The prevalence of von Willebrand disease is 0.6% to 1.3% of the population.

Pathophysiology and Etiology

1. Hereditary (approximately 80% of patients) (Table 48-4).
   a. Autosomal dominant pattern—in rare cases, inherited can see autosomal recessive pattern.
   b. Three types exist—1, 2, and 3:
      i. Type 1—mild-to-moderate reduction in functional normal VWF—accounts for 65% to 80% of affected individuals.
      ii. Type 2—involves expression of functionally abnormal VWF—occurs in 20% to 35% of affected individuals.
      iii. Type 3—absence of VWF—affects 1 in 1 million people.
   c. Those who inherit one copy of the mutated gene will develop type 1 or 2.

Table 48-4 Transmission of Hemophilia

	PROBABILITY OF HEMOPHILIA IN OFFSPRING				
	FEMALE			MALE	
GENOTYPE OF BIOLOGICAL PARENTS	UNAFFECTED (%)	CARRIER (%)	DISEASE (%)	UNAFFECTED (%)	DISEASE (%)
Female carrier/unaffected male	50	50	0	50	50
Noncarrier female/male with hemophilia	0	100	0	100	0
Female carrier/male with hemophilia	0	50	50	50	50

   d. Those who inherit a mutated gene from both biological parents will develop type 3.
   e. May appear in females if a female carrier bears offspring with a male with hemophilia, although this is rare.
2. Spontaneous mutations may occur when the family history is negative for the disease. Although not initially inherited, it can be passed on to the affected person's children.
3. The basic defect is in the intrinsic phase of the coagulation cascade. The blood clotting factors are necessary for the formation of prothrombin activator, which acts as a catalyst in the conversion of prothrombin to thrombin.
   a. When damage to the vessel wall occurs, bleeding starts and platelets are activated to the site of the injury, resulting in platelet aggregation.
   b. Clotting proteins, such as factors VIII and IX, are activated on the surface of the platelets to form a meshlike fibrin clot.
   c. These proteins work in a domino-like reaction known as the coagulation cascade. If the protein is absent, the chain reaction is broken, either preventing clot formation or resulting in slower clot formation.
4. The result is an unstable fibrin clot.
5. Coagulation factors are involved in hemostasis and the formation of clots. Prothrombin time (PTT) is used to measure coagulation factors, including factors VIII and IX.
6. Platelet number and function are normal; therefore, small lacerations and minor hemorrhages are usually not a problem.
7. Patients do not bleed more rapidly; rather, there is delayed or abnormal clot formation.

Clinical Manifestations

1. In majority of patients, hemophilia is diagnosed at birth because of family history, although, in approximately one third of patients, the occurrence of hemophilia represents a new mutation.
2. Approximately 30% of male infants with hemophilia have bleeding with circumcision.
3. In those patients who do not have a family history, diagnosis is often made when the child begins to walk or crawl.
4. Varies in severity, depending on the plasma level of the coagulation factor involved.
   a. Level of less than 1% of normal—severe hemophilia; commonly severe clinical bleeding with minimal or unknown trauma and often experience unprovoked muscle and joint bleeding one to six times monthly (factor level less than 0.01 μ/mL).
   b. Level of 1% to 5% of normal—moderately afflicted; may be free from spontaneous bleeding and may not manifest severe bleeding until trauma occurs (factor level less than 0.02 to 0.05 μ/mL).
   c. Level of 6% to 40% of normal—mildly afflicted; patients usually lead normal lives and bleed only with severe injury or surgery (factor level greater than 0.05 μ/mL).
   d. Degree of severity tends to be constant within a given family. Within an individual, severity does not vary over time unless inhibitor (autoantibody to infused factor) develops.
5. Signs and symptoms of abnormal bleeding include:
   a. History of prolonged bleeding episodes such as after circumcision.
   b. Easily bruised.
   c. Oral bleeding.
   d. Spontaneous soft tissue hematomas.
   e. Hemorrhages into the joints (hemarthrosis)—especially the elbows, knees, and ankles, causing pain, swelling, and limitation of movement.
   f. Hematuria.
   g. Black, tarry stools.
   h. Heavy or long menstrual bleeding, often with blood clots greater than 1 in.
   i. Excessive bleeding from an injury.
   j. Head trauma, resulting in intracranial hemorrhage.

Diagnostic Evaluation

1. PTT and bleeding time—measures clotting ability of factors I, II, VII, and X—normal.
2. Partial thromboplastin time—measures clotting ability of factors VIII, IX, XI, and XII—prolonged.
3. Fibrinogen—assesses patient's ability to form a blood clot.
4. Assays for specific clotting factors—measures levels of factor VIII and IX—abnormal.
5. VWF—helps to diagnose von Willebrand disease and distinguish between types of disease—persons with O type blood have VWF levels 25% less than other blood types.
6. Gene analysis—to detect carrier state, for prenatal diagnosis.

Management

1. Prompt, early, and appropriate treatment is the key to preventing most complications.
2. Replace missing coagulation factor (VIII or IX) via the administration of type-specific coagulation concentrates during bleeding episodes. This is the current standard of care.
   a. *Factor VIII*—75% of the factor is recombinant, which is developed in the laboratory through the use of DNA technology; for control of bleeding episodes, perioperative management of bleeding, and routine prophylaxis in patients with hemophilia A; dosing is IV and based on location and extent of bleeding and patient's clinical condition; not to be used for patients with von Willebrand disease.

b. *Factor IX*—is recombinant and given IV; used for control of bleeding, perioperative management of bleeding, and routine prophylaxis in patients with hemophilia B; for prophylaxis, give 50 IU/kg weekly or 100 IU/kg every 10 days; for minor/moderate bleeding, give 30 to 60 IU/dL and repeat every 48 hours as necessary; for major bleeding, give 80 to 100 IU/dL, repeat in 6 to 10 hours, and then give every 24 hours for 3 days and then every 48 hours until healing is achieved.

3. No viral inactivated concentrate exists for hemophilia C; fresh-frozen plasma is given to supply factor XI.
4. Mild and moderate factor VIII–deficient people with hemophilia and some patients with von Willebrand disease may respond to desmopressin, which causes the release of factor VIII from the endothelial stores. Treatment is started in case of bleeding or before an intervention, that is, dental work. Dosing can be IV to intranasally. IV dosing is 0.3 μg/kg and intranasally 150 μg per nostril. It can be repeated every 12 to 24 hours depending on response. Patients receiving desmopressin should restrict fluids during use to prevent hyponatremia and seizures.
5. Plasma-derived VWF—use dependent on predicted amount of bleeding and intervention to be performed for patients with von Willebrand disease; dosing is concentrate dependent; recombinant von Willebrand concentrate has been developed and has shown increased activity compared to plasma-derived factor. Initial approval for use in children was granted by the Food and Drug Administration (FDA) in 2023.
6. Antifibrinolytics, such as aminocaproic acid and tranexamic acid, are given as adjunctive therapy for dental procedures and for nose and mouth bleeding; it is administered orally.
7. Activated prothrombin complex concentrates that have activated factors VII, IX, and X are used when inhibitors (autoantibodies) have developed to bypass factor VIII or IX.
8. Supportive therapies:
   a. NSAIDs are used to decrease inflammation and arthritic-like pain associated with chronic hemarthroses. They must be used with caution because some types and higher doses interfere with platelet adhesion. Should only be used when prescribed by licensed practitioner who is familiar with bleeding disorders.
   b. Physical therapy to prevent contractures and muscle atrophy. This includes exercise, whirlpool, and icing.
   c. Orthotics to prevent injury to affected joint and to help resolve hemorrhages.
9. Synovectomy—orthopedic surgical intervention to remove damaged synovium in chronically involved joints.
   a. Open procedure provides direct visualization of joint and removal of damaged tissue.
   b. Arthroscopic—visualization and removal of the joint synovium through the use of an arthroscope.
   c. Radionucleotide—instillation of radioisotope P32 into the joint, which removes or stops excessive growth of the synovium, decreases amount of bleeding, and decreases potential for arthritis; done through a needle with x-ray guidance.
10. Gene therapy—much of the research is focused here. One clinical trial allows for the endogenous expression of clotting factor via a viral vector cell administered through autologous hematopoietic stem cells. This would liberate patients from the need for prophylaxis and for IV delivery. It would not be tied to patient adherence and would be a more tolerizing therapy. Other areas of research involve development of tissue factor pathway inhibitors.
11. Patients with bleeding disorders should avoid aspirin and aspirin-containing products, nonsteroidal anti-inflammatories, and blood thinners, such as warfarin and heparin.

Complications

1. Airway obstruction caused by hemorrhage into the neck and pharynx.
2. Joint disease—secondary to repetitive bleeding into the joints, often results in arthritis, and may require joint replacement therapy.
3. Intestinal obstruction caused by bleeding into intestinal walls or peritoneum.
4. Compression of nerves with paralysis caused by hemorrhaging into deep tissues, known as *compartment syndrome.*
5. Intracranial bleeding, resulting in serious neurologic impairments.
6. Inhibitor development—30% of patients with hemophilia A and 2% to 3% of patients with hemophilia B develop inhibitors to factor replacements.
7. Viral infections—risk from plasma-derived factor concentrates—less often now that recombinant forms of factor are available.
8. Death may result from exsanguination after any serious hemorrhage, such as intracranial, airway, or other highly vascular areas.
9. Lifespan—varies based on whether they receive proper treatment; without proper treatment, many die before reaching adulthood; with proper treatment, life expectancy is about 10 years less than those without hemophilia: Children can expect to have a normal life expectancy.

Nursing Assessment

1. Obtain history of and observe for unusual bleeding—ecchymosis, prolonged bleeding from mucous membranes and lacerations, hematomas, hemarthroses, hematuria, and rectal and GI bleeding. Determine time frame of most recent bleeding episode.
2. Obtain history of whether patient has inhibitors and, if so, what their titer is.
3. Assess for acute or chronic bleeding.
4. Priority assessment of joints for swelling, warmth, tenderness, ROM, contractures, and surrounding muscle atrophy.
5. Check for hematuria and bleeding from the mouth, lips, gum, and rectum.
6. Check vision, hearing, and neurologic development.
7. Obtain information on prior treatment with blood products.
8. Assess family resources and coping skills.

Nursing Interventions

Preventing Hypovolemia Through Control of Bleeding

1. Provide emergency care for bleeding.
   a. Apply pressure and cold to the injury site to assist in clot formation. Immobilize and elevate injured area. This should be done especially after venipuncture or injection.
   b. Do not aspirate hematomas or joints.
   c. Suturing and cauterization should be avoided.
2. Immobilize the affected part and elevate above the level of the heart.

3. Recognize early and late signs of a joint bleed. Early signs include tingling and bubbling sensation but no real pain or tightness and pain without visible signs of a bleed. Late signs include swelling at the joint, warmth of the skin to touch, pain when bending or extending the joint, and increased difficulty with mobilization.
4. Administer recombinant factor VIII or factor IX coagulation concentrate.
   a. Administration should be slow IV push; usually 2 to 3 mL/min; consult package inserts.
   b. In the case of head trauma, administer factor replacement immediately and prior to obtaining imaging—waiting to administer factor can have serious neurologic effects.
   c. Cryoprecipitate and fresh-frozen plasma are not recommended because of their lack of viral inactivation treatment. They may be only treatment of choice in some countries.
   d. Stop the transfusion if hives, headaches, tingling, chills, flushing, or fever occurs.
5. Apply fibrinolytic agents to wound for oral bleeding. Popsicles also work for minor mouth bleeding. Do not use fibrinolytic agents for hematuria.
6. Attempt to keep child relaxed and quiet during treatment to decrease pulse and rate of bleeding.
7. Monitor vital signs and treat for shock if child becomes hypotensive.

Providing Protection Against Bleeding

1. For patients with severe hemophilia, administer prophylactic factor IX or XIII bid to three times weekly to prevent spontaneous bleeds.
2. Avoid obtaining rectal temperatures; insert thermometer probe gently and use axillary, oral (if age appropriate), or external ear route.
3. Use soft toothbrush and encourage regular dental checkups.
4. Avoid injections, if possible.
   a. Administer medications orally whenever possible.
   b. SC route is preferred to IM.
   c. Apply pressure to injection site for 10 to 15 minutes. Then apply a pressure dressing with self-adhesive gauze.
5. Maintain a safe environment and teach caregivers safety measures.
   a. Protect child with kneepads, elbow pads, and helmets when riding bicycles.
   b. Use safety belts and straps in high chairs, car seats, and strollers.
   c. Infants should have appropriate padding in cribs or playpen to prevent injury.
   d. Supervise toddlers as they learn to walk.
   e. Remove or pad furniture with sharp corners.
   f. Keep small and sharp objects out of reach.
   g. Check play equipment and outdoor play areas for possible hazards.
   h. Child should wear a medical alert device.
   i. Be aware of safe activities that your child can enjoy, including swimming, biking, and walking.

DRUG ALERT Children with hemophilia should not receive aspirin, compounds containing aspirin, or nonsteroidal anti-inflammatory agents because these medications affect platelet function and prolong bleeding time.

Preserving Mobility

1. Treat hemarthrosis or muscle bleed as soon as possible.
2. Provide supportive care for hemarthrosis.
   a. Immobilize the joint in a position of slight flexion.
   b. Elevate the affected part above the level of the heart.
   c. Factor, if readily available, should be administered before ice is applied to the joint.
3. For severe hemarthroses, continue factor administration at home until joint pain and immobility have resolved.
4. For less severe hemarthroses, begin gentle, passive exercise 48 hours after the acute phase to prevent joint stiffness and fibrosis. Progress to active exercises.
5. Short course of corticosteroids has shown clinical effectiveness in the treatment of hemarthrosis.
6. Physiotherapy is an essential adjunct for joint bleeding.
7. Hydrotherapy can reduce pain and instability in target joints and improve ROM and muscle tone.

Relieving Pain

1. Be aware that increased pain usually means that bleeding continues and further replacement therapy may be needed.
2. Assess for further swelling of joints and limitation of movement.
3. Administer or teach administration of acetaminophen during acute phase. NSAIDs may be used for chronic pain, but cautiously, to prevent interference with platelet function.
4. Administer opioids sparingly, as ordered, for severe, acute pain.
5. If pain persists for a prolonged duration, referral to a Pain Management Center is recommended.

Enhancing Family Coping

1. Acknowledge caregivers' feeling of guilt or anger with regard to diagnosis.
2. Use play therapy to help the young child and siblings adjust to illness.
3. Encourage the caregivers to allow the child to participate in as many normal activities as possible within the realm of safety.
4. Have child wear a medical alert device that also includes clotting factor that is best used in an emergency.
5. Make sure anyone involved in caring for your child is aware of your child's condition.
6. Encourage the child's education. Involve teacher, principal, and assistants in understanding disease process and limitations that need to be enforced for child's safety.
7. Refer to social worker for counseling and identification of resources for financial concerns and emotional support.
8. Encourage avoidance of overprotection. This can place too many restrictions on the child's normal development. This can result in the child becoming overly dependent or becoming defiant and engaging in risky behaviors or activities.
9. Encourage involvement in support group.

Community and Home Care Considerations

1. Perform a home safety survey (inside and outside) to identify potential hazards to the child with hemophilia.
2. Provide teaching and referrals to initiate an infusion therapy program at home when hemorrhage begins.
3. Have child participate in regular exercise program to help strengthen joints, which helps prevent damage or pain from internal bleeding.
4. Make sure that primary health care needs are being met by facilitating the following:
   a. Regular visits to primary care provider for preventive health maintenance.

b. Dental examinations and teeth cleaning every 6 months.
c. All the recommended childhood immunizations, plus hepatitis A, to prevent infection from blood-borne pathogens.

5. Provide education to family and all caregivers about recognizing and treating bleeds appropriately.
6. Provide emotional support through the provision of educational materials, information about support groups, and a list of resources within the community.
7. Educate teachers and other school faculties about the child's special needs.
   a. These children can have permanent mental or physical disabilities from old hemorrhages, necessitating individualized plans.
   b. Avoidance of rough or contact sports and activities.
   c. All injuries must be taken seriously. The school nurse should be notified so that proper first aid and treatment can be initiated.
   d. Although they have a chronic illness, these children have a strong desire to be "normal," with the same opportunities and environmental stimulation as other children.

Family Education and Health Maintenance

1. Review safety measures to prevent or minimize trauma.
2. Encourage education by caregivers to teachers, babysitters, and others involved in child's care so that they can be responsive in an emergency.
3. Advise wearing a medical alert device.
4. Teach emergency treatment for hemorrhage.
   a. Immobilize the part with splints or an elastic compression bandage. (These materials should be immediately available in the home.)
   b. Apply ice packs. Caregivers should keep two or three plastic bags of ice immediately available in the freezer. Popsicles can be used for minor mouth bleeding.
   c. Consult the child's health care provider and initiate additional recommended therapy.
5. Encourage regular medical and dental supervision.
   a. Preventive dental care is important. Soft-bristled or sponge-tipped toothbrushes should be used to prevent bleeding. Factor replacement therapy is necessary for extensive dental work and extractions.
   b. Hepatitis B vaccine is necessary to protect against the rare occurrence of hepatitis B from blood transfusions.
6. Teach healthy diet to avoid obesity, which places additional strain on the child's weight-bearing joints and predisposes to hemarthroses.
7. Assist the caregivers in helping the child to understand the exact nature of the illness as early as possible. Special attention should be given to the signs of hemorrhage, and the child should be told of the need to report even the slightest bleeding to an adult immediately.
8. Advise families that genetic counseling and family planning are available for caregivers and adolescent patients.
9. For additional information and support, refer to National Hemophilia Foundation (*www.hemophilia.org*).

SELECTED READINGS

Aksu, T., & Ünal, Ş. (2023). Iron deficiency anemia in infancy, childhood and adolescence. *Turkish Archives of Pediatrics, 58*(4), 358–362. https://doi.org/10.5152/TurkArchPediatr.2023.23049

Barg, A. A., Levy-Mendelovich, S., Avishai, E., Dardik, R., Misgav, M., Kenet, G., & Livnat, T. (2018). Alternative treatment options for pediatric hemophilia B patients with high-responding inhibitors: A thrombin generation-guided study. *Pediatric Blood and Cancer, 65*(12), e27381. https://doi.org/10.1002/pbc.27381

Behera, B., Subhadarshini, S., Satapathy, J., Mohanty, N., Mishra, D., Mantri, S., Purohit, P., & Patro, M. (2021). Reticulocyte haemoglobin as a diagnostic marker and its response towards oral iron therapy in paediatric iron deficiency anaemia: A feasibility study. *Current Medicine Research and Practice, 11*(2), 78–82. https://doi.org/10.4103/cmrp.cmrp_19_21

Blaney, S. M., Helman, L. J., & Adamson, P. C. (2022). *Pizzo and Poplack's pediatric oncology* (8th ed.). Wolters Kluwer Health.

Booker, S. Q., Baker, T. A., Epps, F., Herr, K. A., Young, H. M., & Fishman, S. (2022). Interrupting biases in the experience and management of pain. *American Journal of Nursing, 122*(9), 48–54. https://doi.org/10.1097/01.NAJ.0000874120.95373.40

Colombatti, R. (2023). Standardizing elements of care in pediatric sickle cell disease centers: The road toward health equity. *Pediatric Blood & Cancer, 70*(1), e30078. https://doi.org/10.1002/pbc.30078

Delimont, N. M., Carlson, B. N., & Nickel, S. (2021). Dental caries are associated with anemia in pediatric patients: A systematic literature review. *Journal of Allied Health, 50*(1), 73–83. PMID: 33646253

Kanter, J., Thompson, A. A., Pierciey, F. J., Hsieh, M., Uchida, N., Leboulch, P., Schmidt, M., Bonner, M., Guo, R., Miller, A., Ribeil, J. A., Davidson, D., Asmal, M., Walters, M. C., & Tisdale, J. F. (2023). Lovo-cel gene therapy for sickle cell disease: Treatment process evolution and outcomes in the initial groups of the HGB-206 study. *American Journal of Hematology, 98*(1), 11–22. https://doi.org/10.1002/ajh.26741

Keam, S. J. (2023). Efanesoctocog Alfa: First approval. *Drugs, 83*(7), 633–638. https://doi.org/10.1007/s40265-023-01866-9

Hon, K. L. E., Tan, Y. W., Leung, K. K. Y., Hui, W. F., Cheung, W. L., & Chung, F. S. (2023). Emergency management of life-threatening anemia in pediatric practice. *Pediatric Emergency Care, 39*(5), 1535–1815. https://doi.org/10.1097/PEC.0000000000002782

Lupu, V. V., Miron, I., Buga, A. M. L., Gavrilovici, C., Tarca, E., Adam Raileanu, A., Starcea, I. M., Cernomaz, A. T., Mocanu, A., & Lupu, A. (2022). Iron deficiency anemia in pediatric gastroesophageal reflux disease. *Diagnostics (Basel), 13*(1), 63. https://doi.org/10.3390/diagnostics13010063

Paulley, L. M., & Duff, E. (2022). Iron deficiency in infants—What nurse practitioners need to know. *The Journal for Nurse Practitioners, 18*(6), 614–617. https://doi.org/10.1016/j.nurpra.2022.03.012

Saultier, P., Guillaume, Y., Demiguel, V., Berger, C., Borel-Derlon, A., Claeyssens, S., Harroche, A., Oudot, C., Rafowicz, A., Trossaert, M., Wibaut, B., Vinciguerra, C., Boucekine, M., Baumstarck, K., Meunier, S., Calvez, T., Chambost, H., FranceCoag PUPs/CoMETH Prophylaxis Study Group, & Hemophilia Treatment Centers of Paris-Necker. (2021). Compliance with early long-term prophylaxis guidelines for severe hemophilia. *Journal of Pediatrics, 234*, 212–219.e3. https://doi.org/10.1016/j.jpeds.2021.02.071

Shimano, K. A., Narla, A., Rose, M. J., Gloude, N. J., Allen, S. W., Bergstrom, K., Broglie, L., Carella, B. A., Castillo, P., de Jong, J. L. O., Dror, Y, Geddis A. E., Huang, J. N., Lau, B. W., McGuinn, C., Nakano, T. A., Overholt, K., Rothman, J. A., Sharathkumar, A., ... Boklan, J. (2021). Diagnostic workup for severe aplastic anemia in children: Consensus of the North American Pediatric Aplastic Anemia Consortium. *American Journal of Hematology, 96*(11), 1491–1504. https://doi.org/10.1002/ajh.26310

Venturieri, M. O., Komati, J. T. S., Lopes, L. H. C., & Sdepanian, V. L. (2019). Treatment with Noripurum EV® is effective and safe in pediatric patients with inflammatory bowel disease and iron deficiency anemia. *Scandinavian Journal of Gastroenterology, 54*(2), 198–204. https://doi.org/10.1080/00365521.2019.1570326

49
Pediatric Immunologic Disorders

IMMUNOLOGIC DISORDERS

Pediatric Human Immunodeficiency Virus/Acquired Immunodeficiency Syndrome

Human immunodeficiency virus (HIV) infection for infants, children, and adolescents is represented by a continuum of immunologic and clinical classifications ranging from no to severe immunologic suppression and asymptomatic to severely symptomatic. *Acquired immunodeficiency syndrome (AIDS)* is the end stage of the continuum. Also see Chapter 25, HIV Infection and AIDS, page 796.

Epidemiology

EVIDENCE BASE UNAIDS. (2023). *Fact sheet world AIDS day*. https://www.unaids.org/en/resources/documents/2023/UNAIDS_FactSheet

Centers for Disease Control and Prevention. (2021). *HIV surveillance report*. Vol. 34. https://www.cdc.gov/hiv/library/reports/hiv-surveillance/vol-34/index.html

1. HIV is a pandemic, affecting people all over the world; the World Health Organization estimated 33.1 to 45.7 million people living with HIV (in 2022).
2. Of the people infected with HIV worldwide, 1.5 million are children under age 15 years (2022). In 2022, approximately 86% of all people living with HIV knew their HIV status, and about 5.5 million people did not know that they were living with HIV.
3. HIV is transmitted through sexual contact with an infected person; through exposure to infected blood and blood components (sharing needles via intravenous [IV] drug use, tattooing, piercing, and unsterilized medical equipment); or from an HIV-infected birthing parent to the baby before or during birth or through breastfeeding.
4. In the United States, sexual acquisition of HIV remains the main mode of transmission. It is estimated that youth aged 13 to 24 years represent the second highest rate of newly acquired HIV.
5. Globally, in 2022, 82% (64% to 98%) of all patients who are pregnant and infected with HIV are treated to prevent vertical transmission.
6. In the United States, prenatally acquired HIV infection has dramatically decreased from about 25% to less than 1% of pediatric cases. Ethnic disparities in HIV diagnosis rates persist but have declined substantially over the last decade.
7. This decrease reflects concerted efforts to provide improved preconception counseling; HIV testing for all patients who are pregnant; initiate the use of combination antiretroviral therapy (cART) as early as possible; with the goal of full viral suppression to the limits of detection; providing prophylaxis medication to the infant; and exclusive formula feeding.
   a. If viral load is suppressed, patients who are infected with HIV can deliver vaginally while continuing to take their oral antiretrovirals during delivery. The HIV-exposed infant will be given 6 weeks of zidovudine as prophylaxis. If the infant is premature, the dose may require modification.
   b. If viral load is not suppressed during delivery (greater than 1,000 copies/mL), additional steps can be taken to reduce the risk of transmission: scheduled cesarean delivery, use of intrapartum IV zidovudine, and use of combination antiretroviral prophylaxis for the infant.
      i. Consultation with a pediatric HIV specialist is highly recommended in cases where cART may be required for the infant.
8. An HIV-infected birthing parent can have a child who is infected and subsequent children who are uninfected. Likewise, one infant in a multiple birth can be infected, whereas the other infant(s) are not.
9. Children born to birthing parents with a high HIV viral load and low $CD4^+$ lymphocyte counts and with severely symptomatic HIV disease are at greater risk for infection.
   a. Infants born to such patients who become infected appear to be at increased risk for more rapid disease progression.
   b. Infants born to people who seroconvert during pregnancy are at an increased risk for becoming infected.

10. With the advent of highly active antiretroviral therapy (HAART), the morbidity and mortality in HIV-infected children has decreased significantly. Thus, in those who have access to medication and who are adherent to therapy, HIV has become a chronic, manageable illness.

EVIDENCE BASE Office of AIDS Research. (2023). *Preventing perinatal transmission of HIV*. https://hivinfo.nih.gov/understanding-hiv/fact-sheets/preventing-perinatal-transmission-hiv#:~:text=Most%20pregnant%20people%20with%20HIV,of%20perinatal%20transmission%20of%20HIV

Lampe, M. (2023). Achieving elimination of perinatal HIV in the United States. *Pediatrics, 151*(5), e2022059604.

Pathophysiology and Etiology

EVIDENCE BASE *Panel on treatment of HIV during pregnancy and prevention of perinatal transmission.* (2023). https://clinicalinfo.hiv.gov/en/guidelines/perinatal/management-infants-diagnosis-hiv-infection-children

American Academy of Pediatrics. (2021). Section 3: Summaries of infectious diseases. In D. Kimberlin, E. Barnett, R. Lynfield, and M. Sawyer (Eds.), *Red book: 2021–2024 report of the committee on infectious diseases* (32nd ed., pp. 453–475). American Academy of Pediatrics.

1. The causative agent is a retrovirus that damages the immune system by infecting and depleting the $CD4^+$ lymphocytes (T4 helper cells). These $CD4^+$ lymphocytes play a central role in the regulation of the immune system.
2. There are also abnormalities in the function of cellular and humoral immunity (B cells, $CD8^+$ cells, natural killer cells, monocytes, macrophages, and specific antibodies).
3. Progressive destruction of the immune system leads to:
   a. Increased incidence of serious bacterial infections, such as bacteremia, bacterial pneumonias, and osteomyelitis.
   b. Opportunistic infections, which commonly include *Pneumocystis jirovecii* pneumonia (PCP), esophageal candidiasis, and *Mycobacterium avium* infection.
   c. More aggressive forms of viral infections, such as severe varicella, disseminated zoster, and cytomegalovirus pneumonitis.
   d. Cancers, especially lymphomas.
   e. Wasting syndromes and encephalopathy.
4. Multisystem organ involvement results in cardiomyopathies; nephropathies; neurologic impairment; gastrointestinal (GI) dysfunction; endocrine disorders; dermatologic manifestations; musculoskeletal abnormalities; ocular impairments; ear, nose, and throat problems; and hematologic disorders.
5. An AIDS diagnosis occurs when a child presents as severely symptomatic (Category C) or with lymphoid interstitial pneumonitis (LIP from Category B) along with severe immunosuppression (see Tables 49-1 and 49-2).
6. Once an AIDS diagnosis is made, it is not reversed even with reconstitution of the immune system and recovery from the opportunistic infection.

Clinical Manifestations of Disease Progression

1. Generalized lymphadenopathy, especially in less common sites, such as epitrochlear and axillary areas.
2. Persistent, recurrent oral candidiasis.
3. Failure to thrive.
4. Developmental delays or loss of previously acquired milestones.
5. Hepatomegaly.
6. Splenomegaly.
7. Persistent diarrhea.
8. Hypergammaglobulinemia or hypogammaglobulinemia (elevated or diminished levels of immunoglobulin [Ig] G, IgM, IgA).
9. Parotitis.
10. Unexplained anemias, thrombocytopenia.
11. Unexplained cardiac or kidney disease.
12. Recurrent mild or serious bacterial infections.

EVIDENCE BASE *Panel on treatment of HIV during pregnancy and prevention of perinatal transmission.* (2023). https://clinicalinfo.hiv.gov/en/guidelines/perinatal/management-infants-diagnosis-hiv-infection-children

Panel on use of antiretroviral agents in the pediatric HIV infection. (2023). https://clinicalinfo.hiv.gov/en/guidelines/pediatric-arv/regimens-recommended-initial-therapy-antiretroviral-naive-children#:~:text=For%20treatment%2Dnaive%20children%2C%20the,strand%20transfer%20inhibitor%2C%20a%20non%2D

Diagnostic Evaluation

1. All pregnant people in the United States should have HIV antibody testing (enzyme–linked immunoassay [ELISA]) as standard of care.

Table 49-1 Pediatric HIV Classification[a]

	CLINICAL CATEGORIES			
IMMUNOLOGIC CATEGORIES	N: NO SIGNS/ SYMPTOMS	A: MILD SIGNS/ SYMPTOMS	B:[B] MODERATE SIGNS/ SYMPTOMS	C:[B] SEVERE SIGNS/ SYMPTOMS
1: No evidence of suppression	N1	A1	B1	C1
2: Evidence of moderate suppression	N2	A2	B2	C2
3: Severe suppression	N3	A3	B3	C3

[a]*Children whose HIV infection status is not confirmed are classified by using the above grid with a letter E (for perinatally exposed) placed before the appropriate classification code (e.g., EN2).*

[b]*Category C and lymphoid interstitial pneumonitis in Category B are reportable to state and local health departments as acquired immunodeficiency syndrome.*

Reprinted from Centers for Disease Control and Prevention. (1994 last reviewed in [2014]). 1994 revised classification system for human immunodeficiency virus infection in children less than 13 years of age. Morbidity and Mortality Weekly Report, 43(RR-12), 1–10. www.cdc.gov/mmwr/preview/mmwrhtml/00032890.htm

Table 49-2 Immunologic Categories Based on Age-Specific CD4+ T-lymphocyte Counts and Percentage of Total Lymphocytes

	AGE OF CHILD					
	YOUNGER THAN AGE 12 MONTHS		AGES 1–5		AGES 6–12	
IMMUNOLOGIC CATEGORY	MM³	(%)	MM³	(%)	MM³	(%)
1: No evidence of suppression	≥1,500	(≥34)	≥1,000	(≥30)	≥500	(≥26)
2: Evidence of moderate suppression	750–1,499	(26–33)	500–999	(22–29)	200–499	(14–25)
3: Severe suppression	<750	(<26)	<500	(<22)	<200	(<14)

Adapted from Centers for Disease Control and Prevention. (2014). Revised surveillance case definitions for HIV infection—United States, 2014. Morbidity and Mortality Weekly Report, 63(RR-3), 1–10.

2. Antibody testing in children less than 18 months of age is not reliable for diagnosis. A positive ELISA test may only be an indication of the presence of circulating maternal antibodies.
3. Virologic assays—HIV RNA or HIV DNA nucleic acid tests (NATs) that directly detect HIV—must be used to diagnose HIV in infants and children less than 18 months of age with perinatal and postnatal HIV exposure. HIV antibody and HIV antigen/antibody tests should not be used. The 2023 Centers for Disease Control and Prevention (CDC) guidelines recommend testing for infants using polymerase chain reaction (PCR) at ages 14 to 21 days, 1 to 2 months, and 4 to 6 months.
4. Residual maternal HIV antibodies may still be present in children 18 to 24 months of age; thus, HIV-RNA or HIV-DNA NATs should be used for diagnosis.
5. After age 24 months, HIV antibody assays can be used for testing because maternal antibodies should not be present by this age. As with adults, a reactive ELISA must be followed by a confirmatory Western blot test.
6. In known infected children or at-risk infants (those born to an HIV-infected birthing parent but whose own status is still indeterminate), computed tomography scanning or magnetic resonance imaging of the head may be indicated if there is evidence of neurologic impairment, falling rate of head growth, or developmental delays or regression.

Management

HIV-Exposed Infant

1. Additional laboratory studies requiring monitoring on the HIV-exposed infant include complete blood count (CBC) with differential (diff) to monitor for anemia and neutropenia and lymphocyte subsets (CD4+ counts), and lactate.

HIV Infected

1. At the time of diagnosis, baseline CD4, HIV RNA (viral load), drug resistance (genotypic and phenotypic resistance should be used) should be performed. Child should have a complete age-appropriate medical history (including immunization history) and physical exam and additional laboratory evaluations for HIV-associated conditions: CBC with differential, chemistry of glucose, liver and renal function, and urinalysis and serologic evaluation for coinfections and immunities. HLA-B*5701 is used to assess potential for abacavir hypersensitivity. In addition, a baseline echocardiogram and chest x-ray should be done and repeated yearly.
2. Child needs ongoing laboratory assessment; CBC with differential, platelet counts, serum chemistries, serial CD4+ counts, and HIV RNA (viral load) should be done every 3 to 6 months (depending on previous results and the stage of disease).
3. Initiation of PCP prophylaxis is indicated when low CD4+ counts occur, with the exception that all infants born to patients infected with HIV should be started on PCP prophylaxis at age 4 to 6 weeks, regardless of their CD4+ count (see Table 49-3).
   a. The first drug of choice is co-trimoxazole.
   b. Pentamidine, atovaquone, and dapsone are alternative choices.
   c. PCP prophylaxis should be discontinued in infants whose infection has been reasonably excluded on the basis of two or more negative viral diagnostic tests performed at greater than 4 weeks and greater than 8 weeks of age. Some experts may choose not to give prophylaxis to infants in whom antenatal and peripartum management has been appropriate and in whom the risk of infection is very low.
   d. Infants confirmed infected should remain on PCP prophylaxis until at least 1 year of age and then reassessed based on their CD4 count.
4. Antiretroviral therapy is recommended for all HIV-infected children less than 1 year of age and in older children who have clinical symptoms of HIV or evidence of immunosuppression regardless of the age of the child or HIV PCR level (viral load). Although new guidelines recommend early initiation of treatment for all HIV-infected individuals, many factors need to be considered for children greater than 1 year of age before starting. Factors such as the severity of disease progression, appropriate medication (availability, cost, dose, formulation, taste, side effects, and complexity of regimen), resistance pattern, and coinfection are but a few.
   a. Clinical trial data from both adults and children have demonstrated that antiretroviral therapy in patients who are symptomatic slows clinical and immunologic disease progression and reduces mortality.

Table 49-3 Recommendations for PCP Prophylaxis and CD4⁺ Monitoring for HIV-Exposed Infants and HIV-Infected Children, by Age and HIV Infection Status

AGE/HIV INFECTION STATUS	PCP PROPHYLAXIS	$CD4^+$ MONITORING
Birth to ages 4–6 wk, HIV exposed	Prophylaxis until determined to be HIV-uninfected or presumptively HIV-uninfected.	1 mo
Ages 4–6 wk to 4 mo, HIV exposed	Prophylaxis	3 mo
Ages 4–12 mo, HIV infected or indeterminate	Prophylaxis	6, 9, and 12 mo
Under ages 4–12 mo, HIV infection reasonably excluded	No prophylaxis	None
Ages 1–5, HIV infected	Prophylaxis if: $CD4^+$ count is <500 cells/L or $CD4^+$ percentage is <15%	Every 3–4 mo
Ages 6–12, HIV infected	Prophylaxis if: $CD4^+$ count is <200 cells/L or $CD4^+$ percentage is <15%	Every 3–4 mo

PCP, Pneumocystis jirovecii pneumonia.
Adapted from Guidelines for the Prevention and Treatment of Opportunistic Infections in Children with and Exposed to HIV. (2023). https://clinicalinfo.hiv.gov/en/guidelines/hiv-clinical-guidelines-pediatric-opportunistic-infections/whats-new?view=full

b. Classes of antiretroviral agents used in children include nucleoside reverse transcriptase inhibitors (NRTIs), protease inhibitors (PIs), nonnucleoside reverse transcriptase inhibitors (NNRTs), fusion inhibitors, chemokine receptor antagonists (CRAs), entry inhibitors (CD4-directed postattachment inhibitors), HIV integrase strand transfer inhibitors, and pharmcokinetic enhancers (boosting agents).
c. Combination therapy is now standard care, using at least three antiretrovirals (ARVs) from at least two drug classes.

5. Adherence is the basis for successful viral suppression; strategies should be developed to encourage adherence. Adherence is essential to prevent viral resistance; particularly, NNRTI resistance develops rapidly with even slight fluctuations in drug levels.
6. Use of IV immunoglobulin is still recommended for HIV-infected children who have had two or more serious bacterial infections within 1 year and for the treatment of HIV-related thrombocytopenia or immunoglobulin deficiency.
7. Use of antifungal drugs, such as nystatin, ketoconazole, fluconazole, itraconazole, and clotrimazole, for persistent or recurrent oral candidiasis.
8. Use of antivirals, such as acyclovir, valacyclovir, ganciclovir, and cidofovir, for suppression or treatment of recurrent viral infections.
9. Aggressive, prompt assessment and treatment of febrile illnesses.
10. Nutritional support.
11. Evaluation and treatment of developmental delays and regression.
12. Adequate pain management in advanced or end-stage disease.
13. Support and interventions for the child and family (including all caregivers) with issues of disclosure, caregiver guilt, long-term care, and bereavement.

DRUG ALERT Test for the presence of ARV drug-resistant virus in both patients who are experienced and those who are naive before initiating ARV combination therapy, thus ensuring the most effective regimen.

DRUG ALERT Lack of adherence to prescribed antiretroviral regimens and subtherapeutic drug levels increase the possibility that a resistant virus will develop. Strict adherence (more than 95%) to combination regimens is critical in ensuring sustained response to treatment.

CLINICAL JUDGMENT Families can find out about clinical treatment trials available for their child by visiting *www.clinicaltrials.gov.*

Complications

1. Untreated or inadequately treated HIV:
   a. Repeated, overwhelming infections and certain cancers, particularly lymphomas.
   b. Hearing loss; tooth and gum disease; acute and chronic ear, nose, and throat infections.
   c. Opportunistic infections.
   d. Reactive airway disease.
   e. Cardiomyopathy.
   f. Failure to thrive, malabsorption, wasting.
   g. Chronic atopic dermatitis and other skin reactions.
   h. Nephropathy.
   i. Neuropathy, myopathy.
   j. Anemia, thrombocytopenia, neutropenia.
   k. Loss of treatment options related to the development of drug resistance.
   l. Developmental delay.
   m. Learning disabilities.
   n. Psychological challenges for children and caregivers, including multiple losses, issues of disclosure, fear, discrimination, stigmatization, and isolation.
   o. Death.
2. Complications of HIV treatment:
   a. NRTIs—anemia, neutropenia, lactic acidosis, pancreatitis, abacavir hypersensitivity reaction, peripheral neuropathy, lipodystrophy/lipoatrophy, renal dysfunction, osteopenia, headache, nausea, potential for vascular dysfunction.

   b. NNRTIs—psychological changes, sleep disturbances/nightmares, neural tube defects (fetal exposure), hepatitis, rash.
   c. PIs—dyslipidemia, GI upset, diarrhea.
   d. Fusion inhibitors—injection site reactions.

DRUG ALERT Because some liquid preparations are unpalatable, nonadherence to the drug regimen is common. Suggestions to overcome this would include using Popsicle just before administration to numb the taste buds, followed by a teaspoon of chocolate/strawberry syrup, jam, or peanut butter immediately after. Speak to a pharmacist about other ways to mask the taste.

Nursing Assessment

1. Review maternal records to identify infants who may be at risk for HIV disease. Infected infants are not easily identifiable by outward appearance.
2. Review records of at-risk or known infected children to determine nutritional status, growth and development, frequency of serious bacterial infections, presence or risk of opportunistic infections, laboratory values, and immunization status.
3. Assess growth, development, lymph nodes, hepatomegaly, splenomegaly, and oropharynx for presence of oral candidiasis and dental caries.
4. Assess the family's understanding of the child's condition, care needs, prognosis, and medical care plan.
5. Assess the family's coping mechanisms, comfort with disclosure issues, and long-term plans for care, including transition plans for the child to an adult care program.
6. Assess the health of primary caregiver and discuss long-term care plans for respite and permanent alternative caregivers (including guardianship issues), as appropriate.
7. Assess the child's understanding of health condition and medications.
8. In children with advanced or end-stage disease, assess the level of pain and discomfort.
9. Assess the child's coping and response to the frequent painful and invasive procedures experienced as part of the ongoing diagnosis and management of the disease.
10. Assess for animal contact.
11. Take a thorough travel history to evaluate risk of coinfections, such as tuberculosis (TB), malaria, or other parasitic infections. Also evaluate potential travel plans, particularly to developing countries.
12. In the adolescent, assess increased at-risk behaviors, such as substance use, piercing, or sexual activity. Also determine methods of birth control, as appropriate.

CLINICAL JUDGMENT Always discuss with the primary caregiver how much the child knows about their own HIV status or about other family members' status. Never assume anyone knows the child's HIV status; other family, friends, daycare, or school; not even the child may know.

DRUG ALERT Some ARVs interact with the effect of birth control pills and may reduce efficacy or increase hormonal-related side effects. *For more information, see* CDC's Update to U.S. Medical Eligibility Criteria for Contraceptive Use, 2020: Updated Recommendations for the Use of Contraception Among Women at High Risk for HIV Infection. Current perinatal guidelines do not restrict the use of efavirenz during pregnancy.

Nursing Interventions

Preventing Infection

EVIDENCE BASE Centers for Disease Control and Prevention. *Recommended immunization schedules for children and adolescents aged 18 or younger, United States 2023.* www.cdc.gov/vaccines/schedules/hcp/child-adolescent.html

1. Monitor viral load, CD4 count, and CBC with differential.
2. Monitor other laboratory values to assess for side effects, that is, significant drop in absolute neutrophil count.
3. Use aseptic techniques when performing invasive procedures.
4. Administer or teach caregiver the importance of giving pharmacologic agents that may help prevent opportunistic infections. See "Management" section.
5. Assess and maintain skin integrity.
6. Monitor immunization status and advocate for completion of all recommended childhood immunizations for children with HIV infection (see guidelines at https://clinicalinfo.hiv.gov/en/guidelines/hiv-clinical-guidelines-pediatric-opportunistic-infections/figure-1-recommended). Also see page 1113 for routine pediatric immunization information based on the CDC. In general, live vaccines should be used with caution in children with HIV infections.
   a. The measles, mumps, rubella (MMR), and varicella vaccines are recommended for HIV-infected children who are not severely immunocompromised.
   b. Oral polio vaccine should be avoided because there is an alternative injectable inactivated polio vaccine available.
   c. Yellow fever vaccine should be avoided unless the risk of exposure is extremely high; consultation with an expert is recommended.
   d. In the United States, the bacille Calmette–Guérin vaccine is also not recommended.
   e. Yearly influenza vaccine and a 3- to 5-year pneumococcal vaccine are also recommended in addition to the standard childhood immunization schedule.
   f. An annual TB skin test should also be administered.
7. Have a high index of suspicion for secondary infection even when clinical manifestations are subtle or absent.
8. Provide appropriate chemoprophylaxis following exposure to communicable diseases.
9. Educate family/patient on the importance of prevention of secondary infections.
   a. Maintain cleanliness of the environment, and teach family members the essentials of environmental sanitation.
   b. Routine handwashing with soap and water.
   c. Oral hygiene and assessment for dental carries.
   d. Skin care to prevent breakdown.
   e. Safe food preparation and clean water use.
   f. Risk associated with handling animals; cats may transmit *toxoplasmosis or bartonella*, birds may transmit *Cryptococcus neoformans* or *M. avium*, and reptiles may transmit Salmonellosis. Good handwashing with soap and water after

handling animals; contact with animal feces should be avoided.
g. Attend Travel Medicine Clinic before traveling, particularly to developing or tropical countries, to prevent infections such as malaria or typhoid.
h. How to use condoms to prevent sexually transmitted infections such as syphilis or chlamydia.

DRUG ALERT Uninfected children living with HIV-infected caregivers or siblings should not receive the oral polio vaccine, but rather the injectable inactivated polio vaccine. This is because of the prolonged shedding of the virus from the live oral vaccine, which may prove to be hazardous for immunocompromised individuals.

Maximizing Adherence to HAART

EVIDENCE BASE Panel on Antiretroviral Therapy and Medical Management of HIV-Infected Children. (2023). *Guidelines for the use of antiretroviral agents in pediatric HIV infection.* https://clinicalinfo.hiv.gov/en/guidelines/pediatric-arv/whats-new

NOTE: Use of ARVs in pediatric patients is evolving rapidly. These guidelines are updated regularly to provide current information. The most recent information is available at https://clinicalinfo.hiv.gov/en

Center for Disease Control and Prevention. (2014). *Recommendations for HIV prevention with adults and adolescents with HIV in the United States, 2014.* https://www.cdc.gov/hiv/guidelines/recommendations/personswithhiv.html

1. Develop a trusting relationship with the patient by maintaining a nonjudgmental attitude to maintain open communication and assist in assessing barriers to adherence.
2. Assess drug readiness and strategies to maximize adherence before initiating therapy.
3. Provide the simplest regimen possible; for example, least number of pills (combination therapies), least often (once daily), based on viral resistance.
4. Stress the need for adherence at every visit.
5. Use several strategies for evaluating adherence (e.g., viral load, pill count, self-reporting, and pharmacy refill checks).
6. Collaborate with patient to determine what reminder tools may work the best (pill box, calendar, stickers, alarm, associating pill-taking with daily routine).

Maintaining Adequate Nutrition

1. Carefully monitor growth parameters (height, weight, head circumference).
2. Consult with a dietitian to develop strategies for nutritional care, including additional calories, nutritional supplements while reducing cholesterol.
3. Teach the family to prepare high-calorie, nutritious meals that are pleasing and acceptable to children.
4. As age appropriate, involve the child in meal planning.
5. Encourage small, frequent meals if the child is experiencing absorption problems.

Maintaining Oral Mucosa and Dental Integrity

1. Include regular examinations of the oral mucosa and teeth in the physical assessment of the child.
2. Administer prescribed antifungal and antiviral therapy.
3. Offer fluids and pureed foods to minimize chewing and facilitate swallowing; avoid highly seasoned or acidic foods.
4. Encourage regular dental hygiene and dental visits.

Minimizing Effects of Diarrhea

1. Monitor for the presence or development of diarrhea.
2. Monitor daily weight when diarrhea is present.
3. Monitor intake and output, and assess skin and mucous membranes for turgor and dryness.
4. Use enteric precautions.
5. Avoid foods that increase intestinal motility.
6. Administer IV hydration, as indicated.
7. Plan a regimen of skin care, including cleansing/blot drying of the anal area and application of ointment or skin barrier cream.
8. Teach the family safe food preparation techniques to minimize contamination of food.
9. Administer medications, as directed, for relief of severe diarrhea and enteric infections.

Detecting and Controlling Fever

1. Monitor for fever, and report any core temperature over 101°F (38.3°C).
2. Institute comfort measures, such as sponge baths, dry clothing and linens, and antipyretics, as ordered.
3. Teach the family how to accurately monitor the child's rectal temperature.
4. Teach the family to promptly report any febrile episode over 101°F rectally.
5. Administer antipyretics.

Promoting Developmental Goals

1. Assess the child's developmental status on a regular basis.
2. Report regression or delay in achieving developmental milestones.
3. Make appropriate referrals for more in-depth developmental evaluation when delays and regression are noted.
4. Teach the family appropriate developmental stimulation activities for their child.
5. Implement recommendations for developmental stimulation (including school-based programs), and assist the family in doing likewise.
6. Facilitate successful transition to adult care (see Box 49-1).

EVIDENCE BASE Ashaba, S., Zanoni, B., Baguma, C., Tushemereirwe, P., Nugaba, G., Kirabira, J., Nansera, D., Maling, S., & Tsai, A. (2023). Challenges and fears of adolescents and young adults living with HIV facing transition to adult HIV care. *AIDS & Behavior, 27*(4), 1189–1198.

Promoting Effective Family Coping

1. Practice within a framework of family-centered care.
2. Assess the family's coping mechanisms, strengths, and weaknesses.
3. Provide emotional support to the family.
4. Refer the family to appropriate community resources for grief counseling and legal assistance (e.g., wills, custody issues).
5. Help the family set realistic goals and expectations for the child.
6. Maintain a nonjudgmental attitude and nonprejudicial approach.
7. Allow the family to use denial as a protective mechanism because this gives them some sense of control.
8. Explain all care and treatment plans to the family.
9. Involve the family in planning for the care and management of their child.

BOX 49-1 Transition to Adult Care

Transition is the purposeful, planned movement of adolescents and young adults with chronic illness/disabilities from child-centered to adult-oriented systems. With the advent of highly active antiretroviral therapy, children with human immunodeficiency virus (HIV) are surviving and living well into adulthood. As they become adults, they are graduating from pediatric health care programs, with caregivers being the child's advocate, to adult programs, where individual care becomes the focus and the young adult becomes their own advocate.

It is imperative for the pediatric health care team to prepare children and families for the changes and challenges of adolescence, with a focus on increased autonomy and self-reliance and independence.

The transition into adolescence is a normal part of growth and development; however, special considerations need to be addressed when caring for a teenager with a chronic illness.

KEY ELEMENTS OF TRANSITION

- Focus the orientation on the future, and keep it proactive and flexible.
- Start as early as possible.
- Build on knowledge about HIV and issues of confidentiality and disclosure.
- Make sure your approach fosters personal and medical interdependence and creative problem solving.
- Provide opportunities for own consultations during clinic visit.
- Have open, honest, age-appropriate sexual health discussions.
- Develop a written transition policy—agreed upon by all members of the multidisciplinary team and target adult services—posted for families and young adults to see.
- Discuss different care models and possible settings in which the young adult can access care as an adult.
- Provide liaison personnel in both pediatric and adult health care centers.
- Coordinate an initial meeting for teen to meet adult care provider and staff.
- Ensure a flexible policy on the timing of events, with anticipation of change.
- Provide an education program for young people and their families that addresses medical, psychosocial, and educational/vocational aspects of care.
- Develop an individualized health care transition plan by age 14, in collaboration with the young adult and their family, and continuously update, as needed.
- Identify a network of relevant community agencies and adult primary and subspecialty care providers.
- Implement a training program for pediatric and adult providers on transition and adolescent issues.
- Provide for appropriate primary preventive care.
- Ensure affordable continuous health and medication insurance coverage.

10. Give strategies and guidance to families regarding *partial truth telling* so they can answer child's questions as honestly as possible.
11. Provide support to new birthing parents who grieve the loss of not being able to breastfeed. Provide strategies on how to deflect questions about the choice not to breastfeed.
12. Encourage caregiver to allow adolescent to start taking increased responsibility for own health care, including individual time alone with health care provider and self-advocacy.
13. Provide family and disclosed patient with hopeful information about the future, such as continuing education or, possibly, getting married and having a family.
14. Refer the family to community resources for home care, daycare of other siblings, transportation services, school-based services, respite care, and hospice.

Strengthening Coping Skills of the Child

EVIDENCE BASE Dantuluri, K., Carlucci, J., Howard, L., Johnson, D., Spencer, H., Desai, N., Garguilo, K., & Wilson, G. (2021). Optimizing disclosure of HIV status to a diverse population of HIV-positive youth at an urban pediatric HIV clinic. *Journal of Adolescent Health, 68*(4), 713–718.

Kidman, R., & Violari, A. (2020). Growing up positive: Adolescent HIV disclosure to sexual partners and others. *AIDS Care, 32*(12), 1565–1572.

1. Introduce the subject of disclosure of diagnosis to the child with the family. Offer the family guidelines as to age-appropriate approaches.
2. Accept that some families may not be able to disclose the nature of the disease to their child, even after much support and guidance.
   a. Explore with families how they want you to address questions the child may present to you.
   b. The illness and its impact can be effectively handled without actually telling the child about the HIV disease or AIDS status, if the family refuses to disclose it.
3. Answer the child's questions as honestly as possible within caregiver constraints that may be present.
4. Actively involve the child in as much of the care as possible, such as by having the child decide where to place the IV line, cleaning off skin for needle insertion, and so forth.
5. Use therapeutic play techniques (age appropriate), such as drawing, playing with dolls, playing with medical equipment, and storytelling, to allow the child to express themselves in less verbal ways.
6. Refer the child and family for counseling if the child's coping skills do not progress or if there appears to be regression in handling the issue of illness and chronic health care needs. Signs indicating possible need for additional in-depth interventions include more acting out by the child, withdrawn behavior, and difficulty in school (either behaviorally or academically).
7. Recommend and facilitate peer support groups.

Minimizing Discomfort

1. Assess for signs of pain in the child. In the infant or nonverbal child, such signs include restlessness, crying, withdrawn behavior, and changes in vital signs.
2. Discuss concerns over pain issues with the primary health care provider and team providing care for the child. Initiate or request referral to a pain management team if the child does not experience relief.
3. Stress to the caregiver or guardian the need for adequate pain management in children; many people do not acknowledge that infants or children suffer from pain and that this needs to be alleviated.
4. Use appropriate techniques to assess the level of pain or discomfort a child is experiencing.

Minimizing Fear

1. Make sure that all painful and invasive procedures are done in a location other than the child's bed in the hospital.
2. Monitor central line if used for venous access. Central line access may be less traumatic over time than repeated peripheral access attempts. Some children with HIV will need long-term, probably lifelong, IV therapies and blood monitoring, and a central line greatly eliminates the pain and anxiety associated with these procedures.
3. Make sure that the biological parent/caregiver realizes that most clinic visits will involve blood tests so that they do not falsely reassure the child that "no needle sticks" will occur.
4. Use diversionary techniques, such as bubble-blowing, for distraction during painful procedures. Practice first with the child, and tell them this is an activity that you will help with during the procedure. Children can also be taught other relaxation techniques.
5. Offer small rewards (such as stickers, small toy items) after painful procedures to reduce anxiety. Such rewards should be given regardless of how the child reacted. The reward is not for "not crying" but acknowledges difficulty in going through painful and invasive procedures on a regular basis.
6. Involve the child in the procedure as much as possible (age appropriate). Such involvement can include selecting a possible site for accessing or receiving IV medications, cleaning the site, or selecting a special bandage for after the procedure. Use topical anesthetic.

Community and Home Care Considerations

1. Assess home environment for resources, such as nutritious foods and safe food preparation; adequate water, heat, electricity, and space; developmentally appropriate toys; and supplies needed for care and hygiene.
2. Assess caregiver's correct administration of medications.
3. Draw blood samples using universal precautions and careful transport of blood and used equipment.
4. Perform developmental assessment periodically.
5. Act as liaison among family, specialists, school officials, and other team members.

Family Education and Health Maintenance

1. Teach families and other caregivers of the child universal precautions. In caring for HIV-infected infants and children, gloves are recommended when handling potentially contaminated body fluids (such as blood) but are not considered necessary for routine diaper-changing unless bloody diarrhea or hematuria exists.
2. Facilitate supply of adequate numbers of latex (or nonlatex, if necessary) gloves to families to use, as indicated.
3. Facilitate education as well as a supply of latex condoms and other forms of birth control for teens who are sexually active or about to become sexually active.
4. Offer guidance as to how to initiate discussion of their child's HIV status with schools and daycare settings. The "need-to-know" principle serves as a guideline when deciding to whom disclosure should be made (generally, the principal, school nurse, and classroom teacher). It is not currently required that schools and daycare centers be advised but is generally encouraged because this alerts the school to notify the caregiver promptly in the event of an outbreak of infectious disease that could pose a threat to the HIV-infected child (such as varicella).
5. Offer guidance to teens about how to initiate disclosure of HIV status to sexual partners or peers. Provide support during the process, and offer to help facilitate the disclosure in the clinical setting.
6. Give families concrete guidelines as to when to notify the health care provider about their child's condition. Signs and symptoms of illness require prompt notification, all fevers over 101°F (38.3°C) should be reported, and any adverse experiences or suspected adverse experiences with medications need prompt reporting.
7. Assess whether the caregivers are receiving care for themselves. Typically, caregivers will neglect their own care to provide for their child. As a result, the caregivers' immune status may become more quickly compromised.
8. Refer families to a social worker or social services agency. Children with HIV may qualify for certain entitlement programs that help with their health care and the family's financial situation. Many states have initiated case management programs for people with HIV.
9. Provide guidance using a childhood chronic illness model that addresses such psychosocial issues as disclosure and caregiver guilt as well as such medical issues as multiorgan involvement and likelihood of exacerbations of a variety of related conditions (e.g., infections and nutritional deficiencies).
10. Assist caregivers in obtaining the latest information regarding treatment protocols for clinical trials. Such information can be obtained through www.clinicaltrials.gov.

Evaluation: Expected Outcomes

- Absolute neutrophil count within normal limits; aseptic technique maintained.
- Maintains medication regimen; keeps follow-up appointments; achieves an undetectable viral load.
- Nutritional intake adequate to meet body requirements; growth curve maintained.
- Oral mucous membranes without ulceration, good dentition.
- Two to three loose stools per day; perianal skin without irritation.
- Afebrile; caregiver demonstrates accurate monitoring of temperature.
- Achieves normal growth patterns as evidenced by height, weight, and developmental tasks.
- Caregivers discuss their feelings about the diagnosis of HIV; family seeks help through community resources.
- Child participates in care, asks questions; adolescent successfully transitions to an adult care program without disruption in care.
- Reports increase in comfort level.
- Practices distraction techniques during procedures; reports reduced fear.

Primary Immunodeficiencies

Primary immunodeficiencies (PIDs), also known as inborn errors of immunity, encompass more than 450 types of disorders that affect distinct components of the innate and adaptive immune systems. The overall incidence of PID is estimated to be 1:20,000. The most common presentation of an immunodeficiency is increased frequency of infections or infections that are unusual or difficult to treat. PID diseases may be undiagnosed or have a significant delay in diagnosis, which can lead to significant end-organ damage from recurrent infections. Increasingly, it is recognized that PID may present in other ways, such as multiple autoimmune or autoinflammatory manifestations, severe allergies, and some types of malignancies.

EVIDENCE BASE Bousfiha, A., Moundir, A., Tangye, S., Picard, C., Jeddane, L., Al-Herz, W., Rundles, C., Franco, J., Holland, S., Klein, C., Morio, T., Oksenhendler, E., Puel, A., Puck, J., Seppanen, M., Somech, R., Su, H., Sullivan, K., Torgerson, T., & Meyts, I. I. (2022). The 2022 update of IUIS phenotypical classification for human inborn errors of immunity. *Journal of Clinical Immunology, 42*(7), 1508–1520.

Pathophysiology and Etiology

EVIDENCE BASE Aghamohammadi, A., Abolhassani, H., Rezaei, N., & Yazdani, R. (Eds.). (2021). *Inborn errors of immunity: A practical guide*. Academic Press.

POPULATION AWARENESS Despite PIDs having genetic mutations in the immune system, patients may present at any age from early infancy to late adulthood.

1. PID diseases are caused by genetic alterations in the immune system that lead to changes in essential immune pathways. Inheritance may be X-linked, autosomal recessive, or autosomal dominant. The genetic mutation may be de novo, with no prior family history.
2. About three quarters of PID diseases are caused by humoral or combined humoral and cellular abnormalities, with the remainder being defects in phagocytic or complement components of the immune system.
3. Risk factors for PID diseases include a family history of immunodeficiency, early infant deaths, caregiver consanguinity, autoimmunity, and increased incidence of lymphoid malignancy in family members.

Clinical Manifestations

1. Hallmark of PID diseases is susceptibility to infection, including recurrent pneumonia, sinusitis, otitis, sepsis, meningitis, recurrent or resistant candidiasis, or infection with an opportunistic organism. Course of infection may be unusual, with a need for intravenous antibiotics and/or hospitalization to clear infections. See Table 49-4.
2. Chronic diarrhea.
3. Nonhealing wounds.
4. Extensive skin lesions.
5. Failure to gain weight or grow normally (failure to thrive).
6. Complications from a live viral vaccine.
7. Unexplained autoimmunity or fevers.
8. Absence or enlargement of lymphoid tissue, including tonsils, spleen, and liver.

Diagnostic Evaluation

Specific Evaluation for Immunodeficiency

1. CBC with diff to look for decreased numbers of lymphocytes and evidence of abnormalities in other cell lines, such as decreased platelets, neutrophils, or hemoglobin.
2. Immunoglobulin levels (IgG, IgA, IgM, and IgE) include total protein and albumin to rule out protein loss.
3. Antibody titers to previously administered vaccines to evaluate the ability to produce functional specific antibodies to infectious agents. Measurement of isoagglutinins (isoantibodies to blood groups) in children older than 2 years.
4. Measurement of the classical (CH50) and alternate pathway (AH50) of the complement system to rule out a complement deficiency.
5. Lymphocyte subset analysis by flow cytometry, including CD3 (total T cells), CD4 (T helper), CD8 (T cytotoxic), CD19 or

Table 49-4 Infections Associated with Subtypes of PID Diseases

TYPE	TYPES OF INFECTIONS	ORGANISMS	OTHER FEATURES
Humoral (B cell)	Sinopulmonary, otitis media, GI, cellulitis, meningitis, osteomyelitis	Encapsulated bacteria: *Haemophilus*, pneumococci, streptococci Parasites: *Giardia lamblia*, *Cryptosporidium* Virus: *Enterovirus*	Autoimmunity GI problems, including malabsorption
Cellular (T cell or combined T and B cells)	Pulmonary, GI, skin	Fungal: *Candida* species, *Pneumocystis jirovecii* Viral: CMV, EBV, RSV, parainfluenza, adenovirus, viral GI disease mycobacterium species	Failure to thrive Oral thrush Skin: rashes, dermatitis Postvaccination disease from live viral vaccines
Phagocytic disorders	Severe skin and visceral infections by common pathogens	Bacteria: *Staphylococcus aureus*, *Pseudomonas* species, *Serratia* species, *Klebsiella* species Fungi: *Candida*, *Nocardia*, *Aspergillus*	Granuloma formation, including granulomatous enteritis Poor wound healing Abscesses Oral cavity infections Anorectal infections
Complement disorders	Meningitis septicemia	*Neisseria* infections: meningococcal, pneumococcal	Rheumatoid disorders: lupus-like syndrome Angioedema

CMV, cytomegalovirus; EBV, Epstein–Barr virus; GI, gastrointestinal; PID, primary immunodeficiencies; RSV, respiratory syncytial virus.

CD20 (B cells), and CD16/56 (natural killer cells) for suspected T cell, B cell, or combined immunodeficiency.
6. Lymphoproliferative assays to assess the cellular function.
7. Measurement of phagocytic oxidative responses (neutrophil oxidative burst index [NOBI] by flow cytometry) if a phagocytic disorder is suggested, such as chronic granulomatous disease.
8. Genetic testing for suspected cause of immunodeficiency.

Other Tests

1. Evaluation for infection, including inflammatory markers (C-reactive protein, sedimentation rate), appropriate cultures, radiologic image of the site of suspected infections.
2. Electrolytes, glucose, urea, creatinine, arterial blood gases, if indicated.
3. Advanced immunologic evaluations, memory T & B cell assays, T-cell repertoire by v-betas, T-cell receptor excision circles (TREC, a measure of mature cells from the thymus).
4. PCR testing for suspected infectious agents if there is concern that the patient may not produce functional antibodies from PI disease.
5. Newborn screen for severe combined immunodeficiency (SCID) by TREC if available.

Management

1. Prompt recognition and treatment of infections. Empiric antibiotic therapy pending culture results should be instituted.
2. May consider preventive antibiotic treatment for some PID diseases.
3. Avoidance of live viral vaccines, as they may be disease-causing in patients with PID.
4. Postexposure infectious prophylaxis may be necessary following exposure to varicella.
5. For suspected T-cell immunodeficiency, blood products must be irradiated to eliminate leukocytes and screened for cytomegalovirus.
6. *Pneumocystis jirovecii* prophylaxis for T-cell immunodeficiencies.
7. Antibody replacement therapy with intravenous or subcutaneous gammaglobulin for combined and antibody deficiencies (X-linked agammaglobulinemia, common variable immunodeficiency, CD40 ligand or CD40 deficiency, selective antibody deficiency, SCID and peritransplant).
8. Immunosuppressive drugs for patients with associated autoimmunity.
9. Stem cell transplant to replace the defective immune system in severe PID diseases (SCID, combined immunodeficiencies, Wiskott–Aldrich syndrome, chronic granulomatous disease, and others). Indications for transplant are constantly expanding, as new genes are identified.
10. Gene therapy is an experimental option for some PID diseases: adenosine deaminase deficiency (a type of SCID), Wiskott–Aldrich syndrome, and chronic granulomatous disease. Uses of gene therapy are continuously expanding.

Complications

1. Organ damage from infection, particularly the lungs, gastrointestinal (GI) tract, and joints.
2. Chronic lung disease (bronchiectasis).
3. Granulomatous lesions in the skin, liver, spleen, and lungs (common variable immunodeficiency and chronic granulomatous disease).
4. GI malabsorption because of infection or from bacterial overgrowth.
5. Autoimmunity.
6. Early death (less than 1 year of age for SCID).
7. Malignancy (especially lymphoma and leukemia).
8. Psychological and social reactions to chronic disease.

Nursing Assessment

1. Focus history on infections, including age of onset, sites, number, frequency, types, duration, and response to treatment.
2. Detailed family history, including focus on unexplained infant deaths, recurrent miscarriages, consanguinity, malignancies, and autoimmunity in other members.
3. Review of immunization record and history to determine complications from vaccines and to ensure that immunizations are given at proper intervals.
4. Focus physical examination on the site of infections, such as lung air entry, as well as vital signs, growth and development, presence or absence of lymphoid tissue, examination of the skin for evidence of candidiasis or other skin abnormalities.
5. Assess the family and child's understanding of the condition, care needs, prognosis, and plan of care.
6. Assess the family's coping mechanisms and resources, particularly for patients that may require stem cell transplant or lifelong treatment with immunoglobulins.

CLINICAL JUDGMENT When considering home gammaglobulin therapy, assess support in the home and the ability of the patient to adhere to treatment.

Nursing Interventions

Preventing Infection

1. Educate families about signs and symptoms of infection that specific PID disease is susceptible to and when to seek health care advice.
2. Administer or teach caregiver to administer prescribed pharmacologic agents, including treatment protocols for gammaglobulin therapy, if indicated.
3. Adhere to infection control policies for protection of severe T-cell immunodeficiencies when hospitalized.
4. Avoid administration of live viral vaccines for suspected PID (oral polio, MMR, varicella, yellow fever, rotavirus, inhaled influenza, and bacilli Calmette-Guérin [BCG] vaccine).
5. Encourage yearly influenza vaccine for patients and family members.
6. Recommend COVID-19 vaccines and consider need for use of monoclonal antibody prophylaxis with tixagevimab and cilgavimab injection.
7. Administer and teach family good infection control techniques, including handwashing and skin care to avoid infection.

DRUG ALERT Live viral vaccines may cause disease if administered to patients with PID diseases, and a diagnosis of PID should be considered in patients presenting with vaccine-derived infections.

Maintaining Adequate Nutrition

1. Carefully monitor growth parameters, including height, weight, and head circumference.
2. Consult with a dietician to develop nutritional plan of care, including adequate caloric intake and caregiver teaching.
3. Administer and teach families to administer supplemental feeds via nasogastric- (NG-) or gastrostomy- (G-)tube if indicated.

Maintaining Oral Mucosa

1. Include assessment of oral mucosa in routine physical assessments.
2. Administer and teach families to administer prescribed antifungal or antiviral medications.
3. Promote good dental hygiene and dental care.

Promoting Therapeutic Regime Management

1. Teach patients and families about prescribed medications and treatments. Review teaching periodically.
2. For patients on gammaglobulin treatment, doses should be adjusted to reflect increased weight, so as to ensure adequate replacement of antibodies. For patients on subcutaneous gammaglobulin, periodically assess patient adherence to infusion protocol and reeducate, as necessary.

Promoting Growth and Development

1. Assess for normal growth and development.
2. Make appropriate referrals for more in-depth developmental assessments, and adhere to treatment programs instituted (important for prolonged admissions, such as bone marrow transplant).
3. Teach the family appropriate developmental activities for their child.
4. Facilitate successful transition to adult care.

Promote Effective Family Coping

EVIDENCE BASE Meyts, I., Bousfiha, A., Duff, C., Singh, S., Lau, Y. L., Condino-Neto, A., Bezrodnik, L., Adli, A., Adeli, M., & Drabwell, J. (2021). Primary immunodeficiencies: A decade of progress and a promising future. *Frontiers in Immunology, 11*, 625753.

1. Assess family coping skills, including strengths and weaknesses.
2. Provide emotional support and counseling, as necessary.
3. Refer the family for genetic counseling, as diagnosis may impact other family members or future pregnancies.
4. Encourage families to allow children to take increased responsibility for their care as they mature.
5. Provide continuous teaching about disease process and treatment. It is particularly important for children diagnosed at very young ages to learn as they grow—lifelong diseases.

Normalizing Family Processes

1. Refer to community resources and support groups.
2. Encourage family and child to verbalize feelings about diagnosis and treatment.
3. Encourage attendance at school, participation in activities, and socialization with peers as much as possible.
4. Encourage caregivers to spend time with siblings and each other, as well as affected child.

Community and Home Care Considerations

1. Assess home environment for resources, such as nutritious foods, developmentally appropriate toys, and supplies needed for care and hygiene.
2. Assess for correct administration and storage, as well as adherence to medications and treatments.
3. Ensure that patient has a community care practitioner.
4. Provide education to school nurses so that individual educational plans are implemented and maintained.

Family Education and Health Maintenance

1. Give families guidelines as to when to notify health care provider about their child's condition. Signs and symptoms of illness require prompt notification, all fevers over 101°F (38.3°C) should be reported, and any adverse experiences or suspected adverse events to medications require prompt reporting.
2. Assess family coping, and refer to social worker or social services, as required.
3. Refer families to immunodeficiency patient support agencies so as to provide ongoing PID disease–specific education to patients and families.

Evaluation and Expected Outcomes

- Reduced incidence of infections.
- Adequate intake for child's age and developmental stage.
- No oral lesions, denies oral discomfort.
- Adherence to treatment regimes.
- Achieves normal growth, as evidenced by height, weight, and developmental tasks.
- Child and family seek appropriate support and resources, as required.
- Child and caregivers verbalize feelings about the illness; include siblings in activities.

CONNECTIVE TISSUE DISORDERS

Juvenile Idiopathic Arthritis

EVIDENCE BASE Martini, A., Lovell, D. J., Albani, S., Brunner, H., Hyrich, K., Thompson, S., & Ruperto, N. (2022). Juvenile idiopathic arthritis. *Nature Reviews Disease Primers, 8*, 5. https://doi.org/10.1038/s41572-021-00332-8

Zaripova, L. N., Midgley, A., Christmas, S. E., Beresford, M. W., Baildam, E. M., & Oldershaw, R. A. (2021). Juvenile idiopathic arthritis: From aetiopathogenesis to therapeutic approaches. *Pediatric Rheumatology Online Journal, 19*(1), 135. https://doi.org/10.1186/s12969-021-00629-8

Juvenile idiopathic arthritis (JIA) has replaced the terms "juvenile chronic arthritis" and "juvenile rheumatoid arthritis" as the commonly agreed-upon terminology to describe arthritis in children. JIA is defined as persistent arthritis for longer than 6 weeks in children ≤16 years of age. It is a heterogeneous disease that has been further classified into several subtypes with similar presentation, clinical features, disease course, and outcomes.

JIA is a chronic disease affecting approximately 1 in 1,000 children. There are epidemiologic differences that are specific to subtype (see Table 49-5, page 1395).

Pathophysiology and Etiology

1. The cause of JIA is unknown. It is likely multifactorial and variable between subtypes. Hypotheses suggest that environmental stimuli trigger disease in genetically predisposed children during a time of susceptibility.
   a. Genetic risk factors—associations with specific human leukocyte antigen (HLA) class I (B27) and class II genes, protein tyrosine phosphatase N22 gene, and interleukin-2 receptor alpha gene have been well established.

Table 49-5 Characteristics of Juvenile Idiopathic Arthritis

ILAR SUBTYPE	OLIGOARTICULAR PERSISTENT EXTENDED	POLYARTICULAR (RF NEGATIVE)	POLYARTICULAR (RF POSITIVE)	SYSTEMIC	ENTHESITIS-RELATED ARTHRITIS	PSORIATIC ARTHRITIS	UNDIFFERENTIATED
% Total patients with JIA	40%–50%	20%–25%	5%	5%–10%	5%–10%	5%–10%	10%
Age of onset	Early childhood; 1–3 yr	2 peaks: 2–4 yr and 6–12 yr	Early adolescence	Throughout childhood	Late childhood and adolescence	2 peaks: 2–4 yr and 9–11 yr	
Sex assigned at birth	F > M	F > M	F > M	F = M	M ≥ F	F ≥ M	
Typical joint involvement	≤4 joints in first 6 mo Large joints: knees, ankles, wrist Extended disease: involves >4 joints after first 6 mo	≥5 joints Symmetric distribution Knees, wrists, ankles TMJ can be affected	≥5 joints Small and large joints Symmetric C-spine and TMJ affected Erosive joint disease	Oligoarticular or Polyarticular distribution Progressive and destructive arthritis	Weight-bearing joints: hip, feet Axial and sacroiliac joint involvement Enthesitis	Asymmetric or symmetric small or large joints Dactylitis Enthesitis	
Laboratory tests	ANA 60%–80% positive	ANA 50% positive	ANA 75% positive RF positive	ANA 5%–10% positive	HLA–B27 positive		
Occurrence of uveitis	Common (30%) Usually asymptomatic	Common (15%)	Rare (<1%)	Rare (<1%)	Symptomatic; acute onset, painful red eye Unilateral	Common (10%)	
Other features	Leg length discrepancies Contractures	Fatigue	Rheumatoid nodules Fever and constitutional signs at onset of disease	Daily quotidian fever ≥2 wk Evanescent rash Lymphadenopathy Hepatosplenomegaly Serositis macrophage activation syndrome is life-threatening complication	Association with inflammatory bowel disease	Nail pits, onycholysis Psoriasis	Does not fulfill criteria for any of the other categories or fulfills criteria for >1 category

ANA, antinuclear antibody; F, person assigned female at birth; HLA, human leukocyte antigen; ILAR, International League for Associations of Rheumatology; JIA, juvenile idiopathic arthritis; M, person assigned male at birth; RF, rheumatoid factor; TMJ, temporomandibular joint.

Adapted with permission from Gowdie, P., & Tse, S. (2012). Juvenile idiopathic arthritis. Pediatric Clinics of North America, 59(2), 301–327, Copyright 2012, with permission from Elsevier.

b. Immune dysregulation of the adaptive and innate immune system. Autoantibodies including antinuclear antibody (ANA); rheumatoid factor (RF); T-lymphocytes and cytokines, tissue necrosis factor (TNF) of adaptive immunity as well as neutrophils and interleukin (IL)-1, IL-6 of innate immunity are present in sera and synovial fluids.
c. Infection as a trigger to immune dysregulation is suspected but has not been clearly established.
d. Hormonal factors.

2. Arthritis is inflammation of one or more synovial joints. Immune complexes trigger the inflammatory response, causing:
   a. The synovium to become thickened from congestion and edema.
   b. Increased production of intra-articular fluid exhibited as a joint effusion. It is not uncommon for synovial cysts to develop (Baker cyst).
   c. Development of periarticular soft tissue edema.
   d. Extension of the inflammatory process to the tendons, tendon sheaths, and entheses.
   e. Weakness and atrophy of muscle surrounding affected joints, leading to flexion contractures.
   f. Growth centers in long bones may undergo either premature epiphyseal closure or accelerated epiphyseal growth. The result is overgrowth or shortening of the affected limb.
3. Long-term disease activity can result in joint destruction and eventual joint failure, necessitating joint replacement.
   a. Degrading enzymes released during synovial inflammation result in chondrolysis and osteolysis; erosion of the articular cartilage and bone.
   b. Following destruction, the overgrowth of granulation tissue may result in the formulation of new cartilage and bone, leading to ankylosis.
   c. Joint destruction is characterized by joint space narrowing, erosions, deformities, subluxation, and ankylosis.
   d. Generalized osteopenia is common, increasing the risk of fracture.

Clinical Manifestations

Clinical manifestations include joint and extra-articular features that vary among subtypes (see Table 49-5, page 1395).

1. The inflamed joint is characterized by four of the five cardinal signs of inflammation: swelling, pain, heat, loss of function. Erythema occurs in some cases.
   a. Joint stiffness in the morning or after prolonged inactivity (gelling) is common.
   b. Pain may not be expressed verbally; the child may alter activities to protect the painful joint.
2. Extra-articular features may include fever, rash, fatigue, weight loss, altered growth, subcutaneous nodules, and uveitis.
   a. Fevers occur in systemic JIA and occasionally at the onset of polyarticular JIA. In systemic JIA, fevers are daily, usually above 102.2°F (39°C), following a quotidian pattern of one or two spikes with a rapid return to baseline and accompanied by a classic salmon-pink rash.
   b. Altered growth includes localized growth abnormalities and poor linear growth.
      i. Overgrowth or undergrowth of bones in sites affected by arthritis result in leg length discrepancy, shortened limbs, and micrognathia and or/retrognathia (receding chin) with arthritis of the temporomandibular joint (TMJ).
      ii. Poor linear growth is attributed to the inhibitory effects chronic inflammation and circulating cytokines have on growth.
   c. Uveitis associated with arthritis is found in 20% to 40% of cases. It is commonly asymptomatic, thus requiring frequent examinations by an eye specialist. An exception is the patient with subtype enthesitis-related arthritis (ERA), who may present with redness, pain, photophobia, headache, and decreased visual acuity.

Diagnostic Evaluation

1. JIA is a diagnosis of exclusion. Laboratory studies cannot exclusively confirm diagnosis. They are used to support diagnosis, measure disease activity, help predict prognoses, and monitor toxicity of therapy.
   a. Elevated erythrocyte sedimentation rate (ESR).
   b. Leukocytosis, thrombocytosis, anemia.
   c. Elevated serum immunoglobulins.
   d. Elevated C-reactive protein.
   e. Presence of ANA, RF, and anticyclic citrullinated peptide (anti-CCP) antibodies. ANA is associated with high incidence of uveitis. Anti-CCP is an early predictor of erosive disease in polyarticular JIA.
2. Radiographic studies.
   a. X-rays early in the progression of the disease show soft tissue swelling, osteopenia, and effusions.
   b. X-rays late in the progression of the disease show erosions, joint space narrowing, boutonniere or swan neck deformity of the fingers, early maturation of cartilage, and subluxations.
   c. Ultrasound for detection of tenosynovitis.
   d. Magnetic resonance imaging (MRI) is most sensitive to detect specific joint disease, including TMJ and sacroiliac.
3. Ophthalmologic examination.
   a. Slit-lamp examination to monitor for uveitis is required within 1 month of diagnosis and every 3 to 12 months, depending on age, presence of ANA, and duration of illness.

Management

1. There is no cure for JIA.
2. Management of JIA should be provided by a multidisciplinary team in a family-centered approach.
3. The primary goal of treatment is to facilitate disease remission off medication.
   a. In the process of working toward remission, other goals of therapy include control pain and maintain range of motion (ROM), muscle strength, and function.
   b. To promote normal growth.
   c. To support normal psychological and social development.
4. Goal attainment requires nonpharmacologic and pharmacologic approaches.
5. Nonpharmacologic approaches to treatment include:
   a. Occupational and physical therapies that employ strength and stretching exercises, splinting, serial casting, orthotics, and thermal modalities to reduce stiffness or pain and to protect function.
   b. Strengthening and aerobic-based exercise are safe in children with JIA. Studies have demonstrated improved physical function and quality of life.
   c. Nutritional and vitamin supplementation are required to promote growth, maintain bone mineralization, and prevent toxicity from medication. Vitamin D, calcium, iron, and folic acid may be prescribed.

d. Orthopedic surgery may be performed to manage joint complications; tendon lengthening for severe contractures; total joint replacements, particularly hips and knees.

6. Pharmacologic therapies are introduced in a systematic stepwise approach targeted to the specific subtypes of JIA. Refer to Table 49-6, page 1398. Recently, a more aggressive progression through the steps is being advocated, as evidence suggests rapid control of inflammation may positively influence prognosis.
   a. Nonsteroidal antiinflammatory drugs (NSAIDS) are the first line of therapy aimed at symptom relief.
   b. Disease-modifying antirheumatic drugs (DMARDs) are second-line immunosuppressive agents that can achieve disease control and influence the course of disease.
   c. Newer biologic agents and the generic equivalents (biosimilars) are selected when DMARDs fail. They target very specific immune responses responsible for inflammation. Biologics offer treatment options for children with refractory arthritis and/or uveitis.
   d. Corticosteroids are potent antiinflammatories used mainly as a bridging therapy until other treatments begin to take effect. Steroids have not been shown to be disease modifying. They can be administered by oral, intramuscular, intravenous, intra-articular, or intraocular route and should be administered at the lowest effective dose. Intra-articular steroid injections are well tolerated, whereas other forms of steroids can lead to serious toxic side effects, including weight gain, edema, acne, fatigue, growth suppression, decreased bone density, hypertension, hyperglycemia, glaucoma, cataracts, and the accompanying psychological sequelae.
7. Children receiving the immunosuppressive therapies used to treat arthritis require special considerations.
   a. Close monitoring for signs of infection.
   b. Screening for tuberculosis (TB) prior to initiation of corticosteroid or biologic therapy. Testing should be repeated for those who have travelled to endemic areas or who have had close contact with visitors from these areas. Steroids can alter the result of tuberculin skin testing; QuantiFERON (QFT) blood testing may be indicated in these cases. Biologic therapy can reactivate latent TB.
   c. Children receiving DMARDs, corticosteroids, or biologics should not receive live vaccines (varicella, measles, mumps, and rubella). When considering treatment with methotrexate, varicella immunization may be recommended prior to starting therapy in susceptible children. In such circumstances, methotrexate cannot be started for 28 days post immunization.
   d. Regular blood monitoring for toxicity, specifically liver and renal.
   e. Regular clinical examinations to assess for adverse effects. In 2010, the Food and Drug Administration (FDA) reported several cases of malignancies in children receiving biologic therapy but, because of the small numbers, were not conclusive. Long-term studies are required. Persistent inflammation also increases the risk of malignancy.
8. The course and outcome of JIA has changed dramatically with early intervention and more successful therapies. However, active disease continues into adulthood in 50% to 70% of children with polyarticular and systemic JIA, 40% to 50% of oligoarticular JIA. Current research in biomarkers, genetics, and immunology to help predict response or nonresponse to therapy choices (treat to target) will guide and advance care within the next decade.

EVIDENCE BASE Unni, J. C., Joseph, R. B., & Bhattad, S. (2020). Drugs in pediatric rheumatology. *Indian Journal of Practical Pediatrics, 22*(3), 262.

Garner, A. J., Saatchi, R., Ward, O., & Hawley, D. P. (2021). Juvenile idiopathic arthritis: A review of novel diagnostic and monitoring technologies. *Healthcare (Basel, Switzerland), 9*(12), 1683. https://doi.org/10.3390/healthcare9121683

El Tal, T., Ryan, M. E., Feldman, B. M., Bingham, C. A., Burnham, J. M., Batthish, M., Bullock, D., Ferraro, K., Gilbert, M., Gillispie-Taylor, M., Gottlieb, B., Harris, J. G., Hazen, M., Laxer, R. M., Lee, T. C., Lovell, D., Mannion, M., Noonan, L., Oberle, E., ... Morgan, E. M. (2022). Consensus approach to a treat-to-target strategy in juvenile idiopathic arthritis care: Report from the 2020 PR-COIN consensus conference. *The Journal of Rheumatology, 49*(5), 497–503. https://doi.org/10.3899/jrheum.210709

Complications

1. Bone and growth changes:
   a. Growth disturbance, short stature.
   b. Osteopenia, osteoporosis.
   c. Cervical spine and TMJ problems (micrognathia/retrognathia).
   d. Leg length discrepancies.
   e. Joint contractures.
2. Psychological and social reactions to illness.
3. Cataracts, glaucoma, or blindness secondary to uncontrolled, chronic uveitis.
4. Pericarditis.
5. Macrophage activation syndrome—a life-threatening complication of systemic JIA characterized by massive activation of T cells and macrophages; features include sustained fever, hepatosplenomegaly, anemia, liver function abnormalities, coagulopathy, encephalopathy, sudden drop in ESR, extreme elevation of ferritin, and marked elevation of D-dimers.

Nursing Assessment

1. History should include a thorough musculoskeletal inquiry, including location, onset, duration of joint pain and stiffness; alleviating and exacerbating factors; activity limitations; medication and other nonpharmacologic treatments used; review of systems to look for associated symptoms and complications of JIA and side effects of medication; most recent ophthalmology examination; immunizations; and TB screening.
2. Physical examination focused on the clinical manifestations of the different subtypes of JIA, including joint and gait assessment, vital signs, growth parameters, and a pain assessment using a developmentally appropriate tool.
3. Gather data for psychosocial assessment, including inquiry into the impact of this chronic, painful disease on the child's self-esteem and coping and the family's coping.

Nursing Interventions

Minimizing Discomfort

1. Administer or teach caregivers/patients to administer medications to reduce inflammation and control pain. When inflammation and pain are controlled, a child is more willing and able to do exercises to improve joint strength and prevent loss of movement.

Table 49-6 Pharmacologic Treatment for Juvenile Idiopathic Arthritis

	MEDICATION	INDICATION	DOSING	ADVERSE EFFECTS	MONITORING	CONSIDERATIONS
NSAIDs	COX-1, COX-2 inhibitors, naproxen, ibuprofen, indomethacin, celecoxib	First-line therapy for all subtypes of JIA; symptom management	PO variable dose frequency	Gastritis; pseudoporphyria; hepatotoxicity; renal toxicity	CBC, liver enzymes, creatinine at baseline then q6 mo	Pseudoporphyria most commonly seen in fair-skinned children
DMARDs	Methotrexate	Second-line therapy for all subtypes except systemic JIA	PO or SC once weekly 15 mg/m^2/dose (maximum 25 mg) Therapeutic effect in 6–12 wk	GI upset; mouth ulcers; hepatotoxicity; teratogenicity	CBC, liver enzymes at baseline, 1 mo then q3–4 mo on stable dose	Provide folate supplement Avoid live vaccines Give VZIG within 96 h for chicken pox exposure Avoid alcohol Avoid pregnancy Avoid interaction with the antibiotics sulfamethoxazole and trimethoprim (bone marrow suppression)
	Sulfasalazine	Oligoarticular JIA; polyarticular JIA; ERA	PO 50 mg/kg/d divided bid. Therapeutic effect in 6–12 wk	GI upset; rash; bone marrow suppression; hepatotoxicity; allergy	CBC, liver enzymes at baseline, then q4–12 wk	Inquire about sulfa allergies Avoid live vaccines Beware of additive hepatotoxicity in combination with methotrexate
	Leflunomide	Oligoarticular; polyarticular	PO once daily 10–20 mg/d Therapeutic effect in 6–12 wk	GI upset; rash; hepatotoxicity; teratogenicity	CBC, liver enzymes at baseline, then q4–12 wk	Use when methotrexate not tolerated Cholestyramine used to enhance elimination Avoid pregnancy Avoid alcohol Avoid live vaccines

Glucocorticoids	Methylprednisolone, prednisone, prednisolone, triamcinolone, hexacetonide	Used for quick antiinflammatory effect or bridging agent for all subtypes of JIA	IV, IM, PO, intra-articular, topical, intraocular for uveitis Dose/frequency depends on route and severity of inflammation	Increased appetite; GI upset; mood changes; hypertension; acne; striae; Cushing syndrome; growth suppression; osteoporosis; hyperglycemia; cataracts; glaucoma	Dependent on route of administration and length of treatment	Monitor BP; urine for glycosuria Annual bone mineral density Delay immunization schedule Give VZIG within 96 h for chicken pox exposure
Biologics	TNF inhibitors: (including biosimilars) Etanercept Infliximab Adalimumab Golimumab	Used when second-line agents fail Effective in treating uveitis	SC (Etanercept, adalimumab) IV (infliximab) Dose/frequency variable Therapeutic effect reported after three doses	Allergic reaction; infection; demyelinating disease; possible risk for malignancy	CBC, liver enzymes, creatinine at baseline, then q3–6 mo Tuberculosis screen prior to start, then yearly	Assess for family history of multiple sclerosis; if positive, then MRI prior to start
	IL inhibitors: Anakinra (IL-1) Canakinumab (IL-1β) Tocilizumab (IL-6)	Systemic JIA Tocilizumab under study for other forms of JIA	Anakinra SC once/day Canakinumab SC q4 wk Tocilizumab IV q2 wk	Injection site or infusion reactions; infection	Tuberculosis screen prior to start, then yearly	Monitor for infection Avoid live vaccines
	T-cell costimulatory modulators: Abatacept	JIA except systemic subtype	IV 10 mg/kg/dose Give at 0, 2 wk, then q4 wk Therapeutic effect reported as early as second infusion	Infection	Tuberculosis screen prior to start, then yearly	Monitor for infection Avoid live vaccines Monitor for infection Avoid live vaccines Avoid pregnancy

BP, blood pressure; CBC, complete blood count; DMARD, disease-modifying antirheumatic drug; ERA, enthesitis-related arthritis; GI, gastrointestinal; IM, intramuscular; IV, intravenous; JIA, juvenile idiopathic arthritis; NSAID, nonsteroidal antiinflammatory drug; PO, oral; SC, subcutaneous, TNF, tissue necrosis factor; VZIG, varicella-zoster immune globulin.

2. Encourage a warm bath or shower to relieve morning stiffness. Use other thermal modalities such as soaking or warm, moist pads or ice packs to soothe inflamed joints. Some children respond to heat and some to cold.
3. Use assistive devices to make mobility and activities of daily living (ADL) easier. Examples include splints; orthotics; special adapters for pencils, doorknobs, or utensils; or Velcro or zipper pulls.

Preserving Joint Mobility

1. Encourage compliance with physical therapy regimen to strengthen muscles and mobilize joints. Assist with ROM exercises, as indicated.
2. Splint joints to maintain proper position (joint extension) and decrease pain and deformity.
3. Encourage prone position with a thin pillow or no pillow and firm mattress.
4. Encourage therapeutic play (swimming, throwing, and bike riding).
5. Encourage child to do own ADL to maintain joint mobility. Refer to occupational therapy for provision of adaptation devices to facilitate completion of daily activities (velcro closures, utensils, and self-care implements with enlarged handles).
6. Schedule rest periods to maximize energy; discourage complete immobilization or lengthy inactivity because they increase stiffness.

Promote Normal Growth and Development

1. Identify developmental tasks appropriate to age of child. Educate caregivers and work with child and family to set goals with necessary adaptations to promote successful achievement.
2. Encourage attendance at school, participation in activities, and socialization with peers as much as possible.
3. Encourage participation in defining treatment plan to engage adherence to help prevent complications.
4. Promote healthy diet; obtain diet history; make referral to dietician, as necessary.
5. Encourage activities to enhance transition activities between ages 12 and 21 years, such as identifying issues, making own appointments, and medication management, including possible administration of injections.

Normalizing Family Processes

1. Refer to community resources and support groups.
2. Encourage child and family to verbalize feelings.
3. Remind caregivers to devote time to other children, themselves, and each other, because the condition affects the whole family.

Family Education and Health Maintenance

1. Educate (consider cultural/language barriers and literacy) and motivate caregivers and child to continue program of treatment at home. This is a chronic disease with an unpredictable course; however, adherence with prescribed treatment is important to improve functional outcome and to allow the child to grow and develop to their full potential.
2. Encourage medication adherence by helping to create a medication calendar or suggesting weekly pill boxes or strategies to reduce side effects such as taking NSAIDs with food or taking methotrexate on the weekends before bed.
3. Encourage open communication with the child's school. The child should receive accommodations such as use of school elevator, two sets of textbooks to avoid having to carry heavy backpack to and from school, use of a computer for difficulties with writing, and allowance to move around during prolonged periods of sitting.
4. Educate the family about the importance of a daily exercise routine to maintain ROM, muscle strength, and function. Periodically reevaluate need for physical and occupational therapy.
5. Provide nutritional counseling to promote a balanced diet, with special attention given to the intake of calcium, vitamin D, folic acid, and iron. Portion control and healthy snacks should be encouraged to prevent obesity.
6. Stress the need for routine follow-up care and ophthalmologic evaluation.
7. Educate families about the special considerations required when their child is receiving immunosuppressive medications: seek prompt medical attention for fever and other signs of infection; child and family members should receive annual influenza vaccine; live vaccinations need to be postponed until child is no longer receiving immunosuppression.
8. Refer family to community agencies such as the Arthritis Foundation (www.arthritis.org).

Evaluation: Expected Outcomes

- Reports decreased pain.
- ROM, muscle strength, and joint function are preserved.
- Growth and development parameters, including psychological and social, are appropriate for age.
- Caregivers seek additional resources.

Systemic Lupus Erythematosus

Systemic lupus erythematosus (SLE) is a systemic multisystem, chronic autoimmune disease that has the potential to affect any organ or organ system. Disease onset in childhood occurs in 10% to 20% of all SLE cases. Although the disease manifestations and disease course of flares and remissions is similar across the life span, patients with pediatric systemic lupus erythematosus (pSLE) have a more severe disease, requiring more aggressive treatment with immunosuppression. The incidence is higher in people assigned female at birth than those assigned male at birth (4.5 to 5:1), with the highest rates in Hispanic, Afro-Caribbean, Aboriginal, and Asian populations.

Pathophysiology and Etiology

1. Cause is unknown. Involves a complex interaction between genetic predisposition and the environment. Etiologic factors include:
   a. Immune system dysregulation of both innate and adaptive immunity.
   b. Genetic susceptibility—associations with certain HLA types, complement deficiencies, and TNF polymorphisms.
   c. Environmental factors.
   d. Hormonal factors—presence of estrogen; low levels of androgens
2. Possible factors that trigger or unmask initial symptoms:
   a. Ultraviolet radiation (ultraviolet B-light)—photosensitivity
   b. Viral infection—herpes family viruses; cytomegalovirus
   c. Stress, extreme fatigue.
   d. Vaccination
   e. Chemical exposure—cigarette smoke, pesticides, heavy metals.
   f. Medications—drug-induced lupus is a lupus-like syndrome that presents after several months of specific

medication use. Complete resolution of symptoms happens weeks to months after discontinuation.

3. SLE is characterized by the production of autoantibodies and the deposition of immune complexes in tissues and organs throughout the body.
   a. Spontaneous hyperactivity of B lymphocytes leads to increased antibody production. Additionally, the life of the B lymphocytes is abnormally prolonged, enhancing antibody production.
   b. These antibodies combine with antigen to form immune complexes, which deposit in tissue.
   c. The immune complexes activate the complement cascade, leading to inflammation (recruitment of inflammatory cells and production of oxidants, proteases, prostaglandins, and cytokines).
   d. Long-term inflammation can lead to irreversible cell destruction and tissue and organ damage.
4. Antiphospholipid syndrome (APS) produces a variety of antibodies against phospholipids and may occur in pSLE. The primary event resulting from APS is thrombolytic in nature.
5. Neonatal lupus erythematosus (NLE) is a separate entity from SLE. It is a disease of the developing fetus and neonate as the result of transplacental passage of maternal autoantibodies (anti-SSA/Ro or anti-SSB/L).
   a. Infant may or may not develop clinical symptoms.
   b. The most common clinical manifestations of NLE are cardiac, dermatologic, hematologic, and hepatic.
   c. The most serious manifestation is congenital heart block (CHB), requiring pacemaker insertion as an infant or child.
   d. The skin, liver, and hematologic symptoms resolve by 1 year of age as the maternal antibodies clear, with few long-term effects.

Clinical Manifestations

The presentation of the manifestations of SLE in children is diverse, involving any organ system and may be gradual or acute.

1. Constitutional symptoms: fever, weight loss, fatigue, loss of appetite.
2. Mucocutaneous disease:
   a. Malar rash (butterfly rash), which is present over the bridge of nose and cheeks, sparing the nasolabial folds; rash may vary from a faint blush to scaly erythematous papules; most often photosensitive. Rash may spread from face and scalp to neck, chest, and extremities. Scarring is rare.
   b. Raynaud phenomenon; triphasic color change of fingers and toes in response to cold; may also be induced by emotions. Tips of nose, ears, and penis may also be affected.
   c. Mucosal ulceration or erythema of hard palate, tongue, or nose. Lesions are usually painless.
   d. Hair loss.
3. Musculoskeletal disease:
   a. Arthritis, most commonly of small joints of hands; rarely associated with erosive disease.
   b. Reduced bone density secondary to both active disease and treatment with steroids.
4. Cardiovascular disease:
   a. Early atherosclerosis—children with lupus have been shown to have unfavorable lipid profiles.
   b. Pericarditis, endocarditis, myocarditis.
5. Renal disease (lupus nephritis):
   a. Nephritis is leading cause of morbidity and mortality; prevalence of 20% to 80% of children with 18% to 50% progressing to end-stage kidney disease.
   b. 80% to 90% develop nephritis within the first year of diagnosis.
   c. Hematuria, proteinuria, and hypertension may be evident.
6. Neuropsychiatric disease:
   a. Central nervous system (CNS) involvement manifested by psychosis (visual and/or auditory hallucinations), depression, headache (severe, unremitting), cerebrovascular disease (stroke), cognitive impairment (worsening school performance), and seizures.
   b. More frequent in children.
7. Hematologic involvement:
   a. Coombs positive autoimmune hemolytic anemia caused by destruction of red cells in the spleen.
   b. Leukopenia involving lymphocytes and neutrophils.
   c. Thrombocytopenia—low platelets can commonly be the initial presentation; immune thrombocytopenic purpura (ITP) can precede lupus by 10 years.
   d. Low complement levels C3 and C4 are an important laboratory measurement of disease activity.
8. Pulmonary involvement with pleural effusion and lupus pneumonitis.

Diagnostic Evaluation

1. Diagnosis is made by both clinical manifestations and specific laboratory findings (see Box 49-2).
2. Laboratory studies:
   a. Autoantibodies, ANA—nonspecific but positive in 90% of people with SLE.
   b. Other antibodies such as anti-ds DNA, anti-Sm, anti-Ro/SSA, anti-La/SSB, anti-ribonucleoprotein (anti-RNP) are all common in SLE. Anti-dsDNA and anti-Sm are highly specific for lupus.
   c. ESR—elevated.
   d. Serum complements studies—decreased.
   e. Complete blood count (CBC)—leukopenia, hemolytic anemia, thrombocytopenia.
   f. Evaluation for APS—elevated prothrombin time, partial thromboplastin time; elevated anti-β2 glycoprotein I antibodies; elevated anticardiolipin antibodies; and elevated dilute Russell viper venom time. The presence of one or more suggests APS and an increased risk for thrombosis.
   g. Serum chemistry and urine studies to detect kidney and other body system involvement.
3. Renal biopsy—verifies lupus nephritis and classification.
4. Electrocardiogram and other cardiac testing.
5. Bone mineral density.

Management

1. There is no cure for SLE. Course is unpredictable, usually progressive, and may terminate in death, if untreated. Therapy is based on the extent and severity of disease. SLE may be classified as:
   a. Mild (fever, arthritis, rash).
   b. Moderate (clinically significant but non–life-threatening involvement of the kidneys or other major organs).
   c. Severe (substantial renal, pulmonary, hematologic, or neurologic disease).

BOX 49-2 Criteria for Diagnosis of Systemic Lupus Erythematosus

According to the American College of Rheumatology, the presence of four or more criteria must be documented to diagnose systemic lupus erythematosus (SLE).

- Malar (butterfly) rash.
- Discoid lupus rash.
- Photosensitivity.
- Oral or nasal mucocutaneous ulcerations.
- Nonerosive arthritis.
- Nephritis[a]:
  - Proteinuria greater than 0.5 g/day.
  - Cellular casts.
- Encephalopathy[a]:
  - Seizures.
  - Psychosis.
- Pleuritis or pericarditis.
- Hemolytic anemia, leukopenia, thrombocytopenia.
- Positive immunoserology[a]:
  - Antibodies to double-stranded DNA.
  - Antibodies to Sm nuclear antigen.
  - Positive finding of antiphospholipid antibodies based on immunoglobulin (Ig)G or IgM anticardiolipin antibodies, lupus anticoagulant, or confirmed false-positive serologic test for syphilis for at least 6 months.
- Positive antinuclear antibody (ANA).

[a]*Any one item satisfies this criterion.*

Source: Aringer, M., Costenbader, K., Daikh, D., Brinks, R., Mosca, M., Ramsey-Goldman, R., Smolen, J. S., Wofsy, D., Boumpas, D. T., Kamen, D. L., Jayne, D., Cervera, R., Costedoat-Chalumeau, N., Diamond, B., Gladman, D. D., Hahn, B., Hiepe, F., Jacobsen, S., Khanna, D., ... Johnson, S. R. (2019). 2019 European League Against Rheumatism/American College of Rheumatology classification criteria for systemic lupus erythematosus. Arthritis & Rheumatology, 71(9), 1400–1412. https://doi.org/10.1002/art.40930

2. Goal of treatment is to control disease activity and to prevent organ damage using the least toxic therapies.
3. Management of SLE should be provided by a multidisciplinary team in a family-centered approach.
4. Nonpharmacologic approaches include:
   a. Nutritional counseling and vitamin supplementation to control disease, promote growth, maintain bone mineralization, and prevent toxicity from medication. Reduced sodium and potassium diets, fluid restrictions for kidney disease. Vitamin D, calcium, iron, and folic acid may be supplemented.
   b. Mental health and social support for the child and family to manage the issues of chronic disease.
   c. Education about sun protection, including avoidance of midday sun, use of protective clothing, application of daily sunscreen 30 minutes prior to going outside.
   d. Vaccination against pneumococcal infection; annual influenza vaccine as well as routine inactivated vaccines.
   e. Regular adequate sleep and exercise.
5. Pharmacologic therapies:
   a. NSAIDs are used to relieve musculoskeletal symptoms, fever, fatigue, and pain. Avoid NSAID use in children with renal insufficiency.
   b. Methotrexate may be used for joint/skin symptoms or as a steroid-sparing agent.
   c. Antimalarials, such as hydroxychloroquine and chloroquine, are used to:
      Relieve joint symptoms and skin rash.
      Manage thrombocytopenia.
      Improve dyslipidemia.
      Maintain remission.
   d. Corticosteroids are required for almost all children with SLE and are administered either orally as prednisone or via intravenous (IV) line as methylprednisolone.
      Low-dose oral steroids are usually used to control arthritis, fever, dermatitis, or serositis.
      High-dose oral or IV steroids are used to treat moderate or severe SLE, especially in the presence of CNS involvement, pulmonary disease, hemolytic anemia, and nephritis.
   e. Immunosuppressive agents—such as azathioprine, cyclophosphamide, cyclosporine, mycophenolate mofetil, tacrolimus, belimumab, and rituximab—are used in severe disease, including nephritis and neuropsychiatric disease.
   f. Treatment of complications with antibiotics, antihypertensives, anticonvulsants, antipsychotics, anticoagulation.
6. Dialysis and renal transplantation as adjunctive therapy for severe lupus nephritis.

DRUG ALERT IV glucocorticoid "pulse" therapy has been known to cause hypertension or hypotension, tachycardia, blurring of vision, flushing, sweating, and metallic taste in the mouth. Close monitoring of temperature, pulse rate, respiratory rate, and blood pressure (BP) is indicated.

Complications

1. Infection—primarily resulting from steroid and immunosuppressive therapy.
2. Renal—hypertension, renal failure.
3. Cardiac—atherosclerosis, myocardial infarction, and valvular disease.
4. Growth disturbance; obesity and short stature secondary to inflammation and steroid therapy.
5. Musculoskeletal—osteopenia/osteoporosis, avascular necrosis, and compression fractures (resulting from steroid therapy).
6. Ocular—cataracts, glaucoma secondary to steroid therapy; retinal toxicity secondary to hydroxychloroquine therapy.
7. Macrophage activation syndrome—a life-threatening complication of SLE.

Nursing Assessment

1. History should include a thorough review of systems aimed at symptoms, complications, and medication side effects; current medications; immunizations; recent ophthalmology examination; auditory/visual hallucinations; and medication adherence.
2. Perform a complete physical examination, focusing on signs that might indicate major organ involvement, including vital signs, growth parameters, and neuromental health assessment.
3. Assess psychosocial status to evaluate child's and family's coping with chronic illness, school performance, and socialization.

Nursing Interventions

Minimizing Fatigue

1. Intersperse periods of rest between activities.
2. Caution to resume school activities slowly. Caregivers should negotiate with the school to implement accommodations to minimize fatigue (i.e., second set of textbooks, rest area, and

extra time to complete assignments). Consider half-days at school until fatigue is diminished. The child may also be a candidate for homeschooling.
3. Maintain good sleep hygiene.

Promoting Comfort

1. Administer or teach caregivers to administer analgesics, NSAIDs, steroids, and other medications, as prescribed. Review medication side effects with family. Provide written medication aids.
2. For child on steroids, monitor for glycosuria, and check blood test results for hyperglycemia, hypokalemia, and hyperlipidemia.
3. Encourage a warm bath or shower to relieve morning stiffness associated with arthritis.
4. Provide diversional activities appropriate for age.

Controlling Fever

1. Monitor temperature every 4 hours and document pattern.
2. Administer or teach caregivers to administer antipyretics, as prescribed; note results.
3. Encourage increased fluids by mouth when feverish. Dress in lightweight clothing.

Protecting From Injury Because of Neuropsychiatric Disease

1. Institute seizure precautions, if indicated.
2. Monitor during seizure and postictal state.
3. Minimize noxious stimuli for patients experiencing hallucinations.
4. Implement safety measures during altered mental state.

Protecting From Adverse Reactions

1. While administering IV glucocorticoid therapy, monitor pulse and BP every 15 minutes for 1 hour and then every 30 minutes for 1 hour.
2. Slow the rate or discontinue infusion if there are significant changes in BP or pulse.
3. Notify the health care provider and continue to monitor vital signs frequently until they return to normal.

Maintaining Urinary Elimination

1. Monitor laboratory tests for signs of renal abnormalities: blood for creatinine, urine for specific gravity, blood, and protein.
2. Monitor intake and output.
3. Monitor BP; watch for development of edema.

Promoting Appropriate Nutritional Intake

1. Allow child to help in selecting and preparing foods. Family members should set an example for healthy diet and consider complying with the same diet plan as has been recommended for the child.
2. Apply topical medication to oral ulcers or give analgesics before meals.
3. Monitor food intake and weight. Consider consultation with a dietician to assist with healthy food choices.
4. Low-sodium and low-potassium diet for those with nephritis and those on high-dose steroid therapy.
5. Encourage food high in calcium and vitamin D to decrease risk of low bone density.

Improving Self-image

1. Encourage contact with peers and family.
2. Allow child to vent feelings about bodily changes and chronic illness.
3. Allow child to be involved in planning care and making decisions.
4. Consider a referral for counseling for adolescents to help with the development of coping strategies, if required.

Family Education and Health Maintenance

1. Teach ways to prevent exacerbations and complications of the disease. Teaching points include:
   a. Get enough rest; try not to overexert.
   b. Minimize stress and anxiety.
   c. Encourage adherence to medication schedule through use of medication calendar, pill boxes; understand adverse medication effects and strategies to reduce them; check with health care provider prior to using over-the-counter drugs or therapies found on the internet.
   d. Avoid contact with people with infectious diseases; get pneumococcal, COVID-19, and flu vaccines; and keep routine immunizations up to date.
   e. Provide nutritional counseling to promote a balanced diet, with special attention given to portion control and the intake of calcium, vitamin D, and, when indicated, iron, potassium, folic acid, and sodium content.
   f. Seek medical attention at times of illness or stress.
   g. Minimize sun exposure through protection with sunscreen, hats, and long clothing.
   h. Recognize warning signs of exacerbation such as fatigue, weight loss, joint pain, hair loss, new rashes, mouth sores, headaches, trouble with concentration, seizures, shortness of breath, chest pain, abdominal pain, fever, and urinary changes.
2. Educate caregivers about normal growth and development, emphasizing issues such as adolescent body image, peer relationships, and the impact of chronic illness on the child and the family.
3. Teach the importance of continual medical follow-up.
   a. Disease management requires frequent reevaluation; medications and laboratory parameters require frequent monitoring to prevent complications and identify disease flares.
   b. Transition to adult care should begin in early adolescence. Teenagers should know their medications; understand their disease; learn to advocate for themselves with their doctor.
4. Advise family that all children with SLE need annual ophthalmologic exams. Those taking hydroxychloroquine require more frequent ophthalmologic evaluation to identify retinal changes early.
5. Refer to agencies such as the Lupus Foundation of America (www.lupus.org).

Evaluation: Expected Outcomes

- Participates in activities with peers without fatigue; attends school full time.
- Reports reduced level of pain.
- Remains afebrile, knows what to do if febrile.
- Seizure precautions maintained.
- No changes in vital signs during glucocorticoid infusion.
- Urine output adequate.
- Appropriate dietary intake, weight stable.
- Compliant with medication regime.
- Prepared for transition to adult care.

Henoch–Schönlein Purpura

Henoch–Schönlein purpura (HSP) is an immune-mediated vasculitis with IgA deposition and subsequent inflammatory reaction around capillaries and arterioles. It is considered a small-vessel vasculitis. HSP can affect the skin, intestines, joints, kidneys, and nervous system. Incidence is higher in people assigned male at birth than in those assigned female at birth (2:1). Onset is generally between ages 3 and 15; it is seen most commonly in winter and can occur in clusters. Higher rate has been noted in those children diagnosed with familial Mediterranean fever.

Pathophysiology and Etiology

1. Cause is unknown; however, theories include an immunologic reaction to a variety of antigenic stimuli, in a genetically prone individual, such as infection (viral, bacterial, or fungal), dietary allergens, insect bites, and drugs.
2. Acute vasculitis develops.
   a. Swelling and edema of capillaries, small venules, and arterioles.
   b. Fibrin is deposited in the glomeruli of the kidney.
3. Vasculitis results in skin manifestations (nonthrombocytopenic palpable purpura), arthritis, gastrointestinal (GI) (abdominal pain, GI bleeding), and renal symptoms.

Clinical Manifestations

1. Rash—sudden onset may precede or follow other manifestations.
   a. Palpable purpura is an essential criterion for diagnosis. Purpura is often preceded by palpable maculopapular erythematous or urticarial rash. Ulcers may also develop.
   b. These lesions range from small petechiae to large ecchymotic areas and progress in color from red to purple to brown until they fade. They do not blanch.
   c. Several stages of the rash may be present at one time.
   d. Rash appears primarily on dependent or pressure-bearing surfaces, including the buttocks, lower back, and extensor aspects of the arms, legs, and face.
   e. Dependent subcutaneous edema over dorsum of hands, feet, scrotum, and periorbital area is common.
2. Arthritis occurs in 50% to 80% of patients, primarily affecting the knee and ankle joints; the wrists, elbows, and finger joints may also be affected, although this is rare.
   a. The arthritis is moderately severe, with painful swelling because of periarticular edema and limitation of motion.
   b. The arthritis is self-limiting, resolving within a few days to a week without permanent sequelae.
3. Orchitis in 2% to 35% of children assigned male at birth.
4. Colicky abdominal pain—from submucosal and subserosal hemorrhage and edema in two thirds of children. May be accompanied by intussusception and GI bleeding.
5. Nausea, vomiting, malaise, low-grade fever.
6. Renal disease—proteinuria and hematuria may develop within 1 month of onset of rash.
7. Rarely, CNS involvement, such as headache, seizure, or cerebral hemorrhage.
8. Symptoms may appear acutely or gradually and vary in intensity and duration.

Diagnostic Evaluation

1. Blood studies (not diagnostic, but support clinical evidence):
   a. IgA may be elevated (more than 50% of cases).
   b. Coagulation studies and platelet count are typically normal in presence of purpura.
   c. ESR and white blood cell (WBC) count may be elevated.
   d. Anemia is possible.
   e. Elevated blood urea nitrogen (BUN) and creatinine with severe kidney involvement.
2. Urine studies show proteinuria, microscopic hematuria, and casts.
3. Stools may show occult or gross blood.
4. Abdominal ultrasound or x-rays may help confirm bowel involvement.

Management

Treatment is primarily symptomatic and supportive. In two thirds of children, HSP resolves within 4 weeks of onset; hydration, rest, and adequate pain relief are the goals of treatment.

1. Bed rest until the child is able to ambulate and can do so without increasing edema of the lower extremities, genital area, and buttocks.
2. Antibiotic therapy if acute episode was preceded by infection, especially streptococcal.
3. Management of complicating abdominal or renal involvement and arthritis.
   a. Steroid use is controversial. Suggested for use if symptoms prevent adequate oral intake or if the child has challenges with ambulation or performing ADL.
   b. Immunosuppressive therapy, such as azathioprine or cyclophosphamide, may be given to stabilize persistent renal involvement (rare).
   c. High-dose immunoglobulin has been recommended for severe cases.
4. Provide comfort measures and analgesics, such as acetaminophen.

Complications

1. Acute nephritis or nephrosis that may lead to chronic nephritis. Ninety percent of children who develop serious renal involvement will do so within 2 months of diagnosis. Less than 5% of cases progress to renal failure.
2. Intussusception (approximately 5% incidence).
3. Significant GI bleeding may require a transfusion (rare).
4. Neurologic vasculitis with headaches, seizures, and neuropathies.

CLINICAL JUDGMENT Be alert for signs of intussusception—sudden onset of paroxysmal, colicky abdominal pain, blood in stools, vomiting, and increasing abdominal distention and tenderness—report immediately.

Nursing Assessment

1. Obtain a complete history. There is some suggestion of allergy to insect bites or medications as a basis for development of the disease. Also controversial is association with streptococci, viruses including COVID-19, and vaccination.
2. Perform physical assessment of renal, integumentary, musculoskeletal, and GI systems and pain scores.
3. Determine impact of illness on the psychosocial well-being of the child and family.

Nursing Interventions

Reducing Discomfort

1. Monitor pain level and location. Use appropriate developmental pain scales to determine level of pain.
2. Administer or teach caregivers to administer pain medications, as prescribed, and monitor child's response.
3. Apply warm or cool compresses to joints or abdomen for 30-minute periods to help soothe painful areas.
4. Provide diversional activities in accordance with the child's age.

Increasing Participation in Activities

1. Monitor completion of daily and diversional activities; offer choice.
2. Alternate activities with rest periods.

Maintaining Skin Integrity

1. Assess skin condition and turgor.
2. Maintain adequate fluids.
3. Provide loose, comfortable clothing.
4. Administer or teach caregivers to administer antipruritics, if necessary.
5. Avoid soap, scratching, or dry skin that may exacerbate rash.

Maintaining Urinary Output

1. Record intake and output, vital signs, weight, urine-specific gravity, and level of edema.
2. Check urine for protein, hematuria, and color; monitor creatinine.
3. Report or teach caregivers to report changes promptly.

Alleviating Fear

1. Allow child and family to verbalize feelings about hospitalization and illness.
2. Monitor anxiety level of child and family. Ensure information is given at the child's level of understanding.
3. Offer realistic encouragement. The long-term outlook is good when renal involvement is minimal.
4. Encourage the family and peers to visit the hospitalized child and bring in familiar items from home.
5. Allow child to make age-appropriate decisions and become involved in planning care.

Family Education and Health Maintenance

1. Reassure the caregivers that symptoms are usually self-limiting.
2. Make sure that caregivers and child understand the disease and the need to report changes in urine or signs of intussusception.
3. Educate the caregivers about the importance of continued care. Long-term follow-up of urinalysis will be necessary to evaluate renal function.

Evaluation: Expected Outcomes

- Reports relief from pain.
- Participates in activity for longer period each day.
- Rash resolved, skin intact.
- Urine output adequate, negative protein.
- Child verbalizes feelings about illness.

Kawasaki Disease

Kawasaki disease (KD) is a common vasculitis of childhood affecting medium and small blood vessels. Coronary arteries are the most common site of damage, giving KD the potential to cause severe morbidity and even death without early diagnosis and treatment. It is characterized by multisystem inflammation, including fever, conjunctivitis, lymphadenopathy, and changes in blood vessels. It is the leading cause of acquired heart disease in children in the United States.

Pathophysiology and Etiology

EVIDENCE BASE Kobayashi, T., Ayusawa, M., Suzuki, H., Abe, J., Ito, S., Kato, T., Kamada, M., Shiono, J., Suda, K., Tsuchiya, K., Nakamura, T., Nakamura, Y., Nomura, Y., Hamada, H., Fukazawa, R., Furuno, K., Matsuura, H., Matsubara, T., Miura, M., & Takahashi, K. (2020). Revision of diagnostic guidelines for Kawasaki disease (6th revised edition). *Pediatrics International, 62*(10), 1135–1138. https://doi.org/10.1111/ped.14326

1. KD is a disease of early childhood, with 85% of affected children under 5 years of age. It occurs in children of all origins, although those of Asian descent have the highest incidence.
2. Etiology is unknown, although most investigators believe the disease is related to an infectious or environmental trigger in a genetically susceptible host. The result is a prolonged immune response targeted at vessel walls of medium and small arteries.
3. Infection as a trigger is supported by the fact that KD is endemic with seasonal fluctuations (winter and early spring). It is further hypothesized that super antigens, proteins present in certain organisms (*Staphylococci*, *Streptococci*, *Mycobacterium*, *Mycoplasma*, Epstein–Barr virus), are responsible for the prolonged inflammation through stimulation of large numbers of T cells.
4. Genetic predisposition to KD is evident in the observations that siblings have a 10-fold higher risk of developing the disease and the children of caregivers who had KD have a twofold increase in risk compared with the general population.
5. Researchers have not found associations between exposure to drugs, environmental toxins, pesticides, chemicals, or heavy metals and KD.
6. KD is a generalized systemic vasculitis involving blood vessels throughout the body. It is thought that marked elevation in the cytokine TNF activates matrix metalloproteinase enzymes capable of breaking down elastin in arterial vessel walls. This breakdown leads to loss of integrity and ballooning and aneurysm formation.
7. Aneurysms, the result of prolonged inflammation, usually develop in the 2nd to 8th week of the illness. The most common site for development is the coronary artery, although other sites may be involved. Early treatment following the recommended protocol of intravenous gamma globulin (IVIG) and aspirin has reduced aneurysm development by 85%.
8. During the COVID-19 pandemic, a new entity similar to KD was described. Multisystem inflammatory syndrome in children (MIS-C) seems to be associated with exposure to the SARS-COV-2 virus. Most illnesses occur 2 to 6 weeks after exposure and resemble signs and symptoms of toxic shock and KD. These children can be seriously ill, requiring intensive care to recover.

EVIDENCE BASE Bultas, M., & Fuller, K. (2021). Multisystem inflammatory syndrome in children and COVID-19 infections. *School Nurse, 36*(6), 341–345.

Waseem, M., Shariff, M., Lim, A., Nunez, J., Narayanan, N., Patel, K., & Tay, E. (2022). Multisystem inflammatory syndrome in children. *Western Journal of Emergency Care, 23*(4), 505–513.

Clinical Manifestations

KD is divided into three phases, each with distinct clinical features. See Figure 49-1.

Acute Phase (First 10 to 14 Days of Illness)

1. During the acute phase, the children exhibit classic signs of inflammation (redness, swelling, and heat) presented as multisystem changes. They appear ill and irritable.

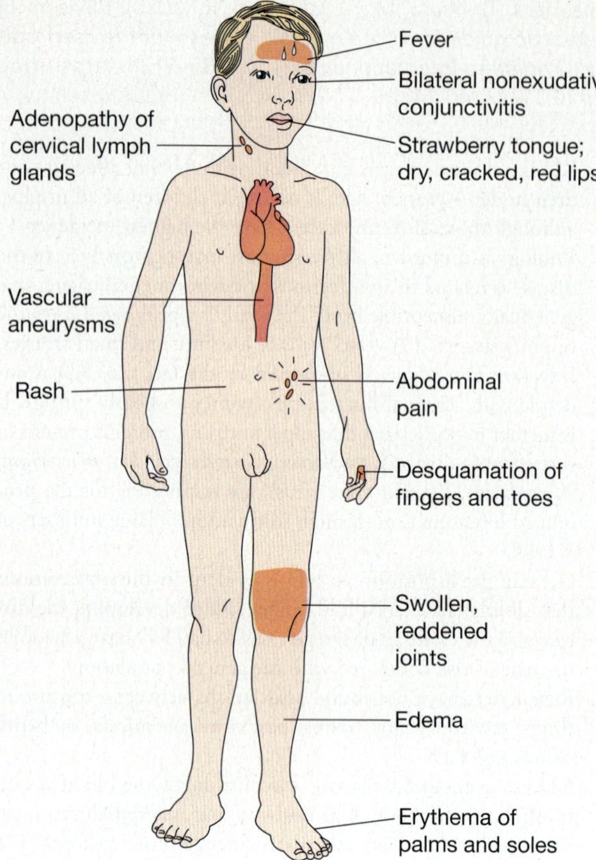

Figure 49-1. Clinical manifestations of acute Kawasaki disease.

2. The diagnostic criteria of KD occur during the acute phase. See Box 49-3. Fever, in addition to four out of five of the other features, is required for diagnosis; not all features occur at a single point in time.
3. Other associated findings:
   a. Cardiovascular—early tachycardia, myocarditis, pericarditis, S3 gallop; reduced contractibility may progress to signs of heart failure.
   b. Aseptic meningitis; anterior uveitis—children extremely irritable; photophobic.
   c. Arthritis—painful; usually large joints; short duration with rapid response to standard treatment for KD.
   d. GI—diarrhea, vomiting, abdominal pain, hepatomegaly, hydrops of the gallbladder.

EVIDENCE BASE McCrindle, B. W., Manlhiot, C., Newburger, J. W., Harahsheh, A. S., Giglia, T. M., Dallaire, F., Friedman, K., Low, T., Runeckles, K., Mathew, M., Mackie, A., Choueiter, N., Pei-Ni, J., Kutty, S., Yetman, A., Raghuveer, G., Pahl, E., Norozi, K., McHugh, K., & Li, J. (2020). Medium-term complications associated with coronary artery aneurysms after Kawasaki disease: A study From the International Kawasaki Disease Registry. *Journal of the American Heart Association, 9*(15), e016440.

Porta, K., & Zammit, C. (2022). Multisystem inflammatory syndrome in children. *JAAPA: Journal of the American Academy of Physician Assistants, 35*(10), 33–37.

BOX 49-3 American Heart Association Diagnostic Features for Kawasaki Disease

Persistent fever for at least 5 days. Fever is high (generally greater than 102.2°F [39°C]). Four out of the following five features:

- Bilateral conjunctival injection.
- Changes of the lips and oral cavity.
- Cervical lymphadenopathy.
- Polymorphous exanthema.
- Changes in the peripheral extremities (swelling of the hands or feet) or perineal area.

Cervical lymphadenopathy; at least one node greater than 1.5 cm; usually unilateral.

Reprinted with permission from McCrindle, B. W., Manlhiot, C., Newburger, J. W., Harahsheh, A. S., Giglia, T. M., Dallaire, F., Friedman, K., Low, T., Runeckles, K., Mathew, M., Mackie, A., Choueiter, N., Pei-Ni, J., Kutty, S., Yetman, A., Raghuveer, G., Pahl, E., Norozi, K., McHugh, K., & Li, J. (2020). Medium-term complications associated with coronary artery aneurysms after Kawasaki disease: A study from the International Kawasaki Disease Registry. Journal of the American Heart Association, 9(15), e016440.

Subacute Phase (11 to 25 Days After Onset of Illness)

1. The classic inflammatory features of the acute phase resolve, and the temperature returns to normal. If treated, many children are asymptomatic. If untreated or unresponsive to treatment, then fever, oral changes, and conjunctivitis may be present until 3rd or 4th week. Arthritis may be present.
2. Desquamation of toes and fingers in classic distribution starting in periungual region.
3. Coronary artery aneurysm is detected.
4. Thrombocytosis peaks at about 14 days.

Convalescent Phase

1. The acute-phase reactants (ESR and platelets) return to normal.
2. The child appears well.
3. Transverse grooves present on fingernails and toenails (Beau lines).
4. Vessels undergo healing, remodeling, fibrosis, and scarring. Preexisting small aneurysms may resolve, and large aneurysms may develop thrombosis, leading to complications, including myocardial infarction, dysrhythmias, or death.

Diagnostic Evaluation

1. There are no specific diagnostic tests for KD. The diagnosis is based on the clinical manifestations occurring in phases. There is a subset of children, usually the very young or old, who do not meet the diagnostic criteria for KD, yet present with prolonged fever and two or three of the features. They are a challenge to diagnose and are the group with the highest risk of developing coronary aneurysms.
2. Although there are no specific laboratory tests, the following may help support diagnosis or rule out other diseases:
   a. CBC—leukocytosis; mild normochromic, normocytic anemia.
   b. Platelet count (from 500,000 to 1 million/mm^3)—increased during 2nd to 4th week of illness.
   c. ESR (usually greater than 40 mm/hour).
   d. C-reactive protein (usually greater than 3.0 mg/dL).
   e. Albumin—low levels associated with more severe and prolonged disease.
   f. Liver enzymes (aspartate transaminase [AST], alanine aminotransferase [ALT])—moderately elevated.

g. Serum lipids—reduced high-density lipoprotein levels; elevated triglyceride and low-density lipoprotein levels during the subacute phase.
3. Lumbar puncture, often performed because of the degree of child's irritability, demonstrates aseptic meningitis; cerebral spinal fluid analysis shows elevated white blood cell count; normal protein; normal glucose.
4. Echocardiogram and electrocardiogram (ECG)—should be performed as soon as the diagnosis is suspected and at 2 weeks and at 6 to 8 weeks after diagnosis. More frequent assessment may be required for complicated cases.
5. Cardiac catheterization and angiocardiography may be required for more complex cardiac abnormalities.

Management

EVIDENCE BASE Gorelik, M., Chung, S. A., Ardalan, K., Binstadt, B. A., Friedman, K., Hayward, K., Imundo, L., Lapidus, S., Kim, S., Son, M. B., Sule, S., Tremoulet, A., Van Mater, H., Yildirim-Toruner, C., Langford, C., Maz, M., Abril, A., Guyatt, G., Archer, A., & Conn, D. (2022). 2021 American College of Rheumatology/Vasculitis Foundation guideline for the management of Kawasaki disease. *Arthritis Care & Research*, *74*(4), 538–548.

1. The goal of treatment is to prevent the long-term sequelae associated with KD by controlling inflammation.
2. The American Heart Association recommends that children with KD should be treated with IVIG and aspirin within 10 days of illness to reduce aneurysm formation. Treatment before day 5 has not shown any effect on coronary outcome and may increase the requirement for a second treatment.
   a. IVIG should be given as a single infusion at a dose of 2 g/kg. Most infusion protocols run very slow, with stepwise increases in rate for a total infusion time of 8 to 12 hours.
   b. Ten to 20% of children will have persistent fever or recurrence of fever within the first 36 hours after treatment with IVIG. Experts agree that these children should be retreated with a single infusion of 2 g/kg.
   c. Aspirin therapy—the antiinflammatory dose of 80 to 100 mg/kg/day divided into four doses is recommended during the acute phase. The length of treatment varies from 24 to 72 hours after fever resolves to 2 weeks. The aspirin is then reduced to antiplatelet dosing of 3 to 5 mg/kg/day, which is continued until laboratory measures of inflammation have returned to normal and the echocardiogram at 6 to 8 weeks shows no sign of coronary aneurysm. Children with aneurysms will continue aspirin for life.
3. In more complicated aneurysms, other anticoagulant and thrombolytic medications may be required.
4. Supportive measures:
   a. Maintain fluid and electrolyte balance.
   b. Give nutritional support.
   c. Provide comfort.
5. Follow-up by pediatric cardiologist with serial echocardiograms/ECGs is necessary to monitor aneurysms and potential arrythmias.

DRUG ALERT Inflammation of the child's heart may compromise the heart's ability to handle the fluid challenge associated with IVIG. The infusion may need to be of longer duration.

DRUG ALERT Risk of Reye syndrome exists for children on aspirin therapy, most often after they develop a viral illness. Families should seek medical attention if the child has altered level of consciousness associated with profuse vomiting.

Complications

1. Coronary aneurysm.
2. Aspirin toxicity.
3. Mortality is less than 0.3%.

Nursing Assessment

1. A thorough history to document data that support the diagnosis of KD; features of KD do not always present simultaneously, nor do all patients have all features.
2. Perform physical examination focusing on clinical features, hydration, and cardiovascular status. Document vital signs, including accurate temperature, BP, heart rate, rhythm, heart sounds, respiratory rate.
3. Perform pain assessment using age-appropriate pain scale.

Nursing Interventions

Reducing Discomfort

1. Offer pain medication on a scheduled basis rather than as needed during acute phase. Monitor pain level and child's response to analgesics.
2. Conjunctivitis and associated uveitis can cause photosensitivity; darken the room; offer sunglasses; apply cool compresses.
3. Use age-appropriate diversional techniques.

Maintaining Cardiac Output

1. Implement continual cardiac monitoring during acute-phase hospitalization.
2. Assess the child for signs of myocarditis and heart failure (tachycardia, gallop rhythm, chest pain, dyspnea, nasal flaring, grunting, retractions, cyanosis, orthopnea, crackles, moist respirations, distended neck veins, edema).
3. Closely monitor intake and output. Calculate fluid balance. Administer oral and IV fluids, as ordered.
4. If administering IVIG, give premedication, as directed, and monitor closely for adverse effects.

DRUG ALERT Infusion of IVIG has been known to cause a precipitous drop in BP, mimicking anaphylaxis. Monitor BP and heart rate at the start of infusion, after 15 and 30 minutes, and then hourly until infusion is complete. Slow the infusion and have patient evaluated for any drop in BP. Give premedication as prescribed to help prevent adverse effects. Make sure medications to treat anaphylaxis are readily available.

Preserving Oral Mucous Membranes

1. Offer and encourage frequent cool liquids (ice chips and ice pops). Avoid acidic, sugary, or carbonated beverages; progress to soft, bland foods.
2. Give mouth care every 1 to 4 hours; use soft toothbrush.
3. Apply balm to dry, cracked lips.

4. Observe the mouth frequently for signs of infection.
5. Monitor food and fluid intake for nutrition appropriate for age.

Improving Skin Integrity

1. Avoid the use of soap to prevent drying; apply emollients to skin, as ordered.
2. Elevate edematous extremities.
3. Use sheepskin, convoluted foam mattress, and smooth sheets.
4. Encourage soft flannel or terry cloth loose-fitting clothing; change damp garments and linens frequently when febrile.
5. Protect peeling skin; observe for signs of infection.

Maintaining Fluid Balance

1. Offer fluids at least every hour when child is awake; monitor and document fluid intake and output.
2. Monitor hydration status by checking skin turgor, daily weight, urine output, presence of tears and moist mucous membranes, and urine-specific gravity.
3. Pay attention to insensible loss during febrile stage. Monitor temperature every 4 to 8 hours and administer antipyretics, as directed. Maintain temperature graph chart.

Reducing Fear

1. Use play therapy (passive and active) to help the child express feelings. Consult a Child Life therapist, as needed.
2. Explain all procedures and treatment plans to the child and family. Encourage the caregivers and child to verbalize their concerns, fears, and questions.
3. Provide respite for caregivers during irritable stage of illness when child may be inconsolable. Provide emotional support, as necessary.
4. Keep family informed of progress, and reinforce information about stages and prognosis.

Family Education and Health Maintenance

1. Advise caregivers to take child's temperature daily for 2 weeks post discharge. Call health practitioner for temperatures over 101°F (38.3°C).
2. Ensure family is aware of plan for follow-up. Emphasize the need for long-term care. Complications can occur during the convalescent period, months after the acute illness.
3. Advise caregivers that IVIG is pooled immunoglobulin. Immunizations, although not harmful, may not mount a protective response after IVIG administration. Live vaccinations are not recommended for 8 to 11 months post treatment. Catch-up vaccinations may be needed.
4. Advocate for compliance with the prescribed level of physical activity. Activity will be restricted if child is receiving anticoagulant therapy or if child has cardiac complications identified on stress testing.
5. Encourage family members to learn cardiopulmonary resuscitation.
6. Teach caregivers to report the possible development of salicylate toxicity—tinnitus, nausea and vomiting, GI distress, blood in stool, and increased respirations.
7. For children without physical activity limitations, educate caregivers that children may be fatigued for several weeks. They may require naps, shorter school days, and special accommodations at school.
8. Provide anticipatory guidance about child's behavior.
   a. Do not overprotect the child.
   b. Discuss regression that often occurs during stresses such as hospitalization and illness.
9. Refer to community organizations such as the American Heart Association (www.heart.org).

Evaluation: Expected Outcomes

- Reports improved comfort level.
- Vital signs stable, no signs of reduced cardiac output.
- Eating and drinking without difficulty, reports no oral discomfort.
- No pain or signs of infection with desquamation.
- Child expresses feelings about illness; caregivers report confidence in ability to manage care.

Adherence to treatment for patients with primary immunologic diseases is challenging owing to the many complex medication regimens and costs that may not be covered by insurance. Nurses should explore patient and caregiver understanding, with recommendations for calendars and computer applications that may prove helpful. If specialized skills are required for administration, initial training and verification on subsequent visits should be required, if necessary. Caregivers and patients should have an understanding of when they should contact their primary care provider or their medical specialist for questions.

SELECTED READINGS

AlGhoozi, D. A., & AlKhayyat, H. M. (2021). A child with Henoch-Schonlein purpura secondary to a COVID-19 infection. *BMJ Case Reports CP, 14*(1), e239910.

Aljaberi, N., Nguyen, K., Strahle, C., Merritt, A., Mathur, A., & Brunner, H. (2021). Performance of the new 2019 European League Against Rheumatism/American College of Rheumatology Classification criteria for systemic lupus erythematosus in children and young adults. *Arthritis Care & Research, 73*(4), 580–585.

Bass, A. R., Chakravarty, E., Akl, E. A., Bingham, C. O., Calabrese, L., Cappelli, L. C., Johnson, S. R., Imundo, L. F., Winthrop, K. L., Arasaratnam, R. J., Baden, L. R., Berard, R., Bridges, S. L., Cheah, J. T. L., Curtis, J. R., Ferguson, P. J., Hakkarinen, I., Onel, K. B., Schultz, G., … Reston, J. (2023). 2022 American College of Rheumatology guideline for vaccinations in patients with rheumatic and musculoskeletal diseases. *Arthritis and Rheumatology, 75*(3), 333–348. https://doi.org/10.1002/art.42386

Carlsson, E., Beresford, M. W., Ramanan, A. V., Dick, A. D., & Hedrich, C. M. (2021). Juvenile idiopathic arthritis associated uveitis. *Children, 8*(8), 646. https://doi.org/10.3390/children8080646

Chang, J. C., Davis, A. M., Klein-Gitelman, M. S., Cidav, Z., Mandell, D. S., & Knight, A. M. (2021). Impact of psychiatric diagnosis and treatment on medication adherence in youth with systemic lupus erythematosus. *Arthritis Care & Research, 73*(1), 30–38.

Cimaz, R., Maioli, G., & Calabrese, G. (2020). Current and emerging biologics for the treatment of juvenile idiopathic arthritis. *Expert Opinion on Biological Therapy, 20*(7), 725–740. https://doi.org/10.1080/14712598.2020.1733524

Costa, A. A., Robba, H. C., Silva, C. A., & Ferreira, J. C. O. (2022). Care provided by nurses to patients with juvenile systemic lupus erythematosus. *Lupus, 31*(3), 367–372.

Foeldvari, I., Maccora, I., Petrushkin, H., Rahman, N., Anton, J., de Boer, J., Calzada-Hernández, J., Carreras, E., Diaz, J., Edelsten, C., Angeles-Han, S. T., Heiligenhaus, A., Miserocchi, E., Nielsen, S., Saurenmann, R. K., Stuebiger, N., Baquet-Walscheid, K., Furst, D., & Simonini, G. (2023), New and updated recommendations for the treatment of juvenile idiopathic arthritis-associated uveitis and idiopathic chronic anterior uveitis. *Arthritis Care & Research, 75*, 975–982. https://doi.org/10.1002/acr.24963

Gamal, S., Fouad, N., Yosry, N., Badr, W., & Sobhy, N. (2021). Disease characteristics in patients with juvenile-and adult-onset systemic lupus erythematosus: A multi-center comparative study. *Archives of Rheumatology, 37*(2), 280–287.

Garg, S., Unnithan, R., Hansen, K. E., Costedoat-Chalumeau, N., & Bartels, C. M. (2021). Clinical significance of monitoring hydroxychloroquine levels in patients with systemic lupus erythematosus: A systematic review and meta-analysis. *Arthritis Care & Research, 73*(5), 707–716.

Gkoutzourelas, A., Bogdanos, D. P., & Sakkas, L. I. (2020). Kawasaki disease and COVID-19. *Mediterranean Journal of Rheumatology, 31*(Suppl 2), 268–274. https://doi.org/10.31138/mjr.31.3.268

Go, E., Van Veenendaal, M., Manlhiot, C., Schneider, R., McCrindle, B. W., & Yeung, R. S. (2021). Kawasaki disease and systemic juvenile idiopathic arthritis—Two ends of the same spectrum. *Frontiers in Pediatrics, 9*, 665815.

Guzman, M., & Hui-Yuen, J. S. (2020). Management of pediatric systemic lupus erythematosus: Focus on belimumab. *Drug Design, Development and Therapy, 14*, 2503–2513.

Hovde, A. M., McFarland, C. A., Garcia, G. M., Gallagher, F., Gewanter, H., Klein-Gitelman, M., & Moorthy, L. N. (2021). Multi-pronged approach to enhance education of children and adolescents with lupus, caregivers, and healthcare providers in New Jersey: Needs assessment, evaluation, and development of educational materials. *Lupus, 30*(1), 86–95.

Jacobi, M., Lancrei, H. M., Brosh-Nissimov, T., & Yeshayahu, Y. (2021). Purpurona: A novel report of COVID-19-related Henoch-Schonlein purpura in a child. *The Pediatric Infectious Disease Journal, 40*(2), e93–e94.

Kallas, R., Li, J., Goldman, D. W., Magder, L. S., & Petri, M. (2022). Trajectory of Damage Accrual in systemic lupus erythematosus based on ethnicity and socioeconomic factors. *The Journal of Rheumatology, 49*(11), 1229–1235.

Lee, J. J., Feldman, B. M., McCrindle, B. W., Li, P., Yeung, R. S., & Widdifield, J. (2023). Evaluating the time-varying risk of hypertension, cardiac events, and mortality following Kawasaki disease diagnosis. *Pediatric Research, 93*(5), 1439–1446. https://doi.org/10.1038/s41390-022-02273-8

Leung, A. K., Barankin, B., & Leong, K. F. (2020). Henoch-Schönlein purpura in children: An updated review. *Current Pediatric Reviews, 16*(4), 265–276.

Mehta, P., Gasparyan, A. Y., Zimba, O., & Kitas, G. D. (2022). Systemic lupus erythematosus in the light of the COVID-19 pandemic: Infection, vaccination, and impact on disease management. *Clinical Rheumatology, 41*(9), 2893–2910.

Reiser, C., Zeltner, N. A., Rettenbacher, B., Baumgaertner, P., Huemer, M., & Huemer, C. (2021). Explaining juvenile idiopathic arthritis to paediatric patients using illustrations and easy-to-read texts: Improvement of disease knowledge and adherence to treatment. *Pediatric Rheumatology, 19*, 158. https://doi.org/10.1186/s12969-021-00644-9

Rife, E., & Gedalia, A. (2020). Kawasaki disease: An update. *Current Rheumatology Reports, 22*, 75. https://doi.org/10.1007/s11926-020-00941-4

Rochette, E., Saidi, O., Merlin, É., & Duché, P. (2023). Physical activity as a promising alternative for young people with juvenile idiopathic arthritis: Towards an evidence-based prescription. *Frontiers in Immunology, 14*, 1119930. https://doi.org/10.3389/fimmu.2023.1119930

Sharma, C., Ganigara, M., Galeotti, C., Burns, J., Berganza, F. M., Hayes, D. A., Singh-Grewal, D., Bharath, S., Sajjan, S., & Bayry, J. (2021). Multisystem inflammatory syndrome in children and Kawasaki disease: A critical comparison. *Nature Reviews Rheumatology, 17*, 731–748. https://doi.org/10.1038/s41584-021-00709-9

Tsoukas, P., & Yeung, R. S. M. (2022). Kawasaki disease and MIS-C share a host immune response. *Nature Reviews Rheumatology, 18*, 555–556. https://doi.org/10.1038/s41584-022-00820-5

Vandevelde, A., & Devreese, K. M. J. (2022). Laboratory diagnosis of antiphospholipid syndrome: Insights and hindrances. *Journal of Clinical Medicine, 11*(8), 2164. https://doi.org/10.3390/jcm11082164. PMID: 35456258. PMCID: PMC9025581.

50 Pediatric Orthopedic Disorders*

ORTHOPEDIC PROCEDURES

See additional online content: Procedure Guidelines 50-1 and 50-2.

Immobilization: Casts, Braces, Splints, and External and Internal Fixators

EVIDENCE BASE Alsaraireh, M., & Elshah, N. F. (2020). Factors that influence the quality of pain management in patients with skin traction. *International Journal of Orthopaedic and Trauma Nursing, 36*, 100713. https://doi.org/10.1016/j.ijotn.2019.100713

Kearney, L., Thompson, J., Zychowicz, M., Shaw, R., & Keyes, S. (2022). The role of patient and parent education in pediatric cast complications. *Orthopedic Nursing, 41*(5), 318–323. https://doi.org/10.1097/NOR.0000000000000878

Casting, bracing, and splinting are all means of immobilizing an injured or diseased body part, primarily bones and musculature. Internal and external fixators have been utilized to provide stability and immobilization of bones, which are fractured or in the process of reconstruction. The length of time for the use of these various devices can vary from a few days to several months. Also see pages 1151, but realize that the management of children who are immobilized requires age-appropriate adaptation and support.

Types of Fixators

1. Fractures that require open reduction, such as those that do not align, include more than one broken area of the bone or involve attaching long bones in reconstructive surgery that can be managed with open reduction internal fixation (ORIF).
2. External fixators involve pins and screws placed through the skin and into the bone to stabilize a fracture. External fixation can include types of traction. They are also used when osteotomies are required or for limb-lengthening procedures.

Complications of Immobilization

1. Peripheral neurovascular compromise.
2. Alteration in skin integrity because of pressure or friction.
3. Loss of efficient use of the affected extremity because of nonadherence.

Traction

Traction is the application of a pulling force to an injured or diseased part of the body or an extremity, whereas a countertraction pulls in the opposite direction. Traction may be used to reduce fractures or dislocations, maintain alignment and correct deformities, decrease muscle spasms and relieve pain, promote rest of a diseased or injured body part, and promote exercise. Advances in nailing and rodding, along with the use of internal and external fixators for fractures and spinal curvatures, have reduced the use of traction overall. Interest in ambulation for children is another consideration when surgeons decide between traction and other methods of immobilization. Currently, traction is still a very viable option, especially for femur and femoral shaft fractures and hip and cervical fractures, but remains an effective process for other immobilization requirements. Types of traction include reference to the mechanism and also specific named types such as Russell or Bryant traction for femoral fractures or halo traction with the use of Crutchfield tongs for stabilization of spinal fractures or injuries. Complications of traction include injury to the cranial nerves and other neurologic injuries.

Types of Traction

1. Manual—direct pulling on the extremity or body part. Usually, it is used to reduce fractures before treatment or immobilization.

*Please note that the term "male" in this chapter refers to a person assigned male at birth, and the term "female" in this chapter refers to a person assigned female at birth.

2. Skin—force is applied directly to the skin by means of traction strips or tapes secured by elastic bandages or by means of traction boots, usually of short-term duration and commonly used in children in whom small amounts of force are required.
3. Skeletal—force is applied to the body part through fixation directly into or through the bone by means of a traction pin or screw. This allows for greater force over longer periods or used when skin traction is not feasible, as in soft tissue injury or damage.
4. Continuous or intermittent—traction forces should be disrupted only in accordance with the health care provider's orders.

Complications of Traction

1. Neurovascular compromise to extremity.
2. Skin and soft tissue injury.
3. Pin or screw tract infection and osteomyelitis (with skeletal traction).

COMMON ORTHOPEDIC DISORDERS IN CHILDREN

See additional online content: Patient Education Guidelines 50-1.

Fractures

A *fracture* is a break or disruption in the continuity of the bone. Fractures in children differ from those in adults because of the differences in anatomy, biomechanics, and physiology of the child's skeleton compared to that of an adult. Involvement of the epiphysis or metaphysis can disrupt the epiphyseal plate, interfering with growth (see Figure 50-1). Fractures are extremely common in children, with an estimated 42% of males and 27% of females sustaining fractures during childhood.

EVIDENCE BASE Farrell, C., Hannon, M., Monuteaux, M., Mannix, R., & Lee, L. K. (2022). Pediatric fracture epidemiology and US emergency department resources utilization. *Pediatric Emergency Care, 38*(7), e1342–e1347. https://doi.org/10.1097/PEC.0000000000002752

Kamienski, M. C. (2020). Pediatric femur fractures. *Orthopaedic Nursing, 39*(2), 107–111. https://doi.org/10.1097/NOR.0000000000000641

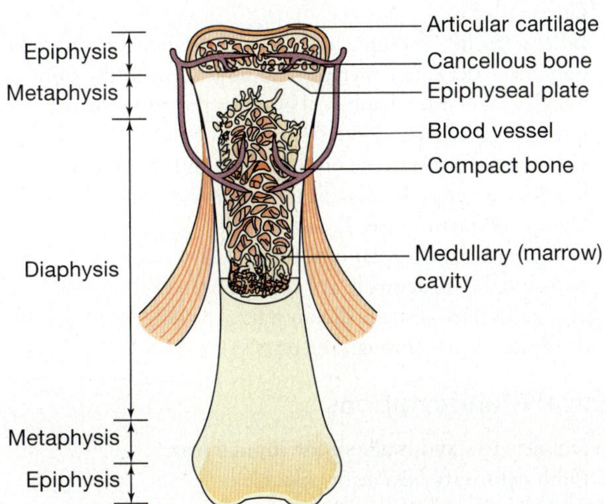

Figure 50-1. Structure of a bone.

Pathophysiology and Etiology

1. Most fractures in children are a result of low-velocity trauma, such as a fall.
   a. Up to the age of 2 years, most fractures are sustained as a result of the child being injured by another person.
   b. Fractures in neonates and infants are commonly the result of child maltreatment, which should be suspected when evaluating and treating fractures in this age group.
2. A bone fractures when the force applied to it exceeds the amount the bone can absorb.
   a. Children's long bones are more resilient than those of adults. They are able to withstand greater deflection without fracturing.
   b. The majority of children who are at risk for long bone fractures are over the age of 1 year.
   c. The bones of children have thick periosteum, as compared to adults, providing a protective membrane to help prevent the incidence of fractures.
3. The involvement of growth plates (epiphyseal plate) is unique to fractures in children. Cartilaginous growth plates are present at each end of the long bones and at one end of metacarpals and metatarsals. The plate is weaker than surrounding ligaments, tendons, and joint capsules and is disrupted before these tissues are injured.
   a. Damage to the growth plate may result in cessation of or a disturbance in bone growth (depending on the extent of damage sustained at the growth plate).
   b. On the other hand, acceleration in bone growth commonly occurs after a fracture in the long bones of children.
4. Children's fractures heal more rapidly than adult fractures. The younger the child, the more rapidly the bone heals.
5. Children's fractures remodel more completely and actively than adult fractures and usually result in less disability and deformity.

Sites of Fractures in Children

EVIDENCE BASE Delgrove, A., Harper, L., Berciaud, S., Laliouli, A., Angelliaume, A., & Lefevre, Y. (2019). Efficacy, pain, and overall patient satisfaction with pediatric upper arm fracture reduction in the emergency department. *Orthopaedics and Traumatology, Surgery and Research, 105*(3), 513–515. https://doi.org/10.1016/j.otsr.2018.10.027

Maharjan, P., Murdock, D., Tielemans, N., Goodall, N., Temple, B., Askin, N., & Wittmeier, K. (2021). Interventions to improve the cast removal experience for children and their families: A scoping review. *Children, 8*(2), 130. https://doi.org/10.3390/children8020130

As children grow, the fracture rate increases, with the peak incidence occurring in early adolescence. Forearm fractures are the most common injury.

Forearm and Wrist Fractures

1. The most common site of fracture in children, occurring more frequently in children older than 5 years.

2. Major categories of classification include fracture dislocations, midshaft fractures, and distal fractures.
3. Most common cause is from a fall on an outstretched arm.

Epiphyseal or Growth Plate Injuries

1. Constitute approximately 15% to 25% of all skeletal injuries in children.
2. The most frequent site of physeal injuries (excluding phalangeal fractures) is the distal radius and ulna.
3. The 11- to 15-year-old age group tends to sustain the majority of physeal injuries to the distal radius and ulna.
4. The mechanism of injury is usually a fall on an outstretched arm.

Clavicle Fractures

1. Frequent site of fracture in children.
2. The shaft of the clavicle is the most common site of injury.
3. A fall on the shoulder or excessive lateral compression of the shoulder as in a difficult vaginal delivery in a newborn is usually the mechanism of injury.
4. Treatment involves support in the form of immobilization with a sling.
5. Reduction of clavicle fractures in children occurs only in instances of extreme displacement.

Humerus Fractures

1. The mechanism of injury for the majority of humeral fractures is a fall onto an outstretched arm or hand.
2. Supracondylar fractures are the most common fractures of the humerus and may be associated with acute vascular injury.
3. Approximately 10% of all humeral fractures occur at the shaft of the humerus; they are usually a result of twisting injuries in infants and toddlers. Direct trauma to the humeral shaft is the most common mechanism of injury in older children.
4. Distal humeral fractures occur more often in the lateral epicondyle than the medial epicondyle.
5. Less than 1% of fractures occur at the proximal humerus.

Spinal Fractures

1. Rare in children.
2. Mechanism of injury is due to significant trauma, such as a fall from a significant height, athletic activities, assault, or pedestrian–motor vehicle accident.
3. Most spinal fractures involve the cervical spine.

Pelvic Fractures

1. Pelvic fractures are uncommon in children and adolescents; they are commonly the result of high-energy trauma or a crush-type injury.
2. Associated injuries are present in approximately 75% of children with pelvic fractures and include hemorrhage and damage to the abdominal wall and pelvic organs.

Hip Fractures

1. Hip fractures in children are uncommon but may occur from motor vehicle accidents, bicycle accidents, falls from significant heights, or child maltreatment (in children under age 3 years).
2. Hip fractures can result in avascular necrosis of the femoral head and damage to the physis resulting in growth arrest, malunion, and nonunion.
3. Pelvic avulsion fractures are more common, especially in males aged 12 to 14 years.

Femur Fractures

1. Common in children. Peak incidence occurs in two age groups—children aged 2 to 3 years and adolescents.
2. Fractures of the femoral shaft (diaphysis) are uncommon in children but are the most common location in this area.
3. Usually the result of high-energy trauma, such as a motor vehicle accident or fall from a significant height; most common cause in children younger than 1 year is child maltreatment.

Tibial Fractures

1. The most common lower extremity fracture in children occurs in the tibial and fibular shaft—constitutes 10% to 15% of all pediatric fractures.
2. Most diaphyseal tibia fractures in children aged 5 to 6 years are nondisplaced or minimally displaced spiral or oblique fractures. A rotational mechanism of injury to the lower leg is the most common cause of tibial fractures in children under age 3 years (toddler's fracture or CAST [childhood accidental spiral tibial]).
3. Greater force is required to injure the tibia in older children; motor vehicle accidents and sports injuries are the most common causes of tibial fractures in children and adolescents.

Ankle Fractures

1. Represent approximately 5% of all pediatric fractures.
2. Involve the growth plate in approximately one of six injuries.
3. Greatest incidence is in males aged 10 to 15 years.
4. Usually the result of direct trauma.
5. Mortise view as well as anteroposterior (AP) and lateral x-rays should be obtained.

Foot Fractures

1. Foot fractures account for approximately 6% of all fractures in children, and 50% of foot fractures occur at the metatarsals.
2. Most metatarsal and phalangeal fractures are nondisplaced.
3. Mechanism of injury is usually a direct or indirect trauma, such as from falls, jumping from heights, object falling on foot, and twisting injuries.

Classification of Fractures

1. Open fractures: Underlying fracture in the bone communicates with an external wound; usually the result of high-energy trauma or penetrating wounds.
2. Closed fractures: underlying fracture with no open wound.
3. Plastic deformation: a bending of the bone in such a manner as to cause a microscopic fracture line that does not cross the bone. When the force is removed, the bone remains bent. Unique to children and most common in the ulna (see Figure 50-2A).
4. Buckle (torus) fractures: fracture on the tension side of the bone near the softer metaphyseal bone; crosses the bone and buckles the harder diaphyseal bone on the opposite side, causing a bulge (see Figure 50-2B).
5. Greenstick fracture: The bone is bent, and the fracture begins but does not entirely cross through the bone (see Figure 50-2C).
6. Complete fractures (see Figure 50-2D):
   a. Spiral—from a rotational force.
   b. Oblique—diagonally across the diaphysis.
   c. Transverse—usually diaphyseal.
   d. Epiphyseal—through the physis.

Clinical Manifestations

1. Inability to stand, walk, or use injured part.
2. Limb deformity (visible or palpable).
3. Ecchymosis.
4. Pain, described as point tenderness.

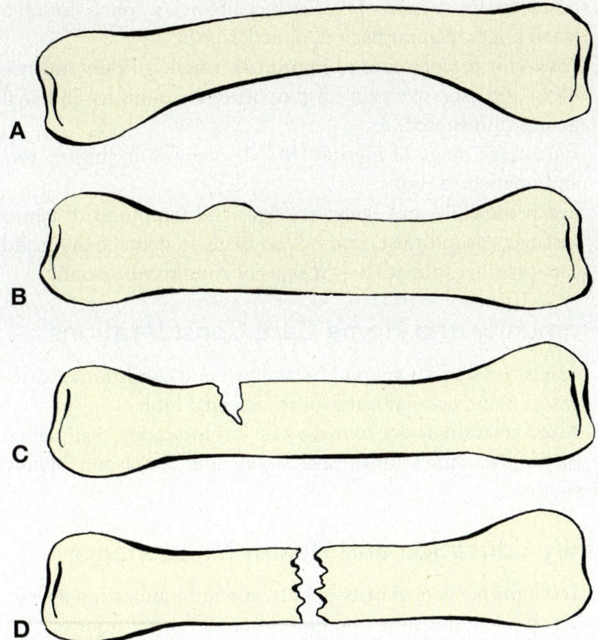

Figure 50-2. Common fractures in children. **(A)** Plastic deformation (bend). **(B)** Buckle (torus). **(C)** Greenstick. **(D)** Complete.

5. History of injury or trauma (may not be the case with pathologic fractures).
6. Spontaneous onset of pain (usually seen with pathologic fractures).
7. Local swelling and marked tenderness.
8. Movement between bone fragments.
9. Crepitus or grating.
10. Muscle spasm.

Diagnostic Evaluation

1. X-rays of suspected limb fractures should include the joint above and below the injury.
   a. Should always include a minimum of two views at 90-degree angles to each other (AP and lateral).
   b. Comparison views of the opposite extremity are frequently needed. They help to distinguish the fracture line from the growth plate.
   c. In some situations, oblique x-rays are warranted to help identify a fracture that is difficult to detect.
2. Further radiologic studies may be indicated in certain instances to evaluate a fracture: ultrasound, tomography, magnetic resonance imaging (MRI), computed tomography (CT) scan, bone scan, and fluoroscopy.
3. Vascular assessment may include the use of:
   a. Doppler studies.
   b. Compartment pressure monitoring.
   c. Angiography.

Management

Treatment is dependent upon the type of fracture, its location, and the age of the child.

1. Treatment may consist of:
   a. Immobilization by cast, splint, external fixator, or brace.
   b. Closed reduction followed by a period of immobilization in a cast or splint.
   c. Open reduction with or without internal fixation and usually followed by a period of immobilization in a cast or splint.
   d. Closed reduction and percutaneous pinning followed by a period of immobilization.
   e. Closed or open reduction and application of an external fixator.
   f. Traction (skin, skeletal) followed by a period of immobilization.
2. Most pediatric fractures heal in 12 weeks or less. Simple fractures that are closed and nondisplaced can heal enough to be free from immobilization within 3 weeks.

Complications

1. Infection and avascular necrosis.
2. Delayed union, nonunion, and malunion.
3. Shortening—epiphyseal arrest (deformities in angulation or limb length).
4. Vascular injuries.
5. Nerve injuries—palsies.
6. Visceral injuries.
7. Tendon and joint injuries.
8. Fat embolism.
9. Compartment syndrome (orthopedic emergency).
10. Osteoarthritis (occurs later).
11. Reflex sympathetic dystrophy.

Nursing Assessment

1. Follow the basic assessment for the trauma patient (see page 924).
2. Obtain history from the child, caregivers, and others to include accident or trauma details, noting the position of the extremity at impact.
3. Perform physical examination for the location of deformity, swelling, ecchymosis, and pain, vital signs, and neurovascular assessment.
4. Assess child's support mechanisms/social situation with consideration of discharge needs.

Nursing Interventions

Also see page 854 for orthopedic surgery.

Promoting Comfort

1. Monitor and assess pain level using an age-appropriate pain scale (e.g., Oucher or FACES scale).
2. Properly position, align, and support the affected body part.
3. Administer analgesics, as indicated, and monitor the effectiveness of analgesia.
4. Use nontraditional methods of pain relief—music therapy, diversionary activities, relaxation techniques, therapeutic touch, and play therapy.

Maintaining Tissue Perfusion

1. Frequently assess perfusion of limb by checking temperature, color, sensation, and pulses.
2. Elevate the extremity above heart level to prevent edema.
3. Encourage movement of digits on the affected limb.
4. Remove compressive bandages (e.g., elastic bandages, splints) that restrict flow of circulation.

Maintaining Skin Integrity

1. Assess for and relieve pressure caused by tight bandages, casts, and splints.

2. Provide periodic cleaning, thorough drying, and lubrication to pressure points if in traction.
3. Encourage frequent position changes as allowed.
4. Assess skin condition on a regular basis.
5. Massage healthy skin around the affected area to stimulate circulation.
6. Protect the skin at risk with special dressings or products (e.g., barrier cream, moisture-permeable dressing).
7. Discourage the use of sticks, pens or pencils, or small toys or other objects to scratch itchy skin.
8. Promote a diet high in protein, carbohydrates, and calcium.

Promoting Effective Coping

1. Assess the child's and caregivers' response to events; provide reassurance and emotional support.
2. Explain condition, treatment, and rehabilitation goals, as indicated.
3. Refer to community-based support agencies (e.g., social services, home care nursing), if indicated.
4. Structure the child's day with routine, activities, and therapy to keep them busy.
5. Encourage the child to express feelings and emotions through writing (e.g., journal), drawing, or play therapy.

Promoting Mobility

1. Encourage exercise of uninvolved limbs regularly throughout the day.
2. Collaborate with physical and occupational therapist to teach appropriate ambulation techniques using aids, such as crutches, walkers, or wheelchairs, as indicated.
3. Teach safety precautions when using an ambulatory aid.

Attaining Independence

1. Assess family situation for ability to care for the child at home.
2. Allow the child to care for self, and participate in care when able.
3. Encourage caregivers and siblings to assist only as needed.
4. Evaluate the child's ability to participate in self-care activities.

Preventing Infection

EVIDENCE BASE Kang, M. S., Park, J., & Kim, J. (2020). Agreement of postoperative pain assessment by parents and clinicians in children undergoing orthopedic surgery. *Journal of Trauma Nursing, 27*(5), 302–309. https://doi.org/10.1097/JTN.0000000000000533

1. Assess wounds, including pin sites, frequently for warmth, erythema, swelling, tenderness, or purulent drainage.
2. Pin site care and the use of dressings are indicated by the orthopedist or institution. A cleansing ritual with chlorhexidine or other antiseptic is beneficial, which includes gentle massage to remove superficial drainage.
3. Report signs of infection.
4. Provide appropriate wound care for open injuries and surgical wounds.
5. Administer antibiotics, as ordered.
6. Encourage the child to eat and maintain good caloric and protein intake to promote healing.
7. Teach good handwashing techniques to the child and caregivers.

Preventing Peripheral Neurovascular Dysfunction

1. Assess the neurovascular status of the affected limb every hour for the first 24 hours (or as indicated by hospital protocol)—compare with unaffected limb.
2. Assess for nerve injury (e.g., abduct all fingers, touch thumb to small finger, plantar flexion, dorsiflexion).
3. Assess for the presence of numbness, tingling, "pins and needles," and excessive pain (disproportionate to injury and analgesia administered).
4. Encourage range of motion (ROM) exercises in fingers, toes, and unaffected limbs.
5. Teach the child and caregivers signs and symptoms of neurovascular compromise, and advise them to contact the health care provider immediately if signs of compromise occur.

Community and Home Care Considerations

1. Assess the skin for signs of breakdown and condition of cast.
2. Assess neurovascular status of the affected limb.
3. Assess traction device to make sure it is intact and maintained.
4. Assess the child's nutritional status and bowel and bladder routine.

Family Education and Health Maintenance

1. Teach proper care of casts, splints, and immobilization devices.
2. Teach safety measures and prevention of further injuries.
   a. Advise the use of bicycle helmets and knee, elbow, and wrist pads.
   b. Emphasize the importance of supervising young children while playing.
   c. Teach safety measures, such as placing gates at stairs and installing top-opening windows on the second floors.
3. Teach the family and child the natural history of fracture healing (e.g., presence of fracture bump, gradual recovery of ROM, predicted time frame for healing).
4. Assess the coping ability of the child and family members and answer questions caregivers may have about the care of their immobilized child.
5. Teach patient and family about care of their child's pin site care and adjustment of screws. Have them do a return demonstration for evaluation of teaching.
6. Teach the child and family about signs and symptoms of infection and whom to contact should an infection occur.

Evaluation: Expected Outcomes

- Reports acceptable level of comfort.
- Extremity warm with good color sensation, pulses, and capillary refill.
- No skin breakdown noted.
- Caregivers comfort the child; the child responds appropriately.
- Uses ambulatory aids and ambulates independently.
- Bathes and feeds self with minimal assistance.
- No fever or signs of infection surrounding wound.
- Denies numbness and tingling.

Osteomyelitis

EVIDENCE BASE Sharma, S. K., Peter, P. P. R., Parashar, A. K., & Arora, S. (2022). Indigenous nutritional intervention for the recovery of a child with osteomyelitis: A clinical anecdote. *International Journal of Orthopedic and Trauma Nursing, 44*, 110902. https://doi.org/10.1016/j.ijotn.2021.100902

Osteomyelitis is a pyogenic infection of the bone and surrounding soft tissues. It occurs mostly in children between ages 3 and 12 years and is primarily a disease of growing bones. Long bones are frequently involved, and the characteristic site of involvement is the metaphyseal region. Males are afflicted two times as frequently as females.

Pathophysiology and Etiology

Etiologic Agents and Risk Factors

1. Microorganisms that cause osteomyelitis vary and are related to the age of the child.
   a. The most commonly identified pathogenic organism in acute osteoarticular infections is *Staphylococcus aureus*, with this organism responsible for about 70% of cases; methicillin-resistant *S. aureus* infections have risen in the past several years.
   b. Group A beta-hemolytic streptococcus, *Enterobacter*, *Escherichia coli*, and *Streptococcus pneumoniae* are other etiologic agents.
   c. Vertebral infections are increasingly a result of gram-negative microorganisms.
2. Classification based on pathogen's mode of entry:
   a. Hematogenous osteomyelitis (through the bloodstream)—occurs primarily in children.
   b. Contiguous osteomyelitis—caused by pathogenic spread from outside the body or by progressive spread of infection from tissue adjacent to the bone.
3. Risk factors include:
   a. Impetigo.
   b. Furunculosis.
   c. Direct trauma to an area adjacent to the site of osteomyelitis.
   d. Infected burns.
   e. Prolonged use of an intravenous (IV) line or intraosseous needle.
   f. Immunizations, especially with *Bacillus* Calmette–Guérin (BCG).
   g. IV drug dependency.
   h. Sickle cell disease.

Pathophysiologic Changes

1. When the site is inoculated, the invading pathogen provokes the following responses:
   a. Inflammatory response.
   b. Pus formation.
   c. Edema.
   d. Vascular congestion.
   e. Leukocyte activity.
   f. Abscess formation.
2. Small terminal vessels thrombose and exudate the bone's canaliculi.
   a. Inflammatory exudate extends into the metaphyseal and marrow cavity and through small metaphyseal openings into the cortex.
3. Exudate reaches the outer surface of the cortex, forming abscesses that lift the periosteum off the underlying bone, disrupting blood vessels and entering the bone through periosteum, thereby causing deprivation of blood supply to the bone. This leads to necrosis and death of the infected bone.
4. Sequestrum or devitalized bone is produced.
5. Intense osteoblastic response is stimulated upon lifting of the periosteum.
6. New bone is laid down by osteoblasts that partially or completely surround infected bone.
7. New bone, also known as *involucrum*, is formed.
8. Exudate escapes into surrounding soft tissue through openings in the involucrum, from which it escapes through the skin via sinus tracts.
9. Acute osteomyelitis is an abrupt onset of inflammation. Failure to halt acute osteomyelitis can lead to chronic osteomyelitis.
10. Chronic osteomyelitis:
    a. Signs and symptoms are usually vague.
    b. Infection is silent between exacerbations.
    c. Small abscesses or fragments containing microorganisms produce occasional flare-ups of acute osteomyelitis.
    d. Inadequate or inappropriate therapy and drug-resistant microorganisms can result in progression of acute osteomyelitis to chronic osteomyelitis.

Clinical Manifestations

1. Infants—involvement of multiple sites within the same bone or in multiple bones.
   a. Acute illness characterized by fever and failure to move the affected limb.
2. Children—usually affects long bones but can affect the pelvis and spine.
   a. Abrupt onset of fever and systemic signs of toxicity.
   b. Swelling, redness, and discrete tenderness over the affected area.
   c. Decreased ability to bear weight as well as decreased ROM of the affected limb.
3. Adolescents (less affected)—affects long bones but may involve vertebrae.
   a. Back pain.
   b. Signs and symptoms described earlier for children.

Diagnostic Evaluation

1. Blood cultures (positive in about 50% of cases) should be obtained before initiation of antibiotic therapy to help identify the causative pathogen.
2. Needle aspiration of soft tissue should be done to identify the causative agent.
   a. Gram stain, culture, and sensitivity of specimen once obtained.
   b. Negative aspirate does not always rule out infection.
3. Complete blood count—marked leukocytosis and low hemoglobin.
4. Erythrocyte sedimentation rate (ESR) and C-reactive protein (CRP)—elevated.
5. X-ray:
   a. Detects deep soft tissue swelling and loss of normal fat planes.
   b. Detects the presence of bone resorption and periosteal new bone formation.
   c. Comparison films of one limb with another can be done.
6. Ultrasound—has become useful for both diagnosis and in guiding aspiration as the ultrasound detects soft tissue changes in periosteum and surrounding soft tissue.
7. Bone scan in children younger than 1 year is required to determine multisite involvement.
   a. Localizes area of skeleton with altered physiology but does not identify the cause.
8. MRI—superior to CT and most useful in showing anatomic detail in many planes as well as detecting pathologic changes within marrow and soft tissues.
9. CT scan—can be used to detect focal areas of bone destruction and to delineate soft tissue abscesses associated with the bone infection.
   a. Unable to detect early stages of osteomyelitis and radiation poses high risk to young children.

Management

1. Aspiration is necessary to confirm the diagnosis of osteomyelitis and to identify the responsible microorganism to treat with the appropriate antibiotic. Aspiration is also needed to determine whether surgical debridement is required.
   a. Aspirated fluid is sent for culture and Gram stain.
2. IV antibiotics:
   a. Broad-spectrum antibiotics such as vancomycin or clindamycin, targeting Gram + organisms until sensitivity is obtained.
   b. Treatment is recommended based on the IV antibiotics for 3 to 6 weeks and based on symptoms and CRP level (there are no established guidelines for the duration of therapy).
   c. May require placement of a central intermittent infusion catheter (e.g., midline or peripherally inserted central catheter [PICC] line).
   d. After a course of IV antibiotics, a switch to oral antibiotic is made.
3. Surgical debridement—helps to stop further tissue destruction, thereby allowing a shorter course of antibiotic therapy.
4. Bed rest and immobilization to help with pain management.

Complications

EVIDENCE BASE Jorda Gómez, P., Vanaclocha, N., Ferras Tarrago, J., Bretón Martínez, J. R., & Blasco Mollá, M. Á. (2020). Osteomyelitis, venous thrombosis, and septic emboli in a pediatric patient: A case report. *Plastic Surgical Nursing, 40*(4), 197–201. https://doi.org/10.1097/PSN.0000000000000332

Complications of osteomyelitis are reported in about 6% of children and include:

1. Chronic osteomyelitis.
2. Pathologic fracture.
3. Growth arrest.
4. Osteonecrosis and avascular necrosis.
5. Recurrence of infection.
6. Septic arthritis.
7. Systemic infection—life-threatening if unrecognized and untreated.
8. Bone or muscle abscess.

Nursing Assessment

1. Obtain a detailed history, including recent infections (ear, tonsils, chest, urinary tract), trauma, and onset of symptoms.
2. Obtain a history of current or recent antibiotic therapy and its effect.
3. Perform physical assessment for signs of primary infection as well as osteomyelitis.
4. Assess coping mechanisms and resources of family.

Nursing Interventions

Maintaining Comfort and Reducing Temperature

1. Assess pain characteristics and use age-appropriate pain measurement tools.
2. Assess temperature every 4 hours and increase fluid intake to prevent dehydration.
3. Maintain rest and immobilization of affected part.
4. Administer analgesics/antipyretics, as indicated, and monitor their effectiveness.

Preventing Complications of Immobility

1. Instruct on allowable activities—generally no weight bearing on the affected limb and remain on bed rest during acute phase.
2. Encourage use and exercise of unaffected limbs and joints through play.
3. Provide ambulatory aids if indicated (e.g., crutches, walker), and instruct on safe and proper use.

Promoting Adherence With Therapeutic Regimen

1. Instruct patient and family on the need for maintaining serum levels of antibiotics after discharge, even after signs and symptoms of infection improve.
2. Initiate appropriate home care referrals for administration and monitoring of IV therapy and wound care.
3. Evaluate response to treatment through periodic laboratory tests (ESR, CRP, serum drug levels if indicated) and follow-up.
4. Teach family about proper maintenance and care of vascular access device (e.g., midline, PICC line).
5. Teach family and patient about oral antibiotic and importance of adherence with therapy.

Community and Home Care Considerations

1. Teach caregivers and child (if appropriate) about signs and symptoms of an infection.
2. Teach caregivers how to prepare the antibiotic for IV administration.
3. Teach caregivers how to administer the IV antibiotic.
4. Teach caregivers about the antibiotic being administered.
5. Teach caregivers and child about maintenance of the vascular access device.
6. Teach caregivers and child how to care for the child's wound.
7. Teach caregivers and child about potential complications after discharge.
8. Assess caregivers' and patient's coping abilities.
9. Reinforce teaching to caregivers on a frequent basis. Employ the use of return demonstrations to assess caregiver ability to administer IV antibiotics and care for their child's wound.
10. Provide the family with the phone number of a nurse whom they may contact for advice or if they have concerns.
11. Ongoing home visits may be necessary to make sure caregivers are comfortable with the child's vascular access device. Coaching about medication administration, maintenance of the device, and wound care can prevent readmission.

Family Education and Health Maintenance

1. Instruct the family on the signs and symptoms of recurrent or chronic infection.
2. Stress the importance of adherence with treatment.
3. Encourage caregivers to seek early medical intervention for subsequent infections.

Evaluation: Expected Outcomes

- Reports reduced pain or no pain.
- Remains afebrile.
- Exercises unaffected limbs.
- Surgical wounds without signs of infection; child and caregivers demonstrate proper techniques for care of IV access device and infusion.

Developmental Dysplasia of the Hip

Developmental dysplasia of the hip (DDH) is the term used to describe abnormalities of the developing hip, including subluxation, dislocation, and dysplasia of the hip joint. DDH may be associated with other congenital anomalies; its incidence is 1 out of every 1,000 live births in the United States. White infants are affected more frequently than Black infants. Bilateral involvement occurs in more than 50% of cases, and the left hip is more frequently involved than the right hip. Females are afflicted four to eight times more frequently than males.

Pathophysiology and Etiology

1. Risk factors include breech birth, firstborn, large infants, oligohydramnios, being a person assigned female at birth, positive family history of DDH, ethnic background, lower limb deformity, torticollis, metatarsus adductus, hip asymmetry, and other congenital musculoskeletal abnormalities.
2. Subluxed hip—maintains contact with the acetabulum, but not fully located within the hip joint.
3. Dislocated hip—no contact between the femoral head and the acetabulum; sometimes located but may be dislocated easily.
4. Dysplasia—acetabulum is shallow or sloping instead of cup shaped (see Figure 50-3).

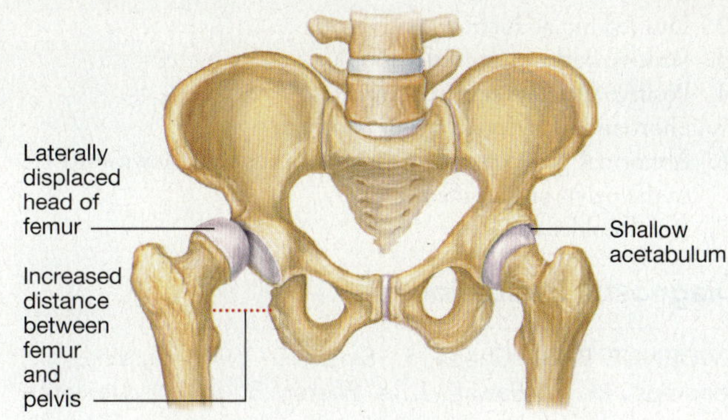

Figure 50-3. Developmental dysplasia of the hip. (Reproduced with permission from Stewart, J. (2017). *Anatomical chart company atlas of pathophysiology* (4th ed.). Wolters Kluwer.)

Clinical Manifestations

Physical findings change as the child ages; the presence of one or more of the following should be noted (see Figure 50-4):

1. Thigh asymmetry or thigh gluteal folds (present in 10% of normal infants).

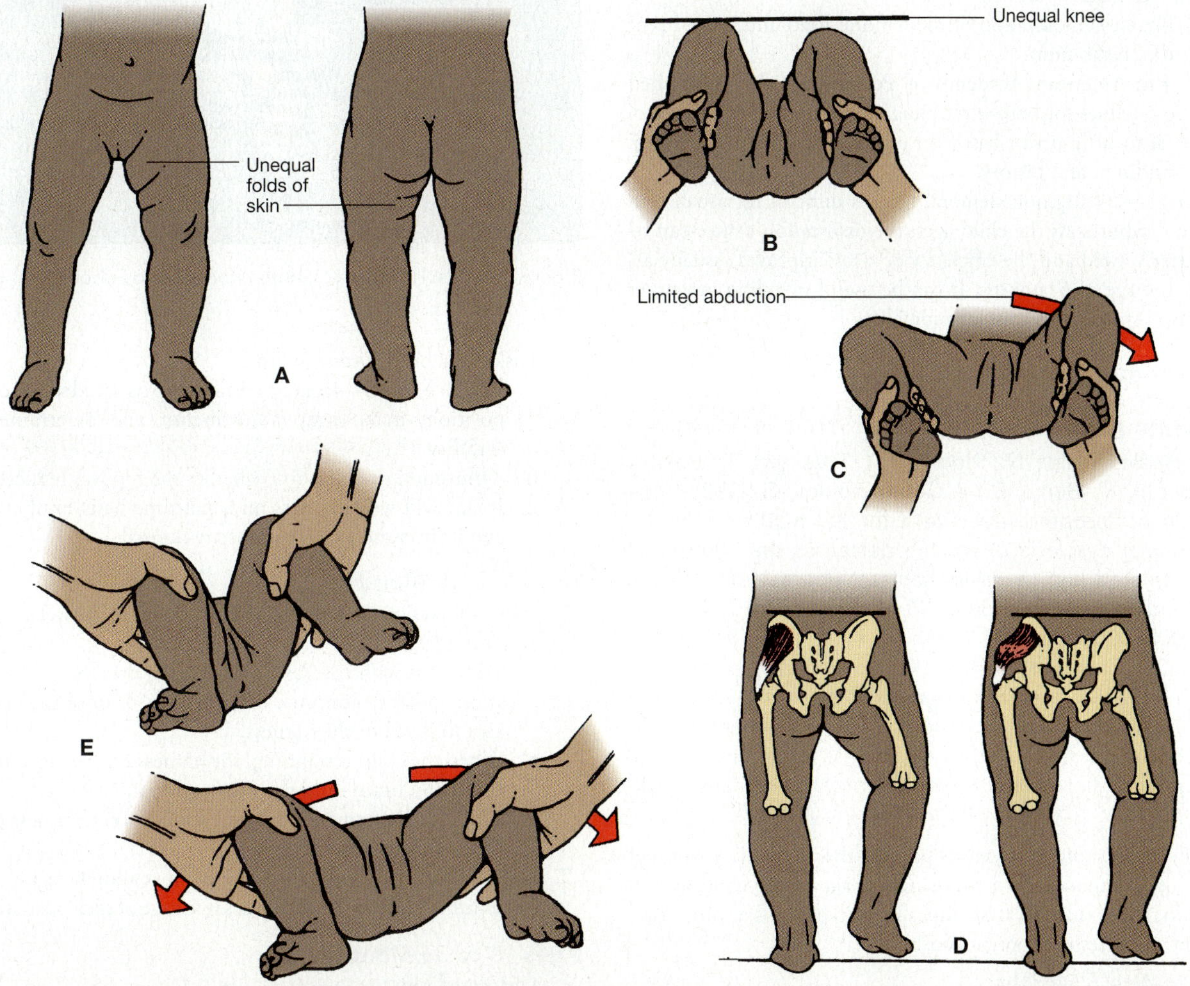

Figure 50-4. Signs of developmental dysplasia of the hip. **(A)** Unequal thigh folds; **(B)** apparent short femur (Galeazzi sign); **(C)** limited abduction of affected hip; **(D)** downward tilt of the pelvis on affected side (Trendelenburg sign); and **(E)** adduction and depression of the femur dislocate hip (Barlow test), and a "click" is felt when dislocated hip is abducted and relocated (Ortolani sign). (Adapted with permission from Jackson, D. B., & Saunders, R. B. [1993]. *Child health nursing.* Lippincott Williams & Wilkins.)

2. Limited hip abduction.
3. Positive Barlow test (dislocation).
4. Positive Ortolani test (reduction).
5. Shortening of affected femur (Galeazzi sign).
6. Abnormal gait patterns—Trendelenburg gait (downward tilt of the pelvis on the affected side).
7. Pain in older children.

Diagnostic Evaluation

EVIDENCE BASE Cheok, T., Smith, T., Wills, K., Wills, K., Jennings, M. P., Rawat, J., & Foster, B. (2023). Universal screening may reduce the incidence of late diagnosis of developmental dysplasia of the hip: A systematic review and meta-analysis. *The Bone & Joint Journal, 105-B*(2), 198–208. https://doi.org/10.1302/0301-620X.105B2.BJJ-2022-0896.R1

Mousavibaygei, S., Karimnia, A., Gerami, M. H., Azadmehr, F., Erfanifam, T., & Ghaedi, A. (2022). An evaluation of clinical and ultrasound results of Pavlik harness treatment for developmental dysplasia of the hip. *Journal of Medicine and Life, 15*(6), 850–853. https://doi.org/10.25122/jml-2021-0289

1. Ultrasound examination (with a skilled technician)—yields a high degree of accuracy in diagnosing DDH in children younger than 6 months.
   a. Enables visualization of the femoral head and outer lip of the acetabulum.
   b. The American Academy of Pediatrics (AAP) published guidelines for both ultrasonography indications and referral to orthopedist based on physical examination, clinical findings, and history.
2. X-rays—cartilaginous femoral head is difficult to visualize in the newborn. As the child ages, the ossification center can be better viewed and the efficiency of x-ray improves, usually after the age of 6 months. It can be useful in ruling out other pelvic, spinal, and femoral anomalies.

Management

EVIDENCE BASE Murphy-Zane, M. S., Carry, P. M., Salton, R. L., Hadley Miller, N., Holmes, K., Freeman, T., Belton, M., Kohuth, B., Burke, D., & Georgopoulos, G. (2023). Application of accepted use criteria for the treatment of developmental dysplasia of the hip decreases the number of infants treated with a Pavlik harness. *Journal of Pediatric Orthopedics, 43*(2), e138–e143. https://doi.org/10.1097/BPO.0000000000002295

Zhou, P., Zhang, J., Dan, T., Xu, T., Kang, X., Hang, Y., & Zhou, Y. (2023). Closed reduction and plaster immobilization: An alternative solution for patients with developmental dysplasia of the hip who failed Pavlik harness treatment. *Journal of Surgery, 93*(3), 663–668. https://doi.org/10.1111/ans.18285

The aim is to restore as closely as possible the anatomic alignment of the hip. Methodology depends on the age of the child at presentation. More than 80% of clinically unstable hips at birth have been shown to resolve spontaneously.

Birth to Age 6 Months

1. Subluxable hips:
   a. Observe for 3 weeks.
   b. If persistent, treat with Pavlik harness (see Figure 50-5).

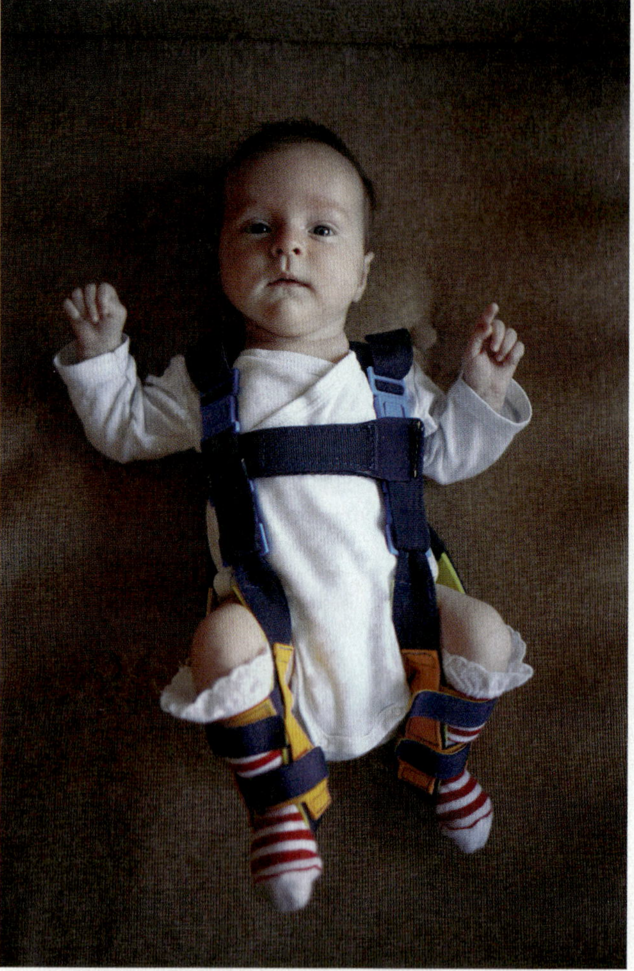

Figure 50-5. Pavlik harness. (Shutterstock/Marko Subotin.)

2. Dislocated or dislocatable hips:
   a. Pavlik harness—frequent follow-up is needed to check position, make strap adjustments, and determine hip stability.
   b. Ultrasound to determine whether the hip was reduced.
   c. Infant will wear harness on a full-time basis until clinical and ultrasound examinations are normal.

Ages 6 to 18 Months

1. Hip subluxation and dislocation in children between ages 6 and 9 months:
   a. Treatment with the Pavlik harness requires frequent evaluation and may continue for 4 months or until the child is able to stand in the harness.
   b. When the child is standing, the harness is exchanged for an abduction brace until the hip is normal.
   c. Closed reduction and hip spica application if harness treatment is unsuccessful.
2. Hip subluxation and dislocation in children ages 9 to 18 months—follow-up continues until age of skeletal maturity.

Ages 18 to 36 Months

1. Dislocated hip:
   a. Closed reduction.
   b. Application of hip spica cast for 3 months to maintain the reduction.

2. Failure of closed reduction and casting:
   a. Open reduction and innominate osteotomy.
   b. Hip spica cast application.
   c. Abduction bracing.
3. Follow-up continues until age of skeletal maturity.

Ages 3 Years and Older

1. Subluxation or dislocation of the hip—treated surgically by open reduction.
2. Follow-up continues until age of skeletal maturity.

Adolescents

1. Acetabular dysplasia:
   a. Use of nonsteroidal anti-inflammatory drugs and an ambulation device (e.g., crutches, cane) to limit weight bearing on the affected limb.
   b. Usually need surgical correction.

Complications

1. Avascular necrosis.
2. Redislocation or subluxation.
3. Loss of ROM.
4. Leg length discrepancy.
5. Early osteoarthritis.
6. Recurrent dislocation or unstable hip.
7. Femoral nerve palsy.
8. Iatrogenic hip dislocation.

Nursing Assessment

1. Obtain a family history, including hip pathology.
2. Obtain an obstetric history for the presence of risk factors, such as breech presentation and firstborn status.
3. Perform a physical assessment for ROM, appearance of Trendelenburg sign, Barlow test, Ortolani test, and examination for asymmetric thigh folds.
4. Assess family's response to the diagnosis.

Nursing Interventions

Also see page 854 for orthopedic surgery.

Promoting Effective Caregiving

1. Explain the condition and treatment in terms the family can understand.
2. Encourage holding the child with abduction of the hips while handling.
3. Advise caregivers to avoid swaddling the infant.
4. Reassure caregivers that effective outcome depends on early intervention and adherence.
5. Demonstrate application of Pavlik harness and make sure that caregivers know and feel comfortable in applying it.
6. Stress the importance of keeping follow-up appointments and strict adherence with prescribed treatment.
7. Provide caregivers with the name and number of a contact person if they have concerns about their child's care.

Maintaining Skin Integrity

See page 1413.

Preventing Complications of Immobility

1. Stimulate the child with games and activities to exercise upper body and feet as able.
2. Turn the child frequently and encourage ambulation as able. Support the head and legs to reposition.
3. Encourage deep breathing exercises at intervals to prevent atelectasis and hypostatic pneumonia. Children can blow bubbles, party favors, and cotton balls across the table as appropriate.
4. Encourage fluids and a high-fiber diet to prevent constipation.

Community and Home Care Considerations

1. An initial home care visit may be required to assess the child in a Pavlik harness.
2. For children in a hip spica cast, see "Community and Home Care Considerations" section under "Fractures."
3. Carefully assess caregiver role development and educate them on normal care of infant as well as special care needed by their child, such as safety measures and positioning.

Family Education and Health Maintenance

1. If the child is to be treated with an abduction splint, explain its purpose and demonstrate its application and removal to the caregivers.
   a. Instruct the caregivers as to if and when the device can be removed.
   b. Instruct the caregivers to check fit of abduction splint at every diaper change.
   c. Allow the caregivers to demonstrate their ability to properly place the device on the child.
   d. Provide the caregivers with written instructions whenever possible.
2. Instruct the caregivers on skin care and to report any skin breakdown or disruption of the cast, brace, or splint.
3. Encourage regular follow-up evaluations and regular health maintenance visits.

Evaluation: Expected Outcomes

- Caregivers hold the child and participate in care (e.g., applying Pavlik harness).
- No perineal skin breakdown.
- Lungs clear with good aeration bilaterally.

Congenital Clubfoot (Talipes Equinovarus)

Clubfoot is a congenital anomaly characterized by a three-part deformity of the foot, consisting of inversion of the heel (hindfoot varus), adduction and supination of the forefoot, and ankle equinus. Clubfoot typically points down and twists inward. The bone, muscle, ligaments, nerves, and blood vessels below the knee may all be displaced. Other congenital disorders of the foot and ankle occur but are less common. Incidence of clubfoot is 1 to 3 in 1,000 live births. It is bilateral in 30% to 50% of afflicted children, and the ratio of occurrence in males to females is 2.5:1.

Pathophysiology and Etiology

1. Equinovarus type (forefoot adduction, about 95% of cases)—foot is plantar flexed (talipes equinus) and inverted (talipes varus; see Figure 50-6).
2. Calcaneovalgus type (reverse clubfoot, about 5% of cases)—foot is dorsiflexed and everted (talipes valgus).
3. Exact etiology is unknown. Suggested theories point to vascular, viral, genetic, anatomic, and environmental factors; may also result from position in utero.

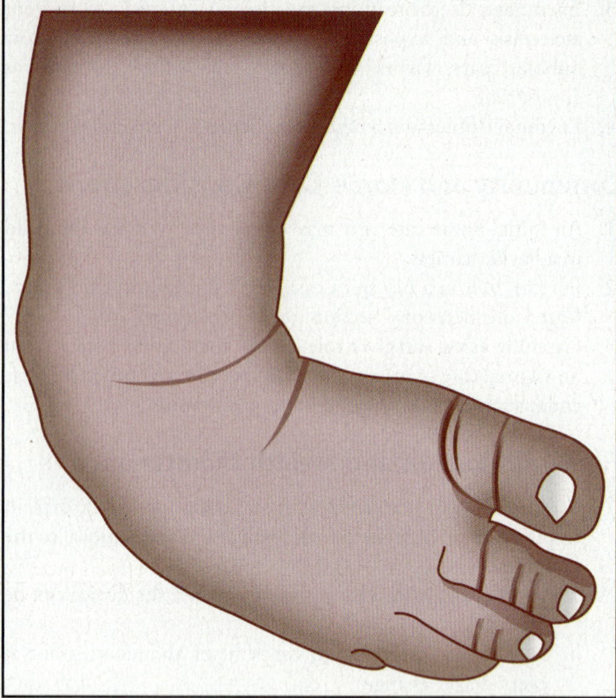

Figure 50-6. Equinovarus-type clubfoot. (Reprinted with permission from Pansky, B., & Gest, T. R. [2011]. *Lippincott concise illustrated anatomy.* Lippincott Williams & Wilkins.)

Clinical Manifestations

1. Deformity usually is obvious at birth with varying degrees of rigidity and ability to correct position. May range from a mild postural clubfoot to severe neuromuscular clubfoot that coexists with various diagnoses, such as arthrogryposis and spina bifida.
2. Deformity becomes fixed if untreated, which can lead to:
   a. Child bearing weight on the lateral border of the foot.
   b. Awkward gait.
   c. Development of callosities and bursae over the lateral side of the foot.

Diagnostic Evaluation

1. Clinical presentation and physical examination.
2. X-rays determine bony anatomy and assess treatment efficiency.

Management

EVIDENCE BASE Inarejos Clemente, E. J., Aparisi Gómez, M. P., Catala March, J., & Restrepo, R. (2023). Ankle and foot deformities in children. *Seminars in Musculoskeletal Radiology, 27*(3), 367–377. https://doi.org/10.1055/s-0043-1766099

Management should begin as soon after birth as possible, with the goal to establish a functional, pain-free foot that can be fit with standard footwear. Despite management, however, the child will always have a small calf and foot on the affected side. Nonoperative management, including manipulation, stretching, and serial casting, is currently the treatment of choice.

1. The Ponseti method is the initial method for treatment and incorporates gentle stretching and manipulation, followed by cast immobilization to promote relaxation and softening of tissues and remodeling of abnormal joint surfaces.
   a. Consists of weekly casting for approximately 6 weeks, followed by an Achilles tenotomy performed under local anesthetic and subsequent wearing of orthotic boots for 23 to 24 hours per day for 3 to 4 months.
   b. Treatment is completed with daytime ankle–foot orthoses (AFOs) and nighttime boots situated on a bar for 2 years.
2. Other nonoperative treatment includes cast changes and foot manipulation, which is usually done on a weekly basis for 6 weeks.
   a. After 6 weeks of weekly manipulation and casting, the foot is then manipulated and casted every 2 weeks.
   b. After the initial period (approximately 3 months of casting), an evaluation is performed to determine whether to continue with manipulation and casting, perform a percutaneous tenotomy, or proceed to use corrective shoes—with or without a Denis–Browne bar or the more recent Wheaton brace or Bebax shoe.
3. Surgical treatment may be required for some children to achieve correction of the deformity; usually performed within the second 6 months of life so that the child is free from postoperative immobilization before beginning walking.
4. Surgical treatment may also be required following nonoperative treatment, consisting of medial plantar release, posterior release, lateral release, or reduction and fixation—depending on the extent of the deformity.
5. The child who presents late or has a recurrent or residual deformity may require an aggressive surgical procedure to stabilize the bony structures and balance the muscle and tendons by a combination of fusions, releases, lengthening, and transfers.
6. Postoperative routines usually include a period of cast immobilization of up to 12 weeks, followed by a brace (AFO) or corrective shoe for a period of 2 to 4 years.

Complications

1. "Rocker bottom" deformity from excessive dorsiflexion and "breaking through" the midtarsal bones.
2. Disturbances in epiphyseal plates from overaggressive manipulation.
3. Recurrent or residual deformity.

Nursing Assessment

1. Obtain a family history of foot deformities.
2. Obtain an obstetric history for risk factors.
3. Perform a physical assessment for the presence of other anomalies and classic foot position and ROM. If late presentation, perform a thorough neurologic examination to rule out causative factors.
4. Assess family coping and resources available for lengthy treatment.

Nursing Interventions

Also see page 854 for orthopedic surgery.

Promoting Effective Caregiving

1. Provide an accurate description of deformity and the importance of treatment in terms the caregivers can understand.
2. Provide an opportunity for caregivers to verbalize questions and concerns.
3. Reinforce causative factors and the fact that it was not anyone's fault that the child has clubfoot.

4. Encourage caregivers to hold and play with the child and participate in care.
5. Provide caregivers with a contact family that has been through the treatment process for support.

Protecting Skin Integrity

1. Assess fit of cast, splint, orthotic device, or special shoes. Advise caregivers that because of rapid growth rate of the infant, the cast or splint may need to be replaced to prevent skin breakdown.
2. Assess and teach assessment of excessive pressure on the skin—redness, excoriation, foul odor from underneath cast, or pain.

Preserving Tissue Perfusion

1. Perform frequent neurovascular assessments after tenotomy and surgery, including color, warmth, sensation, capillary refill, pulses, and presence of pain.
2. Elevate the extremity to prevent edema in the postoperative period.
3. Protect and assess foot for injury.

Relieving Pain

1. Assess for signs of discomfort, such as irritability, crying, poor feeding and sleeping, tachycardia, and increased blood pressure.
2. Administer analgesics regularly for 24 to 48 hours after surgery.
3. Provide comfort measures, such as soft music, pacifier, teething ring, and rocking and cuddling with caregiver.
4. Encourage caregivers to administer analgesics after discharge from hospital (when needed). Discuss dosage and administration and dispel misconceptions about developing a dependence on the drug.

Family Education and Health Maintenance

1. Teach caregivers to remove cast at home before weekly manipulation and recasting by soaking in water and vinegar mixture.
2. Teach the caregivers when orthotic devices may be removed—usually for bathing. Stress that devices must be worn as prescribed.
3. Advise caregivers that infant's sleep may be disturbed initially due to wearing of brace at night and that they may be irritable while awake because of fatigue.
4. Instruct caregivers on providing a safe environment for the ambulatory child.
5. Discuss the importance of long-term and frequent follow-up and assist caregivers with special needs, such as transportation, flexible appointment times, and financing orthotic equipment.
6. Teach caregivers to check color, warmth, capillary refill, movement of toes, and position of cast (make sure cast does not slip to hide the toes).
7. Encourage caregivers to adhere with treatment regimen to achieve the best possible outcome.

Evaluation: Expected Outcomes

- Caregivers hold infant, participating in care.
- No signs of skin breakdown.
- Neurovascular status of affected foot intact.
- Rests and feeds well.

Legg–Calvé–Perthes Disease

Legg–Calvé–Perthes (LCP) disease is a self-limiting condition of the proximal femur characterized by a temporary loss of blood supply, which leads to avascular necrosis of the femoral head. The incidence of LCP is 0.2 to 20 per 100,000 in the general population. It occurs most commonly in children between ages 4 and 8 years. Ratio of occurrence in males to females is 5:1, and it is frequently found in White and Asian individuals. It is bilateral in 10% to 20% of cases. There is a 30% to 40% familial occurrence.

EVIDENCE BASE Galloway, A. M., van-Hille, T., Perry, D. C., Holton, C., Mason, L., Richards, S., Siddle, H. J., & Comer, C. (2020). A systematic review of the non-surgical treatment of Perthes' disease. *Bone and Joint Open, 1*(12), 720–730. https://doi.org/10.1302/2633-1462.112.BJO-2020-0138.R1

Rodríguez-Olivas, A. O., Hernández-Zamora, E., & Reyes-Maldonado, E. (2022). Legg-Calve-Perthes disease overview. *Orphanet Journal of Rare Diseases, 17*(1), 125. https://doi.org/10.1186/s13023-022-02275-z

Pathophysiology and Etiology

General Information

1. Etiology is unknown and may be due to factors such as secondhand smoke, poverty, hyperactivity, delayed bone age, short stature, mechanical dysfunction, and metabolic disorders.
2. Interruption of the vascular supply to the femoral head leads to the death of the bone. Deformity can occur with loss of the spherical nature of the femoral head during the disease process. The disease progresses through four identifiable stages.

Stage I (Avascularity)

1. Spontaneous interruption of the blood supply to the upper femoral epiphysis.
2. Bone-forming cells in the epiphysis die, and the bone ceases to grow.
3. Slight widening of the joint space.
4. Swelling of the soft tissues around the hip.
5. The first stage lasts only a few weeks.

Stage II (Revascularization or Fragmentation)

1. The femoral head is flattened and fragmented. Growth of new vessels supplies the area of necrosis; bone resorption and deposition take place.
2. The new bone lacks strength and pathologic fractures may occur.
3. Abnormal forces on the weakened epiphysis may produce progressive deformity.
4. This stage lasts several months to 1 year.

Stage III (Reossification)

1. The head of the femur gradually reforms.
2. Nucleus of the epiphysis breaks up into a number of fragments with cystlike spaces between them.
3. New bone starts to develop at the medial and lateral edges of the epiphysis, which becomes widened.
4. Dead bone is removed and is replaced with a new bone, which gradually spreads to heal the lesion.
5. This stage lasts 2 to 4 years.

Stage IV (Healing)

1. Without treatment:
   a. Head of the femur flattens and becomes mushroom shaped.
   b. Incongruity between the head of the femur and the acetabulum persists and worsens.
2. With treatment:
   a. Head of the femur remains near spherical.
   b. Acetabulum appears normal.
   c. Width of the neck of the femur is normal.

Clinical Manifestations

1. The child presents with a limp or pain in the hip, may be intermittent initially or may last for several months.
2. Referred pain to knee, inner thigh, and groin—usually with activity and often resolved with rest.
3. Limited abduction and internal rotation of the hip.
4. Mild-to-moderate muscle spasm on rotation of the hip in extension, limited internal rotation flexion, and abduction.
5. Trendelenburg gait—dip on the opposite side of the pelvis when weight bearing on the affected limb.
6. History of related trauma.

Diagnostic Evaluation

1. X-rays (AP and frog leg lateral) allow assessment of the extent of epiphyseal involvement and stage of disease—early findings may be normal.
2. MRI has been useful in detecting infarction but is not accurate in showing the stages of healing.
3. Bone scan is used to help diagnose LCP in the early stage of the disease, where the diagnosis is questionable.
4. Ultrasound may show early joint effusion.
5. Arthrograms may be useful in evaluating sphericity of the femoral head.

Management

EVIDENCE BASE Shaw, K. A., & Herring, J. A. (2023). Skeletal maturity in Legg-Calve-Perthes disease: Significant discrepancy present between the hand and the hip. *Journal of Pediatric Orthopedics, 43*(5), 294–298. https://doi.org/10.1097/BPO.0000000000002368

The goal of management is to preserve and restore the femoral head and to relieve pain.

1. Restore motion—initial relief of synovitis, muscle spasm, and pain in the joint:
   a. Salicylates (with caution) and anti-inflammatory medications.
   b. Limitation of activities and bed rest with or without activity modification.
2. Monitor progress of the disease and make sure the hip remains congruent through serial x-rays.
3. Surgical intervention, now rarely done, may vary but generally involves varus osteotomy, innominate osteotomy, osteotomy of the proximal femur or pelvis, or a combination of these, if the femoral head becomes subluxed or incongruent with the acetabulum before the reparative process.
4. Treatment outcome depends on the age of the child, extent of necrosis, stage of disease at the time of treatment, and congruence of joint with skeletal maturity.

Complications

1. Early degenerative joint disease.
2. Residual deformity.
3. Loss of motion or function of involved hip.
4. Persistent pain and gait disturbance.

Nursing Assessment

1. Obtain a detailed history, including onset of symptoms and characteristics of pain.
2. Perform a physical assessment to include evaluation of gait, ROM, and presence of any contractures.

Nursing Interventions

Also see page 854 for orthopedic surgery.

Promoting Comfort

1. Monitor and assess pain level using age-appropriate pain measurement tool.
2. Instruct the child and caregivers as to which activities can be continued and which to avoid (e.g., contact sports or high-impact sports).
3. Administer analgesics, as indicated, and monitor effectiveness.

Promoting Mobility

1. Encourage activities to maintain ROM (e.g., swimming, bicycle riding).
2. Encourage caregivers to allow activities that involve unaffected body parts within restriction guidelines.
3. Provide equipment to assist with mobility (e.g., wheelchair, walker).

Family Education and Health Maintenance

1. Teach proper care of assistive ambulatory aids and the need to remain adherent with usage.
2. Stress the need to remain active within restrictions and to promote positive body image.
3. Reinforce to the child that they are only temporarily restricted. Stress remaining a positive aspect of activity.
4. Explain the disease process to caregivers and child, emphasizing the importance of adherence with treatment.
5. Allow the child to voice concerns and ask questions about their treatment.
6. Encourage attendance at regular follow-up appointments.

Evaluation: Expected Outcomes

- Pain is adequately managed.
- ROM and function maintained.

Structural Scoliosis

Scoliosis is a lateral curvature of the spine of greater than 10 degrees. The different types of scoliosis vary by age of onset and structure of the spine.

Pathophysiology and Etiology

1. Idiopathic scoliosis—80% of scoliosis in children; possible causes include genetic factors, vertebral growth abnormality, or central nervous system abnormality. Three classifications (based on age at the time of diagnosis) include:
   a. Infantile—birth to age 3 years, less than 1% of all idiopathic scoliosis.
   b. Juvenile—presentation between ages 3 and 10 years or before onset of adolescence.
   c. Adolescent—presentation at adolescence (greater than 10 years):
      i. Partially familial, affects 2% of the population.
      ii. Prevalence for curves greater than 30 degrees is less common—1½ to 3 per 1,000; severe curvatures are rare.
      iii. Progressive curves are more prevalent in females than in males (7:1 females to males for curves greater than 25 degrees). Progression is greatest during adolescent growth spurt, just prior to onset of menses.

2. Congenital scoliosis—congenital malformation of one or more vertebral bodies that results in asymmetric growth.
   a. Type I—failure of vertebral body formation (e.g., isolated hemivertebra, wedged vertebra, multiple wedged vertebrae, multiple hemivertebrae).
   b. Type II—failure of segmentation (e.g., unilateral unsegmented bar, bilateral block vertebra).
   c. Type III—failure of segmentation along with failure of formation.
      i. More than 50% of patients with congenital scoliosis have another associated anomaly commonly associated with other congenital anomalies in other systems (e.g., Klippel–Feil syndrome, genitourinary tract abnormalities, VACTERL syndrome, and others).
3. Neuromuscular scoliosis: can be neuropathic or myopathic, most severe in patients who are nonambulatory. Occurs in children with cerebral palsy, muscular dystrophy, spinal muscular dystrophy, and others.
4. Miscellaneous factors that can cause scoliosis include osteopathic conditions, fractures, arthritic conditions, spinal irradiation, endocrine disorders, postthoracotomy, and nerve root irritation.
5. In all types of scoliosis, the vertebral column develops lateral curvature.
   a. The vertebrae rotate to the convex side of the curve, which rotates the spinous processes toward the concavity.
   b. Vertebrae become wedge shaped.
   c. Disk shape is altered, as are the neural canal and posterior arch of the vertebral body.
6. As the deformity progresses, changes in the thoracic cage increase. Respiratory and cardiovascular compromise can occur in cases of severe progression.
   a. Changes in the thoracic cage, ribs, and sternum lead to further characteristic deformities, such as the "rib hump."
   b. Neurologic compromise in idiopathic scoliosis is rare.

Clinical Manifestations

1. Physical characteristics (see Figure 50-7):
   a. Poor posture.
   b. Increased or decreased thoracic kyphosis or lumbar lordosis.

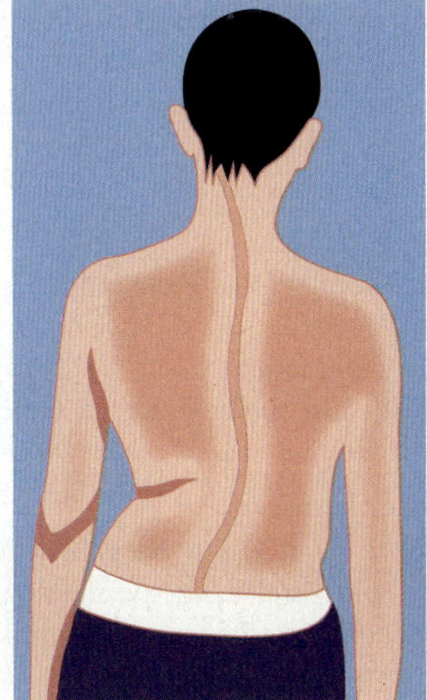
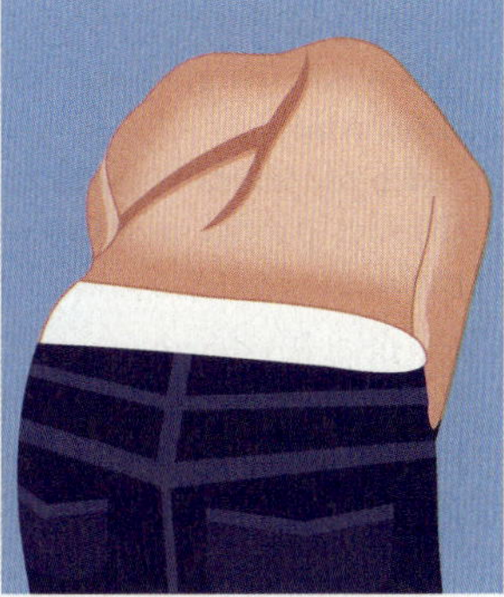

Figure 50-7. Characteristic truncal imbalance and scapular prominence with scoliosis.

   c. Leg length discrepancy.
   d. Shoulder asymmetry.
   e. Scapular prominence.
   f. Truncal imbalance (relationship of trunk over pelvis).
   g. Lump (rib hump) on back.
   h. Uneven waistline.
   i. Uneven breast size.
2. Back pain may be present but is not a routine finding in idiopathic scoliosis.

Diagnostic Evaluation

EVIDENCE BASE Scaturro, D., de Sire, A., Terrana, P., Costantino, C., Lauricella, L., Sannasardo, C. E., Vitale, F., & Mauro, G. L. (2021). Adolescent idiopathic scoliosis screening: Could a school-based assessment protocol be useful for an early diagnosis? *Journal of Back and Musculoskeletal Rehabilitation, 34*(2), 301–306. https://doi.org/10.3233/BMR-200215

1. Thorough history should include onset of menses, recent growth spurt, and family history of scoliosis.
2. Physical examination—the AAP recommends screening for females at ages 10 and 12 years and males at ages 13 and 14 years. Adams forward bending test is used to screen for scoliosis. A scoliometer can be used to measure rotational deformity. Risser classification is used to grade skeletal maturity based on the level of bone ossification and fusion of the iliac crest apophyses.
3. Thorough neurologic evaluation:
   a. Evaluate balance, motor strength, sensation, and reflexes (including abdominal).
   b. Skin examination for café-au-lait spots, axillary freckles, to indicate neurologic problem.
   c. Examination for the presence of a hairy patch or other lesions in the lumbosacral area.
   d. Examination for limb length difference that could cause the appearance of scoliosis.
4. Radiologic assessment of the spine in the upright position, preferably posterior–anterior and lateral views on one long (36-in [91-cm]) plate—shows characteristic curvature.
5. CT scan may be used to further define anatomy. MRI is indicated for all patients with early-onset scoliosis and is often used prior to surgery to rule out other deformities.
6. Pulmonary function tests for those with compromised respiratory status.
7. Clinical photographs to assist with documenting the appearance of the spine over time.
8. Workup for associated renal abnormalities with congenital scoliosis because of a high correlation between the two.

EVIDENCE BASE Zale, C. L., & McIntosh, A. L. (2022). Adolescent idiopathic scoliosis for pediatric providers. *Pediatric Annals, 51*(9), e364–e369. https://doi.org/10.3928/19382359-20220724-01

Management

Goal of management is to stop progression of the existing curve by nonoperative means. When this fails, the goal of operative management should be to correct the scoliosis as much as possible and balance and stabilize the spine by fusion to prevent further progression.

Medical Management

1. Observation—periodic (usually every 6 months) physical and radiographic examinations to detect curve progression.
   a. Child is not skeletally mature.
   b. Curves less than 25 degrees.
2. Brace management—the goal is to prevent progression of the curve.
   a. Requires faithful adherence on the part of the child for success; recommended 23 hours per day.
   b. Some curves progress despite brace wear.
   c. Bracing is for skeletally immature children with curves that are about 25 to 40 degrees.
3. Types of braces include:
   a. Boston orthosis for low thoracic and thoracolumbar curves. This is an underarm molded orthosis.
   b. Milwaukee brace for thoracic or double major curves. Standard brace has neck ring with chin rest.
   c. Charleston bending brace has been tried for nighttime usage in selected patients. Results have been positive in some centers, but widespread acceptance has not occurred.
4. Exercise therapy has been promoted to help maintain flexibility in the spine and prevent muscle atrophy during prolonged bracing by strengthening back muscles.

Surgical Correction

EVIDENCE BASE Tsirikos, A. I., Adam, R., Sutters, K., Fernandes, M., & García-Martínez, S. (2023). Effectiveness of the Boston brace in the treatment of paediatric scoliosis: A longitudinal study from 2010–2020 in a National Spinal Centre. *Healthcare, 11*(10), 1491–1506. https://doi.org/10.3390/healthcare11101491

1. Stabilization of the spinal column is the goal. This is usually accomplished with a spinal fusion and one of several methods of instrumentation.
2. Indications for surgical correction vary, but generally accepted principles include:
   a. Progression of the curve over a short period in a curve greater than 45 degrees despite bracing.
   b. Management with a brace is not possible.
   c. Cosmetic.
3. Surgical approach and techniques may be anterior or posterior with various instrumentation methods.
4. Strategies have evolved from body cast fixation to nonsegmental rods, such as the Harrington; to segmental wire fixation, such as the Luque, Drummond instrumentation, or segmental hook fixation; and Cotrel–Dubousset instrumentation; to current techniques, such as segmental screw fixation.
5. Segmental fixation systems provide a three-dimensional correction of coronal, sagittal, and rotational deformities.
   a. Posterior fusion is the standard approach, which allows correction and instrumentation of the majority of curves and levels.
   b. Stainless or titanium rods with segmental hooks (see Figure 50-8) and pedicle screw fixation are currently the instrumentation systems of choice.
   c. A reduction in the number of vertebrae requiring fusion may be achieved with anterior fusion.
   d. Combined anterior and posterior fusion may be used to correct severe curves.
   e. Perioperative halo-gravity traction may be used in rare cases when the risk of neurologic compromises from rapid correction exists.

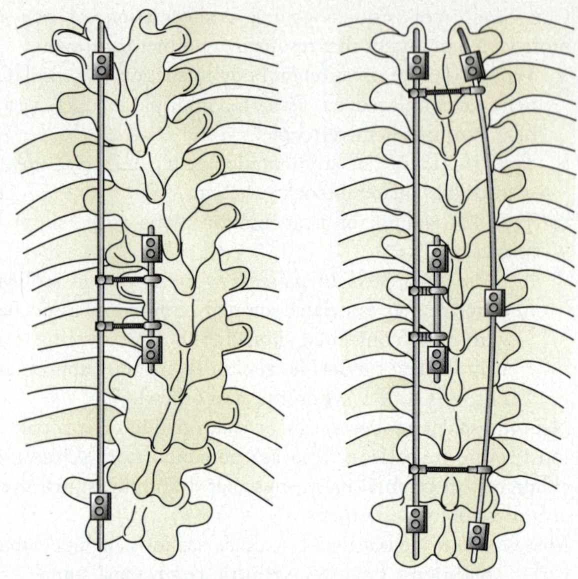

Figure 50-8. Cotrel–Dubousset rods to correct scoliosis. A short distraction rod is linked to a longer one to correct the major curve.

   f. Vertical, expandable prosthetic titanium ribs may be used to lengthen and expand a constricted hemithorax and allow for growth of thoracic spine and rib cage in thoracic insufficiency. Once the child's lungs have fully developed, a spinal instrumentation and fusion can be performed.

Nursing Assessment

1. Assess respiratory, cardiovascular, and neurologic systems.
2. Perform a physical examination in the upright and forward bending positions, and observe physical characteristics, such as leg lengths, gait, hips, shoulders, and overall development.

Nursing Interventions

Also see page 854 for orthopedic surgery.

Promoting Positive Body Image

1. Encourage the child to express feelings and concerns about body image.
2. Encourage the child to express concerns about wearing a brace and offer comfortable options for wearing it and disclosing condition with classmates.
3. Encourage the child to discuss scoliosis with peers, or provide a peer support person to discuss positive outcomes and expected future care.

Preserving Skin Integrity

1. Assess skin integrity and proper fit of brace at every follow-up appointment.
2. Teach proper skin care to patient and family.
3. Instruct patient to wear cotton shirt under brace to avoid rubbing.

Preventing Postoperative Complications

1. Prepare the patient for surgery by teaching deep breathing and coughing exercises and explaining positioning, patient-controlled analgesia, or another method of pain control.
2. Following surgery, encourage frequent logrolling side to side to prevent skin breakdown and respiratory complications. Medicate for pain prior to repositioning and ambulation.

3. Perform frequent neurovascular assessments and monitor vital signs frequently. Encourage early ambulation (1 to 2 days if stable).
4. Monitor drainage or bleeding from incision site.
5. Maintain indwelling urinary catheter as indicated. Monitor intake and output, but remove as soon as possible to prevent urinary infection.
6. Engage physical therapy assistance for patient mobility to be out of bed, sit in chair, and begin ambulation.
7. Active bowel sounds should be present before diet is advanced. Patients should have bowel regimen ordered and adjusted based on stool frequency and consistency. Lack of mobility and opioid use may contribute to constipation.

Promoting Adherence With Treatment

1. Explain scoliosis and the treatment options to the child in a language they can understand.
2. Explain the importance of adhering with treatment and possible outcomes with nonadherence.
3. Encourage the child and family to discuss concerns and questions they may have about scoliosis and the prescribed treatment.
4. Assist with social service referral for financial, transportation, and other needs.

Family Education and Health Maintenance

1. Provide adequate information on condition and treatment.
2. Instruct caregivers to examine brace daily for fit or breakage. Also instruct them to contact orthotist when repairs or adjustments are needed.
3. Teach family to inspect skin for irritation under brace.
4. Ensure that child can be transported safely in vehicles with potential modification in safety restraints.
5. Suggest to the family to discuss child's treatment with teachers and school officials, so the child can receive tutoring or homeschooling to keep up with grade requirements if out for surgery.

Evaluation: Expected Outcomes

- Child makes positive comments about self.
- Skin without signs of breakdown.
- Neurovascular status intact; no bleeding noted; bowel sounds present; pain is adequately managed.
- Wears brace as prescribed, following up as directed.

Slipped Capital Femoral Epiphysis

EVIDENCE BASE Pavone, V., Testa, G., Torrisi, P., McCracken, K. L., Caldaci, A., Vescio, A., & Sapienza, M. (2023). Diagnosis of slipped capital femoral epiphysis: How to stay out of trouble? *Children (Basel), 10*(5), 778–789. https://doi.org/10.3390/children10050778.

Slipped capital femoral epiphysis (SCFE) is the most common hip disorder in adolescents, which occurs in puberty just before the physis (growth plate) closes. It is characterized by a slipping of the epiphysis and metaphysis because of weakening of the perichondral ring of the physis. The epiphysis slips downward and backward. Incidence is 10 per 100,000 and it is three times more common in males than in females. Approximately 20% of patients present with bilateral slips at the time of presentation, and 20% to 30% will develop a contralateral slip within 12 to 18 months of initial slip.

Pathophysiology and Etiology

1. Skeletally immature and obese adolescents are at greatest risk.
2. Left hip is most frequently affected.
3. Exact etiology is unknown; possible risk factors include:
   a. Sedentary lifestyle.
   b. Rapid growth spurt.
   c. Overweight and obesity.
   d. African American ethnicity.
4. Femoral neck slips off the proximal femoral epiphysis and is contained within the acetabulum.
5. Classified by duration of symptoms:
   a. Acute—sudden onset, symptoms for less than 3 weeks.
   b. Chronic—symptoms lasting more than 3 weeks.
6. Approximately 85% of children have stable slips.
7. Because of vague symptoms, diagnosis is often delayed, which can result in complications.

Clinical Manifestations

1. Pain in the groin, medial thigh, or knee (referred pain).
2. Decreased ROM in affected hip.
3. Sudden onset of pain (acute SCFE).
4. Inability to bear weight (acute SCFE).
5. Limp when walking (usually found in chronic cases).
6. Intermittent pain.
7. Trendelenburg gait.
8. External rotation of the lower limb; involved limb may be shortened.

Diagnostic Evaluation

1. X-rays confirm diagnosis—AP and frog leg lateral views.
2. Bone scan—rules out the presence of avascular necrosis.
3. MRI or CT scan—helps to define the extent of slip, used primarily in severe slips.

Management

1. Goal is to prevent progressive slippage and minimize deformity while avoiding necrosis of cartilage (chondrolysis) and avascular necrosis.
2. Treatment is surgical—in situ pinning with one or two screws is usually done within 24 to 48 hours.

Complications

1. Chondrolysis over the femoral head resulting in permanent loss of ROM.
2. Avascular necrosis of the femoral head.
3. Osteoarthritis.

Nursing Assessment

1. Obtain a detailed history, including onset of symptoms and characteristics of pain.
2. Perform a physical assessment and include evaluation of gait and ROM in the hips.

Nursing Interventions

Also see page 854 for orthopedic surgery.

Promoting Comfort

1. Monitor and assess pain level using age-appropriate pain measurement tools.

2. Instruct the child and caregivers as to which activities can be continued and which to avoid (e.g., contact sports, high-impact activities).
3. Administer analgesics, as indicated, and monitor effectiveness.

Promoting Mobility

1. Facilitate bed rest or other activity restrictions, as directed.
2. Provide equipment to assist with mobility (e.g., wheelchair, crutches).

Promoting Diversional Activities

1. Be alert to the needs of adolescents to socialize with peers. Encourage visitation and communication with friends and family.
2. Encourage family to provide books, magazines, games, and electronics for the adolescent to use.
3. Provide support for the family and reinforce the importance of following activity restrictions to prevent permanent damage to the femur.

Family Education and Health Maintenance

1. Teach proper use of mobility devices (e.g., crutches).
2. Stress the need to maintain activity within restrictions and to promote positive body image.
3. Encourage follow-up during active treatment and following surgery. About 25% of children later develop the same condition in the opposite hip, so careful attention must be paid to both legs at follow-up.

Evaluation: Expected Outcomes

- Child reports feeling little or no pain.
- Child follows activity restriction.
- Child maintains socialization with friends and partakes of hobbies in the room.

Many children discharged from the hospital diagnosed with orthopedic conditions will have extensive discharge needs. Families will need support in the transition to home or another aftercare location. It is crucial that they have complete and understandable care instructions on home care, equipment, medications, and follow-up appointments. If arrangements have been made for nursing care in the home, families should be aware of the agency providing services and when they can expect communication regarding care arrangements. Families should have thorough written (and if necessary to assist understanding, pictorial) instructions on signs and symptoms to monitor for that could suggest worsening of status. Families may also need extensive instructions on necessary equipment to ensure safe mobility, including ambulation for the child. Health providers should ensure that the child has safe and appropriate means for transport from the hospital to the home. The bulk of casts and other orthopedic equipment may necessitate changes for car safety as the child may no longer fit in the prior car restraint system. Instructions should include clear understanding of acceptable discharge expectations as many children may be in different phases if a continued surgical repair is necessary. Caregivers should be aware of when and where they should seek further emergency care if the child's condition deteriorates.

SELECTED READINGS

Adulkasem, N., Phinyo, P., Tangadulrat, P., Wongcharoenwatana, J., Ariyawatkul, T., Chotigavanichaya, C., Kaewpornsawan, K., & Eamsobhana, P. (2022). Comparative effectiveness of treatment modalities in severe Legg-Calvé-Perthes disease: Systematic review and network meta-analysis of observational studies. *International Orthopaedics, 46*(5), 1085–1094. https://doi.org/10.1007/s00264-022-05352-x

Ailabouni, R., Zomar, B. O., Slobogean, B. L., Schaeffer, E., Joseph, B., & Mupuri, K. (2022). The natural history of non-operatively managed Legg–Calvé–Perthes' disease. *Indian Journal of Orthopedics, 56*(5), 867–873. https://doi.org/10.1007/s43465-021-00543-x

Berry, J., Glasby, T., Eagan, B., Singer, S., Glader, L., Emara, N., Cox, J., Glotzbecker, M., Crofton, C., Ward, E., Leahy, I., Salem, J., Troy, M., O'Neill, M., Johnson, C., & Ferrari, L. (2020). Pediatric complex care and surgery comanagement: Preparation for spinal fusion. *Journal of Child Health Care, 24*(3), 402–410. https://doi.org/10.1177/1367493519864741

Burkhardt, R., Hecht, C., McNassor, R., & Mistovich, R. (2023). Interventions to reduce pediatric anxiety during orthopaedic cast room procedures: A systematic and critical analysis review. *The Journal of Bone and Joint Surgery Reviews, 11*(2), 1491–1504. https://doi.org/JBJS.RVW.22.00181

Cady, R., Hennessey, T., & Schwend, R. (2022). Diagnosis and treatment of idiopathic congenital clubfoot. *Pediatrics, 149*(2), e2021055555. https://doi.org/10.1542/peds.2021-055555

Davis, R. (2019). Congenital talipes equinovarus: Nursing role for parents and family members. *International Journal of Childbirth Education, 34*(2), 23–26.

Dwan, K., Kirkham, J., Paton, R., Morley, E., Newton, A., & Perry, D. (2022). Splinting for the non-operative management of developmental dysplasia of the hip (DDH) in children under six months of age. *Cochrane Database of Systematic Reviews,* (10), CD012717. https://doi.org/10.1002/14651858.CD012717.pub2

Heath, D., Momtaz, D., Ghali, A., Gibbons, S., & Hogue, G. (2022). Obesity increases time to union in surgically treated pediatric fracture patients. *Journal of American Academy of Orthopedic Surgeons, Global Research & Reviews, 6*(1), e21.00185. https://doi.org/10.5435/JAAOSGlobal-D-21-00185

Hester, G., Nickel, A., Watson, D., Swanson, G., Laine, J., & Bergmann, K. (2021). Improving care and outcomes for pediatric musculoskeletal infections. *Pediatrics, 147*(2), 1–11. https://doi.org/10.1542/peds.2020-0118

Kuhn, A., Troyer, S., & Martus, J. (2022). Pediatric open long-bone fracture and subsequent deep infection risk: The importance of early hospital care. *Children, 9*(8), 1243–1255. https://doi.org/10.3390/children9081243

Lein, G. (2022). Screening for adolescent idiopathic scoliosis: A literature review. *Pediatric Traumatology, Orthopaedics and Reconstructive Surgery, 10*(3), 309–320. https://doi.org/10.17816/PTORS107136

Loder, R., Gunderson, Z., Sun, S., Liu, R., & Novais, E. (2023). Slipped capital femoral epiphysis associated with athletic activity. *Sports Health, 15*(3), 422–426. https://doi.org/10.1177/19417381221093045

Lyons, D. K. (2023). Pediatric osteomyelitis. In J. F. Sarwark & R. L. Carl (Eds.), *Orthopaedics for the newborn and young child* (pp. 285–298). Springer. https://doi.org/10.1007/978-3-031-11136-5_28

Matsumoto, H., Fano, A. N., Quan, T., Akbarnia, B., Blakemore, L., Flynn, J., Skaggs, D., Smith, J., Snyder, B., Sponseller, P., McCarthy, R., Sturm, P., Roye, D., Means, J., & Vitale, M. (2023). Re-evaluating consensus and uncertainty among treatment options for early onset scoliosis: A 10-year update. *Spine Deformity, 11*(1), 11–25. https://doi.org/10.1007/s43390-022-00561-1

Peck, J., Greenhill, D., Morris, W., Do, D., McGuire, M., & Kim, H. (2022). Prolonged non-weightbearing treatment decreases femoral head deformity compared to symptomatic treatment in the initial stage of Legg–Calvé–Perthes disease. *Journal of Pediatric Orthopaedics, 31*(3), 209–215. https://doi.org/10.1097/BPB.0000000000000873

Purcell, M., Reeves, R., & Mayfield, M. (2022). Examining delays in diagnosis for slipped capital femoral epiphysis from a health disparities perspective. *PLoS One, 17*(6), e0269745. https://doi.org/10.1371/journal.pone.0269745

Qureshi, M. A., Keerio, N. H., Hussain, S. S., Amir, H., Saqlain, U. S., Hameed, M. H., Kakar, A., & Noor, S. (2022). Congenital talipes equinovarus (club foot): Overview, and management options. *Journal of Research in Medical and Dental Science, 10*(1), 47–51.

Ravi, M., Fernandez, F., Whitaker, A., & Kaffenberger, J. (2022). Dermatologic complications of orthopedic casts in pediatric patients. *Journal of Pediatric Dermatology, 39*(1), 5–11. https://doi.org/10.1111/pde.14884

Salh, D. A. H., Abdelrahman, K. E., Abdelwahab, A. M., & Algohiny, I. A. I. (2022). Efficacy of single screw fixation for slipped capital femoral epiphysis. *The Egyptian Journal of Hospital Medicine, 88*(1), 3931–3937. https://doi.org/10.21608/EJHM.2022.253075

Salton, R., Carry, P., Freeman, T., Holmes, K., Miller, N., Kohuth, B., Burke, D., Belton, M., Murphy-Zane, M., & Georgopoulos, G. (2022). Twelve-week standard of care protocol longer than median time to normalization among IIc hips treated with Pavlik harness. *Journal of Pediatric Orthopaedics, 31*(4), 313–318. https://doi.org/10.1097/BPB.0000000000000946

van Bergen, C. (2022). Pediatric fractures are challenging from head to toe. *Children, 9*(5), 678. https://doi.org/10.3390/children9050678

51 Pediatric Integumentary Disorders*

BURNS

Management of Burns in Children

Burns are common childhood injuries. They may be caused by heat, electrical energy, or chemicals. Long-term surgical and psychological sequela often follows a serious burn injury and may include reconstruction and issues related to posttraumatic stress disorder. Serious burns may include:

1. Partial-thickness (second-degree) burns of 12% to 15% or more of body surface area.
2. Full-thickness burns.
3. Burns of the face, hands, feet, perineum, or joint surfaces.
4. Electrical and chemical burns.
5. Burns in the presence of other injuries.
6. Any burn that cannot be cared for adequately at home.

Epidemiology

1. Burns are the fourth leading cause of accidental death in children 17 years old and younger, with the highest incidence of burns occurring in children younger than age 5 years.
2. Children at high risk are of lower socioeconomic status and of single parental caregivers. However, any child, supervised or unsupervised, is at risk for a burn injury.
3. Scalds are the leading cause of injury in children, followed by flame burns.
4. Burns from a hot liquid are most common in children younger than age 5.
   a. Tap water temperature above 120°F (48.9°C) (at 130°F [54.4°C]) takes only 30 seconds to produce a full-thickness injury in adult skin—less time in the very young; at 155°F (68.3°C), tap water will cause a full-thickness injury in a child in 1 second.
   b. Child left unsupervised in tub turns on hot water tap.
   c. Child placed in tub of hot water or infant being bathed in a sink in which the temperature of the water has not been tested.
   d. Spilling of hot liquid, such as coffee or tea, on child. Spilling frequently occurs especially when pot handles stick out on top of stove, when hot liquids and foods are removed from microwave oven. Other common circumstances for pediatric burns occur when a child grabs or pulls items from surfaces or when a child is splashed with a hot beverage while being held on the lap of an adult.
   e. Ingestion and aspiration of hot foods and liquids from microwave oven as well as scald burns to skin and palate from hot formula.
5. Burns from open flames:
   a. House fires.
   b. Campfires, bonfires, or fire pits.
   c. Child climbing on stove, resulting in ignited clothing.
   d. Children playing with lighters, especially 3- to 10-year-olds.
   e. Playing or working with gasoline.
   f. Automobile accidents with subsequent fire.
   g. Juvenile fire-setters.
6. Electrical burns in children are not as common but most often caused by:
   a. Child playing with electrical outlets or appliances.
   b. Child playing with extension cords; children commonly bite through the cord.
   c. Child playing on railroad tracks; climbing trees and touching high-tension wires; struck by lightning.
7. Other causes:
   a. Caustic acid or alkali burns, often of the mouth and esophagus.
   b. Chemical burns of the skin—child playing with gasoline or chemical cleaning agents.
   c. Burns inflicted on the child as a result of neglect or abuse (immersion and contact burns are most common).
   d. Smoke inhalation and inhalation from products of combustion of synthetics, such as plastics and rayon, may yield cyanide and formaldehyde.
   e. Radiation burns—sunburn most common, may be secondary to cancer radiation therapy.
   f. Contact burns from touching hot surfaces, such as radiators, woodburning stoves, fireplaces, or open ovens.
   g. Fireworks burns, typically as a result of misuse and lack of adult supervision; may be combined with explosive hand injuries.
   h. Friction burns such as those seen with exercise treadmills in the home.

*Please note that the term "male" in this chapter refers to a person assigned male at birth, and the term "female" in this chapter refers to a person assigned female at birth.

CLINICAL JUDGMENT With combined injury, management of trauma takes precedence over the burn.

Pathophysiology and Etiology

See "burns in adults," page 907.

Clinical Manifestations

Characteristics of Burn Wounds

1. See page 912 for characteristics of superficial, partial-thickness, and full-thickness burns.
2. Electrical burns:
   a. Especially of the mouth in a child younger than age 2 years; may chew or suck on live wire.
   b. Are progressive and may take up to 3 weeks to fully manifest the extent of injury.

Symptoms of Shock

Symptoms of hypovolemic shock are dependent upon the size and thickness of the burn. Hypovolemic shock may develop in large surface size burns within the first 1 to 2 hours of the injury.

1. Rapid pulse and low blood pressure (BP).
2. Subnormal temperature.
3. Pallor, cyanosis, and prostration.
4. Failure to recognize parental caregivers or other familiar people.
5. Poor muscle tone and flaccid extremities.

Upper Respiratory Tract Injury

Causes inflammation or edema of the glottis, vocal cords, and upper trachea and is characterized by symptoms of upper airway obstruction and immediate attention to securing and maintaining the airway takes precedence over the burn injury. Signs of inhalation are:

1. Dyspnea, tachypnea, and hoarseness.
2. Stridor, substernal and intercostal retractions, and nasal flaring.
3. Restlessness, drooling, cough, and increasing hoarseness.
4. Carbonaceous sputum.
5. Facial burns and/or edematous lips.
6. Black nasal or oral secretions.
7. Hypoxemia.
8. History of burn within a closed space.

CLINICAL JUDGMENT Increasing hoarseness, drooling, and stridor are leading indicators for immediate intubation.

Smoke Inhalation

Smoke inhalation may cause no initial symptoms other than mild bronchial obstruction during the initial phase after the burn. Within 6 to 48 hours, the child may develop sudden onset of the following conditions:

1. Bronchiolitis.
2. Pulmonary edema (acute respiratory distress syndrome)—of noncardiac origin.
3. Severe airway obstruction. Larger surface area burns and extensive facial burns increase the risk of airway edema.
4. Delayed damage: up to 7 days after the burn injury.

Suspicious Burns in Children

Mechanism of injury is an important assessment when a burn injury involves a child. If the mechanism of injury seems out of proportion to the injuries of the child, notification to law enforcement is mandated by all nursing practice acts. Be alert for the following characteristics that may require further investigation by law enforcement:

1. Burns that are bilateral and symmetrical and have clearly demarcated lines without splash patterns.
2. Burns with specific patterns of household appliances that may have been used for intentional burns (Iron steam holes, flat irons, etc.)
3. History and physical findings inconsistent with the burn injury.
4. Burn injuries incompatible with child's developmental level.
5. Burn to the buttocks, perineum, or genitals.
6. Burns involving immersion into hot water. Typical findings reveal the back of the knees will be spared of burn injury, with entire feet and lower legs burned.
7. Multiple and new and old burns in different stages of healing.
8. Burns that are circular in nature, likely because of cigarette burns.
9. Presence of other nonburn injuries such as bruises, scrapes, or previous fractures.

Diagnostic Evaluation

Calculation of the Burn Area

1. Rule of nines (used in assessment of the extent of burns in adults) has not been proven to be exact when applied to young children; it may be acceptable to use in child older than age 10 years. It is not recommended for hospital use; the Lund and Browder chart is recommended. Total body surface area (TBSA) is based on age, thus compensating for changes in body surface area that change during growth (see Box 51-1).
   a. During infancy and early childhood, the relative surface area of different parts of the body varies with age.
   b. The younger the child, the greater is the proportion of the surface area constituted by the head and the lesser is the proportion of the surface area constituted by the legs.
2. A rough estimate can be obtained by using the child's hand (palm, with fingers extended), which is equal to 1%. First degree burns (only reddened skin) should not be included in calculations of TBSA.

Categorization of Severity of Burn

1. Total area injured, depth of injury, and location of injury.
2. Age of child.
3. Condition of patient (i.e., level of consciousness). Confusion is the hallmark of an anoxic brain.
4. Medical history (i.e., comorbidities, chronic disease).
5. Additional injuries.

Schematic Classification of Burn Severity

1. Minor burn:
   a. Less than 10% TBSA partial thickness burns (Superficial burns are not used in calculations of TBSA).
2. Moderate burn:
   a. More than 5 to less than 20% TBSA; partial thickness burn.
   b. 2% to 5% TBSA; full thickness burn not involving the eyes, ears, face, genitals, hands, or feet, or circumferential burns.
   c. Burns involving the eyes, ears, face, genitals, hands or feet, or circumferential burns.
3. Major burn:
   a. 20% TBSA or greater; partial thickness burn.
   b. All full thickness burns greater than 10% TBSA for patients greater than 10 years of age, Greater than 5% TBSA of full thickness burns to children less than 10 years of age.

BOX 51-1 The Lund and Browder Chart

Area of Body	Relative Percentage of Body Surface (Varies by Age) 0–1 Yr	1–4 Yr	5–9 Yr	10–15 Yr	Adult	Estimated Percentage of Body Area With: 2nd-degree burns	3rd- and 4th-degree burns
Head	19	17	13	10	7		
Neck	2	2	2	2	2		
Anterior trunk	13	13	13	13	13		
Posterior trunk	13	13	13	13	13		
Right buttock	2	2	2	2	2		
Left buttock	2	2	2	2	2		
Genitalia	1	1	1	1	1		
Right upper arm	4	4	4	4	4		
Left upper arm	4	4	4	4	4		
Right lower arm	3	3	3	3	3		
Left lower arm	3	3	3	3	3		
Right hand	2	2	2	2	2		
Left hand	2	2	2	2	2		
Right thigh	5	6	8	8	9		
Left thigh	5	6	8	8	9		
Right lower leg	5	5	5	6	7		
Left lower leg	5	5	5	6	7		
Right foot	3	3	3	3	3		
Left foot	3	3	3	3	3		
					TOTAL:	+	=

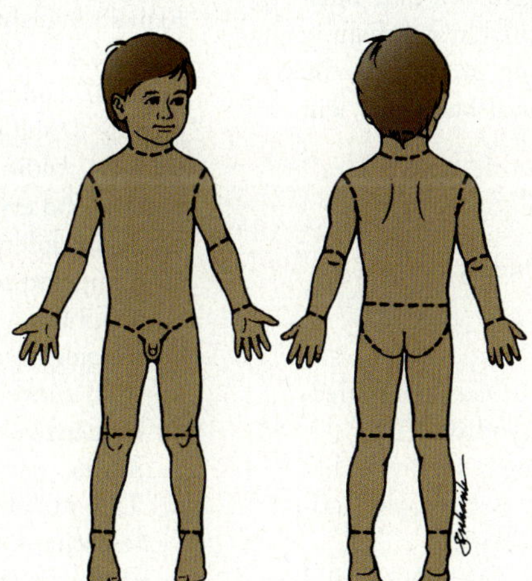

Adapted with permission from Lund, C. C., & Browder, N. C. (1944). The estimation of areas of burns. Surgery, Gynecology and Obstetrics, 79, 352–358.

c. All burns involving the hands, face, eyes, ears, feet, or genitals.
d. All electrical and chemical burns.
e. Complicated burn injuries involving fracture or other major trauma.
f. All poor-risk patients (i.e., head injury, cancer, lung disease, diabetes).

Management

Fluid Resuscitation: Intravenous (IV) Fluid Replacement

Note: Controversy exists regarding fluid resuscitation solution and amount. Not all pediatric patients require fluid resuscitation. Children with burns 15% TBSA or less may be treated with oral rehydration therapies and supplemental maintenance IV fluids.

1. Fluid loss from transcapillary leakage is greatest during the first 12 hours after injury. Fluid loss after 48 hours is due to vaporization of water from the wound.
2. Replacement usually consists of Lactated Ringer (also referred to as Ringers Lactate) solution, an isotonic electrolyte solution. Lactated Ringer solution has a much lower sodium content than 0.9% saline (130 mEq/L vs. 154 mEq/L), has a much higher pH (6.5 vs. 6.0), and has 28 mmol/L of lactate, which is used as a buffering agent.
3. The consensus formula is commonly used to determine the fluid needed for resuscitation for burns greater than 15% TBSA (see page 913). Children up to 30 kg should receive a maintenance containing formula with dextrose to prevent hypoglycemia (5% dextrose or D5LR).
   a. One half of the requirements are given during the first 8 hours.
   b. The remainder is given over the next 16 hours or at a rate adjusted based on clinical presentation of the patient. Fluids should be titrated to meet established resuscitation outcomes.

Burn Treatment

1. Burns are most commonly treated by the closed method. Using the closed method is preferred as it allows children to be more mobile when a burn injury is covered and because they experience less pain.
2. Children should be encouraged to participate with washing off cream whenever possible. A gentle soap or shampoo can be used to wash the nonburned parts of the body and hair. Burned areas are cleaned gently daily with normal saline and gauze.
3. Use pharmaceutical and psychological interventions, unique to each child and appropriate for their developmental stage and comfort needs, to ensure appropriate pain and anxiety management.
4. See page 913 for wound cleaning and debridement, hydrotherapy, topical antimicrobials, surgical management, and burn wound grafting. It is important to use bacitracin ophthalmic ointment on a child's face because touching or rubbing the face may get ointment into the eyes. Topical bacitracin will cause conjunctivitis if it gets into the eyes.

Complications

Vary according to severity of burn injury; commonly occur, especially with severe burn injury.

Acute

1. Infection, burn wound sepsis, pneumonia, urinary tract infection (UTI), and phlebitis, and toxic shock syndrome.
2. Curling (stress) ulcer and GI hemorrhage; rarely seen now that histamine-2 (H_2) blockers are commonly used prophylactically, especially in burns greater than 20% TBSA.
3. Acute gastric dilation, paralytic ileus; occurs especially in child younger than age 2 with greater than 20% injury and develops early in postburn period, lasting 2 to 3 days.
4. Renal failure.
5. Respiratory failure; severe inhalation injury is the insult most likely to cause death.
6. Hypertension.
7. Central nervous system dysfunction.
8. Vascular ischemia.
9. Anxiety and complex pain (acute to chronic presentations).
10. Anemia and malnutrition; may resolve when the burn area is covered.
11. Constipation and fecal impaction.
12. Labile moods secondary to hospitalization, repeated procedures, and changing body image.

Long Term

1. Growth and development delays secondary to malnutrition, hospitalization, and complexities of injury and recovery.
2. Developmental regression.
3. Scarring, disfigurement, and contractures.
4. Impact of psychological trauma.

Nursing Assessment

1. Initially, perform emergency assessment of the burn patient to determine priorities of care.
   a. Airway, breathing, and circulation: airway may be compromised with inhalation injury.
   b. Extent of burn injury.
   c. Additional injuries. (Although establishing a patent airway always comes first, trauma takes precedence over the burn.)
2. Obtain a history of the injury—for example, when the injury occurred; what first aid was given; location of the child; if smoke was present, was child in a closed space; who was supervising the child; what the specific mechanism of injury was; what other factors need to be considered in terms of the context of the injury; and consider if additional injuries may exist.
3. Obtain a complete medical history, including childhood diseases, immunizations (especially tetanus status), current medications, allergies, recent infections, and general health and developmental status.
4. Assess level of pain and emotional status; provide pain relief and reassurance while performing assessment and determining priorities.
5. Subsequently, focus assessment on fluid volume balance, condition of the burn wounds, and signs of infection (burn wound, pulmonary, urinary).
6. Remain vigilant for signs of sepsis. Although not completely supported by all expert clinicians, the American Burn Association 2007 consensus guidelines are the most recent available and provide definitions for sepsis and common infections in burn patients. Additional markers such as procalcitonin, C-reactive protein, and erythrocyte sedimentation rate can be used. Sepsis occurs in children when at least three of the following occur:
   a. Temperature above 102.2°F (39°C) or below 97.7°F (36.5°C).
   b. Progressive tachycardia more than two standard deviations (SD) above age-specific norms.
   c. Progressive tachypnea more than 2 SD above age-specific norms.
   d. Thrombocytopenia (not applicable until 3 days after initial resuscitation) less than 2 SD below age-specific norms.
   e. Hyperglycemia (in the absence of preexisting diabetes mellitus).
      i. Untreated plasma glucose greater than 200 mg/dL.
      ii. Insulin resistance.
   f. Inability to continue enteral feedings for more than 24 hours.
      i. Abdominal distention.
      ii. Enteral feeding intolerance.
      iii. Uncontrollable diarrhea.
7. In addition, it is required that infection be documented by positive culture, pathologic tissue source identified, or clinical response to antimicrobials observed.

EVIDENCE BASE McWilliams, T., Twigg, F., Hendricks, J., Wood, F., Ryan, J., & Keil, A. (2021). The implementation of an infection control bundle within a Total Care Burns Unit. *Burns, 47*(3), 569–575. https://doi.org/10.1016/j.burns.2019.12.012

Williams, F., & Lee, J. (2021). Pediatric burn infection. *Surgical Infections, 22*(1), 54–57. https://doi.org/10.1089/sur.2020.218

Nursing Interventions

Supporting Cardiac Output

1. Be alert to the symptoms of shock that occur shortly after a severe burn—tachycardia, hypothermia, hypotension, pallor, prostration, shallow respirations, and anuria.
2. Monitor the administration of IV fluids because major burns are followed by a reduction in blood volume because of outflow of plasma into the tissues.
3. Maintain and record intake and output to provide an accurate measure of volume.
   a. Record time and amount of all fluids given.
   b. Measure urine output every hour and report diminished output, as ordered (0.5 mL/kg/h is considered minimally acceptable urine output; however, 1 mL/kg/h is preferable).
   c. Check urine specific gravity to determine concentration or dilution.
4. With severe burn injuries and those in the perineal area, insert an indwelling catheter early in care prior to significant swelling.
5. Weigh patient daily to help evaluate fluid balance.
6. Monitor sensorium, pulse, pulse pressure, capillary refill, and blood gas values.
7. Provide a rich oxygen environment to combat hypoxia, as necessary.
8. Monitor electrolyte and hematocrit results as a guide to fluid replacement.
9. Maintain a warm, humidified ambient environment (especially with burns of 20% TBSA) to maintain body temperature and to decrease fluid needs and caloric expenditure.

Preventing Infection

1. Wash hands with antibacterial cleansing agent before and after all patient contact and use appropriate precautions.
   a. Use barrier garments including isolation gown or plastic apron and eye protection—for all care requiring contact with the patient or the patient's bed.
   b. Cover hair and wear mask when wounds are exposed or when performing a sterile procedure.
   c. Use sterile examination gloves for all dressing changes and contact with open wounds. Clean gloves are sufficient for all other patient contact.
2. Be alert for reservoirs of infection and sources of cross-contamination in equipment and assignment of personnel.
3. Observe burn wounds with each dressing change: assess drainage for color, odor, and amount; necrosis; increase in pain; and surrounding erythema, warmth, swelling, and tenderness, which may indicate infection.
4. Administer topical antimicrobials and systemic antibiotics, as ordered.
5. Provide meticulous skin care to prevent infection and promote healing, and to preserve skin integrity of nonburned skin that may be used as donor sites for grafting.
6. Be alert for early signs of septicemia, including changes in mentation, tachypnea, and decreased peristalsis as well as later signs, such as increased pulse, decreased BP, increased or decreased urine output, facial flushing, increased and later decreased temperatures, increasing hyperglycemia, and malaise. Report to health care provider promptly.
7. Obtain urine, sputum, and blood cultures for two or more consecutive temperatures of 103°F (39.4°C) or a single temperature of 104°F (40°C). Additional cultures may be ordered depending on patient condition and institutional policy.
8. Promote optimal personal hygiene for the patient, including daily cleansing of unburned areas, meticulous care of teeth and mouth, shampooing of hair every other day, and meticulous care of IV and urinary catheter sites.
9. Prevent the child from scratching by administering antipruritics and applying protective devices to their hands.
10. Be alert for the development of pneumonia or UTI related to immobility and invasive procedures. Encourage coughing, turning, deep breathing, ambulation, and early discontinuation of indwelling catheter to minimize complications.
11. Ensure that appropriate nutrition and enteral feeding are in place within 6 to 8 hours of injury to prevent translocation of bacteria in the gut.
12. Administer tetanus prophylaxis based on immunization history.
    a. If primary series is complete (or at least three doses of tetanus toxoid are obtained) and last injection was within past 5 years, it is not necessary.
    b. If at least three doses are obtained and last injection was more than 5 years, give tetanus toxoid.
    c. If two or fewer doses are obtained, give tetanus immunoglobulin and tetanus toxoid.

CLINICAL JUDGMENT Even with meticulous skin care, the burn wound is fully colonized in 3 to 5 days. A warm, moist environment becomes an excellent medium for bacterial growth, especially of *Pseudomonas*.

Optimizing Gas Exchange

1. Be alert for and report symptoms of respiratory distress—dyspnea, stridor, tachypnea, restlessness, cyanosis, coughing, increasing hoarseness, and drooling.
2. Younger children, those with larger burn injuries, and those with extensive facial burns are at higher risk of airway compromise from edema.
3. Administer supplemental humidified oxygen as ordered.
4. Monitor arterial blood gas (ABG) levels as necessary.
5. Evaluate the carboxyhemoglobin on ABG results (because of inhalation of carbon monoxide, a product of combustion) and be prepared to support ventilation if signs of hypoxemia and respiratory failure develop.
6. Assist with pulmonary function and bronchoscopy, as indicated.
7. Have intubation supplies readily available. If unable to intubate the child, then tracheostomy may be necessary. If unable to extubate in 14 to 21 days, then may be converted to tracheostomy for continuous pulmonary management. The current trend is to use the earlier time frame.
8. Prevent atelectasis and pneumonia through chest physical therapy, postural drainage, meticulous pulmonary technique, and, if indicated, tracheostomy care.

Ensuring Adequate Nutrition for Healing and Growth Needs

1. Be aware that hypernutrition is important because of the extreme hypermetabolism related to large burn injuries.
   a. Twice the predicted basal metabolic rate in calories, based on ideal weight, may be necessary. Caloric recommendation is 1,800 kcal/m^2 total body surface for maintenance, plus 2,000 kcal/m^2 of burned surface area.
   b. Hypermetabolic state may persist even after the majority of the wounds are grafted or closed.
   c. High caloric intake to support hypermetabolic state; protein synthesis; calories should come from both protein and carbohydrates.
   d. High-protein intake to replace protein lost by exudation; support synthesis of immunoglobulins and structural protein; prevent negative nitrogen balance.
   e. Vitamin and mineral supplement needed, particularly vitamins B and C, iron, and zinc. These may be found in nutritionally complete enteral feedings.
2. Maintain ambient temperature at 82.4°F to 90°F (28°C to 32.2°C) to minimize metabolic expenditure by maintaining core temperature.
3. Minimize anorexia to increase caloric intake.
   a. Offer small amounts of food, perhaps four to five feedings rather than three per day.
   b. Give choice of foods; determine favorites.
   c. Provide high-calorie, high-protein oral or nasogastric (NG) supplementation, as necessary.
   d. Consider long-term use of gastrostomy (G)-tube or nasojejunal (NJ) tube for supplemental nutrition.
   e. Make meals a pleasant time, unassociated with treatments or unpleasant interruptions. Maintain oral intake as much as possible.
4. Monitor dietary adherence to dietary goals and adjust, as needed.
5. Administer total parenteral nutrition, if necessary.
6. Administer serum albumin or fresh frozen plasma to combat hypoalbuminemia when burn area exceeds 20% TBSA.
7. Monitor nutritional status through weight gain, wound healing, serum transferrin, and serum albumin.

Relieving Gastric Dilation and Preventing Stress Ulcer

1. Be alert for the development of gastric distention, especially with burns greater than 20% TBSA, associated injury, or tachypnea.
2. Maintain nothing-by-mouth status if distention or decreased bowel sounds develop.
   - Insert NG tube, as indicated, to prevent vomiting, aspiration, and paralytic ileus.
3. Monitor the return of bowel sounds after NG extubation and before reinstituting oral feeding.
4. Administer H_2 blockers or proton pump inhibitors as ordered to prevent ulcer development.

Promoting Peripheral Perfusion

1. Remove all jewelry and clothing.
2. Elevate extremities.
3. Monitor peripheral pulses hourly. Use Doppler, as ordered.
4. Prepare the patient for escharotomy if circulation is impaired.
5. Avoid tight constrictive dressings.
6. Observe for and report signs of thrombophlebitis or catheter-induced infections.

Facilitating Fluid Balance

1. Titrate fluid intake to achieve clinical goals established by treatment team. The initial resuscitation formula is only a guide.
2. Maintain accurate intake and output records.
3. Weigh the patient per institutional policy. Trending weights should be evaluated at least weekly.
4. Monitor results of serum potassium and other electrolytes.
5. Be alert to signs of fluid overload, especially during initial fluid resuscitation and immediately afterward, when fluid mobilization is occurring.
6. Administer diuretics, as ordered.

Protecting and Reestablishing Skin Integrity

1. Cleanse wounds and change dressings once or twice daily. The size of the burn and the stage of wound healing can be considered when determining the frequency of dressing changes. Use an antimicrobial solution or mild soap and water, rinsing well. Dry gently. This may be done in the hydrotherapy tank, in the bathtub, in the shower, or at the bedside.
2. Perform debridement of dead tissue at this time. May use gauze, scissors, or forceps, as appropriate. Try to limit time to 20 to 30 minutes depending on the patient's tolerance. Additional analgesia may be necessary. Consider having an appropriate time interval to premedicate before debridement for best pain management.
3. Apply topical bacteriostatic agents, as directed. Cream or ointment is applied ⅛-in (3-mm) thick.
4. Dress wounds, as appropriate, using conventional burn pads, gauze rolls, or any combination. Dressings may be held in place, as necessary, with gauze rolls or netting.
5. For grafted areas, use extreme caution in removing dressings; observe for and report serous or sanguineous blebs or purulent drainage. Redress grafted areas according to facility protocol.
6. Observe all wounds daily and document wound status on the patient's record.
7. Promote healing of donor sites by:
   a. Preventing contamination of donor sites that are clean wounds.
   b. Opening to air for drying postoperatively if gauze or impregnated gauze dressing is used. If exudate occurs after the first 24 hours, swab the area for culture and apply an antimicrobial topical cream. If the culture is positive, treatment will be in accord with sensitivities.
   c. Following health care provider's or manufacturer's instructions for care of sites dressed with synthetic materials.
   d. Allowing dressing to peel off spontaneously.
   e. Cleansing healing donor site with mild soap and water when dressings are removed; lubricating site twice daily and as needed.
8. Inspect unburned skin carefully for signs of pressure and breakdown.

Preventing Urinary Infection

1. Maintain closed urinary drainage system and ensure patency. Use a catheter impregnated with an antimicrobial agent whenever possible.
2. Frequently observe color, clarity, and amount of urine.
3. Empty drainage bag per facility protocol.
4. Provide catheter care per facility protocol.
5. Encourage removal of catheter as soon as hourly urine output determinations are not required.

Promoting Stable Body Temperature

1. Be efficient in care; do not expose wounds unnecessarily.
2. Maintain warm ambient temperatures.
3. Use radiant warmers, warming blankets, or adjustment of the bed temperature to keep the patient warm.
4. Obtain urine, sputum, and blood cultures for temperatures above 102°F (38.9°C) rectal or core temperature.
5. Provide a dry top layer for wet dressings to reduce evaporative heat loss.
6. Warm wound cleansing and dressing solutions to body temperature.
7. Use blankets in transporting patient to other areas of the hospital.
8. Administer antipyretics, as prescribed.

Preserving Mobility

1. Make sure that physical and occupational therapy are begun early to facilitate rehabilitation.
2. Child Life Professionals can also assist in making therapy and routines child-friendly, thereby increasing the child's participation and ultimately preserving and improving mobility.
3. Encourage range-of-motion exercises, ambulation, and position changes to minimize joint and skin complications.
4. Position joint in opposite direction of expected contracture. Reassess positioning regularly; reconfigure patient room or positioning of bed or television to encourage different positions if patient is bedridden.
5. Apply splints to aid joint positioning and decrease skin contractures and hypertrophy.
6. Apply pressure garments to aid circulation, protect newly healed skin, and prevent and treat hypertrophic scar formation by promoting dermal collagen fiber growth in parallel direction. Encourage the use of pressure garments for as long as 12 to 18 months after injury, until the healed skin has matured.
7. Medicate for pain before therapy or exercise to minimize discomfort.
8. Use play opportunities to help the child accept the therapy program (e.g., tricycle riding may be used as a form of exercise).

Controlling Pain

EVIDENCE BASE Gillum, M., Huang, S., Kuromaru, Y., Dang, J., Yenikomshian, H., & Gillenwater, T. J. (2022). Nonpharmacologic management of procedural pain in pediatric burn patients: A systematic review of randomized controlled trials. *Journal of Burn Care & Research*, *43*(2), 368–373. https://doi.org/10.1093/jbcr/irab167

Addab, S., Hamdy, R., Thorstad, K., Le May, S., & Tsimicalis, A. (2022). Use of virtual reality in managing paediatric procedural pain and anxiety: An integrative literature review. *Journal of Clinical Nursing*, *31*(21/22), 3032–3059. https://doi.org/10.1111/jocn.16217

1. Assess for signs of pain, such as irritability, crying, increased BP, tachycardia, decreased mobility, and inability to sleep using reliable and valid assessment measures.
2. Use principles of the World Health Organization analgesic ladder using combinations of analgesic where one type is ineffective alone until pain relief is achieved.
   a. Step 1: Nonopioids.
   b. Step 2: Mild opioids.
   c. Step 3: Strong opioids.
3. Acetaminophen has been shown to safely manage background pain in pediatric burns and is considered the first step in managing such pain.
4. Regular nonsteroidal anti-inflammatory drugs should also be prescribed unless contraindicated.
5. Opioid analgesia is the gold standard for burn pain and should be dosed for each individual with concurrent laxative treatment provided. Strong (morphine) opioids should be considered for severe pain. Codeine is no longer recommended for pediatric pain management. Oxycodone may be used for moderate pain.
6. In severe burns, analgesia should be given via IV line because of lack of absorption of IM injections during the emergency phase. Emphasis is on maintaining an alert, reasonably comfortable child. Monitor child closely when using IV opioids and sedatives.
7. Other adjunctive medications, such as antiemetics and sedatives, should be considered to increase comfort and decrease distress.
8. The use of benzodiazepines for continuous infusions in the severely burned child should be approached with caution. Although more research is needed in the pediatric population, there is significant evidence that the development of delirium in mechanically ventilated adult patients is associated with benzodiazepine administration.
9. Use a therapeutic surface to relieve pressure and provide comfort.
10. Maintain warmth and prevent chilling.
11. Provide diversional activities appropriate for age to distract from focus on pain.
12. Teach simple relaxation techniques, such as relaxation breathing and guided imagery.
13. Recognize that fear may exacerbate discomfort; assess anxiety and child temperament. Provide reassurance and empathy. Develop a plan to minimize anxiety and fear. Collaborate with other health care professionals, such as a Child Life therapist.
14. Ensure an adequate sleep routine and establish good sleep hygiene as possible to minimize sleep disturbances.

Addressing Body Image Disturbance

1. Encourage the child to talk about the way they feel and look; let the child set the pace for discussions.
   a. The child may feel guilty and think that the burn is a punishment for some wrong deed.
   b. Small children may be fearful of the appearance of bandages, scars, or pressure garments; offer reassurance.
   c. Encourage the use of play with dolls or puppets, role-playing, or picture drawing to help the child express feelings and fears.
2. Treat the child with warmth and affection and encourage parental caregivers to continually express their love and provide physical and emotional comfort.
3. Support child in viewing self in a mirror when ready and encourage the presence of family members.
4. Encourage early contact with other children. Maintain connections with siblings, friends, and community where possible.
5. Suggest psychiatric consultation and work with psychosocial resources for anticipatory guidance and ongoing adjustment and adaptation to burn injury. Specific requests may be related to heightened anxiety, alterations in mood, or problems manifesting as:
   a. Refusal to eat.
   b. Developmental regression.

c. Resistance to procedures.
d. Aggressive behaviors, excessive sadness, or withdrawal.
e. Increasing isolation or resisting socialization.

6. Advise parental caregivers that returning to home and community routines and separation from the hospital environment, caregivers, and other patients can produce excessive anxiety or disruption in the child's coping.
7. If the child is school age, help prepare for school reentry; contact teacher or discuss with parental caregivers the need to prepare peers for what to expect.
8. Discuss and plan for issues of social reentry, such as responding to questions and stares from strangers and perceived rejection by friends.
   a. Ensure enrollment in an aftercare (follow-up) program, ideally one that is targeted at both child and family adjustment.
   b. Refer to a support group or peer mentor where possible.
   c. Refer to a burn camp—usually this may be the first opportunity for the child to wear a swimsuit after the injury.
9. Initiate family consultation with a plastic surgeon about future scar revision.
10. Encourage the older child to engage in long-term follow-up to address issues of concern as they arise at various developmental stages. Some children and teens may wish to experiment with clothing and consult with a burn cosmetic specialist to enhance appearance and body image.

Reducing Fear and Anxiety

1. Explain procedures, surgeries, and treatments to the child according to age and level of understanding.
2. Allow the child to express fears through puppets, dolls, water play, clay, and drawings.
3. Expect regression because of the physical pain and psychological trauma the child is experiencing.
4. Encourage parental caregivers to stay with a young child as much as possible.
5. Teach parental caregivers how to engage their child to foster development of coping skills.
6. Encourage involvement with treatment plan and self-care activities.

Promoting Effective Caregiving

1. Be alert to signs of depression or stress syndromes in parental caregivers and encourage counseling for them to promote a healthier family.
2. Encourage parental caregivers to assess the effects on siblings at home; they may have needs that are unrecognized or neglected as a result of this crisis.
3. Attempt to have parental caregivers become actively involved in the child's care when they are ready to do so.
   a. Provide training for parental caregivers to effectively participate in treatments and respect their wishes not to participate if the situation is too distressful—the focus for parental caregivers is on their ability to comfort their child.
   b. Advise parental caregivers that their visits and involvement can have a positive effect on the child's survival and recovery.
   c. If the parental caregivers are unable to visit, telephone calls and family photographs are helpful. New technologies like videoconferencing can also be helpful to maintain connections with family and community supports.
4. Give the parental caregivers the opportunity to discuss their feelings.
   a. Parental caregivers commonly express guilt regarding their lack of supervision when the accident occurred.
   b. Typically, burn injury is associated with actual or perceived parental neglect. Remember that this type of injury is sudden and acute, placing the family in a state of crisis.
5. Keep the parental caregivers informed of the child's progress.
   a. Begin initial teaching at admission with supportive words and limited technical information.
   b. Education and orientation to the facility and the burn injury will decrease some anxiety and begin to build rapport on which future support can be based.
   c. Encourage meetings with other parental caregivers who have coped with trauma.
   d. Refer families for aftercare programs intended to support adjustment over time.

Sleep Pattern Disturbance

1. Allow a parental caregiver to stay with the patient.
2. Provide a structured environment. Perform dressing changes, therapy, and meals at the same time daily.
3. Combine interventions so that child can get longest possible intervals of uninterrupted sleep.
4. Minimize noise and lights within the room.
5. Ensure adequate pain relief and comfort measures at bedtime or naptime.

Community and Home Care Considerations

1. Make routine home visits to perform, teach, and supervise burn wound care and rehabilitation program.
2. Inspect the wounds for signs of infection at every visit.
3. Assess coping ability of child and family to care for child and provide psychological support and counseling referrals, as needed.
4. Ensure that parental caregivers can:
   a. Discuss and demonstrate treatments, procedures, and dressing changes.
   b. Obtain equipment necessary to perform treatment at home.
   c. Understand reason for and adverse effects of medications as well as dietary requirements.
   d. Follow up at appropriate intervals with the designated health care provider.
5. Encourage the use of smoke alarms on every floor in the home, a fire extinguisher, and an emergency fire escape plan. Assist parental caregivers to review strategies for childhood safety.

Family Education and Health Maintenance

1. Teach the family that special skin care is necessary after burn injury.
   a. Avoid exposure to sunlight; use sunscreen with sun protection factor (SPF) 30 or higher and apply frequently.
   b. Use pressure garments to prevent hypertrophic scar formation—worn 23 of 24 hours each day for effectiveness for 1 to 2 years depending on the maturation of the scar.
   c. Use lotions and creams to prevent skin from drying, cracking, and itching; topical or oral antihistamines or antipruritics may be necessary to reduce itching.
   d. Burn area has decreased sensation to touch, heat, and pressure; take precautions to prevent injury to the area.
2. Advise the family that adjustment after burn is usually prolonged and challenging. Adjustment can ebb and flow with

developmental stages. Encourage ongoing family and individual psychological and social support.
3. Encourage continued physical therapy to prevent and minimize contractures and preserve function.
4. Monitor outcomes over time in keeping with the Health Outcomes Burn Questionnaire for infants and children 5 years of age and younger; burn size and visible scarring are not predictive of psychological adaptation.
5. Initiate home health, psychiatric referral, physical and occupational therapy, financial assistance, and other referrals, as necessary.
6. Teach parental caregivers and children the prevention of burn injury as well as other safety measures (see page 918).
7. Teach first aid emergency care for burn injury (i.e., cool burned area with cool water, remove clothing, seek medical assistance).
8. Avoid the use of ice in emergency care of burns.
9. Teach children how to stop, drop, and roll if their clothes catch fire, and how to crawl to safety if a fire occurs in the house.

Evaluation: Expected Outcomes

- Absence of shock: stabilization of vital signs and normal serum and electrolyte values.
- Absence of infection: normal laboratory values, clean wound, and normal temperature.
- No respiratory distress: stable vital signs, respiratory status, and ABG levels.
- Adequate nutritional status: weight gain and wound healing.
- No GI complications: normal bowel sounds and ability to tolerate oral feeding.
- Tissue perfusion.
- No signs of fluid overload and weight stable.
- Donor site and burn wounds healing without signs of infection.
- Urine output adequate via catheter.
- Temperature remains below 102°F (38.9°C).
- Improved mobility: involved in play and other activities.
- Minimal discomfort: stable vital signs, verbalization, and involved in play.
- Positive body image: verbalization, socialization, and ability to look in the mirror.
- Relief of fear: able to play and participates in care.
- Effective caregiving: involved in child's care, accurate discussion of child's progress, and treatment plan.
- Sleeping between treatments through the night and napping for 1-hour intervals during the day.

DERMATOLOGIC DISORDERS

Atopic Dermatitis (Infantile and Childhood Eczema)

Atopic dermatitis, the most common cause of eczema in childhood, is a highly pruritic chronic inflammatory skin disorder affecting up to 40% of the pediatric population. Peak prevalence is age 6 months to 8 to 10 years. Many children with atopic dermatitis develop asthma or allergic rhinitis and have a personal or family history of disorders in the atopic triad (allergic rhinitis, asthma, and atopic dermatitis).

Atopic dermatitis (Figure 51-1) has a typical age-related morphology and distribution and a chronic or chronically relapsing nature. The appearance and location of the lesions change with age in a characteristic manner. Atopic dermatitis usually improves or resolves by adolescence but can persist in some form throughout adulthood.

Pathophysiology and Etiology

1. Although it has both immunologic and genetic components, the etiology of atopic dermatitis is unknown. Approximately 80% of children with atopic dermatitis have elevated immunoglobulin (Ig) E levels and increased rates of sensitization to common allergens. Histamine release from basophils is increased, and hyperreactive cutaneous T cells, which secrete proinflammatory cytokines, cause increased Th2 and decreased Th1 cytokine responses. There is also a hereditary component. When both biological parents have a history of atopic dermatitis, there is an 80% chance a child will be affected. When only one biological parent is affected, the prevalence drops to 50%. A number of genes have been tentatively linked to atopic dermatitis.
2. Atopic dermatitis causes breakdown of the stratum corneum, which allows allergens and bacteria to penetrate deeper layers, causing inflammation and possible infection.
3. Atopic dermatitis is known as the "itch that rashes." The skin is dry and becomes pruritic when exposed to common environmental allergens, such as wool; occlusive synthetic fabrics, soaps, and detergents; perspiration; extremes of temperature and humidity; and emotional stress.
4. Food allergies contribute to atopic dermatitis in up to 30% of infants and very young children with moderate to severe disease. Eggs, milk, peanut, soy, wheat, tree nuts, fish, and shellfish account for more than 90% of the reactions. The most common offender is eggs.

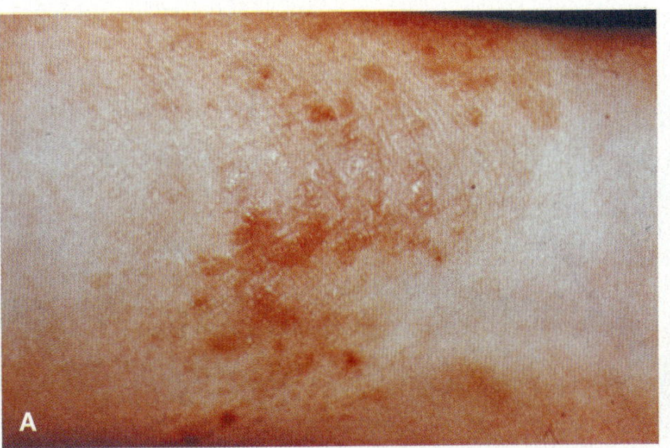

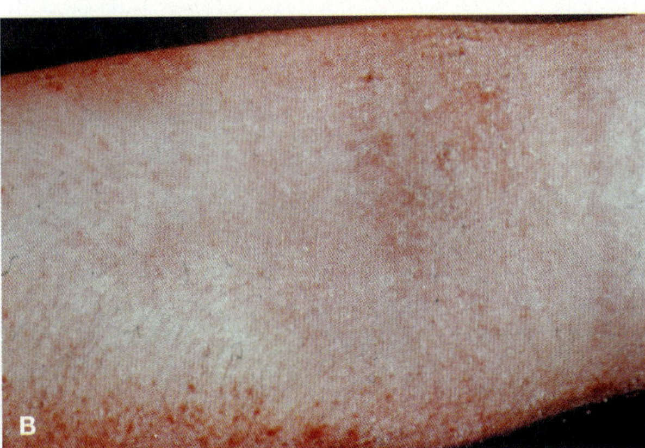

Figure 51-1. **(A)** Acute atopic dermatitis. **(B)** Chronic atopic dermatitis.

BOX 51-2 Clinical Criteria for Atopic Dermatitis

Major Features: Three or More

- Pruritus.
- Eczematous changes.
- Typical and age-specific morphology and location.
- Face, neck, and extensor surfaces in infants/children.
- Flexural lesions in older children/adults.
- Chronicity or chronically relapsing.
- Personal or family history of atopy (allergic rhinitis, asthma, atopic dermatitis).

Minor Features: Three or More

- Early age of onset.
- Elevated serum immunoglobulin E.
- Itching with sweating.
- Intolerance to wool and lipid solvents.
- Immediate (type 1) skin test reactivity.
- Tendency toward skin infections.
- Facial pallor or erythema.
- Food intolerance.
- Xerosis (very dry skin).
- Ichthyosis/palmar hyperlinearity/keratosis pilaris.
- Hand or foot dermatitis.
- Pityriasis alba (white patches on the face).
- Conjunctivitis.
- Severity of symptoms influenced by environmental or emotional factors.

5. One third to one half of children with atopic dermatitis are allergic to house dust mites, animal dander, weeds, and molds.
6. Children with atopic dermatitis are at increased risk for developing allergic rhinitis or asthma, known as the "atopic march" or "atopic triad."

Clinical Manifestations

Age and Distribution of Lesions

See Box 51-2.

Atopic dermatitis is divided into three phases based on the age of the patient and the distribution of the lesions. These are referred to as the infant, childhood, and adult phases.

1. Infant (ages 2 months to 3 years):
   a. The onset is between ages 2 and 6 months. One half of affected infants have spontaneous resolution by age 2 or 3 years.
   b. Characterized by intense itching, erythema, papules, vesicles, oozing, and crusting (see Figure 51-2).
   c. The rash usually begins on the cheeks, forehead, or scalp and then extends to the trunk or extremities in scattered, commonly symmetric patches. The perioral, paranasal, and diaper areas are usually spared (see Figure 51-3).
2. Childhood (ages 4 to 10 years):
   a. Affected people in this age group are less likely to have exudative and crusted lesions. Eruptions are characteristically more dry and papular and commonly occur as circumscribed scaly patches. There is a greater tendency toward chronicity and lichenification.
   b. The typical areas of involvement are the face, including the perioral and paranasal areas, neck, antecubital and popliteal fossae, wrists, and ankles. May have severe pruritus.
3. Adult (puberty to old age):
   a. Predominant areas of involvement include the flexor folds, face, neck, upper arms, back, dorsa of the hands and feet, fingers, and toes.
   b. The eruption appears as thick, dry lesions, confluent papules, and large lichenified plaques. Weeping, crusting, and exudation can occur, but they are usually the result of superimposed external irritation or infection.

Diagnostic Evaluation

1. There is no single clinical, laboratory, or histologic marker that will definitively diagnose atopic dermatitis. It is a clinical diagnosis based on the evaluation of the aggregate of signs, symptoms, stigmata, course, and associated familial findings. The presence of pruritus, recurring symptoms, and age-specific morphology and distribution is the most important diagnostic feature. Several sets of clinical diagnostic criteria have been established; the common criteria include pruritus, eczematous changes, xerosis, and personal or family history of atopy.
2. Although not diagnostic for atopic dermatitis, prick skin testing, patch testing, and radioallergosorbent test may be helpful in the identification of food and aeroallergen triggers in infants and young children with moderate to severe disease. Negative skin prick sensitivity tests eliminate the possibility of IgE-mediated food allergy. Positive tests, which predict 30% to 50% of food allergies, may be useful. To avoid unnecessary dietary restrictions, positive tests can be confirmed by controlled food challenges, elimination diets, or atopy patches.

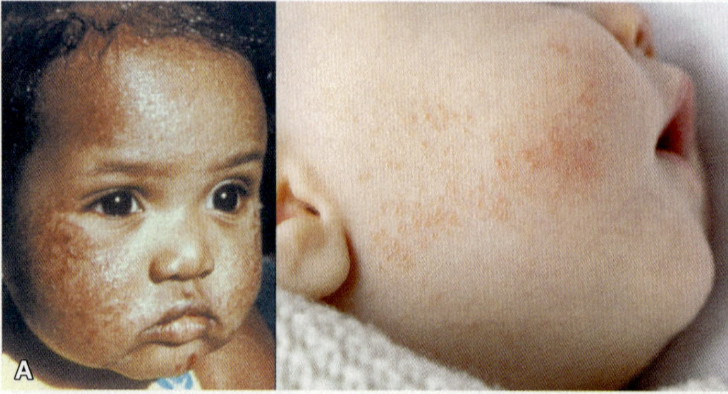

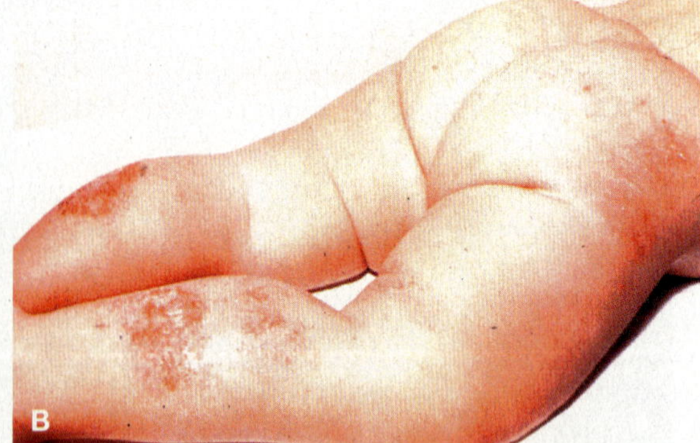

Figure 51-2. Characteristic rash of infant atopic dermatitis of the head **(A)** and of the limbs **(B)**. (**A:** Shutterstock/Olekon.)

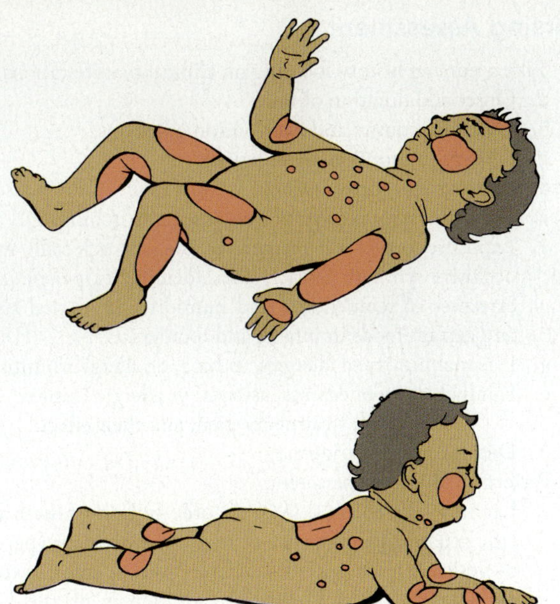

Figure 51-3. Distribution of infant atopic dermatitis occurs primarily on the face but may develop on symmetrical areas of the body. Diaper areas are usually clear.

Management

EVIDENCE BASE Magin, P., & Fisher, K. (2023). Online behavioural interventions for children and young people with atopic eczema: Refining the way forward. *British Journal of Dermatology, 188*(4), 453. https://doi.org/10.1093/bjd/ljac165

Daily skin care is the cornerstone of prevention and treatment, including proper cleansing, frequent moisturizing (at least daily and especially after bathing), trigger avoidance and correct use of medications. Topical medications should be applied directly to damp skin, followed by emollients. Secondary infections should be evaluated and treated promptly.

DRUG ALERT Topical corticosteroids of adequate strength should be used two times per day for a specific length of time, such as 7 to 21 days, to achieve control and avoid adverse effects. Apply the least potent topical corticosteroid that provides adequate control. Group 1 is the most potent class of topical corticosteroids and is avoided in children younger than age 12 because of greater skin absorption and greater risk of side effects. Long-term use of topical corticosteroids can cause striae, cutaneous atrophy, telangiectasia, acne, growth retardation, adrenal suppression, Cushing syndrome, and cataracts.

Although topical corticosteroids, and then topical calcineurin inhibitors (tacrolimus 0.03% ointment and pimecrolimus 1% cream) in the early 2000s, have been the mainstay of medication therapy for atopic dermatitis, the number of medications approved by the U.S. Food and Drug Administration (FDA) to treat atopic dermatitis has grown rapidly since the late 2010s. Perhaps one of the safest topical medications available (the only known adverse effect being application site stinging) is crisaborole ointment, which is FDA-approved for mild-moderate atopic dermatitis in patients aged 3 months and older. Ruxolitinib cream is also FDA-approved for children as young as 12 years old for mild-moderate atopic dermatitis (treatment area should not exceed 20% BSA).

Systemic medications that are FDA-approved for atopic dermatitis in children include dupilumab for patients as young as 6 months old and janus-associated kinase (JAK) inhibitors for patients as young as 12 years old. Administered subcutaneously every 2 to 4 weeks, dupilumab is a monoclonal antibody that decreases inflammation and modulates immune responses via interleukin-4/13 inhibition. Oral JAK inhibitor medications abrocitinib and upadacitinib have been most recently approved for treating atopic dermatitis and found to be especially helpful in lessening the itch experienced by patients.

DRUG ALERT JAK inhibitors have been FDA-approved for use in rheumatic illness for over 20 years and carry boxed warnings (increased risk of serious infection, major adverse cardiovascular events and mortality, malignancy, and thrombosis) related to studies conducted in populations of people older than age 50 with rheumatic illness who smoked and had at least one cardiovascular risk factor. The same degree of risk is not being found in more recent studies with the newer JAK inhibitors in patients with atopic dermatitis. Nonetheless, careful screening prior to treatment, and close monitoring for infection, cardiovascular health, thrombosis, and malignancy throughout the course of therapy, are required.

Complications and nursing implications are similar across populations as discussed in Chapter 29.

EVIDENCE BASE The following websites are excellent resources for factual, reliable information for health care providers, patients, and families.

Pediatric Dermatology Websites:
American Academy of Pediatrics (aap.org)
Contemporary Pediatrics (contemporarypediatrics.com/clinical/dermatology)
International Society of Pediatric Dermatology (ispedderm.com/)
Pediatric Dermatology Research Alliance (https://pedraresearch.org/)
The Society for Pediatric Dermatology (pedsderm.net/)

Acute

1. Open, wet dressings, such as Burow solution, for 1 to 3 days.
2. Avoidance of known allergen or trigger. Atopic dermatitis patients have decreased threshold to irritants.
3. Management of secondary infection.
4. Topical corticosteroids:
   a. Topical corticosteroids are the mainstay of drug therapy. These agents are ranked into seven groups according to potency. Group 1 contains the most potent topical steroids and group 7 the least potent agents. The concentration listed on the medication does not correlate with its potency or safety but is merely a statement of its specific chemical formulation. Adverse effects are related to the potency rating of the compound, the duration of use, and the thickness of the skin to which it is applied.
   b. Group 1 topical corticosteroids are avoided in children younger than age 12 because of greater skin absorption.
5. Oral medications to relieve itching—hydroxyzine, diphenhydramine, or promethazine—often are sedating. Mild sedation may be desirable to allow sleep.

Subacute and Chronic

1. Prevention of dry skin:
   a. Reduce the frequency and duration of bathing.
   b. Use mild soap or hydrophilic cleanser.
   c. Lubricate the skin with emollients. Apply within 3 minutes after exiting bath. Apply over, not under, topical corticosteroids. Newer barrier repair moisturizers contain the skin lipid ceramides and help rebuild/repair skin. (Some over-the-counter products are CeraVe, Cetaphil Restoraderm, and Eucerin Professional Repair.)
   d. Maintain environmental humidity above 40% during winter months.
   e. Tar preparations may be added to bath water; however, they are rarely used because of odor and staining.
2. Avoidance of known allergens or triggers.
3. Management of secondary infection.
4. Topical corticosteroids as described above. Apply the least potent topical corticosteroid that provides adequate control. Topical corticosteroids may be applied under occlusion, which is under plastic wrap to increase absorption, for short-term therapy.
5. Topical immunomodulators, also called *calcineurin inhibitors*, are approved for the short-term and intermittent long-term treatment of subacute and chronic atopic dermatitis for patients age 2 and older when conventional therapies are inadvisable, ineffective, or not tolerated.
   a. Tacrolimus 0.03% ointment and pimecrolimus 1% cream.
   b. These agents do not cause skin atrophy (which corticosteroids may cause) and can be used on the face and neck.
   c. Active viral, bacterial, or fungal skin infections must be cleared before use.
   d. Topical immunomodulators should be discontinued if lymphadenopathy of unknown etiology develops.
6. Phosphodiesterase-4 (PDE4) inhibitor is the newest class of topical medications approved for treatment of mild to moderate atopic dermatitis in patients 2 years and older.
   a. Crisaborole 2% ointment.
   b. Considered relatively safe as the only known adverse effect is application site burning or stinging that resolves after the first 1 to 2 days of use.
   c. No contraindications (except hypersensitivity reaction).

DRUG ALERT The U.S. Food and Drug Administration issued a boxed warning for *calcineurin inhibitors* stating long-term safety has not been established. Although causal relationship has not been proven, rare cases of malignancy (skin and lymphoma) have been reported. Drugs should be used for short-term, second-line therapy for patients over 2 years of age.

Complications

1. Increased risk of secondary infection by bacterial, viral, or fungal agents. Bacterial infections are typically caused by *Staphylococcus aureus*. Rate of infection with methicillin-resistant *S. aureus* is increasing. Infections secondary to papillomaviruses (warts), *Molluscum contagiosum*, herpes simplex, tinea, and candida are more common.
2. Adverse effects from topical corticosteroids (folliculitis, skin atrophy) or topical immunomodulators (local reactions, acne).

Nursing Assessment

1. Take a nursing history focusing on clinical manifestations:
   a. Onset and duration of rash.
   b. Location, course, and distribution of lesions.
   c. Change in morphology of lesions.
   d. Previous episodes of rashes.
   e. Local and systemic symptoms, especially itching.
   f. Exposure to possible allergens or triggers, especially wool, occlusive synthetic fabrics, soaps, detergents, perspiration, extremes of temperature and humidity, emotional stress, and certain foods in infants and toddlers.
   g. Personal history of allergies, asthma, or allergic rhinitis.
   h. Family history of eczema, asthma, or allergic rhinitis.
   i. Medications, treatments tried, and their effect.
   i. Diet for possible triggers.
2. Perform a physical assessment.
   a. Examine the entire skin in an orderly fashion with specific attention to the type of lesion (i.e., macule, papule, or vesicle), its appearance (shape, border, color, texture, and surface), and its distribution (areas of the body involved).
   b. Note associated symptoms, such as scratching, fever, or drainage.
   c. Assess patient for signs of other atopic disorders, including nasal congestion, mouth breathing, cough, or wheezing.
   d. Palpate for lymphadenopathy.
3. Document findings:
   a. Describe skin findings using dermatologic terminology.
   b. Draw pictures to facilitate communication.
   c. Document the presence or absence of associated signs or symptoms.

Nursing Interventions

The nurse may perform the following interventions or teach patient and/or family to do them.

Improving Skin Integrity

1. Reduce inflammation during the acute stage with the topical application of open wet dressings.
   a. Use a soft, lightweight cloth, such as a handkerchief, a thin cloth diaper, or strips of bed sheeting. Do not use gauze (adheres to skin), washcloths, or towels (too heavy). Warm moist pajamas layered under dry pajamas are effective and soothing.
   b. Open wet dressings should be clean. In certain situations, they should be sterile to prevent contamination.
   c. Solutions should be lukewarm or at body temperature to soothe the skin and prevent chilling.
   d. Compresses should be moderately wet, not dripping, and removed after 20 minutes, unless otherwise directed. They should be reapplied three to four times per day.
   e. After the compress, a topical corticosteroid may be applied to further reduce itching and inflammation.
   f. Observe the skin for changes in response to therapy.
2. Prevent dry skin during the subacute and chronic stages.
   a. Decrease the frequency and duration of bathing. Long, hot tub baths should be avoided.
   b. Avoid hot water and harsh soaps. Patients should bathe in lukewarm water using mild soap with a neutral pH (e.g., Dove, Neutrogena); avoid bubble baths; rinse well and pat skin dry with towel.

c. If bath water stings, add 1 cup of table salt.
d. Apply unscented emollients (e.g., Eucerin, Keri, Aquaphor, and Lubriderm) within 3 minutes of bathing, when the skin is still slightly moist. Apply over topical medications. This traps water in the skin. Creams and ointments are more effective than lotions because they are better at preventing evaporation of water from the skin.
e. Some patients may benefit from soaking in a tar bath for 15 to 20 minutes daily, preferably in the evening. Add to bath water as directed. Instructions must include the ability to stain the skin and clothing and cause sunlight sensitivity.
f. For patients with extremely dry skin, clean with a hydrophilic cleanser (e.g., Cetaphil). Apply without water until light foam occurs. Remove by wiping with soft cotton cloth or cleansing tissue.
g. Keep environmental humidity above 40% during winter months. Use a humidifier.
h. Observe the skin for changes in response to therapy.

CLINICAL JUDGMENT Apply unscented emollients to the skin within 3 minutes of bathing when the skin has been patted dry but is still moist to maintain a high level of hydration to the epidermis.

Patient and Caregiver Education to Improve Avoidance of Triggering Factors

1. Follow recommended guidelines related to preventing food allergies.
   a. Encourage breastfeeding during the first 6 months. For infants not breastfed, extensively or partially hydrolyzed formulas (Nutramigen, Alimentum) are preferable to cow's milk formula.
   b. Follow the current American Academy of Pediatrics guidelines related to timing of the introduction of new foods, especially dairy, eggs, peanuts, tree nuts, seafood, and other highly allergenic foods.
2. Eliminate trigger foods for infants and toddlers with known or suspected food allergies.
   a. Observe skin for flare-ups after exposure to potential allergens.
   b. Suggest referral to allergy specialist for infants and young children with moderate to severe atopic dermatitis.
   c. Be aware of the results of skin prick sensitivity, patch testing, or blood testing.
   d. Record known allergens on chart and care plan.
   e. Notify dietary department, caregivers, and school personnel of food allergies.
   f. Consult with dietitian to ensure a balanced diet that excludes identified allergens.
   g. Check food for known allergens before feedings.
   h. Prevent accidental ingestion by informing visitors of food allergies and keeping offending foods from patient.
   i. Teach parental caregivers to read food labels for the elimination of offending food proteins.
   j. Assess adherence to prescribed diet and relief of symptoms.
3. Be aware of environmental triggers.
   a. Maintain a warm climate with moderate humidity and avoid exposure to excessive heat and cold or humidity extremes.
   b. Dress child in soft, lightweight cotton clothing and avoid wool and occlusive synthetic fabrics. A new type of nonirritating, antimicrobial fabric impregnated with silver is useful as a sleep garment. Infants should not be allowed to crawl on wool carpeting.
   c. Participation in strenuous athletic activities that promote sweating. Activities should be modified according to the needs of the child. Swimming in chlorinated pools might be soothing for some children while drying and irritating for others.
   d. Irritating/harsh soaps, perfumes, detergents, chemicals, and fabric softeners.
   e. Bathing in hot water.
   f. Smoking around child.
   g. Avoid harsh soap and hot water. Avoid fabric softeners. Use fragrance-free and dye-free detergents.
   h. Discourage smoking in child's presence.
4. Try to alleviate stress.
   a. Encourage parental caregivers to stay with young child as much as possible.
   b. Involve child in age-appropriate diversional activities.

Controlling Pruritus

1. Apply topical medications as ordered by the health care provider.
   a. Assess for possible contraindications to medication before use. Check skin for active viral, bacterial, or fungal infection and for lymphadenopathy.
   b. Apply a thin layer of topical medication to the affected skin two to four times per day, as directed by the health care provider. Use only for the duration prescribed.
   c. Do not apply to wet or occluded skin.
   d. Apply emollients over top of medication.
   e. Observe for possible adverse effects including burning, itching, and erythema at application site and from long-term use of topical medications such as striae, cutaneous atrophy, telangiectasia, and acne because of topical corticosteroid use.
2. Note scratching and apply age-appropriate interventions to address avoidance of scratching.
3. Consider interventions such as cool compresses and bleach baths as described above.
4. Administer prescribed oral antipruritic medications, monitor for side effects, and provide related medication teaching as needed.

Preventing Secondary Infection

1. Discourage and prevent scratching per interventions described above.
2. Assess and treat secondary infection.
   a. Observe the skin for signs of bacterial, viral, or fungal infection (discharge, oozing, crusts, increased redness, fever). Report any positive findings.
   b. Administer medications, as prescribed.
   c. Loosen exudate and crusts with water or wet dressings, unless otherwise specified.
   d. Note changes in the skin in response to therapy.

Family Education and Health Maintenance

1. Teach patient and family to avoid potential triggering factors.
2. Use fragrance-free and dye-free detergents and soaps.

3. Bathe/shower in tepid water and apply emollients immediately after bathing. The child should bathe/shower after swimming and exposure to other irritants or triggering factors.
4. Avoid stressful situations, when possible.
5. Follow the American Academy of Pediatrics guidelines related to the introduction of new and solid foods.
6. Make sure that the child and/or family know to avoid common triggers, prevent dry skin, recognize signs of flares or secondary infection, apply topical medications, and follow up for routine appointments.
7. Recommend consultation with dermatology specialist for children with severe or persistent atopic dermatitis.
8. Provide resources for additional information from the following websites:
   a. American Academy of Dermatology (*www.aad.org*).
   b. American Academy of Pediatrics (*www.aap.org*).
   c. National Eczema Society (*www.eczema.org*).
9. Stress the importance of regular health maintenance examinations, immunizations, and preventive practices.

Table 51-1 Common Pediatric Skin Problems

DISORDER/ORGANISM	CLINICAL MANIFESTATIONS

Impetigo
Bacterial infectious disease affecting the superficial layers of the skin and characterized by the formation of vesicles, honey-colored crusts, or bullae.
Etiology and incidence:
• Caused by *Staphylococcus aureus* and *Streptococcus pyogenes.* Occurs most commonly when personal hygiene is poor.
• Common in children younger than age 10.
• Spread by close contact—easily conveyed from person to person via hands, nasal discharge, shared towels and toys, plastic wading pools in summer—when water is not replaced and no disinfectant is used; highly contagious.
• An abrasion of the skin may serve as a portal of entry.
Diagnosis:
• Usually clinical.
• Rarely, a culture of the lesion's exudate is indicated to confirm the diagnosis.
	• Incubation period is 1–10 d.
	• Lesion first appears as pink–red macules that quickly change to vesicles, which, in turn, rupture, develop crusts, and leave a temporary superficial erythematous area.
	  • Bullous (neonate and older child)—large, thin-roofed blisters break to form thin, light-brown crusts. Lesions may occur anywhere on the body but are more common on the face, axillae, and groin.
	  • Crusted (preschool age—seen more commonly in summer on exposed body parts)—lesions appear with thick, yellow crusts; skin around crusts is red and weeping with satellite lesions.
	• Regional lymphadenopathy is common with secondary infection of insect bites, eczema, poison ivy, and scabies.
	• Autoinoculation is the major cause of spreading.
	• Pruritus may occur.

Ringworm of the Scalp (Tinea Capitis)
(See page 900 for ringworm of the body [Tinea corporis])
A fungal infection of the scalp and hair follicles
Etiology and incidence:
• Most ringworm of the scalp is caused by *Trichophyton tonsurans. Microsporum canis* and *Microsporum audouinii* are also causative agents.
• Is seen primarily in children before puberty (usually ages 3–10).
• May be spread through child-to-child contact as well as through the common use of towels, pillows, combs, brushes, and hats. Cats and dogs may also be the source of the infection.
Diagnosis:
Hair or skin scrapings for microscopic evaluation or fungal culture, obtained by rubbing a swab or toothbrush over the affected area.
Differential diagnosis:
• Tinea amiantacea, lichen planopilaris, and perifolliculitis capitis abscedens et suffodiens must be ruled out clinically or histologically. Woods lamp inspection has limited benefit.
	• The lesions appear on the scalp in a variety of ways:
	  • One or more patchy areas of dandruff-like scaling with little or extensive alopecia (hair loss).
	  • One or more discrete areas of alopecia with tiny broken hairs.
	  • Numerous discrete pustules or excoriations with little alopecia.
	  • A kerion or boggy, tender, inflammatory mass that produces edema and pustules.
	• Pruritus usually occurs in the involved area.

CLINICAL JUDGMENT Advise family that fresh water (pond, lake, river) should be avoided if child has breaks in skin integrity, because of risk of infection.

Evaluation: Expected Outcomes

- Skin intact with minimal erythema and lichenification.
- Names common triggers and avoidance measures.
- Verbalizes less itching and less scratching observed.
- No signs of secondary infection.

Other Dermatologic Disorders

See Table 51-1.

TREATMENT/PREVENTION	NURSING CONSIDERATIONS

Based on etiology and type of infection.
• Gently wash affected area with soap and water three times per day.
• Crusts and debris can be removed from the affected area by gentle soaking or wet compresses. Use tap water, normal saline, or 1:20 Burow solution.
Note: If indicated, obtain drainage or debris for culture before antibiotics are provided.
• Apply topical antibacterial medication, such as bacitracin or mupirocin ointment or retapamulin.
• Systemic antibiotics (cephalosporins, erythromycin, or dicloxacillin) if widespread or recurrent.
• Methicillin-resistant *S. aureus* infection is common.
• Prevention—close contact with other children should be avoided until 24 h after treatment is initiated.
	• Assess the child's skin condition and document the location and appearance of lesions. Note new lesions.
	• Initiate and teach measures to prevent the spread of infection.
	  • Engage in frequent handwashing. Use separate towels.
	  • Daily bathing with soap and water. Regular laundering for contaminated bed linens, towels, and clothing.
	  • Observe drainage and secretion precautions for 24 h after the start of therapy.
	  • Isolate the child from direct contact with other children (school or day care) until 24 h after treatment has started.
	  • Trim fingernails and toenails. Apply small amount of bacitracin or mupirocin ointment under the fingernails to prevent the spread of infection.
	  • Engage the child in diversional activities to discourage scratching.
	• Be aware that the patient with streptococcal impetigo has an increased risk of acute glomerulonephritis.

• Micronized griseofulvin—an antifungal antibiotic that is administered orally, 15–20 mg/kg/day (maximum 1 g) in a single dose with a high-fat food for 4–12 wk. Some children may require higher doses or micronized griseofulvin 20–25 mg/kg/day or ultramicronized griseofulvin 5–10 mg/kg/day (maximum 750 mg).
• Topical antifungal medicines are not effective. Selenium sulfide lotion 2.5% used twice per week decreases fungal shedding and may curb the spread of infection.
• Treatment should be continued for 2 wk after clinical resolution.
• Treatment with oral itraconazole, oral terbinafine, or oral fluconazole is effective, but only terbinafine has been approved by the U.S. Food and Drug Administration (FDA) for this disorder.
	• Assess the scalp for characteristic lesions.
	• Administer or teach the patient and family to administer medications as prescribed.
	• Be aware of adverse effects, such as headache, heartburn, nausea, epigastric discomfort, diarrhea, urticaria, photosensitivity, and possible granulocytopenia caused by griseofulvin.
	• Griseofulvin is absorbed more efficiently with a fatty meal. Children can be given the medicine once per day with ice cream or peanut butter.
	• Liver function monitoring may be required for prolonged treatment (greater than 6 mo) or for children with baseline abnormal liver function.
	• Teach the child and family methods to prevent further episodes.
	  • Teach general hygiene measures—regular shampooing and bathing.
	  • Advise them to avoid sharing hats, combs, brushes, pillows.
	  • Routine cleaning of heavily contaminated articles, such as pillowcases, sheets, towels, hats, bike helmets, combs, brushes.
	  • All family members and close contacts should be screened for tinea infections. The child's school should be notified to facilitate the screening of classmates.
	• Hair loss is usually temporary, except in some cases with a kerion, when the hair follicles may have been destroyed.
	• Child may attend school after treatment has been initiated. Hats are not necessary.

(*continued*)

Table 51-1 Common Pediatric Skin Problems (*continued*)

Pediculosis

Infestation of humans by lice.

Etiology:

- Three types of lice affect human beings:
  - *Pediculosis capitis* (head lice)—commonly infests school-age children.
  - *Pediculosis corporis* (body lice)—rare in the United States.
  - *Pediculosis pubis* (pubic or crab lice)—common in sexually active adolescents or adults—can be found on pubic hair, chest hair, axillary hair, eyebrows, eyelashes, and beards.
- Each type of louse generally remains in the area designated by its name.
  - Lice are transmitted by personal contact with people harboring them or through contact with articles that temporarily harbor them (clothing or bed linens).
  - Head and pubic lice are not health hazards or signs of uncleanliness. Only body lice can transmit disease.

Diagnosis:

- Identification of lice or their eggs with the naked eye confirmed by using a hand lens or microscope.
- In active infection of head or pubic lice, nits and eggs are found on the hair shaft within 1 cm of the skin and are difficult to remove.
- Body lice and their eggs are found in the seams of undergarments.

- Itching in the area affected is the primary symptom of pediculosis. Scratch marks may be evident in these areas. However, not all affected people itch.
- Other signs of infestation are pillows or clothing that looks unusually dirty.
- Infested scalp areas may become secondarily infected from scratching.
- Crusts, lice, nits, eggs, and dirt may combine to cause a foul odor and matted hair.
- Body lice may produce minute red lesions.

Scabies

A disease of the skin produced by the burrowing action of a parasitic mite in the epidermis, resulting in irritation and the formation of burrows, vesicles, or pustules.

Etiology:

- The mite, *Sarcoptes scabiei*, is the cause of this disorder.
- Occurs in people of all socioeconomic levels, regardless of personal hygiene standards.
- Is transmitted by direct skin contact with infected people or by indirect contact through soiled bed linens, clothing.

Diagnosis:

- Identification of a mite, ova, or feces from skin scrapings.
- Often based on clinical presentation.

- Itching, particularly at night, is the primary symptom. The onset of itching is usually insidious.
- Secondary skin infection is common and may confuse the diagnosis.
- Systemic manifestations are absent, unless they result from the secondary infection.
- The burrow, a gray or white, tortuous, threadlike line, is seen most commonly in older children and adults between the fingers, in the wrists, in the axillary and buttock folds, along the belt line, on the male genitalia, on the female breasts, and on the knees, elbows, and ankles.
- In infants and small children, the lesions may occur on any part of the body and are usually widespread. Vesicles on the palms and soles are characteristic.
- Incubation period in children without previous exposure is 4–6 wk.

- Pediculosis capitis and pediculosis pubis may be treated with a one time application of 0.9% topical Spinosad for pediculosis for children greater than 6 months of age and scabies for children 4 years of age and older. Over the counter agents, such as permethrin or natural pyrethrin based products. Natural pyrethrin based products may be reapplied 7-10 days later.
- For infestation of eyelashes by crab lice, petroleum jelly applied twice daily to the eyelashes for 8–10 d is effective.
- Pediculicides are not necessary for the treatment of pediculosis corporis. Washing infested clothing and linens, where the lice harbor, in hot water and machine drying (on hot cycle) is adequate.
- Because pediculicides kill lice shortly after application, the detection of living lice on scalp inspection 24 h or more after treatment suggests incorrect use, reinfection, or resistance. Immediate retreatment with a different pediculicide followed by a second application 7 d later is recommended.
- A dry-on, suffocation-based pediculicide (DSP) lotion applied and then blown dry with a hair dryer weekly for up to 3 wk effectively treats 95% of head lice. The hair can be shampooed 8 h after application. The lotion is not visible and the hair can be styled.
- Studies of the efficacy of suffocation of lice by the application of occlusive agents, such as petroleum jelly, olive oil, or mayonnaise, have not been performed. Cotrimoxazole and ivermectin have been shown to be effective, but neither is approved by the FDA as a pediculicide.
- "No nit" policies requiring children to be free from nits for the return to school do not reduce transmission and are not recommended.
- Shaving head is not necessary.

- Administer or teach administration of antiparasitic as directed. Natural pyrethrin-based products work best on dry hair. Avoid shampoo, cream rinses, and conditioners before application.
- Although both pyrethrins and permethrin are quite safe, limit exposure to the skin by rinsing the hair in a sink rather than the shower and use cool water to minimize absorption from vasodilation.
- Removal of nits with a fine-tooth comb may be attempted for aesthetic reasons or to decrease diagnostic confusion. However, mechanical removal of nits after treatment does not prevent spread.
- Inspect the scalp (or have the family inspect the scalp) 24–48 h after treatment to see what lice remain. The presence of large lice may mean that the treatment was ineffective or that the lice are resistant.
- Provide appropriate teaching for the family to prevent recurrences.
  - Wash clothing, bed linens, and towels in hot water and machine dry (on hot cycle). Temperature above 128.3°F (53.5°C) for 5 min will kill lice and eggs. Dry cleaning or simply storing contaminated articles in a well-sealed plastic bag for 10 d is also effective.
  - Teach children not to share combs, brushes, headgear or hats. Combs and brushes can be disinfected by soaking in hot water for 10 min or washing with a pediculicide shampoo.
  - Environmental insecticide sprays are not helpful. Vacuuming carpets and car seats is a safe alternative.
  - Household, other close contacts, and classmates of the child with head lice should be screened for parasites and treated if affected. Prophylactic treatment of head lice is unnecessary and may increase resistance. Notify the child's school or day care so classmates can be screened.
  - Children should be allowed back to school or day care the morning after their first treatment. "No nit" policies for the return to school are unnecessary.
  - Prophylactic treatment of all sexual contacts of adolescents and adults with pubic lice is warranted because of the high coinfection rate.

- Application of a scabicide to the skin:
- The drug of choice is 5% permethrin. Alternative drugs are lindane 1% and crotamiton. Permethrin should be removed after 8–14 h by bathing, lindane after 8–12 h, and crotamiton after 48 h.
  - Lindane can cause neurotoxicity from absorption through the skin. It should be avoided in children younger than age 2, people with known seizures, pregnant and lactating people, and those with extensive dermatitis.
- Infected children and adults should apply the scabicidal lotion or cream on the entire body from the neck down. The entire head, neck, and body of infants and young children should be treated. Bathing immediately before treatment should be avoided.
- Oral ivermectin at 200 μg/kg/dose is not FDA-approved but has been shown to be effective.

- People caring for affected children should wear gloves.
- Contagion is unlikely 24 h after treatment. Children may return to school or day care.
- Teach the patient and family to launder all clothing, bed linens, and towels used by the patient during the 4 d prior to therapy with hot water and hot drying cycle to kill mites. Clothing that cannot be laundered can be stored in a plastic bag for 1 wk. Further environmental disinfection is rarely necessary.
- Itching may continue 2–3 wk after successful therapy because of a hypersensitivity reaction to the mites. The use of oral antihistamines and topical corticosteroids can help relieve symptoms.
- All household and close contacts should be treated prophylactically and at the same time to prevent reinfection. Caregivers with prolonged skin-to-skin contact with patients who are infected may also benefit from prophylactic treatment. Manifestations of scabies can occur as late as 2 mo after exposure.

(continued)

Table 51-1 Common Pediatric Skin Problems (*continued*)

DISORDER/ORGANISM	CLINICAL MANIFESTATIONS
Oral Candidiasis (Thrush)	
Oral candidiasis is a mycotic stomatitis characterized by the appearance of white plaques on the oral mucous membranes, gums, and tongue. (Chronic mucocutaneous candidiasis may be associated with endocrine diseases or immunodeficiency disorders or use of systemic antibiotic or inhaled corticosteroids.) *Etiology*: • Caused by *Candida albicans*. • Maternal vulvovaginitis is the primary source of neonatal thrush. Evaluate for endocrine diseases or immunodeficiency disorders if thrush occurs after 6 mo of life or is chronic. • Nipples, pacifiers may be reservoirs.	• The infant develops small plaques on the oral mucous membranes, tongue, or gums. These plaques look like curds of milk but cannot be wiped out of the mouth. • Most infants with thrush appear to have little pain or discomfort, unless the case is severe and there are erosion and ulceration of the mucosa. • The mouth may be dry. • Occasionally, the infant may appear to have some difficulty swallowing or may eat less vigorously. • Enteric infection is usually associated with oral thrush.
Diaper Dermatitis	
Candidal diaper dermatitis—a rash characterized by bright red, sharply circumscribed but moist patches with pustular satellite lesions. *Etiology*: • 80% of diaper rashes present for 3 or more days are caused by *Candida albicans*. • Most commonly seen in infants and toddlers who wear diapers. • May be associated with oral candidiasis.	• Buttock rash consisting of erythematous maculopapular eruption with perianal distribution. • Generally causes discomfort, especially with wetting and cleanings. Lesions last approximately 2 wk, desquamate, and resolve without scarring.

TREATMENT/PREVENTION	NURSING CONSIDERATIONS
• Topical administration of nystatin in suspension three to four times daily is the treatment of choice. Apply ½ doses to each side of the mouth after feeding. • Retain in the mouth as long as possible before swallowing. Allow the child to swallow any medication to treat any lesions along the GI tract. • Clotrimazole troches can be used in children older than age 3. • Amphotericin B, clotrimazole, ketoconazole, fluconazole, and newer antifungal agents are used for candidiasis resistant to nystatin. Not all of these drugs are approved for use in infants and children.	• Recognize the appearance of thrush. • Be aware of the infant or child who is particularly susceptible to the development of this condition, especially typical infants younger than age 6 mo, low-birth-weight infants, immunocompromised or debilitated hosts, and people on prolonged, broad-spectrum antibiotics. • Teach parental caregivers to inspect the child's mouth before every feeding for the presence of thrush and report the appearance of thrush.

• Keep the affected area clean and dry by frequent diaper changes.
• Clean the skin with water-based, alcohol-free baby wipes with a pH of 5.5 or with water.
• Use disposable diapers with sodium polyacrylate polymers in the diaper core that form a gel when hydrated to keep liquid away from the skin or a breathable diaper.
• Topical application of nystatin, clotrimazole, or miconazole cream or ointment after gentle cleaning of the affected area. If no improvement in 2 d, consider nonadherence, failure to relieve aggravating factors, or need for a different drug.
• Nystatin may be given orally if rash is persistent.
• Burow solution compresses for severe inflammation or vesiculation.
• Low-potency topical corticosteroids for short-term use may be added.
	• Teach parental caregivers the general principles of prevention.
	  ◦ Change diaper as soon as possible after wetting or soiling. Prolonged contact of feces with the skin promotes the development of candidal diaper dermatitis. Check diaper frequently (every 3–4 h). Encourage use of disposable diapers.
	  ◦ Wash the entire diaper area with warm water or use water-based, alcohol-free baby wipes.
	  ◦ If using cloth diapers, use a second hot rinse when washing diapers to neutralize ammonia produced when infant urinates; use vinegar, Borax, or Diaparene in wash.
	  ◦ Avoid powder and oil, which tend to clog pores and cake on skin, retaining bacteria.
	  ◦ Avoid occlusive plastic coverings and tightly pinned or double diapers, all of which tend to increase production and retention of body heat and moisture.
	  ◦ Allow the infant to go without a diaper for short periods to leave area open to air.
	• Diaper rashes present for 3 or more days should be evaluated by a health care provider.

SELECTED READINGS

American Academy of Pediatrics. (2021). *Treatment of atopic dermatitis.* https://www.aap.org/en/patient-care/atopic-dermatitis/treatment-of-atopic-dermatitis/

American Burn Association. (2023). *Advanced burn life support provider manual.* Author.

Apet, R., Prakash, L., Shewale, K., Jawade, S. & Dhamecha, R. (2023). Treatment Modalities of Pediculosis Capitis: A Narrative Review. *Cureus, 15*(9), e45028. https://doi.org/10.7759/cureus.45028.

Brar, K., Singh, A., De Guzman, N., & Aquino, M. (2023). Atopic dermatitis: Diagnosis, disparity, and management in children of color. *NASN School Nurse, 38*(2), 56–61. https://doi.org/10.1177/1942602X221147033

Cameron, M. (2023). JAK inhibitor safety: What did ORAL Surveillance really teach us? *The Dermatologist, 31*(2), 28–32. https://www.hmpgloballearningnetwork.com/site/thederm/cover-story/jak-inhibitor-safety-what-did-oral-surveillance-really-teach-us

Cartotto, R., Johnson, L., Rood, J., Lorello, D., Matherly, A., Parry, I., Romanowski, K., Wiechman, S., Bettencourt, A., & Carson, J. (2023). Clinical practice guideline: Early mobilization and rehabilitation of critically ill burn patients. *Journal of Burn Care & Research, 44*(1), 1–15. https://doi.org/10.1093/jbcr/irac008

Dollani, L., & Marathe, K. (2020). Impetigo/staphylococcal scalded skin disease. *Pediatrics in Review, 41*(4), 210–212. https://doi.org/10.1542/pir.2018-0206

Drabick, Z., Driscoll, I., & Nguyen, D. (2022). Evaluation of a stress ulcer prophylaxis protocol in an burn intensive care unit. *Journal of Burn Care & Research, 43*(Supplement_1), S156–S157. https://doi.org/10.1093/jbcr/irac012.257

Dunk, A., Broom, M., Fourie, A., & Beeckman, D. (2022). Clinical signs and symptoms of diaper dermatitis in newborns, infants, and young children: a scoping review. *Journal of Tissue Viability, 31*(3), 404–415. https://doi.org/10.1016/j.jtv.2022.03.003

Fishbein, A., Silverberg, J., Wilson, E., & Ong, P. (2021). Update on atopic dermatitis: Diagnosis, severity assessment, and treatment selection. *The Journal of Allergy and Clinical Immunology in Practice, 8*(1), 91–101. https://doi.org/10.1016/j.jaip.2019.06.044

Hattier, G., Talasila, S., & Cohen, B. (2022). Looking at the spectrum of diaper dermatitis. *Contemporary Pediatrics, 39*(7), 27–31. https://www.contemporarypediatrics.com/view/looking-at-the-spectrum-of-diaper-dermatitis

Herndon, D. (2017). *Total burn care* (5th ed.). Elsevier.

James, W. D., Elston, D., & Treat, J. (2020). *Andrews' diseases of the skin clinical dermatology* (13th ed.). W.B. Saunders.

Jeschke, M., Kamolz, L.-P., & Shahrokhi, S. (Eds.). (2021). *Burn care and treatment: A practical guide* (2nd ed.). Springer Publishing.

Johnson, M. (2020). Impetigo. *Advanced Emergency Nursing Journal, 42*(4), 262–269. https://doi.org/10.1097/TME.0000000000000320

Kassem, R., Shemesh, Y., Nitzan, O., Azrad, M., & Peretz, A. (2021). Tinea capitis in an immigrant pediatric community: A clinical signs-based treatment approach. *BMC Pediatrics, 21*(1), 1–8. https://doi.org/10.1186/s12887-021-02813-x

Kawalec, A., & Pawlas, K. (2021). The impact of burn wound cooling on chosen parameters of burns in children. *Burns, 47*(5), 1222–1223. https://doi.org/10.1016/j.burns.2020.01.016

Khan, L. (2022). Molluscum and tinea and warts, oh my! *Pediatric Annals, 51*(1), e2–e5. https://doi.org/10.3928/19382359-20211209-02

Kouchek, M., Coltani, S., Memarian, A., & Aghakhani, K. (2023). Etiology and prognosis in burning of children and adolescents during 2009-2019. *Online Journal of Health & Allied Sciences, 22*(1), 1–5. https://www.ojhas.org/issue85/2023-1-4.html

Lizano-Diez, I., Naharro, J., & Zsolt, I. (2021). Indirect costs associated with skin infectious disease in children: A systematic review. *BMC Health Services Research, 21*(1), 1–11. https://doi.org/10.1186/s12913-021-07189-3

Merceron, T., William, R., Ingram, W., & Abramowicz, S. (2021). Epidemiology and management of pediatric head and neck burns: An institutional review. *American Surgeon, 87*(5), 741–746. https://doi.org/10.1177/0003134820952828

National Center for Injury Prevention and Control & Centers for Disease Control and Prevention. (2023). *Injury prevention & control.* https://webappa.cdc.gov/sasweb/ncipc/leadcause.html

National Eczema Association. (2023). *Atopic dermatitis in children.* https://nationaleczema.org/eczema/children/atopic-dermatitis/

Nolt, D., Moore, S., Yan, A., & Melnick, L. (2022). Head lice. *Pediatrics, 150*(4), e2022059282. https://doi.org/10.1542/peds.2022-059282

Ogbuefi, N., & Kenner-Bell, B. (2021). Common pediatric infestations: Update on diagnosis and treatment of scabies, head lice, and bed bugs. *Current Opinion in Pediatrics, 33*(4), 410–415. https://doi.org/10.1097/MOP.0000000000001031

Ozlu, O., & Basaran, A. (2022). Infections in patients with major burns: A retrospective study of a burn intensive care unit. *Journal of Burn Care Research, 43*(4), 926–930. https://doi.org/10.1093/jbcr/irab222

Paller, A. S., & Mancini, A. J. (2021). *Hurwitz clinical pediatric dermatology* (6th ed.). Elsevier.

Puthumana, J., Ngaage, L., Borrelli, M., Rada, E., Caffrey, J., & Rasko, Y. (2021). Risk factors for cooking-related burn injuries in children, WHO global burn registry. *Bulletin of the World Health Organization, 99*(6), 439–445. https://doi.org/10.2471/BLT.20.279786

Schachner, L., Torrelo, A., Grada, A., Micali, G., Kwong, P., Scott, G., Benjamin, L., Gonzalez, M., Andriessen, A., Eberlein, T., & Eichenfield, L. (2020). Treatment of impetigo in the pediatric population: Consensus and future directions. *Journals of Drugs in Dermatology, 19*(3), 281–290. https://doi.org/10.36849/JDD.2020.4679

Silverberg, J., Barbarot, S., Gadkari, A., Simpson, E., Weidinger, S., Paola Mina-Osorio, P., Rossi, A., Brignoli, L., Saba, G., Guillemin, I., Fenton, M., Auziere, S., & Eckert, L. (2021). Atopic dermatitis in the pediatric population: A cross-sectional, international epidemiologic study. *Annals of Allergy, Asthma and Immunology, 126*(4), 417–428.e2. https://doi.org/10.1016/j.anai.2020.12.020

Sobowale, K., Clayton, A., & Smith, M. (2021). Diaper need is associated with pediatric care use: An analysis of a nationally representative sample of parents of young children. *Journal of Pediatrics, 230*, 146–151. https://doi.org/10.1016/j.jpeds.2020.10.061

Taylor, M., Brizuela, M., & Raja, A. (n.d.). *Oral candidiasis.* In: *StatPearls* [Internet]. StatPearls Publishing. Updated March 19, 2023. https://www.ncbi.nlm.nih.gov/books/NBK545282/

Thompson, R., Westbury, S., & Slape, D. (2021). Paediatrics: How to manage scabies. *Drugs in Context, 10*, 2020-12-3. https://doi.org/10.7573/dic.2020-12-3

Trotter, Z., Foster, K., Khetarpal, S., & Sinha, M. (2020). Age-based characteristics of pediatric burn injuries from outdoor recreational fires. *Journal of Burn Care Research, 41*(6), 1198–1201. https://doi.org/10.1093/jbcr/iraa064

Tully, C., Amatya, K., Batra, N., Inverso, H., & Burd, R. S. (2022). Parent resilience after young child minor burn injury. *Families, Systems & Health, 40*(3), 322–331. https://doi.org/10.1037/fsh0000703

Unal, D., & Hazir, M., (2022). Airway management in pediatric patients with burn contractures of the face and neck. *Journal of Burn Care & Research, 43*(5), 1186–1202. https://doi.org/10.1093/jbcr/irac016

Vassantachart, J., Florentino, A., & Admani, S. (2021a). Lice infestations in the pediatric population. *Journal of the Dermatology Nurses' Association, 13*(5), 284–287. https://doi.org/10.1097/JDN.0000000000000636

Vassantachart, J., Florentino, A., & Admani, S. (2021b). Scabies infestations in the pediatric population. *Journal of the Dermatology Nurses' Association, 13*(6), 301–304. https://doi.org/10.1097/JDN.0000000000000653

52 Developmental Disabilities*

OVERVIEW AND ASSESSMENT

The spectrum of developmental disabilities is a group of interrelated neurodevelopmental disorders that may be chronic. Such disorders can include intellectual disabilities, autism, learning impairments, communication disorders, mental health disorders that interfere with learning and communication, and attention-deficit disorders. These conditions are suspected or noticed at varying stages during childhood. Some conditions, such as Down syndrome, can be recognized prenatally or at birth; other conditions, such as cerebral palsy or autism, may not present themselves until the child fails to meet typical developmental milestones. This phenomenon makes the nurse's role in developmental assessment crucial. The pediatric nurse—who understands that the development of the child occurs in an orderly, predictable manner and who knows what the milestones should be—may be the first person to recognize the alteration and communicate the concern to the parental caregiver or pediatrician. Because there are many confusing and overlapping characteristics for many of these conditions, it is important for the health care provider and family to refer to clinicians who are experienced and knowledgeable in typical and atypical child development to arrive at an accurate diagnosis and coordinate an appropriate care plan. Nurses can play a significant role in supporting the family in navigating the complex needs of many of these disorders.

When a known condition exists, the nurse should be aware of the predisposing health issues associated with the condition and the resources available to promote optimal growth and development of the child within the family.

CLINICAL JUDGMENT Typical child development is predictable and sequential. The nurse who is knowledgeable about typical development may be the first person to raise the question that a developmental disability exists.

Signs of Developmental Delay

Criteria for Referral

Communication and Feeding

1. Feeding difficulties—weak sucking or poor coordination of suck–swallowing to sustain typical weight gain.
2. No social smile by age 4 months.
3. No babbling (*ga-ga, da-da*) by age 9 months.
4. No *mama* and *dada* (specific) by age 14 months.
5. No name of object (one word) by age 14 months.
6. At least 10 words by age 18 months (not just repeating).
7. Combines words (e.g., *me outside, more milk*) and uses pronouns by age 24 months.
8. Regression in language or social responses at any age.
9. Unresponsive to name.

CLINICAL JUDGMENT Do not simply reassure the family that typical development "should" or "probably will" develop. Make sure that the child is referred for an appropriate evaluation to properly assess the suspected delay and establish a diagnosis, if possible. In the presence of a developmental delay, a comprehensive vision and hearing evaluation should also be included.

Motor Delay

1. Asymmetrical movements and poor tone are noted.
2. Not rolling over by age 6 months.
3. Not sitting by age 9 months.
4. Not walking by age 15 months.
5. Not stair climbing by age 2 years.

See Chapter 36 for typical pediatric growth and development.

*Please note that the term "male" in this chapter refers to a person assigned male at birth, and the term "female" in this chapter refers to a person assigned female at birth.

Care of the Child With a Developmental Disability

Nursing Assessment

1. Review the child's record, including the prenatal and birth history to determine existing health problems that may cause or affect the developmental disability. Always rule out a vision or hearing impairment.
2. Review the family history, if available, to determine if there are any family members with a history of developmental disabilities. If possible, assess when parental caregivers and siblings of the patient reached specified developmental milestones.
3. Assess the family's understanding of the diagnosis and the ramifications. The following affect the parental caregivers' ability to assimilate information provided: their experiences, cultural beliefs, attitudes toward disabilities, cognitive ability, stage of grief, and their own health. It will be necessary to repeat the information. (For example, a patient who has just given birth to a child with Down syndrome may have difficulty processing much information shortly after the birth.) If possible, provide the family with written information that reinforces verbal information given at the visit. Provide culturally appropriate resources, with careful consideration of information overload. Additional information and resources may be better introduced at subsequent visits.
4. Determine the developmental age of the child. The pediatric nurse should be familiar with typical developmental milestones (see Chapter 36, page 1083), noting the child's strengths and areas presenting challenges, for example, the communication skills are at a 12-month level and the gross motor skills are at a 36-month level. Children who are found to be functioning at one half or less of their chronological age have a moderate to severe developmental delay.
5. Administer a developmental tool such as the Clinical Adaptive Test–Clinical Linguistic Auditory Milestone Scales (CAT–CLAMS). It is a reliable tool that nurses can be trained to use to assess cognitive and communicative development in children at the 1- to 36-month developmental level. It has been found to be more sensitive than the Denver Developmental Screening Scale because language development is the best early predictor of cognitive abilities.
6. Assess the functional level of the child. The WeeFIM is a tool used to track functional independence in children. It has had multiple revisions and is reliable and valid. It uses the following categories to describe function: completely dependent, needs some physical assistance, can physically perform the task but needs verbal cues and coaching, and completely independent. Functional areas to assess include:
   a. Feeding.
   b. Grooming and bathing.
   c. Dressing.
   d. Mobility.
   e. Problem-solving.
   f. Communication.
7. Assess parental caregivers' perception of the child's development level and the appropriateness of parental expectations. Use such questions as, "Do you have any concerns regarding things your child is doing or should be doing?" "Is your child progressing like your other children have?"
8. Assess parental caregiver–child interaction. Observe and explore bonding and attachment, ability to set appropriate limits, management of behavioral problems, and methods of discipline.
9. Assess the need for additional resources, such as financial aid, transportation, and counseling, for long-term support of child and family.

CLINICAL JUDGMENT Be aware of the diversity of cultural norms that may affect developmental milestones.

EVIDENCE BASE Mert, S., & Kosgeroglu, N. (2022). Meeting the care needs of people with intellectual and developmental disabilities and their families through the Model of Nursing Based on Activities of Living. *Journal of Intellectual Disabilities, 26*(3), 687–703. https://doi.org/10.1177/17446295211010023

Manion, A., Alfieri, N., & Golbeck, E. (2023). Improved confidence, competence, and knowledge in child-focused APN clinicians following participation in infant motor development course. *Journal of Pediatric Healthcare, 37*(4), 457. https://doi.org/10.1016/j.pedhc.2023.04.008

Nursing Interventions

Promoting Adjustment

1. Allow the parental caregivers access to the infant at all possible times to promote bonding when parental caregivers appear ready.
2. Focus on the positive aspects of the infant and serve as a role model for handling and stimulating.
3. Be cognizant of the grieving process (loss of the anticipated and planned-for "typical child") that families experience when a diagnosis is made, and be aware that spouses can be at different stages.
4. Accept all questions and reactions nonjudgmentally, offering verbal and written explanations in appropriate language.
5. Provide the family a quiet place to discuss their questions with each other and someone knowledgeable about the condition (primary care provider, clinical nurse specialist) to support their concerns.
6. Offer the family the option to take advantage of counseling. A social worker or psychologist can help families deal with immediate reactions. Many parental caregivers benefit from continuous or periodic support of counseling professionals.

CLINICAL JUDGMENT Children with developmental disabilities and chronic illness are at greater risk for experiencing divorce of their caregivers, child abuse, and neglect than the general population.

Strengthening the Role of the Family

1. Help the family to realize what strengths they have in caring for their child. The role of the parental caregivers is critical; a nurturing, loving environment gives the child the best chance at maximizing potential. An individual who grows up at home has markedly higher adaptive abilities and an increased life span compared with those raised in residential care facilities.
2. Enlist the help of family and siblings who can offer valuable support to the parental caregivers and child and assist with stimulation activities. Including siblings in the care can help them feel needed and involved, thus strengthening the family.

3. If sibling issues arise, suggest family counseling to address the needs of all family members. (Such issues could include a sibling without an illness or disability resenting the extra time and attention the parental caregivers spend on the child with the illness/disability).
4. Identify resources available to the family, such as support groups, early intervention programs, specialty clinics, pediatrician or primary health care provider, respite care, financial support programs, and advocacy groups for individuals with developmental disabilities.
5. For those parental caregivers concerned with their long-term ability to care for the child, explore with them their options of family assistance, community resources, foster care, adoption, and residential placement in a nonjudgmental manner.
6. Ensure that the family has adequate respite services to prevent exhaustion and mental fatigue.

Establishing Effective Feeding Techniques

EVIDENCE BASE DeGuzman, P. B., Huang, G., Lyons, G., Snitzer, J., & Keim-Malpass, J. (2021). Rural disparities in early childhood well child visit attendance. *Journal of Pediatric Nursing, 58*, 76–81. https://doi.org/10.1016/j.pedn.2020.12.005

Govender, V., Naidoo, D., & Govender, P. (2021). Developmental delay in a resource-constrained environment: Screening, surveillance and diagnostic assessment. *South African Family Practice, 63*(1, Part 2), 1–4. https://doi.org/10.4102/safp.v63i1.5306

1. Be aware that the presence of hypotonia, as in children with many genetic syndromes and metabolic disorders, or hypertonia, as in children with cerebral palsy, can interfere with feeding by compromising sucking and swallowing.
2. Demonstrate proper feeding positioning, with the infant's head elevated, and encourage the parental caregivers to always hold the infant during feedings with their head elevated and supported in arms.
3. Try different nipples, bottles, and feeding positions to find the easiest option for the infant to use without leakage or danger of aspiration.
4. Allow adequate time for feeding and increase frequency of feedings if infant tires easily.
5. Offer support and guidance for breastfeeding. Refer to lactation consultant, if needed.
6. Consider referral for a feeding evaluation to a speech therapist or to an occupational therapist who has experience working with children and families.
7. Be aware of and anticipate the need for initiation of tube feeding (nasogastric or gastrostomy) so that early referral and education of the parental caregivers about feeding options can be discussed.
8. Assess for signs of feeding intolerance and gastroesophageal reflux disease, which is common in children with hypotonia; implement management strategies to optimize feeding and minimize risk of aspiration, such as upright position after feedings.
9. Frequently assess growth (length or height, weight, and head circumference) to ensure adequate dietary intake, and be aware that growth in children with neurologic impairment and genetic syndromes may be slower or limited in relation to the general pediatric population and standard growth charts.
10. Monitor bowel and elimination patterns of children with neurologic impairment, especially those with generalized hypotonia, as they are at risk for poor gastric motility and constipation. Dietary measures, such as increased fiber and fluid intake, or pharmacologic agents to promote adequate elimination may be needed.

Promoting Optimum Growth and Development

1. Refer parental caregivers to the early intervention program administered by their county so that they can take advantage of the educational and support services available for children from birth to age 3 years.
2. If the condition is identified after age 3 years, refer parental caregivers to the school district in which they reside.
3. Help the parental caregivers to understand the concept of developmental age and to identify the functional level of the child.
4. Determine whether there is consistency between the developmental age of the child and their degree of independence. Cognitive and physical limitations may interfere with emerging independence; however, parental caregivers may "baby" or overindulge a child who has a disability.
5. Work with parental caregivers to set reasonable expectations and to break down tasks into simple, achievable steps. Care should be taken not to address too many areas at one time so as not to overwhelm the family.
6. Use appropriate discipline and behavior modification techniques, such as extinction, time-out, and reward, to achieve cooperation and success.
7. Demonstrate and encourage play with the child at the appropriate level to provide stimulation and work toward achieving developmental milestones.
8. Provide parental caregivers with information and links to community, regional, or national associations for children with special needs, and refer to support groups. These resources are frequently found online and can be easily accessed to provide an ongoing source of information and support to families.
9. Ensure that the child's physical well-being is optimized to promote optimal development and self-esteem. Any congenital anomalies should be considered for repair (i.e., orthopedic, cardiac, craniofacial), and attention should be paid to dental health and restorative orthodontic procedures that can improve facial appearance.
10. Consider any pertinent cultural and ethnic impact on health care.

Providing Opportunities to Develop Social and Self-care Skills

1. Be aware that feeding, toileting, dressing, and grooming are important aspects of socialization and development of self-esteem. These tasks should be taught in a developmentally appropriate manner to children with a focus on maximizing independence. Many adaptive devices are available, and an occupational therapist can guide families in effective techniques to help children with developmental disabilities master these important self-care skills.
2. Make parental caregivers aware that recreational and leisure-time experiences are valuable in building social skills and self-esteem. Rehearse and role-play desirable social behaviors—such as waving goodbye, saying "hello," taking turns, saying "please" and "thank you," and responding to their name—will help build social confidence and acceptance within the child's peer group.

3. Offer suggestions that will be enjoyable and developmentally appropriate for the child. Interaction with developmentally delayed and neurotypical peers is desirable. The Special Olympics is one example of an adaptive program. Local programs are also available in many areas such as unified sports teams that include all interested students without regard to developmental level.
4. Praise the child for participation in activities, regardless of whether the child succeeds.

Maintaining Safety

1. When handling the infant, provide adequate support with a firm grasp because the infant may be floppy because of poor muscle tone.
2. If hypotonia is accompanied by poor head control and neck strength, position the infant to prevent aspiration should vomiting occur.
   a. Support the infant with a diaper roll, if needed, to maintain position.
   b. Change the infant's position frequently.
   c. Continuously check the environment for the safety needs of the child.
3. Be aware that hypotonia can also lead to increased heat loss as more surface area is exposed; therefore, infants may need close attention paid to swaddling and environmental control to maintain thermoregulation.
4. Advise the parental caregivers to:
   a. Maintain appropriate surveillance of the child when cooking or when they are exposed to other potential hazards that they may be able to get into but not understand.
   b. Help the child to read words, such as *danger* and *stop*, as well as to recognize sign shapes/colors representing these commands.
   c. Teach the child how to call out to ask for help.
   d. Teach the child to say no to strangers.
   e. Teach the child appropriate and socially acceptable sexual behaviors to prevent exploitation.
   f. Provide sex education in a way the child and adolescent can understand, offering practical information about anatomy, physical development, contraception, and consent.
5. Ensure that parental caregivers have the knowledge and resources to transport their child safely.

CLINICAL JUDGMENT Teach caregivers to base safety needs on the developmental, not the chronological, age of the child.

Family Education and Health Maintenance

1. Remind the parental caregivers to recognize the child's routine health care needs and maintain regular follow-up with a primary care provider.
   a. Immunizations.
   b. Regular dental checkups.
   c. Vision and hearing examinations.
   d. Anticipatory guidance related to developmental stages, safety, behavior, and transition planning.
2. Provide guidance and support to parental caregivers with their child's multidimensional treatment plan. Make sure they know whom to contact when problems arise. Encourage them to develop and maintain information, including a calendar, to keep track of agencies, subspecialists, and professionals who will be involved with their child. It should include business cards, names, addresses, phone numbers, appointment dates, health providers' orders, and insurance information.
3. Teach parental caregivers the benefits of a therapeutic home environment.
   a. Develop optimum sleeping, eating, working, and playing routines.
   b. Ensure adequate nutrition.
   c. Divide tasks and expectations into small, manageable parts. Give only one or two instructions at a time.
   d. Set firm but reasonable limits on behavior and carry through with consistent discipline expectations for parental caregivers and other adults who are providing consistent child care.
   e. Avoid situations that cause excessive excitement, stimulation, or fatigue. Maintain a consistent schedule, if possible.
   f. Provide an energy outlet through physical activity and outdoor play. Also provide a vocal outlet by encouraging the child to discuss the events of the day, feelings they are currently experiencing, or what they would like to do in the future (tomorrow's plans).
   g. Channel the need for movement into safe, appropriate activities.
4. Discuss preparation for independent living, when appropriate.
   a. Help the parental caregivers identify areas of home responsibilities that may be delegated to the child with a cognitive impairment.
   b. Guide development of social skills that will be an asset to later vocational life.
   c. Help the child to develop a set of attitudes and behaviors that will increase motivation.
   d. Refer for vocational assistance to ARC (formerly Association of Retarded Citizens) or other rehabilitative agencies.
   e. Begin planning for transition from pediatric care providers to adult providers well in advance of when eligibility for services will run out to ensure appropriate provider(s) can be established in a timely way and to avoid gaps in health care.
5. As warranted by the diagnosis, refer for genetic consultation for information about genetics of the disorder, risk in subsequent pregnancies (biological parents), risk to biological offspring (patient), or risk to other biological relatives.

EVIDENCE BASE Tyler, C. V., Jr., & McDermott, M. (2021). Transitioning young adults with an intellectual or other developmental disability to adult healthcare. *Exceptional Parent, 51*(10), 21–23. https://www.epmagazine.com/blog/transitioning-young-adults-with-an-intellectual-or-other-developmental-disability-to-adult-healthcare

Evaluation: Expected Outcomes

- Parental caregivers hold infant frequently and seek information from health care provider.
- Family members feed, assist with care, and bond with child.
- Parental caregivers and health care providers monitor nutrition, growth, and development closely, with ongoing assessment of most effective feeding techniques and management of any feeding-related problems.
- Parental caregivers describe developmental level of child and have realistic goals for attainment of next milestones in collaboration with their health care team and occupational, speech, and physical therapists.

- Parental caregivers seek out support and resources that enable them to share their experience in raising a child with special needs and gain information needed to optimize the child's developmental and health outcomes throughout childhood.
- Child remains safe through careful handling and appropriate supervision.

DEVELOPMENTAL DISABILITIES

Cognitive Developmental Delay

Cognitive developmental delay, also known as *intellectual disability*, refers to the most severe, general lack of cognitive and problem-solving skills. The American Association on Intellectual and Developmental Disabilities defines intellectual disability as a disability characterized by significant limitations both in intellectual functioning and in adaptive behavior, which covers many everyday social and practical skills. This disability originates before the age of 18 years. There are many causes and a wide range of impairments. Up to 7.7 million people in the United States have at least a mild developmental disability that impacts their daily functioning. One in six children (or about 15%) aged 3 through 17 years have one or more developmental disabilities.

Pathophysiology and Etiology

1. No identifiable organic or biologic cause can be found for 50% of children with cognitive delays.
2. Identifiable causes include:
   a. Genetic causes, such as Down syndrome, Fragile X syndrome, Angelman syndrome, and inborn errors of metabolism such as phenylketonuria (PKU).
   b. Congenital anomalies, including brain malformations, hydrocephalus, and microcephaly.
   c. Intrauterine influences, such as alcohol and drug exposure, congenital infections, and teratogens.
   d. Perinatal trauma—birth hypoxia and intracranial hemorrhage.
   e. Postnatal trauma—acquired brain injury from falls, automobile accidents, near drownings, and child abuse (shaken baby syndrome).
   f. Postnatal infections and diseases (meningitis, encephalitis, sepsis, hypoxia, brain tumors).
   g. Environmental exposure to toxins such as lead, environmental deprivation, and neglect.
3. The malfunctioning brain is poorly understood in most cases, but physiologic alterations identified in some cases include:
   a. Congenital brain malformations, brain tissue damage, or underdevelopment of the brain as shown by results of computed tomography (CT) scan or magnetic resonance imaging (MRI).
   b. Biochemical errors or errors of metabolism, in which an absence of an enzyme or hormone produces atypical brain function or formation, as in PKU or hypothyroidism.
4. IQ is 75 or below; a person with an IQ in this range has mild or severe intellectual disability, encompassing both cognitive and functional abilities.
   a. The more severe types of intellectual developmental disability tend to be diagnosed in early infancy, especially when they coexist with an identifiable syndrome or congenital anomaly.
   b. Milder forms of intellectual developmental disability tend to be diagnosed in the preschool years, when language and behavioral concerns call attention to slower development.
5. Limitations in adaptive ability occur in communication, self-care, home living, social skills, community use, self-direction, health and safety, functional academics, leisure, and work.

Clinical Manifestations

Developmental delays (failure to achieve age-appropriate skills) are evident to some degree in almost all areas.

Infancy

1. "Poor feeder"—a weak or uncoordinated suck results in poor breast- or bottle-feeding, leading to poor weight gain.
2. Delayed or decreased visual alertness and curiosity with poor visual tracking of the face or objects.
3. Decreased or lack of auditory response.
4. Decreased spontaneous activity or asymmetric activity.
5. Delayed head and trunk control.
6. Floppy (hypotonic) or spastic (hypertonic) muscle tone.

CLINICAL JUDGMENT Although 75% of individuals with intellectual developmental disabilities have no physical signs, they typically achieve motor milestones at a slower rate.

Toddler

1. Delayed independent sitting, crawling, pulling to stand, and independent ambulation.
2. Delayed communication—failure to develop receptive and expressive language milestones. Almost 50% of children with intellectual developmental disability are identified after age 3 years, when speech delays manifest themselves.
3. Failure of the child to make progress or show interest in the area of independence in self-feeding, dressing, and toilet training may reflect cognitive impairment.
4. Short attention span and distractibility.
5. Behavioral disturbances.
6. Decreased muscle coordination.

Diagnostic Evaluation

Federal law (PL 94-142, Education for All Handicapped Children, and PL 101-476, Individuals with Disabilities Education Act [IDEA]) ensures that each child with a delay or suspected of having a delay has a comprehensive evaluation by a multidisciplinary team. Part C of PL 105-17 calls for the creation of statewide, coordinated, multidisciplinary interagency programs for the provision of early intervention services. Each state has its own definitions and organizational framework to provide these services. No single test can diagnose intellectual developmental disabilities. The multidisciplinary evaluation should be individually tailored to the child.

1. Rule out sensory deficits by assessment of vision and hearing, even if neonate hearing screen was normal.
2. Medical evaluation should include prenatal history, developmental history, sequential developmental assessments, family history including genetic assessment, and physical examination. The positive findings determine the direction of the individual evaluation and any diagnostic testing.
   a. Unusual appearance (dysmorphic features) warrants evaluation by a genetic specialist.

b. History consistent with loss of developmental milestones and positive family history warrant workup for presence of an inborn error of metabolism (diagnosed by blood, urine, or DNA analysis), other genetic disorders, or environmental exposures such as lead poisoning.
c. Children with macrocephaly, microcephaly, or neurologic anomalies may require imaging studies, such as CT scan or MRI.
d. Electroencephalogram (EEG) is indicated for children with seizures.

3. Psychological testing (appropriate tests selected by a developmental specialist such as a child psychologist):
   a. The Bayley Scales are used to assess children of various ages. This test is weighted on nonlanguage items and is used to assess fine motor skills, gross motor skills, language skills, and visual problem-solving.
   b. The McCarthy Scale offers a "general cognitive index" that is roughly equivalent to an IQ score.
   c. The Stanford-Binet Intelligence Scale is used to test the mental abilities of children aged 2 and older.
   d. The Wechsler Preschool and Primary Scale of Intelligence-Fourth Edition (WPPSI-IV) measures mental age of children 2 years and 6 months to 7 years and 7 months.
   e. The Wechsler Intelligence Scale for Children-Fifth Edition (WISC-V) tests children whose functional age is above a 6-year level.
   f. The Vineland Scale tests social-adaptive abilities—self-help skills, self-control, interaction with others, and cooperation; the Adaptive Behavior Scale is similar to Vineland but also measures adjustment.

Complications and Associated Findings

1. Seizure disorders.
2. Cerebral palsy.
3. Sensory deficits.
4. Communication disorders (speech and language).
5. Neurodevelopmental disorders.
6. Psychiatric illness.
7. Specific learning disabilities.
8. Emotional and behavioral problems (self-injury, hyperactivity, aggression).

Management

1. An interdisciplinary team evaluation by a developmental pediatrician, clinical psychologist, and counselor is usually the initial step in the management of mental delays. This type of evaluation can be obtained through a state or private diagnostic and evaluation center, public school, or university-affiliated program.
2. Associated medical problems, such as seizures, feeding difficulties and poor nutrition, sensory deficits, or dental problems, must be treated to allow the child to maximize their potential.
3. If a treatable cause is identified, such as an inborn error of metabolism, a therapeutic diet can be instituted. Hypothyroidism can be treated with thyroid hormone.
4. A family assessment is essential to address:
   a. Financial stressors—financial aid may be available through social security, Medicaid, or state and local programs to help families with children with developmental delays.
   b. Family functioning and coping abilities.
   c. Support for parental caregivers, siblings, and extended family.
   d. Respite services.
   e. Support groups.
   f. Recreational programs, such as the Special Olympics and summer camps.
   g. Identification of other affected or at-risk people and the need for genetic counseling for recurrence risk.
5. The initial evaluation usually leads to recommendations for more targeted evaluations, such as physical therapy, occupational therapy, and social work assessment.

See "Care of the Child With a Developmental Disability" section, page 1448.

Down Syndrome

EVIDENCE BASE Shaw, D., Bar, S., & Champion, J. D. (2021). The impact of developmental behavioral pediatrics in a population of children with Down syndrome. *Journal of Pediatric Nursing*, *57*, 38–42. https://doi.org/10.1016/j.pedn.2020.10.019

Down syndrome was first described in 1866. Also referred to as trisomy 21, it is the most common genetic cause of intellectual disability. According to the National Down Syndrome Society, the incidence of this error in cell division is about 1 in 772 live births, about 5,100 infants each year. Down syndrome occurs when an individual has a full or partial extra copy of chromosome 21. Each child with Down syndrome has a unique set of genes, besides the effects of the extra genes on chromosome 21, and the child will need individualized evaluation. The most common life experience of a child with Down syndrome is to live with the family, participate in infant stimulation and preschool programs, and attend school while receiving support from special education services. Adults with Down syndrome can function in supported employment or supervised programs. These adults may live in small residential group homes, with their families or in environments with supervision. Life expectancy depends on the presence of medical complications; when there are no complications, life expectancy is slightly shorter than average, approximately 60 years.

Pathophysiology and Etiology

See Table 52-1.

Clinical Manifestations and Associated Problems

1. Characteristic facies—brachycephaly; oblique palpebral fissures; epicanthal folds; flat nasal bridge; protruding tongue; small, low-set ears; and simian crease of palms (see Figure 52-1).
2. Congenital heart anomalies (seen in up to 50% of infants with Down syndrome, compared with 0.8% in the general population), most commonly ventricular septal defects and patent ductus arteriosus.
3. Mental delays.
4. Hypotonia.
5. Growth retardation.
6. Dry, scaly skin.
7. Table 52-2, pages 1455 to 1456, provides a comprehensive list of potential problems that occur with Down syndrome. Some are identified at birth; others arise and cause difficulties later in the life cycle. Percentages are listed that represent occurrence within the Down syndrome population.

Table 52-1 Selected Genetic Disorders

DISORDER AND INCIDENCE	CHARACTERISTICS	ETIOLOGY AND RECURRENCE RISKS	CONSIDERATIONS AND COMMENTS
Chromosomal Disorders			
Autosomal			
Down syndrome (Trisomy 21) 1 in 772 neonates; incidence increases with advanced maternal age (e.g., risk at maternal age 25 is 1 in 1,250; at age 35, 1 in 400; at age 45, 1 in 30)	Brachycephaly: oblique palpebral fissures; epicanthal folds; Brushfield spots; flat nasal bridge; protruding tongue; small, low-set ears; clinodactyly; simian crease; congenital heart defects; hypotonia; intellectual disability; growth retardation; dry, scaly skin; increased risk for childhood leukemia and early-onset Alzheimer disease	• Extra copy of number 21 chromosome (total of three copies). • 94% of cases are trisomy (karyotype 47, +21) for three distinct number 21 chromosomes because of nondisjunction (failure of chromosomal separation during meiosis); recurrence risk 1%, plus maternal age-related risk if older than age 35. • 4% of cases have a translocation—the extra number 21 is attached to another chromosome, usually a number 13 or number 14; half of these translocations are new occurrences, and the other half are inherited from a biological parent. • 2% of cases are mosaic—affected individual has two different cell lines, one with the normal number of chromosomes and the other cell line trisomic for the number 21 chromosome; because of a postconception error in chromosomal division during mitosis.	• Recurrence risk for biological parents of affected are dependent on one or more of the following: chromosomal type of disorder, maternal age, parental karyotype, family history, and sex of transmitting parent and other chromosome involved (if translocation). • May demonstrate nuchal thickening prenatally on ultrasound examination. • Associated with moderate intellectual disability. • No phenotypic differences between trisomy Down syndrome and translocation Down syndrome. • Chromosome analysis should be performed on all persons with Down syndrome. • Prenatal maternal serum screening can adjust risk for the pregnancy. See page 969 for nursing care.
Sex Chromosome			
Turner syndrome (45, X) 1 in 2,500 female births	Webbing of neck and short stature; lymphedema of hands and feet as neonate; congenital cardiac defects (especially coarctation of the aorta); low posterior hairline; cubitus valgus; widely spaced nipples; underdeveloped breasts; immature internal genitalia (e.g., streak ovaries); primary amenorrhea; learning disabilities	• About 50% because of a nondisjunctional error during meiosis (karyotype 45, X); 20% are mosaic because of nondisjunction during mitosis; 30% have two X chromosomes, but one is functionally inadequate (e.g., because of presence of abnormal gene); generally a sporadic occurrence.	• Webbing of neck and short stature may be detected prenatally by ultrasound. • Early diagnosis enhances optimal health care management (e.g., planning for administration of growth hormone therapy, estrogen replacement). • Psychosocial implications associated with short stature, delayed onset of puberty. • Infertility associated with ovarian dysgenesis; oocyte donation and adoption are generally the only options for having children. See page 1328.
Microdeletion/Microduplication			
Fragile X syndrome 1 in 4,000 to 1 in 7,000 for male births and 1 in 6,000 to 1 in 11,000 for female births.	Motor delays; hypotonia; speech delay and language difficulty; hyperactivity; classic features including long face, prominent ears, and macroorchidism manifest around puberty; autism (about 7% of males); intellectual disability in most males; learning disabilities in most affected females	• Mutation in the FMR-1 gene, represented as a large DNA expansion of a normally present trinucleotide. • Carrier mother of an affected male has a 50% risk for future affected males and 50% chance of transmitting the FMR-1 X chromosome to a daughter who would be a carrier, may be unaffected, or manifest features associated with the fragile X syndrome and has a 50% chance of transmitting that gene to future offspring.	• Expansion of DNA in the region of the gene that houses a CpG island results in methylation of the DNA resulting in the gene being "shut down," and the protein normally made by the gene is not made resulting in the phenotype. Testing involves DNA analysis to characterize the size of the DNA expansion. Testing for methylation status of the DNA increases sensitivity. • Phenotypic expression of this gene in males and females is variable; genetic mechanisms determining expression of this gene are very complicated. • Fragile X should be considered in the differential diagnosis of any male with intellectual disability who is undiagnosed; it is the most common intellectual disability in males.

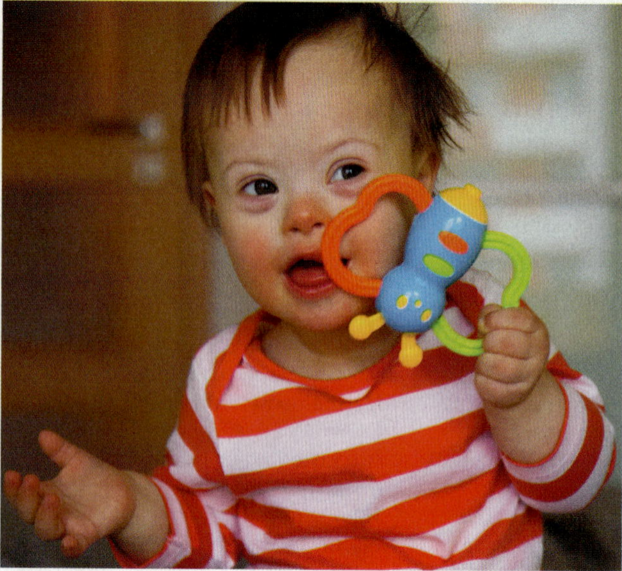

Figure 52-1. A young child with Down syndrome. (Shutterstock/Tatiana Diuvbanova.)

Diagnosis and Management

1. See "Care of the Child With a Developmental Disability" section, page 1448, for a general approach to assessment.
2. See Table 52-2, pages 1455 to 1456, for specific conditions requiring medical management related to Down syndrome, such as otolaryngologic, endocrine, orthopedic, gastrointestinal, and cardiac problems.
3. Alternative therapies—nutritional and supplemental vitamin therapy for Down syndrome remains controversial and effects have not been medically proven.

Considerations for Adult Patients With Down Syndrome

EVIDENCE BASE Fuca, E., Costanzo, F., Ursumando, L., Celestini, L., Scoppola, V., Mancini, S., Valentini, D., Villani, A., & Vicari, S. (2022). Sleep and behavioral problems in preschool-age children with Down syndrome. *Frontiers in Psychology, 13*, 943516. https://doi.org/10.3389/fpsyg.2022.943516

Infants born with Down syndrome today are expected to live well into their sixth decade of life. Adults with Down syndrome experience accelerated aging and have a higher incidence of dementia. Other medical problems more prevalent in this population include spinal and neck problems, pulmonary hypertension, hypothyroidism, testicular cancer, sleep apnea, and dermatologic problems. Mental health disorders can include depression and obsessive–compulsive disorder. Annual health examinations are crucial, and every attempt should be made to find a health care provider who is comfortable with these patients and knowledgeable of the specific health maintenance concerns.

Fragile X Syndrome

Fragile X syndrome is the second most common identifiable cause of intellectual developmental disability, as well as the most common inherited cause. About 80% of males with fragile syndrome demonstrate intellectual disabilities compared with about one third of females. The fragile X phenotype is nonspecific and commonly becomes more apparent with age; therefore, diagnosis usually is not made until middle childhood or later. This syndrome can cause a wide range of cognitive and behavioral characteristics, ranging from mild to severe. Chromosome analysis reveals that the long arm of the X chromosome is constricted and appears fragile, but this cannot be detected in all cases; thus, deoxyribonucleic acid (DNA) analysis is preferred for diagnosis. Fragile X is more common in males, occurring in 1 in 4,000 to 7,000 males and 1 in 6,000 to 11,000 females. Genetic counseling and testing of family members are necessary to evaluate recurrence risks.

Pathophysiology and Etiology

See Table 52-1.

Clinical Manifestations and Associated Problems

1. Mild to moderate developmental delays (IQ range 41 to 88).
2. Elongated face, prominent ears, macrocephaly, high-arched palate, dental crowding, epicanthal folds (fold of the skin on either side of the nose), hypertelorism (increased distance between the eyes), and flattened nasal bridge.
3. Macroorchidism (enlarged testicles) after puberty.
4. Delay in both expressive and receptive language and perseverative or repetitive speech.
5. Delay in adaptive behavior skills.
6. Autistic-like communication disorders.
7. Attention deficit and hyperactivity.
8. Self-stimulating and self-injurious behaviors such as hand biting.
9. Associated problems, including mitral valve prolapse, seizures, joint laxity or hyperextensibility, and feeding problems.
10. Adult patients may develop tremors and ataxia.
11. Females are at risk for premature ovarian failure and early menopause.

Diagnosis and Management

1. See "Care of the Child With a Developmental Disability" section, page 1448, for a general approach to management.
2. See Table 52-3, for specific medical issues related to fragile X syndrome.

Turner Syndrome

Turner syndrome is a genetic disorder found in females. The incidence of this syndrome is approximately 1 in 2,000 female live births. The most severe phenotype occurs in approximately 50% of females with the absence of an X chromosome. There are typically mosaic variations seen with Turner syndrome, and the clinical effects can vary between individuals. It is important to note that most people with Turner syndrome will present with short stature and/or ovarian failure, but the other syndrome characteristics may not be present or may be present in mild form, causing a delay in diagnosis. The cognitive impairments and phenotype can be nonspecific in early childhood, and a diagnosis is commonly not made until failure of pubertal development is noted.

Pathophysiology and Etiology

See Table 52-1.

Table 52-2 Medical Issues Related to Down Syndrome (DS)

POTENTIAL PROBLEMS	EVALUATION	MANAGEMENT
Congenital heart malformations (i.e., AV canal, VSD, PDA, and tetralogy of Fallot) (40%)	• Observe for color changes, pulse, and respiratory rate at rest and with stress. Assess tolerance of feeding for early tiring or frequent interruptions in feeding. Echocardiogram is usually done during neonatal period on all infants with DS.	• Early identification and treatment can prevent heart failure and decompensation or poor growth. Medical or surgical intervention correction has minimized mortality from simple cardiac anomalies.
Congenital GI malformations (12%) • Pyloric stenosis • Duodenal atresia, tracheoesophageal fistula	• Observe for coughing or vomiting, especially with feeding: bile-stained vomitus suggests lower tract anomalies; partially digested contents suggest upper tract problem. Observe bowel movements and for abdominal distention. • Radiographic studies are done.	• GI reflux (spillage of material from the esophagus into the trachea) can cause arching during feedings, poor weight gain, chronic respiratory problems, allergy and asthma symptomatology, pneumonia, and aspiration. Medication management and, if needed, surgical intervention can occur in the early neonatal period.
Hypothyroidism (10%–20%)	• Monitor for weight gain, hair loss, lethargy, short stature, voice changes, and depression (can develop at any time over life cycle). Neonatal screening includes T_3, TSH, and T_4 biannually.	• Thyroid hormone replacement.
Visual anomalies • Refractive errors (70%) • Strabismus (50%) • Nystagmus (35%) • Cataracts (3%)	• Observe for indication of vision problems, such as head tilt or poor visual tracking. Use Teller activity as a visual screen tool for those who cannot cooperate with Snellen chart. • Positive findings in the first year of life warrant immediate referral to ophthalmologist. All individuals should be seen by a pediatric ophthalmologist (or one who is skilled in evaluating children) at age 1, and vision evaluations should continue throughout life.	• Undetected visual deficits can cause failure to achieve developmental milestones and cause permanent loss of vision.
Hearing anomalies (60%–90%): • Mild to moderate conductive hearing loss • Enlarged adenoids • Sleep apnea	• Assess for curiosity and response to sounds of varying quality. Auditory brain stem response assesses hearing in infants. Sound field testing for children older than age 1 year. • Tympanometry to assess middle ear function.	• Narrow ear canals and subtle immunodeficiencies can cause chronic middle ear infections. Enlarged adenoids can cause upper airway obstruction, especially during sleep. • Treatment can range from antibiotics for simple otitis media to myringotomy tubes, adenoidectomy, or hearing loss.
Hypotonia of infants (100%)	• Observe for floppiness, poor head control, and poor oral motor function. Infant should be placed on abdomen periodically while being observed and monitored for potential for suffocation.	• Physical, occupational, and speech therapy. Adaptive equipment gives extra support to the head and neck when handling neonate. Always keep head elevated for at least 1 h after meals. Change position regularly.
Atlanto-occipital and atlantoaxial subluxation (dislocation of the upper spine because of joint laxity) (15%)	• Assess for head tilt; increasing clumsiness, limping, or refusal to walk; and weakness of the arms. X-ray of cervical spine to evaluate for atlantoaxial dislocation at age 2 and then every 5 yr during childhood. Precise measurements are taken to document alignment of the skull and vertebrae. Shifting of the two can cause compression and neurologic damage. Participation in Special Olympics and other activities that may require neck flexion should warrant a baseline evaluation.	• If present, participation in contact sports and gymnastics is contraindicated. In severe cases, surgery to fuse the vertebrae and occiput and stabilize the spinal column.
Gait anomalies (15%)	• Monitor for onset of limp, leg length discrepancy. Hip x-rays can document dislocation or subluxation.	• Physical therapy and, sometimes, orthopedic surgery are necessary.
Failure to thrive	• Monitor growth on DS growth chart. Monitor feedings for length of feeding, feeding schedule, loss of feeding by vomiting, or poor seal on nipple. Monitor type of formula and caloric content.	• Nutritionist can advise on formula adjustments. Therapists can help with positioning and types of nipples used to counteract effects of weak sucking reflex and large, protruding tongue.

(continued)

Table 52-2 Medical Issues Related to Down Syndrome (DS) (continued)

POTENTIAL PROBLEMS	EVALUATION	MANAGEMENT
Short stature (100%)	• Plot growth on DS growth chart. Monitor stages of puberty. Delayed puberty may warrant further investigation.	• Use of human growth hormone may be considered; this is still controversial.
Obesity (50%)	• Monitor thyroid hormone levels. Serial monitoring of weight. Monitor for amount of exercise and caloric intake.	• Overindulgence by adults or use of food in behavior management increases risk of overeating. Lack of social involvement leads to decreased activity. Behavior modification is necessary.
Malocclusions (60%–100%)	• Assess for malocclusions, periodontal disease, and delayed eruption of teeth. Regular dental checkups begin at age 1 yr or when teeth erupt.	• Encourage good oral hygiene with proper toothbrushing.
Intellectual disability with varying degrees from mild to moderate (100%)	• Routine developmental assessment using standardized tools of measurement.	• Special education and training.
Alzheimer disease after age 40 (15%–30%)	• Assess for decreased cognitive function and loss of memory. MRI or CT scan shows areas of plaque.	• Increased supervision is needed.
Seizures (6%)	• Onset of seizures is seen primarily during adolescence and middle age.	• Neurologic evaluation and appropriate antiseizure medications.
Other problems • Communication disorders • Alopecia (10%) • Leukemia (1%)		

AV, atrioventricular; CT, computed tomography; GI, gastrointestinal; MRI, magnetic resonance imaging; PDA, patent ductus arteriosus; T3, triiodothyronine; T4, levothyroxine; TSH, thyroid-stimulating hormone; VSD, ventricular septal defect.

Clinical Manifestations and Associated Problems

1. The most prevalent characteristics of Turner syndrome include:
   a. Short stature, webbed neck, low posterior hairline, and edema of the hands and feet (see Figure 52-2).
   b. Congenital cardiac anomalies.
   c. Broad chest with inverted or underdeveloped nipples.
   d. Immature reproductive organs, delayed puberty, and primary amenorrhea.
   e. Hypothyroidism, obesity, type II diabetes, osteoporosis, and fractures in adulthood.
   f. Learning disabilities.
2. Associated problems include:
   a. Coarctation of the aorta and idiopathic hypertension.
   b. Hearing loss—conductive or sensorineural.
   c. Obesity and glucose intolerance.
   d. Feeding problems.
   e. Renal anomalies.

Diagnosis and Management

1. See "Care of the Child With a Developmental Disability" section, page 1448, for a general approach to assessment.
2. See Table 52-4, for specific medical issues related to Turner syndrome.
3. Diagnosis may occur prenatally through an amniocentesis, with genetic testing, or any time after birth. A preliminary diagnosis may be made based on physical characteristics. This should then be confirmed by genetic testing. A diagnosis is often not made until there is a failure to begin menstruation.

Fetal Alcohol Spectrum Disorder

Fetal alcohol spectrum disorder (FASD) is a significant problem. Children with FASD have a wide range of physical, mental, behavioral, and/or learning disabilities that put them at risk. FASD is the leading known preventable cause of intellectual developmental disabilities in developed countries.

Pathophysiology and Etiology

1. According to the National Institute on Alcohol Abuse and Alcoholism of the National Institutes of Health (NIH), the prevalence of FASD in the general population ranges from 0.2 to 1.5 cases per 1,000 children and 2% to 5% for the entire continuum of FASD. It is caused by use or misuse of alcohol during pregnancy. The alcohol ingested by the pregnant person passes easily across the placenta to the fetus.
   a. There is no "safe" level of alcohol use during pregnancy; a pregnant person who drinks any amount of alcohol is at risk.
   b. Larger amounts of alcohol and binge drinking appear to cause more significant risk to the fetus.
   c. Alcohol use in the first trimester is most problematic.

Table 52-3 Medical Issues Related to Fragile X Syndrome

POTENTIAL PROBLEMS	EVALUATION	MANAGEMENT
Hypotonia of infancy	• Assess ability to control the head and assume upright posture. • Assess feeding for efficient suck and coordination of suck/swallow.	Physical therapy, stimulation program, feeding adaptations.
Seizures (20% of cases)	• Assess for muscle tremors, deviation of the eyes to one side, rhythmic jerking of the body, and loss of consciousness.	Referral to a neurologist for diagnosis and anticonvulsants to treat seizures.
Mitral valve prolapse (80% of males)	• Assess dyspnea, cyanosis, and murmur. Echocardiogram to evaluate valve function.	Antibiotics for prophylaxis before invasive procedures to prevent endocarditis. Treatment of heart failure; surgical repair may be necessary.
Self-stimulating behavior	• Rule out source of pain (i.e., otitis media, tooth pain) that may be causing behavior. Rule out sensory deficits.	Behavior management techniques: focus on replacing undesirable behaviors with purposeful, meaningful ones, with emphasis on positive reinforcement and extinguishing negative reinforcement.
Hyperactivity, attention deficits	• Assess activity of attention span within the context of the developmental age of the child.	Behavior management and special educational techniques.
Discipline problems	• Assess social skills.	Males tend to do best in self-contained classrooms for children with similar degrees of intellectual disability.
Communication disorders	• Assess language development (usually weakest area of development).	Speech–language therapy can be beneficial.
Poor auditory memory; auditory reception	• Assess how child lets needs be known: cries, gestures, single words, or sentences.	Speech therapy, behavior modification.
Cognitive dysfunction • Short-term memory deficits • Poor problem-solving skills • Functional limitations in self-care	• Assess for appropriateness of educational placement and child's reaction to situation.	Specialized training and education, assisted living.

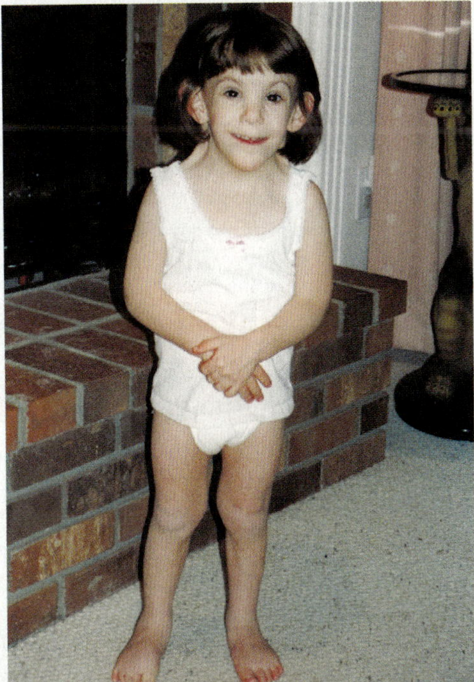

Figure 52-2. A 3-year-old child with Turner syndrome. Note the webbed neck.

Clinical Manifestations and Associated Problems

EVIDENCE BASE Geier, D. A., & Geier, M. R. (2022). Fetal alcohol syndrome and the risk of neurodevelopmental disorders: A longitudinal cohort study. *Brain and Development, 44*(10), 706–714. https://doi.org/10.1016/j.braindev.2022.08.002

Whittingham, L., & Coons-Harding, K. (2021). Connecting people with people: Diagnosing persons with fetal alcohol spectrum disorder using telehealth. *Journal of Autism and Developmental Disorders, 51*(4), 1067–1080. https://doi.org/10.1007/s10803-020-04607-z

1. Intrauterine growth delay.
2. Decreased muscle tone and poor coordination.
3. Delayed development and problems in three or more major areas: cognitive, speech, motor, or social skills.
4. Hyperactivity and attention deficits.
5. Vision or hearing problems.
6. Heart anomalies such as ventricular septal defect or atrial septal defect.
7. Craniofacial anomalies, including narrow, small eyes with large epicanthal folds, small head, small upper jaw, smooth groove in the upper lip, and smooth and thin upper lip.

Table 52-4 Medical Issues Related to Turner Syndrome

POTENTIAL PROBLEMS	EVALUATION	MANAGEMENT
Congenital heart malformations: • Increased incidence of left-sided heart anomalies • Aortic valve anomalies • Coarctation of the aorta	Observe for color changes, pulse, and respiratory rate at rest and with stress. Monitor blood pressure. Assess tolerance of feeding for early tiring or frequent interruptions in feeding. An electrocardiogram should be done in the neonatal period. A yearly echocardiogram or magnetic resonance imaging should also be done.	Early identification and treatment can prevent secondary problems. If needed, prophylactic antibiotic for subacute bacterial endocarditis. Referral to a cardiologist.
Renal and renovascular anomalies: • Horseshoe kidney • Duplicated renal pelvis • Vascular anomalies	Renal sonogram should be done to rule out anomalies. Routine urinalysis and culture to screen for urinary tract infection and glycosuria.	Referral to a nephrologist if a renal anomaly is present. Monitor for the development of diabetes mellitus.
Edema in the hands and feet	Edema may persist for months or may recur; if recurrence, monitor for renal or cardiac causes.	—
Dysmorphic features: webbed neck, face, and ears	Parental caregivers may elect plastic surgery to minimize the visible anomalies.	Enhances the socialization of females with Turner syndrome in school. May need additional support or therapy.
Nutrition: failure to thrive in the infant period and obesity in childhood	Infants may have inefficient sucking and swallowing reflexes. Monitor growth utilizing a Turner syndrome growth chart.	Nutrition counseling and encouragement of exercise to maintain appropriate weight.
Hearing loss	Hearing loss may be conductive or sensorineural. Routine screening should be performed.	Otitis media should be treated aggressively to minimize potential hearing loss.
Short stature and failure to develop secondary sex characteristics	—	Endocrine therapy may be indicated for growth and development. Hormonal therapy may enhance the development of secondary sex characteristics.
Infertility	Ovaries are not developed. Usually no need for testing.	Infertility is generally expected in Turner syndrome. Infertility techniques may be able to assist with childbearing.
Hypothyroidism	Periodic laboratory testing.	Thyroid hormone replacement therapy.
Behavioral problems, learning disabilities	—	Behavioral management. Special education.
Strabismus	If detected, referral to an ophthalmologist is recommended.	Patching or surgical repair.
Cognitive function	Average to slightly below-average intelligence. Problem areas include spatial perception and math functions.	Special education.

8. The average IQ is 65, with a range from 20 to 120, with many of these children qualifying for special education services.
9. Many will go on to have disrupted school progress, criminal offenses, and alcohol- and drug-related problems.

Diagnosis and Management

1. Diagnosis is usually made with history and clinical presentation. Ultrasounds during pregnancy may show physical features. Brain imaging studies (CT and MRI) may be performed later to document neuroanomalies.
2. Management includes evaluation and regular monitoring of growth and nutrition. Ongoing management of symptoms related to other medical issues is a priority.
3. Nurses should be knowledgeable of educational and community resources that may be necessary for the child to reach their maximum potential. See "Care of the Child With a Developmental Disability" section, page 1448.

PERVASIVE DEVELOPMENTAL DISORDER OR AUTISM SPECTRUM DISORDER

Autism spectrum disorders (ASDs) refer to a group of pervasive developmental disorders, including autism, Asperger disorder (AD), and disorders noted as pervasive developmental disorder, not otherwise specified. This disorder has been identified in 1 in 36 children.

Autism

EVIDENCE BASE Sappok, T., Heinrich, M., & Bohm, J. (2020). The impact of emotional development in people with autism spectrum disorder and intellectual developmental disability. *Journal of Intellectual Disability Research, 64*(12), 946–955. https://doi.org/10.1111/jir.12785

Syriopoulou-Delli, C. (2023). Quality of life in people with intellectual and developmental disability, autism: Advances in practice and research. *International Journal of Developmental Disabilities, 69*(3), 359–361. https://doi.org/10.1080/20473869.2023.2205287

Autism is a complex neurobiologic developmental disorder that most typically appears during the first 2 years of life. The diagnosis of autism is based on a persistent deficit in social communication and social interaction across multiple contexts as manifested in the time of examination or by history. Autism is a lifelong disorder defined by the individual's interactive difficulties, which can range from mild to severely impaired. It is four to five times more common in males than in females, but affected females tend to be more severely impaired.

Approximately 50% of people with autism are cognitively impaired, with a wide range of potential IQs. Autism is seen in approximately 1% of the population worldwide.

Pathophysiology and Etiology

1. A clear cause has not been identified; however, evidence suggests a genetic predisposition, but no specific mutation has been identified.
2. Studies have shown that measles, mumps, and rubella vaccine do *not* cause autism. Likewise, thimerosal, a preservative found in many vaccines, does *not* cause autism.
3. Before diagnosis, parental caregivers may be initially concerned about their infant's social interactions, delayed or unusual speech development, and reactions to various stimuli (i.e., tactile defensiveness).
4. Individuals with ASD have neuroanatomic differences, including small neuron cell size, increased cell packing, relative macrocephaly, and large third ventricles.

Clinical Manifestations

1. In general, the features present with the diagnosis include problems with social interactions, communication, and language skills.
2. Patients with autism have anomalies in relating to people, objects, and events. They have atypical responses to sensory stimuli, usually sound.
3. The stereotypical behaviors of autism are restricted and repetitive, like the commonly known symptom of echolalic speech.

Diagnosis and Management

EVIDENCE BASE Carter, E. W., Carlton, M. E., & Travers, H. E. (2020). Seeing strengths: Young adults and their siblings with autism or intellectual disability. *Journal of Applied Research in Intellectual Disabilities, 33*(3), 574–583. https://doi.org/10.1111/jar.12701

Siman-Tov, A., & Sharabi, A. (2023). Differences between typically-developing brothers & sisters of individuals with developmental disabilities. *Journal of Child and Family Studies, 32*(5), 1559–1570. https://doi.org/10.1007/s10826-023-02574-4

1. Early diagnosis leads to earlier interventions, resulting in improved outcomes for these children.
2. The two major diagnostic challenges in the evaluation of ASD include making the differential diagnosis and searching for the etiologic disorder associated with ASD (fragile X syndrome is the most common known single-gene cause of ASD).
3. Comprehensive standardized assessment tools specific for ASD usually require specialized training; these tools include Childhood Autism Rating Scale (CARS), Diagnostic Interview of Social and Communication Disorders (DISCO), Autism Diagnostic Interview (ADI), Autism Diagnostic Interview Schedule (ADIS), and Checklist for Autism in Toddlers (CHAT).
4. Alternative treatments such as nutrition and vitamin therapy are being investigated, but no definitive research has been conclusive to date.
5. Many children with ASD also have psychiatric comorbidities with such conditions as obsessive–compulsive disorder, attention-deficit/hyperactivity disorder (ADHD), depression, mood disorders, and Tourette syndrome. These conditions can be challenging to diagnose, because it may be difficult to assess the child with communication and behavioral problems. Indeed, health care providers need to be vigilant in screening and monitoring for these comorbidities to ensure optimal functioning of the child with ASD.
6. Treatment is focused on management of symptoms. Medications may be helpful in treating some of the more disruptive behavioral symptoms. The most commonly used medications include select serotonin reuptake inhibitors, atypical antipsychotic/neuroleptics, stimulants, and alpha agonists.
7. Medical comorbidities are also common in children with ASD, including seizure disorders, sleep disturbances, GI disorders, and dental problems. As with psychiatric comorbidities, health care providers need to be vigilant in their assessment, as it can improve behavior and functioning of the child with ASD.
8. A multidisciplinary team—including primary care provider; medical subspecialists; occupational, speech, and physical therapists; and educational specialist—is essential for optimal care. See "Care of the Child With a Developmental Disability" section, page 1448.

Childhood Disintegrative Disorder

Childhood disintegrative disorder follows a period of typical development. This typical developmental period may last from ages 2 to 10 years, with the most common age of onset being 3 and 4 years of age. The child begins to experience a significant loss of previously acquired skills. Areas that may be affected include expressive and receptive language, social skills or adaptive behavior, bowel and bladder control, and motor skills. The loss of these skills generally reaches a point at which they do not disintegrate further. At such point, some limited improvements may be seen. This condition differs from autism in the pattern of onset, course, and outcome.

Pathophysiology and Etiology

Etiology is unknown. Childhood disintegrative disorder appears to be more common in males. The incidence of this disorder is rare.

Diagnosis and Management

See "Care of the Child With a Developmental Disability" section, page 1448, for a general approach to assessment.

Asperger Disorder

Asperger disorder is considered a milder form of autism and is characterized by poor peer relationships, lack of empathy, and the tendency to be overfocused on certain topics.

AD is one of several developmental disabilities associated with typical intelligence. Academic and functional underachievement in the preschool and school-age child with typical intelligence is the common picture. Proper diagnosis, utilizing a cooperative team effort from several individuals, is imperative to develop an individualized treatment plan.

Pathophysiology and Etiology

The etiology is unknown. AD is commonly not diagnosed until the child reaches school age. The prevalence estimates vary widely with many individuals never being formally diagnosed.

Clinical Manifestations

1. Child does not seek spontaneous interpersonal interactions.
2. Average to above-average intelligence and development of typical language skills with regard to vocabulary and grammar.
3. No significant delays in the areas of cognitive development, development of age-appropriate self-help skills, adaptive behavior, and curiosity about the environment.
4. Limited range of interests, strict adherence to routines and rituals, and repetitious motor movements or sequences.
5. May have obsessional interests and appear "eccentric" to others.

Diagnosis and Management

1. Complete medical review, family history, and physical examination, including vision and hearing assessment and neurologic evaluation, to rule out other disorders.
2. Genetic evaluation and counseling to identify the presence of recurrence risks.
3. Psychological testing to determine the exact nature of cognitive and perceptual dysfunctions.
4. Behavioral and social assessment.
5. Assessment of academic performance.
6. MRI and other testing to determine underlying neurologic anomaly, if appropriate.
7. Occupational and physical therapy and speech and language evaluations, as necessary.
8. School evaluation—involves IQ testing and achievement testing (teacher's input is also essential).
   a. The focus of a school evaluation is to determine eligibility for services. Most school systems will provide services only when moderate to severe problems exist.
   b. It may be necessary for the family to provide remediation for problems considered mild or outside of the educational setting.
9. Because the disorder may include health manifestations as well as behavioral and educational implications, the school nurse should be prepared to provide guidance on complex management.

EVIDENCE BASE Hayden, N. K., Hastings, R. P., & Bailey, T. (2023). Behavioural adjustment of children with intellectual disability and their sibling is associated with their sibling relationship quality. *Journal of Intellectual Disability Research*, 67(4), 310–322. https://doi.org/10.1111/jir.13006

Pervasive Developmental Disorder, Not Otherwise Specified

Pervasive developmental disorder, not otherwise specified (PDD-NOS) is no longer used. PDD-NOS, previously one of several distinct subtypes of autism, is now encompassed within the single diagnosis of ASD. A diagnosis may be made at a later date because of the appearance of additional manifestation. The *Diagnostic and Statistical Manual of Mental Disorders, Fifth Edition, Text Revision (DSM-5-TR)* notes that individuals with a well-established diagnosis of autistic disorder, AD, or pervasive developmental disorder, not otherwise specified, should be given the diagnosis of ASD. This suggests that there is a spectrum of developmental disorders with common features, which may range widely in severity and represent a range of genetically influenced impairments.

ATTENTION DISORDERS AND LEARNING DISABILITIES

Attention disorders and learning disabilities are separate but overlapping problems and may need specific approaches based on the nature of the disability. An estimated 5% to 10% of children have attention-deficit disorder (ADD); learning disabilities may also be present. Almost 9 of 10 children with attention-deficit/hyperactivity disorder (ADHD) received school support, including school accommodations and help in the classroom.

Pathophysiology and Etiology

1. Multiple hypotheses exist because the exact causes are unknown; they may be genetic.
   a. A family trait—other members of the family have similar difficulties.
   b. Characteristic of inborn errors of metabolism.
   c. Sex chromosome anomalies commonly exhibit these traits.
2. Not shown to be associated with a history of birth trauma or brain damage.
3. Exposure to prenatal and postnatal factors that might adversely affect brain development and function—lead, alcohol, cocaine, central nervous system (CNS) infections, low birth weight, and prematurity.
4. May coexist with other disabling conditions, such as spina bifida, cerebral palsy, or seizure disorders.
5. May have biomedical, emotional, social, and environmental components.
6. ADD is an alteration in the response-inhibition mechanisms of the brain controlled by the frontal cortex and reticular activating system and alteration in neurotransmitter.
7. Learning disabilities—authorities are investigating anomalies in the parietal lobe of the brain and in the central visual pathways located in the occipital lobe.
8. Although emotional and environmental factors play a role, serotonin deficiency may serve as a physiologic basis for these disorders.

Attention Disorders

EVIDENCE BASE Burack, J. A., Friedman, S., Lessage, M., & Brodeur, D. (2023). Re-visiting the "mysterious myth of attention deficit": A systematic review of the recent evidence. *Journal of Intellectual Disability Research*, 67(3), 271–288. https://doi.org/10.1111/jir.12994

Attention disorders are characterized by a cluster of symptoms, including developmentally inappropriate short attention span, impulsivity, and distractibility. The classification system identifies three subtypes of attention disorders: predominantly inattentive, predominantly hyperactive–impulsive, and combined. Attention disorders are more common in males than in females by a ratio of 3:1. Females are much more likely to have inattentive type, showing more symptoms of attention deficit rather than hyperactivity.

There is no specific laboratory test or radiographical test that can diagnose attention disorders. The best way to diagnose attention disorders is through careful history from parental caregivers, child, and teachers; use of standardized questionnaires or rating scales; and observation. There are a number of behavior rating scales that are used to establish the diagnosis of ADD and ADHD. Examples of rating scales include the Conners Rating Scale, the Brown Attention-Deficit Disorder Scale for Children and Adolescents, and the Vanderbilt ADHD Rating Scale.

Clinical Manifestations and Diagnostic Evaluation

General Behavior

EVIDENCE BASE Salari, N., Hoorman, A., Abdoli, N., Rahmani, A., Shiri, M. H., Hashemian, A. H., Akbari, H., & Mohammadi, M. (2023). The global prevalence of ADHD in children and adolescents: A systematic review and meta-analysis. *Italian Journal of Pediatrics*, *49*(1), 48. https://doi.org/10.1186/s13052-023-01456-1

Behavior varies slightly based on the child's age. Some impairments across the life span can include:

1. Childhood: Needs for special education, grade retention, classroom behavior management issues, and behavioral difficulties at home and other settings.
2. Adolescence: School failure and dropout, social difficulties with peer relationships, substance use (in untreated), high comorbidity with other psychiatric disorders, and involvement in juvenile criminal activities.
3. Adult: Fewer employment possibilities and frequent job hopping; high risk of tobacco, drug, and alcohol use; high risk of motor vehicle accidents; marital problems and higher divorce rates; and increased incidence of criminal activity.

Diagnostic Criteria for ADHD

The *Diagnostic and Statistical Manual of Mental Disorders, Fifth Edition*, Text Revision (*DSM-5-TR*) outlines diagnostic criteria for ADHD. In this edition, the core symptoms reflect how the disorder presents in school-age children, as well as in older adolescents and adults. Examples of questions to be considered include:

1. Does the child often fidget with hands or feet or squirm in seat?
2. Does the child have difficulty remaining seated when required to do so?
3. Is the child easily distracted by extraneous stimuli?
4. Does the child have difficulty awaiting their turn in games or group situations?
5. Does the child often blurt out answers to questions before they have been completed?
6. Does the child often have difficulty following instructions from others?
7. Does the child have difficulty sustaining attention in tasks or play activities?
8. Does the child often shift from one uncompleted activity to another?
9. Does the child have difficulty playing quietly?
10. Does the child often talk excessively?
11. Does the child often interrupt or intrude on others?
12. Does the child often not seem to listen to what is being said to them?
13. Does the child often lose things necessary for tasks or activities at school or at home?
14. Does the child often engage in physically dangerous activities without considering possible consequences?

Management

Multidisciplinary Approach

A multidisciplinary approach, including environmental and behavioral approaches, is the treatment of choice.

Pharmacologic Treatment

1. CNS stimulants are generally effective for 70% to 80% of children with attention disorders.
   a. Effective in decreasing motor activities and increasing attention span and concentration, thereby allowing the child to be more available to learn.
   b. Medications generally include stimulant medications, but nonstimulant medications may also be effective, especially in adults. Examples include methylphenidate, dextroamphetamine, amphetamine, lisdexamfetamine, and atomoxetine.
2. Adverse effects:
   a. Insomnia may result from increased dosage or if administered too late in the day.
   b. Anorexia, weight loss, hair loss, and temporary growth retardation.
   c. Increased pulse and respiratory rates, nervousness, nausea, and stomachache.
   d. Altered effects of many antiseizure drugs and tricyclic antidepressants.
   e. Do not cause euphoric effect or dependency in children.

Nursing Responsibilities and Family Education

1. Administer the drug before breakfast and lunch (sustained-release forms may not require a second dose).
2. Work with school system to make sure that the lunch dose is given if prescribed.
3. Consider "drug holidays" during vacations and on weekends to monitor effectiveness and the need for a dosage change; this is especially recommended at the start of each academic school year.
4. "Drug holidays" may be difficult in the older adolescent population because the medication may be necessary for optimal functioning in employment and while driving motor vehicles.
5. Children without cardiac disease who receive stimulant therapy are not at increased risk of cardiovascular (CV) events compared with the general population, so cardiac evaluations are not routinely ordered. If a focused history and physical examination suggest the possible presence of CV disease, appropriate evaluation should be initiated, and cardiology consultation should be considered, before starting pharmacotherapy of ADHD.
6. Stimulant drugs are not usually given to children younger than the age of 6 years.
7. The child is usually started on a small dose, which is gradually increased until the desired response is achieved.
8. Evaluate the child's response to the drug by direct observation and consultation with others, such as parental caregivers and teachers.

DRUG ALERT Stimulant drugs for attention disorders should be used in conjunction with a comprehensive therapeutic regimen (e.g., behavioral modification) and not as the sole method of treatment. Stimulant drugs require monitoring and feedback from the parental caregivers and teachers who directly observe the effects.

Learning Disabilities

Difficulties with academic achievement fall under a broad category of learning disabilities. The cause or influencing factors can be biomedical, developmental, behavioral, emotional, social, environmental, family issues, or, frequently, a combination of multiple factors. The problem may be in the area of reading, math, written expression, motor skills, and communication disorders. ADD, anxiety, and behavioral disorders must be ruled out.

Clinical Manifestations

1. Signs of learning disabilities include:
    a. School achievement significantly lower than predicted based on developmental age.
    b. Perceptual–motor impairments.
    c. Emotional lability.
    d. Speech and language disorders.
    e. Coordination deficits.
2. There can be a wide range of cognitive ability from mild intellectual disability to above-average intelligence.

Areas of Learning Disabilities

Auditory Perception

Auditory perception is characterized by difficulty distinguishing between similar sounds or words. This includes the inability to process the sounds into words that have a meaning at a rapid enough rate to be able to follow conversations.

Visual Perception

Visual perception difficulties involve problems interpreting what is seen. This may include problems recognizing shapes and positions of letters or words. Depth perception may pose a problem to some children with visual perception disorders.

Integrative Processing

Integrative processing disabilities encompass, to varying degrees, the inability to sequence events or facts, comprehend abstract ideas or implied meanings, and organize learned information and apply it to what has been previously acquired.

Memory

Disabilities generally affect short-term memory, which stores information that has just been perceived for a brief period before it is either discarded or stored in long-term memory.

Expressive Language

An *expressive language* disorder affects the child's verbal communication. Characteristics depend on the child's age and the severity of the disorder. Language skills in terms of vocabulary, grammatical content, fluency, and language formulation can be affected.

Motor

Motor disabilities can affect either gross motor or fine motor muscle groups. A disability affecting the gross motor development can cause children to be "clumsy." These children have a tendency to fall or bump into things and have difficulty running and playing sports. Fine motor disabilities affect muscles for detailed tasks, such as writing, using scissors, and painting.

Management and Special Teaching Strategies

1. For visual perceptual deficit—present material verbally; use hands-on experience; tape-record teaching sessions.
2. For auditory perceptual deficit—provide materials in written form; use pictures; provide tactile learning.
3. For integrative deficit—use multisensory approaches; print directions while you verbalize them; use calendars and lists to organize tasks and activities.
4. For motor and expressive deficits—break down skills and projects into their multiple component parts; verbally describe the component parts; provide extra time to perform; allow the child to type work rather than use cursive writing.
5. For highly distractible child—provide a structured environment; have child sit in the front of the class; place child away from doors or windows; decrease clutter on their desk.

CRITICAL JUDGMENT Historically, preschool and kindergarten screening tools have not been accurate in predicting learning disabilities; tests of language and memory are better predictors.

Resources and Support Groups

Agencies that may provide information, support, and additional resources include:

The ARC of the United States (formerly Association for Retarded Citizens of the United States)
2000 Pennsylvania Avenue NW, Suite 500 Washington, DC 20006
(800) 433-5255
www.thearc.org

Autism Society
6110 Executive Boulevard, Suite 305
Rockville, Maryland 20852
(800) 328-8476
www.autism-society.org

Children and Adults with Attention Deficit/Hyperactivity Disorder (CHADD)
4221 Forbes Blvd. Suite 720
Lanham, MD 20706
(301) 306-7070
www.chadd.org

Council for Learning Disabilities
11184 Antioch Road
P.O. Box 405
Overland Park, KS 66210
(913) 491-1011
www.cldinternational.org

The Joseph P. Kennedy Jr. Foundation
1133 19th Street NW, 11th floor
Washington, DC 20036
(202) 393-1250
www.jpkf.org

Learning Disabilities Association of America
4156 Library Road, #1
Pittsburgh, PA 15234-1349
(412) 341-1515
www.ldanatl.org

National Down Syndrome Congress
30 Mansell Court, Suite 108
Roswell, GA 30076
(800) 232-NDSC (6372)
www.ndsccenter.org

National Down Syndrome Society
8 E 41st Street, 8th floor
New York, New York 10017
(800) 221-4602
www.ndss.org

National Fragile X Foundation
1012 14th Street NW, Suite 500
Washington, DC 20005
(800) 688-8765
https://fragilex.org

SELECTED READINGS

American Psychiatric Association. (2022). *Diagnostic and statistical manual of mental disorders* (5th ed. rev.). Author.

Becerra, M. A. (2022). Closing the diagnostic gap: Early autism spectrum disorder screening for every child. *Health & Social Work, 47*(2), 87–91. https://doi.org/10.1093/hsw/hlac008

Farnsworth, E. M., Cordle, M., & Sullivan, A. L. (2022). Predictors of kindergarten-reading performance for children with special needs: Do intervention intensity and service provider matter? *Children & Society, 36*(5), 806–820. https://doi.org/10.1111/chso.12540

Fontil, L., Gittens, J., Beaudoin, E., & Sladeczek, I. E. (2020). Barriers to and facilitators of successful early school transitions for children with autism spectrum disorders and other developmental disabilities: A systematic review. *Journal of Autism and Developmental Disorders, 50*(6), 1866–1881. https://doi.org/10.1007/s10803-019-03938-w

Freeman, M., Crawford, A., Gough, L., Rianto, M., Yakubov, R., Rampton, G., Fitzgerald, E., Fang, H., & Di Rezze, B. (2022). Examining the development and utilization of infection control policies to safely support adults with intellectual and developmental disabilities in congregate living settings during COVID-19. *Canadian Journal of Public Health, 113*(6), 918–929. https://doi.org/10.17269/s41997-022-00674-0

Giesbrecht, G. F., Lebel, C., Dennis, C. L., Silang, K., Xie, E. B., Tough, S., McDonald, S., & Tomfohr-Madsen, L. (2023). Risk for developmental delay among infants born during the COVID-19 pandemic. *Journal of Developmental and Behavioral Pediatrics, 44*(6), e412–e420. https://doi.org/10.1097/DBP.0000000000001197

Hofmann, V., & Muller, C. M. (2022). Challenging behaviour in students with intellectual disabilities: The role of individual and classmates' communication skills. *Journal of Intellectual Disability Research, 66*(4), 353–367. https://doi.org/10.1111/jir.12922

Jensen, M. L., & Vamosi, M. (2023). The association between nonpharmacological interventions and quality of life in children with attention deficit hyperactivity disorder: A systematic review. *Journal of Child and Adolescent Psychiatric Nursing, 36*(2), 114–123. https://doi.org/10.1111/jcap.12402

Munsell, E. G. S., McConnell, H., & Coster, W. J. (2023). Adolescents' perspectives on learning to manage the responsibilities of adulthood. *American Journal of Occupational Therapy, 77*(5), 7705345010. https://doi.org/10.5014/ajot.2023.050228

Olusanya, B. O., Smythe, T., Ogbo, F. A., Nair, M. K. C., Scher, M., & Davis, A. C. (2023). Global prevalence of developmental disabilities in children and adolescents: A systematic umbrella review. *Frontiers in Public Health, 11*, 1122009. https://doi.org/10.3389/fpubh.2023.1122009

Roth, M., & Drucker, R. (2021). Nutritional requirements for children with special needs. *Exceptional Parent, 51*(2), 34–36. https://reader.mediawiremobile.com/epmagazine/issues/206939/viewer?page=35

Stehouwer, N., Sawaya, A., Shaniuk, P., & White, P. (2021). Consultation needs for young adults with intellectual and developmental disabilities admitted to an adult tertiary care hospital: Implications for inpatient practice. *Journal of Pediatric Nursing, 60*, 288–292. https://doi.org/10.1016/j.pedn.2021.07.029

Vancampfort, D., Van Damme, T., Firth, J., Stubbs, B., Schuch, F., Suetani, S., Arkesteyn, A., & Van Biesen, D. (2022). Physical activity correlates in children and adolescents, adults, and older adults with an intellectual disability: A systematic review. *Disability and Rehabilitation, 44*(16), 4189–4200. https://doi.org/10.1080/09638288.2021.1909665

Part Four

Psychiatric Nursing

53 Problems of Mental Health*

ANXIETY-RELATED DISORDERS

Anxiety Disorders

EVIDENCE BASE American Psychiatric Association. (2022). *Diagnostic and statistical manual of mental disorders: Fifth edition, text revision: DSM-5-TR* (5th ed.). Author.

Amaral, R. I., Weston, F. C. L., Hirakata, V. N., Paz, A. A., & Wesner, A. C. (2022). Effectiveness and efficacy of therapeutic interventions performed by nurses for anxiety disorders: A systematic review. *Journal of the American Psychiatric Nurses Association, 28*(4), 283–294. https://doi.org/10.1177/10783903211068105

Anxiety disorders are the most common of all psychiatric disorders. An individual with one of these disorders experiences physiologic, cognitive, and behavioral symptoms of anxiety. The physiologic manifestations are related to the "fight, flight, or freeze" response and result in cardiovascular, respiratory, neuromuscular, and gastrointestinal (GI) stimulation. The cognitive symptoms include subjective feelings of apprehension, uneasiness, fear, uncertainty, or dread. Behavioral manifestations include irritability, restlessness, pacing, crying, sighing, and complaints of tension and nervousness. The common theme among anxiety disorders is that the individual experiences a level of anxiety that interferes with functioning in personal, occupational, and social areas. Note: *Obsessive–compulsive disorder is no longer classified as an anxiety disorder. It is considered part of the class of body dysmorphic and hoarding disorders, which are not covered in this book because of space constraints; however, anxiety is a key feature.*

Classification

1. Panic disorder.
2. Agoraphobia.
3. Specific phobia.
4. Social anxiety disorders.
5. Generalized anxiety disorder.
6. Anxiety disorder because of a general medical condition.
7. Substance-induced anxiety disorder.
8. Anxiety disorder not otherwise specified.

Pathophysiology and Etiology

The underlying etiology of anxiety disorders as well as any of the psychiatric disorders is complex, having multiple factors that interact. Therefore, it is essential to examine the biochemical, genetic, psychosocial, and sociocultural factors.

Biochemical Factors

1. The limbic system, which is called the *emotional brain*, regulates emotional responses. Anxiety disorders are associated with abnormalities within this system (including the frontal cortex, hypothalamus, amygdala, hippocampus, brainstem, and the autonomic nervous system).
2. Neurotransmitters and their specific receptor sites function to transmit inhibiting or stimulating messages across the synapses between nerve cells in the brain. Abnormalities in the neurotransmitters or the receptor sites have been associated with multiple psychiatric disorders, including anxiety disorders.
3. Norepinephrine is a stimulating neurotransmitter, which is released as part of the fight, flight, or freeze acute stress response and is associated with the cardiovascular and respiratory effects of anxiety. Serotonin is a neurotransmitter that regulates multiple responses, including sleep and alertness and sensations of hunger and satiation. Genetic variation resulting in a decrease in the number of select serotonin receptors (particularly 1A) may be associated with the development of panic disorder.
4. Panic disorders may be related to the reception of a false signal from the brain that there is a shortage of oxygen or an increase in carbon dioxide (suffocation alarm theory). Those who have panic attacks have also been reported to have higher levels of norepinephrine.
5. Positron emission tomography (PET) and computed tomography (CT) scanning have shown abnormalities in glucose

*Please note that the term "male" in this chapter refers to a person assigned male at birth, and the term "female" in this chapter refers to a person assigned female at birth.

metabolism in the frontal and prefrontal cortex and the basal ganglia of the brains of individuals with panic disorder.

Genetic Factors

1. First-degree biological relatives of individuals with panic disorder have a four to seven times greater risk of developing this disorder. Twin studies demonstrate a higher concordance rate for monozygotic than dizygotic twins.
2. Approximately 20% of first-degree biological relatives of people with agoraphobia also have agoraphobia.
3. Approximately 25% of first-degree biological relatives with generalized anxiety disorder are also affected by generalized anxiety disorder.

Psychosocial Factors

1. Psychodynamic theory describes unconscious conflicts having early childhood origin and resulting from unconscious wishes and drives. These conflicts cause guilt and shame, which lead to anxiety and associated symptoms.
2. Interpersonal theory implicates early relationships, which directly affect development of self-concept and self-esteem. Individuals with poor self-concept and decreased self-esteem have increased susceptibility to anxiety-related disorders.
3. Behavioral theory describes anxiety and associated symptoms as a conditioned response to internal and external stressors.
4. Cognitive theory describes faulty thinking patterns that lead to an individual's misperceiving events affecting self, the future, and the world. These faulty thinking patterns contribute to the subjective experience of anxiety.

Sociocultural Factors

1. Anxiety disorders and ritualistic behaviors are commonly seen in high-technology societies.
2. There is a higher incidence of anxiety disorders in urban communities than in rural communities.

Clinical Manifestations

Generalized Anxiety Disorder

1. A pattern of worrying or anxiety that results in increased autonomic activity persisting for a period of at least 6 months.
2. An examination and history would reveal symptoms from the following three of four categories:
   a. Motor (e.g., trembling, restlessness, inability to relax, and fatigue).
   b. Autonomic hyperactivity (e.g., sweating, palpitations, cold clammy hands, urinary frequency, lump in the throat, pallor or flushing, increased pulse, and rapid respirations).
   c. Apprehensiveness (e.g., worry, dread, fear, rumination, insomnia, and inability to concentrate).
   d. Hypervigilance (e.g., feeling edgy, scanning the environment, and distractibility).

Panic Disorder

1. The presence of recurrent unexpected anxiety attacks for at least 1 month with a sudden onset of feelings of intense apprehension and dread.
2. These feelings result in sympathetic activation that manifests through the appearance of at least four of the following symptoms: chest discomfort or pain, dyspnea, palpitations, syncope, diaphoresis, trembling, hot or cold flashes, and dizziness.

Phobias

1. A phobia is a persistent irrational fear of an object or situation that the person may recognize as being unreasonable.
2. Exposure to the feared object or situation may result in a panic attack.
3. An example is agoraphobia, which is a fear of being alone in open or public places where escape might be difficult.

Diagnostic Evaluation

1. Measurement tools for anxiety:
   a. Hamilton Anxiety Rating Scale (HAM-A).
   b. State–Trait Anxiety Inventory (STAI).
   c. General Anxiety Disorder-7 (GAD-7).
   d. Beck Anxiety Inventory (BAI).
2. Measurement tools for panic disorders:
   a. Panic Disorder Severity Scale (PDSS).
   b. Sheehan Panic Disorder Scale (SPS).
3. Sodium lactate infusion or carbon dioxide inhalation will likely produce a panic attack in a person with panic disorder.
4. Increased arousal may be measured through studies of autonomic functioning (i.e., heart rate, electromyography, sweat gland activity) in a person with post traumatic stress disorder (PTSD).
5. Dexamethasone suppression test (DST) may be used to demonstrate heightened glucocorticoid feedback in individuals with PTSD.
6. Measurement tools for dissociation:
   a. Dissociative Experiences Scale (DES-II).
   b. Dissociative Disorders Interview Schedule (DDIS).

Management

EVIDENCE BASE Rosenthal, L. D., Burchum, J. R., & Rosenthal, L. D. (2021). *Lehne's pharmacotherapeutics for advanced practice nurses and physician assistants*. Elsevier.

Walter, H. J., Bukstein, O. G., Abright, A. R., Keable, H., Ramtekkar, U., Ripperger-Suhler, J., & Rockhill, C. (2020). Clinical practice guideline for the assessment and treatment of children and adolescents with anxiety disorders. *Journal of the American Academy of Child & Adolescent Psychiatry, 59*(10), 1107–1124. https://doi.org/10.1016/j.jaac.2020.05.005

1. Various levels and sites of care can be provided: psychiatric inpatient, outpatient, or home care. Most care is provided on an outpatient basis. Site of care is based on many factors, including the degree of disability of the affected individual, community services available, and insurance and managed care considerations. Generally, the recommended treatment is a combination of drugs and psychotherapy, along with education of the individual and family.
2. Psychoeducational strategies:
   a. Relaxation techniques.
   b. Progressive muscle relaxation.
   c. Guided imagery or visualization exercises.
   d. Stress management.
   e. Assertiveness training.
3. Psychotherapy:
   a. Psychodynamic—assists people in understanding their experiences by identifying unconscious conflicts and developing effective coping behaviors.
   b. Behavioral—focuses on the individual problematic behavior and works to modify or extinguish the behavior. One form of behavioral therapy effective in the management of phobic disorders is systematic desensitization.

c. Cognitive—assists patient to question faulty thought patterns (reframing) and examine alternatives. In the treatment of PTSD and dissociative disorders, reframing is used to help the patient view self as a survivor rather than a nonsurvivor.
d. Hypnotherapy—can be used as part of therapy for those suffering dissociative disorders.
e. Support group therapy—useful in providing a supportive and psychoeducational approach for patients with anxiety or dissociative disorders.
4. Somatic therapies:
a. Biofeedback—relaxation through biofeedback is achieved when a person learns to control physiologic mechanisms that are not ordinarily within one's awareness. Awareness and control are accomplished by monitoring body processes, including muscle tone, heart rate, and brain waves.
b. Psychopharmacologic—traditionally, drugs used to treat anxiety-related disorders were those that would increase gamma-aminobutyric acid (GABA) (benzodiazepines), regulate serotonin and/or norepinephrine levels (antidepressants), or reduce physiologic effects of anxiety by causing peripheral beta-adrenergic blockade (beta-adrenergic blockers). Currently, antidepressants are prescribed as first-line treatment for managing several anxiety-related disorders because of their safety and tolerability (see Table 53-1).

Complications

1. Undiagnosed medical reasons for anxiety could lead to physical deterioration and a delay in obtaining appropriate medical care. It is important to screen for coexisting medical illness.
2. If panic and phobic disorders are left untreated, they can lead to increasing social withdrawal and isolation, which may severely impair the person's social and work life.
3. Undiagnosed or untreated PTSD or acute stress disorder can lead to substance use or dependence, aggressive or violent behavior, and, possibly, suicide.
4. If a person with a dissociative disorder goes untreated, aggressive behavior may develop toward self or others. Such behaviors may include assaults, depression, PTSD, psychoactive substance use disorder, rape, self-mutilation, and suicide attempts.

Nursing Assessment

1. Assess psychological, physiologic, cognitive, and behavioral symptoms.
a. Defense mechanisms or coping measures used.
b. Mood.
c. Suicide risk.
d. Thought content and process.
e. Severity of subjective experience of anxiety.
f. Understanding of specific disorder.
2. Explore social functioning.
a. Ability to function in social and work situations.
b. Impact of symptoms on patient relationships, especially work and family relationships.
c. Diversional and recreational behavior.
d. Identification of stressors related to self-concept, role performance, life values, social status, and support systems.
e. Benefits (primary and secondary gains) and risks of the presenting symptoms.

Table 53-1 Dosage and Adverse Reactions of Antianxiety Drugs

DRUG: CLASS/GENERIC NAME	ADULT THERAPEUTIC DOSAGE RANGE (mg/d)	ADVERSE REACTIONS
Benzodiazepines		**For all benzodiazepines:**
Alprazolam	0.25–4	• Drowsiness, sedation, and dizziness
Chlordiazepoxide	15–100	• Possibility of dependence
Clonazepam	0.25–2	
Clorazepate	15–60	
Diazepam	4–40	
Lorazepam	1–10	
Oxazepam	30–120	
Tetracyclic Agent		
Mirtazapine	15–45	• Somnolence, increased appetite, weight gain, dry mouth, constipation
Selective Serotonin Reuptake Inhibitors (SSRIs)		
Citalopram	20–40	• Nausea, dry mouth, diarrhea, fatigue, drowsiness, ejaculatory delay, impotence
Duloxetine	40–120	• Nausea, dry mouth, dizziness, constipation, diarrhea, fatigue, increased sweating
Escitalopram	10–20	• Nausea, ejaculatory delay, impotence
Fluoxetine	20–80	• Delayed orgasm, headache, nervousness, insomnia, anxiety, tremor, dizziness, nausea, diarrhea, anorexia, dry mouth
Fluvoxamine	50–300	• Nausea, vomiting, drowsiness, anorexia, constipation, tremor, insomnia
Paroxetine	12.5–50	• Nausea, dry mouth, headache, somnolence, insomnia, diarrhea, constipation, tremor

Nursing Interventions

Reducing Symptoms of Anxiety

1. Help patient identify anxiety-producing situations and plan for such events.
2. Assist patient to develop assertiveness and communication skills.
3. Practice stress reduction techniques with patient.
4. Teach patient to monitor for objective and subjective manifestations of anxiety.
   a. Tachycardia, tachypnea.
   b. Signs and symptoms associated with autonomic stimulation—perspiration, difficulty concentrating, insomnia.
5. Promote the use of stress reduction techniques in managing symptoms of anxiety.
6. Encourage patient to verbalize feelings of anxiety.
7. Administer prescribed anxiolytics to decrease anxiety level.

DRUG ALERT Benzodiazepines are associated with tolerance and dependence and are appropriate for short-term use. Withdrawal symptoms may occur when drug is abruptly discontinued. Gradual dosage reduction is necessary. Overdose or taking benzodiazepines with alcohol or other central nervous system (CNS) depressants can cause respiratory depression requiring emergency intervention.

Improving Concentration

1. Use short, simple sentences when communicating with patient.
2. Maintain a calm, serene manner.
3. Use adjuncts to verbal communication, such as visual aids and role-playing, to stimulate memory and retention of information.
4. Teach relaxation techniques to diminish distress that interferes with concentration ability.

Increasing Social Interaction

1. Encourage discussion of reasons for and feelings about social isolation.
2. Help patient identify specific causes and situations that produce anxiety that inhibits social interaction.
3. Recommend participation in programs directed at specific conflict areas, skill building, and learning coping skills. Such programs may focus on assertiveness skills, body awareness, managing multiple role responsibilities, and stress management.

Encouraging Independence

1. Identify secondary benefits, such as decreased responsibility and increased dependency, that inhibit patient's move to independence.
2. Provide experiences in which patient can be successful.
3. Explore alternative methods of meeting dependency needs.
4. Explore beliefs that support a helpless or dependent mode of behavior.
5. Teach and role-play assertive behaviors in specific situations.
6. Provide instruction in decision-making skills, allowing opportunities for practice and rehearsal of techniques in role-play situations.
7. Assist patient to improve skills based on performance.
8. Encourage family members to avoid fostering dependency.

Strengthening Identity

1. Develop an honest, nonjudgmental relationship with patient.
2. Establish open communication.
3. Teach patient containment techniques to assist in coping with the painful memories becoming conscious (e.g., visualizing a safe environment, recall of past successes in dealing with anxiety, focusing on slowing of physiologic responses).

Reducing Harm From Behavior

1. Encourage patient to set limits on ritualistic behavior as part of established treatment plan.
2. Assist patient in listing all objects and places that trigger anxiety as part of exposure–response prevention program.
3. Use cognitive strategies, such as reframing, to assist patient in placing thoughts and feelings in a different perspective.
4. Participate as member of treatment team in establishing program for systematic desensitization.
5. Intervene as needed and obtain emergency assistance when patient is in immediate danger.
6. Minimize environmental stimuli. Use clear, simple language.
7. Monitor and assess patient for safety.

Community and Home Care Considerations

1. Patients with anxiety-related disorders are generally treated in an outpatient setting. Many of these patients may not see a mental health professional but will be treated by their family health care provider, utilizing pharmacologic therapy. Nurses who encounter patients taking prescribed drugs for anxiety should assess effectiveness and patient knowledge base regarding the safe use of these drugs. Patients should be encouraged to utilize anxiety reduction techniques.
2. Because anxiety disorders will affect family functioning, the nurse should provide support for the family, including teaching family members about the disorder and treatment measures.
3. Patients may elect to utilize alternative and complementary therapies to obtain relief from symptoms. Advise patients not to use nutritional supplement or "natural" remedy, such as St. John wort or kava kava, without discussing it with a health care provider; many drug interactions exist.
4. Several community support groups are available to provide patient with continued support. Patient may also be able to learn further techniques for the management of anxiety through participation in these programs. Such programs may also provide patient with an opportunity to practice previously learned skills in a supportive environment.

CLINICAL JUDGMENT Medication monitoring for effectiveness and adverse reactions is of utmost importance to keep the patient safe, reduce inpatient admission and readmission, and improve outcomes. Be aware that cost may affect adherence, and some medications (such as antidepressants) require a period of 2 to 3 weeks until a desired effect is seen.

Family Education and Health Maintenance

1. Teach patient and family members about anxiety.
   a. Define anxiety and differentiate it from fear.
   b. Explain the causes of anxiety.
   c. Identify events that can trigger anxiety.
   d. Identify relevant signs and symptoms of anxiety.
2. Describe the drug regimen, including significant action, adverse effects, dosage considerations, and any food or drug interactions.
3. Identify, describe, and practice deep muscle relaxation techniques, relaxation breathing, imagery, and other relaxation therapies (see page 62).

4. Teach family to give positive reinforcement for the use of healthy behaviors.
5. Teach family not to assume responsibilities or roles normally assigned to patient.
6. Teach family to give attention to patient, not patient's symptoms.
7. Teach alternative ways to perform activities of daily living (ADLs) if physical or emotional disability inhibits function and performance.
8. For additional information and support, refer to agencies such as the Anxiety and Depression Association of America (https://adaa.org).
9. Many websites provide support for individuals and family members. Some examples include Agoraphobics Building Independent Lives, www.anxietysupport.org (for sufferers from anxiety disorders), and the National Alliance on Mental Illness, www.nami.org.

Evaluation: Expected Outcomes

- Identifies stressors and demonstrates normal heart rate, respirations, sleep pattern, and subjective feelings of anxiety.
- Demonstrates improved concentration and thought processes through improved ability to focus, think, and solve problems.
- Reports increased participation and enjoyment in family- and community-related events.
- Reports going to work, keeps appointments.
- Uses coping strategies in situations that are anxiety provoking.
- Does not injure self or others.

Stress- and Trauma-Related Disorders

EVIDENCE BASE American Psychiatric Association. (2022). *Diagnostic and statistical manual of mental disorders: Fifth edition, text revision: DSM-5-TR* (5th ed.). Author.

Ortega, V. A., Mercer, E. M., Giesbrecht, G. F., & Arrieta, M. C. (2021). Evolutionary significance of the neuroendocrine stress axis on vertebrate immunity and the influence of the microbiome on early-life stress regulation and health outcomes. *Frontiers in Microbiology, 12,* 634539. https://doi.org/10.3389/fmicb.2021.634539

Stress- and traumatic-related disorders are characterized by exposure to a traumatic or stressful event. These disorders were previously classified underneath the umbrella of anxiety orders, primarily because of the association of fear and anxiety with responses to the exposure event. Over time, it has become apparent that the responses to stressful events can result in variable symptomology and distress. As a result, a category of stress-related disorders was created. These disorders still share a significant number of features with anxiety and related disorders, primarily the expression of fear.

Classification

1. Acute stress disorder.
2. PTSD.
3. Reactive attachment disorder.
4. Disinhibited social engagement disorder.
5. Adjustment disorders.

Pathophysiology and Etiology

Fear responses lead to activation of the amygdala and other parts of the brain involved with the interpretation of environmental stimuli. This leads to a condition response to events that may share features with the original event. This results in hypervigilance as the individual remains alert for events that pose a danger. Sympathetic hyperarousal results from exposure to events triggering the fear response.

Biochemical Factors

1. GABA is an inhibitory neurotransmitter that normally acts to decrease anxiety responses. An individual who genetically produces lower amounts of GABA may have an increased likelihood of developing anxiety- or stress-related disorders (e.g., PTSD).
2. Suppression of cortisol through administration of dexamethasone has been associated with PTSD, suggesting heightened glucocorticoid feedback sensitivity.

Genetic Factors

1. Reduced hippocampal volumes are believed to contribute vulnerability to PTSD.
2. Deficits in the expression of a protein (FKBP5) associated with immune responses are found to be related to stress disorders.
3. Variants in a gene that regulates the breakdown of catecholamines may lead to prolonged catecholamine activity, increasing the risk for the development of stress-related disorders.

Clinical Manifestations

1. Conscious or unconscious efforts to avoid stimuli related to the triggering event lead to hypervigilance and avoidant behaviors.
2. Signs and symptoms may include elements of dissociation manifesting as flashbacks.
3. Affect and emotions often appear negative, and the individual could display a sense of numbness, a lack of emotional responses, feelings of depersonalization or derealization, a feeling of confusion, and a loss of memory for aspects of the original event.

Acute Stress and Posttraumatic Stress Disorders

1. Acute stress and PTSD share several symptoms, with the major difference between the two conditions being the time frame in which symptoms develop.
2. For acute stress, symptoms develop within 1 month of the traumatic event and last for 2 days to 3 weeks, whereas for PTSD, the symptoms are more enduring and have lasted for at least 1 month at the time of diagnosis.
3. During the initial traumatic event, the individual needs to have displayed an initial response of horror, accompanied by intense feelings of helplessness to meet criteria for each of these disorders.
4. Both disorders share a cluster of dissociative symptoms with attempts to avoid stimuli associated with the original trauma while also reexperiencing intrusive memories and recollections of the traumatic event.
5. An examination and history would elicit findings that would include three or more of the following: a sense of numbness, a lack of emotional responses, feelings of depersonalization or derealization, a feeling of confusion, and a loss of memory for aspects of the original event.
6. A trauma response may occur when the individual is presented with stimuli associated with or similar to the original traumatic event. This may include sympathetic activation, hypervigilance, increased anxiety, and a pattern of reexperiencing the event through intrusive dreams or flashbacks. Increased sympathetic activation associated with anxiety is demonstrated through insomnia, difficulty concentrating, feelings of restlessness, and hypervigilance.

Note: Personality disorders are a class independent of stress- and trauma-related disorders. However, a history of trauma can play a role in personality disorders (such as borderline personality disorder). Personality disorders involve long-term maladaptive patterns of thoughts and behaviors that are unhealthy and inflexible, resulting in problems with relationships, emotional regulation, work activities, social activities, and adaptive coping skills. History of trauma is a key feature. Note that full coverage of personality disorders is beyond the scope of this book.

Reactive Attachment Disorder

A stress-related disorder occurring in children younger than 5 years of age. Believed to result from environments characterized by emotional or social neglect. Situations in which the primary caregiver has frequently changed are also related to the development of the condition through a lack of opportunities for the child to learn appropriate social relations. The child exhibits a lack of emotional engagement with others, manifesting as decreased interaction with adults and reduced responsiveness to attempts from adults to engage or comfort the child.

For diagnostic evaluation, management, and the nursing process, see pages 1467-1469.

Dissociative Disorders

Dissociative disorders are conditions in which the anxiety associated with a stressful or traumatic event induces a subjective feeling of being not connected to one's body or to reality. These conditions are viewed as unconscious defense mechanisms that result in a disorder when the ability to function in social or work environments is significantly impaired because of feelings of dissociation. These conditions were previously grouped under the umbrella of anxiety disorders but are now considered a separate but interrelated diagnostic category.

EVIDENCE BASE American Psychiatric Association. (2022). *Diagnostic and statistical manual of mental disorders: Fifth edition, text revision: DSM-5-TR* (5th ed.). Author.

Gatus, A., Jamieson, G., & Stevenson, B. (2022). Past and future explanations for depersonalization and derealization disorder: A role for predictive coding. *Frontiers in Human Neuroscience, 16*, 744487.

Classification/Clinical Manifestations

1. Depersonalization/derealization disorder—a persistent or recurrent experience of feeling detached from oneself. A common sensation is of being an outside observer of one's body. This experience can cause significant impairment in daily function.
2. Dissociative amnesia—one or more episodes of inability to recall important information, usually of a traumatic or stressful nature.
3. Dissociative identity disorder—previously known as *multiple personality disorder*, this disorder is evidenced by the presence of two or more distinct identities, each with its own patterns of relating, perceiving, and thinking. At least two of these identities take control of the person's behavior.

Pathophysiology

1. Associated with traumatic events, often in childhood.
2. Individual responds by "splitting off" or dissociating the self from the memory of the trauma.
3. Dissociative identity disorder may result from severe physical, sexual, or psychological abuse in early childhood.

For diagnostic evaluation, management, and the nursing process, see pages 1467-1469.

Somatic Symptoms and Related Disorders

EVIDENCE BASE American Psychiatric Association. (2022). *Diagnostic and statistical manual of mental disorders: Fifth edition, text revision: DSM-5-TR* (5th ed.). Author.

Roenneberg, C., Henningsen, P., & Hausteiner-Wiehle, C. (2020). [Chronic pain syndromes and other persistent functional somatic symptoms]. *Der Nervenarzt, 91*(7), 651–661. https://doi.org/10.1007/s00115-020-00917-w

Somatic symptoms and related disorders are characterized by physical symptoms that cannot be explained by known *physical mechanisms*. These disorders have in common the belief that physical symptoms are real despite evidence to the contrary. The affected individual experiences changes or loss in physical function. The physical symptoms are not under the individual's voluntary control. Significant impairment occurs in social or occupational functioning.

Classification

1. Somatic symptom disorder.
2. Factitious disorder.
3. Conversion disorder.
4. Illness anxiety disorder.
5. Somatic symptom and related disorder not otherwise specified.

Pathophysiology and Etiology

The underlying etiology of somatoform disorders is difficult to define. The following factors may interact in the individual with these disorders.

Biochemical Factors

1. An individual with a somatoform disorder may experience high levels of physiologic arousal (increased awareness of somatic sensations).
2. The phenomenon of alexithymia, or deficient communication between brain hemispheres, may result in difficulty expressing emotions directly, and therefore, distress may be expressed as physical symptoms.
3. The concept of somatosensory amplification—in which there is the tendency to experience a wide range of benign bodily sensations that are intense, intrusive, noxious, and disruptive—may be related to the development of somatoform disorders.

Genetic Factors

1. Somatization disorder has been found to have a 10% to 20% frequency in first-degree female biological relatives of females with this disorder.
2. Twin studies have validated some increased risk in conversion disorder in monozygotic twins.
3. The genetic basis for other somatoform disorders is not well established.

Psychosocial Factors

1. Psychodynamic theory—the psychological source of ego conflict is denied and finds expression through displacement

of anxiety onto physical symptoms. Both primary gain (anxiety relief) and secondary gains (increased dependence and relief from normal responsibilities) are common to these disorders.
2. Behavioral theory—the child learns from caregiver to express anxiety through somatization; secondary gains reinforce symptoms.
3. Cognitive theory—the individual has cognitive distortions in which benign symptoms are magnified and interpreted as serious disease.
4. Family theory—a family system that is overly enmeshed may utilize dysfunction in one person as a means to handle anxiety. In such families, the individual may not see self as a separate and distinct person; instead, the person may view themself as an extension of the family.

Sociocultural Factors

1. Incidence of somatoform disorders is highest in rural populations and in low socioeconomic groups.
2. Somatic symptoms are more common in cultures that view direct expression of emotions as unacceptable.
3. Females may experience certain chronic pain conditions more commonly than males (this may have more of a cultural than a genetic basis).

Clinical Manifestations

Somatic disorders are psychiatric conditions that manifest in the appearance of, or preoccupation with, symptoms that reflect medical illnesses or injuries. For the diagnosis of these conditions to be made, other physical health issues must be ruled out. As with other mental health conditions, these problems lead to problems with the ability to perform necessary ADLs.

Somatic Symptom Disorder

1. This disorder is characterized by presentation of at least one somatic symptom (pain, fatigue, etc.) that is distressing in nature or leads to a significantly impairment in daily function.
2. The individual displays recurrent and intrusive thoughts or behaviors related to the symptom.
3. A significant level of anxiety may occur.
4. The symptoms must manifest over a period of 6 months, although they may not be constant during that period.
5. Based on the number of symptoms, the disorder may be classified as mild, moderate, or severe.

Factitious Disorder

1. The individual fakes or otherwise falsifies the signs or symptoms of a disease or injury.
2. The falsified disease may be physical or psychological.
3. The individual claims to be ill or impaired to others.

Conversion Disorder

1. With this condition, the individual develops symptoms compatible with a neurologic disorder.
2. Examples include loss of vision, deafness, peripheral neuropathy, or bladder and bowel dysfunction. Some patients may exhibit paralysis or seizure activity.
3. These symptoms cannot be associated with a physical illness for the diagnosis of this disorder.

Illness Anxiety Disorder

1. A fixed preoccupation the individual has is a serious medical condition.
2. This belief often persists despite medical tests or procedures that do not find any physical condition.
3. The condition must exist for at least 6 months; however, the nature of the preoccupation may change during that time.
4. This preoccupation often leads to significant problems with daily function.

Diagnostic Evaluation

1. Individuals with somatic disorders will likely present in the medical rather than the psychiatric setting because of their belief that the problems are medical.
2. The individual should receive a thorough medical evaluation (if possible, avoiding repeating tests that have already had negative results).
3. The diagnosis of somatoform disorder will be made after a thorough medical evaluation in which no organic basis for the symptoms is found.

Management

1. Level and setting of care to be provided are determined. In general, the individual will be treated on an outpatient basis, unless a risk for self-harm and/or suicide is present.
2. Referral to psychiatric treatment may be rejected by the individual with a somatoform disorder; therefore, the goal of management is to maintain a long-term relationship with a specific health care provider to prevent patient from seeking multiple providers with multiple recommendations for testing, treatments, and drugs.
3. Psychotherapy:
   a. Psychodynamic—assist the individual to express conflicts and emotions verbally rather than displacing them onto physical symptoms.
   b. Behavioral—establish a program whereby adaptive behavior is reinforced and illness behaviors do not receive secondary gains.
   c. Cognitive—restructure belief system that perpetuates illness-related behaviors.
   d. Family therapy—assist family members to define appropriate boundaries and support patient in increasing self-responsibility.
4. Somatic therapies: Psychopharmacologic drugs may be used to treat patients with somatic disorders, depending on the underlying and comorbid psychiatric illnesses.
5. Mood disorders, especially depression, are a common comorbid problem in individuals with somatic disorders. Antidepressant drugs may be used to treat the mood disorder.

Complications

1. A patient with a known history of a somatic disorder may have a coexisting medical condition that could go undiagnosed. Careful screening is essential to rule out medical problems.
2. Increased risk of suicide and substance use disorder is possible in patient with an untreated somatic disorder.

Nursing Assessment

1. Assess physical complaints.
   a. Current and past history as well as duration of problems.
   b. Diagnostic testing completed.
   c. Number of health care providers consulted.

d. Types and amounts of drugs as well as whether self-medicating (over the counter) or prescribed.

2. Assess psychological processes.
   a. Perception of illness and current stressors.
   b. Self-concept and body image.
   c. Personal short- and long-term treatment goals.
   d. Motivation for receiving treatment.
   e. Mood.
   f. Suicide risk.
3. Explore social functioning (see page 1468).

Nursing Interventions

Encouraging Recognition of Anxiety

1. Discuss current life stressors in the areas of social, occupational, and family functioning.
2. Assist patient to identify anxiety-producing situations and plan coping strategies.
3. Avoid focus on physical symptoms (after appropriate screening to rule out physical etiology).
4. Maintain focus on feelings and emotional responses rather than on somatic symptoms.

Improving Coping

1. Teach and reinforce problem-solving approach to stressors.
2. Practice the use of stress reduction techniques with patient.
3. Encourage the use of support groups.
4. Set limits on maladaptive coping behaviors in a matter-of-fact manner.
5. Decrease reinforcement of secondary gains for physical symptoms.
6. Help patient identify and use positive means to meet emotional needs.
7. Maintain transparent, empathetic, and coping-oriented therapeutic approach.

Community and Home Care Considerations

1. Encourage patient to cooperate with referrals for psychiatric or psychotherapy treatments.
2. Promote patient attendance and participation at community support groups.
3. Teach patient and family the importance of remaining with one health care provider to ensure continuity of care.
4. Focus on patient's strengths and capabilities rather than on disability.

Family Education and Health Maintenance

1. Teach patient and family about the relationship between stressors, anxiety, and physical symptoms.
2. Family should expect person to function despite physical symptoms; doing things and making decisions for patient will increase dependent behaviors.
3. Encourage family therapy, which may be helpful to clarify roles, communication, and expectations.

Evaluation: Expected Outcomes

- Verbalizes anxiety about specific problems rather than expressing anxiety with physical symptoms.
- Makes decisions on own; demonstrates less dependence on family and friends.

MOOD DISTURBANCES

Depressive Disorders

Depressive disorders are considered mood disorders. A mood is a sustained emotion that, when extreme, affects the person's view of the world. Mood disorders are characterized by disturbances in feelings, thinking, and behavior. These disorders may occur on a continuum ranging from severe depression to severe mania (hyperactivity). A depressive illness is painful and can be psychophysiologically debilitating. Depression is much more than just sadness; it affects the way one feels about the future and can alter basic attitudes about the self. A depressed person can become so despairing as to express hopelessness. When moods become severe or prolonged or interfere with a person's interpersonal or occupational functioning, this may signal a mood disorder.

Pathophysiology and Etiology

The exact causes for depressive disorders have not been established. These disorders are thought to result from complex interactions among various factors.

Biochemical Factors

1. Biogenic amine theory proposes that there is a norepinephrine and serotonin deficiency in individuals with a depressive disorder. Changes in the quantity and sensitivity of receptor sites for these neurotransmitters may also be important.
2. Kindling theory describes a process whereby external environmental stressors activate internal physiologic stress responses, which trigger the first depressive episode. Subsequent episodes can occur with less stress in response to the electrophysiologic sensitivity that was established in the brain from the initial episode.
3. Neuroendocrine dysfunction:
   a. Hypothalamic–pituitary–adrenal axis dysfunction may be present in some individuals. Abnormalities include increased cortisol levels, resistance of cortisol to suppression by dexamethasone, and blunted adrenocorticotropin hormone response to corticotropin-releasing factor.
   b. Subclinical hypothyroidism has been associated with depression, especially in females.
   c. Dysfunction of circadian rhythms has been theorized related to depression. Abnormal sleep electroencephalograms (EEGs) have been demonstrated in many individuals. Increased early morning awakening is common, as are multiple nighttime awakenings.

Genetic Factors

1. Risk of developing a mood disorder is 1½ to 3 times greater in individuals with a first-degree biological relative with a mood disorder.
2. Twin studies reveal a higher rate of concordance in monozygotic twins than in dizygotic twins.
3. Mood states are associated with activation of several neuroendocrine pathways within the central and peripheral nervous systems. These pathways involve several neurochemical processes that involve activation of a particular binding protein identified as cyclic AMP response-binding protein 1 (CREB-1). Genetic profiles of individuals with depression have found evidence that genes involved in the cellular signaling pathways utilizing CREB-1 are associated with major depression. There then may be alleles (coding genes) that are related to the development of mood disorder.

4. Genetic variation in a certain region of the serotonin transporter gene (*5-HTT*) has been found to interact with the perception of stressful events (possibly through neuroendocrine pathways) to produce higher levels of depression and suicidality than in individuals without this variation.
5. Although genetic evidence has supported conceptualizations of neurochemical and biologic alteration in the development of mood and other psychiatric disorders, no one single gene or factor has appeared to emerge as the main culprit. Most likely, several genes and disposing factors are involved. Possible genes include *5-HTT*, brain-derived neurotrophic growth factor, and the monoamine oxidase A.

Medical Factors

1. Many drugs have the adverse effect of depression, including hormones, cardiovascular drugs, psychotropic drugs, and anti-inflammatory and antiulcer drugs.
2. Clinically significant depressive symptoms are detected in approximately 12% to 36% of individuals with a nonpsychiatric general medical condition.

Psychosocial Factors

1. Psychodynamic theory describes the occurrence of a significant loss (object loss) that is associated with anger and aggression, which is turned inward and leads to negative feelings about self. The negative feelings about the self, including shame and guilt, then lead to depression.
2. Life events and environmental stress, such as loss of a family member through death, divorce, or separation; lack of social support; and significant health problems have all been associated with the onset of depression.
3. Cognitive theory describes how faulty thought patterns, including negative distortions of life experiences, produce negative self-evaluation, pessimistic thinking, and hopelessness.
4. Learned helplessness theory posits that a person who internalizes the belief that an unwanted event is their own fault and that nothing can be done to avoid or change it is prone to developing depression.

Clinical Manifestations

EVIDENCE BASE American Psychiatric Association. (2022). *Diagnostic and statistical manual of mental disorders: Fifth edition, text revision: DSM-5-TR* (5th ed.). Author.

Rush, A. (2023). Unipolar major depression in adults: Choosing initial treatment. *UpToDate*. Retrieved January 28, 2023, from https://www.uptodate.com/contents/unipolar-major-depression-in-adults-choosing-initial-treatment

Depression

1. A major depressive disorder reflects a level of depression that persists over a 2-week period.
2. The severity of depression may be classified as mild, moderate, or severe depending on the number of symptoms.
3. Certain qualifying terms can be used that indicate whether the depression is associated with a change in the seasons (with seasonal pattern) or follows the birth of an infant (with peripartum onset).
4. Should delusions or hallucinations exist, the depression would be said to have psychotic features.
5. Major depression results in a significant change in the ability to work or participate in social activities.
6. Physical examination and history findings should reveal at least five or more symptoms that include the following:
   a. Depressed mood, fatigue.
   b. Insomnia or an increased need for sleep.
   c. Lack of interest in pleasurable activities (anhedonia).
   d. Recent gain or loss of weight that represents at least 5% of body weight.
   e. Feelings of worthlessness.
   f. Inability to concentrate or make decisions.
   g. Suicidal ideation.

Persistent Depressive Disorder

1. A chronic, less intense level of depressed mood characterized by the same symptoms as seen in major depression and that lasts for at least 2 years in adults, at least 1 year in children and adolescents. Previously known as *dysthymia*.
2. A major distinguishing feature is that depression does not alter the ability to participate in social or work-related functions to the extent of major depressive disorder.

Diagnostic Evaluation

1. Rating scales of depression—to determine the presence and severity of the problem:
   a. Zung Depression Scale.
   b. Hamilton Depression Rating Scale (HAM-D).
   c. Beck Depression Inventory (BDI).
   d. The Patient Health Questionnaire (PHQ-9).
2. Laboratory studies:
   a. Thyroid function tests and thyrotropin-releasing hormone stimulation test—to detect underlying hypothyroidism, which may cause depression.
   b. Dexamethasone suppression test (DST)—to evaluate depression that may be responsive to antidepressant or electroconvulsive therapy (ECT).
   c. A 24-hour urinary 3-methoxy-4-hydroxyphenylglycol (MHPG)—may show slightly lower level in unipolar depression than in bipolar depression.
3. Polysomnography—an increase in the overall amount of rapid eye movement (REM) sleep and shortened REM latency period in patients with major depression.
4. Additional diagnostic tests to evaluate physical conditions, such as computed tomography (CT) scan or magnetic resonance imaging (MRI), complete blood count (CBC), chemistry panel, rapid plasma reagin (RPR), human immunodeficiency virus (HIV) test, EEG, vitamin B_{12} and folate levels, and toxicology studies.

Management

1. Patients may receive treatment in acute inpatient psychiatric hospitals or in the community in an outpatient program. Decision about treatment setting is made according to the severity of patient's illness, with primary concern being the risk of self-harm and/or suicide as well as the presence of symptoms that are severely disabling.
2. Inpatient treatment is directed toward drug management and supportive psychotherapy using milieu management.
3. Somatic therapies:
   a. Psychopharmacologic: Antidepressant drugs may be used to treat depression; they increase serotonin and norepinephrine and may reduce symptoms (see Table 53-2, page 1475).

Table 53-2 Dosage and Adverse Reactions of Antidepressant Drugs

DRUG: CLASS/GENERIC NAME	ADULT THERAPEUTIC DOSAGE RANGE (mg/d)	ADVERSE REACTIONS
Tricyclic Agents		
Amitriptyline	25–300	*For all tricyclic and tetracyclic agents:* • Possibility of triggering a manic episode in patients with bipolar • Anticholinergic effects. Dry mouth, constipation, blurred vision, urine retention • Sedative effects • Autonomic effects: orthostatic hypotension, sweating, palpitations, and increased blood pressure • Cardiac effects: tachycardia, T-wave flattening, prolonged QT interval • Twitch, extrapyramidal movement effects
Clomipramine	25–250	
Desipramine	25–300	
Doxepin	50–300	
Imipramine	25–300	
Nortriptyline	75–150	
Protriptyline	15–60	
Trimipramine	75–200	
Tetracyclic Agent		
• Mirtazapine	15–45	*See tricyclic agents:* • Somnolence, increased appetite, weight gain, dry mouth, constipation
Bicyclic Agent		
Venlafaxine	37.5–375	• Nervousness, weight loss, dizziness, hypertension
Desvenlafaxine	50–100	• Nausea, headache, dry mouth, insomnia, fatigue, dizziness
SSRIs		
Citalopram	20–40	• Nausea, dry mouth, diarrhea, fatigue, drowsiness, ejaculatory delay, impotence
Duloxetine	40–120	• Nausea, dry mouth, dizziness, constipation, diarrhea, fatigue, increased sweating
Escitalopram	10–20	• Nausea, ejaculatory delay, impotence
Fluoxetine	20–80	• Delayed orgasm, headache, nervousness, insomnia, anxiety, tremor, dizziness, nausea, diarrhea, anorexia, dry mouth
Fluvoxamine	50–300	• Nausea, vomiting, drowsiness, anorexia, constipation, tremor, insomnia
Paroxetine	12.5–50	• Nausea, dry mouth, headache, somnolence, insomnia, diarrhea, constipation, tremor
Sertraline	50–200	• Insomnia, diarrhea, nausea, weight loss
Vilazodone	10–40	• Nausea, vomiting, insomnia, diarrhea
MAOIs		
Isocarboxazid	10–60	For all MAOIs: • Orthostatic hypotension, weight gain, edema, insomnia, sexual dysfunction, myoclonus, muscle pains, paresthesia, anticholinergic effects • Food and beverages containing tyramine in combination with MAOIs as well as combining sympathetic drugs with an MAOI can cause hypertensive crisis.
Phenelzine	45–90	
Tranylcypromine	10–60	
Selegiline	6–12	
Dibenzoxazepine Agent		
Amoxapine	100–400	• Dizziness, orthostatic hypotension, reflex tachycardia, extrapyramidal movement disorders
Unicyclic Agent		
Bupropion	200–450	• Dry mouth, constipation, headache, insomnia, restlessness, agitation, menstrual irregularities, increased seizure risk
Triazolopyridine Agent		
Trazodone	150–600	• Sedation, orthostatic hypotension, dizziness, headache, nausea, priapism
Phenylpiperazine Agent		
Nefazodone	200–600	• Orthostatic hypotension, anxiety, nervous tremor, agitation
Combination Therapies		
Amitriptyline and chlordiazepoxide	2.5–5 /10–25	• Blurred vision, dizziness, drowsiness, fatigue, tremor
Fluoxetine and olanzapine	6–12 /25–50	• Dry mouth, fatigue, somnolence, increased appetite, and increased weight
Perphenazine and amitriptyline	2–4 /10–25	• Extrapyramidal reactions are possible because of the presence of perphenazine.

MAOI, monoamine oxidase inhibitor; SSRI, selective serotonin reuptake inhibitor.

   b. ECT may be used to treat severe depression that is unresponsive to antidepressant drugs.
   c. Ultraviolet light therapy may be recommended for depression that occurs during fall and winter months (seasonal affective disorder).
4. Patient may select complementary and alternative treatments. The use of herbal supplements, especially St. John wort, is a popular alternative for antidepressant drugs. However, the use of nutritional or herbal supplements should be discussed with the health care provider because of the potential for drug interactions.
5. Psychotherapy:
   a. *Psychodynamic therapy* helps patient to become aware of unconscious anger directed toward object loss and "work through" these feelings to alleviate depression.
   b. *Cognitive therapy* is the recommended psychotherapeutic approach for depression. This approach includes identifying and challenging the accuracy of patient's negative thought patterns and encouraging behaviors designed to counteract depressive symptoms.
   c. *Family therapy* assists patient and family members in developing a sense of self that is separate from that of the family as a whole. The patient is then encouraged to take responsibility for their own actions.

DRUG ALERT Antidepressant drugs have many interactions, which may lead to serotonin syndrome, a state of excessive serotonin in the synaptic cleft. Symptoms include insomnia, confusion, agitation, hyperreflexia, involuntary movements, and hypotension. Hypertensive crisis can occur if patients take a monoamine oxidase inhibitor antidepressant in combination with a sympathomimetic drug, or if they eat excessive amounts of foods that are high in tyramine.

Complications

1. An undiagnosed medical condition causing depressive symptoms could lead to physical deterioration and delay in obtaining appropriate treatments.
2. Untreated depressive illness can increase the risk for suicide.
3. Use of alcohol or recreational drugs for self-medication to numb dysphoric feelings.

CLINICAL JUDGMENT During the first 60 days of antidepressant therapy, children and young adults (those under age 24) are at increased risk for suicidal thinking and behavior. The Food and Drug Administration has issued boxed warnings of this risk for most antidepressants. Those taking these medications require additional monitoring and supervision during this period. The evidence does not support the need for this type of monitoring in those over age 24.

EVIDENCE BASE Boland, R. J., Verduin, M. L., & Ruiz, P. (Eds.). (2022). Depressive Disorders. In *Kaplan & Sadock's Synopsis of Psychiatry* (12th ed., pp. 379–400). Lippincott Williams & Wilkins.

Nursing Assessment

1. Assess posture and affect for:
   a. Poor or slumped posture.
   b. Appearance of being older than stated age.
   c. Facial expression of sadness, dejection.
   d. Episodes of weeping.
   e. Anhedonia—inability to experience pleasure.
2. Assess thought processes:
   a. Identify the presence of suicidal thoughts.
   b. Poor judgment, indecisiveness.
   c. Impaired problem-solving, poor concentration.
   d. Negative thoughts.
   e. Presence of psychosis.
3. Explore feelings for:
   a. Anger and irritability.
   b. Anxiety, guilt.
   c. Worthlessness.
   d. Helplessness, hopelessness.
4. Assess physical behavior for:
   a. Psychomotor agitation or retardation.
   b. Vegetative signs of depression.
      i. Change in eating patterns.
      ii. Change in sleeping patterns.
      iii. Change in elimination patterns.
      iv. Change in level of interest in sex.
      v. Change in personal hygiene.
5. Assess for evidence of "masked depression":
   a. Hypochondriasis.
   b. Psychosomatic disorders.
   c. Compulsive gambling.
   d. Compulsive overwork.
   e. Accident proneness.
   f. Eating disorders.
   g. Substance use disorder.
6. Assess for risk of suicide. All individuals who identify as having a mental illness, especially those who are depressed, should be assessed for harm to self or others. Refer for crisis intervention if they are deemed at risk.

Nursing Interventions

Strengthening Coping and Sense of Hope

1. Initiate interaction with patient at a regularly scheduled time.
2. Be clear and honest about your own feelings related to patient's behavior.
3. Encourage verbal expression of feelings.
4. Validate feelings that are appropriate to the situation.
5. Explore with patient what is producing and maintaining the feeling of depression.
6. Encourage patient to identify events that cause unpleasant emotional responses.
7. Assess significant losses patient has experienced.
8. Identify cultural and social factors that may contribute to how patient copes with loss and feelings.
9. Assess patient's support network.

Maintaining Safety

1. Assess current suicide risk.
2. Implement appropriate level of observation based on a focused suicide assessment (e.g., constant observation or 15-minute checks).
3. Explain observation precautions to patient.
4. Remove harmful objects from patient's possession and assess environmental safety of the patient's room and unit.
5. Encourage patient to create a personalized safety plan with staff assistance.
6. Monitor the need to revise the level of observation.

7. Provide additional structure by keeping patient involved in therapeutic and psych rehabilitative activities.

Encouraging Participation in Activities of Daily Living

1. Collaborate with occupational and physical therapists to determine patient's functional capacity to accomplish activities of daily living (ADLs).
2. If patient cannot accomplish ADLs independently, provide hygiene activities in collaboration with the patient.
3. Acknowledge and reinforce patient's efforts to maintain appearance; do not rush the patient when self-care is slow.
4. Reinforce what patient can do rather than what patient cannot do without assistance.
5. Remain with patient during mealtimes to determine the level of need for assistance or cueing in the ability to eat.

Facilitating Sleep

1. Determine patient's past and current sleep patterns and sleep hygiene.
2. Ask what strategies patient has already used to improve sleep and elicit which ones have been successful.
3. Consider decreasing the amount of daytime sleep by encouraging participation in an activity.
4. Discuss alternative methods for facilitating sleep:
   a. Avoid caffeine and nicotine.
   b. Avoid emotionally charged or upsetting discussions before bedtime.
   c. Avoid exercise 30 minutes to 1 hour before bed.
   d. Increase physical activity within functional limits.
   e. Use relaxation techniques.
   f. Try a warm bath or warm milk.
5. Administer prescribed drugs that cause sleepiness at bedtime; avoid giving drugs that cause insomnia at night.

Community and Home Care Considerations

1. Mood disorders tend to be chronic, with acute episodes that may require inpatient treatment. In the home or community setting, patient will require ongoing monitoring regarding the use of drugs as well as support and education in terms of the disorder.
2. Community health care providers, including nurses, must be aware of the need for primary and secondary prevention programs directed at education as well as early case finding and prompt treatment.

Family Education and Health Maintenance

1. Instruct patient and family members about symptoms of depression.
2. Instruct patient and family members about the purpose of antidepressant drugs, effects, adverse effects, and their management and how to recognize early signs and symptoms of relapse.
3. Instruct patient and family members about the effect of a depressive disorder on the family system.
4. Provide patient and family members with written material on coping with depression.
5. Provide patient and family members with information about appropriate community-based programs and support groups. Contact the National Foundation for Depressive Illness (www.depression.org).
6. Provide patient and family members with information about the Suicide and Crisis Lifeline number (https://988lifeline.org/).

Evaluation: Expected Outcomes

- Reports improvement in mood and increased interest in daily living.
- Remains free from self-harm.
- Accomplishes ADLs in an independent manner.
- Obtains a minimum of 5 hours of uninterrupted sleep.

Bipolar and Related Disorders

Bipolar disorders, also considered *mood disorders*, include the occurrence of depressive episodes and one or more elated mood episodes. An elated mood can include a range of affect, from normal mood to hypomania to mania. In the most intense presentation, the person with bipolar disorder experiences altered thought processes, which can produce bizarre delusions.

Pathophysiology and Etiology

Genetic Factors

1. Twin studies reveal a concordance rate of 65% in monozygotic twins for bipolar disorder.
2. Risk of developing bipolar disorder is increased 4% to 24% in first-degree biological relatives of people with bipolar disorder.
3. Current research indicates that defective genes located within chromosomes 18 and 21 may be related to bipolar disorder.

Biochemical Factors

1. Patients with bipolar disorders may have lower plasma norepinephrine, urinary MHPG, and platelet serotonin uptake and higher red blood cell/plasma lithium rates than do unipolar populations.
2. Pathology of the limbic system, basal ganglia, and hypothalamus is proposed to contribute to the development of mood disorders.

Psychosocial Factors

1. Psychosocial stressors appear to have an important role early in the illness, in concert with the electrical kindling and behavioral sensitization models.
2. Mania and hypomania have been viewed by psychoanalytic theorists as a defense against depression.

Clinical Manifestations

EVIDENCE BASE American Psychiatric Association. (2022). *Diagnostic and statistical manual of mental disorders: Fifth edition, text revision: DSM-5-TR* (5th ed.). Author.

Groves, S. J., Douglas, K. M., Milanovic, M., Bowie, C. R., & Porter, R. J. (2021). Systematic review of the effects of evidence-based psychotherapies on neurocognitive functioning in mood disorders. *The Australian and New Zealand Journal of Psychiatry, 55*(10), 944–957. https://doi.org/10.1177/00048674211031479

Mood disorders are often characterized by varying degrees of mania that can alternate with periods of depression. The distinguishing characteristic between forms of bipolar disorder is the degree of mania, with or without the signs of depression. Mania is an elevation of mood that persists for at least 1 week.

Bipolar I Disorder

1. Physical examination and history findings for bipolar I disorder are the presence of a single manic episode generally

without the individual also meeting the criteria for a major depressive episode.
2. Severity of the disorder can be classified as mild, moderate, or severe depending on the number of symptoms present.
3. A mixed episode refers to the symptoms of mania and depression coexisting across the course of 1 week.
4. Mania is characterized by a cluster of at least three symptoms across the course of at least 1 week that result in a disruption in daily function. These behaviors can include the following:
   a. Excessive or pressured speech.
   b. Difficulty in maintaining concentration or focus.
   c. A reduced need for sleep and an increase in either goal-directed or pleasure-seeking behaviors.

Bipolar II Disorder

1. In bipolar II disorder, there has been an episode of hypomania along with an episode of major depression.
2. Hypomania is a less intense form of mania (increased energy does not result in significant changes in functional ability) with duration of at least 4 days, but less than a week.

Cyclothymic Disorder

1. A chronic alteration in mood that persists over a 2-year period during which there are several episodes of hypomania and depressed mood, but no episodes of major depression.
2. In children and adolescents, a 1-year time frame is used.
3. During the 2 years, symptoms cannot have abated for more than 2 months.

Diagnostic Evaluation

1. Rating scale assessment tools:
   a. Young Mania Rating Scale (YMRS).
   b. Manic State Rating Scale (MSRS).
2. There appear to be no laboratory features that distinguish major depressive episodes found in major depressive disorder from those in bipolar I or bipolar II disorder.
3. Complete psychophysiologic examination.
4. Complete assessment to rule out medical conditions.

Management

EVIDENCE BASE Carvalho, A. F., Firth, J., & Vieta, E. (2020). Bipolar disorder. *New England Journal of Medicine, 383*(1), 58–66. https://doi.org/10.1056/nejmra1906193

1. Patients may receive treatment in acute inpatient psychiatric hospitals or in the community in an outpatient program. The decision about the treatment setting is made according to the severity of patient's illness, including the degree of mania or depression as well as the risk of self-harm or harm to others.
2. Inpatient treatment is directed toward drug management as well as supportive psychotherapy to alleviate the acute manic symptoms.
3. Pharmacologic treatment for acute mania and bipolar disorder consists of:
   a. Lithium carbonate.
   b. Anticonvulsants, such as carbamazepine and valproate, for mood-stabilizing properties.
   c. Neuroleptic agents, such as risperidone, for acute psychotic thinking.
   d. Benzodiazepines, such as clonazepam or lorazepam, for acute agitation.
   e. Combination therapies, often incorporating an antipsychotic (perphenazine or olanzapine) along with an antidepressant (amitriptyline or fluoxetine). Another approach involves combining a benzodiazepine (chlordiazepoxide) with an antidepressant (amitriptyline) to combat comorbid depression and anxiety.
4. Psychotherapy is used as described in the section related to depression.
5. Psychiatric home care nursing to facilitate adherence to drug regimens and therapeutic interventions.
6. Community-based support group participation.

DRUG ALERT Patients taking lithium can develop toxicity related to elevated levels in the blood; therefore, lithium blood levels must be monitored periodically. Initial therapy requires daily monitoring until a safe, therapeutic level is attained; weekly and then monthly monitoring is then recommended. Lithium toxicity is related to decreased serum sodium levels and inadequate hydration. Therefore, patients taking lithium must have normal sodium intake and drink 2 L of water daily.

Complications

1. Untreated bipolar disorder can lead to physical exhaustion.
2. Poor judgment and risk-taking behavior can lead to financial problems.
3. Alcohol and drug use problems can develop and cause disruption in the family.
4. Concurrent medical conditions may be exacerbated.

Nursing Assessment

1. Assess mood for stability; range of affect, from elation to irritability to severe agitation; laughing, joking, and talking continuously; uninhibited familiarity with interviewer.
2. Assess behavior for constant activity, starting many projects but finishing few, mild-to-severe hyperactivity, spending large sums of money, increased appetite, indiscriminate sexual behavior, minimal to no sleeping, outlandish or bizarre dress, poor concentration.
3. Assess thought processes for flight of ideas; pressured speech, usually with content that is sexually explicit; clang associations (sound of word, rather than its meaning, directs subsequent associations); delusions; hallucinations.

Nursing Interventions

Improving Impulse Control and Decreasing Disturbed Thoughts

1. Assess patient's degree of distorted thinking.
2. Redirect patient when you are unable to follow thought processes.
3. Use brief explanations.
4. Remain consistent in approach and expectations.
5. Frequently orient patient to reality; speak in a clear, simple manner.
6. Provide patient with a relaxing area with decreased environmental stimulation.
7. Assist patient with a gradual and progressive integration into the social environment while observing for behavioral changes that indicate readiness for participation in further activities.

Improving Sleep Pattern

1. Establish a distraction-free environment at bedtime.
2. Help patient avoid the intake of caffeine and nicotine.

3. Administer prescribed drugs, as ordered, and monitor patient's response.

Improving the Effect of Bipolar Illness on Family

1. Assess family's external support network and encourage participation in family therapy and support groups.
2. Assess communication and boundaries within family.
3. Observe and assess interaction patterns within family and discuss their influence on patient and family functioning.
4. Provide patient and family with information about bipolar disorder and the treatment plan, prognosis, and aftercare plan.

Ensuring Adequate Nutrition

1. Maintain accurate documentation of food and fluid intake.
2. Offer small, frequent meals of high-calorie foods. Include foods that patient likes and that can be eaten "on the move."
3. Serve patient meals in a low-stimulus environment.
4. Monitor patient's serum electrolyte and albumin levels and weigh patient every other day.
5. Monitor patient's vital signs.

Family Education and Health Maintenance

1. Instruct patient and family about bipolar illness, including symptoms of relapse.
2. Instruct patient and family members about psychopharmacologic treatment, including its purpose, effects, adverse effects, and management.
3. Advise patient and family members about community-based support groups or health care agencies that are relevant to their care.
4. For additional information, refer to organizations such as the National Association on Mental Illness (www.nami.org).

Evaluation: Expected Outcomes

- Improved thought processes demonstrated by clear sentences with no evidence of flight of ideas and completion of simple tasks.
- Sleeps for at least 5 hours at night.
- Family members verbalize realistic, goal-directed thinking related to patient's abilities, recovery, and control of condition.
- No weight loss noted.

THOUGHT DISTURBANCES (PSYCHOTIC DISORDERS)

Schizophrenia, Schizophreniform, and Delusional Disorders

Schizophrenia, schizophreniform, and delusional disorders are conditions in which there is a disruption of thought process and/or perception. These conditions are often defined by the presence of psychotic symptoms. Psychotic symptoms are produced by a loss of ego boundaries or a gross impairment in reality testing, which includes prominent hallucinations and delusions, disorganized speech, and grossly disorganized or catatonic behavior. Schizophrenia can be classified as having positive or negative symptoms, although most patients have a mixture. The positive symptoms include hallucinations, delusions, loose associations, and bizarre or disorganized behavior. The negative symptoms include restricted emotion (flat affect), anhedonia (lack of interest in pleasurable activities), avolition (lack of motivation or initiative), alogia (lack of speech or content), and social withdrawal.

Pathophysiology and Etiology

The exact cause of these disorders remains unclear. The current consensus is that they result from complex interactions among various factors.

Schizophrenia, Schizophreniform Disorder

1. Genetic factors:
   a. Studies of monozygotic twins reveal a 50% concordance rate with a 15% rate with dizygotic twins.
   b. If one biological parent is affected with schizophrenia, a 12% rate is demonstrated in the children; having two biological parents with the disorder increases the risk to 35% to 39%.
   c. Research is focused on a number of different genes that may be related to the development of schizophrenia. An increased risk of schizophrenia is seen in individuals with genetic variation in the catechol-*O*-methyltransferase gene, which is involved in the manufacture of an enzyme that metabolizes neurotransmitters. Other current candidate genes include *GRM3*, *DISC1*, dysbindin, and neuregulin.
2. Biochemical and structural brain factors:
   a. Dopamine hypothesis—hyperactivity in the dopaminergic system, possibly because of receptor neurons that are functionally hyperactive.
   b. Norepinephrine, serotonin, glutamate, and gamma-aminobutyric acid (GABA) may also play a role in modulating the symptoms of schizophrenia.
   c. Endogenous dysfunction of *N*-methyl-D-aspartate receptor–mediated neurotransmission could lead to the development of schizophrenia.
   d. Neuroanatomic studies—cerebral ventricular enlargement; sulcal enlargement; cerebellar atrophy; decreased cranial, cerebral, and frontal size; abnormalities in basal ganglia; structural abnormalities at the cellular level, particularly in the limbic and periventricular regions.
   e. Functional and metabolic studies—regional cerebral blood flow studies demonstrated hypofrontality: Patients with schizophrenia were unable to increase blood flow to their frontal lobes during a task thought to increase frontal lobe functions; positron emission tomography (PET) studies also consistently found evidence for a biological relative hypofrontality.
   f. Electrophysiologic studies—electroencephalographic (EEG) findings in patients with schizophrenia demonstrated decreased alpha and increased delta activity; changes in evoked potential studies and amplitude reduction may occur in responses reflecting selective attention and stimulus evaluation. P300 response (reduced amplitude to unexpected stimuli using auditory and visual parameters) is the most pronounced and prolonged. This defect leads to information or sensory overload and an inability to "screen out" irrelevant stimuli.
   g. Research evidence supports speculation that schizophrenia is a neurodevelopmental disorder that may result from brain injury occurring early in life and interfering with normal developmental events.
3. Psychosocial factors:
   a. Psychodynamic theory proposes that the essential feature of schizophrenia is a result of dysfunction in interpersonal relationships because of a withdrawal of the libido into the self.
   b. Interpersonal theory proposes that the lack of a warm, nurturing relationship in the early years of life contributes

to the lack of self-identity, reality misperception, and relationship withdrawal that is apparent in the disorder.

c. Family theory related to the role of the family in the development of schizophrenia has not been validated by research. An area of family functioning that has been implicated is increased relapse risks in families characterized by highly expressed emotion. This characteristic is described as emotional overinvolvement along with hostile and critical feedback.

Delusional Disorder

1. Little has been established about the etiology of delusional disorders.
2. There is no demonstrated genetic linkage.
3. It is possible that psychosocial stressors have a role in the etiology of delusional disorders in some people. This is illustrated in some of the rarer conditions, such as shared psychotic disorder.

Clinical Manifestations

EVIDENCE BASE American Psychiatric Association. (2022). *Diagnostic and statistical manual of mental disorders: Fifth edition, text revision: DSM-5-TR* (5th ed.). Author.

Faden, J., & Citrome, L. (2023). Schizophrenia: One name, many different manifestations. *The Medical Clinics of North America*, *107*(1), 61–72. https://doi.org/10.1016/j.mcna.2022.05.005

Thought disorders are characterized by the appearance of positive and negative symptomatology. *Positive symptomatology* refers to the presence of delusions or hallucinations, whereas negative is the lack of personality traits that should normally be present. A lack of affect, interest in daily activities, and an inability to attend to daily hygiene or self-care reflect negative symptomatology. Distinguishing between the various thought disorders requires careful attention to the presence and duration of positive and negative symptomatology. As with other psychiatric disorders, the symptoms must be severe enough to alter daily function.

Schizophrenia

Previously schizophrenia was classified into five different forms. Currently, for diagnosis, the individual must display at least one positive symptom.

1. Positive symptoms include delusional thinking, disorganized speech, and hallucinations.
2. Symptoms must be present for at least 1 month with a total duration of illness for a period of at least 6 months. The 6-month period may include periods of active symptoms and remission.
3. Symptoms must lead to a significant disruption of the individual's ability to function in social or social settings, or impact the ability to attend activities of daily living (ADLs).
4. The diagnosis may indicate whether this is an acute episode or if the individual is in remission.
5. Severity can be rated on a five-point scale, ranging from 0 to 4. A rating of 4 would indicate the presence of severe and active symptoms, while 0 indicates that symptoms are not currently present.

Schizophreniform Disorder

1. The primary difference between schizophreniform disorder and schizophrenia is a period of symptom duration of less than 6 months but more than 1 month.
2. Those with this disorder can appear schizophrenic with the presence of positive and/or negative symptomatology.
3. Diagnostic criteria include delusions, hallucinations, and patterns of disorganized behavior or speech along with negative symptoms.

Schizoaffective Disorder

1. A psychiatric condition in which there is a comorbid thought and mood disorder.
2. Those with this disorder may display signs and symptoms of depression or mania along with the positive and negative symptoms of schizophrenia.

Other Psychotic Disorders

1. Delusional disorders encompass nonbizarre delusions of at least 1-month duration but no positive or negative symptoms of schizophrenia present.
2. Psychotic disorder, because of a general medical disorder, contains prominent hallucinations that may last longer than the course of the underlying disorder.
3. Brief psychotic disorders contain one or more of the following: delusions, disorganized speech, grossly disorganized or catatonic behavior, hallucinations. Duration is at least 1 day and less than 1 month, then return to previous level of functioning.
4. Shared psychotic disorder occurs in an individual with an already established delusion who develops another delusion similar to another's in the context of a close relationship with that person.
5. Substance-induced psychotic disorder contains prominent hallucinations and delusions associated with substance intoxication or withdrawal, but not exclusively during the course of underlying drug use.

Diagnostic Evaluation

1. Clinical diagnosis is developed on historical information and thorough mental status examination.
2. No laboratory findings have been identified that are diagnostic of schizophrenia.
3. Routine battery of laboratory tests may be useful in ruling out possible organic etiologies, including complete blood count (CBC), urinalysis, liver function tests, thyroid function tests, rapid plasma reagin (RPR), human immunodeficiency virus (HIV) test, serum ceruloplasmin (rules out an inherited disease, Wilson disease, in which the body retains excessive amounts of copper), PET scan, computed tomography (CT) scan, and magnetic resonance imaging (MRI).
4. Rating scale assessment:
   a. Scale for the Assessment of Negative Symptoms (SANS).
   b. Scale for the Assessment of Positive Symptoms (SAPS).
   c. Brief Psychiatric Rating Scale (BPRS).
   d. Positive and Negative Symptoms Scale (PANSS).

Management

EVIDENCE BASE Wagner, E., Siafis, S., Fernando, P., Falkai, P., Honer, W. G., Röh, A., Siskind, D., Leucht, S., & Hasan, A. (2021). Efficacy and safety of clozapine in psychotic disorders—A systematic quantitative meta-review. *Translational Psychiatry*, *11*(1), 487. https://doi.org/10.1038/s41398-021-01613-2

Schizophrenia and Schizophreniform Disorder

1. Patients may receive treatment in inpatient settings or in community-based outpatient programs or psychiatric home care. The level of care depends on the severity of symptoms and the risk of harm to self and others.
2. These disorders generally require long-term treatment; therefore, a case management approach is important to coordinate multiple services.
3. Pharmacologic therapy with either the typical or atypical neuroleptics (antipsychotics) is the mainstay of treatment (see Table 53-3).
   a. The typical neuroleptics have multiple adverse effects that require careful management (see Table 53-4, page 1482).
   b. The atypical neuroleptics have fewer adverse effects and may also be more effective in decreasing the negative symptoms of schizophrenia.

Table 53-3 Dosage and Adverse Reactions of Antipsychotic Drugs

DRUG: CLASS/GENERIC NAME	ADULT THERAPEUTIC DOSAGE RANGE (mg/d)	ADVERSE REACTIONS
Butyrophenone		
Haloperidol	6–40	Extrapyramidal adverse effects are common. Decreased incidence of orthostatic hypotension as compared with phenothiazines.
Aliphatic Phenothiazine		
Chlorpromazine	200–1,000	Orthostatic hypotension, sedation, dry mouth, extrapyramidal adverse effects, agranulocytosis, ocular changes
Piperidine Phenothiazine		
Thioridazine	200–800	Sedation, orthostatic hypotension, fewer extrapyramidal symptoms than other phenothiazines
Piperazine Phenothiazine		
Fluphenazine Perphenazine Trifluoperazine	5–40 8–64 15–40	Extrapyramidal symptoms and lower incidence of orthostatic hypotension than with other phenothiazines
Dibenzoxazepine		
Loxapine	30–100	Extrapyramidal adverse effects, hypotension, dizziness
Thioxanthene		
Thiothixene	15–50	Extrapyramidal adverse effects, hypotension, tachycardia, insomnia
Atypical Antipsychotics		Extrapyramidal adverse effects can occur with the use of any of the atypical antipsychotics, although the incidence of occurrence usually is less than that seen with other classes of antipsychotic medications. Use of atypical antipsychotics can place an individual at risk for metabolic syndrome, which involves a cluster of risk factors for cardiovascular disease such as dyslipidemia, weight gain, type 2 diabetes, and hypertension.
Aripiprazole	10–30	Headache, anxiety, insomnia, nausea, vomiting, dizziness, and drowsiness
Asenapine	5–10	Extrapyramidal adverse effects, drowsiness, oral hypoesthesia, weight gain
Clozapine	150–600 (requires careful titration)	Seizure, agranulocytosis (obtain weekly white blood cell count), hypotension, tachycardia, cardiac dysrhythmia, drowsiness, sedation, increased salivation
Iloperidone	12–24	Extrapyramidal adverse effects, orthostatic hypotension, weight gain
Lurasidone	40–160	Extrapyramidal adverse effects primarily akathisia and pseudoparkinsonism, nausea, somnolence.
Olanzapine	5–20	Orthostatic hypotension, tachycardia, drowsiness, agitation, akathisia, constipation
Paliperidone	3–12	Extrapyramidal adverse effects, tremor, muscle stiffness
Pimozide	1–10	Orthostatic hypotension, tachycardia, drowsiness, sedation, akathisia, akinesia
Quetiapine	300–800	Orthostatic hypotension, tachycardia, drowsiness, dizziness, dry mouth
Risperidone	2–8	Orthostatic hypotension, tachycardia, drowsiness, dizziness, dry mouth
Ziprasidone	20–160	Dysrhythmia, drowsiness, dizziness, nausea, restlessness, constipation

Table 53-4 Management of Adverse Effects of Neuroleptic Drugs

SYMPTOM	MANAGEMENT
Orthostatic hypotension	Assess for orthostatic blood pressure changes and dizziness and teach the patient: • When rising from bed or chair, get up slowly. • Sit at side of bed for a few minutes, dangling legs. • Do ankle pumps before standing. • Once standing, move slowly. • Do not twist or turn quickly. • Use assistive devices, handrails, canes, walkers when necessary for functional deficits. • Do not drive or operate machinery when dizzy.
Peripheral Anticholinergic Effects	
Dry mouth and nose, blurred vision, constipation, urine retention	*Dry mouth:* • Brush teeth after each meal with a fluoridated toothpaste. • Rinse mouth frequently. • Limit caffeinated or alcoholic drinks because they can be dehydrating. • Stop smoking because of the irritation of oral mucosa. • Suck on sugarless candy or gum; avoid sugared candy to decrease the risk of fungal infections and dental caries. • Avoid dry or spicy foods. • Drink fluids between meals unless on a specific fluid restriction. • Avoid acidic beverages because of potential irritation. • Use dressing, juices, or sauces (if allowed) to moisten food. *Constipation:* • Drink fluids (within prescribed limits set by health care provider). • Eat roughage: fruits, vegetables (raw leafy types) to increase bulk and help soften stool. • Eat dried fruits, such as prunes or dates, for laxative effect. • Maintain activity level within functional limits. • Consult with health care provider to determine appropriate use of over-the-counter laxatives or stool softeners. *Urine retention:* • Void at regular intervals. • Ensure privacy.
Metabolic Effects of Antipsychotics	
Metabolic syndrome	Monitor weight. Monitor blood glucose. Monitor BP. Monitor cholesterol levels.
Extrapyramidal Adverse Effects	
Short term	
Akathisia: symptoms of anxiety, agitation; compulsive, restless movement.	• Reassure patient. • Consider reducing dosage. • Consider switching patient to another class of antipsychotic. • Consider treating symptoms with benzodiazepine, beta-blocker, or anticholinergic medications.
Akinesia: weakness (hypotonia), fatigue, painful muscles, anergy (lack of energy), absence of movement	• Assess functional ability. • Dose reduction or cessation should improve movement if problems are due to akinesia vs. psychotic symptoms.
Acute dystonia: spasm of muscles of tongue, face, neck, and back; oculogyric crises, head–neck stiffness, myoclonic twitches, laryngeal–pharyngeal dystonia	• Consider prophylaxis with anticholinergic medications. • Treat with IM or IV anticholinergics, as prescribed.
Parkinsonian effects: bradykinesia, mask-like facies, tremor, rigidity, shuffling gait, drooling, cogwheeling, stooped posture.	• Treat with anticholinergics, as prescribed. • Discontinue antipsychotic, as directed.

Table 53-4 Management of Adverse Effects of Neuroleptic Drugs (*continued*)

Long term	
Tardive dyskinesia: a delayed effect of neuroleptic drugs usually occurring after 6 mo of treatment involving abnormal, involuntary, irregular, oral–facial dyskinesias and choreoathetoid movements of the muscles of the head, limbs, and trunk	• Complete regular objective rating/assessment of the movement disorder. • Reduce antipsychotic dosage, consider discontinuation of neuroleptic and anticholinergic drugs. • Consider treating symptoms with benzodiazepines. • Consider clozapine or risperidone, or other second-generation antipsychotic. • Comprehensive medical psychiatric assessment necessary with close monitoring of movement disorder.

BP, blood pressure; IM, intramuscular; IV, intravenous.

c. Pharmacologic therapy with both the typical and atypical neuroleptics can include the use of long-acting, or depot, injections. The use of such injections is increasing. Some of the available psychopharmacologic drugs in long-acting depot formulations include aripiprazole, aripiprazole lauroxil, haloperidol, fluphenazine, olanzapine, paliperidone, and risperidone. These formulations provide more feasible adherence for patients, because one dose will last for weeks or months at a time.

4. Psychosocial treatments (social skills training, ADL instruction).
5. Supportive therapy that is reality oriented and pragmatic.
6. Family therapy.
7. Psychoeducational individual, group, and family support.
8. Support groups in the community.
9. Community-based partial hospitalization programs.
10. Psychiatric home care nursing.
11. Vocational and social skills education.

Delusional Disorder

1. Neuroleptic drugs have demonstrated some success in reducing the intensity of the delusion.
2. Individual psychotherapy.
3. Hospitalization for comprehensive assessment for diagnostic purposes or if suicidal or homicidal.

Complications

1. If left undiagnosed, untreated, or ineffectively treated, schizophrenia can lead to profound inability to function, a shorter average lifespan, homelessness, and a greater risk of suicide.
2. Neglect of other medical conditions; therefore, complications because of untreated medical illness are common.
3. Depression and thoughts of harm to self or others.
4. Substance use or dependency.

Nursing Assessment

Assess for positive symptoms of schizophrenia. These symptoms reflect atypical mental activity and are usually present early in the first phase of the schizophrenic illness.

Alterations in Thinking

1. Delusion—false, fixed belief that is not amenable to change by reasoning. The most frequent elicited delusions include the following:
   a. Ideas of reference.
   b. Delusions of grandeur.
   c. Delusions of jealousy.
   d. Delusions of persecution.
   e. Somatic delusions.
2. Loose associations—lack of association between different ideas resulting in disorganized thoughts.
3. Neologisms—made up of words that are usually nonsensical and unrecognizable but have a special meaning to the person with delusion.
4. Concrete thinking—an overemphasis on small or specific details and an impaired ability to abstract.
5. Echolalia—meaningless repetition of words just spoken by another person.
6. Clang associations—words associated with similarity of sound rather than meaning. A meaningless rhyming of a word.
7. Word salad—a mixture of words that have little or no logical connection and are incomprehensible and meaningless to the listener.

Alterations in Perceiving

1. Hallucinations—sensory perceptions that have no external stimulus. The most common are auditory, followed by visual and, less frequently, gustatory, olfactory, and tactile.

   Auditory command hallucinations commonly occur in individuals with schizophrenia. Command hallucinations instruct patients to act in specific ways that can range from benign (e.g., hearing voices telling the patient to shut the door) to serious and life-threatening (e.g., hearing voices telling the patient to hurt themselves or others).
2. Loss of ego boundaries—lack a sense of their body and how they relate to the environment.
   a. Depersonalization is a nonspecific feeling or sense that a person has lost their identity or is unreal.
   b. Derealization is the perception by a person that the environment has changed.

Alterations in Behavioral Responses

1. Bizarre behavioral patterns.
   a. Motor agitation and restlessness.
   b. Automatic obedience or robot-like movement.
   c. Negativism.
   d. Stereotyped behaviors.
   e. Stupor.
   f. Waxy flexibility (allowing another person to reposition extremities).
2. Agitated or impulsive behavior.
3. Negative symptoms of schizophrenia that reflect a deficiency of mental functioning:
   a. Alogia—lack of speech.
   b. Anergia—inability to react.
   c. Anhedonia—inability to experience pleasure.
   d. Avolition—lack of motivation or initiation.
   e. Poor social functioning.

   f. Poverty of speech.
   g. Social withdrawal.
   h. Thought blocking.
4. Associated symptoms of schizophrenia:
   a. Substance use or dependence.
   b. Depression.
   c. Alterations in reality.
   d. Violent or aggressive behavior.
   e. Water intoxication.
   f. Withdrawal.
   g. Anosognosia, leading patient to not take medicine.

Nursing Interventions

Strengthening Differentiation Between Delusions and Reality

1. Provide patient with honest and consistent feedback in a nonthreatening manner.
2. Avoid challenging the content of patient's delusions and behaviors.
3. Administer drugs, as prescribed, while monitoring and documenting patient's response to the drug regimen.
4. Use simple and clear language when speaking with patient.
5. Explain all procedures, tests, and activities to patient before starting them, and provide written or video material for learning purposes.

Promoting Socialization

1. Encourage patient to talk about feelings in the context of a trusting, supportive relationship.
2. Allow patient time to reveal delusions to you without engaging in a power struggle over the content or the reality of the delusions.
3. Use a supportive, empathic approach to focus on patient's feelings about troubling events or conflicts.
4. Provide opportunities for socialization and encourage participation in group activities.
5. Be aware of patient's personal space and use touch judiciously.
6. Help patient to identify behaviors that alienate significant others and family members.

Improving Activity Tolerance

1. Assess patient's response to the prescribed antipsychotic drug.
2. Assess for side effects of psychotropic medication. Perform the Abnormal Involuntary Movement Scale (AIMS), as needed.
3. Collaborate with patient and occupational and physical therapy specialists to assess patient's ability to perform ADLs.
4. Collaborate with patient to establish a daily, achievable routine within physical limitations.
5. Teach strategies to manage adverse effects of antipsychotic drug that affect patient's functional status, including:
   a. Change positions slowly.
   b. Gradually increase physical activities.
   c. Limit overdoing it in hot, sunny weather.
   d. Use sun precautions.
   e. Use caution in activities if extrapyramidal symptoms develop.

Improving Coping With Thoughts and Feelings

1. Encourage patient to express feelings.
2. Focus on patient's feelings and content of thoughts.
3. Provide honest perceptions of reality and feedback about symptoms and behaviors.
4. Encourage patient to explore adaptive behaviors that increase abilities and success in socializing and accomplishing ADLs.
5. Decrease environmental stimuli.

Ensuring Safety

1. Monitor patient for behaviors that indicate increased anxiety and agitation.
2. Collaborate with patient to identify anxious behaviors as well as the causes.
3. Assess for the presence of command hallucinations.
4. Tell patient that you will help with maintaining behavioral control.
5. Establish consistent limits on patient's behaviors and clearly communicate these limits to the patient, family members, and health care providers.
6. Secure all potential weapons and articles from patient's room and the unit environment that could be used to inflict an injury to self or others.
7. To prepare for possible continued escalation, form a psychiatric emergency assist team and designate a leader to facilitate an effective and safe aggression management process.
8. Determine the need for external control, including seclusion or restraints. Communicate the decision to patient and put plan into action.
9. Frequently monitor patient within the guidelines of facility's policy on restrictive devices and assess patient's level of agitation.
10. When the patient's level of agitation begins to decrease and self-control is regained, establish a behavioral agreement that identifies specific behaviors that indicate self-control against a reescalation of agitation.

Community and Home Care Considerations

1. Patients may require supportive housing such as transitional living halfway houses, group or foster homes, and board and care homes. Supervision and drug management are important areas of concern for the nurse working in the community.
2. Psychosocial rehabilitation approach may be used in the community setting, where skills necessary for independent living are taught. Patient who has been symptomatic since early adulthood may not have learned these skills. The nurse working in the community setting may work as a member of the treatment team using this approach.

Family Education and Health Maintenance

1. Instruct patient and family members on the disease process and how to recognize and cope with relapse symptoms.
2. Instruct patient and family members about the uses, actions, and adverse effects of the prescribed drugs.
3. Provide instruction on when to notify the primary care provider regarding adverse drug effects or increased disease symptomatology.
4. Instruct patient and family about community resources, support groups, and possible use of psychiatric home care nursing.
5. For additional information and support, refer patient and family to agencies as such the Brain and Behavior Research Foundation (www.bbrfoundation.org) or *Schizophrenia*. The National Alliance on Mental Illness (www.nami.org) has a 24-hour helpline 800-950-6264.

Evaluation: Expected Outcomes

- Exhibits improved reality orientation, concentration, and attention span, as demonstrated through speech and behavior.
- Communicates with family and staff in a clear manner without evidence of loose, dissociated thinking.
- Independently maintains personal hygiene without fatigue.

- Attends group activities.
- Remains free from harm and violence to self or others.

NEUROCOGNITIVE DISORDERS

Delirium, Dementia, and Amnestic Disorders

Neurocognitive disorders reflect states in which cognitive impairment is the primary issue. This category encompasses specific disorders that produce either temporary or permanent neuronal damage, resulting in psychological or behavioral dysfunction, such as delirium, dementia, and amnestic disorder, as described in *Diagnostic and Statistical Manual of Mental Disorders, Fifth Edition, Text Revision* (*DSM-5-TR*). Although *dementia* is recognized as a term reflecting chronic disruption, the preferred diagnosis is neurocognitive disorder.

Delirium is an acute disturbance of consciousness and a change in cognition that develops over a brief period and is often reversible. *Dementia or neurocognitive disorder* is a chronic, progressive disturbance involving multiple cognitive deficits, including memory impairment. Impairment can be classified as mild or major based on the degree of cognitive decline and whether symptoms interfere with daily function. For major neurocognitive disorder, symptoms must interfere with the ability of the individual to be independent in activities of daily living (ADLs). *Amnestic disorder* is characterized by memory impairment in the absence of other significant cognitive impairments.

Pathophysiology and Etiology

Delirium

Can be caused by numerous pathophysiologic conditions. Some of the major possibilities include the following:

1. Central nervous system (CNS) pathology: head trauma, hypertensive cerebral changes, seizures, tumors.
2. Endocrinopathies: hyperthyroidism or hypothyroidism, hyperparathyroidism or hypoparathyroidism.
3. Hypoxemia.
4. Hypothermia or hyperthermia.
5. Substance intoxication or abstinence and withdrawal states.
6. Exposure to certain metals, toxins, or drugs.
7. Metabolic: diabetic acidosis, hypoglycemia, acid–base imbalances.
8. Hepatic encephalopathy.
9. Thiamine deficiency.
10. Postoperative states.
11. Psychosocial stressors: relocation stress, sensory deprivation or overload, sleep deprivation, immobilization.

Mild or Major Neurocognitive Disorder (Dementia)

1. Neurodegenerative disease—psychotic features may occur:
   a. Alzheimer disease.
   b. Lewy body disease.
   c. Vascular disease.
2. Infection-related dementias:
   a. Acquired immunodeficiency syndrome.
   b. Chronic meningitis.
   c. Creutzfeldt-Jakob disease.
   d. Progressive multifocal leukoencephalopathy.
   e. Postencephalitic dementia syndrome.
   f. Syphilis.
   g. Subacute sclerosing panencephalitis.
   h. Tuberculosis.
3. Subcortical degenerative disorders:
   a. Huntington disease.
   b. Parkinson disease.
   c. Wilson disease.
   d. Thalamic dementia.
4. Hydrocephalic dementias.
5. Vascular dementias.
6. Traumatic conditions, such as posttraumatic encephalopathy and subdural hematoma.
7. Neoplastic dementias:
   a. Glioma.
   b. Meningioma.
   c. Meningeal carcinomatosis.
   d. Metastatic deposits.
8. Inflammatory conditions, such as sarcoidosis, systemic lupus erythematosus, and temporal arteritis.
9. Toxic conditions, such as alcohol-related syndrome and iatrogenic dementias (anticonvulsant, anticholinergic, antihypertensive, psychotropic drugs).
10. Metabolic disorders:
    a. Anemias.
    b. Deficiency states (minerals and vitamins).
    c. Cardiac or pulmonary failure.
    d. Hepatic encephalopathy.
    e. Porphyria (deficiency in enzymes involved in heme synthesis).
    f. Uremia.
11. Genetic factors:
    a. Familial Alzheimer disease is associated with abnormal genes on chromosomes 1, 14, and 21, particularly with genes located on these chromosomes (1 and 14) that encode for amyloid precursor protein, which leads to the accumulation of the amyloid beta-peptide in plaques.
    b. A specific cholesterol-bearing protein, apolipoprotein E4 (Apo E4), is found on chromosome 19 twice as often in people with Alzheimer disease as in the general population.
12. Biochemical and brain structural factors:
    a. The neurotransmitter acetylcholine has been implicated in terms of relative deficit or receptor abnormalities as related to Alzheimer disease.
    b. Autopsy findings reveal the presence of brain changes, that is, the presence of amyloid plaques and neurofibrillary tangles associated with nerve cell destruction.
    c. Additional areas of investigation include the following:
       i. Slow viral infection.
       ii. Autoimmune processes.
       iii. Head trauma.

Amnestic Disorder

1. Posttraumatic amnesia: Head trauma is the most common cause of amnesia.
2. Poststroke amnesia: damage to the fornix or hippocampus.
3. Neoplasms.
4. Anoxic states.
5. Herpes simplex encephalitis.
6. Hypoglycemic states.
7. Epileptic seizures.
8. Electroconvulsive therapy (ECT).
9. Substance induced.

Clinical Manifestations

See Table 53-5.

Table 53-5 Clinical Manifestations of Neurocognitive Disorders

DISORDER	CLINICAL MANIFESTATIONS
Delirium	
Severe impairment in functioning	• Fluctuating levels of awareness • Clouding of consciousness (confused and disoriented) • Perceptual disturbances (illusions and hallucinations) • Memory, especially recent memory, is disturbed. • Alteration in sleep–wake cycle • EEG changes • Abrupt onset may last about 1 wk. • Reversible when underlying cause has been treated
Dementia (Neurocognitive Disorder)	
Severe impairment in functioning	• Slow, insidious onset • Impaired long- and short-term memory • Deterioration of cognitive abilities—judgment, abstract thinking • Often irreversible, based on cause • Personality changes • No or slow EEG changes
Amnestic Syndrome	
Moderate-to-severe impairment in functioning	• Impairment in short- and long-term memory • Inability to learn new material • Remote memory better than that of recent events • Confabulation • Apathy, lack of initiative • Emotionally bland

EEG, electroencephalogram.

Diagnostic Evaluation

Various diagnostic tests may be done to determine the cause. A comprehensive neuropsychiatric evaluation must be completed to make an accurate diagnosis.

1. Basic laboratory examination, including CBC with differential, chemistry panel (including blood urea nitrogen, creatine, and ammonia), arterial blood gas values, chest x-ray, toxicology screen (comprehensive), thyroid function tests, and serologic tests for syphilis.
2. Additional tests may include computed tomography (CT) scan, magnetic resonance imaging (MRI), additional blood chemistries (heavy metals, thiamine, folate, antinuclear antibody, and urinary porphobilinogen), lumbar puncture, positron emission tomography (PET)/single-photon emission CT scans.
3. Complete mental status examination.
4. Comprehensive physical examination.

Management

EVIDENCE BASE Bogdan, A., Manera, V., Koenig, A., & David, R. (2020). Pharmacologic approaches for the management of apathy in neurodegenerative disorders. *Frontiers in Pharmacology, 10,* 1581. https://doi.org/10.3389/fphar.2019.01581

Delirium

1. Treatment generally occurs in acute hospital-based setting where the goal is diagnosis to identify specific reversible causes of the delirium so that treatment is focused on ameliorating the causative factors.
2. Pharmacologic therapy is dependent on underlying causes. Additional drugs may be used that are directed toward the reduction of the acute symptoms of delirium, including:
   a. Benzodiazepines, such as lorazepam, for substance withdrawal states.
   b. Neuroleptics, such as risperidone and haloperidol, for agitation.
   c. Combined administration of haloperidol and lorazepam for agitated and psychotic symptomatology.
3. Environmental management:
   a. Safe, structured environment.
   b. Orientation facilitated by clocks, calendars, and other visual cues.
4. Family teaching about the nature of the disorder.
5. Family participation in the treatment plan to assist in the management of behavior.

Dementia

1. Treatment is generally community focused; the goal of treatment is to maintain the quality of life as long as possible despite the progressive nature of the disease. Effective treatment is based on:
   a. Diagnosis of primary illness and concurrent psychiatric disorders.
   b. Assessment of auditory and visual impairment.
   c. Measurement of the degree, nature, and progression of cognitive deficits.
   d. Assessment of functional capacity and ability for self-care.
   e. Family and social system assessment.
2. Environmental strategies to assist in maintaining the safety and functional abilities of patient as long as possible.
3. Pharmacologic therapy used for the person with Alzheimer disease is directed toward the use of anticholinesterase drugs to slow the progression of the disorder by increasing the relative amount of acetylcholine. Available drugs include donepezil, galantamine, and rivastigmine. An *N*-methyl-D-aspartic acid (NMDA) receptor antagonist memantine may be provided in an attempt to improve cognition (see Table 53-6). Other drugs may be used for behavioral control and symptom reduction.
   a. Agitation management: neuroleptic drugs, antipsychotic drugs, benzodiazepines.
   b. Psychosis: neuroleptic drugs.
   c. Depression: select antidepressants such as citalopram, duloxetine, escitalopram, fluoxetine, fluvoxamine, paroxetine, and mirtazapine; ECT.
4. Hypertension management in vascular dementia is important in reducing the severity of symptoms.
5. Family education is a treatment strategy because statistics indicate that family caregivers provide care for patients with

Table 53-6 Dosage and Adverse Reactions of Drugs Used in the Treatment of Dementia

DRUG: CLASS/GENERIC/TRADE NAME	ADULT THERAPEUTIC DOSAGE RANGE (mg/d)	ADVERSE REACTIONS
Cholinesterase Inhibitors		
Donepezil	5–23	Nausea, diarrhea, anorexia, fatigue
Galantamine	8–24	Nausea, diarrhea, dizziness, fatigue
Rivastigmine	6–13.3	Nausea, vomiting, anorexia, dizziness
NMDA Receptor Antagonist		
Memantine	5–21	Fatigue, dizziness, headache

NMDA, N-methyl-D-aspartic acid.

Alzheimer disease in 7 out of 10 cases. The family and the treatment team collaborate in the delivery of care.

Complications

1. Without accurate diagnosis and treatment, dementia resulting from another disease states may result in permanent cognitive deficits.
2. Falls with serious orthopedic or cerebral injuries.
3. Self-inflicted injuries.
4. Aggression or violence toward self, others, or property.
5. Wandering events, in which the person can get lost and potentially suffer exposure, hypothermia, injury, and even death.
6. Serious depression is demonstrated in caregivers who receive inadequate support.
7. Caregiver stress and burden may result in patient neglect or abuse.

Nursing Assessment

See Table 53-7.

1. Assess the onset and characteristics of symptoms (determine type and stage of disorder).
2. Establish cognitive status using standard measurement tools.
3. Determine self-care abilities.
4. Assess threats to physical safety (e.g., wandering, poor reality testing).
5. Assess the affect and emotional responsiveness.
6. Assess the ability and level of support available to caregivers.

Nursing Interventions

Improving Communication

1. Speak slowly and use short, simple words and phrases.
2. Consistently identify yourself and address the person by name at each meeting.
3. Focus on one piece of information at a time. Review what has been discussed with patient.
4. If patient has vision or hearing disturbances, have their wear prescription eyeglasses or a hearing device.
5. Keep environment well lit.
6. Use clocks, calendars, seasonal decorations, and familiar personal effects in patient's view.
7. If patient becomes verbally aggressive, identify and acknowledge feelings.
8. If patient becomes aggressive, shift the topic to a safer, more familiar one.
9. If patient becomes delusional, acknowledge feelings, and reinforce reality. Do not attempt to challenge the content of the delusion.

Promoting Independence in Self-care

1. Assess and monitor the patient's ability to perform ADLs.
2. Encourage decision-making regarding ADLs as much as possible.
3. Label clothes with patient's name, address, and telephone number.
4. Use clothing with elastic and Velcro for fastenings rather than buttons or zippers, which may be too difficult for patient to manipulate.

Table 53-7 Nursing Assessment for Delirium, Dementia, and Amnestic Disorder

	DELIRIUM	DEMENTIA	AMNESTIC DISORDER
Onset	Acute	Slow, insidious	Sudden
Course	Usually brief	Progresses over years	Transient or chronic
Mood	Fearfulness, anxiety, irritability	Mood labile, personality traits accentuated	Apathy, agitation, emotional blandness, shallow range of affective expression
Perception	Auditory, visual, tactile hallucinations; illusions	Hallucinations not a prominent feature	No hallucinatory experiences
Memory	Short-term memory impaired	Short-term memory deficit followed by long-term memory deficit	Impaired ability to learn new information; unable to recall previously learned information or past events
Communication	Slurred speech; confabulation	Normal—early stage: progressive aphasia and confabulation	Confabulation

5. Monitor food and fluid intake.
6. Weigh patient weekly.
7. Provide food that the patient can eat while moving.
8. Sit with patient during meals and assist by cueing.
9. Initiate a bowel and bladder program early in the disease process to maintain continence and prevent constipation or urine retention.

Ensuring Safety

1. Discuss restriction of driving when recommended.
2. Assess patient's home for safety: Remove throw rugs, label rooms, and keep the house well lit.
3. Assess community for safety.
4. Alert neighbors about patient's wandering behavior.
5. Alert police and have current pictures taken.
6. Provide patient with a medical alert device.
7. Install complex safety locks on doors to outside or basement.
8. Install safety bars in bathroom.
9. Closely observe patient while they are smoking.
10. Encourage physical activity during the daytime.
11. Give patient a card with simple instructions (address and phone number) in case they get lost.
12. Use nightlights.
13. Install alarm and sensor devices on doors.

Improving Socialization

1. Provide magazines with pictures as reading and language abilities diminish.
2. Encourage participation in simple, familiar group activities, such as singing, reminiscing, doing puzzles, and painting.
3. Encourage participation in simple activities that promote the exercise of large muscle groups.

Preventing Violence and Aggression

1. Respond calmly and do not raise your voice.
2. Remove objects that might be used to harm self or others.
3. Identify stressors that increase agitation.
4. Distract patient when an upsetting situation develops.

Community and Home Care Considerations

1. Multidisciplinary team approach is important, along with collaboration among professionals in nursing, medicine, psychiatry, nutrition, social work, pharmacy, and rehabilitative specialties.
2. Nurses involved in community care need to utilize case-finding approach as well as provide long-term support for family members involved in caregiving.
3. Adult day care and respite care may be utilized to provide the level of care needed by patient as well as allow the family to continue to maintain normal functioning.

Family Education and Health Maintenance

1. Instruct family about the process of the disorder, whether delirium, dementia, or amnestic disorder.
2. Instruct family about safety measures, environmental supports, and effective interventions for common symptoms to provide care in the home.
3. Instruct about and refer family members to community-based groups (adult day care centers, senior assessment centers, home care, respite care, and family support groups).
4. For additional information and support, refer to the Alzheimer's Association (www.alz.org) or the National Institutes of Health, the National Institute on Aging, the Alzheimer's Disease Education and Referral Center (800-438-4380; https://www.nia.nih.gov/health/alzheimers). For information on caregiving tips and advice with referral to local community groups, consult Today's Caregiver (https://caregiver.com) or AlzOnline Caregiver Support Online (800-677-1116; http://alzonline.phhp.ufl.edu).

Evaluation: Expected Outcomes

- Demonstrates decreased anxiety and increased feelings of security in supportive environment.
- Maintains maximum degree of orientation and self-care within the level of ability.
- Safety precautions and close surveillance maintained, no injury.
- Attends group activities, sings, exercises with group.
- Decreased occurrence of acting-out behaviors.

SUBSTANCE-RELATED DISORDERS

Substance Use Disorder

The use of alcohol and other psychoactive substances has become an endemic problem throughout all levels of society. In terms of substance use, a substance can be defined as a prescribed drug, an illegal drug, or a substance used in an unintended manner to produce mood or mind-altering effects (e.g., inhalants, glues, or steroids). Continued substance use may arise unintentionally from the initial use of a substance for its approved purpose. The individual commonly faces not only the psychological ramifications of a substance-related disorder but also physiologic consequences resulting from substance use.

Current criteria for diagnosing substance use disorder recognize elements of dependence. The criteria reflect dynamics of inability to control the use of a substance, use in situations that may put the individual at risk, and a centering of daily activities around the use or obtaining of a substance. These criteria reflect a pattern of use that has led to the development of one or more life problems.

Classification

EVIDENCE BASE American Psychiatric Association. (2022). *Diagnostic and statistical manual of mental disorders: Fifth edition, text revision: DSM-5-TR* (5th ed.). Author.

Dugosh, K., & Cacciola, J. (2022). Substance use disorders: Clinical assessment. *UpToDate*. Retrieved January 28, 2023, from https://www.uptodate.com/contents/substance-use-disorders-clinical-assessment

A substance use disorder includes elements of use and possible dependence within the criterion. The defining characteristic of a disorder is when there is impairment of ability to perform social roles in the home, school, or work setting. Substance use can occur in relation to the use of any of 10 categories of substance: caffeine, tobacco, opioids, alcohol, hallucinogens, sedatives, stimulants, anxiolytics, inhalants, and hypnotics. In addition, the severity of substance use can be specified as mild, moderate, or severe based on the number of symptoms present.

- Substance (specify) use.
- Substance (specify)-induced disorders.
- Substance (specify) intoxication.

Several disorders can be induced through the use of a particular substance; in such cases, the symptoms cannot be explained by another condition or disorder and are related to substance use. Such substance-induced disorders include the following:

- Substance-induced intoxication.
- Substance-induced withdrawal.
- Substance- or medication-indicated mental health disorders.

Dual diagnosis is defined as the presence of a substance-related diagnosis along with another psychiatric disorder.

Pathophysiology and Etiology

As with the development of other psychiatric conditions and disorders, the development of substance-related disorders reflects a complex interaction of biological, genetic, sociologic, and psychological factors. Several theoretical approaches have been developed to describe the process of use and dependence.

Biochemical Factors

1. Dopamine is one of the primary neurotransmitters within the central nervous system (CNS) and is known to be involved in the integration of environmental stimuli with physiologic responses. Cannabis, cocaine, and alcohol increase the dopamine level, thereby producing a strong association between physiologic effects and behavior.
2. Dopamine is also involved in CNS pathways that mediate feelings of pleasure. Opioids indirectly increase dopamine activity by modulation of the mesolimbic system, leading to reinforcement of substance use.
3. Neurons in the mesolimbic system can become sensitized to the presence of amphetamine and cocaine. Such sensitization is the reverse of tolerance, with the development of an enhanced neuronal response upon repeated exposure. These responses appear to be associated with the development of substance dependence.

Genetic Factors

1. Alcohol use disorder is strongly associated with a familial history of the condition. In these individuals, a genetic disposition to alcohol use disorder combines with a learning environment in which the patient develops certain beliefs about the use of a substance and its effects. The presence of genetic disposition, in the absence of a biological parent's alcohol use disorder, does not result in a significantly higher risk of alcohol use disorder than in those individuals without such disposition. These findings provide support for models focusing on genetic and environmental interaction in the etiology of substance use.
2. Genetic variation in gene regulation resulting in lower levels of serotonin in the CNS may be associated with the development of alcohol use disorder.

Psychosocial Factors

1. An individual learns to use substances in certain situations with certain expectations as to the effects of the substance (e.g., relaxation, disinhibition). As the individual experiences the desired effects, this may reinforce the desire to use the substance.
2. Use may begin with an attempt to fit in with a larger peer group as a means of boosting self-esteem.
3. Substances may be used to relieve anxiety or as a means of coping with other traumatic events (self-medication).

Sociocultural Factors

1. Societies around the world use psychoactive substances for several reasons. The individual learns the approved use of the substance within the societal or familial structure and may consider such use to be appropriate.
2. The society in which an individual resides may consider dependence on certain substances to be a minor issue, thereby providing a justification for continued use.

Clinical Manifestations

EVIDENCE BASE American Psychiatric Association. (2022). *Diagnostic and statistical manual of mental disorders: Fifth edition, text revision: DSM-5-TR* (5th ed.). Author.

Substance Abuse and Mental Health Services Administration. (2020). *Treatment Improvement Protocol 26: Treating substance use disorders in older adults.* Pep 20-02-01-011: Substance Abuse and Mental Health Services Administration.

Substance Abuse and Mental Health Services Administration. (2020). *Evidence-Based Resource Guide: Treatment of stimulant use disorders.* Pep 20-06-01-011: Substance Abuse and Mental Health Services Administration.

Overview

1. Substance use disorder is characterized by a loss of control.
2. A pattern of substance use must be sustained over a period of 12 months and impair ADLs.
3. Whether the pattern is one of steady or binge use, activities related to substance use must interfere with daily functioning, in terms of time off work or curtailing of social activities to provide more time to participate in, or recover from, substance use.
4. A differentiating factor between misuse and dependence is that dependence is characterized by the development of tolerance with the appearance of substance-specific withdrawal symptomatology in the absence of use.

CLINICAL JUDGMENT The complications of substance use such as injuries and liver disease may be treated in the hospital, but the underlying substance use may not be known or addressed by the medical staff. Nurses should monitor for the presence of substance use and withdrawal symptoms during and following hospitalization so that the medical condition does not worsen, and appropriate referrals can be made.

Substance Use

Physical examination and history findings compatible with substance use include at least one of the following:

1. Continued use even in the face of an inability to meet major life obligations.
2. Use in situations that pose a danger of harm to self or others (i.e., driving while intoxicated).
3. Continued use regardless of legal issues associated with use (e.g., continued driving while intoxicated after suspension of a license) or continued use after the development of problems in social relationships (e.g., an impending divorce brought about by substance use).

Substance Dependence

Physical examination and history findings include meeting at least three diagnostic criteria, which include the following:

1. Tolerance to substance-related effects.
2. Withdrawal in the absence of the substance.
3. Unsuccessful attempts to reduce or halt use.

4. Cutting down or avoiding social obligations or work responsibilities to spend time in substance-related activity (e.g., obtaining, using, recovering from).
5. Continued use despite the development of significant life problems (e.g., loss of job).

Diagnostic Evaluation

A number of tools have been designed to assess for the presence of substance-related disorders in specific populations (e.g., adolescents, pregnant individuals). The tool used should be specific to the patient being assessed.

1. Measurement tools for alcohol use or dependence:
   a. CAGE: alcohol screening questionnaire.
   b. Michigan Alcohol Screening Test (MAST).
   c. Alcohol Use Disorders Identification Test (AUDIT).
2. Measurement tools for other substance use and dependence:
   a. CAGE-AID: a version of the CAGE alcohol screening questionnaire adapted to include drug use.
   b. Drug Abuse Screening Tool (DAST).
   c. Screening, Brief Intervention, and Referral to Treatment (SBIRT).
3. Laboratory testing of blood, saliva, sweat, and hair for the presence of a substance or metabolite. The period of effective measurement varies based on the procedure and the substance.
4. States of drug intoxication or withdrawal can be identified through the presence of physiologic and behavioral symptoms associated with the use of a particular substance.
5. Additional screening and testing are recommended for the presence of other disease conditions or illnesses (human immunodeficiency virus [HIV], hepatitis) that may have resulted from risk-taking behavior while under the influence of substances or may have resulted from the physiologic effects of the substance (as in cardiac dysrhythmia in the case of cocaine use).

Management

For the treatment of substance overdose and alcohol-related delirium, see Chapter 35, pages 1027 to 1029.

1. The management of substance use includes outpatient and inpatient treatment modalities. Inpatient modalities include programs of detoxification and therapy sessions designed to aid in the recognition of a substance-related disorder. Outpatient therapies include support groups, continued therapy sessions, and the use of pharmacologic drugs to aid in the maintenance of sobriety.
2. Initial detoxification is typically provided through inpatient hospitalization. Detoxification protocols are unique to each substance. Benzodiazepine taper is utilized during detoxification from alcohol. The treatment of cocaine withdrawal may include administration of prescribed drugs that can reduce craving, such as amantadine or bromocriptine. The treatment of heroin withdrawal generally involves transdermal clonidine along with oral administration, as necessary.
3. Drugs may also be used in the treatment of alcohol use.
   a. Disulfiram is used as aversion therapy. It leads to the accumulation of acetaldehyde in the blood system, causing flushing, tachycardia, vomiting, nausea, and chest pain if alcohol is consumed.
   b. A nonaversion therapy, acamprosate sodium, may be used in attempts to ensure abstinence from alcohol. It interacts with the gamma-aminobutyric acid (GABA) neurotransmitter system to restore balance between neuronal excitation and inhibition.
   c. Topiramate, an anticonvulsant, may reduce craving for alcohol. Clinical trials have demonstrated that ondansetron may aid in reducing drinking.
4. Drug therapy in the treatment of opiate withdrawal includes several classes.
   a. Administration of an opioid antagonist, such as naloxone and naltrexone, reverses the effects of opioids. Injectable sustained-release formulations of naltrexone may also be used.
   b. Outpatient detoxification is typically focused on the administration of the opioid agonist, methadone, or levo-alpha-acetylmethadol, a longer lasting formulation, to substitute for the illicit drug.
   c. Another opioid agonist, buprenorphine, is available in the outpatient treatment of opioid dependency. An injectable form is used in the treatment of chronic pain. It is also available in sublingual and transdermal formulations and often blended with naloxone to prevent euphoria from intravenous injection of oral formulations.
5. Psychosocial support using 12-step or other treatment programs such as Rational Recovery.
6. Psychoeducational therapy to understand triggers of substance use and prevention of relapse.
7. Family support and educational groups.

Complications

1. The physiologic complications of substance-induced disorders are specific to the substance involved. Physiologic complications can also result from exposure to other substances (e.g., talcum powder, strychnine) that are mixed with cocaine or heroin.
2. Psychological complications include increased potential for risk-taking and suicidal behavior.
3. Individuals under the influence of substances are more likely to experience automobile or other accidents.
4. Suicide rates increase in the presence of substance use. This includes accidental overdose related to the substance.
5. The physiologic complications or consequences associated with alcohol use involve each organ system and include the development of gastrointestinal (GI) ulcers, liver disease, malnutrition, anemia, and dehydration.
6. Complications associated with the use of cocaine or amphetamines include cardiac dysrhythmia, seizures, dehydration, and acute renal failure. Mood lability and psychosis are commonly associated with the use of amphetamines and cocaine.
7. Heroin use can result in respiratory complications and the development of infectious disease through the sharing of needles. Endocarditis, skin abscesses, and other infectious sequelae may result.
8. The use of 3,4-methylenedioxymethamphetamine (Ecstasy) can have complications like those associated with amphetamine use. Research has also demonstrated the effects on short- and long-term memory through neurotoxic effects on serotonergic pathways, with possible additional effects on dopamine pathways in the CNS.

Nursing Assessment

1. Assess physiologic stability:
   a. Elevated or decreased blood pressure.
   b. Cardiac abnormalities.

   c. Confusion, memory deficits, ataxia, nystagmus (Wernicke encephalopathy, a thiamine deficiency).
   d. Lasting memory deficits (Korsakoff amnestic disorder).
   e. Lung congestion or diminished breath sounds.
   f. Fever.
   g. Mood lability.
2. Assess for evidence of medical complications:
   a. Hepatic disease.
   b. Renal disease.
   c. Anemia.
   d. Sexually transmitted infection.
   e. Anxiety and depression.
3. Identify risk-taking behaviors:
   a. Participation in criminal activities.
   b. Sexual activity and behaviors, including the use of protective devices.
   c. Motor vehicle violations.
   d. Participation in hazardous sports or activities.
4. Gather information regarding substance use:
   a. Substances used and amounts.
   b. Method of use (e.g., injection, inhalation).
   c. Previous attempts to reduce or stop use.
   d. Prior history of withdrawal symptoms.
   e. Longest previous period of sobriety.
   f. Prior treatment programs attended.
   g. Familial history of substance use.
   h. Precipitating events to substance use.
5. Examine coping mechanisms and behaviors:
   a. Denies presence of a substance-related problem.
   b. Does not recognize the presence of physical or emotional health problems.
   c. Blames others for the presence of problems.
   d. Uses substance in stress-provoking situations.
   e. Justifies use of substance.
   f. Prior psychiatric history.
6. Monitor for withdrawal symptoms:
   a. Agitation, mood lability, paranoia, or mania (cocaine, amphetamines).
   b. Dehydration, nutritional deficiencies, hallucinations, seizures, GI disturbances (alcohol and other substances).
   c. Nausea, vomiting, flulike symptoms, diarrhea, and muscle pain (opioids).

Nursing Interventions

Facilitate Recognition of Substance-Related Disorder

1. Approach patient in a direct, nonjudgmental manner.
2. Assess the patient's level of knowledge about substance.
3. Have patient identify situations preceding substance use.
4. Discuss consequences of substance use.
5. Reinforce desire for change.

Encourage Participation of Family and Significant Others

1. Provide support to family and significant others while acknowledging substance-related disorder of patient.
2. Encourage family to attend supportive and educational group meetings.
3. Have family members identify effects of substance use on family functioning.
4. Discuss role relationships with family that may be related to substance-seeking behavior.

Ensuring Safety

1. Monitor patient for symptoms of substance withdrawal.
2. Provide prescribed medications, as indicated, for the treatment of withdrawal symptomatology.
3. Educate patient on relationship between symptoms and substance use.
4. Monitor hydration and nutritional status.
5. Reduce the level of stimulation, as appropriate.
6. Assess for the presence of agitation or mood lability.

Enhancing Coping Strategies

1. Aid in identifying triggers to use.
2. Have patient develop a list of personal strengths.
3. Help patient develop an understanding of dependence as an illness.
4. Assist patient in developing alternative coping strategies through participation in role-playing activities and groups.
5. Identify alternative methods of participating in social situations without resorting to use of substance.
6. Reinforce need for ongoing attendance of support group meetings.

Community and Home Care Considerations

1. Assist in resource finding for inpatient or outpatient program. Provide referral and information about community-based programs and activities that can aid in the maintenance of sobriety. The individual may benefit from placement in a residential treatment program or halfway house that provides supportive services and continued programs of treatment in a community setting.
2. Assist in educating and encouraging adherence to drug therapy regimen. Provide information about medication therapy, as appropriate, including known adverse effects and means of obtaining prescribed drugs, as necessary (e.g., methadone).

Family Education and Health Maintenance

1. Instruct patient and family about adverse physiologic and psychological effects of substance use.
2. Discuss health maintenance practices to minimize potential effects of substance use (e.g., vitamin use, proper diet).
3. Explain the potential for injury from risk-taking behaviors.
4. Reinforce the need for aftercare groups and activities.
5. For general information and support, consult agencies such as the National Institute on Drug Abuse, National Institutes of Health (www.drugabuse.gov), or the National Institute on Alcohol Abuse and Alcoholism, National Institutes of Health (www.niaaa.nih.gov). General information can also be obtained from Substance Abuse & Mental Health Services Administration (https://www.samhsa.gov) or Alcoholics Anonymous (www.aa.org).

Evaluation: Expected Outcomes

- Acknowledges the presence of a substance-related disorder.
- Identifies negative effects of substance use on family, work, and other relationships.
- Describes negative effects of substance use on physical and emotional health.
- Continues to attend treatment programs, refrains from substance use.

CHILD AND ADOLESCENT DISORDERS

Children and adolescents can develop the same psychiatric disorders seen in adult populations, such as major depression, bipolar disorder, and substance-related disorders. In addition, children and adolescents face several developmental and age-specific mental health issues. A child faced with a traumatic situation may engage in a pattern of destructive or deviant behavior. Working with such a child can be frustrating to both health care personnel and caregivers. The intent of this section is to provide a brief overview of a select group of mental health issues specific to pediatric populations. For further information, the reader is strongly encouraged to seek out texts and materials dedicated to pediatric mental health and child development.

EVIDENCE BASE American Psychiatric Association. (2022). *Diagnostic and statistical manual of mental disorders: Fifth edition, text revision: DSM-5-TR* (5th ed.). Author.

Harden, K. P., Engelhardt, L. E., Mann, F. D., Patterson, M. W., Grotzinger, A. D., Savicki, S. L., Thibodeaux, M. L., Freis, S. M., Tackett, J. L., Church, J. A., & Tucker-Drob, E. M. (2020). Genetic associations between executive functions and a general factor of psychopathology. *Journal of the American Academy of Child & Adolescent Psychiatry, 59*(6), 749–758. https://doi.org/10.1016/j.jaac.2019.05.006

Sadock, B., & Sadock, V. (2020). *Kaplan and Sadock's concise textbook of child and adolescent psychiatry.* Wolters Kluwer.

Psychiatric disorders specific to child populations, as defined by the *Diagnostic and Statistical Manual of Mental Disorders, Fifth Edition, Text Revision* (*DSM-5-TR*), include the following:

1. Attentional deficit and autism spectrum disorders (see Chapter 52, pages 1458 to 1463).
2. Behavioral disorders.
   a. Conduct disorder.
   b. Oppositional defiant disorder.
3. Elimination disorders.
   a. Encopresis—incontinence of feces not caused by organic process.
   b. Enuresis—involuntary voiding during sleep; may be physiologic during early childhood.

Other psychiatric disorders already discussed in this chapter may appear in childhood and adolescence and persist into adulthood. Eating disorders commonly begin during the adolescent years and continue well into adulthood (see Chapter 16, page 558).

Behavioral Disorders

Conduct disorder and oppositional defiant disorder may arise in children of all ages. The most significant difference between the two is that in conduct disorder, the child or adolescent is violating societal norms and rules. With oppositional defiant disorder, the child or adolescent is displaying disruptive and negative behavior primarily toward authority figures, without violation of societal norms.

Pathophysiology and Etiology

The development of a psychiatric disorder commonly reflects a complex interaction of several etiologic factors.

1. Twin studies have provided some evidence that conduct disorder may have a genetic predisposition.
2. Other genetic studies have indicated that regions located on chromosomes 2 and 19 may be associated with the development of conduct disorder.
3. These predisposing genetic factors most likely interact with environmental influences, such as household violence, neglect, and other situational variables, in contributing to the development of behavioral or attentional disorders.

Clinical Manifestations

1. Conduct disorder is a pattern of persistent behavior during which the individual violates either the rights of another person or accepted societal norms. Behavioral criteria incorporate four possible domains, across which three or more behaviors must be observed within a 12-month period:
   a. Aggression toward people or animals (threatening behaviors, physical cruelty, initiating of physical confrontations, or weapon use).
   b. Aggression toward property (intentional fire-setting or destruction of property).
   c. Theft or deceitfulness (breaking into property of others, stealing of items).
   d. Violation of rules (before age 13), such as staying out late at night, regardless of caregiver instruction; running away from home; and absence from school.
2. If the individual does not violate societal norms but engages in a pattern of hostile, defiant, and negative behavior toward authority figures or adults in general, oppositional defiant disorder may be considered. This pattern of behavior must endure for at least 6 months, during which time at least four of the following behaviors are exhibited:
   a. Frequently loses temper.
   b. Often argues with adults.
   c. Often refuses to comply with, or defies, rules.
   d. Often blames others for behavior or mistakes.
   e. Intentionally provokes others on a frequent basis.
   f. Often appears easily annoyed or irritated by others.
   g. Often appears angry or resentful toward others.
   h. Frequently engages in spiteful and vindictive behavior.
3. The behavioral disorders have been found to have a significant degree of comorbidity. These disorders may also coexist with attention deficits such as attention-deficit/hyperactivity disorder (ADHD).

Diagnostic Evaluation

1. The evaluation of a child and adolescent ideally incorporates information from patient, caregivers, other family members, and teachers.
2. Evaluation should also include a detailed physical and nutritional assessment.
3. Depending on the patient's age, play activities may be incorporated into the interview to facilitate trust and patient expression. Younger children may be more capable of depicting family dynamics and their own feelings through play or art.

Management

1. Care of the individual with a behavioral disorder may initially involve treatment in a structured inpatient program that incorporates many behavioral modification techniques, including a level system, a token economy, and close monitoring.
2. Residential or partial hospitalization treatment programs may also be employed.

3. Treatment of a behavioral disorder includes family therapy, caregiver and patient education, and, ideally, teacher interaction. Family counseling and education are essential aspects of any treatment modality.
4. Drugs may be employed in the treatment program, based on the presence of comorbidities and behavioral severity.

Nursing Interventions

Interventions should be selected that encourage the verbal expression of feelings and provide alternatives to destructive behavior. Interventions should also be included that address caregiver education. Interventions to be considered include the following:

1. Aid patient in identifying events that trigger inappropriate behavioral responses.
2. Assist patient in developing communication skills.
3. Teach alternative behaviors and methods of expression.
4. Provide consistent limits and consequences for inappropriate behaviors.
5. Provide positive feedback for appropriate behaviors.
6. Monitor behavior for violence directed toward self or others.
7. Utilize role-play to practice alternative behavioral responses.
8. Teach caregiving skills to primary caregivers.
9. Teach caregivers appropriate limit setting, and emphasize the need to clearly state expectations.

Evaluation: Expected Outcomes

- Reduction in frequency and intensity of outbursts while interacting with others.
- Uses alternative coping strategies in situations in which they would previously have been angered or engaged in destructive behavior.
- Attends school on a consistent basis.
- Does not injure self or others

SELECTED READINGS

American Psychological Association. (2023). *APA dictionary of psychology*. American Psychological Association. https://dictionary.apa.org/

Barnes, M. D., Hanson, C. L., Novilla, L. B., Magnusson, B. M., Crandall, A. C., & Bradford, G. (2020). Family-centered health promotion: Perspectives for engaging families and achieving better health outcomes. *INQUIRY: The Journal of Health Care Organization, Provision, and Financing, 57*, 1-6. https://doi.org/10.1177/0046958020923537

Bighelli, I., Wu, H., Hansen, W., Priller, J., Davis, J. M., Salanti, G., & Leucht, S. (2023). Metabolic side effects in persons with schizophrenia during mid- to long-term treatment with antipsychotics: A network meta-analysis of Randomized Controlled Trials. *World Psychiatry, 22*(1), 116–128. https://doi.org/10.1002/wps.21036

Burschinski, A., Schneider-Thoma, J., Chiocchia, V., Schestag, K., Wang, D., Siafis, S., Bighelli, I., Wu, H., Hansen, W. P., Priller, J., Davis, J. M., Salanti, G., & Leucht, S. (2023). Metabolic side effects in persons with schizophrenia during mid- to long-term treatment with antipsychotics: A network meta-analysis of randomized controlled trials. *World Psychiatry, 22*(1), 116–128. https://doi.org/10.1002/wps.21036

Costantini, L., Costanza, A., Odone, A., Aguglia, A., Escelsior, A., Serafini, G., Amore, M., & Amerio, A. (2021). *A breakthrough in research on depression screening: From validation to efficacy studies. Acta Bio-medica: Atenei Parmensis, 92*(3), e2021215.

Goes, F. S. (2023). Diagnosis and management of bipolar disorders. *British Medical Journal, 381*, e073591.

Halter, M. J. (2022). *Varcarolis' foundations of Psychiatric-Mental Health Nursing: A clinical approach* (9th ed.). Elsevier.

Hausteiner-Wiehle, C., & Hungerer, S. (2020). Factitious disorders in everyday clinical practice. *Deutsches Ärzteblatt International, 117*, 452–459. https://doi.org/10.3238/arztebl.2020.0452

Lenouvel, E., Chivu, C., Mattson, J., Young, J. Q., Klöppel, S., & Pinilla, S. (2022). Instructional Design Strategies for teaching the mental status examination and psychiatric interview: A scoping review. *Academic Psychiatry, 46*(6), 750–758. https://doi.org/10.1007/s40596-022-01617-0

McCutcheon, R. A., Marques, T. R., & Howes, O. D. (2020). Schizophrenia—An overview. *JAMA Psychiatry, 77*(2), 201. https://doi.org/10.1001/jamapsychiatry.2019.3360

McWhirter, L., Ritchie, C., Stone, J., & Carson, A. (2020). Functional cognitive disorders: A systematic review. *The Lancet Psychiatry, 7*(2), 191–207.

MedlinePlus, National Library of Medicine. (2023). *Personality disorders. MedlinePlus*. https://medlineplus.gov/personalitydisorders.html

Mughal, A. Y., Devadas, J., Ardman, E., Levis, B., Go, V. F., & Gaynes, B. N. (2020). A systematic review of validated screening tools for anxiety disorders and PTSD in low to middle income countries. *BMC Psychiatry, 20*(1), 338. https://doi.org/10.1186/s12888-020-02753-3

Rudenstine, S., Espinosa, A., & Kumar, A. (2020). Depression and anxiety subgroups across alcohol use disorder and substance use in a National Epidemiologic Study. *Journal of Dual Diagnosis, 16*(3), 299–311. https://doi.org/10.1080/15504263.2020.1784498

Silveira, K., Garcia-Barrera, M. A., & Smart, C. M. (2020). Neuropsychological impact of trauma-related mental illnesses: A systematic review of clinically meaningful results. *Neuropsychology Review, 30*(3), 310–344. https://doi.org/10.1007/s11065-020-09444-6

Sousa, S., Teixeira, L., & Paúl, C. (2020). Assessment of major neurocognitive disorders in primary health care: Predictors of individual risk factors. *Frontiers in Psychology, 11*, 1413. https://doi.org/10.3389/fpsyg.2020.01413

Zhao, X., & Zhang, Z. (2020). Risk factors for postpartum depression: An evidence-based systematic review of systematic reviews and meta-analyses. *Asian Journal of Psychiatry, 53*, 102353. https://doi.org/10.1016/j.ajp.2020.102353

Appendix A
Diagnostic Studies and Interpretation*†

Table A-1 Reference Ranges—Hematology and Coagulation

	NORMAL ADULT REFERENCE RANGE		
LABORATORY TEST	**CONVENTIONAL UNITS**	**SI UNITS**	**CLINICAL SIGNIFICANCE**
Bleeding Time	3–10 min	3–10 min	• Prolonged in thrombocytopenia, defective platelet function, and aspirin therapy
D-Dimer	<250 ng/mL	<0.5 mg/L	• Increased in disseminated intravascular coagulation, malignancy, and arterial and venous thrombosis
Erythrocyte Count			
Males	4,100,000–5,800,000/mm^3	4.1–5.8 × 10^{12}/L	• Increased in severe diarrhea and dehydration, polycythemia, acute poisoning, and pulmonary fibrosis • Decreased in all anemias in leukemia and after hemorrhage, when blood volume has been restored
Females	3,770,000–5,280,000/mm^3	4.7–5.28 × 10^{12}/L	
Erythrocyte Indices			
Mean corpuscular volume (MCV)	79–97 μm^3	79–97 fL	• Increased in macrocytic anemia; decreased in microcytic anemia
Mean corpuscular hemoglobin (MCH)		26.6–33 pg	• Increased in macrocytic anemia; decreased in microcytic anemia
Mean corpuscular hemoglobin concentration (MCHC)	31.5–35.7 g/dL	Concentration fraction: 0.31.5–0.35.7	• Decreased in severe hypochromic anemia
Erythrocyte Sedimentation Rate (ESR)—Westergren Method			
Males <50 yr	<15 mm/h	<15 mm/h	• Increased in tissue destruction, whether inflammatory or degenerative; during menstruation and pregnancy; and in acute febrile diseases
Males ≥50 yr	<20 mm/h	<20 mm/h	
Females <50 yr	<20 mm/h	<20 mm/h	
Females ≥50 yr	<30 mm/h	<30 mm/h	
Hematocrit			
Males	37.5%–51%	Volume fraction: 0.36–0.51	• Decreased in severe anemia, anemia of pregnancy, and acute massive blood loss • Increased in erythrocytosis of any cause and in dehydration or hemoconcentration associated with shock
Females	34%–46.6%	Volume fraction: 0.34–0.46	

(continued)

*Please note that the term "male" in this appendix refers to a person assigned male at birth, and the term "female" in this appendix refers to a person assigned female at birth.
† Laboratory values may vary according to the techniques used in different laboratories.

Table A-1 Reference Ranges—Hematology and Coagulation (*continued*)

LABORATORY TEST	NORMAL ADULT REFERENCE RANGE: CONVENTIONAL UNITS	NORMAL ADULT REFERENCE RANGE: SI UNITS	CLINICAL SIGNIFICANCE
Hemoglobin			
Males	12.6–17.7 g/dL	7.82–10.98 mmol/L	• Decreased in various anemias, in pregnancy, in severe or prolonged hemorrhage, and with excessive fluid intake • Increased in polycythemia, chronic obstructive pulmonary disease, failure of oxygenation due to heart failure, and normally in people living at high altitudes
Females	11.1–15.9 g/dL	6.89–9.87 mmol/L	
Leukocyte Count			
Total	3,400–10,800 μL	3.4–10.8 × 10^9/L	• Total is elevated in acute infectious diseases, predominantly in the neutrophilic fraction with bacterial diseases, and in the lymphocytic and monocytic fractions in viral diseases • Elevated in acute leukemia, following menstruation, and following surgery or trauma • Eosinophils elevated in collagen disease, allergy, and intestinal parasitosis • Depressed in aplastic anemia, in agranulocytosis, and by toxic chemotherapeutic agents used in treating malignancy
Basophils	0–1%		
Eosinophils	1%–6%		
Lymphocytes	20%–40%		
Monocytes	2%–10%		
Neutrophils	40%–75%		
Platelet Count	140,000–400,000/μL	140–400 × 10^9/L	• Increased in malignancy, myeloproliferative disease, rheumatoid arthritis, and postoperatively; about 50% of patients with unexpected increase of platelet count will be found to have a malignancy • Decreased in thrombocytopenic purpura, acute leukemia, and aplastic anemia and during cancer chemotherapy
Reticulocytes	0.5%–1.5% of red blood cells		• Increased with any condition stimulating increase in bone marrow activity (infection, blood loss [acute and chronically following iron therapy in iron deficiency anemia], and polycythemia vera) • Decreased with any condition depressing bone marrow activity, acute leukemia, and late stage of severe anemias

Table A-2 Reference Ranges—Serum, Plasma, and Whole Blood Chemistries

LABORATORY TEST	NORMAL ADULT REFERENCE RANGE: CONVENTIONAL UNITS	NORMAL ADULT REFERENCE RANGE: SI UNITS	CLINICAL SIGNIFICANCE: INCREASED	CLINICAL SIGNIFICANCE: DECREASED
Alkaline Phosphatase Adults	40–150 IU/L	40–150 IU/L	• Conditions reflecting increased osteoblastic activity of bone • Rickets • Hyperparathyroidism • Hepatic disease	• Malnutrition • Cretinism • Severe anemia • Celiac disease
Alanine Aminotransferase (ALT)	5–40 IU/L	5–40 IU/L	• Liver disease • Muscle trauma • Muscle injury	• Azotemia • Chronic dialysis
Aspartate Aminotransferase (AST)	5–40 IU/L	5–40 IU/L	• Same as ALT	

Table A-2 Reference Ranges—Serum, Plasma, and Whole Blood Chemistries (*continued*)

	NORMAL ADULT REFERENCE RANGE		CLINICAL SIGNIFICANCE	
LABORATORY TEST	CONVENTIONAL UNITS	SI UNITS	INCREASED	DECREASED
Bilirubin				
Total	0.1–1.2 mg/dL	2–20 µmol/L	• Hemolytic anemia (indirect) • Biliary obstruction and disease • Hepatocellular damage (hepatitis) • Pernicious anemia • Hemolytic disease of the newborn	
Direct (conjugated)	0.1–0.2 mg/dL	0–4 µmol/L		
Indirect (unconjugated)	0.1–1 mg/dL	1.7–17.1 µmol/L		
Calcium	8.6–10.3 mg/dL	2.15–2.57 mmol/L	• Tumor or hyperplasia of parathyroid • Hypervitaminosis D • Multiple myeloma • Nephritis with uremia • Malignant tumors • Sarcoidosis • Hyperthyroidism • Skeletal immobilization • Excess calcium intake: milk-alkali syndrome	• Hypoparathyroidism • Diarrhea • Celiac disease • Vitamin D deficiency • Acute pancreatitis • Nephrosis • After parathyroidectomy
Carbon Dioxide, Venous	22–30 mEq/L	22–30 mmol/L	• Respiratory acidosis (CO_2 retention) • Metabolic alkalosis (vomiting)	• Respiratory alkalosis (hyperventilation) • Metabolic acidosis (diabetic ketoacidosis)
Chloride	98–106 mEq/L	98–106 mmol/L	• Nephrosis • Nephritis • Urinary obstruction • Cardiac decompensation • Anemia	• Diabetes • Diarrhea • Vomiting • Pneumonia • Heavy metal poisoning • Cushing syndrome • Intestinal obstruction • Febrile conditions
Creatinine	0.7–1.4 mg/dL	62–124 µmol/L	• Renal insufficiency, muscle disease • Chronic renal disease	• Advanced liver disease
Glucose				
Fasting	60–99 mg/dL	3.3–6.05 mmol/L	• Diabetes • Cushing disease • *Note:* 100–126 is impaired fasting glucose; >126 fasting is diagnostic for diabetes	• Hyperinsulinism/insulinemia • Addison disease • Insulin therapy
Postprandial (2 h)	65–140 mg/dL	3.58–7.7 mmol/L		
Potassium (K)	3.5–5 mEq/L	3.5–5 mmol/L	• Renal failure • Acidosis • Cell lysis • Tissue breakdown or hemolysis	• Gastrointestinal losses • Diuretic administration
Protein, Total	6–8 g/dL	60–80 g/L	• Hemoconcentration • Shock • Multiple myeloma (globulin fraction) • Chronic infections (globulin function) • Liver disease (globulin)	• Malnutrition • Hemorrhage • Loss of plasma from burns • Proteinuria
Albumin	3.5–5 g/dL	35–50 g/L		
Globulin	1.5–3 g/dL	15–30 g/L		
Sodium	135–145 mEq/L	135–145 mmol/L	• Hemoconcentration • Diabetes insipidus	• Diuretic therapy • Water intoxication
Urea Nitrogen, Blood (BUN)	10–20 mg/dL	3.6–7.2 mmol/L	• Acute glomerulonephritis • Obstructive uropathy • Mercury poisoning • Nephrotic syndrome	• Severe hepatic failure • Pregnancy

SELECTED ABBREVIATIONS USED IN APPENDICES

CONVENTIONAL UNITS

- kg = kilogram
- g = gram
- mg = milligram
- µg = microgram
- µµg = micromicrogram
- ng = nanogram
- pg = picogram
- dL = 100 milliliters
- mL = milliliter
- mm^3 = cubic millimeter
- fL = femtoliter
- mM = millimole
- nM = nanomole
- mOsm = milliosmole
- mm = millimeter
- µm = micron or micrometer
- mm Hg = millimeters of mercury
- U = unit
- mU = milliunit
- µU = microunit
- mEq = milliequivalent
- IU = International Unit
- mIU = milliInternational Unit

SI UNITS

- g = gram
- L = liter
- mol = mole
- mmol = millimole
- µmol = micromole
- nmol = nanomole
- pmol = picomole

Appendix B
Conversion Tables

Table B-1 Metric Units and Symbols

QUANTITY	UNIT	SYMBOL	EQUIVALENT
Length	Millimeter	mm	1,000 mm = 1 m
	Centimeter	cm	100 cm = 1 m
	Decimeter	dm	10 dm = 1 m
	Meter	m	1,000 m = 1 km
Volume	Cubic centimeter	cc or cm^3	1,000 cc = 1 liter
	Milliliter	ml or mL	1,000 mL = 1 liter
	Cubic decimeter	dm^3	1,000 dm^3 = 1 m^3
	Liter	L	1,000 L = 1 m^3
Mass	Microgram	µg	1,000 µg = 1 mg
	Milligram	mg	1,000 mg = 1 g
	Gram	g	1,000 g = 1 kg
	Kilogram	kg	1,000 kg = 1 metric ton (t)

To convert from pounds to kilograms, divide by 2.2.
To convert from kilograms to pounds, multiply by 2.2.

Table B-2 Celsius (Centigrade) and Fahrenheit Temperature Formulas

To convert °F to °C: Subtract 32, then divide by 1.8. Example: 97°F – 32 = 65, 65 divided by 1.8 = 36°C.
To convert °C to °F: Multiply by 1.8, then add 32. Example: 37°C × 1.8 = 66.6, 66.6 + 32 = 98.6°F.

Table B-3 Sample Conversions of Pounds and Ounces to Grams*

POUNDS	OUNCES															
	0	1	2	3	4	5	6	7	8	9	10	11	12	13	14	15
0	—	28	57	85	113	142	170	198	227	255	283	312	340	369	397	425
1	454	482	510	539	567	595	624	652	680	709	737	765	794	822	850	879
2	907	936	964	992	1,021	1,049	1,077	1,106	1,134	1,162	1,191	1,219	1,247	1,276	1,304	1,332
3	1,361	1,389	1,417	1,446	1,474	1,503	1,531	1,559	1,588	1,616	1,644	1,673	1,701	1,729	1,758	1,786
4	1,814	1,843	1,871	1,899	1,928	1,956	1,984	2,013	2,041	2,070	2,098	2,126	2,155	2,183	2,211	2,240
5	2,268	2,296	2,325	2,353	2,381	2,410	2,438	2,466	2,495	2,532	2,551	2,580	2,608	2,637	2,665	2,693
6	2,722	2,750	2,778	2,807	2,835	2,863	2,892	2,920	2,948	2,977	3,005	3,033	3,062	3,090	3,118	3,147

1 ounce = approximately 30 g.

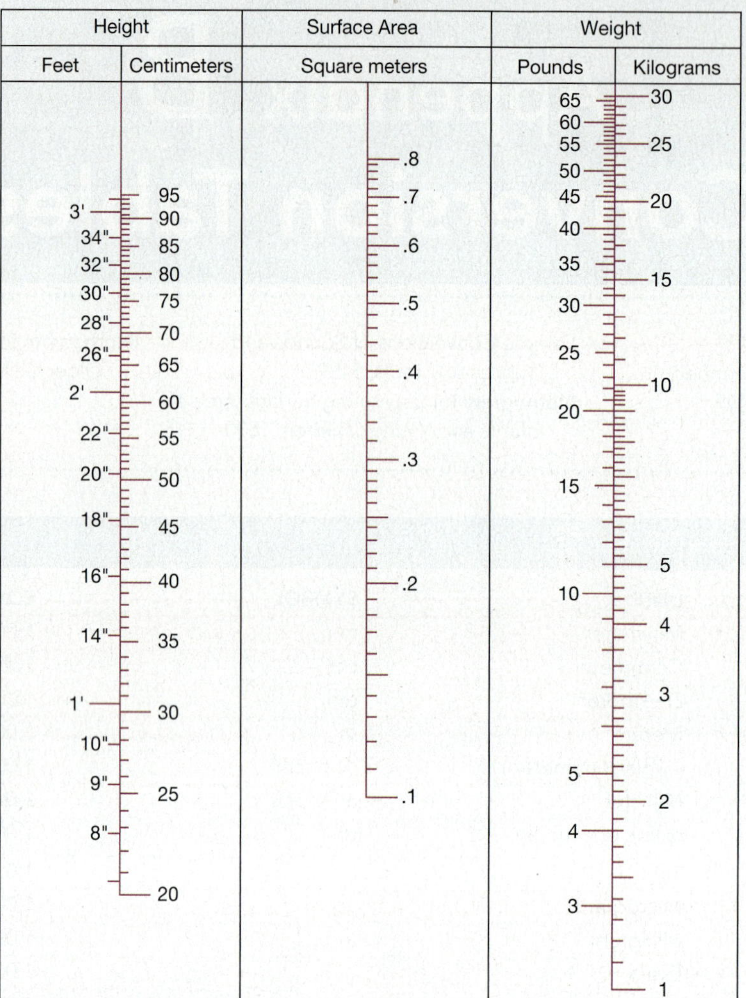

Figure B-1. Nomogram for estimating surface area of infants and young children. To determine the surface area of the patient, draw a straight line between the point representing the patient's height on the left vertical scale and the point representing the patient's weight on the right vertical scale. The point at which this line intersects the middle vertical scale represents the surface area in square meters. (LifeART image copyright (c) 2025 Lippincott Williams & Wilkins. All rights reserved)

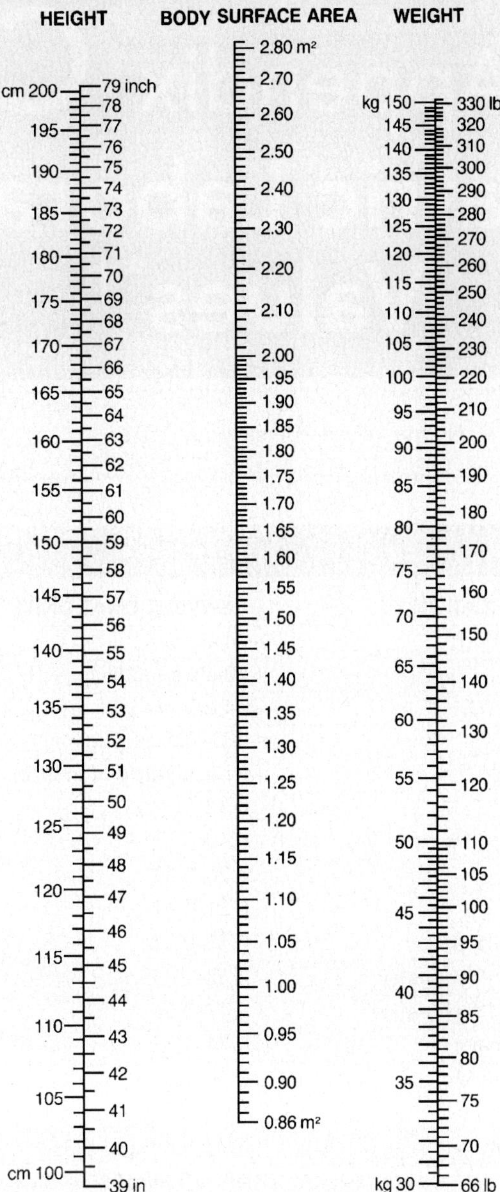

Figure B-2. Nomogram for estimating surface area of older children and adults. To determine the surface area of the patient, draw a straight line between the point representing the patient's height on the left vertical scale and the point representing the patient's weight on the right vertical scale. The point at which this line intersects the middle vertical scale represents the surface area in square meters. (Reprinted with permission from Knapp, R. (2020). *Hemodynamic monitoring made incredibly easy!* (4th ed., unnumbered image on p. 108). Wolters Kluwer.)

Appendix C
Pediatric Laboratory Values*†

Table C-1 Blood Chemistries

LABORATORY TEST	QUALIFICATION	CONVENTIONAL UNITS	SI UNITS
Carbon Dioxide (CO_2) Content	Cord blood	14–22 mmol/L	14–22 mmol/L
	Child	20–24 mmol/L	20–24 mmol/L
	Adult	24–30 mmol/L	24–30 mmol/L
Chloride	—	100–107 mEq/L	100–107 mmol/L
Creatinine (Serum)	**Age (yr)**	**Range, mg/dL (μmol/L)**	
	0–14 d	0.32–0.92	
	15 d to <2 yr	0.10–0.36	
	2 to <5 yr	0.20–0.43	
	5 to <12 yr	0.31–0.61	
	12 to <15 yr	0.45–0.81	
	15 to <19 yr (male)	0.62–1.08	
	15 to <19 yr (female)	0.49–0.84	
	Adult (male)	0.74–1.35	
	Adult (female)	0.59–1.04	
Potassium	Preterm	3.0 -6.0 mEq/L	3.0-6.0 mmol/L
	Newborn	3.7-5.9 mEq/L	3.7-5.9 mmol/L
	Infant	4.1–5.3 mEq/L	4.2–5.3 mmol/L
Sodium	Premature	130–140 mEq/L	130–140 mmol/L
	Older	135–148 mEq/L	135–148 mmol/L
Urea Nitrogen	—	7–22 mg/dL	2.5–7.9 mmol/L

*Please note that the term "male" in this appendix refers to a person assigned male at birth, and the term "female" in this appendix refers to a person assigned female at birth.
† Laboratory values may vary according to the techniques used in different laboratories.

Table C-2 Normal Values—Hematology

AGE	HEMOGLOBIN (G/DL) MEAN (–22 SD)	HEMATOCRIT (%) MEAN (–22 SD)	MEAN CORPUSCULAR VOLUME (FL) MEAN (–22 SD)	MEAN CELL HEMOGLOBIN CONCENTRATION (G/DL RBC) MEAN (–22 SD)	RETICULOCYTE COUNT (%)	WHITE BLOOD CELL/MM^3 × 100 MEAN (–2 SD)	PITS (10^3/MM^3) MEAN (±2 SD)
26–30 Weeks' Gestation*	13.4 (11)	41.5 (34.9)	118.2 (106.7)	37.9 (30.6)	—	4.4 (2.7)	254
28 Weeks' Gestation	14.5	45	120	31	(5–10)	—	(180–327)
32 Weeks' Gestation	15	47	118	32	(3–10)	—	275
Term† (Cord)	16.5 (13.5)	51 (42)	108 (96)	33 (30)	(3–7)	18.1 (9–30)‡	290
1–3 Days	18.5 (14.5)	56 (45)	108 (95)	33 (29)	(1.8–4.6)	18.9 (9.4–34)	290
2 Weeks	16.6 (13.4)	53 (41)	105 (88)	31.4 (28.1)	—	11.5 (5–20)	192
1 Month	13.9 (10.7)	44 (33)	101 (91)	31.8 (28.1)	(0.1–1.7)	10.8 (5–19.5)	252
2 Months	11.2 (9.4)	35 (28)	95 (84)	31.8 (28.3)	—	—	—
6 Months	12.6 (11.1)	36 (31)	76 (68)	35 (32.7)	(0.7–2.3)	11.9 (6–17.5)	—
6 Months to 2 Years	12 (10.5)	36 (33)	78 (70)	33 (30)	—	10.6 (6–17)	(150–350)
2–6 Years	12.5 (11.5)	37 (34)	81 (75)	34 (31)	(0.5–1.0)	8.5 (5–15.5)	(150–350)
6–12 Years	13.5 (11.5)	40 (35)	86 (77)	34 (31)	(0.5–1.0)	8.1 (4.5–13.5)	(150–350)
12–18 Years							
Male	14.5 (13)	43 (36)	88 (78)	34 (31)	(0.5–1.0)	7.8 (4.5–13.5)	(150–350)
Female	14 (12)	41 (37)	90 (78)	34 (31)	(0.5–1.0)	7.8 (4.5–13.5)	(150–350)

*Values are from fetal samplings.

†Younger than age 1 mo, capillary Hb exceeds venous: age 1 h, 3.6 g difference; age 5 d, 2.2 g difference; age 3 wk, 1.1 g difference.

‡Mean (95% confidence limits).

Reprinted with permission from Kleinman, K., McDaniel, L., & Molloy, M. (2021). The Harriet land handbook (22nd ed.). Elsevier, permission conveyed through Copyright Clearance Center, Inc

Appendix D
Guide to General Pain Management

OVERVIEW AND ASSESSMENT

Types of Pain

1. Somatic pain—caused by direct tumor involvement of sensory receptors in cutaneous and deep tissues.
   a. Usually described as dull, sharp, aching, and throbbing; usually constant and localized.
   b. Most common somatic pain is bone pain caused by metastasis.
   c. Can usually be controlled with nonsteroidal anti-inflammatory drugs (NSAIDs) or oral opioids.
2. Neuropathic pain.
   a. Results from nerve injury or compression.
   b. Includes phantom pain and postherpetic neuralgia.
   c. Described as burning, shooting, electric, and lancinating (it can be constant or sporadic).
   d. Usually associated with paresthesia.
   e. Treatment usually includes combinations of antidepressants, anticonvulsants, and opioids.
3. Visceral pain.
   a. Usually described as deep, dull, aching, squeezing, or pressure sensation. It can be vague or ill-defined and can be referred to cutaneous sites, making it difficult to differentiate from somatic pain.
   b. Usually caused by abnormal stretching of smooth muscle walls, ischemia of visceral muscle, and serosal irritation.
   c. Can be treated with oral opioids or surgery to remove the cause.

Other Clinical Manifestations

1. Fatigue from sleep disturbances—most patients have not slept for extended periods.
2. Loss of appetite and weight loss.
3. Anxiety and depression.
4. Change in self-concept and quality of life.

Pain Assessment

1. Screen for pain at each visit. Evaluate objectively the nature of the patient's pain, including location, duration, quality, and impact on daily activities. Pain self-assessment is the most reliable guide to both the cause of the pain and the effectiveness of pain treatment.
   a. Explore pain interventions that have been used and their effectiveness.
   b. Determine whether the intensity of the pain correlates with the prescribed analgesic.
2. Assess patient history and physical examination findings and laboratory values to differentiate expected pain from pain due to a new problem, a complication, or worsening of the underlying process.
3. Use a pain intensity scale of 0 (no pain) to 10 (worst possible pain) or other pain scale as appropriate. Take careful history of prior and present medications, response, and adverse effects.
   a. Ask the patient, "On a scale of 0 to 10, what would be your pain rating, if 0 means no pain and 10 means the worst pain you can imagine?"
4. Assess relief from medications and duration of relief. (Use the same measuring scale every time.) Reevaluate the pain frequently. In acute pain, analgesia should decrease pain as the condition improves due to healing or if other treatment is given, such as physical therapy or radiation therapy. In cases of pain from an untreatable progressive disease or chronic untreatable pain, the patient may not get satisfactory pain relief from typical dosages of pain medication. These patients are frequently managed by a pain specialist and may require substantially higher dosages.

MANAGEMENT OF PAIN

EVIDENCE BASE Tavernier, J. R. (2022). Combating the opioid epidemic through nurse use of multimodal analgesia: An integrative literature review. *AJN American Journal of Nursing, 122*(5), 20–32.

McCabe, C., Feeney, A., Basa, M., Eustace-Cook, J., & McCann, M. (2023). Nurses' knowledge, attitudes and educational needs towards acute pain management in hospital settings: A meta-analysis. *Journal of Clinical Nursing, 32*(15/160), 4325–4336.

Principles of Pain Management

1. The goal of pain management is complete relief of pain.
2. Placebos are never indicated for the treatment of pain.
3. Physical dependence and tolerance commonly occur; patients may require escalating doses of medications to control pain.
4. It is essential that health care providers do not confuse dependency with tolerance. Dependency is an unrelated medical disorder with behavioral components. With patients who are reluctant to take medications, the nurse should stress that higher doses of medication will not make the patient dependent on the medication.
5. Multimodal therapies are often most effective, utilizing several classes of medication, and adding nonpharmacologic therapies. Cognitive behavioral therapies and transcutaneous elective nerve stimulation can be effective adjuncts to pharmacologic therapies.

Pharmacologic Management

Nonopioid Analgesics

1. Acetaminophen—a centrally acting analgesic; does not have anti-inflammatory or antiplatelet activities. May be effective for children and adults as a component of a multimodal therapy.
2. Nonsteroidal anti-inflammatory drugs (NSAIDs).
   a. Produce analgesia by decreasing levels of inflammatory mediators such as prostaglandins at the site of tissue injury.
   b. Suppress platelet function, decrease creatinine clearance, and interfere with the protective effect of prostaglandins on the gastric mucosa.
   c. Used to treat mild to moderate pain; examples include ibuprofen, 400 to 800 mg PO tid; nabumetone, 500 to 1,000 mg PO bid; indomethacin, 25 to 50 mg PO tid.
   d. COX-2 inhibitors are NSAIDs that are somewhat selective for cyclooxygenase 2 (COX-2) compounds, present in most tissues but less present than COX-1 in gastric mucosa. COX-2 is induced in response to inflammation and converts arachidonic acid to prostaglandin. COX-2 inhibitors inhibit prostaglandins at the site of inflammation but cause less gastrointestinal (GI) irritation and bleeding. Examples include celecoxib 100 to 200 mg PO bid or meloxicam 7.5 to 15 mg PO bid.
3. Corticosteroids—may decrease inflammation and edema associated with acute musculoskeletal injuries, rheumatologic conditions, and tumor invasion in cancer.
   a. Examples include dexamethasone, 4 to 10 mg PO qd (dosage varies); prednisone, 5 to 60 mg PO qd (dosage varies).
4. Bisphosphonates—used for lytic bone lesions to prevent fractures and may help control bone pain. Examples include zoledronic acid, 4 mg intravenous (IV) every 3 to 4 weeks; pamidronate, 90 mg IV every 4 weeks.
5. Anticonvulsants and antidepressants for neuropathic pain—used to enhance the effect of opioids. Examples include amitriptyline, 25 to 100 mg PO every h.s. (may cause drowsiness); gabapentin, 300 to 600 mg qid to tid; pregabalin, 100 to 300 mg/day.

Opioid Analgesics

1. Oral route is preferred unless the patient cannot swallow or absorb medications through the GI tract. Doses should be adjusted to achieve pain relief with an acceptable level of adverse effects.
2. Most important to administer on a schedule rather than on an as-needed basis.
3. Optimal treatment approach is to treat with long-acting drugs to control baseline pain, paired with short-acting drugs, as needed, for breakthrough pain.
4. Oral opioids—primary course of treatment for moderate to severe pain; produce analgesia by binding to specific opiate receptors in the brain and spinal cord.
   a. Short-acting opioids—may be used for breakthrough pain, with relief lasting 3 to 4 hours. Examples include morphine, oxycodone, or hydromorphone.
   b. Long-acting opioids—should be equivalent to daily dose of short-acting opiates. Examples include morphine and oxycodone. Should be prescribed every 8 to 12 hours.
   c. Fentanyl—transdermal patch applied to the skin that is changed every 3 days. The peak effect is delayed for up to 3 days after applying. Should be used for patients with stable opioid requirements.
5. Parenteral administration of opioids is used for patients who cannot tolerate oral opioids or who are in an acute pain crisis.
   a. Patient-controlled analgesia (PCA)—administered by either subcutaneously (SC) or IV route using a computer-assisted drug delivery system.
   b. SC infusion of morphine should not exceed 5 mL/hour.
6. Intraspinal administration of opiates for management of acute or chronic pain:
   a. A catheter is placed into spinal epidural or subarachnoid (intrathecal) space.
   b. Catheter may be placed percutaneously and sutured in site or tunneled subcutaneously to the abdominal wall and exteriorized, or the pump system may be implanted.
   c. Catheter is positioned as near as possible to the spinal segment where the pain is projected.
   d. Preservative-free sterile morphine or other analgesic or local anesthetic drug is injected into the system at specified intervals.
   e. May be delivered by PCA pump or by continuous or intermittent infusion.
   f. Spinally administered local anesthetics produce their effects predominantly by action on axons of spinal nerve roots; produce long-lasting pain relief with relatively low doses with little or no blunting of patient's level of responsiveness.
   g. Complications of intraspinal administration include respiratory depression, urine retention, pruritus, infection, leakage, technical problems, and development of tolerance.

Nursing Interventions

1. Base the initial analgesic choice on the patient's report of pain.
2. Administer drugs orally whenever possible; avoid intramuscular (IM) injection.
3. Administer analgesia "around the clock" (i.e., at regular prescribed intervals) rather than as needed.
4. Convey the impression that the patient's pain is understood and that the pain can be controlled.
5. Use alternative measures to relieve pain such as guided imagery, relaxation, and biofeedback.
6. Provide ongoing support and open communication. It is estimated that 40% of cancer survivors experience persistent pain.

7. Assess for side effects of medication.
   a. Respiratory depression is a potentially life-threatening adverse effect of opioids; be alert for shallow respirations and hypoxemia in patients who are opioid naive.
   b. Constipation is expected with opioids and is treated prophylactically.
   c. Nausea is usually transitory and controllable with prophylactic antiemetics.
   d. Sedation is common initially and is transitory.

CLINICAL JUDGEMENT Ensure that opioid reversal agent is readily available for emergency use if respiratory distress or unresponsiveness occurs. Prescriptions for opioids should be accompanied by prescriptions for naloxone. Ensure that any patient going home with opioid therapy has naloxone nasal inhalation solution or prefilled syringe for injection available and caregivers know how to use it.

8. Suggest referral to a pain specialist for intractable pain.
9. Ensure that the least effective dose is used for the shortest amount of time and that refills are not given without repeated assessment.
10. Assess the risk of adverse effects of opioids used in pain management and incorporate universal precautions to minimize misuse, dependency, and adverse consequences.
11. Follow specific state regulations that allow access to medical cannabis or cannabinoids for patients with chronic pain, if such treatment is prescribed.

Index

Note: Page numbers with b indicate boxes; those with f indicate figures; and those with t indicate tables.

A

B

C

D

E

F

H

J

K

L

N

O

P

T

V